HARRISON'S Volume 2
PRINCIPLES OF INTERNAL MEDICINE

THIRTEENTH EDITION

EDITORS OF PREVIOUS EDITIONS

THIRTEENTH EDITION

HARRISON'S
PRINCIPLES
OF
INTERNAL
MEDICINE

Volume 2

Editors

KURT J. ISSELBACHER, A.B., M.D.

Mallinckrodt Professor of Medicine, Harvard Medical School; Physician and Director, Cancer Center, Massachusetts General Hospital, Boston

EUGENE BRAUNWALD, A.B., M.D., M.A. (Hon.), M.D. (Hon.)

Hersey Professor of the Theory and Practice of Physic, Harvard Medical School; Chairman, Department of Medicine, Brigham and Women's Hospital, Boston

JEAN D. WILSON, M.D.

Charles Cameron Sprague Distinguished Chair and Professor of Internal Medicine; Chief, Division of Endocrinology and Metabolism, The University of Texas Southwestern Medical Center, Dallas

JOSEPH B. MARTIN, M.D., Ph.D., F.R.C.P. (C), M.A. (Hon.)

Professor of Neurology and Chancellor, University of California, San Francisco

ANTHONY S. FAUCI, M.D.

Director, National Institute of Allergy and Infectious Diseases; Chief, Laboratory of Immunoregulation; Director, Office of AIDS Research, National Institutes of Health, Bethesda

DENNIS L. KASPER, M.D.

William Ellery Channing Professor of Medicine, Harvard Medical School; Chief, Division of Infectious Diseases, Beth Israel Hospital; Co-Director, Channing Laboratory, Brigham and Women's Hospital, Boston

McGraw-Hill, Inc.
Health Professions Division

New York St. Louis San Francisco Colorado Springs Auckland Bogotá Caracas Hamburg Lisbon London
Madrid Mexico Milan Montreal New Delhi Paris San Juan São Paulo Singapore Sydney Tokyo Toronto

Note: Dr. Fauci's work as editor and author was performed outside the scope of his employment as a U.S. government employee. This work represents his personal and professional views and not necessarily those of the U.S. government.

HARRISON'S
PRINCIPLES OF INTERNAL MEDICINE
Thirteenth Edition

1 2 3 4 5 6 7 8 9 0   DOW DOW   9 8 7 6 5 4

Foreign Language Editions
CHINESE (Twelfth Edition)—McGraw-Hill Book Company-Singapore, © 1994
FRENCH (Twelfth Edition)—Flammarion, © 1992
GERMAN (Tenth Edition)—Schwabe and Company, Ltd., © 1986
GREEK (Twelfth Edition)—Parissianos, © 1994 (est.)
ITALIAN (Twelfth Edition)—McGraw-Hill Libri Italia S.r.l. © 1992
JAPANESE (Eleventh Edition)—Hirokawa, © 1991
PORTUGUESE (Twelfth Edition)—Editora Guanabara Koogan, S.A., © 1992
SPANISH (Twelfth Edition)—McGraw-Hill/Interamericana de Espana, © 1992

This book was set in Times Roman by Monotype Composition Company. The editors were J. Dereck Jeffers and Stuart D. Boynton. The indexer was Irving Tullar; the production supervisor was Roger Kasunic; the designer was Marsha Cohen; R. R. Donnelley & Sons Company was printer and binder.

Library of Congress Cataloging-in-Publication Data

Harrison's principles of internal medicine—13th ed./editors,
   Kurt J. Isselbacher . . . [et al.]
      p.   cm.
   Includes bibliographical references and index.
   ISBN 0-07-032370-4 (1-vol. ed.) : 98.00 — ISBN 0-07-911169-6 (2 vol. ed. set) : 127.00 — ISBN 0-07-032371-2 (bk. 1). — ISBN 0-07-032372-0 (bk. 2)
    1. Internal medicine.   I. Harrison, Tinsley Randolph, 1900–
II. Isselbacher, Kurt J.   III. Title: Principles of internal medicine.
   [DNLM: 1. Internal Medicine.   WB 115 P957 1994]
RC46.H333 1994
616—dc20
DNLM/DLC
for Library of Congress
                                      93-47393
                                      CIP

A SALUTE TO ROBERT G. PETERSDORF

By The Editors Of Harrison's.

We dedicate this thirteenth edition of *Harrison's Principles of Internal Medicine* to Robert G. Petersdorf. Dr. Petersdorf became an editor of Harrison's in 1968 for the preparation of the sixth edition and served as Editor-in-Chief of the tenth edition. He was a powerful force for seven editions and more than 20 years in establishing the pivotal role of this book in the education of students, residents and practitioners of medicine.

Dr. Petersdorf is a graduate of Brown University and of Yale University Medical School. His graduate training included residencies in medicine at Yale and at the Peter Bent Brigham Hospital and a research fellowship at Johns Hopkins. As Chair of the Department of Medicine at the University of Washington he fashioned one of the truly great departments of internal medicine in the nation, with well-balanced and great strengths in education, clinical care, and research. His interests and contributions broadened steadily and he served successively as the first President of the newly merged Brigham and Women's Hospital in Boston, as Vice Chancellor for Health Sciences and Dean of the School of Medicine, University of California, San Diego, and most recently as President of the Association of American Medical Colleges.

Dr. Petersdorf has, from the beginning of his career, made notable and outstanding contributions in a number of areas in the field of Infectious Disease. He carried out a series of classic studies on the pathogenesis of fever, on pneumococcal meningitis and infective endocarditis, and on the chemoprophylaxis and epidemiology of gram-negative infections, especially of the urinary tract.

NOTICE

Medicine is an ever-changing science. As new research and clinical experience broaden our knowledge, changes in treatment and drug therapy are required. The editors and the publisher of this work have checked with sources believed to be reliable in their efforts to provide information that is complete and generally in accord with the standards accepted at the time of publication. However, in view of the possibility of human error or changes in medical sciences, neither the editors, nor the publisher, nor any other party who has been involved in the preparation or publication of this work warrants that the information contained herein is in every respect accurate or complete. Readers are encouraged to confirm the information contained herein with other sources. For example and in particular, readers are advised to check the product information sheet included in the package of each drug they plan to administer to be certain that the information contained in this book is accurate and that changes have not been made in the recommended dose or in the contraindications for administration. This recommendation is of particular importance in connection with new or infrequently used drugs. Readers should also consult their own laboratories for normal values.

ABBREVIATED CONTENTS

CONTENTS

PART SIX
INFECTIOUS DISEASE

Section 1: Basic Considerations in Infectious Disease

Section 2: Clinical Syndromes—Community Acquired

Section 3: Clinical Syndromes—Nosocomial Infections

Section 4: Bacterial Disease: General Considerations

Section 5: Diseases Caused by Gram-Positive Bacteria

Section 6: Diseases Caused by Gram-Negative Bacteria

PART SEVEN
DISORDERS OF THE CARDIOVASCULAR SYSTEM

Section 1: Disorders of the heart

* Deceased

PART THIRTEEN
ENDOCRINOLOGY AND METABOLISM

Section 1: Endocrinology

**PART FOURTEEN
NEUROLOGIC DISORDERS**

COLOR PLATES

ATLAS OF DERMATOLOGY *Stephen F. Templeton / Thomas J. Lawley*

1 Common skin diseases and lesions

A1-1 Acne vulgaris **A1-2** Acne rosacea **A1-3** Psoriasis **A1-4** Atopic dermatitis **A1-5** Dyshidrotic ezcema **A1-6** Seborrheic dermatitis **A1-7** Stasis dermatitis **A1-8** Allergic contact dermatitis **A1-9** Lichen planus **A1-10** Pityriasis rosea **A1-11** Vitiligo **A1-12** Alopecia areata **A1-13** Urticaria **A1-14** Epidermoid cysts **A1-15** Seborrheic keratoses **A1-16** Keloids **A1-17** Cherry hemangiomas

2 Cutaneous neoplasms

A2-18 Actinic keratoses **A2-19** Keratoacanthoma **A2-20** Basal cell carcinoma **A2-21** Squamous cell carcinoma **A2-22** Kaposi's sarcoma **A2-23** Mycosis fungoides **A2-24** Non-Hodgkin's lymphoma **A2-25** Metastatic carcinoma

3 Pigmented lesions—benign and malignant

A3-26 Nevus **A3-27** Dysplastic nevi **A3-28** Superficial spreading melanoma **A3-29** Lentigo maligna melanoma **A3-30** Nodular melanoma **A3-31** Acral lentiginous melanoma

4 Infectious disease and the skin

A4-32 Impetigo contagiosa **A4-33** Folliculitis **A4-34** Erysipelas **A4-35** Herpes simplex **A4-36** Varicella **A4-37** Herpes zoster **A4-38** Verrucae **A4-39** Molluscum contagiosum **A4-40** Oral hairy leukoplakia **A4-41** Pseudomembranous oral candidiasis **A4-42** Tinea corporis **A4-43** Tinea cruris **A4-44** Tinea versicolor **A4-45** Scabies **A4-46** Erythema chronicum migrans **A4-47** Rocky Mountain spotted fever **A4-48** Disseminated gonococcemia **A4-49** Fulminant meningococcemia **A4-50** Primary syphilis **A4-51** Secondary syphilis **A4-52** Secondary syphilis **A4-53** Condylomata lata **A4-54** Chancroid **A4-55** Condylomata acuminata

5 Immunologically mediated skin disease

A5-56 Systemic lupus erythematosus **A5-57** Discoid lupus erythematosus **A5-58** Dermatomyositis **A5-59** Dermatomyositis **A5-60** Scleroderma **A5-61** Scleroderma **A5-62** Erythema multiforme **A5-63** Erythema nodosum **A5-64** Vasculitis **A5-65** Pemphigus vulgaris **A5-66** Dermatitis herpetiformis **A5-67** Bullous pemphigoid

6 Skin manifestations of internal disease

A6-68 Acanthosis nigricans **A6-69** Pretibial myxedema **A6-70** Sarcoid **A6-71** Neurofibromatosis **A6-72** Coumarin necrosis **A6-73** Pyoderma gangrenosum

ATLAS OF ENDOSCOPIC FINDINGS

A7-1 Normal esophagus **A7-2** Peptic regurgitant esophagitis **A7-3** Ulcerated squamous cell carcinoma **A7-4** Moniliasis of the esophagus **A7-5** Barrett's metaplasia of the esophagus with an adenocarcinoma **A7-6** Normal body of the stomach with rugal folds **A7-7** Large, benign lesser curve gastic ulcer **A7-8** Gastric polyp **A7-9** Arteriovenous malformation of the gastric mucosa **A7-10** Normal pylorus **A7-11** Normal duodenal bulb **A7-12** Duodenal ulcer **A7-13** Normal papilla of Vater **A7-14** Periampullary carcinoma **A7-15** Endoscopic papillotomy **A7-16** Normal colon **A7-17** Colonic adenomatous polyp **A7-18** Multiple small colonic adenomatous polyps **A7-19** Colon adenocarcinoma **A7-20** Crohn's colitis **A7-21** Severe ulcerative colitis **A7-22** Kaposi's sarcoma involving the colon **A7-23** Colonic varices **A7-24** Normal appearing ileal pouch

ATLAS OF FUNDOSCOPIC EXAMINATION

A8-1 Normal optic nerve and retina **A8-2** Central retinal artery occlusion **A8-3** Central retinal vein occlusion **A8-4** Early papilledema **A8-5** Drusen of the optic nerve head **A8-6** Anterior ischemic optic neuropathy **A8-7** Primary optic atrophy **A8-8** Angioid streaks **A8-9** Retinitis pigmentosa **A8-10** Band keratopathy **A8-11** Glaucomatous optic disk with secondary atrophy **A8-12** Diabetic retinopathy with microaneurysms **A8-13** Proliferative diabetic retinopathy **A8-14** Cytomegalovirus retinitis in AIDS **A8-15** Retinal arteriovenous malformation in the Wyburn-Mason syndrome **A8-16** Kayser-Fleischer ring in Wilson's disease.

ATLAS OF HEMATOLOGY

A9-1 Normal blood smear **A9-2** Megaloblastic anemia **A9-3** Liver disease **A9-4** Iron deficiency anemia **A9-5** Thalassemia intermedia **A9-6** Sickle cell anemia **A9-7** Traumatic hemolysis **A9-8** Spur cell anemia **A9-9** Uremia **A9-10** Hereditary spherocytosis **A9-11** Immunohemolytic anemia **A9-12** Myeloid metaplasia **A9-13** Normal granulocyte (A); normal monocyte and lymphocyte (B) **A9-14** Normal eosinophil (A); basophil (B) **A9-15** Normal granulocyte precursors in marrow **A9-16** Neutrophils with toxic granulation **A9-17** Band with Döhle body **A9-18** Hypersegmentation **A9-19** Chediak-Higashi anomaly (A); Pelger-Huët anomaly (B) **A9-20** Reactive lymphocytes **A9-21** Chronic granulocytic leukemia **A9-22** Leukemic cell in acute promyelocytic leukemia **A9-23** Chronic lymphocytic leukemia **A9-24** Leukemic cells in acute lymphoblastic leukemia **A9-25** Hodgkin's disease **A9-26** Non-Hodgkin's nodular lymphoma **A9-27** Multiple myeloma

LIST OF CONTRIBUTORS

ELIAS ABRUTYN, M.D.

Professor and Associate Chairman, Medicine, and Vice-Dean for Veterans Affairs, Medical College of Pennsylvania; Chief, Infectious Diseases, Veterans Administration Medical Center, Philadelphia

RAYMOND D. ADAMS, B.A., M.A., M.D., M.A. (Hon.), D.Sc. (Hon.), M.D. (Hon.)

Bullard Professor of Neuropathology, Emeritus, Harvard Medical School; Consultant Neurologist, Massachusetts General Hospital; Emeritus Director, Eunice K. Shriver Research Center, Boston; Médicin Adjoint L'Hôpital, Cantonale de Lausanne, Lausanne

MICHAEL J. AMINOFF, M.D.

Professor of Neurology; Director, Clinical Neurophysiology Laboratories, University of California, San Francisco

MICHAEL A. APICELLA, M.D.

Professor and Head, Department of Microbiology, University of Iowa College of Medicine, Iowa City

GORDON LEE ARCHER, M.D.

Professor of Medicine and Microbiology/Immunology and Chairman, Division of Infectious Diseases, Medical College of Virginia, Virginia Commonwealth University, Richmond

ARTHUR K. ASBURY, M.D.

Ruth Wagner Van Meter and J. Ray Van Meter Professor of Neurology; Vice Dean for Research, University of Pennsylvania School of Medicine and Hospital of the University of Pennsylvania, Philadelphia

K. FRANK AUSTEN, M.D.

Theodore Bevier Bayles Professor of Medicine, Harvard Medical School; Chairman, Department of Rheumatology and Immunology, Brigham and Women's Hospital, Boston

ROBERT AUSTRIAN, M.D., D.Sci. (Hon.)

John Herr Musser Professor and Chairman Emeritus, Department of Molecular and Cellular Engineering, University of Pennsylvania School of Medicine, Philadelphia

BERNARD BABIOR, M.D., Ph.D.

Head, Division of Biochemistry, Department of Molecular and Experimental Medicine and Member, Division of Hematology and Oncology, Department of Medicine, Scripps Clinic and Research Foundation, La Jolla

KAMAL F. BADR, M.D.

Professor of Medicine, Emory University; Chief, Division of Nephrology, Atlanta Veteran's Medical Center; Attending Physician, Emory University Hospital, Atlanta

DONALD S. BAIM, M.D.

Associate Professor of Medicine, Harvard Medical School; Chief, Interventional Cardiology Section, Beth Israel Hospital, Boston

ANN SULLIVAN BAKER, M.D.

Associate Professor of Medicine, Harvard Medical School; Director, Infectious Diseases Service, Massachusetts Eye and Ear Infirmary; Physician, Infectious Disease Service, Massachusetts General Hospital, Boston

ANDREA BALLABIO, M.D.

Associate Professor, Institute for Molecular Genetics and Human Genome Center, Baylor College of Medicine, Houston

KENNETH J. BART, M.D., M.P.H.

Director, National Vaccine Program, Office of the Assistant Secretary of Health, Department of Health and Human Services, Rockville

ROBERT C. BAST, Jr., M.D.

R. Wayne Rundle Professor of Medicine and Director, Duke Comprehensive Cancer Center, Duke University Medical Center, Durham

M. FLINT BEAL, M.D.

Associate Professor of Neurology, Harvard Medical School; Assistant Neurologist, Massachusetts General Hospital, Boston

ARTHUR L. BEAUDET, M.D.

Professor, Institute for Molecule Genetics and Departments of Pediatrics and Cell Biology, Baylor College of Medicine; Investigator, Howard Hughes Medical Institute, Houston

JOHN E. BENNETT, M.D.

Head, Clinical Mycology Section, Laboratory of Clinical Investigation, National Institute of Allergy and Infectious Diseases, National Institutes of Health, Bethesda

ANDREW BERCHUCK, M.D.

Associate Professor, Division of Gynecologic Oncology, Duke University Medical Center, Durham

MICHAEL S. BERNSTEIN, M.D.

Assistant Professor of Medicine and Anesthesia, Division of Pulmonary and Critical Care Medicine, University of California at San Francisco Medical Center, San Francisco

DANIEL G. BICHET, M.D.

Associate Professor of Medicine, University of Montreal; Director, Clinical Research Unit, Hôpital du Sacre-Coeur de Montréal, Montreal

DAVID R. BICKERS, M.D.

Professor and Chairman, Department of Dermatology, Case Western Reserve University School of Medicine; Director, Department of Dermatology, University Hospitals of Cleveland, Cleveland

EDWIN L. BIERMAN, M.D.

Professor of Medicine and Head, Division of Metabolism, Endocrinology and Nutrition, University of Washington School of Medicine, Seattle

NEIL R. BLACKLOW, M.D.

Richard M. Haidack Professor of Medicine and Chairman, Department of Medicine, University of Massachusetts Medical School, Worcester

MARTIN J. BLASER, M.D.

The Addison B. Scoville Professor of Medicine; Director, Division of Infectious Diseases and Professor of Microbiology and Immunology, Vanderbilt University School of Medicine; Staff Physician, Veterans Affairs Medical Center, Nashville

JEAN L. BOLOGNIA, M.D.

Associate Professor of Dermatology, Department of Dermatology, Yale University School of Medicine, New Haven

LAWRENCE F. BORGES, M.D.

Associate Professor of Surgery (Neurosurgery), Harvard Medical School; Associate Visiting Neurosurgeon, Massachusetts General Hospital, Boston

RICHARD C. BOUCHER, Jr., M.D.

Professor of Medicine and Director, Division of Pulmonary Diseases, Critical Care and Occupational Medicine, University of North Carolina at Chapel Hill; University of North Carolina Hospitals, Chapel Hill

AUBREY E. BOYD III, M.D.

Professor of Medicine and Neuroscience; Chief, Division of Endocrinology, Diabetes, Metabolism and Molecular Medicine, New England Medical Center, Boston

WALTER G. BRADLEY, D.M., F.R.C.P.

Professor and Chairman, Department of Neurology, University of Miami School of Medicine, Miami

HUGH R. BRADY, M.D., Ph.D., F.R.C.P.I.

Assistant Professor of Medicine, Harvard Medical School; Chief, Renal Section, Brockton/West Roxbury Veteran's Affairs Medical Center; Associate Physician, Brigham and Women's Hospital, Boston

DAVID L. BRAFF, M.D.

Professor of Psychiatry, University of California at San Diego; Director of Psychiatry, UCSD Medical Center, San Diego

KENNETH D. BRANDT, M.D.

Professor of Medicine and Head, Rheumatology Division, Indiana University School of Medicine, Indianapolis; Director, Multipurpose Arthritis and Musculoskeletal Diseases Center, Indiana University School of Medicine, Indianapolis

EUGENE BRAUNWALD, A.B., M.D., M.A. (Hon.), M.D. (Hon.), Sc.D. (Hon.)

Hersey Professor of the Theory and Practice of Medicine, Harvard Medical School; Chairman, Department of Medicine, Brigham and Women's Hospital, Boston

IRWIN M. BRAVERMAN, M.D.

Professor, Department of Dermatology, Yale University School of Medicine, New Haven

JAMES L. BREELING, M.D.

Associate Chief, Medical Service, West Roxbury VA Medical Center, Boston

JOEL G. BREMAN, M.D., D.T.P.H.

Deputy Chief, Malaria Branch, Division of Parasitic Diseases, National Center for Infectious Diseases, Centers for Disease Control and Prevention, Atlanta; Visiting Lecturer, Harvard School of Public Health, Boston

BARRY M. BRENNER, M.D., A.M. (Hon.), D.Sc. (Hon.), D.M.Sc. (Hon.)

Samuel A. Levine Professor of Medicine, Harvard Medical School; Senior Physician and Director, Renal Division, Brigham and Women's Hospital, Boston

KENNETH R. BRIDGES, M.D.

Assistant Professor of Medicine, Harvard Medical School; Brigham and Women's Hospital, Boston

KAREN THATCHER BRITTON, M.D., Ph.D.

Professor of Psychiatry, University of California at San Diego, La Jolla

CLAIRE V. BROOME, M.D.

Associate Director for Science, Centers for Disease Control and Prevention, Atlanta

MARTIN M. BROWN, M.A., M.D., M.R.C.P.

Senior Lecturer in Neurology, St. George's Hospital Medical School, London

MICHAEL S. BROWN, M.D.

Paul J. Thomas Professor, Department of Molecular Genetics, The University of Texas Southwestern Medical Center, Dallas

ROBERT H. BROWN, Jr., M.D., D.Phil.

Associate Professor, Harvard Medical School; Associate Neruologist and Director, Cecil B. Day Laboratory for Neuromuscular Research, Massachusetts General Hospital, Boston

H. FRANKLIN BUNN, M.D.

Professor of Medicine, Harvard Medical School; Senior Physician and Director, Hematology Research, Brigham and Women's Hospital, Boston

RONALD M. BURDE, M.D.

Isidor Tachna Professor and Chairman, Department of Ophthalmology; Ophthalmologist and Neuro-ophthalmologist, Albert Einstein College of Medicine/Montefiore Medical Center, New York

JOAN R. BUTTERTON, M.D.

Clinical and Research Fellow, Infectious Diseases Unit, Massachusetts Gneral Hospital, Boston

STEPHEN B. CALDERWOOD, M.D.

Associate Professor of Medicine, Harvard Medical School; Chief, Infectious Diseases Unit, Massachusetts General Hospital, Boston

CHARLES B. CARPENTER, M.D.

Professor of Medicine, Harvard Medical School; Director, Laboratory of Immunogenetics and Transplantation, Brigham and Woman's Hospital, Boston

BRUCE R. CARR, M.D.

Paul C. MacDonald Professor and Director, Division of Reproductive Endocrinology, Department of Obstetrics and Gynecology, The University of Texas Southwestern Medical Center, Dallas

VERNE S. CAVINESS, Jr., M.D., Ph.D.

Joseph P. and Rose F. Kennedy Professor of Child Neurology and Mental Retardation, Harvard Medical School; Chief, Pediatric Neurology Service, Massachusetts General Hospital, Boston

WALLACE A. CLYDE, Jr., M.D.

Professor of Pediatrics and Microbiology, University of North Carolina, Chapel Hill

FREDRIC L. COE, M.D.

Professor of Medicine and Physiology and Chief, Nephrology Program, University of Chicago Pritzker School of Medicine, Chicago

ALAN S. COHEN, M.D.

Distinguished Professor of Medicine and Rheumatology; Director, Arthritis Center at Boston University School of Medicine, Boston University School of Medicine, Boston

WILSON COLUCCI, M.D.

Associate Professor of Medicine, Harvard Medical School; Physician, Brigham and Women's Hospital

PATRICIA C. COME, M.D.

Associate Professor of Medicine, Harvard Medical School; Harvard Community Health Plan, Boston

JOEL D. COOPER, M.D.

Professor of Surgery and Head, Section of General Thoracic Surgery, Washington University School of Medicine; Barnes Hospital, St. Louis

MAX D. COOPER, M.D.

Professor of Medicine, Pediatrics and Microbiology and Howard Hughes Medical Institute Investigator, University of Alabama at Birmingham, Birmingham

LAWRENCE COREY, M.D.

Professor of Laboratory Medicine, Microbiology and Medicine, University of Washington, Seattle

MARK A. CREAGER, M.D.

Associate Professor of Medicine, Harvard Medical School; Director, Vascular Diagnostic Laboratory, Brigham and Women's Hospital, Boston

RONALD G. CRYSTAL, M.D.

Webster Professor of Medicine, Cornell University Medical College; Attending Physician, New York Hospital; Chief, Division of Pulmonary and Critical Care Medicine, New York Hospital-Cornell Medical Center, New York

JOHN J. CUSH, M.D.

Associate Professor of Internal Medicine, Rheumatic Diseases Division University of Texas Southwestern Medical Center at Dallas, Dallas

CHARLES A. CZEISLER, Ph.D., M.D.

Associate Professor of Medicine, Harvard Medical School; Physician and Director, Laboratory for Circadian and Sleep Disorders Medicine, Brigham and Women's Hospital, Boston

THOMAS M. DANIEL, M.D.

Professor of Medicine and International Health, Center for International Health, CWRU School of Medicine, Cleveland

GILBERT H. DANIELS, M.D.

Associate Professor of Medicine, Harvard Medical School; Physician and Co-Director, Thyroid Clinic, Massachusetts General Hospital, Boston

ROBERT B. DAROFF, M.D.

Gilbert W. Humphrey Professor and Chairman, Department of Neurology, Case Western Reserve University School of Medicine; Director, Department of Neurology, University Hospitals of Cleveland; Neurology Service, Cleveland Veteran's Administration Medical Center, Cleveland

JOHN R. DAVID, M.D.

Richard Pearson Strong Professor and Chairman, Department of Tropical Public Health, Harvard School of Public Health, Boston

CHARLES EDWARD DAVIS, M.D.

Professor of Pathology and Medicine, School of Medicine, University of California, San Diego; Director, Microbiology Laboratory, UCSD Medical Center, San Diego

KENNETH DAVIS, M.D., F.A.C.R.

Professor of Radiology, Harvard Medical School; Department of Neuroradiology, Massachusetts General Hospital, Boston

ROBERT L. DERESIEWICZ, M.D.

Instructor in Medicine, Harvard Medical School; Associate Physician, Brigham and Women's Hospital, Boston

ROBERT J. DESNICK, Ph.D., M.D.

Professor and Chairman, Department of Human Genetics, Mount Sinai School of Medicine; Attending Physician, Mount Sinai Hospital, New York

MARC A. DICHTER, M.D., Ph.D.

Professor of Neurology and Pharmacology, University of Pennsylvania School of Medicine and Graduate Hospital, Philadelphia

JULES L. DIENSTAG, M.D.

Associate Professor of Medicine, Harvard Medical School; Associate Physician, Massachusetts General Hospital, Boston

ALAN R. DIMICK, M.D.

Professor of Surgery, University of Alabama at Birmingham; Director, Burn Center, University of Alabama Hospital, Birmingham

CHARLES A. DINARELLO, M.D.

Professor of Medicine, Tufts University School of Medicine; Division of Geographic Medicine and Infectious Diseases, New England Medical Center, Boston

ROBERT G. DLUHY, M.D.

Associate Professor of Medicine, Harvard Medical School; Associate Program Director of the Clinical Research Center, Brigham and Women's Hospital, Boston

RAPHAEL DOLIN, M.D.

Charles A. Dewey Professor of Medicine; Chair, Department of Medicine, University of Rochester School of Medicine and Dentistry, Rochester

DANIEL B. DRACHMAN, M.D.

Professor of Neurology and Neurosciences and Director, Neuromuscular Unit, The Johns Hopkins University School of Medicine, Baltimore

JEFFREY M. DRAZEN, M.D.

Parker B. Francis Professor of Medicine, Harvard Medical School; Chief, Pulmonary Division, Brigham and Women's and Beth Israel Hospitals, Boston

JOHANNA T. DWYER, D.Sc., R.D.

Professor of Medicine and Community Health, Tufts University School of Medicine; Professor of Nutrition, Tufts University School of Nutrition; Senior Scientist, USDA Human Nutrition Research Center on Aging, Tufts University; Director, Frances Stern Nutrition Center, New England Medical Center Hospital, Boston

VICTOR J. DZAU, M.D.

William G. Irwin Professor of Medicine and Chief, Division of Cardiovascular Medicine, Stanford University School of Medicine; Stanford University Hospital, Stanford

BARRY I. EISENSTEIN, M.D.

Professor of Medicine, Indiana University School of Medicine; Vice President, Lilly Research Laboratories, Indianapolis

VIRGINIA L. ERNSTER, Ph.D.

Professor and Chair, Department of Epidemiology and Biostatistics, University of California, San Francisco

KENNETH H. FALCHUK, M.D.

Associate Professor of Medicine, Harvard Medical School; Physician, Brigham and Women's Hospital, Boston

FERRIC C. FANG, M.D.

Assistant Professor of Medicine and Pathology, University of Colorado Health Sciences Center; Director, Clinical Microbiology Laboratory, University Hospital, Denver

ANTHONY S. FAUCI, M.D.

Director, National Institute of Allergy and Infectious Diseases; Chief, Laboratory of Immunoregulation; Director, Office of AIDS Research, National Institutes of Health, Bethesda

MURRAY J. FAVUS, M.D.

Professor of Medicine, Sections of Endocrinology and Nephrology, Department of Medicine, University of Chicago Pritzker School of Medicine, Chicago

THOMAS F. FERRIS, M.D.

Nesbitt Professor and Chairman, Department of Medicine, University of Minnesota; University of Minnesota Hospital and Clinics, Minneapolis

BERNARD N. FIELDS, M.D.

Adele Lehman Professor of Microbiology and Molecular Genetics, Professor of Medicine and Chairman, Department of Microbiology and Molecular Genetics, Harvard Medical School, Boston

HOWARD L. FIELDS, M.D., Ph.D.

Professor of Neurology and Physiology and Vice Chairman, Department of Neurology, University of California, San Francisco

GREGORY A. FILICE, M.D.

Associate Professor of Medicine and Chief, Infectious Disease Section, University of Minnesota VA Medical Center, Minneapolis

ROBERT W. FINBERG, M.D.

Associate Professor of Medicine, Harvard Medical School; Chief, Laboratory of Infectious Diseases, Dana-Farber Cancer Institute, Boston

STUART C. FINCH, M.D.

Professor of Medicine, University of Medicine and Dentistry of New Jersey-Robert Wood Johnson Medical School and the Cooper Hospital/University Medical Center, Camden

J. STEPHEN FINK, M.D.

Associate Professor, Harvard Medical School; Assistant Neurologist, Massachusetts General Hospital, Boston

DANIEL W. FOSTER, M.D.

Donald W. Seldin Distinguished Chair in Internal Medicine and Chairman, Department of Internal Medicine, The University of Texas Southwestern Medical Center, Dallas

MICHAEL M. FRANK, M.D.

Professor and Chairman, Department of Pediatrics, Duke University Medical Center; Professor of Medicine, Department of Medicine, Duke University Medical Center, Durham

ARNOLD S. FREEDMAN, M.D.

Assistant Professor of Medicine, Harvard Medical School; Division of Tumor Immunology, Dana-Farber Cancer Institute, Boston

STANLEY D. FREEDMAN, M.D.

Clinical Professor of Medicine, University of California at San Diego; Head, Division of Infectious Diseases, Scripps Clinic and Research Foundation, La Jolla

MICHAEL FREISSMUTH, M.D.

Lecturer, Department of Pharmacology, University of Vienna, Vienna

GERALD H. FRIEDLAND, M.D.

Director, AIDS Program, Yale University School of Medicine, New Haven

HARVEY MICHAEL FRIEDMAN, M.D.

Chief, Infectious Disease Division, Department of Medicine, University of Pennsylvania School of Medicine, Philadelphia

LAWRENCE S. FRIEDMAN, M.D.

Associate Professor of Medicine, Harvard Medical School; Associate Physician, Massachusetts General Hospital, Boston

PAUL J. FRIEDMAN, M.D.

Professor of Radiology, University of California, San Diego

WILLIAM F. FRIEDMAN, M.D.

J.H. Nicholson Professor of Pediatrics (Cardiology) and Executive Chairman, Department of Pediatrics, University of California, Los Angeles School of Medicine; University of California, Los Angeles Medical Center, Los Angeles

LAWRENCE A. FROHMAN, M.D.

Edmund F. Foley Professor and Head, Department of Medicine, University of Illinois at Chicago, Chicago

ROBERT F. GAGEL, M.D.

Professor of Medicine and Chief of Endocrinology Section, The University of Texas, M.D. Anderson Cancer Center, Houston

JOHN I. GALLIN, M.D.

Director, Division of Intramural Research, National Institute of Allergy and Infectious Diseases, National Institutes of Health, Bethesda

ROBERT C. GALLO, M.D.

Chief, Laboratory of Tumor Cell Biology, National Cancer Institute, National Institutes of Health, Bethesda

MARC B. GARNICK, M.D.

Associate Clinical Professor of Medicine, Dana-Farber Cancer Institute and Harvard Medical School; Vice President for Clinical Development, Genetics Institute, Cambridge

JEFFREY A. GELFAND, M.D.

Sara Murray Jordan Professor and Vice Chairman, Department of Medicine, Tufts University School of Medicine; Associate Physician-in-Chief, New England Medical Center, Boston

JAMES L. GERMAN III, M.D.

Professor of Pediatrics, Cornell University Medical College; Director, Laboratory of Human Genetics, New York Blood Center, New York

BRUCE C. GILLILAND, M.D.

Professor of Medicine, Professor of Laboratory Medicine and Adjunct Professor of Microbiology, and Associate Dean, Clinical Affairs, University of Washington School of Medicine, Seattle

ALFRED G. GILMAN, M.D., Ph.D.

Raymond Willie Distinguished Chair in Molecular Neuropharmacology; Department of Pharmacology, The University of Texas Southwestern Medical Center, Dallas

SID GILMAN, M.D.

Professor and Chairman, Department of Neurology, University of Michigan, Ann Arbor

RICHARD J. GLASSOCK, M.D.

Professor and Chairman, Department of Internal Medicine, University of Kentucky College of Medicine, Lexington

ROBERT M. GLICKMAN, M.D.

Herrman Ludwig Blumgart Professor of Medicine, Harvard Medical School; Physician-in-Chief, Beth Israel Hospital, Boston

MARK A. GOLDBERG, M.D.

Assistant Professor of Medicine, Harvard Medical School; Associate Physician, Brigham and Women's Hospital, Boston

ARY GOLDBERGER, M.D.

Associate Professor of Medicine, Harvard Medical School; Physician, Beth Israel Hospital, Boston

DAVID W. GOLDE, M.D.

Professor of Medicine, Cornell University Medical College; Professor of Molecular Pharmacology and Therapeutics, Sloan-Kettering Division of the Cornell Graduate School of Medical Sciences; Member, Attending Physician, and Head, Division of Hematologic Oncology, Memorial Sloan-Kettering Cancer Center, New York

LEE GOLDMAN, M.D.

Professor of Medicine, Harvard Medical School; Vice-Chairman, Department of Medicine and Chief, Division of Clinical Epidemiology, Brigham and Women's Hospital, Boston

JOSEPH L. GOLDSTEIN, M.D.

Paul J. Thomas Professor and Chairman, Department of Molecular Genetics, The University of Texas Southwestern Medical Center, Dallas

RAJ K. GOYAL, M.D.

Rabb Professor of Medicine, Harvard Medical School; Chief, Division of Gastroenterology, Beth Israel Hospital, Boston

JOHN W. GRAEF, M.D.

Associate Clinical Professor of Pediatrics, Harvard Medical School; Director, The Lead/Toxicology Clinic, The Children's Hospital, Boston

HARRY B. GREENBERG, M.D.

Professor of Medicine and Microbiology and Immunology, Stanford University Medical Center, Stanford

NORTON J. GREENBERGER, M.D., M.A.C.P.

Peter T. Bohan Professor and Chairman, Department of Medicine, University of Kansas Medical Center, Kansas City

JOHN S. GREENSPAN, B.D.S, Ph.D., F.R.C.Path.

Professor and Chairman, Department of Stomatology, University of California School of Dentistry, San Francisco

JAMES E. GRIFFIN, M.D.

Professor of Internal Medicine, The University of Texas Southwestern Medical Center, Dallas

J. McLEOD GRIFFISS, M.D.

Professor of Lab Medicine and Medicine, University of California at San Francisco VA Medical Center, San Francisco

ROBERT C. GRIGGS, M.D.

Edward A. and Alma Vollertsen Rykenboer Professor of Neurophysiology, Professor of Neurology and Medicine, and Chairman, Department of Neurology, University of Rochester School of Medicine and Dentistry, University of Rochester Medical Center, Rochester

WILLIAM GROSSMAN, M.D.

Dana Professor of Medicine, Harvard Medical School; Chief, Cardiovascular Division, Beth Israel Hospital, Boston

JOHN H. GROWDON, M.D.

Professor of Neurology, Harvard Medical School; Neurologist and Director, Memory Disorders Unit, Massachusetts General Hospital, Boston

SUBHASH C. GULATI, M.D., Ph.D.

Associate Professor of Medicine, Cornell University Medical College; Associate Member and Associate Attending Physician, Memorial Sloan-Kettering Cancer Center, New York

VLADIMIR HACHINSKI, M.D.

Richard and Beryl Ivey Professor and Chairman, Department of Clinical Neurological Sciences, University of Western Ontario, University Hospital, London, Ontario

BEVRA HANNAHS HAHN, M.D.

Professor of Medicine, Department of Medicine; Chief of Rheumatology, University of California, Los Angeles, Los Angeles

ROBERT I. HANDIN, M.D.

Associate Professor of Medicine, Harvard Medical School; Director, Hematology Oncology Division, Brigham and Women's Hospital, Boston

H. HUNTER HANDSFIELD, M.D.

Professor of Medicine, University of Washington School of Medicine; Director, STD Control Program, Seattle-King County Department of Public Health, Seattle

STEPHEN L. HAUSER, M.D.

Betty Anker Fife Professor and Chairman, Department of Neurology, University of California, San Francisco

BARTON F. HAYNES, M.D.

Director, Arthritis Center; Chief, Division of Rheumatology and Immunology; Frederic M. Hanes Professor of Medicine; Director, Basic Research, Center for AIDS Research, Duke University School of Medicine, Durham

STEVEN C. HERBERT, M.D.

Associate Professor of Medicine, Harvard Medical School; Physician, Brigham and Women's Hospital, Boston

I. CRAIG HENDERSON, M.D.

Professor of Medicine; Chief of Medical Oncology; Director, Clinical Oncology Program, Moffitt-Long Hospitals, San Francisco

CHARLES B. HIGGINS, M.D.

Professor of Radiology and Chief, Magnetic Resonance Imaging, University of California School of Medicine, San Francisco

RAYMOND L. HINTZ, M.D.

Professor of Pediatrics and Head, Division of Pediatric Endocrinology, Stanford University School of Medicine, Stanford

MARTIN S. HIRSCH, M.D.

Professor of Medicine, Harvard Medical School; Massachusetts General Hospital, Boston

FRED HOCHBERG, M.D.

Associate Professor of Neurology, Harvard Medical School; Neurologist, Massachusetts General Hospital, Boston

GARY S. HOFFMAN, M.D.

Chairman, Department of Rheumatic and Immunologic Diseases, Cleveland Clinic Foundation, Cleveland

JOHN H. HOLBROOK, M.D.

Professor of Internal Medicine, University of Utah School of Medicine, Salt Lake City

MICHAEL F. HOLICK, Ph.D., M.D.

Professor of Medicine, Physiology and Dermatology; Chief of Endocrinology, Diabetes and Metabolism; Director of the General Clinical Research Center, Boston University School of Medicine, Boston

KING K. HOLMES, M.D., Ph.D.

Professor of Medicine and Director, Center for AIDS and Sexually Transmitted Diseases, University of Washington School of Medicine, Seattle

RANDALL K. HOLMES, M.D., Ph.D.

Chairman, Department of Microbiology and Immunology, Uniformed Services University of the Health Sciences, Bethesda

THOMAS H. HOSTETTER, M.D.

Professor of Medicine, University of Minnesota School of Medicine; Director, Division of Renal Disease, University Hospital, Minneapolis

LYN J. HOWARD, B.M., D.Ch., F.R.C.P.

Professor of Medicine and Associate Professor of Pediatrics; Head, Division of Clinical Nutrition, Albany Medical College, Albany

HOWARD HU, M.D., M.P.H., Sc.D.

Assistant Professor of Medicine, Harvard Medical School; Associate Physician, Channing Laboratory, Brigham and Women's Hospital, Boston

GARY W. HUNNINGHAKE, M.D.

Professor of Internal Medicine and Director, Pulmonary and Critical Care Medicine, University of Iowa College of Medicine, Iowa City

EDWARD P. INGENITO, M.D., Ph.D.

Assistant Professor of Medicine, Harvard Medical School; Director, Medical Intensive Care Unit, Brigham and Women's Hospital, Boston

ROLAND H. INGRAM, Jr., M.D.

Professor of Medicine, Emory University School of Medicine; Chief of Medicine, Emory-Crawford Long Hospital, Atlanta

CHARLES E. IRWIN, Jr., M.D.

Professor of Pediatrics; Director, Division of Adolescent Medicine, Department of Pediatrics School of Medicine, University of California, San Francisco, San Francisco

KURT J. ISSELBACHER, M.D.

Mallinckrodt Professor of Medicine, Harvard Medical School; Physician and Director, MGH Cancer Center, Massachusetts General Hospital, Boston

MARK E. JOSEPHSON, M.D.

Professor of Medicine, Harvard Medical School; Director, Harvard-Thorndike Electrophysiology Institute and Arrhythmia Service, Beth Israel Hospital, Boston

LEWIS L. JUDD, M.D.

Mary Gilman Marston Professor and Chairman, Department of Psychiatry, University of California at San Diego, La Jolla

LEE M. KAPLAN, M.D., Ph.D.

Assistant Professor of Medicine, Harvard Medical School; Assistant in Medicine, Gastrointestinal Unit, Massachusetts General Hospital, Boston

DENNIS L. KASPER, M.D.

William Ellery Channing Professor of Medicine, Harvard Medical School; Chief, Division of Infectious Diseases, Beth Israel Hospital; Co-Director, Channing Laboratory, Brigham and Women's Hospital, Boston

LLOYD H. KASPER, M.D.

Professor of Medicine, Neurology and Microbiology, Dartmouth Medical School, Hanover

SATISH KATHPALIA, M.D., F.A.C.P.

Associate Professor of Medicine, University of Illinois School of Medicine; Attending Physician, Renal Division, Department of Medicine, Michael Reese Hospital and Medical Center, Chicago

DONALD KAYE, M.D.

Klinghoffer Professor and Chairman, Department of Medicine, The Medical College of Pennsylvania, Philadelphia

GERALD T. KEUSCH, M.D.

Professor of Medicine and Chief, Division of Geographic Medicine and Infectious Diseases, New England Medical Center Hospitals, Boston

MICHAEL B. KIMMEY, M.D.

Associate Professor of Medicine and Director of GI Endoscopy, University of Washington School of Medicine, Seattle

LOUIS V. KIRCHHOFF, M.D.

Associate Professor of Internal Medicine and Staff Physician, Department of Veterans Affairs Medical Center, Iowa City

J. PHILLIP KISTLER, M.D.

Associate Professor of Neurology, Harvard Medical School; Associate Neurologist and Director of Stroke Service, Massachusetts General Hospital, Boston

HARVEY G. KLEIN, M.D.

Chief, Department of Transfusion Medicine, Clinical Center, National Institutes of Health, Bethesda

JAMES P. KNOCHEL, M.D.

Professor of Internal Medicine, The University of Texas Southwestern Medical Center; Chairman, Department of Medicine, Presbyterian Hospital, Dallas

HOWARD K. KOH, M.D.

Associate Professor of Dermatology, Medicine, and Public Health; Co-Director, Skin Oncology Program; Director, Cancer Prevention and Control Center, Boston University Schools of Medicine and Public Health, Boston

ANTHONY KOMAROFF, M.D.

Professor of Medicine, Harvard Medical School; Director, Division of General Medicine, Brigham and Women's Hospital, Boston

STANLEY J. KORSMEYER, M.D.

Professor, Howard Hughes Medical Institute, Washington University School of Medicine, Saint Louis

WILLIAM J. KOVACS, M.D.

Associate Professor of Medicine, Division of Endocrinology, Vanderbilt University School of Medicine, Nashville

STEPHEN M. KRANE, M.D.

Persis, Cyrus, and Marlow B. Harrison Professor of Medicine, Harvard Medical School; Physician and Chief, Arthritis Unit, Massachusetts General Hospital, Boston

DONALD KUFE, M.D.

Professor of Medicine, Harvard Medical School and Dana-Farber Cancer Institute, Boston

HELENA KUIVANIEMI, M.D., Ph.D.

Research Assistant Professor, Department of Biochemistry and Molecular Biology, Jefferson Medical College of Thomas Jefferson University, Philadelphia

J. THOMAS La MONT, M.D.

Chief, Section of Gastroenterology, The University Hospital, Boston

LEWIS LANDSBERG, M.D

Irving S. Cutter Professor and Chairman, Department of Medicine, Northwestern University Medical School; Physician-in-Chief, Northwestern Memorial Hospital, Chicago

H. CLIFFORD LANE, M.D.

Clinical Director, National Institute of Allergy and Infectious Diseases, National Institutes of Health; Chief, Clinical Molecular Retrovirology Section, Laboratory of Immunoregulation, National Institute of Allergy and Infectious Diseases, NIH, Bethesda

THOMAS J. LAWLEY, M.D.

Professor and Chairman, Department of Dermatology, Emory University School of Medicine, Atlanta

ALEXANDER R. LAWTON III, M.D.

Edward C. Stahlman Professor in Pediatric Physiology and Cell Metabolism; Professor of Pediatrics and Microbiology; Head, Division of Pediatric Immunology and Rheumatology, Vanderbilt University School of Medicine, Nashville

J. MICHAEL LAZARUS, M.D.

Associate Professor of Medicine, Harvard Medical School; Senior Physician and Director of Clinical Services, Nephrology Division, Brigham & Women's Hospital, Boston

ROBERT SAMUEL LEBOVICS, M.D., F.A.C.S.

Chief, Otolaryngology, National Institute on Deafness and Other Communication Disorders, National Institutes of Health, Bethesda

RICHARD T. LEE, M.D.

Assistant Professor of Medicine, Harvard Medical School; Director, Noninvasive Cardiac Laboratory, Brigham and Women's Hospital, Boston

PHILLIP I. LERNER, M.D.

Professor of Medicine, Case Western Reserve University School of Medicine; Chief, Division of Infectious Diseases, The Mount Sinai Medical Center, Cleveland

NORMAN G. LEVINSKY, M.D.

Wade Professor and Chairman, Department of Medicine, Boston University School of Medicine; Physician-in-Chief, Boston City Hospital and Boston University Medical Center Hospital, Boston

MATTHEW E. LEVISON, M.D.

Professor of Medicine and Chief, Division of Infectious Diseases, Medical College of Pennsylvania, Philadelphia

RICHARD W. LIGHT, M.D.

Professor of Medicine, University of California, Irvine; Physician, Veterans Administration Hospital, Long Beach

CHRISTOPHER H. LINDEN, M.D., F.A.C.E.P.

Associate Professor of Medicine; Associate Director, Toxicology Service and Associate Clinical Director, Department of Emergency Medicine, University of Massachusetts Medical Center, Worcester

PETER E. LIPSKY, M.D.

Professor of Internal Medicine and Microbiology; Director, Rheumatic Diseases Division; Director, Harold C. Simmons Arthritis Research Center, The University of Texas Southwestern Medical Center at Dallas, Dallas

LEO X. LIU, M.D., D.T.M.H.

Assistant Professor of Medicine, Harvard Medical School; Division of Infectious Diseases, Department of Medicine, Beth Israel Hospital, Boston

BERNARD LO, M.D.

Professor of Medicine; Director, Program in Medical Ethics; Co-Director, Robert Wood Johnson Clinical Scholars Program; Physician, Moffitt-Long Hospitals, University of California, San Francisco

RICHARD M. LOCKSLEY, M.D.

Associate Professor of Medicine and Microbiology and Immunology and Chief, Division of Infectious Diseases, Department of Medicine, University of California, San Francisco

DAN L. LONGO, M.D.

Director, Biological Response Modifiers Program, Division of Cancer Treatment, National Cancer Institute, Frederick Cancer Research and Development Center, Frederick

FREDERICK H. LOVEJOY, Jr., M.D.

William Berenberg Professor of Pediatrics, Harvard Medical School; Associate Physician-in-Chief, The Children's Hospital, Boston

SHEILA A. LUKEHART, Ph.D.

Research Associate Professor, Department of Medicine, Division of Infectious Diseases, University of Washington School of Medicine, Seattle

LAWRENCE C. MADOFF, M.D.

Assistant Professor of Medicine, Harvard Medical School; Channing Laboratory, Brigham and Women's Hospital; Division of Infectious Diseases, Beth Israel Hospital, Boston

JAMES HARVEY MAGUIRE, M.D.

Associate Professor of Medicine, Harvard Medical School; Physician, Brigham and Women's Hospital, Boston

HENRY J. MANKIN, M.D.

Edith M. Ashley Professor of Orthopaedic Surgery, Harvard Medical School; Chief, Orthopaedic Services, Massachusetts General Hospital, Boston

JOSEPH B. MARTIN, M.D., Ph.D., F.R.C.P. (C), M.A. (Hon.)

Professor of Neurology and Chancellor, University of California, San Francisco

JOEL B. MASON, M.D.

Assistant Professor, Divisions of Clinical Nutrition and Gastroenterology; Scientist, USDA Human Nutrition Research Center on Aging, Tufts University, Boston

HENRY MASUR, M.D.

Chief, Critical Care Medicine Department, National Institutes of Health, Bethesda

ROBERT J. MAYER, M.D.

Professor of Medicine and Clinical Director, Department of Medicine, Dana-Farber Cancer Institute, Boston

JOHN D. McCONNELL, M.D.

Associate Professor of Surgery, Division of Urology, The University of Texas Southwestern Medical Center, Dallas

E. R. McFADDEN, Jr., M.D.

Argyl J. Beams Professor of Medicine and Director, Division of Pulmonary and Critical Care Medicine, Case Western Reserve University School of Medicine, Cleveland

JAMES E. McGUIGAN, M.D.

Chairman, Department of Medicine, University of Florida College of Medicine, Gainesville

NANCY K. MELLO, Ph.D.

Professor of Psychology, Department of Psychiatry (Neuroscience), Harvard Medical School, Boston; Co-Director, Alcohol and Drug Abuse Research Center, McLean Hospital, Belmont

JERRY R. MENDELL, M.D.

Professor and Chairman, Department of Neurology, The Ohio State University College of Medicine, Columbus

JOHN MENDELSOHN, M.D.

Winthrop Rockefeller Chair in Medical Oncology and Chairman, Department of Medicine, Memorial Sloan-Kettering Cancer Center

JACK H. MENDELSON, M.D.

Professor of Psychiatry (Neuroscience), Harvard Medical School, Boston; Co-Director, Alcohol and Drug Abuse Research Center, McLean Hospital, Belmont

RICHARD A. MILLER, M.D.

Associate Professor of Medicine, University of Washington School of Medicine; Chief, Infectious Disease Section, Seattle VA Medical Center, Seattle

JOHN D. MINNA, M.D.

Professor of Medicine and Pharmacology and Director, Simmons Cancer Center, The University of Texas Southwestern Medical Center, Dallas

JEROME H. MODELL, M.D.

Professor of Anesthesiology, College of Medicine, University of Florida; Senior Associate Dean for Clinical Affairs; Associate Vice President for University of Florida Health Science Center Affiliations, Gainesville

J. P. MOHR, M.D.

Sciarra Professor of Clinical Neurology, College of Physicians and Surgeons of Columbia University Neurological Institute, New York

STEPHEN MORSE, Ph.D.

Director, Division of Sexually Transmitted Diseases Laboratory Research, National Center for Infectious Diseases, Centers for Disease Control and Prevention, Atlanta

KENNETH M. MOSER, M.D.

Professor of Medicine, School of Medicine, University of California at San Diego; Director, Pulmonary/Critical Care Division, UCSD Medical Center, San Diego

ARNOLD M. MOSES, M.D.

Professor of Medicine and Director, Clinical Research, Unit, State University of New York Health Science Center, Syracuse

HARALAMPOS M. MOUTSOPOULOS, M.D.

Professor and Head of Medicine, Department of Internal Medicine, University of Ioannina Medical School, Ioannina, Greece

ROBERT F. MUNFORD, M.D.

Professor of Internal Medicine and Microbiology, University of Texas Southwestern Medical Center, Dallas

DANIEL M. MUSHER, M.D.

Chief, Infectious Disease Section, Veterans Affairs Medical Center; Professor of Medicine and Professor of Microbiology and Immunology, Baylor College of Medicine, Houston

ROBERT J. MYERBURG, M.D.

Professor of Medicine and Physiology and Director, Division of Cardiology, University of Miami School of Medicine, Miami

LEE M. NADLER, M.D.

Professor of Medicine, Harvard Medical School; Division of Tumor Immunology, Dana-Farber Cancer Institute, Boston

THEODORE ELLIOT NASH, M.D.

Senior Scientist, Laboratory of Parasitic Diseases, National Institutes of Health, Bethesda

LAURENCE NEEDLEMAN, M.D.

Associate Professor of Radiology and Associate Director, Division of Diagnostic Ultrasound, Thomas Jefferson University Hospital, Philadelphia

THOMAS B. NUTMAN, M.D.

Senior Investigator, Laboratory of Parasitic Diseases, National Institute of Allergy and Infectious Diseases, National Institutes of Health, Bethesda

JOHN OATES, M.D.

Professor and Chairman, Department of Medicine, Vanderbilt University School of Medicine; Physician-in-Chief, Vanderbilt University Hospital, Nashville

JERROLD M. OLEFSKY, M.D.

Professor of Medicine and Head, Division of Endocrinology and Metabolism, School of Medicine, University of California at San Diego, La Jolla

ANDREW B. ONDERDONK, Ph.D.

Associate Professor of Pathology, Harvard Medical School; Director, Clinical Microbiology Laboratory, Brigham and Women's Hospital, Boston

STUART H. ORKIN, M.D.

Leland Fikes Professor of Pediatric Medicine, Harvard Medical School; Children's Hospital, Boston

ROBERT A. O'ROURKE, M.D.

Charles Conrad Brown Distinguished Professor of Medicine, The University of Texas Health Science Center at San Antonio; Director of Cardiology, The University of Texas Health Science Center Teaching Hospitals, San Antonio

DARWIN L. PALMER, M.D.

Professor of Medicine and Chief, Division of Infectious Diseases, University of New Mexico School of Medicine, Albuquerque

JOSEPH E. PARRILLO, M.D.

James B. Herrick Professor of Medicine, Rush Medical College; Chief, Section of Cardiology; Chief, Section of Critical Care Medicine and Medical Director, Rush Heart Institute, Rush-Presbyterian-St. Luke's Medical Center, Chicago

RICHARD C. PASTERNAK, M.D.

Assistant Professor of Medicine, Harvard Medical School; Director of Preventive Cardiology and Cardiac Rehabilitation, Massachusetts General Hospital, Boston

PETER L. PERINE, M.D.

Professor of Epidemiology, Center for AIDS and STD, University of Washington, Seattle; Professor of Tropical Public Health and Medicine Emeritus, Uniformed Services University of the Health Sciences, Bethesda

ELIOT A. PHILLIPSON, M.D.

Sir John and Lady Eaton Professor of Medicine and Chair, Department of Medicine, University of Toronto; Physician-in-Chief, Mount Sinai Hospital, Toronto

GERALD B. PIER, Ph.D.

Associate Professor of Medicine, Harvard Medical School; Channing Labatory, Brigham and Women's Hospital, Boston

DANIEL K. PODOLSKY, M.D.

Associate Professor of Medicine, Harvard Medical School; Chief, Gastrointestinal Unit, Massachusetts General Hospital, Boston

RONALD J. POLINSKY, M.D.

Senior Associate Director, Human Pharmacology, Drug Safety Department, Sandoz Research Institute, Sandoz Pharmaceuticals Corporation, East Hanover, New Jersey

RONALD E. POLK, Pharm.D.

Professor of Pharmacy and Medicine, School of Pharmacy, Medical College of Virginia, Virginia Commonwealth University, Richmond

MATTHEW POLLACK, M.D.

Professor of Medicine, Uniformed Services University of the Health Sciences, F. Edward Hebert School of Medicine, Bethesda

JOHN T. POTTS, Jr., M.D.

Jackson Professor of Clinical Medicine, Harvard Medical School; Physician-in-Chief, Massachusetts General Hospital, Boston

LAWRIE W. POWELL, M.D.

Professor of Medicine, The University of Queensland; Director, Queensland Institute of Medical Research, Brisbane

DARWIN J. PROCKOP, M.D.

Professor and Chairman, Department of Biochemistry and Molecular Biology, Jefferson Medical College of Thomas Jefferson University; Director, Jefferson Institute of Molecular Medicine, Philadelphia

AMY PRUITT, M.D.

Assistant Professor of Neurology, University of Pennsylvania School of Medicine and Graduate Hospital, Philadelphia

LOUIS J. PTÁČEK, M.D.

Department of Neurology, The University of Utah School of Medicine, Salt Lake City

JOEL M. RAPPEPORT, M.D.

Professor of Medicine, Yale University School of Medicine; Director, Bone Marrow Transplantation Program, Yale New Haven Hospital, New Haven

NEIL H. RASKIN, M.D.

Professor of Neurology, University of California, San Francisco

C. GEORGE RAY, M.D.

Professor and Chairman, Department of Pediatrics, St. Louis University School of Medicine, St. Louis

SHARON LEE REED, M.D.

Associate Professor of Pathology and Medicine and Associate Director, Microbiology Laboratory, Division of Infectious Diseases, UCSD Medical Center, San Diego

ANTONIO J. REGINATO, M.D.

Head, Division of Rheumatology; Professor of Medicine, Cooper Hospital/University Medical Center, University of Medicine and Dentistry of New Jersey/Robert Wood Johnson Medical School at Camden, Camden

RICHARD C. REICHMAN, M.D.

Professor of Medicine and Head, Infectious Disease Unit, University of Rochester School of Medicine and Dentistry, Rochester

NEIL M. RESNICK, M.D.

Assistant Professor of Medicine, Harvard Medical School; Chief, Division of Gerontology, Brigham and Women's Hospital; Geriatric Research Education and Clinical Center, Brockton-West Roxbury Veterans Administration Medical Center, Boston

HERBERT Y. REYNOLDS, M.D.

Chairman, Department of Medicine and J. Lloyd Huck Professor of Medicine, The Pennsulvania State University; University Hospital, The Milton S. Hershey Medical Center, Hershey

STUART RICH, M.D.

Professor of Medicine and Chief, Section of Cardiology, University of Illinois at Chicago College of Medicine, Chicago

GARY S. RICHARDSON, M.D.

Instructor in Medicine, Harvard Medical School; Associate Physician, Brigham and Women's Hospital, Boston

HAL B. RICHERSON, M.D.

Professor of Internal Medicine, University of Iowa College of Medicine; University of Iowa Hospitals and Clinics, Iowa City

JAMES M. RICHTER, M.D.

Assistant Professor of Medicine, Harvard Medical School; Chief, Gastrointestinal Clinic, Massachusetts General Hospital, Boston

R. PAUL ROBERTSON, M.D.

Professor of Medicine and Cell Biology; Director, Division of Diabetes, Endocrinology and Metabolism, University of Minnesota, Minneapolis

ALLAN H. ROPPER, M.D.

Professor of Neurology, Tufts University School of Medicine; Chief, Division of Neurology, St. Elizabeth's Medical Center, Boston

IRWIN H. ROSENBERG, M.D.

Professor of Medicine, Nutrition and Physiology; Director, USDA Human Nutrition Research Center on Aging, Tufts University, Boston

LEON E. ROSENBERG, M.D.

President, Bristol-Myers Squibb Pharmaceutical Research Institute, Princeton

WENDELL F. ROSSE, M.D.

Florence Reynaud McAlister Professor of Medicine and Medical Research, Duke University School of Medicine; Duke University Medical Center, Durham

DANIEL ROTROSEN, M.D.

Medical Office, Laboratory of Host Defenses, National Institute of Allergy and Infectious Diseases, National Institutes of Health, Bethesda

JODI ROY, M.S., R.D.

Frances Stern Nutrition Center, New England Medical Center Hospital, Boston

ARTHUR H. RUBENSTEIN, M.D.

Lowell T. Coggeshall Professor; Chairman, Department of Medicine, University of Chicago Pritzker School of Medicine, Chicago

JEREMY N. RUSKIN, M.D.

Associate Professor of Medicine, Harvard Medical School; Director, Cardiac Arrhythmia Service, Massachusetts General Hospital, Boston

ARTHUR I. SAGALOWSKY, M.D.

Professor of Urology and Surgical Director of Renal Transplantation, The University of Texas Southwestern Medical Center, Dallas

MATTHEW SAMORE, M.D.

Instructor in Medicine, Harvard Medical School; New England Deaconess Hospital, Boston

JAY P. SANFORD, M.D.

Professor of Internal Medicine, University of Texas Southwestern Medical School; Dean Emeritus, Uniformed Services University of the Health Sciences, Dallas

DAVID A. SCHEINBERG, M.D., Ph.D.

Chief, Leukemia Service, Memorial Sloan-Kettering Cancer Center, New York

I. HERBERT SCHEINBERG, M.D.

Senior Lecturer in Medicine, College of Physicians and Surgeons, Columbia University; Senior Research Associate, St. Luke's/Roosevelt Hospital, New York

W. MICHAEL SCHELD, M.D.

Professor of Internal Medicine and Neurosurgery and Associate Chair for Residency Programs, University of Virginia School of Medicine, Charlottesville

ALAN L. SCHILLER, M.D.

Irene Heinz Given and John LaPorte Given Professor and Chairman of Pathology, Mount Sinai School of Medicine; Chairman of Pathology, The Mount Sinai Hospital, New York

ROBERT T. SCHOOLEY, M.D.

Professor of Medicine and Head, Infectious Disease Division, University of Colorado Health Sciences Center, Denver

JOHN SPEER SCHROEDER, M.D.

Professor of Medicine (Cardiology), Stanford University School of Medicine; Stanford Hospital, Stanford

ANNE SCHUCHAT, M.D.

Medical Epidemiologist, Meningitis and Special Pathogens Branch, Division of Bacterial and Mycotic Diseases, National Center for Infectious Diseases, Centers for Disease Control and Prevention, Atlanta

MARC A. SCHUCKIT, M.D.

Professor of Psychiatry, School of Medicine, University of California at San Diego; Director, Alcohol Research Center, San Diego Veteran's Administration Medical Center, La Jolla

PETER H. SCHUR, M.D.

Professor of Medicine, Harvard Medical School; Department of Rheumatology, Brigham and Women's Hospital, Boston

DAVID S. SEGAL, Ph.D.

Professor of Psychiatry, University of California at San Diego, La Jolla

JULIAN I. SEIFTER, M.D.

Associate Professor of Medicine, Harvard Medical School; Physician, Brigham and Women's Hospital, Boston

ANDREW P. SELWYN, M.D.

Associate Professor of Medicine, Harvard Medical School; Director of Cardiac Catheterization, Brigham and Women's Hospital, Boston

PETER A. SELWYN, M.D., M.P.H.

Associate Professor of Internal Medicine, Epidemiology and Public Health, and Associate Director, AIDS Program, Yale University School of Medicine, New Haven

MARY-ANN SHAFER, M.D.

Professor of Pediatrics; Associate Director, Division of Adolescent Medicine, Department of Pediatrics, School of Medicine, University of California, San Francisco

GORDON C. SHARP, M.D.

Curators' Professor and Michael Einbender Distinguished Professor of Medicine; Director, Division of Immunology and Rheumatology; Director, Arthritis Center; Director, Missouri Arthritis Rehabilitation Research and Training Center; Associate Chairman for Research, Department of Internal Medicine, University of Missouri-Columbia School of Medicine; Director, Antinuclear Antibody Laboratory, University of Missouri Hospital & Clinics, Columbia

ELIZABETH M. SHORT, M.D.

Associate Chief Medical Director for Academic Affairs, Department of Veteran's Affairs, Washington, DC

GEORGE R. SIBER, M.D.

Associate Professor of Medicine, Harvard Medical School; Director, Massachusetts Public Health Biologic Laboratories, Jamaica Plain

WILLIAM SILEN, M.D.

Johnson and Johnson Professor of Surgery, Harvard Medical School; Surgeon-in-Chief, Beth Israel Hospital, Boston

FRED E. SILVERSTEIN, M.D.

Professor of Medicine and Director, Gastrointestinal Endoscopy Fellowship Training, University of Washington School of Medicine, Seattle

KARL L. SKORECKI, M.D., F.R.C.P.(C)

Director, Division of Nephrology, Department of Medicine and Pediatrics, University of Toronto, Toronto

THOMAS L. SLAMOVITZ, M.D.

Professor and Vice Chairman, Department of Ophthalmology and Professor of Neurology and Neurosurgery, Albert Einstein College of Medicine/Montefiore Medical Center, New York

CHRISTOPHER A. SLAPAK, M.D.

Assistant Professor of Medicine, Harvard Medical School and Dana-Farber Cancer Institute, Boston

JAMES B. SNOW, JR., M.D.

Director, National Institute on Deafness and Other Communication Disorders, National Institutes of Health, Bethesda

ARTHUR J. SOBER, M.D.

Associate Professor of Dermatology, Harvard Medical School; Associate Chief of Dermatology, Massachusetts General Hospital, Boston

FRANK E. SPEIZER, M.D.

Edward H. Kass Professor of Medicine, Harvard Medical School; Co-Director, Channing Laboratory, Brigham and Women's Hospital, Boston

ANDREW SPIELMAN, SD

Professor of Tropical Public Health, Harvard School of Public Health, Boston

WALTER E. STAMM, M.D.

Professor of Medicine, University of Washington School of Medicine; Head, Infectious Diseases, Harborview Medical Center, Seattle

ALLEN C. STEERE, M.D.

Professor of Medicine and Chief, Rheumatology/Immunology, New England Medical Center and Tufts University School of Medicine, Boston

ROBERT S. STERN, M.D.

Professor, Department of Dermatology, Beth Israel Hospital, Boston

DENNIS L. STEVENS, M.D., Ph.D.

Professor of Medicine, University of Washington School of Medicine, Seattle; Chief, Infectious Diseases, VA Medical Center, Boise

GENE H. STOLLERMAN, M.D.

Professor of Medicine and Public Health, Boston University; University Hospital, Boston

RICHARD M. STONE, M.D.

Assistant Professor of Medicine, Harvard Medical School and Dana-Farber Cancer Institute, Boston

STEPHEN E. STRAUS, M.D.

Chief, Laboratory of Clinical Investigation, National Institute of Allergy and Infectious Diseases, National Institutes of Health, Bethesda

DAVID H.P. STREETEN, M.D.

Professor of Medicine and Head, Section of Endocrinology, State University of New York Health Science Center, Syracuse

ROBERT A. SWERLICK, M.D.

Associate Professor, Department of Dermatology, Emory University School of Medicine, Atlanta

RUP TANDAN, M.D., M.R.C.P.

Associate Professor of Neurology, University of Vermont College of Medicine; Attending Neurologist, Medical Center Hospital of Vermont, Burlington

JOEL D. TAUROG, M.D.

Associate Professor, Department of Internal Medicine and Investigator, Harold C. Simmons Arthritis Research Center, The University of Texas Southwestern Medical Center; Attending Physician, Parkland Memorial Hospital, Sale Lipshy University Hospital, Veterans Administration Medical Center, Dallas

BAYU TEKLU, M.D.

Professor and Chairman, Department of Internal Medicine, College of Medicine, King Saud University, Abha Branch; Consultant Physician, Asir Central Hospital, Saudi Arabia

STEPHEN F. TEMPLETON, M.D.

Assistant Professor of Dermatology and Pathology, Emory University School of Medicine, Atlanta

E. DONNALL THOMAS, M.D.

Professor of Medicine Emeritus, University of Washington; Member, Fred Hutchinson Cancer Research Center, Seattle

LUCY STUART TOMPKINS, M.D.

Associate Professor of Medicine (Infectious Diseases and Geographic Medicine) and Microbiology and Immunology, Stanford University School of Medicine; Director, Clinical Microbiology Laboratory, Stanford University Medical Center, Stanford

PHILLIP P. TOSKES, M.D.

Professor of Medicine and Chief, Division of Gastroenterology, University of Florida, Gainesville

GERARD TROMP, M.D.

Research Assistant Professor, Department of Biochemistry and Molecular Biology, Jefferson Medical College of Thomas Jefferson University, Philadelphia

E. P. TRULOCK, M.D.

Associate Professor of Medicine, Washington University School of Medicine; Barnes Hospital, St. Louis

KENNETH L. TYLER, M.D.

Associate Professor of Neurology, Medicine and Microbiology, University of Colorado Health Sciences Center; Chief, Neurology Service, VA Medical Center, Denver

DAVID VALLE, M.D.

Professor of Pediatrics and Molecular Biology and Genetics, Johns Hopkins University School of Medicine; Investigator, Howard Hughes Medical Institute, Baltimore

MAURICE VICTOR, M.D.

Professor of Medicine (Neurology), Dartmouth Medical School, Hanover; Distinguished Physician of the Veterans Administration, White River Junction

JAMES F. WALLACE, M.D.

Professor of Medicine, University of Washington School of Medicine; Associate Physican-in-Chief, University of Washington Medical Center, Seattle

RICHARD J. WALLACE, Jr., M.D.

Chairman, Department of Microbiology, University of Texas Health Center, Tyler

PETER D. WALZER, M.D.

Professor of Medicine, University of Cincinnati College of Medicine; Chief, Infectious Disease Section, VA Medical Center, Cincinnati

LEONARD WARTOFSKY, M.D.

Professor of Medicine and Physiology, Uniformed Services University of the Health Sciences; Chairman, Department of Medicine, Washington Hospital Center, Washington, DC

CARL V. WASHINGTON, Jr. M.D.

Assistant Professor of Dermatology, Emory University School of Medicine, Atlanta

STEVEN E. WEINBERGER, M.D.

Associate Professor of Medicine, Harvard Medical School; Associate Chairman for Education, Department of Medicine, and Clinical Director, Pulmonary and Critical Care Division, Beth Israel Hospital, Boston

LOUIS WEINSTEIN, M.D., Ph.D.

Senior Physician (Emeritus), Department of Medicine, Brigham and Women's Hospital

ROBERT A. WEINSTEIN, M.D., F.A.C.P.

Professor of Medicine and Program Director, Joint University of Illinois/University of Chicago Infectious Disease Fellowship Training Program, Department of Medicine, Michael Reese Hospital and Medical Center, Chicago

PETER F. WELLER, M.D.

Associate Professor of Medicine, Harvard Medical School; Division of Infectious Diseases, Department of Medicine, Beth Israel Hospital, Boston

MICHAEL R. WESSELS, M.D.

Associate Professor of Medicine, Harvard Medical School; Associate Physician, Beth Israel Hospital; Division of Infectious Diseases, Channing Laboratory, Brigham and Women's Hospital, Boston

NICHOLAS J. WHITE, M.B., B.S., B.Sc., M.R.C.P.

Wellcome Mahidol University, Oxford Tropical Medicine Research Programme, Faculty of Tropical Medicine, Mahidol University, Bangkok

RICHARD J. WHITLEY, M.D.

Loeb Eminent Scholar in Pediatrics and Professor of Pediatrics, Medicine and Microbiology, University of Alabama at Birmingham, Birmingham

GRANT R. WILKINSON, Ph.D.

Professor of Pharmacology, Vanderbilt University School of Medicine, Nashville

GORDON H. WILLIAMS, M.D.

Professor of Medicine, Harvard Medical School; Chief, Endocrine-Hypertension Division, Brigham and Women's Hospital, Boston

JEAN D. WILSON, M.D.

Charles Cameron Sprague Distinguished Chair and Professor of Internal Medicine; Chief, Division of Endocrinology and Metabolism, The University of Texas Southwestern Medical Center, Dallas

BRUCE U. WINTROUB, M.D.

Professor and Chairman, Department of Dermatology, University of California at San Francisco; Associate Dean, UCSF/Mt. Zion Medical Center, San Francisco

SHELDON M. WOLFF, M.D.

Endicott Professor and Chairman, Department of Medicine, Tufts University School of Medicine; Physician-in-Chief, New England Medical Center, Boston

BEVERLY WOO, M.D.

Assistant Professor of Medicine, Harvard Medical School; Physician, Brigham and Women's Hospital, Boston

ALASTAIR J. J. WOOD, M.B.Ch.B., FRCP (Edin)

Professor of Medicine and Professor of Pharmacology, Vanderbilt University School of Medicine; Attending Physician, Vanderbilt University Hospital, Nashville

THEODORE E. WOODWARD, M.D., M.A.C.P.

Professor of Medicine Emeritus, University of Maryland School of Medicine and Hospital, Baltimore

ROBERT L. WORTMANN, M.D.

Professor and Chairman, Department of Medicine, East Carolina University School of Medicine; Chief Medical Service, Pitt County Memorial Hospital, University Medical Center of Eastern Carolina-Pitt County, Greenville

SHIRLEY H. WRAY, M.D., Ph.D., F.R.C.P.

Associate Professor of Neurology, Harvard Medical School; Director, Unit for Neurovisual Disorders, Department of Neurology, Massachusetts General Hospital, Boston

PAUL W. WRIGHT, M.D.

Professor of Family Practice, University of Texas Health Center, Tyler

JOSHUA WYNNE, M.D.

Professor of Internal Medicine and Chief, Division of Cardiology, Wayne State University School of Medicine; Chief, Section of Cardiology, Harper Hospital, Detroit

KIM B. YANCEY, M.D.

Senior Investigator, Dermatology Branch, National Cancer Institute, National Institutes of Health, Bethesda

JAMES B. YOUNG, M.D.

Professor of Medicine, Northwestern University Medical School; Attending Physician, Northwestern Memorial Hospital, Chicago

DORI F. ZALEZNIK, M.D.

Assistant Professor of Medicine, Harvard Medical School; Hospital Epidemiologist, Beth Israel Hospital, Boston

PREFACE

Since the first edition of *Harrison's Principles of Internal Medicine* was published nearly 50 years ago, each subsequent edition has built upon the solid clinical foundation and scientific advances occurring in the interim. In the present 13th edition of *Harrison's*, the Editors have extensively revised the text to reflect important advances in our understanding of the biology and pathophysiology of disease and at the same time to build appropriate links between the extraordinary advances in basic science and clinical medicine, and to emphasize these advances while retaining those facts which, while not new, remain clinically useful and important. Every chapter in the 13th edition has been revised or substantially rewritten, and major new ones have been added. In this preface, we cannot describe all of these revised sections. However, we would like to call to the reader's attention some of the most important ones:

Part One, "Introduction to Clinical Medicine," contains new chapters dealing with medical ethics and the impact of social factors on disease, including the effects of age, gender, genetic background, geography, and ethnic origin. These factors importantly influence the incidence and clinical expression of human disease. Examples of women's health issues discussed in Chap. 5 include screening for ischemic heart disease and discussions of osteoporosis and immunologically mediated diseases in women. Important medical disorders during pregnancy are dealt with in a new Chap. 6. A new Chap. 8, "Geriatric Medicine," describes age-related changes in each organ system and their clinical consequences. There is also a detailed discussion of the management of common geriatric conditions, including intellectual impairment, mobility, incontinence, and iatrogenic drug reactions. Two timely chapters (9 and 10) focus on cost awareness and the quantitative aspects of medicine.

Part Two, "Cardinal Manifestations of Disease," remains the mainstay of this edition, and serves as a comprehensive introduction to clinical medicine. Major patient symptoms are reviewed by organ systems and correlated with specific disease states—the basis of differential diagnosis. The 13th edition also contains chapters on headache, back and neck pain, fever, including fever of unknown origin, and disturbances of smell, taste, and hearing. There is an entirely new and extensively rewritten chapter on diarrhea and constipation, as well as a completely new chapter on jaundice.

Part Three, "Genetics and Disease," has been extensively updated, including a new chapter on genes and neoplasia.

Part Four, "Clinical Pharmacology" and Part Five, "Clinical Nutrition," have been reorganized and updated. The chapters on clinical pharmacology include principles of drug therapy and a new chapter on adverse reactions to drugs. Up-to-date coverage of the physiology and pharmacology of the autonomic nervous system explores its key role in many disease states and the various ways in which drugs interact with this system. Included here also is an updated chapter on G proteins and the regulation of second messengers.

Coverage of nutrition in clinical medicine encompasses nutritional requirements, the assessment of nutritional status, important eating disorders such as anorexia nervosa and bulimia, and obesity. New discussions are presented on diet therapy, including enteral and parenteral nutrition.

A primarily etiologically oriented review in Part Six, "Infectious Disease," has been extensively revised and updated under the aegis of our new editor, Dennis L. Kasper. Here the reader will find the latest approaches to the diagnosis, prevention, and treatment of bacterial, viral, and fungal infections and parasitic infestations. New chapters include "Infections (Excluding AIDS) in Injection Drug Users," "Infections in the Immunocompromised Host," and "Infec-

tions of Skin, Muscle, and Soft Tissues." There have also been major revisions of chapters covering host-organism interaction, the laboratory diagnosis of infectious diseases, septicemia and septic shock, nosocomial infections, and molecular mechanisms of bacterial pathogenesis. There is an important and up-to-date chapter on the human retroviruses.

We believe that the chapter on HIV disease and AIDS by Anthony S. Fauci and H. Clifford Lane is one of the most comprehensive and up-to-date treatises on AIDS. It covers the areas from the natural history and epidemiology to a scholarly treatise on the immunopathogenic mechanisms of HIV disease. In addition, the chapter contains both an organ system by organ system approach as well as an infection breakdown of the major complications of HIV disease.

The core of *Harrison's*, disorders of the organ systems, encompasses Parts Seven through Fourteen, and includes succinct accounts of the pathophysiology of the major human diseases, with emphasis on disease manifestations, diagnostic procedures, differential diagnosis, and treatment strategies. This comprehensive review of organ system disorders includes new chapters on electrocardiography, with excellent new illustrations on the electrocardiographic recognition of acute myocardial infarction. There are updated chapters on cystic fibrosis, lung transplantation, glomerulopathies associated with multisystem diseases, acid-peptic disease (with special focus on *H. pylori*), acute and chronic hepatitis, and liver transplantation.

The section on hematology and oncology includes chapters on oncogenes and tumor suppressor genes, with thorough discussions of p53, the tumor suppressor gene most commonly lost or mutated in human cancers. There is an important new chapter on cancer therapy, with emphasis on immunotherapy and the potential role of gene therapy. There are also new chapters on disorders affecting multiple endocrine systems, porphyrias, and gout. The chapter on diabetes includes a discussion of the impact of tight control on the development of diabetic complications.

In the Part Fourteen, "Neurological Diseases," there are new chapters on the impact of neurobiology on both neurology and psychiatry. There is also a detailed tabulation of the recent molecular genetic discoveries in neurology. There are new chapters on clinical electrophysiology, demyelinating diseases like multiple sclerosis, bacterial meningitis and brain abscess, viral diseases of the central nervous system, and disorders of the autonomic nervous system. For the first time there is a chapter on chronic fatigue syndrome, an entity which has created great interest because of its relationship to psychosomatic medicine.

Finally, Part Fifteen, "Environmental and Occupational Hazards," has been expanded and reorganized.

In the 12th edition of *Harrison's*, the editors decided to identify laboratory data using the International System (SI) of units for clinical laboratory values, plus the conventional system of laboratory nomenclature used in most hospitals in the United States. We felt this was important, since SI units are in frequent use in many countries other than the United States. In the 12th edition and in the present 13th edition, we have listed the SI units first and the conventional units in parentheses for all measurements except blood pressure, which is given only in millimeters of mercury, and for those measurements in which the numbers are the same for both systems. As the readers of the medical literature may be aware, in 1992 the *New England Journal of Medicine*, having previously endorsed SI units, decided to "retreat" to the use of only conventional units. However, the *Harrison's* editors have concluded that, at least for the 13th edition, we should continue to use the SI units, with conventional units in parentheses. In most instances, the interconversion between SI and conventional units is straightforward. However, it is imperative that readers consult their own laboratory for normal values. Perhaps the greatest potential danger inherent in the existence of the two systems is in the interpretation of plasma glucose and plasma calcium levels, but caution should be observed in the interpretation of all laboratory values.

In view of the requirements for continuing education for licensure and relicensure, as well as the emphasis on certification and recertification, a revision of the *Pre-Test Self-Assessment and Review* will be published with this edition. It consists of several hundred questions based on *Harrison's*, along with answers and explanations for the answers. In addition, the *Companion Handbook* that was pioneered as a supplement to the 11th edition of *Harrison's* is being updated and will appear shortly.

One of the strengths of *Harrison's* is the close-knit relationship among the editors. In that context, we are delighted to welcome as a new editor Dr. Dennis L. Kasper, who possesses great depth and expertise in all aspects of infectious diseases. Dr. Kasper is Chief of the Infectious Diseases Division at the Beth Israel Hospital in Boston and serves as Co-Director of the Channing Laboratory, which is associated with the Brigham and Women's Hospital. He is also Professor of Medicine at the Harvard Medical School. We welcome Dr. Kasper as both a new editor and distinguished colleague.

We also wish to express our appreciation to our many associates and colleagues, who, as experts in their fields, have helped us with constructive criticism and helpful suggestions: Robert Alpern, Jon Astor, JudyAnn Bigby, Troyen Brennan, Neil A. Breslau, Bruce Bristrian, Charles Carpenter, Richard Davey, William Dec, William P. Dillon, Robert Dluhy, Jeffrey Drazen, Stuart J. Eisendrath, Judy Falloon, Christopher Fanta, Robert A. Fishman, David W. Foster, Patricia Fraser, Jonas Galper, Alan M. Gelb, Donald Goldmann, Stephen Goldring, Linnie Golightly, Christine Grady, James E. Griffin, Rachel Haft, Robert Handin, Seigo Izumo, Joseph H. Keffer, Arthur Kleinman, Anthony Komaroff, H. Clifford Lane, Russell K. Laros, Jr., Richard M. Locksley, Joseph Loscalzo, Carlos Luciano, James Maguire, Robert Mayer, Walter O'Donnell, Tristram G. Parslow, Dolores M. Peterson, Lynn Peterson, Michael Polis, Kenneth Ryan, Frank Sacks, Jay P. Sanford, Paul Sax, Michael Seiden, Egilius Spierings, Christopher Stowell, Daniel Vlock, Robert Walker, Steven Weinberger, Michael Wessels, Alison Wichman and Edward Yeh.

This book could not have been edited without the dedicated help of our coworkers in the editorial offices of the individual editors. We are especially indebted to: Dorothy Binford, Marie Bullock, Martha Cassin, Hilda Gardner, Christy K. Gonzales, Brenda H. Hennis, Leslie LaPiana, Julie McCoy, Jaylyn Olivo, Lucy Renzi, Kathryn A. Saxon, and Elin Woodger.

Finally, we continue to be indebted to two outstanding members of the McGraw-Hill organization: J. Dereck Jeffers, Editor-in-Chief, and Stuart Boynton, Development Editor. They are an effective team who have given the editors constant encouragement and sage advice, and have been of enormous help in bringing this edition to fruition in a timely manner.

THE EDITORS

PART EIGHT

DISORDERS OF THE RESPIRATORY SYSTEM

212 APPROACH TO THE PATIENT WITH DISEASE OF THE RESPIRATORY SYSTEM

EUGENE BRAUNWALD

As in other branches of medicine, a careful and detailed history and physical examination are the cornerstones for establishing an accurate diagnosis in patients with disorders of the respiratory system. In addition, the roentgenographic examination occupies a particularly important role in the evaluation of patients with lung disease. Since abnormalities of the respiratory system are frequently a manifestation of a systemic process, a comprehensive evaluation of the patient's entire health status is essential. For example, the presence of a pulmonary lesion on x-ray may be due to metastatic disease with the primary tumor elsewhere, and hemoptysis may be due to a disorder of hemostasis. Diffuse pulmonary infiltrative disease may be secondary to diffuse scleroderma (Chap. 286), and multiple pulmonary cavities may be a manifestation of Wegener's granulomatosis (Chap. 291). All the so-called collagen vascular diseases may have prominent pulmonary manifestations. Carcinoma of the lung (Chap. 227) may be accompanied by prominent extrathoracic manifestations, which may overshadow the pulmonary lesion. These include myopathy, peripheral neuropathy, hypertrophic pulmonary osteoarthropathy, and a variety of endocrine and metabolic manifestations, including Cushing's syndrome, the carcinoid syndrome, a hyperparathyroid-like picture, inappropriate secretion of antidiuretic hormone, gonadotropin (Chap. 327), and increased frequency of pulmonary infections. Patients with AIDS frequently have pulmonary manifestations. These include pneumonia caused by *Pneumocystis carinii* (Chap. 178), commonly an "AIDS defining" illness. Other manifestations include Kaposi's sarcoma involving the tracheobronchial tree and pulmonary infection with a variety of organisms, including *Mycobacterium tuberculosis*, *Mycobacterium avium* complex, histoplasmosis, cryptococcosis, coccidioidomycosis, and cytomegalovirus.

HISTORY In eliciting the history of patients with pulmonary disease, it must be appreciated that an increasing fraction of the population is exposed to materials which are potentially toxic to the lung (Chap. 219). The history must therefore contain a detailed *occupational and personal history* with a description of exposure to hazards such as asbestos, coal, silica, beryllium, bagasse, iron oxide, tin oxide, cotton dust, titanium oxide, silver, nitrogen dioxide, animals, moldy hay, air conditioners, and furnace humidifiers. It is useful to construct a work history, which includes the patient's duties, duration of exposure, use of protective devices, and the occurrence and nature of illness in fellow workers. The occupational history should include information on a job-by-job basis as well as the military service. Contact with both wild and domestic animals may result in pulmonary symptoms, such as bronchospasm in subjects allergic to pets or, less commonly, acute pneumonitis in patients with psittacosis, tularemia (Chap. 122), or Q fever. Because it is such an important risk factor for many forms of lung disease, a history of tobacco consumption, especially cigarette smoking, must be sought

and should be quantified, generally in "pack-years." The habits of the patient with pulmonary disease must be explored. Aspiration pneumonia and pneumococcal and *Klebsiella* pneumonia are often seen in alcoholics; lung abscess occurs in intravenous drug abusers.

A history of intravenous drug abuse or of sexual relations with individuals at high risk for AIDS (Chap. 279) should be obtained, especially in patients with a pulmonary infiltrate and fever. A record of the patient's *previous residence* is of considerable importance in the diagnosis of histoplasmosis (the south and midwestern United States; Chap. 162), coccidioidomycosis (the southwestern United States; Chap. 163), tropical eosinophilia, and South American blastomycosis. For example, pulmonary mass lesions in patients in the Mediterranean Basin may be due to hydatid cysts, hemoptysis in patients from central China may be caused by paragonimiasis (Chap. 184), and in Egypt cor pulmonale frequently results from schistosomiasis (Chap. 183).

It is especially important to elicit a history of *drug exposure* in patients with unexplained pulmonary disease, since essentially every class of drugs can produce pulmonary toxicity (Chap. 218), and all parts of the respiratory apparatus can be affected, including the alveoli, tracheobronchial tree, mediastinum, pleural cavities, pulmonary vessels, respiratory muscles, and the medullary respiratory center. Examples include the interstitial infiltrative diseases caused by amiodarone, bleomycin, cyclophosphamide, methotrexate, nitrofurantoin, and sulfonamides; noncardiogenic pulmonary edema caused by heroin; bronchospasm caused by beta-adrenergic blockers, cholinergic drugs, and nonsteroidal anti-inflammatory drugs; pulmonary vasculitis from intravenous drug abuse; cough and pulmonary thromboembolism in women receiving oral contraceptives; (drug-induced) systemic lupus erythematosus with pleural involvement caused by hydralazine and procainamide; and respiratory depression caused by aminoglycoside antibiotics, opiates, and trimethaphan.

The *family history* should consider pulmonary diseases which may be genetic, such as cystic disease of the lung, pulmonary emphysema due to α_1-antitrypsin deficiency (Chap. 223), cystic fibrosis (Chap. 222), asthma (Chap. 217), hereditary telangiectasia, Kartagener's syndrome, and alveolar microlithiasis, as well as infections due to the tubercle bacilli and fungi where exposure to involved family members is important.

Dyspnea is a cardinal manifestation of diseases involving the respiratory and cardiovascular systems (Chap. 31). A detailed examination of both organ systems is therefore mandatory in every patient with this symptom. Dyspnea secondary to cardiac disease is often recognized by the presence of other evidence of heart failure, such as cardiac enlargement, gallop rhythms, and cardiac murmurs. It may be difficult to differentiate paroxysmal nocturnal dyspnea due to pulmonary edema of cardiac origin from nocturnal attacks of bronchial asthma and from chronic pulmonary disease with pooling of the secretions in the recumbent position, but a detailed description of the circumstances in which this symptom occurs is most useful. Dyspnea also is a common functional complaint, and an important clue in the identification of this form is the observation that shortness of breath often occurs at rest and is relieved during exertion; the opposite is the case in patients in whom this symptom is secondary to disease of the lungs or heart. Equally important in the differential diagnosis is a careful elucidation of the relationship of dyspnea to other symptoms such as angina pectoris (favoring ischemic heart disease) or cough with expectoration (favoring pulmonary disease).

Patients with diseases involving the respiratory system also may present with *chest pain* which is frequently caused by inflammation of the pleura, occurring in pneumonia, pulmonary thromboembolism, tuberculosis, and malignancy (Chap. 12). Pleuritic pain is usually localized to one side of the chest and is related to respiration and to movements of the thorax. Lesions confined to the pulmonary parenchyma do not produce pain, while diseases involving the organs in the mediastinum (Chap. 228) may cause local discomfort. Pain also may originate in or be referred to the chest wall; it may be due to intercostal neuritis, as in herpes zoster, or to compression of the intercostal nerves as they leave the spinal cord. Such pain is often superficial in character and may be intensified by coughing or straining. Thoracic pain also may be due to myositis, costochondral disturbances, myocardial ischemia, pericarditis, esophageal disease, and aortic dissection and aneurysm (Chap. 12). The most common causes of pain related to respiration are disorders of the chest wall, pleurisy, intercostal neuritis, and costochondral disease. The last condition characteristically causes chest pain intensified by palpation. A major task is to distinguish chest pain due to abnormalities of the bronchopulmonary system from that due to myocardial ischemia (see Chap. 12).

Cough and *expectoration* are also cardinal features of pulmonary disease (Chap. 30). Few patients can describe the severity of cough or quantity of expectoration reliably, and it is therefore desirable for the physician to inspect a 24-h collection of sputum. Cough is often precipitated by foreign materials irritating nerve endings in airways and is frequently caused by inflammation of the bronchi; the latter may be persistent (as in patients with a cigarette cough and chronic bronchitis) or acute (as in a variety of viral and bacterial infections). The time of occurrence of the cough and the character and quantity of expectorated material may point to the diagnosis. For example, bronchiectasis, lung abscess, and necrotizing pneumonia can produce purulent sputum which may have an offensive odor or be streaked with blood (Chaps. 220 and 221). In pulmonary edema, the sputum is pink, frothy, and watery (Chap. 31). Mucoid (translucent, viscid, shiny, white or gray) or mucopurulent (mucoid with flecks of yellow or green pus) sputum is characteristic of acute and chronic bronchitis. Sputum is bloody or rusty in pneumococcal pneumonia; it is thick, gelatinous, brick red, and laced with pus in *Klebsiella* pneumonia. Paroxysmal cough also may be the presenting feature in patients with bronchial asthma, in whom physical examination may or may not reveal wheezing respirations and squeaking musical sounds (Chap. 217); indeed unexplained cough may be caused by asthma. Paroxysmal cough occurs frequently in patients with left ventricular failure, in whom it generally occurs at night and in the recumbent position

(Chap. 195). Pulmonary tuberculosis (Chap. 130), though less common than previously, remains a common cause of chronic cough, as does primary neoplasm of the lung (Chap. 227). A change in the character of a chronic cough, unaccompanied by an acute infection, should alert the physician to the need to carry out a detailed examination.

Hemoptysis is often a frightening symptom (Chap. 30). Faint streaking of the sputum with blood may be observed in acute infections of the respiratory tract. However, many patients with bloody sputum have serious disease, such as pulmonary thromboembolism, tuberculosis, critical mitral stenosis, neoplasm of the lung, lung abscess, or bronchiectasis. In all instances it is necessary to exclude sources of blood in the nasopharynx and bleeding of gastric or esophageal origin. The character of the bloody expectorate should be defined, since it may be helpful in identifying the underlying disease process. Sputum which is frankly bloody without mucus or pus may be due to pulmonary thromboembolism (Chap. 226). When pus is present, pneumonia, bronchiectasis, or lung abscess should be considered. Dilute, pink, frothy sputum is observed in acute pulmonary edema (Chap. 31).

PHYSICAL EXAMINATION A careful examination of the thorax, including inspection, palpation, percussion, and auscultation, often provides the clue to the diagnosis of many common pulmonary disorders (Table 212-1). Abnormalities such as small or moderate amounts of fluid in the alveoli or in the mediastinum, bronchospasm, and pleural effusions can sometimes be detected more accurately by physical examination than by chest roentgenography or other imaging techniques. Tracheal deviation can be readily recognized on physical examination and may be observed in obstruction of a major bronchus and in atelectasis. A meticulous *general physical examination* is mandatory in patients with disorders of the respiratory system. Enlarged lymph nodes in the cervical and supraclavicular regions should be sought. Disturbances of mentation or even coma occurs in patients with acute carbon dioxide retention and hypoxemia. Telltale stains on the fingers point to heavy cigarette smoking; infected teeth and gums may occur in patients with aspiration pneumonitis and lung abscess; characteristic cutaneous lesions may point to sarcoidosis (Chap. 292), collagen vascular disease, Wegener's granulomatosis, Kaposi's sarcoma, and berylliosis, all of which may have prominent pulmonary manifestations. Clubbing of the fingers or, when advanced, osteoarthropathy (Chap. 299) may suggest carcinoma (Chap. 227) or suppurative disease (Chap. 220) of the lung, chronic hypoxemia, as occurs in patients with chronic bronchitis (Chap. 223), pulmonary arteriovenous fistula, or congenital heart disease with right-to-left shunt (Chap. 199). However, clubbing also occurs in some patients with biliary cirrhosis, regional enteritis, and ulcerative colitis. A careful search for infection in the teeth, gums, tonsils, or sinuses is

TABLE 212-1 Physical findings in some common pulmonary disorders

Disorder	Inspection	Palpation	Percussion	Auscultation
Bronchial asthma (acute attack)	Hyperinflation; use of accessory muscles	Impaired expansion; decreased fremitus	Hyperresonant; low diaphragm	Prolonged expiration; inspiratory and expiratory wheezes
Pneumothorax (complete)	Lag on affected side	Absent fremitus	Hyperresonant or tympanitic	Absent breath sounds
Pleural effusion (large)	Lag on affected side	Decreased fremitus; trachea and heart shifted away from affected side	Dullness or flatness	Absent breath sounds
Atelectasis (lobar obstruction)	Lag on affected side	Decreased fremitus; trachea and heart shifted toward affected side	Dullness or flatness	Absent breath sounds
Consolidation (pneumonia)	Possible lag or splinting on affected side	Increased fremitus	Dullness	Bronchial breath sounds; bronchophony; pectoriloquy; crackles

SOURCE: JF Murray, in *Textbook of Respiratory Medicine*, JF Murray, JA Nadel (eds), p 449.

recommended in patients suspected or known to have bronchiectasis or lung abscess.

Neurologic findings which may provide a clue to the presence of pulmonary disease include headache, drowsiness, papilledema, and other evidence of increased intracranial pressure which may occur in patients with pulmonary disease who have hypoxemia and hypercapnia. Vascular collapse is a late complication of carbon dioxide retention and is characterized by hypotension, flushed skin, sweating, and tachycardia. A detailed examination of the cardiovascular system (Chap. 187) is mandatory in patients suspected of having respiratory disease and in patients with unexplained dyspnea, cough, or cyanosis because of the frequent difficulty of differentiating disorders of the respiratory and cardiovascular systems.

DIAGNOSTIC TESTS   The *roentgenographic examination* of the chest represents the cornerstone of the diagnostic workup of the patient with suspected pulmonary disease, and it is the integration of the information obtained from the clinical examination and the roentgenogram which often provides the key to diagnosis. Every effort must be made to obtain past chest x-rays. Unfortunately, physical examination of the chest has been deemphasized, largely because of the recognition of the enormous value of imaging techniques.

Chest roentgenograms obtained in the lateral decubitus position frequently reveal small pleural effusions not evident in the upright posture. A number of other potentially important abnormalities may be associated with normal roentgenograms. These include solitary lesions less than 6 mm in diameter, acute pulmonary thromboembolism without infarction, early interstitial pneumonia, diffuse granulomatous disease such as miliary tuberculosis, interstitial disease such as scleroderma and systemic lupus erythematosus, bronchiectasis, acute chronic bronchitis, mild to moderate emphysema, endobronchial masses only partially obstructing the airways, and the majority of instances of hypoventilation due to disorders of the central nervous system or neuromuscular disease. On the other hand, gross abnormalities of thoracic structure; pulmonary, mediastinal, and pleural masses; parenchymal consolidation; cysts; cavities; and abnormalities of the pulmonary vascular bed are all detected reliably by roentgenography.

An abnormal chest roentgenogram may be the presenting feature in an asymptomatic patient. In such circumstances, the physician must make every effort to obtain earlier films in order to determine whether the lesion is new or old. Computed tomography, magnetic resonance imaging, thoracic ultrasound, angiocardiography, and pulmonary scintigraphy (Chap. 215) are additional imaging modalities which may be helpful in establishing a diagnosis in a patient with an abnormality on the plain chest roentgenogram.

A variety of other diagnostic procedures are helpful in the workup of the patient with known or suspected pulmonary disease. These are discussed in Chap. 216 and include skin tests for tuberculosis, histoplasmosis, and a variety of other fungal infections, scratch or intradermal tests to detect atopic reactions, appropriate serum complement fixation tests, and examination and culture of the sputum, pleural fluid, and bronchial washings. Bronchoscopy, bronchial brushings, and bronchoscopic biopsy have been greatly facilitated by the development of the fiberoptic bronchoscope. Mediastinoscopy, scalene node and mediastinal node biopsy, and pleural and lung biopsy (open or via transcutaneous needle) also may be instrumental in establishing a diagnosis in an otherwise asymptomatic patient. Particularly important points which must be investigated in the history of the asymptomatic patient with an abnormality discovered on a routine chest roentgenogram include exposure to individuals with tuberculosis, a history of behavior placing the patient at high risk for developing AIDS, previous tuberculin and fungal skin tests, residence in or visits to areas where fungal disease is endemic, a history of smoking and of exposure to dusts, and symptoms of systemic disease such as fever, sweat, fatigue, and weight loss.

Physiologic (lung function) studies (Chap. 214) are of limited value in establishing an etiologic diagnosis in the patient with pulmonary diseases but are occasionally diagnostic in the asthmatic with a normal examination who demonstrates reversible airflow obstruction or bronchial hyperresponsiveness. These studies are, however, very helpful in assessing the physiologic consequences of disorders of the respiratory system and chest wall, as well as in following the effects of their progression or remission and treatment. Simple functional tests, such as observing the patient climb a flight of stairs, may detect gross disablement.

In the approach to a patient with pulmonary disease, consideration must be given to the observation that substantial changes in the relative incidence of disease affecting the respiratory system have taken place in the United States during the past three decades. The prevalence of chronic infectious disorders such as lung abscess and bronchiectasis have decreased. Tuberculosis declined only to resurge when two susceptible populations, patients with AIDS and immigrants from Southeast Asia, increased. Patients with chronic bronchitis and with emphysema now survive longer and form an increasing fraction of patients with chronic respiratory disease, as do patients with environmental lung disease and with drug-induced pulmonary disease. Modern intercontinental travel has increased the appearance in the western world of parasitic infestations of the lung. Also, the reduction of immunologic competence which occurs in patients with AIDS and in diabetics as well as in the treatment of patients with a variety of malignancies and those receiving immunosuppressive drugs has led to an increasing incidence of opportunistic infections of the lungs with a variety of microorganisms rarely pathogenic in the past.

REFERENCES

FISHMAN AP (ed): *Update: Pulmonary Diseases and Disorders*. New York, McGraw-Hill, 1992

HOLLAND WW: Chronic respiratory diseases. J Epidemiol Community Health 47:4, 1993

JAAKKOLA MS et al: Respiratory symptoms in young adults should not be overlooked. Am Rev Respir Dis 147:359, 1993

MURRAY JF: History and physical examination in *Textbook of Respiratory Medicine*, JF Murray, JA Nadel (eds). Philadelphia, Saunders, 1988, pp 431–451

BAUM GL, WOLINSKY E: *Textbook of Pulmonary Diseases*, 4th ed. Boston, Little, Brown, 1989

---

213   IMPACT OF CELL AND MOLECULAR BIOLOGY ON PULMONARY DISEASE

RONALD G. CRYSTAL

The major function of the lung is to exchange gases with the environment. As such, its essential role is mechanical—to bring the ambient air into close proximity to the output of the right heart, permitting efficient gas exchange at little energy cost. The traditional methods used to assess the lung in health and disease reflect this role, with chest x-rays used to evaluate lung anatomy and physiologic tests to assess lung function. These approaches define the type and extent of lung abnormalities associated with various categories of lung disease, but they give little insight into the pathogenic processes.

These traditional methods have now been supplemented with the disciplines of cell and molecular biology. For this to become a reality, it was first necessary to have access to sufficient numbers of purified cellular and extracellular components of the lung so that they could be evaluated in vitro. Two developments made this possible: (1) techniques permitting the purification and in vitro culture of lung inflammatory and parenchymal cells; and (2) the use of the fiberoptic bronchoscope to sample the components of the epithelial surface of the lung by bronchoalveolar lavage and epithelial brushing.

The adaptation of tissue culture techniques to lung cells made it possible to study purified human lung alveolar macrophages and T lymphocytes, as well as lung parenchymal cells including bronchial and alveolar epithelial cells, endothelial cells, and mesenchymal cells.

Bronchoalveolar lavage (BAL) is a simple extension of fiberoptic bronchoscopy and typically yields 1 to 3 mL of epithelial lining fluid containing 10 to 30 $\times$ 10^6 inflammatory cells from normal individuals and up to 200 $\times$ 10^6 cells from subjects with chronic inflammatory diseases. Both the extracellular and cellular components can be assessed by the techniques of cellular and molecular biology.

Epithelial brushing is also an extension of fiberoptic bronchoscopy and permits assessment of the surface epithelium of the large airways. Typically, 7 to 10 $\times$ 10^5 bronchial epithelial cells are recovered per brush, and several samples can be obtained from each individual, permitting ready assessment of gene expression in the airway epithelium.

Four disorders will be discussed to illustrate how these techniques have led to major advances in the understanding of human lung disease: idiopathic pulmonary fibrosis, chronic beryllium disease, alpha$_1$ antitrypsin deficiency, and cystic fibrosis.

IDIOPATHIC PULMONARY FIBROSIS (IPF) IPF is a chronic inflammatory fibrotic disorder localized to the lower respiratory tract and characterized by an alveolitis dominated by alveolar macrophages and neutrophils and, to a lesser extent, lymphocytes and eosinophils (see Chap. 224). The disease usually presents as dyspnea on exertion, the chest x-ray shows diffuse reticulonodular infiltrates, and analysis of lung function reveals restrictive abnormalities. Evaluation of the inflammatory cells recovered by BAL led to the concept that the cell responsible for directing the process of scar formation is the alveolar macrophage, a cell that normally defends the alveolar structures by phagocytosing infectious agents and particulates. In IPF, for reasons not completely understood but likely related to immune complexes formed in the local milieu, the alveolar macrophages express several genes that code for potent polypeptide mediators capable of recruiting fibroblasts and signaling them to proliferate. The consequence is that fibroblasts are abundant in the milieu of chronic damage. Since fibroblasts secrete a collagenous extracellular matrix, more collagen, i.e., a scar, forms.

Among the polypeptide mediators released by alveolar macrophages of IPF patients is fibronectin, a 220-kDa dimeric glycoprotein that interacts with the connective tissue matrix and with specific receptors on fibroblasts. Studies of fibronectin gene expression in alveolar macrophages demonstrate that fibronectin mRNA levels correlate with fibronectin release. Indeed, alveolar macrophages recovered from IPF patients contain more fibronectin mRNA than do alveolar macrophages of normals (Fig. 213-1A and B).

Perhaps the most potent alveolar macrophage "growth factor" is platelet-derived growth factor (PDGF), a glycoprotein that in human alveolar macrophages is composed of dimers of A and B chains or homodimers of A or B chains. The genes for the A and B chains of PDGF are on different chromosomes and are modulated independently. Interestingly, the B chain is encoded by the c-sis gene, a cellular proto-oncogene on chromosome 22 with close homology to the v-sis gene, a transforming viral oncogene. Alveolar macrophages recovered from the lower respiratory tract of individuals with IPF express c-sis mRNA transcripts, and the PDGF protein product of the c-sis gene is released by these cells at a level fourfold greater than by normal macrophages (Fig. 213-1C). Thus, in this disease, a gene homologous to a viral oncogene is expressed in an exaggerated fashion in one site (the lower respiratory tract) and contributes to a localized proliferation of mesenchymal cells and eventual organ fibrosis. Importantly, glucocorticoid therapy (the conventional treatment) does not affect PDGF release by the macrophages. Consequently, it is no surprise that most IPF patients continue to deteriorate even when treated in this fashion.

CHRONIC BERYLLIUM DISEASE Multiple exposures to airborne beryllium dusts, salts, or fumes can result, in susceptible individuals, in a chronic interstitial lung disorder characterized by the accumulation of lymphocytes and mononuclear phagocytes and the formation of noncaseating granulomas in the lower respiratory tract (see Chap. 219). The alveolitis is dominated by alveolar macrophages and T lymphocytes, activated CD4+ helper-inducer T cells, characteristic of the T cells in sites of chronic, delayed-type hypersensitivity reactions (Fig. 213-2A). Most noteworthy, the lung T cells proliferate in response to beryllium and do so to a greater extent than do blood T cells from the same individual, i.e., the antigen-specific T cells are compartmentalized to the site of the disease (Fig. 213-2B). Furthermore, the lung T cells proliferating in response to beryllium are confined to the helper-inducer subset and the extent of the proliferative response is modulated by subsets of the DP class of the MHC locus. The proliferative response of these lung T cells is truly beryllium-specific in that the cells do not proliferate in response to other metal salts or to typical recall antigens such as tetanus toxoid or streptokinase.

Together, these observations define chronic beryllium disease as a chronic hypersensitivity disease in which beryllium-primed lung CD4+ T cells play a central role in its pathogenesis. Beryllium presumably acts as an antigen by combining (as a hapten) with one or more proteins. However, since chronic beryllium disease develops in only a small proportion of those exposed to the agent, individual susceptibility must play a major role in determining who is at risk. Recent evidence suggests the HLA DP locus plays a major role in this process. The proliferative response of lung T cells to beryllium provides a diagnostic tool to identify individuals with this disorder, thus obviating the need for chemical analysis of the lung parenchyma.

ALPHA$_1$ ANTITRYPSIN DEFICIENCY Alpha$_1$ antitrypsin (α1AT) deficiency is a hereditary disorder characterized by reduced serum levels of α1AT, an antiprotease that provides the major defense for the lower respiratory tract against the ravages of neutrophil elastase, a powerful destructive protease. The loss of this protective screen of the fragile alveolar walls results in emphysema (Chap. 223).

The emphysema is the result of a variety of mutations in the α1AT gene on chromosome 14 (Fig. 213-3A). The two parental α1AT genes are codominantly expressed and together define the α1AT level in serum. The gene is pleomorphic with approximately 75 known alleles, of which at least 20 can cause a clinically relevant deficiency state. Most normal α1AT alleles are classified as M-type. Most α1AT is synthesized by liver hepatocytes; the enzyme is a typical secretory glycoprotein that is translated on the rough endoplasmic reticulum (RER), glycosylated in the cisternae of the RER, translocated to the Golgi, and then secreted (Fig. 213-3B). The two most common "deficiency" mutations are Z (exon V, Glu^{342} GAG $\rightarrow$ Lys AAG) and S (exon III, Glu^{264} GAA $\rightarrow$ Val GTA).

The Z mutation, carried by 1 in 50 Caucasians of European descent, causes hepatocytes of homozygotes to secrete only 10 to 15 percent of the normal amount of α1AT. Because the Glu^{342} $\rightarrow$ Lys substitution reverses the charge at this residue, the Z-type α1AT molecules aggregate in the RER, less α1AT is translocated to the Golgi and subsequently secreted, and hence α1AT deficiency results.

The S mutation, carried by up to 1 in 25 persons, causes a different derangement of α1AT processing. The hepatocytes degrade an increased proportion of the newly synthesized α1AT, resulting in less α1AT for secretion and hence the deficiency state. However, the relative "deficiency" associated with the S allele is less than that associated with Z. Consequently, S homozygotes are not at risk for emphysema, but SZ heterozygotes are at mild risk.

Z homozygotes have reduced α1AT in the lung and hence have a deficient screen against proteolytic attack by neutrophil elastase (Fig. 213-3C). While S homozygotes also have reduced α1AT levels, the amount is sufficient to afford protection, i.e., the "threshold" protective level is between that of S and Z homozygotes. Based on this concept, strategies to prevent the emphysema associated with α1AT deficiency have focused on augmenting the protective screen of the lower respiratory tract with α1AT. In this regard, intravenous administration of 60 mg/kg body weight of α1AT once a week results in α1AT serum levels sufficient to maintain lung levels above that

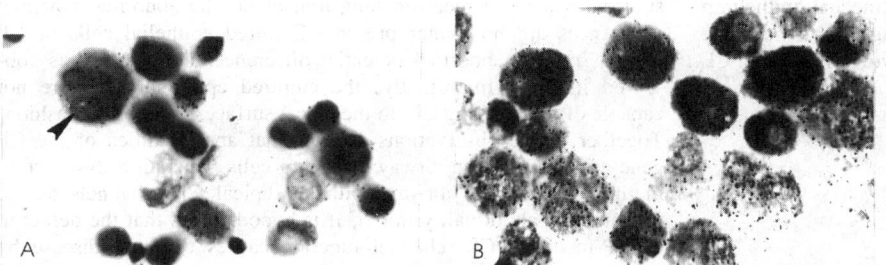

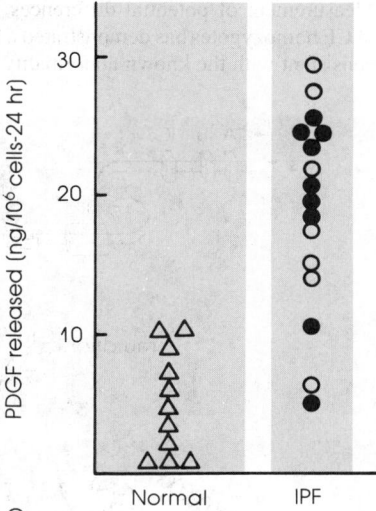

FIGURE 213-1 Exaggerated expression of alveolar macrophage genes coding for polypeptide mediators that modulate fibroblast accumulation in the alveolar walls of patients with idiopathic pulmonary fibrosis. *A*. Example of in situ hybridization analysis of fibronectin mRNA transcripts in alveolar macrophages of a normal individual. The mRNA transcripts in macrophages recovered by bronchoalveolar lavage were assessed with a ^{35}S-labeled fibronectin antisense cRNA probe and autoradiography. The grains above the macrophage (arrow) indicate fibronectin mRNA transcripts ($\times 500$). *B*. Similar to panel *A*, but with alveolar macrophages of a patient with IPF. On the average, there are twofold more fibronectin mRNA transcripts per macrophage than in normals ($\times 500$). *C*. Spontaneous exaggerated release of PDGF by alveolar macrophages recovered from the lower respiratory tract of individuals with IPF. Macrophages recovered by bronchoalveolar lavage were cultured for 24 h. Supernatants were evaluated for the presence of PDGF using a specific immunoassay. Each symbol represents one individual. For the IPF patients, closed circles represent untreated patients and open circles represent those receiving prednisone. Note that therapy has no effect on the release of this potent mediator.

necessary to provide sufficient antielastase protection to the alveoli, i.e., augmentation therapy reverses the biochemical abnormalities at the site of the target organ and thus is a rational approach to prevent the emphysema. Based on these concepts, weekly augmentation therapy is now the standard treatment for α1AT deficiency.

CYSTIC FIBROSIS (CF) CF is an autosomal recessive disorder of exocrine glands characterized in lung by accumulation of thick mucus, chronic bacterial infections, and chronic obstructive lung disease associated with severe bronchiectasis and parenchymal derangements (see Chap. 222). It is the most common lethal genetic disorder affecting Caucasian populations, with a heterozygote frequency of 1 in 20 to 25 individuals.

The gene causing CF, called the *cystic fibrosis transmembrane conductance regulator* (CFTR) gene, was localized to within approximately 300 kb in the q21-31 region of chromosome 7, using the technique of "chromosome walking" (Fig. 213-4*A*). Extensive analysis of the CFTR gene has led to the identification of more than 200 mutations, most in the 27 coding exons of the 250-kb gene. One mutation, an in-phase deletion of the codon for Phe^{508}, is responsible for 50 to 80 percent of all CF alleles.

The sequence of the CFTR gene predicts that it codes for a protein of 168 kDa that spans the plasma membrane and contains two domains capable of binding adenosine triphosphate and one domain that is phosphorylated. The CFTR protein has been clearly shown to function as a cAMP-regulated Cl$^-$ secretory channel on the apical surface of epithelial cells, although it may serve other functions as well. With mutations of the CFTR gene the cell has insufficient CFTR function, a fact relevant to the pathogenesis of the disease (Fig. 213-4*B*).

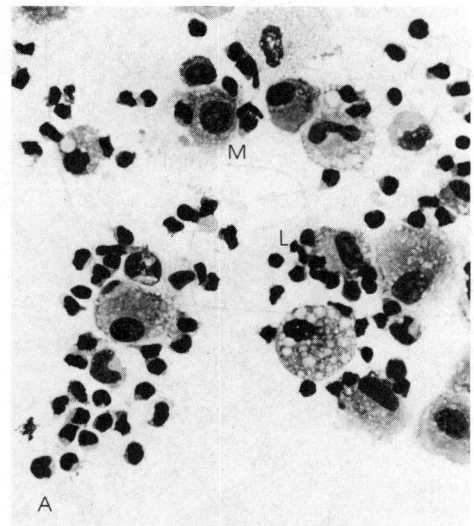

FIGURE 213-2 Beryllium-specific inflammatory processes in the lower respiratory tract of individuals with chronic beryllium disease. *A*. Inflammatory cells recovered by bronchoalveolar lavage of an individual with chronic beryllium disease. The alveolitis is dominated by lymphocytes (L) and alveolar macrophages (M) ($\times 500$). Flow cytometric analysis with appropriate monoclonal antibodies demonstrates that the lymphocytes are predominantly CD4+ helper-inducer T lymphocytes. *B*. In vitro proliferation of blood and lung T lymphocytes of patients with chronic beryllium disease and normals in response to beryllium. The data are presented as a stimulation index (values >1 represent proliferation above control) and each symbol represents one individual. Normal blood and lung T cells rarely proliferate in response to beryllium. In contrast, lung, but not blood, T cells from individuals with chronic beryllium disease respond briskly to beryllium, with the CD4+ helper-inducer T cells dominating the proliferative response.

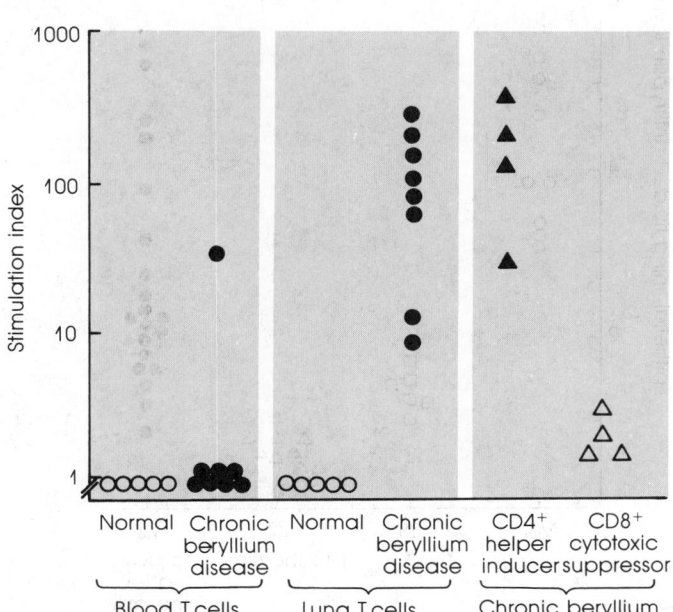

Measurement of potential differences across the tracheal epithelium of CF homozygotes has demonstrated a higher voltage than in normals, consistent with the known abnormality in electrolyte transport. In CF

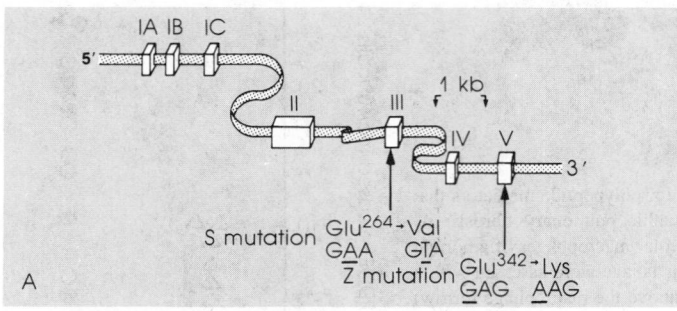

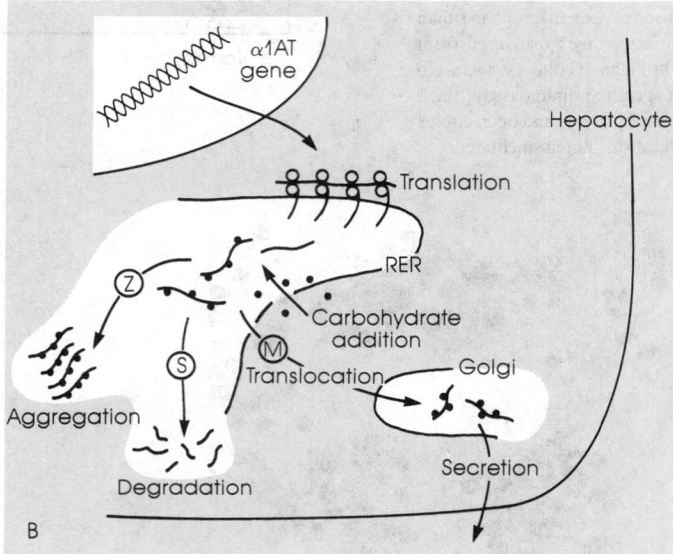

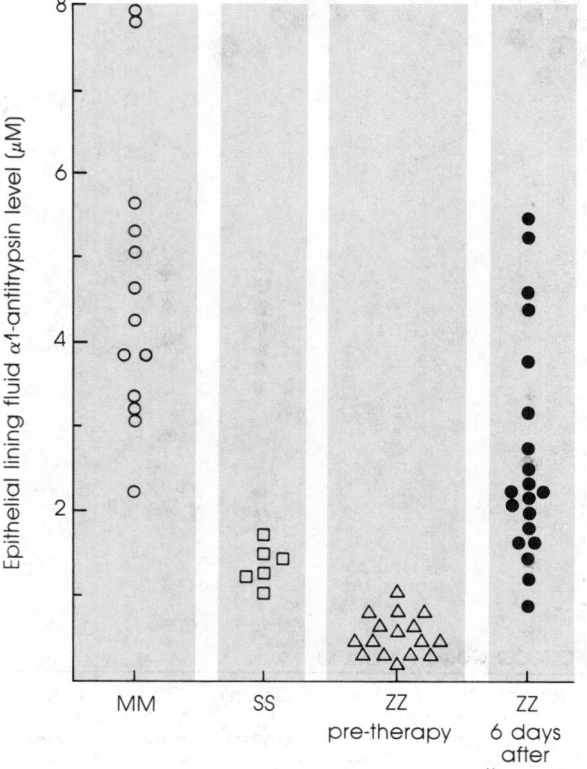

subjects who have received lung transplants the abnormal potential differences are no longer present. Cultured epithelial cells of CF patients exhibit abnormal potential differences similar to those observed in vivo. Importantly, the cultured epithelial cells are not capable of transporting Cl^- to the apical surfaces in a normal fashion. Together, these observations suggest that abnormalities of the CF gene are expressed in airway epithelial cells, causing a dysfunction in the regulation of airway epithelial apical Cl^- channels as the fundamental abnormality in CF. It is hypothesized that the defect in cAMP-mediated Cl^- channel function causes CF lung disease by modifying the quantity and composition of the airway epithelial fluid. Presumably, such changes alter the composition of mucus and thus interfere with mucociliary clearance mechanisms, resulting in chronic infection, inflammation, and derangement of the airways.

Based on this fundamental knowledge, there has been rapid progress in the development of strategies to treat the respiratory manifestations of CF by transferring the normal CFTR cDNA directly into the airway epithelium in vivo. This can be accomplished using a recombinant replication-deficient adenovirus vector to carry the normal cDNA into airway cells. Animal studies with brushing of the airway epithelium to recover the genetically modified cells have demonstrated the feasibility of this strategy and human studies will soon begin.

OTHER DISEASES   There are additional pulmonary disorders in which the application of cell and molecular biology methods has provided insight.

1 In the *pneumoconioses* (see Chap. 219), energy-dispersive x-ray analysis and electron diffraction methods permit identification and quantification of specific inorganic dusts in lung tissue and alveolar macrophages recovered by BAL. These methods provide new diagnostic techniques and new insights into the relationship of particle retention, host defense, and disease susceptibility associated with the chronic inhalation of inorganic dusts.

2 Despite the characteristic skin anergy in individuals with *sarcoidosis*, evaluation of T cells in the lower respiratory tract of patients with active disease has lead to the concept that sarcoid is a disease of heightened cellular immunity, with T cells responding to specific antigens in an exaggerated fashion at sites of disease (see Chap. 292).

3 The use of specific DNA probes now permits definitive diagnosis of *lung infection* previously very difficult to identify, including infection caused by various mycobacteria, fungi, and viruses. For example, in individuals seropositive for human immunodeficiency virus (HIV) infection (see Chap. 279), but without evidence of lung involvement, the HIV genome can be detected in lung inflammatory cells using HIV-specific DNA primers and the polymerase chain reaction.

4 *Pulmonary histiocytosis X* (eosinophilic granuloma of the lung) can be diagnosed using bronchoalveolar lavage and a monoclonal antibody (OKT6) specific for Langerhans cells (see Chap. 224).

FIGURE 213-3   Pathogenesis and therapy of alpha$_1$ antitrypsin (α1AT) deficiency. *A.* Schematic of the 12.2-kb, 7-exon (I_A-I_C, II-V) α1AT gene. The two most common mutations of the normal M gene are S and Z. *B.* Synthesis and secretion of α1AT by hepatocytes. The normal M α1AT mRNA protein is translated on the rough endoplasmic reticulum (RER), carbohydrates are added, the molecule is translocated to the Golgi and secreted. The Z mutation results in aggregation of newly synthesized α1AT in the RER while the S mutation results in degradation. *C.* Consequences of mutations in the α1AT gene at the level of the alveoli. Shown are α1AT levels in alveolar epithelial lining fluid recovered by bronchoalveolar lavage. Each symbol represents a single individual. S and Z homozygotes have "deficient" amounts of α1AT in the lung, with the level for Z homozygotes below the threshold levels necessary to protect the lung. With once-weekly intravenous augmentation therapy with purified human α1AT, the lung epithelial lining fluid α1AT level of Z homozygotes is restored above the protective threshold, thus protecting the lung from emphysema.

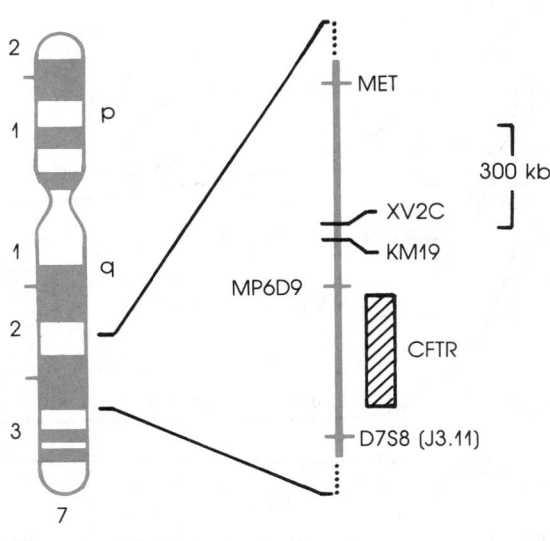

A

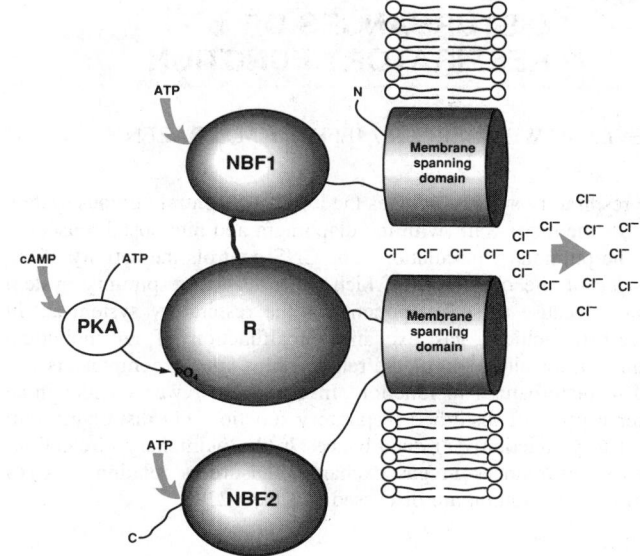

B

FIGURE 213-4   Current concepts of the molecular and biologic abnormalities associated with cystic fibrosis (CF). *A.* Localization of the cystic fibrosis transmembrane conductance regulator (CFTR) gene. Shown at the left is a representation of chromosome 7; the CF gene is localized to region q21-31. At the right is an expanded view of the region between the locus for the proto-oncogene MET and the genomic marker D7S8 (J3.11); XV2C, KM19, and MP6D9 are other marker regions of DNA containing polymorphisms useful in haplotype analysis. Chromosomal mapping localized the CFTR gene to a 250-kb region between the markers MP6D9 and D7S8. Even before the gene was identified with DNA probes, analysis of genomic DNA could accurately predict the inheritance of CF, permitting family planning. Now, specific probes have made accurate diagnosis rapid and simple. *B.* Schematic of the CFTR protein on the apical (air) membrane of an airway epithelial cell. In vivo measurements of electric potentials in the tracheal epithelium together with in vitro studies of cultured airway epithelial cells have shown that the CFTR protein functions as a cAMP-regulated Cl⁻ channel on the apical surface of the epithelial cell. The CFTR protein has three intracytoplasmic domains, nucleotide binding fold 1 (NBF1), a regulatory (R) region, and nucleotide-binding fold 2 (NBF2). Phosphokinase A (PKA), ATP, and cAMP play central roles in regulatory CFTR function. With mutations in the CFTR gene, the cells have insufficient CFTR function. This can be corrected by directed transfer of the normal CFTR cDNA to the epithelial cells of individuals with CF.

5 In the *respiratory distress syndrome of the newborn*, immature alveolar type II cells do not produce sufficient surfactant to maintain alveolar stability, leading to lung collapse. The control of surfactant biosynthesis in alveolar type II cells has been delineated using cell culture techniques, strategies have been developed to accelerate the expression of the surfactant system using pharmacologic agents, and the biochemical nature of surfactant has been fully defined. This definition has led to cloning of the apoproteins of surfactant, allowing in vitro reconstitution of an artificial surfactant for use in therapy.

6 In *asthma*, cell biology methodologies have led to the identification of a broad armamentarium of naturally occurring mediators that likely play a role in the pathogenesis of reversible airway disease, and several genes related to these mediators have been cloned and characterized (see Chap. 217).

7 Capitalizing on the identification, cloning, and in vitro production of a variety of potent "inflammatory" polypeptides, much attention has been given to the concept that mediators such as tumor necrosis factor play a role in modulating the parenchymal dysfunction characteristic of the respiratory failure of *adult respiratory distress syndrome*.

Finally, the recognition that it is the high concentration of DNA that gives purulent mucus its thick, sticky properties led to the cloning of human recombinant DNase I as a therapeutic agent. When given by aerosol to individuals with cystic fibrosis, there is improvement in lung function as the airways are opened and a decrease in the incidence of airway infections.

CONCLUSIONS   The application of modern cell and biology methods to investigate human disease depends on the capacity to obtain appropriate biologic materials relevant to the pathogenesis of the disease. For most diseases, the relevant biologic material must be obtained directly from the target organ, and this is a difficult task for internal organs. Utilizing cell culture techniques and the fiberoptic bronchoscope to gain access to the epithelial surface of the lung, many pulmonary disorders can now be investigated by the techniques of cell and molecular biology. As a consequence there has been a remarkable advance in the understanding of the pathogenesis of a variety of lung disorders and for several new insights into therapy.

REFERENCES

ADACHI K et al: Evaluation of fibronectin gene expression by *in situ* hybridization: Differential expression of the fibronectin gene among populations of human alveolar macrophages. Am J Pathol 138:193, 1988

BOST T et al: Increased TNF-alpha and IL6 mRNA expression by alveolar macrophages in chronic beryllium disease. Chest 103:138S, 1993

COUTELLE C et al: Gene therapy for cystic fibrosis. Arch Dis Child 68:437, 1993

CRYSTAL RG: α1-Antitrypsin deficiency, in *Update: Pulmonary Disease and Disorders*, AP Fishman (ed). New York, McGraw-Hill, 1992, pp 19–35

————: Gene therapy strategies for pulmonary disease. Am J Med 1992:92 (suppl 6A):44 S–52 S

CRYSTAL RG et al: Interstitial lung disease of unknown cause: Disorders characterized by chronic inflammation of the lower respiratory tract. N Engl J Med 310:154, 235, 1984

HUBBARD RC, CRYSTAL RG: Vulnerability of the lung to proteolytic injury, in *The Lung: Scientific Foundations*, RG Crystal et al (eds). New York, Raven, 1991, pp 2059–2072

HUBBARD RC et al: A preliminary study of aerosolized recombinant human DNase therapy in the treatment of cystic fibrosis. N Engl J Med 326:812, 1992

MARTINET Y et al: Exaggerated spontaneous release of a platelet-derived growth factor by alveolar macrophages from patients with idiopathic pulmonary fibrosis. N Engl J Med 317(4):202, 1987

ROSENFELD MA et al: *In vivo* transfer of the human cystic fibrosis transmembrane conductance regulator gene to the airway epithelium. Cell 68:143, 1992

SALTINI C et al: Chronic pulmonary berylliosis: Maintenance of the alveolitis by proliferation of beryllium-specific helper T-cells. N Engl J Med 230:1103, 1989

SFERRA TJ, COLLINS FS: The molecular biology of cystic fibrosis. Annu Rev Med 44:133, 1993

WEWERS MD et al: Replacement therapy for alpha 1-antitrypsin deficiency associated with emphysema. N Engl J Med 316:1055, 1987

214   DISTURBANCES OF RESPIRATORY FUNCTION

STEVEN E. WEINBERGER / JEFFREY M. DRAZEN

The respiratory system includes the lungs, the central nervous system (CNS), the chest wall (with the diaphragm and intercostal muscles), and the pulmonary circulation. The CNS controls the activity of the muscles of the chest wall, which serve as the respiratory system pump. Because these components of the respiratory system act in concert to achieve gas exchange, malfunction of an individual component or alteration of the relationships among components can lead to disturbances in function. In this chapter we consider three major aspects of disturbed respiratory function: (1) disturbances in ventilatory function, (2) disturbances in the pulmonary circulation, and (3) disturbances in gas exchange. Disorders relating to CNS control of ventilation are discussed in Chap. 229.

DISTURBANCES IN VENTILATORY FUNCTION

Ventilation is the process whereby the lungs replenish the gas within the alveoli. Measurements of ventilatory function in common diagnostic use consist of quantification of the gas volume contained within the lungs under certain circumstances and the rate at which gas can be expelled from the lungs. Two measurements of lung volume commonly used for respiratory diagnosis are total lung capacity (TLC) and residual volume (RV). The former is the volume of gas contained within the lungs after a maximal inspiration, whereas the latter is the volume of gas remaining within the lungs at the end of a maximal expiration. The volume of gas that is exhaled from the lungs in going from TLC to RV is called the *vital capacity* (VC) (Fig. 214-1).

Common clinical measurements of airflow are obtained from maneuvers in which the subject inspires to TLC and then forcibly exhales to RV. Three measurements are commonly made from a volume-time recording, i.e., a spirogram, obtained during such a forced expiratory maneuver: (1) the volume of gas exhaled during the first second of expiration (forced expiratory volume in 1 s, or FEV_1), (2) the total volume exhaled (forced vital capacity, or FVC), and (3) the average expiratory flow rate during the middle 50 percent of the vital capacity (forced expiratory flow between 25 and 75 percent of the vital capacity, or $FEF_{25-75\%}$, also called maximal midexpiratory flow rate, or MMFR) (Fig. 214-2).

PHYSIOLOGIC FEATURES   The lungs are elastic structures containing collagen and elastic fibers which resist expansion. In order

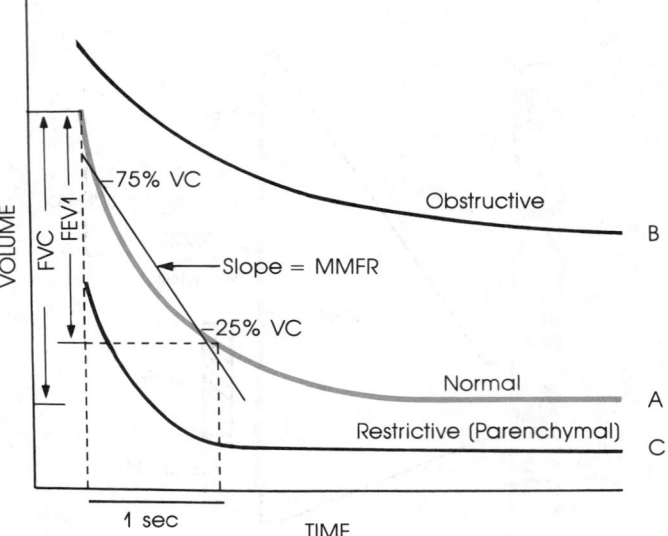

FIGURE 214-2   Spirographic tracings of forced expiration, comparing a normal tracing (*A*) and tracings in obstructive (*B*) and parenchymal restrictive (*C*) disease. Calculations of FVC, FEV_1, and $FEF_{25-75\%}$ are shown only for the normal tracing. Since there is no measure of absolute starting volume with spirometry, the curves are artificially positioned to show the relative starting lung volumes in the different conditions.

for normal lungs to contain air, they must be distended by either a positive internal pressure, i.e., within the airways and alveolar spaces, or a negative external pressure, i.e., outside the lung. The relationship between the volume of gas contained within the lungs and the distending pressure (transpulmonary pressure, or P_{TP}, defined as internal pressure minus external pressure) is described by the pressure-volume curve of the lungs (Fig. 214-3A).

The chest wall is also an elastic structure, with properties similar to that of an expandable and compressible spring. The relationship between the volume enclosed by the chest wall and the distending pressure for the chest wall is described by the pressure-volume curve of the chest wall (Fig. 214-3B). For the chest wall to assume a volume different from its resting volume, the internal or external pressures acting on it must be altered.

At functional residual capacity (FRC), defined as the volume of gas in the lungs at the end of a normal exhalation, the lungs are partially inflated, so their elastic recoil exerts a force tending to empty the lungs. At the same time, chest wall volume is such that its elastic recoil promotes outward expansion. Functional residual capacity occurs at the lung volume at which the tendency of the lungs to contract is opposed by the equal and opposite tendency of the chest wall to expand (Fig. 214-3C).

In order for the lungs and the chest wall to achieve a volume other than the resting volume or FRC, either the pressures acting on them can be changed passively, e.g., with a mechanical ventilator delivering positive pressure to the airways and alveoli, or the respiratory muscles can actively oppose the tendency of the lungs and the chest wall to return to FRC. During inhalation to volumes above FRC, the inspiratory muscles must actively overcome the tendency of the respiratory system to decrease volume back to FRC. During active exhalation below FRC, expiratory muscle activity must overcome the tendency of the respiratory system to increase volume back to FRC. At TLC, the maximal force applied by the inspiratory muscles to expand the lungs is primarily opposed by the inward recoil of the lungs. As a consequence, the major determinants of TLC are the stiffness of the lungs and inspiratory muscle strength. If the lungs become stiffer, i.e., less compliant, TLC is decreased. If the lungs become less stiff, i.e., more compliant, TLC is increased. If the inspiratory muscles are significantly weakened, they are less able to overcome the inward elastic recoil of the lungs, and TLC is lowered.

FIGURE 214-1   Lung volumes, shown by block diagrams (*left*) and by a spirographic tracing (*right*). TLC = total lung capacity; VC = vital capacity; RV = residual volume; IC = inspiratory capacity; ERV = expiratory reserve volume; FRC = functional residual capacity; V_T = tidal volume. (*From Weinberger.*)

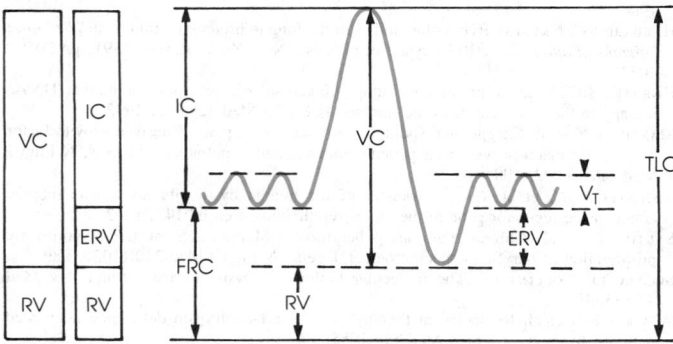

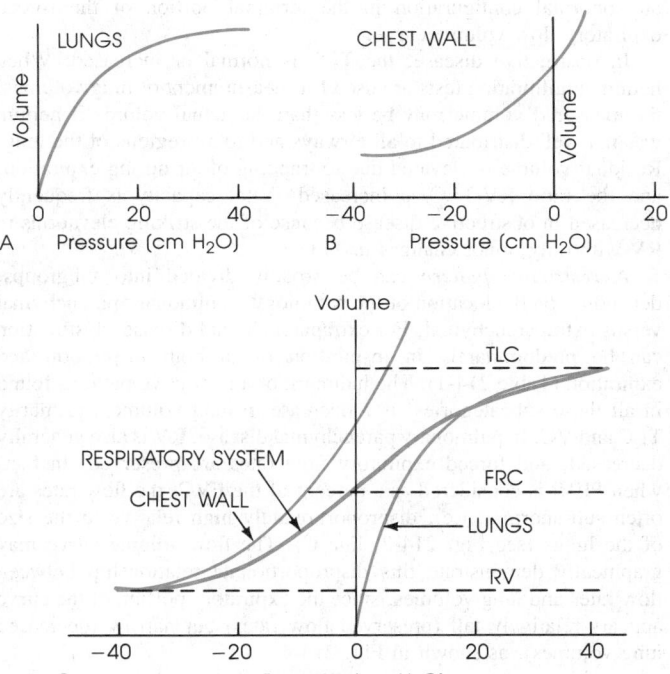

FIGURE 214-3 *A.* Pressure-volume curve of the lungs. *B.* Pressure-volume curve of the chest wall. *C.* Pressure-volume curve of the respiratory system, showing the superimposed component curves of the lungs and the chest wall. RV = residual volume; FRC = functional residual capacity; TLC = total lung capacity. (*From Weinberger.*)

At RV, the force exerted by the expiratory muscles to decrease lung volume further is balanced by the outward recoil of the chest wall, which becomes extremely stiff at low lung volumes. Two factors influence the volume of gas contained within the lungs at RV. The first is the ability of the subject to exert a prolonged expiratory effort, which is related to muscle strength and to the ability to overcome sensory stimuli from the chest wall. The second is the ability of the lungs to empty to a small volume. In normal lungs, as P_{TP} is lowered, lung volume decreases. In lungs with diseased airways, as P_{TP} is lowered, flow-limitation or airway closure can limit the amount of gas that is expired. Consequently, either weak chest wall muscles or intrinsic airways disease can result in an elevation in measured RV.

Dynamic measurements of ventilatory function are made by having the subject inhale to TLC and then perform a forced expiration to RV. If a subject performs a series of such expiratory maneuvers using increasing muscular intensity, expiratory flow rates will increase until a certain level of effort is reached. Beyond this level, additional effort will not result in an increment in forced expiratory flow rates; this phenomenon is known as the *effort independence* of forced expiratory flow. The physiologic mechanisms determining the flow rates during this effort-independent phase of forced expiratory flow have been shown to be the elastic recoil of the lung, the airflow resistance of the airways between the alveolar zone and the physical site of flow limitation, and the airway wall compliance at the site of flow limitation. Physical processes which decrease elastic recoil, increase airflow resistance, or increase airway wall compliance decrease the flow rate that can be achieved at any given lung volume. Conversely, processes that increase elastic recoil, decrease resistance, or stiffen airway walls increase the flow rate that can be achieved at any given lung volume.

MEASUREMENT OF VENTILATORY FUNCTION Ventilatory function is measured under static conditions for determination of lung volumes and under dynamic conditions for determination of forced expiratory flow rates. VC, expiratory reserve volume (ERV), and inspiratory capacity (IC) (see Fig. 214-1) are measured by having the patient breathe into and out of a spirometer, a device capable of

measuring expired or inspired gas volume while plotting volume as a function of time. Other volumes, specifically RV, FRC, and TLC, cannot be measured in this way because they include the volume of gas present within the lungs even after a maximal expiration. Two techniques are commonly used to measure these volumes: helium dilution or body plethysmography. In the helium-dilution method, the subject repeatedly breathes in and out from a reservoir with a known volume of gas containing a trace amount of helium. The helium is diluted by the gas previously present in the lungs and is not absorbed into the pulmonary circulation. From knowledge of reservoir volume and initial and final helium concentrations, the volume of gas present within the lungs can be calculated. With the helium-dilution method, the volume of gas present within the lungs may be underestimated if there are slowly communicating airspaces, such as bullae. In this situation, lung volumes can be more accurately measured with a body plethysmograph, a sealed box in which the patient sits while panting against a closed mouthpiece. Because there is no airflow into or out of the plethysmograph, pressure changes within the thorax during panting cause compression and rarefaction of gas within the lungs and simultaneous rarefaction and compression of gas within the plethysmograph. By measuring pressure changes in the plethysmograph and at the mouthpiece, the volume of gas present within the thorax can be calculated by using Boyle's law.

Lung volumes and measurements made during forced expiration are interpreted by comparing the values measured with the values expected based on the age, height, sex, and race of the patient (see Appendix). Regression curves have been constructed based on data obtained from large numbers of normal, nonsmoking individuals without any evidence of lung disease. Predicted values for a given patient can then be obtained by using the patient's age and height in the appropriate regression equation; different equations are used depending on the patient's race and gender. Because some variability among normal individuals is to be expected, values between 80 and 120 percent of predicted have traditionally been considered normal. Increasingly, calculated percentiles are used in determining normality. Specifically, values of individual measurements falling below the fifth percentile are considered below the lower limits of normal.

The normal ratio FEV_1/FVC is approximately 0.75 to 0.80, although this value does fall somewhat with advancing age. The $FEF_{25-75\%}$ is often considered a more sensitive measurement of early airflow obstruction, particularly in small airways. However, this measurement must be interpreted cautiously in the patient with abnormally small lungs (low TLC and VC). Then, less volume is exhaled during forced expiration, and the $FEF_{25-75\%}$ may appear abnormal when compared with the predicted value for the patient's age, height, race, and gender, even though it is normal relative to the size of the patient's lungs.

It is also a common practice to plot expiratory flow rates against lung volume (rather than against time); the close linkage of flow rates to lung volumes produces a typical *flow-volume curve* (Fig. 214-4). In addition, the spirometric values mentioned above can be calculated from the flow-volume curve. Commonly, flow rates during a maximal inspiratory effort performed as rapidly as possible are plotted as well, making the flow-volume curve into a *flow-volume loop*. At TLC, before expiratory flow starts, the flow rate is zero; once forced expiration has begun, a high peak flow rate is rapidly achieved. As expiration continues and lung volume approaches RV, the flow rate falls progressively, in a nearly linear fashion as a function of lung volume for a person with normal lung function. During maximal inspiration from RV to TLC, inspiratory flow is most rapid at the midpoint of inspiration, so the inspiratory portion of the loop is U-shaped or saddle-shaped. The flow rates achieved during maximal expiration can be analyzed quantitatively by comparing the flow rates at specified lung volumes with the predicted values or qualitatively by analyzing the shape of the descending limb of the expiratory curve.

Assessing the strength of respiratory muscles is an additional part of the overall evaluation of some patients with respiratory dysfunction. When a patient exhales completely to RV and then tries to inspire

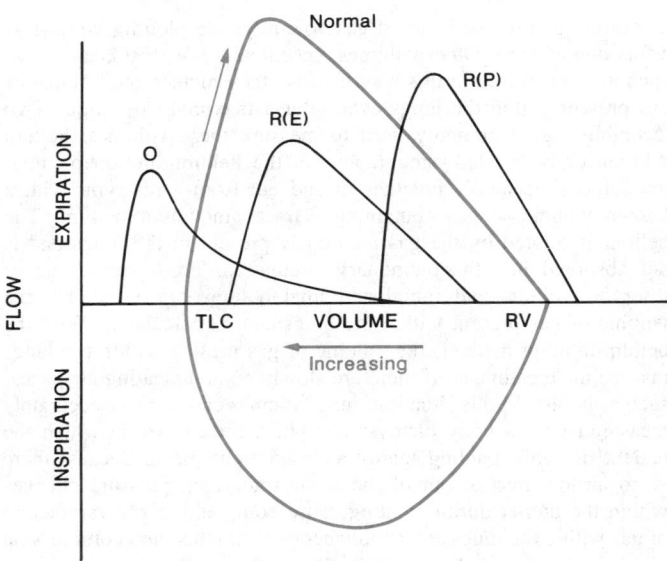

FIGURE 214-4   Flow-volume curves in different conditions: O = obstructive disease; R(P) = parenchymal restrictive disease; R(E) = extraparenchymal restrictive disease with limitation in inspiration and expiration. Forced expiration is plotted in all conditions; forced inspiration is shown only for the normal curve. TLC = total lung capacity; RV = residual volume. By convention, increasing lung volume is to the left on the abscissa. The arrow alongside the normal curve indicates the direction of expiration from TLC to RV.

maximally against an occluded airway, the pressure that can be generated is called the *maximal inspiratory pressure* (MIP). On the other hand, when a patient inhales to TLC and then tries to expire maximally against an occluded airway, the pressure generated is called the *maximal expiratory pressure* (MEP). In the proper clinical setting, these studies may provide useful information regarding the cause of abnormal lung volumes and the possibility that respiratory muscle weakness may be causally related to the lung volume abnormalities.

PATTERNS OF ABNORMAL FUNCTION   The two major patterns of abnormal ventilatory function, as measured by static lung volumes and spirometry, are restrictive and obstructive patterns. In the *obstructive pattern*, the hallmark is a decrease in expiratory flow rates. With fully established disease, the ratio FEV_1/FVC is decreased, as is the $FEF_{25-75\%}$ (see Fig. 214-2, line *B*). The expiratory portion of the flow-volume loop demonstrates decreased flow rates for any given lung volume. Nonuniform emptying of airways is reflected by a coved (concave upward) configuration of the curve (see Fig. 214-4). With early obstructive disease, which originates in the small airways, FEV_1/FVC may be normal; the only abnormalities noted on routine testing of pulmonary function may be a depression in $FEF_{25-75\%}$ and

an abnormal configuration in the terminal portion of the forced expiratory flow-volume curve.

In obstructive disease, the TLC is normal or increased. When helium equilibration tests are used for measurement of lung volumes, the measured volume may be less than the actual volume if helium was not well distributed to all airways and to all regions of the lung. Residual volume is elevated due to trapping of air during expiration, and the ratio RV/TLC is increased. Vital capacity is frequently decreased in obstructive disease because of the striking elevations in RV with only minor changes in TLC.

A *restrictive pattern* can be broadly divided into subgroups, depending on the location of the pathology—pulmonary parenchymal versus extraparenchymal. For extraparenchymal disease, dysfunction can be predominantly in inspiration or in both inspiration and expiration (Table 214-1). The hallmark of a restrictive pattern, found in all these subcategories, is a decrease in lung volumes, primarily TLC and VC. In pulmonary parenchymal disease, RV is also generally decreased, and forced expiratory flow rates are preserved. In fact, when FEV_1 is considered as a percent of the FVC, the flow rates are often supranormal, i.e., disproportionately high relative to the size of the lungs (see Fig. 214-2, line *C*). The flow-volume curve may graphically demonstrate this disproportionate relationship between flow rates and lung volumes, since the expiratory portion of the curve appears relatively tall (preserved flow rates) but narrow (decreased lung volumes), as shown in Fig. 214-4.

In the extraparenchymal pattern characterized by *inspiratory dysfunction*, due to either inspiratory muscle weakness or a stiff chest wall, adequate distending forces are prevented from being exerted on an otherwise normal lung. As a result, achieved TLC values are less than predicted, RV is often not significantly affected, and expiratory flows are preserved. If inspiratory muscle weakness is the cause of this pattern, then MIP is decreased. In the extraparenchymal pattern characterized by *inspiratory and expiratory dysfunction*, the ability to expire to a normal RV is also limited, either because of expiratory muscle weakness or a deformed chest wall that is abnormally rigid at volumes below FRC. Consequently, RV is often elevated, unlike the pattern observed in the other restrictive subcategories. The ratio FEV_1/FVC is variable and depends on expiratory muscle strength. If expiratory muscle strength is significantly decreased, then MEP is decreased, the ability to expire rapidly is impaired, and FEV_1/FVC may be decreased even though there is no airflow obstruction. If expiratory muscle strength is normal but the chest wall is abnormally stiff below FRC, then FEV_1/FVC is normal or increased.

CLINICAL CORRELATIONS   In Table 214-1, the expected alterations in ventilatory function as indicated by pulmonary function testing are summarized. One reason to establish a ventilatory diagnosis is to categorize the functional disorder. This in turn can provide diagnostic information as outlined in Table 214-2. Note that lung disease can be present without abnormal ventilatory function, but the presence of specific diagnostic findings is an aid in differential diagnosis.

TABLE 214-1   Alterations in ventilatory function

	TLC	RV	VC	FEV₁/FVC	MIP	MEP
Obstructive	N to ↑	↑	↓	↓ *	N	N
Restrictive						
Pulmonary parenchymal	↓	↓	↓	N to ↑	N	N
Extraparenchymal— inspiratory	↓	N to ↓	↓	N	↓ /N†	N
Extraparenchymal— inspiratory + expiratory	↓	↑	↓	Variable	↓ /N†	↓ /N†

* Mild obstructive (small airways) disease may have ↓ FEF₂₅₋₇₅% with normal FEV₁/FVC.
† ↓ if due to respiratory muscle weakness; N if due to chest wall stiffness.
NOTE: N = normal; for other abbreviations, see text.

TABLE 214-2 Common respiratory diseases by diagnostic categories

OBSTRUCTIVE

Asthma
Chronic obstructive lung disease (chronic bronchitis, emphysema)
Bronchiectasis
Cystic fibrosis
Bronchiolitis

RESTRICTIVE—PARENCHYMAL

Sarcoidosis
Idiopathic pulmonary fibrosis
Pneumoconiosis
Drug- or radiation-induced interstitial lung disease

RESTRICTIVE—EXTRAPARENCHYMAL

Neuromuscular
  Diaphragmatic weakness/paralysis
  Myasthenia gravis*
  Guillain-Barré syndrome*
  Muscular dystrophies*
  Cervical spine injury*
Chest wall
  Kyphoscoliosis
  Obesity
  Ankylosing spondylitis*

* Can have inspiratory and expiratory limitation (see text).

DISTURBANCES IN THE PULMONARY CIRCULATION

PHYSIOLOGIC FEATURES The pulmonary vasculature must handle the entire output of the right ventricle, approximately 5 L/min in a normal adult at rest. The comparatively thin-walled vessels of the pulmonary arterial system provide relatively little resistance to flow and are capable of handling this large volume of blood at low perfusion pressures compared with those of the systemic circulation. The normal mean pulmonary artery pressure of 15 mmHg is much less than the normal mean aortic pressure of approximately 95 mmHg. Regional blood flow within the lung is dependent on hydrostatic forces. In the upright person, pulmonary arterial pressure is lowest at the apex of the lung and highest at the lung bases. As a result, in the upright position, perfusion is least at the apex and greatest at the lung bases. When cardiac output increases, as occurs during exercise, the pulmonary vasculature is capable of recruiting previously unperfused vessels and distending underperfused vessels. As a result, the pulmonary vascular system is capable of handling the increase in flow with a decrease in pulmonary vascular resistance, so the increment in mean pulmonary arterial pressure, even with a three- to four-fold increase in cardiac output, is small.

METHODS OF MEASUREMENT Assessment of circulatory function within the pulmonary vasculature depends on measuring pulmonary vascular pressures and cardiac output. Clinically, these measurements are commonly made in intensive care units capable of invasive monitoring and in cardiac catheterization laboratories. With a flow-directed pulmonary arterial (Swan-Ganz) catheter, pulmonary arterial and pulmonary capillary wedge pressures can be measured directly, and cardiac output can be obtained by the thermodilution method. Pulmonary vascular resistance can then be calculated according to the equation

$$PVR = 80(PAP - PCW)/CO$$

where PVR = pulmonary vascular resistance (dyn·s/cm^5)
    PAP = mean pulmonary arterial pressure (mmHg)
    PCW = pulmonary capillary wedge pressure (mmHg)
      CO = cardiac output (L/min)

The normal value for pulmonary vascular resistance is approximately 50 to 150 dyn·s/cm^5.

MECHANISMS OF ABNORMAL FUNCTION (See also Chap. 225) Pulmonary vascular resistance may increase by a variety of mechanisms. Pulmonary arterial and arteriolar vasoconstriction is a prominent response to alveolar hypoxia. Pulmonary vascular resistance also increases if intraluminal thrombi or proliferation of smooth muscle within vessel walls diminishes the luminal cross-sectional area. If small pulmonary vessels are destroyed, either by scarring or by loss of alveolar walls, the total cross-sectional area of the pulmonary vascular bed diminishes, and pulmonary vascular resistance increases. When pulmonary vascular resistance is elevated, pulmonary arterial pressure rises to maintain normal cardiac output or cardiac output falls if pulmonary arterial pressure does not increase.

CLINICAL CORRELATIONS Disturbances in function of the pulmonary vasculature as a result of primary cardiac disease, either congenital heart disease or conditions which elevate left atrial pressure such as mitral stenosis, are beyond the scope of this chapter and are discussed in Chaps. 191 and 201, respectively. Instead, the focus will be on the pulmonary vasculature as its function is affected by diseases primarily involving the respiratory system, including the pulmonary vessels themselves.

All diseases of the respiratory system causing hypoxemia are potentially capable of increasing pulmonary vascular resistance, since alveolar hypoxia is a very potent stimulus for pulmonary vasoconstriction. The more prolonged and intense the hypoxic stimulus, the more likely it is that a significant increase in pulmonary vascular resistance and pulmonary hypertension will result. In practice, patients with hypoxemia caused by chronic obstructive lung disease, interstitial lung disease, chest wall disease, and the obesity hypoventilation–sleep apnea syndrome are particularly prone to developing pulmonary hypertension. If there are additional structural changes in the pulmonary vasculature secondary to the underlying process, these will increase the likelihood of developing pulmonary hypertension.

With diseases directly affecting the pulmonary vessels, a decrease in the cross-sectional area of the pulmonary vascular bed is primarily responsible for increased pulmonary vascular resistance, while hypoxemia generally plays a lesser role. In the case of recurrent pulmonary emboli, parts of the pulmonary arterial system are occluded by intraluminal thrombi originating in the systemic venous system. With primary pulmonary hypertension (Chap. 225) or with pulmonary vascular disease secondary to scleroderma, the small pulmonary arteries and arterioles are affected by a generalized obliterative process that narrows and occludes these vessels. Pulmonary vascular resistance increases, and significant pulmonary hypertension often results.

DISTURBANCES IN GAS EXCHANGE

PHYSIOLOGIC FEATURES The primary functions of the respiratory system are to remove the appropriate amount of CO_2 from blood entering the pulmonary circulation and to provide adequate O_2 to blood leaving the pulmonary circulation. In order for these functions to be carried out properly, there must be adequate provision of fresh air to the alveoli for delivery of O_2 and removal of CO_2 (ventilation), adequate circulation of blood through the pulmonary vasculature (perfusion), adequate movement of gas between alveoli and pulmonary capillaries (diffusion), and appropriate contact between alveolar gas and pulmonary capillary blood (ventilation-perfusion matching).

A normal individual at rest inspires approximately 12 to 16 times per minute, each breath having a tidal volume of approximately 500 mL. A portion (approximately 30 percent) of the fresh air inspired with each breath does not reach the alveoli but remains in the conducting airways of the lung. This component of each breath, which is not generally available for gas exchange, is called the *anatomic dead space component*. The remaining 70 percent reaches and rapidly mixes with the gas resident in the alveolar zone and can participate in gas exchange. In this example, total ventilation each minute is approximately 7 L, composed of 2 L/min of dead space ventilation and 5 L/min of alveolar ventilation. In certain diseases, some alveoli are ventilated but not perfused so that additional ventilation beyond that portion related to the anatomic dead space is wasted. If total dead space ventilation is increased but total minute ventilation is unchanged, then alveolar ventilation must fall correspondingly.

Gas exchange is dependent on alveolar ventilation rather than total minute ventilation, as outlined below. The partial pressure of CO_2 in arterial blood (Pa_{CO_2}) is directly proportional to the amount of CO_2 produced per minute ($\dot{V}_{CO_2}$) and inversely proportional to alveolar ventilation ($\dot{V}_A$), according to the relationship

$$Pa_{CO_2} = 0.863 \times \dot{V}_{CO_2}/\dot{V}_A$$

where $\dot{V}_{CO_2}$ is expressed in mL/min, $\dot{V}_A$ in L/min, and Pa_{CO_2} in mmHg. At fixed $\dot{V}_{CO_2}$, when alveolar ventilation increases, Pa_{CO_2} falls, and when alveolar ventilation decreases, Pa_{CO_2} rises. Maintaining a normal level of O_2 in the alveoli (and consequently in arterial blood) also depends on provision of adequate alveolar ventilation to replenish alveolar O_2. This principle will become more apparent from consideration of the alveolar gas equation below.

Diffusion of O_2 and CO_2 Both O_2 and CO_2 diffuse readily down their respective concentration gradients through the alveolar wall and pulmonary capillary endothelium. Under normal circumstances, this process is rapid, and equilibration of both gases is complete within one-third of the transit time of erythrocytes through the pulmonary capillary bed. Even in disease states in which diffusion of gases is impaired, it is unlikely to be so severe that equilibration of the CO_2 and O_2 is not reached. Consequently, a diffusion abnormality rarely results in arterial hypoxemia at rest. If erythrocyte transit time in the pulmonary circulation is shortened, as occurs with exercise, and diffusion is impaired, then diffusion limitation may contribute to hypoxemia. Exercise testing can often demonstrate such physiologically significant abnormalities due to impaired diffusion. Even though diffusion limitation rarely makes a clinically significant contribution to resting hypoxemia, clinical measurements of what is known as *diffusing capacity* (see below) can be a useful measure of the integrity of the alveolar-capillary membrane.

Ventilation-perfusion matching In addition to the absolute levels of alveolar ventilation and perfusion, gas exchange is critically dependent on the proper matching of ventilation and perfusion. The spectrum of possible ventilation-perfusion ($\dot{V}/\dot{Q}$) ratios within an alveolar-capillary unit ranges from zero, in which ventilation is totally absent and the unit behaves as a shunt, to infinity, in which perfusion is totally absent and the unit behaves as dead space. The P_{O_2} and P_{CO_2} of blood leaving each alveolar-capillary unit depend on the gas tension (blood and air) entering that unit and on the $\dot{V}/\dot{Q}$ ratio of that particular unit. At one extreme, when an alveolar-capillary unit has a $\dot{V}/\dot{Q}$ ratio of 0 and behaves as a shunt, blood leaving the unit has the composition of mixed venous blood entering the pulmonary capillaries, i.e., $P\bar{v}_{O_2} \approx 40$ mmHg and $P\bar{v}_{CO_2} \approx 46$ mmHg. At the other extreme, when an alveolar-capillary unit has a high $\dot{V}/\dot{Q}$ ratio, it behaves almost like dead space, and the small amount of blood leaving the unit has partial pressures of O_2 and CO_2 ($P_{O_2} \approx 150$ mmHg, $P_{CO_2} \approx 0$ mmHg while breathing room air) approaching the composition of inspired gas.

In the ideal situation, all alveolar-capillary units have equal matching of ventilation and perfusion, i.e., with a ratio of approximately 1 when each is expressed in L/min. However, even in the normal individual, some $\dot{V}/\dot{Q}$ mismatching is present, since there is normally a gradient of blood flow from the apices to the bases of the lungs. Moreover, there is a similar gradient of ventilation from the apices to the bases, but the gradient is less marked for ventilation than for perfusion. As a result, ventilation-perfusion ratios are higher at the lung apices than at the lung bases. Therefore, blood coming from the apices has a higher P_{O_2} and lower P_{CO_2} than blood coming from the bases. The net P_{O_2} and P_{CO_2} of the resulting mixture of blood coming from all areas of the lung is a flow-weighted average of the individual components, which takes into account the relative amount

of blood from each unit and the O_2 and CO_2 *content* of blood coming from each unit. Because of the sigmoid shape of the oxyhemoglobin dissociation curve (see Fig. 302-4, p. 1697), it is important to distinguish between the partial pressure and the content of O_2 in blood. Hemoglobin is almost fully saturated at a P_{O_2} of 60 mmHg, and little additional O_2 is carried by hemoglobin even with substantial elevations of P_{O_2} above 60 mmHg. On the other hand, significant O_2 desaturation of hemoglobin occurs once P_{O_2} falls below 60 mmHg and onto the steep descending limb of the curve. As a result, blood coming from regions of the lung with a high $\dot{V}/\dot{Q}$ ratio, a high P_{O_2}, but only a small elevation in O_2 content cannot compensate for blood coming from regions with a low $\dot{V}/\dot{Q}$ ratio, a low P_{O_2}, and a significant decrease in O_2 content. Although $\dot{V}/\dot{Q}$ mismatching can influence P_{CO_2}, this effect is less marked and often is overcome by an increase in overall minute ventilation.

MEASUREMENT OF GAS EXCHANGE Arterial blood gases
The most commonly used measures of gas exchange are the partial pressures of O_2 and CO_2 in arterial blood, i.e., Pa_{O_2} and Pa_{CO_2}, respectively. These partial pressures do not measure directly the quantity of O_2 and CO_2 in blood but rather the driving pressure for the gas in blood. The actual quantity or content of each of these gases in blood depends on the solubility of the gas in plasma and the ability of any component of blood to react with or to bind the gas of interest. Since hemoglobin is capable of binding large amounts of O_2, oxygenated hemoglobin is the primary form in which O_2 is transported in blood. The actual content of O_2 in blood therefore depends both on the hemoglobin concentration and on the Pa_{O_2}. The Pa_{O_2} determines what percentage of hemoglobin is saturated with O_2, based on the position on the oxyhemoglobin dissociation curve. Oxygen content in normal blood (at 37°C, pH 7.4) can be determined by adding the amount of O_2 dissolved in plasma to the amount bound to hemoglobin, according to the equation

$$O_2 \text{ content} = 1.34 \times [\text{hemoglobin}] \times \text{saturation} + 0.0031 \times P_{O_2}$$

since each gram of hemoglobin is capable of carrying 1.34 mL O_2 when fully saturated, and the amount of O_2 that can be dissolved in plasma is proportional to the P_{O_2}, with 0.0031 mL O_2 dissolved per deciliter of blood per mmHg P_{O_2}. In arterial blood, the amount of O_2 transported dissolved in plasma (approximately 0.3 mL O_2 per deciliter of blood) is trivial compared with the amount bound to hemoglobin (approximately 20 mL O_2 per deciliter of blood).

Most commonly, P_{O_2} is the measurement used to quantitate the adequacy of oxygenation of arterial blood. Direct measurement of O_2 saturation in arterial blood by oximetry is also important in selected clinical conditions. For example, in patients with carbon monoxide exposure, carbon monoxide preferentially displaces O_2 from hemoglobin, essentially making a portion of hemoglobin unavailable for binding to O_2. In this circumstance, carbon monoxide saturation is high and O_2 saturation is low, even though the driving pressure for O_2 to bind to hemoglobin, reflected by P_{O_2}, is normal. Measurement of O_2 saturation, in order to determine O_2 content, is also important when mixed venous blood is sampled from a pulmonary arterial catheter to calculate cardiac output by the Fick technique. In mixed venous blood, the P_{O_2} is normally about 40 mmHg, but small changes in P_{O_2} may reflect relatively large changes in O_2 saturation.

A useful calculation in the assessment of oxygenation is the alveolar-arterial O_2 difference ($PA_{O_2} - Pa_{O_2}$), commonly called the *alveolar-arterial O_2 gradient* (or A–a gradient). This calculation takes into account the fact that alveolar and, hence, arterial P_{O_2} can be expected to change depending on the level of alveolar ventilation, reflected by the arterial P_{CO_2}. When a patient hyperventilates and has a low P_{CO_2} in arterial blood and alveolar gas, alveolar and arterial P_{O_2} will rise; conversely, hypoventilation and a high P_{CO_2} are accompanied by a decrease in alveolar and arterial P_{O_2}. These changes in arterial P_{O_2} are independent of abnormalities in O_2 transfer at the alveolar-capillary level and reflect only the dependence of alveolar P_{O_2} on the level of alveolar ventilation.

In order to determine the alveolar-arterial O_2 difference, the alveolar P_{O_2} (PA_{O_2}) must first be calculated. The equation most commonly used for this purpose, a simplified form of the alveolar gas equation, is

$$PA_{O_2} = FI_{O_2} \times (P_B - P_{H_2O}) - Pa_{CO_2}/R$$

where FI_{O_2} = fractional concentration of inspired O_2 (≈ 0.21 when breathing room air)

P_B = barometric pressure (approximately 760 mmHg at sea level)

P_{H_2O} = water vapor pressure (47 mmHg when air is fully saturated at 37°C)

R = respiratory quotient (the ratio of CO_2 production to O_2 consumption, usually assumed to be 0.8)

If the preceding values are substituted into the equation for the patient breathing air at sea level, the equation becomes

$$PA_{O_2} = 150 - 1.25 \times Pa_{CO_2}$$

The alveolar-arterial O_2 difference can then be calculated by subtracting measured Pa_{O_2} from calculated PA_{O_2}. In a healthy young person breathing room air, the $PA_{O_2} - Pa_{O_2}$ is normally less than 15 mmHg; this value increases with age and may be as high as 30 mmHg in elderly patients.

Adequacy of CO_2 elimination is measured by the partial pressure of CO_2 in arterial blood, i.e., Pa_{CO_2}. A more complete understanding of the mechanisms and chronicity of abnormal levels of P_{CO_2} also requires measurement of pH and/or bicarbonate (HCO_3^-), since P_{CO_2} and the patient's acid-base status are so closely intertwined (see Chap. 46).

Pulse oximetry Because measurement of Pa_{O_2} requires arterial puncture and provides intermittent rather than continuous data about the patient's oxygenation, it is not ideal for close monitoring of unstable patients. Over the past several years, an alternative method for assessing oxygenation, pulse oximetry, has become readily available in many clinical settings. The pulse oximeter measures oxygen saturation (rather than Pa_{O_2}) using a probe usually clipped over a patient's finger. The device measures absorption of two wavelengths of light by hemoglobin in pulsatile, cutaneous arterial blood. Because of differential absorption of the two wavelengths of light by oxygenated and nonoxygenated hemoglobin, the percentage of hemoglobin that is saturated with oxygen, i.e., the Sa_{O_2}, can be calculated and displayed instantaneously.

Although the pulse oximeter has been a major advance in the noninvasive, continuous monitoring of oxygenation, there are several issues and potential problems that should be recognized when this device is used. First, the clinician must be aware of the relationship between oxygen saturation and tension as shown by the oxyhemoglobin dissociation curve (see Fig. 302-4 on p. 1697). Because the curve becomes relatively flat above an arterial P_{O_2} of 60 mmHg (corresponding to Sa_{O_2} = 90 percent), the oximeter is relatively insensitive to changes in Pa_{O_2} above this level. In addition, the position of the curve and therefore the specific relationship between Pa_{O_2} and Sa_{O_2} may change depending on factors such as temperature, pH, and the erythrocyte concentration of 2,3-DPG. Second, when cutaneous perfusion is decreased, e.g., with low cardiac output or use of vasoconstrictors, the signal from the oximeter may be less reliable or even unobtainable. Third, other forms of hemoglobin, such as carboxyhemoglobin and methemoglobin, are not distinguishable when only two wavelengths of light are used. The reported values for Sa_{O_2} by the pulse oximeter are not reliable in the presence of significant amounts of either of these forms of hemoglobin. In contrast, the device used to measure oxygen saturation in samples of arterial blood, called the CO-oximeter, uses at least four wavelengths of light and is capable of distinguishing oxyhemoglobin, reduced hemoglobin, carboxyhemoglobin, and methemoglobin. Finally, the clinician must remember that the often-used goal of $Sa_{O_2} \geq 90$ percent does not indicate anything about CO_2 elimination and therefore does not ensure a clinically acceptable P_{CO_2}.

Diffusing capacity The ability of gas to diffuse across the alveolar-capillary membrane is ordinarily assessed by the diffusing capacity of the lung for carbon monoxide (DL_{CO}). In this test, a small concentration of carbon monoxide (0.3%) is inhaled, usually in a single breath that is held for approximately 10 s. The carbon monoxide is diluted by the gas already present in the alveoli and is also taken up by hemoglobin as the erythrocytes course through the pulmonary capillary system. The concentration of carbon monoxide in exhaled gas is measured, and DL_{CO} is calculated as the quantity of carbon monoxide absorbed per minute per mmHg pressure gradient from the alveoli to the pulmonary capillaries. The value obtained for DL_{CO} depends on the alveolar-capillary surface area available for gas exchange and on the pulmonary capillary blood volume. In addition, the thickness of the alveolar-capillary membrane, the degree of $\dot{V}/\dot{Q}$ mismatching, and the patient's hemoglobin level will affect the measurement. Because of this effect of hemoglobin levels on DL_{CO}, the measured DL_{CO} is frequently corrected to take the patient's hemoglobin level into account. The value for DL_{CO}, ideally corrected for hemoglobin, can then be compared with a predicted value, based either on age, height, and gender or on the alveolar volume (VA) at which the value was obtained. Alternatively, the DL_{CO} can be divided by VA and the resulting value for DL_{CO}/VA compared with a predicted value.

MECHANISMS OF HYPOXEMIA AND HYPERCAPNIA Arterial blood gases Hypoxemia is a common manifestation of a variety of diseases affecting the lungs or other parts of the respiratory system. The broad clinical problem of hypoxemia is often best characterized according to the underlying mechanism. The four basic mechanisms of hypoxemia are (1) decrease in inspired P_{O_2}, (2) hypoventilation, (3) shunt, and (4) $\dot{V}/\dot{Q}$ mismatching. Hypoxemia due to decreased diffusion occurs only under selected clinical circumstances and is not usually included among the general categories of hypoxemia. Determining the underlying mechanism for hypoxemia depends on measurement of the Pa_{CO_2}, calculation of $PA_{O_2} - Pa_{O_2}$, and knowledge of the response to supplemental O_2. A flowchart summarizing the approach to the hypoxemic patient is found in Fig. 214-5.

Decrease in the inspired P_{O_2} and hypoventilation both cause hypoxemia by lowering PA_{O_2} and therefore Pa_{O_2}. In each case, gas exchange at the alveolar-capillary level occurs normally, and $PA_{O_2} - Pa_{O_2}$ is not elevated. Hypoxemia due to decreased inspired P_{O_2} can be diagnosed by knowledge of the clinical situation. Inspired P_{O_2} is lowered either because the patient is at a high altitude, where barometric pressure is low, or, much less commonly, because the patient is breathing a gas mixture containing less than 21% O_2. The hallmark of hypoventilation as a cause of hypoxemia is an elevation in Pa_{CO_2}. This is associated with an increase in PA_{CO_2} and a fall in PA_{O_2}. When hypoxemia is due purely to a low inspired P_{O_2} or to alveolar hypoventilation, $PA_{O_2} - Pa_{O_2}$ is normal. If $PA_{O_2} - Pa_{O_2}$ and Pa_{CO_2} are both elevated, then an additional mechanism, such as $\dot{V}/\dot{Q}$ mismatching or shunt, is contributing to hypoxemia.

Shunting is a cause of hypoxemia when desaturated blood effectively bypasses oxygenation at the alveolar-capillary level. This occurs either because of a structural problem that allows desaturated blood to bypass the normal site of gas exchange or because perfused alveoli are not ventilated. Shunting is associated with an elevation in the $PA_{O_2} - Pa_{O_2}$. When shunting is an important contributing factor to hypoxemia, the lowered Pa_{O_2} is relatively refractory to improvement by supplemental O_2.

Finally, the largest clinical category of hypoxemia is $\dot{V}/\dot{Q}$ mismatching. With $\dot{V}/\dot{Q}$ mismatching, regions with low $\dot{V}/\dot{Q}$ ratios contribute blood with a low P_{O_2} and a low O_2 content. Corresponding regions with high $\dot{V}/\dot{Q}$ ratios contribute blood with a high P_{O_2}. However, because blood is already almost fully saturated with a normal P_{O_2}, elevation of the P_{O_2} to a high value does not significantly increase O_2 saturation or content and therefore cannot compensate for the reduction of O_2 saturation and content in blood coming from regions with a low $\dot{V}/\dot{Q}$ ratio. When $\dot{V}/\dot{Q}$ mismatch is the primary cause of hypoxemia, $PA_{O_2} - Pa_{O_2}$ is elevated, and P_{CO_2} is generally

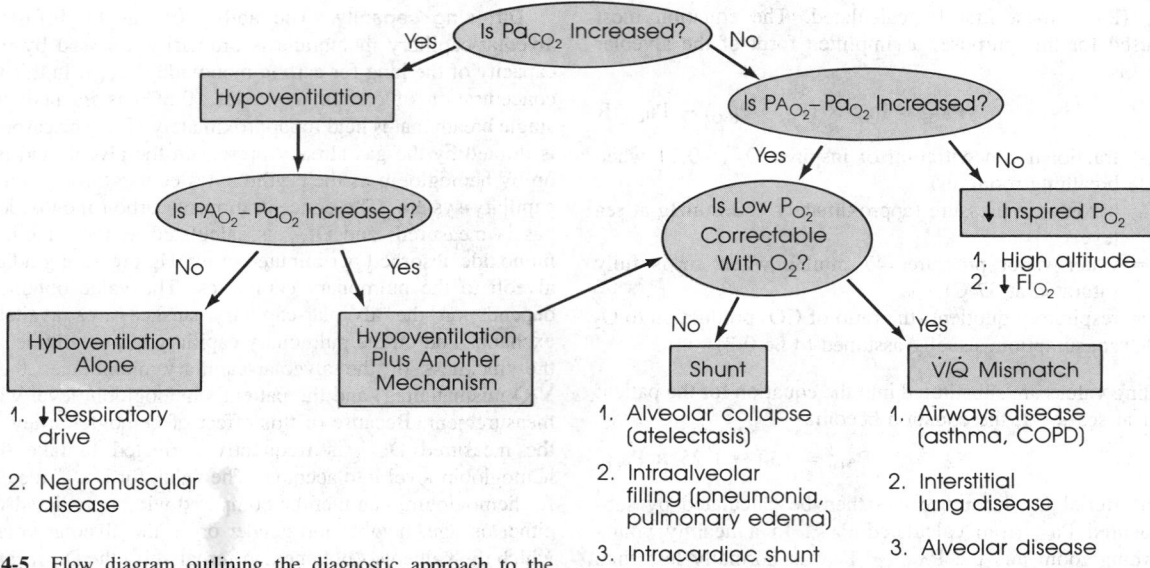

FIGURE 214-5 Flow diagram outlining the diagnostic approach to the patient with hypoxemia ($Pa_{O_2} < 80$ mmHg). $PA_{O_2} - Pa_{O_2}$ is usually < 15 mmHg for subjects ≤ 30 years old and increases ~ 3 mmHg per decade after age 30.

normal. Supplemental O_2 corrects the hypoxemia by raising the P_{O_2} in blood coming from regions with a low $\dot{V}/\dot{Q}$ ratio; this response distinguishes hypoxemia due to $\dot{V}/\dot{Q}$ mismatch from that due to true shunt.

The essential mechanism underlying all cases of hypercapnia is inadequate alveolar ventilation for the amount of CO_2 produced. It is conceptually useful to characterize CO_2 retention further, based on a more detailed examination of the potential contributing factors. These include (1) increased CO_2 production, (2) decreased ventilatory drive ("won't breathe"), (3) malfunction of the respiratory pump or increased airways resistance, making it more difficult to sustain adequate ventilation ("can't breathe"), and (4) inefficiency of gas exchange (increased dead space or $\dot{V}/\dot{Q}$ mismatch) necessitating a compensatory increase in overall minute ventilation. In practice, more than one of these mechanisms is commonly responsible for hypercapnia, since increased minute ventilation is capable of compensating for increased CO_2 production and for inefficiencies of gas exchange.

Diffusing capacity Although abnormalities in diffusion are rarely responsible for hypoxemia, clinical measurement of diffusing capacity is frequently used to assess the functional integrity of the alveolar-capillary membrane, which includes the pulmonary capillary bed. Diseases solely affecting the airways generally do not lower DL_{CO}, whereas diseases affecting alveolar walls or the pulmonary capillary bed will have an effect on DL_{CO}. Even though DL_{CO} is a useful marker to assess whether disease affecting the alveolar-capillary bed is present, an abnormal DL_{CO} does not necessarily imply that diffusion limitation is responsible for hypoxemia in a particular patient.

CLINICAL CORRELATIONS Useful clinical correlations can be made with the mechanisms underlying hypoxemia (see Fig. 214-5). A lowered inspired P_{O_2} contributes to hypoxemia either at high altitude or if the concentration of inspired O_2 is less than 21%. The latter problem occurs if a patient receiving anesthesia or ventilatory support is inadvertently given a gas mixture to breathe containing less than 21% O_2 or if O_2 is consumed from ambient gas, as can occur during smoke inhalation from a fire. The primary feature of hypoventilation as a cause of hypoxemia is an elevation in arterial P_{CO_2}. The clinical correlations with hypoventilation are discussed in Chap. 229.

Shunt as a cause of hypoxemia can reflect transfer of blood from the right to the left side of the heart without it ever entering the pulmonary circulation, as occurs with an intracardiac shunt. This problem occurs most commonly in the setting of cyanotic congenital

heart disease, when an interatrial or interventricular septal defect is associated with pulmonary hypertension, so that shunting is in the right-to-left rather than the left-to-right direction. Shunting of blood through the pulmonary parenchyma is most frequently due to disease causing absence of ventilation to perfused alveoli. This can occur if the alveoli are atelectatic or if they are filled with fluid, as in pulmonary edema (both cardiogenic and noncardiogenic) or with extensive intraalveolar exudation of fluid due to pneumonia. Less commonly, vascular anomalies with arteriovenous shunting in the lung can cause hypoxemia. These anomalies can be hereditary, as found with hereditary hemorrhagic telangiectasia (Osler-Rendu-Weber syndrome), or acquired, as in pulmonary vascular malformations secondary to hepatic cirrhosis, which are similar to the commonly recognized cutaneous vascular malformations ("spider hemangiomas").

Ventilation-perfusion mismatch is the most common cause of hypoxemia clinically. Most of the processes affecting either the airways or the pulmonary parenchyma are distributed unevenly throughout the lungs and do not necessarily affect ventilation and perfusion equally. Some areas of lung may have good perfusion and poor ventilation, whereas others may have poor perfusion and relatively good ventilation. Important examples of airways diseases in which $\dot{V}/\dot{Q}$ mismatch causes hypoxemia are asthma and chronic obstructive lung disease. Parenchymal lung diseases causing $\dot{V}/\dot{Q}$ mismatch and hypoxemia include interstitial lung disease and pneumonia.

Clinically important alterations in CO_2 elimination range from excessive ventilation and hypocapnia to inadequate CO_2 elimination and hypercapnia. These clinical problems are discussed in Chap. 229.

Diffusing capacity Measurement of DL_{CO} may be useful for assessing disease affecting the alveolar-capillary bed or the pulmonary vasculature. In practice, three main categories of disease are associated with lowered DL_{CO}: interstitial lung disease, emphysema, and pulmonary vascular disease. With interstitial lung disease, scarring of alveolar-capillary units diminishes the area of the alveolar-capillary bed as well as pulmonary blood volume. With emphysema, alveolar walls are destroyed, so the surface area of the alveolar-capillary bed is again diminished. In patients with disease causing a decrease in the cross-sectional area and volume of the pulmonary vascular bed, such as recurrent pulmonary emboli or primary pulmonary hypertension, DL_{CO} is commonly diminished.

Diffusing capacity may be elevated if pulmonary blood volume is increased, as may be seen in congestive heart failure. However, once interstitial and alveolar edema ensue, the net DL_{CO} depends on the opposing influences of increased pulmonary capillary blood volume elevating DL_{CO} and pulmonary edema decreasing it. Finding an elevated DL_{CO} may be useful in the diagnosis of alveolar hemorrhage, such as in Goodpasture's syndrome. Hemoglobin contained in erythrocytes within the alveolar lumen is capable of binding carbon monoxide, so the exhaled carbon monoxide concentration is diminished and the measured DL_{CO} is increased.

REFERENCES

AMERICAN THORACIC SOCIETY: Lung function testing: Selection of reference values and interpretative strategies. Am Rev Respir Dis 144:1202, 1991

CLARK JS et al: Noninvasive assessment of blood gases. Am Rev Respir Dis 145:220, 1992

CRAPO RO, FORSTER RE II: Carbon monoxide diffusing capacity. Clin Chest Med 10:187, 1989

GIBSON GJ: Standardised lung function testing. Eur Respir J 6:155, 1993

QUANJER PH et al: Lung volumes and forced ventilatory flows. Report Working Party Standardization of Lung Function Tests, European Community for Steel and Coal. Official Statement of the European Respiratory Society. Eur Respir J Suppl 16:5, 1993

SOCIETY OF CRITICAL CARE MEDICINE: A model for technology assessment applied to pulse oximetry. Crit Care Med 21:615, 1993

WEINBERGER SE: *Principles of Pulmonary Medicine*, 2d ed. Philadelphia, Saunders, 1992

WEST JB: *Respiratory Physiology: The Essentials*, 4th ed. Baltimore, Williams & Wilkins, 1990

215   IMAGING IN PULMONARY DISEASE

PAUL J. FRIEDMAN

Radiologic examination of the lungs and pleura has grown beyond the capability—great as it is—of the plain chest radiograph and includes the imaging modalities of computed tomography, nuclear magnetic resonance, ultrasound, and nuclear medicine. This chapter will focus on their applications in relation to the traditional chest film.

THE BASIC PRINCIPLES OF CLINICAL IMAGING

Problem-based imaging   The first step in ordering a radiologic examination is to define the problem clearly enough to indicate what new information needs to be provided by an imaging study.

Consultation   The next step is to decide if a plain chest radiograph (CR) will suffice, whether special radiographic views are necessary, or if the problem demands more expensive and time-consuming techniques. In this era of growing specialization, rapidly changing technology, and cost consciousness, it is increasingly important to get radiologic consultation for this step.

Getting the results   The value of a radiographic report often depends on whether the radiologist was aware of the question being asked. It has been shown that radiologic interpretation is far more accurate when an appropriate history is provided. Even with a relevant history, the false-negative error rate (the "misses") is 30 to 40 percent, on average, when measured in controlled situations. It is therefore important to (1) provide a history, (2) read the report carefully but skeptically, (3) look at the films yourself, and (4) review them with a radiologist.

Screening   Ordering a routine posteroanterior (PA) and lateral CR is an exception to problem-based imaging, but admission films are needed only if there is suspicion of cardiac or pulmonary disease. Periodic health examinations do not require a CR unless there is a relevant history or physical finding.

OCCUPATIONAL HEALTH SCREENING   Evaluating the extent of lung damage from exposure to coal or silica dust has been achieved by standardized CR, with an ingenious scoring system for pneumoconiosis. Health risks from exposure to asbestos dust are currently monitored by radiography, though with improved industrial hygiene the expected plaques are more rare and pulmonary fibrosis from asbestos is unusual. Occupational exposures to agents more likely to cause asthma than pneumoconiosis should not be monitored by CR.

APPLICATIONS OF IMAGING TECHNOLOGY, NEW AND OLD

Variations on chest radiography   Chest radiologists uniformly agree that the technique of choice is high kilovoltage (>120 kVp), with a stationary scatter-absorbing grid, and a wide-latitude film-screen combination (more shades of gray, less black-and-white). Many new techniques are under development, from improved x-ray–sensitive fluorescent screens, to Xerox-like methods of transferring latent images from solid-state receivers, to electronic scanning, digitization, and storage of radiographic images. These new technologies allow computer manipulation of the images to compensate for exposure problems, speed image retrieval from archives, and allow their electronic transmission to other clinical sites. However, available displays lack the fine detail of the conventional chest radiograph.

Portable films   Though necessary in many cases, the portable CR is deficient in detail resolution, latitude, and penetration and fails to show the normal gravitational gradient necessary for physiologic interpretation. It also has increased geometric distortion, more lung is obscured by heart or diaphragm, and it does not provide a lateral view. Because of these technical limitations, replacement of the conventional film-screen combination by photo-stimulable phosphor plates will be most acceptable and potentially useful at the bedside.

Lateral decubitus or prone positions may be useful in bedside radiography to show parts of the lung otherwise obscured by effusion; the lateral decubitus and other horizontal-beam films are good for demonstrating pneumothorax or fluid levels in the lung or pleural space. Portable radiographic examinations are also useful in assessing the positions of tubes and catheters commonly used in the intensive care unit.

Conventional tomography   Essentially obsolete for chest work, tomography is rarely used even for studying the hilar regions; far more information can be obtained about the hilar structures and the adjacent mediastinum from computed tomography (CT) or magnetic resonance (MR) imaging. Screening the lungs for metastases, formerly a major application of conventional tomography, is better done with CT. Conventional tomography should be used only in facilities where more advanced technology is not available.

COMPUTED TOMOGRAPHY

The x-ray absorption of each point (pixel) in a cross section of the body can be calculated by measuring the absorption of many fine x-ray beams at many angles within the plane of the cross section. The calculated absorption coefficients are displayed as radiographic densities with far more shades of gray than possible with CR (Fig. 215-1). CT eliminates the superimposition of structures that makes CR anatomy so difficult, and though the images are "noisy," there is less problem with CT than with CR in detecting an abnormality because of obscuration by normal structures. However, a set of images is needed to encompass the chest, since each represents only the information in a 1-cm thick transverse cross section. Each set of data is collected during suspended respiration, taking 1 to 2 s, and requires patient cooperation in taking and holding a comparable breath each time for good results. The new generation of "spiral" CT scanners collect data for several serial sections continuously, greatly reducing the problem of missing parts of the lung because of inconsistent inspiratory efforts.

MEDIASTINAL CT   After less than two decades of use in the chest, CT is well established as the diagnostic procedure of choice for studying the mediastinum (see Fig. 215-1*B*). The most common

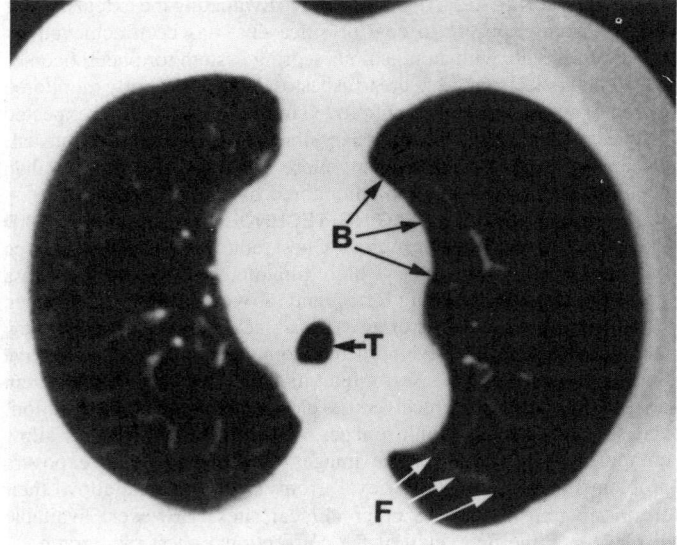

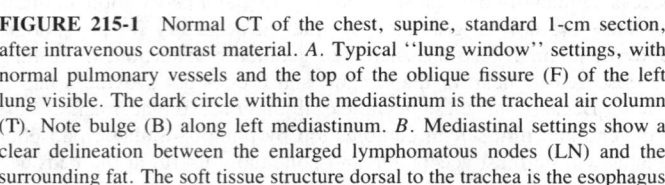

A

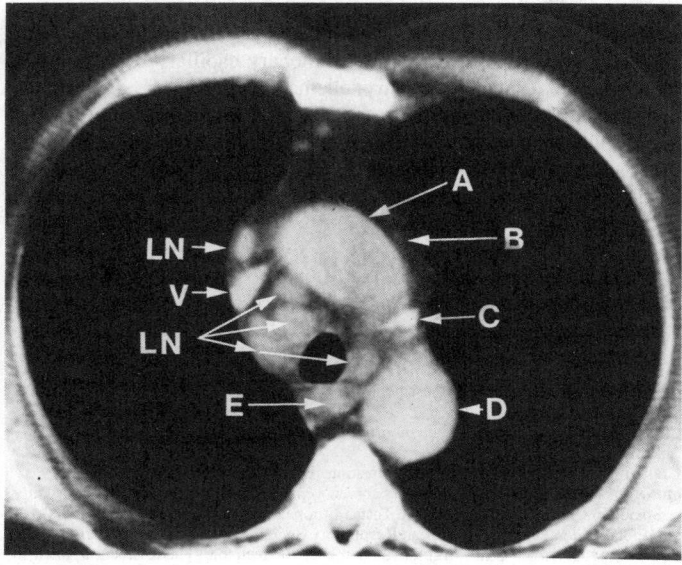

B

FIGURE 215-1 Normal CT of the chest, supine, standard 1-cm section, after intravenous contrast material. *A*. Typical "lung window" settings, with normal pulmonary vessels and the top of the oblique fissure (F) of the left lung visible. The dark circle within the mediastinum is the tracheal air column (T). Note bulge (B) along left mediastinum. *B*. Mediastinal settings show a clear delineation between the enlarged lymphomatous nodes (LN) and the surrounding fat. The soft tissue structure dorsal to the trachea is the esophagus

(E). The major vessels visible are the superior vena cava (V) and ascending (A) and descending (D) aorta; small veins are also seen in the fat in front of the spine behind the esophagus, and ventrally, behind the sternum, as well as in the generous layer of subcutaneous fat. The calcification (C) is a plaque in the aortic arch rather than a calcified lymph node. The mediastinal bulge (B) alongside the ascending aorta on the left is simply mediastinal fat, not an enlarged node.

use is the assessment of lymph node size in the staging of lung cancer (Chap. 227). Enlarged nodes require biopsy for diagnosis, since enlargement caused by acute inflammation cannot be confidently distinguished from that caused by metastasis on CT (or MR) images. The false-negative error rate of CT is significantly greater than that of mediastinoscopy, but CT is still useful in screening patients being considered for cancer surgery if mediastinoscopy is not planned.

Lumps and bumps of the mediastinum detected on CR are readily analyzed using CT. Mediastinal cysts, tumors, fat, and calcification are readily distinguished because of the good density resolution. CT is also excellent for distinguishing vascular from nonvascular structures and for recognizing vascular anatomic variants or aneurysms.

CONTRAST MATERIAL   There is no consensus about the indications for using intravenous contrast material in chest CT. Some institutions use contrast material universally and may even use the high dose–rapid infusion method known as *dynamic CT*. Others use contrast material regularly in studies of vessels or tumors but not for routine lung cancer staging. Injection of traditional hypertonic contrast material adds to the cost and risk of the study, since allergic and idiosyncratic reactions occur regularly. Serious reactions are uncommon, however, and death occurs no more than about once in every 40,000 intravenous injections. Newer low-osmolar agents are less toxic but are still several times as expensive.

CT OF THE PLEURA   CT imaging resolves complex abnormalities which might involve the lung or pleura or both. For example, the diagnosis of bronchopleural fistula requires distinguishing pleural pockets from lung abscesses or cysts. The solid and fluid components of a pleural collection, which are the same density on CR, can be usefully distinguished on CT.

Tumors of the pleura are demonstrated in the transverse plane much more clearly than on CR, where they are hard to distinguish from inflammatory pleural thickening. The true extent of malignant mesothelioma or metastatic adenocarcinoma is therefore best shown on CT. An asbestos-related application is the detection of pleural plaques and calcifications (Chap. 219). Though routine health screening of asbestos-exposed workers relies on the posteroanterior CR,

sometimes it is necessary to use the much greater sensitivity of CT to detect pleural plaques or the characteristic small pleural calcifications.

HIGH-RESOLUTION CT OF THE LUNG AND AIRWAYS   Since CR has such excellent resolution and shows air/tissue density differences so well, this application of CT has been the slowest to develop. The geometric resolution of ordinary CT is nearly tenfold less than CR, but high-resolution (HRCT) technique brings it up to within a factor of two or three. HRCT uses a thin image plane, usually 1 to 2 mm instead of the conventional 10 mm, to reduce volume averaging of densities and a higher contrast or edge-enhancing image reconstruction. The result is comparable with a pathologist's naked-eye view of a slice of lung. The trade-off is that the number of these thin slices that can be made is limited by radiation exposure, which precludes covering the entire lung; HRCT is used to sample the lung, like a noninvasive biopsy.

The trachea and main bronchi are shown well in cross section (see Fig. 215-2), and CT shows the mediastinal extent of endobronchial lesions, though longitudinal images of the trachea would be more useful clinically. Intrinsic tumors or deformity from other mediastinal primary or secondary neoplasms are demonstrable but are not an indication for CT unless endoscopy is contraindicated. HRCT has much greater sensitivity for bronchial abnormality (thickening, dilatation, mucoid impaction) than CR. HRCT has essentially replaced bronchography in screening for surgical bronchiectasis (Chap. 221), missing only minimal or localized cylindrical bronchiectasis.

Details of both airspace and interstitial lung diseases can be demonstrated well by HRCT. Characteristic changes have been described in many diffuse diseases such as carcinomatosis, interstitial fibrosis (see Fig. 215-3), eosinophilic granuloma, sarcoidosis, bronchiolitis, and emphysema. HRCT can reveal subtle interstitial fibrosis of asbestosis before it is evident on the chest film, and a delicate ground glass pattern of partial alveolar filling, such as in *Pneumocystis carinii* pneumonia, can be seen when the chest film still appears normal. The distribution and amount of emphysema can be assessed readily, and early destructive changes can be detected before pulmonary function tests become abnormal.

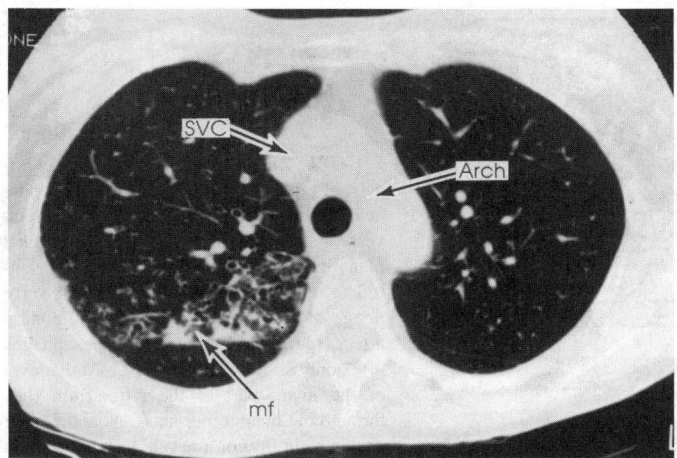

FIGURE 215-2   High-resolution CT, supine, 1.5-mm section, with edge-sharpening technique and standard "lung window." Patient has bronchiectasis in posterior segment of right upper lobe. The ring shadows and irregular patchy light regions just ventral to the major fissure (mf) represent, respectively, the dilated, thick-walled bronchi and patchy bronchopneumonia. An opacity was visible on the chest radiograph but the abnormal bronchi could not be perceived. Major vessels bulging the mediastinal shadow are the superior vena cava (SVC) and aortic arch (Arch). The left lung shows normal bronchi and vessels at this level.

The clinical indications for HRCT thus fall into two broad categories: first, to confirm the presence, extent, or activity of suspected interstitial, airspace, or airway disease, and second, to show the detailed pathology underlying an ambiguous radiographic pattern, enabling differential diagnosis of these several kinds of disease.

LIMITED CT STUDIES   CT scans of the chest initially were complete, top to bottom, without and with contrast injection. With greater awareness of the capabilities of CT, studies of a limited part of the chest, using regular or HRCT technique and no contrast, should play an increasing role. Their cost can be substantially less than a full scan, hardly more than adding oblique views to a routine CR. Confusing CR findings can often be resolved rapidly using limited CT studies, in preference to waiting a few costly hospital days for the diagnosis to become clear. CT densitometry is useful in determining the presence or absence of calcification in solitary pulmonary nodules.

FIGURE 215-3   High-resolution CT, prone, 1.5 mm section, with edge-sharpening image processing, shown as a light "lung window." Chronic interstitial fibrosis with severe honeycombing: a graphic portrayal, comparable to looking directly at a lung specimen. HRCT can show detailed gross pathologic findings in many lung diseases, with great sensitivity for alveolar filling, for interstitial alterations of various kinds, and for emphysema. *(Courtesy of I. Feuerstein.)*

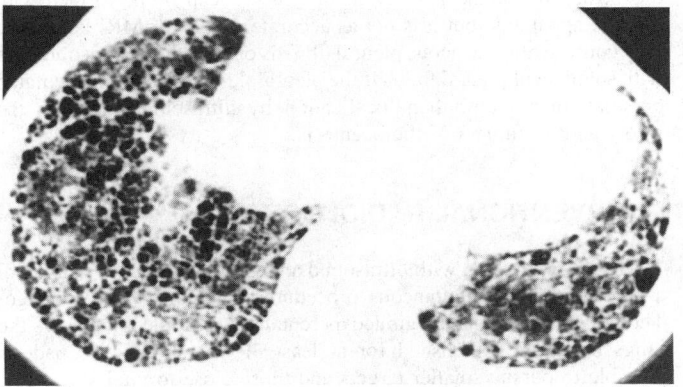

MAGNETIC RESONANCE IMAGING

Nuclear magnetic resonance is a property of atomic nuclei with an odd number of nucleons, of which the most abundant in the body is hydrogen. While in a strong magnetic field, the alignment of these spinning nuclei can be changed with a superimposed radio-frequency signal, and the rate at which they return to alignment with the field ("relaxation") can be measured by their emission of a faint signal. There are two kinds of relaxation rates, which are functions of the atomic and chemical environment of each nucleus, and therefore they differ in different tissues.

By ingenious use of gradients, relaxation rates can be measured simultaneously at many points within a three-dimensional volume, which allows them to be shown as a set of gray scale images, either in the transverse, coronal, or sagittal plane. The timing of the imposed radio-frequency signal determines which of the relaxation rates predominates, and therefore the constructed images have different shades of gray for the same tissue, though the underlying anatomic structure is unchanged. At this time, there is only limited standardization of technique, especially since optimal differentiation of specific abnormalities requires different machine settings.

Transverse MR images look much like CT images except for the different substitutions of light and dark for different tissues (Fig. 215-4). For example, fat is darker than water on CT but is the brightest tissue on "T_1-weighted" MR images. Water (e.g., cerebrospinal fluid) becomes as bright as fat on T_2-weighted MR images (see Fig. 215-4). The values T_1 and T_2 are the half-times of the relaxation rates mentioned above and are therefore a property of the tissue itself. The flexibility of eliciting and displaying the two relaxation rates provides MR images with even more effective tissue characterization contrast than CT.

Though the protons in blood have a strong MR signal because of the atomic environment of the iron and should therefore appear bright, flowing blood is seen as black, a signal void, on images. During the pause after the radio-frequency signal is triggered, while waiting to measure relaxation signals, the blood containing the altered protons has time to flow out of the plane of interest and is replaced by blood that is emitting no signal. Therefore, normal blood vessels as well as bronchi appear black on MR images (see Fig. 215-4), but the distinction between nodes and vessels in the hilar regions is greatly facilitated when compared with CT. There are artifactual signals from blood vessels, however, when blood flow is slow, notably on scans gated to diastole in the cardiac cycle (which are essential for studying the heart and hilar regions of the mediastinum) and on multisection simultaneous scans, when altered protons from one section may arrive at another level just in time for their signal to be detected. Newer methods of "fast scanning" result in images with flowing blood giving a bright image as in an angiogram.

MR scanning has important limitations compared with CT. A wide variety of artifacts complicate the interpretation of MR images, and the images are also noisier and less uniform than those of CT. The geometric resolution of whole-body scans is inferior to that of CT, though superficial small regions can be shown with superb detail using special surface antennae to detect the faint relaxation signals. The advantage of being able to display sections in any planar direction is weakened by the necessity (at present) of leaving a gap between the image slices. The collection of data (except with fast-scan techniques) requires several minutes, which means that there are breathing artifacts in addition to those from cardiac motion. The narrow magnet tunnel into which the patient is inserted promotes claustrophobia, and the changes in the magnetic field cause a distressing noise. Ferromagnetic materials, including those in the patient, cannot be brought into the magnet room safely, for they will fly toward the center of the magnet. Other metal in the patient will merely ruin the image in its vicinity. Finally, the cost of MR scanning is substantial, approximately twice that of a contrast CT.

MR APPLICATIONS   Gated cardiac studies are of great interest (Chap. 191) but are outside the scope of this discussion. The spine

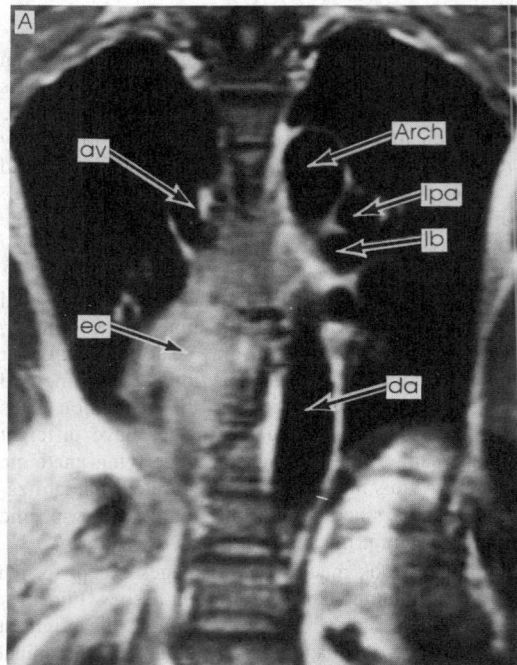

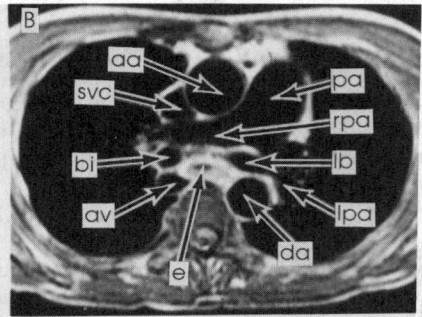

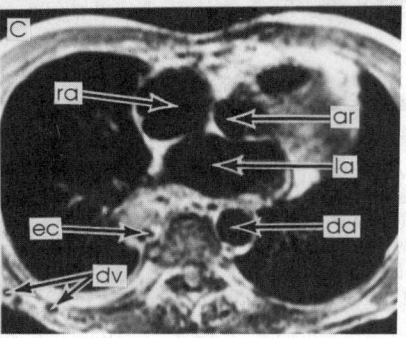

FIGURE 215-4 Magnetic resonance images of a patient with a bulky lower esophageal carcinoma (EC). Both bronchi and blood vessels show a signal void. *A*. The coronal plane image intersecting the tumor just ventral to the vertebral column. *B*. Transverse image at the level of the right pulmonary artery (rpa), where the wall of the esophagus (e) is only slightly thickened. *C*. At the level of the lower part of the left atrium (la), through the main tumor mass. Note the large azygos vein (av) on images *A* and *B* and the dilated chest wall veins (dv) on image *C*, raising a question of obstruction of the inferior vena cava. No distinct adenopathy is seen. Other anatomic structures seen include the ascending and descending aorta (aa, da), aortic root (ar) and arch (Arch), main and left pulmonary arteries (pa, lpa), bronchus intermedius (bi), left main bronchus (lb), and right atrium (ra).

can be displayed with the perspective of an anatomic diagram because of the availability of sagittal projections. This enables MR scanning to be particularly useful in questions of paraspinal, intraspinal, or intraosseous tumor. Tumors in the mediastinum can be analyzed by their T_1 and T_2 properties, but the ability to distinguish inflammatory enlargement of nodes from that of tumor has not been realized. As noted, MR imaging is more sensitive than CT for distinguishing nonvascular tissue in the complex hilar regions and in the central portions of the lung (see Fig. 215-4) but is probably less satisfactory in the mediastinum. Detection of intravascular pulmonary emboli or thrombi has been demonstrated experimentally, but clinical application is still limited.

Use of sagittal and coronal or oblique images of the mediastinum facilitates study of the arteries, so MR scanning of the aorta is the preferred noninvasive way to detect aortic dissection or aneurysm (Chap. 210). These projections should be ideal for studying the trachea, but the trachea and bronchi are poorly displayed, with an artifactual narrowing of the lumen. The staging of lung cancer by mediastinal scanning has about the same effectiveness using MR as CT.

SPECTROSCOPY   When chemists use MR to analyze mixtures and determine chemical structure, they study many nuclei in addition to hydrogen. Only hydrogen is sufficiently abundant in the body to provide enough signal to form images, but other substances can be quantitated in a large volume that would be unsuitable for imaging. The most important is phosphorus, which has different resonant frequencies in its various molecular positions as part of ATP, AMP, creatine phosphate, inorganic phosphorus, etc. A limited number of relatively abundant cellular metabolites also can be measured by detecting protons with specific resonance values, if the strong proton signal from water is suppressed. Metabolic processes can therefore be monitored by in vivo MR spectroscopy, a research technique of potential future clinical application.

NUCLEAR MEDICINE IMAGING

Injected or inhaled radioisotopes (radionuclides) incorporated into carefully chosen substances can provide anatomic, physiologic, and pathologic information from their distribution and disposition, as revealed on gamma camera images. Nuclear medicine remains the primary technique for the clinical problem of pulmonary thromboembolism (Chaps. 216 and 226) and the regional functional assessment of obstructive lung diseases.

ULTRASOUND IN THE CHEST

Imaging with ultrasound requires the computerized reconstruction of series of echoes of high-frequency sound emitted at various angles from a piezoelectric crystal transducer. The echoes arise as the radiating sound encounters surfaces of different acoustic impedance at right angles to its path. Ultrasound does not pass through air or bone, so the lungs themselves and the ribs are major limitations on its usefulness in the chest. A fluid collection such as a cyst or abscess will be echo-free, or *sonolucent*, unless it has debris in it and will transmit sound to make deeper echoes without attenuation. In solid tissues, the signal is attenuated as the sound is absorbed, so the echoes become weaker as their depth in the tissue increases. Air-containing lung has no echo beyond the pleural interface at its surface, although consolidated lung may look like solid tissue.

APPLICATIONS   The principal application of ultrasonography in the mediastinum is cardiac, discussed in detail in Chap. 190, including the detection of pericardial fluid and cysts. Bronchogenic cysts, in their most common subcarinal location, also may be confirmed to be fluid-containing by ultrasound. The most common pulmonary application is detection of fluid or pus in the pleural space. For diagnosis, ultrasound is convenient, since it can be performed with bedside apparatus, but it is not as accurate as CT (or MR) because it may confuse homogeneous pleural fibrosis or pulmonary consolidation with sonolucent pleural fluid. If the pleural fluid collection is loculated or small in amount, then localization by ultrasound enhances the safety and usefulness of thoracentesis.

INTERVENTIONAL RADIOLOGY

Advances in imaging with ultrasound and CT have brought with them a renaissance of percutaneous procedures for biopsy and drainage. Though fluoroscopically guided percutaneous needle biopsy of the lungs has been established for at least 30 years, CT has made it possible to pursue smaller targets and those close to vital structures.

Under CT control, needle biopsy of the mediastinum can replace mediastinoscopy, particularly when inoperability is being established by biopsy of enlarged nodes.

A more recent interventional innovation is drainage of pleural effusions, pneumothorax, and empyema in the thorax, and abscesses in the abdomen by catheters inserted over guidewires that have been introduced through percutaneous needles using techniques originally developed for angiography. The fluid or air pocket is localized and the needle position confirmed using ultrasound or CT, the specific technique depending on the ease with which the fluid can be delineated with ultrasound. Even lung abscesses can be drained percutaneously. Transcatheter embolization with particulate matter, coils, or detachable balloons has become widely used in the treatment of massive hemoptysis and arteriovenous malformations of the lung. Considerable savings are achieved in risk, pain, recovery time, and cost by avoiding major surgery with these methods.

REFERENCES

BERGIN CJ et al: Magnetic resonance imaging of lung parenchyma. J Thorac Imaging 8:12, 1993

DOBBINS JT et al: Threshold perception performance with computed and screen-film radiography: Implications for chest radiography. Radiology 183:179, 1992

FRIEDMAN PJ: Lung cancer staging: Efficacy of CT. Radiology 182:307, 1992

NAIDICH DP et al: Hemoptysis: CT-bronchoscopic correlations in 58 cases. Radiology 177:357, 1990

NAIDICH DP et al: *Computed Tomography and Magnetic Resonance of the Thorax.* New York, Raven, 1991

WEBB WR et al: *High-Resolution CT of the Lung.* New York, Raven, 1992

WHITE CS et al: Imaging in lung cancer. Semin Oncol 20:142, 1993

216 DIAGNOSTIC PROCEDURES IN RESPIRATORY DISEASES

KENNETH M. MOSER

In seeking a definitive diagnosis in the patient with respiratory disease, a wide choice of diagnostic procedures is available. These procedures vary considerably, not only in diagnostic reliability and specificity but also in terms of the discomfort, hazard, and cost to the patient. Hence, an orderly sequence of test selection is mandatory. This sequence should begin with procedures involving little risk and cost and, only if necessary, move on to those that entail greater expense as well as higher morbidity and potential mortality.

NONINVASIVE PROCEDURES

RADIOGRAPHIC PROCEDURES (See also Chap. 215) The *chest roentgenogram* serves two major roles in the search for a diagnosis in the patient with respiratory disease: *detector* and *guide.* Occasionally, in its role as a detector, the routine chest roentgenogram initiates the diagnostic search by disclosing an abnormality in an asymptomatic individual. However, routine chest roentgenography (e.g., as an element of all hospital admissions) is neither necessary nor cost-effective. Therefore, more commonly, it detects pulmonary involvement in someone already ill. Rarely, detection may coincide with diagnosis, e.g., in spontaneous pneumothorax or when a radiopaque foreign body has been aspirated.

Far more frequently, however, the roentgenogram, having detected potential disease, provides a guide to the selection of subsequent diagnostic procedures. Many radiographic findings are quite characteristic of certain diseases. A number of radiographic patterns are sufficiently repetitive to warrant descriptive names, such as bilateral hilar adenopathy, solitary pulmonary nodule, diffuse interstitial infiltrate, alveolar filling pattern, multinodular lesion, and honeycomb lung. Thus, a particular radiographic finding, combined with other pertinent data, often permits establishment of a reasonable list of possible diagnoses. For example, the radiographic detection of bilateral hilar adenopathy in an asymptomatic, 26-year-old black male immediately places sarcoidosis at the top of the list. A chest roentgenogram disclosing upper lobe cavities in a febrile male whose brother recently was admitted to a tuberculosis sanitarium would make tuberculosis the most likely entity. Or a "diffuse interstitial" infiltrate—for which more than 100 causes exist—may yield a prompt diagnosis of varicella pneumonia when combined with the classic skin lesions. A diffuse alveolar filling process in an HIV-positive patient suggests *Pneumocystis carinii* pneumonitis (PCP). Multinodular lesions, with some cavitating, in a patient with sinusitis and red cell casts on urinalysis makes Wegener's granulomatosis a primary diagnostic possibility. However, no radiographic pattern is sufficiently specific to *establish* a diagnosis. Lung cancer (primary and metastatic) can present many radiographic patterns, as can both infectious and noninfectious lung disorders. For example, cardiogenic pulmonary edema may present as a perihilar or diffuse alveolar filling pattern, as an interstitial process, and, rarely, as a lobar infiltrate or interlobar collection of fluid ("pseudotumor")—all with or without a pleural effusion.

In some instances, special radiographic techniques may provide valuable diagnostic insights.

Fluoroscopy allows visualization of the thoracic contents in a dynamic rather than static manner and also permits a wide range of special views. It also indicates whether a lesion is pulsatile, what its precise location in the thorax is, whether the hemidiaphragms move normally, i.e., whether they are fixed or move paradoxically, and how various zones of the lung behave during inspiration and expiration. Thus, fluoroscopy, a relatively inexpensive procedure, can define whether a radiographic density is actually in a rib or in the pleura rather than in the parenchyma; and may distinguish between a unilateral hyperlucent lung due to emphysema (mediastinum shifts toward the normal lung on expiration) or to unilateral pulmonary arterial obstruction (no shift).

Thoracic *computed tomography* (CT) has essentially replaced standard tomography (laminography, planigraphy). Both techniques provide a sequence of images, each representing a "slice of the lung" at a different depth. Ordinarily, "cuts" are made at 0.5- to 1.0-cm distances through the areas of interest. These procedures can identify a number of features that are not appreciated on the "routine" roentgenogram, including calcium in a solitary nodule (which if diffuse or in concentric rings signifies a benign etiology); a cavity within a mass lesion; and the presence of hilar, paratracheal, and subcarinal node enlargement. The CT scan is particularly useful in the definition of pleural disease (e.g., differentiating fluid from tumor; identifying calcium in asbestos-exposed individuals); with contrast injections, in differentiating tissue masses from vascular structures; and in identifying small parenchymal nodules. However, to some extent, the sensitivity of CT is a mixed blessing because it is still not known how many "normal" individuals have pleural or parenchymal abnormalities by CT and how these small, benign, hitherto undetected lesions can be distinguished from neoplastic lesions. The CT scan is also proving useful in the detection of interstitial lung disease not apparent (or equivocal) on routine chest roentgenogram and in quantifying emphysematous changes.

Magnetic resonance (MR) imaging remains, in terms of its value in pulmonary diseases, an investigational technique. It has potential value in achieving fine definition of mediastinal lesions, pleural lesions, and, perhaps, in defining embolic occlusion of major pulmonary arteries.

SKIN TESTS Having arrived at a tentative list of diagnostic possibilities based on the history, physical examination, and radiographic appearance, the physician should move to other procedures.

One of the simplest, least costly, and most commonly overlooked is the application of *skin tests* with specific antigens. Antigens are now available to assist in the diagnosis of tuberculosis, histoplasmosis, coccidioidomycosis, blastomycosis, trichinosis, toxoplasmosis, and aspergillosis. These tests vary with respect to sensitivity and cross-reactivity, and attention to scrupulous technique in performance and interpretation is vital. Also, some antigens (e.g., histoplasmosis) may confound serologic tests performed subsequently. A positive skin test indicates only that the antigen has been encountered previously by the host; it does not, regardless of reaction intensity, imply active disease. Furthermore, drugs or diseases that depress cell-mediated immunity (e.g., prednisone, cyclophosphamide, lymphomas, sarcoidosis, HIV infection, disseminated tuberculosis, or coccidioidomycosis) may cause skin anergy. Indeed, a negative battery of skin tests, if it incorporates antigens such as mumps, streptokinase-streptodornase, *Trichophyton*, and *Candida*, suggests that a cause of skin anergy should be sought.

SEROLOGIC TESTS   These relatively inexpensive tests also may be useful in the diagnosis of histoplasmosis, blastomycosis, coccidioidomycosis, toxoplasmosis, *Mycoplasma* pneumonia, Legionnaires' disease, a variety of other infectious diseases involving the lungs, and certain immunologically mediated lung diseases (e.g., lupus erythematosus, Wegener's granulomatosis). Often, more extensive diagnostic procedures can be avoided if appropriate serologic tests are obtained. However, there is substantial interinstitutional variability with respect to the sensitivity, specificity, and types of serologic tests available. Therefore, their appropriate use requires close interaction with the responsible laboratory. Serologic testing for HIV status, of course, has become an important element in the evaluation of patients with a variety of pulmonary lesions.

SPUTUM EXAMINATION   Another rapid, innocuous, and inexpensive diagnostic procedure is *sputum examination*. It is important that the specimen contain sputum, not saliva, the latter being identified by the presence of squamous (mouth) rather than epithelial (bronchial) cells. The gross nature of the sputum—color, odor, and the presence of blood—may provide valuable clues; e.g., foul sputum suggesting anaerobic pulmonary infection, and blood, in any amount, indicating an abnormality that mandates further investigation. Carefully stained smears of the sputum should be examined next, for these may disclose the causative organism in many bacterial pneumonias, tuberculosis, *Pneumocystis* pneumonia, and in some fungus infections. Sputum eosinophilia can suggest the presence of reversible airway disease responsive to glucocorticoids; hemosiderin-laden macrophages suggest the possibility of Goodpasture's syndrome. Often valuable time is lost because the sputum smear is not examined and results of culture are awaited instead. Sputum samples can be obtained from patients who are not coughing by having them inhale a heated mixture of a mildly irritative solution that induces cough. Such induced samples have been particularly useful in the diagnosis of *P. carinii* pneumonia and in obtaining cytologic specimens for the diagnosis of carcinoma of the lung (Chap. 227). Careful handling of such specimens and interpretive expertise heavily determine the diagnostic yield.

Culture of expectorated sputum (spontaneous or induced) has fallen into disrepute because of uncertain yield and, particularly, because of frequent and unavoidable contamination by the oropharyngeal bacterial flora. Although such cultures are invaluable for identification of organisms responsible for tuberculous and fungus infections, their utility in detection of other bacterial agents responsible for pulmonary infection is often uncertain and can be misleading, particularly in patients who are immunocompromised, intubated, or receiving antimicrobial therapy. Blood cultures may be useful in certain contexts, particularly in AIDS patients with *Mycobacterium avium-intracellulare* (MAI) infections in whom sputum examinations are often negative.

Beyond such standard approaches to obtaining material for culture, five procedures, described below, are now gaining wide acceptance because they limit oropharyngeal contamination and/or can be used to obtain representative samples of lung secretions from the area of

lung involvement: (1) catheter-brush sampling, (2) bronchoalveolar lavage, (3) transtracheal aspiration, (4) transbronchial lung biopsy, and (5) percutaneous needle aspiration of the lung.

PULMONARY FUNCTION TESTS (See also Chap. 214)   Certain "patterns" of derangement in spirometric tests, arterial blood gases, diffusing capacity, and other functional parameters are particularly suggestive of certain pulmonary diseases. For example, diffuse interstitial fibrotic diseases of the lungs (Chap. 224) produce a "restrictive" spirometric defect, reduced pulmonary compliance, a reduced diffusing capacity, and an alveolar-arterial oxygen tension difference that is widened at rest and widens further with exercise. Emphysema (Chap. 223) characteristically causes expiratory obstruction, lung hyperinflation, decreased static elastic recoil (increased compliance), and a reduced diffusing capacity.

PULMONARY SCINTIPHOTOGRAPHY   Scintiphotographs of intrathoracic structures are obtained by a variety of "scanning" devices that record the pattern of intrathoracic radioactivity after intravenous injection or inhalation of gamma-emitting radionuclides. Direct photographic or computer-derived images, or digital data, reflecting radionuclide distribution are used for diagnostic purposes. The most commonly used images are those that reflect the distribution of pulmonary blood flow (perfusion) and ventilation. Such scans have multiple diagnostic applications. For example, a normal perfusion scan excludes the diagnosis of acute pulmonary embolism (Chap. 226). When perfusion scans showing defects are combined with ventilation scans, ventilation-perfusion patterns are provided that assist in the diagnosis of parenchymal lung diseases and vascular occlusive disorders, including pulmonary embolism.

Another type of scan involves intravenous injection of radionuclides that have an affinity for intrathoracic inflammatory and neoplastic tissues. Gallium 67 is the most useful of such radionuclides now available. Concentration of such agents, defined by scanning, may permit detection of neoplastic or inflammatory disease in the lungs or mediastinal lymph nodes. Uptake by the lungs may, in some patients, reflect the intensity of inflammatory activity associated with diffuse interstitial pneumonitis, sarcoidosis, and granulomatous infections. Inapparent extrapulmonary foci of granulomatous or neoplastic diseases also may be detected by body scanning.

New radionuclides continue to emerge that, when complexed with such materials as platelets, white blood cells (e.g., indium 111), fibrinogen, and certain monoclonal antibodies, may allow imaging of intrathoracic vessels, thrombi, inflammation, and neoplasms. Tomographic and other image-processing methods are emerging that may further extend the value of these techniques.

All the above procedures involve minimal risks and discomfort to the patient. Where applicable, these approaches should be considered before the more invasive techniques discussed below are employed, unless the condition of the patient demands immediate diagnosis.

INVASIVE PROCEDURES

BRONCHOSCOPY   The primary objectives of bronchoscopy include direct visualization of the tracheobronchial tree, including abnormalities such as tumors or granulomatous lesions; biopsy of suggestive or obvious endobronchial lesions; and lavage, brushing, or biopsy of lung regions for cultural and cytologic examinations. Both the *diagnostic reach of* and *accessibility to* bronchoscopy have been expanded by the flexible fiberoptic bronchoscope (FOB). This can be understood best by comparing the FOB with the "standard" rigid bronchoscope.

The rigid bronchoscope is a wide-bore metal tube that incorporates a lighted mirror-lens system. The FOB is composed of fiberoptic bundles that provide both illumination and visualization pathways. One or more small channels with a diameter of 1 to 3 mm traverse the FOB, through which instruments can be passed, fluids delivered, and suction applied. The rigid bronchoscope comes in various external diameters limited only by the feasibility of introducing the rigid device orally and through the larynx. Biopsy and other procedures can be carried out through the rather capacious interior of the rigid tube. The FOB also is available in various external diameters, but all are substantially smaller than rigid bronchoscopes (since no "wall" exists in the FOB). The distal tip of the FOB can be *flexed* easily to 90° and usually to 130° or more from the vertical.

Thus, the rigid bronchoscope permits visualization only of lobar bronchi and the orifices of some segmental bronchi. The flexible, smaller FOB extends the range of *view* to all segmental and subsegmental bronchi and the range for *biopsy and sampling* to the pulmonary parenchyma itself. A biopsy forceps, catheter, or brush passed through the FOB can be directed well beyond the tip of the bronchoscope itself, permitting *transbronchial lung biopsy*, *brushings*, or *aspiration of secretions* for culture and cytologic examination from the most distal regions of the lung. Indeed, both forceps and brush can reach and perforate the pleura, leading to pneumothorax. Therefore, when the lesion being approached is distal, fluoroscopic guidance is essential. Not only does this permit placement of the FOB, forceps, catheter, or brush directly into the area of interest but also it ensures that the pleura will not be inadvertently reached and punctured. The FOB also allows *regional* lung lavage to obtain materials for cytologic examination and culture. Specially designed catheters (see below) placed through the FOB are quite useful in obtaining representative, noncontaminated secretions for culture, thus avoiding the problems mentioned previously with expectorated sputum.

Thus, the FOB has sharply increased the limited diagnostic reach previously available with rigid bronchoscopy. Equally important, the FOB has made bronchoscopy more available to the physician and more acceptable to the patient. The performance of rigid bronchoscopy requires the supine position for peroral insertion of the device; can be performed safely by a relatively few trained physicians; and is often carried out under general anesthesia in an operating room. Therefore, it has been a procedure requiring significant preparation and hence delay. Fiberoptic bronchoscopy can be performed in the sitting or supine position, as the FOB is easily inserted transnasally; can be performed by a large number of trained pulmonary specialists as well as surgeons; usually requires only local anesthesia; and can be performed safely on the wards, in diagnostic rooms equipped with a "dentist-type" chair, and in intensive care units. The FOB can be used easily in intubated patients on ventilators with simple "side-arm" adapters attached to the endotracheal tube. Therefore, when bronchoscopy is indicated, it is not surprising that fiberoptic bronchoscopy is now commonly the first choice. The roomier rigid bronchoscope is now usually reserved for situations in which the small biopsy-suction channel in the FOB may be inadequate (e.g., for removal of large foreign bodies, for laser surgery). The FOB also has a widening range of therapeutic applications including aspiration or lavage of secretions in patients with airway obstruction or atelectasis due to retained secretions; obstruction of bleeding areas of the lung, with a wedged FOB itself or with a balloon catheter passed via the FOB, in patients who are poor surgical risks; removal of small foreign bodies; and placement of radionuclides in tumors. Transtracheal needle aspiration of paratracheal and subcarinal nodes also can be performed via the FOB, a procedure which is particularly useful in the staging of carcinoma of the lung.

FOB has assumed a particularly important role in diagnostic appraisal of patients with AIDS and pulmonary involvement. If induced sputa do not provide a diagnosis, bronchoalveolar lavage (BAL) specimens often do. For example, *Histoplasma capsulatum*, cryptococcal antigen, or cytomegalovirus may be recovered in BAL samples.

The hazards of bronchoscopy are modest but should be recognized. In addition to the risk of general anesthesia, which rigid bronchoscopy usually requires, they can include hypoxemia, laryngospasm, bronchospasm, pneumothorax, and, of course, bleeding following biopsy. Proper management before, during, and after bronchoscopy should prevent most of these complications. There is no absolute contraindica-

tion to FOB. Even in the presence of massive hemoptysis, FOB with appropriate precautions can yield useful information. Patients with bronchospasm (or a history of bronchospasm) are at particular risk of acute enhancement of spasm and should be approached after good preparation and with resources for intubation-ventilation at hand. The primary contraindication to both rigid and fiberoptic bronchoscopy is the same: performance by inexperienced personnel. Lack of experience sharply reduces diagnostic and therapeutic yield while increasing risks.

BRONCHOGRAPHY In this method, radiopaque material is instilled into the tracheobronchial tree via a catheter or bronchoscope. In most situations in which bronchography was used in the past (e.g., for the diagnosis of bronchiectasis), it has been replaced by chest CT.

TRANSTRACHEAL, CATHETER-BRUSH, AND PERCUTANEOUS NEEDLE ASPIRATION OF THE LUNG All three of these procedures are used to obtain material for culture and microscopic examination. In the case of culture, all three techniques bypass the oropharyngeal flora, though transtracheal aspiration is the least certain in this regard.

Transtracheal aspiration involves needle puncture of the cricothyroid membrane, insertion of a plastic cannula, and instillation of a saline solution, followed by suctioning of a sample. The procedure cannot be performed in intubated patients; contamination rates are high in previously intubated patients or those who have aspirated oropharyngeal contents. Because the procedure entails risks, although these are minimized by meticulous technique and experience, clear indications for its use should exist. These include apparent pulmonary infections in patients who are unable to cough, in whom cough is nonproductive, or in whom there has been a lack of response to therapy based on smears or cultures from expectorated sputum.

In these same contexts, *catheter-brush devices* specially designed with a distal plug to avoid oropharyngeal contamination can be used. These are manipulated (through an FOB or without it) under fluoroscopic guidance into the involved lung area. The distal absorbable plug is then ejected, and the inner brush or catheter advanced for sampling. Finally, an alternative procedure is direct percutaneous aspiration, which can be performed using a small (23- or 25-gauge), thin-walled, *noncutting* needle. The needle, connected to a syringe, is introduced percutaneously into the area of the lung of interest; 2 to 3 mL saline is injected and then aspirated into the syringe and the needle withdrawn. Both the catheter-brush and needle approaches are high-yield, low-contamination procedures. In experienced hands, the risks are low, consisting chiefly of pneumothorax and bleeding. Patients should be carefully monitored for both.

The presence of a hemorrhagic diathesis is a relative contraindication to all three of the above procedures.

BRONCHOALVEOLAR LAVAGE This procedure is usually performed by lightly wedging a fiberoptic bronchoscope in distal airways, gently irrigating the air spaces beyond with saline, and analyzing the cells obtained. A "liquid biopsy" of the contents of the distal air spaces is obtained. The procedure has value in the diagnosis of *P. carinii* pneumonia and other infections, in alveolar proteinosis, and in some patients with interstitial pneumonitis of uncertain cause. Maximum diagnostic yield requires careful techniques and expert sample processing.

THORACENTESIS AND PLEURAL BIOPSY (See also Chap. 228) Thoracentesis should be performed to obtain pleural fluid in all pleural effusions of uncertain etiology and may be indicated for relief of symptoms in some patients with effusion of known cause. In effusions of uncertain cause, closed (needle) pleural biopsy should be performed as part of the same procedure.

When pleural fluid is small in amount or when its presence or location is uncertain from routine or lateral decubitus roentgenograms, performance of the thoracentesis and biopsy under fluoroscopic, ultrasound, or CT scan guidance enhances both yield and safety. Although utilizing such special procedures adds patient expense, the yield and/or safety gains justify their use in this context. Pleural fluid obtained should be examined for specific gravity, white blood cell count and differential, protein and glucose concentrations, lactic acid dehydrogenase (LDH), pH, P_{CO_2} (sample collected anaerobically), and amylase. Gram stain, cultures, and exfoliative cytologic specimens should be obtained, and, in some instances, rheumatoid factor and complement levels are measured. The gross appearance of the fluid, the quantity obtained, and the precise location of the thoracentesis should be recorded. A pleural fluid LDH above 200 IU, a pleural fluid/serum protein ratio greater than 0.5, and a pleural fluid/serum LDH ratio greater than 0.6 all indicate that an "exudative" rather than "transudative" process is present. A low pH (<7.20) often indicates that an empyema, probably requiring tube drainage, is present. Specific diagnostic findings in pleural fluid may include the opalescent, pearly fluid characteristic of chylothorax; positive smears or cultures for tuberculosis or other infections; a marked elevation of amylase indicative of effusion secondary to pancreatitis or a ruptured esophagus; and the very low glucose values often seen in effusions associated with rheumatoid arthritis.

As already noted, closed (needle) pleural biopsy should follow thoracentesis whenever the diagnosis is uncertain. It is important to leave some fluid in the pleural space as this makes biopsy easier and safer. Bleeding, pneumothorax, and bronchopleural fistula induced by cutting through the visceral pleura are all more likely in the absence of fluid, and a satisfactory biopsy specimen is less likely to be obtained. Several special needles are available for biopsy of the parietal pleura. All have a cutting edge and some device for retaining the biopsy. The needle is inserted into the pleural effusion, then withdrawn until it is seated on the parietal pleura, from which a biopsy is obtained with the cutting edge. Usually, three biopsies are taken from different sites at the same session. Care should be exercised to place the needle in a position least likely to impinge on the intercostal vessels. All fluid to be used for diagnosis should be removed before biopsy as postbiopsy bleeding may obscure the true character of the fluid.

Pleuroscopy   This is another procedure available for assisting in the diagnosis and management of pleural lesions. Insertion of rigid or flexible devices through intercostal trocars allows direct visualization of the pleural space. Aspiration of fluid, biopsy of pleural lesions or lung, and other types of intervention are possible.

Thoracoscopy   Although this procedure requires anesthesia and a degree of lung collapse, seems likely to replace alternative procedures for inspecting and sampling the pleura (e.g., open pleural biopsy through a limited thoracotomy and, in certain instances, closed needle biopsy). Use of miniaturized cameras allows excellent visualization of the pleural space and the lung. Rapid technical advances are likely to make this procedure widely applicable to the diagnosis and management of pleural and certain parenchymal diseases. Not only pleural biopsy but also lung biopsy can be performed, and in the hands of experienced physicians, such procedures as pleural abrasion or scarification and bullectomy are feasible in selected patients.

PULMONARY AND BRONCHIAL ANGIOGRAPHY   Visualization of the pulmonary arteries by *pulmonary angiography* is achieved by direct, rapid injection of radiopaque materials into the main pulmonary artery or its branches, preferably via cardiac catheterization. Nonionic radiopaque materials, although more expensive, reduce the frequency and severity of unwanted respiratory and hemodynamic responses (e.g., cough, elevation in pulmonary arterial pressure). Multiple, large films can be obtained by an automatic filmchanger, or motion picture or video film (cineangiography) can be used. If visualization of smaller pulmonary vessels is required, magnification techniques can be used. Digital subtraction pulmonary angiography, providing computer-derived images of digital data, may allow imaging of the larger pulmonary arteries with contrast injected more proximally (into superior or inferior vena cava or peripheral vein) or at lower concentrations; however, motion artifacts limit its sensitivity and specificity. Angiography is frequently used to detect pulmonary emboli and a variety of congenital and acquired lesions of the pulmonary vessels. The procedure carries some risk, particularly in

patients with pulmonary hypertension; but with appropriate precautions and experienced personnel that risk is extremely small.

Angioscopy, an experimental technique for direct visualization of the right cardiac chambers and pulmonary arterial system, can be accomplished by insertion of a fiberoptic device via a peripheral vein. The diagnostic role of this procedure in embolic and other disorders remains to be defined. To date it has been useful in defining which patients with chronic embolic pulmonary emboli may be candidates for thromboendarterectomy.

Bronchial arteriography is of value to identify and control (embolotherapy) otherwise obscure bleeding sites in the lungs. Transarterial placement of a catheter into the orifices or parent vessels of bronchial arteries can be accomplished by experienced operators. Radiopaque material is then injected so that these arteries can be visualized. If a bleeding site is identified, emboli can be injected via the catheter as a means for halting hemoptysis.

MEDIASTINOSCOPY AND MEDIASTINOTOMY   Another favored site for biopsy is the lymph nodes in the mediastinum. Because they receive lymphatic drainage from the lungs, these nodes often disclose intrathoracic diseases such as carcinoma, granulomatous infections, and sarcoidosis. As noted above, transtracheal needle aspiration of mediastinal nodes via the FOB is one approach to such nodes. Another is mediastinoscopy, which involves insertion of a lighted mirror-lens system, much like a bronchoscope, through an incision at the base of the neck anteriorly. The instrument is advanced under visual control into the mediastinum, where inspection and biopsy can be carried out. Because of its higher yield of diagnostic lymph nodes, mediastinoscopy has virtually replaced biopsy of the *scalene fat pad* for nodes of interest on the right side of the mediastinum. However, for anatomic reasons, mediastinoscopy on the left is less satisfactory and more hazardous. Nodes in this location are usually approached through a limited left anterior thoracotomy (mediastinotomy). Needle aspiration, mediastinoscopy, and mediastinotomy are low-risk, high-yield procedures. They are invaluable in the "staging" of patients with known or suspected pulmonary malignancy.

LUNG BIOPSY   Finally, if the diagnosis still remains unclear, biopsy of the lung may be required. Again, "closed" and "open" approaches are available. Closed biopsies are of three types: transbronchial, aspiration, and "cutting needle." Transbronchial biopsy, carried out through the fiberoptic bronchoscope, is a highly useful procedure, particularly since larger forceps have been introduced and the taking of multiple biopsies during one procedure has become routine.

However, when lesions are small and/or anatomically located beyond the reach of the FOB, direct aspiration needle biopsy is often more rewarding. *Aspiration* biopsy, mentioned previously, provides cytologic material but does not actually obtain a specimen of lung whose architecture can be examined, a feature that may be necessary to establish a diagnosis. Various "cutting" needles are available that do provide a "core" of the involved lung. However, this approach has waned in popularity because of the high incidence of pneumothorax and bleeding, occasional deaths due to air embolism, and the small size of the biopsy specimen, which may limit diagnostic interpretation. Fluoroscopic or CT guidance is essential in all these closed approaches, and they are contraindicated if pulmonary hypertension or a hemorrhagic diathesis is present.

Open-lung biopsy, requiring thoracotomy, is the final diagnostic resort. It is, however, a relatively safe procedure even in patients with respiratory failure, hemorrhagic diathesis, or pulmonary hypertension if meticulous surgical and anesthetic techniques are observed. Direct visualization allows selection of an optimum biopsy site, and of course, a specimen of adequate size is obtained. To what extent thoracoscopic lung biopsy may replace lung biopsy via thoracotomy remains to be identified. In selecting among these closed and open options, consideration of local expertise in their performance is a key factor.

All specimens obtained by biopsy should be both cultured and processed for pathologic examination.

REFERENCES

BORDOW RA, MOSER KM: *Manual of Clinical Problems in Pulmonary Medicine.* 3d ed. Boston, Little, Brown, 1991

DAVIS SD et al: MR imaging of pleural effusions. J Comp Assist Tomog 14:192, 1990

DURTSCHI MB: Use of thoracoscopy in clinical practice. Am J Surg 165:592, 1993

GIBSON SP: A prospective audit of the value of fibre optic bronchoscopy in adults admitted with community acquired pneumonia. Respir Med 87:105, 1993

HASLAM PL: Bronchoalveolar lavage. Semin Respir Med 6:55, 1984

HULL RD, RASKOB GE: Low probability lung scan findings: A need for change. Ann Intern Med 114:142, 1991

KUWANO K et al: The diagnosis of mild emphysema: Correlation of computed tomography and pathology scores. Am Rev Respir Dis 141:169, 1990

MILLER NL, MILLER RR: Computed tomography of chronic diffuse infiltrative lung disease. Am Rev Respir Dis 142:1205, 1440, 1990

PEARSON FG: Staging of the mediastinum. Role of mediastinoscopy and computed tomography. Chest 103:346S, 1993

PIOPED INVESTIGATORS: Value of the ventilation-perfusion scan in prospective investigations of pulmonary embolism diagnosis. JAMA 263:2753, 1990

SULAVIK SB et al: Recognition of distinctive patterns of 67-Ga distribution in sarcoidosis. J Nucl Med 31:1909, 1990

TURNER-WARWICK M, HASLAM PL: The value of serial bronchoalveolar lavage in assessing the clinical progress of patients with cryptogenic fibrosing alveolitis. Am Rev Respir Dis 135:26, 1987

217   ASTHMA

E. R. McFADDEN, JR.

DEFINITION   Asthma is a disease of airways that is characterized by increased responsiveness of the tracheobronchial tree to a multiplicity of stimuli. Asthma is manifested physiologically by a widespread narrowing of the air passages, which may be relieved spontaneously or as a result of therapy, and clinically by paroxysms of dyspnea, cough, and wheezing. It is an episodic disease, acute exacerbations being interspersed with symptom-free periods. Typically, most attacks are short-lived, lasting minutes to hours, and after them the patient seems to recover completely clinically. However, there can be a phase in which the patient experiences some degree of airway obstruction daily. This phase can be mild, with or without superimposed severe episodes, or much more serious, with severe obstruction persisting for days or weeks, a condition known as *status asthmaticus*. In unusual circumstances, acute episodes can terminate fatally.

PREVALENCE AND ETIOLOGY   Asthma is a very common disorder, and it is estimated that 4 to 5 percent of the population of the United States is affected. Similar figures have been reported from other countries. Bronchial asthma occurs at all ages but predominantly in early life. About one-half of the cases develop before age 10, and another third occur before age 40. In childhood, there is a 2:1 male/female preponderance, which equalizes by age 30.

From an etiologic standpoint, asthma is a heterogeneous disease. It is useful for epidemiologic and clinical purposes to classify asthma by the principal stimuli that incite or are associated with acute episodes. However, it is important to emphasize that this distinction may often be artificial, and the response of a given subclassification usually can be initiated by more than one type of stimulus. With this reservation in mind, one can describe two broad groups: allergic and idiosyncratic.

Allergic asthma is often associated with a personal and/or family history of allergic diseases such as rhinitis, urticaria, and eczema; positive wheal-and-flare skin reactions to intradermal injection of extracts of airborne antigens; increased levels of IgE in the serum; and/or positive response to provocation tests involving the inhalation of specific antigen.

A significant segment of the asthmatic population will present with negative family or personal histories of allergy, negative skin tests, and normal serum levels of IgE and therefore cannot be classified on the basis of defined immunologic mechanisms. These we term *idiosyncratic*. Many of these will develop a typical symptom complex upon contracting an upper respiratory illness. The initial insult may be little more than a common cold, but after several days the patient begins to develop paroxysms of wheezing and dyspnea that can last for days to months. These individuals should not be confused with persons in whom the symptoms of bronchospasm are superimposed on chronic bronchitis or bronchiectasis (see Chap. 223).

Unfortunately, many patients will not clearly fit into either of the preceding categories but will fall into a mixed group with features of each. In general, those patients whose onset of disease is in early life will tend to have a strong allergic component to their illness, while those who develop their asthma late tend to be nonallergic or to have mixed etiologies.

PATHOGENESIS OF ASTHMA   The common denominator underlying the asthmatic diathesis is a nonspecific hyperirritability of the tracheobronchial tree. In asthmatics it correlates well with the clinical features of the illness. When airway reactivity is high, lung function becomes more unstable, symptoms are more severe and persistent, the acute response to bronchodilators is larger, and the amount of therapy required to control the patient's complaints increases. In addition, the magnitude of diurnal fluctuations in lung function becomes greater, and the patient tends to awaken at night or in the early morning with breathlessness.

In both normal and asthmatic subjects, airway reactivity is known to rise following viral infections of the respiratory tract and exposure to oxidant air pollutants such as ozone and nitrogen dioxide. Viruses have more profound consequences, and following a seemingly trivial upper respiratory tract infection, airway responsivity may remain elevated for many weeks. In contrast, with exposure to ozone, airway reactivity remains high for only a few days. Allergens can cause airway responsiveness to rise within minutes and to remain elevated for weeks. If the dose of antigen is high enough, acute episodes of obstruction may occur daily for a prolonged period of time following a single exposure.

A number of causes have been postulated for the increased airway reactivity of asthma; however, the basic mechanism remains unknown. The most popular hypothesis at present is that of airway inflammation. Following exposure to an initiating stimulus, mediator containing such cells as mast cells, basophils, and macrophages can be activated to release a variety of inflammatory compounds which produce direct effects on airway smooth muscle and capillary permeability, thereby evoking an intense local reaction which can then be followed by a more chronic one. The latter may be brought about by the release of chemotactic factors which recruit cellular elements to the site of injury. In addition, it is thought that the acute and chronic effects of mediator release and cellular infiltration may result in epithelial damage with involvement of neural endings within the airways and the activation of an axon reflex. In this fashion, an essentially local phenomenon can be amplified to have widespread effects throughout the tracheobronchial tree.

The stimuli that interact with airway responsiveness and incite acute episodes of asthma can be grouped into seven major categories: allergenic, pharmacologic, environmental, occupational, infectious, exercise-related, and emotional.

Allergens   Allergic asthma is dependent on an IgE response controlled by T and B lymphocytes and activated by the interaction of antigen with mast cell–bound IgE molecules. Most of the allergens that provoke asthma are airborne, and in order to induce a state of sensitivity, they must be reasonably abundant for considerable periods of time. Once sensitization has occurred, however, the patient can then exhibit exquisite responsivity so that minute amounts of the offending agent can produce significant exacerbations of the disease. Immunologic mechanisms appear to be causally related to the development of asthma in 25 to 35 percent of all cases and contributory in perhaps another third. Higher prevalences have been suggested, but it is difficult to know how to interpret the data because of confounding factors. Allergic asthma is frequently seasonal, and it is most often observed in children and young adults. A nonseasonal form may result from allergy to feathers, animal danders, dust mites, molds, and other antigens present continuously in the environment. Exposure to antigen typically produces an immediate response in which airway obstruction develops in minutes and then resolves. In 30 to 50 percent of patients, a second wave of bronchoconstriction, the so-called late reaction, develops 6 to 10 h later. In a minority, only a late reaction occurs. It was formerly thought that the late reaction was essential to the development of the increase in airway reactivity that follows antigen exposure. Recent data show this not to be the case.

PATHOGENESIS The mechanism by which an inhaled antigen provokes an acute episode of asthma is unknown but seems to depend, in part, on antigen-antibody interactions on the surface of pulmonary mast cells with the subsequent generation and release of the mediators of immediate hypersensitivity. Current postulates hold that very small antigenic particles penetrate the lung's defenses and come in contact with mast cells that are interdigitating with the epithelium at the luminal surface of the central airways. (No mechanism has yet been proposed that explains how antigen can contact the mast cells in the submucosa.) The subsequent elaboration of mediators then produces the sequence outlined above. The mediators released—histamine; bradykinin; the leukotrienes C, D, and E; platelet-activating factor; prostaglandins PGE_2, $PGF_{2\alpha}$, and PGD_2, and thromboxane A_2—produce an intense inflammatory reaction with bronchoconstriction, vascular congestion, and edema formation. In addition to their ability to produce prolonged contraction of airway smooth muscle and mucosal edema, the leukotrienes also produce some of the other pathophysiologic features of asthma, such as increased mucus production and impaired mucociliary transport. The chemotactic factors elaborated (eosinophil and neutrophil chemotactic factors of anaphylaxis and leukotriene B_4) bring eosinophils, platelets, and polymorphonuclear leukocytes to the site of the reaction. One of the most important of these may be the eosinophil; when activated, these cells can produce leukotriene C_4 and platelet-activating factor and thereby contribute directly to airway narrowing and edema. They also can cause mast cells to release histamine and chemotactic factors which could set up a self-sustaining cycle in which additional secondary effector cells including more eosinophils are brought to the site of the reaction. Equally important, degranulation of eosinophils can release major basic protein and eosinophil cationic protein into the airways, thus causing cilia to stop beating and disrupting mucosal integrity with exfoliation of cells into the bronchial lumen in the form of Creola bodies.

While the preceding theories concerning pathogenesis are attractive, translation of the cellular events into precise pathophysiologic sequences is difficult and incomplete. For example, mediators per se cannot explain the whole picture, for they have been found in the blood of individuals with mast cell diseases such as cold-induced and cholinergic-induced urticaria and the airways of atopic nonasthmatics. Since these individuals were devoid of any lower respiratory illness or complaints, the alleged mediators of asthma appear to need a unique substrate upon which to exhibit their effects. Similarly, the inflammatory cells believed to be important in asthma are also found in the airways of atopic nonasthmatics, raising the possibility that they are merely nonspecific markers of atopy rather than specific indices of asthma.

Pharmacologic stimuli The drugs most commonly associated with the induction of acute episodes of asthma are aspirin, coloring agents such as tartrazine, beta-adrenergic antagonists, and sulfiting agents. The typical aspirin-sensitive respiratory syndrome primarily affects adults, although the condition may be seen in childhood. This problem usually begins with perennial vasomotor rhinitis that is followed by a hyperplastic rhinosinusitis with nasal polyps. Progressive asthma then appears. On exposure to even very small quantities of aspirin, affected individuals typically develop ocular and nasal congestion and acute, often severe episodes of airway obstruction. The prevalence of aspirin sensitivity in asthmatic subjects varies from

study to study, but many authorities feel that 10 percent is a reasonable figure. There is a great deal of cross reactivity between aspirin and other nonsteroidal anti-inflammatory compounds. Indomethacin, fenoprofen, naproxen, zomepirac sodium, ibuprofen, mefenamic acid, and phenylbutazone are particularly important in this regard. On the other hand, acetaminophen, sodium salicylate, choline salicylate, salicylamide, and propoxyphene are well tolerated. The exact frequency of cross reactivity to tartrazine and other dyes in aspirin-sensitive asthmatic subjects is also controversial, and again, 10 percent is the commonly accepted figure. This peculiar complication of aspirin-sensitive asthma is particularly insidious, however, in that tartrazine and other potentially troublesome dyes are widely present in the environment and may be unknowingly ingested by sensitive patients.

Patients with aspirin sensitivity can be desensitized by daily administration of the drug. Following this form of therapy, cross tolerance also develops to other nonsteroidal anti-inflammatory agents. The mechanism by which aspirin and other such drugs produce bronchospasm is unknown but may be related to aspirin-induced preferential generation of leukotrienes. Immediate hypersensitivity does not seem to be involved.

Beta-adrenergic antagonists regularly produce airway obstruction in asthmatics as well as in others with heightened airway reactivity and should be avoided in such individuals. Even the selective $beta_1$ agents have this propensity, particularly at higher doses. In fact, even the local use of $beta_1$ blockers in the eye for the treatment of glaucoma has been associated with worsening asthma.

Sulfiting agents, such as potassium metabisulfite, potassium and sodium bisulfite, sodium sulfite, and sulfur dioxide, which are widely used in the food and pharmaceutical industry as sanitizing and preservative agents, also can produce acute airway obstruction in sensitive individuals. Exposure usually follows ingestion of food or beverages containing these compounds, e.g., salads, fresh fruit, potatoes, shellfish, and wine. Exacerbation of asthma has been reported following the use of sulfite-containing topical ophthalmic solutions, intravenous glucocorticoids, and some inhalational bronchodilator solutions. The incidence and mechanism of action of this phenomenon are unknown. When suspected, the diagnosis can be confirmed by either oral or inhalational provocations.

Environment and air pollution (See Chap. 219) Environmental causes of asthma are usually related to climatic conditions that promote the concentration of atmospheric pollutants and antigens. These conditions tend to develop in heavy industrial or densely populated urban areas and are frequently associated with thermal inversions or other situations associated with stagnant air masses. In these circumstances, although the general population can develop respiratory symptoms, patients with asthma and other respiratory diseases tend to be more severely affected. The air pollutants known to have this effect are ozone, nitrogen dioxide, and sulfur dioxide. The last needs to be present in high concentrations and produces its greatest effects during periods of high ventilation.

Occupational factors (See Chap. 219) Occupation-related asthma is a significant health problem, and acute and chronic airway obstruction has been reported to follow exposure to a large number of compounds used in many types of industrial processes. Bronchoconstriction can result from working with, or exposure to, *metal salts* (e.g., platinum, chrome, and nickel), *wood and vegetable dusts* (e.g., oak, western red cedar, grain, flour, castor bean, green coffee bean, mako, gum acacia, karay gum, and tragacanth), *pharmaceutical agents* (e.g., antibiotics, piperazine, and cimetidine), *industrial chemicals and plastics* (e.g., toluene diisocyanate, phthalic acid anhydride, trimellitic anhydride, persulfates, ethylenediamine, para-phenylenediamine, and various dyes), *biologic enzymes* (e.g., laundry detergents and pancreatic enzymes), and *animal and insect dusts, serums, and secretions*. It is important to recognize that exposure to sensitizing chemicals, particularly those used in paints, solvents, and plastics, also can occur during leisure or non-work-related activities.

The underlying mechanisms for this airway obstruction appear to be three in number: (1) in some cases the offending agent results in the formation of a specific IgE, and the cause seems immunologic (the immunologic reaction can be immediate, late, or dual); (2) materials being employed, in other cases, cause a direct liberation of bronchoconstrictor substances; and (3) work-related irritant substances, in still other cases, directly or reflexly stimulate the airways of either latent or frank asthmatics. With occupational exposures, other than those which give an immediate and dual immunologic reaction, the patients give a characteristic cyclic history. They are well when they arrive at work, and symptoms develop toward the end of the shift, progress after leaving the work site, and then regress. Absence from work during weekends or vacation periods brings about a remission. Frequently, there are similar symptoms in fellow employees.

Infections Respiratory infections are the most common of the stimuli that evoke acute exacerbations of asthma. Well-controlled investigations have demonstrated that respiratory viruses and not bacteria or allergy are the major etiologic factors. In young children, the most important infectious agents are respiratory syncytial virus and parainfluenza virus. In older children and adults, rhinovirus and influenza virus predominate as pathogens. Simple colonization of the tracheobronchial tree is insufficient to evoke acute episodes of bronchospasm, and attacks of asthma occur only when symptoms of an ongoing respiratory tract infection are, or have been, present. The mechanism by which viruses induce asthma is unknown, but it is probable that the resulting inflammatory changes in the airway mucosa alter host defenses and make the tracheobronchial tree more susceptible to exogenous stimuli. Supporting evidence for this concept is derived from the fact that the airway responsiveness of even normal (nonasthmatic) subjects to nonspecific stimuli is transiently increased after a viral infection. Increased airway responsiveness, associated with cough and rarely wheezing, can last from 2 to 8 weeks after the infection in both normal individuals and asthmatics.

Exercise Exercise is one of the most common precipitants of acute episodes of asthma. This stimulus differs from other naturally occurring provocations such as antigen or viral infections in that it does not evoke any long-term sequelae nor does it change airway reactivity. Initiation of bronchospasm by exercise is probably operative to some extent in every asthmatic patient, and in some it may be the only trigger mechanism that will produce symptoms. When such patients are followed for sufficient periods of time, they often develop recurring episodes of airway obstruction independent of exercise; thus the onset of this problem frequently can serve as the first manifestation of the full-blown asthmatic syndrome. There is a significant interaction among the ventilation achieved by the exercise task, the temperature, and water content of the inspired air and the magnitude of the postexertional obstruction. Thus, for the same inspired air conditions, running will produce a more severe attack of asthma than will walking. Conversely, for a given task, the inhalation of cold air during its performance will markedly enhance the response, while warm, humid air will blunt or abolish it. Consequently, activities such as ice hockey, cross-country skiing, or ice skating are more provocative than is swimming in an indoor heated pool. The mechanism by which exercise produces obstruction may be related to a thermally produced hyperemia and engorgement of the microvasculature of the bronchial wall and does not appear to involve smooth-muscle contraction.

Emotional stress Abundant objective data exist which demonstrate that psychological factors can interact with the asthmatic diathesis to worsen or ameliorate the disease process. The pathways and nature of the interactions are complex but have been shown to be operational to some extent in almost half the patients studied. Changes in airway caliber seem to be mediated through modification of vagal efferent activity, but endorphins also may play a role. The most frequently studied variable has been that of suggestion, and the weight of current evidence is that it can be quite an important influence in selected asthmatics. When psychically responsive individuals are given the appropriate suggestion, they can actually decrease or increase the pharmacologic effects of adrenergic and cholinergic

stimuli on their airways. The extent to which psychological factors participate in the induction and/or continuation of any given acute exacerbation is unknown but probably varies from patient to patient and in the same patient from episode to episode.

PATHOLOGY In a patient who has died of acute asthma, the most striking feature of the lungs at necropsy is their gross overdistention and failure to collapse when the pleural cavities are opened. When the lungs are cut, numerous gelatinous plugs of exudate are found in the majority of the bronchial branches down to the terminal bronchiole. Histologic examination shows hypertrophy of the bronchial smooth muscle, hyperplasia of mucosal and submucosal vessels, mucosal edema, denudation of the surface epithelium, pronounced thickening of the basement membrane, and eosinophilic infiltrates in the bronchial wall. In asthmatic patients who die from trauma and causes other than asthma itself, mucous casts, basement membrane thickening, and eosinophilic infiltrates are frequently observed. In both situations there is an absence of any of the well-recognized forms of destructive emphysema. It is now recognized that infiltration of the mucosa and submucosa with eosinophils and other inflammatory cells, as well as epithelial damage and denudation, exist in airway biopsies from asymptomatic asthmatics. These findings, in concert with those in airway mediator levels, have given rise to the construct that asthma is a chronic inflammatory disease.

PATHOPHYSIOLOGY The pathophysiologic hallmark of asthma is a reduction in airway diameter brought about by contraction of smooth muscle, vascular congestion, edema of the bronchial wall, and thick tenacious secretions. The net result is an increase in airway resistance, decreased forced expiratory volumes and flow rates, hyperinflation of the lungs and thorax, increased work of breathing, alterations in respiratory muscle function, changes in elastic recoil, abnormal distribution of both ventilation and pulmonary blood flow with mismatched ratios, and altered arterial blood gases. Thus, although asthma is considered to be primarily a disease of airways, virtually all aspects of pulmonary function are compromised during an acute attack. In addition, in very symptomatic patients there frequently is electrocardiographic evidence of right ventricular hypertrophy and pulmonary hypertension. When a patient presents for therapy, his or her forced vital capacity tends to be ≤50 percent of normal. The 1-s forced expiratory volume (FEV_1) averages 30 percent or less of predicted, while the maximum and minimum midexpiratory flow rates are reduced to 20 percent or less of expected. In keeping with the alterations in mechanics, the associated air trapping is substantial. In acutely ill patients, residual volume (RV) frequently approaches 400 percent of normal, while functional residual capacity doubles. The patients tend to report that their attacks have ended clinically when their RV has fallen to 200 percent of its predicted value and when the FEV_1 rises to 50 percent.

Hypoxia is a universal finding during acute exacerbations, but frank ventilatory failure is relatively uncommon, being observed in 10 to 15 percent of patients presenting for therapy. Most asthmatics have hypocapnia and a respiratory alkalosis. In acutely ill patients, the finding of a normal arterial carbon dioxide tension tends to be associated with quite severe levels of obstruction. Consequently, when found in a symptomatic individual, it should be viewed as impending respiratory failure and treated as such. Equally, the presence of metabolic acidosis in the setting of acute asthma heralds severe obstruction. Usually, there are no clinical counterparts to the derangements in blood gases. Cyanosis is a very late sign. Hence a dangerous level of hypoxia can go undetected. Likewise, the signs which are attributable to carbon dioxide retention, such as sweating, tachycardia, and wide pulse pressure, or to acidosis, such as tachypnea, do not tend to be of great value in predicting the presence of hypercapnia or hydrogen ion excess in individual patients, for they are too frequently seen in anxious patients with more moderate disease to be of much use. Thus trying to judge the state of an acutely ill patient's ventilatory status on clinical grounds alone can be extremely hazardous and should not be relied on with any confidence. Arterial blood gas tensions, therefore, must be measured.

CLINICAL FEATURES   The symptoms of asthma consist of a triad of dyspnea, cough, and wheezing, the last often being regarded as the *sine qua non*. In its most typical form, asthma is an episodic disease, and all three symptoms coexist. At the onset of an attack, patients experience a sense of constriction in the chest, often with a nonproductive cough. Respiration becomes audibly harsh, and wheezing in both phases of respiration becomes prominent, expiration becomes prolonged, and patients frequently have tachypnea, tachycardia, and mild systolic hypertension. The lungs rapidly become overinflated, and the anteroposterior diameter of the thorax increases. If the attack is severe or prolonged, there may be a loss of adventitial breath sounds, and wheezing becomes very high pitched. Further, the accessory muscles become visibly active, and frequently, a paradoxical pulse will develop. These two signs have been found to be extremely valuable in indicating the severity of the obstruction. In the presence of either, pulmonary function tends to be significantly more impaired than in its absence. It is important to note that the development of a paradoxical pulse and accessory muscle use depends on the generation of large negative intrathoracic pressures. Thus, if the patient's breathing is shallow, these signs could be absent even though obstruction is quite severe. The other signs and symptoms of asthma imperfectly reflect the physiologic alterations that are present, so much so that if one relies on the loss of subjective complaints, or even the sign of wheezing, as being the end point at which therapy for an acute attack should be terminated, an enormous reservoir of residual disease is missed.

Termination of the episode is frequently marked by a cough producing thick, stringy mucus which often takes the form of casts of the distal airways (Curschmann's spirals) and, when examined microscopically, often shows eosinophils and Charcot-Leyden crystals. In extreme situations, wheezing may markedly lessen or even disappear completely, cough may become extremely ineffective, and the patient may begin a gasping type of respiratory pattern. These findings imply extensive mucous plugging and impending suffocation. Ventilatory assistance by mechanical means may be required. Atelectasis due to inspissated secretions may occasionally occur with asthmatic attacks. Other complications such as spontaneous pneumothorax and/or pneumomediastinum are rare.

Less typically, a patient with asthma may complain of intermittent episodes of nonproductive cough or exertional dyspnea. Unlike other asthmatics, when these patients are examined during their symptomatic periods, they tend to have normal breath sounds but may wheeze after repeated forced exhalations and/or may show dynamic ventilatory impairments when tested in the laboratory. In the absence of both, a bronchoprovocation may be required to make the diagnosis.

DIFFERENTIAL DIAGNOSIS   The differentiation of asthma from other diseases associated with dyspnea and wheezing is usually not difficult, particularly if the patient is seen during an acute episode. The physical findings and symptoms listed above and the history of periodic attacks are quite characteristic. A personal or family history of allergic diseases such as eczema, rhinitis, or urticaria is valuable contributory evidence. An extremely common feature of asthma is nocturnal awakening with dyspnea and/or wheezing. In fact, this phenomenon is so prevalent that its absence makes one doubt the correctness of the diagnosis. *Upper airway obstruction by tumor* or *laryngeal edema* can occasionally be confused with asthma. Typically, such a patient will present with stridor, and the harsh respiratory sounds can be localized to the area of the trachea. Diffuse wheezing throughout both lung fields is usually absent. However, differentiation can sometimes be difficult, and indirect laryngoscopy or bronchoscopy may be required. Asthma-like symptoms have been described in patients with glottic dysfunction. These individuals narrow their glottis during inspiration and expiration and produce episodic attacks of severe airway obstruction. Occasionally they will develop carbon dioxide retention. However, unlike asthma, the arterial oxygen tension is well preserved, and the alveolar-arterial gradient for oxygen narrows during the episode and does not widen, as is the case with lower airway obstruction. To establish the diagnosis of glottic dysfunction,

the glottis should be examined when the patient is symptomatic. A normal examination at this time excludes the diagnosis; normal findings during asymptomatic periods do not.

Persistent wheezing localized to one area of the chest in association with paroxysms of cough indicates *endobronchial disease* such as foreign-body aspiration, neoplasms, or bronchial stenosis.

The signs and symptoms of *acute left ventricular failure* can occasionally mimic asthma, but the findings of moist basilar rales, gallop rhythms, blood-tinged sputum, and other signs of heart failure (Chap. 195) allow the appropriate diagnosis to be reached.

Recurrent episodes of bronchospasm can occur with *carcinoid tumors* (Chap. 276), *recurrent pulmonary emboli* (Chap. 226), and *chronic bronchitis* (Chap. 223). In the last there are no true symptom-free periods, and one can usually obtain a history of chronic cough and sputum production as a background upon which acute attacks of wheezing are superimposed. Recurrent emboli, particularly in young women on oral contraceptives, can be very difficult to separate from asthma. Frequently, these patients will present with episodes of breathlessness, particularly on exertion, and they can sometimes wheeze. Pulmonary function studies may show evidence of peripheral airway obstruction (Chap. 214), and when these changes are present, lung scans also may be abnormal. The therapeutic response to bronchodilators, discontinuation of the contraceptives, and institution of anticoagulant therapy may be helpful, but pulmonary angiography may be necessary in order to establish the correct diagnosis.

Eosinophilic pneumonias (Chap. 218) are often associated with asthmatic symptoms, as are various chemical pneumonias and exposures to insecticides and cholinergic drugs. Bronchospasm can occasionally be a manifestation of *systemic vasculitis* with pulmonary involvement.

DIAGNOSIS   The diagnosis of asthma is established by demonstrating reversible airway obstruction. *Reversibility* is traditionally defined as a 15 percent or greater increase in FEV_1 following two puffs of a beta-adrenergic agonist. When the presenting spirometry is normal, the diagnosis can be made by showing heightened airway responsiveness to challenges with histamine, methacholine, or isocapnic hyperventilation of cold air. Once the diagnosis is confirmed, the course of the illness and the effectiveness of therapy can be followed by measuring peak expiratory flow rates (PEFR) at home and/or the FEV_1 in the laboratory. Positive wheal-and-flare reactions to skin tests can be demonstrated to various allergens, but such findings do not necessarily correlate with the intrapulmonary events. Sputum and blood eosinophilia and measurement of serum IgE levels are also helpful but are not specific for asthma. Chest roentgenograms showing hyperinflation are also nondiagnostic.

THERAPY   Elimination of the causative agent(s) from the environment of an allergic asthmatic is the most successful means available for treating this condition (for details on avoidance, see Chap. 282). Desensitization or immunotherapy with extracts of the suspected allergens has enjoyed widespread favor, but controlled studies are limited and have not proved it to be highly effective.

Drug treatment   The drugs used in the treatment of asthma may be grouped conveniently into five categories: beta-adrenergic agonists, methylxanthines, glucocorticoids, mast cell stabilizing agents, and anticholinergics. Inhibitors of mediator synthesis and mediator-receptor antagonists are currently undergoing clinical trials.

ADRENERGIC STIMULANTS   The drugs in this category consist of the catecholamines, resorcinols, and saligenins. These agents are analogues and produce airway dilatation through stimulation of beta receptors with the resultant formation of cyclic AMP. They also decrease release of mediators and improve mucocilliary transport. The catecholamines in widespread clinical use are epinephrine, isoproterenol, isoetharine, rimiterol, and hexoprenaline. The last two are not available in the United States. As a group, these compounds are short-acting and effective only by inhalational or parenteral routes. Epinephrine and isoproterenol are not beta$_2$-selective and have considerable chronotropic and inotropic cardiac effects. Epinephrine also has substantial alpha-stimulating effects. The usual dose is

0.3 to 0.5 mL of a 1:1000 solution administered subcutaneously. Isoproterenol is devoid of alpha activity and is the most potent agent of this group. It is usually administered in a 1:200 solution by inhalation. Isoetharine is the most beta$_2$-selective compound of this class, but it is a relatively weak bronchodilator. It is employed as an aerosol and supplied as a 1% solution. The pharmacologies of hexoprenaline and rimiterol are similar to that of isoetharine.

The commonly used resorcinols are metaproterenol, terbutaline, and fenoterol, and the most widely known saligenin is albuterol, or salbutamol. With the exception of metaproterenol, these drugs are highly selective for the respiratory tract and virtually devoid of significant cardiac effects except in high doses. Their major side effect is tremor. They are active by all routes of administration, and because their chemical structures allow them to bypass the metabolic processes used to degrade the catecholamines, their effects are long-lasting, exceeding 6 h in many studies. Differences in potency and duration between agents can be eliminated by adjusting doses and/or administration schedules.

Inhalation is the preferred route of administration because it increases the bronchial selectivity of these drugs and allows maximal bronchodilation to occur with fewer side effects. This is true not just in maintenance therapy but also during the treatment of severe acute obstruction. In the past it was fashionable to treat episodes of severe asthma with intravenous sympathomimetics such as isoproterenol. This approach no longer appears justifiable. Isoproterenol infusions clearly can induce myocardial damage, and even the beta$_2$-selective agents such as terbutaline and albuterol, when given intravenously, offer no advantages over the inhaled route.

METHYLXANTHINES Theophylline and its various salts are medium-potency bronchodilators that work through an undefined mechanism. It was formerly thought that these drugs increased cyclic AMP by the inhibition of phosphodiesterase; however, the available evidence does not support this concept. The therapeutic plasma concentrations of theophylline lie between 10 and 20 μg/mL, but the dose required to achieve this level varies widely from patient to patient owing to differences in the metabolism of the drug. Theophylline clearance, and thus dosage requirements, is decreased substantially in neonates and the elderly and those with acute and chronic hepatic dysfunction, cardiac decompensation, and cor pulmonale. Clearance is also decreased during febrile illnesses. Clearance is increased in children. In addition, a number of important drug interactions can alter theophylline metabolism. Clearance falls with the concurrent use of erythromycin and troleandomycin, allopurinol, cimetidine, and propranolol. It rises with cigarettes, marijuana, phenobarbital, and phenytoin or any other drug that has the capability of inducing hepatic microsomal enzymes.

For maintenance therapy, long-acting theophylline compounds are available and are usually given twice per day or once daily. The dose is adjusted on the basis of the clinical response with the aid of serum theophylline levels. Single-dose administration in the evening may reduce nocturnal symptoms. In contrast to the large number of oral compounds, aminophylline is the only compound available for intravenous use. The recommendations for intravenous therapy in children aged 9 to 16 and young adult smokers not currently receiving theophylline products are as follows: A loading dose of 6 mg/kg is given, followed by an infusion of 1.0 mg/kg per hour for the next 12 h and then 0.8 mg/kg per hour thereafter. In nonsmoking adults, older patients, and those with cor pulmonale, congestive heart failure, and liver disease, the loading dose remains the same, but the maintenance dose is reduced to between 0.1 and 0.5 mg/kg per hour. In those patients already receiving theophylline, the loading dose is frequently withheld or in extreme situations given in a reduced amount at 0.5 mg/kg.

The most common side effects of theophylline are nervousness, nausea, vomiting, anorexia, and headache. At plasma levels greater than 30 μg/mL there is a risk of seizures and cardiac arrhythmias.

GLUCOCORTICOIDS Glucocorticoids are not bronchodilators, and their major use in asthma is in reducing airway inflammation. Steroids are most beneficial in acute illness, when severe airway obstruction is not resolving or is worsening despite intense optimal bronchodilator therapy, and in chronic disease, when there has been failure of a previously optimal regimen with frequent recurrences of symptoms of progressive severity.

The dose that one should use is a matter of debate. The available data indicate, however, that very high doses do not offer advantage over more conventional amounts. For example, 6 mg/kg per day of hydrocortisone has been shown to produce the same effects as 80 mg/kg per day in status asthmaticus, and 15 to 20 mg of methylprednisolone every 6 h has the same consequences as doses eight to ten times greater. In most acute situations, the intravenous administration of 4 mg/kg of hydrocortisone (or equivalent) as a loading dose, followed several hours later by an infusion regulated to deliver 3 mg/kg every 6 h seems adequate. It should be emphasized that the effects of steroids in acute asthma are not immediate and may not be seen for 6 h or more after their initial administration. Consequently, it is mandatory to continue vigorous bronchodilator therapy during this interval. After 24 to 72 h, depending on response, the patient can be switched to oral agents. A usual starting point is 40 to 60 mg prednisone as a single daily morning dose. The amount can then be reduced by half every third to fifth day. More rapid tapering frequently results in recurrent obstruction. In situations in which it appears that continued steroid therapy will be needed, an alternate-day schedule should be instituted to minimize side effects. This is particularly important in children, since continuous corticosteroid administration interrupts growth. Long-acting preparations such as dexamethasone should not be used in this approach, for they defeat the purpose of alternate-day schedules by causing prolonged suppression of the pituitary-adrenal axis.

Several inhaled steroids of high topical potency are available and greatly facilitate the withdrawal of oral agents. They are also useful in reducing airway reactivity and as an alternative to oral glucocorticoids in situations where asthma symptoms are escalating. The effects of inhaled steroids are dose-dependent. If symptoms are not readily controlled, some have advocated increasing the dose to two or more times conventional recommendations. While this course of action diminishes the need for oral glucocorticoids, it carries with it the risk of greater side effects. In addition to thrush and dysphonia, the increased systemic absorption of larger doses of inhaled steroids has been reported to produce adrenal suppression, cataract formation, decreased growth in children, interference with bone metabolism, and purpura.

MAST CELL STABILIZING AGENTS Cromolyn sodium and nedocromil sodium are not bronchodilators. Their major therapeutic effects are the inhibition of degranulation of mast cells, thereby preventing the release of the chemical mediators of anaphylaxis.

Cromolyn and nedocromil, like the inhaled steroids, improve lung function, reducing symptoms and lower airway reactivity in asthmatics. They are most efficacious in atopic patients who have either seasonal disease or are experiencing perennial stimulation of their airways. To produce their effects, a therapeutic trial of two puffs daily for 4 to 6 weeks is frequently necessary. Unlike steroids, nedocromil and cromolyn, when given prophylactically, will block the acute obstructive effects of exposure to antigen, industrial chemicals, exercise, and cold air. With antigen, the late response is also abolished. Hence a patient who has intermittent exposure to either antigenic or nonantigenic stimuli that provoke acute episodes of asthma need not use these drugs continuously. Rather, such individuals can readily be protected by only taking cromolyn or nedocromil 15 to 20 minutes before contact with the precipitant.

ANTICHOLINERGICS Anticholinergic drugs, such as atropine sulfate, produce bronchodilation in patients with asthma, but their use is limited by systemic side effects. Nonabsorbable quaternary ammonium congeners (atropine methylnitrate and ipratropium bromide) have been found to be both effective and free of untoward effects. They may be of particular benefit for patients with coexistent heart disease, in whom use of methylxanthines and beta stimulants may be dangerous. There is some evidence that addition of anticholinergics may enhance the bronchodilation achieved by sympathomimetics, but the effect is not large. The major disadvantages of the anticholinergics are that they are slow to act (60 to 90 min may be required before peak bronchodilation is achieved) and they are only of modest potency.

MISCELLANEOUS It has been suggested that steroid-dependent patients might benefit from the use of immunosuppressant agents such as methotrexate or gold salts. The effects of these agents on steroid dosage and disease activity are minor, and side effects can be considerable. Consequently, this form of treatment can only be viewed as experimental. Opiates, sedatives, and tranquilizers should be absolutely avoided in the acutely ill asthmatic because the risk of depressing alveolar ventilation is great and respiratory arrest has been reported to occur shortly after their use. Admittedly most individuals are anxious and frightened, but experience has shown that they can be calmed equally well by the physician's presence and reassurances. Beta-adrenergic blockers and parasympathetic agonists are contraindicated because they can cause marked deterioration in lung function.

Expectorants and mucolytic agents have enjoyed great vogue in the past, but they do not add significantly to the treatment of the acute or chronic phases of this disease. Mucolytic agents such as acetylcysteine may actually produce bronchospasm when administered to susceptible asthmatics. This can be overcome by aerosolizing them in solution with a beta-adrenergic agent. The use of intravenous fluids in the treatment of acute asthma also has been advocated. There is little evidence to indicate that this adjunct hastens recovery.

SPECIAL INSTRUCTIONS The treatment of patients with asthma who have coexisting conditions such as heart disease or pregnancy does not differ materially from that outlined above. Inhaled therapy with beta₂-selective and anti-inflammatory agents is the mainstay. The doses of adrenergics administered should be the lowest possible quantities required to produce the desired therapeutic effects.

FRAMEWORK FOR MANAGEMENT Emergency situations The most efficacious form of treatment for acute episodes of asthma are aerosolized beta₂ agonists. These drugs provide three to four times more relief than intravenous aminophylline. In emergency situations, they can be given every 20 minutes by hand-held nebulizer for three doses. Thereafter, the frequency can be reduced to every 2 h until the attack has subsided. Aminophylline can be added to the regimen after the first hour in an attempt to speed resolution.

Acute episodes of bronchial asthma represent one of the most common respiratory emergencies seen in the practice of medicine, and it is essential that the physician recognize which episodes of airway obstruction are life-threatening and which patients demand what level of care. This can be readily accomplished by assessing selected clinical parameters in combination with measures of expiratory flow and gas exchange. The presence of a paradoxical pulse, use of accessory muscles, and marked hyperinflation of the thorax signify severe airway obstruction, and failure of these signs to remit within short order following aggressive therapy mandates objective monitoring of the patient using arterial blood gases and the peak expiratory flow rate (PEFR) or FEV_1.

In general, there is a direct correlation between the severity of the obstruction with which the patient presents and the time that it takes to resolve it. Those individuals with the most impairment typically require the most extensive therapy for resolution. If the PEFR or FEV_1 is equal to or less than 20 percent of predicted on presentation and does not double within an hour of receiving the preceding therapy, the patient is likely to require extensive treatment including glucocorticoids before the obstruction dissipates. In such circumstances, if the clinical signs of a paradoxical pulse and accessory muscle use are diminishing, and/or if PEFR is increasing, there is no need to change medications or doses. One need only to continue to follow the patient. If, however, PEFR is falling or the magnitude of the pulsus paradoxicus is increasing, serial measures of arterial blood gases are required as well as a reconsideration of the therapeutic modalities being employed. If the patient has hypocarbia, one can

afford to continue the current approaches a while longer. On the other hand, if the Pa_{CO_2} is within the normal range or is elevated, the patient should be monitored in an intensive care setting, and therapy should be intensified in order to reverse or arrest the patient's respiratory failure.

Chronic treatment The goal of chronic therapy is to achieve a stable, asymptomatic state with the best pulmonary function possible. As in the acute situation, first-line therapy should be a beta₂ agonist by inhalation. In patients who have difficulty coordinating inhalation with activation of a metered-dose inhaler, a spacing device should be incorporated. If nocturnal complaints continue, a long-acting theophylline compound given at night may be included.

In patients with persistent symptoms and unstable lung function despite adequate bronchodilator therapy, treatment with inhaled steroids and/or mast cell stabilizing agents should be instituted. Since these agents frequently take weeks to lower airway reactivity, it may be efficacious to start a short but intense course of oral glucocorticoids to speed the remission. During this process, PEFR should be monitored and medication adjustments should be based on objective changes in lung function as well as the patient's symptoms. Once the asthma has stabilized, there should be a systematic reduction in medication, beginning with the most toxic, to find the minimum required to maintain the patient's well-being.

PROGNOSIS AND CLINICAL COURSE The mortality from asthma is small. The most recent figures indicate less than 5000 deaths per year out of a population of approximately 10 million patients at risk. Death rates, however, appear to be rising in inner-city areas where there is limited availability of health care.

Information on the clinical course of asthma suggests a good prognosis for 50 to 80 percent of all patients, particularly those whose disease is mild and develops in childhood. The number of children still having asthma 7 to 10 years after the initial diagnosis varies from 26 to 78 percent, with an average of 46 percent; however, the percentage who continue to have severe disease is relatively low (6 to 19 percent).

Unlike other airway diseases such as chronic bronchitis, asthma is not progressive. Although there are reports of patients with asthma developing irreversible changes in lung function, these individuals frequently have comorbid stimuli such as cigarette smoking that could account for these findings. Even when untreated, asthmatics do not continuously move from mild to severe disease with time. Rather, their clinical course is characterized by exacerbations and remissions. Some studies suggest that spontaneous remissions occur in approximately 20 percent of those who develop the disease as adults and 40 percent or so can be expected to improve with less frequent and severe attacks as they grow older.

REFERENCES

AMERICAN THORACIC SOCIETY: Guidelines for the Evaluation of impairment/disability in patients with asthma. Am Rev Respir Dis 147:1056, 1993
BURR ML: Epidemiology of asthma. Monogr Allergy 31:80, 1993
HOLGATE S: Mediator and cytokine mechanisms in asthma. Thorax 48:103, 1993
KALINER MA, MCFADDEN ER JR: Bronchial asthma, in *Immunological Diseases*, M Samter et al (eds). Boston, Little Brown, 1988, pp 1067–1118
KEMP JP: Approaches to asthma management. Realities and recommendations. Arch Intern Med 153:805, 1993
MCFADDEN ER JR: Pulmonary structure, physiology and clinical correlates in asthma, in *Allergy: Principles and Practice*, E Middleton et al (eds). St Louis, Mosby, 1993
——, GILBERT IA: Asthma. N Engl J Med 327:1928, 1992
SHEFFER AL, TAGGART VS: The National Asthma Education Program. Expert panel report guidelines for the diagnosis and management of asthma. Med Care 31:MS20, 1993
SKORODIN MS: Pharmacotherapy for asthma and chronic obstructive pulmonary disease. Current thinking, practices, and controversies. Arch Intern Med 153:814, 1993
WARDLAW AJ: The role of air pollution in asthma. Clin Exp Allergy 23:81, 1993

218 HYPERSENSITIVITY PNEUMONITIS AND EOSINOPHILIC PNEUMONIAS

GARY W. HUNNINGHAKE / HAL B. RICHERSON

HYPERSENSITIVITY PNEUMONITIS

Hypersensitivity pneumonitis (HP), or extrinsic allergic alveolitis, is an immunologically induced inflammation of the lung parenchyma, involving alveolar walls and terminal airways, secondary to repeated inhalation of a variety of organic dusts and other agents by a susceptible host. In contrast to many of the other interstitial lung diseases, the cause of this interstitial and alveolar filling disease is known. The prevalence of HP is unknown but varies with the environmental exposure and the antigen involved. The prevalence of farmer's lung among Wisconsin dairy farmers has been reported as 42 per 100,000. The diagnosis of HP requires a constellation of clinical, radiographic, physiologic, pathologic, and immunologic criteria, each of which is rarely pathognomonic alone, and the preferred treatment is avoidance of the causative antigen when practical.

ETIOLOGY   Agents implicated as causes of HP include those listed in Table 218-1. Many cases of HP occurring in various occupations involve exposure to similar agents, particularly the thermophilic actinomycetes. The common sources of causative antigens are "moldy" hay, silage, or grain; pet birds; and heating, cooling, and humidification systems. Simple chemicals, such as isocyanates, may also cause hypersensitivity pneumonitis.

PATHOGENESIS   The finding that precipitating antibodies against extracts of moldy hay were demonstrable in most patients with farmer's lung led to the early conclusion that HP was an immune-complex-mediated reaction. Subsequent investigations of HP in human beings and animal models provided evidence for the importance of cell-mediated hypersensitivity. The very early (acute) reaction is characterized by an increase in polymorphonuclear leukocytes in the alveoli and small airways. This early lesion is followed by an influx of mononuclear cells into the lung and the formation of granulomas. The latter lesion appears to be a classic delayed hypersensitivity reaction to repeated inhalation of antigen and adjuvant-active materials.

Bronchoalveolar lavage (Chap. 216) in patients with HP consistently demonstrates an increase in T lymphocytes in lavage fluid (a finding that is also observed in patients with other granulomatous lung disorders). Patients with recent or continual exposure to antigen may also have an increase in polymorphonuclear leukocytes in lavage fluid. Increased numbers of mast cells have also been reported. In most patients examined during recovery from acute disease, the T lymphocytes in lavage fluid are predominantly the CD8+ T-cell subset. In patients with very recent exposure to antigen, however, the numbers of CD4+ T cells may increase in lavage fluid. Similar findings may be present in similarly exposed, asymptomatic individuals. These observations suggest that there is an active modulation of granuloma formation in the lung by immunoregulatory T cells in this disorder.

CLINICAL PRESENTATION   The *clinical picture* is that of an interstitial pneumonitis, although it varies from patient to patient and is related to the frequency and intensity of exposure to the causative

---

TABLE 218-1   Selected examples of hypersensitivity pneumonitis (HP)

Disease	Antigen	Source of antigen
Bagassosis	Thermophilic actinomycetes	"Moldy" bagasse (sugar cane)
Bird fancier's, breeder's, or handler's lung	Parakeet, budgerigar, pigeon, chicken, turkey proteins	Avian droppings or feathers
Cephalosporium HP	Contaminated basement (sewage)	*Cephalosporium*
Cheese washer's lung	*Penicillium casei*	Moldy cheese
Chemical worker's lung	Isocyanates	Polyurethane foam, varnishes, lacquer, foundry casting
Coffee worker's lung	Coffee bean dust	Coffee beans
Compost lung	*Aspergillus*	Compost
Detergent worker's disease	*Bacillus subtilis* enzymes	Detergent
Familial HP	*Bacillus subtilis*	Contaminated wood dust in walls
Farmer's lung	Thermophilic actinomycetes*	"Moldy" hay, grain, silage
Fish meal worker's lung	Fish meal dust	Fish meal
Furrier's lung	Animal fur dust	Animal pelts
Hot tub lung	*Cladosporium* sp.	Mold on ceiling
Humidifier or air-conditioner lung (ventilation pneumonitis)	*Aureobasidium pullulans* or other microorganisms	Contaminated water in humidification and forced-air air-conditioning systems
Japanese summer house HP	*Trichosporon cutaneum*	House dust? Bird droppings
Laboratory worker's HP	Male rat urine	Laboratory rat
Lycoperdonosis	*Lycoperdon* puffballs	Puffball spores
Malt worker's lung	*Aspergillus fumigatus* or *A. clavatus*	Moldy barley
Maple bark disease	*Cryptostroma corticale*	Maple bark
Miller's lung	*Sitophilus granarius* (wheat weevil)	Infested wheat flour
Mushroom worker's lung	Thermophilic actinomycetes,* other	Mushroom compost
Paulis HP	Paulis reagent	Laboratory reagent
Pituitary snuff taker's lung	Animal proteins	Heterologous pituitary snuff
Potato riddler's lung	Thermophilic actinomycetes,* *Aspergillus*	"Moldy" hay around potatoes
Sauna taker's lung	*Aureobasidium* sp., other	Contaminated sauna water
Sequoiosis	*Aureobasidium, Graphium* sp.	Redwood sawdust
Streptomyces albus HP	*Streptomyces albus*	Contaminated fertilizer
Suberosis	Cork dust mold	Cork dust
Tap water lung	Unknown	Contaminated tap water
Thatched roof disease	*Saccharomonospora viridis*	Dried grasses and leaves
Tobacco worker's disease	*Aspergillus* sp.	Mold on tobacco
Winegrower's lung	*Botrytis cinerea*	Mold on grapes
Wood trimmer's disease	*Rhizopus* sp., *Mucor* sp.	Contaminated wood trimmings
Woodman's disease	*Penicillium* sp.	Oak and maple trees
Woodworker's lung	Wood dust; *Alternaria*	Oak, cedar, and mahogany dusts; pine and spruce pulp

* Thermophilic actinomycetes species include *Micropolyspora faeni, Thermoactinomyces vulgaris, T. saccharrii, T. viridis,* and *T. candidus.*

antigen and perhaps other host factors. The presentation can be *acute, subacute,* or *chronic.* In the *acute form,* symptoms such as cough, fever, chills, malaise, and dyspnea may occur 6 to 8 h after exposure to the antigen and usually clear within a few days if there is no further exposure to antigen. The *subacute form* often appears insidiously over a period of weeks marked by cough and dyspnea and may progress to cyanosis and severe dyspnea requiring hospitalization. In some patients, a subacute form of the disease may persist after an acute presentation of the disorder, especially if there is continued exposure to antigen. In most patients with the acute or subacute form of HP, the symptoms, signs, and other manifestations of HP disappear within days, weeks, or months if the causative agent is no longer inhaled. Transformation to a chronic form of the disease may occur in patients with continued antigen exposure, but the frequency of such progression is uncertain. The *chronic form* may also present as a gradually progressive interstitial disease associated with cough and exertional dyspnea without a prior history consistent with acute or subacute manifestations. Such a gradual onset frequently occurs with low-dose exposure to the antigen.

DIAGNOSIS Following acute exposure to antigen, neutrophilia and lymphopenia are frequently present. Eosinophilia is not a feature. All forms of the disease may be associated with elevations in erythrocyte sedimentation rate, C-reactive protein, rheumatoid factor, and serum immunoglobulins. Antinuclear antibodies are rarely present.

Examination for *serum precipitins* against suspected antigens, such as those listed in Table 218-1, is an important part of the diagnostic workup and should be performed on any patient with interstitial lung disease, especially if a suggestive exposure history is elicited. If found, precipitins indicate sufficient exposure to the causative agent for generation of an immunologic response. The diagnosis of HP is not established solely by the presence of precipitins, however, as precipitins are found in sera of many individuals exposed to appropriate antigens who demonstrate no other evidence of HP. False-negative results may occur because of poor-quality antigens or an inappropriate choice of antigens. Extraction of antigens from the patient's environment may at times be helpful.

No specific or distinctive *chest roentgenogram* occurs in HP. It can be normal even in symptomatic patients. The acute or subacute phase may be associated with poorly defined, patchy, or diffuse infiltrates or with discrete, nodular infiltrates. In the chronic phase, the chest x-ray usually shows a diffuse reticulonodular infiltrate. Honeycombing may eventually develop as the condition progresses. Abnormalities rarely seen in HP include pleural effusion or thickening, and hilar adenopathy. High-resolution chest computed tomography (CT) has been reported to show a characteristic constellation of abnormalities, providing support for an otherwise uncertain clinical diagnosis, although no pathognomonic CT features of HP have been described.

Pulmonary function studies in all forms of HP typically show a restrictive pattern with loss of lung volumes, impaired diffusion capacity, decreased compliance, and an exercise-induced hypoxemia. A resting hypoxemia may be found. Functional abnormalities may gradually increase in severity or may occur rapidly following acute or subacute exposure to antigen. As the chronic stage progresses, changes consistent with airway obstruction may become increasingly prominent.

Bronchoalveolar lavage is used in some centers to aid in diagnostic evaluation, and the characteristic features of the lavage fluid are described above.

Lung biopsy may be indicated in patients without sufficient other criteria to make a definitive diagnosis. The initial biopsy procedure is usually a transbronchial biopsy. In some patients, an open-lung biopsy may be necessary, as this procedure will provide adequate material for pathologic studies whereas transbronchial biopsy may not. Although the histopathology is distinctive, it may not be pathognomonic of HP. When the biopsy is taken during the active phase of disease, typical findings include an interstitial alveolar infiltrate consisting of plasma cells, lymphocytes, and occasional eosinophils and neutrophils, usually with accompanying granulomas. Interstitial fibrosis may be present but most often is mild in earlier stages of the disease. Some degree of bronchiolitis is found in about half the cases, whereas vasculitis is not a feature of the disorder. The triad of mononuclear bronchiolitis, interstitial infiltrates of lymphocytes and plasma cells, and single, nonnecrotizing, and randomly scattered parenchymal granulomas without mural vascular involvement is consistent with but not specific for HP.

The lack of standardized, nonirritating antigens and of proven controlled protocols makes *skin testing* and *inhalational challenge* useful only for research purposes. Similarly, *in vitro tests of cell-mediated (delayed) hypersensitivity* have not been shown to consistently correlate with clinical HP and have no place in the routine diagnostic workup.

In summary, the diagnosis in most cases is established by (1) consistent history, physical findings, pulmonary function tests, and chest x-ray; (2) exposure to a recognized antigen; and (3) finding an antibody to that antigen. In a few circumstances, bronchoalveolar lavage and/or lung biopsy may be needed. Provocation tests are research procedures and are not indicated.

DIFFERENTIAL DIAGNOSIS Chronic HP may often be difficult to distinguish from a number of other interstitial lung disorders such as idiopathic pulmonary fibrosis, interstitial lung disease associated with a collagen vascular disorder, and drug-induced lung diseases. A negative history for use of appropriate drugs and no evidence of a systemic disorder usually exclude the presence of drug-induced lung disease or a collagen vascular disorder. Bronchoalveolar lavage often shows predominance of neutrophils in idiopathic pulmonary fibrosis and a predominance of CD4+ lymphocytes in sarcoidosis. The diagnosis of sarcoidosis is also favored by hilar lymph node involvement or evidence of multisystem involvement. In some patients, a lung biopsy may be required to differentiate chronic HP from other interstitial diseases.

The lung disease associated with acute or subacute HP may clinically resemble other disorders that present with systemic symptoms and recurrent pulmonary infiltrates. These disorders include the collagen vascular disorders, drug-induced lung disease, allergic bronchopulmonary aspergillosis, and other eosinophilic pneumonias. Eosinophilic pneumonia is often associated with asthma and is typified by peripheral eosinophilia; neither of these is a feature of HP. Allergic bronchopulmonary aspergillosis is sometimes confused with HP because of the presence of precipitating antibodies to *Aspergillus fumigatus.* It is an obstructive rather than a restrictive lung disease, however, that is associated with allergic (atopic) asthma.

The term *inorganic dust toxic syndrome* has been applied to a condition often mistaken for HP; it follows heavy exposure to organic dusts and is characterized by transient fever and muscle aches, with or without respiratory symptoms. Serum precipitins are absent, and the chest x-ray is usually normal.

Massive exposure to moldy silage may result in a syndrome termed *pulmonary mycotoxicosis* or *atypical farmer's lung* with fever, chills, and cough and the presence of pulmonary infiltrates within a few hours of exposure. No previous sensitization is required, and precipitins are absent to *Aspergillus,* the suspected causative agent.

TREATMENT Because effective treatment depends largely on avoiding the antigen, identification of the causative agent and its source is essential. This is usually possible if the physician takes a careful environmental and occupational history or, if necessary, visits the patient's environment.

The simplest way to avoid the incriminated agent is to remove the patient from the environment or the source of the agent from the patient's environment. This recommendation cannot be taken lightly when it completely changes the life-style or livelihood of the patient. In many cases, however, the source of exposure (birds, humidifiers) can easily be removed. If occupational exposure is involved, an initial attempt can be made at antigen avoidance maneuvers least disruptive to the patient's livelihood, which usually means avoiding areas associated with heavy exposure and wearing an appropriate mask. This will not suffice for small-molecular-weight agents such as isocyanates, which require elaborate filtration devices. Pollen masks, personal dust respirators, airstream helmets, and ventilated helmets with a supply of fresh air are increasingly efficient means of purifying inhaled air. If symptoms recur or physiologic abnormalities progress in spite of these measures, then more effective measures to avoid antigen exposure must be pursued.

Compromises with environmental control pertain primarily to the acute, recurrent, transient clinical form of HP and must be accompanied by careful follow-up. Subacute forms are ordinarily the result of a heavy, sustained exposure. The chronic form typically results from low-grade or recurrent exposure over many months to years, and the lung disease may already be partially irreversible. These patients should be advised to avoid completely all possible contact with the offending agent, although follow-up studies of farmer's lung and bird fancier's lung have found resolution of the disease despite continued exposure in some patients.

Patients with the *acute*, recurrent form of HP usually recover without need for glucocorticoids. *Subacute* HP may be associated with severe symptoms and marked physiologic impairment and may continue to progress for several days despite hospitalization. Urgent establishment of the diagnosis and prompt institution of glucocorticoid treatment are indicated in such patients. Such therapy may also hasten recovery in patients with lesser involvement. Prednisone at a dosage of 1 mg/kg per day or its equivalent is continued for 7 to 14 days and then tapered over the ensuing 2 to 6 weeks at a rate that depends on the patient's clinical status.

Patients with *chronic* HP may gradually recover without therapy following environmental control. In many patients, however, a trial of prednisone may be useful to obtain maximal reversibility of the lung disease. Following initial prednisone therapy (1 mg/kg per day for 2 to 4 weeks), the drug is tapered to the lowest dosage that will maintain the functional status of the patient. Many patients will not require or benefit from long-term therapy if there is no further exposure to antigen. Available studies report no effect of glucocorticoid therapy on long-term prognosis of farmer's lung.

EOSINOPHILIC PNEUMONIAS

Eosinophilic pneumonias are composed of distinct individual syndromes characterized by eosinophilic pulmonary infiltrates and, commonly, peripheral blood eosinophilia. Since Loeffler's initial description of a transient, benign syndrome of migratory pulmonary infiltrates and peripheral blood eosinophilia of unknown cause, this group of disorders has been enlarged to include several diseases of both known and unknown etiology (Table 218-2). These diseases may be considered as examples of hypersensitivity lung disease but are not to be confused with hypersensitivity pneumonitis (extrinsic allergic alveolitis) in which eosinophilia is not a feature.

When an eosinophilic pneumonia is associated with bronchial asthma, it is important to determine if the patient has extrinsic (allergic, atopic) asthma and has wheal-and-flare skin reactivity to

---

TABLE 218-2 Eosinophilic pneumonias

ETIOLOGY KNOWN

Allergic bronchopulmonary aspergillosis
Parasitic infestations
Drug reactions

IDIOPATHIC

Loeffler's syndrome
Chronic eosinophilic pneumonia
Allergic granulomatosis of Churg and Strauss
Hypereosinophilic syndrome

TABLE 218-3 Diagnostic features of allergic bronchopulmonary aspergillosis (ABPA)

MAIN DIAGNOSTIC CRITERIA

1 Bronchial asthma
2 Pulmonary infiltrates
3 Peripheral eosinophilia ($> 1000/\mu L$)
4 Immediate wheal-and-flare response to *Aspergillus fumigatus*
5 Serum precipitins to *A. fumigatus*
6 Elevated serum IgE
7 Central bronchiectasis

OTHER DIAGNOSTIC FEATURES

1 History of brownish plugs in sputum
2 Culture of *A. fumigatus* from sputum
3 Elevated IgE (and IgG) class antibodies specific for *A. fumigatus*

Aspergillus allergens. If so, other criteria should be sought for diagnosis of *allergic bronchopulmonary aspergillosis* (ABPA) (Table 218-3). *A. fumigatus* is the most common cause, although other *Aspergillus* species have also been implicated. ABPA has been reported to complicate cystic fibrosis. The chest roentgenogram in ABPA may show transient, recurrent infiltrates or may suggest the presence of proximal bronchiectasis. High-resolution chest CT is a sensitive, noninvasive technique for the recognition of proximal bronchiectasis. The bronchial asthma of ABPA likely involves an IgE-mediated hypersensitivity, whereas the bronchiectasis associated with this disorder is thought to result from a deposition of immune complexes in proximal airways. Adequate treatment usually requires the long-term use of systemic glucocorticoids.

Tropical eosinophilia is usually caused by filarial infection; however, eosinophilic pneumonias also occur with other parasites such as *Ascaris, Ancyclostoma* species, *Toxocara* species, and *Strongyloides stercoralis*. Tropical eosinophilia due to *Wuchereria bancrofti* or *W. malayi* occurs most commonly in southern Asia, Africa, and South America, and is treated successfully with diethylcarbamazine.

Drug-induced eosinophilic pneumonias are typified by acute reactions to nitrofurantoin, which may begin 2 h to 10 days after nitrofurantoin is started, with symptoms of dry cough, fever, chills, and dyspnea; an eosinophilic pleural effusion accompanying patchy or diffuse pulmonary infiltrates may also occur. Other drugs associated with eosinophilic pneumonias include sulfonamides, penicillin, chlorpropamide, thiazides, tricyclic antidepressants, hydralazine, mephenesin, mecamylamine, nickel carbonyl vapor, gold salts, isoniazid, para-aminosalicylic acid, and others. Treatment consists of withdrawal of the incriminated drugs and the use of glucocorticoids, if necessary.

The idiopathic eosinophilic pneumonias consist of a group of diseases of varying severity. *Loeffler's syndrome* is a benign, acute eosinophilic pneumonia characterized by migrating pulmonary infiltrates and minimal clinical manifestations. *Acute eosinophilic pneumonia* has been described as an acute febrile illness of less than 7 days' duration, severe hypoxemia, pulmonary infiltrates, and no history of asthma. *Chronic eosinophilic pneumonia* presents with significant systemic symptoms including fever, chills, night sweats, cough, anorexia, and weight loss of several weeks to months' duration. The chest x-ray frequently shows peripheral infiltrates that have been described as a photographic negative of pulmonary edema. Some patients also have bronchial asthma, which is of the intrinsic or nonallergic type. Dramatic clearing of symptoms and chest x-rays is often noted within 48 h after initiation of glucocorticoid therapy.

Allergic angiitis and granulomatosis of Churg and Strauss is a multisystem vasculitic disorder that frequently involves the skin, kidney, and nervous system in addition to the lung (Chap. 291). The disorder may occur at any age and favors persons with a history of bronchial asthma. The asthma often is progressive until the onset of fever and exaggerated eosinophilia, at which time the symptoms of asthma may ease. The illness may be fulminating and the prognosis grave unless treated aggressively with glucocorticoids and immuno-suppressive therapy.

The hypereosinophilic syndrome is characterized by presence of over 1500 eosinophils per microliter of peripheral blood for 6 months or longer; lack of evidence for parasitic, allergic, or other known causes of eosinophilia; and signs or symptoms of multisystem organ dysfunction. Consistent features are blood and bone marrow eosinophilia with tissue infiltration by relatively mature eosinophils. The organs affected typically include the heart, lungs, liver, spleen, skin, and nervous system. Therapy of the disorder consists of glucocorticoids and/or hydroxyurea plus therapy as needed for cardiac dysfunction, which is frequently responsible for much of the morbidity and mortality in this syndrome.

REFERENCES

Hypersensitivity pneumonitis

GRAMMER LC, PATTERSON R: Occupational immunologic lung disease. Ann Allergy 58:151, 1987

HANSELL DM, MOSKOVIC E: High-resolution computed tomography in extrinsic allergic alveolitis. Clin Radiol 43:8, 1991

IMBEALT B. CORMIER Y: Usefulness of inhaled high-dose corticosteroids in allergic bronchopulmonary aspergillosis. Chest 103:1614, 1993

KOKKARINEN JI et al: Recovery of pulmonary function in farmer's lung. A five-year follow-up study. Am Rev Respir Dis 147:793, 1993

MARX JJ et al: Cohort studies of immunologic lung disease among Wisconsin dairy farmers. Am J Ind Med 18:263, 1990

PITCHER WD: Hypersensitivity pneumonitis. Am J Med Sci 300:251, 1990

RICHERSON HB: Unifying concepts underlying the effects of organic dust exposures. Am J Ind Med 17:139, 1990

———— et al: Guidelines for the clinical evaluation of hypersensitivity pneumonitis. J Allergy Clin Immunol 84:839, 1989

Eosinophilic pneumonias

ALLEN JN et al: Acute eosinophilic pneumonia as a reversible cause of noninfectious respiratory failure. N Engl J Med 321:569, 1989

GREENBERGER PA, PATTERSON R: Allergic bronchopulmonary aspergillosis: A model of bronchopulmonary disease with defined serologic, radiologic, pathologic and clinical findings from asthma to fatal destructive lung disease. Chest 91:165S, 1987

HUTCHESON PS et al: Variability in parameters of allergic bronchopulmonary aspergillosis in patients with cystic fibrosis. J Allergy Clin Immunol 88:390, 1991

ROSENOW EC III et al: Drug-induced pulmonary disease: An update. Chest 102:239, 1992

219 ENVIRONMENTAL LUNG DISEASES

FRANK E. SPEIZER

This chapter provides perspectives on ways to assess pulmonary diseases for which environmental causes are suspected. This assessment is important because removal of the patient from a harmful environment is often the only intervention that might prevent further significant deterioration or lead to improvement in a patient's condition. Furthermore, the identification of an environmentally associated disease in a single patient may lead to primary preventive strategies in other similarly exposed people who have not yet developed disease. Unless the physician specifically considers environmental exposures, these diseases and their causes will go undetected.

The exact magnitude of the problem is unknown, but there is no question that large numbers of people are at risk of developing serious respiratory disease as a result of occupational or environmental exposures. For example, recent estimates suggest that approximately 2.3 million workers have been exposed to crystalline silica or asbestos dust in mining and nonmining industries. If only 5 percent (a conservative estimate) of these workers are to suffer from respiratory

disease as a result of their exposure, this represents more than 100,000 individuals in the United States.

Although industries are required to spend substantial amounts of capital in efforts to protect their workers, occupationally related respiratory diseases continue to occur. These diseases are often attributed to exposures in the distant past at a time when we were not aware of the risk incurred and the need for worker protection to the degree that we are today. We have, as a society, elected to pay compensation to affected individuals, and the physician is often called on to judge not only the physical condition of such a patient but also the degree to which the illness can be related to, or aggravated by, a particular occupational exposure.

HISTORY AND PHYSICAL EXAMINATION The patient history is of paramount importance in assessing any potential occupational or environmental exposure. Often one is dealing with potential exposures in industries or environmental settings in which the physician has little personal experience. The physician must therefore ask the patient to describe a suspected environmental exposure in detail.

Inquiry into specific work practices should include questions about specific contaminants involved, the availability and use of personal respiratory protection devices, the size and ventilation of workspaces, the numbers of other workers potentially at risk of exposure, and whether other coworkers have similar complaints. In addition, the patient must be questioned about alternative sources for potentially toxic exposures, including hobbies or other environmental exposures at home. Short-term exposures to potential toxic agents in the distant past also must be considered. This information can be best elicited by a detailed occupational history which inquires about every job (beginning even with part-time jobs during schooling) and about the nature of the work, the materials handled, and the duration and chronologic years of employment (see Chap. 394).

Many people are aware of the potential hazards in their workplaces, and many states require that employees be informed about potentially hazardous exposures. These requirements include the provision of specific educational materials (including Material Safety Data Sheets), personal protective equipment and instructions in their use, and information on environmental control procedures. Reminders posted in the workplace may warn workers about hazardous substances. Protective clothing, lockers, and shower facilities may be considered necessary parts of the job. However, even in these more progressive industries, the introduction of new processes, particularly when related to the use of new chemical compounds, may change exposure significantly, and often only the employee on the production line is aware of the change. For the physician who regularly sees patients from a particular industry, a visit to the work site can be very instructive. Alternatively, physicians can request inspections by appropriate federal and/or state authorities through which clinically relevant exposure information can be obtained.

The physical examination of patients with environmentally related lung diseases may help to determine the nature and severity of the pulmonary condition. Unfortunately, the pulmonary response to most injurious agents is the development of a limited number of nonspecific physical signs. These findings do not point to the specific causative agent, and other types of information must be used to arrive at an etiologic diagnosis.

PULMONARY FUNCTION TESTS AND CHEST RADIOGRAPH The use of pulmonary function tests and radiographic examinations of the chest can provide insight into the nature of the exposures which have led to the current condition of the patient and the level of impairment. Many mineral dusts produce characteristic alterations in the mechanics of breathing and lung volumes which clearly indicate a restrictive pattern (Chaps. 214 and 224). Exposures to a number of organic dusts or chemical agents capable of producing occupational asthma result in pronounced obstructive patterns of pulmonary dysfunction that may be reversible (Chap. 217). Standardized approaches for measuring the mechanics of breathing and diffusion across the alveolar membrane (Chap. 214) have been proposed for screening large industrial groups. Measurement of change in forced expiratory volume (FEV$_1$) before and after a working shift can be used to detect an acute inflammatory or bronchoconstrictive response. An acute decrement of FEV$_1$ over the Monday work shift is a characteristic feature of cotton textile workers with byssinosis.

For many years the chest radiograph has been used to detect and monitor the pulmonary response to mineral dusts. To provide a standardized method of recording judgments about the kind and severity of radiographic abnormalities, the International Labour Organization (ILO) International Classification of Radiographs of Pneumoconioses was developed. The ILO scheme involves classifying chest radiographs according to the nature and size of opacities seen and the extent of involvement of the parenchyma. Although useful for screening large numbers of workers, the procedure lacks specificity and may over- or underestimate the functional impact of pneumoconiosis. With dusts causing rounded, regular opacities, such as in coal worker's pneumoconiosis, the degree of involvement on the chest radiograph may be extensive, while pulmonary function may be only minimally impaired. In contrast, in pneumoconiosis causing linear, irregular opacities, as seen in asbestosis, the radiograph may lead to underestimation of the severity of the impairment. It is possible to have a history of exposure, moderately reduced forced vital capacity (FVC), and a reduced diffusion in asbestosis with a relatively normal chest radiograph. The radiographic findings of irregular or linear opacities are simply more difficult to separate from normal markings until relatively late in the disease. When shadows become large (radiographic lesions greater than 1 cm in diameter), the condition is termed *complicated pneumoconiosis*, sometimes called *progressive massive fibrosis* (PMF). For the individual patient with a history of exposure, conventional computed tomography (CT) and high-resolution computed tomography (HRCT) have improved the sensitivity of identifying diffuse parenchymal abnormalities of the lung. The procedures have been shown to provide earlier detection of silicosis and asbestosis.

Other diagnostic procedures of use in identifying environmentally induced lung disease include evaluating heavy metal concentrations in urine (arsenic in smelter workers, cadmium in battery plant workers); bacteriologic studies (tuberculosis in medical care personnel, anthrax in wool sorters); fungal studies (coccidioidomycosis in southwestern farm workers, histoplasmosis in poultry or pigeon handlers); or serologic studies (psittacosis in pet shop workers or owners of sick birds, Q fever in tanners or slaughterhouse workers). Ultimately, a lung biopsy may be required both to make a morphologic diagnosis of the underlying pulmonary disease and to attempt to identify the specific etiologic agent.

MEASUREMENT OF EXPOSURE If reliable environmental sampling data are available, these sources of information should be used in assessing a patient's exposure. Since many of the chronic diseases result from exposure over many years, current environmental measurements should be combined with work histories to arrive at estimates of past exposure. However, the dose of any environmental agent is a complex interaction of chemical reaction, both at the emission source and in the ambient atmosphere, and physiologic factors, including ventilation rate and depth, which may affect transport and deposition of aerosols and gases in the lung. Even in acute conditions, when monitoring of exposure may be possible, little may be known about the actual dose received by the lung. Most of the research on health effects of air pollutants (discussed later in this chapter) has relied on fixed-station monitoring of outdoor air, often at locations somewhat distant from the residences of the people being studied. In addition, most people spend less than 20 percent of their time outdoors. Efforts to determine the penetration rate of outdoor contaminants into the indoors suggest that these penetration rates are highly pollutant specific. Therefore, outdoor measurements can be used only in a relative sense, and they cannot be relied on to estimate actual dose.

In situations where individual exposure to specific agents has been determined, either in a work setting or for ambient air pollutants, transport of these agents through the airways may be an important factor affecting dose. Highly soluble gases such as sulfur dioxide are absorbed in the upper airway and presumably produce their effects by reflex response to sensitive neural fibrils in the trachea or larger airways. In contrast, nitrogen dioxide, which is less soluble, may reach the bronchioles and alveoli in sufficient quantities to result in an acute life-threatening disease in farmers exposed even briefly to the gas evolved from moldy hay in silos (silo filler's disease).

Particle size and chemistry of air contaminants also must be considered. Particles above 10 to 15 μm, because of their settling velocities in air, do not penetrate beyond the upper airways. These larger particles are often referred to as "fugitive dusts" and include pollens, other windblown dusts, and dusts resulting from mechanical industrial processes. They have little or no role in chronic respiratory disease except as possibly related to cancer (see below).

Particles below 10 μm in size are created by the burning of fossil fuels or high-temperature industrial processes resulting in condensation products from gases, fumes, or vapors. These particles are divided into two size fractions on the basis of their chemical characteristics. Particles approximately 2.5 to 10 μm (coarse-mode fraction) contain crustal elements, such as silica, aluminum, and iron. These particles mostly deposit relatively high in the tracheobronchial tree. Particles less than approximately 2.5 μm (fine-mode fraction or accumulation mode) contain sulfates, nitrates, and organic compounds. The deposition of the fine-mode particles is more often in the terminal bronchioles and alveoli. The smallest particles, those less than 0.1 μm in size, remain in the airstream and deposit in the lung only on a random basis as they come into contact with the alveolar walls through thermal forces and/or Brownian movement.

Besides the size characteristics of particles and the solubility of gases, the actual chemical composition, mechanical properties, and immunogenicity or infectivity of inhaled material determine in large part the nature of the diseases found among exposed persons.

OCCUPATIONAL EXPOSURES AND PULMONARY DISEASE

INORGANIC DUSTS Asbestos exposure Except in localized regions with single industrial exposures, such as coal-mining or granite-quarrying regions, the most frequent inorganic dust–related chronic pulmonary diseases are associated with industries using *asbestiform fibers. Asbestos* is a generic term for several different mineral silicates, including chrysolite, amosite, anthophyllite, and crocidolite. Besides mining, milling, and manufacturing of asbestos products, the exceptional thermal and electric insulation properties of asbestos led to its widespread use in construction, leading to exposure of pipe fitters, boiler makers, and other workers in the building trades. In addition, asbestos was used in the manufacture of fire-smothering blankets and safety garments, as filler for plastic materials, in cement and floor tiles, and in friction materials, such as brake and clutch linings.

Exposure to asbestos is not limited to persons who directly handle the material. Cases of asbestos-related diseases have been encountered in individuals with only moderate exposure, such as the painter or electrician who works alongside the insulation worker in a shipyard or the housewife who does no more than shake out and wash her husband's work clothes. Community exposure has probably resulted from the use of asbestos-containing material sprayed on steel girders in many large buildings as a safety feature to prevent buckling in case of fire. Clusters of cases of mesothelioma have been noted in the neighborhood of an asbestos plant in London and in the communities near asbestos mines in South Africa.

Asbestos was first used extensively in the 1940s. Starting in 1975 it has been mostly replaced with man-made mineral fibers, such as fiberglass or slag wool. However, asbestos is still used in the manufacture of brake linings and remains as pipe and boiler insulation in hundreds of thousands of workplaces and homes. Despite current regulations mandating adequate training for any worker potentially exposed to asbestos, exposure probably continues among inexperienced demolition workers. The major health effects from exposure to asbestos are pulmonary fibrosis (asbestosis) and cancers of the respiratory tract and pleura and, rarely, peritoneum.

Asbestosis is a diffuse interstitial fibrosing disease of the lung which is directly related to the intensity and duration of exposure. Except for a history of exposure to asbestos (generally in a work setting), asbestosis resembles the other forms of diffuse interstitial fibrosis (Chap. 224). Usually at least 10 years of moderate to severe exposure has occurred before the disease becomes manifest.

Physiologic studies reveal a restrictive pattern with a decrease in lung volumes. Flow rates are commonly reduced less than would be predicted on the basis of the volume reduction. An early sign of severe disease may be a reduction in diffusing capacity.

Pulmonary fibrosis may occur following sufficient exposure to any of the asbestiform fiber types. The fibrotic lesions do not appear to relate to either shape or chemical composition of any fiber type. Recent studies indicate that during phagocytosis of the asbestos fiber, the membrane of the macrophage is damaged, which results in the release of lysosomes containing enzymes which may act to damage the lung parenchyma. The clinical manifestations are typical of those physical findings in any patient with pulmonary fibrosis (Chap. 224).

The chest radiograph can be used to determine a number of manifestations of asbestos exposure, as well as to identify specific lesions. Past exposure is specifically indicated by pleural plaques, which are characterized by either thickening or calcification along the parietal pleura, particularly along the lower lung fields, the diaphragm, and the cardiac border. Without additional manifestations, pleural plaques imply only exposure, not pulmonary impairment. Benign pleural effusions may occur, particularly in patients with abestosis, but are not necessarily restricted to those with overt disease. The fluid is sterile but may be a serous or blood-stained exudate and may occur bilaterally. The effusion may be slowly progressive or may resolve spontaneously.

The radiographic diagnosis of asbestosis depends on the presence of irregular or linear opacities, usually first noted in the lower lung fields and spreading into the middle and upper lung fields as the disease progresses. An indistinct heart border or a "ground glass" appearance in the lung fields is seen in some cases. As the fibrotic changes in the parenchyma begin to coalesce, the patient develops obliteration of entire acinar units with eventual formation of the classical honeycombed lung, which appears on chest radiographs as coarse infiltrates with small (about 7- to 10-μm) air spaces. In cases in which the x-ray changes are less obvious, HRCT may show distinct changes of subpleural curvilinear lines 5 to 10 cm in length which appear to be parallel to the pleural surface. No specific therapy is available in the management of patients with asbestosis. The supportive care is that of any patient with diffuse interstitial fibrosis from any cause.

In general, newly diagnosed cases will have resulted from exposure levels that were present many years before and, in spite of the patients' having left the industry, are attributable to that former exposure. Since the patient may be eligible for compensation within a specific time frame after the diagnosis of an asbestos-related disease is made, the physician making the diagnosis should be certain to inform the patient promptly. On occasion, the physician may have reason to suspect ongoing exposure from a patient's current job description or actual monitoring data. In such cases, federal or state health authorities may need to be notified. Present-day occupational safety and health regulations, if followed properly, protect workers from exposure. Because the association of smoking and asbestos exposure increases the risk of developing lung cancer (see below), it is extremely important to advise patients with such exposure histories to stop smoking.

Lung cancer (Chap. 227), either squamous cell or adenocarcinoma, is the most frequent cancer associated with asbestos exposure. The excess frequency of lung cancer in asbestos workers is associated with a minimum lapse of 15 to 19 years between first exposure and development of the disease. Persons with more exposure are at greater risk of disease. In addition, there appears to be a significant multiplicative effect which leads to a far greater risk of lung cancer in persons who are cigarette smokers and have asbestos exposure than would be expected by taking the sum of both risks. Efforts to consider these high-risk individuals for special surveillance studies, including sputum cytologic examinations and repeated chest x-rays as frequently as every 4 to 6 months, suggest that cancers can be detected at an earlier stage and that the survival of these patients may be prolonged.

Mesotheliomas (Chap. 228), both pleural and peritoneal, also are associated with asbestos exposure. In contrast to lung cancer, there does not appear to be any association with smoking. Relatively short-term exposures of 1 to 2 years or less occurring some 20 to 25 years in the past have been associated with the development of mesotheliomas (which stresses the point of obtaining a complete environmental exposure history). The risk for this type of tumor peaks 30 to 35 years after initial exposure. Although approximately 50 percent of mesotheliomas metastasize, the tumor generally is locally invasive, and death usually results from local extension. Most patients present with effusions that may obscure the underlying pleural tumor. In contrast to other causes of effusion, because of the restriction placed on the chest wall, no shift of mediastinal structures toward the opposite chest will be seen. The major diagnostic problem is differentiation from peripherally spreading pulmonary adenocarcinoma or adenocarcinoma metastatic to pleura from an extrathoracic primary site. Although a needle biopsy may be diagnostic, an open biopsy is often necessary and even when performed may not provide a definitive diagnosis of the origin of the tumor.

One concern in making a definitive diagnosis of a mesothelioma relates to potential compensation to the survivors of a patient with this usually fatal disease. Since epidemiologic studies have shown that more than 80 percent of mesotheliomas may be associated with asbestos exposure, documented mesothelioma in a worker with occupational exposure to asbestos may be compensable in many parts of the United States.

Other naturally occurring asbestiform material (e.g., erionite, a fibrous zeolite) induces mesotheliomas in test animals and has been associated with an excess incidence of lung cancer and mesotheliomas in a population in central Turkey exposed to it in volcanic rock. Man-made mineral fibers (MMMF) have similar physiochemical properties to naturally occurring asbestiform fibers. However, recent studies of exposure suggest that if excess risks of lung cancer do occur, they are less than with naturally occurring fibers. To date, no cases of mesotheliomas from MMMF without exposure to asbestos has been reported. Part of the difficulty in assessing the effects of MMMF is that they have been used for relatively shorter periods and generally at lower exposure levels than for asbestos. Thus concern for worker protection needs to be maintained.

Silicosis   In spite of the technical adequacy of existing protective equipment, *free silica* (SiO_2), or crystalline quartz, is still a major occupational hazard. In the United States, estimates of potential numbers of exposed workers range between 1.2 to 3 million people. The major occupational exposures include mining, stone cutting, abrasive industries, foundry workers, packers of silica flour, and quarrying, particularly of granite. Most often the progressive pulmonary fibrosis (silicosis) occurs in a dose-response fashion after many years of exposure.

Workers exposed to sandblasting in confined spaces, tunneling through rock with high quartz content (15 to 25 percent), and engaged in the manufacture of abrasive soaps may develop acute silicosis with as little as 10 months' exposure. The disease may be rapidly fatal in less than 2 years despite the worker being removed from exposure. A radiographic picture of profuse miliary infiltration or consolidation is characteristic of acute silicosis.

In long-term, relatively less intense exposure, radiographic changes of rounded, small opacities in the upper lobes with retraction and hilar adenopathy classically appear after 15 to 20 years of exposure. Calcification of hilar nodes may occur in as many as 20 percent of cases and produces the characteristic "eggshell" pattern. These changes may be preceded by or be associated with a reticular pattern of irregular densities which are uniformly present throughout the upper lung zones.

The nodular fibrosis may be progressive in the absence of further exposure, with coalescence and formation of nonsegmental conglomerates of irregular masses in excess of 1 cm in diameter. These masses become quite large and are characteristic of progressive massive fibrosis (PMF). Significant functional impairment with both restrictive and obstructive components may be associated with this form of silicosis. In the late stages of the disease ventilatory failure may develop. In more subtle cases, CT may be helpful both in identifying nodules which are preferentially located in the posterior aspect of the upper lobes, as well as in identifying larger opacities and more coalescence than might be noted on regular chest x-rays. Patients with silicosis are at greater risk of acquiring *Mycobacterium tuberculosis* infections (silicotuberculosis), as well as atypical mycobacterial infections, although tuberculosis is not always involved in the progression of the disease to PMF. Because the frequency with which tuberculosis has been found at autopsy in patients with PMF exceeds considerably the frequency of premorbid diagnosis, treatment for tuberculosis is indicated in any patient with silicosis and a positive tuberculin test.

Other less hazardous silicates include fuller's earth, kaolin, mica, diatomaceous earths, silica gel, soapstone, carbonate dusts, and cement dusts. The production of fibrosis in workers exposed to these agents is believed to be related to either the free silica content of these dusts or, for substances which contain no free silica, to the potentially large dust loads to which these workers may be exposed.

Other silicates, including *talc dusts*, may be contaminated with asbestos and/or free silica. Accidental exposure to significant quantities of talc may result in an acute syndrome with cough, cyanosis, and labored breathing (acute talcosis). Severe progressive fibrosis with respiratory failure may ensue within a few years. Far more common is the fibrosis and/or pleural or lung cancer associated with chronic exposure in rubber workers who use commercial talc as a lubricant in tire molds. Pure talc does not produce fibrosis; thus it is difficult to sort out whether the effects are due to the contamination of commercial talc by asbestos or by free silica.

Coal worker's pneumoconiosis (CWP)   *Coal dust* is associated with CWP, which has enormous social, economic, and medical significance in every nation in which coal mining is an important industry. Simple radiographically identified CWP is seen in 12 percent of all miners and in as many as 50 percent of anthracite miners with more than 20 years' work on the coal face. The prevalence of disease is lower in workers in bituminous coal mines. Since much of the western U.S. coal is bituminous, CWP is less prevalent in that region.

Much of the symptomatology associated with simple CWP appears to be similar and additive to the effects of cigarette smoking on the development of chronic bronchitis and obstructive lung disease (Chap. 223). In the early stages of simple CWP, radiographic abnormalities consist of small, irregular opacities (reticular pattern). With prolonged exposure, one sees small, rounded, regular opacities, 1 to 5 mm in diameter (nodular pattern). Calcification is generally not seen, although approximately 10 percent of older anthracite miners have calcified nodules.

Complicated CWP is manifested by the appearance on the chest radiograph of nodules ranging from 1 cm in diameter to the size of an entire lobe, generally confined to the upper half of the lungs. This condition, considered a form of PMF, is accompanied by a significant reduction in diffusing capacity and with premature mortality. In contrast to patients with silicosis, only a relatively small percentage of underground miners with simple CWP (5 to 15 percent, depending on the type of coal) develop PMF.

The mechanism whereby PMF occurs in CWP is not fully understood. Several hypotheses have been proposed, including (1) sufficient free silica is present in the dust, (2) normal clearance mechanisms are unable to clear the excessive dust loads, (3) an interplay occurs between an intrinsic immunologic mechanism and the dust and/or damaged lung tissue, and (4) atypical reactions to *Mycobacterium tuberculosis* occur. As previously described, PMF in silicosis is associated with prolonged duration and high intensity of exposure to free silica. Heavy exposure to carbon particles free of silica occurs in carbon black, graphite, and charcoal workers. The prolonged exposure of these workers may result in sufficient accumulation of carbon in the lung to produce PMF. The mechanism appears to relate to a breakdown of the clearance capacity of the airways.

Caplan's syndrome, which includes seropositive rheumatoid arthritis with characteristic PMF, is consistent with an immunopathologic mechanism. The syndrome was first described in coal miners but subsequently has been found in a number of pneumoconioses. Similarly, the high prevalence of antinuclear antibodies in sandblasting workers with silicosis and the elevation of gamma globulin levels in silicotic individuals suggest an immunologic mechanism. Although mycobacterial infections are found more often in coal miners than PMF is found in silicotic patients, tuberculosis does not appear to be associated with most of the cases of PMF in coal miners.

Berylliosis   Beryllium may produce an acute pneumonitis or, far more commonly, a chronic interstitial pneumonitis. Unless one inquires specifically about occupational exposures to beryllium in the manufacture of alloys, ceramics, high-technology electronics, and, before the 1950s, the production of fluorescent lights, one may miss entirely the etiologic relationship to an occupational exposure. Nonspecific pulmonary function tests may be normal or may indicate evidence of restrictive disease. Between 2 and 15 years of exposure, depending on its intensity, is required for the disease to become manifest. On open lung biopsy, granulomatous formation similar to that seen in sarcoidosis (Chap. 292) may make differentiation impossible unless tissue levels of beryllium are measured.

Rarely, other hard metals, including aluminum powders, chromium, cobalt, titanium dioxide, and tungsten, may produce an interstitial pneumonitis.

Other inorganic dusts   Other dusts are considered *nuisance dusts* because their major impact seems to be reduction in visibility and irritation of eyes, ears, nasal passages, and other mucous membranes. If they penetrate to the lower airways, they do not affect the architecture of the terminal bronchioles or acinar spaces or destroy collagen. Generally, clinical effects are reversible. Pulmonary function tests are usually normal unless another disease process coexists. If radiodense, macular collections of these dusts may produce striking radiographic pictures which are so characteristic that patients with a history of significant exposure are easily diagnosed as having the condition which bears the name reflecting the nature of the dust. Examples are iron and iron oxides from welding or silver finishing (*siderosis*); tin oxide used in metallurgy, color stabilization, printing, and the manufacture of porcelain, glass, and fabric (*stannosis*); and barium sulfate used as a catalyst for organic reactions, drilling mud components, and electroplating (*baritosis*). Other metal dusts producing similar radiodense pictures include *cerium dioxide* and *antimony salts*.

Most of the inorganic dusts discussed thus far are associated with the production of either dust macules or interstitial fibrotic changes in the lung. Another set of dusts (see Table 219-1), along with some of the dusts previously discussed, is associated with chronic mucous hypersecretion (chronic bronchitis), with or without reduction of expiratory flow rates. These conditions may be caused by cigarette smoking, and any effort to attribute some component of the disease to occupational and environmental exposures must take cigarette smoking into account. Most studies suggest an additive effect of dust exposure and smoking. The pattern of the effect is similar to that of cigarette smoking, suggesting that small airways may be the initial

TABLE 219-1 Selected occupational dusts believed to be associated with mucous hypersecretion and/or obstructive airway disease and other respiratory diseases*

Agent (exposure)	Mucous hyper-secretion	Obstruction	Other conditions†
INORGANIC DUSTS			
Antimony (storage batteries, solder, ceramics, glass, plastics)	X		P
Arsenic (manufacture of pesticides, pigments, glass, alloys)	X		C
Barium and compounds including BaO, BaSO$_4$, BaCO$_3$ (catalyst, drilling mud, electroplating)	X		P
Cadmium dust (electroplating, battery manufacture, welding, smelting, aluminum soldering)	X	X	P
Cement dust (construction trades, manufacture of cement blocks)	X	X	
Chromium and CrO$_3$, CrF$_2$ (corrosion inhibitor pigment, metallurgy, electroplating)	X		C
Coal dust (mining)	X		P
Coke oven emissions (retort house, coke ovens)	X	X	P, C
Graphite (steelmaking, lubricants, pencils, paints, stove polish)	X	X	P
Iron dust (steel and nonferrous foundry workers, welding)	X	X	P
Mica (insulation, roofing shingles, oil refining, rubber manufacturing)	X		P
Phosphorus, elemental chlorides, sulfides (manufacture of fireworks, agricultural chemicals, insecticides, pesticides)	X	X	
Rock dusts (miners, tunnelers, quarry workers)	X		P
Vanadium pentoxide (welding electrodes, additive to steel, by-product in ash from oil burning)	X	X	
ORGANIC DUSTS (see Chap. 218)			
Cotton dust, flax, hemp (manufacture of yarns for linen, rope, cotton; ginning, cottonseed crushing; waste fiber processing)	X	X	
Grain dusts (farmers, workers in grain elevators, barge and grain ship crewmembers)	X	X	
Moldy hay (farmers, other animal attendants)	X		HP

* The table excludes agents associated with asthma as the primary disease (see Chap. 217).
† Other conditions include hypersensitivity pneumonitis (HP), pneumoconiosis (P), and cancers (C).
NOTE: X indicates that mucous hypersecretion or obstruction are associated with exposure.

site of pathologic response to those cases associated with the development of obstructive lung disease. Cigarette smoke is usually the more noxious agent, and dust effects may be discernible only in nonsmokers.

ORGANIC DUSTS Some of the specific diseases associated with organic dusts are discussed in detail in the chapters on asthma (Chap. 217) and hypersensitivity pneumonitis (Chap. 218). Many of these diseases are named for the specific setting in which the disease is

found, e.g., farmer's lung, malt worker's disease, or mushroom worker's disease. Occupational and other environmental exposures must be sought when these conditions are suspected. Often the temporal relation of symptoms to exposure furnishes the best evidence for the diagnosis. Three occupational groups are singled out for discussion because they represent the largest proportion of people affected by the diseases resulting from organic dusts.

Cotton dust (byssinosis) Estimates of the number of exposed persons in the United States vary, but probably over 800,000 persons are exposed occupationally to cotton, flax, or hemp in the production of yarns for cotton, linen, and rope making. Although this discussion focuses on cotton, the same syndrome to a somewhat lesser degree has been reported in exposure to flax, hemp, and jute.

Although cotton dust–related disease was first described in the seventeenth century, it is only in the last 40 years that the disease has been recognized as a worldwide problem in the textile industry. Exposure occurs throughout the manufacturing process but is most pronounced in those portions of the factory involved with the treatment of the cotton prior to spinning—i.e., blowing, mixing, and carding (straightening of fibers). Cases reported from spinning rooms are believed to be due to secondary contamination from carding rooms. Recent attempts to control dust levels by use of exhaust hoods, general increases in ventilation, and wetting procedures in some settings have been highly successful. However, respiratory protective equipment appears to be required during certain operations to prevent workers from being exposed to levels of dust that exceed the current U.S. cotton dust standard.

Byssinosis is characterized clinically as occasional (early stage) and then regular (late stage) chest tightness toward the end of the first day of the workweek (Monday chest tightness). In epidemiologic studies, depending on the level of exposure in the carding room air, up to 80 percent of employees may show a significant drop in their FEV$_1$ over the course of a Monday shift.

Initially the symptoms do not recur on subsequent days of the week. However, in 10 to 25 percent of workers the disease may be progressive, with chest tightness recurring or persisting throughout the workweek. After more than 10 years of exposure, workers with recurrent symptoms are more likely to have an obstructive pattern on pulmonary function testing. These higher grades of impairment are seen in workers exposed both to high levels of dust and for greater durations. There is an additive effect of cotton dust exposure plus cigarette smoking. The highest grades of impairment are generally seen in smokers.

Treatment in the early stages of the disease is directed toward reversing the bronchospasm with bronchodilators; however, the chest tightness appears at least in part to relate to histamine release, and antihistamines have been shown to lessen the anticipated fall in FEV$_1$ the first day of the week. Clearly, reduction of dust exposure is of primary importance. All workers with persistent symptoms or significantly reduced levels of pulmonary function should be moved to areas of lower risk of exposure. Regular surveillance of pulmonary function in the industry has made it easier to identify affected persons. Persons with reduced pulmonary function, a personal history of respiratory allergy, and positive history of continued cigarette smoking should be considered at increased risk of developing byssinosis in association with working in the cotton industry.

Grain dust Although the exact number of workers at risk in the United States is not known, at least 500,000 people work in grain elevators, and over 2 million farmers are potentially exposed. The presentation of disease in grain elevator employees or workers in flour or feed mills is virtually identical to the characteristic finding in cigarette smokers, i.e., persistent cough, mucus hypersecretion, wheeze and dyspnea on exertion, and reduced FEV$_1$ and FEV$_1$/FVC ratio (Chap. 214).

Dust concentrations in grain elevators vary greatly but appear to be in excess of 10,000 μg/m^3, with approximately one-third of the particles by weight being in the respirable range. The effect of grain dust exposure is additive to that of cigarette smoking, with approximately 50 percent of workers who smoke having symptoms. Among nonsmoking grain elevator operators, approximately one-quarter have mucus hypersecretion, about five times the number that would be expected in unexposed nonsmokers. However, evidence of obstruction on pulmonary function studies is observed only in workers who smoke. It is not clear if this results from an enhancement of cigarette smoking effect in exposed workers or if smokers are more susceptible to the effects of grain dust.

Farmer's lung This condition results from exposure to moldy hay containing spores of thermophilic actinomycetes that produce a hypersensitivity pneumonitis (Chap. 218). There are few good population-based estimates of the frequency of occurrence of this condition in the United States. However, among farmers in Great Britain, the rate of disease ranges from approximately 10 to 50 per 1000. The prevalence of disease varies in association with rainfall, which determines the amount of fungal growth, and with differences in agricultural practices related to turning and stacking hay.

The patient with acute farmer's lung presents 4 to 8 h after exposure with fever, chills, malaise, cough, and dyspnea without wheezing. The history of exposure is obviously essential to separate this disease from similar symptoms that might occur in influenza or pneumonia. In the chronic form of the disease, the history of repeated attacks after similar exposure is important to separate this syndrome from other causes of patchy fibrosis, e.g., sarcoidosis.

A wide variety of other organic dusts are associated with the occurrence of hypersensitivity pneumonitis (Chap. 218). For those patients who present with hypersensitivity pneumonitis, specific and careful inquiry about occupations, hobbies, or other home environmental exposures will, in most cases, reveal the source of the etiologic agent.

ASSESSMENT OF DISABILITY Significant reduction of dust levels in coal mines has resulted from federal legislation, enacted in the United States in 1969, which requires that respirable dust levels in underground mines be reduced to less than 2000 μg/m^3. This same legislation authorized payment to coal miners (or their survivors) totally disabled by CWP. The criteria for disability from CWP remain unclear and arbitrary. Much of the difficulty relates to the inability to determine in an individual with simple CWP what proportion of an observed respiratory impairment is related to coal dust and what proportion is due to cigarette smoking. The laws as currently interpreted suggest that to be eligible for payment of a claim, one need only show that an underlying condition (i.e., chronic bronchitis with obstruction, presumably due to cigarette smoking) is aggravated by CWP. Thus it becomes critical that physicians involved in occupational lung disease claim cases be aware of detailed exposure histories of their patients, in terms of both occupational exposures and other environmental exposures (cigarette smoking). In addition, these physicians must understand that the extent to which the level of physiologic impairment incapacitates an individual may not be the sole criterion for determining disability. To assess disability properly may require input not only from physicians but also from experts in ergonomics and vocational rehabilitation, lawyers, and employer and employee representatives.

TOXIC CHEMICALS Exposure to toxic chemicals affecting the lung generally occurs in the form of gases and vapors. A common accident is one in which the victim is trapped in a confined space where the chemicals have accumulated to toxic levels. In addition to the specific toxic effects of the chemical, the victim will often sustain considerable anoxia, which can play a dominant role in determining whether the individual survives.

Table 219-2 lists a variety of toxic agents which can produce acute and sometimes life-threatening reactions in the lung. All these agents in sufficient concentrations have been demonstrated, at least in animal studies, to affect the lower airways and disrupt alveolar architecture, either acutely or as a result of chronic exposure. Some of these agents may be generated acutely in the environment. For example, when plastics burn, a number of compounds, including hydrogen cyanide and hydrochloric acid, may be formed and released. The effects and

treatment of exposure to these toxic gases are discussed elsewhere (Chap. 395).

Firefighters and fire victims are at risk of *smoke inhalation*, a numerically important cause of acute cardiorespiratory failure. Smoke inhalation kills more fire victims than does thermal injury. Carbon monoxide poisoning with resulting significant hypoxemia can be life-threatening (Chap. 395). Firefighters may inappropriately use the "blackness" of the smoke to indicate the degree to which incomplete combustion and, thus, elevation of carbon monoxide levels are present. The use of synthetic materials (plastic, polyurethanes), which, when burned, may release a variety of other toxic agents, must be considered when evaluating smoke inhalation victims. Exposed victims may suffer some degree of lower respiratory tract inflammation, similar to that seen with exposure to other irritant gases, e.g., chlorine. Severe cases may develop pulmonary edema.

Firefighters and victims also may be exposed to large quantities of particulate smoke. Significant long-term effects are not clearly associated with this particulate exposure except as related to the production of irritating effects on the upper airways. Studies attempting to demonstrate either an increased risk of cardiovascular events, presumably from recurrent exposure to carbon monoxide, or excess incidence of chronic respiratory disease from repeated smoke inhalation are inconclusive, partly because of the difficulties in measuring exposure. Recent studies suggest increased airways responsiveness in firefighters with repeated episodes of smoke inhalation.

Some agents used in the manufacture of synthetic materials such as plastics, polyurethanes, and other polymers have resulted in some workers being sensitized to extremely low levels of *isocyanates, aromatic amines*, or *aldehydes*. Repeated exposure to these agents causes some workers to develop chronic cough and sputum production, asthma, or episodes of low-grade fever and malaise. Occasionally, as in byssinosis, these symptoms occur early in the workweek but usually recur without workweek periodicity. In the case of exposure to diisocyanate in the production of polyurethane, chronic and persistent asthma in selected individuals appears to result from exposure to concentrations well below the recognized industrial standard. Methods to identify susceptible individuals are needed. At present, challenge testing is being used to determine if a given patient is sensitive. These challenges can be carried out in special environmental chambers where the physician can simulate the work exposure. Alternatively, nonspecific challenges with either pharmacologic agents, such as methacholine and histamine, or isocapneic cold air breathing are being used to identify patients with hyperreactive airways. The usefulness of this nonspecific approach as a method to screen potential sensitive workers has yet to be established.

An unusual route of exposure occurs in *polymer fume fever*. Polymers, notably fluorocarbons, which at normal temperatures produce no reaction, may be transmitted from a worker's hands to his or her cigarettes. Upon burning the cigarette, the polymer is volatilized, and the inhaled agent causes a characteristic syndrome of fever, chills, malaise, and occasionally mild wheezing. The same condition occurs in workers exposed to heated polymers without cigarette use. The syndrome is obviously controlled by proper attention to hygiene in the workplace. A similar self-limited, influenza-like syndrome—*metal fume fever*—results from acute exposure to fumes or smoke of zinc, copper, magnesium, and other volatilized metals. The syndrome may begin several hours after work and resolves within 24 h, only to return on repeated exposure. A proper occupational history should make the diagnosis evident.

ENVIRONMENTAL RESPIRATORY CARCINOGENS Historically, it has been the astute clinician who has recognized a higher incidence of malignant tumors associated with certain environmental exposures. When these observations are linked to an occupational setting, they must be pursued by epidemiologic studies of relatively large groups of both current and former workers. Often the concentration and/or exact nature of the substances contained in the putative exposures cannot be determined. Rarely, the possibility that a substance can play an etiologic role in cancer is supported by observing

TABLE 219-2 Selected common toxic chemical agents

Agents	Selected exposures	Acute effects from high or accidental exposure	Chronic effects from relatively low exposure
Acid fumes; H_2SO_4, HNO_3	Manufacture of fertilizers, chlorinated organic compounds, dyes, explosives, rubber products, metal etching, plastics	Mucous membrane irritation, followed by chemical pneumonitis 2–3 days	No data
Ammonia	Refrigeration, petroleum refining, manufacture of fertilizers, explosives, plastics, and other chemicals	Same as for acid fumes	Chronic bronchitis
Cyanides	Electroplating, extraction of gold or silver, manufacture of mirrors, fumigants, photo supplies	Increase in respiratory rate followed by respiratory arrest, lactic acidosis, pulmonary edema, death	No data
Diazomethane	Methylating agent for acid compounds; laboratory workers	Violent coughing, dyspnea, wheezing, pulmonary edema	No data
Formaldehyde	Manufacture of resins, leathers, rubber, metals, and woods; laboratory workers, embalmers; emission from urethane foam insulation	Same as for acid fumes	Cancers in one species of animals; no data on humans
Halides (Cl, Br, F)	Bleaching in pulp, paper, textile industry; manufacture of chemical compounds; synthetic rubber, plastics, disinfectant, rocket fuel, gasoline	Mucous membrane irritation, pulmonary edema; possible reduced FVC 1–2 yrs after exposure	Dryness of mucous membrane, epistaxis, dental fluorosis, tracheobronchitis
Hydrogen sulfide	By-product of many industrial processes, oil, other petroleum processes and storage	Low exposure: conjunctival irritation; higher: respiratory paralysis similar to cyanides	Chronic bronchitis, recurrent pneumonitis
Isocyanates (TDI, HDI, MDI)	Production of polyurethane foams, plastics, adhesives, surface coatings	Mucous membrane irritation, dyspnea, cough, wheeze, pulmonary edema	Upper respiratory tract irritation, cough, asthma, allergic alveolitis
Nitrogen dioxide	Silage, metal etching, explosives, rocket fuels, welding, by-product of burning fossil fuels	Cough, dyspnea, pulmonary edema may be delayed 4–12 h; possible result from acute exposure: bronchiolitis obliterans in 2–6 wks	Emphysema in animals, ?chronic bronchitis
Ozone	Arc welding, flour bleaching, deodorizing, emissions from copying equipment, photochemical air pollutant	Mucous membrane irritant, pulmonary hemorrhage and edema, reduced pulmonary function transiently in children and adults exposed to summer haze	Chronic eye irritation
Phosgene	Organic compound, metallurgy, volatization of chlorine-containing compounds	Delayed onset of bronchiolitis and pulmonary edema	Chronic bronchitis
Phthalic anhydride	Manufacture of resin esters, polyester resins, thermoactivated adhesives	Nasal irritation, cough	Asthma, chronic bronchitis
Sulfur dioxide	Manufacture of sulfuric acid, bleaches, coating of nonferrous metals, food processing, refrigerant, burning of fossil fuels, wood pulp industry	Mucous membrane irritant, epistaxis	?Chronic bronchitis

that a few cases of a very rare tumor in a particular group represent "an epidemic." Examples of this are nasal sinus and lung cancer in nickel workers, angiosarcomas of the liver in vinyl chloride workers, and adenocarcinomas of the nose in woodworkers.

Only in those few cases in which animal studies have been carried out can one confirm that a given suspected agent is really a carcinogen. For example, bis(chloromethyl) ether (BCME) has been shown to produce tumors in animals and oat cell cancer of the lung in humans. In this particular case, BCME, used as a chemical intermediary in the manufacture of a number of organic compounds, was known to produce tumors in animals almost before the substance was introduced into industry. (This case is one of the prime examples of why federal legislation was enacted in the United States in the 1970s to control the release of toxic substances, particularly new chemicals.)

In addition to the asbestos trades, other occupational exposures associated with either proven or suspected respiratory carcinogens include acrylonitrile, arsenic compounds, beryllium (animal studies only), BCME, chromium, coke ovens (exposure to polycyclic hydrocarbons), iron oxide, isopropyl oil (nasal sinuses), mustard gas, the various ores used to produce pure nickel, talc (possible asbestos

contamination in both mining and milling), vinyl chloride, welding, wood used in woodworking (nasal cancer only), and uranium. The occurrence of excess cancers in uranium miners raises the possibility that there exists a large number of workers at risk by virtue of exposure to similar radiation hazards. This includes not only workers involved in processing uranium, up to and including its use in nuclear power plants and in military nuclear hardware, but also workers exposed in underground mining operations where radon daughters may be emitted from rock formations. In the latter case, the levels of exposure are generally considered to be relatively low; however, specific consideration must be given to the possibility of excess exposure for any hard rock miner.

GENERAL ENVIRONMENTAL EXPOSURES

AIR POLLUTION Dramatic and disastrous episodes of air pollution inversion have been documented in many industrialized centers in the world. Each of these episodes has been associated with excess acute mortality in the very old, the very young, and those with chronic cardiopulmonary diseases. The most dramatic event was the London fog of 1952, in which approximately 4000 excess deaths occurred over a 2-week period following 5 days of severe cold and dense fog. Similar episodes in the United States, although less dramatic in terms of total deaths, occurred in Donora, Pennsylvania, in 1948, and in New York City in the 1960s. In these episodes, generally associated with cold temperature and air stagnation, patients with underlying cardiopulmonary disease were most severely affected.

In addition to significant excess mortality during these episodes, a large number of people required medical care for cardiorespiratory complaints. Subsequent follow-up studies failed to implicate these episodic disasters in the etiology of chronic respiratory disease in adults. On the other hand, many epidemiologic studies of both international and regional differences in the prevalences of chronic respiratory disease suggest that long-term exposures in polluted areas in the early to middle part of the twentieth century were associated with excess chronic respiratory disease.

In 1970, the U.S. government established air quality standards for several pollutants believed to be responsible for excess cardiorespiratory diseases. Primary standards regulated by the Environmental Protection Agency (EPA) designed to protect the public health with an adequate margin of safety exist for sulfur dioxide, particulates <10 μm in size, nitrogen dioxide, ozone, lead, and carbon monoxide. These standards were updated in 1990 based on additional health effects data. The standards vary in their averaging times and levels, in part related to the differences in the known physiologic responses and epidemiologic evidence for each pollutant.

Pollutants are generated from both stationary sources (power plants and industrial complexes) and mobile sources (automobiles), and none of the pollutants occur in isolation. Thus, except for the change in carboxyhemoglobin from carbon monoxide exposure, it becomes extremely difficult to relate any specific health effect to any single pollutant. Furthermore, pollutants may be changed by chemical reactions after being emitted. For example, reducing agents, such as sulfur dioxide and particulate matter from a power plant stack, may react in air to produce acid sulfates and aerosols, the precursors of acid rain, which can be transported long distances in the atmosphere. Oxidizing substances, such as oxides of nitrogen and oxidants from automobile exhaust, may react with sunlight to produce ozone. Although originally a problem confined to the southwestern part of the United States, in recent years, at least during the summertime, elevated ozone and acid aerosol levels can occur throughout the United States. Both acute and chronic effects of these exposures are currently under investigation.

The symptoms and diseases associated with air pollution are the same as the nononcogenic conditions commonly associated with cigarette smoking. In addition, respiratory illness in early childhood has been associated with chronic exposure to only modestly elevated levels of SO$_2$ and respirable particles. It is not known whether persistent chronic exposure to a relatively constant level of pollutant(s) and recurrent short-term peak exposures which average to the same mean level have different effects. One can only advise the individual with significant cardiopulmonary impairment to stay indoors during periods when pollution exceeds current standards.

INDOOR EXPOSURE Because of increased concern about energy costs, efforts to become energy efficient have led to reduced air exchange rates in indoor environments. The effects of these efforts have been to increase exposures to a variety of air contaminants heretofore not considered important.

Until relatively recently, little attention was given to the effects of *passive cigarette smoking.* Several studies have shown that the respirable particulate load in any household is directly proportional to the number of cigarette smokers living in the home. Increases in prevalence of respiratory illnesses and reduced levels of pulmonary function measured with simple spirometry have been found in children of smoking parents in a number of studies. Although a modest increase in the risk of lung cancer is found in the aggregate of studies,

the long-term consequences in terms of nononcogenic respiratory diseases are unknown.

A novel source of indoor exposure to *formaldehyde* results from the curing process involved in the placement of urea-formaldehyde insulating foam or in several wood products used in modern furniture and the construction of mobile homes. Natural "degassing" of formaldehyde occurs during the first few months after the foam has been blown into the walls, with concentrations of formaldehyde as high as 5 ppm rapidly dropping off to less than 0.1 ppm. Chronic exposure to low levels of urea-formaldehyde (generally less than 1 ppm) may result if the foam is improperly installed. Patients apparently sensitive to concentrations of formaldehyde generally well below 1 ppm will complain of upper airway irritation with occasional epistaxis and sore throats. Lower respiratory complaints, such as chest pain and wheeze, however, are uncommon, and often the most disturbing complaints are mild memory and mood disorders. Formaldehyde is a proven animal carcinogen. Whether it causes cancer in humans is not established.

Radon gas is believed to be a risk factor for lung cancer. The main radon product (radon 222) is a gas that results from the decay series of uranium 238, with the immediate precursor being radium 226. The amount of radium in earth materials determines how much radon gas will be emitted. Outdoors, the concentrations are trivial. Indoors, levels are dependent on the ventilation rate and the size of space into which the gas is emitted. Levels associated with excess lung cancer risk may be present in as many as 10 percent of the houses in the United States. Where smoking exists in the household, the problem is potentially greater, since the molecular size of radon particles allows them to readily attach to smoke particles that are inhaled. Fortunately, technology is available for assessing and reducing the level of exposure.

PORTAL OF ENTRY The lung is a primary source of entry into the body for a number of toxic agents that affect other organ systems. For example, the lung is a route of entry for benzene (bone marrow), carbon disulfide (cardiovascular and nervous systems), cadmium (kidney), and metallic mercury (kidney, central nervous system). Thus, in any disease state of obscure origin, it is important to consider possible inhaled environmental agents. Such consideration can sometimes furnish the clue needed to identify a specific external cause for a disorder that might otherwise be labeled "idiopathic."

REFERENCES

BALAAN MR et al: Clinical aspects of coal workers' penumononiosis and silicosis. Occup Med 8:19, 1993

BECKLAKE MR et al: The relationship between acute and chronic airway responses to occupational exposures. Curr Pulmonol 9:25, 1988

BERRY G: Prediction of mesothelioma, lung cancer, and asbestosis in former Wittenoom asbestos workers. Br J Ind Med 48:793-802, 1991

COCHRANE AL, MOORE FA: A 20-year follow-up of men aged 55–64 including coal miners and foundry workers in Stavley. Br J Ind Med 37:226, 1980

Guidelines for the Use of International Labour Office Classification of Radiographs of Pneumoconiosis. Occupational Safety and Health Sciences 22 (Revised 1980). Geneva, ILO, 1980

LAPP NL, CASTRANOVA V: How silicosis and coal workers' pneumoconioses develop— a cellular assessment. Occup Med 8:35, 1993

LARUNERYS RR: Occupational toxicology, in *Casarett and Doull's Toxicology, The Basic Science of Poison,* 3d ed, CD Kloassen, MD Amden, J Doull (eds). New York, MacMillan, 1986, chap 29

LEONARD JF, TEMPLETON PA: Pulmonary imaging techniques in the diagnosis of occupational interstitial lung disease, in *Occupational Medicine: State of the Art Reviews,* vol 7, no 2, WS Beckett, R Bascon (eds). Philadelphia, Hanley and Belfus, 1992, pp 241–260

MULLOY KB et al: Use of chest radiographs in epidemiological investigations of pneumoconioses. Br J Ind Med 50:273, 1993

PARKES WR: *Occupational Lung Disorders,* 2d ed. London, Butterworth, 1982

RAFFLE PAB: Occupational cancer and occupational asthma, in *Hunter's Diseases of Occupations,* PAB Raffle et al (eds). Boston, Little, Brown, 1987, chaps 24 and 25

ROGGLI VL et al: Asbestos fiber type in malignant mesothelioma: An analytical scanning electron microscopic study of 94 cases. Am J Ind Med 23:605, 1993

SAMET JM, SPENGLER JD: *Indoor Air Pollution: A Health Perspective,* Baltimore, Johns Hopkins, 1991, chaps 2 and 15

SHERSON D, LANDER F: Morbidity of pulmonary tuberculosis among silicotic and nonsolicotic foundry workers in Denmark. J Occup Med 32:110-113, 1990

220   PNEUMONIA, INCLUDING NECROTIZING PULMONARY INFECTIONS (LUNG ABSCESS)

MATTHEW E. LEVISON

Pneumonia is an infection of the pulmonary parenchyma. Various bacterial species, mycoplasmas, chlamydiae, rickettsiae, viruses, fungi, and parasites can cause pneumonia. Thus pneumonia is not a single disease, but a group of specific infections, each with a different epidemiology, pathogenesis, clinical presentation, and clinical course. Identification of the etiologic microorganism is of primary importance, since this is the key to appropriate antimicrobial therapy. However, because of the serious nature of the infection, patients generally need to be started on antimicrobial therapy immediately, often before laboratory confirmation of the causative agent. The specific microbial etiology remains elusive in about a third of patients, e.g., when no sputum is available for examination, the blood cultures are sterile, and there is no pleural fluid. Serologic confirmation, of necessity, requires weeks for formation of specific antibody.

The initial choice of antimicrobial therapy is often empirical, based on the setting in which the infection was acquired, the clinical presentation, patterns of abnormality on chest radiography, stains of sputum or other infected body fluids, and knowledge of current patterns of susceptibility to antimicrobial agents. After the etiologic agent is identified, specific antimicrobial therapy can be chosen.

DEFENSE MECHANISMS   The lung is a complex structure composed of aggregates of units that are formed by the progressive branching of the airways. Approximately 80 percent of the cells lining the central airways are ciliated, pseudostratified, columnar epithelial cells, with the percentage decreasing in peripheral airways. Each ciliated cell contains about 200 cilia that beat in coordinated waves about 1000 times per minute, with a fast forward stroke and a slower backward recovery. Ciliary motion is also coordinated between adjacent cells so that each wave is propagated toward the oropharynx. The cilia are covered by a liquid film, about 5 to 10 μm thick, that is composed of two layers. The outer, or gel, layer is viscous and traps deposited particles. The cilia beat in the less viscous inner, or sol, layer. During the forward stroke, the tips of the cilia just touch the viscous gel and propel it toward the oropharynx. During recovery, the cilia move entirely within the low-resistance sol layer. Ciliated cells are interspersed with mucus-secreting cells in the trachea and bronchi, but not in the bronchioles.

The alveolar walls, from blood to air, consist of the capillary endothelium that lines the network of anastomotic capillaries, the capillary basement membrane, the interstitial tissue, the alveolar basement membrane, the alveolar lining epithelial cells (which are either flattened type I pneumocytes that cover 95 percent of the alveolar surface or rounded, granular surfactant-producing type II pneumocytes), and epithelial lining fluid. The epithelial lining fluid contains surfactant, fibronectin, and immunoglobulin, which may opsonize or, in the presence of complement, lyse microbial pathogens that are deposited on the alveolar surface. Loosely attached to the lining cells or lying free within the lumen are the alveolar macrophages, lymphocytes, and a small number of polymorphonuclear leukocytes.

The normal lower respiratory tract is sterile, despite being adjacent to enormous numbers of microorganisms that reside in the oropharynx and being exposed to environmental microorganisms in the inhaled air. Sterility of the lower respiratory tract is the result of efficient filtering and clearance mechanisms.

Infectious particles deposited on the squamous epithelium of distal nasal surfaces normally are removed by sneezing, while those deposited on the more proximal ciliated surfaces are swept posteriorly in the mucus lining into the nasopharynx, where they are swallowed or expectorated. Reflex closure of the glottis and cough protect the lower respiratory tract. Those particles deposited on the tracheobronchial surface are swept by ciliary motion toward the oropharynx. Infectious particles that bypass defenses in the airways and are deposited on the alveolar surface are cleared by phagocytic cells and humoral factors. Alveolar macrophages are the major phagocytes in the lower respiratory tract. Some phagocytosed microorganisms are killed by the phagocyte's oxygen-dependent systems, lysosomal enzymes, and cationic proteins. Other microorganisms can evade microbicidal mechanisms and persist within the macrophage. For example, *Mycobacterium tuberculosis* persists within the lysosome, while *Legionella* resides within intracellular inclusions that fail to fuse with lysosomes. Intracellular pathogens can then be transported to the ciliated surfaces and into the oropharynx or via the lymphatics to regional lymph nodes. The alveolar macrophages process and present microbial antigens to the lymphocyte and also secrete cytokines (e.g., tumor necrosis factor and interleukin 1) that modulate the immune process in T and B lymphocytes. Cytokines facilitate the generation of an inflammatory response, activate alveolar macrophages, and recruit additional phagocytes and other immunologic factors from plasma. The inflammatory exudate is responsible for many of the local signs of pulmonary consolidation and systemic manifestations of pneumonia, such as fever, chills, myalgias, and malaise.

TRAMSMISSION   Microbial pathogens may enter the lung by one of several routes.

Aspiration of organisms that colonize the oropharynx   Most pulmonary pathogens originate in the oropharyngeal flora. Aspiration of these pathogens is the most common mechanism for production of pneumonia. Normal individuals transiently carry in the nasopharynx at various times during the year common pulmonary pathogens, including *Streptococcus pneumoniae*, *S. pyogenes*, *M. pneumoniae*, *Haemophilus influenzae*, and *Moraxella catarrhalis*. The sources of anaerobic pulmonary pathogens, such as *Porphyromonas gingivalis*, *Prevotella melaninogenica*, *Fusobacterium nucleatum*, *Actinomyces* spp., spirochetes, and anaerobic streptococci, are the gingival crevice and dental plaque, which contain more than 10^{11} colony-forming units (CFU) of microorganisms per gram. The frequency of aerobic gram-negative bacillary colonization of the oropharyngeal mucosa, which is unusual in normal patients (<2 percent), increases with hospitalization, worsening debility, severity of underlying illness, alcoholism, diabetes, and advanced age and may be a consequence of increased salivary proteolytic activity, which destroys fibronectin, a glycoprotein coating the surface of the mucosa. Fibronectin is the receptor for the normal gram-positive flora of the oropharynx. Loss of fibronectin exposes the receptors on the epithelial cell surface for aerobic gram-negative bacilli. The source of aerobic gram-negative bacilli may be either the patient's own stomach, which can become colonized with these organisms as a consequence of an increase in gastric pH with atrophic gastritis or following use of H-2 blocking agents or antacids, contaminated respiratory equipment, hands of health care workers, or contaminated food and water. Nasogastric tubes can facilitate transfer of gastric bacteria to the pharynx.

About 50 percent of normal adults aspirate oropharyngeal secretions into the lower respiratory tract during sleep. Aspiration occurs more frequently and may be more severe in individuals with an impaired level of consciousness (e.g., alcoholics, drug abusers, patients following seizures, strokes, or general anesthesia), neurologic dysfunction of the oropharynx, and swallowing disorders or mechanical impediments (e.g., nasogastric or endotracheal tubes). Pneumonia is a more likely outcome if the aspirated material is large in volume or contains virulent microbial flora or foreign bodies, such as aspirated food or necrotic tissue. The presence of an impaired cough reflex or mucociliary or alveolar macrophage dysfunction increases the risk of pneumonia.

Inhalation of infectious aerosols   Deposition of inhaled particles within the respiratory tract is primarily determined by particle size. Particles over 10 μm are deposited largely in the nose and upper airways. Particles less than 3 to 5 μm in diameter, also called *airborne* *droplet nuclei*, that contain one or perhaps two microorganisms fail to settle out by gravity and remain suspended in the atmosphere for long periods unless removed by ventilation or by filtration in the lungs of an individual breathing the contaminated air. These infectious aerosols are small enough to bypass host defenses in the upper respiratory tract and airways. More particles are deposited in small bronchioles and alveoli as particle size decreases below 5 μm. One inhaled particle of appropriate size may be sufficient to reach the alveolus and initiate infection. Examples of pneumonia typically acquired by inhalation of infectious aerosols include tuberculosis, influenza, legionellosis, psittacosis, histoplasmosis, and Q fever.

Hematogenous dissemination from an extrapulmonary site of infection   Hematogenous dissemination to the lung, usually with *Staphylococcus aureus*, occurs in patients, such as intravenous drug abusers, who have either right- or left-sided bacterial endocarditis or in patients with intravenous catheter infections. *Fusobacterium* infections of the retropharyngeal tissues (Lemierre's syndrome, i.e., retropharyngeal abscess and jugular venous thrombophlebitis) also disseminate to the lungs.

Two additional routes for transmission of bacteria to the lungs are direct inoculation as a result of either tracheal intubation or stab wounds of the chest and contiguous spread from an adjacent site of infection.

PATHOLOGY   The pneumonic process may involve primarily the interstitium or the alveoli. Involvement of an entire lobe is called *lobar pneumonia*. When the process is restricted to alveoli contiguous to bronchi, it is called *bronchopneumonia*. Confluent bronchopneumonia may be indistinguishable from lobar pneumonia. The classification of pneumonias is best based on the causative microorganism whenever possible rather than on these anatomic characteristics, as was formerly done.

EPIDEMIOLOGY   The patient's living circumstances, occupation, travel history, pet or animal exposure, disease in the patient's contacts, and knowledge of the epidemic curve of community outbreaks are useful clues to the microbial etiology of the infection (Table 220-1).

The relative frequency of various pulmonary pathogens varies with the setting in which the infection was acquired, e.g., community, nursing home, or hospital. In patients hospitalized with community-acquired pneumonia, the most frequent pathogens are *S. pneumoniae*, *H. influenzae*, *Chlamydia pneumoniae*, and *L. pneumophila*. *M. pneumoniae*, which usually causes mild illness, is common among nonhospitalized patients with community-acquired pneumonia. In contrast, enteric gram-negative bacilli and *Pseudomonas aeruginosa*, uncommon causes of community-acquired pneumonia, are estimated to account for over 50 percent and *S. aureus* over 10 percent of hospital-acquired pneumonia. The relative frequencies of pathogens in pneumonia acquired in nursing homes fall somewhere in between those of community- and hospital-acquired pneumonias, with enteric gram-negative bacilli and *P. aeruginosa* being more common among nursing home residents than among patients who acquire pneumonia in noninstitutional settings.

TABLE 220-1   Microbial pathogens that cause pneumonia

Community-acquired	Hospital-acquired
Mycoplasma pneumoniae	Enteric gram-negative bacilli
Streptococcus pneumoniae	*Pseudomonas aeruginosa*
Haemophilus influenzae	*Staphylococcus aureus*
Chlamydia pneumoniae	Oral anerobes
Legionella pneumophila	
Oral anaerobes	
Moraxella catarrhalis	
Pneumocystis carinii	
Nocardia spp.	
Influenza virus, cytomegalovirus, respiratory syncytial virus, measles virus, herpes zoster virus	
Histoplasma, Coccidioides, Blastomyces	

Oral anaerobes, frequently in combination with aerobic bacterial flora, such as viridans streptococci, are causes of community-acquired pneumonia and anaerobic lung abscess in patients who are prone to aspiration. Edentulous persons, who have lower numbers of oral anaerobes, are less likely to develop pneumonia due to anaerobes. When the etiology of the pneumonia has been studied in unselected patients hospitalized with community-acquired pneumonia by methods that use strict anaerobic bacteriology and that avoid contamination of lower respiratory tract secretions by oral flora, anaerobic bacteria have been found to account for as many as 20 to 30 percent of cases. In hospital-acquired pneumonia, anaerobes are the pathogens, with or without aerobic copathogens, in about a third of patients. However, in the case of hospital-acquired pneumonia, the aerobic copathogens are frequently virulent microorganisms in their own right, such as enteric gram-negative bacilli, *P. aeruginosa*, and *S. aureus*.

Age is another important predictor of the infecting agent in pneumonia—*Chlamydia trachomatis* and respiratory syncytial virus being common in infants under 6 months of age, *H. influenzae* in those between 6 months and 5 years, *M. pneumoniae* and *C. pneumoniae* in young adults, and *H. influenzae, L. pneumophila*, and *M. catarrhalis* in the elderly with chronic lung disease.

The season of the year and geographic location are other predictors. The frequency of influenza as a cause of both community-acquired and institutionally acquired pneumonia increases in the winter months. Influenza causes an increase in frequency of secondary bacterial pneumonias due to *S. pneumoniae, S. aureus*, and *H. influenzae*. Influenza outbreaks in a community tend to be explosive and widespread, with many secondary cases of influenza as a result of the short incubation period of several days and high communicability. Legionellosis also occurs in explosive outbreaks if large numbers of susceptible people are exposed to an infectious aerosol; however, no secondary cases occur, as a result of low communicability. *Mycoplasma* can cause outbreaks, usually in relatively closed populations, such as military bases, colleges, or households, but because of the long incubation period of 2 to 3 weeks and relatively low communicability, *Mycoplasma* infection moves through the community slowly, affecting another person as the first is recovering. In communities where human immunodeficiency virus type 1 (HIV-1) infection is endemic, *Pneumocystic carinii* and *M. tuberculosis* assume a more prominent role as causes of community-acquired pneumonia. Histoplasmosis, blastomycosis, and coccidioidomysis have specific geographic distributions, and *C. psittaci* produces illness in bird handlers.

CLINICAL MANIFESTATIONS   Community-acquired pneumonias   Traditionally these have been thought to present as two different syndromes, the typical and atypical presentations. Although recent data suggest that these two syndromes may be less distinct than was once thought, the characteristics of the clinical presentation may, nevertheless, have some diagnostic value.

The "typical" pneumonia syndrome is characterized by sudden onset of fever, cough productive of purulent sputum, and possibly pleuritic chest pain; signs of pulmonary consolidation (dullness, increased fremitus, egophony, bronchial breath sounds, and rales) may be found on physical examination in areas of radiographic abnormality. The typical pneumonia syndrome is usually caused by the most common bacterial pathogen of community-acquired pneumonia, *S. pneumoniae*, as well as other bacterial pathogens, such as *H. influenzae* and mixed oral anaerobes and aerobes.

The "atypical" pneumonia syndrome is characterized by a more gradual onset, dry cough, prominence of extrapulmonary symptoms (such as headache, myalgias, fatigue, sore throat, nausea, vomiting, and diarrhea), and abnormalities on chest radiographs despite minimal signs of pulmonary involvement on physical examination, other than rales. Atypical pneumonia is classically produced by *M. pneumoniae* but also can be caused by *L. pneumophila, C. pneumoniae*, oral anaerobes, and *P. carinii*, as well as *S. pneumoniae* and the less frequently encountered pathogens *C. psittaci, Coxiella burnetii, Francisella tularensis, Histoplasma capsulatum*, and *Coccidioides immitis. Mycoplasma* pneumonia (see Chap. 139) may be complicated by erythema multiforme, hemolytic anemia, bullous myringitis, encephalitis, and tranverse myelitis. *Legionella* (see Chap. 113) frequently produces deterioration in mental status, renal and hepatic abnormalities, and marked hyponatremia; the mycoses frequently produce erythema nodosum. In *C. pneumoniae* pneumonia (see Chap. 140), sore throat, hoarseness, and wheezing are relatively common. The atypical pneumonia syndrome in a patient with a history of behaviors that place them at risk of HIV infection suggests *Pneumocystis* infection. These patients may have concurrent infection with other opportunistic pathogens, such as oral thrush due to *Candida albicans* or extensive perineal ulcers due to herpes simplex virus.

Certain viruses also produce pneumonia that is usually characterized by an atypical presentation, i.e., chills, fever, dry, nonproductive cough, and predominance of extrapulmonary symptoms. Primary viral pneumonia can be caused by influenza, usually as part of a community outbreak in winter; respiratory syncytial virus infection in children or immunosuppressed individuals; measles and varicella, accompanied by their characteristic rashes; and cytomegalovirus infection in patients immunocompromised by HIV infection or therapy given for organ transplantation. Influenza, measles, and varicella can in addition predispose to secondary bacterial pneumonia as a result of destruction of the mucociliary barrier of the airways. Secondary bacterial infection may either follow the viral infection without interruption or be separated by several days of transient symptomatic relief. Bacterial infection may be heralded by sudden worsening of the patient's clinical course, with persisting or renewed chills, fever, and cough productive of purulent sputum, possibly accompanied by pleuritic chest pain.

The patient's underlying disease may be characterized by specific immunologic or inflammatory defects that predispose to pneumonia due to specific pathogens. For example, patients who have severe hypogammaglobulinemia (<200 mg/dL) are at risk of infection with encapsulated bacteria, such as *S. pneumoniae* and *H. influenzae.* HIV-infected patients also may have ineffective antibody formation, which predisposes to infection with these encapsulated bacteria. Severe neutropenia (<500 neutrophils per microliter) increases risks for infection due to *P. aeruginosa,* Enterobacteriaceae, *S. aureus,* and, if neutropenia is prolonged, *Aspergillus.* Those HIV-infected patients with circulating CD4+ lymphocyte counts of less than 500 per microliter are at risk of *M. tuberculosis;* with counts of less than 200 per microliter, *P. carinii, Histoplasma capsulatum,* and *Cryptococcus neoformans;* with counts of less than 50 per microliter, *Mycobacterium avium-intracellulare* and cytomegalovirus. Glucocorticoid therapy increases the risk of tuberculosis and nocardiosis. Nocardiosis (see Chap. 126) is frequently complicated by metastatic lesions to the skin and central nervous system. Signs of pulmonary consolidation, cough, and sputum production may be absent in patients unable to mount an inflammatory response, such as those with agranulocytosis. The major manifestations in these patients may be limited to fever, tachypnea, agitation, and altered mental status. Elderly or severely ill patients may fail to develop fever.

Nosocomial pneumonias Patients with nosocomial pneumonia often present a diagnostic challenge. The usual criteria, which include new or progressive pulmonary infiltrates, purulent tracheobronchial secretions, fever, and leukocytosis, are frequently unreliable in these patients who often have preexisting pulmonary disease, endotracheal tubes that irritate the tracheal mucosa, or multiple other problems likely to produce fever and leukocytosis. Patients with hematogenous *S. aureus* pneumonia may present with only fever and dyspnea. In these patients, the inflammatory response is initially confined to the pulmonary interstitium. Cough, sputum production, and signs of pulmonary consolidation occur only after infection extends into the bronchi. These patients are usually gravely ill, with intravascular infection as well as pneumonia, and may present with signs of endocarditis, e.g., cardiac murmurs, Janeway lesions, Osler nodes, and petechiae.

Anaerobic pneumonia and lung abscess Although aspirated oral anaerobes can initially produce an infiltrative process, ultimately

they produce putrid sputum, tissue necrosis, and pulmonary cavities. The clinical course of an anaerobic, polymicrobial abscess in about three-quarters of patients is indolent and mimics that of a pulmonary tuberculosis, i.e., cough, shortness of breath, chills, fever, night sweats, weight loss, pleuritic chest pain, and blood-streaked sputum for several weeks or more. In other patients the disease may present more acutely. Patients with anaerobic abscesses are usually prone to aspiration of oropharyngeal contents and have periodontal disease. One of the oral anaerobes, *Actinomyces* spp., produces a chronic, fibrotic necrotizing process that crosses tissue planes and may involve the pleural space, ribs, vertebrae, and subcutaneous tissue with eventual discharge of sulfur granules (macroscopic bacterial masses) through the skin (empyema necessitatis).

DIAGNOSIS Radiography Chest radiographs can confirm the presence and location of the pulmonary infiltrate; assess the extent of the pulmonary infection; detect the presence of pleural involvement, pulmonary cavitation, or hilar lymphadenopathy; and gauge response to antimicrobial therapy. However, chest radiographs may be normal in patients who are unable to mount an inflammatory response (e.g., those with agranulocytosis) or early in an infiltrative process (e.g., hematogenous *S. aureus* pneumonia, *Pneumocystis* pneumonia in patients with AIDS).

Anatomic localization of the inflammatory process as visualized in chest radiographs occasionally has diagnostic implications. Most pulmonary pathogens produce focal lesions. Multicentric distribution suggests hematogenous infection, in which case remote infections, such as endocarditis or thrombophlebitis, should be sought. Hematogenous pneumonia, which results from septic embolization in patients with thrombophlebitis or right-sided endocarditis or from bacteremia in patients with left-sided endocarditis, appears on the chest radiograph as multiple areas of pulmonary infiltration that subsequently may cavitate. Diffuse distribution suggests *P. carinii,* cytomegalovirus, measles, or herpes zoster virus, the later two pathogens being diagnosed by the characteristic rash that always accompanies the pneumonia. Pleurisy and hilar nodal enlargement are unusual with *Pneumocystis* and cytomegalovirus pneumonia; their presence suggests another etiology. Diffuse lesions in immunocompromised patients also suggests possible legionellosis, tuberculosis, histoplasmosis, or *Mycoplasma* or disseminated *Strongyloides* infection.

Cavities occur when necrotic material is discharged into communicating airways, which results in either necrotizing pneumonia (multiple small cavities, each <2 cm in diameter in one or more bronchopulmonary segments or lobes) or lung abscess (one or more cavities >2 cm in diameter). Oral anaerobes, *S. aureus, S. pneumoniae* serotype III, aerobic gram-negative bacilli, *M. tuberculosis,* or fungi and certain noninfectious conditions can produce tissue necrosis and cavities (Table 220-2). In contrast, *H. influenzae, M. pneumoniae,* viruses, and most other serotypes of *S. pneumoniae* almost never cause cavities. Apical disease, with or without cavities, suggests reactivation tuberculosis. Anaerobic abscesses are located in dependent, poorly ventilated, and poorly draining bronchopulmonary segments, which characteristically have air-fluid levels, unlike the well-ventilated, well-drained upper lobe cavities caused by *M. tuberculosis,* an obligate aerobe. Air-fluid levels also may be present in cavities

---

TABLE 220-2   Causes of pulmonary cavities

INFECTIOUS

Bacteria: Oral anaerobes (*Bacteroides* spp., fusobacteria, *Actinomyces* spp., anaerobic and microaerophilic cocci), enteric aerobic gram-negative bacilli, *P. aeruginosa, Legionella* spp., *S. aureus,* type III *S. pneumoniae, M. tuberculosis, Nocardia* spp.
Fungi: *Histoplasma capsulatum, Coccidioides immitis Blastomyces* spp.

NONINFECTIOUS

Neoplasms, Wegener's granulomatosis, infarction, infected bullae and cysts

due to other infectious causes of pulmonary necrosis. *Mucor* and *Aspergillus* invade blood vessels and cause pleural-based, wedge-shaped areas of pulmonary infarction; these infarcts may subsequently cavitate.

In the patient with an uncomplicated course, chest radiographs need not be repeated before discharge, since resolution of infiltrates may take up to 6 weeks after initial presentation. However, patients who do not respond clinically, who have a pleural effusion on admission, who are suspected of postobstructive pneumonia, or who are infected with certain pathogens (e.g., *S. aureus,* aerobic gram-negative bacilli, or oral anaerobes) need more intensive surveillance. At times, computed tomography (CT) may be especially helpful to distinguish different processes, e.g., pleural effusion versus underlying pulmonary consolidation, hilar adenopathy versus pulmonary mass, or pulmonary abscess versus empyema with an air-fluid level.

Sputum examination Examination of the sputum remains the mainstay in evaluation of a patient with acute bacterial pneumonia. Unfortunately, expectorated material is frequently contaminated by potentially pathogenic bacteria that colonize the upper respiratory and, at times, the lower respiratory tract without actually causing disease. This contamination reduces the specificity of any lower respiratory tract specimen. In addition, it has been estimated that the usual laboratory processing methods yield the pulmonary pathogen in less than 50 percent of expectorated sputum samples in patients with bacteremic pneumonia. This loss of sensitivity may be due to misinterpretation of the alpha-hemolytic colonies of *S. pneumoniae* as nonpathogenic alpha-hemolytic streptococci ("normal flora"), overgrowth of the cultures by more hardy colonizing organisms, or loss of more fastidious organisms due to slow transport or improper processing. In addition, certain very common pulmonary pathogens, such as anaerobes, *Mycoplasma, Chlamydia, Pneumocystis,* mycobacteria, fungi, and *Legionella,* cannot be cultured by routine methods.

Since expectorated material is routinely contaminated by oral anaerobes, the diagnosis of anaerobic pulmonary infection is frequently putative. Confirmation requires culture of anaerobes from pulmonary secretions that are uncontaminated by oropharyngeal secretions, which in turn requires that pulmonary secretions be obtained by special techniques, such as transtracheal aspiration, transthoracic lung puncture, and protected brush via bronchoscopy. These procedures are invasive and usually are withheld, unless the patient fails to respond to empirical therapy.

Gram's stain of sputum specimens, screened initially under low-power magnification ($10\times$ objective and $10\times$ eyepiece) to determine the degree of contamination with squamous epithelial cells, is of utmost diagnostic importance. In patients with the typical pneumonia syndrome who produce purulent sputum, the sensitivity and specificity of the Gram's stain of sputum minimally contaminated by upper respiratory tract secretions (>25 polymorphonuclear leukocytes and <10 epithelial cells per low power field) in identifying the pathogen as *S. pneumoniae* are 62 and 85 percent, respectively. The Gram's stain in this case is more specific and probably more sensitive than the accompanying sputum culture. The finding of mixed flora on Gram's stain of an uncontaminated sputum specimen suggests an anaerobic infection. Acid-fast stains of sputum should be done when mycobacterial infection is suspected. Examination of Giemsa-stained expectorated respiratory secretions from patients with AIDS has given satisfactory results for the diagnosis of *Pneumocystis* pneumonia when examined by experienced pathologists. The sensitivity of sputum examination has been increased by the use of monoclonal *Pneumocystis* antibodies and diminished by prior prophylactic use of inhaled pentamidine. Examination of wet preparations of sputum can be diagnostic for blastomycosis. Sputum can be examined for *Legionella* by staining directly with fluorescent antibody, but this test has a relatively high frequency of false-negative results. Sputum also should be cultured for *Legionella* on special media. A highly sensitive and specific urinary antigen test is available to detect *L. pneumophila* serogroup 1, which accounts for about 70 percent of *L. pneumophila* infection, in patients with pneumonia.

TABLE 220-3 Criteria for hospitalization of patients with pneumonia

1 Elderly (>65 years of age)
2 Significant comorbidity, e.g., renal, heart, or lung disease; diabetes mellitus; neoplasm; immunosuppression
3 Leukopenia (<5000 white blood cells per microliter) unattributable to a known condition
4 Suspected cause of pneumonia is *S. aureus,* gram-negative bacilli, or anaerobes
5 Suppurative complications, e.g., empyema, arthritis, meningitis, endocarditis
6 Failure of outpatient management
7 Inability to take oral medication
8 Tachypnea (>30 beats/min), tachycardia (>140 beats/min); hypotension (<90 mmHg systolic); hypoxemia (arterial P_{O_2} < 60 mmHg); acute alteration of mental status

---

In the initial evaluation of a patient with pneumonia, several blood cultures should be obtained, and if empyema is a clinical consideration, diagnostic thoracentesis is indicated. Bacteremia or positive pleural fluid cultures are generally considered diagnostic for the organisms causing the pneumonia. However, bacteremia and empyema each occur in fewer than 10 to 30 percent of patients with pneumonia. Serologic studies are sometimes helpful in defining the etiology of certain types of pneumonia, although serologic diagnosis, being delayed by the necessity to demonstrate at least a fourfold rise in convalescent phase antibody titer, is usually retrospective. A single elevated *Legionella* antibody titer of ≥1:128 suggests acute legionellosis.

Expectorated sputum is usually easily collected in patients with a vigorous cough but may be scant in those with an atypical syndrome, in the elderly, and in those with altered mental status. If the patient is not producing sputum and can cooperate, respiratory secretions should be induced with ultrasonic nebulization of 3% saline. An attempt to obtain lower respiratory secretions by passage of a catheter through the nose or mouth rarely achieves the desired results in an alert patient and is discouraged; usually the catheter can be found coiled in the oropharynx.

In some patients who do not require hospitalization (see Table 220-3), the need to establish an accurate microbial diagnosis may not be crucial, and empirical therapy can be started on clinical and epidemiologic evidence alone. This also may be the case with hospitalized patients who are not severely ill and who are unable to produce an induced sputum specimen. Use of more invasive procedures to establish a microbial diagnosis carries risks that must be weighed against potential benefits. However, the decision to initiate empirical therapy without evaluation of induced sputum should be undertaken with caution and always supplemented by several blood cultures in hospitalized patients. The ability to understand the cause (see Table 220-4) of a poor response to empirical antimicrobial therapy may be compromised by the lack of an initial sputum culture.

The sensitivities and specificities of invasive procedures described below for obtaining pulmonary material vary with different types of immunocompromised patients, different types of pulmonary lesions, and prior exposure to therapeutic or prophylactic antimicrobial agents.

TABLE 220-4 Factors involved in poor response to empirical antimicrobial therapy

Incorrect microbiologic diagnosis.
Inappropriate antimicrobial agent or dosing regimen.
Drug hypersensitivity or other adverse effect, e.g., *Clostridium difficile* colitis.
Infectious complication: empyema, metastatic spread, superinfection.
Atelectasis, parapneumonic effusion, phlebitis.
Poor host defenses, e.g., endobronchial obstruction, life-threatening comorbidity.

Transtracheal aspiration (TTA), popular several decades ago, is rarely performed today. Although the sensitivity of the procedure is high (approaching 90 percent), the specificity is low. Material, which is obtained from a catheter inserted through the cricothyroid cartilage and advanced toward the carina, is not contaminated by upper respiratory tract secretions but can contain organisms that colonize the tracheobronchial tree without necessarily being the cause of the pneumonia. Significant morbidity and even mortality have attended its use. TTA, which is contraindicated in patients with a bleeding diathesis, may cause infection at the puncture site and severe subcutaneous and mediastinal emphysema in patients who are coughing vigorously.

Percutaneous transthoracic lung puncture uses a skinny (small-gauge) needle that is advanced into the area of pulmonary consolidation with CT guidance. The procedure requires patient cooperation, good hemostasis, and the ability to tolerate pulmonary hemorrhage or pneumothorax that may be associated with the procedure. Patients on mechanical ventilation cannot undergo lung puncture because of the high incidence of complicating pneumothorax.

Fiberoptic bronchoscopy, safe and relatively well-tolerated, has become the standard invasive procedure to obtain lower respiratory tract secretions when indicated in seriously ill or immunocompromised patients with complex or progressive pneumonia. It allows direct vision of the lower airways. Specimens obtained by bronchoscopy should be stained with Gram's, acid-fast, *Legionella* direct fluorescent antibody, and Gomori's methenamine silver stains and cultured for routine aerobic and anaerobic bacteria, *Legionella*, mycobacteria, and fungi. Sampling is done with a protected double-sheathed brush (PSB), by bronchoalveolar lavage (BAL), or by transbronchial biopsy (TBB) at the site of pulmonary consolidation. The PSB sample is usually contaminated by oropharyngeal flora; quantitative cultures must be performed of the 1 mL of sterile culture medium in which the brush is placed after withdrawal from the inner catheter to differentiate contamination (<1000 CFU/mL) from infection (≥1000 CFU/mL). The results of PSB have shown high specificity and sensitivity, especially in patients who have not received antibiotics before culture. BAL is usually performed with 150 to 200 mL of sterile, nonbacteriostatic saline. Quantitative bacteriology of the BAL sample has given results similar to those of PSB. Gram's stain of the cytocentrifuged BAL specimen can serve as an immediate guide to antimicrobial therapy while awaiting results of cultures.

Open lung biopsy is needed most commonly in the immunocompromised patient with progressive pneumonia when bronchoscopically obtained specimens have been unrevealing. Limitations on performance of an open lung biopsy include hypoxemia and a bleeding diathesis, which may supervene while the physician is deciding whether to do this procedure. Results of an open lung biopsy are considered diagnostic because of the large tissue sample. Its diagnostic yield is highest in focal lesions, whereas bronchoscopic evaluation is most useful in diffuse lesions.

DECISION TO HOSPITALIZE Use of hospital services is costly and at times hazardous to the patient (e.g., risk of nosocomial infections). Hospitalization should be justified by the patient's poor functional status or social support system that would compromise care at home, poor prognostic factors, unstable vital signs, or need for intensive nursing care or specialized diagnostic procedures. Guidelines for hospitalization are given in Table 220-3. Discharge from the hospital should be guided by similar considerations.

TREATMENT Community-acquired pneumonia: Outpatient management Most community-acquired pneumonias in otherwise healthy adults do not require hospitalization. Since it is often not feasible to make a microbial diagnosis in an office setting, oral antimicrobial therapy frequently is empirical (see Table 220-5). The pathogen in such a situation is likely to be *Mycoplasma*, the pneumococcus, or *C. pneumoniae*. In older patients with chronic respiratory disease, *L. pneumophila*, *H. influenzae*, or *M. catarrhalis* also should be considered. In patients at risk of aspiration, oral anaerobes are an additional consideration. There is no oral therapy that has a reliable spectrum encompassing all these pathogens (see Table 220-5). Many experts still recommend penicillin V (500 mg every 6 h) or amoxicillin (500 mg every 8 h) for 7 to 10 days for community-acquired pneumonia with a "typical" presentation in younger outpatients without preexisting disease, since the pneumococcus is the most common pathogen. Second-generation cephalosporins (e.g., cefuroxime axetil, 500 mg every 8 h), doxycycline (100 mg every 12 h), and erythromycin (500 mg every 6 h) are alternative choices. Trimethoprim-sulfamethoxazole is not active against up to 10 percent of strains of *S. pneumoniae*, and ciprofloxacin has only borderline in vitro activity against pneumococci. For the past decade, pneumococcal isolates in other countries frequently have been reported to be erythromycin-resistant; recently, such resistance also has been reported in 10 to 20 percent of pneumococcal isolates from certain centers in the United States as well. These strains are resistant to other macrolides, such as clarithromycin and azithromycin, and are also more likely to be resistance to many other commonly used oral antibiotics. Pneumococcal strains resistant to multiple antibiotics, including penicillin, are not a problem in most of the United States at present. The Centers for Disease Control and Prevention (CDCP), Respiratory Diseases Branch, has reported that of 567 isolates of *S. pneumoniae* from normally sterile body sites submitted during the period for October 1991 through September 1992 in the national pneumococcal surveillance, 5.3 percent were resistant to erythromycin (MIC ≥ 2 μg/mL). The emergence of such strains, however, would require changes in antibiotic recommendations and deserves close scrutiny.

In older patients or adult outpatients with preexisting respiratory disease and "typical" presentation of community-acquired pneumonia and in whom ß-lactamase–producing pathogens, such as *H. influenzae* or *M. catarrhalis*, are common, amoxicillin plus clavulanate, a ß-lactamase inhibitor, doxycycline, or cefuroxime axetil can be used. Erythromycin has poor activity against *H. influenzae*. In comparison to erythromycin, two new oral antibiotics related to erythromycin, azithromycin (500 mg as a single dose on the first day and 250 mg once daily for 4 more days) and clarithromycin (500 mg twice daily for 7 to 10 days), have equal or greater potency against many lower respiratory pathogens and much less frequent gastrointestinal intolerance. Although more costly than erythromycin, these new macrolides may come to replace erythromycin for therapy of community-acquired pneumonia in outpatients if pneumococcal resistance to macrolides does not become a widespread problem.

TABLE 220-5 Empirical oral antimicrobial therapy for outpatient management of community-acquired pneumonia

Pathogen	Penicillin G	Amoxicillin/clavulanate	Cefuroxime	Trimethoprim-sulfamethoxazole	Doxycycline	Erythromycin	Ciprofloxacin
S. pneumoniae	+	+	+	±	+	+*	±
H. influenzae	−	+	+	+	+	±	+
M. catarrhalis	−	+	+	+	+	+	+
Anaerobes	±	+	±	−	−	−	−
M. pneumoniae	−	−	−	−	+	+	+
C. pneumoniae	−	−	−	−	+	+	+
L. pneumophila	−	−	−	±	±	+	±

* 10 to 20 percent of strains recently have been reported to be resistant to macrolides in some locations in the United States (−, ineffective; +, effective).

Doxycycline, erythromycin, and ciprofloxacin are active against *M. pneumoniae* and *C. pneumoniae* and can be used in younger adults with an "atypical" presentation. Although erythromycin is the drug of choice for legionellosis, doxycycline, trimethoprim-sulfamethoxazole, and ciprofloxacin are alternative agents that have been used successfully according to anecdotal reports. Duration of therapy for *Mycoplasma* and *Legionella* infections is 2 to 3 weeks, the longer duration frequently recommended to prevent relapse. The optimal duration of therapy for *C. pneumoniae* infection is unknown but also probably is 2 to 3 weeks.

Pneumonia due to anaerobes can be treated with clindamycin (300 mg every 6 h or 450 mg every 8 h for 7 to 10 days), amoxicillin (500 mg every 8 h) combined with metronidazole (500 mg every 6 h), or amoxicillin/clavulanic acid (500 mg every 8 h). Metronidazole has inadequate activity against microaerophilic gram-positive cocci and must be supplemented by a ß-lactam agent that conpensates for this deficit in coverage.

Community-acquired pneumonia: Inpatient management Patients who have community-acquired pneumonia and are ill enough to be hospitalized (see Table 220-3) must have a prompt microbiologic evaluation, with the Gram's stained sputum and knowledge of the current antimicrobial sensitivities of the pulmonary pathogens in the local geographic area guiding empirical therapy, as outlined in Tables 220-6 and 220-7. Parenteral antimicrobial therapy in the hospitalized patient is usually mandatory. Lack of sputum production, an "atypical" clinical presentation, diffuse radiographic infiltrates in a patient with a rapidly progressive, downhill course, and poor response to prior empirical therapy are some of the reasons to use invasive procedures to detect the pulmonary pathogen, especially in the immunocompromised patient. Although broad-spectrum antibacterial therapy should be started while undertaking a full evaluation in severely ill patients with a rapidly progressing process, these empirical regimens cannot encompass all the possible pathogens without producing unnecessary toxicity and expense. Indeed, in immunocompromised patients, including those with neutropenia or HIV infection, the number of microbial as well as noninfectious causes of pulmonary disease is large and increasing. Since failure to specifically treat the causative agent can be rapidly fatal in these patients, a diagnosis should be sought aggressively so that optimal therapy can be started promptly.

Penicillin or ampicillin remains the drug of choice for suspected pneumococcal pneumonia in the United States. Penicillin resistance among pneumococci (screened with use of a 1-μg oxacillin disk) has become a worldwide problem; it is still unusual in most of the United States (4.1 percent nationwide for 1987–1988), although Alaska had a rate of 25.8 percent in 1987–1988. Data from the CDCP, Respiratory Diseases Branch, indicate that of 567 isolates from normally sterile body sites submitted during the period from October 1991 through September 1992 in the national pneumococcal surveillance, 6.9 percent had some level of resistance to penicillin (MIC > 0.1 μg/mL) and 1.2 percent had high-level resistance (MIC > 1.0 μg/mL). However, one study has reported an alarming increase in resistance (20.1 percent) in 1990–1991 in the United States, although most of

TABLE 220-7 Dosage of antimicrobial agents for pneumonia in hospitalized patients*

Drug	Dosage
Ampicillin/sulbactam	3 g IV every 6 h
Aztreonam	2 g IV every 8 h
Cefazolin	1–2 g IV every 8 h
Cefotaxime, ceftizoxime	1–2 g IV every 8–12 h
Ceftazidime	2 g IV every 8 h
Ceftriaxone	1–2 g IV every 12–24 h
Cefuroxime	750 mg IV every 8 h
Ciprofloxacin	400 mg IV or 750 mg PO every 12 h
Clindamycin	600–900 mg IV every 8 h
Erythromycin	0.5–1.0 g IV every 6 h
Gentamicin (or tobramycin)	5 mg/kg in three equally divided dose IV every 8h
Imipenem	500 mg IV every 6 h
Metronidazole	500 mg IV or PO every 8 h
Nafcillin	2 g IV every 4 h
Penicillin G	1 million units IV every 4–6 h
Ticarcillin/Clavulanate	3.1 g IV every 4 h
Vancomycin	1 g IV every 12 h

* Dosage must be modified in patients with renal failure. Guidelines on duration of therapy for each pathogen are given in the text of this chapter and in individual chapters on infecting agents.

the 524 strains had minimal inhibitory concentrations (MICs) between 0.1 and 1.0 μg/mL penicillin. Penicillin-resistant stains also may be resistant to other groups of antimicrobial agents. Nevertheless, MICs of cefotaxime, ceftriaxone, imipenem, and vancomycin are lower than those of penicillin or ampicillin and most other ß-lactam antibiotics for penicillin-resistant strains. However, some strains with intermediate resistance to penicillin (MIC 0.25 to 1 μg/mL) have been reported recently to have high-level resistance to second- and third-generation cephalosporins. Although there are no good studies on the treatment of pneumonia due to penicillin-resistant strains, high-dose intravenous penicillin G (e.g., 10 to 20 million units daily) is probably adequate therapy for pneumonia due to strains exhibiting intermediate resistance to penicillin. High-level penicillin resistance (MIC 2 to 16 μg/mL) has been unusual in the United States, but the frequency of high-level penicillin resistance among the pencillin-resistant strains may approach 50 percent of isolates in some European countries. Effectiveness of high-dose intravenous penicillin for pneumonia due to these highly resistant strains is unknown, but anecdotal reports suggest that cefotaxime or ceftriaxone may be adequate. Since all penicillin-resistant strains are sensitive to vancomycin, initial therapy should include this antibiotic for patients with pneumococcal pneumonia who live in regions where penicillin resistance is common and are severely ill or have significant comorbidity.

If the sputum Gram's stain is not interpretable or not available, either a second- or third-generation cephalosporin plus metronidazole or ampicillin plus sulbactam is an adequate empirical regimen, unless *Legionella* or *Chlamydia* is the likely pathogen, in which case erythromycin should be added to the regimen. With rapid clinical improvement, therapy can be switched from intavenous to oral agents to complete a 7- to 10-day course if antimicrobial agents are available

TABLE 220-6 Empirical antimicrobial therapy for the management of hospitalized patients with community-acquired pneumonia

Pathogen	Penicillin G	First-generation cephalosporin	Second- or third-generation cephalosporin	Metronidazole	Trimethoprim-sulfamethoxazole	Erythromycin	Ampicillin/sulbactam
S. pneumoniae	+	+	+	−	±	+ *	+
S. aureus	−	+	+	−	+	−	+
H. influenzae	−	−	+	−	+	±	+
M. catarrhalis	−	−	+	−	+	+	+
Anaerobic gram-positive cocci	+	+	+	+	−	−	+
Anaerobic gram-negative bacilli	−	−	−	+	−	−	+
C. pneumoniae	−	−	−	−	−	+	−
L. pneumophila	−	−	−	−	±	+	−

* 10 to 20 percent of strains recently have been reported to be resistant to macrolides in some locations in the United States (−, ineffective; +, effective).

that are readily absorbed after oral administration to achieve tissue levels above the MIC. The presence of *S. aureus*, aerobic gram-negative bacilli, or suppurative complications requires a more prolonged course of therapy. Legionellosis should be treated with 1 g erythromycin, IV, every 6 h for 3 weeks, to prevent relapses; rifampin should be added in critically ill patients with legionellosis. Anaerobic lung abscess should be treated with the regimens suggested for aspiration pneumonia until a chest radiograph (taken at 2-week intervals) is clear or shows only a small, stable scar. Therapy is prolonged for 6 weeks or more to prevent relapse, although shorter courses of therapy are probably sufficient for most patients. Surgery is rarely required for lung abscess; indications for surgery include massive hemoptysis and neoplasm. Supportive measures include supplemental oxygen, intravenous fluids, assistance in clearing secretions, fiberoptic bronchoscopy, and ventilatory support, if necessary. Caution should be exercised in bronchoscopic drainage of large, fluid-filled lung abscesses because of potential sudden, massive spillage of large collections of pus into the airways.

Patients with risk factors for HIV infection and an atypical pneumonia syndrome should be evaluated for *Pneumocystis* infections because of its frequency as an index diagnosis in HIV infection and its potential severity. Tuberculosis, as well as other causes of atypical pneumonia in these patients, must be excluded as part of the evaluation. Initial empirical therapy can be either trimethoprim-sulfamethoxazole (15 to 20 mg/kg of trimethoprim daily in four divided doses IV or PO) or pentamidine (3 to 4 mg/kg daily IV), and therapy is continued for 3 weeks in confirmed cases of *Pneumocystis* infection. Although some data suggest that trimethprim-sulfamethoxazole may be more effective than ·pentamidine, further studies directly comparing the two agents are needed. The frequency and severity of adverse effects of both drugs are thought by most to be equivalent. Addition of glucocorticoids (prednisone, 40 mg twice daily followed by a tapering dose) early in the course of *Pneumocystis* pneumonia in patients with an arterial $P_{O_2} < 70$ mmHg decreases the need for mechanical ventilation and improves survival and functional status. Prophylaxis for recurrent *Pneumocystis* pneumonia must be started at the end of therapy.

Institutionally acquired pneumonia Pneumonia acquired in institutions such as nursing homes or hospitals is frequently caused by enteric gram-negative bacilli, *P. aeruginosa*, or *S. aureus*, with or without oral anaerobes. Again, antimicrobial therapy should be guided by Gram's stain of sputum (see Tables 220-7 and 220-8) and knowledge of the prevalent nosocomial pathogens and curent in vitro antimicrobial sensitivity patterns of these nosocomial pathogens in the particular institution. An aggressive diagnostic approach is needed

in some circumstances, especially for the immunocompromised patient, as outlined above.

S. aureus acquired in some institutions is frequently methicillin-resistant. Such strains are resistant to all ß-lactam antibiotics and can be resistant to clindamycin, erythromycin, and the fluoroquinolones. Only vancomycin is predictably active against these organisms and should be added to an empirical regimen when methicillin-resistant organisms are possibly the cause of pneumonia.

Pneumonia due to gram-negative bacilli in the institutionalized patient when multiantibiotic resistance is not a problem can be treated initially with a ß-lactam active against *P. aeruginosa* (ceftazidime, ticarcillin/clavulanate, aztreonam, or imipenem) or a parenterally administered fluoroquinolone (ciprofloxacin or ofloxacin). Ticarcillin/clavulanate is preferred as an empirical antibiotic over other penicillins with activity against *P. aeruginosa*, such as piperacillin, which, although more potent against *P. aeruginosa*, is not sufficiently active against *Klebsiella pneumoniae*, a relatively common pathogen. Amipicillin/sulbactam, the other parenterally administered ß-lactam antibiotic/ß-lactamase inhibitor combination, does not have activity against many nosocomial pathogens, such as *P. aeruginosa*, *Enterobacter* spp., and *Serratia* spp., and therefore is inappropriate for empirical therapy of nosocomial pneumonia.

In seriously ill patients, especially those infected with *P. aeruginosa*, use of a ß-lactam/aminoglycoside combination for bactericidal synergy is prudent. Combinations of ß-lactam plus aminoglycoside are also used to broaden the spectrum of antibacterial activity for the possibility of infection with resistant pathogens, to treat polymicrobial infection, and to prevent emergence of antimicrobial resistance. Combinations of ß-lactams or aminoglycosides with a fluoroquinolone are not expected to exhibit an enhancement of the already rapid bactericidal activity of the fluoroquinolone alone; nevertheless, they are expected to broaden the spectrum and perhaps prevent the emergency of resistance. Fluoroquinolone plus either a ß-lactam or an aminoglycoside could be used in institutions where there is a greater expectation for infection with a fluoroquinolone-resistant nosocomial pathogen, e.g., *Acinetobacter calcoaceticus*, or with organisms that frequently exhibit emergence of resistance on therapy, e.g., *P. aeruginosa*.

Pneumonia due to possible coinfection with aerobic gram-negative bacilli and anaerobes, as reflected by a polymicrobial flora on Gram's stain of sputum, may usually be treated with any of the following regimens: (1) ceftazidime plus metronidazole or clindamycin, (2) aztreonam or a fluoroquinolone plus clindamycin, and (3) imipenem alone or ticarcillin/clavulanate. The regimens that contain a ß-lactam agent usually also should include an aminoglycoside (see Table 220-8).

Production of chromosomally encoded, inducible ß-lactamases by some aerobic gram-negative bacilli, including *Serratia marcescens*, *E. cloacae*, *Citrobacter freundii*, *Morganella morganii*, *P. aeruginosa*, and *Acinetobacter calcoaceticus*, has important implications for therapy of nosocomial pneumonia in institutions where these organisms are common nosocomial pathogens. Antibiotic resistance in these pathogens has been attributed to two related mechanisms: inducible production of chromosomally encoded ß-lactamases and selection of mutants that have lost a gene that controls expression of ß-lactamase production. The control gene represses ß-lactamase production in the absence of a ß-lactam agent and allows ß-lactamase production in the presence of a ß-lactam agent. This group of organisms has a relatively high mutation rate for loss of this control gene, and loss of the gene results in continuous production of large amounts of ß-lactamase (stable derepression). The derepressed mutants are resistant to third-generation cephalosporins, aztreonam, and broad-spectrum penicillins. These chromosomally encoded, inducible ß-lactamases are not inhibited by clavulanic acid or sulbactam.

Selection by the ß-lactam antibiotic of the derepressed mutants present in the dense bacterial populations of infected pulmonary tissue at the initiation of antibiotic therapy apparently accounts for emergence of resistance during therapy, which is especially a problem in severely

---

TABLE 220-8 Empirical antimicrobial therapy of institutionally acquired pneumonia based on Gram's stain of sputum

Presumptive *S. aureus*	Nafcillin or vancomycin*	
Presumptive Enteric gram-negative bacilli or *P. aeruginosa*	1 Ceftazidime	±Aminoglycoside
	2 Ticarcillin/clavulanate	±Aminoglycoside
	3 Aztreonam	±Aminoglycoside
	4 Imipenem†	±Aminoglycoside
	5 Fluoroquinolone†	±Aminoglycoside or β-lactam
Mixed flora	1 Ceftazidime + clindamycin (or metronidazole) ± aminoglycoside‡	
	2 Ticarcillin/clavulanate ± aminoglycoside‡	
	3 Aztreonam + clindamycin (or metronidazole§) ± Aminoglycoside‡	
	4 Imipenem† ± Aminoglycoside‡	
	5 Fluoroquinolone† + clindamycin (or metronidazole‡,§) ± aminoglycoside or β-lactam‡	

* If methicillin-resistant *S. aureus* is present in the institution, use vancomycin; otherwise, use an antistaphylococcal β-lactam, e.g., nafcillin or cefazolin.
† Use when chromosomal, inducible β-lactamase producers are endemic in the institution.
‡ Add vancomycin if methicillin-resistant *S. aureus* is present in the institution.
§ Metronidazole must be combined with vancomycin or another antimicrobial that covers microaerophilic and anaerobic gram-positive cocci.

compromised patients whose defective host defenses are unable to control the growth of at first few resistant mutants. The only ß-lactam agent that maintains activity against the derepressed mutants is imipenem. Ciprofloxacin and aminoglycosides may retain activity against these mutants. Trimethoprim-sulfamethoxazole also may remain active against these gram-negative bacilli, except *P. aeruginosa*, which is inherently resistant. Some clinicians have questioned the efficacy of aminoglycosides alone in the therapy of gram-negative bacillary pneumonia. The poor clinical efficacy has been attributed to low levels of aminoglycoside in bronchial secretions and loss of antimicrobial activity due to the relatively acidic purulent secretions, the anaerobic conditions in infected lung, and, in the case of *P. aeruginosa*, the presence of the divalent cations calcium and magnesium. The nephrotoxicity and ototoxicity of aminoglycosides lead to underdosing with these agents. These problems are compounded by unpredictable pharmacokinetics that necessitate measurement of serum levels of aminoglycosides. If multiantibiotic-resistant nosocomial organisms are likely to be pathogens in severely compromised patients, the only reliable empirical agents are fluoroquinolones and imipenem, unless resistance to these drugs is also endemic in the institution. Up-to-date knowledge of antimicrobial sensitivities of nosocomial pathogens and use of preventive practices are mandatory.

Amantidine (200 mg/d in most adults and 100 mg/d in persons over 65 years of age) is effective for prevention of influenza A infection in the unimmunized patients during an influenza A outbreak and for therapy (for 5 to 7 days) of early influenza A infection. Ribavirin is effective for respiratory syncytial virus infection. Intravenous acyclovir (5 to 10 mg/kg every 8 h for 7 to 14 days) is appropriate for varicella pneumonia. Relatively high doses of intravenous immunoglobulin combined with either ganciclovir (2.5 mg/kg every 12 h for 20 days, then 5 mg/kg once daily for 5 days a week for 20 more doses) may be effective for cytomegalovirus pneumonitis.

PREVENTION Prevention of pneumonia involves either decreasing the likelihood of encountering the pathogen or strengthening the host's response once the pathogen is encountered. The former method can include use of face masks by persons dealing with affected patients, use of negative-pressure isolation rooms for patients with contagious tuberculosis or with pneumonia spread by the aerosol route, prompt institution of effective chemotherapy for contagious patients, or use of therapy to correct conditions that facilitate aspiration. The latter method includes use of chemoprophylaxis or immunization of patients at risk. Chemoprophylaxis may be administered to patients who have encountered or are likely to encounter the pathogen before they become symptomatic (amantidine during a community outbreak of influenza A, INH for tuberculosis, trimethoprim-sulfamethoxazole for pneumocystosis) or administered to patients who are likely to have a recurrence following recovery from a symptomatic episode (trimethoprim-sulfamethoxazole for pneumocystosis in patients with HIV infection). Gastric acidity is a major factor that prevents colonization of the gastrointestinal tract by nosocomial gram-negative bacillary pathogens. To prevent stress ulceration, it is preferable to use sucralfate, which maintains gastric acidity, rather than H-2 blocking agents. Vaccines (see Chaps. 82, 101, and 112) are available for immunization against the following pulmonary pathogens: *S. pneumoniae, H. influenzae* type B, influenza viruses A and B, and measles virus. Influenza and pneumococcal vaccines are strongly recommended for those over 65 years of age and persons of any age who are at risk of adverse consequences of influenza or pneumonia because of underlying conditions. Pneumococcal, hemophilus, and influenza vaccines are recommended for HIV-infected patients who are still capable of responding to a vaccine challenge. The currently available 23-valent pneumococcal vaccine covers 88 percent of the serotypes causing systemic disease as well as 8 percent of related serotypes. The increasing prevalence of multiantibiotic resistance of pneumococci makes immunization of high-risk individuals with the pneumococcal vaccine of utmost importance. Immune serum globulin is available for replacement therapy in those patients with congenital or acquired hypogammaglob-

ulinemia. Prevention of nosocomial pneumonia requires good infection-control practices, judicious use of broad-spectrum antimicrobial agents, and maintenance of patients' gastric acidity.

REFERENCES

CRAVEN DE et al: Nosocomial pneumonia in the 1990s: Update of epidemiology and risk factors: Semin Respir Infect 5:157, 1990

FANG GD et al: New and emerging etiologies for community-acquired pneumonia with implications for therapy. Medicine 69:307, 1990

FINE MJ: Pneumonia in the elderly: The hospital admission and discharge decisions. Semin Respir Infect 65:303,1990

HAHN DL et al: Association of *Chlamydia pneumoniae* (strain TWAR) infection with wheezing, asthmatic bronchitis and adult-onset asthma. JAMA 266:225, 1991

JACOBS MR: Treatment and diagnosis of infections caused by drug-resistant *Streptoccocus pneumoniae*. Clin Infect Dis 15:119, 1992

LEVISON ME, BUSH L: Pharmacodynamics of antimicrobial agents: Bactericidal and postantibiotic effects. Infect Dis Clin North Am 3:415, 1989

——— et al: Clindamycin compared with penicillin for the treatment of anaerobic lung abscess. Ann Intern Med 98:466, 1983

LEVISON, ME (ED): The pneumonias. Clinical approaches to infectious diseases of the lower respiratory tract. Boston, John Wright. PSG Inc, 1984.

LORBER B, SWENSON RM: Bacteriology of aspiration pneumonia: A prospective study of community and hospital acquired cases. Ann Intern Med 81:329, 1974

RIES K et al: Transtracheal aspiration in pulmonary infection. Arch Intern Med 133:453, 1974

RILEY RL: Airborne infection. Am J Med 57:466, 1974

SANDERS CC, SANDERS WE JR: Clinical significance of inducible beta-lactamase in gram-negative bacteria. Eur J Clin Microbiol 6:435, 1987

SHELHAMER JH et al: NIH conference: Respiratory disease in the immunosuppressed patient. Ann Intern Med 117:415, 1992

VERGHESE A, BERK SL: Bacterial pneumonia in the elderly. Medicine 62:271, 1982

WOODHEAD MA et al: Prospective study of the aetiology and outcome of pneumonia in the community. Lancet 1:671, 1987

221 BRONCHIECTASIS AND BRONCHOLITHIASIS

STEVEN E. WEINBERGER

BRONCHIECTASIS

DEFINITION Bronchiectasis is an abnormal and permanent dilatation of bronchi. It may be either focal, involving airways supplying a limited region of pulmonary parenchyma, or diffuse, involving airways in a more widespread distribution. Although this definition is based on pathologic changes in the bronchi, diagnosis is often suggested by the clinical consequences of chronic or recurrent infection in the dilated airways and the associated secretions that pool within these airways.

PATHOLOGY The bronchial dilatation of bronchiectasis is associated with destructive and inflammatory changes in the walls of medium-sized airways, often at the level of segmental or subsegmental bronchi. The normal structural components of the wall, including cartilage, muscle, and elastic tissue, are destroyed and may be replaced by fibrous tissue. The dilated airways frequently contain pools of thick, purulent material, while more peripheral airways are often occluded by secretions or obliterated and replaced by fibrous tissue. Additional microscopic features include bronchial and peribronchial inflammation and fibrosis, ulceration of the bronchial wall, squamous metaplasia, and mucous gland hyperplasia. The parenchyma normally supplied by the affected airways is abnormal, containing varying combinations of fibrosis, emphysema, bronchopneumonia, and atelectasis. As a result of the inflammation, vascularity of the bronchial wall increases, with associated enlargement of the bronchial arteries and anastomoses between the bronchial and pulmonary arterial circulations.

Three different patterns of bronchiectasis were described by Reid in 1950. In *cylindrical bronchiectasis* the bronchi appear as uniformly dilated tubes that end abruptly at the point that smaller airways are obstructed by secretions. In *varicose bronchiectasis* the affected bronchi have an irregular or beaded pattern of dilatation resembling varicose veins. In *saccular (cystic) bronchiectasis* the bronchi have a ballooned appearance at the periphery, ending in blind sacs without recognizable bronchial structures distal to the sacs.

ETIOLOGY AND PATHOGENESIS Bronchiectasis is a consequence of inflammation and destruction of the structural components of the bronchial wall. Infection is the usual cause of the inflammation, but on occasion airway injury is due to a toxin or an immune response. Secondary factors may perpetuate inflammation and impair mucociliary clearance, thereby promoting further infection. Microorganisms such as *Pseudomonas aeruginosa* and *Haemophilus influenzae* produce pigments, proteases, and other toxins that injure the respiratory epithelium and impair mucociliary clearance. The host inflammatory response, although protective on the one hand, also induces epithelial injury, largely as a result of mediators released from neutrophils. For example, serine proteases with elastolytic activity and oxygen-derived free radicals can produce additional damage to bronchial epithelium and further impair mucociliary clearance. As protection against infection is compromised, the dilated airways become more susceptible to colonization and growth of bacteria. Thus, a reinforcing cycle can result, with inflammation producing airway damage, impaired clearance of microorganisms, and further infection, which then completes the cycle by inciting more inflammation.

Infectious causes Infection, either as a single severe event or as a recurrent problem, is the trigger for bronchial wall inflammation and destruction in most cases. When a single episode of infection is responsible, the host usually does not have underlying compromise of local or systemic defense mechanisms. Rather, the characteristics of the infectious agent and the severity of the inflammatory response are presumably the important features.

A wide variety of infectious agents can initiate bronchiectasis. In the past, bronchiectasis during childhood was often a complication of measles or pertussis; these are now rare causes, the result of effective immunization. At present, adenovirus and influenza virus are the main viruses that cause bronchiectasis in association with lower respiratory tract involvement. Although not as common as in the preantibiotic era, virulent bacterial infections, especially with potentially necrotizing organisms such as *Staphylococcus aureus*, *Klebsiella*, and anaerobes, remain important causes of bronchiectasis when antibiotic treatment of a pneumonia is not given or is significantly delayed. Tuberculosis can produce bronchiectasis by a necrotizing effect on pulmonary parenchyma and airways and indirectly as a consequence of airway obstruction from bronchostenosis or extrinsic compression by lymph nodes. Nontuberculous mycobacteria are frequently associated with bronchiectasis, but usually as secondary infections or colonizing organisms rather than as primary pathogens. Mycoplasmal and necrotizing fungal infections are rare causes.

Impaired host defense mechanisms are often involved in the predisposition to recurrent infections. A localized structural defect may impair clearance of microorganisms and secretions from the affected airway(s), or a systemic defect may predispose to infection that potentially affects more than one region of lung.

The major cause of localized impairment of host defenses is endobronchial obstruction. Bacteria and secretions cannot be cleared adequately from the obstructed airway, which develops recurrent or chronic infection. Although primary lung cancer is the most common cause of endobronchial obstruction, it is an infrequent cause of bronchiectasis, since either the involved area is removed surgically or the disease progresses before bronchiectasis becomes an important problem. Slowly growing endobronchial neoplasms such as carcinoid tumors are more commonly associated with bronchiectasis. Foreign body aspiration is another important cause of endobronchial obstruction, particularly in children. Airway obstruction can also result from bronchostenosis, from impacted secretions, or from extrinsic compression by enlarged lymph nodes.

Generalized impairment of pulmonary defense mechanisms occurs with immunoglobulin deficiency, primary ciliary disorders, or cystic fibrosis. Infections and bronchiectasis are therefore often more diffuse. With panhypogammaglobulinemia, the best described of the immunoglobulin disorders associated with recurrent infection and bronchiectasis, patients often also have a history of sinus or skin infections. Selective IgA deficiency can be associated with bronchiectasis, frequently with coexisting deficiency of IgG subclasses (especially IgG2 or IgG4).

The primary disorders associated with ciliary dysfunction are termed *primary ciliary dyskinesia*. Numerous defects are encompassed under this category, including structural abnormalities of the dynein arms, radial spokes, and microtubules. The cilia become dyskinetic, their coordinated, propulsive action is diminished, and bacterial clearance is impaired. The clinical effects include recurrent upper and lower respiratory tract infections, such as sinusitis, otitis media, and bronchiectasis. Because normal sperm motility also depends on proper ciliary function, males are generally infertile (see also Chap. 48). Approximately half of patients with primary ciliary dyskinesia fall into the subgroup of *Kartagener's syndrome*, in which situs inversus accompanies bronchiectasis and sinusitis. It has been hypothesized that ciliary motility is necessary for proper rotation of the viscera during embryogenesis, so that visceral rotation is random when normal ciliary motion is lost.

In cystic fibrosis (see Chap. 222), the tenacious secretions in the bronchi are associated with impaired bacterial clearance, resulting in colonization and recurrent infection with a variety of organisms, particularly mucoid strains of *P. aeruginosa* but also *Staphylococcus aureus*, *H. influenzae*, *Escherichia coli*, and *P. cepacia*. Additional respiratory tract complications in cystic fibrosis include recurrent pneumothoraces, sinusitis, and nasal polyps. Males are generally infertile due to atresia of the vas deferens.

Noninfectious causes Some cases of bronchiectasis are associated with exposure to a toxic substance that incites a severe inflammatory response. Examples include inhalation of a toxic gas such as ammonia or aspiration of acidic gastric contents, though the latter problem is often also complicated by aspiration of bacteria. An immune response in the airway may also trigger inflammation, destructive changes, and bronchial dilatation. This mechanism is presumably responsible at least in part for bronchiectasis with allergic bronchopulmonary aspergillosis (ABPA), which is due to an immune response to *Aspergillus* organisms that have colonized the airway. Bronchiectasis accompanying ABPA often involves proximal airways and is associated with mucoid impaction. Bronchiectasis also occurs rarely in ulcerative colitis and rheumatoid arthritis, but it is not known whether an immune response triggers airway inflammation in these patients.

Bronchiectasis is a potential complication of uncommon disorders affecting airway cartilage. In *Williams-Campbell syndrome*, thought to be a congenital, perhaps inherited deficiency in bronchial cartilage of medium-sized airways, the affected airways may dilate. In *tracheobronchomegaly (Mounier-Kuhn syndrome)*, an acquired defect in components of the airway wall, including cartilage, elastic tissue, and muscle, is thought to be responsible for dilatation of the trachea and bronchi.

Other causes of bronchiectasis have also been described. In *Young's syndrome*, defined as obstructive azoospermia, men have normal spermatogenesis but obstruction of the epididymis by inspissated secretions. Approximately 20 to 30 percent of these patients also have bronchiectasis by an unknown mechanism. In *alpha₁-antitrypsin deficiency*, the usual respiratory complication is the early development of panacinar emphysema, but affected individuals may occasionally have bronchiectasis. In the *yellow nail syndrome*, which is due to hypoplastic lymphatics, the triad of lymphedema, pleural effusion, and yellow discoloration of the nails is accompanied by bronchiectasis in approximately 40 percent of patients. Finally, some cases of atelectasis and pulmonary fibrosis are associated with bronchial dilatation due to increased traction on the airways from the surrounding pulmonary parenchyma. Theoretically, the term bronchiectasis should not be used for the latter cases unless there is also destruction of components of the airway wall, which may be due to secondary infection in the involved airways.

CLINICAL MANIFESTATIONS Patients typically present with persistent or recurrent cough and purulent sputum production. Hemoptysis occurs in 50 to 70 percent of cases and can be due to bleeding from friable, inflamed airway mucosa. More significant, even massive bleeding is often a consequence of bleeding from hypertrophied bronchial arteries.

When a specific infectious episode initiates bronchiectasis, patients may describe a severe pneumonia followed by chronic cough and sputum production. Alternatively, patients without a dramatic initiating event often describe the insidious onset of symptoms. In some cases, patients are either asymptomatic or have a nonproductive cough, often associated with "dry" bronchiectasis in an upper lobe. Dyspnea or wheezing generally reflects either widespread bronchiectasis or underlying chronic obstructive pulmonary disease. With exacerbations of infection, the amount of sputum increases, the appearance becomes more purulent and often more bloody, and patients may become febrile. Such episodes may be due solely to exacerbations of the airway infection, but associated parenchymal infiltrates sometimes reflect an adjacent pneumonia.

Physical examination of the chest overlying an area of bronchiectasis is quite variable. Any combination of crackles, rhonchi, and wheezes may be heard, all of which reflect the damaged airways containing significant secretions. As with other types of chronic intrathoracic infection, clubbing may be present. Patients with severe, diffuse disease, particularly those with chronic hypoxemia, may have associated cor pulmonale and right ventricular failure.

Other nonpulmonary complications of bronchiectasis are now seen infrequently, largely because of better antibiotic control of the bacterial infections within the bronchiectatic airways. For example, brain abscess presumably results from septicemia, and amyloidosis can result from chronic infection and inflammation.

RADIOGRAPHIC AND LABORATORY FINDINGS Though the chest radiograph is important in the evaluation of suspected bronchiectasis, the findings are often nonspecific. At one extreme, the radiograph may be normal with mild disease. Alternatively, patients with saccular bronchiectasis may have prominent cystic spaces, either with or without air-liquid levels, corresponding to the dilated airways. These may be difficult to distinguish from enlarged airspaces due to bullous emphysema or from regions of honeycombing in patients with severe interstitial lung disease. Other findings are due to dilated airways with thickened walls, which result from peribronchial inflammation. Because of decreased aeration and atelectasis of the associated pulmonary parenchyma, these dilated airways are often crowded together in parallel. When seen longitudinally, the airways appear as "tram tracks"; when seen in cross-section, they produce "ring shadows." Because the dilated airways may be filled with secretions, the lumen may appear dense rather than radiolucent, producing an opaque tubular or branched tubular structure.

Bronchography, which involves coating the airways with a radioopaque, iodinated lipid dye instilled through a catheter or bronchoscope, can provide excellent visualization of bronchiectatic airways. However, this technique has largely been replaced by computed tomography (CT), which also provides an excellent view of dilated airways as seen in cross-sectional images. With the advent of high-resolution CT scanning, in which the images are 1.5 mm thick, the sensitivity for detecting bronchiectasis has improved even further.

Examination of sputum often reveals an abundance of neutrophils and colonization or infection with a variety of possible organisms. Although common bacterial pathogens such as *Streptococcus pneumoniae* and *H. influenzae* may be present, a number of other organisms are seen frequently. *P. aeruginosa* is particularly common, and may be a clue to the presence of previously unsuspected bronchiectasis. Other organisms include *Staph. aureus*, anaerobes, and nontubercu-

lous (atypical) mycobacteria. Appropriate staining and culturing of sputum often provides a guide to antibiotic therapy.

Additional evaluation is aimed at diagnosing the cause for the bronchiectasis. When bronchiectasis is focal, fiberoptic bronchoscopy may reveal an underlying endobronchial obstruction. In other cases, upper lobe involvement may be suggestive of either tuberculosis or ABPA. With more widespread disease, measurement of sweat chloride levels for cystic fibrosis, structural or functional assessment of nasal or bronchial cilia or sperm for primary ciliary dyskinesia, and quantitative assessment of immunoglobulins may explain recurrent airway infection. In an asthmatic person with proximal bronchiectasis or other historical features to suggest ABPA, skin testing, serology, and sputum culture for *Aspergillus* are helpful in confirming the diagnosis.

Pulmonary function tests may demonstrate airflow obstruction as a consequence of diffuse bronchiectasis or associated chronic obstructive lung disease. Bronchial hyperreactivity, e.g., to methacholine challenge, and some reversibility of the airflow obstruction with inhaled bronchodilators are relatively common for reasons not well defined. Other laboratory evaluation is often relatively nonspecific. For example, as a result of chronic infection within the thorax, patients may develop the normocytic, normochromic anemia of chronic disease.

TREATMENT Therapy has four major goals: (1) elimination of an identifiable underlying problem; (2) improved clearance of tracheobronchial secretions; (3) control of infection, particularly during acute exacerbations; and (4) reversal of airflow obstruction. Appropriate treatment should be instituted when a treatable cause is found, for example, treatment of hypogammaglobulinemia with immunoglobulin replacement, tuberculosis with antituberculous agents, and ABPA with glucocorticoids.

Secretions are typically copious and thick and contribute to the symptoms. Chest physical therapy with vibration, percussion, and postural drainage frequently helps patients with copious secretions. Mucolytic agents to thin secretions and allow better clearance are controversial. Data from a recent study utilizing iodinated glycerol in chronic obstructive lung disease have led to increasing interest in the use of mucolytics in the treatment of bronchiectasis.

Chronic or recurrent bacterial infections cause much of the morbidity of bronchiectasis. Antibiotics have an important role in management, but which antibiotic should be given and the frequency and duration of administration are not well established. For patients with infrequent exacerbations characterized by an increase in quantity and purulence of the sputum, antibiotics are commonly used only during acute episodes. Although choice of an antibiotic may be guided by Gram's stain and culture of sputum, empiric coverage (e.g., with ampicillin, amoxicillin, trimethoprim-sulfamethoxazole, or cefaclor) is often given initially. When *P. aeruginosa* is present, oral therapy with a quinolone or parenteral therapy with an aminoglycoside or third-generation cephalosporin may be appropriate. In patients with chronic purulent sputum despite short courses of antibiotics, more prolonged courses, e.g., with oral amoxicillin or inhaled aminoglycosides, or intermittent but regular courses of single or rotating antibiotics have been used.

Bronchodilators to improve obstruction and aid clearance of secretions are particularly useful in patients with airway hyperreactivity and reversible airflow obstruction. Although surgical therapy was common in the past, more effective antibiotic and supportive therapy has largely replaced surgery. However, when bronchiectasis is localized and the morbidity is substantial despite adequate medical therapy, surgical resection of the involved region of lung should be considered.

Complications present additional treatment issues. When massive hemoptysis, often originating from the hypertrophied bronchial circulation, does not resolve with conservative therapy, including rest and antibiotics, therapeutic options are either surgical resection or bronchial arterial embolization. Although resection may be successful if disease is localized, embolization is preferable with widespread disease. When embolization is performed by an experienced interventional radiologist, accidental embolization of a spinal artery with resulting spinal cord infarction, a serious complication of bronchial artery embolization, is rare. In patients with extensive disease, chronic hypoxemia and cor pulmonale may indicate the need for long-term supplemental oxygen. For selected patients who are disabled despite maximal therapy, lung transplantation is a therapeutic option.

BRONCHOLITHIASIS

Broncholithiasis is defined as the presence of one or more calcified stones within the tracheobronchial tree. These stones usually result from erosion of a calcified lymph node into an adjacent bronchus; less common causes are fragmentation and erosion of calcified tracheobronchial cartilage into the airway and calcification of aspirated foreign material. Eroding calcified lymph nodes are most frequently due to granulomatous infection, including histoplasmosis, tuberculosis, and coccidioidomycosis.

Manifestations include cough with expectoration of calcified material (lithoptysis), hemoptysis, and pneumonia or atelectasis secondary to obstruction of the airway with calcified material. Rarely, calcified material may also erode into the esophagus or the aorta, causing fistula formation between these structures and the airway.

Chest radiography often demonstrates one or more calcified densities representing calcified lymph nodes or the actual stone(s) within the airway lumen. Movement or disappearance of a calcified focus on chest radiograph is particularly suggestive of the diagnosis. Endobronchial obstruction may cause atelectasis, consolidation, or bronchiectasis involving the lung distal to the obstruction. The relationship between calcified material and an airway is best visualized noninvasively with CT scanning. Distortion and inflammatory changes of the airway may be demonstrated by fiberoptic bronchoscopy; calcified material within the lumen or adherent to the wall of the airway may also be seen.

Treatment is not always necessary, as symptoms may be minimal or the broncholiths may be spontaneously expectorated. Endoscopic removal of the calcified stones is sometimes possible with the rigid bronchoscope, which affords better airway control than does the fiberoptic bronchoscope and the use of larger instruments for retrieving stones. Surgical resection may be required for massive or recurrent hemoptysis, obstruction with recurrent infection, or fistula formation.

REFERENCES

Bronchiectasis

BARKER AF, BARDANA EJ JR: Bronchiectasis: Update of an orphan disease. Am Rev Respir Dis 137:969, 1988

COLE PJ: Inflammation: A two-edged sword—the model of bronchiectasis. Eur J Respir Dis 69(suppl 147):6, 1986

CURRIE DC, GARBETT ND et al: Double-blind randomized study of prolonged higher-dose oral amoxycillin in purulent bronchiectasis. Q J Med 76:799, 1990

DAVIS AL, SALZMAN SH: Bronchiectasis, in Chronic Obstructive Pulmonary Disease, NS Cherniack (ed). Philadelphia, Saunders, 1991, pp 316-338

GREENSTONE M, RUTMAN A et al: Primary ciliary dyskinesia: Cytological and clinical features. Q J Med 67:405, 1988

MURRAY JF: New presentations of bronchiectasis. Hosp Pract 26:55, 1991

PANG J, CHAN HS et al: Prevalence of asthma, atopy, and bronchial hyperreactivity in bronchiectasis: A controlled study. Thorax 44:948, 1989

TRUCKSIS M, SWARTZ MN: Bronchiectasis: A current view. Curr Clin Top Infect Dis 11:170, 1991

WESTCOTT JL: Bronchiectasis. Radiol Clin N Amer 29:1031, 1991

Broncholithiasis

CONCES DJ JR, TARVER RD et al: Broncholithiasis: CT features in 15 patients. Am J Radiol 157:249, 1991

DIXON GF, DONNERBERG RL et al: Advances in the diagnosis and treatment of broncholithiasis. Am Rev Respir Dis 129:1028, 1984

TRASTEK VF, PAIROLERO PC et al: Surgical management of broncholithiasis. J Thorac Cardiovasc Surg 90:842, 1985

222   CYSTIC FIBROSIS

RICHARD C. BOUCHER

Cystic fibrosis (CF) is a monogenetic disorder that presents as a multisystem disease. The first signs and symptoms typically occur in childhood, but nearly 3 percent of patients are diagnosed as adults. Due to improvements in therapy, more than 25 percent of patients reach adulthood and more than 9 percent live past the age of 30. Thus, CF is no longer only a pediatric disease, and internists must be prepared to recognize and treat its many complications. The disease is characterized by chronic airways infection that ultimately leads to bronchiectasis and bronchiolectasis, exocrine pancreatic insufficiency, abnormal sweat gland function, and urogenital dysfunction.

PATHOGENESIS   Genetic basis   CF is an autosomal recessive disease resulting from mutations in a gene located on chromosome 7. The prevalence of CF varies with the ethnic origin of a population. CF is detected in approximately 1 in 2500 live births in the Caucasian population of North America and northern Europe, 1 in 17,000 live births of African-Americans, and 1 in 90,000 live births of the Asian population of Hawaii. The most common mutation in the CF gene is a 3-base-pair deletion that results in an absence of phenylalanine at amino acid position 508 (ΔF_{508}) of the CF gene protein product, known as the CF transmembrane regulator (CFTR). The large number of other mutations identified in the CF gene (>200) makes it unfeasible to use DNA diagnostic technologies for identifying heterozygotes in populations at large, and no physiologic measurements allow heterozygote detection.

CFTR protein (See Fig. 213-4, p. 1151)   The CFTR protein is a single polypeptide chain containing 1480 amino acids that appears to function as a cyclic AMP-regulated Cl^- channel. The fully processed form of CFTR is found in the plasma membrane in normal epithelia (Fig. 222-1). Biochemical studies indicate that the ΔF_{508} mutation leads to improper processing and intracellular degradation of the CFTR protein. Thus absence of CFTR protein at appropriate cellular sites may be a part of the pathophysiology of CF. However, other mutations in the CF gene produce CFTR proteins that are fully processed but are nonfunctional at the appropriate cellular sites.

Epithelial dysfunction (See also Chap. 213)   The epithelia affected by CF exhibit different functions in their native state; i.e., some are volume-absorbing (airways and intestinal epithelia), some are salt-absorbing but not volume-absorbing (sweat duct), whereas others are volume-secretory (pancreas). Given this diverse array of native activities, it should not be surprising that CF produces very different effects on patterns of electrolyte and water transport. However, the unifying concept is that all affected tissues express abnormal cAMP-regulated Cl^- channel activity.

ORGAN-SPECIFIC PATHOPHYSIOLOGY   Lung   The diagnostic biophysical hallmark of CF is the raised transepithelial electric potential difference (PD) detected in airway epithelia. The transepithelial PD reflects components of both the rate of active ion transport and the resistance to ion flow of the superficial epithelium. CF airway epithelia exhibit both raised transport rates (Na^+) and decreased ion permeability (Cl^-) (Fig. 222-2). The Cl^- transport defect appears to be the result of abnormal regulation of Cl^- transport. CF epithelia do not respond to beta-adrenergic agonists or agonists that activate protein kinase C with Cl^- secretion as normal airway epithelia do. This failure to regulate cellular Cl^- transport is a direct consequence of mutations in the CFTR protein. An important observation is that there is an alternative Cl^- channel expressed in airway epithelia. This channel is different from CFTR and is regulated by intracellular Ca^{2+} levels or by extracellular triphosphate nucleotides, e.g., UTP. This channel can substitute for CFTR with regard to net Cl^- transport and may be a potential therapeutic target.

Raised Na^+ absorption is a feature of CF airway epithelia. Na^+ transport abnormalities in CF are not a widespread feature of the

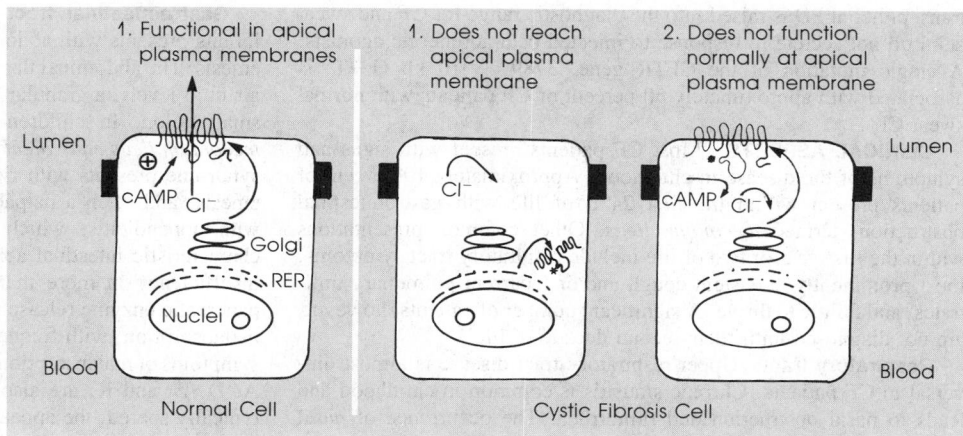

FIGURE 222-1 Cellular metabolism of the CFTR protein. In a normal cell (*left*), CFTR is synthesized in the rough endoplasmic reticulum (RER), glycosylated in the Golgi apparatus, and functions as a Cl^- channel when located in the plasma membrane. Two possible outcomes of mutations in the CF gene are shown (*right*). (1) If a mutation disturbs protein folding, e.g., the ΔF_{508} mutation, CFTR is degraded intracellularly so that no protein is transported to the plasma membrane. (2) With other mutations, the abnormal protein is processed and trafficks to the plasma membrane but functions abnormally at that site.

CF epithelial phenotype and appear confined to volume-absorbing epithelia. The mechanisms for Na^+ hyperabsorption reflect in part an increase in apical cell membrane Na^+ channel activity. It is not yet known how the abnormal CF gene product, CFTR, produces the Na^+ transport defect.

The central hypothesis of CF airways pathophysiology has been that the abnormal Na^+ and Cl^- transport rates produce secretions that are dehydrated and poorly cleared. The unique predisposition of CF airways to chronic infection by *Staphylococcus aureus* and *Pseudomonas aeruginosa* raises the issue that other as yet undefined abnormalities in airway surface liquids also may contribute to the failure of lung defense.

Gastrointestinal tract The gastrointestinal effects of CF are diverse. In the exocrine pancreas, it appears that the absence of the CFTR Cl^- channel in the apical membrane of pancreatic ductal epithelia impairs the function of an apical membrane $Cl^--HCO_3^-$ exchanger to effect net secretion of bicarbonate and Na^+ (by a passive process) into the duct. The failure to secrete $Na^+-HCO_3^-$ and water leads to retention of enzymes in the pancreas and ultimately destruction of virtually all pancreatic tissue. In CF the intestinal epithelium, because of the lack of Cl^- and water secretion, has an impaired ability to flush the secreted mucins and other macromolecules from intestinal crypts. Ultimately, this process can lead to obstruction of both the small and large intestines. In the hepatobiliary system, defective hepatic ductal salt (Cl^-) and water secretion causes retention

of biliary secretions and focal biliary cirrhosis and bile duct proliferation in approximately 25 to 30 percent of CF patients. The inability of the CF gallbladder epithelium to secrete salt and water can lead to both chronic cholecystitis and cholelithiasis.

Sweat gland CF patients secrete nearly normal volumes of sweat into the sweat acinus but are unable to absorb NaCl from sweat as it moves through the sweat duct. The defect in ductal function represents the inability to absorb Cl^- across the Cl^--impermeable CF ductal epithelia.

DIAGNOSIS Because of the large number of CF mutations, DNA analysis is not used for primary diagnosis. The diagnosis of CF rests on a combination of clinical criteria and analyses of sweat Cl^- values. The values for the Na^+ and Cl^- concentration in sweat vary with age, but typically in adults a Cl^- concentration of >70 mEq/L discriminates between CF patients and patients with other lung disease.

It is likely that DNA analyses will be performed increasingly in CF patients. Comprehensive genotype-phenotype relationships have not been established sufficiently for prognosis. A relationship between ΔF_{508} homozygosity and pancreatic insufficiency has been established, but no predictive relationship holds for ΔF_{508} homozygosity and lung disease. DNA diagnosis has not been used for newborn screening of CF patients.

Between 1 and 2 percent of patients with the clinical syndrome of CF have normal sweat Cl^- values. In most of these patients, the nasal

FIGURE 222-2 Comparison of ion transport properties of normal (*left*) and CF (*right*) airway epithelia. The vectors describe routes and magnitudes of Na^+ and Cl^- transport. The normal basal pattern for ion transport is absorption of Na^+ from the lumen via an amiloride-sensitive Na^+ channel. This process is accelerated in CF. The capacity to initiate cAMP-mediated Cl^- secretion

is diminished in CF airway epithelia due to absence/dysfunction of the CFTR Cl^- channel. An alternative Cl^- channel (Cl_a^-), regulated by Ca^{2+} and extracellular nucleotides, is expressed in some but not all epithelia affected by CF. The Na^+, K^+-ATPase that provides the energy for both the Na^+ and Cl^- transport is shown on the basolateral surface.

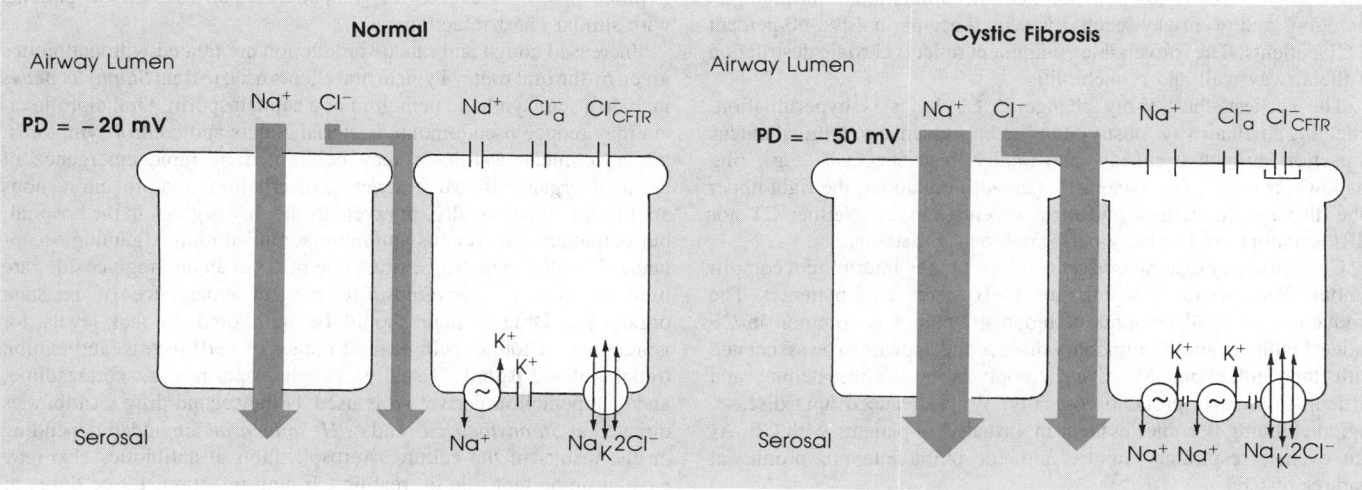

transepithelial PD is raised into the diagnostic range for CF and sweat acini do not secrete in response to injected beta-adrenergic agonists. A single mutation of the CFTR gene, 3789 + 10 kb G→T, is associated with approximately 50 percent of CF patients with normal sweat Cl⁻.

CLINICAL ASPECTS Most CF patients present with signs and symptoms of the disease in childhood. Approximately 10 percent of patients present within the first 24 h of life with gastrointestinal obstruction, termed *meconium ileus*. Other common presentations within the first year or two of life include respiratory tract symptoms, most prominently persistent cough and/or recurrent pulmonary infiltrates, and failure to thrive. A significant number of patients, however, are not diagnosed until their second decade of life.

Respiratory tract Upper respiratory tract disease is almost universal in CF patients. Chronic sinusitis is common in childhood and leads to nasal obstruction and rhinorrhea. The occurrence of nasal polyps approaches 15 to 20 percent and often requires surgery.

In the lower respiratory tract, the first symptom of CF is cough. With time the cough becomes continuous and produces viscous, purulent, often greenish colored sputum. Inevitably, periods of clinical stability are interrupted by "exacerbations," defined by increased cough, weight loss, increased sputum volume, and decrements in pulmonary function. Typically these exacerbations are treated with intravenous antibiotics (see below) with recovery of most lung function. Over the course of years, the exacerbations become more frequent and the recovery of lost lung function less complete, leading to respiratory failure.

CF patients exhibit a characteristic sputum microbiology. *Haemophilus influenzae* and *S. aureus* are often the first organisms recovered from samples of lung secretions in newly diagnosed CF patients. *P. aeruginosa* is typically cultured from lower respiratory tract secretions thereafter. After repetitive antibiotic exposure, *P. aeruginosa*, often in a mucoid form, is usually the predominant organism recovered from sputum and may be present as several strains with different antibiotic sensitivities. *P. cepacia* has been recovered from CF sputum and is pathogenic. Patient-to-patient spread of this organism indicates that infection control in the hospital should be practiced. Other gram-negative rods recovered from CF sputum include *Klebsiella*, *Proteus*, and *Escherichia coli*, also in mucoid forms. Up to 50 percent of CF patients have *Aspergillus fumigatus* in their sputum, and up to 10 percent of these patients exhibit the syndrome of allergic bronchopulmonary aspergillosis. *Mycobacterium tuberculosis* is rare in CF patients. However, 10 to 20 percent of adult CF patients have sputum cultures positive for nontuberculous mycobacteria, and in some patients these microorganisms are associated with disease.

The first lung function abnormalities observed in CF children, increased RV/TLC ratios, suggest that small airways disease is the first functional lung abnormality in CF. As the disease progresses, both reversible and irreversible changes in FVC and FEV_1 are noted. The reversible component reflects accumulation of intraluminal secretions and/or airway reactivity, which occurs in 40 to 60 percent of CF patients. The irreversible component reflects chronic destruction of the airway wall and bronchiolitis.

The earliest chest x-ray change in CF lungs is hyperinflation, reflecting small airways obstruction. Later, evidence of luminal mucus impaction, bronchial cuffing, and finally, bronchiectasis, e.g., ring shadows, is noted. For reasons that are still unknown, the right upper lobe displays the earliest and most severe changes. Neither CT nor MRI scanning are routinely performed on CF patients.

CF pulmonary disease is associated with many intermittent complications. Pneumothorax is common (>10 percent of patients). The production of small amounts of blood in sputum is common in CF patients with advanced pulmonary disease and appears to be associated with lung infection. Massive hemoptysis is life-threatening and difficult to localize bronchoscopically. With advanced lung disease, digital clubbing becomes evident in virtually all patients with CF. As late events, respiratory failure and cor pulmonale are prominent features of CF.

Gastrointestinal tract The syndrome of meconium ileus in infants presents with abdominal distention, failure to pass stool, and emesis. The abdominal flat plate can be diagnostic with small intestinal air fluid levels, a granular appearance representing meconium, and a small colon. In children and young adults, a syndrome termed *meconium ileus equivalent* or distal intestinal obstruction occurs. The syndrome presents with right lower quadrant pain, loss of appetite, emesis, and often a palpable mass. The syndrome can be confused with appendicitis, which occurs frequently in CF patients. The characteristic intestinal abnormalities are complicated by pancreatic insufficiency in more than 90 percent of CF patients. Insufficient pancreatic enzyme release yields the typical pattern of protein and fat malabsorption, with frequent, bulky, foul-smelling stools. Signs and symptoms of malabsorption of fat-soluble vitamins, including vitamins A, D, E, and K, are also noted. Because pancreatic beta cells are typically spared, the appearance of hyperglycemia and a requirement for insulin is a late finding in CF and occurs in only a small percentage of patients.

Genitourinary system Late onset of puberty is common in both males and females with CF. The delayed maturational pattern is likely secondary to the effects of chronic lung disease and inadequate nutrition on reproductive endocrine function. More than 95 percent of male patients with CF are azoospermic, reflecting obliteration of the vas deferens. Twenty percent of CF women are infertile due to effects of chronic lung disease on the menstrual cycle and thick, tenacious cervical mucus that blocks sperm migration. More than 90 percent of completed pregnancies produce viable infants, and CF women are generally able to breast-feed infants normally.

TREATMENT The major objectives of therapy for CF are to promote clearance of secretions and control infection in the lung, provide adequate nutrition, and prevent intestinal obstruction. Ultimately, gene therapy may be the treatment of choice.

Lung disease At present, the techniques for clearing pulmonary secretions are a combination of breathing exercises and chest percussion. A number of pharmacologic agents for increasing mucus clearance are being tested. *N*-Acetyl-cysteine has not been shown to have clinically significant effects on mucus clearance and/or lung function. However, agents that degrade the high concentrations of DNA in CF sputum, e.g., human recombinant DNAse, appear to be effective in decreasing sputum viscosity and increasing airflow during short-term administration. Experimental drugs aimed at restoring salt and water content of secretions, e.g., amiloride and triphosphate nucleotides, appear promising.

More than 95 percent of CF patients die of complications resulting from lung infection. Antibiotics are the principal agents available for treating lung infection, and their use should be guided by sputum culture results. Early intervention with antibiotics is useful, and long courses of treatment are the rule. Because of increased total-body clearance and volume of distribution of antibiotics in CF patients, the required doses are higher for CF patients than for non-CF patients with similar chest infections.

Increased cough and mucus production are treated with antibiotics given by the oral route. Typical oral agents used to treat *Staphylococcus* include a semisynthetic penicillin or a cephalosporin. Oral ciprofloxacin may reduce pseudomonal bacterial counts and control symptoms, but its clinical usefulness may be limited by rapid emergence of resistant organisms. More severe exacerbations require intravenous antibiotics. Traditionally, intravenous therapy is given in the hospital, but outpatient intravenous antibiotic administration is gaining acceptance. Usually, two drugs, often one of them an aminoglycoside, are used to treat *P. aeruginosa* to prevent emergence of resistant organisms. Drug dosage should be monitored so that levels for gentamicin or tobramycin peak at ranges of ~10 μg/mL and exhibit troughs of <2 μg/mL. Usually, a cephalosporin, e.g., ceftazadime, and/or a penicillin derivative is used as the second drug. Antibiotics directed at *Staphylococcus* and/or *H. influenzae* are added depending on the results of the culture. Aerosolization of antibiotics also may have an important role in treating CF lung infection. Large doses of aminoglycosides (600 mg tobramycin twice daily) via aerosol are optimal. Aerosol administration also permits other drugs, e.g., colistin, to be utilized that are ineffective by the intravenous route.

Inhaled beta-adrenergic agonists can be useful to control airways constriction. They achieve a short-term increase in airflow, but long-term benefit has not been shown. Inhaled anticholinergics provide an alternative. Oral steroids are not first-line agents for controlling airways constriction and are of no use in improving the nonreversible component of lung function. Steroids may be useful for treating allergic bronchopulmonary aspergillosis.

A number of pulmonary complications require acute interventions. Atelectasis is best treated with chest physiotherapy and antibiotic therapy. Pneumothoraces involving 10 percent or less of the lung can be observed. The use of chest tubes to expand collapsed, diseased lung often requires long periods of time, and sclerosing agents should be used with caution because of limitations for subsequent lung transplantation. Small-volume hemoptysis requires no specific therapy other than treatment of lung infection and assessment of coagulation and vitamin K status. If massive hemoptysis occurs, bronchial artery embolization can be successful. The most ominous complications of CF are respiratory failure and cor pulmonale. The most effective conventional therapy for these conditions is vigorous medical management of the lung disease. Ultimately, the only effective treatment for respiratory failure in CF is lung transplantation. The 2-year survival for lung transplantation exceeds 50 percent, and deaths in transplant patients result principally from graft rejection, often involving obliterative bronchiolitis. The transplanted lungs do not develop a CF-specific phenotype.

Gastrointestinal disease Maintenance of adequate nutrition is critical for the health of the CF patient. Most (>90 percent) of CF patients benefit from pancreatic enzyme replacement. Capsules generally contain between 4000 and 24,000 units of lipase. The dose of enzymes should be adjusted on the basis of weight gain, abdominal symptomatology, and character of stools. Replacement of fat-soluble vitamins is also required. Hyperglycemia most often becomes manifest in the adult. Principles for treating other causes of nonketotic hyperglycemia should be employed.

For treatment of acute obstruction due to meconium ileus equivalent, megalodiatrizoate or other hypertonic radiocontrast materials delivered by enema to the terminal ileum are utilized. For control of symptoms, adjustment of pancreatic enzymes and the supplementation of intake by salt solutions containing osmotically active agents, e.g., propyleneglycol, are utilized. Hepatic and gallbladder complications are treated as for non-CF patients. End-stage liver disease can be treated by transplantation, which has a 2-year survival rate exceeding 50 percent.

Psychosocial factors CF imposes a tremendous burden on patients. Health insurance, career options, family planning, and life expectancy become major issues, thus assisting patients with the psychosocial adjustments required by CF is critical.

REFERENCES

AITKEN ML et al: Recombinant human DNAse inhalation in normal subjects and patients with cystic fibrosis: A phase 1 study. JAMA 267:1947, 1992

AITKEN ML, FIEL SB: Cystic fibrosis. Dis Mon 39:1, 1993

BEAR CE et al: Purification and functional reconstitution of the cystic fibrosis transmembrane conductance regulator (CFTR). Cell 68:809, 1992

CHENG SH et al: Defective intracellular transport and processing of CFTR is the molecular basis of most cystic fibrosis. Cell 63:827, 1990

HARRIS A, ARGENT BE: The cystic fibrosis gene and its product CFTR. Semin Cell Biol 4:37, 1993

KNOWLES MR et al: Activation by extracellular nucleotides of chloride secretion in the airway epithelia of patients with cystic fibrosis. N Engl J Med 325:533, 1991

O'LOUGHLIN EV et al: Abnormal epithelial transport in cystic fibrosis jejunum. Am J Physiol 260:G758, 1991

SFERRA TJ, COLLINS FS: The molecular biology of cystic fibrosis. Annu Rev Med 44:133, 1993

WALTERS S et al: Demographic and social characteristics of adults with cystic fibrosis in the United Kingdom. Brit Med J 306:549, 1993

223 CHRONIC BRONCHITIS, EMPHYSEMA, AND AIRWAYS OBSTRUCTION

ROLAND H. INGRAM, JR.

Chronic bronchitis and emphysema are two distinct processes, most often present in combination in patients with chronic airways obstruction. The diagnosis of chronic bronchitis is made by history, chronic airways obstruction is assessed physiologically, and emphysema can be diagnosed with certainty in most instances only by histologic examination of sections of whole lung fixed at inflation. Although the relationships among clinical characteristics, physiologic derangements, and morphologic changes have been studied for many years, reasonably certain and uniform clinical criteria are still not available. Definitions and classifications have evolved, but these are not universally accepted. Nonetheless, the following definitions along with brief qualifications and descriptions are currently used by most persons involved in the diagnosis, treatment, and epidemiology of the chronic obstructive airways syndromes.

DEFINITIONS *Chronic bronchitis* is a condition associated with excessive tracheobronchial mucus production sufficient to cause cough with expectoration for at least 3 months of the year for more than 2 consecutive years. Several subclassifications have been proposed. *Simple chronic bronchitis* describes a condition characterized by mucoid sputum production. *Chronic mucopurulent bronchitis* is characterized by persistent or recurrent purulence of sputum in the absence of localized suppurative diseases such as bronchiectasis. Since there may or may not be obstruction as assessed by the use of the forced expiratory vital capacity maneuver, *chronic bronchitis with obstruction* deserves a separate classification. There is a further subset of patients with chronic bronchitis and obstruction who experience severe dyspnea and wheezing in association with inhaled irritants or during acute respiratory infections. Such patients are said to have *chronic infective asthma* or *chronic asthmatic bronchitis*. Since there is considerable but not complete reversibility of airflow obstruction with bronchodilator treatment and abatement of inflammation, and since hyperresponsiveness of airways to nonspecific stimuli is seen in this group of patients, confusion is possible between patients with this condition and those with asthma who may also have *chronic airways obstruction* (Chap. 217). The differentiation is based mainly on the history of the clinical illness. The patient with chronic asthmatic bronchitis has a long history of cough and sputum production with a later onset of wheezing, whereas the asthmatic with chronic obstruction gives a long history of wheezing with later onset of chronic productive cough.

Emphysema is defined as distention of the air spaces distal to the terminal bronchiole with destruction of alveolar septa. *Chronic obstructive lung disease* is defined as a condition in which there is chronic obstruction to airflow due to chronic bronchitis and/or emphysema (see below). Although the degree of obstruction may be less when the patient is free from respiratory infection and may improve somewhat with bronchodilator drugs, significant obstruction is always present.

PREVALENCE Approximately 20 percent of adult males have chronic bronchitis, yet only a minority of these are clinically disabled. According to all surveys, males are more often affected than females. With increased cigarette smoking in women, however, the prevalence of bronchitis in them is increasing. Although cigarette smoking is the single most important etiologic factor, occupational and environmental exposures are now receiving more attention, mainly as additive to the effects of cigarette smoking (Chap. 219).

Although CT scanning can detect emphysema, this tool cannot be used for population screening. Hence the incidence data are derived solely from postmortem surveys. It is rare to find adult lungs completely free of emphysema. There is a distinct increase in the extent of emphysema in the fifth decade, with further increases through the seventh decade and little increase after that. Approximately two-thirds of adult males and one-fourth of females (most without recognized dysfunction) will have well-defined emphysema, which is often limited in extent. Therefore, the majority of those with emphysema will not have had disability or even symptoms associated with it. The situation is analogous to atherosclerosis in that the morphologic changes are far more frequent than the clinical manifestations attributable to the changes.

PATHOLOGY *Chronic bronchitis* is associated with hyperplasia and hypertrophy of the mucus-producing glands found in the submucosa of large cartilaginous airways. Quantitation of this anatomic change, known as the *Reid index*, is based on the ratio of the thickness of the submucosal glands to that of the bronchial wall. In persons without a history of chronic bronchitis, the mean ratio is 0.44 with a standard deviation $\pm$ 0.09, whereas in those with such a history the mean ratio is 0.52 $\pm$ 0.08. Although a low index is *rarely* associated with symptoms and a high index is commonly associated with symptoms during life, there is a great deal of overlap. Therefore, many persons will have morphologic changes in large airways without having had chronic bronchitis.

Perhaps more important than the abnormalities in large airways are the changes often found in the small noncartilaginous airways. Goblet cell hyperplasia, mucosal and submucosal inflammatory cells, edema, peribronchial fibrosis, intraluminal mucus plugs, and increased smooth muscle are characteristic findings in small airways. The frequency of these latter findings in relation to premortem clinical and functional status has not been determined. However, in lungs from patients with chronic obstructive lung disease which have been studied at postmortem, the major site of airflow obstruction has been shown to be in the small airways.

Emphysema is classified according to the pattern of involvement of the gas-exchanging units (acini) of the lung distal to the terminal bronchiole. Although several morphologic patterns have been described, the two most important in the context of this discussion are those involving the respiratory bronchioles and alveolar ducts in the center of the acinus (centriacinar emphysema) and those involving the entire acinus (panacinar emphysema). Quite often both morphologic patterns are present in a single lung of a patient dying from chronic obstructive lung disease, although one type may predominate over the other.

With centriacinar emphysema the distention and destruction are mainly limited to the respiratory bronchiole and alveolar ducts, with relatively less change peripherally in the acinus. Because of the large functional reserve in the lung, many units must be involved in order for overall dysfunction to be detectable. The centrally destroyed regions of the acinus have a high ventilation/perfusion ratio because the capillaries are missing yet ventilation continues. This results in increased wasted ventilation (Vd/Vt), while the peripheral portions of the acinus have crowded and small alveoli with intact, perfused capillaries giving a low ventilation/perfusion ratio. This results in wasted blood flow to give a high alveolar-arterial P_{O_2} difference ($PA_{O_2} - Pa_{O_2}$) (Chap. 214). Mild degrees of centriacinar emphysema, often limited to the lung apices, are extremely common in lungs from persons above age 50 and are practically considered a normal finding.

Panacinar emphysema involves both the central and peripheral portions of the acinus, which results, if the process is extensive, in a reduction of the alveolar-capillary gas exchange surface and loss of elastic recoil properties. When emphysema is severe, it may be difficult to distinguish between the two types which most often coexist in the same lung.

CONTRIBUTORY FACTORS **Smoking** Cigarette smoking is the most commonly identified correlate with both chronic bronchitis during life and extent of emphysema at postmortem. Experimental studies have shown that prolonged cigarette smoking impairs ciliary movement, inhibits function of alveolar macrophages, and leads to hypertrophy and hyperplasia of mucus-secreting glands; massive

exposure in dogs can produce emphysematous changes. In addition to these chronic effects, it is probable that smoke inhibits antiproteases and causes polymorphonuclear leukocytes to release proteolytic enzymes acutely. Inhaled cigarette smoke can produce an acute increase in airways resistance due to vagally mediated smooth-muscle constriction, presumably by way of stimulating submucosal irritant receptors. The relationship of such recurrent episodes of acute bronchial constriction to the development and progression of chronic airways obstruction is uncertain. Recent studies, however, indicate that increased airways responsiveness is associated with more rapid progression in those with chronic airways obstruction.

It is now well established that some young asymptomatic smokers have anatomic and functional changes in small airways without there being a diminution in the forced expiratory volume in 1 s. However, flow rates at or below the mid-vital capacity range are often diminished in persons with mild small-airways obstruction. It has been shown that obstruction of small airways is the earliest demonstrable mechanical defect in young cigarette smokers and that the obstruction may disappear completely after cessation of smoking. Although smoking cessation does not result in complete reversal of more pronounced obstruction, there is a significant slowing of the decline in lung function in all smokers who give up cigarettes. In effect, it is never too late to quit smoking cigarettes.

Not only is cigarette smoking the most common single factor leading to chronic airways obstruction, it also adds to the effects of every other contributory factor to be discussed below.

Air pollution The incidence and mortality rates of both chronic bronchitis and emphysema may be higher in heavily industrialized urban areas. Exacerbations of bronchitis are clearly related to periods of heavy pollution with sulfur dioxide (SO_2) and particulate matter. While nitrogen dioxide (NO_2) can produce small-airways obstruction (bronchiolitis) in experimental animals exposed to high concentrations, there are no data convincingly implicating NO_2, at even the highest pollutant levels, in the pathogenesis or worsening of airways obstruction in humans (Chap. 219).

Occupation Chronic bronchitis is more prevalent in workers who engage in occupations exposing them to either inorganic or organic dusts or to noxious gases. Epidemiologic surveys have succeeded in demonstrating an accelerated decline in lung function in many such workers—e.g., workers in plastics plants exposed to toluene diisocyanate and carding room workers in cotton mills (Chap. 219)—suggesting that their occupational exposure contributes to their future disability.

Infection Morbidity, mortality, and frequency of acute respiratory illnesses are higher in patients with chronic bronchitis. Many attempts have been made to relate these illnesses to infection with viruses, mycoplasmas, and bacteria. However, only the rhinovirus is found more often during exacerbations; that is to say, pathogenic bacteria, mycoplasmas, and viruses other than rhinovirus are found just as often between as during exacerbations. It is intuitively appealing to assign some role to respiratory infections in the pathogenesis and progression of chronic obstructive lung disease, and although this question is under study, there has been no conclusion to date. Epidemiologic studies, however, implicate acute respiratory illness as one of the major factors associated with the etiology as well as the progression of chronic airways obstruction. It has been shown that cigarette smokers may either transitorily develop or worsen small-airways obstruction in association with even mild viral respiratory infections. There is also some evidence that severe viral pneumonia early in life may lead to chronic obstruction, predominantly in small airways.

Familial and genetic factors Familial aggregation of chronic bronchitis has been well demonstrated in the past. Recent surveys have shown that children of smoking parents may experience more frequent and severe respiratory illnesses and have a higher prevalence of chronic respiratory symptoms. In addition, nonsmokers who remain in the presence of cigarette smokers (passive smokers) have increased blood levels of carbon monoxide which indicate that they are significantly exposed to smoke. Another well-documented form of indoor air pollution relates to the use of natural gas for cooking. The role of such pollution, however, remains controversial. Thus a part of the familial aggregation may be related to home air pollution. However, some studies of monozygotic twins have suggested some genetic predisposition to the development of chronic bronchitis independent of personal or familial smoking habits and other indoor air pollution. The exact genetic mode of transmission, if it exists at all, is uncertain.

The protease inhibitor α_1-antitrypsin is an acute-phase reactant, and normally the serum levels rise in association with many inflammatory reactions and with estrogen administration. Either deficient or absent serum levels of α_1-antitrypsin are found in some patients with the early onset of emphysema. By use of the techniques of acid starch gel and immunoelectrophoresis, genetic typing of the protease inhibitor (Pi) types has been possible. Most members of the normal population have two M genes, designated as Pi type MM, and have serum α_1-antitrypsin levels in excess of 2.5 g/L. Several genes are associated with alterations in levels of serum α_1-antitrypsin, but the most common ones associated with emphysema are the Z and S genes. Individuals who are homozygous ZZ or SS have serum levels often near 0 but always less than 0.5 g/L and develop severe panacinar emphysema in the third and fourth decades of life. The panacinar process predominates at the lung bases. Progressive dyspnea with minimal cough characterizes the clinical presentation, although chronic bronchitis is prominent in smokers. Given that α_1-protease inhibitors can be chemically synthesized or biologically produced in significant quantities and can be shown with intravenous infusion to restore the protease-antiprotease balance in liquid lavaged from the lungs of ZZ patients, it has been suggested that replacement therapy with α_1-antitrypsin should be of value in preventing the development of emphysema in these patients. Since replacement therapy was available before efficacy had been assessed, a prospective, randomized trial has not been possible. Through a national registry, a natural history study is underway from which it might be possible to evaluate the effects of therapy if the treated and untreated groups turn out to be sufficiently comparable at entry.

The MZ and MS heterozygotes have intermediate levels of serum α_1-antitrypsin (i.e., between 0.5 and 2.5 g/L); hence the genetic expression is that of an autosomal codominant allele. It is a matter of some controversy whether the heterozygous state is associated with lung function abnormalities. Published studies are in direct conflict on this point, and further data are needed to be certain. The matter is of some importance, since the heterozygous state is common, with incidence estimates varying between 5 and 14 percent of the general population.

The precise way in which antitrypsin deficiency produces emphysema is unclear. In addition to inhibition of trypsin, α_1-antitrypsin is an effective inhibitor of elastase and several other proteolytic enzymes. There is experimental evidence that the structural integrity of lung elastin depends on this antienzyme, which protects the lung from proteases released from leukocytes. It is tempting to speculate that recurrent inflammatory reactions related to infection and pollutants play some role in pathogenesis by calling forth leukocytes whose released proteases are uninhibited and are free to cause the damage.

The role of proteolytic enzymes in the induction of emphysema is not restricted to patients with α_1-antitrypsin deficiency. Evidence is accumulating that proteolytic enzymes derived from neutrophilic leukocytes and alveolar macrophages can produce emphysema even in subjects with normal circulating levels of antiproteases. It is possible that local concentrations of proteolytic enzymes may exceed the inhibitory capacity of antiproteases, that some proteases present are not susceptible to the available antiproteases, or that some of the proteolytic enzymes may be physically inaccessible to the antiprotease activity. The ultimate clinical utility of exogenously produced protease inhibitors currently under development will undoubtedly depend on which of the protease-antiprotease interactions predominates in the production of emphysema. Reduction of endogenous elastase release

from leukocytes in the lung has been achieved by colchicine (0.6 mg/d orally) in a randomized, placebo-controlled trial in ex-smokers with chronic airways obstruction. Current smokers showed no such reductions. An assessment of the clinical efficacy of this inexpensive and nontoxic form of therapy in ex-smokers must await a large, prospective clinical trial.

PATHOPHYSIOLOGY   On the basis of the use of flow rates from forced expiratory vital capacity maneuvers and more sophisticated measures of airways resistance and elastic recoil properties of the lung, it has become clear that both chronic bronchitis and emphysema can exist without evidence of obstruction. However, by the time a patient begins to experience dyspnea as a result of these processes, obstruction is always demonstrable. Since chronic bronchitis and emphysema are usually combined, it might appear fruitless to determine the role of each in producing an individual patient's disability. However, one process may dominate over the other, and to the extent that inflammatory airways disease, secretions, and bronchospasm are present, there are therapeutic possibilities with some hope for improvement. Therefore, it is of value to understand the mechanisms of airways obstruction in order to guide therapy and anticipate results.

Both chronic bronchitis and emphysema result in airways narrowing. In addition to the primary airways processes of chronic bronchitis, loss of elastic recoil of the lung in emphysema accounts for a decrease in airways caliber through loss of radial traction on airways. Narrowing of airways is often associated with both an increase in airways resistance and a diminution in maximal expiratory flow rates.

There are occasions in which a normal or only slightly elevated airways resistance is accompanied by low maximal expiratory flow rates. Under such circumstances, an increase in the dynamic collapsibility of intrathoracic airways during forced exhalation is a possible explanation. Also in this context, the elastic recoil pressure of the lung must be considered in a slightly different way. In addition to providing radial support to airways during quiet breathing, the elastic recoil properties of the lung serve as a major determinant of maximal expiratory flow rates. The static recoil pressure of the lung is the difference between alveolar and intrapleural pressure. During forced exhalations, when alveolar and intrapleural pressures are high, there are points in the airway at which bronchial pressure equals pleural pressure. Flow does not increase with higher pleural pressure after these points become fixed so that the effective driving pressure between alveoli and such points is the elastic recoil pressure of the lung (Fig. 223-1). Hence maximal expiratory flow rates represent a complex and dynamic interplay between airways caliber, elastic recoil pressures, and collapsibility of airways. As a direct consequence of the altered pressure-airflow relationships, the work of breathing is increased in bronchitis and emphysema. Since flow-resistive work is flow rate–dependent, there is a disproportionate increase in the work of breathing with increased ventilation.

The designated subdivisions of the lung volume outlined in Chap. 214 are abnormal to varying degrees in both bronchitis and emphysema. The residual volume (RV) and functional residual capacity (FRC) are almost always higher than normal. Since the normal FRC is the volume at which the inward recoil of the lung is balanced by the outward recoil of the chest wall, loss of elastic recoil of the lung would clearly result in a higher static FRC. In addition, prolongation of expiration in association with obstruction would lead to a dynamic increase in FRC if inspiration is initiated before the respiratory system reaches its static balance point. Elevations of total lung capacity (TLC) are frequent. The exact cause is uncertain, but increases in TLC are often found in association with decreases in the elastic recoil of the lung. The vital capacity is frequently decreased, yet significant airways obstruction can be present with a normal to near-normal vital capacity.

The consequences of the airways and parenchymal processes are far more extensive than just the mechanical alterations discussed above. Maldistribution of inspired gas and blood flow is always

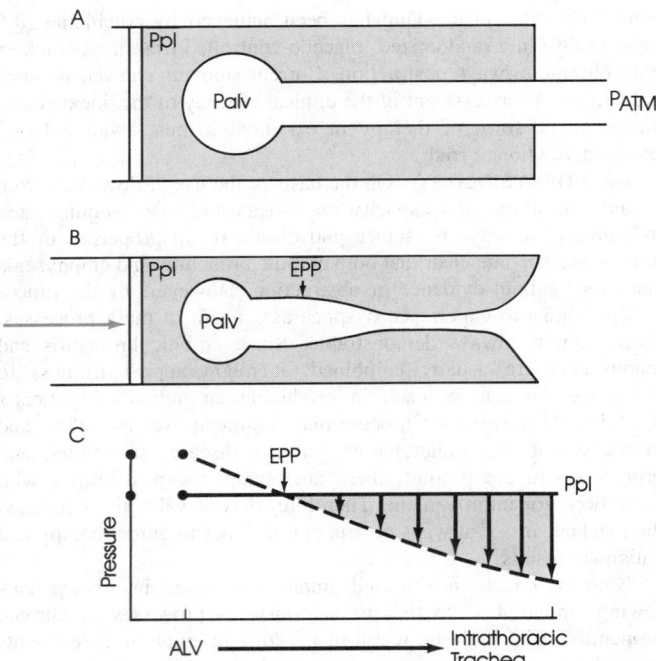

FIGURE 223-1 *A.* A schematic diagram of the lung and intrathoracic airways with no airflow. The alveolar pressure (Palv) is greater than pleural pressure (Ppl) by an amount equal to the elastic recoil pressure of the lung (Pel)—i.e., Palv is the algebraic sum of Ppl + Pel. With no airflow Palv = P atmospheric, and for all of the intrathoracic airways, pressure outside is less than the pressure inside due to the Pel. *B.* The same schematic lung during forced exhalation when pleural pressure becomes quite positive. Palv is still greater than Ppl by an amount equal to Pel. However, there is a pressure drop along the airway associated with flow, and at some point Ppl equals local bronchial pressure (so-called equal pressure point, EPP). Mouthward from this point, Ppl exceeds local bronchial pressure and hence acts to compress the airways. *C.* Pressure within the airways from alveoli to the intrathoracic trachea is shown as a dashed line (---) and Ppl is shown as a constant (———). Therefore, the driving pressure from alveoli to EPP is equal to Pel, and a decrease in Pel (i.e., loss of elastic recoil) would mean a smaller driving pressure and smaller flow rates.

present to some extent. When the mismatching is severe, impairment of gas exchange is reflected in abnormalities of arterial blood gases. There are regions of the lung with ventilation in excess of perfusion which increase the wasted ventilation ratio (that is, Vd/Vt; Chap. 214). At a normal resting CO_2 production, the net effective alveolar ventilation, as reflected by the arterial P_{CO_2}, may be excessive, normal, or insufficient depending on the relationship of the overall minute volume to the wasted ventilation ratio. The net contribution of regions with perfusion in excess of ventilation can be assessed by either estimating or measuring the alveolar-arterial P_{O_2} difference (that is, $PA_{O_2} - Pa_{O_2}$; Chap. 214). In chronic bronchitis and emphysema, there are some degree increases in both wasted ventilation and wasted blood flow.

The clinical manifestations depend, in large part, on the ventilatory response to the disordered lung function. Some patients, at the cost of extremely high effort of breathing and chronic dyspnea, will maintain a strikingly increased minute volume, which results both in a normal to low arterial P_{CO_2}, despite the high Vd/Vt, and a relatively high arterial P_{O_2}, despite the high difference, $PA_{O_2} - Pa_{O_2}$. Other patients with only modest increases in effort of breathing and less dyspnea will maintain a normal to only moderately elevated minute volume at the cost of accepting a high arterial P_{CO_2} and a severely depressed arterial P_{O_2}.

Factors which account for clear differences in ventilatory responses between patients have been studied and debated for years. The bulk of available evidence suggests that those patients who maintain relatively normal or low arterial P_{CO_2} levels are those with an increased ventilatory drive relative to their blood gas values and those who chronically maintain high arterial P_{CO_2} and lower P_{O_2} levels have a diminished ventilatory drive in relation to their more severely deranged blood gas values. It is not at all certain whether individual differences are accounted for by variations in peripheral or central chemoreceptor sensitivity or through other afferent pathways. Perhaps of more immediate value is the fact that patients with predominant emphysema are either normally or excessively responsive both to hypercapnia and to exercise, whereas those with predominant bronchitis are less responsive to both, despite similar degrees of airways obstruction by spirometry.

The pulmonary circulation malfunctions not only in terms of regional distribution of blood flow but in terms of abnormal overall pressure-flow relationships. There is often mild to severe pulmonary hypertension at rest with further increases disproportionate to cardiac output elevations during exercise. A reduction in the total cross-sectional area of the pulmonary vascular bed can be attributed to anatomic changes and constriction of vascular smooth muscle in pulmonary arteries and arterioles as well as destruction of alveolar septa with loss of capillaries. Rarely does loss of capillaries alone lead to severe pulmonary hypertension with cor pulmonale, except as a near-terminal event. Of more importance is the constriction of pulmonary vessels in response to alveolar hypoxia. The constriction is reversible upon increase in alveolar P_{O_2} with therapy. There is a synergism between hypoxia and acidosis which assumes importance during episodes of acute or chronic respiratory insufficiency. Chronic hypoxia leads not only to pulmonary vascular constriction but also to secondary erythrocytosis. The latter, although not proved to be a significant contributor to pulmonary hypertension, could add an unfavorable rheologic load. As discussed in Chap. 204, the chronic afterload on the right ventricle leads to hypertrophy and, in association with disordered blood gases, ultimately to failure.

CLINICAL-FUNCTIONAL CORRELATIONS   Dyspnea and impairment of physical work capacity are characteristic only of severe to moderately severe airways obstruction. There is considerable variation among patients, and those with predominant emphysema have greater dyspnea and restriction of physical activity with lesser degrees of obstruction than those in whom chronic bronchitis predominates. The majority of patients have functionally mixed disease, will usually experience exertional dyspnea when the forced expiratory volume in 1 s (FEV_1) falls below 50 percent of that predicted, and will have dyspnea at rest when the FEV_1 is less than 25 percent of that predicted. In addition to dyspnea at rest, carbon dioxide retention and cor pulmonale frequently occur when the FEV_1 falls to 25 percent of that predicted. However, those with predominant bronchitis often have carbon dioxide retention and cor pulmonale with FEV_1 values above 25 percent of normal, in contrast to patients with predominant emphysema, whose FEV_1 usually falls well below that level before the onset of carbon dioxide retention and cor pulmonale. With a respiratory infection, small changes in the degree of obstruction can make a large difference in symptoms and gas exchange. Thus small therapeutic gains have rewarding results.

In general, the more severe the obstruction, the poorer the prognosis. Despite the general relationship, 20 to 30 percent of patients with severe obstruction and carbon dioxide retention will survive beyond 5 years.

CLINICAL SYNDROMES   It is clear that the clinical presentation can vary in severity from simple chronic bronchitis without disability to the severely disabled state with chronic respiratory failure. From a practical standpoint, it is well to consider that any symptom or any measurable abnormality may foreshadow the development of severe disabling disease; hence cessation of smoking and avoidance of environmental irritants and toxins are to be advised. However, the advice to modify behavior and life patterns is rarely taken, and most physicians are called on to categorize and treat patients with fully developed, chronic airways obstruction. Thus the approach taken here is to describe two polar opposite types of fully developed, chronic

TABLE 223-1 Chronic obstructive lung disease: Salient features of the two types

	Predominant emphysema	Predominant bronchitis
Age at time of diagnosis, y	60±	50±
Dyspnea	Severe	Mild
Cough	After dyspnea starts	Before dyspnea starts
Sputum	Scanty, mucoid	Copious, purulent
Bronchial infections	Less frequent	More frequent
Respiratory insufficiency episodes	Often terminal	Repeated
Chest film	"Hyperinflation" ± bullous changes, small heart	Increased bronchovascular markings at bases, large heart
Chronic Pa_{CO_2}, mmHg	35–40	50–60
Chronic Pa_{O_2}, mmHg	65–75	45–60
Hematocrit, %	35–45	50–55
Pulmonary hypertension:		
Rest	None to mild	Moderate to severe
Exercise	Moderate	Worsens
Cor pulmonale	Rare, except terminally	Common
Elastic recoil	Severely decreased	Normal
Resistance	Normal to slight increase	High
Diffusing capacity	Decreased	Normal to slight decrease

obstructive pulmonary disease with the realization that the majority of patients will have some features of both types. The salient features of each type are outlined in Table 223-1.

Predominant emphysema These patients often give a long history of exertional dyspnea with minimal cough which is productive of only small amounts of mucoid sputum. Mucopurulent exacerbations in association with infections are not frequent. The body build is asthenic with evidence of weight loss. The patient appears distressed with obvious use of accessory muscles of respiration which serve to lift the sternum in an anterosuperior direction with each inspiration. There is tachypnea with a relatively prolonged expiration through pursed lips, or expiration is begun with a grunting sound. While sitting, these patients often lean forward, extending the arms to brace themselves. The neck veins may be distended during expiration, yet they collapse briskly with inspiration. The lower intercostal spaces retract with each inspiration, and by palpation the lower lateral chest wall can be felt to move inward. The percussion note is hyperresonant, and by auscultation the breath sounds are diminished, with faint, high-pitched rhonchi heard toward the end of expiration. The cardiac impulse, if at all visible, is seen only in the xiphoid and subxiphoid regions, and cardiac dullness is either absent or severely reduced. By palpation there is frequently a sustained forward and downward right ventricular impulse in the subxiphoid region, and a presystolic gallop accentuated during inspiration is commonly heard.

The arterial P_{O_2} is often in the mid-70s (mmHg), and the P_{CO_2} is low to normal. Because of the maintained increase in minute volume and the maintenance of arterial P_{O_2} sufficient to nearly saturate hemoglobin, these patients have been referred to as "pink puffers." Their increased ventilatory drive probably accounts for their relatively preserved oxygenation and lack of hypercapnia; however, this increased drive with attendant increases in ventilation undoubtedly contributes to the severity of their dyspnea.

The TLC and RV are invariably increased, the vital capacity is low, and the maximal expiratory flow rates are diminished. The elastic recoil properties of the lung are severely impaired, and in direct proportion to this impairment, the capacity of the lung to transfer carbon monoxide is lowered.

On radiographic examination the diaphragms are low and flattened, the bronchovascular shadows do not extend to the periphery of the lung, and the cardiac silhouette is lengthened and narrowed. These findings in association with a large retrosternal translucency on lateral

chest radiographs are interpreted as hyperinflation, which correlates well with increases in TLC and loss of elastic recoil. Peripheral attenuation of bronchovascular markings and increased retrosternal lucency correlate best with subsequent postmortem demonstration of extensive and severe emphysema which is predominantly of the panacinar type. Computed tomography (CT) has been shown to localize and quantitate emphysema. However, determining the localization of such regions most often is of little practical value, and the overall quantitative assessments from elastic recoil properties and carbon monoxide transfer are just as good. Hence CT scans are not ordinarily employed for this purpose.

It is fortunate that the patient with predominant emphysema is less prone to mucopurulent relapses than is the patient with predominant bronchitis, since such relapses frequently lead to severe respiratory failure and death. That is to say, right-sided heart failure and hypercapnic respiratory failure are often terminal events in those patients with predominant emphysema. In the absence of such relapses, the clinical course is characterized by severe and progressive dyspnea for which little can be done. The physician's role is to seek out and treat any factor that is possibly reversible and strive to avoid pollutants and infections.

Predominant bronchitis The patient with predominant bronchitis usually has an impressive history of cough and sputum production for many years with an immodest history of cigarette smoking. Initially the cough is present only in the winter months, and the patient is apt to seek medical attention, if at all, only during the more severe of the frequent mucopurulent relapses. Over the years the cough progresses from hibernal to perennial, and mucopurulent relapses increase in frequency, duration, and severity. After beginning to experience exertional dyspnea, the patient often seeks medical help and will be found to have a severe degree of obstruction. Occasionally, such a patient will seek out a physician only after the onset of peripheral edema secondary to overt right ventricular failure. More rarely the initial medical contact is made by family members who present the physician with a deeply cyanotic, edematous, and stuporous patient with acute respiratory insufficiency.

The patient with predominant bronchitis is often overweight and cyanotic. There is usually no apparent distress at rest, the respiratory rate is normal or only slightly increased, and there is no apparent usage of accessory muscles. The chest percussion note is normally resonant, and by auscultation, one can usually hear coarse rhonchi and wheezes which change in location and intensity after a deep and productive cough. There may be a sustained heave along the lower left sternal border which indicates right ventricular hypertrophy. In the presence of right ventricular failure there are often an early diastolic gallop and occasionally a holosystolic murmur, both of which are accentuated by inspiration. The latter finding is indicative of functional tricuspid regurgitation which is frequently accompanied by neck vein distention characterized by large *v* waves and brisk *y* descents. With right ventricular failure the cyanosis deepens and peripheral edema becomes prominent. Clubbing of the digits is unusual.

With or without right ventricular failure, the minute volume is only slightly increased due to an overall diminution in ventilatory drive which modulates the level of dyspnea. However, failure to increase minute volume greatly in the face of significant proportions of wasted ventilation and blood flow results in severely deranged arterial blood gases, with arterial P_{CO_2} values which are chronically increased to the range of the high 40s to low 50s (mmHg). The lowered P_{O_2} produces desaturation of hemoglobin, serves to stimulate erythropoiesis, and results in hypoxic pulmonary vasoconstriction. Desaturation and erythrocytosis combine to produce the cyanosis, and hypoxic pulmonary vasoconstriction accentuates the right-sided heart failure. Because of cyanosis and edema secondary to heart failure, such patients have been referred to as "blue bloaters." It has been proposed, with some supporting data, that one of the pathophysiologic events in blue bloaters is the occurrence of repeated episodes of severe nocturnal oxygen desaturation in association with episodes of sleep apnea or periods of worsening hypoventilation. Such sleep-related ventilatory events worsen the degree of pulmonary hypertension and secondary erythrocytosis.

The TLC is often normal, and there is a moderate elevation of RV. The vital capacity is mildly diminished, and maximal expiratory flow rates are invariably low. The elastic recoil properties of the lung are normal or only slightly impaired, and the capacity of the lung to transfer carbon monoxide is either normal or minimally decreased.

On radiographic examination the diaphragms are well rounded, the bronchovascular markings are increased in the lower lung fields, and the cardiac silhouette is somewhat enlarged. In association with right ventricular failure the cardiac silhouette enlarges further, pulmonary arteries become more prominent, and an antigravity distribution of perfusion is apparent.

Despite well-planned management (see below) the patient with predominant bronchitis may experience many episodes of respiratory failure from which recovery is frequent with proper therapy (see later). The ability to recover from such repeated episodes in these patients is in striking contrast to the frequently fatal outcome of such events in those with predominant emphysema. Ultimately, the lungs at postmortem will be found to have severe bronchitic changes in both large and small airways and only moderate emphysema, predominantly of the centriacinar variety.

It should be reemphasized that the preceding syndromes are described as polar ends of a continuous spectrum of clinical features. Hence most patients will have some characteristics of each syndrome. Recognizing and understanding the pathophysiologic bases for these aids in the planning of appropriate management strategies for each patient.

PRINCIPLES OF MANAGEMENT   Intelligent management must be based on as complete knowledge as possible of the degree of obstruction, the extent of disability, and the relative reversibility of the patient's illness. To the extent that obstructive processes in the airways are contributory, there is a chance for treatment to be effective. Since emphysema is an irreversible process, prevention of progression and avoidance of acute insults constitute the main approach. History, physical examination, and chest radiographs should be supplemented by tests of lung function performed during a symptomatically stable period. Ideally, complete spirometry, plethysmographic lung volumes, transfer of carbon monoxide, arterial blood gases, and lung elastic recoil properties should be measured. Spirometry and lung volumes should be remeasured after the administration of bronchodilators in order to assess the degree of acutely reversible airways obstruction. Failure to see an acute change with bronchodilator drugs does not rule out the possibility of improvement with more prolonged administration of these agents. In instances in which the degree of exertional dyspnea appears to be disproportionately greater than the degree of obstruction, measurements of blood gases, minute volume, CO_2 production, and O_2 consumption during exercise are indicated in order to determine whether impaired lung function is sufficient to account for the symptoms. After the initial assessment, the physician has some idea of the relative emphasis to be placed on patient education, rehabilitative and preventive measures, and direct therapeutic interventions in management of the patient and the illness.

Smoking and the environment   Cessation of smoking is the only certain means of influencing the progression of the chronic obstructive airways syndromes, and although such behavior modification is most effective at early stages of the disease processes, it is effective in slowing the rate of decline in lung function, even when such function is severely compromised. In the instances in which occupational or environmental exposures are thought to play a significant role, change of occupation or relocation of dwelling is advisable. The validity of such advice should be considered carefully, since the impact on both the patient and the family is likely to be great. A simpler environmental change is that of eliminating aerosol sprays such as deodorants, hair sprays, and insecticides from the household. Hair sprays have been shown to produce acute airways responses even in normal subjects.

Other preventive measures include yearly vaccination against the common or expected influenza virus strains. The patient need be given pneumococcal polysaccharide vaccine only once in a lifetime due to prolonged effectiveness of the immune response. However, if an earlier vaccine was used that contained only 14 capsular antigen types, revaccination with the current 23-valent vaccine is probably advisable.

Respiratory infections   Infections cannot be totally avoided, and the patient should be made aware that increasing purulence, viscosity, or volume of secretions signals the onset of an infection which should be treated early. The most common pathogenic bacteria found are *Haemophilus influenzae* and *Streptococcus pneumoniae*. As mentioned above, however, the role of such bacteria is in question, since they are just as often isolated during periods of relative clinical quiescence. Nonetheless, a broad-spectrum antibiotic should be given for a 7- to 10-day course. It is practical to have the patient keep a 7- to 10-day supply of antibiotics at home and to begin treatment at the onset of symptoms. In Great Britain it is common practice to give continuous antibiotic therapy during winter months in order to prevent mucopurulent relapses. Although there is evidence that viruses are frequent causes of mucopurulent relapses, clinical studies have shown that the standard antibiotic regimens decrease the duration and severity of infective episodes unrelated to culturable bacterial pathogens. Microscopic examination and culture of sputum are indicated if there are chills, fever, or chest pain or if purulence fails to respond to usually administered antibiotics.

Exercise and nutrition   It has been shown repeatedly that exercise programs, although not accompanied by measurable improvement in lung function, result in increased exercise tolerance and an improved sense of well-being. The improvement is usually task-specific, so most physicians advise walking in preference to the use of special apparatus, such as stationary bicycles. Arm exercise is poorly tolerated; the necessary muscles required for breathing are also recruited for the exercise task and hence are doing double duty.

If malnutrition (body weight less than 85 percent of ideal) is present, oral dietary supplements can result in improved muscle strength, less fatigability, and lessening of breathlessness. A carefully taken dietary history and elimination of other serious causes for low body weight and weight loss should precede the start of any major nutritional supplement effort. As with exercise programs, there is not a direct and measurable effect on lung function from treating malnutrition, yet subjective relief and objective improvement in strength and exercise performance have been of great benefit in such patients.

Bronchodilator drugs   These are often quite helpful in alleviating symptoms, especially in those patients who respond to them acutely in the laboratory. These drugs form three categories: the methylxanthines, sympathomimetics with strong beta$_2$-adrenergic-stimulating properties, and anticholinergics. The ethylene diamine salt of theophylline (aminophylline), the most commonly used methylxanthine, can be given orally or parenterally; in addition to bronchodilatation, it stimulates respiration and has cardiotonic and diuretic properties. Oral theophylline preparations vary greatly in their intestinal release and rate of absorption. There is extreme variability in rates of absorption, degradation, and secretion among patients. In those patients who, with standard doses, either fail to benefit or show signs of toxicity, theophylline blood levels should be measured. Measurements at expected peak absorption and just before the subsequent dose will allow adjustment of dose. Blood levels between 10 and 20 mg/L should be maintained. Side effects such as insomnia and nervousness are frequent when levels are in the therapeutic range. Nausea, vomiting, tachyarrhythmias, and seizures are seen mainly when blood levels exceed 20 mg/L. Parenteral administration of theophylline is rarely indicated in the chronic obstructive syndromes, except during episodes of respiratory failure, when agents cannot be given orally. Selective beta$_2$-stimulating drugs such as albuterol and metaproterenol can be given both orally and by aerosol with fewer cardiac side effects than are experienced with isoproterenol. Orally and parenterally administered beta$_2$ agonists are effective but are associated with greater tremulousness and cardiovascular side effects than result from inhaled agents. The latter can be most conveniently given in metered-dose inhalers at two to four puffs four to six times a day. Collecting chambers or spacers may improve the reliability of deposition of these agents. Anticholinergic agents such as atropine have been avoided in the past because of their tendency to desiccate secretions; however, ipratropium bromide, an anticholinergic agent in metered-dose inhaler form, is an effective bronchodilator in chronic bronchitic patients. It is considered by many to be the bronchodilator of choice for these patients.

Corticosteroids   The use of systemic glucocorticoids is, at our present state of knowledge, based on very little scientific data from properly controlled clinical trials. Since these agents have time- and dose-related side effects that vary from deleterious to catastrophic, the almost invariable subjective benefit must be supported by objective measurements. There is little room for doubt in the minds of physicians that some patients respond well, even dramatically, to these agents in both objective and subjective terms. The real problem is how to select those patients most likely to benefit. Eosinophilia in the sputum, rather than in the blood, appears in some instances to identify that subgroup in advance. However, the best guidelines are, first, to try these agents only after maximal bronchodilator and bronchopulmonary drainage measures have been tried without success; second, to begin prednisone 30 mg once per day; third, to confirm the objective change in terms of spirometry and gas exchange, stopping these agents if no objective benefit is seen; and fourth, to decrease to the smallest dose that will maintain the improved level of function. The role, if any, of inhaled glucocorticoid agents for these patients, in contrast to asthmatic patients, has not been established in the syndromes with chronic obstruction.

Bronchopulmonary drainage should be maintained in patients with hypersecretion. If the coughing mechanism is ineffective or if paroxysms of coughing are exhausting, postural drainage is often a useful adjunct. Although liquefaction of secretions by means of orally administered expectorants or aerosol delivery of mucolytic agents is an appealing idea, it has never been shown by properly designed trials to be more effective than simple maintenance of total-body hydration.

Intermittent positive pressure breathing (IPPB) devices were formerly advocated for home management. The various rationales included diminution in the work of breathing, promotion of broncho-pulmonary drainage, and more efficient delivery of bronchodilator drugs. The first of the rationales has been shown to have no basis in fact, and the goals of the last two have been shown to be as well accomplished by postural drainage and use of less elaborate aerosol generators. Hence the use of IPPB for home management cannot be justified.

Treatment of hypoxia and erythrocytosis   When arterial hypoxia is persistent and severe (Pa$_{O_2}$ of 55 to 60 mmHg) in association with cor pulmonale (see Chap. 204) and signs of right heart failure, continuous oxygen therapy is indicated. If the Pa$_{O_2}$ is persistently < 55 mmHg, with or without cor pulmonale, continuous oxygen supplementation also should be prescribed. The available data indicate that supplemental oxygen improves both exercise tolerance and neuropsychological function and alleviates pulmonary hypertension and right heart failure. In patients with severe hypoxemia, the need for hospitalization occurs less frequently and life span is lengthened by the use of supplemental oxygen.

Since most patients with chronic airways obstruction, especially those with features of predominant bronchitis, can be shown to decrease their Pa$_{O_2}$ values significantly during sleep, most prominently during the REM phase, nocturnal oxygen administration has been suggested. While the rationale is clear and the results quite good, a cooperative clinical trial that compared nocturnal with continuous O$_2$ supplementation in severely hypoxic patients found that continuous O$_2$ administration was associated with a significantly lower mortality rate. Patients in both treatment groups experienced neuropsychological

and hemodynamic benefits. Thus supplemental nocturnal oxygen is better than none, but continuous oxygen is better than nocturnal in such severely ill patients. Those patients not requiring continuous oxygen therapy may require supplementation during air travel. Even with modern pressurization, cabin altitudes may reach the equivalent of 8000 ft, at which the Pa$_{O_2}$ may fall by 25 mmHg below that found at sea level. Hence oxygen supplementation during prolonged flights should be considered for patients with sea level Pa$_{O_2}$ values in the mid-70s.

Secondary erythrocytosis with the hematocrit in excess of 50 percent is most easily viewed as a mechanism allowing greater oxygen delivery to compensate for the chronically lowered arterial P$_{O_2}$; hence improvement in oxygenation through improved lung function or by oxygen administration is the most physiologic means to reverse erythrocytosis. Since erythrocytosis results in elevation of blood viscosity at all shear rates, the proposal has been made that pulmonary vascular hypertension is aggravated by its presence. Although no study has demonstrated an objective improvement in hemodynamics, lung mechanics, or gas exchange at rest following phlebotomy, ventilatory and cardiovascular function during exercise improve. Some patients who complain of headaches and a sense of head fullness show a favorable subjective response to periodic phlebotomy when the hematocrit is in excess of 55 percent. In support of this subjective improvement is the demonstration that, following phlebotomy, cerebral blood flow, previously diminished, returns toward normal.

Other measures   Despite employing all the foregoing measures, some patients remain severely incapacitated. For these patients, lung transplantation can return them to both a functional and comfortable state (see Chap. 232). Criteria for transplanting such patients are being evolved in the several centers performing this procedure. Medical directors of such programs should be consulted if the possibility of a lung transplant is being considered.

There are two therapeutic interventions well short of lung transplantation that have been proposed repeatedly by a few investigators and that remain extremely controversial. It cannot be denied that some supporting data exist; the counterintuitive nature of the interventions and the absence of controlled trials preclude their wide acceptance. These are (1) bilateral carotid body resection and (2) periodic use of negative pressure ventilation. The initial rationale for bilateral carotid body resection was to relieve dyspnea by diminishing the ventilatory responsiveness to hypoxemia and hypercapnia, which would present its own set of dangers. Several studies have shown improved lung mechanics and exercise performance after the procedure. Use of negative pressure ventilation for periods up to 8 h/d for 2 consecutive days has been shown to improve gas exchange, muscle strength, and ventilatory responsiveness for several subsequent days.

ACUTE RESPIRATORY FAILURE

DIAGNOSIS   Although it may be strongly suspected on clinical grounds, the firm diagnosis of acute respiratory failure in chronic airways obstruction is based on measurements of arterial blood gas (Pa$_{O_2}$, Pa$_{CO_2}$) and pH values that must be interpreted in relation to the patient's chronic status. Since many patients will have chronically lowered Pa$_{O_2}$ levels and increased Pa$_{CO_2}$ values, the diagnosis is based on the degree of change from the usual state of the individual patient. With regard to oxygenation, an acute decrease in Pa$_{O_2}$ from a usual mid-70 range to the low 60s (mmHg) is just as indicative of acute respiratory failure as is an acute drop from a chronic mid-50 range to the mid-40s (mmHg). Thus a drop in Pa$_{O_2}$ equal to or greater than 10 to 15 mmHg indicates acute failure.

Since renal compensation for chronic hypercapnia results in adjustment of arterial pH to near-normal values, the acuteness of the increase in Pa$_{CO_2}$ can often be judged by the pH, unless there is a concomitant metabolic acidemia. As a practical guide, any level of hypercapnia associated with an arterial pH value less than 7.30 should be considered as acute respiratory failure.

PRECIPITATING FACTORS Increases in volume, viscosity, and/or purulence of secretions, presumably due to infection of the tracheobronchial tree, are the most common antecedents of acute respiratory failure in chronic obstructive lung disease. Increasing airways obstruction with airways inflammation and secretion, especially in association with a relatively blunted ventilatory drive, leads to worsening hypoxia and increasing CO_2 retention. Agitation, insomnia, and increasing dyspnea with impending respiratory failure are occasionally treated, mistakenly, with either sedatives or narcotics, and these, too, may precipitate frank respiratory failure. In fact, depressant drugs which impair ventilatory drive should be avoided at all times in patients with severe chronic obstructive lung disease. Major episodes of air pollution also can lead to respiratory failure, and the physicians responsible for patients with severe bronchitis and emphysema should be alert to these environmental events.

Pneumonia, thromboembolism, left ventricular failure, and pneumothorax occasionally precipitate acute respiratory failure and are extremely difficult to detect unless considered and specifically sought. As a minimum, chest radiographs, electrocardiograms, and sputum examinations should be obtained in addition to arterial blood gas measurements in all patients with respiratory failure.

TREATMENT OF RESPIRATORY FAILURE The treatment of respiratory failure consists of two simultaneous processes: (1) maintaining acceptable levels of oxygenation and ventilation and (2) treatment of infection, removal of secretions, and reversal of any airways constriction present.

Management of hypoxia These patients *need* oxygen when they are severely hypoxic, and while fears of respiratory depression due to the removal of the hypoxic respiratory stimulus are realistic, O_2 must be used, yet in the smallest concentration possible, to give a Pa_{O_2} in the mid-50 range while the patient's Pa_{CO_2}, pH, and clinical status are carefully monitored. It is best to begin with only modest increases in FI_{O_2} to approximately 0.24 (cf. air at 0.21), which can be accomplished using nasal prongs with O_2 flows at 1 to 2 L/min or, more precisely, with the use of a 0.24 Venturi mask. These latter masks, based on Bernoulli's principle, deliver a fixed concentration of O_2 irrespective of the O_2 flow rate by entraining air in direct proportion to O_2 flow rate. They are high-flow masks (oxygen plus air entrained from the room), each designed for a specific FI_{O_2} (0.24, 0.28, 0.35, 0.40). Even small increases in Pa_{O_2} when starting from low levels result in significant increases in arterial oxygen content due to the shape of the oxygen-hemoglobin saturation curve over this range (Chap. 302).

With improved oxygenation some patients will concomitantly increase their Pa_{CO_2} values. The standard explanation has been that this increase is due to the removal of the hypoxic drive to ventilation leading to further hypoventilation. While this is the most important mechanism, recent data indicate that worsening ventilation-perfusion relationships (Chap. 214) occur with O_2 treatment. This is attributed to reversal of hypoxic pulmonary arterial constriction in the more initially hypoxic, less well ventilated regions, which in turn leads to decreased perfusion of initially less hypoxic, better ventilated regions. The result is an increase in the wasted ventilation ratio (Vd/Vt; Chap. 214) leading to a smaller effective alveolar ventilation. In either case, the FI_{O_2} should be increased as little as possible to achieve a Pa_{O_2} in the mid-50 range. Some increase in Pa_{CO_2} can be expected and should not cause alarm if the patient is alert. The majority of patients can be managed in this conservative way with excellent results. However, occasionally, large increases in Pa_{CO_2} occur and lead to stupor and coma. This can be explained by CO_2-induced cerebral vascular dilatation with increased intracranial pressure, including the development of papilledema, combined with the effect of hypercapnia and hypoxia on cerebral function. It must be emphasized that if stupor and coma supervene, stopping the administration of oxygen is the *worst possible* course of action. When CO_2 narcosis is present, respirations are sufficiently depressed from the CO_2 itself that the patient will no longer respond to the rapidly worsening hypoxia, and fatal arrhythmias, generalized seizures, and death may ensue. The

only alternative is to intubate the trachea and provide mechanical ventilatory support. Mechanical ventilators are described in Chap. 231.

Once mechanical ventilation has been instituted, the tidal volume and frequency should be set to decrease gradually the Pa_{CO_2} only down to the chronically elevated level rather than attempt to decrease it to or below a normal value. Since such patients have renal compensation for their chronic hypercapnia, Pa_{CO_2} values at or below the normal level result in significant alkalemia which in turn can lead to severe tachyarrhythmias and generalized seizures.

Control of infection, bronchoconstriction, and secretions As mentioned above, maintaining oxygenation and ventilation serves to buy time while secretion removal, bronchial dilatation, and treatment of infection are instituted. Removal of secretions is accomplished by urging the patient to cough or by passing suction catheters into the trachea which, in addition to removing secretions that are present, stimulate cough that brings more secretions up to the region of the catheter tip. The advantage, if any, from the use of mucolytic agents in this process has yet to be demonstrated. However, beta$_2$-adrenergic bronchodilating agents have been shown to increase the rate of transport of particles by the mucociliary blanket, and, thus, in addition to bronchodilatation, such agents should improve the clearance of airway secretions. Postural drainage and chest percussion are other often-used adjuncts that have been shown, especially when secretions are voluminous, to improve tracheobronchial clearance, to increase sputum volume beyond that produced by cough, and to reduce airways obstruction.

Bronchodilatation with aminophylline given orally or by infusion and beta$_2$-adrenergic agonists and anticholinergics by inhalation has assumed a prominent role in treatment of acute respiratory failure in chronic airways obstruction. In addition to bronchodilatation these agents improve bronchopulmonary clearance and may help induce diuresis and hemodynamic improvement when there is cor pulmonale with heart failure (Chap. 204). Unless there is clearly an acute pneumonia, the use of antibiotics is more controversial in the setting of acute respiratory failure than in mucopurulent relapses without failure. Nonetheless, broad-spectrum antibiotics, if no single agent is suspected or isolated, or erythromycin, if legionellae or mycoplasmas are suspected, should be added to the regimen.

Management of complications Complications arising in the course of treatment for acute respiratory failure are cardiac arrhythmias, most often multifocal supraventricular tachycardias, left ventricular failure, pulmonary emboli, and gastrointestinal hemorrhage from stress ulceration. Cardiac arrhythmias resulting from rapid decreases in oxygenation or increases in pH due to overventilation can be readily avoided. However, when giving multiple drugs having cardiotonic properties, the question always arises as to whether the arrhythmias are related to these. Keeping serum theophylline levels in the 10 to 20 mg/L range and using relatively selective beta agonists, such as isoetharine or albuterol by inhalation, can minimize these effects.

Left ventricular failure, usually attributable to coronary atherosclerosis with acute myocardial infarction, systemic hypertension, or aortic valvular disease, is difficult to detect in the presence of cor pulmonale. Fortunately, improving lung function and oxygenation most often reverse the pulmonary hypertension and right ventricular failure (Chap. 204) and induce a brisk diuresis. If signs of congestive failure persist or worsen after providing adequate oxygenation, consideration must be given to left ventricular failure; an assessment in such patients is best made through echocardiography or radioventriculography, since the usual physical and radiographic findings are obscured in such patients. Only in the presence of adequate gas exchange and only with either the firm demonstration of, or strong clinical suspicion of, left ventricular failure should digitalis be used. Diuretic agents should also be reserved for left ventricular failure. They almost invariably produce hypokalemic, hypochloremic metabolic alkalemia that results in depression of ventilatory drive and interference with removal from mechanical ventilatory support.

Pulmonary emboli are suspected to be common in the setting of acute respiratory failure and are extremely difficult to detect since the lung scan is totally nonspecific and signs of cor pulmonale fluctuate in concert with the degree of lung dysfunction. Hence low-dose heparin prophylaxis should be used to prevent this complication. Gastrointestinal hemorrhage commonly complicates acute respiratory failure and is thought to be due to stress ulceration of the gastric mucosa. Awareness of this complication enhances the ability to detect it and act quickly. Antacids, coating agents such as sucralfate, nasogastric suction, and/or cimetidine have been used to diminish the frequency.

Weaning from mechanical ventilation For those patients who have required mechanical ventilatory support, the process of removal from that support is largely empirical. In general, improving gas exchange and lung mechanics along with alertness and responsiveness of the patient signal that the support can be removed. Data such as maximal voluntary inspiratory mouth pressures greater than 20 cmH$_2$O, vital capacity greater than 10 mL/km of body weight, and spontaneous tidal volume greater than 5 mL/kg of body weight are reassuring. However, many patients can be removed from such support with lesser values than these.

Failure to maintain gas exchange after removal of mechanical ventilatory support can usually be explained. *First* on the list is the continued administration or persistence of sedative and tranquilizing drugs that may have been prescribed earlier for agitation. These should be discontinued and time allowed for their metabolism. *Second* is the possibility that the endotracheal tube is of small bore and imposes a resistive load. If so, it should be replaced by a larger one. *Third* is worsening airways obstruction and accumulation of secretions; continued bronchial dilatation and airway suctioning avoid these. *Fourth* is a metabolic alkalemia, with or without diuretic therapy, that should be treated with potassium chloride. *Fifth* is having maintained, while on mechanical ventilation, a Pa$_{O_2}$ and Pa$_{CO_2}$ that are too high and too low, respectively. This can be avoided by using an Fi$_{O_2}$ just sufficient to keep the Pa$_{O_2}$ around 60 mmHg and using the assist mode with small enough tidal volumes to keep the Pa$_{CO_2}$ at the expected chronic level (i.e., that associated with a normal or slightly low arterial pH) before discontinuing mechanical support. *Sixth* is poor nutrition, hypokalemia, or neuromuscular disease, making the patient too weak to maintain breathing or resulting in fatigue of the respiratory muscles. Nutrition, of course, is a longer range problem that should be anticipated, while hypokalemia is often handled along with the metabolic alkalemia. Muscle fatigue, especially diaphragmatic, has received a great deal of attention. From a practical standpoint, paradoxical (inward) movement of the upper abdomen with inspiration is the key clinical finding. Experimental evidence suggests that therapeutic levels of aminophylline or beta$_2$ agonists, such as fenoterol, reverse the manifestations of fatigue, but the role of respiratory stimulants continues to be debated and the data to be inconclusive. In those patients with severely blunted ventilatory drive and improving lung function, stimulants may be tried cautiously. If there is severe metabolic alkalemia, acetazolamide can be tried as a stimulant while chloride replacement is being carried out. Medroxyprogesterone, a central stimulant, or almitrine, a peripheral chemoreceptor stimulant, appear to be safe and, in some instances, effective. Hypothyroidism is a metabolic condition with neuromuscular consequences and is difficult to detect in this clinical setting. Thus any prolonged and difficult weaning process should lead to the assessment of thyroid function.

PROGNOSIS On the average, data collected on large populations demonstrate a slow and relentless diminution in ventilatory function in patients with chronic airways obstruction. Although slow, the decrement in function with time far exceeds the rate of change seen with normal aging. In general, the likelihood of episodes of acute respiratory failure increases when the FEV$_1$ falls below 25 percent of predicted normal values. Although the in-hospital mortality rate averages 30 percent for a single episode and the 5-year survival rate after the initial episode of respiratory failure averages only 15 to 20 percent, the clinical syndrome is extremely important in determining

both the short- and long-range prognosis. As noted above, those patients with predominant emphysema have a poorer prognosis after the onset of respiratory failure than do those with predominant bronchitis. In either case long-term oxygen treatment in those with severe hypoxemia results in prolongation of life and improvement in the quality of life.

BULLOUS EMPHYSEMA Confluent air spaces with diameters in excess of 1 cm are occasionally congenital but most often are found in association with generalized emphysema or progressive fibrotic processes. Gradual increases in size of such air spaces (or bullae) result from traction applied by regions with better elastic recoil properties, and such regions lose volume as the bullae become enlarged. If disability is severe, if the bulla is extremely large, and if either lobar gas sampling or ventilation and perfusion scans demonstrate that sufficient function remains in the nonbullous regions, surgical excision of the bulla may lead to functional improvement. Usually, however, improvement is relatively transitory because other emphysematous regions gradually enlarge into bullae after surgery.

VARIANTS OF EMPHYSEMA In addition to the centriacinar and panacinar forms of emphysema described above, other structural patterns have been described but are functionally less important. Often there is overdistention and alveolar septal destruction in lung regions surrounding scar tissue (paracicatricial or scar emphysema) or along the borders of the acinus (paraseptal emphysema). The latter form, when it occurs at the visceral pleural surface, may predispose to episodes of spontaneous pneumothorax (Chap. 228). Infants rarely develop a check valve mechanism in a lobar bronchus which leads to rapid and life-threatening overdistention (congenital lobar emphysema). Unilateral emphysema may be an incidental radiographic finding (Macleod's or Swyer-James's syndromes). Since, in this condition, the airways are normal in number and structure but the alveoli are reduced in number, this form of unilateral emphysema has been attributed to disease occurring before the age of 8 years when alveoli are normally increasing in number. Overdistention and alveolar septal destruction are not present, and so this condition does not fit the definition of true emphysema. Most often the pulmonary artery on the affected side is hypoplastic. Although usually an incidental finding, the affected lung may become repeatedly infected so that surgical excision may be indicated.

MISCELLANEOUS DIFFUSE OBSTRUCTIVE SYNDROMES *Bronchiolitis obliterans* is a term applied to widespread inflammatory and fibrotic obstruction of small airways. Initially this syndrome was thought to be restricted to those persons who had suffered severe viral infections in childhood, particularly those due to parainfluenza virus. However, recently this syndrome has also been described in adult patients with rheumatoid arthritis. The response to bronchodilator treatment is poor, as would be expected from the histopathologic findings, and fatal respiratory failure often ensues within 2 years. There have been reports suggesting a relationship between penicillamine therapy and the development of bronchiolitis obliterans in patients with rheumatoid arthritis; however, it is clear that this syndrome can develop in patients who have never received penicillamine.

A syndrome with similar histopathology has been described in recipients of autologous bone marrow transplants. Although most often interstitial pneumonitis and fibrosis are sequelae, it has been documented that some patients develop a bronchiolitis obliterans picture. It appears that the development of this process occurs most often in the setting of a chronic graft-versus-host syndrome; however, it is clear that diffuse airways obstruction has developed without evidence of this syndrome in bone marrow recipients.

Cystic fibrosis in the adult with chronic airways obstruction is discussed elsewhere (Chap. 222).

REFERENCES

BERG BW et al: Oxygen supplementation during air travel in patients with chronic obstructive lung disease. Chest 101:638, 1992

CAMPBELL EJ, SENIOR RM: Emphysema, in *Update: Pulmonary Diseases and Disorders*, AP Fishman (ed). New York, McGraw-Hill, 1992, pp 37–52

CRYSTAL RG: α₁-Antitrypsin deficiency, in *Update: Pulmonary Diseases and Disorders*, AP Fishman (ed). New York, McGraw-Hill, 1992, pp 19–36

DUNN WF et al: Oxygen-induced hypercarbia in obstructive pulmonary disease. Am Rev Respir Dis 144:526, 1991

FERNANDEZ E et al: Sustained improvement in gas exchange after negative pressure ventilation for 8 hours per day on 2 successive days in chronic airflow limitation. Am Rev Respir Dis 144:390, 1991

JOSEPHSON GD et al: Airway obstruction. New modalities in treatment. Med Clin North Am 77:539, 1993

KIM WD et al: Centrilobular and panlobular emphysema in smokers. Am Rev Respir Dis 144:1385, 1991

KING TE JR: Bronchiolitis obliterans. Lung 169:S159, 1991

ORR PH et al: Randomized placebo-controlled trials of antibiotics for acute bronchitis: A critical review of the literature. J FAM Pract 36:507, 1993

REID LM: Chronic obstructive pulmonary diseases, in *Pulmonary Diseases and Disorders*, 2d ed, AP Fishman (ed). New York, McGraw-Hill Book Co, 1988, pp 1247–1272

SKWARSKI K et al: Predictors of survival in patients with chronic obstructive pulmonary disease treated with long-term oxygen therapy. Chest 100:1522, 1991

STOCKLEY RA: Alpha-1-antitrypsin and the pathogenesis of emphysema. Lung 169:S205, 1991

WHIPP BJ et al: Physiologic changes following bilateral carotid-body resection in patients with chronic obstructive pulmonary disease. Chest 101:656 1992

YANAI M et al: Site of airway obstruction in pulmonary disease: Direct measurement of intrabronchial pressure. J Appl Physiol 72:1016 1992

---

224   INTERSTITIAL LUNG DISEASES

HERBERT Y. REYNOLDS

The interstitial lung diseases (ILDs) are a heterogeneous group of conditions that involve the alveolar walls and perialveolar tissue. The ILDs are nonmalignant and are not caused by any defined infectious agents. Although an acute phase of illness may occur, the onset is often insidious, and the disease is usually chronic in duration. The initial response of the host to the disease process is inflammation in the air spaces and alveolar walls, causing an acute phase of intraluminal and mural alveolitis. If the disease is chronic and smoldering, inflammation will spread to adjacent portions of the interstitium and vasculature and eventually produce interstitial fibrosis. The resultant scarring and distortion of lung tissue leads to significant derangement of gas exchange and ventilatory function. Inflammation also can involve the conducting airways, and bronchiolitis obliterans associated with an organizing pneumonia is probably part of the spectrum of an ILD.

This diverse group of diseases has many features in common, including similarity of symptoms, comparable appearance of chest radiographs, consistent alterations in pulmonary physiology, and typical histologic features. However, ILDs have been difficult to classify because approximately 180 known individual diseases are characterized by interstitial lung involvement, either as primary disease or as a significant part of a multiorgan process, as occurs in the collagen vascular diseases. The chest radiograph is of limited aid in classification because it can have a similar appearance in many of the ILDs as well as in other unrelated lung diseases. One useful approach for classification is to separate ILDs into two groups, those with known causes and those with unknown causes; each of these groups can be divided into subgroups according to the presence or absence of histologic evidence of granulomas in interstitial or vascular areas (Table 224-1). For each ILD there may be an acute phase, and there is usually a chronic one as well.

Among the ILDs of known cause, the largest group comprises occupational and environmental inhalant exposures; these include diseases due to inhalation of inorganic dusts (Chap. 219), organic dusts, and various irritative or noxious gases (Chap. 218). The number of ILDs of unknown cause is also very large. The major ones within

TABLE 224-1   Major categories of alveolar and interstitial inflammatory lung diseases (ILDs)

Known cause	Unknown cause
LUNG RESPONSE: ALVEOLITIS, INTERSTITIAL INFLAMMATION, AND FIBROSIS	
Asbestos	Idiopathic pulmonary fibrosis
Fumes, gases	Collagen vascular diseases
Drugs (antibiotics) and chemotherapy drugs	Systemic lupus erythematosus, rheumatoid arthritis, ankylosing spondylitis,
Radiation	systemic sclerosis, Sjögren's syndrome,
Aspiration pneumonia	polymyositis-dermatomyositis
Residual of adult respiratory distress syndrome	Pulmonary hemorrhage syndromes
	Goodpasture's syndrome, idiopathic pulmonary hemosiderosis
	Pulmonary alveolar proteinosis
	Lymphocytic infiltrative disorders (lymphocytic interstitial pneumonitis associated with collagen vascular diseases)
	Eosinophilic pneumonias
	Lymphangioleiomyomatosis
	Amyloidosis
	Inherited diseases
	Tuberous sclerosis, neurofibromatosis, Niemann-Pick disease, Gaucher's disease, Hermansky-Pudlak syndrome
	Gastrointestinal or liver diseases (Crohn's disease, primary biliary cirrhosis, chronic active hepatitis, ulcerative colitis)
	Graft vs. host disease (bone marrow transplantation)
LUNG RESPONSE: AS ABOVE BUT WITH GRANULOMA	
Hypersensitivity pneumonitis (organic dusts)	Sarcoidosis
Inorganic dusts: beryllium silica	Langerhans cell granulomatosis (eosinophilic granuloma)
	Granulomatous vasculitides
	Wegener's granulomatosis, allergic granulomatosis of Churg-Strauss, lymphomatoid granulomatosis
	Bronchocentric granulomatosis

this category are idiopathic pulmonary fibrosis (IPF), sarcoidosis, and the ILD often associated with collagen vascular disorders. ILD secondary to inorganic dust exposure usually can be recognized if the occupational history is pursued. For the myriad (see Table 224-1) of other diffuse ILDs, however, a precise diagnosis is obtained with difficulty, usually only after interpretation of an open-lung biopsy specimen; most of these diseases are relatively rare.

Although the initiating agent(s) or circumstances of the various ILDs may be diverse, and many are unknown, the immunopathogenic responses of lung tissue are limited, so the initial mechanisms of injury, the development of alveolitis, and the attempts at repair sometimes leading to fibrosis will have common features. Idiopathic pulmonary fibrosis is discussed as the prototype ILD, since it is encountered relatively frequently and much of the recent research on mechanisms of lung fibrosis has focused on this disease.

IDIOPATHIC PULMONARY FIBROSIS (IPF)

Many patients who present with nonproductive cough, progressive dyspnea, a chest radiograph showing lower lung zone reticulonodular shadows, and pulmonary function tests showing a restrictive pattern (Chap. 214) will be said to have IPF after the diagnostic evaluation is completed. This condition is also known as *cryptogenic fibrosing alveolitis*. Although the terms *idiopathic* and *cryptogenic* mean that the etiologic agent is unknown, this is not a nebulous "wastebasket" diagnosis or just a diagnosis of exclusion but rather a well-defined clinical entity.

IMMUNOPATHOGENESIS   Several parts of the alveolar structure are affected in IPF, including the alveolar walls lined with type I and type II pneumocytes and the interstitial supporting structure composed of mesenchymal cells, especially fibroblasts and myofibroblasts, collagen, and various adhesive proteoglycans. The capillary endothelium also may be involved. The disease process does not affect the upper or conducting airways, but bronchiolitis of respiratory bronchioles may be present and alveolar units are always involved.

Normally, overlying or interspersed in the alveoli are a variety of immune cells, including alveolar macrophages, dendritic macrophages, interstitial monocytes, lymphocytes, and inflammatory cells, such as polymorphonuclear leukocytes (PMNs) and eosinophils. The cellular content of normal bronchoalveolar lavage (BAL) fluid consists of approximately 80 percent alveolar macrophages, 10 percent lymphocytes (of which 70 percent are T lymphocytes), 1 to 5 percent B lymphocytes or plasma cells, 1 to 3 percent polymorphonuclear leukocytes, and 1 percent eosinophils. In the lymphocyte population, the ratio of CD4 T helper and CD8 T suppressor/cytotoxic cells is about 1.5.

In the earliest, reversible forms of alveolar injury, "leakiness" of the alveolar type I cells and the adjacent capillary endothelial cells occurs, causing alveolar and interstitial edema and the formation of intraalveolar hyaline membranes. With persistence of the disease, increased alveolar-capillary permeability and desquamation of intraalveolar cells (alveolitis), mural inflammation, and interstitial fibrosis are present on biopsy. This process is also reflected in the composition of cells and enzymes recovered in BAL fluid (Table 224-2) and in cellular components present in lung biopsy tissue. The presence and severity of the disease process are spotty in distribution; a continuum of inflammatory and fibrotic changes can be found throughout the affected lung. Fibrosis follows from an organization of inflammatory exudate within the airspaces in which fibroblasts beneath the type I epithelium proliferate and increase their production of fibronectin and collagen.

Depicted in Fig. 224-1 are immunopathogenic mechanisms that interconnect the intraalveolar (luminal) and alveolar mural tissue with the interstitial space and capillary vascular areas. Although the inciting agent or stimulus is unknown, it is likely an antigen that can initiate an immunoglobulin response. This is reflected by an increased ratio

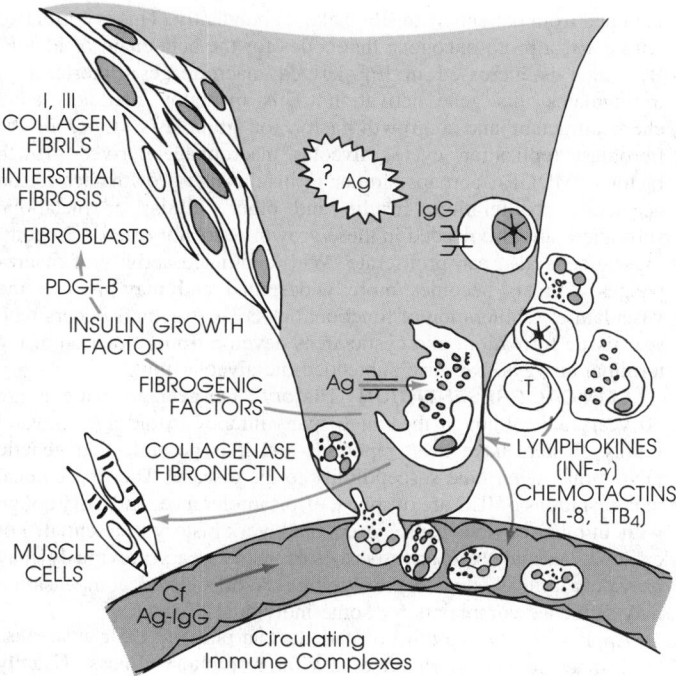

FIGURE 224-1 Immunologic mechanisms within the alveolar space, alveolar walls, and interstitium that can lead to inflammation and eventual fibrosis. The focus is the alveolar macrophage, which is activated, possibly by an immune complex and an as yet unidentified antigen (Ag). Through mediators such as chemotaxins, the macrophage attracts PMNs and other cells from the circulation to the alveolar space, or it can initiate fibrogenesis with various mediators that can stimulate fibroblasts and muscle cells to proliferate. Interstitial fibrosis may result. Abbreviations: IL-8 (interleukin 8), LTB$_4$ (leukotriene B$_4$), INF-γ (interferon γ), PDGF-B (platelet-derived growth factor). *(After Reynolds, HY: Idiopathic interstitial pulmonary fibrosis: Contribution of bronchoalveolar lavage analysis. Chest 89:139, 1986.)*

TABLE 224-2 Cellular and immunologic changes in various IPF specimens

BLOOD

IgG (IgG1,3) elevated, immune complexes, cryoglobulins
Serologic titers (low)
T lymphocytes (sensitized to type I collagen)

BRONCHOALVEOLAR FLUID

Alveolitis characterized by increased percentage of PMNs (20%) and eosinophils (2–4%), but lymphocytes may be increased also (20%)
Alveolar macrophages: activated macrophages and their secretory components are numerous:
    Chemotaxins to attract PMNs and muscle cells (IL-8, with mRNA for IL-8 expressed in macrophages, and leukotriene B$_4$)
    Plasminogen activator
    Macrophage-derived growth factor (or insulin-like growth factor)
    Fibronectin
    Platelet-derived growth factor B (expressed by c-*sis* oncogene)
Steroid receptors increased; mitotic index increased
Collagenase (PMN origin)
Antioxidant glutathione decreased
IgG increased (G3, G1 subclasses)
Immune complexes detectable
IgG-releasing cells present
Histamine elevated
Surfactant protein A reduced

LUNG TISSUE

Interstitial inflammation
Plasma cells, muscle cells, fibroblasts increased
Collagen synthesis increased
Fibrosis but no granuloma
Bronchiolitis obliterans can develop

of IgG subclasses IgG1 and G3, an increased number of IgG-releasing cells, and perhaps the formation of immune complexes. Recently, serum antibody against hepatitis C antigen was detected in about 20 percent of patients with IPF; most of these did not have antecedent hepatitis. Speculation continues that a viral etiology is probable for many cases of IPF.

An increased number of macrophages, which are activated phagocytes capable of producing many cytokines that affect other lung cells, is a hallmark of the alveolitis. These macrophage cytokines or mediators can operate in two directions. First, through the production of chemotaxins, which include leukotriene B$_4$ and interleukin 8, inflammatory cells such as PMNs and eosinophils are attracted into the alveoli. IPF lung macrophages express increased mRNA for IL-8, which correlates with the percent of PMNs in BAL fluid. An increased percentage of PMNs (20 percent or more) and eosinophils (1 to 4 percent) in the profile of BAL cells is usual in IPF. Lymphocytes are not usually increased, unless the IPF is part of a collagen vascular disease. Enzymes or oxidant radicals from inflammatory cells and histamine may cause local injury or alter the permeability of type I cells. Conversely, the antioxidant glutathione is deficient in the BAL fluid, further impairing neutralization of oxidants. Second, macrophages are also capable of secreting substances that stimulate mesenchymal cells. For fibroblasts to replicate in the interstitium and in the alveolar walls, they must be primed to enter the G$_1$ phase of a growth cycle to proliferate.

Several products from alveolar macrophages can participate in these steps. Platelet-derived growth factor B (PDGF-B) is a chemoattractant for mesenchymal cells and a stimulus for fibroblasts to change from resting cells to cells entering G$_1$. Although PDGF-B is not produced by normal monocytes or macrophages, alveolar macrophages obtained from patients with IPF make it abundantly. This is correlated with c-*sis*, a proto-oncogene that codes for the beta chain of PDGF-B, which is increased in IPF-derived macrophages. Interferon γ up-regulates this gene activation. This mediator also acts as a chemoattractant and a growth factor for fibroblasts. Later in the fibroblast replication cycle, alveolar macrophage–derived growth factor (AMDGF), perhaps similar to insulin-like growth factor, can accelerate proliferation. Insulin and other cellular or metabolic substances are also needed in these growth-regulatory steps. Smooth-muscle cells also can proliferate. With continued activity of macrophages, fibrosis becomes more widespread and may involve the vasculature. Obliteration of functional alveolar structures occurs with scar tissue formation, and cystic areas develop from retraction of the terminal airways that once subtended the alveolar unit.

CLINICAL PRESENTATION **History** On average, patients are 50 years old, although the range spans infancy to old age. Several family clusters have been reported, and it is possible that genetic factors may determine susceptibility to the disease. The first clinical manifestations of ILD are dyspnea, effort intolerance, and a dry cough without other obvious cause. A detailed work history is essential. For example, casual exposure to asbestos many years previously may provide a crucial clue to the etiology. Work-related compensation may influence complaints for some individuals.

Approximately one-third of patients can pinpoint their awareness of dyspnea to the aftermath of a viral respiratory illness. Usually months or years elapse between the onset of exertional dyspnea and its progression perhaps to the point of breathlessness at rest. Dyspnea and frequent coughing are often accompanied by other constitutional symptoms such as fatigue, anorexia, weight loss, and arthralgias.

Physical findings Initially, the physical examination may not be revealing, and auscultation of the chest may be normal. As the disease advances, dry crackles, or coarse crackles on inspiration, are usually heard at the lung bases. There may be tachypnea at rest, cyanosis, and clubbing of the fingers and toes, usually without hypertrophic osteoarthropathy. In later stages, cor pulmonale (Chap. 204) is evident, with findings of pulmonary hypertension, such as an accentuated pulmonic second sound or a right-sided lift, and eventually signs of right-sided heart failure. The right ventricular ejection fraction determined by radionuclide ventriculography is often depressed in the face of normal left ventricular performance.

LABORATORY AND DIAGNOSTIC TESTS **Imaging studies** The chest radiograph usually reveals a pattern of diffuse reticulonodular markings, prominent in the lower lung zones. Several radiographic patterns can be seen which correlate roughly with the duration of the disease. Early, a hazy "ground glass" appearance of the lower lung fields coincides with the stage of acute alveolitis. Later, curvilinear shadows predominate and may coalesce into nodular infiltrates. With end-stage disease, the linear opacities are seen in all lung fields, the lung fields appear contracted, and ring-shaped opacities resulting from cystic and bronchiectatic changes are obvious, creating the *honeycombed* or *swiss cheese* appearance of the lung. Biopsy-proven forms of diffuse IPF occur occasionally (about 14 percent) in patients with normal chest radiographs despite significant exercise intolerance, abnormal pulmonary function tests (including a reduced diffusing capacity), and dry crackles.

High-resolution computed tomographic (CT) scanning is a sensitive means of documenting tissue infiltration and the presence of bronchiectasis or pleural changes. It can distinguish between early cellular changes and more advanced fibrosis, emphasizing the inhomogeneous distribution of disease in IPF.

Laboratory examination The erythrocyte sedimentation rate is usually elevated, circulating immune-complex titers and serum immunoglobulin levels may be increased, and cryoimmunoglobulins may be present. Serologic tests to screen for collagen vascular diseases are necessary to exclude these diagnoses. Although serum rheumatoid factor, antinuclear antibodies, depressed levels of complement, and other parameters of autoimmune diseases may be detected in approximately 10 percent of patients with IPF, the titers are generally quite low.

Lung function tests In patients with advanced disease, reductions in total lung capacity, vital capacity, and residual volume are found (Chap. 214). Usually, evidence of airway obstruction is minimal and the FEV_1/FVC ratio is normal or increased. A restrictive respiratory functional pattern is usually present, reflecting the stiff, noncompliant lungs characteristic of IPF and its common aftermath, fibrosis. There is usually resting arterial hypoxemia, but the carbon dioxide tension is normal or decreased. Blood pH is normal. The alveolar-arterial oxygen gradient during exercise is elevated, and exercise tolerance is reduced. The carbon monoxide diffusing capacity is usually reduced by 30 to 50 percent. Changes in these variables are useful in monitoring the course of the illness and in assessing the effectiveness of treatment. However, current or former cigarette smoking in IPF patients can alter lung function to misrepresent the extent of restriction and/or obstruction if both emphysema and interstitial fibrosis are present; this has implications and raises caution for evaluating lung function in these patients. Diffusing capacity (DL_{CO}) becomes a more important test in this assessment.

Bronchoscopy Direct investigation of the airways by fiberoptic bronchoscopy is part of the evaluation, and four to six transbronchial biopsies are taken to obtain lung tissue for diagnosis. These provide a sufficient quantity of tissue for a definitive pathologic diagnosis in approximately one-fourth of all cases of IPF. In some diffuse granulomatous interstitial diseases, such as sarcoidosis (Chap. 292), transbronchial biopsy will provide a tissue diagnosis in about 80 percent of cases. Bronchoscopy also permits bronchoalveolar lavage, which provides useful information about cells and proteins in the airways that generally correlates with histologic changes in the interstitial and alveolar tissues. An analysis of BAL fluid and cells can reveal a number of changes in IPF (see Table 224-2).

Lung biopsy The importance of an adequate sample of lung tissue to permit a full histologic evaluation, good microbial cultures, immunofluorescence and electron-microscopic studies, and analysis of inorganic substances cannot be overemphasized. Therefore, if a transbronchial biopsy does not yield sufficient tissue for a confident diagnosis, open-lung biopsy should be considered. It is prudent to substantiate a tissue diagnosis before embarking on immunosuppressive therapy with its attendant complications.

DIAGNOSTIC APPROACH AND STAGING OF DISEASE ACTIVITY Following the clinical examination, chest radiograph (or high-resolution chest CT scan), pulmonary function tests [lung volumes, FEV_1/FVC, and diffusing capacity (Chap. 214)], and arterial blood gas determination measuring desaturation under exercising conditions, the functional disability from the lung disease can be estimated. However, a histologic analysis of lung tissue should be made before the disease is diagnosed definitively. Fiberoptic bronchoscopy is usually the first invasive procedure and is important for ruling out infection, malignancy, and other specific diseases. Although transbronchial biopsy has a lower diagnostic yield in IPF than in sarcoidosis and other granulomatous diseases, it is nevertheless a useful, low-risk procedure with a 20 to 30 percent success rate for obtaining an adequate sample for a confident pathologic diagnosis. BAL for cellular and protein analysis may be useful in judging the nature of alveolar inflammation and immunologic activity (see Table 224-2). However, the value of the periodic use of BAL analysis to monitor disease activity or its response to therapy has not been established. Use of gallium 67 lung scanning does not add more diagnostic accuracy or help with monitoring activity.

If the diagnosis is still in doubt after the bronchoscopy and related procedures, an open-lung biopsy should be considered. The referring physician and the thoracic surgeon should cooperate in choosing the most representative area of the lung for biopsy, and the proper microbial cultures and immunologic studies should be obtained.

THERAPY Treatment is usually offered to patients with IPF, even to patients with advanced fibrotic disease. About 2 weeks after the open-lung biopsy, a trial of oral prednisone can be instituted in a dose of 1 mg/kg daily and continued for 8 to 12 weeks. If lung disease shows objective improvement, the dose is tapered to a maintenance level. Should the disease not respond or be progressive, the dosage of prednisone can be increased, but immunosuppression with cyclophosphamide should be considered. Cyclophosphamide is given at a dose of about 1.0 mg/kg daily (50 to 75 mg) with the patient continuing on a daily maintenance dose of oral prednisone (0.25 mg/kg). The dosages of cyclophosphamide may be increased as necessary by 50-mg increments at 7- to 10-day intervals. The objective is to reduce the white blood cell count to approximately half the normal baseline value, causing a distinct drop in the total blood lymphocyte count. However, a minimum count of 1000 polymorphonuclear leukocytes per microliter should be maintained.

Use of high-dose, pulsed glucocorticoids does not offer special advantages over daily dosing. Azathioprine has been used in place of cyclophosphamide. Other agents such as colchicine, penicillamine, and cyclosporine have not been evaluated thoroughly.

Several other measures may help respiratory function. It is imperative that patients discontinue cigarette smoking. Since there is frequently a marked drop in Pa_{O_2} with exercise, supplemental oxygen therapy may be useful, sometimes using transtracheal catheter oxygen delivery, which can reduce oxygen requirements and help with the logistics of supplying high-flow therapy. As the pulmonary vascular bed is destroyed by progressive fibrosis, pulmonary hypertension and cor pulmonale can develop; right-sided congestive heart failure can be difficult to control. Judicious use of diuretics is advised. Adequate oxygenation is probably the best treatment for right-sided heart failure (Chap. 204). Some patients also may develop obstruction to airflow and wheezing and coughing which may respond to bronchodilators. Infection may occur during immunosuppressive therapy and should be treated promptly and aggressively. Prophylactic use of pneumococcal and influenza vaccines is indicated. If refractory disease limited to the chest is present, the possibility of lung transplantation should be considered. Success with single-lung transplantation for ILD makes this therapy a reality for some patients. Selection criteria, contraindications, and availability of organs must be discussed candidly with patients so as not to create unrealistic expectations.

INDIVIDUAL FORMS OF ILD

ILD ASSOCIATED WITH COLLAGEN VASCULAR DISORDERS
In these diseases, various pulmonary structures can be affected, especially the pleura, so that ILD is but one manifestation of intrathoracic involvement and often a minor part of the multiorgan process. Analysis of BAL fluid and cells from patients with ILD associated with rheumatoid arthritis and systemic sclerosis is similar to that found in IPF (see Table 224-2) and suggests similar pathogenetic mechanisms for fibrosis. A lymphocytic alveolitis may accompany some cases of ILD in rheumatoid disease and may predict a better response to immunosuppressive therapy.

Systemic lupus erythematosus (SLE) (See Chap. 284) About half of patients with SLE ultimately develop overt lung disease. Pleuritis, pleural effusion(s), and acute pneumonitis are the most frequent forms of lung disease, while a chronic, progressive ILD is uncommon. It is important to exclude pulmonary infection. Although pleuropulmonary involvement may not be evident clinically, pulmonary function testing, particularly the diffusing capacity for carbon monoxide, reveals abnormalities in many patients.

Rheumatoid arthritis (See Chap. 285) A variety of pulmonary manifestations can occur, including pleural disease (pleural effusion and subpleural nodules), parenchymal nodular infiltrates associated with pneumoconiosis in miners (Caplan's syndrome), and diffuse interstitial fibrosis. The ILD can develop before joint disease becomes evident, particularly in men, and is accompanied by high titers of rheumatoid factor. Rarely, upper airway obstruction can occur from arthritis of the cricoarytenoid joint. Patients with rheumatoid arthritis who are receiving treatment with methotrexate or gold may develop

ILD that represents a drug hypersensitivity, which must be differentiated from a preexisting or developing ILD associated with the underlying disease. Penicillamine therapy in patients with rheumatoid arthritis has been implicated as a cause of bronchiolitis obliterans.

Ankylosing spondylitis (See Chap. 289) Bilateral upper lobe fibrosis, which can be complicated by fibrocavitary disease, may develop late in the course.

Systemic sclerosis (See Chap. 286) Radiographic evidence of lung involvement develops in a majority of patients, but its severity or progression is variable. Because distal esophageal motor dysfunction is present in many patients, reflux with regurgitation and chronic aspiration is common. In addition, cutaneous scleroderma can involve the anterior chest wall and abdomen, causing restrictive lung function.

Sjögren's syndrome (See Chap. 288) General dryness and lack of airways secretions cause the major problems of hoarseness, cough, and bronchitis. Presence of an ILD in these patients may signify a lymphocytic infiltrate in lung tissue which can behave as a low-grade lymphoma.

Polymyositis and dermatomyositis (See Chap. 384) Although ILD is reported to occur in only 5 to 10 percent of patients, its presence is more common in the subgroup of patients with an anti-Jo-1 antibody that is directed to tRNA synthetase. Weakness of respiratory muscles contributing to aspiration pneumonitis is a common occurrence.

SYNDROMES OF ILD WITH PULMONARY HEMORRHAGE Recurrent hemoptysis, dyspnea, and hypoxemia in the presence of a chest radiographic pattern of diffuse alveolar opacities should raise the possibility of alveolar hemorrhage. An association between vasculitis involving the kidney (lung-renal syndromes) or other organ systems should be investigated. Alveolar hemorrhage occurs rarely in all collagen vascular disorders, but it is described most often with systemic lupus erythematosus. It can occur with systemic vasculitis and is described as an initial presentation of Wegener's granulomatosis; with Behçet's disease, in which aneurysm formation and rupture of small muscular arteries are manifestations of necrotizing vasculitis; in allergic Churg-Strauss granulomatosis; in Henoch-Schönlein purpura syndrome; and in essential (mixed) cryoimmunoglobulinemia. Exposure to the toxic aerosol trimellitic anhydride may cause alveolar hemorrhage. Serologic tests for antinuclear antibody, anti-glomerular basement membrane antibody, and complement to document a vasculitis and immunologic disorder are the first steps, but renal biopsy and possibly lung biopsy may be required for a definitive diagnosis. Some specific syndromes in this category will be discussed next.

Goodpasture's syndrome (See Chap. 241) Pulmonary hemorrhage and glomerulonephritis are the features of this disease in which most patients have antibodies to renal glomerular and lung alveolar basement membranes.

Idiopathic pulmonary hemosiderosis Diffuse alveolar hemorrhage can occur in the absence of other organ involvement or an obvious immunologic cause and is therefore a diagnosis of exclusion after considering the many causes of alveolar bleeding associated with collagen vascular and vasculitic diseases. A lung biopsy is usually necessary to document the lack of inflammatory injury in the lung tissues and to exclude other diseases with confidence. The clinical course can be variable, ranging from recurrent and fulminant with development of progressive interstitial fibrosis to minimal disease that may remit without sequelae. Children and young adults are usually affected. Glucocorticoid treatment is useful for control of bleeding acutely but is not a predictable long-term remedy for keeping the disease suppressed and preventing recurrence.

PULMONARY ALVEOLAR PROTEINOSIS Similar clinical symptoms and the general appearance of the chest radiograph, showing diffuse alveolar consolidation and/or nodular shadows typically radiating from the hilar regions, place pulmonary alveolar proteinosis (PAP) in the ILD category. Histologically, the alveoli are filled with granular material that stains with periodic acid Schiff reagent, but they exhibit no inflammation and have relatively normal septal structure. Strictly speaking, then, PAP is an intraalveolar process which resembles, but is not, an ILD. Because the proteinaceous response can be associated with inhaled dust exposure (silica and aluminum), malignancy, and chronic infection, termed *secondary PAP*, these disorders should be differentiated from primary PAP by lung biopsy. The intraalveolar material is a combination of surfactant phospholipid produced by type II pneumocytes and of other proteins and immunoglobulins found in alveolar lining fluid. The cytoplasm of alveolar macrophages appears engorged with inclusions (lamellar bodies). The "stuffed" macrophages with large phagolysosomes have diminished microbial killing capacity in vitro, but lung infections with unusual organisms are not frequent. Whole-lung lavage(s) will provide relief to many patients with dyspnea and progressive deterioration of arterial oxygenation and also may provide long-term benefit.

LYMPHOCYTIC INFILTRATIVE DISORDERS   This is a group of disorders that feature lymphocyte and plasma cell infiltration of the lung parenchyma and either are benign or can behave as low-grade lymphomas. Within the spectrum of chronic interstitial pneumonias, a subset has been described with lung histology that shows diffuse interstitial infiltration with lymphocytes and plasma cells. In some of these patients, an autoimmune disease or dysproteinemia exists. However, lymphocytic interstitial pneumonia (LIP) is probably not a distinct entity, belongs within the IPF group, and can be associated with Sjögren's syndrome. LIP has been reported in patients, particularly children, with AIDS.

Included among these disorders is immunoblastic lymphadenopathy, also termed *angioimmunoblastic lymphadenopathy*, which usually is a fulminant lymphoma-like disease that may have an element of ILD in some cases. *Lymphomatoid granulomatosis* can be included, but its granulomatous response also places it with the granulomatous ILDs (see Table 224-1).

EOSINOPHILIC PNEUMONIAS (See Chap. 218)   These pneumonias encompass a spectrum of diseases in which lung hypersensitivity plays a role and in which a specific cause may or may not be identified. For example, with extrinsic asthma and exposure to fungal antigens, allergic bronchopulmonary mycosis can develop; filarial and other parasitic infections can cause tropical pulmonary eosinophilia; many common drugs can induce eosinophilic pneumonia. Chronic eosinophilic pneumonia has features that make it difficult to distinguish from IPF and other forms of progressive ILD. The disease, which more commonly affects older females, has several radiologic characteristics that are helpful in diagnosis: (1) a peripheral pattern of dense lung infiltrates that appear to cross anatomic lobar boundaries with sparing of the central lung regions, (2) regression but reappearance of infiltrates in the same lung locations, and (3) extreme sensitivity of the infiltrates (and disease symptoms) to modest doses of oral glucocorticoids. The diagnosis can be established by lung biopsy, which shows an eosinophilic inflammatory process.

LYMPHANGIOLEIOMYOMATOSIS   Immature smooth-muscle cells can proliferate in lung tissue around and throughout bronchial, vascular, and lymphatic structures, causing local obstruction or creating constricting lesions that develop into cysts. Lymphatics and lymph nodes in other organs are also usually affected. Because this disorder occurs predominantly in females of reproductive age, an association between estrogens and the disease is probable. Pulmonary symptoms consist of dyspnea, cough, and hemoptysis; a more overt presentation occurs with spontaneous pneumothorax, which can be recurrent, or with chylous effusion. In addition, the chest radiograph shows reticulonodular shadows and small cyst-like areas or honeycombing throughout the lung fields. In contrast to most forms of ILD, lung volumes are normal or increased, as is also the case with Langerhans cell granulomatosis (see below). Therapy for progressive lung disease has not been particularly effective. Pneumothoraces and effusions may require chemical or surgical pleurodesis. Treatment with progesterone combined with ovariectomy has been used. Lung transplantation may be considered for some patients.

AMYLOIDOSIS (See Chap. 281)   Deposits of amyloid in the form of plaques or nodules can develop at all sites of the respiratory tract. Tracheal and endobronchial mucosal plaques or incidental parenchymal nodules can be difficult to diagnose clinically, but they usually coexist with extrapulmonary manifestations of primary or, less commonly, secondary amyloidosis. Lung biopsy is necessary for definitive diagnosis. As part of primary systemic amyloidosis or a plasma cell dyscrasia, an ILD may occur from amyloid deposits in alveolar septa and associated blood vessels, producing dyspnea, radiographic findings of diffuse reticulonodular shadows, and restrictive pulmonary function.

INHERITED DISORDERS ASSOCIATED WITH ILD   Pulmonary infiltrates and respiratory symptoms typical of mild ILD can develop in related family members and in several inherited diseases. These include the phacomatoses (Chap. 378) tuberous sclerosis and neurofibromatosis and the lysosomal storage diseases (Chap. 349), such as Niemann-Pick disease and Gaucher's disease. The *Hermansky-Pudlak syndrome* is an autosomal recessive disorder in which granulomatous colitis and ILD may occur. It is characterized by oculocutaneous albinism, bleeding diathesis from platelet dysfunction, and the accumulation of a chromolipid, lipofuscin material in cells of the reticuloendothelial system. The pulmonary fibrosis is similar to IPF, but the alveolar macrophages may contain cytoplasmic ceroid-like inclusions.

GASTROINTESTINAL AND LIVER DISEASE   Rarely, inflammatory bowel disease and chronic hepatitis may be associated with a mild form of ILD. Crohn's disease, which has a number of similarities with sarcoidosis, also may be accompanied by asymptomatic lymphocytic alveolitis.

GRAFT-VERSUS-HOST DISEASE (GVHD) (See Chap. 313)   Some degree of GVHD occurs in all patients receiving bone marrow transplantation. However, in about 10 percent a chronic phase may ensue with the onset of dry cough, mucositis, dyspnea, and airflow obstruction in the small airways, as demonstrated by pulmonary function testing. Chest radiographs reveal peribronchiolar infiltrates, and lung biopsy shows focal areas of interstitial infiltration with a mixture of lymphocytes and PMNs. The lesions are consistent with bronchiolitis; no vasculitis is present. Some recipients of heart-lung transplants also develop bronchiolitis. Bronchiolitis in chronic GVHD may stabilize and disappear or may be progressive and fatal. Treatment includes increasing the doses of the immunosuppressive drugs together with bronchodilators and antibiotics. Infection, especially with viral agents, is a common complication.

ILD WITH A GRANULOMATOUS RESPONSE IN LUNG TISSUE OR VASCULAR STRUCTURES   Inhalation of organic dusts, which causes hypersensitivity pneumonitis, or of inorganic particles such as silica, which causes alveolitis and elicits a granulomatous inflammatory reaction leading to ILD, produces diseases of known etiology (see Table 224-1) that are discussed in Chaps. 218 and 219. Sarcoidosis (Chap. 292) is prominent among granulomatous diseases of *unknown cause* in which ILD is an important feature.

Langerhans cell granulomatosis (eosinophilic granuloma or histiocytosis X) (See Chap. 58)   This condition is being recognized with increasing frequency and may account for about 1 to 5 percent of ILD of unknown etiology. Previously, the proliferation of tissue macrophages (histiocytes) was thought to be characteristic of this disease that affects the lung, bones, and viscera. Now it is recognized that the precursor cell is the *dendritic cell*, which has potent stimulatory and accessory cell immune function, is normally found in the interstitium and alveolar septal areas, and is distinctly different from a tissue macrophage. The dendritic cell can evolve into the Langerhans cell, characterized by a specific CD1a surface antigen that reacts with a monoclonal antibody identified as T_6 and by intracytoplasmic organelles seen by electron microscopy that are called X bodies or Birbeck granules. Langerhans cells can be identified in skin and are present in bronchiolar epithelium of normal lung. Cigarette smoking or a similar irritant seems to be a stimulus for their proliferation. An increased number of these cells can be recovered in BAL from normal smokers, patients with bronchoalveolar carcinoma, and patients with IPF. However, in Langerhans cell granulomatosis of the lung, 3 percent or more of the BAL cells may be so identified, which greatly exceeds the percentage found in these other disorders. However, the Langerhans cells are not pathognomonic for this disease. The number of alveolar macrophages is also increased. Early in the disease a focus of Langerhans and surrounding inflammatory cells can be found adjacent to respiratory and terminal bronchioles, causing bronchiolitis. Later, alveolar structures are involved in progressive interstitial inflammation and fibrosis. In advanced disease, lung histology does *not* reveal the discrete typical granulomas that are found in sarcoidosis and hypersensitivity pneumonitis, nor are eosinophils greatly increased—two reasons that the prior appellation "eosinophilic granuloma" was really a misnomer.

The pulmonary form of this disease occurs in young and middle-aged adults, usually males, and in those who use tobacco heavily; it may remain focal or involve one or several bony sites (long bones, spine, skull, or jaw). Occasionally, multifocal disease can affect the posterior pituitary gland, causing diabetes insipidus, a condition that is termed *Hand-Schüller-Christian disease*. In infants, *Letterer-Siwe disease* is a more fulminant visceral form of this disorder that mimics a malignant lymphoma. In adults, the presenting symptoms and signs do not distinguish this disease from other forms of ILD unless signs of a bone lesion exist. A spontaneous pneumothorax may herald the disease. Chest radiographs will show diffuse micronodular shadows and cystic spaces, sparing the costophrenic angles and preserving lung volume, as occurs in lymphangioleiomyomatosis. Pulmonary function tests may disclose a combination of obstructive and restrictive defects. As the disease progresses, greater airway obstruction may develop, and the chest radiograph can resemble that in advanced chronic obstructive lung disease. Treatment involves a mandatory cessation of tobacco use, which may cause the pulmonary disease to stabilize or regress. Glucocorticoids usually are not helpful. Penicillamine has been used in an attempt to prevent fibrosis with variable success. Local bone lesions may require irradiation treatment. For patients with increasing symptoms of airway obstruction, supportive therapy and bronchodilators may be tried, but their success has been modest.

Granulomatous vasculitis (See Chap. 291) Certain forms of vasculitis, accompanied by a granulomatous response, can involve the respiratory tract as part of a multiorgan process or can occasionally be localized to the respiratory tract, as occurs with a predominantly pulmonary form of Wegener's granulomatosis in which glomerulonephritis may not be prominent. It is very important to differentiate these conditions from lymphomatoid granulomatosis. Allergic angiitis and the granulomatosis of Churg and Strauss are forms of granulomatous vasculitis affecting many organs but especially the lungs; a history of asthma and the presence of eosinophilia are distinguishing features.

Lymphomatoid granulomatosis (See Chaps. 58 and 291) This involves primarily the lungs and less frequently the skin, central and peripheral nervous systems, and kidneys with an infiltration of lymphocytoid, plasma-like cells and macrophages creating a necrotic granulomatous inflammatory reaction, especially in or near blood vessels. The disease can progress as a lymphoproliferative disorder and evolve into malignant lymphoma in as many as 50 percent of patients. Treatment of lymphomatoid granulomatosis with glucocorticoids and cyclophosphamide may induce a remission, and if this occurs, subsequent relapse and development of lymphoma are not likely.

BRONCHOCENTRIC GRANULOMATOSIS In contrast to the necrotizing granulomatous reaction in lung vessels, i.e., angiocentric vasculitis, granulomatous destruction of bronchioles occurs in this condition. There is usually associated parenchymal inflammation causing ILD. Eosinophils can be present if asthma and hypersensitivity to fungal antigens within the bronchi have occurred. In other cases without these associated conditions, hypersensitivity to other microbial antigens is postulated. Bronchocentric granulomatosis must be differentiated from hypersensitivity pneumonitis caused by inhalation of organic dusts (see Chaps. 218 and 219).

REFERENCES

Idiopathic pulmonary fibrosis

DU BOIS RM: Idiopathic pulmonary fibrosis. Annu Rev Med 44:441, 1993
CHERNIACK RM et al: Current concepts in idiopathic pulmonary fibrosis: A road map for the future. Am Rev Respir Dis 143:680, 1991
EPLER GR et al: Bronchiolitis obliterans with organizing pneumonia. N Engl J Med 312:152, 1985
LYNCH JP: Neutrophilic alveolitis in idiopathic pulmonary fibrosis. Am Rev Respir Dis 145:1433, 1992
PIQUET PF: Cytokines involved in pulmonary fibrosis. Int Rev Exp Pathol 34:173, 1993

Other interstitial lung diseases

ADAMSON D et al: Successful treatment of pulmonary lymphangiomyomatosis with oophorectomy and progesterone. Am Rev Respir Dis 132:916, 1985
CHAN CK et al: Small-airways disease in recipients of allogenic bone marrow transplants. Medicine 66:327, 1987
FAUCI AS et al: Lymphomatoid granulomatosis—prospective clinical and therapeutic experience over 10 years. N Engl J Med 306:68, 1982
HANCE AJ et al: Pulmonary and extrapulmonary manifestations of Langerhans cell granulomatosis (histiocytosis X). Semin Respir Med 9:349, 1988
HELMERS R et al: Pulmonary manifestations associated with rheumatoid arthritis. Chest 100:235, 1991
KARIMAN K et al: Pulmonary alveolar proteinosis: Prospective clinical experience in 23 patients for 15 years. Lung 162:223, 1984
MILLER KS et al: Lung disease associated with progressive systemic sclerosis. Am Rev Respir Dis 141:301, 1990
REYNOLDS HY: Bronchoalveolar lavage. Am Rev Respir Dis 135:250, 1987
———: Immunologic system in the respiratory tract. Physiol Rev 71:1117, 1991
SIBILLE Y et al: Macrophages and polymorphonuclear neutrophils in lung defence and injury. Am Rev Respir Dis 141:471, 1990
SPECKS U et al: Granulomatous vasculitis. Rheum Dis Clin North Am 16:377, 1990
TAZELAAR HD et al: Interstitial lung disease in polymyositis and dermatomyositis. Am Rev Respir Dis 141:727, 1990
TRULOCK EP et al: The Washington University–Barnes Hospital experience with lung transplantation. JAMA 266:1943, 1991

225 PRIMARY PULMONARY HYPERTENSION

STUART RICH

Primary pulmonary hypertension is an uncommon disease characterized by increased pulmonary artery pressure and pulmonary vascular resistance without an obvious cause. The diagnosis can be made only after all causes of pulmonary hypertension have been excluded. There is a female-to-male preponderance (1.7:1), with patients most commonly presenting in the third and fourth decades, although the age range is from infancy to greater than 60 years. Because the predominant symptom of primary pulmonary hypertension is dyspnea, which can have an insidious onset in an otherwise healthy person, the disease is typically diagnosed late in its course. By that time, the clinical and laboratory findings of severe pulmonary hypertension are usually present.

PATHOLOGY The histopathology of primary pulmonary hypertension is not pathognomonic for the disease but is observed in pulmonary hypertension from a variety of causes. The majority of patients have a primary pulmonary arteriopathy which incorporates the features of plexogenic and thrombotic arteriopathies.

Medial hypertrophy associated with concentric laminar intimal fibrosis and plexiform lesions (plexogenic arteriopathy) is characteristically found in younger women, whereas eccentric intimal fibrosis with medial hypertrophy, fibroelastic intimal pads in the arteries and arterioles, and scattered evidence of old recanalized thrombi appearing as fibrous webs (thrombotic arteriopathy) appear to affect men and women equally. In most patients, some features of both patterns of vascular changes can be found. The common pathogenetic denominator appears to be an undefined injury to the pulmonary vascular endothelium, which results in (1) an impaired ability to maintain a relaxed state of vasomotor tone and (2) a conversion to a procoagulant state within the pulmonary arteriolar bed that disposes to the development of in situ thrombosis. The types of vascular changes noted are likely determined by the nature of the injury to the pulmonary vascular endothelium and/or its duration, the patient's gender, and underlying genetic predisposition. The recent findings of primary pulmonary hypertension in patients infected with the human immunodeficiency virus (HIV), as well as the high frequency of antinuclear antibodies, implicates an abnormality of the immune system in the development of pulmonary hypertension in some patients. The association of primary pulmonary hypertension with cirrhosis and portal hypertension, while statistically significant, remains unexplained.

Pulmonary venoocclusive disease   This is a distinct pathologic entity, found in less than 10 percent of patients with primary pulmonary hypertension. Histologically, it is manifest by widespread intimal proliferation and fibrosis of the intrapulmonary veins and venules, occasionally extending to the arteriolar bed. The pulmonary venous obstruction explains the increased pulmonary capillary wedge pressure observed in patients with advanced disease. These patients may develop orthopnea that can mimic left ventricular failure.

Pulmonary capillary hemangiomatosis   This is a rare form of primary pulmonary hypertension. Histologically, it is characterized by infiltrating thin-walled blood vessels that are widespread throughout the pulmonary interstitium and walls of the pulmonary arteries and veins. These patients often have hemoptysis as a clinical feature.

CLINICOPATHOLOGIC CONSIDERATIONS   It is difficult to distinguish the pathologic subsets of primary pulmonary hypertension on clinical grounds, since the symptoms are similar and the severity of pulmonary hypertension is comparable in all types. The perfusion lung scan is often abnormal, with a diffuse patchy pattern that seems to reflect widespread arteriolar thrombosis. Patients with pulmonary venoocclusive disease, along with abnormal perfusion scans, may have increased bronchovascular markings at the lung bases on chest radiograph. Patients with pulmonary capillary hemangiomatosis may have fluffy-appearing infiltrates in the lung fields, abnormal perfusion scans, and a uniquely abnormal appearance of the pulmonary angiogram revealing areas of increased vascularity at the lung periphery.

ETIOLOGY   By definition, the underlying cause of primary pulmonary hypertension is unknown. Insight into possible mechanisms was provided from the experience in Europe in the late 1960s in which the number of patients with unexplained pulmonary hypertension increased with the introduction of aminorex fumarate, an amphetamine-like drug used for appetite suppression. Use by susceptible individuals caused development of chronic pulmonary hypertension, the mechanism possibly pulmonary vasoconstriction from endothelial injury. Histologically, features of plexogenic and thrombotic pulmonary arteriopathy have been described. The median survival of patients with pulmonary hypertension from aminorex was almost three times longer than that of patients with primary pulmonary hypertension. While some patients improved when the aminorex was discontinued, others had a progressive downhill course, even though the causative agent had been withdrawn.

Pregnancy and oral contraceptives had been proposed as etiologic factors, but this has not been substantiated by other studies. Their frequent association is more likely related to the prevalence of primary pulmonary hypertension in young women.

PATHOPHYSIOLOGY   The underlying hemodynamic derangement in primary pulmonary hypertension is an increased resistance to pulmonary blood flow. Early in the disease there is a marked elevation in pulmonary artery pressure with relatively normal cardiac function. Over time the cardiac output becomes progressively reduced rather than the pulmonary artery pressure becoming progressively increased. Initially, the pulmonary arteries may respond to vasodilators, but as the disease progresses, the elevated pulmonary vascular resistance becomes fixed. The pulmonary capillary wedge pressure remains normal until the late stages, when it tends to rise in response to impaired diastolic filling of the left ventricle due to the altered configuration of the intraventricular septum. Eventually, as the right

ventricle fails, the right atrial and right ventricular end-diastolic pressures rise in an attempt to compensate for the myocardial depression that has developed in response to chronic severe right ventricular pressure overload.

Pulmonary function is usually normal in primary pulmonary hypertension, although a mild restrictive pattern (see Chap. 214) is sometimes seen. Hypoxemia is common and is believed to be due to a mismatch between pulmonary ventilation and perfusion, magnified by a low cardiac output. Occasional patients with a patent foramen ovale may develop right-to-left shunting, which also can contribute to systemic arterial desaturation.

DIAGNOSIS   A thorough diagnostic evaluation to look for all potential causes should be undertaken (see Fig. 225-1 and Table 225-1). The history usually reveals the gradual onset of shortness of breath with effort, progressing until the patient is dyspneic with minimal activity. The average duration from symptom onset until diagnosis is 2.5 years. Other common symptoms are fatigue, angina pectoris which likely represents right ventricular ischemia, syncope, near syncope, and peripheral edema. Approximately 7 percent of the cases are familial with the features of an autosomal dominant defect with variable expression.

The physical examination is characteristic. Increased jugular venous pressure, a reduced carotid pulse, and an easily palpable right ventricular lift are typical. Most patients have an increased pulmonic component of the second heart sound and right-sided third and fourth heart sounds. Tricuspid and pulmonic regurgitation and peripheral cyanosis and edema may be noted. Clubbing is not a feature.

The chest x-ray generally shows enlarged central pulmonary arteries and clear lung fields. The electrocardiogram usually reveals right axis deviation and right ventricular hypertrophy. The echocardiogram demonstrates right ventricular enlargement, a reduction in left ventricular cavity size, and abnormal septal configuration consistent

FIGURE 225-1   An algorithm for the workup of a patient with unexplained pulmonary hypertension. (*Adapted with permission from S Rich.*)

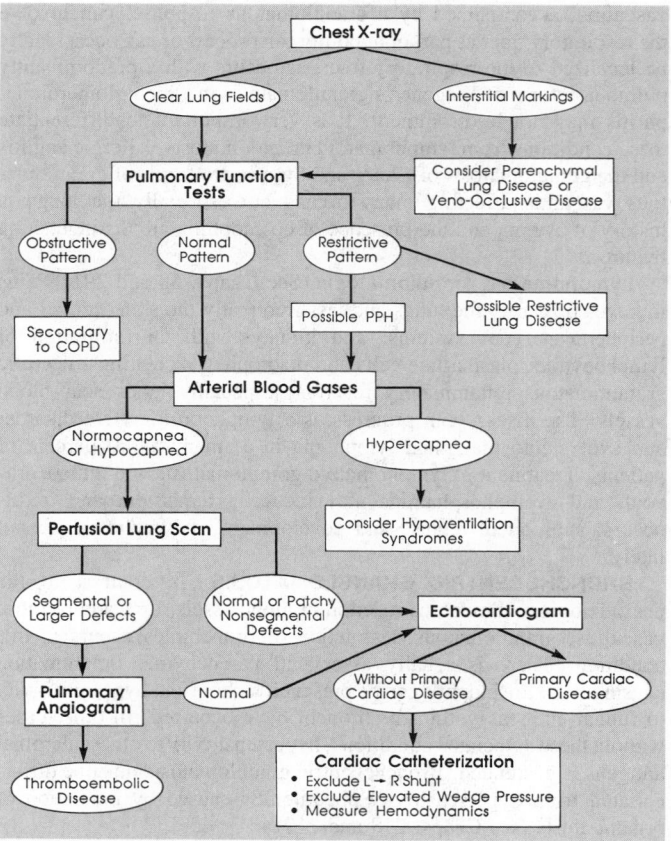

TABLE 225-1 Secondary causes of chronic pulmonary hypertension

Persistent fetal circulation
Congenital heart disease
Valvular heart disease
Primary myocardial disease
Pulmonary thromboembolic disease
Obstructive lung disease
Interstitial lung disease
Arterial hypoxemia with hypercapnea
Collagen vascular disease
Parasitic disease involving the lung
Sickle cell anemia
Intravenous drug abuse
Granulomatous lung disease
Chronic liver disease
Pulmonary artery stenosis
Pulmonary venous hypertension
Aminorex fumarate ingestion

SOURCE: From S Rich, Prog Cardiovasc Dis 31:205, 1988; used with permission.

with right ventricular pressure overload. Doppler studies have revealed a marked dependence on atrial systole for ventricular filling. This would imply that atrial fibrillation could result in inadequate left ventricular filling and might be one cause for sudden death, since no patient with primary pulmonary hypertension and atrial fibrillation has been described. A mild restrictive pattern on pulmonary function tests is consistent with pulmonary hypertension and does not necessarily indicate restrictive lung disease. Hypoxemia, hypocapnia, and an abnormal diffusing capacity for carbon monoxide are almost invariable findings. Evidence of airways obstruction suggests a secondary etiology for the pulmonary hypertension. A perfusion lung scan may be normal or abnormal with multiple diffuse patchy filling defects of a nonsegmental nature and not suggestive of pulmonary thromboembolism. If the lung scan reveals perfusion defects of a segmental or subsegmental nature, a pulmonary angiogram must be done. Severe pulmonary hypertension in a patient with a high-probability lung scan should suggest a chronic process and not acute pulmonary embolism, since the nonconditioned right ventricle is unable to generate high systolic pressures acutely in the face of pulmonary thromboembolism. Chronic thromboembolic obstruction of the large pulmonary arteries (Chap. 226) can mimic primary pulmonary hypertension but can be amenable to treatment with surgical thromboendarterectomy. Defining the precise location and extent of the clots is imperative for surgical removal.

There is risk in performing pulmonary angiography in patients with primary pulmonary hypertension, particularly in the presence of right ventricular failure with elevated right ventricular end-diastolic pressure. In these patients it is recommended that selective or subselective injections with smaller amounts of contrast material be made to minimize the risks, and the use of low-osmolar, nonionic contrast material also may diminish risk. One mechanism for cardiac arrest in this setting is hypotension and bradycardia that may be vagally mediated; the pretreatment of selected patients with 1 mg atropine is also advocated.

Cardiac catheterization is mandatory to characterize the disease and exclude an underlying cardiac shunt as the cause. The use of balloon-flotation catheters, especially those with removable guidewires, can facilitate right heart catheterization, which can be technically difficult. A right-to-left shunt might be attributable to a patent foramen ovale, but any left-to-right shunting implies the presence of a congenital defect. Although it may be difficult to obtain an accurate pulmonary capillary wedge pressure tracing in some patients, the wedge pressure is not falsely elevated. If recordings suggest that the wedge pressure is increased, left heart catheterization also should be performed to exclude mitral stenosis or increased left ventricular end-diastolic pressures as the cause. Although the diagnostic evaluation of these patients can be hazardous, experience from a national multicenter study revealed no mortality or serious morbidity in more

than 300 patients whose evaluation included pulmonary angiography and cardiac catheterization. It is not necessary to perform an open lung biopsy in these patients to make an accurate diagnosis. If the diagnostic evaluation is undertaken as outlined, a correct diagnosis will almost always be made.

On occasion a patient may have marked elevations in pulmonary artery pressure and a relatively mild disease that is known to cause pulmonary hypertension. It would be a mistake to characterize these patients as having primary pulmonary hypertension on the belief that the pulmonary hypertension is out of proportion to the underlying associated condition. Since the pulmonary vascular bed has variable vasoreactivity, these cases probably reflect an exaggerated pulmonary vasoconstrictive response to the associated condition. Thus severe pulmonary hypertension can coexist with mild chronic obstructive pulmonary disease, small intracardiac shunts, mild mitral stenosis, and even ischemic heart disease. The distinction, however, is important because the treatment of pulmonary hypertension should always be focused toward the underlying cause.

NATURAL HISTORY The natural history of primary pulmonary hypertension is unknown because initially the disease is largely asymptomatic. Several series have reported a mean survival of 2 to 3 years for patients from the time of diagnosis. Few patients survive more than 10 years. Functional class is a strong predictor of survival, since patients who are functional class II and III have a mean survival of 3.5 years compared with those who are functional class IV, in whom the mean survival is 6 months. The cause of death is usually right ventricular failure or sudden death; sudden death appears to be a late feature of the disease. Increased right atrial pressure above 15 mmHg and reduced cardiac index below 2 $(L/min)/m^2$ are hemodynamic predictors of a poor prognosis.

MANAGEMENT The treatment of primary pulmonary hypertension, while still unsatisfactory, has improved considerably. Because the pulmonary vascular resistance increases dramatically with exercise, patients should be cautioned against participating in activities that demand increased physical stress. The use of digoxin remains controversial, since no studies have documented a benefit or detriment. Diuretic therapy may relieve dyspnea and peripheral edema and may be useful in reducing right ventricular volume overload in the presence of tricuspid regurgitation.

The main focus of therapy is vasodilator drugs. For vasodilators to have sustained beneficial effects, they must lower the pulmonary artery pressure along with the pulmonary vascular resistance while preserving systemic blood pressure. Calcium channel antagonists, when given in high doses (e.g., nifedipine 120 to 240 mg/d or diltiazem 540 to 900 mg/d*) that are titrated to the hemodynamic response, can produce dramatic reductions in pulmonary artery pressure and pulmonary vascular resistance associated with improvement in symptoms, regression of right ventricular hypertrophy, and improved survival. However, less than half the patients with primary pulmonary hypertension respond to this regimen. In addition, it is unknown whether the response depends on the histologic subtype, but the therapy appears to be more successful in patients who are diagnosed early and have less advanced disease. None of the other classes of vasodilator drugs that have been investigated, including beta-adrenergic agonists, alpha-adrenergic blockers, smooth-muscle vasodilators, nitrates, and angiotensin-converting enzyme inhibitors, has shown similar sustained effectiveness.

The administration of vasodilators can have serious acute and chronic adverse effects. The most common response is a reduction in pulmonary vascular resistance, manifest by an increased cardiac output, without a reduction in the mean pulmonary artery pressure. This results in increased stroke work of the right ventricle, which can result in worsening of ventricular function and precipitate right ventricular failure over time. In addition, maintenance of adequate systemic blood pressure is crucial, since right ventricular coronary

* These agents have not been approved for the treatment of primary pulmonary hypertension by the U.S. Food and Drug Administration.

blood flow is already compromised due to the loss of the normal gradient for myocardial perfusion between the aorta and right ventricle. Vasodilator drugs can provoke acute right ventricular ischemia, and deaths have been reported. For these reasons, the pharmacologic evaluation of primary pulmonary hypertension should always be undertaken with direct monitoring of systemic and pulmonary arterial pressures and cardiac output.

Prostacyclin† has been employed intravenously as a treatment of patients who fail to respond to calcium channel antagonists. Preliminary studies have shown that patients receiving prostacyclin have an improvement in exercise tolerance and a reduction in mortality. The mechanism by which prostacyclin exhibits its effects are unclear. The side effects of prostacyclin, which include flushing, jaw pain, bloating, and diarrhea, are generally tolerated by most patients. Whether the use of prostacyclin will be limited to patients with advanced disease who are waiting organ transplantation or as a chronic therapy remains to be determined.

Anticoagulant therapy also has been advocated based on the evidence that thrombosis in situ is common. One retrospective study and one prospective study have demonstrated that the anticoagulant warfarin increases the survival of patients with primary pulmonary hypertension, and thus consideration for its use should be given to all patients. The dose of warfarin is generally titrated to achieve an increase in INR of 1.5 to 2.5 of control. Anticoagulants should not be expected to cause regression of the disease and result in any substantial change in symptoms.

Patients who fail to respond to vasodilator drugs should be considered as possible candidates for heart-lung or lung transplantation (Chaps. 196 and 232). Single lung transplantation is the preferred operation, since it has been shown that patients with primary pulmonary hypertension who receive a single lung have a substantial reduction in the pulmonary artery pressure and a marked amelioration of symptoms, even in the face of preexisting right ventricular dysfunction and failure. It is also a simpler operation with a shorter waiting time than heart-lung transplantation. The operation is best reserved for patients who are in the advanced stages of the disease, in whom it may be predicted that survival is likely to be less than 1 year. Recurrence of disease has not been reported in any patient with primary pulmonary hypertension who has undergone single lung or heart-lung transplantation.

REFERENCES

D'ALONZO GE et al: Survival in patients with primary pulmonary hypertension: Results from a national prospective study. Ann Intern Med 115:343, 1991

FUSTER V et al: Primary pulmonary hypertension: Natural history and the importance of thrombosis. Circulation 70:580, 1984

PACKER M: Vasodilator therapy for primary pulmonary hypertension. Ann Intern Med 103:258, 1985

PASQUE MK et al: Single-lung transplantation for pulmonary hypertension: Three-month hemodynamic follow-up. Circulation 84:2275, 1991

PIETRA GG et al: Histopathology of primary pulmonary hypertension: A qualitative and quantitative study of pulmonary blood vessels from 58 patients in the National Heart, Lung and Blood Institute Primary Pulmonary Hypertension Registry. Circulation 80:1198, 1989

RICH S: Primary pulmonary hypertension. Prog Cardiovasc Dis 31:205, 1988

—— et al: High-dose calcium blocking therapy for primary pulmonary hypertension: Evidence for long-term reduction in pulmonary artery pressure and regression of right ventricular hypertrophy. Circulation 76:135, 1987

—— et al: Primary pulmonary hypertension: A national prospective study. Ann Intern Med 107:216, 1987

—— et al: The effect of high doses of calcium-channel blockers on survival in primary pulmonary hypertension. N Engl J Med 327:76, 1992

—— et al: Pulmonary hypertension from chronic pulmonary thromboembolism. Ann Intern Med 108:425, 1988

RUBIN LJ et al: Treatment of primary pulmonary hypertension with continuous intravenous prostacyclin (epoprosternol): Results of a randomized trial. Ann Intern Med 112:485, 1990

---

226 PULMONARY THROMBOEMBOLISM

KENNETH M. MOSER

Pulmonary thromboembolism (PTE) is a leading cause of morbidity and mortality and can appear in many clinical contexts. Epidemiologic surveys indicate that PTE is responsible for more than 50,000 deaths in the United States annually. However, available data suggest that less than 10 percent of all pulmonary emboli result in death. Thus the incidence of fatal plus nonfatal emboli probably exceeds 500,000 annually. This overall incidence seems verified by autopsy statistics. Evidence of recent or old embolism is detected in 25 to 30 percent of routine autopsies; with special techniques, this figure exceeds 60 percent. Even these data underestimate incidence, since many emboli resolve without trace and are not found at postmortem examination. The high incidence of PTE at autopsy contrasts sharply with the incidence of antemortem diagnosis. Available information suggests that an antemortem diagnosis has been made in only 10 to 30 percent of all cases in which old or recent embolism is demonstrated at autopsy.

The incidence of embolism does not appear to be decreasing, despite advances in diagnosis and prophylaxis. This apparent paradox is likely explained by medical advances, e.g., higher survival in trauma patients, the increase in "open heart," orthopedic (e.g., hip replacement), and other medical and surgical procedures, particularly among patients in older age groups, and more widespread use of indwelling catheters. Thus there is an expanding population at high risk for developing venous thrombosis.

VENOUS THROMBOSIS

PATHOGENESIS Available data indicate that more than 95 percent of pulmonary emboli arise from thrombi in the deep venous system of the lower extremities. Furthermore, it appears that the larger leg veins (popliteal vein and above) are by far the most common source of those pulmonary emboli which reach clinical attention. Thrombi occurring in the right cardiac chambers or in other veins account for the remainder, but are uncommon unless some inciting factor is present, such as indwelling catheters or intracavitary pacing wires. In situ pulmonary arterial thrombosis is rare. Thus embolism should be viewed as a *complication* of deep venous thrombosis (DVT) in the lower extremity veins. Finally, some 90 percent of the deaths due to embolism occur within an hour or two—before a diagnostic-therapeutic plan can be implemented. These facts have several important implications with respect to PTE: (1) prevention of DVT is the most effective approach to prevention of, and death due to, embolism; (2) prompt treatment of DVT may limit the frequency of embolism; and (3) techniques which identify the patient at high risk of DVT and allow prompt diagnosis are the key to reduction of embolic risk.

The three factors which promote DVT (and, therefore, embolic risk), as defined by Virchow in the nineteenth century, are stasis, abnormalities of the vessel wall, and alterations in the blood coagulation system. Coagulation alterations have been studied extensively, but as yet there is no reliable test for a state of "hypercoagulability," i.e., a test which will predict the risk of DVT. However, there is a growing list of conditions in which thrombotic risk is increased: deficiencies of antithrombin III, protein C, protein S, and components of the fibrinolytic system; presence of a lupus anticoagulant; and homocystinuria. However, such discrete abnormalities are uncommon in the population that develops DVT and are usually discovered after the event. Therefore, the risk of DVT is best assessed by recognizing the presence of known "clinical" risk factors. Conditions associated with a high risk of venous thromboembolism include any surgical

---

† This drug is currently available as an Investigational New Drug only.

procedure requiring 30 min or more of general anesthesia, the postpartum period, left and right ventricular failure, fractures or injuries or surgical procedures involving the lower extremities, chronic deep venous insufficiency of the legs, prolonged bed rest, carcinoma, obesity, and the use of estrogens.

NATURAL HISTORY In the contexts noted above, deep venous thrombi usually develop in the region of a venous valve. Platelets aggregate, forming a nidus (white thrombus), followed by development of a large fibrin (red) thrombus. The process is apparently a rapid one; large, extensive thrombi can develop within minutes. Growth occurs by continued fibrin and platelet accretion. Beyond formation, two processes may contribute to resolution: fibrinolysis and organization. Fibrinolysis may result in complete resolution within hours to several days. Any remaining thrombus undergoes organization, leaving behind a fibrotic zone that becomes reendothelialized. Valves are often rendered incompetent by this process, and modest or extensive luminal narrowing may occur. Once thrombus growth has halted, available data indicate that fibrinolysis/organization reaches a stable state in 7 to 10 days. It is during the first few days after formation, therefore, that embolic risk is highest.

DETECTION The clinical diagnosis of DVT is difficult and, indeed, unreliable. DVT is frequently present in the absence of clinical signs (e.g., pain, heat, swelling), and it is absent in 50 percent of patients in whom clinical signs or symptoms suggest its presence. Therefore, a number of diagnostic tests have been developed. The gold standard is *ascending contrast venography*. The application of this test is often limited by technical and logistic considerations, however, and repetitive venography is impractical. Among available noninvasive techniques, two have been well-validated against venography: (1) impedance plethysmography (IPG), which detects venous outflow obstruction, is highly sensitive to acute above-knee thrombosis but fails to detect many below-knee thrombi, and (2) the radiofibrinogen method, which is very sensitive to thrombus formation in calf veins and lower thigh veins but not sensitive to thrombi which form in the upper thigh or above. Unfortunately, radiolabeled fibrinogen is no longer available for clinical use. Doppler ultrasound ("duplex") studies are widely used. However, the criteria employed to interpret this test have not been standardized, the sensitivity and specificity of the technique have been poorly validated against venography, and the test is quite operator-dependent. Other methodologies employing radionuclides (attached to platelets, monoclonal antibodies directed against fibrin or platelet components) are under investigation.

PROPHYLAXIS Application of IPG and radiofibrinogen leg scanning has provided insights into the relative risks of DVT (and, therefore, PTE) in various patient populations. Such data, in turn, have led to recommendations for an escalating intensity of prophylaxis based on degree of risk. Four safe and effective prophylactic options have been validated: low-dose heparin, warfarin, intermittent venous compression devices, and combinations of either anticoagulant drug with the compression devices. Patients in the low- and or moderate-risk categories should receive either low-dose heparin (5000 units subcutaneously every 12 h) or intermittent venous compression (by devices which compress the calf, or calf and thigh, approximately once per minute). Patients in these categories include those undergoing major surgery (defined as any procedure requiring general anesthesia for 30 min or more), patients immobilized for any reason, patients with myocardial infarction and congestive heart failure, and women delivered by cesarean section. If heparin cannot be used (e.g., neurosurgery, spinal cord injury), compression devices alone can be applied. Patients at high risk include those with pelvic or lower extremity injury or surgery (e.g., hip/knee replacement). In these patients, combinations of compressive devices plus either heparin or warfarin are warranted. A prior history of DVT or PTE places any patient in the high-risk category. With these multiple options available, some prophylaxis is available for almost every patient at risk of DVT. In patients with severe trauma in whom no other option exists, prophylactic placement of an inferior vena caval filter can be considered.

NATURAL HISTORY OF PULMONARY EMBOLISM

THE ACUTE EVENTS The immediate result of thromboembolism is complete or partial obstruction of the pulmonary arterial blood flow to the distal lung. This obstruction leads to a series of pathophysiologic events which can be categorized as the "respiratory" and "hemodynamic" consequences of PTE.

Respiratory consequences Embolic obstruction produces a zone of the lung which is ventilated but not perfused—an intrapulmonary "dead space" (Chap. 214). Because it cannot participate in the process of gas exchange, ventilation of this nonperfused area is "wasted," in the functional sense. A potential consequence of embolic obstruction is constriction of the air spaces and airways in the affected lung zone. This pneumoconstriction, which might be viewed as a homeostatic mechanism to reduce wasted ventilation, appears to be due to the marked bronchoalveolar hypocapnia that results from cessation of pulmonary capillary blood flow, because it is abolished by inhalation of carbon dioxide–enriched air. While it occurs in animal experiments in which a double-lumen tube separates the ventilation from each lung, it probably occurs very rarely in patients who inhale dead space air (rich in carbon dioxide) into embolized lung zones.

Another disturbance caused by embolic obstruction—loss of alveolar surfactant—does not occur immediately. This surface-active lipoprotein is required to maintain alveolar stability. In its absence, alveolar collapse occurs. Cessation of pulmonary capillary blood flow leads to reduction in surfactant within 2 or 3 h, which becomes severe at 12 to 15 h. Frank atelectasis—the morphologic expression of alveolar instability—can be detected 24 to 48 h after interruption of blood flow.

Arterial hypoxemia is a common, though by no means universal, consequence of PTE. Several mechanisms can contribute to hypoxemia: ventilation-perfusion disturbances, cardiac failure with a lowered mixed venous P_{O_2} (widened arteriovenous difference), and obligatory perfusion through hypoventilated lung zones. Such obligatory perfusion develops because elevation of pulmonary arterial pressure due to embolic obstruction can overcome the vasoconstriction normally present in hypoventilated lung zones.

Hemodynamic consequences The primary hemodynamic consequence of thromboembolic obstruction is a reduction in the cross-sectional area of the pulmonary arterial bed. This loss of vascular capacity increases the resistance to pulmonary blood flow, which, if marked, leads to pulmonary hypertension and acute failure of the right ventricle. Tachycardia and often a decline in cardiac output also occur.

The factors that determine the severity of these hemodynamic changes have been the subject of continued debate. There is agreement that the *extent of embolic obstruction* is a key factor. However, the reserve capacity of the pulmonary arteriocapillary bed is so extensive that more than 50 percent of the vascular area must be obstructed before significant elevation in pulmonary arterial pressure results. Because pulmonary hypertension occurs in some patients with occlusion of lesser extent, investigators have searched for reflex or humoral vasoconstrictor mechanisms associated with embolism. Despite a long and careful search for such mechanisms, their extent and frequency in human PTE remains unknown. Hence some workers maintain that the degree of embolic obstruction itself is the only determinant of hemodynamic impairment. They suggest that instances of apparent disparity between the extent of embolism and clinical response reflect only clinical underestimation of the magnitude of the embolism. Other investigators, however, have presented compelling evidence to support the occurrence of pulmonary vasoconstriction with embolism. Some have demonstrated that constriction is associated with obstruction of the smaller, but not the larger, pulmonary arterial vessels. According to another hypothesis, serotonin or thromboxane, known pulmonary vasoconstrictive-bronchoconstrictive substances, are released from platelets and coat fresh emboli as they lodge in the pulmonary tree. This thesis introduces the attractive concept that an embolus might be regarded, in part, as a packet with pharmacologic, as well as obstructive, potential. A consensus view is that while the extent of embolism is a key factor, humoral and/or reflex influences probably operate in certain patients and compromise the pulmonary circulation to a greater extent than might be expected on an anatomic basis alone.

The cardiopulmonary status of the patient prior to embolism is also critical in determining the clinical severity of embolism. A small embolus may have limited impact on an otherwise healthy individual but may have serious consequences in someone with advanced cardiac or pulmonary disease.

Both experimental and clinical studies have established that infarction—death of lung tissue—rarely accompanies embolic occlusion. It is likely that less than 10 percent of emboli in humans lead to infarction. That infarction rarely follows embolism should occasion little surprise. The lung has three avenues for obtaining oxygen: the pulmonary arterial circulation, the bronchial arterial circulation, and the airways. Thus infarction occurs infrequently, and its appearance usually is associated with compromise of bronchial arterial flow and/or airways to the involved area. Such compromise is promoted by the existence of other cardiac or pulmonary diseases, such as left ventricular failure, mitral stenosis, and chronic obstructive lung disease. Thus infarction may occur in 30 percent or more of such patients, while it is quite rare in individuals who are free of cardiopulmonary disease.

BEYOND THE ACUTE STATE   The vast majority of pulmonary emboli resolve, and resolve rather quickly. Resolution of fresh emboli begins within the first few days and is well advanced in 10 to 14 days. As in DVT, two mechanisms promote restoration of vascular patency: the fibrinolytic system and the process of organization. However, the fibrinolytic system appears capable of more rapid dissolution of emboli than of venous thrombi.

The availability of these two efficient mechanisms raises the question why all emboli do not resolve. There may be some impairment of the intrinsic fibrinolytic system. The emboli may have been well organized prior to their lodgment in the lung so that they are subject to neither fibrinolytic attack nor further organization. Alternatively, some emboli may be recurrent, so their failure to resolve is more apparent than real.

Another important element of the natural history of thromboembolism is the development of bronchial arterial collateral circulation. If pulmonary arterial obstruction persists, bronchial arterial flow increases substantially over a period of several weeks, restoring flow to the capillary bed. With the return of flow, surfactant production is restored, so that alveolar stability is regained and atelectasis resolves.

DIAGNOSTIC FEATURES

Studies of patients with venous thrombosis of the thigh veins (popliteal and above) have demonstrated that *asymptomatic* embolism, often of substantial magnitude, occurs in some 40 to 60 percent. In those who do develop symptoms, and *sudden onset of unexplained dyspnea is the most common, often the only, symptom of pulmonary embolism. Pleuritic chest pain and hemoptysis are present only when infarction has occurred* and, because bland embolism rarely leads to infarction, are usually absent. With extensive embolism, severe substernal oppressive discomfort may be present, probably due to right ventricular ischemia. Patients also may present with syncope, suggesting a neurologic disorder. Other "occult" presentations in which embolism should be considered include repetitive bouts of otherwise unexplained supraventricular tachyarrhythmias, sudden onset or worsening of congestive heart failure (see Chap. 195); sudden deterioration in the patient with chronic obstructive lung disease, and as an alternative to the diagnosis of "psychic" (anxiety-associated) hyperventilation. The most reliable symptom, however, is breathlessness. Severe, persistent dyspnea is an ominous sign, for it usually indicates extensive embolic occlusion.

PHYSICAL EXAMINATION   Findings on physical examination, like the history, may be deceptively normal. Examination of the lungs may disclose a few atelectatic rales; localized wheezes rarely are heard. A pleural friction rub or evidence of pleural effusion will not be present unless infarction has occurred.

On cardiac examination, the single consistent finding is tachycardia. Only in the rare cases of massive embolism will signs such as a right ventricular gallop, a palpable "lift" over the right ventricle (along the left sternal border), a loud pulmonary closure sound, or prominent *a* waves in the jugular venous pulse be found. A scratchy systolic ejection-type murmur may be heard in the pulmonic area. Also, a systolic or continuous murmur accentuated by inspiration may be audible over the lung fields. These murmurs appear to be generated by turbulence of flow in vessels partially obstructed by emboli, since they disappear after resection or resolution of emboli. They should be carefully sought in any patient suspected of having PTE. Wide, fixed splitting of the second heart sound may be present. This indicates extensive embolic obstruction and implies both severe pulmonary hypertension and right ventricular failure. As embolic resolution occurs, this finding disappears. Absence of an accentuated pulmonic closure sound is not a reliable guide to the severity of PTE, since when embolism is sufficiently massive to reduce cardiac output, pulmonary arterial pressure falls and the pulmonary closure sound may be normal or diminished.

The detection of *deep venous thrombosis* qualifies as an excellent clue to the diagnosis of embolism, but its absence does not exclude embolism, because the entire venous thrombus may embolize. Even when sought with diligence, *clinical* evidence of thrombophlebitis is found in less than half of patients with PTE. *Fever* in patients with pulmonary embolism is uncommon without complicating infection or infarction. With infarction, fever of 37.5 to 38.5°C (oral) is the rule, but temperature elevations to 39°C or above may occur, making the differentiation between pulmonary infarction and infection difficult.

On clinical grounds alone, then, a firm diagnosis of embolism cannot be made; the clinical *suspicion* of embolism requires confirmation by laboratory studies (Fig. 226-1).

LABORATORY STUDIES   Routine laboratory studies contribute little toward the diagnosis. Leukocytosis and elevation of the sedimentation rate are rarely present in the absence of infarction. A variety of other blood tests, such as assay for specific fibrinopeptides, fibrin degradation products such as D-dimer, or enzymes, have been proposed; none has been shown to be diagnostically sensitive or specific.

Aside from tachycardia, the *electrocardiogram* is normal in most patients. With extensive embolization, there may be evidence of acute pulmonary hypertension (rightward shift of the QRS axis, a tall, peaked P wave), and ST-T changes indicative of right ventricular strain (Chap. 189). These changes are often transient, lasting minutes to hours, but when persistent, they suggest severe pulmonary vascular obstruction.

The *chest roentgenogram* may show a parenchymal infiltrate and evidence of a pleural effusion if *infarction* has occurred. Characteristically, the infiltrates caused by infarction abut against the pleura. However, their shape varies, and they do not usually appear until 12 to 36 h after the embolism has occurred. The effusion, which often precedes the infiltrate, is characteristically small. Thoracentesis usually, but by no means invariably, yields hemorrhagic fluid, with the characteristics of an exudate.

The radiographic findings with embolism alone are more subtle. Elevation of the hemidiaphragm may occur. *Differences in diameter between vessels that should be of equivalent size* should raise the suspicion of embolism. For example, embolic obstruction of the right main pulmonary artery can lead to dilation of the left main pulmonary artery because that vessel must accept the entire pulmonary flow. There may be *abrupt "cutoff"* of a vessel; i.e., as the vessel is traced distally, it suddenly disappears. Clot has the same radiodensity as blood, accounting for the proximal shadow; the absence of flow

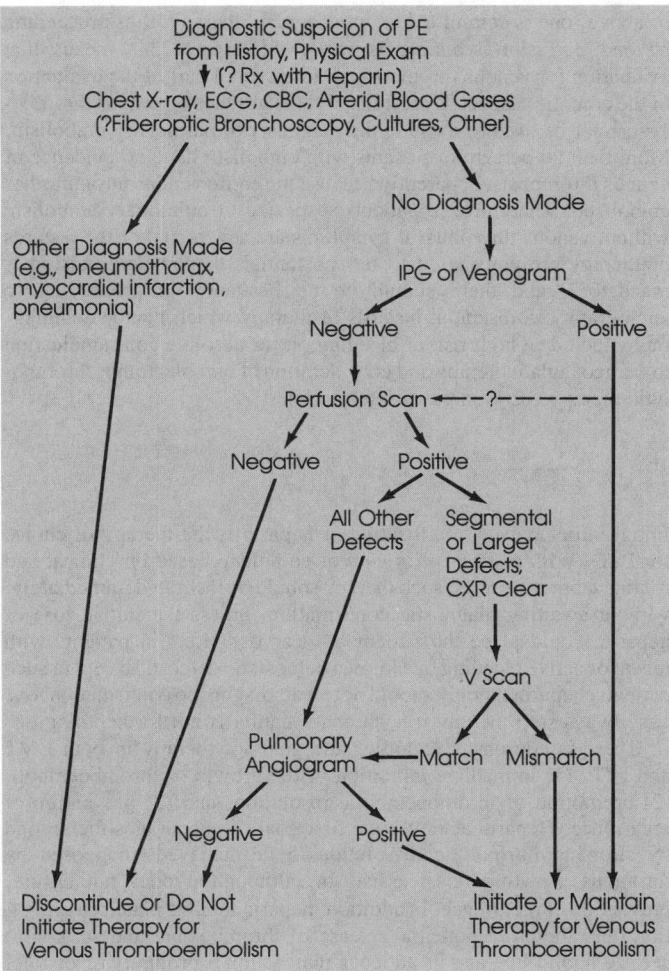

FIGURE 226-1 Flowchart used in diagnosis of pulmonary embolism (PE). IPG, impedance plethysmogram; V scan, ventilation scan.

beyond the clot explains the sudden radiographic "disappearance" of the vessel.

Organization of a clot within a pulmonary artery may lead to retraction of the vessel's walls and a so-called rattail configuration, in which the vessel is relatively normal proximally and suddenly tapers to a sharp point. Finally, there may be *abnormal radiolucency* in some lung zones due to absent or decreased flow. Such abnormally lucent areas (the "Westermark sign"), indicative of proximal arterial obstruction, are best appreciated by examining comparable areas in the two lung fields.

Even in embolization without infarction, the roentgenogram may show small infiltrates, which appear in about 24 h and reflect atelectasis secondary to surfactant depletion. They are not associated with effusion, may fail to touch a pleural surface, and disappear without the linear scarring characteristic of infarction. It should be emphasized that a *normal chest roentgenogram does not exclude the diagnosis of PTE.* Indeed, a *normal* chest roentgenogram is the *most common* finding in embolic disease.

Echo-Doppler studies Standard transthoracic echo-Doppler studies may suggest the diagnosis of embolism by demonstrating right ventricular enlargement, thrombi "trapped" in the right atrium or ventricle, an elevated pulmonary artery pressure, or echogenic densities in the right main pulmonary artery. Transesophageal echocardiography may provide a better view of embolic material in the right main, and rarely the proximal left main, pulmonary artery, but more distal emboli are not reliably detected.

CT with contrast and MRI CT "cuts" through the right and left main pulmonary arteries, with contrast injection, may identify

centrally placed emboli, but as with echo techniques, more distal emboli (which are the most common) cannot be reliably detected. The value of MRI techniques for embolic detection remains uncertain.

Arterial blood gases Massive embolism is commonly associated with arterial hypoxemia, hypocapnia, and respiratory alkalosis. In addition, the difference between alveolar P_{CO_2} and arterial P_{CO_2} ($PA_{CO_2} - Pa_{CO_2}$) may be widened owing to the increase in alveolar dead space (Chap. 214). However, a normal Pa_{O_2} does not exclude the diagnosis.

The laboratory tests discussed thus far are often negative in PTE, and most are relatively nonspecific. Therefore, it is usually necessary to proceed to two more definitive techniques: pulmonary perfusion and ventilation radiophotoscans and the pulmonary angiogram.

Pulmonary perfusion and ventilation scintigraphy Perfusion scintiphotographs (photoscans) are obtained by gamma-camera imaging of the distribution of intravenously injected gamma-emitting radionuclides. The most commonly used radionuclides are microspheres or macroaggregates of albumin (MAA), labeled with a gamma-emitting isotope such as technetium 99m. The radioactive particles, 50 to 100 μm in diameter, are trapped in the pulmonary capillary bed because the pulmonary capillaries approximate 10 μm in diameter. Alternatively, xenon 133 gas, dissolved in saline solution, may be used, but patients must hold their breath. The distribution of labeled particles entrapped in capillaries, or of xenon 133 evolved from them, accurately depicts the distribution of pulmonary blood flow.

The camera-generated perfusion image can be recorded on radiographic film, on special photographic film, on videotape, or projected on to a television screen. Normal scans exhibit homogeneous distribution of radioactivity, smooth margins, and a configuration which corresponds to the normal anatomy of the lungs. Any deviation from these characteristics requires explanation because it represents an abnormality in blood flow distribution.

The perfusion lung photoscan is quite valuable in the diagnosis of embolism. A properly performed perfusion scan which is *normal* excludes the diagnosis of clinically significant pulmonary embolism, as indicated by reports of the excellent outcomes of persons suspected of embolism, who had normal scans and who were not treated (so long as DVT also was absent). On the other hand, a scan demonstrating zones of absent or sharply decreased radioactivity in the patient whose other findings are compatible with PTE keeps the diagnosis of embolism among the possibilities. Scanning is simple, safe, and rapid. It can be repeated to define the resolution, or recurrence, of obstructive vascular phenomena. Like any laboratory test, however, the photoscan must be applied and interpreted with care. It is important, for example, to obtain multiple scan views because lesions not apparent in one view may be easily detected in others. Furthermore, the lung photoscan demonstrates only abnormalities of the *distribution of blood flow.* It does not provide anatomic information.

Many disorders other than PTE are associated with abnormalities in the distribution of pulmonary blood flow. Any disease process, such as pneumonia, atelectasis, or pneumothorax, which reduces the ventilation of a lung zone will decrease its perfusion. Parenchymal diseases, such as emphysema, sarcoidosis, bronchogenic carcinoma, and tuberculosis, can all produce scan defects. Therefore, an abnormal perfusion defect lacks specificity. One approach to enhancing specificity is the performance of a ventilation scan, best achieved by having patients breathe a radioactive gas such as xenon 127 or xenon 133.

To assist in deciding whether a ventilation scan may be useful and when pulmonary angiography is required, two factors should be considered: the size of the perfusion defect(s) and the chest roentgenographic findings. If all defects are subsegmental in size *or* if all defects (of any size) are limited to areas of roentgenographic infiltration, ventilation scanning will not be useful, and pulmonary angiography is required if a definitive diagnosis is necessary. If defect(s) are segmental or larger in size, and one or more are in areas clear by x-ray, a ventilation scan should be done. If the radioactive gas enters ("washes in") and is cleared ("washes out") from the

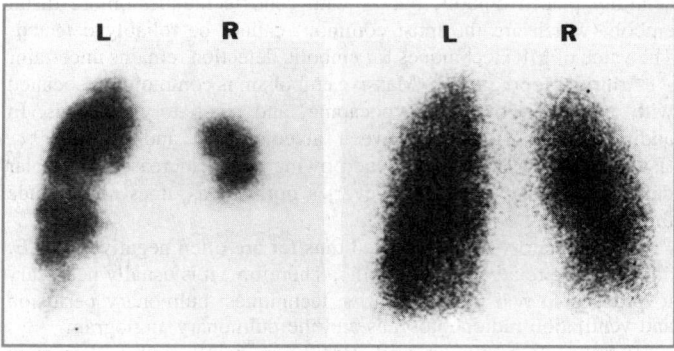

FIGURE 226-2 Perfusion scan (*left*), posterior view, shows multiple segmental and larger perfusion defects in right upper and lower lobes, left lower lobe, and lingula. Ventilation scan (*right*) is normal at equilibrium. Xenon 133 washed in and out normally. Multiple emboli were confirmed angiographically.

area(s) of perfusion defect(s), this "mismatch" of ventilation and perfusion is characteristic of vascular obstruction (Fig. 226-2). Pulmonary vascular obstruction is present in 90 percent or more of patients with this pattern. However, if ventilation is also abnormal (i.e., ventilation-perfusion "match" is present), no reliable diagnostic conclusion can be reached; pulmonary angiography is required. (It may not be required if DVT is present and already mandates therapy.) In some centers, ^{99m}Tc-DTPA particles are used for ventilation studies; this approach provides multiple views but does not allow "washout" evaluation.

In summary, three basic scan patterns emerge: normal, "diagnostic" (which others call "high probability"), and "nondiagnostic" (which others call "intermediate or low probability"). Patients in this last category require pulmonary angiography to establish or exclude the diagnosis of embolism.

Pulmonary angiography   This is the only established means for providing anatomic information about the pulmonary vasculature. Radiopaque material is injected, preferably through a cardiac catheter advanced into the pulmonary artery. Cardiac catheterization and angiography require specialized personnel and a reasonable period for preparation and performance, and they entail more risk than the procedures discussed above. However, angiography provides a visual image of the pulmonary vessels, and catheterization can provide potentially important hemodynamic data (pulmonary artery and wedge pressures, cardiac output). Interpretive limitations of angiography are of two types: (1) *Injection artifacts* may occur which suggest absence of flow to a vessel. Injection should be repeated whenever the question of such artifacts exists. (2) Interpretive errors also may be a consequence of *not looking for the proper type of defect*. There are only two findings diagnostic of acute embolism. One is the *abrupt "cutoff"* of a vessel at the point of embolic impaction. However, complete embolic obstruction is uncommon. Therefore, *filling defects* are the most frequent finding; i.e., the embolus creates a "negative" shadow as the radiopaque material flows around it. The major contraindication to angiography is the absence of personnel who are experienced in both performing the procedure and interpreting the results. Serious diagnostic errors are commonplace if optimal techniques are not used or the complexities of interpretation are not appreciated. However, the risks of angiography are low in experienced hands. Injection of large boluses of contrast medium into the main pulmonary artery should be avoided in favor of small injections into vessels supplying lung regions identified as abnormal on the perfusion scan.

How far one should proceed down the diagnostic pathway outlined above depends on many factors, the major ones being the presence or absence of documented venous thrombosis, the severity of the patient's symptoms, and the hazards of contemplated therapy. In each condition, there is a need for precise diagnosis. If IPG or venography already has documented deep venous thrombosis of the popliteal vein

or above, one is committed to anticoagulant therapy; thus proceeding beyond perfusion scanning is rarely necessary. This means that evaluation for venous thrombosis is an essential part of the evaluation of the embolic suspect. Unfortunately, the absence of venous thrombosis cannot be used to exclude the diagnosis of pulmonary embolism. More than 20 percent of patients with embolism have no evidence of venous thrombosis, apparently because the entire venous thrombus has embolized. Therefore, in patients suspected of pulmonary embolism without venous thrombus, if symptoms are severe and/or the hazards of therapy are considered to be substantial, diagnostic precision is mandatory, and there should be no hesitancy in proceeding to angiography. Substantial hazards of therapy which mandate angiography include a high risk of bleeding on, or absolute contraindication to, anticoagulant therapy and consideration of embolectomy, thrombolytic therapy, or vena caval interruption.

TREATMENT

Initial intravenous administration of heparin is the therapy of choice for PTE. With a strong *suspicion* of embolism based on clinical and routine laboratory tests, such therapy should be instituted immediately, without awaiting diagnostic confirmation, unless the initial dose of heparin would place the patient at clear risk (i.e., in patients with recent or active bleeding or a known hemostatic defect). Except in such patients, heparin therapy should not await diagnostic confirmation; one can always stop therapy if such confirmation is not forthcoming.

There is consensus regarding the goals of therapy in both DVT and PTE: (1) immediate inhibition of the growth of thromboemboli, (2) promotion of thromboembolic resolution, and (3) prevention of recurrence. Heparin achieves the first goal, it encourages the second by allowing fibrinolytic dissolution to be achieved unopposed by thrombus growth, and it assists in, although it does not ensure, prevention of recurrence. In addition, heparin inhibits platelet aggregation (and therefore potential release of thromboxane and serotonin) at the embolic site, and its anticoagulant action is promptly reversible.

There is *not* consensus, however, regarding (1) heparin regimens which best combine safety and efficacy, (2) the need for, and type of, tests for monitoring coagulation behavior during heparin therapy, (3) how long, and with what agents, antithrombotic therapy should be maintained, or (4) in which patients thrombolytic therapy should antedate antithrombotic therapy.

REGIMENS   In DVT, three methods of heparin administration have been advocated by various investigators: continuous intravenous, intermittent intravenous, and intermittent subcutaneous. Continuous intravenous heparin is usually given in a dose of approximately 1000 units per hour. Intermittent intravenous heparin is commonly given in a dose of approximately 5000 units every 4 h or 7500 units every 6 h. Subcutaneous heparin has been recommended at a dose of 5000 units every 4 h, 10,000 units every 8 h, or 20,000 units every 12 h. Studies exist which indicate that each of these regimens is more efficacious, safer, or both. Therefore, at this time, one can conclude only that *each* of these regimens (which approximate 30,000 to 40,000 units per 24 h) represents an acceptable treatment regimen. Despite such apparent comparability, the continuous intravenous regimen, delivered by an infusion pump, is by far the most popular in the United States. *Intramuscular* injection of heparin is to be avoided because hematomas will develop. (Indeed, *all* intramuscular injections should be avoided during anticoagulant therapy.)

It also should be recognized that there is a growing consensus that DVT that remains confined to the calf veins need *not* be treated with anticoagulant therapy. No increase in morbidity or mortality has been reported among patients in this category who are not treated. However, since 15 to 20 percent of calf-limited thrombi will extend to the popliteal veins and above during a 10- to 12-day period, such patients *must* be followed by serial IPG (or, perhaps, ultrasound) tests until this period has elapsed. If they cannot be followed in this manner, they should be treated.

In PTE, the same options for heparin therapy exist. The only additional question is whether an initial large intravenous bolus (10,000 to 20,000 units) should be given to inhibit the aggregation (and release reaction) of platelets adherent to the embolus. Most experts advocate such a dose, with one of the "standard" regimens being started 2 to 4 h later.

MONITORING The value of clotting times (CT), partial thromboplastin times (PTT), or other coagulation tests to monitor the safety and efficacy of heparin remains controversial. With regard to safety, the risk of hemorrhage (the principal complication of heparin therapy) is not clearly related to coagulation test alterations; rather, it appears related to such factors as the coexistence of other diseases associated with bleeding risk (gastric or duodenal ulcer, coagulopathies, uremia) and advanced age. Likewise, achievement of the desired effect of heparin (cessation of thrombus growth in vivo) has not been related consistently to coagulation tests. Therefore, it is questionable whether monitoring with such tests is superior to empiric use of one of the regimens described above. While animal investigations have disclosed that maintaining the PTT above 1.5 times control does prevent growth of venous thrombi, data are not available documenting this in human patients. If done improperly or poorly timed, the CT or PTT tests are worthless and may be misleading. Furthermore, even with continuous intravenous therapy, the CT and PTT may vary substantially during a 24-h period. Despite these vagaries, a majority of experts currently recommend attempting to keep the CT or PTT, measured *just prior* to the next intermittent dose, at or above 1.5 times the baseline CT or PTT and at 1.5 to 2.0 times control with continuous infusion.

DURATION OF THERAPY In DVT, full anticoagulant protection is usually maintained for 7 to 10 days, the rationale being that this is the period required for dissolution and/or organization of the thrombus. In PTE, for the same reasons, a similar duration of therapy is advised. Bed rest is indicated only until cardiopulmonary or leg symptoms subside. Carefully applied elastic support hose should be used (to encourage venous flow) as soon as leg pain, if present, subsides and the patient is ambulated.

During and beyond the acute phase there are several options for achieving proper anticoagulant protection. In deciding among these options, it should be recognized that the major question being addressed is: Does the patient need continued protection against the risk of *recurrent* DVT (and, therefore, PTE)? If the risk factor(s) that precipitated the acute episode of DVT-PTE is (are) no longer present, the patient is asymptomatic, and the IPG is normal, it is acceptable to reduce heparin to a lower dose starting on day 7, ambulate the patient, and, if no symptoms develop, discontinue heparin on day 9 or 10. If these criteria are not met, as is the case in most patients, prolonged prophylactic therapy is warranted. Two options exist for such prophylaxis. The most common one is to initiate a prothrombinopenic agent (e.g., warfarin) as soon as the decision for long-term protection is made. Often, this can be done on day 2 or 3 of heparin therapy. Prothrombinopenic drugs are not suitable for initial therapy in thromboembolism because their onset of action is too slow. Their only role is in maintaining anticoagulant protection for prolonged periods. If they are initiated early in the acute treatment course, the patient must be "in range," as defined by a prothrombin time of 1.5 to 1.8 times the control time for at least 3 days *before heparin is discontinued.* A second option for long-term protection is the use of self-injected subcutaneous heparin. Current data suggest that a dose of 7500 to 10,000 units every 12 h is adequate, is well-tolerated, and need not be monitored with coagulation tests.

There is no consensus regarding the period for which anticoagulant protection should be maintained beyond hospital discharge because firm data on this point are lacking. If *reversible* risk factors are present (e.g., immobilization after a leg fracture), therapy should be continued until the risk factors present have resolved. If the risk factors present are nonreversible (e.g., severe left and/or right ventricular failure), if the IPG remains positive, or if major lung scan defects persist at discharge, empiric decisions are made. At a minimum, 3 months of therapy seems wise, because recurrence is relatively common during this period. Beyond 3 months, however, continuation depends on the balance among specific risk factors exhibited by the patient, IPG results, lung scan results, and the risks of continued therapy. In some instances, this balance may warrant lifetime maintenance on anticoagulant drugs.

Thrombolytic therapy The place of thrombolytic (fibrinolytic) agents (Chap. 202) in the management of acute venous thromboembolism remains to be defined. There is no question that available first-generation agents (streptokinase, urokinase), the second-generation agents (tissue plasminogen activator, tPA), and potential third-generation agents can hasten the resolution of venous thrombi and pulmonary emboli. They do not replace antithrombotic therapy. When used, thrombolytic agents must be followed by a standard course of antithrombotic therapy. Despite extensive study, it has not been established that such agents alter short- or long-term morbidity, mortality, or recurrence rates among patients with DVT or PTE. These drugs, despite high fibrin specificity in the case of tPA, are associated with hemorrhagic risk in patients who have had, or require, any invasive procedure (e.g., vein puncture, arterial puncture, angiography, Swan-Ganz catheterization) and in patients with localized vascular lesions due to recent operation, trauma, or concomitant disease (e.g., peptic ulcer, stroke). If thrombolytic agents prove to have a therapeutic advantage, it would appear to be (1) in patients with extensive, large-vein DVT (e.g., iliofemoral) and (2) in patients with massive embolism and persistent systemic hypotension despite appropriate supportive measures (oxygen, pressor infusions).

Surgical therapy for DVT (thrombectomy) is now rarely considered because the results have not been encouraging. In PTE, surgical therapy should be reserved for those patients in whom heparin therapy is deemed inadequate or impractical. Anticoagulant therapy may be contraindicated by the presence of a bleeding diathesis, or the patient may be in such critical condition that it is felt unwise to await a response to medical therapy. In such instances, *venous interruption* and *pulmonary embolectomy* should be considered.

The objective of venous interruption is to prevent immediate recurrence of embolism from lower extremity venous thrombi. While multiple ligation and clipping procedures have been used in the past, these have been largely supplanted by the use of filters placed in the inferior vena cava by a transvenous approach (jugular, femoral veins). Ligation of the inferior vena cava has been abandoned because it requires surgery, obstructs venous return acutely, and encourages rapid collateral vein formation which bypasses the ligation. Clips require surgery for placement, may obstruct caval flow, and may thrombose. The filters, typified by the Greenfield filter, which has been the most widely used in recent years, are inserted transvenously, do not obstruct caval flow, protect against emboli greater than 2 mm in diameter, and are rarely subject to thrombosis.

There are two major indications for placement of a caval filter: (1) as a lifesaving procedure in patients with massive embolism who could not tolerate an embolic recurrence and (2) to prevent embolism in patients with documented venous thrombosis in whom anticoagulant therapy is contraindicated.

There is one instance, however, in which caval ligation may be the therapy of choice: septic thrombophlebitis of pelvic origin with multiple septic pulmonary emboli. If these patients do not respond promptly to a heparin-antibiotic regimen, they may die unless caval (and left ovarian vein) ligation is carried out.

Two criteria should be met before emergency pulmonary embolectomy is performed: (1) there must be evidence of severe hemodynamic compromise due to embolism, particularly sustained systemic hypotension, which is not responsive to supportive measures, and (2) the personnel and equipment required for embolectomy carried out with the aid of cardiopulmonary bypass must be available. Even with these criteria satisfied, it now appears likely that management of such patients by alternative approaches (e.g., placement of a caval filter plus heparin therapy, thrombolytic therapy) will be associated with lower mortality rates than is emergency embolectomy.

SPECIAL CONSIDERATIONS   Total resolution of emboli does not always occur. Why in some patients (perhaps 0.1 percent) emboli fail to resolve is not yet known. However, if residual vascular obstruction is substantial, the patient may present, months or years after the actual embolic events, with dyspnea and pulmonary hypertension of uncertain cause, often with right ventricular failure. Such patients commonly are misdiagnosed, for months or years, as having asthma, chronic lung disease, primary pulmonary hypertension, or cor pulmonale of unclear etiology, particularly if, as is commonly the case, the initial pulmonary embolic event went unrecognized.

Such patients should be studied by appropriate techniques, since emboli in the main or lobar arteries can be surgically removed (thromboendarterectomy), allowing cure of this otherwise fatal form of pulmonary hypertensive disease. This entity, once an autopsy curiosity, is more common than previously appreciated. More than 400 patients have been reported to have undergone thromboendarterectomy. Because surgical mortality is heavily conditioned by the severity of right ventricular dysfunction at the time of operation, early recognition is important. A follow-up lung scan after diagnosed massive embolism may help in this regard.

PROGNOSIS IN PULMONARY EMBOLISM   The prognosis of the patient with pulmonary embolism *in whom therapy is promptly instituted* is excellent. As stated at the outset of this chapter, less than 1 embolic event in 10 is lethal. The majority of these deaths occur suddenly and can be avoided only by prophylaxis (see above). The remainder appear to be due to embolic extension or recurrence, which therapy can moderate. Thus, for patients who survive long enough to reach medical attention and receive heparin, the outlook is quite good. Morbidity following embolism is uncommon, since embolic resolution is the rule, and very few patients develop the pulmonary hypertensive problem noted above.

Limited reliable data are available regarding recurrence rates in the months and years after a single embolic event (with or without prolonged postembolic anticoagulant therapy). In the absence of risk factors or a positive IPG, recurrence appears to be uncommon, but more precise data are needed.

Whether the therapeutic approaches discussed here will be altered by new agents, such as low-molecular-weight heparin, heparinoids, and newer thrombolytic agents, remains to be seen. However, in the case of low-molecular-weight heparin, data are appearing which suggest that once-daily subcutaneous injections of fixed doses, without monitoring, may someday become the "standard regimen" for both DVT and PTE.

NONTHROMBOTIC EMBOLISM

Because the lung vasculature serves as a filter of the venous circulation, it is the recipient of diverse materials which can gain entry into venous blood, including bone marrow, foreign bodies, parasites, and tumor cells. The most frequently encountered form of nonthrombotic embolism is *fat embolism*. This dramatic and controversial entity follows the introduction of neutral fat into the venous circulation, most commonly after bone trauma or fracture (marrow fat), but occasionally after trauma to adipose tissue or liver infiltrated by fat. The clinical sequence is characteristic. After a latent period of 12 to 36 h or more, during which the patient is asymptomatic, sudden cardiopulmonary and neurologic deterioration appears. Mental aberrations, delirium, and coma develop. Dyspnea, tachypnea, and tachycardia occur, and the chest roentgenographic and physiologic components of the "adult respiratory distress syndrome" appear (see Chap. 230). Anemia and thrombocytopenia are common, as are petechiae on the upper thorax and arms. The pathogenesis of the syndrome is not clear, but it seems likely that two events occur: release of free fatty acids (by action of lipases on the neutral fat), which induces a toxic vasculitis, followed by platelet-fibrin thrombosis, and actual obstruction of small pulmonary arteries by macroaggregates of fat. Several forms of therapy have been proposed (e.g., corticosteroids, heparin, ethanol), but none has proved effective. Treatment remains supportive, and the mortality rate is high.

Another dramatic form of nonthrombotic embolism is *amniotic fluid embolism*. This occurs during both spontaneous delivery and cesarean section. Sudden and massive obstruction of the pulmonary microvasculature occurs, leading to shock and, often, death. With survival of the initial phase of the disease, the picture of disseminated intravascular coagulation appears. The syndrome is due to the entrance of a significant quantity of amniotic fluid into the venous circulation. This fluid is a potent thromboplastic agent which induces thrombosis in the pulmonary vasculature and elsewhere. The fluid also contains particulates which lodge in the lung. Treatment consists of supportive measures.

Nonembolic pulmonary arterial obstruction due to *vasculitis* has become a common problem among intravenous drug users. This vasculitis, caused by the drugs per se or materials (e.g., talc) mixed with the drugs, can induce thrombosis. This entity may be difficult to distinguish from PTE. Repetitive episodes may lead to irreversible and severe pulmonary hypertension. Other forms of vasculitis (e.g., Takayasu's arteritis) also may obstruct the large pulmonary arteries and mimic pulmonary embolism, as may primary pulmonary artery sarcomas and fibrosing mediastinitis.

REFERENCES

CARSON JL et al: The clinical course of pulmonary embolism. N Engl J Med 326:1240, 1992

HIRSH J: Oral anticoagulant drugs. N Engl J Med 324:1865, 1991

———: Heparin. N Engl J Med 324:1565, 1991

HOMMES DW et al: Subcutaneous heparin compared with continuous intravenous heparin administration in the initial treatment of deep vein thrombosis: A meta-analysis. Ann Intern Med 116:279, 1992

HUISMAN MV et al: Utility of impedance plethysmography in the diagnosis of recurrent deep vein thrombosis. Arch Intern Med 148:681, 1988

HULL RD, RASKOB GE: Low probability lung scan findings: A need for change. Ann Intern Med 114:142, 1991

——— et al: Subcutaneous low-molecular-weight heparin compared with continuous intravascular heparin in the treatment of proximal-vein thrombosis. N Engl J Med 326:975, 1992

——— et al: Pulmonary angiography, ventilation lung scanning and venography for clinically suspected pulmonary embolism in the abnormal perfusion scan. Ann Intern Med 98:891, 1983

KAKKAR VV et al: Prevention of post-operative embolism by low-dose heparin: An international multicenter trial. Lancet 2:45, 1975

LENSING AW et al: Detection of deep vein thrombosis by real-time B-mode ultrasonography. N Engl J Med 320:342, 1989

LINDBLAD B et al: Autopsy-verified pulmonary embolism in a surgical department: Analysis of the period from 1951 to 1988. Br J Surg 78:849, 1991

MERCANDETTI A et al: Influence of perfusion and ventilation scans on therapeutic decision-making and outcome among embolic suspects. West J Med 142:208, 1985

MOSER KM, FEDULLO PF: Venous thromboembolism: Three simple decisions. Chest 83:117, 256, 1983

——— et al: Chronic major vessel thromboembolic pulmonary hypertension. Circulation 81:1735, 1990

———: Venous thromboembolism: State of the art. Ann Rev Respir Dis 141:235, 1990

NIH CONSENSUS CONFERENCE: Prevention of venous thrombosis and pulmonary embolism. JAMA 256:744, 1986

PALEVSKI HI, FISHMAN AP: Diagnosis and treatment of pulmonary embolism and deep venous thrombosis, in *Update: Pulmonary Diseases and Disorders*, AP Fishman (ed). McGraw-Hill, New York, 1992, pp 451–464

PIOPED INVESTIGATIONS: Value of the ventilation/perfusion scan in acute pulmonary embolism: Results of the prospective investigation of pulmonary embolism diagnosis (PIOPED). JAMA 263:2753, 1990

RITTOO D et al: Role of transesophageal echocardiography in diagnosis and management of central pulmonary artery thromboembolism. Am J Cardiol 71:1115, 1993

SALZMAN EW et al: Intraoperative external pneumatic calf compression to afford long-term prophylaxis against deep vein thrombosis in urologic patients. Surgery 87:239, 1980

227   NEOPLASMS OF THE LUNG

JOHN D. MINNA

Each year, primary carcinoma of the lung affects more than 100,000 males and 50,000 females in the United States, most of whom die within 1 year of diagnosis, making it the leading cause of cancer death. The peak incidence of lung cancer occurs between ages 55 and 65 years. The overall incidence is increasing, causing the age-adjusted lung cancer death rate to double every 15 years. However, the effects of antismoking efforts begun 10 to 20 years ago have finally started to be seen in a flattening of the incidence rate of lung cancer in white males, while, unfortunately, the rate in females is still increasing. At the time of diagnosis, only 20 percent of all lung cancer patients will have local disease, while 25 percent will have disease spread to regional lymph nodes, and 55 percent will have distant metastatic cancer. Even in those patients with supposedly localized disease, overall 5-year survival is only 30 percent for males and 50 percent for females, and this survival rate has not changed significantly over the past 20 years. Thus primary carcinoma of the lung is a major health problem with a generally grim prognosis. However, an orderly approach to diagnosis, staging, and treatment based on knowledge of the clinical behavior of lung cancer allows selection of the best therapy for either potential cure or optimal palliation of individual patients. This approach should be multidisciplinary, involving interaction of internists, chest physicians, medical, radiation, and surgical oncologists, pathologists, and supportive care personnel.

PATHOLOGY

The histologic classification of primary lung neoplasms recommended by the World Health Organization in 1977 should be used. Four major cell types make up 95 percent of all primary lung neoplasms. These are *squamous* or *epidermoid carcinoma*, *small cell* (also called *oat cell*) *carcinoma*, *adenocarcinoma* (including bronchioloalveolar), and *large cell* (also called *large cell anaplastic*) *carcinoma*. The remainder include combined epidermoid and adenocarcinomas, carcinoids, bronchial gland tumors (including cylindromas and mucoepidermoid tumors), and mesotheliomas, as well as rarer tumor types. The various cell types have different natural histories and responses to therapy, and thus a correct histologic diagnosis by an experienced pathologist is the first step to correct treatment. In the past 10 years, for unknown reasons, the incidence of adenocarcinoma is rising, while that of epidermoid cancer is falling.

Major treatment decisions are made on the basis of the crucial distinction between histologic classification of a tumor as a small cell carcinoma or one of the non-small cell varieties (which include epidermoid, adenocarcinoma, large cell carcinoma, bronchioloalveolar carcinoma, and mixed versions of these). Some of these distinctions are summarized in Tables 227-1 and 227-2. In general, small cell carcinoma has spread beyond the bounds of resectional surgery at the time of presentation and is primarily managed with chemotherapy with or without radiotherapy. In contrast, non-small cell cancers found to be localized at the time of presentation should be considered for a curative attempt with either surgery or radiotherapy. Further, the response of non-small cell cancers to chemotherapy usually is not dramatic, making such therapy less important in metastatic disease than it is in nearly all small cell lung cancer patients.

Ninety percent of patients with lung cancer of all histologic types are cigarette smokers, while the rare nonsmoking patient who develops lung cancer usually has adenocarcinoma. However, in nonsmokers with adenocarcinoma involving the lung, the possibility of other primary sites should be considered. Epidermoid and small cell cancers

TABLE 227-1   Incidence, frequency of metastases, and surgical resectability of the major lung cancer histologic types

Cell type	Incidence, %*	Necropsy frequency of distant metastases when clinically localized, %[†]	Resectability rate (AJC study), %[‡]	5-Year survival after curative resection, %
Non-small cell carcinoma				
Epidermoid	17	17	60	37
Adenocarcinoma	40	40	38	27
Large cell carcinoma	15	14	38	27
Small cell carcinoma	25	63	11	<1

* Recent incidence figures reflect an increase in adenocarcinomas. In addition, 3 percent of tumors are mixtures of other types. The incidence of lung cancer with bronchioalveolar components is increasing (>5 percent) and is included in this 3 percent and with the adenocarcinomas.
[†] Determined from autopsy studies of patients dying of causes other than cancer within 30 days following an apparent curative surgical resection.
[‡] AJC = American Joint Committee Study for Cancer Staging and End Results Reporting, indicating percentage of cases thought to undergo a curative resection.
SOURCE: Adapted from DC Ihde et al, 1992.

usually present as central masses with endobronchial growth, while adenocarcinomas and large cell cancers tend to present as peripheral nodules or masses with pleural involvement. Epidermoid and large cell cancers cavitate in approximately 20 percent of cases. Bronchioloalveolar carcinoma can present as a single mass, a diffuse, multinodular lesion, or as a fluffy infiltrate.

ETIOLOGY

The large majority of lung cancers are caused by carcinogens and tumor promoters ingested via cigarette smoking. Overall, the relative risk of developing lung cancer is increased about 13-fold by active smoking and about 1.5-fold by long-term passive exposure to cigarette smoke. Probably there is a cocarcinogenic effect of smoking and industrial or environmental pollutants such as radon gas from natural sources in the ground. There is a dose-response relationship between the lung cancer death rate and the total amount (often expressed in "cigarette pack-years") of cigarettes smoked, such that the risk is increased 60- to 70-fold for the man smoking two packs a day for 20 years compared with the nonsmoker. Conversely, the chance of developing lung cancer decreases with cessation of smoking but may never return to the nonsmoker level. The increase in lung cancer in women is also associated with a rise in cigarette smoking. As a preventive measure, efforts to get persons to stop smoking are mandatory. However, this is extremely difficult because the smoking habit represents a powerful addiction to nicotine. Therefore, it is of vital importance to prevent people from starting to smoke. This requires new efforts targeted at children, since addiction to cigarettes has occurred by the late teen years.

The poor prognosis for most patients with lung cancer requires the continued performance of well-designed clinical trials to test new forms of therapy. These include further adjuvant and neoadjuvant trials combined with surgery and radiotherapy; prospective testing of tumor sensitivity in vitro to drugs, radiation therapy, and biologic response modifiers; tests of anti-growth factor therapy; and application of newer methods for early detection. The key intervention remains prevention, and broad antismoking efforts must continue. Recently, chemoprevention trials with agents such as retinoic acid have started. The detection of genetic lesions predisposing to malignancy in airway epithelial cells would be a major step forward in focusing preventive efforts, providing intermediate endpoints, molecular early diagnosis, and eventually targeting therapy at the products that make lung cancer cells malignant.

TABLE 227-2 Comparison between small cell and non-small cell lung cancers

	Small cell	Non-small cell
Histology	Scant cytoplasm; small hyperchromatic nuclei with fine chromatin pattern; nucleoli indistinct; diffuse sheets of cells	Abundant cytoplasm; pleomorphic nuclei with coarse chromatin pattern; nucleoli often prominent; glands or squamous architecture
General neuroendocrine properties:		
Dense core granules	Present	Absent*
L-Dopa decarboxylase activity	High	Absent
Chromogranin	Present	Absent
Synaptophysin	Present	Absent
Neuron-specific enolase	High	Low
Creatine kinase BB isozyme	High	Low
Leu-7, HNK-1 antigens	Present	Absent
Peptide hormone production:		
Gastrin-releasing peptide gene products	Present	Absent
Other neuropeptides	ACTH, AVP, calcitonin, ANF	PTH
Other markers:		
HLA, β_2-microglobulin	Absent/low	Present
Intermediate filament pattern	"SCLC"	"Non-SCLC"
Neurofilaments	Present	Absent
Opioid receptors	Present	Present
Nicotine receptors	Present	Present
EGF receptors	Low or absent	Present
Mucin	Absent	Present in adenocarcinomas
Surfactant associate proteins	Absent	Often present
Carcinoembryonic antigen	Present	Present
Cytogenetics and mutations:		
3p deletions	Present ~100%	Present in >90%
rb gene mutations	Present in ~100%	Present in >20%
p53 mutations	Present in >90%	Present in >50%
Other deletions (see text)	Present	Present
ras mutations	<1%	~30%
myc family overexpression	>50%	>50%
Response to radiotherapy	Objective shrinkage in 80–90%; often complete response	Objective shrinkage in 30–50%; uncommonly complete
Response to combination chemotherapy:		
Overall regression rate	90%	30–40%
Complete regression rate	50%	5%
Overall 5-year survival rates	5%	8%

* Ten percent of non-small cell lung cancers have populations of cells expressing neuroendocrine markers, and these are best demonstrated by immunohistochemical stains.

While human lung cancer is not thought of as a genetic disease, a variety of molecular genetic studies have shown that lung cancer cells have acquired a number of genetic lesions including activation of dominant oncogenes and inactivation of tumor suppressor or recessive oncogenes (Chap. 317). In fact, it appears that to become clinically evident, lung cancer cells have to accumulate a large number

(perhaps 10 or more) of such lesions. For the dominant oncogenes, these include point mutations in the coding regions of the *ras* family of oncogenes (particularly in the K-*ras* gene in adenocarcinoma of the lung) and amplification, rearrangement, and/or loss of transcriptional control of *myc* family oncogenes (c-, N-, and L-*myc*), with changes in c-*myc* found in non-small cell cancers while changes in all *myc* family members are found in small cell lung cancer. Tumor mutations in *ras* genes are associated with poor prognosis in non-small cell lung cancer, while tumor amplification of c-*myc* is associated with poor prognosis in small cell lung cancer.

For the recessive oncogenes (*tumor suppressor genes*), cytogenetic and restriction fragment length polymorphism (RFLP) analyses have shown deletions (allele loss) involving chromosome regions 1p, 1q, 3p14, 3p21, 3p24-25, 3q, 5q (familial polyposis gene cluster), 9p (interferon gene cluster), 11p, 13q14 (retinoblastoma, *rb*, gene), 16q, and 17p13 (*p53* gene), as well as other sites. There appear to be several candidate recessive oncogenes on chromosome 3p which are involved in nearly all lung cancers. The *p53* and *rb* genes are both mutated in more than 90 percent of small cell lung cancers, while *p53* is mutated in more than 50 percent and *rb* in more than 20 percent of non-small cell lung cancers. Mutations in the familial polyposis and interferon gene clusters are also common. The large number of genetic lesions in clinically evident cancer has prompted a search for these mutations in lung tissue before classic cytopathologic evidence of malignancy can be found, to provide for molecular early diagnosis and as intermediate endpoints in prevention efforts, including chemoprevention treatment.

The large number of lesions shows that lung cancer, like other common epithelial malignancies, is a multistep process likely to involve both carcinogens (causing initiation by mutagenesis) and tumor promoters (allowing the outgrowth of cells with genetic lesions). Prevention can be directed at both processes. Cell biologic studies have shown that lung cancer cells both produce a large number of peptide hormones and express receptors for these hormones, which thereby can act to stimulate tumor cell growth in an "autocrine" fashion. Nicotine potentially plays a very central role in lung cancer pathogenesis. Highly carcinogenic derivatives of nicotine are formed in cigarette smoke. Smoking is tied to nicotine addiction, and nicotine gum and patches are now widely used to help persons to stop smoking. Lung cancer cells of all histologic types express receptors for nicotine that are very similar to nicotinic acetylcholine receptors. Thus it is possible that nicotine itself could be directly involved in lung cancer pathogenesis.

While lung cancer does not have a clear pattern of Mendelian inheritance, there are several indications of a potential for familial association. These include inherited mutations in *rb* (patients with retinoblastomas living to adulthood) and *p53* (Li-Fraumeni syndrome) genes; studies that show that first-degree relatives of lung cancer probands have a significantly (two- to threefold) excess risk of lung cancer or other cancers, many of which are not smoking-related; and a strong risk of developing lung cancer has been shown to be linked with the development of chronic obstructive pulmonary disease. Finally, several studies have proposed an association between P450 enzyme phenotype or genotype with the development of lung cancer, the most prominent being inheritance of the high-debrisoquine metabolic phenotype [P450 enzyme 2D6 on chromosome 22 (see Chap. 66)] associated with a six- to tenfold increased risk of lung cancer.

CLINICAL MANIFESTATIONS AND MODE OF PRESENTATION

Lung cancer gives rise to signs and symptoms from local tumor growth, invasion or obstruction of adjacent structures, growth in regional nodes via lymphatic spread, growth in distant metastatic sites after hematogenous dissemination, or as a remote effect (paraneoplastic syndrome). The latter usually results from peptide hormone secretion by the tumor or immunologic cross reaction between tumor and normal tissue antigens. Appropriate identification of these signs and symptoms as tumor-related will guide further evaluation and therapy and be of prognostic importance.

If programs screening asymptomatic patients are excluded, 5 to 15 percent of patients are detected while asymptomatic, usually on a routine chest radiograph, while the vast majority of patients present with some sign or symptom. Signs and symptoms secondary to central or endobronchial growth of the primary tumor include cough, hemoptysis, wheeze and stridor, dyspnea, and pneumonitis (fever and productive cough) from obstruction. Signs and symptoms secondary to the peripheral growth of the primary tumor include pain from pleural or chest wall involvement, cough, dyspnea on a restrictive basis, and symptoms of lung abscess resulting from tumor cavitation. Signs and symptoms related to the regional spread of tumor in the thorax by contiguity or by metastasis to regional lymph nodes include tracheal obstruction, esophageal compression with dysphagia, recurrent laryngeal nerve paralysis with hoarseness, phrenic nerve paralysis with elevation of the hemidiaphragm and dyspnea, and sympathetic nerve paralysis with Horner's syndrome (enophthalmus, ptosis, miosis, and ipsilateral loss of sweat). *Pancoast's* (or *superior sulcus tumor) syndrome* results from local extension of a tumor (usually epidermoid) growing in the apex of the lung with involvement of the eighth cervical and first and second thoracic nerves, with shoulder pain which characteristically radiates in the ulnar distribution of the arm, often with radiologic destruction of the first and second ribs. Often Horner's syndrome and Pancoast's syndrome will coexist. Other problems of regional spread include *superior vena cava syndrome* from vascular obstruction; pericardial and cardiac extension with resultant tamponade, arrhythmia, or cardiac failure; lymphatic obstruction with resultant pleural effusion; and lymphangitic spread through the lungs with hypoxemia and dyspnea. In addition, bronchioloalveolar carcinoma can spread transbronchially, producing tumor growing along multiple alveolar surfaces with resultant impairment of oxygen transfer, respiratory insufficiency, dyspnea, hypoxemia, and production of large amounts of sputum.

Extrathoracic metastatic disease is found at autopsy in over 50 percent of patients with epidermoid carcinoma, 80 percent of patients with adeno- and large cell carcinoma, and over 95 percent of patients with small cell cancer. These autopsy studies have found lung cancer metastases in virtually every organ system. Thus the majority of lung cancer patients eventually need therapy to palliate symptoms. Common clinical problems related to extrathoracic metastatic lung cancer include brain metastases with neurologic deficits; bone metastases with pain and pathologic fractures; bone marrow invasion with cytopenias or leukoerythroblastosis; liver metastases causing biochemical liver dysfunction, biliary obstruction, and pain; lymph node metastases in the supraclavicular region and occasionally in the axilla and groin; and spinal cord compression syndromes from epidural or bone metastases.

Paraneoplastic syndromes are common in lung cancer patients and may be the presenting finding or first sign of recurrence. In addition, paraneoplastic syndromes may mimic metastatic disease and, unless detected, lead to inappropriate palliative rather than curative treatment. Often the paraneoplastic syndrome may be relieved with successful treatment of the tumor, and tumor treatment is the basis for correcting such syndromes. In some cases the pathophysiology of the paraneoplastic syndrome is known, particularly when a hormone with biologic activity is secreted by a tumor (Chap. 327). However, in many cases the pathophysiology is unknown. *Systemic symptoms* of anorexia, cachexia, weight loss (seen in 30 percent of patients), fever, and suppressed immunity are paraneoplastic syndromes of unknown etiology. *Endocrine syndromes* are seen in 12 percent of patients and have the best understood pathophysiology, including hypercalcemia and hypophosphatemia resulting from ectopic parathyroid hormone or PTH-related peptide production by epidermoid cancer, hyponatremia with the syndrome of inappropriate secretion of antidiuretic hormone or possibly atrial natriuretic factor by small cell cancer, and ectopic secretion of ACTH by small cell cancer,

which usually results in additional electrolyte disturbances, especially hypokalemia, rather than the changes in body habitus seen in Cushing's syndrome from a pituitary adenoma.

Skeletal–connective tissue syndromes include clubbing in 30 percent (usually non-small cell) and hypertrophic pulmonary osteoarthropathy in 1 to 10 percent (usually adenocarcinomas) with periostitis and clubbing giving pain, tenderness, and swelling over the affected bones and a positive bone scan. *Neurologic-myopathic syndromes* are seen in only 1 percent of patients but are dramatic and include the myasthenic *Eaton-Lambert syndrome* and retinal blindness with small cell cancer, while peripheral neuropathies, subacute cerebellar degeneration, cortical degeneration, and polymyositis are seen with all lung cancer types. Many of these are caused by autoimmune responses such as the development of antivoltage-gated calcium channel antibodies in the Eaton-Lambert syndrome. *Coagulation and thrombotic and hematologic manifestations* occur in 1 to 8 percent of patients and include migratory venous thrombophlebitis (*Trousseau's syndrome*), nonbacterial thrombotic (marantic) endocarditis with arterial emboli, disseminated intravascular coagulation with hemorrhage, and anemia, granulocytosis, and leukoerythroblastosis. *Cutaneous manifestations* such as dermatomyositis and acanthosis nigricans are uncommon (1 percent or less), as are the *renal manifestations* of nephrotic syndrome or glomerulonephritis (1 percent or less).

DIAGNOSIS AND STAGING

EARLY DIAGNOSIS Screening persons at high risk (males over 45 years of age smoking 40 or more cigarettes per day) for lung cancer with sputum cytologies and chest radiographs every 4 months has shown a prevalence rate of lung cancer in asymptomatic patients of 4 to 8 cases per 1000 persons. With follow-up screening, 4 new cases of lung cancer are found per 1000 persons followed per year. These lung cancers are detected 72 percent of the time by radiographs alone and 20 percent by cytology alone, while 6 percent are detected by both methods. In contrast to nonscreened patients, 90 percent of these screened patients who develop lung cancer are asymptomatic, 62 percent have resectable lung cancer, and 53 percent of all the new cases are postoperative stage I (see below) with a 5-year survival probability of 45 percent. However, in a large, multi-institutional, prospective, randomized trial there was no difference in the survival rate between the screened and the nonscreened group of smoking males 45 years of age or older. This was because of the presence of clinically silent and undetected metastases in the majority of patients even when primary tumors were detected at a very early stage.

ESTABLISHING A TISSUE DIAGNOSIS OF LUNG CANCER Once signs, symptoms, or screening studies suggest lung cancer, it is necessary to establish a tissue diagnosis of malignancy, determine the histologic cell type, and stage the patient for appropriate treatment. In the initial evaluation of each patient, tumor tissue should be obtained so that a histologic diagnosis of cancer and tumor cell type can be firmly made. Distinction of small cell from non-small cell lung cancer is crucial and is often difficult in cytology preparations. Therefore, cytologic diagnoses from washings or needle aspirates should be reserved for very high risk patients or patients relapsing with cancer after initial treatment. Tumor tissue can be obtained from a bronchial biopsy or transbronchial forceps biopsy at fiberoptic bronchoscopy; from node biopsy at mediastinoscopy; from the operative specimen at the time of definitive surgical resection; from percutaneous biopsy of an enlarged lymph node, soft tissue mass, lytic bone lesion, bone marrow, or pleural lesion; or from an adequate cell block from a malignant pleural effusion.

STAGING PATIENTS WITH LUNG CANCER Lung cancer staging consists of two parts: first, a determination of the location of tumor (anatomic staging) and, second, an assessment of a patient's ability to withstand various antitumor treatments (physiologic staging). For example, in a patient with non-small cell lung cancer, it is crucial to

TABLE 227-3   TNM classification of lung cancer using the new International Staging System (ISS)

PRIMARY TUMOR (T)

T0	No evidence of a primary tumor.
TX	Occult cancer seen in bronchial washing cytologies but not seen on x-ray or fiberoptic bronchoscopy.
TIS	Carcinoma in situ.
T1	Tumor ≤3 cm in greatest dimension, surrounded by lung or visceral pleura, and without evidence of invasion proximal to a lobar bronchus at bronchoscopy. (Uncommon superficial tumors of any size with invasive components limited to the bronchial wall that extend proximal to the main bronchus are also classified as T1.)
T2	Tumor >3 cm in greatest dimension *or* a tumor of any size that either invades the visceral pleura or has associated atelectasis–obstructive pneumonitis extending to the hilar region. At bronchoscopy, the proximal extent of demonstrable tumor must be within a lobar bronchus or at least 2 cm distal to the carina. Any associated atelectasis or obstructive pneumonitis must involve less than an entire lung.
T3	A tumor of any size with direct extension into the chest wall (including superior sulcus tumors), diaphragm, mediastinal pleura, or pericardium without involving heart, great vessels, trachea, esophagus, or vertebral body *or* a tumor in the main bronchus within 2 cm of the carina without involving the carina.
T4	A tumor of any size with invasion of the mediastinum or involving heart, great vessels, trachea, esophagus, vertebral body, or carina *or* the presence of a malignant pleural effusion. (Pleural effusions that are not bloody and not exudative with several negative cytopathologic examinations are not scored as a malignant effusion for staging purposes.)

REGIONAL LYMPH NODES (N)

N0	No demonstrable metastasis to regional lymph nodes.
N1	Metastasis to lymph nodes in the peribronchial or ipsilateral hilar region, or both, including direct extension.
N2	Metastasis to ipsilateral mediastinal or subcarinal lymph nodes.
N3	Metastasis to contralateral mediastinal, contralateral hilar, ipsilateral or contralateral scalene, or supraclavicular lymph nodes.

DISTANT METASTASIS (M)

M0	No known distant metastasis.
M1	Distant metastasis present with site specified (e.g., brain).

STAGE GROUPING USING THE NEW ISS

Occult carcinoma	TX	N0	M0
Stage 0	TIS	Carcinoma in situ	
Stage I	T1	N0	M0
	T2	N0	M0
Stage II	T1	N1	M0
	T2	N1	M0
Stage IIIa	T3	N0	M0
	T3	N1	M0
	T1–3	N2	M0
Stage IIIb	Any T	N3	M0
	T4	Any N	M0
Stage IV	Any T	Any N	M1

SOURCE: Adapted from CF Mountain, 1988.

TABLE 227-4   Pretreatment staging procedures for lung cancer patients

ALL PATIENTS

Complete history & physical examination
   Determination of performance status and weight loss
   Ear, nose, and throat examination
Complete blood count with platelet determination
Serum electrolytes, glucose, calcium, phosphorus, renal and liver function tests
Electrocardiogram
Skin test for tuberculosis
Chest x-ray
Computed tomography scan of brain, chest, abdomen, and radionuclide scan of bone if any of the above studies suggest presence of tumor metastasis in these organs
X-rays of suspicious bony lesions detected by scan or symptom
Barium swallow radiographic examination if esophageal symptoms exist
Pulmonary function studies and arterial blood gas measurements if signs or symptoms of respiratory insufficiency are present
Biopsy of accessible lesions suspicious for cancer if a histologic diagnosis is not yet made or if treatment or staging decisions would be based on whether or not a lesion contained cancer

PATIENTS PRESENTING WITH NO OBVIOUS CONTRAINDICATION TO CURATIVE SURGERY OR RADIOTHERAPY

All above and:

Fiberoptic bronchoscopy with washings, brushings, and biopsy of suspicious areas
Pulmonary function tests and arterial blood gas measurements
Coagulation tests
Computed tomographic scans of brain, chest, and abdomen
If surgical resection is planned: surgical evaluation of the mediastinum at mediastinoscopy or at thoracotomy
If the patient is a poor surgical risk or a candidate for curative radiotherapy: Transthoracic fine-needle aspiration biopsy or transbronchial forceps biopsy of peripheral lesions if material from routine fiberoptic bronchoscopy is negative

PATIENTS PRESENTING WITH DISEASE THAT IS NOT CURABLE BY EITHER SURGERY OR RADIOTHERAPY*

For non-small cell lung cancer or unknown, all under "All Patients" and:

Fiberoptic bronchoscopy if indicated by hemoptysis, obstruction, pneumonitis, or no histologic diagnosis of cancer
Biopsy of accessible lesions suspicious for tumor to obtain a histologic diagnosis or if therapy would be altered by finding of tumor
Transthoracic fine-needle aspiration biopsy or transbronchial forceps biopsy of peripheral lesions if fiberoptic bronchoscopy is negative and no other material exists for a histologic diagnosis
Diagnostic and therapeutic thoracentesis if a pleural effusion is present

For proven small cell lung cancer, all under "All Patients" and:

Fiberoptic bronchoscopy with washings and biopsy
Chest, abdomen, and brain CT scans useful but not mandatory
Bone marrow aspiration and biopsy

* Patients with non-small cell lung cancer and extrathoracic metastatic disease, malignant pleural effusion, or intrathoracic disease beyond the bounds of a tolerable radiotherapy port.

---

determine if the tumor can be resected by a standard surgical procedure such as a lobectomy or pneumonectomy (determination of *resectability*) based on the anatomic stage of the tumor and whether the patient could tolerate such a surgical procedure (determination of *operability*) based on the cardiopulmonary condition of the patient.

Non-small cell lung cancer   The TNM international stage system (ISS) developed by the American Joint Committee (AJC) on End Results Reporting, and modified by an international commission, should be used in non-small cell lung cancer, particularly in preparing patients for curative attempts with surgery or radiotherapy (Table 227-3). The various T (tumor size), N (regional node involvement), and M (presence or absence of distant metastasis) factors are combined to form different stage groups, and in addition, there is a group covering occult carcinoma detected on screening cytology exam with no other evidence of tumor (Table 227-3).

Small cell lung cancer   A simple two-stage system adapted from the Veterans Administration Lung Cancer Study Group is used. In this two-stage system, *limited-stage disease* (about 30 percent of all small cell cancer patients) is defined as disease confined to one hemithorax and regional lymph nodes (including mediastinal, contralateral hilar, and usually ipsilateral supraclavicular nodes), while *extensive-stage disease* (about 70 percent of all patients) is defined as disease beyond this. Employed in staging are clinical studies such as physical examination, x-rays, scans, and bone marrow examination. In part, the definition of *limited stage* relates to whether the known tumor can be encompassed within a tolerable radiation therapy port. Thus contralateral supraclavicular nodes, recurrent laryngeal nerve involvement, and superior vena caval obstruction can all be limited-stage disease. However, cardiac tamponade, malignant pleural effusion, and bilateral pulmonary parenchymal involvement are generally scored as extensive-stage disease because of the size of the radiation therapy port required to cover all known disease.

GENERAL STAGING PROCEDURES   (See Table 227-4)   All lung cancer patients should have a complete history and physical examination, with evaluation of all other medical problems and a determination of performance status and weight loss, both of which have great prognostic value. An ear, nose, and throat examination is also necessary because of the frequent occurrence of second cancers in this area. While not done in every patient, fiberoptic bronchoscopy remains a cornerstone of lung cancer staging and follow-up, providing material for pathologic examination and information on tumor size, location, degree of bronchial obstruction, and recurrence.

Chest roentgenograms are needed to evaluate tumor size and nodal involvement, and it is very useful to obtain old x-ray films for comparison. Computed tomography (CT) scans (chest and abdomen) are now widely used in the staging and follow-up of lung cancer patients. CT scans are of use in non-small cell lung cancer in preoperative staging to detect mediastinal nodes and pleural extension and occult abdominal disease (e.g., liver and adrenal glands), as well as in the planning of curative radiation therapy to allow design of fields to encompass all known tumor volume while avoiding as much normal tissue as possible. However, definitive characterization of mediastinal nodal involvement should depend on histologic proof when planning curative treatment. Likewise, unless the CT-detected abnormalities are unequivocal, malignancy of suspicious abdominal lesions should be confirmed by procedures such as fine-needle aspiration if the patient would otherwise be considered for curative treatment. In small cell lung cancer, CT scans are used for chest radiation treatment planning and assessing the response to chemotherapy and radiation therapy. In following patients after surgery or radiotherapy, procedures which can make interpretation of conventional chest x-rays difficult, CT scans can provide good evidence of tumor recurrence.

If signs or symptoms suggest organ involvement by tumor, appropriate CT or radionuclide scans (e.g., brain, liver, or bone) are performed, as well as radiographs of any suspicious bony lesions. Any accessible lesions suspicious for cancer should be biopsied if a histologic diagnosis has not already been made or if treatment decisions would be based on whether or not the lesion contained cancer.

In patients presenting with a mass lesion on chest x-ray and no obvious contraindications to a curative approach with surgery or radiotherapy after the initial evaluation, the mediastinum must be investigated. Approaches vary between different centers and include performing chest CT scan and mediastinoscopy (right-sided tumors) or lateral mediastinotomy (left-sided lesions) on all patients and proceeding directly to thoracotomy with staging of the mediastinum. In patients presenting with disease confined to the chest but not resectable, thus making them candidates for curative radiotherapy, other tests are done as indicated to evaluate specific symptoms. In patients presenting with non-small cell cancer that is not curable by either surgery, radiotherapy, or their combination, all the general procedures are done plus fiberoptic bronchoscopy as indicated to evaluate hemoptysis, obstruction, or pneumonitis, as well as diagnostic-therapeutic thoracentesis with cytologic examination if fluid is present.

STAGING OF SMALL CELL LUNG CANCER Pretreatment staging for patients with histologically documented small cell lung cancer includes the initial general lung cancer evaluation as well as fiberoptic bronchoscopy with washings and biopsies to determine the tumor extent before therapy; brain CT scan, since 10 percent of patients have metastases; bone marrow biopsy and aspiration, since 20 to 30 percent of patients have tumor in the bone marrow; and CT (liver) and radionuclide scans (bone) if symptoms or other findings are suggestive of disease involvement in these areas. Chest and abdominal CT scans are very useful but not mandatory to evaluate and follow tumor response to therapy. CT-directed liver biopsy may be performed if other findings are suggestive but not diagnostic of the presence of tumor in the liver and if tumor involvement there would alter the planned therapy.

If signs or symptoms of spinal cord compression or leptomeningitis develop at any time in lung cancer patients of any histologic type, a myelogram or magnetic resonance scan and examination of the cerebrospinal fluid cytology are performed to determine the need for local therapy to the site of compression (usually with radiotherapy) and for intrathecal chemotherapy (usually with methotrexate) if malignant cells are detected. In addition, a brain CT scan is performed to search for brain metastases that are often associated with spinal cord or leptomeningeal metastases.

DETERMINATION OF RESECTABILITY AND OPERABILITY In patients with non-small cell lung cancer, the following are major contraindications to curative attempts by surgery or radiotherapy alone using standard treatment methods: extrathoracic distant metastases, superior vena cava syndrome, vocal cord and, in most cases, phrenic nerve paralysis, malignant pleural effusion, cardiac tamponade, tumor within 2 cm of the carina (not curable by surgery but potentially curable by radiotherapy), metastasis to the contralateral lung, bilateral endobronchial tumor (potentially curable by radiotherapy), metastasis to the supraclavicular lymph nodes, lymph node metastasis in the contralateral mediastinum (potentially curable by radiotherapy), involvement of the main stem pulmonary artery. While a histologic diagnosis of small cell lung cancer is usually highly correlated with other findings of unresectability, if all other findings suggest the potential for resection, this option should be considered. This is usually encountered in small peripheral small cell lung cancer lesions (see below).

PHYSIOLOGIC STAGING Patients with lung cancer often have cardiopulmonary and other problems related to chronic obstructive pulmonary disease as well as other medical problems. To improve their preoperative condition, correctable problems (e.g., anemia, electrolyte and fluid disorders, infections, and arrhythmias) should be addressed, smoking stopped, and appropriate chest therapy instituted. Since it is not always possible to predict whether a lobectomy or pneumonectomy will be required until the time of operation, a conservative approach is to restrict resectional surgery to patients who could potentially tolerate a pneumonectomy. In addition to nonambulatory performance status, a myocardial infarction within the past 3 months is a contraindication to thoracic surgery because 20 percent of patients will die of reinfarction alone, while an infarction in the past 6 months is a relative contraindication. Other major contraindications include uncontrolled major arrhythmias, maximum breathing capacities of less than 40 percent predicted, an FEV_1 of less than 1 L, CO_2 retention (which is more serious than hypoxemia), and severe pulmonary hypertension. Recommending surgery when the FEV_1 is 1.1 to 2.4 L requires careful judgment, while an FEV_1 of over 2.5 L will usually permit a pneumonectomy. In patients with borderline pulmonary status or a question of pulmonary hypertension, split pulmonary function testing by ventilation-perfusion lung scans can define physiologic operability. The activity from quantitative scans is summed for each lung in the anterior and posterior views, and the ratio of the normal to total lung activity is multiplied by the FEV_1. Pneumonectomy usually is physiologically tolerable if this predicted value is greater than 1 L.

TREATMENT

After a histologic diagnosis is obtained and appropriate anatomic and physiologic staging studies are completed, the overall treatment approach to patients with lung cancer may be formulated (Table 227-5).

NON-SMALL CELL LUNG CANCER: LOCALIZED DISEASE In patients with non-small cell lung cancer of stages I and II (see Table 227-3) who can tolerate operation, the treatment of choice is pulmonary resection. In stage IIIa cases with favorable age, cardiopulmonary function, and anatomy, resection also should be considered. If a complete resection is possible, the 5-year survival rate for N1 disease is about 50 percent, while it is about 30 percent for N2 disease. However, only 20 percent of all patients who have N2 disease are technically resectable, and in most cases these resectable patients

TABLE 227-5 Summary of treatment approach to lung cancer patients

NON-SMALL CELL LUNG CANCER

Resectable (stages I, II, IIIa, and selected T3, N2 lesions)
  Surgery
  Radiotherapy for "nonoperable" patients
  Postoperative radiotherapy for N2 disease
Nonresectable (N2 and M1)
  Confined to chest: high-dose chest radiotherapy (RT) if possible
  Extrathoracic: RT to symptomatic local sites; chemotherapy (CT) (for
    good-performance-status patients, with evaluable lesions)

SMALL CELL LUNG CANCER

Limited stage (good performance status)
  Combination chemotherapy + chest RT
Extensive stage (good performance status)
  Combination chemotherapy
Complete tumor responders (all stages)
  Prophylactic cranial RT
Poor-performance-status patients (all stages)
  Modified-dose combination chemotherapy
  Palliative RT

ALL PATIENTS

Radiotherapy for brain metastases, spinal cord compression, weight-bearing
  lytic bony lesions, symptomatic local lesions (nerve paralyses, obstructed
  airway, hemoptysis in non-small cell lung cancer and in small cell cancer
  not responding to chemotherapy)
Appropriate diagnosis and treatment of other medical problems and
  supportive care during chemotherapy
Encouragement to stop smoking
Entrance into clinical trial, if eligible

are discovered to have N2 disease only at thoracotomy. Patients with contralateral or bilateral positive mediastinal (N3) nodes, extracapsular nodal involvement, or fixed nodes are not currently considered resectable. New approaches to convert patients from unresectable to resectable status include chest wall resections for direct extension of tumor, tracheal sleeve pneumonectomy, and sleeve lobectomy for lesions near the carina. Neoadjuvant (preoperative) chemotherapy, while experimental, gives tumor response rates of 50 to 60 percent and converts many responding patients to resectability. Video-assisted thoracic surgery (VATS) via thoracoscopy is being evaluated.

The extent of resection is a matter of surgical judgment based on findings at exploration. In general, conservative resection that encompasses all known tumor gives survival equal to that obtained with more extensive procedures. However, recent data from the Lung Cancer Study Group show that lobectomy is superior to wedge resection in terms of reducing local recurrences. Thus lobectomy is preferred to pneumonectomy and wedge resection, while wedge resections and segmentectomies are reserved for patients with poor pulmonary reserve and small peripheral lesions. Approximately 43 percent of all lung cancer patients will undergo thoracotomy. Of these, 76 percent will have a definitive resection, 12 percent will only be explored for disease extent, and 12 percent will have a palliative procedure with known disease left behind. The fraction of long-term survivors following definitive surgical therapy is remarkably consistent throughout major centers performing lung cancer surgery in the United States. Approximately 30 percent of all patients resected for cure survive 5 years, and 15 percent survive 10 years. The 30-day hospital mortality following pulmonary resection at major centers is also very consistent, 3 percent for lobectomy and 6 percent for pneumonectomy. As a function of postoperative treatment stage, the 5-year survival data are (1) epidermoid: stage I, 54 percent, stage II, 35 percent, stage IIIa N0–N1, 19 percent, stage IIIa N2, 13 percent, and (2) adenocarcinoma and large cell carcinoma: stage I, 51 percent, stage II, 18 percent, stage IIIa N0–N1, 10 percent, stage IIIa N2, 2 percent. Thus the majority of patients who were initially thought to have a "curative" resection ultimately died of metastatic disease (usually within 2 years of surgery).

MANAGEMENT OF OCCULT AND STAGE 0 CARCINOMAS

When sputum cytology screening indicates malignant cells but a normal chest radiograph is found (TX tumor stage), the lesion must be localized. Over 90 percent can be localized by meticulous examination of the bronchial tree with a fiberoptic bronchoscope under general anesthesia and collection of a series of differential brushings and biopsies. Often carcinoma in situ or multicentric lesions are found in these patients. Current recommendations are for the most conservative surgical resection, allowing removal of the cancer and conservation of lung parenchyma even if the bronchial margins are positive for carcinoma in situ. The 5-year overall survival for these occult cancers is approximately 60 percent. Close follow-up of these patients is indicated because of the high incidence of second primary lung cancers (approximately 5 percent per patient per year). A new approach to in situ or multicentric lesions uses systemically administered hematoporphyrin (which localizes to tumors and sensitizes them to light) followed by bronchoscopic phototherapy.

SOLITARY PULMONARY NODULE When a patient presents with an asymptomatic, solitary pulmonary nodule (defined as an x-ray density completely surrounded by normal aerated lung, with circumscribed margins, of any shape, usually 1 to 6 cm in greatest diameter), a decision to resect or follow the nodule must be made. Approximately 35 percent of all such lesions in adults will be malignant, the majority being primary lung cancer, while less than 1 percent are malignant in nonsmoking patients under 35 years of age. A complete history, including a smoking history, physical examination, routine laboratory tests, fiberoptic bronchoscopy, and old chest x-rays are obtained. If no diagnosis is immediately apparent, the following risk factors would all argue strongly in favor of proceeding with resection to establish a histologic diagnosis: history of cigarette smoking; age 35 years or older; a relatively large-sized lesion; lack of calcification; chest symptoms; associated atelectasis, pneumonitis, or adenopathy; and growth of the lesion compared with old x-rays. At present, only two radiographic criteria are strongly reliable for benignity of a solitary pulmonary nodule: lack of growth over a period greater than 2 years and certain characteristic patterns of calcification. Calcification alone does not exclude malignancy. However, a dense central nidus, multiple punctate foci, and "bull's eye" (granuloma) and "popcorn ball" (hamartoma) calcifications are all highly suggestive of a benign lesion.

When old x-rays are not available and the characteristic calcification patterns are absent, the following approach is reasonable: Nonsmoking patients under 35 years can be followed with serial chest x-rays every 3 months for 1 year and then yearly. If any significant growth is found, a histologic diagnosis is needed. For patients over age 35 and all patients with a smoking history, a histologic diagnosis must be made. This can occur either at the time of nodule resection or, if the patient is a poor operative risk, via transthoracic fine-needle biopsy. Some institutions would use preoperative fine-needle aspiration on all such lesions; however, all positive lesions will have to proceed to resection, and negative cytologic findings will in most cases have to be confirmed by histology on a resected specimen. While much has been made of sparing patients an operation, the high probability of finding a malignancy (particularly in smokers over age 35) and the excellent chance for surgical cure when the tumor is small both suggest an aggressive approach to these lesions.

RADIOTHERAPY Those patients who are stage III, as well as those with stages I and II disease who refuse surgery or appear not to be candidates for pulmonary resection for medical reasons, should be considered for radiation therapy with curative intent. The decision to administer high-dose and potentially curative radiotherapy is based on the extent of disease and the volume of the chest that requires irradiation. Patients with distant metastases, positive supraclavicular nodes, pleural effusion, or cardiac involvement are generally not considered for such curative radiation treatment. The median survival for unresectable patients with non-small cell lung cancer localized to the chest undergoing primary radiotherapy with curative intent is less than 1 year. However, 6 percent of these patients are alive at 5 years and cured when treated with radiotherapy alone. In addition to potential cure, radiotherapy, by controlling the primary tumor, may increase the quality and length of life of noncured patients. Treatment usually involves midplane doses of 55 to 60 Gy (5500 to 6000 rad), and the major concern is the amount of lung parenchyma and other organs in the thorax included within the treatment plan, including the spinal cord, heart, and esophagus. Patients with a major degree of underlying pulmonary disease may have to have the treatment plan compromised because of the deleterious effect of radiation on pulmonary function. Recent studies suggest that continuous fraction radiotherapy be given. The development of radiation pneumonitis is proportional to the dose of radiation and volume of lung incorporated within the radiation field. The full clinical syndrome (dyspnea, fever, and radiographic infiltrate corresponding to the treatment port) occurs in 5 percent of cases. Acute radiation esophagitis occurs during treatment but usually is self-limited, while spinal cord injury should be avoided by careful treatment planning. Twice-daily fractionated chest radiotherapy may achieve high doses and avoid toxicity.

COMBINED-MODALITY THERAPY Recent randomized trials have shown survival benefit for adjuvant chemotherapy given after surgical resection. However, this will have to be confirmed before adjuvant chemotherapy after surgery or radiotherapy is recommended for general use. While many centers give high-dose postoperative radiation if postoperative staging documents nodal disease, its efficacy has not been established. However, a randomized trial of postoperative radiotherapy, while showing improved local tumor control, did not show survival benefit.

Carcinomas of the superior pulmonary sulcus producing *Pancoast's syndrome* are often treated with combined radiotherapy and surgery. These patients should have the usual preoperative staging procedures, including mediastinoscopy and CT scans to determine tumor extent and neurologic examination with electromyography to document neurologic findings. Often a histologic diagnosis is not made, and with the constellation of tumor location and pain distribution, the diagnostic accuracy for cancer is better than 90 percent. If mediastinoscopy is negative, two curative approaches may be used in treating a Pancoast's syndrome tumor. In the first, preoperative irradiation [30 Gy (3000 rad) in 10 treatments] is given to the area followed by an en bloc resection of the tumor and involved chest wall 3 to 6 weeks later. At 3 years, survival figures of 42 percent for epidermoid and 21 percent for adeno- and large cell carcinomas have been reported. The second approach involves radiotherapy alone in curative doses and standard fractionation with similar survival to combined-modality therapy reported.

Data have now appeared suggesting a high frequency of brain metastases as isolated sites of relapse in patients with adenocarcinoma of the lung otherwise cured by surgery or radiotherapy. While there is no proven role for "prophylactic" cranial irradiation, it is not unreasonable to follow potentially cured, asymptomatic adenocarcinoma patients with frequent brain CT scans to detect such recurrence at the earliest possible time so that radiotherapy can be given.

DISSEMINATED NON-SMALL CELL LUNG CANCER The 70 percent of patients who have unresectable non-small cell cancer have a poor prognosis. For example, median survivals of 34, 25, 17, 8, and 4 weeks are seen for patients with performance status scores of 0 (asymptomatic), 1 (symptomatic, fully ambulatory), 2 (in bed < 50 percent of the time), 3 (in bed > 50 percent of the time), and 4 (bedridden), respectively. Standard medical management, the judicious use of pain medications, and the appropriate use of radiotherapy form the cornerstone of management. Patients whose primary tumors are causing symptoms such as bronchial obstruction with pneumonitis, hemoptysis, or upper airway or superior vena caval (SVC) obstruction should, in general, have radiotherapy to the primary tumor. The case for prophylactic treatment of the asymptomatic patient is to prevent major symptoms from occurring within the thorax. However, if the patient can be followed closely, deferring treatment until the development of symptoms is appropriate. Usually a course of 30 to 40 Gy (3000 to 4000 rad) over 2 to 4 weeks is given to the

tumor. The frequencies of relief by radiation therapy of intrathoracic symptoms are hemoptysis, 84 percent; SVC syndrome, 80 percent; dyspnea, 60 percent; cough, 60 percent; atelectasis, 23 percent; and vocal cord paralysis, 6 percent. Other symptoms of metastatic disease treated with radiotherapy include cardiac tamponade (treated with pericardiocentesis and radiation therapy to the entire cardiac silhouette), painful bony metastases (with relief in 66 percent of cases), brain or spinal cord compression, and brachial plexus involvement. Usually, with brain and cord compression, dexamethasone (25 to 100 mg total per day in four divided doses) is also given and then rapidly tapered to the lowest dosage which relieves neurologic symptoms.

The key to effective palliation is to detect the complication and begin radiotherapy at the earliest possible time. Pleural effusions are common and are usually treated with thoracentesis as needed, but without radiotherapy. If they recur and are symptomatic, chest tube drainage with a sclerosing agent such as intrapleural doxycycline is used. First, the chest cavity is completely drained. Xylocaine 1% is instilled (15 mL), followed by 50 mL normal saline. Then 500 to 750 mg doxycycline HCl is dissolved in 100 mL normal saline, and this is injected via the chest tube. The chest tube is clamped for 4 h if tolerated, and the patient is rotated onto different sides to distribute the sclerosing agent. Then 24 to 48 h later the chest tube is pulled when there is little drainage (usually less than 100 mL per 24 h). Recently, video-assisted thoracoscopy has been used to drain and treat large malignant effusions. Symptomatic intrabronchial lesions that recur after surgery or radiotherapy, or the development of such lesions in patients with severely compromised pulmonary function, are difficult to treat with conventional therapy. However, neodymium-YAG (yttrium-aluminum-garnet) laser therapy administered via a flexible fiberoptic bronchoscope (usually under general anesthesia) can provide palliation to 80 to 90 percent of patients even when the tumor has relapsed after radiotherapy. In addition, patients can be retreated with YAG laser therapy.

Chemotherapy The use of chemotherapy for non-small cell lung cancer requires careful judgment to balance potential benefits and toxicity. However, recent results suggest modest survival benefits from such combination chemotherapy. Approximately 30 to 40 percent of patients will have objective tumor response to combination chemotherapy. However, a complete clinical regression of tumor (a *complete response*) occurs in less than 5 percent of cases. Those patients whose tumors respond to chemotherapy have significantly longer survivals (around 30 to 40 weeks median survival) compared with those patients who do not respond to therapy (10 to 20 weeks median). The problem is that the responding patients also have better prognostic features (such as good performance status), and it is difficult to separate the effect of these on survival from that of chemotherapy. However, in patients with good performance status, response to chemotherapy is also associated with prolonged survival and, in some cases, relief of symptoms. Nevertheless, such combination chemotherapy can have severe side effects, including treatment-related mortality. Thus, in those patients with non-small cell lung cancer who desire chemotherapy, it is reasonable to give chemotherapy if the patient is fully ambulatory, has an evaluable tumor mass (to follow response to therapy), has not received prior chemotherapy, and is able to understand and accept the potential benefits and toxicities from such therapy. The chemotherapy should be delivered by an experienced physician or medical oncologist, who should use one of the published standard regimens, such as etoposide + cisplatin. Finally, all eligible patients should be encouraged to enter clinical trials.

SMALL CELL LUNG CANCER Untreated patients with small cell lung cancer have median survivals of only 6 to 17 weeks, while patients treated with combination chemotherapy have median survivals of 40 to 70 weeks. Thus the correct integration of chemotherapy with or without radiotherapy or surgery is the cornerstone of the treatment of small cell cancer. The goal of treatment is to obtain a complete clinical regression of tumor documented by repeating the initial positive staging procedures, particularly fiberoptic bronchoscopy with washings and biopsy. The initial response, determined 6 to 12 weeks after the start of therapy, predicts both median and long-term survival and potential cure. Patients obtaining a complete clinical regression of tumor survive longer than patients with only partial regression (tumor shrinkage of more than 50 percent of visible disease with no sign of tumor progression elsewhere), who in turn survive longer than patients with no response. In addition, all long-term (over 3 years) survivors come from the complete response group.

Following initial staging, patients are grouped into the limited or extensive disease stages and classified as being physiologically able or not able to tolerate combination chemotherapy or combined-modality chemoradiotherapy. The overall mortality rate from initial combination chemotherapy even in these selected patients is about 5 percent at major centers. This figure is comparable with the operative mortality rate for pulmonary resection and indicates the need for physiologic staging of patients before chemotherapy. Such therapy should be reserved for ambulatory patients with no prior chemotherapy or radiotherapy, no other major medical problems, and adequate heart, liver, renal, and bone marrow function. The arterial P_{O_2} on room air should be above 6.6 kPa (50 mmHg), and there should be no CO_2 retention. All patients with some or more of these limitations must have their initial chemoradio- or chemotherapy modified to prevent undue toxicity. In all patients the chemoradiotherapy must be coupled with supportive care for infectious, hemorrhagic, and other medical complications. This induction period is best supervised by a medical oncologist. Meticulous attention to the details of therapy and the day-to-day management of the patient through the initial 6 to 12 weeks of treatment is essential if therapy-related mortality is to be kept low.

Chemotherapy   A variety of effective combination chemotherapy regimens have been reported for small cell lung cancer, including CAV (cyclophosphamide + doxorubicin + vincristine), CAVP-16 (cyclophosphamide + doxorubicin + VP-16), and VP-16 (etoposide) + cisplatin. At present, there is no evidence that any one regimen is better than another if adequate drug dosages and schedules are used. The initial combination chemotherapy often results in moderate to severe granulocytopenia (e.g., granulocyte counts less than 500 to 1500 per microliter) and thrombocytopenia (platelets less than 50,000 to 100,000 per microliter). Following the initial *induction* therapy, patients should be restaged to determine if they have entered a *complete clinical remission*, indicated by complete disappearance of all clinically evident lesions and paraneoplastic syndromes, or a *partial remission*, or have *no response* or tumor progression (seen in 10 percent of patients or less). Following this, *maintenance* chemotherapy is given to responding patients for periods of 6 to 12 months in 3-, 4-, or 6-week cycles, depending on the chemotherapy regimen used. Appropriate drug dose modifications are made to keep the white blood count above 2000 per microliter and the platelet count above 50,000 per microliter. The patients are restaged between 6 and 12 months, depending on the individual regimens; if they are still in a complete remission, chemotherapy is stopped. The value of more prolonged chemotherapy is not documented. Patients with a partial tumor regression are generally kept on chemotherapy until the time of objective tumor progression and then switched to new chemotherapy (either with known activity or on an experimental protocol). Patients not responding or with objective tumor progression should be switched to new chemotherapy, preferably with a non-cross-resistant combination in an attempt to get an objective tumor response.

Radiotherapy   High-dose [40 Gy (4000 rad)] radiotherapy to the whole brain should be given to patients with documented brain metastases. Prophylactic cranial irradiation (PCI) may be given to patients with complete responses, since this will significantly decrease the development of brain metastases (occurring in 60 to 80 percent of patients living 2 or more years who do not receive such prophylactic radiotherapy), but such prophylactic therapy has not been shown to prolong survival. Because some studies indicate possible deficits in cognitive ability that could be related to PCI, long-term quality of life after PCI needs to be further studied. In the case of symptomatic,

progressive lesions in the chest or at other critical sites, if radiotherapy has not yet been given to these areas, it may be administered in full doses [e.g., 40 Gy (4000 rad)] to the chest tumor mass].

There are definite toxicities of both an acute and chronic nature that should be expected with combined-modality chemoradiotherapy, particularly if chemo- and radiotherapy are given concurrently. However, retrospective analyses of long-term survivors and analyses of local failures in the chest following chemotherapy alone suggest that chest radiotherapy is of benefit, and thus it is currently recommended for limited-stage patients. Patients should be selected (limited-stage disease with PS 0–1 and initial good pulmonary function) such that radiotherapy can be given in full doses and in a manner that will not sacrifice too much lung. The radiation oncologist must be prepared to deliver tailored radiotherapy with shaping of fields during treatment, much the same as is done for Hodgkin's disease. Several centers employing twice-daily radiotherapy with concomitant etoposide + cisplatin chemotherapy have reported good results with respect to local tumor control and toxicity. In extensive-stage disease, the routine use of initial chest radiotherapy usually is not advocated. However, in favorable patients (e.g., those with PS 0–1, good pulmonary function, and only one site of extensive disease), radiotherapy can be considered. In all patients, if chemotherapy is inadequate to relieve local tumor symptoms, a course of radiotherapy can be added.

Several centers around the world have reported potential cure rates of 15 to 25 percent for limited-stage disease and 1 to 5 percent for extensive-stage disease. Overall, approximately 50 percent of patients with limited-stage and 30 percent with extensive-stage disease will enter a complete remission, and 90 to 95 percent of all patients will have some objective tumor shrinkage (complete or partial response). These responses increase the median survival from 2 to 4 months for untreated patients to 10 to 12 months for extensive-stage and 14 to 18 months for limited-stage patients. In addition, most patients have relief of their tumor-related symptoms and improvement of performance status. However, the maintenance of good performance status by the patient while receiving outpatient chemotherapy requires judgment and skill on the part of the medical oncologist delivering the chemotherapy so as to avoid undue therapeutic toxicity. New treatments such as new drug combinations, very intensive initial or "reinduction" therapy with autologous bone marrow infusion, as well as novel forms of combining chemo- and radiotherapy and surgery should all be reserved for approved clinical protocols.

While surgical resection is not routinely recommended for small cell lung cancer, occasional small cell cancer patients will either meet the usual AJC requirements for resectability (stage I or II with negative mediastinal nodes) or only have a histologic diagnosis made on review of the resected surgical specimen. Such patients have been reported to have high cure rates (above 25 percent) if adjuvant combination chemotherapy is used. Thus such uncommon, resectable small cell lung cancer patients are candidates for combined-modality surgery and chemotherapy.

BENIGN LUNG NEOPLASMS

The benign neoplasms of the lung, representing less than 5 percent of all primary tumors, include bronchial adenomas and hamartomas (90 percent of such lesions) and a group of very uncommon neoplasms (chondromas, fibromas, lipomas, hemangiomas, leiomyomas, teratomas, pseudolymphomas, and endometriosis). The diagnostic and primary treatment approach is basically the same for all these neoplasms. They can present as central masses causing airway obstruction, cough, hemoptysis, and pneumonitis with or without x-ray findings but be accessible to fiberoptic bronchoscopy. Alternatively, they can present without symptoms as solitary pulmonary nodules and thus will be evaluated as part of a solitary pulmonary nodule workup. In all cases, the extent of surgery must be determined at operation, and a conservative procedure with appropriate reconstructions is usually performed.

BRONCHIAL ADENOMAS Bronchial adenomas (80 percent of which are central) are slowly growing intrabronchial lesions that represent 50 percent of all benign pulmonary neoplasms. Eighty to ninety percent are carcinoids, 10 to 15 percent are adenocystic tumors (or cylindromas), and 2 to 3 percent are mucoepidermoid tumors. Adenomas present in patients 15 to 60 years old (average age 45) as intrabronchial lesions and are often symptomatic for several years. Patients may have chronic cough, recurrent hemoptysis, or obstruction with atelectasis, lobar collapse, or pneumonitis and abscess formation. Bronchial carcinoids, which usually follow a benign course, and small cell lung cancers, which are highly malignant, are both derived from the same normal bronchial epithelial component, the Kulchitsky cell. This cell is part of the amine precursor uptake and decarboxylation (APUD) system. Carcinoids, like small cell lung cancers, may secrete other hormones such as ACTH or arginine vasopressin and thus cause paraneoplastic syndromes which resolve with resection. In addition, bronchial carcinoids when metastatic (usually to the liver) may produce the carcinoid syndrome, with cutaneous flush, bronchoconstriction, diarrhea, and cardiac valvular lesions (see Chap. 276), which small cell lung cancer does not. Occasionally, pathologists may have difficulty in distinguishing carcinoids from small cell lung cancers. Carcinoid tumors appearing more aggressive histologically (referred to as *atypical carcinoids*) metastasize in 70 percent of cases to regional nodes, liver, or bone, compared with only a 5 percent metastasis rate of carcinoids with typical histology.

Bronchial adenomas of all types, because of their endobronchial and often central location, are usually visible via fiberoptic broncho-scopy, and tissue for histologic diagnosis is obtained in this manner. Because they are hypervascular, they can bleed profusely after bronchoscopic biopsy, and this should be anticipated. Bronchial adenomas must be dealt with as potentially malignant and thus require removal not only for symptom relief but also because they can be locally invasive or recurrent, potentially can metastasize, or may produce paraneoplastic syndromes. Surgical excision is the primary treatment for all types of bronchial adenomas. The extent of surgery is determined at operation and should be as conservative as possible. Often bronchotomy with local excision, sleeve resection, segmental resection, or lobectomy is sufficient. Five-year survival rates following surgical resection are 95 percent, decreasing to 70 percent if regional nodes are involved. The treatment of metastatic pulmonary carcinoids is currently unclear because they can either be indolent, growing slowly over several years, or behave more like small cell lung carcinoma. Assessment of the tempo and histology of the disease in the individual patient is necessary to determine if and when chemotherapy or radiotherapy is indicated.

HAMARTOMAS Pulmonary hamartomas have a peak incidence at age 60 and are more frequent in men than in women. Histologically, they contain normal pulmonary tissue components (smooth muscle and collagen) in a disorganized fashion. They are usually peripheral, clinically silent, and benign in their behavior. While it would be advantageous to avoid thoracotomy in these older patients, unless the radiographic findings are pathognomonic of hamartoma with "popcorn" calcification, the lesions will usually have to be resected for diagnosis, particularly if the patient is a smoker.

METASTATIC PULMONARY TUMORS

The lung is frequently the site of metastatic disease from primary cancers outside the lung. Usually such metastatic disease is considered incurable. However, two special situations may arise. First is the development of a solitary pulmonary shadow on chest x-ray in a patient known to have an extrathoracic neoplasm. This may represent a metastasis or a new primary lung cancer. Because the natural history of lung cancer is worse than for most other primary tumors, it is wise to approach the single pulmonary nodule in a patient with a known extrathoracic tumor as though the nodule were a primary lung cancer, particularly if the patient is over 35 years of age and a smoker. This

means a vigorous evaluation looking for other sites of active cancer and, if none are found, surgical resection of the nodule. Second, multiple pulmonary nodules may be resected for cure as well. This is usually recommended if, after careful staging, (1) the patient can tolerate the contemplated pulmonary resection, (2) the primary tumor has been definitively and successfully treated, and (3) all known metastatic disease can be encompassed by the projected pulmonary resection. The key is selection and screening of patients to exclude patients with uncontrolled primary tumors and extrapulmonary metas-tases. Primary tumors whose pulmonary metastases have been success-fully resected for cure include osteogenic and soft tissue sarcomas; colon, rectal, uterine, cervix, and corpus tumors; head and neck, breast, testis, and salivary gland cancer; melanoma; and bladder and kidney tumors. Five-year survival rates of 20 to 30 percent have been found in carefully selected patients, and the most dramatic results have been seen in osteogenic sarcomas, where resection of pulmonary metastases (sometimes requiring several thoracotomies) is becoming a standard curative treatment approach.

REFERENCES

BENOWITZ NL: Pharmacologic aspects of cigarette smoking and nicotine addiction. N Engl J Med 319:1318, 1988

CARBONE DP, MINNA JD: The molecular genetics of lung cancer. Adv Intern Med 37:145, 1991

GINSBERG RJ et al: Cancer of the lung: Non-small cell lung cancer, in *The Principles and Practice of Oncology*, 4th ed, VT DeVita et al (eds). Philadelphia, Lippincott, 1992

————, RUBENSTEIN L, FOR THE LCSG: Patients with T1N0 non-small cell lung cancer: Local recurrence increase with limited resection. Lung Cancer 7(suppl):83,1991

HENDERSON BE et al: Toward the primary prevention of cancer. Science 254:1131, 1991

IHDE DC, MINNA JD: Non-small cell lung cancer: I. Biology, diagnosis, and staging. Curr Probl Cancer 15:63, 1991

————, ————: Non-small cell lung cancer: II. Treatment. Curr Probl Cancer 15:107, 1991

———— et al: Cancer of the lung: Small cell lung cancer, in *The Principles and Practice of Oncology*, 4th ed, VT DeVita et al (eds). Philadelphia, Lippincott, 1992

LUNG CANCER STUDY GROUP: Effects of postoperative mediastinal radiation on completely resected stage II and stage III epidermoid cancer of the lung. N Engl J Med 315:1377, 1986

MACK M et al: The present role of thoracoscopy in the diagnosis and treatment of diseases of the chest. Ann Thorac Surg 54:403, 1992

MANSSON I: Treatment of malignant pleural effusion with doxycycline. Scand J Infect Dis Suppl 53:29, 1988

MOUNTAIN CF: Prognostic implications of the International Staging System for Lung Cancer: A new international staging system for lung cancer. Semin Oncol 15:236, 1988

————: Value of the new TNM staging system for lung cancer. Chest 96:475, 1989

THE HEALTH CONSEQUENCES OF SMOKING: Nicotine Addiction. A report of the Surgeon General. Washington, DC, Dept Health and Human Services, 1988

228 DISORDERS OF THE PLEURA, MEDIASTINUM, AND DIAPHRAGM

RICHARD W. LIGHT

DISORDERS OF THE PLEURA

STRUCTURE AND FUNCTION The pleural space lies between the lung and chest wall and normally contains a very thin layer of fluid. The pleural space with its thin layer of liquid serves as a coupling system between the lung and chest wall. The serous membrane covering the lung parenchyma is called the *visceral pleura*, while the serous membrane covering the chest wall, the diaphragm, and the mediastinum is called the *parietal pleura*.

PLEURAL EFFUSION A patient has a pleural effusion when there is an excess amount of fluid in the pleural space. More than 1 million cases of pleural effusion occur annually in the United States.

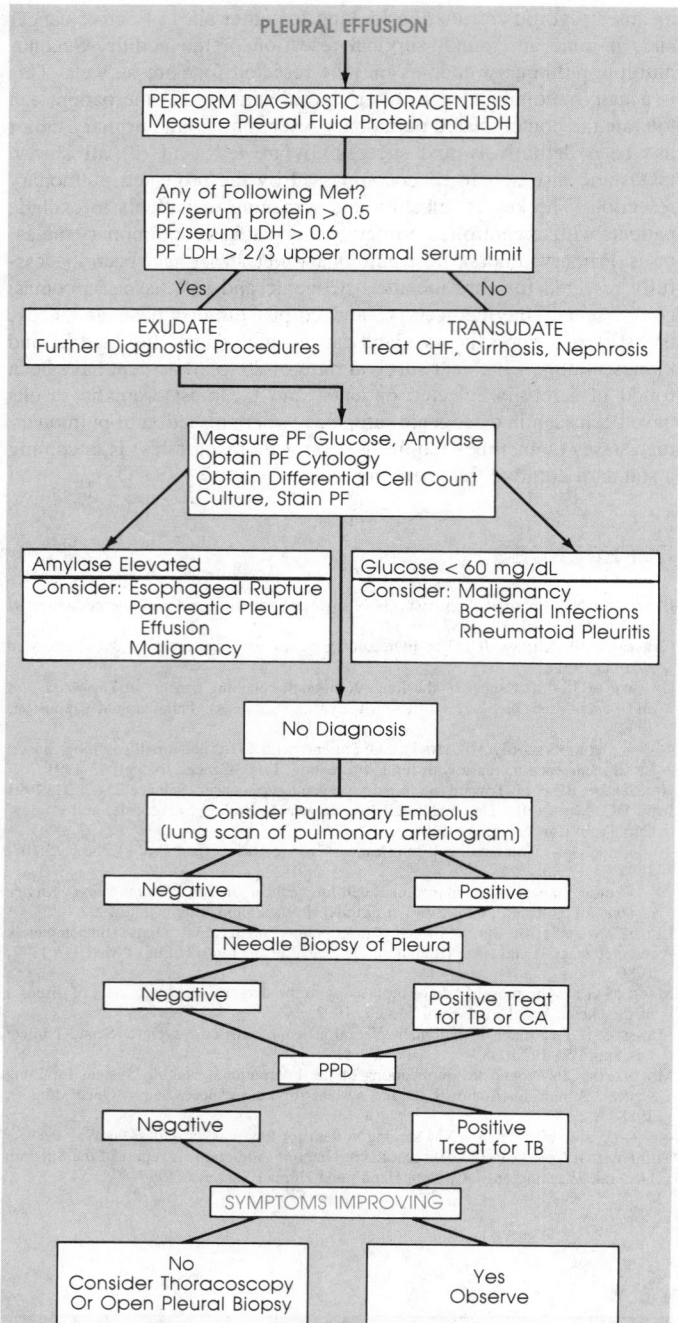

FIGURE 228-1   Approach to the diagnosis of pleural effusions.

TABLE 228-1   Differential diagnoses of pleural effusions

TRANSUDATIVE PLEURAL EFFUSIONS

A Congestive heart failure
B Pericardial disease
C Cirrhosis
D Nephrotic syndrome
E Peritoneal dialysis
F Superior vena cava obstruction
G Myxedema
H Pulmonary emboli
I Urinothorax

EXUDATIVE PLEURAL EFFUSIONS

A Neoplastic diseases
   1 Metastatic disease
   2 Mesothelioma
B Infectious diseases
   1 Bacterial infections
   2 Tuberculosis
   3 Fungal infections
   4 Viral infections
   5 Parasitic infections
C Pulmonary embolization
D Gastrointestinal disease
   1 Esophageal perforation
   2 Pancreatic disease
   3 Intraabdominal abscesses
   4 Diaphragmatic hernia
   5 After abdominal surgery
   6 Endoscopic variceal sclerotherapy
E Collagen-vascular diseases
   1 Rheumatoid pleuritis
   2 Systemic lupus erythematosus
   3 Drug-induced lupus
   4 Immunoblastic lymphadenopathy
   5 Sjögren's syndrome
   6 Wegener's granulomatosis
   7 Churg-Strauss syndrome
F Post-cardiac injury syndrome
G Asbestos exposure
H Sarcoidosis
I Uremia
J Meigs' syndrome
K Yellow nail syndrome
L Drug-induced pleural disease
   1 Nitrofurantoin
   2 Dantrolene
   3 Methysergide
   4 Bromocriptine
   5 Procarbazine
   6 Amiodarone
M Trapped lung
N Radiation therapy
O Electrical burns
P Hemothorax
Q Iatrogenic injury
R Ovarian hyperstimulation syndrome
S Chylothorax

Etiology   Pleural fluid accumulates when pleural fluid formation exceeds pleural fluid absorption. Normally, fluid enters the pleural space from the capillaries in the parietal pleura and is removed via the lymphatics situated in the parietal pleura. Fluid also can enter the pleural space from the interstitial spaces of the lung via the visceral pleura or from the peritoneal cavity via small holes in the diaphragm. The lymphatics have the capacity to absorb 20 times more fluid than is normally formed. Accordingly, a pleural effusion may develop when there is excess pleural fluid formation (from the parietal pleura, the interstitial spaces of the lung, or the peritoneal cavity) or when there is decreased fluid removal by the lymphatics.

Diagnostic approach   When a patient is found to have a pleural effusion, an effort should be made to determine the cause (Fig. 228-1). There are many different causes of pleural fluid accumulation

(Table 228-1). The first step is to determine whether the patient has a transudative or an exudative pleural effusion. A *transudative* pleural effusion occurs when *systemic factors* that influence the formation and absorption of pleural fluid are altered. The leading causes of transudative pleural effusions in the United States are left ventricular failure (~500,000 per year), pulmonary embolism (~75,000 per year), and cirrhosis (~50,000 per year). An *exudative* pleural effusion occurs when *local factors* that influence the formation and absorption of pleural fluid are altered. The leading causes of exudative pleural effusions are bacterial pneumonia (~300,000 per year), malignancy (~200,000 per year), viral infection (~100,000 per year), and pulmonary embolism (~75,000 per year). The primary reason to make this differentiation is that additional diagnostic procedures are indicated only with exudative effusions to define the cause of the local disease.

Transudative and exudative pleural effusions are distinguished by measuring the lactate dehydrogenase (LDH) and protein levels in the pleural fluid. Exudative pleural effusions meet at least one of the following criteria, whereas transudative pleural effusions meet none:

1 Pleural fluid protein/serum protein >0.5
2 Pleural fluid LDH/serum LDH >0.6
3 Pleural fluid LDH more than two-thirds normal upper limit for serum

If a patient has an exudative pleural effusion, the following tests on the pleural fluid should be obtained: description of the fluid, glucose level, amylase level, differential cell count, microbiologic studies, and cytology.

Effusion due to heart failure The most common cause of a pleural effusion is congestive heart failure with left ventricular failure. The effusion occurs because the increased amounts of fluid in the lung interstitial spaces exit in part across the visceral pleura. This overwhelms the capacity of the lymphatics in the parietal pleura to remove fluid. The effusions are usually bilateral and roughly the same size. A diagnostic thoracentesis should be performed if the effusions are not bilateral and comparable in size, if the patient is febrile, or if the patient has pleuritic chest pain to verify that the patient has a transudative effusion. Otherwise the patient is best treated with diuretics. If the effusion persists despite diuretic therapy, a diagnostic thoracentesis should be performed. Diuretic therapy for a few days does not significantly change the biochemical characteristics of the pleural fluid.

Hepatic hydrothorax Pleural effusions occur in approximately 5 percent of patients with cirrhosis and ascites. The predominant mechanism is the direct movement of peritoneal fluid through small holes in the diaphragm into the pleural space. The effusion is usually right-sided and frequently is large enough to produce severe dyspnea. If medical management does not control the ascites and the effusion, there are no good alternatives. Consideration can be given to inserting a peritoneal-venous shunt, thoracotomy with surgical repair of the leak, or tube thoracostomy with the injection of a sclerosing agent.

Parapneumonic effusion A parapneumonic effusion is any pleural effusion associated with bacterial pneumonia, lung abscess, or bronchiectasis. These effusions are probably the most common exudative pleural effusion in the United States at this time. The term *complicated parapneumonic effusion* is used to refer to those effusions that require tube thoracostomy for their resolution. An *empyema* is pus in the pleural space, and this term is reserved for effusions on which the Gram stain of the pleural fluid is positive.

Patients with aerobic bacterial pneumonia and pleural effusion present with an acute febrile illness consisting of chest pain, sputum production, and leukocytosis. Patients with anaerobic infections present with a subacute illness with weight loss, a brisk leukocytosis, mild anemia, and a history of some factor that predisposes them to aspiration. Although aerobic bacteria are responsible for many more cases of pneumonia than are anaerobic bacteria, positive cultures on pleural fluid are roughly equally divided between the two different types of bacteria.

The possibility of a parapneumonic effusion should be considered whenever a patient with a bacterial pneumonia is initially evaluated. The presence of free pleural fluid can be demonstrated with a lateral decubitus radiograph. If the free fluid separates the lung from the chest wall by more than 10 mm on the decubitus radiograph, a diagnostic thoracentesis should be performed. The purpose of this diagnostic thoracentesis is to determine whether or not chest tubes should be inserted.

Any of the following is an indication for tube thoracostomy in patients with parapneumonic effusion:

1 The presence of gross pus in the pleural space
2 Organisms visible on Gram stain of the pleural fluid
3 Pleural fluid glucose level of less than 50 mg/dL
4 Pleural fluid pH below 7.00 and 0.15 units lower than arterial pH

There should be no delay in its performance because a free-flowing parapneumonic effusion can become loculated within a matter of hours.

If the pleural fluid is loculated and is not adequately drained with one chest tube, either streptokinase, 250,000 units, or urokinase, 100,000 units, should be injected intrapleurally to dissolve the fibrin membranes which create the loculations. If the pleural drainage is inadequate after the intrapleural thrombolytic therapy, a decortication should be performed. If the patient is too sick to tolerate a decortication, then an open drainage procedure can be done.

Effusion secondary to malignancy Malignant pleural effusions secondary to metastatic disease are the second most common type of exudative pleural effusion (~200,000 per year). The three tumors that cause approximately 75 percent of all malignant pleural effusions are lung carcinoma (30 percent), breast carcinoma (25 percent), and tumors of the lymphoma group (20 percent). Most patients complain of dyspnea which is frequently out of proportion to the size of the effusion. The pleural fluid is an exudate, and its glucose level may be reduced if the tumor burden in the pleural space is high.

The diagnosis is usually made via cytology of the pleural fluid. If the initial cytologic examination is negative, then a needle biopsy of the pleura with repeat cytology is indicated. If there is still no diagnosis, thoracoscopy is likely to provide the diagnosis if the patient has malignancy. At the time of thoracoscopy, talc or some similar agent should be instilled into the pleural space to effect a pleurodesis.

Patients with a malignant pleural effusion are treated symptomatically for the most part, since the presence of the effusion indicates disseminated disease and most malignancies associated with pleural effusion are not curable with chemotherapy. The only symptom that can be attributed to the effusion itself is dyspnea. If the patient's lifestyle is compromised by dyspnea, and if the dyspnea is relieved with a therapeutic thoracentesis, then one of the following procedures should be performed: (1) tube thoracostomy with the instillation of a sclerosing agent such as bleomycin, 60 IU, or minocycline, 5 to 10 mg/kg, (2) thoracoscopy with pleural abrasion or the insufflation of talc, or (3) insertion of a pleuroperitoneal shunt.

Mesothelioma Malignant mesotheliomas are primary tumors which arise from the mesothelial cells that line the pleural cavities. Most cases of malignant mesothelioma are related to asbestos exposure. Patients with mesothelioma present with chest pain and shortness of breath. The chest radiograph reveals a pleural effusion, generalized pleural thickening, and a shrunken hemothorax. Usually either thoracoscopy or open pleural biopsy is necessary to establish the diagnosis. Various treatment modalities, including radical surgery, chemotherapy, and radiation therapy, have been tried, but none has been proven to be more effective than symptomatic therapy. It is recommended that chest pain be treated with opiates and that shortness of breath be treated with oxygen and/or opiates.

Effusion secondary to pulmonary embolization The diagnosis most commonly overlooked in the differential diagnosis of a patient with an undiagnosed pleural effusion is pulmonary embolism. Dyspnea is reported by more than 80 percent of patients and is usually greater than one would expect from a similar-sized effusion with a different cause.

There is nothing characteristic about the pleural fluid associated with pulmonary embolization, and it can be either transudative or exudative. The diagnosis is suggested by lung scanning and/or pulmonary arteriography. Treatment of the patient with a pleural effusion secondary to pulmonary embolism is the same as for any patient with pulmonary emboli. If the pleural effusion increases in size with treatment, the patient probably has recurrent emboli or another complication such as a hemothorax or a pleural infection.

Tuberculous pleuritis In many parts of the world, the most common cause of an exudative pleural effusion is tuberculosis, but in the United States this is relatively uncommon. Tuberculous pleural effusions are thought to be due primarily to a hypersensitivity reaction to tuberculous protein in the pleural space. Patients with tuberculous pleuritis present with fever, weight loss, dyspnea, and/or pleuritic chest pain. The pleural fluid is an exudate with predominantly small lymphocytes. The diagnosis is usually established by the demonstration of granulomas on needle biopsy of the pleura. Adequate treatment consists of isoniazide, 300 mg/d, plus rifampin, 600 mg/d, for 6 months.

Effusion secondary to viral infection   Viral infections are probably responsible for a sizable percentage of undiagnosed exudative pleural effusions. In many series, no diagnosis is established for approximately 20 percent of exudative effusions, and these effusions resolve spontaneously with no long-term residua. The importance of these effusions is that one should not be too aggressive in trying to establish a diagnosis for the undiagnosed effusion, particularly if the patient is improving clinically.

AIDS   Pleural effusions are uncommon in such patients. The most common cause is Kaposi's sarcoma, followed by parapneumonic effusion. Other common causes are tuberculosis, cryptococcosis, and lymphoma. Pleural effusions are very uncommon with *Pneumocystis carinii* infection.

Chylothorax   A chylothorax occurs when the thoracic duct is disrupted and chyle accumulates in the pleural space. The most common cause of chylothorax is trauma, but it also may result from tumors in the mediastinum. Patients with chylothorax present with dyspnea, and the chest radiograph reveals a large pleural effusion. Thoracentesis reveals milky fluid, and biochemical analysis reveals a triglyceride level which is usually above 110 mg/dL. Patients with chylothorax and no obvious trauma should have a lymphangiogram and a mediastinal computed tomographic (CT) scan to assess the mediastinum for lymph nodes. The treatment of choice for most chylothoraces is implantation of a pleuroperitoneal shunt. Patients with chylothoraces should not undergo tube thoracostomy with prolonged chest tube drainage because this will lead to malnutrition and immunologic incompetence.

Hemothorax   When a diagnostic thoracentesis reveals bloody pleural fluid, a hematocrit should be obtained on the pleural fluid. If the hematocrit is greater than 50 percent that of the peripheral blood, the patient has a hemothorax. Most hemothoraces are the result of trauma; other causes include rupture of a blood vessel or tumor. Most patients with hemothorax should be treated with tube thoracostomy. Placing a chest tube allows continuous quantification of bleeding. If the bleeding emanates from a laceration of the pleura, apposition of the two pleural surfaces is likely to stop the bleeding. If the pleural hemorrhage exceeds 200 mL/h, consideration should be given to thoracotomy.

Miscellaneous causes of pleural effusion   There are many other causes of pleural effusion (see Table 228-1), and space precludes an in-depth discussion of these multiple entities. Key features of some of these conditions are as follows: If the pleural fluid amylase level is elevated, the diagnosis of esophageal rupture or pancreatic disease is likely. If the patient is febrile, has predominantly polymorphonuclear cells in the pleural fluid, and has no parenchymal abnormalities, an intraabdominal abscess should be considered. The diagnosis of lupus pleuritis is best made by demonstrating an elevated antinuclear antibody (ANA) level in the pleural fluid. The diagnosis of an asbestos pleural effusion is one of exclusion. Benign ovarian tumors can produce ascites and a pleural effusion (Meigs' syndrome). Several drugs can cause pleural effusion, and the associated fluid is usually eosinophilic. Many pleural effusions follow from medical manipulations such as abdominal surgery, coronary artery bypass surgery, endoscopic variceal sclerotherapy, radiation therapy, or the intravascular insertion of central lines.

PNEUMOTHORAX   Pneumothorax is the presence of gas in the pleural space. A *spontaneous* pneumothorax is one that occurs without antecedent trauma to the thorax. A *primary spontaneous* pneumothorax occurs in an individual without underlying lung disease, while a *secondary spontaneous* pneumothorax occurs in an individual with underlying lung disease. A *traumatic* pneumothorax results from penetrating or nonpenetrating chest injuries. A *tension* pneumothorax is a pneumothorax in which the pressure in the pleural space is positive throughout the respiratory cycle.

Primary spontaneous pneumothorax   Primary spontaneous pneumothoraces are usually due to rupture of apical pleural blebs. These are small cystic spaces, seldom exceeding 1 to 2 cm in diameter, which lie within or immediately under the visceral pleura. These pneumothoraces most commonly occur in tall, thin individuals. Primary spontaneous pneumothoraces occur almost exclusively in smokers, which suggests that the patients indeed do have subclinical lung disease. Approximately 50 percent of individuals who have an initial primary spontaneous pneumothorax will have a recurrence. The initial recommended treatment for primary spontaneous pneumothorax is simple aspiration. If the lung does not expand with aspiration, or if the patient has a recurrent pneumothorax, tube thoracostomy with instillation of a sclerosing agent such as minocycline is indicated. Thoracoscopy or thoracotomy with pleural abrasion is almost 100 percent successful in preventing recurrences.

Secondary spontaneous pneumothorax   Most secondary spontaneous pneumothoraces are due to chronic obstructive pulmonary disease, but pneumothoraces have been reported with virtually every lung disease. Pneumothorax in patients with lung disease is more life-threatening than it is in normal individuals because of the lack of pulmonary reserve in patients with lung disease. Nearly all patients with secondary spontaneous pneumothorax should be treated with tube thoracostomy and the instillation of a sclerosing agent. Patients with either primary or secondary spontaneous pneumothoraces who have a persistent air leak or an unexpanded lung after 6 days of tube thoracostomy should be subjected to open thoracotomy.

Traumatic pneumothorax   Traumatic pneumothoraces can result from both penetrating and nonpenetrating chest trauma. Traumatic pneumothoraces should be treated with tube thoracostomy. If a hemopneumothorax is present, one chest tube should be placed in the superior part of the hemithorax to evacuate the air, and another should be placed in the inferior part of the hemithorax to remove the blood. Iatrogenic pneumothorax is a type of traumatic pneumothorax which is becoming more common. The leading causes are transthoracic needle aspiration, thoracentesis, and the insertion of central intravenous catheters. The treatment differs according to the degree of distress and can be observation, supplemental oxygen, aspiration, or tube thoracostomy.

Tension pneumothorax   Tension pneumothorax usually occurs during mechanical ventilation or resuscitative efforts. The positive pleural pressure is life-threatening both because ventilation is severely compromised and because the positive pressure is transmitted to the mediastinum, which results in decreased venous return to the heart and reduced cardiac output.

Difficulty in ventilation during resuscitation or high peak inspiratory pressures during mechanical ventilation strongly suggest the diagnosis. The diagnosis is made by physical examination of the patient, which reveals an enlarged hemithorax with no breath sounds and shift of the mediastinum to the contralateral side. Tension pneumothorax must be treated as a medical emergency. If the tension in the pleural space is not relieved, the patient is likely to die from inadequate cardiac output or marked hypoxemia. A large-bore needle should be inserted into the pleural space through the second anterior intercostal space. If large amounts of gas escape from the needle after insertion, the diagnosis is confirmed. The needle should be left in place until a thoracostomy tube can be inserted.

DISORDERS OF THE MEDIASTINUM

The mediastinum is the region between the pleural sacs. It is separated into three compartments. The *anterior mediastinum* extends from the sternum anteriorly to the pericardium and brachiocephalic vessels posteriorly. It contains the thymus gland, the anterior mediastinal lymph nodes, and the internal mammary arteries and veins. The *middle mediastinum* lies between the anterior and posterior mediastina and contains the heart; the ascending and transverse arches of the aorta; the venae cavae; the brachiocephalic arteries and veins; the phrenic nerves; the trachea, main bronchi, and their contiguous lymph nodes; and the pulmonary arteries and veins. The *posterior mediastinum* is bounded by the pericardium and trachea anteriorly and the vertebral column posteriorly. It contains the descending thoracic aorta, esophagus, thoracic duct, azygos and hemiazygos veins, and the posterior group of mediastinal lymph nodes.

MEDIASTINAL MASSES The most common abnormality of the mediastinum is a mass. The first step in evaluating a mediastinal lesion is to place it in one of the three mediastinal compartments, since each compartment has different characteristic lesions. The most common lesions in the anterior mediastinum are thymomas, lymphomas, teratomatous neoplasms, and thyroid masses. The most common masses in the middle mediastinum are vascular masses, lymph node enlargement from metastases or granulomatous disease, and pleuropericardial and bronchogenic cysts. In the posterior mediastinum, neurogenic tumors, meningoceles, meningomyeloceles, gastroenteric cysts, and esophageal diverticula are commonly found.

The diagnostic approach to disorders of the mediastinum may be divided into imaging techniques (CT scans, magnetic resonance imaging, radionuclide studies, and intravenous contrast studies) and procedures for obtaining tissue samples (needle aspiration, mediastinoscopy, thoracoscopy, and open biopsy). CT scan of the mediastinum is the most valuable imaging technique and is probably the only imaging technique that should be done. Magnetic resonance imaging (MRI) appears to have no distinct advantages over CT in imaging the mediastinum. Barium studies of the gastrointestinal tract are indicated in many patients with posterior mediastinal lesions, since hernias, diverticula, and achalasia are readily diagnosed in this manner. A iodine 131 nuclear medicine scan can efficiently establish the diagnosis of intrathoracic goiter.

A definite diagnosis can be obtained with mediastinoscopy or anterior mediastinotomy in many patients with masses in the anterior or middle mediastinal compartments. A diagnosis can be established without thoracotomy via percutaneous fine needle aspiration biopsy of mediastinal masses in any of the mediastinal compartments. Video-assisted thoracoscopy will probably be used in the future to make the diagnosis in many instances.

ACUTE MEDIASTINITIS Most cases of acute mediastinitis are either due to esophageal perforation or occur after median sternotomy for cardiac surgery. Patients with esophageal rupture are acutely ill with chest pain and dyspnea due to the mediastinal infection. The esophageal rupture can occur spontaneously or as a complication of esophagoscopy or the insertion of a Blakemore tube. Appropriate treatment is exploration of the mediastinum with primary repair of the esophageal tear and drainage of the pleural space and the mediastinum.

The incidence of mediastinitis following median sternotomy is 0.4 to 5.0 percent. Patients most commonly present with wound drainage. Other presentations include sepsis or a widened mediastinum. The diagnosis is usually established with mediastinal needle aspiration. Treatment includes immediate drainage, debridement, and parenteral antibiotic therapy, but the mortality still exceeds 20 percent.

CHRONIC MEDIASTINITIS The spectrum of chronic mediastinitis ranges from granulomatous inflammation of the lymph nodes in the mediastinum to fibrosing mediastinitis. Most cases are due to tuberculosis or histoplasmosis, but sarcoidosis, silicosis, and other fungal diseases are at times causative. Patients with granulomatous mediastinitis are usually asymptomatic. Those with fibrosing mediastinitis usually have signs of compression of some mediastinal structure such as the superior vena caval syndrome, large airway obstruction, phrenic or recurrent laryngeal nerve paralysis, or obstruction of the pulmonary artery or proximal pulmonary veins. In most cases, mediastinal exploration is necessary to distinguish benign mediastinitis from malignant processes. No medical or surgical therapy has been demonstrated to be effective for mediastinal fibrosis, but the patient should be treated for tuberculosis if smears or cultures demonstrate tuberculous organisms.

PNEUMOMEDIASTINUM With this condition there is gas in the interstices of the mediastinum. The three main causes are (1) alveolar rupture with dissection of air into the mediastinum, (2) perforation or rupture of the esophagus, trachea, or main bronchi, and (3) dissection of air from the neck or the abdomen into the mediastinum. The symptoms associated with pneumomediastinum range from none to severe. Typically, there is severe substernal chest pain with or without radiation into the neck and arms. The physical examination usually reveals subcutaneous emphysema in the suprasternal notch and *Hamman's sign*, which is a crunching or clicking noise synchronous with the heartbeat and best heard in the left lateral decubitus position. The diagnosis is confirmed with the chest radiograph. Usually no treatment is required, but the mediastinal air will be absorbed faster if the patient inspires high concentrations of oxygen. If mediastinal structures are compressed, the compression can be relieved with needle aspiration.

DISORDERS OF THE DIAPHRAGM

The diaphragm is the principal muscle of breathing and moves like a piston within the cylinder of the thoracic cavity.

DIAPHRAGMATIC PARALYSIS The presence of bilateral diaphragmatic paralysis almost always causes severe morbidity in adults. The most common causes include high spinal cord injury, thoracic trauma (including cardiac surgery), multiple sclerosis, anterior horn disease, and muscular dystrophy. Most patients with severe diaphragmatic weakness will present with hypercapnic respiratory failure, frequently complicated by cor pulmonale and right ventricular failure, atelectasis, and pneumonia.

The degree of diaphragmatic weakness is best quantitated by measuring transdiaphragmatic pressures. Normally, this pressure is greater than $100 \, cmH_2O$. The treatment of choice is assisted ventilation for all or part of each day. This may be accomplished without tracheostomy using a rocking bed, corset-type positive-pressure wrap, nasal continuous positive pressure, or a negative-pressure ventilation. If the nerve to the diaphragm is intact, diaphragmatic pacing may be a viable alternative. If the paralysis occurs during open heart surgery, recovery frequently occurs, but it may take 6 months or more.

Unilateral paralysis of the diaphragm is much more common than is bilateral paralysis. The most common cause is nerve invasion from malignancy, usually a bronchogenic carcinoma. If the patient does not have malignancy, then usually no cause for the paralysis is found. The diagnosis is suggested by finding an elevated hemidiaphragm on the chest roentgenogram. Confirmation is best established with the "sniff test." When a patient is observed with fluoroscopy while sniffing, the paralyzed diaphragm will move paradoxically upward with the sniff due to the negative intrathoracic pressure. Patients with a unilateral paralyzed diaphragm are usually asymptomatic. Their vital capacity and total lung capacity are each reduced about 20 percent. If a patient has a mediastinal mass in conjunction with the diaphragmatic paralysis, further workup should be done. However, if the patient is asymptomatic with a normal chest radiograph, no invasive procedures are warranted.

HICCUP A hiccup is an involuntary spasm of the inspiratory muscles followed by an abrupt closure of the glottis. Hiccups are usually precipitated by irritation of the diaphragm, most commonly due to gastric distention or inflammation following rapid or excessive eating or drinking. Although hiccups usually are of short duration, if they persist, they may be very distressing. Patients with troublesome hiccups should first be asked to rapidly swallow 1 teaspoon of dry white granulated sugar. If this is ineffective, the stomach can be decompressed with a nasogastric tube, which also provides pharyngeal irritation. Pharmacologic agents that at times are curative are chlorpromazine, 10 to 20 mg every 4 to 6 h, or quinidine, 200 mg four times a day orally. As a last resort, a phrenic nerve can be blocked with bupivacaine or interrupted surgically.

REFERENCES

BERKMAN N, KRAMER MR: Diagnostic tests in pleural effusion—an update. Postgrad Med J 69:12, 1993

LIGHT RW: *Pleural Diseases*. Philadelphia, Lea & Febiger, 1990

MILES DW, KNIGHT RK: Diagnosis and management of malignant pleural effusion. Cancer Treat Rev 19:151, 1993

MULLER NL: Imaging of the pleura. Radiology 186:297, 1993

———: Pleural diseases. Dis Mon 28:266, 1992

PISTOLESI M et al: Pleural liquid and solute exchange. Am Rev Respir Dis 140:825, 1989

THOMAS CR JR, BONOMI PD: Mediastinal tumors. Curr Opin Oncol 3:335, 1991

229   DISORDERS OF VENTILATION

ELIOT A. PHILLIPSON

HYPOVENTILATION

DEFINITION AND ETIOLOGY   Alveolar hypoventilation exists by definition when arterial P_{CO_2} (Pa_{CO_2}) increases above the normal range of 37 to 43 mmHg, but in clinically important hypoventilation syndromes Pa_{CO_2} is generally in the range of 50 to 80 mmHg. Hypoventilation disorders can be acute or chronic. The acute disorders, which represent life-threatening emergencies, are discussed in Chap. 230; this chapter deals with chronic hypoventilation syndromes.

Chronic hypoventilation can result from numerous disease entities (Table 229-1), but in all cases the underlying mechanism involves a defect in either the metabolic respiratory control system, the respiratory neuromuscular system, or the ventilatory apparatus. Disorders associated with impaired respiratory drive, defects in the respiratory neuromuscular system, some chest wall disorders such as obesity, and upper airway obstruction produce an increase in Pa_{CO_2}, despite normal lungs, because of a reduction in overall minute volume of ventilation and hence in alveolar ventilation. In contrast, most disorders of the chest wall and disorders of the lower airways and

lungs may produce an increase in Pa_{CO_2}, despite a normal or even increased minute volume of ventilation, because of severe ventilation-perfusion mismatching that results in net alveolar hypoventilation.

Several hypoventilation syndromes involve combined disturbances in two elements of the respiratory system. For example, patients with chronic obstructive pulmonary disease may hypoventilate not simply because of impaired ventilatory mechanics but also because of a reduced central respiratory drive, which can be inherent or secondary to a coexisting metabolic alkalosis (related to diuretic and steroid therapy).

PHYSIOLOGICAL AND CLINICAL FEATURES   Regardless of cause, the hallmark of all alveolar hypoventilation syndromes is an increase in alveolar P_{CO_2} (PA_{CO_2}) and therefore in Pa_{CO_2} (Fig. 229-1). The resulting respiratory acidosis eventually leads to a compensatory increase in plasma HCO_3^- concentration and a decrease in Cl^- concentration. The increase in PA_{CO_2} produces an obligatory decrease in PA_{O_2}, resulting in hypoxemia. If severe, the hypoxemia manifests clinically as cyanosis and can stimulate erythropoiesis and induce secondary polycythemia. The combination of chronic hypoxemia and hypercapnia also may induce pulmonary vasoconstriction, leading eventually to pulmonary hypertension, right ventricular hypertrophy, and congestive heart failure. The disturbances in arterial blood gases are typically magnified during sleep because of a further reduction in central respiratory drive. The resulting increased nocturnal hypercapnia may cause cerebral vasodilation leading to morning headache; sleep quality also may be severely impaired, resulting in morning fatigue, daytime somnolence, mental confusion, and intellectual impairment. Other clinical features associated with hypoventilation syndromes are related to the specific underlying disease (see Table 229-1).

DIAGNOSIS   Investigation of the patient with chronic hypoventilation involves several laboratory tests that will usually localize the disorder to either the metabolic respiratory control system, the neuromuscular system, or the ventilatory apparatus (Fig. 229-2). Defects in the control system impair responses to chemical stimuli, including ventilatory, occlusion pressure, and diaphragmatic electromyographic (EMGdi) responses. During sleep, hypoventilation is usually more marked, and central apneas and hypopneas are common. However, because the behavioral respiratory control system (which is anatomically distinct from the metabolic control system), the neuromuscular system, and the ventilatory apparatus are intact, such patients can usually hyperventilate voluntarily, generate normal

TABLE 229-1   Chronic hypoventilation syndromes

Mechanism	Site of defect	Disorder
Impaired respiratory drive	Peripheral and central chemoreceptors	Carotid body dysfunction, trauma Prolonged hypoxia Metabolic alkalosis
	Brainstem respiratory neurons	Bulbar poliomyelitis, encephalitis Brainstem infarction, hemorrhage, trauma Brainstem demyelination, degeneration Chronic drug administration Primary alveolar hypoventilation syndrome
Defective respiratory neuromuscular system	Spinal cord and peripheral nerves	High cervical trauma Poliomyelitis Motor neuron disease Peripheral neuropathy
	Respiratory muscles	Myasthenia gravis Muscular dystrophy Chronic myopathy
Impaired ventilatory apparatus	Chest wall	Kyphoscoliosis Fibrothorax Thoracoplasty Ankylosing spondylitis Obesity-hypoventilation
	Airways and lungs	Laryngeal and tracheal stenosis Obstructive sleep apnea Cystic fibrosis Chronic obstructive pulmonary disease

SOURCE: Phillipson, in Murray and Nadel (eds), pp. 1831–1840, with permission.

FIGURE 229-1   Physiologic and clinical features of alveolar hypoventilation. (*After Phillipson.*)

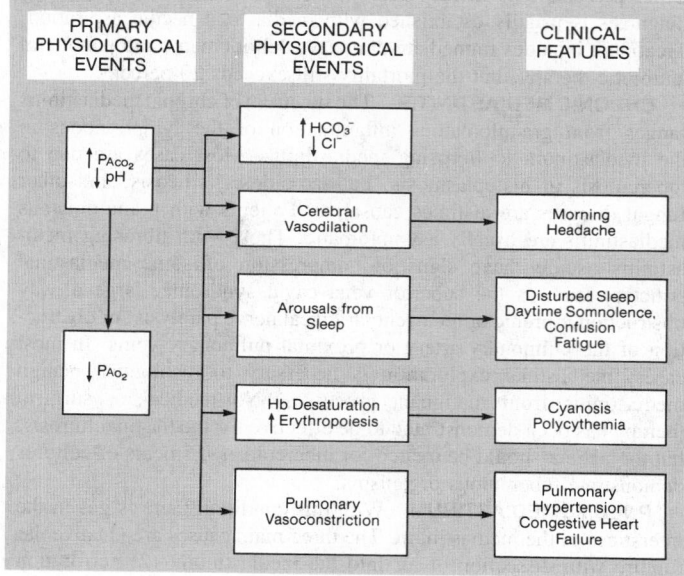

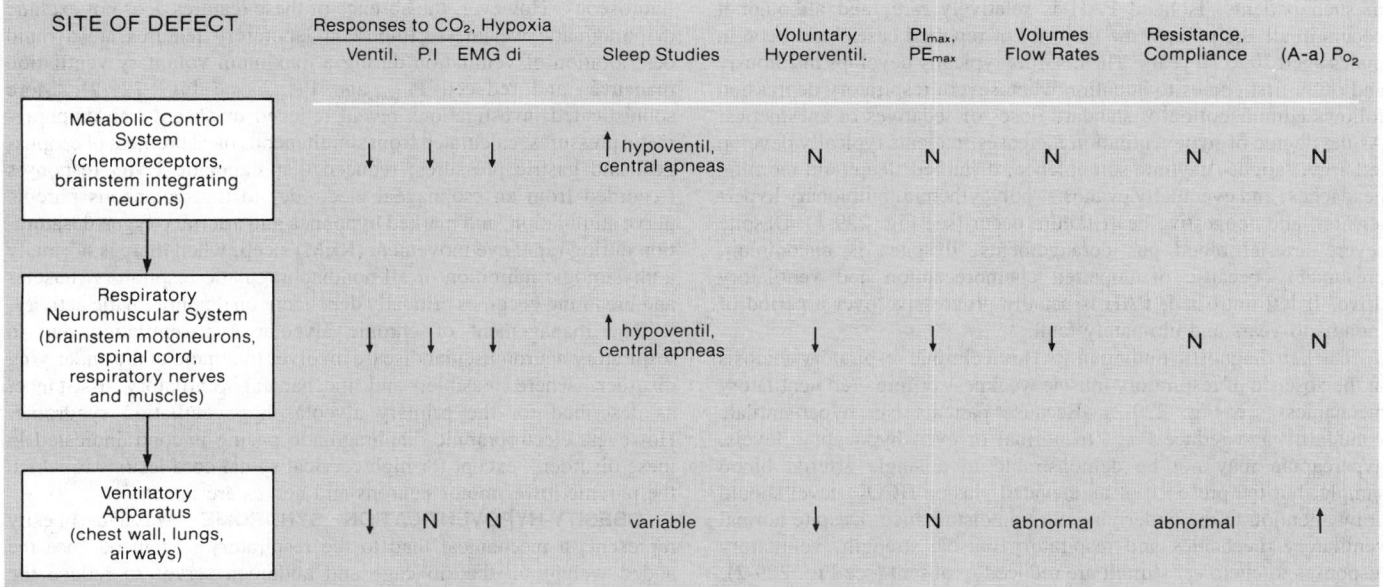

FIGURE 229-2 Pattern of laboratory test results in alveolar hypoventilation syndromes, based on the site of defect. Ventil = ventilation; P.1 = mouth pressure generated after 0.1 s of inspiration against an occluded airway; EMGdi = diaphragmatic EMG; PI_{max}, PE_{max} = maximum inspiratory or expiratory pressure that can be generated against an occluded airway; (A − a)P_{O_2} = alveolar-arterial P_{O_2} difference; N = normal. Defects in the metabolic control system impair central respiratory drive in response to chemical stimuli (CO_2 or hypoxia); therefore responses of EMGdi, P.1, and minute volume of ventilation are reduced and hypoventilation during sleep is aggravated. In contrast, tests of voluntary respiratory control, muscle strength, lung mechanics, and gas exchange [(A − a)P_{O_2}] are normal. Defects in the respiratory neuromuscular system impair muscle strength; therefore all tests dependent on muscular activity (voluntary or in response to metabolic stimuli) are abnormal, but lung resistance, lung compliance, and gas exchange are normal. Defects in the ventilatory apparatus usually impair gas exchange. Because resistance and compliance are also impaired, all tests dependent on ventilation (whether voluntary or in response to chemical stimuli) are abnormal; in contrast, tests of muscle activity or strength that do not involve airflow (that is, P.1, EMGdi, PI_{max}, PE_{max}) are normal. *(After Phillipson.)*

inspiratory and expiratory muscle pressures (PI_{max}, PE_{max}, respectively) against an occluded airway, generate normal lung volumes and flow rates on routine spirometry, and have normal respiratory system resistance and compliance and a normal alveolar-arterial P_{O_2} [(A − a) P_{O_2}] difference. Patients with defects in the respiratory neuromuscular system also have impaired responses to chemical stimuli but in addition are unable to hyperventilate voluntarily or to generate normal static respiratory muscle pressures, lung volumes, and flow rates. However, at least in the early stages of the disease the resistance and compliance of the respiratory system and the alveolar-arterial oxygen difference are normal.

In contrast to patients with disorders of the respiratory control or neuromuscular systems, patients with disorders of the chest wall, lungs, and airways typically demonstrate abnormalities of respiratory system resistance and compliance and have a widened (A − a)P_{O_2}. Because of the impaired mechanics of breathing, routine spirometric tests are abnormal, as is the ventilatory response to chemical stimuli. However, because the neuromuscular system is intact, tests that are independent of resistance and compliance are usually normal, including tests of respiratory muscle strength and of respiratory control that do not involve airflow.

TREATMENT The management of chronic hypoventilation must be individualized to the patient's particular disorder, circumstances, and needs and should include measures directed toward the underlying disease. Coexistent metabolic alkalosis should be corrected, including elevations of HCO_3^- that are inappropriately high for the degree of chronic hypercapnia. Administration of supplemental oxygen is effective in attenuating hypoxemia, polycythemia, and pulmonary hypertension but can aggravate CO_2 retention and the associated neurologic symptoms. For this reason, supplemental oxygen must be prescribed judiciously and the results monitored carefully. Pharmacologic agents that stimulate respiration (particularly progesterone) are of benefit in some patients, but generally, results are disappointing.

Most patients with chronic hypoventilation related to impairment of respiratory drive or neuromuscular disease eventually require mechanical ventilatory assistance for effective management. When hypoventilation is severe, treatment may be required on a 24-h basis, but in most patients ventilatory assistance only during sleep produces dramatic clinical improvement and lowering of daytime Pa_{CO_2}. In patients with reduced respiratory drive but intact respiratory lower motor neurons, phrenic nerves, and respiratory muscles, diaphragmatic pacing through an implanted phrenic electrode can be very effective. However, for patients with defects in the respiratory nerves and muscles, electrophrenic pacing is contraindicated. Such patients can usually be managed effectively with either intermittent negative-pressure ventilation in a cuirass or intermittent positive-pressure ventilation delivered through a tracheostomy or nose mask. For patients who require ventilatory assistance only during sleep, positive-pressure ventilation through a nose mask is the preferred method because it obviates a tracheostomy and avoids the problem of upper airway occlusion that can arise in a negative-pressure ventilator.

Hypoventilation related to restrictive disorders of the chest wall (see Table 229-1) also can be managed effectively with nocturnal intermittent positive-pressure ventilation through a nose mask or tracheostomy. Nocturnal ventilatory assistance also has been advocated for patients with hypercapnic chronic obstructive lung disease as a means of alleviating possible chronic respiratory muscle fatigue, but the efficacy of such an approach has yet to be confirmed.

HYPOVENTILATION SYNDROMES

PRIMARY ALVEOLAR HYPOVENTILATION Primary alveolar hypoventilation (PAH) is a disorder of unknown cause characterized by chronic hypercapnia and hypoxemia in the absence of identifiable neuromuscular disease or mechanical ventilatory impairment. The disorder is thought to arise from a defect in the metabolic respiratory control system, but few neuropathologic studies have been reported in such patients. Isolated PAH is relatively rare, and although it occurs in all age groups, the majority of reported cases have been in males aged 20 to 50 years. The disorder typically develops insidiously and often first comes to attention when severe respiratory depression follows administration of standard doses of sedatives or anesthetics. As the degree of hypoventilation increases, patients typically develop lethargy, fatigue, daytime somnolence, disturbed sleep, and morning headaches, and eventually cyanosis, polycythemia, pulmonary hypertension, and congestive heart failure occur (see Fig. 229-1). Despite severe arterial blood gas derangements, dyspnea is uncommon, presumably because of impaired chemoreception and ventilatory drive. If left untreated, PAH is usually progressive over a period of months to years and ultimately fatal.

The key diagnostic finding in PAH is a chronic respiratory acidosis in the absence of respiratory muscle weakness or impaired ventilatory mechanics (see Fig. 229-2). Because patients can hyperventilate voluntarily and reduce Pa_{CO_2} to normal or even hypocapnic levels, hypercapnia may not be demonstrable in a single arterial blood sample, but the presence of an elevated plasma HCO_3^- level should draw attention to the underlying chronic disturbance. Despite normal ventilatory mechanics and respiratory muscle strength, ventilatory responses to chemical stimuli are reduced or absent (see Fig. 229-2), and breath-holding time may be markedly prolonged without any sensation of dyspnea.

Patients with PAH maintain rhythmic respiration when awake, although the level of ventilation is below normal. However, during sleep there is typically a further deterioration in ventilation with frequent episodes of central hypopnea or apnea, a disturbance that has been termed *Ondine's curse*.

PAH must be distinguished from other central hypoventilation syndromes that are secondary to underlying neurologic disease of the brainstem or chemoreceptors (see Table 229-1). This distinction requires a careful neurologic investigation for evidence of brainstem or autonomic disturbances. Unrecognized respiratory neuromuscular disorders, particularly those which produce diaphragmatic weakness, are often misdiagnosed as PAH. However, such disorders can usually be suspected on clinical grounds (see below) and can be confirmed by the finding of reduced voluntary hyperventilation, as well as Pl_{max} and PE_{max}.

Some patients with PAH respond favorably to respiratory stimulant medications and to supplemental oxygen. However, the majority eventually require mechanical ventilatory assistance. Excellent long-term benefits can be achieved with diaphragmatic pacing by electrophrenic stimulation or with negative- or positive-pressure mechanical ventilation. The administration of such treatment only during sleep is sufficient in most patients.

RESPIRATORY NEUROMUSCULAR DISORDERS Several primary disorders of the spinal cord, peripheral respiratory nerves, and respiratory muscles produce a chronic hypoventilation syndrome (see Table 229-1). Hypoventilation usually develops gradually over a period of months to years and often first comes to attention when a relatively trivial increase in mechanical ventilatory load (such as mild airways obstruction) produces severe respiratory failure. In some of the disorders (such as motor neuron disease, myasthenia gravis, and muscular dystrophy), involvement of the respiratory nerves or muscles is usually a later feature of a more widespread disease. In other disorders, respiratory involvement can be an early or even isolated feature, and hence the underlying problem is often not suspected. Included in this category are the postpolio syndrome [a form of chronic respiratory insufficiency that develops 20 to 30 years following recovery from poliomyelitis (Chap. 375)], the myopathy associated with adult acid maltase deficiency, and idiopathic diaphragmatic paralysis.

Generally, respiratory neuromuscular disorders do not result in chronic hypoventilation unless there is significant weakness of the diaphragm. Distinguishing features of bilateral diaphragmatic weakness include orthopnea, paradoxical movement of the abdomen in the supine posture, and paradoxical diaphragmatic movement under fluoroscopy. However, the absence of these features does not exclude diaphragmatic weakness. Important laboratory features are a rapid deterioration of ventilation during a maximum voluntary ventilation maneuver and reduced Pl_{max} and PE_{max} (see Fig. 229-2). More sophisticated investigations reveal reduced or absent transdiaphragmatic pressures, calculated from simultaneous measurement of esophageal and gastric pressures; reduced diaphragmatic EMG responses (recorded from an esophageal electrode) to transcutaneous phrenic nerve stimulation; and marked hypopnea and arterial oxygen desaturation during rapid eye movement (REM) sleep, when there is normally a physiologic inhibition of all nondiaphragmatic respiratory muscles and breathing becomes critically dependent on diaphragmatic activity.

The management of chronic alveolar hypoventilation due to respiratory neuromuscular disease involves treatment of the underlying disorder, where feasible, and mechanical ventilatory assistance, as described for the primary alveolar hypoventilation syndrome. However, electrophrenic diaphragmatic pacing is contraindicated in these disorders, except for high cervical spinal cord lesions in which the phrenic lower motor neurons and nerves are intact.

OBESITY-HYPOVENTILATION SYNDROME Massive obesity represents a mechanical load to the respiratory system because the added weight on the rib cage and abdomen serves to reduce the compliance of the chest wall. As a result, the functional residual capacity (i.e., end-expiratory lung volume) is reduced, particularly in the recumbent posture. An important consequence of breathing at a low lung volume is that some airways, particularly those in the lung bases, may be closed throughout part or even all of each tidal breath, resulting in underventilation of the lung bases and widening of the $(A - a)P_{O_2}$. Nevertheless, in the majority of obese subjects, central respiratory drive is increased sufficiently to maintain a normal Pa_{CO_2}. However, a small proportion of obese subjects develop chronic hypercapnia, hypoxemia, and eventually polycythemia, pulmonary hypertension, and right-sided heart failure. Those patients who also develop daytime somnolence have been designated as having the *Pickwickian syndrome* (see Chap. 29). In many such patients, obstructive sleep apnea is a prominent feature, and even in those patients without sleep apnea, sleep-induced hypoventilation is an important element of the disorder and contributes to its progression. Most patients demonstrate a decrease in central respiratory drive which may be inherent or acquired, and many have mild to moderate degrees of airflow obstruction, usually related to smoking. Based on these considerations, several therapeutic measures can be of considerable benefit, including weight loss, cessation of smoking, elimination of obstructive sleep apnea, and enhancement of respiratory drive by medications such as progesterone.

SLEEP APNEA *Sleep apnea* is defined as an intermittent cessation of airflow at the nose and mouth during sleep. By convention, apneas of at least 10 s duration have been considered important, but in most patients the apneas are 20 to 30 s in duration and may be as long as 2 to 3 min. There is uncertainty as to the minimum number of apneas that should be considered clinically important, although by the time most patients come to attention they have at least 10 to 15 events per hour of sleep.

Sleep apneas have been classified into three types: central, obstructive, and mixed. In central sleep apnea (CSA) the neural drive to all the respiratory muscles is transiently abolished. In contrast, in obstructive sleep apnea (OSA) airflow ceases despite continuing respiratory drive because of occlusion of the oropharyngeal airway. Mixed apneas, which consist of a central apnea followed by an obstructive component, are a variant of OSA.

OBSTRUCTIVE SLEEP APNEA Pathogenesis The definitive event in OSA is occlusion of the upper airway usually at the level of the oropharynx (Fig. 229-3). The resulting apnea leads to progressive asphyxia until there is a brief arousal from sleep, whereupon airway patency is restored and airflow resumes. The patient then returns to sleep, and the sequence of events is repeated, often up to 400 to 500 times per night.

The immediate factor leading to collapse of the upper airway in

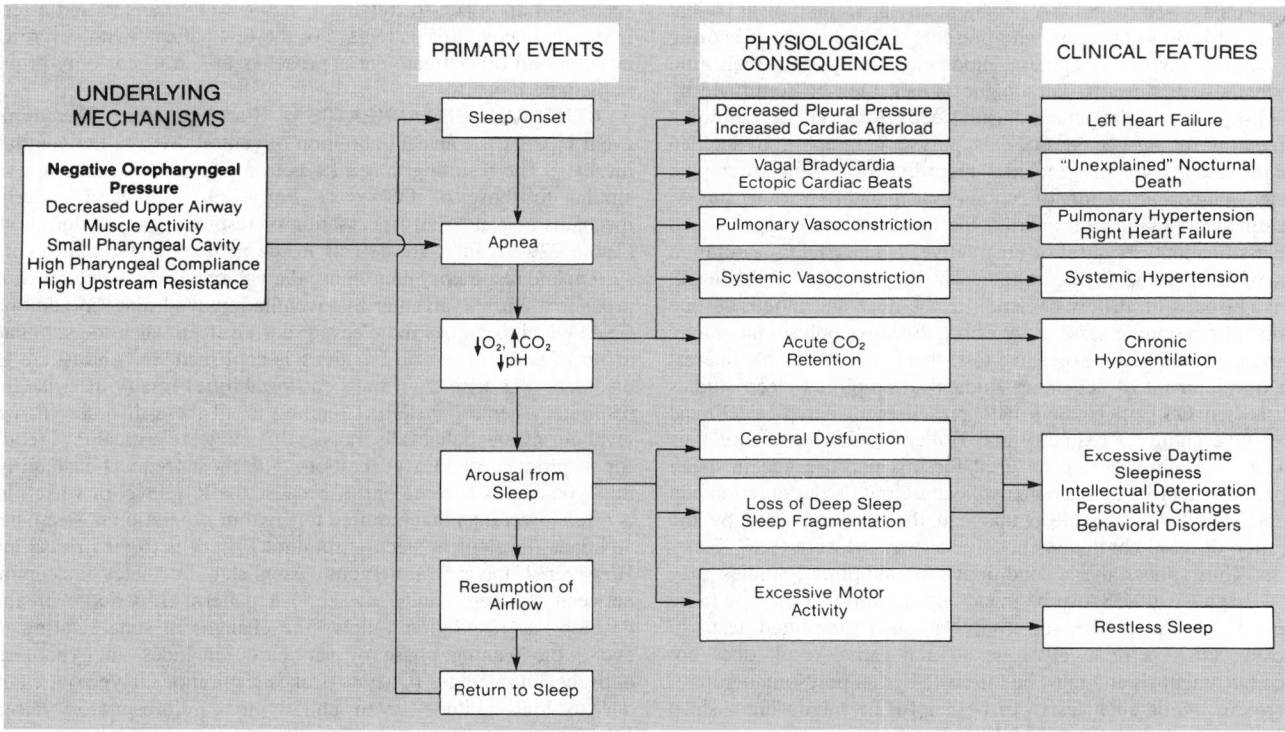

FIGURE 229-3 The primary sequence of events, underlying mechanisms, physiologic responses, and clinical features of obstructive sleep apnea. *(From EA Phillipson, Med North Am 23: 2314, 1982.)*

OSA is the generation of a critical subatmospheric pressure during inspiration that exceeds the ability of the airway dilator and abductor muscles to maintain airway stability (see Fig. 229-3). Sleep plays a permissive but crucial role by reducing the activity of the muscles of the upper airways. Alcohol is frequently an important cofactor because of its selective depressant influence on these muscles. In most patients the patency of the airway is also compromised structurally and therefore predisposed to occlusion. In a minority of patients the structural compromise is due to obvious anatomic disturbances, such as adenotonsillar hypertrophy, retrognathia, and macroglossia. However, in the majority of patients the structural defect is simply a subtle reduction in airway size that can often be appreciated clinically as "pharyngeal crowding" and that can usually be demonstrated by imaging and acoustic reflection techniques. Obesity frequently contributes to the reduction in size of the upper airways. Snoring, a high-frequency vibration of the palatal and pharyngeal soft tissues that results from the decrease in size of the upper airway lumen, may aggravate the narrowing by producing edema of the soft tissues. More sophisticated studies also demonstrate a high airway compliance—i.e., the airway is "floppy" and therefore prone to collapse. In some patients, a high upstream (i.e., nasal) resistance contributes to collapse of the upper airway by increasing the subatmospheric pressure generated in the pharynx during inspiration.

Pathophysiologic and clinical features The narrowing of the upper airways during sleep, which predisposes to OSA, inevitably results in snoring. In most patients, snoring antedates the development of obstructive events by many years. However, the majority of snoring individuals do not have an OSA disorder; hence, in the absence of other symptoms, snoring alone does not warrant an investigation for OSA.

The recurrent episodes of nocturnal asphyxia and of arousal from sleep that characterize OSA lead to a series of secondary physiologic events, which in turn give rise to the clinical complications of the syndrome (see Fig. 229-3). The most common manifestations are neuropsychiatric and behavioral disturbances that are thought to arise from the fragmentation of sleep and loss of slow-wave sleep induced by the recurrent arousal responses. Nocturnal cerebral hypoxia also

may play an important role. The most pervasive manifestation is excessive daytime sleepiness. OSA is now recognized as a leading cause of daytime sleepiness and has been implicated as an important risk factor for motor vehicle accidents. Indeed, several studies have demonstrated two to three times more automobile accidents in patients with OSA compared with other drivers. Other related symptoms include intellectual impairment, memory loss, personality disturbances, and impotence.

The other major manifestations are cardiorespiratory in nature and are thought to arise from the recurrent episodes of nocturnal asphyxia (see Fig. 229-3). Most patients demonstrate a cyclical slowing of the heart during the apneas to 30 to 50 beats per minute, followed by a tachycardia of 90 to 120 beats per minute during the ventilatory phase. A small number of patients develop severe bradycardia with asystoles of 8 to 12 s duration or dangerous tachyarrhythmias, including unsustained ventricular tachycardia. The presence of such arrhythmias has led to the notion that OSA may result in sudden death during sleep, but firm corroborative data are lacking. Several epidemiologic studies have implicated OSA as a risk factor for the development of systemic hypertension, myocardial ischemia and infarction, stroke, and premature death. However, because these studies were cross-sectional or retrospective in design, the natural history of OSA remains largely undefined. OSA also markedly aggravates left ventricular failure in patients with underlying heart disease. This complication is probably due to the combined effects of increased left ventricular afterload during each obstructive event, secondary to increased negative intrathoracic pressure (see Fig. 229-3), recurrent nocturnal hypoxemia, and chronically elevated sympathoadrenal activity. Treatment of OSA in such patients often results in dramatic improvement in left ventricular function. Finally, a small proportion of patients with OSA (10 to 15 percent) develop pulmonary hypertension, right ventricular failure, polycythemia, and chronic hypercapnia and hypoxemia. All such patients have evidence of sustained daytime hypoxemia in addition to the nocturnal ventilatory disturbance, usually as a result of reduced ventilatory drive and/or diffuse airways obstruction. Most of these patients are obese and sleepy and are therefore said to have the *Pickwickian syndrome.*

Diagnosis   Although OSA occurs at any age, the typical patient is a male aged 30 to 60 years who presents with a history of snoring and excessive daytime sleepiness, moderate obesity, and often mild to moderate hypertension. The diagnosis can often be confirmed by direct observation of the patient during sleep. However, the definitive investigation for suspected OSA is polysomnography, a detailed overnight sleep study that includes recording of (1) electrographic variables that permit the identification of sleep and its various stages, (2) ventilatory variables that permit the identification of apneas and their classification as central or obstructive, (3) arterial O_2 saturation by ear oximetry, and (4) heart rate. The key diagnostic finding in OSA is episodes of airflow cessation at the nose and mouth despite evidence of continuing respiratory effort. Because polysomnography is a time-consuming and expensive test, there is considerable interest in the development of screening studies or simplified sleep studies for suspected OSA in patients who present with a typical clinical picture. Overnight ear oximetry and Holter monitoring (continuous electrocardiography) have been used for this purpose and in many such patients clearly demonstrate cyclical arterial O_2 desaturation and brady/tachycardia during sleep that can then be abolished by the application of nasal continuous positive airway pressure (see "Treatment"). Thus, under these conditions, the simplified studies may allow a diagnosis of OSA to be made and nonsurgical therapy to be prescribed. However, the sensitivity of such simplified tests in diagnosing OSA is relatively low, so a negative result does not exclude the diagnosis and must be followed by full polysomnography. Furthermore, while such tests can be helpful in diagnosing a sleep apnea disorder, they are not useful in identifying or excluding other possible causes of daytime sleepiness (narcolepsy, periodic leg movements during sleep, nonrestorative sleep syndromes, phase-shift disorders) that may coexist with sleep apnea.

Treatment   Several approaches to treatment of OSA have been advocated, based on an understanding of the mechanisms underlying the disorder (Table 229-2). The specific choice of treatment depends largely on the severity of OSA. Mild to moderate OSA can often be managed effectively by modest weight reduction, avoidance of alcohol, improvement of nasal patency, and avoidance of sleeping in the supine posture. In some patients with more severe OSA, tricyclic medications, particularly protriptyline (20 to 30 mg at bedtime), have been beneficial. The role of nocturnal supplemental oxygen in managing OSA is uncertain but is generally not satisfactory. The most widely used treatments in moderate to severe OSA are uvulopalatopharyngoplasty and nasal continuous positive airway pressure (CPAP) during sleep. Uvulopalatopharyngoplasty is a surgical procedure designed to increase the pharyngeal lumen by resecting redundant soft tissue. When applied to unselected patients with OSA, it produces long-term benefits in only about 50 percent. More recent attempts to select patients based on the specific site of upper airway occlusion have yielded a higher success rate. Nasal CPAP, which prevents upper airway occlusion by splinting the pharyngeal airway with a positive pressure delivered through a nose mask, is currently the most successful approach to treatment, being well-tolerated and effective in over 80 percent of patients. For the few patients with severe OSA in whom all other treatment approaches fail, tracheostomy provides immediate relief.

CENTRAL SLEEP APNEA (CSA)   Pathogenesis   The definitive event in CSA is transient abolition of central drive to the ventilatory muscles. The resulting apnea leads to a primary sequence of events similar to those of OSA (see Fig. 229-3). Several underlying mechanisms can result in cessation of respiratory drive during sleep (Table 229-3). First are defects in the metabolic respiratory control system and respiratory neuromuscular apparatus. Such defects usually produce a chronic alveolar hypoventilation syndrome (in addition to CSA) which becomes more severe during sleep when the stimulatory effect of wakefulness on breathing is abolished. In contrast are CSA disorders that arise from transient instabilities in an otherwise intact respiratory control system. Common to all these disorders is a P_{CO_2} level during sleep that falls transiently below the critical P_{CO_2} required for respiratory rhythm generation. The most frequent instability of this type occurs at sleep onset, because the P_{CO_2} level of wakefulness is often lower than that required for rhythm generation in sleep; hence an apnea develops at sleep onset until P_{CO_2} rises to the critical level. However, if the central nervous system state fluctuates at sleep onset between "asleep" and "awake," a pattern of periodic breathing develops as respiration follows the changes in state. During each cycle, the waning phase of ventilation includes an hypopnea or outright central apnea (Cheyne-Stokes respiration). Hypoxia, whether due to high altitude or to underlying cardiorespiratory disease, enhances the tendency to periodic breathing and CSA because of the associated hyperventilation that may drive P_{CO_2} levels during wakefulness well below the critical value required for respiratory rhythm generation during sleep. Hyperventilation due to CNS disease or to lung congestion secondary to heart failure produces periodic breathing and CSA by a similar mechanism. Circulatory slowing secondary to cardiac failure also may induce ventilatory instability by prolonging the time lag between changes in blood gas values by ventilation and the detection of those changes by the peripheral and central chemoreceptors (Chap. 195). Consequently, the ventilatory system overshoots the mark before reversing direction, resulting in periodic breathing that frequently includes central apneas.

Pathophysiologic and clinical features   Many healthy individuals demonstrate a small number of central apneas during sleep, particularly at sleep onset and in REM sleep. These apneas are not associated with any physiologic or clinical disturbances. In patients with clinically important CSA, the primary sequence of events that characterizes the disorder leads to prominent physiologic and clinical consequences (see Fig. 229-3). In those patients whose CSA is a component of an alveolar hypoventilation syndrome, daytime hypercapnia and hypoxemia are usually evident, and the clinical picture is dominated by a history of recurrent respiratory failure,

---

TABLE 229-2   Management of obstructive sleep apnea (OSA)

Mechanism	Mild to moderate OSA	Severe OSA
↑ Upper airway muscle tone	Avoidance of alcohol, sedatives	Tricyclics
↑ Upper airway lumen size	Weight reduction Avoidance of supine posture Oral prosthesis	Uvulopalatopharyngoplasty
↓ Upper airway subatmospheric pressure	Improved nasal patency	Nasal continuous positive airway pressure
Bypass occlusion		Tracheostomy

SOURCE: Phillipson, in Murray and Nadel (eds), pp. 1841–1860, with permission.

TABLE 229-3   Mechanisms underlying central sleep apnea

Underlying mechanism	Clinical example
Defects in metabolic control system or respiratory muscles	Primary and secondary central alveolar hypoventilation syndromes Respiratory muscle weakness
Transient instabilities in central respiratory drive	Sleep onset Hyperventilation-induced hypocapnia Hypoxia (high altitude, pulmonary disease) Cardiovascular disease, pulmonary congestion CNS disease Prolonged circulation time
Inhibition of central respiratory drive by upper airway reflexes	Esophageal reflux Aspiration Upper airway collapse

SOURCE: Phillipson, in Murray and Nadel (eds), pp 1841–1860, with permission.

polycythemia, pulmonary hypertension, and right-sided heart failure. Complaints of sleeping poorly, morning headache, and daytime fatigue and sleepiness are also prominent. In contrast, in patients whose CSA results from an instability in respiratory drive, the clinical picture is dominated by features related to sleep disturbance, including recurrent nocturnal awakenings, morning fatigue, and daytime sleepiness.

Diagnosis Initially, many patients with CSA are suspected clinically of having OSA because of a history of snoring, sleep disturbance, and daytime sleepiness. However, obesity and hypertension are less prominent in CSA than in OSA. Definitive diagnosis of CSA requires a polysomnographic study, with the *key observation being recurrent apneas that are not accompanied by respiratory effort.* Measurements of transcutaneous P_{CO_2} are particularly useful in CSA. Those patients with a defect in respiratory control or neuromuscular function typically demonstrate an elevated P_{CO_2} that tends to increase progressively during the night, particularly during REM sleep. In contrast, patients with instabilities in the respiratory control system often demonstrate a mild degree of hypocapnia, which is an integral pathogenetic feature of their disorder (see above).

Treatment The management of patients whose CSA is a component of an alveolar hypoventilation syndrome is essentially the same as management of the underlying hypoventilation disorder. Management of patients whose CSA arises from an instability of respiratory drive is more problematic. Patients with hypoxemia usually respond favorably to nocturnal supplemental oxygen. Others have responded to acidification with acetazolamide, and recent reports indicate a good response to nasal CPAP (as for OSA). The precise mechanism by which CPAP abolishes central apneas is not clear but probably involves a small increase in Pa_{CO_2} as a result of the added expiratory mechanical load.

HYPERVENTILATION AND ITS SYNDROMES

DEFINITION AND ETIOLOGY Alveolar hyperventilation exists when Pa_{CO_2} decreases below the normal range of 37 to 43 mmHg. *Hyperventilation* is not synonymous with *hyperpnea*, which refers to an increased minute volume of ventilation without reference to Pa_{CO_2}. Although hyperventilation is frequently associated with dyspnea, patients who are hyperventilating do not necessarily complain of shortness of breath; and conversely, patients with dyspnea need not be hyperventilating.

Numerous disease entities can be associated with alveolar hyperventilation (Table 229-4), but in all cases the underlying mechanism involves an increase in respiratory drive. Thus hypoxemia drives ventilation by stimulating the peripheral chemoreceptors, and several pulmonary disorders and congestive heart failure drive ventilation by stimulating afferent vagal receptors in the lungs and airways. Low cardiac output and hypotension stimulate the peripheral chemoreceptors and inhibit the baroreceptors, both of which increase ventilation. Metabolic acidosis, a potent respiratory stimulant, excites both the peripheral and central chemoreceptors and increases the sensitivity of the peripheral chemoreceptors to coexistent hypoxemia. Hepatic failure also can produce hyperventilation, presumably as a result of metabolic stimuli acting on the peripheral and central chemoreceptors.

Several neurologic disorders are thought to drive ventilation through the behavioral respiratory control system. Included in this category are psychogenic or anxiety hyperventilation and severe cerebrovascular insufficiency, which may interfere with the inhibitory influence normally exerted by cortical structures on the brainstem respiratory neurons. Rarely, disorders of the midbrain and hypothalamus induce hyperventilation, and it is conceivable that fever and sepsis also cause hyperventilation through effects on these structures. Several drugs cause hyperventilation by stimulating the central or peripheral chemoreceptors or by direct action on the brainstem respiratory neurons. Chronic hyperventilation is a normal feature of pregnancy and results from the effects of progesterone and other hormones acting on the respiratory neurons.

TABLE 229-4 Hyperventilation syndromes

Hypoxemia
 A High altitude
 B Pulmonary disease

Pulmonary disorders
 A Pneumonia
 B Interstitial pneumonitis, fibrosis, edema
 C Pulmonary emboli, vascular disease
 D Bronchial asthma
 E Pneumothorax

Cardiovascular disorders
 A Congestive heart failure
 B Hypotension

Metabolic disorders
 A Acidosis (diabetic, renal, lactic)
 B Hepatic failure

Neurologic disorders
 A Psychogenic or anxiety hyperventilation
 B Central nervous system infection, tumors

Drug-induced
 A Salicylates
 B Methylxanthine derivatives
 C Beta-adrenergic agonists
 D Progesterone

Miscellaneous
 A Fever, sepsis
 B Pain
 C Pregnancy

PHYSIOLOGIC AND CLINICAL FEATURES Because hyperventilation is associated with increased respiratory drive, muscle effort, and minute volume of ventilation, the most frequent symptom associated with hyperventilation is dyspnea. However, there is considerable discrepancy between the degree of hyperventilation, as measured by Pa_{CO_2}, and the degree of associated dyspnea. In patients whose hypocapnia is associated with alkalemia, neurologic symptoms may be present, including dizziness, visual impairment, syncope, and seizure activity (secondary to cerebral vasoconstriction); parasthesias, carpopedal spasm, and tetany (secondary to decreased free serum calcium); and muscle weakness (secondary to hypophosphatemia). Severe alkalemia also can induce cardiac arrhythmias and evidence of myocardial ischemia. Patients with a primary respiratory alkalosis are also prone to periodic breathing and central sleep apnea (see "Central Sleep Apnea").

DIAGNOSIS In most patients with a hyperventilation syndrome, the cause is readily apparent on the basis of history, physical examination, and knowledge of coexisting medical disorders (see Table 229-4). In patients in whom the cause is not clinically apparent, investigation begins with arterial blood gas analysis, which establishes the presence of alveolar hyperventilation (decreased Pa_{CO_2}) and its severity. Equally important is the arterial pH, which generally allows the disorder to be classified as either a primary respiratory alkalosis (elevated pH) or a primary metabolic acidosis (decreased pH). Also of importance is the Pa_{O_2} and calculation of the $(A - a)P_{O_2}$, since a widened alveolar-arterial oxygen difference suggests a pulmonary disorder as the underlying cause. The finding of a reduced plasma HCO_3^- level establishes the chronic nature of the disorder and points toward an organic cause. Measurements of ventilation and arterial or transcutaneous P_{CO_2} during sleep are very useful in suspected psychogenic hyperventilation, since such patients do not maintain the hyperventilation during sleep.

The disorders that most frequently give rise to unexplained hyperventilation are pulmonary vascular disease (particularly chronic or recurrent thromboembolism) and psychogenic or anxiety hyperventilation. Hyperventilation due to pulmonary vascular disease is associated with exertional dyspnea, a widened $(A - a)P_{O_2}$ and maintenance of hyperventilation during exercise. In contrast, patients with psychogenic hyperventilation typically complain of dyspnea at rest and not during mild exercise and of the need to sigh frequently.

They are also more likely to complain of dizziness, sweating, palpitations, and paresthesias. During mild to moderate exercise, their hyperventilation tends to disappear and $(\text{A} - \text{a})\text{P}_{O_2}$ is normal, but heart rate and cardiac output may be increased relative to metabolic rate.

TREATMENT   Alveolar hyperventilation is usually of relatively minor clinical consequence and therefore is generally managed by appropriate treatment of the underlying cause. In the few patients in whom alkalemia is thought to be inducing significant cerebral vasoconstriction, parasthesias, tetany, or cardiac disturbances, inhalation of a low concentration of CO_2 can be very beneficial. For patients with disabling psychogenic hyperventilation, careful explanation of the basis of their symptoms can be reassuring and is often sufficient. Others have benefited from beta-adrenergic antagonists or an exercise program. Specific treatment for anxiety may also be indicated.

REFERENCES

CHERNIACK NS, LONGOBARDO GS: Abnormalities in respiratory rhythm, in *Handbook of Physiology*, section 3: *The Respiratory System*, vol 2, *Control of Breathing*, NS Cherniack, JG Widdicombe (eds). Bethesda, Md, Am Physiol Soc, 1986, pp 729–749

FAIRBANKS DN: Uvulopalatopharyngoplasty: Strategies for success and safety. Ear Nose Throat J 72:46, 1993

FUJITA S: Obstructive sleep apnea syndrome: Pathophysiology, upper airway evaluation and surgical treatment. Ear Nose Throat J 72:77, 1993

HUDGEL DW, CHERNIACK NS: Sleep and breathing, in *Update: Pulmonary Diseases and Disorders*, AP Fishman (ed). New York, McGraw-Hill, 1992, pp 249–262

PHILLIPSON EA: Hypoventilation syndromes, in *Textbook of Respiratory Medicine*, JF Murray, JA Nadel (eds). Philadelphia, Saunders, 1988, chap 84, pp. 1831–1840

———: Sleep disorders, in *Textbook of Respiratory Medicine*, JF Murray, JA Nadel (eds). Philadelphia, Saunders, 1988, chap 85, pp 1841–1860

———, BRADLEY TD (eds): Breathing disorders in sleep. *Clin Chest Med* 13:(3)383, 1992

230   ADULT RESPIRATORY DISTRESS SYNDROME

ROLAND H. INGRAM, JR.

Adult respiratory distress syndrome (ARDS) is a descriptive term that has been applied to many acute, diffuse infiltrative lung lesions of diverse etiologies when they are accompanied by severe arterial hypoxemia. The term was chosen because of several clinical and pathologic similarities between such acute illnesses in adults and the neonatal respiratory distress syndrome. However, in the neonatal form, immaturity of alveolar surfactant production and a highly compliant chest wall are primarily involved in the pathophysiology, whereas in the adult form, alveolar surfactant changes are secondary to the primary process and the chest wall is not compliant. Despite the large number of causes (Table 230-1), the clinical characteristics, respiratory pathophysiologic derangement, and current techniques for supportive management of these acute abnormalities are remarkably similar. It has been argued that the "lumping" of such processes of different etiologies obscures the unique features of each in terms of pathogenesis, prevention, and specificity of treatment. However, irrespective of cause, there are many common features at the onset of respiratory failure. The conditions listed do not always lead to respiratory failure, and specific treatment of the underlying processes will often be different. The most common cause of ARDS is sepsis; therefore, that etiology and its pathogenesis will be the focus of this chapter. The reader is urged to refer to the appropriate sections of this text for the special characteristics of other causes. Several causative factors can come into play during the course of ARDS; for example, respiratory failure in association with acute pancreatitis can

TABLE 230-1   Conditions which may lead to the adult respiratory distress syndrome

1 Diffuse pulmonary infections (e.g., viral, bacterial, fungal, *Pneumocystis*)
2 Aspiration (e.g., gastric contents with Mendelson's syndrome, water with near drowning)
3 Inhalation of toxins and irritants (e.g., chlorine gas, NO_2, smoke, ozone, high concentrations of oxygen)
4 Narcotic overdose pulmonary edema (e.g., heroin, methadone, morphine, dextropropoxyphene)
5 Nonnarcotic drug effects (e.g., nitrofurantoin)
6 Immunologic response to host antigens (e.g., Goodpasture's syndrome, systemic lupus erythematosus)
7 Effects of nonthoracic trauma with hypotension
8 In association with systemic reactions to processes initiated outside the lung (e.g., gram-negative septicemia, hemorrhagic pancreatitis, amniotic fluid embolism, fat embolism)
9 After cardiopulmonary bypass ("pump lung," "postperfusion lung")

be complicated by a bacterial pneumonia, which, in turn, can lead to a sepsis syndrome (see below). ARDS then becomes the pulmonary manifestation of a systemic disorder associated with diffuse endothelial injury and increased capillary permeability in multiple organ systems.

PATHOPHYSIOLOGY   Regardless of the initiating process, ARDS is invariably associated with increased liquid in the lungs. It is a form of pulmonary edema, although distinct from cardiogenic pulmonary edema because pulmonary capillary pressure is not elevated (Chap. 31). Since hydrostatic pressures are not elevated, there is increased permeability of the alveolocapillary membranes that occurs via direct chemical injury in the case of inhaled toxic gases or aspirated acid or indirectly through activation and aggregation of formed elements of the blood within pulmonary capillaries. In association with sepsis, bacterial endotoxins (gram-negative bacteria) or exotoxins (gram-positive bacteria) stimulate monocytic phagocytes and polymorphonuclear leukocytes to adhere to endothelial surfaces and undergo a respiratory burst to inflict oxidant injury and release mediators of inflammation such as leukotrienes, thromboxanes, and prostaglandins. The monocytic phagocytes, mainly macrophages in the alveoli and those lining the vasculature, also release oxidants, mediators, cytokines, and a series of degradative enzymes and peptides that directly damage endothelial and alveolar surfaces and cause polymorphonuclear leukocytes to release their lysosomal enzymes. Initially, the injury to the alveolocapillary membrane results in leakage of liquid, macromolecules, and cellular components from the blood vessels into the interstitial space and, with increasing severity, into the alveoli.

The increasing vascular permeability to proteins (decreased reflection coefficient σ, discussed in Chap. 31) leaves the hydrostatic gradient unopposed so that even mild elevations in capillary pressures (due to increased intravenous fluid loads and cardiac dysfunction characteristic of sepsis) greatly increase interstitial and alveolar edema. Alveolar collapse occurs secondary to the effect of the alveolar liquid, especially its fibrinogen, that interferes with normal surfactant activity and the possible impairment of further surfactant production by injury to the granular pneumocytes. Fibrinolytic mechanisms that would normally clear the alveoli are inhibited, and their deficiency can lead to hyaline membranes that may act as a matrix for fibrogenesis. Though radiographically diffuse, the regional dysfunction is nonhomogeneous; it leads to severe ventilation-perfusion imbalance and the shunting of blood through regions in which alveoli are collapsed or filled with liquid and fibrin. The lungs become less compliant—i.e., stiffen because of interstitial edema, alveolar collapse, and increase in surface forces. Because of the decreased compliance, large inspiratory pressures must be generated by the respiratory muscles, so the work of breathing is elevated. The large mechanical load may lead to fatigue of the muscles of breathing with resulting diminution in tidal volumes and worsening gas exchange. Both hypoxemia and the stimulation of receptors in the stiff lung parenchyma cause an increase in respiratory frequency, decrease in tidal volume, and deterioration in gas exchange.

PATHOLOGY In the absence of specific demonstrable pathogens, the pathology is remarkably similar among the various conditions leading to ARDS, since the lung has a limited number of ways in which it reacts to a large number of injuries. Grossly, the lungs are heavy, edematous, and nearly airless with regions of hemorrhage, atelectasis, and consolidation. By light microscopy, there is edema and cellular infiltration of interalveolar septa and interstitial spaces surrounding airways and blood vessels, atelectasis and hyaline membranes in many regions, engorgement of vessels with red blood cells, and aggregates of platelets and polymorphonuclear leukocytes along with interstitial and alveolar hemorrhage. In addition to loss of alveolar type I pneumocytes, both hyperplasia and dysplasia of the granular (type II) pneumocytes are often present.

If the illness has been prolonged beyond 10 days, there is often a surprising amount of fibrosis in addition to the acute changes. In instances of recovery and subsequent death from another cause, significant interstitial fibrosis and emphysematous changes may be found in the lung. Many patients, however, will recover completely and have normal pulmonary function with no respiratory symptoms. Hence aggressive clinical management is both indicated and often rewarding.

CLINICAL CHARACTERISTICS At the time of initial injury and for several hours thereafter, the patient may be free of respiratory symptoms or signs. The earliest sign often is an increase in respiratory frequency followed shortly by dyspnea. Arterial blood gas measurement in the earlier period will disclose a depressed P_{O_2} despite a decreased P_{CO_2} so that the alveolar-arterial difference for oxygen (Chap. 214) is increased. At this early stage, administration of oxygen results in a significant increase in the arterial P_{O_2}. The brisk rise in P_{O_2} indicates that ventilation-perfusion mismatching and, possibly, diffusion impairment account for the widened alveolar-arterial P_{O_2} difference $[(A - a)P_{O_2}]$ initially. Physical examination may be unremarkable, although a few fine inspiratory rales may be audible. Radiographically, the lung fields may be clear or demonstrate only minimal and scattered interstitial infiltrates. With progression, the patient becomes cyanotic and increasingly dyspneic and tachypneic. Rales may become more prominent and easily heard throughout both lung fields along with regions of tubular breath sounds; the chest radiograph demonstrates diffuse, extensive bilateral interstitial and alveolar infiltrates (Fig. 230-1). At this point, hypoxemia cannot be corrected simply by increasing the oxygen concentration of the inspired gas, and mechanical ventilatory support must be started. Right-to-left shunting of blood through collapsed or filled alveoli becomes the major mechanism for arterial hypoxemia at this more advanced stage. In contrast to ventilation-perfusion mismatching and diffusion impairment, with right-to-left shunts, $(A - a)P_{O_2}$ remains high with breathing of pure oxygen. Positive end-expiratory pressure (PEEP) serves to increase lung volume, which in turn opens collapsed alveoli and decreases shunting. With further progression, and if mechanical ventilator and PEEP therapy are delayed, the combination of increasing tachypnea and decreasing tidal volumes results in alveolar hypoventilation, a rising P_{CO_2}, and worsening hypoxemia; these represent an ominous constellation of findings.

When there is evidence of infection, most commonly intraabdominal, renal, or lung; the presence of tachycardia (>90 beats per minute), tachypnea (>20 breaths per minute), either fever (>38.3°C) or hypothermia (<35.5°C), and some combination of alteration in mental status, lactic acidemia, oliguria (<0.5 mL/kg for more than 1 h); and an elevated alveolar-arterial P_{O_2}, the criteria for the sepsis syndrome are met. It is at this point that many immunologic and pharmacologic interventions directed against bacterial products, cytokines, oxidants, and arachidonic acid metabolites are being tried.

If the syndrome progresses to frank ARDS with hypotension and multiorgan failure, which occurs in a large percentage of cases of the sepsis syndrome, the mortality rate is exceedingly high despite supportive measures.

SUPPORTIVE MANAGEMENT OF HYPOXEMIC RESPIRATORY FAILURE The brief description given above contains the salient

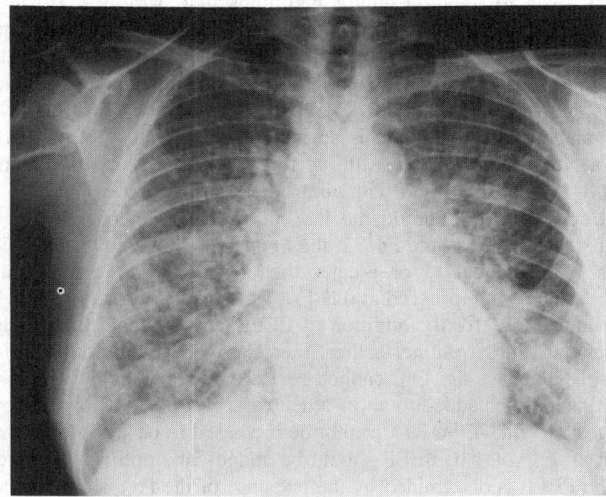

FIGURE 230-1 A standard posteroanterior chest radiograph from a patient with the adult respiratory distress syndrome secondary to a severe viral pneumonitis. Such a diffuse radiographic change is typical of all conditions listed in Table 230-1 when they are severe enough to cause acute hypoxemic respiratory failure. A similar radiographic picture is also seen in pulmonary edema due to left ventricular failure (Chap. 31). Often in such acutely ill patients, the radiograph must be taken with a portable unit and the film exposed from the anterior direction. Both the anteroposterior exposure and the failure to take a deep inspiration result in an apparent enlargement of the cardiac silhouette which further obscures the reliable detection of left ventricular failure.

principles of management, integrated with the clinical events that lead to escalation of therapeutic interventions. Implicit in that description is that the simplest method and the lowest inspired fraction of oxygen (FI_{O_2}) should be used to give the desired result. The oxyhemoglobin dissociation curve gives some guide to the most desirable level of Pa_{O_2}. At a P_{O_2} of 60 mmHg, hemoglobin is approximately 90 percent saturated. Therefore, a reasonable objective is to achieve that Pa_{O_2}, since higher levels add little to oxygenation and introduce the risk of oxygen toxicity to the lung. In contrast to respiratory failure complicating chronic airways obstruction (Chap. 223), depression of ventilation is not an important factor in hypoxemic respiratory failure.

There are multiple means for delivering O_2, in order of increasing effectiveness: soft nasal prongs, simple face masks, and face masks with inspiratory reservoir bags. The effective FI_{O_2} (that is actually entering the trachea) will be determined by the concentration of O_2 delivered from the tank or wall device, its flow rate, and the minute ventilation of the patient. In the hypoxemic form of respiratory failure, it is reasonable to start with moderate flow rates (5 to 10 L/min of 100% O_2) and monitor arterial blood gases, adjusting flow rates and O_2 concentrations depending on results.

Mechanical ventilatory support If adequate oxygenation cannot be maintained with these less invasive measures, endotracheal intubation is needed and mechanical ventilatory support should be instituted (see Chap. 231). The rationale behind mechanical ventilatory support in a patient who is hyperventilating is *not* to increase ventilation but to increase mean lung volume, thereby opening previously closed airways and improving oxygenation. This is accomplished by using large tidal volumes (approximately 10 to 15 mL/kg of lean body weight) at a slower breathing rate (12 to 15 breaths per minute) than the spontaneous one of the patient. Most often, at this juncture, the respiratory system is sufficiently stiff that high inflation pressures are required and a volume-cycled ventilator (in contrast to the pressure-cycled ones) is needed. If the patient makes expiratory efforts during the inflation cycle, peak inspiratory pressures will increase, possibly enough to activate the high-pressure pop-off valve, which results in delivery to the patient of a smaller tidal volume than selected. Under these circumstances during controlled ventilation, consideration is often given to sedation and/or neuromuscular paralysis. However, an alternative is to institute synchronized intermittent mandatory ventilation (SIMV). In the SIMV mode, the patient is allowed to breathe spontaneously with periodic delivery of mandatory breaths that are synchronized with spontaneous inspiratory efforts. If the spontaneous breathing rate is so rapid that expiratory efforts occur before the mandatory breath is fully delivered, sedation and/or paralysis should be used with controlled ventilation.

Use of PEEP   Should the Pa_{O_2} be greater than 60 mmHg, the next step is to lower the Fi_{O_2}. If the Fi_{O_2} can be lowered to 0.6 or less with a Pa_{O_2} equal to or greater than 60 mmHg, the mechanical ventilation should proceed at that Fi_{O_2} as long as necessary. There are two indications for the addition of PEEP, the rationale for which is to increase lung volume further, thereby opening previously closed alveoli. First, if the Fi_{O_2} cannot be lowered to or below 0.6, then PEEP should be added to allow a decrease of the Fi_{O_2} below the toxic range. Second, if the Pa_{O_2} cannot be increased to or above 60 mmHg with an Fi_{O_2} of 1.0, PEEP should be added. The optimal magnitude of the PEEP is determined by the response of the Pa_{O_2} and the extent of the cardiovascular alterations resulting from the higher pressure. The major alteration is a decrease in cardiac output due to two mechanisms. First, increased intrapleural pressures serve to impede venous return directly, an effect which is, to a variable extent, offset by peripheral venoconstriction. Second, increases in lung volume may increase pulmonary vascular resistance, leading to increased pressure and dilatation of the right ventricle, which in turn displaces the interventricular septum toward the left. This displacement decreases left ventricular diastolic compliance; hence less filling leads to smaller stroke volumes. An additional mechanism for decreased diastolic filling of the ventricles is direct compression of the heart by the stiffened lung. The optimal levels of PEEP are those associated with the greatest delivery of O_2 to the body; the latter is the product of cardiac output and arterial oxygen content.

Patients who are critically ill may simultaneously develop both deterioration of arterial oxygenation, due to increased lung fluid and/or a fall in mixed venous oxygen levels, and precarious hemodynamics, due to the pressure effects of mechanical ventilation and/or cardiac dysfunction with either a contracted or an expanded intravascular volume. Ventilator adjustments (see Chap. 231) are not often helpful because higher inflation pressures reflect worsening lung function. In this situation of falling blood pressure, urinary output, and arterial oxygenation, the decision to expand intravascular volume by infusion or to decrease it by diuresis is difficult. Body-weight change is rarely a reliable indicator of blood volume, since there is often fluid retention from positive intrathoracic pressures produced by the ventilator (see Chap. 231) plus "third space" fluid sequestration, especially with sepsis. Nor is physical examination of much help, since rales are usual in any case and portable anteroposterior chest radiographs do not allow accurate assessment of subtle changes in cardiac size. Therefore, a flow-directed right heart balloon-tipped (Swan-Ganz) catheter is often used for monitoring pulmonary arterial and capillary wedge pressures and measuring changes in cardiac output by the thermodilution technique. Recognition of overdamping and accelerative artifacts in the pulmonary arterial pressure signal and learning the criteria for true wedging are essential if serious misinterpretations are to be avoided. Even with accurate pressure measurements, there is an additional precaution that must be taken with regard to interpretation of intrathoracic vascular pressures referenced to atmosphere when PEEP is being used. If pleural pressure is greater than atmospheric pressure, as is most often the case with PEEP, the transmural (i.e., intravascular minus pleural) pressure will be overestimated and could lead to errors in both assessment and management. Since the lungs are stiff, only a portion of the applied PEEP is transmitted to the pleural space. A reasonable estimate of the transmural pressure is gained by examining vascular pressures just before inflation and subtracting from these pressures an amount equal to one-half the value of PEEP. In view of the leaky alveolocapillary membrane, it is best to keep the pulmonary capillary wedge pressure

as low as is compatible with a reasonable cardiac output, arterial pressure, and urinary output. Inotropic and selective vasoactive agents (e.g., dopamine) have been used with some success to achieve this but require careful monitoring to assess effects and adjust doses.

Mixed venous blood P_{O_2} values have long been considered to indicate the adequacy of oxygen delivery relative to demand. A low value (e.g., <20 mmHg) surely indicates that there is tissue hypoxemia irrespective of measured cardiac output and Pa_{O_2}. However, a high value does not exclude serious tissue hypoxia, especially in gram-negative septicemia, in which systemic low-resistance shunts can develop and leave several capillary beds underperfused.

Body position also may affect the degree of arterial oxygenation. Although patients with ARDS have diffuse lung disease, there may be some regional variation in the extent of disease such that one side is more severely involved than the other. In this instance, the less involved lung should be the more dependent one when the patient is in a lateral position. Since the distribution of pulmonary blood flow is so heavily determined by gravity (Chap. 214), having the more involved lung, with its minimal ventilation, in the more dependent position results in a measurable increase in intrapulmonary shunting which may be manifested by a striking fall in Pa_{O_2}. The possible contribution of a positional effect on arterial oxygenation should always be considered before escalating therapeutic interventions.

Occasionally, PEEP must be gradually increased to levels in excess of 20 cmH_2O in an attempt to maintain arterial oxygenation. At these high levels of PEEP there may be a paradoxic decrease in Pa_{O_2}. The explanation for this paradox is as follows: High levels of PEEP may not open some of the closed airways but will overdistend those alveolar units already open. Overdistention of units increases the vascular resistance in these regions and results in more blood perfusing regions with closed airways, thereby increasing the degree of shunt. The only alternative is to decrease PEEP to a level associated with the greatest delivery of oxygen to the body (product of cardiac output and arterial oxygen content).

High inflation pressures, the necessity of which indicate severe lung dysfunction, have been shown to directly damage the alveolar capillary membrane in the experimental setting. Based on the clinical suspicion that high inflation pressures also might compound the lung injury in ARDS, attempts have been made to remove CO_2 by extracorporeal perfusion techniques, thereby allowing the use of smaller tidal volumes and pressures from the ventilator. The clinical value of this approach has not yet been established.

In the situations where maximal PEEP with an Fi_{O_2} of 1.0 does not supply sufficient oxygen, the possibility of utilizing extracorporeal membrane oxygenators (ECMO) has been both considered and tried. Despite the logical appeal of this form of supportive therapy, a randomized, large prospective study of ECMO therapy has demonstrated that while it can support gas exchange, there is no effect on survival in acute hypoxemic respiratory failure.

Inactivation and decreased production of surfactant undoubtedly contribute to the gas exchange and mechanical abnormalities of the lung. Replacement of surfactant in ARDS, using either bovine sources or a synthetic phospholipid in combination with a recombinant human protein, is being assessed in clinical trials. Given the unresolved issues of optimal delivery systems, doses, intervals of administration, and appropriateness of end points, an early and clear answer is not likely.

Strategies in the management of sepsis causing ARDS   (See also Chap. 83)   Identification of the source of infection and the organism(s) responsible is necessary for proper antibiotic therapy. If there is a localized source of sepsis requiring surgical drainage, this must be accomplished quickly. Although the surgical mortality is high, failure to drain a purulent focus leads to an almost uniformly fatal outcome.

The range of implicated bacterial products, endogenously produced mediators, cytokines, peptides, enzymes, and oxidants gives a rationale for many interventions designed to interrupt the injurious processes. Most strategies only represent reasonable postulates, others are backed by limited experiments, several are subjects of current trials, and very few, if any, have been tested clinically and found to be both practical and useful. A major problem is that the sequence of events and the relative role of each participant are not clear. The most logical intervention, in the case of gram-negative sepsis, is the administration of antibodies to endotoxin, since endotoxin release appears to initiate the cascade of tissue injury. The human monoclonal IgM antibody, HA-1A, which binds to endotoxin, prevents death in laboratory animals and appears to modify the clinical outcome only in the bacteremic subset of patients with sepsis. Given the delay in establishing the presence of bacteremia and the apparent need for early treatment, most patients with sepsis would be treated needlessly and at great expense. Guidelines for the use of this expensive therapy are in the process of being established.

COMPLICATIONS Increasing severity of the clinical illness and continued radiographic progression in association with the primary process often obscure complications that arise during the course of acute hypoxemic respiratory failure. The development of *left ventricular failure* is a good example of a common, easily missed complication. This is so because all patients are likely to have diffuse rales and rhonchi, even without left ventricular failure, and these sounds also serve to make it difficult to detect gallop rhythms. An additional difficulty is that portable chest films are taken in the anteroposterior direction, often at less than full lung inflation, so the cardiac silhouette appears enlarged. As a consequence, the ordinary physical and radiographic assessments are not always reliable. With deterioration, therefore, left ventricular failure should be suspected; it is helpful to insert a Swan-Ganz catheter (see above) which can be used to monitor pulmonary arterial pressure continuously and intermittently to assess pulmonary capillary wedge pressure and oxygen content of mixed venous blood.

With a diffuse radiographic pattern, a secondary bacterial infection is easily overlooked; therefore, frequent sputum smears and cultures should be obtained, especially when there is fever. With many conditions—e.g., gram-negative septicemia, acute hemorrhagic pancreatitis, and "shock lung"—there may be associated *disseminated intravascular coagulation*, which leads to gastrointestinal and intrapulmonary hemorrhage. Frequent monitoring of platelet count, fibrinogen level, and partial thromboplastin and prothrombin times is helpful in the early detection of this complication and in guiding treatment.

Bronchial obstruction by endotracheal or tracheostomy tubes is common. When these tubes are too long or poorly anchored, they may slide into one main bronchus, usually the right one because of its less angulated origin from the trachea. The tube then blocks ventilation of the other main bronchus, and atelectasis may ensue. This event usually causes abrupt deterioration in the patient with respiratory failure. It is detected readily by physical examination, which reveals the absence of breath sounds over the occluded lung. The tube should immediately be pulled back slowly if this complication is suspected. In the course of treating ARDS with mechanical ventilators and high inflation pressures, *pneumothorax* or *pneumomediastinum* may develop and may be impossible to detect except radiologically. Occasionally, the presence of subcutaneous emphysema provides a clinical clue. Any deterioration should lead to consideration of this complication, repetition of the chest radiograph, and immediate institution of treatment of pneumothorax, if present. If deterioration is sudden, *tension pneumothorax* should be suspected; if physical signs are present, a pleural catheter should be inserted immediately without radiographic confirmation. High oxygen concentrations (>0.60) for prolonged periods can produce both the lesions and the clinical picture of ARDS. Therefore, the *minimal* oxygen concentration associated with acceptable arterial oxygenation should always be used.

Discontinuation of mechanical ventilatory support The ability of the patient to maintain adequate gas exchange without the support of a mechanical ventilator is most often heralded by a decreasing $F_{I_{O_2}}$ requirement, smaller inflation pressures for mandatory or assisted breathing, and a fall in spontaneous respiratory rate (see Chap. 231).

PROGNOSIS Given the diversity of the etiologies and the frequency of associated diseases, it is difficult, if not impossible, to give meaningful prognostic figures for ARDS. If all recently published series are taken together, the mortality rate is between 50 and 60 percent. This represents an improved survival rate over the nearly 100 percent mortality rate of a few years ago and is a result of the application of modern treatment techniques described above. If ARDS is due to drug overdose, the mortality rate is low; if associated with shock, the chances of a fatal outcome are much greater. Multiple organ system failure (e.g., renal, hepatic) supervenes when there is an extrapulmonic source of sepsis in need of surgical drainage, and almost all such patients die despite maximal support of the respiratory and cardiovascular systems. Other etiologies and associated diseases fall between these two extremes. The following factors appear to be associated with a poor outcome: an increase in $(A - a)P_{a_{O_2}}$, requiring increasing inspired O_2 concentrations and PEEP; decreasing compliance, requiring greater inflation pressures; either low or falling colloid osmotic pressures; and the onset of systemic arterial hypotension not responding to intravascular volume replacement.

In survivors with previously normal lung function, the long-term prognosis for recovery appears to be remarkably good. Lung volumes and arterial blood gases have been shown to return to normal levels within 4 to 6 months after respiratory failure. There are instances, however, when the fibrotic residua are sufficiently great that complete recovery is unlikely.

REFERENCES

ALBELDA SM: The alveolar-capillary barrier in adult respiratory distress syndrome, in *Update: Pulmonary Diseases and Disorders*, AP Fishman (ed). New York, McGraw-Hill, 1992, pp 197–212

BERNARD GR: *N*-Acetylcysteine in experimental and clinical acute lung injury. Am J Med Suppl 30:54S, 1991

BONE RC et al: Adult respiratory distress syndrome: Sequence and importance of development of multiple organ failure. Chest 101:320, 1992

———: Gram-negative sepsis: Background, clinical features, and intervention. Chest 100:802, 1991

FISER DH: Adult respiratory distress syndrome. Pediatr Rev 14:163, 1993

GREGORY TJ et al: Surfactant chemical composition and biophysical activity in acute respiratory distress syndrome. J Clin Invest 88:1976, 1991

HYERS TM et al: Tumor necrosis factor levels in serum and bronchoalveolar lavage fluid of patients with the adult respiratory distress syndrome. Am Rev Respir Dis 144:268, 1991

INGRAM RH, BRAUNWALD E: Pulmonary edema: Cardiogenic and noncardiogenic, in *Heart Disease*, E Braunwald (ed). Philadelphia, Saunders, 1992, p 551

MARINI JJ: Recent advances in mechanical ventilation, in *Update: Pulmonary Diseases and Disorders*, AP Fishman (ed). New York, McGraw-Hill, 1992, pp 401–418

MARTIN TR et al: The function of lung and blood neutrophils in patients with the adult respiratory distress syndrome: Implications for the pathogenesis of lung infections. Am Rev Respir Dis 144:254, 1991

METZ C, SIBBALD WJ: Anti-inflammatory therapy for acute lung injury: A review of animal and clinical studies. Chest 100:1110, 1991

MORRIS P, BERNARD GR: Adult respiratory distress syndrome: Strategies to provide support and enhance oxygen delivery. Postgrad Med 90:163, 1991

PATTISHALL EN, LONG WA: Surfactant treatment of adult respiratory distress syndrome, in *Update: Pulmonary Diseases and Disorders*, AP Fishman (ed). New York, McGraw-Hill, 1992, pp 225–236

PETTY TL et al: Contemporary clinical trials in acute respiratory distress syndrome. Chest 101:550, 1992

RANIERI VM et al: Effects of positive end-expiratory pressure on alveolar recruitment and gas exchange in patients with the adult respiratory distress syndrome. Am Rev Respir Dis 144:544, 1991

SEEGER W et al: Alveolar surfactant and adult respiratory distress syndrome. Pathogenetic role and therapeutic prospects. Clin Investig 71:177, 1993

WEST JB, MATHIEU-COSTELLO O: Stress failure of pulmonary capillaries: Role in lung and heart disease. J Appl Physiol 70:1731, 1991

ZIEGLER EJ et al: Treatment of gram-negative bacteremia and septic shock with HA-1A human monoclonal antibody against endotoxin. N Engl J Med 324:429, 1991

231   MECHANICAL VENTILATORY SUPPORT

EDWARD P. INGENITO / JEFFREY M. DRAZEN

Ventilators are medical devices that provide external mechanical support of the ventilatory function of the respiratory system. They are considered a mainstay of physiologic supportive care; they provide ventilatory support to patients through episodes of respiratory failure as the underlying disease process is definitively treated.

INDICATIONS FOR MECHANICAL VENTILATION

Respiratory failure is the primary indication for initiation of mechanical ventilation. It is important to distinguish among the various forms of respiratory failure because the therapeutic goals of mechanical ventilation differ depending on which form is present.

Hypoxemic respiratory failure most commonly results from pulmonary conditions such as severe pneumonia, pulmonary edema, pulmonary hemorrhage, and respiratory distress syndrome causing ventilation-perfusion ($\dot{V}/\dot{Q}$) mismatch. Hypoxemic respiratory failure is present when arterial oxygen saturations of less than 90 percent are observed despite an inspired oxygen fraction of greater than 0.6. The goal of ventilator treatment in this setting is to provide adequate arterial oxygen saturation.

Hypercarbic respiratory failure results from disease states causing either a decrease in minute ventilation or an increase in physiologic dead space such that, despite adequate total minute ventilation, alveolar ventilation is inadequate to meet metabolic demands. Common clinical conditions associated with hypercarbic respiratory failure include neuromuscular diseases, such as myasthenia gravis, ascending polyradiculopathy, and myopathies, as well as diseases that cause respiratory muscle fatigue due to increased workload, such as asthma, chronic obstructive pulmonary disease, and restrictive lung disease. *Acute* hypercarbic respiratory failure is present when arterial P_{CO_2} values exceed 50 mmHg and the arterial pH is below 7.30 (Chap. 46). *Chronic* hypercarbic respiratory failure is characterized by arterial P_{CO_2} values of greater than 50 mmHg and an arterial pH above 7.30.

Mechanical ventilation generally should be instituted in acute hypercarbic respiratory failure. In contrast, the decision to institute mechanical ventilation when components of both acute and chronic hypercarbic respiratory failure are present depends on blood gas parameters and clinical evaluation. In particular, if a patient is not in respiratory distress and is not mentally impaired by CO_2 accumulation, it is not mandatory to initiate mechanical ventilation while other forms of treatment are being administered. The goal of ventilator treatment in hypercarbic respiratory failure is to normalize arterial pH through changes in carbon dioxide tensions. Hypoxemic and hypercarbic respiratory failure may coexist in a given individual; in such cases, the indications for and goals of mechanical ventilation are similar to those in these two individual entities.

Accepted therapeutic applications of mechanical ventilation include controlled hyperventilation to reduce cerebral blood flow in patients with increased intracranial pressure or to improve pulmonary hemodynamics in patients with postoperative pulmonary hypertension. Mechanical ventilation also has been used to reduce the work of breathing in patients with congestive heart failure, especially in the presence of myocardial ischemia. In addition to being used in established respiratory failure, ventilator support is indicated in conjunction with endotracheal intubation to prevent aspiration of gastric contents in otherwise unstable patients during gastric lavage for suspected drug overdose or during upper gastrointestinal endoscopy. In the critically ill patient, intubation and mechanical ventilation are indicated before essential diagnostic or therapeutic studies if it appears that respiratory failure may occur during these maneuvers.

PHYSIOLOGIC ASPECTS OF MECHANICAL VENTILATION

Most modern mechanical ventilators function by providing warmed and humidified gas to the airway opening in conformance with various specific volume, pressure, and time patterns. The ventilator serves as the energy source for inspiration, replacing the muscles of the diaphragm and chest wall. Expiration is passive, driven by the recoil of the lungs and chest wall; at the completion of inspiration, internal ventilator circuitry vents the airway to atmospheric pressure or a specified level of positive end-expiratory pressure (PEEP).

PEEP helps maintain alveolar patency in the presence of destabilizing factors and therefore reverses hypoxemia and atelectasis by improving $\dot{V}/\dot{Q}$ matching. PEEP levels between 0 and 5 cmH$_2$O are generally safe and effective; higher levels are recommended only in the management of significant refractory hypoxemia unresponsive to increments in inspired oxygen content up to an inspired oxygen content ($F_{I_{O_2}}$) of 0.6.

ESTABLISHING AN AIRWAY   A cuffed endotracheal tube must be inserted to allow positive-pressure ventilators to deliver conditioned gas, at pressures above atmospheric pressure, to the lungs in a controlled fashion. If neuromuscular paralysis is to be induced during intubation, the use of agents whose mechanism of action includes depolarization at the neuromuscular junction, such as succinylcholine chloride, should be avoided in patients with renal failure, tumor lysis syndrome, crush injuries, or medical conditions associated with elevated serum potassium levels because these agents may elevate the serum potassium to potentially lethal levels. Opiates and benzodiazepines can have a deleterious effect on hemodynamics in patients with depressed cardiac function or low systemic vascular resistance and should be used cautiously in this setting. Morphine can promote histamine release from tissue mast cells and may worsen bronchospasm in asthmatics; fentanyl, sufentanil, and alfentanil are acceptable alternatives to morphine. Ketamine may increase systemic arterial pressure as well as intracranial pressure and has been associated with dramatic hallucinatory responses; it should be used with caution in patients with hypertensive crisis, increased intracranial pressures, or a history of psychiatric disorders.

VENTILATOR MODE   This setting specifies the manner in which ventilator breaths are triggered, cycled, and limited; commonly used modes of mechanical ventilation are given in Table 231-1. The *trigger*, either an inspiratory effect or a time-based signal, defines what the ventilator senses to initiate an assisted cycle. This trigger may be either an inspiratory effort or a time-based signal. *Cycle* refers to the factors that determine end inspiration. For example, in volume-cycled ventilation, inspiration ends when a specific tidal volume is delivered to the patient. Other types of cycling include pressure cycling, time cycling, and flow cycling. *Limiting factors* are operator-specified values, such as airway pressure, that are monitored by internal ventilator circuitry throughout the respiratory cycle; if the specified values are exceeded, inspiratory flow is immediately stopped and the ventilator circuit vented to atmospheric pressure or the specified PEEP.

Assist control mode ventilation (ACMV)   This mode is patient/time triggered, volume cycled, and pressure limited. An inspiratory cycle is initiated either by the patient's inspiratory effort or, if no patient effort is detected within a specified time window, by a timer signal within the ventilator. Every breath delivered consists of the full operator-specified tidal volume. Ventilatory rate is determined either by the patient or by the operator-specified backup rate, whichever is of higher frequency (Fig. 231-1A). ACMV is the recommended mode for initiation of mechanical ventilation because it ensures a backup minute ventilation in the absence of an intact respiratory drive and allows for synchronization of the ventilator cycle with the patient's inspiratory effort.

TABLE 231-1 Clinical characteristics of commonly used modes of mechanical ventilation

Independent variables (set by user)	Dependent variables (monitored by user)	Trigger/cycle limit	Advantages	Disadvantages	Initial settings
ASSIST/CONTROL MODE VENTILATION (ACMV)					
FI_{O_2} Tidal volume Ventilator rate Level of PEEP Inspiratory flow pattern Peak inspiratory flow Pressure limit	Peak airway pressure, Pa_{O_2}, Pa_{CO_2} Mean airway pressure I/E ratio	Patient/timer Pressure limit	Timer backup Patient-vent synchrony Patient controls minute ventilation	Not useful for weaning Potential for dangerous respiratory alkalosis	$FI_{O_2} = 1.0^*$ $V_t = 10-15$ mL/kg $f = 12-15$/min PEEP $= 0-5$ cmH$_2$O Inspiratory flow $= 60$ L/min
SYNCHRONIZED INTERMITTENT MANDATORY VENTILATION (SIMV)					
Same as for ACMV	Same as for ACMV	Same as for ACMV	Timber backup useful for weaning	Potential dysynchrony	Same as for ACMV
CONTINUOUS POSITIVE AIRWAY PRESSURE (CPAP)					
FI_{O_2} Level of CPAP	Tidal volume Rate, flow pattern Airway pressure Pa_{O_2}, Pa_{CO_2}, I/E ratio	No trigger Pressure limit	Allows assessment of spontaneous function Helps prevent atelectasis	No backup	$FI_{O_2} = 0.5-1.0^*$ CPAP $= 5-15$ cmH$_2$O
PRESSURE-CONTROL VENTILATION (PCV)					
FI_{O_2} Inspiratory pressure level Ventilator rate Level of PEEP Pressure limit I/E ratio	Tidal volume Flow rate, pattern Minute ventilation; Pa_{O_2}, Pa_{CO_2}	Timer/patient Timer/pressure limit	System pressures regulated Useful for barotrauma treatment Timer backup	Requires heavy sedation Not useful for weaning	$FI_{O_2} = 1.0^*$ PC $= 20-40$ cmH$_2$O PEEP $= 5-10$ cmH$_2$O $f = 12-15$/min I/E $= 0.7/1-4/1$
PRESSURE-SUPPORT VENTILATION (PSV)					
FI_{O_2} Inspiratory pressure level PEEP Pressure limit	Same as for PCV + I/E ratio	Inspiratory flow Pressure limit	Ensures synchrony Good for weaning	No timer backup	$FI_{O_2} = 0.5-1.0^*$ PS $= 10-30$ cmH$_2$O 5 cmH$_2$O usually the level used PEEP $= 0-5$ cmH$_2$O

*FI_{O_2} is usually set to 1.0 initially, unless there is a specific clinical indication to minimize FI_{O_2}, such as history of chemotherapy with bleomycin. Once adequate oxygenation is documented by blood gas analysis, FI_{O_2} should be decreased in decrements of 0.1 to 0.2 as tolerated, until the lowest FI_{O_2} required for an Sa_{O_2} of greater than 90 percent is achieved.

A number of potential problems can arise when ACMV is used. In patients with tachypnea due to nonrespiratory, nonmetabolic factors such as anxiety, pain, or airway irritation, respiratory alkalemia may develop and may trigger myoclonus or seizures. Dynamic hyperinflation (so-called auto-PEEP) may occur if the patient's respiratory mechanics are such that inadequate time is available for complete exhalation between inspiratory cycles. Auto-PEEP can limit venous return and decrease cardiac output. ACMV is not effective for weaning patients from mechanical ventilation because it provides full ventilator assistance on each patient-initiated breath.

Synchronized intermittent mandatory ventilation (SIMV) This mode is similar to ACMV in that it is dually patient/time triggered, volume cycled, and pressure limited. The major difference between SIMV and ACMV is that in the former the patient is allowed to breathe spontaneously, i.e., without ventilator assist, between delivered ventilator breaths. However, at a frequency determined by the operator, mandatory breaths are delivered in synchrony with the patient's inspiratory efforts. If the patient fails to initiate a breath, the ventilator delivers a fixed-tidal-volume breath and resets the internal timer for the next inspiratory cycle (see Fig. 231-1B). SIMV differs from ACMV in that only the preset number of breaths is ventilator-assisted.

SIMV allows patients with an intact respiratory drive to exercise inspiratory muscles between assisted breaths. This characteristic makes SIMV a useful mode of ventilation for both supporting and weaning intubated patients. SIMV may be difficult to use in patients with tachypnea because they may attempt to exhale during the ventilator-programmed inspiratory cycle. When this occurs, the airway pressure may exceed the inspiratory pressure limit, the ventilator-assisted breath will be aborted, and minute volume may drop below that programmed by the operator. In this setting, if the tachypnea is in response to respiratory or metabolic acidosis, a change to ACMV will increase minute ventilation and help normalize the pH while the underlying process is further evaluated. If the tachypnea is in response to a stimulus other than acidosis, the addition of sedative medications is appropriate while the underlying processes are further evaluated.

Continuous positive airway pressure (CPAP) This is not a true support-mode ventilation, since all ventilation occurs through the patient's spontaneous efforts. The ventilator provides fresh gas to the breathing circuit with each inspiration and charges the circuit to a constant, operator-specified pressure that can range from 0 to 20 cmH$_2$O (see Fig. 231-1C). CPAP is used to assess extubation potential in patients who have been effectively weaned and are requiring little ventilator support and in patients with intact respiratory system function who require an endotracheal tube for airway protection.

Pressure-control ventilation (PCV) This form of ventilation is time triggered, time cycled, and pressure limited. During the inspiratory phase, a given pressure is imposed at the airway opening, and the pressure remains at this user-specified level throughout inspiration (Fig. 231-2A). Since inspiratory airway pressure is specified by the operator, tidal volume and inspiratory flow rate are *dependent* rather than *independent* variables and are not user specified. PCV is

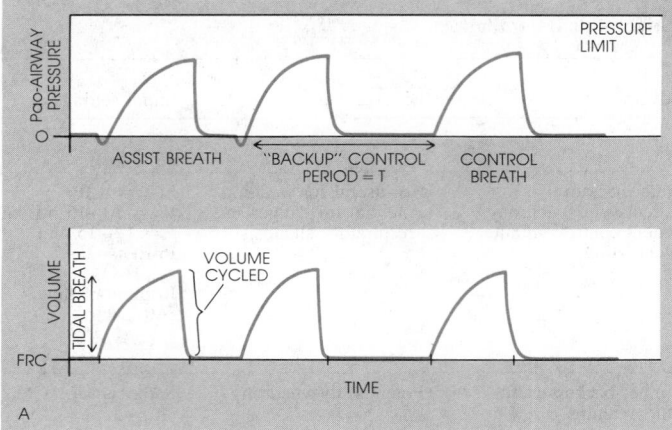

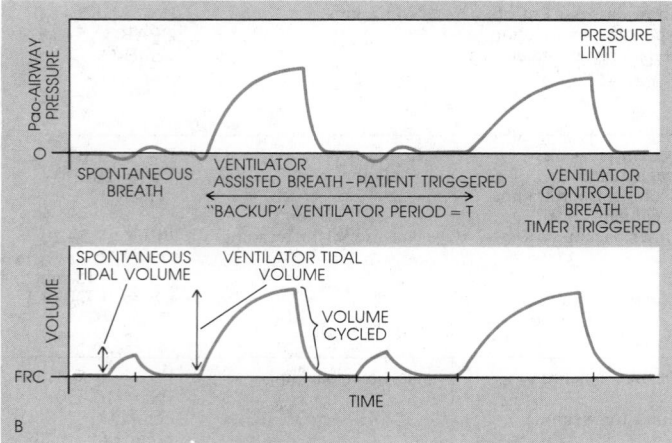

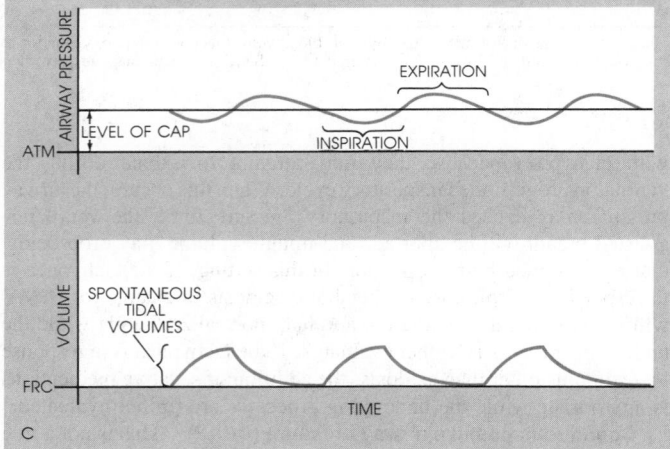

FIGURE 231-1 *A*. Airway pressure and lung volume versus time profile during ACMV. Assisted breaths are triggered by the patient's effort. Controlled breaths are triggered by the ventilator timer. Every breath, whether triggered by the patient or by the timer, is a complete volume-cycled breath, with airway pressure as a dependent variable. The pressure limit is set above the peak inspiratory pressure.

B. Airway pressure and lung volume versus time profiles during SIMV. Spontaneous breaths occur between patient-triggered assisted breaths and timer-triggered breaths. The tidal volume of the spontaneous breaths is determined by the patient's effort and lung impedance. Assisted and controlled breaths are volume cycled.

C. Airway pressure and lung volume versus time profiles during CPAP. Breathing is spontaneous, and no ventilator assist is provided. The spontaneous profile is superimposed on an elevated mean airway pressure that the user specifies.

the preferred mode of ventilation for patients with documented barotrauma, since airway pressures can be limited, and for postoperative thoracic surgical patients, in whom the shear forces across a fresh suture line should be limited. When using PCV, minute ventilation and tidal volume must be monitored; minute ventilation is altered through changes in rate or in the pressure-control value.

The major practical limitation of PCV is patient-ventilator asynchrony related to its time-cycled and time-triggered characteristics. Since PCV requires that the patient passively accept ventilator breaths, most patients require heavy sedation to be maintained on this ventilatory mode, which may be hazardous in the hemodynamically unstable patient.

Modified versions of PCV designed to improve patient-ventilator synchrony are available on some newer ventilators. The first type is patient/time-triggered, time-cycled, and pressure-limited PCV, where every breath initiated by the patient is pressure-assisted with concurrent time-cycled pressure-assist backup. In second type of PCV, a mandatory number of synchronized, patient-triggered, time-cycled, and pressure-limited PCV breaths are provided with time-cycled backup, and spontaneous breathing can occur between mandatory breaths. These two modified versions of PCV are the pressure-assisted equivalents of ACMV and SIMV. Because they are dually patient and timer triggered, these modified versions of PCV are better tolerated than standard PCV and can be employed safely without heavy sedation.

Pressure-support ventilation (PSV) This form of ventilation is patient triggered, flow cycled, and pressure limited; it is specifically designed for use in the weaning process. During PSV, the inspiratory phase is terminated when inspiratory airflow falls below a certain level; in most ventilators this flow rate cannot be adjusted by the operator. When PSV is used, patients receive ventilator assist only when the ventilator detects an inspiratory effort (see Fig. 231-2*B*). PSV also can be used in combination with SIMV to ensure volume-cycled backup for patients whose respiratory drive is depressed either spontaneously or as a result of various therapeutic maneuvers. However, when backup ventilation is provided, the usefulness of PSV as a weaning aid is partially vitiated.

PSV is well tolerated by most patients who are being weaned: PSV parameters can be set in such a way as to provide full or nearly full ventilatory support and can be withdrawn slowly over a period of days in a systematic fashion to gradually load the respiratory muscles.

COMPLICATIONS OF MECHANICAL VENTILATION

Endotracheal intubation and positive-pressure mechanical ventilation have direct and indirect effects on several organ systems, including the lung and upper airways, the cardiovascular system, and the gastrointestinal system. Pulmonary complications include barotrauma, nosocomial pneumonia, oxygen toxicity, tracheal stenosis, and deconditioning of respiratory muscles. *Barotrauma,* which occurs when high pressures (i.e., greater than 50 cmH$_2$O) disrupt lung tissue, is clinically manifest by interstitial emphysema, pneumomediastinum, subcutaneous emphysema, or pneumothorax. Although the former conditions may resolve simply by reducing airway pressures, clinically significant pneumothorax, as indicated by hypoxemia, decreased lung compliance, and hemodynamic compromise, requires tube thoracostomy.

Patients intubated for longer than 72 h are at high risk for *nosocomial pneumonia* as a result of aspiration from the upper airways via small leaks around the endotracheal tube cuff; the most common organisms responsible for this condition are enteric gram-negative rods, *Staphylococcus aureus,* and anaerobic bacteria. Because the endotracheal tube and upper airways of patients on mechanical ventilation are commonly colonized with bacteria, the diagnosis of nosocomial pneumonia requires "protected brush" bronchoscopic sampling of airway secretions coupled with quantitative microbiologic techniques to differentiate colonization from infection.

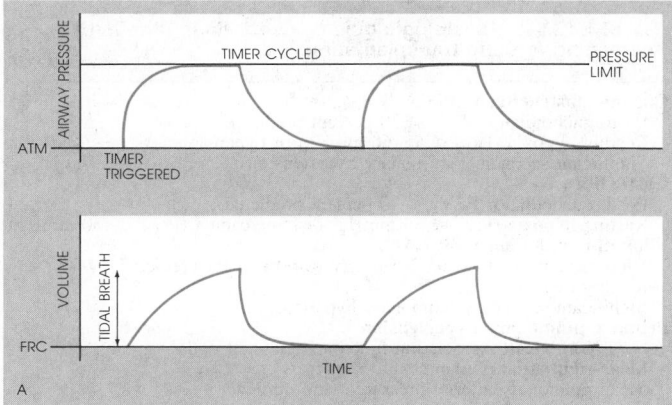

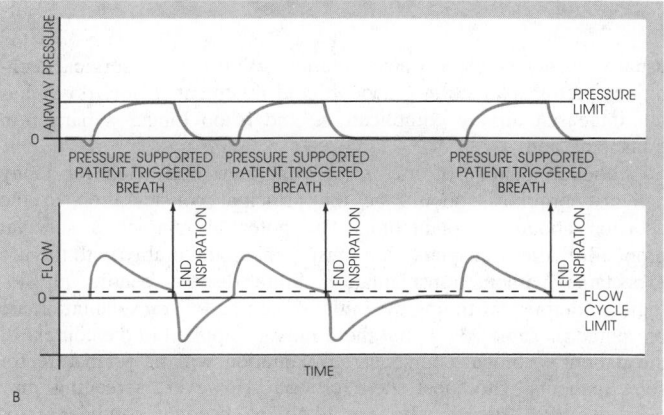

FIGURE 231-2 *A.* Airway pressure and lung volume versus time profiles during PCV. All breaths are timer triggered, timer cycled, and pressure limited. Peak airway pressure is set by the operator, and tidal volume is a dependent variable. The profiles shown here display the pressure limit as slightly higher than pressure-control level. This need not be the case, but it is appropriate to set the pressure limit only slightly above the pressure-control level when using this mode of ventilation for management of the patient with barotrauma.

B. Airway pressure and airway flow versus time profiles during PSV. All breaths are patient triggered and flow cycled. Inspiration is cycled off when the inspiratory flow drops below a predetermined threshold internally set in the ventilator circuit. In the example shown, the pressure limit is slightly greater than the pressure-support level. Since each can be set independently, this need not be the case.

Oxygen toxicity is a potential complication when an FI_{O_2} of 0.6 or greater is required for more than 72 h. The condition can be prevented in some cases through the use of PEEP to allow for FI_{O_2} values to go below 0.6 while primary therapy for the underlying condition is instituted. Although oxygen toxicity is thought to result from the effects of oxygen free radicals on the lung interstitium, the therapeutic use of antioxidants such as superoxide dismutase, catalase, selenium, and vitamin E remains experimental.

Hypotension resulting from elevated intrathoracic pressures with decreased venous return is almost always responsive to intravascular volume repletion. In patients judged to have hypotension or respiratory failure on the basis of alveolar edema, hemodynamic monitoring with a pulmonary arterial catheter may be of value in optimizing oxygen delivery via manipulation of intravascular volume, FI_{O_2}, and PEEP levels.

Gastrointestinal effects of positive-pressure ventilation include *stress ulceration* and *mild to moderate cholestasis.* It is common practice to provide prophylaxis with H-2 receptor antagonists or sucralfate for stress-related ulcers. Mild cholestasis (i.e., total bilirubin values ≤ 4.0) attributable to the effects of increased intrathoracic

pressures on portal vein pressures is common and generally self-limited. Cholestasis of a more severe degree should not be attributed to a positive-pressure ventilation response and is more likely due to a primary hepatic process. Additional complications, including malnutrition, decubitus ulcers, muscle deconditioning, venous thrombosis, and depression, are common and require appropriate treatment.

WEANING FROM MECHANICAL VENTILATION

Removal of mechanical ventilator support requires that a number of criteria be met. Upper airway function must be intact for a patient to remain extubated but is difficult to assess in the intubated patient. Therefore, if a patient can breathe on his or her own through an endotracheal tube but develops stridor or recurrent aspiration once the tube is removed, upper airway dysfunction or an abnormal swallowing mechanism should be suspected and plans for achieving a stable airway developed. An intact cough when respiratory secretions are suctioned is a good indicator of a patient's ability to mobilize secretions. Respiratory drive and chest wall function are assessed by observation of respiratory rate, tidal volume, inspiratory pressure, and vital capacity. The weaning index, defined as the ratio of breathing frequency to tidal volume (breaths per minute per liter), has been shown to be both sensitive and specific for predicting the likelihood of successful extubation. When this ratio is less than 105 with the patient breathing without mechanical assistance through an endotracheal tube, successful extubation is likely. An inspiratory pressure of more than -30 cmH$_2$O and a vital capacity of greater than 10 mL/kg are considered indicators of acceptable chest wall and diaphragm function. Alveolar ventilation is generally adequate when systemic arterial P_{CO_2} is less than or equal to 45 mmHg, and arterial oxygen saturations greater than 90 percent can be achieved with an FI_{O_2} of less than 0.5 and a PEEP of 5 cmH$_2$O or less. Although many patients may not meet all criteria for weaning, the likelihood that a patient will tolerate extubation without difficulty increases as more criteria are met.

Many approaches to weaning patients from ventilator support have been advocated. T-piece and CPAP weaning are best tolerated by patients who have undergone ventilation for brief periods and require little respiratory muscle reconditioning, while SIMV and PSV are best for patients who have been intubated for extended periods and require gradual respiratory-muscle reconditioning.

T-piece weaning involves brief spontaneous breathing trials with supplemental oxygen. These trials are usually initiated for 5 min/h followed by a 1-h interval of rest. T-piece trials are increased in 5- to 10-min increments until the patient can remain ventilator independent for periods of several hours. Extubation can then be attempted. CPAP weaning is similar to T-piece weaning except that trials of spontaneous breathing are conducted on the ventilator in CPAP mode.

Weaning by means of SIMV/IMV involves gradually tapering the mandatory backup rate in increments of 2 to 4 breaths per minute while monitoring blood gas parameters and respiratory rates. Rates of greater than 25 breaths per minute upon withdrawal of mandatory ventilator breaths generally indicate respiratory muscle fatigue and the need to combine periods of exercise with periods of rest. Exercise periods are gradually increased until a patient remains stable on SIMV at 4 breaths per minute or less without needing rest at higher SIMV rates. A CPAP or T-piece trial can then be attempted before planned extubation.

PSV, as described in detail above, is used primarily for weaning from mechanical ventilation. PSV is usually initiated at a level adequate for full ventilator support (PSV$_{max}$); i.e., PSV is set slightly below the peak inspiratory pressures the patient requires during volume-cycled ventilation. The level of pressure support is then gradually withdrawn in increments of 5 cmH$_2$O until a level is reached at which the respiratory rate increases to 25 breaths per minute. At this point, intermittent periods of higher-pressure support are alternated with periods of lower-pressure support to provide muscle reconditioning without causing diaphragmatic fatigue. Gradual withdrawal of PSV continues until the level of support is just adequate to overcome the resistance of the endotracheal tube (approximately 5 cmH$_2$O). At that point, support can be discontinued and the patient extubated.

REFERENCES

COHEN IL et al: Mechanical ventilation for the elderly patient in intensive care. Incremental changes and benefits. JAMA 269:1025, 1993

HINSON JR, MARINI JJ: Principles of mechanical ventilator use in respiratory failure. Annu Rev Med 43:341, 1992

INGENITO EP, DRAZEN JM: Mechanical ventilators, in *Principles of Critical Care*, JB Hall, GA Schmidt, LDH Wood (eds). New York, McGraw-Hill, 1992, pp 142–154

PHAM LH et al: Diagnosis of nonsocomial pneumonia in mechanically ventilated patients: Comparison of a plugged telescoping catheter with the protected specimen brush. Am Rev Respir Dis 143:1055, 1991

RANIERI VM et al: Physiologic effects of positive end-expiratory pressure in patients with chronic obstructive pulmonary disease during acute ventilatory failure and controlled mechanical ventilation. Am Rev Respir Dis 147:5, 1993

YANG KL, TOBIN MJ: A prospective study of indexes predicting the outcome of trials of weaning from mechanical ventilation. N Engl J Med 324:1445, 1991

232   LUNG TRANSPLANTATION

E. P. TRULOCK / JOEL D. COOPER

During the last decade transplantation became a therapeutic option for patients with end-stage lung disease, and activity in lung transplantation has increased exponentially since 1989. Worldwide, more than 1800 lung transplants had been reported through March 1993, and in the United States 534 lung transplants were recorded in 1992 alone. The number of patients awaiting lung transplantation has also been increasing rapidly, and by the end of 1992 the U.S. waiting list had almost 1000 registrants. The 1-year and 2-year actuarial survival rates are 68 percent and 60 percent respectively, for the cumulative experience in the St. Louis International Lung Transplant Registry, but these results have been exceeded at some centers.

INDICATIONS   Patients with a variety of end-stage lung diseases have undergone transplantation. The most common diagnoses have been chronic obstructive pulmonary disease, antitrypsin deficiency emphysema, idiopathic pulmonary fibrosis, cystic fibrosis, and primary pulmonary hypertension, but a smaller number of patients with other diseases have also received lung transplants. Controversial indications include systemic diseases with predominantly pulmonary involvement and interstitial lung diseases caused by chemotherapy or radiotherapy for a previous neoplasm.

Recipient selection   Potential recipients should have clinically and physiologically severe lung disease with a poor prognosis for survival in spite of optimal medical management, but should have no other health problems that would either jeopardize the success of the operation or limit life expectancy after transplantation. Specific recipient selection criteria vary somewhat among centers. In general, candidates should have normal left ventricular function without significant coronary artery disease and no significant dysfunction of other vital organs. They should be ambulatory and in acceptable nutritional condition, and they should have a satisfactory psychosocial profile and history of compliance with medical management.

Other considerations include the patient's age, prior thoracic surgical history, and glucocorticoid therapy. Typical age limits are ~50 to 55 years for bilateral lung transplantation and ~60 to 65 years for single lung transplantation. The technical difficulties and operative risks of lung transplantation in patients with prior thoracic procedures are variable; however, diagnostic open lung biopsy, tube thoracostomy with or without chemical pleurodesis for pneumothorax, or lobectomy

TABLE 232-1   Physiologic guidelines for timing the initial screening for lung transplantation

Chronic obstructive pulmonary disease
Postbronchodilator FEV$_1$ < 30 percent predicted
Resting hypoxia (Pa$_{O_2}$ < 55–60 mmHg) or hypercapnia
Significant secondary pulmonary hypertension
Cystic fibrosis
Postbronchodilator FEV$_1$ < 30 percent predicted
Resting hypoxia (Pa$_{O_2}$ < 55 mmHg) or hypercapnia (Pa$_{CO_2}$ > 50 mmHg)
Idiopathic pulmonary fibrosis
Vital capacity or total lung capacity < 60 percent predicted
Resting hypoxia
Significant secondary pulmonary hypertension
Primary pulmonary hypertension
New York Heart Association functional class III or IV
Mean right atrial pressure > 10 mmHg
Mean pulmonary arterial pressure > 50 mmHg
Cardiac index < 2.5 (L/min)m^2

usually do not preclude transplantation. With current surgical techniques pretransplantation glucocorticoid treatment in low doses has not increased airway complications and is no longer a barrier to transplantation.

Although quality of life is an important motivation for many patients, prognosis should be the principal consideration in the decision about transplantation. The potential recipient's survival probability after transplantation must compare favorably with the life expectancy without transplantation. Some disease-specific, physiologic guidelines for timing the initial screening for transplantation are presented in Table 232-1, but these must be applied in the context of the patient's clinical course. Transplantation will be premature for some patients who meet these criteria. However, screening may help identify patients who are likely to become candidates for transplantation in the future.

Donor-recipient matching   Blood group compatibility and lung size, within reasonable tolerance, are the only factors that are routinely matched between the donor and recipient. When possible, cytomegalovirus (CMV) seronegative recipients should be transplanted with lungs from a CMV seronegative donor to prevent serious posttransplant CMV infection, but this strategy is often impractical because of the shortage of donor organs. Prospective histocompatibility matching has not been used in lung transplantation, and its impact on graft and patient survival have yet to be studied thoroughly.

PROCEDURES AND RESULTS   Both combined heart-lung and isolated lung transplantation have been performed for many end-stage lung diseases. Heart-lung transplantation should be reserved for those situations which require cardiac replacement, e.g., Eisenmenger's syndrome with a surgically uncorrectable cardiac abnormality (Chap. 196). Cor pulmonale alone does not necessitate cardiac transplantation because right ventricular function can recover when the afterload is normalized by lung transplantation. Bilateral lung transplantation is mandatory for patients with generalized bronchiectasis and chronic pulmonary infection. Either bilateral or single lung transplantation can be utilized for most other diseases, but single lung transplantation maximizes the use of the limited supply of donor lungs.

Regardless of the type of operation, lung transplantation improves lung function in patients with restrictive or obstructive disease and alleviates pulmonary hypertension in patients with pulmonary vascular disease. Exercise performance and quality of life are enhanced; supplemental oxygen is unnecessary; and normal daily activities, including most occupations, can be resumed.

POSTTRANSPLANT MANAGEMENT AND COMPLICATIONS   As an allograft the lung has been vulnerable to three major complications: bronchial anastomotic dehiscence and stenosis, acute and chronic rejection, and infection. Deaths soon after lung transplantation have been caused primarily by technical and cardiac complications of the operation, but mortality beyond the first postoperative month has been related to rejection and infection.

Anastomotic dehiscence and stenosis The bronchial circulation to the donor lung is severed during extraction, and after implantation the donor bronchus is dependent on retrograde blood flow from the pulmonary circulation until other collaterals develop. Although surgically reestablishing the bronchial supply to the donor lung is possible, the technique is complex and has not been widely used.

Endoscopically visible signs of airway ischemia or small defects in the anastomosis are not unusual, but the majority of these require no intervention and resolve without sequelae. Significant stenosis or dehiscence still occurs in ~10 to 20 percent of cases but can be managed by dilation and/or stent placement. Fatal airway complications are very rare with current surgical techniques.

Rejection Most recipients have early episodes of acute rejection, and 25 percent or more develop late, chronic rejection. Acute rejection can occur as early as three days and as late as several years after transplantation. Clinical features include cough, dyspnea, fever, adventitious lung sounds, radiographic infiltrates, and deterioration in oxygenation and pulmonary function. The chest radiograph, however, is normal or unchanged in three-fourths of episodes occurring more than 1 month after transplantation. Because the presentation of acute pulmonary rejection is nonspecific, bronchoscopy with transbronchial lung biopsy is useful to distinguish rejection from infection. The clinical utility of bronchoalveolar lavage is limited to the diagnosis of infection.

Standard treatment for acute rejection is high-dose methylprednisolone. Glucocorticoid therapy is sufficient to reverse most episodes, but refractory acute rejection can be treated with antilymphocyte globulin, antithymocyte globulin, or OKT3 monoclonal antibody.

Chronic rejection is a clinicopathologic syndrome characterized physiologically by airflow limitation and histologically by obliterative bronchiolitis and a variable degree of vascular sclerosis. Both antecedent acute rejection and CMV pneumonia appear to be risk factors. It is the most problematic late complication and the leading cause of late mortality and morbidity. With current immunosuppressive drug regimens and surveillance protocols, approximately 25 to 40 percent of long-term survivors are affected by chronic rejection.

Chronic rejection may develop as early as 2 months and as late as several years after transplantation, but the mean time to onset is 8 to 12 months. The most frequent presentation mimics an upper respiratory tract infection or bronchitis, but the onset may be more insidious. The diagnosis is based on the clinical, physiological, and pathologic features. The evolution of new or worsening airflow limitation is strongly suggestive of rejection. Transbronchial lung biopsy is less sensitive and less specific for chronic rejection than for acute rejection.

Chronic rejection is treated by augmenting the immunosuppressive therapy with glucocorticoids or the antilymphocyte agents. Beneficial results have been achieved with these, but the relapse rate has been high.

Infection The lung as an allograft is particularly vulnerable to infection. The lower respiratory tract of brain-dead, ventilator-dependent donors is often colonized with nosocomial organisms, and these potential pathogens are transmitted with the donor lung. After transplantation the normal pulmonary defense mechanisms are breached at many levels. Mucociliary clearance is diminished, and, because the transplanted lung is denervated, the cough reflex is depressed. Moreover, some of the antimicrobial functions of alveolar macrophages may be impaired. Bacterial, fungal, viral, and protozoal infections have all occurred, but the most common problems have been bacterial pneumonia and CMV pneumonia.

Purulent bacterial bronchitis and bronchopneumonia occur frequently in the early posttransplant period; gram negative, nosocomial bacteria and staphylococci are the predominant organisms. Because of the high risk of bacterial pneumonia in the perioperative period, antibiotic therapy should be directed at any potential pathogens isolated from respiratory specimens. Bacterial pneumonia is also a significant problem during long-term follow-up. Gram-negative organisms are responsible for most cases, but other community-acquired pathogens also contribute.

CMV pneumonia is the most frequent opportunistic pulmonary infection after lung transplantation. The risk and severity of infection are related to the CMV serologic status of the donor and recipient. First episodes of CMV pneumonia usually occur between 3 weeks and 4 months after lung transplantation. The clinical presentation is almost indistinguishable from allograft rejection, and the diagnosis should be confirmed by histology and virology. Most episodes respond to treatment with ganciclovir, but relapses are not uncommon.

Herpes simplex tracheobronchitis and pneumonitis occur occasionally, and other respiratory viruses are sometimes isolated and may be important depending on the clinical circumstances. Colonization with *Candida* species is common, particularly in the early posttransplant period, but invasive infection is infrequent. Subsequently, *Aspergillus* is the principal fungal pathogen. Pneumonias caused by other agents are unusual after lung transplantation. *Pneumocystis carinii* infection has been almost eliminated by prophylaxis, and *Nocardia* has not been problematic. Only a few cases of tuberculous or nontuberculous mycobacterial infections have been recorded.

Recurrence of the original disease The native disease has recurred in the allograft in some recipients with sarcoidosis. Other diseases have not recurred; however, the posttransplant follow-up of most recipients is relatively short compared to the natural history of their underlying diseases.

REFERENCES

AMERICAN THORACIC SOCIETY: Lung transplantation. Report of the ATS workshop on lung transplantation. Am Rev Respir Dis 147:772, 1993

GROSSMAN RF, MAURER JR (eds): Pulmonary considerations in transplantation. Clinics Chest Med 11(2):195, 1990

PATTERSON GA, COOPER JD (eds): *Lung Transplantation.* Chest Surgery Clin North Amer 3(1):1, 1993

TRULOCK EP: Management of lung transplant rejection. Chest 103:1566, 1993

PART NINE

DISORDERS OF THE KIDNEY AND URINARY TRACT

233 APPROACH TO THE PATIENT WITH DISEASES OF THE KIDNEYS AND URINARY TRACT

FREDRIC L. COE / BARRY M. BRENNER

Diseases of the kidneys and urinary tract frequently give rise to consistent arrays or clusters of clinical signs, symptoms, and laboratory findings called *syndromes*. Syndromes are useful diagnostically because each has fewer causes than the individual clinical signs and symptoms it contains. For example, any injured capillary bed from glomerulus to urethral meatus can cause hematuria, but only glomerular injury also can cause heavy albuminuria and erythrocyte casts (Chap. 44), and only a few of the diseases that injure the glomerular capillaries enough to cause hematuria and proteinuria also cause a rapid fall in glomerular filtration rate. Routine clinical evaluation is often sufficient to suggest that a particular syndrome may be present (Table 233-1), but additional laboratory measurements beyond the routine, as well as radiologic and/or urologic evaluation and sequential clinical observations, are usually required to establish the diagnosis. This chapter presents the general features of the syndromes, lists the clinical and laboratory data required for their recognition, and outlines the diseases that cause them. Succeeding chapters describe the diseases and their treatment in detail.

ACUTE (ARF) AND RAPIDLY PROGRESSIVE RENAL FAILURE (RPRF) Whether the glomerular filtration rate falls over days (acute renal failure) or weeks (rapidly progressive renal failure) is a useful distinction, because the causes of these two syndromes are somewhat different (Tables 233-1 and 233-2). For example, acute tubular

TABLE 233-1 Initial clinical and laboratory data base for defining major syndromes in nephrology

Syndromes	Important clues to diagnosis	Findings which are common but not of diagnostic value	Location of discussion of diseases causing syndrome
Acute or rapidly progressive renal failure	Anuria Oliguria Documented recent decline in GFR	Hypertension, hematuria Proteinuria, pyuria Casts, edema	Chaps. 236, 240, 242, 243, 246
Acute nephritis	Hematuria, RBC casts Azotemia, oliguria Edema, hypertension	Proteinuria Pyuria Circulatory congestion	Chaps. 239, 240, 241
Chronic renal failure	Azotemia for > 3 months Prolonged symptoms or signs of uremia Symptoms or signs of renal osteodystrophy Kidneys reduced in size bilaterally Broad casts in urinary sediment	Hematuria, proteinuria Casts, oliguria Polyuria, nocturia Edema, hypertension Electrolyte disorders	Chaps. 235, 237
Nephrotic syndrome	Proteinuria > 3.5 g per 1.73 m^2 per 24 h Hypoalbuminemia Hyperlipidemia Lipiduria	Casts Edema	Chaps. 236, 241
Asymptomatic urinary abnormalities	Hematuria Proteinuria (below nephrotic range) Sterile pyuria, casts		Chap. 240
Urinary tract infection	Bacteriuria > 10^5 colonies per milliliter Other infectious agent documented in urine Pyuria, leukocyte casts Frequency, urgency Bladder tenderness, flank tenderness	Hematuria Mild azotemia Mild proteinuria Fever	Chap. 90
Renal tubule defects	Electrolyte disorders Polyuria, nocturia Symptoms or signs of renal osteodystrophy Large kidneys Renal transport defects	Hematuria "Tubular" proteinuria Enuresis	Chaps. 242, 244
Hypertension	Systolic/diastolic hypertension	Proteinuria Casts Azotemia	Chaps. 34, 209, 243
Nephrolithiasis	Previous history of stone passage or removal Previous history of stone seen by x-ray Renal colic	Hematuria Pyuria Frequency, urgency	Chap. 245
Urinary tract obstruction	Azotemia, oliguria, anuria Polyuria, nocturia, urinary retention Slowing of urinary stream Large prostate, large kidneys Flank tenderness, full bladder after voiding	Hematuria Pyuria Enuresis, dysuria	Chap. 246

TABLE 233-2 Syndromes produced by diseases of the kidneys and urinary tract

Diseases (Chap.)	ARF	RPRF	AN	CRF	NS	AUA
			Syndromes			
Bilateral arterial occlusion (243)	T					
Acute tubular necrosis (236)	T					
Bilateral acute renal vein thrombosis (243)	T					
Acute uric acid nephropathy (242)	T					
Hypovolemia (236)	T					
Cardiovascular collapse (236)	T					
Acute bilateral upper tract obstruction (206)	T					
Hypercalcemic nephropathy (242)	T			O		
Hemolytic uremic syndrome (243)	T	O	O			
Acute urinary retention (246)	T					
Malignant nephrosclerosis (243)	T	O				
Essential mixed cyroimmunoglobulinemia (241)	T	O	O	O	O	
Nephrotoxic drugs and chemicals (236, 242)	T			O		
Oxalate nephropathy (242)	T			O		
Cortical necrosis (236)	T			O		
Postpartum glomerulosclerosis (236)	T			O		
Hypersensitivity nephropathy (242)	T		O			P,H,L
Scleroderma (243)	T					P
Idiopathic rapidly progressive GN (240)	O	T	T		R	
Goodpasture's syndrome (240)	O	T	T	O		P,H
Non-Goodpasture's anti-GBM disease (240)	O	T	T	O		P,H
Acute bacterial endocarditis or visceral sepsis (240)		T	T	O	O	
Microscopic polyarteritis nodosa (241, 243)		T	T			
Wegener's granulomatosis (241, 243)		T	T			
Allergic granulomatosis (291)		T	T			
Acute radiation nephritis (242)		T	T			P
Poststreptococcal glomerulonephritis (240)		R	T	O	R	P,H
Nonstreptococcal postinfectious GN (240)		R	T	R	R	P,H
Macroscopic polyarteritis nodosa (275, 241, 243)				T		P,H
Diffuse proliferative lupus nephritis (241)	R	O	R	T	O	P,H,L
Chronic radiation nephritis (242)				T	O	
Balkan nephropathy (242)				T		P*,H
Analgesic nephropathy (242)				T		L,H
Heavy metals (lead, cadmium, mercury) (242, 396)				T		P*
Cystinosis (242)				T		P*
Chronic obstructive uropathy (246)				T		H
Adult polycystic renal disease (244)				T		H,P
Medullary cystic renal disease (244)				T		
Gouty nephropathy (242)				T		
Minimal change disease (240)					T	
Idiopathic membranous nephropathy (240)				O	T	P,H
Membranoproliferative glomerulonephritis (240)		R	O	O	T	P,H
Renal amyloidosis (241)				O	T	P
Membranous lupus nephropathy (241)				O	T	P
Renal vein thrombosis (243)	O			O	T	
Rheumatoid arthritis (241)					T	
Congenital nephrotic syndrome (241)				O	T	
Dermatomyositis (240)					T	
Dermatitis herpetiformis (240)				O	T	
Medullary sponge kidney (244)						T:H
Nephrolithiasis (239)						T:H
Neoplasms (247)						T:H
Arteriolar nephrosclerosis (243)				O		T:P
Waldenström's macroglobulinemia (241)	O					T:P
Multiple myeloma (241)	O	O		O	O	T:P
Reflux nephropathy (90, 243)				O	O	T:P
Diabetic nephropathy (241, 337)				O	O	T:P
Toxemia of pregnancy (6, 243)						T:P
Orthostatic proteinuria (240)						T:P
Sarcoid nephropathy (241)						T:P
Hypokalemic nephropathy (242)						T:P
Berger's (IgA) nephropathy (240)	R	R	O	O	O	T:H,P
Henoch-Schönlein purpura (241)		O	O	R	O	T:H,P
Fabry's disease (241)				O		T:H,P
Alport's syndrome (241)				O		T:H,P
Sickle cell nephropathy (241)				O	R	T:H,P
Subacute bacterial endocarditis (85)						T:H,P
Minimal and mesangial lupus nephritis (241)						T:P,H
Mesangial proliferative GN (240)				R	O	T:P,H
Mixed connective tissue disease (241)					R	T:P,H
Chronic glomerulonephritis (237)				O		T:P,H
Nail patella syndrome (241)				R		T:P,H
Focal glomerulosclerosis (240)		R	O	O	O	T:P,H,L
Focal and segmental lupus nephritis (241)				O	O	T:P,H,L
Sjögren's syndrome (241)						T:L,P
Urinary and renal infection (90)						T:L,H

NOTE: T, typical presentation; O, occurs frequently, but not invariably; R, occurs rarely; P*, tubular proteinuria; P, proteinuria; H, hematuria; L, leukocyturia; ARF, acute renal failure; RPRF, rapidly progressive renal failure; AN, acute nephritis; CRF, chronic renal failure; NS, nephrotic syndrome; AUA, asymptomatic urinary abnormality.

necrosis, from sepsis, nephrotoxic materials, shock, or other cause (see Chap. 236), is the usual cause of acute renal failure, whereas extracapillary proliferative (crescentic) glomerulonephritis, due to immunologic injury or to vasculitis, is an important cause of rapidly progressive, but not acute, renal failure (Chap. 240).

Proof for the existence of either syndrome requires serial determination of the glomerular filtration rate (GFR), blood urea nitrogen, or serum creatinine level. Anuria or oliguria (Chap. 44) strongly suggest acute renal failure, since life cannot be sustained for long with such inadequate renal function. Symptoms and signs of uremia of recent onset suggest rapidly progressive or acute renal failure but also could result from chronic renal failure that has only recently become life-threatening. Although edema, hypertension, and abnormalities of electrolytes and the urine sediment (Table 233-1) are frequent in acute and rapidly progressive renal failure, they occur in other syndromes as well and are not specific.

The causes of these two important syndromes number about 36, but only 18 (indicated by T, Table 233-2) typically cause acute renal failure, and 8 cause rapidly progressive renal failure. Urinary obstruction, acute tubular necrosis, some forms of vasculitis, major renal vascular accidents, and endogenous and exogenous nephrotoxins are the usual causes of acute renal failure. Vasculitis and crescentic glomerulonephritis are the main causes of rapidly progressive renal failure. Hemolytic-uremic syndrome, malignant nephrosclerosis, and essential mixed cryoimmunoglobulinemia occasionally present as rapidly progressive renal failure. Idiopathic rapidly progressive glomerulonephritis—the prototype of a disease that produces rapidly progressive renal failure—sometimes causes acute renal failure. Chronic renal failure may occur in some patients with diseases that typically cause acute renal failure. Nevertheless, despite some variability of disease presentations, the finding of acute or rapidly progressive renal failure narrows the range of causes.

ACUTE NEPHRITIS (AN) A number of diseases involve the glomeruli and, to a generally lesser extent, the tubules in an acute but transient inflammatory process, manifested clinically by acute reduction in GFR, rapidly progressive renal failure, and salt and water retention. Expansion of the extracellular volume, if marked, causes hypertension, pulmonary vascular congestion, and facial and peripheral edema (Chap. 240). Since the causes of this syndrome all can damage the glomerular wall enough to permit red blood cells and plasma proteins to enter the urinary space and appear in the urine, gross or microscopic hematuria, red blood cell casts, and proteinuria are necessary for the diagnosis of acute nephritis, and their absence suggests other diagnoses. Acute nephritis is a transient inflammatory process, so its clinical and laboratory manifestations wax and wane over days to weeks. Many of the diseases that cause acute nephritis also cause acute or rapidly progressive renal failure (see Table 233-2).

The fact that many diseases produce both acute nephritis and acute or rapidly progressive renal failure, some produce only acute nephritis, and some produce acute or chronic renal failure without acute nephritis is useful in diagnosis. Only two diseases, poststreptococcal glomerulonephritis and nonstreptococcal postinfectious glomerulonephritis, typically cause acute nephritis alone, and only three of the diseases that typically cause acute renal failure, idiopathic rapidly progressive glomerulonephritis, Goodpasture's syndrome, and non-Goodpasture's anti-glomerular basement membrane (anti-GBM) disease, also cause acute nephritis (see Table 233-2). On the other hand, most of the diseases that cause acute nephritis also cause rapidly progressive renal failure.

Acute glomerulonephritis following infection with group A streptococci is the prototype of a disease that causes acute nephritis alone (Chap. 240). Immune complexes deposit in the subepithelial region of the glomerular capillary wall, between the basement membrane and the visceral epithelial cells that separate the membrane from the urinary space, and provoke an intense but transient inflammatory process. GFR falls but returns to normal within weeks to months in most patients. Deposition of immune complexes is also believed to

be the cause of acute nephritis following other bacterial and viral infections and of lupus nephritis, membranoproliferative glomerulonephritis, Henoch-Schönlein purpura, and Berger's disease, i.e., IgA nephropathy. That the typical presentations of the last four diseases are chronic renal failure, nephrotic syndrome, and asymptomatic urinary abnormalities illustrates the weakness of relationships between pathogenesis and final clinical manifestations.

Renal biopsy is usually required for the evaluation of patients with acute nephritis, whether or not acute or rapidly progressive renal failure is also present. The usual histologic picture is proliferative glomerulonephritis, often with extracapillary crescent formation, but prognosis and treatment are influenced strongly by the precise histologic and ultrastructural pattern, as well as the types of immune complexes and immunoglobulins deposited in the renal tissues.

CHRONIC RENAL FAILURE (CRF) Chronic renal failure results from progressive and irreversible destruction of nephrons, regardless of cause (Chap. 237). This diagnosis implies that GFR is known to have been reduced for at least 3 to 6 months (see Table 233-1). Often a gradual decline in GFR occurs over a period of years. Proof of chronicity is also provided by the demonstration of bilateral reduction of kidney size by scout film, ultrasonography, intravenous pyelography, or tomography. Other findings of long-standing renal failure, such as renal osteodystrophy or symptoms of uremia, also help to establish this syndrome. Several laboratory abnormalities are often regarded as reliable indicators of chronicity of renal disease, such as anemia, hyperphosphatemia, or hypocalcemia, but these are not specific (Chap. 235). In contrast, the finding of broad casts in the urinary sediment (Chap. 44) is specific for chronic renal failure, the wide diameters of these casts reflecting the compensatory dilatation and hypertrophy of surviving nephrons. Proteinuria is a frequent but nonspecific finding, as is hematuria. Chronic obstructive uropathy, polycystic and medullary cystic diseases, analgesic nephropathy, and the inactive end stage of any chronic tubulointerstitial nephropathy are conditions in which the urine often contains little or no protein, cells, or casts even though nephron destruction has progressed to chronic renal failure.

When ARF occurs in the presence of CRF, the acute component must be evaluated as if CRF were not present, because the acute component is potentially reversible. In most instances, depletion of extracellular fluid volume is the cause of acute deterioration of renal function, but urinary tract obstruction, drug-induced nephrotoxicity, or exacerbation of underlying renal disease also may be responsible (Chap. 237).

NEPHROTIC SYNDROME (NS) This diagnosis previously implied that a patient excretes more than 3.5 g protein per 1.73 m^2 surface area per 24 h, the proteinuria consists mainly of albumin, and that the patient has reduced serum albumin, edema, and hyperlipidemia (Table 233-1). Massive proteinuria alone has now come to define the syndrome, since this finding connotes serious renal disease whether or not the protein losses lead to hypoalbuminemia, lipid disturbances, or edema (Chap. 44). Provided the proteins in the urine are not paraproteins readily excreted by the normal kidney (e.g., immunoglobulin light chains in multiple myeloma), massive proteinuria is invariably a sign of injury to the glomeruli.

Common causes of the nephrotic syndrome include minimal change disease, idiopathic membranous glomerulopathy, focal glomerulosclerosis, and diabetic glomerulosclerosis (Chaps. 240 and 241). Because these diseases typically cause less inflammation than those that cause acute nephritis, the urine contains fewer cellular elements, and acute changes in GFR and urine volume are uncommon. Hematuria may occur in some forms of nephrotic syndrome, however, especially chronic membranoproliferative glomerulonephritis (Chap. 240). The presence of cellular or granular casts should suggest lupus nephritis (Chap. 241) or acute nephritis associated with massive proteinuria, such as essential mixed cryoimmunoglobulinemia, acute bacterial endocarditis, visceral sepsis, and Henoch-Schönlein purpura (see Table 233-2).

ASYMPTOMATIC URINARY ABNORMALITIES (AUA)   As indicated in Table 233-2, mild microscopic hematuria, pyuria, and casts or less than 3.5 g protein per 1.73 m² surface area per 24 h may be present in the urine of a patient with no evidence of other nephrologic syndromes. By exclusion, these patients belong to the syndrome of asymptomatic urinary abnormalities. Isolated hematuria or proteinuria, or unexplained pyuria, are the most frequent abnormalities in this syndrome.

Isolated hematuria, without proteinuria or casts, may be the sole clue to the presence of neoplasm, stone, or infection (e.g., tuberculosis) in any part of the urinary tract (Chaps. 44, 239, 245, and 247). Isolated hematuria also may arise from renal papillae in analgesic and sickle cell nephropathies (Chaps. 242 and 243). Persistent isolated hematuria often requires intravenous pyelography, cystoscopy, and, occasionally, renal arteriography to identify the source of bleeding. *Nephronal hematuria*, in which casts contain red blood cells or hemoglobin pigment, indicates damage to the nephron (Chap. 44). It occurs without proteinuria, mainly in benign recurrent hematuria and Berger's disease (Chap. 240). *Nephronal hematuria and proteinuria* occur together in many renal diseases that may lead to chronic renal failure (Chap. 237). In general, the combination of nephronal hematuria and proteinuria suggests a worse prognosis than either alone.

Isolated proteinuria, without red blood cells or other formed elements in the urinary sediment, is characteristic of many renal diseases which manifest little or no inflammatory reaction within the glomeruli (e.g., diabetes mellitus, amyloidosis). Less than nephrotic-range proteinuria is common in mild forms of all the diseases that can cause overt nephrotic syndrome (Chaps. 240 and 241). ''Tubular'' proteinuria (Chap. 44) is the rule in cystinosis; in intoxication from cadmium, lead, or mercury; and in the peculiar Balkan nephropathy localized to a small region along the Danube River (Chap. 242).

Pyuria (leukocyturia) also may be a sole urinary abnormality and may reflect infection or inflammation of the lower urinary tract rather than parenchymal renal disease. Nevertheless, prominent pyuria can occur in any inflammatory disease of the kidneys, especially tubulointerstitial nephritis, lupus nephritis, pyelonephritis, and renal transplant rejection, but usually in association with mild proteinuria or hematuria. The finding of leukocyte casts (Chap. 44) establishes the kidney as the site of the inflammatory reaction.

Pyuria associated with urine that is sterile on routine bacteriologic culture presents a special problem. Causes of ''sterile pyuria'' include (1) recent bacterial urinary infection being treated with antibiotics, (2) glucocorticoid therapy, (3) acute febrile episodes, (4) cyclophosphamide administration, (5) pregnancy, (6) renal transplant rejection, (7) genitourinary trauma, and (8) prostatitis and cystourethritis. Leukocytes from vaginal secretions may contaminate the urine, so a midstream, clean-catch urine sample should be collected to substantiate a urinary origin. Pyuria associated with proteinuria, nephronal hematuria (Chap. 44), or casts usually signifies inflammatory disease of the renal glomeruli, tubules, interstitium, or microcirculation, and evaluation should focus not on the pyuria but on the nature of the renal disease.

Persistent sterile pyuria that cannot be ascribed to any of the foregoing causes has a narrow differential diagnosis. Unusual infections, such as tuberculosis, fungi, atypical mycobacteria, *Haemophilus influenzae*, anaerobic bacteria, fastidious bacteria that grow only on enriched media, and L forms, all must be sought. Intravenous pyelography may be needed to detect causes such as urinary tract calculi, papillary necrosis, and renal infiltration by lymphoma or myeloma cells. The latter is usually suspected because of other evidence of myeloma or lymphoma, for both rarely involve only the kidneys. If all tests are negative, cystoscopy may reveal cystitis or trigone inflammation.

URINARY TRACT INFECTION (UTI)   This syndrome is defined by the demonstration in urine of pathogenic organisms, either bacteria, tubercle bacilli, or fungi (Chap. 90). When urine is obtained for culture, the condition under which the urine is collected must minimize contamination from external surfaces. Women should void into a wide-mouthed sterile container after preliminary cleansing of the vulva with a moist, sterile gauze pledget. In men, midstream collection is usually adequate. Bacterial colony counts of 10⁵ organisms per milliliter or greater in urine generally indicate urinary tract colonization and infection. Levels above 10² colonies per milliliter are sufficient to indicate infection in symptomatic patients (Table 233-1) and in urine samples obtained by suprapubic aspiration or bladder catheter (Chap. 242). When the urinary tract is anatomically normal, *Escherichia coli* is the usual pathogen. After prolonged antibiotic treatment of persistent infections, particularly when urinary drainage is impaired or stones are present, *Klebsiella*, *Enterobacter*, and *Proteus* species predominate.

As discussed in Chap. 90, a positive urine culture need not imply that an organism is producing tissue inflammation or injury. In some patients, tissue effects may be trivial; in others, injury may occur even though symptoms or urinary abnormalities are not present at the time of evaluation. When bacteriuria is associated with tissue inflammation or injury, clinical manifestations usually depend on the site(s) involved. Dysuria, frequency, urgency, and suprapubic tenderness are common symptoms of bladder and urethral inflammation (Chap. 44 and Table 233-1). Prostatitis also leads to frequency, dysuria, and urgency, and the prostate may be boggy and tender on rectal examination. Flank pain, chills, fever, nausea and vomiting, hypotension from sepsis, and leukocyte casts all suggest true renal parenchymal infection, i.e., pyelonephritis; their absence, however, does not exclude pyelonephritis.

RENAL TUBULE DEFECTS (RTD)   This syndrome encompasses a large number of acquired and hereditary disorders, all of which tend to affect tubules more than glomeruli. Hereditary anatomic defects, including polycystic renal disease, medullary cystic disease, and medullary sponge kidney, are readily detected by intravenous pyelography, which is usually performed because of hematuria, bacteriuria, flank pain, or unexplained azotemia (Chap. 244).

Defects in tubule transport functions, on the other hand, tend not to be associated with prominent renal anatomic defects and arise either as inherited traits (Chap. 244) or during the course of acquired renal disease (Chap. 242). In general, these functional defects impair secretion and/or reabsorption of electrolytes and organic solutes or limit urinary concentrating and diluting ability (see Table 233-1). Typical manifestations of such functional disturbances include polyuria and nocturia (Chap. 44), metabolic acidosis (Chap. 46), and various disorders of fluid and electrolyte balance (Chap. 45). Such defects are defined by direct physiologic measurements; their elucidation requires a sound understanding of normal renal physiology.

HYPERTENSION (H)   Hypertension implies that the average of a series of reliable blood pressure measurements exceeds 140 mmHg systolic or 90 mmHg diastolic (see Table 233-1). The pathogenetic mechanisms, clinical and laboratory manifestations, and therapeutic approaches are discussed in detail elsewhere (Chaps. 34 and 209). In addition, a number of renal complications of hypertension are reviewed in Chap. 243, as is the entity of renal artery stenosis, an infrequent but potentially curable cause of hypertension.

NEPHROLITHIASIS (N)   This syndrome is recognized with certainty when a stone is passed, visualized by x-ray, or removed at surgery or cystoscopy (see Table 233-1 and Chap. 245). Less certain, but suggestive, evidences of nephrolithiasis include renal colic, painful hematuria, or unexplained pyuria, dysuria, and urinary frequency (Chap. 44). Colic varies in its symptomatology but usually begins suddenly in one flank, radiates downward toward the groin, and is excruciatingly painful.

Most renal stones are composed of calcium, uric acid, cystine, or struvite (magnesium ammonium phosphate). All are radiopaque except for uric acid stones and are therefore visible by routine abdominal radiography. Uric acid stones appear as radiolucent filling defects and can be mistaken for tumor or blood clot.

URINARY TRACT OBSTRUCTION (UTO)   Documentation of the various structural or functional causes of urinary tract obstruction usually requires radiologic or surgical visualization. The manifestations of obstruction, which initiate the search for its causes, are numerous (see Table 233-1) and are reviewed in Chap. 246. Anuria in an adult is almost always due to obstruction of bladder outflow. Less commonly, blockage of upper urinary drainage from both kidneys or from a solitary functioning kidney accounts for total or near-total cessation of urine flow. A large bladder after voiding is a sign of outflow obstruction, usually due to urethral stricture, tumor, stone, neurogenic causes, or prostatic hypertrophy. Nocturia, frequency and overflow incontinence, and slowing or hesitancy of micturition also suggest outflow obstruction (Chap. 44). Upper tract obstruction often produces few manifestations. When it is incomplete or unilateral, urine volume may be normal or even elevated because of a loss of renal concentrating ability. Urinary stasis secondary to obstruction predisposes to recurrent urinary tract infection or chronic obstruction to progressive loss of renal function (Table 233-2).

REFERENCES

Coe FL, Bushinsky DA: Clinical and laboratory assessment of patients with renal and urinary tract disease, in *Clinical Nephrology*, BM Brenner, F Coe, FC Rector Jr (eds). Philadelphia, Saunders, 1987, p 1

Levey AS et al: Laboratory assessment of renal disease: Clearance, urinalysis and renal biopsy, in *The Kidney*, BM Brenner, FC Rector Jr (eds). Philadelphia, Saunders, 1991, p 919

Rosenberg ME, Hostetter TH: Proteinuria, in *The Kidney*, DW Seldin, G Giebisch (eds). New York, Raven, 1992, p 3039

234 IMPACT OF CELLULAR AND MOLECULAR BIOLOGY ON NEPHROLOGY

KARL L. SKORECKI / DANIEL G. BICHET / BARRY M. BRENNER

Like other branches of medicine, nephrology is being transformed by advances in molecular cell biology and recombinant DNA technology. Molecular cloning strategies now provide clinicians and investigators with erythropoietin, atrial natriuretic peptides, and endothelins—potent gene products whose availability (indeed, whose existence, in the case of the endothelins) was not imagined a decade ago. Advances also have been made in the cloning and sequencing of DNA constructs that encode various transport proteins; in unraveling the interplay of second messengers, G proteins, and intracellular calcium transients; in linking abnormalities of genotype with phenotype, as in autosomal dominant polycystic kidney disease and various oncogene-associated renal neoplasms; and in understanding the regulatory elements governing the immune response. This chapter will address several of these issues to illustrate the advances in nephrology made possible by these technologies.

MOLECULAR DETERMINANTS OF NEPHRON DEVELOPMENT AND FUNCTION Normal renal function depends on the axial organization of individual nephron segments. Beyond the glomerulus, the filtrate is processed by as many as 20 functional tubule segments, each containing distinct cells and each characterized by distinct functions. Key processes in the development and maintenance of coordinated function of nephron segments include (1) expression of the polarized epithelial cell phenotype, (2) epithelial cell migration and branching, (3) orderly segregation of the specialized cell types comprising each nephron segment, and (4) apposition at the proximal nephron of a highly specialized microcirculatory element (the glomerular capillary tuft) capable of generating large volumes of a nearly ideal (protein-free) ultrafiltrate. Many disorders of kidney function can now be understood in terms of disruptions of the molecular determinants of these processes either during renal development or in the response to nephron injury.

Molecular determinants of the polarized epithelial cell phenotype and epithelial morphogenesis Vectorial transport of solute is characteristic of all tubule segments and reflects cell polarity, the signature feature of epithelial cells. The polarized epithelial cell is characterized by distribution of plasma membrane proteins into distinct apical and basolateral domains and the polarized distribution of cytoplasmic organelles and structural proteins comprising the cellular cytoskeleton. In general, apical membrane proteins subserve functions of regulated solute and water transport to and from the tubule lumen, while basolateral membrane proteins facilitate cell-cell contact and adhesion and participate in generation of ion gradients and signal reception and transduction (Fig. 234-1).

In the developing kidney, a key step in the differentiation of precursor cells of the metanephros to an epithelial lineage capable of expressing the polarized epithelial phenotype involves induction as the result of cell contact with the ureteric bud. This process is analogous to induction of mesoderm by ectoderm and endoderm in *Xenopus*; fibroblast growth factor, members of the *wnt* gene family, and *activins* (relatives of TGF-β) are possible candidates in the induction process. Once induced, expression of the polarized epithelial phenotype depends either on cell-cell or cell-substratum (e.g., tubule basement membrane) contact. Cell surface molecules that are expressed with development of the polarized epithelial phenotype and that mediate such contact include the calcium-dependent cell adhesion molecule *E-cadherin* (cell-cell contact) and the matrix protein *laminin* (cell-substratum contact). Cell-cell contact promotes the formation of highly developed junctional complexes that link the cytoskeletons of adjacent cells to facilitate cell-cell communication. Soon after cell-cell or cell-substratum contact, the component of the cell membrane exposed to the lumen adopts distinctive characteristics in terms of lipid composition (rich in glycosphingolipids and depleted in phosphatidylcholine) relative to the basolateral membrane and serves as a site for insertion of specialized apical transport proteins. This targeting is a function of both the epithelial phenotype and sorting signals intrinsic to the targeted proteins. The formation of tight junctions segregates the proteins of the apical from the basolateral membrane and serves as a barrier to lateral diffusion of phospholipids of the outer leaflet of the apical membrane.

Another characteristic of the polarized epithelial phenotype is that no transport protein resides in both the apical and basolateral membranes at the same time within the same cell. Indeed, it is the coordinated expression and function of proteins in the basolateral membrane (e.g., Na^+, K^+-ATPase) with proteins on the apical membrane (e.g., Na^+ channels and Na^+-H^+ antiporter of the proximal tubule) that allow vectorial transepithelial transport (e.g., reabsorption of sodium and water) to occur. Acquired loss of epithelial polarity occurs in at least two kidney diseases, namely acute tubular necrosis (ATN) and autosomal dominant polycystic kidney disease. The disturbances in fluid and solute reabsorption in these disorders highlight the importance of the polarized epithelial phenotype to nephron function.

Some molecules of mesenchymal origin that appear to be responsible for cell migration, branching tubulogenesis, and other components of epithelial morphogenesis necessary for nephron organization have been identified. Three such factors are *hepatocyte growth factor* (and its receptor the *met* oncogene), *nerve growth factor*, and *epimorphin*. Interruption of the expression or function of these factors disrupts epithelial morphogenesis. Expression of these or related factors is believed to contribute to orderly repair following acute tubule cell injury.

Molecular determinants of specialized function of nephron segments Segmentation of nephrons depends on establishing demarcated boundaries for expression of genes that define a given cellular phenotype. This orderly segmental pattern of gene expression

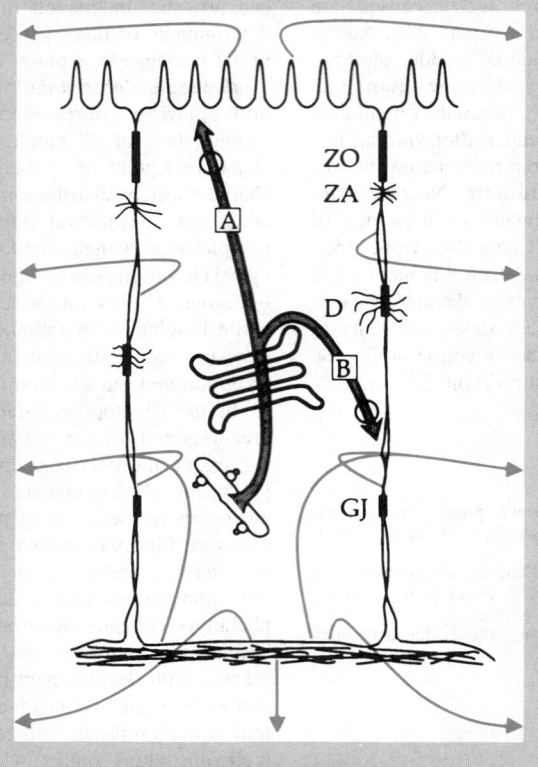

Functions

Apical plasma membrane
- *regulation of nutrient and water uptake*
- *regulated secretion (pathway A)*
- *protection*

Lateral plasma membrane
- *cell contact and adhesion*
- *cell communication*

Basal-lateral membrane
- *signal reception and transduction*
- *generation of ion gradients*
- *constitutive secretion (pathway B)*

Basal membrane
- *cell-substratum contact*

Components

Apical plasma membrane
- *Hydrolases*
- *Amiloride - sensitive Na^+ Channel*
- *Na^+-dependent Transporters*
- *Cl^- channel*
- *H^+-ATPase*
- *Proteins linked via glycosyl - phosphatidylinositol*
- *Glycolipids*

Lateral plasma membrane
- *Cell Adhesion Molecules*
- *Junctional Complex:*
  Zonula occludens (ZO)
  Zonula adherens (ZA)
  Desmosomes (D)
  Gap junctions (GJ)

Basal-lateral membrane
- *Anion Channel (Cl^-/HCO_3^- exchanger)*
- *Na^+,K^+-ATPase*
- *Growth factor receptors*
- *Hormone and Neurotransmitter receptors*
- *Transduction systems associated with receptors*

Basal membrane
- *Basement Membrane Receptors*

Basement membrane
- *Laminin, Type IV Collagen, Proteoglycans*

FIGURE 234-1 In polarized epithelial cells, the apical plasma membrane faces the lumen and is responsible for the absorption of ions and nutrients via ion channels and transporters. In secretory epithelial cells, the apical plasma membrane is also the site of regulated secretion (pathway A). The lateral plasma membrane participates in cell-cell contact, mediated by specialized components of the junctional complex. Tight junctions [zonula occludens (ZO)] serve as a paracellular barrier between lumen and interstitium. Cell-cell contact is initially influenced by cell adhesion molecules and maintained by belt [zonula adherens (ZA)] and spot desmosomes (D). Intercellular communication is facilitated by gap junctions (GJ), specialized channels that make possible the exchange of small solutes. The basal plasma membrane is attached to the basement membrane via specific receptors for laminin, type IV collagen, and proteoglycans. Proteins and receptors localized to the basolateral plasma membrane are involved in solute transport and signal transduction and participate in constitutive secretion (pathway B). (*After E Rodriguez-Boulan and WJ Nelson, Science 245:719, 1989. Copyright 1989 by the AAAS.*)

is reminiscent of the expression of homeobox genes that determine body segmentation in *Drosophila* and other species. Indeed, analogues of homeobox genes (including the *pax-2* member of the paired-box gene family) may play a causal role in mammalian kidney development.

The specialization of nephron segments in the mature kidney is well characterized at the functional level, and efforts have been made to isolate and identify genes encoding the proteins that subserve these specialized functions. *Expression cloning* has been a powerful tool to identify several of these genes and characterize their protein products. This technique involves the introduction (e.g., microinjection) of fractionated messenger RNA (mRNA) into an expression system (e.g., *Xenopus* oocyte), followed by screening of the test system for the new appearance of the function of interest (e.g., sodium-dependent glucose transport). This approach allows the isolation of a gene or genes on the basis of a given specialized functional activity prior to identification of the protein that subserves the function.

Another strategy to clone specific genes of interest to nephron function takes advantage of patterns of homology of conserved sequences (consensus motifs) for molecules that share common functions or interactions and are therefore part of a large gene family. With this approach, genes have been cloned that encode novel receptor tyrosine kinases, such as members of the fibroblast growth factor

receptor family, that appear to be of importance in tubulogenesis. The genes encoding several receptors that act by coupling to G proteins and novel members of the G-protein family itself also have been cloned in this way.

As a result of these and other strategies, functional differentiation of distinct renal cells can be defined in terms of the expression of identified or candidate genes that provide the molecular basis for nephron segment specialization. Table 234-1 provides a number of examples in which the isolation of cDNAs has yielded insight into the physiology or pathobiology of individual nephron segments.

GLOMERULUS   In vivo micropuncture and cell physiologic studies of cultured cells of glomerular origin (endothelial, epithelial, mesangial) suggest that circulating and locally produced vasoactive hormones and growth factors regulate glomerular hemodynamics on a moment-to-moment basis and control cell growth and matrix elaboration long term. Alterations in this system occur in both acute and chronic forms of glomerular injury. For example, the basis for an autocrine loop of mesangial cell origin has been identified in which platelet-derived growth factor (PDGF) interacts with its receptor during normal glomerulogenesis. Reactivation of this autocrine loop in experimental glomerular injury promotes mesangial cell proliferation and glomerular vasoconstriction. Indeed, the infusion of a blocking antibody to PDGF in an animal model of mesangial proliferative glomerulonephritis

TABLE 234-1 Examples of nephron proteins whose cDNAs have been cloned

Nephron segment	Protein
Glomerulus	Endothelins
	Nitric oxide synthase (type I)
	Receptors for angiotensin (vascular subtype), parathormone, vasopressin (vascular subtype), endothelins, thromboxane A_2, prostaglandin E_2, prostacyclin, catecholamines, PDGF-β chain, epidermal growth factor, and fibroblast growth factor
Proximal tubule	Vasopressin-insensitive water channel
	Nonvascular type angiotensin receptor
	Sodium-dependent glucose cotransporters (SGLT-1 and SGLT-2)
	Sodium-hydrogen exchanger
	Sodium-phosphate cotransporter
	Amino acid transport protein (D-2)
Loop of Henle	Epidermal growth factor
	Sodium-potassium-chloride cotransporter
	Chloride channel
	K_{ATP} channel
	Tamm-Horsfall protein
Distal nephron, and collecting tubule	Vasopressin receptor (antidiuretic subtype)
	Vasopressin sensitive water channel
	Bradykinin
	Thiazide-sensitive Na-Cl cotransporter
	H-ATPase (32-kDa subunit)
	Dihydropyridine-sensitive calcium channel (CaCh4)
	Sodium-calcium exchanger
	K_{ATP} channel
	Sodium channel
	Urodilatin
	Insulin-like growth factor I
	Aldose reductase

inhibits mesangial cell proliferation, suggesting a potential therapy for glomerulonephritis. Similarly, identification by expression cloning of the cDNA clones encoding the vascular type vasopressin (V_1) and angiotensin II (AT_1) receptors and the thromboxane A_2 receptor extend the tools needed to clarify the role of these vasoactive mediators in glomerular disease states. Of particular interest in the case of angiotensin II, molecular probes (e.g., cDNAs encoding renin, angiotensin-converting enzyme, and the angiotensin II receptor) have been utilized to confirm the existence of a self-contained intrarenal renin-angiotensin system capable of modulating glomerular hemodynamics. Molecular identification of endothelin and its receptor antedated functional characterization. The latter revealed that interaction of this peptide of endothelial origin and its mesangial cell receptor results in glomerular vasoconstriction and glomerular cell proliferation in normal and disease states. An example of the latter includes the contribution of augmented endothelin release to acute cyclosporine nephrotoxicity.

Signals downstream from these vasoconstrictor and growth promoting receptors (endothelin, angiotensin II, and V_1 vasopressin) are transduced by several intracellular proteins whose cDNAs or genes have been cloned. These include the G_q member of the G-protein family, phospholipase-C β, protein kinase C isozymes, and the inositol trisphosphate receptor. The concerted actions of these signaling proteins mediate calcium- and protein kinase–mediated responses that eventuate in glomerular response to these hormones. Although the glomerulus is not usually considered in terms of ion transport or channel properties, membrane depolarization and calcium influx control glomerular hemodynamics by contractile mesangial cells of the glomerular microcirculation.

Three vasodilator systems have been identified in the glomerular microcirculation. The first involved identification of cDNAs encoding the phospholipase A_2 and cyclooxygenase proteins involved in the elaboration of vasodilatory eicosanoids and their receptors. The second was identification of cDNA clones encoding components of the synthetic pathway for production of nitric oxide from its precursor L-arginine in glomerular endothelial cells. The third was elucidation

of subclasses of receptors for atrial natriuretic peptides (ANP) and of ANP degradative enzymes, which provide a molecular basis for understanding heterogeneous pharmacologic responses to atrial natriuretic peptides in different sodium-retaining states. In all cases, elucidation of the molecules involved in synthesis, action, or degradation of vasodilator components provides the basis for development of therapeutic strategies to treat renal vasoconstriction (e.g., hypertension, cyclosporine toxicity).

Several approaches, including development of transgenic mice, have been applied to elucidate the basis of various forms of glomerular injury. Expression of *Thy-1*, a member of the immunoglobulin gene superfamily, in transgenic mice causes proteinuric glomerular disease characterized by mesangial cell proliferation and dense subendothelial deposits. The pathogenetic role of PDGF was elucidated, as noted above in the rodent counterpart of this form of immune-mediated glomerular injury. A reverse approach has involved insertional inactivation of native genes, which in the case of one transgenic mouse line, caused the nephrotic syndrome. It will now be possible to clone and identify the gene whose inactivation caused the disease. Glomerular cells from transgenic mice have been perpetuated as immortalized cell lines in culture, thereby facilitating their functional and molecular characterization.

Several candidate genes involved in glomerular cell hypertrophy and genes responsible for the production and degradation of extracellular matrix components have been identified and characterized. These include the genes encoding TGF-β and its receptor, specific collagen subtypes, a tissue inhibitor of metalloproteinase, and others. In the case of the TGF-β receptor, cloning of the cDNA revealed its function as a receptor serine/threonine kinase. The availability of probes for the mRNAs encoding these proteins and cytokines, which mediate glomerular injury, will make possible new approaches to the interpretation of information obtained from renal biopsy specimens. In particular, in situ hybridization and quantitative PCR processing of biopsy specimens with appropriate probes will allow more accurate diagnosis, improve understanding of pathogenesis, and suggest therapies for the management of glomerular disease.

PROXIMAL TUBULE Physiologic studies in isolated, perfused, proximal tubule segments led to the identification of apical and basolateral transporters that account for the functional characteristics of each segment. Perhaps the best characterized are the apical sodium-dependent glucose transporter and sodium-hydrogen antiporter. Together, these transporters are responsible for most transcellular transport of sodium in the earliest portions of the proximal tubule. The cDNA encoding the sodium-hydrogen antiporter was first cloned on the basis of the importance of this protein in the regulation of intracellular pH in all cells of the body, and the formation gleaned from this expression cloning was applied to the corresponding protein that mediates transcellular sodium and bicarbonate reabsorption in the proximal tubule. Expression cloning also was used to identify the cDNA encoding a family of sodium-dependent glucose transporters in a variety of epithelial cell systems. Lessons learned from cloning of the sodium-hydrogen antiporter and the sodium-dependent glucose transporter are enabling investigators to clone cDNAs for other sodium gradient–dependent transport systems in the renal proximal tubule (e.g., other sugars, amino acids, phosphate, sulfate, and organic metabolites). It is probable that molecular probes derived from other systems (e.g., red blood cell water channel; muscle and hepatic sodium-independent glucose carrier, red cell band 3 anion exchanger) will clarify some of the ambiguities as to the nature of the transport systems that contribute to overall transcellular solute and water uptake in the proximal tubule.

Identification of one of the members of the *multidrug resistance gene family* (*MDR1*) in the apical membrane of the proximal tubule utilized the reverse approach, in which molecular investigation antedated and motivated physiologic and pathophysiologic studies. The 170-kDa glycoprotein product of this gene mediates resistance to a wide variety of cationic hydrophobic cytotoxic drugs in cancer cells, presumably through an ATP-dependent drug-pumping efflux mechanism. Localization of this protein in the apical membrane of the proximal tubule implies a role in the transport of a naturally occurring substrate whose identification may shed light on the physiologic role of the pump.

The activity of transporters in each of the proximal tubule segments is regulated by input from a number of receptors in the basolateral membrane, such as the angiotensin II receptor and the parathyroid hormone receptor. cDNA clones encoding both receptors have been isolated. Transmembrane signal-transduction systems (G proteins coupled to the regulation of ion channels via lipoxygenase product intermediates) are also present on the apical membrane.

LOOP OF HENLE   The countercurrent mechanism responsible for production of urine of varying osmolality depends on the differential axial expression of solute transporters and membrane permeabilities to water, urea, and ions. This pattern of expression of transporters and permeabilities defines each of the limbs of the loop of Henle. Several aspects of the function of the loop of Henle await clarification. For example, the thin ascending limb of Henle has the highest chloride permeability reported in the nephron. Physiologic studies have not been able to distinguish whether this permeability reflects predominantly a paracellular or transcellular route of chloride movement. Similarly, the principal, if not only, conductance in the basolateral membrane of cells of the thick ascending limb of Henle is a chloride conductance. It is likely that analysis of the characteristics of proteins that mediate chloride channel conductance in other systems will provide the clues or probes to enhance our understanding of chloride movement in the thin and thick ascending limb of Henle and in other nephron segments. Identification of the cystic fibrosis gene product as a chloride channel has increased interest in identification of genes encoding chloride channels in the nephron. However, to date, no cystic fibrosis gene homologues have been identified in the nephron.

Attempts are also underway to identify the proteins of the apical Na-K-2Cl cotransporter of the thick ascending limb of Henle. The cloning of the vasopressin V_2 receptor gene (see below) will make it possible to define the regulatory role of vasopressin in modulating activity of this transporter in the medullary thick ascending limb of Henle. The ascending limb of Henle is also a major site for production of epidermal growth factor (EGF). The precursor molecule (pre-pro-EGF) is inserted as an integral transmembrane glycoprotein into the apical membrane. The mature EGF is sheared off the luminal side and excreted into the urine. Excretion of EGF in the urine is decreased in acute renal failure. Furthermore, infusion of EGF accelerates recovery of injured cells in experimental models of ATN. EGF and its receptors are also present in vascular and glomerular sites in the kidney, where they are thought to regulate eicosanoid production. It is of interest that the most abundant normally secreted urinary protein, Tamm-Horsfall protein, which is also produced in the ascending limb of Henle, shows a high degree of structural homology with pre-pro-EGF. Although the Tamm-Horsfall protein cDNA has been cloned, the physiologic function of the protein and the significance of its urinary excretion remain to be delineated.

DISTAL AND COLLECTING TUBULE SEGMENTS   The portion of the nephron beyond the macula densa contains at least 5 cell types (distal cell proper, connecting tubule cell, principal cell, and two configurations of intercalated cells) and at least 11 segments (4 in the distal tubule and 7 in the collecting tubule), as defined by morphologic and functional markers. It is at the connecting tubule that the demarcation of cells of ureteric bud (mesonephric) origin from cells of metanephric origin occurs, and beyond this demarcation the nephron displays branching tubulogenesis.

In a few instances genes and their proteins have been isolated whose differential expression defines the characteristics for a given segment or cell type. These include, among others, receptors for mineralocorticoid, ANP, and vasopressin. The vasopressin receptor in this case is the V_2 receptor coupled to adenylate cyclase and to the antidiuretic response. An unique cloning strategy based on the expression of adenylate cyclase responsiveness was used to identify V_2 receptor genomic DNA. Since the expression of the V_2 receptor is relatively restricted to the kidney, the gene encoding this molecule is a candidate for the potential identification of kidney-specific transcription activating factors. In addition, isolation of the V_2 receptor gene has permitted the molecular examination of hereditary disorders of water conservation (see below). V_1 receptors coupled to calcium signaling and prostaglandin production are also present in the collecting tubule, but the functional role remains to be determined.

The unique transport properties of the collecting tubule segments reflect the expression of highly specialized channels and/or transport proteins coupled with tight junctions capable of sustaining the highest transtubular solute gradients and epithelial resistances found along the nephron. Much attention is now focused on cloning the genes encoding these highly specialized transport elements, with the greatest emphasis on those proteins whose functional characteristics have been best defined, e.g., vasopressin-sensitive water and urea channels (principal cell of cortical and medullary collecting tubule), apical sodium and potassium channels (principal cell of cortical collecting tubule), and H^+-ATPase and chloride-bicarbonate exchanger of intercalated cells. Progress has been made in the case of the water channel, utilizing strategies based on homology with the erythrocyte water channel. This approach, combined with expression cloning, has made it possible to identify the vasopressin-insensitive water channel in the proximal tubule of the nephron and may make it possible to identify the collecting tubule water channel responsible for the antidiuretic response to vasopressin.

MOLECULAR GENETICS OF SELECTED DISORDERS OF KIDNEY FUNCTION (See Table 234-2)   The strategies involved in the characterization of the genetic defects responsible for hereditary renal disease will probably also find application in defining other renal illnesses.

Alport's syndrome   In X-linked Alport's syndrome, ultrastructural and immunostaining defects in the glomerular basement membrane implicated an alteration in a structural protein, type IV collagen, as the cause of the glomerular defect. The product of the human *COL4A5* gene is the a5 (IV) collagen chain, which is a specific component of glomerular basement membrane. This gene, which maps to the same region of the X chromosome long arm as does

TABLE 234-2   Hereditary diseases of renal function and their chromosomal loci

Disease	Gene product	Locus
Renal cell carcinoma/ von Hippel–Lindau syndrome		3p25–p26
Osteopetrosis–renal tubular acidosis–cerebral calcification syndrome	Carbonic anhydrase II	8q22
Tuberous sclerosis		9q11–q22
Fructose intolerance	Fructose-1-phosphate aldolase B	9q22
Nail-patella syndrome		9q34
Wilms' tumor		11p13
Vitamin D–dependent rickets, type 2	1,25(OH)$_2$ vitamin D receptor	12
Hemodialysis-related amyloidosis		15q21–q22
Adult dominant polycystic kidney disease		16p13.3
Urolithiasis (2,8- dihydroxyadenine)	Adenosine phosphoribosyl- transferase	16q24
Diabetes insipidus		20
Hypophosphatemia		Xp22
Hypomagnesemia		Xp22
Fabry's disease		Xq22
Alport's syndrome		Xq22–q25
Lowe oculocerebrorenal syndrome		Xq25
Lesch-Nyhan syndrome	Hypoxanthine-guanine phosphoribosyl- transferase	Xq26–q27.2
Congenital nephrogenic diabetes insipidus		Xq28–qter
Proximal renal tubular acidosis		X
Pseudohypoparathyroidism		X

Alport's syndrome (q22–q25), has 51 coding exons spread over 100 kilobases of genomic DNA. Since the first *COL4A5* mutations were described in 1990, additional mutations have been identified, and attempts have been made to correlate phenotypes with the various point mutations, deletions, and insertions. To date, no clear genetic differences have been identified between juvenile-onset and adult-onset end-stage Alport's syndrome.

X-linked nephrogenic diabetes insipidus As noted above, the antidiuretic hormone arginine vasopressin (AVP) activates specific V_2 receptors on basolateral surfaces of renal collecting tubule cells. Subsequent stimulation of the Gs-protein/adenylate cyclase system promotes insertion of water channels into the luminal membrane and thereby facilitates reabsorption of water and excretion of concentrated urine. In congenital nephrogenic diabetes insipidus, the kidneys fail to respond to vasopressin, and physiologic studies implicated a defect in the V_2 receptor. The gene for nephrogenic diabetes insipidus has been assigned to the q28–qter portion of the X chromosome long arm by linkage and functional studies. Furthermore, the V_2 receptor gene colocalizes to the same region. A deletion and two separate point mutations in the V_2 receptor gene have been detected in three independent families with the disease, and it is likely that defects in the V_2 receptor gene are responsible for abnormal water conservation in most. In both Alport's syndrome and nephrogenic diabetes insipidus, prenatal diagnosis and detection of carrier females at risk are now possible. Also, understanding of the relation between the nature of these molecular defects and phenotypic expression may lead to the design of appropriate therapies.

Autosomal dominant polycystic kidney disease (ADPKD) and molecular mechanisms of cyst formation ADPKD is a single-gene disorder that affects approximately 1 in 100 whites and leads to end-stage renal disease. Affected individuals also have an increased incidence of subarachnoid hemorrhage, due to berry aneurysms, and cystic manifestations in other organs, especially liver and pancreas. Up to 10 percent of patients who undergo renal replacement therapy in North America have this disorder. The biochemical defect has not been identified. Demonstration of linkage with the α chain of hemoglobin and more than 10 other genetic markers made it possible to assign the principal (>95 percent) locus for ADPKD mutations (designated PDK_1) to chromosome 16 (16p13.3). Twenty-three genes, each larger than 65 kilobases have been identified in the PDK_1 region.

Mutations at other loci also can produce renal cystic disease. Accordingly, information concerning the molecular basis of cyst formation will facilitate screening of candidate mutations. One possibility is a defect in the molecular determinants of epithelial cell polarity; Na^+, K^+-ATPase is localized to the apical membranes of cells in the epithelial lining of cysts form ADPKD kidneys, in contrast to the typical location in the basolateral membrane of renal cells in adjacent normal tubules in the same kidney. The reversal of polarity is not specific to Na^+, K^+-ATPase, since several other basolateral proteins, including EGF receptor, ankyrin, fodrin, and E-cadherin, are also mis-sorted to the apical surface. By contrast, other proteins, including the band 3 anion transporter, gp 330 antigen, laminin, and type IV collagen, are located normally in cystic epithelia.

Wilms' tumor and other renal malignancy syndromes Wilms' tumor, an embryonal malignancy of the kidney, affects approximately 1 in 10,000 infants and children. In 1971, Knudson proposed a mechanism to account for both the sporadic and hereditary forms of retinoblastoma and the relative occurrence of multiple, bilateral tumors in the two groups, a unifying hypothesis that also applies to Wilms' tumors. It is based on the concept of the tumor suppressor gene: Somatic cells homozygous for mutations that interfere with a tumor gene product have proliferative advantages that lead to clonal overgrowth. Cells heterozygous for such a mutation behave normally because tumor suppressor activity encoded by the "normal" gene is sufficient to suppress proliferation. In other words, since tumor suppressor mutations are recessive, two mutations at the same locus are required for tumor formation—the "two hit" hypothesis. The Wilms' tumor gene (*wt*1) has been characterized. All or part of *wt*1

polypeptides have features characteristic of transcription regulatory factors (including zinc finger domains). The tumor suppressor gene *wt*1 on chromosome 11 (p13) is expressed at high levels in the glomeruli of the kidney, the gonadal ridge of the developing gonad, Sertoli cells of the testes, and the epithelial and granulosa cells of the ovary, suggesting a developmental role in the genital system in addition to the kidney. Such a role might explain the 10-fold higher incidence of hypospadias and cryptorchidism among patients with bilateral Wilms' tumor compared with the general population. In the WAGR syndrome, Wilms' tumor (W), congenital aniridia (A), genitourinary malformations (G), and mental retardation (R) often coexist. This constellation of anomalies defines a cluster of genes within 11p13 that appears to be important in the development of the iris, kidney, urogenital tract, and brain. Of these, *wt*1 is a recessive oncogene. A consistent chromosome 3p deletion and loss of heterozygosity has been reported in sporadic cases of renal cell carcinoma and in renal carcinoma associated with the von Hippel–Lindau syndrome. A candidate tumor suppressor gene responsible for the renal malignancies in the Von Hippel-Lindau syndrome has been identified by positional cloning. Characterization of the product of this gene will provide insight into the mechanisms for the regulation of growth and differentiation of the renal epithelium.

REFERENCES

ALPER SL, LODISH HF: Molecular biology of renal function, in *The Kidney*, 4th ed, BM Brenner, FC Rector Jr (eds). Philadelphia, Saunders, 1991, pp 132–163

BARKER DF et al: Identification of mutations in the COL4A5 collagen gene in Alport syndrome. Science 248:1224, 1990

BRENNER BM: Determinants of epithelial differentiation and early nephrogenesis in the developing kidney. J Am Soc Nephrol 1:127, 1990

KOVACS G et al: Consistent chromosome 3p deletion and loss of heterozygosity in renal cell carcinoma. Proc Natl Acad Sci USA 85:1571, 1988

LATIF F et al: Identification of the Von Hippel-Lindau disease tumor suppressor gene. Science 260:1317, 1993

PELLETIER J et al: Germline mutations in the Wilms' tumor suppressor gene are associated with abnormal urogenital development in Denys-Drash syndrome. Cell 67:437, 1991

REEDERS S: Multilocus polycystic disease. Genetics 1:235, 1992

ROSENTHAL W et al: Molecular identification of the gene responsible for congenital nephrogenic diabetes insipidus. Nature 359 (6392):233, 1992

235 DISTURBANCES OF RENAL FUNCTION

BARRY M. BRENNER / STEVEN C. HEBERT

Near constancy of the composition of the internal environment, including the volume, tonicity, and compartmental distribution of the body fluids, is essential to survival. With day-to-day variations in amount and composition of food and fluids, preservation of the internal environment requires the excretion of these substances (and/or their by-products) in amounts that balance the quantities ingested. Although losses from skin, lungs, and intestine contribute to this excretory capacity, the greatest responsibility for solute and water excretion is borne by the kidneys.

The kidneys operate primarily to maintain the composition and volume of the *extracellular* fluid compartment. The continuous exchange of water and solutes across all cell membranes, however, permits the kidneys to contribute indirectly to the regulation of the volume, composition, and tonicity of the *intracellular* fluids as well. To accomplish these tasks, physiologic mechanisms enable the individual to excrete excesses of water and nonmetabolized solute contained in the diet, as well as the nonvolatile end products of nitrogen metabolism, such as urea and creatinine. By contrast, when faced with deficits of water and/or any of the other major constituents of the body fluids, renal excretion of these substances can be curtailed, reducing the likelihood of volume or solute depletion. The purpose of this chapter is to review the excretory functions of the kidney and to examine the way these functions are affected by disease.

MECHANISMS OF RENAL EXCRETORY FUNCTION WITH NORMAL AND REDUCED NEPHRON MASS

The volume of urine excreted per day (about 1.5 L, or roughly 1 mL/min) is the small residuum of two large, and in many ways opposing, processes—namely, *ultrafiltration* of 180 L or more fluid per day (approximately 125 mL/min) across glomerular capillaries on the one hand and, on the other, *reclamation* (or *reabsorption*) of more than 99 percent of this ultrafiltrate by transport processes in the renal tubules. Under resting conditions, about 20 percent of the cardiac output passes through the kidneys, which comprise less than 1 percent of body weight. Hence, per unit weight of tissue, the rate of blood flow to the kidneys is greater than that to heart, brain, or liver.

GLOMERULAR ULTRAFILTRATION Urine formation begins with the elaboration of a protein-free ultrafiltrate of plasma across the walls of the glomerular capillaries. The rate of ultrafiltration (glomerular filtration rate, GFR) is determined by three factors: (1) the balance of pressures acting across the capillary wall (the glomerular capillary hydrostatic and Bowman's space oncotic pressures tend to favor filtration, while glomerular capillary oncotic and Bowman's space hydrostatic pressures tend to retard it), (2) the rate at which plasma flows through the glomeruli, and (3) the permeability and the total surface area of the filtering capillaries. A decrease in GFR can be expected when (1) glomerular hydrostatic pressure is reduced (as in hypotension), (2) tubule (hence Bowman's space) hydrostatic pressure is increased (ureteral or bladder neck obstruction), (3) plasma oncotic pressure rises to high levels (hemoconcentration due to dehydration, multiple myeloma, or other dysproteinemias), (4) renal (hence glomerular) blood and plasma flow are decreased (circulatory collapse, heart failure), and (5) permeability and/or total filtering surface area is reduced (acute or chronic glomerulonephritis).

Despite the high rate of water movement across the glomerular capillary wall, all but the smallest plasma proteins are normally excluded from passage through this barrier. Molecules the size of inulin (approximately 5200 mol wt) or smaller normally appear in glomerular urine in the same concentrations as in plasma water, whereas the transport of substances of increasingly greater size diminishes progressively, approaching very low values as the size of albumin is approached. The *glomerular capillary basement membrane* and the *slitlike diaphragms* that connect adjacent epithelial cell foot processes on the glomerular capillary wall (see Fig. 44-1) serve as major barriers to protein filtration. In addition, *electrostatic factors* also retard the filtration of plasma proteins, especially albumin. The albumin molecule behaves as a polyanion in physiologic solution and is therefore retarded by the anionic glycoproteins in the glomerular wall. With disruption of these mechanical and electrostatic barriers, as in many forms of glomerular injury (see Chaps. 239 to 241), large quantities of plasma proteins gain access to the urine.

BIOLOGIC CONSEQUENCES OF SUSTAINED REDUCTIONS IN GFR Measurement of total GFR of both kidneys is a sensitive index of overall renal excretory function. When renal excretory function is impaired, either acutely or chronically, one or more determinants of GFR in affected nephrons is altered unfavorably so that total GFR declines. The magnitude of decline is determined by the sum of the impairments of function of individual glomeruli. Initially, the effect of such impairments in single-nephron GFR (SNGFR), no matter how small, is to reduce the total rate of excretion of water and solutes in the glomerular ultrafiltrate. In the steady state, these reduced rates of filtration, when accompanied by comparably reduced rates of excretion, lead to *retention* and *accumulation* of the unexcreted substances in the body fluids. Further reduction in GFR augments the degree to which these substances are retained.

Figure 235-1 depicts the major response to these impairments in

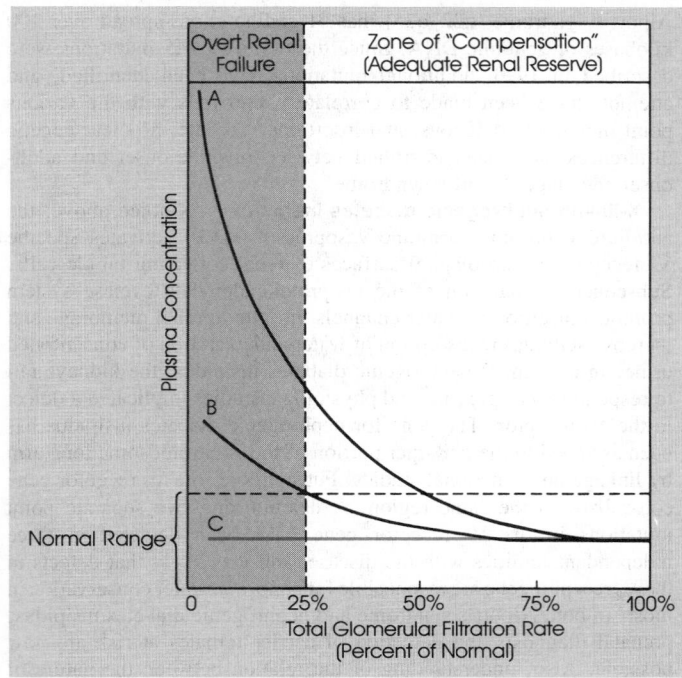

FIGURE 235-1 Representative patterns of adaptation for different types of solutes in body fluids in chronic renal failure. (*After NS Bricker et al, in Brenner and Rector, 4th ed.*)

filtration. The degree of reduction in total GFR is plotted on the abscissa, expressed as a percentage of normal (100 percent). For the various solutes normally contained in glomerular filtrate, three general types of response are common. Curve A describes the pattern with substances such as creatinine and urea which normally depend largely on glomerular filtration for excretion into the urine; i.e., urinary excretion is not appreciably influenced by secretion. Therefore, as GFR falls, plasma levels of creatinine, urea, and other substances normally excreted largely by filtration rise progressively, albeit in the nonlinear manner illustrated.

The clinical course of chronic renal failure (CRF) usually also conforms to the pattern described by curve A. Patients with CRF usually pass from a long asymptomatic period of "compensation" to a more accelerated and clinically symptomatic terminal phase. In other words, chronic forms of renal injury that lead to inexorable destruction of nephron mass usually lead to progressive but modest elevations in creatinine and urea levels in plasma but not to levels beyond the range of normal, despite loss of as much as 50 percent of total GFR. With further loss of nephron mass and further reduction in GFR, however (even though the rate of nephron destruction may not be accelerated), the limits of renal reserve are exceeded, and continued accumulation of curve A–type solutes leads to elevated plasma concentrations (see Fig. 235-1). Because these retained solutes are believed to exert "toxic" effects on all organ systems, manifestations of CRF now become overt. As a result, for patients with reduced renal mass, even small additional decrements in total GFR may spell the difference between "compensation" and overt uremia.

The accumulation of curve A–type solutes with progressive renal failure continues until external balance is achieved, i.e., until acquisition and/or production rates and excretion rates are exactly matched. In the case of creatinine, for example, assuming a constant rate of creatinine production, a 50 percent reduction in GFR results in an approximate doubling of the plasma creatinine concentration. The latter restores the filtered load of creatinine (i.e., GFR × plasma creatinine concentration) to normal, and the urinary excretion rate again is equivalent to creatinine production. Unfortunately, since no mechanism exists for augmenting creatinine excretion beyond this level, elimination of retained creatinine is not possible, and plasma concentration remains twice normal. With progressive reduction in GFR, plasma creatinine levels continue to rise, due both to the recent loss of nephron excretory function and to the retention associated with earlier nephron destruction (see Fig. 235-1). *In practice, so long as the net rates of acquisition and production (i.e., liver function and muscle mass) remain reasonably constant, the inverse relationship between plasma concentrations of solutes such as creatinine and urea and GFR is sufficiently reliable and predictable to allow plasma levels of the solutes to serve as clinical indexes of GFR.*

In contrast to solutes of the curve A type, plasma levels of phosphate, urate, and potassium (K^+) and hydrogen (H^+) ions usually do not rise until GFR falls to a small percentage of normal. With progressive renal failure this pattern of response (curve B in Fig. 235-1) reflects the participation of tubule transport mechanisms in the excretion of these substances. In other words, *as GFR declines, the tubules facilitate the excretion of greater fractions of the filtered load of these solutes, either by enhancing net secretion and/or by diminishing net reabsorption.* Plasma levels of curve B–type solutes, therefore, rise less than those of curve A because, with progressive reduction in GFR, *excretion rate per nephron* and, therefore, *fractional excretion* both increase. Eventually, however, enhanced fractional excretion can no longer offset the reduction in the filtered load of these solutes caused by a diminished GFR, and plasma levels rise (see Fig. 235-1). For urate, phosphate, and K^+, at least, increased fractional excretion serves to maintain normal plasma levels until GFR falls to less than one-fourth of normal.

Finally, for certain solutes, such as sodium chloride (NaCl), concentrations in plasma remain normal throughout the course of CRF, despite continued ingestion of these substances in normal amounts (curve C in Fig. 235-1). The compensation represents a fundamental adaptation to renal injury. To illustrate the magnitude of the adaptation involved, it is useful to compare the excretion of Na^+ in a normal individual (GFR of 125 mL/min) with that in advanced renal insufficiency (GFR of 2 mL/min). Both subjects are allowed to ingest a diet containing 7 g salt per day (120 mmol Na^+). With a normal serum Na^+ concentration of 140 mmol/L, external Na^+ balance is normally achieved by excreting approximately 0.5 percent of the filtered load. By contrast, for external balance to be maintained in the patient with CRF, fractional excretion of Na^+ must rise to 30 percent. *In other words, external balance for Na^+ demands that the same quantity of Na^+ (120 mmol) be excreted into the urine each day in the subject with CRF as in the normal subject.* Given the drastic reduction in GFR in CRF, external balance can be achieved only by transformation of the Na^+ reabsorptive processes in surviving tubules so that a progressively larger fraction of the filtered load of Na^+ escapes reabsorption and appears in final urine. In short, *the rate of excretion of Na^+ per surviving nephron increases in inverse proportion to the composite GFR of surviving nephrons.*

MECHANISMS OF TUBULE TRANSPORT WITH NORMAL AND REDUCED NEPHRON MASS   Loss of renal function with progressive renal disease is usually attended by distortion of renal morphology and architecture. Despite this structural disarray, glomerular and tubule functions often remain as closely integrated (i.e., *glomerulotubular balance*) as in the normal organ, at least until the final stages of CRF. A fundamental feature of this *intact nephron hypothesis* is that following loss of nephron mass, renal function is due primarily to the operation of surviving healthy nephrons, while the diseased nephrons cease functioning. Despite progressive nephron destruction, many of the mechanisms that control solute and water balance differ only quantitatively, and not qualitatively, from those that operate normally. The most important of these are considered below.

Tubule transport of sodium chloride and water   Most of the filtered water and Na^+ salts are reabsorbed by the tubules, leaving small and variable amounts, equivalent on average to the quantities ingested, to reach the final urine. About two-thirds of the glomerular ultrafiltrate is reabsorbed in the *proximal tubule* with little change in

the osmolality or Na^+ concentration of the unreabsorbed fraction (Fig. 235-2). In other words, fluid reabsorption in the proximal tubule is nearly *isosmotic* and is coupled to the active transport of Na^+. Since Cl^- and HCO_3^- are the primary anions in the extracellular fluid, most of the filtered Na^+ is reabsorbed with these anions. In the early convoluted portion of the proximal tubule, bicarbonate is the principal anion accompanying the reabsorption of sodium. This process occurs via a Na^+/H^+ exchange mechanism at the luminal brush border and is dependent on carbonic anhydrase. Glucose, amino acids, and other organic solutes (e.g., lactate) are also extensively reabsorbed in the proximal convoluted tubule by a cotransport process that links the cellular entry of these organic substrates with Na^+. Three processes appear to operate in parallel to couple water (i.e., volume) absorption with solute absorption. First, given the remarkably high water permeability of this nephron segment, very small transepithelial osmolality differences, i.e., *luminal hypotonicity* on the order of 2 to 3 mosmol, produced by solute absorption, could drive volume absorption. Second, due to the *preferential* absorption of HCO_3^- and organic solutes in the early portions of the proximal tubule, the concentrations of these substances decrease while that of Cl^- increases along the proximal tubule. Volume absorption would occur if the rate of Na^+ and Cl^- diffusion down their respective electrochemical gradients were more rapid than the back diffusion of sodium bicarbonate into the lumen. Finally, an *effective osmotic gradient* would be established (despite equal macroscopic osmolalities of luminal and peritubular fluids) if the effective osmolality of Cl^- in the lumen were greater than that for bicarbonate in the peritubular fluid.

The rate of reabsorption of fluid from proximal convoluted tubules and peritubular interstitium is sensitive to *physical factors*, i.e., the hydrostatic and colloid osmotic (or oncotic) pressures across the walls of the peritubular capillaries. Because the plasma proteins in glomerular capillaries are concentrated by ultrafiltration, there is a marked rise in the oncotic pressure along the glomerular capillary network. This step-up in plasma oncotic pressure is transmitted largely unchanged to the peritubular capillaries, via the efferent arterioles. These resistance vessels cause a substantial drop in hydrostatic pressure, however, so that when the plasma reaches the peritubular capillaries, oncotic pressure greatly exceeds hydrostatic pressure. These *Starling forces* are therefore oriented in an *uptake mode*, in contrast to the *filtration mode* at the glomerulus, where hydrostatic pressure exceeds oncotic pressure. The extent to which oncotic pressure exceeds hydrostatic pressure in the peritubular capillary network modulates the overall rate of reabsorption of fluid by the proximal tubules. Therefore, when peritubular oncotic pressure falls or hydrostatic pressure rises, uptake of fluid by these capillaries is reduced. As a result, fluid is retained in the interstitial space, altering the hydrostatic pressure in the space and ultimately retarding the egress of fluid from the lateral intercellular channels. Without an adequate route of drainage, fluid in the channels leaks back into the tubule lumen and diminishes *net fluid reabsorption* by this tubule segment. The opposite occurs in states in which peritubular oncotic pressure increases (increased filtration fraction) or hydrostatic pressure decreases (enhanced efferent arteriolar tone). Under these circumstances, peritubular capillary uptake of reabsorbate is augmented, leading ultimately to *enhanced net fluid reabsorption* by the proximal tubule.

In contrast to the proximal tubule, active outward transport of NaCl from tubule lumen to peritubular blood has not been established for the *thin ascending limb of Henle's loop*. However, passive outward salt transport does occur, as indicated in Fig. 235-2. In the next segment of the nephron, the *medullary thick ascending limb of Henle*, the concentration of NaCl is reduced below that at the beginning of this segment. Here Cl^- absorption occurs by an active process involving a furosemide-sensitive $Na^+:K^+:2Cl^-$ cotransport mechanism in the luminal membrane, with one-half of Na^+ absorption proceeding passively, driven by the lumen-positive transepithelial voltage. Since the ascending limb of Henle is impermeable to water, net NaCl reabsorption generates hypotonic tubule fluid and gives rise

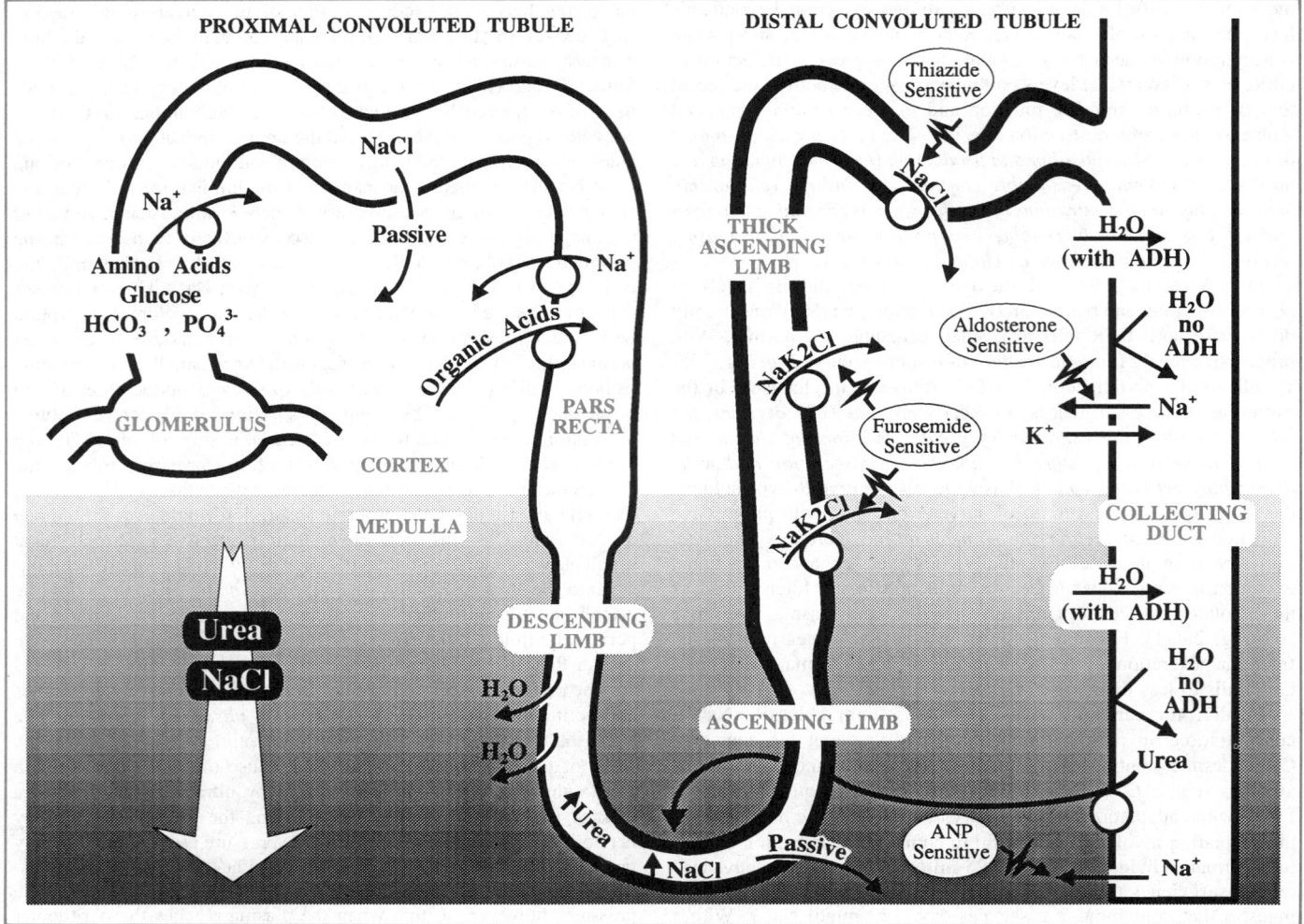

FIGURE 235-2 Transport functions of the various anatomic segments of the mammalian nephron. Fluid reabsorption across the proximal tubule is isosmotic and accounts for reabsorption of approximately two-thirds of the filtered Na^+ and H_2O. The major portions of the filtered HCO_3^-, amino acids, glucose, and phosphate are reabsorbed in the early proximal convoluted tubule. Reabsorption of glucose and amino acids is coupled to Na^+ transport and thereby generates a negative potential difference within the tubule lumen. At the same time, HCO_3^- is reabsorbed by a nonelectrogenic mechanism, via H^+ secretion. The active transport of these solutes results in transepithelial concentration and effective osmotic pressure gradients promoting H_2O flow across the proximal tubule, into the peritubular capillaries. The rise in tubule fluid Cl^- concentration is a necessary reciprocal consequence of the decreased luminal HCO_3^- concentration. The resultant high concentration of Cl^- becomes an important force for the outward passive transport of Cl^- down its concentration gradient, resulting in a lumen-positive potential difference in the late proximal convoluted tubule. The pars recta of the proximal tubule is capable of active electrogenic transport of Na^+ independent of organic solute transport. Under normal conditions, approximately one-third of the glomerular filtrate enters the descending limb of Henle's loop. Because the thin descending limb is incapable of active outward NaCl transport and is characterized by low permeability to Na^+ but high H_2O permeability, H_2O is abstracted passively as the fluid approaches the bend of Henle's loop. Hypertonic fluid

with a greater NaCl concentration but lower urea concentration than the surrounding medullary interstitium thus enters the thin ascending limb of Henle, which is largely impermeable to H_2O and urea but highly permeable to NaCl. This permits passive diffusion of NaCl outward. Active NaK_2Cl transport across the water-impermeable thick ascending limb of Henle allows for separation of solute and water. In consequence, tubule fluid becomes dilute and the medullary interstitium hypertonic.

Irrespective of the final osmolality of the urine, the fluid that enters the distal convoluted tubule is always hypoosmotic. This segment exhibits active Na^+ reabsorption. All but the terminal portion of the distal convoluted tubule is water-impermeable, even in the presence of ADH. Aldosterone exerts its effect in this segment by enhancing Na^+ reabsorption, which is variably coupled to K^+ and H^+ secretion. The cortical and papillary portions of the collecting duct are sites where ADH exerts its principal effect. The permeability of these segments to H_2O in the absence of ADH is very low but can be greatly enhanced in the presence of ADH. These segments are also characterized by active Na^+ reabsorption, which appears to depend on the presence of mineralocorticoid. In the absence of ADH, the collecting tubule is water impermeable so that hypotonic tubule fluid courses through it. However, in the presence of ADH, water is avidly reabsorbed here, resulting in hypertonic final urine. Sites of action of furosemide and thiazide diuretics and of aldosterone and atrial natriuretic peptide (ANP) are shown.

to the high NaCl concentration of the outer medullary interstitium (see Fig. 235-2). In certain animals, vasopressin (AVP or ADH) enhances NaCl absorption but not water permeability in the medullary portion of the thick ascending limb, but whether this occurs in human beings is uncertain.

The fluid leaving the thick ascending limb of Henle is normally low in NaCl concentration, a condition largely independent of the

organism's diet or state of hydration. In the *distal convoluted tubule*, water reabsorption is variable, depending on the state of hydration or, more specifically, on the presence or absence of AVP in plasma. In the absence of AVP, this and more distal nephron segments are impermeable to water, so the hypotonic fluid entering this segment is excreted as *dilute urine*. Indeed, continued salt reabsorption along the distal convoluted tubule, a process that can be initiated by thiazide diuretics, results in further dilution of the urine. In the presence of AVP, the permeability of the late portion of this segment to water increases, and as a result, the osmolality of the tubule fluid rises to a value close to that of plasma. NaCl continues to be reabsorbed from the tubule lumen, against moderately steep chemical and electrical gradients. The reabsorption of NaCl at this site is enhanced by *aldosterone*.

The *cortical collecting tubule* possesses a low permeability to water in the absence of AVP, whereas permeability increases in the presence of the hormone. The sensitivity of this segment to AVP appears to be more pronounced than that of the distal convoluted tubule. As with the distal convoluted tubule, the cortical collecting tubule is capable of active reabsorption of NaCl.

The terminal segment of the distal nephron is the highly branched *papillary collecting duct*. Continued electrolyte transport in this segment results in the large ion concentration differences that normally exist between urine and plasma. As in the cortical collecting tubule, Na$^+$ transport appears to be active, since reabsorption proceeds against sizable electrochemical gradients. The rate of Na$^+$ transport in this segment depends on the load of Na$^+$ delivered from more proximal segments and is affected by aldosterone. The permeability to water also increases markedly in the presence of AVP.

Effects of reduced nephron mass on sodium chloride transport in surviving nephrons With reductions in nephron mass, the remaining healthy or less damaged nephrons may hypertrophy so that GFR is increased toward normal. For example, a patient with a unilateral nephrectomy loses one-half of the nephron mass, and GFR is reduced by 50 percent at the time of surgery. However, within several months, GFR may return to 80 percent of the preoperative value for two kidneys. This requires that the blood flow, GFR, and transport functions of individual remaining nephrons increase above normal. This "compensatory hypertrophy" is evident by the large glomeruli and tubules observed on histologic sections and by increases in many of the biochemical processes associated with tubule transport (e.g., Na$^+$,K$^+$-ATPase). Similar hypertrophic changes occur in nephrons from kidneys damaged by other processes (e.g., glomerulonephritis); however, as nephron damage progresses, the hypertrophy of single nephrons can no longer make up for the magnitude of nephron loss, and GFR falls.

With progressive destruction, *maintenance of external balance for NaCl requires that fractional salt excretion increase as GFR decreases*. Several mechanisms contribute to this adaptive increase in fractional excretion. With losses of functioning nephron units, peritubular capillary hydrostatic and oncotic pressures are probably altered in directions that serve to suppress proximal tubule reabsorption of NaCl and water. For example, a rise in peritubular capillary hydrostatic pressure, which tends to inhibit net proximal fluid reabsorption, might be anticipated with hypertension, a common feature of renal insufficiency. Similarly, peritubular oncotic pressure probably declines with renal injury, owing both to reductions in filtration fraction and to hypoalbuminemia. Aldosterone, normally an important determinant of Na$^+$ reabsorption in distal portions of the nephron, is probably not a major factor responsible for reducing fractional Na$^+$ reabsorption, since levels in plasma are rarely reduced in CRF. Furthermore, external Na$^+$ balance is preserved in bilaterally adrenalectomized, uremic dogs maintained on fixed doses of mineralocorticoid. Yet another factor contributing to the suppression of fractional NaCl reabsorption in CRF may relate to the retention of solutes as GFR declines. In addition to urea and creatinine, *organic acids* (including *hippurates*) also accumulate. These substances are normally excreted by both filtration and tubule secretion; the latter process involves a carrier-mediated organic acid transport system in proximal tubule epithelia. When GFR is reduced and plasma levels of these organic acids increase, sufficient fluid may accompany their secretion into the proximal tubule lumen (by osmosis) to diminish net fluid reabsorption and even favor net fluid secretion. Evidence for this mechanism derives from studies in which uremic sera induced net fluid secretion in isolated proximal tubules of rabbits in vitro.

Several factors that regulate NaCl transport across the tubules also may participate in the enhanced fractional excretion of salt in renal insufficiency. Atrial natriuretic peptide is released from the cardiac atria in response to plasma volume expansion and atrial distention. This hormone effects a natriuresis by reducing net sodium reabsorption through complementary actions on active collecting duct Na$^+$ transport and on physical factors within the adjacent vasa recta. In addition, prostaglandin E reduces NaCl reabsorption from the thick ascending limb. Since prostaglandin E production per nephron appears to rise in renal insufficiency, the local action of this prostaglandin also may contribute to natriuresis in the setting of reduced renal mass. Finally, other inhibitors of ion transport appear in uremic serum, including an inhibitor(s) of the Na$^+$,K$^+$-ATPase. This factor(s) has not been fully characterized, and whether it represents an adaptation for maintenance of homeostasis or an unregulated accumulation of a toxin is also uncertain.

Serum and urine from patients with uremia contain factors capable of inhibiting NaCl transport across frog skin, toad bladder, and rat renal tubule. Accumulation of natriuretic factors in uremia may not be without cost; the "trade-off" for maintenance of external Na$^+$ balance is the possibility of abnormalities occurring in Na$^+$ transport across cell membranes, which often occurs in advanced renal insufficiency (see Chap. 237).

The obligatory high rate of solute excretion per surviving nephron (so-called osmotic diuresis due to urea and other retained solutes) also contributes to enhancing fractional NaCl excretion, much as occurs in normal subjects following administration of nonreabsorbable solutes such as mannitol. Finally, certain forms of CRF tend to be associated with unusually large salt losses in urine. These *salt-wasting nephropathies* include chronic pyelonephritis and other tubulointerstitial diseases (see Chap. 242) as well as polycystic and medullary cystic diseases. These disorders have in common greater destruction of medullary and interstitial than cortical and glomerular portions of the renal parenchyma. Preferential impairment of tubule reabsorptive function, rather than a primary reduction in GFR, may, therefore, underlie the salt-losing tendency in these disorders. Clinical derangements that alter renal handling of NaCl in CRF (including hypo- and hypervolemia, hypertension, etc.) are considered in Chap. 237.

Effects of reduced nephron mass on water reabsorption in surviving nephrons As with NaCl, there is a progressive increase in the fractional excretion of water with advancing renal insufficiency so that external water balance can be maintained even with a total GFR of 5 mL/min or less. The adaptations in the handling of water by the diseased kidney are of importance in the urinary concentrating defect and, hence, the polyuria and nocturia seen commonly in CRF (see Chap. 44). To appreciate the mechanisms involved, the responses of a normal and a uremic subject in maintaining external water balance need to be compared. Assuming that both subjects ingest the same diet and the same amount of fluid, total solute and volume excretion in each subject should be identical as well. If the *obligatory solute load* to be excreted in each is 600 mmol/d (600 mosmol/d), and urine osmolality is 300 mmol/kg water (300 mosmol/kg), a urine volume of 2 L/d will be required to excrete the total solute. If GFR in normal and uremic subjects is 180 and 4 L/d, respectively, urinary volume excretion of 2 L/d represents excretion of slightly more than 1 percent of the filtered water in the normal individual, compared with 50 percent in the uremic subject. Since the range of urine osmolalities that the diseased kidney can achieve [250 to 350 mmol/kg (250 to 350 mosmol/kg)] is narrower than in the normal [40 to 1200 mmol/kg (40 to 1200 mosmol/kg)], the individual with normal function is able to excrete the obligatory daily solute load of 600 mmol (600 mosmol) in as little as 500 mL urine per day or as much as 15 L/d, compared with the narrower range in renal insufficiency, from about 1.7 to 2.4 L/d.

In CRF, the limited ability to concentrate the urine usually correlates with other measures of impaired renal function. Isosthenuria is therefore a nearly universal finding when GFR falls below 25 mL/min. At this level of GFR and below, urine osmolality does not rise even with supraphysiologic doses of vasopressin, suggesting that the concentrating defect is related both to loss of diseased nephrons and to impaired concentrating ability in surviving nephrons. As has been discussed, with diminution in functioning nephron mass, there is a concurrent increase in fractional excretion of a number of solutes. As a consequence, solute diuresis per nephron obligates a nearly isosmotic amount of water and prevents the elaboration of either hypotonic or hypertonic urine. Disease-induced abnormalities of the architecture of the renal medulla (loops of Henle, vasa recta), aberrations in renal medullary blood flow, and defective transport of NaCl in the ascending limb of Henle also contribute to this defect in urine concentration. Finally, uremia per se may impair the responsiveness of terminal nephron segments to vasopressin.

Since patients with renal insufficiency are unable to excrete concentrated urine, they must have access to adequate amounts of water to ensure the excretion of total daily solute loads. For this reason, restriction of fluid intake may be hazardous in patients with CRF. Likewise, impairment of diluting capacity may prevent many patients from excreting large amounts of ingested fluids. The consequences of the abnormal water excretion patterns in CRF, including the tendencies to development of hypo- and hypernatremia, are considered in Chaps. 45 and 237.

Tubule transport of phosphate with normal and reduced nephron mass Under normal physiologic conditions, about 80 to 90 percent of the filtered load of phosphate is reabsorbed, mainly in the proximal tubule. *Parathyroid hormone* (*PTH*), by augmenting phosphate excretion via inhibition of this proximal reabsorptive process (Chap. 356), plays a key role in phosphate homeostasis. When dietary phosphate intake increases, a *transient* rise in plasma phosphate concentration is usually observed. This results in a similarly transient reduction in the plasma ionized calcium concentration (due largely to calcium phosphate deposition in bone), which, in turn, stimulates PTH secretion. By enhancing fractional phosphate excretion, PTH restores external phosphate balance and normophosphatemia. This then enables plasma ionized calcium levels to return to normal, thereby removing the stimulus to PTH release and restoring the phosphate control system to the original steady state.

With advancing renal disease and constant dietary intake of phosphate, external phosphate balance is achieved by progressive reduction in fractional phosphate reabsorption. Enhanced PTH secretion is an important determinant of this phosphaturic response. With each succeeding decrement in GFR, the total amount of phosphate filtered by surviving glomeruli is reduced, leading to transient retention of phosphate and, therefore, a rise (albeit small) in the phosphate concentration in extracellular fluid, including plasma. This rise in plasma phosphate concentration leads to a reciprocal small decline in plasma ionized calcium concentration and a corresponding increase in PTH secretion. Although the phosphaturic response of surviving tubules to this elevation in circulating PTH restores plasma phosphate and, therefore, calcium levels to normal (at least in the "compensated" stage of CRF described by the relatively flat portion of curve *B* in Fig. 235-1), the biologic cost of this return to normophosphatemia and normocalcemia is a *persistent elevation in the plasma PTH level*. With successive decrements in GFR, each stage in this overall process is repeated, but at an ever-increasing cost, namely, *progressive elevation in the circulating level of PTH*.

Alterations in vitamin D metabolism also contribute to the elevated PTH levels in renal failure. The kidneys are normally the major site of *metabolic conversion of vitamin D to its active metabolites*. As discussed in Chap. 356, vitamin D, synthesized in skin or acquired from foods, undergoes initial hydroxylation in the liver to form 25-hydroxyvitamin D [25(OH)D]. The kidney is the site of a second important hydroxylation, formation of 1,25-dihydroxyvitamin D [1,25(OH)$_2$D]. This activated form of vitamin D acts directly on the parathyroid gland to suppress PTH secretion as well as to enhance intestinal calcium and phosphate absorption and promote resorption of these ions from bone. In addition, 1,25(OH)$_2$D probably opposes the phosphaturic action of PTH in the renal tubule by augmenting,

rather than diminishing, phosphate reabsorption. With advancing renal disease, reduction in renal mass causes vitamin D hydroxylation to be impaired; phosphate retention also suppresses this reaction. Not only are the circulating levels of 1,25(OH)$_2$D diminished in uremia, but the receptors that mediate its action within the parathyroid cells are also diminished. These two effects disinhibit parathyroid hormone secretion and thereby increase circulating PTH levels. Reduction in circulating 1,25(OH)$_2$D levels, by suppressing calcium absorption from gut, contributes to the development of the hypocalcemia and PTH excess of CRF (see Chap. 237).

At least two additional processes are thought to contribute to elevated PTH levels in renal failure. One relates to the skeletal resistance to the calcemic effect of PTH in uremia. This resistance necessitates a higher level of circulating PTH to effect an increment in serum calcium concentration. The other derives from the finding that reductions in renal mass impair the ability of the kidneys to degrade circulating PTH. The fact that phosphate conforms more to a curve *B*– than curve *C*–type solute in Fig. 235-1 indicates that these forms of adaptation are limited; ultimately, phosphate retention occurs when GFR falls below about 25 mL/min.

Since PTH exerts major biologic effects on bone, as well as renal tubules, the external balance of phosphate in CRF is achieved at the expense of elevated PTH levels, which, in turn, account for many of the bone changes of renal osteodystrophy (i.e., *secondary hyperparathyroidism*; see Fig. 237-1). In support of this *trade-off hypothesis*, when dietary phosphate intake is reduced in proportion to the reduction in GFR in animals with CRF, external balance of phosphate no longer requires augmentation of fractional phosphate excretion in surviving nephrons. Accordingly, circulating PTH levels no longer rise, and the bone changes of secondary hyperparathyroidism are diminished, if not prevented.

Hydrogen and bicarbonate transport with normal and reduced nephron mass As discussed in Chap. 46, the pH of extracellular fluid is normally maintained within a narrow range (7.36 to 7.44) despite day-to-day variations in the quantity of acids entering the body fluids from dietary and metabolic sources (approximately 1 mmol H$^+$ per kilogram of body weight per day). These acids consume both intracellular and extracellular buffers, of which bicarbonate (HCO$_3^-$) is the most important in the intracellular compartment. Such buffering minimizes the changes in pH. The HCO$_3^-$ buffer system would be of little long-term benefit were it not for homeostatic mechanisms, however, since with unrelenting acquisition of nonvolatile acids from dietary and metabolic sources, buffering capacity would ultimately be exhausted, culminating in fatal acidosis. The kidneys normally function to prevent this possibility by *regenerating* HCO$_3^-$ and, thereby, maintaining the concentration of HCO$_3^-$ in the plasma. In addition to generating HCO$_3^-$, the kidneys also *reclaim* the HCO$_3^-$ in the glomerular ultrafiltrate. This reabsorptive process takes place largely in the proximal tubule and is virtually complete below a critical serum HCO$_3^-$ concentration—the threshold concentration—which in humans is normally about 26 mmol/L, identical to the concentration of HCO$_3^-$ in plasma. As a consequence, urinary wastage of HCO$_3^-$ is prevented. Alternatively, when plasma HCO$_3^-$ rises above this threshold, reabsorption becomes less complete, and the excess HCO$_3^-$ escapes into the final urine, returning the plasma HCO$_3^-$ to the threshold level. Despite reabsorption of all the filtered HCO$_3^-$, metabolic acidosis would still ensue if HCO$_3^-$ consumed in buffering nonvolatile strong acids were not constantly regenerated.

The *reabsorption* of filtered HCO$_3^-$ in the proximal tubule occurs by the following mechanism. In proximal tubule cells, H$^+$, formed by the splitting of water into H$^+$ and OH$^-$, is secreted into the tubule lumen, very likely in exchange for Na$^+$. The OH$^-$ ion, under the influence of *carbonic anhydrase*, combines with CO$_2$ to form HCO$_3^-$, which moves across the peritubular cell membrane via an electrogenic Na(HCO$_3$)$_2$ cotransporter to enter the extracellular HCO$_3^-$ pool. The H$^+$ secreted into the tubule lumen combines with a filtered HCO$_3^-$, forming H$_2$CO$_3$. Dehydration of the latter in the proximal tubule lumen leads to the formation of CO$_2$, which also diffuses from lumen to peritubular blood. As a result, *a filtered HCO₃⁻ ion is reclaimed.* Secreted H⁺ ions are also free to combine with non-HCO₃⁻ buffers (e.g., phosphate or ammonia) in the tubule fluid and are excreted in these forms in the final urine. HCO_3^-, the other original product of the breakdown of H_2CO_3, formed within the tubule cell, enters the peritubular blood, and *an HCO₃⁻ ion is regenerated.*

Hydrogen ions in the urine are bound primarily to filtered buffers (e.g., phosphate) in an amount (the so-called titratable acid) equivalent to the amount of alkali required to titrate the pH of the urine to the pH of blood. It is usually not possible, however, to excrete all the daily acid load as titratable acid alone. Metabolism of glutamine by proximal tubule cells to form ammonium (i.e., ammoniagenesis) serves as an additional mechanism for bicarbonate regeneration. Glutamine metabolism forms not only NH_4^+ (i.e., NH_3 plus H⁺) but also HCO_3^- which is transported across the proximal tubule (HCO_3^- regeneration). The generated NH_4^+ must be excreted in urine for this process to be effective in bicarbonate regeneration. The excretion of ammonium involves secretion by proximal tubule cells (possibly on the Na:H exchanger as $Na^+:NH_4^+$), generation of high medullary interstitial NH_4^+ concentration by an elaborate countercurrent multiplication/exchange system, and finally, secretion of the interstitial NH_4^+ by the collecting duct by a combination of H⁺ secretion and passive NH_3 diffusion. *Ammoniagenesis* is responsive to the acid-base needs of the individual. When faced with an acute acid burden and an increased need for HCO₃⁻- regeneration, the rate of renal ammonia synthesis increases sharply.

The quantity of hydrogen ions excreted as titratable acid and NH_4^+ is equal to the quantity of HCO_3^- regenerated in tubule cells and added to the plasma. Under steady state conditions, the quantity of net acid excreted into the urine (the sum of titratable acid and NH_4^+ minus HCO_3^-) must equal the quantity of acid gained by the extracellular fluid from all sources. Metabolic acidosis and alkalosis result when this delicate balance is perturbed, the former the result of *insufficient* net acid excretion and the latter due to *excessive* acid excretion.

Progressive loss of renal function usually causes little or no change in arterial pH, plasma bicarbonate concentration, or arterial carbon dioxide tension (P_{CO_2}) until GFR falls below 50 percent of normal. Thereafter, all three quantities tend to decline as *metabolic acidosis* ensues. In general, the metabolic acidosis of CRF is not due to overproduction of endogenous acids but is largely a reflection of the reduction in renal mass, which limits the amount of NH_3 (and therefore HCO_3^-) that can be generated. Although surviving nephrons are probably capable of generating supernormal quantities of NH_3 *per nephron*, the diminished nephron population causes overall NH_3 production to be reduced to an extent inadequate to permit sufficient buffering of H⁺ in urine. Although patients with CRF may acidify the urine normally (i.e., urine pH as low as 4.5), the defect in NH_3 production limits total daily acid excretion to 30 to 40 mmol, or one-half to two-thirds the quantity of nonvolatile acid formed in the same time period. Metabolic acidosis is the inevitable consequence of this positive balance for H⁺, which in most patients with stable CRF is relatively mild and nonprogressive (arterial pH of approximately 7.33 to 7.37).

Given this substantial daily accumulation of H⁺ and the typically stable and nonprogressive nature of the resulting acidosis, including the observed relative constancy of the plasma HCO_3^- concentration (albeit at reduced levels of 14 to 20 mmol/L), it follows that some large tissue source of buffering must account for the stability of the acidosis in CRF. Bone is the likely candidate, in view of its large reservoir of alkaline salts (calcium phosphate and calcium carbonate). Dissolution of this buffer source probably contributes to the osteodystrophy of CRF (see Fig. 237-1).

Although the acidosis of CRF is due to the reduction in total renal mass and is therefore tubular in origin, it nevertheless depends to a large extent on the level of GFR. When GFR is reduced to only a moderate extent (i.e., to about 50 percent of normal), retention of anions, principally sulfates and phosphates, is not pronounced, so as the plasma HCO_3^- level falls owing to tubule dysfunction, retention of Cl^- by the kidneys leads to the development of *hyperchloremic acidosis.* At this stage, therefore, *the anion gap is normal.* With further reduction in GFR and more pronounced azotemia, however, retention of phosphates, sulfates, and other *unmeasured* anions is the rule, and plasma Cl^- concentration falls to normal levels despite the reduction in plasma HCO_3^- concentration. *A moderate to large anion gap therefore develops.*

Tubule potassium transport with normal and reduced nephron mass   As with H⁺, the concentration of K⁺ in extracellular fluid is normally maintained within a relatively narrow range, 4 to 5 mmol/L. Ninety-five percent or more of total-body K⁺ is in the intracellular fluid compartment, where the intracellular concentration is approximately 160 mmol/L. Normal individuals maintain external K⁺ balance by excreting into the urine an amount of K⁺ per day equivalent to the amount ingested, minus the relatively small amounts lost in stool and sweat. K⁺ is freely filtered at the glomerulus, although the amount excreted usually represents no more than about 20 percent of the quantity filtered. The great bulk of the filtered K⁺ is *reabsorbed* in the early portions of the nephron, about two-thirds in the proximal tubule, and an additional 20 to 25 percent in the loop of Henle. A K⁺ *secretory process* operates in the distal tubule and terminal nephron segments. This process is largely dependent on Na⁺ reabsorption and the accompanying lumen-negative voltage creating an electrical gradient across the tubule wall, favoring K⁺ secretion into the lumen of distal tubule and collecting duct.

The ability to maintain external K⁺ balance and normal plasma K⁺ concentration until relatively late in the course of CRF is a consequence primarily of a progressive increase in fractional excretion of K⁺. Greatly enhanced rates of K⁺ secretion occur in distal portions of surviving tubules. The augmented secretion rate of aldosterone contributes to enhanced tubule secretion of K⁺. In addition, both the increased distal tubule flow rates in residual functioning nephrons due to the osmotic diuresis and the enhanced luminal electronegativity created by the increased concentration of highly impermeable anions such as phosphate and sulfate enhance K⁺ excretion. Aldosterone also stimulates net entry of K⁺ into the lumen of the colon, a mechanism known to be enhanced in CRF. More detailed discussions of the abnormalities in K⁺ homeostasis in acute and chronic forms of renal failure are given in Chaps. 236 and 237.

REFERENCES

Brenner BM: Nephron adaptation to renal injury or ablation. Am J Physiol 249:F324, 1985

———— et al: Diverse biological actions of atrial natriuretic peptide. Physiol Rev 70:665, 1990

————, Rector FC Jr (eds): *The Kidney*, 4th ed. Philadelphia, Saunders, 1991

Feinfeld DA, Sherwood LM: Parathyroid hormone and 1,25(OH)₂D₃ in chronic renal failure. Kidney Int 33:1049, 1988

Kaji D, Kahn T: Na⁺-K⁺ pump in chronic renal failure. Am J Physiol 252:F785, 1987

Maxwell MH et al: *Clinical Disorders of Fluid and Electrolyte Metabolism*, 4th ed. New York, McGraw-Hill, 1987

Warnock DG: Uremic acidosis. Kidney Int 34:278, 1988

236   ACUTE RENAL FAILURE

HUGH R. BRADY / BARRY M. BRENNER

Acute renal failure (ARF) is characterized by rapid decline in glomerular filtration rate (hours to weeks) and retention of nitrogenous waste products. This syndrome occurs in approximately 5 percent of all hospital admissions and up to 30 percent of admissions to intensive care units. Oliguria (urine output <400 mL/d) is frequent (~50 percent) but not invariable. ARF is usually asymptomatic and is diagnosed when screening of hospitalized patients reveals a recent increase in serum blood urea nitrogen (BUN) and creatinine. ARF may complicate a wide range of diseases which for purposes of diagnosis and management are conveniently divided into three categories: (1) disorders of renal hypoperfusion in which the kidney is intrinsically normal (*prerenal azotemia, prerenal ARF*) (~55 percent), (2) diseases of the renal parenchyma (*renal azotemia, intrinsic renal ARF*) (~40 percent), and (3) acute obstruction of the urinary tract (*postrenal azotemia, postrenal ARF*) (~5 percent). Although usually reversible, ARF is a major cause of in-hospital morbidity and mortality due to the serious nature of the underlying illnesses and the high incidence of complications.

ETIOLOGY AND PATHOPHYSIOLOGY Prerenal azotemia (prerenal ARF)

This is responsible for half of cases. This syndrome is due to a functional response to renal hypoperfusion and is rapidly reversible upon restoration of renal blood flow and glomerular ultrafiltration pressure. Renal parenchymal tissue is not damaged; indeed, kidneys from individuals with prerenal azotemia function well when transplanted into recipients with normal cardiovascular function. However, severe or prolonged hypoperfusion may lead to ischemic renal parenchymal injury and intrinsic renal azotemia. Prerenal azotemia can complicate a variety of hemodynamic disturbances, including hypovolemia, low cardiac output, systemic vasodilatation, and selective renal vasoconstriction (Table 236-1).

Intravascular volume depletion sufficient to cause ARF may result from hemorrhage (e.g., surgical, traumatic, gastrointestinal), burns, dehydration, gastrointestinal fluid losses (e.g., vomiting, diarrhea, surgical drainage), urinary tract fluid losses (e.g., drug-induced or osmotic diuresis), or sequestration of fluid in extravascular compartments (e.g., peritonitis, pancreatitis, trauma, burns, or severe hypoalbuminemia). Prerenal azotemia also may occur when *"effective" arterial blood volume* is decreased despite normal or expanded intravascular volume. "Effective" hypovolemia may complicate *low cardiac output states* (e.g., myocardial, valvular, or pericardial disease, complicated arrhythmias) and diseases characterized by *systemic vasodilatation* (e.g., sepsis, vasodilator therapy, anesthesia, anaphylaxis).

True or "effective" hypovolemia leads to a fall in mean arterial pressure that is detected as reduced stretch by arterial (e.g., carotid sinus) and cardiac baroreceptors. The latter trigger a series of neurohumoral responses designed to maintain arterial pressure. These include activation of the sympathetic nervous system and renin-angiotensin-aldosterone system and release of vasopressin (AVP; ADH) and endothelin. Norepinephrine, angiotensin II, AVP, and endothelin cause vasoconstriction in musculocutaneous and splanchnic vascular beds, reduce salt loss through sweat glands, stimulate thirst and salt appetite, and promote renal salt and water retention. As a result, cardiac and cerebral perfusion is preserved relative to that of other "less essential" organs. Several renal responses combine to maintain glomerular perfusion and filtration in this setting. Stretch receptors in afferent arterioles, in response to a reduction in perfusion pressure, trigger relaxation of arteriolar smooth-muscle cells and vasodilatation (autoregulation). Biosynthesis of vasodilator renal prostaglandins (e.g., prostacyclin, prostaglandin E_2) and nitric oxide is also enhanced, and these compounds preferentially dilate afferent arterioles. In addition, angiotensin II induces preferential constriction of efferent arterioles, probably by virtue of the increased density of angiotensin II receptors at this location. As a result, intraglomerular pressure is preserved, and the fraction of renal plasma filtered by glomeruli (filtration fraction) is increased. During severe hypoperfusion, however, these responses prove inadequate, and ARF ensues.

Drugs that interfere with the adaptive responses may convert compensated renal hypoperfusion into overt prerenal azotemia or trigger progression of prerenal azotemia to intrinsic renal azotemia (see below). Consequently, inhibitors of renal prostaglandin biosynthesis (*cyclooxygenase inhibitors*) or of angiotensin-converting enzyme activity (*ACE inhibitors*) should be used with caution in high-renin

---

TABLE 236-1 Classification and major causes of acute renal failure

PRERENAL FAILURE

Hypovolemia
  Hemorrhage, burns, dehydration
  Gastrointestinal fluid loss: vomiting, surgical drainage, diarrhea
  Renal fluid loss: diuretics, osmotic diuresis (e.g., diabetes mellitus), adrenal insufficiency
  Sequestration of fluid in extravascular space: pancreatitis, peritonitis, trauma, burns, hypoalbuminemia
Low cardiac output
  Diseases of myocardium, valves, and pericardium, arrhythmias, tamponade
  Other: pulmonary hypertension, pulmonary embolus, positive pressure mechanical ventilation
Increased renal systemic vascular resistance ratio
  Systemic vasodilatation: sepsis, antihypertensives, afterload reducers, anesthesia, anaphylaxis
  Renal vasoconstriction: hypercalcemia, norepinephrine, epinephrine, cyclosporine, amphotericin B
  Cirrhosis with ascites
Renal hypoperfusion with impairment of renal autoregulatory responses
  Cyclooxygenase inhibitors, angiotensin-converting enzyme inhibitors
Hyperviscosity syndrome (rare)
  Multiple myeloma, macroglobulinemia, polycythemia

INTRINSIC ACUTE RENAL FAILURE

Renovascular obstruction (bilateral or unilateral: one functioning kidney)
  Renal artery obstruction: atherosclerotic plaque, thrombosis, embolism, dissecting aneurysm, vasculitis
  Renal vein obstruction: thrombosis, compression
Diseases of glomeruli or renal microvasculature
  Glomerulonephritis and vasculitis
  Hemolytic uremic syndrome, thrombotic thrombocytopenic purpura, disseminated intravascular coagulation, toxemia of pregnancy, accelerated hypertension, radiation nephritis, scleroderma, systemic lupus erythematosus
Acute tubular necrosis
  Ischemia: as for prerenal azotemia (hypovolemia, low cardiac output, renal vasoconstriction, systemic vasodilatation), obstetrical complications (abruptio placentae, postpartum hemorrhage)
  Toxins: exogenous—contrast, cyclosporine, antibiotics (e.g., aminoglycosides, amphotericin B), chemotherapeutic agents (e.g., cisplatin), organic solvents (e.g., ethylene glycol), acetaminophen, illegal abortifacients; endogenous—rhabdomyolysis, hemolysis, uric acid, oxalate, plasma cell dyscrasia (e.g. myeloma)
Interstitial nephritis
  Allergic: antibiotics (e.g., beta-lactams, sulfonamides, trimethoprim, rifampin), cyclooxygenase inhibitors, diuretics, captopril
  Infection: bacterial (e.g., acute pyelonephritis, leptospirosis), viral (e.g., CMV), fungal (e.g., candidiasis)
  Infiltration: lymphoma, leukemia, sarcoidosis
  Idiopathic
Intratubular deposition and obstruction
  Myeloma proteins, uric acid, oxalate, acyclovir, methotrexate, sulfonamides
Renal allograft rejection

POSTRENAL FAILURE (OBSTRUCTION)

Ureteric
  Calculi, blood clot, sloughed papillae, cancer, external compression (e.g. retroperitoneal fibrosis)
Bladder neck
  Neurogenic bladder, prostatic hyperplasia, calculi, cancer, blood clot
Urethra
  Stricture, congenital valve, phimosis

---

states associated with renal vasoconstriction and hypoperfusion. ACE inhibitors should be used with special caution in patients with bilateral renal artery stenosis or unilateral stenosis in a solitary functioning kidney. Under these circumstances, glomerular perfusion and filtration may be exquisitely dependent on the actions of angiotensin II. Angiotensin II preserves glomerular filtration pressure distal to stenoses by increasing systemic arterial pressure and by triggering selective constriction of efferent arterioles. ACE inhibitors blunt these responses and precipitate ARF, usually reversible, in approximately 30 percent of such patients. Indeed, while patients with renal artery stenosis are particularly prone to develop ARF following therapy with ACE inhibitors, severe systemic hypotension from any cause can compromise glomerular filtration in this setting.

Other pharmacologic agents that can induce *primary intrarenal vasoconstriction* and ARF, particularly in the setting of mild hypovolemia, include radiocontrast agents, cyclosporine, amphotericin B, epinephrine, norepinephrine, and high doses of dopamine. Hypercalcemia may compromise glomerular filtration in a similar manner. *Sepsis* due to gram-negative endotoxin-producing organisms can cause systemic vasodilatation in the presence of intense intrarenal vasoconstriction.

ARF may complicate hepatic failure (hepatorenal syndrome) due to cirrhosis or other *liver diseases,* including malignancy, hepatic resection, and biliary obstruction. Intrarenal vasoconstriction and avid sodium retention are early responses under these circumstances and may precede alterations in systemic hemodynamics. In addition, patients with liver disease complicated by portal hypertension and ascites usually have increased plasma volume but "effective" hypovolemia due to systemic vasodilatation and pooling of blood in the portal circulation. Azotemia may develop slowly as hepatic failure progresses or may be precipitated in compensated patients by hemodynamic insults such as hemorrhage, paracentesis, or administration of diuretics, vasodilators, or cyclooxygenase inhibitors. ARF may progress relentlessly in hepatic failure even in the presence of satisfactory plasma volume and blood pressure, possibly as a result of ongoing intrarenal vasoconstriction, hypoperfusion, and ischemia. It must be remembered, however, that patients with liver disease also can develop other forms of ARF (e.g., sepsis, nephrotoxic medications) and that a diagnosis of hepatorenal syndrome should be made only after exclusion of other causes.

Intrinsic renal azotemia (intrinsic renal ARF) This can complicate many disorders that affect the renal parenchyma (see Table 236-1). Most cases are caused either by ischemia secondary to renal hypoperfusion (ischemic ARF) or toxins (nephrotoxic ARF). Since ischemic and nephrotoxic ARF are frequently associated with necrosis of tubule epithelial cells, this syndrome is often referred to as *acute*

tubular necrosis (ATN). Unfortunately, the terms *intrinsic renal ARF* and *ATN* are often used interchangeably, but this is inappropriate because some parenchymal diseases (e.g., vasculitis, glomerulonephritis, interstitial nephritis) can cause ARF without tubule cell necrosis. Furthermore, the pathologic term *ATN* is frequently inaccurate even in ischemic or nephrotoxic ARF because tubule cell necrosis may not be present in >20 to 30 percent of cases.

ISCHEMIC ARF As noted above, prerenal azotemia and ischemic ARF can represent a spectrum of the same disease. They differ in that ischemic ARF, in contrast to prerenal azotemia, does not resolve rapidly upon restoration of normal renal perfusion. Renal hypoperfusion from any cause (see Table 236-1) may lead to ischemic ARF if severe enough to overwhelm renal autoregulatory and neurohumoral defense mechanisms (see above). Ischemic ARF occurs most frequently after cardiovascular surgery, trauma, hemorrhage, sepsis, or dehydration. This syndrome also may complicate mild forms of true or "effective" hypovolemia, particularly in patients receiving cyclooxygenase or ACE inhibitors or with renovascular disease.

Postulated mechanisms by which renal hypoperfusion and ischemia impair glomerular filtration include (1) reduction in glomerular perfusion and filtration (previously called *vasomotor nephropathy*), (2) obstruction of urine flow in tubules by cells and debris (including casts) derived from ischemic tubule epithelium, and (3) backleak of glomerular filtrate through ischemic tubule epithelium (Fig. 236-1). In addition, neutrophil activation within the renal vasculature and neutrophil-mediated cell injury may contribute.

Glomerular filtration is flow-dependent, and intrarenal vasoconstriction impairs GFR and compromises renal oxygenation. Ischemia of renal endothelial cells may cause a sustained fall in renal blood flow, glomerular ultrafiltration pressure, and surface area by blocking production of endothelial cell–derived vasodilators (e.g., nitric oxide, prostacyclin) and/or release of endothelial cell–derived vasoconstric-

FIGURE 236-1 Proposed pathophysiology of ischemic acute renal failure.

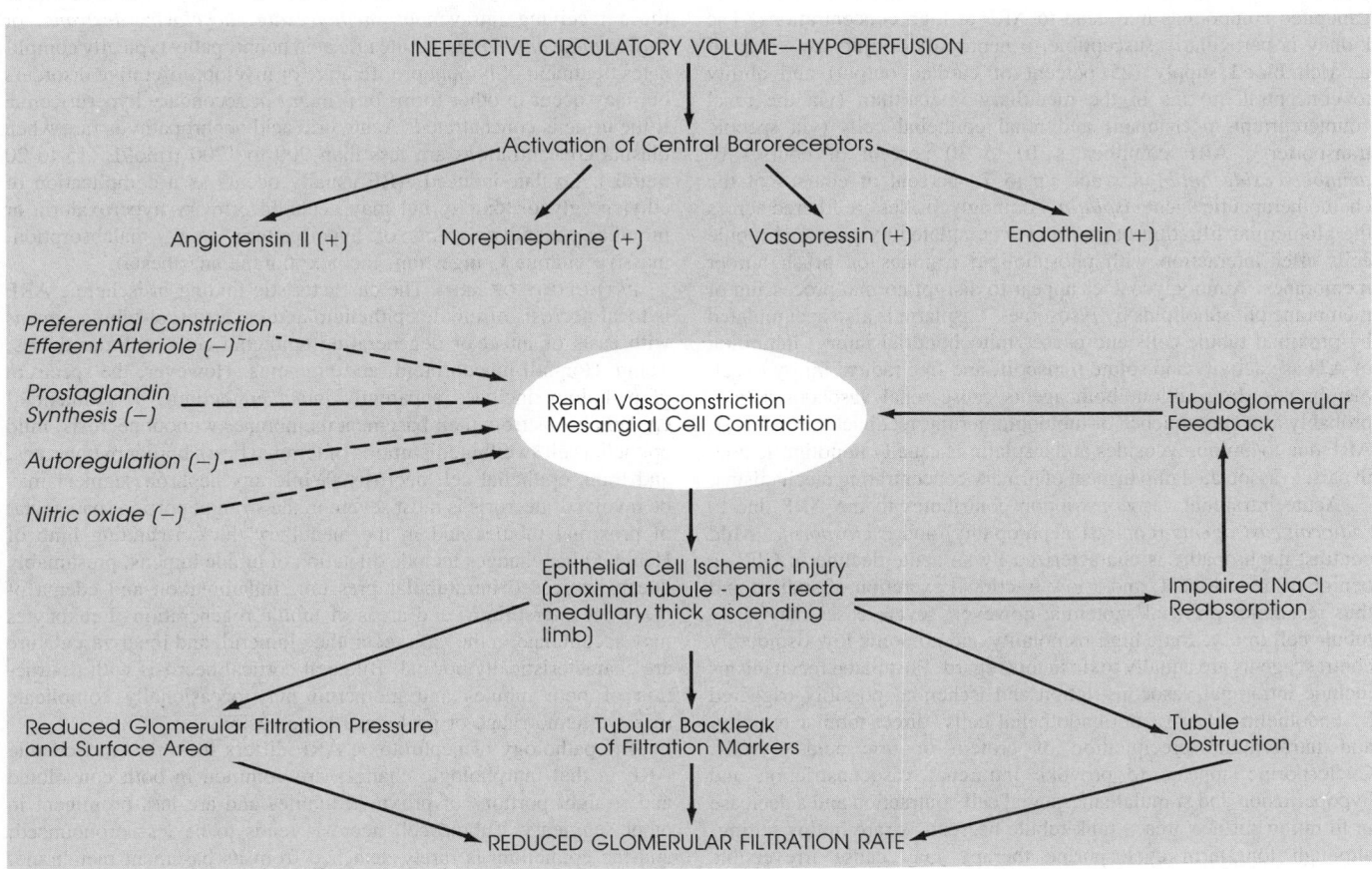

tors (e.g., endothelin). Renal hypoperfusion leads to ischemia of renal tubule cells, particularly the terminal straight portion of proximal tubules (pars recta) and the thick ascending limb of the loop of Henle. These segments traverse the corticomedullary junction and outer medulla, regions of the kidney that are relatively hypoxic compared with the renal cortex, even in health, because of the unique countercurrent arrangement of the vasculature. Furthermore, proximal tubules and thick ascending limb cells have greater oxygen requirements than other renal cells because of high rates of active (ATP-dependent) sodium transport. Proximal tubule cells may be prone to ischemic injury because they rely exclusively on mitochondrial oxidative phosphorylation (oxygen-dependent) for ATP synthesis and cannot generate ATP from anerobic glycolysis. Cellular ischemia causes alterations in energetics, ion transport, and membrane integrity that ultimately lead to cell necrosis. These include depletion of ATP, inhibition of active transport of sodium and other solutes, impairment of cell volume regulation and cell swelling, cytoskeletal disruption, accumulation of intracellular calcium, altered phospholipid metabolism, free radical formation, and peroxidation of membrane lipids. While epithelial cell function is impaired during ischemia, free radical–mediated injury may be most severe during reperfusion and reoxygenation. Necrotic tubule epithelium may permit backleak of filtered solutes, including creatinine, urea, and other nitrogenous waste products, thus rendering glomerular filtration ineffective. In addition, necrotic tubule cells may slough into tubule lumens, obstruct urine flow, increase intratubular pressure, and impair further formation of glomerular filtrate.

Epithelial cell injury per se causes secondary intrarenal vasoconstriction by a process termed *tubuloglomerular feedback*. Specialized epithelial cells in the macula densa region of distal tubules detect increases in distal salt (probably chloride) delivery due to impaired reabsorption by proximal nephron segments and in turn stimulate constriction of adjacent afferent arterioles and further compromise glomerular perfusion and filtration.

NEPHROTOXIC ARF   This may complicate administration of diverse pharmacologic agents (see Table 236-1). In addition, endogenously generated compounds may lead to ARF at high concentrations. The kidney is particularly susceptible to nephrotoxic injury by virtue of its rich blood supply (25 percent of cardiac output) and ability to concentrate toxins in the medullary interstitium (via the renal countercurrent mechanism) and renal epithelial cells (via specific transporters). ARF complicates 10 to 30 percent of courses of *aminoglycoside antibiotics* and up to 70 percent of courses of the chemotherapeutic agent *cisplatin*. Aminoglycosides are filtered across the glomerular filtration barrier and accumulated by proximal tubule cells after interaction with phospholipid residues on brush border membranes. Aminoglycosides appear to disrupt normal processing of membrane phospholipids by lysosomes. Cisplatin is also accumulated by proximal tubule cells and causes mitochondrial injury, inhibition of ATPase activity and solute transport, and free radical injury to cell membranes. In addition, both agents cause renal vasoconstriction, probably as a consequence of tubuloglomerular feedback (see above). ARF due to aminoglycosides and cisplatin is usually nonoliguric due, in part, to associated impairment of urinary concentrating mechanisms.

Acute intrarenal vasoconstriction contributes to the ARF due to *radiocontrast agents* (contrast nephropathy) and *cyclosporine*. Mild contrast nephropathy is characterized by an acute decline in GFR, a benign urine sediment, and a low fractional excretion of sodium and thus resembles prerenal azotemia; however, severe cases may show tubule cell injury. Ionic high-osmolality and nonionic low-osmolality contrast agents are equally toxic in this regard. Postulated mechanisms include intrarenal vasoconstriction and ischemia, possibly triggered by endothelin release from endothelial cells, direct tubular toxicity, and intraluminal precipitation of protein or uric acid crystals. Cyclosporine appears to provoke intrarenal vasoconstriction and hypoperfusion and stimulate mesangial cell contraction and a decrease in filtration surface area. Frank tubule necrosis is rare in this setting, although long-term cyclosporine therapy may cause irreversible

renal impairment as a consequence of chronic medullary ischemia. *Amphotericin* causes dose-related ARF by inducing intense renal vasoconstriction and via direct toxicity to proximal and distal tubule cells. Chronic renal failure, hypovolemia, concomitant exposure to other toxins, and old age predispose patients to most forms of nephrotoxic injury. In addition, diabetes mellitus and multiple myeloma are risk factors for acute contrast agent nephropathy.

Rhabdomyolysis and *hemolysis* can cause ARF, particularly in hypovolemic or acidotic individuals. Rhabdomyolysis and myoglobinuric ARF may occur with traumatic crush injury, muscle ischemia (e.g., arterial insufficiency, muscle compression, cocaine overdose), seizures, excessive exercise, heat stroke or malignant hyperthermia, alcoholism, and infectious (e.g., influenza, legionella) or metabolic disorders (e.g., hypokalemia, hypophosphatemia, or myophosphorylase or phosphofructokinase deficiency). ARF due to hemolysis is seen most commonly following blood transfusion reactions. The mechanisms by which rhabdomyolysis and hemolysis impair GFR are unclear, since neither hemoglobin nor myoglobin is nephrotoxic when injected into laboratory animals. Myoglobin and hemoglobin or other compounds released from muscle or red blood cells may cause ARF via direct toxic effects on tubule epithelial cells or by inducing intratubular cast formation. Hypovolemia or acidosis may contribute to ARF in this setting by promoting intranephronal cast formation. In addition, hemoglobin and myoglobin inhibit nitric oxide and may trigger intrarenal vasoconstriction and ischemia in patients with borderline renal hypoperfusion.

Intratubular obstruction may play an important role in ARF in several diseases. Casts containing filtered immunoglobulin light chains and other urine proteins, including Tamm-Horsfall protein produced by thick ascending limb cells, may cause ARF in patients with plasma cell dyscrasias (myeloma-cast nephropathy). High urine salt concentrations and low urine pH appear to promote this process. However, the correlation between cast formation and renal insufficiency is poor in myeloma, suggesting that light chains may be toxic to tubule epithelial cells. Intratubular obstruction also may cause ARF in patients with severe *hyperuricosuria* or *hyperoxaluria* or in those receiving intravenous *methotrexate*, *acyclovir*, *dextrans*, or *sulfonamide antibiotics*. Acute uric acid nephropathy typically complicates treatment of lymphoproliferative or myeloproliferative disorders but may occur in other forms of primary or secondary hyperuricemia if the urine is concentrated. Acute uric acid nephropathy is rare when plasma concentrations are less than 900 to 1200 µmol/L (15 to 20 mg/dL). Oxalate-induced ARF usually occurs as a complication of ethylene glycol toxicity but may occur in primary hyperoxaluria or in other secondary forms of hyperoxaluria (e.g., malabsorption, massive vitamin C ingestion, methoxyflurane anesthesia).

PATHOLOGY OF ARF   The characteristic finding in ischemic ARF is focal necrosis of tubule epithelium and occlusion of tubule lumens with casts of intact or degenerating epithelial cells, cellular debris, Tamm-Horsfall mucoprotein, and pigments. However, the spectrum of pathology includes apparently intact epithelium, detachment of epithelial cells from their basement membranes without necrosis, mild epithelial cell swelling, disruption of luminal brush border membranes, and frank epithelial cell necrosis. While any nephron segment may be involved, necrosis is most severe in the straight portion (pars recta) of proximal tubules and in the medullary thick ascending limb of Henle. Other changes include dilatation of tubule lumens, presumably due to increased intratubular pressure, inflammation and edema of the renal interstitium, and areas of tubule regeneration. Leukocytes may accumulate in the vasa recta; the glomeruli and renal vasculature are characteristically normal. Bilateral cortical necrosis with destruction of both tubules and glomeruli may occasionally complicate massive hemorrhage or prolonged hypotension.

The pathology of nephrotoxic ARF differs from that in ischemic ARF in that morphologic changes are common in both convoluted and straight portions of proximal tubules and are less prominent in other segments. Tubule cell necrosis tends to be less pronounced, and the epithelium is rarely detached from its basement membrane.

Indeed, renal biopsy specimens may be normal in nephrotoxic ARF even in the presence of epithelial cell dysfunction. Proximal tubule myeloid bodies, characteristic, albeit nonspecific, findings in amino-glycoside-induced ARF, are electron-dense lamellar structures that reflect accumulation of cell membrane phospholipids in lysosomes and likely result from abnormal intracellular phospholipid processing. Their role in the pathogenesis of aminoglycoside nephrotoxicity is uncertain.

COURSE OF ISCHEMIC AND NEPHROTOXIC ARF   Most cases of ischemic or nephrotoxic ARF are characterized by three distinct phases. The *initiation phase* is the period from initial exposure to the causative insult to development of established ARF. Restoration of renal perfusion or elimination of nephrotoxins during this phase may reverse or limit the renal injury. The early initiation phase is usually identified retrospectively, since serum creatinine does not rise until GFR is reduced by 40 percent or more. In milder renal injury, the decline in GFR is counterbalanced by an increase in creatinine secretion into the tubule lumen. During the *maintenance phase* (average 7 to 14 days), the GFR is depressed, and metabolic consequences of ARF may develop. A *recovery phase* in most patients is characterized by tubule cell regeneration and a gradual return of GFR to or toward normal. The recovery phase may be complicated by diuresis (*diuretic phase*) due to excretion of retained salt and water and other solutes, continued use of diuretics, and/or delayed recovery of epithelial cell function (solute and water reabsorption) relative to glomerular filtration.

INTRINSIC RENAL AZOTEMIA FROM OTHER CAUSES   Other diseases of the renal vasculature, glomeruli, and interstitium may lead to ARF (see Table 236-1). Acute obstruction of renal arteries or veins (e.g., thrombosis) may cause an abrupt decline in GFR if bilateral or if unilateral in patients with a solitary functioning kidney. Patients with advanced atherosclerosis may develop ARF spontaneously, following trauma, or after manipulation of the aorta or renal arteries due to embolization of cholesterol crystals to the renal vasculature. Choles-terol crystals lodge in small and medium-sized arteries and incite a giant cell and fibrotic reaction in the vessel wall with narrowing or obstruction of the lumen. Atheroembolic ARF is usually irreversible. Other diseases of the renal microvasculature that may cause intrinsic renal azotemia include acute glomerulonephritis and vasculitis, hemo-lytic-uremic syndrome (HUS), thrombotic thrombocytopenic purpura (TTP), disseminated intravascular coagulation (DIC), malignant hy-pertension, toxemia of pregnancy, scleroderma, and radiation injury. These disorders are characterized by either immune or physical injury to vessel walls, thrombotic microangiopathy, or both. Occlusion of renal arteries, arterioles, or glomerular capillaries leads to glomerular hypoperfusion and a fall in GFR. Pharmacologic agents may cause ARF by triggering allergic interstitial nephritis, characterized by infiltration of the interstitial space by macrophages, lymphocytes, plasma cells, polymorphonuclear leukocytes, and other inflammatory cells and interstitial edema. Common causes of allergic interstitial nephritis include antibiotics (e.g., penicillins, cephalosporins, trimeth-oprim, sulfonamides, rifampicin), nonsteroidal anti-inflammatory drugs, captopril, and diuretics (see Table 236-1). Occasionally, ARF may complicate interstitial nephritis due to infections, neoplasia, or infiltrative processes.

Pregnancy is associated with an increased risk of ARF, although the incidence has decreased with improvements in obstetric care. Azotemia is usually triggered by ischemic (e.g., abruptio placentae, postpartum hemorrhage) or nephrotoxic (illegal abortifacients) renal injury or toxemia of pregnancy. In addition, the postpartum period may be complicated by ARF and thrombotic microangiopathy.

Postrenal azotemia   Urinary tract obstruction accounts for ap-proximately 5 percent of ARF. Since one kidney has sufficient clearance capacity to excrete nitrogenous waste products, ARF from obstruction either requires obstruction between the external urethral meatus and bladder neck, bilateral ureter obstruction, or unilateral ureter obstruction in a patient with one functioning kidney. Bladder neck obstruction is the most common cause and may be due to

prostatic disease (e.g., hyperplasia, neoplasia, or infection), neuro-genic bladder, or anticholinergic drugs. Less common causes include blood clots, calculi, and urethritis with spasm. Ureteric obstruction may result from intraluminal obstruction (e.g., calculi, blood clots, sloughed renal papillae), infiltration of the ureteric wall (e.g., neoplasia), or external compression (e.g., retroperitoneal fibrosis, neoplasia or abscess, inadvertent surgical ligature). During the early stages of obstruction (hours to days), continued glomerular filtration leads to increased intraluminal pressure upstream to the obstruction, eventuating in gradual distension of proximal ureter, renal pelvis, and calyces and a fall in GFR. While acute obstruction may cause an initial increase in renal blood flow, arteriolar vasoconstriction supervenes and leads to a further decline in glomerular filtration.

CLINICAL FEATURES AND DIFFERENTIAL DIAGNOSIS   Pa-tients with azotemia should be assessed to determine if renal failure is acute or chronic. An acute process is established if review of laboratory records reveals a recent rise in BUN and serum creatinine, but previous measurements are usually not available. Findings that suggest chronic renal failure include anemia, neuropathy, and radio-logic evidence of renal osteodystrophy or small scarred kidneys (see Chap. 237). However, anemia also may complicate ARF (see below), and renal size may be normal or increased in chronic renal disease (e.g., diabetic nephropathy, amyloid, polycystic kidney disease). Once a diagnosis of ARF is established, appropriate management relies on elucidation of the cause of ARF and requires careful clinical assessment, including review of presenting symptoms, drug history and hospital course, physical examination and urinalysis, appropriate laboratory tests and renal imaging techniques, and occasional renal biopsy.

Clinical assessment   *Prerenal azotemia* should be suspected in patients suffering an elevation in serum creatinine following hemorrhage, excessive gastrointestinal or urinary fluid loss, or exten-sive burns, particularly if access to fluids is restricted (e.g., as in comatose or obtunded patients or those on mechanical ventilation). Supportive evidence includes thirst, orthostatic hypotension and tachycardia, reduced jugular venous pressure, decreased skin turgor, dry mucous membranes, and reduced axillary sweating. Nursing and pharmacy records should be reviewed for evidence of a decline in urine output and body weight and recent use of cyclooxygenase or ACE inhibitors. Clinical examination may reveal stigmata of chronic liver disease and portal hypertension (e.g., palmar erythema, jaundice, telangiectasia, caput medusae, splenomegaly, ascites), cardiac failure (e.g., peripheral edema, hepatic congestion, elevated jugular venous pressure, bibasilar lung crackles, gallop rhythm, cold extremities), or other causes of "effective" hypovolemia (see Table 236-1). Invasive hemodynamic monitoring (central venous and/or Swan-Ganz catheterization) may be necessary in complicated cases. Definitive diagnosis of prerenal azotemia can only be made when restoration of renal perfusion results in prompt resolution of ARF.

Intrinsic renal azotemia due to ischemia is likely in patients with ARF following prolonged or severe renal hypoperfusion complicating hypovolemic or septic shock or major surgery. However, a significant fall in arterial blood pressure occurs in the latter setting in less than half of patients with clinical and biochemical features of ischemic ARF. The likelihood of ischemic ARF is increased further if ARF persists despite restoration of renal perfusion. Diagnosis of nephrotoxic ARF requires review of the history and of pharmacy, nursing, and radiology records for nephrotoxic medications or radiocontrast agents. ARF after cancer chemotherapy suggests a diagnosis of tumor lysis syndrome and acute urate nephropathy, although other considerations include prerenal azotemia due to emesis or diarrhea and direct nephrotoxicity of chemotherapeutic or antimicrobial agents. Rhabdo-myolysis is suggested by a recent history of seizures, excessive exercise, alcohol or drug abuse, or muscle tenderness or limb ischemia on physical examination.

While ischemic and nephrotoxic ARF account for most intrinsic renal azotemia, patients should be assessed for other renal parenchymal diseases. Flank pain may be prominant following acute renal artery or vein occlusion and in acute pyelonephritis and acute necrotizing glomerulonephritis. Subcutaneous nodules, livedo reticularis, bright orange retinal arteriolar plaques, and digital ischemia despite palpable pedal pulses suggest atheroembolization. ARF in association with oliguria, edema, hypertension, and an "active" urine sediment (nephritic syndrome) suggests acute glomerulonephritis or vasculitis and should prompt a search for secondary causes (e.g., systemic lupus erythematosus, bacterial endocarditis, cryoglobulinemia). However, this constellation of findings may occur in patients with other diseases of the renal microvasculature (e.g., HUS, TTP, hypertensive nephrosclerosis, toxemia of pregnancy). HUS and TTP are considerations in patients with a history of infective diarrhea or upper respiratory tract infection and physical evidence of easy bruising, anemia, or neurologic deficit. Malignant hypertension is a likely cause in patients with moderate or severe hypertension and evidence of hypertensive injury to other organs (e.g., left ventricular hypertrophy and failure, hypertensive retinopathy and papilledema, neurologic dysfunction). Fever, arthralgias, and a pruritic erythematous rash suggest allergic interstitial nephritis, although systemic features of hypersensitivity are frequently absent.

Postrenal azotemia may be asymptomatic if obstruction develops slowly. Alternatively, suprapubic or flank pain may be present if there is acute distension of the bladder, renal collecting system, and capsule, respectively. Colicky flank pain radiating to the groin suggests acute ureteric obstruction. Prostatic disease should be suspected in men with a history of nocturia, frequency, and hesitancy and an enlarged or indurated prostate on rectal examination. Neurogenic bladder is likely in patients receiving anticholinergic medications (e.g., tricyclic antidepressants) or with physical evidence of neurologic disease and autonomic insufficiency (e.g., paralysis, abnormal rectal sphincter tone). Bladder distension may be evident on abdominal percussion and palpation. Definitive diagnosis of postrenal azotemia usually relies on judicious use of radiologic investigations and rapid improvement in renal function following relief of obstruction.

Urinalysis   Assessment of urine volume is relatively unhelpful in evaluating ARF. Complete anuria suggests complete urinary tract obstruction but may complicate prerenal or intrinsic renal azotemia (e.g., renal artery occlusion, proliferative glomerulonephritis, bilateral cortical necrosis). Wide fluctuations in urine output suggest intermittent obstruction, and patients with partial urinary tract obstruction may have polyuria due to secondary impairment of urine concentrating mechanisms.

In contrast, examination of the sediment and supernatant of a centrifuged urine specimen is valuable in distinguishing among prerenal, intrinsic renal, and postrenal azotemia and in elucidating the etiology of intrinsic renal azotemia. Urine sediment should be inspected for casts, hematuria, pyuria, and crystals. In prerenal azotemia, the sediment is characteristically acellular and may contain transparent hyaline casts ("bland," "benign," "inactive" urine sediment). Hyaline casts are formed in concentrated urine from normal constituents of urine, principally Tamm-Horsfall protein that is normally secreted by epithelial cells of the loop of Henle. Postrenal azotemia also may have an inactive sediment, although hematuria and pyuria are common with intraluminal obstruction and prostatic disease. Pigmented "muddy brown" granular casts and casts containing tubule epithelial cells are characteristic of tubule necrosis and suggest ischemic or nephrotoxic ARF. They are usually found in association with microscopic hematuria and mild "tubular" proteinuria (<1 g/d); the latter reflects impaired reabsorption and processing of filtered proteins by injured proximal tubule cells. Casts may be absent in 20 to 30 percent of patients with ischemic or nephrotoxic ARF and are not requisite for diagnosis. Indeed, there is a poor correlation between the functional renal impairment and the urinalysis in these conditions. Red blood cell casts indicate acute glomerular injury. Dysmorphic red blood cells are more common in the urine of patients with glomerular injury but are less specific than red cell casts. Urine sediment abnormalities are variable in diseases involving preglomerular blood vessels (e.g., HUS, TTP, atheroembolic disease, vasculitis

involving medium-sized or large vessels) and range from benign to frankly nephritic. White cell casts and nonpigmented granular casts suggest interstitial nephritis, and the broad granular casts of chronic renal disease are probably due to interstitial fibrosis and dilatation of tubules. Eosinophiluria (between 1 and 50 percent of urine leukocytes) is common (~90 percent) in drug-induced allergic interstitial nephritis when studied using Hansel's stain. Wright's stain is less sensitive (~20 percent) in this regard. Eosinophiluria is, however, only 85 percent specific for allergic interstitial nephritis, and similar eosinophiluria can occur in atheroembolization, ischemic and nephrotoxic ARF, proliferative glomerulonephritis, pyelonephritis, cystitis, and prostatitis. Uric acid crystals (pleomorphic in shape) may be seen in urine in prerenal azotemia but suggest acute urate nephropathy if present in abundance. Oxalate (envelope-shaped) and hippurate (needle-shaped) crystals suggest ethylene glycol toxicity.

Increased urine protein excretion, characteristically <1 g/d, is common in ischemic or nephrotoxic ARF and reflects both failure of reabsorption of filtered protein and excretion of cellular debris ("tubular" proteinuria). Proteinuria of >1 g/d suggests injury to the glomerular ultrafiltration barrier ("glomerular" proteinuria) or excretion of myeloma light chains. The latter are not detected by conventional dipsticks (which detect albumin) and must be sought by other means (e.g., sulfosalicylic acid test, immunoelectrophoresis). Marked proteinuria is also frequent (~80 percent) with allergic interstitial nephritis triggered by cyclooxygenase inhibitors. These patients have interstitial inflammation and a glomerular lesion almost identical to minimal change glomerulonephritis. A similar syndrome has occurred with other agents, including ampicillin, rifampicin, and interferon-α. Hemoglobinuria or myoglobinuria should be suspected if urine is strongly positive for hemoglobin by dipstick but contains few red cells and if the supernatant of centrifuged urine is also positive for free hemoglobin. Hemolysis and rhabdomyolysis can usually be differentiated by inspection of plasma. The latter is pink in hemolysis but usually not in rhabdomyolysis, since free hemoglobin is a larger molecule than myoglobin, is protein-bound, and is filtered slowly by the kidney. Bilirubinuria may provide a clue to the presence of hepatorenal syndrome.

Renal failure indices   Analysis of urine and blood biochemistry are useful in distinguishing prerenal from intrinsic renal azotemia (Table 236-2). Estimation of the fractional excretion of sodium (FeNa) relates sodium clearance to creatinine clearance. Sodium is reabsorbed avidly from glomerular filtrate in prerenal azotemia in an attempt to restore intravascular volume but not in ARF because of tubular

---

TABLE 236-2   Urine diagnostic indices in separation of prerenal from intrinsic renal azotemia

Diagnostic index	Prerenal azotemia	Intrinsic renal azotemia
Fractional excretion of sodium (%)* $\dfrac{U_{Na} P_{Cr}}{P_{Na} U_{Cr}} \times 100$	<1	>1
Urine sodium concentration (mmol/L)	<10	>20
Urine creatinine to plasma creatinine ratio	>40	<20
Urine urea nitrogen to plasma urea nitrogen ratio	>8	<3
Urine specific gravity	>1.018	<1.012
Urine osmolality (mmol/kg H₂O)	>500	<250
Plasma BUN/creatinine ratio (mg/dL)	>20	<10–15
Renal failure index* $\dfrac{U_{Na}}{U_{Cr}/P_{Cr}}$	<1	>1
Urinary sediment	Hyaline casts	Muddy brown granular casts

* Most sensitive indices

epithelial cell injury. In contrast, creatinine is reabsorbed less efficiently than sodium in both conditions. Consequently, patients with prerenal azotemia typically have an FeNa concentration of <1.0 percent (frequently <0.01 percent), while in patients with ischemic or nephrotoxic ARF the FeNa is usually >1.0 percent. The renal failure index (RFI) (see Table 236-2) provides similar information, since variations in serum sodium concentration are relatively small. Urine sodium concentration is a less sensitive index for distinguishing prerenal azotemia from ischemic and nephrotoxic ARF. Similarly, indices of urinary concentrating ability such as urine specific gravity, urine osmolality, urine to plasma creatinine or urea ratios, and serum urea nitrogen to creatinine ratio are of limited value, particularly in elderly subjects, in whom urine concentrating mechanisms are frequently impaired, while sodium reabsorption is preserved.

FeNa may occasionally be >1.0 percent in prerenal azotemia in patients receiving diuretics or with bicarbonaturia (accompanied by sodium to maintain electroneutrality), underlying chronic renal failure complicated by salt wasting, or adrenal insufficiency. In contrast, approximately 15 percent of patients with nonoliguric ischemic or nephrotoxic ARF have an FeNa concentration of <1.0 percent, which likely reflects a milder form of renal injury (intermediate syndrome). This syndrome has been described in patients with ARF from a variety of causes, including ischemia, aminoglycosides, radiocontrast agents, rhabdomyolysis, hemolysis, burns, sepsis, and hepatorenal syndrome. Under these circumstances, epithelial cell damage is probably localized to the corticomedullary junction and outer medulla with relative preservation of function in other sodium-transporting segments. The FeNa concentration is usually <1.0 percent in ARF due to urinary tract obstruction, glomerulonephritis, and diseases of the renal vasculature; other parameters must therefore be used to distinguish these conditions from prerenal azotemia.

Laboratory investigations Analysis of serial measurements of serum creatinine may be useful in differential diagnosis. Prerenal azotemia is frequently characterized by rapid fluctuations in creatinine that parallel changes in hemodynamic function. Serum creatinine rises rapidly (apparent within 24 to 48 h) in ARF following renal ischemia, atheroembolization, and radiocontrast exposure, three possibilities in patients undergoing emergency cardiac or aortic angiography and surgery. Peak creatinine levels in contrast nephropathy are usually observed after 3 to 5 days and return to normal within 5 to 7 days. In contrast, creatinine levels typically peak later (7 to 10 days) in ischemic ARF and atheroembolic disease. ARF usually resolves over the next 7 to 14 days in ischemic ARF but may be irreversible in atheroembolic disease. With many tubule epithelial cell toxins (e.g., aminoglycosides, cisplatin) the initial elevation of serum creatinine levels is characteristically delayed until the second week of therapy and probably reflects the need for accumulation of these agents within cells before overt injury is apparent biochemically.

Hyperkalemia, hyperphosphatemia, hypocalcemia, and elevations in serum uric acid and creatine kinase (MM isoenzyme) levels suggest rhabdomyolysis. Hyperuricemia of >900 μmol/L (>15 mg/dL) in association with hyperkalemia, hyperphosphatemia, and increased circulating levels of lactate dehydrogenase (LDH) may indicate acute urate nephropathy. Severe hypercalcemia from any cause can induce ARF. Elevated serum anion and osmolal gaps (measured serum osmolality minus calculated osmolality) suggest ethylene glycol toxicity, and severe anemia in the absence of hemorrhage suggests hemolysis, multiple myeloma, or thrombotic microangiopathy (e.g., HUS, TTP, toxemia, DIC, accelerated hypertension, SLE, scleroderma, radiation injury). Other laboratory findings of thrombotic microangiopathy include thrombocytopenia, dysmorphic red blood cells on peripheral blood smear, and elevated circulating levels of LDH. Systemic eosinophilia suggests allergic interstitial nephritis, atheroembolic disease, or polyarteritis nodosa. Depressed complement levels and high titers of anti-glomerular basement membrane antibodies, antineutrophil cytoplasmic antibodies, antinuclear antibodies, circulating immune complexes, or cryoglobulins are helpful with suspected glomerulonephritis or vasculitis.

Radiology Imaging of the urinary tract by ultrasonography, computed tomography (CT), or magnetic resonance (MR) imaging is recommended in most patients with ARF to exclude obstructive uropathy. While pelvicalyceal dilatation is usual with urinary tract obstruction (98 percent sensitivity), dilatation may not be observed during the initial period of obstruction or with obstruction due to ureteric encasement (e.g., retroperitoneal fibrosis, neoplasia). Retrograde or anterograde pyelography should be used for definitive diagnosis when these possibilities are considered likely and may be employed for precise localization of obstruction in other cases. Ultrasonography, CT, and MR imaging also provide a measure of renal size and cortical thickness that is useful in distinguishing ARF from chronic renal disease. A plain film of the abdomen is useful with suspected nephrolithiasis. Doppler ultrasonography and MR flow imaging appear promising for assessment of patency of renal arteries and veins in suspected vascular obstruction, but contrast angiography is required for definitive diagnosis.

Renal biopsy This is usually performed when prerenal and postrenal failure have been excluded and the cause of intrinsic renal azotemia is unclear. Biopsy is particularly useful when clinical assessment, urinalysis, and laboratory investigation suggest diagnoses other than ischemic or nephrotoxic injury that may respond to specific therapy. Examples include anti-glomerular basement membrane disease and other forms of necrotizing glomerulonephritis, vasculitis, HUS and TTP, and allergic interstitial nephritis.

COMPLICATIONS ARF impairs renal excretion of sodium, potassium, and water; divalent cation homeostasis; and urinary acidification mechanisms. As a result, ARF is frequently complicated by intravascular volume overload, hyponatremia, hyperkalemia, hyperphosphatemia, hypocalcemia, hypermagnesemia, and metabolic acidosis. In addition, patients are unable to excrete nitrogenous waste products and may develop the uremic syndrome (see Chap. 237). In general, the severity of complications mirrors the degree of renal impairment and the catabolic state.

Intravascular volume overload is a consequence of diminished salt and water excretion, especially in oliguric or anuric individuals. While milder forms are characterized by rales, increased venous pressure, peripheral edema, and increased body weight, severe volume expansion may precipitate life-threatening pulmonary edema. Volume overload is a particular problem in patients receiving multiple intravenous medications, sodium bicarbonate for correction of acidosis, or enteral or parenteral nutrition. *Hypertension* is uncommon (~15 percent) and usually mild in ischemic or nephrotoxic ARF. Moderate or severe hypertension suggests hypertensive nephrosclerosis, glomerulonephritis, renal artery stenosis, or other diseases of the renal vasculature. Excessive fluid ingestion or inappropriate administration of water can cause *hyponatremia*, which, if severe, can lead to cerebral edema.

Hyperkalemia is common. Serum potassium typically rises by 0.5 mmol/L per day in oliguric and anuric patients due to impaired excretion. Metabolic acidosis may exacerbate hyperkalemia by promoting potassium efflux from cells. Hyperkalemia may be particularly severe in patients with rhabdomyolysis, hemolysis, and tumor lysis syndrome. Mild hyperkalemia (<6.0 mmol/L) is usually asymptomatic. Higher levels are associated with ECG abnormalities, including peaked T waves, prolongation of PR intervals, P-wave flattening, widening of the QRS complex, and left axis deviation. These ECG changes may herald the onset of life-threatening cardiac arrhythmias, including bradycardia, heart block, ventricular tachycardia or fibrillation, and asystole. In addition, hyperkalemia may cause neuromuscular dysfunction, including paresthesias, hyporeflexia, weakness, ascending flaccid paralysis, and respiratory failure. *Hypokalemia* is rare in ARF by may complicate nonoliguric aminoglycoside, cisplatin, or amphotericin B nephrotoxicity, presumably reflecting profound epithelial cell injury.

Metabolism of dietary protein yields between 50 and 100 mmol/d of fixed nonvolatile acids that are normally excreted by the kidneys. Consequently, ARF is often complicated by *metabolic acidosis* and an increased serum anion gap. Acidosis may be particularly severe when endogenous acid production is increased by other mechanisms (e.g., diabetic or fasting ketoacidosis; lactic acidosis complicating generalized tissue hypoperfusion, liver disease, or sepsis; metabolism of ethylene glycol). *Metabolic alkalosis* is infrequent in ARF but may occur following overzealous correction of acidosis with bicarbonate or loss of gastric acid by vomiting or therapeutic aspiration. Mild asymptomatic *hyperuricemia* 700 to 900 mmol/L (12 to 15 mg/dL) is common since uric acid is cleared from blood by glomerular filtration and secretion by proximal tubule cells. Higher levels suggest increased uric acid production, such as after treatment of myeloproliferative or lymphoproliferative disorders (see above).

Mild *hyperphosphatemia* is almost invariable in ARF. Severe hyperphosphatemia occurs in highly catabolic patients or following rhabdomyolysis, hemolysis, or tumor lysis. Metastatic deposition of calcium phosphate can lead to *hypocalcemia*, particularly when the product of serum calcium (mg/dL) and phosphate (mg/dL) concentrations exceeds 70. Other factors that contribute to hypocalcemia include tissue resistance to the actions of PTH and reduced levels of 1,25-dihydroxyvitamin D. Hypocalcemia is usually asymptomatic, possibly due to the counterbalancing effects of acidosis on neuromuscular excitability. However, hypocalcemia can be symptomatic with rhabdomyolysis or acute pancreatitis or following treatment of acidosis with bicarbonate. Manifestations of hypocalcemia include perioral paresthesias, muscle cramps, seizures, hallucinations and confusion, and prolongation of the QT interval and nonspecific T-wave changes on ECG (also see Chap. 357). Chvostek's sign (contraction of facial muscles upon tapping of jaw over facial nerve) and Trousseau's sign (carpopedal spasm following occlusion of arterial blood supply to the arm for 3 min by a blood pressure cuff) are indices of latent tetany in high-risk patients. Mild asymptomatic *hypermagnesemia* is usual in oliguric ARF due to impaired excretion of ingested magnesium (dietary magnesium, magnesium-containing laxatives or antacids). *Hypomagnesemia* occasionally complicates nonoliguric cisplatin and amphotericin B nephrotoxicity and likely reflects injury to the thick ascending limb of loop of Henle, the principal site for magnesium reabsorption. Manifestations of magnesium deficiency include neuromuscular instability, cramps, seizures, and cardiac arrhythmias; most cases are asymptomatic.

Anemia develops rapidly in ARF and is usually mild and multifactorial in origin. Contributing factors include impaired erythropoiesis, hemolysis, bleeding, hemodilution, and reduced red cell survival time. Prolongation of the *bleeding time* and *leukocytosis* are also common. The former may result from thrombocytopenia, platelet dysfunction, and/or clotting factor abnormalities (e.g., factor VIII dysfunction), and leukocytosis usually reflects sepsis, stress response, or other concurrent illness. *Infection* is the dread complication, occurring in 50 to 90 percent of ARF and accounting for up to 75 percent of deaths. It is unclear if ARF causes a defect in host immune responses or whether the high incidence of infection reflects repeated breaches of mucocutaneous barriers (e.g., intravenous cannulae, mechanical ventilation, bladder catheterization). *Cardiac complications* include arrhythmias, myocardial infarction, and pulmonary embolism. While these events may reflect primary cardiac disease, abnormalities in myocardial contractility and excitability may be triggered or aggravated by intravascular volume overload, acidosis, hyperkalemia, and other complications of azotemia. The increased incidence of pulmonary embolism probably reflects immobilization. Mild *gastrointestinal bleeding* (10 to 30 percent) is usually due to stress ulceration of gastric or small intestinal mucosa. Alterations in *neurologic* function may be due to the uremic syndrome, metabolic complications, impaired excretion of psychotropic medications, or primary neurologic disease.

Protracted ARF is associated with development of the *uremic syndrome* (see Chap. 237). Manifestations of the uremic syndrome include pericarditis, pericardial effusion, and cardiac tamponade; gastrointestinal complications such as anorexia, nausea, vomiting, and ileus; and neuropsychiatric disturbances such as lethargy, confusion,

stupor, coma, agitation, psychosis, asterixis, myoclonus, hyperreflexia, restless leg syndrome, focal neurologic deficit, and seizures.

A vigorous diuresis during the *recovery phase* may lead to intravascular volume depletion and delayed recovery of renal function. *Hypernatremia* also may complicate recovery if water losses via hypotonic urine are not replaced. *Hypokalemia, hypomagnesemia, hypophosphatemia,* and *hypocalcemia* occur rarely during this period. Mild hypercalcemia during recovery may be a consequence of transient hyperparathyroidism or may be due to mobilization of sequestered calcium from injured muscle.

MANAGEMENT   Prevention   Many cases of ARF can be prevented if cardiovascular function and intravascular volume are protected and exposure to nephrotoxic drugs is minimized in high-risk situations. Renal function may be protected in patients receiving aminoglycoside antibiotics or cyclosporine if serum drug concentrations are monitored and drug doses adjusted accordingly. Diuretics, cyclooxygenase, ACE inhibitors, and other vasodilators should be used with caution in patients with suspected true or "effective" hypovolemia or renovascular disease. Hypovolemia also should be avoided in patients receiving nephrotoxic medications, since renal hypoperfusion potentiates the toxicity of most of these agents. Allopurinol limits uric acid generation in patients at high risk for acute urate nephropathy, while forced diuresis and alkalinization of urine may attenuate renal injury due to uric acid, methotrexate, or rhabdomyolysis. *N*-acetylcysteine limits acetaminophen-induced renal injury if given within 24 h of ingestion, and dimercaprol, a chelating agent, may prevent heavy metal nephrotoxicity. Ethanol inhibits ethylene glycol metabolism to oxalic acid and other toxic metabolites and is an important adjunct to hemodialysis in the emergency management of this intoxication.

Specific therapies   By definition, *prerenal azotemia* is rapidly reversible upon correction of the primary hemodynamic abnormality, and *postrenal azotemia* resolves upon relief of obstruction. There are no specific therapies for established *intrinsic renal ARF* due to ischemia or nephrotoxicity. Management of these disorders should focus on elimination of the causative hemodynamic abnormality or toxin, avoidance of additional insults, and prevention and treatment of complications. Treatment of other causes of intrinsic renal azotemia varies according to the underlying pathology.

Treatment of *prerenal azotemia* due to hypovolemia varies depending on the fluid lost. Hypovolemia due to hemorrhage should be corrected with packed red blood cells in saline, while isotonic saline is usually appropriate replacement for plasma loss (e.g., burns, pancreatitis). Urinary and gastrointestinal fluid losses vary in composition but are usually hypotonic. Accordingly, initial replacement is with hypotonic solutions (e.g., 0.45% saline), and subsequent therapy should be based on measurements of the volume and ionic content of excreted or drained fluids. Serum potassium and acid-base status should be monitored. Potassium replacement is rarely required unless sodium bicarbonate is administered for moderate or severe metabolic acidosis. Cardiac failure may require aggressive management with antiarrhythmic drugs, inotropic agents, preload- and afterload-reducing agents, and/or mechanical aids such as intraaortic balloon pumps. Invasive hemodynamic monitoring may be required to guide therapy when clinical assessment of cardiovascular function and intravascular volume may be unreliable.

Fluid management may be particularly difficult in patients with ARF and cirrhosis with ascites. While ARF in this context usually results from combined intrarenal vasoconstriction and systemic vasodilation, systemic arterial hypovolemia may be a contributory factor in patients taking diuretics for control of ascites. The role of hypovolemia in this setting must be assessed by administration of a fluid challenge. Fluids should be administered slowly, and patients must be monitored closely because ascites formation may worsen and/or pulmonary edema may develop in nonresponders. Paracentesis usually can be used to drain large volumes of ascitic fluid without deterioration in renal function if albumin is administered simultaneously. Indeed, large-volume paracentesis may afford an increase in GFR possibly by lowering intraabdominal pressure and improving flow in renal veins. Shunting of ascitic fluid from the peritoneum to a central vein (peritoneojugular shunt, LeVeen or Denver shunts) is an alternative approach in refractory cases. This maneuver also may cause a transient improvement in GFR and sodium excretion, probably because the increase in central blood volume stimulates release of atrial natriuretic peptides and inhibits secretion of aldosterone and norepinephrine.

A variety of therapeutic agents have been tried in *ischemic* and *nephrotoxic ARF*. These include strategies to increase renal blood flow and urine flow (e.g., low-dose dopamine, atrial natriuretic peptide, mannitol, loop-blocking diuretics), relieve tubule obstruction (e.g., mannitol, loop-blocking diuretics), reduce epithelial cell swelling (e.g., mannitol), reduce epithelial cell ATP and oxygen requirements by inhibiting ion transport (e.g., loop-blocking diuretics), replenish cellular ATP levels (MgATP), scavenge oxygen free radicals (e.g., superoxide dismutase, catalase, mannitol), prevent accumulation of intracellular calcium (e.g., calcium channel blockers), and stimulate cellular regeneration (e.g., amino acid infusions). While many of these and other agents (e.g., glycine infusion, epidermal growth factor, growth hormone) afford some benefit in experimental models of ischemic or nephrotoxic ARF, they have been either ineffective or too toxic for use in humans.

Acute renal failure due to *other intrinsic renal diseases* such as acute glomerulonephritis or vasculitis may respond to glucocorticoids, alkylating agents, and/or plasmapheresis depending on the primary pathology. Glucocorticoids appear to hasten remission in some cases of allergic interstitial nephritis. Antiplatelet agents, plasma exchange, and plasma infusion are useful in treatment of HUS and TTP. Aggressive control of systemic arterial pressure is of paramount importance in limiting renal injury in the nephrosclerosis of malignant hypertension, toxemia of pregnancy, and other vascular diseases. Hypertension and ARF due to scleroderma may be exquisitely sensitive to treatment with ACE inhibitors.

Management of *postrenal azotemia* requires close collaboration among nephrologist, urologist, and radiologist. Obstruction of the urethra or bladder neck usually can be relieved temporarily by transurethral or suprapubic placement of a bladder catheter while the obstructing lesion is identified and treated. Similarly, ureteric obstruction may be treated initially by percutaneous catheterization of the dilated ureteric pelvis or ureter; indeed, obstructing lesions (e.g., calculus, sloughed papilla) often can be removed percutaneously or bypassed (e.g., carcinoma) by insertion of a ureteric stent. Most patients experience an appropriate diuresis for several days following relief of obstruction; approximately 5 percent develop a transient salt-wasting syndrome that may require administration of intravenous saline to maintain blood pressure.

Supportive measures   Since intravascular volume overload, hyperkalemia, hyperphosphatemia, and metabolic acidosis are almost invariable in oliguric ARF, preventive measures should be taken from the time of diagnosis (Table 236-3). Prescription of nutrition should be designed to maintain caloric balance and minimize catabolism. In addition, doses of drugs excreted via the kidney must be adjusted for the degree of renal impairment.

Following correction of intravascular volume deficits, salt and water intake should be adjusted to match losses (urinary, gastrointestinal, drainage sites, insensible losses). *Intravascular volume overload* usually can be managed by restriction of salt and water intake and by use of diuretics. Indeed, there is no rationale for administration of diuretics in ARF other than to treat this complication. High doses of loop-blocking diuretics such as furosemide (up to 400 mg IV) or bumetanide (up to 10 mg IV) may be required in patients who fail to respond to conventional doses. Diuretic therapy should be discontinued in resistant patients to avoid complications such as deafness. Continuous intravenous infusion of low doses of dopamine (2 to 5 μg/kg per min) may promote salt and water excretion by increasing renal blood flow and GFR and by inhibiting sodium reabsorption in the proximal tubule. However, the role of dopamine remains to be established, since renal responses are variable under these circumstances. Ultrafil-

TABLE 236-3   Supportive treatment of intrinsic acute renal failure

Complication	Therapy
Intravascular volume overload	Salt (1–2 g/d) and water (usually <1 L/d) restriction Diuretics (usually loop blockers) Ultrafiltration or dialysis
Hyponatremia	Restriction of water intake
Hyperkalemia	Restriction of dietary K^+ Eliminate K^+ supplements and K^+-sparing diuretics Potassium-binding ion-exchange resins Glucose (50 mL of 50% dextrose) and insulin (10 units regular) Sodium bicarbonate (usually 50–100 mmol) Calcium gluconate (10 mL of 10% solution over 5 min) Dialysis
Metabolic acidosis	Restriction of dietary protein Sodium bicarbonate (maintain serum bicarbonate >15 mmol/L) Dialysis
Hyperphosphatemia	Restriction of dietary phosphate intake Phosphate binding agents (calcium carbonate, aluminum hydroxide)
Hypocalcemia	Calcium carbonate (if symptomatic or if sodium bicarbonate to be administered) Calcium gluconate (10–20 mL of 10% solution)
Hypermagnesemia	Discontinue Mg^{2+}-containing antacids
Hyperuricemia	Treatment usually not necessary if < 900 mmol/L (<15 mg/dL)
Nutrition	Restriction of dietary protein (−0.5 g/kg/d) Carbohydrate (−100 g/d) Enteral or parenteral nutrition (if recovery prolonged)
Drug dosage	Adjust doses for degree of renal impairment
Indications for dialysis	Clinical evidence (symptoms or signs) of uremia Intractable intravascular volume overload Hyperkalemia or severe acidosis resistant to conservative measures

tration or dialysis may be employed for volume reduction when conservative measures fail. *Hyponatremia* usually can be corrected by restriction of water intake. Conversely, *hypernatremia* is treated by administration of water or hypotonic saline solutions.

Mild *hyperkalemia* (<5.5 mmol/L) should be managed initially by restriction of dietary potassium intake and elimination of potassium supplements and potassium-sparing diuretics. Moderate hyperkalemia (5.5 to 6.5 mmol/L) in patients without clinical or electrocardiographic evidence of hyperkalemia usually can be controlled by administration of potassium-binding ion exchange resins such as sodium polystyrene sulfonate (15 to 30 g q 3–4 h) together with sorbitol (50 to 100 mL of 20% solution) by mouth or as a retention enema. Loop diuretics also increase potassium excretion in diuretic-responsive patients. Emergency measures should be employed in patients with serum potassium values of greater than 6.5 mmol/L and in all patients with ECG abnormalities or clinical features of hyperkalemia. Intravenous insulin (10 units of regular insulin) and glucose (50 mL of 50% dextrose) promote potassium shift into cells within 30 to 60 min, a benefit that lasts for several hours. Sodium bicarbonate (1 ampule, 44.6 mmol IV over 5 min) also promotes rapid (onset <15 min, duration 1 to 2 h) shift of potassium into the intracellular space. Since sodium polysterene sulfonate and sodium bicarbonate carry an obligatory sodium load, these compounds should be used judiciously in oliguric patients to avoid intravascular volume overload. Calcium gluconate (10 mL of 10% solution IV over 5 min) antagonizes the cardiac and neuromuscular effects of hyperkalemia and is a valuable emergency measure while other agents reduce serum potassium concentration. Dialysis is indicated if hyperkalemia is resistant to these measures.

Metabolic acidosis does not require treatment unless serum bicarbonate concentration falls below 15 mmol/L. More severe acidosis can be corrected by either oral or intravenous bicarbonate administration. Initial rates of replacement should be based on estimates of bicarbonate deficit and adjusted thereafter according to serum levels. Patients should be monitored for complications of bicarbonate administration, including metabolic alkalosis, hypocalcemia, hypokalemia, volume overload, and pulmonary edema. *Hyperphosphatemia* usually can be controlled by restriction of dietary phosphate intake and oral administration of agents (e.g., aluminum hydroxide or calcium carbonate) which reduce absorption of phosphate from the gastrointestinal tract. *Hypocalcemia* does not usually require treatment unless severe, such as with rhabdomyolysis or pancreatitis or following administration of bicarbonate. *Hyperuricemia* is usually mild in ARF [<900 mmol/L (<15 mg/dL)] and does not require intervention.

Nutritional management requires collaboration among physicians, nurses, and dieticians. The objective during the maintenance phase of ARF is to provide sufficient calories to avoid catabolism and starvation ketoacidosis while minimizing production of nitrogenous waste. This is best achieved by restricting dietary protein intake to approximately 0.5 g/kg of body weight per day of protein of high biologic value (i.e., rich in essential amino acids) and to provide most calories in the form of carbohydrate (approximately 100 g/d). Management of nutrition is easier in nonoliguric patients and after institution of dialysis. Parenteral alimentation has been claimed to improve prognosis, but a consistent benefit has not been demonstrated.

Anemia may neccessitate blood transfusion or administration of erythropoietin. Uremic bleeding usually responds to desmopressin, correction of anemia, estrogens, or dialysis. *Doses of drugs* which are excreted by the kidney must be adjusted for the degree of renal impairment. Antacids appear to reduce the incidence of *gastrointestinal hemorrhage* and may be more potent than H-2 blockers in this regard. Febrile patients must be investigated aggressively for *infection* and may be given broad-spectrum antibiotics while awaiting identification of specific organisms. Meticulous care of intravenous cannulas, catheters, and other invasive devices is mandatory. Unfortunately, prophylactic antibiotics do not appear to reduce the incidence of infection in these high-risk patients.

Dialysis   Dialysis does not appear to hasten recovery in ARF. Early studies which suggested that early dialysis therapy improved prognosis have not been confirmed. Indeed, hemodialysis may potentially exacerbate renal hypoperfusion, since transient hypotension is a common complication. Accordingly, dialysis is reserved for treatment of symptoms or signs of uremia and management of volume overload, hyperkalemia, or acidosis refractory to conservative therapy. The type of dialysis (peritoneal dialysis, hemodialysis) and prescription depend on individual requirements. Peritoneal dialysis is effected through a temporary intraperitoneal catheter, and vascular access for short-term hemodialysis is usually achieved using a double-lumen catheter inserted into the subclavian, internal jugular, or femoral vein. Slow continuous arteriovenous hemofiltration and dialysis are alternative modalities for patients who do not tolerate conventional short-term dialysis and in whom peritoneal dialysis is not possible (e.g., after abdominal surgery). Ultrafiltration of plasma, without dialysis, may be used for intractable volume overload in patients without symptomatic uremia. Although many patients recover from ARF, a few (<5 percent) require long-term renal replacement therapy. With this in mind, every effort should be made to preserve veins (i.e., avoid venepuncture) on the nondominant arm of patients with severe ARF, since these may be required for chronic hemodialysis access (arteriovenous fistula) at a later date.

OUTCOME AND LONG-TERM PROGNOSIS   The mortality rate from ARF approximates 50 percent and has changed little over the last 30 years. However, mortality rates vary depending on the cause: ~15 percent in obstetrical patients, ~30 percent in toxin-related

ARF, and ~60 percent following trauma or major surgery. Oliguria (<400 mL/d) at presentation and a rise in serum creatinine of greater than 260 μmol/L (3 mg/dL) are associated with a poor prognosis and probably reflect the extent of renal parenchymal damage and severity of the underlying disease. Mortality rates are higher in older, debilitated patients and those with multiple organ failure. With proper management, death usually results from primary diseases and rarely from uremia per se. Most patients who survive an episode of ARF recover sufficient renal function to live normal lives. However, half have subclinical impairment of glomerular filtration and urinary concentrating or acidification mechanisms or residual scarring on renal biopsy. Approximately 5 percent never recover function, presumably due to complete cortical necrosis, and require therapy with long-term dialysis or transplantation. An additional 5 percent have progressive decline in renal function following an initial recovery phase, probably due to hyperfiltration and subsequent sclerosis of remnant glomeruli (see Chap. 237). Progression to chronic renal failure may be observed more often following ARF as life-expectancy increases.

REFERENCES

ANDERSON RJ, SCHRIER RW: Acute tubular necrosis, in *Diseases of the Kidney*, RW Schrier, CW Gottschalk (eds). Boston, Little, Brown, 1988, p 1413

BRENNER BM, LAZARUS JM (eds). *Acute Renal Failure*, 3d ed. New York, Churchill Livingstone, 1993

BREZIS M et al: Acute renal failure, in *The Kidney*, 4th ed, BM Brenner, FC Rector Jr (eds). Philadelphia, Saunders, 1991, p 993

LIEBERTHAL W, LEVINSKY NG: Acute clinical renal failure, in *The Kidney, Physiology and Pathophysiology*, 2d ed, DW Seldin, G Giebisch (eds). New York, Raven, 1992, p 3181

OLSEN S: Acute tubular necrosis and toxic renal injury, in *Renal Pathology with Clinical and Functional Correlations*, CC Tisher, BM Brenner (eds). Philadelphia, Lippincott, 1989, p 656

---

237   CHRONIC RENAL FAILURE

BARRY M. BRENNER / J. MICHAEL LAZARUS

In contrast to the capacity of the kidney to regain function following acute renal injury, discussed in the preceding chapter, renal injury of a more sustained nature is often not reversible but leads to progressive destruction of nephron mass. Despite successful treatment of hypertension, urinary tract obstruction and infection, and systemic disease, many forms of renal injury progress inexorably to chronic renal failure (CRF). Reduction of renal mass causes structural and functional hypertrophy of remaining nephrons. This "compensatory" hypertrophy is due to adaptive hyperfiltration mediated by increases in glomerular capillary pressures and flows. Eventually, these adaptations prove "maladaptive" in that they predispose to glomerular sclerosis, an enhanced functional burden on less affected glomeruli, leading in turn to their ultimate destruction.

Glomerulonephritis, in its several forms, was the most common initiating cause of chronic renal failure in the past. Possibly because of more aggressive treatment of glomerulonephritis and because of changing practices in patient acceptance of end-stage renal disease programs, diabetes mellitus and hypertension are now the leading causes of chronic renal failure (see Fig. 237-1). These and other progressive forms of renal disease are considered in detail in the remaining chapters of this section. Irrespective of cause, the eventual impact of severe reduction in nephron mass is an alteration in function of virtually every organ system in the body. *Uremia* is the term generally applied to the clinical syndrome that results from profound loss of renal function. Although the cause(s) of the syndrome remain unknown, the term *uremia* was adopted originally because of the

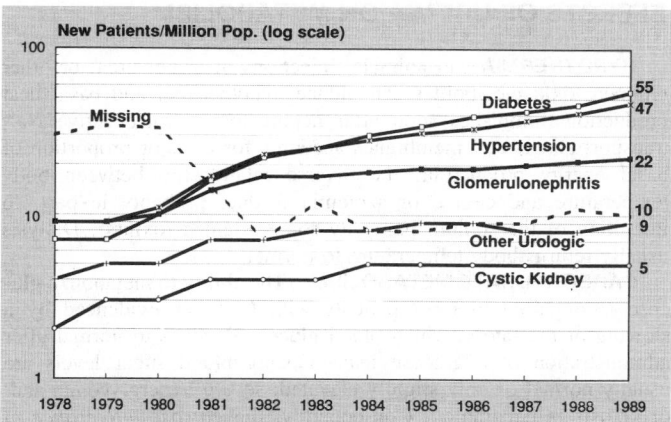

FIGURE 237-1 Incidence rates per million population of treated chronic renal failure by five major primary disease groups (diabetes mellitus, hypertension, glomerulonephritis, cystic kidney, other urologic), 1978–1989. Unadjusted, semilog scale; Medicare patients only.

presumption that the abnormalities result from retention in the blood of urea and other end products of metabolism normally excreted in the urine. But the term *uremia* represents more than renal excretory failure alone. A host of metabolic and endocrine functions normally subserved by the kidney are also impaired, and the inexorable course to renal failure is often accompanied by malnutrition; impaired metabolism of carbohydrates, fats, and proteins; and defective utilization of energy. Therefore, *uremia* refers generally to the constellation of signs and symptoms associated with CRF, regardless of cause.

The presentation and severity of signs and symptoms of uremia vary from patient to patient, depending, at least in part, on the magnitude of the reduction in functioning renal mass and the rapidity with which renal function is lost. As discussed in Chap. 235, in the relatively early stage of CRF [i.e., when total glomerular filtration rate (GFR) is reduced to levels about 35 to 50 percent of normal], overall renal function is sufficient to maintain the patient symptom-free, although renal reserve is diminished. At this stage, biosynthetic, excretory, and other regulatory functions of the kidney are generally well maintained. At a somewhat later stage in the course of CRF (GFR about 20 to 35 percent of normal), *azotemia* occurs, and initial manifestations of renal insufficiency usually appear. Although patients are relatively asymptomatic at this stage, renal reserve is diminished sufficiently that sudden stress, such as intercurrent infection, urinary tract obstruction, dehydration, or administration of a nephrotoxic drug, may compromise renal function still further, often leading to signs and symptoms of overt uremia. With further loss of nephron mass (GFR below 20 to 25 percent of normal), the patient develops *overt renal failure.* Uremia may be viewed as the final stage in this inexorable process, when many of or all the untoward manifestations of CRF become evident clinically. In this chapter the causes and characteristics of the disturbances of the various organ systems in CRF will be considered.

PATHOPHYSIOLOGY AND BIOCHEMISTRY OF UREMIA

The finding that sera from patients with uremia exert toxic effects in a variety of biologic test systems has motivated a diligent search to identify the responsible toxin(s). The most likely candidates as toxins in uremia are the *by-products of protein and amino acid metabolism.* Unlike fats and carbohydrates, which are eventually metabolized to carbon dioxide and water, substances that are easily excreted even in uremic subjects via lungs and skin, the products of protein and amino acid metabolism depend largely on the kidneys for excretion. A vast number of such products have been identified, with urea being

quantitatively the most important. *Urea* represents some 80 percent or more of the total nitrogen excreted into the urine. The *guanidino compounds* are the next most abundant of the nitrogenous end products of protein metabolism and include substances such as guanidine, methyl- and dimethylguanidine, creatinine, creatine, and guanidino-succinic acid. As with urea, guanidines are derived, at least in part, from urea cycle amino acids. Other metabolic products that are possible uremic toxins include *urates and other end products of nucleic acid metabolism, aliphatic amines,* a variety of *peptides,* and finally, several *derivatives of the aromatic amino acids tryptophan, tyrosine, and phenylalanine.* The role of these various substances in the pathogenesis of the uremic syndrome is unclear. Uremic symptoms correlate only in a rough and inconsistent way with concentrations of urea in blood. Nevertheless, although probably not a major cause of overt uremic toxicity, urea may account for some of the clinical abnormalities, including anorexia, malaise, vomiting, and headache. On the other hand, elevated levels of plasma *guanidinosuccinic acid,* by interfering with activation of platelet factor III by adenosine diphosphate (ADP), contribute to the impaired platelet function in CRF. *Creatinine,* generally regarded as a nontoxic substance, may cause adverse effects following conversion to metabolites such as sarcosine and methylguanidine. The extent to which these substances, as well as *creatine,* a metabolic precursor of creatinine, and the other compounds cited above, are of importance in the pathogenesis of uremic toxicity remains to be established.

Nitrogenous compounds of larger molecular weight are also retained in CRF. A toxic role for these substances has been suggested because of the impression that patients treated with intermittent peritoneal dialysis are less troubled with neuropathy than patients maintained on chronic hemodialysis, despite higher levels of urea and creatinine in blood in the former group. Since the clearance of small molecules depends mainly on blood and dialysate flow rates, which are higher with hemodialysis, whereas clearance of larger molecules depends more on membrane surface area and time, which are greater with peritoneal dialysis, this latter therapy may be a more effective means of removing substances of larger molecular weight. However, a multicenter study examining clearance of small versus middle-sized molecular substances, dialysis time, and morbidity indicated that urea or other small-molecular-weight substances play a more important role in determining uremic symptoms. The role of "middle" molecules in the uremic syndrome remains speculative.

Not all middle-sized molecules accumulate in uremic plasma because of decreased renal excretion alone. The kidney normally *catabolizes* a number of circulating plasma proteins and polypeptides; with reduced renal mass, this capacity may be impaired greatly. Furthermore, plasma levels of many polypeptide hormones [including parathyroid hormone (PTH), insulin, glucagon, growth hormone, luteinizing hormone, and prolactin] rise with renal failure, often markedly so, not only because of impaired renal catabolism but also because of enhanced secretion. Of these, excessive PTH may be an important uremic "toxin" because of its adverse effect on several organ systems. The consequences of high circulating levels of PTH and other hormones in chronic renal failure are considered below and in Chap. 235.

EFFECTS OF UREMIA ON CELLULAR FUNCTIONS

Alterations in the composition of intracellular and extracellular fluids in CRF are believed to be a consequence, at least in part, of *defective ion transport* across cell membranes generally, with retained uremic toxins possibly mediating these alterations in transmembrane ion transport. Integrity of cellular volume and composition depends to a large extent on the active outward transport of Na^+ from cell interior to exterior, the resulting intracellular fluid being relatively low in Na^+ and high in K^+, whereas the reverse is true for extracellular fluid. Active Na^+ transport is metabolically costly, accounting for a major fraction of basal energy utilization and oxygen consumption.

The consequences of this efflux of Na^+ from cells include (1) the generation of a resting electrical potential difference across the cell membrane (with this transcellular voltage oriented so that cell interior is electronegative to cell exterior) and (2) a mechanism for enhancing the influx of K^+ into cells.

In animals, partial inhibition of this active efflux mechanism for Na^+ across cell membranes leads to alterations in body composition and cell functions similar to those in erythrocytes, leukocytes, skeletal muscle, and other tissues of uremic subjects. These include increased and decreased intracellular concentrations of Na^+ and K^+, respectively, and reduction in magnitude of the transcellular voltage. These alterations are largely reversed by efficient hemodialysis and, for erythrocytes at least, are recreated when cells from normal subjects are incubated in uremic serum. Other derangements also have been implicated as causes for altered body composition in uremia. For example, *Na^+- and K^+-stimulated ATPase activity* is decreased in erythrocytes and brain from uremic patients and animals, respectively. Whether the uremic "toxins" that account for these derangements in cellular function represent abnormally retained products of metabolism that fail to be excreted or normal substances present in increased quantities in response to reduced renal mass remains unknown. *Parathyroid and natriuretic hormones*, examples of this category of substances, are discussed in this context in Chap. 235.

EFFECTS OF UREMIA ON WHOLE-BODY COMPOSITION

What is the impact of these disturbances in active transcellular Na^+ transport on the organism? From the pathophysiologic considerations already discussed, CRF is likely to lead to abnormally high intracellular Na^+ concentrations and hence to osmotically induced overhydration of cells, whereas these same cells are relatively deficient in K^+. With the development of malaise, anorexia, nausea, vomiting, and diarrhea, patients with CRF may eventually develop protein-calorie malnutrition and negative nitrogen balance, often with profound losses of lean body mass and fat deposits. Owing to the concomitant tendency for salt and water retention, these losses often go unnoticed until the late stages of CRF. Whereas a large fraction of the increase in total-body water in uremia is the result of expansion of intracellular volume, extracellular volume expansion also occurs. With initiation of intermittent hemodialysis or renal transplantation, there is often an immediate loss of body weight, due primarily to correction of this overhydration. With successful transplantation, the initial diuresis is followed by a period of weight gain, due to restoration of lean body mass and fat deposits to preillness levels. For patients on chronic dialysis, the anabolic response is less dramatic, even when therapy is regarded as optimal, involving mainly reaccumulation of fat deposits. The failure to restore lean body mass to normal with chronic dialysis may reflect insufficient intake of calories and protein, which, in adequately dialyzed patients, should be maintained at levels of 150 kJ/kg (35 kcal/kg) and 1.0 to 1.4 g/kg of body weight per day, respectively.

Deficits in intracellular K^+ concentration in CRF may result from inadequate intake (poor diet or overzealous K^+ restriction by the physician), excessive losses (vomiting, diarrhea, diuretics), reduction of Na^+- and K^+-stimulated ATPase, or a combination of these. In addition to promoting losses of K^+ into urine (which may be substantial if urine volume remains relatively normal in uremic subjects), the high levels of plasma aldosterone often seen in CRF also may augment net secretion of K^+ into the colon, thereby contributing to K^+ losses in stool or diarrheal fluids. Despite deficits in intracellular K^+, serum K^+ is usually normal or high in CRF, owing most often to metabolic acidosis, which induces an efflux of K^+ from cells. Uremic patients are also relatively resistant to the action of insulin (see below), which normally enhances K^+ uptake by skeletal muscle.

EFFECTS OF UREMIA ON METABOLISM

HYPOTHERMIA   In animals, injections of urine, urea, or other retained toxic metabolites can induce hypothermia, and basal heat production diminishes soon after nephrectomy. Since active Na^+ transport across cell membranes accounts for a major proportion of basal energy production, the inverse relationship between body temperature and degree of azotemia is due, probably in part, to inhibition of the sodium pump by some retained toxin(s). Dialysis usually returns body temperature to normal.

CARBOHYDRATE METABOLISM   The ability to metabolize glucose is impaired in most patients with CRF, as evidenced by a slowing of the rate at which blood glucose declines to normal after administration of a glucose load. Fasting blood sugar levels are usually normal or only slightly elevated; severe hyperglycemia and/or ketosis is uncommon. Consequently, the *glucose intolerance of CRF* usually does not require specific therapy (hence the term *azotemic pseudodiabetes*). Because insulin depends to a large extent on the kidney for its removal from plasma and degradation, circulating insulin levels in plasma are slightly to moderately increased in most fasting uremic subjects, and levels in excess of normal are usually demonstrable after a glucose load. The response to intravenous insulin in patients with CRF is also impaired, and the rate of utilization of glucose by peripheral tissues is diminished. The glucose intolerance of uremia results largely from this peripheral resistance to the action of insulin. Other possible factors contributing to glucose intolerance include intracellular deficits of potassium, metabolic acidosis, increased levels of glucagon, catecholamines, growth hormone, and prolactin, as well as the myriad of potentially toxic metabolites retained in CRF. In true insulin-dependent diabetics, there is often a decrease in insulin requirement with progressive azotemia, a phenomenon not related solely to decreased caloric intake.

NITROGEN AND LIPID METABOLISM   Since the capacity to eliminate the nitrogenous end products of protein catabolism is reduced, CRF may be regarded as a state of *protein intolerance*. As discussed above, retention of the end products of nitrogen metabolism is a dominant cause of the signs and symptoms of uremic toxicity.

Hypertriglyceridemia and decreased high-density lipoprotein cholesterol are common in uremia, whereas cholesterol levels in plasma are usually normal. Whether uremia accelerates triglyceride production by the liver and intestine is unknown. The enhancement of lipogenesis by insulin may contribute to increased triglyceride synthesis. In addition, the rate of removal of triglycerides from the circulation, which depends in large part on the enzyme *lipoprotein lipase*, is depressed in uremia, an effect not corrected appreciably by hemodialysis. The high incidence of premature atherosclerosis in patients on chronic dialysis (see "Cardiovascular and Pulmonary Abnormalities" below) may be related in part to these abnormalities in lipid metabolism.

CLINICAL ABNORMALITIES IN UREMIA

Chronic renal failure is associated with a constellation of signs and symptoms with or without reduced urine output but always with elevation in serum urea nitrogen and creatinine concentrations. As pointed out in Chap. 235, elevations of serum urea nitrogen and creatinine occur late in the course of renal failure. Differentiation between acute and chronic renal failure can be difficult. The history is often most helpful, particularly if normal renal function existed prior to a sudden recent insult. The laboratory findings and physical examination may not be helpful in the differentiation. The usual hallmark of chronic renal failure is reduced kidney size on ultrasound, abdominal scout film, or pyelogram. In the absence of small kidneys, renal biopsy may be necessary for diagnosis.

As noted earlier, CRF leads to disturbances in function of every organ system. With the application of chronic dialysis, the incidence and severity of these disturbances are modified so that where modern medicine is practiced, the overt and florid manifestations of uremia have largely disappeared. Unfortunately, however, even optimal dialysis therapy is not a panacea, because, as indicated in Table 237-1, some disturbances resulting from impaired renal function fail to respond fully, while others progress despite dialysis treatment. Furthermore, as with many complex therapeutic modalities, dialysis may cause unique abnormalities not seen prior to initiation of therapy; these abnormalities should be viewed as complications of dialysis.

FLUID, ELECTROLYTE, AND ACID-BASE DISORDERS (See also Chaps. 45 and 46) **Sodium and volume homeostasis** In most patients with stable CRF, total-body Na^+ and water content are increased modestly, although extracellular fluid (ECF) volume expansion may not be apparent. With ingestion of excessive amounts of salt and water, however, control of excess volume becomes an important consideration. In general, excessive *salt* ingestion contributes to, or aggravates, congestive heart failure, hypertension, ascites, and edema. On the other hand, hyponatremia and weight gain are the consequence of excessive ingestion of *water*, abnormalities that in most patients are relatively mild or asymptomatic. In most patients, daily intake of fluid equal in volume to urine volume per day plus about 500 mL usually maintains the serum Na^+ concentration at normal levels. Hypernatremia is relatively infrequent in CRF. In the edematous patient with CRF not on dialysis, diuretics and modest restriction of salt and water intake are the mainstays of therapy.

In volume-expanded dialysis patients, management should include ultrafiltration and restriction of salt and water intake between dialyses.

Patients with CRF have impaired renal mechanisms for conserving Na^+ and water (see Chap. 235). When an *extrarenal* cause for increased fluid loss is present (e.g., vomiting, diarrhea, fever), these patients are prone to develop ECF volume depletion, with dryness of mouth and other mucous membranes, dizziness, syncope, tachycardia, decreased filling of jugular veins, orthostatic hypotension, and vascular collapse. Depletion of extracellular fluid volume typically results in deterioration of residual renal function and, in the previously stable and asymptomatic patient with mild CRF, signs and symptoms of overt uremia. Cautious fluid repletion usually restores extracellular and intravascular volumes to normal and often returns renal function to stable levels.

Potassium homeostasis Derangements in K^+ balance (see Chaps. 45 and 235) are occasionally documented by laboratory analysis in patients with CRF but are rarely responsible for clinical symptoms unless GFR is below 5 mL/min or unless an endogenous (hemolysis, trauma, infection) or exogenous (stored blood, K^+-containing medications) K^+ load is administered. Despite progression of renal failure, most patients maintain normal serum K^+ concentrations until the final stages of uremia. This ability to sustain K^+ balance with advancing renal failure is due to adaptations in the renal distal tubules and colon, sites where aldosterone and other factors serve to enhance K^+ secretion (see Chap. 235). Not surprisingly,

---

TABLE 237-1 Clinical abnormalities in uremia*

FLUID AND ELECTROLYTE DISTURBANCES

Volume expansion and contraction (I)
Hypernatremia and hyponatremia (I)
Hyperkalemia and hypokalemia (I)
Metabolic acidosis (I)
Hyperphosphatemia (I)
Hypocalcemia (I)

ENDOCRINE-METABOLIC DISTURBANCES

Renal osteodystrophy (I or P)
Osteomalacia (D)
Aluminum-induced
Vitamin D–deficient osteomalacia (I)
Secondary hyperparathyroidism (I or P)
Carbohydrate intolerance (I)
Hyperuricemia (I or P)
Hypothermia (I)
Hypertriglyceridemia (P)
Protein-calorie malnutrition (I or P)
Impaired growth and development (P)
Infertility and sexual dysfunction (P)
Amenorrhea (P)
Dialysis (beta$_2$-microglobulin, amyloid) arthropathy (D)

GASTROINTESTINAL DISTURBANCES

Anorexia (I)
Nausea and vomiting (I)
Uremic fetor (I)
Gastroenteritis (I)
Peptic ulcer (I or P)
Gastrointestinal bleeding (I, P, or D)
Hepatitis (D)
Refractory ascites on hemodialysis (D)
Peritonitis (D)

CARDIOVASCULAR AND PULMONARY DISTURBANCES

Arterial hypertension (I or P)
Congestive heart failure or pulmonary edema (I)
Pericarditis (I)

Cardiomyopathy (I or P)
Uremic lung (I)
Accelerated atherosclerosis (P or D)
Hypotension and arrhythmias (D)

DERMATOLOGIC DISTURBANCES

Pallor (I)[†]
Hyperpigmentation (I, P, or D)
Pruritus (P)
Ecchymoses (I or P)
Uremic frost (I)

NEUROMUSCULAR DISTURBANCES

Fatigue (I)[†]
Sleep disorders (P)
Headache (I or P)
Impaired mentation (I)[†]
Lethargy (I)[†]
Asterixis (I)
Muscular irritability (I)
Peripheral neuropathy (I or P)
Restless legs syndrome (I or P)
Paralysis (I or P)
Myoclonus (I)
Seizures (I or P)
Coma (I)
Muscle cramps (D)
Dialysis disequilibrium syndrome (D)
Dialysis dementia (D)
Myopathy (P or D)

HEMATOLOGIC AND IMMUNOLOGIC DISTURBANCES

Normocytic, normochromic anemia (I)[†]
Microcytic (aluminum-induced) anemia (D)
Lymphocytopenia (P)
Bleeding diathesis (I or D)
Increased susceptibility to infection (I or P)
Splenomegaly and hypersplenism (P)
Leukopenia (D)
Hypocomplementemia (D)

---

* Virtually all abnormalities in this table are completely reversed in time by successful renal transplantation. The response of these abnormalities to hemo- or peritoneal dialysis therapy is more variable. (I) denotes an abnormality that usually improves with an optimal program of dialysis and related therapy. (P) denotes an abnormality that tends to persist or even progress, despite an optimal program. (D) denotes an abnormality that develops only after initiation of dialysis therapy.
† Improves with dialysis and erythropoietin (EPO) therapy.

oliguria, or disruption of key adaptive mechanisms, can lead to *hyperkalemia* and its potentially ominous effects on cardiac function. Antikaliuretic drugs such as spironolactone, triamterene, or amiloride should be used with extreme caution in chronic renal failure. Likewise, angiotensin-converting enzyme inhibitors and beta blockers may cause hyperkalemia. In the transplanted patient, cyclosporine is another common cause of increased serum potassium. Hyperkalemia in CRF also may be induced by abrupt lowering of arterial blood pH, since acidosis is associated with efflux of K^+ from intracellular to extracellular fluids. A useful index of the magnitude of this hydrogen-potassium exchange is that for every 0.1-unit change in blood pH, there will be a reciprocal change in serum K^+ concentration of approximately 0.6 mmol/L. Correction of acidosis-induced hyperkalemia with sodium bicarbonate is the treatment of choice. Intravenous insulin and dextrose are useful in lowering serum potassium acutely, while the ion exchange resin sodium polystyrene sulfonate is useful in longer-term control of hyperkalemia. When hyperkalemia persists in the absence of excessive K^+ intake, oliguria, or acute acidosis, the possibility of *hyporeninemic hypoaldosteronism* should be considered. Patients with this syndrome have reduced circulating levels of renin and aldosterone in the plasma and often have diabetes mellitus.

Hypokalemia due to diminished ability of the kidneys to conserve K^+ is uncommon in most forms of CRF. When hypokalemia occurs in these patients, poor dietary K^+ intake, usually in association with excessive diuretic therapy or gastrointestinal losses, is likely to be the underlying cause. When hypokalemia occurs as a result of primary K^+ wasting in urine, it may represent a solitary renal reabsorptive defect or, more commonly, may be associated with other solute transport abnormalities, as in Fanconi's syndrome, renal tubular acidosis, or other forms of hereditary or acquired tubulointerstitial diseases (see Chaps. 242 and 244). The clinical consequences and management of hypokalemia and hyperkalemia are discussed in Chap. 45.

Metabolic acidosis   With advancing renal failure, total daily acid excretion and buffer production fall below the level needed to maintain external balance of hydrogen ions. Metabolic acidosis is the inevitable result, and the mechanisms involved are considered in Chap. 235. In most patients with stable renal insufficiency, administration of 20 to 30 mmol/d sodium bicarbonate or sodium citrate corrects the acidosis. In response to a sudden acid challenge (whether from an endogenous or exogenous source), however, patients with CRF are susceptible to acidosis, which requires more substantial quantities of alkali for correction. Administration of sodium must be carried out with careful attention to volume status.

Phosphate, calcium, and bone   As discussed in Chap. 235, hypocalcemia in chronic renal failure results from the impaired ability of the diseased kidney to synthesize 1,25-dihydroxyvitamin D [$1,25(OH)_2D$], the active metabolite of vitamin D (Fig. 237-2). Absorption of calcium in the gut is impaired when circulating levels of this active metabolite are low. Also, serum phosphate concentration begins to rise when GFR falls below about 25 percent of normal. Calcium deposition in bone is dependent on the availability of phosphate; retention of phosphate in plasma, therefore, facilitates calcium entry into bone and contributes to the hypocalcemia and elevation of plasma PTH levels in CRF. Finally, in advanced CRF, the ability of PTH to mobilize calcium salts from bone may be altered. Despite hypocalcemia, tetany is rare unless patients are treated with large amounts of alkali.

Overproduction of parathyroid hormone, disordered vitamin D metabolism, chronic metabolic acidosis, and excessive fecal losses of calcium all contribute to the bone diseases in uremia (see Fig. 237-2). *Renal* and *metabolic osteodystrophy* are terms that

FIGURE 237-2   Pathogenesis of bone diseases in chronic renal failure.

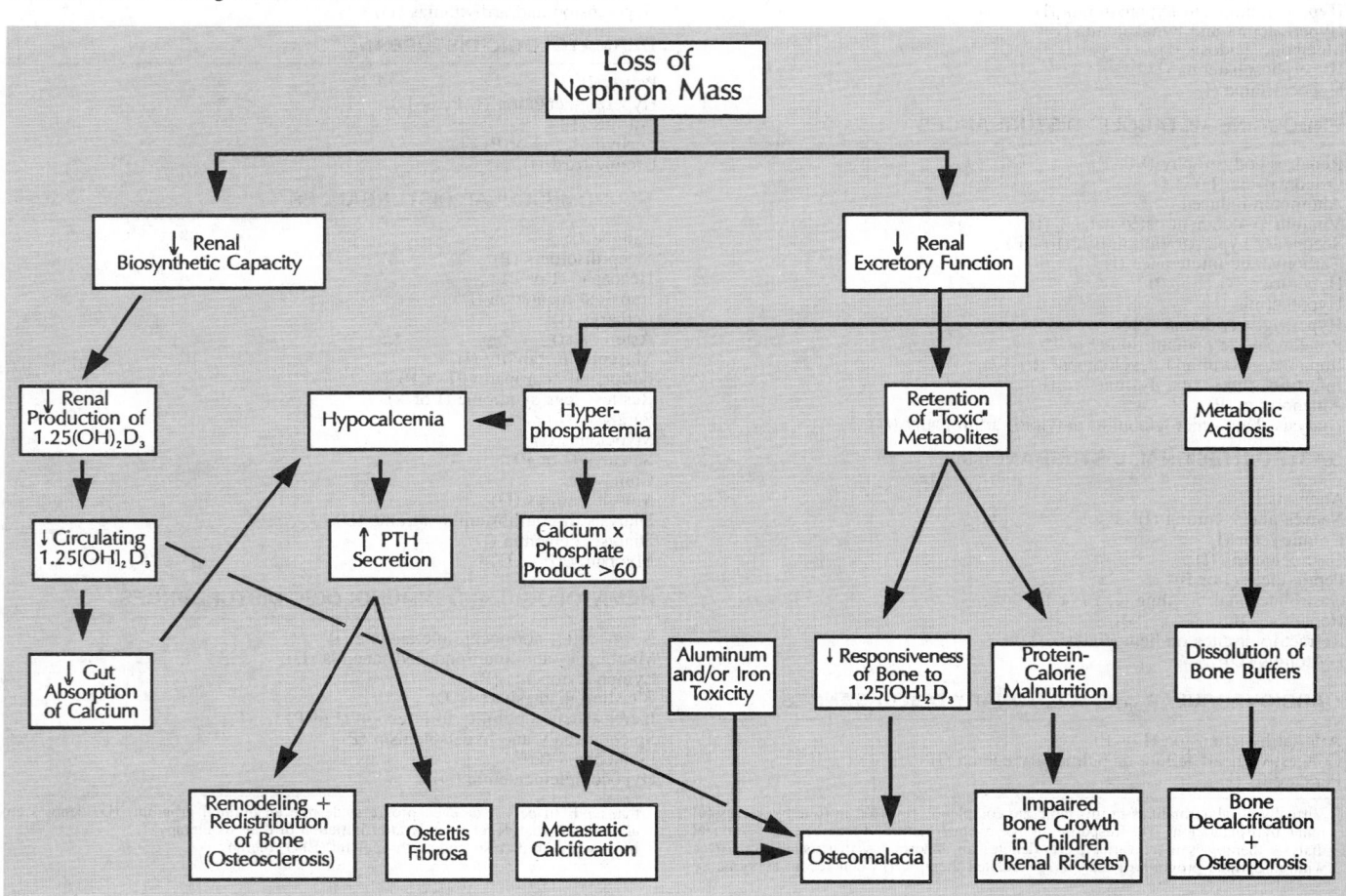

encompass a number of skeletal abnormalities, including osteomalacia, osteitis fibrosa cystica, osteosclerosis, and, in children especially, impaired bone growth. Although clinical symptoms of bone disease are present in less than 10 percent of predialysis patients with advanced renal failure, radiologic and histologic abnormalities are observed in, respectively, about 35 and 90 percent. In patients treated by dialysis for several years, bone disease is a major cause of morbidity. Renal osteodystrophy is more common in children than in adults, and especially in patients with slowly progressive renal insufficiency. On radiologic examination, three types of lesions can be identified: (1) changes analogous to those of nutritional rickets, namely, widened osteoid seams at the growth margin of bones (so-called renal rickets), (2) the bone changes of *secondary hyperparathyroidism* (*osteitis fibrosa cystica*), characterized by osteoclastic bone resorption and subperiosteal erosions, especially of the phalanges, long bones, and distal ends of the clavicles, and (3) *osteosclerosis*, often best evidenced by enhanced bone density in the upper and lower margins of vertebrae, producing the so-called rugger jersey spine.

Osteomalacia can be secondary to decreased availability of $1,25(OH_2)D$ or to deposition of aluminum in the calcification fronts. The sources are aluminum in dialysate and aluminum-containing phosphate-binding agents. In aluminum-induced osteomalacia, the serum level of parathyroid hormone is usually low and that of calcium is often high. With osteitis fibrosa cystica and osteomalacia, there is a tendency to spontaneous fractures which are often slow to heal. The ribs are most commonly involved. Painful joints may occur due to calcium deposition in bursa and other periarticular structures. Bone pain may occur in the absence of fractures. When bone pain is severe, a proximal *myopathy* often coexists, giving rise to gait abnormalities and to impairment of ambulation. The incidence of *aseptic necrosis of the hip* is increased in renal transplant recipients, probably related to chronic glucocorticoid therapy, secondary hyperparathyroidism, and altered vitamin D metabolism. In CRF there is a tendency to *extraosseous*, or *metastatic, calcification* when the calcium-phosphate product is very high. Medium-sized blood vessels; subcutaneous, articular, and periarticular tissues; myocardium; eyes; and lungs are common sites of metastatic calcification. An arthropathy is associated with deposition of amyloid or beta$_2$ microglobulin. The cause is unknown but may be related to elevated levels of cytokines in chronic dialysis patients.

Management of renal osteodystrophy includes reduction in dietary phosphate through the use of a restricted phosphate diet as well as phosphate-binding agents. Calcium carbonate is the preferred phosphate-binding agent, but in some circumstances a combination of aluminum hydroxide and calcium carbonate is necessary. Dialysate calcium, oral calcium, aluminum hydroxide, and calcitriol must be properly balanced to maintain the serum phosporus at approximately 1.4 mmol/L (4.5 mg/dL) and the serum calcium at approximately 2.5 mmol/L (10 mg/dL) in an attempt to improve osteitis fibrosa cystica, osteomalacia, and myopathy. Treatment should be initiated early in chronic renal failure so that secondary hyperparathyroidism and bone disease may be prevented. It is particularly important to keep the calcium-phosphorous product in the normal range to avoid metastatic calcification or any possible role of these substances in progressive renal failure.

Other solutes Other derangements in CRF include *hyperuricemia* and *hypermagnesemia*. Uric acid retention is a common feature of CRF but rarely leads to symptomatic gout. Hypophosphatemia is usually a consequence of overzealous oral administration of phosphate-binding gels. Because serum magnesium levels tend to rise in CRF, magnesium-containing antacids and cathartics should be avoided.

CARDIOVASCULAR AND PULMONARY ABNORMALITIES
Fluid retention in uremia often results in congestive heart failure and/or pulmonary edema. A unique form of pulmonary congestion and edema may occur even in the absence of volume overload and is associated with normal or mildly elevated intracardiac and pulmonary wedge pressures. This entity, characterized radiologically by perihilar vascular congestion giving rise to a "butterfly wing" distribution, is due to increased permeability of the alveolar capillary membrane. This low-pressure pulmonary edema, as well as cardiopulmonary abnormalities associated with circulatory overload, usually responds promptly to vigorous dialysis.

Hypertension is the most common complication of end-stage renal disease. When it is not present, the patient either has a salt-wasting form of renal disease (e.g., polycystic or medullary cystic disease or chronic pyelonephritis), is receiving antihypertensive therapy, or is volume-depleted, the last condition usually being due to excessive gastrointestinal fluid losses or overzealous diuretic therapy. Since fluid overload is the major cause of hypertension in uremia, the normotensive state can usually be restored by dialysis. Nevertheless, some patients remain hypertensive despite rigorous salt and water restriction and ultrafiltration because of hyperreninemia. In approximately 30 percent of patients on chronic erythropoietin therapy, the severity of hypertension is increased. In most cases, routine antihypertensive drug therapy is effective. A minority develop *accelerated or malignant hypertension*, manifested by markedly elevated systolic and diastolic pressures, severe hyperreninemia, encephalopathy, seizures, retinal changes, and papilledema. Drugs such as diazoxide, minoxidil, captopril, enalapril, and nitroprusside, along with control of extracellular volume, generally control such hypertension.

Pericarditis, once a common complication of CRF, is now infrequent because of early initiation of dialysis. Retained metabolic toxins are thought to be the cause of *pericarditis*. The unusual occurrence of pericarditis in the well-dialyzed patient is usually due to viral infection or systemic disease.

The clinical presentation of pericarditis in uremic subjects is generally similar to that of other etiologies (Chap. 206), except that effusions are usually hemorrhagic. Treatment with intensive dialysis is recommended, and systemic anticoagulation should be avoided to minimize the occurrence of hemorrhagic tamponade. In some patients, pericardiocentesis with intrapericardial instillation of air or glucocorticoids is effective for pericardial tamponade. Pericardiectomy should be considered if more conservative treatment fails.

Chronically dialyzed patients have a high incidence of *accelerated atherosclerosis*, leading to coronary, cerebral, and peripheral vascular manifestations. Causes for these complications include hypertension, hyperlipidemia, glucose intolerance, chronic high cardiac output, and metastatic vascular and myocardial calcification.

HEMATOLOGIC ABNORMALITIES *Normochromic, normocytic anemia* occurs regularly and contributes to the symptomology in CRF. Erythropoiesis is depressed in CRF, due both to the effects of retained toxins on bone marrow and to diminished biosynthesis of erythropoietin by the diseased kidney or to the presence of erythropoietin inhibitors. The administration of recombinant human erythropoietin (EPO) results in a dramatic increase in hematocrit and hemoglobin, suggesting that reduced serum erythropoietin is perhaps the more important of these factors. The anemia of chronic uremia also may be due in part to aluminum intoxication, which causes a microcytic anemia, fibrosis of the bone marrow due to hyperparathyroidism, and occasionally, inadequate replacement of folic acid. *Hemolysis* is due to an extracorpuscular defect, since survival of erythrocytes from normal subjects is reduced when these cells are transfused into uremic patients and erythrocytes from patients with CRF have relatively normal survival times when transfused into normal individuals. Gastrointestinal and chronic dialyzer *blood loss* contributes to anemia, as does *hypersplenism* in the occasional patient. Blood loss is exaggerated in hemodialysis patients because of the need for heparin during dialysis.

EPO is available for patients with advanced renal insufficiency and those on maintenance dialysis. Hematocrits of 30 to 36 vol% are attained in a high percentage of patients. In patients on dialysis, improved cardiovascular function, mental status, and energy level associated with the increased hematocrit enhanced the quality of life. The administration of 25 to 50 U/kg body weight three times per week is a reasonable starting dose. Dosage increases after 8 to 12 weeks may be warranted with careful monitoring of hematocrit.

Transfusions may contribute to suppression of erythropoiesis in CRF and, due to increased risk of hepatitis and hemosiderosis, should be avoided unless anemia fails to respond to EPO. Failure to respond to EPO is usually related to iron deficiency but may in part be due to aluminum-induced microcytosis or marrow fibrosis. Parenteral or oral iron therapy is indicated in patients with documented iron deficiency. Folic and ascorbic acids and the soluble B vitamins should be given to offset chronic losses of these substances via dialysis. Hemochromatosis is an uncommon complication since the introduction of EPO therapy.

Abnormal hemostasis is also common in CRF, characterized by a tendency to abnormal bleeding and bruising. Bleeding from the surgical wounds or spontaneously into the gastrointestinal tract, pericardial sac, and intracranial vault, in the form of subdural hematoma or intracerebral hemorrhage, is of greatest concern. Prolongation of bleeding time, decreased platelet factor III activity, abnormal platelet aggregation and adhesiveness, and impaired prothrombin consumption contribute to the clotting defects. The abnormality in factor III correlates with increased plasma levels of guanidinosuccinic acid and can largely be corrected by dialysis. Prolongation of the bleeding time is common even in the well-dialyzed patient. Abnormal bleeding times and coagulopathy in renal failure may be reversed with desmopressin, cryoprecipitate, conjugated estrogens, and blood transfusions, as well as by use of EPO.

Changes in leukocyte formation and function in uremia lead to *enhanced susceptibility to infection.* Lymphocytopenia and atrophy of lymphoid structures occur, whereas neutrophil production is relatively unimpaired. Nevertheless, function of all leukocyte cell types may be affected adversely by uremic serum. Decreased chemotaxis causes impairment of acute inflammatory response and decreased delayed hypersensitivity. There is a tendency for uremic patients to have less fever in response to infection. Leukocyte function also may be impaired in patients with CRF because of coexisting acidosis, hyperglycemia, protein-calorie malnutrition, and serum and tissue hyperosmolarity (due to azotemia). Mucosal barriers to infection also may be defective, and in dialysis patients, vascular access devices are common portals of entry for pathogens, particularly staphylococci. Glucocorticoids and immunosuppressive drugs add further to the risk of infection. Leukopenia is a common transient finding in patients exposed to cellophane-derived membranes during dialysis (Chap. 238).

NEUROMUSCULAR ABNORMALITIES Subtle disturbances of central nervous system function, including inability to concentrate, drowsiness, and insomnia, are among early symptoms of uremia. Mild behavioral changes, loss of memory, and errors in judgment soon follow and may be associated with neuromuscular irritability, including hiccups, cramps, and fasciculations and twitching of muscles. Asterixis, myoclonus, and chorea are common in terminal uremia, as are stupor, seizures, and coma. Many of these neuromuscular complications of severe uremia resolve with dialysis, although nonspecific EEG abnormalities may persist.

Peripheral neuropathy is common in advanced CRF. Initially, sensory nerve involvement exceeds motor, lower extremities are involved more than the upper, and the distal portions of the extremities more than proximal. The "restless legs syndrome" is characterized by ill-defined sensations of discomfort in the feet and lower legs and frequent leg movement. If dialysis is not instituted soon after onset of sensory abnormalities, motor involvement follows, including loss of deep tendon reflexes, weakness, peroneal nerve palsy (foot drop), and eventually, flaccid quadriplegia. Accordingly, evidence of peripheral neuropathy is a firm indication to initiate dialysis or transplantation.

Two types of neurologic disturbances appear to be unique to patients on chronic dialysis. *Dialysis dementia* is seen in patients who have been on dialysis for a number of years and is characterized by speech dyspraxia, myoclonus, dementia, and eventually seizures and death. Aluminum intoxication is probably a major contributor to this syndrome. Other factors (viral infection?) probably play a role, since only a small percent of patients with aluminum exposure develop the syndrome. *Dialysis disequilibrium*, occurs during the first few dialyses, in association with rapid reduction of blood urea levels. Nausea, vomiting, drowsiness, headache, and even convulsions have been attributed to the more rapid (dialysis-induced) pH change and reduction in osmolality of extracellular than intracellular fluids within the cranium, leading to cerebral edema and raised intracranial pressure.

GASTROINTESTINAL ABNORMALITIES Anorexia, hiccups, nausea, and vomiting are common, early manifestations of uremia. Carefully monitored protein restriction in the diet may be useful to slow progression of renal insufficiency if initiated early. Protein restriction is also useful in diminishing nausea and vomiting late in the course. Protein restriction should not, of course, be implemented in those patients with protein-calorie malnutrition. *Uremic fetor*, a uriniferous odor to the breath, derives from the breakdown of urea in saliva to ammonia and is often associated with unpleasant taste sensation. Mucosal ulcerations leading to blood loss can occur at any level of the gastrointestinal tract in very late stages of CRF—so-called uremic gastroenteritis. Peptic ulcer disease occurs in as many as one-fourth of uremic subjects. Whether this incidence is related to increased gastric acidity, hypersecretion of gastrin, or secondary hyperparathyroidism is unknown. Most gastrointestinal symptoms, except those related to peptic ulcer disease, improve with dialysis. Idiopathic ascites is seen rarely in patients on chronic dialysis, presumably secondary to fluid overload and/or chronic passive hepatic congestion. Patients with chronic renal failure, particularly those with polycystic kidney disease, have an increased incidence of diverticulosis. Viral hepatitis is more common in patients on chronic dialysis (see Chap. 238).

ENDOCRINE-METABOLIC DISTURBANCES The disturbances in parathyroid function, glucose tolerance, and insulin metabolism, as well as the lipid, protein-calorie, and other nutritional abnormalities of uremia, have already been considered. Pituitary, thyroid, and adrenal functions are relatively normal, often despite abnormalities in circulating thyroxine, growth hormone, aldosterone, and cortisol levels. In women, estrogen levels are low, and amenorrhea and inability to carry pregnancies to term are early manifestations of uremia. While menses frequently reappear after chronic dialysis is initiated, successful pregnancies are rare. In men with CRF, including those on chronic dialysis, impotence, oligospermia, and germinal cell dysplasia are common, as are reduced plasma testosterone levels. As with growth, sexual maturation is often impaired in adolescent children, even among those on chronic dialysis.

DERMATOLOGIC ABNORMALITIES The skin shows many abnormalities. This is not surprising in view of anemia (pallor), defective hemostasis (ecchymoses and hematomas), calcium deposition and secondary hyperparathyroidism (pruritus, excoriations), dehydration (poor skin turgor, dry mucous membranes), and the general cutaneous consequences of protein-calorie malnutrition. A sallow, yellow cast may reflect the combined influences of anemia and retention of a variety of pigmented metabolites, or *urochromes*. In advanced uremia, urea concentrations in sweat may reach sufficiently high levels that, after evaporation, a fine white powder can be found on the skin surface—so-called uremic (urea) frost. Although many of these cutaneous abnormalities improve with dialysis, *uremic pruritus* is usually resistant to most systemic and topical therapies. Hemochromatosis causes a slate-gray–bronze discoloration of the skin and is common in the dialysis patient who has received multiple transfusions.

CONSERVATIVE MANAGEMENT OF PROGRESSIVE RENAL FAILURE

Treatment directed to specific organ system abnormalities has been discussed in the preceding paragraphs. Principles of dialysis and transplant therapy are discussed in Chap. 238. Conservative (nondialytic, nontransplant) therapy is instituted early to control symptoms, minimize complications, prevent long-term sequelae, and slow the progression of renal insufficiency. The level of renal function should be ascertained at periodic intervals, and any reversible component that may be present should be corrected. In patients with slowly progressive renal failure, urine output is usually well maintained. Blood urea nitrogen and serum creatinine levels correlate only roughly with symptoms and are poor measures of glomerular filtration rate (GFR) (see Chap. 235). The inverse of serum creatinine (1/CR) was previously considered to be a more accurate measure of renal function and to be useful in comparing the effects of treatments that may affect renal failure progression. However, 1/CR is no more accurate than serum creatinine determination alone. Creatinine clearance (urine to plasma creatinine concentration ratio × volume of urine per minute) tends to overestimate GFR, while calculated urea clearance often underestimates GFR. By averaging simultaneously determined creatinine and urea clearances, a reasonably accurate estimation of GFR can therefore be obtained. More exact measures of GFR by isotope clearance techniques require injection of radioisotope and accurate collection of urine specimens at timed intervals over a 2- to 4-h period, usually by an experienced technician. Of those available, the iothalamate clearance (Glofil) is the most useful clinically.

Prerenal factors, such as volume depletion, decreased cardiac output, and renal artery stenosis, and postrenal components, such as urethral or ureteric obstruction, may exacerbate chronic renal insufficiency and must be identified and corrected. Hypertension, urinary tract infections, nephrolithiasis, structural abnormalities of the urinary tract, or those forms of glomerulonephritis that respond to immunosuppressive therapy also should be treated aggressively. Preventive aspects include avoidance of nephrotoxic drugs and radiopaque agents in the patient with compromised renal function.

Modification of diet is an important aspect of conservative therapy. Early restriction of sodium may be important in the treatment of hypertension. As renal insufficiency progresses, foods high in phosphate and potassium content should be restricted. Reduction of dietary protein content reduces anorexia, nausea, and vomiting and, if initiated early (GFR > 40 to 50 mL/min), may retard progression of renal disease. Adults should receive no less than 0.6 g protein per kilogram of body weight per day to avoid negative nitrogen balance. Protein diets of 0.28 to 0.60 g protein per kilogram per day must be supplemented with essential ketoamino acid therapy, allowing utilization of urea as a source of nonessential nitrogen. Preliminary results from a multicenter study (modification of diet in renal disease) sponsored by the U.S. National Institutes of Health/Health Care Financing Administration suggest that control of hypertension may be as important as control of the protein content of the diet. Completion of this study should make it possible to define the usefulness of protein restriction and aggressive treatment of hypertension in slowing progression. Preliminary data from other studies suggest a particularly beneficial role for angiotensin-converting enzyme (ACE) inhibitors. Hyperkalemia and compromised renal function (in the presence of renal artery stenosis) are not uncommon complications of these drugs. Combination therapy of ACE inhibitors with diuretics, calcium channel blockers, or beta-adrenergic blockers may be necessary to control hypertension.

Correction of electrolyte imbalance, e.g., use of sodium bicarbonate or calcium carbonate to correct metabolic acidosis and bicarbonate, dextrose-insulin combinations, or sodium-potassium exchange resins for treatment of hyperkalemia, may be necessary in more advanced uremia. Hypermagnesemia, hyperamylasemia, hypertriglyceridemia, and mild carbohydrate intolerance generally do not require or are not amenable to treatment. Hyperuricemia should be treated if gout develops. Mild hyperuricemia alone does not require therapy. Treatment of anemia has been discussed above. Secondary hyperparathyroidism may accentuate progression of renal failure. Whether this is due to hyperphosphatemia, an elevated calcium-phosphorus product, or parathyroid hormone itself is not clear. Nonetheless, vigorous efforts using phosphate-binding agents, calcium supplements, and vitamin D (dihydrotachysterol or calcitriol) to maintain appropriate serum calcium and phosphorous levels are often effective in sup-

pressing parathyroid levels, preventing severe bone disease, and perhaps even in slowing the progression of renal insufficiency. To avoid visceral and vascular calcification, the calcium-phosphorus product (conventional laboratory units) should be kept at less than 60. Dietary restrictions of sodium, potassium, phosphate, and protein often prove unacceptable to patients. Consequently, when the complications of uremia worsen despite conservative management, dialysis and/or transplantation are the remaining options for long-term life support.

REFERENCES

ANDERSON S, BRENNER BM: Progressive renal disease: A disorder of adaptation. Q J Med 70:185, 1989

ANDRESS DL et al: Intravenous calcitriol in the treatment of refractory osteitis fibrosa of chronic renal failure. N Engl J Med 321:274, 1989

ATTMAN PO, ALAUPOVIC P: Lipid abnormalities in chronic renal insufficiency. Kidney Int 39(suppl 31):S16, 1991

ESCHBACH JW et al: Recombinant human erythropoietin in anemic patients with end-stage renal disease: Results of phase III multicenter clinical trial. Ann Intern Med 111:992, 1989

FRASER CL, ARIEFF AI: Nervous system complications in uremia. Ann Intern Med 109:143, 1988

GLASSOCK RJ: Nutrition, immunology and renal disease. Kidney Int 24(suppl 16):S194, 1983

HAKIM RM, LAZARUS JM: Biochemical parameters in chronic renal failure. Am J Kidney Dis 11:238, 1988

KLEINMAN KS et al: The use of recombinant human erythropoietin in the correction of anemia in predialysis patients and its effect on renal function: a double-blind, placebo-controlled trial. Am J Kidney Dis 14:486, 1989

PERRONE RD et al: Utility of radioisotope filtration markers in chronic renal insufficiency: Simultaneous comparison of ^{125}I-iothalamate, ^{99m}Tc-DPTA, and insulin. Am J Kidney Dis 16:224, 1990

POWELL D et al: Toxins and inhibitors in chronic renal failure. Am J Kidney Dis 7:292, 1986

WALSER M et al: Reciprocal creatinine slopes often give erroneous estimates of progression of chronic renal failure. Kidney Int Suppl. 27:S81, 1989

238 DIALYSIS AND TRANSPLANTATION IN THE TREATMENT OF RENAL FAILURE

CHARLES B. CARPENTER / J. MICHAEL LAZARUS

Dialysis and transplantation prolong the lives of patients with renal insufficiency. The approach to treatment in acute renal failure is different than in chronic renal failure because of the irreversible nature of the latter. Conservative medical management and dialysis are the mainstays of therapy for acute renal failure. Obviously, transplantation is not a treatment for this group of patients.

The term *end-stage renal disease* (ESRD) is used by government agents such as HCFA and has come to be synonymous with the late stages of chronic renal failure. Initially, patients with ESRD are managed with conservative therapy, but eventually they require hemodialysis, peritoneal dialysis, or transplantation. Because of limited success with each of these modalities, chronic renal failure should be approached with the concept of moving from one form of therapy to another as indicated by the degree of success and incidence of complications with each.

Therapy for renal failure should be initiated when serious complications, as noted in Chaps. 235 and 237, will be prevented, but not when the patient is completely asymptomatic. The advanced complications of uremia should be avoided by early treatment. Early dialysis is appropriate in patients with acute renal failure in whom resumption of renal function can be expected and in patients with chronic renal failure who have a good immunologic match with a related donor and are to be transplanted without prior long-term dialysis. In the remainder of patients, the clinical judgment to move from conservative treatment to dialysis or transplantation is determined by the patient's quality of life and whether or not the benefits of treatment outweigh the risks. The correlation of uremic symptoms with renal function varies from patient to patient depending on the cause of renal disease (earlier onset of symptoms in subjects with diabetes mellitus), muscle mass (large, muscular patients tolerate high levels of azotemia), diet, nutritional status, and coexisting conditions. Therefore, it is ill-advised to assign a certain "usual" level of blood urea nitrogen, serum creatinine, or glomerular filtration rate to the need to start dialysis. Treatment with dietary protein restriction and aggressive control of hypertension, as described in Chap. 237, may prolong the time before dialysis and/or transplantation are required but should be carried out only if complications of such therapy do not worsen morbidity and mortality. For example, malnutrition is a major factor in mortality in dialysis patients.

Selection of patients to receive dialysis and/or transplantation is a matter of some debate. Because of the reversible nature of acute renal failure, *all* patients with this diagnosis should be supported with dialysis, at least for some period of time, to allow return of renal function. In patients with irreversible or chronic renal failure, criteria for selection for transplantation are generally more stringent than those for dialysis and are guided by the possibility of complications related to immunosuppressive therapy. Table 238-1 lists considerations in the selection of a recipient for a human renal allograft. Transplantation should be undertaken only when conservative treatment has failed, when there are no reversible elements in the renal failure, and when the patient is too ill to be maintained comfortably with the usual methods of treatment. However, morbidity is less if transplantation is performed before the patient is critically ill. Transplantation should not be utilized in an attempt to salvage patients from failure to thrive on dialysis.

The recipient should be free of life-threatening extrarenal complications such as cancer, severe coronary artery disease, and cerebrovascular disease. Provided that diffuse vascular involvement is not present, diabetes mellitus is not a contraindication. Oxalosis may recur in relatively short order in a transplanted kidney and is generally a contraindication for transplantation. Although advanced age may be a limiting factor, it is advanced "physiologic" rather than chronologic age that contraindicates transplantation. In general, patients reach a "physiologic" limit at approximately age 60 to 65 years, when the incidence of complications due to glucocorticoids becomes much higher. Although abnormalities of the bladder and urethra present additional hazards, successful renal allografts have been placed in individuals with these abnormalities by prior constitution of an artificial bladder (i.e., ileal conduit) into which the donor ureter is placed. Patients with any disease process that may be aggravated by glucocorticoids, cyclosporine, azathioprine, or other immunosup-

pressive agents or any patient with coexisting medical conditions so severe that the risks of operation and drug therapy are high should not be offered transplantation.

Criteria for treatment with hemodialysis or peritoneal dialysis are more liberal because dialysis has less morbidity than transplantation in older patients in those with the aforementioned medical complications. Because of the cost of these programs, some have suggested that entry be restricted in those of advanced age. Such decisions, based on moral, social, and economic issues, continue to generate debate. In general, nearly all patients are accepted if they or their families desire prolongation of life. The physician should inform the patient of the likelihood of success and review the complications and untoward effects. The patient and family should be given an estimate of prognosis and expected quality of life. In most areas of the world, the cost of medical care for chronic renal failure is borne by government. In the United States, the mechanism of coverage is by Medicare, with all patients eligible regardless of age.

PREPARATION FOR THERAPY OF ESRD

While conservative measures as described in Chap. 237 are being carried out, it is important to prepare the patient with an intensive educational program, explaining the likelihood and timing of complete renal failure and the various forms of therapy available. The more knowledgeable patients are concerning hemodialysis, peritoneal dialysis, and transplantation, the easier and more appropriate will be their decisions at a later time. With hemodialysis, the major method of obtaining blood for treatment is from an arteriovenous fistula. Since these devices often take months to develop, prophylactic placement of a fistula in a patient planning for hemodialysis is important in minimizing future complications of circulatory access. For those who select peritoneal dialysis (continuous ambulatory peritoneal dialysis— CAPD; or continuous cyclic peritoneal dialysis—CCPD), placement of the peritoneal catheter does not require preparation, and therapy can be instituted when uremic signs and symptoms develop. In those who may perform home dialysis or undergo transplantation, early education of family members for selection and preparation as a home dialysis helper or a related donor for transplantation should occur before the onset of symptomatic renal failure. In those patients who have a good antigenic match with a willing donor, transplantation without intervening hemodialysis or peritoneal dialysis should be considered. Approximately 25 percent of patients receiving renal transplants at our institution do so without having had prior dialysis. In considering related-donor transplantation, the risk of unilateral nephrectomy, including development of proteinuria and hypertension, should be considered. As discussed below, the success rate of cadaver-donor transplantation has improved sufficiently that this form of therapy should be considered both by the patient and by potential donors. Early referral of patients to ESRD programs will allow education of the patient and family and preparation for an appropriate therapy. Table 238-2 illustrates the distribution of treatment modalities based on age, sex, race, and disease etiology in the United States.

DIALYSIS Hemodialysis Hemodialysis employs the process of diffusion across a semipermeable membrane to remove unwanted substances from the blood while adding desirable components. A constant flow of blood on one side of the membrane and a cleansing solution dialysate on the other allow removal of waste products in a fashion similar to that of glomerular filtration. By altering the composition of the dialysate, the method of exposure of blood and dialysate (geometry of the dialyzer), the type and surface area of dialysis membrane, and the frequency and duration of exposure (the dialysis prescription), patients without renal function can be maintained in a relatively healthy state. Hemodialysis equipment consists of three components—the blood delivery system, the composition and delivery system of the dialysate, and the dialyzer itself (Fig. 238-1). Blood is pumped to the dialyzer by a roller pump

---

TABLE 238-1   Contraindications to kidney transplantation

ABSOLUTE CONTRAINDICATIONS

Reversible renal involvement
Ability of conservative measures to maintain useful life
Advanced forms of major extrarenal complications (cerebrovascular or coronary disease, neoplasia)
Active infection
Active glomerulonephritis
Previous sensitization to donor tissue

RELATIVE CONTRAINDICATIONS

Age
Presence of vesical or urethral abnormalities
Iliofemoral occlusive disease
Psychiatric problems
Oxalosis

TABLE 238-2 Treatment Modality Summary by age,* sex, race, and primary diagnosis, December 31, 1989

Patient characteristics	Percent[†]			
	With a functioning transplant	Receiving center hemodialysis	Receiving home hemodialysis	Receiving CAPD/CCPD
Total	25.0	58.0	1.6	9.0
Age 20	55.5	19.0	0.6	12.8
20–44	44.0	39.1	1.5	8.3
45–64	23.3	59.0	1.9	9.2
65 +	2.7	81.8	1.4	9.1
Male	28.0	55.3	1.7	8.6
Female	21.3	61.2	1.5	9.5
Native American	23.2	61.3	3.2	9.8
Asian	27.7	61.5	0.9	7.0
Black	13.3	74.1	1.0	6.8
White	30.4	51.0	1.8	10.1
Diabetes mellitus	18.9	66.1	1.0	10.5
Hypertension	12.2	75.2	1.2	8.5
Glomerulonephritis	35.8	47.4	1.9	9.9

* Age on December 31, 1989.
† Percents add to almost 100; the remainder includes other and unknown dialysis.
SOURCE: U.S. Renal Data System, *USRDS 1991 Annual Data Report*, The National Institutes of Health, National Institute of Diabetes and Digestive and Kidney Diseases, Bethesda, Md., August 1991.

through lines with appropriate equipment to measure flow and pressures within the system; blood flow should be approximately 300 to 450 mL/min. Negative hydrostatic pressure on the dialysate side of the system can be manipulated to achieve desirable fluid removal, so-called ultrafiltration. Dialysis membranes have differing ultrafiltration coefficients (i.e., fluid removed per millimeters of mercury pressure per minute), the selection of which, along with the hydrostatic pressure changes, determines fluid removal. The dialysate is delivered to the dialyzer from a storage tank or proportioning system which manufactures dialysate on-line. In most systems, dialysate passes once across the membrane, countercurrent to blood flow at a rate of 500 mL/min. The composition of the dialysate is similar to plasma water but may be altered depending on need. The dialysate potassium is varied most often, but the sodium, calcium, and acetate or bicarbonate are usually decided in each dialysis unit. Table 238-3 outlines the range of formulas available. The principal dialyzer in use in the United States is the hollow fiber or capillary dialyzer, in which membrane material is spun into fine capillaries, thousands of which are packed into bundles with blood flowing through the capillaries while dialysate is circulated on the outside of the fiber bundle.

With current dialysis techniques, most patients require between 9 and 12 h of dialysis per week, equally divided into several sessions. The time depends on body size, residual renal function, dietary intake, complicating illnesses, and degree of anabolism or catabolism. The time, frequency of treatments, type and size of dialyzer, and dialysate composition, blood, or dialysate flow may all be altered to accomplish

FIGURE 238-1 Schema for hemodialysis.

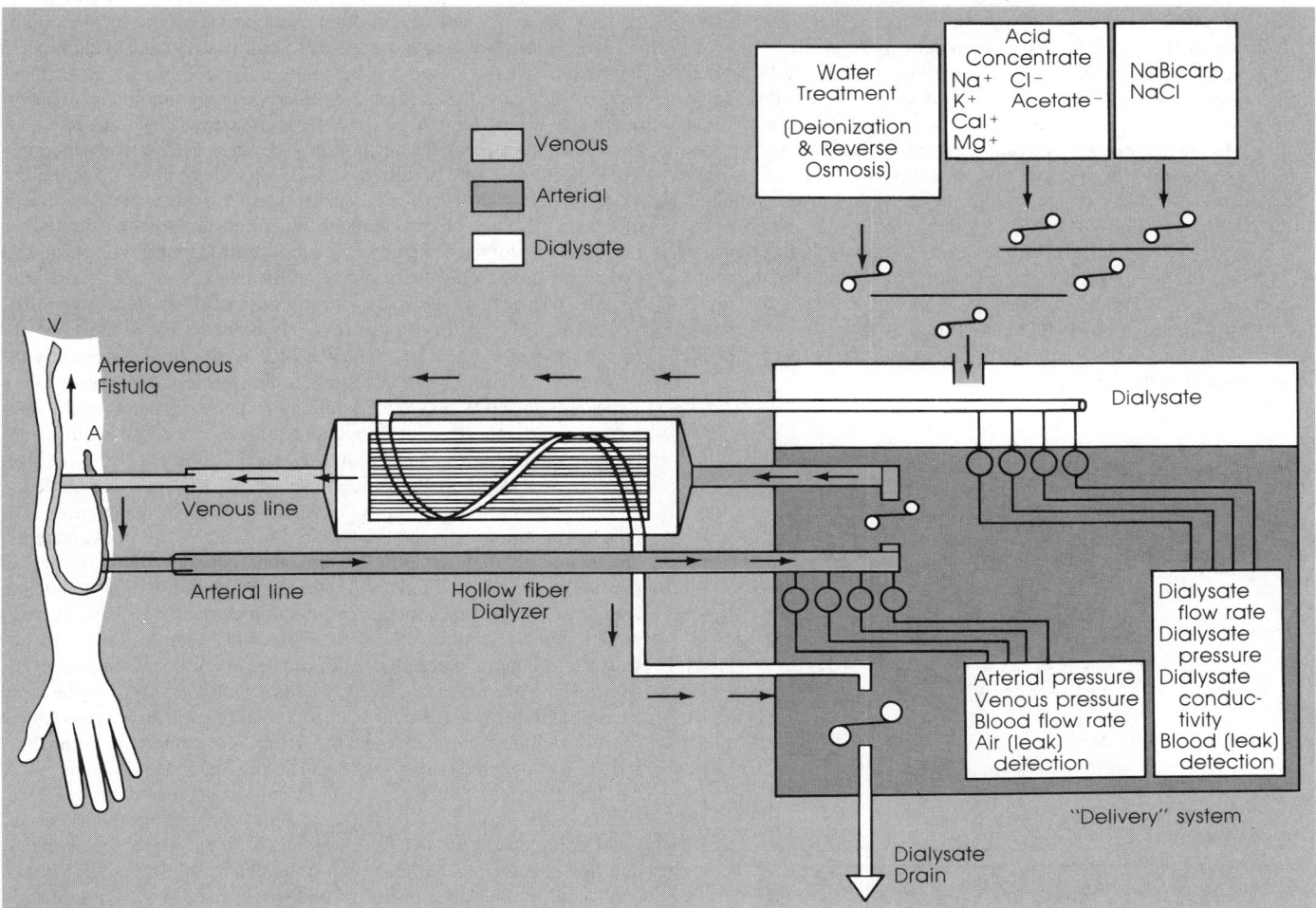

TABLE 238-3   Range of dialysis components available

Component	mmol/L
Sodium	138–145
Potassium	0–4.0
Calcium	2.0–3.5
Magnesium	0.4–1.0
Bicarbonate	30–37
Chloride	100–107

specific needs (see Fig. 238-2). The type of membrane and surface area (size) are determinants of ultrafiltration and clearance and are important in the immunologic (i.e., biocompatible) response by the patient. Cuprahane (Cupra-ammonium cellophase) and cellulose acetate are "tighter" membranes with less diffusive and ultrafiltration capabilities and less biocompatibility. Polyacrylnitrile (PAN), poly-methylmethacrylate (PMNA), and polysulphone are porous (high flux), biocompatible, and more expensive. Kinetic modeling, utilizing urea generation and protein catabolic rates, provides a more definite dialysis prescription. Urea kinetic modeling is based on the assumption that the body is a single pool. The term KT/V (K = clearance, T = dialysis time, and V = volume of distribution of the patient) is a dimensionless measure of treatment used in urea kinetic modeling. By determining each of these components, one can measure the adequacy of treatment as well as determine the protein catabolic rate (PCR), which is a measure of catabolism and, by inference, nutrition. An acceptable KT/V is 1.0 to 1.2, while the PCR should be approximately 1.2 g/kg per day. A simpler measure—the percent reduction of urea during each treatment (URR or PRU)—correlates well with KT/V. Based on these studies, an acceptable PRU or URR during each treatment is approximately 65 percent. The development of bicarbonate dialysis, variable sodium delivery, high-flux or ultraefficient membranes, and urea kinetic modeling has resulted in reductions in dialysis time. Clinical trials of this so-called high-flux, short-time dialysis are underway. Reduction of dialysis time without documentation of adequacy of treatment is associated with an increased morbidity and mortality. In addition to hemodialysis, a new method of treatment has been developed for the patient with acute renal failure. Slow continuous ultrafiltration (SCUF) or continuous arteriovenous hemodialysis (CAVHD) are techniques that employ high-efficiency dialyzers with cardiac-generated blood flow (via a cannulated femoral artery) along with very slow dialysate flow rates. This therapy is useful in the unstable, acute renal failure patient, has essentially replaced acute peritoneal dialysis in the ICU, and is often preferable to intermittent hemodialysis.

FIGURE 238-2 Factors in the development of the uremic syndrome and considerations in its treatment.

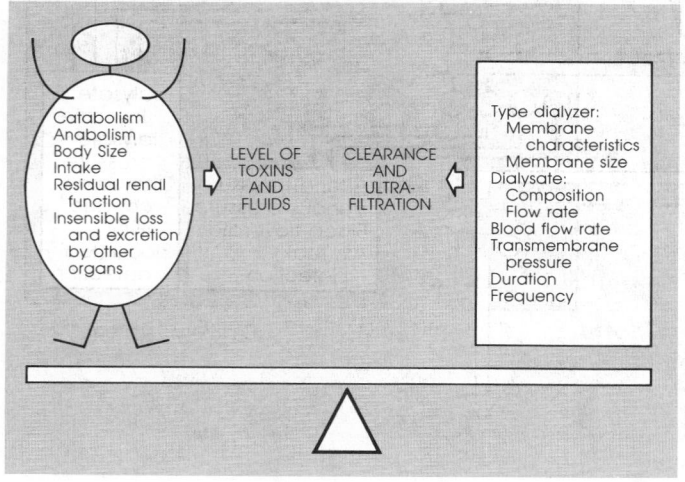

COMPLICATIONS OF HEMODIALYSIS   Many complications of chronic dialysis are related to underlying disease or those uremic conditions not reversed by dialytic therapy. These and other related problems of hemodialysis are discussed in Chap. 237. The Achilles' heel of hemodialysis is access to the circulation. The development of the arteriovenous shunt made chronic dialysis possible. This device had a high failure rate because of infection and thrombosis and led in 1966 to the development of the arteriovenous (AV) fistula. The fistula is preferably created from a native vein, but a prosthetic conduit (extended polytetrafluoroethylene) subcutaneously placed between an artery and a nearby vein may be utilized. Cannulation of arteriovenous fistulas with 15- to 16-gauge needles allows blood flow sufficient to carry out hemodialysis. Unfortunately, infection, thrombosis, and aneurysm formation also occur in the arteriovenous fistula, particularly in prosthetic devices. There is a relatively high incidence of septicemia and septic embolization associated with shunt and fistula infection; the most common infecting agent is *Staphylococcus aureus*.

Depression and altered self-image are common psychiatric problems. The rapid flux in osmolality may cause a dialysis disequilibrium syndrome consisting of confusion, clouding of consciousness, and seizures. In addition, rapid changes in electrolytes (particularly potassium) may lead to arrhythmia during dialysis. Hypotension during hemodialysis is due to many factors—the size of the extracorporeal circulation, degree of ultrafiltration, change in serum osmolality, presence of autonomic neuropathy, concomitant use of antihypertensive agents, removal of catecholamines, or infusion of acetate (used as the dialysate buffer), which is a cardiac depressant and vasodilator. Careful estimation of the extracellular fluid to be removed and use of isolated ultrafiltration and higher-sodium dialysate are helpful in preventing hypotension. In addition, many dialysis units now use bicarbonate as the dialysate buffer rather than acetate. Syndromes of dialysis dementia and osteomalacia may be secondary to aluminum contamination of dialysate water or result from oral intake of aluminum hydroxide. An increased incidence of HBsAg (hepatitis B surface antigen) antigenemia is related to decreased immunologic integrity and an increased transfusion rate. Patients with chronic antigenemia are usually asymptomatic and have little derangement of liver function. There is a higher rate of non-A, non-B hepatitis and cytomegalovirus infection, but these, too, are usually of mild degree. As mentioned in Chap. 237, use of recombinant human erythropoietin (EPO) has reduced or eliminated the need for blood transfusion in hemodialysis patients, thus reducing the risk of hepatitis. In addition, use of hepatitis vaccine has decreased the incidence of hepatitis B. Occurrence of non-A, non-B hepatitis (hepatitis C) is of unknown signficance in dialysis patients; however, evidence of hepatic disease secondary to hepatitis C is important in the consideration for renal transplantation. Patients with AIDS may have a rapidly progressive nephropathy and have poor prognosis with or without dialysis. Because of this and because of the high incidence of AIDS in IV drug abusers who also have heroin nephropathy, the presence of HIV-positive patients is common in dialysis units. Based on clinical experience and recommendations from the Centers for Disease Control, these patients are treated in dialysis units as are other patients with no special precautions. It is extremely important however, that all patients receive universal precautions for infection control. Mechanical and/or iatrogenic complications, such as hemolysis, air embolus, blood leaks, and contaminated dialysate, are less common with improved equipment. Membrane-induced adverse reactions may occur, as exemplified by complement-mediated leukopenia and hypoxemia. More prominent symptoms, such as back and chest pain, bronchospasm, and anaphylaxis, rarely occur in this reaction. Elaboration of cytokines, specifically IL-1, IL-6, and tumor necrosis factor (TNF), occurs with exposure of blood to some dialysis membranes. Simulation of the complement and cytokine systems likely plays a role in anorexia and hypercatabolism in hemodialysis patients. These cytokines also contribute to the development of dialysis-induced amyloid arthropathy—consisting of carpal tunnel syndrome, cystic degeneration of the cervical spine and femoral head and neck, and an infiltrating shoulder lesion. Use of the more biocompatible synthetic membranes—PAN, PMMA, and polysulphone—may have a beneficial effect in this regard. These membranes, as mentioned earlier, are expensive, however. Reuse of dialyzers, which occurs in approximately 68 percent of dialysis patients, will make their use feasible. Heparin, necessary during the hemodialysis procedure to prevent clotting in the lines and dialyzer, may lead to complications such as subdural hematoma and retroperitoneal, gastrointestinal, pericardial, and pleural hemorrhage. Recognition of the risks and modification of the dose of heparin reduce these complications. One of the major concerns in long-term dialysis patients is mortality related to myocardial infarction and cerebral vascular accidents. This is likely due to the preexistence and continuation of common risk factors in the uremic patient, such as hypertension, hyperlipidemia, vascular calcification due to hyperparathyroidism, and high cardiac output due to anemia or other factors. Control of hypertension is essential and can be accomplished in about 80 percent of dialysis patients with ultrafiltration and reduction of extracellular volume to the point of mild hypotension—so-called dry weight. For those in whom this is not possible because of cardiac or cerebral disease or who do not respond to ultrafiltration, use of hypertensive medications is warranted. Peripheral dilator agents and beta-adrenergic blockers seem to aggravate hypotension and must be used with care in the dialysis patient. ACE inhibitors and calcium channel blocking drugs cause less hypotension but in any case should be administered after the dialysis procedure. Hypercholesterolemia is uncommon in dialysis patients, while hypertriglyceridemia and decreased high-density lipoproteins are often seen. Hypocholesterolemic agents, such as lovastatin or gemfibrozil, are indicated when hypertriglyceridemia is accompanied by hypercholesterolemia. Hyperparathyroidism can often be controlled by binding phosphate with calcium carbonate along with use of calcitriol. Prevention of a calcium-phosphorous product greater than 60 will prevent vascular calcification. As mentioned earlier, EPO has virtually eliminated anemia.

The potential for complications should cause the physician to evaluate the risk/benefit ratio with dialysis before proceeding. Advantages of hemodialysis are the relatively short treatment time and minimal interruption of life-style between treatments. It is more efficient than peritoneal dialysis, allowing rapid changes in abnormal serum values. Hemodialysis can be performed in the home, but the patient requires an assistant during treatment. Hemodialysis is the most widely utilized form of dialysis.

Peritoneal dialysis Peritoneal dialysis, like hemodialysis, may be performed in various settings and with several techniques. In patients with acute renal failure, intermittent peritoneal dialysis has largely been replaced by intermittent hemodialysis or CAVHD. Chronic peritoneal dialysis was attempted in the late 1940s but was impractical until development of a permanent peritoneal catheter—the Tenckhoff catheter. Use of this indwelling catheter and closed continuous-cycle dialysate delivery equipment led to treatment protocols with which patients were treated two to three times per week for a total of 30 to 40 h (intermittent peritoneal dialysis—IPD) to achieve clearances and fluid removal similar to those of hemodialysis. In 1978, the concept of continuous peritoneal lavage with prolonged dwell times led to the development of CAPD, which differs from intermittent peritoneal dialysis in that patients instill fluid into the peritoneal cavity, seal the catheter, continue in an ambulatory mode, and every 4 to 6 h empty the peritoneal cavity and replace the dialysate. This technique generally utilizes 2-L containers of dialysate and obviates the need for dialysis equipment. Modification using a cyclic dialysate delivery device to exchange dialysate during the night and chronic dwelling of fluid during the waking hours (CCPD) is acceptable to some patients.

IPD or CCPD may be performed in a center or at home (usually overnight), while CAPD can be performed anywhere. As with hemodialysis, the composition of the dialysate can be modified for individual needs. The major difference in peritoneal dialysate formulas is in the amount of dextrose used as an osmotic agent (1.5, 2.5, or

4.25 g/dL). Advantages of peritoneal dialysis are avoidance of heparinization and vascular surgery and a slower clearance rate (helpful for some cardiovascular patients). It is more amenable to self-treatment. Disadvantages include the longer treatment time (intermittent or continuous involvement). It should not be used in patients with extensive abdominal surgery or pulmonary disease. Inadequate clearance may occur in patients with scleroderma, vasculitis, malignant hypertension, or peritoneal disease. Complications include catheter tunnel infection, peritonitis, protein loss with malnutrition, hypertriglyceridemia, hypercholesterolemia, obesity, and inguinal and abdominal hernias. Determination of adequacy of treatment by CAPD or CCPD is not as easy as with hemodialysis (see Table 238-2).

RESULTS Of new patients with ESRD, approximately 35 to 50 percent are physically and psychologically suitable for transplantation. Many are on hemodialysis and peritoneal dialysis awaiting availability of a kidney. An acutely ill or medically complicated patient will likely undergo dialysis in a hospital dialysis unit or intensive care unit, while stable patients may be dialyzed as outpatients or at home. Most centers attempt to have patients participate in their own care, so-called self-dialysis. Home dialysis (either hemodialysis or peritoneal) is preferable for many because of self-reliance and freedom from hospital or center schedules. Patient motivation is the primary factor in selection of home or in-center self-dialysis. Dialysis in the hospital setting is most expensive, while home dialysis with a nonpaid family assistant or alone (peritoneal dialysis only) is less expensive than in-center dialysis. Despite absence of equipment, peritoneal dialysis is as expensive as home hemodialysis because of the cost of dialysate and of hospitalization related to peritonitis. The total amount of Medicare payments for ESRD (covering hemodialysis, peritoneal dialysis, and transplantation) in the year 1991 was $3 billion, substantially greater than anticipated at the initiation of the ESRD program in 1973. This cost reflects an increasing number of recipients, not an increasing cost per patient, which, in fact, has been reduced over the past 20 years.

The mean age for patients on dialysis is 62 years. This number continues to rise also, partly because nephrosclerosis and eventual renal failure from other parenchymal diseases occur in older patients but more likely because the selection process favors transplantation in younger patients.

Approximately 10 to 20 percent of patients with chronic renal failure are totally rehabilitated by dialysis, and another 30 to 40 percent of nondiabetic patients may be rehabilitated to a functional status even if they are not employed. Twenty percent of patients will be returned to a level of function not considered rehabilitated but able to care for themselves. The remainder (approximately 20 percent) are dependent on support from others. Diabetics, who have rehabilitation and survival rates lower than those of nondiabetic patients, make up much of the latter two groups. Mortality rates vary, depending on the age of the patient and the disease process(es) involved. Yearly gross mortality rates of patients in the ESRD program in the United States have increased from 20 percent in 1982 to approximately 24 percent in 1990. This increase in mortality may be due to case-mix factors, i.e., acceptance in recent years of older patients with a higher incidence of comorbid conditions such as diabetes mellitus, nephrosclerosis, coronary artery disease, peripheral vascular disease, and pulmonary and hepatic disease. Others have suggested that treatment has become inadequate for a number of reasons. Clinical studies are underway to determine the causes of this increased mortality and to improve rehabilitation and quality of life. In patients less than 45 years of age and with no complicating medical illnesses, mortality with hemodialysis, peritoneal dialysis, or transplantation is below 5 percent per year.

TRANSPLANTATION

Transplantation of the human kidney is frequently appropriate for the treatment of advanced chronic renal failure. Worldwide, tens of thousands of such procedures have been performed. When azathioprine and prednisone are used as immunosuppressive drugs, the results with properly matched familial donors are superior to those with organs from cadaveric donors, namely, 75 to 90 percent compared with 50 to 60 percent graft survival rates at 1 year. When antilymphocyte globulins (ALG) are added to the treatment regimens in some centers, the results with cadaveric donors approach those with living related donors, at least for the first 2 years after transplantation. Cyclosporine has also improved 1-year cadaveric survival rates to the 80 percent range when used along with prednisone in place of azathioprine and ALG. With all therapies, the rate of graft loss from rejection is much slower after the first year, although occasionally acute irreversible rejection may occur after many months of good function. This is especially likely if the patient neglects to take the immunosuppressive drugs. Results in recent years have improved with regard to patient morbidity and mortality rates, the latter declining to less than 5 percent in a number of centers. This improvement is the result of a tendency on the part of transplant teams to decrease immunosuppressive therapy so that in the case of severe rejection the kidney rather than the patient is lost. Second and even third transplants can be performed, and the overall results show a 10 to 20 percent reduction in expected survival compared with first transplants; cyclosporine therapy does not erase the increased risk of rejecting subsequent transplants, however. Overall, transplantation returns the majority of patients to a near-normal life-style.

DONOR SELECTION Donors can be cadavers or volunteer blood-related living donors. Living volunteer donors should be normal on physical examination and of the same major ABO blood group, because crossing major blood group barriers prejudices survival of the allograft. It is possible, however, to transplant a kidney of a type O donor into an A, B, or AB recipient. Selective renal arteriography should be performed on donors to rule out the presence of multiple or abnormal renal arteries, because the surgical procedure is difficult and the ischemic time of the transplanted kidney long when vascular abnormalities exist. Cadaveric donors should be free of malignant neoplastic disease because of possible transmission to the recipient.

In the United States, a coordinated national system (United Network for Organ Sharing) of computerized information about and logistic support for the transportation of cadaver kidneys to suitable recipients is under development. It is now possible to remove cadaver kidneys and to maintain them for over 48 h on cold pulsatile perfusion or simple flushing and cooling. This permits adequate time for typing, cross-matching, transportation, and selection problems to be solved.

TISSUE TYPING AND CLINICAL IMMUNOGENETICS Matching for antigens of the HLA major histocompatibility gene complex (Chap. 64) is the ideal criterion for selection of donors for renal allografts. Each mammalian species has a single chromosomal region that encodes the strong, or major, transplantation antigens, and this region on the human sixth chromosome is called *HLA*. Other antigens, called ''minor,'' may nevertheless play crucial roles, especially the ABH(O) blood groups and endothelial antigens that are not shared with lymphocytes. Evidence for designation of HLA as the genetic region encoding major transplantation antigens comes from the success rate in living related donor renal and bone marrow transplantation, with superior results in HLA-identical sibling pairs. Nevertheless, 5 to 10 percent of HLA-identical renal allografts are rejected, often within the first weeks after transplantation. These failures probably represent states of prior sensitization to non-HLA antigens. Non-HLA antigens are relatively weak and therefore suppressible by conventional immunosuppressive therapy. Once priming has occurred, however, secondary responses are much more refractory to treatment. In fact, ABH incompatibilities are hazardous because of the presence of natural anti-A and anti-B antibodies in recipients and the normal expression of A and B blood group substances on endothelium.

Living related donors From 1962 to 1982 when azathioprine was the main immunosuppressive drug, living related donors provided superior graft survivals. Among first-degree relatives, the general level of expected graft success was in direct proportion to matching

for 2, 1, or no HLA haplotypes, as defined by HLA serologic typing and the presence or absence of a proliferative response in the mixed-lymphocyte response (MLR) (Chap. 64). HLA-incompatible siblings did slightly better than the overall average with cadaveric donors (50 to 60 percent at 1 year), while HLA semi-identicals (haploidentical) were in the 70 to 75 percent range. Intrafamilial MLRs among haploidenticals were found to be a measure of responsiveness. Low-responder donor-recipient pairs had a 1-year graft survival rate of 90 percent, while vigorous responders were at the level of 55 percent unless donor-specific blood transfusions were given to eliminate this disadvantage. The MLR is a relatively imprecise technique, but MLR reactivity with a specific donor was more predictive of graft outcome than serologic typing for HLA-A, -B, -C, or -DR antigens. Improvements in serologic and DNA-based techniques (Chap. 64) have made the MLR test unnecessary for most related-donor cases.

Cyclosporine has altered the assumption that living related donors are generally superior to cadaveric donors, because in most series cadaveric results now rival the 80 percent 1-year result attained with haploidentical relatives. One must now weigh the choices in light of the availability of organs and waiting times on dialysis rather than on the initial rate of graft success. Long-term survival rates, however, are not improved. With either azathioprine or cyclosporine, the half-life estimated after the first year is 25 to 30 years with HLA-identical donors, 11 to 12 years with haploidentical donors, and 7 to 9 years with cadaveric donors. The major advantage of cyclosporine over azathioprine, therefore, is in the initial results at 1 to 2 years for cadaveric transplantation and not in the rate of graft loss thereafter.

Concern has been expressed regarding the potential risk to a volunteer kidney donor of premature renal failure after several years of increased blood flow and hyperfiltration per nephron in the remaining kidney. There are a few reports of the development of hypertension, proteinuria, and even lesions of focal segmental sclerosis in donors under long-term follow-up. Difficulties in donors followed for 15 or more years are unusual, however, and it may be that having a single kidney becomes significant only when another condition, such as hypertension, is superimposed. In this regard, it is desirable to consider the risk of development of type I diabetes mellitus in a family member who is a potential donor to a diabetic renal failure patient. Anti-insulin and anti-islet antibodies should be measured, and glucose tolerance tests should be performed in such cases to rule out a prediabetic state. The acceptance of living unrelated donors (spouses, distant relatives, close friends) has been debated as a means to improve the supply of organs and to shorten the waiting period on dialysis. Since volunteer donors who are not matched for one or both HLA haplotypes present as strong a tissue barrier as randomly matched cadaveric donors, they cannot be expected to provide, on average, as reliable a source for long-functioning grafts as a well-matched cadaveric organ. Actual data on this matter are conflicting. It is illegal in the United States to purchase organs for transplantation.

HLA matching and cadaveric donors The question of whether matching of HLA antigens in unrelated donor-recipient pairs would approximate the high initial success rates and slow rates of subsequent graft loss with HLA-identical sib pairs could not be answered until the late 1980s when reliable class II histocompatibility (DR) typing became widely available. With the 1-year success rate now at 80 to 85 percent for first cadaveric grafts, it is difficult to see an early improvement related to matching when small series of cases are compiled, especially, as is often the case, when the reporting centers have a very small fraction of well-matched cases. Now that pooled data on several thousands of cadaveric renal transplants from all over the world are available, the HLA-matching effect can be clearly seen, especially in the long-term survival figures. It is shown in Fig. 238-3 that there is an overall beneficial effect of HLA matching in first cadaveric grafts. When compared with HLA-identical transplants, where the 1-year graft survival rate is 95 percent and the subsequent half-life is 25 years, one-HLA-haplotype–matched family donor transplants and no-antigen–mismatched cadaveric cases have 1-year survival rates of 85 percent with an 11- to 12-year half-life. With

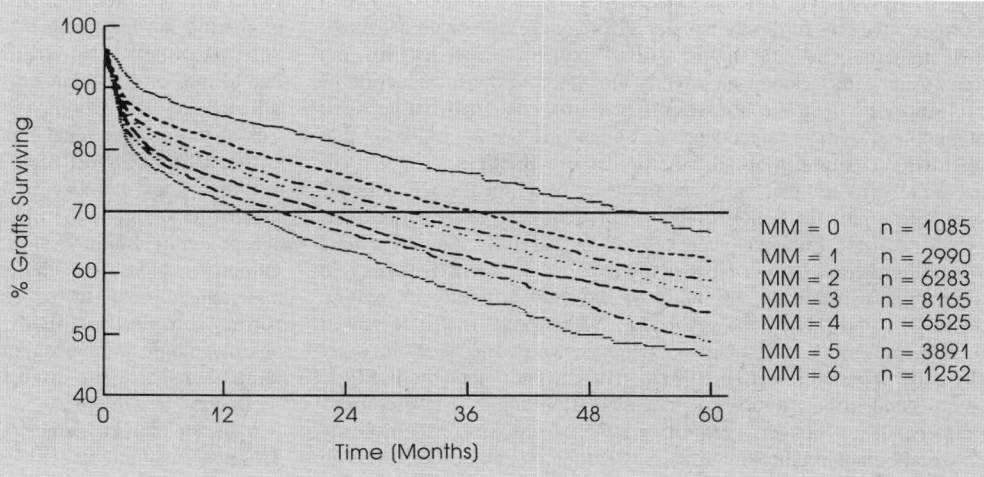

FIGURE 238-3 Survival of over 30,000 first cadaveric renal transplants over 5 years after transplantation. The transplants were performed in more than 200 centers around the world between 1982 and 1989. Cyclosporine was used in virtually all cases. The curves for each HLA matching grade are shown, according to the number of mismatches (MM) for HLA-A, -B, and -DR antigens. Since each individual has two genes for each locus, there is a potential for up to six mismatches. The overall effect of matching in this international Collaborative Transplant Study stratifies according to the mismatch grade (weighted regression, $p < 0.0001$) *(From Opelz.)*

increasing numbers of mismatches for cadaveric donors, the 1-year survival rate declines from 80 to 70 percent, and the half-life decreases from 9 to 7 years. The survival rates at the 10-year mark are projected to range from 50 (zero mismatches) to 30 percent (six mismatches). Many centers report 1-year graft survival rates in the 85 to 90 percent range for all renal transplants, possibly the result of heavy initial immunosuppression, but the subsequent half-lives are similar to those above. The contribution of the HLA locus to the matching effect is strongest for DR, moderate for B, and weak for A. Repeat transplants, following rejection of first grafts, do less well by about 15 to 20 percent; in these cases, the benefits of HLA matching are even more striking, while cyclosporine adds relatively little. The United Network for Organ Sharing requires that donor-recipient pairs with a ''six-antigen match'' for HLA-A, -B, and -DR be matched on a nationwide basis, while sharing for lesser degrees of match is voluntary. A 20 to 30 percent rate of DR-compatible cadaveric transplants has been achieved by some organ-sharing systems. With the waiting list in the United States having some 18,000 potential recipients and 8000 donors each year, matching grades approaching these rates and higher are possible if transplant centers are willing to share organs on this basis.

Presensitization   A positive cross match of recipient serum with donor T lymphocytes representing anti-HLA class I is usually predictive of an acute vasculitic event termed *hyperacute* rejection. Patients making such antibodies, detected by testing against a surrogate panel of normal lymphocytes, were previously thought to be at high risk for accelerated, if not hyperacute, rejection, even when the donor-specific cross match was negative. That this is no longer so can be attributed to greater efforts in monitoring patients on dialysis and in defining not only the presence or absence of antibodies but also the HLA antigens to which they are directed. Patients with anti-HLA antibodies can be safely transplanted if careful cross matching is performed. Patients sustained by hemodialysis often show fluctuating antibody titers and specificity patterns, sometimes, but not always, temporally related to receipt of blood transfusions. At the time of assignment of a cadaveric kidney, cross matches are performed with more than one highly reactive serum, and the previously analyzed antibody specificities are also taken into account. Anti-HLA antibody responses do not necessarily recur several months later when the incompatible antigen is given in a blood-product transfusion. Indeed, it seems relatively safe to ignore positive cross matches with sera kept in storage for several months as long as recent sera are negative. Data on this point are conflicting, showing either no risk or a 15 percent increased risk of early graft loss if only the stored serum samples older than 6 months are reactive with donor cells. The loss of anamnesis to HLA by chronic dialysis patients may result from development of specific unresponsiveness due to suppressor cell activation or from anti-idiotypic immunity. Low-titer presensitization

to antigens expressed on B lymphocytes, but not T lymphocytes, is not a contraindication to transplantation. Some of these antibodies are anti-DR, while others are non-HLA IgM antibodies active in the cold and at room temperature but apparently not relevant to graft survival. High-titer (>1:4) anti-DR antibodies have been related to early graft rejection in a few reported cases. A cross match performed by fluorescence techniques on a flow cytometer may be useful in sensitized patients.

Endothelial-monocyte system   In some cases of unexpected accelerated rejection, antibodies with reactivity to renal endothelium and blood monocytes have been found, both in the circulation and in eluates from rejected grafts. Practical aspects of typing and cross matching for this non-HLA system are difficult. Second transplants following rapid loss of the first graft seem to be particularly at risk.

Overview of transplantation immunogenetics   In addition to the ABH(O) blood groups, the important histocompatibility antigens presently known are HLA-A, -B, -C, -DR, and the endothelial-monocyte system (Table 238-4). Major primary immunogenicity lies in the DR antigens, while A, B, C, and endothelial-monocyte antigens provide the major targets for effector IgG and, in the case of A, B, and C, at least, for killer T lymphocytes. Hence the current emphasis is on A, B, and C cross matching and DR matching, although HLA-B compatibility adds to the DR-matching effect. The predictive accuracy of class I typing is improved by defining HLA-A and -B antigens using the best-quality serologic typing, while for class II antigens studies of polymorphisms at the level of DNA sequences are most reliable (Chap. 64).

Blood transfusions   At a time when it appeared that transfusion-induced sensitization against a random lymphocyte panel was predictive of a high graft failure rate, a number of transplantation units undertook a policy of withholding blood from as many dialysis patients as possible. The clinical need for blood was found to be less than originally thought, especially in nonnephrectomized patients, and avoidance of possible exposure to hepatitis also was a consideration. The overall experience with the nontransfused patients was the opposite to what had been predicted: Such patients were at the *highest*

TABLE 238-4   Histocompatibility in renal transplantation

Relative importance of typing and cross matching for serologically defined antigens

Antigens	Typing (antigen matching)	Cross matching
Class I (HLA-A, -B, -C)	+ +	+ + +
Class II (HLA-DR)	+ + +	−
Endothelial-monocyte (non-HLA)	? −	+ + +

risk for graft failure. Since the early 1980s, however, there has been a progressive loss of the transfusion effect, with little or no detriment now remaining in the nontransfused patients. The loss of the transfusion effect cannot be directly attributed to the introduction of cyclosporine, since the transfusion effect had declined before large numbers of patients received this agent. It seems unlikely that worldwide changes in blood bank processing practices are involved. It is most likely that the overall level of clinical management, particularly in recognition and prompt treatment of rejection, has played a role. Indeed, when looked at carefully, some centers withholding transfusions have noted increased rejection activity in their nontransfused patients but have not had difficulty in treating them. One study shows, however, that graft survival is still decreased in that subset of nontransfused patients who also have an early clinically apparent rejection episode. The current practice to use little or no blood in preparation for transplantation comes at a propitious time because of concerns regarding HIV transmission. The efficacy of recombinant erythropoietin in sustaining red blood cell mass in chronic renal failure patients further reduces the clinical need for blood transfusions.

IMMUNOLOGY OF REJECTION   Knowledge of the immunology of tissue transplantation stems largely from animal experimentation. However, enough evidence has accumulated in humans, particularly in kidney transplantation, to indicate that the evidence is similar, though not identical, for the different species. The immunologic mechanisms are not qualitatively different from those found in other areas of immunology (Chap. 277). Early rejection is associated with T lymphocytes having direct specificity against donor antigens. These may be cytotoxic cells (CD8+ or CD4+) or cells that mediate delayed hypersensitivity (CD4+); however, significant numbers of B lymphocytes, null cells, natural killer (NK) cells, and macrophages appear in the early infiltrate, and cells capable of mediating antibody-dependent cell-mediated cytotoxicity (ADCC) are also present (Fig. 238-4). Many of the B lymphocytes produce immunoglobulins. The spectrum of cellular and humoral response and graft injury is quite varied, depending on specific genetic differences between donor and recipient and states of presensitization. The greater the degree of presensitization, the more likely it is that one will find antibody-mediated vascular lesions. All the processes shown in Fig. 238-4 are possible, but their relative contribution varies from case to case. Further dissection of the heterogeneity of the human allograft response utilizing techniques for the identification of lymphocyte subsets is adding to the value of graft biopsy as a guide to therapy and prognosis. Monitoring of peripheral blood lymphocyte subsets utilizing monoclonal antibodies to functionally related surface molecules, such as CD4 (T helper cells) and CD8 (T suppressor/cytotoxic cells), has been related to the degree of rejection activity in some surveys, but the CD4/CD8 ratio has not always been meaningful. Part of the problem may lie in the fact that these subsets are not as uniquely related to function as originally believed. Indeed, the principal role of the CD4 molecule is to promote interaction of T cells with class II HLA molecules on antigen-presenting cells, and similarly, CD8 interacts with class I HLA (see Chap. 277). Finally, the cytokine mediators of the cellular immune response IL-1 to IL-4, IL-6, TNF, and IFN γ) are involved in the control and expression of the alloimmune rejection response. For example, T cell production of IFN γ causes increased expression of HLA antigens on endothelial cells. In normal immunobiology this effect may be to promote more efficient presentation of foreign antigen, while in transplantation it enhances the immunogenicity of the vascularized transplant. Also, IL-2, the major growth factor for expansion of effector T cells, is the product of a major subset of CD4 cells, while other CD4 cells produce B cell growth factors, such as IL-4.

The failure of transplanted kidneys after several years of adequate function is said to be due to "chronic rejection." In such kidneys, the development of nephrosclerosis, with proliferation of the vascular intima of renal vessels, and intimal fibrosis, with marked decrease in the lumen of the vessels, takes place (Fig. 238-5). The result is renal ischemia, hypertension, tubular atrophy, interstitial fibrosis, and glomerular atrophy with eventual renal failure. It is not established, however, whether slow deterioration of graft function over years is due to the same mechanisms in all cases. Except for the established influence of HLA incompatibility, little is known about the pathogenesis of progressive renal failure in transplanted patients.

IMMUNOSUPPRESSIVE TREATMENT   When histocompatibility differences exist between donor and recipient, it is necessary to modify or suppress the immune response to enable the recipient to accept a graft. Immunosuppressive therapy, in general, suppresses all immune responses, including those to bacteria, fungi, and even malignant tumors. In the 1950s when clinical renal transplantation began, sublethal total-body irradiation was employed. Currently, pharmacologic immunosuppression is safer. Agents to suppress the immune response are discussed in the following paragraphs.

Drugs   *Azathioprine*, an analogue of mercaptopurine, was for two decades the keystone to immunosuppressive therapy in humans. This agent can inhibit synthesis of DNA, RNA, or both. Because cell division and proliferation are a necessary part of the immune response to antigenic stimulation, suppression by this agent may be mediated by the inhibition of mitosis of immunologically competent lymphoid cells, interfering with synthesis of DNA. Alternatively, immunosuppression may be brought about by blocking the synthesis of RNA (possibly messenger RNA), inhibiting processing of antigens prior to lymphocyte stimulation. This drug has little effect in suppressing a secondary immune response, however. Therapy with azathioprine is generally instituted 2 days prior to transplantation in the recipient of a living-donor kidney and on the day of transplantation in the case of a cadaveric-donor kidney recipient at a level of 4 mg/kg per day. The drug is later tapered to levels of 1.5 to 3 mg/kg per day as long as the allograft functions. Because the drug is rapidly metabolized by the liver, its dosage need not be varied directly in relation to renal function, even though renal failure results in retention of the metabolites of azathioprine. Some patients are unusually sensitive to this drug, particularly when renal function is compromised, and reduction in dosage is required because of leukopenia and occasionally thrombocytopenia. Excessive amounts of azathioprine also may cause jaundice, anemia, and alopecia. If it is essential to administer allopurinol concurrently, the azathioprine dose must be reduced, since inhibition of xanthine oxidase delays degradation. This combination is best avoided.

Glucocorticoids are important adjuncts to immunosuppressive therapy. Of all the agents employed, prednisone has effects that are easiest to assess, and in large doses it is effective for the reversal of rejection. In general, 30 to 40 mg prednisone is given immediately prior to or at the time of transplantation, and the dosage is gradually reduced. The side effects of the glucocorticoids, particularly impairment of wound healing and predisposition to infection, make it desirable to taper the dose as rapidly as possible in the immediate postoperative period. Customarily, methylprednisolone, 0.5 to 1.0 g intravenously, is administered immediately upon diagnosis of beginning rejection and continued once daily for 3 days. When the drug is effective, the results are usually apparent within 96 h. Such "pulse" doses are less effective in chronic rejection. Most patients whose renal function is stable after 6 months or a year do not require large doses of prednisone; maintenance doses of 10 to 20 mg/d are the rule. Many patients tolerate an alternate-day course of steroids without an increased risk of rejection.

A major effect of steroids is on the monocyte-macrophage system, preventing the release of IL-6 and IL-1. Lymphopenia after large doses of glucocorticoids is primarily due to sequestration of recirculating blood lymphocytes to lymphoid tissue.

Cyclosporine is a fungal peptide with potent immunosuppressive activity. It appears to have a preferential effect on early activation of helper-inducer T lymphocytes, thereby sparing suppressor T cell responses. Although it works alone, cyclosporine is more effective in conjunction with glucocorticoids. Since cyclosporine blocks production of IL-2 by helper-inducer (CD4+) T cells, its combination with

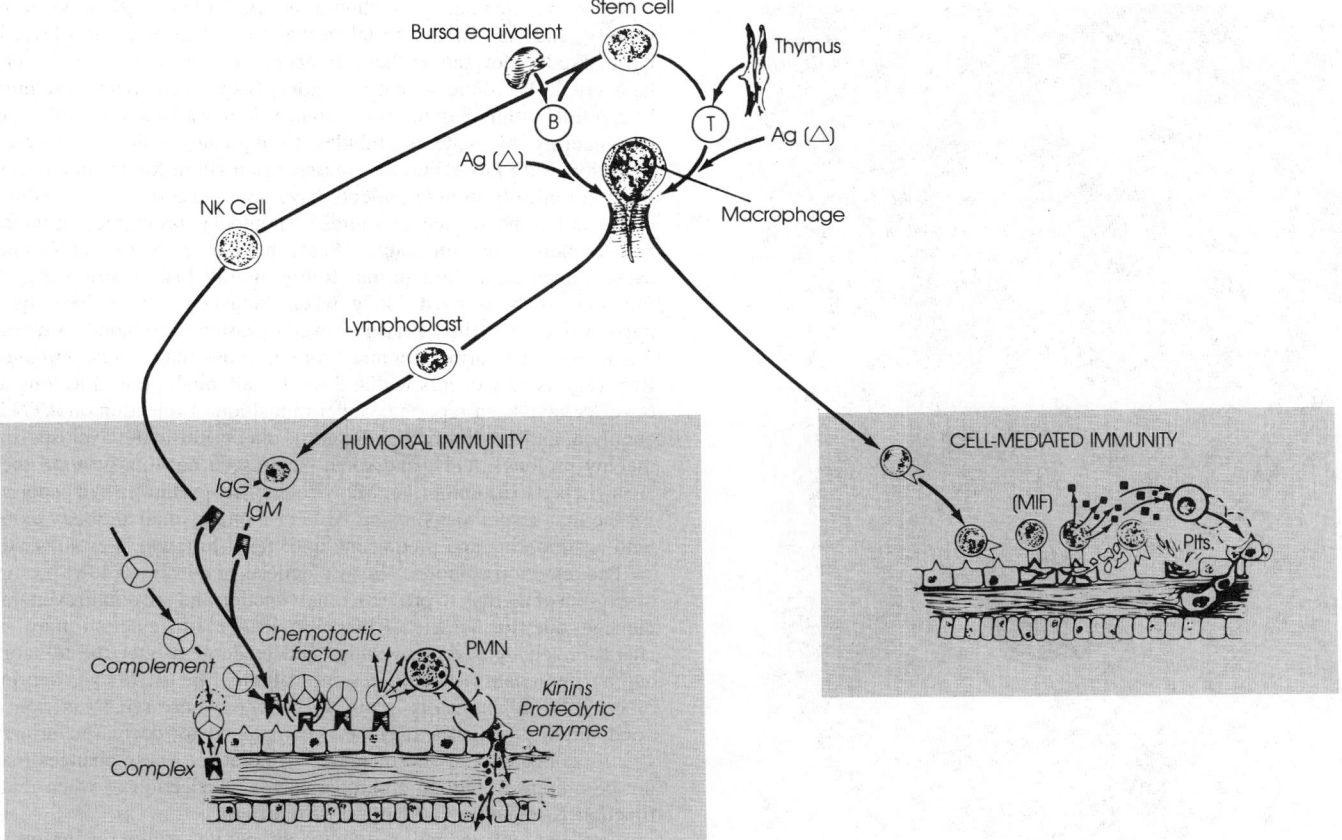

FIGURE 238-4 Overall scheme of the development of effector mechanisms in graft rejection. A set of bone marrow precursor stem cells is selected in the thymus gland to become mature thymus-derived (T) lymphocytes which are clonally determined to recognize non-self antigens (Δ) presented as fragments bound to self major histocompatibility molecules. These antigen-presenting structures are on the surfaces of macrophages, dendritic cells, and B lymphocytes. In transplantation, major histocompatibility antigens, such as HLA, may be recognized directly as the antigen-presenting molecules present in the grafted tissues or as fragments of donor HLA presented by recipient antigen-presenting cells. In avian species, but not in mammals, an anatomic site called the *bursa of Fabricius* provides the differentiating stimuli for maturation of B lymphocytes from bone marrow precursors. B lymphocytes with immunoglobulin receptors for a given antigen (Δ) proliferate and differentiate by a process of somatic mutation of immunoglobulin genes and selection by antigen for further growth. They begin to secrete IgM and, subsequently, IgG, IgE, and IgA. The response matures with help from T lymphocytes, which includes elaboration of the cytokines IL-4, IL-5, and IL-2. The proliferative phases of T and B lymphocyte response are illustrated by the lymphoblast.

Humoral immunity produces tissue injury following binding of immunoglobulins to tissue and, in particular, to the endothelium of a transplanted organ. Complement activation and chemotaxis of polymorphonuclear cells (PMN) are common in "hyperacute" rejection lesions when recipients have antidonor antibodies. Cell-mediated immunity is principally mediated by T lymphocytes bearing receptors for tissue antigens. These cells receive a major degree of help initially from macrophages that secrete the cytokines IL-6 and IL-1. Expanded populations of graft-specific T lymphocytes exert tissue damage by a delayed type hypersensitivity mechanism or by direct cytotoxic "killer" mechanisms. As noted in text, the T lymphocyte CD4 or CD8 phenotypes indicate whether the target antigens are HLA class II or class I, respectively.

The principal growth factor for T lymphocytes is an autocrine product, IL-2. Other T cell products include cytokines, such as interferon γ and tumor necrosis factor, which increase the pace of tissue injury. Activated macrophages can add nonspecifically to the inflammatory process. Natural killer cells (NK) play a minor role; however, they, along with other cells that bear receptors for the Fc portion of immunoglobulin, can provide cell-mediated target damage after fixation to IgG molecules previously bound to grafted cells (antibody-dependent cell-mediated cytotoxicity—ADCC). Any of these mechanisms can result in vascular occlusion by platelet aggregation and thrombosis (see also Fig. 64-5).

steroids is expected to produce a double block in the macrophage $\rightarrow$ IL-1 $\rightarrow$ T cell $\rightarrow$ IL-2 sequence. As noted, clinical results with several thousands of renal transplants have been impressive. Of its toxic effects (nephrotoxicity, hepatotoxicity, hirsutism, tremor, gingival hyperplasia), only nephrotoxicity presents a serious management problem and is discussed further below.

Antibodies to lymphocytes When serum from animals made immune to host lymphocytes is injected into the recipient, a marked suppression of cellular immunity to the tissue graft results. The action on cell-mediated immunity is greater than on humoral immunity. A globulin fraction of serum (antilymphocyte globulin—ALG) is the agent generally employed. For use in humans, peripheral human lymphocytes, thymocytes, or lymphocytes from spleens or thoracic duct fistulas have been injected into horses, rabbits, or goats to produce antilymphocyte serum, from which the globulin fraction is then separated. Although ALG or ATG (antithymocyte globulin) is unquestionably effective in prolonging grafts in animals, its efficacy in the transplantation of human tissue is less clear, since it varies from source to source. Heterologous antibody against defined T lymphocyte subsets, in the form of mouse antihuman monoclonal antibody, may offer a more precise form of therapy. OKT3, in common clinical use, is such an antibody. It is directed to the CD3 molecules which form a portion of the T cell antigen-receptor complex; hence CD3 is expressed on all mature T cells. CD4 or CD8 molecules also form part of the fully activated cluster of molecules, and monoclonal antibodies to these offer the potential for more selective

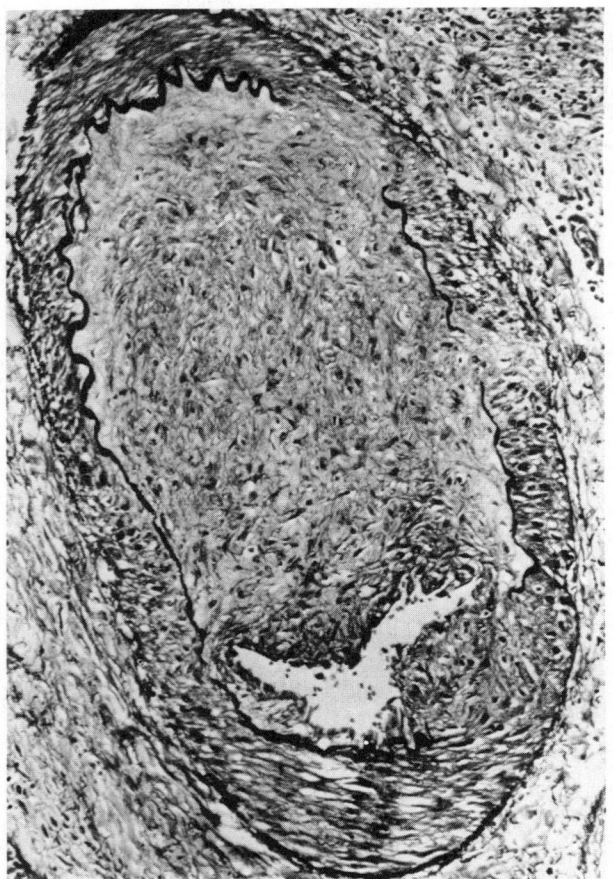

FIGURE 238-5 Biopsy of the renal cadaveric allograft illustrating oblitera-tive endarteritis. Loss of the media is associated with intimal thickening. The elastic tissue shows dissolution of the elastica. The evidence for arteritis with subsequent thrombosis is typically the gaps in the elastica and media. The intimal thickening probably represents organization of a thrombus formed in response to the arteritis. (*From GJ Dammin, JP Merrill, in Structural Basis for Renal Disease, EL Becker (ed), New York, Hoeber-Harper, 1968.*)

targeting of T cell subsets. Another approach to more selective therapy is to target the 55-kDa beta chain of the IL-2 receptor, expressed only on T cells that have been recently activated. When the antibody is administered during the first 10 days after transplantation, a temporary protection from rejection is obtained. Clinical trials of genetically engineered "humanized" monoclonal antibodies are in progress. This approach offers the possibility of improved clearance and destruction of the targeted lymphocytes and reduced potential for development of human antimouse antibodies (HAMA). The latter response limits the efficacy of monoclonal antibody therapy. The destruction of targeted cells also can be improved by conjugation of antibodies with a cellular toxin, such as ricin.

Other techniques   Thoracic duct lymph drainage, removal of thymus or spleen, and local irradiation of the transplanted kidney have been abandoned. Fractional total-lymph-node irradiation (TLI), as employed in the therapy of Hodgkin's disease, is under investi-gation.

CLINICAL COURSE AND MANAGEMENT OF THE RECIPIENT
Bilateral nephrectomy at some point prior to transplantation is performed for a specific cause but not as a routine. Hypertension which is difficult to control or infection involving the end-stage kidneys are the two most common indications. Nephrectomized patients maintain a much lower hematocrit, but this is no longer considered a disadvantage because of the availability of recombinant EPO. Nephrectomy per se does not appear to affect the survival of subsequent renal allografts.

Adequate hemodialysis should be performed within 48 h of surgery, and care should be taken that the serum potassium level is not markedly elevated so that intraoperative cardiac arrhythmias can be averted. The diuresis that commonly occurs postoperatively must be carefully monitored; in some instances it may be massive, reflecting the inability of ischemic tubules to regulate sodium and water excretion; with large diureses, massive potassium losses may occur. Most chronically uremic patients have some excess of extracellular fluid, and some degree of diuresis should be promoted, provided hemodynamics remain stable. Acute tubular necrosis (ATN) may cause immediate oliguria or may follow an initial short period of graft function. ATN is most likely when cadaveric donors have been hypotensive or if the interval between cessation of blood flow and organ harvest (warm ischemic time) is more than a few minutes. Recovery usually occurs within 3 weeks, although periods as long as 6 weeks have been reported. Superimposition of rejection on ATN is common, and the differential diagnosis may be difficult. Cyclosporine therapy prolongs ATN, and some patients do not diurese until they are switched to azathioprine. Many centers avoid starting cyclosporine for the first several days, using ALG or a monoclonal antibody along with azathioprine and prednisone until renal function is established.

The rejection episode   Early diagnosis of rejection allows prompt institution of therapy to preserve renal function and prevent irreversible damage due to fibrosis. Clinical evidence of rejection may be characterized by fever, swelling, and tenderness over the allograft and by significant reduction in urine volume. The use of cyclosporine blunts such inflammatory signs. In patients whose renal function is good initially, oliguria may be accompanied by decreased urinary sodium concentration and increased osmolarity. These changes may not be present in the more chronic stages of rejection or when renal function is impaired at the onset of rejection.

Arteriography and radioactive iodohippurate sodium renograms of the transplanted kidney may be useful in ascertaining changes in the renal vasculature and in renal blood flow, even in the absence of urinary flow. Diagnostic ultrasound is the procedure of choice to rule out urinary obstruction or to confirm the presence of perirenal collections of urine, blood, or lymph. When renal function has been good initially, a rise in the serum creatinine level and a decrease in the creatinine clearance is the most sensitive and reliable indicator of possible rejection and may be the only sign.

Cyclosporine may cause deterioration in renal function in a manner similar to a rejection episode. In fact, rejection processes tend to be more indolent with cyclosporine, and the only way to make a diagnosis may be by renal biopsy. Cyclosporine has an afferent arteriolar constrictor effect on the kidney and, in addition, may produce permanent vascular and interstitial injury after sustained high-dose therapy. There is no universally accepted lesion(s) which makes a diagnosis of cyclosporine toxicity, although interstitial fibrosis and thickening of arteriolar walls have been noted by some. Basically, if the biopsy does not reveal moderate and active cellular rejection activity, the serum creatinine will most likely respond to a reduction in cyclosporine dose. Blood levels of drug can be useful if very high or very low but do not correlate precisely with renal function. If rejection activity is present in the biopsy, appropriate therapy is indicated.

OKT3 monoclonal antibody, given intravenously for 10 to 14 days, is effective in more than 90 percent of first rejections, although it is less effective if methylprednisolone pulses have failed and in cases of severe recurrent rejection activity. A major problem with OKT3 is that severe systemic reactions may be produced during the first day or two of therapy. Chills, fever, hypotension, and headache are the direct result of the antibody effects on the targeted T cells, most likely related to the known potential of OKT3 to activate T cells nonspecifically. If the antibody is administered to overhydrated oliguric patients, pulmonary edema may be induced. These reactions are not characteristic of other monoclonal antibodies, such as those to the IL-2 receptor. Recurrent or rebound rejection activity may require additional therapy. In such circumstances, methylprednisolone may be effective even though it failed initially. Second courses of OKT3 may be given in spite of antimouse antibodies generated in response to the first course if the titers are low and the human antibodies are not directed to the combining-site region (idiotype) of the OKT3.

Management problems Modification of the usual clinical manifestations of infection by immunosuppressive therapy is a major problem in the posttransplant period. The major toxic effect of azathioprine is bone marrow suppression, while cyclosporine has no marrow effects. They both may predispose to unusual opportunistic infections, however. The signs and symptoms of infection may be masked and distorted, and fever without obvious cause is common. Only after days or weeks will it become apparent that it has a viral or fungal origin. Bacterial infections are most common during the first month after transplantation. The importance of blood cultures in such patients cannot be overemphasized, because systemic infection without obvious foci is frequent, although wound infections with or without urinary fistulas are most common. Particularly ominous are rapidly occurring pulmonary lesions, which may result in death within 5 days of onset. When these become apparent, immunosuppressive agents should be discontinued, except for maintenance doses of prednisone. Aggressive diagnostic procedures, including transbronchial and open lung biopsy, are frequently indicated. In the case of *Pneumocystis carinii* (Chap. 178) infection, trimethoprim-sulfamethoxazole is the treatment of choice; amphotericin B has been used effectively in systemic fungal infections. Prophylaxis against *P. carinii* with daily low-dose trimethoprim-sulfamethoxazole is very effective. Involvement of the oropharynx with *Candida* (Chap. 166) may be treated with local nystatin. Small doses (a total of 300 mg) of amphotericin given over a period of 2 weeks may be effective in refractory oral candidiasis. *Aspergillus* (Chap. 167), *Nocardia* (Chap. 126), and cytomegalovirus (CMV) (Chap. 146) infections also occur. CMV is a common and dangerous infection in transplant recipients. It does not generally appear until the end of the first posttransplant month. Active CMV infection is sometimes associated, or occasionally confused, with rejection episodes. Patients at highest risk for severe CMV disease are those without anti-CMV antibodies who receive a graft from a CMV antibody–positive donor (15 percent mortality). Serial intravenous administration of high-titer CMV immune globulin is effective in reducing this risk. Prophylactic use of acyclovir and other antiviral agents is under study. Treatment of active CMV disease with ganciclovir is generally effective. Severe CMV disease is common after treatment with OKT3, and concurrent treatment with ganciclovir during OKT3 administration appears to be effective for prophylaxis of CMV activation. The complications of glucocorticoid therapy are well known and include gastrointestinal bleeding, impairment of wound healing, osteoporosis, diabetes mellitus, cataract formation, and hemorrhagic pancreatitis. The treatment of jaundice in transplant patients should include cessation of azathioprine or cyclosporine if hepatitis or drug toxicity is suspected. It is surprising that cessation of azathioprine or cyclosporine therapy in such circumstances often does not result in rejection of a graft, at least for several weeks. Antiplatelet agents and anticoagulants, although effective in theory, have not been successful in the prevention of the chronic vascular lesion. Persistent elevation of serum creatinine levels above 220 μmol/L (2.5 mg/dL) in patients on cyclosporine is an indication for dose reduction, particularly if cyclosporine blood levels are elevated. Some centers convert patients from cyclosporine to azathioprine after 6 to 12 months, but some patients have rejection episodes, and some of those lose their grafts. The alternative to conversion is to use lower doses of cyclosporine indefinitely. The risk of long-term cumulative toxicity to the kidney now seems to be low. Reduction of cyclosporine is best accomplished by routine use of "triple therapy," in which the following dose levels are used for maintenance after 6 to 8 months: cyclosporine, 3 to 5 mg/kg of body weight per day; azathioprine, 1.0 to 1.5 mg/kg per day; prednisone, 0.15 to 0.20 mg/kg per day. Many patients do well on cyclosporine and prednisone in these dose ranges, without azathioprine. In general, minimal or no

rejection during the first 6 months after transplantation is a predictor of safety in reducing immunosuppression therapy over subsequent months to years.

Despite the potential teratogenic effects of immunosuppressive agents, both women and men have become parents after transplantation. The incidence of congenital abnormalities in the offspring is not increased.

Glomerular lesions Even identical twins, who do not require immunosuppression, may develop glomerular lesions after transplantation. Glomerular lesions occur in 10 to 15 percent of allografts, even when the original disease was accidental removal of a solitary kidney. The pathogenesis is related to a chronic rejection process. In other cases the lesions resemble those of the original disease. The recurrence of the nephrotic syndrome with "nil disease" in transplanted kidneys whose recipient's original nil disease had progressed to renal failure with focal sclerosis, and the recurrence in renal allografts of the classic lesions of IgA nephropathy and of membranoproliferative glomerulonephritis with electron-dense deposit disease are examples. In the last of these, the incidence of recurrence has been reported to be as high as 30 to 40 percent. In most instances, the recurrence of the original renal lesions represents no threat to the immediate prognosis, and a primary diagnosis of glomerulonephritis is rarely a contraindication to transplantation.

Malignancy The incidence of tumors in patients on immunosuppressive therapy is 5 to 6 percent, or approximately 100 times greater than that in the general population of the same age range. The most common lesions are cancer of the skin and lips and carcinoma in situ of the cervix, as well as lymphomas, such as non-Hodgkin's lymphomas. The risks are increased in proportion to the total immunosuppressive load administered.

Other complications *Hypercalcemia* after transplantation may indicate failure of hyperplastic parathyroid glands to regress. Aseptic necrosis of the head of the femur is probably due to preexisting hyperparathyroidism, with aggravation by glucocorticoid treatment. With improved management of calcium and phosphorus metabolism during chronic dialysis, the incidence of parathyroid-related complications has fallen dramatically.

Hypertension may be caused by (1) native kidneys, (2) rejection activity in the transplant, (3) renal artery stenosis, if an end-to-end anastomosis was constructed with an iliac artery branch, and (4) renal cyclosporine toxicity. The latter may improve with reduction in cyclosporine dose. Whereas angiotensin-converting enzyme inhibitors may be useful, calcium channel blockers are frequently more effective in cyclosporine-treated patients.

Chronic hepatitis, particularly when due to hepatitis B virus, can be a progressive, fatal disease over a decade or so. Patients who are persistently HBsAg-positive are at higher risk, according to some studies, but the presence of hepatitis C is also a concern when one embarks on a course of immunosuppression in a transplant recipient.

Both chronic dialysis and renal transplant patients have a higher incidence of death from myocardial infarction and stroke than in the population at large, and this is particularly true in diabetics. Contributing factors are hypertension and hypertriglyceridemia. Increased low-density lipoprotein cholesterol and depressed high-density lipoprotein cholesterol concentrations may be exaggerated after transplantation and require treatment.

REFERENCES

BARTLETT RH et al: Continuous arteriovenous hemofiltration: Improved survival in surgical acute renal failure? Surgery 100:400, 1986

DAUGIRDAS JT: Dialysis hypotension: A hemodynamic analysis. Kidney Int 39:233, 1991

HERBELIN A et al: Influence of uremia and hemodialysis on circulating interleukin-1 and tumor necrosis factor α. Kidney Int 37:116, 1990

INSTITUTE OF MEDICINE SPECIAL REPORT: The Medicare end-stage renal disease program. N Engl J Med 324:1143, 1991

LOWRIE EG et al: Effect of the hemodialysis prescription on patient morbidity. N Engl J Med 305:1176, 1981

Lowrie EG, Lew NL: Death risk in hemodialysis patients: The predictive value of commonly measured variables and an evaluation of death rate differences between facilities. Am J Kidney Dis 15:458, 1990

Nolph KD: Continuous ambulatory peritoneal dialysis as long-term treatment for end-stage renal disease. Am J Kidney Dis 17:154, 1991

Novello AC: Ethical, social, and financial aspects of end stage renal disease, in *The Kidney*, 4th ed, B Brenner, F Rector (eds). Philadelphia, Saunders, 1991, p 2424

Opelz G: HLA matching should be utilized for improving kidney transplant success rates. Transplant Proc 23:46, 1991

Palder SB et al: Vascular access for hemodialysis: Patency rates and results of revision. Ann Surg 202:235, 1985

Ramos EL et al: Clinical aspects of renal transplantation, in *The Kidney*, 4th ed, B Brenner, F Rector (eds). Philadelphia, Saunders, 1991, p 2361

Strom TB, Carpenter CB: Immunobiology of kidney transplantation, in *The Kidney*, 4th ed, B Brenner, F Rector (eds). Philadelphia, Saunders, 1991, p 2336

Teehan BP et al: A quantitative approach to the CAPD prescription. Peritonal Dialysis Bulletin, July-September 1985, p 152

Teraska PI (ed): *Clinical Transplants 1991*. Los Angeles, UCLA Tissue Typing Laboratory, 1991

239   IMMUNOPATHOGENIC MECHANISMS OF RENAL INJURY

RICHARD J. GLASSOCK / BARRY M. BRENNER

Immunologic events play an important role in many forms of renal injury, especially those involving the glomerular circulation. While investigation of animal models of disease has provided insight into these immunologic processes, the specific etiologic factors and pathogenetic pathways in human disease are incompletely understood.

Immune renal injury may be broadly divided into the initiating events and the processes that mediate tissue injury. The initiating events can be further categorized according to the site of the immune interaction (e.g., within the tissue or organ affected or within the general circulation) or according to the nature of the aberrant immune response (e.g., humoral or cell-mediated immunity).

The mechanisms for development of autoreactivity to self-antigens (autoimmunity) have been only partially elucidated but involve a failure of processes that maintain self-tolerance. Environmental factors, such as drugs and microbial organisms, interact with a predisposing genetic milieu in the pathogenesis of autoimmune disorders. Many conditions associated with the development of autoreactivity are associated with specific genes within the major histocompatability (HLA) complex on chromosome 6. Circulating antibody derived from an expanded B cell clone may react with its respective glomerular antigen in situ to initiate a cascade of events ultimately leading to structural and/or functional alterations in the glomerular circulation. The antigen may be an intrinsic constituent of the kidney or one that has been bound or "planted" in the renal tissue by virtue of a particular biochemical or immunologic affinity. Depending on the nature of the antigen, this category of injury is often referred to as an *antitissue antibody–mediated* or an *in situ immune-complex–mediated disease*. The intrinsic (native) antigens may be either insoluble, slowly renewable components of the extracellular matrix (e.g., basement membrane) or a soluble component of the cell intimately associated with the matrix components. On the other hand, bound or "planted" antigens can be derived from diverse sources, both endogenous and exogenous. The reaction of circulating antibody with an intrinsic or planted antigen can give rise to a variety of structural alterations and immunohistochemical features, as discussed below.

Antibody also may react with soluble intrinsic or extrinsic antigens in the general circulation, giving rise to macromolecular aggregates of antigen and antibody of varying size (i.e., circulating immune complexes). These immune complexes may localize and deposit in a variety of organs and tissues, including the kidney, and thereby invoke injury. This mechanism is often referred to as *circulating immune-complex disease*. Unlike antitissue antibody disease, the pathogenetic immune complexes need not bear any special immunochemical relationship with renal structures; indeed, the kidney is best viewed as passively damaged by immune events occurring outside the kidney. Immune-complex–induced disease can give rise to a variety of structural and immunohistochemical defects.

Cell-mediated processes independent of humoral immunity were originally believed to play only minor roles in renal injury. However, based on animal experiments, several disorders not readily explainable by an antibody-dependent mechanism may be caused by aberrant T cell–dependent events. Furthermore, even in disorders believed to be primarily due to antibody-dependent mechanisms, T cell–mediated renal injury may be an important component. In distinction to antibody-dependent mechanisms, the precise nature of the antigen and the details of the cellular interactions responsible for tissue injury still remain to be resolved in cell-mediated processes. Both antibody-dependent and cell-mediated reactions to the same antigen may occur simultaneously, since both reactions are activated concomitantly in most immune events.

Although antibodies, immune complexes, and activated cells can injure tissue independently, the outcome of immune-mediated renal injury is to a great extent conditioned by the secondary mediator systems called into play. These mediator systems also can be broadly divided into humoral and cellular categories (Table 239-1). Humoral mediators are derived from circulating precursor proteins or through the *de novo* synthesis of peptides or lipids. Complement and coagulation proteins are examples of the former, and vasoactive peptides, cytokines, growth factors, and eicosanoids are examples of the latter. Polymorphonuclear leukocytes, eosinophils, monocytes, macrophages, and platelets constitute the cellular mediators of injury. Through interaction with humoral mediators (e.g., complement, cytokines, platelet-activating factor), they are activated and release local factors that enhance tissue injury (e.g., toxic oxygen radicals, membrane-bound procoagulants, cationic proteins, enzymes, growth factors, and interleukins). The activation of cells also induces the expression on the cell surface of molecules that enhance their adhesion to vascular endothelium, thus promoting their migration and localization within sites of tissue injury. Both humoral and cell mediators can directly influence renal hemodynamics, capillary wall permeability, and tubular function. Complement activation can lead to the release of chemoattractant peptides and permeability factors and result in cytolysis or functional alterations of glomerular cells. Localized coagulation can further interfere with cell or organ function. Infiltrating leukocytes, called forth by complement-dependent or complement-independent mechanisms, can foster the local production of toxic oxygen radicals and promote the release of cytokines, growth factors, and degradative enzymes. Platelet activation and aggregation promote thrombosis and release mitogenic and growth factors locally. Monocytes and macrophages release interleukins, eicosanoids, and

TABLE 239-1   Mediators of glomerular injury

Soluble	Cellular
Complement components (C3, C5b-C9)	Polymorphonuclear leukocytes
Coagulation proteins (fibrinogen)	Monocytes (macrophages)
Cytokines (IL-1, IL-2, IL-6), tumor necrosis factor, interferon	Lymphocytes (T cells), platelets
Growth factors (transforming growth factor, platelet-derived growth factor)	
Platelet-activating factor	
Eicosanoids (prostaglandins, thromboxane, leukotrienes, lipoxins)	
Vasoactive peptides and amines (angiotensin, histamine)	
Reactive oxygen species	

procoagulant factors. Many of these mediator systems are held in check by naturally occurring inhibitors, e.g., toxic oxygen radical scavengers or enzyme inhibitors.

The mediators utilized for injury vary according to the nature of the immunologic attack and the site of the immune interaction. The final outcome of disease, i.e., complete healing or progressive disease, depends both on the initiating events and on the nature, intensity, and degree of the mediator response. Thus a single initiating event can lead to a self-limited injury that heals without defect or a relentlessly progressive disease that eventually destroys the tissue or organ. T cells and/or macrophages, either or both, are major participants in cell-mediated immune injury. T cells can be involved in the direct cytolysis of glomerular cells or, by virtue of the release of cytokines, may call forth a cascade of supporting cells or molecules. Immunologic specificity is conferred by the ability of T cell receptors to react with an antigenic peptide presented by the major histocompatibility complex molecule on other cells such as macrophages. Because all the elements necessary for a cell-mediated immune response are present within the kidney, indeed within the glomerulus itself, there is no requirement for delivery of sensitized, activated T cells from the circulation, although such activation is likely in many renal diseases. Finally, even with subsidence of the initiating immune events and quiescence of the inflammatory process, ongoing damage can be perpetuated by nonimmune, noninflammatory factors such as hypertension, vascular disease, atherosclerotic events at the microvascular level, or maladaptive processes arising from attempts to compensate for the loss of functioning nephron mass. These nonimmune factors may constitute an important determinant of the outcome of an immune-mediated renal injury.

ANTITISSUE ANTIBODY–INDUCED GLOMERULAR INJURY
Anti-basement membrane antibody disease The classic prototype of an antitissue antibody–mediated renal disease is that produced by reaction of a circulating autoantibody (usually of the IgG isotype) with a fixed, native, insoluble basement membrane antigen, often called *anti-basement membrane antibody disease*. The antigen involved in the classic variety involving the glomerulus is a product of a gene on chromosome 2 that encodes a noncollagenous lobular domain on the alpha-3 chain of type IV collagen. This domain is involved in the cross-linking of type IV basement membrane collagen and is in glomerular and tubular basement membranes and in other organs, such as the lung. Reaction of antibody with lung basement membrane antigens may give rise to pulmonary hemorrhage. *Goodpasture's disease* is defined by the presence of anti-basement membrane autoantibody to the noncollagenous domain of type IV collagen, pulmonary hemorrhage, and often glomerulonephritis. *Goodpasture's syndrome*, on the other hand, may be more broadly defined as any circumstance where pulmonary hemorrhage and glomerular injury are found concomitantly. The production of autoantibodies to particular basement membrane epitopes is the characteristic that defines Goodpasture's disease. Immunohistochemically, this disorder is characterized by linear deposits of IgG along the glomerular capillary wall. Ready access of this site to inflammatory mediators both of a cellular and humoral nature explains the participation of leukocytes, platelets, complement, and coagulation in the resultant immune injury. Other basement membrane constituents, such as laminin, intactin, and heparan sulfate proteoglycan, also could be targets of an antitissue antibody response, but such reactions provoking disease are rare in humans.

Antibody to non-basement membrane antigens The glomerulus is a complex structure composed of cellular (endothelial, mesangial, and epithelial cells) and matrix elements. Cell-surface antigens of the cellular elements can serve as targets for antitissue antibody responses. One of these, the so-called Heymann antigen, evokes a particular form of renal disease. The reaction of a circulating autoantibody with a high-molecular-weight glycoprotein (Gp330) in the clatherin-coated endocytotic pits of visceral epithelial cells results in the formation of immune complexes in situ. Presumably, IgG autoantibodies percolate through the glomerular basement membrane,

where they encounter their respective antigen on the surface of the visceral epithelial cells. An in situ immune complex is formed and shed into the surrounding subepithelial space. Newly synthesized antigen continually reacts with newly arriving antibody, and the immune complexes eventually grow to an ultrastructurally visible size, forming the subepithelial, electron-dense immune deposits characteristic of the disorder. Eventually, new basement membrane synthesis leads to thickening of the capillary wall. In this instance, the location of the immune reaction diminishes the opportunity for cellular mediators to participate, but soluble mediators, such as complement, cause functional alterations in the capillary wall, particularly enhanced permeability.

Mesangial cells also may be damaged by antibody- and complement-dependent processes, but because of the location of the immune events, greater involvement of other cells, such as monocytes and platelets, may occur.

Antibodies reacting with planted glomerular antigens Circulating endogenous or environmental substances with special affinity for glomerular structures, including the glomerular capillary wall or mesangium, may deposit in these structures and thus act as a "planted" antigen. An antibody or cellular response to these planted nonglomerular or extrinsic antigens could result in disease as a result of the formation of antigen-antibody complexes in situ. The pattern of disease produced depends on the sites of the planted antigen and the nature of the immune response. Examples of such planted antigens thus far described include certain drugs, plant lectins, cationized plasma proteins, aggregated immunoglobulins, and deoxyribonucleic acid. Experimental models of this sequence have been described, but there is little definitive information regarding comparable mechanisms in humans.

CIRCULATING IMMUNE-COMPLEX DISEASE (See Chap. 283)
The deposition in the kidney of immune complexes formed in the circulation accounts for many diseases of the kidney for which there is clear evidence of participation of some immunologic process. In this category, an immunogenic replicating or nonreplicating substance arises in the circulation either from an endogenous (autologous) or exogenous (environmental) source. An antibody response to the antigen while the antigen remains in the circulation leads to the formation of an aggregate of antigen and antibody known as a *circulating immune complex*. The complement system plays an important role in the transport and removal of circulating immune complexes, and defects in the complement system may predispose to the deposition and accumulation of immune complexes at various tissue sites, including the glomerulus. Activated complement components, particularly C1q and C3b, interfere with the precipitation of immune complexes or solubilize preformed immune complexes, thus preventing their deposition as insoluble aggregates. Circulating immune complexes containing bound C3b are transported to the mononuclear phagocyte system (liver, spleen) via the erythrocyte CR1 receptor. Such transport and delivery favor uptake and degradation of immune complexes by the mononuclear phagocyte system. A small fraction of circulating immune complexes may escape removal by the mononuclear phagocyte system and instead be trapped by vascular structures, including the glomeruli. Circulating immune complexes trapped in these sites have the capability of evoking inflammation utilizing many of the mediator systems described above. One of the best-studied examples of this circulating immune-complex disease involving a nonreplicating antigen is serum sickness, which results from the acute or chronic administration of an immunogenic, soluble, heterologous, foreign serum protein (see Fig. 283-1). A small portion of the immune complexes localize within the glomerular mesangium; in the walls of peripheral capillaries; and in joints, heart valves, choroid plexus, splenic sinusoids, and larger blood vessels, particularly at sites of turbulent flow. Once deposited, these complexes evoke an inflammatory response at the site of deposition.

Although this formulation presupposes that immune complexes form within the circulation and then are deposited in vascular structures, immune complexes may form in the extravascular (intersti-

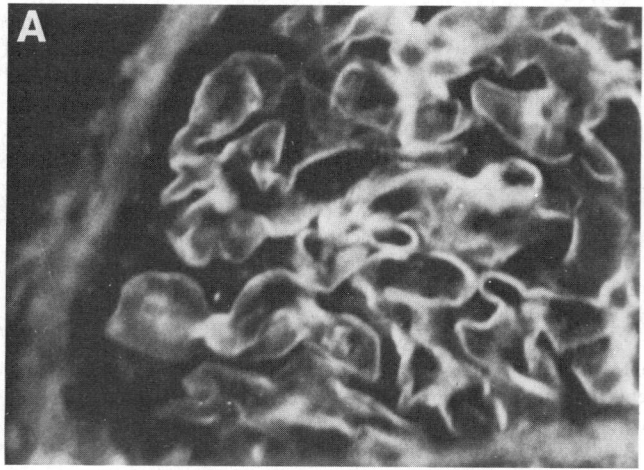

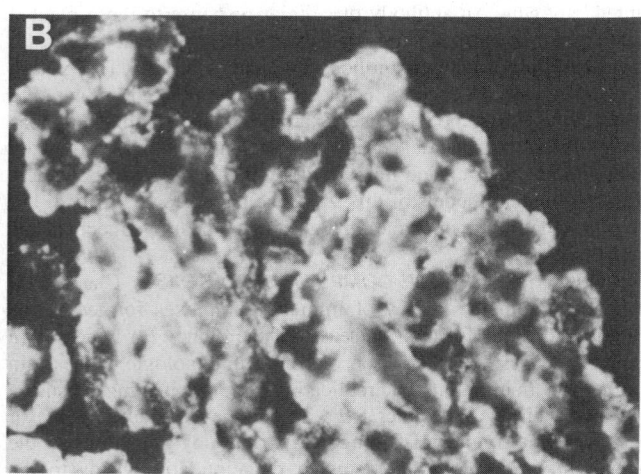

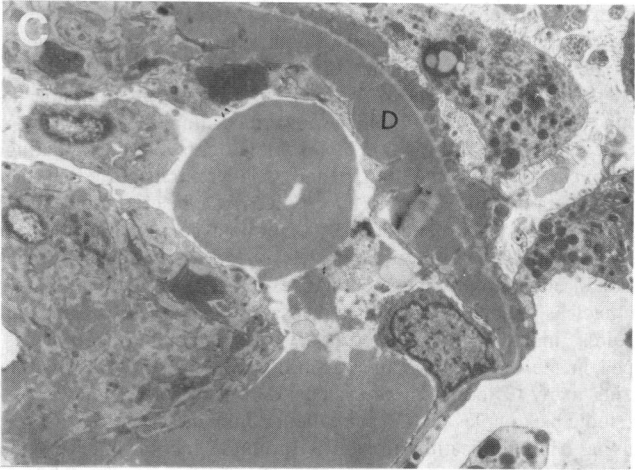

FIGURE 239-1 *A.* Immunofluorescence photomicrograph of a portion of a glomerulus from a patient with anti-glomerular basement membrane antibody–mediated glomerular injury. Note the linear deposits (fluorescein-labeled antihuman IgG). *B.* Immunofluorescence photomicrograph of a portion of a glomerulus from a patient with immune-complex–mediated (in situ or circulating) glomerular injury. Note the irregular, granular deposits (fluorescein-labeled antihuman IgG). *C.* Electron micrograph of a portion of a glomerular capillary from a patient with immune-complex–mediated glomerular injury. Note the electron-dense deposits, *D.*

tial) compartment by virtue of diffusion into this fluid compartment of cell-derived antigens and circulating antibody. Such a phenomenon may explain the deposition of immune complexes in the interstitial areas of the kidney, with relative sparing of the glomerular circulation. Regardless of the nature of the antibody or antigen or the particular circumstances surrounding the immunologic events, a clue to the presence of immune-complex deposition or in situ formation is the morphologic pattern found when tissues are examined by immunofluorescence or electron-microscopic techniques. Granular, discontinuous, and irregular deposits of Ig, often in conjunction with complement components, are found by immunofluorescence (Fig. 239-1*B*), whereas electron-dense deposits are seen by electron microscopy (Fig. 239-1*C*). As indicated above, such deposits are not proof of origin in the circulation, since the formation of immune complexes in situ may produce similar deposits, particularly on the subepithelial aspect of the glomerular capillary wall. Sometimes these deposits acquire a definite substructure, but for the most part they are rather homogeneous. The deposits may develop in several locations within the glomerulus: beneath the epithelial cells (subepithelial), within the basement membrane (intramembranous), beneath the endothelium (subendothelial), and within the mesangial matrix. Immune complexes also may localize in the peritubular capillary network. The reason for localization at these different sites may involve factors such as size or charge of the complexes, receptors for the Fc or complement components within glomerular structures, or local hemodynamic events. The deposits appear to increase in size by cross-linking and aggregation, and glomerular cells may participate in their removal. The persistence of deposits is related to the rate of formation balanced by the activity of removal systems. Ig itself in a circulating immune complex trapped in the glomerular circulation may behave as a planted antigen, either via the idiotypic determinants in the antigen-binding sites of antibody or via the Fc portions evoking an anti-immunoglobulin (rheumatoid factor) response. The roles played by anti-idiotype antibody or rheumatoid factor in the evolution of glomerular lesions in immune-complex–mediated disease is not clear. Once deposited in glomeruli, circulating immune complexes evoke local inflammatory and functional changes, which at least for the glomerular circulation may be relatively independent of complement or polymorphonuclear leukocytes. Infiltrating monocytes may play a critical role in mediating glomerular injury. In situ formation of an immune complex in the subepithelial space may not be associated with the accumulation of inflammatory cells. The morphologic lesions which result from immune-complex deposition may vary considerably from diffuse proliferative to nonproliferative membranous or sclerosing lesions. Coagulation, platelet aggregation, cellular infiltration with cytokine and growth factor release, and release of vasoactive amines may participate in determining the pattern of morphologic response.

The *exogenous* antigens involved in circulating immune-complex–mediated disease are derived chiefly from infectious agents such as bacteria, viruses, or parasites. Replication of the organism provides a continuing source of antigen. The best-studied examples of these in humans are *infective endocarditis, leprosy, syphilis, hepatitis B,* and *malaria.* The endogenous antigens involved in human disease vary considerably and include *DNA, thyroglobulin, autologous immunoglobulins, erythrocyte stroma, renal tubule antigens,* and *tumor-specific* or *tumor-associated* antigens.

CELL-MEDIATED IMMUNITY IN GLOMERULAR AND TUBULOINTERSTITIAL DISEASES Monocytes (macrophages) and T cells participate actively in both the initiation and mediation of glomerular and tubulointerstitial injury. These cells are present in large numbers in the glomerulus and interstitium in many forms of glomerulonephritis and tubulointerstitial nephritis. Interference with the accumulation of these cells within the kidney may ameliorate the clinical and morphologic manifestations of disease. Recruitment of these cells to the sites of injury involves complement components, various cytokines, chemoattractant lipids, and adhesion molecules. The mechanisms by which these cells induce injury is not clear. Macrophages probably exert their deleterious effect in an immunologically nonspecific fashion by releasing cytokines (e.g., interleukin 1, tumor necrosis factor, interleukin 6), growth factors (transforming growth factor, platelet-derived growth factor), proteolytic enzymes, and reactive oxygen species. T cells may exert a damaging effect in an immunologically specific fashion by recognizing foreign antigens presented in association with class II major histocompatibility complex molecules and subsequently by direct cytolysis. In addition, T cells may participate in injury by elaborating factors that promote the infiltration of tissue by other damaging cells, such as macrophages. T cells also may promote fibrogenesis directly. Little is known about the specific nature of the T cell effector and the autoantigens that cause cell-mediated immunity in human disease. Glomerular diseases that lack the typical hallmarks of antibody-mediated disease, such as immunoglobulin deposits, are candidates for cell-mediated mechanisms. Minimal change disease associated with idiopathic nephrotic syndrome is such a candidate disease, and T cells may play a role in this disorder. The rejection of renal allografts and several forms of hypersensitivity interstitial nephritis are probably dependent on cell-mediated immunity.

COMPLEMENT-ASSOCIATED GLOMERULAR INJURY Although there is little evidence that complement activation, independent of antitissue antibody or circulating immune complexes, can bring about glomerular injury, there are certain associations between complement and renal disease. The clinicopathologic entity known as *idiopathic membranoproliferative glomerulonephritis* (see also Chap. 240) may be associated with serum complement deposition within glomeruli suggestive of involvement of the alternative pathway of complement activation, perhaps independent of immune-complex deposition. These patterns are not necessarily unique to this group of disorders, since they also may be observed in postinfectious glomerulonephritides and in certain collagen-vascular diseases.

In *idiopathic membranoproliferative glomerulonephritis*, particularly the subset known as *dense deposit disease*, serum C3 levels are depressed; C4, C1, and C2 levels tend to be normal; and C3 may be deposited in glomeruli without Ig (see also Chap. 240). In addition, an autoantibody (an immunoconglutinin) to alternative pathway C3 convertase is frequently found in the circulation. This autoantibody reacts with a conformational neoantigen of the alternative pathway C3 convertase and stabilizes this enzyme from the influence of C3b inactivator and the inhibitor protein $\beta_1 H$ in a fashion similar to properdin. As a result, sera containing this autoantibody are capable of inducing C3 cleavage in vitro by permitting the assembly of a stable fluid-phase C3 convertase. This antibody is also known as *C3 nephritic factor* (C3NeF) and was first described in patients with glomerulonephritis and persistent depression of C3 levels.

The relationship between these aberrations in the complement pathway and glomerular injury is uncertain. No experimental models of persistent activation of the alternative pathway are associated with glomerulonephritis; thus glomerular injury may be a closely associated but unrelated phenomenon, perhaps genetically determined. The recognition that certain structural genes for complement components (C2, C4) are closely associated with the major histocompatibility complex provides a potential explanation for the association of disease susceptibility with defects in biosynthesis of complement proteins. On the other hand, persistent hypocomplementemia may interfere with the normal removal processes for environmental antigens such as viruses. Such a defect might favor the persistence of these antigens in the circulation and enhance the likelihood of formation of circulating immune complexes. The discovery that C3 and its degradation products (primarily C3b) are able to solubilize aggregates of antigen and antibody may provide an additional explanation for the occurrence of immune-complex disease in association with defects of complement synthesis or activation.

REFERENCES

COUSER WG: Mechanisms of glomerular injury in immune complex disease. Kidney Int 28:569, 1985

GLASSOCK RJ (ed): A primer in renal immunology. Semin Nephrol 12:377, 1992
GLOTZ D, DRUET P: Immune mechanisms of glomerular damage, in *Oxford Textbook of Clinical Nephrology*, S Cameron et al (eds). Oxford, Oxford University Press, 1991, pp 240–262
WILSON CB: The renal response to immunological injury, in *The Kidney*, 4th ed, BM Brenner, FC Rector Jr (eds). Philadelphia, Saunders, 1991, pp 1062–1181
WILSON CB (ed): Immunopathology of renal disease, in *Contemporary Issues in Nephrology*, vol 18. New York, Churchill Livingstone, 1988, pp 1–297

240   THE MAJOR GLOMERULOPATHIES

RICHARD J. GLASSOCK / BARRY M. BRENNER

Alterations of the structural and functional integrity of the glomerular capillary circulation are often associated with hematuria, proteinuria, reduced glomerular filtration rate (GFR), and hypertension. Five major glomerulopathic syndromes are recognized: *acute glomerulonephritis, rapidly progressive glomerulonephritis, chronic glomerulonephritis, the nephrotic syndrome*, and *asymptomatic urinary abnormalities*. This chapter deals with diseases in which the kidney is either the sole or the predominant organ involved (i.e., the primary glomerulopathies) or is involved as a complication of infection or drug exposure. Glomerular injury associated with multisystem disorders is discussed in Chap. 241.

ACUTE GLOMERULONEPHRITIS

The causes of acute glomerulonephritis (AGN) are given in Table 240-1. The "acute nephritic syndrome" consists of the abrupt onset of *hematuria* and *proteinuria*, often accompanied by *azotemia* (i.e., reduced GFR) and renal *salt and water retention*. If GFR is reduced markedly, oligoanuria may be present (see also Chap. 236). Salt and water retention leads to circulatory congestion, hypertension, and edema. Hematuria is likely the consequence of migration of erythrocytes across damaged glomerular and/or peritubular capillary walls leading to the presence of erythrocytes in tubule fluid in the early part of the nephron. Proteinuria is the consequence of a loss of anionic charges of the capillary wall (charge-selective defect) or the appearance of glomerular capillaries with larger-than-normal pore radius, permitting large plasma protein molecules to traverse the glomerular filter. Glomerular filtration rate is reduced because of infiltration of the capillaries by inflammatory cells or by expansion of the number of intrinsic glomerular cells, which thereby reduce filtering surface area. Alternatively, the filtering surface area could be functionally decreased due to the local elaboration of vasoactive compounds capable of

---

TABLE 240-1   Causes of acute glomerulonephritis

Infectious diseases
 A Poststreptococcal glomerulonephritis*
 B Nonstreptococcal postinfectious glomerulonephritis
  1 Bacterial: infective endocarditis,* "shunt nephritis," sepsis,* pneumococcal pneumonia, typhoid fever, secondary syphilis, meningococcemia
  2 Viral: hepatitis B, infectious mononucleosis, mumps, measles, varicella, vaccinia, echovirus, and coxsackievirus
  3 Parasitic: malaria, toxoplasmosis
Multisystem diseases: systemic lupus erythematosus,* vasculitis,* Henoch-Schönlein purpura,* Goodpasture's disease
Primary glomerular diseases: membranoproliferative glomerulonephritis, Berger's disease (IgA nephropathy),* "pure" mesangial proliferative glomerulonephritis
Miscellaneous: Guillain-Barré syndrome, radiation of Wilms's tumor, diphtheria-pertussis-tetanus vaccine, serum sickness

---

* Most common causes.

reversibly contracting mesangial cells (e.g., angiotensin II, leukotrienes), thereby leading to a reduction in the number of perfused glomerular capillaries. Proliferation of visceral or parietal cells admixed with infiltrating cells (monocytes) and polymerized fibrin may obliterate Bowman's space, further impeding filtration. Fluid retention is due both to decreased glomerular filtration rate and to persistence of avid distal nephron salt and water reabsorption. Extracellular and intravascular fluid volumes are expanded by salt and fluid retention.

The edema of acute glomerulonephritis tends to appear initially in areas of low tissue pressure, such as the *periorbital* areas, but may subsequently progress to involve dependent portions of the body and lead to *ascites* and/or *pleural effusions. Circulatory congestion* is manifested by an increase in systemic and pulmonary vascular pressures, and a normal or increased cardiac output. If pulmonary capillary pressure rises above the opposing plasma oncotic pressure pulmonary edema may ensue. *Arterial diastolic hypertension* is the consequence of extracellular fluid volume expansion, enhanced cardiac output, and modest increases in peripheral vascular resistance. Plasma renin activity, aldosterone, and the sympathetic nervous system are relatively suppressed. Hypertension may be accompanied by encephalopathy, particularly in young children.

The extent and severity of urinary abnormalities in AGN vary. Gross (macroscopic) *hematuria* is the most common and is often described as smoky-, coffee-, or cola-colored urine. Lesser degrees of hematuria may go unrecognized by the patient or parent; for this reason, the features of fluid retention and hypertension may be ascribed erroneously to other illnesses if examination of the urine sediment is omitted from the initial evaluation. Hematuria is often, but not invariably, accompanied by the excretion of *red cell casts*. The erythrocytes in the urinary sediment are characteristically small, distorted, fragmented, and hypochromic (dysmorphic hematuria). Leukocyturia and leukocyte casts may indicate the presence of inflammation in the glomerulus and interstitium. The degree of *proteinuria* varies according to the nature and severity of the underlying glomerular lesions. Rarely, protein excretion rates are within the normal range, but generally they are between 0.5 and 3 g/d. If proteinuria is marked and sustained, the nephrotic syndrome may appear (see below).

The short-term evolution of acute glomerulonephritis depends upon the underlying glomerular lesions and their treatment. For example, in infective endocarditis resolution of urinary findings and improved renal function may occur rapidly after control of the bacteremia by antimicrobials. Within a week or so of onset, most patients with poststreptococcal acute glomerulonephritis begin to experience spontaneous resolution of fluid retention and hypertension. Urinary abnormalities often take longer to resolve. A few patients with the acute nephritic syndrome will develop a rapidly progressive form of renal failure (i.e., rapidly progressive glomerulonephritis, discussed below). The long-term outlook for patients with AGN is also considered below. Renal biopsy is useful in characterizing the nature of the underlying lesion but need not be done in every case.

ACUTE POSTSTREPTOCOCCAL GLOMERULONEPHRITIS
Clinical features and diagnosis This disorder is the archetype of AGN. Poststreptococcal glomerulonephritis (PSGN) follows in the wake of *pharyngeal* or *cutaneous infection* with one of a limited number of strains of *group A β-hemolytic streptococci.* These "nephritogenic" streptococci may be identified by serotyping of a cell wall antigen (M protein). Among outbreaks of infection with proved "nephritogenic" strains of streptococci the PSGN attack rate is relatively uniform. Among families, asymptomatic episodes of PSGN exceed symptomatic episodes by a factor of 3 or 4 to 1. Immunity to M protein is type-specific, long-lasting, and protective. Repeated episodes of PSGN are therefore unusual. Outbreaks of pharyngeal infection–associated PSGN are commonest in children aged 6 to 10. AGN following cutaneous streptococcal infection is commonly associated with poor personal hygiene, overcrowding, and concomitant cutaneous disease, such as scabies infestation. Seasonal

and geographic variations in prevalence of PSGN are more marked for pharyngeal- than for cutaneous-associated disease.

An important feature is the existence of a *latent period* between the earliest manifestations of infection and the onset of signs and symptoms of nephritis. Following pharyngeal infections the latent period usually is 6 to 10 days. Cutaneous infections are associated with longer latent periods, averaging about 2 weeks. Signs of glomerular inflammation occurring at the same time as, or shortly after, infection usually indicate *exacerbation* of a preexisting glomerular disease such as Berger's disease (IgA nephropathy).

The diagnosis of PSGN rests upon the demonstration of at least two of the following three features: (1) A group A β-hemolytic streptococcus of a potentially nephritogenic strain is found in a throat or skin lesion. (2) An immune response to one or more of the streptococcal *exoenzymes*, including antistreptolysin O (ASO), antistreptokinase (ASK), anti-deoxyribonuclease B (ADNAase B), antinicotinyl adenine dinucleotidase (ANADase), or antihyaluronidase (AH). ASO responses are typically brisk in pharyngeal infections but often absent in cutaneous infection, whereas AH, ADNAase, and ANADase responses occur after the latter. Testing for multiple antibody responses and serial determinations are necessary to achieve a diagnostic accuracy of 90 percent. Early antimicrobial therapy may prevent the antibody response to exoenzymes and render throat cultures negative but may not prevent the development of PSGN; this makes accurate serologic diagnosis difficult or impossible; (3) A transient decline in the serum concentration of the C3 component of complement, with a return to normal within 8 weeks after the first signs of renal disease. Other complement components (i.e., C1q and C4) are less frequently depressed. In addition to these laboratory features it is desirable to document a latent period appropriate to the infection. Furthermore, the patient should not have any known preexisting renal disease.

The erythrocyte sedimentation rate is usually elevated, while C-reactive protein and rheumatoid factor are generally normal or undetectable. Cryoglobulinemia may be transiently detected. Mild anemia and hypoalbuminemia, both largely dilutional in origin, may occur. Severe hypoalbuminemia may develop if heavy proteinuria is prolonged. Excretion rates of urinary protein in excess of 3.5 g/d occur in less than 20 percent of hospitalized patients. Proteinuria is of a nonselective character and frequently contains high concentrations of fibrin-degradation products and C3 protein, particularly during the diuretic phase. Hyponatremia, hyperchloremia, hyperkalemia, and metabolic acidosis may be seen in azotemic or oliguric patients, especially those with free access to water or potassium. Plasma renin activity and aldosterone secretion rates are low, reflecting suppression secondary to expanded plasma volume and/or hyperkalemia with elevated levels of atrial natriuretic peptide. Urinary sodium concentration is usually low, reflecting avid salt reabsorption in the distal nephron. Abdominal films reveal normal or enlarged kidneys. The chest x-ray may be normal or reveal a slightly enlarged heart, often accompanied by pulmonary congestion. The electrocardiogram may reveal nonspecific T-wave abnormalities. Rheumatic fever rarely coexists with acute PSGN.

The differential diagnosis of PSGN includes other infectious or primary renal diseases which may produce an identical acute nephritic syndrome (Table 240-1). Multisystem diseases such as systemic lupus erythematosus, Henoch-Schönlein purpura, and vasculitis may present initially as acute nephritis (Chap. 241). Predominantly nonglomerular diseases, including thrombotic thrombocytopenic purpura, hemolytic-uremic syndrome, atheroembolic renal disease, and acute hypersensitivity interstitial nephritis may also present the features of the acute nephritic syndrome (Chaps. 242 and 243).

Pathology and pathogenesis Renal biopsies early in the course reveal *diffuse, endocapillary proliferative glomerulonephritis.* Infiltration of glomeruli with polymorphonuclear leukocytes and monocytes is common. The glomerular capillary walls are usually thin and delicate and free of necrosis. Occasional discrete proteinaceous deposits projecting from the outer aspects of the capillary wall toward the urinary space (humps) may be recognized by light microscopy and coincide with the electron-dense deposits seen by electron microscopy. Segmental extracapillary proliferation (crescents) may involve a few glomeruli, but diffuse and extensive circumferential crescent formation is uncommon except among a subset presenting with severe and rapidly progressive acute renal failure (see section below on rapidly progressive glomerulonephritis). Extraglomerular vessels and tubulointerstitial areas are usually normal. Red blood cells are frequent in the lumens of distal tubules, where they form red blood cell casts.

By immunofluorescence microscopy, granular deposits of IgG are seen in peripheral capillary loops and mesangium, nearly always accompanied by C3 and less commonly by C1q and C4 (Chap. 239). Several patterns of Ig and/or C3 deposition have been described. Extensive involvement of the peripheral capillary loops with deposits may be associated with a poorer prognosis, while deposits exclusively involving the mesangium usually indicate a more benign outcome. The precise nature of the antigen-antibody systems involved remains unknown. Most likely the antigen is derived from the streptococcal organism. The profile of altered serum complement components described above, and the prominent C3 deposition in glomeruli are suggestive of involvement of the alternative pathway of complement activation (Chap. 239).

Course and treatment The ultimate *prognosis* for PSGN differs between sporadic and epidemic forms and between adults and children. *Epidemic* forms of the disease in *children* have a favorable short- and long-term prognosis. Few patients die of complications of renal failure, and nearly all experience a spontaneous resolution of signs within a week after the onset of illness. Abnormalities in the urinary sediment and protein excretion subside slowly in the ensuing months; in a few cases, several years elapse before the urinary sediment is consistently normal. Among children with PSGN during epidemics of streptococcal infection, and in whom preexisting chronic glomerular disease was absent, long-term follow-up has revealed little or no evidence of progression to chronic renal disease. A small percentage may develop extensive crescentic glomerulonephritis with its progressive course. The site of the streptococcal infection, the type of M protein, the severity of abnormalities of complement or urinary sediment, or the extent of the rise in antibody response to exoenzymes have little bearing on the prognosis. Prolonged and persistent heavy proteinuria and/or abnormal GFR imply unfavorable outcome. *Sporadic* cases of PSGN among *children* may have more serious long-term consequences. After the subsidence of the acute disease, some children develop slowly progressive glomerular capillary obliteration (glomerulosclerosis), reduced GFR, and hypertension; after several decades, end-stage renal failure from chronic glomerulonephritis may result. The persistence of proteinuria is the rule in such cases.

The prognosis for *adults* with PSGN is less favorable than for children. The reason for this difference is poorly understood. Although the overall prognosis for PSGN in *epidemics* seems good, *sporadic* PSGN in adults is associated with lasting and/or progressive deterioration in renal function in one-third to one-half of cases. This may take the form of persistent proteinuria and/or hematuria or of slowly progressive glomerulosclerosis and renal failure, often accompanied by hypertension. This evolution is more likely when the initial disease is unusually severe. Whether milder forms of sporadic PSGN can lead to chronic disease is an unresolved issue (see "Chronic Glomerulonephritis" below).

The *treatment* of acute PSGN is supportive. It is reasonable to recommend bed rest until the signs of glomerular inflammation and circulatory congestion (primarily hypertension) subside, but prolonged inactivity is of no benefit in the healing process. Fluid retention, circulatory congestion, and edema may be treated with sodium and fluid restriction or loop diuretics. Diuresis alone often ameliorates mild to moderate hypertension. If severe hypertension is present, vasodilator drugs such as nitroprusside, nifedipine, hydralazine, or diazoxide may be useful. Encephalopathy and pulmonary congestion generally improve with lowering of blood pressure and the relief of circulatory overload. Digitalis should be avoided except in well-documented organic heart disease with congestive failure. Treatment with ion exchange resins and/or dialysis may be required for severe oliguria, fluid overload, and hyperkalemia. Mild protein restriction is desirable for azotemic patients. A 7- to 10-day course of antimicrobials (e.g., penicillin or erythromycin) should be given if streptococcal infection is documented. Long-term chemoprophylaxis is not indicated. Glucocorticoids and cytotoxic drugs are not of value.

NONSTREPTOCOCCAL ACUTE POSTINFECTIOUS GLOMERULONEPHRITIS Clinical features and diagnosis A wide variety of infectious illnesses other than those caused by group A β-hemolytic streptococci may also be associated with AGN (Table 240-1). These include *bacteremic states* and various *viral* and *parasitic* diseases. Ordinarily these diseases can be diagnosed by the presence of typical extrarenal clinical features or by bacteriologic or serologic findings. Infective endocarditis, sepsis of other types, typhoid fever, infectious mononucleosis, acute viral hepatitis (hepatitis B), falciparum malaria, and toxoplasmosis are infectious diseases capable of evoking AGN. Circulating immune complexes play an important role in the pathogenesis of AGN in these diseases. Chronic or subacute bacteremic states are frequently associated with depression of serum complement components C1q, C4, and C3, elevated levels of rheumatoid factor, circulating cryoimmunoglobulins, and positive tests for circulating immune complexes. Control of infection usually results in the resolution of glomerular inflammation, although rapidly progressive or chronic glomerulonephritis may ensue.

RAPIDLY PROGRESSIVE GLOMERULONEPHRITIS

Transient azotemia, often associated with oliguria, is common in AGN. A diuresis usually follows within days or a few weeks, and GFR returns to normal. On the other hand, some cases of AGN are characterized by a rapidly progressive form of renal failure, which often develops abruptly and displays little tendency for spontaneous or complete recovery. The clinical term *rapidly progressive glomerulonephritis* (*RPGN*) is often applied to this group to connote the development of renal failure in weeks to months, rather than years or decades, as is typical of chronic glomerulonephritis (see below). Extensive *extracapillary* (*crescentic*) *glomerulonephritis* is the pathologic lesion are often found in RPGN, but other lesions may include segmental or diffuse necrotizing glomerulonephritis.

RPGN can arise in one of four clinical settings (Table 240-2): (1) as a complication of an acute or subacute infectious disease, (2) as a renal complication of multisystem diseases, (3) in association with the use of certain drugs, and (4) as a primary glomerular disease in which the kidney is the sole organ affected by the disease process and in which extrarenal manifestations are the result of disturbances of renal function. In the latter circumstance RPGN can arise de novo or be superimposed on another primary glomerular disease process. RPGN occurring as a primary glomerular disease will be discussed here, while that arising secondary to infectious diseases, multisystem diseases, or drugs will be considered in Chap. 241. The term "idiopathic" RPGN is also applied to this latter group of disorders, by some despite the fact that the pathogenesis is understood.

IDIOPATHIC RAPIDLY PROGRESSIVE GLOMERULONEPHRITIS Clinical features and diagnosis This group of disorders affects individuals in a broad age distribution and has a predilection for males. Wide geographic differences in prevalence have been noted, and outbreaks ("miniepidemics") may occur. Some patients have had exposure to volatile hydrocarbons, but there is little evidence to support a cause-and-effect relationship. While a flulike or viral prodrome may occur, frank arthritis, sinusitis, otitis, skin rash, neuritis, or encephalopathy are uncommon and are more in keeping with a multisystem disease. Symptoms of weakness, nausea, and vomiting (indicative of azotemia) usually dominate the clinical picture. Oliguria, abdominal or flank pain, and hemoptysis may also be present (see "Goodpasture's Disease," Chap. 241). The blood pressure is

TABLE 240-2 Causes of rapidly progressive glomerulonephritis

INFECTIOUS DISEASES

A Poststreptococcal glomerulonephritis*
B Infective endocarditis*
C Occult visceral sepsis
D Hepatitis B infection (with vasculitis and/or cryoimmunoglobulinemia)

MULTISYSTEM DISEASES

A Systemic lupus erythematosus*
B Henoch-Schönlein purpura*
C Systemic necrotizing vasculitis (including Wegener's granulomatosis) and microscopic polyarteritis*
D Goodpasture's disease*
E Essential mixed (IgG/IgM) cryoimmunoglobulinemia
F Malignancy
G Relapsing polychondritis
H Rheumatoid arthritis (with vasculitis)

DRUGS

A Penicillamine*
B Hydralazine
C Allopurinol (with vasculitis)
D Rifampin

PRIMARY GLOMERULAR DISEASE

A Idiopathic or primary crescentic glomerulonephritis*
  1 Type I—with linear deposits of Ig .
    (anti-glomerular basement membrane antibody–mediated)
  2 Type II—with granular deposits of Ig (immune-complex–mediated)
  3 Type III—with few or no immune deposits of Ig ("pauci-immune")
    a Antineutrophil-cytoplasmic-antibody-associated (renal-limited microscopic polyarteritis)
    b Antineutrophil-antibody–negative
  4 Type IV—combinations of types I and IIIa
B Superimposed on another primary glomerular disease
  1 Mesangiocapillary (membranoproliferative glomerulonephritis)* (especially type II)
  2 Membranous glomerulonephritis*
  Berger's disease (IgA nephropathy)*

* Most common.

normal or modestly elevated. Urinalysis typically reveals dysmorphic hematuria and red cell casts, but relatively benign urine sediment rarely may be present. Proteinuria is always present and may be massive. Other biochemical features of the nephrotic syndrome are uncommon, probably because of the rapidity of disease development and concomitant reduction in GFR. Proteinuria is typically nonselective, and fibrin degradation products are found in urine. Azotemia develops early and tends to progress at a rapid rate. Other clinical and laboratory features relate to the underlying pathology and pathogenesis.

Pathology and pathogenesis Idiopathic or primary RPGN is not a homogeneous disease. By light microscopy the characteristic abnormality in the kidneys is *extensive extracapillary proliferation*, i.e., *crescents* often associated with segmental or diffuse necrotizing lesions of the glomerular capillaries. The extent and degree of glomerular involvement vary; however, among patients with rapid deterioration of renal function it is usual for more than 70 percent of glomeruli to be involved with circumferential crescents. Endocapillary proliferation, if prominent, suggests the presence of infection. Segmental or diffuse endocapillary necrosis suggests underlying vasculitis. Fibrin-related antigens are nearly always demonstrable within the crescents by special stains or by immunofluorescence. Gaps or focal discontinuities in the glomerular basement membrane (GBM) and/or Bowman's capsule are observed in association with crescents.

Variations in the underlying pathogenetic mechanisms responsible for RPGN are illustrated by immunofluorescence studies of renal biopsies and by serologic studies for the presence of various autoantibodies. In approximately 5 to 20 percent of cases, *linear deposits* of IgG indicate involvement of *anti-GBM antibodies*. Circulating anti-GBM antibodies can be demonstrated by indirect immunofluorescence, hemagglutination, or radioimmunoassay techniques. Patients in this subgroup tend to have normal serum complement levels and a tendency to develop hemoptysis (see also "Goodpasture's Disease," Chap. 241). These patients frequently are HLA-DR2 antigen–positive. About 15 to 30 percent of cases have findings of *immune-complex–mediated disease*, namely, *granular deposits* of immunoglobulin by immunofluorescence microscopy and electron-dense deposits by electron microscopy. This mechanism of RPGN tends to occur in older individuals, to produce more constitutional symptoms, and to result in more disturbances of the complement pathways than does anti-GBM antibody–mediated disease. Hemoptysis may also occur, but circulating anti-GBM antibodies are absent. C3 levels may be decreased. The remainder of cases of RPGN reveal scanty or no immunoglobulins or complement by immunofluorescence ("pauci-immune"); their pathogenesis is unknown. However, circulating autoantibodies to neutrophil (and monocyte) cytoplasmic antigens can frequently (about 70 to 80 percent) be demonstrated (see also Chap. 243). Because similar autoantibodies are also found in various systemic vasculitides, primarily microscopic polyarteritis, this group of disorders may be a renal form of vasculitis limited to the kidney. On rare occasions, antiglomerular basement membrane and antineutrophil cytoplasmic autoantibodies develop simultaneously or sequentially in patients with crescentic glomerulonephritis.

Uncommonly, other idiopathic (primary) glomerular diseases may be complicated by a rapidly progressive glomerulonephritis accompanied by extensive crescent formation. These glomerular diseases include mesangiocapillary (membranoproliferative) glomerulonephritis, Berger's disease (IgA nephropathy), and membranous glomerulonephritis (Table 240-2). The pathogenetic mechanisms underlying this complication vary. Lung hemorrhage may be observed in RPGN. This subject is covered in greater detail in the section on Goodpasture's Disease in Chap. 241.

Course and treatment The prognosis for preservation of renal function is poor. Patients with crescent formation in 70 percent or more of glomeruli or oliguria or severe reduction in GFR (less than 5 mL/min) at the time of presentation and those with an anti-GBM antibody–mediated process have the worst prognosis. Although advances in treatment are changing the outlook, as many as one-half require maintenance hemodialysis within 6 months of onset. Exceptional patients with crescentic glomerulonephritis have a more protracted illness. Spontaneous resolution is uncommon, except among patients with infection as the basis for formation of antigen-antibody complexes, where removal of antigen can take place.

Glucocorticoids, in the form of "pulses" of parenteral methylprednisolone in high doses, and daily oral prednisone, often combined with *cytotoxic agents* (azathioprine or cyclophosphamide), have yielded varying success, particularly in the patients with granular or minimal Ig deposits in glomeruli, especially in association with vasculitis. Since few controlled studies have yet been conducted, however, it is difficult to ascertain the value of these regimens. Nonetheless, more than two-thirds of patients treated with several "pulses" of intravenous methylprednisolone have experienced improvement in renal function often sufficient to avoid the necessity of dialysis. The addition of *anticoagulants* (heparin or warfarin sodium) and antithrombotic agents (dipyridamole, sulfinpyrazone) seems rational on the basis of evidence for involvement of the coagulation process in the genesis of crescent formation. However, evidence of benefit from such therapies in animals with experimentally induced crescentic glomerulonephritis is inconsistent, in part because of variations in the severity of the disease models, the timing of treatment, and the nature of the anticoagulant or antithrombotic agent used. Anticoagulants may be hazardous in advanced renal failure or with pulmonary hemorrhage. *Intensive plasma exchange* (plasmapheresis—2 to 4 L of plasma daily or three times weekly), combined with glucocorticoids and cytotoxic agents, has been employed. Encouraging long-term results have been obtained in patients revealing linear Ig deposits in glomeruli (anti-GBM antibody–mediated disease), providing therapy is begun *before* renal failure has progressed to require dialysis support. A beneficial effect of intensive plasma exchange combined with immunosuppressive agents has also been claimed in patients with RPGN who do not demonstrate evidence of anti-GBM antibody production. Such benefit has been observed primarily in patients who have progressed to dialysis-dependent renal failure. High dose glucocorticoids and immunosuppressive therapy seem to be sufficient for the majority of patients in this category who have not progressed to dialysis-dependent renal failure.

Renal biopsy assessment of the nature, severity, and potential reversibility of disease is a vital aspect of evaluation of patients suspected of having rapidly progressive glomerulonephritis. Such biopsies should be performed early in the course. Despite aggressive therapy, many patients with oliguria do poorly. Treatment must be individualized, and because dialysis therapy and/or transplantation are available to most patients, one should probably err on the side of a conservative approach, unless compelling evidence of potential reversibility is present.

RPGN may recur after renal transplant. At present it seems prudent to recommend that, after initiating dialysis, a period of 3 to 6 months be allowed to elapse before undertaking renal transplantation in patients who have circulating anti-GBM antibodies. There is no convincing evidence that bilateral nephrectomy in advance of transplantation reduces the risk of recurrent disease in the transplant.

THE NEPHROTIC SYNDROME

The nephrotic syndrome (NS) is characterized by *albuminuria, hypoalbuminemia, hyperlipidemia,* and *edema.* These abnormalities are consequences of excessive glomerular leakage of plasma proteins into the urine (see also Chaps. 33 and 44). The defects in the charge- or size-selective barriers of the glomerular capillary wall that underline the excessive filtration of plasma proteins can arise as a consequence of a variety of disease processes, including immunologic disorders, toxic injuries, metabolic abnormalities, biochemical defects, and vascular disorders. Thus, nephrotic syndrome is a common end point of a variety of disease processes that alter the permeability properties of the glomerular capillary wall. *Proteinuria* is the hallmark of the nephrotic state. Arbitrarily, total urinary protein excretion rates in excess of 3.5 g per 1.73 m² surface area per day [or urinary protein concentration of greater than 0.4 mg/mmol (3.5 mg/mg) creatinine] are considered to be in the nephrotic range, primarily because proteinuria of this magnitude is seldom observed in tubulointerstitial and vascular diseases of the kidney. Sustained heavy proteinuria is often, but not invariably, accompanied by *hypoalbuminemia.* Excessive urinary losses, increased renal catabolism, and inadequate hepatic synthesis of albumin all contribute to depression of plasma albumin. The resulting decrease in plasma oncotic pressure leads to a disturbance in the Starling forces across peripheral capillaries. Intravascular fluid migrates into the interstitial tissue (i.e., *edema*), particularly in areas of low tissue pressure. These disturbances are postulated to lead to "underfilling" of the circulation which in turn initiates a series of homeostatic adjustments designed to correct the deficit in effective plasma volume. These include activation of the renin-angiotensin-aldosterone system, enhanced vasopressin secretion, stimulation of the sympathetic nervous system, and perhaps an alteration in the secretion or renal response to atrial natriuretic peptide. These and other poorly understood adjustments lead to renal sodium and water retention, primarily because of avid reabsorption in distal nephron segments, resulting in unrelenting edema. In this formulation the kidney is viewed as responding maladaptively to a disturbance in effective arterial volume. However, the "underfilling" scenario may not be the complete explanation for salt and water retention in nephrotic syndrome. In fact, measurements of plasma volume, renin, and aldosterone, and determination of the events underlying renal salt and water reabsorption have documented heterogeneity in the pathophysiology of fluid volume homeostasis in nephrotic syndrome.

Some patients have expanded intravascular fluid volume and suppressed renin-aldosterone axis, presumably mediated by primary, non-aldosterone-dependent renal salt and fluid retention, resembling the pathophysiology of acute nephritis (see above). These patients often, but not invariably, have some decrease in GFR and structural glomerular lesions. At the other end of the spectrum are patients with overt hypovolemia, hyperreninemia, and avid secondary renal salt retention. Serum albumin levels are low, *extracellular* fluid volume is expanded, and edema is usually present in both groups. As expected, the magnitude of edema correlates with the degree of depression of plasma albumin (and thereby plasma oncotic pressure); however, the relationship is inexact, perhaps reflecting a component of primary renal sodium and water retention in many patients.

The diminished plasma oncotic pressure also appears to stimulate hepatic lipoprotein synthesis, and *hyperlipidemia* is a frequent accompaniment of the nephrotic state. Low-density lipoproteins and cholesterol are elevated most frequently, but as the plasma oncotic pressure falls further, very low density lipoproteins and triglycerides also increase. Excessive urinary losses of plasma protein factors regulating lipoprotein synthesis or disposal may also contribute to the hyperlipidemic state. Whether these lipid abnormalities contribute to accelerated atherosclerosis remains controversial. Lipid bodies (fatty casts, oval fat bodies) commonly appear in the urine.

Urine losses of plasma proteins other than albumin are also of importance. Loss of thyroxine-binding globulin may produce abnormalities in thyroid function tests, including a low thyroxine and an enhanced resin triiodothyronine uptake. Loss of cholecalciferol-binding protein may lead to vitamin D deficiency and secondary hyperparathyroidism and may contribute to the hypocalcemia and hypocalciuria seen commonly. Enhanced urinary excretion of transferrin may produce an iron-resistant microcytic, hypochromic anemia. Zinc and copper deficiency may result from urinary losses of metal-binding proteins. A hypercoagulable state frequently accompanies severe nephrotic syndrome [serum albumin less than 20 g/L (2 g/dL)]. A variety of factors contribute to the enhanced tendency to thrombosis in nephrotic patients including deficiencies in antithrombin III (due to urine losses), reduced levels or activity of protein C or protein S, hyperfibrinogenemia, impaired fibrinolysis, enhanced platelet aggregation, and hyperlipidemia.

Some patients develop severe IgG deficiency, in part due to urinary losses and hypercatabolism. Low-molecular-weight complement components may also be lost in the urine and contribute to defects in the opsonization of bacteria. Various drug-binding proteins (chiefly albumin) may be decreased, altering the pharmacokinetics and toxicity of many drugs. Electrophoresis of serum reveals, in addition to diminished albumin levels, increases of alpha and beta globulins.

COMPLICATIONS AND MANAGEMENT OF THE NEPHROTIC SYNDROME *Edema* should be managed cautiously and conservatively. Overly vigorous diuresis with potent loop diuretics may result in an abrupt decline in effective plasma volume as the deficit in plasma oncotic pressure may preclude rapid mobilization of the extracellular fluid into the intravascular compartment. This is more likely to occur if plasma volume is diminished and may lead to further reduction in GFR, worsening azotemia, and postural hypotension. Severe extracellular volume depletion may predispose to the development of renal failure, but acute reversible renal failure may also develop even when plasma volume is normal or increased. Renal edema, intratubular obstruction from proteinaceous casts, and alterations in glomerular water permeability have been suggested to account for these episodes. The temptation to administer concentrated salt-poor albumin should be resisted, as nearly all the administered protein will be excreted in 24 to 48 h, so that any beneficial effect on plasma oncotic pressure will be transient. In addition, the increase in filtered protein may have adverse effects on the kidney or the response to therapy (e.g., diuretics). However, such treatment may be necessary in severely hypoalbuminemic patients suffering from profound postural symptoms or refractory anasarca.

The treatment of *hyperlipidemia* is frequently unsuccessful, and its influence on morbidity and mortality is uncertain. Colestipol, probucol, and lovastatin can all cause modest (25–40%) decrements in plasma total cholesterol in patients with nephrotic hyperlipidemia. Whether such treatment reduces risk for atherosclerosis and ischemic heart or cerebral disease is not proven. Nevertheless, most clinicians believe that an attempt should be made to lower cholesterol levels.

The *thromboembolic complications* of NS are reasonably common, including spontaneous peripheral venous and/or arterial, pulmonary arterial, and renal venous occlusions. *Renal vein thrombosis* (RVT), either unilateral or bilateral, is a particularly distressing complication. In the past, this was regarded as a cause rather than a consequence of NS, a conclusion no longer held. Certain glomerular lesions are more likely than others to be associated with RVT. These include membranous or membranoproliferative glomerulonephritis, and amyloidosis. Features suggestive of *acute* RVT include unilateral or bilateral flank or loin pain, gross hematuria, left-sided varicocele, widely fluctuating GFR and urinary protein excretion rates, and asymmetry of renal size and/or function. *Chronic* forms of RVT are commonly asymptomatic. Scalloping of the ureters (due to collateral circulation) and evidence of pulmonary emboli and/or infarction (Chap. 243) may occur in chronic RVT.

Some advocate an aggressive approach in nephrotic syndrome due to lesions associated with inherently high prevalence of RVT (e.g., membranous glomerulonephritis), routinely employing selective renal venous angiography. If RVT is detected, long-term (optimal duration unknown) anticoagulants are prescribed. Such an approach might prevent serious embolic complications, but since the risk of pulmonary embolism is not known, although probably low, the benefit-risk relationship of this approach cannot be determined. A more conservative approach has also been advocated in which renal venous angiography is performed only in those patients with a pulmonary embolism (e.g., symptoms, compatible laboratory findings, and a high-probability ventilation-perfusion scan or pulmonary angiogram) and who have no evidence of deep venous thrombosis in the lower extremities. Since such patients would receive anticoagulant therapy in any case, the value of localizing the site of thrombosis is not established. Intermediate probability ventilation-perfusion scans in asymptomatic nephrotic patients are likely to have limited value, since subsegmental defects in perfusion may be observed even in the absence of renal vein or lower extremity deep venous thrombosis. These changes could be due to in situ pulmonary arterial thrombosis. The risk of renal vein thrombosis or deep venous thrombosis is increased primarily in patients with a very low serum albumin level [e.g., less than 20 g/L (2 g/dL)]. The presence of a thromboembolic complication is usually regarded as a clear indication for long-term oral anticoagulation. The effectiveness of heparin may be impaired by concomitant antithrombin III deficiency, a factor required for the heparin-induced antithrombin effect.

High-protein diets are frequently prescribed; however, the main effect of increasing dietary protein is to increase urinary protein excretion, and the effect on serum albumin levels is modest. Furthermore, such diets are difficult to manage with concomitant salt restriction and, at least theoretically, could aggravate the progression of an underlying structural glomerular lesion. An alternative approach is to prescribe modest protein restriction (e.g., 0.6 g/kg body weight per day), particularly in azotemic patients; some also advocate adding a supplementary amount of dietary protein equal to urinary protein losses. Dietary protein should be of high biologic value and can be supplemented with amino acids. Plasma albumin and transferrin concentrations and urinary protein excretion rates should be monitored to evaluate the effect of diet on nutritional status. Correction of transport protein deficiencies is not feasible. Supplemental vitamin D might be desirable if deficiency is present. In rare circumstances, profound protein malnutrition or other complications of massive proteinuria may justify ablation of renal function by medical or surgical means.

A classification of the causes of nephrotic syndrome is provided in Table 240-3. The multisystemic, heredofamilial, neoplastic, and

---

TABLE 240-3　Causes of the nephrotic syndrome

PRIMARY GLOMERULAR DISEASES*

A　Minimal change disease*
B　Mesangial proliferative glomerulonephritis[†]
C　Focal and segmental glomerulosclerosis*
D　Membranous glomerulonephritis*
E　Membranoproliferative glomerulonephritis*
　　1　Type I
　　2　Type II
　　3　Other variants
F　Other uncommon lesions
　　1　Crescentic glomerulonephritis
　　2　Focal and segmental proliferative glomerulonephritis[d]
　　3　Fibrillary and/or immunotactoid glomerulonephritis

SECONDARY TO OTHER DISEASES

A　Infections: poststreptococcal glomerulonephritis,* endocarditis, "shunt nephritis," secondary syphilis, leprosy, hepatitis B,* HIV infection and AIDS, infectious mononucleosis, malaria, schistosomiasis, filariasis
B　Drugs: organic gold; inorganic, organic, and elemental mercury; penicillamine; "street" heroin, nonsteroidal anti-inflammatory agents,* probenecid; captopril; Tridione; mesantoin; perchlorate; antivenom; antitoxins; contrast media
C　Neoplasia: Hodgkin's disease, lymphomas, leukemia, carcinomas, melanoma, Wilms's tumor
D　Multisystem: systemic lupus erythematosus,* Henoch-Schönlein purpura,* vasculitis, Goodpasture's disease, dermatomyositis, dermatitis herpetiformis, amyloidosis,* sarcoidosis, Sjögren's syndrome, rheumatoid arthritis, mixed connective tissue disease
E　Heredofamilial: diabetes mellitus,* Alport's syndrome, sickle cell disease, Fabry's disease, nail-patella syndrome, lipodystrophy, lecithin-cholesterol acyltransferase deficiency, congenital nephrotic syndrome
F　Miscellaneous: preeclamptic toxemia, thyroiditis, myxedema, malignant obesity, renovascular hypertension, chronic interstitial nephritis with vesicoureteric reflux, chronic allograft rejection,* bee stings

* Most common.
† Includes Berger's disease (IgA nephropathy).

---

metabolic causes are discussed in Chap. 241. The primary (idiopathic) glomerular diseases associated with nephrotic syndrome, as well as the diseases secondary to infectious or drug causes, are considered below.

IDIOPATHIC NEPHROTIC SYNDROME　This diagnosis is arrived at by exclusion of known causes such as infections, drug exposure, malignancy, multisystem disease, or hereditary disorders. The exclusion of these disorders may, at times, prove difficult since they may exist in covert forms (especially cancer and hepatitis B). The idiopathic forms are further classified according to the morphologic features on renal biopsy (Table 240-4). Performance of a renal biopsy, at least among adults, is required for the accurate classification of idiopathic NS, for the formulation of a rational plan of treatment, and for the estimation of the likelihood of subsequent progressive to renal failure. Children need not always be subjected to renal biopsy since clinical study can often lead to accurate diagnosis.

Minimal change disease　In the past this lesion was called *lipoid nephrosis, nil lesion*, or *foot process disease*. In this form of idiopathic NS, although little or no alterations of the glomerular capillaries are demonstrable by light microscopy (hence the designation "minimal change"). Although mild degrees of hypercellularity of the glomerulus may be observed, the glomeruli are of normal size in contradistinction to focal sclerosis (see below). *Diffuse epithelial foot process effacement*[1] is evident by electron microscopy. Immunofluorescence microscopy reveals absent or irregular and nonspecific deposits of immunoglobulin and complement components (chiefly IgM and C3). Minimal change disease is the most frequently encountered form of idiopathic NS in children, accounting for more than 70 to 80 percent of cases diagnosed before the age of 16. Peak prevalence is between 6 and 8 years. This lesion is not rare in adults, representing 15 to 20 percent

---

[1] The term "fusion" is often used to describe these changes in foot processes, although true fusion of cell membranes does not occur.

TABLE 240-4 Idiopathic nephrotic syndrome: selected features of underlying primary glomerular lesions

Lesion	Morphology*			Approximate prevalence in children/ adults, %	Common clinical/ lab features	Response to therapy[†]	Likelihood of maintaining renal function[‡]
	LM	IFM	EM				
Minimal change disease	Normal or very mild proliferation	Negative–trace IgM	Foot process fusion, no deposits	70–80/15–20	Highly selective proteinuria,[§] *normal* C3, decreased IgG, increased IgM	Steroids + + Cytotoxic drugs + (cyclophosphamide, chlorambucil) Cyclosporine + + Levamisole + Frequent relapses	95 +
Mesangial proliferative	Diffuse mesangial proliferation	Negative or variable mesangial IgM, IgG, C3[¶]	Mesangial deposits	15–20/5–10	Hematuria, *normal* C3	Steroids± Cytotoxic drugs (?)	80 (?)
Focal and segmental glomerulosclerosis (with hyalinosis)	Focal and segmental sclerosis and hyalinosis	Focal and segmental IgM, C3	Foot process fusion, sclerosis, hyalinosis, lipid deposits	10/10–20	Hematuria, leukocyturia, poorly selective proteinuria, *normal* C3	Steroids + Cytotoxic drugs + Cyclosporine +	45–50
Membranous glomerulonephritis	Thick capillary wall, spikes of BM material	Diffuse granular capillary wall IgG, ±C3	Subepithelial deposits	<5/30–40	Variable protein selectivity, *normal* C3, renal vein thrombosis	Steroids± Cytotoxic drugs + Intravenous IgG (?) Cyclosporine (?)	70 +
Membranoproliferative glomerulonephritis							
Type I	Mesangial proliferation interposition, lobular change	Diffuse C3; variable IgG, IgM	Subendothelial deposits	8/<5	Hematuria, *reduced* C3 (intermittent)	Steroids (?) Anticoagulants (?) Cytotoxic drugs (?) Antithrombotics +	50
Type II	Mesangial proliferation interposition	C3 capillary wall and mesangial nodules	Intramembranous deposits	3/<5	Hematuria, *reduced* C3 (persistent), +C3NF	Steroids − Cytotoxic drugs −	40

* LM = light microscopy, IFM = immunofluorescence microscopy, EM = electron microscopy, BM = basement membrane.
† Response to therapy: + + = highly responsive, + = variably responsive, ± = occasionally responsive, − = unresponsive.
‡ Percent of patients maintaining sufficient renal function to obviate need for chronic dialysis or transplantation within 5 years.
§ Protein selectivity = differential protein clearance, e.g., IgG/transferrin clearance ratio. Highly selective = <0.1, moderately selective = 0.11 to 0.20, poorly selective = >0.20.
¶ IgA deposits are seen in Berger's disease, IgA nephropathy.
NOTE: C3NF = C3 nephritic factor.

of idiopathic NS in patients over age 16. There is a slight predilection for males. Typically patients present with overt NS, normal blood pressure, normal or slightly reduced GFR, and a "benign" urinary sediment. Varying degrees of microscopic hematuria are found in up to 20 percent of cases. Urinary protein is typically highly selective in children (e.g., it contains principally albumin and minimal amounts of high-molecular-weight plasma proteins such as IgG, alpha$_2$ macroglobulin, or C3) but is variable in adults. The pattern of protein excretion indicates a major "charge-selective" defect in permselectivity. Fibrin split products and C3 are absent in the urine. Serum levels of complement components are normal, except for a slight reduction in C1q. IgG concentrations are often depressed during relapse, whereas IgM levels are modestly increased, both during remission and relapse. Some cases may have associated allergic diathesis (e.g., to milk, pollens, etc.), a history of recent immunization, or upper respiratory infection. The histocompatibility antigen HLA-B12 is more prevalent when minimal change disease is associated with atopy, indicating a possible genetic predisposition to this disease. Thromboembolic manifestations occur, but renal vein thrombosis is uncommon.

Spontaneous remissions and relapses of heavy proteinuria may occur in 30 to 40 percent of untreated patients. Interestingly, an identical lesion is encountered in patients with Hodgkin's disease in whom NS develops, suggesting a role for lymphocytes in its pathogenesis. Except for patients who develop focal and segmental sclerosing lesions (see below), a progressive decline in GFR does not occur. Acute renal failure is rare. In the preantibiotic era infection

with encapsulated organisms (e.g., pneumococci) was a leading cause of death, but now the mortality rate is low, and most deaths are associated with complications of treatment rather than the disease itself. Rarely, acute renal failure may occur even without profound hypovolemia. The mechanism is obscure but could relate to tubular obstruction from heavy proteinuria or interstitial edema or severe glomerular epithelial cell effacement. The renal failure is often responsive to glucocorticoids and diuretics.

Since the etiology and pathogenesis are unknown, treatment is empirical and symptomatic. Glucocorticoids enhance the natural tendency for this disease to undergo spontaneous remission. Daily or alternate-day therapy seems to be equally effective; the latter is associated with fewer complications. Daily prednisone or prednisolone (60 mg/m^2 surface area in children, 1 to 1.5 mg/kg body weight in adults) for 4 weeks, followed by alternate-day prednisone (35 to 40 mg/m^2 in children, 1 mg/kg in adults) for 4 additional weeks is a regimen for initial treatment of this disorder. While initial therapy with high dose intravenous methylprednisolone (1.0 g/d for 3 to 6 doses) may accelerate the development of remission, a higher relapse rate also occurs.

Over 95 percent of children (less than age 16) with minimal change disease respond with a complete disappearance of proteinuria within 8 weeks of the institution of prednisone therapy. Because of the high probability of minimal change disease in children, many pediatricians treat without an initial renal biopsy. A complete steroid response in such circumstances is indicative of underlying minimal change disease in children.

On the other hand, only about 50 percent of adults with minimal change disease respond within 8 weeks of instituting prednisone therapy, with a maximum response often not attained until 20 to 24 weeks from initiation of treatment. Patients over the age of 40 seem to be less responsive than those under the age of 40. Ultimately the overall response rate in adults with minimal change disease is only slightly less than that in children. The delayed response to glucocorticoids in adults could be due, in part, to the lower doses of prednisone relative to the doses used in children. Because of the likelihood of a lesion other than minimal change disease and the fact that some other lesions (e.g., focal sclerosis) may also sometimes respond to glucocorticoids, a steroid-responsive adult patient with idiopathic nephrotic syndrome cannot be assumed to have minimal change disease.

Among both adults and children, 50 to 60 percent of patients with minimal change disease relapse during the tapering or after the cessation of therapy. Too rapid withdrawal of glucocorticoids seems to encourage relapse. Spontaneous remissions tend to be more stable with a low frequency of relapse. A relapse during the tapering phase of glucocorticoid therapy or shortly after the discontinuance of therapy defines the steroid-dependent state. Frequent relapses (more than three per year) may require repetitive treatment with steroids and may be associated with exogenous Cushing's syndrome. Such patients can ordinarily be identified within 12 to 18 months after steroid treatment. Relapses may be treated with the initial regimen but with more gradual withdrawal of prednisone and with low maintenance doses of 5 to 10 mg daily or on alternate days for 3 to 6 months.

A patient with multiple relapses may benefit by a brief course of cyclophosphamide 2 to 3 mg/kg body weight per day or chlorambucil 0.1 to 0.2 mg/kg body weight per day for 8 to 10 weeks preferably begun after a steroid-induced remission. The frequently relapsing patient has a lower likelihood of a prolonged relapse-free interval after such therapy. Such patients seem to have fewer relapses if therapy with cytotoxic drugs (e.g., cyclophosphamide or chlorambucil) is extended to 12 weeks. Overall, only about half of frequently relapsing patients with minimal change disease treated with cyclophosphamide or chlorambucil remain free of disease after 5 years. Among children with minimal change disease the frequency of relapses declines with age. However, cytotoxic agents have adverse effects on bone marrow, the gonads and urinary bladder. Careful monitoring of hematologic and urinary findings is mandatory. They may also be oncogenic. Since they may augment infectious diseases, particularly measles, varicella, tuberculosis, and fungal disease, appropriate precautions should be taken in patients at risk. Azathioprine, previously believed to be ineffective in minimal change disease, will require reevaluation because of anecdotal reports of slow but eventual disappearance of proteinuria in patients with minimal change disease and steroid-sensitive or steroid-dependent nephrotic syndrome treated for 6 months to 1 year with azathioprine 2 to 2.5 mg/kg body weight per day. Cyclosporine in doses of 4 to 6 mg/kg body weight per day induces remissions of nephrotic syndrome in about 70–80% of patients treated for 8 to 10 weeks; however, relapses upon discontinuance of this agent are common. Prolonged therapy (over 4 to 6 months) may be associated with nephrotoxicity. Further controlled trials are needed before this nephrotoxic agent can be recommended for routine use. Cyclosporine may prove to be valuable for steroid-dependent patients who continue to relapse despite cyclophosphamide or chlorambucil therapy or who become steroid unresponsive. Levamisole, an immuno-stimulatory agent, is also capable of inducing remissions in steroid-responsive or steroid-dependent minimal change disease but seldom results in a lasting cure of proteinuria.

The use of cytotoxic agents should be reserved for patients who develop complications of steroid therapy. The long-term prognosis of patients with the minimal change lesion is excellent; 15-year survival is in excess of 90 percent, but a few develop renal failure as a consequence of focal sclerosing glomerular lesions (see below) in association with acquired resistance to glucocorticoid therapy.

Mesangial proliferative glomerulonephritis   The lesion is characterized by a moderate diffuse increase in the cellularity of the glomerular capillary bed. The peripheral glomerular capillary walls are thin and delicate, and extracapillary proliferation is not seen. The precise nature of the proliferating cells is not clearly understood but may represent combinations of proliferating mesangial cells, endothelial cells, and infiltrating mononuclear cells. Glomerular involvement is usually reasonably uniform, although there may be segmental accentuation of hypercellularity. Necrosis of glomerular tufts is absent. Deposits of proteinaceous material, if seen, are confined to the mesangial areas. Interposition of mesangial cells and cytoplasm into the periphery of the glomerular capillary wall does not occur. By immunofluorescence, a variety of patterns are observed. If granular IgA deposits in the mesangium predominate, accompanied by C3 and fibrin-reactive antigens but not the early acting components of the complement cascade, then the lesion is categorized as IgA nephropathy, or Berger's disease (see below). Other patterns of immunofluorescence include a predominance of IgM deposits in a granular pattern diffusely throughout the mesangium, isolated mesangial C3 deposits, scattered mesangial IgG deposits, and no immunoglobulin or complement deposits. Thus, mesangial proliferative glomerulonephritis is a heterogeneous group of glomerular diseases. Some patients with this morphologic lesion may in fact represent resolving postinfectious glomerulonephritis, hereditary nephritis, or other multisystem diseases such as Henoch-Schönlein purpura, vasculitis, or systemic lupus erythematosus. Electron-microscopic findings are nonspecific. Occasionally small electron-dense paramesangial deposits may be observed. The findings of large electron-dense deposits in the mesangium in association with the morphologic appearance of mesangial proliferative glomerulonephritis should heighten the suspicion of a multisystem disease or IgA nephropathy.

This lesion accounts for approximately 5 percent of idiopathic nephrotic syndrome in adults and 5 to 10 percent in children. It is more common in older children and young adults. Males are affected slightly more often than females. Hematuria, either gross or microscopic, is common. Loin pain, bilateral or unilateral, may be seen in the idiopathic disorder but is more frequent in patients who have underlying IgA nephropathy. Laboratory features are not distinctive. Renal function may be modestly decreased or normal at diagnosis. Complement component levels are most often normal. IgG levels may be reduced, and IgA levels may be increased. Anti-streptolysin O titers are usually normal. Proteinuria is most often nonselective. The pathogenesis is almost certainly the result of diverse pathogenetic processes. The presence of mesangial immunoglobulin deposits and circulating immune complexes in some patients suggests an immune-complex pathogenesis, although the antigen(s) is unknown.

Among adult patients with nephrotic syndrome and moderate to severe diffuse mesangial proliferation, there is a tendency for persistence of proteinuria and progression to renal insufficiency. This is particularly true if lesions of focal and segmental glomerular sclerosis are superimposed on the mesangial proliferative lesion at the initial biopsy. Patients with milder forms of mesangial proliferative glomerulonephritis, particularly when unassociated with mesangial immunoglobulin deposition or superimposed focal and segmental glomerulosclerosis may follow a more benign course. Some patients, particularly children, behave in a fashion similar to those with the minimal change lesion. Since renal biopsies from patients with the minimal change lesion may display mild degrees of glomerular hypercellularity, the benign course may indicate that they have the minimal change lesion with more prominent mesangial proliferation rather than a separate disorder classifiable under the heading of mesangial proliferative glomerulonephritis. Well-developed mesangial proliferative lesions, particularly in association with mesangial IgM deposits, tend to be unresponsive to glucocorticoid therapy and to evolve over time into focal and segmental glomerular sclerosis. Patients with mesangial proliferative glomerulonephritis who have remission of proteinuria following treatment with glucocorticoids tend to do well, with little inclination toward progressive renal insufficiency. Exacerbations and remissions of proteinuria may occur. Steroid-unresponsive patients with persistent nephrotic syndrome progress at variable rates to renal insufficiency. The role of adjunctive cytotoxic therapy (cyclophosphamide, chlorambucil, or azathioprine) has not yet been established in this disorder.

Because of the variable pathogenesis and the relative rarity of this disorder, long-term prospective studies of natural history and therapy have not been conducted. Many patients, particularly those with mild degrees of proliferation and a remitting course following glucocorticoids, have a benign prognosis. Other patients, particularly those with steroid unresponsiveness and superimposed focal and segmental glomerulosclerosis on the initial biopsy, have a poor prognosis, often developing renal failure 5 to 10 years after diagnosis.

Focal and segmental glomerulosclerosis with hyalinosis (focal sclerosis)   This lesion is characterized by sclerosis and hyalinosis of some, but not all, glomeruli (hence the term *focal*). Among affected glomeruli, only a portion of the glomerular tuft is abnormal (hence, *segmental*). Enlargement of the less-affected glomeruli is characteristic of the idiopathic lesion. There is a predilection for these lesions initially to affect the *juxtamedullary glomeruli* and to be associated with progressive tubulointerstitial damage. By immunofluorescence, granular and nodular deposits of IgM and C3 are found in the segmental sclerosing lesion. By electron microscopy, focal basement membrane collapse and denudation of epithelial surfaces are noted. All glomeruli, even those unaffected by sclerosis or hyalinosis, reveal diffuse epithelial foot process effacement. Visceral epithelial cell vacuolization is common. This lesion accounts for about 10 to 15 percent of cases of idiopathic NS among children and is more common in adults, particularly between the ages of 16 and 30. Males are affected more often than females. Focal sclerosis may represent a stage in the evolution of a subgroup of patients with minimal change disease or ''pure'' mesangial proliferative glomerulonephritis (see above). In more than two-thirds of cases of focal sclerosis overt NS is present at diagnosis; the remainder have proteinuria in the nonnephrotic range. Hypertension, reduced GFR, abnormal tubule function, and abnormal urinary sediment (leukocyturia, hematuria) occur commonly. Focal sclerosis may have clinical and laboratory features indistinguishable from either minimal change disease, mesangial proliferative glomerulonephritis, or membranous glomerulopathy (see below). Proteinuria is nearly always nonselective or becomes so on follow-up. Fibrin degradation products and C3 may be present in the urine. Serum levels of C3 are normal and IgG levels are reduced, but not as severely as in minimal change disease. Similar lesions may be seen in association with heroin abuse, vesicoureteral reflux, human immunodeficiency virus infection and acquired immunodeficiency syndrome, massive obesity, solitary kidney, and renal allograft rejection and may complicate other primary glomerular diseases in the late stages. The occurrence of focal and segmental glomerulosclerosis in remnant glomeruli after extensive renal ablation has led to the suggestion that glomerular hypertrophy hyperfiltration (or some hemodynamic determinant thereof) may play a causative role in pathogenesis. The attendant lipid abnormalities (e.g., hypercholesterolemia) may also contribute to the progressive nature of the underlying lesion. Abnormalities in the prevalence of HLA antigens have not been consistently described. Renal vein thrombosis is uncommon.

There is little tendency for spontaneous remission, except among children. GFR declines, albeit at variable rates. A subset of patients with focal sclerosis, heavy proteinuria (i.e., greater than 15 to 20 g/d), and profound hypoalbuminemia progress rapidly to end-stage renal failure, occasionally in a few months.

The cause and pathogenesis of focal sclerosis are unknown. A variety of mechanisms have been postulated including immunologic, toxic, biochemical, and hemodynamic disturbances. A systemic process is suggested by the high prevalence of recurrent disease in renal allografts (30 to 40 percent).

Although few prospective trials have been conducted, a decline in proteinuria concomitant with glucocorticoid therapy and a lowered risk of progressive renal failure among patients with complete or partial remission of proteinuria suggest that steroids exert a beneficial effect on the disorder. Indeed, between 20 and 40 percent of patients treated with either alternate-day or daily prednisone in a fashion similar to that described for minimal change disease experience complete or partial remissions of proteinuria. If such remissions persist following reduction of steroid dosage, significant protection from progressive renal failure may be provided. The response of patients who have already developed renal insufficiency is less favorable. Cytotoxic drugs, such as cyclophosphamide, may be of value in patients who are fully or partially steroid responsive, but controlled trials have been disappointing. An aggressive approach with high-dose methylprednisolone given in reducing doses over many months combined with oral cyclophosphamide has given encouraging results, but prospective trials are needed. Cyclosporine, in doses of 4 to 6 mg/kg body weight per day combined with alternate-day oral prednisone will induce partial or complete remissions in 50 to 60 percent of steroid-responsive patients, but remissions are seen in only 15 to 20 percent of steroid-unresponsive patients. The effect seems to be dependent on continuous administration of the agent. Prolonged therapy, over 4 to 6 months, may be associated with nephrotoxicity, especially in patients with impaired renal function and those with tubular atrophy and/or interstitial fibrosis on initial renal biopsy. Further control trials are needed to determine the proper place of cyclosporine and related agents in the management of focal sclerosis. Angiotensin-converting enzyme inhibitors or other antihypertensive agents with antiproteinuric effects (e.g., diltiazem) may be useful in patients with heavy proteinuria and/or moderately impaired renal function even if hypertension is absent or mild. Such therapy may slow progression of the disease, but this has not yet been proven. Hyperlipidemia, often severe, is characteristic of focal sclerosis and probably deserves aggressive therapy with hypolipidemic agents such as lovastatin. At least half of patients with persistent heavy proteinuria develop end-stage renal failure or die of intercurrent illnesses within 10 years of diagnosis. The rate at which renal failure develops is inversely related to the magnitude of proteinuria. Patients who excrete more than 10 g/d develop end-stage renal failure in approximately 3 years. The prognosis is worse for those with azotemia or hypertension at diagnosis. This lesion commonly recurs in renal allografts, occasionally within a few hours of transplantation, suggesting as its cause a humoral factor. Repeated recurrence in subsequent transplants is the rule.

Membranous glomerulonephritis   This lesion is characterized by irregular, discontinuous proteinaceous deposits along the outer (or subepithelial) aspect of the glomerular capillary wall. These deposits contain IgG and sometimes C3 and later-acting complement components (C5b–C9). The deposits also appear dense by electron microscopy. Unlike focal sclerosis, *all glomeruli are involved uniformly.* At an early stage all glomeruli may appear normal by light microscopy, but as the disease progresses, immune deposits coalesce, and new basement membrane-like material is produced, causing the capillary wall to thicken. Eventually, increased amounts of basement membrane material project toward the urinary space, giving the appearance of ''spikes.'' There is little proliferation of capillary endothelial or mesangial cells, although mesangial sclerosis may occur in advanced cases. Tubulointerstitial atrophy and vascular lesions are other late manifestations. The cause and pathogenesis of the idiopathic disorder are unknown, but the in situ formation of immune complexes in the subepithelial space is suggested by the similarity of the human disorder to experimental models.

This disorder accounts for 30 to 40 percent of cases of idiopathic NS in adults but is rare in children. In over 80 percent of cases the nephrotic syndrome is overt. In the remainder only isolated proteinuria is found. Men are affected more often than women. Blood pressure, GFR, and urinary sediment tend to be normal early in the course, making it difficult to distinguish membranous glomerulonephritis from minimal change disease on clinical grounds. Urinary protein selectivity is variable. The excretion of C5b–C9 antigens in the urine may indicate the formation of subepithelial immune deposits. Serum complement components are normal, but IgG levels are depressed. Membranous glomerulonephritis may develop in association with systemic lupus erythematosus (Chap. 241), certain chronic infections (e.g., malaria, hepatitis B), solid tumors (e.g., melanoma and cancer of the lung and colon), or exposure to heavy metals (gold, mercury) or drugs (penicillamine, captopril). Since these causes may be covert at the time of presentation a careful search for these causes is warranted in every case of membranous glomerulonephritis. Renal vein thrombosis is frequent (see above).

Spontaneous complete remissions of NS are common in children and occur in 20 to 40 percent of adults. Progressive renal failure is seen in only 20 to 30 percent of patients, usually 3 or more years after diagnosis and often in association with proteinuria over 5 g/d. Steroid treatment does not greatly influence the development of lasting complete remissions, but may temporarily reduce proteinuria to nonnephrotic levels. A long-term beneficial effect of steroids is unlikely since most prospective trials have not demonstrated benefit. On the other hand, randomized trials and case control studies have demonstrated a beneficial effect both on proteinuria and renal function of combinations of glucocorticoids and cytotoxic agents. The safest and most effective regimen is not known, but protocols involving daily oral prednisone and cyclophosphamide for 6 months to 1 year or sequential cycles of intravenous methylprednisolone, oral prednisone, and oral chlorambucil both appear to be effective. Nevertheless, since the overall long-term prognosis for patients with idiopathic membranous glomerulonephritis is favorable, a conservative approach to treatment is generally recommended. Parameters to identify patients likely to develop progressive renal insufficiency include male sex, older age at onset, hypertension, elevated serum creatinine at discovery, severe hyperlipidemia, proteinuria greater than 10 g/d. Renal biopsy findings often do not aid in the determination of prognosis, but advanced glomerular capillary wall alterations, segmental sclerosis, interstitial fibrosis, and tubular atrophy all indicate a poor prognosis. Patients with features associated with a poor prognosis may be candidates for an aggressive therapeutic approach. Delay of such an aggressive approach (e.g., combined cytotoxic agents and glucocorticoids) until *after* renal impairment is progressive is advocated by some investigators. Indeed, since one third or more of patients with membranous glomerulonephritis enter into a spontaneous remission, an initial aggressive approach may unnecessarily treat some patients destined to have a favorable course in the absence of intervention. On the other hand, if a delay to await progression prejudices against a response to therapy, then too long a delay of therapy may be inadvisable. Treating patients with adverse prognostic indicators initially makes sense, while a wait-and-see approach seems to be advisable for the majority with features compatible with a benign outcome. As indicated above, slowly progressive renal functional impairment occurs almost exclusively in patients with persistent proteinuria in the nephrotic range. Such renal failure seldom develops within 3 to 4 years of diagnosis. However, on occasion patients may have a more rapidly progressive course. The rapid decline of renal function in membranous glomerulonephritis suggests a complicating drug-induced interstitial nephritis, acute renal vein thrombosis, or superimposed crescentic glomerulonephritis. Within 10 years of diagnosis, however, 10 to 20 percent of patients die of intercurrent illness or end-stage renal failure. The majority of survivors have complete or partial remission of proteinuria. A few patients have developed superimposed RPGN. The lesion may recur or develop de novo in renal allografts.

Membranoproliferative glomerulonephritis This disorder is characterized by proliferation of mesangial cells, often with segmental or diffuse interposition of these cells or their cytoplasm into peripheral capillary loops. Mesangial matrix synthesis is increased as well. The glomerular capillary wall is irregularly thickened, by virtue of the mesangial extensions and the attendant synthesis of basement

membrane–like material. This group of disorders is also known as *mesangiocapillary* or *lobular glomerulonephritis*. Immunofluorescence and electron-microscopic patterns reflect heterogeneous mechanisms of pathogenesis. In the *type I* lesion, subendothelial electron-dense deposits are present, C3 is deposited in a granular pattern indicative of immune-complex pathogenesis, and IgG and the early components of complement may or may not be present. In the *type II* lesion the lamina densa of the GBM is transformed into an electron-dense character, giving rise to the term *dense deposit disease*. Basement membranes in Bowman's capsules and in tubules are similarly affected. C3 is found irregularly in the GBM and in granules or rings in the mesangium. Small amounts of Ig (typically IgM) are present, but the early complement components are absent from the deposits. Properdin deposition is variable. Additional ultrastructural variants, based upon location of deposit and basement membrane changes, have been described.

Membranoproliferative glomerulonephritis, types I and II, is found in about 5 percent of idiopathic NS in children, particularly between the ages of 8 to 16 years, and somewhat less commonly in adults. Type I accounts for at least two-thirds of cases. Males and females are affected equally. In 50 to 75 percent of patients, a full-blown NS is present, often with features of AGN. In the remainder, proteinuria in the nonnephrotic range is nearly always accompanied by microscopic hematuria. Blood pressure and GFR are frequently abnormal, and the urinary sediment is active. Functional abnormalities of the renal tubules are common. Urinary protein selectivity is usually poor; fibrin degradation products and C3 are found in the urine. Serum C3 levels are reduced in the majority of cases. The early acting complement components C1q, C4, and C2 are often normal, especially in type II disease. This pattern may be indicative of activation of the alternate complement pathway (see Chap. 239). C3 nephritic factor (C3NF) is often found in the serum of patients with type II, especially if the C3 level is quite low. Circulating immune complexes are found in type I. Lesions similar to type I membranoproliferative glomerulonephritis may also be found in SLE, hemolytic-uremic syndrome, transplant rejection, chronic hepatitis B antigenemia, and "shunt" nephritis. Renal vein thrombosis may occur. Type II nephritis may be associated with partial lipodystrophy.

Spontaneous remissions are uncommon. Long-term, alternate-day prednisone therapy (0.3 to 0.5 mg/kg body weight every other day) may delay the progression of the disease. Treatment regimens that combine steroids and cytotoxic agents are not of proven value. Anticoagulants and inhibitors of platelet aggregation (acetylsalicylic acid plus dipyridamole) may have a long-term beneficial effect. The course is progressive, and approximately half of patients die or develop end-stage renal failure within 10 years of the diagnosis. The prognosis for type II lesions seems somewhat worse than for type I. Type II disease almost invariably recurs in the transplanted kidney but does not always result in the premature loss of the allograft.

Other forms of idiopathic nephrotic syndrome In a small percentage of adults and children with idiopathic NS other lesions are encountered on renal biopsy. These include *crescentic glomerulonephritis* and *focal* and *segmental proliferative glomerulonephritis*. The pathogenetic mechanisms for these lesions vary. For example, some cases of focal and segmental glomerulonephritis may have extensive mesangial IgA deposits and fit into the category of Berger's disease (see below). Serum C3 levels are usually normal. The clinical characteristics, natural history, and response to treatment of these lesions are not well defined. Hematuria is common and may be recurrent. Proteinuria tends to be nonselective. Spontaneous remissions of NS are uncommon. Since no controlled studies have been conducted, it is not possible to evaluate the effectiveness of treatment. *Crescentic glomerulonephritis* is likely to have a poor prognosis, whereas mesangial and focal and segmental proliferative glomerulonephritis have a more favorable long-term outlook. Another group of lesions may be encountered in older patients presenting with nephrotic syndrome often accompanied by hematuria and impaired renal function. These lesions, *fibrillary glomerulonephritis* and *immunotactoid* *glomerulopathy*, are characterized by fibrillary or microtubular deposits in the glomerular capillaries resembling amyloid. However, such deposits are Congo red negative and contain variable amounts of immunoglobulin, sometimes of restricted heavy chain isotype. These lesions may represent an unusual form of dysproteinemia or paraproteinemia, although as yet systemic abnormalities are rare and plasma cell or lymphocytic malignancies are not seen. Treatment is generally unsatisfactory, and many patients, particularly those with persisting heavy proteinuria, progress to renal failure.

NEPHROTIC SYNDROME CAUSED BY INFECTIOUS AGENTS, DRUGS, OR CHEMICALS   Table 240-3 lists the common infectious and drug-related causes of NS. In many instances, NS abates following cure of the infection or withdrawal of the offending medication. In patients receiving gold therapy for rheumatoid arthritis or in those exposed to inorganic, organic, or elemental mercury or to penicillamine, membranous glomerulonephritis is usually the lesion responsible for NS. Minimal lesions and interstitial nephritis are seen with *nonsteroidal anti-inflammatory agents*. Human immunodeficiency viral infection with or without full-blown AIDS may be associated with nephrotic syndrome and progressive renal failure. The renal lesion is quite distinctive and consists of focal sclerosis, interstitial nephritis, microscopic transformation of the proximal and distal tubules, and tubuloreticular inclusions (see Chap. 279). NS is known to follow immunization and antiserum treatment of tetanus or snakebite and to occur in situations associated with atopy.

ASYMPTOMATIC URINARY ABNORMALITIES

This group of patients has *proteinuria in the nonnephrotic range and/ or hematuria*, initially unaccompanied by edema, reduced GFR, or hypertension. Abnormalities are often discovered incidentally and may be persistent or recurrent. In some this syndrome is a phase in the natural history of other glomerulopathic syndromes, especially nephrotic syndrome or chronic glomerulonephritis. Common glomerular disorders that present as asymptomatic proteinuria and/or hematuria are listed in Table 240-5. The heredofamilial and multisystem diseases are discussed in Chap. 241. The presence of dysmorphic erythrocytes and/or red cell casts indicates a glomerular cause for the hematuria.

IDIOPATHIC RENAL HEMATURIA (See also Chap. 44)   **Berger's disease (IgA nephropathy)**   This disorder was first described by Berger and Hinglais in 1968 and is characterized by recurrent gross or microscopic hematuria. The diagnosis depends on the finding of prominent IgA deposits in the mesangium by immunofluorescence microscopy. Berger's disease is the most common cause of recurrent hematuria of glomerular origin. It most commonly affects older children and young adults, mostly males. It is common in certain Native American tribes. Typically, episodes of macroscopic hematuria are associated with minor flulike illnesses or vigorous exercise. Vague constitutional symptoms may be present, but skin rash, arthritis, and abdominal pain are absent. Urine protein excretion rates are usually less than 3.5 g/d; protein excretion is normal or mildly increased. The nephrotic syndrome develops occasionally. In some patients a self-limited and reversible form of acute renal failure may occur. Such episodes are frequently preceded by an upper respiratory infection and accompanied by bouts of macroscopic hematuria. Thus, these patients resemble those with acute poststreptococcal glomerulonephritis. On rare occasions, patients present with malignant hypertension. Blood pressure, GFR, and serum albumin are usually normal early in the disease. Serum IgA levels are increased in about 50 percent of cases, and serum complement component levels remain normal. IgA-fibronectin complexes, IgA rheumatoid factor, IgA antineutrophil cytoplasmic autoantibodies, and low-titer antinuclear antibodies may also be found. Biopsy of the skin of forearm sometimes reveals dermal capillary deposits of IgA, C3, and fibrin but not early acting complement components or IgA secretory fragments. Similar skin biopsy findings are encountered in Henoch-Schönlein purpura (Chap. 241). Indeed, Berger's disease may be a monosymptomatic form of Henoch-Schönlein purpura.

Renal biopsy reveals a spectrum of changes, but diffuse mesangial proliferative or focal and segmental proliferative glomerulonephritis is found most often. In some cases glomerular morphology may be normal by light microscopy; uncommonly, crescents are found particularly during episodes of macroscopic hematuria and impaired renal function. The distinguishing feature is the finding by immunofluorescence microscopy of *diffuse mesangial deposition of IgA*, often accompanied by lesser amounts of IgG, C3, and properdin, but not by C1q or C4. Fibrin reactive antigens are common in the mesangium or in association with crescents if the latter are present. The pathogenesis of IgA nephropathy is unknown, but the systemic character of the IgA deposits (skin and glomerular capillaries), the presence of circulating IgG and IgA complexes in the majority, and its similarity to Henoch-Schönlein purpura suggest that it is an immune-complex–mediated disease. The nature and source of the antigen are unknown.

The prognosis is variable, but the disease tends to progress slowly. Spontaneous remissions develop in less than 5 percent of adults but more commonly in children. Approximately 50 percent of patients develop end-stage renal failure within 25 years of diagnosis. Self-limited acute renal failure may develop, particularly following upper respiratory infections. Hematuria and biopsy findings of moderate crescent formation (less than 50 percent glomerular involvement and tubular abnormalities) are common in this setting. Azotemia, hypertension, or proteinuria in the nephrotic range are associated with a poor prognosis. At present, there is no evidence that therapy influences the natural history, although intermittent glucocorticoid therapy or broad-spectrum antibiotics may reduce the frequency of episodes of gross hematuria. Glucocorticoids may also result in remissions of proteinuria in those patients with mild glomerular abnormalities by light microscopy. High-dose intravenous methylprednisolone, cytotoxic drugs, and plasma exchange may be useful for patients with rapidly progressive glomerulonephritis with extensive crescents (greater than 50 percent glomerular involvement). IgA nephropathy recurs in the transplanted kidney in approximately 30 to 40 percent of cases. Such recurrences seldom result in loss of renal function but may be associated with hematuria.

Other primary renal hematurias   Some cases of recurrent hematuria do not exhibit the typical immunofluorescence seen in Berger's disease. This group is poorly defined, and the cause and pathogenesis

---

TABLE 240-5   Glomerular causes of asymptomatic urinary abnormalities

Hematuria with or without proteinuria
  A Primary glomerular diseases
     1 Berger's disease (IgA nephropathy)*
     2 Membranoproliferative glomerulonephritis
     3 Other primary glomerular hematurias accompanied by ''pure'' mesangial proliferation, focal and segmental proliferative glomerulonephritis, or other lesions
     4 ''Thin basement membrane'' disease*
  B Associated with multisystem or heredofamilial diseases
     1 Alport's syndrome and other ''benign'' familial hematurias*
     2 Fabry's disease
     3 Sickle cell disease
  C Associated with infections
     1 Resolving poststreptococcal glomerulonephritis*
     2 Other postinfectious glomerulonephritides*
Isolated nonnephrotic proteinuria
  A Primary glomerular diseases
     1 ''Orthostatic'' proteinuria*
     2 Focal and segmental glomerulosclerosis*
     3 Membranous glomerulonephritis*
     4 Berger's disease (IgA nephropathy)
  B Associated with multisystem or heredofamilial diseases
     1 Diabetes mellitus*
     2 Amyloidosis*
     3 Nail-patella syndrome
     4 Leaitin-cholesterol acyltransferase deficiency
     5 Von Gierke's disease

* Most common.

are varied. Some may represent resolving acute glomerulonephritis or early examples of membranoproliferative or hereditary glomerulonephritis (Alport's syndrome, see Chap. 241). A common morphologic lesions is focal and segmental or diffuse mesangial proliferative glomerulonephritis, although mild and nonspecific changes may also be observed. Immunofluorescence studies reveal varying degrees of immunoglobulin and/or complement component deposition (principally IgM and/or C3) in the mesangium. Some show linear deposits of IgG, suggesting a possible anti-GBM antibody pathogenesis. Electron microscopy may reveal dense deposits in the mesangium. Overall, these patients have an excellent prognosis, with frequent spontaneous permanent remissions of recurrent hematuria. Progressive renal insufficiency is unusual. Because of the benign prognosis no treatment is indicated. In some cases, exceptionally thin basement membranes may be demonstrated by electron microscopy (thin basement membrane nephropathy). Such patients may have persistent microscopic hematuria and may have a family history of hematuria. The prognosis tends to be benign, but progression has been described.

ISOLATED NONNEPHROTIC PROTEINURIA OF GLOMERULAR ORIGIN (See also Chap. 44)   Mild to moderate proteinuria (i.e., greater than 150 mg but less than 2.0 g/d), unaccompanied by abnormalities in the urinary sediment or evidence of hypertension or reduced renal function, is common. Such patients may display other features of heredofamilial or multisystem diseases, including diabetes mellitus, amyloidosis, rheumatoid arthritis, or cancer. The abnormality may be persistent or evanescent. Proteinuria may occur primarily in the upright posture (*orthostatic proteinuria*) or both in recumbent and erect positions (*constant proteinuria*). Fixed and reproducible orthostatic proteinuria has a benign prognosis and frequently disappears with time. Renal biopsies reveal normal glomeruli or trivial alterations of dubious significance. On the other hand, persistent and constant proteinuria may indicate more serious disease, and renal biopsies often reveal a structural lesion. Some of the lesions have been discussed in the context of idiopathic nephrotic syndrome. Other patients have an unsuspected disease such as amyloidosis or diabetes mellitus. In the remainder, the lesions are trivial and nonspecific, and the long-term significance is uncertain. In primary glomerular diseases, so long as urinary protein excretion remains modest (less than 2.0 g/d), the prognosis is excellent, and deterioration of renal function is relatively uncommon. Renal biopsy is not commonly undertaken in patients with persistent, isolated nonnephrotic proteinuria, as determining morphology seldom leads to specific therapy and adds information chiefly of a prognostic nature. Since patients with proteinuria more than 2.0 g/d are more likely to have lesions that progress, many nephrologists limit renal biopsies to this latter group of patients.

CHRONIC GLOMERULONEPHRITIS

The syndrome of chronic glomerulonephritis (CGN) is characterized chiefly by *persistent urinary abnormalities* (e.g., proteinuria and/or hematuria) and by *slowly progressive impairment of renal function*, eventuating in hypertension, contracted, granular kidneys, and end-stage renal failure. With the possible exception of the minimal change lesion associated with idiopathic nephrotic syndrome (see above) all the disorders described in this chapter and in Chap. 241 can lead eventually to CGN. The pathophysiology of CGN in the context of renal failure is described in Chaps. 235 and 237.

The structural alterations may be categorized as *proliferative* (including mesangial, endo- and/or extracapillary proliferative glomerulonephritis, and focal and segmental proliferative glomerulonephritis), *sclerosing* (including focal and diffuse glomerular sclerosis), and *membranous*. Such lesions are found in most patients with CGN. In the remainder, the lesions are not readily categorized morphologically and are often referred to as *chronic "nonspecific" glomerulonephritis*.

The clinical characteristics of the specific lesions are described in other sections of this chapter. The etiologic and pathogenetic origins

of chronic nonspecific glomerulonephritis are heterogeneous. Complicating vascular disease contributes to the glomerular obliteration. Some patients with chronic nonspecific glomerulonephritis may have had an earlier unrecognized episode of acute PSGN.

The detection of CGN usually occurs in one of several ways: (1) the incidental finding of abnormal urine, impaired renal function, or hypertension during multiphasic screening of asymptomatic individuals; (2) the result of the insidious onset of symptoms or signs of renal disease, especially anemia and hypertension; or (3) after an exacerbation of glomerulonephritis, usually during the course of viral or bacterial illness. In advanced stages, the separation of CGN from other causes of renal failure may be difficult; however, the presence of symmetrically contracted kidneys, moderate to heavy proteinuria, abnormal urinary sediment (especially red blood cell casts), and x-ray evidence of normal pyelocalyceal systems suggest CGN.

The evolution of CGN varies, depending upon the underlying disease and the presence of complications, especially hypertension. Many years may elapse from the discovery of an abnormal urine sediment until the development of end-stage renal failure. Because hypertension is common and clinical and laboratory findings are nonspecific, many patients are diagnosed as having "essential hypertension" and secondary arteriolonephrosclerosis. Nevertheless, many, if not most, patients with essential "nonmalignant" hypertension who develop progressive renal insufficiency have an underlying renal parenchymal disease (including primary forms of glomerulonephritis such as IgA nephropathy). Renal biopsy is necessary to define the underlying glomerular lesion. The principal advantage of a morphologic evaluation is to determine prognosis rather than therapy.

Treatment is supportive and symptomatic. The management of specific lesions is discussed in greater detail in the relevant sections of this chapter. Hypertension and urinary tract infections should be treated vigorously, taking care to avoid nephrotoxic agents. Diuretics should be employed only as adjuncts to antihypertensive management or to deal with edema. Rigorous salt or potassium restriction is usually unnecessary and may be hazardous. In the absence of congestive heart failure or marked hypoalbuminemia, severe edema is rare until the terminal phases. Protein and phosphate restriction may slow the rate of progression of renal failure (see Chap. 237).

REFERENCES

D'amico G: The commonest glomerulonephritis in the world. IgA Nephropathy. Quart J Med 64:769, 1987

Cameron JS, Glassock RJ (eds): *The Nephrotic Syndrome*. New York, Marcel Dekker, 1988

Donadio JV et al: Idiopathic membranous nephropathy. Kidney Int 33:708

Glassock RJ et al: Primary glomerular disease, in *The Kidney*, 4th ed, BM Brenner, FC Rector Jr (eds). Philadelphia, Saunders, 1991, pp 1182–1279

Rees AJ, Cameron JS: Crescentic glomerulonephritis, in *Oxford Textbook of Clinical Nephrology*, J Cameron et al (eds). Oxford, Oxford University Press, 1992, pp 408–437

241   GLOMERULOPATHIES ASSOCIATED WITH MULTISYSTEM DISEASES

RICHARD J. GLASSOCK / BARRY M. BRENNER

Glomerular injury may be a prominent feature of diseases that affect multiple organs and systems. By and large, the etiologies of these diseases are unknown, but aberrant immunologic processes, neoplasia, metabolic disturbances, and biochemical abnormalities are believed to be dominant factors in their pathogenesis. These processes lead to alterations in glomerular structure and function. Some of the glomerular lesions are specific for the underlying disease (e.g., amyloidosis, Fabry's disease, nodular diabetic glomerulosclerosis); however, the majority are nonspecific. Proteinuria results from defects in the charge- and/or size-selective glomerular permeability barriers. Reductions in glomerular filtration rate develop because of loss of filtration surface area in individual nephrons or because of a decline in the total number of nephrons or both. Although extrarenal manifestations are often useful in establishing a diagnosis, some may present with predominant or exclusive renal involvement and only covert extrarenal manifestations.

IMMUNOLOGICALLY MEDIATED MULTISYSTEM DISEASES

SYSTEMIC LUPUS ERYTHEMATOSUS (See also Chap. 284) Systemic lupus erythematosus (SLE) is the archetype of an immunologically mediated multisystem disease and is representative of the multisystem diseases in which renal involvement is common. The cause of SLE is unknown; however, genetic factors and abnormal immune responsiveness probably interact to produce the disease. The principal mechanism for tissue injury in SLE appears to be the deposition of circulating immune complexes, although other mechanisms also play a role, including antitissue antibody and in situ immune-complex formation (see Chap. 239). The circulating immune complexes may be composed of a variety of endogenous antigens combined with autoantibodies. DNA (single-stranded and double-stranded) is a major antigenic component of immune complexes, but other nuclear or cytoplasmic antigens also may be involved. The prevalence of clinical renal involvement in SLE ranges from as low as 35 percent to more than 90 percent in different series. Manifestations of renal disease range from mild abnormalities of the urinary sediment (predominantly hematuria) to massive proteinuria and from chronic indolent glomerulonephritis to a fulminant inflammatory process leading to rapidly progressive renal failure.

The diagnosis and extrarenal manifestations of SLE are described in Chap. 284. This section will deal with the renal involvement. Although extrarenal features usually lead to the correct diagnosis, SLE may present initially with predominant renal manifestations. Morphologic evidence of renal involvement may exist with or without clinical manifestations of renal disease. If immunofluorescence and electron-microscopic studies of renal tissue are performed, abnormalities are present in virtually every patient with SLE. The abnormal glomerular morphologic lesions in SLE form a spectrum based on correlative light- and electron-microscopic and immunofluorescence studies of renal biopsies.

Minimal lupus glomerular lesion This pattern is characterized by few or no changes by light microscopy. Immunofluorescence studies reveal moderate immunoglobulin and complement deposits exclusively in mesangium. Scattered electron-dense deposits are found in mesangium by electron microscopy. Clinical manifestations may include mild proteinuria and microscopic hematuria. Nephrotic syndrome is uncommon. Glomerular filtration rate (GFR) is almost always normal. Serologic manifestations vary depending on the activity of extrarenal disease. Antibodies to DNA are usually present in low titer, and levels of C3 and C4 may be decreased, especially if dermatitis is severe. Immune complexes also may be detected in skin lesions.

Mesangial lupus glomerulonephritis This pattern is characterized by mild to moderate diffuse mesangial cell proliferation and/or mesangial sclerosis. Immunofluorescence studies reveal immunoglobulins (IgG, IgM, and IgA) and complement components (C1q, C4, and C3) deposited in a granular pattern principally in the mesangium. By electron microscopy, electron-dense deposits are confined to the mesangium. This morphologic appearance present in the absence of clinical renal disease or associated with minor abnormalities in the urinary sediment and modest proteinuria. Nephrotic syndrome and hypertension occasionally may be present. GFR is almost always normal. Mesangial lupus glomerulonephritis may be the initial renal involvement in SLE, from which other patterns evolve. Associated serologic abnormalities depend on the degree of extrarenal activity. These include increased levels of antibody to native double-stranded DNA (dsDNA); depressed serum levels of C3, C4, and C1q; and detectable levels of circulating immune complexes (CIC) (Table 241-1).

Focal and segmental lupus glomerulonephritis This pattern is characterized by focal and segmental cellular proliferation, often associated with necrosis, superimposed on diffuse mesangial hypercellularity. Granular deposits of immunoglobulins and complement involve both the mesangium and occasional glomerular capillary loops. By electron microscopy, dense subendothelial deposits are found in the mesangium and in some peripheral capillary loops. Clinical and laboratory evidence of renal injury is more common than in mesangial lupus glomerulonephritis. Nephrotic syndrome may occur in 10 to 20 percent of patients, but in general, GFR is well preserved. This lesion may persist, resolve, or progress to diffuse proliferative lupus glomerulonephritis. Serologic features of active disease are often present in untreated patients.

Diffuse proliferative lupus glomerulonephritis This pattern is characterized by diffuse mesangial and endothelial cell proliferation that may include extensive peripheral capillary wall interposition of mesangial cells. In addition, focal cellular necrosis, hematoxylinophilic bodies, fibrinoid necrosis, and "wire loops" (capillaries with a thickened appearance owing to subendothelial deposits) may be present. Extensive extracapillary proliferative (crescentic) glomerulonephritis, vasculitis, and interstitial nephritis also may be found

TABLE 241-1 Serologic findings in selected multisystem diseases

Disease	C3	C4	FANA	Anti-dsDNA	Anti-GBM	ANCA	Cryo-Ig	CIC	Other
Systemic lupus erythematosus	↓↓	↓↓	+++	++	−	±	++	+++	↑ IgG, RF++
Goodpasture's disease	−	−	−	−	+++	+	−	±	−
Henoch-Schönlein purpura	−	−	−	−	−	−	±	++	↑ IgA, IgA RF
Polyarteritis	↓↑	↓↑	+	±	+	+++	++	+++	↑ IgG
Wegener's granulomatosis	↓↑	−	−	−	−	+++	±	++	−
Cryoimmunoglobulinemia	↓	↓↓↓	−	−	−	−	+++	++	RF+++
Multiple myeloma	−	−	−	−	−	−	±	−	↑ IgG, IgA, IgE, IgD, MC
Waldenström's macroglobulinemia	−	−	−	−	−	−	−	−	↑ IgM
Amyloidosis	−	−	−	−	−	−	−	−	Ig, MC

NOTE: C3 = C3 component of complement; Ig = immunoglobulin levels; FANA = fluorescent antinuclear antibody assay; anti-dsDNA = antibody to double-stranded (native) DNA; anti-GBM = antibody to glomerular basement membrane antigens; cryo-Ig = cryoimmunoglobulin; CIC = circulating immune complexes; ANCA = anti-neutrophil cytoplasmic antibody; RF = Rheumatoid factor; MC = monoclonal; − = normal; + = occasionally slightly abnormal; ++ = often abnormal; +++ = severely abnormal.

occasionally. Varying chronic lesions include focal and segmental glomerulosclerosis, fibrocellular crescents, interstitial fibrosis, tubular atrophy, and nephroangiosclerosis. Granular deposits of immunoglobulins and complement components are extensive and involve the mesangium and nearly every capillary loop. Electron microscopy reveals widespread subendothelial and mesangial electron-dense deposits as well as occasional intramembranous or subepithelial deposits. Most patients have an active urinary sediment, heavy proteinuria, and progressive impairment of renal function; occasionally, clinical evidence of renal involvement is lacking. In the untreated patient, evidence of serologic activity is usually present, including depressed serum C3 and C4 concentrations, high levels of precipitating and complement-fixing antibody to dsDNA, cryoimmunoglobulinemia, and circulating immune complexes. This lesion is associated with an ominous prognosis, although vigorous treatment may modify the course (see below).

Membranous lupus glomerulonephritis   This pattern is nearly identical with that described for idiopathic membranous glomerulonephritis (Chap. 240), except that mesangial deposits and mesangial proliferation are more frequent. The glomerular capillary wall is thickened due to the presence of immunoglobulin and complement-containing electron-dense deposits in the subepithelial space, often associated with a spikelike basement membrane reaction. Nearly all patients have heavy proteinuria and the nephrotic syndrome. Although GFR may be normal initially, many patients ultimately develop progressive renal failure. A focal and segmental or diffuse proliferative lesion may be superimposed on the basic membranous lesions. These histologic findings confer a more ominous prognosis (see below). Serologic features of SLE may or may not be present at the time of diagnosis of this nephropathy. Antibody to dsDNA tends to be nonprecipitating and of low titer. Some patients with membranous lupus glomerulonephritis may be erroneously categorized as having idiopathic membranous glomerulopathy (see Chap. 240). Measurements of the level of antibody to dsDNA or of serum complement levels and biopsies of skin for dermal-epidermal deposits of Ig ("lupus band test") may be helpful for diagnosis in such cases.

Sclerosing or end-stage lupus glomerulonephritis   This pattern is characterized by obliterative and sclerosing lesions of the glomeruli and probably represents a late stage of proliferative lesions. Immunofluorescence studies may be only weakly positive for immunoglobulins; subendothelial deposits are infrequent. Hypertension and impaired renal function are common. Serologic parameters of activity of SLE may or may not be present.

Prognosis and treatment   The prognosis and treatment of SLE with renal involvement depend on the nature of the underlying renal lesion, the degree of renal functional impairment, and perhaps the activity and chronicity of renal lesions as disclosed by renal biopsy. Patients with milder forms of renal disease (e.g., minimal or mesangial lupus glomerulonephritis) tend to do well if treatment is directed toward control of the extrarenal manifestations of the disease. Glucocorticoids in modest doses, salicylates, or antimalarials are usually sufficient. Potent nonsteroidal, anti-inflammatory agents may cause functional depression of GFR and should be used with caution in patients with known renal involvement. Serologic parameters, including anti-dsDNA and complement components (C3, C4), should be followed serially. Fluorescent antinuclear antibody tests have little value in prognosis or in following the effectiveness of treatment. A return to normal values for antibody to dsDNA and/or complement components is a favorable sign; however, persistently abnormal serologic features do not necessarily indicate worsening or progressive renal involvement, especially in patients with active extrarenal manifestations. For patients with mild lesions, 85 percent or more can be expected to survive at least 10 years. Patients with membranous lupus glomerulonephritis uncomplicated by superimposed focal or diffuse proliferative lesions and who receive treatment directed primarily at the extrarenal features also have favorable long-term prognosis. On the other hand, patients with extensive focal or diffuse proliferative lupus glomerulonephritis or combined membranous and proliferative lesions do less well and, therefore, warrant a more aggressive approach toward ameliorating the renal disease. High-dose, long-term oral glucocorticoid therapy, although capable of improving extrarenal signs of active disease and reducing the acute inflammatory component of the renal lesions, is not an altogether satisfactory regimen for lupus nephritis. Such treatment is associated with a high prevalence of side effects and may not prevent progression of chronic lesions. High-dose, short-term intravenous methylprednisolone is effective in reducing signs of systemic and renal activity of the disease, especially in patients with recent deterioration. Adjunctive use of cytotoxic agents (azathioprine, cyclophosphamide, or chlorambucil) exerts a steroid-sparing effect and may prevent progression of chronic lesions, particularly among those with mild chronic lesions prior to therapy. The optimal regimen has not yet been established; however, intermittent intravenous cyclophosphamide (500 to 1000 mg/m^2 of surface area monthly for 6 to 12 months) plus low-dose oral prednisone (0.5 mg/kg of body weight per day) and combinations of azathioprine or cyclophosphamide with low-dose oral prednisone appear to be relatively safe and more effective than glucocorticoids alone in selected patients with severe proliferative lesions. Because prospective, randomized trials have involved only small numbers of patients, it is premature to adopt any particular regimen as the treatment of choice. Even combinations of azathioprine and low-dose prednisone may exert an overall beneficial effect in certain patients. Little is gained by using a combined steroid-cytotoxic approach in patients with advanced renal failure due to progressive glomerular capillary obliteration and sclerosis. These patients are best treated with dialysis and/or transplantation. Reports claiming efficacy of combined intensive plasma exchange and immunosuppressive therapy for severe glomerulonephritis have not been substantiated in a randomized, prospective trial. Such treatment therefore cannot be recommended for the *routine* management of patients with severe and progressive glomerular disease. However, anecdotal reports of dramatic recovery from extrarenal manifestations (e.g., central nervous system lupus) consequent to the use of intensive plasma exchange plus immunosuppression have appeared. Since, from time to time, patients with systemic lupus erythematosus may develop a syndrome closely resembling thrombotic thrombocytopenic purpura, the beneficial effect of intensive plasma exchange may be the consequence of an alteration in thrombotic microangiopathy rather than control of an active immunologically mediated process.

Serologic studies, especially serial measurements of antibody to dsDNA and complement components (C3, C4), may be useful in assessing patients under therapy. Return of these parameters to normal usually indicates satisfactory control of disease and that drug dosage can be safely diminished. These measurements also can be monitored to guide more aggressive therapy when appropriate. However, too heavy reliance on serologic parameters of activity should be discouraged. The correlation between clinical activity and serologic disturbances is poor, at least among patients receiving therapy with steroids and immunosuppressive agents.

Overall, long-term prognosis for patients with SLE and renal involvement has greatly improved. The degree to which changes in methods of diagnosis, serologic monitoring, or treatment are responsible is unknown. End-stage renal failure develops in 15 to 25 percent of patients with diffuse proliferative nephritis within 10 years of initiating therapy with aggressive regimens, such as low-dose alternate-day glucocorticoids combined with oral or intravenous cytotoxic agents. The degree of renal functional impairment and its response to therapy are the most powerful clinical predictors of outcome. Whether the information gleaned from renal biopsy adds to the prognosis is not clear. Cerebral involvement and infectious complications of therapy are now major causes of morbidity and mortality in SLE. Patients with SLE seem to do well on regular chronic dialysis; moreover, as uremia develops, some patients experience remissions of extrarenal activity. In transplanted patients, recurrence of SLE in the renal allograft is uncommon. Thus patients with SLE and nephritis are satisfactory candidates for both dialysis and transplantation.

GOODPASTURE'S SYNDROME The term *Goodpasture's syndrome* refers to the combination of alveolar hemorrhage and glomerular hemorrhage. Such clinical manifestations occur in a wide variety of disorders, including anti-basement membrane antibody–mediated nephritis (often referred to as *Goodpasture's disease*), systemic necrotizing vasculitis, microscopic polyarteritis, Wegener's granulomatosis, mixed essential cryoimmunoglobulinemia, Henoch-Schönlein purpura, and systemic lupus erythematosus. In addition, hemoptysis can occur with *Legionella* infection and interstitial nephritis, and renal vein thrombosis accompanying nephrotic syndrome can produce pulmonary emboli with infarction and hemoptysis. Thus two broad categories of this syndrome can be described: those in which production of an autoantibody to basement membrane antibodies can be documented (so-called Goodpasture's disease) and a heterogeneous group unassociated with anti-basement membrane antibody production. This section will deal with Goodpasture's disease as mediated by antibody to basement membrane antigens. The cause is unknown. Goodpasture's disease may appear at any age and typically affects young men. However, the frequency may be increasing in women.

Pulmonary hemorrhage may be covert and easily overlooked or severe and life-threatening. The initial manifestations of pulmonary involvement are cough, shortness of breath, and hemoptysis. Hilar pulmonary infiltrates may be seen by chest x-ray, and hypoxia is frequent. With marked intraalveolar hemorrhage, pulmonary carbon monoxide uptake is increased, and the pulmonary clearance of radioactive carbon monoxide is depressed. Pulmonary iron sequestration may be documented by scanning of the lungs with ^{59}Fe. Hemosiderin-laden macrophages may be seen in the sputum, but this is a nonspecific finding. Iron-deficiency anemia may result if pulmonary bleeding is prolonged and severe. A history of recent inhalation of volatile hydrocarbons or of viral influenza may be obtained. Cocaine inhalation also can provoke lung hemorrhage. Cigarette smoking increases the risk of alveolar bleeding in patients with anti-basement membrane antibody–mediated disease. Fever, arthralgias, and other systemic symptoms are mild or absent at the time of presentation. Other disorders in which renal disease is associated with pulmonary (alveolar) hemorrhage can ordinarily be differentiated from Goodpasture's disease by their extrarenal features and by typical serologic findings (see Table 241-1).

The glomeruli in Goodpasture's disease range from normal or nearly normal to focal proliferative and necrotizing glomerulonephritis; most often there is extensive extracapillary proliferation (crescents). Rapidly progressive renal failure is a common feature, although patients may initially have normal renal function and mild abnormalities in the urinary sediment. Immunofluorescence studies of renal biopsy material reveal the typical *linear deposits* of IgG (or rarely IgA) anti-basement membrane antibody, often but not necessarily always accompanied by C3 deposition. Electron-microscopic studies do not reveal electron-dense deposits.

Circulating antibody to glycopeptide antigens related to the noncollagenous domains on type IV (basement membrane) collagen are found in over 90 percent of cases if sera are examined early in the course by a sensitive immunoassay (see Table 241-1). The level of circulating antibody does not correlate well with the severity of the renal or pulmonary manifestations. Measurements of circulating antibody are of diagnostic value and have little or no prognostic significance. Serum complement components are nearly always normal, and circulating immune complexes and cryoimmunoglobulins are absent. On occasion, antineutrophil cytoplasmic autoantibodies may be found or develop subsequent to the initial diagnosis, often in association with systemic features of vasculitis. About 80 to 85 percent of patients are HLA-DR2 antigen–positive.

The course is variable. Patients surviving an initial bout of severe hemoptysis may undergo long-term remissions or may have repeated bouts of pulmonary hemorrhage. Mild forms of glomerular injury may not progress, and the principal clinical problems may be related to recurrent hemoptysis. The diagnosis in such patients may be confused with idiopathic pulmonary hemosiderosis. More commonly, the renal disease is progressive, sometimes fulminant, leading to oliguric renal failure in weeks or months (i.e., rapidly progressive glomerulonephritis).

Life-threatening pulmonary hemorrhage may respond temporarily to high doses of parenteral methylprednisolone (10 to 15 mg/kg of body weight) given over short periods. The effectiveness of such therapy in reversing extensive crescentic glomerular lesions is not established. Anticoagulants are contraindicated in the face of active pulmonary hemorrhage. Intensive plasma exchange in combination with cytotoxic drugs and modest doses of glucocorticoids has been associated with dramatic remissions of pulmonary hemorrhage and improvement of the glomerular lesions. This is particularly true if treatment is initiated early in patients with relatively acute disease in whom dialysis is not yet required for therapy of renal failure. The duration and frequency of plasma exchanges depend on the response of the patient and the changes in levels of circulating antibody to glomerular basement membrane antigens, but daily or every other day exchanges are recommended for the first week or two. Renal biopsy is helpful in guiding the management, but even in the presence of extensive crescent formation, responses may be satisfactory. If irreversible glomerular obliteration, extensive interstitial fibrosis, and tubular atrophy are found, especially in the oliguric patient requiring dialysis with long-standing disease, plasma exchange offers little hope for improving the renal lesion. Such patients are best managed by regular hemodialysis and/or transplantation. Although recurrences may develop, the diagnosis is not a contraindication to transplantation as long as the procedure is delayed until levels of circulating anti-basement membrane antibody decrease to undetectable levels. Long-term therapy is usually not required. Glucocorticoids and immunosuppressive agents may be withdrawn gradually after approximately 6 months of treatment with careful monitoring of clinical features and of anti-glomerular basement membrane and antineutrophil cytoplasmic autoantibody levels. Relapses are uncommon but may at times be due to the emergence of antineutrophil autoantibody–associated vasculitis. In patients with severe initial disease, persistent proteinuria and slowly progressive renal failure may ensue unrelated to anti-basement membrane antibody production (see below).

HENOCH-SCHÖNLEIN PURPURA (See also Chap. 315) This disorder is characterized by nonthrombocytopenic purpura, arthralgias, abdominal pain, and glomerulonephritis. Although usually a disease of children, typical disease may be seen in adults of any age. Renal involvement is common and is manifested chiefly by hematuria and proteinuria. In some instances, renal involvement is severe, leading to rapidly progressive glomerulonephritis or nephrotic syndrome. The onset of the disease may resemble acute postinfectious glomerulonephritis. Serum complement component levels are usually normal. Serum IgA levels are increased in about half the patients (see Table 241-1), and IgA rheumatoid factor, IgA-containing immune complexes, or IgA-fibronectin complexes can be detected in 50 to 80 percent. Renal biopsy reveals a spectrum of abnormalities. Mild diffuse mesangial cell proliferation and/or focal and segmental proliferative glomerulonephritis is most common when bouts of macroscopic hematuria and proteinuria are present. More severe and diffuse proliferative glomerulonephritis, sometimes accompanied by extracapillary proliferation (crescents), arises in patients with heavy proteinuria and/or rapidly diminishing GFR. Characteristically, immunofluorescence studies reveal mesangial and peripheral capillary granular deposits of IgA, IgG, C3, and fibrinogen but not C1q, C4, or IgA secretory piece. Similar immunofluorescence findings are present in the dermal capillaries of biopsies of involved and uninvolved skin. Electron microscopy reveals electron-dense deposits principally in the mesangium. These findings suggest that Henoch-Schönlein purpura is due to circulating IgA-containing immune complexes but that the nature of the antigen and the antibody reactivity of the IgA are unknown. Although food allergies and upper respiratory infections may be present, there is no clear-cut etiologic relationship. *Berger's disease* (IgA nephropathy, Chap. 240) may represent a monosymptomatic form of Henoch-Schönlein purpura.

The diagnosis is ordinarily not difficult when the typical clinical features are present. The differential diagnosis includes SLE, polyarteritis, infective endocarditis, postinfectious glomerulonephritis, and essential cryoimmunoglobulinemia.

The course is usually benign; however, progressive renal failure may occur. Renal biopsy is a useful prognostic tool. Patients with persistent urinary abnormalities may experience deterioration of renal function several years after diagnosis. Treatment is symptomatic. There is no convincing evidence that glucocorticoid or immunosuppressive therapy is beneficial for the renal lesion, although these treatments may ameliorate extrarenal features. Patients with rapidly progressive (crescentic) glomerulonephritis benefit from intensive plasma exchange combined with immunosuppressive drugs (see Chap. 240).

SYSTEMIC NECROTIZING VASCULITIS (See also Chap. 291) Glomerular involvement is common in the heterogeneous group of disorders that result from widespread inflammatory and necrotizing lesions of blood vessels. Several variations are recognized, including microscopic polyarteritis (hypersensitivity angiitis), macroscopic polyarteritis (periarteritis nodosa), Wegener's granulomatosis, allergic angiitis and granulomatosis (Churg-Strauss syndrome), rheumatoid vasculitis, temporal arteritis, and Takayasu's arteritis. Henoch-Schönlein purpura and SLE also can be considered examples of vasculitis. Many patients with glomerulonephritis accompanying systemic necrotizing vasculitis have characteristic extrarenal findings such as cutaneous palpable purpura, necrotizing skin lesions, pulmonary infiltrates, upper airway or sinus lesions, mononeuritis multiplex, fever, and wasting. Hypertension is frequent in polyarteritis nodosa but may be absent in hypersensitivity vasculitis and Wegener's granulomatosis. Necrotizing pulmonary infiltrates, upper airway disease, sinusitis, and otitis characterize the Wegener's granulomatosis variant. Laboratory findings, often nonspecific, include anemia, mild leukocytosis, eosinophilia, and markedly elevated erythrocyte sedimentation rate. Autoantibodies to cytoplasmic antigens present in polymorphonuclear leukocytes have been reported in a high percentage of patients with Wegener's granulomatosis and microscopic polyarteritis, as well as in some patients with polyarteritis nodosa and the Churg-Strauss syndrome. Because of the presence of these autoantibodies, many regard this latter disorder as a renal-limited form of microscopic polyarteritis. In addition, such autoantibodies also may coexist with anti-basement membrane autoantibodies (see "Goodpasture's syndrome" and Table 241-1). The detection of such autoantibodies is helpful in establishing the nature of the underlying disease in patients suspected of having vasculitis. Renal biopsies are a poor means of establishing the diagnosis, since they frequently reveal segmental or diffuse necrotizing glomerulonephritis with or without crescents in the absence of any extraglomerular vascular involvement. Lung biopsies more frequently reveal the typical granulomatous necrotizing vasculitis characteristic of Wegener's granulomatosis. Sural nerve biopsies may be useful in establishing the diagnosis of vasculitis in patients presenting with mononeuritis multiplex.

The prognosis is generally poor for patients with systemic necrotizing vasculitis, especially in the absence of treatment; however, aggressive management with glucocorticoids combined with oral cyclophosphamide has been associated with improvement in overall prognosis. Among the antineutrophil cytoplasmic autoantibody–positive subset of patients with vasculitis, a relapse may be predicted by rising titer or reappearance of autoantibody. Some patients with fulminant glomerulonephritis secondary to systemic necrotizing vasculitis in which severe glomerular involvement is accompanied by extensive crescent formation and rapidly progressive dialysis-dependent renal failure may benefit from combined therapy involving plasma exchange, glucocorticoids, and intravenous or oral cyclophosphamide. The long-term prognosis for such patients remains uncertain, since extrarenal involvement and/or complications of immunosuppressive treatment may ultimately be fatal. Late-onset renal failure associated with hypertension and persistent proteinuria may be due to nonimmune

processes and can be ameliorated with aggressive angiotensin converting enzyme inhibitor therapy.

MISCELLANEOUS IMMUNOLOGICALLY MEDIATED MULTISYSTEM DISEASES   Mixed connective tissue disease (MCTD) In this disorder (see also Chap. 287) renal disease is uncommon and, if present, mild. Clinical manifestations include hematuria and proteinuria and occasionally nephrotic syndrome. Pathologically, membranous or membranoproliferative glomerulonephritis is seen. The prognosis is generally favorable. Glucocorticoid therapy often results in improvement of the glomerular lesions.

Rheumatoid arthritis Several forms of glomerular injury may occur in rheumatoid arthritis (Chap. 285). Secondary amyloidosis is present in 5 to 10 percent of patients with long-standing arthritis. Nephrotic syndrome may arise as a complication of either gold or penicillamine therapy (see Chap. 240). In addition, the kidney may share in the vasculitis seen occasionally in severe rheumatoid arthritis. Finally, patients with rheumatoid arthritis (untreated with gold or penicillamine) may develop a mild proliferative or membranous glomerulonephritis which resembles lesions seen in SLE. Proteinuria, sometimes with nephrotic syndrome, is the principal clinical feature of such lesions. Prolonged and excessive use of analgesics may lead to renal papillary necrosis.

Other disorders *Sjögren's syndrome* (Chap. 288) may be associated with nephrotic syndrome due to membranous or membranoproliferative glomerulonephritis (type I) or, more frequently, interstitial nephritis. *Sarcoidosis* is rarely complicated by membranous glomerulonephritis. *Partial or total lipodystrophy* may be associated with membranoproliferative glomerulonephritis (type II, dense deposit disease) (see Chap. 240). Complement abnormalities consist of depressed C3 levels, normal C1q and C4 levels, and circulating C3 nephritic factor.

Chronic liver disease may be complicated by glomerular disease. The nephrotic syndrome may appear in the course of *chronic active hepatitis* associated with persistent hepatitis B surface antigenemia (see below). Glomerular lesions include membranous membranoproliferative (type I) glomerulonephritis. Immunofluorescence studies in such patients reveal granular deposits of immunoglobulins, complement components, and hepatitis B viral antigens, indicating an immune-complex disease. Serum C3 levels are often reduced, and tests for circulating immune complexes and cryoimmunoglobulins are frequently positive. Occasionally, patients with little clinical evidence of liver disease develop distinct glomerular lesions secondary to chronic hepatitis B infection. *Acute viral hepatitis* may be associated with transient hematuria or proteinuria and may resemble other postinfectious glomerulonephritides (see Chap. 240). Severe *chronic liver disease* (cirrhosis) may be associated with diffuse glomerulosclerosis. Few clinical manifestations of glomerular disease are found. Prominent mesangial IgA deposits, of unknown pathogenic significance, have been noted in patients with cirrhosis.

MULTISYSTEM DISEASES ASSOCIATED WITH PARAPROTEINEMIA AND NEOPLASIA

ESSENTIAL (MIXED) CRYOIMMUNOGLOBULINEMIA This disorder is associated with circulating cold-precipitable immunoglobulins (cryoimmunoglobulins), usually consisting of polyclonal IgG and monoclonal IgM; the latter possesses rheumatoid factor activity. Purpura, necrotizing skin lesions in cold-exposed areas, arthralgias, fever, and hepatosplenomegaly are common. Hepatitis B infection and other occult fungal, bacterial, or viral infections may be found to underlie this syndrome. Circulating cryoimmunoglobulins are also found in chronic infections and probably represent circulating immune complexes with unusual physical properties. Glomerular disease results from the precipitation of the polyclonal cryoimmunoglobulin in the glomerular capillaries and may result in acute renal failure, rapidly progressive (crescentic) glomerulonephritis, or the nephrotic syndrome. Serum complement, particularly the C4, components are depressed (see Table 241-1). Pathologically, a diffuse proliferative glomerulonephritis with extensive monocyte infiltration is seen with findings consistent with the deposition of the circulating cryoimmunoglobulin. Eradication of the underlying infection, if possible, is of value in treatment. Intermittent intravenous ''pulses'' of methylprednisolone and intensive plasma exchange, accompanied by the administration of oral glucocorticoids and cytotoxic agents, have been of some value in severe cases.

MONOCLONAL GAMMOPATHIES *Multiple myeloma* (Chap. 280) may be associated with several types of glomerular injury. Amyloidosis (Chap. 281) (see below) occurs in 10 to 15 percent of patients with multiple myeloma. Lesions resembling those in cryoimmunoglobulinemia also may develop. Proteinuria and the nephrotic syndrome are common. In addition, a tubulointerstitial lesion (myeloma kidney) consisting of large, laminated intratubular casts, tubule cell atrophy, interstitial fibrosis, and inflammation is common in patients with multiple myeloma and acute or chronic renal failure. *Light chain nephropathy* is characterized by deposits of monoclonal Ig light chains (usually the kappa chain) along the glomerular and tubular basement membranes and by lesions resembling nodular diabetic glomerulosclerosis. The urine typically contains large amounts of the monoclonal light chains, but serum electrophoresis may reveal only hypogammaglobulinemia. Treatment with glucocorticoids and alkylating agents may be beneficial. *Waldenström's macroglobulinemia* may cause acute renal failure when the IgM paraprotein precipitates in glomerular capillaries as ''thrombi.'' Intensive plasma exchange and therapy with alkylating agents may be beneficial. Hyperviscosity may cause functional alterations in GFR. Renal amyloidosis is uncommon. *Benign monoclonal gammopathies* are seldom associated with glomerular complications, except for mild asymptomatic proteinuria and, rarely, nephrotic syndrome.

AMYLOIDOSIS (See also Chap. 281) This disorder may occur in the absence of systemic disease (primary amyloidosis), may be secondary to chronic inflammatory processes (e.g., rheumatoid arthritis, osteomyelitis, paraplegia), multiple myeloma, or other neoplastic diseases, or may occur in a hereditary form (e.g., in association with familial Mediterranean fever). All forms may affect the glomeruli.

Primary amyloidosis commonly affects the kidneys and usually occurs in older age groups. Proteinuria, often of nephrotic proportions, is the most common manifestation of renal involvement. The urine sediment tends to be benign. The degree of proteinuria is not necessarily related to the extent of glomerular deposition of amyloid. Enlarged kidneys may be present in patients with well-preserved renal function, but this is a nonspecific finding. The blood pressure is normal unless advanced uremia is present. Typical pathologic features include hypocellular glomeruli infiltrated with amorphous deposits that stain with Congo red and exhibit green birefringence under polarized light. The fibrillar nature of the amyloid deposits can be readily demonstrated by electron microscopy. Immunofluorescence studies reveal amorphous deposits of immunoglobulin and/or monoclonal light chains and complement in glomeruli. Similar findings also may occur in another disorder discussed in Chap. 240, fibrillary or immunotactoid glomerulonephritis. In the latter disorder, the deposits are Congo red–negative, and the fibrils are larger. Renal vein thrombosis may complicate the course of amyloidosis.

Renal amyloidosis is a progressive disease for which there is no established treatment. Remissions may occur in secondary amyloidosis if the cause can be eliminated. Remissions in primary amyloidosis are exceedingly rare; a few reports describe remissions following the use of combinations of melphalan and glucocorticoids. Colchicine is of value in prevention of amyloidosis in familial Mediterranean fever. Overall, the 5-year survival for patients with primary amyloidosis is less than 20 percent. Azotemia, persistent nephrotic syndrome, and myocardial involvement confer an even more ominous prognosis.

NEOPLASTIC DISEASE Glomerular alterations may develop with a variety of neoplastic diseases. *Carcinomas*, especially adenocarcinoma of lung, colon, stomach, and breast, may be accompanied by glomerular lesions resembling idiopathic membranous glomerulonephritis, although, on occasion, minimal change lesions, crescentic or focal and segmental proliferative glomerulonephritis, or even amyloidosis may be present. Nephrotic syndrome is the most common clinical renal manifestation, and approximately 5 to 10 percent of patients with idiopathic nephrotic syndrome associated with membranous glomerulonephritis harbor an underlying malignancy. However, among patients over age 60 at diagnosis of membranous glomerulonephritis, as many as 20 percent may have underlying neoplastic disease. Successful treatment of the tumor, especially by surgical means, may lead to remission of the renal manifestation. Presumably the glomerular lesions arise because of the deposition of circulating immune complexes that are composed of tumor antigen and antitumor antibody.

Lymphomas and leukemias also may give rise to glomerular abnormalities. Hodgkin's disease is associated with the findings of idiopathic nephrotic syndrome (minimal change disease). Other glomerular lesions may include membranous glomerulonephritis, focal proliferative and sclerosing glomerulonephritis, and amyloidosis. The mechanism of the association of Hodgkin's disease with minimal change disease may involve an underlying T cell abnormality. Proteinuria may wax and wane with fluctuations in the clinical activity of the Hodgkin's disease. Remissions may be produced by local irradiation of involved lymph nodes or by systemic chemotherapy.

METABOLIC, BIOCHEMICAL, AND HEREDITARY DISORDERS

DIABETIC NEPHROPATHY (See also Chap. 337) Diabetes mellitus affects the structure and function of the kidney in many ways. The term *diabetic nephropathy* encompasses all the lesions occurring in the kidneys of patients with diabetes mellitus. These lesions include *glomerulosclerosis* (diffuse or nodular), *arterionephrosclerosis, chronic interstitial nephritis, papillary necrosis,* and various tubular lesions. Diabetic nephropathy is associated with a variety of clinical syndromes, including mild asymptomatic proteinuria, nephrotic syndrome, progressive renal failure (acute, rapidly progressive, or chronic), and hypertension. Glomerular lesions are particularly common and account for the majority of abnormal clinical findings referable to the kidney. *Diffuse diabetic glomerulosclerosis* (diffuse intercapillary glomerulosclerosis) is the most common lesion and can be identified in the vast majority of diabetic patients regardless of the presence of abnormal clinical findings referable to the kidney. This lesion consists of a diffuse increase in the volume of mesangial matrix accompanied by an increased width of the glomerular basement membrane. Various exudative lesions, such as capsular drops and fibrin caps, also may be present. Hyaline arteriosclerosis, particularly of the efferent arteriole, is also common. Taken together, these lesions suggest the diagnosis of diabetes mellitus, but individually they are not specific. *Nodular glomerulosclerosis* (Kimmelstiel-Wilson lesion), on the other hand, is reasonably specific for diabetes mellitus. This lesion consists of PAS-positive, laminated, intercapillary nodules on a background of an increase in mesangial matrix. At the periphery of the nodules, open glomerular capillary loops are found. The nodules are relatively acellular, in contrast to the cellular lesions of membranoproliferative glomerulonephritis. As noted above, *light chain nephropathy* may evoke a similar lesion. The pathogenesis of diffuse or nodular diabetic glomerulosclerosis is poorly understood but involves the deleterious effect of the diabetic milieu on matrix biosynthesis and turnover and hemodynamic alterations of the glomerular circulation.

The principal clinical manifestation of diabetic glomerular disease is proteinuria. Initially, only small amounts of albumin (15 to 40 μg/min) are excreted, particularly following exercise (microalbuminuria). This amount of albumin excretion is undetectable by routine screening methods. Under ordinary circumstances, microalbuminuria develops within 10 to 15 years of the onset of hyperglycemia and usually progresses within 3 to 7 years to overt proteinuria and clinical diabetic nephropathy. With "tight" control of hyperglycemia and/or rigorous control of elevated blood pressure, the development of microalbuminuria may be prevented or reversed. With time, the quantity of protein excreted usually increases and may progress to an overt nephrotic syndrome. Glomerular filtration rate is initially elevated and subsequently falls toward normal coincident with the onset of overt proteinuria. The urinary sediment is typically benign, although microhematuria and/or pyuria also may be present if a complicating urinary tract infection or papillary necrosis is present. Hypertension develops as microalbuminuria appears and as GFR falls from supernormal levels but is seldom of malignant proportions. When hypertension is severe or abrupt in onset, one should suspect a complicating atherosclerotic renal arterial stenosis. Typically, plasma renin activity is normal or decreased. Acquired hyporeninemic hypoaldosteronism with persistent hyperkalemia and mild hyperchloremic metabolic acidosis is common. Once azotemia develops, the disease progresses at variable rates, but GFR declines, on average, about 10 to 15 mL/min per year. End-stage renal failure usually develops within 5 to 7 years of the onset of overt proteinuria and clinical nephropathy depending on therapeutic intervention and compliance. Despite poor control of hyperglycemia, only about 50 to 60 percent of insulin-dependent diabetic patients develop clinical nephropathy. The factors that protect the remaining patients from renal failure are unknown but seem to be related to the propensity for the development of hypertension. Patients with non-insulin-dependent diabetes mellitus also may develop clinical nephropathy.

Until the cause of diabetes mellitus is established, prevention of the glomerulopathy will not be feasible. If the abnormal diabetic milieu is responsible for the vascular complications (including glomerular disease), as some have suggested, then very precise regulation of blood sugar (e.g., meticulous attention to diet, exercise, and insulin dosage and servofeedback devices for insulin administration) may be effective in reducing the development of nephropathy. During the microalbuminuric phase, tight metabolic control slows the rate of increase in albumin excretion, as does lowering the arterial blood pressure and dietary protein restriction. Once the nephropathy has reached the stage of overt proteinuria, aggressive management of hypertension will slow the rate of loss of renal function, but strict control of blood sugar does not seem to retard the rate of progression once overt nephropathy (proteinuria >500 mg/d) has emerged. Patients with end-stage renal failure due to diabetic nephropathy are not ideal candidates for long-term dialysis because of concomitant multiple organ dysfunction secondary to widespread arteriovascular disease. Mortality rates among diabetics on chronic dialysis are about three times higher than among similarly treated nondiabetics of comparable age. Renal transplantation may be successful in the younger diabetic, especially if a living related donor is available. The overall success rate is somewhat less than in the nondiabetic population owing to the adverse effects of extrarenal vascular involvement (e.g., coronary artery disease), but transplantation is a viable alternative to dialysis in selected patients. Recurrence of typical diabetic glomerular lesions has been documented in renal allografts, but thus far, progressive loss of GFR secondary to recurrent disease seems to be uncommon.

ALPORT'S SYNDROME   This disorder consists of sensorineural deafness associated with hereditary nephritis. Renal disease manifests itself at an early age, principally as recurrent hematuria. Men are more frequently and more severely affected than women. Slowly progressive renal insufficiency in men commonly terminates in end-stage renal disease in the second to third decade. There is no clear-cut relationship between the onset or severity of the hearing abnormality and the extent of renal disease. Other associated abnormalities include two related ophthalmologic complications, spherophakia and lenticonus, as well as thrombopenia, hyperprolinemia, and

cerebral dysfunction. Family studies have indicated autosomal dominant or X-linked modes of inheritance with variable expressivity. The pathogenesis may be due to defective synthesis of components of glomerular and tubular basement membranes. The gene responsible for the X-linked variety has been mapped to a particular site on the X chromosome (Xq21.2–q22.1) and appears to encode for the synthesis of a unique chain (alpha 5) in type IV collagen.

The pathologic features detected by light microscopy are nonspecific, and a diagnosis cannot be established by optical microscopy alone. Both glomerular and interstitial lesions are present. Focal and diffuse glomerular proliferation, with segmental sclerosis, is common. Interstitial foam cells are nonspecific findings. Electron microscopy reveals thinning, splitting, and delamination of both glomerular and tubular basement membranes, thought by some to be specific for the syndrome. Immunofluorescence studies fail to reveal deposits of immunoglobulins or complement components. The autoantibody to basement membrane antigens found in patients with Goodpasture's disease does not react with the glomeruli of some patients with Alport's syndrome. Treatment is supportive; glucocorticoids and cytotoxic agents are ineffective. The disease is not known to recur following transplantation. (See also Chap. 351).

FABRY'S DISEASE (See also Chap. 349)   This disorder, angiokeratoma corporus diffusum, is an X-linked inborn error of glycosphingolipid metabolism that leads to the accumulation of neutral glycosphingolipids in many tissues including the kidney. A milder disease may develop in heterozygous females. Manifestations are more frequent in hemizygous males and include angiokeratomas involving the lower trunk, scrotum, and buttocks; acroparesthesia; corneal opacities; tortuous retinal veins; and premature coronary and cerebral ischemic disease. Renal manifestations include hematuria and modest proteinuria, often associated with slowly progressive renal failure. Light-microscopic findings include foamy alterations of the epithelial cells of the glomerulus due to the accumulation of lipid. Electron microscopy reveals intracellular rounded laminated bodies ("myelin figures"). The disorder is untreatable unless replacement of the deficient enzyme can be ensured; successful renal transplantation may partially correct the enzyme deficiency.

NAIL-PATELLA SYNDROME   This autosomal dominant disease is characterized by dystrophic nails, absence of one or both patellae, iliac horns, and renal disease. The renal manifestations include isolated proteinuria and hematuria and occasionally the nephrotic syndrome. Progressive renal failure is uncommon. Glomerular lesions are nonspecific by light microscopy, but electron microscopy reveals a characteristic moth-eaten appearance of the glomerular basement membrane associated with intramembranous collagen fibrils. The prognosis is generally favorable. No treatment is known.

CONGENITAL NEPHROTIC SYNDROME   This autosomal recessive trait is characterized by the development of nephrotic syndrome at the time of or shortly after birth. It occurs with highest frequency in families of Finnish origin. Affected individuals have very large placentas, low birth weight, anasarca, polycythemia, and initially normal GFRs. Levels of alpha fetoprotein are increased in amniotic fluid and maternal serum. Proteinuria is marked and nonselective. Nephrotic syndrome appearing several months after birth is usually due to other causes, especially minimal change disease or focal glomerular sclerosis (Chap. 240). Congenital syphilis and congenital toxoplasmosis may produce similar syndromes and must be excluded. Pathologically, microcystic transformation of the cortical nephrons results from proximal tubular dilatation. Glomerular changes are nonspecific. The anionic charge density on glomerular basement membrane is reduced. Extensive effacement of the foot processes and sclerosis of the glomerular tufts are seen by electron microscopy. Immunofluorescence findings are nonspecific. The course is progressive, and few patients survive the first year of life. Treatment is ineffective. Death is usually due to inanition, infection, or renal failure. A few patients may survive long enough to be considered for renal transplantation.

SICKLE CELL DISEASE (See also Chap. 306) This disorder is an autosomal trait characterized by an abnormal hemoglobin (hemoglobin S). Glomerular lesions occur occasionally in homozygous disease. The medulla is affected, leading to impairment of concentrating ability and potassium and acid excretion and, occasionally, to papillary necrosis. Rarely, patients develop mainly glomerular lesions, either membranous or membranoproliferative glomerulonephritis, accompanied by proteinuria and a nephrotic syndrome. Immunofluorescence studies demonstrate glomerular deposition of immunoglobulin and complement in a granular pattern suggesting immune-complex–mediated disease. The course in patients with the glomerulopathy of sickle cell disease is often relentless, leading to end-stage renal disease. No treatment is known to be effective. Transplantation is occasionally successful.

LECITHIN:CHOLESTEROL ACYLTRANSFERASE DEFICIENCY (See also Chap. 344) This autosomal recessive trait leads to absence of the enzyme in plasma that catalyzes the conversion of lecithin and cholesterol to lysolecithin and cholesteryl ester. Multiple lipoprotein abnormalities develop, including absence of α and pre-β lipoproteins, hypertriglyceridemia, accumulation of abnormal lipoproteins, and increased plasma-esterified cholesterol. Corneal opacities, anemia, hyperuricemia, proteinuria, and progressive renal failure are characteristic. Foam cells are present in bone marrow and glomeruli, and a picture resembling focal and segmental glomerulosclerosis may evolve. Treatment is generally ineffective, but plasma or blood transfusions may transiently correct the disorder. Renal failure has been corrected by renal transplantation, but recurrence of disease in allografts may occur.

VON GIERKE'S DISEASE (See also Chap. 350) Glycogen storage disease secondary to glucose-6-phosphatase deficiency (Von Gierke's disease) causes renal manifestations. Patients with this autosomal recessive disorder are of short stature and have poorly developed skeletal muscles. Hypoglycemia may precipitate convulsions in childhood. The kidneys are enlarged, and a Fanconi-like syndrome with aminoaciduria, glycosuria, and phosphaturia may be present. Renal insufficiency is associated with moderate proteinuria and with focal and segmental glomulerulosclerosis. Hyperuricemia may cause gout. The kidneys and liver are uniformly enlarged.

DRUG-INDUCED GLOMERULAR DISEASE Many drugs have been associated with the development of glomerular disease; however, it is usually difficult to establish a direct cause and effect relationship. In a few situations the association is clear-cut, and reexposure has led to recurrence of disease. A partial listing of these drugs is provided in Table 241-2. Certain *heavy metals* (Hg, Au) and their inorganic salts or organic compounds may produce membranous glomerulonephritis and nephrotic syndrome. Removal of the drug is not invariably associated with resolution. *Sulfhydryl compounds* (penicillamine, captopril) also may cause membranous or proliferative glomerulonephritis. The risk of developing a renal complication following

penicillamine or gold therapy for rheumatoid arthritis is influenced by genes in the major histocompatibility complex. *Nonsteroidal anti-inflammatory agents* may produce nephrotic syndrome (minimal change disease), interstitial nephritis, and acute renal failure. *Probenecid, trimethadione*, or *paramethadione* may be associated with nephrotic syndrome and a variety of glomerular lesions, including minimal change disease and membranous glomerulonephritis. *Heroin* abuse may be associated with focal and segmental glomerulosclerosis that may progress to nephrotic syndrome and progressive renal failure. *Intravenous amphetamine abuse* may be associated with systemic necrotizing vasculitis. Chronic hepatitis B infection may be involved in the development of glomerular lesions in association with intravenous drug abuse. Allopurinol, hydralazine, and rifampin may cause vasculitis and/or crescentic glomerulonephritis.

INFECTION-RELATED GLOMERULAR DISEASES

As discussed in Chap. 240, a wide variety of infectious agents have been implicated in glomerular diseases, and a similarly broad array of clinical features and morphologic patterns of glomerular injury can complicate infectious disease. Acute glomerulonephritis, particularly that due to beta-hemolytic streptococcal infection is dealt with in detail in Chap. 240. *Infective endocarditis, visceral sepsis, salmonellosis, pneumococcal pneumonia, meningococcemia*, and *gonococcemia* have all been associated from time to time with glomerulonephritis, most typically a proliferative lesion associated with features of the acute nephritic syndrome. *Syphilis*, both congenital and secondary, may evoke the nephrotic syndrome with a proliferative or membranous lesion. Parasitic diseases such as *malaria, toxoplasmosis, schistosomiasis*, and *filariasis* also may produce proteinuria of the nephrotic syndrome or a picture resembling acute glomerulonephritis. Many acute viral diseases, including *hepatitis B, Epstein-Barr, measles*, and *varicella* infections, also may be associated with a transient glomerulonephritis. On the other hand, chronic viral diseases, such as *hepatitis B* and *human immunodeficiency virus* (HIV) infections, may evoke heavy proteinuria and nephrotic syndrome accompanied by progressive renal failure. Hepatitis B infection is most often associated with membranous glomerulonephritis. Serologic markers of chronic infection such as persistent hepatitis B surface or e antigen are present. Low C3 levels and cryoimmunoglobulins also may be present. Features of liver disease may be minimal. The long-term prognosis is poor. Glucocorticoids may worsen liver disease. Therapy with recombinant interferon-α and low doses of glucocorticoids may be beneficial. HIV infection seems to evoke a particular pattern of glomerular disease, most often in black men (see Chap. 279). Focal glomerulosclerosis, tubulointerstitial nephritis, microcystic changes in tubules, giant casts, and intracytoplasmic inclusions are commonly observed. Heavy proteinuria is associated with progressive renal failure. Kidney size is usually normal or increased. The renal lesion may be more severe than other manifestations of HIV infection. Therapy is usually ineffective, but treatment of the infection with antimetabolities, such as zidovudine or related agents, may retard the rate of progression of disease. Remissions are rare, and rapid development of end-stage renal failure is the rule.

TABLE 241-2 Drugs associated with glomerular lesions

Elemental, inorganic, or organic mercury compounds
Organic gold compounds
Penicillamine
Captopril
Heroin
Amphetamines
Probenecid
Oxazoladinedione derivatives (e.g., trimethadione)
Antivenoms and antitoxins
Sulfonamides
Vaccinations
Allopurinol
Hydralazine
Rifampin
Nonsteroidal anti-inflammatory agents

REFERENCES

ATKINS CL et al: Alport syndrome, in *Disease of the Kidney*, 4th ed, RW Schrier, CW Gottschalk (eds). Boston, Little, Brown, 1988, pp 617–641

AUSTIN HA et al: Therapy of lupus nephritis: Controlled trial of prednisone and cytotoxic drugs. N Engl J Med 314:1004, 1989

GLASSOCK RJ et al: Secondary glomerular diseases, in *The Kidney*, 4th ed, BM Brenner, FC Rector Jr (eds). Philadelphia, Saunders, 1991, pp 1280–1368

SAVAGE COS et al: Microscopic polyarteritis: Presentation, pathology and prognosis. Q J Med 56:467, 1985

242 TUBULOINTERSTITIAL DISEASES OF THE KIDNEY

THOMAS H. HOSTETTER / BARRY M. BRENNER

An etiologically diverse group of renal diseases can be distinguished from those considered in Chaps. 240 and 241 because the histologic and functional abnormalities involve the tubules and interstitium to a greater degree than the glomeruli and renal vasculature (see Table 242-1). Both clinically and histologically, these disorders can be divided into acute and chronic forms. The chronic group may be due to sustained insults by a factor or factors that initially cause acute disease or to a slower, progressive, cumulative insult without an identifiable acute episode. Morphologically, acute forms of these disorders are characterized by interstitial edema, often associated with cortical and medullary infiltration by polymorphonuclear leukocytes

and patchy areas of tubule cell necrosis. In more chronic forms, interstitial fibrosis predominates, inflammatory cells are typically mononuclear, and abnormalities of the tubules tend to be more widespread, as evidenced by atrophy, luminal dilatation, and thickening of tubule basement membranes. In the past, the diagnosis of chronic pyelonephritis (see Chap. 90) was almost universally applied when these chronic tubulointerstitial abnormalities were found. It is now apparent that only a small proportion of these lesions result from infection. Nonbacterial factors, including exogenous toxins and metabolic and immunologic derangements, constitute the major pathogenic mechanisms. Because of the nonspecific nature of the histology, particularly in chronic tubulointerstitial diseases, biopsy specimens rarely provide a specific diagnosis. The urine sediment is also unlikely to be diagnostic, except in allergic forms of acute tubulointerstitial disease, in which eosinophils may predominate in the urinary sediment.

Defects in renal function often accompany these alterations of tubule and interstitial structure (see Table 242-2). Proximal tubule dysfunction may be manifested as selective reabsorptive defects leading to hypokalemia, aminoaciduria, glycosuria, phosphaturia, uricosuria, or bicarbonaturia (proximal or type II renal tubular acidosis; see Chap. 244). In combination, these defects constitute the *Fanconi syndrome*. Protein excretion is usually modest, rarely exceeding 2 g/d. The excreted proteins are typically of low molecular weight and include beta$_2$ microglobulin, lysozyme, and immunoglobulin light chains. Defective proximal tubule reabsorption of these readily filtered small proteins accounts for their augmented excretion. Tubule sodium reabsorption also may be deranged in patients with advanced tubulointerstitial diseases, predisposing to salt wasting and hypovolemia. One or more of these reabsorptive defects are commonly encountered with heavy metal poisoning, multiple myeloma, and other diffuse tubulointerstitial processes.

Defects in urinary acidification and concentrating ability often represent the most troublesome of the tubule dysfunctions encountered in patients with tubulointerstitial disease. Hyperchloremic metabolic acidosis often develops at a relatively early stage in the course. Patients with this finding generally elaborate urine of maximal acidity (pH of 5.3 or less). In such patients the defect in acid excretion is usually caused by a reduced capacity to generate and excrete ammonia due to the reduction in renal mass. Preferential damage to the collecting ducts, as in amyloidosis or chronic obstructive uropathy, also may predispose to distal or type I renal tubular acidosis, characterized by high urine pH (>5.5) during spontaneous or NH_4Cl-induced metabolic acidosis. Patients with tubulointerstitial diseases affecting medullary and papillary structures predominantly also may evidence concentrating defects, with resultant nocturia and polyuria.

TABLE 242-1 Principal causes of tubulointerstitial disease of the kidney

TOXINS

Exogenous toxins
  Analgesic nephropathy*
  Lead nephropathy (see Chap. 396)
  Miscellaneous nephrotoxins (e.g., antibiotics, cyclosporine, radiographic contrast media, heavy metals)*†
Metabolic toxins
  Acute uric acid nephropathy (see Chap. 347)
  Gouty nephropathy (see Chap. 347)*
  Hypercalcemic nephropathy (see Chap. 357)
  Hypokalemic nephropathy (see Chap. 45)
  Miscellaneous metabolic toxins (e.g., hyperoxaluria, cystinosis, Fabry's disease)

NEOPLASIA

Lymphoma (see Chap. 34)
Leukemia (see Chap. 310)
Multiple myeloma (see Chap. 280)*

IMMUNE DISORDERS

Hypersensitivity nephropathy*†
Sjögren's syndrome (see Chap. 288)
Amyloidosis (see Chap. 281)
Transplant rejection (see Chap. 238)†
Tubulointerstitial abnormalities associated with glomerulonephritis (see Chaps. 240 and 241)
AIDS (see Chap. 279)

VASCULAR DISORDERS (see Chaps. 236 and 243)

Arteriolar nephrosclerosis*
Atheroembolic disease
Sickle cell nephropathy
Acute tubular necrosis*†

HEREDITARY RENAL DISEASES

Hereditary nephritis (Alport's syndrome) (see Chaps. 241 and 351)
Medullary cystic disease (see Chap. 244)
Medullary sponge kidney (see Chap. 244)
Polycystic kidney disease (see Chap. 244)

INFECTIOUS INJURY (see Chap. 90)

Acute pyelonephritis*†
Chronic pyelonephritis

MISCELLANEOUS DISORDERS

Chronic urinary tract obstruction (see Chap. 246)*
Vesicoureteral reflux*
Radiation nephritis

* Common.
† Typically acute.

TABLE 242-2 Transport dysfunctions of tubulointerstitial disease

Defect	Cause(s)
Reduced GFR*	Obliteration of vasculature and obstruction of tubules
Fanconi syndrome or competent defects	Damage to proximal tubular reabsorption of glucose, amino acids, phosphate, and bicarbonate
Hyperchloremic acidosis*	1. Reduced ammonia production 2. Inability to acidify the collecting duct fluid (distal renal tubular acidosis) 3. Proximal bicarbonate wasting
Tubular or small-molecular-weight proteinuria*	Failure of proximal tubule protein reabsorption
Polyuria, isothenuria*	Damage to medullary tubules and vasculature
Hyperkalemia*	Potassium secretory defects including aldosterone resistance
Salt wasting	Distal tubular damage with failure of sodium reabsorption

* Common

The impairment in maximal concentration is typically unresponsive to the administration of vasopressin and hence is a form of nephrogenic diabetes insipidus. Analgesic nephropathy and sickle cell disease are prototypes of this form of injury.

Although the major structural defects originate in the tubules and interstitium, progressive reduction in glomerular filtration rate (GFR) is a functional accompaniment of most, if not all, forms of tubulointerstitial damage, reflecting secondary injury to glomeruli and other elements of the renal microcirculation. Indeed, oliguric acute renal failure may be caused by acute forms of tubulointerstitial disease, and about a third of patients with chronic renal insufficiency suffer from a primary chronic tubulointerstitial disease.

TOXINS

The renal tubules and interstitium are prone to toxic injury. Although the kidneys constitute less than 1 percent of total body mass, they receive approximately 20 percent of the cardiac output, and 90 percent or more of renal blood flow is distributed to the renal cortex. Exposure of tubules and interstitium of the renal cortex to circulating toxins is therefore greater than is that of most other tissues. Transport processes in renal tubules contribute further to the intrarenal accumulation of toxins, enhancing local concentrations of noxious agents. The urinary concentrating mechanism also can establish high levels of toxins within medullary and papillary portions of the kidney, predisposing these regions to chemical injury. Finally, the relatively acid pH of the fluid within most nephron segments may affect the ionization characteristics of potentially toxic compounds and thereby influence local concentration and solubility. Although these processes render the kidney vulnerable to toxic injury, the role of nephrotoxins in renal damage often goes unrecognized because the manifestations of such injury are usually nonspecific in nature and insidious in onset. Diagnosis largely depends on a history of exposure to a certain toxin, a difficult matter because exposure may be occult. Particular attention should be paid to the occupational history, as well as to an assessment of exposure—current and remote—to drugs, especially antibiotics and analgesics. The recognition of a potential association between a patient's renal disease and exposure to a nephrotoxin is crucial, because, unlike many other forms of renal disease, progression of the functional and morphologic abnormalities associated with toxin-induced nephropathies may be prevented, and even reversed, by eliminating additional exposure.

EXOGENOUS TOXINS Analgesic nephropathy Individuals who ingest large quantities of analgesic drugs are prone to develop tubulointerstitial damage and papillary necrosis. Indeed, in Australia, Switzerland, and Sweden, analgesic abuse is one of the most common causes of chronic renal failure, and it is an important cause in the United States as well. While aspirin, phenacetin, and acetaminophen (the metabolite of phenacetin) may alone or in combination induce chronic renal disease, epidemiologic studies incriminate phenacetin and acetaminophen as the more injurious combination. Chronic ingestion of aspirin without these other compounds seems to be an uncommon cause of serious renal damage.

Morphologically, analgesic nephropathy is characterized by papillary necrosis and tubulointerstitial inflammation. At an early stage, damage to the vascular supply of the inner medulla (vasa recta) leads to a local interstitial inflammatory reaction and, eventually, to papillary ischemia, necrosis, fibrosis, and calcification. Destruction of papillae usually precedes extension of the tubulointerstitial abnormalities to the renal cortex and, therefore, occurs before renal size and GFR are reduced significantly. Although papillary necrosis is a common finding in patients with the nephropathy of analgesic abuse, necrosis of papillae also may occur in patients with chronic pyelonephritis, diabetes mellitus, sickle cell disease, and obstructive uropathy. The susceptibility of the renal papillae to damage by phenacetin is believed to be related to the establishment of a renal gradient for its acetominophen metabolite, resulting in papillary tip

concentrations tenfold higher than those in renal cortex. Hydration dissipates this gradient and may explain the protective effect of this maneuver in preventing phenacetin-induced papillary necrosis in animals. Aspirin in these analgesic compounds contributes to renal injury by uncoupling oxidative phosphorylation in renal mitochondria and by inhibiting the synthesis of renal prostaglandins, which are potent endogenous renal vasodilator hormones. Both effects of aspirin favor hypoxia in renal tissues and therefore enhance the susceptibility of the inner medulla to nephrotoxic injury.

Analgesic nephropathy occurs some three to five times more commonly in women than in men. A direct relationship exists between the total amount of analgesic compounds ingested and the degree of renal impairment. The intake of 1.0 g phenacetin per day for 1 to 3 years or the total ingestion of 2 kg phenacetin in combination with other analgesics appears to represent minimum requirements for the development of analgesic nephropathy. In such patients, renal function usually declines gradually, in association with chronic necrosis of papillae and diffuse tubulointerstitial damage to the renal cortex. Occasionally, papillary necrosis may be associated with hematuria and even renal colic owing to obstruction of a ureter by necrotic tissue. More than half of patients with analgesic nephropathy have pyuria, which, if persistently associated with sterile urine, provides an important clue to the diagnosis. Nonetheless, active pyelonephritis may coexist in patients with analgesic nephropathy. Proteinuria, if present, is typically mild (less than 1 g/d). Patients with analgesic nephropathy are usually unable to generate maximally concentrated urine, reflecting the underlying medullary and papillary damage. An acquired form of distal renal tubular acidosis may contribute to the development of *nephrocalcinosis*. The occurrence of anemia out of proportion to the degree of azotemia also may provide a clue to the diagnosis of analgesic nephropathy. Occult gastrointestinal bleeding (usually secondary to analgesic-induced gastritis) and, in an occasional patient, hemolysis (particularly in those with glucose-6-phosphate dehydrogenase deficiency) contribute to the anemia. Vague abdominal complaints, nonspecific headaches, and arthralgias are common. Moderate hypertension is also common and progresses to a malignant phase in only a small minority. When analgesic nephropathy has progressed to renal insufficiency, the kidneys usually appear bilaterally shrunken on intravenous pyelography, and the calyces are deformed. A "ring sign" on the pyelogram is pathognomonic of papillary necrosis and represents the radiolucent sloughed papilla surrounded by the radiodense contrast material in the calyx. Transitional cell carcinoma may develop in the urinary pelvis or ureters as a late complication of analgesic abuse.

Every effort must be made to convince the patient who ingests excessive analgesics to discontinue this hazardous practice. When renal damage is at an early stage, cessation of abuse usually arrests the progression of the nephrotoxic process; not infrequently, overall renal function improves with time. With continued abuse, however, progressive renal damage leads invariably to chronic renal failure.

Lead nephropathy (See also Chap. 396) Children and adults with lead intoxication often develop a chronic tubulointerstitial renal disease. In children, lead poisoning usually results from ingestion of lead-based paints (pica). The oxide of lead liberated from paint or present in the vapor arising from the welding of metals covered with lead-based paint may be inhaled in substantial quantities, thereby constituting an industrial form of exposure in adults. Alcohol, illegally distilled in an apparatus constructed from automobile radiators (so-called moonshine), is another cause of lead poisoning. Tubule transport processes enhance the accumulation of lead within renal cells, particularly in the proximal convoluted tubule, leading to cell degeneration, mitochondrial swelling, and eosinophilic intranuclear inclusion bodies rich in lead. In addition to tubule degeneration and atrophy, lead nephropathy is associated with ischemic changes in the glomeruli, fibrosis of the adventitia of small renal arterioles, and focal areas of cortical scarring. Eventually, the kidneys become atrophic. In addition to progressive azotemia, abnormalities of tubule function may occur, particularly *renal glycosuria* and *aminoaciduria*. Urinary excretion of lead, bile pigments, and porphyrin precursors, such as δ-aminolevulinic acid, coproporphyrin, and urobilinogen, may be increased. Patients with chronic lead nephropathy are characteristically *hyperuricemic*, a consequence of enhanced reabsorption of filtered urate. Acute gouty arthritis (so-called saturnine gout) occurs in about 50 percent of patients with lead nephropathy, in striking contrast to other forms of chronic renal failure in which gout is rare (also see Chap. 347). Hypertension is also a complication. Therefore, in any patient with slowly progressive renal failure, atrophic kidneys, gout, and hypertension, the diagnosis of lead intoxication should be considered. In addition, patients with chronic lead poisoning often complain of abdominal colic and have evidence of anemia, peripheral neuropathy, and encephalopathy. The diagnosis may be suspected by finding elevated serum levels of lead. However, because blood levels may not be elevated even in the presence of a toxic total-body burden of lead, the quantitation of lead excretion following infusion of the chelating agent calcium disodium edetate is a more reliable indicator of serious lead exposure. Urinary excretion of more than 0.6 mg/d of lead is indicative of overt or potential toxicity. Treatment includes removing the patient from the source of exposure and augmenting lead excretion with a chelating agent such as calcium disodium edetate.

Miscellaneous nephrotoxins   Use of lithium salts for manic-depressive illness has been associated with tubulointerstitial disease. The most frequent clinical finding is a mild to moderate nephrogenic diabetes insipidus resulting in polyuria and polydipsia. It is unclear whether long-term lithium therapy produces irreversible chronic tubulointerstitial lesions and impairment of GFR. Though some patients develop histologic evidence of such injury, there are only rare reports of chronic renal insufficiency attributable to this agent. In any case, renal function should be followed in patients taking this drug, and caution should be exercised if lithium is employed in patients with underlying renal disease.

The immunosuppressant cyclosporine causes both acute and chronic renal injury. The acute injury and the use of cyclosporine in transplantation are discussed in Chap. 238. The chronic injury is a progressive decline in GFR with mild proteinuria and arterial hypertension. Hyperkalemia is a relatively common complication and results in part from tubule resistance to aldosterone. Hypomagnesemia due to urinary magnesium wasting is less common but can cause hypocalcemia. The histologic changes in renal tissue comprise patchy interstitial fibrosis and tubular atrophy. In addition, the intrarenal vasculature often demonstrates hyalinosis, and focal segmental glomerular sclerosis can be present as well. Indeed, renal vasoconstriction induced by the drug appears to be a major mechanism of the renal injury. In patients receiving this drug for renal transplantation, chronic rejection and recurrence of the primary disease may coincide with chronic cyclosporine injury, and on clinical grounds, distinction among these may be difficult. Whether the chronic injury can be prevented by dose reduction is uncertain. However, use of the lowest doses of cyclosporine consistent with adequate immunosuppression appears to mitigate nephrotoxicity. In addition, treatment of any associated arterial hypertension may lessen renal injury.

Many agents that commonly lead to acute renal failure are also capable of producing tubulointerstitial injury (see Chap. 236). These include antibiotics (e.g., aminoglycosides, amphotericin B), radiographic contrast agents, various hydrocarbons (e.g., carbon tetrachloride), and heavy metals (e.g., mercury, cadmium, and bismuth).

METABOLIC TOXINS   Acute uric acid nephropathy (See also Chap. 347)   Acute overproduction of uric acid and extreme hyperuricemia often lead to a rapidly progressive renal insufficiency, so-called acute uric acid nephropathy. This tubulointerstitial disease is usually seen in patients given cytotoxic drugs for the treatment of lymphoproliferative or myeloproliferative disorders but also may occur in these patients before such treatment is begun. The pathologic changes are largely the result of deposition of uric acid crystals in the kidneys and their collecting systems, leading to partial or complete obstruction of collecting ducts, renal pelvis, or ureter. Since obstruction is often

bilateral, patients typically show the clinical course of acute renal failure, characterized by oliguria and rapidly rising serum creatinine concentration. In the early phase uric acid crystals can be found in urine, usually in association with microscopic or gross hematuria. Peak serum uric acid levels vary but are almost always above 1200 μmol/L (20 mg/dL) and may even exceed 3500 μmol/L (60 mg/dL).

Prevention of hyperuricemia in patients at risk by treatment with allopurinol in doses of 200 to 800 mg/d prior to cytotoxic therapy reduces the danger of acute uric acid nephropathy. Once hyperuricemia develops, however, efforts should be directed to preventing deposition of uric acid within the urinary tract. Increasing urine volume with potent diuretics (furosemide or mannitol) effectively lowers intratubular uric acid concentrations, and alkalinization of the urine to pH 7 or greater with sodium bicarbonate and/or a carbonic anhydrase inhibitor (acetazolamide) enhances uric acid solubility. If these efforts, together with allopurinol therapy, are ineffective in preventing acute renal failure, dialysis should be instituted to lower the serum uric acid concentration as well as to treat the acute manifestations of uremia. The combination of conservative therapy and hemodialysis allows most patients with acute uric acid nephropathy to survive acute renal failure and ultimately recover renal function.

Gouty nephropathy (See also Chap. 347)   Patients with less severe but prolonged forms of hyperuricemia are predisposed to a more chronic tubulointerstitial disorder, often referred to as *gouty nephropathy*. Since other conditions associated with hyperuricemia, such as hypertension, nephrolithiasis, pyelonephritis, and even lead poisoning, may contribute to renal damage, the effect of chronic hyperuricemia per se on renal function is unclear. Nevertheless, the severity of renal involvement correlates with the duration and magnitude of the elevation of the serum uric acid concentration. Histologically, the distinctive feature of gouty nephropathy is the presence of crystalline deposits of uric acid and monosodium urate salts in kidney parenchyma. These deposits are believed to represent the primary pathogenic process in gouty nephropathy, with intraluminal crystallization of uric acid taking place in distal tubules and collecting ducts where urine pH is generally quite low and where uric acid concentrations are considerably in excess of levels in plasma. These deposits not only cause intrarenal obstruction but also incite an inflammatory response, leading to lymphocytic infiltration, foreign-body giant cell reaction, and eventual fibrosis, especially of medullary and papillary regions of the kidney. Bacteriuria and pyelonephritis occur in about one-fourth of cases, presumably as complications of intrarenal urinary stasis. Since patients with gout frequently suffer from hypertension and hyperlipidemia, degenerative changes of the renal arterioles may constitute a striking feature of the histologic abnormality, often out of proportion to other morphologic defects. Clinically, gouty nephropathy is an insidious cause of renal insufficiency. Early in its course, GFR may be near normal, often despite focal morphologic changes in medullary and cortical interstitium, proteinuria, and diminished urinary concentrating ability. Whether reducing serum uric acid levels with allopurinol exerts a beneficial effect on the kidney remains to be demonstrated. Although such undesirable consequences of hyperuricemia as gout and uric acid stones respond well to allopurinol, use of this drug in asymptomatic hyperuricemia has not been shown to improve renal function consistently. On the other hand, uricosuric agents such as probenecid, which may increase uric acid stone production, clearly have no role in the treatment of renal disease associated with hyperuricemia.

Hypercalcemic nephropathy (See also Chap. 357)   Chronic hypercalcemia, as occurs in primary hyperparathyroidism, sarcoidosis, multiple myeloma, vitamin D intoxication, or metastatic bone disease, can cause tubulointerstitial damage and progressive renal insufficiency. The earliest renal lesion induced by hypercalcemia is a focal degenerative change in renal epithelia, primarily in collecting ducts, distal convoluted tubules, and loops of Henle. Tubule cell necrosis leads to nephron obstruction and stasis of intrarenal urine, favoring local precipitation of calcium salts and infection. Dilatation and atrophy of tubules eventually occur, as do interstitial fibrosis, mononuclear leukocyte infiltration, and interstitial calcium deposition (nephrocalcinosis). Calcium deposition also may occur in glomeruli and the walls of renal arterioles. Clinically, the most striking defect is an inability to concentrate the urine maximally, resulting in polyuria and nocturia. Defective transport of chloride in the ascending limb of Henle's loop is responsible, at least in part, for this concentrating defect. Additionally, reduced collecting duct responsiveness to vasopressin may contribute to this abnormality. Reductions in GFR and renal blood flow also occur, both in acute severe hypercalcemia and with prolonged hypercalcemia of lesser severity. Distal renal tubular acidosis and sodium and potassium wasting also have been described in these chronic states. Eventually, uncontrolled hypercalcemia leads to severe tubulointerstitial damage and overt renal failure. Urinalysis is rarely a clue to the presence of hypercalcemic renal failure, but abdominal x-rays may demonstrate nephrocalcinosis as well as nephrolithiasis, the latter due to the hypercalciuria which often accompanies hypercalcemia. Treatment for hypercalcemic nephropathy consists of reducing the serum calcium concentration toward normal and correcting the primary abnormality of calcium metabolism. The management of hypercalcemia is discussed in Chap. 357. Prognosis for recovery of renal function depends on the severity of the renal lesion at the time hypercalcemia is corrected. Renal dysfunction of acute hypercalcemia may be completely reversible. Gradual, progressive renal insufficiency related to chronic hypercalcemia, however, may not improve with correction of the calcium disorder. Nonetheless, every effort should be made to return serum calcium concentration to normal to minimize further loss of renal function.

Hypokalemic nephropathy (See also Chap. 45)   Disturbances of renal structure and function occur commonly in patients with moderate to severe potassium depletion of at least several weeks' duration. Histologically, renal epithelial cells are often seen to contain numerous vacuoles, most marked in proximal and, to a lesser extent, distal convoluted tubules. These findings usually disappear with potassium repletion. Glomeruli are reduced in size and may become sclerotic, while larger blood vessels are usually uninvolved. Whether prolonged or recurrent potassium deficiency results in irreversible tubulointerstitial fibrosis, scarring, and atrophy is unresolved. Loss of urinary concentrating ability is the most commonly encountered functional defect. In animals this urinary concentrating abnormality is preceded by a period of primary polydipsia. The reduced concentrating capacity which eventually develops is due, at least in part, to defective operation of the countercurrent multiplier system. Elevated rates of intrarenal prostaglandin synthesis also may contribute to this concentrating defect, since prostaglandins antagonize the hydroosmotic action of antidiuretic hormone on collecting-duct epithelium. Nocturia, polyuria, and polydipsia are frequently encountered in patients with chronic potassium depletion, although, occasionally, patients with severe hypokalemia have no complaints referable to the urinary tract. Patients with hypokalemic nephropathy may have an enhanced susceptibility to pyelonephritis. The polydipsia is probably due to both the impaired renal concentrating ability and a primary disorder of the thirst mechanism, which is believed to be a common feature of chronic potassium depletion. Urinalysis often reveals no abnormalities except for mild proteinuria. Serum creatinine and urea nitrogen concentrations usually remain within normal limits. Treatment should be directed at repleting body potassium stores and correcting the primary process responsible for potassium loss. With correction of body potassium, functional and histologic abnormalities of the kidneys usually disappear, although maximal urinary concentrating ability may not return to normal for several months.

Miscellaneous metabolic toxins   Urinary oxalate, derived from the metabolism of glycine and, to a variable extent, from ingested oxalate, may deposit as insoluble intratubular calcium oxalate crystals and result in chronic tubulointerstitial damage in patients with hereditary or acquired forms of *hyperoxaluria*. *Cystinosis* and *Fabry's disease* are other hereditary depositional disorders affecting the renal tubules and interstitium (see Chaps. 241, 244, and 245).

RENAL PARENCHYMAL DISEASE ASSOCIATED WITH EXTRARENAL NEOPLASM

In addition to being the site of origin of several benign and malignant neoplasms (see Chap. 247), the kidneys are frequently affected by neoplasms arising outside the urinary tract. Except for the glomerulopathies associated with lymphomas and several solid tumors (see Chap. 241), the renal manifestations of primary extrarenal neoplastic processes are confined mainly to the interstitium and tubules. Although metastatic renal involvement by solid tumors is unusual, the kidneys are often invaded by neoplastic cells in various lymphomas and leukemias and in multiple myeloma. In postmortem studies of patients with *lymphoma*, renal involvement is found in approximately half. The involvement may be focal, in the form of multiple discrete nodules, or diffuse, with lymphomatous infiltration throughout the renal parenchyma. Diffuse infiltration is seen most commonly in lymphomas other than Hodgkin's disease. There may be flank pain related to massive renal infiltration, and x-rays may show enlargement of one or both kidneys. Renal insufficiency occurs in a minority of cases, and overt uremia is rare. Treatment of the primary disease may improve renal function in these cases.

The kidneys are also commonly involved in various forms of *leukemia*. At postmortem examination, bilateral renal involvement is present in approximately 50 percent of cases. As with lymphoma, uremia is rarely, if ever, a consequence of leukemic infiltration of the kidneys. The kidneys also can be involved in leukemias because of the associated high incidence of hyperuricemia, hypercalcemia, and lysozymuria. The myelogenous leukemias, particularly of the monocytic type, may be complicated by tubule defects involving potassium and magnesium wasting.

In contrast, infiltration of the kidneys with *myeloma* cells is infrequent (see also Chap. 280). When it occurs, the process is usually focal, so renal insufficiency from this cause is also uncommon. The more usual lesion is *myeloma kidney*, characterized histologically by atrophic tubules, many with eosinophilic intraluminal casts, and numerous multinucleated giant cells within tubule walls and in the interstitium. The frequent occurrence of myeloma kidney in patients with Bence Jones proteinuria has suggested a causal relation. Bence Jones proteins are thought to cause myeloma kidney through direct toxicity to renal tubule cells. In addition, Bence Jones proteins may precipitate within the distal nephron where the high concentrations of these proteins and the acid composition of the tubule fluid favor intraluminal cast formation and intrarenal obstruction. Indeed, positive immunofluorescence staining for immunoglobulin light chains can often be demonstrated in casts found in myeloma kidneys. Occasionally, acute renal failure occurs after intravenous pyelography in patients with multiple myeloma and is believed to result from the further precipitation of Bence Jones proteins induced by dehydration prior to radiographic study. Dehydration of the patient with myeloma in preparation for intravenous pyelography should therefore be avoided. Multiple myeloma also may affect the kidneys indirectly. Hypercalcemia or hyperuricemia may lead to the nephropathies described above. Proximal tubule disorders are also seen occasionally, including type II proximal renal tubular acidosis and the Fanconi syndrome. Additionally, intrarenal deposits of *amyloid* (see below) may contribute to impaired excretory function.

IMMUNE DISORDERS

HYPERSENSITIVITY NEPHROPATHY   An acute diffuse tubulointerstitial reaction may result from hypersensitivity to a number of drugs. First reported after the use of sulfonamides, acute tubulointerstitial damage is now seen most often with the antibiotic *methicillin*, although *ampicillin, penicillin, cephalothin, phenindione, thiazides, furosemide*, and nonsteroidal anti-inflammatory drugs also have been implicated. Of note, the tubulointerstitial nephropathy which develops in some patients taking nonsteroidal anti-inflammatory drugs may be associated with nephrotic-range proteinuria and histologic evidence of minimal change glomerulopathy. Grossly, the kidneys are usually enlarged. Histologically, the glomeruli appear normal. The principal pathologic abnormalities are in the interstitium of the kidney, which reveals pronounced edema and infiltration with polymorphonuclear leukocytes, lymphocytes, plasma cells, and, in some cases, large numbers of eosinophils. If the process is severe, tubule cell necrosis and regeneration also may be apparent. Immunofluorescence studies either have been unrevealing or have demonstrated a linear pattern of immunoglobin and complement deposition along tubule basement membranes. In a few cases of methicillin-induced acute tubulointerstitial disease, circulating anti-tubule basement membrane antibodies also have been found, suggesting that autoantibody formation may have been induced by the penicilloyl hapten of methicillin (by conjugation of hapten with tubule basement membrane proteins, thereby altering the native antigenicity of the basement membrane). In cases associated with nonsteroidal anti-inflammatory drugs, a role for cell-mediated immunity has been proposed, since renal infiltration by both T and B lymphocytes has been observed with a relative predominance of cytotoxic T cells. Evidence for an immunologic basis for these various drug-related nephropathies also derives from the facts that the onset of nephropathy does not appear to be dose-related, often follows a second exposure to the drug presumed to be responsible for the renal injury, and often is associated with increased levels of serum IgE. In the case of methicillin, the patients usually develop evidence of renal injury after about 2 weeks of drug administration. Hematuria, fever, skin rash, and eosinophilia are prominent. Many patients develop azotemia which typically resolves after withdrawal of the offending 'drug. Proteinuria and pyuria often accompany the hematuria, and occasionally eosinophils are found in the urine sediment. The clinical picture may be confused with acute glomerulonephritis, but when acute azotemia and hematuria are accompanied by eosinophilia, skin rash, and a history of drug exposure, a hypersensitivity reaction leading to acute tubulointerstitial nephritis should be regarded as the leading diagnostic possibility. Discontinuation of the drug usually results in complete reversal of the renal injury; rarely, renal damage may be irreversible. Glucocorticoids have been used, but their value has not been established.

SJÖGREN'S SYNDROME (See also Chap. 288) Keratoconjunctivitis sicca, or Sjögren's syndrome, is an immunologic disorder characterized by dryness of mucous membranes and mononuclear cell infiltration of salivary and lacrimal glands; it is often seen in patients with rheumatoid arthritis. When the kidneys are involved, the predominant histologic findings are those of chronic tubulointerstitial disease. Interstitial infiltrates are composed primarily of lymphocytes, causing the histology of the renal parenchyma in these patients to resemble that of the salivary and lacrimal glands. Renal functional defects include diminished urinary concentrating ability and distal (type I) renal tubular acidosis. Urinalysis may show pyuria (predominantly lymphocyturia) and mild proteinuria.

AMYLOIDOSIS (See also Chaps. 241 and 281) Glomerular pathology usually predominates and leads to heavy proteinuria and azotemia. However, tubule function also may be deranged, giving rise to a nephrogenic diabetes insipidus and to distal (type I) renal tubular acidosis. In several cases these functional abnormalities correlated with peritubular deposition of amyloid, particularly in areas surrounding vasa rectae, loops of Henle, and collecting ducts. Bilateral enlargement of the kidneys, especially in a patient with massive proteinuria and tubule dysfunction, should raise the possibility of amyloid renal disease.

HIV INFECTION (See also Chap. 279) Chronic renal disease occurs in a fraction of patients infected with HIV. This complication usually presents with nephrotic proteinuria and a rapid decline in renal function and may precede overt AIDS. Glomerular abnormalities include focal and segmental glomerular sclerosis, and tubulointerstitial changes include tubular dilation with cystic change, epithelial cell vacuolization, and mononuclear cell infiltrates. Uncertainty exists

whether direct infection of renal cells by the virus or some indirect immune reaction is responsible for the renal disease. Some renal abnormalities result from associated nephrotoxic insults including intravenous drug abuse and multiple exposure to nephrotoxic antibiotics. In addition, the accumulated effects of multiple septic episodes, such as infectious granulomatous cytomegalovirus inclusions, and Kaposi's sarcoma obviously are secondary to the compromised immune state and should not be considered HIV-specific renal disease. The prevalence of the specific HIV-related renal lesion appears to be variable. The reason for this disparity is uncertain. However, black patients with HIV are especially at risk for renal complications, and the variations in reported prevalence of renal disease in HIV infection may, in part, reflect different racial distributions among the HIV-infected populations studied.

TUBULOINTERSTITIAL ABNORMALITIES ASSOCIATED WITH GLOMERULONEPHRITIS A number of primary glomerulopathies also may be associated with damage to tubules and interstitium. Pathogenically, the extraglomerular component in these renal disorders often involves the same mechanisms responsible for the more pronounced glomerular injury. For example, in more than half of patients with the nephropathy of systemic lupus erythematosus, deposits of immune complexes can be identified in tubule basement membranes, usually accompanied by an interstitial mononuclear inflammatory reaction. Similarly, in many patients with glomerulonephritis associated with anti-glomerular basement membrane antibody, the same antibody is reactive against tubule basement membranes as well.

MISCELLANEOUS DISORDERS

VESICOURETERAL REFLUX (See also Chaps. 90 and 246) Normally, the junction of the terminal ureter with the urinary bladder provides a competent sphincter so that during micturition urine leaves the bladder only via the urethra. However, when the function of the ureterovesical junction is impaired, urine may reflux into the ureters due to the high intravesical pressure that develops during voiding. Clinically, reflux is often detected on the voiding and postvoiding films obtained during intravenous pyelography, although voiding cystourethrography may be required for definitive diagnosis. Bladder infection may ascend the urinary tract to the kidneys through incompetent ureterovesical sphincters. Not surprisingly, therefore, reflux is often discovered in patients with acute and/or chronic urinary tract infections. In children particularly, reflux of minor degree may disappear with standard therapy of intercurrent urinary infection. With more severe degrees of reflux, characterized by dilatation of ureters and renal pelves, progressive renal damage often appears, and although active infection also may be present, uncertainty exists as to the necessity of infection in producing the scarred kidney of reflux nephropathy. In contrast to those with other forms of chronic tubulointerstitial disease, patients with renal insufficiency and scarring due to reflux often demonstrate substantial proteinuria. Indeed, in such cases glomerular lesions similar to those of idiopathic focal glomerulosclerosis (Chap. 240) are often present in addition to the changes of chronic tubulointerstitial disease. Surgical correction of reflux is usually necessary only with the more severe degrees of reflux since renal damage correlates with the extent of reflux. Obviously, if extensive glomerulosclerosis already exists, urologic repair may no longer be warranted.

RADIATION NEPHRITIS Renal dysfunction can be expected to occur if 23,000 Gy (2300 rad) or more of x-ray irradiation is administered to both kidneys during a period of 5 weeks or less. Histologic examination of the kidneys reveals hyalinized glomeruli, atrophic tubules, extensive interstitial fibrosis, and hyalinization of the media of renal arterioles. Radiation-induced renal ischemia is believed to be the main pathogenic factor responsible for the tubulointerstitial damage, which may not become evident clinically for months after completion of radiation. The presentation of acute radiation nephritis includes rapidly progressive azotemia, moderate to malignant hypertension, anemia, and proteinuria which may reach the nephrotic range. More than 50 percent progress to chronic renal failure. A more insidious form is characterized by slower development of azotemia, anemia, and nephrotic syndrome. Malignant hypertension may follow unilateral renal irradiation and resolve with ipsilateral nephrectomy. Radiation nephritis has all but vanished because of heightened awareness of its pathogenesis by radiotherapists.

REFERENCES

ADLER SG et al: Hypersensitivity phenomena and the kidney: Role of drugs and environmental agents. Am J Kidney Dis 5:75, 1985

ARANT BS: Reflux nephropathy. Kidney 21:19, 1989

BENNET WM: Lead nephropathy. Kidney Int 28:218, 1985

———, DEBROE ME: Analgesic nephropathy. A preventable renal disease. N Engl J Med 320, 1269, 1989

——— et al: Tubulointerstitial disease and toxic nephropathy, in The Kidney, 4th ed, BM Brenner, FC Rector Jr (eds). Philadelphia, Saunders 1991

BOTON R et al: Prevalence, pathogenesis, and treatment of renal dysfunction associated with chronic lithium therapy. Am J Kidney Dis 10:329, 1987

CAMERON JS: Immunologically mediated interstitial nephritis: Primary and secondary. Adv Nephrol 18:207, 1989

MURRAY T, GOLDBERG M: Chronic interstitial nephritis: Etiologic factors. Ann Intern Med 82:453, 1975

MYERS BD et al: The long-term course of cyclosporine-associated chronic nephropathy. Kidney Int 33:590, 1988

RAO TKS: Clinical features of human immunodeficiency virus associated nephropathy. Kidney Int 40(suppl 35):S-13, 1991

SANDLER DP et al: Analgesic use and chronic renal disease. N Engl J Med 320:1238, 1989

243 VASCULAR INJURY TO THE KIDNEY

KAMAL F. BADR / BARRY M. BRENNER

Adequate delivery of blood to the glomerular capillary network is crucial for glomerular filtration and overall salt and water balance. Thus, in addition to the threat to the viability of renal tissue, vascular injury to the kidney may compromise the maintenance of body fluid volume and composition. Involvement of the renal vessels by atherosclerotic, hypertensive, embolic, inflammatory, and hematologic disorders is usually a manifestation of generalized vascular pathology. The morphologic and clinical responses to these insults and the unique renal vasculopathy associated with the toxemias of pregnancy are considered in this chapter.

THROMBOEMBOLIC DISEASES OF THE RENAL ARTERIES

Thrombosis of the major renal arteries or their branches is an important cause of deterioration of renal function, especially in the elderly. It is often difficult to diagnose and therefore requires a high index of suspicion. Thrombosis may occur as a result of intrinsic pathology in the renal vessels (posttraumatic, atherosclerotic, or inflammatory) or as a result of emboli originating in distant vessels, most commonly fat emboli, emboli originating in the left heart (mural thrombi following myocardial infarction, bacterial endocarditis, or aseptic vegetations), or "paradoxical" emboli passing from the right side of the circulation via a patent foramen ovale or atrial septal defect. Emboli are bilateral in 15 to 30 percent of cases.

The clinical presentation is variable, depending on the time course and the extent of the occlusive event. Acute thrombosis and infarction, such as follows embolization, may result in sudden onset of flank pain and tenderness, fever, hematuria, leukocytosis, nausea, and vomiting. If infarction occurs, renal enzymes may be elevated, namely aspartate aminotransferase (AST), lactic dehydrogenase (LDH; most reliable), and alkaline phosphatase, which rise and fall in the order

TABLE 243-1 Clinical presentations of ischemic renal disease

1 Acute renal failure
2 Progressive azotemia in a patient with known renovascular hypertension (usually on medical therapy)
3 Unexplained progressive azotemia in an elderly patient with or without refractory hypertension
4 Hypertension and azotemia in a renal transplant patient

listed. Urinary LDH and alkaline phosphatase also may increase after infarction. Renal function deteriorates acutely, leading in bilateral thrombosis to acute oliguric renal failure. More gradual (i.e., atherosclerotic) occlusion of a single renal artery may go undetected. A spectrum of clinical presentations lies between these two extremes (Table 243-1). Hypertension usually follows renal infarction and results from renin release in the peri-infarction zone. Hypertension is usually transient but may be persistent. Diagnosis is established by renal arteriography.

Management of *acute* renal arterial thrombosis includes surgical intervention, anticoagulant therapy, conservative and supportive therapy, and control of hypertension. The choice of treatment depends mainly on (1) the condition of the patient, in particular the patient's ability to withstand major surgery, and (2) the extent of renovascular occlusion and amount of renal mass at risk of infarction. In general, supportive care and anticoagulant therapy are indicated in unilateral disease. In bilateral thrombosis, medical and surgical therapies yield comparable results. Twenty-five percent of patients die during the acute episode, usually from extrarenal complications. In *chronic* ischemic renal disease, surgical revascularization is more likely to preserve and improve renal function and to control the hypertension (see below).

ATHEROEMBOLIC DISEASE OF THE RENAL ARTERIES

Atheroembolic disease typically results from multiple showers of cholesterol-containing microemboli dislodged from atheromatous plaques in large arteries. Such emboli occlude small (150- to 200-μm diameter) vessels in the kidney and in other organs (retina, brain, pancreas, muscles, skin, and extremities). It usually occurs in an elderly individual with atherosclerotic disease elsewhere and usually follows aortic surgery or renal or coronary arteriography. Spontaneous atheroembolic disease has been reported. Manifestations include deterioration of renal function (sudden or gradual), mild proteinuria, microscopic hematuria, and leukocyturia. Urine volume may remain normal or fall to oliguric levels depending on severity. Renal ischemia can induce or exacerbate preexisting hypertension.

Antemortem diagnosis of atherosclerotic renal emboli is difficult. The demonstration of cholesterol emboli in the retina is helpful, but a firm diagnosis is established only by demonstration of cholesterol crystals in the smaller arteries and arterioles in renal biopsy or autopsy specimens. These also may be seen in asymptomatic skeletal muscle or skin. No specific treatment is available.

RENAL VEIN THROMBOSIS
Thrombosis of one or both main renal veins (RVT) occurs in a variety of settings (Table 243-2). The pathogenesis is not always clear, particularly when it occurs in so-called hypercoagulable states such as may develop in pregnant women, users of oral contraceptives, subjects with nephrotic syndrome, or

TABLE 243-2 Conditions associated with renal vein thrombosis

1 Trauma
2 Extrinsic compression (lymph nodes, aortic aneurysm, tumor)
3 Invasion by renal cell carcinoma
4 Dehydration (infants)
5 Nephrotic syndrome
6 Pregnancy or oral contraceptives

dehydrated infants. Nephrotic syndrome accompanying membranous glomerulopathy and certain carcinomas seems to predispose to the development of RVT, which occurs in 10 to 50 percent of patients with these disorders. RVT may exacerbate preexisting proteinuria but is infrequently the cause of the nephrotic syndrome.

The clinical manifestations depend on the severity and abruptness of its occurrence. Acute cases occur typically in children and are characterized by sudden loss of renal function, often accompanied by fever, chills, lumbar tenderness (with kidney enlargement), leukocytosis, and hematuria. Hemorrhagic infarction and renal rupture may lead to hypovolemic shock. In young adults RVT is usually suspected from an unexpected and relatively acute or subacute deterioration of renal function and/or exacerbation of proteinuria and hematuria in the appropriate clinical setting (underlying nephrotic syndrome, trauma, pregnancy, oral contraceptive use). In cases of gradual thrombosis, usually occurring in the elderly, the only manifestation may be recurrent pulmonary emboli or development of hypertension. A Fanconi-like syndrome and proximal renal tubular acidosis have been described.

The definitive diagnosis can only be established through selective renal venography with visualization of the occluding thrombus. Treatment consists of anticoagulation, the main purpose of which is prevention of pulmonary embolization, although some authors have also claimed improvement in renal function and proteinuria. Encouraging reports have appeared concerning the use of streptokinase. Spontaneous recanalization with clinical improvement also has been observed. Anticoagulant therapy is more rewarding in the acute thrombosis seen in younger individuals. Nephrectomy is advocated in infants with life-threatening renal infarction. Thrombectomy is effective in some cases.

RENAL ARTERY STENOSIS Stenosis of the main renal artery and/or its major branches accounts for 2 to 5 percent of hypertension. The common cause in the middle-aged and elderly is an atheromatous plaque at the origin of the renal artery. In younger women, stenosis is due to intrinsic structural abnormalities of the arterial wall caused by a heterogeneous group of lesions termed *fibromuscular dysplasia*.

Renal artery stenosis should be suspected when hypertension develops in a previously normotensive individual over 50 years of age or in the young (under 30 years) with suggestive features: symptoms of vascular insufficiency to other organs, high-pitched epigastric bruit on physical examination, symptoms of hypokalemia secondary to hyperaldosteronism (muscle weakness, tetany, polyuria), and metabolic alkalosis. If renovascular hypertension is suspected, a positive captopril test, which has a sensitivity and specificity of greater than 95 percent, constitutes an excellent screening procedure to assess the need for more invasive radiographic evaluation. The test relies on the exaggerated increase in plasma renin activity (PRA) following administration of captopril to patients with renovascular hypertension as compared with those with essential hypertension. It is considered positive when all the following criteria are satisfied: stimulated PRA of 12 (μg/L)/h, absolute increase in PRA of 10 (μg/L)/h or more, and increase in PRA of greater than 150 percent [or 400 percent if baseline PRA is less than 3 (μg/L)/h]. In the appropriate clinical setting, particularly in the presence of a positive captopril test, digital subtraction renal arteriography should be performed. This procedure obviates the need for cannulation of the arterial system and has a low incidence of false-positive (5 percent) and false-negative (10 percent) results. The most definitive diagnostic procedure is bilateral arteriography with repeated bilateral renal vein and systemic renin determinations. If renal vein renin measurements from the two kidneys differ by a factor of 1.5:1 or more (higher value from the affected kidney) in a patient with radiographic unilateral renal artery stenosis, the chance of cure of hypertension by surgical reconstruction is almost 90 percent, particularly if renal vein renin level from the unaffected kidney is equal to or less than systemic levels (suppressible). A ratio of less than 1.5:1, however, does not exclude the diagnosis of renovascular hypertension, particularly in the presence of bilateral disease. Two diagnostic modalities for the noninvasive

evaluation of significant renal artery stenosis are duplex scanning (sensitivity 95 percent, specificity 90 percent) and magnetic resonance angiography (sensitivity 100 percent for lesions with ≥50 percent stenosis, specificity 92 percent).

The aims of treatment are control of the blood pressure and restoration of perfusion to the ischemic kidney. In general, it is now firmly established that interventional therapy (i.e., surgery or angioplasty) is superior to medical therapy, which, while controlling blood pressure, does little to salvage renal mass lost to ischemic injury. Success rates with percutaneous transluminal angioplasty in young patients with fibromuscular dysplasia are 50 percent cure and 30 percent improvement in blood pressure control. Angioplasty is best suited for noncalcified, segmental short lesions and is also useful in some elderly patients who are poor surgical risks. About half of elderly individuals with reduced renal function as a result of renal arterial stenosis improve following angioplasty or surgery, even when preintervention arteriography shows little evidence of cortical perfusion. Despite the risks associated with surgery, long-term follow-up studies demonstrate an advantage of surgery over angioplasty both with regard to the incidence of restenosis and to the preservation or improvement in GFR.

Renal artery stenosis, particularly if atherosclerotic, is a progressive disease that may lead to gradual and silent loss of renal functional tissue. Compensatory contralateral hypertrophy may maintain renal function until affected by superimposed pathologic processes, at which time azotemia supervenes. Even if angioplasty or surgery fail to return blood pressure to normal, these procedures usually render medical therapy easier.

HEMOLYTIC UREMIC SYNDROME (HUS) AND THROMBOTIC THROMBOCYTOPENIC PURPURA (TTP) (See also Chap. 240) HUS and TTP, consumptive coagulopathies characterized by microangiopathic hemolytic anemia and thrombocytopenia, have a particular predilection for the kidney and the central nervous system, the latter especially in TTP. The kidneys of patients with HUS or TTP often exhibit a "flea-bitten" appearance, the result of multiple cortical hemorrhagic infarcts. The major sites of pathology are the small renal arteries and afferent arterioles, which are nearly occluded as a result of marked intimal hyperplasia (particularly in TTP) and fibrin deposits in the subintimal regions. When the vasoocclusive process is extensive, bilateral cortical necrosis may occur. In addition, arteriolar microaneurysms, glomerular infarction, or nonspecific focal changes may be seen. In keeping with the focal nature of the vascular lesions, patchy areas of interstitial edema, tubular necrosis, and, eventually, fibrosis occur. By immunofluorescence staining, complement components and immunoglobulins may be demonstrated in the arterioles, and fibrinogen deposits are present in arteries, arterioles, and glomerular capillary loops.

Several mechanisms have been implicated in the etiology of the intravascular coagulopathy seen in HUS and TTP, including induction of a generalized Shwartzman phenomenon by microorganisms or endotoxin, genetic predisposition, and deficiency of platelet antiaggregatory substance(s) (e.g., prostacyclin). Some patients improve following exchange transfusion or plasmapheresis, suggesting accumulation of an as yet unidentified toxin.

Renal failure is common in both HUS and TTP, usually manifested by oligoanuria (more severe in HUS), azotemia, mild proteinuria, microscopic and/or gross hematuria, and cylindruria. Patients with HUS have more severe renal failure, often marked by oligoanuria and hypertension and commonly progressing to chronic renal failure. The prognosis in HUS is better in children than in adults. In TTP, the course of which may span days to months, renal failure is usually less severe. The overall prognosis, however, remains poor in view of the severe central nervous system involvement.

In the management of TTP, high-dose glucocorticoids and plasma exchange often provide complete remission or cure. Plasma exchange should be initiated as early as possible, and the treatment cycles can be repeated if thrombocytopenia recurs. Splenectomy and antiplatelet therapy also have been used with varying degrees of success in TTP patients. The success of plasma exchange in adult HUS is less well established than in TTP.

ARTERIOLAR NEPHROSCLEROSIS Whether hypertension is "essential" or of known etiology, persistent exposure of the renal circulation to elevated intraluminal pressures results in development of intrinsic lesions of the renal arterioles (hyaline arteriolosclerosis) that eventually lead to loss of function (nephrosclerosis). Nephrosclerosis is divided into two distinct entities: "benign" and "malignant" (or accelerated).

Benign arteriolar nephrosclerosis Benign arteriolar nephrosclerosis is seen in patients who are hypertensive for an extended period of time (blood pressure more than 150/90 mmHg) but whose hypertension has not progressed to a malignant form (described below). Such patients, usually in the older age group, are often discovered to be hypertensive on routine physical examination or as a result of nonspecific symptomatology (e.g., headaches, weakness, palpitations).

Kidney size is normal to reduced, with loss of cortical mass leading to a fine granularity. Although the larger arteries may show atherosclerotic changes, the characteristic pathology is in the afferent arterioles, which have thickened walls due to deposition of homogeneous eosinophilic material (hyaline arteriolosclerosis). This material is composed of plasma proteins and fats that have been deposited in the arteriolar wall due to injury to the endothelium, probably secondary to the elevated intraluminal hydraulic pressure. Narrowing of vascular lumina results, with consequent ischemic injury to glomeruli and tubules.

Nephrosclerosis accompanying long-standing systemic arterial hypertension is only one manifestation of a generalized process affecting the cardiovascular system. Physical examination, therefore, may reveal changes in retinal vessels (arteriolar narrowing and/or flame-shaped hemorrhages), cardiac hypertrophy, and possibly signs of congestive heart failure. Renal disease may manifest as a mild to moderate elevation of serum creatinine concentration, microscopic hematuria, and/or mild proteinuria. In general, clinical evaluation does not reveal significant renal abnormalities. More specialized examination may disclose elevated urinary albumin excretion, tapering and loss of caliber of intrarenal vessels on arteriography, and an exaggerated natriuresis in response to a fluid challenge. Patients with benign nephrosclerosis maintain a near-normal GFR despite a reduction in renal blood flow.

Malignant arteriolar nephrosclerosis Patients with long-standing benign hypertension or patients not known to be hypertensive previously may develop malignant hypertension characterized by a sudden (accelerated) elevation of blood pressure (diastolic often above 130 mmHg) accompanied by papilledema, central nervous system manifestations, cardiac decompensation, and acute progressive deterioration of renal function. The absence of papilledema does not rule out the diagnosis in a patient with markedly elevated blood pressure and rapidly declining renal function. The kidneys are characterized by a flea-bitten appearance resulting from hemorrhages in surface capillaries. Histologically, two distinct vascular lesions can be seen. The first, affecting arterioles, is fibrinoid necrosis, i.e., infiltration of arteriolar walls with eosinophilic material including fibrin. There is thickening of vessel walls and, occasionally, an inflammatory infiltrate (necrotizing arteriolitis). The second lesion, involving the interlobular arteries, is a concentric hyperplastic proliferation of the cellular elements of the vascular wall with deposition of collagen to form a hyperplastic arteriolitis (onion-skin lesion). Fibrinoid necrosis occasionally extends into the glomeruli, which also may undergo proliferative changes or total necrosis. Most glomerular and tubular changes are secondary to ischemia and infarction. The sequence of events leading to the development of malignant hypertension is poorly defined. Two pathophysiologic alterations appear central in its initiation and/or perpetuation: (1) increased permeability of vessel walls to invasion by plasma components, particularly fibrin, which activates clotting mechanisms leading to a microangiopathic hemolytic anemia, thus perpetuating the vascular pathology, and (2) activation of the renin-angiotensin-aldosterone system at some point in the

disease process, which contributes to the acceleration and maintenance of blood pressure elevation and, in turn, to vascular injury.

Malignant hypertension is most likely to develop in a previously hypertensive individual, usually in the third or fourth decade of life. There is a higher incidence among men, particularly black men. The presenting symptoms are usually neurologic (dizziness, headache, blurring of vision, altered states of consciousness, and focal or generalized seizures). Cardiac decompensation and renal failure appear thereafter. Renal abnormalities include a rapid rise in serum creatinine, hematuria (at times macroscopic), proteinuria, and red and white blood cell casts in the sediment. Nephrotic syndrome may be present. Elevated plasma aldosterone levels cause hypokalemic metabolic alkalosis in the early phase. Uremic acidosis and hyperkalemia eventually obscure these early findings. Hematologic indices of microangiopathic hemolytic anemia (i.e., schistocytes) are often seen.

Control of hypertension is the principal goal of therapy for both benign and malignant forms. The time of initiation of therapy, its effectiveness, and patient compliance are crucial factors in arresting the progression of benign nephrosclerosis. Untreated, most of these patients succumb to the extrarenal complications of hypertension. In contrast, malignant hypertension is a medical emergency; its natural course includes a death rate of 80 to 90 percent within 1 year of onset, almost always due to uremia. Supportive measures should be instituted to control the neurologic, cardiac, and other complications of acute renal failure, but the mainstay of therapy is prompt and aggressive reduction of blood pressure, which, if successful, can reverse all complications in the majority of patients. Presently, 5-year survival is 50 percent, and some patients have evidence of partial reversal of the vascular lesions and a return of renal function to near-normal levels.

SCLERODERMA (PROGRESSIVE SYSTEMIC SCLEROSIS) Renal vascular involvement in scleroderma is characterized by a distinctive lesion of the small arteries (diameters of 150 to 500 μm) consisting of intimal proliferation, medial thinning, and increased collagen deposition in the adventitial layer. Fibrinoid changes in the walls of afferent arterioles and microinfarcts may occur. Glomerular changes are generally nonspecific and secondary to ischemic damage. Tubules are often atrophic. As part of a generalized increase in vasomotor tone, a vasospastic (Raynaud-like) phenomenon at the level of the renal vasculature contributes to the renal insufficiency. Reduction in renal blood flow is the major mechanism underlying the deterioration in kidney function, being present in 80 percent of patients, even in the absence of other clinical abnormalities. As vascular narrowing progresses, hypertension, azotemia, and proteinuria eventually develop. Plasma renin rises in response to sustained renal ischemia. The resulting hypertension causes further renal injury and may play a role in the intimate destruction of nephrons. As more and more nephrons are lost to the combined insults of ischemia and hypertension, development of azotemia heralds a particularly grim prognosis. Proteinuria, usually mild, is a consequence of ischemic and hypertensive glomerular injury.

Although the majority of patients with scleroderma present with extrarenal manifestations, renal involvement is eventually manifested in half of patients followed for up to 20 years. Renal involvement can present in one of two ways, depending on whether malignant hypertension is superimposed on the renal pathology: (1) *Persistent urinary abnormalities* with or without hypertension tend to follow an indolent course with mild proteinuria, occasional casts, cellular elements in the urinary sediment, and a propensity for development of hypertension. Azotemia is absent initially, but when it develops, dialysis is required within 1 year. (2) *Scleroderma renal crisis* is a rapid deterioration in renal function, usually accompanied by malignant hypertension, oliguria, fluid retention, microangiopathic hemolytic anemia, and central nervous system involvement. It may occur in patients with previously undemonstrable or slowly progressive renal disease. Untreated, it leads to chronic renal failure within days to months.

The prognosis of scleroderma renal disease is generally poor, particularly following the onset of azotemia. Aggressive antihypertensive therapy may be effective in delaying the progression of renal failure. In scleroderma renal crisis, prompt treatment with beta blockers, minoxidil, and particularly angiotensin I converting enzyme (ACE) inhibitors may reverse acute renal failure. The effect of these interventions on renal function over the long term is uncertain.

SICKLE CELL NEPHROPATHY (See also Chap. 241)   Sickle cell disease causes renal complications that arise mainly as a result of sickling of red blood cells in the microvasculature. The hypertonic and relatively hypoxic environment of the renal medulla, coupled with the slow blood flow in the vasa recta, favors the sickling of red blood cells, with resultant local infarction (papillary necrosis). Functional tubule defects in patients with sickle cell disease are likely the result of partial ischemic injury to the renal tubules.

In addition to the intrarenal microvascular pathology described above, young patients with sickle cell disease are characterized by renal hyperperfusion, glomerular hypertrophy, and hyperfiltration. Many of these individuals eventually develop a glomerulopathy leading to proteinuria (present in as many as 30 percent) and, in some, the nephrotic syndrome. Mild azotemia and hyperuricemia also can develop, but advanced renal failure and uremia are rare. Although an immunologic basis for the glomerulopathy of sickle cell disease has been proposed, hemodynamically mediated renal injury, resulting from intrarenal hyperperfusion and glomerular hyperfiltration, may be the major pathogenetic mechanism. Nephron loss secondary to ischemic injury also contributes to the development of azotemia in these patients.

The renal complications of sickle cell disease include the following: *Cortical infarcts* can cause loss of function, persistent hematuria, and perinephric hematomas. *Papillary infarcts*, demonstrated radiographically in 50 percent of patients with sickle trait, lead to an increased risk of bacterial infection in the scarred renal tissues and functional tubule abnormalities. Painless gross hematuria occurs with a higher frequency in sickle trait than in sickle cell disease and likely results from infarctive episodes in the renal medulla. *Functional tubule abnormalities* such as nephrogenic diabetes insipidus result from marked reduction in vasa recta blood flow, combined with ischemic tubule injury. This concentrating defect places these patients at increased risk of dehydration and, hence, sickling crises. The concentrating defect also occurs in individuals with sickle trait. Other tubule defects involve potassium and hydrogen ion excretion, occasionally leading to hyperkalemic metabolic acidosis and a defect in uric acid excretion which, combined with increased purine synthesis in the bone marrow, results in hyperuricemia. Glomerulopathy is an established consequence of sickle cell disease and is due to a combination of hemodynamically mediated glomerular injury referred to earlier and to an immune-complex glomerulonephritis in which tubule epithelial antigens, released into the circulation during episodes of ischemic injury, provoke an antibody response leading to immune-complex deposition in the glomeruli. Proteinuria is the chief manifestation of sickle cell glomerulopathy and may reach nephrotic proportions.

TOXEMIAS OF PREGNANCY (See also Chap. 6)   Renal function is "reset" at a higher level during normal pregnancy. Renal plasma flow (RPF) and glomerular filtration rate (GFR) both increase by 30 to 50 percent. Therefore, serum creatinine levels above 70 μmol/L (0.8 mg/dL) or blood urea nitrogen (BUN) levels above 4.6 mmol/L (13 mg/dL) are abnormal in pregnant women and should be investigated. Systolic and diastolic blood pressures decrease by an average of 10 to 15 mmHg below pregravid values. A diastolic pressure above 75 mmHg during the second trimester or above 85 mmHg during the third trimester is therefore abnormal. Vasodilation in the uterine, renal, and cutaneous beds, vasodilator prostaglandin release from the uteroplacental unit, and a decrease in arteriolar sensitivity to angiotensin II all play a role in the decline of blood pressure during pregnancy.

Preeclampsia-eclampsia   The toxemia syndrome, usually occurring in the third trimester of primigravidas, includes hypertension, proteinuria, edema, consumptive coagulopathy, sodium retention, hyperreflexia (preeclampsia), and, if uncontrolled, convulsions (eclampsia). In pure preeclampsia (i.e., not superimposed on previously existing hypertensive or renal disease), the primary sites of pathology are the glomerular endothelial cells. These cells show marked swelling due to an increase in cytoplasmic volume with vacuolization (endotheliosis) and encroach on the vascular lumen, rendering the enlarged glomeruli ischemic. The glomerular basement membrane and the extraglomerular blood vessels are intact. The pathogenesis is unknown. Coagulation abnormalities, hormonal factors, uteroplacental ischemia, and immune mechanisms have all been implicated. The mechanisms mediating the hypertension are also not understood. Despite sodium retention, intravascular volume is contracted as compared with pregravid values. An increased sensitivity to angiotensin II is the basis for the "roll-over test" (an increase in diastolic blood pressure of 20 mmHg or more upon changing the patient's position from lateral recumbent to supine, presumably due to alterations in circulating angiotensin levels). In the supine position, the reduction in venous return due to compression by the gravid uterus increases circulating levels of angiotensin II. This results in a hypertensive response in preeclamptic patients, who are hyperresponsive to angiotensin II, but not in normal women, in whom pregnancy leads to a relative resistance to the pressor effects of this hormone.

A diagnosis of preeclampsia-related hypertension can be made when repeated measurements over a 4- to 6- h period show a blood pressure of 140/85 mmHg or more. The rise in blood pressure tends to be more severe at night. When preeclampsia occurs in a previously hypertensive patient, a rapid acceleration of the blood pressure elevation is accompanied by an increase in proteinuria, oliguria, edema, and coagulopathy. This is a life-threatening syndrome and tends to recur with future pregnancies. In addition to proteinuria, which correlates with the severity of the renal lesion, GFR and RPF are depressed. In view of the preexisting high levels, however, GFR in preeclamptic women often remains above nonpregnant levels. Uric acid clearance also falls, resulting in hyperuricemia. In the postpartum period, these patients are particularly susceptible to the development of "postpartum renal failure," which is thought to be a form of adult HUS.

Management consists of bed rest in a quiet environment and control of neurologic manifestations and blood pressure, the former with magnesium sulfate and the latter usually with vasodilators such as hydralazine and methyldopa. Diuretics are avoided. The ultimate "treatment" is delivery, which should be induced if fetal maturity is adequate or if life-threatening coagulopathy or renal failure occur. The long-term prognosis is generally favorable.

Development of acute renal failure/preeclampsia in a pregnant woman should alert the physician to potential preexisting renal disease and/or hypertension. The latter is particularly likely if systolic blood pressure is greater than 200 mmHg. Hypertension and preexisting proteinuria tend to worsen in 50 percent of women during pregnancy. In addition, these abnormalities may be unmasked during pregnancy as the first manifestations of an underlying glomerulopathy. Conversely, patients with established underlying renal disease should be followed closely during pregnancy with monthly measurements of 24-h urinary protein excretion and GFR. Sudden deterioration should raise suspicion of superimposed preeclampsia. There is no convincing evidence that pregnancy has an adverse effect on the long-term outcome of immunologic glomerular diseases or diabetic nephropathy. In all situations, control of blood pressure should be the primary therapeutic goal in view of its established beneficial effects on the progression of renal injury.

Bilateral cortical necrosis   Acute bilateral cortical necrosis is associated with septic abortions, abruptio placentae, and preeclampsia. Coagulation in cortical vessels and arterioles leads to renal tissue necrosis. Anuria and renal failure ensue and may be irreversible. In other cases, renal function returns partially, but on long-term follow-up most patients slowly progress to uremia.

VASCULITIS (See also Chap. 241) The kidney is commonly involved in systemic disorders in which necrotizing inflammatory injury to vessels is a primary feature. Several lines of evidence point toward an immunologic pathogenesis for the vasculitides, the prototype of which is periarteritis nodosa (PAN).

Periarteritis nodosa In PAN, arcuate and intralobular arteries are primarily involved. Acute lesions are characterized by destruction of the internal elastic lamina, segmental fibrinoid necrosis of the intima and/or the entire vessel wall, intense intra- and periarterial leukocytic infiltration, and occasional aneurysmal dilatation of the vessel wall (demonstrable radiographically). Fibroblast proliferation leads eventually to occlusion and obliteration of vessel lumina. These vascular changes typically lead to glomerular ischemia, occasionally associated with proliferative changes in the glomerular tufts and juxtaglomerular apparatus. Progression to acute necrotizing crescentic glomerulonephritis may occur.

Clinically, renal involvement in PAN is often associated with hypertension (renin-mediated) which at times progresses to a severe or malignant form. Hematuria, microscopic or gross, also can occur as a result of ischemia, hypertensive renal injury, or glomerulonephritis. Proteinuria is usually mild, and the urinary sediment contains all the formed elements (red and white blood cells, renal epithelial cells, and their respective casts). Nephrotic syndrome is uncommon. Acute renal failure occurs in approximately 10 percent of cases and is usually the result of malignant hypertension and/or the development of rapidly progressive crescentic glomerulonephritis. The diagnosis of PAN can be established by documenting the typical arterial lesions in biopsy material from involved organs (testes, muscle, skin). Renal biopsy seldom shows the arterial lesions but may reveal focal or diffuse crescentic glomerulonephritis. Renal and celiac arteriography, however, frequently demonstrates characteristic aneurysmal dilatation of the involved arteries.

Untreated, PAN is generally progressive, causing death from renal failure, gastrointestinal bleeding, or other extrarenal catastrophes. Encouraging therapeutic results have been obtained with glucocorticoid therapy in combination with cytoxic agents (cyclophosphamide or azathioprine) and plasma exchange. In addition, hypertension should be controlled. Early initiation of antihypertensive therapy prolongs survival in more than 90 percent of patients and causes complete remission in 20 percent. Allergic granulomatosis (Churg-Strauss syndrome), a variant of PAN, is similar in its renal manifestations but also causes immediate-type hypersensitivity reactions, including primary pulmonary involvement, asthma, and eosinophilia.

Hypersensitivity angiitis (microscopic form of PAN) Hypersensitivity angiitis is an acute fulminant form of necrotizing vasculitis in which the characteristic pathologic finding is an intense leukocytic infiltration of the smaller renal vessels (arterioles, venules, capillaries) with or without fibrinoid necrosis. Thus the pathology is more often limited to the glomerular vessels (including the afferent and postglomerular arterioles). The infiltrating leukocytes fragment as they invade the vessel walls, giving rise to the term *leukocytoclastic angiitis*. Endothelial proliferative changes are also seen, and in severe cases the pathologic picture may be indistinguishable from crescentic (rapidly progressive) glomerulonephritis. Immunofluorescence staining may reveal IgG and IgM in the mesangium. In contrast to the subacute or chronic course of PAN, hypersensitivity angiitis is characterized by rapid onset of renal failure. Urinalysis reveals proteinuria (at times reaching nephrotic range), hematuria, and casts. Microangiopathic hemolytic anemia and systemic eosinophilia are often present. Hypertension, however, is characteristically absent or mild. Uremia leads to death in the majority. Treatment regimens are similar to those for PAN, but the response to glucocorticoids appears to be more favorable in this disease than in PAN.

Other vasculitides in which renal involvement is present include

Wegener's granulomatosis (in which the renal lesion is primarily in the form of a necrotizing glomerulitis) and Takayasu's arteritis, which may involve the main renal arteries and their branches (see Chap. 291).

REFERENCES

BARRÉ P et al: Successful treatment with streptokinase of renal vein thrombosis associated with oral contraceptive use. Am J Nephrol 6:316, 1986

BERLAND LL et al: Renal artery stenosis: Prospective evaluation of diagnosis with color duplex US compared with angiography. Radiology 174:421, 1990

EKNOYAN G, RIGGS SA: Renal involvement in patients with thrombotic thrombocytopenic purpura. Am J Nephrol 6:117, 1986

HAKIM RM et al: Successful management of thrombocytopenia, microangiopathic anemia, and acute renal failure by plasmapheresis. Am J Kidney Dis 3:170, 1985

HOFFMAN U et al: Role of duplex scanning for the detection of atheroslerotic renal artery disease. Kidney Int 39:1232, 1991

HOLLENBERG NK: The treatment of renovascular hypertension: Surgery, angioplasty, and medical therapy with converting enzyme inhibitors. Am J Kidney Dis 1(suppl):52, 1987

JACOBSON HR: Ischemic renal disease: An overlooked clinical entity? Kidney Int 34:729, 1988

KASHGARIAN M: Pathology of small blood vessels in hypertension. Am J Kidney Dis 5:A104, 1985

KIM D: Abdominal aorta and renal artery stenosis: Evaluation with MR angiography. Radiology 174:727, 1990

LINDHEIMER MD, BAYLIS C (eds): Renal function and disease in pregnancy: An international symposium. Am J Kidney Dis 9:243, 1987

LLACH F: *Renal Vein Thrombosis*. New York, Futura, 1983

MATERSON BJ: Special uses for captopril. Am J Kidney Dis 1(suppl):88, 1987

MULLER FB et al: The captopril test for identifying renovascular disease in hypertensive patients. Am J Med 80:6333, 1986

RATLIFFE N: Renal vascular disease: Pathology of large blood vessel disease. Am J Kidney Dis 5:A93, 1985

WORKING GROUP ON RENOVASCULAR HYPERTENSION: Final Report: Detection, evaluation, and treatment of renovascular hypertension. Arch Intern Med 147:820, 1987

244   HEREDITARY TUBULAR DISORDERS

FREDRIC L. COE / SATISH KATHPALIA

POLYCYSTIC RENAL DISEASE IN ADULTS

ETIOLOGY AND PATHOLOGY This disorder is found in 1 in 500 autopsies and 1 in 3000 hospital admissions and accounts for approximately 10 percent of end-stage renal failure. Inheritance is autosomal dominant and is linked in most families to the alpha-hemoglobin gene complex and the phosphoglycerate kinase genes on the short arm of chromosome 16. The cortex and medulla of both kidneys are usually filled with thin-walled, spherical cysts, ranging from millimeters to centimeters in diameter, that enlarge the organs and interfere with function, presumably by compressing the nephrons and causing localized obstruction. The cysts are lined by a low cuboidal epithelium and contain straw-colored fluid that becomes hemorrhagic with trauma or infection. The intervening renal parenchyma may be normal or show changes of nephrosclerosis or interstitial nephritis.

CLINICAL FEATURES Symptoms usually begin in the third or fourth decades. Common symptoms include flank pain, gross and microscopic hematuria, especially after trauma, and nocturia due to impaired concentrating ability. Ten percent of patients pass renal calculi whose composition and pathogenesis have not been well studied. Stones and blood clots can cause renal colic. The kidneys are usually palpable and asymmetric and have a knobby surface. Hypertension develops in 75 percent of patients, and progression to chronic renal failure is usual (Table 244-1).

TABLE 244-1 Renal tubule defects

Disease	Renal morphologic abnormalities	Functional abnormalities	Mode of Inheritance*	Associated abnormalities
Adult polycystic disease	Cortical and medullary cysts	Chronic renal failure	AD	Hepatic cysts, intracranial aneurysms
Infantile polycystic disease	Distal tubule and collecting duct cysts	Renal failure in the newborn	AR	Intrahepatic bile duct abnormalities
Childhood polycystic disease	Medullary ductal ectasia	Variable chronic renal failure	AR	Hepatic fibrosis and portal hypertension
Medullary sponge kidneys	Ectatic ducts of Bellini	Nephrocalcinosis	AD + S	None
Medullary cystic disease, recessive	Distal tubule and collecting duct cysts	Chronic renal failure, <20 yr salt wasting, polyuria	AR	Variable retinal degeneration (renal retinal dysplasia)
Medullary cystic disease, dominant	Same	Chronic renal failure, >20 yr salt wasting, polyuria	AD	None
Bartter's syndrome	Hyperplasia of juxtaglomerular and medullary interstitial cells	Hypokalemia, high renin and aldosterone levels, polyuria	AR	None
Liddle's syndrome	None	Hypokalemia, low aldosterone levels	AR	None
Familial nephrogenic diabetes insipidus	None	Vasopressin-resistant renal concentrating defect	XL	None
Renal tubular acidosis, type 1	Papillary nephrocalcinosis	Inability to lower urine pH normally, reduced acid excretion	AD	Periodic paralysis, hypokalemia, non-anion-gap metabolic acidosis, growth retardation, rickets
Renal tubular acidosis, type 2	None	Reduced bicarbonate reabsorption	AR AD XL	Non-anion-gap metabolic acidosis, growth retardation rickets, Fanconi syndrome
Renal tubular acidosis, type 4	Underlying renal disease	Reduced proton and potassium secretion	ACQ	Azotemia
X-linked hypophosphatemia	None	Reduced phosphate reabsorption, hypophosphatemia	XL	Rickets, osteomalacia, normal serum 1,25(OH)$_2$D
Vitamin D–dependent rickets, type 1	None	Defective renal 1,25(OH)$_2$D production	AR	Rickets, osteomalacia, low serum 1,25(OH)$_2$D
Vitamin D–dependent rickets, type 2	None	Defective cell, 1,25(OH)$_2$D receptors	AR	Rickets, osteomalacia, high serum 1,25(OH)$_2$D, variable alopecia
Oncogenic osteomalacia	None	Reduced phosphate reabsorptions, hypophosphatemia	ACQ	Osteomalacia; mesenchymal tumors; cancer of the prostate or lung
Renal glucosuria	None	Reduced glucose reabsorption	AD	None
Isolated hypouricemia	None	Reduced urate reabsorption	AR	Variable hypercalciuria, bone demineralization
Cystinuria	Cystine stones	Reduced reabsorption of dibasic amino acids	AR	Short stature
Hartnup disease	None	Reduced reabsorption of mono-amino and carboxylic amino acids	AR	Pellagra-like rash, ataxia, delirium
Iminoglycinuria	None	Reduced reabsorption of proline, hydroxyproline, and glycine	AR	None
Adult Fanconi syndrome	Swan neck deformity of the proximal tubule	Reduced proximal tubule reabsorption of bicarbonate, glucose, uric acid, phosphate, and amino acids	AR	Rickets, osteomalacia, acidosis, dwarfism, low serum potassium
Lowe's syndrome (oculocerebrorenal syndrome)	Same	Same	XL	Ocular and cerebral malformations

* AR, autosomal recessive; AD, autosomal dominant; XL, X-linked; ACQ, acquired; S, sporadic.

Proteinuria rarely exceeds 2 g/d. Urinary infection occurs at some time in most patients, usually as a consequence of instrumentation and renal calculi; women are infected more frequently than men. Erythrocytosis may occur because of high erythropoietin levels; in other patients hematuria may cause blood loss anemia.

Acute renal failure can result from infection, ureteral obstruction due to clots or stone, or sudden angulation of a ureter by a cyst. Azotemia progresses slowly in the absence of these complications. Patients with end-stage renal failure tend to have higher hematocrits than patients with other renal diseases. Fluid overload is infrequent because of a tendency for renal salt wasting.

Hepatic cysts occur in about 30 percent of patients. Hepatic function is usually normal, and the liver cysts can be asymptomatic, cause epigastric discomfort or biliary colic, or become infected. Cysts also may occur in the spleen, pancreas, lungs, ovaries, testes, epididymis, thyroid, uterus, broad ligament, and bladder. Subarachnoid hemorrhage from intracranial aneurysm causes death or neurologic injury in about a tenth of patients, but routine cerebral arteriography is not warranted. Mitral valve prolapse (25 percent) and mitral, aortic, and tricuspid valve incompetence occur more often than in control groups.

DIAGNOSIS Palpable kidneys, hypertension, and abnormalities of urine in asymptomatic individuals may be the only manifestations. Excretory or retrograde urography typically shows large kidneys with elongated pelvises and flat calyces indented by cysts. Ultrasonography and radioisotopic renal scanning can both demonstrate the cysts quite well. Gray scale sonography is preferable to intravenous pyelography for screening individuals at risk, especially when genetic counseling is desired. Computed tomography may be useful.

TREATMENT Superimposed renal damage such as is produced by analgesics, obstruction, urinary infection, nephrotoxic antibiotics, and hypertension must be guarded against. Dehydration and inadequate intake of sodium chloride (less than 100 mmol/d) should be avoided. The management of chronic renal failure is simplified because fluid overload is not a usual problem and the hypertension usually responds to treatment, but the cysts can cause special problems, such as pain, bleeding, infection, or ureteral obstruction. Puncture of cysts, and in some instances even nephrectomy, may be necessary.

POLYCYSTIC RENAL DISEASE IN INFANTS AND CHILDREN

CLINICAL FEATURES The *infantile form* is manifest at birth by diffusely enlarged kidneys, renal failure, and maldevelopment of intrahepatic bile ducts. The *childhood form* consists of medullary ductal ectasia, which is usually asymptomatic, congenital hepatic fibrosis, and portal hypertension. Both conditions are rare, and both are inherited as autosomal recessive traits. Renal failure develops frequently in both forms, but death in the childhood form is usually due to hepatic disease.

MORPHOLOGY In the infantile form, the distal tubules and collecting ducts are dilated into elongated cysts that are arranged in a radial fashion, particularly in the cortex, and make the kidneys large and spongy. In the childhood form, cysts are fewer, cortical collecting ducts are less involved, and the kidneys are not as large. Small intrahepatic bile ducts are irregularly dilated, and large interconnecting spaces, lined by hyperplastic epithelium, fill the portal areas. There is portal fibrosis rather than dilatation and proliferation of small bile ducts, and portal hypertension is the rule by late childhood.

DIAGNOSIS AND TREATMENT Infantile polycystic kidneys may cause dystocia. At birth they do not function and cause oliguric renal failure, respiratory distress, hypertension, and congestive heart failure. Intravenous pyelography may reveal a mottled appearance with variable retention of contrast material in cysts that corresponds to dilated cortical and medullary collecting ducts. On retrograde urography the calyces are blunted, and pyelotubular reflux may be seen. In the childhood type the intravenous pyelogram may suggest medullary sponge kidney, because medullary tubular ectasia is prominent. Renal failure and chronic infection are common.

MEDULLARY SPONGE KIDNEY

PATHOLOGY The ducts of Bellini, i.e., the terminal collecting ducts that reach the ends of the papillae and drain the urine into the renal pelvis, are dilated to cystic proportions and may contain calcium oxalate calculi. The kidneys are asymmetric, and the more abnormal kidney is usually the larger. One or more medullary cysts are found near the tip of each involved papilla, and calculi form in the terminal collecting ducts in or proximal to the cysts (Fig. 244-1). Parenchymal alterations are secondary to intrarenal obstruction. The cysts are lined by cuboidal and, sometimes, by pseudostratified and stratified squamous epithelium.

CLINICAL DIAGNOSIS AND TREATMENT Medullary sponge kidney is present in 1 in 200 unselected intravenous pyelograms. Although most cases are sporadic, autosomal dominant inheritance has been described. The disease has a bimodal pattern of appearance, the first in adolescence and the second during the third and fourth decades. Calculi, infection, and hematuria occur in 60, 35, and 30 percent of patients, respectively. Papillary nephrocalcinosis due to clusters of stones in cysts is common. Hypercalciuria occurs in about half of stone-forming patients but is equally common in other forms of calcium stone disease (Chap. 245). Hypertension is no more common than in the general population. Renal failure is rare, unless nephrolithiasis and/or renal infections are severe.

The diagnosis is made by intravenous urography. The magnitude of pyelotubular backflow varies from a simple papillary blush to tubular ectasia at the tips of the papillae. Small pyramidal cysts and nephrocalcinosis are frequent, and papillary concretions are obscured by the urographic contrast medium. Ectatic collecting ducts are difficult to fill during retrograde pyelography, and the contrast material remains separate from papillary concretions in the cysts.

Asymptomatic patients require no treatment except advice to avoid dehydration and thereby reduce the risk of stone formation. The cause of stones should be sought and treated conventionally, while infection and urologic consequences of stones should be treated as described in Chap. 245. Medullary sponge kidneys are vulnerable to infection, and urologic instrumentation should therefore be minimized.

MEDULLARY CYSTIC DISEASE (NEPHRONOPHTHISIS COMPLEX)

ETIOLOGY Several hereditary medullary cystic diseases have similar morphology but different patterns of inheritance. The recessive form is associated with renal failure before 20 years of age (early-

FIGURE 244-1 *A.* Radiographic appearance of medullary sponge kidney. Abdominal flat plate reveals multiple bilateral calcifications. *B.* Radiographic contrast material accumulates in the dilated and cystic terminal collecting ducts and obscures the calcifications.

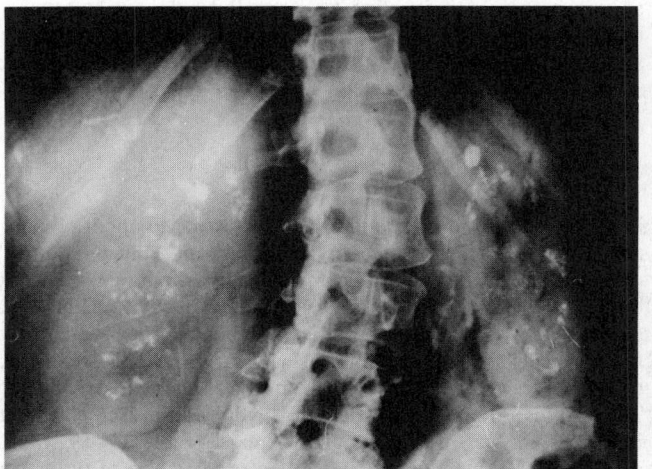

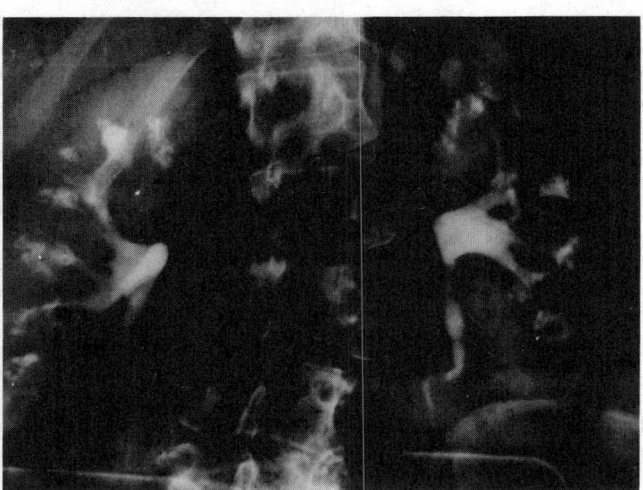

A

B

onset type), whereas the dominant form causes renal failure only after the second decade (adult-onset type). When renal disease is associated with retinal degeneration (renal retinal dysplasia), inheritance is recessive, and renal failure occurs during adult life.

PATHOLOGY   In both forms, most of the cysts are in the medulla and corticomedullary region and involve the collecting ducts and distal convoluted tubules. Cysts have a low, frequently atrophic, epithelium and range in size from micrometers to millimeters. The kidneys usually are asymmetrically scarred and shrunken. Both tubular atrophy and periglomerular fibrosis are present, but the former is more severe. In advanced cases, glomeruli become sclerotic and hyalinized, cortical fibrosis and cellular interstitial infiltration appear, and the histology resembles that of chronic interstitial nephritis.

DIAGNOSIS AND TREATMENT   Concentrating ability, acid excretion, and sodium conservation are defective as might be expected from a lesion that damages distal segments of the nephron. Polyuria, progressive renal failure, stunted growth, severe anemia, hyperchloremic metabolic acidosis, and poor sodium conservation are common. In adults, the inability to conserve sodium may cause salt-wasting that resembles adrenal insufficiency but is unresponsive to mineralocorticoids. Hypertension is a terminal event. The urinalysis is normal at first, but proteinuria may develop. On intravenous pyelography, the kidneys are small, scarred, and without calcification. The calyces are distorted by cysts in the corticomedullary area.

High sodium and water intake and alkali replacement for acidosis are needed. Treatment of infections, anemia, hypertension, and other aspects of end-stage renal failure are as discussed in Chap. 237. Genetic counseling may be helpful in family planning and in selection of an unaffected related donor for renal transplantation.

BARTTER'S SYNDROME

Bartter's syndrome consists of hypokalemia due to renal potassium wasting, elevated plasma renin activity and aldosterone secretion, normal blood pressure, hyporesponsiveness of blood pressure to infused angiotensin II, and hyperplasia of the granular cells of the juxtaglomerular apparatus of the kidney. Weakness or periodic paralysis and polyuria occur because of potassium depletion. Hypomagnesemia may be present. Hyperplasia of renal medullary interstitial cells, which produce prostaglandins PGE and PGF, and elevated PGF_2 production have been described. Inheritance is autosomal recessive, and manifestations commonly begin in childhood.

PATHOGENESIS   The main defect seems to be reduced NaCl reabsorption by the thick ascending limb of Henle's loop (TAHL). Volume depletion stimulates aldosterone production and raises serum aldosterone levels, and the combination of high aldosterone levels and increased delivery of NaCl and water to the distal nephron causes kaliuresis and hypokalemia. Magnesuria and hypomagnesemia occur, perhaps because TAHL is a main site for magnesium reabsorption and because hypomagnesemia enhances kaliuresis. Hypokalemia further increases aldosterone production by stimulating release of prostaglandins E_2 and I_2, which promote increased secretion of renin. Both angiotensin II and aldosterone increase renal kallikrein, which increases plasma bradykinin. The normal blood pressure reflects an interaction between the vasodepressor actions of PGE_2 and bradykinin and elevated angiotensin II. Bartter's syndrome may be mimicked by magnesium deficiency, diuretic use, or vomiting. Magnesium depletion causes kaliuresis; diuretics cause potassium and volume depletion; vomiting causes renal potassium wasting and volume depletion.

Excessive production of PGE_2 resulting from hypokalemia, a stimulator of PGE_2 synthesis, may be a secondary consequence. In some cases blockade of PGE_2 production with indomethacin lowers renin levels and restores vascular response to angiotensin II infusion but does not reduce potassium wasting.

TREATMENT   The dietary intake of sodium chloride and potassium should be liberal; potassium supplements may be required.

Aldosterone antagonists (spironolactone) can prevent potassium wasting, though sodium intake must be increased. Inhibition of prostaglandin synthesis with indomethacin, ibuprofen, or aspirin has varying success, as indicated above. Beta-adrenergic blockade may lower renin production.

LIDDLE'S SYNDROME (PSEUDOHYPERALDOSTERONISM)

This rare inherited disorder is characterized by hypertension, hypokalemic alkalosis, and negligible aldosterone secretion. It appears to be due to an unusual tendency of distal tubules or collecting ducts to conserve sodium and excrete potassium despite the virtual absence of aldosterone. No other biochemical abnormalities have been described. However, transport rates of sodium in red blood cells are altered. These patients respond to 100 mg/d of triamterene (Chap. 195), a diuretic agent that blocks sodium channels in the distal tubule.

X-LINKED NEPHROGENIC DIABETES INSIPIDUS (DI)

In affected males the distal tubules and collecting ducts are unresponsive to vasopressin because of an X-linked recessive disorder, and there is variable expressivity in heterozygous females. Affected individuals excrete large volumes of hypotonic urine even when plasma osmolality and vasopressin concentration are high. Polyuria, polydipsia, and hypertonic dehydration after restriction of fluid intake result from renal tubular insensitivity to vasopressin (AVP) (also see Chap. 333). Unresponsiveness to vasopressin in this disorder is due to mutations that impair the function of the vasopressin receptor (see Chap. 234). Other hereditary tubular defects such as juvenile nephronophthisis, medullary cystic and polycystic diseases, cystinosis, and congenital or acquired chronic urinary tract obstruction also can cause vasopressin-resistant (nephrogenic) DI, but in these syndromes the characteristic features of the underlying disorder are also present.

Affected infants easily become dehydrated, hypernatremic, and hyperthermic, and damage of the central nervous system, including mental retardation, may result. In the absence of dehydration, overall renal function is normal. On intravenous pyelography the renal pelvis, ureters, and bladder are dilated, as in all forms of DI, because of massive diuresis.

Oral hydration usually is adequate treatment except during early infancy, when hypotonic parenteral fluids may be required. Vasopressin and its synthetic analogues are ineffective, but diuretic agents such as hydrochlorothiazide reduce polyuria. This drug inhibits NaCl reabsorption in the distal convoluted tubule, thereby reducing production of free water. In addition, hydrocholorothiazide produces a diuresis, causes contraction of extracellular fluid volume, and in turn, stimulates reabsorption of NaCl and water in the proximal tubule and limits their delivery to the TAHL. Sodium restriction enhances its effect.

RENAL TUBULAR ACIDOSES (RTA)

In these disorders renal excretion of acid is reduced out of proportion to reduction of GFR. Metabolic acidosis results, but in contrast to renal failure the anions that accompany surplus hydrogen ions in the blood, such as sulfate and phosphate, are excreted normally and are unavailable to balance the fall in serum bicarbonate. Therefore, the kidneys reabsorb chloride in unusually large amounts, and serum chloride rises to preserve electroneutrality in the extracellular fluid. The result is *hyperchloremic acidosis*, and the unmeasured anion gap is normal. At least four types of RTA exist (Table 244-2). Types 1 and 2 are often hereditary. Type 3 is a rare mixture of types 1 and 2. Type 4 is acquired and is associated with either hyporeninemic

TABLE 244-2 Comparison of three types of renal tubular acidosis*

Finding	Type 1	Type 2	Type 4
Non-anion-gap acidosis	Yes	Yes	Yes
Minimum urine pH	>5.5	<5.5	<5.5
% filtered HCO_3 excreted	<10	>15	<10
Serum potassium	Low	Low	High
Fanconi syndrome	No	Yes	No
Stones/nephrocalcinosis	Yes	No	No
Daily acid excretion	Low	Normal	Low
Ammonium excretion	High for pH	Normal	Low for pH
Daily HCO_3 replacement needs	<4 mmol/kg	>4 mmol/kg	<4 mmol/kg

* HCO_3, bicarbonate. Type 3 renal tubular acidosis is a rare form of a mixture of types 1 and 2.

hypoaldosteronism or tubular hyporesponsiveness to mineralocorticoids.

TYPE 1 (DISTAL) RTA Sporadic cases occur, but autosomal dominant inheritance is usual. The kidney does not lower urine pH normally, either because the collecting ducts permit excessive back-diffusion of hydrogen ions from lumen to blood or because they fail to transport hydrogen ions against a steep pH gradient. Since titration of urine buffers and diffusion trapping of NH_4^+ in the tubules both depend on a low intraluminal pH, excretion of acid is deficient. However, urine ammonium excretion is as high or higher than in normal people whose urine is equally alkaline. Urinary concentration and potassium conservation also tend to be impaired.

Chronic acidosis lowers tubule reabsorption of calcium, causing renal hypercalciuria and mild secondary hyperparathyroidism. The hypercalciuria, alkaline urine, and low levels of urine citrate, which normally complexes about 40 percent of urine calcium, cause calcium phosphate stones and nephrocalcinosis. Growth in children is stunted because of rickets; this growth defect responds to amelioration of the acidosis with sodium bicarbonate or other alkali. In the adult, osteomalacia occurs. In both children and adults, bone disease may result, in part, from acidosis-induced loss of bone mineral and inadequate production of 1,25-dihydroxyvitamin D_3 [1,25(OH)$_2$D$_3$]. Since the kidney does not conserve potassium or concentrate the urine normally, polyuria and hypokalemia occur. With the stress of an intercurrent illness, acidosis and hypokalemia can be life-threatening.

The diagnosis is suggested by osteomalacia or rickets, hyperchloremic acidosis associated with alkaline urine, and calcium phosphate stones or nephrocalcinosis. To prove that the urine pH cannot be lowered normally, the oral ammonium chloride (NH_4Cl) loading test should be carried out: 0.1 g (1.9 mmol) NH_4Cl per kilogram of body weight is administered, and blood and urine pH are followed with time. Although systemic acidosis worsens, urine pH does not fall below 5.5. Urinary tract infection must not be present during this test because bacteria may possess urease, which hydrolyzes urea to ammonia and produces an alkaline urine. When hyperchloremic acidosis is severe and the urine is grossly alkaline, the test is unnecessary.

A confusing situation may occur when type 1 RTA results from nephrocalcinosis due to hereditary idiopathic hypercalciuria. In this circumstance, stones may be composed of calcium phosphate, but hypokalemia and metabolic acidosis are absent; urine pH is high and does not fall below 5.5 after NH_4Cl administration. *Incomplete RTA* is a common term for this circumstance. Other hereditary diseases that cause RTA, such as medullary sponge kidney, galactosemia, Ehler-Danlos syndrome, Fabry's disease, and hereditary elliptocytosis, can be excluded by clinical findings. The relatives of patients with type 1 RTA should be screened for this treatable disorder.

Treatment Sodium bicarbonate tablets (10 grains = 7.2 mmol base) and Shohl's solution (1 mmol base per milliliter, as Na and K citrate) are both convenient for treatment; the dose should be 0.5 to 2.0 mmol/kg of body weight in four or five divided doses daily. The total dose of alkali should be raised until acidosis and hypercalciuria are both eliminated, and the patients should be followed by measurements of serum chloride and CO_2 content and of urine calcium excretion approximately twice yearly. Potassium supplementation is normally not required. Requirements for alkali usually rise during intercurrent illnesses but are usually below 4 mmol/kg of body weight per day. Incomplete RTA is best treated using thiazide diuretics as in ordinary idiopathic hypercalcemia (Chap. 245).

TYPE 2 (PROXIMAL) RTA Proximal RTA usually occurs as part of a generalized disorder of proximal tubule function. It can be a transient disorder of infancy that disappears in childhood. The pathophysiology is the same whether isolated or part of a generalized disorder. Bicarbonate reabsorption in the proximal tubule is defective, and renal bicarbonate wasting occurs at a normal concentration of plasma bicarbonate. As plasma bicarbonate falls, the filtered load drops to a level that the defective tubule can reabsorb. Then the urine is free of bicarbonate and has a low pH. Potassium wasting and hypokalemia occur, especially when supplementary alkali is given, because bicarbonate is excreted in the urine partly as the potassium salt. Hypercalciuria is moderate, and stone formation is rare. During the NH_4Cl loading test, urine pH falls below 5.5.

Treatment is often not required. When acidosis is severe, bicarbonate must be given in large amounts daily, often >4 mmol/kg of body weight, and even up to 10 mmol/kg per day, because bicarbonate is rapidly excreted in the urine. Another approach is to use a thiazide diuretic and a low-salt diet, which induce mild volume depletion and enhance proximal bicarbonate reabsorption, thereby reducing the required dose. Potassium supplements are needed during treatment because excessive sodium bicarbonate reaches the distal nephron, where much of the sodium is exchanged for potassium, which is then lost in the urine.

TYPE 4 RTA Some patients have a form of renal tubular acidosis that differs from types 1 and 2 and has been called type 4. They have metabolic acidosis without an elevation of the anion gap but differ from type 1 patients in having an acid urine during periods of severe acidosis (see Table 244-2) and from type 2 patients in having low urine excretion of bicarbonate and a daily alkali requirement of <4 mmol/kg of body weight. They differ from both types 1 and 2 in having a high serum potassium and a low urine ammonia excretion. They have neither Fanconi syndrome nor stone disease. Because potassium and hydrogen excretion are abnormal, such patients are considered to have generalized distal nephron dysfunction due either to intrinsic renal disease or to abnormal aldosterone levels. Hyperkalemia worsens acidosis by suppressing renal production of ammonia, which is the most important urinary buffer, and thereby limiting acid excretion.

Most patients with type 4 renal tubular acidosis have hyporeninemic hypoaldosteronism; plasma levels of renin and aldosterone are subnormal, even during extracellular volume depletion. Diabetic nephropathy, nephrosclerosis from hypertension, and chronic tubulointerstitial nephropathies are the usual causes. Hyperkalemia and acidosis can be treated with replacement doses of mineralocorticoid such as fludrocortisone, 0.1 to 0.2 mg/d; some require 0.3 to 0.5 mg/d, suggesting tubule unresponsiveness to the hormone. Furosemide also can improve the hyperkalemia and acidosis, provided salt intake is sufficient to prevent extracellular volume contraction.

A less common condition is *mineralocorticoid-resistant hyperkalemia;* hyperkalemia and acidosis do not improve despite mineralocorticoid treatment. This occurs in occasional patients with renal disease who also have severe salt wasting, as a consequence of distal nephron damage. Plasma renin and aldosterone levels are elevated, and extracellular fluid volume depletion may occur. Treatment requires salt and alkali, but mineralocorticoid supplements are not necessary. Other patients with mild acidosis have no evidence of renal disease and do not waste salt in the urine. Plasma renin and aldosterone levels are low, but hyperkalemia and acidosis do not respond to mineralocorticoid treatment. The cause is thought to be increased distal tubule permeability to chloride ion; sodium chloride reabsorption is elevated, the potential across the distal tubule epithelium is presumed to be below normal, potassium secretion is reduced because it is driven by the transepithelial voltage, hyperkalemia causes acidosis by suppressing ammonia production, and extracellular volume expansion from sodium chloride absorption suppresses renin and aldosterone levels and causes hypertension. The main evidence for this formulation is that infusion of sodium bicarbonate or sodium sulfate raises potassium excretion to normal or supranormal levels. Treatment is with thiazide diuretics or low-sodium diet.

Primary mineralocorticoid deficiency from diseases of the adrenals also causes hyperkalemia and acidosis. Evaluation and treatment of adrenal disorders is discussed in Chap. 335.

VITAMIN D DISORDERS

X-LINKED HYPOPHOSPHATEMIA (See also Chaps. 234 and 358) Reduced tubular reabsorption of phosphate by the proximal tubule and hypophosphatemia occur in this X-linked dominant disease, which is also termed *renal phosphate leak*. Patients may be asymptomatic but are usually short and have rachitic bones; the legs are particularly short and deformed, and osteomalacia develops in adult life. Bone age and dentition are retarded, and the teeth are poorly developed. The skull becomes deformed, and the maxillofacial region may be abnormal. Overgrowth of bone at sites of muscular attachment can limit movement or compress nerves. Bony abnormalities are less common in women. Serum alkaline phosphatase is elevated, serum parathyroid is normal or high, serum calcium is usually normal, and urinary calcium excretion is normal or low.

The hypophosphatemia arises in part from decreased tubular reabsorption of phosphate and increased fractional excretion of phosphate. Intestinal absorption of calcium and phosphate may be decreased in untreated patients and increased during treatment with vitamin D. Although glycinuria and mild glucosuria may occur, most patients exhibit only a defect in excretion of phosphate. Absence of hyperchloremic acidosis and a normal serum calcium concentration help to exclude RTA, malabsorption, and nutritional rickets.

Treatment requires oral neutral phosphate, 1 to 4 g/d, in divided doses, and either calcitriol or some other form of vitamin D. Bony deformities require orthopedic management, but corrective surgery, except for genu valgum, should be postponed until active growth is completed.

VITAMIN D–DEPENDENT RICKETS TYPE 1 (See also Chaps. 234 and 358) Also known as *hereditary pseudovitamin D–deficiency rickets*, this disease is inherited as an autosomal recessive trait. Defective production of $1,25(OH)_2D_3$ by the kidneys, perhaps because of a genetic defect in 25-hydroxycholecalciferol 1α-hydroxylase, is probably the basis for the disease. However, the dose of calcitriol required to heal rickets is higher than that for vitamin D–deficiency rickets, suggesting an attenuated response to, or excessive degradation of, $1,25(OH)_2D_3$.

Rickets usually begins before 2 years of age. Serum calcium is low, parathyroid hormone and alkaline phosphatase levels are high, and plasma phosphorus is variable. Urinary calcium is decreased, fecal calcium is increased, and tubular phosphate reabsorption is reduced. Serum levels of $1,25(OH)_2D$ are undetectable. Aminoaciduria and hyperchloremic acidosis can occur, but urinary cyclic AMP increases normally in response to PTH infusion.

The 1α-hydroxylated metabolites of vitamin D bypass the enzyme defect and produce a dramatic healing of rickets. Vitamin D is also effective, but oral calcium, 0.5 to 2.0 g/d, is needed as well. The need for vitamin D persists throughout life. Calcitriol is the drug of choice, but one must watch for hypercalcemia.

VITAMIN D–DEPENDENT RICKETS TYPE 2 Like type 1, this autosomal recessive disease causes rickets, hypocalcemia, hypophosphatemia, and secondary hyperparathyroidism. Serum levels of $1,25(OH)_2D$ are elevated, and treatment with additional $1,25(OH)_2D$ does not increase the serum calcium level or heal the bone disease

even though it can reduce serum levels of parathyroid hormone. Generalized alopecia is often present and may be either a linked defect or the result of the mineral disorder. The disorder is due to mutations that impair the function of the $1,25(OH)_2D_3$ receptor (also see Chaps. 234 and 329). Treatment with a high dose of calcitriol and mineral supplements may achieve healing of bone, but relapse may occur despite continued treatment.

ONCOGENIC OSTEOMALACIA Mesenchymal tumors, usually benign, can cause renal phosphate wasting similiar to that of X-linked hypophosphatemic rickets, with resulting osteomalacia. Carcinoma of the prostate and oat cell carcinoma of the lung also have caused this syndrome. The disease almost always occurs in adults and develops gradually, over years. The tumors occur mainly in the extremities, head, nose, and mandible, in close association with bone. Their removal cures the phosphate wasting and leads to healing of the osteomalacia.

RENAL GLUCOSURIA (See Chap. 353.)

ISOLATED HYPOURICEMIA (See also Chap. 353.)

There is a defect in proximal tubular reabsorption of sodium urate in this autosomal recessive trait. Hypouricemia also can occur in the Fanconi syndrome, Hartnup disease, and Wilson's disease. Uric acid clearance is high, and urine oxypurine levels are normal, excluding hereditary xanthinuria. Patients are asymptomatic except for occasional uric acid nephrolithiasis. No treatment is needed except the avoidance of dehydration. Coexistent hypercalciuria and decreased bone density have been described in a few patients, who may have a related disease.

SELECTED DISORDERS OF AMINO ACID TRANSPORT

HARTNUP DISEASE (See also Chap. 353) In this rare autosomal recessive disorder, renal and intestinal transport of monoamino-monocarboxylic amino acids is defective. An erythematous, scaly rash appears after exposure to sunlight, and episodic cerebellar ataxia, emotional instability, delirium, and aminoaciduria occur. The prevalence is 1 in 15,000 newborns.

Dietary monoamino-monocarboxylic amino acids undergo bacterial degradation in the intestinal lumen. At the same time, they are lost in the urine. Inadequate tryptophan availability limits nicotinamide synthesis and leads to secondary pellagra (see Chap. 77). Decreased absorption and urine loss of the other monoamino-monocarboxylic amino acids can cause generalized malnutrition.

The diagnosis is based on demonstration of massive urine losses of alanine, serine, threonine, asparagine, glutamine, valine, leucine, isoleucine, phenylalanine, tyrosine, tryptophan, histidine, glycine, and citrulline. Hypouricemia may occur. Renal function is otherwise normal. Most patients respond to treatment with oral nicotinamide, 40 to 200 mg/d, and a high-protein diet to compensate for amino acid malabsorption and loss. The ultimate prognosis is good, and the disease often improves with age.

FAMILIAL IMINOGLYCINURIA (See also Chap. 353) This autosomal recessive trait is characterized by excessive urinary excretion of proline, hydroxyproline, and glycine despite normal plasma levels of these amino acids, probably because of deletion or alteration of a membrane transport protein of the renal tubule cells. The patients are asymptomatic. Iminoglycinuria can occur in normal newborn infants up to 3 months of age.

FANCONI SYNDROME

Fanconi syndrome is a constellation of transport defects in the proximal tubule involving amino acids, monosaccharides, sodium, potassium, calcium, phosphate, bicarbonate, uric acid, and proteins. Generalized aminoaciduria, glucosuria, salt wasting, hypercalciuria, hypophosphatemia, proximal renal tubular acidosis, hypouricemia, and tubular proteinuria (Chap. 44) may result. Fanconi syndrome can be secondary to diseases such as cystinosis, tyrosinemia, galactosemia, fructose intolerance, glycogen storage disease (type 1), Wilson's disease, familial nephrosis, and hereditary amyloidosis. Lowe's (or oculocerebrorenal) syndrome is an X-linked recessive form of the Fanconi syndrome associated with ocular and cerebral abnormalities.

An autosomal recessive disease, *adult Fanconi syndrome*, occurs in the absence of any systemic disorder. The term *adult* is misleading because cases are recognized in childhood, but no abnormalities are apparent at birth. Dwarfism and hypophosphatemic rickets occur along with the laboratory abnormalities of Fanconi syndrome. Renal failure is rare, and the prognosis is good when the systemic manifestations are treated. Typically, there is a "swan-neck" deformity and cellular atrophy of the initial portion of the proximal tubule which is probably the anatomic basis of this tubular disorder. The associated defects in the transport of water, sodium, potassium, acid, and phosphate excretion often require treatment. Water, sodium, and potassium intake must be liberal, and phosphate supplements may be needed. Metabolic acidosis can be corrected by the administration of alkali. Vitamin D helps promote bone healing. Glucosuria, uricosuria, and tubular proteinuria do not require treatment.

CYSTINURIA (See Chap. 353.)

REFERENCES

BERGERON M, SCRIVER CR: Pathophysiology of renal hyperaminoacidurias and glycouria, in *The Kidney*, DW Seldin, G Giebisch (eds). New York, Raven, 1992, p 2947

BERNSTEIN J, KISSANE JM: Hereditary disorders of the kidney: Part 1. Parenchymal defects and malformations. Perspect Pediatr Pathol 1:117, 1973

BUCKALEW VM JR: Calcium nephrolithiasis and renal tubular acidosis, in *Disorders of Bone and Mineral Metabolism*, FL Coe, MJ Favus (eds). New York, Raven, 1992, p 729

CANTANI A et al: Familial juvenile nephronophthisis: A review and differential diagnosis. Clin Pediatr 25:90, 1986

COE FL, PARKS JH: Calcium phosphate stones and renal tubular acidosis, in *Nephrolithiasis: Pathogenesis and Treatment*. Chicago, Year Book, 1988, chap 5

ECONS MJ, DREZNER MK: Bone disease resulting from inherited disorders of renal tubule transport and vitamin D metabolism, in *Disorders of Bone and Mineral Metabolism*, FL Coe, MJ Favus (eds). New York, Raven, 1992, p 935

GABOW PA et al: Polycystic kidney disease: Prospective analysis of nonazulemic patients and family members. Ann Intern Med 101:238, 1984

GARRICK R et al: Bartter's syndrome: A unifying hypothesis. Am J Nephrol 5:379, 1985

HUSSACK KF et al: Echocardiographic findings in autosomal dominant polycystic kidney disease. N Engl J Med 319:907, 1988

LEVEY AS et al: Occult intracranial aneurisms in polycystic kidney disease. N Engl J Med 308:986, 1983

LEVY HL: Hartnup disorder, in *The Metabolic Basis of Inherited Disease*, 6th ed, CR Scriver et al (eds). New York, McGraw-Hill, 1989, chap 101, p 2515

LIBBER S et al: Treatment of nephrogenic diabetes insipidus with prostaglandin synthesis inhibitors. J Pediatr 108:35, 1986

LIDDLE GW et al: A familial renal disorder simulating primary aldosteronism but with negligible aldosterone secretion. Trans Assoc Am Phys 76:199, 1963

MORRIS RC, IVES HE: Inherited disorders of the renal tubule, in *The Kidney*, BM Brenner, FC Rector Jr (eds). Philadelphia, Saunders, 1991, p 1596

RASMUSSEN H, TENENHOUSE HT: Hypophosphatemias, in *The Metabolic Basis of Inherited Disease*, 6th ed, CR Scriver et al (eds). New York, McGraw-Hill, 1989, chap 105, p 2581

REEDERS ST: Genetic abnormalities of renal function, in *The Kidney*, DW Seldin, G Giebisch (eds). New York, Raven, 1992, p 3085

REEVES WB, ANDREOLI TE: Nephrogenic diabetes insipidus, in *The Metabolic Basis of Inherited Disease*, 6th ed, CR Scriver et al (eds). New York, McGraw-Hill, 1989, chap 78, p 1985

SCHWAB SJ et al: Renal infections in autosomal dominant polycystic kidney disease. Am J Med 82:714, 1987

SIRIS ES et al: Tumor-induced osteomalacia. Am J Med 82:307, 1987

TOFUKU Y et al: Hypouricemia due to renal urate wasting: Two types of tubular transport defects. Nephron 30:39, 1982

245 NEPHROLITHIASIS

FREDRIC L. COE / MURRAY J. FAVUS

TYPES OF STONES

Calcium salts, uric acid, cystine, and struvite ($MgNH_4PO_4$) are the basis of most kidney stones in the western hemisphere. Calcium oxalate and calcium phosphate stones make up 75 to 85 percent of the total (Table 245-1) and may be admixed in the same stone. Calcium phosphate in stones is usually hydroxyapatite [$Ca_5(PO_4)_3OH$] or, less commonly, brushite ($CaHPO_4 \cdot H_2O$).

Calcium stones are more common in men; the average age of onset is the third decade. Most persons who form a single calcium stone eventually form another, and the intervals between successive stones shorten or remain constant. The average rate of new stone formation in patients who have had a previous stone is about one stone every 2 or 3 years. Calcium stone disease is frequently familial.

In the urine, calcium oxalate monohydrate crystals (whewellite) usually grow as biconcave ovals that resemble red blood cells in shape and size but may occur in a larger, "dumbbell" form. In polarized light the crystals appear bright against a dark background with an intensity that is dependent on orientation, a property known as *birefringence*. Calcium oxalate dihydrate crystals (weddellite) are bipyramidal and only weakly birefringent. Apatite crystals do not exhibit birefringence and appear amorphous because the actual crystals are too small to be resolved by light microscopy. Brushite produces elongated lathlike (narrow, long, rectangular) crystals.

Uric acid stones (see Table 245-1) are radiolucent and are also more common in men. Half of patients with uric acid stones have gout; uric acid lithiasis is usually familial whether or not gout is present. In urine, uric acid crystals are red-orange in color because they adsorb the pigment uricine. Anhydrous uric acid produces small crystals that appear amorphous by light microscopy. They are indistinguishable from apatite crystals, except for their birefringence. Uric acid dihydrate tends to form teardrop-shaped crystals as well as flat, square plates; both are strongly birefringent. Uric acid gravel appears like red dust, and the stones are also orange or red on some occasions. *Cystine stones* are uncommon (see Table 245-1), are lemon yellow, and sparkle; radiopacity is due to the sulfur content. Cystine crystals appear in the urine as flat, hexagonal plates.

Struvite ($MgNH_4PO_4$) *stones* are common (see Table 245-1) and potentially dangerous. These stones occur mainly in women and result from urinary tract infection with urease-producing bacteria, usually *Proteus* species. The stones can grow to a large size and fill the renal pelvis and calyces to produce a "staghorn" appearance. They are radiopaque and have a variable internal density. In urine, struvite crystals are rectangular prisms said to resemble coffin lids.

MANIFESTATIONS OF STONES

As stones grow on the surfaces of the renal papillae or within the collecting system, they need not produce symptoms. Asymptomatic stones may be discovered during the course of radiographic studies undertaken for unrelated reasons. Stones rank, along with benign and malignant neoplasms, renal cysts, and genitourinary tuberculosis, among the common causes of isolated hematuria. Much of the time, however, stones break loose and enter the ureter or occlude the ureteropelvic junction, causing pain and obstruction.

STONE PASSAGE A stone can traverse the ureter without symptoms, but passage usually produces pain and bleeding. The pain begins gradually, usually in the flank, but increases over the next 20 to 60 min to become so severe that narcotic drugs may be needed for its control. The pain may remain in the flank or spread downward and anteriorly toward the ipsilateral loin, testis, or vulva. Pain that

TABLE 245-1   Major causes of renal stones

Stone type and causes	Percent of all stones*	Percent occurrence of specific causes*	Ratio of men to women	Etiology	Diagnosis	Treatment
Calcium stones	75–85		2:1 to 3:1			
Idiopathic hypercalciuria		50–55	2:1	Hereditary (?)	Normocalcemia, unexplained hypercalciuria[†]	Thiazide diuretic agents
Hyperuricosuria		20	4:1	Diet	Urine uric acid >750 mg per 24 h (women), >800 mg per 24 h (men)	Allopurinol or diet
Primary hyperparathyroidism		5	3:10	Neoplasia	Unexplained hypercalcemia	Surgery
Distal renal tubular acidosis		Rare	1:1	Hereditary	Hyperchloremic acidosis, minimum urine pH >5.5	Alkali replacement
Intestinal hyperoxaluria		~1–2	1:1	Bowel surgery	Urine oxalate >50 mg per 24 h	Cholestyramine or oral calcium loading
Hereditary hyperoxaluria		Rare	1:1	Hereditary	Urine oxalate and glycolic or l-glyceric acid increased	Fluids and pyridoxine
Idiopathic stone disease		20	2:1	Unknown	None of the above present	Oral phosphate, fluids
Uric acid stones	5–8					
Gout		~50	3:1 to 4:1	Hereditary	Clinical diagnosis	Alkali to raise urine pH
Idiopathic		~50	1:1	Hereditary (?)	Uric acid stones, no gout	Allopurinol if daily urine uric acid above 1000 mg
Dehydration		?	1:1	Intestinal, habit	History, intestinal fluid loss	Alkali, fluids, reversal of cause
Lesch-Nyhan syndrome		Rare	Men	Hereditary	Reduced hypoxanthine-guanine phosphoribosyltransferase level	Allopurinol
Malignant tumors		Rare	1:1	Neoplasia	Clinical diagnosis	Allopurinol
Cystine stones	1		1:1	Hereditary	Stone type; elevated cystine excretion	Massive fluids, alkali, D-penicillamine if needed
Struvite stones	10–15		2:10	Infection	Stone type	Antimicrobial agents and judicious surgery

* Values are percent of patients who form a particular type of stone and who display each specific cause of stones.
† Urine calcium above 300 mg per 24 h (men), 250 mg per 24 h (women), or 4 mg/kg per 24 h either sex. Hyperthyroidism, Cushing syndrome, sarcoidosis, malignant tumors, immobilization, vitamin D intoxication, rapidly progressive bone disease, and Paget's disease all cause hypercalciuria and must be excluded in diagnosis of idiopathic hypercalciuria.

migrates downward indicates that the stone has passed to the lower third of the ureter, but if the pain does not migrate, the position of the stone cannot be predicted. A stone in the portion of the ureter within the bladder wall causes frequency, urgency, and dysuria that may be confused with urinary tract infection. Hematuria is usual with passage of a stone.

OTHER SYNDROMES   **Staghorn calculi**   Struvite, cystine, and uric acid stones often grow too large to enter the ureter. They gradually fill the renal pelvis and may extend outward through the infundibula to the calyces themselves.

Nephrocalcinosis   Calcium stones grow on the renal papillae. Most break loose and cause colic, but they may remain in place so that multiple papillary calcifications are found by x-ray, a condition termed *nephrocalcinosis*. Papillary nephrocalcinosis is common in hereditary distal renal tubular acidosis and in other types of severe hypercalciuria. In medullary sponge kidney disease (see Chap. 244) calcification may occur in dilated distal collecting ducts.

Sludge   Sufficient uric acid or cystine in the urine may plug both ureters with precipitate. Calcium oxalate crystals do not do this because less than 100 mg oxalate usually is excreted daily in the urine even in severe hyperoxaluric states, compared with 1000 mg uric acid in patients with hyperuricosuria and 400 to 800 mg cystine in patients with cystinuria. Calcium phosphate crystals can render the urine milky but do not plug the urinary tract.

INFECTION   Although urinary tract infection is not a direct consequence of stone disease, it can occur after instrumentation and surgery of the urinary tract, which are frequent in the treatment of stone disease. Stone disease and urinary infection can enhance the seriousness of one another and interfere with treatment. Obstruction of an infected kidney by a stone may lead to sepsis and extensive damage of renal tissue, since it converts the urinary tract proximal to the obstruction into a closed, or partially closed, space that can

become an abscess. On the other hand, infection due to bacteria that possess the enzyme urease can cause stones composed of struvite.

ACTIVITY OF STONE DISEASE   *Active disease* means that new stones are forming or that preformed stones are growing. Sequential radiographs of the renal areas are needed to document the growth or appearance of new stones and to ensure that passed stones are actually newly formed, not preexistent ones.

PATHOGENESIS OF STONES

Urinary stones usually arise because of the breakdown of a delicate balance. The kidneys must conserve water, but they also must excrete materials that have a low solubility. These two opposing requirements must be balanced during adaptation to diet, climate, and activity. The problem is mitigated to some extent by the fact that urine contains substances that inhibit crystallization of calcium salts and others that bind calcium in soluble complexes. These protective mechanisms are less than perfect. When the urine becomes supersaturated with insoluble materials, because excretion rates are excessive and/or because water conservation is extreme, crystals form and may grow and aggregate to form a stone.

SUPERSATURATION   In a solution in equilibrium with crystals of calcium oxalate, the product of the chemical activities of the calcium and oxalate ions in the solution is termed the *equilibrium solubility product*. If the crystals are removed, and if either calcium or oxalate ions are added to the solution, the activity product increases, but the solution may remain clear; no new crystals form. Such a solution is *metastably supersaturated*. If new calcium oxalate seed crystals are now added, they will grow in size. Ultimately, the activity product reaches a critical value at which a solid phase begins to develop spontaneously. This value is called the *upper limit of* *metastability*, or the *formation product*. Stone growth in the urinary tract requires a urine that, on average, is above the equilibrium solubility product. Persistence of a stone requires an average activity product at least equal to the solubility product. Excessive supersaturation is common in stone formation.

Calcium, oxalate, and phosphate form many stable soluble complexes among themselves and with other substances in urine, such as citrate. As a result, their free ion activities are below their chemical concentrations and can be measured only by indirect techniques. Reduction in ligands such as citrate can increase ion activity without changing total urinary calcium. Urine supersaturation can be increased by dehydration or by overexcretion of calcium, oxalate, phosphate, cystine, or uric acid. Urine pH is also important; phosphate and uric acid are weak acids that dissociate readily over the physiologic range of urine pH. Alkaline urine contains more urate and dissociated phosphate, favoring deposits of sodium hydrogen urate, brushite, and apatite. Below a urine pH of 5.5, uric acid crystals (pK 5.47) predominate, whereas phosphate crystals are rare. The solubility of calcium oxalate, on the other hand, is not influenced by changes in urine pH. Measurements of supersaturation in a pooled 24-h urine sample probably underestimate the risk of precipitation. Transient dehydration or postprandial bursts of overexcretion may cause values considerably above average.

NUCLEATION **Homogeneous nucleation** In urine that is supersaturated with respect to calcium oxalate, these two ions form clusters. The higher the supersaturation, the larger and more numerous are the clusters. Most small clusters eventually disperse because the internal forces that hold them together are too weak to overcome the random tendency of ions to move away. Clusters of over 100 ions can remain stable because attractive forces balance surface losses. Once they are stable, nuclei can grow at levels of supersaturation below that needed for their creation. The formation product marks the point at which stable nuclei become frequent enough to create a permanent solid phase.

Heterogeneous nucleation If a supersaturated urine is seeded with preformed nuclei of a crystal that is similar in structure to calcium oxalate, calcium and oxalate ions in solution will bind to the crystal's surface as they would on a seed crystal of calcium oxalate itself. The organized growth of one crystal on the surface of another is called *epitaxial growth*, and the seeding of a supersaturated solution by foreign nuclei is called *heterogeneous nucleation*. Sodium hydrogen urate, uric acid, and hydroxyapatite crystals can serve as heterogeneous nuclei that permit calcium oxalate stones to form even though urine calcium oxalate supersaturation never exceeds the metastable limit.

INHIBITORS OF CRYSTAL GROWTH AND AGGREGATION Stable nuclei must grow and aggregate to produce a stone of clinical significance. Urine contains potent inhibitors of both these processes for calcium oxalate and calcium phosphate but not for uric acid, cystine, or struvite. Inorganic pyrophosphate is a potent inhibitor that appears to affect calcium phosphate more than calcium oxalate crystals. Other urine components that appear to be glycoproteins inhibit the growth of calcium oxalate crystals. Slowing of crystal growth increases the apparent upper limit of metastability because the critical growth of ion clusters into stable nuclei is hindered. As a consequence of the presence of these inhibitors, crystal growth in urine is slow compared with growth in simple salt solutions, and the upper limit of metastability is higher. Urine citrate also may inhibit crystal growth or nucleation.

EVALUATION AND TREATMENT OF PATIENTS WITH NEPHROLITHIASIS

Most patients with nephrolithiasis have remediable metabolic disorders that cause stones and can be detected by chemical analyses of serum and urine. A practical outpatient evaluation consists of three 24-h urine collections, each with a corresponding blood sample; measurements of serum and urine calcium, uric acid and creatinine, urine oxalate and

citrate, and serum electrolytes should be made. When possible, the composition of kidney stones should be determined because treatment depends on stone type (see Table 245-1). No matter what disorders are found, every patient should be counseled to avoid dehydration and to drink six to eight glasses of water daily. Since treatment is prolonged, the use of medications must be justified by the activity and severity of stone disease and the importance of protection against new stones.

The management of stones already present in the kidneys or urinary tract requires a combined medical and surgical approach. The specific treatment depends on the location of the stone, the extent of obstruction, the function of the affected and unaffected kidneys, the presence or absence of urinary tract infection, the progress of stone passage, and the risk of operation or anesthesia given the clinical state of the patient. In general, severe obstruction, infection, intractable pain, and serious bleeding are indications for removal of a stone.

In the past, stones were removed by operation or by passing a flexible basket retrograde up the ureter from the bladder during cystoscopy. There are now three alternatives. Extracorporeal lithotripsy causes the in situ fragmentation of stones in the kidney, renal pelvis, or proximal ureter by exposing them to shock waves. The patient is submerged in a water tank, the kidney with the stone is centered at the focal point of parabolic reflectors, and high-intensity shock waves are created by high-voltage discharge. The waves are focused by the reflectors so that they pass through the patient and fracture the stone as they pass. After multiple discharges, most stones are reduced to powder that moves through the ureter into the bladder. Larger fragments are removed by cystoscopy. Percutaneous ultrasonic lithotripsy requires the passage of a rigid cystoscope-like instrument into the renal pelvis through a small incision in the flank. Stones can be disrupted by a small ultrasound transducer, and fragments can be removed directly. The last method is endoscopic passage of an ultrasonic transducer into the ureter via a cystoscope; ureteral stones that are inaccessible to extracorporeal or percutaneous lithotripsy can be fragmented and removed. These various forms of lithotripsy have largely replaced pyelolithotomy and ureterolithotomy.

CALCIUM STONES **Idiopathic hypercalciuria** (See also Chap. 357) This condition appears to be hereditary, and its diagnosis is straightforward (see Table 245-1). In some patients, primary intestinal hyperabsorption of calcium causes transient postprandial hypercalcemia that suppresses secretion of parathyroid hormone. The renal tubules are deprived of the normal stimulus to reabsorb calcium at the same time that the filtered load of calcium is increased. In other patients, reabsorption of calcium by the renal tubules appears to be defective, and secondary hyperparathyroidism is evoked by urinary losses of calcium. Renal synthesis of 1,25-dihydroxyvitamin D is increased, enhancing intestinal absorption of calcium. In the past, the separation of "absorptive" and "renal" forms of hypercalciuria was used to guide treatment. However, these may not be distinct entities but the extremes of a continuum of behavior. Hypercalciuria contributes to stone formation by raising urine saturation with respect to calcium oxalate and calcium phosphate.

Thiazide diuretics lower urine calcium in both types of hypercalciuria and are effective in preventing the formation of stones. The drug effect requires slight contraction of the extracellular fluid volume, and massive use of NaCl reduces its therapeutic effect. Potassium citrate is useful to prevent hypokalemia and raise urine citrate; the latter lowers urine calcium ion levels.

Hyperuricosuria About 20 percent of calcium oxalate stone formers are hyperuricosuric, primarily because of an excessive intake of purine from meat, fish, and poultry. The mechanism of stone formation probably is heterogeneous nucleation of calcium oxalate by crystals of sodium hydrogen urate or uric acid. A low purine diet is desirable but difficult for many patients to achieve. The alternative is allopurinol, usually 100 mg bid.

Primary hyperparathyroidism (See also Chap. 357) The diagnosis of this condition is established by documenting that hypercalcemia that cannot be otherwise explained is accompanied by inappropriately elevated serum concentrations of parathyroid hormone. Hypercalciuria, usually present, raises the urine supersaturation of calcium phosphate and/or calcium oxalate (see Table 245-1). Prompt diagnosis is important because parathyroidectomy should be carried out before renal damage occurs.

Distal renal tubular acidosis (See also Chap. 244)   The defect in this condition seems to reside in the distal nephron, which cannot establish a normal pH gradient between urine and blood, leading to hyperchloremic acidosis. The minimum urine pH in response to an oral challenge with NH_4Cl, 1.9 mmol/kg of body weight, is above 5.5. Hypercalciuria, an alkaline urine, and a low urine citrate level cause supersaturation with respect to calcium phosphate. Calcium phosphate stones form, nephrocalcinosis is common, and osteomalacia or rickets may occur. Renal damage is frequent, and glomerular filtration rate falls gradually. Treatment with supplemental alkali reverses hypercalciuria and limits the production of new stones. The usual dose of sodium bicarbonate is 0.5 to 2.0 mmol/kg of body weight per day in four to six divided doses. An alternative is Shohl's solution, which contains citrate and citric acid. In incomplete renal tubular acidosis (RTA), systemic acidosis is absent, but urine pH cannot be lowered below 5.5 after an exogenous acid load such as ammonium chloride. Incomplete RTA may develop in some patients who form calcium oxalate stones because of idiopathic hypercalciuria; the importance of the RTA in producing stones in this situation is uncertain, and thiazide treatment is a reasonable alternative. Some patients with incomplete RTA form calcium phosphate stones because of low urine citrate and an alkaline urine and are best treated with alkali as if RTA were complete.

Hyperoxaluria   Overabsorption of dietary oxalate and consequent oxaluria, i.e., so-called intestinal oxaluria, is one consequence of fat malabsorption (Chap. 254). The latter can be caused by a variety of conditions, including bacterial overgrowth syndromes, chronic disease of the pancreas and biliary tract, jejunoileal bypass in treatment of obesity, or ileal resection for inflammatory bowel disease. With fat malabsorption, calcium in the bowel lumen is bound by fatty acids instead of oxalate, which is left free for absorption in the colon. Delivery of unabsorbed fatty acids and bile salts to the colon may injure the colonic mucosa and enhance oxalate absorption. Dietary excess of oxalate, ascorbic acid loading, and hereditary hyperoxaluric states are less common causes of hyperoxaluria. Ethylene glycol intoxication and methoxyflurane also can cause oxalate overproduction and hyperoxaluria. Hyperoxaluria from any cause can produce tubulointerstitial nephropathy (Chap. 242) and lead to stone formation.

The oxalate-binding resin cholestyramine at a dose of 8 to 16 g/d, correction of fat malabsorption, and a low-fat diet are effective treatments for oxaluria secondary to intestinal absorption. Calcium lactate, 8 to 14 g/d, which precipitates oxalate in the gut lumen, is an alternative form of therapy. There is no treatment for primary hyperoxaluria, the result of an enzymatic defect involving the metabolism of the precursor of oxalate that is inherited as an autosomal recessive (also see Chap. 352). A high fluid intake, phosphate, and pyridoxine (200 mg/d) are recommended, but irreversible renal failure secondary to recurrent stone formation usually occurs before age 20.

Idiopathic calcium lithiasis   At least 20 percent of patients have no obvious cause for stones (see Table 245-1). The best treatment appears to be a high fluid intake so that the urine specific gravity remains at 1.005 or below throughout the day and night. Oral phosphate at a dose of 2 g phosphorus daily may lower urine calcium and increase urine pyrophosphate and thereby reduce the rate of recurrence. Orthophosphate causes mild nausea and diarrhea initially, but tolerance may improve with continued intake. Thiazide treatment to reduce calcium excretion and allopurinol to diminish uric acid output also may be helpful.

URIC ACID STONES   These stones form because the urine becomes supersaturated with undissociated uric acid, uric acid that is protonated at its N-9 position. In gout, idiopathic uric acid lithiasis, and dehydration, the average pH is usually below 5.4 and often below 5.0. Undissociated uric acid therefore predominates and is soluble in urine only in concentrations of 100 mg/L. Concentrations above this level represent supersaturation that causes crystals and stones to form. Hyperuricosuria, when present, increases supersaturation, but urine of low pH can be supersaturated with undissociated uric acid even though the daily excretion rate is normal. Myeloproliferative syndromes, chemotherapy of malignant tumors, and the Lesch-Nyhan syndrome cause such massive production of uric acid and consequent hyperuricosuria that stones and uric acid sludge form even at a normal urine pH. Plugging of the renal collecting tubules by uric acid crystals can cause acute renal failure.

The two goals of treatment are to raise urine pH and to lower excessive urine uric acid excretion to less than 1 g/d. Supplemental alkali, 1 to 3 mmol/kg of body weight per day, should be given in three or four evenly spaced, divided doses, one of which should be given at bedtime. The form of the alkali may be important. Potassium citrate may reduce the risk of calcium salts crystallizing when urine pH is increased, whereas sodium citrate or sodium bicarbonate may increase the risk. If the overnight urine pH is below 5.5, the evening dose of bicarbonate may be raised, or 250 mg acetazolamide added at bedtime. With massive overexcretion of uric acid, doses of allopurinol above 300 mg daily may be needed. Treatment with allopurinol should be instituted prior to chemotherapy of highly cellular tumors, since massive hyperuricosuria can be expected. Alkali treatment must be avoided if hypercalciuria is also present.

CYSTINURIA AND CYSTINE STONES (See also Chap. 352)   In this disorder, proximal tubular and jejunal transport of the dibasic amino acids cystine, lysine, arginine, and ornithine are defective, and excessive amounts are lost in the urine. Clinical disease is due solely to the insolubility of cystine, which forms stones.

Pathogenesis   Cystinuria probably occurs because of defective transport of amino acids by the brush borders of renal tubule and intestinal epithelial cells. Cystine, lysine, arginine, and ornithine appear to share a common renal transport pathway, since infusion of lysine decreases tubular reabsorption of the other three. However, cystine is also transported by a separate transport mechanism, because cystinuria and dibasic aminoaciduria can occur independently. The intestinal defects are not similar in all patients who are homozygous for cystinuria, and the extent of aminoaciduria in individuals who are heterozygous carriers of the defect varies from family to family. Three types of inheritance have been described (see Chap. 352).

Diagnosis and treatment   Cystine stones are formed only by patients with cystinuria, but 10 percent of stones in cystinuric patients do not contain cystine; therefore, every stone former should be screened for the disease. The sediment from a first morning urine specimen in many patients with homozygous cystinuria reveals typical flat hexagonal platelike cystine crystals. Cystinuria also can be detected using the urine sodium nitroprusside test. The test is positive with 75 to 125 mg cystine per gram of creatinine, a concentration lower than that in the urine of patients with cystinuria but above the levels in normal urine. Because the test is sensitive, it is positive in many asymptomatic heterozygotes for cystinuria. A positive nitroprusside test or the finding of cystine crystals in the urine sediment should be evaluated by measurement of daily cystine excretion. Normal adults excrete 40 to 60 mg cystine per gram of creatinine, heterozygotes usually excrete less than 300 mg/g, and homozygotes almost always excrete above 250 mg/g.

Treatment consists of a high fluid intake, even at night. Daily urine volume should exceed 3 L. Raising urine pH with alkali is helpful, provided the urine pH exceeds 7.5. Because side effects are frequent, penicillamine, which forms the soluble disulfide cysteine-penicillamine, should be used only when fluid loading and alkali therapy are ineffective. Mercaptopropinylglycine has been used to dissolve renal calculi by perfusion of the renal pelvis and has been given by mouth to prevent stones. Low-methionine diets have not proved to be practical for clinical use.

STRUVITE STONES   These stones are a result of urinary infection with bacteria, usually *Proteus* species, which possess urease, an enzyme that degrades urea to NH_3 and CO_2. The NH_3 hydrolyzes to

NH_4^+ and raises pH, usually to 8 or 9. The CO_2 hydrates to H_2CO_3 and then dissociates to CO_3^{2-} which precipitates with calcium as $CaCO_3$. The NH_4^+ precipitates PO_4^{3-} and Mg^{2+} to form $MgNH_4PO_4$. The result is a stone of calcium carbonate admixed with struvite. Struvite does not form in urine in the absence of infection, because NH_4^+ concentration is low in urine that is alkaline in response to physiologic stimuli. Chronic *Proteus* infection can occur because of impaired urinary drainage, urologic instrumentation or surgery, and especially with chronic antibiotic treatment, which can favor the dominance of *Proteus* in the urinary tract.

Treatment Methenamine mandelate, which lowers urine pH and liberates formaldehyde, is used for chronic suppression of infection when a stone is present. More extreme lowering of urine pH with chronic administration of NH_4Cl may retard stone growth but also may raise urine calcium level and promote the formation of calcium oxalate stones. Antimicrobial treatment is best reserved for dealing with acute infection and for maintenance of a sterile urine after surgery, in the hope of preventing recurrence or minimizing stone growth. Surgery may be appropriate for severe obstruction, pain, bleeding, or intractable urinary infection. Since stones can regrow from any infected fragment which is left behind, recurrences following operation are quite common. In some centers it is possible to irrigate the renal pelvis and calyces with Renacidin, a solution that dissolves struvite, using a catheter passed through a cutaneous flank incision into the kidney.

REFERENCES

COE FL, PARKS JH: *Nephrolithiasis: Pathogenesis and treatment*. Chicago, Year Book, 1988
———et al: Effect of low calcium diet on urine calcium excretion, parathyroid function, and serum 1,25(OH)$_2$D$_3$ levels in patients with idiopathic hypercalciuria and in normal subjects. Am J Med 72:25, 1982
COE FL, FAVUS MJ: Disorders of stone formation, in *The Kidney*, 4th ed, BM Brenner, FC Rector Jr (eds). Philadelphia, Saunders, 1991, p 1728
LEMANN J JR: Pathogenesis or idiopathic hypercalciuria and nephrolithiasis, in *Disorders of Bone and Mineral Metabolism*, FL Coe, MJ Favus (eds). New York, Raven, 1992, p 685
LINGEMAN JF: Mechanisms of stone disruption and dissolution, in *Disorders of Bone and Mineral Metabolism*, FL Coe, MJ Favus (eds). New York, Raven, 1992, p 625
NAKAGAWA Y et al: Purification and characterization of the principal inhibitors of calcium oxalate monohydrate crystal growth in human urine. J Biol Chem 258:12594, 1983
NEWMAN DM et al: Long-term follow-up of 1,900 ESWL treatments, in *Shock Wave Lithotripsy*, JE Lingeman, DM Newman (eds). New York, Plenum, 1988
RESNICK MI, PAK CYC: *Urolithiasis*. Philadelphia, Saunders, 1991
SMITH LH: Urolithiasis, in *Diseases of the Kidney*, 4th ed, RW Schrier, CW Gottschalk (eds). Boston, Little, Brown, 1988, p 785
STRAUSS AL et al: Factors that predict relapse of calcium nephrolithiasis during treatment. Am J Med 72:25, 1982

---

246 URINARY TRACT OBSTRUCTION

JULIAN L. SEIFTER / BARRY M. BRENNER

Obstruction to the flow of urine, with attendant stasis and elevation in urinary tract pressure, impairs renal and urinary conduit functions and is a common cause of acute and chronic renal failure. With early relief of obstruction, the defects in function usually disappear completely. However, chronic obstruction may produce permanent loss of renal mass (renal atrophy) and excretory capability, as well as enhanced susceptibility to local infection and stone formation. Early diagnosis and prompt therapy are therefore essential to minimize the otherwise devastating effects of obstruction on kidney structure and function.

ETIOLOGY Obstruction to urine flow can result from *intrinsic* or *extrinsic mechanical blockade* as well as from *functional defects* not associated with fixed occlusion of the urinary drainage system.

Mechanical obstruction can occur at any level of the urinary tract, from the renal calyces to the external urethral meatus. Normal points of narrowing, such as the ureteropelvic and ureterovesical junctions, bladder neck, and urethral meatus, are common sites of obstruction. When blockage is above the level of the bladder, unilateral dilatation of the ureter (*hydroureter*) and renal pyelocalyceal system (*hydronephrosis*) occur; lesions at or below the level of the bladder cause bilateral involvement.

Common forms of obstruction are listed in Table 246-1. In childhood, *congenital malformations*, including marked narrowing of the ureteropelvic junction, anomalous (retrocaval) location of the ureter, and posterior urethral valves, predominate. The latter defect is the most common cause of bilateral hydronephrosis in boys. Children also may have bladder dysfunction secondary to congenital urethral stricture, urethral meatal stenosis, or bladder neck obstruction. In adults, urinary tract obstruction is due mainly to *acquired defects*. Pelvic tumors, calculi, and urethral stricture predominate. Ligation of, or injury to, the ureter during pelvic or colonic surgery can lead to hydronephrosis which, if unilateral, may remain relatively silent and undetected. *Schistosoma haematobium* and genitourinary tuberculosis are infectious causes of ureteral obstruction. Obstructive uropathy also may result from extrinsic neoplastic (carcinoma of cervix or colon, retroperitoneal lymphoma) or inflammatory disorders. One such inflammatory disorder is retroperitoneal fibrosis, a process of unknown cause seen most commonly in middle-aged men, which occasionally leads to bilateral ureteral obstruction. Retroperitoneal fibrosis must be distinguished from other retroperitoneal causes of ureteral obstruction, particularly lymphomas and pelvic neoplasms.

Functional impairment of urine flow usually results from disorders that involve both the ureter and bladder. Common functional lesions include neurogenic bladder, often with adynamic ureter, and vesicoureteral reflux. Reflux of urine from bladder to ureter(s) is more

TABLE 246-1 Common mechanical causes of urinary tract obstruction

Ureter	Bladder outlet	Urethra
CONGENITAL		
Ureteropelvic junction narrowing or obstruction	Bladder neck obstruction	Posterior urethral valves
Ureterovesical junction narrowing or obstruction	Ureterocele	Anterior urethral valves
Ureterocele		Stricture
Retrocaval ureter		Meatal stenosis
		Phimosis
ACQUIRED INTRINSIC DEFECTS		
Calculi	Benign prostatic hyperplasia	Stricture
Inflammation	Cancer of prostate	Tumor
Trauma	Cancer of bladder	Calculi
Sloughed papillae	Calculi	Trauma
Tumor	Diabetic neuropathy	Phimosis
Blood clots	Spinal cord disease	
Uric acid crystals	Anticholinergic drugs and alpha-adrenergic antagonists	
ACQUIRED EXTRINSIC DEFECTS		
Pregnant uterus	Carcinoma of cervix, colon	Trauma
Retroperitoneal fibrosis	Trauma	
Aortic aneurysm		
Uterine leiomyomata		
Carcinoma of uterus, prostate, bladder, colon, rectum		
Retroperitoneal lymphoma		
Accidental surgical ligation		

common in children than in adults and may result in severe unilateral or bilateral hydroureter and hydronephrosis. Abnormal insertion of the ureter into the bladder is the most common cause of vesicoureteral reflux in children. Reflux in the absence of urinary tract infection or bladder neck obstruction usually does not lead to renal parenchymal damage and often resolves spontaneously as the child matures. Surgical reinsertion of the ureter into the bladder is indicated if reflux is severe and unlikely to improve spontaneously if renal function deteriorates or if urinary tract infections recur despite chronic antimicrobial therapy. Hydronephrosis, usually more marked on the right than on the left, is common in pregnancy, due both to ureteral compression by the enlarged uterus and to functional effects of progesterone.

CLINICAL FEATURES   The pathophysiology and clinical features of urinary tract obstruction are summarized in Table 246-2. *Pain* is the symptom which most commonly provokes the need for medical attention. The pain of urinary tract obstruction is due to distention of the collecting system or renal capsule. The severity of the pain is influenced more by the rate at which distention develops than by the degree of distention. Acute supravesical obstruction, as from a stone lodged in a ureter (Chap. 245), is associated with excruciatingly severe pain, usually called *renal colic*. This pain is relatively steady and continuous, with little fluctuation in intensity, and often radiates to the lower abdomen, testes, or labia. By contrast, more insidious causes of obstruction, such as chronic narrowing of the ureteropelvic junction, may produce little or no pain yet result in total destruction of the affected kidney. Flank pain which occurs only with micturition is pathognomonic of vesicoureteral reflux.

Azotemia develops in urinary tract obstruction when overall excretory function is impaired. This may occur in the setting of bladder outlet obstruction, bilateral renal pelvic or ureteric obstruction, or unilateral disease in a patient with a solitary functioning kidney. Complete bilateral obstruction should be suspected when acute renal failure is accompanied by anuria. Any patient with renal failure otherwise unexplained or with a history of nephrolithiasis, hematuria, diabetes mellitus, prostatic enlargement, pelvic surgery, trauma, or tumor should be evaluated for urinary tract obstruction.

Symptoms of *polyuria* and *nocturia* commonly accompany chronic partial urinary tract obstruction and result from impaired renal concentrating ability. This defect usually does not improve with administration of vasopressin and is therefore a form of acquired nephrogenic diabetes insipidus. Disturbances in sodium chloride transport in the ascending limb of Henle and, in azotemic patients, the osmotic (urea) diuresis per nephron lead to decreased medullary hypertonicity and hence a concentrating defect. Partial obstruction, therefore, may be associated with increased rather than decreased urine output. Indeed, wide fluctuations in urine output in a patient with azotemia should always raise the possibility of intermittent or partial urinary tract obstruction. If fluid intake is inadequate, severe dehydration and hypernatremia may develop. Hesitancy and straining to initiate the urinary stream, postvoid dribbling, urinary frequency, and (overflow) incontinence are common with obstruction at or below the level of the bladder (see Chap. 44).

In addition to loss of urinary concentrating ability and azotemia, partial bilateral urinary tract obstruction often results in other derangements of renal function, including *acquired distal renal tubular acidosis, hyperkalemia*, and *renal salt wasting*. These defects in tubule function are often accompanied by renal tubulointerstitial damage. Morphologic abnormalities appear early in the course of obstruction; initially the interstitium becomes edematous and infiltrated with mononuclear inflammatory cells. With continued obstruction, the interstitium becomes fibrotic; scarring and atrophy of the papillae and medulla occur and precede these processes in the cortex.

The possibility of urinary tract obstruction must always be considered in patients with urinary tract infections or urolithiasis. Urinary stasis encourages the growth of organisms as well as the formation of crystals, especially magnesium ammonium phosphate (struvite). *Hypertension* is frequent in acute and subacute unilateral obstruction and is usually a consequence of increased release of renin by the involved kidney. Chronic unilateral or bilateral hydronephrosis, in the presence of extracellular volume expansion or other renal disease, may result in significant hypertension. *Polycythemia*, an infrequent complication of obstructive uropathy, is probably secondary to increased erythropoietin production by the obstructed kidney.

DIAGNOSIS   A history of difficulty in voiding, pain, infection, or changes in urinary volume is common. Evidence for distention of the kidney or urinary bladder often can be obtained by palpation and percussion of the abdomen. A careful rectal examination may reveal enlargement or nodularity of the prostate, abnormal rectal sphincter tone, or a rectal or pelvic mass. The penis should be inspected for evidence of meatal stenosis or phimosis. In the female, vaginal, uterine, and rectal lesions responsible for urinary tract obstruction are usually revealed by inspection and palpation.

Urinalysis and examination of the urine sediment may reveal hematuria, pyuria, and bacteriuria. Often, however, the urine sediment is normal, even when obstruction leads to marked azotemia and extensive structural damage. An abdominal scout film should be obtained to evaluate the possibility of nephrocalcinosis or a radiopaque stone at any level of the urinary collecting system. As indicated in Fig. 246-1, if urinary tract obstruction is suspected, abdominal ultrasonography should be performed to evaluate renal and bladder size, as well as pyelocalyceal contour. If these structures are not distended, functionally significant urinary tract obstruction can safely be excluded in differential diagnosis. Abdominal ultrasound also may detect an obstructing pelvic mass.

Intravenous pyelography is indicated if an obstructive abnormality is revealed by ultrasound. If the patient is not azotemic, a standard dose of contrast medium usually provides adequate information. With renal insufficiency, however, high-dose (drip-infusion) pyelography with nephrotomography is usually required for adequate visualization. In the presence of obstruction, the appearance time of the nephrogram is often delayed but eventually becomes more dense than normal because of slow tubular fluid flow rate which results in enhanced water reabsorption by the nephrons and greater concentration of contrast medium within tubules. The kidney involved by an acute

TABLE 246-2   Pathophysiology of bilateral ureteral obstruction

Hemodynamic effects	Tubule effects	Clinical features
ACUTE		
↑ Renal blood flow ↓ GFR ↓ Medullary blood flow ↑ Vasodilator prostaglandins	↑ Ureteral and tubule pressures ↑ Reabsorption of Na$^+$, urea, water	Pain (capsule distention) Azotemia Oliguria
CHRONIC		
↓ Renal blood flow ↓ ↓ GFR ↑ Vasoconstrictor prostaglandins ↑ Renin-angiotensin production	↓ Medullary osmolarity ↓ Concentrating ability Structural damage; parenchymal atrophy ↓ Transport functions for Na$^+$, K$^+$, H$^+$	Azotemia Hypertension ADH-insensitive polyuria Natriuresis Hyperkalemic, hyperchloremic acidosis
RELEASE OF OBSTRUCTION		
Slow ↑ in GFR (variable)	↓ Tubule pressure ↑ Solute load per nephron (urea, NaCl) Natriuretic factors present	Postobstructive diuresis Potential for volume depletion and electrolyte imbalance (Na$^+$, K$^+$, PO$_4^{2-}$, Mg^{2+} excretion)

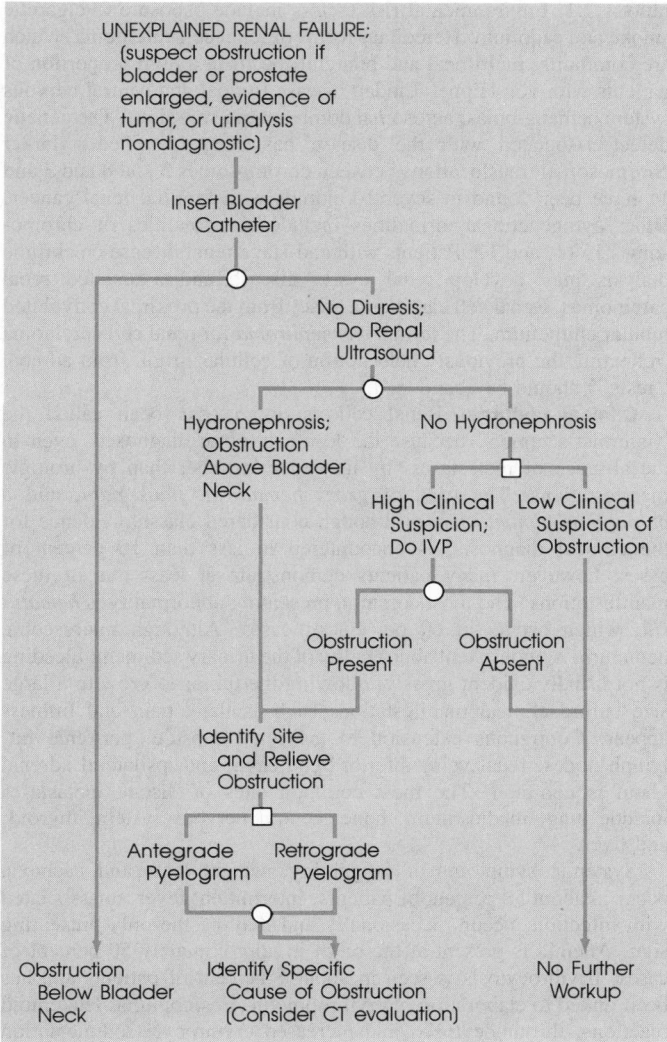

UNEXPLAINED RENAL FAILURE;
(suspect obstruction if
bladder or prostate
enlarged, evidence of
tumor, or urinalysis
nondiagnostic)

Insert Bladder
Catheter

No Diuresis;
Do Renal
Ultrasound

Hydronephrosis;
Obstruction
Above Bladder
Neck

No Hydronephrosis

High Clinical
Suspicion;
Do IVP

Low Clinical
Suspicion of
Obstruction

Obstruction
Present

Obstruction
Absent

Identify Site
and Relieve
Obstruction

Antegrade
Pyelogram

Retrograde
Pyelogram

Obstruction
Below Bladder
Neck

Identify Specific
Cause of Obstruction
(Consider CT evaluation)

No Further
Workup

FIGURE 246-1 Diagnostic approach for urinary tract obstruction in unexplained renal failure. Circles represent diagnostic procedures, and squares indicate clinical decisions based on available data. CT, computed tomography; IVP, intravenous pyelogram.

obstructive process is usually slightly enlarged, and there is dilatation of the calyces, renal pelvis, and ureter above the obstruction. The ureter, however, is not tortuous, as is the case when the obstruction is chronic. In comparison with the nephrogram, the pyelogram may be extremely faint, especially if the dilated renal pelvis is voluminous, causing dilution of the contrast medium. The radiographic study should be continued until the site of obstruction is determined or the contrast medium is excreted. Radionuclide scans define less anatomic detail than intravenous pyelography and, like the pyelogram, are of limited value when renal function is poor. Nonetheless, such scans are sensitive for the detection of obstruction and provide a substitute test in some patients at high risk for reaction to intravenous contrast dyes.

Patients suspected of having intermittent ureteropelvic obstruction (whether functional or mechanical) should have radiologic evaluation while they are in pain, since a normal pyelogram is commonly seen during asymptomatic periods. Hydration or mannitol infusion often helps to provoke a symptomatic attack. Voiding cystourethrography is of great value in the diagnosis of vesicoureteral reflux and bladder neck and urethral obstructions. Patients with obstruction at or below the level of the bladder exhibit thickening, trabeculation, and diverticula of the bladder wall. Postvoiding films reveal residual urine. If

these radiographic studies fail to provide adequate information for diagnosis, endoscopic visualization by the urologist often permits precise identification of lesions involving the urethra, prostate, bladder, and ureteral orifices. To facilitate visualization of a suspected lesion in a ureter or renal pelvis, *retrograde* or *antegrade pyelography* should be attempted. These diagnostic studies may be preferable to the intravenous pyelogram in the azotemic patient, in whom poor excretory function precludes adequate visualization of the collecting system. Furthermore, intravenous pyelography carries the risk of contrast-induced renal failure in patients with renal insufficiency, diabetes mellitus, and multiple myeloma, particularly when performed under conditions of dehydration. For these reasons, retrograde and antegrade pyelography may offer advantages over the intravenous approach in the diagnostic evaluation of the azotemic patient. The retrograde approach involves catheterization of the involved ureter under cystoscopic control, while the antegrade technique necessitates placement of a catheter into the renal pelvis via a needle inserted percutaneously under ultrasonic or fluoroscopic guidance. While the antegrade approach carries the added advantage of providing immediate decompression of a unilateral obstructing lesion, many urologists initially attempt the retrograde approach and resort to the antegrade method only when attempts at retrograde catheterization are unsuccessful or when cystoscopy or general anesthesia is contraindicated.

Computed tomography is useful in the diagnosis of specific intraabdominal and retroperitoneal causes of obstruction but is less practical as an initial test to establish the presence of obstruction. Magnetic resonance imaging also may be useful in the identification of specific obstructive causes.

TREATMENT AND PROGNOSIS An individual with any form of urinary tract obstruction complicated by infection requires relief of obstruction as soon as possible to prevent development of generalized sepsis and progressive renal damage. On a temporary basis, depending on the site of obstruction, drainage is often satisfactorily achieved by nephrostomy, ureterostomy, or ureteral, urethral, or suprapubic catheterization. The patient with acute urinary tract infection and obstruction should be given appropriate antibiotics based on in vitro bacterial sensitivity and ability of the drug to concentrate in the kidney and urine. Treatment may be required for 3 to 4 weeks. Chronic or recurrent infections in an obstructed kidney with poor intrinsic function may necessitate nephrectomy. When infection is not present, immediate surgery often is not required, even in the presence of complete obstruction and anuria (because of the availability of dialysis), at least until acid-base, fluid and electrolyte, and cardiovascular status are restored to normal. Nevertheless, the site of obstruction should be ascertained as soon as feasible, in part because of the possibility that sepsis may occur and necessitate prompt urologic intervention. Elective relief of obstruction is usually recommended in patients with urinary retention, recurrent urinary tract infections, persistent pain, or progressive loss of renal function. Infrequently, mechanical obstruction can be alleviated by nonsurgical means, as with radiation therapy for retroperitoneal lymphoma. Likewise, functional obstruction secondary to neurogenic bladder may be decreased with the combination of frequent voiding and cholinergic drugs. The approach to obstruction secondary to renal stones is discussed in Chap. 245.

With relief of obstruction, the *prognosis* regarding return of renal function depends largely on whether irreversible renal damage has occurred. When obstruction is not relieved, the course will depend mainly on whether the obstruction is complete or incomplete, bilateral or unilateral, and whether urinary tract infection is also present. Complete obstruction with infection can lead to total destruction of the kidney within days. In dogs, relief of complete obstruction of 1 and 2 weeks' duration restores glomerular filtration rate to 60 and 30 percent of normal, respectively; after 8 weeks of obstruction, recovery does not occur. Nevertheless, in the absence of definitive evidence of irreversibility, every effort should be made to decompress in the hope of restoring renal function at least partially.

In patients undergoing cystectomy for bladder cancer, the ileal conduit is the currently preferred urinary diversionary procedure. This approach is preferable to ureterosigmoidostomy, a procedure complicated by a high incidence of ureteral obstruction, reflux, hypokalemic metabolic acidosis, pyelonephritis, and neoplasms developing at the ureteral anastomotic site.

POSTOBSTRUCTIVE DIURESIS Relief of bilateral, but not unilateral, complete urinary tract obstruction commonly leads to a postobstructive diuresis, characterized by polyuria, which may be massive. The urine is usually hypotonic and may contain a large amount of sodium chloride. The natriuresis is due, at least in part, to the excretion of retained urea, which acts as a poorly reabsorbable solute and diminishes salt and water reabsorption in the tubules (osmotic diuresis). The increase in intratubular pressure very likely also contributes to the impairment in net sodium chloride reabsorption, especially in the terminal nephron segments. Natriuretic factors (other than urea) also may accumulate during uremia induced by obstruction and depress salt and water reabsorption when urine flow is reestablished. In the majority of patients this diuresis is physiologic, resulting in the *appropriate* excretion of the excesses of salt and water retained during the period of obstruction. When extracellular volume and composition return to normal, the diuresis usually abates spontaneously. Therefore, replacement of urinary losses should serve only to prevent hypovolemia, hypotension, or disturbances in serum electrolyte concentrations. Occasionally, iatrogenic expansion of extracellular volume, secondary to administration of excessive quantities of intravenous fluids, is responsible for, or sustains, the diuresis observed in the postobstructive period. Replacement of no more than two-thirds of urinary volume losses per day is usually effective in avoiding this complication. In a rare patient, however, relief of obstruction may be followed by urinary salt and water losses severe enough to provoke profound dehydration and vascular collapse. In these patients, an intrinsic defect in tubule reabsorptive function is probably responsible for the marked diuresis. Appropriate therapy in such patients includes intravenous administration of large quantities of salt-containing solutions to replace sodium and volume deficits.

REFERENCES

GILLENWATER JY: The pathophysiology of urinary obstruction, in *Campbell's Urology*, 6th ed, PC Walsh et al (eds). Philadelphia, Saunders, 1992, pp 499–532

HARRIS RH, YARGER WE: The pathogenesis of post-obstructive diuresis. J Clin Invest 56:880, 1975

KAYE AD, POLLACK HM: Diagnostic imaging approach to the patient with obstructive uropathy. Semin Nephrol 2:55, 1982

WILSON DR: Renal function during and following obstruction. Ann Rev Med 28:329, 1977

————: Urinary tract obstruction, in *Diseases of the Kidney*, 4th ed, RW Schrier, SW Gottschalk (eds). Boston, Little, Brown, 1988, p 715

YARGER WE: Urinary tract obstruction, in *The Kidney*, 4th ed, BM Brenner, FC Rector Jr (eds). Philadelphia, Saunders, 1991, p 1768

---

247 TUMORS OF THE URINARY TRACT

MARC B. GARNICK / BARRY M. BRENNER

TUMORS OF THE KIDNEY

RENAL CELL CARCINOMA Renal cell carcinoma (renal adenocarcinoma, formerly "hypernephroma") accounts for 85 percent of all primary renal neoplasms. Approximately 25,000 new cases are diagnosed annually, with 10,000 deaths in the United States. The peak age incidence is between 55 and 60 years; the male-to-female ratio is 2:1. Environmental risk factors include exposure to cigarette smoke and cadmium. Hereditary forms of renal cell carcinoma, which are commonly multifocal and bilateral, occur in a high proportion of patients with von Hippel–Lindau disease (retinal and central nervous system hemangiomas, autosomal dominant transmission). The genetic defect associated with the disease has been identified. Marker chromosomal translocations between chromosomes 3 and 8 and 3 and 11 have been found in several kindreds with familial renal cancer. Other cytogenetic abnormalities include abnormalities of chromosomes 1, 11, and 17. Patients with end-stage renal disease on chronic dialysis may develop renal cystic disease and associated renal carcinomas. Renal cell carcinoma arises from the proximal convoluted tubular epithelium. The term *hypernephroma* for renal cell carcinoma (reflecting the previously held notion of cellular origin from adrenal "rests") should be abandoned.

Clinical features Renal cell carcinoma has been called the "internist's tumor" because the lesion is often diagnosed, even in the absence of metastases, by its *systemic* rather than by urologic manifestations. The triad of *gross hematuria, flank pain*, and a *palpable abdominal mass*, although considered classic evidence for the clinical diagnosis, is encountered in less than 10 percent of cases; however, many patients demonstrate at least one of these manifestations. The most common presenting abnormality is *hematuria*, which occurs in 60 percent of cases. Although microscopic hematuria is a consistent abnormality of the urinary sediment, bleeding is not usually evident grossly, allowing the tumor to grow to a large size before clinical manifestations such as flank pain and fullness appear. Contiguous extension to the renal capsule, perirenal fat, lymph nodes, renal vein, inferior vena cava, and ipsilateral adrenal gland is common. The most common sites of distant metastases include lung, mediastinum, bone, central nervous system, thyroid, and liver.

Systemic symptoms of fatigability, weight loss, and cachexia occur in about 50 percent of patients. Intermittent fever, unassociated with infection, occurs occasionally and may be the only presenting sign. Anemia is present at the onset in approximately 50 percent of cases. Erythrocytosis is seen in about 5 percent of patients and has been linked to elaboration of erythropoietin. Eosinophilia, leukemoid reactions, thrombocytosis, and increased erythrocyte sedimentation rate also occur. Renal cell carcinomas may produce hormones or hormone-like substances, including parathyroid hormone and prostaglandins (which may lead to hypercalcemia), prolactin (galactorrhea), renin (hypertension), gonadotropins (feminization and masculinization), and glucocorticoids (Cushing's syndrome). In vascular tumors, intrarenal arteriovenous fistulas may predispose to high-output congestive heart failure. Tumor invasion of the renal vein and inferior vena cava may result in the development of abrupt, symptomatic left varicocele and lower extremity edema, respectively. Hepatic vein occlusion by tumor, with or without vena caval obstruction, may lead to hepatosplenomegaly and ascites. Disturbances in liver function (elevated alkaline phosphatase, hypoalbuminemia, and prolonged prothrombin time) are sometimes found in patients without demonstrable liver metastases and are often reversed following removal of the primary tumor.

Diagnosis (Fig. 247-1) Although intrarenal calcifications and/or alterations in renal contours on the abdominal scout film may suggest the presence of a renal cell carcinoma, *intravenous pyelography* (IVP) with *nephrotomography* is the primary examination by which most renal masses are detected and evaluated. The major task is to differentiate cystic lesions from renal neoplasms. Splaying, distortion, or nonvisualization of the collecting system and distorted renal outlines suggest cancer. Nephrotomography provides clear delineation of renal borders and further aids in distinguishing cystic from solid lesions. *Ultrasonography* has improved the ability to distinguish cysts from renal neoplasms. When combined with nephrotomography, the accuracy of ultrasonography in diagnosing a benign cyst approaches 97 percent. If a cystic lesion on IVP, combined with a benign-appearing sonolucent cystic lesion on ultrasound, is found in an asymptomatic

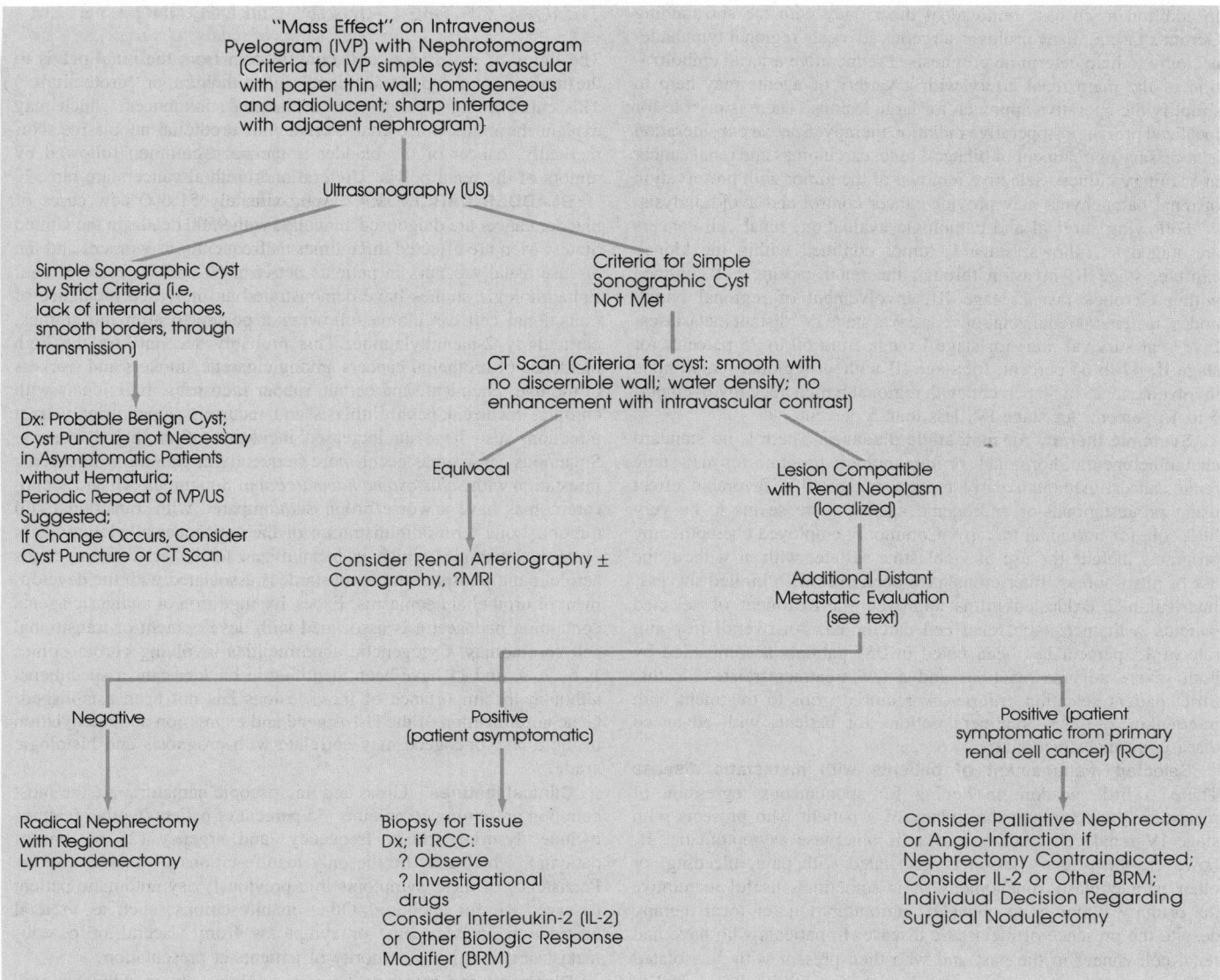

FIGURE 247-1   Diagnostic evaluation for renal mass.

patient without hematuria, cyst puncture is probably unnecessary. Repeat IVP or ultrasound should then be performed periodically, initially every year and then, if no change has occurred during the interval, less often.

If diagnostic accuracy beyond 97 percent is required, or if there are changes on repeat IVP or ultrasound, needle aspiration with evaluation of the aspirated fluid for cytology can be performed. The finding of clear yellow fluid or negative cytology usually supports the diagnosis of a simple cyst. Aspiration of cloudy or bloody fluid usually demands a surgical diagnosis, even though the cytology may be negative for cancer. A renal cystogram following aspiration can sometimes provide additional valuable information. Although renal cell carcinoma may coexist within a simple cyst, this is rare.

If the IVP or ultrasound examination demonstrates a lesion which does not satisfy the criteria for a benign, simple cyst, *computed tomography* (CT) is the next modality employed. CT is comparable and possibly superior to selective renal arteriography in both diagnosing and staging renal cell carcinoma. In addition, CT is equivalent to selective renal arteriography in the determination of renal vein involvement and superior to arteriography in determining whether regional nodes are enlarged (representing either tumor or hyperplasia) and/or the liver is involved. CT is the preferred modality for the diagnosis and staging of renal cell carcinoma. Thus selective renal

arteriography is not necessarily needed preoperatively. If, however, the findings on CT are equivocal or additional definition of vascular anatomy is required, renal arteriography should complement CT studies. Magnetic resonance imaging (MRI) also has been used extensively in the evaluation of renal masses. Its role compared to CT scanning is being defined; MRI may provide information for preoperative tumor staging, including nodal anatomy, perirenal fat involvement, adjacent organ extension, and renal vein involvement with thrombosis.

OTHER STUDIES   Evaluation of urinary cytology is not useful in the diagnosis of renal adenocarcinomas. Retrograde pyelography may be a useful adjunct for opacifying the collecting systems that are not filled by standard IVP and may suggest the diagnosis of transitional cell carcinoma of the renal pelvis. In patients who present with hematuria and a renal mass, cystoscopy is an important adjunct to exclude the coexistence of an unsuspected urothelial tumor, such as carcinoma of the bladder. If the diagnosis of renal cell carcinoma is likely, the patient should then undergo routine chest x-ray, bone scan, and liver function studies in addition to the abdominal CT to evaluate other potential sites of tumor spread.

Staging, primary treatment, and prognosis   If there is no evidence of metastatic disease following the preoperative evaluation, the treatment of choice for renal cell carcinoma is radical nephrectomy.

In addition to en bloc removal of the kidney with the surrounding Gerota's fascia, many urologic surgeons advocate regional lymphadenectomy to help determine prognosis. Preoperative arterial embolization of the main renal artery with a variety of agents may help to simplify the operative approach for large lesions. There is no role for localized pre- or postoperative radiation therapy. Special consideration is necessary in treatment of bilateral renal carcinomas and renal cancer in a solitary kidney. Selective removal of the tumor with preservation of renal parenchyma may provide cancer control and avoid dialysis.

Following surgical and pathologic evaluation, renal cell cancers are staged as follows: stage I, tumor confined within the kidney capsule; stage II, invasion through the renal capsule but confined within Gerota's fascia; stage III, involvement of regional lymph nodes, ipsilateral renal vein, or vena cava; stage IV, distant metastases. Five-year survival rates for stage I range from 60 to 75 percent; for stage II, 47 to 65 percent; for stage III without regional lymph node involvement, 25 to 50 percent; with regional lymph node involvement, 5 to 15 percent; for stage IV, less than 5 percent.

Systemic therapy for metastatic disease　There is no standard chemotherapeutic, hormonal, or immunologic program for metastatic renal cancer. Although early reports suggested a favorable effect using progestational or androgenic agents, there seems to be very little role for hormonal therapy. Commonly employed chemotherapy programs include the use of vinblastine sulfate, with or without the use of nitrosoureas. Interferons have been used with limited success. Interleukin 2 (Aldesleukin) is approved for treatment of selected patients with metastatic renal cell carcinoma. An overall response rate of 15 percent has been noted in 255 patients accompanied by both severe adverse reactions and a few treatment-related deaths. Strict patient selection criteria are required prior to treatment with interleukin 2. Other treatment options for patients with advanced disease are investigational.

Selected management of patients with metastatic disease　There is little wisdom in hoping for spontaneous regression of metastases by removing the kidney of a patient who presents with stage IV renal cell carcinoma who is otherwise asymptomatic. If, however, the primary lesion is associated with pain, bleeding, or other paraneoplastic phenomena, it is sometimes useful to remove the primary tumor or to consider angioinfarction for local therapy despite the presence of metastatic disease. In patients who have had renal cell cancer in the past and who then present with an isolated pulmonary or central nervous system metastasis, it is often useful to resect these metastases. Generally, patients selected for surgical nodulectomy have been disease-free for at least 1 year from the original diagnosis to the time of metastatic development and have tumors with a slow doubling time. On occasion, radiation therapy may offer palliation for painful bony lesions and may relieve an obstructed bronchus or ureter.

MISCELLANEOUS TUMORS OF THE KIDNEY　In children, Wilms' tumor (nephroblastoma) is the most common cancer of the kidney. These tumors respond well to multimodality therapy, including surgery, radiation, and combination chemotherapy, usually with dactinomycin and vincristine. Metastatic lesions to the kidney occur commonly in patients with lung and breast cancer and melanoma. Kidney involvement with malignant lymphoma, too, is common; however, functional renal abnormalities from parenchymal involvement are unusual.

Benign renal tumors are usually recognized as incidental findings at autopsy. CT scanning may suggest the presence of an angiomyolipoma, especially in patients with tuberous sclerosis. Surgery should always be considered when radiographic studies are equivocal. In addition, on occasion, benign lesions can cause persistent hematuria and, like the renal oncocytoma, can undergo malignant degeneration. These lesions are usually managed with nephrectomy when detected clinically. In newborns and infants, mesoblastic nephroma (fetal hamartoma) is the most common benign tumor and is successfully treated by simple nephrectomy.

TUMORS OF THE URINARY COLLECTING SYSTEM

The lining of the urinary collecting system from the renal pelvis to the urethra is made up of transitional cell epithelium, or "urothelium." This entire lining is subject to carcinogenic influences, which may explain the multicentric characteristics of urothelial neoplasms. Numerically, cancer of the bladder is the most common followed by tumors of the renal pelvis. Ureteral and urethral cancers are rare.

BLADDER CARCINOMA　Approximately 51,600 new cases of bladder cancer are diagnosed annually, with 9500 deaths in the United States. Men are affected three times as frequently as women, and the disease usually occurs in patients between 60 and 70 years of age. Epidemiologic studies have demonstrated an increased incidence of transitional cell carcinoma following exposure to aromatic amines, particularly 2-naphthylamine. This probably accounts for the high incidence of urothelial cancers among cigarette smokers and workers in the dye, chemical, and certain rubber industries. Individuals with chronic, recurrent nephrolithiasis and recurrent upper urinary tract infections also have an increased incidence of urothelial cancers. Squamous carcinomas occur more frequently in patients with chronic infestation with *Schistosoma haematobium*. Squamous cell and adenocarcinomas have a worse prognosis compared with transitional cell tumors. Long-term administration of the anticancer alkylating agent cyclophosphamide, which is metabolized to the active compounds acrolein and phosphoramide mustard, is associated with the development of urothelial neoplasms. Excessive ingestion of analgesic agents containing phenacetin is associated with development of transitional cell carcinomas. Cytogenetic abnormalities involving chromosomes 1, 5, 7, 9, and 11 have been identified in bladder cancer specimens, although the importance of these lesions has not been established. Gene amplification of the H-*ras* gene and expression and methylation in the c-*myc* oncogene may correlate with prognosis and histologic grade.

Clinical features　Gross and microscopic hematuria are the most common presenting complaints (75 percent of patients); other features include dysuria, urinary frequency, and urgency (25 percent of patients), which may be the only manifestations of bladder cancer. Persistence of these symptoms in a previously asymptomatic patient deserves careful attention. Other manifestations, such as ureteral obstruction, pelvic pain, or symptoms from visceral or osseous metastases, occur in a minority of patients at presentation.

Diagnosis and staging　Urinary cytology, obtained by examination of bladder washing, catheterized urine or voided urine, IVP, and cystoscopic evaluation with tumor biopsies and selected mucosal biopsies, as well as bimanual examination under anesthesia, are the mainstays for diagnosis of bladder cancer. Findings on IVP that suggest a bladder carcinoma include unilateral or bilateral ureteral obstruction with hydronephrosis, filling defect, or lack of distensibility of the bladder. Additional staging information may be obtained with abdominal or pelvic CT scanning. Following endoscopic resection of a bladder neoplasm, the depth of penetration into the bladder wall is assessed. If additional staging procedures, including physical examination, chest x-ray, and routine serum chemistries, are within normal limits, the patient is clinically staged, based on the cystoscopic biopsy, as having either *superficial* or *invasive* disease. Additional information about perivesical extension or nodal metastases can be obtained at the time of cystectomy and indicates the true pathologic stage of disease. A substantial number of patients who are clinically staged endoscopically as having muscle-invasive disease will have occult lymphatic or distant metastases if surgically staged at the time of cystectomy. Such occult micrometastatic disease indicates systemic involvement and accounts for the high percentage of patients who eventually develop distant metastatic disease despite treatment of the primary bladder lesion.

Treatment　Bladder cancer can be subdivided conceptually as being *superficial, invasive,* or *metastatic. Superficial carcinoma* of the bladder includes patients with carcinoma in situ, mucosal involvement (stage 0), or submucosal involvement (stage A). These patients are generally treated with endoscopic resection and selected bladder biopsies with repeat cystoscopic evaluations every 3 to 6 months. Approximately 50 to 70 percent of these patients have a superficial recurrence (limited to the mucosa or submucosa) within a period of 3 years following initial diagnosis. Patients with superficial recurrences are then often treated with intravesical therapies, including thiotepa, doxorubicin, mitomycin, bacillus Calmette-Guérin (BCG), or interferons, in addition to cystoscopic resection. BCG is most effective in treating carcinoma in situ of the urinary bladder. Other modalities include laser therapy applied directly to superficial lesions and photodynamic therapies in which hematoporphyrin derivatives, administered intravesically, can help localize superficial carcinomas. The use of intravesical therapy in selected instances may decrease the number of superficial recurrences and prolong relapse-free intervals.

An additional 12 percent with initial superficial disease eventually develop progressive disease into the bladder muscularis (stage B) and perivesical fat (stage C) or metastatic disease to lymph nodes (stage D1), bone, or other viscera (stage D2). Alternatively, patients may present initially with invasive or metastatic disease.

INVASIVE DISEASE These patients generally have extension of tumor into the muscle and/or perivesical fat. Traditional treatments are cystectomy (radical or simple) or radiation therapy. Preoperative radiation therapy followed by cystectomy does not provide survival benefit as compared with cystectomy alone. Five-year survival rates are approximately 50 percent with such treatments. The majority of these patients die of distant metastatic disease despite radical surgery or radiation rather than from local recurrences. In addition, the use of multimodality therapy, including chemotherapy with radiation therapy, may spare individuals with invasive disease radical cystectomy. Surgical techniques, utilizing portions of the small bowel as bladder reservoirs, have enhanced the quality of life in individuals undergoing radical cystectomy. Such procedures allow continent urinary diversion (e.g., Koch pouch, Indiana pouch, or Mainz pouch), thus eliminating the need for an external ostomy appliance. Many clinical studies today utilize systemic chemotherapy prior to definitive surgery or radiation therapy in attempts to "control" suspected systemic micrometastatic disease, as well as to improve control of the primary lesion. Preliminary data are encouraging.

METASTATIC DISEASE For patients who have distant metastatic disease in lymph nodes, viscera, or bone, the use of systemic chemotherapy has produced responses from 30 to 70 percent of patients but usually not lasting more than 6 months. Following the development of metastatic disease, most patients die within 2 years. The most active agents include cisplatin, methotrexate, doxorubicin, cyclophosphamide, and vinblastine, and combinations of these agents have on occasion produced meaningful and durable remissions. Myelosuppression, a common toxicity of chemotherapy programs, can be ameliorated with concurrent administration of erythropoietin.

TRANSITIONAL CELL CANCER OF THE RENAL PELVIS Renal pelvic tumors account for approximately 10 percent of all primary renal cancer. Nearly 90 percent are transitional cell carcinomas. In addition to the etiologic associations implicated for bladder carcinoma, renal pelvic tumors also occur with analgesic abuse nephropathy. These patients are usually middle-aged women with a psychiatric history or chronic headaches who ingest >3 kg of analgesics over years.

Most patients present with painless gross hematuria. Ureteral obstruction and pain secondary to clots are unusual. The diagnosis is suggested by IVP, which may demonstrate an obstructed, poorly functioning, or nonvisualized kidney or filling defects in a visualized kidney, and a positive urinary cytology. Cystoscopy and retrograde pyelography with brush biopsy generally establish the nature and location of the renal pelvic or ureteral tumor. For low-grade, low-stage tumors, conservative treatment with local excision and preservation of the kidney parenchyma is associated with favorable 5-year survival rates. For high-stage, high-grade lesions, the treatment of choice is radical nephroureterectomy and removal of the cuff of the bladder containing the ipsilateral ureteral orifice. This operative approach is dictated by the high likelihood of recurrence in the ureteral stump and orifice if not removed. In addition, routine follow-up with cystoscopies and urinary cytologies are mandatory to help detect the subsequent development of metachronous bladder carcinomas and/or contralateral ureteral and renal pelvic tumors. Five-year survival rates range from 10 to 50 percent. Although chemotherapy programs employed for bladder cancer have been used for patients with metastatic transitional cell carcinoma of the renal pelvis, the overall results are not as successful.

REFERENCES

BRODSKY G, GARNICK MG: Renal tumors in the adult patient, in *Renal Pathology*, CC Tisher, BM Brenner (eds). Philadelphia, Lippincott, 1989, p 1467

CHISHOLM GD, ROY RR: The systemic effects of malignant renal tumors. Br J Urol 43:687, 1971

CRONAN J, ZEMAN RK: Renal mass imaging: The internist's role. Am J Med 81:1026, 1986

CRONIN RE et al: Renal cell carcinoma: Unusual systemic manifestations. Medicine 55:291, 1976

GARNICK MB (ed): Genitourinary cancer, in *Contemporary Issues in Clinical Oncology*, vol 5. New York, Churchill Livingstone, 1985

HRICAK H: Detection and staging of renal neoplasms: A reassessment of MR imaging. Radiology 166:643, 1988

KALISH LA et al: A determination of appropriate endpoints in assessing efficacy of intravesical therapies in superficial bladder cancer. J Clin Oncol 5:2004, 1987

RAGHAVAN D et al: Biology and management of bladder cancer. N Engl J Med 322:1129, 1990

RIESELBACH RE, GARNICK MB (eds): *Cancer and the Kidney*. Philadelphia, Lea & Febiger, 1982

SAROSKY MF, LAMM DL: Long-term results of intravesical BCG therapy for superficial bladder cancer. J Urol 142:719, 1989

SEE WA, WILLIAMS RD: Tumors of the kidney, ureter and bladder. West J Med 156:523, 1992

STERNBERG CN et al: M-VAC (methotrexate, vinblastine, doxorubicin, and cisplatin) for advanced transitional cell carcinoma of urothelium. J Urol 139:461, 1988

WEST WH et al: Constant infusion recombinant interleukin-2 in adoptive immunotherapy of advanced cancer. N Engl J Med 316:898, 1987

section 1 **Disorders of the alimentary tract**

248 APPROACH TO THE PATIENT WITH GASTROINTESTINAL DISEASE

KURT J. ISSELBACHER / DANIEL K. PODOLSKY

BIOLOGIC CONSIDERATIONS The mucosal surface of the gastrointestinal tract is composed of a remarkably dynamic population of epithelial cells that are highly developed in their capacity for transmembrane absorption and secretion. These secretory and absorptive abilities facilitate the essential function of the digestive tract in digestion and nutrient uptake, which must be accomplished while maintaining the barrier between the host and potentially harmful pathogens and mutagens in the lumen. The latter is accomplished through both the physical integrity of the intact mucosal surface and the extensive population of resident immune cells.

The intestinal surface itself also contains the distinctive M cells that serve to sample the antigenic milieu of the lumen. The predominance of suppressor lymphocytes within the surface epithelial layer (intraepithelial lymphocytes) suggests that dampening of the body's response to the enormous number of potentially antigenic substances in the lumen is necessary to prevent the constant and unrestrained activation of immune and inflammatory processes. Conversely, the presence of large numbers of helper lymphocytes as well as other cellular effectors of immune response in the lamina propria and submucosa attests to a large armamentarium ready to respond when surface defenses have been breached. No doubt the concentration of so many immune cells capable of attracting and activating inflammatory cells predisposes to the numerous inflammatory conditions to which the gastrointestinal tract is subject.

The mucosal surface of the gastrointestinal tract is also remarkable for the very rapid turnover of the epithelial cell population. It is likely that the epithelium turns over in its entirety every 24 to 72 h. This may permit rapid restitution of a functional cell population following an acute insult and may reduce the risk of malignancy through loss of cells affected by the many potential and actual mutagens in the luminal contents. Nevertheless, this proliferative potential must inherently create the setting for neoplastic disorders, which are so common to the gastrointestinal tract. Another fundamental feature of gastrointestinal mucosa is the spatial segregation of the proliferative compartment from the terminally differentiated cells. This is true throughout the gastrointestinal tract but is most apparent in the small intestine where a gradient of differentiation exists from the depths of the crypts of Lieberkühn to the villus tip. This organization is important in understanding the histology and pathophysiology of many mucosal disorders, e.g., nontropical sprue.

In view of the important secretory and absorptive activities of mucosal surface, diseases of the gastrointestinal tract may result in clinical consequences secondary to the physical disruption of the mucosal layer (e.g., blood loss, fluid loss, pathogenic invasion) or nutritional derangements due to impaired digestion and nutrient absorption. In focal or localized disease processes the former predominate, whereas the latter may be especially prominent in disorders that affect extensive areas of the gastrointestinal tract in a diffuse manner.

While the essential role of the gastrointestinal tract is the absorption of nutrients and excretion of the products is in large part accomplished at the luminal surface, these processes are also dependent on the deeper muscular layers for the coordinated propulsion of food through the lumen. The complexity of both local and distant neural and endocrine factors that contribute to the regulation of intestinal motility is only now becoming fully appreciated. Disruption of normal motility is quite common, with functional bowel complaints affecting as many as 15 percent of adults. Alterations in frequency of bowel movements, abdominal distention, abdominal pain, and nausea, individually or in varying combinations, may result from dysmotility. In addition, structural lesions may also indirectly lead to symptoms through their impact on motility involving some or all regions of the gastrointestinal tract. These range from the *direct* effects of an obstructing lesion to the *indirect* actions of substances released by a primary mucosal disorder (e.g., inflammatory mediators such as arachidonic acid metabolites that also affect smooth-muscle activity).

Although valid unifying generalizations can be made about the gastrointestinal tract in its entirety, the spectrum of diseases affecting this system and their clinical manifestations are significantly related to the constituent organ(s) involved. Thus, esophageal disorders predominantly manifest through their relationship to swallowing, while gastric disorders are dominated by features relating to acid secretion, and disease of the small and large intestine by disruption of nutrition and alterations of bowel movements. Similarly, diseases of the related ancillary organs, the exocrine pancreas and the hepatobiliary system, present characteristic clinical challenges. Finally, it should be remembered that in addition to intrinsic disease, the gastrointestinal tract may be affected by systemic disorders. These include vascular, inflammatory, infectious, and neoplastic conditions leading to focal or diffuse structural lesions. Metabolic and endocrine abnormalities as well as drugs can disrupt normal bowel motility.

CLINICAL CONSIDERATIONS **History** A thorough clinical history is almost uniformly reliable in directing the clinician's attention to appropriate diagnostic considerations in the patient with gastrointestinal symptoms. The most common complaints resulting from disorders involving the gastrointestinal tract include pain, and alteration in bowel habit, especially diarrhea and constipation. Among these, *abdominal pain* is the most frequent and variable and may reflect a broad spectrum of problems from the least threatening to the most urgent. In conjunction with an estimation of its intensity, initial distinction should be made between pain of acute onset and more chronic discomfort. Pain of abrupt onset is often encountered in serious illness requiring urgent intervention, while a history of chronic discomfort may typically be related to an indolent disorder. However, change in the pattern or character of pain may be equally important, signifying progression of a problem of initial mild onset (either recent or chronic) to a more critical stage. Ascertaining the location (upper or lower, localized or diffuse), character (sharp, burning, cramping), and relationship of the pain to meals will often provide significant insight into the most important diagnostic considerations. If eating produces the symptom, the clinician should determine whether the discomfort occurs while eating (as in esophageal disorders and abdominal angina), shortly after the meal (as often occurs in biliary tract disease), or 30 to 90 min later (as typically seen in peptic disease). Pain that is not affected by eating suggests a process outside of the bowel lumen, such as an abscess, peritonitis, pancreatitis, and some malignancies. Conversely, identification of factors that relieve the symptom is also helpful, e.g., relief with eating or antacids is characteristic of peptic ulcer disease or gastritis. Relationship of the discomfort to bowel movement, especially in association with an altered bowel habit, should focus attention on a disorder of the small or large bowel such as inflammatory bowel disease.

Alterations in bowel habit can result from either disruption of normal intestinal motility or significant structural pathology. A thorough determination of the temporal evolution of the change and the nature of the alteration in conjunction with other constitutional symptoms such as weight loss, fever, or anorexia is important. Temporary variation in bowel habit in association with some life stress and in the absence of signs of systemic illness is suggestive of the common "irritable bowel syndrome," especially when the alteration varies between diarrhea and constipation. Small pellet-like stools are often described by the patient. Associated symptoms of bloating, nausea, and "gas" are also common. This diagnosis can essentially be made on the basis of a thorough history and physical examination and very limited laboratory testing, which exclude structural disease. In contrast, the onset of worsening constipation in an adult with previously regular habits, especially when accompanied by systemic symptoms such as weight loss, suggests the possible presence of an underlying obstructing process, particularly malignancy. If diarrhea is present, one should determine the average number of stools, their consistency, their pattern, and if any blood is present. Although *diarrhea* refers to an increased frequency of movements, patients will often use the term to describe loose or watery stools primarily. The occurrence of nocturnal or true bloody diarrhea almost always reflects structural rather than functional bowel disease. A pungent odor or the presence of undigested meat in the movement are suggestive of pancreatic insufficiency. An alteration in color can be seen in cholestasis or steatorrhea (light-colored) or hemorrhage (melenic to maroon or bright red). Mucus in the movement is usually a sign of functional bowel syndrome, while pus is more strongly suggestive of infectious or inflammatory disease. Less common but more dramatic are the symptoms of acute gastrointestinal bleeding, including hematemesis, melena, and hematochezia, which usually leads to prompt efforts to find medical attention but should always be solicited by the clinician.

In the evaluation of male patients, especially those with diarrhea, a tactful inquiry into sexual activity is essential. Homosexual males are at increased risk for a large variety of gastrointestinal disorders as well as AIDS, which may first manifest itself with gastrointestinal symptoms. Finally, careful attention must be given to a general medical history with an emphasis on any medications or nonprescription drugs that may have been used. Thyroid and other metabolic disorders, especially those affecting calcium metabolism, can cause a variety of gastrointestinal symptoms. Unless asked, patients may forget to mention that they take aspirin almost daily for headache, and this may account for occult blood found in the stool. The use of daily laxatives may explain chronic diarrhea.

Physical examination, endoscopy, and radiology All of the cardinal methods of examination are helpful in evaluating the patient with gastrointestinal symptoms. *Inspection* may disclose signs of cholestasis or nutritional deficiencies. An abnormal contour of the abdomen or inspection of the perianal region may manifest signs of a mass or a draining fistula. *Auscultation* is also important. A succussion splash can be elicited in the patients with symptoms of gastric outlet obstruction. The absence of bowel sounds or alteration in pitch can lead to recognition of an evolving ileus or an obstructing process. A bruit may also be appreciated where there are symptoms of ischemic bowel disease. Careful *palpation* of the abdomen is especially important in detecting tenderness and masses, which in the appropriate clinical setting will lead to the recognition of cholecystitis, regional enteritis, periappendiceal abscess, and many other disorders. Findings on abdominal palpation will often be complemented by *percussion*, which is essential to assessing liver and spleen size.

Elicitation of rebound tenderness, either direct or referred, after removal of the examining hand provides an important clue to localized or more generalized peritonitis characteristic of many abdominal emergencies, including a perforated viscus, intraabdominal abscess, or tissue infarction. The clinician should be particularly alert to these signs in patients with severe pain of abrupt onset. Typically, the patient will remain immobile to avoid the accentuation of pain that may follow even slight movement and jarring of the abdomen. This contrasts with the sometimes frantic efforts to find a position of comfort in patients with severe pain deriving from visceral disease, e.g., pancreatitis or intestinal ischemia. In these disorders, the absence of findings on palpation of the abdomen may be in striking contrast to the evident distress of the patient. Only with progression of the process to tissue destruction (e.g., necrotizing pancreatitis or intestinal infarction) and secondary peritonitis will the abdominal examination prove remarkable, often in concert with striking signs of systemic illness including hemodynamic instability. In addition to the examination of the abdomen, a carefully performed digital rectal examination is also essential. In the patient with complaints of incontinence the integrity of the sphincter can be assessed. Most importantly, masses intrinsic to the rectum as well as abnormalities in the pelvis or the pouch of Douglas may only be detected by this examination, and the presence or absence of frank or occult blood in the stool is always important diagnostic information. Sigmoidoscopy should be viewed as a routine extension of the physical examination in the patient with diarrhea or other alteration in bowel habit as well as in the patient with known or suspected blood loss from the lower bowel. This procedure, which can be performed with either the rigid sigmoidoscope or a flexible fiberoptic instrument, allows for direct inspection of the rectosigmoid mucosa permitting detection of cancers and polyps in this segment that may well be missed by barium x-rays. Inflammatory changes of the mucosa can help identify the patient with infectious dysentery or other forms of colitis, most notably ulcerative colitis. The findings of edema, granularity, and diffuse friability (easily induced mucosal bleeding) as well as superficial ulcerations are characteristic in the latter disorder. Fresh stool samples for microbiologic studies and superficial mucosal biopsies obtained at the time of sigmoidoscopy can also yield crucial diagnostic information.

Definitive demonstration or exclusion of structural lesions of the gastrointestinal tract, particularly the great majority of disorders that primarily affect mucosal surface, can often not be accomplished by physical examination alone. Many disorders of the upper or lower gastrointestinal tract are accessible to inspection through fiberoptic instruments. As a result, endoscopic studies are supplanting conventional contrast x-ray studies for many clinical problems, both because of the heightened precision of these diagnostic tools and the opportunity in many instances to accomplish a meaningful therapeutic intervention as an adjunct to the acquisition of diagnostic information. However, it should be emphasized that *no procedure should be considered routine* and used indiscriminately; there must be a rational basis for its use in the individual patient. These techniques are discussed in detail in Chap. 250. Upper gastrointestinal endoscopy permits evaluation of the esophagus, stomach, and duodenum and, with specially designed instruments, the proximal jejunum. When the clinical history warrants a diagnostic examination of the upper gastrointestinal tract for a structural lesion, endoscopic examination is preferable to radiologic study in most patients when the choice is available. Side-viewing scopes permit inspection and cannulation of the ampulla of Vater facilitating retrograde cholangiopancreatography. The colonoscope can be used to visualize the entire colon and often the terminal ileum, resulting in more accurate diagnosis of inflammatory bowel disease and mass lesions. Frequently colonic polyps can be removed at the time of initial colonoscopic identification.

Endoscopic techniques are relatively precise in defining many problems, but the limitations of these tools as well as the continued advantages of x-ray studies in some situations should be recognized. Endoscopic tools are not useful in assessing gastrointestinal (GI) motility, which may be more accurately gauged by barium studies. In addition, some areas, notably the small intestine, remain relatively inaccessible to fiberoptic instruments. In hospitals where endoscopy is not feasible, the upper GI series and barium enema remain good diagnostic modalities for the upper and lower GI tract especially when air-contrast techniques are employed. However, they should generally be avoided in the patient with GI bleeding or suspected bowel obstruction. In addition the physician must exercise judgment in preparing the patient for these studies, recognizing that cathartics may markedly worsen the condition of a patient with obstructing lesions or colitis.

Although endoscopy has obviated the need for many conventional GI x-rays, other radiologic imaging modalities have assumed a crucial role in the approach to the patient with gastrointestinal symptoms. These techniques include ultrasound (US), computed tomography (CT), and magnetic resonance imaging (MRI). The application of these tools to the liver and biliary tract is discussed in Chap. 262. Both US and CT are useful in the delineation of abdominal masses. CT, though more expensive, is often more effective in the evaluation of the lower abdomen, where inflammatory masses in patients with Crohn's disease or complications of diverticular disease may be accurately imaged. However, US is an effective and generally less expensive tool for the evaluation of the right upper quadrant including the gall bladder and biliary tract. These techniques are often complementary in the evaluation of pancreatic disease. In combination with Doppler analysis, US can be used to assess the patency and direction of blood flow in the portal vein in the patient with advanced liver disease. MRI may permit exquisitely accurate information on the anatomic extent of invasive rectal cancers and blood flow in patients with vascular disorders, but the full range of its uses in GI disorders remains to be delineated. More-sophisticated CT and MRI equipment can actually permit the performance of digital angiography without the invasive catheterization necessary in conventional visceral angiography.

Finally, one must emphasize that the optimal use of endoscopic and radiologic imaging techniques also depends on the recognition that each modality has inherent limitations. Only the clinician can determine whether the information is sufficient to establish or exclude a diagnosis in a patient with relevant historical and/or physical findings and a negative or nondiagnostic study. Was the preparation of the patient or the examination of sufficient quality to have detected an abnormality if present? Was the examiner aware of the important diagnostic considerations, and was the study adapted to address those concerns? Conversely only the physician can determine whether irregularities found in diagnostic studies are indeed causally related to the patient's symptoms. This judgment usually relies upon a sound understanding of the biologic basis of gastrointestinal disorders.

DIAGNOSTIC APPROACHES   Abdominal pain   Determination of the cause of abdominal pain remains an imposing clinical challenge. As noted above, a spectrum of disorders from the acute and catastrophic to the chronic and indolent causes abdominal pain. Furthermore, differential diagnostic considerations may encompass diseases extrinsic to the gastrointestinal tract per se including disorders of the genitourinary tract (e.g., pelvic inflammatory disease) and the peritoneum as well as alterations of the various constituents of the GI tract. The history and physical examination are essential guides to a sensible diagnostic approach to the broad potential array of disorders causing abdominal pain. The primary goal to be achieved through initial approaches to the patient is the distinction between an urgent problem requiring expeditious delineation and nonacute disorders. In the former, initial clinical impressions based on the history and physical examination can be further refined through routine laboratory tests such as a complete blood test and differential as well as plain films of the abdomen. Particular features will dictate the appropriateness of urgent US or CT examination or the need to proceed directly with emergency exploratory laparotomy. In the patient with a longstanding and relatively stable problem, diagnostic evaluation is undertaken in a more considered time frame. The clinician may be able to reasonably establish a functional basis for the complaint on the strength of the history and physical examination alone. Radiologic contrast studies, other imaging modalities (e.g., US, CT), or endoscopic examination may be appropriate to exclude or identify the gamut of disorders discussed above. If all these approaches prove inadequate to determine the cause of the patient's symptoms, more unusual causes of abdominal pain may have to be excluded through specific urine or blood tests (e.g., porphyrins).

Problems of swallowing   The approach should be as follows:

1 *Thorough determination of the nature of dysphagia.* Is the difficulty primarily in swallowing liquids, solids, or both? The location of the difficulty from the patient's perspective and presence or absence of accompanying odynophagia are important to ascertain. These historical clues are complemented by careful visual and neurologic examination of the oropharynx when appropriate.

2 *Routine esophageal x-rays* in the upright and lateral or Trendelenburg position. The horizontal views are essential for demonstration of the swallowing mechanism, unaided by gravity, and of the esophagogastric junction. For details of the pharyngoesophageal area cineradiography is necessary because of the rapidity with which the contrast medium passes through. Hiatus hernia is extremely common (in 15 to 35 percent of persons over 50) and often asymptomatic unless spontaneous reflux of gastric contents can be demonstrated to occur repeatedly. Careful attention is usually needed to detect lower esophageal rings or webs, which may be visible as indentations in the barium column only from a limited angle.

3 *Esophagoscopy.* This procedure is desirable to describe lesions suggested by x-ray or, if the lesion is unsuspected, to obtain biopsies from masses or abnormal mucosa and to obtain washings for exfoliative cytologic study. The diagnoses of peptic esophagitis and Barrett's esophagus are made endoscopically. Endoscopy is the most sensitive technique for identifying esophageal or gastric varices, although they are seldom important in the absence of hemorrhage. Fiberoptic instruments with US probes at their tip may ultimately become established as the most useful diagnostic tools for particular problems of the esophagus (and other sites of the GI tract), but instruments remain costly and continue to undergo significant technological evolution so that the ultimate role of so-called endosonography remains uncertain.

4 *Manometric studies* of the upper esophagus, particularly in conjunction with cineradiography. At present, this procedure offers the best differential between disorders primarily in the central nervous system, primary pharyngeal muscular disease, and cricopharyngeal dystonia. Manometry of the lower esophagus is useful in the diagnosis of diffuse esophageal spasm, achalasia, and infiltrative diseases that can alter esophageal motility.

Peptic or digestive disorders   The approaches to these disorders include:

1 *Insertion of a nasogastric tube.* This is used to establish whether significant gastric retention (more than 75 mL of gastric contents

in the fasting state) exists and whether there is acid, bile, blood, or other material in these contents. If pyloric obstruction or gastric atony is present, the tube is used to maintain suction while the patient's electrolyte and fluid balance is restored to normal; the stomach is kept as clean as possible so that reliable diagnostic investigation may be carried out.

2 *Upper intestinal endoscopy.* This procedure is most helpful in identifying the diffuse mucosa in gastritis or, together with biopsy and brushings for cytology, in differentiating between peptic and neoplastic ulcerating lesions. It may identify a specific bleeding site in clinical situations where several potential bleeding sites could exist, such as in the patient with portal hypertension. In addition, it may be possible to cauterize or otherwise intervene to control hemorrhage with the endoscope (e.g., injections of vasoconstricting agents such as epinephrine). The frequent association of gastritis with *Helicobacter pylori* in patients with nonulcer dyspepsia, as well as in those with actual peptic ulceration, has been well documented, even if its true role in the pathogenesis of these disorders remains uncertain. Nevertheless, at this time, *H. pylori* infection can be most reliably documented in the individual patient by endoscopy and biopsy. Endoscopy can detect a number of potential sources of upper GI bleeding which are often missed by x-ray studies (e.g., erosive gastritis, Mallory-Weiss syndrome). Gastroscopy is particularly helpful in inspecting the postoperative stomach, especially in detecting stomal ulceration or so-called alkaline reflux gastritis. The first and second portions of the duodenum can also be routinely examined with the fiberoptic gastroscope, and important information about ulcers and other lesions can be obtained by this procedure. Radiologic studies may be useful when endoscopy is not readily available or in the assessment of suspected motility disorders (e.g., gastroparesis). In addition, radiologic examination may be preferred when there are contraindications to safe endoscopy.

3 *Gastric acid secretory studies.* Though not routinely necessary, these are useful in the diagnosis of the Zollinger-Ellison syndrome or atrophic gastritis and for determination of completeness of vagotomy. Suspected gastric carcinoma is better diagnosed directly through gastroscopy and biopsy than indirectly through acid secretory studies (achlorhydria). These studies should not be obtained for the routine diagnosis of uncomplicated duodenal ulcer. There is no convincing evidence that acid studies are useful in determining the type of surgery for duodenal ulcer.

Obstructive and vascular disorders of the small intestine
When intestinal problems present as obstructive syndromes, the plain x-ray of the abdomen is the most important diagnostic adjunct to careful physical examination. Patterns of dilatation of individual loops of intestine may be characteristic, as in volvulus or acute pancreatitis; erect and decubitus views will often show fluid levels in the affected segments. Motility disorders of the small intestine (temporary ileus or chronic intestinal pseudoobstruction) may also present with obstructive symptoms and similar x-ray findings but must be managed medically without surgical intervention. Air under the diaphragm is diagnostic of a perforated viscus; air in the portal vein usually results from intestinal necrosis secondary to mesenteric vascular occlusion. The diagnostic accuracy of the plain x-ray in all types of intestinal obstruction is about 75 percent. In patients with symptoms of incomplete obstruction, the radiographic small-bowel series will often be diagnostic in defining the site and degree of obstruction. Infrequently, in this setting, all conventional x-ray studies are unremarkable. In such cases, the radiologist may perform a small-bowel enteroclysis study by passing a special tube into the proximal jejunum; the rapid instillation of barium through the tube will distend the intestine and often reveal subtle lesions missed by other tests.

Vascular diseases of the small intestine are among the most difficult diseases to diagnose. In chronic mesenteric ischemia, radiographic, endoscopic, and laboratory tests are usually normal. Early in the course of acute mesenteric ischemia, the plain film of the abdomen may be unremarkable despite complaints of severe abdominal pain. In these settings, prompt mesenteric angiography is essential in confirming the diagnosis of vascular disease.

Inflammatory and neoplastic diseases of small and large intestine   Patients with these conditions are usually identified by history, physical examination, and careful examination of the stools for exudate and blood. Examination of fresh stool samples for common bacterial pathogens and parasites by laboratories skilled in these techniques is important in identifying or excluding infectious causes of diarrhea, particularly in the patient with colitis. Sigmoidoscopy is valuable in identifying mucosal and neoplastic lesions of the lower 25 cm of the colon. The mucosal surface of the entire colon and terminal ileum can be examined directly and biopsied through the fiberoptic sigmoidoscope or colonoscope. The radiologic examination of the small intestine is highly reliable in identifying the prestenotic and stenotic lesions of Crohn's disease. In the colon a single barium enema examination in a well-prepared patient has a diagnostic accuracy of 80 to 85 percent; the addition of air-contrast technique brings the accuracy up over 90 percent, but none of these figures is meaningful if the patient is poorly prepared for the examination, and the cecal area is hard to examine adequately because of its anatomy. Colonoscopy may be preferable for its greater accuracy and the capability to remove the vast majority of polyps as well as to obtain preoperative tissue confirmation in the patient who probably has cancer. The immunologic assay for the carcinoembryonic antigen has not proved to be specific for colonic cancer; nevertheless, it does contribute to the detection of residual or recurrent disease in postoperative patients.

Peroral biopsy of the small intestine and forceps biopsy of the rectosigmoid are of considerable importance in revealing mucosal disease. Rectal biopsy is an excellent means of demonstrating amyloidosis, schistosomiasis, and amebiasis. Submucosal disease is not seen in these superficial biopsies. Hirschsprung's disease is histologically diagnosed by a deep surgical biopsy of the lower part of the rectum.

Malabsorption syndromes   Malabsorption may be suspected on the basis of history and physical examination and is confirmed by examination of the stools. Radiologic examination is of general help in ruling out local lesions and suggesting motor and secretory dysfunction, but it is rarely diagnostic unless an abnormal small-bowel mucosa or fistulas between intestine and stomach are demonstrated.

The tests useful in the diagnosis of malabsorption are discussed in Chap. 254. A simple screening test for excessive fat in the stools can be accomplished by the microscopic examination of a stool specimen stained with Sudan. Chemical analysis of 3-day stool collection for fat, with the patient on a standard diet, is used to establish the diagnosis of steatorrhea. The D-xylose absorption test is about 90 percent accurate in separating mucosal disease from pancreatic insufficiency. Peroral biopsy of the small intestine via the endoscope or a specialized biopsy device is of value in the diagnosis of celiac disease, and it may show the less common infiltrations of the mucosa by amyloid or bacterial mucoproteins (Whipple's disease). Leakage of protein into the intestinal lumen may cause hypoproteinemia and can be demonstrated by the recovery in stools of the serum protein α_1-antitrypsin or intravenously administered markers such as albumin labeled with iodine or chromium isotopes.

Pancreas   The pancreas is difficult to study directly because of its anatomic location and relative inaccessibility. Calcification of the pancreas on a plain abdominal film is highly suggestive of chronic pancreatitis and may be associated with fat malabsorption. Pancreatic exocrine insufficiency can be documented by intubation of the duodenum and collection of pancreatic juice after stimulation with secretin or a test meal. Abdominal US and CT are the best radiographic means of searching for pancreatic enlargement (see Chaps. 273 and 274). Both techniques may also be used to guide needle biopsies of the pancreas and may provide sufficient diagnostic information to obviate the need for exploratory surgery. The pancreatic duct can be cannulated via the fiberoptic duodenoscope and visualized by the injection of radiographic dye. Visualization of the duct may be helpful in the diagnosis of pancreatic pseudocysts, carcinoma, or chronic pancreatitis.

REFERENCES

JOHNSON LR et al: *Physiology of the Gastrointestinal Tract*, 2d ed. New York, Raven, 1987

SLEISENGER MH, FORDTRAN JS: *Gastrointestinal Disease*, 4th ed. Philadelphia, Saunders, 1989

YAMADA T et al: *Textbook of Gastroenterology*, Philadelphia, Lippincott, 1991

---

249 IMPACT OF CELLULAR AND MOLECULAR BIOLOGY ON GASTROINTESTINAL DISEASE

DANIEL K. PODOLSKY / KURT J. ISSELBACHER

In recent years, broad progress in biochemistry, cellular biology, and molecular biology has led to a better understanding of basic processes and in some instances their molecular alteration in gastrointestinal and liver diseases. This has been paralleled by newer approaches to diagnosis and treatment, increasingly dominated by medical rather than surgical interventions. While not attempting to describe all the recent advances in the cellular biology and molecular biology of the gastrointestinal tract, this chapter summarizes a number of those discoveries which are having an impact on the approach to the diagnosis and management of gastrointestinal disease.

CELL SURFACE RECEPTORS FOR SPECIFIC LIGANDS (NEU-ROTRANSMITTERS AND HORMONES) A seminal insight of the past two decades is the role of cell surface receptors in causing functional changes in response to diverse stimuli following binding of specific ligands. From this appreciation of receptor-ligand interaction has come the ability to develop agents that mimic ligands. If the agent binds and activates the receptor, agonist activity is observed; if it binds to but does not stimulate the receptor because it is structurally different from the natural ligand, antagonist activity results. The potential importance of this insight for the approach to disorders of the gastrointestinal tract is apparent when one considers how H-2 receptor antagonists have revolutionized the treatment of peptic ulcer disease.

The major functional properties of the gastrointestinal tract, including motility, secretion, absorption, growth, and proliferation, can be modulated by a variety of stimuli acting through cell surface receptors. The ligands capable of achieving important effects in this way include small amino acid derivatives (e.g., classical neurotransmitters), nucleotide derivatives (e.g., adenosine), and small to medium-sized peptides. While these regulatory ligands can be produced by any cell type, most are produced by neural and endocrine cellular elements.

As classically defined for endocrine hormone production and action, receptor-specific ligands may be released at a distance from the cellular targets expressing the receptor or close to its cellular targets, as in neural transmission. It is now recognized that some peptides, including many which modulate proliferation in the gastrointestinal tract, bind to receptors on the same cells as produce the growth factor (*autocrine* regulation) or to receptors on adjacent or nearby cells (*juxtacrine* and *paracrine* regulation, respectively).

The structural features of many important receptors in the gastrointestinal tract have been elucidated (Fig. 249-1). Most are members of a relatively small number of protein families. Within these families,

FIGURE 249-1 Cell surface receptors in the gastrointestinal tract. Three structurally distinct classes of cell surface receptors are especially important: (1) tyrosine kinase receptor, characterized by a single membrane-spanning domain of receptor in which the ligand binds to the extracellular domain and induces a tyrosine kinase activity present on either the intracellular portion of the same protein or present on another protein closely associated with the receptor (the latter kinase a member of the so-called nonreceptor tyrosine kinase family related to *src*); (2) ligand-gated ion channel receptors formed by the association of four or five separate subunits, each with approximately four membrane-spanning domains in which ligand binding alters the influx of specific ions through the channel formed by the subunits to result in a cellular response; and (3) single-chain receptors, which encompass seven membrane-spanning domains whose biologic activity following ligand binding is effected through interaction with a G protein complex. Examples of each class of receptor which play an important role in the gastrointestinal tract are indicated. (*After Logsdon.*)

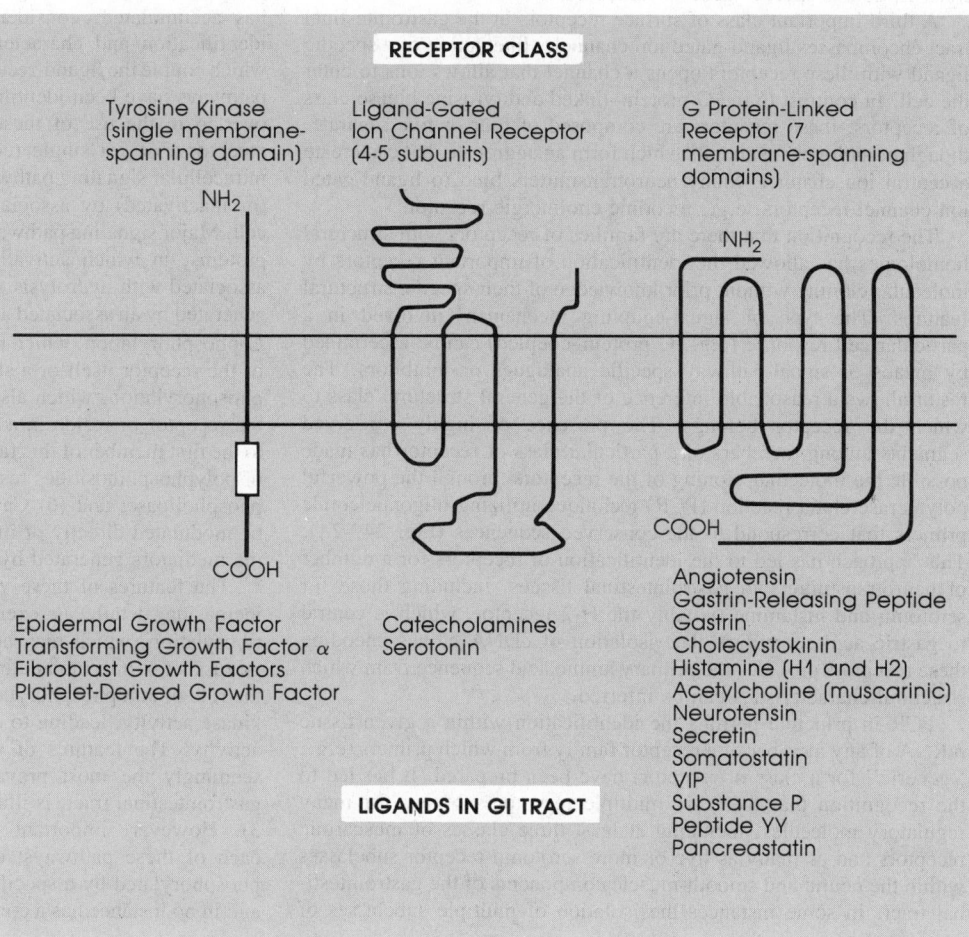

RECEPTOR CLASS

Tyrosine Kinase (single membrane-spanning domain)

Ligand-Gated Ion Channel Receptor (4-5 subunits)

G Protein-Linked Receptor (7 membrane-spanning domains)

NH₂

COOH

Epidermal Growth Factor
Transforming Growth Factor α
Fibroblast Growth Factors
Platelet-Derived Growth Factor

Catecholamines
Serotonin

Angiotensin
Gastrin-Releasing Peptide
Gastrin
Cholecystokinin
Histamine (H1 and H2)
Acetylcholine (muscarinic)
Neurotensin
Secretin
Somatostatin
VIP
Substance P
Peptide YY
Pancreastatin

LIGANDS IN GI TRACT

individual members share significant structural similarities and mechanisms of signal transduction whereby ligand-receptor binding ultimately leads to changes in cellular function. Many receptors transmit an intracellular signal through association with guanosine triphosphate–binding proteins that possess GTPase activity. These *G protein–linked receptors* have seven membrane-spanning domains, and there is significant amino acid sequence similarity in the membrane-spanning domains of different receptors. This receptor class includes receptors for many nonpeptide neurotransmitters as well as many peptide ligands of the neuroendocrine network.

A second class of receptors in the gastrointestinal tract contains a single membrane-spanning domain and depends on tyrosine phosphorylation for signal transduction. Typically, these receptors are composed of a large extracytoplasmic domain and an intracellular cytoplasmic tail of varying length. In many instances, the cytoplasmic domain itself exhibits tyrosine kinase activity, generating an intracellular signal following ligand binding. In some receptor complexes, the tyrosine kinase activity may be present in a discrete cytoplasmic protein (nonreceptor tyrosine kinase) which associates with the receptor. In most instances, members of this class of receptor can phosphorylate specific residues within their own cytoplasmic domain, resulting in attenuation of receptor activity and thus a degree of autoregulation. Within the gastrointestinal tract, receptors of this class include those for various growth-regulatory peptides (e.g., epidermal growth factor, transforming growth factor α, insulin, and insulin-like growth factors). Other classes of receptors create an intracellular signal through either phosphokinase or phosphatase activities. Still other receptors are complexed to protein kinase C or enzymes which modulate the production of polyphosphinositides and related substances. The final effector steps in these pathways themselves may be quite diverse, including changes in membrane characteristics or the state of intramembrane proteins, changes in structural proteins, altered translation of mRNA, and/or, most important, changes in transcription of specific genes within the nucleus.

A third important class of surface receptors in the gastrointestinal tract encompasses ligand-gated ion channels. Interaction of a specific ligand with these receptors opens a channel that allows ions to enter the cell. In contrast to the G protein–linked and tyrosine kinase class of receptors, these receptors are composed of four or five separate, though homologous, subunits which form an aggregate that can create a central ion channel. Many neurotransmitters bind to ligand-gated ion channel receptors, e.g., nicotinic cholinergic receptors.

The recognition that there are families of receptors with structural homologies has allowed the identification of important receptors by molecular cloning without prior knowledge of their specific structural features. The type of signal-coupling mechanism involved in a particular cell response (e.g., G protein–coupled) can be ascertained by means of signal-pathway–specific analogues or inhibitors. The result allows a reasonable inference of the general structural class to which the receptor belongs. The presence of highly conserved segments among members of a particular class of receptor has made possible the molecular cloning of the receptors through the powerful polymerase chain reaction (PCR) technique utilizing oligonucleotide primers that correspond to the conserved sequences (Fig. 249-2A). This approach has led to the identification of receptors for a number of neurotransmitters in gastrointestinal tissues, including those for serotonin and histamine (notably the H-2 receptor, which is central to gastric acid secretion). The isolation of cDNA clones encoding these receptors provides the primary amino acid sequence from which structural characteristics can be inferred.

PCR in principle permits the identification within a given tissue mRNA of any member of a receptor family from which primers (e.g., ''generic'' for a class of receptor) have been prepared. It has led to the recognition that there are multiple receptor subtypes for many regulatory molecules, including at least three classes of muscarinic receptors and as many as five or more serotonin receptor subclasses within the neural and smooth-muscle components of the gastrointestinal tract. In some instances the isolation of multiple subclasses of

structurally distinct receptors could be anticipated either from ligand-binding studies or by variability in the functional responses of different cells to different ligand congeners. In other instances the heterogeneity was unanticipated and has led to the appreciation of previously unrecognized distinctions in the functional effects of a ligand at different sites within the gastrointestinal tract. The importance of these insights into neurotransmitter and hormone receptors extends beyond giving us an expanded understanding of the physiology of these tissues, promising to help development of therapeutic agents that can selectively target one of the functional properties of a broadly important regulatory molecule such as acetylcholine or serotonin.

An alternative approach utilizing different molecular biologic techniques has allowed the characterization of other important receptors in the gastrointestinal tract (Fig. 249-2B). In these approaches, transfection of DNA-encoding genes expressed in a gastrointestinal tissue into a mammalian cell line capable of transcribing and translating that genetic information leads to the presence of the specific receptor on those cells which receive a segment of DNA encoding the receptor of interest. These cells can be identified by their acquired ability to bind the peptide of interest. The transfected DNA responsible for the appearance of specific peptide binding in the recipient cells can be reisolated and the features of the receptor evaluated by determination of its nucleotide sequence and in turn its amino acid sequence. This powerful approach has been effective in the study of receptors for diverse hormones, including gastrin and cholecystokinin.

It is likely that, by these approaches, the receptors of many or all of the known important regulatory peptides within the gastrointestinal tract will soon be identified and characterized. Most important, determination of the structural features of receptors, including those elements responsible for specific ligand binding, may facilitate rational design of agents that will either inhibit or augment the effects of regulatory hormones and other molecules.

SIGNAL TRANSDUCTION AND GENE REGULATION (See also Chap. 69)   As knowledge of the structure of cell surface receptors has accumulated, considerable advances have been made in the identification and characterization of the intracellular mechanisms which couple the ligand-receptor binding to cellular response. Multiple pathways have been identified. In many instances there is significant overlap in the use of these pathways in association with different receptors; i.e., a single receptor may interact with more than one intracellular signaling pathway, and a given pathway may be activated (or inactivated) by association with different receptors in a single cell. Major signaling pathways include (1) those utilizing GTP-binding proteins, in which activation/inactivation of signal transduction is associated with hydrolysis of GTP to GDP; (2) those utilizing cAMP generated by an associated adenyl cyclase activity; (3) serine/threonine O-phosphorylation, which may be effected by the cytoplasmic portion of the receptor itself or a structurally discrete kinase; (4) tyrosine O-phosphorylation, which also may be found as an intrinsic activity of the receptor or reside in a nonreceptor tyrosine kinase (homologous to the first member of this family to be identified, c-*src*); (5) generation of polyphosphinositides resulting from the other protein kinase C and phospholipase; and (6) Ca^{2+}, whose intracellular concentration can be modulated directly or indirectly by a variety of factors, including the mediators generated by other signaling pathways.

The features of these various pathways have been elucidated in increasing detail, as exemplified by (1) the key role of ADP-ribosylation, which may be specifically inactivated by subunit B of pertussis toxin in modulating G protein–dependent signaling, and (2) the role of autophosphorylation of receptors by their intrinsic tyrosine kinase activity, leading to downregulation of the activated receptor's activity. The features of the G protein receptor-effector complex, seemingly the most prevalent receptor complex paradigm in the gastrointestinal tract, is illustrated in Fig. 249-3 (and also in Fig. 69-3). However, important details remain to be understood about each of these pathways; e.g., the full range of substrate proteins phosphorylated by a specific receptor kinase has not been delineated and in no instance has a complete sequence of events been determined

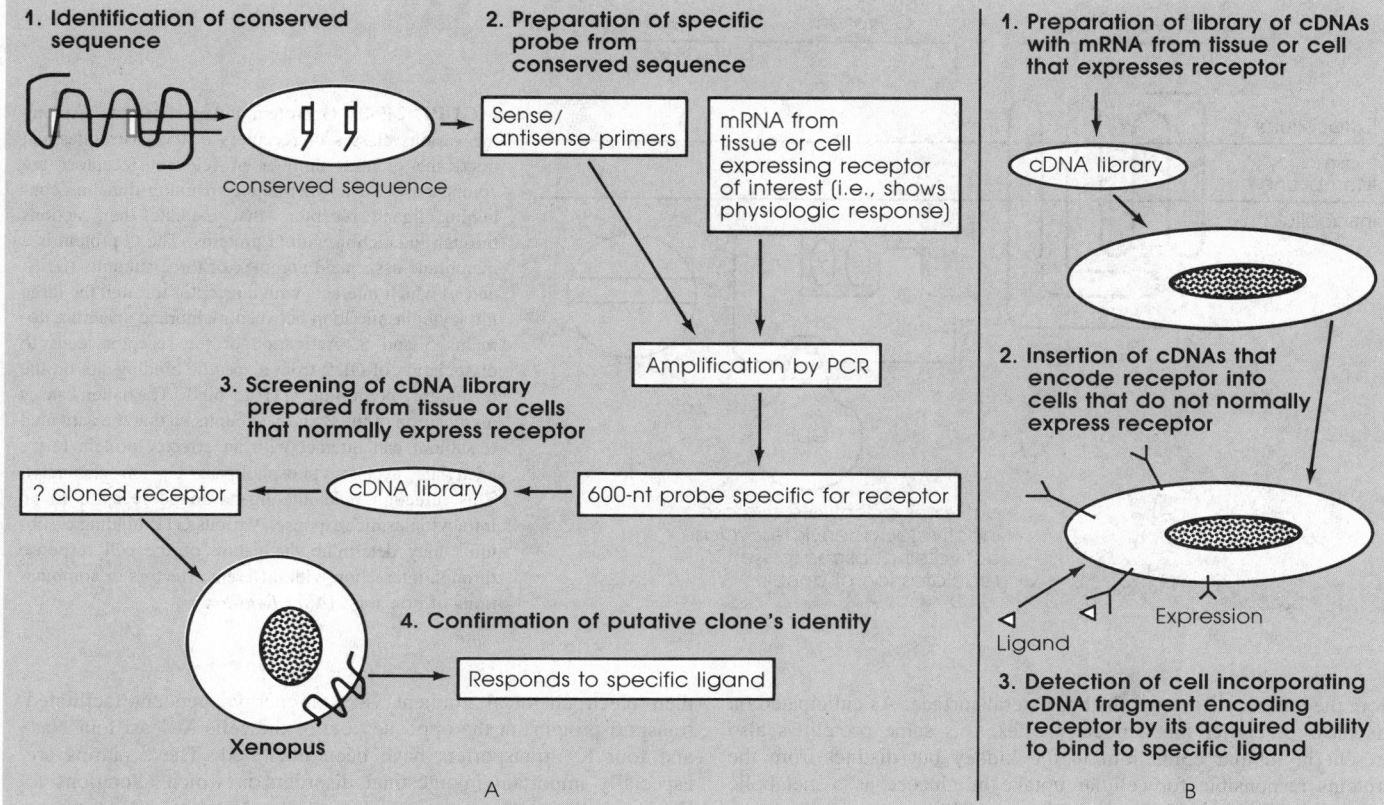

FIGURE 249-2 Experimental strategies for the isolation of specific receptors. *A*. Molecular cloning on the basis of structural conservation. Within receptor classes the amino acid sequence is highly similar in particular regions (e.g., within each corresponding membrane-spanning domain in the G-coupled receptor family). With a nucleotide primer based on these sequences and utilizing the polymerase chain reaction and mRNA from a tissue or cell known to express the receptor of interest, a nucleotide probe is obtained. The amplified probe, which will encompass sequences unique to the specific receptor, can then be used to identify clones within a cDNA library which encode the receptor protein. The validity of the isolated cDNA clones can be tested by introducing the DNA by a vector into a cell that does not bear the receptor and watching for responsiveness to the appropriate ligand. *B*. Molecular cloning on the basis of ligand binding. Complementary DNA is prepared from mRNA obtained from a tissue or cell known to express a specific receptor. The DNA is introduced (transfected) into mammalian cells capable of transcribing and translating introduced genetic material (designated an *expression cloning system*). The cells within this system that receive the DNA encoding the specific receptor can be identified by the specific binding of radioactively labeled ligand to their cell surface.

through which receptor activation leads to alteration in gene transcription in the nucleus. Nonetheless, it has been possible to determine the key signaling pathways involved in many cellular responses to important stimuli in the gastrointestinal tract through a variety of approaches, including the use of selective inhibitors to block cellular responses, e.g., pertussis toxin blockade of pancreatic response to secretin.

Progress in this area has been especially important in understanding the mechanism of toxin-mediated injury of many gastrointestinal tract pathogens, including cholera, *Clostridium difficile*, enterotoxigenic *E. coli*, and *Shigella*. These insights, in conjunction with studies of basic mechanisms of nutrient and electrolyte transport (see below), provide a rational basis for development of several important therapies, as exemplified by oral-based rehydration solutions. Studies of pathways involving receptors, signal transduction, and eventual alteration in gene transcription have served as a foundation for insights into the molecular basis of tumor formation in the gastrointestinal tract, particularly the colon (see below). This progress follows from the recognition that these pathways are utilized by various growth stimuli, including peptide growth factors, and the appreciation that alteration of any step in this pathway which converts one component to its growth-activating state will lead to a tonic growth stimulus with a high potential for promoting neoplasia. Thus corresponding oncogenes have been found for each component of these pathways.

CARRIER AND TRANSPORT PROTEINS/ION PUMPS Absorption and secretion are the central functions of the gastrointestinal tract and its accessory organs. At the cellular level, these functions are accomplished through specialized proteins which transport nutrients, ions (and corresponding passive movement of water), and other special molecules across the epithelial cells which form the mucosal surface throughout the gastrointestinal tract. Over the past few years, molecular biologic approaches building on insights gained through earlier biochemical studies have finally led to identification and direct characterization of various transport proteins.

Molecular cloning of the genes encoding nutrient transport proteins has been accomplished by approaches similar to those useful in the molecular cloning of surface receptors. Injection of mRNA or a DNA copy from enterocytes or other cells into cells which normally do not express a given transporter (typically the large egg cells of the frog, *Xenopus laevis*) can be used to verify that the sample encodes the protein of interest by the appearance of the transport activity in the injected cells. These approaches, in conjunction with conventional biochemical techniques, have demonstrated active Na^+-coupled glucose uptake at the microvillar membrane in the initial process of concerted absorption of glucose. Five structurally distinct glucose transport proteins have been identified that are expressed by various tissues, including two proteins (designated GLUT2 and GLUT5) responsible for the efficient facilitated transport of this key nutrient

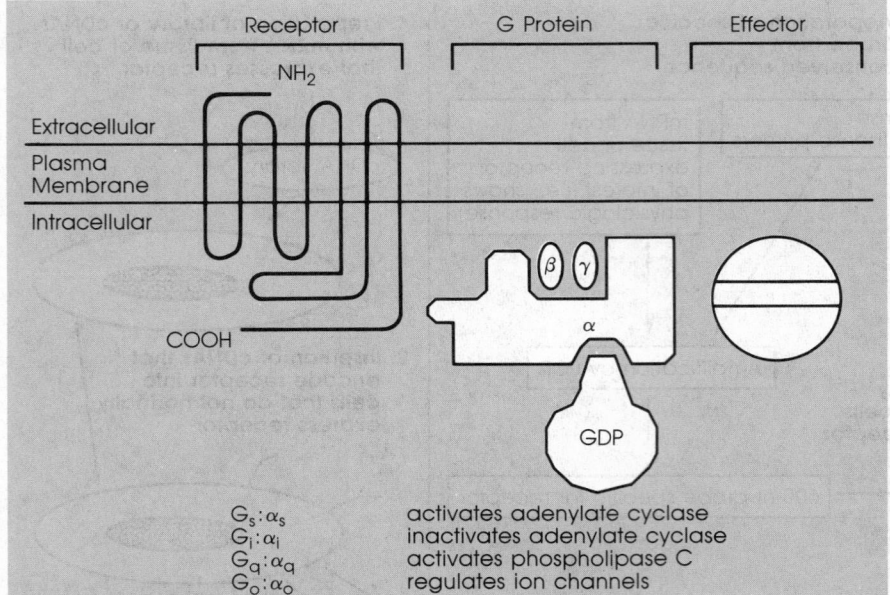

FIGURE 249-3   G protein–linked receptors. Among the various classes of receptors in the gastrointestinal tract, the greatest number of relevant receptors are composed of seven membrane-spanning domains containing ligand receptors that mediate their actions through interaction with G proteins. The G protein is a membrane-associated complex of three subunits (α, β, and γ) which interacts with a receptor through the large intracytoplasmic loop between membrane-spanning domains 5 and 6. Activation of the receptor leads to dissociation of GDP from a specific binding site on the α subunit, permitting GTP to bind. The latter causes dissociation of the β and γ subunits so that the activated α subunit can interact with an effector protein (e.g., adenylate cyclase, phospholipase C, ion channels). This infection links the ligand-bound receptor to an intracytoplasmic response. Various GTP-binding α subunits may determine the nature of the cell response through interaction with different effectors or combinations of effectors. (*After Logsdon.*)

from the enterocyte through its basolateral surface. As anticipated on the basis of earlier biochemical studies, this same protein is also present in tubular epithelium in the kidney but distinct from the proteins responsible for cellular uptake of glucose as a metabolic substrate in liver, skeletal muscle, brain, and other tissues.

With the molecular cloning of both types of glucose transporters, key structural features have become apparent, including the presence of 12 membrane-spanning domains which can form a channel through which the hexose traverses the lipid bilayer. This has provided a coherent view of the mechanisms responsible for glucose absorption through energy-dependent sodium-coupled glucose at the microvillar surface and the transfer of the absorbed glucose from the enterocyte by the non-energy-dependent facilitated transporters present at the basolateral surface. The transport proteins for other mono-, di-, and trisaccharides have been isolated by similar approaches, and it is likely these techniques also will allow characterization of amino acid transporters to yield a comprehensive understanding of the molecular basis of the absorption of the major nutrients.

Different approaches have led to an appreciation of the absorption of fatty acids liberated from dietary triglyceride by lipase from luminal micelles and their reesterification and association with apoprotein within the enterocyte prior to secretion as chylomicrons from the basolateral surface. Molecular cloning has identified the features of the fatty acid–binding protein present within enterocytes which is essential to this process as well as the nature of the apoproteins necessary for chylomicron formation. Interestingly, the intestinal form of the apoprotein (apoB48) is distinguished from its hepatocyte counterpart (apoB100) by the presence of a distinctive stop codon in the gene generating a protein truncated at its carboxy terminus. Molecular cloning techniques also have led to the identification and characterization of the binding and transport proteins which are necessary for the uptake of key vitamins such as vitamin B_{12} and folate.

Considerable progress has been made in understanding the fundamental basis of electrolyte uptake and secretion, which are essential functions throughout the gastrointestinal tract. Biochemical studies have provided kinetic characterization of the energy-dependent transport of the key cations Na^+, K^+, and H^+ as well as the important anions Cl^- and HCO_3^-. In general, active transport is accomplished against electrochemical concentration gradients through the hydrolysis of ATP by ion-coupled ATPases. Transport of ions across epithelial cells is completed by the passive movement of intracellular ions down

their electrochemical gradient via non-energydependent facilitated transport proteins at the opposite pole of the cell. At least four Na^+ and four K^+ transporters have been identified. These pumps are especially important in intestinal disorders in which alterations in fluid and electrolyte secretion play a role. Notably, all causes of diarrhea may ultimately be related to excess net secretion of Cl^- and secondary net water movement. Conversely, an awareness that one of the most abundant pumps for Na^+ couples uptake of this cation with glucose forms the mechanistic rationale for fluid replacement in cholera and other so-called secretory diarrheal states (see Chaps. 39 and 254). Another indication of the therapeutic importance of understanding ion transport is made evident by the characterization of the H^+ pump (actually an H^+, K^+ ATPase) present at the parietal cell canalicular membrane in gastric mucosa which generates gastric acid secretion. Targeting of agents to block this pump (e.g., omeprazole) has proven an especially effective approach to control gastric acid secretion in the treatment of acid-dependent disorders, including reflux esophagitis and the Zollinger-Ellison syndrome (see Chaps. 251 and 252).

CELLULAR AND MOLECULAR BASIS OF DIGESTION AND SECRETION   Extensive studies using both sophisticated morphologic and biochemical techniques have led to a detailed understanding of the structural basis of the highly specialized features of the enterocyte essential for its function in the digestion and absorption of nutrients and maintenance of mucosal integrity in the face of a complex mixture of potentially noxious substances in the lumen. These features include an extensive array of apical microvilli formed by several proteins (actin, myosin, fimbrin, talin, and others) which are coupled by a circumferential ring containing actomyosin linked to tight junctions at the lateral surface near the apical pole. These tight junctions between adjacent enterocytes provide the barrier necessary to maintain the integrity of the mucosa. The molecular details of most of the proteins which form these tight junctions have yet to be elucidated. It is possible that alterations in the structure and function of these tight junctions play a role in disorders of the gastrointestinal tract.

The enterocyte also makes an important contribution to mucosal immune function through the secretion of IgA into the lumen. Molecular approaches have clarified some features of the pathway responsible for secretion of IgA. These include uptake of dimeric IgA produced by plasma cells in the lamina propria by a specific receptor which is itself a member of the immunoglobulin protein superfamily on the basolateral surface of the enterocyte. Subsequently, the receptor-IgA complex is internalized and transported within the cell to the apical surface, where the dimer, in association with a fragment of the IgA receptor–designated secretory component resulting from proteolytic cleavage, is secreted into the lumen. These advances will undoubtedly serve as a foundation for understanding the mechanistic basis of the protective role of secretory IgA.

MOLECULAR CHARACTERIZATION OF VIRAL PATHOGENS

Many of the most important disorders of the gastrointestinal tract and liver are the result of viral infection. Molecular biologic approaches have been especially productive in advancing understanding of common viral hepatitides, including infection resulting from hepatitis A, B, C, D, and E viruses. Molecular characterization has led to improved understanding of the pathogenesis of hepatitis B virus infection. The molecular sequence of the entire hepatitis B virus genome has been determined. Beyond the important information that molecular approaches have yielded in understanding the structure of HBV, these advances have facilitated the development of valuable vaccines by recombinant techniques. The impact of molecular biology on progress in the understanding, diagnosis, and treatment of viral hepatitis is considered in detail in Chap. 266.

BENIGN AND MALIGNANT NEOPLASIA

Significant advances have been made in the understanding of tumorigenesis in the colon and liver using the tools of molecular biology. These observations include the detection of a variety of oncogenes among different colon tumors, both benign polyps and cancers, e.g., *ras* and *src*. However, additional insights have resulted from the study of the relatively rare familial adenomatous polyposis which have served to illuminate molecular mechanisms of neoplasia essential to the more common sporadic colon cancer. Using genetic markers scattered throughout the genome in combination with the technique of restriction-fragment length polymorphism, it was possible to assess whether a tumor contained both parenteral alleles for each genetic marker. This led to the demonstration that this familial disorder was associated with the germline loss of a copy of a presumptive tumor suppressor gene on the long arm of chromosome 5. Similar loss of allelic heterogeneity at other loci including chromosomes 17p and 18q also has been found in various sporadic tumors. The specific genes at these various sites whose loss is related to tumor formation have been identified and found to encode a variety of different types of protein products, including a presumptive cell adhesion molecule and a nuclear transcription factor (p53). Familial forms of colon cancer have been found to be associated with a germline mutation of a specific tumor suppressor gene (see Chap. 257).

While it is likely that other genetic alterations, including activation of oncogenes and inactivation of tumor suppressor genes, will be found to contribute to the development of some colonic neoplasia (and tumors at other sites of the gastrointestinal tract), important general concepts have already emerged from these observations. Malignant tumor formation appears to result from the accumulation of a critical aggregate number of genetic alterations rather than from a specific combination or order of genetic changes. The various genes which may be altered in different tumors encode diverse protein products. Variability in the biologic characteristics of tumors in different individuals (e.g., early invasion versus rapid local expansion) may be related to the profile of the genetic alterations. Many of these same genetic loci, especially those encoding oncogenes, have been implicated in the development of malignancies in the esophagus, stomach, pancreas, and liver. The interface between inherited genetic alterations and acquired mutations resulting from environmental factors has been highlighted by the study of hepatocellular carcinoma. In addition to the appreciation of the potential role of HBV acting as an insertional mutagen due to integration of the virus into the host genome, molecular analysis of hepatocellular carcinoma has shown mutation of a tumor suppressor gene with a chemical carcinogen. Thus aflatoxin, a chemical present in foodstuffs contaminated with *Aspergillus*, which has long been implicated by epidemiologic studies, has been demonstrated to be associated with a specific mutation of

the p53 tumor suppressor gene in some hepatocellular carcinomas in South Africa and China.

LABORATORY DIAGNOSIS AND FUTURE THERAPEUTIC APPROACHES

The techniques of cellular and molecular biology in conjunction with new insights into specific diseases have already yielded powerful new diagnostic tools which aid the clinician. PCR, a technique which can detect even a single copy of a specific DNA molecule, has made possible a marked increase in the sensitivity and specificity of diagnostic detection of viral and other infectious agents. The development of monoclonal antibodies emerging from progress in cellular biologic studies has provided reagents for both serologic diagnosis and more precise morphologic analysis through immunohistochemistry and immunocytochemistry. The latter is occasionally essential in the determination of the origin of a seemingly undifferentiated tumor, particularly lymphomas of the gastrointestinal tract. In situ hybridization, a technique in which specific mRNA rather than protein can be localized within cells, promises to further enhance this capability. Finally, molecular probes encoding specific gene sequences or sequences linked with disease-associated loci are making possible genetic screening for inherited disorders (e.g., familial adenomatous polyposis) in members of affected kindreds. Although the HLA alleles which could be evaluated by specific antisera or monoclonal antibodies have been helpful in determining inheritance of disorders which are linked to these genes on chromosome 6 (e.g., hemochromatosis), disease-related genes elsewhere can only be assessed through markers scattered throughout the genome, which is feasible with collections of DNA probes.

One of the most profound outgrowths of recombinant DNA techniques is the identification and production of important regulatory proteins. A large network of cytokines, broadly defined as proteins that affect the functional characteristics of target cell populations, has been identified as the product of lymphocytes, monocytes, and other cell populations. Cytokines affect processes as diverse as immune activation, cell proliferation, fibrosis, and other functions. Recombinant interferons, a class of cytokines, have made these immunomodulatory proteins available for the treatment of chronic viral hepatitis. Recombinant forms of several other cytokines such as interleukin 1 receptor antagonist, macrophage inhibitory proteins, and transforming growth factor β are being explored for their effects on various inflammatory conditions of the gastrointestinal tract. In addition, considerable interest has focused on a number of growth factors, members of this cytokine network, for their potential importance in facilitating healing of mucosal ulceration and adaptation following resection or infarction of large segments of intestine. It is possible that growth factors may be employed to facilitate intestinal reconstitution following high-dose chemotherapy or radiation treatment for malignancy in a manner similar to the use of stem cell factors to restore hematopoietic function.

The most important impact of advances in molecular biology on gastrointestinal disease may ultimately lie in gene therapy, the introduction of DNA sequences with sustained function to correct an aberration or absence of a relevant gene. The liver will be an important target organ for these innovative approaches both because of its central role in the metabolic processes affected by many inherited disorders and because of the feasibility of targeting DNA to the hepatocytes. The use of DNA coupled to glycoproteins specifically taken up by hepatocyte has already demonstrated the feasibility of introducing DNA sequences with subsequent production of functional proteins (albumin, HMG CoA-reductase). While a number of significant hurdles remain, it is likely that the ability to introduce genetic information in a stable fashion into hepatocytes and other cells will lead to fundamentally new approaches to the treatment of disease of the liver and gastrointestinal tract as well as more systemic disorders.

REFERENCES

CADENA DL et al: Receptor tyrosine kinases. FASEB J 6:2332, 1992

ESCHER JC et al: Molecular basis of lactase levels in adult humans. J Clin Invest 89:480, 1992

GANTZ I et al: Molecular cloning of a gene encoding the histamine H2 receptor. Proc Natl Acad Sci USA 88:429, 1991

HIGUCHI K et al: Human apoliprotein B (apoB) mRNA: Identification of two distinct apoB mRNAs, an mRNA with the apoB-100 sequence and an apoB mRNA containing a premature in-frame translational stop codon, in both liver and intestine. Proc Natl Acad Sci USA 85:1772, 1988

KOPIN AS et al: Expression cloning and characterization of the canine parietal cell gastrin receptor. Proc Natl Acad Sci USA 89:3605, 1992

LOGSDON CD: Receptors: Cell and molecular biology. Reg Peptide Lett 3:37, 1991

TAYLOR GR, FARMERY SM: Single gene disorders affecting the gastrointestinal tract. Gut 34:433, 1993

WILSON JM et al: Hepatocyte-directed gene transfer in vivo leads to transient improvement of hypercholesterolemia in low density lipoprotein receptor-deficient rabbits. J Biol Chem 267:963, 1992

250   GASTROINTESTINAL ENDOSCOPY

MICHAEL B. KIMMEY / FRED E. SILVERSTEIN

Fiberendoscopes have revolutionized the examination of the gastrointestinal tract. Because of the flexibility of the fiberoptic bundles and the controllability of the instrument tip, the operator can steer the instrument around multiple bends under visual control. A channel permits passage of a variety of endoscopic tools such as biopsy forceps, cytology brushes, wash tubes, and electrocautery snares. The viewing window and the light at the instrument's distal end can be washed free of obscuring material. Fluid can be aspirated from hollow organs, and air can be insufflated as needed to improve visualization. The videoendoscope is a modification of the fiberendoscope in which a charge-coupled device on the distal tip of the instrument transmits the image onto a TV screen. This system is being used increasingly because it permits storage, analysis, and transmission of the endoscopic images.

The usefulness of fiberendoscopy in diagnosing gastrointestinal disease is well established. Shallow lesions such as erosions or healing ulcers are missed by single-contrast x-ray but not by endoscopy. The brilliant success of polypectomy via the colonoscope has led to the development of other endoscopic therapeutic techniques such as endoscopic sphincterotomy; endoscopic therapy is now a recognized alternative to surgery in many situations.

Although esophagogastroduodenoscopy (EGD) is not a procedure for the occasional operator, it is widely available in both inpatient and outpatient settings. It is a relatively easy procedure to perform technically, but training and continued experience are necessary for optimal diagnostic accuracy. The more complex procedures such as colonoscopy and endoscopic retrograde cholangiopancreatography (ERCP) require special dexterity, a substantial investment of time for learning, and constant practice to maintain adequate skill; they are probably best accomplished by subspecialists. Complications are most frequent when the operator is inexperienced.

A history and physical examination should be done before any endoscopic procedure. Special care is taken in patients with significant cardiac or pulmonary disease; blood clotting parameters should be checked in those with a history of excessive bleeding. Patients with prosthetic heart valves and those with a history of bacterial endocarditis should receive antibiotic prophylaxis. Contraindications to endoscopy in most situations include the inability of the patient to cooperate or give informed consent, an unstable cardiac or pulmonary condition, and an unstable neck prior to upper endoscopy. Intestinal perforation is also a contraindication to any endoscopic procedure.

Most patients and endoscopists prefer to use conscious sedation for endoscopic procedures other than flexible sigmoidoscopy and some screening upper endoscopies. After insertion of an intravenous catheter, a benzodiazepine such as diazepam or midazolam is titrated to light sedation. Supplementation with a narcotic such as meperidine also may be useful. Adequate monitoring of vital signs and oxygen saturation is important, as is the availability of resuscitation equipment.

Topical pharyngeal anesthesia with a gargle or spray of lidocaine or similar anesthetic is useful prior to upper endoscopic procedures.

UPPER GASTROINTESTINAL ENDOSCOPY   The tip of a forward-viewing endoscope is placed at the cricopharyngeal sphincter of the esophagus, and the patient is encouraged to swallow while gentle pressure is exerted. Small amounts of air are passed through the endoscope to visualize the esophageal lumen. The endoscope is then passed under direct vision into the stomach. The gastric body and antrum are carefully examined. The instrument tip is retroflexed to view the gastric cardia, the fundus, and the whole lesser curvature. The pylorus is traversed, and the first and second portions of the duodenum are visualized. The examination is repeated as the instrument is withdrawn. Visualized lesions can be recorded on photographs or videotape. Biopsies and brush cytologic examinations can be obtained from suspicious areas.

EGD is a relatively safe procedure in experienced hands. Several large surveys suggest a risk of serious complications during diagnostic EGD of approximately 1 in 500 and a risk of death of approximately 1 in 10,000. The risks are higher in emergency procedures and in the elderly or seriously ill. In a survey of patients examined by endoscopy during bleeding, 1 in 200 had serious complications and 1 in 700 died from the procedure. The main causes of mortality were cardiopulmonary complications and perforations by the instrument. Endoscopy is preferred over x-ray in the urgent diagnosis of gastrointestinal illness in women who might be pregnant.

Gastroesophageal reflux disease   Esophagitis is one of the most common diseases of the upper gastrointestinal tract (see Chap. 251). Esophageal pain may be confused with cardiac disease, or esophagitis may present as painless blood loss. Because esophagitis usually involves only the superficial mucosa, it cannot be diagnosed by routine single-contrast radiography. At endoscopy, friable mucosa, linear erosions, and ulcerations are clearly visible. Not every patient with heartburn requires esophagoscopy, but the procedure is indicated if the patient complains of dysphagia; if an x-ray shows a stricture, a mass, or an ulcer; if symptoms persist despite therapy; or if antireflux surgery is contemplated. Patients over age 40 with significant complaints of heartburn for over 10 years should be considered for endoscopy to detect Barrett's esophagus.

The squamous mucosa of the esophagus is more vulnerable to peptic digestion than is the columnar epithelium of the stomach. Thus esophagitis is located on the squamous side of the esophagogastric junction and is most severe in the distal esophagus, where the squamous mucosa is most exposed to regurgitated acid and pepsin from the stomach. Discrete peptic ulceration of the esophagus is uncommon.

A short area of esophagitis or a stricture can be seen even in the upper esophagus. This is explained by progressive replacement of distal eroded squamous mucosa with metaplastic epithelium, which is more resistant to peptic digestion (Barrett's epithelium). This finding can be documented by biopsy. Such epithelium is more prone to malignant transformation and, therefore, may merit regular surveillance with esophagoscopy and biopsy every 12 to 24 months. Flow cytometry also may prove useful in the early detection of abnormal cell DNA populations (e.g., polyploidy). If dysplasia is present, more frequent surveillance may be indicated to detect early carcinoma.

Esophagitis may progress to scarring and stricture formation. The endoscopic appearance of a benign stricture is characteristic but not diagnostic; a malignancy should be ruled out by biopsy and cytologic brushing before medical treatment is undertaken with dilation and antacids. The whole length of the stricture should be sampled. Endoscopy is also indicated to biopsy the rim of an esophageal ulcer to rule out cancer.

Dilations of difficult strictures are best initiated by passing a flexible-tipped guidewire via the biopsy channel of the endoscope through the stricture under direct vision. The endoscope can then be withdrawn over the wire, which serves as a guide for passage of progressively larger polyvinyl dilators through the stricture under fluoroscopic control. An alternative technique utilizes balloon catheters passed via the endoscope channel or over a guidewire through the stricture. The balloon is inflated under endoscopic and/or fluoroscopic guidance to dilate the stricture.

Peptic ulcer Esophagogastroduodenoscopy is more accurate than upper gastrointestinal x-ray in detecting ulcers. It has been suggested that x-ray be abandoned entirely in favor of endoscopy for detecting ulcers. This makes sense when the source of acute upper gastrointestinal bleeding is sought and urgent surgical intervention is being considered. However, in the workup of the patient with less pressing ulcer complaints, a double-contrast upper gastrointestinal x-ray is still often used as the initial diagnostic test. The greater expense and discomfort of endoscopy are justified if the x-ray is equivocal or suggests that the ulcer is malignant, if the x-ray is negative but the clinical picture suggests peptic ulceration, or if the patient is about to be operated on for ulcer. Patients with duodenal ulcers shown by x-ray or with classic ulcer deformities of the duodenal bulb do not require endoscopy for diagnosis if the presenting symptoms are characteristic and if the symptomatic response to antiulcer treatment is good. Screening endoscopy using small-diameter endoscopes without sedation is a reasonable alternative to contrast x-rays as the initial diagnostic test in the symptomatic patient.

There are some situations in which x-ray reveals ulcers missed by endoscopy, e.g., ulcers in hourglass constrictions of the stomach or in small, incompletely visualized duodenal bulbs. Fiberendoscopy is especially useful in visualizing postbulbar ulcers, giant duodenal ulcers, and stomal ulceration after partial gastrectomy, all of which can be missed by x-ray. Endoscopy may be of use in determining the cause of gastric outlet obstruction.

In the enthusiasm for fiberendoscopy one must not forget that visual interpretation of gross pathology is subjective—one observer's ulcer is another's erosion. An erosion is confined to the mucosa and heals without a trace, whereas an ulcer is deeper and usually implies a chronic recurrent disease. Endoscopically, erosions are superficial, small, and multiple; ulcers are deeper and larger and tend to be solitary. As indicated above, visualized lesions can readily be recorded as photographs or on videotape.

Cancer The endoscopic appearance of upper gastrointestinal cancer may seem obvious, especially if there is a mass growing into the lumen. On the other hand, malignant ulcers, infiltrative carcinomas, or small early carcinomas are frequently impossible to diagnose by their gross appearance. Six to eight biopsies should be taken from the rim of a gastric ulcer to exclude malignancy. Experience and skill in choosing the biopsy site improves the accuracy. A cytologic examination of lavage or brush specimen adds to the diagnostic accuracy in all areas of the upper gastrointestinal tract (see Chap. 253).

In most patients, gastric ulcers should be assessed for healing by endoscopy after 12 weeks of antiulcer therapy. Persistent ulcers should be biopsied if they were not biopsied at the time of the initial diagnosis or they should be rebiopsied if they are not healing. Some patients with a low likelihood of malignancy, for example, a young person taking anti-inflammatory drugs, can be assessed for healing radiographically. Duodenal ulcers are rarely malignant and therefore do not need to be assessed for healing following therapy in most circumstances.

Primary gastric lymphoma can mimic benign gastric ulcer or adenocarcinoma on gastroscopy or x-ray. It can be diagnosed by biopsy or cytology, although the accuracy is not as high as in adenocarcinoma. The diagnosis of lymphoma is aided by special studies of fresh, unfixed biopsy specimens to detect a clonal population of lymphocytes.

If a polypoid lesion of the stomach is covered by mucosa that appears normal by gastroscopy, the likelihood of malignancy is very small. Such lesions are often intramural, subepithelial benign tumors such as leiomyomas or pancreatic rests. Biopsies of such lesions are usually not diagnostic. Lesions over 2 cm in diameter can be evaluated by endoscopic ultrasonography, a technique that combines diagnostic ultrasound with endoscopy. Polyps covered by abnormal-appearing mucosa can be benign or malignant. Random biopsy can miss carcinoma within a polyp. If technically feasible, polyps should therefore be removed in their entirety by snare cautery for histologic examination. If over 2 cm in diameter, they are more likely to contain cancer (see Chap. 253). Large polyps may require surgical excision.

Ampullary carcinoma may be diagnosed by biopsy during duodenoscopy, although a prior endoscopic sphincterotomy may increase diagnostic yield. Other primary duodenal malignancies are very rare. Extensions from pancreatic or biliary tract cancer are difficult to diagnose because the tumor may not have extended into the mucosa and may therefore not be accessible for endoscopic biopsy or cytologic examination. In these secondary tumors, diagnosis must depend on some combination of echography, computed tomography, and ERCP with cytologic examination of ductal strictures.

Upper gastrointestinal bleeding (See also Chap. 41) Endoscopy within the first 12 to 24 h of an upper gastrointestinal hemorrhage can be very helpful in planning rational therapy by visualizing the bleeding source. Superficial lesions not visible by x-ray may be seen (esophagitis, Mallory-Weiss tear, erosive gastritis, stress ulcer, and telangiectasia). Lesions that are visible by x-ray may not be the source of bleeding. Endoscopy can determine the actual bleeding site and degree of bleeding. For example, visualization of a spurting artery which is flooding the stomach indicates massive ongoing bleeding requiring prompt therapeutic intervention. Several studies have shown that the demonstration at endoscopy of any bleeding whatsoever or a nonbleeding vessel or sentinel clot in the ulcer base makes rebleeding more likely. The diagnostic accuracy of emergency endoscopy in upper gastrointestinal bleeding approaches 90 percent.

Every patient having endoscopy for upper gastrointestinal bleeding merits a complete endoscopic examination of the esophagus, stomach, and duodenum. Finding a potential bleeding lesion is not proof that this is the source of hemorrhage unless active bleeding is seen. Up to 50 percent of patients with esophageal varices can be shown endoscopically to be bleeding from another source such as erosive gastritis, duodenal ulcer, or gastric ulcer. Occasionally it is not possible to diagnose the exact lesion that is bleeding, but localizing the area of bleeding can be very helpful; for example, bright red arterial blood may be seen pouring into the stomach from the duodenum when the esophagus and stomach are relatively free of blood.

There are three controversial areas. First, *do all bleeders need endoscopy?* Endoscopy is indicated in all patients who may require surgery because of continual bleeding or rebleeding because selection of the type of operation depends on what lesion is bleeding. Although 85 percent of upper gastrointestinal bleeders stop spontaneously, it is impossible to predict which ones will; therefore, endoscopy is recommended for most bleeders. Second, *how early should endoscopy be performed in the acutely bleeding patient?* Most studies suggest that the diagnostic accuracy of EGD remains high for the first 12 to 24 h after the bleeding episode. All would agree that it is desirable to delay endoscopy until vital signs have been stabilized after adequate blood replacement. Upper endoscopy is usually performed during waking hours at a time during the first day of bleeding when the patient's vital signs are stable and when the full endoscopic team is available. Emergency endoscopy at night should be reserved for those patients with continued massive bleeding or rebleeding requiring an immediate decision regarding surgery or other treatment. If the patient is exsanguinating, endoscopy can follow induction of anesthesia just preceding surgery. Thus the patient's airway is protected by an endotracheal tube. Finally, *does endoscopy affect the clinical outcome?* Earlier studies that did not use endoscopic therapy suggest that it does not. Recent studies of the endoscopic treatment of bleeding lesions with heater probes and bipolar probes suggest that these methods are safe and reduce blood requirements, need for surgery, and mortality in some patients with bleeding ulcers.

Injection therapy of bleeding lesions is another therapeutic modality used to stop bleeding. Injection of a dilute solution of epinephrine alone or followed by injection of either alcohol or a sclerosing agent often stops active bleeding from peptic ulcers. Injection of various sclerosing solutions into or next to esophageal varices is effective treatment for stopping active variceal bleeding. Alternatively, rubber band ligation of varices at endoscopy has been shown to stop bleeding. Repeated injection sclerotherapy or band ligation to achieve variceal eradication produces results comparable to portacaval shunting in terms of mortality, although rebleeding after endoscopic therapy may necessitate further endoscopic intervention or shunting.

Emergency and therapeutic endoscopy is not for the inexperienced. It requires considerable technical skill and interpretive experience and the best available instruments.

Percutaneous endoscopic gastrostomy   The placement of feeding or decompression gastrostomy tubes can be facilitated with the use of an endoscope. Under sedation, the endoscope's light within the stomach is used to identify a suitable location for a gastrostomy in the left upper quadrant of the abdomen. A needle is introduced into the stomach percutaneously, and then a snare passed through the endoscope is used to capture a wire or suture placed through the needle. A feeding tube is advanced over the wire into the stomach. Feedings are begun the following day. Hospitalization time and morbidity and mortality of operative gastrostomy are reduced.

Patients with transfer dysphagia secondary to strokes and degenerative neurologic disorders benefit the most from percutaneous endoscopic gastrostomy. Other indications include dysphagia produced by head and neck neoplasms and the inability to eat secondary to diffuse cerebral injury. Patients with severe gastroparesis can be fed through a jejunal feeding tube placed through the gastrostomy and then directed through the pylorus. Simultaneous gastric decompression is possible through a separate lumen in the gastrostomy.

Palliation of esophageal carcinoma   Patients with dysphagia caused by malignant esophageal strictures usually cannot be cured by esophagectomy. Surgical resection and radiation therapy are often chosen for palliation of dysphagia in this situation. The endoscopist also can help palliate these patients when radiation therapy has failed or when surgical risks are too great.

Dilation of malignant strictures is usually possible with polyvinyl dilators passed over an endoscopically placed guidewire. It may improve the patient's swallowing initially, but more definitive therapy is usually needed. This can be in the form of laser ablation or by placement of a prosthesis or stent. Tumor within the esophageal lumen can be destroyed by application of Nd:YAG laser energy using a laser waveguide placed through the biopsy channel of the endoscope. Alternatively, after stricture dilation, large-caliber stents can be placed over a dilator. When the dilator is removed, the stent lumen is available for the passage of food. Stenting is especially useful in the palliation of malignant tracheoesophageal fistulas.

Other indications   Upper endoscopy is usually substituted for x-ray in the urgent diagnosis of gastrointestinal illness in *pregnancy*. Patients with *dysphagia* merit esophagoscopy because the cause is frequently organic and may be missed by x-ray. Dysphagia caused by esophageal dysmotility is best diagnosed by manometry or cineradiography in addition to endoscopy. *Painful swallowing* (odynophagia), especially in immunosuppressed or diabetic patients, may merit esophagoscopy because biopsy and brushings of the involved esophageal wall may reveal monilial, herpetic, or cytomegalovirus infections. Soon after ingestion of a corrosive agent, if there is no indication of wall necrosis, limited and gentle esophagoscopy is useful in evaluating the severity of injury. Many impacted foreign bodies can be removed from the esophagus or stomach with a snare or forceps; sharp foreign bodies are usually best removed by pulling them into the lumen of a rigid tubular esophagoscope or into a protective overtube around a fiberoptic endoscope. Careful esophagoscopy after removal of an esophageal foreign body is important to determine whether there is an underlying lesion which caused the impaction (e.g., cancer, benign stricture, peptic esophagitis).

In the postoperative stomach, gastroscopy is especially useful in detecting carcinoma, recurrent ulceration, retrograde intussusception,

and stomal stricture. Several European studies indicate a definite threat of carcinoma developing in the gastric stump 10 to 20 years after a Billroth II gastrectomy. The diagnosis of such postoperative carcinomas may require many biopsies of seemingly normal mucosa near the anastomosis. Studies of the natural history of this condition in the United States do not suggest a similar high incidence of postoperative carcinoma.

When the duodenal bulb shows reddening or nodularity, many endoscopists diagnose *duodenitis*. There is little evidence to suggest that this picture is of significance. On the other hand, diffuse and bleeding erosions of the duodenal bulb merit a diagnosis of *erosive duodenitis*, especially after ingestion of mucosal irritants such as aspirin. A nodular or narrow duodenum will occasionally yield granulomas on biopsy, indicative of Crohn's disease.

ENDOSCOPIC RETROGRADE CHOLANGIOPANCREATOGRAPHY   ERCP involves placing a side-viewing instrument in the descending duodenum. The papilla of Vater is cannulated, contrast medium is injected, and the pancreatic ducts and hepatobiliary tree are visualized radiographically. Skilled operators can visualize 90 to 95 percent of pancreatic ducts and 90 percent of biliary ducts.

ERCP is performed on an x-ray table after sedation and induction of duodenal hypotonia with atropine or glucagon. The pancreatic duct is gently filled throughout its entire length with 2 to 5 mL of contrast material with constant fluoroscopic monitoring (Fig. 250-1A). Injection is continued until the first side branches are seen, and overfilling is avoided. By insertion of the cannula at a more acute cephalad angle, the common bile duct and the whole biliary tract including the gallbladder are visualized (Fig. 250-1B).

ERCP is a safe procedure when performed by an experienced operator. Asymptomatic amylase elevations occur in 30 to 40 percent of patients after pancreatography and are rarely of clinical significance. Pancreatitis occurs in less than 5 percent of patients but is usually benign and self-limited. In a nationwide survey of complications, the morbidity rate was 3 percent and mortality rate 0.2 percent. The main serious complication is retention of nonsterile contrast material proximal to an obstructed duct, causing cholangitis or pancreatic sepsis. Patients suspected of having bile duct obstruction are started on systemic antibiotics prior to the ERCP. Furthermore, if bile duct or pancreatic duct obstruction is first revealed by ERCP, antibiotic coverage is indicated to reduce the incidence of bacteremia; such patients should be drained, if possible, either with endoscopic therapy (papillotomy, stents, nasobiliary drains, etc.) or surgically within 36 h.

Retrograde cholangiography   This procedure is especially useful in patients with persistent jaundice the cause of which cannot be established by conventional diagnostic methods. The important differential diagnosis is between obstructive and nonobstructive jaundice. When the cause of jaundice is unclear, approximately 15 percent of patients thought to have nonobstructive jaundice prove to have extrahepatic biliary obstruction requiring surgery or endoscopic therapy, and conversely, the same percentage of patients thought to have obstructive jaundice prove to have an open ductal system by ERCP and can be spared unnecessary intervention.

Remediable causes of obstructive jaundice which can be diagnosed by retrograde cholangiography include common duct stones (Fig. 250-1C) and benign and malignant strictures. In jaundiced patients with suspected primary liver disease, such as primary biliary cirrhosis, ERCP can assure that no operable obstruction is being missed.

In addition to ERCP, other methods of visualizing the biliary tree in the jaundiced patient include *percutaneous transhepatic cholangiography* (PTC), in which contrast material is injected from the exterior via a needle into the intrahepatic bile ducts under fluoroscopic control, and the noninvasive methods of *ultrasound*, *computed tomography* (CT), and radionuclide biliary scintigraphy (see Chap. 262). Most physicians first use ultrasound or CT to see whether the biliary ducts are dilated and to seek the cause of the patient's jaundice (stones, pancreatic mass, etc.). The radionuclide scan will determine if the cystic duct and bile ducts are patent. Direct visualization is undertaken if the diagnosis is not established. PTC is

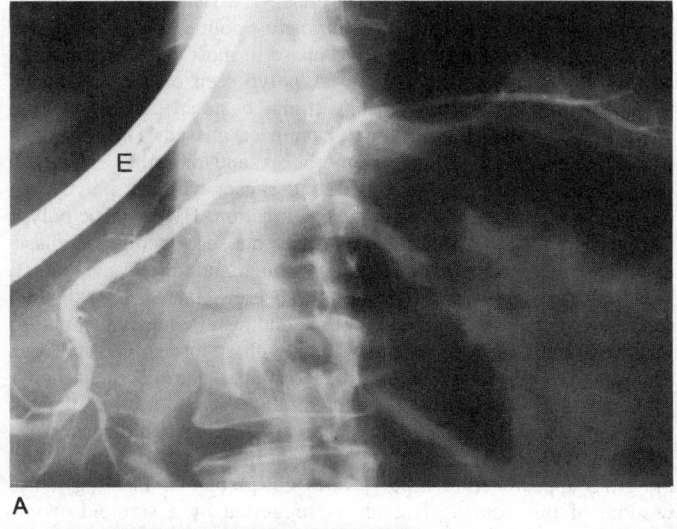

A

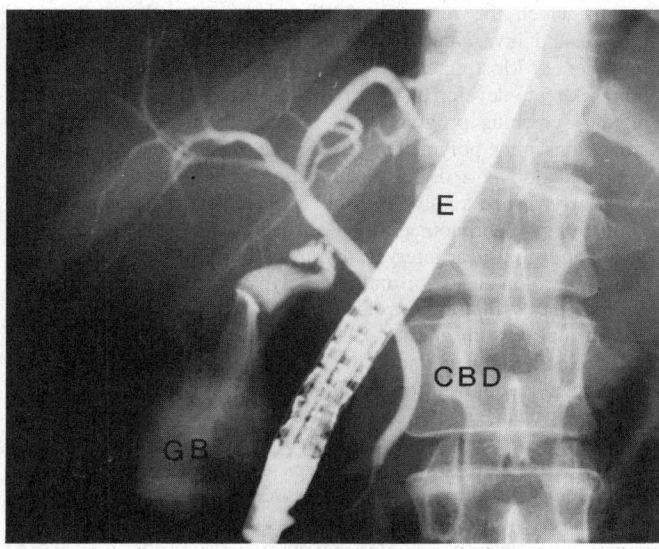

B

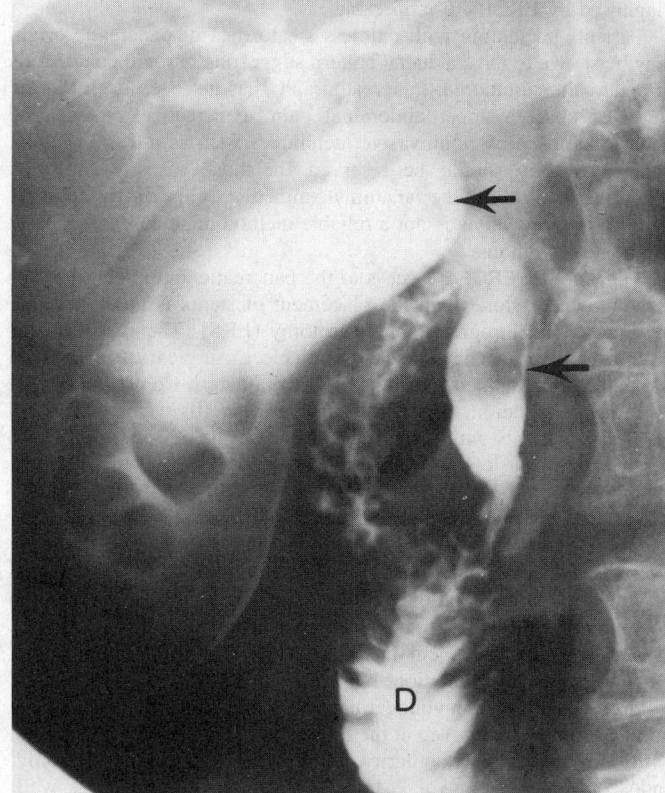

C

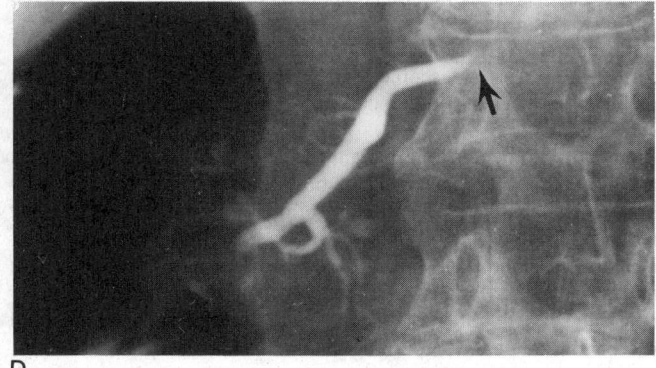

D

FIGURE 250-1 *A*. A tapering pancreatic duct of normal caliber is seen and may be compared to the endoscope (E) 1 cm in diameter. *B*. Normal cholangiogram. The diameter of the common duct (CBD) is normal. The intrahepatic ducts branch normally, and the gallbladder (GB) can be seen. The endoscope (E) is seen in the duodenum. *C*. Several stones (*arrows*) can be seen in an obstructed, dilated common duct. The gallbladder also contains several stones. Regurgitated contrast material is seen in the duodenum (D). *D*. The sharp cutoff (*arrow*) of the pancreatic duct is caused by a carcinoma of the body of the pancreas. *(Courtesy of Dr. Charles Rohrmann.)*

often attempted first if an intrahepatic or proximal bile duct obstruction is suggested by imaging tests. ERCP is used first if distal obstruction is suspected. Advantages of the endoscopic approach are that the papilla and the pancreatic duct are seen (in addition to the biliary ducts) and that therapy can be performed with endoscopic sphincterotomy or drainage when appropriate. In the event of a technical failure or incomplete information resulting from either ERCP or PTC, the other technique is tried. This approach detects most lesions requiring surgical intervention.

ERCP or PTC also can be useful in patients with biliary pain, cholangitis, or impaired liver function after previous biliary surgery. Remediable postoperative lesions such as strictures can be discovered and sometimes treated endoscopically. Should endoscopic therapy fail, their precise anatomy is outlined so that reoperation is less difficult. Biliary manometry also can be performed in this setting to

diagnose sphincter of Oddi dysfunction. A perfused catheter is placed into the sphincter via the endoscope, and pressures are recorded. A high basal sphincter pressure may predict a beneficial effect of sphincterotomy.

Retrograde pancreatography Patients with recurrent or chronic pancreatitis may merit retrograde pancreatography to seek a lesion which can be approached endoscopically or surgically, such as localized pancreatitis in the tail or ductal pathology amenable to endoscopic stenting or surgical drainage.

Patients with symptoms, signs, or laboratory findings suggesting pancreatic carcinoma may have pancreatograms suggesting malignancy with a narrowed, encased, or sharply "cut off" pancreatic duct (Fig. 250-1*D*). Differentiation of such pancreatic ductal findings from benign inflammatory disease can be difficult. Cytologic examination of pancreatic duct brushings obtained during ERCP may prove helpful.

Unfortunately, most patients with symptomatic pancreatic cancer diagnosed by ERCP are inoperable.

Patients presenting with painless steatorrhea of pancreatic origin may be shown to have a ductal pattern suggesting chronic pancreatitis or pancreatic carcinoma. Pancreatography has not been useful in the study of obscure upper abdominal pain. Pancreatic cysts can be better diagnosed by noninvasive techniques such as ultrasound, and pancreatography should be reserved for those cases where it is desirable to outline the anatomy immediately prior to surgery. Pancreatography alone is not a reliable method of screening for early pancreatic carcinoma.

Therapeutic ERCP   Access to the pancreatic and biliary tree for the removal of stones and the placement of stents is made possible by endoscopic retrograde sphincterotomy (ERS). The pancreatic or biliary sphincter mechanism is cut using electrosurgical current passed through a wire attached to the ERCP catheter. Complications of bleeding, perforation, pancreatitis, and cholangitis occur in about 8 percent of patients with a resulting mortality rate of approximately 1 percent. The role of pancreatic sphincterotomy in the management of pancreatic stones and strictures is evolving; however, biliary sphincterotomy is now an established therapy for several conditions.

Common bile duct stones in patients with prior cholecystectomy are successfully removed from the bile duct after ERS by experienced operators 90 percent of the time. Small stones are pulled into the duodenum with a balloon catheter or after being captured by a basket. Stones larger than 1.5 cm in diameter may be difficult to extract without prior fragmentation by 'mechanical or other techniques. Common duct stones in younger patients with intact gallbladders have traditionally been removed at the time of cholecystectomy. However, with the increasing popularity of laparoscopic cholecystectomy, endoscopic stone removal is being utilized in this setting as well. Older patients with increased surgical risks can sometimes be managed with ERS and stone extraction alone; cholecystectomy can be delayed or avoided entirely. ERS is also assuming an increasing role in the initial treatment of patients with acute cholangitis and severe biliary pancreatitis. Early endoscopic stone removal in both these settings has been shown to reduce complications associated with these conditions.

Patients with benign and malignant bile duct strictures may benefit from the endoscopic placement of biliary stents after ERS. Benign strictures frequently remain dilated following removal of stents that have been left in place for several months. Patients with either pancreatic carcinoma or cholangiocarcinoma resulting in obstructive jaundice can be palliated effectively by placement of a plastic or metal biliary stent. Stents usually occlude after 3 to 6 months and must be exchanged if recurrent jaundice or cholangitis develops. Strictures involving the hilum of the liver (see Chap. 272) are difficult to palliate endoscopically; stents sometimes must be placed into both sides of the liver. These patients may require additional percutaneous radiologic procedures to achieve adequate biliary drainage.

COLONOSCOPY   The interior of the entire length of the colon from anus to cecum can be visualized by the experienced colonoscopist. This is one of the most significant diagnostic and therapeutic applications of fiberoptic endoscopy because it can diagnose potentially curable colonic cancers missed by other techniques and remove potentially precancerous adenomatous polyps.

Most initial colonoscopies are performed to investigate findings on an abnormal barium enema or to elucidate the cause of gastrointestinal bleeding. The ability to examine the whole colon is also useful in the management of some patients with inflammatory bowel disease and in patients with a strong family history of colon polyps or cancer.

Patients are prepared for colonoscopy with laxatives and tap water enemas or by a total-gut lavage with a nonabsorbable electrolyte solution.

The main complications of colonoscopy are hemorrhage and perforation (morbidity rate is 0.5 to 1.3 percent; mortality rate is 0.02 percent). The complication rate for polypectomy is 1 to 2 percent. Diverticular or ischemic disease and prior irradiation make the procedure more difficult and hazardous. The risk of perforation is also increased in the patient with very active colitis, and colonoscopy should be avoided during the acute phase in most circumstances.

Polyps (See also Chap. 257)   A polyp seen on barium enema merits colonoscopy for two reasons: It may be an artifact or a cancer, and a second polyp or cancer may have been missed. The polyp can usually be excised, with lower morbidity and mortality rates than with surgery. The best way to rule out cancer within a polyp is to remove it completely for histologic examination. Hyperplastic polyps do not become malignant; colonic polyps that show benign neoplasia histologically may become malignant (tubular and villous adenomas). The risk of neoplastic polyps being cancerous increases with their size. The risk is also higher in villous adenomas. Pedunculated polyps with cancer confined to the mucosa and with an uninvolved stalk can be cured by removal with an electrocautery snare during colonoscopy. Thus most colonoscopists will remove all polyps more than 0.5 cm in diameter. Polyps smaller than 0.5 cm in diameter should be biopsied or removed because more than 50 percent may be adenomatous, and the gross appearance of a polyp does not predict its histology. The wisdom of this course of action is suggested by a sigmoidoscopic study in which the removal of all polyps reduced the expected incidence and invasiveness of subsequent cancers in the anatomic area screened. Most agree that the patient with adenomatous polyps is more likely to develop another polyp or cancer and therefore merits a regular screening program. The optimal frequency of follow-up examinations after polypectomy is not yet established. The current recommendation is a digital examination and stool test for occult blood yearly. When a polyp is discovered, the entire colon should be examined for synchronous polyps or cancer. This should probably be repeated at 3- to 5-year intervals and more frequently in patients with a history of colon cancer or multiple polyps. If stools are positive for occult blood or symptoms develop, immediate evaluation is indicated.

Abnormal barium enema   All filling defects on barium enema merit evaluation by colonoscopy. If the lesion is a pedunculated polyp, it can be removed for histologic examination; if its appearance suggests a cancer, it can be biopsied for histologic confirmation. When a polyp or a carcinoma is found, the remainder of the colon should be screened for additional polyps and synchronous carcinoma. This avoids multiple colotomies to search for a second lesion and reduces surgical morbidity. Some lesions diagnosed as a mass by x-ray may not be present on colonoscopy or are due to lesions such as a polyp rather than a cancer.

Narrowing by x-ray   Determining the cause of segmental narrowing may be difficult by x-ray. Colonoscopy often permits this and also can help one differentiate adenocarcinoma from inflammation secondary to ischemia, irradiation, diverticular disease, or Crohn's colitis. Even the most classic "apple-core" lesion indicated by x-ray may be covered by normal mucosa at colonoscopy, suggesting an extrinsic inflammatory lesion. In 10 to 30 percent of patients, narrowed segments present on x-ray are not visualized during colonoscopy, probably because they are areas of temporary spasm. Such findings avoid unnecessary operations.

Chronic bleeding (x-ray and sigmoidoscopy negative)   This is a common indication for colonoscopy. The x-ray is more likely to miss a lesion when single contrast is used rather than air contrast. The cause of bleeding is found in approximately 40 percent of such patients from such sources as adenomatous polyp, adenocarcinoma, and inflammatory bowel disease. If no bleeding source is found, a search may be appropriate for an upper gastrointestinal source with an upper gastrointestinal x-ray or upper endoscopy.

Inflammatory bowel disease   Colonoscopy is not routinely indicated in patients with inflammatory bowel disease. Colonoscopy may help in the initial diagnosis, especially in differentiating Crohn's colitis from ulcerative colitis. It can aid the surgeon in assessing the activity and extent of the disease before surgery. Colonoscopy can help in the evaluation of radiographic abnormalities suggesting cancer, such as strictures, polyps, or masses. Colonoscopy may be indicated in patients with ulcerative colitis of more than 10 years' duration because of the increased risk of carcinoma; it is hoped that repeated colonoscopies will serve to detect these malignancies while the lesions are still curable. The optimal frequency of colonoscopy in such patients is not yet established. If an expert gastrointestinal pathologist finds high-grade dysplasia in colonic biopsies in a patient with long-standing ulcerative colitis, most would consider this to be an indication for colectomy. Colonoscopy is contraindicated in patients with toxic megacolon, very active disease, or a possible intestinal perforation.

Other indications The flexible sigmoidoscope is replacing the rigid 25-cm sigmoidoscope for routine screening because it can be passed to 40 to 60 cm with minimal preparation, less discomfort, and a higher diagnostic yield. After segmental colonic resection for carcinoma, colonoscopy may detect early mucosal recurrence and differentiate it from benign anastomotic strictures or bleeding suture granulomas. Colonoscopy is occasionally used during laparotomy to assist the surgeon in ruling out other lesions. The colonoscope can be advanced to the cecum rapidly with the surgeon's assistance and additional polyps removed without colotomy. Colonoscopy is useful in the management of selected patients with lower gastrointestinal bleeding. Patients with severe active bleeding are often managed with radionuclide-labeled red blood cell scans followed immediately, if active bleeding is present, by selective angiography. Colonoscopic visualization in this setting is difficult because of excessive luminal blood. If the labeled red blood cell scan is negative, colonic lavage with a balanced electrolyte solution followed in several hours by colonoscopy may identify the bleeding site. Bleeding polyps may be removed by snare electrocautery. Endoscopic hemostatic therapy may be useful in other bleeding lesions such as angiodysplasia.

Colonoscopy is usually not necessary for the diagnosis of familial polyposis because affected family members can be diagnosed by periodic flexible sigmoidoscopy. Carcinoma is a great threat in those familial polyposis syndromes which produce many adenomatous polyps (familial polyposis and Gardner's syndrome); in these conditions, polypectomy is useful for diagnosis, but colectomy is the only treatment which prevents development of carcinoma. These patients are also at risk of developing duodenal and periampullary cancer and should probably undergo periodic surveillance with a side-viewing duodenoscope.

CONSCIOUS DIAGNOSTIC LAPAROSCOPY The potentials for laparoscopy in conscious patients have not been as fully appreciated in North America as they have been in other countries, where it is used widely. This procedure has extremely low mortality and morbidity rates in experienced hands. The instrument usually used for laparoscopy is a rigid tube with a lens system that provides a superb view. Under local anesthesia, pneumoperitoneum is gradually induced with air or nitrous oxide.

Much of the exterior of the liver, gallbladder, spleen, peritoneum, diaphragm, and pelvic organs can be clearly visualized. Portions of the colon and small bowel also can be seen. Lesions can be biopsied under direct vision and any resultant bleeding controlled by electrocoagulation.

Laparoscopy may permit one to make a difficult diagnosis without resorting to laparotomy by biopsying localized hepatic disease under direct vision. Laparoscopy can often help differentiate nonobstructive from obstructive jaundice and also may enable staging of malignant disease without laparotomy.

REFERENCES

CELLO JP et al: Endoscopic sclerotherapy versus portacaval shunt in patients with severe cirrhosis and acute variceal hemorrhage: Long-term follow-up. N Engl J Med 316:11, 1987

COOK DJ et al: Endoscopic therapy for acute nonvariceal upper gastrointestinal hemorrhage: A meta-analysis. Gastroenterology 102:139, 1992

HAGGITT RC et al: Prognostic factors in colorectal carcinomas arising in adenomas: Implications for lesions removed by endoscopic polypectomy. Gastroenterology 89:328, 1985

JENSEN DM, MACHICADO GA: Diagnosis and treatment of severe hematochezia: The role of urgent colonoscopy after purge. Gastroenterology 95:1569, 1988

LAI ECS et al: Endoscopic biliary drainage for severe acute cholangitis. N Engl J Med 326:1582, 1992

LAINE L: Multipolar electrocoagulation in the treatment of active upper gastrointestinal tract hemorrhage. N Engl J Med 316:1613, 1987

NAVEAU S et al: Endoscopic Nd-YAG laser therapy as palliative treatment for esophageal and cardial cancer: Parameters affecting long-term outcome. Dig Dis Sci 35:294, 1990

REID BJ etal: Flow cytometric and histologic progression to malignancy in Barrett's esophagus: Prospective endoscopic surveillance of a cohort. Gastroenterology 102:1212, 1992

SILVERSTEIN FE, TYTGAT GNJ: Atlas of Gastrointestinal Endoscopy. Philadelphia, Saunders, 1987

SIVAK MV: Gastroenterologic Endoscopy. Philadelphia, Saunders, 1987

251 DISEASES OF THE ESOPHAGUS

RAJ K. GOYAL

The two major functions of the esophagus are the transport of the food bolus from the mouth to the stomach and the prevention of retrograde flow of gastrointestinal contents. The transport function is achieved by peristaltic contractions (see Chap. 37). Retrograde flow is prevented by the two esophageal sphincters, which remain closed between swallows. The upper esophageal sphincter remains closed by the elastic properties of its wall and by tonic contraction of the cricopharyngeus and inferior pharyngeal constrictor muscles due to continuous neural excitation of the lower motor neurons which innervate these muscles via motor end plates. The opening of the upper sphincter is due to inhibition of contraction of the cricopharyngeus and inferior pharyngeal constriction and forward displacement of the larynx by the suprahyoid muscles. In contrast, the lower esophageal sphincter remains closed largely because of its intrinsic myogenic tone. The lower esophageal sphincter is innervated by preganglionic parasympathetic fibers in the vagus nerve and postganglionic inhibitory and excitatory neurons in the wall of the esophagus that cause its relaxation and contraction, respectively. The neurotransmitters of the inhibitory nerves are vasoactive intestinal peptide (VIP) and nitric oxide. The antireflux function of the lower esophageal sphincter is supplemented by the diaphragmatic crura which surround the sphincter. A reflex decrease in the lower sphincter pressure occurs during the belching reflex and gastric distention. Fatty meals, smoking, and beverages with a high xanthine content (tea, coffee, cola) also cause a reduction in sphincter pressure. Many hormones and neurotransmitters can modify lower sphincter pressure. Cholinergic muscarinic (M-2 receptor) agonists, alpha-adrenergic agonists, gastrin, pancreatic polypeptide, substance P, and prostaglandin $F_{2\alpha}$ cause contraction; in contrast, nicotine, beta-adrenergic agonists, dopamine, cholecystokinin, secretin, VIP, calcitonin-gene–related peptide (CGRP), adenosine, and nitric oxide and nitric oxide donors such as nitrates cause relaxation of the sphincter. These effects are mediated by actions on the inhibitory intramural neurons or on the sphincter muscle directly. Effects of many of these agents are pharmacologic rather than physiologic.

SYMPTOMS

DYSPHAGIA See Chap. 37.

ESOPHAGEAL PAIN *Heartburn*, or pyrosis, is characterized by burning retrosternal discomfort that may move up and down the chest like a wave. When severe, it may radiate to the sides of the chest, neck, and angles of the jaw. Heartburn is a characteristic symptom of reflux esophagitis and may be associated with regurgitation or a feeling of warm fluid climbing up the throat. It is aggravated by bending forward, straining, or lying recumbent and is worse after meals. It is relieved by upright posture, by swallowing of saliva or water, or, more reliably, by antacids. Heartburn appears to be produced by heightened mucosal sensitivity and can be reproduced by infusion of dilute (0.1 N) hydrochloric acid (Bernstein test) or neutral hyperosmolar solutions into the esophagus.

Odynophagia, or painful swallowing, is characteristic of nonreflux esophagitis, particularly monilial and herpes esophagitis. Odynophagia also may occur with peptic ulcer of the esophagus (Barrett's ulcer), carcinoma with periesophageal involvement, caustic damage of the esophagus, and esophageal perforation. Odynophagia is unusual in uncomplicated reflux esophagitis. Crampy chest pain associated with impaction of a food bolus should be distinguished from odynophagia.

Atypical chest pain other than heartburn and odynophagia occurs in influx esophagitis or esophageal motility disorders such as diffuse esophageal spasm. This may occur spontaneously or during a meal. Chest pain due to periesophageal involvement caused by carcinoma or peptic ulcer may be constant and agonizing. Sometimes different types of esophageal pains exist together in the same patient, and frequently patients are not able to describe the pain accurately enough to allow its classification. Esophageal disease is a common cause of noncardiac atypical chest pain. However, many of these patients have nonspecific esophageal motor abnormalities. The cause-and-effect relationship of the nonspecific esophageal motor abnormalities and the atypical chest pain is unclear. Many of these patients have behavioral abnormalities, psychosomatic disorders, depression, anxiety, panic reactions, and other somatization disorders.

REGURGITATION   *Regurgitation* is the effortless appearance of gastric or esophageal contents in the mouth. In distal esophageal obstruction and stasis, as in achalasia or a large diverticulum, the regurgitated material consists of tasteless mucoid fluid or undigested food. Regurgitation of sour or bitter-tasting material occurs in severe gastroesophageal reflux and is associated with incompetence of both the upper and lower esophageal sphincters. Regurgitation may result in laryngeal aspiration, with spells of coughing and choking that awaken the patient from sleep, and aspiration pneumonia. Water brash is reflex salivary hypersecretion which occurs in response to peptic esophagitis; it should not be confused with regurgitation.

DIAGNOSTIC TESTS

RADIOLOGIC STUDIES   Barium swallow with fluoroscopy and esophagogram is the most widely used test for diagnosis of esophageal disease and can be used to evaluate both structural and motor disorders. The pharynx is examined to detect stasis of barium in the valleculae and piriform sinuses and regurgitation of barium into the nose and tracheobronchial tree. Since the oropharyngeal phase of swallowing lasts no more than a second, videofluoroscopy may be necessary to permit detection and analysis of abnormalities of oral and pharyngeal function. Spontaneous reflux of barium from the stomach into the esophagus should be sought in patients with suspected reflux esophagitis. Esophageal peristalsis is best studied in the recumbent position, since in the upright position the passage of most of the barium occurs by gravity alone. A double-contrast esophagogram, obtained by coating the esophageal mucosa with barium and distending the esophageal lumen with air using effervescent granules, is particularly useful in demonstrating mucosal ulcers and early cancers. Figures 251-1 and 251-2 illustrate the radiographic appearance of some esophageal disorders.

ESOPHAGOSCOPY   Fiberoptic esophagogastroduodenoscopy is described in Chap. 250. Esophagoscopy is the direct method of establishing the cause of mechanical dysphagia and of identifying mucosal lesions, such as superficial ulcers and esophagitis, which may not be identified by the usual barium swallow. In the presence of marked luminal narrowing, examination can be achieved by using a smaller-caliber endoscope, although on occasion a stricture must be dilated prior to a complete endoscopic examination. Transendoscopic biopsies are useful in diagnosing carcinoma, reflux esophagitis, or other mucosal diseases. Obtaining cells by scraping the mucosa with a Teflon brush during endoscopy may enable the cytologist to detect carcinoma.

ESOPHAGEAL MOTILITY   The study of esophageal motility entails simultaneous recording of pressures from different sites in the esophageal lumen. This is usually done with a train of three to four water-filled catheters connected to pressure transducers. The assembly is passed by mouth or nose through the esophagus into the stomach

FIGURE 251-1   Radiographic appearance of some motor disorders of the pharynx and esophagus. (1) Pharyngeal paralysis with tracheal aspiration (arrow). (2) Cricopharyngeal achalasia. Note the prominent cricopharyngeus, which is recognized by its smoothness and location in the posterior wall. (3) Diffuse esophageal spasm. Note typical corkscrew appearance of the lower part of the esophagus. (4) Achalasia showing dilated esophageal body with air-fluid level and closed lower esophageal sphincter. (5) Muscular (contractile) lower esophageal ring. Note a symmetric contraction in 5A that has disappeared in 5B, obtained during the same examination. (6) Scleroderma esophagus showing dilated esophagus with a stricture in 6A and reflux of barium from the stomach into the esophagus in 6B. *(Courtesy of Dr. Harvey Goldstein.)*

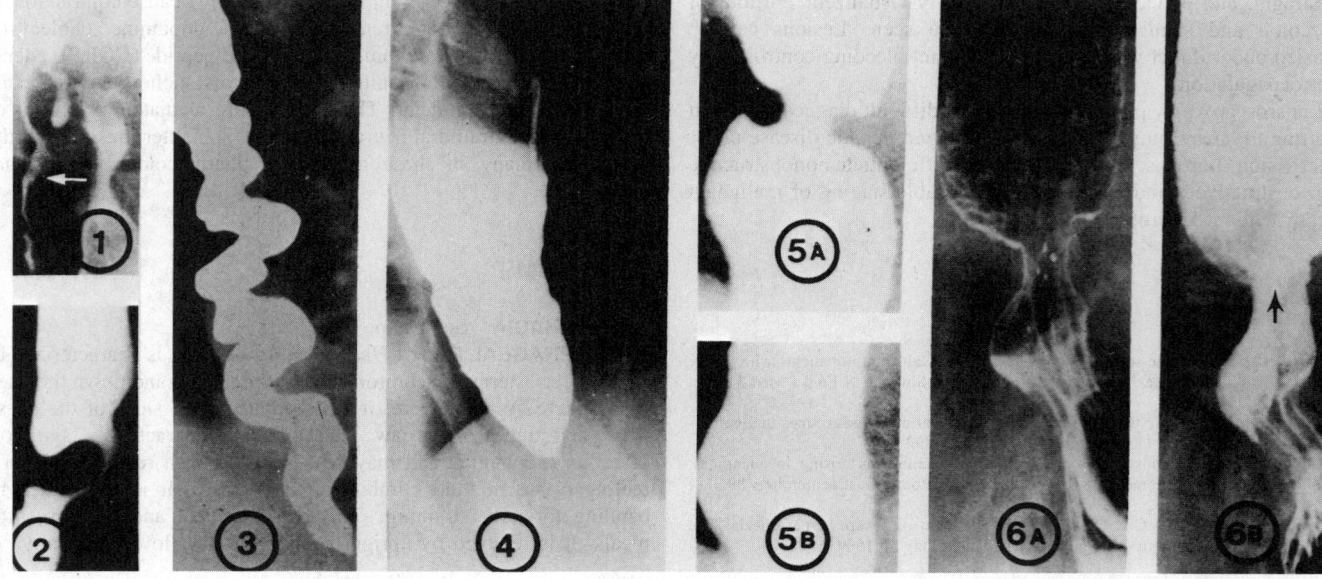

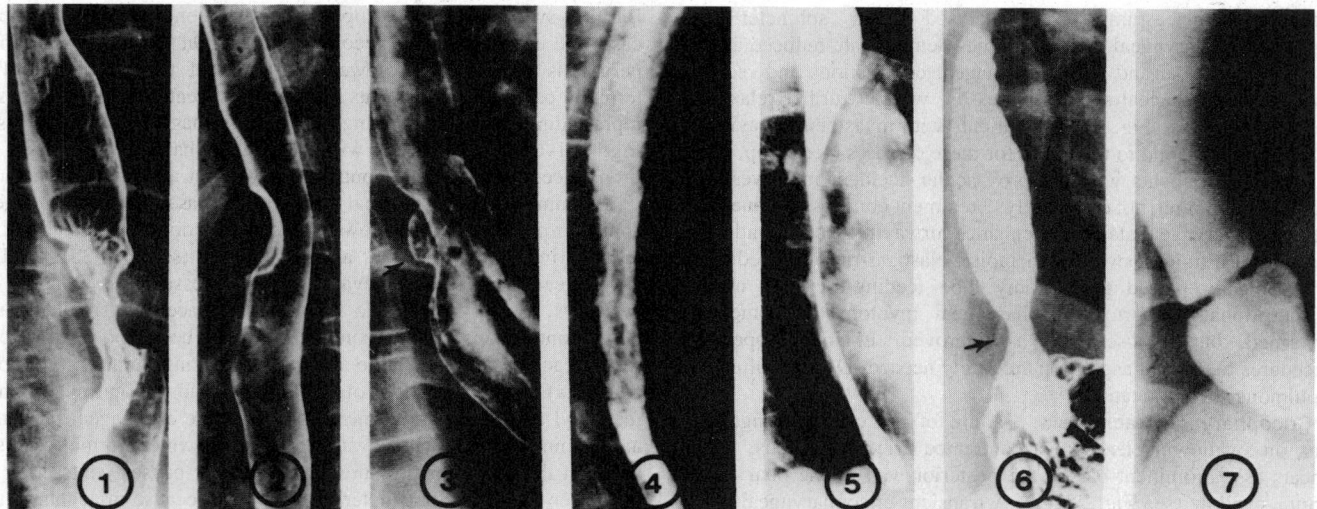

FIGURE 251-2 Selected structural lesions of the esophagus. (1) Carcinoma of the esophagus with typical annular narrowing with overhanging margins and destruction of the mucosa. (2) Leiomyoma of the esophagus with smooth filling defect and right angles of origin from the esophageal wall. (3) Esophageal ulcer in columnar-cell-lined esophagus (Barrett's esophagus). (4) Monilial esophagitis with irregular plaquelike filling defects. (5) Long stricture secondary to lye ingestion. (6) Peptic stricture, short and tubular, with associated hiatus hernia. (7) Mucosal lower esophageal mucosal (Schatzki) ring. Thin weblike annular constriction at the esophagogastric junction is associated with a small hiatal hernia. *(Courtesy of Dr. Harvey Goldstein.)*

and then gradually withdrawn 1 cm at a time until pressures from each centimeter of the esophagus and pharynx are recorded in between and during swallows. The upper and lower esophageal sphincters appear as zones of high pressure that relax on swallowing. The pharynx and esophageal body normally show peristaltic waves with each swallow.

Esophageal motility studies are very helpful in the diagnosis of achalasia, diffuse esophageal spasm and its variants, scleroderma, and other motor disorders of the esophagus, as well as neuromuscular disorders of the upper esophagus and pharynx (Fig. 251-3) but are of no value in the diagnosis of mechanical dysphagia. In patients with reflux esophagitis, esophageal manometry is useful in quantitating lower esophageal competence and providing information on the status of the esophageal body motor activity. The information obtained by manometry is quantitative and cannot be obtained by barium swallow or endoscopy.

Special tests for the evaluation of reflux esophagitis are described later.

MOTOR DISORDERS

STRIATED MUSCLE   Pharyngeal paralysis   Pharyngeal paralysis is characterized by dysphagia, nasal regurgitation, and tracheobronchial aspiration during swallowing. It occurs in a variety of neuromuscular disorders (see Table 37-2). Some of these disorders also may involve laryngeal and orofacial muscles. When the suprahyoid muscles are also paralyzed, the upper sphincter does not open with swallowing, leading to paralytic achalasia of the upper esophageal sphincter and severe dysphagia.

Barium swallow, oropharyngography, and cineradiography reveal stasis of barium in the valleculae and piriform sinuses, nasal and

FIGURE 251-3 Motility patterns in selected esophageal and pharyngeal disorders. In normal subjects, the upper and lower esophageal sphincters (UES and LES) appear as zones of high pressure. With a swallow (indicated by ↑), pressure in the sphincters falls and a contraction wave starts in the pharynx and progresses down the esophagus. In scleroderma, the lower part of the esophagus (smooth muscle) shows reduced amplitude of contractions, which may be peristaltic or simultaneous in onset, and hypotension of the lower sphincter. In achalasia, the lower part of the esophagus shows reduced amplitude of contractions that are simultaneous in onset. In contrast to scleroderma, the lower esophageal sphincter in achalasia is hypertensive and fails to relax in response to a swallow. In diffuse esophageal spasm, the lower part of the esophagus shows simultaneous onset, large amplitude, long duration, repetitive contractions. In polymyositis, the smooth-muscle part of the esophagus is normal. The skeletal muscle part shows reduced amplitude of contractions. The upper esophageal sphincter is hypotensive and may not relax normally on swallowing due to associated weakness of the suprahyoid muscles.

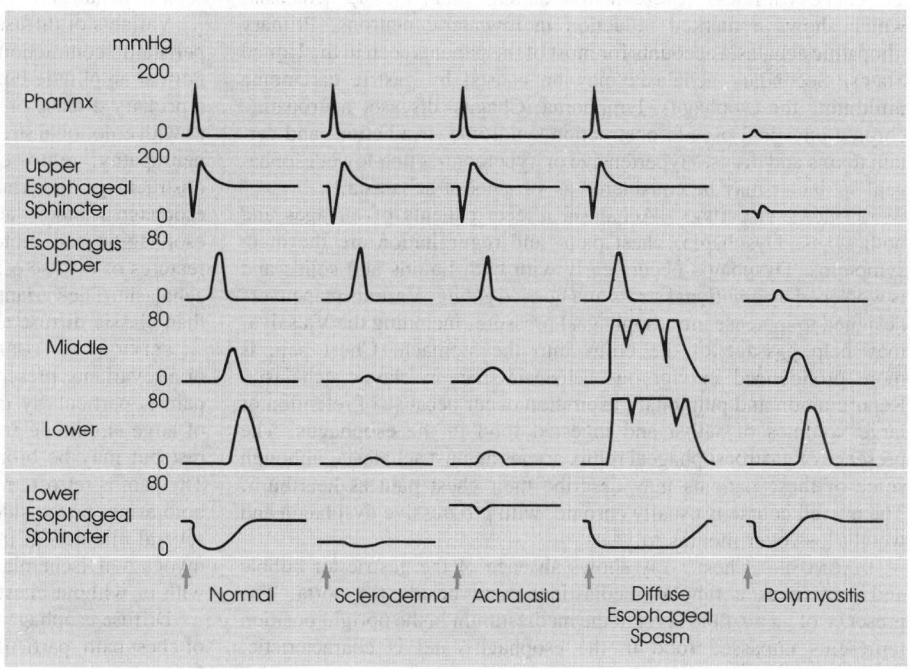

tracheobronchial aspiration, and closed upper sphincter (see Fig. 251-1). Pharyngeal motility studies demonstrate reduced amplitude of pharyngeal and upper esophageal contractions and reduced basal upper esophageal sphincter pressure without further relaxation on swallowing (see Fig. 251-3). Patients with myasthenia gravis and polymyositis respond to treatment for these diseases (see Chap. 386). Dysphagia in patients with cerebrovascular accident improves with time, although often not completely. Treatment consists of maneuvers to reduce pharyngeal stasis and enhance airway protection under the direction of a trained swallow therapist. Nasogastric tube feeding or endoscopically placed gastrostomy tube feeding may be needed for nutritional support. Cricopharyngeal myotomy is sometimes performed, but its usefulness is unproved. Extensive operative procedures to prevent aspiration are rarely needed. Death is often due to pulmonary complications.

Cricopharyngeal achalasia   Failure of the cricopharyngeus to relax on swallowing leads to a contracted cricopharyngeus, which appears as a prominent bar on the posterior wall of the pharynx on barium swallow (see Fig. 251-1). A transient cricopharyngeal bar is seen in up to 5 percent of subjects without dysphagia undergoing upper gastrointestinal studies; it can be produced in normal subjects during a Valsalva maneuver. When contraction is persistent, patients may complain of food sticking in their throats. Cricopharyngeal myotomy may be helpful, but it is contraindicated in the presence of gastroesophageal reflux because in such patients this procedure may lead to pharyngeal and pulmonary aspiration.

Globus pharyngeus   A sensation of a constant lump in the throat but with no difficulty during swallowing occurs especially in subjects with emotional disorders, particularly in women. Barium studies are normal, but manometry may show a hypertensive upper sphincter. Treatment is primarily one of reassurance.

SMOOTH MUSCLE   Achalasia   Achalasia is a motor disorder of the esophageal smooth muscle in which the lower esophageal sphincter is hypertensive and does not relax properly with swallowing, and the normal peristalsis of the esophageal body is replaced by abnormal contractions. Based on the changes in the esophageal body, achalasia can be of two types: In *classic achalasia* simultaneous contractions of small amplitude occur, while in *vigorous achalasia* contractions are simultaneous in onset, large in amplitude, and repetitive, resembling those seen in diffuse esophageal spasm.

PATHOPHYSIOLOGY   The underlying abnormality is defective innervation of the smooth-muscle portion of the esophageal body and the lower esophageal sphincter. Pathologically, vigorous achalasia is associated with less severe neural damage than classic achalasia, which shows a marked reduction in myenteric neurons. Primary idiopathic achalasia accounts for most of the patients seen in the United States. Secondary achalasia may be caused by gastric carcinoma infiltrating the esophagus, lymphoma, Chagas' disease, neuropathic chronic intestinal pseudo-obstruction syndrome, irradiation, and certain toxins and drugs. Hypertensive or hypercontracting lower esophageal sphincter may be considered as variants of achalasia.

CLINICAL FEATURES   Achalasia affects patients of all ages and both sexes. Dysphagia, chest pain, and regurgitation are the main symptoms. Dysphagia occurs early with both liquids and solids and is worsened by emotional stress and hurried eating. Various maneuvers designed to increase intraesophageal pressure, including the Valsalva, may help passage of the bolus into the stomach. Chest pain is more pronounced in vigorous achalasia than in classic achalasia. Regurgitation and pulmonary aspiration occur because of retention of large volumes of saliva and ingested food in the esophagus. The presence of gastroesophageal reflux argues against achalasia, although some of these patients may describe their chest pain as heartburn. The overall course is usually chronic, with progressive dysphagia and weight loss over months to years.

DIAGNOSIS   Chest x-ray shows absence of the gastric air bubble and sometimes a tubular mediastinal mass beside the aorta. The presence of an air-fluid level in the mediastinum in the upright position represents unpassed food in the esophagus and is characteristic.

Barium swallow shows esophageal dilatation, and in advanced cases the esophagus may become sigmoid. On fluoroscopy, normal peristalsis is lost in the lower two-thirds of the esophagus. The terminal part of the esophagus shows a persistent beaklike narrowing representing the nonrelaxing lower esophageal sphincter [see Fig. 251-1(2)]. In patients with vigorous achalasia, there may be pronounced nonperistaltic contractions without a dilated esophagus.

Manometry shows normal or elevated basal lower esophageal sphincter pressure and swallow-induced relaxation which is absent or reduced in degree, duration, and consistency (see Fig. 251-3). The esophageal body shows elevated resting pressure. In response to swallows, primary peristaltic waves are replaced by simultaneous-onset contractions. These contractions may be of poor amplitude (classic achalasia) or of large amplitude and long duration (vigorous achalasia). Administration of the cholinergic muscarinic agonist mecholyl causes a marked increase in baseline esophageal pressure, and administration of cholecystokinin (CCK), which normally causes a fall in the sphincter pressure, paradoxically causes contraction of the lower esophageal sphincter. This occurs because in achalasia the neurally transmitted inhibitory effect of CCK is absent due to the loss of inhibitory neurons. Endoscopy is helpful in excluding the secondary causes of achalasia, particularly gastric carcinoma.

TREATMENT   Medical treatment using soft foods, sedatives, nitrates, and anticholinergic drugs is usually unsatisfactory. Nitrates and calcium channel antagonists such as nifedipine have been used with some success. The best available therapy involves balloon dilation to reduce the basal lower esophageal sphincter pressure by tearing muscle fibers. In experienced hands this technique is effective in about 85 percent of patients. Perforation and bleeding are potential complications. Heller's extramucosal myotomy of the lower sphincter, in which the circular muscle layer is incised, is equally effective. Reflux esophagitis and peptic stricture (more often with myotomy than with balloon dilation) may follow successful treatment.

Diffuse esophageal spasm and related motor disorders   Diffuse esophageal spasm is a motor disorder of the esophageal smooth muscle characterized by multiple spontaneous contractions and by swallow-induced contractions that are of simultaneous onset, large amplitude, long duration, and repetitive occurrence. Variants show some but not all of these motor abnormalities.

PATHOPHYSIOLOGY   The pathogenesis of the various abnormalities of peristalsis in diffuse esophageal spasm is not known. Histopathologic studies show patchy neural degeneration localized to nerve processes rather than the prominent degeneration of nerve cell bodies seen in achalasia.

Variants of diffuse esophageal spasm, such as large amplitude but peristaltic contractions (sometimes called "nutcracker" esophagus) or normal amplitude but simultaneous contractions, frequently occur as a primary disease or in association with a variety of diseases as well as with emotional stress and aging. Collagen vascular disease, diabetic neuropathy, reflux esophagitis, irradiation esophagitis, esophageal obstruction, and cholinergic and anticholinergic drugs can cause esophageal motor abnormalities. The relationship between reflux esophagitis and motor abnormalities is controversial. Overlapping features of diffuse esophageal spasm and achalasia occur in vigorous achalasia. The variant syndromes are more frequent in clinical practice than classic diffuse esophageal spasm.

CLINICAL FEATURES   The symptomatic patient with diffuse spasm or its variants presents with chest pain, dysphagia, or both. Chest pain is particularly marked in patients with esophageal contractions of large amplitude and of long duration. Chest pain usually occurs at rest but may be brought on by swallowing or by emotional stress. The pain is retrosternal; it may radiate to the back, sides of the chest, both arms, or the sides of the jaw and may last for a few seconds to several minutes. It may be acute and severe, mimicking the pain of myocardial ischemia. Dysphagia for solids and liquids may occur with or without chest pain.

Diffuse esophageal spasm must be differentiated from other causes of chest pain, particularly ischemic heart disease with atypical angina.

Often a complete cardiac workup is done before the esophageal etiology is seriously considered. The presence of dysphagia in association with pain should point to the esophagus as the site of disease. Symptoms of esophageal spasm should be carefully distinguished from those of reflux esophagitis; the two may coexist.

DIAGNOSIS Barium swallow shows that normal sequential peristalsis below the aortic arch is replaced by uncoordinated simultaneous contractions that produce the appearance of curling or multiple ripples in the wall, sacculations, and pseudodiverticula—the "corkscrew" esophagus [see Fig. 251-1(3)]. Sometimes an esophageal contraction obliterates the lumen, and barium is pushed away in both directions. The lower esophageal sphincter opens normally.

Manometry reveals the characteristic prolonged large amplitude and repetitive contractions of simultaneous onset in the lower part of the esophagus (see Fig. 251-3). Only one or two of these abnormalities may be present in variants of diffuse spasm. Because the abnormalities may be episodic, manometry may be normal at the time of the study; therefore, several techniques are used in attempts to provoke esophageal spasm. Cold swallows produce chest pain but do not produce spasm on manometric studies. Solid boluses and pharmacologic agents, particularly edrophonium, induce both chest pain and motor abnormalities. However, there is a poor correlation between induction of pain and motility changes. Ergonovine can induce motor abnormalities but also may cause coronary artery spasm and therefore should not be used. Overall, the usefulness of pharmacologic provocative tests is limited.

TREATMENT Anticholinergics are usually of limited value. Agents that relax smooth muscle such as sublingual nitroglycerin (0.3 to 0.6 mg) or longer-acting agents such as isosorbide dinitrate (2.5 to 10 mg sublingually before meals) and nifedipine (10 to 20 mg before meals) may be helpful in some cases. Esophageal dilation with mercury-filled rubber dilators may produce symptomatic relief by distending the lower esophagus or by a placebo effect. Reassurance and tranquilizers are helpful in allaying patients' apprehension. Balloon dilation is sometimes attempted but can be hazardous in inexperienced hands. In severe cases resistant to all therapy, a longitudinal myotomy of esophageal circular muscle is performed; it relieves pain in up to two-thirds of patients.

Scleroderma involving the esophagus The esophageal lesions in systemic sclerosis consist of atrophy of the smooth-muscle contraction, manifested by weakness in the lower two-thirds of the esophageal body and incompetence of the lower esophageal sphincter. The esophageal wall is thin and atrophic and may exhibit areas of patchy fibrosis. Patients usually present with dysphagia to solids. Liquids may cause dysphagia when the patient is in the recumbent position. Some patients present with heartburn and regurgitation due to gastroesophageal reflux and esophagitis, which in turn may lead to stricture formation and more pronounced dysphagia. Barium swallow shows dilation and loss of peristaltic contractions in the middle and distal portions of the esophagus. The lower esophageal sphincter is patulous, and gastroesophageal reflux may occur freely (see Fig. 251-1). Mucosal changes from esophageal ulceration may be detected, and esophageal stricture may be present. Motility studies show marked reduction in the amplitude of smooth-muscle contractions, which may be peristaltic or nonperistaltic. Lower esophageal sphincter resting pressure is subnormal, but sphincter relaxation is normal (see Fig. 251-3). Esophageal motor abnormalities are frequently found in patients with Raynaud's syndrome alone. Currently, there is no effective treatment for the motor difficulty. Reflux esophagitis and its complications should be treated aggressively, as described under reflux esophagitis.

INFLAMMATORY DISORDERS

GASTROESOPHAGEAL REFLUX AND ESOPHAGITIS Reflux esophagitis consists of esophageal mucosal damage from reflux of gastric or intestinal contents into the esophagus. Depending on the causative agent, it is referred to as peptic, bile, or alkaline esophagitis.

Pathophysiology Three considerations involved in the pathophysiology of reflux esophagitis are (1) the pathogenesis of the esophageal reflux episode, (2) the cumulative, or net, esophageal reflux, and (3) the pathogenesis of esophagitis.

Two conditions must be met for a *reflux episode* to occur: The gastrointestinal contents must be "ready" to reflux, and the antireflux mechanism at the lower end of the esophagus must be compromised. Gastrointestinal contents are most likely to reflux (1) when gastric volume is increased (after meals, with pyloric obstruction or gastric stasis syndrome, and in acid hypersecretory states), (2) when the gastric contents are located near the gastroesophageal junction (due to recumbency or bending), and (3) when gastric pressure is increased (with obesity, pregnancy, ascites, or tight binders or girdles).

The normal antireflux mechanisms consist of the lower esophageal sphincter (LES) and the anatomic configuration of the gastroesophageal junction. Reflux occurs only when the LES–gastric pressure gradient is lost. It can be caused by increased intragastric pressure or a transient or sustained decrease in the sphincter tone itself. The decrease in sphincter tone may be due to muscle weakness or possibly to neurally mediated inappropriate sphincter relaxation. The secondary causes of LES incompetence include scleroderma-like diseases, a myopathic type of chronic intestinal pseudo-obstruction syndrome, pregnancy, smoking, smooth-muscle relaxants (such as beta-adrenergics, aminophylline, nitrates, and calcium channel blockers), destruction of the sphincter by surgical resection, myotomy or balloon dilation, and esophagitis. Abnormal activity of the diaphragmatic crural muscle which surrounds the esophageal hiatus in the diaphragm and changes the anatomic configuration of the esophagogastric junction, as in hiatal hernia, also predisposes to gastroesophageal reflux.

The *net*, or *cumulative, esophageal reflux*, i.e., the amount and duration of refluxed noxious material remaining in the esophagus, is dependent on (1) the amount of refluxed material per episode, (2) the frequency of reflux episodes, (3) the rate of clearing of the esophagus by gravity and peristaltic contraction, and (4) neutralization of gastric acid by salivary secretion.

Esophagitis is a complication of reflux, and it develops when the mucosal defenses that normally counteract the effect of injurious agents on the esophageal mucosa succumb to the onslaught of the refluxed acid pepsin or bile. *Mild esophagitis* is manifested by microscopic changes of mucosal infiltration with granulocytes or eosinophils, hyperplasia of basal cells, and elongation of dermal pegs. It can occur with or without endoscopic abnormalities. *Erosive esophagitis* shows endoscopically visible damage to the mucosa in the form of marked redness, friability, bleeding, superficial linear ulcers, and exudates. *Peptic stricture* results from fibrosis that causes constriction of the esophageal lumen. The fibrosis is predominantly submucosal, but it may involve the whole wall. Peptic strictures occur in about 10 percent of patients with reflux esophagitis. Short peptic strictures caused by spontaneous reflux are usually 1 to 3 cm long and are present in the distal esophagus near the squamocolumnar junction (see Fig. 251-2). Long and tubular peptic strictures can result from persistent vomiting or prolonged nasogastric intubation. Replacement of the squamous epithelium of the esophagus by columnar epithelium *(Barrett's esophagus)* also may result from reflux esophagitis. Columnar cell–lined esophagus may be further complicated by peptic ulcer or peptic stricture high up in the lower or midesophagus, and by adenocarcinoma in 2 to 5 percent of cases. Adenocarcinoma frequently occurs in areas adjoining the squamous mucosa. Barrett's esophagitis also may occur as a result of esophageal mucosal damage due to chemotherapy.

Clinical features Heartburn is the characteristic symptom and is produced by the contact of refluxed material with the inflamed esophageal mucosa. Angina-like or atypical chest pain may occur in some patients, while others may experience no heartburn or chest pain. Dysphagia suggests development of peptic stricture. In peptic strictures, the usual history is of several years of heartburn preceding dysphagia. However, in one-third of patients dysphagia may be the presenting symptom. Rapidly progressive dysphagia and weight loss may indicate development of adenocarcinoma in Barrett's esophagus. Bleeding occurs due to mucosal erosions or Barrett's ulcer. Reflux in the absence of esophagitis is usually asymptomatic. Severe reflux may reach the pharynx and mouth and result in laryngitis, morning hoarseness, and pulmonary aspiration. Recurrent pulmonary aspiration can cause aspiration pneumonia, pulmonary fibrosis, or chronic asthma.

Diagnosis   Evaluation of reflux esophagitis is designed to assess the presence and severity of reflux, nature of refluxant, presence and severity of esophagitis, and pathophysiology of reflux. History, barium swallow, esophagoscopy, mucosal biopsy, esophageal motility, and a variety of special tests are utilized.

The *presence of reflux* is suggested by history. Spontaneous reflux from the stomach into the esophagus on barium examination suggests advanced reflux. Reflux of barium induced by stressful maneuvers is not very helpful, however, because of the high incidence of false-positive and false-negative results. Scintiscan using ^{99m}Tc-sulfur colloid has been used to quantitate gastroesophageal reflux. Several tests that utilize the recording of esophageal luminal pH with a small pH electrode have been proposed to detect and quantitate reflux of gastric acid. In these tests, the pH electrode is swallowed, positioned in the stomach, gradually withdrawn across the LES, and then fixed at 5 cm above the sphincter. In the standard acid reflux test, a diagnosis of reflux can be made by failure of the pH to rise as the electrode enters the esophagus and by a decrease in esophageal pH with straining maneuvers. Quantitative information on acid reflux is obtained by ambulatory long-term (24-h) esophageal pH recording. The pH recordings are helpful only in the evaluation of acid reflux. The presence of bile or alkaline reflux is suggested by the occurrence of reflux symptoms in the absence of gastric acid and by the demonstration of bile in the aspirate of esophageal reflux.

The *presence and complications of reflux esophagitis* are assessed by barium swallow, esophagoscopy, mucosal biopsy, and the Bernstein test. Barium swallow is usually normal in uncomplicated esophagitis but may reveal the complication of stricture or ulcer formation. A high esophageal peptic stricture, deep ulcer, and adenocarcinoma suggest complications of Barrett's esophagus. Uncomplicated Barrett's esophagus is not diagnosed reliably by barium studies. Esophagoscopy may reveal the presence of erosive esophagitis, distal peptic stricture, or columnar cell–lined lower esophagus with or without a proximally located peptic stricture, ulcer, or adenocarcinoma. Esophagoscopy may be normal in many patients with esophagitis; in such patients, mucosal biopsies and the Bernstein test are helpful. The mucosal biopsies should be obtained at least 5 cm above the LES because esophageal mucosal changes of chronic esophagitis are quite frequent in the most distal esophagus in otherwise normal subjects. False-positive and false-negative results occur in approximately 10 percent of biopsies. Patients with Barrett's esophagus will show columnar mucosa lining the esophagus which may be of gastric fundic, cardiac, or specialized type. The Bernstein test consists of an infusion of solutions of 0.1 N HCl and normal saline into the esophagus. It is useful in diagnosing reflux esophagitis which is not endoscopically obvious. In patients with reflux esophagitis, infusion of acid, but not of saline, reproduces the symptoms of heartburn. Infusion of acid in normal subjects usually produces no symptoms. Reflux esophagitis should be included in the differential diagnosis of chest pain, esophagitis, upper gastrointestinal bleeding, and dysphagia.

The *causative and predisposing factors* are assessed by history, esophageal motility, and esophageal clearance studies. Esophageal motility studies may provide useful quantitative information on the competence of the LES and of esophageal motor function. Barium swallow and scintiscans can be used to study esophageal clearance. An esophageal acid clearance test using a pH electrode quantifies the number of swallows necessary to clear the esophagus of 10 mL of instilled dilute 0.1 N HCl.

Full diagnostic evaluation is not necessary in every patient with reflux esophagitis. In transient and mild cases with a clear-cut history of reflux esophagitis, a therapeutic trial may be sufficient. In persistent cases and when the diagnosis is not clear, barium swallow, esophagoscopy, and esophageal motility with pH monitoring are indicated.

Patients with angina-like chest pain in whom coronary artery disease has been excluded may be investigated by the Bernstein test, 24-h ambulatory esophageal pH recording, and motility recording. Most of these patients are found to have reflux esophagitis, while a few have specific esophageal motor disorders. It also should be remembered that reflux esophagitis and nonspecific esophageal motility disorders may frequently coexist with coronary artery disease.

Treatment   The goals of treatment are to decrease gastroesophageal reflux, renders the refluxate harmless, improve esophageal clearance, and protect the esophageal mucosa. These goals can be achieved by certain general measures and specific drug treatments. The management of uncomplicated cases generally includes weight reduction, sleeping with elevation of the head of the bed by about 4 to 6 in with blocks, and elimination of factors that increase abdominal pressure. Patients should avoid smoking, fatty foods, coffee, chocolate, alcohol, mint, orange juice, ingestion of large quantities of fluids with meals, and certain medications (such as anticholinergic drugs, calcium channel blockers, and other smooth-muscle relaxants). In mild cases, H-2 blocking agents (cimetidine 300 mg, ranitidine 150 mg, or famotidine 20 mg at bedtime) or antacids to neutralize acidity are usually successful.

In moderate to severe cases, the preceding measures are more strictly enforced. H-2 blockers are used in higher doses (cimetidine, 300 mg qid; ranitidine, 150 mg bid; famotidine, 20 mg bid). A protective agent such as sucralfate (1-g chewable tablet, 1 h before meals) is useful in some cases. If the patient does not respond fully, a prokinetic agent such as metoclopramide, 10 mg 30 min before meals and at bedtime, domperidone, or cisapride is prescribed to raise sphincter pressure, hasten gastric emptying, and improve esophageal clearance. (Domperidone and cisapride have not yet been approved for use in the United States.) Inhibition of H^+, K^+-ATPase, the parietal cell pump that is responsible for acid secretion, with omeprazole (20 to 40 mg tablet, daily) is very effective in resistant cases. If a complete response is not achieved, gastric juice pH should be checked to verify patient compliance or underlying acid hypersecretory state. Reflux esophagitis requires prolonged therapy for 3 to 6 months or longer if the disease recurs quickly. Patients with reflux esophagitis with complications such as Barrett's esophagus (with or without a deep ulcer) should be treated vigorously. Patients who have an associated peptic stricture are treated with dilators to relieve dysphagia in addition to vigorous treatment for reflux. To detect and treat high-grade dysplasia and early adenocarcinoma, close follow-up with periodic endoscopic biopsies is indicated every 2 years or so in patients without evidence of dysplasia; patients with dysplasia require more frequent surveillance.

Antireflux surgery, in which the gastric fundus is wrapped around the esophagus (fundoplication), increases the lower sphincter pressure and should be considered in resistant and complicated cases of reflux esophagitis that do not fully respond to medical therapy or in patients for whom long-term medical therapy is not desirable. In the ideal candidates for fundoplication, motility studies should show persistently inadequate lower sphincter pressure but normal peristaltic contractions in the esophageal body.

Patients with alkaline esophagitis are treated with general antireflux measures and neutralization of bile salts with cholestyramine, aluminum hydroxide, or sucralfate. Sucralfate is particularly useful in these cases, since it also serves as a surface protector.

INFECTIOUS ESOPHAGITIS   With the recent increase in immunodeficiency states, infectious esophagitis has become increasingly important. Infectious esophagitis can be due to viral, bacterial, fungal, or parasitic organisms. In severely immunocompromised patients, multiple organisms may coexist.

Viral esophagitis (See also Chap. 143) *Herpes simplex virus* (HSV) type I may occasionally cause esophagitis in the immunocompetent person, but either type I or type II may afflict patients who are immunosuppressed. These patients complain of the acute onset of chest pain, odynophagia, and dysphagia. Bleeding may occur in severe cases, and systemic manifestations such as nausea, vomiting, fever, chills, and mild leukocytosis may be present. The persistent infection may lead to superinfection of denuded esophageal mucosa with fungi or bacteria. Herpes vesicles on the nose and lips sometimes provide a clue to the diagnosis. Barium swallow is inadequate to detect early lesions and cannot reliably distinguish HSV from other types of infections. Endoscopy shows vesicles and small, discrete, punched-out superficial ulcerations with or without fibrinous exudate. In later stages there is diffuse erosive esophagitis caused by enlargement and coalescence of the ulcers. Mucosal cells from biopsy of the edge of an ulcer or cytologic smear show ballooning degeneration, ground glass change in the nuclei with eosinophilic intranuclear inclusions (Cowdry type A), and giant cell formation on routine stains. Culture becomes positive within days and is helpful in diagnosis. For prophylaxis in a severely immunocompromised host, acyclovir, 800 mg orally twice daily or 250 mg/m^2 of body surface area every 12 h intravenously, is recommended. For treatment of esophagitis, intravenous therapy, 250 mg/m^2 every 8 h, is usually initiated. As swallowing improves, the therapy is changed to 200 to 400 mg orally five times daily. Symptoms usually resolve in 1 week, but large ulcerations may take longer to heal. Foscarnet may be useful if acyclovir resistance occurs. These patients also may have reflux esophagitis, which may worsen the symptoms and add to complications.

Varicella-zoster virus (VZV) sometimes produces esophagitis in children with chickenpox and adults with herpes zoster. Esophageal VZV also can be the source of disseminated VZV infection in the absence of skin involvement. In an immunocompromised host, VZV esophagitis causes vesicles and confluent ulcers and usually resolves spontaneously, but it may cause necrotizing esophagitis in a severely compromised host. On routine histology of mucosal biopsies or cytology specimens, VZV is difficult to distinguish from HSV, but the distinction can be made immunohistologically or on culture. Acyclovir is effective in prevention and treatment of esophagitis, but much higher doses are needed than those for HSV.

Cytomegalovirus (CMV) infections occur only in the immunocompromised patient. CMV is usually activated from a latent stage or may be acquired from blood product transfusions. CMV lesions initially appear as serpiginous ulcers in an otherwise normal mucosa. These may coalesce to form giant ulcers, particularly in the distal esophagus. The virus involves submucosal fibroblasts and endothelial cells of the blood vessels but not the epithelial cells.

Patients present with painful swallowing, chest pain, hematemesis, nausea, and vomiting. Barium swallow may show nonspecific abnormalities or large esophageal ulcers. Diagnosis requires endoscopy and biopsies of the center of the ulcer. Mucosal brushings are not useful. Routine histology shows intranuclear and small intracytoplasmic inclusions in large fibroblasts and endothelial cells of blood vessels. Immunohistology with monoclonal antibodies to CMV and in situ hybridization of CMV DNA can be performed on centrifugation culture and are useful for early diagnosis. Ganciclovir (DHPG), 5 mg/kg every 12 h intravenously, is the treatment of choice. Foscarnet can be used in resistant cases. Therapy is continued until healing, which may take weeks to months.

Human immunodeficiency virus (HIV) may be associated with a self-limited syndrome of acute esophageal ulceration associated with oral ulcers and a maculopapular skin rash. This syndrome occurs in homosexual men coincident with both HIV seroconversion and the inversion of the T lymphocyte helper/suppressor ratio. Electron microscopy of affected tissue reveals retrovirus-like particles that are different from CMV or HSV.

Bacterial esophagitis *Bacterial esophagitis* is unusual, but esophagitis caused by *Lactobacillus* and beta-hemolytic streptococci

has been described in the immunocompromised host. In profoundly granulocytopenic patients and in patients with cancer, bacterial esophagitis is often missed because it is commonly present with other organisms, including viruses and fungi, and because bacteria are difficult to identify on routine histology. In patients with AIDS, infection with *Cryptosporidium* and *Pneumocystis carinii* may cause nonspecific inflammation and *Mycobacterium tuberculosis* may cause deep ulcerations of the distal esophagus.

Candida **esophagitis** Many *Candida* species are normal commensals in the throat but become pathogenic and produce esophagitis in immunodeficiency states. These include HIV; malignant neoplasms (particularly lymphoma and leukemia); treatment with immunosuppressive agents, glucocorticoids, and broad-spectrum antibiotics; diabetes mellitus; hypoparathyroidism; systemic lupus erythematosus; hemoglobinopathy; corrosive esophageal injury; and esophageal stasis. Occasionally, monilial *Candida* esophagitis occurs in the absence of any of the above predisposing factors. Patients may be asymptomatic or complain of odynophagia and dysphagia. Oral thrush or other evidence of mucocutaneous candidiasis may be absent. Rarely, *Candida* esophagitis may be complicated by esophageal bleeding, perforation, and stricture or by systemic invasion. Barium swallow may be normal or may show multiple nodular filling defects of various sizes (see Fig. 251-2). Large nodular defects may resemble clusters of grapes. Endoscopy shows small yellow-white raised plaques with surrounding erythema in mild disease. In extensive disease, confluent linear and nodular plaques are seen. Diagnosis is made by demonstration of yeast or hyphae forms in the smear of plaques and exudate stained with Gram's, periodic acid–Schiff, or silver stains. Biopsies are usually not positive. Culture is not useful in diagnosis but may be helpful in confirming the species and, if needed, the drug sensitivities of the yeast (see Chap. 168). In normal or minimally immunocompromised patients, nystatin or clotrimazole is often successful. Nystatin is used as an oral suspension (100,000 units per milliliter) in doses of 10 to 20 mL every 6 h; clotrimazole (10-mg tablet) is to be sucked five times a day. Ketoconazole (200 to 400 mg in a single oral dose) is effective treatment; the higher dose is used in the severely immunocompromised host. The bioavailability of ketoconazole is severely reduced at increased gastric pH; therefore, it should not be used concurrently with gastric acid suppression therapy or in achlorhydric subjects. Fluconazole (200 mg on the first day, followed by 100 mg daily) is the preferred treatment because its absorption is not affected by high gastric pH. Poorly responsive patients are treated with amphotericin, 10 to 15 mg as an intravenous infusion for 6 h daily for a total dose of 300 to 500 mg. Miconazole and amphotericin lozenges are currently not available in the United States. The treatment is for 7 to 10 days followed by nystatin, clotrimazole, ketoconazole, or fluconazole for as long as the host resistance remains low.

OTHER TYPES OF ESOPHAGITIS *Radiation esophagitis* is a common occurrence during radiation treatment for lung, mediastinal, or esophageal carcinoma. The frequency and severity of esophagitis increase with the amount of radiation to the area and the subsequent use of certain chemotherapeutic agents such as doxorubicin, bleomycin, cyclophosphamide, and cisplatin. Dysphagia and odynophagia are the main symptoms and may last several weeks to several months after the conclusion of therapy. The esophageal mucosa becomes erythematous, edematous, and friable. Superficial erosions coalesce to form larger superficial ulcers. Submucosal fibrosis and degenerative changes in the blood vessels, muscles, and myenteric neurons may be present. The treatment is relief of pain with viscous lidocaine during the acute phase, while indomethacin may lessen the radiation damage. Esophageal stricture may develop and require dilation. *Corrosive esophagitis* occurs following ingestion of caustic agents, such as strong alkalies or acids. When severe, corrosive injury may lead to esophageal perforation, bleeding, and death. Steroids have not been shown to be useful in acute corrosive esophagitis. Healing is usually associated with stricture formation. Caustic strictures are usually long and rigid (see Fig. 251-2) and generally require dilation with dilators passed over a guidewire through the stricture. *Pill-induced esophagitis* is associated with the ingestion of certain pills and accounts for many cases of erosive esophagitis. Antibiotics such as doxycycline, tetracycline, and clindamycin account for over half the cases. Other commonly prescribed pills that cause esophageal injury include aspirin, potassium chloride, ferrous sulfate, quinidine, alprenolol, and various steroidal and nonsteroidal anti-inflammatory agents. Pill esophagitis can be prevented by washing pills down with copious amounts of fluids. *Sclerotherapy* for bleeding esophageal varices usually produces transient retrosternal chest pain and dysphagia due to edema, inflammation, and deranged motility. Esophageal ulcer, stricture, hematoma, or perforation may occur. *Esophagitis associated with mucocutaneous and systemic diseases* is usually associated with blister and bulla formation, epithelial desquamation, and thin, weblike or dense esophageal strictures. Esophageal involvement is indicated by development of odynophagia and dysphagia. Pemphigus vulgaris and bullous pemphigoid form intraepithelial and subepithelial bullae, respectively, and can be distinguished by a specific immunohistology. They are both characterized by sloughing of epithelium or esophageal casts. Glucocorticoid treatment is usually effective. Dystrophic epidermolysis bullosa is an inherited disease that presents in childhood in which local trauma is associated with bulla formation and scarring. Cicatricial pemphigoid, Stevens-Johnson syndrome, and toxic epidermolysis bullosa can produce esophageal bullous lesions and strictures requiring gentle dilation. Graft-versus-host disease occurs in patients who have received allogeneic bone marrow transplants and is associated with generalized desquamation and esophageal strictures. Behçet's disease and eosinophilic gastroenteritis may involve the esophagus and may respond to steroid therapy. Crohn's disease and an erosive lichen planus also can involve the esophagus, and Crohn's disease may cause inflammatory strictures, sinus tract, filiform polyps, and fistulas in the esophagus.

OTHER ESOPHAGEAL DISORDERS

DIVERTICULA Diverticula are outpouchings of the wall of the esophagus. *Zenker's diverticula* appear in the natural weakness in the posterior hypopharyngeal wall and cause halitosis and regurgitation of saliva and food particles consumed several days previously. When they become large and filled with food, they can compress the esophagus and cause dysphagia or complete obstruction. Nasogastric intubation and endoscopy should be performed with utmost care in these patients, since the two may cause perforation of the diverticulum. *Midesophageal diverticula* may be caused by traction from old adhesions or by propulsion associated with esophageal motor abnormalities. *Epiphrenic diverticula* may be associated with achalasia. Small or medium-sized diverticula and midesophageal and epiphrenic diverticula are usually asymptomatic. *Diffuse intramural diverticulosis* of the esophagus is due to dilation of the deep esophageal glands. This may lead to chronic candidiasis or a stricture high up in the esophagus. These patients may present with dysphagia. Symptomatic Zenker's diverticula are treated by cricopharyngeal myotomy with or without diverticulectomy. Very large symptomatic esophageal diverticula are removed surgically. When they are associated with motor abnormalities, distal myotomy is performed. Strictures associated with diffuse intramural diverticulosis are treated with rubber dilators.

WEBS AND RINGS Weblike constrictions of the esophagus are usually congenital or inflammatory in origin. Asymptomatic hypopharyngeal webs are demonstrated in up to 10 percent of normal individuals. When concentric, they cause intermittent dysphagia to solids. Symptomatic hypopharyngeal webs with iron-deficiency anemia in middle-aged women constitute *Plummer-Vinson syndrome*. The clinical importance of this syndrome is uncertain. Midesophageal webs are rare. *Lower esophageal mucosal ring* (Schatzki ring) is a thin, weblike constriction located at the squamocolumnar mucosal junction at or near the border of the lower esophageal sphincter (see

Fig. 251-2). It invariably produces dysphagia when the diameter is less than 1.3 cm. The dysphagia to solids is the only symptom, and it is usually episodic. Asymptomatic rings may be present in about 10 percent of normal individuals. Lower esophageal ring is one of the common causes of dysphagia. Symptomatic webs and mucosal lower esophageal ring are easily treated by dilation. *Lower esophageal muscular ring* (contractile ring) is located proximal to the site of mucosal rings and may represent the abnormal uppermost segment of the lower esophageal sphincter. These rings are characterized by a change in size and shape from one time to another (see Fig. 251-1). They also may cause dysphagia and should be differentiated from peptic strictures, achalasia, and lower esophageal mucosal ring. They are treated by dilation.

HIATAL HERNIA *Hiatal hernia* is a herniation of a part of the stomach into the thoracic cavity through the esophageal hiatus in the diaphragm. *Sliding hiatal hernia* is one in which the gastroesophageal junction and fundus of the stomach slide upward. A sliding hernia may result from weakening of the anchors of the gastroesophageal junction to the diaphragm, longitudinal contraction of the esophagus, or increased intraabdominal pressure. Small sliding hernias can be demonstrated commonly during barium studies if intraabdominal pressure is increased. Their incidence increases with age; in the sixth decade of life the prevalence of such hernias is around 60 percent. It is unlikely that a small sliding hiatal hernia by itself produces any clinical symptoms, but it plays a role in the pathogenesis of reflux esophagitis. *Paraesophageal hernia* is one in which the esophagogastric junction remains fixed in its normal location and a pouch of stomach is herniated beside the gastroesophageal junction through the esophageal hiatus. A paraesophageal or mixed paraesophageal and sliding hernia may become incarcerated and strangulate. This situation is manifested by acute chest pain, dysphagia, and a mediastinal mass and requires prompt operative treatment. A herniated gastric pouch may cause dysphagia and may be the site of gastritis and ulceration causing chronic blood loss. A large paraesophageal hernia should be surgically repaired because of a high rate of complications.

MECHANICAL TRAUMA *Esophageal rupture* may be caused by (1) iatrogenic damage from instrumentation of the esophagus or external trauma, (2) increased intraesophageal pressure associated with forceful vomiting or retching (this is also called *spontaneous rupture* or *Boerhaave's syndrome*), or (3) diseases of the esophagus such as corrosive esophagitis, esophageal ulcer, and neoplasm. The site of perforation is variable and depends on the cause. Instrumental perforation usually occurs in the pharynx or in the lower esophagus. The esophageal perforation often occurs just above the diaphragm in the posterolateral wall. Esophageal perforation causes severe retrosternal chest pain that may be worsened by swallowing and breathing. Free air enters the mediastinum and spreads to neighboring structures and causes palpable subcutaneous emphysema in the neck, mediastinal crackling sounds on auscultation, and pneumothorax. With time, secondary infection supervenes, and mediastinal abscess and pleuropulmonary suppurative complications may develop. Esophageal perforation associated with vomiting usually deposits gastric contents in the mediastinum and causes severe mediastinal complications. On the other hand, instrumental perforation may be clinically mild and free of severe complications. Spontaneous rupture of the esophagus may mimic myocardial infarction, pancreatitis, or ruptured abdominal viscus. Symptoms of chest pain may be mild, particularly in the elderly. Mediastinal emphysema may develop late. X-ray of the chest shows abnormalities in the majority of patients but computed tomographic scan of the chest is more sensitive in detecting mediastinal air. Diagnosis is confirmed by swallow of radiopaque contrast material. Treatment includes esophageal and gastric suction and parenteral broad-spectrum antibiotics. Surgical drainage and repair of the laceration should be performed as soon as possible. In patients with terminal carcinoma, surgical repair may not be feasible, and those with minor instrumental perforation can be treated conservatively. Extensive corrosive damage may require esophageal diversion and subsequent excision of the damaged portion of the esophagus.

Mucosal tear (Mallory-Weiss syndrome)   This is usually caused by vomiting and retching, and it usually involves the gastric mucosa near the squamocolumnar mucosal junction but also may involve the esophageal mucosa. Patients present with upper gastrointestinal bleeding that may be severe. In most patients bleeding ceases spontaneously; continued bleeding may respond to vasopressin therapy or angiographic embolization. Surgery is rarely needed.

Intramural hematoma   Emetogenic injury, particularly in patients with bleeding abnormalities, can cause bleeding between the mucosa and muscle layers of the esophagus. The patients develop sudden dysphagia. Diagnosis is made by barium swallow and computed tomographic scan. Spontaneous resolution usually occurs.

FOREIGN BODIES   Foreign bodies may lodge in the cervical esophagus just beyond the upper esophageal sphincter, around the aortic arch, or above the lower esophageal sphincter. Impaction of a bolus of food, particularly a piece of meat or bread, may occur when the esophageal lumen is narrowed due to stricture, carcinoma, or a lower esophageal ring. Acute impaction causes complete inability to swallow and severe chest pain. Both foreign bodies and food boluses may be removed endoscopically. Use of meat tenderizer to facilitate passage of an obstructed meat bolus is to be discouraged because of potential esophageal perforation and aspiration pneumonia.

REFERENCES

ANDERSON KD et al: A controlled trial of corticosteroids in children with corrosive injury of the esophagus. N Engl J Med 323:637, 1990

BOTT S et al: Medication-induced esophageal injury: Survey of the literature. Am J Gastroenterol 82:758, 1987

CONNOLLY GM: Oesophageal symptoms, their causes, treatment, and prognosis in patients with acquired immune deficiency syndrome. Gut 30:1033, 1989

DODDS WJ: The pathogenesis of gastroesophageal reflux disease. AJR 151:49, 1988

GOYAL RK, CRIST JR: Chest pain of esophageal etiology. Hosp Prac 23:15, 1988

HETZEL DJ et al: Healing and relapse of severe peptic esophagitis after treatment with omeprazole. Gastroenterology 95:903, 1988

McDONALD GB et al: Esophageal infections in immunosuppressed patients after marrow transplantation. Gastroenterology 88:1111, 1985

ORLANDO RC: Esophageal epithelial defense against acid injury. J Clin Gastroenterol 13:51, 1991

RICHTER JE et al: Esophageal chest pain: Current controversies in pathogenesis, diagnosis, and therapy. Ann Intern Med 110:66, 1989

SARTON S et al: Barrett's esophagus after chemotherapy with cyclophosphamide, methotrexate, and S-fluorouracil (CMF): An iatrogenic injury. Ann Intern Med 114:210, 1991

SHAPIRO J, GOYAL RK: Disorders of the upper esophageal sphincter, in *The Larynx: A Multidisciplinary Approach*, M Fried (ed). Boston, Little, Brown, 1988, pp 293–317

SIMON D et al: Treatment options for AIDS-related esophageal and diarrheal disorders. Am J Gastroenterol 87:274, 1992

SPECHLER SJ, GOYAL RK: Barrett's esophagus. N Engl J Med 315:362, 1986

—— et al: Comparison of medical and surgical therapy for complicated gastroesophageal disease in veterans. N Engl J Med 326:786, 1992

252   PEPTIC ULCER AND GASTRITIS

JAMES E. McGUIGAN

Peptic ulcer is a term used to refer to a group of ulcerative disorders of the upper gastrointestinal tract involving principally the most proximal portion of the duodenum and the stomach, which have in common the participation of acid-pepsin in their pathogenesis. The major forms of common peptic ulcer are duodenal ulcer and gastric ulcer, both of which are chronic diseases. Ulcer associated with the Zollinger-Ellison syndrome, caused by gastrin-releasing islet cell tumors (gastrinomas), is also considered a form of peptic ulcer. The term has also been used in reference to gastric or duodenal ulcers associated with stress or drug ingestion.

Although our present knowledge of the cause of peptic ulcer is incomplete, available information supports a crucial role for acid-pepsin. Ulcer development or resistance to ulceration depends on the balance between *aggressive factors* (principally secreted gastric acid and pepsin) and factors that comprise *mucosal defense* or *mucosal resistance* to ulceration. Peptic ulcer results when the aggressive effects of acid-pepsin outweigh the protective effects of gastric or duodenal mucosal defense. Considering the extraordinarily corrosive character of acid-pepsin, why do not all humans develop peptic ulcer? The normal capacity of gastric and proximal duodenal mucosa to resist the corrosive effects of acid and pepsin is unique in the body. It is not shared by other tissues—hence the susceptibility of the esophageal mucosa to injury from refluxed gastric juice, the frequent ulceration of the small intestine when attached surgically to actively secreting gastric mucosa, and corrosion of the skin predictably produced with gastrocutaneous fistulas.

Much has been learned about mechanisms regulating gastric acid secretion and factors which appear important in development of peptic ulcer. Consideration of gastric physiology provides an understanding of some etiologic elements as well as a rational basis for treatment and prevention of peptic ulcer.

GASTRIC PHYSIOLOGY RELATED TO PEPTIC ULCER

AGGRESSIVE FACTORS: ACID AND PEPSINS   The gastric mucosa possesses an extraordinary capacity to secrete acid. Parietal cells (oxyntic cells), interspersed along the course of mucosal glands of the body and fundus of the stomach, secrete hydrochloric acid by a process involving oxidative phosphorylation. Parietal cells secrete hydrogen ions at a concentration about 3 million times that found in blood. The estimated concentration of HCl secreted directly by parietal cells is approximately 160 mM. Each secreted hydrogen ion (H^+) is accompanied by a chloride ion (Cl^-). With each increase in hydrogen ion secretion, there is a reciprocal decrease in sodium ion secretion. For each hydrogen ion secreted into the gastric lumen, one bicarbonate ion (HCO_3^-) is released into the gastric venous circulation, accounting for the *alkaline tide*, a direct reflection of the magnitude of gastric H^+ secretion. Bicarbonate is released from carbonic acid generated from carbon dioxide by parietal cell carbonic anhydrase. The final step in hydrogen ion secretion is accomplished by a proton pump mechanism involving a specific hydrogen-potassium adenosine triphosphatase (H^+,K^+-ATPase) located in the apical microvillus membrane and tubovesicular apparatus of the parietal cell. This H^+,K^+-ATPase exchanges hydrogen for potassium across the microvillus membrane.

Multiple *chemical*, *neural*, and *hormonal* factors participate in regulation of gastric acid secretion. *Acid secretion is stimulated* by gastrin and by postganglionic vagal fibers via muscarinic cholinergic receptors on parietal cells. Gastrin, the most potent known stimulant of gastric acid secretion, is contained in and released into the circulation from cytoplasmic secretory granules of gastrin cells (G cells) which are scattered singly or in small clusters among the epithelial lining cells of the middle and deeper portions of the antral pyloric glands. Gastrin release is inhibited by somatostatin and stimulated by the neuropeptide gastrin-releasing peptide. Gastrin in tissues and in the circulation exists in several molecular forms (Fig. 252-1). The principal form of gastrin in gastric antral mucosa (and in gastrinoma) is heptadecapeptide gastrin (G-17), which contains 17 amino acid residues, the active site region being the carboxyl-terminal tetrapeptide amide (Try-Met-Asp-Phe-NH$_2$). Gastrin II is the form in which the tyrosyl residue at position 12 is sulfated, and gastrin I is the nonsulfated form. G-17 accounts for more than 90 percent of gastrin in antral mucosa. Approximately two-thirds of serum gastrin is a larger molecular species of gastrin, which contains 34 amino acids (G-34). Although G-17 has a shorter half-life than G-34, circulating G-17 is approximately as potent as G-34 in stimulating gastric acid secretion.

Gastrin is also present in duodenal mucosa, with its highest

Big Gastrin (G34)	⌐Glu-Leu-Gly-Pro-Gln-Gly-Pro-Pro-His-Leu-Val-Ala-Asp-Pro-Ser-Lys-Lys--Gln-Gly-Pro-Trp-Leu-Glu-Glu-Glu-Glu-Glu-Ala-Tyr*-Gly-Trp-Met-Asp-Phe-NH₂
Heptadecapeptide Gastrin (G 17)	⌐Glu-Gly-Pro-Trp-Leu-Glu-Glu-Glu-Glu-Glu-Ala-Tyr*-Gly-Trp-Met-Asp-Phe-NH₂
Minigastrin (G 14)	Trp-Leu-Glu-Glu-Glu-Glu-Glu-Ala-Tyr*-Gly-Trp-Met-Asp-Phe-NH₂
C-Terminal Pentapeptide	Gly-Trp-Met-Asp-Phe-NH₂

FIGURE 252-1 Amino acid sequences of selected gastrin peptides, all of which contain the common C-terminal pentapeptide amide. (*Tyrosyl is sulfated in gastrin II and nonsulfated in gastrin I molecules.)

concentration in the most proximal duodenum (approximately 10 percent of antral concentration). The mucosal concentration of gastrin and the proportion of G-17 decrease with progression down the duodenum. The effects of gastrin and vagal stimulation on gastric acid secretion are intimately interrelated. Vagal stimulation increases gastric acid secretion by cholinergic stimulation of parietal cell secretion, by stimulating release of gastrin into the circulation, and by lowering the parietal cell threshold for response to circulating gastrin concentrations. Certain vagal branches or fibers also inhibit gastrin release.

The gastric mucosa contains large amounts of histamine. Histamine is contained in cytoplasmic granules of mast cells, which are nonepithelial (interstitial) in location, and enterochromaffin-like (ECL) cells, epithelial endocrine cells distributed singly in the oxyntic glands, often in direct contact with parietal cells. For many years, views differed on the importance of histamine in stimulating gastric acid secretion; some suggested that histamine was the "final common pathway" for cholinergic and gastrin stimulation of parietal cell acid secretion. Others were skeptical about any role for histamine in the acid secretory process. Interest in the role of histamine in acid secretion was renewed by discovery of H-2 receptor antagonists which inhibit competitively the action of histamine on H-2 receptors (located on gastric parietal, cardiac atrial, and uterine smooth-muscle cells). These drugs exert negligible effects on H-1 receptors, which are inhibited readily by conventional antihistamines (H-1 receptor antagonists). H-2 receptor antagonists (e.g., cimetidine, ranitidine, famotidine, nizatidine) inhibit basal acid secretion as well as secretion in response to feeding, gastrin, histamine, hypoglycemia, or vagal stimulation. Most data support the conclusions that (1) histamine plays an important role in stimulating gastric acid secretion and (2) histamine acts in concert with gastrin and cholinergic activity on parietal cells, but that (3) there is still uncertainty as to whether histamine is the final common effector molecule in stimulation of parietal cell secretion. The basolateral membranes of parietal cells contain receptors for histamine, gastrin, and acetylcholine, which stimulate acid secretion, and for prostaglandins and somatostatin, which inhibit acid secretion. Parietal cell histamine, gastrin, and somatostatin receptors are members of the seven-membrane spanning class of G protein–coupled receptors. Gastrin stimulates gastric acid secretion by direct stimulation of parietal cells and by stimulating histamine release by ECL cells. Histamine stimulates gastric acid secretion by increasing parietal cell cyclic adenosine monophosphate (AMP), thereby activating cyclic AMP–dependent protein kinase(s). Gastrin and acetylcholine, which do not stimulate cyclic AMP production, stimulate acid secretion by increasing parietal cell cytosolic calcium.

The major physiologic stimulus for gastric acid secretion is ingestion of food. Traditionally, regulation of gastric acid secretion has been classified into three phases—cephalic, gastric, and intestinal. This classification is of some value in analyzing factors that participate in regulation of gastric acid secretion. The *cephalic phase* encompasses the gastric acid secretory response to the sight, smell, taste, and anticipation of food. The *gastric phase* is induced by food in the stomach. The *intestinal phase* is due to the entry or presence of food within the lumen of the small intestine. Although these three phases are convenient for considering the diverse contributions to gastric

acid secretion, each phase is complex and not due necessarily to a single stimulatory control mechanism.

The cephalic phase, which includes cortical and hypothalamic components, is mediated primarily by vagal activation, which increases gastric acid secretion principally by direct stimulation of parietal cells and to a lesser extent by promoting gastrin release. The gastric phase results from stimulation of chemical and mechanical receptors in the gastric wall by luminal contents. Mechanical distention of the stomach stimulates gastric acid secretion but results in little, if any, gastrin release; this mechanical effect is inhibited by atropine and appears to be mediated by vagal reflexes. Food in the stomach promotes gastric acid secretion by increasing gastrin release. It is principally the *protein* and especially the *products of protein digestion* contained in the meal that have this effect; oral glucose and fat cause slight increases in serum gastrin but do not stimulate gastric acid secretion. Food in the proximal small intestine stimulates the intestinal phase of gastric acid secretion. A peptone meal (partially hydrolyzed meat protein) in the small intestine stimulates gastric acid secretion but not gastrin release. Food in the small intestine may induce release of an intestinal hormone(s) (distinct from gastrin) that stimulates gastric acid secretion. Increases in circulating amino acids, absorbed from the small intestine, also may contribute to the intestinal phase of gastric acid secretion. *Basal* or *interdigestive gastric acid secretion* can be considered to be a *fourth phase* of acid secretion. This phase is unrelated to feeding, reaches its peak around midnight and its lowest point about 7 A.M., and neural pathways are probably most important in its regulation.

Ingestion of both caffeine-containing and caffeine-free *coffee* stimulates gastric acid secretion, and both stimulate gastrin release. Ingestion of *ethanol* and ethanol-containing beverages stimulates gastric acid secretion. Intravenous ethanol stimulates gastric acid secretion, suggesting that both systemic and local mechanisms are involved.

Intravenous *calcium* stimulates gastric acid secretion and produces minimal increases in serum gastrin levels. Oral calcium has been reported to stimulate gastric acid secretion directly, i.e., without an increase in serum calcium or gastrin concentrations. Except in patients who harbor gastrinomas, hypercalcemia is not usually associated with gastric acid hypersecretion or with increases in serum gastrin.

Inhibition of gastric acid secretion can be produced by several mechanisms. Acid secretion may be inhibited by acid in the stomach or duodenum, by hyperglycemia, or by hypertonic fluids or fat in the duodenum. Reduction of the intragastric pH to 3.0 produces partial inhibition of gastrin release; further reduction to pH 1.5 or below blocks completely release of gastrin to almost all stimuli. *Somatostatin* appears to play an important role in this acid-induced feedback-control inhibition of gastrin release. Somatostatin inhibits gastrin release by its local (paracrine) effects on gastrin cells. Somatostatin-containing antral mucosal endocrine cells (D cells) have cytoplasmic processes which extend to neighboring gastrin cells. In addition, cytoplasmic processes of somatostatin cells in oxyntic glands extend to direct intimate contact with parietal cells and other cells. Somatostatin reduces gastric acid secretion by inhibiting gastrin release and by directly inhibiting parietal cell secretion. Acid in the duodenum decreases gastric acid secretion by the stomach, most likely by stimulating release into the circulation of intestinal peptides that inhibit gastric acid secretion. *Secretin*, a linear polypeptide (27 amino acids) related structurally to glucagon, is capable of inhibiting gastric acid secretion. Secretin is released from endocrine cells (S cells) in the mucosa of the proximal small intestine in response to mucosal acidification. Fat in the duodenum also inhibits gastric acid secretion; gastric inhibitory peptide (GIP) has been proposed as a candidate for this enterogastrone action; however, this effect of GIP remains to be proven. The mechanisms by which hyperglycemia or intraduodenal hyperosmolality inhibit gastric acid secretion are not known. Additional small intestinal mucosal peptides possessing the capacity to inhibit gastric acid secretion include vasoactive intestinal peptide (VIP), enteroglucagon, neurotensin, peptide YY, and urogastrone. *Vasoactive intestinal peptide*, a neuropeptide and putative neurotransmitter, is unlikely to inhibit gastric acid secretion as a circulating hormone since, although released in response to feeding, it is inactivated during its portal passage through the liver. *Enteroglucagon* is composed of oxyntomodulin (glucagon with an 8 amino acid carboxyl-terminal extension) and glicentin (oxyntomodulin with a 32 amino acid amino-terminal extension). *Neurotensin*, oxyntomodulin, and *peptide YY* are released from the small intestine in response to luminal lipid perfusion. *Urogastrone* is structurally and functionally identical to epidermal growth factor. The extent to which these peptides contribute to the physiologic regulation of gastric acid secretion has not been defined.

The proteolytic effects of *pepsins* in concert with the corrosive properties of secreted gastric acid are the integral components which account for the tissue injury that produces peptic ulcer. Gastric acid catalyzes the cleavage of inactive pepsinogen molecules, converting them to proteolytically active pepsins, and also provides the appropriate low pH required for pepsin activity. Activity of pepsins is maximal at pH approximately 2.0 and is reduced substantially above pH 4.0. Pepsins are denatured and irreversibly inactivated at neutral or alkaline pH. A variety of pepsinogens and their respective pepsins are present in gastric juice. Pepsinogens (and their corresponding active pepsins) have been classified by immunochemical techniques as either PG I (pepsinogens 1 through 5) or PG II (pepsinogens 6 and 7). Pepsinogen I is found in chief and mucous cells in the body and fundus of the stomach. Pepsinogen II is located in cells of the pyloric glands, Brunner's glands of the duodenum, mucous cells of the gastric cardiac glands, and the same cells in which PG I is found. Both PG I and PG II are present in plasma, whereas only PG I is detected in urine. In general, there is a direct correlation between PG I serum concentrations and maximal gastric acid secretion. Most agents which stimulate gastric acid secretion also stimulate pepsinogen secretion. Cholinergic action is particularly potent in promoting pepsinogen secretion. Although it inhibits gastric acid secretion, secretin stimulates pepsinogen secretion.

In addition to secretion of hydrochloric acid, parietal cells also secrete *intrinsic factor*. Agents which stimulate gastric acid secretion also lead to secretion of intrinsic factor.

MUCOSAL DEFENSE The mechanisms whereby the normal stomach and duodenum resist the corrosive effects of acid-pepsin (i.e., *mucosal resistance* to injury or *mucosal defense*) have not been defined completely. However, a variety of factors have been identified which contribute to and are considered to comprise mucosal defense.

Gastric mucus is important in mucosal defense and in preventing peptic ulceration. Gastric mucus is secreted by mucous cells of the gastric mucosal epithelium and gastric glands. Mucus secretion is stimulated by mechanical or chemical irritation and by cholinergic stimulation. Gastric mucus is present in two phases: in gastric juice in a soluble phase and as an insoluble mucus gel layer, approximately 0.2 mm in thickness, which coats the mucosal surface of the stomach. Normally the mucus gel is secreted constantly by gastric mucous epithelial cells and is continuously solubilized by pepsins secreted into the gastric lumen. Gastric mucus is a large polymeric glycoprotein (2×10^6 mol wt) containing four subunits connected by disulfide bridges. Depolymerization of the glycoprotein subunits of mucus, by peptic digestion or disruption of disulfide bonds, renders the glycoprotein incapable of forming or maintaining the gel. When intact, this mucus gel serves as an unstirred water layer which slows ionic diffusion but is much more impermeable to penetration by macromolecules such as pepsins (34,000 mol wt). Pepsin molecules secreted into the gastric lumen are denied reentry by the intact mucus gel, thereby potentially protecting mucosal cells from proteolytic injury. Gel thickness is increased by prostaglandins of the E series and reduced by nonsteroidal anti-inflammatory drugs (NSAIDs), including aspirin. Gastric mucus glycoproteins also contain antigenic determinants used to classify AB(H) blood group substances. Approximately three-fourths of the population secrete gastric juice containing these AB(H) substances, and such individuals are referred to as *secretors*.

Bicarbonate ions, secreted by nonparietal gastric epithelial cells, enter the mucus gel, contributing to the development of a microenvironment in the gel with a substantial hydrogen ion gradient between the zone of the gel facing the gastric lumen (pH 1 to 2) and the zone in contact with the gastric mucosal cells (pH 6 to 7). As an unstirred water layer, the mucus gel slows hydrogen ion diffusion back toward the gastric mucosal surface, allowing buffering by bicarbonate within the gel. Gastric bicarbonate secretion is stimulated by calcium, certain prostaglandins of the E and F series, cholinergic agents, and dibutyryl cyclic guanosine monophosphate. It is inhibited by NSAIDs, including aspirin, and by acetazolamide, alpha-adrenergic agents, and ethanol.

Normally, the gastric epithelial cell luminal surfaces and intercellular tight junctions provide an almost completely impermeable *gastric mucosal barrier* to back-diffusion of hydrogen ions from the lumen; this barrier appears to be an important component of mucosal resistance to acid-peptic injury. The barrier can be interrupted by bile acids, salicylates, ethanol, and weak organic acids, thereby permitting back-diffusion of hydrogen ions from lumen into gastric tissues. This may cause cell injury, release of histamine from mast cells, further stimulation of acid secretion, damage to small blood vessels, mucosal hemorrhage, and erosion or ulceration. Interruption of the gastric mucosal barrier appears to contribute to the hemorrhagic erosive gastritis associated with salicylate or ethanol ingestion and with other forms of gastric mucosal injury. Because of its high rate of metabolic activity and substantial oxygen requirements, maintenance of normal *blood flow* to the gastric mucosa is an essential component of mucosal resistance to injury. Decreased mucosal blood flow, accompanied by back-diffusion of luminal hydrogen ions, is important in producing gastric mucosal damage.

Prostaglandins are abundant in the gastric mucosa. Various prostaglandins, particularly those of the E series, have been shown to inhibit gastric mucosal injury caused by a wide variety of agents. Endogenous prostaglandins are important elements constituting mucosal defense. They stimulate secretion of gastric mucus and gastric and duodenal mucosal bicarbonate, which buffer a substantial portion of secreted gastric acid. Prostaglandins participate in the maintenance of gastric mucosal blood flow and in the integrity of the gastric mucosal barrier. Prostaglandins promote epithelial cell renewal in response to mucosal injury.

MEASUREMENT OF GASTRIC ACID SECRETION Since HCl secretion by the stomach is important in producing peptic ulcer, measurement of basal and stimulated gastric acid secretion may be of value in the clinical assessment of some patients with peptic ulcer. The range of values for normal subjects is extremely broad and overlaps substantially with those for patients with duodenal ulcer, gastric ulcer, and even the Zollinger-Ellison syndrome. Mean basal acid output (BAO) in normal males without known ulcer disease is about 1.5 to 2.0 mmol/h. In general, basal and stimulated acid outputs in females are approximately two-thirds to three-fourths those found in males. In duodenal ulcer patients, mean basal acid output average from 4 to 6 mmol/h, again with wide variation. Patients with gastric ulcer tend to have acid secretory rates that are normal or often slightly less than those for normal subjects.

Measurement of gastric acid output is not helpful in the diagnosis or exclusion of peptic ulcer and clearly is not necessary in most ulcer patients. However, it is of value in selected clinical situations. Detection of gastric acid hypersecretion is important when the Zollinger-Ellison syndrome is suspected. Measurement of gastric output is useful to detect achlorhydria, as in patients with pernicious anemia. Since patients with benign gastric ulcer virtually always secrete some acid, pentagastrin-fast achlorhydria in a patient with a gastric ulcer is almost always associated with malignancy. Measurement of gastric acid secretion is indicated in the search for the cause of ulcer recurrence after peptic ulcer surgery. It is also of value in patients in whom hypergastrinemia has been identified, in order to distinguish between clinical conditions characterized by gastric acid hypersecretion or achlorhydria.

To measure gastric acid output, a radiopaque gastric tube is passed so that its tip is located in the most dependent portion of the stomach. With the patient reclining or semirecumbent on the left side, the tube position is verified by fluoroscopy. Gastric contents are aspirated and discarded. Secretions are then collected in four consecutive 15-min intervals to determine the 1-h basal acid output. Secretion volume and acid concentration (titrated with sodium hydroxide to pH 7.0 or calculated by formula from the pH of the aspirated gastric juice) are measured, and acid output is expressed in millimoles per hour.

A variety of substances have been used to stimulate maximal acid output (MAO) by the stomach. These include *histamine*; *betazole* (Histalog), a structural analogue of histamine; and *pentagastrin* (Peptavlon). Histamine, the first standard stimulant used for gastric acid secretory testing, requires simultaneous administration of an antihistamine (H-1 receptor antagonist) to inhibit systemic side effects. Betazole possesses fewer undesirable side effects than histamine and does not require concomitant administration of an antihistamine. Pentagastrin (N-*tert*-butyloxycarbonyl-β-Ala-Trp-Met-Asp-Phe-NH$_2$) contains the biologically active carboxyl-terminal tetrapeptide amide portion of gastrin and is the preferred agent to stimulate maximal acid secretion. Following collection of basal acid secretion, gastric juice is collected for four additional consecutive 15-min periods after the subcutaneous injection of pentagastrin (6 μg/kg). MAO is expressed as millimoles of acid aspirated during the 1 h after pentagastrin administration. Peak acid output (PAO) is calculated by combining the two highest consecutive 15-min acid outputs following pentagastrin injection and multiplying by 2.

DUODENAL ULCER

Duodenal ulcer is characteristically a chronic and recurrent disease. These ulcers are usually deep and sharply demarcated. They penetrate through the mucosa and submucosa, often into the muscularis propria. This is in contrast to erosions, which are superficial and limited to the mucosa. The ulcer floor contains no intact epithelium and usually consists of a zone of eosinophilic necrosis resting on a base of granulation tissue surrounded by variable amounts of fibrosis. The ulcer bed may be clear or may contain blood or a proteinaceous exudate with entrapped erythrocytes and acute and chronic inflammatory cells. More than 95 percent of duodenal ulcers occur in the first portion of the duodenum, and approximately 90 percent of those are located within 3 cm of the junction of the pyloric and duodenal mucosa. Duodenal ulcers are usually round or oval, but they may be irregular or elliptic. They are usually less than 1 cm in diameter. Rarely, duodenal ulcers are extremely large (3 to 6 cm in diameter) and may be mistaken radiographically for the entire duodenal bulb. These giant ulcers often escape radiologic detection and are usually identified by endoscopy, at surgery, or at postmortem examination.

The absolute prevalence of duodenal ulcer is not known. It is estimated to occur in from 6 to 15 percent of the population. This variation in estimates may be explained by differences in populations examined, study designs, diagnostic methods (e.g., endoscopy versus radiologic examination), and actual changes occurring in the frequency of duodenal ulcer. During the past 40 years, the frequency of duodenal ulcer (and its complications) has been decreasing in the United States

and England, especially in males. The reasons for this reduction are not known. Duodenal ulcers now appear to be approximately as common in males as in females. Best current estimates suggest that approximately 10 percent of the population has clinical evidence of duodenal ulcer at some time in their lives. The natural history of duodenal ulcer is that of spontaneous healing and recurrence; about 60 percent of healed duodenal ulcers recur within 1 year, and 80 to 90 percent recur within 2 years.

ETIOLOGY AND PATHOGENESIS   Much is now known concerning factors that contribute to the development of duodenal ulcer, but we do not completely understand all aspects of its pathogenesis. It is clear that acid secretion by the stomach is required for production of a duodenal ulcer. However, all the factors which render the acid-secreting subject susceptible to duodenal ulceration have not been defined completely. Though as a group duodenal ulcer patients secrete more acid than normal, from one-half to two-thirds of them have acid secretory rates (BAO and MAO) within the normal range. Duodenal ulcer patients have approximately 1.9 billion parietal cells, with a maximum capacity of approximately 42 mmol gastric acid secreted per hour; this is in contrast to 1.0 billion parietal cells and 22 mmol/h secretion rate for nonduodenal ulcer subjects (mean approximate values). However, variations in both groups are so large that most duodenal ulcer patients fall within the normal range. As a group, in response to stimulation duodenal ulcer patients also have comparable increases in gastric secretion of pepsin and in serum PG I levels. Peptic ulcer develops when there is an unfavorable balance between acid-pepsin secretion and mucosal defense; in the pathogenesis of duodenal ulcer, evidence favors the importance of absolute or, in most instances, relative gastric hypersecretion. In contrast, for gastric ulcer, defective mucosal defense appears to be the major contributing factor.

Fasting *serum gastrin* concentrations are normal in duodenal ulcer patients. However, in many duodenal ulcer patients more gastrin is released into the circulation in response to a protein-containing meal than by normal subjects. Duodenal ulcer patients also have greater gastric acid secretory responses to administered gastrin than do nonulcer subjects. In duodenal ulcer patients, intragastric acid may be less effective in inhibiting gastrin release and further gastric acid secretion. Duodenal ulcer patients tend to empty their stomachs more rapidly than do nonduodenal ulcer patients. This phenomenon, when coupled with relative gastric acid hypersecretion, may contribute to a greater rate of acid delivery to the first part of the duodenum (the primary location of ulceration) in patients with duodenal ulcer. Acidification of the proximal duodenum in patients with duodenal ulcer results in less secretion of bicarbonate into the lumen by duodenal mucosal cells than in nonulcer subjects.

Genetic factors appear to be important. Duodenal ulcers are approximately three times as common in first-degree relatives of duodenal ulcer patients as in the general population. Patients with duodenal ulcers have an increased frequency of blood group O and of the nonsecretor status [those who do not secrete AB(H) blood group antigens in their gastric juice], but these associations are weak. An increased incidence of HLA-B5 antigen has been reported in white male subjects with duodenal ulcer.

Cigarette smoking has been associated with increased duodenal ulcer frequency, decreased response to therapy, and increased duodenal ulcer mortality. Cigarette smoking does not increase gastric acid secretion. It has been suggested that the increased incidence of duodenal ulcer among cigarette smokers may be due to inhibition of pancreatic bicarbonate secretion (an endogenous neutralizer of secreted gastric acid) by nicotine or cigarette smoke and/or by accelerated emptying of gastric acid into the duodenum.

The incidence of duodenal ulcer also has been reported to be increased in patients with chronic renal failure, alcoholic cirrhosis, renal transplantation, hyperparathyroidism, systemic mastocytosis, and chronic obstructive pulmonary disease. Antibodies to herpes simplex have been reported to be higher in titer and more frequent in sera of patients with duodenal ulcer than in normals.

The importance of *psychological factors* in the pathogenesis of duodenal ulcer remains controversial. Contrary to earlier views, there is no single, characteristic duodenal ulcer personality. Chronic anxiety and psychological stress may, however, be factors in exacerbation of ulcer activity. There is some evidence that patients with duodenal ulcer may view stress more negatively than nonulcer subjects. No differences have been identified in the frequency of duodenal ulcer among different socioeconomic classes or occupation groups.

HELICOBACTER PYLORI Gastric colonization with *Helicobacter pylori* has been reported in 90 to 95 percent of patients with duodenal ulcer and in 60 to 70 percent of patients with gastric ulcer. Healthy persons less than 30 years of age have prevalence rates of gastric colonization with *H. pylori* of approximately 10 percent. Gastric colonization increases with age, with those over age 60 having colonization rates approximating their age. Most patients with gastric colonization by *H. pylori* never develop ulceration and remain asymptomatic. Rates are increased with deprived socioeconomic circumstances as well as in custodial institutions and have been reported to be increased in black and Hispanic Americans. *H. pylori* is a spiral, gram-negative bacillus with multiple flagella with preference for a microaerophilic environment. *H. pylori* does not invade tissues. The organism resides in the mucus gel coating the epithelial cells, with a minor proportion of *H. pylori* directly adherent to the epithelial cells. Most *H. pylori*–infected persons have neutrophils in the lamina propria and epithelial glands and an increase in chronic inflammatory cells in the lamina propria. Colonization of *H. pylori* in the duodenum is restricted to areas of gastric metaplasia and is found in metaplastic gastric epithelium in the duodenal bulb of most patients with duodenal ulcer. *H. pylori* has been shown to be the cause of several forms of acute and chronic gastritis (see "Gastritis," below). *H. pylori* has been proposed as an important factor in the pathogenesis of duodenal ulcer. Evidence is mounting in support of this proposal. However, it remains to be established whether *H. pylori* is an important cause of duodenal ulcer, a potential contributing or modifying factor, or, and less likely, its presence reflects an extremely frequent commensal association.

CLINICAL FEATURES Epigastric pain is by far the most frequent symptom of duodenal ulcer. The pain is often described as sharp, burning, or gnawing. Alternatively, the pain may be ill-defined, boring, or aching or may be perceived as abdominal pressure or fullness or as a hunger sensation. In approximately 10 percent of patients the pain is located to the right of the epigastrium. The pain of duodenal ulcer characteristically occurs from 90 min to 3 h after eating. It frequently awakens the patient at night. Pain on awakening before breakfast is sufficiently rare in patients with duodenal ulcer as to challenge the diagnosis. The pain is usually relieved within a few minutes by food or antacids. Symptoms tend to be recurrent and episodic. The severity of pain varies widely from patient to patient. Duodenal ulcers recur often in the absence of pain. Episodes of pain may persist for periods of several days to weeks or months. Periods of remission usually last from weeks to years and are almost always longer than the episodes of pain. In some patients the disease is more aggressive, with frequent and persistent symptoms and/or development of complications. Pain relief with antacids or food is believed to result from acid neutralization. Ingestion of food leads to transient partial neutralization of gastric acid, which is followed by gastrin release and resultant stimulation of acid secretion. With subsequent gastric emptying and increasing gastric acid secretion, a sufficiently low pH is achieved in the stomach and first portion of the duodenum that pain results. Acid-induced pain in patients with duodenal ulcer is believed to be due to (1) acid stimulation of chemical receptors and/or (2) alterations in gastric motility.

Changes in the character of ulcer pain may signal the development of complications. For example, ulcer pain which becomes constant, is no longer relieved by food or antacids, or radiates to the back or to either upper quadrant may herald *penetration* of the ulcer (often posteriorly into the pancreas). Pain associated with duodenal ulcer which is accentuated, rather than relieved, by food and/or is accom-panied by vomiting often indicates *gastric outlet obstruction*. Abrupt, severe, or generalized abdominal pain is characteristic of free ulcer *perforation* into the peritoneal cavity. Weight loss, in the absence of some degree of gastric outlet obstruction, is unusual. Duodenal ulcer may cause acute gastrointestinal *hemorrhage*, with vomiting of blood or "coffee grounds" material or with the passage of black, tarry stools or even frankly red blood, if the bleeding is massive. More commonly, blood loss with duodenal ulcer is more subtle, with occult blood loss detected by stool examination or by variable degrees of anemia which may be accompanied by iron deficiency.

It is important to emphasize that *many patients with active duodenal ulcer have no ulcer symptoms*. This leads to a significant, although not precisely quantifiable, underestimate of duodenal ulcer frequency in the population. Prospective studies using upper gastrointestinal endoscopy suggest that approximately half of duodenal ulcer recurrences are without symptoms. Endoscopic studies also show a lack of good correlation among ulcer activity, symptom resolution, and ulcer healing. The absence of ulcer-type pain does not exclude dudoenal ulcer as a potential cause for acute or chronic gastrointestinal hemorrhage, gastric outlet obstruction, or abrupt ulcer perforation.

On *physical examination*, epigastric tenderness is by far the most frequent abnormal finding. The area of tenderness is usually in the midline, often midway between the umbilicus and the xiphoid process. In approximately 20 percent of patients the tender area is to the right of the midline. Acute free ulcer perforation into the peritoneal cavity often produces a rigid, boardlike abdomen, usually with generalized rebound tenderness. Initially, auscultation of the abdomen may reveal hyperactive bowel sounds which, with clinical progression, may diminish or disappear. Patients with gastric outlet obstruction caused by a duodenal or pyloric channel ulcer may have a "succussion splash" produced by fluid and air in the distended stomach. Tachycardia and/or hypotension, in some instances demonstrable only by orthostatic maneuvers, may result from acute duodenal ulcer hemorrhage. Cutaneous and mucosal pallor may reflect anemia from acute or chronic blood loss.

Only 5 percent of duodenal ulcers are located distal to the duodenal bulb, and most of those are in the immediate postbulbar portion of the first part of the duodenum. Postbulbar ulcer pain may be located in the right upper quadrant and may radiate to the back. Obstruction and hemorrhage are more frequent with postbulbar ulcers than with those in the duodenal bulb. Most immediate postbulbar ulcers, i.e., within 2 cm of the duodenal bulb, are of the common duodenal ulcer variety. Ulceration located in or beyond the second portion of the duodenum suggests the Zollinger-Ellison syndrome.

The pyloric channel, which is 1 to 2 cm in length, is the narrowest portion of the gastric outlet. Because of their gastric acid secretory characteristics and clinical features, pyloric channel ulcers are classi-fied with duodenal rather than with gastric ulcers. Ulcers in this location often produce symptoms similar to those of a duodenal ulcer; however, symptoms tend to be less responsive to food and antacids. In patients with pyloric channel ulcers, food may accentuate rather than relieve ulcer pain and may produce vomiting due to partial gastric outlet obstruction. In general, surgery is required more frequently for pyloric channel ulcers than for those in the duodenal bulb.

DIAGNOSIS Barium examination of the upper gastrointestinal tract is of value in identifying duodenal ulcer and is still the most com-mon initial method used to establish the diagnosis. The proportion of ulcers identified radiographically depends on the skill, persistence, en-thusiasm, and diagnostic criteria of the radiologist. Using conventional single-contrast barium techniques, 70 to 80 percent of duodenal ul-cers found at endoscopy can be identified by x-ray examination. With double-contrast barium examinations, it is possible to detect about 90 percent of duodenal ulcers. On x-ray, the typical duodenal ulcer ap-pears as a discrete crater in the proximal portion of the duodenal bulb. Marked deformity of the duodenal bulb, common in patients with chronic recurrent duodenal ulcer, may make radiographic identification of the ulcer difficult or impossible (Figs. 252-2 and 252-3).

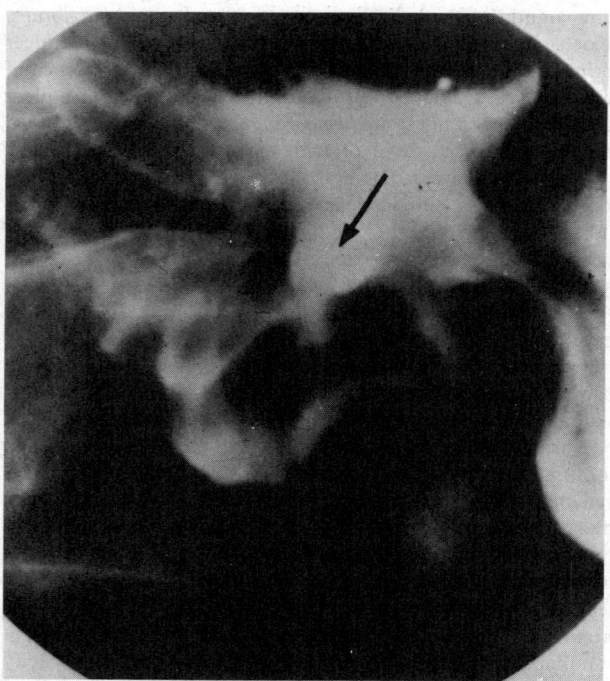

FIGURE 252-2   Deformed duodenal bulb with ulcer crater.

Endoscopic examination of the upper gastrointestinal tract has facilitated accurate diagnosis of duodenal ulcer. Endoscopy is not required for diagnosis of duodenal ulcer when it has been identified by barium radiographic examination. Endoscopy may be of greatest value, however, (1) in detecting duodenal ulcer suspected in the absence of a radiographically demonstrable ulcer, (2) in patients with

FIGURE 252-3   Distortion of the duodenal bulb with "cloverleaf" deformity.

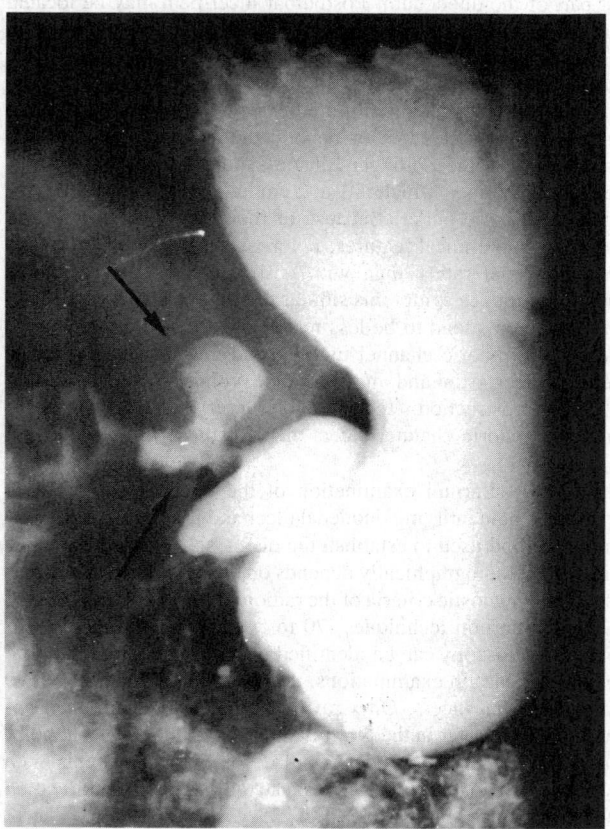

radiographic deformity and uncertainty regarding ulcer activity, (3) in identifying ulcers too small or too superficial to be recognized by x-ray, and (4) in identifying (or excluding) an ulcer as the source of active gastrointestinal hemorrhage. Endoscopy permits direct visualization and photographic documentation of the character of the ulcer—its size, shape, and location—and may provide a reference base for assessment of ulcer healing.

Measurement of gastric acid secretion is not necessary in the assessment of most patients with suspected or confirmed duodenal ulcer. Determination of the serum gastrin level is recommended in those patients in whom surgery is planned or gastrinoma is considered. Epigastric pain readily relieved by food or antacids strongly suggests duodenal ulcer. However, even after careful radiographic and endoscopic examination many patients with these ulcer-like symptoms have no evidence of ulcer; this has led to the term *nonulcer dyspepsia*. Although symptoms are similar, it is uncertain whether this entity is related to peptic ulcer.

MEDICAL TREATMENT   Major objectives of duodenal ulcer therapy are relief of pain and acceleration of ulcer healing. Prevention of ulcer recurrence and complications is an additional important objective. In the past, enthusiasm has been expressed for virtually every kind of treatment ever tried for duodenal ulcer. Conclusions regarding the effectiveness of therapy were obscured by spontaneous healing of duodenal ulcer, an intrinsic component of the natural history of the disease, and by imprecise methods used to assess ulcer activity. Therapeutic agents shown to be effective which are currently available and recommended for consideration in treatment of duodenal ulcer are discussed below.

Antacids   For many decades, antacids have been a major form of treatment for duodenal ulcer. Prospective endoscopic studies conducted only relatively recently verified the effectiveness of antacids in accelerating duodenal ulcer healing. Many types of antacids are available for use in treatment of duodenal ulcer. The ideal antacid should be potent in neutralizing gastric acid, inexpensive, not adsorbed from the gastrointestinal tract, and contain negligible amounts of sodium. It should be sufficiently palatable to be tolerated with repeated dosage and should be free from side effects. Individual antacids differ substantially in their capacities to neutralize acid, their sodium contents, their absorption properties, and their potential adverse effects. Although the ideal antacid is yet to be developed, a number of preparations are available that can be used effectively in treatment of patients with duodenal ulcer.

The most widely used antacid preparations are mixtures of aluminum hydroxide and magnesium hydroxide, in some instances with additional agents. *Aluminum hydroxide* neutralizes hydrochloric acid with the production of aluminum chloride and water. Use of aluminum hydroxide tends to produce constipation. Aluminum binds phosphate within the gut lumen, thereby facilitating phosphate excretion. As a consequence, prolonged and regular use of aluminum hydroxide may induce systemic phosphate depletion with resultant weakness, malaise, and anorexia. Phosphate depletion is probably restricted to, and should be considered in, those patients with phosphate-poor diets, e.g., dietary deficiency with chronic alcoholism or other states of reduced dietary protein intake. *Magnesium hydroxide* is a potent antacid which neutralizes hydrochloric acid, producing magnesium chloride and water. Magnesium hydroxide may produce loose stools. This laxative effect and the constipating effects of aluminum hydroxide can be overcome by using antacids which contain these agents in combination. From 5 to 10 percent of magnesium in magnesium hydroxide is absorbed by the small intestine. Magnesium is excreted by the kidney, and hypermagnesemia, which is not a problem with normal renal function, develops in a small number of patients with renal insufficiency who are treated with magnesium-containing antacids. *Magnesium trisilicate*, which is included in various antacid mixtures, is a slow-acting weak antacid.

Calcium carbonate is a potent and inexpensive antacid. In neutralizing acid, it is converted to calcium chloride in the stomach. Approximately 10 percent of calcium ingested as calcium carbonate is absorbed from the proximal small intestine. Calcium carbonate is unique among antacids in that its ingestion is followed by stimulation of gastrin acid secretion ("acid rebound"). This is due to the direct action of calcium in stimulating parietal cell acid secretion and, perhaps to a lesser extent, to calcium-mediated stimulation of gastrin release. Chronic excessive calcium carbonate administration may be associated with the milk-alkali syndrome, producing elevations of serum calcium, phosphate, urea nitrogen, creatinine, and bicarbonate levels. These patients may develop renal calcinosis and progressive renal insufficiency. Because of its potential adverse effects, calcium carbonate is not recommended for use as an antacid for primary treatment of patients with peptic ulcer.

Sodium bicarbonate is a potent, rapidly acting, inexpensive antacid. However, because of its tendency to induce systemic alkalosis and its high sodium content, it should not be used as an antacid in the treatment of peptic ulcer.

Acceptance of the crucial role of acid in the pathogenesis of duodenal ulcer has provided a rational basis for the use of antacids in the treatment of patients with duodenal ulcer. In a controlled endoscopic study, 4 weeks of treatment with a potent magnesium and aluminum hydroxide antacid mixture increased the rate of duodenal ulcer healing. Ulcer healing occurred in 45 percent of patients receiving placebo and in 78 percent of those treated with 30 mL antacid (144 mmol) given 1 and 3 h after meals and at bedtime. It has been proposed that variably smaller and less frequent doses also may achieve satisfactory ulcer healing.

H-2 receptor antagonists It had been known for many years that conventional antihistamines, which block the actions of histamine on smooth muscle of blood vessels, gut, or bronchi, do not inhibit histamine-stimulated gastric acid secretion. This observation led to the development of specific classes of histamine antagonists for different types of histamine receptors. The gastric parietal cell receptor for histamine has been classifed as an H-2 receptor and that blocked by classic antihistamines as an H-1 receptor. H-2 receptor antagonists are potent inhibitors of basal (unstimulated) and stimulated gastric acid secretion. H-2 receptor antagonists exhibit some structural similarities to histamine and to each other, with variations in ring structures and side chains (see Fig. 252-4). H-2 receptor antagonists are safe and effective in accelerating healing and reducing recurrence of duodenal ulcer. Healing rates for H-2 receptor antagonists are similar to those described above for antacids. Compliance appears superior. Daily maintenance doses of H-2 receptor antagonists (one-half the therapeutic dose) reduce duodenal ulcer recurrence by 50 to 70 percent. At the present time, H-2 receptor antagonists are the therapeutic agents used most frequently in the management of patients with duodenal ulcer.

Cimetidine was the first H-2 receptor antagonist developed and has been used extensively in the treatment of duodenal ulcer. Cimetidine is related structurally to histamine (Fig. 252-4), sharing the same imidazole ring, but bearing an extended side chain containing a cyanoguanidine group. Much information regarding the actions of H-2 receptor antagonists was obtained in the detailed characterization of the actions of cimetidine. Cimetidine (300 mg) was shown to inhibit basal acid secretion by more than 80 percent and meal-stimulated acid secretion by approximately 70 percent. It strikingly reduced acid secretory responses to histamine, caffeine, insulin, hypoglycemia, and gastrin. Cimetidine was shown to be effective in promoting endoscopically verified duodenal ulcer healing. Initially, the oral dose of cimetidine recommended and used in treatment of duodenal ulcer was 300 mg four times daily, with meals and at bedtime. More recently, 400 mg cimetidine twice each day (morning and bedtime) or 800 mg once daily (at bedtime) has been shown to be equally effective. The 800-mg bedtime dose is recommended. Treatment of active duodenal ulcer with cimetidine is continued for periods from 4 to 8 weeks. In patients with healed duodenal ulcer, prolonged administration of cimetidine (400 mg at bedtime) has been shown to reduce substantially the frequency of duodenal ulcer recurrence.

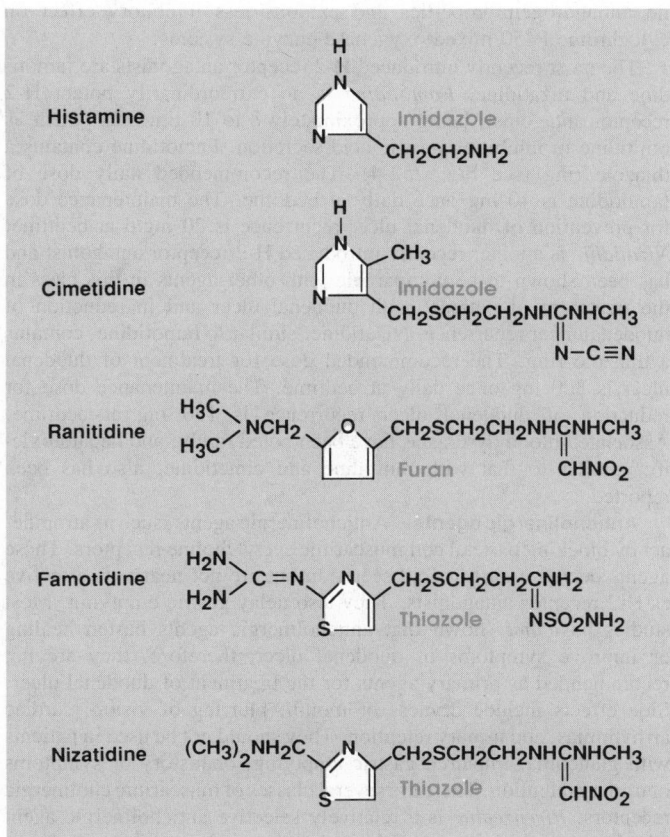

FIGURE 252-4 Chemical structures of histamine and the H-2 receptor antagonists cimetidine, rantidine, famotidine, and nizatidine. Note the similarities and differences in the ring structures, including the imidazole ring shared by histamine and cimetidine, the furan ring in ranitidine, and the thiazole ring in famotidine and nizatidine.

Considering the enormous number of patients who have been treated with cimetidine, few serious adverse effects have been experienced. Slight and reversible increases in serum aminotransferase and creatinine levels may occur. Reversible confusional states have been reported in a small number of severely ill patients with preexisting hepatic-renal functional impairment. Brief increases in serum prolactin have been found after intravenous and oral cimetidine. Cimetidine has been shown to inhibit some cytochrome P450 hepatic microsomal enzyme systems and therefore may increase blood levels, duration of action, and pharmacologic effects of drugs metabolized by those systems. Tender gynecomastia due to the weak antiandrogenic effect of cimetidine has been reported in patients with the Zollinger-Ellison syndrome requiring and treated with extremely large doses for months to years.

Ranitidine, the second H-2 receptor antagonist made available for use, is prescribed frequently in the treatment of patients with duodenal ulcer. Ranitidine does not share the imidazole ring of histamine but rather is a substituted aminomethylfuran (see Fig. 252-4). On a molar basis, ranitidine is about six times as potent as cimetidine in inhibiting gastric acid secretion. Cimetidine and ranitidine have similar half-lives, approximately 1.5 to 2 h. They both appear to be effective in accelerating healing of duodenal ulcer and in reducing duodenal ulcer recurrence. The initial recommended dose of ranitidine for treatment of duodenal ulcer was 150 mg twice each day; 300 mg at bedtime has been found to be equally effective. The maintenance dose for reducing duodenal ulcer recurrence is 150 mg once a day at bedtime. Ranitidine may increase levels of serum AST and ALT (previously designated SGOT and SGPT). There have been occasional reports of reversible hepatitis with ranitidine administration. It appears to have no antiandrogen properties and exhibits less inhibitory effect on cytochrome P450 mixed oxygenase enzyme systems.

The most recently introduced H-2 receptor antagonists are famotidine and nizatidine. *Famotidine* is an extraordinarily potent H-2 receptor antagonist, being approximately 8 to 10 times as potent as ranitidine in inhibiting gastric acid secretion. Famotidine contains a thiazole ring (see Fig. 252-4). The recommended daily dose of famotidine is 40 mg once daily at bedtime. The maintenance dose for prevention of duodenal ulcer recurrence is 20 mg/d at bedtime. *Nizatidine* is another recently introduced H-2 receptor antagonist and has been shown to be comparable with other agents in this class in the treatment of patients with duodenal ulcer and in reduction of duodenal ulcer recurrence. Nizatidine, similar to famotidine, contains a thiazole ring. The recommended dose for treatment of duodenal ulcer is 300 mg once daily at bedtime. The maintenance dose for reduction of duodenal ulcer recurrence is 150 mg at bedtime. Associated blood dyscrasias have been noted rarely, and hepatotoxicity, similar to that with ranitidine and cimetidine, also has been reported.

Anticholinergic agents   Anticholinergic agents, such as atropine, act by blocking parietal cell muscarinic acetylcholine receptors. These agents decrease gastric acid secretion but are not nearly as effective as H-2 receptor antagonists. They also delay gastric emptying. Most studies have *not* shown that anticholinergic agents hasten healing or improve symptoms of duodenal ulcer; therefore, they are not recommended as primary agents for the treatment of duodenal ulcer. Side effects include dryness of mouth, blurring of vision, cardiac arrhythmias, and urinary retention. They should not be used in patients with glaucoma, impaired gastric emptying, or history or symptoms of urinary retention. There are several classes of muscarinic cholinergic receptors. *Pirenzepine* is a relatively selective anticholinergic agent which is more specific in inhibiting gastric acid secretion with fewer side effects than other anticholinergic agents. Pirenzepine, not yet available for prescribing in the United States, has been reported to be effective in treatment of duodenal ulcer. It may prove useful as primary therapy or as adjunctive therapy in duodenal ulcer patients.

Coating agents   Several drugs that act neither by neutralization nor by inhibition of gastric acid secretion have been used in treatment of duodenal ulcer. Among these is *sucralfate*, a complex polyaluminum hydroxide salt of sucrose sulfate. Sucralfate becomes highly polar at acid pH and binds to the ulcer bed for up to 12 h, whereas relatively little binds to intact gastric or duodenal mucosa. It is believed that adherence of sucralfate to granulation tissue impedes diffusion of H$^+$ to the base of the ulcer. In addition, sucralfate binds bile acids and pepsins and may therefore reduce their injurious effects. Sucralfate may increase endogenous tissue prostaglandins and thereby increase mucosal defense. It is only minimally absorbed, with less than 5 percent appearing in the urine. Sucralfate appears to be similar to antacids and H-2 receptor antagonists in its effectiveness in the treatment of duodenal ulcer and in prevention of duodenal ulcer recurrence. The recommended dose of sucralfate is 1 g 1 h before each meal and at bedtime. *Colloidal bismuth* compounds also aid ulcer healing. They form (in an acid medium) a bismuth-protein coagulant which is believed to protect the ulcer from acid-pepsin digestion. Colloidal bismuth compounds have little acid-neutralizing effect and do not reduce gastric acid secretion. These compounds inhibit pepsin activity, bind to the gastric mucus gel layer, and may prevent diffusion of hydrogen ions. They stimulate gastric mucosal secretion of prostaglandins, bicarbonate, and glycoprotein mucus. Bismuth-containing compounds also may be of value in the treatment of duodenal ulcer because of their effects on *H. pylori*, a bacterium which is responsible for some forms of gastritis (see "Gastritis," below) and which, as noted previously, has been proposed as a potential pathogenetic factor in the etiology of duodenal ulcer. Colloidal bismuth compounds are the only class of antiulcer drugs that eradicate *H. pylori* and the gastritis associated with its colonization. Several duodenal ulcer clinical trials have shown good healing rates of duodenal ulcer in patients treated with colloidal bismuth subcitrate

as well as with various triple-therapy combinations of colloidal bismuth compounds, metronidazole, and other antibiotics, e.g., tetracycline or amoxicillin. In those therapeutic trials, eradication of *H. pylori* was associated with ulcer healing and recolonization with ulcer recurrence. Triple therapy results in 80 to 90 percent *H. pylori* eradication at 1 month. Several studies have shown greatly reduced rates of recurrence of duodenal ulcer following ulcer healing by treatment with colloidal bismuth or colloidal bismuth and antibiotic combinations when compared with treatment with H-2 receptor antagonists. When ulcers recurred, they were associated with gastric recolonization with *H. pylori*.

Prostaglandins   A variety of *prostaglandins*, particularly those of the E series (PGE$_1$ and PGE$_2$), have been shown to be effective in clinical trials in the treatment of duodenal ulcer, with healing rates approximately comparable to those achieved with antacid therapy and H-2 receptor antagonists. Their mechanism of action is believed to be twofold: (1) they reduce basal and stimulated gastric acid secretion, and (2) they enhance mucosal resistance to tissue injury. Exogenous prostaglandins exert the following actions important in enhancing mucosal defense: PGEs (1) stimulate gastric mucus secretion, (2) stimulate gastric and duodenal bicarbonate secretion, (3) maintain or increase gastric mucosal blood flow, (4) maintain the gastric mucosal barrier to back-diffusion of H$^+$, and (5) stimulate mucosal cell restitution. Although comparable with weaker H-2 receptor antagonists in inhibiting gastric acid secretion and in ulcer healing, PGEs are not approved in the United States for treatment of duodenal ulcer. Misoprostol, a PGE$_1$ analogue, is effective in preventing ulcers caused by nonsteroidal anti-inflammatory drugs (NSAIDs).

Proton pump inhibition   The final phase of hydrogen ion secretion by parietal cells is accomplished by an enzyme (H$^+$,K$^+$-ATPase) which serves as a proton pump, exchanging hydrogen for potassium. The H$^+$,K$^+$-ATPase is located in the apical membrane and tubulovesicular apparatus of parietal cells. The luminal surface of the transmembrane enzyme is exposed ot the gastric luminal acid pH. *Omeprazole*, a specific inhibitor of parietal cell H$^+$,K$^+$-ATPase, has been shown to be extraordinarily potent in decreasing gastric acid secretion. Omeprazole, a substituted benzimidazole (Fig. 252-5) binds to the H$^+$,K$^+$-ATPase, irreversibly inactivating the enzyme. Omeprazole, a weak base, is a prodrug that becomes concentrated in an acid environment (below pH 4) generating an active sulfur group which forms a covalent disulfide bond with the H$^+$,K$^+$-ATPase, thereby denaturing and inactivating the enzyme. Omeprazole completely blocks basal and stimulated acid secretion. It produces prolonged inhibition of gastric acid secretion, with acid secretory recovery requiring synthesis of new enzyme. The maximum effect of omeprazole occurs within 2 h, with 50 percent of maximum inhibition at 24 h and the duration of inhibition persisting for up to 72 h. With once-daily dosing a plateau is reached after 4 days, and after discontinuance, gastric acid secretory activity returns gradually over 3 to 5 days.

Omeprazole is approved and effective for treatment of duodenal ulcer, erosive esophagitis, and gastric acid hypersecretory states, including the Zollinger-Ellison syndrome. Omeprazole is recommended for treatment of duodenal ulcer at a dose of 20 mg daily in the morning before breakfast for periods from 4 to 8 weeks.

FIGURE 252-5   Chemical structure of omeprazole, a substituted benzimidazole which inhibits gastric acid secretion by inhibition of H$^+$,K$^+$-ATPase located on the tubovesicular apparatus and apical membranes of parietal cells.

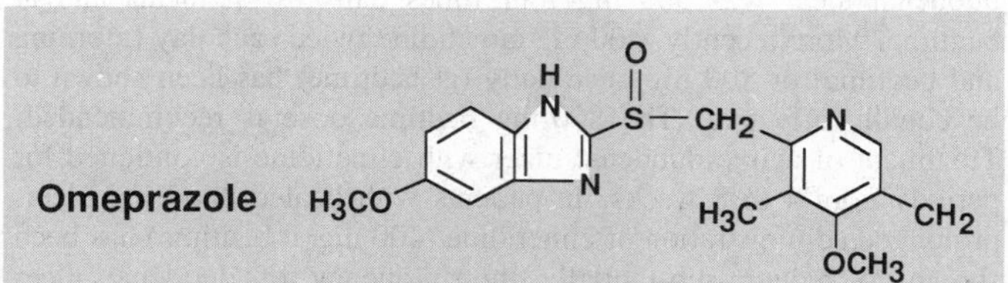

Omeprazole

Omeprazole administration is associated with small to moderate increases in serum gastrin secondary to its effect on gastric acid secretion. Serum gastrin levels return to pretreatment levels within 2 weeks after drug discontinuance. Hyperplasia of gastric mucosal ECL cells and carcinoid tumors due to striking hypergastrinemia in rats receiving omeprazole have not been reported in humans.

DIET   With little or no justification, many different diet programs have been used for treatment of patients with duodenal ulcer. There is no evidence that bland diets reduce gastric acid secretion, promote healing, or relieve symptoms of duodenal ulcer. Similarly, soft diets or diet free of spices or fruit juices have not been proven of benefit. Although traditionally milk and cream were prescribed in the treatment of ulcer patients, there is no evidence that they benefit ulcer healing. They may contribute to development of the milk-alkali syndrome and may accelerate atherogenesis. Many physicians recommend that patients with duodenal ulcer avoid coffee, with or without caffeine, and other caffeine-containing beverages because of their effects on gastric secretion. It also may be desirable to restrict alcohol intake in these patients. It is reasonable to suggest that if patients experience symptoms after ingestion of certain foods, these foods should be avoided.

GENERAL THERAPEUTIC CONSIDERATIONS   How does one integrate the large amount of available information concerning treatment of duodenal ulcer in selecting a therapeutic program for individual patients? There are several reasonable alternatives: Effective therapy may be based on neutralization of gastric acid by antacids, on inhibition of gastric acid secretion by antisecretory agents, or on local actions of some other agents. There is no evidence that combinations of these drugs are required in the treatment of duodenal ulcer. The various classes of agents appear to be comparably effective in accelerating duodenal ulcer healing. In general, although side effects differ from group to group, these are all safe and effective drugs. Most duodenal ulcers will heal within 4 to 6 weeks of treatment with each of these groups of agents. It is seldom necessary to continue treatment of active duodenal ulcer for more than 8 weeks.

There is not yet general agreement concerning which patients should receive prolonged maintenance therapy to reduce the frequency of duodenal ulcer recurrence. Most physicians do not initiate maintenance treatment after the first (uncomplicated) episode of duodenal ulcer activity. Maintenance therapy is often recommended in patients with frequent, especially severe, duodenal ulcer recurrences; in those with previous, especially recurrent, duodenal ulcer complications; and perhaps in those with troublesome ulcer disease and other medical conditions which would make ulcer complications or surgery particularly hazardous. Maintenance therapy, when recommended, is usually continued for at least 1 year. Elimination of cigarette smoking, in most studies, appears to facilitate ulcer healing and may reduce duodenal ulcer recurrence. There is no evidence that dietary manipulation plays an important role in duodenal ulcer treatment.

GASTRIC ULCER

The peak incidence for gastric ulcer is in the sixth decade, approximately 10 years later than for duodenal ulcer. Slightly more than half of gastric ulcers occur in males. Although clinically recognized duodenal ulcer is decreasing, hospitalization for gastric ulcer has stabilized and may be increasing. Gastric ulcers are deep, penetrating beyond the mucosa of the stomach, and are similar histologically to duodenal ulcer, but usually with more extensive gastritis surrounding the ulcer. Almost all benign gastric ulcers are found immediately distal to the junction of the antral mucosa with the acid-secreting mucosa of the body of the stomach. The location of this junction is variable, especially on the lesser gastric curvature. In general, antral mucosa extends approximately two-thirds of the way up the lesser curvature and one-third of the way up the greater curvature of the stomach. Benign gastric ulcers are rare in the fundus of the stomach. Benign gastric ulcers are virtually always accompanied by antral gastritis with variable amounts of mucosal atrophy. Gastritis may be present or absent with gastric ulcers associated with aspirin and other nonsteroidal anti-inflammatory drugs; they are usually located in the antrum, but they are not confined to the junction of the antral and parietal cell mucosa.

ETIOLOGY AND PATHOGENESIS   Acid-pepsin appears to be important in the pathogenesis of gastric ulcer; however, in contrast to duodenal ulcer, gastric ulcer patients generally have acid secretory rates that are normal or reduced compared with nonulcer subjects. True achlorhydria (in response to pentagastrin stimulation) almost never occurs in patients with benign gastric ulcer. Ten to twenty percent of patients with gastric ulcers also have duodenal ulcers. Patients with both duodenal and gastric ulcers tend to have acid secretory patterns that parallel those of duodenal ulcer. Patients with pyloric channel ulcers have acid secretory rates and clinical patterns similar to those found with common duodenal ulcer.

Most evidence supports the primary importance of defective gastric mucosal resistance and/or direct gastric mucosal injury in the pathogenesis of gastric ulcer. Unlike duodenal ulcer, serum gastrin levels are increased in a significant proportion of gastric ulcer patients, but increases are limited to those with gastric acid hyposecretion. Gastric emptying has been shown to be delayed in gastric ulcer. Regurgitation of duodenal contents, especially those containing bile, may induce gastric mucosal injury and subsequent gastric ulceration by interruption of the gastric mucosal barrier with resultant back-diffusion of secreted hydrogen ions. Nonsteroidal anti-inflammatory drugs (NSAIDs) are responsible for a large proportion of gastric ulcers. This is believed to be due primarily to reduced mucosal defense produced by inhibition of synthesis of gastric mucosal prostaglandins.

CLINICAL FEATURES   As with duodenal ulcer, epigastric pain is the most common symptom; however, it is less typical than in patients with duodenal ulcer. Some gastric ulcer patients experience no relief of pain with eating. Pain may actually be precipitated or accentuated by food, and symptom relief with antacids is less consistent than with duodenal ulcers. Gastric ulcers tend to heal but then recur, often in the same location. Recognizable episodes of recurrent gastric ulcer activity are, in general, less frequent than those of duodenal ulcer. The precise incidence of gastric ulcer is not known, since many gastric ulcer patients are asymptomatic. Although duodenal ulcer is identified clinically more frequently than gastric ulcer, most autopsy studies show an equal or greater proportion of gastric ulcers. This may be due in part to acute preterminal events but also may reflect the often asymptomatic clinical course of gastric ulcer. Whereas in duodenal ulcer patients nausea and vomiting almost always indicate gastric outlet obstruction, in patients with gastric ulcer they may occur in the absence of mechanical obstruction. Weight loss may occur due to anorexia or aversion of food due to discomfort produced by eating.

Hemorrhage is a common complication, occurring in approximately 25 percent. Mortality is greater in patients with gastric ulcer than in those with duodenal ulcer. Gastric perforation occurs less frequently than hemorrhage. Mortality with gastric ulcer perforation is approximately three times that with duodenal ulcers. Increased mortality is due in part to the increased age of gastric ulcer patients but also may result from uncertainty and delay in diagnosis and from greater soilage of the peritoneum with gastric ulcer perforation. Gastric outlet obstruction may develop when ulcers are in the pyloric channel or in the most distal antrum but is rare with ulcer in other parts of the stomach.

DIAGNOSIS   The history is of value in suspecting gastric ulcer, but it is not as characteristic as in duodenal ulcer. The two major methods for diagnosis are barium examination and endoscopy. Gastric ulcer usually can be identified by barium examination, with an accuracy approximating 80 percent. NSAID-associated gastric ulcers are frequently more superficial and are less often identified radiographically. Both benign and malignant gastric ulcers are more common on the lesser than on the greater curvature (Fig. 252-6). Radiation of

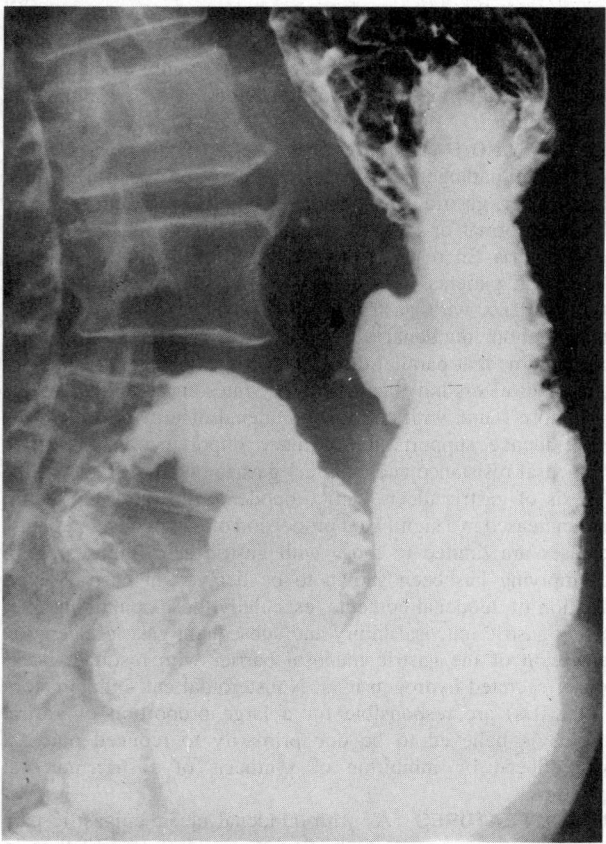

FIGURE 252-6 Benign lesser curvature gastric ulcer. Note ulceration beyond the projected margins of the stomach and the collar of edema.

gastric mucosal folds from the margin of the ulcer crater suggests a benign lesion. Large gastric ulcers, i.e., those greater than 3 cm in diameter, are more often malignant than smaller ones. An ulcer within a mass, as defined radiographically, also suggests malignancy. Approximately 4 percent of gastric ulcers which appear benign radiographically prove to be malignant (by endoscopic biopsy or at surgery). Because of false-positive and false-negative errors, radiographic appearance cannot be used as the sole criterion for the benign or malignant nature of a gastric ulcer.

Endoscopic visualization of the ulcer allows definition of its size, location, and, by biopsy, its histologic characteristics. To exclude malignancy at gastroscopy, a total of at least six biopsies are obtained from the inner margin of the ulcer and from the ulcer bed. If accurate cytology is available, brushings of the ulcer should be obtained prior to biopsy. By application of combined radiographic, endoscopic, and histologic techniques, distinguishing malignant from benign gastric ulcers should be possible with more than 95 percent confidence.

Gastric ulcer with pentagastrin-fast achlorhydria is rare. When it occurs, it almost always indicates gastric carcinoma. However, most patients with gastric carcinoma (about two-thirds to three-fourths) are capable of secreting gastric acid, but usually less than normal.

MEDICAL TREATMENT In general, with whatever medical treatment modality is selected, gastric ulcers tend to heal more slowly than duodenal ulcers, and the healing response rates are somewhat less than those for duodenal ulcer. Larger gastric ulcers take longer to heal than smaller ones. *Antacids* are effective in gastric ulcer treatment. However, since acid hypersecretion is not characteristic of the disease, smaller doses of antacid may be required than for treatment of duodenal ulcer. *H-2 receptor antagonists* and *sucralfate* are approximately as effective as antacid therapy. The dosage schedules for these drugs are similar to those for duodenal ulcer.

Anticholinergic agents have been recommended by some physi-

cians. However, because of substantial side effects of anticholinergic drugs, their tendency to reduce gastric emptying (which is already impaired in these patients), the fact that gastric ulcer patients are often older and therefore more susceptible to the complications of these agents, and the lack of evidence for their benefit, the use of anticholinergic drugs in gastric ulcer treatment does not appear justified. Some studies have suggested that hospitalization and/or cessation of smoking are of benefit in gastric ulcer healing.

Since salicylates and other NSAIDs have been associated with the development of gastric ulcers, patients with gastric ulcer should not ingest these. Alcohol, because of its injurious effects on the gastric mucosa, probably also should be avoided. Milk and cream, as well as bland or homogenized diets, have not been shown to be of value in treatment. In general, it is probably sufficient to recommend that patients consume a diet of their own choice. Since coffee (caffeine-containing or caffeine-free) and other caffeine-containing liquids stimulate gastric acid secretion, it may be desirable to avoid these beverages.

Gastric ulcers are present in approximately 15 percent (10 to 30 percent) of patients receiving chronic NSAID treatment, with a smaller increase in the prevalence of duodenal ulcer. Patients at high risk for ulcer while on NSAIDs include patients of advanced age, females, those on high-dose and protracted-use NSAIDs, those undergoing simultaneous NSAID and glucocorticoid administration, and those with severe intercurrent disease. *Misoprostol*, a PGE_1 analogue, in doses of 100 μg or 200 μg four times a day, has been shown to reduce NSAID-associated gastric ulcer by approximately 75 and 95 percent, respectively. For ulcer prevention in high-risk patients requiring NSAID treatment, misoprostol is administered with gradual increases in dose, beginning at 100 μg/d and increasing, as tolerated, to the full dose of 200 μg four times a day. Gradual increments of 100 μg/d at 1- or 2-week intervals are suggested because of abdominal cramping and/or diarrhea which occasionally may be experienced with abrupt initiation of the full dose.

Carbenoxalone has been used in many countries (though not available in the United States) in the treatment of gastric ulcer. This drug, a hydrolytic product of glycyrrhizic acid (derived from licorice), has been shown to decrease symptoms and increase the rate of gastric ulcer healing. Carbenoxalone, which does not decrease gastric acid secretion, increases the life span of gastric mucosal epithelial cells as well as the secretion and viscosity of gastric mucus. Carbenoxalone possesses aldosterone-like effects, producing sodium and water retention. Its side effects and availability of effective alternatives have led to its decreased use.

Benign gastric ulcers should heal completely within 3 months of vigorous therapy. The failure of gastric ulcer to decrease satisfactorily in size and to heal with medical treatment has been used to suggest gastric malignancy. The following is suggested as one reasonable scheme to monitor gastric ulcer healing. Upper gastrointestinal barium examination or gastroscopy is suggested after 4 weeks of treatment, at which time definite healing of benign gastric ulcers should be demonstrable; i.e., the diameter of most ulcers should be reduced by more than 50 percent. If not, malignancy must be suspected, and endoscopy, exfoliative cytology, and biopsies of the ulcer should be performed. If no malignancy is identified, medical therapy should be continued. If the ulcer has not healed completely at 8 weeks, endoscopic examination should be repeated in another month, at which time most benign gastric ulcers should have healed. Apparently complete healing does not guarantee the benign nature of a gastric ulcer, since approximately 70 percent of gastric ulcers eventually found to be malignant will undergo significant (albeit usually incomplete) healing with medical treatment.

COMPLICATIONS AND SURGERY FOR PEPTIC ULCER

Surgery is reserved for patients with complications of peptic ulcer and for those who do not respond to vigorous and attentive medical treatment. Complications include hemorrhage, obstruction, and perforation.

Hemorrhage occurs in approximately 15 percent of patients with duodenal ulcers; a recurrence of bleeding is estimated to occur in about 40 percent of patients with an initial hemorrhage. Hemorrhage due to NSAID-associated ulcer occurs particularly frequently in the absence of prior peptic ulcer symptoms (approximately 50 percent). In most patients hemorrhage from peptic ulcer responds satisfactorily to medical management, including gastric suction and antacid or H-2 receptor antagonist administration.

Free *perforation* into the peritoneal cavity occurs in approximately 6 percent of patients with duodenal ulcer. Five to ten percent of these patients will have had no recognizable ulcer symptoms prior to perforation. Simultaneous hemorrhage occurs in approximately 10 percent of patients with duodenal ulcer perforation; mortality is greatly increased in this group. Duodenal ulcers, especially those located posteriorly, may penetrate into adjacent structures, most often the pancreas, frequently resulting in increased serum amylase levels. Less commonly, duodenal ulcers penetrate the liver, biliary tract, or colon.

Gastric outlet *obstruction* occurs in 2 to 4 percent of patients admitted to the hospital with duodenal or pyloric channel ulcers. Symptoms include abdominal bloating, nausea, vomiting, and weight loss. These patients usually have had ulcer symptoms for many years and often obstructive symptoms for several months.

Failure to respond satisfactorily to medical treatment requires consideration of surgery. The true incidence of lack of ulcer healing with vigorous medical programs is not known. It is clear that, especially with currently available drugs, the vast majority of patients with peptic ulcer can be treated successfully without surgery.

Decisions regarding surgery for patients with complications of peptic ulcer must be individualized. Risks of surgery must be balanced against risks of the disease. The patient's discomfort, costs of medical care and hospitalization, and time lost from work must be examined in relation to the morbidity and possible mortality associated with surgery and anesthesia, risks of recurrent ulcer, and long-term postoperative sequelae. The skill and experience of the surgeon must be weighed as major factors in considering operation.

SURGERY FOR DUODENAL ULCER   No single surgical procedure has been accepted universally as the most satisfactory duodenal ulcer operation. At present, the most commonly performed surgical procedures are *vagotomy with antrectomy*, *vagotomy with pyloroplasty*, and *parietal cell vagotomy* (also referred to as *proximal gastric* or *superselective vagotomy*) without a gastric drainage procedure.

With truncal vagotomy with antrectomy, the vagal trunks are transected, the antrum is removed, and gastrointestinal continuity is reestablished by anastomosis of the remaining stomach with the proximal duodenum (Billroth I anastomosis) or with a loop of the jejunum (Billroth II anastomosis). Vagotomy with antrectomy is an effective procedure with a low recurrence rate (approximately 1 percent). Morbidity and mortality with vagotomy with antrectomy are variable depending on patient selection and the skill of the surgeon but are probably slightly greater than with vagotomy with pyloroplasty.

When vagotomy with pyloroplasty is selected, pyloroplasty is performed to facilitate gastric drainage after truncal or selective vagotomy. Vagotomy is performed to inhibit vagal stimulation of gastric acid secretion. It does not inhibit gastrin release; in fact, release of gastrin is enhanced after vagal interruption. Three types of vagotomy are now used in the surgical treatment of duodenal or pyloric channel ulcer, namely *truncal vagotomy*, *selective vagotomy*, and *parietal cell vagotomy*. Pyloroplasty with truncal vagotomy is associated with approximately 1 percent mortality. Ulcer recurrence during the 5 years after surgery is about 5 to 8 percent. With selective vagotomy only the branches of the vagus that supply the stomach are transected, preserving the vagal innervation of other abdominal viscera. Selective vagotomy has been found by some surgeons to result in a more complete vagotomy, less ulcer recurrence, and fewer postvagotomy complications than truncal vagotomy. Parietal cell vagotomy denervates only the acid-secreting portion of the stomach,

sparing the branches of the vagus that innervate the antrum, which makes a gastric drainage procedure (e.g., pyloroplasty) unnecessary. Both immediate and late postoperative complications are less common with parietal cell vagotomy than with truncal vagotomy, and reductions in acid secretion are similar to those achieved with truncal or selective vagotomy. Mortality with parietal cell vagotomy is less than 1 percent. Most studies indicate that, with experience, recurrence is comparable to that of other forms of vagotomy with pyloroplasty. This procedure, which is being used with increasing frequency, appears to be a safe and effective surgical therapy.

SURGERY FOR GASTRIC ULCER   Surgical treatment is required for gastric ulcer patients who do not respond satisfactorily to medical therapy or who develop complications similar to those described for duodenal ulcer. With the available diagnostic accuracy of careful radiographic examination, endoscopy, biopsy of the ulcer margins, and exfoliative cytology, it is rarely necessary to operate because of uncertainty regarding the malignant or benign nature of the ulcer. The recommended surgical procedure for the treatment of gastric ulcer is antrectomy with gastroduodenal (Billroth I) anastomosis. It is not necessary to perform a vagotomy when antrectomy is performed for gastric ulcer (not located in the pyloric channel).

CONDITIONS AFTER PEPTIC ULCER SURGERY

Modern surgery for peptic ulcer is effective in the treatment of ulcer complications and in the prevention of ulcer recurrence. However, numerous postoperative sequelae and syndromes may occur.

RECURRENT ULCERATION   Recurrent ulceration has been reported in approximately 5 percent of all patients after surgery for peptic ulcer. Approximately 95 percent of these recurrences follow surgery for duodenal ulcer disease. The risk of recurrent ulcer is 3 to 10 percent after surgery for duodenal ulcer and approximately 2 percent after gastric ulcer surgery. Recurrence is more common after vagotomy with pyloroplasty and after parietal cell vagotomy than after vagotomy with antrectomy. When ulcers occur after partial gastric resection, the ulcer is usually located at the anastomosis (stomal or marginal ulcer) or immediately distal to it in the small intestine. Abdominal pain is the most common symptom in patients with a stomal ulcer. The pain is usually epigastric but is often not characteristic of common duodenal ulcer. It is usually, but not always, relieved by meals or antacids and, in general, tends to be more persistent and progressive than that observed with unoperated duodenal ulcer. Hemorrhage or anemia due to blood loss, nausea and vomiting from obstruction, weight loss, or symptoms from perforation may occur. The development of a stomal ulcer after duodenal ulcer surgery usually indicates that an incomplete vagotomy was performed. Inadequate gastric resection, when performed without vagotomy, also may result in stomal ulceration. Additional causes for recurrent ulcer include an excessively long jejunal afferent loop, an inadvertently performed gastroileal or gastrocolic anastomosis, poor gastric drainage, and ingestion of ulcerogenic drugs (especially NSAIDs). Less commonly, a marginal ulcer may be caused by acid hypersecretion secondary to gastrinoma or a retained antrum.

Radiographic examination with barium is of limited diagnostic value and identifies only from 50 to 60 percent of stomal ulcerations. Surgical deformity at the anastomotic site often may mimic stomal ulcer in its absence or conceal it when present. When suspected, endoscopic examination is required to identify stomal ulceration. Medical treatment with antacids is almost always unsatisfactory in patients with stomal ulcer. H-2 receptor antagonists have been reported to induce healing of stomal ulcers. The long-term effectiveness of these agents on stomal ulcers and prevention of their recurrence remain to be established. Surgery is usually necessary for treatment of ulcer recurrence, and it is usually successful. In patients with ulcer recurrent after surgery, provocative testing with measurement of serum gastrin is needed to identify or exclude gastrinoma (see below).

RECURRENT ULCER DUE TO RETAINED ANTRUM Recurrent ulcers have been described in a small number of patients after antrectomy with gastrojejunostomy (Billroth II anastomosis) in which the antral resection was not complete. In these patients, the distal antrum, inadvertently not resected, remains in continuity with the duodenum after surgery. These patients usually develop or continue to have gastric acid hypersecretion due to gastrin release by the residual antral mucosa which is no longer is contact with gastric acid, the normal inhibitor of gastrin release. Fasting serum gastrin levels in these patients may be normal to moderately increased. Patients with retained antrum can be distinguished from those with gastrinoma by intravenous injection of secretin and measurements of serum gastrin levels. Gastrinoma patients exhibit substantial increases in serum gastrin (>200 pg/mL increase), whereas those with retained antrum exhibit decreased serum gastrin levels, stay the same, or show slight increases after secretin administration. These patients can be treated successfully by surgical removal of the remaining antrum.

AFFERENT LOOP SYNDROMES Patients with partial gastric resection with gastrojejunostomy (Billroth II anastomosis) may experience abdominal bloating and pain 20 min to 1 h after eating, frequently followed by nausea and vomiting. The vomitus often contains large amounts of bile. Characteristically, the bloating and abdominal discomfort are relieved by vomiting. This type of afferent loop syndrome, which is uncommon, is believed to be caused by distention of an incompletely draining afferent intestinal loop by pancreatic and biliary secretions, which are stimulated by eating. Serum amylase levels may be mildly or moderately increased. Because of partial obstruction, it is often difficult to demonstrate the afferent loop by barium meal examination. Treatment is surgical correction of the incomplete afferent loop obstruction and, in some instances, revision to a gastroduodenal anastomosis.

A second form of afferent loop dysfunction is that due to stasis with bacterial overgrowth within the afferent loop. These patients may exhibit the same characteristics as those found with other forms of small intestinal bacterial overgrowth or blind loop syndromes (see Chap. 254) e.g., malabsorption, especially of fat and vitamin B_{12}. Correction of the afferent loop bacterial overgrowth syndrome can be accomplished by surgical revision of the afferent loop.

BILE REFLUX GASTRITIS After peptic ulcer surgery, a small proportion of patients experience early satiety, abdominal discomfort, and vomiting, which is believed due to reflux of duodenal contents into the stomach. Endoscopic examination usually reveals regurgitated bile in the stomach and diffuse gastritis, often involving the entire gastric remnant. Various terms assigned to this entity include *alkaline reflux gastritis*, *bile reflux gastritis*, *duodenogastric reflux*, and *bilious vomiting*. The mechanisms or materials contained in the refluxed intestinal contents accounting for these symptoms have not been defined. Although the term *bile reflux gastritis* has been used, there is no certainty that regurgitated bile is responsible for the syndrome. Administration of cholestyramine, intended to bind bile acids and facilitate their excretion, has not been proven of benefit in this disorder. Some surgeons have reported successful treatment of bile reflux gastritis by diversion of duodenal contents from proximity to the stomach with a roux-en-Y anastomosis.

DUMPING SYNDROME Following peptic ulcer surgery, some patients experience an assortment of vasomotor symptoms after eating. These include palpitation, tachycardia, light-headedness, diaphoresis, and, less frequently, postural hypotension. Abdominal discomfort and vomiting also may occur. The vasomotor symptoms, referred to as the *early dumping syndrome*, are usually experienced within 30 min after eating and are believed to result from rapid emptying of hyperosmolar gastric contents into the proximal small intestine. This leads to a shift of fluid into the gut lumen and produces intestinal distention and contraction of plasma volume. Additional proposed mechanisms for these symptoms include stimulation of autonomic reflexes secondary to small intestinal distention and/or release of hormones from the gut in response to rapid entry of gastric contents into the duodenum or jejunum.

The *late dumping syndrome* refers to a symptom complex comprising dizziness, light-headedness, palpitation, diaphoresis, confusion, and, in rare instances, syncope occurring 90 min to 3 h after eating. The symptoms can often be precipitated by meals rich in simple carbohydrates, especially sucrose. The syndrome appears to be caused by hypoglycemia due to insulin release stimulated by abrupt increases in blood glucose secondary to rapid emptying of sugar-containing meals into the proximal small intestine.

Both forms of the dumping syndrome are treated by dietary measures. These include limitation of simple sugar-continuing liquids and solids (sweets), elimination of liquids at mealtime, and frequent small meals. Most patients have not been benefited from surgical procedures such as creation of reversed jejunal loops and isoperistaltic jejunal interposition.

POSTVAGOTOMY DIARRHEA A significant number of patients experience diarrhea after peptic ulcer surgery, especially with procedures including truncal vagotomy. Diarrhea has been estimated to occur in 20 to 30 percent of patients after truncal vagotomy with drainage, in 10 to 20 percent with selective vagotomy and drainage, and in only 1 to 8 percent of those with parietal cell vagotomy (without drainage). Diarrhea usually occurs within 2 h of eating. Although the mechanism is not clear, interruption of vagal fibers to the abdominal viscera appears important in production of the diarrhea. The surgical drainage procedure, pyloroplasty or antrectomy, removes the pyloric regulatory emptying mechanism. Rapid emptying of gastric contents into the small intestine, resulting in increased fluid volume within the intestinal lumen due to the osmotic action of the meal, also may contribute to the diarrhea.

HEMATOLOGIC COMPLICATIONS Intrinsic factor secreted by gastric parietal cells is necessary for active absorption of vitamin B_{12} by the distal ileum. Patients after total gastrectomy invariably develop malabsorption of vitamin B_{12} and should receive monthly intramuscular injections of vitamin B_{12} (50 to 100 μg) indefinitely. Megaloblastic anemia due to vitamin B_{12} deficiency is rare after partial gastric resection; however, reduced serum vitamin B_{12} levels have been observed in about 14 percent of these patients. Even more rarely, vitamin B_{12} deficiency may be produced by bacterial overgrowth in a stagnant afferent loop following Billroth II anastomosis. Gastritis in the remaining stomach develops in more than 60 percent of duodenal ulcer patients after vagotomy with antrectomy or vagotomy with pyloroplasty. This may result in decreased vitamin B_{12} absorption. Inasmuch as the stomach secretes intrinsic factor approximately 100 times in excess of need, peptic ulcer patients treated with partial gastric resection do not develop vitamin B_{12} deficiency secondary to the amount of stomach resected. (In addition, the resected portion of the stomach is almost always principally antrum, which contains few parietal cells.) However, after peptic ulcer surgery, patients may develop decreased serum vitamin B_{12} levels as a result of reduced absorption of food-bound vitamin B_{12}; these patients will often have normal absorption of free vitamin B_{12}, as used in the Schilling test. The precise mechanism of the malabsorption of food-bound vitamin B_{12} is not known. It may be due in part to rapid emptying of gastric contents, with reduced efficiency of intrinsic factor binding of vitamin B_{12}. Anemia after peptic ulcer surgery also may result from deficiency produced by malabsorption of iron or folate. A combined deficiency of vitamin B_{12}, iron, and folate is common in patients with anemia following partial or subtotal gastric resection. Iron deficiency is the most common single hematologic defect after peptic ulcer surgery and may result from either blood loss (e.g., with persistent or recurrent ulcers) or iron malabsorption. Patients with gastric resection who malabsorb dietary iron have normal absorption of iron salts; therefore, they will respond favorable to treatment with therapeutic oral iron preparations. Folate deficiency may result from either reduced dietary intake or impaired folate absorption. Except for anemia from blood loss caused by early recurrent ulcer, development of anemia after peptic ulcer surgery is gradual, usually occurring over several years.

The nature of the anemia after ulcer surgery should be clarified by determination of the red blood cell morphology and by measurements of serum iron, folate, and vitamin B_{12}. Iron or folate deficiency should be treated by oral replacement. Vitamin B_{12} deficiency should be treated with monthly intramuscular injections of the vitamin.

OSTEOMALACIA AND OSTEOPOROSIS Osteoporosis and osteomalacia are common after partial or complete gastrectomy but occur rarely after vagotomy with pyloroplasty. Osteomalacia is extremely frequent following gastrojejunostomy or Billroth II anastomosis. These bone changes are believed to result from malabsorption of calcium and vitamin D. Patients may develop bone pain and have pathologic fractures. The incidence of bone fractures in men following gastric resection has been estimated to be almost twice that of control subjects of similar age. Reduced bone density identified by x-ray requires years to develop. Patients with osteomalacia usually have increased levels of serum alkaline phosphatase and may have reduced serum calcium concentrations. These patients should be treated by supplemental oral vitamin D and calcium. The frequency of osteoporosis and osteomalacia after partial or complete gastrectomy is sufficiently great to justify treatment with vitamin D and calcium indefinitely, especially in females, following gastric resection.

GENERAL MALABSORPTION (See also Chap. 254) Mild, chemically demonstable steatorrhea is common in patients after ulcer surgery. Weight loss is more common after partial gastric resection (approximately 60 percent of patients) than with vagotomy without resection. The major cause of weight loss is reduced food intake. On a 100-g fat diet, loss of stool fat seldom exceeds 15 g/d (normal individuals less than 7 g/d). The causes of maldigestion and malabsorption after peptic ulcer surgery include rapid gastric emptying, reduced dispersion of food in the stomach, reduced bile concentrations in the gut lumen, increased rate of transit of the meal through the small intestine, and reduced or delayed pancreatic secretory responses to feeding. Steatorrhea and weight loss, sometimes accompanied by vitamin B_{12} malabsorption, may develop as a result of bacterial overgrowth, especially in patients with afferent loop bacterial stasis. Overt symptoms and other manifestations of malabsorption appearing after surgery for peptic ulcer also may be due to other preexisting conditions, including latent celiac sprue and chronic pancreatitis.

CARCINOMA AFTER PARTIAL GASTRECTOMY Several studies have documented an increased incidence of adenocarcinoma of the stomach in duodenal ulcer patients following partial gastric resection and after vagotomy and drainage without resection. This usually develops 10 or more years after ulcer surgery. The possibility of carcinoma of the stomach should be considered when abdominal symptoms, which may be similar to or distinct from those due to the original ulcer, appear many years after apparently successful surgery.

ZOLLINGER-ELLISON SYNDROME (GASTRINOMA)

In 1955, Zollinger and Ellison described the syndrome that bears their names, which consists of ulcer disease of the upper gastrointestinal tract, marked increases in gastric acid secretion, and non-beta islet cell tumors of the pancreas.

ETIOLOGY AND PATHOGENESIS Zollinger and Ellison, in their original description of the syndrome, suggested that the ulcer disease in these patients resulted from release of a secretagogue from these tumors into the circulation which accounted for the often enormously increased rates of gastric acid secretion. Their proposal proved correct when in 1960 extracts of Zollinger-Ellison (Z-E) tumors were shown to stimulate gastric acid secretion. Subsequently, it was found that these pancreatic islet cell tumors contained gastrin and that there were large amounts of this hormone in the circulation producing the pathophysiologic characteristics of the syndrome. These gastrin-containing tumors are therefore now called *gastrinomas*.

Gastrinomas have been reported most often within the pancreas. Pancreatic gastrinomas may vary in size from 1 mm to more than 20 cm in diameter. Multiple primary tumors are common. From one-half to two-thirds of patients have multiple gastrinomas. Pancreatic gastrinomas are most common in the head of the pancreas. In more

than half of Zollinger-Ellison patients harboring gastrinomas the tumors cannot be identified at surgery. There is recent evidence that with careful search when gastrinomas are located they are found as frequently (or perhaps more frequently) in the wall of the duodenum as in the pancreas. Duodenal gastrinomas, approximately 50 percent of which are solitary, are usually found in the submucosa of the first or second parts of the duodenum. Gastrinomas also have been located less commonly in other sites, including the hilum of the spleen and rarely in the stomach. Gastrinomas have been found in lymph nodes in proximity to the pancreas, proximal duodenum, and spleen in the absence of demonstrated primary tumors. These probably represent local metastases from undiscovered duodenal wall gastrinomas. Approximately 90 percent of gastrinomas are found within an anatomic triangle (the gastrinoma triangle) which is comprised of the junction of the cystic and common bile ducts superiorly, the junction of the second and third portions of the duodenum inferiorly, and the junction of the pancreatic body and neck medially. In unusual instances, the Z-E syndrome has resulted from gastrinomas originating from remote organs, e.g., parathyroid and ovarian tumors. About two-thirds of gastrinomas are histologically or biologically malignant. Malignant gastrinomas usually grow slowly; however, a small portion may be rapidly invasive and may metastasize early and widely. Metastasis is most often to regional lymph nodes and liver; spread also may be to peritoneal surfaces, spleen, bone, skin, or mediastinum. Gastrinomas have light-microscopic similarities to carcinoid tumors and may be mistaken for these tumors, especially when gastrinomas arise from the mucosa of the small intestine or stomach. Pancreatic islet cell hyperplasia occurs in approximately 10 percent of patients with the Z-E syndrome. Hyperplasia of the islets, accompanying recognized or unidentified gastrinoma, appears to be an association or a consequence, rather than a cause, of excess gastrin release, since gastrin is not present in the hyperplastic tissue.

In an estimated 20 to 60 percent of patients with the Z-E syndrome the gastrinoma is a component of the multiple endocrine neoplasia type 1 (MEN 1) syndrome, an autosomal dominant disorder with a high degree of penetrance and great variability in expressivity. The MEN 1 locus is on chrosomome 11. Patients with MEN 1 may have clinically recognized hyperplasia, adenomas, or carcinoma involving, in order of frequency, the parathyroid glands, pancreatic islets, and pituitary. Hyperparathyroidism has been reported in 87 percent of patients with MEN 1 syndrome, and gastrinoma has been reported in approximately half of them (see Chap. 343). However, there is accumulating evidence that when carefully sought for there is probably involvement of all three organs in all patients with MEN 1, although it is frequently without overt clinical expression. Gastrinomas in non-MEN 1 patients are considered to be sporadic. Multiple gastrinomas are usually present in patients with MEN 1 and are usually smaller than sporadic gastrinomas. Gastrinomas with MEN 1 are located more frequently in the wall of the duodenum than in the pancreas. Patients, including those with duodenal gastrinomas, usually have multiple pancreatic islet cell tumors, most of which are not gastrinomas.

In most gastrinomas, approximately 80 to 95 percent of gastrin is in the form of heptadecapeptide gastrin (G-17), with most of the remainder being G-34. In contrast, approximately two-thirds of circulating gastrin in gastrinoma patients is G-34; most of the remainder is G-17. However, smaller amounts of even larger forms of gastrin and smaller gastrin fragments can be detected in the serum. When examined carefully, almost all gastrin-secreting islet cell tumors are found to contain multiple hormones that are usually clinically silent. These have included, among others, ACTH, glucagon, melanocyte-stimulating hormone, parathyroid hormone, growth hormone releasing factor (GRF), insulin, pancreatic polypeptide, and vasoactive intestinal peptide. Of these, ACTH is the most common; it is found in approximately 30 percent of gastrinomas. Cushing's syndrome with increased serum ACTH levels has been reported in 8 percent of 75 Z-E patients. ACTH-releasing gastrinomas are often aggressively malignant. In contrast, ACTH may be released by pituitary tumors in patients with MEN 1, in whom symptoms of Cushing's syndrome are generally mild and gastrinomas are usually not metastatic. Approximately one-third of patients with gastrinomas have increases in serum concentrations of *pancreatic polypeptide*.

The parietal cell mass is substantially expanded to from three to six times normal secondary to the trophic effects of circulating gastrin on parietal cells. Small, multicentric, noninvasive carcinoid tumors have been identified in the gastric mucosa of patients with the Z-E syndrome. These tumors and associated focal areas of enterochrom-affin-like (ECL) cell hyperplasia are believed to result from substantial and sustained hypergastrinemia. They also have been found in the gastric mucosa of patients with pernicious anemia and achlorhydria, who have striking increases in serum gastrin in the range of those found with gastrinoma.

While the true incidence of the Z-E syndrome is not known, estimates are that it accounts for 0.1 to 1 percent of peptic ulcers. The Z-E syndrome may occur at any age, but initial manifestations occur most commonly between the ages 30 and 60.

CLINICAL FEATURES   From 90 to 95 percent of patients with gastrinomas develop ulceration of the gastrointestinal tract at some point during the course of their disease. Profound gastric acid hypersecretion is found in most, but not all, patients. Especially early in the course of the disease, symptoms are usually similar to those of patients with typical peptic ulcer. However, ulcer symptoms may be more fulminant, progressive, and persistent and, in general, respond poorly to usual medical and surgical peptic ulcer treatment programs. The anatomic site of the ulcers in patients with gastrinoma is similar, but not identical, to that of patients with common types of peptic ulcer. About 75 percent of gastrinoma patients have ulcers in the first portion of the duodenum or in the stomach; these are usually single but may be multiple. When multiple ulcers occur, they are frequently located not only in the first portion of the duodenum, the site of common duodenal ulcer, but also in the remainder of the duodenum or even the jejunum. In one large series, 14 percent of the ulcers were in the duodenum beyond its first portion and 11 percent in the jejunum.

Diarrhea occurs in about 40 percent of patients, and about 7 percent of patients with gastrinoma have diarrhea in the absence of ulcer disease. The diarrhea is due to the outpouring of large amounts of hydrochloric acid into the proximal duodenum and can be reduced or eliminated by aspiration of gastric juice. The excessive acid has been shown to reduce the pH of the contents of the proximal and distal jejunum to as low as 1 and 3.6, respectively. Inflammatory changes may be produced in the mucosa of the small intestine secondary to the injurious effect of large amounts of acid and pepsin. Steatorrhea, which is less common than diarrhea, results from inactivation of pancreatic lipase by large concentrations of acid in the proximal small intestine and from decreases in luminal bile acids. The decrease in intraluminal bile acid concentration is caused by precipitation of the major bile acids at low pH. This leads to impaired micelle formation, which, in turn, reduces intestinal absorption of fatty acids and monoglycerides (see Chap. 254). Vitamin B_{12} malabsorption, not correctable by addition of intrinsic factor, has been detected in some patients with the Z-E syndrome. Although gastric secretion of intrinsic factor appears normal, the reduced pH within the gut interferes with intrinsic factor–mediated vitamin B_{12} absorption. This can be corrected by neutralization of the intestinal contents. The mechanisms by which low pH in the gut interferes with intrinsic factor action is not known.

DIAGNOSIS   The presence of gastrinoma should be suspected in patients with a compatible clinical history, especially in those with marked acid hypersecretion. More than 90 percent of gastrinoma patients have basal gastric acid outputs (BAO) that exceed 15 mmol/h. In some instances, the basal output may be greater than 150 mmol/h. However, there is substantial overlap in rates of gastric acid secretion among patients with gastrinoma, those with duodenal ulcer, and normal subjects. Gastrinoma patients often have BAO rates that are greater than 60 percent of those induced by maximal stimulation (MAO). In most normal subjects and duodenal ulcer patients, basal

acid secretory rates are less than 60 percent of maximal secretion. However, because of frequent exceptions in patients with gastrinomas and common duodenal ulcers, the use of the BAO/MAO ratio is of no value in the certain identification of patients with gastrinoma.

Some radiographic features may suggest the diagnosis of the Z-E syndrome. Large mucosal folds may be demonstrated most prominently in the stomach but also in the duodenum and, in some instances, the jejunum. The lumen of the stomach and small intestine often contains large amounts of fluid. Radiographic features of most ulcers in these patients, except when they are distal in location, are similar to those of common peptic ulcer. Gastrinomas are difficult to localize. In almost half of patients with clinical and laboratory evidence, the tumors cannot be identified at surgery. Selective arteriography identifies gastrinomas in approximately one-third of patients with clinical and biochemical evidence of the Z-E syndrome. Computed tomography (CT) identifies gastrinomas in 30 percent and ultrasound in 15 percent of patients with the Z-E syndrome. Use of both selective arteriography and CT has been reported to identify 44 percent of gastrinomas in Z-E patients and 80 percent of those located at surgery. Endoscopic retrograde pancreaticoduodenography has not proved to be of assistance in the diagnosis or exclusion of pancreatic gastrinomas. A small number of duodenal wall gastrinomas have been identified and confirmed histologically by duodenoscopy.

The diagnosis in a patient with clinical features consistent with the Z-E syndrome depends on the demonstration of *increased serum gastrin levels* by radioimmunoassay. Fasting serum gastrin levels in normal subjects and patients with typical duodenal ulcer average approximately 20 to 50 pg/mL and usually do not exceed 150 pg/mL. Patients with gastrinoma almost always have fasting serum gastrin levels that are greater than 200 pg/mL and have been found as high as 450,000 pg/mL. Approximately half these patients have fasting serum gastrin levels that are less than 1000 pg/mL (an approximate mean value for serum gastrin for patients with gastrinoma).

Several provocative tests have been used to evaluate patients with possible gastrinoma, especially those who do not exhibit pronounced hypergastrinemia (i.e., serum gastrin > 1000 pg/mL). These tests utilize measurements of serum gastrin levels in response to intravenous secretin injection, calcium infusion, or ingestion of a standard test meal.

In the *secretin injection test*, secretin (Kabi secretin, 2 units per kilogram) is given intravenously over 30 to 60 s. Gastrin is measured in serum samples obtained immediately before injection of secretin, at 2 and 5 min after secretin, and at 5-min intervals thereafter for a total of 30 min. In normal individuals and patients with common duodenal ulcer, secretin produces no change, small reductions, or small increases in serum gastrin levels. In contrast, in gastrinoma patients, intravenous secretin induces substantial increases in serum gastrin. The serum gastrin levels increase promptly by at least 200 pg/mL, usually at 5 min (and virtually always by 10 min), and then gradually decrease toward or to preinjection levels by 30 min. In the *calcium infusion test*, serum samples for gastrin measurements are obtained before and at 30-min intervals for 4 h after initiation of a constant 3-h intravenous infusion of calcium gluconate (5 mg calcium per kilogram per hour). In gastrinoma patients, serum gastrin concentrations usually increase above the basal serum gastrin level by more than 400 pg/mL. The third provocative test involves the *feeding of a standard meal*: Gastrin is measured in serum samples obtained before the meal and at 15-min intervals after it for 90 min. This test has been used to attempt to distinguish between patients with gastrinoma and those with hypergastrinemia and gastric acid hypersecretion due to antral gastrin cell hypertrophy or hyperplasia.

The secretin injection test is by far the most valuable provocative test in identifying gastrinoma patients. Positive serum gastrin responses to intravenous secretin are found in more than 95 percent of patients with gastrinoma. Using the criteria suggested, substantial increases in serum gastrin following secretin injection have been detected only rarely in nongastrinoma patients. Reduced gastric acid secretion, achlorhydria or profound hypochlorhydria, is by far the most common cause of hypergastrinemia. For this reason, gastric acid secretion should be measured before consideration of the secretin injection test. Exaggerated release of gastrin in response to calcium infusion is found in more than 80 percent of gastrinoma patients; however, this exaggerated response to calcium infusion occurs in some nongastrinoma patients with hypergastrinemia (e.g., with achlorhydria). Enhanced gastrin release with calcium infusion is rarely observed in gastrinoma patients in the absence of the abnormally large gastrin release in response to secretin. Since the calcium infusion test does not add significantly to the sensitivity or specificity of the secretin injection test, and since calcium infusion is potentially more hazardous, it is usually not necessary or recommended.

In a very small proportion of duodenal ulcer patients (much less than 1 percent), gastric acid hypersecretion may be accompanied by increased serum gastrin levels due to hyperfunction and/or hyperplasia of antral gastrin cells (G cells). These patients can be distinguished from those with gastrinoma by the secretin injection and meal stimulation tests. In patients with this antral gastrin cell abnormality, intravenous secretin does not produce large increases in serum gastrin characteristic of gastrinoma. Some authors have reported increases in serum gastrin concentrations greater than 200 percent after test meals in patients with gastrin cell hypertrophy or hyperplasia, suggesting that this may be of value distinguishing these patients from those with gastrinoma. Other authors more recently have found similarly large amounts of gastrin released into the sera of patients with gastrinomas, suggesting that the meal-stimulated test is of limited value in distinguishing between patients with antral gastrin cell hyperplasia and those with gastrinoma.

TREATMENT In general, patients with Z-E syndrome are resistant to those medical therapies and surgical procedures designed for and usually effective in treating common peptic ulcer. Antacids may produce transient symptom relief but rarely, if ever, induce ulcer healing or sustained relief of symptoms. Incomplete gastric resection (with or without vagotomy) or pyloroplasty with vagotomy is frequently followed by prompt and often fulminant ulcer recurrence. In the past, many patients with gastrinoma had multiple surgical procedures, particularly in those instances in which the diagnosis was not established initially. Mortality was reported to be lowest in patients with the Z-E syndrome in whom gastrectomy was the initial gastric surgery. This led to the conclusion that when surgery was required in gastrinoma patients, total gastrectomy was the surgical procedure of choice.

Development of effective drugs to reduce acid secretion and more precise diagnostic techniques to locate gastrinomas have increased substantially the therapeutic options. The key to management in these patients is individualization of treatment, since patients with the Z-E syndrome are highly heterogeneous with respect to clinical manifestations and extent of disease. As with many other predominantly malignant tumors, the ideal treatment is removal of the gastrinoma.

H-2 receptor antagonists are effective in reducing gastric acid secretion, producing symptom relief, and inducing ulcer healing in patients with the Z-E syndrome. *Cimetidine* was the first H-2 receptor antagonist used successfully in the treatment of these patients. Improvement in clinical symptoms, decreases in gastric acid output, and ulcer healing were found in 80 to 85 percent. Administration of cimetidine was required at 4- to 6-h intervals, with total daily doses usually four to eight times those used in the treatment of common duodenal ulcer. More recently, *ranitidine, famotidine,* and *nizatidine* also have been shown effective in treatment of patients with the Z-E syndrome. These H-2 receptor antagonists require comparable increases in dosage when compared with doses used in treatment of common duodenal ulcer. When instituted, H-2 receptor antagonist therapy must be continued indefinitely, since even temporary discontinuance is usually followed by ulcer recurrence. Ulcers fail to respond or recur while on treatment with H-2 receptor antagonists in approximately 25 percent of patients with the Z-E syndrome. The dose of H-2 receptor antagonist required to maintain a satisfactory

reduction in gastric acid secretion can be assessed by measuring the basal gastric acid output during the hour immmediately prior to the next anticipated dose of the drug; the goal is to reduce gastric acid output to less than 10 mmol/h at that time.

Omeprazole, the parietal cell H^+,K^+-ATPase inhibitor, is the most effective drug and agent of choice in reducing gastric acid secretion and in healing ulcer in Z-E patients, including those with ulcers resistant to treatment with H-2 receptor antagonists. As a function of potency and dosage, the effectiveness of omeprazole can be prolonged and sustained. The usual initial daily recommended dose of omeprazole is 60 mg in a single dose administered in the morning before breakfast. The dose is adjusted to maintain gastric acid secretion to less than 10 mmol/h during the hour immediately before the next dose is due. Twice a day dosing is recommended if the patient requires 100 mg or more omeprazole per day. Some Z-E patients, in whom gastrinomas could not be identified or removed surgically, have been treated with parietal cell vagotomy, which has reduced or, in a few instances, eliminated the dose of H-2 receptor antagonist required in these patients.

Treatment for patients with the Z-E syndrome should be individualized. In selecting the best therapy, the biologic behavior of the tumor and the clinical manifestations in each patient must be taken into consideration. Early studies indicated that morbidity and mortality in patients with the Z-E syndrome were due principally to complications of severe ulcer disease. However, with earlier diagnosis, effective antiulcer treatment, and longer follow-up, more frequent consequences of the malignant properties of gastrinoma are now recognized. Approximately 50 percent of patients with the Z-E syndrome in whom the gastrinoma has not been removed will die from malignant invasion by the tumor. Complete *surgical resection of the tumors*, when possible, represents *optimal treatment in patients with gastrinoma*. Complete surgical removal of gastrinoma, with cure, has been achieved in approximately 25 percent of patients with the Z-E syndrome. Successful resection of tumor in Z-E patients with sporadic gastrinoma or with gastrinoma with MEN I requires thorough abdominal exploration and recognition and removal of multiple gastrinomas when found, including those in the wall of the duodenum and other extrapancreatic sites. Gastrinoma in lymph nodes and metastatic to the liver should be removed when safe and possible.

Treatment with omeprazole is indicated in the period during which the diagnosis is being established, while the location and extent of the tumor are being determined, and also as treatment prior to anticipated surgery. At present, omeprazole is certainly indicated for patients who are unsatisfactory candidates for surgery, in those who refuse surgery, and in those in whom surgical removal of the tumor is not possible. Patients with aggressively invasive gastrinoma have been treated with streptozotocin and 5-fluorouracil, in some instances combined with doxorubicin, in attempts to reduce tumor bulk and associated symptoms. Success with chemotherapy is limited, with only an initial response of approximately 40 percent and no complete responses. When metastatic and/or otherwise nonresectable gastrinoma is present, control of the ulcer disease may be achieved in most instances by treatment with omeprazole or, rarely, when required, by total gastric resection. There is no convincing evidence that tumor progression is usually influenced by gastrectomy.

STRESS ULCERS AND EROSIONS

A number of acute ulcerative lesions of the gastrointestinal tract are distinct clinically from chronic peptic ulcer. Among these are the acute upper gastrointestinal erosions and ulcers often observed in patients with shock, massive burns, sepsis, and severe trauma. These are often referred to as *stress erosions* and *ulcers*. These lesions, which are frequently multiple, are most common in the acid-secreting portion of the stomach, but they also may occur in the antrum and duodenum.

These erosions and superficial ulcers are extremely frequent and occur in about 80 to 90 percent of patients with massive injuries and burns. The most common clinical finding in these patients is painless gastrointestinal hemorrhage. Blood loss is usually minimal but may be substantial and life-threatening. Erosions develop most frequently approximately 24 h after trauma. Small amounts of blood loss may be detected in the first 24 to 48 h after trauma. However, when massive hemorrhage occurs, it is usually more than 2 or 3 days after the acute insult. Acute stress ulcers and erosions should be suspected when there is evidence of upper gastrointestinal bleeding in patients with severe injuries, burns, infections, and/or shock. The diagnosis is best established by upper gastrointestinal endoscopy. Erosions are usually too superficial to be recognized by barium examination of the upper gastrointestinal tract.

Many theories have been proposed to explain stress-associated acute mucosal ulceration. Mucosal ischemia and tissue injury from gastric acid appear to be important in their production. There is usually no evidence of acid hypersecretion; however, the lesions cannot be produced in experimental animals in the absence of acid. Most evidence supports the conclusion that ischemia of the gastric mucosa, which has enormous oxygen requirements, is the most important element in producing stress erosions and ulceration.

Treatment of acute stress ulcerations and erosions is principally preventive. In high-risk patients, the frequency of stress ulcerations can be diminished by vigorous use of antacids or H-2 receptor antagonists. When medical therapy fails to arrest bleeding, surgical approaches have included pyloroplasty with vagotomy and total gastrectomy.

The term *Cushing's ulcer* has been applied to acute ulcer of the upper gastrointestinal tract associated with intracranial injury or increases in intracranial pressure, e.g., with brain tumors or subdural hematoma. These ulcers may involve the stomach, proximal duodenum, or esophagus and frequently lead to hemorrhage or perforation. They do not differ histologically from acute stress ulceration. However, unlike stress ulcers, Cushing's ulcers are frequently associated with gastric acid hypersecretion. Treatment includes correction of increased intracranial pressure, when possible, and the usual measures for treatment of acute erosions and ulcerations, including vigorous therapy with antacids or H-2 receptor antagonists.

DRUG-ASSOCIATED ULCERS AND EROSIONS

Gastric and duodenal ulcers have been described following administration of many drugs. Aspirin is associated with an increased incidence of gastric ulcer and, to a lesser extent, duodenal ulcer and is a frequent cause of hemorrhagic erosive gastritis. Gastric mucosal injury, similar to that produced by aspirin, also has been observed in patients treated with a variety of other NSAIDs (e.g., indomethacin, ibuprofen, naproxen, tolmetin, sulindac, piroxicam, diflunisal, fenoprofen, and others). Several mechanisms by which salicylates and other NSAIDs induce gastric ulcer and erosions have been proposed. Aspirin and other NSAIDs are directly toxic to the gastric mucosa, and they deplete protective endogenous mucosal prostaglandins by inhibiting prostaglandin synthesis (see "Gastritis," below). Aspirin and other NSAIDs may contribute to development of gastric ulcer by interruption of the gastric mucosal barrier, permitting back-diffusion of hydrogen ions that may injure the gastric mucosa. They reduce gastric mucus secretion and gastric and duodenal bicarbonate secretion and may increase gastric acid secretion. Depletion of mucosal prostaglandins also impairs epithelial cell reconstitution after injury.

Administration of glucocorticoids has been reported and is commonly assumed to be associated with ulcer disease of the upper gastrointestinal tract. The association is controversial, supported by some data and rejected by other data.

GASTRITIS

Gastritis is *inflammation of the gastric mucosa*. Gastritis is not a single disease. Rather, it is a group of disorders that have inflammatory

changes in the gastric mucosa in common but that have different clinical features, histologic characteristics, and pathogeneses. Several classifications have been used for consideration of gastritis. In general, these classifications have been based on (1) the acuteness or chronicity of the clinical manifestations, (2) the histologic features characterizing the gastritis, (3) the anatomic distribution of the gastritis, or, in some instances, (4) the proposed pathogenesis of each of the two principal varieties of chronic gastritis. Based on the *clinical features* of the gastritis, the two principal forms, which constitute very different clinical entities, are *acute gastritis* and *chronic gastritis*. Different types of chronic gastritis exhibit histologic features which permit their classification according to the presence or absence of mucosal atrophy associated with the gastritis and the anatomic distribution of the gastritis or atrophy in the gastric mucosa.

In this section the major clinical forms of acute gastritis and chronic gastritis will be addressed, including reference to the histologic features of the major forms of gastritis. Attention also will be directed to additional specific forms of gastritis.

ACUTE GASTRITIS A principal, and certainly the most dramatic, form of acute gastritis is *acute hemorrhagic gastritis*, which is also referred to as *acute erosive gastritis*. These terms reflect the bleeding from the gastric mucosa almost invariably found in this form of gastritis and the characteristic loss of integrity of the gastric mucosa (erosion) that accompanies the inflammatory lesion. Gross examination in hemorrhagic gastritis shows edema, mucosal friability, erosions, and sites of bleeding with extravasation of blood into the mucosa and the lumen of the stomach. Gastric erosions and sites of hemorrhage may be distributed diffusely throughout the gastric mucosa or localized to the body or antrum of the stomach. They are often placed linearly on the crests of the gastric folds.

Histologic examination of the gastric mucosa reveals infiltration of the lamina propria with mononuclear cells and polymorphonuclear leukocytes with extravasation of blood in the mucosa, distorting the glandular structures. Proteinaceous exudate containing polymorphonuclear leukocytes may be present in gastric glands. Gastric erosions, by definition, are limited to the mucosa and do not extend beneath the muscularis mucosa. Acute erosive gastritis may accompany deeper, more focal lesions, which represent acute ulcers and may extend to and through all layers of the gastric wall.

Etiology and pathogenesis Acute erosive gastritis may develop without apparent explanation but is more likely to occur in several specific clinical circumstances. Erosive gastritis is usually associated with serious illness or with various drugs. Erosive gastritis has been estimated to occur in up to 80 to 90 percent of critically ill hospitalized patients. It is found most often in patients in medical or surgical intensive care units with severe trauma; major surgery; hepatic, renal, or respiratory failure; shock; massive burns; or severe infections with septicemia. Acute erosive gastritis associated with these severe illnesses is often referred to as *stress-induced gastritis*. The contributions of all mechanisms responsible for erosive gastritis in critically ill patients have not been defined completely. However, important factors appear to include ischemia of the gastric mucosa, acid diffusion from the gastric lumen into gastric mucosal tissues, and, perhaps in some forms, bile acids and/or other duodenal-pancreatic secretions refluxed into the gastric lumen. Mucosal ischemia and acid in the gastric lumen are clearly crucial elements in the etiopathogenesis of stress-induced gastritis. Septic shock with resulting mucosal ischemia produces gastric erosions in experimental animals. During such experimentally induced shock, the intramural pH of the gastric mucosa falls precipitously when the gastric lumen is irrigated with HCl; this produces severe hemorrhagic lesions. The decrease in intramural pH results from diffusion of luminal hydrogen ions, which damage the gastric mucosa. With neutral pH irrigation, the fall in intramural pH is much less, and gastric lesions are minimal. Counteracting the effects of acid by vigorous and continuous treatment with antacids or by inhibiting secretion with H-2 receptor antagonists has been effective in reducing the hemorrhagic complications of acute erosive gastritis in critically ill patients.

Various agents are known to injure the gastric mucosa. These include aspirin and other NSAIDs, bile acids, pancreatic enzymes, and ethanol. These agents disrupt the gastric mucosal barrier, which under normal conditions impedes the back-diffusion of hydrogen ions from the gastric lumen to the mucosa (despite and against an enormous H^+ concentration gradient). The most common and very important cause of drug-associated acute erosive gastritis is ingestion of aspirin or other NSAIDs. As indicated above, these drugs inhibit gastric mucosal cyclooxygenase activity, thereby reducing the synthesis and tissue levels of endogenous mucosal prostaglandins, which play important roles in mucosal defense. This reduction in tissue prostaglandins is thought to be a principal, but perhaps not the exclusive, mechanism by which aspirin and other NSAIDs damage the gastric mucosa. It is possible that aspirin may injure small vessels in the gastric mucosa by inhibition of prostacyclin in their walls or by inhibition of synthesis of thromboxane by platelets. An additional proposed mechanism for aspirin-induced gastrointestinal mucosal injury is via the effects of sodium salicylate, the product of aspirin metabolism found in the circulation, which is toxic to mitochondrial respiration and oxidative phosphorylation of cells. This may produce endothelial and epithelial cell injury with hemorrhage into the tissues or vascular thrombosis by endothelial cell disruption. Acid in the gastric lumen appears crucial to the production of salicylate-associated injury to the gastric mucosa.

Ethanol damage to the gastric mucosa is associated principally with subepithelial hemorrhages with surrounding edema and only slight to moderate increases in mucosal inflammatory cells. The mechanism by which alcohol injures the gastric mucosa is uncertain. Suggestions include cell injury due to its inherent lipophilic and lipolytic properties and/or interruption of the gastric mucosal barrier or direct damage to small mucosal blood vessels.

Clinical features Bleeding from the gastric mucosa with acute gastritis may range from abrupt and dramatic upper gastrointestinal hemorrhage to the most subtle blood loss, perhaps detected only by the presence of occult blood in the stool or development of mild, asymptomatic, and unexplained anemia. Except for possible consequences of blood loss, erosive gastritis is usually asymptomatic. However, less common symptoms may include epigastric or upper abdominal pain, nausea, and vomiting. Pain is much less common with erosive gastritis than with ulcer disease; in fact, painless gastrointestinal hemorrhage is frequently the only clinical manifestation. Physical examination is often normal in patients with acute hemorrhagic gastritis. However, they may have upper abdominal tenderness or evidence of blood loss such as pallor, tachycardia, and hypotension. When they occur, white blood cell count abnormalities, such as leukocytosis or leukopenia, more often reflect the associated serious illness than the gastritis.

Diagnosis The presence of erosive gastritis is usually first suspected by detection of blood in the stool or in the gastric aspirate. The diagnosis is best established by upper gastrointestinal endoscopy, which reveals mucosal hemorrhages, friability and congestion, erosions, and, in some instances, superficial or deep ulcerations which, when present, are usually in the fundus or body of the stomach. Radiographic examination is much less reliable than endoscopy in detecting acute hemorrhagic-erosive gastritis.

Treatment Treatment should be directed to prevention of erosive gastritis, treatment of the associated disease, withdrawal of the offending agent, and general supportive measures, as required, including maintenance of oxygen, blood volume, and fluid and electrolyte requirements. Hourly antacid administration (e.g., 30 mL of an aluminum-magnesium hydroxide liquid preparation) and/or administration of an H-2 receptor antagonist (usually intravenously) have been shown to be effective in reducing the frequency of hemorrhagic gastritis in critically ill patients. These drugs should be used in doses and frequencies sufficient to maintain the pH of gastric contents constantly above 4. Although proven of value in prevention, it is less certain that they are effective in treatment of acute hemorrhagic gastritis. However, a similar therapeutic program with antacids or H-2 receptor antagonists does seem reasonable and generally is advised. Sucralfate also has been used in treatment.

Most patients with acute hemorrhagic gastritis respond favorably during vigorous treatment by the measures indicated. Acute hemorrhagic gastritis tends to improve as the patient's clinical condition improves. Because of the rapid cell renewal and restitutive properties of the gastric mucosa, lesions of acute hemorrhagic gastritis may disappear, both endoscopically and histologically, within 48 h of an acute event. However, occasionally, further measures are required in attempts to arrest persistent life-threatening blood loss. These have included embolization or vasopressin infusion of the left gastric artery. Uncommonly, surgery is required for relentless hemorrhage. Vagotomy with pyloroplasty with oversewing of focal bleeding ulcerations has been used with limited success, and rarely, total gastrectomy is required. Morbidity and mortality with surgery are very great, usually reflecting the severity of their associated illnesses. Surgery should not be performed unless absolutely necessary.

ENTEROPATHIC EROSIVE GASTRITIS Enteropathic erosive gastritis is a rare clinical entity with multiple erosions of the gastric mucosa found in the absence of recognized precipitating factors. These patients may have anorexia, nausea, vomiting, or poorly defined upper abdominal discomfort. Less commonly they show evidence of gastrointestinal blood loss or weight loss. Endoscopic examination is usually required to establish the diagnosis. Erosions, which may be few or numerous, are usually located on the crests of the folds but may be found in any portion of the gastric mucosa. Gastric biopsies are performed primarily to exclude other abnormalities, e.g., gastric lymphoma, carcinoma, and Crohn's disease. Erosions usually heal completely and may or may not return. The cause is not known, nor are there accepted principles for specific recommendations for therapy.

ACUTE GASTRITIS ASSOCIATED WITH *H. PYLORI* *H. pylori* is a short (0.2 to 0.5 μm in length), spiral-shaped, microaerophilic gram-negative bacillus responsible for certain forms of acute and chronic gastritis. Gastric colonization also has been associated with duodenal and gastric ulcer (see "Peptic Ulcer," above). With gastric colonization, *H. pylori* are found in the deep portions of the mucus gel layer that coats the gastric mucosa and between the mucus gel layer and the apical surfaces of the gastric mucosal epithelial cells. They also may be located in the regions of the tight junctions between adjacent mucosal epithelial cells. *H. pylori* may adhere to the luminal surfaces of gastric epithelial cells, but they do not invade the gastric mucosa.

H. pylori is the cause, or at least the principal cause, of a form of gastritis that has been designated *active chronic gastritis*. *H. pylori* is associated with active chronic gastritis in virtually 100 percent of patients. Active chronic gastritis is characterized by dense infiltration of the lamina propria of the gastric mucosa with invasion of the epithelial cell layer by polymorphonuclear leukocytes. The mucosal surface is usually intact, without erosions or hemorrhagic lesions. When erosions do occur, they are usually small and limited to the superficial epithelial cell layer. There is poor correlation between the histologic abnormalities and the endoscopic appearance of the mucosa; endoscopy may reveal subtle abnormalities, or more often, the endoscopic appearance is totally normal. Histologic abnormalities are associated with positive culture for *H. pylori*, and the degree of histologic abnormality, in general, parallels the number of organisms that can be identified. The more active the gastritis, reflected by mucosal infiltration with polymorphonuclear leukocytes, the greater the likelihood that *H. pylori* will be found. Healing of the gastritis occurs when the organism is eradicated and cultures become negative. Spontaneous disappearance of *H. pylori* has not been noted. Active chronic gastritis with *H. pylori* colonization has been observed to persist in gastric mucosal biopsies of untreated patients for years.

H. pylori can be identified in gastric mucosal samples by histologic examination, culture, urease activity, and endonuclease analysis. On stained tissue sections, *H. pylori* is Giemsa-positive and faintly hematoxylin-positive. The organisms can be cultured successfully from biopsy material but usually not from gastric secretions. *H. pylori* produces large amounts of urease. The rapid urease test of gastric biopsy material is a relatively simple and reliable method for presumptive identification of *H. pylori*. The biopsy urease test involves use of a urea-containing broth in which the gastric biopsy is placed. A positive test results in an increase in pH, with the phenol red indicator turning from light orange to red within 5 min. The test is inexpensive, with sensitivity of at least 90 percent and specificity approaching 100 percent. A urea breath test using ^{13}C or ^{14}C also has been developed for identifying *H. pylori*. Antibodies (IgG and IgA) to *H. pylori* have been identified in sera of individuals with *H. pylori* colonization. There is a high degree of correlation between these serum antibodies and histologic gastritis.

H. pylori produces a variety of proteins which appear to mediate or facilitate its damaging effects on the gastric mucosa. The urease produced by *H. pylori* catalyzes the hydrolysis of urea to yield ammonia and carbon dioxide. This provides a more alkaline microenvironment that protects *H. pylori* from the effects of gastric acid, which prevents gastric colonization by other bacteria. The urease results in damage to gastric mucosal epithelial cells by the hydroxide ions generated by the equilibration of water with ammonia. *H. pylori* produces surface proteins that are chemotactic for human neutrophils and monocytes and secretes a proinflammatory platelet-activating factor, as well as urease, which is also proinflammatory. *H. pylori* activates monocytes which express HLA-DR and interleukin 2 receptors on their cell surfaces and produce superoxides, interleukin 1, and tumor necrosis factor α. *H. pylori* produces proteases and phospholipases which degrade the glycoprotein-lipid complex of the mucus gel layer. This reduces the thickness and viscosity of the gastric protective mucus gel overlying the gastric mucosal epithelial cells in spite of increased mucus synthesis and secretion. *H. pylori* also produces an adhesin which facilitates the attachment of the bacterium to gastric epithelial cells.

At initiation of infection by *H. pylori*, there may be transient increased gastric acid secretion; however, this is often followed by hypochlorhydria which lasts for several months, followed by return to approximate preinfection acid secretory rates within 1 year. By retrospective examination, *H. pylori* were demonstrated in gastric mucosal biopsy specimens obtained from volunteers participating in gastric secretory studies who developed epidemic gastritis, with reductions in rates of gastric acid secretion. *H. pylori* infection may be associated with increased serum gastrin levels and normal gastric acid secretion; with eradication of *H. pylori*, serum gastrin levels return to normal, implying interruption of the acid-mediated feedback control mechanism regulating gastrin release by *H. pylori*. In patients with *H. pylori* infection, gastric mucosal somatostatin levels are reduced and inversely correlated with gastric luminal ammonia. This suggests somatostatin deficiency as the mechanism responsible for enhanced gastrin release in patients with *H. pylori* infection. This probably also explains increased gastrin release in response to feeding and decreased gastric mucosal somotostatin reported in duodenal ulcer patients (see ''Peptic Ulcer,'' above).

H. pylori has been cultured from antral biopsy specimens in 90 to 100 percent of patients with duodenal ulcer, 60 to 70 percent with gastric ulcer, and about 50 percent of patients with nonulcer dyspepsia. *H. pylori* is also frequent in asymptomatic individuals considered to be otherwise well. In such asymptomatic individuals endoscopic examination has usually appeared normal, in spite of the histologic evidence of gastritis and *H. pylori*. It has not been proven that *H. pylori* gastritis produces symptoms. Nor has it been proven that *H. pylori* is responsible for symptoms in patients with nonulcer dyspepsia.

Colloidal bismuth compounds have been shown to eradicate *H. pylori* from gastric mucosa. Eradication may be due to antibacterial effects or to binding or coating of the organism. However, bismuth alone results in only approximately 10 percent long-term eradication. Amoxicillin (or other antibiotics), bismuth subsalicylate, and metronidazole have each been used singly or in combination for periods of from 1 week to 2 months to eradicate *H. pylori*. Therapy with

metronidazole, 250 mg three times a day, and bismuth, 525 mg (in the form of Pepto-Bismol) four times a day, eradicates the organism in 75 percent of patients for up to 12 months. Eradication of *H. pylori* results in disappearance of inflammatory changes. When recolonization of the organism occurs after treatment, it is usually with the same bacterial subtype and is associated with recurrence of gastritis.

CHRONIC GASTRITIS   The inflammatory cell infiltrate in chronic gastritis consists predominantly of lymphocytes and plasma cells. Polymorphonuclear leukocytes and eosinophils may be present in small numbers but do not predominate. Chronic gastritis is often patchy and irregular in distribution.

Histologic classification   Chronic gastritis has been classified descriptively on the basis of several characteristic histologic abnormalities. In its evolution, chronic gastritis initially involves the superficial and glandular areas of the gastric mucosa and progresses to glandular destruction, which may be followed by a profound reduction in gland number (atrophy) and/or gland metaplasia.

Superficial gastritis is that form of gastritis with inflammatory changes in the lamina propria of the superficial mucosa, with cellular infiltration and edema separating the gastric glands. Superficial gastritis appears to represent the initial stage in the development of chronic gastritis. With superficial gastritis, the inflammatory cell infiltrate is limited to the lamina propria of the upper (epithelial) half of the gastric mucosa, and the glands are preserved. There may be a decrease in mucus in glandular mucous cells and in mitotic figures in cells of the glands.

Atrophic gastritis is the next stage in the developmental chronology of chronic gastritis. In atrophic gastritis, the inflammatory infiltrate extends to the deep portions of the mucosa. There is progressive distortion and destruction of the glands, which become separated by the inflammatory process. Atrophic gastritis usually begins in the antrum and extends proximally into the body and fundus of the stomach. Atrophic gastritis is followed by the development of the final stage of chronic gastritis, which is *gastric atrophy*. With gastric atrophy, there is a profound loss of the glandular structures, which are now separated widely by connective tissue, with a greatly reduced or absent inflammatory infiltrate. The mucosa is thin, often revealing the prominence of its underlying vessels by endoscopic examination.

As chronic gastritis progresses, there may be changes in the morphology of the gastric glandular elements. *Intestinal metaplasia* is the term used to describe the conversion of gastric glands to the appearance of small intestinal mucosal glands containing goblet cells. Intestinal metaplasia may be patchy or extensive in the gastric mucosa. With *pseudopyloric gland metaplasia* the glands of the body of the stomach assume the appearance of antral pyloric glands. Pseudopyloric metaplasia may occur with either atrophic gastritis or gastric atrophy.

Chronic gastritis: Types A and B   The two major forms of chronic gastritis have been classified as types A and B based on their distributions in the gastric mucosa coupled with implications regarding their pathogenesis.

Type A gastritis is the less common form of chronic gastritis; it characteristically involves the body and fundus of the stomach, with relative sparing of the antrum. This is the form of gastritis that may lead to pernicious anemia. The frequent presence of antibodies to parietal cells and to intrinsic factor in sera of patients with Type A gastritis and pernicious anemia has suggested an immune or autoimmune pathogenesis for this form of gastritis. Antibodies to parietal cells have been shown to be cytotoxic for gastric mucosal cells. Cell-mediated immune mechanisms also have been proposed to participate in gastric mucosal cell injury in pernicious anemia and related forms of type A gastritis. Antibodies to parietal cells have been found in sera of approximately 90 percent of patients with pernicious anemia and in more than half of other patients with type A gastritis. Relatives of patients with pernicious anemia have a higher than normal frequency of serum antibodies to parietal cells, atrophic gastritis, and reduced gastric acid secretion. In control populations, parietal cell antibodies may be found in up to 20 percent of individuals over age 60 and in approximately 20 percent of all patients with hypoparathyroidism, Addison's disease, and vitiligo. About 50 percent of patients with pernicious anemia have antibodies to thyroid antigens, and approximately 30 percent of patients with thyroid disease have circulating antibodies to parietal cells. Serum antibodies to intrinsic factor are more specific than parietal cell antibodies and are present in about 40 percent of patients with pernicious anemia.

In patients with pernicious anemia, the gastric parietal cell–containing glands are invariably destroyed, accounting for their inability to secrete hydrochloric acid. Since, in human beings, parietal cells also secrete intrinsic factor, there is failure to absorb vitamin B_{12} actively, with resulting hematologic and/or neurologic consequences characteristic of pernicious anemia.

Type B gastritis is much the more common form of chronic gastritis. In younger patients type B gastritis principally involves the antrum, whereas in older patients the entire stomach is affected. This transition is estimated to require about 15 to 20 years. The incidence of chronic gastritis, most of it type B gastritis, increases with age, reaching 78 percent in individuals over age 50 and virtually 100 percent after age 70.

A large number of studies from various parts of the world have established that *H. pylori* is the agent responsible for type B gastritis. Chronic gastritis with *H. pylori* infection and/or persistence is associated with reduced gastric acid secretion. Eradication of *H. pylori* produces improvement in histologic findings; when treatment is stopped, inflammatory changes recur, and organisms reappear. These observations have supported the conclusion that type B gastritis is caused by chronic bacterial infection by *H. pylori*. Gastric colonization with *H. pylori* is found in virtually all patients with chronic superficial gastritis, with fewer bacteria demonstrable with progress to atrophic gastritis. *H. pylori* are few in number or rarely demonstrated with severe gastric atrophy. Chronic reflux of pancreatic-biliary secretions, bile acids and lysolecithin in particular, also has been proposed as a potential contributing factor in the production of type B chronic gastritis.

Gastric acid secretion is reduced in both type A and type B chronic gastritis. In general, the reduction in gastric acid secretion, which is complete in patients with pernicious anemia, is proportionate to the severity of parietal cell destruction and mucosal atrophy in the body and fundus of the stomach. Serum gastrin levels are usually elevated substantially in patients with pernicious anemia and are in approximately the same range as those of patients with the Z-E syndrome (gastrinoma). Since the antral mucosa is relatively spared, the antral gastrin-containing cells, deprived of feedback control normally exercised by acid in the stomach, release gastrin continuously. Serum gastrin levels are also often similarly elevated in patients with type A gastritis with achlorhydria or profound hypochlorhydria who do not have pernicious anemia. Patients with type B gastritis have fasting serum gastrin levels that are highly variable, not consistently elevated, and often in the normal range. A small portion of patients with type B gastritis have serum antibodies to gastrin, leading some to propose an autoimmune mechanism for this form of gastritis. Alternatively, and probably more likely, these antibodies may represent responses to the inflammatory process rather than contributing factors.

There is no persuasive evidence that acute gastric mucosal injury associated with stress, with ethanol, or with aspirin or other NSAIDs progresses to chronic gastritis. Acute gastritis caused by *H. pylori* appears to be the form of acute gastritis in which there is sufficient information to support progression to a chronic form of gastritis, i.e., type B chronic gastritis.

Diagnosis   Biopsy provides the most reliable means of identifying and classifying gastritis. Caution must be exercised in the interpretation of a single gastric mucosal biopsy. The patchy and irregular distribution of the gastritis may lead to substantial sampling error. Therefore, several biopsies of suspected areas, when safe and possible, are recommended.

Treatment   No specific treatment is required for type A or type B chronic gastritis with or without mucosal atrophy. The only form that requires specific treatment is pernicious anemia, the most complete expression of type A gastritis. Vitamin B_{12} deficiency in these patients, resulting from malabsorption of vitamin B_{12} secondary to destruction of parietal cells in the body and fundus of the stomach, requires indefinite regular parenteral vitamin B_{12} administration.

MÉNÉTRIER'S DISEASE   *Ménétrier's disease* is a clinical entity characterized by large tortuous gastric mucosal folds. The abnormalities in Ménétrier's disease may be localized or diffuse throughout the stomach. Prominent mucosal folds are often most conspicuous in the gastric body and fundus. Histologic inflammation is not a component of this disease. Therefore, it is not a form of gastritis. The primary pathologic feature is thickening of the gastric mucosa due to hyperplasia of surface and glandular mucous cells, which replace most of the chief and parietal cells. Pits of the gastric glands elongate and may become extremely tortuous. The lamina propria may contain an increased number of lymphocytes. Intestinal metaplasia may be present.

The most common symptom is epigastric pain. Anorexia, nausea, vomiting, and weight loss are less frequent. Gastric bleeding is unusual and, when present, is due to superficial mucosal erosions. Uncommonly, gastric ulcer or gastric carcinoma may develop in these patients. Patients often develop a protein-losing gastropathy resulting in hypoalbuminemia and edema. Gastric acid secretion is usually reduced or may be absent. Barium examination of the upper gastrointestinal tract reveals the large gastric folds, which are readily confirmed by endoscopic examination. The diagnosis is best established by deep mucosal biopsy (and cytology) to exclude gastric malignancy. The depth of these lesions and the disconcerting prominence of the folds may require a surgical full-thickness biopsy to exclude lymphoma or infiltrating carcinoma.

Anticholinergic agents and H-2 receptor antagonists have been reported to decrease protein loss in patients with Ménétrier's disease. Treatment includes a high-protein diet, when required, to replace protein losses. If present, ulcers should be treated as described previously for common gastric ulcer. Severe disease with persistent substantial protein loss may require total gastrectomy.

GASTRITIS DUE TO CORROSIVE AGENTS   Ingestion of a variety of corrosive chemicals can cause severe damage to the gastric mucosa. Because of its anatomic location, the antrum is a frequent site for such injury. Ingested substances which are particularly injurious to the gastric mucosa include strong acids (e.g., hydrochloric acid, sulfuric acid) or strong alkali (e.g., sodium hydroxide). Depending on dose and concentration, these agents can cause injury ranging from mild inflammation to extensive tissue necrosis. With alkali ingestion (especially lye), the esophagus is particularly susceptible to severe injury, necrosis, and potential subsequent stricture. The stomach, especially the antrum, is more susceptible to acute injury from ingestion of strong acid. With ingestion of these corrosive substances, patients may describe burning of the mouth, throat, and retrosternal area. Epigastric pain and vomiting often signal gastric injury. Hemorrhage and/or perforation may occur. Treatment of strong acid ingestion includes dilution with water, followed by antacids and supportive therapy as required. Neutralization of ingested lye by administrated acid is not recommended.

INFECTIOUS GASTRITIS   Infectious causes of gastritis, other than that associated with gastric *H. pylori* colonization, are unusual. *Phlegmonous gastritis*, a rare form of bacterial gastritis, is a life-threatening disease with extensive infiltration of the gastric wall, tissue necrosis, and manifestations of generalized sepsis. Responsible infectious agents include, among others, streptococci, staphylococci, *Proteus* species, and *Escherichia coli*. Treatment includes appropriate intravenous antibiotics and necessary supportive care with fluid and electrolyte replacement as required. Lack of response to therapy may require gastrectomy. Additional infectious causes of gastritis may be found in immunocompromised patients. Gastric erosions may be produced by herpes simplex virus. Typical intranuclear inclusions of cytomegalovirus, with positive cultures, have been found by endoscopic gastric biopsy in some immunocompromised patients.

This has been interpreted to represent disseminated cytomegalovirus infection.

EOSINOPHILIC GASTRITIS   *Eosinophilic gastritis* may occur as isolated involvement of the stomach or as a component of eosinophilic gastroenteritis. Eosinophilic gastritis is characterized by extensive eosinophilic infiltration of the wall of the stomach, usually with circulating eosinophilia. Biopsy reveals extensive eosinophilic infiltration which may involve all coats of the stomach or may be limited to mucosa, submucosa, or muscular regions of the gastric wall. The antrum is involved more frequently than the gastric body or fundus. There may be prominent antral mucosal folds with edema and mucosal thickening, uncommonly leading to gastric outlet obstruction. Epigastric pain, which may be accompanied by nausea and vomiting, is the most frequent symptom. These patients usually respond favorably to treatment with glucocorticoids. Rarely, surgery is required to establish the diagnosis or for relief of obstructive symptoms.

GRANULOMATOUS GASTRITIS   A number of generalized diseases, some of which are infectious, can involve the stomach, producing *granulomatous gastritis.* Crohn's disease, as in the small intestine, may produce gastric ulceration, granulomatous infiltration, and/or scarring with stricture formation. Its distinction from other gastric lesions requires biopsy at the time of endoscopic examination. Less common infectious causes of granulomatous disease of the stomach include, among others, histoplasmosis, candidiasis, syphilis, and tuberculosis. Rarely, idiopathic granulomatous gastritis and eosinophilic granulomas also involve the stomach. In patients with granulomatous disease of the stomach, multiple biopsies and cytology are usually required to establish the diagnosis and to exclude malignancy. If the diagnosis is not established by biopsy at endoscopy, surgical exploration may be required.

GASTRITIS AND PRIOR GASTRIC SURGERY   Variable amounts of gastritis almost always occur in the remaining stomachs of patients treated surgically by partial gastrectomy and, to a somewhat lesser extent, after vagotomy with pyloroplasty. Gastritis is especially common and often severe after gastrojejunal (Billroth II) anastomosis.

Gastric surgery appears to accelerate the development of gastritis, with progressive loss of parietal cells in the gastric remnant after surgery. Most patients are asymptomatic; however, a small proportion develop mild or severe symptoms, most commonly epigastric pain, nausea, and vomiting. This form of gastritis has been referred to as *alkaline gastritis* or *bile reflux gastritis.* It has been assumed, but not proven, that gastritis results from reflux of pancreaticobiliary secretions. Endoscopic examination often reveals a beefy red and sometimes friable gastric mucosa. Abnormalities may be limited to mucosa in the region of the anastomosis or may involve all remaining gastric mucosa. Bile is often seen in the gastric remnant. Biopsies of involved mucosa at endoscopy show variable degrees of acute and/or chronic gastritis. Gastric acid secretion is usually decreased.

Managing patients with severe symptoms is very difficult. Various therapeutic approaches have been used with limited, if any, success. These have included cholestyramine, H-2 receptor antagonists, sucralfate, antacids, and pancreatic enzyme replacement. Surgery, which is sometimes successful, is Roux-en-Y, which diverts pancreaticobiliary secretions away from the gastric remnant. Nonsurgical modalities should be exhausted before proceeding with attempts to treat this disease by surgery.

REFERENCES

Peptic ulcer

BARDHAN KD et al: Double-blind comparison of cimetidine and placebo in the maintenance and healing of chronic duodenal ulceration. Gut 20:158, 1979

CRYER B, FELDMAN M: Effects of nonsteroidal anti-inflammatory drugs on endogenous gastrointestinal prostaglandins and therapeutic strategies for prevention and treatment of nonsteroidal anti-inflammatory drug-induced damage. Arch Intern Med 152:1145, 1992

GRAHAM DY et al: Effect of treatment of *Helicobacter pylori* infection on the long-term recurrence of gastric or duodenal ulcer: A randomized, controlled study. Ann Intern Med 116:705, 1992

GREGORY RA et al: Amino acid constitution of two gastrins isolated from Zollinger-Ellison variety. N Engl J Med 278:1308, 1968

MATON PN et al: Cushing's syndrome in patients with the Zollinger-Ellison syndrome. N Engl J Med 315:1, 1986

MCARTHUR KE et al: Treatment of acid-peptic diseases by inhibition of gastric H+,K+-ATPase. Annu Rev Med 37:97, 1986

MCGUIGAN JE, TRUDEAU WL: Differences in rates of gastrin release in normal persons and patients with duodenal ulcer. N Engl J Med 288:64, 1973

――――, ――――: Immunochemical measurement of elevated levels of gastrin in the serum of patients with pancreatic tumors of the Zollinger-Ellison variety. N Engl J Med 278:1308, 1968

PETERSON WL: *Helicobacter pylori* and peptic ulcer disease. Curr Concepts Nutr 324:1043, 1991

PIPELEERS-MARICHAL M et al: Gastrinomas in the duodenums of patients with multiple endocrine neoplasia type 1 and the Zollinger-Ellison syndrome. N Engl J Med 322:723, 1990

PISEGNA JR et al: Effects of curative gastrinoma resection on gastric secretory function and antisecretory drug requirement in the Zollinger-Ellison syndrome. Gastroenterology 102:767, 1992

PEURA DA, JOHNSON LF: Cimetidine for prevention and treatment of gastroduodenal lesions in patients in an intensive care unit. Ann Intern Med 103:173, 1985

RICHARDSON CT: Sucralfate. Ann Intern Med 97:269, 1982

VINAYEK R et al: Famotidine in the therapy of gastric hypersecretory states. Am J Med 81:49, 1986

―――― et al: Zollinger-Ellison syndrome: Recent advances in the management of the gastrinoma. Gastroenterol Clin North Am 19:197, 1990

WOLFE MM, SOLL AH: The physiology of gastric acid secretion. N Engl J Med 319:1707, 1988

Gastritis

BLASER MJ: Hypotheses on the pathogenesis and natural history of *Helicobacter pylori*–induced inflammation. Gastroenterology 102:720, 1992

DOIG P et al: Production of a conserved adhesin by the human gastroduodenal pathogen *Helicobacter pylori.* J Bacteriol 174:2539, 1992

HENTSCHEL E et al: Effect of ranitidine and amoxicillin plus metronidazole on the eradication of *Helicobacter pylori* and the recurrence of duodenal ulcer. N Engl J Med 328:308, 1993

KANEKO H et al: *Helicobacter pylori* infection induces a decrease in immunoreactive somatostatin concentrations of human stomach. Dig Dis Sci 37:409, 1992

LEE SP: The mode of action of colloidal bismuth subcitrate. Scand J Gastroenterol 26(suppl 185):1, 1991

MAJ UEH et al: Surface proteins from *Helicobacter pylori* exhibit chemotactic activity for human leukocytes and are present in gastric mucosa. J Exp Med 175:517, 1992

ROBERT A: Cytoprotection by prostaglandins. Gastroenterology 77:761, 1979

SEARCY CM, MALAGELADA JR: Ménétrier's disease and idiopathic hypertrophic gastropathy. Ann Intern Med 100:565, 1984

TAKEUCHI KD: Role of pH gradient of mucus in protection of gastric mucosa. Gastroenterology 84:331, 1983

VANE JR: Inhibition of prostaglandin synthesis as a mechanism for aspirin-like drugs. Nature 23:232, 1971

253   NEOPLASMS OF THE ESOPHAGUS AND STOMACH

ROBERT J. MAYER

ESOPHAGEAL CANCER

INCIDENCE AND ETIOLOGY   In the United States, cancer of the esophagus is a relatively uncommon but extremely lethal malignant condition. It is estimated that the diagnosis was made in 11,300 Americans in 1993, leading to 10,200 deaths. Worldwide, the incidence of esophageal cancer varies strikingly. It occurs frequently within a so-called Asian esophageal cancer belt extending from the southern shore of the Caspian Sea on the west to northern China on the east and encompassing parts of Iran, Central Asia, Afghanistan, Siberia, and Mongolia. Additionally, high-incidence "pockets" of the disease are present in such disparate locations as Finland, Iceland, Curaçao, southeastern Africa, and northwestern France. In North America and western Europe, the disease is far more common in blacks than whites, greater in males than females, appearing most frequently after age 50, and appearing to be an illness associated with lower socioeconomic classes.

A variety of causative factors have been implicated in the

TABLE 253-1 Some etiologic factors believed to be associated with esophageal cancer

Excess alcohol consumption
Cigarette smoking
Other ingested carcinogens
  A Nitrates (converted to nitrites)
  B Smoked opiates
  C Fungal toxins in pickled vegetables
Mucosal damage from physical agents
  A Hot tea
  B Lye ingestion
  C Radiation-induced strictures
  D Chronic achalasia
Host susceptibility
  A Esophageal web with glossitis and iron deficiency (i.e., Plummer-Vinson or Paterson-Kelly syndrome)
  B Congenital hyperkeratosis and pitting of the palms and soles (i.e., tylosis palmaris et plantaris)
? Dietary deficiencies—molybdenum, zinc, vitamin A
? Celiac sprue
Chronic gastric reflux (i.e., Barrett's esophagus)—for adenocarcinoma

development of the disease (Table 253-1). In the United States, 80 to 90 percent of esophageal cancer cases are believed attributable to excess consumption of alcohol and/or a long-standing history of cigarette smoking. The relative risk increases with either the amount of tobacco smoked or alcohol consumed. The consumption of whiskey is seemingly linked to a higher incidence than the consumption of wine or beer. The development of esophageal cancer has also been associated with the ingestion of other carcinogens such as nitrites, smoked opiates, and fungal toxins in pickled vegetables, as well as with mucosal damage caused by such physical insults as long-term exposure to extremely hot tea, the ingestion of lye, radiation-induced strictures, and chronic achalasia. The presence of an esophageal web in association with glossitis and iron deficiency (i.e., Plummer-Vinson or Paterson-Kelly syndrome) and congenital hyperkeratosis and pitting of the palms and soles (i.e., tylosis palmaris et plantaris) have each been linked with esophageal cancer, as have dietary deficiencies of molybdenum, zinc, and vitamin A. The risk for esophageal cancer may be slightly greater in individuals with celiac sprue and is definitely increased in the presence of chronic gastric reflux (i.e., Barrett's esophagus). In contrast to other esophageal cancers, neoplasms arising from Barrett's esophagus afflict white individuals far more commonly than blacks.

CLINICAL FEATURES Approximately 15 percent of esophageal cancers occur in the upper third of the esophagus ("cervical esophagus"), 50 percent in the middle third, and 35 percent in the lower third. More than 85 percent of esophageal tumors are squamous cell carcinomas, arising from the squamous epithelium which lines the lumen of the esophagus. Adenocarcinomas, while far less frequent, develop more commonly from columnar epithelium which may appear dysplastic in the distal esophagus in association with chronic gastric reflux (i.e., Barrett's esophagus). These malignancies have the biologic behavior of gastric rather than esophageal cancers. Attempts at endoscopic and cytologic screening for carcinoma in patients with Barrett's esophagus, while effective as a means of detecting high-grade dysplasia, have not yet been proven beneficial in positively influencing the prognosis in individuals found to have a carcinoma. It should be noted that squamous cell carcinomas and adenocarcinomas of the esophagus cannot be distinguished radiographically or endoscopically.

Progressive dysphagia and weight loss of short duration are the initial symptoms in the vast majority of patients. Dysphagia initially occurs with solid foods and gradually progresses to include semisolids and liquids. By the time these symptoms develop, the disease is usually incurable since difficulty in swallowing does not occur until 60 percent or more of the esophageal circumference is infiltrated with cancer. Dysphagia may be associated with pain on swallowing (odynophagia), pain radiating to the chest and/or back, regurgitation

or vomiting, and aspiration pneumonia. The disease most commonly spreads to adjacent and supraclavicular lymph nodes, liver, lungs, and pleura. Tracheoesophageal fistulas may develop as the disease advances, leading to severe suffering. As with other squamous cell carcinomas, hypercalcemia occasionally may occur in the absence of osseous metastases. This is believed to result from a tumor-secreted protein structurally analogous to a portion of parathyroid hormone.

DIAGNOSIS Routine, contrast radiographs effectively identify esophageal lesions of sufficient size to cause symptoms. In contrast to benign esophageal leiomyomata which result in esophageal narrowing with preservation of a normal mucosal pattern, esophageal carcinomas characteristically cause ragged, ulcerating changes in the mucosa in association with deeper infiltration, producing a picture resembling achalasia. Smaller, potentially resectable tumors are often poorly visualized despite technically adequate esophagograms. Because of this, esophagoscopy should be performed in all patients suspected of having an esophageal abnormality in order to visualize the tumor and to obtain histopathologic confirmation of the diagnosis. Since the same population of patients at risk for esophageal carcinoma (i.e., smokers and drinkers) also has a high rate of cancers of the lung and head and neck region, endoscopic inspection of the larynx, trachea, and bronchi also should be considered. A thorough examination of the fundus of the stomach (by retroflexing the endoscope) is imperative as well. Endoscopic biopsies of esophageal tumors fail to recover malignant tissue in one-third of cases because the biopsy forceps cannot penetrate deeply enough through normal mucosa pushed in front of the carcinoma. Cytologic examination of tumor brushings frequently complements standard biopsies and should be performed routinely. The extent of tumor spread to the mediastinum and paraaortic lymph nodes should also be assessed by computed tomography (CT) scans of the chest and abdomen.

TREATMENT The prognosis for patients with esophageal carcinoma is poor. Less than 5 percent of patients are alive 5 years after the initial diagnosis, leading many physicians to focus management efforts solely on symptomatic control. Surgical resection of all gross tumor (i.e., total resection) is feasible in only 40 percent of cases, with residual tumor cells frequently present at the resection margins. Such esophagectomies have been associated in the past with a postoperative mortality rate in excess of 20 percent due to anastomotic fistulas, subphrenic abscesses, and respiratory complications; more recent reports suggest far better tolerance and diminished morbidity from these surgical procedures. Less than 20 percent of patients who survive a total resection can be expected to be alive after 5 years. The therapeutic outcome following the administration of primary radiation therapy (5500 to 6000 cGy) is not dissimilar to that of radical surgery, sparing patients perioperative morbidity but often resulting in less satisfactory palliation of obstructive symptoms. The evaluation of chemotherapeutic agents in patients with esophageal carcinoma has been hampered by ambiguity in the definition of "response" (i.e., benefit) and the debilitated physical condition of many treated individuals. Nonetheless, significant reductions in the size of measurable tumor masses have been reported in 15 to 25 percent of patients given single-agent treatment and in 30 to 60 percent of patients treated with drug combinations which include cisplatin. Recent therapeutic efforts have been directed at utilizing combination chemotherapy and radiation therapy as the initial therapeutic approach, either alone or followed by an attempt at operative resection. Although the preliminary results of these experiences have been encouraging, it remains to be determined whether such an intensive multimodality approach will increase the cure rate.

For the incurable, surgically unresectable patient with esophageal cancer, dysphagia, malnutrition, and the management of tracheoesophageal fistulas loom as major issues. Approaches to palliation of these cancer-related complications include repeated endoscopic dilatation, the surgical placement of a gastrostomy or jejunostomy for hydration and feeding, and the surgical insertion of a polyvinyl prosthesis to bypass the tumor. Endoscopic fulguration of the obstructing tumor with lasers appears to be the most promising of these techniques.

TUMORS OF THE STOMACH

GASTRIC ADENOCARCINOMA   Incidence and epidemiology
For reasons which remain uncertain, the incidence and mortality rates for gastric cancer have decreased markedly during the past 60 years. In 1930, gastric cancer represented the leading cause of cancer-related deaths among American men by a factor of two, while the disease in women ranked just behind tumors of the uterine cervix and breast. During the ensuing years, the mortality rate from gastric cancer in the United States has dropped in men from 28 to 5.3 per 100,000 population, while in women, the rate has decreased from 27 to 2.3 per 100,000. Nonetheless, it was estimated in 1993 that 24,000 new cases of stomach cancer were diagnosed in the United States and that 13,600 Americans died of the disease. The decreased incidence in gastric cancer in the United States is also reflected worldwide. The incidence of gastric cancer varies widely among different countries, being comparatively high in Japan, China, Chile, and Ireland; however, a decrease in both incidence and mortality has occurred in these areas as well.

Epidemiologic surveys have suggested the risk of gastric cancer to be greater among lower socioeconomic classes. Furthermore, migrants from high- to low-incidence nations appear to maintain their susceptibility to gastric cancer while the risk for their offspring more closely approximates that of the new homeland. These findings suggest that an environmental exposure, probably beginning early in life, is related to the development of gastric cancer with dietary carcinogens considered the most likely factor(s).

Pathology   Approximately 90 percent of stomach cancers are adenocarcinomas with 10 percent due to non-Hodgkin's lymphomas and leiomyosarcomas. Gastric adenocarcinomas may be subdivided into two categories: a *diffuse type* in which cell cohesion is absent, resulting in individual cells infiltrating and thickening the stomach wall without forming a discrete mass; and an *intestinal type* characterized by cohesive neoplastic cells forming glandlike tubular structures. The diffuse carcinomas occur more often in younger patients, develop throughout the stomach including the cardia, result in a loss of distensibility of the gastric wall (so-called linitis plastica or "leather bottle" appearance), and are associated with a far more ominous prognosis. Intestinal-type lesions are frequently ulcerative, more commonly appear in the antrum and lesser curvature of the stomach, and are often preceded by a prolonged precancerous process. While the incidence of diffuse carcinomas is similar in most populations, the intestinal type tends to predominate in the high-risk geographic regions mentioned earlier and is less likely to be found in areas where the frequency of gastric cancer is declining. Thus, different etiologic factor(s) may be involved in these two subtypes. In the United States, the distal stomach is the site of origin of about half of gastric cancers. Approximately 20 percent of these tumors arise in the lesser curvature, 25 percent in the cardia, and only 3 to 5 percent in the greater curvature. More than 10 percent of gastric carcinomas involve the entire stomach.

Etiology   The relationship between dietary patterns and the development of gastric carcinoma has been extensively investigated. The long-term ingestion of high concentrations of nitrates in dried, smoked, and salted foods appears to be associated with a higher risk. The nitrates are thought to be converted to carcinogenic nitrites by bacteria (Table 253-2). Such bacteria may be introduced exogenously through the ingestion of the partially decayed foods which are consumed in abundance worldwide by the lower socioeconomic classes. Bacteria such as *helicobacter pylori* may also appear endogenously, possibly as a result of a lack or loss of gastric acidity. This may occur when acid-producing cells of the gastric antrum have been surgically removed 15 to 20 years previously at the time of a partial gastrectomy to control benign peptic ulcer disease or when achlorhydria, atrophic gastritis, and even pernicious anemia develop in the elderly. Serial endoscopic examinations of the stomach in patients with atrophic gastritis have documented replacement of the usual gastric mucosa by intestinal-type cells. This process of intestinal

TABLE 253-2   Dietary factors as a cause of gastric carcinoma*

Sources of nitrate-converting bacteria

Exogenous
  A Bacterially contaminated food
  B Frequent in lower socioeconomic classes who have higher incidence of the disease
  C Diminished by improved food preservation and refrigeration
  D ? *Helicobacter pylori* infection
Endogenous
  A Decreased gastric acidity
  B Prior gastric surgery (antrectomy)—15 to 20 year latency period
  C Atrophic gastritis and/or pernicious anemia
  D ? Prolonged exposure to histamine-2-receptor antagonists

*Hypothesis: Dietary nitrates are converted to carcinogenic nitrites by bacteria

metaplasia may lead to cellular atypia and eventual neoplasia. Since the declining incidence of gastric cancer in the United States is primarily a reflection of a decline in distal, ulcerating, intestinal-type lesions, it is conceivable that better food preservation and the availability to all socioeconomic classes of refrigeration for food storage have resulted in a decrease in the dietary ingestion of exogenous bacteria. It remains uncertain whether the iatrogenic achlorhydria induced by the widespread, prolonged use of parietal cell histamine antagonists will result in a future increase in intestinal-type gastric cancer.

Several additional etiologic factors have been associated with gastric carcinoma. Gastric ulcers and adenomatous polyps have occasionally been so linked, but data regarding a cause-and-effect relationship are unconvincing. The inadequate clinical distinction between benign gastric ulcers and small ulcerating carcinomas may, in part, account for this presumed association. The presence of extreme hypertrophy of gastric rugal folds (i.e., Ménétrier's disease), giving the impression of polypoid lesions, has been associated with a striking frequency of malignant transformation; such hypertrophy, however, does not represent the presence of true adenomatous polyps. Individuals with blood group A have been reported to have a higher incidence of gastric cancer than persons with blood group O; it is possible that this observation is related to differences in the mucous secretion of the various ABO blood groups, thereby leading to greater or lesser mucosal protection from carcinogens. No association has been identified between duodenal ulcers and gastric cancer.

Clinical features   Gastric cancers, when superficial and surgically curable, usually produce no symptoms. As the tumor becomes more extensive, patients may complain of an insidious upper abdominal discomfort varying in intensity from a vague, postprandial fullness to a severe, steady pain. Anorexia, often with slight nausea, is very common but is not the usual presenting complaint. Weight loss may eventually be observed and nausea and vomiting are particularly prominent with tumors of the pylorus; dysphagia may be the major symptom caused by lesions of the cardia. There are no early physical signs of the disease, and the finding of a palpable abdominal mass generally indicates long-standing growth and, all too often, regional extension.

Gastric carcinomas spread by direct extension through the gastric wall to the perigastric tissues, occasionally adhering to adjacent organs such as the pancreas, colon, or liver. The disease also spreads via lymphatics or by seeding of peritoneal surfaces. Metastases to intraabdominal and supraclavicular lymph nodes may occur frequently as may metastatic nodules to the ovary (Krukenberg's tumor), periumbilical region ("Sister Mary Joseph node") or to the peritoneal cul-de-sac (Blumer's shelf); malignant ascites may also develop. The liver is the most common site for hematogenous spread of tumor.

The presence of iron-deficiency anemia in men and occult blood in the stool of both sexes should mandate a search for an occult lesion in the gastrointestinal tract. Such a careful assessment is of particular importance in patients having atrophic gastritis or pernicious anemia. Unusual clinical features associated with gastric adenocarcinomas include migratory thrombophlebitis, microangiopathic hemolytic anemia, and acanthosis nigricans.

Diagnosis A double-contrast radiographic examination is the simplest diagnostic procedure for the evaluation of a patient with epigastric complaints. The use of double-contrast techniques helps to detect small lesions by improving mucosal detail. The stomach should be distended at some time during every radiographic examination since decreased distensibility may be the only indication of a diffuse infiltrative carcinoma. Although gastric ulcers can be detected fairly early, it may be impossible to distinguish benign from malignant lesions. The anatomic location of an ulcer is not in itself an indication of the presence or absence of a cancer.

Radiographic demonstrations of benign-appearing gastric ulcers presents special problems. Some physicians believe that gastroscopy is not mandatory if the radiographic features are typically benign, if complete healing can be visualized by x-ray within 6 weeks, and if a follow-up contrast radiograph several months later is normal. However, many feel that gastroscopic biopsy and brush cytology are required for all patients with a gastric ulcer in order to exclude a malignancy. The identification of malignant gastric ulcers prior to their penetration into surrounding tissues is crucial since the curability of such early lesions when limited to the mucosa or submucosa, even in the United States, is greater than 80 percent. Since gastric carcinomas are difficult to distinguish clinically or radiographically from gastric lymphomas, endoscopic biopsies should be made as deeply as possible due to the submucosal location of lymphoid tumors.

Treatment Surgical removal of the complete tumor with resection of adjacent lymph nodes offers the only chance for cure. However, this is possible in less than one-third of patients. In general, a subtotal gastrectomy represents the treatment of choice for patients with distal carcinomas while total or near-total gastrectomies are required for more proximal tumors. The prognosis following complete surgical resection is adversely influenced by the degree of tumor penetration into the stomach wall, regional lymph node involvement, vascular invasion, and abnormal DNA content (i.e. aneuploidy), characteristics found in the vast majority of American patients. As a result, the probability of survival after 5 years for the 25 to 30 percent of patients in the United States able to undergo a complete resection of a gastric cancer is approximately 25 percent for distal tumors and less than 10 percent for proximal tumors, with continued tumor recurrences being observed for at least 8 years following surgery. In the absence of ascites or extensive hepatic or peritoneal metastases, however, even the patient who is believed to be surgically incurable should be offered an attempt at resecting the primary lesion since the reduction of residual tumor offers the best form of palliation and may enhance the probability of subsequent benefit if chemotherapy and/or radiation therapy are administered.

Gastric adenocarcinoma is a relatively radioresistant tumor, requiring doses of external beam irradiation in excess of the tolerance of surrounding structures such as bowel mucosa and spinal cord if adequate control of the primary tumor is to be achieved. As a result, the major role of radiation therapy in patients with gastric cancer has been limited to palliation of pain. Controlled trials have indicated that radiation therapy alone after a complete resection does not prolong survival. In the setting of surgically unresectable disease limited to the epigastrium, comparative studies have shown that patients treated with 3500 to 4000 cGy did not live longer than similar patients not receiving radiotherapy; however, survival was prolonged slightly when 5-fluorouracil (5-FU) was given concomitantly with radiation therapy. In this clinical setting, the 5-FU may well be functioning as a radiosensitizer.

The administration of combinations of cytotoxic drugs to patients with advanced gastric carcinoma has been associated with reductions of greater than 50 percent in measurable tumor masses ("partial responses") in 30 to 50 percent of cases, providing significant benefit to individuals who respond to treatment. Such drug combinations have generally included 5-FU and doxorubicin together with mitomycin-C, cisplatin, or high doses of methotrexate. Despite this encouraging

response rate for a malignant condition once thought untreatable, complete disappearances of tumor masses remain uncommon, the partial responses are transient, and the overall impact of such multidrug therapy on survival has been a source of debate. The use of prophylactic (i.e., adjuvant) chemotherapy following the complete resection of a gastric cancer as a means of eradicating clinically undetectable micrometastases and improving the potential for cure has generally proven to be unsuccessful. The role of such adjuvant treatment as well as preoperative ("neoadjuvant") chemotherapy should be considered investigational.

PRIMARY GASTRIC LYMPHOMA Primary lymphoma of the stomach is relatively uncommon, comprising about 7 percent of gastric malignancies and about 2 percent of all lymphomas. It is however, the most frequent extranodal location for lymphoma. The disease is difficult to distinguish clinically from gastric adenocarcinoma; both tumors are most often detected during the sixth decade of life, present with epigastric pain, early satiety, and generalized fatigue, and are usually characterized by ulcerations with a ragged, thickened mucosal pattern demonstrated by contrast radiographs. The diagnosis of lymphoma of the stomach may occasionally be made through cytologic brushings of the gastric mucosa, but usually requires a biopsy at the time of gastroscopy or laparotomy. The failure of gastroscopic biopsies to detect lymphoma should not be interpreted as being conclusive since superficial biopsies may miss the more deeply situated lymphoid infiltrate. The macroscopic pathology of gastric lymphoma may also mimic adenocarcinoma, either as a bulky ulcerated lesion localized in the corpus or antrum or as a diffuse process spreading throughout the entire gastric submucosa and even extending into the duodenum. Microscopically, the vast majority of gastric lymphoid tumors are non-Hodgkin's lymphomas of B-cell origin; Hodgkin's disease involving the stomach is extremely uncommon. Histologically, these tumors may range from well-differentiated, superficial processes (mucosa-associated lymphoid tissue, "MALT") to high-grade, large cell lymphomas. Gastric lymphomas spread initially to regional lymph nodes (often to Waldeyer's ring) and may then disseminate.

Primary gastric lymphoma is a far more treatable disease than adenocarcinoma of the stomach, underscoring the need for making the correct diagnosis. All detectable tumor can be removed in over two-thirds of patients by some type of a subtotal gastrectomy. The prognosis in such patients is encouraging with 5-year survival rates of 40 to 60 percent having been reported. The best prognosis seems to be associated with those gastric lymphomas having small, single lesions, more differentiated histologies, and absence of spread to adjacent lymph nodes. While postoperative radiation therapy to the abdomen has been employed in the past, even when all obvious disease has been resected, the value of such a practice is open to serious question since the majority of recurrences develop in anatomic sites distant from the epigastrium and outside the fields of radiation treatment. Combination chemotherapy, which has proved to be highly effective in the management of disseminated non-Hodgkin's lymphoma including the diffuse large cell subtype, has gained favor as an adjunct to surgery, particularly when regional lymph node involvement is present. In the past, such drug therapy was not considered to be a substitute for surgery, even if the lymphoma were localized, since the rapid destruction of lymphoma masses by chemotherapy occasionally led to life-threatening hemorrhage. The results of recent clinical trials, however, have suggested that the probability for such bleeding may be relatively small and that drug treatment alone may be adequate to eradicate the lymphoma. If widespread disease is discovered at the time of laparotomy, combination chemotherapy should be utilized.

GASTRIC (NONLYMPHOID) SARCOMA Leiomyosarcomas are the most common of this group of gastric malignancies and comprise approximately 1 to 3 percent of all gastric neoplasms. They most frequently involve the anterior and posterior walls of the gastric fundus and often ulcerate and bleed. Even those lesions which appear benign on histologic examination may behave in a malignant fashion.

Leiomyosarcomas rarely invade adjacent viscera and characteristically do not metastasize to lymph nodes but may spread to the liver and lungs. The treatment of choice is surgical resection. Combination chemotherapy should be reserved for patients with metastatic disease.

REFERENCES

Esophageal cancer

BLOT WJ et al: Rising incidence of adenocarcinoma of the esophagus and gastric cardia. JAMA 265:1287, 1991

BOYCE HW: Palliation of advanced esophageal cancer. Semin Oncol 11:186, 1984

FORASTIERE AA et al: Preoperative chemoradiation followed by transhiatal esophagectomy for carcinoma of the esophaghus. Final report. J Clin Oncol 11;1118, 1993

HAGIWARA A et al: Endoscopic local injection of a new drug delivery format of pleomycin for superficial esophageal cancer. A pilot study. Gastroenterology 104:1037, 1993

HERSKOVIC A et al: Combined chemotherapy and radiotherapy compared with radiotherapy alone in patients with cancer of the esophagus. N Engl J Med 326:1593, 1992

KELSEN D: Chemotherapy of esophageal cancer. Semin Oncol 11:159, 1984

LIGHTDALE CJ, WINAWER SJ: Screening diagnosis and staging of esophageal cancer. Semin Oncol 11:101, 1984

POPLIN E et al: Combined therapies for squamous-cell carcinoma of the esophagus, a Southwest Oncology Group Study (SWOG - 8037). J. Clin Oncol 5:622, 1987

REID BJ et al: Endoscopic biopsy can detect high-grade dysplasia or early adenocarcinoma in Barrett's esophagus with grossly recognizable neoplastic lesions. Gastroenterology 94:81, 1988

SCHOTTENFELD D: Epidemiology of cancer of the esophagus. Semin Oncol 11:92, 1984

SKINNER DB: Surgical treatment for esophageal carcinoma. Semin Oncol 11:136, 1984

Gastric tumors

BEDIKIAN AY et al: The natural history of gastric cancer and prognostic factors influencing survival. J Clin Oncol 2:305, 1984

CORREA P: Human gastric carcinogenesis: a multistep and multifactorial process—First American Cancer Society award lecture on cancer epidemiology and prevention. Cancer Res 52:6735, 1992

DOUGLASS HO, NAVA HR: Gastric adenocarcinoma—management of the primary disease. Semin Oncol 12:32, 1985

GOHMANN JJ, MACDONALD JS: Chemotherapy of gastric cancer. Cancer Invest 7:39, 1989

HABER DA, MAYER RJ: Primary gastrointestinal lymphoma. Semin Oncol 15:154, 1988

KELSEN D: Adjuvant therapy of upper gastrointestinal tract cancers. Semin Oncol 18:543, 1991

KURTZ RC, SHERLOCK P: The diagnosis of gastric cancer. Semin Oncol 12:11, 1985

LANGMAN MJS: Antisecretory drugs and gastric cancer. Br Med J 290:1850, 1985

LIGHT JD et al: Gastrointestinal sarcomas. Semin Oncol 15:181, 1988

NANUS DM et al: Flow cytometry as a predictive indication in patients with operable gastric cancer. J Clin Oncol 7:1105, 1989

PARSONETT J et al: *Helicobacter pylori* infection and the risk of gastric carcinoma. N Engl J Med 325:1127, 1991

POWELL J, McCONKEY CC: Increasing incidence of adenocarcinoma of the gastric cardia and adjacent sites. Brit J Cancer 62:440, 1990

SEVERSON RK, DAVIS S: Increasing incidence of primary gastric lymphoma. Cancer 66:1283, 1990

TERSMETTE AC et al: Meta-analysis of the risk of gastric stump cancer: detection of high risk patient subsets for stomach cancer after remote partial gastrectomy for benign conditions. Cancer Res 50:6486, 1990

254 DISORDERS OF ABSORPTION

NORTON J. GREENBERGER / KURT J. ISSELBACHER

MECHANISMS OF ABSORPTION

Diseases of the small intestine are frequently accompanied by alterations in intestinal function, and clinically, this impaired function is seen as the malabsorption syndrome. In order to obtain a better appreciation of the derangements which occur in the many disorders of intestinal function, the processes of normal absorption will first be reviewed.

It is important to distinguish between digestion and absorption, since an increased loss of nutrients in the stool may be a reflection of a derangement of either process. Digestion involves the breakdown or hydrolysis of nutrients to smaller molecules in order to prepare the ingested substances for absorption, or transport across the intestinal cell. It will be recalled that most of the digestive process is initiated in the stomach by acid and pepsin and is continued in the upper small intestine primarily by the action of pancreatic enzymes such as lipase, amylase, and trypsin. As a result of these digestive actions carbohydrates are broken down to monosaccharides and disaccharides, proteins to peptides and amino acids, and fats to monoglycerides and fatty acids. In the adult it is in this form that nutrients are, to a large extent, transported across the epithelial surface of the intestinal cell.

ANATOMIC AND PHYSIOLOGIC FACTORS The intestine has an enormous surface area. This can be attributed in large part to its length, which in the adult is more than 4 m, and to the foldings of the surface plicae. At the light-microscopic level, the villi of the small intestine provide additional surface area, which is further augmented by the presence of microvilli (approximately 2×10^8 per square centimeter) on the outer, or brush border, region of epithelial cells. Thus the total absorptive area of the small intestine is enormous.

Motility (contractility) of the bowel is an important process which permits nutrients to remain in intimate contact with the intestinal cells and possibly influences the continued movement of the nutrients *into* and along the absorbing channels, such as the lymphatics. Two types of motility aid in this process: the gross motility of the intestine itself and the motility of individual villi. Entrance of the nutrients into the general circulation is achieved via the capillaries into the portal system or via the lacteals into the intestinal lymphatics.

TYPES OF ABSORPTION (See also Chap. 39)   Four mechanisms have been considered to be important in the transport of substances across the intestinal cell membrane, namely, active transport, passive diffusion, facilitated diffusion, and endocytosis.

Active transport involves the transport of a substance across the cell against an electric or chemical gradient; this process requires energy, is carrier-mediated, and is subject to competitive inhibition. *Passive diffusion* is the opposite of this process; energy is not required, transport is with (rather than against) the electric or chemical gradient, the process is not carrier-mediated, and it does not show properties of competitive inhibition. Thus active transport may be viewed as "uphill" transport, whereas passive diffusion is equivalent to "downhill" transport. *Facilitated diffusion* is similar to passive diffusion except that such a process shows evidence of being carrier-mediated and frequently subject to competitive inhibition.

Endocytosis is a process akin to phagocytosis. By this mechanism, nutrients (soluble or particulate) upon entering the cell are surrounded by the components of the outer plasma cell membrane. In the intestinal tract, endocytosis occurs in the neonatal period and, contrary to earlier belief, also occurs to a limited extent in the adult. While quantitatively limited, it appears to account, at least in part, for uptake of antigens.

SITES OF ABSORPTION   While many substances are absorbed throughout the length of the small intestine, certain nutrients tend to be absorbed more in one region than in others. The proximal intestine is a major area for the absorption of iron, calcium, water-soluble vitamins, and fat (monoglycerides and fatty acids). Sugars are absorbed in the proximal intestine as well as the midintestine. While the amino acids appear to be absorbed primarily in the middle of the small intestine, or jejunum, some absorption also occurs in the upper and lower areas. The distal small intestine appears to be the *major* absorptive area for bile salts and vitamin B_{12}. As is emphasized below, this is of clinical significance in circumstances where there has been removal or disease of the ileum.

The colon is important for the absorption of water and electrolytes, a process which occurs predominantly in the cecum. Although the rectum is not a usual site for absorption of ingested nutrients, drugs introduced by rectum may be absorbed there. Thus drugs introduced by this route, such as salicylates or steroids, may have systemic as well as local effects.

ABSORPTION OF SPECIFIC NUTRIENTS Carbohydrate absorption Much of the carbohydrate we ingest is in the form of starch, a complex polysaccharide consisting of many hexose units (attached either in a 1,4 or 1,6 linkage). By the action of salivary and pancreatic amylase, starch is hydrolyzed to oligosaccharides and then to disaccharides (mostly maltose). While monosaccharides such as glucose are readily absorbed, disaccharides are not. Disaccharides are split enzymatically into their component sugars by disaccharidases (or oligosaccharidases) located in the microvilli of intestinal epithelial cells. The two types of disaccharidases are β-galactosidases (lactase) and α-glucosidases (sucrase, maltase). By the action of these enzymes, lactose is split into glucose and galactose, sucrose into glucose and fructose, and maltose into two molecules of glucose. The resultant monosaccharides are then transported through the cell into the portal circulation. Most disaccharides are hydrolyzed so rapidly by brush border enzymes that the capacity of the transport mechanism is exceeded and some monosaccharides diffuse back into the intestinal lumen. Lactose, however, is hydrolyzed at a slower rate, and thus lactose hydrolysis is the rate-limiting step in lactose absorption.

Sugars such as glucose and galactose are absorbed by an active transport mechanism. Glucose (and galactose) entry into the cell is largely coupled to sodium ions (so-called symport); both sodium and glucose appear to bind to the hexose carrier in the microvillus membrane. Energy is required for the movement of glucose into the cell, which seems largely to come from the sodium pump and the Na^+,K^+-ATPase of the basolateral membrane (see below).

Protein and amino acid absorption Dietary proteins are initially subject to degradation in the stomach by pepsin. However, complete hydrolysis is largely achieved by the action of pancreatic trypsin and chymotrypsin, as well as by other endopeptidases and exopeptidases such as carboxypeptidase. By these enzymatic processes, oligopeptides, dipeptides, and amino acids are formed. Just as there are disaccharidases in mucosal cells to digest disaccharides, there are also oligopeptidases to split small peptides. Dipeptidases are located in the cytoplasm as well as on the microvilli. Dipeptides are absorbed more rapidly than amino acids, and presumably their uptake involves a separate mechanism. Thus digestion of proteins to amino acids occurs in three locations: intestinal lumen, brush border, and cytoplasm of mucosal cells. As indicated above, contrary to earlier beliefs, proteins also can be absorbed by the adult intestine. Although quantitatively limited, protein absorption can be immunologically significant.

Most naturally occurring amino acids are L-amino acids, and these are subject to a number of different transport processes. *Neutral* amino acids share a common carrier mechanism; thus amino acids such as tryptophan and alanine show competitive inhibition. Among the *dibasic* amino acids which appear to have a distinct transport

mechanism are arginine, ornithine, and lysine. The neutral amino acid cystine shares this mechanism. There is a separate transport system for *glycine* and the *imino acids* proline and hydroxyproline. There is also a transport system for *dicarboxylic* acids such as glutamic and aspartic acids. Therefore, in genetic disorders such as cystinuria, one will find impaired absorption not only of cystine but also of arginine, ornithine, and lysine. Similarly, in Hartnup disease, a defect in the transport of neutral amino acids (especially of tryptophan, phenylalanine, histidine) is found. In these genetic disorders, uptake and absorption of dipeptides is normal (see Chap. 353).

Absorption of amino acids is rapid in the duodenum and jejunum but slow in the ileum. As in the case of carbohydrates, sodium ions are necessary for the entry of these acids and the energy needed for their concentration within the cell. Some amino acids have affinity for more than one mechanism. For example, glycine may be transported by both the neutral and imino acid transport systems.

Fat absorption (Fig. 254-1) Most of the ingested dietary fats are in the form of long-chain triglycerides. These triglycerides contain both saturated fatty acids (such as palmitic and stearic) and unsaturated fatty acids (such as oleic and linoleic). The particle size of the fat is decreased largely by the churning action of the stomach. The entry of fat into the duodenum, plus the presence of acid, causes release of secretin and cholecystokinin, which in turn leads to a stimulation of the flow of bile and pancreatic juice.

ROLE OF PANCREATIC LIPASE The hydrolysis of triglycerides by pancreatic lipase is a complex process involving lipase, colipase, and bile salts. Pancreatic lipase binds to the oil-water interface of an emulsified triglyceride substrate. The detergent properties of bile salts permit pancreatic lipase to gain access to water-insoluble lipids. One of the important functions of bile salts is to clear the oil-water interface of dietary fat from proteins of exogenous and endogenous origin, thus making it available for pancreatic lipolysis. Colipase, a protein present in pancreatic juice, is also essential for the action of lipase; its function is to anchor the lipase close to the surface of the triglyceride droplet. All three components, i.e., pancreatic lipase, colipase, and bile salts, form a *ternary complex* which generates lipolytic products that diffuse away from the complex and are absorbed. With colipase present, lipase remains at the interface and forms 2-monoglycerides and fatty acids, which are the major end products of triglyceride hydrolysis. Less than 5 percent of ingested fat remains in the form of diglycerides and triglycerides. Without colipase, bile acids would actually wash pancreatic lipase away from the interface, and the hydrolytic rate of triglycerides would be reduced.

FIGURE 254-1 Scheme of intestinal digestion, absorption, esterification, and transport of dietary triglycerides. TG = triglycerides; FA = fatty acids; MG = monoglycerides; BS = bile salts.

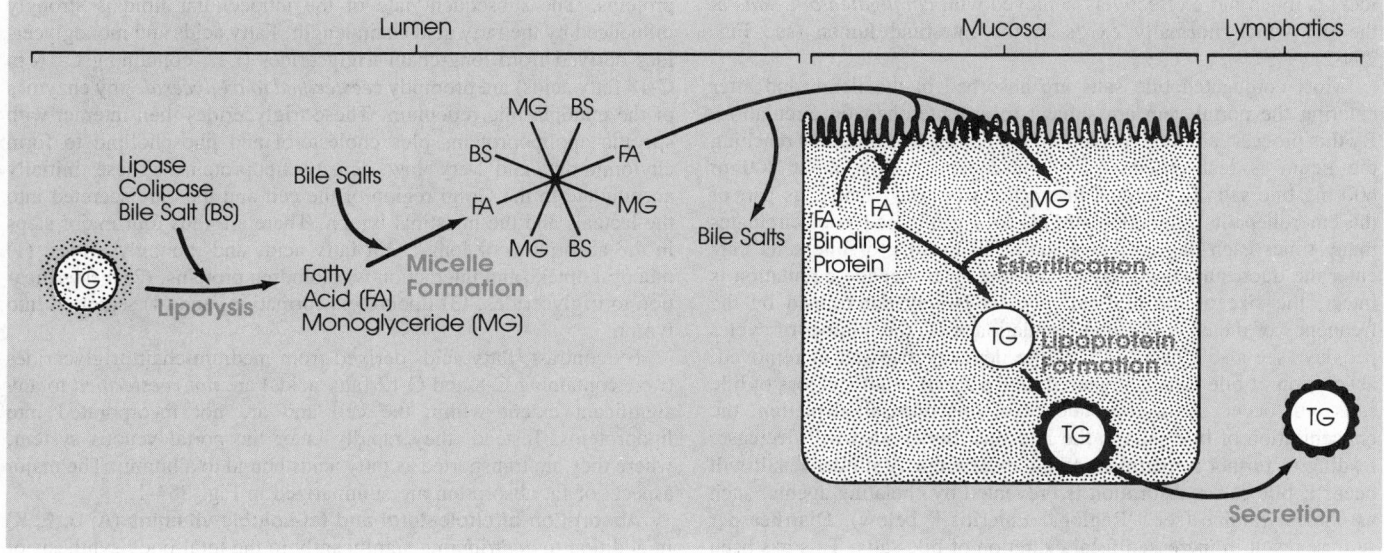

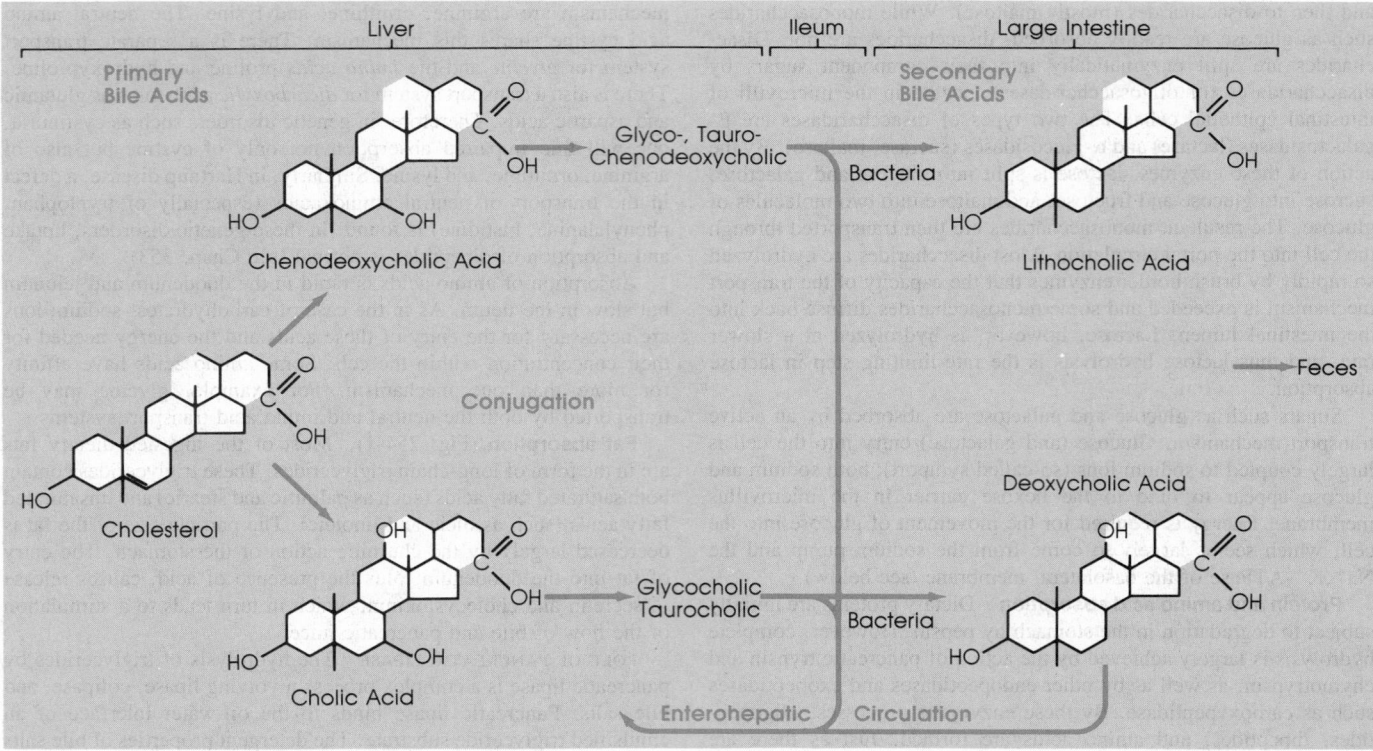

FIGURE 254-2 Scheme of hepatic and intestinal metabolism of bile salts and the enterohepatic circulation (from ileum to liver). Note that bacteria lead to the formation of secondary bile acids; of the latter, only deoxycholic acid is absorbed to any appreciable extent.

ROLE OF BILE SALTS (Fig. 254-2) Bile salts play an important role in the digestion and absorption of fat. They are synthesized in the liver (approximately 200 to 600 mg daily) from cholesterol and excreted in the bile in the form of their glycine or taurine conjugates. In humans the principal bile acids excreted are conjugates of cholic and chenodeoxycholic acid. Bile salts are good detergents, because they have both polar (hydrophilic) and nonpolar (hydrophobic) groups. During digestion, the concentration of conjugated bile salts in the lumen is in the range of 5 to 15 μmol/mL, and at these concentrations the bile salts aggregate to form *micelles*. Fatty acids and monoglycerides enter these micelles, forming mixed micelles. An emulsion of triglyceride is turbid; mixed micelles containing bile salts, fatty acids, and monoglycerides are clear solutions. The formation of *mixed micelles*, and hence the solubilization of fatty acids and monoglycerides, is much more effectively achieved with *conjugated bile salts* at the pH which normally exists in the intestinal lumen (see Fig. 254-2).

Most conjugated bile salts are absorbed in the ileum and after entering the portal vein are subject to an enterohepatic circulation. By this process, about 90 percent of the conjugated bile salts reaching the ileum is reabsorbed. As a consequence, only about 200 to 600 mg bile salts is excreted in the feces per day, while, as part of the enterohepatic circulation, the 3- to 4-g bile salt pool circulates many times each day so that actually 20 to 30 g of bile salts may enter the duodenum each day. When the enterohepatic circulation is intact, the size of the bile salt pool is largely determined by the frequency of the enterohepatic circulation, i.e., the number of cycles per day (see also Chap. 272). If the ileum is diseased or removed, absorption of bile salts is impaired, and a significant fecal loss of bile salts will occur. As a consequence of this bile salt depletion, the concentration of bile salts in the intestinal lumen also will decrease, leading to further impairment of fat absorption. A similar result will occur if bile salt reabsorption is prevented by chelating agents, such as cholestyramine (see "Regional Enteritis," below). Diarrhea per se may result in increased fecal excretion of bile salts. This has been demonstrated both in normal subjects in whom diarrhea has been induced and in patients with chronic idiopathic diarrhea.

INTRAMUCOSAL ASPECTS OF FAT ABSORPTION (Fig. 254-1) After the hydrolysis of fatty acids to monoglycerides and their interaction with bile salts to form mixed micelles, the lipids pass through an "unstirred" water layer covering the cell surface. The mixed micelles apparently do not enter the cell, but instead the component fatty acids and monoglycerides are released from the micellar phase and then enter the cell by diffusion. In aqueous duodenal contents, large bile salt mixed micelles saturated with products of lipolysis coexist with larger liquid crystal liposomes of the same lipids saturated with free fatty acids and mixed bile salts. These phases are interconvertible, and both may be important in fat digestion and absorption. Upon entry into the mucosal cell, fatty acids interact with specific binding proteins. The subsequent fate of the intracellular lipid is strongly influenced by the fatty acid chain length. Fatty acids and monoglycerides derived from long-chain triglycerides (i.e., containing C-16 to C-18 fatty acids) are promptly *reesterified to triglycerides* by enzymes of the endoplasmic reticulum. These triglycerides then interact with specific apolipoproteins plus cholesterol and phospholipid to form chylomicrons and very low density lipoproteins. These initially accumulate in the Golgi region of the cell and then are secreted into the lacteals and the intestinal lymph. There are thus four major steps in the absorption of long-chain fatty acids and monoglycerides: (1) mucosal uptake and interaction with binding proteins, (2) reesterification to triglycerides, (3) lipoprotein formation, and (4) secretion into lymph.

By contrast, fatty acids derived from medium-chain triglycerides (i.e., containing C-8 and C-12 fatty acids) are *not reesterified* to any significant extent within the cell and are not incorporated into lipoproteins. Instead, they rapidly enter the portal venous system, where they are transported as fatty acids bound to albumin. The major aspects of fat absorption are summarized in Fig. 254-1.

Absorption of cholesterol and fat-soluble vitamins (A, D, E, K)
In addition to contributing significantly to the total-body synthesis of

cholesterol, the intestine also plays an active role in the absorption of cholesterol and its esters. Within the lumen, cholesterol esters from the bile and diet are hydrolyzed by a pancreatic esterase. There is also a separate cholesterol esterase in the intestinal microvilli which completes this hydrolysis. As a result, only free cholesterol enters the intestinal cell. However, just as in the case of long-chain fatty acids, much of the cholesterol is reesterified and is then secreted primarily into lymph.

The absorption mechanisms of the fat-soluble vitamins A, D, E, and K are not well understood. The intestine is able to convert β-carotene into vitamin A. The vitamin A thus formed or absorbed from the lumen is esterified in the mucosa primarily with palmitic acid, transported in the chylomicrons of the lymph, and stored as retinol palmitate in the liver. The other lipid-soluble vitamins also appear in lymph chylomicrons, but esterification with fatty acids does not appear to be necessary for their transport.

Water and sodium absorption (See also Chap. 39)   The mechanisms responsible for fluid absorption differ in the jejunum, ileum, and colon. There are two pathways by which water and ions cross the intestinal mucosa: the paracellular and transcellular pathways. Individual intestinal mucosa cells are joined near their apex by a "tight junction," and ions and water traverse this *paracellular* pathway during absorption and secretion. The tight junction pathway contains aqueous-filled channels or pores. Such intercellular spaces are closed in the resting state and dilated during absorption. Considerable evidence has accumulated indicating that pumps and carriers are involved in intestinal water and solute transport. For example, in the ileum, Na^+ enters in exchange for H^+, and Cl^- enters in exchange for HCO_3^-. Sodium entry into the cell also occurs coupled with glucose via the glucose-sodium carrier in the microvillus membrane. Inside the cell, the Na^+ pump located in the basolateral membrane actively transports Na^+ out of the mucosal cell and into the intercellular space. *Transcellular* transport requires passage of ions through two membrane barriers, i.e., the apical brush border plasma membrane and the basolateral membrane. After Na^+ and Cl^- are transported across the brush border membrane into the cell, Na^+ is pumped across the basolateral membrane and Cl^- either follows passively or is also pumped into the intercellular space. The Na^+,K^+-ATPase is present in the basolateral but not in the brush border membrane and is the biochemical mediator of this pump. Bulk water movement obviously influences the movement of Na^+, K^+, and Cl^-. This "solvent drag" effect is explained by two mechanisms: (1) solutes may be caught in a moving stream of water and transported across a membrane, and (2) water movement results in increased concentration of solute on the side of the membrane from which water was transported, which causes solute to diffuse through the direction of flow. Diarrhea can be simply defined as impaired net absorption of water and electrolytes by the small intestine or colon. Some mechanisms producing diarrhea are listed in Table 254-1.

Calcium absorption   Calcium is actively transported by the small intestine, and this process is intimately linked to the active form of vitamin D_3, namely, 1,25-dihydroxycholecalciferol. The role of two other intestinal cell proteins, calcium-binding protein and calmodulin, in the absorption of calcium remains unclear. Recent studies indicate that calcium is absorbed to the same extent from various calcium salts (carbonate, citrate, gluconate, lactate, and acetate) and from milk in healthy subjects; an average of 32 percent of the ingested calcium was absorbed from the various sources.

Iron absorption   The formation of soluble iron complexes is important for maintaining intraluminal iron in an absorbable form. Gastric acid facilitates the chelation of inorganic iron with substances such as ascorbic acid, sugars, amino acids, and bile; these macromolecular complexes then remain soluble in the more alkaline duodenum and jejunum. With the average western diet the iron intake averages 15 to 25 mg/d; iron absorption averages 0.5 to 1.0 mg/d in men and 1.0 to 2.0 mg/d in women during their reproductive years. Iron is actively transported by the small intestine, and the duodenum is the principal site of iron absorption. The transferrin receptor and also

TABLE 254-1   Some mechanisms in the production of diarrhea

SECRETORY DIARRHEA

A Secretory agents associated with adenylate cyclase system
   1 Enterotoxin-producing bacteria (*Vibrio cholerae, Escherichia coli*)
   2 Methylxanthines (caffeine, theophylline)
   3 Prostaglandins
   4 Vasoactive intestinal peptide (VIP)
   5 Dihydroxy bile acids (affect colon primarily; effects seen after ileal resection)
B Secretory agents *not associated* with adenylate cyclase system
   1 Glucagon, secretin, cholecystokinin-pancreozymin, serotonin, calcitonin, gastrin inhibitory polypeptide (GIP)
   2 Some laxatives* (ricinoleic acid, bisacodyl, phenolphthalein, dioctyl sodium sulfosuccinate)
   3 Bacterial enterotoxins (*Shigella, Staphylococcus aureus, Clostridium perfringens*)
C Mucosal injury, altered cell permeability
   1 *Salmonella, Shigella*, invasive *E. coli*, gastroenteritis viruses
   2 Celiac sprue
   3 Inflammatory bowel disease (ulcerative colitis, regional enteritis)
D Neoplasms with or without hormone production
   1 Gastrinoma (gastrin)
   2 Carcinoid syndrome (serotonin, prostaglandins)
   3 Medullary carcinoma of thyroid (calcitonin, prostaglandins)
   4 Pancreatic cholera syndrome (? VIP)
   5 Villous adenoma
E Medications
   1 Diuretics
   2 Theophylline
   3 Colchicine
   4 Prostaglandins (misoprostol)
   5 Azodisalicylate
F Congenital
   1 Microvillus inclusion disease
   2 Congenital chloridorrhea

OSMOTIC DIARRHEA

A Impaired carbohydrate absorption
   1 Disaccharidase deficiency (lactose or sucrose-isomaltose intolerance)
   2 Glucose-galactose malabsorption
B Nonabsorbable osmotically active agents (lactulose, sorbitol, mannitol, dietetic foods)
C Laxative ingestion or abuse
   1 Saline purgatives (magnesium phosphate, magnesium hydroxide–containing antacids)
D Postoperative disorders
   1 Vagotomy and pyloroplasty*
   2 Gastrojejunostomy* (Billroth I and II)

MOTILITY DISORDERS

A Laxative abuse*
B Irritable bowel syndrome
C Diverticular disease of the colon
D Diabetic diarrhea with visceral neuropathy
E Hyperthyroidism

* Multiple mechanisms involved in production of diarrhea.

duodenal ferritin in small intestinal mucosal cells appear to have a regulatory/inhibitory role in iron absorption. The absorption of elemental iron in humans and animals involves at least two distinct steps: (1) mucosal uptake of iron from the lumen and (2) mucosal transfer of iron to the plasma. Much of the iron entering the mucosal cell is not transferred to the plasma but remains trapped within the cell and is excreted into the lumen when the cell is shed. Iron lost by this mechanism seems to vary inversely with body iron stores. However, this mucosal regulatory mechanism can be overcome when pharmacologic doses of iron are ingested. Hemoglobin iron is also absorbed by human subjects depending on body requirements for iron; the heme is split from globin in the lumen and absorbed as an intact metalloporphyrin. Organic iron in the form of hemoglobin is absorbed more effectively than iron from cereals and vegetables. The absorption of inorganic iron is increased by ascorbic acid. Similarly, the presence of anemia, liver injury, pregnancy, idiopathic hemochromatosis, or a portacaval shunt may result in increased iron absorption.

Conversely, the prior ingestion of large doses of iron and the presence in the lumen of phosphates, carbonates, and phytates may lead to decreased absorption of inorganic iron. Impaired absorption of iron is frequent in disorders (such as celiac sprue) which involve the duodenal mucosa.

Water-soluble vitamins   *Vitamin B_{12} absorption* is discussed in Chap. 304. In the case of *folic acid absorption*, it should be emphasized that folates exist in food conjugated with glutamyl peptides. These *polyglutamates* must be deconjugated (by folic deconjugase) to monoglutamates for absorption to occur. Certain drugs (such as oral contraceptives, sulfasalazine, diphenylhydantoin, trimethoprim, and pyrimethamine) inhibit the absorption of dietary folate and hence can cause folate deficiency. Sulfasalazine, for example, competitively inhibits three enzymes important in the intestinal metabolism of folate, i.e., dihydrofolate reductase, methylene tetrahydrofolate reductase, and serine transhydroxymethylase. Thiamine and riboflavin appear to be absorbed by passive diffusion.

TESTS USEFUL IN THE DIAGNOSIS OF MALABSORPTION
Most of the tests useful in the diagnosis of malabsorption indicate the presence of abnormal absorptive or digestive function, and only a few tests may suggest a specific diagnosis. Accordingly, it is frequently necessary to employ a combination of tests to establish a diagnosis. To illustrate the use of various tests, the characteristic findings in celiac sprue, an example of a primary malabsorptive disorder, and pancreatic insufficiency, an example of impaired digestion, are compared in Table 254-2.

Stool fat   The qualitative examination of the stool for undigested muscle fibers, neutral fat, and split fat is a simple and reliable screening test for steatorrhea. The finding of an increased number of muscle fibers indicates impaired intraluminal digestion. Properly performed, the qualitative microscopic examination of a stool specimen with the Sudan III stain is of value and correlates well with the quantitative determination of fecal fat. The latter remains the most reliable measurement of steatorrhea. A normal fecal fat excretion is less than 6 g for 24 h, or greater than 94 percent coefficient of fat absorption. It has been demonstrated that diarrhea itself can induce mild secondary steatorrhea. When the quantitative fecal fat test is used in patients with diarrhea, mild abnormalities (up to 14 g/d) are not specific for a primary defect in fat digestion or absorption, i.e., they may represent false-positive results.

Although not used frequently, oral [^{14}C]triolein can be used as an effective test for fat absorption. During the digestive process, the triolein is hydrolyzed, and the labeled glycerol is absorbed and metabolized by the liver. The $^{14}CO_2$ produced is exhaled and can then be measured hourly (for 6 h) in the expired air. Normally, more than 3.5 percent of the administered label [0.185 MBq (5 μCi)] appears in the breath per hour.

Xylose absorption   In the most commonly employed test of carbohydrate absorption, the patient ingests 25 g D-xylose. A 5-h urine xylose excretion of 26 mmol (4.0 g) or greater is considered normal. Low values may be obtained in patients with ascites, intestinal bacterial overgrowth, or renal insufficiency, after administration of certain drugs (e.g., aspirin, indomethacin), and most commonly if the urine collection is incomplete. To prevent difficulties in interpreting the test, it is advisable to determine the blood xylose level 2 h after ingestion of xylose. A blood xylose level of 2 mmol/L (30 mg/dL) or greater indicates normal absorption of D-xylose. An abnormal D-xylose absorption test is found most frequently in disorders affecting the mucosa of the proximal small intestine, such as celiac sprue and tropical sprue.

Gastrointestinal x-ray studies   All patients with malabsorption should have radiographic examinations of the small intestine and, in many cases, of the esophagus, stomach, and colon as well. Occasionally, the latter two examinations may provide important clues to the presence of such disorders as celiac sprue, scleroderma, Zollinger-Ellison syndrome, regional enteritis, ulcerative colitis, and intestinal fistulas. Traditional radiographic findings suggesting a diagnosis of

malabsorption include flocculation of barium within fluid-filled loops causing fragmentation and segmentation of the barium column. However, these patterns are no longer demonstrated reliably in small-bowel series because of widespread use of barium products that contain a nonflocculating suspension of micropulverized barium sulfate. In celiac sprue, the most consistent abnormalities are thickened and nodular duodenal folds and dilatation of the small bowel. However, these findings are nonspecific and may be found in several of the disorders listed in Table 254-3. Some representative examples of abnormal small-bowel radiographs are shown in Fig. 254-3.

Small-intestinal biopsy   The most commonly used instrument for obtaining peroral biopsy specimens from the small intestine is the upper gastrointestinal endoscope, which has largely superseded the use of the Crosby, Carey, and Ross-Moore capsules. Examination of small-bowel biopsy specimens has proved to be of considerable value in the differential diagnosis of malabsorptive disorders. Table 254-3 lists disorders associated with abnormalities in intestinal biopsies, and Fig. 254-4 depicts some illustrative lesions.

Schilling test for vitamin B_{12} absorption   The Schilling test is valuable in the differential diagnosis of malabsorption and is frequently carried out in three stages: (1) without intrinsic factor, (2) with intrinsic factor, and (3) after a course of treatment with antibiotics or anti-inflammatory drugs. Since vitamin B_{12} is absorbed primarily in the distal ileum, an abnormal Schilling test may indicate a pathologic condition of the distal small bowel. In disorders affecting the terminal ileum, such as regional enteritis and lymphomas, the first- and second-stage Schilling tests are frequently abnormal. The ileal receptor site appears to be damaged in these disorders, and the impaired absorption of B_{12} is not corrected by the addition of intrinsic factor or the use of antibiotics. However, the Schilling test may normalize after treatment with prednisone or sulfasalazine. The Schilling test also may be useful in establishing a diagnosis of abnormal bacterial overgrowth of the small bowel, which may be present in disorders such as blind loop syndrome, scleroderma, and multiple small-bowel diverticula (see below). In the blind loop syndrome, for example, the bacteria can actually take up vitamin B_{12} with resultant impaired absorption of B_{12}. Under these conditions, the first-stage Schilling test is frequently abnormal, as is the second stage. After appropriate antibiotic treatment, the Schilling test usually returns to normal. Vitamin B_{12} absorption is frequently abnormal in patients with exocrine pancreatic insufficiency (see Chap. 274).

Secretin and other pancreatic tests   The secretin test, secretin cholecystokinin test, intraduodenal perfusion with essential amino acids, and bentiromide test, which may be useful in establishing a diagnosis of pancreatic insufficiency, are discussed in detail in Chap. 273.

Serum calcium, albumin, cholesterol, magnesium, and iron   Abnormal serum calcium, albumin, cholesterol, magnesium, and iron values may be found in several malabsorptive disorders. The primary value of such tests is to suggest that abnormal intestinal absorptive function may be present. These tests are usually of limited value in the *differential diagnosis* of malabsorption but, if abnormal, may be helpful in supporting this diagnosis.

Serum carotenes, vitamin A, and prothrombin time   Absorption of the fat-soluble vitamins A, D, K, and E is frequently impaired in patients with steatorrhea. Measurements of serum carotene and vitamin A levels are useful as screening tests for malabsorption. However, other tests not only are more sensitive but often give more specific information than the serum carotene and vitamin A levels. The blood prothrombin time is an important test, since patients with malabsorption may present with abnormal bleeding due to vitamin K deficiency. If the decreased prothrombin activity is due to malabsorption, it should be readily correctable with parenteral vitamin K.

Breath tests   The bile acid breath test utilizing [^{14}C]cholylglycine is a reasonably reliable screening test for bacterial overgrowth syndromes. Approximately two-thirds of patients with a positive small-bowel culture will have an abnormal bile acid breath test.

TABLE 254-2 Tests useful in the diagnosis of malabsorptive disorders

Test	Normal values	Malabsorption (celiac sprue)	Maldigestion (pancreatic insufficiency)	Comment
I Quantitative determination of stool fat	<6 g per 24 h: >95% coefficient of fat absorption	>6 g per 24 h	>6 g per 24 h	Best test for establishing presence of steatorrhea
II Carbohydrate absorption				
A D-Xylose absorption (25-g oral dose)	5-h urinary excretion >26 mmol (>4.5 g); peak blood level >2.0 mmol/L (>30 mg/dL)	↓	Normal	A good screening test for carbohydrate absorption
III Small-intestine x-rays		Malabsorption pattern	Normal or minimal malabsorption pattern; occasionally pancreatic calcification	
IV Blood tests				
A Serum calcium	2.2–2.7 mmol/L (9–11 mg/dL)	Frequently ↓	Usually normal	
B Serum albumin	35–55 g/L (3.5–5.5 g/dL)	Frequently ↓	Usually normal	Decreased levels of both serum albumin and globulins should raise the question of protein-losing enteropathy
C Serum cholesterol	3.90–6.45 mmol/L (150–250 mg/dL)	↓	Frequently ↓	Usually decreased in disorders associated with significant steatorrhea
D Serum iron	14–24 μmol/L (80–150 μg/dL)	Frequently ↓	Normal	Low values may reflect decreased body iron stores
E Serum magnesium	0.6–1.0 mmol/L (1.2–2.0 mEq/L)	Frequently ↓	Usually normal	
F Serum zinc	12–20 μmol/L	Frequently ↓	Usually normal	Decreased levels common in malnutrition, cirrhosis, and malabsorption
G Serum carotenes	>100 IU/dL	↓	Usually ↓	Fairly satisfactory screening tests for malabsorption
H Serum vitamin A	>100 IU/dL	↓		
I Prothrombin time	70–100%; 12–15 s	Frequently ↓	Frequently ↓	
V Small intestinal mucosal biopsy		Abnormal	Normal	A specific diagnosis can be established in a small number of disorders (see text)
VI Urine tests				
A Vitamin B₁₂ absorption	>8% urinary excretion in 48 h	Frequently ↓	Frequently ↓	Useful in determining whether vitamin B_{12} malabsorption is due to gastric or small-intestinal disorders
B Urine 5-hydroxyindole-acetic acid (5-HIAA)	10–47 μmol per 24 h (2–9 mg per 24 h)	↑	Normal	Slightly increased level (12–16 mg per 24 h) characteristically found in celiac sprue
VII Breath tests				
A Breath H₂ (after 50 g lactose)	Minimal breath H_2	May be ↑	Normal	Secondary to lactase deficiency (see text)
B Breath H₂ (after 10 g lactulose)	Minimal breath H_2	May be normal or ↓	Normal	Early peak in bacterial overgrowth; can be used to determine intestinal transit time
C Breath ¹⁴CO₂ (after [¹⁴C]xylose)	Minute amounts $^{14}CO_2$	May be ↓	Usually normal	Increased in bacterial overgrowth
D Glycocholic acid metabolism (oral glycine-1-[¹⁴C]glycocholate)	<1% of dose excreted $^{14}CO_2$ in 4 h	Normal	Normal	Increased $^{14}CO_2$ excretion with bacterial overgrowth or bile acid malabsorption (due to ileal resection or inflammatory disease)
	<4% of dose excreted in stools	Normal	Normal	Increased fecal excretion of ^{14}C in bile acid malabsorption
E [¹⁴C]Triolein absorption (breath test)	>3.5% of dose as breath $^{14}CO_2$ per hour	Decreased	Decreased	Correlates well with chemical stool fat; recently introduced test
VIII Miscellaneous				
A Bacteria (culture)	<10³ organisms per milliliter	Normal	Normal	>10⁵ organisms per milliliter indicates bacterial overgrowth
B Secretin test	Volume >1.8 (mL/kg)/h Bicarbonate concentration >80 mmol/L	Normal	Abnormal	See discussion of pancreatic insufficiency in Chaps. 273 and 274
C Bentiromide test	Urine excretion arylamines ≥50%	May be abnormal	Abnormal	See discussion of pancreatic disease in Chaps. 273 and 274

However, in patients with suspected malabsorption of bile acids, the test is rather insensitive without the additional determination of fecal bile acid excretion. The excretion of breath hydrogen after ingestion of lactose is a sensitive, specific, and noninvasive test for detecting lactase deficiency. Lactulose and [¹⁴C]xylose breath tests for bacterial overgrowth also have been found helpful.

PATHOPHYSIOLOGIC BASIS FOR SYMPTOMS AND SIGNS IN MALABSORPTIVE DISORDERS The common symptoms and signs found in malabsorptive disorders are listed in Table 254-4. The most frequent symptoms are those of malnutrition, weight loss, and diarrhea. However, in each of the clinical settings listed in Table 254-4, it is important to consider the cause of the malabsorption.

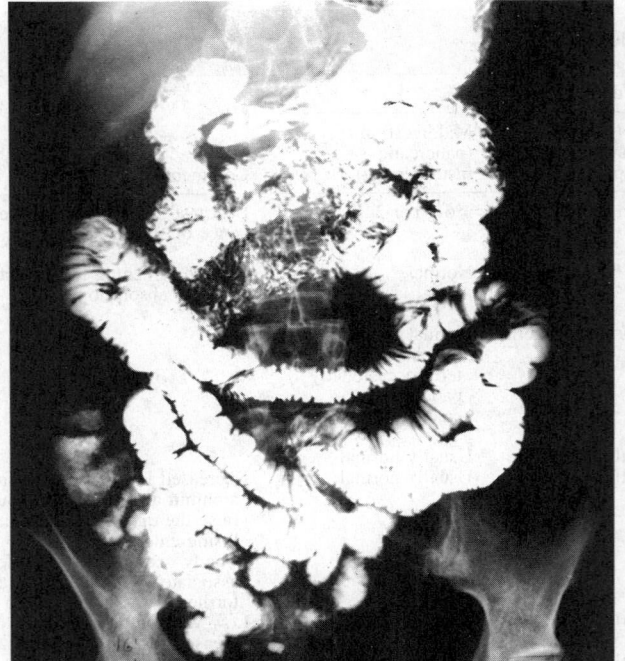

A

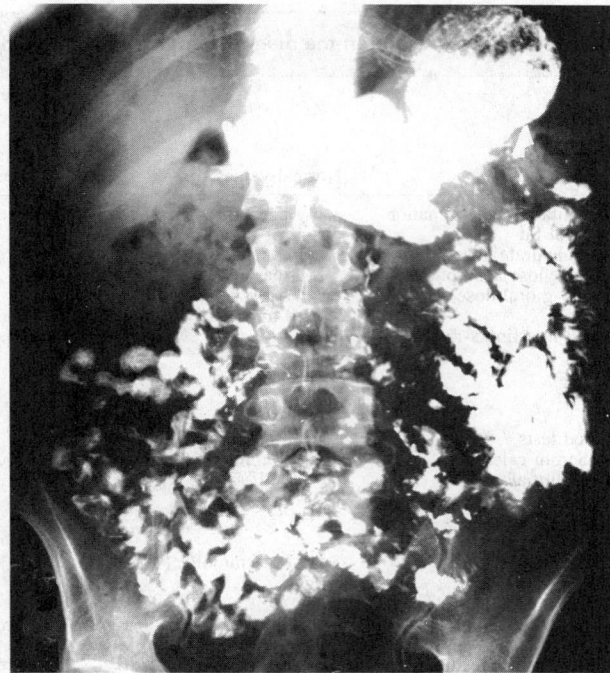

B

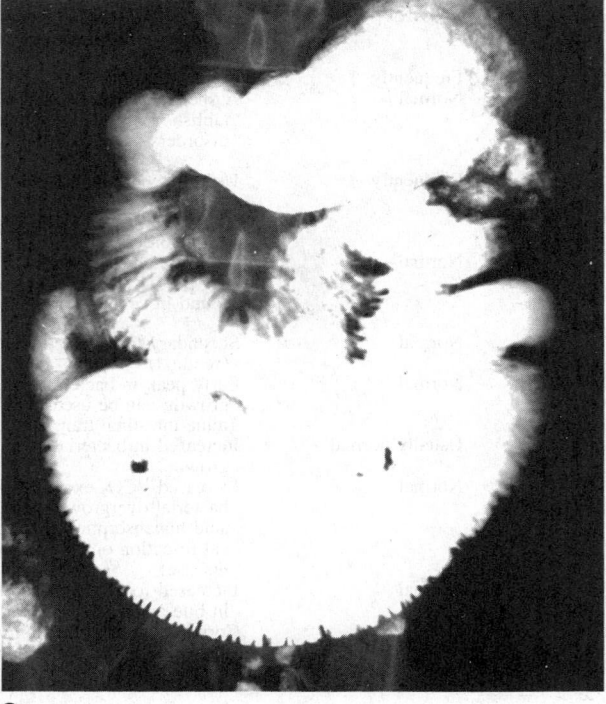

C

FIGURE 254-3   *A*. X-ray of a normal small intestine showing good mucosal pattern. *B*. Intestinal x-ray of a patient with celiac sprue. Note dilatation of small bowel, lack of mucosal markings, and segmentation and clumping of barium. *C*. Intestinal x-ray of patient with obstructed lymphatics due to Köhlmeier-Degos disease, with "accordion-pleated" pattern (*lower edge*).

DISORDERS OF MALABSORPTION (See Table 254-5)

INADEQUATE DIGESTION   Liver and biliary tract disease   It is not generally appreciated that patients with acute or chronic liver disease may develop malabsorption due to impaired intraluminal digestion. Steatorrhea has been described in acute viral hepatitis,

chronic extrahepatic biliary tract obstruction, primary biliary cirrhosis, and postnecrotic and nutritional cirrhosis. Absorption of D-xylose and vitamin B_{12} is usually normal, and small-intestinal mucosal biopsy specimens are generally unremarkable. The steatorrhea associated with liver and biliary tract disease is thought to be due to impaired

---

TABLE 254-3   Disorders asscoiated with abnormalities in small-bowel biopsy specimens

BIOPSY HAS DIAGNOSTIC VALUE (DIFFUSE LESIONS)

A Whipple's disease: Lamina propria infiltrated with macrophages containing PAS-positive glycoproteins
B Abetalipoproteinemia: Villus structure normal; epithelial cells vacuolated due to excess fat
C Agammaglobuinemia: Flattened or absent villi; increased lymphocyte infiltration; absence of plasma cells

BIOPSY MAY HAVE DIAGNOSTIC VALUE (PATCHY LESIONS)

A Intestinal lymphoma: Infiltration of lamina propria and submucosa with malignant cells
B Intestinal lymphangiectasia: Dilated lacteals and lymphatics in lamina propria; clubbed villi
C Eosinophilic enteritis: Diffuse or patchy eosinophilic infiltration in lamina propria and mucosa
D Amyloidosis: Presence of amyloid confirmed by special stains
E Regional enteritis: Noncaseating granulomas
F Parasitic infestations: Parasitic invasion of mucosa; adherence of trophozoites to mucosal surface, as in giardiasis
G Systemic mastocytosis: Mast cell infiltration of lamina propria

BIOPSY IS ABNORMAL BUT NOT DIAGNOSTIC

A Celiac sprue: Shortened or absent villi; hypertrophied crypts; damaged surface epithelium; mononuclear infiltrate
B "Collagenous" sprue: Indistinguishable from celiac sprue; extensive subepithelial collagen deposition
C Tropical sprue: Lesion similar to celiac sprue with shortened or absent villi; lymphocyte infiltration
D Folate deficiency: Shortened villi; megalocytosis; decreased mitoses in crypts
E Vitamin B_{12} deficiency: Similar to folate deficiency
F Acute radiation enteritis: Similar to folate deficiency
G Systemic scleroderma: Fibrosis around Brunner's glands
H Bacterial overgrowth syndromes: Patchy damage to villi and increased lymphocyte infiltration

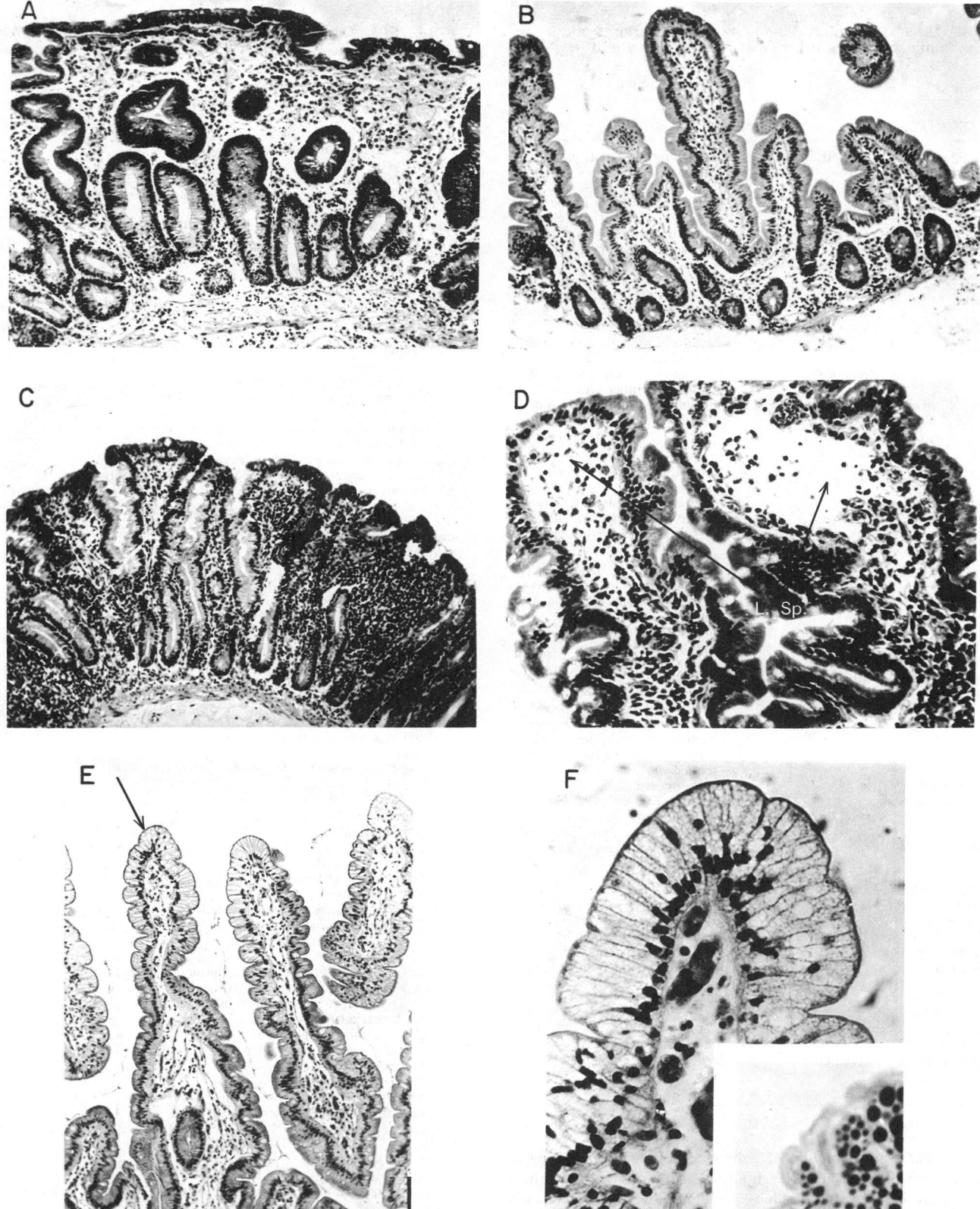

FIGURE 254-4 Typical peroral intestinal biopsies. *A*. Jejunal mucosa of patient with celiac sprue. Note virtual absence of villi, elongated crypts (some cut in cross section), mononuclear infiltrate, cuboidal instead of columnar epithelium on top of villi (300×). *B*. Biopsy from the same patient as in *A*, after 9 months on a gluten-free diet. Note reappearance of villi with normal-appearing columnar cells and reduction in infiltrate and crypt height (300×). *C*. Biopsy from patient with agammaglobulinemia. The features bear a striking resemblance to those of celiac sprue. There is a marked mononuclear infiltration, some of it in aggregates (200×). *D*. Close-up of villi of patient with protein-losing enteropathy. Note broadened and dilated tips, and lymphatic spaces (*arrows*). (450×). *E*. Intestinal biopsy from patient with abetalipoproteinemia. The villus tips have a "lacy" appearance (*arrow*) due to retained fat (300×). *F*. High-power micrograph of villus in *E*. Vacuoles are filled with lipid (750×). Insert shows dark-staining (osmium) lipid droplets in mucosal cells (osmium counterstained with Giemsa; 800×).

TABLE 254-4 Pathophysiologic basis for symptoms and signs in malabsorptive disorders

Symptom or sign	Pathophysiology
GASTROINTESTINAL	
Generalized malnutrition and weight loss	Malabsorption of fat, carbohydrate, and protein → loss of calories
Diarrhea	Impaired absorption or increased secretion of water and electrolytes; unabsorbed dihydroxy bile acids and fatty acids → decreased absorption of water and electrolytes; excess load of fluid and electrolytes presented to the colon may exceed its absorptive capacity
Flatus	Bacterial fermentation of unabsorbed carbohydrate
Glossitis, cheilosis, stomatitis	Deficiency of iron, vitamin B_{12}, folate, and other vitamins
Abdominal pain	Distention or inflammation of bowel
GENITOURINARY	
Nocturia	Delayed absorption of water, hypokalemia
Azotemia, hypotension	Fluid and electrolyte depletion
Amenorrhea, ↓ libido	Protein depletion and "caloric starvation" → secondary hypopituitarism
HEMATOPOIETIC	
Anemia	Impaired absorption of iron, vitamin B_{12}, and folic acid
Hemorrhagic phenomena	Vitamin K malabsorption → hypoprothrombinemia
MUSCULOSKELETAL	
Bone pain	Protein depletion → impaired bone formation → osteoporosis Calcium malabsorption → demineralization of bone → osteomalacia
Osteoarthropathy	Cause uncertain
Tetany, paresthesias	Calcium malabsorption → hypocalcemia; magnesium malabsorption → hypomagnesemia
Weakness	Anemia: electrolyte depletion (hypokalemia)
NERVOUS SYSTEM	
Night blindness	Impaired absorption vitamin A → vitamin A deficiency
Xerophthalmia	Vitamin A deficiency
Peripheral neuropathy	Vitamin B_{12}, thiamine deficiency
SKIN	
Eczema	Cause uncertain
Purpura	Vitamin K deficiency
Follicular hyperkeratosis and dermatitis	Deficiency of vitamin A, zinc, essential fatty acids, and other vitamins

TABLE 254-5 Classification of the malabsorption syndromes

Inadequate digestion
 A Postgastrectomy steatorrhea*
 B Deficiency or inactivation of pancreatic lipase
  1 Exocrine pancreatic insufficiency
   a Chronic pancreatitis
   b Pancreatic carcinoma
   c Cystic fibrosis
   d Pancreatic resection
  2 Ulcerogenic tumor of the pancreas (Zollinger-Ellison syndrome, gastrinoma)*
Reduced intestinal bile salt concentration (with impaired micelle formation)
 A Liver disease
  1 Parenchymal liver disease
  2 Cholestasis (intrahepatic or extrahepatic)
 B Abnormal bacterial proliferation in the small bowel
  1 Afferent loop stasis
  2 Strictures
  3 Fistulas
  4 Blind loops
  5 Multiple diverticula of the small bowel
  6 Hypomotility states (diabetes, scleroderma, intestinal pseudoobstruction)
 C Interrupted enterohepatic circulation of bile salts
  1 Ileal resection
  2 Ileal inflammatory disease (regional ileitis)
 D Drugs (by sequestration or precipitation of bile salts)
  1 Neomycin
  2 Calcium carbonate
  3 Cholestyramine
Inadequate absorptive surface
 A Intestinal resection or bypass
  1 Mesenteric vascular disease with massive intestinal resection
  2 Regional enteritis with multiple bowel resections
  3 Jejunoileal bypass
 B Gastroileostomy (inadvertent)
Lymphatic obstruction
 A Intestinal lymphangiectasia
 B Whipple's disease
 C Lymphoma
Cardiovascular disorders
 A Constrictive pericarditis
 B Congestive heart failure
 C Mesenteric vascular insufficiency
 D Vasculitis
Primary mucosal absorptive defects
 A Inflammatory or infiltrative disorders
  1 Regional enteritis*
  2 Amyloidosis
  3 Scleroderma*
  4 Lymphoma*
  5 Radiation enteritis
  6 Eosinophilic enteritis
  7 Tropical sprue
  8 Infective enteritis (e.g., salmonellosis)
  9 Collagenous sprue
  10 Nonspecific ulcerative jejunitis
  11 Mastocytosis
  12 Dermatologic disorders (e.g., dermatitis herpetiformis)
 B Biochemical or genetic abnormalities
  1 Celiac sprue (gluten-induced enteropathy)
  2 Disaccharidase deficiency
  3 Hypogammaglobulinemia
  4 Abetalipoproteinemia
  5 Hartnup disease
  6 Cystinuria
  7 Monosaccharide malabsorption
Endocrine and metabolic disorders
 A Diabetes mellitus*
 B Hypoparathyroidism
 C Adrenal insufficiency
 D Hyperthyroidism
 E Ulcerogenic tumor of the pancreas (Zollinger-Ellison syndrome, gastrinoma)*
 F Carcinoid syndrome

* Malabsorption caused by multiple defects.

hepatic synthesis or excretion of conjugated bile salts, resulting in impaired formation of micellar lipid. In addition to steatorrhea, patients with liver disease may have impaired absorption of vitamin D and calcium, resulting in severe metabolic bone disease. This is particularly common in patients with primary biliary cirrhosis. Skeletal roentgenograms may show increased porosity of bone, cortical thinning, vertebral compression, and spontaneous pathologic fractures. Patients with alcohol-induced liver disease also may have exocrine pancreatic insufficiency. Accordingly, pancreatic function should be evaluated in patients with liver disease and malabsorption.

Postgastrectomy malabsorption The presence of a malabsorption syndrome has been documented frequently in patients after subtotal gastrectomy. Steatorrhea is more common with a Billroth II than a Billroth I type of anastomosis. Usually the fat loss is minimal, ranging from 7 to 10 g per 24 h. Patients with gross steatorrhea usually have impaired intraluminal fat digestion due to several factors: (1) With a Billroth II anastomosis the duodenum is bypassed, and there is a decreased entry of stomach contents into the proximal duodenum (i.e., afferent loop). This leads to a decreased stimulus for the release of *secretin* and *cholecystokinin-pancreozymin* from the duodenum and may result in a depressed pancreatic enzyme response. (2) There may be *inadequate mixing* of the pancreatic enzymes and bile salts secreted into the proximal duodenum with the gastric contents entering the jejunum. (3) There may be *stasis* of intestinal contents in the afferent loop, resulting in abnormal bacterial proliferation in the proximal small bowel. This in turn may lead to abnormalities in bile salt metabolism (see "Malabsorption Due to Bacterial Overgrowth of the Small Bowel, Pathophysiology," below). (4) The presence of maldigestion may lead to *protein depletion*, which in turn may produce further impairment in pancreatic function. (5) The *loss of the reservoir function of the stomach* may result in decreased intestinal transit time. Perhaps the most important factor is rapid gastric emptying, which results in low luminal concentrations of digestive secretions for the first 60 to 80 min after a meal. Such a disorder has been described in patients with subtotal gastrectomy and duodenostomy (Billroth I), gastrojejunostomy (Billroth II), and truncal vagotomy and pyloroplasty (V&P). That gastric emptying rates are somewhat slower in patients with V&P may account for the overall less severe nutritional deficiencies in such patients. In some patients, treatment with pancreatic enzymes may lead to significant improvement. Specimens of duodenal or jejunal fluid should be obtained for culture of both aerobic and anaerobic organisms and appropriate antibiotic therapy instituted if there is evidence of abnormal bacterial overgrowth (colony count of greater than 10^7 per milliliter of jejunal fluid). Because the duodenum is the principal site of absorption of iron and calcium, in patients with a Billroth II anastomosis, impaired absorption of calcium and iron also may develop. Occult metabolic bone disease occurs frequently in this setting.

INADEQUATE ABSORPTIVE SURFACE (SHORT BOWEL SYNDROME) Extensive intestinal resection often results in the short bowel syndrome. The most common disorders resulting in short bowel syndrome are (1) massive intestinal resection following a vascular insult to the small intestine, (2) regional enteritis with multiple bowel resections, and (3) jejunoileal bypass for morbid obesity. In general, the absorption of nutrients will be influenced by the extent and site of small bowel resected, the presence of the ileocecal valve, and adaptation of the remaining small bowel. Resection of 40 to 50 percent of the small bowel is usually well tolerated, provided the proximal duodenum, the distal half of the ileum, and the ileocecal valve are spared. By contrast, resection of the ileum and the ileocecal valve alone may induce severe diarrhea and malabsorption, even though less than 30 percent of the small intestine is resected.

Several measures are important in the management of short bowel syndrome: (1) The diet should contain at least 2500 kcal and consist primarily of carbohydrate and protein, with fat restricted to less than 40 g/d. A fat-restricted diet is effective in reducing diarrhea, presumably because there is decreased production of hydroxy fatty acids from long-chain fats. Such hydroxy fatty acids, in essence, are cathartics and increase net secretion of water and electrolytes by the colon as well as the small bowel. (2) It is often necessary to provide vitamin and mineral supplements, which usually include K^+, Cl^-, Mg^{2+}, Ca^{2+}, trace metals (Zn, Cd, Mn), iron, folate, vitamin B_{12}, other vitamins (A, D, E, K, B_1, B_2, B_6, biotin), and essential fatty acids. (3) Specific drugs (e.g., belladonna alkaloids, diphenoxylate, loperamide, and codeine) which decrease intestinal motility and prolong mucosal contact time are helpful in controlling diarrhea. These agents also decrease ileostomy outputs. (4) A bile salt–sequestering agent such as cholestyramine blunts the effects of bile salts, which stimulate net secretion of water and electrolytes by the colon. (5) Patients with short bowel syndrome may have gastric acid hypersecretion which is often transient and which results in dilution of pancreatic secretions as well as inactivation of pancreatic enzymes. Under these conditions, a histamine H-2 receptor antagonist is useful because it will suppress gastric acid secretion and decrease the volume of fluid entering the proximal small bowel, thus leading to an increased

concentration of pancreatic enzymes. In addition, supplemental pancreatic enzyme therapy may be required. (6) A bypassed colon can be used to receive infusions of fluid and electrolytes, since a portion of the colon can still absorb 1000 to 1500 mL fluid per day. (7) Octreotide, the long-acting somatostatin analogue, reduces digestive secretions (biliary, pancreatic, succus entericus) and thus may ameliorate diarrhea. Finally, (8) total parenteral nutrition is frequently required during the first 6 months after massive intestinal resection until some degree of adaptation has occurred. Such patients also may require long-term parenteral hyperalimentation with a silicone rubber catheter in the superior vena cava, and this can be done at home.

For a discussion of regional enteritis see Chap. 255.

MALABSORPTION DUE TO BACTERIAL OVERGROWTH OF THE SMALL BOWEL The proximal small intestine is usually bacteriologically sterile because of three factors: (1) the acid milieu of the stomach, (2) intestinal peristalsis, which sweeps bacteria to the distal small bowel, and (3) secretion into the lumen of the intestine of immunoglobulins, which may serve as coproantibodies. When bacteria are isolated from the upper small bowel, they are frequently contaminants transported from the mouth and upper respiratory tract, and the colony count rarely exceeds 10^4 per milliliter of jejunal fluid. The major mechanism limiting the growth of bacteria in the small intestine is normal peristalsis. Any disorder leading to impaired intestinal motility may result in abnormal stasis of intestinal contents with ineffective mechanical cleansing of bacteria. This, in turn, may lead to abnormal bacterial proliferation and malabsorption. Several malabsorptive disorders have been associated with bacterial overgrowth of the small bowel, and these are listed in Table 254-6.

Pathophysiology Bacterial overgrowth may result in changes in bile salt metabolism, and these are believed directly and indirectly to account for the steatorrhea. First, bacteria (especially anaerobic gram-positive bacteria) may lead to the intraluminal deconjugation of bile salts with a consequent production of free bile acids. In contrast to conjugated bile salts, unconjugated bile salts may be absorbed in the proximal small bowel by nonionic diffusion, resulting in decreased intraluminal concentrations of bile salts in the jejunum. Second, the decreased bile salt concentrations, the increase of unconjugated bile salts, and the decrease of the conjugated salts all serve to contribute to impaired intraluminal micelle formation and hence fat malabsorption. In addition to abnormalities in bile salt metabolism, intestinal

---

TABLE 254-6 Causes of intestinal bacterial overgrowth (intestinal colonization)

Structural abnormalities producing stasis of intestinal contents
  A Multiple small-bowel diverticula
  B Strictures
    1 Regional enteritis*
    2 Radiation enteritis*
    3 Occlusive vascular disease: vasculitis
  C Billroth II subtotal gastrectomy with afferent loop stasis*
  D Multiple laparotomies resulting in adhesions and partial small-bowel obstruction
Fistulas
  A Gastrocolic, gastroileal, jejunoileal, jejunocolic
Motor abnormalities resulting in intestinal hypomotility
  A Scleroderma*
  B Amyloidosis*
  C Diabetes mellitus*
  D Hypothyroidism
  E Vagotomy
  F Intestinal pseudoobstruction (see Table 254-7)
Miscellaneous
  A Hypogammaglobulinemia*
  B Nodular lymphoid hyperplasia
  C Pancreatic insufficiency
  D Gastric hypochlorhydria/achlorhydria
    1 Subtotal gastrectomy
    2 Pernicious anemia
    3 Prolonged use of H-2 receptor antagonists

* No underlying disorder detected.

mucosal lesions have been demonstrated in patients with intestinal stasis. Such lesions are often patchy in distribution, and the histologic appearance ranges in severity from minimal changes in villous architecture to severe lesions with virtual absence of villi. The cause of these lesions is unclear; possible causes include damage caused by bacterial invasion, bacterial toxins, or metabolic products such as unconjugated bile salts. In this regard, certain bacteria such as *Bacteroides* elaborate proteases which solubilize brush border proteins and destroy disaccharidases such as sucrase and maltase. The impaired absorption of vitamin B_{12} is not related to the disturbed bile salt metabolism but appears to be due to uptake of vitamin B_{12} by microorganisms.

Many of the preceding abnormalities in bile salt metabolism may be reversed by appropriate antibiotic therapy. When such treatment is instituted, unconjugated bile salts in the jejunal fluid decrease, an increase in the micellar lipid phase occurs, and steatorrhea diminishes or disappears. In addition, significant improvement in the absorption of vitamin B_{12} occurs with broad-spectrum antibiotics such as tetracycline.

Clinical manifestations Breath tests, i.e., tests with ^{14}C-labeled bile acid, [^{14}C]xylose, and lactulose, are useful screening tests for malabsorption syndrome due to abnormal bacterial overgrowth of the small intestine. The 2-h 50-g glucose breath hydrogen test reliably predicts the presence of bacterial overgrowth; a positive test is characterized by a rise in breath hydrogen of at least 12 parts per million (ppm) within 2 h of a 50-g glucose challenge *and* a high fasting breath hydrogen level of at least 15 ppm. A definitive diagnosis is established by demonstrating larger numbers of microorganisms (greater than 10^5 per milliliter) and a polymicrobial flora in cultures of duodenal or jejunal fluid. Other clinical features include the following: (1) steatorrhea of a moderate degree, usually in the range of 15 to 30 g fecal fat per 24 h, (2) macrocytic anemia with a megaloblastic bone marrow, (3) impaired absorption of vitamin B_{12} which is not corrected by intrinsic factor, and (4) correction of steatorrhea and impaired vitamin B_{12} absorption by antibiotic therapy. Absorption of D-xylose, peroral small-intestinal biopsy specimens, and other tests of absorptive function (see Table 254-2) may be normal in these patients. A single course or intermittent courses (2 to 3 weeks per month) of therapy with antibiotics such as tetracycline, ampicillin, metronidazole, or trimethoprim-sulfamethoxazole are usually given.

Chronic intestinal pseudoobstruction (See also Chap. 257) Chronic intestinal pseudoobstruction is a heterogeneous syndrome with a variety of causes (Table 254-7). Primary or idiopathic intestinal

---

TABLE 254-7 Causes of chronic intestinal pseudoobstruction

PRIMARY: IDIOPATHIC

A Visceral myopathy
B Visceral neuropathy

SECONDARY

A Collagen vascular disease
 1 Scleroderma
 2 Dermatomyositis/polymyositis
 3 Systemic lupus erythematosus
B Amyloidosis
C Endocrine disorders
 1 Hypothyroidism
 2 Diabetes mellitus
D Neurologic diseases
 1 Chagas' disease
E Paraneoplastic visceral neuropathy
 1 Small cell lung carcinoma
F Drugs
 1 Chronic narcotic use (narcotic bowel syndrome)
 2 Tricyclic antidepressants
G Miscellaneous
 1 Jejunal diverticulosis
 2 Jejunoileal bypass

---

pseudoobstruction is a chronic illness characterized by recurrent episodes of intestinal obstruction in which all known causes of mechanical obstruction and other illnesses known to produce intestinal pseudoobstruction have been excluded. In addition to abnormalities in small-bowel motility, derangements in esophageal, gastric, and colonic motility also have been described. The primary clinical manifestations are nausea and vomiting, abdominal pain, distention, constipation, diarrhea, and urinary tract symptoms. Patients typically exhibit prolonged transit of chyme along the gastrointestinal tract, especially the small bowel, where pressure activity patterns are markedly disordered. Oral cisapride accelerates gastric emptying, normalizes intestinal transit, and improves propulsive small-bowel activity in patients with pseudoobstruction. Octreotide also may prove to be useful. Malabsorption secondary to stasis of intestinal contents with resultant abnormal bacterial proliferation in the small bowel is frequently present.

Tropical sprue Tropical sprue is a malabsorptive disorder of unknown cause affecting residents of or visitors to tropical regions. Both epidemic and endemic forms of the disease have been recognized. Tropical sprue may have its onset months or even years after a patient has returned from the tropics. The etiology of the disorder has not been elucidated, but it might well result from one or more of the following: (1) a nutritional deficiency, (2) a transmissible infectious microorganism, and (3) a toxin elaborated by a microorganism or contained in the diet. It is of interest that coliform organisms, shown to produce an enterotoxin causing fluid secretion, have been isolated from the jejunum of tropical sprue patients but not from other patients with bacterial overgrowth of the proximal small bowel. Anorexia, diarrhea, weight loss, symptoms of anemia, sequelae of nutritional deficiency (see Table 254-4), and abdominal distention are common findings. Patients are frequently deficient in iron as well as vitamin B_{12} and folate. Laboratory studies usually reveal anemia (megaloblastic in 60 percent of cases) and impaired absorption of fat, xylose, and vitamin B_{12}. Malabsorption of at least two nutrients is considered essential for the diagnosis. Jejunal biopsy classically reveals shortened and thickened villi, increased crypt depth, and increased infiltration of mononuclear cells in the lamina propria and epithelium (see Table 254-3). However, these biopsy findings are not specific, and the lesion may be patchy; in addition, interpretation is difficult because "control" biopsies from asymptomatic residents in the same tropical region are often considered abnormal when compared with normal biopsies from patients in temperate zones. Such histologic findings have been termed *tropical jejunitis*. Treatment with vitamin B_{12}, folate, and antibiotics have all been effective in inducing a remission. A short course, i.e., 2 to 4 weeks, of combined therapy with a sulfonamide or tetracycline and folic acid is usually given. Occasional patients require more prolonged antibiotic therapy.

Scleroderma Although there are numerous reports of small-intestinal involvement in scleroderma, frank malabsorption has been reported in only one-third of patients. Malabsorption is due to two key factors: (1) impaired intestinal motility and jejunal pseudodiverticulosis leading to relative stasis of intestinal contents and hence bacterial overgrowth and (2) involvement of the intestinal wall by the disease. In some cases, abnormal bacterial proliferation in the upper small bowel can be documented, and in these patients antibiotic therapy may result in decreased steatorrhea, gain in weight, and increased absorption of vitamin B_{12}. In the intestinal wall there also may be extensive deposition of collagen, especially in the muscular mucosa, submucosa, and muscularis externa, with significant muscle atrophy. Studies of duodenal myoelectric activity in scleroderma revealed absence of migrating motor complexes in the basal state and decreased excitability of the bowel to mechanical stimuli such as distention and humoral stimuli such as pentagastrin and secretin. This motor dysfunction is an important factor in the dilatation, atony, and stasis of intestinal contents in scleroderma. Therapy with the somatostatin analogue octreotide has stimulated intestinal motility, reduced bacterial overgrowth, and ameliorated obstructive gut symptoms.

Malabsorption in AIDS Diarrhea and weight loss occur frequently in patients with AIDS. These symptoms are often due to enteric infections or small-intestinal Kaposi's sarcoma. The jejunal mucosa is often abnormal in patients infected with HIV, and such abnormalities can be masked by an opportunistic infection. However, such symptoms can be due to malabsorption, which has been well documented in patients with AIDS in whom identifiable enteric infections and intestinal involvement with Kaposi's sarcoma have been excluded. The presence of malabsorption in these patients has been documented by steatorrhea and abnormal D-xylose absorption tests. Serum zinc levels may be decreased. In addition, small-bowel biopsy specimens have revealed dense infiltration of mononuclear cells and histiocytes. Microorganisms also have been identified in the mucosa.

DISORDERS ASSOCIATED WITH LYMPHATIC OBSTRUCTION
Whipple's disease This is a rare disorder characterized clinically by arthralgia, abdominal pain, diarrhea, progressive weight loss, dilated lacteals in the bowel wall, and impaired intestinal absorption. Wasting, low-grade fever, increased skin pigmentation, and peripheral lymphadenopathy are frequently present. In addition, central nervous system manifestations, including confusion, memory loss, focal cranial nerve signs, nystagmus, and ophthalmoplegia, may be present. Laboratory examination usually reveals the presence of steatorrhea, impaired xylose absorption, abnormal small-bowel x-rays, hypoalbuminemia, and anemia. Hypoalbuminemia is due to excessive loss of serum albumin into the gastrointestinal tract as well as impaired synthesis of albumin.

The diagnosis is established by demonstrating the presence in the mucosa of macrophages containing large cytoplasmic granules which give a brilliant magenta stain with the periodic acid Schiff reagent (PAS). Such macrophages also may be seen in other tissues such as lymph nodes, spleen, or liver. The finding of PAS-positive macrophages in the lamina propria is not specific for Whipple's disease, but virtual replacement of most cellular elements in the lamina propria by these macrophages has been seen only in this disorder. In addition to the PAS-positive macrophages, jejunal biopsies frequently show dilated lymphatics and some degree of blunting of the intestinal mucosal villi.

Electron-microscopic studies have revealed the presence of rod-shaped structures (or bacilliform bodies) 0.3 by 1.5 to 2.5 μm within and adjacent to the macrophages in the lamina propria as well as within epithelial cells and polymorphonuclear leukocytes. The bacterium has not been cultured but has been identified as a gram-negative actinomycete with distinct morphologic characteristics and thus named *Tropheryma whippelii*. It is of particular interest that after treatment of the patient with antibiotics the bacilliform bodies decrease or disappear together with a decrease in the number of PAS-positive macrophages. In addition, the reappearance of the bacteria often heralds the onset of a clinical relapse after antibiotics have been withdrawn.

Whipple's disease at one time was thought to be invariably fatal. However, it is now clear that therapy with antibiotics will usually induce a clinical remission. In a few cases there has been complete reversal of the histologic abnormalities in the jejunal mucosa, and some of these cases have been followed for more than 10 years. Patients with Whipple's disease should be treated with antibiotics such as trimethoprim-sulfamethoxazole for at least 1 year. Treatment with tetracycline alone or penicillin alone is not adequate initial therapy; relapse rates with these drugs are approximately 40 percent. The most important parameter for following the disease and predicting its course is the presence or absence of bacilli in sections of small-bowel biopsies.

Intestinal lymphoma Steatorrhea is a manifestation of *primary* intestinal lymphoma. The disease occurs predominantly in men, and the mean age of onset of symptoms is about 50 years. The diagnosis should be suspected in patients with malabsorption with the following findings: (1) a malabsorption syndrome in which clinical and biopsy features resemble those of celiac sprue but in which there is an incomplete response to a gluten-free diet, (2) the presence of

abdominal pain and *fever*, and (3) signs and symptoms of intestinal obstruction. The usual stigmata of generalized lymphoma are frequently absent. Hepatomegaly, splenomegaly, palpable abdominal masses, and peripheral adenopathy are usually not found. Lymphangiography and CT scanning may reveal abnormal intraabdominal nodes. The diagnosis can be established by laparotomy and often may be made by thorough examination of multiple mucosal biopsy specimens obtained perorally. There may be a total absence of villi or lesser degrees of blunting and shortening of the villi. In contrast to celiac sprue, the lamina propria is usually massively infiltrated with lymphoid cells. Malignancy may be diagnosed by demonstrating lymphoid cells with the cytologic features of malignancy, the presence of reticulum cells outside germinal centers, and infiltration and destruction of crypts by pleomorphic lymphoid cells. Some patients elaborate or secrete a fragment of the heavy chain of IgA immunoglobulins (α-*chain disease*). The latter is probably a variant of intestinal lymphoma.

The mechanism of malabsorption in intestinal lymphoma may be related to several factors: (1) diffuse involvement of the small-intestinal mucosa, (2) involvement of the bowel wall with lymphatic obstruction, and (3) localized stenosis with stasis of intestinal contents and bacterial overgrowth. It should be emphasized that it is often difficult, by clinical and morphologic features alone, to distinguish celiac sprue from intestinal lymphoma. Indeed, there is evidence to suggest that lymphoma may develop as a late complication of celiac sprue.

The course of intestinal lymphoma has ranged from 4 months to 4 years from the onset of symptoms. Perforation, bleeding, and intestinal obstruction are common terminal complications. There is insufficient evidence to determine whether radiation therapy, chemotherapy, or localized surgical resection modifies the natural course of the disease.

CARDIOVASCULAR DISORDERS Steatorrhea has been described in patients with chronic congestive heart failure, superior mesenteric artery insufficiency, and constrictive pericarditis. Abnormal dilated mucosal lymphatics and excessive enteric loss of protein have been demonstrated in patients with constrictive pericarditis. The mechanism of steatorrhea in patients with chronic heart failure remains uncertain. It might be due to congestion and edema of the mucosa, mucosal hypoxia, or abnormalities in pancreatic function. Although pronounced steatorrhea is uncommon in congestive heart failure, these patients are frequently anorectic, and a low fat intake could mask a latent steatorrhea. Steatorrhea is quite infrequent in patients with vasculitis and is thought to be due to segmental infarction of the small bowel in addition to intestinal ischemia.

DEFECTS IN MUCOSAL FUNCTION

INFLAMMATORY OR INFILTRATIVE DISORDERS **Regional enteritis** The clinical features of regional enteritis are described in Chap. 255. Malabsorption in regional enteritis may result from several factors: (1) interruption of the enterohepatic circulation of bile salts by ileal disease or resection, (2) deconjugation of bile salts due to bacterial overgrowth, in turn related to strictures and/or fistulas, (3) active inflammatory bowel disease causing impaired mucosal cell function, (4) inadequate absorptive surface resulting from intestinal resection or fistulas, and (5) severe protein depletion producing impaired exocrine pancreatic function. Active ileal disease and/or ileal resection resulting in an interrupted enterohepatic circulation of and deficiency of conjugated bile salts appears to be the major factor responsible for steatorrhea as well as impaired absorption of vitamin B_{12}. Small-bowel absorptive function has been correlated with the extent of ileal disease or resection. When the length of ileal dysfunction exceeds 90 to 100 cm, virtually all patients will have steatorrhea and vitamin B_{12} malabsorption. After intestinal resection, the functional capacity of the remaining small bowel will depend on the site and extent of resection as well as the presence of residual inflammatory disease. Massive intestinal resection usually results in impaired absorption of all food constituents. When the malabsorption is due to strictures and blind loops as a result of previous surgical therapy, antibiotic therapy may be helpful, but surgical removal of these areas is usually necessary for long-term improvement. With diffuse inflammatory disease, a florid malabsorption syndrome may occur with steatorrhea, hypocalcemia, impaired vitamin B_{12} absorption, and hypoalbuminemia due to increased enteric protein loss. Treatment with sulfasalazine, glucocorticoids, and other immunosuppressive drugs may be beneficial (see Chap. 255).

After *ileal resection*, patients frequently have bothersome diarrhea. This appears to be due to *interruption of the enterohepatic circulation* whereby increased amounts of bile salts reach the colon, where they interfere with water and electrolyte absorption and thus have a cathartic effect. The *bile salt–induced diarrhea* after ileal resection may respond to treatment with cholestyramine, an exchange resin which binds bile salts and causes them to lose their biochemical effect on the bowel. Patients with ileal resection of less than 100 cm and fecal fat excretion less than 20 g/d show the best symptomatic response to cholestyramine, usually at a dose of 4 g tid.

Chronic nongranulomatous ulcerative jejunoileitis This disorder is characterized by abdominal pain, weight loss, fever, diarrhea, steatorrhea, hypoalbuminemia, and protein-losing enteropathy. Clinical features mimic those found in both regional enteritis and celiac sprue. Indeed, the intestinal lesion may be indistinguishable from celiac sprue. However, exclusion of gluten from the diet does not result in any benefit. Glucocorticoid treatment has resulted in transient improvement, but long-term effects are unpredictable.

Amyloidosis This disorder is discussed in detail in Chap. 281.

Radiation injury to the small bowel Extensive morphologic damage of the small-intestinal mucosa often follows normal or excessive abdominal irradiation. These changes include a decrease in crypt mitoses, marked shortening of the villi, megalocytosis of epithelial cells, and inflammatory cell infiltration of the lamina propria. This may be associated with transient diarrhea and impaired intestinal absorption. However, restoration of normal intestinal architecture is usually complete within 2 weeks after cessation of therapy. Persistent diarrhea and malabsorption may develop shortly after x-ray therapy, or there may be a latent period of several years before the onset of diarrhea. Steatorrhea, ranging from 10 to 40 g/d, has been observed frequently, but impaired absorption of calcium, iron, D-xylose, or vitamin B_{12} is less common. In some patients, intestinal strictures due to vasculopathy and ischemia may develop following irradiation, and thus stasis of intestinal contents and abnormal bacterial proliferation may occur. In others, intestinal lymphangiectasia, presumably due to lymphatic obstruction, has been documented. Diarrhea and malabsorption may be refractory to all methods of management. Treatment with antibiotics, pancreatic enzymes, gluten-free diet, adrenal glucocorticoids, and opiates has met with but limited success.

Eosinophilic enteritis Eosinophilic gastroenteritis is a disorder of the stomach, small bowel, and colon of unknown etiology characterized by peripheral blood eosinophilia and eosinophilic infiltration of the gut wall but without evidence of vasculitis. The clinical manifestations, usually recurrent, are protean and relate to the site of gastrointestinal tract involvement. Three main patterns have been identified: (1) Predominant mucosal disease manifested by iron-deficiency anemia, hypoalbuminemia due to protein-losing enteropathy, and mild steatorrhea. Patients in this group often present with a malabsorption syndrome and a history of intolerance to specific foods. (2) Predominant muscle layer disease characterized by marked thickening and rigidity of the stomach and proximal small bowel with obstructive symptoms and radiologic features of pyloric narrowing and obstruction. The obstructive form of eosinophilic gastroenteritis accounts for half the cases reported since 1970. Accordingly, eosinophilic enteritis should be considered in the differential diagnosis of gastric outlet obstruction, diffuse small-bowel disease, and ileocolitis. Indeed, eosinophilic enteritis often mimics regional enteritis. (3) Predominant subserosal disease in which the cardinal manifestation is ascites with marked eosinophilia in the ascitic fluid. Although the

preceding classification based on tissue layer of major involvement is useful in understanding the principal manifestations, it should be emphasized that multiple clinical forms, e.g., ascites (serosal involvement) and obstruction (muscular involvement), also occur.

Previous reports have emphasized food allergy and mucosal features of this disease. However, food sensitivity is related to symptoms in less than 20 percent of patients. In such patients, fasting serum IgE levels are often elevated, and challenge with offending foods frequently evokes symptoms of abdominal pain and diarrhea in addition to a marked increase in serum IgE levels. In most patients with eosinophilic enteritis, however, immunologic studies, including serum immunoglobulins, serum complement, lymphocyte quantitation, and lymphocyte response to nonspecific mitogens, reveal no abnormalities. Thus both IgE-mediated and IgE-dependent mechanisms may be operative in different patients with eosinophilic gastroenteritis. Several nonreaginic factors influence peripheral blood and tissue eosinophilia. It seems clear that evidence of allergy or food sensitivity is often absent and is not required for the diagnosis of eosinophilic enteritis. In addition, even in patients with food allergies, elimination diets are frequently ineffective, and such patients may require prolonged glucocorticoid therapy to remain well. Surgical treatment for relief of obstructive symptoms and glucocorticoids are the mainstays of therapy.

Dermatitis and malabsorption A malabsorption syndrome, usually mild, has been reported in patients with a variety of dermatologic disorders, including psoriasis, eczematoid dermatitis, and dermatitis herpetiformis. Proximal intestinal mucosal abnormalities are almost invariably found in patients with dermatitis herpetiformis. In one study, 21 of 22 patients had lesions ranging in severity from a completely "flat" to an almost normal intestinal mucosa. The mucosal lesions were often patchy in distribution. Clinical and laboratory evidence of significant malabsorption was infrequent, possibly due to the limited length of small intestine involved in this skin disorder. While the skin lesions of dermatitis herpetiformis respond to sulfone, the gut lesions do not. By contrast, in some patients with blunted and flattened intestinal mucosal lesions and steatorrhea, there may be a striking improvement in villous architecture and regression of steatorrhea after withdrawal of gluten from the diet without improvement in the skin lesions. Further, in patients with dermatitis herpetiformis and a morphologically normal small-intestinal mucosa, administration of a high-gluten diet may result in blunted and flattened mucosal lesions indistinguishable from those of celiac sprue. As in the latter disease, an increased frequency of HLA-A1 and HLA-B8 is also seen. These observations raise the interesting question as to whether certain patients with dermatitis herpetiformis and a malabsorption syndrome have latent celiac sprue.

BIOCHEMICAL OR GENETIC ABNORMALITIES **Celiac sprue** Celiac sprue is a disorder characterized by malabsorption, abnormal small-bowel structure, and intolerance to gluten, a protein found in wheat and wheat products. It has been appropriately referred to as *gluten-induced enteropathy*. Celiac disease in children and celiac sprue in adults are probably one and the same disorder with the same pathogenesis.

There are insufficient data to provide an accurate estimation of the incidence of celiac sprue in any population. This is largely because the severity of the disease varies greatly, and individuals may have typical mucosal change and yet have no overt symptoms. Seventy percent of the cases in most reported series are women. The incidence in siblings appears to be many times higher than that in the general population, and it has been suggested that sprue may be inherited through a dominant gene of incomplete penetrance. Celiac sprue patients have an increased frequency of serum histocompatibility antigens, particularly of the HLA-DR3 and HLA-DQw2 types. The HLA-DR3 phenotype has been found in 70 to 90 percent of sprue patients as compared with 20 to 25 percent in normal subjects. The HLA antigens may be linked to immune response genes which may determine the immunologic recognition of certain substances (see Chap. 64). It has been suggested that such genetic factors may predispose to immunologic tolerance of dietary proteins such as the peptides in gluten or to the production of pathogenic antigluten antibodies which could result in binding of gluten to epithelial cells with subsequent tissue damage. The discordance for celiac sprue among HLA-identical siblings and some identical twins raises the question of whether an additional susceptibility gene (or genes) not yet identified is required for the development of celiac sprue.

PATHOPHYSIOLOGY Gluten and the related substance gliadin are high-molecular-weight proteins found especially in wheat. The alcohol-soluble fraction of gluten consists of glutamine-rich gliadin polypeptides, which can be fractionated into γ, β, δ, and α subgroups; peptides from all four gliadin subgroups are toxic and induce the intestinal lesion when administered to celiac sprue patients in remission. The exact mechanism for this effect is not clear, but two theories have been proposed, namely, a "toxic" and an immunologic theory. One possible mechanism is that patients with celiac sprue lack a specific mucosal peptidase so that gluten or its larger glutamine-containing peptides are not effectively hydrolyzed to smaller peptides (i.e., dipeptides or amino acids). As a consequence, "toxic" peptides might accumulate in the mucosa. It has been demonstrated that patients with celiac sprue in remission will develop steatorrhea and typical mucosal changes when they are given gluten. Similar results will occur with the administration of peptide hydrolysates containing at least eight amino acids with a terminal glutamine residue. It has been shown that when gluten is instilled into the *ileum* of celiac sprue patients, histologic changes begin to occur within hours. This does not occur in the *upper jejunum*, suggesting that the effect is immediate and local rather than systemic. After noxious gluten fractions damage surface absorptive cells, the damaged cells are sloughed rapidly from the mucosal surface into the gut lumen. To compensate for this, cell proliferation increases, crypts undergo hypertrophy, and cell migration accelerates to replace the damaged and sloughed epithelial cells. This more rapid than normal epithelial cell renewal can be reversed by a gluten-free diet. The intestinal mucosa of patients with celiac sprue shows many enzyme alterations, including decreased levels of disaccharidases, alkaline phosphatase, and peptide hydrolases, as well as impaired ability to digest gluten peptides. However, these abnormalities usually revert toward normal after successful treatment with a gluten-free diet. There is additional evidence supporting the concept of toxicity of gluten and gluten breakdown products in celiac sprue. First, gliadin, especially the A-gliadin moiety, is toxic to sprue mucosa maintained in organ culture, causing ultrastructural changes and depression of disaccharidase activity. Second, sprue mucosa hydrolyzes a specific fraction of a gliadin digest (i.e., fraction 9) in a defective manner, and fraction 9 is selectively toxic to sprue mucosa. Third, specific fractions of gluten fed to celiac sprue patients cause transient alterations in mucosal histology and depression of disaccharidase activity, but full recovery is observed in 72 h. The rapid onset of these changes and prompt recovery are consistent with a direct toxic effect. Despite intensive study, however, no persistent, specific, or selective peptidase or other enzyme deficiency has been demonstrated.

It also has been suggested that gluten or gluten metabolites may initiate an *immunologic reaction* in the intestinal mucosa. Alternatively, the interaction of T lymphocytes with crypt epithelium may be a primary event in the pathogenesis of the intestinal lesion. The presence of a mononuclear inflammatory cell infiltrate in the lamina propria of the mucosa, the beneficial response to glucocorticoid drugs, the finding of abnormal antibodies to gliadin in the serum of celiac sprue patients, the synthesis of increased amounts of antigliadin antibody by sprue mucosa maintained in organ culture, and the elaboration of lymphokines such as migration inhibitory factor (MIF) by sprue mucosa incubated with gliadin have all been cited as evidence in support of this hypothesis. However, there is still no definitive evidence indicating that an abnormal (immune) mechanism is important in initiating or perpetuating this disease process.

A possible role for adenovirus serotype 12 (Ad12) in the pathogenesis of celiac sprue has been proposed based on two observations: (1) homology of amino acid sequences between a portion of A-gliadin and a viral-encoded protein (E16) produced by Ad12, and (2) patients with untreated celiac sprue have a much higher frequency of antibodies to Ad12 compared with treated celiac sprue patients and controls. Other studies, however, have not demonstrated a strikingly higher prevalence of previous infection with type 12 adenovirus among a cohort of celiac sprue patients compared with persons without the disease. Nonetheless, these observations are in accord with the hypothesis that there must be an *environmental* factor as well as a *genetic predisposition* to explain why only certain people develop celiac sprue. Despite intensive studies, there is not yet enough information to integrate the distinctive dietary, immunologic, and genetic features of celiac sprue into a clear understanding of the pathogenesis of the disease.

Jejunal biopsy specimens from patients with celiac sprue usually show a characteristic lesion. There is blunting and flattening of the mucosal surface, with villi either absent or broad and short. The crypts are elongated, and there is generally a dense infiltration of inflammatory cells in the lamina propria. The surface epithelium is altered with a sparse brush border, cuboidal rather than the normal columnar cells, and infiltration of inflammatory cells in the epithelial layer. These changes are usually most severe in the proximal small bowel, presumably because this area of the bowel is exposed to the highest gluten concentration. The typical morphologic changes illustrated in Fig. 254-4 are characteristic of celiac sprue but are not specific. Similar changes have been described in other conditions, including lymphoma, tropical sprue, and hypogammaglobulinemia associated with malabsorption. Many biochemical abnormalities have been demonstrated in mucosal biopsy specimens from celiac sprue patients. Impaired esterification of fatty acids to triglycerides, decreased uptake of amino acids, and decreased activity of intestinal disaccharidases (especially lactase) have been well documented. The latter observation may account for the high incidence of milk intolerance in untreated celiac sprue patients or those in relapse. However, the greater abundance of undifferentiated crypt cells may be important, since crypt cells normally have a lower capacity for nutrient uptake than do villus cells.

Since the mucosa is damaged and altered in patients with celiac sprue, there may be *decreased release of pancreatotropic hormones* (secretin and cholecystokinin, i.e., CCK). This results in decreased stimulation of the pancreas with lower than normal intraluminal levels of pancreatic enzymes in response to a meal. In addition, the gallbladder appears to be resistant to the action of cholecystokinin, resulting in absent or minimal contractions of the gallbladder, in turn leading to sequestration of bile salts in an inert gallbladder. These two defects may result in impaired intraluminal digestion of fat and protein, which will be superimposed on the defect in intestinal transport caused by a damaged mucosa.

Diarrhea is common in celiac sprue patients and is due to a number of factors, including *impaired absorption* of salt and water by duodenum and jejunum, net *secretion* of water and electrolytes by an abnormally permeable jejunal mucosa, and net colonic secretion of water and electrolytes induced by unabsorbed fatty acids and hydroxy fatty acids. However, the distal small intestine in celiac sprue has the ability to adapt to the damage and loss of absorptive capacity in the proximal small intestine. Indeed, increased ileal absorption of sodium, chloride, and water has been demonstrated in celiac sprue patients.

CLINICAL FEATURES Most patients with celiac sprue will have a typical malabsorption syndrome characterized by weight loss, abdominal distention and bloating, diarrhea, steatorrhea, and abnormal tests of absorptive function. The characteristic alterations in tests of intestinal absorption are outlined in Table 254-2. It should be emphasized, however, that some sprue patients may present with isolated abnormalities which initially do not suggest the diagnosis of celiac sprue. Thus a patient may be admitted for investigation of iron-deficiency anemia without apparent blood loss or of abnormal bleeding due to hypoprothrombinemia but may not have diarrhea or overt steatorrhea. Likewise, sprue patients may present with puzzling metabolic bone disease without diarrhea or steatorrhea. Such patients usually complain of bone pain and tenderness and frequently are found to have extensive demineralization of bone, compression deformities, kyphoscoliosis, and Milkman's fractures. Emotional disturbances are common in these patients, and many individuals with a diagnosis of weight loss initially considered related to severe anxiety and depression are subsequently found to have celiac sprue. In each of the preceding clinical settings, the diagnosis of celiac sprue should be considered in the differential diagnosis. In addition to dermatitis herpetiformis, there are established associations between celiac sprue and diabetes mellitus, selective IgA deficiency, primary sclerosing cholangitis, primary biliary cirrhosis, ulcerative colitis, and perhaps most important, lymphocytic or microscopic colitis (see Chaps. 255 and 268).

Since there is no specific diagnostic test, three criteria should be met in order to establish a definite diagnosis of celiac sprue: (1) evidence of malabsorption, (2) an abnormal small-bowel (jejunal) biopsy showing blunting and flattening of the villi along with changes in the surface epithelium, and (3) clinical, biochemical, and histologic improvement after institution of a gluten-free diet. In equivocal cases, the patient can be challenged with 30 to 50 g gluten orally, and if this promptly results in increased diarrhea and steatorrhea, the diagnosis of gluten-induced enteropathy is established. It should be emphasized that tests of intestinal absorption may reveal abnormalities which range from very minimal alterations to severe changes. Abnormalities in absorption tests have been shown to correlate reasonably well with the length of small-bowel involvement and to a lesser extent with the severity of the proximal lesion. Antigliadin antibodies have been widely used in the screening of celiac disease. In a study using this test, candidates for jejunal biopsy were selected from 328 first-degree relatives of 128 adult celiac patients. Twenty-one turned out to be positive for antigliadin antibodies, and in 13 jejunal histology was consistent with celiac disease. Antiendomysial antibody also seems to be a promising test. Thus, antigliadin and antiendomysial antibody testing appear to be valuable methods for the screening of celiac disease among family members. Relatives with positive tests may be regarded as subjects with latent celiac disease. A possible variant of celiac sprue is *collagenous* sprue. In this disorder, small-bowel biopsy specimens characteristically reveal a blunted and flattened mucosa and large masses of eosinophilic hyaline material in the lamina propria. In one study of 349 jejunal biopsy specimens from 145 patients with celiac sprue, 45 (31 percent) showed basement membrane thickening often associated with collagen deposition, but dense collagen deposition was found in only 11 patients. Fatal, unremitting malabsorption developed in 4 of the latter patients. These observations suggest that collagenous membrane thickening is a fairly frequent finding in jejunal biopsies from patients with sprue but that dense collagen deposits are an unusual feature and may indicate a poor prognosis.

TREATMENT   Despite the uncertainties concerned with the diagnosis of celiac sprue, approximately 80 percent of the patients improve after institution of a *gluten-free diet*. Symptomatic improvement usually occurs within a few weeks, but improvement in tests of absorptive function and small-bowel histologic characteristics may not occur for months. It has been repeatedly demonstrated that strict adherence to a gluten-free diet more consistently results in improvement than does suboptimal gluten restriction. Nevertheless, even with strict diet adherence, some cases show little improvement in intestinal histologic features. Patients with celiac sprue treated with glucocorticoids but continuing a normal gluten-containing diet have shown symptomatic improvement as well as improvement in intestinal histology and tests of intestinal absorptive function. The mechanism by which glucocorticoids protect the mucosa from the effects of gluten is not clear.

If a patient with celiac sprue does not respond to a gluten-free diet, other possibilities or complicating factors must be considered: (1) the diagnosis is incorrect, (2) the patient is not adhering strictly to the diet, (3) there may be another concurrent disease, such as

pancreatic insufficiency, (4) the patient may have ulceration of the jejunum or ileum, (5) lactase deficiency may be present with resultant milk intolerance, (6) the patient may have collagenous sprue, (7) the patient may have developed intestinal lymphoma, a disease which appears to occur more frequently in patients with sprue than in the general population, and (8) the patient may have developed lymphocytic or microscopic colitis. Finally, it should be emphasized that a small number of patients show a markedly delayed response to a gluten-free diet, with significant improvement occurring only after 24 to 36 months of therapy. Approximately 50 percent of patients with refractory sprue respond to glucocorticoids; such patients also may require parenteral hyperalimentation.

Systemic mastocytosis   Some evidence of malabsorption occurs in 30 percent of patients with systemic mastocytosis. Malabsorption is usually not severe and is manifested primarily as minimal or moderate steatorrhea and impaired absorption of D-xylose and vitamin B_{12}. Small-bowel biopsy specimens typically show moderate blunting of villi and mast cell infiltration.

Disaccharidase deficiency syndromes   As indicated above, the hydrolysis of disaccharides occurs on or within the brush border (microvilli) of intestinal epithelial cells by specific disaccharidases located there. As would be anticipated, both primary (genetic or familial) and secondary (acquired) deficiencies of these disaccharidases have been observed.

LACTASE DEFICIENCY IN THE ADULT   Instances of isolated deficiency of mucosal lactase occur; they are associated with symptoms of lactose intolerance. Since lactose is the principal carbohydrate of milk, such individuals show milk intolerance with symptoms of abdominal cramps, bloating or distention, and diarrhea. Similar symptoms will occur following the ingestion of lactose. The symptoms are due to the fact that lactose when not hydrolyzed is not absorbed, and its osmotic effect in the lumen leads to shifts of fluid into the intestinal tract. The pH of the stool also will decrease because of the production of lactic acid and short-chain fatty acids from the fermentation of lactose by colonic bacteria. Although primary intestinal lactase deficiency seems to be hereditary, lactose or milk intolerance may not become clinically evident until puberty or late adolescence. There are significant racial differences in the incidence of this entity. It would appear that about 5 to 15 percent of the adult white population shows intestinal lactase deficiency, but in black Americans, Bantus, and Orientals, the incidence has been reported as high as 80 to 90 percent.

The diagnosis may be suspected when one obtains a history of gastrointestinal symptoms following milk ingestion. It should be emphasized that the ingestion of only moderate amounts of lactose, e.g., 5 to 12 g or the amount contained in 100 to 240 mL milk, often results in symptoms. Bloating, cramps, and flatulence, but not diarrhea, are usually produced with ingestion of small to moderate amounts of lactose. The vast majority of lactose-intolerant patients are aware that they are milk-intolerant and avoid milk. That these symptoms are not due to allergic reactions to the proteins in milk (i.e., milk allergy or hypersensitivity) can be demonstrated by performing a lactose tolerance test. This test consists of administering an oral dose of lactose (usually from 0.75 to 1.5 g/kg of body weight) and obtaining serial blood samples for measurements of blood glucose. In a positive test, intestinal symptoms occur, and the blood glucose increases less than 1.1 mmol/L (20 mg/dL) above the fasting level. However, false-positive and false-negative tests occur in 20 percent of normal subjects because the test is influenced by gastric emptying and glucose metabolism. Measurement of breath hydrogen after ingestion of 50 g lactose is a more sensitive and specific test. The rationale for this test is that hydrogen is released from unabsorbed lactose by colonic bacteria, and breath hydrogen excretion subsequently rises. The test is noninvasive and is not influenced by gastric emptying or metabolic factors. Approximately 70 percent of patients with primary lactose intolerance will respond to a lactose-restricted diet, while the remaining 30 percent will not because of an underlying irritable bowel syndrome.

Acquired lactase deficiency is often seen in association with a variety of gastrointestinal diseases, in many of which there is histologic evidence of mucosal damage. The disorders in which lactose intolerance and lactase deficiency may occur include celiac and tropical sprue, regional enteritis, viral and bacterial infections of the intestinal tract, giardiasis, abetalipoproteinemia, cystic fibrosis, and ulcerative colitis. Patients with both primary and acquired (secondary) lactase deficiency are often able to tolerate yogurt because the latter contains bacterial-derived lactases.

DEFICIENCY OF OTHER DISACCHARIDASES Damage to the intestinal mucosa may produce decreased levels of other disaccharidases, such as sucrase-isomaltase, but usually these are not as depressed as lactase, and symptoms of specific intolerance, such as sucrose intolerance, are uncommon. There are instances of primary and apparently hereditary sucrose intolerance, but these always occur in association with sucrase-isomaltase deficiency. Sucrase-isomaltase deficiency, while not as frequent as lactase deficiency, is nonetheless an important cause of diarrhea, bloating, and cramping abdominal pain in children. Such patients are often unable to adhere to a low-sucrose diet. Thus the observation that the symptoms of sucrose malabsorption can be ameliorated by the simple expedient of ingesting viable yeast cells is of considerable practical importance.

Hypogammaglobulinemia Malabsorption may be associated with hypogammaglobulinemia or agammaglobulinemia. The hypogammaglobulinemia may be of the congenital or the acquired type, with the onset in either childhood or adulthood. When malabsorption has been noted, it has included impaired absorption of fat, D-xylose, and vitamin B_{12}. Peroral intestinal biopsy may reveal changes comparable with those seen in celiac sprue, but often one finds a more striking mononuclear infiltrate giving a nodular appearance to the mucosa both microscopically and macroscopically. Diarrhea and steatorrhea may precede or follow the development of hypogammaglobulinemia, and these may worsen during infections and subside after the infection is controlled with antibiotics. Intestinal infestation with *Giardia lamblia* is common in hypogammaglobulinemic patients. Meticulous collection and culture of intestinal fluids have revealed excessive numbers of anaerobic bacteria in the small bowel of some patients with hypogammaglobulinemia. However, the relationship between such overgrowth with anaerobes and diarrhea and steatorrhea remains to be clarified. Arthritis, resembling rheumatoid arthritis, and thymoma also have been described in patients with this syndrome. In some patients improvement in diarrhea and malabsorption may occur spontaneously, whereas in others improvement may follow treatment with a gluten-free diet, glucocorticoids, antibiotics, injections of gamma globulin, and cholestyramine. These forms of therapy have not been uniformly successful. Although transient improvement is common, complete cessation of symptoms is distinctly unusual.

The relationship between hypogammaglobulinemia and malabsorption remains obscure. There is no evidence to date indicating that excessive enteric loss of gamma globulin or alteration of the intestinal microflora occurs, but abnormalities in IgA metabolism may be important in this syndrome. This immunoglobulin is the predominant one in the intestinal mucosa and is found in many exocrine secretions, including tears, saliva, gastric juice, and intestinal juice. A few patients have been described with malabsorption and selective deficiency of IgA.

Abetalipoproteinemia See Chap. 344.

Hartnup disease, cystinuria See Chap. 353.

ENDOCRINE AND METABOLIC DISORDERS **Diabetes mellitus** The occurrence of diarrhea and steatorrhea in patients with diabetes mellitus has been well documented. When steatorrhea accompanies diabetes, it may be due to the presence of (1) exocrine pancreatic insufficiency, (2) coexistent celiac sprue, (3) abnormal bacterial proliferation in the proximal small bowel, or (4) severe and uncontrolled diabetes per se (e.g., so-called diabetic diarrhea). Patients falling into the first three categories will usually respond in a satisfactory manner to treatment with pancreatic extracts, a gluten-free diet, and antibiotics, respectively. The pathogenesis of diarrhea

and steatorrhea in patients in the fourth category remains poorly understood, and the response to various forms of therapy has been quite variable. It has been demonstrated that patients with diabetic diarrhea and steatorrhea may have involvement of the autonomic nervous system with degenerative changes in the sympathetic and parasympathetic nerves and ganglia. In some patients, bacterial overgrowth in the stomach and proximal small bowel may occur and contribute to the diarrhea and steatorrhea.

The clinical features in patients with diarrhea and steatorrhea due to diabetes per se seem to be fairly uniform. Diabetes usually develops at a young age and is often severe and difficult to control. There is a distinct predominance of males. Several signs of autonomic neuropathy are usually present, including postural hypotension, anhydrosis, impotence, and bladder irregularities. Peripheral vascular disease and peripheral neuropathy are also common. Gastrointestinal x-rays may show delayed gastric emptying and disordered transit through the small bowel. Peroral small-bowel biopsy specimens are normal. Tests of intestinal absorptive function are normal except for steatorrhea and azotorrhea. There has been no consistent response to therapy with pancreatic extracts, gluten-free diet, or glucocorticoids. When bacterial overgrowth is present, broad-spectrum antibiotics may be helpful. Clonidine has proved useful in patients with large-volume diarrhea not responding to dietary measures and anticholinergics.

Hypoparathyroidism Steatorrhea has been documented in several patients with idiopathic hypoparathyroidism. In addition to hypocalcemia, impaired absorption of D-xylose and vitamin B_{12}, decreased serum iron values, and abnormal small-intestinal roentgenograms have been demonstrated in some cases. In such patients the serum phosphorus level is elevated (due to the hypoparathyroidism) rather than low (as in primary malabsorption). The cause of malabsorption in this disorder is unclear.

Adrenal insufficiency Although there are few studies on fat excretion in adrenal insufficiency in human beings, malabsorption, especially of fat, appears to occur more frequently than has been generally appreciated. Patients with adrenal insufficiency have been found to have steatorrhea which is corrected by therapy with adrenal glucocorticoids.

Hyperthyroidism There are few detailed studies on intestinal absorptive function in patients with hyperthyroidism. Mild to moderate steatorrhea and hypoalbuminemia have been reported, but absorption of D-xylose and vitamin B_{12} is frequently normal. Steatorrhea usually remits after successful treatment of hyperthyroidism. Clinical studies suggest that steatorrhea in hyperthyroidism is not due to any defect of pancreatic, biliary, or small-intestinal mucosal function but is a result of hyperphagia with ingestion of unusually large amounts of fat occurring in association with rapid gastric emptying and intestinal transit.

Ulcerogenic tumor of the pancreas (Zollinger-Ellison syndrome) The clinical features of ulcerogenic tumor of the pancreas are described in Chap. 252. Malabsorption is frequently found in this disease. The acidification and dilution of intestinal contents caused by gastric acid hypersecretion leads to major disturbances in fat digestion and absorption. Impaired formation of micellar lipid due to inactivation of pancreatic lipase is probably the major factor in the production of steatorrhea. Other factors contributing to fat malabsorption in this disorder include (1) precipitation of glycine-conjugated bile salts due to low intraluminal pH, (2) alteration of the intestinal mucosa with ulceration and metaplasia, and (3) impaired fatty acid esterification and chylomicron formation.

Carcinoid syndrome (See also Chap. 276) Although diarrhea is common in the carcinoid syndrome, malabsorption with significant steatorrhea is unusual. In many of the cases of carcinoid syndrome with steatorrhea there has been a prior intestinal resection (usually ileal), and in these cases the resection is the important factor in the cause of steatorrhea. However, direct involvement of the bowel wall and mesentery by the carcinoid tumor has been well documented. That abnormalities in serotonin metabolism also may be important is suggested from the decrease in the steatorrhea observed in some of these patients when treated with the antiserotonin drug methysergide. Although side effects may occur, for control of diarrhea and steatorrhea, patients may be given a trial of 8 to 12 mg methysergide per day.

PROTEIN-LOSING ENTEROPATHY   The gastrointestinal tract has been shown to play a significant role in the metabolism and physiologic degradation of plasma proteins. The exact magnitude of the normal gastrointestinal protein loss in human beings has remained unclear, but studies with labeled albumin have suggested that between 10 and 20 percent of the normal turnover of albumin may be accounted for by enteric protein loss. However, under certain pathologic conditions, excessive gastrointestinal protein loss may develop. An extensive number of disorders have been found to be associated with intestinal protein loss. Some of these are listed in Table 254-8.

Pathophysiology   Several mechanisms have been proposed for the passage of plasma proteins across the gastrointestinal mucosa, both normally and in certain disease states. First, plasma proteins may pass into the gastrointestinal tract through an inflamed or ulcerated mucosa and account for the protein loss occasionally seen in regional enteritis and ulcerative colitis. Second, plasma protein loss may occur as a result of disordered mucosal cell structure. For example, patients with celiac sprue have abnormal villous structure and surface epithelium, and these changes could facilitate the diffusion of plasma protein between the cells. Third, in the presence of increased lymphatic pressure, there may be increased passage of plasma proteins into the lumen via the intercellular spaces of the mucosal epithelium. This might be expected to occur in disorders in which there is granulomatous or neoplastic involvement of lymphatics. Fourth, dilated lymph vessels in the mucosa may rupture through the surface epithelium, discharging their contents into the intestinal lumen. This is thought to be important in the pathogenesis of steatorrhea and hypoproteinemia

TABLE 254-8   Disorders associated with protein-losing enteropathy

STOMACH

A Gastric carcinoma
B Giant hypertrophy of the gastric mucosa
C Atrophic gastritis
D Postgastrectomy syndrome

SMALL INTESTINE

A Intestinal lymphangiectasia
B Celiac sprue
C Tropical sprue
D Regional enteritis
E Whipple's disease
F Lymphoma
G Intestinal tuberculosis
H Acute infectious enteritis
I Scleroderma
J Jejunal diverticulosis
K Allergic gastroenteropathy

COLON

A Colonic neoplasm
B Ulcerative colitis
C Granulomatous colitis
D Megacolon

HEART

A Congestive heart failure
B Constrictive pericarditis
C Interatrial septal defect
D Primary cardiomyopathy

MISCELLANEOUS

A Esophageal carcinoma
B Gastrocolic fistula
C Agammaglobulinemia
D Nephrosis

in patients with idiopathic intestinal lymphangiectasia (see ''Intestinal Lymphangiectasia,'' below).

Several techniques have been developed for the detection and quantitation of gastrointestinal protein loss. In the past these have primarily involved the use of intravenously administered radiolabeled macromolecules such as ^{125}I-labeled serum albumin, ^{51}CrCl$_3$, ^{51}Cr-labeled albumin, and indium 111. ^{111}In-labeled transferrin and ^{51}CrCl$_3$ (which rapidly become attached to circulating transferrin) are the compounds available commercially for clinical use. After the intravenous administration of 0.93 to 1.11 MBq (25 to 30 μCi) of the labeled compound to normal subjects, between 0.1 and 0.7 percent of the administered radioactivity is recovered in the stool over a 4-day period. Patients with excessive enteric protein loss may excrete from 2 to 40 percent of the injected radioactive label versus 0.1 to 0.7 percent in normal subjects. False-positive results may be obtained if the stool specimen is contaminated with urine. There is also a reliable and sensitive *nonisotopic* method to measure intestinal protein loss which involves the measurement of α_1-antitrypsin (AT). This serum enzyme, which has the same molecular weight as albumin (50,000), is resistant to proteolysis and when leaked into the intestinal lumen is not degraded. One can easily measure AT in serum and stool by radial immunodiffusion in order to obtain AT loss in stool (normal loss is less than 2.6 mg/g of stool) or intestinal clearance of AT (normal is less than 13 mL/d). Results using AT as a marker of intestinal protein loss correlate well with the more cumbersome and costly isotopic methods. Random fecal AT assays also can be used as a simple screening method for enteric protein loss.

The rate of albumin synthesis and degradation can be determined using intravenously administered radioiodinated albumin and measuring the decline in radioactivity in the serum. Such studies carried out in patients with protein-losing enteropathies have demonstrated a reduced circulating (intravascular) and total-body pool of albumin, a normal or increased rate of albumin synthesis, markedly shortened albumin survival, and increased fecal protein loss. Whereas normal subjects catabolize 5 to 10 percent of their intravascular albumin pool each day (the fractional catabolic rate), patients with excessive enteric protein loss may have fractional catabolic rates of 50 to 60 percent.

Studies utilizing radioiodinated immunoglobulins have demonstrated a decreased intravascular globulin pool and increased fractional catabolic rate. However, the synthesis of IgG is usually normal, suggesting that a decreased level of IgG and increased enteric protein loss are not potent stimuli for IgG synthesis. The increase in fractional catabolic rate is comparable for albumin, IgG, and IgM immunoglobulins, further suggesting that there is bulk loss of plasma proteins into the intestinal tract and not a selective loss of certain proteins. The finding of decreased globulins often is an ancillary aid in excluding renal, cardiac, and hepatic causes of hypoalbuminemia.

Abnormalities in albumin and globulin metabolism in patients with a protein-losing enteropathy may be reversed or diminished within a few months after the institution of appropriate therapy. It is obviously important that a specific etiologic diagnosis should be established in all patients with treatable disorders, who may be expected to have a remission induced by the appropriate therapy for the underlying disease. The intestinal protein loss in patients with celiac sprue, Whipple's disease, constrictive pericarditis, regional enteritis, ulcerative colitis, and Ménétrier's disease has been ameliorated by therapy appropriate to the underlying disorder.

Intestinal lymphangiectasia   PATHOPHYSIOLOGY   The disorder intestinal lymphangiectasia is characterized by increased enteric loss of protein, hypoproteinemia, edema, lymphocytopenia, malabsorption, and abnormal dilated lymphatic channels in the small intestine. The high incidence of chylous effusions and abnormal peripheral, retroperitoneal, and thoracic lymphatics indicates that intestinal lymphangiectasia is part of a generalized congenital disorder of the lymphatic system. It has been suggested that the hypoplastic visceral lymphatic channels result in obstruction to lymph flow, with the subsequent development of increased intestinal lymphatic pressure. This, in turn, may lead to dilated lymphatic vessels throughout the small-bowel wall and mesentery. Hypoproteinemia and steatorrhea are thought to be due to rupture of the dilated lymphatic vessels with discharge of lymph into the bowel lumen. In adults, approximately 1500 mL lymph, containing 70 g fat and 50 g albumin, passes through the thoracic duct each day. The leakage of a small amount of this lymph might be expected to result in considerable loss of protein and fat into the intestinal lumen. In addition, absorption of dietary long-chain triglycerides stimulates lymph flow, and this may increase further the retrograde leakage of intestinal lymph into the lumen. Three lines of evidence support the concept of intestinal leakage of lymph in intestinal lymphangiectasia: (1) chylous fluid has been recovered from the duodenum in these patients, (2) retrograde passage of contrast material from retroperitoneal lymphatics into the duodenum and jejunum has been documented, and (3) significant steatorrhea may persist in patients after institution of a completely fat-free diet, suggesting an increased enteric loss of endogenous fat present in lymph.

CLINICAL FEATURES   The disease affects primarily children and young adults. All patients have edema, which may be asymmetric because of hypoplastic peripheral lymphatics. Chylous effusions and diarrhea are common symptoms. The primary laboratory finding is hypoproteinemia with decreased serum levels of albumin, immunoglobulins IgG, IgA, and IgM, transferrin, and ceruloplasmin. Despite moderate to severe hypogammaglobulinemia, there does not appear to be an increased incidence of pyogenic bacterial infections. In addition, circulating antibody response to challenge with *Brucella* and typhoid antigens is normal. Steatorrhea is usually mild, although in some instances fat loss may be as much as 40 g/d. Some patients have hypocalcemia and impaired absorption of vitamin B_{12}. Lymphocytopenia (due to the loss of lymphocytes in lymph) is common, with lymphocyte counts ranging from 400 to 1000 per milliliter (normal: 1500 to 4000 per milliliter). This is associated with abnormal delayed hypersensitivity, as evidenced by prolonged homograft survival and impaired cutaneous responsiveness to antigens such as mumps and monilia.

Small-bowel roentgenograms are frequently abnormal, showing changes of mucosal edema and a malabsorption pattern. Lymphangiograms may demonstrate hypoplastic peripheral and visceral lymphatics with the absence of groups of retroperitoneal lymph nodes. Specimens of jejunal mucosa characteristically reveal dilated and telangiectatic lymphatic vessels in the lamina propria and submucosa. The villi may be club-shaped because of distortion from grossly dilated lymphatics (see Fig. 254-4). Such changes in the intestinal mucosa may be reversed after appropriate therapy. The diagnosis of intestinal lymphangiectasia is therefore established by (1) small-intestinal biopsy and (2) demonstration of increased enteric protein loss using radioactive macromolecules.

TREATMENT   A low-fat diet, by decreasing lymph flow, usually results in significant improvement with decreased fecal fat excretion, decreased enteric protein loss, increased serum calcium and albumin levels, and an increased half-life of injected ^{125}I-labeled albumin. Similar results may be obtained by the substitution of medium-chain triglycerides (MCT) for dietary long-chain triglycerides, since MCT are transported as medium-chain fatty acids by the portal vein rather than via the lymph.

REFERENCES

ARRANZ E, FERGUSON A: Intestinal antibody pattern in celiac disease: Occurrence in patients with normal jejunal biopsy histology. Gastroenterology 104:1263, 1993

CHERNER JA et al: Gastrointestinal dysfunction in systemic mastocytosis. A prospective study. Gastroenterology 95:657, 1988

CHIN JS et al: Paraneoplastic visceral neuropathy as a cause of severe gastrointestinal motor dysfunction. Gastroenterology 95:1279, 1988

CORAZZA G et al: Gliadin immune reactivity is associated with overt and latent enteropathy in relatives of celiac patients. Gastroenterology 102:1517, 1992

FERGUSON A et al: Clinical and pathological spectrum of coeliac disease—acitve, silent, latent, potential. Gut 34:150, 1993

FINE KD et al: Diagnosis of magnesium-induced diarrhea. N Engl J Med 324:1012, 1991

———, FORDTRAN JS: The effect of diarrhea on fecal fat excretion. Gastroenterology 102:1936, 1992

FLORENT C et al: Intestinal clearance of α_1-antitrypsin: A sensitive method for the detection of protein-losing enteropathy. Gastroenterology 81:777, 1981

GASKIN KJ et al: Colipase and maximally activated pancreatic lipase in normal subjects and patients with steatorrhea. J Clin Invest 69:368, 1982

GILLIN JS et al: Malabsorption and mucosal abnormalities of the small intestine in the acquired immunodeficiency syndrome. Ann Intern Med 102:619, 1985

HAMMER HF et al: Carbohydrate malabsorption: Its measurement and its contribution to diarrhea. J Clin Invest 86:1936, 1990

HARMS HK: Enzyme substitution therapy with the yeast saccharomyces cerevisial in congenital sucrase-isomaltase deficiency. N Engl J Med 316:1306, 1987

KAGNOFF M et al: Evidence for the role of human intestinal adenovirus in the pathogenesis of coeliac disease. Gut 28:5, 1987

KEINATH RD et al: Antibiotic treatment and relapse in Whipple's disease. Long term followup of 88 patients. Gastroenterology 88:1867, 1985

KERLIN P, WONG L: Breath hydrogen testing in bacterial overgrowth of the small intestine. Gastroenterology 95:982, 1988

KHOURI MR et al: Sudan stain of fecal fat: New insight into an old test. Gastroenterology 96: 421, 1989

KLIPSTEIN FA: Tropical sprue in travelers and expatriates living abroad. Gastroenterology 80:590, 1981

LOUGHRAN TP et al: T-cell intestinal lymphoma associated with celiac sprue. Ann Intern Med 104:44, 1986

LUBY LD et al: Lactulose/mannitol test: An ideal screen for celiac disease. Gastroenterology 96:79, 1989

MARSH M: Gluten: Major histocompatability complex, and the small intestine. Gastroenterology 102:330, 1992

PETERS TJ, BJARNASON I: Coeliac syndrome: Biochemical mechanisms and the missing peptidase hypothesis revisited. Gut 25:913, 1984

RELMAN DA et al: Identification of the uncultured bacillus of Whipple's disease. N Engl J Med 327:293, 1992

SCHILLER LR et al: Studies on the prevalence and significance of radiolabeled bile acid malabsorption in a group of patients with idiopathic chronic diarrhea. Gastroenterology 92:151, 1987

SLEIKH MS et al: Gastrointestinal absorption of calcium from milk and calcium salts. N Engl J Med 317:532, 1987

STANGHELLINI V: Chronic idiopathic intestinal pseudo-obstruction: Clinical and intestinal manometric findings. Gut 28:5, 1987

TRIER JS: Medical progress: Celiac sprue. N Engl J Med 325:1709, 1991

VAN ELBURG RM et al: Intestinal permeability in patients with coeliac disease and relatives of patients with coeliac disease. Gut 34:354, 1993

255   INFLAMMATORY BOWEL DISEASE (Ulcerative colitis and Crohn's disease)

ROBERT M. GLICKMAN

DEFINITION   *Inflammatory bowel disease* (IBD) is a general term for a group of chronic inflammatory disorders of unknown cause involving the gastrointestinal tract. Since there are no pathognomonic features or specific diagnostic tests, in a strict sense, these disorders remain diagnoses of exclusion. Their features are sufficiently characteristic, however, to permit accurate diagnosis in the majority of cases. Chronic IBD may be divided into two major groups, chronic nonspecific *ulcerative colitis* and *Crohn's disease*. The original description of the disease by Crohn, Ginzberg, and Oppenheimer in 1932 localized the disease to segments of ileum. However, the same process may involve the buccal mucosa, esophagus, stomach, and duodenum, as well as the jejunum and ileum. Crohn's disease of the small bowel is also known as *regional enteritis*. In addition, a similar inflammatory picture may occur in the colon, either alone or with accompanying small-intestinal involvement. In most instances, this form of colitis can be distinguished clinically and pathologically from ulcerative colitis and is also referred to as *Crohn's disease of the colon*. *Granulomatous colitis* is a less accurate term because only a portion of cases exhibit granulomas. Clinically these disorders are characterized by recurrent inflammatory involvement of intestinal segments with diverse clinical manifestations often resulting in a chronic, unpredictable course.

EPIDEMIOLOGY   The epidemiologic and etiologic considerations in ulcerative colitis and Crohn's disease share many features in common and will be discussed together. These diseases are more common in whites than in blacks and Orientals with an increased incidence (three- to sixfold) in Jews compared with non-Jews. Both sexes are equally affected.

The incidence and prevalence of the two diseases differ slightly, with most studies showing ulcerative colitis to be more common. When analyzed in western Europe and the United States, ulcerative colitis (including ulcerative proctitis) has an incidence of approximately 6 to 8 cases per 100,000 population and an estimated prevalence of approximately 70 to 150 cases per 100,000 population. Estimates of the incidence of Crohn's disease (colonic plus small bowel) are approximately 2 cases per 100,000 population; the prevalence is estimated at 20 to 40 per 100,000 population. Many believe the incidence of Crohn's disease (especially colonic) to be increasing. In western Europe and North America, the incidence and prevalence of Crohn's disease have been increasing five times faster than for ulcerative colitis.

While peak occurrence of both diseases is between the ages of 15 and 35, it has been reported in every decade of life. A familial incidence of IBD has been recorded with estimates that 2 to 5 percent of persons with Crohn's disease or ulcerative colitis will have one or more relatives affected. There is no specificity, however, for a given form of IBD within a given family. Such epidemiologic clustering of cases could argue for either genetic or common environmental influences on the development of these diseases (see below). It has been suggested that there is a probable hereditary basis for these disorders plus a strong environmental component.

ETIOLOGY AND PATHOGENESIS   While the cause of ulcerative colitis and Crohn's disease remains unknown, certain features of these diseases have suggested several areas of possible importance. These include familial or genetic, infectious, immunologic, and psychological factors.

Inflammatory bowel disease is more common in whites, occurs with an increased frequency in Jews, and exhibits some familial clustering. This suggests that there may be a *genetic* predisposition to the development of the disease. An increased incidence of Crohn's disease in monozygotic twins provides strong evidence for a genetic component. A search for genetic markers which might be of value in identifying susceptible individuals has not identified any single marker (i.e., histocompatibility antigen) in patients with inflammatory bowel disease.

The chronic inflammatory nature of these diseases has prompted a continuing search for a possible *infectious* cause. Despite numerous attempts to find known bacterial, fungal, or viral agents, none has thus far been isolated. Preliminary reports of isolates of cell wall variants of *Pseudomonas* or of transmissible agents producing cytopathic effects in tissue culture have yet to be confirmed. Efforts to produce specific granulomatous tissue reactions with filtrates from Crohn's disease tissue have yielded conflicting and nonreproducible results. As discussed below, many infectious agents can produce *acute* colitis or ileitis; however, there is no evidence that these agents are involved in *chronic* inflammatory bowel disease.

The theory that an *immune* mechanism may be involved is based on the concept that the extraintestinal manifestations which may accompany these disorders (e.g., arthritis, pericholangitis) may represent autoimmune phenomena and that therapeutic agents, such as glucocorticoids and azathioprine, may exert their effects via immunosuppressive mechanisms. Patients with inflammatory bowel disease may have *humoral antibodies* to colon cells, bacterial antigens such as *Escherichia coli*, lipopolysaccharide, and foreign proteins such as cow's milk protein. In general, the presence and titer of these antibodies do not correlate with disease activity. It is likely that these antigens gain access to immunocompetent cells secondary to epithelial damage. In addition, IBD has been described in association with agammaglobulinemia as well as IgA deficiency, casting further doubt on the pathogenetic role of humoral antibodies. *Immune complexes* also have been invoked to explain extraintestinal manifestations of IBD. While there are well-defined examples of tissue injury resulting from immune complexes, studies utilizing specific detection tech-

niques have failed to demonstrate an increased frequency of immune complexes in patients with IBD.

Associated abnormalities of *cell-mediated immunity* include cutaneous anergy, diminished responsiveness to various mitogenic stimuli, and decreases in the number of peripheral T cells. Since many of these changes may revert to normal when the disease is quiescent, it is likely that they are secondary phenomena. Many associated abnormalities of cell-mediated immunity have been described in the mucosa of patients with IBD. They include increased mucosal IgG cells, as well as changes in subsets of T cells, suggesting antigenic stimulation. Activation of mucosal immune cells results in a complex expression of cytokines which may contribute to the mucosal inflammatory response. In addition, noncytokine inflammatory mediators such as prostaglandin and thromboxane products are elevated in the mucosa of patients with IBD and are further stimuli for the inflammatory response. Several recent animal models of IBD, including a transgenic rat model which expresses human HLA-B27, a mouse deficient in interleukin 2, and the spontaneous chronic colitis of the cotton-top tamarin, also may shed important insights into the pathogenesis of IBD. Thus far, however, none of the altered immunologic findings has been specific for either ulcerative colitis or Crohn's disease.

The *psychological* features of patients with inflammatory bowel disease also have been stressed. It is not uncommon for these diseases to present initially or to flare in association with major psychological stresses such as the loss of a family member. It has been suggested that patients with IBD have a characteristic personality which renders them susceptible to emotional stresses which in turn may precipitate or exacerbate their symptoms. While there is little evidence directly relating possible emotional factors to the etiology of inflammatory bowel disease, there is little doubt that a chronic disease of unknown cause affecting individuals in the prime of their life often results in feelings of anger, anxiety, and some degree of depression. These reactions are undoubtedly important factors in modifying the course of these diseases and in the response to therapy.

PATHOLOGY   In ulcerative colitis there is an inflammatory reaction primarily involving the colonic mucosa. Grossly, the colon appears ulcerated, hyperemic, and usually hemorrhagic (Fig. 255-1). A striking feature of the inflammation is that it is *uniform* and *continuous* with no intervening areas of normal mucosa. The rectum is usually involved (95 percent of cases), and the inflammation extends proximally in a continuous fashion but for a variable distance. When

FIGURE 255-1   Ulcerative colitis. Resected colon with portion of terminal ileum. The specimen showed uniform inflammation, erythema, and hemorrhage and a normal terminal ileum.

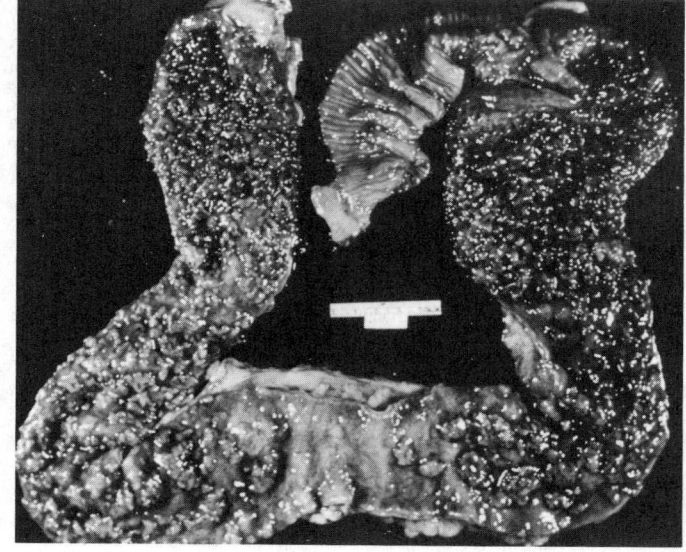

there is involvement of the entire colon, there may be minimal involvement of a few centimeters of the terminal ileum, referred to as "backwash ileitis." This involvement never leads to the thickening and narrowing characteristic of Crohn's disease. The surface mucosal cells as well as the crypt epithelium and submucosa are involved in an inflammatory reaction with neutrophilic infiltration (Fig. 255-2A). This progresses to epithelial damage with loss of surface epithelial cells resulting in multiple ulcerations. Infiltration of the crypts with neutrophils results in characteristic (but not specific) small crypt abscesses and their eventual destruction. There also may be loss of crypt epithelium with a loss of goblet (mucus-producing) cells and submucosal edema. With repetitive cycles of inflammation, mild submucosal fibrosis develops. Regenerative activity is evidenced by irregular crypt epithelium often showing bifurcation at the base of the crypts. It is important to stress that, unlike Crohn's disease, deeper layers of the bowel beneath the submucosa usually are not involved. In severe ulcerative colitis, as seen with toxic megacolon, the bowel wall may become extremely thin, the mucosa denuded, and inflammation extending to the serosa, leading to dilatation and subsequent perforation.

Recurrent inflammation may lead to characteristic features of chronicity. Fibrosis and longitudinal retraction result in shortening of the colon. Loss of the normal haustral pattern leads radiologically to a smooth, "lead-pipe" appearance of the colon. Regenerating islands of mucosa surrounded by areas of ulceration and denuded mucosa appear as "polyps" protruding into the lumen of the colon. However, these protrusions are inflammatory in nature and not neoplastic and are therefore called *pseudopolyps* (Fig. 255-2B).

With long-standing ulcerative colitis, the surface epithelium may show features of *dysplasia*. Changes of nuclear and cellular atypia are thought to represent a premalignant change occurring in the setting of long-standing ulcerative colitis. Marked dysplasia in colonic biopsies in the setting of long-standing colitis is associated with a significant risk of a coexistent carcinoma elsewhere in the colon and may influence the decision to advise colectomy.

Crohn's disease, in contrast to ulcerative colitis, is characterized by chronic inflammation extending through *all layers of the intestinal wall* and involving the mesentery as well as regional lymph nodes. Whether or not the small bowel or colon is involved, the basic pathologic process is the same.

The earliest pathologic changes in Crohn's disease are poorly defined, since surgery is usually not electively undertaken early in the course of the disease. At laparotomy, the terminal ileum appears hyperemic and boggy, with mesentery and mesenteric lymph nodes swollen and reddened. At this early stage, the bowel wall, although edematous, is usually pliable. While some patients with this initial presentation will subsequently develop typical regional enteritis, a significant number will recover completely. This acute form of ileitis will undoubtedly be shown to have diverse causes. Indeed, a significant number of patients with this presentation have been shown to be infected with *Yersinia enterocolitica*, an organism capable of producing a self-limited, acute inflammatory ileitis.

As the disease progresses, the gross appearance assumes a characteristic picture. The bowel appears greatly thickened and leathery with the lumen narrowed (Fig. 255-3). This characteristic stenosis can occur in any portion of the intestine and may be associated with varying degrees of intestinal obstruction. The mesentery appears greatly thickened, fatty, and often extends over the serosal surface of the bowel in characteristic finger-like projections. The appearance of the mucosa is variable, depending on the severity and stage of the disease, but it may appear relatively normal in sharp contrast to ulcerative colitis. In more advanced cases, the mucosa has a nodular, "cobblestoned" look. This is the result of submucosal thickening and mucosal ulceration, often linear in the long axis of the bowel at the base of mucosal folds. These ulcerations may penetrate into the submucosa and muscularis and coalesce to form intramural channels which become manifested as fistulas and fissures.

There are other morphologic features distinguishing Crohn's disease from ulcerative colitis. In Crohn's disease, the disease is often *discontinuous;* severely involved segments of bowel are separated from each other by "skip areas" of apparently normal bowel. In approximately 50 percent of Crohn's disease of the colon, the rectum may be spared. In sharp contrast, in ulcerative colitis the involvement is contiguous and the rectum is almost always involved. In addition, in Crohn's disease the transmural inflammatory process, involving serosa and mesentery, also accounts for the characteristic fistula and abscess formation. As a result of serosal inflammation, adjacent loops of small intestine may become adherent and matted together by a fibrinous peritoneal reaction, leading to a palpable mass, most often in the right lower quadrant. Fistula formation may occur between adherent loops of intestine, colon, or other adjacent organs such as the bladder or vagina. Fistulous tracts also may lead to the skin or end blindly within the peritoneum or retroperitoneum, surrounded by adherent loops of bowel and inflammatory tissue. Fistula formation is not seen in ulcerative colitis.

Microscopically, granulomas are most helpful in distinguishing Crohn's disease from other forms of inflammatory bowel disease; they do not occur in ulcerative colitis. They may be seen in rectal or colonoscopic biopsies (Fig. 255-2D). While granulomas are a helpful finding when present, it is the chronic inflammation involving all layers of the intestinal wall which is most characteristic.

In most series reporting the distribution of Crohn's disease, approximately 30 percent will involve the small intestine (usually the terminal ileum) without colonic disease, 30 percent with only colonic involvement, and 40 percent with ileocolic involvement usually of the ileum and right colon. In a small number of patients (mostly children and adolescents) there may be diffuse and extensive ulceration of the jejunum and ileum.

While there often are sufficient features to permit distinction between ulcerative colitis and Crohn's disease of the colon (Table 255-1), in 10 to 20 percent of cases this distinction may not be possible.

CLINICAL FEATURES

ULCERATIVE COLITIS The major symptoms of ulcerative colitis are bloody diarrhea and abdominal pain, often with fever and weight loss in more severe cases. With mild disease, there may be one or two semiformed stools containing little blood and with no systemic manifestations. In contrast, the patient with severe disease may have frequent liquid stools containing blood and pus, complain of severe cramps, and demonstrate symptoms and signs of dehydration, anemia, fever, and weight loss. With predominantly rectal involvement, constipation rather than diarrhea may be present, and tenesmus may be a major complaint. On occasion, intestinal symptoms may be overshadowed by fever, weight loss, or one of the extracolonic manifestations of the disease (see below).

The physical findings in ulcerative colitis are usually nonspecific; there may be some abdominal distention or tenderness along the course of the colon. In mild cases, the general physical examination will be normal. Extracolonic manifestations include arthritis, skin changes, or evidence of liver disease. Fever, tachycardia, and postural hypotension are usually associated with more severe disease. The laboratory findings are often nonspecific and usually reflect the degree and severity of bleeding and inflammation. There may be anemia which reflects chronic disease as well as iron deficiency from chronic blood loss. Leukocytosis with a left shift and an elevated sedimentation rate are often seen in the severely ill, febrile patient. Electrolyte abnormalities, especially hypokalemia, reflect the degree of diarrhea. Hypoalbuminemia is common with extensive disease and usually represents luminal protein loss through an ulcerated mucosa. An elevated alkaline phosphatase level may indicate associated hepatobiliary disease (see below).

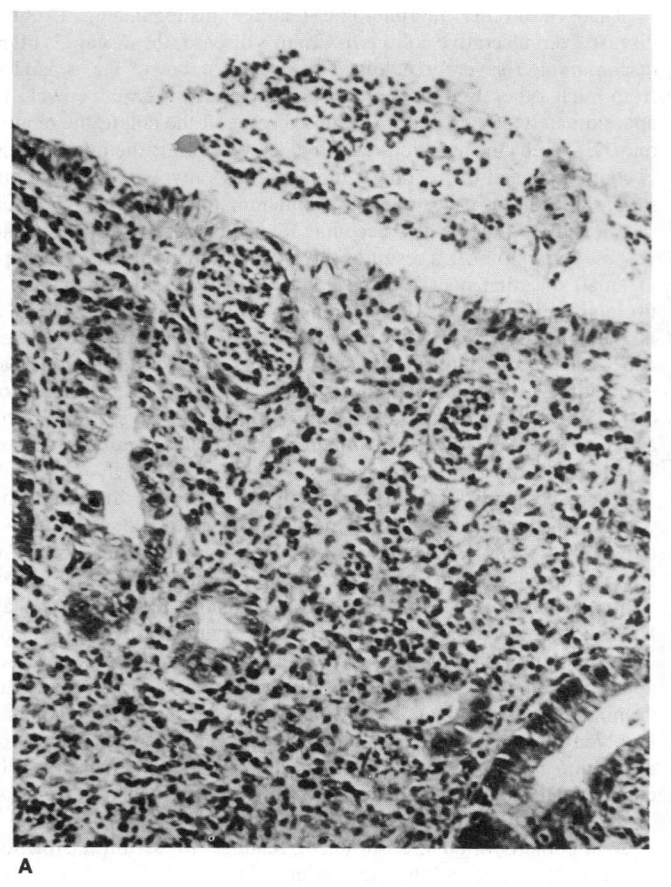

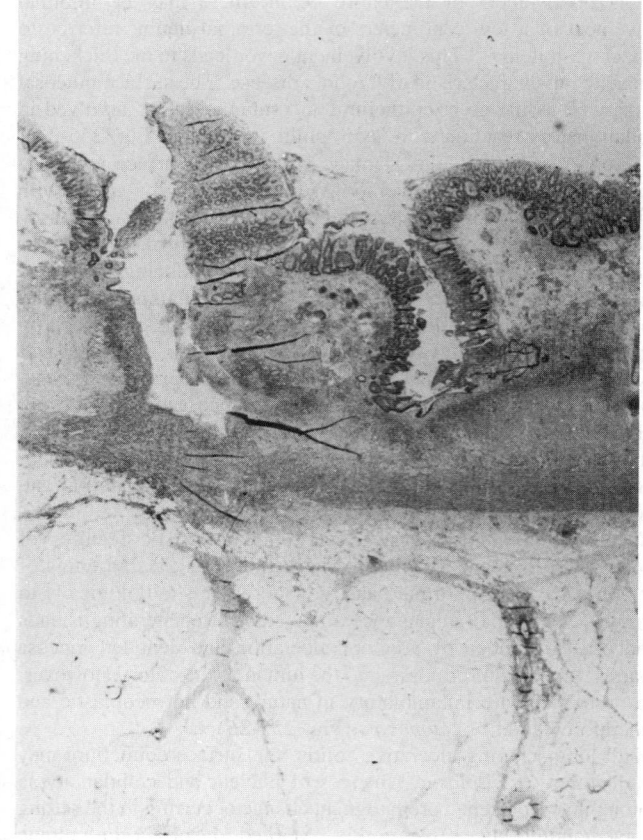

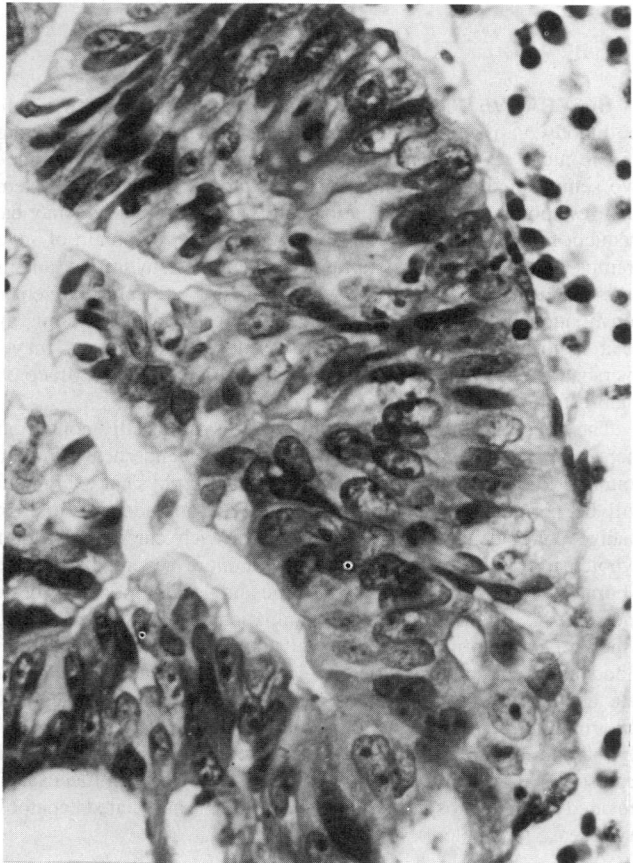

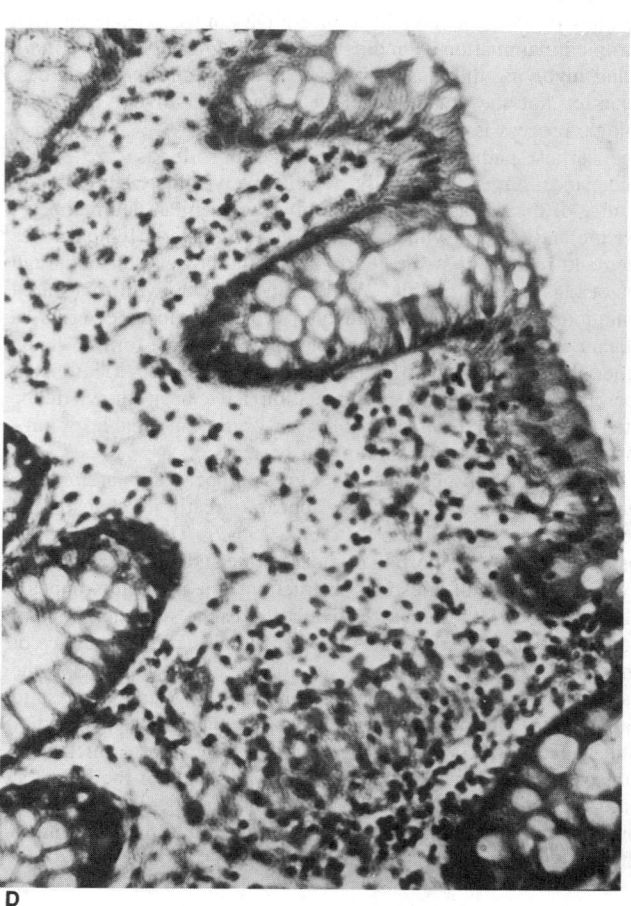

The clinical course of ulcerative colitis is variable. The majority of patients will suffer a relapse within 1 year of the first attack, reflecting the recurrent nature of the disease. There may, however, be prolonged periods of remission with only minimal symptoms. In general, the severity of symptoms reflects the extent of colonic involvement and the intensity of the inflammation. At one end of the spectrum are patients who present with limited involvement of the rectum (ulcerative proctitis) or rectum and sigmoid (ulcerative proctosigmoiditis). Consistent with this limited colonic involvement, the disease is usually mild, with minimal systemic or extracolonic manifestations, although ulcerative proctitis may on occasion be therapeutically difficult, with protracted bleeding and tenesmus. The major symptoms are rectal bleeding and tenesmus. Most of these patients, especially those with only rectal involvement, will not develop more extensive disease. In the remainder, the disease may extend proximally with variable involvement. Perhaps 85 percent of patients with ulcerative colitis will have mild to moderate disease of an intermittent nature and can be managed without hospitalization. In approximately 15 percent of patients, the disease assumes a more fulminant course, involves the entire colon, and presents with severe bloody diarrhea and systemic signs and symptoms. The patients are at risk to develop toxic dilatation and perforation of the colon (described below) and represent a medical emergency.

CROHN'S DISEASE   As discussed above, the basic pathologic features of Crohn's disease are the same whether the disease involves the small bowel or colon. The clinical presentation, however, will largely reflect the anatomic location of the disease and to some degree will predict which complications of the disease may develop. The clinical features of ulcerative colitis and Crohn's disease are compared in Table 255-1.

The major clinical features of Crohn's disease are fever, abdominal pain, diarrhea often without blood, and generalized fatigability. There may be associated weight loss. With *colonic involvement*, diarrhea and pain are the most frequent symptoms. Rectal bleeding is distinctly less common than with ulcerative colitis and reflects (1) sparing of the rectum in many patients and (2) the transmural nature of the disease with only irregular mucosal involvement. There may be associated severe anorectal complications such as fistulas, fissures, and perirectal abscess. Such features may antedate the clinical onset of colitis and should always raise the suspicion of associated Crohn's disease. With recurrent perirectal inflammation, the anal canal may be thickened, and perianal fistulas or scarring may be present. With extensive colonic involvement, dilatation of the colon may occur. However, since Crohn's disease often results in a thickened colonic wall, this is less common with Crohn's disease than with ulcerative colitis. Extracolonic manifestations (discussed below), particularly arthritis, are seen more commonly with colonic than with small-bowel Crohn's disease (regional enteritis).

With involvement of the *small bowel*, there may be additional presenting signs and symptoms. Typically, the disease has its onset in a young adult with a history of fatigue, variable weight loss, right lower quadrant discomfort or pain, and diarrhea. Low-grade fever, anorexia, nausea, and vomiting also may be present. The abdominal pain may be steady and localized to the right lower quadrant or may assume a colicky or crampy pattern, reflecting variable degrees of intestinal stenosis. The diarrhea is often moderate, usually without gross blood; if there is no rectal involvement, tenesmus is absent. Physical examination at this time often reveals right lower quadrant

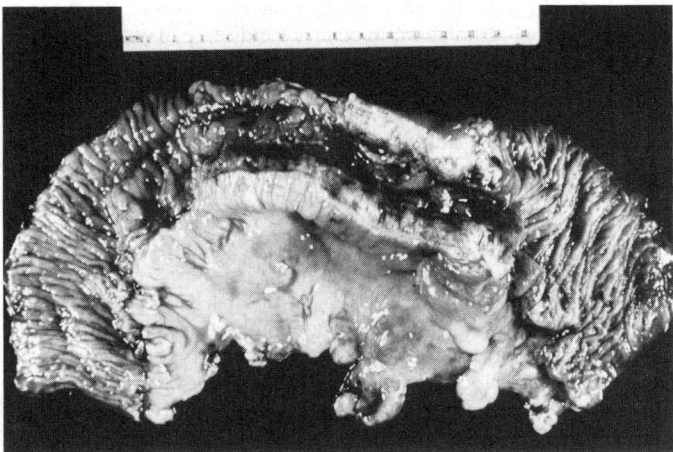

FIGURE 255-3 Regional enteritis. Resected specimen of terminal ileum demonstrates thickened bowel wall and chronically inflamed mucosa. Note the relatively sharp demarcation of the diseased segment with grossly normal mucosa on either side.

tenderness with an associated fullness or mass reflecting adherent loops of bowel. At this time the patient may have mild anemia, mild to moderate leukocytosis, and an elevated sedimentation rate.

Since acute ileitis may have an abrupt onset with fever, leukocytosis, and right lower quadrant pain, the clinical picture may be indistinguishable from acute appendicitis. The diagnosis can be made only at laparotomy, when the characteristic beefy red terminal ileum, boggy mesenteric fat, and succulent mesenteric lymph nodes indicate that appendicitis alone could not produce this picture.

While the symptoms of diarrhea and abdominal pain will usually alert the clinician to the possibility of regional enteritis, other symptoms may dominate the clinical presentation. In children and the aged, fever of undetermined origin and unexplained weight loss may be prominent and initially may cause one to suspect underlying

FIGURE 255-2 Colonic biopsies in inflammatory bowel disease. *A.* Ulcerative colitis. The surface mucosa is destroyed and the submucosa is diffusely infiltrated with polymorphonuclear leukocytes. Crypt abscesses are also present. *B.* Pseudopolyp. Regenerating island of mucosa with adjacent area of ulceration. *C.* Ulcerative colitis. Severe dysplasia occurring in long-standing chronic ulcerative colitis. Note atypical changes in the nuclei and marked palisading of nuclei of the crypt epithelium. *D.* Crohn's disease of the colon. Note the relatively intact mucosa with a solitary granuloma in the lamina propria.

TABLE 255-1   Pathologic and clinical features of IBD

	Ulcerative colitis	Crohn's disease
PATHOLOGIC		
Segmental	0	+ +
Transmural involvement	+ / −	+ +
Granulomas	0	+ / + + (50%)
Fibrosis	+	+ +
Fissuring, fistulas	+ / −	+ +
Mesenteric fat, lymph node involvement	0	+ +
CLINICAL		
Diarrhea	+ +	+ +
Rectal bleeding	+ +	+
Abdominal pain	+	+ +
Palpable mass	0	+ +
Fistulas	+ / −	+ +
Strictures	+	+ +
Small bowel involvement	+ / − ("backwash ileitis")	+ +
Rectal involvement	+ + (95%)	+ / + + (50%)
Extracolonic disease	+	+
Toxic megacolon	+	+ / −
Recurrence after colectomy	0	+
Malignancy (with long-standing disease)	+	+ / −

NOTE: 0 = never; + / − = rare; + = occasional; + + = frequent, common.

malignancy. In some patients, the first manifestation of the disease may be intestinal obstruction; in others, the disease may present with fistula formation in the form of perianal sepsis or urinary tract infection resulting from an enterovesical fistula. Similarly, right ureteral obstruction and hydronephrosis may occur due to external compression of the ureter by a right lower quadrant inflammatory mass. On occasion, often in the setting of extensive small-bowel involvement, features of malabsorption may be prominent. These features, along with anorexia and the catabolic effects of the chronic inflammatory process, may combine to produce striking degrees of weight loss.

The complications of the disease are often local, resulting from intestinal inflammation and involvement of adjacent structures.

Intestinal obstruction is a frequent complication, occurring in 20 to 30 percent of patients during the course of the disease. In the initial stages, the obstruction usually is due to the acute inflammation and edema of the involved intestinal segment, usually the terminal ileum. However, as the disease progresses and fibrosis develops, obstruction may be due to a fixed narrowing of the bowel.

Fistula formation is a frequent complication of chronic regional enteritis as well as Crohn's disease of the colon. Fistulas may occur between contiguous segments of intestine; they also may burrow into the retroperitoneal spaces and present as cutaneous fistulas or indolent abscesses. In a significant number of patients, the first indication of the disease may be the presence of persistent rectal fissures, a perirectal abscess, or a rectal fistula. Although uncommon, pneumaturia should raise the suspicion of enterovesical fistula and is often associated with a persistent urinary tract infection.

Since Crohn's disease is a transmural disease with the bowel wall greatly thickened, free *intestinal perforation* is uncommon. In a small number of cases, however, it may be the presenting feature, and the disease is first discovered at the time of laparotomy for a perforated viscus. The passage per rectum of bright red blood should alert one to the possible coexistence of rectal involvement (i.e., ileocolitis). Crohn's disease also may involve the *stomach* and *duodenum*. The involvement is usually of the antrum and/or the first and second portions of the duodenum. Symptoms may include pain mimicking peptic ulcer disease. Later in the course of the disease, chronic scarring may produce gastric outlet or duodenal obstruction.

There are increasing reports of *small-bowel* and *colonic malignancy* developing in the setting of long-standing Crohn's disease. Although the risk of developing malignancy is statistically increased, the complication is uncommon when compared with the frequency of malignancy in ulcerative colitis (see below). As in other chronic inflammatory diseases, patients with long-standing Crohn's disease may rarely develop secondary *amyloidosis*, which may manifest itself with hepatosplenomegaly or significant proteinuria. The presence of extensive ileal disease, resulting in *bile salt malabsorption*, is associated with a decreased bile salt pool and an increased lithogenicity of bile (see Chap. 254). Up to 30 percent of patients with extensive ileal disease will develop gallstones. Also, in the setting of ileal disease and an intact colon there is increased colonic absorption of dietary oxalate with resultant hyperoxaluria and the development of *urinary oxalate stones*. Dehydration due to diarrhea is an additional predisposing factor in renal stone formation.

DIAGNOSIS

The diagnosis of IBD should be entertained in all patients presenting with diarrhea or bloody diarrhea, persistent perianal sepsis, and abdominal pain. There may be atypical presentations such as fever of unexplained origin in the absence of bowel symptoms or with extracolonic manifestations such as arthritis or liver disease antedating or overshadowing the bowel involvement. Since Crohn's disease also may involve the small intestine, it should be considered in the differential diagnosis of all types of malabsorption syndromes, intermittent intestinal obstruction, and abdominal fistulas.

The laboratory examination is usually nonspecific and reflects the extent and severity of the inflammatory reaction. In addition, when Crohn's disease involves the small bowel, laboratory features of malabsorption may be present. There may be a variable degree of anemia, from occult blood loss or the effect of chronic inflammation on the bone marrow. Folate or vitamin B_{12} malabsorption also may contribute to the anemia. While the Schilling test may be abnormal in patients with extensive ileal disease, frank macrocytic anemia due to vitamin B_{12} malabsorption alone is unusual, attesting to the marked efficiency of ileal absorption of the vitamin. When there is significant diarrhea, electrolyte abnormalities (hypokalemia, hypomagnesemia) may be prominent. Hypocalcemia may reflect extensive mucosal involvement and malabsorption of vitamin D. Hypoalbuminemia may result from amino acid malabsorption as well as from protein-losing enteropathy. Variable degrees of steatorrhea may result from bile salt depletion and mucosal damage. Mild abnormalities of liver function (especially an increased serum alkaline phosphatase) may reflect the development of a fatty liver in the malnourished patient or a coexisting early sclerosing cholangitis. Significant jaundice is unusual. Proteinuria may reflect secondary amyloidosis, a rare complication.

Sigmoidoscopy and *radiologic* studies of the bowel are most important in establishing the diagnosis of inflammatory bowel disease. Sigmoidoscopy must be performed in all patients presenting with chronic diarrhea and in all instances of rectal bleeding. While meticulous air-contrast barium enema examination of the perfectly prepared colon may disclose the earliest mucosal changes in either ulcerative colitis or Crohn's disease (see below), a conventional barium enema examination is often "normal" in early disease. Direct visualization of the colonic mucosa combined with biopsy is the most sensitive way of determining whether rectal inflammation is present. It can often be performed without prior enema preparation in the patient actively having diarrhea. The goal of sigmoidoscopy is to establish *whether* mucosal inflammation is present and not necessarily to determine its full *extent* at the initial examination. Thus, if sigmoidoscopic changes are encountered within the first 8 to 10 cm, it is not necessary to pass the instrument to its full length, which may cause discomfort when the bowel is acutely inflamed. In ulcerative colitis, findings include a loss of mucosal vascularity, diffuse erythema, friability of the mucosa, and often an exudate consisting of mucus, blood, and pus. Mucosal friability and uniform involvement are characteristic. Once diseased mucosa is encountered (usually in the rectum), there are no areas of intervening normal mucosa before the proximal extent of the disease is reached. Ulceration is shallow, may be small or confluent, but invariably occurs in segments of active colitis. Full colonoscopic examination of the colon in ulcerative colitis is not indicated in the acutely ill patient. Rectal biopsy may corroborate mucosal inflammation. With more chronic disease, the mucosa may show a granular appearance, and pseudopolyps may be present.

Endoscopic examination of the colon is also of value in the diagnosis of colonic Crohn's disease. The findings are of ulcerations which may be tiny, aphthous erosions or deep, longitudinal fissures. They usually occur in segments of otherwise normal mucosa. Since the mucosa is not uniformly involved, friability and diffuse granularity, which are hallmarks of ulcerative colitis, are not characteristic of Crohn's colitis. Rather, a cobblestone appearance, which is a coarse irregularity of the mucosal surface, reflects submucosal inflammation and is characteristic of Crohn's disease. Pseudopolyps, edema, and strictures may be seen in Crohn's colitis as well as in ulcerative colitis. Colonic mucosal biopsy reveals granulomas in 30 to 50 percent of specimens taken from involved areas. Features such as crypt abscesses, infiltration with inflammatory cells, or ulcerations are nonspecific but compatible features. Since skip areas and rectal sparing are characteristic of Crohn's disease, colonoscopy may be superior to sigmoidoscopy in the evaluation of Crohn's disease. Colonoscopic examination is also indicated when Crohn's disease appears only to involve the small bowel. Ileal biopsy may be feasible, and coexisting colonic involvement occurs in a significant number of cases. Perianal inflammatory lesions as well as areas of rectal disease seen at endoscopy will often show granulomatous inflammation. Rectal biopsy of seemingly uninvolved areas also may show microscopic evidence of granulomatous inflammation in only 5 to 15 percent of patients.

The *radiologic evaluation* of the bowel provides essential information in the diagnosis of IBD. Barium enema, in ulcerative colitis, may reveal the extent of the disease and help define associated features such as stricture, pseudopolyposis, or carcinoma. The earliest features seen in ulcerative colitis are irritability and incomplete filling due to associated inflammation. Fine ulcerations may be seen at this time as serrations along the contour of the bowel producing a hazy margin (Fig. 255-4). The ulcerations may become deeper and with more fulminant disease produce a grossly ragged and irregular contour. Polypoid defects appear as a result of edematous mucosa between ulcerations. The diffuse pattern of ulceration is best seen on the evacuation film or on air-contrast barium enema. In the chronic stage of the disease (Fig. 255-5), the characteristic features are shortening of the bowel, depression of the flexures, narrowing of the bowel lumen, and rigidity. The bowel has a symmetric, ahaustral, tubular appearance with a decreased mucosal pattern. Although strictures are uncommon, when they occur, they have a concentric lumen with fusiform tapering margins. Eccentricity should raise the suspicion of an associated carcinoma.

Barium enema examination in Crohn's disease of the colon has features which usually distinguish it from ulcerative colitis. Features characteristic of Crohn's disease include rectal sparing, the presence of skip lesions, and the finding of small ulcerations occurring on small irregular nodules. The small ulcerations often extend to produce longitudinal ulcers (Fig. 255-6) and transverse fissures which in reality are limited sinus tracts. These may extend into adjacent tissues to produce fistulas. Irregular thickening and fibrosis may lead to stricture formation, which may be multiple. In 10 to 15 percent of cases the disease may uniformly involve the entire colon, making differentiation from ulcerative colitis more difficult. Reflux of barium into the

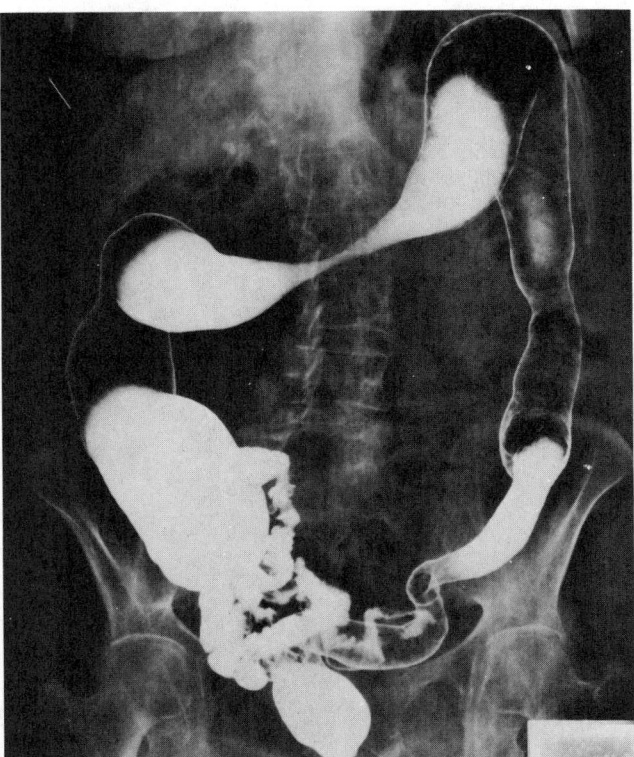

FIGURE 255-5 Chronic ulcerative colitis. Note the loss of haustrations and the fusiform stricture in the transverse colon. *(Courtesy of R Gold, Columbia Presbyterian Medical Center.)*

terminal ileum during barium enema may reveal characteristic ileal changes of regional enteritis.

When Crohn's disease involves the small intestine, the terminal ileum is most characteristically involved with features similar to colonic involvement. Careful x-ray examination of the small bowel may demonstrate loss of mucosal detail and rigidity of involved segments resulting from submucosal edema or stenosis. The submucosal inflammation may lead to the characteristic radiologic cobblestoned appearance of the mucosa (Fig. 255-7), and fistulous tracts may be seen, especially in the ileocecal area (Fig. 255-8). Involvement of the stomach and duodenum usually appears radiologically as stiffening and infiltration of the mucosa and can mimic an infiltrative tumor. If such an appearance is due to regional enteritis, there is almost always coexistent involvement of either the jejunum or ileum. In Crohn's disease, computed tomographic (CT) imaging of the abdomen may be of value in the evaluation of thickened, separated bowel loops and to help distinguish thickened, matted loops (phlegmon) from intraabdominal abscess.

While barium studies often provide information on the pattern and extent of inflammatory bowel disease, caution must be exercised in obtaining these studies in the acutely ill patient with severe colitis, in whom barium study and the bowel cleansing which precedes it may result in a worsening of the disease and can precipitate toxic dilatation of the colon.

Fiberoptic colonoscopy has added greatly to the diagnosis of colonic inflammatory bowel disease. Areas formerly beyond the reach of the sigmoidoscope can now be directly visualized and biopsy material obtained. Early in the course of colonic inflammation, endoscopic examination and biopsy are the most sensitive techniques to demonstrate mucosal involvement. Polypoid lesions, strictures, and unclear x-ray features can usually be fully defined. Periodic colonoscopic examination and biopsy are being used increasingly in cancer surveillance in patients with long-standing inflammatory bowel disease (see below).

FIGURE 255-4 Acute ulcerative colitis, air-contrast study. Note the diffuse fine ulceration of the entire colon, producing serration along the contour of the bowel. *(Courtesy of R Gold, Columbia Presbyterian Medical Center.)*

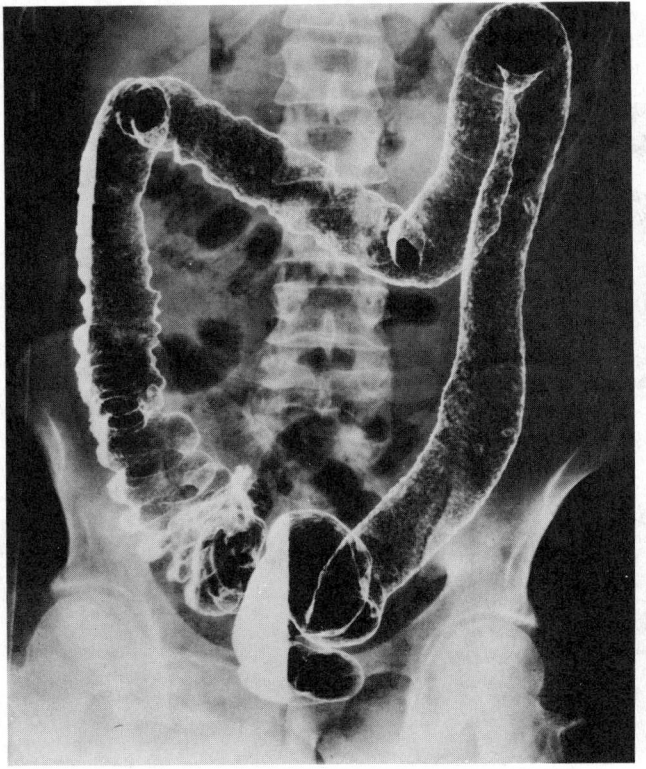

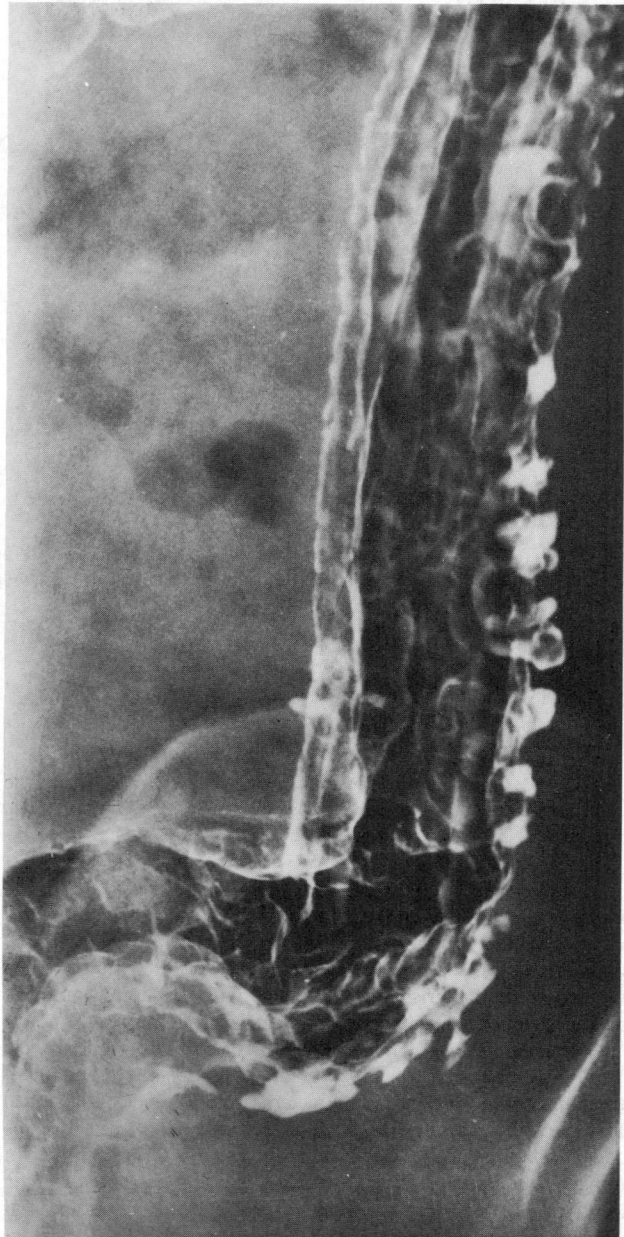

FIGURE 255-6   Crohn's colitis. Air-contrast study.

DIFFERENTIAL DIAGNOSIS

Many entities must be considered in the differential diagnosis in IBD. The focus of the differential diagnosis in large measure will be determined by the presenting features of the disease. When *rectal bleeding* is the presenting complaint, a colonic source should be considered. While *hemorrhoids* are commonly found, they must be considered a tentative source of bleeding until sigmoidoscopy and barium enema have eliminated other colonic lesions. Colonic *neoplasms* (carcinoma, adenomatous polyps) also may present with rectal bleeding and can usually be diagnosed by barium enema with subsequent sigmoidoscopic or colonoscopic biopsy. It should be remembered that carcinoma may complicate long-standing colitis. Rectal bleeding from *colonic diverticula* or *arteriovenous malformations* usually presents no problem in differential diagnosis, since radiologic and endoscopic features of inflammatory bowel disease are absent. *Radiation proctitis*, which may present as a localized area of colitis, is usually found in the setting of pelvic irradiation. The onset

may, however, occur at variable (months to years) periods of time after irradiation. Characteristic features on sigmoidoscopy include mucosal atrophy and telangiectasia along with friability and small ulcerations. A colitis sometimes indistinguishable from ulcerative colitis may occur in Behçet's syndrome and is associated with aphthous oral ulceration, uveitis, and urethritis.

Acute colitis may be caused by a variety of *infectious* agents (Chap. 87). Often presenting with bloody diarrhea, infectious colitis may be difficult to distinguish from IBD at initial presentation, and severe cases may present with colonic dilatation mimicking toxic megacolon. Rectal biopsy in infectious colitis shows marked polymorphonuclear infiltration with pronounced edema and relative sparing of the crypts, features which may distinguish it from idiopathic inflammatory bowel disease. A listing of these agents is given in Table 255-2.

Amebiasis may present with bloody diarrhea and at sigmoidoscopy may be indistinguishable from idiopathic ulcerative colitis. A history of recent foreign travel or homosexual exposure would be important. Amebic serologies may be of value, although initial positive titers may indicate prior infection of indeterminate age. Since specific amebicidal therapy is necessary to eradicate this infection and corticosteroids may be detrimental, every effort should be made to exclude this diagnosis in appropriate individuals via serologic titers and careful examination of colonic secretions and biopsies. Acute *bacillary dysentery* may be caused by *Shigella* and *Salmonella* or *Campylobacter*, all easily diagnosed by stool culture. *Yersinia enterocolitis*, which may present as acute ileitis, also can produce a self-limited colitis, sometimes with granulomatous reaction. Infectious agents may cause acute proctitis indistinguishable from idiopathic ulcerative proctitis. Such infections, often seen in homosexuals, may be due to herpes simplex virus, *gonorrhea, lymphogranuloma venereum* (LGV), *cytomegalovirus, Isospora,* or *Treponema pallidum,* as well as *amebiasis.* In homosexual men, non-LGV strains of *Chlamydia* have been shown to produce a granulomatous proctitis closely resembling Crohn's disease of the rectum.

Pseudomembranous colitis (antibiotic-associated colitis) is caused by a necrolytic toxin elaborated by *Clostridium difficile*, which under certain circumstances proliferates within the bowel. Most often the

FIGURE 255-7   Crohn's ileocolitis. Note the nodularity and ulceration of the terminal ileum and the deformity of the cecum.

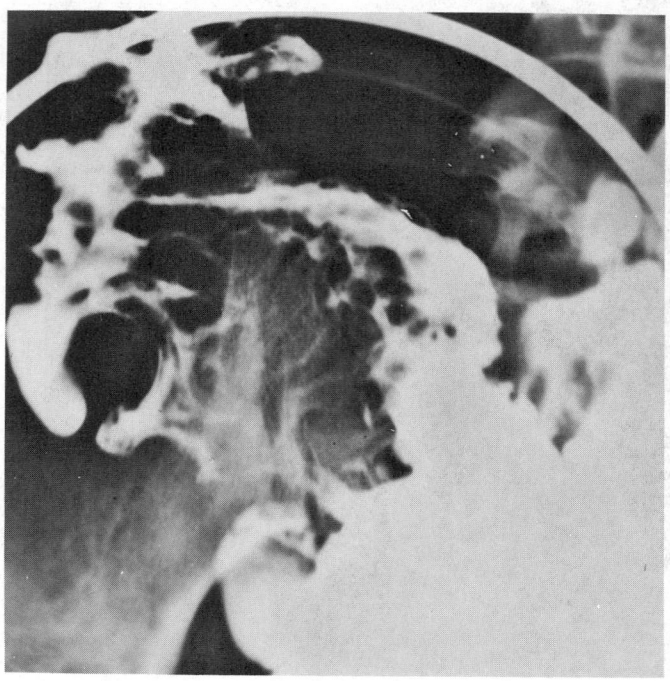

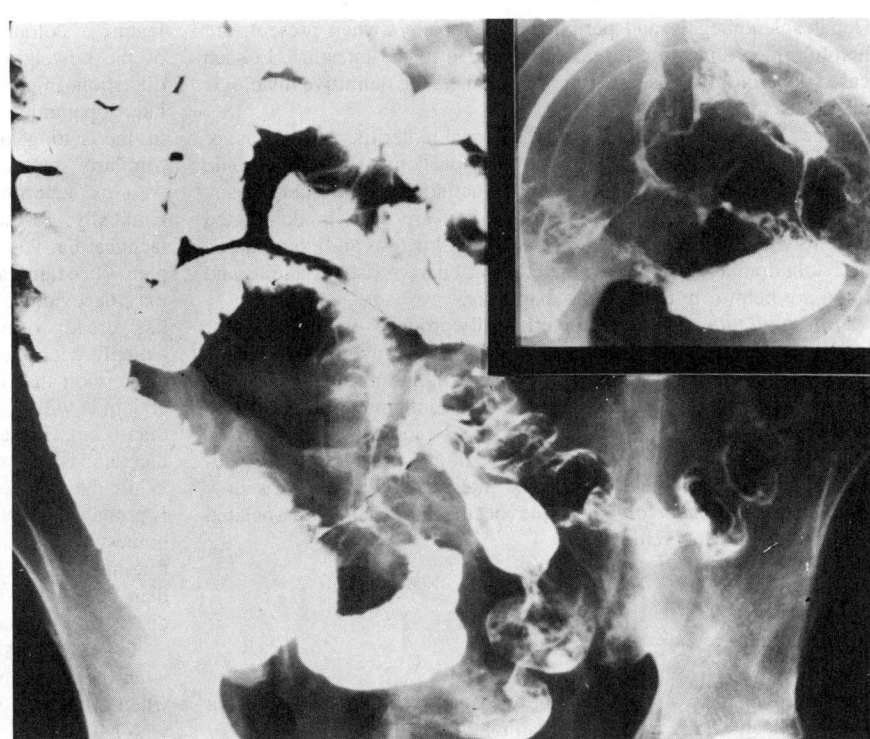

FIGURE 255-8 Regional enteritis. X-ray showing fistulas between loops of bowel. Insert is a compression film of this area; note fistulas between adjacent loops of bowel.

disease is a result of antibiotic therapy which presumably upsets the normal ecologic balance of the bowel flora and permits *C. difficile* to proliferate. Almost every antibiotic has been implicated, although cases related to the use of vancomycin or aminoglycosides are rare. Most often diarrhea is profuse and watery, although bloody diarrhea occurs in 5 percent of cases. Characteristic lesions are seen on sigmoidoscopy and appear as multiple, discrete yellowish plaques which on biopsy show features of acute inflammation and ulceration with a pseudomembrane of fibrin and necrotic material. On occasion, lesions may be beyond reach of the sigmoidoscope and require colonoscopy. Diagnosis is best made by detecting *C. difficile* toxin in the stool. Treatment is initially directed at eradicating *C. difficile* organisms from the stool. Vancomycin (250 mg PO qid for 7 to 14 days) is the treatment of choice for more severely ill patients and should produce clinical improvement within 5 days. Since vancomycin therapy is expensive, alternative therapies have been proposed. The use of metronidazole (500 mg PO qid for 7 to 14 days) has been shown to be equally effective as vancomycin. Alternatively, bacitracin (20,000 units qid for 7 to 14 days) is also quite effective. With all forms of therapy, relapse rates (15 to 30 percent) have been observed and may require a subsequent course of therapy to eradicate the organism. On occasion, infectious causes of colitis will be superimposed on ulcerative colitis or Crohn's disease. In this case, once the acute infection has subsided, symptoms and inflammatory mucosal changes may persist, raising the possibility of associated idiopathic IBD. Similar considerations apply to the patient with IBD who uncommonly may develop associated *pseudomembranous* colitis. The finding of *C. difficile* toxin in the stool and subsequent treatment will serve to clarify this presentation.

Abdominal pain in association with rectal bleeding, especially in the older age group, may be due to *ischemic colitis* and be most difficult to distinguish from inflammatory bowel disease, especially Crohn's disease. Because of an excellent collateral circulation, the rectum is usually spared. Radiologic features are often characteristic, showing submucosal edema or hemorrhage (thumb printing) which typically resolves spontaneously over several weeks.

Inflammatory bowel disease may be difficult to distinguish from functional diarrhea early in the course of disease. The presence of constitutional symptoms such as fatigue, fever, weight loss, and

nocturnal diarrhea, coupled with laboratory features of anemia, elevated erythrocyte sedimentation rate, or occult blood in the stool, should alert the clinician to the possibility of IBD. Similarly, finding leukocytes in a stained stool specimen points to an inflammatory basis for the diarrhea. In all cases, stool cultures and parasitologic examination of the stool are required to rule out enteric bacterial pathogens or amebiasis. In the *irritable bowel syndrome*, sigmoidoscopy, rectal biopsy, and barium enema examination are all normal.

Once the diagnosis of idiopathic IBD has been established, the distinction between ulcerative colitis and Crohn's disease of the colon is usually possible. Differential diagnostic features are shown in Table 255-1.

With small-intestinal involvement (regional enteritis), the differential diagnosis should include disorders presenting with intraabdominal abscesses, fistulas, intestinal obstruction, and malabsorption. The finding of associated colonic involvement in patients with ileal disease will often serve to distinguish Crohn's disease from other ileal disorders. With diffuse involvement of the jejunum and ileum, regional enteritis must be distinguished from *nongranulomatous ulcerative jejunoileitis*. Abdominal pain and diarrhea are prominent features of this disorder, and weight loss, malabsorption, and hypoproteinemia tend to be more prominent than in regional enteritis. Small-bowel biopsy shows a more diffuse lesion with flattened villi (similar to celiac sprue), infiltration of the lamina propria, and mucosal ulceration. *Abdominal lymphoma* may likewise present with clinical and radiologic features difficult to distinguish from regional enteritis.

TABLE 255-2   Microbiologic causes of colitis

Shigella
Salmonella
Amebiasis
Yersinia
Campylobacter
Lymphogranuloma venereum (LGV)
"Non-LGV" *Chlamydia*
Gonorrhea
Pseudomembranous colitis (*Clostridium difficile* toxin)
Tuberculosis

Hepatosplenomegaly and peripheral adenopathy, when present, are helpful clues, but often disease is confined to the intestine. In such cases, laparotomy is usually required to make the definitive histologic diagnosis.

The advanced presentation of regional enteritis with areas of stenosis and draining fistulas also may be confused with *chronic fungal infection of the bowel*, including actinomycosis, aspergillosis, and blastomycosis. These infections often are seen in debilitated patients with impaired host defenses. Fungal skin tests and examination of fistula drainage and biopsy material for characteristic granules and fungi are helpful in making the diagnosis.

Intestinal tuberculosis characteristically produces stenotic lesions, usually in the terminal ileum, also often involving the contiguous cecum and ascending colon. Unlike regional enteritis, skip areas are unusual. Histologically, the granulomatous inflammation seen with *Mycobacterium tuberculosis* infection may be indistinguishable from regional enteritis; acid-fast stains and cultures are required. Fortunately, in western countries primary intestinal tuberculosis is now rare; when intestinal involvement does occur, it invariably is associated with pulmonary tuberculosis.

COMPLICATIONS OF INFLAMMATORY BOWEL DISEASE

The complications of IBD may be classified as local, which are a direct reflection of mucosal inflammation and its extension, or systemic (Table 255-3). Local complications of IBD such as fistulas, abscesses, and strictures have been described above. In addition, perforation, toxic dilatation, and the development of carcinoma may complicate both ulcerative colitis and Crohn's disease.

PERFORATION   Intestinal perforation can occur in severe ulcerative colitis since with extensive ulceration the bowel wall may become extremely thin. The clinical features are those of acute peritonitis with signs of peritoneal inflammation and the demonstration of free air under the diaphragm on upright film of the abdomen. These are an indication for immediate colectomy.

Toxic dilatation of the colon may occur in Crohn's colitis but is more common in ulcerative colitis. This complication can best be considered as a severe form of ulcerative colitis with the additional

---

TABLE 255-3   Some systemic complications of inflammatory bowel disease

Nutritional and metabolic
  Weight loss, ↓ muscle mass, growth retardation (children)
  Electrolyte deficiency (K^+, Ca^{2+}, Mg^{2+})
  Hypoalbuminemia (↓ nutrition, protein-losing enteropathy)
  Anemia (chronic disease, iron deficiency; rarely folate or vitamin B_{12} deficiency in Crohn's disease)
  Bile salt deficiency with ileal disease (steatorrhea and fat-soluble vitamin deficiency; ↑ colonic oxalate absorption → renal stones; ↑ lithogenicity of bile → gallstones)
Musculoskeletal
  Peripheral arthralgia, arthritis
  Ankylosing spondylitis, sacroileitis
  Granulomatous myositis (rare)
Hepatobiliary disease
  Fatty liver
  Cholelithiasis
  Pericholangitis, biliary cirrhosis (rare)
  Sclerosing cholangitis
  Bile duct carcinoma
  Chronic active hepatitis and cirrhosis
Skin and mucous membrane
  Erythema nodosum
  Pyoderma gangrenosum
  Aphthous stomatitis
  Crohn's disease of buccal mucosa, gingiva, vagina
Eye
  Iritis, uveitis, episcleritis
Venous thrombosis and thromboembolism (hypercoagulability, dehydration, stasis)

---

feature of colonic dilatation. It is thought that the neuromuscular tone of the bowel is affected by the severe inflammation, resulting in dilatation. Injudicious use of hypomotility agents (codeine, diphenoxylate, loperamide, paregoric, anticholinergic agents) to treat diarrhea in the setting of acute colitis can precipitate this complication. Similarly, cathartic preparation and barium enema examination as well as superimposed hypokalemia may be contributing factors. Clinically, features of severe colitis are present with high fever, tachycardia, volume depletion, electrolyte imbalance, and abdominal pain. On examination, the patient appears toxic, and colonic dilatation may be evident. There is abdominal tenderness, and if perforation has already occurred, peritoneal signs are present. Diarrhea may actually decrease markedly due to colonic atony, creating the false impression that the colitis is clinically improved. Plain film of the abdomen will show colonic dilatation with the colonic diameter more than 6 cm. There may be air in the wall of the colon, and irregular, ulcerated islands of mucosa may be silhouetted against the air shadow. While the transverse colon is the most common site of dilatation, this is probably largely positional, since with the patient supine this is the highest portion of the colon. This presentation of colitis represents a true medical emergency and is associated with a mortality of greater than 30 percent if perforation has occurred. Appropriate therapy is discussed below.

CARCINOMA AND INFLAMMATORY BOWEL DISEASE   There is an increased incidence of carcinoma in patients with chronic IBD when compared with the general population, especially in patients who have more extensive mucosal involvement (i.e., pancolitis) and those who have had their disease for extended periods of time. Cumulative risk of cancer begins to rise 10 years after the disease is diagnosed. While the incidence of cancer varies with the patient population studied, it is estimated that the overall incidence of cancer is 0.5 to 1 percent per year after 10 years. It has been estimated that with pancolitis there is a risk of cancer of 12 percent at 15 years, 23 percent at 20 years, and 42 percent at 24 years, although estimates in community-based practices have been lower, with the probability that colon cancer will develop in patients with pancolitis being 10 percent at 26 years. In children, the risk of cancer appears to rise more sharply after the first 10 years of disease, perhaps reflecting the higher incidence of pancolitis in children. Patients with ulcerative proctitis (disease limited to rectum) have no increased risk of cancer. Malignancy developing in Crohn's disease of the colon or small bowel is less well documented, but the incidence of both small- and large-bowel malignancy is increased compared with the general population. However, it is lower than in ulcerative colitis, perhaps because less mucosa is often chronically involved with Crohn's disease than with ulcerative colitis.

The development of colon carcinoma arising in the setting of IBD demonstrates important differences when compared with carcinoma arising in a noncolitic population. Clinically, many of the earlier warning signs of a colonic neoplasm (i.e., rectal bleeding, change in bowel habits) will be difficult to interpret in the setting of colitis. In colitic patients, the distribution of carcinomas is more uniform throughout the colon than in noncolitic patients; in the latter the majority of carcinomas are in the rectosigmoid, within reach of the sigmoidoscope. In colitis patients, the tumors are more often multiple, flat, and infiltrating and appear to have a higher grade of malignancy. There is some evidence to suggest that these features may reflect the younger age at which they occur rather than the associated colitis. Further adding to the difficulty in diagnosis is the frequent occurrence of mucosal irregularities, ulcerations, and pseudopolyps, making a small carcinoma difficult to diagnose radiologically or endoscopically.

Efforts have been directed toward devising effective screening procedures to detect carcinoma developing in the setting of IBD. Carcinoembryonic antigen (CEA) may be elevated nonspecifically in ulcerative colitis and therefore is of limited value. Periodic barium enemas and/or sigmoidoscopy or colonoscopy have been suggested, but interpretation is sometimes hampered by abnormalities related to the colitis itself. The addition of colonic mucosal biopsy may add a significant dimension. It was originally suggested that a generalized precancerous lesion may be present in high-risk patients with colitis who either harbor an occult malignancy or who will develop cancer. Subsequent studies in patients with long-standing colitis showed that if severe dysplasia was present, there was approximately a 50-percent chance that an associated malignancy was present in those patients who subsequently came to colectomy. Complicating these findings was the fact that dysplastic changes were found in rectal biopsies only 60 percent of the time, making colonoscopy with multiple biopsies desirable. In addition, in some patients not undergoing colectomy, dysplasia was not a consistent finding on subsequent biopsies. While more information is needed on the prognostic significance and reproducibility of finding dysplastic changes on mucosal biopsy, it seems prudent to examine patients with colonic IBD of greater than 8 to 10 years' duration with colonoscopy and multiple mucosal biopsies at regular intervals. The frequency of such examinations has not been established, with recommendations varying from 6 months to 2 years. If severe dysplasia is found, then confirmation at less than 6-month intervals seems prudent. While most authorities would not advise "prophylactic" colectomy in the patient with long-standing colitis with mild or moderate dysplasia, the finding of severe dysplasia may well identify a subgroup who already harbor an occult carcinoma or who are at high risk of its development. There can be no uniform recommendation for this small group of patients, but many physicians will advise colectomy in this setting.

EXTRAINTESTINAL MANIFESTATIONS OF INFLAMMATORY BOWEL DISEASE

There are a variety of nonintestinal symptoms and signs which may be associated with IBD and occur in both ulcerative colitis and Crohn's disease (see Table 255-3). Since some of these manifestations may not coincide with or may overshadow the underlying bowel disease, they may on occasion pose difficult diagnostic problems. Their cause is currently unknown.

Joint manifestations occur in 25 percent of patients with IBD. These may range from arthralgia only to an acute arthritis with painful, swollen joints.

The nondeforming arthritis is mono- or polyarticular and often migratory. Knees, ankles, and wrists are most commonly involved, but any joint may be affected. Joint fluid, if aspirated, reveals findings of an acute arthritis without crystals or evidence of infection. Tests for specific forms of arthritis (rheumatoid factor, antinuclear antibody, and LE factor) are negative. Typically, the arthritis correlates with activity of the underlying bowel disease. Rarely, peripheral arthritis may truly antecede clinical bowel symptoms. Arthritis is found more commonly in patients with colonic than with small-bowel involvement alone (regional enteritis).

In contrast, the central arthritis or ankylosing spondylitis associated with IBD is unrelated to the activity of the underlying bowel disease. It may antedate the bowel disease by years and persist after surgical or medical remission of the disease has been achieved. Symptoms are of low backache and stiffness with eventual limitation of motion. This may be associated with sacroileitis as well. X-rays usually reveal characteristic changes. In contrast to the peripheral arthritis, there is a strong association of HLA-B27 with ankylosing spondylitis, whether or not IBD is present.

Like the peripheral arthritis, *skin manifestations* are more common with colonic disease. They occur in about 15 percent of patients, and when present, the severity correlates with activity of the bowel disease. *Erythema nodosum* may be seen and heals without scarring. *Pyoderma gangrenosum*, an ulcerating lesion often occurring on the trunk, is relatively painless and may heal with scarring. In the rare patient, the lesion may persist even after colectomy for ulcerative colitis. *Aphthous ulcers* resemble "canker sores" of the mouth, and in approximately 5 to 10 percent of patients they are present during periods of active disease and then resolve. Their cause is unknown, and they are treated symptomatically. *Ocular manifestations* such as episcleritis, recurrent iritis, and uveitis occur in approximately 5 percent of patients and may represent a severe manifestation of the disease. In general, their activity parallels the course of the bowel disease, and the lesions may respond dramatically when colectomy is done for other indications.

Abnormalities of *liver function* are common in IBD. In the severely ill, malnourished patient, mild abnormalities of serum aminotransferases and alkaline phosphatase are often seen and represent nonspecific focal hepatitis or fatty infiltration. Factors favoring fatty infiltration of the liver in the severely ill patient are poor nutrition and often concomitant steroid therapy. The lesion is not progressive and resolves with disease remission. *Pericholangitis* is characterized histologically by portal tract inflammation, some bile ductular proliferation, and concentric fibrosis around bile ductules. Some authorities feel that this lesion represents the intrahepatic form of sclerosing cholangitis. Most often, the lesion is clinically insignificant, and its sole manifestation is an elevated serum alkaline phosphatase level. It is usually nonprogressive and requires no therapy. Rarely, there may be an apparent progression to cirrhosis of either the postnecrotic or biliary type. Uncommonly, patients with IBD may develop *sclerosing cholangitis* (Chap. 272), a chronic inflammation of unknown cause involving the extrahepatic and intrahepatic bile ducts which may produce varying degrees of extrahepatic biliary obstruction. Corticosteroids and immunosuppressive therapy are not beneficial. Reversal of the disease after colectomy is an inconsistent result and should not form the sole indication for colectomy. Cholangiocarcinoma, arising in the extrahepatic biliary tree, has an increased incidence in patients with chronic ulcerative colitis. Such patients will present with extrahepatic biliary obstruction which must be distinguished from sclerosing cholangitis. Finally, *chronic active hepatitis* which may progress to *cirrhosis* may be seen in IBD, although the exact relationship between these disorders is unknown. The evaluation and therapy are similar to the disease occurring in noncolitic patients. There is no clear evidence that colectomy influences the course of this form of liver disease.

TREATMENT

In general, the treatment of ulcerative colitis and Crohn's disease shares certain common principles. Initial treatment of all forms of uncomplicated IBD is primarily medical, and the principles of medical therapy are similar. Surgery is reserved for (1) specific complications and (2) intractability of disease. There are certain important differences, however, between ulcerative colitis and Crohn's disease; namely, the response to drug therapy may differ, complications often differ, and the prognosis after surgical therapy is not the same.

ULCERATIVE COLITIS   Medical therapy   Once the diagnosis is established, the severity of the disease must be assessed. Mild ulcerative colitis, including ulcerative proctitis, can usually be treated on an ambulatory basis. It should be noted that on occasion, disease, although limited to the rectum, may be severe. More severe disease, especially at initial presentation, is best treated in a hospital setting. The disease can worsen rapidly, and the course of a given attack cannot be predicted at the outset. The aims of therapy are to control the inflammatory process and replace nutritional losses. A certain degree of improvement usually follows intravenous correction of fluid and electrolyte disturbances. Blood transfusions may be required in severe anemia, especially when there is continued active bleeding. Agents to control diarrhea (diphenoxylate, loperamide, codeine, anticholinergics) should be used with extreme caution for fear of precipitating colonic dilatation and toxic megacolon. The decision to institute specific nutritional replacement therapy will be determined by the nutritional status of the patient and whether a protracted clinical course can be anticipated. In the severely ill patient, even clear liquids orally may stimulate colonic activity, and it is often wise to give the patients nothing by mouth. In this setting, intravenous alimentation, either peripheral or central, has been used as interim nutritional replacement therapy (see Chap. 76). While there is no evidence that intravenous alimentation is effective as primary therapy, it is an important component of a treatment program. In the less severely ill patients able to tolerate fluids by mouth, the use of elemental oral diets may be beneficial, providing supplemental nutrition with low fecal volume. While milk is not contraindicated in ulcerative colitis, diarrhea will be exacerbated if there is an associated lactase deficiency.

The principal drugs used in the therapy of ulcerative colitis are the *anti-inflammatory agents, sulfasalazine* (Azulfidine), and *adrenal glucocorticoids.* Sulfasalazine consists of a sulfonamide (sulfapyridine) moiety chemically bound to a salicylate (5-aminosalicylate); it undergoes bacterial cleavage in the colon. The liberated sulfapyridine is efficiently absorbed and largely excreted in the urine; the liberated 5-aminosalicylate, believed to be the active component, remains largely in the colon and is excreted in the stool. The salicylate moiety is thought to exert its action through inhibition of prostaglandin synthesis. While most physicians are familiar with the use of sulfasalazine to prevent recurrences of ulcerative colitis, it is less well appreciated that this agent is effective in the therapy of acute ulcerative colitis of mild to moderate severity. Therapeutic doses of 4 to 6 g/d are required. The drug is usually started at a dose of 500 mg bid and then increased daily or every other day by 1 g until the therapeutic dose is achieved. Topical preparations of 5-aminosalicylate (mesalamine) given as an enema are effective in the control of distal proctocolitis. Several preparations of oral 5-aminosalicylate (encapsulated in a pH-sensitive slow-release form or as two molecules of 5-aminosalicylate conjugated to each other as a dimer) are also effective.

In the severely ill patient who may not tolerate oral medication and for whom a more rapid time frame of therapy is often desired, initial therapy is begun with glucocorticoids. While ACTH is equally effective when given in equivalent dosages and by comparable routes of administration, most physicians seldom use ACTH. The choice is one of individual preference; oral prednisone (45 to 60 mg/d) is usually employed initially. In the severely ill patient, parenteral administration of corticosteroids (i.e., intravenous prednisolone, 45 to 60 mg/d) is preferable to avoid the uncertainty of adequate oral absorption. Improvement is usually noted after 7 to 10 days of such therapy by a reduction in fever, decrease in bloody diarrhea, and improvement in appetite.

After initial improvement, low-roughage oral feedings can be resumed. At this point, the dose of steroids can be tapered. There is no specific schedule for tapering glucocorticoids. The guiding principle, however, is that once clinical remission is achieved, there is no evidence that chronic steroid administration favorably influences the long-term outlook of the disease or that recurrences can be prevented by chronic steroid therapy. In practice, steroid therapy can be tapered and discontinued over a 2- to 3-month period after discharge. In some patients (10 to 15 percent), efforts to completely eliminate steroids may be associated with a flare of the disease, and low to moderate steroids (10 to 15 mg prednisone daily) may be required to suppress disease activity. This should not be confused with the prophylactic administration of steroids to patients in remission but rather represents incompletely responsive disease. Once the acutely ill patient is taking oral feedings, sulfasalazine should be added as described above in a daily dose of 2 g. Controlled trials have shown that this dose of sulfasalazine, when administered chronically to patients with ulcerative colitis, is effective in decreasing the frequency of relapses and should be continued chronically after glucocorticoids have been discontinued. Patients with glucose phosphate dehydrogenase deficiency or those exhibiting severe allergic reactions to the drug unfortunately cannot be maintained on it. Patients who exhibit intolerance for the drug (headache, nausea) or mild skin allergic reactions can be treated with formulations of 5-aminosalicylate (see above), thus avoiding allergic reactions due to sulfa. Targeted systems for the delivery of the active moiety, 5-aminosalicylate (mesalamine), provide a number of options for the physician. Mesalamine enemas

are effective topical therapy for distal ulcerative colitis and are necessary to maintain remission. Oral formulations of 5-aminosalicylate (see above) also can be employed in patients intolerant of sulfasalazine who prefer oral to topical therapy.

The use of immunosuppressive therapy with drugs such as azathioprine is less well established in ulcerative colitis. As a single agent in the therapy of acute ulcerative colitis, the drug is ineffective. However, the drug may be added to the regimen at a dose of 1.5 to 2.0 mg/kg when glucocorticoids fail or when the steroid dose needed to reduce inflammation is too high. It is desirable to monitor the blood count and observe the patient carefully for infection. Azathioprine also may have a limited role as a "steroid-sparing agent" in the patient with chronic ulcerative colitis who must be maintained on corticosteroids to control disease activity. Cyclosporine, a potent immunosuppressive agent, also has been found to be beneficial in severely ill patients, with marked improvement in this group of patients otherwise requiring colectomy. In these patients, the limited use of cyclosporine may be indicated.

Toxic megacolon is a major complication of severe ulcerative colitis which requires rapid, intensive management, best carried out jointly by the internist or gastroenterologist and surgeon. Once the diagnosis is established, prompt and vigorous use of intravenous fluids, electrolyte replacement therapy, and blood transfusions are indicated. Because of the fear of perforation and high likelihood that bacteremia and occult perforation have occurred, many physicians institute broad-spectrum antibiotic coverage after appropriate cultures have been obtained. The patient is given nothing by mouth, and nasogastric suction is often instituted. Full intravenous corticosteroid therapy is also begun. Majority opinion favors an initial period of medical stabilization for the first 24 to 48 h. If significant objective improvement has not occurred, and if perforation seems imminent, emergency colectomy should be carried out. While it is certainly true that some patients, under maximal medical therapy, may slowly improve and thus avoid colectomy, the risk of this course of action must be considered carefully. If perforation occurs, mortality rates rise sharply, approaching 50 percent in those who subsequently go on to colectomy.

At the other end of the spectrum is the patient with mild ulcerative colitis, limited to the rectum or rectosigmoid, who is managed on an ambulatory basis. Therapy is started with sulfasalazine, 0.5 to 1.0 g four times a day with meals. Alternatively, in the sulfa-allergic patient, 5-aminosalicylate enemas or oral 5-aminosalicylate preparations can be substituted. If rectal symptoms such as tenesmus are prominent, topical steroids in the form of small enemas may produce marked improvement. The equivalent of 100 mg hydrocortisone (20 mg prednisone) in 60 to 100 mL saline is used as a bedtime enema. On occasion, the use of steroid foam preparations may be better tolerated in the patient with severe tenesmus. Retention enemas have been shown to deliver medication as far as the descending colon, and absorption of steroid is small (10 to 20 percent). If large doses of rectal steroids are required for control, it is preferable to use oral prednisone at a moderate dosage (20 mg/d).

Psychotherapy   The elements of trust and mutual understanding combined with the compassion and expertise of the physician are essential in the therapy of any chronic disease and are particularly important in the long-term management of patients with inflammatory bowel disease. Often these patients are intelligent young adults who are frequently resentful of a disease affecting them during the most productive years. Through the vigorous participation of the physician, many patients are able to lead reasonably stable and productive lives. More formal psychiatric assistance may be required in the chronically ill patient, in particular children or adolescents, or in the elderly, in whom severe depressive reactions are common. This is particularly true when colectomy is being advised and in the emotional adjustment which must be made after colectomy.

Pregnancy and ulcerative colitis   While many physicians are apprehensive about the management and prognosis of ulcerative colitis in the pregnant patient, the outcome for the patient and the fetus is excellent. In general, the pregnancy is not threatened by coexistent colitis, with no increase in stillbirths or premature deliveries when compared with the general population. When patients with inactive colitis become pregnant, approximately 50 percent may have an exacerbation of their disease, with some clustering of these flares during the first trimester and in the postpartum period. The therapy of ulcerative colitis during pregnancy is largely the same as in the nonpregnant patient. Sulfasalazine is used to treat mild to moderate disease, since there is no evidence that the drug is harmful to the fetus or leads to increased incidence of fetal malformations. Women with inactive colitis who enter a pregnancy on maintenance sulfasalazine should be continued on the drug to protect the mother during the postpartum period from a relapse of disease. Corticosteroids should be used in the same dosage and for the same indications as in the nonpregnant patient. Immunosuppressive agents should not be used during pregnancy.

Thus it is clear that the patient with colitis can realistically plan to have a family. It is prudent, however, to bring active disease under control before pregnancy is undertaken to ensure the most optimal physical and emotional setting for the pregnancy. Similar conclusions apply to the management of Crohn's disease during pregnancy.

Surgical therapy Approximately 20 to 25 percent of patients with ulcerative colitis will require colectomy during the course of their disease. A major indication for colectomy is failure to respond to intensive medical management. Such patients, although not showing colonic dilatation, may fail to improve after 7 to 10 days of optimal medical therapy. Fever, persistent bloody diarrhea, and severe fatigue may persist, and consideration should be given to semielective colectomy. Elective colectomy may be performed in patients whose disease remains chronically active and who require continuous corticosteroid administration. Such patients are at risk of developing the complications of chronic steroid therapy. After colectomy, these patients often feel more energetic and usually gain back weight to their preillness level. As discussed above, the patient with long-standing colitis is at high risk for colonic cancer. While most authorities do not advise "prophylactic" colectomy in the patient with quiescent disease, the finding of marked dysplasia on colonoscopic biopsies done as a part of a surveillance program should make the physician think seriously about advising colectomy.

The decision to advise colectomy in other than emergency circumstances is difficult for both patient and physician. Many patients have an understandable reluctance to undergo colectomy and have difficulty in conceptualizing life with an ileostomy. In most metropolitan centers there are ileostomy groups who visit patients preoperatively and can provide answers to many practical questions. It is also desirable for the patient to be visited by a nurse familiar with stoma care to instruct the patient on the practical aspects of handling the ileostomy.

While total proctocolectomy with permanent ileostomy has been the standard surgical procedure for almost all patients undergoing colectomy, several alternative approaches may be desirable. The *continent ileostomy* is an ileal loop reservoir fashioned under the skin with a nipple valve to prevent spilling of ileal contents. Ileal effluent collects in this reservoir, which must be emptied with a soft rubber catheter. Only a small stoma is externally visible, thus eliminating an external ileostomy appliance. Problems with leakage and frequent revisions have made this procedure less attractive. There is great enthusiasm for ileal-rectal anastomosis with an internal ileal pouch created to act as a reservoir. This often produces a highly satisfactory result, with continence and five to seven stools per day. Complications such as pouchitis or the need for surgical revision seem less frequent than with the continent ileostomy. The procedure is an excellent alternative for those patients who will not accept an ileostomy.

CROHN'S DISEASE The medical management of colonic Crohn's disease is similar in most respects to that of ulcerative colitis. In a multicenter study (National Cooperative Crohn's Disease Study), sulfasalazine was shown to be effective in the therapy of active colonic disease. Glucocorticoids also were efficacious but less so than with small-bowel involvement. The indications and dosages of these medications are similar to those for ulcerative colitis. Since in Crohn's disease intraabdominal sepsis can result from fistula or abscess formation, corticosteroids must be used with caution, and constant attention is required to detect evidence of sepsis, which can be masked by these agents. In general, the disease is less explosive in onset, and although toxic dilatation and perforation can occur, they are less common than in ulcerative colitis. The principles of management are the same. Because of the indolent nature of the disease, the response to therapy is often less complete than in ulcerative colitis, and the disease tends to progress despite apparent clinical inactivity. It may be more difficult to achieve a clinical remission and to withdraw steroids completely. As in ulcerative colitis, controlled studies have shown no benefit to continuing steroids after remission, since the frequency of recurrence is not altered by prophylactic steroid therapy. Disappointingly, sulfasalazine did not decrease recurrence rates in Crohn's disease.

While response to therapy of the initial attack of Crohn's colitis may be satisfactory, many patients continue to have persistently active disease. This may express itself as progressive weight loss, diarrhea, and deterioration of general health. Perianal disease with predominantly left-sided colonic involvement (fistula formation and perirectal abscesses) may constitute a recurrent problem. In one controlled study, *metronidazole* (20 mg/kg per day in divided dosage) resulted in marked improvement in 10 of 18 patients with chronic perineal fistulas associated with Crohn's disease. It is not clear whether the drug is active because of its antibacterial properties or through another mechanism. It is possible that this drug may prove to be of value in the therapy of the perineal complications of Crohn's disease before surgical therapy is attempted. The role of immunosuppressive therapy in the treatment of Crohn's disease has become better established in recent years. The use of 6-mercaptopurine or azathioprine (1.5 to 2.0 mg/kg) has been shown to decrease activity, close or decrease the activity of fistulas, exert a steroid-sparing effect, and may decrease relapse rate if used as maintenance therapy. Often, adding these drugs to a maximal program in the nonresponding patient produces beneficial results. However, a beneficial response may take 3 to 4 months.

The management of Crohn's disease of the small intestine (regional enteritis) is similar to that for colonic Crohn's disease, and as noted, many patients have concomitant small- and large-bowel disease. Several additional considerations are pertinent, however. *Intestinal obstruction* is not uncommonly a presenting feature with ileal involvement. Initially, this may be secondary to acute inflammation and will respond to corticosteroids. With recurrent involvement and the development of fibrosis, steroid therapy is less effective, and surgical decompression is required. *Nutritional problems* often are more severe with involvement of the small intestine than with colonic involvement alone. Added to the general catabolic nature of the disease may be loss of absorptive surface, which may result from progressive involvement or because of surgical resection. Refinements in the technique of parenteral alimentation have made it possible to provide a patient's total daily caloric intake intravenously for a period of weeks or even months (see Chap. 76). Parenteral alimentation has been employed with increasing frequency in the severely ill patient as a means of placing the gastrointestinal tract "at rest" and in preparing the malnourished patient for surgery. With this approach, the disease may become quiescent, and the drainage from fistulas may decrease. However, disease activity frequently recurs when oral feedings are resumed. On occasion, prolonged intravenous alimentation, administered at home, may be required when oral feedings are not effective or in children exhibiting severe growth failure associated with Crohn's disease. Most often it is possible to design a dietary program of oral supplementation to nourish the patient adequately.

In patients with extensive small-bowel involvement or in those with a short bowel resulting from extensive intestinal resection, supplementation of electrolytes, minerals, and vitamins will be required. Extensive ileal disease or resection often results in diarrhea induced by bile salts and in malabsorption; cholestyramine may be needed to control the diarrhea, and medium-chain triglycerides may need to be added to reduce fat malabsorption (see Chap. 254). In patients with stenotic segments of intestine, a low-residue (low-fiber) diet should be recommended. A lactose-free diet should be instituted if there is an associated lactase deficiency. Other dietary modifications have not been shown to have any beneficial effect on the primary disease process. Patients should be encouraged to eat a nutritious, appealing diet of their own choosing. *Surgical therapy* is generally reserved for the complications of Crohn's disease rather than as a primary form of therapy. In contrast to ulcerative colitis, more patients with Crohn's disease will require surgery in the chronic management of the disease. Approximately 70 percent of patients will require at least one operation during the course of their disease. Although each case and situation must be individualized, in general, surgery may be required (1) for persistent or fixed bowel narrowing or obstruction, (2) for symptomatic fistula formation to the bladder, vagina, or skin, (3) for persistent anal fistulas or abscesses, and (4) for intraabdominal abscesses, toxic dilatation of the colon, or perforation. In contrast to ulcerative colitis, where colectomy is curative, in Crohn's disease surgical resection of the small or large intestine is followed by a high rate of recurrence. With resection of segments of small bowel or ileum and reanastomosis, a recurrence rate of 50 to 75 percent over a 5-year period is not unusual. Recurrence of disease is invariably proximal to the created anastomosis. When total colectomy and ileostomy are performed for Crohn's disease of the colon without significant small-intestinal involvement, recurrence rates are lower, varying from 10 to 30 percent. Despite these recurrences, most patients do not develop a short bowel syndrome and usually can expect significant improvement. Faced with the possibility of recurrent disease, many physicians are reluctant to advise surgery in Crohn's disease, except for the type of clear-cut complications described above. Alternatively, patients with persistently active disease may require chronic maintenance on unacceptably high levels of corticosteroids and with the appreciable risk of steroid side effects. Just as a failure of medical therapy should lead to colectomy in ulcerative colitis, it should be the conclusion in the patient with Crohn's colitis without major small-bowel involvement. While in this setting there is also a definite rate of recurrence, such recurrences are often not disabling. When extensive small-bowel disease is present, surgical therapy is often not feasible and should only be reserved for specific disease complications. In selected patients, limited surgical procedures (strictureplasty) can be employed to open highly strictured areas and avoid further resective surgery.

The therapy of Crohn's disease in children presents special problems, since normal growth and development may be retarded in the presence of active disease. In addition to conventional drug therapy, intensive nutritional therapy or the judicious use of surgery may be required.

PROGNOSIS

The overall prognosis of IBD has been favorably affected by the use of corticosteroids and sulfasalazine, as well as by supportive techniques such as intravenous alimentation. In *acute* ulcerative colitis, these therapeutic modalities can result in a remission in almost 90 percent of patients. The mortality of an initial acute attack is approximately 5 percent. Poor prognostic factors and an increased mortality rate are likely when there is total colonic involvement, when the onset occurs over age 60, and when toxic megacolon develops.

The long-term prognosis of *chronic* ulcerative colitis is more difficult to assess due to the variable and intermittent nature of the disease and improvements in therapy. Left-sided colitis and ulcerative proctitis have a very favorable prognosis and probably no increase in mortality; similarly, the long-term prognosis for extensive colitis has improved greatly. Older studies suggested a poor prognosis for extensive colitis, with less than 50 percent of patients surviving 15 years after onset. More recent observations (longest follow-up 11

years) show a 10-year mortality rate of between 5 and 10 percent for severe first attacks (excluding toxic megacolon). Approximately 75 percent of patients will experience relapses, and 20 to 25 percent will require colectomy. The problem of carcinoma developing in the setting of long-standing chronic ulcerative colitis is an important factor in determining the long-term prognosis of ulcerative colitis. As discussed above, periodic surveillance with colonoscopy and multiple biopsies to detect dysplastic changes are indicated to detect a high-risk group for which to advise colectomy.

The prognosis for Crohn's disease is not as favorable as for ulcerative colitis. An exception is *acute regional enteritis*, often discovered during laparotomy for suspected appendicitis; this has an excellent prognosis. More than two-thirds of such patients may show no subsequent evidence of regional enteritis, and this form of acute ileitis may well be due to *Yersinia* infection (see above). Prevailing surgical opinion favors a conservative approach in this situation, and in most instances operative resection is not advised.

In the majority of patients with Crohn's disease, the course is chronic and intermittent regardless of the site of involvement. The disease responds less well to medical therapy with time, and over two-thirds of patients develop complications requiring surgery at some point in their disease. In contrast to ulcerative colitis, where mortality appears greatest early in the disease, in Crohn's disease the mortality rate increases with the duration of the disease and probably ranges from 5 to 10 percent. Most deaths occur from peritonitis and sepsis. As indicated above, following surgery, patients with Crohn's disease often have recurrence and relapses. Nevertheless, the therapy of Crohn's disease will result in reasonably stable and productive lives for most Crohn's disease patients.

REFERENCES

General

Kirsner JB, Shorter RG (eds): *Inflammatory Bowel Disease*, 3d ed. Philadelphia, Lea & Febiger, 1988

Podolsky DK: Inflammatory bowel disease. N Engl J Med 325:928, 1991

Sleisenger MH, Fordtran JS (eds): *Gastrointestinal Diseases*, 4th ed. Philadelphia, Saunders, 1989

Stenson WF, MacDermott RP: Inflammatory bowel disease, in *Textbook of Gastroenterology*, T Yamada et al (eds). Philadephia, Lippincott, 1991

Etiology and diagnostic aspects

Blaser MJ, Reller LB: *Campylobacter* enteritis. N Engl J Med 305:1444, 1981

Goldberg HI et al: Computed tomography in the evaluation of Crohn's disease. Am J Roent 140:277, 1983

Greenstein AJ et al: The extraintestinal complications of ulcerative colitis and Crohn's disease: A study of 700 patients. Medicine 55:401, 1976

Jess P: Acute terminal ileitis: A review of recent literature on the relationship to Crohn's disease. Scand J Gastroenterol 16:321, 1981

MacDermott RP, Stenson WF: Alterations of the immune system in ulcerative colitis and Crohn's disease. Adv Immunol 42:285, 1988

Quinn TC et al: *Chlamydia trachomatis* proctitis. N Engl J Med 305:195, 1981

Surawicz CM, Belic L: Rectal biopsy helps to distinguish acute self limited colitis from idiopathic inflammatory bowel disease. Gastroenterology 86:104, 1984

Van Trappen G et al: *Yersinia* enteritis and enterocolitis: Gastroenterological aspects. Gastroenterology 72:220, 1977

Therapy of inflammatory bowel disease

Azad Khan AK et al: Optimum dose of sulphasalazine for maintenance treatment in ulcerative colitis. Gut 12:232, 1980

Brandt LJ et al: Metronidazole therapy for perineal Crohn's disease: A follow-up study. Gastroenterology 83:383, 1982

Collins RH et al: Colon cancer in ulcerative colitis. Gastroenterology 94:1089, 1988

Donaldson RM Jr: Management of medical problems in pregnancy: Inflammatory bowel disease. N Engl J Med 312:1616, 1985

Ekbom A et al: Ulcerative colitis and colorectal cancer. N Engl J Med 323:1228, 1990

Fabricius PJ et al: Crohn's disease in the elderly. Gut 26:461, 1985

Farmer RG et al: Long-term follow-up of patients with Crohn's disease. Relationship between clinical pattern and prognosis. Gastroenterology 88:1818, 1985

Gaginella TS, Walsh RE: Sulfasalazine: Multiplicity of action. Dig Dis Sci 37:801, 1992

Kelts DG et al: Nutritional basis of growth failure in children and adolescents with Crohn's disease. Gastroenterology 76:720, 1979

Lennard Jones JE et al: Cancer in colitis: Assessment of the individual risk by clinical and histological criteria. Gastroenterology 73:1280, 1977

Pemberton JH et al: Ileal pouch—Anal anastomosis for chronic ulcerative colitis. Long-term results. Ann Surg 206:504, 1987

PEPPERCORN MA: Advances in drug therapy for inflammatory bowel disease. Ann Intern Med 112:50, 1990

PRESENT DH et al: 6-Mercaptopurine in the management of inflammatory bowel disease: short- and long-term toxicity. Ann Intern Med 111:641, 1989

RANSOHOFF DF et al: Ulcerative colitis and colon cancer: Problems in analyzing the diagnostic usefulness of mucosal dysplasia. Dis Colon Rectum 28:383, 1985

RIDDELL RH et al: Dysplasia in inflammatory bowel disease. Hum Pathol 14:931, 1983

SANDBORN WJ et al: Ulcerative colitis disease activity following treatment of associated primary sclerosing cholangitis with cyclosporin. Gut 34:242, 1993

SCHROEDER KW et al: Coated oral 5-aminosalicylate acid therapy for mild to moderately active ulcerative colitis. A randomized study. N Engl J Med 317:1625, 1987

SUGITA A et al: Colorectal cancer in ulcerative colitis: Influence of anatomical extent and age at onset in colitis-cancer interval. Gut 32:169, 1991

URSING B et al: A comparative study of metronidazole and sulfasalazine for active Crohn's disease. The Cooperative Crohn's Disease Study in Sweden. Gastroenterology 83:550, 1982

256   DISEASES OF THE SMALL AND LARGE INTESTINE

J. THOMAS LaMONT / KURT J. ISSELBACHER

SYMPTOMS OF INTESTINAL DISEASE

SYMPTOMS OF SMALL-INTESTINAL DISEASE   The major clinical manifestations of small-bowel disease are *motility disturbances*, abdominal *pain* and *distention*, gastrointestinal *bleeding*, and *malabsorption*.

Altered intestinal peristalsis is a common manifestation of a variety of diseases. The presentation may be one of decreased motility, such as paralytic ileus resulting from metabolic disturbance or peritonitis, or intestinal obstruction caused by tumors, adhesions, volvulus, or intussusception (Chap. 258). Diarrhea frequently accompanies small-bowel disease (Chap. 39) resulting from direct mucosal involvement by inflammatory or infiltrative lesions (sprue, regional enteritis). The associated malabsorption of fat and bile salts is an important factor in the pathogenesis of diarrhea in these conditions (Chaps. 39 and 254).

Abdominal pain due to small-intestinal disease is usually periumbilical or supraumbilical and often poorly localized. With obstruction, pain is classically described as intermittent or colicky. Visceral pain arises from distention or stretching of the intestinal wall or from inflammation of the overlying parietal peritoneum. As the intestine becomes progressively dilated with loss of muscular tone, the colicky nature of the pain may become less apparent. Acute inflammation of the small intestine which involves the visceral or parietal peritoneum is associated with steady, aching pain, usually located directly over the inflamed area, and may be accompanied by guarding and rebound tenderness if the parietal peritoneum is involved. *Gastrointestinal bleeding* due to small-bowel disease may be detected as occult bleeding or, less commonly, brisk hemorrhage. In general, bleeding from the stomach or small intestine causes black or tarry stool (melena), while bleeding from the colon causes passage of red blood or clots. Obviously, the appearance of blood in the stool depends not only on site of bleeding but also on the rate of the hemorrhage and the rapidity of transit; thus localization of the bleeding site by stool appearance alone may be misleading.

An important clue to the presence of small-bowel disease is the presence of fat malabsorption. With extensive mucosal damage or lymphatic obstruction, the presenting symptoms may relate to any of the features of a malabsorption syndrome or protein-losing enteropathy (Chap. 254) and should direct attention to the small intestine.

SYMPTOMS OF COLONIC DISEASE   The major symptoms of colonic disease are *alteration in bowel habit, rectal bleeding*, and *pain*. Alteration in bowel habit implies a change from previous patterns of defecation; hence a detailed history is important. Most normal individuals have one to three movements of well-formed

stools each day. *Diarrhea* means the passage of watery or loose stools usually with increased frequency, while *constipation* implies infrequent passage of hard, dry stools; *obstipation* is the absence of spontaneous bowel movements. A persistent change in bowel habit, particularly in older individuals with no previous irregularity, is usually an important early symptom of organic disease of the colon and should never be labeled *functional* unless a thorough diagnostic evaluation is negative. The appearance of the stool also may provide important diagnostic clues. Blood coating the exterior of a formed stool implies a lesion in the anal canal or rectum, while blood admixed with the feces indicates a bleeding source higher in the colon. Brisk hemorrhage from the colon or distal small intestine results in passage of fresh blood, called *hematochezia*. This may appear as fresh blood and clots if the lesion is in the left colon or darker, maroon-colored blood if the bleeding source is in the right colon.

Pain resulting from colonic disease is usually localized to either of the lower abdominal quadrants, as opposed to pain of small-intestinal origin, which is localized to the periumbilical area or higher. Rectal pain is often felt deep in the pelvis, while pain in the anal canal is accurately localized to the perineum. The mechanisms of colonic pain are similar to those in other intestinal viscera (see Chap. 13). Distention from gas or fluid causes crampy or colicky pain from stretching of the muscle layers and resulting contraction or spasm. Pain of this type is often relieved by passage of flatus or stool. Pain also may result if the colonic wall is inflamed or infiltrated by tumor. Acute colonic inflammation which involves the visceral or parietal peritoneum produces sharply localized pain, which may be accompanied by abdominal guarding and rebound tenderness. An important symptom of rectal disease is *tenesmus*, or painful straining at stool, with a sensation of incomplete emptying after defecation. This symptom can be caused by retention of stool in the rectum, by tumors of the rectum which simulate retained stools, or by colonic inflammation.

DIAGNOSTIC PROCEDURES

PHYSICAL EXAMINATION   Careful *examination* of the abdomen may disclose a mass or fistula associated with inflammatory or neoplastic disease, localized tenderness, or abdominal distention resulting from ileus or intestinal obstruction. The physical examination and findings in the patient with acute abdominal pain are discussed in Chap. 13.

Thorough examination also may reveal extraintestinal findings associated with small-intestinal diseases. Thus buccal pigmentation or telangiectasia may indicate coexistent small-bowel polyposis or intestinal telangiectasia and may clarify episodes of abdominal pain or chronic bleeding. Similarly, evidence of iritis, arthritis, or erythema nodosum may suggest the presence of inflammatory bowel disease.

Perhaps the most important part of the physical examination in the diagnosis of colonic diseases is the *digital rectal examination*. This procedure should never be omitted for reasons of modesty or fear of embarrassment because it is essential in the diagnosis of perianal, sphincteric, and ampullary lesions; prostatic and uterine abnormalities; and even small rectal masses. A metastatic tumor may be felt in the perirectal tissues as a shelflike deformity (Blumer's shelf), especially anteriorly above the prostate. The fecal material on the glove should be immediately tested with guaiac-impregnated cards for occult blood. Approximately one-half of all rectal carcinomas lie within reach of the index finger, and omission of the rectal examination may delay diagnosis and worsen the prognosis.

STOOL EXAMINATION   Abnormal stools constitute important objective evidence of colonic disease. Stools should be examined by the physician as soon as possible after defecation for the presence of visible blood on the surface or within the specimen. A small sample should be tested for occult blood. Microscopic examination of fresh stool is important in the diagnosis of parasitic diseases, particularly in amebic colitis when motile trophozoites can be seen in fresh, warm stool suspensions. Stool suspensions also can be stained with a drop of methylene blue for polymorphonuclear leukocytes, which indicate the presence of an acute inflammatory exudate, such as occurs in ulcerative colitis, amebic colitis, and bacillary dysentery. Fixed and stained slides of stool also may reveal amebas and other parasites, while stool culture is essential for the diagnosis of bacillary dysentery. Sudan III stain of stool is a useful screening test for steatorrhea.

BARIUM STUDIES   The considerable length of the small intestine (some 4 to 7 m in the adult) makes *radiologic studies* of the small bowel of prime importance, and these studies usually form the basis for the diagnosis of small-bowel diseases. *Small-bowel x-rays* are not usually part of a routine upper gastrointestinal series and must be specifically requested. In view of the length of the small bowel and wide variations in transit time, it is essential to provide the radiologist with as much information as possible, since the precise nature of the problem may determine various technical aspects of the examination. Enteroclysis is a specialized small-bowel barium study during which barium is infused rapidly via a nasogastric tube into the jejunum. This technique allows distention of bowel loops and rapid filling of the entire small intestine, thus avoiding the problems of inadequate distention and poor transit sometimes encountered in routine small-bowel barium studies. Enteroclysis is indicated in patients with suspected small-bowel lesions not visualized by ordinary barium studies.

Barium enema is a useful diagnostic tool for the identification of certain colonic diseases, including diverticulosis and its complications, motility disturbances, and displacement of the colon by extrinsic lesions. Barium enema is also useful for detection of loss of haustral markings in chronic ulcerative colitis and for diagnosis of intestinal fistulas. Fiberoptic colonoscopy is more accurate for the diagnosis of early changes of inflammatory bowel disease or for detection of colonic neoplasms. Colonoscopy offers the additional advantage of allowing biopsy of suspicious lesions and removal of most polyps.

SIGMOIDOSCOPY   The technique of fiberoptic sigmoidoscopy is not difficult to master, and with practice, the discomfort to the patient is minimal. The availability of flexible fiberoptic sigmoidoscopes now makes it possible to examine the lower 40 to 60 cm of the colon, compared with the 25-cm limit of the rigid sigmoidoscope. Flexible sigmoidoscopy is generally less painful than rigid sigmoidoscopy. Because approximately half of all colorectal neoplasms lie in the distal 50 cm of the bowel, sigmoidoscopy is an important diagnostic tool. It should be stressed that a rectal carcinoma can be missed on routine barium enema yet easily visualized and biopsied through the sigmoidoscope. Furthermore, the earliest changes of ulcerative colitis may not be demonstrated radiographically but may be obvious through the sigmoidoscope. Rectal biopsy is easily and painlessly accomplished through the instrument and is associated with minimal morbidity except in the presence of bleeding disorders.

COLONOSCOPY   See Chap. 250.

MESENTERIC ANGIOGRAPHY   Angiography is helpful in the diagnosis of two conditions: intestinal ischemia and gastrointestinal hemorrhage. Patients suspected of having acute intestinal ischemia from arterial embolus as well as chronic ischemia (intestinal angina) should undergo angiography to locate the site of blockage. Angiography may be diagnostic in some patients with acute gastrointestinal blood loss, especially when bleeding exceeds 0.5 mL/min.

RADIONUCLIDE BLEEDING SCAN   Bleeding from the small or large bowel can be localized in certain circumstances by radionuclide scanning of the abdomen after intravenous injection of technetium 99m sulfur colloid or autologous red cells labeled with the same agent (Fig. 256-1). If the patient is bleeding at a rate of 0.1 to 0.5 mL/min or greater, the location of radioactivity in the abdomen may indicate the source of bleeding. This diagnostic approach usually requires confirmation by another diagnostic modality such as angiography or endoscopy. The radionuclide bleeding scan is noninvasive, a particular advantage in older patients with bleeding from the small bowel or colon. The bleeding scan is not recommended in patients with suspected bleeding from the esophagus, stomach, or duodenum, who are best studied by upper endoscopy.

DISORDERS OF INTESTINAL MOTILITY

A major function of the intestinal tract is to propel the intestinal contents (food, secretions, chyme, feces) from stomach toward anus. Abnormalities of motility comprise the most common intestinal diseases: diverticulosis, megacolon, constipation, and irritable bowel syndrome. Although these conditions share a common abnormality, i.e., dysmotility, their clinical features are quite diverse.

DIVERTICULOSIS   Diverticula may be either congenital or acquired and may affect either the small or large intestine. Congenital diverticula are herniations of the entire thickness of intestinal wall, while the more common acquired diverticula consist of herniations of the mucosa through the muscularis, generally at the site of a nutrient artery.

Small-intestinal diverticula   Diverticula may occur in any portion of the small intestine; however, with the exception of Meckel's diverticulum, the most common locations are in the duodenum and jejunum. Most often diverticula are asymptomatic and discovered incidentally on upper gastrointestinal x-rays. On occasion, however, they may cause symptoms either because of their anatomic proximity to other structures or rarely from inflammation or bleeding.

Duodenal diverticula arise singly from the medial surface of the second portion of the duodenum. In most patients, they cause no symptoms. Rarely, they may present as acute diverticulitis with abdominal pain, fever, gastrointestinal bleeding, or, most rarely, perforation. Periampullary diverticula are occasionally associated with cholangitis or pancreatitis. Jejunal diverticula, while less common,

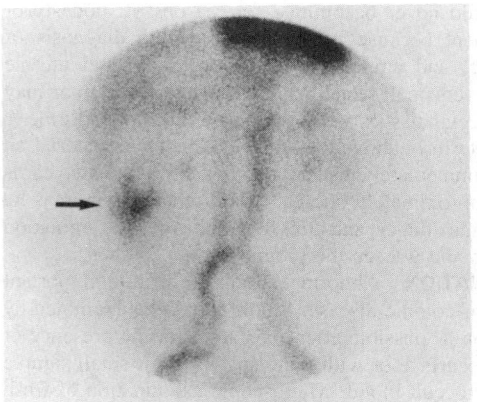

10 min

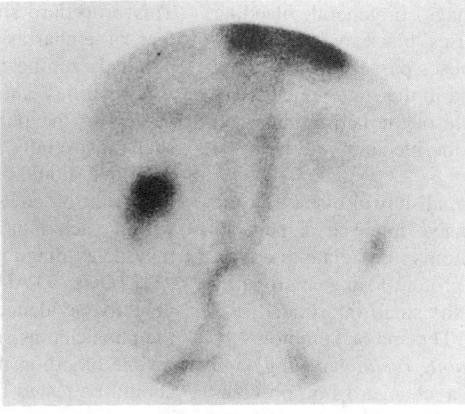

30 min

FIGURE 256-1 Radionuclide bleeding scan using intravenous injection of technetium-labeled autologous red cells. Ten minutes after injection, a blush appears in the right abdomen over the cecum (*arrow*). Thirty minutes after injection, the blush has increased in intensity. The cardiac blood pool is noted at the top. Surgery revealed a bleeding diverticulum in the cecum.

also may be the site of acute inflammation, bleeding, or perforation with resulting abscess or peritonitis.

Multiple jejunal diverticula may be associated with a malabsorption syndrome related to bacterial overgrowth within the diverticula, similar to other situations where intestinal stasis (i.e., blind loops) permits bacterial proliferation. The consequences of bacterial proliferation with resultant mucosal damage, deconjugation of bile salts, and vitamin B_{12} malabsorption are discussed in Chap. 254.

Meckel's diverticulum, a persistent omphalomesenteric duct, is the most frequent congenital anomaly of the digestive tract, occurring in approximately 2 percent of autopsied adults. The diverticulum is wide-mouthed, about 5 cm long, and arises from the antimesenteric border of the ileum, usually within 100 cm of the ileocecal valve. The sac may be lined with normal ileal mucosa (approximately 50 percent) or contain gastric, duodenal, pancreatic, or colonic mucosa. While rarely symptomatic after age 5, Meckel's diverticulum may produce hemorrhage, inflammation, and obstruction in children and teenagers.

Hemorrhage occurs almost exclusively before age 10 and invariably results from peptic ulceration of ileal mucosa adjacent to a Meckel's diverticulum lined with gastric mucosa. The diagnosis may be established by isotope scanning of the abdomen after injection of technetium, which is taken up by the ectopic gastric mucosa in the diverticulum. False-negative and false-positive Meckel's scans are not uncommon; thus other clinical and laboratory features must be assessed carefully before recommending surgery. In older children and young adults, inflammation of the diverticulum may mimic acute appendicitis. Mechanical obstruction also may occur if the diverticulum intussuscepts into the lumen of the bowel or twists on a fibrous remnant of the omphalomesenteric duct which extends from the diverticulum to the abdominal wall. The treatment of any of these complications of Meckel's diverticulum is surgical excision.

Colonic diverticula Diverticula of the colon are herniations or saclike protrusions of the mucosa through the muscularis, at the point where a nutrient artery penetrates the muscularis. Diverticula occur most commonly in the sigmoid colon and decrease in frequency in the proximal colon. They increase with age, and the incidence ranges between 20 and 50 percent in western populations over age 50. The exact mechanism for their formation is unknown but may be related to an increase in intraluminal pressure. Thickening of the muscle coat of the colon in most patients with diverticula suggests that herniations of mucosa are caused by increased pressure produced by colonic muscle contractions. The rarity of colonic diverticula in underdeveloped nations in contrast to their frequent occurrence in western countries has led to the speculation that diverticula result from the highly refined western diet, which is deficient in dietary fiber or roughage. It is proposed that such diets result in decreased fecal bulk, narrowing of the colon, and an increase in intraluminal pressure in order to move the smaller fecal mass. The role of dietary fiber in the etiology and treatment of diverticular disease remains to be determined.

Colonic diverticula are usually asymptomatic and are an incidental finding on barium enema or colonoscopy. The major complications of inflammation, both acute and chronic, and hemorrhage occur in only a small percentage of individuals with diverticulosis. Since diverticulosis is quite common in older patients, one must avoid the temptation of attributing pain or bleeding to the diverticula unless other conditions, especially colonic neoplasm, have been excluded.

Diverticulitis Inflammation can occur in or around the diverticular sac. The cause of diverticulitis is probably mechanical, related to retention in the diverticula of undigested food residues and bacteria, which may form a hard mass called a *fecalith*. This compromises the blood supply to the thin-walled sac (made up solely of mucosa and serosa) and renders it susceptible to invasion by colonic bacteria. The inflammatory process may vary from a small intramural or pericolic abscess to generalized peritonitis. Some attacks are accompanied by minimal symptoms and seem to heal spontaneously. Studies of resected specimens indicate that most perforations of the diverticular

sac are small and result in inflammation of the sac itself and the adjacent serosal surface. Diverticulitis occurs more often in men than in women and three times as often in the left as in the right colon. This suggests that diverticulitis may be related to the higher intraluminal pressures and the more solid fecal material in the sigmoid and descending colon.

Acute colonic diverticulitis is a disease of variable severity characterized by fever, left lower quadrant abdominal pain, and signs of peritoneal irritation—muscle spasm, guarding, rebound tenderness. Rectal examination may reveal a tender mass if the area of inflammation is close to the rectum. Although constipation may not have been noted prior to onset of the illness, the inflammation around the colon often results in some degree of acute constipation or obstipation. Rectal bleeding, usually microscopic, is noted in 25 percent of cases; it is rarely massive. Polymorphonuclear leukocytosis is common. Complications include free perforation, which results in acute peritonitis, sepsis, and shock, particularly in the elderly. The perforation may be walled off by adherent omentum or neighboring structures such as the bladder or small bowel. Abscess formation or fistulas then occur as the inflammatory mass burrows into other organs. Severe pericolitis may cause a fibrous stricture around the bowel which can be associated with colonic obstruction and may mimic a neoplasm.

DIAGNOSIS During the acute phase of diverticulitis, barium enema and sigmoidoscopy may be hazardous, since contrast material or air under pressure may lead to rupture of an inflamed diverticulum and convert a walled-off inflammatory lesion to a free perforation. These examinations are usually safe after adequate treatment and healing of the diverticulitis. The radiologic findings on barium enema suggestive of diverticulitis are leakage of barium from a diverticular sac, stricture formation, and the presence of a pericolic inflammatory mass. In many patients, the distortion caused by inflammation prevents a clear distinction between cancer and diverticulitis. In these cases, colonoscopy or surgical excision may be required for accurate diagnosis. Abdominal CT scan may be useful in demonstrating the presence of a pericolic abscess.

TREATMENT Most patients with acute diverticulitis should be hospitalized for bowel rest, intravenous fluids, and broad-spectrum antibiotics. Repeated attacks of diverticulitis in the same area generally require surgical resection. Severe attacks with acute peritoneal signs, suspected abscess, or perforation require intravenous antibiotics directed against gram-negative anaerobic bacteria, followed by surgical drainage or resection. The usual procedure is a diverting colostomy with resection of the involved colon; reanastomosis is then performed at a second operation.

Painful diverticular disease without diverticulitis Some patients with diverticulosis develop recurrent left lower quadrant colicky pain without clinical or pathologic evidence of acute diverticulitis. They often have bouts of alternating constipation and diarrhea, and the pain may be relieved by defecation or passage of flatus. These features suggest the coexistence of the irritable bowel syndrome (see below). Examination during a bout of pain reveals tenderness of the sigmoid colon, but signs of peritoneal inflammation such as rebound tenderness, muscle guarding, fever, and leukocytosis are absent. Barium enema shows typical diverticula without evidence of inflammation and stricture, plus a "sawtooth" irregularity of the lumen reflecting muscle hypertrophy and spasm. In some patients the pain is severe enough to warrant observation in a hospital and restriction of food, since feeding aggravates the pain by causing colonic contraction. Anticholinergics, which reduce sigmoid contractions, and mild sedation are usually all that is required. After recovery, the patient should be started on a high-residue diet or given a bulk laxative such as hemicellulose, unprocessed bran, or psyllium extract. Surgical excision is usually not indicated unless acute diverticulitis or its complications occur.

Hemorrhage from diverticula Massive hemorrhage from colonic diverticula is one of the most common causes of hematochezia in patients over age 60. This complication of diverticulosis is caused by erosion of a vessel by a fecalith within the diverticular sac. The bleeding is painless and not accompanied by signs or symptoms of diverticulitis. Most cases of mild or moderate hemorrhage stop spontaneously with bed rest and blood transfusion. Localization of bleeding can be obtained by bleeding scan or angiography. In patients with severe hemorrhage, mesenteric angiography can be both diagnostic in localizing the bleeding site and therapeutic, since vasoconstrictive drugs or artificial blood clot infused intraarterially can sometimes effectively control hemorrhage. Colonoscopy is also useful in evaluating acute hematochezia, and the endoscopist may be able to cauterize angiodysplasias (see Chap. 41). The location of bleeding diverticula demonstrated at angiography on several series has been more commonly in the right colon, particularly the ascending colon, in contrast to the sigmoid colon, where diverticula are more numerous.

MEGACOLON   Megacolon, or giant colon, is characterized by massive distention of the colon, usually accompanied by severe constipation or obstipation. This condition can be either congenital or acquired and is seen in all age groups. Acute toxic megacolon is a severe complication of chronic ulcerative colitis (see Chap. 255).

Aganglionic megacolon (Hirschsprung's disease)   This is a congenital disorder which becomes manifest in early infancy, occurring more frequently in males, and is often familial. These infants have massive abdominal distention, absent bowel movements, and impaired nutrition due to chronic obstruction of the colon. In some individuals with less severe symptoms the disease may not be diagnosed until adolescence or early adulthood. The inability to defecate is caused by the absence of ganglion cells (Meissner's and Auerbach's plexuses) in a small segment of the distal colon, usually near the anus. This aganglionic segment is unable to relax to permit passage of stool, causing the normal colon proximal to it to become greatly dilated. On rectal examination, the ampulla is empty of feces and the anal sphincter is normal. Barium enema reveals a narrowed segment in the rectosigmoid area, with massive dilatation above. Diagnosis is made by full-thickness surgical biopsy under anesthesia and demonstration of absent ganglion cells in the diseased segment. In most patients the aganglionic segment is in the rectosigmoid colon; in rare instances the lesion may involve more proximal bowel or even the entire colon. The treatment of choice is a pull-through procedure in which normally innervated colon is anastomosed to the distal rectum just above the internal sphincter, thus bypassing the contracted aganglionic segment and restoring normal defecation.

Chronic idiopathic megacolon   This condition, also called *psychogenic megacolon*, has its onset later in childhood, usually at the time toilet training begins. It is characterized by severe chronic constipation and distention, and in contrast to Hirschsprung's disease, digital examination reveals the rectal ampulla to be invariably distended with feces. Barium enema shows the entire colon to be distended with stools, no narrowed segment is seen, and rectal biopsy discloses the normal complement of ganglion cells in Auerbach's plexus. Treatment is based on education in normal bowel habits, but a long course of enemas or large doses of mineral oil may be required until the patient acquires more normal bowel movements.

Acquired megacolon   In Central and South America, infection with *Trypanosoma cruzi* (Chagas' disease) can result in destruction of the ganglion cells of the colon, producing a clinical picture similar to congenital megacolon, except that the onset is in adult life rather than childhood. A number of other diseases are associated with megacolon in adults. Patients with schizophrenia or depression, particularly institutionalized patients, may have obstipation and massive colonic dilatation. Severe neurologic disorders, including cerebral atrophy, spinal cord injury, and parkinsonism, also may cause megacolon. Myxedema, infiltrative diseases such as amyloidosis, and scleroderma also can reduce colonic motility and produce marked colonic distention. Narcotic drugs, particularly morphine and codeine, can cause severe constipation, especially when administered to bedridden patients. Digital rectal examination of adults with acquired megacolon reveals a rectum distended with feces, as opposed to the empty rectum in aganglionic megacolon. Treatment is aimed

at the underlying disease, as well as the careful use of enemas and cathartics.

INTESTINAL PSEUDOOBSTRUCTION   Intestinal pseudoobstruction is an acute or chronic motility disorder characterized by distention or dilatation of the small and large intestine. Abdominal pain, nausea, and vomiting may lead to diagnostic confusion with mechanical obstruction, but as the name of this condition implies, the underlying cause is not obstruction but rather a severe dysmotility resulting in distention. Pseudoobstruction may be primary or secondary and acute or chronic. In primary or idiopathic pseudoobstruction, no other contributing condition can be identified, and the motility disorder is attributed to abnormalities of sympathetic innervation or of the muscle layers of the intestine. Secondary pseudoobstruction may result from scleroderma, diabetes, amyloidosis, neurologic diseases, drugs, or sepsis.

Chronic or intermittent secondary pseudoobstruction   Numerous medical conditions can cause chronic dilatation of the large and small bowel. Some of these may involve the intestinal smooth muscle, such as scleroderma, dermatomyositis, amyloidosis, or muscular dystrophy. Endocrine disorders, including myxedema and diabetes mellitus, may result in chronic distention, which in the diabetic results from autonomic visceral neuropathy. Chronic neurologic diseases, including Parkinson's disease and stroke, may be complicated by chronic pseudoobstruction; in these patients drugs and relative immobility are contributing features. Finally, psychotic patients (especially those who are institutionalized) may suffer from prolonged megacolon.

The symptoms of chronic secondary pseudoobstruction are chronic or intermittent constipation, crampy abdominal pain, anorexia, and bloating. Gastric distention and disordered swallowing may be present. Abdominal x-rays reveal gaseous distention of the large and small bowel and occasionally of the stomach. Air fluid levels are unusual and should raise the possibility of mechanical obstruction. Upper gastrointestinal series and barium enema do not reveal specific abnormalities of the intestine such as tumor, stricture, or volvulus. The presence of an autoimmune disorder or endocrinopathy may require confirmation by serologic or blood tests; biopsy may be needed as in amyloidosis or muscular dystrophy.

The treatment of chronic intestinal pseudoobstruction is made difficult by the complexity and chronicity of the underlying systemic disease. Patients with scleroderma may respond to broad-spectrum antibiotics if intestinal bacterial overgrowth is suspected. Metoclopramide may benefit gastric dysmotility in the diabetic. Discontinuation of psychotropic or anti-Parkinson drugs occasionally may result in improvement. Cathartics and enemas may be required to relieve fecal impaction, and the regular use of stool softeners and a high-fiber diet may help prevent recurrences.

Idiopathic intestinal pseudoobstruction   This term encompasses patients with signs and symptoms of pseudoobstruction in whom no systemic disease can be identified. The typical patient has recurrent attacks of abdominal pain and distention with nausea and vomiting. The small intestine is primarily involved, and chronic constipation is much less frequent than in secondary pseudoobstruction. Steatorrhea secondary to bacterial overgrowth of the small intestine is common and may lead to chronic diarrhea and malnutrition. Many patients exhibit abnormalities of motility in the esophagus and urinary bladder, in addition to the small and large intestine. Neuromuscular defects have been described in patients with this syndrome, including abnormalities of the mesenteric plexus and myopathy of the intestinal and urinary bladder smooth muscle (so-called hollow visceral myopathy). Elevated prostaglandin E levels have been reported in some patients. Treatment of idiopathic pseudoobstruction is unsatisfactory. Surgery to relieve "obstruction" is to be avoided, since the condition is often worsened by abdominal surgery. Medical therapy with metoclopramide and cholinergic agents has been unsuccessful. Nutritional support in the form of low-residue elemental diets or parenteral hyperalimentation may be helpful. Unfortunately, the lack of effective therapy and the progressive nature of the illness make the prognosis of idiopathic pseudoobstruction rather unfavorable. Death from malnutrition and steatorrhea are common. The long-term impact of total parenteral nutrition on this disease is not yet clear.

Acute intestinal pseudoobstruction This entity, sometimes referred to as *Ogilvie's syndrome*, is characterized by acute intestinal dilatation involving primarily the colon but occasionally also the small intestine. As in other forms of pseudoobstruction, the clinical features are difficult to distinguish from mechanical obstruction. The patient may complain of colicky lower abdominal pain and acute constipation. Examination reveals a distended, tympanitic abdomen, with reduced or absent bowel sounds. Localized tenderness over the distended colon is common, but diffuse abdominal tenderness, rigidity, or rebound tenderness are unusual. Abdominal films reveal massive dilatation of the colon and small intestine, occasionally with the presence of air fluid levels. The cecum, being the most capacious part of the colon, is often massively dilated and tender. The onset of these symptoms usually occurs in patients who have recently undergone severe surgical or medical stress such as major surgery, myocardial infarction, sepsis, or respiratory failure. Patients with acute pseudoobstruction are frequently on respirators, have received narcotics or sedatives, and have metabolic and electrolyte disturbances.

Management of acute pseudoobstruction requires careful correction of fluid and electrolyte abnormalities, intubation of the stomach or small intestine for decompression, and avoidance of drugs which depress intestinal motility. Barium enema may be hazardous because of the risk of perforating the already dilated bowel. Decompressive colonoscopy is beneficial in some patients, and cecostomy may be required in some patients with massive cecal dilatation. The outcome depends in large part on the prognosis of the associated medical or surgical conditions. Patients who recover from the underlying medical or surgical conditions usually have a return of normal colonic function.

IRRITABLE BOWEL SYNDROME The irritable bowel syndrome (IBS) is the most common gastrointestinal disease in clinical practice, and although not a life-threatening illness, it causes great distress to those afflicted and feelings of helplessness and frustration for the physician attempting to treat it. The patient with IBS may present with one of *three clinical variants*. Patients with so-called spastic colitis complain primarily of chronic abdominal pain and constipation. A second group has chronic intermittent diarrhea, often without pain. Some patients have both features and complain of alternating constipation and diarrhea.

IBS is characterized by chronic intermittent symptoms, including recurrent abdominal pain, usually in the left lower quadrant; altered frequency of defecation with hard stools (constipation) or watery stools (diarrhea); stool urgency; a sense of incomplete evacuation; feeling of abdominal distention; and excess flatus.

Two pathophysiologic abnormalities appear to underlie these symptoms: altered intestinal motility and increased visceral perception. Patients with diarrhea have accelerated transit of fecal material through the ascending and transverse colon, while patients with constipation have overall delays in colonic transit. Small-bowel motility patterns are also abnormal in conscious IBS patients but not during sleep, suggesting that altered gut motility may result, in part, from central nervous system input.

Heightened visceral perception in IBS patients has been demonstrated by excessive sensitivity to balloon distention in the ileum, colon, and rectum. This increased sensitivity to distention is accompanied by development of increased reflex intestinal motor activity. It is thought that these findings may explain the frequent complaints of gaseous distention in IBS patients, even though the volume of intestinal gas in these patients does not differ from that in normal individuals.

Evidence of significant psychological disturbances may be seen in some patients with IBS. Depression, hysteria, and obsessive-compulsive traits are common, and psychological stress frequently triggers an exacerbation of symptoms. Some female patients give a history of childhood sexual abuse. It should be noted, however, that increased intracolonic pressure has been observed in normal volunteers during acute stress. This suggests that psychological stress may be a nonspecific trigger of symptoms in IBS, as is the case in many other illnesses of diverse etiology.

Clinical features IBS is a disease of young or middle-aged adults; the female-to-male ratio is 4:1. The predominant feature is a history of chronic constipation, diarrhea, or both occurring *intermittently* for months or years. The diarrhea is usually worse in the morning upon arising or after breakfast. After the passage of three or four loose stools with excessive mucus, the patient may feel well for the remainder of the day. Diarrhea throughout the day or especially nocturnal diarrhea is most unusual. The diarrhea may last for weeks or months and then disappear spontaneously for variable periods of time. Some patients describe "pencil-like," pasty stools rather than diarrhea.

Another typical presentation is that of chronic abdominal pain with constipation or with alternating constipation and diarrhea. These patients describe intermittent crampy lower abdominal pain, often over the sigmoid colon, which is usually relieved by passage of flatus or stool. The patient may describe excessive bloating which is not discernible to the physician. A variety of other complaints, such as heartburn, excessive bloating, back pain, weakness, faintness, and palpitations, are frequent in patients with IBS. The pain may occasionally be in the right upper quadrant, or midepigastric pain may lead to diagnostic confusion with biliary tract or peptic ulcer disease.

Physical examination reveals these patients to be anxious, but significant abdominal tenderness or distention is unusual. A tender sigmoid full of feces may be palpated in the left lower quadrant. Sigmoidoscopy may reveal a prominent vascular pattern, muscle spasm, or excess mucus, but the mucosa itself is normal.

The *diagnosis* of IBS is suggested by the chronic intermittent nature of symptoms without obvious signs of physical deterioration, the relation of symptoms to environment or emotional stress, and the exclusion of other conditions. The evaluation should include a careful history, complete physical examination, and stool examination for occult blood, parasites, and pathogenic bacteria. In some patients, colonoscopy will be necessary to exclude inflammation or neoplasia. Barium enema may reveal spasticity of the sigmoid, accentuated haustra, and a tubular appearance to the descending colon. Lactase deficiency may masquerade as IBS and should be excluded by a trial of milk restriction, a lactose tolerance test, or a lactose breath hydrogen test (see Chap. 254). Thyrotoxicosis is easily confused with IBS and should be excluded by appropriate laboratory studies. Endometriosis also can cause altered bowel habit and pelvic pain.

Treatment of the IBS requires both skill and patience. It is important that the patient be reassured that this condition normally does not lead to the development of chronic inflammatory bowel disease (i.e., ulcerative colitis) or colonic malignancy. It is also important for both the patient and the physician to realize that the condition is chronic, and while it may be alleviated, it cannot be cured. The patient should be encouraged to adapt to the symptoms so as to minimize their impact on life-style. The physician should not imply that the symptoms are largely emotional or psychological in origin, since this is usually rejected by the patient. It is appropriate, however, to emphasize the relationship between psychological stress and the onset of severity of symptoms, since this may allow the patient to better deal with the disease. After the diagnosis is established, frequent x-rays and endoscopies are not necessary; general physical examinations, hemograms, and stool examinations for occult blood, however, should be carried out at regular intervals.

Drug treatment is aimed at altering the abnormal colonic motility in this disease. Patients with constipation may respond to an increase in dietary bulk in the form of unprocessed bran or psyllium bulk laxatives. Mild sedation with tranquilizers may be indicated, and anticholinergic drugs such as dicyclomine are useful in some patients. Troublesome diarrhea may respond to diphenoxylate or loperamide. Unfortunately, no specific drug or dietary regimen affords good relief in all patients, and thus a number of therapeutic maneuvers need to be tried.

CHRONIC CONSTIPATION   The mechanism of defecation is discussed in Chap. 39. Chronic constipation is widespread in western society, with approximately 10 percent of the population taking laxatives on a regular basis. Most cases of chronic constipation arise from habitual neglect of afferent impulses, failure to initiate defecation, and accumulation of large, dry fecal masses in the rectum. This voluntary suppression of the call to stool may arise during the period of toilet training in childhood or later in life because of a sense of social impropriety, unaccustomed surroundings, uncomfortable toilet facilities, or illnesses which require confinement to bed. Chronic constipation is much more common in women, with onset typically in late adolescence or early adulthood. As constant distention of the rectum with feces becomes chronic, the patient grows less aware of rectal fullness. Bowel movements become progressively more difficult, and painful hemorrhoids or anal fissures reinforce suppression of the urge to defecate. To avoid these problems, the patient begins the chronic use of laxatives or enemas, without which defecation becomes impossible.

Treatment   The physician should make every attempt to educate the patient about the chain of events which has led to chronic constipation. Attempts should be made to alter patterns of many years' duration, and the patient must recognize the importance of responding to, rather than suppressing, the urge to defecate. It is helpful to initiate a routine whereby defecation is attempted at a given time each day. In most individuals the call to stool occurs in the morning after breakfast. Physical exercise such as a brisk walk just before attempts at defecation may be helpful. Patients are instructed to increase dietary bulk with foods rich in fiber, such as green vegetables and unprocessed cereal grains, or by the regular use of bulk laxatives, such as hemicellulose, psyllium extract, and powdered unprocessed bran. The success of such a regimen depends to some extent on the duration of symptoms. Elderly patients with long-standing constipation and reliance on enemas or laxatives are more resistant to these measures than younger patients whose bowel patterns are less established. Moreover, poor muscle tone, reduced physical activity, and increased incidence of other medical conditions make the problem more difficult in the older age group. Bedridden elderly patients often develop severe constipation and even fecal impaction unless preventive measures are taken. This applies not only to patients with previous constipation but also to those with regular bowel movements prior to their confining illness. Regular administration of stool softeners, bulk laxatives, or mild cathartics is necessary until full ambulation and a normal diet are resumed. The onset of fecal impaction in bedridden patients is heralded by a feeling of rectal distention, urgency of defecation, or tenesmus. Occasionally, the fecal impaction will result in low-grade chronic obstruction with dilatation and increased fluid content proximal to the impaction; "paradoxical diarrhea" may thus occur as fluid moves past the obstructing fecal mass. This situation will be aggravated if antidiarrheal drugs are given because the underlying constipation will be worsened. The appropriate maneuver is to disimpact the rectum manually or to administer gentle enemas if the impaction is beyond the reach of the finger.

VASCULAR DISORDERS OF THE INTESTINE

Ischemia is the end result of interruption or reduction of the blood supply of the intestine. However, the clinical manifestations of intestinal ischemia range from mild chronic symptoms to catastrophic episodes, depending on the segment involved, the degree of involvement, and the rapidity of the process, and the clinician should be aware of this spectrum of manifestations (Table 256-1). The gut derives its arterial blood supply from the celiac axis and the superior and inferior mesenteric arteries. The small intestine is supplied by the celiac and superior mesenteric arteries; the colon is supplied by

TABLE 256-1   Patterns of intestinal ischemia

Condition	Etiology	Clinical features	Management
Mesenteric artery embolus	Arterial embolus associated with atrial fibrillation or rheumatic heart disease	Acute central abdominal pain, shock, peritonitis	Immediate angiography and embolectomy if possible
Abdominal angina	Atherosclerosis of celiac and superior mesenteric arteries	Chronic postprandial pain, weight loss	Angiography and surgery in selected cases
Ischemia colitis	Low-flow state	Acute lower abdominal pain, rectal bleeding	Sigmoidoscopy; surgery only for peritonitis

branches of the superior and inferior mesenteric arteries. A rich network of anastomotic vessels and the possible development of collateral circulation determine the clinical picture of acute or chronic intestinal arterial insufficiency.

MESENTERIC ISCHEMIA AND INFARCTION   Acute small-intestinal ischemia may be classified as *occlusive* or *nonocclusive*. Occlusion may result from arterial thrombus or embolus of the celiac or superior mesenteric arteries or from venous occlusion in the same distribution. Arterial embolus occurs most commonly in patients with chronic or recurrent atrial fibrillation, artificial heart valves, or valvular heart disease, while arterial thrombosis is associated with extensive atherosclerosis or low cardiac output. Venous occlusion is quite rare and is occasionally seen in women taking oral contraceptives. Approximately one-half of patients with mesenteric ischemia do not have a definite occlusion of a major vessel, a condition referred to as *nonocclusive* ischemia. The exact cause of nonocclusive disease is obscure; systemic arterial hypotension, cardiac arrhythmias, prolonged heart failure, digitalis therapy, dehydration, and endotoxemia have been suggested as contributing factors.

The outstanding clinical feature of acute mesenteric ischemia is severe abdominal pain, often colicky and periumbilical at the onset, later becoming diffuse and constant. Vomiting, anorexia, diarrhea, and constipation are also frequent but of little diagnostic help. Examination of the abdomen may reveal tenderness and distention. Bowel sounds are often normal even in the face of severe infarction. Some patients have a surprisingly normal abdominal examination in spite of severe pain. Mild gastrointestinal bleeding is often detected by guaiac examination of stool, but gross hemorrhage is unusual except in ischemic colitis (see below). A typical laboratory finding is a pronounced polymorphonuclear leukocytosis. Late in the course of the disease (24 to 72 h), gangrene of the bowel occurs with diffuse peritonitis, sepsis, and shock. Abdominal plain films in patients with mesenteric ischemia may reveal air fluid levels and distention. Barium study of the small intestine reveal nonspecific dilatation, poor motility, and evidence of thick mucosal folds ("thumbprinting") (Fig. 256-2).

Acute mesenteric ischemia is a grave condition with a high morbidity and mortality. Patients suspected of having acute arterial embolus should undergo immediate celiac and mesenteric angiography to localize the embolus, followed by embolectomy. Restoration of normal circulation may allow complete recovery if performed before irreversible necrosis or gangrene has occurred. Unfortunately, infarction and transmural necrosis are frequently found at surgery, necessitating resection. Arterial or venous thrombosis is not generally amenable to surgical removal of the thrombus, and resection of the affected bowel is required. Similarly, patients with nonocclusive ischemia are not candidates for corrective vascular surgery (as major vessels are patent). These individuals often have extensive necrosis of the small or large intestine because of the widespread nature of the ischemic event. The decision to operate on patients with suspected mesenteric ischemia is a difficult one because the typical patient is a poor surgical risk owing to advanced age, dehydration, sepsis, and other serious medical conditions.

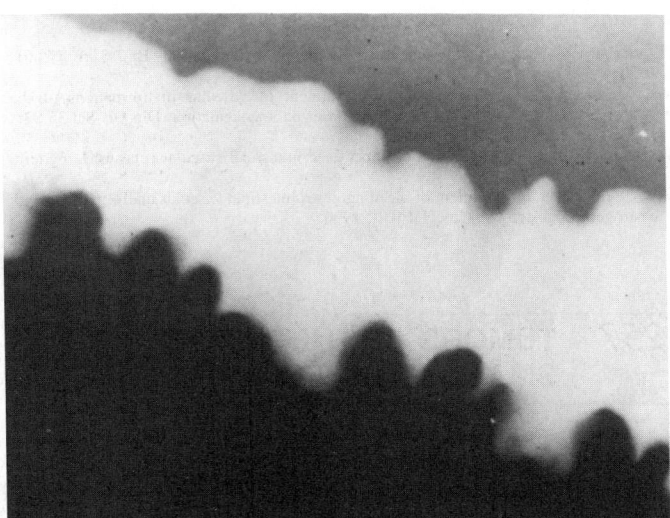

FIGURE 256-2 Barium enema showing ''thumbprinting'' or submucosal edema of the inferior margin of the transverse colon, in a patient with acute ischemic colitis.

Chronic arterial insufficiency may precede acute vascular insufficiency, producing so-called abdominal angina. As in angina pectoris, the pain of chronic mesenteric insufficiency occurs under conditions of increased demand for splanchnic blood flow. The patient complains of intermittent dull or cramping midabdominal pain 15 to 30 min after a meal, lasting for several hours postprandially. Significant weight loss is primarily due to a decreased food intake; however, chronic intestinal ischemia also may produce mucosal damage and malabsorption, which in turn aggravates the weight loss. Since abdominal angina may progress to bowel infarction, serious consideration should be given to performing arteriographic studies to confirm the diagnosis in those patients who are candidates for abdominal vascular surgery. The only definitive treatment is vascular surgery or balloon angioplasty to remove the thrombus or the construction of bypass arterial grafts to the ischemic bowel.

A number of systemic conditions are associated with *vasculitis* of the large and small arteries supplying the intestine. Most often these disorders can be recognized by the associated extraintestinal manifestations, as in polyarteritis nodosa, lupus erythematosus, dermatomyositis, Henoch-Schönlein purpura (allergic vasculitis), and rheumatoid vasculitis. When larger arteries are involved, as in polyarteritis nodosa, the picture of acute intestinal infarction is similar to that of embolic or atherosclerotic vascular occlusion. Often the involvement of smaller vessels leads to areas of intramural hemorrhage and edema resulting in abdominal pain, variable degrees of intestinal obstruction, and bleeding. Barium enema may show ''thumbprinting'' and ''spiculation'' due to localized edema, hemorrhage, and ulceration. In many instances, treatment of the underlying disorder may lead to regression of symptoms. If signs of an acute abdomen develop, surgical exploration is usually indicated.

Intramural small-intestinal hemorrhage may occur with vasculitis, trauma, or impaired coagulation, especially in patients receiving anticoagulants. The clinical and radiologic features resemble those seen with vasculitis and local mucosal hemorrhage.

ISCHEMIC COLITIS   Ischemia of the colon most often affects the elderly population because of the greater frequency of vascular disease in that group. Ischemic colitis is almost always a nonocclusive disease, that is, obstruction of major arteries is not seen. Shunting of blood away from the mucosa may contribute to this condition, but the mechanism of ischemia is not known.

The clinical picture depends on the degree of ischemia and the rate of its development. In *acute fulminant ischemic* colitis, the major manifestations are severe lower abdominal pain, rectal bleeding, and hypotension. Dilatation of the colon and physical signs of peritonitis

are seen in severe cases. Plain abdominal films may reveal thumbprinting from submucosal hemorrhage and edema. Barium enema is hazardous in the acute situation because of the risk of perforation. Sigmoidoscopy or colonoscopy may detect ulcerations, friability, and bulging folds from submucosal hemorrhage. Angiography is not helpful in the management of patients with presumed ischemic colitis because a remediable occlusive lesion is very rarely found. Surgical resection may be required in some patients with fulminant ischemic colitis to remove gangrenous bowel; others with lesser degrees of ischemia may respond to conservative medical management.

Subacute ischemic colitis, the most common clinical variant of ischemic colonic disease, produces lesser degrees of pain and bleeding, often occurring over several days or weeks. The left colon may be involved, but the rectum is usually spared because of collateral blood flow, a distinguishing feature from acute ulcerative colitis. Barium enema reveals edema, cobblestoning, thumbprinting, and occasionally superficial ulceration. Angiography is not indicated because almost all cases are nonocclusive. Occasionally, *stricture formation* may follow a bout of ischemic colitis or may present de novo without a history of antecedent pain or bloody diarrhea. Most cases of nonocclusive ischemic colitis resolve in 2 to 4 weeks and do not recur. Surgery is not required except for obstruction secondary to postischemic stricture.

ANGIODYSPLASIA OF THE COLON   These are vascular ectasias (not neoplasms) which occur in the right colon of many older individuals and may cause bleeding (see Chap. 41). Angiodysplasia is a degenerative lesion consisting of dilated, distorted, thin-walled vessels lined by vascular endothelium. Angiodysplasia may result from partial obstruction of the submucosal venous plexus by the tension generated in the cecal wall during muscular contraction. Aortic stenosis occurs in some patients and may cause chronic ischemia of the colon that leads to angiodysplasia. Grossly, angiodysplasias look similar to spider angiomas of the skin and appear as star-shaped branching vessels in the submucosa measuring from 2 mm to 1 cm in diameter. The lesions are usually multiple and are found primarily in the cecum and ascending colon, but in some patients they may be distributed from the stomach to rectum.

Cecal angiodysplasia is important because of the likelihood of bleeding, either massively or chronically. In patients over age 60, approximately one-quarter of colonic bleeding episodes are secondary to angiodysplasia. The diagnosis is easiest to establish by colonoscopy, which allows treatment by electrocautery or injection with sclerosant. Some patients with massive uncontrolled bleeding or multiple sites of angiodysplasia may require right hemicolectomy. Angiodysplasias also may respond to chronic estrogen-progesterone therapy.

ANORECTAL PROBLEMS

HEMORRHOIDS   The internal hemorrhoidal plexus of veins is located in the submucosal space above the valves of Morgagni. The anal canal separates it from the external hemorrhoidal venous plexus, but the two spaces communicate under the anal canal, the submucosa of which is attached to underlying tissue to form the interhemorrhoidal depression. Whenever the internal hemorrhoidal plexus is enlarged, there is associated increase in supporting tissue mass, and the resultant venous swelling is called an *internal hemorrhoid*. When veins in the external hemorrhoidal plexus become enlarged or thrombosed, the resultant bluish mass is called an *external hemorrhoid*.

Both types of hemorrhoids are very common and are associated with increased hydrostatic pressure in the portal venous system, such as during pregnancy, straining at stool, or with cirrhosis. When internal hemorrhoids enlarge, pain is not a usual feature until the situation is complicated by thrombosis, infection, or erosion of the overlying mucosal surface. Most persons complain of bright red blood on the toilet tissue or coating the stool, with a feeling of vague anal discomfort. The discomfort is increased when the hemorrhoid enlarges or prolapses through the anus; prolapse is often accompanied by edema and sphincteric spasm. Prolapse, if not treated, usually becomes chronic as the muscularis stays stretched, and the patient complains of constant soiling of underclothing with very little pain. Prolapsed hemorrhoids may be infected or thrombosed; the overlying mucous membrane may bleed profusely from the trauma of defecation.

External hemorrhoids, because they lie under the skin, are quite often painful, particularly if there is a sudden increase in their mass. These episodes result in a tender blue swelling at the anal verge due to thrombosis of a vein in the external plexus and need not be associated with enlargement of the internal veins. Since the thrombus usually lies at the level of the sphincteric muscles, anal spasm often occurs.

The diagnosis of internal and external hemorrhoids is made by inspection, digital examination, and direct vision through the anoscope and proctoscope. Since such lesions are very common, they must not be regarded as the cause of rectal bleeding or chronic hypochromic anemia until a thorough investigation has been made of the more proximal gastrointestinal tract. Acute blood loss can occasionally be attributed to internal hemorrhoids. Chronic anemia or occult blood in the stool in the presence of large but not definitely bleeding hemorrhoids requires a search for a polyp, cancer, or ulcer.

Most hemorrhoids respond to conservative therapy such as sitz baths or other forms of moist heat, suppositories, stool softeners, and bed rest. Internal hemorrhoids which remain permanently prolapsed are best treated surgically; milder degrees of prolapse or enlargement with pruritus ani or intermittent bleeding can be handled successfully by banding or injection of sclerosing solutions. External hemorrhoids which become acutely thrombosed are treated by incision, extraction of the clot, and compression of the incised area following clot removal. No surgical procedure should be carried out in the presence of acute inflammation of the anus, ulcerative proctitis, or ulcerative colitis. Proctoscopy or colonoscopy should always be performed before a patient is subjected to hemorrhoidectomy.

ANAL INFLAMMATION   Perianal inflammatory lesions may be primary or may be associated with inflammatory bowel disease or diverticular disease, as mentioned above. Anal *fissures* are superficial erosions of the anal canal which usually heal rapidly with conservative therapy. Anal *ulcers* are more chronic and deep and give symptoms largely as the result of painful spasm of the external anal sphincter during and after defecation. Bleeding may occur with either fissure or ulcer; healing of the ulcer often is associated with a hypertrophied anal papilla and some degrees of anal contracture. *Fistula in ano*, a tract leading from the rectal lumen to the perianal skin, usually results from local crypt abscesses. The fistula is a chronically inflamed canal made up of fibrous tissue surrounding granulation tissue, the lumen of which may be difficult to demonstrate. Perirectal *abscesses* often represent the tracking down into the anal area of purulent material escaping from the rectosigmoid; diverticulitis, Crohn's disease, ulcerative colitis, or previous surgery may be the underlying cause. Fistulas between the rectum and vagina or the rectum and bladder represent serious complications of granulomatous, septic, or malignant disorders and require the patient to be hospitalized for definitive diagnostic and therapeutic procedures.

REFERENCES

Disorders of motility

COLEMONT LJ, CAMILLERI M: Chronic intestinal pseudo-obstruction: Diagnosis and treatment. Mayo Clin Proc 64:60, 1989

DROSSMAN DA, THOMPSON WG: The irritable bowel syndrome: Review and a graduated multicomponent treatment approach. Ann Intern Med 116:1009, 1992

PRESTON DM, LENNARD-JONES JE: Severe chronic constipation of young women: Idiopathic slow transit constipation. Gut 27:41, 1986

Diverticular diseases

BRIAN JE, STAIR JM: Non-colonic diverticular disease. Surg Gynecol Obstet 161:189, 1985

STEFANSSON T et al: Increased risk of left sided colon cancer in patients with diverticular disease. Gut 34:499, 1993

THOMPSON WG, PATEL DG: Clinical picture of diverticular disease of the colon. Clinics Gastrol 15:903, 1986

Intestinal ischemia and angiodysplasia

CLAVIEN PA: Diagnosis and management of mesenteric infarction. Br J Surg 77:601, 1990

NAVEAU S et al: Long-term results of treatment of vascular malformations of the gastrointestinal tract by neodynium YAG laser photocoagulation. Dig Dis Sci 35:821, 1990

SARGEANT IR et al: Laser ablation of upper gastrointestinal vascular ectasias: Long term results. Gut 34:470, 1993

VAN CUTSEM E et al: Treatment of bleeding gastrointestinal vascular malformations with oestrogen-progesterone. Lancet 1:953, 1990

257   TUMORS OF THE LARGE AND SMALL INTESTINE

ROBERT J. MAYER

COLORECTAL CANCER

INCIDENCE   Cancer of the large bowel is second only to lung cancer as a cause of cancer death in the United States. Approximately 152,000 new cases were anticipated in 1993, resulting in 57,000 deaths. The incidence and mortality rates for this extremely common malignant condition have not changed substantially in males during the past 40 years, although, for some reason, a slight decrease in the mortality rate has appeared in females. Colorectal cancer generally occurs in individuals 50 years of age or older.

ETIOLOGY AND RISK FACTORS (Table 257-1)   **Diet**   The etiology for most cases of large-bowel cancer appears to be related to environmental factors. The disease occurs more often in upper socioeconomic populations who live in urban areas. Epidemiologic studies in various countries have documented a direct correlation between mortality from colorectal cancer and per capita consumption of calories, meat protein, and dietary fat and oil as well as elevations in the serum cholesterol concentration and mortality from coronary artery disease. Any geographic variations in incidence do not appear to be related to genetic differences, since migrant groups tend to assume the large-bowel cancer incidence rates of their adopted countries. Furthermore, population groups such as Mormons and Seventh Day Adventists, whose lifestyle and dietary habits differ somewhat from those of their neighbors, have significantly lower-than-expected incidence and mortality rates for colorectal cancer, while the appearance of colorectal cancer has increased in Japan since that nation has adopted a more "western" diet. It is therefore assumed that dietary patterns influence the development of colorectal cancer. At least two hypotheses have been proposed to explain this relationship, neither of which is fully satisfactory.

ANIMAL FATS   Based on the association of colorectal cancer with hypercholesterolemia and coronary artery disease as well as the increased incidence of large-bowel tumors in geographic areas where meat is a dietary staple, it has been suggested that the ingestion of animal fats leads to an increased proportion of anaerobes in the gut microflora, resulting in the conversion of normal bile acids into

TABLE 257-1   Risk factors for the development of colorectal cancer

Diet
  ? Animal fat
  ? Fiber
Hereditary syndromes (autosomal dominant inheritance)
  Polyposis coli
  Non-polyposis syndrome
Inflammatory bowel disease
Streptococcus bovis bacteremia
Ureterosigmoidostomy

carcinogens. This provocative hypothesis is supported by several reports of increased amounts of fecal anaerobes in the stools of patients with colorectal cancer. However, there are conflicting data from population studies relating fat intake to the risk for colon cancer and from unsuccessful attempts at altering the profile of fecal microflora through short-term alterations in diet. Any definitive assessment of the animal fat concept must await a prospective survey of a defined population, correlating carefully obtained and periodically updated dietary histories with quantitative cultures of stool microflora, and determining the incidence of colorectal cancer in these individuals over a 10 to 20 year period of time.

FIBER The observation that South African Bantus ingest a diet far higher in roughage, produce more frequent, bulkier stools, and have a lower incidence of large-bowel cancer than their American and European counterparts led to the proposal that the higher rate of colorectal cancer in western society is in large part the result of a low intake of dietary fiber. This theory suggests that dietary fiber accelerates intestinal transit time, thereby reducing the exposure of colonic mucosa to potential carcinogens and diluting these carcinogens because of enhanced fecal bulk. Such a proposition appears somewhat simplistic when subjected to careful scrutiny. Although an enhanced fiber intake increases fecal bulk, there has been no consistent evidence that a higher fiber intake actually shortens the transit time of stool. Additionally, despite the generally higher fiber intake in low-incidence countries, the environmental differences between developing and industrialized nations are myriad and include such other important dietary variables as meat and fat consumption. Finally, a diet low in fiber may lead to chronic constipation and such associated conditions as diverticulosis. If a low fiber diet alone were a significant factor in colorectal cancer, individuals having diverticulosis should be at higher risk for the development of large-bowel tumors; this does not appear to be the case.

OTHER Emerging data suggest that the risk for the development of colorectal cancer may be diminished by calcium supplements or aspirin. It is thought that dietary calcium may inactivate bowel carcinogens through the formation of insoluble soaps. In support of this concept are (1) the finding that supplementary dietary calcium reduced the proliferation of colonic epithelial cells in familial colon cancer kindreds and (2) the results of a survey of the dietary habits of a cohort of about 2000 men over a 19-year period, suggesting that the risk of colonic cancer decreased with increased oral intake of calcium.

Aspirin, an inhibitor of arachidonic acid metabolism, inhibits the growth of chemically induced colon tumors in rodents. A recent survey suggested that human colon cancer mortality might be reduced by the regular use of aspirin although it remains uncertain whether such a reduction was the result of prevention or earlier detection. Confirmation of this observation through a prospective trial will be required before routine use of aspirin as a form of chemoprevention can be recommended.

Thus, while the weight of epidemiologic evidence implicates diet as being the major etiologic factor for colorectal cancer, no single foodstuff has been sufficiently identified as being a causative or protective agent to justify specific recommendations for widespread changes in eating habits.

Hereditary factors and syndromes As many as 25 percent of patients with colorectal cancer may have a family history of the disease, suggesting a hereditary predisposition. Such inherited large-bowel cancers can be divided into two main groups: the well-studied but uncommon polyposis syndromes and the less well defined nonpolyposis syndromes (Table 257-2).

Polyposis coli (i.e., familial polyposis of the colon) is a rare condition characterized by the appearance of thousands of adenomatous polyps throughout the large bowel. The condition is transmitted in an autosomal dominant manner; the occasional patients with no family history are thought to have developed the polyposis due to a spontaneous mutation. Molecular studies have associated polyposis coli with a deletion in the long arm of chromosome 5 (*APC* gene). It has been hypothesized that the loss of this genetic material (i.e., allelic loss) results in the absence of tumor-suppressor genes whose protein products would normally inhibit neoplastic growth. The presence of soft tissue, bony tumors, and ampullary cancers in addition to the colonic polyps characterizes a subset of polyposis coli known as *Gardner's syndrome*, while the appearance of malignant tumors of the central nervous system accompanying polyposis coli defines *Turcot's syndrome*. The colonic polyps in all these conditions are rarely present prior to puberty but are generally evident in affected individuals by age 25. If left surgically untreated, colorectal cancer will develop in almost all patients prior to age 40. Polyposis coli has been studied intensively and appears to result from a defect in the colonic mucosa leading to an abnormal proliferative pattern and an impaired ability for cellular repair following exposure to radiation or ultraviolet light. Once the multiple polyps that constitute polyposis coli are detected, patients should have a total colectomy. It remained unclear in the past (*A*) whether the optimal operative approach in such a clinical setting was to resect the entire colon and rectum, requiring the young patient to have a permanent ileostomy, or to perform an ileoproctostomy. While the latter procedure retained the distal rectum and anal sphincter, it placed the patient at continued risk for the development of cancer in the rectal remnant and necessitated semiannual or annual proctoscopic surveillance. The development of the ileoanal anastomotic technique allows removal of the entire bowel while retaining the anal sphincter and appears to be the best treatment. (*B*) The offspring of patients with polyposis coli, who are often prepubertal when the diagnosis is made in the parent, have a 50 percent risk for the eventual development of this premalignant disorder and should be carefully screened by annual flexible sigmoidoscopy until age 35. Testing for occult blood in the stool is an inadequate screening maneuver. Unfortunately, no disease-specific screening technique is generally available for the children of polyposis coli patients, although radioautographic measurements of colonic mucosal proliferation have been utilized with apparent efficacy in a small number of patients at highly specialized medical centers. Conceivably, molecular probes for the *APC* gene will prove to be useful in this regard in the future.

The hereditary predisposition for colorectal cancer in families

TABLE 257-2 Hereditable (autosomal dominant) gastrointestinal polyp syndromes

Syndrome	Distribution of polyps	Histologic type	Malignant potential	Associated lesions
Familial colonic polyposis	Large intestine	Adenoma	Common	None
Gardner's syndrome	Large and small intestines	Adenoma	Common	Osteomas, fibromas, lipomas, epidermoid cysts, ampullary cancers
Turcot's syndrome	Large intestine	Adenoma	Common	Brain tumors
Non-polyposis syndrome	Large intestine	Adenoma	Common	Endometrial tumors
Peutz-Jeghers syndrome	Small and large intestines, stomach	Hamartoma	Rare	Mucocutaneous pigmentation; tumors of the ovary, breast, pancreas, endometrium
Juvenile polyposis	Large and small intestines, stomach	Hamartoma rarely progressing to adenoma	Rare	Various congenital abnormalities

having no history of polyposis coli, the so-called hereditary nonpolyposis colorectal cancer syndrome, has received increased attention since the identification of several kindreds who displayed risks as high as 50 percent for the development of a colonic malignancy. These lesions involved the proximal large bowel in an unusually high frequency. Such families frequently include patients having multiple primary cancers, with the association of colorectal and endometrial adenocarcinomas being especially prominent in women. The trait for cancer appears to be transmitted in an autosomal dominant manner, possibly involving an abnormality in chromosome 2, and the median age for the appearance of an adenocarcinoma is about age 45, 15 to 20 years below the usual age for the general population. The offspring of such predisposed patients should undergo intensive screening, consisting of triannual colonoscopies, from age 25.

Inflammatory bowel disease (See also Chap. 255) Large-bowel cancer represents a not infrequent complication in patients with long-standing inflammatory bowel disease. The development of a neoplasm appears to occur more commonly in patients with ulcerative colitis than in those with granulomatous colitis, but such an impression may result in part from the occasional difficulty in differentiating these two conditions. The risk of colorectal cancer in a patient with inflammatory bowel disease is relatively small during the initial 10 years following the onset of the disease, but then appears to increase at a rate of approximately 0.5 to 1.0 percent per year. Actuarially derived cumulative cancer rates in such symptomatic patients have ranged from 8 to 30 percent after 25 years. The risk is generally considered to be higher in younger patients with pancolitis.

Cancer surveillance in patients with inflammatory bowel disease is unsatisfactory. Symptoms such as bloody diarrhea, abdominal cramping, and obstruction, which may signal the appearance of a tumor, are similar to the complaints of patients whose underlying disease is flaring. In patients with a history of inflammatory bowel disease lasting 15 years or more who continue to experience exacerbations, the surgical removal of the colon can significantly reduce the risk for cancer and also eliminate the target organ for the underlying chronic gastrointestinal disorder. The value of such surveillance techniques as colonoscopy with mucosal biopsies and brushings for less symptomatic individuals with chronic inflammatory bowel disease is uncertain. The purpose of such procedures has been the identification of premalignant mucosal dysplasia, thereby justifying surgical intervention. The lack of uniformity regarding the pathologic criteria that characterize dysplasia and the absence of data that such surveillance reduces the development of lethal cancers, however, has made this costly practice an area of controversy.

Other high-risk conditions STREPTOCOCCUS BOVIS BACTEREMIA For unknown reasons, individuals who develop endocarditis or septicemia from this fecal bacteria seem to have a high incidence of occult colorectal tumors and, possibly, upper gastrointestinal cancers as well. Endoscopic or radiographic screening appears advisable.

URETEROSIGMOIDOSTOMY There is a 5 to 10 percent incidence of colon cancer 15 to 30 years after ureterosigmoidostomy to correct congenital extrophy of the bladder. Neoplasms characteristically are found at a site distal to the ureteral implant where colonic mucosa is chronically exposed to both urine and feces.

POLYPS The majority of colorectal cancers, regardless of etiology, are believed to arise from adenomatous polyps. A polyp is a grossly visible protrusion from the mucosal surface and may be classified pathologically as a nonneoplastic hamartoma (*juvenile polyp*), a hyperplastic mucosal proliferation (*hyperplastic polyp*), or an adenomatous polyp. Only adenomas are clearly premalignant and only a minority of such lesions ever develop into cancer. Population-screening studies and autopsy surveys have revealed that adenomatous polyps may be found in the colons of about 30 percent of middle-aged or elderly people. Based on this prevalence and the known incidence of colorectal cancers, it appears that less than 1 percent of polyps ever become malignant. Most polyps produce no symptoms and remain clinically undetected. Occult blood in the stool may be found in less than 5 percent of patients with such lesions.

A number of molecular changes have been described in the DNA obtained from adenomatous polyps, dysplastic lesions, and polyps containing microscopic foci of tumor cells (i.e., *carcinoma in situ*). Consistent with the multistep process leading to cancer, a series of alterations has been observed, often beginning with a specific mutation in the *ras* proto-oncogene followed by deletions in chromosomes 5, 18, and 17 (see Chap. 63, Fig. 63-9). The loss of genetic material on the short arm of chromosome 17 appears to be associated with activation of a gene leading to the production of transformation-associated protein p53. Thus, the altered proliferative pattern of the colonic mucosa (which results in the progression to a polyp and then to a carcinoma) may involve the mutational activation of an oncogene followed by and coupled with the loss of genes which normally suppress tumorigenesis. Based on this model, it is believed that neoplasia develops only in those polyps in which all of these mutational events take place.

Clinically, the probability of an adenomatous polyp becoming a cancer is dependent upon the gross appearance of the lesion, its histologic features, and its size. Adenomatous polyps may be pedunculated (i.e., extending from adjacent bowel on a stalk) or sessile (i.e., flat). Cancers develop more frequently in sessile polyps. Histologically, adenomatous polyps may be tubular, villous (i.e., papillary), or tubulovillous. Villous adenomas, which are predominantly sessile in appearance, become malignant more than three times as often as tubular adenomas. The likelihood that any polypoid lesion in the large bowel contains invasive cancer is related to the size of the polyp, being negligible (<2 percent) in lesions smaller than 1.5 cm, intermediate (2 to 10 percent) in lesions 1.5 to 2.5 cm in size, and substantial (>10 percent) in lesions larger than 2.5 cm.

Following the detection of an adenomatous polyp, the entire large bowel should be visualized endoscopically or radiographically since synchronous lesions are present in approximately one-third of cases. Colonoscopy should then be repeated periodically, even in the absence of a previously documented malignancy, since such patients have a 30 to 50 percent probability of developing another adenoma and are at a higher-than-average risk for developing a colorectal carcinoma. Adenomatous polyps are thought to require more than 5 years of growth before becoming clinically significant; therefore, colonoscopy need not be carried out more frequently than every 3 years.

SCREENING The rationale for colorectal cancer screening programs is that the earlier detection of localized, superficial neoplasms in asymptomatic individuals will increase the surgical cure rate. Screening strategies have been based on the assumption that more than 60 percent of such early lesions are located in the rectosigmoid, making them accessible to rigid proctosigmoidoscopy. For unexplained reasons, however, there has been a consistent decrease during the past several decades in the proportion of large-bowel cancers arising in the rectum with a corresponding increase in the more proximal descending colon. As such, the potential for rigid proctosigmoidoscopy to detect a sufficient number of occult neoplasms to make the procedure cost-effective has been questioned. Nonetheless in support of periodic rigid proctosigmoidoscopic examination is a case-control study reporting a reduction in mortality from a distal large bowel cancer in individuals who had undergone such screening. The availability of flexible, fiberoptic sigmoidoscopes, permitting trained operators to visualize the colon for up to 60 cm, should further enhance cancer detection and resolve this issue.

Most programs directed at the early detection of colorectal cancers have focused on digital rectal examinations and testing stool for the presence of occult blood. The digital examination should be part of any routine physical evaluation in adults older than age 40, serving as an effective screening test for prostate cancer in men, a component of the pelvic examination in women, and as an inexpensive maneuver for the detection of masses in the rectum. The development of the Hemoccult test has greatly facilitated the potential to detect occult fecal blood. Unfortunately, even when performed optimally, the Hemoccult test has major limitations as a screening technique. Approximately 50 percent of patients with documented colorectal cancers have a negative fecal Hemoccult test, consistent with the intermittent bleeding pattern of these tumors. When random cohorts of asymptomatic persons have been tested, 2 to 4 percent have Hemoccult-positive stools. Colorectal cancers have been found in only 5 to 10 percent of these "test-positive" cases, with benign polyps being detected in an additional 20 to 30 percent. Consequently, a colorectal neoplasm will *not* be found in the majority of asymptomatic individuals with occult blood in their stool. Nonetheless, persons found to have Hemoccult-positive stool routinely undergo further medical evaluation that includes sigmoidoscopy, barium enema, and/or colonoscopy—procedures that not only are uncomfortable and expensive, but also are associated with a low but finite risk for significant complications. The added cost of these studies would appear justifiable if the minority of patients found to have occult neoplasms because of Hemoccult screening could be shown to have an improved prognosis and prolonged survival. Prospectively controlled trials addressing this issue are ongoing. One of these studies, conducted at the University of Minnesota, involving more than 46,000 participants, reported a statistically significant reduction in mortality from colorectal cancer for individuals undergoing annual screening. However, this benefit only emerged after more than 13 years of follow-up and was extremely expensive to achieve since all positive tests (the majority of which were falsely positive) were followed by colonoscopy.

Screening techniques for large-bowel cancer in asymptomatic persons remain unsatisfactory. Recommendations from governmental and private agencies are conflicting. At present, the American Cancer Society suggests annual digital rectal examinations beginning at age 40, annual fecal Hemoccult screening beginning at age 50, and sigmoidoscopy (preferably flexible), every 3 to 5 years, beginning at age 50 for asymptomatic individuals having none of the high-risk factors for colorectal cancer. More effective techniques for screening are needed, perhaps taking advantage of the molecular changes which have been described in these tumors. An analysis for specific *ras* proto-oncogene mutations from DNA recovered from stool in patients with a history of colorectal cancer represents an initial step in this direction.

CLINICAL FEATURES   Presenting symptoms   Symptoms vary with the anatomic location of the tumor.

Since stool is relatively liquid as it passes through the ileocecal valve into the right colon, neoplasms arising in the cecum and ascending colon may become quite large, significantly narrowing the bowel lumen, without resulting in any obstructive symptoms or noticeable alterations in bowel habits. Lesions of the right colon commonly ulcerate, leading to chronic, insidious blood loss without a change in the appearance of the stool. Consequently, patients with tumors of the ascending colon often present with symptoms such as fatigue, palpitations, and even angina pectoris and are found to have a hypochromic, microcytic anemia indicative of iron deficiency. Since the cancer may bleed intermittently, however, a random test for the presence of occult blood in the stool may be negative. As a result, the unexplained presence of iron-deficiency anemia in any adult (with the possible exception of a premenopausal, multiparous woman) mandates a thorough endoscopic and/or radiographic visualization of the entire large bowel (Fig. 257-1).

Since stool becomes more concentrated as it passes into the transverse and descending colon, tumors arising there tend to impede the passage of stool, resulting in the development of abdominal cramping, occasional obstruction, and even perforation. Radiographs of the abdomen often reveal characteristic annular, constricting lesions ("apple-core" or "napkin-ring") (Fig. 257-2).

Neoplasms arising in the rectosigmoid often are associated with hematochezia, tenesmus, and narrowing in the caliber of stool; nonetheless, anemia is an infrequent finding. While these symptoms may lead patients and their physicians to suspect the presence of hemorrhoids, the development of rectal bleeding and/or altered bowel habits demands a prompt digital rectal examination and proctosigmoidoscopy.

Staging, prognostic factors, patterns of spread   The prognosis

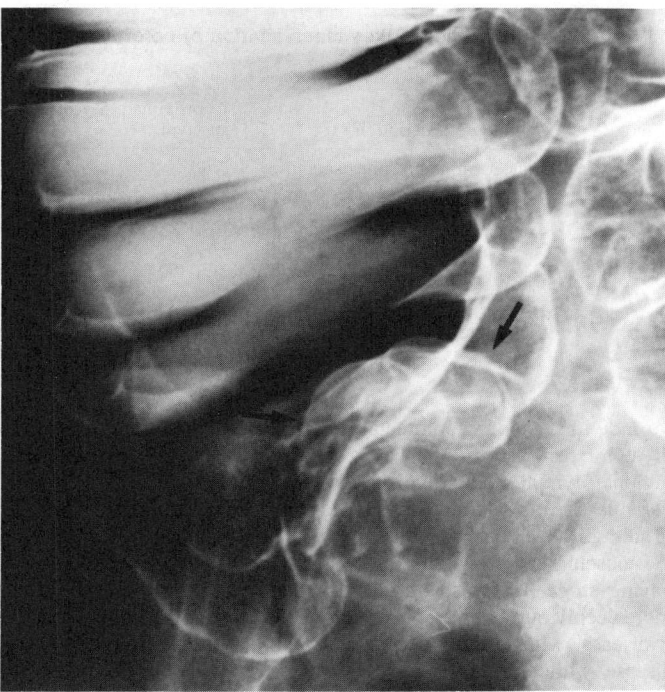

FIGURE 257-1   Double-contrast air-barium enema revealing a sessile tumor of the cecum in a patient with iron-deficiency anemia and guaiac-positive stool. The lesion at surgery was a stage B adenocarcinoma.

FIGURE 257-2   Annular, constricting adenocarcinoma of the descending colon. This radiographic appearance is referred to as an "apple-core" lesion and is always highly suggestive of malignancy.

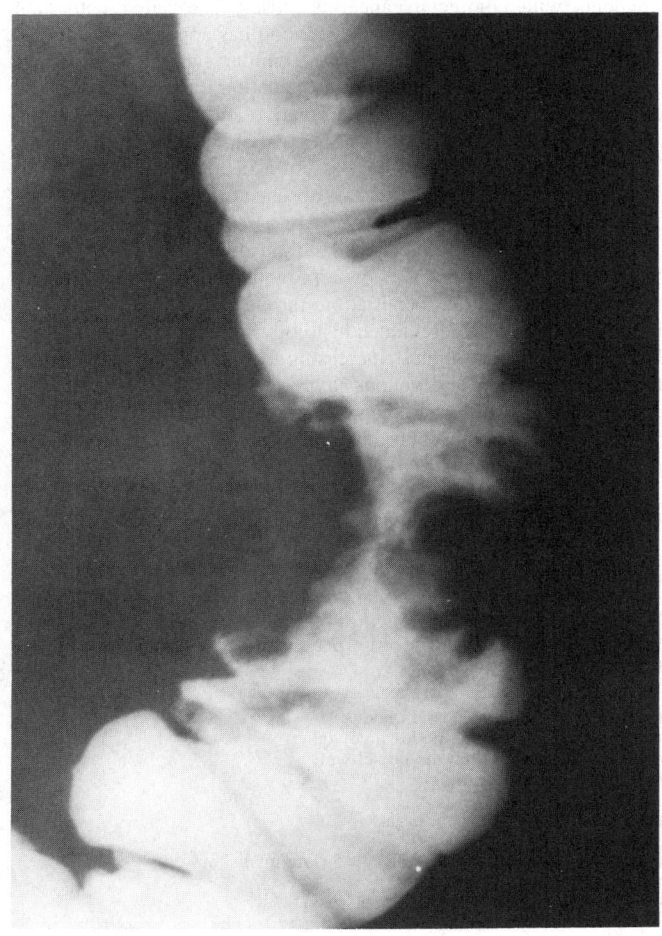

TABLE 257-3 Modified Dukes classification of colorectal cancer

Stage	Pathologic description	Approximate 5-year survival, %
A	Cancer limited to mucosa and submucosa	>90
B_1	Cancer extends into muscularis	85
B_2	Cancer extends into or through serosa	70–85
C	Cancer involves regional lymph nodes	30–60
D	Distant metastases (i.e., liver, lung, etc.)	5

for individuals having colorectal cancer is closely related to the depth of tumor penetration into the bowel wall and the presence of both regional lymph node involvement and distant metastases. These variables are incorporated into the staging system introduced by Dukes (Table 257-3). Patients with superficial lesions not penetrating into the muscularis or involving regional lymph nodes are designated as having *stage A* disease; those individuals whose tumors penetrate more deeply but without spread to lymph nodes are said to have *stage B* disease (with lesions restricted to the muscularis termed *stage B_1* disease while lesions involving the serosa classified as *stage B_2* disease); regional lymph node involvement defines *stage C* disease; and metastatic spread to sites such as liver, lung, or bone indicates *stage D* disease. Unless gross evidence of metastatic disease is present, it is impossible to accurately determine disease stage prior to surgical resection and pathologic analysis of the operative specimens.

Most recurrences after a surgical resection of a large-bowel cancer occur within the first 4 postoperative years, making the 5-year mark a fairly reliable indicator of cure. The likelihood for 5-year survival in patients with colorectal cancer is closely associated with their Dukes stage (Table 257-3). That likelihood has appeared to improve during the past several decades when similar surgical stages have been compared. The most plausible explanation for this improvement appears to be more thorough intraoperative and pathologic staging. In particular, more exacting attention to pathologic detail has revealed that the prognosis following the resection of a colorectal cancer is not related merely to the presence or absence of regional lymph node involvement but may be more precisely assessed by the number of involved lymph nodes (i.e., 1 to 4 lymph nodes versus >5 lymph nodes). Other predictors of a poor prognosis after a total surgical resection include tumor penetration through the bowel wall into pericolic fat, poorly differentiated histology, perforation and/or tumor adherence to adjacent organs (increasing the risk for an anatomically adjacent recurrence), and venous invasion by tumor (Table 257-4). Regardless of the clinicopathologic stage, a preoperative elevation of the plasma carcinoembryonic antigen (CEA) titer is suggestive of eventual tumor recurrence. The presence of abnormal DNA content (i.e., aneuploidy) and specific chromosomal deletions (i.e., so-called allelic loss) in tumor cells, as determined by flow cytometry and

restriction fragment length polymorphism analysis respectively, appears to predict a higher risk for metastatic spread. In contrast to most other carcinomas and sarcomas, the prognosis in individuals with colorectal cancer is *not* influenced by the size of the primary lesion when adjusted for nodal involvement and histologic differentiation.

Cancers of the large bowel generally spread to regional lymph nodes or to the liver via the portal venous circulation. The liver represents the most frequent visceral site of metastatic dissemination; it is the initial site of distant spread in one-third of recurring colorectal cancers and eventually becomes involved in greater than two-thirds of such patients at the time of death. In general, colorectal cancer rarely metastasizes to the lungs, supraclavicular lymph nodes, bone, or brain without prior spread to the liver. A major exception to this rule occurs in patients having primary tumors in the distal rectum, from where tumor cells may spread through the paravertebral venous plexus, escaping the portal venous system and thereby reaching the lungs or supraclavicular lymph nodes without hepatic involvement. The median survival after the detection of distant metastases may range from 6 to 9 months (hepatomegaly, liver abnormalities) to 24 to 30 months (small liver nodule initially identified by elevated CEA level and subsequent CT scan).

TREATMENT Total resection of tumor represents optimal management when a malignant lesion is endoscopically or radiographically detected in the large bowel. An evaluation for the presence of metastatic disease, including a thorough physical examination, a chest radiograph, biochemical assessment of liver function, and a plasma CEA level, should be performed prior to surgery. When possible, a colonoscopy of the entire large bowel should be performed to identify synchronous neoplasms and/or polyps. The detection of metastases should not preclude surgery in patients with tumor-related symptoms such as gastrointestinal bleeding or obstruction, but may often result in a less radical operative procedure being carried out. At the time of laparotomy, the entire peritoneal cavity should be examined with the liver, pelvis, and hemidiaphragm being thoroughly inspected and the full length of the large bowel being carefully palpated. Following recovery from a complete resection, patients should be carefully observed for 5 years by semiannual physical examinations and yearly blood chemistries. If a complete colonoscopy was not performed preoperatively, this should be carried out within the first several postoperative months. Some authorities favor obtaining plasma CEA levels at 3-month intervals because of the sensitivity of this test as a marker for otherwise undetectable tumor recurrence. Subsequent endoscopic or radiographic surveillance of the large bowel, probably at triannual intervals, is indicated, since patients who have been cured of one colorectal cancer have a 3 to 5 percent probability of developing an additional bowel cancer during their lifetime and a risk in excess of 15 percent for the development of adenomatous polyps. Anastomotic (i.e., "suture-line") recurrences are infrequent in colorectal cancer patients, if the surgical resection margins were adequate and free of tumor.

Radiation therapy to the pelvis is generally recommended for patients with rectal cancer because of the 30 to 40 percent probability of regional recurrences following complete surgical resection of stages B and C tumors, especially if they have penetrated through the serosa. This alarmingly high rate of local disease recurrence is believed to be due to the fact that the contained anatomic space within the pelvis limits the extent of the resection and because the rich lymphatic network of the pelvic side wall immediately adjacent to the rectum facilities the early spread of malignant cells into surgically inaccessible tissue. Prospectively randomized trials have indicated that the prophylactic use of radiation therapy, either pre- or postoperatively, reduces the likelihood of pelvis recurrences but does not appear to prolong survival. Preoperative radiotherapy is clearly indicated for patients with large, potentially unresectable rectal cancers, since such anatomically fixed lesions may shrink sufficiently to permit subsequent surgical removal.

Chemotherapy in patients with advanced colorectal cancer has proven to be of only marginal benefit. Since its introduction into

TABLE 257-4 Poor prognostic predictors following total surgical resection

Tumor spread to regional lymph nodes
Number of regional lymph nodes involved
Tumor penetration through the bowel wall
Poorly differentiated histology
Perforation
Tumor adherence to adjacent organs
Venous invasion
Preoperative elevation of CEA titer (>5.0 ng/mL)
Aneuploidy
Specific chromosomal deletion (allelic loss)

clinical trials more than 25 years ago, 5-fluorouracil (5-FU) remains the most effective treatment for this disease. It is as useful when given alone as when combined with other drugs, but is associated with only a 15 to 20 percent likelihood of reducing measurable tumor masses by 50 percent or more (i.e., partial response). While the probability for tumor response appears to be somewhat greater for patients with liver metastases when such chemotherapy is infused directly into the hepatic artery as compared to a peripheral vein, intraarterial treatment is costly and toxic and does not appear to prolong survival. The results of recent studies have suggested that the concomitant administration of folinic acid (also known as leucovorin or citrovorum factor) will improve the efficacy of 5-FU in patients with advanced colorectal cancer, presumably by enhancing the binding of 5-FU to its target enzyme, thymidylate synthase, thereby increasing the suppression of DNA synthesis and accompanying cytotoxicity. The majority of randomized trials have indicated a threefold improvement in the likelihood of partial response when folinic acid is combined with 5-FU; however, the effect on survival appears marginal and the optimal dose-schedule remains to be defined.

The value of postoperative chemotherapy and/or radiation therapy has been assessed in patients with stages B and C cancers as a means of eradicating clinically undetectable micrometastases and thereby increasing the probability for cure. The weight of evidence from more than 12 prospectively randomized trials in patients who have undergone the resection of a colon cancer suggests that the use of such prophylactic chemotherapy (i.e., including 5-FU given alone or in combination with other cytotoxic drugs) does not reduce the recurrence rate or prolong survival. However, the results of two clinical studies have indicated that the administration of adjuvant 5-FU with an anthelmintic agent, levamisole, to patients with stage C cancers, leads to a decrease in the likelihood of recurrence and a modest improvement in survival. The levamisole is thought to act in this therapeutic setting as a nonspecific immunomodulator. In contrast, in patients who have undergone the resection of a rectal cancer, data from controlled studies indicate that postoperative radiation therapy when combined with chemotherapy appears to reduce the likelihood of regional recurrences and increase the potential for cure. It has been postulated that the chemotherapy, believed to be ineffective when given prophylactically for patients with colon lesions, acts as a radiation sensitizer when given to individuals who have been operated upon for rectal cancer, thereby enhancing the biologic effect of the radiotherapy.

TUMORS OF THE SMALL INTESTINE

Small-bowel tumors comprise only 3 to 6 percent of gastrointestinal neoplasms. Because of their rarity, a correct diagnosis is often delayed. Abdominal symptoms are usually vague and poorly defined, and conventional radiographic studies of the upper and lower intestinal tract are often normal. Small-bowel tumors should be considered in the following situations: (1) recurrent, unexplained episodes of crampy abdominal pain; (2) intermittent bouts of intestinal obstruction, especially in the absence of inflammatory bowel disease or prior abdominal surgery; (3) intussusception in the adult; and (4) evidence of chronic intestinal bleeding in the presence of negative conventional radiographs. A careful small-bowel barium study is the diagnostic procedure of choice; the diagnostic accuracy may be improved by infusing barium through a nasogastric tube placed into the duodenum (enteroclysis).

BENIGN TUMORS In general, the histology of benign small-bowel tumors is difficult to predict on clinical and radiologic grounds alone. The symptomatology of benign tumors is not distinctive, with pain, obstruction, and hemorrhage being the most frequent symptoms. These tumors are usually discovered during the fifth and sixth decades of life, more often in the distal rather than the proximal small intestine. The most common benign tumors are adenomas, leiomyomas, lipomas, and angiomas.

Adenomas These tumors include those of the islet cells and Brunner's glands as well as polypoid adenomas. *Islet cell adenomas* are occasionally located outside the pancreas; the associated syndromes are discussed in Chap. 338. *Brunner's gland adenomas* are not truly neoplastic but represent a hypertrophy or hyperplasia of submucosal duodenal glands. These appear as small nodules in the duodenal mucosa that secrete a highly viscous alkaline mucus. Most often this is an incidental radiographic finding not associated with any specific clinical disorder.

Polypoid adenomas (See Table 257-2) Approximately 25 percent of benign small-bowel tumors are polypoid adenomas. They may present as single polypoid lesions or, less commonly, as papillary villous adenomas. As in the colon, the sessile or papillary form of the tumor is sometimes associated with a coexistent carcinoma. Occasionally, patients with Gardner's syndrome (a variant of polyposis coli) may develop premalignant adenomas in the small bowel; such lesions are generally in the duodenum. Multiple polypoid tumors may occur throughout the small bowel (and occasionally the stomach and colorectum) in the Peutz-Jeghers syndrome. The polyps are usually hamartomas (juvenile polyps) having a low potential for malignant degeneration. Mucocutaneous melanin deposits as well as tumors of the ovary, breast, pancreas, and endometrium are also associated with this autosomal dominant condition.

Leiomyomas These neoplasms arise from smooth-muscle components of the intestine and are usually intramural, affecting the overlying mucosa. Ulceration of the mucosa may cause gastrointestinal hemorrhage of varying severity. Cramping, intermittent abdominal pain is frequently encountered.

Lipomas These tumors occur with greatest frequency in the distal ileum and at the ileocecal valve. They have a characteristic radiolucent appearance, are usually intramural and asymptomatic, but may on occasion be associated with bleeding.

Angiomas While not true neoplasms, these lesions are important because they frequently cause intestinal bleeding. They may take the form of telangiectasia or hemangiomas. Multiple intestinal telangiectasia occur in a nonhereditary form confined to the gastrointestinal tract or as part of the hereditary Osler-Rendu-Weber syndrome. Vascular tumors may also take the form of isolated hemangiomas, most commonly in the jejunum. Angiography, especially during bleeding, is the procedure of choice in evaluating these lesions.

MALIGNANT TUMORS While infrequent in appearance, small-bowel malignancies occur in patients with long-standing regional enteritis and celiac sprue as well as in individuals with AIDS. In contrast to benign tumors, malignant tumors of the small bowel are frequently associated with fever, weight loss, anorexia, bleeding, and a palpable abdominal mass. After ampullary carcinomas (many of which arise from biliary or pancreatic ducts), the most frequently occurring small-bowel malignancies are adenocarcinomas, lymphomas, carcinoid tumors, and leiomyosarcomas.

Adenocarcinomas The most common primary cancers of the small bowel are adenocarcinomas, which account for about 50 percent of the malignant tumors. These neoplasms occur with highest frequency in the distal duodenum and proximal jejunum, where they tend to ulcerate and cause hemorrhage or obstruction. Radiologically, they may be confused with chronic duodenal ulcer disease or with Crohn's disease if the patient has long-standing regional enteritis. The diagnosis is best made by endoscopy and biopsy under direct vision. Surgical resection is the treatment of choice.

Lymphomas Lymphomatous involvement of the small bowel may be primary or secondary. A diagnosis of a primary intestinal lymphoma requires histologic confirmation of a lymphoproliferative neoplasm in a clinical setting in which palpable adenopathy and hepatosplenomegaly are absent and there is no evidence of lymphoma on a chest radiograph, CT scan, peripheral blood smear, or on bone marrow aspiration and biopsy. In general, symptoms referable to the small bowel are present, usually accompanied by an anatomically discernible lesion. Secondary lymphoma of the small bowel refers to involvement of the intestine by a lymphoid malignancy extending from involved retroperitoneal lymph nodes and hence is a manifestation of a generalized systemic neoplasm (see Chap. 317).

Primary intestinal lymphoma comprises 25 percent of malignancies of the small bowel. Essentially all these neoplasms are non-Hodgkin's lymphomas, most frequently having a diffuse, large-cell (i.e., "high-grade") histology. Intestinal lymphoma involves the ileum more frequently than the jejunum, which, in turn, is more commonly affected than the duodenum, a pattern which mirrors the relative amount of normal lymphoid cells in these anatomic areas. The risk of small-bowel lymphoma is increased in patients with a prior history of malabsorptive conditions (e.g., celiac sprue), regional enteritis, and depressed immunologic function due to congenital immunodeficiency syndromes, prior organ transplantation, autoimmune disorders, or AIDS.

The development of localized or nodular masses that narrow the lumen results in periumbilical pain (made worse by eating) as well as weight loss, vomiting, and occasional intestinal obstruction. The diagnosis of small-bowel lymphoma may be suspected by the appearance on contrast radiographs of patterns such as infiltration and thickening of mucosal folds, mucosal nodules, areas of irregular ulceration, or stasis of contrast material. The diagnosis can be confirmed by surgical exploration and resection of involved segments. Intestinal lymphoma may occasionally be diagnosed by peroral intestinal mucosal biopsy, but since the disease mainly involves the lamina propria, full-thickness surgical biopsies are usually required.

Resection of the tumor constitutes the initial treatment modality. While postoperative radiation therapy has been offered to some patients following such a total resection, most authorities favor short-term systemic treatment with combination chemotherapy. The frequent presence of widespread intraabdominal disease at the time of diagnosis and the occasional multicentricity of the tumor often make a total resection impossible. Combination chemotherapy would appear to be appropriate management for these patients as well. The probability of sustained remission or cure is approximately 75 percent in patients with localized disease, but 25 percent or less in individuals with unresectable lymphoma.

A unique form of small-bowel lymphoma, diffusely involving the entire intestine, was first described in oriental Jews and Arabs and is referred to as immunoproliferative small intestinal disease (IPSID), Mediterranean lymphoma, or alpha-heavy chain disease. The typical presentation includes chronic diarrhea and steatorrhea associated with vomiting and abdominal cramps; clubbing of the digits may be observed as well. A curious feature in many patients with IPSID is the presence in the blood and intestinal secretions of an abnormal IgA which contains a shortened alpha-heavy chain and is devoid of light chains. It is suspected that the abnormal alpha chains are produced by plasma cells infiltrating the small bowel. The clinical course of patients with IPSID is generally one of exacerbations and remissions, with death frequently resulting from either progressive malnutrition and wasting or the development of an aggressive lymphoma. Chemotherapy and radiation therapy have been ineffective.

Carcinoid tumors   Among the more common epithelial tumors of the small intestine are carcinoid tumors. They arise from argentaffin cells of the crypts of Lieberkühn and are found from the distal duodenum to the ascending colon, areas embryologically derived from the midgut. More than 50 percent of intestinal carcinoids are found in the distal ileum, with the majority congregating in close proximity to the ileocecal valve. Most intestinal carcinoids are asymptomatic and of low malignant potential, but invasion and metastases may occur, leading to the carcinoid syndrome (Chap. 276).

Leiomyosarcomas   Large, bulky tumors, leiomyosarcomas often are greater than 5 cm in diameter and may be palpable on abdominal examination. Bleeding, obstruction, and perforation are common.

CANCERS OF THE ANUS

Cancers of the anus account for 1 to 2 percent of the malignant tumors of the large bowel. The majority of such lesions arise in the anal canal which is defined as the anatomic area extending from the anorectal ring to a zone approximately halfway between the pectinate (or dentate) line and the anal verge. Carcinomas arising proximal to the pectinate line (i.e., in the transitional zone between the glandular mucosa of the rectum and the squamous epithelium of the distal anus) are known as basaloid, cuboidal, or cloacogenic tumors; approximately one-third of anal cancers have this histologic pattern. Malignancies arising distal to the pectinate line have a squamous cell histology, ulcerate more frequently, and represent approximately 55 percent of anal cancers. The prognosis for patients with basaloid and squamous cell cancers of the anus is identical when corrected for tumor size and the presence or absence of nodal spread.

Anal cancers occur most commonly in individuals with a prior history of chronic anal irritation. Such irritation may result from condylomata accuminata (i.e., viral lesions thought to be caused by papilloma virus infection), perianal fissures and/or fistulas, chronic hemorrhoids, and leukoplakia. The risk for anal cancer appears to be increased among homosexual males, presumably due to trauma related to anal intercourse. There presently are no data to indicate that anal cancers are AIDS-related tumors associated with direct infection by the human immunodeficiency virus. Anal cancers occur most commonly in middle-aged individuals, develop more frequently in women than men, and are most often associated with bleeding, pain, the sensation of a perianal mass, and perianal pruritus at the time of diagnosis.

Until recently, radical surgery (abdominal-perineal resection with lymph node sampling and a permanent colostomy) was the treatment of choice for this tumor type. The probability of survival 5 years following such a procedure ranged from 55 to 70 percent in the absence of spread to regional lymph nodes and decreased to less than 20 percent if nodal involvement was present. However, an alternative therapeutic approach combining external beam radiation with concomitant chemotherapy has resulted in biopsy-proven disappearance of all tumor in more than 80 percent of patients whose initial lesion was less than 3 cm in size. Tumor recurrences have occurred in less than 10 percent of these patients. Thus, it appears that approximately 70 percent of patients with anal cancers can be cured with nonoperative treatment and that disfiguring surgery should be reserved for the minority of individuals who are found to have residual tumor after being managed initially with radiation combined with chemotherapy.

REFERENCES

Colorectal cancer
Etiology and risk factors

AALTONEN LA et al: Clues to the pathogenesis of familial colorectal cancer. Science 260:812, 1993

BELL SM et al: Prognostic value of p53 overexpression and c-Ki *ras* gene mutations in colorectal cancer. Gastroenterology 104:57, 1993

COLLINS RH JR et al: Colon cancer, dysplasia, and surveillance in patients with ulcerative colitis. N Engl J Med 316:1654, 1987

EKBOM A et al: Increased risk of large-bowel cancer in Crohn's disease with colonic involvement. Lancet 336:357, 1990

————: Ulcerative colitis and colorectal cancer. A population-based study. N Engl J Med 323:1228, 1990

HAGGITT RC, REID BJ: Hereditary gastrointestinal polyposis syndromes. Am J Surg Path 10:871, 1986

HAMILTON SR: The molecular genetics of colorectal neoplasia. Gastroenterology 105:3, 1993

KINZLER KW et al: Identification of a gene located at chromosome 5q21 that is mutated in colorectal cancers. Science 251:1366, 1991

LIPKIN M, NEWMARK H: Effect of added dietary calcium on colonic epithelial cell proliferation in subjects at high risk for familial colonic cancer. N Engl J Med 313:1381, 1985

LYNCH HT et al: Hereditary colorectal cancer. Semin Oncol 18:337, 1991

NEUGUT AI et al: Dietary risk factors for the incidence and recurrence of colorectal adenomatous polyps. A case-control study. Ann Intern Med 118:91, 1993

TALAMONTI MS et al: Increase in activity and level of pp60^{c-src} in progressive stages of human colorectal cancer. J Clin Invest 91:53, 1993

THUN MJ et al: Aspirin use and reduced risk of fatal colon cancer. N Engl J Med 325:1593, 1991

VOGELSTEIN B et al: Genetic alterations during colorectal-tumor development. N Engl J Med 319:595, 1988

WANG L et al: Mutation in the *nm23* gene is associated with metastasis in colorectal cancer. Cancer Res 53:717, 1993

WILLETT WC et al: Relation of meat, fat, and fiber intake to the risk of colon cancer in a prospective study among women. N Engl J Med 323:1664, 1990

Polyps

CANNON-ALBRIGHT LA et al: Common inheritance of susceptibility to colonic adenomatous polyps and associated colorectal cancers. N Engl J Med 319:533, 1988

FENOGLIO-PREISER CM, HUTTER RVP: Colorectal polyps: Pathological diagnosis and clinical significance. Cancer 35:322, 1985

O'BRIEN MJ et al: the National Polyp Study. Patient and polyp characteristics associated with high-grade dysplasia in colorectal adenomas. Gastroenterology 98:371, 1990

Screening

AHLQUIST DA et al: Accuracy of fecal occult blood screening for colorectal neoplasia. A prospective study using hemoccult and hemoquant tests. JAMA 269:1262, 1993

ALLISON et al: Hemoccult screening in detecting colorectal neoplasm: sensitivity, specificity and predictive value. Ann Inter Med 112:328, 1990

DUDOUET B et al: Presence of villin tissue specific cytoskeletal protein in sera of patients and an initial clinical evaluation of its value for the diagnosis and follow-up of colorectal cancers. Cancer Res 50:438, 1990

KNIGHT KK et al: Occult blood screening for colorectal cancer. JAMA 261:586, 1989

MANDEL JS et al: Screening for fecal occult blood reduces mortality from colorectal cancer: Results from the Minnesota Colon Cancer Control Study. N Engl J Med, in press

NEUGUT AI, PITA S: Role of sigmoidoscopy in screening for colorectal cancer: A critical review. Gastroenterology 95:492, 1988

RANSOHOFF DF, LANG CA: Screening for colorectal cancer. N Engl J Med 325:37, 1991

RANSOHOFF DF, LANG CA: Sigmoidoscopic screening in the 1990's. JAMA 269:1278, 1993

SELBY JV et al: A case-control study of screening sigmoidoscopy and mortality from colorectal cancer. N Engl J Med 326:653, 1992

SIDRANSKY D et al: Identification of *ras* oncogene mutations in the stool of patients with curable colorectal tumors. Science 256:102, 1992

SIMON JB: Occult blood screening for colorectal carcinoma: A critical review. Gastroenterology 88:820, 1985

WINAWER SJ et al: Randomized comparison of surveillance intervals after colonoscopic removal of newly diagnosed adenomatous polyps. N Engl J Med 328:901, 1993

Clinical features

GASTROINTESTINAL TUMOR STUDY GROUP: Adjuvant therapy of colon cancer—results of a postoperatively randomized trial. N Engl J Med 310:737, 1984

KERN SE et al: Allelic loss in colorectal carcinoma. JAMA 261:3099, 1989

WANEBO JH et al: Preoperative carcinoembryonic antigen level as a prognostic indicator in colorectal cancer. N Engl J Med 229:448, 1978

WITZIG TE et al: DNA ploidy and cell kinetic measurements as predictors of recurrence and survival in stages B$_2$ and C colorectal adenocarcinoma. Cancer 68:879, 1991

Treatment

FUCHS CS, MAYER RJ: Adjuvant chemotherapy for colon and rectal cancer. Semin Rad Oncol 3:29, 1993

GASTROINTESTINAL TUMOR STUDY GROUP: Prolongation of the disease-free interval in surgically treated rectal carcinoma. N Engl J Med 312:1465, 1985

KROOK JE et al: Effective surgical adjuvant therapy for high risk rectal cancer. N Engl J Med 324:709, 1991

MAYER A et al: The prognostic significance of proliferating cell nuclear antigen, epidermal growth factor receptor and *mdr* gene expression in colorectal cancer. Cancer 71:2454, 1993

MAYER RJ: Chemotherapy for metastatic colorectal cancer. Cancer 70:1414, 1992

MOERTEL CG et al: Levamisole and fluorouracil for adjuvant therapy of resected colon carcinoma. N Engl J Med 322:352, 1990

NIH CONCENSUS CONFERENCE: Adjuvant therapy for patients with colon and rectal cancer. JAMA 264:1444, 1990

Tumors of the small intestine

HABER DA, MAYER RJ: Primary gastrointestinal lymphoma. Semin Oncol 15:154, 1988

SINDELAR WF: Cancer of the small intestine, in *Cancer: Principles and Practice of Oncology*, VT DeVita Jr et al (eds), 3d ed. Philadelphia, Lippincott, 1989, pp 875–894

Anal cancer

DALING JR et al: Sexual practices, sexually transmitted diseases, and the incidence of anal cancer. N Engl J Med 317:973, 1987

LEICHMAN L et al: Cancer of the anal canal: Model for preoperative adjuvant combined modality therapy. Am J Med 78:211, 1985

PALEFSKY JM et al: Anal intraepithelial neoplasia and anal papilloma virus infection among homosexual males with group IV HIV disease. JAMA 263:2911, 1990

SISCHY B et al: Definitive irradiation and chemotherapy for radiosensitization in management of anal carcinoma: Interim report in Radiation Therapy Oncology Group study no. 8314. J Natl Cancer Inst 81:850, 1989

258 ACUTE INTESTINAL OBSTRUCTION

WILLIAM SILEN

ETIOLOGY AND CLASSIFICATION Intestinal obstruction may be *mechanical* or *nonmechanical* (resulting from neuromuscular disturbances which produce either *adynamic* or *dynamic ileus*). The causes of mechanical obstruction of the lumen are conveniently divided into (1) lesions *extrinsic* to the intestine, e.g., adhesive bands, internal and external hernias, (2) lesions *intrinsic* to the wall of the intestine, e.g., diverticulitis, carcinoma, regional enteritis, and (3) obturation of the lumen, e.g., gallstone obstruction, intussusception. Clinically, however, it is most useful to consider whether the obstructive mechanism involves the small or large intestine, because the causes, symptoms, and treatments are different (see below). Adhesions and external hernias are the most common causes of obstruction of the small intestine, constituting 70 to 75 percent of cases of this type. Adhesions, however, almost never produce obstruction of the colon, whereas carcinoma, sigmoid diverticulitis, and volvulus, in that order, are the most common causes and together account for about 90 percent of the cases.

Adynamic ileus is probably the most common overall cause of obstruction. The development of this condition is mediated via the hormonal component of the sympathoadrenal system. Adynamic ileus may occur after any peritoneal insult, and its severity and duration will be dependent to some degree on the type of peritoneal injury. Hydrochloric acid, colonic contents, and pancreatic enzymes are among the most irritating substances, whereas blood and urine are less so. Adynamic ileus occurs to some degree after any abdominal operation; it usually lasts 2 to 3 days after most operative procedures. Retroperitoneal hematomas, particularly associated with vertebral fracture, commonly cause severe adynamic ileus, and the latter may occur with other retroperitoneal conditions, such as ureteral calculus or severe pyelonephritis. Thoracic diseases, including lower-lobe pneumonia, fractured ribs, and myocardial infarction, frequently produce adynamic ileus, as do electrolyte disturbances, particularly potassium depletion. Finally, intestinal ischemia, whether the result of vascular occlusion or intestinal distention itself, may perpetuate an adynamic ileus. *Spastic* or *dynamic ileus* is very uncommon and results from extreme and prolonged contraction of the intestine. It has been observed in heavy metal poisoning, uremia, porphyria, and extensive intestinal ulcerations. Primary intestinal pseudoobstruction (see Chap. 256) is a chronic motility disorder which frequently mimics mechanical obstruction. Unnecessary operations in such patients should be avoided.

PATHOPHYSIOLOGY Distention of the intestine is caused by the accumulation of gas and fluid proximal to and within the obstructed segment. Between 70 and 80 percent of intestinal gas consists of swallowed air, and because this is composed mainly of nitrogen, which is poorly absorbed from the intestinal lumen, removal of air by continuous gastric suction is a useful adjunct in the treatment of intestinal distention. The accumulation of fluid proximal to the obstructing mechanism results not only from ingested fluid, swallowed saliva, gastric juice, and biliary and pancreatic secretions but also from interference with normal sodium and water transport. During the first 12 to 24 h of obstruction, there is a marked depression of flux from lumen to blood of sodium and consequently water in the distended proximal intestine. After 24 h, there is movement of sodium and water into the lumen, contributing further to the distention and fluid losses. Intraluminal pressure rises from a normal of 2 to 4 cmH$_2$O to 8 to 10 cmH$_2$O. During peristalsis, when simple obstruction or a "closed loop" is present, pressures reach 30 to 60 cmH$_2$O. Closed-loop obstruction of the small intestine results when the lumen is occluded at two points by a single mechanism such as a hernial ring or adhesive band, thus producing a closed loop whose blood supply is often obstructed at the same time. Strangulation of the loop itself is thus common in association with marked distention proximal to the involved loop. A form of closed-loop obstruction is encountered when complete obstruction of the colon exists in the presence of a competent ileocecal valve (85 percent of individuals). Although the blood supply of the colon is not entrapped within the obstructing mechanism, distention of the cecum is extreme because of its greater diameter (LaPlace's law), and impairment of the intramural blood supply is considerable with consequent gangrene of the cecal wall, usually anteriorly. Necrosis of the small intestine may occur by the same mechanism of interference with intramural blood flow when distention is extreme, but this sequence is uncommon in the small intestine. Once impairment of blood supply occurs, bacterial invasion supervenes, and peritonitis develops. The systemic effects of extreme distention include elevation of the diaphragm with restricted ventilation and subsequent atelectasis. Venous return via the inferior vena cava also may be impaired.

The loss of fluids and electrolytes may be extreme and, unless replacement is prompt, leads to hemoconcentration, hypovolemia, renal insufficiency, shock, and death. Vomiting, accumulation of fluids within the lumen by the mechanisms described above, and the sequestration of fluid into the edematous intestinal wall and peritoneal cavity as a result of impairment of venous return from the intestine all contribute to massive loss of fluid and electrolytes, especially potassium. As soon as significant impedance to venous return is present, the intestine becomes severely congested, and blood begins to seep into the intestinal lumen. Blood loss may reach significant levels when long segments of intestine are involved.

SYMPTOMS   *Mechanical small-intestinal obstruction* is characterized by cramping midabdominal pain which tends to be more severe the higher the obstruction. The pain occurs in paroxysms, and the patient is relatively comfortable in the intervals between the pains. Audible borborygmi are often noted by the patient simultaneously with the paroxysms of pain. The pain may become less severe as distention progresses, probably because motility is impaired in the edematous intestine. When strangulation is present, the pain is usually more localized and may be steady and severe without a colicky component, a fact that often causes delay in diagnosis of obstruction. Vomiting is almost invariable, and it is earlier and more profuse the higher the obstruction. The vomitus initially contains bile and mucus and remains as such if the obstruction is high in the intestine. With low ileal obstruction, the vomitus becomes feculent, i.e., orange-brown in color with a foul odor, which results from the overgrowth of bacteria proximal to the obstruction. Singultus is common. Obstipation and failure to pass gas by rectum are invariably present when the obstruction is complete, although some stool and gas may be passed spontaneously or after an enema shortly after onset of the complete obstruction. Diarrhea is occasionally observed in partial obstruction. Blood in the stool is rare but does occur in cases of intussusception. Other than some minor but inconsistent differences in pain patterns noted above, the symptoms of strangulating obstructions cannot be distinguished from those of nonstrangulating obstructions.

Mechanical colonic obstruction produces colicky abdominal pain similar in quality to that of small-intestinal obstruction but of much lower intensity. Complaints of pain are occasionally absent in stoic elderly patients. Vomiting occurs late, if at all, particularly if the ileocecal valve is competent. Paradoxically, feculent vomitus is very rare. A history of recent alterations in bowel habits and blood in the stool is common because carcinoma and diverticulitis are the most frequent causes. Constipation becomes progressive, and obstipation with failure to pass gas ensues. Acute symptoms may develop over a period of a week. Cecal volvulus more closely resembles obstruction of the small intestine clinically, whereas patients with sigmoid volvulus more typically have the picture of colonic obstruction in which marked distention predominates, with relatively less pain.

In *adynamic ileus*, colicky pain is absent, and only discomfort from distention is evident. Vomiting may be frequent but is rarely profuse. It usually consists of gastric contents and bile and is almost never feculent. Complete obstipation may or may not occur. Singultus is common.

PHYSICAL FINDINGS   *Abdominal distention* is the hallmark of all forms of intestinal obstruction. It is least marked in cases of obstruction high in the small intestine and most marked in colonic obstruction. Early, especially in closed-loop strangulating small-bowel obstruction, distention may be barely perceptible or absent. Tenderness and rigidity are usually minimal; the temperature is rarely above 37.8°C (100°F) in nonstrangulating obstruction of the small and large intestine. Contrary to popular belief, the same is true of strangulating obstruction until very late, a fact that has often resulted in unfortunate delay in treatment. Signs and symptoms of shock also occur *very late* in strangulating obstruction. The appearance of shock, tenderness, rigidity, and fever often means that there has been contamination of the peritoneum with infected intestinal content. The presence of a palpable abdominal mass usually signifies a closed-loop strangulating small-bowel obstruction because the tense fluid-filled loop is the palpable lesion. Auscultation may reveal loud, high-pitched borborygmi coincident with the colicky pain, but this finding is often absent late in strangulating or nonstrangulating obstruction. A quiet abdomen does not eliminate the possibility of obstruction, nor does it necessarily establish the diagnosis of adynamic ileus.

LABORATORY AND X-RAY FINDINGS   Leukocytosis, with shift to the left, usually occurs when strangulation is present, but a normal white blood cell count does not exclude strangulation. Elevation of the serum amylase level is encountered occasionally in all forms of intestinal obstruction, especially the strangulating variety.

The x-ray is extremely valuable but under certain circumstances also may be misleading. In nonstrangulating complete small-bowel obstruction, x-rays are almost completely reliable. Distention of fluid- and gas-filled loops of small intestine usually arranged in a "stepladder" pattern with air-fluid levels and an absence or paucity of colonic gas are pathognomonic (Fig. 258-1). These findings, however, are absent in slightly over half the cases of strangulating small-bowel obstruction, especially early in the disease. A general haze due to peritoneal fluid and sometimes a "coffee bean"-shaped

FIGURE 258-1 Acute mechanical obstruction of small intestine (upright film). Note air-fluid levels, marked distention of bowel loops, and absence of colonic gas.

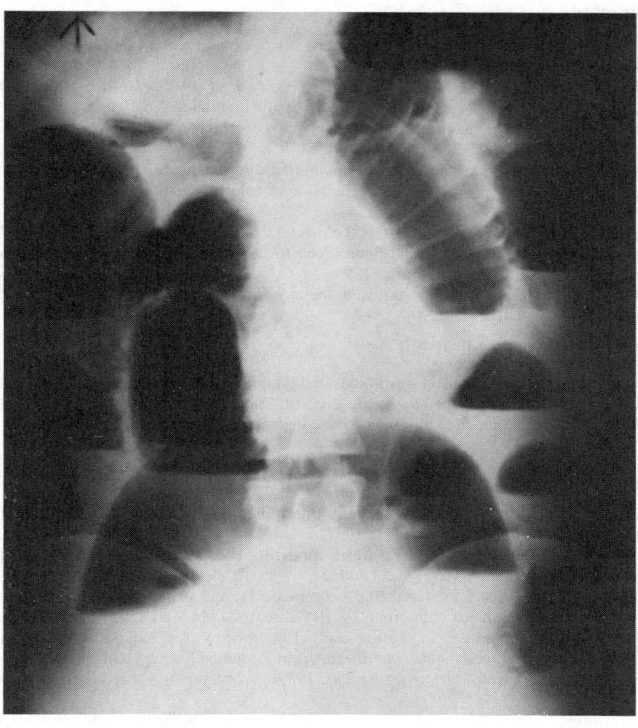

mass are seen in strangulating obstruction. Occasionally, the films are normal, but when symptoms are consistent with obstruction of the small intestine, a normal film should suggest strangulation. Roentgenographic differentiation of partial mechanical small-bowel obstruction from adynamic ileus may be impossible because gas is present in both the small and large intestines; however, colonic distention is usually more prominent in adynamic ileus. A radiopaque dye given by mouth is useful in making this distinction.

Colonic obstruction with a competent ileocecal valve is easily recognized because distention with gas is mainly confined to the colon. Barium enema, sigmoidoscopy, or colonoscopy, depending on the suspected site of obstruction, is usually advisable to determine the nature of the lesion, except when concomitant perforation is suspected, a rare occurrence. Sigmoidoscopy may be therapeutic in cases of sigmoid volvulus. When the ileocecal valve is incompetent, the films resemble those of partial small-bowel obstruction or adynamic ileus, and barium enema or colonoscopy is necessary to establish the correct diagnosis. Barium given by mouth is perfectly safe when obstruction is in the small intestine, since the barium sulfate does not become inspissated in this location. *Barium should never be given by mouth to a patient with possible colonic obstruction* until that possibility has been excluded by barium enema.

PROGNOSIS AND TREATMENT **Small-intestinal obstruction** The overall mortality rate for obstruction of the small intestine is about 10 percent, even under the most optimal conditions. While the mortality rate for nonstrangulating obstruction is as low as 5 to 8 percent, that for strangulating obstruction has been reported to be between 20 and 75 percent. Well over half the deaths from small-bowel obstruction occur in those with strangulation; however, the latter constitute only one-fourth to one-third of the cases. Careful studies indicate that the clinical, laboratory, and x-ray findings are not reliable in distinguishing strangulating from nonstrangulating obstruction when obstruction is complete. Complete obstruction is suggested when there has been a total cessation in the passage of gas or stool per rectum and when gas is absent in the distal intestine by x-ray. Since strangulating small-bowel obstruction is always complete, operation should always be undertaken in such patients after suitable preparation. Prior to operation, fluid and electrolyte balance should be restored and decompression instituted by means of a nasogastric tube. Replacement of potassium is especially important because intake is nil and losses in vomitus are large. Six to eight hours of preparation may be necessary. During this period, broad-spectrum antibiotics are indicated if strangulation is felt to be likely, but operation should not be delayed unless there is unequivocal clinical and roentgenographic evidence of resolution of the obstruction during the period of preparation. Attempts to pass a long tube into the small intestine usually fail while putting the patient through uncomfortable, unproductive manipulations which delay appropriate fluid replacement and decompression. *There are probably few, if any, indications for the use of a long intestinal tube.* Procrastination of operation because of improvement in well-being of the patient during resuscitation and gastric decompression usually leads to unnecessary and hazardous delay in proper treatment. Purely nonoperative therapy is safe only in the presence of incomplete obstruction and is best utilized in patients with (1) repeated episodes of partial obstruction, (2) recent postoperative partial obstruction, and (3) partial obstruction following a recent episode of diffuse peritonitis.

Colonic obstruction The mortality rate for colonic obstruction is about 20 percent. As in small-bowel obstruction, nonoperative treatment is contraindicated unless the obstruction is incomplete. Occasionally, but not always, when the obstruction is incomplete, nonoperative therapy may result in sufficient decompression that a definitive operative procedure can be undertaken at a later date. This usually can be accomplished by discontinuation of all oral intake and perhaps by nasogastric suction, although attempts to decompress a *completely* obstructed colon by intubation are almost invariably futile. A long intestinal tube will not decompress an obstructed colon with a competent ileocecal valve. When obstruction is complete, early

operation is mandatory, especially when the ileocecal valve is competent; cecal gangrene is likely if the cecal diameter exceeds 10 cm on plain abdominal film. For obstruction on the left side of the colon, the most common site, preliminary operative decompression by cecostomy or transverse colostomy followed by definitive resection of the primary lesion has been the treatment of choice. Recently, primary resection of obstructing left-sided lesions with on-table washout of the colon has been accomplished safely. For a lesion of the right or transverse colon, primary resection and anastomosis can be performed safely because distention of the ileum with consequent discrepancy in size and hazard in suture are not present.

Adynamic ileus This type of ileus usually responds to nonoperative continuous decompression and adequate treatment of the primary disease. The prognosis is usually good. Recently, successful decompression of severe colonic ileus has been accomplished by colonoscopy, but this should be avoided if tenderness in the right lower quadrant suggests possible cecal gangrene. Rarely, adynamic colonic distention may become so great that cecostomy is required if cecal gangrene is feared. Spastic ileus usually responds to treatment of the primary disease.

REFERENCES

BECKER WF: Acute adhesive ileus: A study of 412 cases with particular reference to the abuse of tube decompression in treatment. Surg Gynecol Obstet 95:472, 1952

BULKLEY GB et al: Intraoperative determination of small intestinal viability following ischemic injury: Prospective controlled trial of two adjuvant methods (Doppler and fluorescein) compared with standard clinical judgement. Ann Surg 193:628, 1981

COHN I, ATIK M: Strangulation obstruction: Closed loop studies. Ann Surg 153:94, 1961

DUBOIS A et al: Postoperative ileus: Physiopathology, etiology and treatment. Ann Surg 178:781, 1973

GOUGH IR: Strangulating adhesive small bowel radiographs. Br J Surg 65:431, 1978

HOFSETTER SR: Acute adhesive obstruction of the small intestine. Surg Gynecol Obstet 152:141, 1981

JACKSON BR: The diagnosis of colonic obstruction. Dis Colon Rectum 25:603, 1982

NOLAN DJ: Barium examination of the small intestine. Gut 22:682, 1981

SHIELDS R: The absorption and secretion of fluid and electrolytes by the obstructed bowel. Br J Surg 52:774, 1965

SILEN W: *Cope's Early Diagnosis of the Acute Abdomen,* 18th ed. London, Oxford, 1991

259 ACUTE APPENDICITIS

WILLIAM SILEN

INCIDENCE AND EPIDEMIOLOGY The maximum incidence of acute appendicitis occurs in the second and third decades of life. While the disease may be encountered at any time of life, it is relatively rare at the extremes of age. Males and females are equally affected, except between puberty and age 25, when males predominate in a 3:2 ratio. Perforation is relatively much more common in infancy and in the aged, during which periods mortality rates are highest. The mortality rate has decreased steadily in Europe and the United States from 8.1 per 100,000 of the population in 1941 to less than 1 per 100,000 in 1970 and subsequently. The absolute incidence of the disease also decreased by about 40 percent between 1940 and 1960 but since then has remained unchanged. Although various factors such as changing dietary habits, altered intestinal flora, and better nutrition and intake of vitamins have been suggested to explain the reduced incidence, the exact reasons have not been elucidated. The overall incidence of appendicitis is much lower in underdeveloped countries, especially parts of Africa, and in lower socioeconomic groups.

PATHOGENESIS The primary pathogenetic hallmark has always been thought to be luminal obstruction. While obstruction can be identified in 30 to 40 percent of cases, recent studies have shown that ulceration of the mucosa is the initial event in the majority. The causation of the ulceration is unknown, although a viral etiology has been postulated. Recently, it has been suggested that infection with *Yersinia* organisms may cause the disease, since high complement fixation titers have been found in as many as 30 percent of cases of proven appendicitis 1 week after operation. Whether the inflammatory reaction attendant with ulceration is sufficient to obstruct the tiny appendiceal lumen even transiently is not clear. Obstruction, when present, is most commonly caused by a fecalith, which results from accumulation and inspissation of fecal matter around vegetable fibers. Enlarged lymphoid follicles associated with viral infections (e.g., measles), inspissated barium, worms (e.g., pinworms, *Ascaris*, and *Taenia*), and tumors (e.g., carcinoid or carcinoma) also may obstruct the lumen. Secretion of mucus distends the organ, which has a capacity of only 0.1 to 0.2 mL, and luminal pressures rise as high as 60 cmH$_2$O. Luminal bacteria multiply and invade the appendiceal wall as venous engorgement and subsequent arterial compromise result from the high intraluminal pressures. Finally, gangrene and perforation occur. If the process evolves slowly, adjacent organs such as the terminal ileum, cecum, and omentum may wall off the appendiceal area so that a localized abscess will develop, whereas rapid progression of vascular impairment may cause perforation with free access to the peritoneal cavity. Subsequent rupture of primary appendiceal abscesses may produce fistulas between the appendix and bladder, small intestine, sigmoid, or cecum. Occasionally, acute appendicitis may be the first manifestation of Crohn's disease. While chronic infection of the appendix with tuberculosis, amebiasis, and actinomycosis may occur, a useful clinical aphorism states that *chronic appendiceal inflammation is not usually the cause of prolonged abdominal pain of weeks' or months' duration.* In contrast, it is clear that recurrent acute appendicitis does occur, often with complete resolution of inflammation and symptoms between attacks. Recurrent acute appendicitis may become more frequent as antibiotics are dispensed more freely.

CLINICAL MANIFESTATIONS The history and sequence of symptoms are among the most important diagnostic features of appendicitis. The initial symptom is almost invariably *abdominal pain* of the visceral type, resulting from appendiceal contractions or distention of the lumen. It is usually poorly localized in the periumbilical or epigastric region. There is often an accompanying urge to defecate or pass flatus, neither of which relieves the distress. This visceral pain is mild, often cramping, and rarely catastrophic in nature, usually lasting 4 to 6 h, but it may not be noted by stoic individuals or by some patients during sleep. As inflammation spreads to the parietal peritoneal surfaces, the pain becomes somatic, steady, and more severe, aggravated by motion or cough, and usually located in the *right lower quadrant*. *Anorexia* is so frequent that the presence of hunger should arouse serious suspicion of the diagnosis of acute appendicitis. *Nausea* and *vomiting* occur in 50 to 60 percent of cases, but vomiting is rarely profuse and protracted. The development of nausea and vomiting before the onset of pain is extremely rare. Change in bowel habit is of little diagnostic value, since any or no alteration may be observed, although the presence of diarrhea caused by an inflamed appendix in juxtaposition to the sigmoid may cause serious diagnostic difficulties. Urinary frequency and dysuria occur if the appendix lies adjacent to the bladder. The typical sequence of symptoms (poorly localized periumbilical pain followed by nausea and vomiting with subsequent shift of pain to the right lower quadrant) occurs in only 50 to 60 percent of patients, and some variations are considered below.

Physical findings vary with time after onset of the illness and according to the location of the appendix, which may be situated deep in the pelvic cul-de-sac, in the right lower quadrant in any relation to the peritoneum, cecum, and small intestine, in the right upper quadrant (especially during pregnancy), or even in the left lower quadrant. *The diagnosis cannot be established unless tenderness can be elicited.* While tenderness is sometimes absent in the early visceral stage of the disease, it ultimately always develops and is found in any location corresponding to the position of the appendix. Abdominal tenderness may be completely absent if a retrocecal or pelvic appendix is present, in which case the sole physical finding may be tenderness in the flank or on rectal or pelvic examination. Percussion, rebound tenderness, and referred rebound tenderness are often, but not invariably, present; they are most likely to be absent early in the illness. Flexion of the right hip and guarded movement by the patient are due to parietal peritoneal involvement. Hyperesthesia of the skin of the right lower quadrant and a positive psoas or obturator sign are often late findings and are rarely of diagnostic value. When the inflamed appendix is in close proximity to the anterior parietal peritoneum, muscular rigidity is present yet is often minimal early. The temperature is usually normal or slightly elevated [37.2 to 38°C (99 to 100.5°F)], but a temperature above 38.3°C (101°F) should always suggest the presence of perforation. Tachycardia is commensurate with the elevation of the temperature. Rigidity and tenderness become more marked as the disease progresses to perforation and localized or diffuse peritonitis. Distention is rare unless severe diffuse peritonitis has developed. The alleged disappearance of pain and tenderness just prior to perforation is extremely unusual. A mass may develop if localized perforation has occurred but usually will not be detectable before 3 days after onset of the disease. Earlier presence of a mass suggests carcinoma of the cecum or Crohn's disease. Perforation is rare before 24 h after onset of symptoms, but the rate may be as high as 80 percent after 48 h.

Laboratory examination does not establish the diagnosis because the latter is based primarily on clinical grounds. Although moderate leukocytosis of 10,000 to 18,000 cells per microliter is frequent (with a concomitant shift to immature cells), the absence of leukocytosis does not eliminate the possibility of acute appendicitis. Leukocytosis of greater than 20,000 cells per microliter should alert the clinician to the probability of perforation. Anemia and blood in the stool suggest a primary diagnosis of carcinoma of the cecum, especially in elderly individuals. The urine may contain a few white or red blood cells without bacteria if the appendix lies close to the right ureter or bladder.

Urinalysis is most useful, however, in excluding genitourinary conditions which may mimic acute appendicitis. X-rays are rarely of value except when an opaque fecalith (5 percent of patients) is observed in the right lower quadrant (especially in children) together with other clinical findings consistent with appendicitis. Consequently, there is no routine need to obtain films of the abdomen unless there is a possibility of other conditions such as intestinal obstruction or ureteral calculus. In some patients in whom symptoms are either recurrent or more prolonged, a careful barium enema may disclose an extrinsic defect on the medial wall of the cecum or a calcified fecalith. The diagnosis also may be established by the ultrasonic demonstration of an enlarged and thick-walled appendix, but if the appendix cannot be seen, the diagnosis cannot be excluded. Ultrasound is most useful to exclude ovarian cysts, ectopic pregnancy, or tuboovarian abscess.

While the typical historical sequence and physical findings are present in 50 to 60 percent of cases, it is obvious that a wide variety of atypical patterns of disease are encountered, especially at the age extremes and during pregnancy. The 70 to 80 percent incidence of perforation and generalized peritonitis in infants under 2 years of age is dramatic testimony to the importance of the history in the early detection of the disease. Any infant or child with diarrhea, vomiting, and abdominal pain is highly suspect. Fever is much more common in this age group, and abdominal distention is often the only physical finding. In the elderly, pain and tenderness are often obtunded, and thus the diagnosis is frequently delayed. A 30 percent incidence of perforation in patients over 70 attests to the importance of this delay. Elderly patients often present themselves initially with a slightly painful mass (a primary appendiceal abscess) or sometimes appear with adhesive intestinal obstruction 5 or 6 days after a previously undetected perforated appendix. Appendicitis occurs about once in every 1000 pregnancies and is the most common extrauterine condition requiring abdominal operation. The diagnosis may be missed or delayed because of the frequent occurrence of mild abdominal discomfort and nausea and vomiting during pregnancy. During the last trimester, when the mortality rate from appendicitis is highest, uterine displacement of the appendix to the right upper quadrant and laterally leads to confusion in diagnosis because pain and tenderness are similarly displaced.

DIFFERENTIAL DIAGNOSIS   A listing of the differential diagnoses of acute appendicitis would produce an encyclopedic compendium of all conditions which cause abdominal pain, since appendicitis may simulate any of these diseases. Diagnostic accuracy is about 75 to 80 percent for experienced clinicians and must be based solely on the clinical criteria outlined above. It is probably better to err slightly in the direction of overdiagnosis, since delay is associated with perforation and increased morbidity and mortality. In unperforated appendicitis, the mortality rate is 0.1 percent, little more than that associated with general anesthesia; for perforated appendicitis, there is an overall mortality of 3 percent, a figure that increases to 15 percent in the elderly. In doubtful cases, 4 to 6 h of observation is always more beneficial than harmful, however. The most common conditions discovered at operation when acute appendicitis is erroneously diagnosed are, in rough order of frequency, mesenteric lymphadenitis, no organic disease, acute pelvic inflammatory disease, ruptured graafian follicle or corpus luteum cyst, and acute gastroenteritis. In addition, acute cholecystitis, perforated ulcer, acute pancreatitis, acute diverticulitis, strangulating intestinal obstruction, ureteral calculus, and pyelonephritis frequently present diagnostic difficulties.

It is useful to consider separately some of the more common and difficult diagnostic possibilities, especially in the female. Differentiation of *pelvic inflammatory disease* from acute appendicitis may be virtually impossible. Gram-negative intracellular diplococci on cervical smear are not pathognomonic unless *Neisseria gonorrhoeae* can be cultured. Pain on movement of the cervix is not specific and may occur in appendicitis if perforation has occurred or if the appendix lies adjacent to the uterus or adnexa. *Rupture of a graafian follicle* (mittelschmerz) occurs at midcycle with spill of blood and fluid to produce pain and tenderness more diffuse and usually of a less severe degree than in appendicitis. Fever and leukocytosis are usually absent. *Rupture of a corpus luteum cyst* is identical clinically to rupture of a graafian follicle but develops about the time of menstruation. The presence of an adnexal mass, evidence of blood loss, and a positive pregnancy test help differentiate *ruptured tubal pregnancy*, but a negative pregnancy test is present when tubal abortion has occurred. *Twisted ovarian cyst* and *endometriosis* occasionally are difficult to distinguish from appendicitis. In all these female conditions, ultrasonic examination of the pelvis and laparoscopy may be of great value.

Acute mesenteric lymphadenitis is the appellation usually given when enlarged, slightly reddened lymph nodes at the root of the mesentery and a normal appendix are encountered at operation in a patient who usually has right lower quadrant tenderness and a somewhat higher temperature than most patients with acute appendicitis. Whether this is a single, discrete entity is unclear, since the causative factor is not known. It has been recognized recently that some of these patients have infection with *Yersinia pseudotuberculosis* or *Y. enterocolitica*, in which case the diagnosis can be established by culture of the mesenteric nodes or by serologic titers (see Chap. 123). The diagnosis is essentially impossible clinically, although retrospectively there often appears to have been more diffuse pain and tenderness. Children seem to be affected more frequently than adults. Operation should be undertaken unless there is rapid resolution of all symptoms and findings. *Acute gastroenteritis* usually causes profuse watery diarrhea, often with nausea and vomiting, but without localized findings. Between cramps, the abdomen is completely relaxed. In *Salmonella* gastroenteritis, the abdominal findings are similar, although the pain may be more severe and more localized, and fever and chills are common. The occurrence of similar symptoms among other members of the family may be helpful. When the diagnosis of acute pelvic appendicitis with perforation has been

missed, gastroenteritis is the most common previous working diagnosis. Persistent abdominal or rectal tenderness should eliminate the diagnosis of gastroenteritis. *Regional enteritis* (Crohn's disease) is usually associated with a more prolonged history, often with previous exacerbations regarded by the patient or physician as episodes of gastroenteritis unless the diagnosis has been established previously. *Meckel's diverticulitis* usually cannot be distinguished from acute appendicitis but is very rare.

TREATMENT   Cathartics and enemas should be avoided if appendicitis is under consideration, and antibiotics should not be administered when the diagnosis is in question, since they will only mask the presence or development of perforation. The treatment is early operation and appendectomy as soon as the patient can be prepared. Appendectomy has been successfully accomplished laparoscopically, but the exact role of this treatment, especially in cases of rupture, has not been clarified. Preparation rarely takes more than 1 to 2 h in early appendicitis but may require 6 to 8 h in cases of severe sepsis and dehydration associated with late perforation. The *only* circumstance in which operation is *not* indicated is the presence of a palpable mass 3 to 5 days after the onset of symptoms. Should operation be undertaken at that time, a phlegmon rather than a definitive abscess will be found, and complications from dissection of such a phlegmon are frequent. Such patients treated with broad-spectrum antibiotics, parenteral fluids, and rest usually show resolution of the mass and symptoms within 1 week. *Interval appendectomy* can and should be done safely 3 months later. Should the mass enlarge or the patient become more toxic, drainage of the abscess is necessary. The complications of subphrenic, pelvic, or other intraabdominal abscesses usually follow perforation with generalized peritonitis and can be avoided by early diagnosis of the disease.

REFERENCES

BOLTON JP: Assessment of the value of the white cell count in management of suspected acute appendicitis. Br J Surg 62:906, 1975

BUTLER C: Surgical pathology of acute appendicitis. Hum Pathol 12:870, 1981

GUERRANT RL, BOBAK DA: Bacterial and protozoal gastroenteritis. N Engl J Med 32:327, 1991

HOFFMAN J, RASMUSSEN OO: Aids in the diagnosis of acute appendicitis. Br J Surg 76:774, 1989

KOEPSELL TD et al: Factors affecting perforation in acute appendicitis. Surg Gynecol Obstet 153:508, 1981

PUVLAERT JBCM: A prospective study of ultrasonography in the diagnosis of appendicitis. N Engl J Med 317:666, 1987

RAVAL B et al: Use of computed tomography in appendicitis: Technique, findings, and pitfalls. J Comput Tomogr 11:17, 1987

SCHWERK WB et al: Ultrasonography in the diagnosis of acute appendicitis: A retrospective study. Gastroenterology 97:630, 1989

260 DISEASES OF THE PERITONEUM AND MESENTERY

KURT J. ISSELBACHER / J. THOMAS LaMONT

ACUTE PERITONITIS   Peritonitis is a localized or generalized inflammatory process of the peritoneum that may appear in both acute and chronic forms. In the acute form, the motor activity of the intestine is decreased, and the intestinal lumen becomes distended with gas and fluid. Fluid accumulates as a result of failure to reabsorb the 7 or 8 L normally secreted daily into the lumen and absorbed from the distal small bowel and colon. Because of accumulation of fluid in the peritoneal cavity as well as decreased oral intake, rapid depletion of the plasma volume with impaired cardiac and renal function may occur.

Etiology *Bacterial* peritonitis may be due to entry of bacteria into the peritoneal cavity from a perforation in the gastrointestinal tract or from an external penetrating wound. *Chemical* peritonitis results from spillage of pancreatic enzymes, gastric acid, or bile as a result of injury or perforation of the intestine or biliary tract. *Sterile* peritonitis occurs in patients with systemic lupus erythematosus, porphyria, and familial Mediterranean fever during attacks of their disease.

The most common causes of bacterial peritonitis are appendicitis, perforations associated with diverticulitis, peptic ulcer, gangrenous gallbladder, and gangrenous obstruction of the small bowel from adhesive bands, incarcerated hernia, or volvulus. Any lesion leading to the escape of intestinal bacteria may be a source, including a perforating carcinoma, foreign body, and ulcerative colitis. The peritoneal cavity is remarkably resistant to contamination, and unless continuing contamination occurs, the peritonitis remains localized. Patients with alcoholic cirrhosis and ascites have an increased susceptibility to *spontaneous* bacterial peritonitis, usually from enteric pathogens. This complication occurs in the absence of recognizable perforation of a viscus and may be due to leakage of bacteria through the intestinal wall (see Chap. 268).

Clinical features The cardinal manifestations of peritonitis are acute abdominal pain and tenderness. The location of the pain and tenderness depends on the underlying cause and whether the inflammation is localized or generalized. In *localized* peritonitis, as seen in uncomplicated appendicitis or diverticulitis, the physical findings are limited to the area of inflammation. With widespread peritoneal inflammation there is *generalized* peritonitis with diffuse abdominal tenderness and rebound. Rigidity of the abdominal wall is a common finding in peritonitis and may be localized or generalized.

Peristalsis may be present initially but usually disappears as the illness progresses and bowel sounds disappear. Hypotension, tachycardia, oliguria, and leukocytosis, with cell counts greater than 20,000 cells per microliter, are common, especially in generalized peritonitis. Plain abdominal films may reveal dilatation of the large and small bowel with edema of the small-bowel wall, as evidenced by the distance between adjacent loops of gas-filled small intestine. Diagnostic paracentesis is sometimes valuable in determining the nature of the exudate as well as whether bacteria can be demonstrated or cultured.

GONOCOCCAL PERITONITIS This usually involves an extension of gonococcal infection from a primary focus in the female reproductive tract. The signs of inflammation usually are limited to the pelvis, but there may be findings of a mild generalized peritonitis. Occasionally, the patient has right upper quadrant pain and tenderness caused by gonococcal perihepatitis involving the liver capsule and adjacent peritoneum (Fitz-Hugh–Curtis syndrome; see also Chap. 110).

STARCH PERITONITIS An acute granulomatous peritonitis can develop in some patients as a foreign-body reaction to cornstarch used to powder surgical gloves. The clinical picture is that of acute abdominal pain and fever 10 to 30 days after an abdominal operation. The diagnosis can be made by paracentesis and demonstration of starch granules in monocytes. However, most patients are reexplored because of the fear of abscess or bacterial peritonitis, with the finding of foreign-body granuloma studding the peritoneum.

PSEUDOMYXOMA PERITONEI This is a rare condition resulting from rupture of a mucocele of the appendix, a mucinous ovarian cyst, or mucin-secreting intestinal or ovarian adenocarcinoma. The abdomen becomes filled with masses of jelly-like mucus. Occasionally, with removal of the mucocele or the ovarian cyst and most of the myxomatous material, a cure may ensue. In other cases, however, the mucoid material recurs, leading to progressive wasting and eventual death. Colloid carcinoma arising from the stomach or colon with peritoneal implants may resemble pseudomyxoma at laparotomy. The course of this type of highly malignant tumor is one of rapid cachexia and early death. The diagnosis usually can be made by the appearance of many highly malignant cells in the peritoneal implants.

CANCER OF THE PERITONEUM Aside from mesothelioma, which in most patients is caused by previous exposure to asbestos, cancer of the peritoneum is usually secondary to a neoplasm within the abdomen, most commonly of the stomach and ovary. This type of metastatic malignancy is invariably associated with progressive ascites with a high specific gravity and high protein content, often with large numbers of red blood cells or even gross blood. The diagnosis is established by demonstrating malignant cells in the fluid. The clinical progress of this malignant spread can sometimes be arrested by installations of radioactive gold, nitrogen mustard, or chloroquine.

FAMILIAL MEDITERRANEAN FEVER See Chap. 293.

PNEUMATOSIS CYSTOIDES INTESTINALIS This is a condition in which multiple gas-filled blebs or cysts accumulate in the intestinal wall beneath the serosal surface of the bowel. The exact source of the gas has not been explained satisfactorily. In some instances, this disease is associated with specific ulceration of the intestinal mucosa, in particular peptic ulcer with outlet obstruction. Cysts in the wall of the small bowel are seen as an occasional complication of mesenteric vascular occlusion. In the large bowel, these cysts are usually benign, may be seen with a variety of other disorders, and usually disappear over time.

There are no specific physical findings secondary to the pneumatosis, and the diagnosis is made either by x-ray or at laparotomy. Occasionally, the subserosal cysts may rupture, resulting in pneumoperitoneum.

CHYLOUS ASCITES This term refers to the accumulation of chyle (intestinal lymph) in the peritoneal cavity. The condition is sometimes associated with chylothorax. The fluid in the peritoneal cavity appears milky or creamy because of the presence of chylomicrons. This fat may be demonstrated microscopically by staining with Sudan III and may be removed by acidification of the fluid followed by extraction with ether. The chyle (lipid) will then go into the ether phase. Many conditions may be associated with the cloudy or milky-appearing peritoneal fluid, so-called pseudochylous ascites. The milky or turbid appearance is usually due to the presence of protein and desquamated cells. The turbidity of this fluid will not be removed with the ether but will clear with addition of alkali.

The causes of chylous ascites include (1) penetrating or nonpenetrating trauma that damages the main duct in the lymphatic system within the abdomen, (2) intestinal obstruction if it is associated with rupture of a major lymphatic channel, (3) congenital lymphangiectasia, (4) malignant disease or tuberculous infection that obstructs the intestinal lymphatics, (5) filariasis, or (6) cirrhosis.

The sudden accumulation of chyle in the peritoneal cavity often results in abdominal pain, signs of peritoneal irritation, and leukocytosis. These symptoms gradually subside, leaving the patient with a distended but nontender, fluid-filled abdomen. Lymphangiography is of value in determining the location of the leak or site of obstruction to the lymphatic channels. The course depends upon the underlying etiologic factors.

MESENTERIC LIPODYSTROPHY This is a rare disorder usually affecting middle-aged women and characterized pathologically by infiltration of the mesentery with lipid-laden macrophages and fibrous tissue. These patients present with ill-defined abdominal pain and occasionally an abdominal mass. The diagnosis is made at laparotomy by demonstration of thick fibrofatty masses at the root of the mesentery with retraction and distortion of the bowel loops.

REFERENCES

KIPFER RE et al: Mesenteric lipodystrophy. Ann Intern Med 80:582, 1974
LIMBER GK et al: Pseudomyxoma peritonei. Ann Surg 1978:587, 1973
PRESS OW et al: Evaluation and management of chylous ascites. Ann Intern Med 96:358, 1982
SCHWARTZ SI et al: *Principles of Surgery*, 5th ed. New York, McGraw-Hill, 1989
TITO L et al: Spontaneous bacterial peritonitis. Hepatology 8:27, 1988
WARSHAW AL: Diagnosis of starch peritonitis by paracentesis. Lancet 2:1054, 1972
YAMADA T et al (eds): *Textbook of Gastroenterology*. Philadelphia, Lippincott, 1991

section 2 Liver and biliary tract disease

261	**APPROACH TO THE PATIENT WITH LIVER DISEASE**

KURT J. ISSELBACHER / DANIEL K. PODOLSKY

BIOLOGIC CONSIDERATIONS An understanding of diseases of the liver and their clinical manifestations can be derived from a knowledge of fundamental normal hepatic structure and function. An appreciation of anatomic aspects of the liver and biliary tree from the gross level to that of the individual hepatocyte and other cellular constituents is needed to understand the spectrum of clinical manifestations of liver disease. The dual blood supply, unique to the liver and including the portal venous system, makes the liver an intermediate filter for most of the venous drainage of the abdominal viscera. This often leads to secondary hepatic involvement in a number of extrahepatic diseases and makes the liver a relatively common site of solid tumor metastases. Furthermore, an appreciation of the relevant anatomy, especially that of the portal venous system, is important in understanding clinically important manifestations of portal hypertension, a common complication of chronic liver disease when scarring and regeneration lead to distortion of the intrahepatic microvasculature. These anatomic considerations lead the clinician to look for evidence of splenic enlargement and hypersplenism, gastrointestinal bleeding, accumulation of ascites, and signs of portal-systemic encephalopathy. Certainly an understanding of the anatomy of the biliary tract from canaliculus to common bile duct is integral to understanding the basis and sequelae of obstructive jaundice. While inflammation of the gallbladder may lead to fever and pain, choledocholithiasis will cause biliary colic as well as jaundice. Diffuse processes affecting the intrahepatic ducts, such as primary sclerosing cholangitis, will lead to cholestasis and its attendant symptoms, while a focal process affecting a single branch of the biliary tree, such as a neoplasm, usually will not.

The structural organization at a level intermediate between the gross anatomic and the cellular also contributes to the clinical patterns seen with disorders of the liver. While various concepts have been offered, the most useful is that of the traditional liver lobule. Blood emanates from the portal venules at the periphery and passes through the hepatic sinusoids to the central vein. The portal venules, terminal bile ductules, and hepatic arterioles are arranged in a *triad*. Appreciation of this organization and the presence of concentric zones of function within the lobule explain distinct patterns of injury such as the centrilobular injury resulting from ischemia. These structural features no doubt also provide the basis for the relative preservation of hepatocellular function in many disorders that can lead to significant portal hypertension, such as schistosomiasis and biliary cirrhosis.

As important as the anatomic features are in understanding liver disease, many liver disorders and their manifestations can only be appreciated in the context of the functional complexity of the liver at the cellular level. As detailed in Chap. 264, the hepatocyte plays an important role in diverse general metabolic processes that may be deranged as a consequence of liver disease. In addition, this metabolic diversity leads to hepatic involvement in many inborn errors of metabolism, including a wide variety of storage diseases, and less well-understood disorders of iron metabolism (hemosiderosis and hemochromatosis) and copper homeostasis (Wilson's disease).

Some other functional aspects also should be emphasized. The hepatocyte modifies numerous endogenous (e.g., bilirubin) and exogenous (e.g., alcohol, acetaminophen) potentially toxic compounds through oxidation, reduction, and conjugation carried out by several enzymes of the endoplasmic reticulum. Conjugation of substrates generally facilitates their hepatic excretion, converting water-insoluble substances to water-soluble derivatives. It is therefore not surprising that parenchymal liver disease may lead to either conjugated or unconjugated hyperbilirubinemia and jaundice. Metabolic modifications may significantly alter the pharmacologic activity of drugs through formation of derivatives with either decreased or enhanced activity. These metabolic processes may create intermediates which are toxic to the liver itself. This explains the selective susceptibility of the liver to the toxicity of carbon tetrachloride, acetaminophen, and, most important, alcohol, which is converted to acetaldehyde.

Additional functions of the hepatocyte that may have significant clinical ramifications include the production of a variety of soluble proteins for secretion into the circulation and the presence of receptors specific for various circulating ligands. The latter is a property shared with the Kupffer cell, which fulfills much of its function as a constituent of the reticuloendothelial system by clearing a number of serum glycoproteins through asialoglycoprotein receptor–mediated endocytosis. There is evidence to suggest that some of the substances taken up by this endocytotic mechanism may subsequently pass to and through the hepatocyte to complete an enterohepatic circulation. Carcinoembryonic antigen (CEA) is a glycoprotein and tumor-associated marker which is handled in this manner, leading to artifactual elevations in hepatobiliary disease. In contrast to the Kupffer cell, the spectrum of ligands taken up by hepatocytes via specific receptors is much broader. In addition to ligands targeted for lysosomal degradation, the hepatocyte possesses receptors for ligands which are metabolically active after their uptake and dissociation from their receptors. These include transferrin-bound iron and, most important, low-density lipoprotein (LDL), which contributes to regulation of overall body cholesterol metabolism. Disruption of lysosomal degradation of specific ligands in hereditary storage disease leads to hepatomegaly and a variety of infiltrative disorders. Disruption of the nonlysosomal endocytotic pathway ligands can lead to systemic disorders. It is not clear whether specific receptors or other hepatocyte membrane components play a role in the relative or absolute tropism of infectious agents (particularly the hepatitis viruses) which account for a large proportion of both acute and chronic liver disease. However, the relative selectivity of the hepatitis viruses (A, B, C, E, and indirectly D) for the hepatocyte is essential in understanding the clinical features of the illnesses caused by these agents, which derive from the extent of hepatocyte destruction, largely due to immune destruction rather than direct cytopathic effects of the virus. At the same time, the hepatocyte may be infected by less strictly organotropic agents including other viruses (e.g., Epstein-Barr virus) and a wide variety of bacterial and parasitic organisms. The vascular supply of the liver leads to its frequent involvement in disseminated infections.

A final feature of hepatocyte cell biology that contributes to the expression of liver disease is the potential for proliferation and regeneration. Although few mitotic figures are seen in normal hepatic parenchyma, rapid regeneration involving both proliferation and cellular hypertrophy occurs following hepatic resection in experimental animals and humans. The capacity for hepatocellular regeneration is evident in the complete recovery which usually occurs following fulminant hepatitis (due either to viral or toxic agents) if the patient can be sustained through the period of acute injury. Architecturally disordered regeneration in concert with fibrosis is an essential factor in the development of cirrhosis and leads both to disruption of blood flow through the hepatic parenchyma and to uneven hepatocellular function due to distortion of normal lobular structure. Although the mechanisms which control hepatocyte proliferation after hepatocellular loss are incompletely understood, evidence suggests that a complex balance of various peptide growth factors plays an important role.

CLINICAL CONSIDERATIONS In approaching the patient with known or suspected liver disease, consideration of the patient's problem in the context of a few salient questions permits the clinician to focus on the most important diagnostic possibilities and the severity of the illness. Is the problem primarily hepatocellular or cholestatic? Was the onset of the illness abrupt or gradual? Has the problem led to clinically significant impairment of normal hepatocellular function, such as signs of altered mentation or coagulopathy? Are there signs or symptoms of portal hypertension? Important and reliable clues which address these questions often may be obtained from a careful history and physical examination.

Clinical history A number of historic features may distinguish cholestatic and hepatocellular disease processes. A history of marked right upper quadrant pain or previous indigestion suggests cholelithiasis, cholecystitis, or choledocholithiasis, whereas vague, nagging discomfort suggests hepatocellular or infiltrative disease with hepatomegaly causing pain due to distention of Glisson's capsule. Additional important symptoms which should be elicited include pruritus, jaundice, anorexia, weight loss, and fever. Complaints of easy bruising or mental confusion by the patient (or family) should be regarded as ominous signs of either fulminant acute or advanced chronic liver disease.

Family history is important with respect to jaundice, anemia, splenectomy, or cholecystectomy; a positive history may be helpful in diagnosing hemolytic anemia, congenital or familial hyperbilirubinemia, or gallstones. In Wilson's disease (hepatolenticular degeneration), there may be a family history of tremor or neurologic abnormalities. *Occupation* should be reviewed in detail, and *environmental factors* need to be examined. Note should be made of the use of any medications or exposure to known or putative toxins such as carbon tetrachloride, beryllium, or vinyl chloride. The patient should be asked about travel to other countries, especially to areas where hepatitis may be endemic. Careful questioning regarding alcohol intake is important in most cases. Since the alcoholic often denies or understates the amounts consumed, it may be desirable to check the validity of the history with relatives or close friends.

Contact with jaundiced patients (especially intimate or sexual relations) should be noted. If the patient has had any *injections*, hepatitis B or C infection may be the underlying disease. Injections include blood tests, blood or plasma transfusions, tattooing, and dental treatment. Postoperative jaundice may be due to the anesthetic, especially after multiple uses of halothane, or to impaired hepatic excretory function resulting from relative hypoxemia of liver cells during the operative or postoperative period.

As suggested, the *onset of the illness* should be noted. The relatively abrupt onset of nausea, anorexia, and aversion to smoking followed by progressive jaundice suggests viral hepatitis. A gradual development of jaundice associated with pruritus suggests cholestasis. Intermittent right upper quadrant abdominal pain followed by cholestatic jaundice points to gallstone disease, while the gradual onset of painless jaundice with weight loss is suggestive of tumor, such as carcinoma of the head of the pancreas. Jaundice associated with fever and chills makes cholangitis and extrahepatic biliary obstruction likely possibilities. The awareness of progressive abdominal swelling,

perhaps first noticed because of tightness of clothing, suggests ascites, which may be due to malignancy or an insidious first manifestation of cirrhosis. The patient with hepatitis generally feels ill, and dark urine and light stools occur before the appearance of scleral or skin icterus. In cholestatic hepatitis, the patient may feel relatively well and complain only of symptoms due to the obstruction, such as pruritus.

Physical examination Jaundice is looked for in the sclera as well as the skin. Pallor indicative of anemia may be a reflection of hemolysis, cirrhosis, or neoplasm. Significant cachexia, especially of the extremities, may be associated with cancer or cirrhosis. In the cirrhotic patient, one should look for stigmas of alcohol abuse such as parotid and lacrimal gland enlargement and Dupuytren's contracture, as well as other features of cirrhosis, such as gynecomastia, testicular atrophy, and diminished axillary or pubic hair.

The *skin examination* may reveal ecchymoses due to prothrombin deficiency or purpura due to thrombocytopenia. *Palmar erythema* or *spider angiomas* may reflect acute or chronic liver disease. Spider angiomas are usually found above the umbilicus and especially on the face, neck, shoulders, forearms, and dorsum of the hands. The presence of a few spider angiomas is not abnormal in women, especially during pregnancy. However, their appearance in men is always abnormal and should be carefully searched for. In chronic cholestasis, *scratch marks, finger clubbing*, and *xanthoma* of the eyelids and extensor surfaces of the tendons of the wrists and ankles may be found. A *slate color* to the skin due to increased iron or bronze discoloration resulting from melanin deposition should suggest the presence of hemochromatosis.

Evaluation of the *mental state* and *neurologic function* is important. Slight deterioration of the intellect and minimal personality changes may suggest hepatocellular disease or the presence of portal-systemic venous shunts, but care must be taken to exclude other causes such as neurologic disease. The presence of flapping tremor of the hands (asterixis) may be found in association with portal-systemic encephalopathy or impending hepatic coma.

Abdominal examination may reveal ascites, which, together with dilated periumbilical veins, suggests cirrhosis and extensive portal collateral circulation. If additional features of liver disease are lacking, malignancy must be considered more seriously. A very large, nodular, and rock-hard liver suggests the presence of hepatoma or hepatic metastases. Careful percussion is necessary to evaluate the size of a nonpalpable liver. A small liver may indicate cirrhosis (especially postnecrotic); a small liver which diminishes in size suggests severe hepatitis or massive hepatic necrosis. In the alcoholic, fatty infiltration and cirrhosis often produce a uniform enlargement of the liver. The liver edge is tender in hepatitis, in congestive heart failure, and occasionally in malignant disease and with alcoholism (especially "alcoholic hepatitis").

A palpable, enlarged gallbladder (Courvoisier's sign) suggests extrahepatic biliary obstruction, often due to pancreatic cancer. A tender gallbladder and positive Murphy's sign suggest cholelithiasis or choledocholithiasis. A palpable spleen may indicate hepatitis or cirrhosis; significant splenomegaly may be a reflection of portal hypertension.

Abdominal auscultation may reveal the presence of a venous hum over dilated collateral veins radiating from the umbilicus, the so-called caput medusae. In advanced cirrhosis this venous hum is virtually diagnostic of significant portal hypertension. A bruit may sometimes be heard over large regenerating nodules in cirrhosis and occasionally over hepatomas and metastatic nodules in the liver. A friction rub occasionally may be heard over hepatomas and metastatic liver nodules.

Serum assays for biochemical markers of liver disease are an integral part of the proper evaluation of liver and biliary tract disease. In general, the serum bilirubin level is measured to confirm the presence and severity of jaundice and determine the extent of bilirubin conjugation. Aminotransferase (transaminase) elevations reflect the severity of active hepatocellular damage, though not necessarily the

TABLE 261-1 Classification of liver disease

PARENCHYMAL

I Hepatitis (viral, drug-induced, toxic, ischemic)
   A Acute
   B Chronic (persistent or active)
II Cirrhosis
   A Alcoholic (portal, nutritional, Laennec's cirrhosis)
   B Postnecrotic
   C Biliary
   D Hemochromatosis
   E Rare types (e.g., Wilson's disease, galactosemia, cystic fibrosis of pancreas, alpha$_1$-antitrypsin deficiency)
III Infiltrations
   A Glycogen
   B Fat (neutral fat, cholesterol, gangliosides, cerebrosides)
   C Amyloid
   D Lymphoma, leukemia
   E Granuloma (e.g., sarcoidosis, tuberculosis, idiopathic)
IV Space-occupying lesions
   A Hepatoma, metastatic tumor
   B Abscess (pyogenic, amoebic)
   C Cysts (polycystic disease, *Echinococcus*)
   D Gummas
V Functional disorders associated with jaundice
   A Gilbert's syndrome
   B Crigler-Najjar syndrome
   C Dubin-Johnson and Rotor syndromes
   D Cholestasis of pregnancy and benign recurrent cholestasis

HEPATOBILIARY

I Extrahepatic biliary obstruction (by stone, stricture, or tumor)
II Cholangitis (septic, primary biliary cirrhosis, primary sclerosing cholangitis, drug, toxic)

VASCULAR

I Chronic passive congestion and cardiac cirrhosis
II Hepatic vein thrombosis (Budd-Chiari syndrome)
III Portal vein thrombosis
IV Pylephlebitis
V Arteriovenous malformations
VI Venocclusive disease

aggregate severity of liver injury (e.g., transaminase levels may actually decline with near-complete hepatic parenchymal destruction), while alkaline phosphatase elevations are found with cholestasis and hepatic infiltrates. Serum albumin level and the prothrombin time are used as indexes of hepatic synthetic function. These and other tests are reviewed in Chaps. 42 and 263.

The further evaluation of patients with hepatobiliary disease should be individualized depending on the history, physical findings, and initial screening laboratory tests. Hepatocellular disease such as hepatitis is often sufficiently clear that only serologic tests are needed. Nonetheless, in many patients, computed tomography (CT), ultrasound, scintiscans, magnetic resonance imaging (MRI), or liver biopsy may be needed to determine the nature of the liver disease. When hepatic tumors are suspected, CT, ultrasound, MRI, or scintiscan may be performed followed by liver biopsy or laparoscopy for a more specific diagnosis. When biliary obstruction is suspected, the first examination is usually an ultrasound study to determine the size of the bile ducts, whether gallstones are present, or whether there is the suggestion of a mass in the head of the pancreas. Frequently, more information is needed, and thus a cholangiogram, performed through the endoscope or through percutaneous puncture under ultrasound or CT guidance, should be obtained.

CLASSIFICATION OF LIVER DISEASE No single classification of the various types of liver disease is entirely satisfactory because in many instances the etiology and pathogenetic mechanism are obscure. As a consequence, one finds an abundance of labels and names applied to hepatic disorders. Some individuals use the term *hepatitis* to imply viral infection; others, simply to connote evidence of hepatic inflammation. The often used words *acute, subacute,* and

chronic are ambiguous. *Chronicity* should refer to continuing or recurrent disease (i.e., duration). *Activity* should refer to evidence of the presence of perpetuation of liver cell injury; this is most readily identified by serum transaminase elevations and by the degree of hepatocellular necrosis on biopsy.

Because of the difficulties involved in defining the etiology of many types of liver disease, in most instances the process is best defined and described by an examination of the morphologic character of the lesion. Therefore, a *morphologic classification* of liver disease, as outlined in Table 261-1, appears at present more practical than one based on etiology.

REFERENCES

Millward-Sadler GH et al: *Wright's Liver and Biliary Disease*, 3d ed. London, Saunders, 1992

Sherlock S, Dooley J: *Diseases of the Liver and Biliary System*, 9th ed., Oxford, Blackwell, 1993

Zakim D, Boyer TD: *Hepatology: A Textbook of Liver Disease*, 2d ed. Philadelphia, Saunders, 1990

262 HEPATOBILIARY IMAGING

LAWRENCE S. FRIEDMAN / LAURENCE NEEDLEMAN

Selection of appropriate imaging techniques for the liver and biliary tract in a given patient depends on the particular clinical problem and on an understanding of the uses and limitations of each technique; in many situations, two or more imaging methods may provide complementary and useful information. In determining the optimal studies, communication between the clinician and the radiologist is essential.

PLAIN ABDOMINAL RADIOGRAPHS AND BARIUM STUDIES OF THE GASTROINTESTINAL TRACT Standard plain films of the abdomen provide little diagnostic information about the hepatobiliary system. They may permit a rough estimation of hepatic size and detection of splenic enlargement or gross ascites. Their major value is in demonstrating *calcified lesions*, including gallstones (about 15 percent are radiopaque) and intrahepatic lesions such as echinococcal cysts, calcified granulomas due to previous tuberculosis or histoplasmosis, or, rarely, tumors or vascular lesions. Plain abdominal x-rays may also demonstrate *air in the biliary tract*, as may occur after endoscopic papillotomy or with a biliary-enteric fistula, either surgical or as a result of inflammation or erosion of a stone from the gallbladder into the intestine. Emphysematous cholecystitis is associated with air in the wall of the gallbladder as a result of severe inflammation. Air seen in a branching pattern extending to the periphery of the liver is usually within portal venous branches and associated with serious inflammatory processes in the intestine.

A barium swallow may demonstrate large esophageal varices in patients with portal hypertension, but the sensitivity is only about 50 percent and endoscopy is more sensitive for the detection of varices.

ULTRASONOGRAPHY Ultrasonography has the advantages of relatively low cost, portability, and safety, as ionizing radiation is not required. Ultrasound imaging depends on small differences in the acoustic properties of soft tissue. Short pulses (1 μs) of high-frequency sound (3 to 10 million Hz) are transmitted into the patient; at each interface between tissues of different acoustic properties, a small portion of the energy is reflected back to the transducer, which also acts as a receiver. With *B-mode*, or *gray-scale*, ultrasound scanning, ultrasound reflections are displayed as shades of gray; cross-sectional, transverse, longitudinal, or oblique images of organs can be produced depending on the orientation of the transducer. With *real-time* ultrasonography, scanning is so rapid that a continuously changing ("real time") image is displayed, thus permitting a survey of the abdominal anatomy in a short period of time and demonstration of physiologic tissue movements, such as arterial pulsations. The major limitation of ultrasonography is its inability to penetrate bone or air, including bowel gas, which may limit complete examination of abdominal organs. In general, tissue penetration of ultrasound decreases as resolution increases.

Ultrasonography is the preferred initial method for imaging the gallbladder and biliary tree (Fig. 262-1). It is sensitive and specific (>95 percent) for the detection of *cholelithiasis*, and, unlike oral cholecystography, is not limited by the presence of jaundice or dye allergy in the patient. Ultrasonography is also highly sensitive for detecting a *dilated biliary tract* in patients with cholestasis and may indicate whether the site of obstruction is in the intra- or extrahepatic ducts. The cause of biliary obstruction, such as a mass lesion in the head of the pancreas or porta hepatis, may also be detected by ultrasonography, although the area around the distal common bile duct may be obscured by bowel gas.

Ultrasonography is also a primary screening examination for hepatic disease, which may be suspected because of symptoms, hepatomegaly, abnormal liver function tests, jaundice, or the suspicion of a mass lesion (Fig. 262-2). In general, *focal hepatic lesions* are better visualized than diffuse parenchymal disease such as fatty liver, hepatitis, or cirrhosis. Hepatic masses as small as 1 cm may be detected, and cystic lesions or abscesses can be distinguished from solid lesions, although the nature of a solid hepatic mass (adenoma, hepatocellular carcinoma, metastasis, hemangioma, etc.) may not be identified. Nevertheless, a specific diagnosis may be facilitated by percutaneous "thin"-needle biopsy of hepatic lesions under ultrasound guidance, and insertion of a catheter under ultrasound guidance may permit nonoperative drainage of an abscess. Other uses of ultrasonography include detection of ascites when the physical examination is equivocal, demonstration of portal vein thrombosis in patients with bleeding gastroesophageal varices, and evaluation of patency of portosystemic shunts in patients with recurrent variceal bleeding after shunt surgery. Ultrasonography is usually the first

FIGURE 262-1   Sonogram showing dilated bile ducts due to pancreatic carcinoma. The diameter of the extrahepatic bile ducts is 1.2 cm measured anterior to the portal vein (between asterisks). The site of maximal dilatation is 2.0 cm in the distal common bile duct (between arrows).

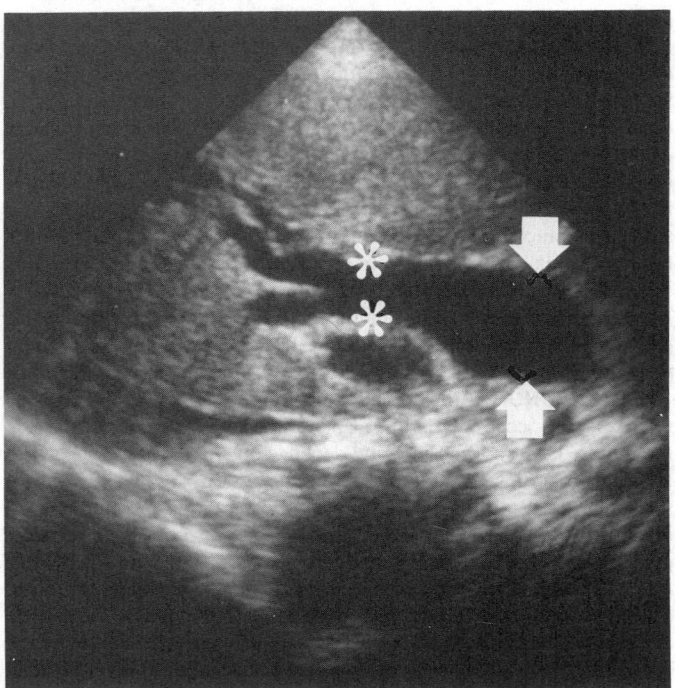

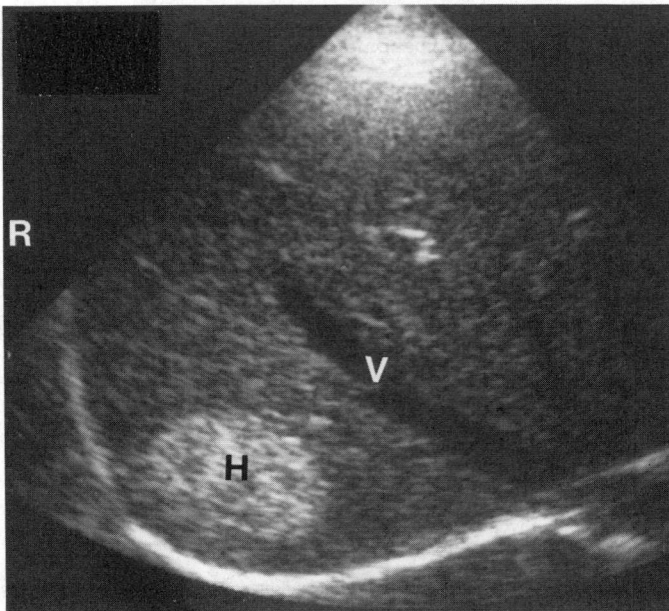

FIGURE 262-2   Sonogram showing an echogenic mass which represents a hemangioma (H) in the posterior right lobe of the liver lateral to the right hepatic vein (V). R = right side of the patient.

imaging study performed in patients with hepatic dysfunction after liver transplantation to look for a biliary leak or vascular occlusion.

Doppler ultrasonography, which may be enhanced by color imaging, allows detection of the presence and direction of blood flow based on changes in the frequency of back-scattered ultrasound waves caused by the movement of blood and is useful in detecting vascular occlusions, such as portal or hepatic vein occlusion. *Intraoperative ultrasonography* involves the application of the ultrasound transducer to the exposed liver at surgery, thereby increasing the sensitivity of detecting occult hepatic metastases. *Endosonography* involves the attachment of an ultrasound transducer to the tip of an endoscope to permit ultrasonographic imaging from within the bowel lumen, thereby minimizing the obscuring effects of bowel gas. Compared to conventional imaging techniques, endosonography permits more precise determination of the depth of tumor invasion through the bowel wall and improved detection of gastroesophageal varices and early pancreatic lesions, especially pancreatic islet cell tumors.

COMPUTED TOMOGRAPHY   Because computed tomographic (CT) scans can detect very small differences in the attenuation of x-rays, structures not visible on conventional radiographs can be identified. With current CT scanning techniques, the radiation dose received by the patient is similar to that of diagnostic procedures such as barium enema. The identification of anatomic structures can be facilitated by the administration of an oral contrast agent to define the bowel lumen and an intravenous contrast agent to enhance blood vessels and tissues. In general, anatomic definition is more complete with CT scanning than with ultrasonography, and CT scanning has the additional advantage that obesity and intestinal gas do not reduce the quality of the examination. However, a paucity of fat in malnourished patients or children may limit the resolution of the CT image. The disadvantages of CT scanning are radiation exposure and cost. In many instances, CT scanning is reserved for patients in whom ultrasonography is technically difficult or inconclusive.

CT scanning before and after intravenous administration of a contrast agent is an excellent method of evaluating *hepatic masses*. Cystic lesions are readily identified, and abscesses can usually be distinguished from tumors (Fig. 262-3). Masses as small as 1 cm can usually be identified by CT scanning, and, as with ultrasonography, the lesions can be biopsied under CT guidance. Intravenous administra-

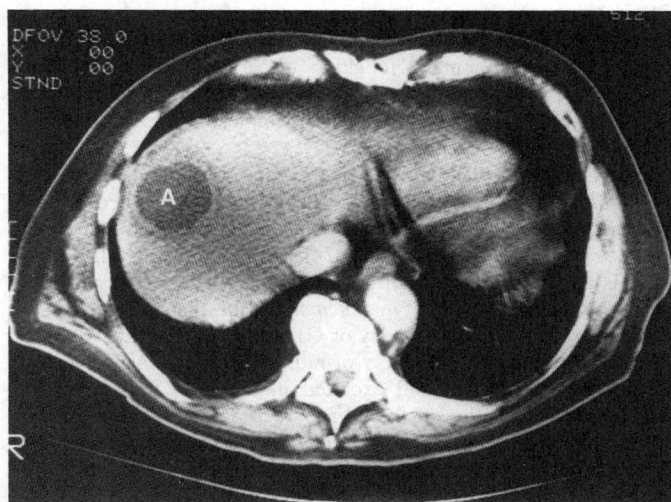

FIGURE 262-3 CT scan with contrast showing a low attenuation mass (A) in the dome of the liver, which represents an amebic abscess. R = right side of the patient.

tion of a contrast agent may result in enhancement of a primary or secondary tumor relative to the surrounding liver, and certain lesions, such as a cavernous hemangioma, may show a pattern of enhancement that is characteristic enough to confirm the diagnosis. Invasion of blood vessels by tumor may also be demonstrated in this way. *CT portography*, in which CT scanning follows injection of contrast into an angiographic catheter placed directly into the superior mesenteric artery, further enhances the sensitivity of detecting mass lesions in the liver. CT scanning has had an increasing role in the evaluation of diffuse liver disease, such as cirrhosis, which may be suggested by shrinkage and nodularity of the liver and associated portosystemic collaterals. Characteristic CT findings may also be associated with *fatty infiltration* of the liver, in which the density of the liver is significantly reduced (Fig. 262-4), and *hemochromatosis* or *secondary iron overload*, in which the density of the liver is increased and an estimate of hepatic iron concentration may be made.

Although CT scanning is nearly as accurate as ultrasonography in detecting cholelithiasis or dilated bile ducts, ultrasonography is usually the preferred initial test because of its availability, lack of risk,

and lower cost. However, CT scanning is more accurate than ultrasonography in identifying the level and cause of biliary obstruction. CT scanning may also be used to define the extent of carcinoma of the gallbladder or pancreas.

MAGNETIC RESONANCE IMAGING Magnetic resonance imaging (MRI) detects the density of protons in tissue water and lipids and their relaxation times. Because hydrogen nuclei (protons) have an odd number of particles, they behave like magnets when placed in a strong magnetic field. In MRI, protons aligned in a magnetic field are subjected to a brief pulse of weak radio waves, the frequency of which (termed the *resonant frequency*) is related mathematically to the externally applied magnetic field. The pulse of radio waves causes the protons to change their direction of spin and alignment. After the radio wave pulse, the protons return to their original orientation and emit energy with the same radio frequency as that absorbed. Imaging may be accomplished by the detection and analysis of proton density, the T1 relaxation time (a measure of the rate at which the nuclei realign themselves in the magnetic field), or the T2 relaxation time (a measure of the rate at which the emitted radio frequency energy decays). Each method produces a slightly different type of image. The choice of imaging technique depends on the contrast resolution needed for a particular organ. In general, because the magnetic environments of protons in fat, intracellular water, and extracellular water differ, MRI provides sharp contrast differentiation of tissues containing varying amounts of water or fat. MRI is also an excellent method of detecting blood flow.

In addition to excellent contrast resolution between normal and abnormal tissues, advantages of MRI include the lack of ionizing radiation and the ability to image in transverse, longitudinal, coronal, or even oblique planes. Its disadvantages include cost, slow imaging time that results in blurred images due to respiration and peristalsis, and limitations imposed by a strong magnetic field, such as the inability to study patients with pacemakers and other metallic devices.

The range of applications of MRI and its role relative to other imaging modalities are continually evolving. MRI of *mass lesions* of the liver appears to have greater sensitivity than CT scanning; however, like CT scanning, MRI cannot reliably distinguish primary from metastatic tumors (Fig. 262-5). Hepatic abscesses can be detected readily, although on occasion it may be difficult to distinguish abscesses from tumors with necrotic centers. MRI is the technique of choice in the detection of hemangiomas, which have an appearance sufficiently characteristic to permit differentiation from hepatic malignancy. Whereas its value in diffuse parenchymal liver disease such

FIGURE 262-4 CT scan showing fatty infiltration of the liver. Note that the attenuation of the liver is lower than that of the spleen (S). The more highly attenuated linear structures of the liver (arrows) are the intrahepatic vessels. St = stomach filled with orally administered barium contrast agent.

FIGURE 262-5 Magnetic resonance (MR) image of the liver showing three hepatic metastases (arrows) with higher signal than the surrounding liver. R = right side of the patient, K = kidney.

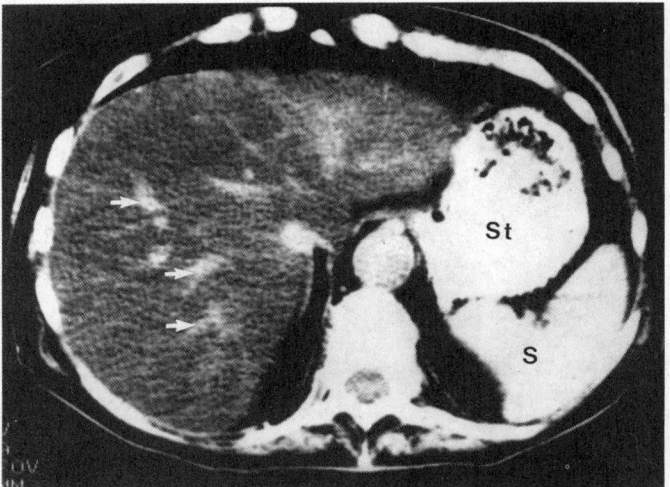

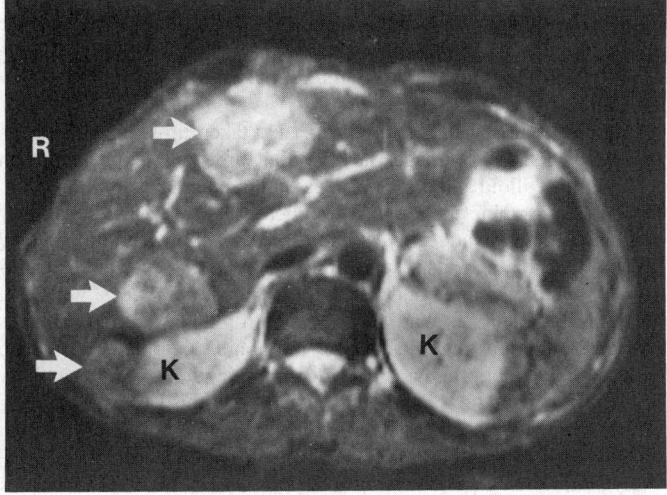

as hepatitis or cirrhosis is still under investigation, MRI can distinguish a regenerating nodule in a cirrhotic liver from a tumor. MRI can also serve as a useful noninvasive method for the diagnosis and monitoring of iron and copper deposition in hemochromatosis, secondary iron overload, or Wilson's disease. A modification of MRI *(proton spectroscopic imaging)*, in which the image of fat is subtracted from the image of water, can identify fatty liver and may be used to quantify hepatic fat content. Because rapidly flowing blood is often signal-free on MRI, blood vessels can be distinguished without the need for a contrast agent in most cases; thus, MRI may be useful in assessing the surgical resectability of vascular tumors or detecting hepatic vein occlusion (Budd-Chiari syndrome).

The gallbladder and bile ducts can be demonstrated by MRI, and cholelithiasis and cholecystitis can be detected; however, MRI currently offers no advantages over other imaging techniques. Although gallstones in the common bile duct are not detected by MRI, other causes of bile duct obstruction, such as pancreatitis or pancreatic carcinoma, may be identified.

Currently, MRI is based on hydrogen, which is the most abundant nucleus in the body and very sensitive to MR. *MR spectroscopy* also permits imaging based on other isotopes, such as phosphorus 31, with the ability to permit study of the metabolic state of normal and diseased organs.

RADIOISOTOPE SCANNING　A variety of radioisotopes can be used to study the anatomy and function of the liver and biliary system. After injection into a peripheral vein, the radioisotope is extracted by the liver and excreted in the bile. A scintillation (gamma) camera produces an image by detecting the radiation emitted during the decay of the radioisotope. Depending on the information desired, radioisotopes can be chosen that are taken up by hepatic parenchymal cells, Kupffer cells, or neoplastic and inflammatory cells or that are rapidly excreted in bile. Many previously available radioisotopes such as ^{198}gold or ^{75}selenomethionine are no longer in use. Because radioisotope scanning of the liver seldom provides a precise diagnosis, it has largely been replaced by ultrasonography and CT scanning for first-line imaging. However, radioisotope scanning of the biliary tract is an important tool in the investigation of acute cholecystitis.

Technetium 99m–labeled sulfur colloid scanning　The most commonly used radiopharmaceutical for anatomic evaluation of the liver is ^{99m}Tc-labeled sulfur colloid, which is taken up by reticuloendothelial (Kupffer) cells in the liver. Such scanning can be used to assess the size and shape of the liver. Any disease process that results in replacement of Kupffer cells, including *primary and metastatic tumors*, *cysts*, and *abscesses*, produces a "cold" area in the hepatic scintigram. Lesions greater than 2 to 3 cm in diameter can be reliably detected. Because of impaired blood flow and reticuloendothelial function, *diffuse hepatic disease*, such as hepatitis and cirrhosis, may result in decreased or patchy uptake of radiocolloid with preferential uptake by the bone marrow and spleen, particularly when portal hypertension is present. Occasionally, the irregular uptake of radiocolloid in cirrhosis results in the falsely positive appearance of hepatic filling defects. *Obstruction of the hepatic veins* (Budd-Chiari syndrome) may result in preferential uptake of radiocolloid by the caudate lobe of the liver.

Indium (^{111}In)-labeled colloids are also taken up by Kupffer cells and may be used to image the liver but are more expensive than ^{99m}Tc-sulfur colloid and expose the patient to a greater radiation dose. Newer scintigraphic techniques designed to improve the sensitivity of liver imaging include *single photon emission computed tomography* (SPECT), which permits visualization of the cross-sectional distribution of a radioisotope, and *positron emission tomography* (PET), which utilizes isotopes that decay by positron emission and provides information about regional blood flow and alterations in tissue metabolism. Scintigraphy following the injection of radioactively labeled antibody to tumor antigens has shown promise in distinguishing benign from malignant liver masses.

Gallium scanning　^{67}Gallium citrate accumulates in tissues actively synthesizing protein and is taken up by *tumors and abscesses*.

On scanning, the lesion appears as an area of increased activity, or "hot spot." Imaging with this agent may be useful in detecting hepatocellular carcinomas, Hodgkin's disease, some non-Hodgkin's lymphomas, and melanomas, although nonspecific uptake of gallium by the liver, bone marrow, and gastrointestinal tract limits the reliability of gallium scanning.

Tagged blood cell scanning　Intravenous injection of *autologous white blood cells* labeled with ^{111}In increases the specificity of radioisotope scanning for the detection of hepatic (and abdominal) *abscesses*. Similarly, *autologous red blood cells* or circulating proteins such as albumin or transferrin labeled with ^{111}In or ^{99m}Tc provide a sensitive method of identifying *hemangiomas* that are detected as mass lesions by ultrasonography or CT scanning (Fig. 262-6).

Biliary scanning　A variety of radiopharmaceuticals are rapidly cleared by hepatocytes and excreted in the bile, thus permitting scintigraphic evaluation of the biliary tract. The first agent used for this purpose was ^{131}I-rose bengal, which, because of its high radiation dose, has been replaced by agents that can be labeled with ^{99m}Tc. The most widely used agents are *N*-substituted iminoacetic acids (HIDA, PIPIDA, DISIDA), which concentrate in the bile even when serum bilirubin levels are elevated. Biliary scanning is used most often in evaluating patients with suspected *acute cholecystitis*, in whom visualization of the gallbladder excludes obstruction of the cystic duct and hence acute cholecystitis (Fig. 262-7). Persistent nonvisualization of the gallbladder over several hours with normal visualization of the liver, bile ducts, and intestine indicates a diagnosis of acute cholecystitis with 95 percent accuracy. False-positive results may occur in patients receiving parenteral nutrition or narcotics and those with hepatitis. Biliary scanning is less accurate in patients with chronic cholecystitis, in whom delayed visualization of the gallbladder is frequent. However, biliary scanning may be useful in identifying *cholestasis, acute and chronic biliary obstruction, bile leaks, biliary-enteric fistulas*, and *choledochal cysts*.

ORAL CHOLECYSTOGRAPHY　Although the use of oral cholecystography declined markedly with the advent of ultrasonography, the recent development of nonsurgical approaches to the treatment of cholelithiasis (e.g., extracorporeal shock wave lithotripsy and oral dissolution therapy with chenodeoxycholic or ursodeoxycholic acid) has led to a resurgence of interest in oral cholecystography. The test is simple and inexpensive. It involves radiographic assessment of gallbladder opacification 14 to 16 h after oral administration of iopanoic acid or 10 to 12 h after oral administration of sodium tyropanoate, both of which are concentrated in the gallbladder after intestinal absorption and hepatic excretion. A second dose of dye may need to be administered to as many as 15 to 25 percent of

FIGURE 262-6　^{99m}Tc-labeled autologous red blood cell scan of the hemangioma shown in Fig. 262-2. S = spleen, K = kidney.

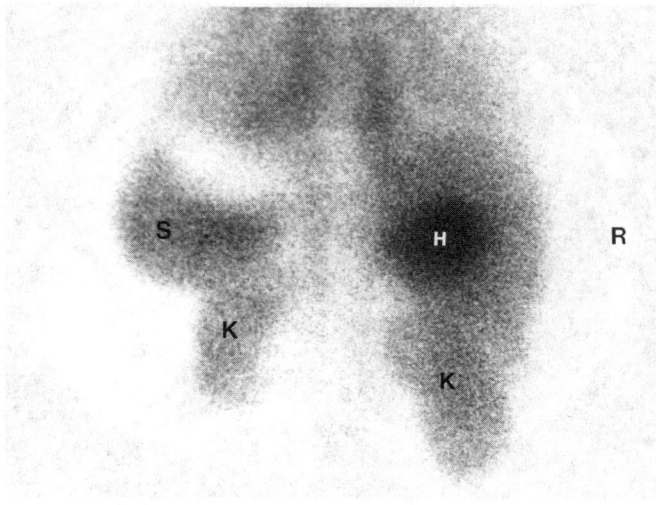

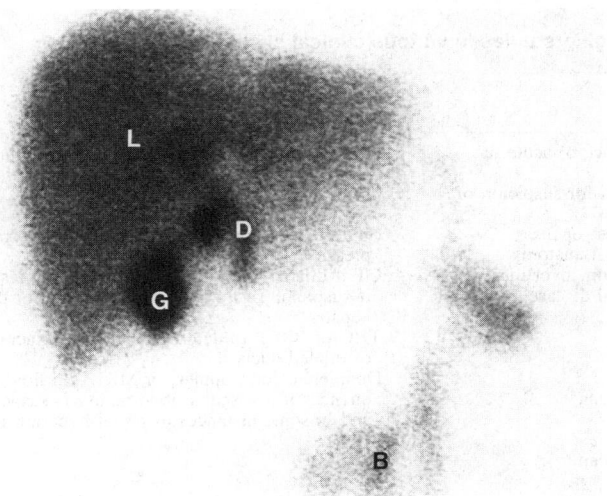

A

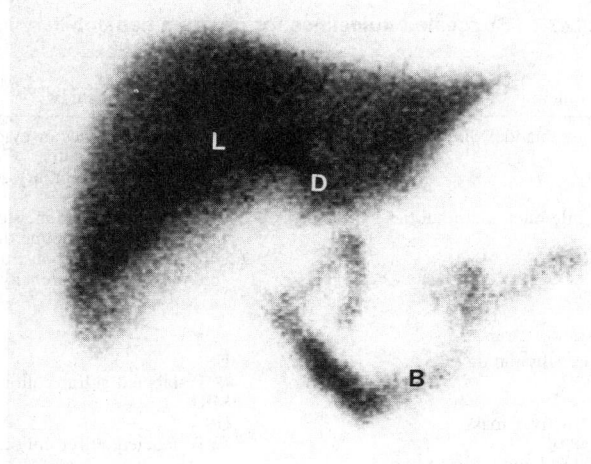

B

FIGURE 262-7 *A*. Hepatobiliary scan using ^{99m}Tc-DISIDA in a normal person showing uptake in the liver (L), gallbladder (G), bile ducts (D), and bowel (B) with patency of the cystic duct and biliary system. *B*. Abnormal hepatobiliary scan showing radioisotope in the liver (L), bile ducts (D), and bowel (B) but not in the gallbladder. This is due to an obstructed cystic duct (with a patent common bile duct) due to acute cholecystitis.

persons in whom gallbladder opacification is not achieved after a single dose.

Nonvisualization of the gallbladder indicates *gallbladder disease* with nearly 95 percent certainty, whereas normal visualization excludes gallbladder disease with 97 percent certainty. Failure of the gallbladder to opacify may also result from patient noncompliance, intestinal malabsorption, and liver disease; the gallbladder will not visualize when the serum direct bilirubin level is greater than 34 μmol/L (2 mg/dL). Oral cholecystography is as sensitive as ultrasonography in the overall detection of gallbladder disease (stones, polyps, adenomyomatosis, cholesterolosis, cholecystitis), although ultrasonography is more sensitive in detecting stones per se. However, oral cholecystography is more accurate in determining the *number and size of stones* and, unlike ultrasonography, can demonstrate *cystic duct patency*, factors that are important in determining a patient's suitability for nonoperative gallstone therapy.

CHOLANGIOGRAPHY In the past, *intravenous cholangiography*, in which contrast dye is administered as a bolus by peripheral vein, was the principal radiographic technique to visualize the bile ducts. Because of a high rate of serious reactions to the dye, the lack of bile duct visualization when the serum bilirubin level was above 42 μmol/L (2.5 mg/dL), and the development of more effective radiologic techniques to visualize the bile ducts, intravenous cholangiography has become obsolete.

Percutaneous transhepatic cholangiography (THC) This technique involves the direct percutaneous injection, via a "thin" (22-gauge) needle, of contrast dye into bile ducts in the liver under fluoroscopic guidance. When intrahepatic ducts are dilated, the success rate of duct opacification approaches 100 percent, but when the intrahepatic ducts are not dilated, as in primary sclerosing cholangitis, the success rate is around 90 percent and multiple attempts may be required. Serious complications occur in no more than 3 percent of cases and include hemorrhage, bile peritonitis, and sepsis.

THC may be used to determine the cause of *biliary obstruction* or *cholestasis* and is of particular value in evaluating the potential surgical resectability of proximal cholangiocarcinomas. In addition, biliary biopsies and cytologic brushings may be obtained and strictures may be balloon-dilated via a catheter inserted through the THC tract. In patients with biliary obstruction who are poor operative risks, an external drain may be left in place to permit biliary decompression or an internal stent (endoprosthesis) may be placed to relieve obstruction.

Endoscopic retrograde cholangiopancreatography (ERCP) (See Chap. 250) This technique uses fiberoptic endoscopy to visualize the ampulla of Vater and guide the insertion of a catheter through the ampulla for the selective injection of contrast material into the common bile and pancreatic ducts, which are then imaged radiologically (see Chap. 250). The success rate for cannulation depends on the experience of the endoscopist and can approach 95 percent or more; unlike THC, successful biliary cannulation does not depend on a dilated bile duct. Serious complications may occur in about 5 percent of cases and include pancreatitis and cholangitis.

Using THC, ERCP, or both, the biliary system can be visualized in nearly all patients. ERCP is preferable when the bile ducts are not dilated and when an *ampullary*, *pancreatic*, or *distal bile duct lesion* is suspected. In patients with *choledocholithiasis*, ERCP permits sphincterotomy and stone extraction. Additionally, ERCP may permit ampullary biopsy, pancreatic or biliary ductal brushings for cytologic examination, balloon dilation of a stricture, placement of a nasobiliary drain to decompress an obstructed biliary system, and insertion of a stent to relieve biliary obstruction caused by tumors. ERCP can also be used for *manometric measurements of the sphincter of Oddi*, a potentially valuable technique in the diagnosis of papillary stenosis and ampullary spasm.

ANGIOGRAPHY Angiography is required less often now than in the past for evaluating the hepatobiliary system. Nevertheless, newer contrast agents, improved techniques of vascular catheterization, and the development of therapeutic applications make angiography of value in certain situations. Selective cannulation of the hepatic artery or one of its branches may be helpful in distinguishing certain *vascular lesions* of the liver, including hemangiomas, adenomas, focal nodular hyperplasia, hemangioendotheliomas, and hepatocellular carcinomas (Fig. 262-8). Angiography may be particularly valuable in assessing the *surgical resectability* of an isolated hepatic lesion or in identifying a vascular occlusion after liver transplantation. In planning portosystemic shunt surgery, angiography is an excellent imaging technique to define portal venous anatomy and assess the patency of the vessels to be used. The portal venous system may be examined on the venous phase of celiac and superior mesenteric arteriography or after direct injection of contrast into the portal venous system via a splenic or transhepatic route. Hepatic venography and hemodynamic measurements, including wedged hepatic venous pressures, can be obtained concurrently (see Chap. 268). Therapeutic applications of angiography include *embolization* of bleeding vessels, arteriovenous fistulas, or certain highly vascular or inoperable tumors, and nonsurgical creation of a *portosystemic shunt* via a transjugular approach (transjugular intrahepatic portosystemic shunt, or TIPS).

Although no algorithm for hepatobiliary imaging tests will satisfy

TABLE 262-1   Suggested guidelines for ordering hepatobiliary imaging studies in various clinical situations

Clinical problem	Initial imaging study	Supplemental imaging studies (if necessary)
Suspected gallbladder disease	US to detect stones or evidence of acute or chronic cholecystitis	OCG to assess gallbladder function and number of stones
	Nuclear medicine biliary scan for suspicion of acute cholecystitis	CT if abscess suspected
Suspected bile duct abnormalities	US to detect dilatation, stones, or mass	CT to detect stones or cause of extrinsic compression
	THC or ERCP to define ductal anatomy	
Jaundice	US to detect biliary obstruction, liver masses, or obvious hepatic parenchymal disease	CT if dilated ducts to detect obstructing lesion or if suspicion of a mass in the pancreas or porta hepatis
		THC or ERCP to determine site and exact cause of dilated ducts
Hepatic parenchymal disease	US	Doppler, color Doppler, or MRI with flow sequences if a vascular abnormality is suspected and in some instances of portal hypertension
	^{99m}Tc-labeled sulfur colloid scan	
	MRI	
Screening for liver mass	US	MRI
	^{99m}Tc-labeled sulfur colloid scan	
Characterizing known liver mass		
Suspicion of malignancy	US- or CT-directed biopsy	CT portogram
		MRI
		Intraoperative US
Suspicion of benign lesion (hemangioma, regenerative nodule, focal nodular hyperplasia, adenoma)	MRI (after detection on US or CT)	Angiography
	Nuclear medicine scan (e.g., ^{99m}Tc-labeled red blood cell scan for suspected hemangioma)	US- or CT-directed biopsy
Suspicion of abscess	US or CT	Nuclear medicine abscess scan (gallium or ^{111}In-labeled white blood cell scan)
	US- or CT-directed aspiration	

NOTE: US, ultrasound; OCG, oral cholecystogram; CT, computed tomography; THC, transhepatic cholangiography; ERCP, endoscopic retrograde cholangiopancreatography; MRI, magnetic resonance imaging; Tc, technetium; In, indium.

all clinical scenarios, broad guidelines for the sequential use of these tests are offered in Table 262-1. In general, techniques that are less invasive and less expensive should be considered before those that are more invasive and more expensive, but the choice of specific tests may depend as well on availability and local expertise.

FIGURE 262-8   Arterial phase of a selective hepatic angiogram showing a hepatocellular carcinoma as a hypervascular mass (outlined by arrows) with many irregular and corkscrew-shaped tumor vessels in the right lobe of the liver.

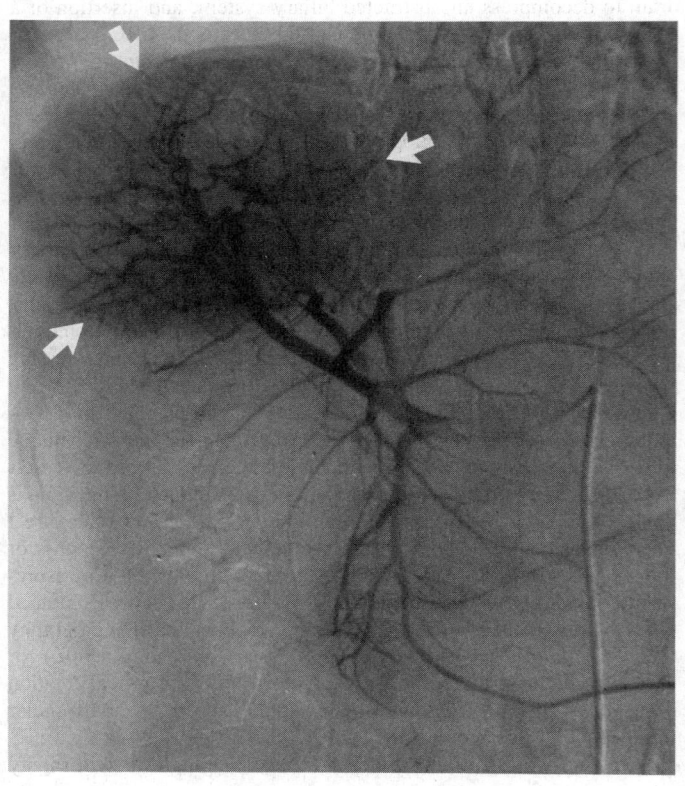

REFERENCES

BENNETT WF, BOVA JG: Review of hepatic imaging and a problem-oriented approach to liver masses. Hepatology 12:761, 1990

BERNARDINO ME (ed): Imaging of the liver and biliary tree. Rad Clin North Am 29:1129, 1991

COUNCIL ON SCIENTIFIC AFFAIRS, AMERICAN MEDICAL ASSOCIATION: Magnetic resonance imaging of the abdomen and pelvis. JAMA 261:420, 1989

FERRUCCI JT: Liver tumor imaging: Current concepts. AJR 155:473, 1990

——— et al: Advances in hepatobiliary radiology. Radiology 168:3198, 1988

MARTON KI, DOUBILET P: How to image the gallbladder in suspected cholecystitis. Ann Intern Med 109:722, 1988

MITCHELL DG: Focal manifestations of diffuse liver disease at MR imaging. Radiology 185:1, 1992

NABI HA, DOERR RJ: Radiolabeled monoclonal antibody imaging (immunoscintigraphy) of colorectal cancers: Current status and future perspectives. Am J Surg 163:448, 1992

ROTHSCHILD MA, ORATZ M: Hepatic imaging. Semin Liv Dis 9:1, 1989

SHERLOCK S, DOOLEY J: *Diseases of the Liver and Biliary System*, 9th ed. Oxford, Blackwell, 1993

STARK DD, BRADLEY WG: *Magnetic Resonance Imaging*. St Louis, Mosby Year Book, 1991

263   DIAGNOSTIC TESTS IN LIVER DISEASE

DANIEL K. PODOLSKY / KURT J. ISSELBACHER

The diversity of normal liver functions and the disruption of these functions by the spectrum of disorders which may affect the liver preclude the use of any single test as a reliable measure of overall liver function. Many disease processes may lead to severe impairment of some liver functions, while others remain entirely unaffected. Since no battery of tests is universally applicable, those most appropriate to a given clinical problem must be selected, their potential value and risks considered, and the results interpreted in relation to the clinical findings.

In assessing the severity and course of liver disease, the physician should be guided by several practical principles. The tests selected should (1) assess different parameters of liver function, (2) be used *serially* in order to evaluate the evolution or course of the disease, and (3) be interpreted within the total clinical context, with recognition that any single laboratory test may be fallible.

BLOOD TESTS OF LIVER FUNCTION   (See Table 263-1)

BILIRUBIN   Bilirubin metabolism and its assessment are discussed in detail in Chaps. 42 and 265. Spectrophotometric determinations of serum bilirubin in the clinical laboratory measure two pigment fractions: (1) the water-soluble conjugated fraction that gives a *direct reaction* with the diazo reagent and consists largely of conjugated bilirubin (as the mono- and diglucuronide) and (2) the lipid-soluble *indirect-reaction* fraction (total minus direct) that represents primarily unconjugated bilirubin. The serum of normal adults (when measured by the van den Bergh reaction) contains less than 4.2 μmol/L (0.25 mg/dL) direct-reacting bilirubin and 17 μmol/L (1 mg/dL) or less of total bilirubin. Studies with high-performance liquid chromatography (HPLC) suggest that even these levels may be artifactually high in normal persons (see Chap. 42).

Conjugated hyperbilirubinemia with elevated direct- and indirect-reacting material indicates impairment of secretion into the bile, while unconjugated hyperbilirubinemia reflects impaired conjugation. The latter is found in a limited number of processes, including such nonhepatic conditions as hemolytic anemia and ineffective erythropoiesis (increased pigment load) and a few hepatic disorders, principally Gilbert's syndrome or the relatively rare Crigler-Najjar syndrome. Although measurement of both the direct and total serum bilirubin will determine whether the patient has predominantly unconjugated or conjugated hyperbilirubinemia, this distinction is of limited usefulness, since the majority of hepatobiliary disorders lead to conjugated hyperbilirubinemia. In most instances, fractionation of serum bilirubin does not distinguish cholestasis due to parenchymal disease from that arising from biliary tract processes.

Bilirubin appears in the urine only after it is converted to a water-soluble form; generally this involves conjugation with polar glucuronide groups which enhance water solubility. Rapid assessment of bilirubinuria is possible using commercially available dipsticks and may be helpful as an initial screening measure. Bilirubinuria occurs with even minimal degrees of jaundice and may be detected before jaundice is evident. Its usefulness is otherwise quite limited. Urobilinogen, a product of luminal bacterial metabolism of bilirubin, is reabsorbed from the bowel and secreted in the urine. Complete bile duct obstruction blocks excretion of bilirubin into the gut and results in disappearance of urobilinogen from the urine. Assessment of urobilinogen in a freshly collected 2-h urine specimen by the Watson method (normal values 0.2 to 1.2 units) may distinguish biliary tract obstruction from parenchymal dysfunction, but this test has been largely superseded by newer methods.

SERUM ENZYME ASSAYS   A number of serum enzymes have been used to distinguish and assess hepatocellular injury and biliary tract dysfunction or obstruction. All have inherent limitations in sensitivity and specificity, and none truly distinguishes these processes definitively. Elevations in enzyme activities also may be seen in association with nonhepatic disorders. Nevertheless, with proper and careful interpretation, a number of serum enzymes provide important clinical tools.

Aminotransferases (transaminases)   Assays of many serum enzymes have been proposed as indicators of hepatocellular damage. Of these, aspartate aminotransferase (AST, SGOT) and alanine aminotransferase (ALT, SGPT) activities have proven most useful. These enzymes catalyze the transfer of the γ-amino groups of aspartate and alanine, respectively, to the γ-keto group of ketoglutarate, leading to the formation of oxaloacetic acid and pyruvic acid. In contrast to ALT, which is found primarily in the liver, AST is present in many tissues, including heart, skeletal muscle, kidney, and brain, and is thus somewhat less specific as an indicator of liver function. The source of serum AST and ALT in the normal person [less than 0.58 μkat/L (35 U/L)] is unclear, and the mechanism responsible for clearance of these enzymes is uncertain. In the hepatocyte, ALT is found exclusively in the cytosol, while different isoenzymes of AST exist in mitochondria and the cytosol. Although elevated serum levels of AST or ALT may be observed in a variety of nonhepatic diseases, notably in myocardial infarction and skeletal muscle disorders, these disorders can usually be distinguished clinically from liver disease. Conversely, uremia may lead to spuriously low aminotransferase values.

Serum AST and ALT are elevated to some extent in nearly all liver disorders. Highest levels are found in association with conditions causing extensive hepatic necrosis, such as severe viral hepatitis, toxin-induced liver injury, or prolonged circulatory collapse. Lesser elevations are encountered in mild acute viral hepatitis as well as in both diffuse and focal chronic liver diseases (e.g., chronic active hepatitis, cirrhosis, and hepatic metastases). However, the absolute levels of aminotransferases correlate poorly with severity of liver injury or prognosis, and serial determinations are usually most helpful. Thus, in the patient with massive hepatic necrosis, there may be marked elevations in the early phase (i.e., 24 to 48 h), but by the time the patient is tested 3 to 5 days later, the levels may be in the range of 3.34 to 5.8 μkat/L (200 to 350 U/L). It is noteworthy that in severe alcoholic hepatitis one commonly finds only modest increases in these enzymes (generally less than 5.0 μkat/L). Minimal elevations of AST and ALT (less than 1.67 μkat/L) also may be found in association with biliary tract obstruction; higher levels suggest the development of cholangitis with resultant hepatic cell necrosis.

In general AST and ALT levels parallel each other, with a couple of exceptions. In alcoholic hepatitis the AST/ALT ratio may be greater than 2; this appears to result from a reduction in hepatic ALT content due to a deficiency in the cofactor pyridoxine-5-phosphate. An increase in the ratio of AST/ALT (>1) also can be seen occasionally in patients with the fatty liver associated with pregnancy.

Alkaline phosphatase   Human serum contains several forms of alkaline phosphatase, a plasma membrane–derived enzyme of uncertain physiologic function which hydrolyzes synthetic phosphate esters at pH 9. These activities arise from bone, intestine, liver, and placenta. A number of different assays have been developed which utilize different substrates.

In the absence of bone disease or pregnancy, elevated levels of alkaline phosphatase activity usually reflect impaired biliary tract function. The increased levels reflect increased synthesis of the enzyme by hepatocytes and biliary tract epithelium rather than regurgitation of enzyme due to obstruction. Bile acids may play a role both by inducing synthesis and by promoting solubilization of the membrane-associated enzyme activity.

Slight to moderate increases in alkaline phosphatase (1 to 2 times normal) occur in many patients with parenchymal liver disorders such as hepatitis and cirrhosis; transient increases may occur in all types

TABLE 263-1   Abnormalities shown by tests of liver function

Test	Type of liver disease	
	Obstructive	Parenchymal
AST and ALT (SGOT and SGPT)	↑	↑ – ↑↑↑
Alkaline phosphatase	↑↑↑	↑
Albumin	N	↓ – ↓↓↓
Prothrombin time	N– ↑ *	↑ – ↑↑↑
Bilirubin	N– ↑↑↑	N– ↑↑↑
γ-Glutamyl transpeptidase (GGT)	↑↑↑	N– ↑↑↑
5'-Nucleotidase	↑ – ↑↑↑	N– ↑

* Correctable with parenteral vitamin K if elevated.

NOTE: N, normal: ↑, elevated; ↓, decreased.

of liver disease. However, the most striking increases in alkaline phosphatase (3 to 10 times normal) occur with extrahepatic biliary tract (mechanical) obstruction or with intrahepatic (functional) cholestasis, as in drug-induced cholestasis or primary biliary cirrhosis. Conversely, it is unusual for the serum alkaline phosphatase to remain normal when there is obstructive jaundice, and a normal enzyme level argues strongly against the presence of cholestasis. The alkaline phosphatase is usually mildly elevated in metastatic or infiltrative liver disease (e.g., leukemia, lymphoma, and sarcoid). The enzyme may be elevated in the presence of incomplete biliary obstruction or when there is obstruction of only one hepatic duct, conditions in which the serum bilirubin is often normal or only slightly elevated. Serum alkaline phosphatase is also elevated in nonhepatic disorders, most notably in some bone disorders (e.g., Paget's disease, osteomalacia, and metastases to bone) and sometimes with malignancy. Occasionally, tumors produce an alkaline phosphatase which is identical or similar to the placental form, the so-called Regan isoenzyme.

Although one can usually make a reasonable assessment as to whether an elevation of the alkaline phosphatase is of hepatic or nonhepatic origin, several methods can distinguish the different isoenzymes, facilitating resolution of any uncertainty. In contrast to that derived from bone, the hepatic isozyme is stable to treatment with heat (56°C for 15 min) or urea. These enzymes also can be separated by electrophoresis, but this is usually impractical. Parallel determination of serum 5'-nucleotidase activity is also helpful; an increase of both 5'-nucleotidase and alkaline phosphatase is consistent with an hepatobiliary source of the enzyme elevation. Even after correction for age and sex (higher levels being found in the young and in older women), isolated elevations in alkaline phosphatase may occasionally be encountered in adults with no apparent disease.

5'-Nucleotidase, leucine aminopeptidase, and γ-glutamyltranspeptidase   *5'-Nucleotidase* catalyzes the hydrolysis of phosphate from the 5' position of the pentose component of the nucleotide. Although tissue distribution is widespread, elevations are generally associated with hepatobiliary disease. The principal value of the 5'-nucleotidase measurement is to confirm the hepatic origin of an elevated alkaline phosphatase level in children or pregnant women or in those settings where coincident bone disease may be present. However, 5'-nucleotidase levels do not always parallel alkaline phosphatase in liver disease, and lack of elevation does not exclude an hepatic source of elevated serum alkaline phosphatase.

γ-Glutamyltranspeptidase   GGT catalyzes the transfer of the γ-glutamyl group from peptides such as glutathione to other amino acids and may play a role in amino acid transport. It is found throughout the hepatobiliary system as well as in other tissues. In liver disease, GGT correlates with alkaline phosphatase levels and is the most sensitive indicator of biliary tract disease. However, elevations of GGT are nonspecific and may be associated with pancreatic, cardiac, renal, and pulmonary disorders as well as with diabetes and alcoholism. This enzyme may be increased by agents which induce microsomal enzymes, and it has been suggested as a potential marker of alcoholism. However, overall lack of specificity has limited its clinical usefulness.

Other enzymes   Measurement of total serum lactic dehydrogenase (LDH) or its isoenzymes is usually not helpful in diagnosis of liver disease because of this enzyme's nearly ubiquitous body distribution. Moderate LDH elevations are common in acute viral hepatitis, cirrhosis, and metastatic carcinoma to the liver. Biliary tract disease also may produce slight elevations. Marked elevations of LDH in association with abnormal results of other liver function tests may reflect a hematologic malignancy such as lymphoma. Numerous other dehydrogenases (e.g., isocitrate dehydrogenase, sorbitol dehydrogenase, and glutamate dehydrogenase) have been used or proposed as markers of liver disease, but none appears to offer significant diagnostic improvement over standard aminotransferase determinations. Elevation of serum ornithine carbamyl transferase (OCT), a urea cycle enzyme present only in liver and intestine, occurs primarily

in liver disease, but its lack of association with any specific type of liver disease has limited its diagnostic usefulness.

SERUM PROTEINS   Extensive liver injury may lead to *decreased* blood levels of albumin, prothrombin, fibrinogen, and other proteins synthesized exclusively by hepatocytes. In contrast to measurements of serum enzymes, serum protein levels reflect liver synthetic function rather than just cell injury. Three important caveats should be remembered regarding interpretation of serum protein levels: (1) they are neither early nor sensitive indicators of liver disease (because of the extent of hepatic reserve and their half-life, see below), (2) they are of little value in the differential diagnosis of liver disease, and (3) decreases in their serum levels are not specific for liver disease.

Albumin and globulin   Albumin is quantitatively the most important serum protein synthesized by the liver; the normal serum value ranges from 35 to 55 g/L (see Chap. 264). Albumin has a fairly long half-life (14 to 20 days) with less than 5 percent turnover daily; it is therefore not a good indicator of acute or mild liver injury. Furthermore, there is a substantial reserve of hepatic albumin synthesis; thus adequate synthesis may continue until there is extensive hepatocellular injury. Serum levels are influenced by a variety of nonhepatic factors, most notably nutritional status, hormonal factors, and plasma oncotic pressure. Routes of degradation in health remain undefined, but nonhepatic conditions may lead to depressed serum albumin levels mainly due to excessive loss despite adequate synthetic function (e.g., nephrotic syndrome or protein-losing enteropathy). Nonetheless, reduction in the serum albumin levels provides an excellent indication of the severity of chronic liver disease. In the patient with ascites, an increased volume of distribution as well as an absolute reduction in protein synthesis may contribute to hypoalbuminemia.

Serum globulins are a heterogeneous group of proteins whose production in a variety of tissues is influenced by a number of factors. Serum globulins (normal 20 to 35 g/L) include alpha and beta globulins as well as serum immunoglobulins, the latter largely accounting for the gamma fraction. Serum globulins are often diffusely elevated in association with chronic liver disease and in other nonhepatic disorders. In cirrhosis, varying degrees of hyperglobulinemia may occur; this may reflect increased stimulation of the peripheral reticuloendothelial compartment due to shunting of antigens past the liver and impaired clearance by hepatic Kupffer cells. Although some have suggested that elevations in different globulin fractions as assessed by electrophoretic or other means may have a differential diagnostic value, this remains a largely unfulfilled promise. Similarly, the albumin/globulin ratio has no physiologic significance.

Clotting factors   The liver synthesizes six coagulation factors: fibrinogen (factor I), prothrombin (factor II), and factors V, VII, IX, and X. With the exception of factor V, production of functional proteins requires the presence of the cofactor vitamin K. Because most of these factors are normally present in excess concentrations, impaired coagulation is usually seen only in severe liver disease. Abnormalities of these factors can be most efficiently determined by the one-stage *prothrombin time*, which measures the rate of prothrombin conversion to thrombin in the presence of thromboplastin and calcium and requires the integrity of most of the vitamin K–dependent clotting factors (see Chap. 57). Factor VII is the rate-limiting factor in this pathway and thus has the greatest influence on the prothrombin levels. The prothrombin time is dependent on normal hepatic synthesis of clotting factors and sufficient intestinal uptake of vitamin K. Absorption of this fat-soluble vitamin itself requires adequate dietary intake and normal function of intestinal mucosa and biliary secretion. Severe acute or chronic parenchymal liver injury may lead to prolongation of the prothrombin time due to impaired synthesis of the clotting proteins. Because these proteins have a shorter half-life than that of albumin, the prothrombin time may be an earlier indicator than serum albumin level of severe liver injury. In both acute and chronic hepatocellular injury, an increase in the prothrombin time serves as an ominous prognostic sign. Because vitamin K is a fat-soluble vitamin, prolongation of the prothrombin time can result from vitamin K malabsorption, which may occur with cholestasis due to biliary tract disease or due to fat malabsorption (steatorrhea) of any cause (e.g., pancreatic insufficiency). Poor dietary intake, antibiotic therapy, and use of warfarin-type anticoagulants are additional causes of a prolonged prothrombin time, owing to deficiencies of active vitamin K. These processes can be distinguished from hepatic synthetic failure by demonstrating normalization of the prothrombin time (within 24 to 48 h) after parenteral injections of vitamin K. The *partial thromboplastin time*, which reflects the activities of fibrinogen, prothrombin, and factors V, VIII, IX, X, XI, and XII, also may be prolonged in severe liver disease. Clotting functions should be assessed in all patients with liver disease prior to any surgical procedure, including liver biopsy (see Chaps. 57 and 315).

BLOOD AMMONIA Ammonia is elevated in the blood of some patients with either acute or chronic liver disease. Although influenced by a number of factors (summarized in Chap. 264), elevations in blood ammonia reflect disruption of the pathways of urea synthesis by which the liver detoxifies amine groups. A markedly elevated blood ammonia usually reflects severe hepatocellular necrosis. Cirrhotic patients, especially those with endogenous or surgically created portal-systemic shunting, often have varying degrees of hyperammonemia and hepatic encephalopathy. However, there is only a rough correlation between blood ammonia levels and the degree of hepatic encephalopathy; some patients will function normally with a twofold elevation, while others will be stuporous at the same concentration. Ammonia levels may increase before the onset of coma; similarly, they may return to normal some 48 to 72 h before improvement of the neurologic status.

SERUM LIPIDS AND LIPOPROTEINS AND BILE ACIDS Abnormalities in serum lipids and lipoproteins are sensitive but nonspecific indicators of liver diseases. Acute parenchymal liver disease is commonly associated with increased plasma triglycerides, decreased cholesterol esters, and abnormal lipoproteins. The absence of alpha and prebeta bands with a concomitant increase in the beta fraction is typical of acute viral hepatitis. Less marked but more persistent abnormalities are found in patients with chronic parenchymal disease reflecting deficiencies in lecithin:cholesterol acyltransferase (LCAT) and hepatic triglyceride lipase. Either intra- or extrahepatic cholestasis may lead to an increase in unesterified cholesterol and in serum phospholipids.

Removal of bile acids from portal blood is impaired in liver disease because of parenchymal damage and portal-systemic shunts; there also may be reentry of bile acids into blood from injured hepatocytes or an obstructed biliary tract. Although there are a variety of techniques for measuring serum bile acids, these determinations are not yet of proven value for routine clinical use.

IMMUNOLOGIC AND OTHER TESTS

A number of immunologic derangements may be seen in liver disease. Antimitochondrial antibodies are found in 85 to 90 percent of patients with primary biliary cirrhosis. These antibodies appear to be directed against components of the pyruvate dehydrogenase complex and other related mitochondrial enzyme complexes. In this test, serum is incubated with rabbit hepatocytes. The presence of antimitochondrial antibodies can then be assessed after subsequent staining with a fluorescein-tagged second antibody. However, this marker is not entirely specific and is occasionally found in patients with chronic active hepatitis and drug-induced hepatitis. Its primary value is in helping to distinguish primary biliary cirrhosis from extrahepatic biliary obstruction. In chronic active hepatitis, the *lupus erythematosus–cell test* (LE-cell test) may be positive, and *antinuclear antibodies* as well as *anti-smooth-muscle antibodies* may be present (see Chap. 284). Alpha fetoprotein is of value in the diagnosis of hepatocellular carcinoma (see Chap. 269). Measurements of serum alpha$_1$-antitrypsin and ceruloplasmin should be performed in infants with cirrhosis or

hepatitis since they may reflect alpha$_1$-antitrypsin deficiency or Wilson's disease, respectively (see Chaps. 270 and 348).

Studies assessing iron stores are essential in the evaluation of those patients suspected of hemochromatosis on clinical grounds, those exhibiting compatible nonspecific abnormal liver function tests results (e.g., unexplained mild to moderate elevation of aminotransferase), or those with evidence of liver disease, early or advanced, of uncertain cause. Routine tests include iron, total serum iron-binding capacity (TIBC), and ferritin. Hemochromatosis is associated with elevated levels of both iron and TIBC and an increased ratio of iron/TIBC, typically >90 percent, consistent with a high degree of saturation of iron-binding capacity. While elevated levels of saturation may be seen in many chronic systemic illnesses, the overall level of iron and TIBC will be diminished. Serum levels of ferritin, the intrahepatic ion storage protein, are typically markedly elevated in hemochromatosis. Somewhat less pronounced increases may be seen in other forms of liver injury, including alcoholic liver disease and other diseases (e.g., lymphoma). Particular confusion may arise in distinguishing secondary hemosiderosis, most commonly seen in alcoholics but also encountered in patients receiving numerous transfusions (e.g., sickle cell anemia), from primary idiopathic hemochromatosis by these initial serum determinations. Diagnosis often ultimately requires percutaneous liver biopy or other more specific tests (see Chap. 345).

OTHER DIAGNOSTIC PROCEDURES **Percutaneous needle biopsy of the liver** Percutaneous needle biopsy is a safe, simple, and valuable method for the diagnostic evaluation of liver disease. *Diffuse parenchymal disorders* such as cirrhosis, hepatitis, and drug reactions may be diagnosed with remarkable accuracy. In *disseminated focal diseases* (such as granulomas or tumor infiltrates), serial sections may demonstrate characteristic lesions.

Biopsy is performed under local anesthesia, usually with the Menghini (aspiration), Klatskin, or Vim-Silverman (cutting) needle, by either a transpleural or subcostal approach. If the operator is skillful and patients are carefully selected, morbidity should be quite low and limited to occasional postbiopsy pain or vasovagal reactions.

Some of the most frequent indications for needle biopsy are (1) unexplained hepatomegaly or hepatosplenomegaly, (2) cholestasis of uncertain cause, (3) persistently abnormal liver function tests, (4) suspected systemic or infiltrative diseases such as sarcoidosis, miliary tuberculosis, or fever of unknown origin, and (5) suspected primary or metastatic liver tumor. Percutaneous liver biopsy may be performed either for diagnostic purposes or to evaluate the extent and severity of a known disease process. However, other new and improved noninvasive diagnostic methods have obviated the need for biopsy in many circumstances, and thus biopsy should be performed only when information from these other techniques is inadequate.

Needle biopsy should not be performed if (1) the patient is unable to cooperate, (2) clinical or laboratory evidence indicates impaired hemostasis (prothrombin time prolonged by 3 s or more over control, thrombocytopenia less than 80 to 100 × 10^9 platelets per liter, or partial thromboplastin time or bleeding time prolonged), (3) there is infection of the right pleural space or septic cholangitis, (4) tense ascites is present, with risk of continued leakage of ascitic fluid, (5) compatible blood is not available for transfusion in case of hemorrhage, (6) high-grade biliary obstruction is suspected and there is an increased risk of bile peritonitis, or (7) a vascular lesion is suspected. In patients in whom a percutaneous biopsy cannot be performed safely due to impaired hemostasis or ascites, biopsy can sometimes be carried out by a transjugular approach, in which the tissue is obtained via the hepatic vein and any bleeding occurs directly into the vascular space. With the increasing use of CT scan and ultrasonography, it is possible to perform "directed" aspiration biopsies of isolated lesions with very thin needles. Aspirated material can be used for cytology (tumors) and culture (abscesses) but is often inadequate for assessment of liver architecture.

Laparoscopy and laparotomy (peritoneoscopy) See Chap. 250.

REFERENCES

FERRUCCI JT JR et al: Advances in hepatic radiology. Radiology 168:3198, 1988

MOSS, AA et al Hepatic tumors: Magnetic resonance and CT appearance. Radiology 150:191, 1984

ROTHSCHILD MA et al: Serum albumin. Hepatology 8:385, 1988

SABESIN SM: Cholestatic lipoproteins. Their pathogenesis and significance. Gastroenterology 83:704, 1982

ZAKIM D, BOYER TD: *Hepatology, A Textbook of Liver Disease*, 2d ed. Philadelphia, Saunders, 1990

————, ORATZ M: Hepatic imaging. Semin Liv Dis 9:1, 1989

264   DERANGEMENTS OF HEPATIC METABOLISM

DANIEL K. PODOLSKY / KURT J. ISSELBACHER

The liver plays a central role in the maintenance of metabolic homeostasis. It is therefore not surprising that the development of clinically important liver disease is accompanied by diverse manifestations of disordered metabolism. Although some functions are more sensitive than others, the liver has considerable reserve capacity, so minimal or even moderate cell injury may not be reflected by measurable metabolic changes. However, a variety of defects may be seen, depending on the nature and extent of the initial insult.

The biochemical functions in which the liver plays a major role include (1) the intermediate metabolism of amino acids and carbohydrates, (2) synthesis and degradation of proteins and glycoproteins, (3) metabolism and degradation of drugs and hormones, and (4) regulation of lipid and cholesterol metabolism. The derangements of these functions are discussed in connection with their occurrence in various forms of parenchymal liver disease. Alterations of bilirubin, bile salt, and porphyrin metabolism are discussed elsewhere (Chaps. 41, 254, and 346).

Metabolic derangements are most evident in the patient with advanced liver disease, and the manifestations are similar regardless of the initial etiologic insult. To a varying degree, similar abnormalities are observed in patients with severe chronic hepatitis, micronodular cirrhosis, and postnecrotic cirrhosis. Since the many functions of the liver may be affected to varying degrees in individual patients, no single test effectively measures the overall state of liver function. The proper interpretation of liver function tests is discussed in Chap. 263.

CARBOHYDRATE METABOLISM   The liver functions to maintain normal levels of blood sugar by a combination of glycogenesis, glycogenolysis, glycolysis, and gluconeogenesis. These pathways are regulated by a number of hormones, including insulin, glucagon, growth hormone, and certain catecholamines. Although it has been presumed that exquisite sensitivity of the hepatocytes to insulin is responsible for the uptake of an oral glucose load by the liver, there are also data that have challenged the importance of insulin-mediated glucose uptake by the hepatocyte. In the fasting state, the liver contributes to glucose homeostasis by glycogenolysis and gluconeogenesis in response to hypoinsulinemia and hyperglucagonemia. Maintenance of normal blood glucose levels through gluconeogenesis is ultimately related to catabolism of muscle protein, which provides the necessary amino acid precursors, especially alanine. In a complementary fashion, in the postprandial state, the liver directs alanine and branched-chain amino acids to the peripheral tissues, where they are then incorporated into muscle protein. These reciprocal pathways form a glucose-alanine shuttle which is modulated by ambient changes in the hormones mentioned above (Fig. 264-1). While it has been presumed that synthesis of glycogen and fatty acid in the postprandial state arises from direct conversion of glucose, there are data to suggest that, in fact, these pathways are *indirect*, with products deriving from three-carbon metabolites of glucose or other gluconeogenic compounds such as lactate, fructose, and alanine.

Abnormalities of glucose homeostasis are common in cirrhosis (Table 264-1). Most frequently, hyperglycemia and glucose intolerance are observed. Glucose intolerance is associated with normal or increased levels of plasma insulin (except in patients with hemochromatosis), suggesting that insulin resistance rather than insulin deficiency may be responsible. One of the factors that may play a role in the apparent insulin resistance is an absolute decrease in the liver's ability to metabolize a glucose load because of a decrease in functioning hepatocellular mass. There is also evidence that response to insulin is diminished due to both receptor and postreceptor defects in hepatocytes of patients with cirrhosis. In addition, both hyperinsulinemia and hyperglucagonemia may be present due to decreased hepatic clearance of this hormone resulting from portalsystemic shunting. In patients with hemochromatosis, insulin levels, however, may indeed be low due to pancreatic iron deposition and sometimes concomitant diabetes mellitus. Patients with cirrhosis also may have elevated serum lactate levels, reflecting the decreased capacity of the liver to utilize lactate for gluconeogenesis.

Hypoglycemia, although more common in acute fulminant hepatitis, also may be seen with end-stage cirrhosis. Glycogen in the liver accounts for 5 to 7 percent of the normal tissue weight. Because the capacity of the liver to store glycogen is limited (approximately 70 g) and glucose consumption continues at a constant rate (approximately 150 g/d), hepatic glycogen stores are depleted after 1 day of fasting. Hypoglycemia in end-stage cirrhosis may be due to decreased hepatic glycogen stores, diminished glucagon responsiveness, or decreased capacity to synthesize glycogen due to extensive parenchymal destruction.

AMINO ACID AND AMMONIA METABOLISM   Through a variety of anabolic and catabolic processes, the liver is the major site of amino acid interconversion. Amino acids utilized for hepatic protein synthesis are derived from dietary protein, metabolic turnover of endogenous protein (primarily from muscle), and direct synthesis in the liver. Most of the amino acids entering the liver via the portal vein are catabolized to urea (except for the branched-chain amino acids leucine, isoleucine, and valine). A lesser amount is released into the general circulation as free amino acids, and these may play an important role in the glucose-alanine cycle mentioned above. In addition, amino acids are utilized for the synthesis of liver intracellular proteins, plasma proteins, and special compounds such as glutathione, glutamine, taurine, carnosine, and creatine. Disruption of normal amino acid metabolism may be reflected in altered plasma amino acid concentrations. In general, levels of aromatic amino acids normally metabolized by the liver (as well as methionine) are elevated, while those of the branched-chain amino acids, largely utilized by skeletal muscle, tend to be normal or depressed. It has been suggested that an alteration in the ratio of these two types of amino acids plays a role in the development of hepatic encephalopathy (see below), but there is not agreement on this concept.

Hepatic catabolism or degradation of amino acids involves two major reactions: transamination and oxidative deamination. In transamination, an amino group of an amino acid is transferred to a keto acid. This process is catalyzed by aminotransferases, which are found in very high amounts in liver but are also present in other tissues, such as kidney, muscle, heart, lung, and brain. Glutamic-oxaloacetic acid transaminase (aspartate aminotransferase, AST) has been studied most extensively, and increased levels are found in the serum secondary to various types of liver injury (e.g., acute viral and drug-induced hepatitis). As a result of transamination, amino acids can enter the citric acid cycle and then function in the intermediary metabolism of carbohydrates and lipids. Most of the nonessential amino acids are also synthesized in the liver by transamination. Oxidative deamination, which results in conversion of amino acids to keto acids (and ammonia), is catalyzed by L-amino acid oxidase with two exceptions: Glycine oxidation is catalyzed by glycine oxidase, and glutamic oxidation is catalyzed by glutamic dehydrogenase. With severe liver damage (e.g., massive hepatic necrosis), utilization of amino acids is impaired, free amino acids in the

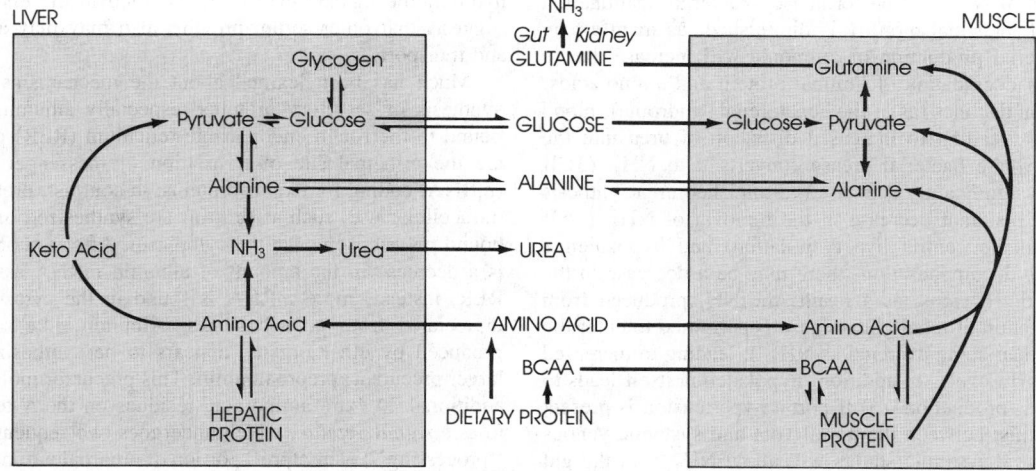

FIGURE 264-1 Carbohydrate-protein exchange between muscle and liver. After an overnight fast there is net release of amino acids by muscle (predominantly alanine and glutamine). These are derived from transamination of pyruvate, degraded amino acids, and glucose. Branched-chain amino acids (BCAA) are particularly important as a source of nitrogen for alanine synthesis. Alanine is utilized for gluconeogenesis by the liver, and urea is formed as a by-product. The main sites of glutamine uptake are the kidney and gut, where

it is used for ammonia production and as a possible source of energy, respectively. Following ingestion of dietary protein, skeletal muscle goes into an anabolic phase; there is selective hepatic escape and muscle uptake of dietary BCAA, reduced muscle output of alanine and glutamine, and a reduced rate of hepatic gluconeogenesis. Hepatic tissue protein also goes into an anabolic phase following protein ingestion. (*Modified with permission from AS Tavill in Wright et al.*)

bloodstream increase, and an "overflow" type of aminoaciduria may occur.

Urea production is intimately related to the metabolic pathways outlined above, providing a means for disposal of ammonia, the toxic product of nitrogen metabolism. Disruption of this process is of particular clinical importance in the patient with severe acute and chronic liver disease. The fixation of amino acid–derived NH_3 in the form of urea is carried out via the Krebs-Henseleit cycle. The final step of this cycle, the formation of urea by arginase, is irreversible. In advanced liver disease, urea synthesis is often depressed, leading to an accumulation of NH_3, usually with a significant reduction in blood urea nitrogen (BUN), an ominous sign of liver failure. This finding may be obscured by superimposed renal impairment, which often develops in patients with severe hepatic failure. Urea is mostly excreted by the kidney, but approximately 25 percent will diffuse into the intestine, where it is converted to NH_3 by bacterial urease. The intestinal production of ammonia also occurs from the bacterial deamination of unabsorbed amino acids and of protein derived from the diet, exfoliated cells, or blood in the gastrointestinal tract.

Gut NH_3 is absorbed and transported to the liver via the portal vein, where it is again converted to urea. The kidney also produces varying amounts of NH_3, largely by the deamination of glutamine.

The contributions of the gut and kidney to ammonia synthesis have important implications for the management of the hyperammonemic state frequently seen in patients with advanced liver disease, usually in association with portal-systemic shunting of blood.

While the exact chemical mediators of hepatic encephalopathy remain unknown and may include endogenous benzodiazepine compounds, elevated levels of blood NH_3 generally correlate with the degree of encephalopathy, although approximately 10 percent of such patients have normal levels of blood ammonia. In addition, therapeutic measures that reduce serum NH_3 levels also usually lead to clinical improvement. The several mechanisms known to lead to increased blood NH_3 levels in patients with cirrhosis are illustrated in Fig. 264-2 and include the following: (1) If there is excessive nitrogenous material in the intestine (from bleeding or dietary protein),

FIGURE 264-2 Major factors (steps 1 to 4) influencing the level of blood ammonia. In cirrhosis with portal hypertension, venous collaterals allow ammonia to bypass the liver (step 5), permitting the entry of ammonia into the systemic circulation (portal-systemic shunting).

TABLE 264-1	Alteration of glucose metabolism in cirrhosis

FACTORS LEADING TO HYPERGLYCEMIA

Decreased hepatic glucose uptake
Decreased hepatic glycogen synthesis
Hepatic resistance to insulin
Portal-systemic glucose shunting
Peripheral insulin resistance
Hormonal abnormalities (serum)
  ↑ Glucagon
  ↓ Cortisol
  ↑ Insulin (↓ in hemochromatosis)

FACTORS LEADING TO HYPOGLYCEMIA

Decreased gluconeogenesis
Decreased hepatic glycogen content
Hepatic resistance to glucagon
Poor oral intake
Hyperinsulinemia secondary to portal-systemic shunting

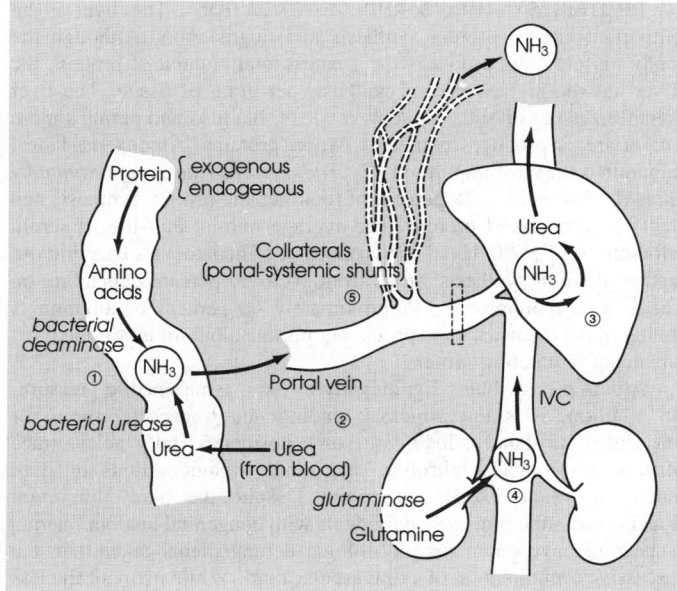

excessive amounts of NH_3 will be formed by bacterial deamination of amino acids. If intestinal motility is diminished, as manifest by constipation, bacterial production of ammonia will increase due to prolonged time for degradation of luminal protein and amino acids. (2) If renal function declines (as in the hepatorenal syndrome), blood urea nitrogen rises, leading to increased diffusion of urea into the intestinal lumen, where bacterial urease converts it to NH_3. (3) If hepatic function is significantly depressed, diminished urea synthesis may occur with a resultant decrease in the removal of NH_3. (4) If alkalosis (often due to central hyperventilation) and hypokalemia accompany hepatic decompensation, there may be a decrease in the renal availability of H^+ ions; as a result, the NH_3 produced from glutamine by the action of renal glutaminase is permitted to enter the renal vein (rather than being excreted as NH_4^+), leading to increased peripheral blood NH_3 levels. In addition, hypokalemia itself leads to increased renal NH_3 production. (5) If portal hypertension is present and anastomoses exist between the portal vein and systemic venous channels, these portal-systemic shunts will allow NH_3 from the gut to bypass hepatic detoxification, leading to elevated blood NH_3 levels. Thus, with portal-systemic shunting of blood, elevated NH_3 levels may develop with relatively modest hepatocellular dysfunction. It is unclear what effects these same factors may have on other compounds which may play a role in the development of hepatic encephalopathy.

An additional factor important in determining whether a given NH_3 level in the blood will be detrimental to the central nervous system is the blood pH. The more alkaline the pH, the more toxic a given level of NH_3 is likely to be. At 37°C, the pK of NH_3 is 8.9; this is close enough to the pH' of blood that minor changes in pH can affect the NH_4^+/NH_3 ratio. Because un-ionized NH_3 crosses membranes more readily than NH_4^+ ions, alkalosis favors the entry of ammonia into the brain (with subsequent changes in cell metabolism) by shifting the equilibrium of the following reaction to the right

$$NH_4^+ + OH^- \rightleftharpoons NH_3 + HOH$$

As a result, alkalosis not only increases peripheral blood NH_3 levels by renal mechanisms but also increases tissue levels by influencing the diffusion of NH_3 across membranes. Similarly, alterations in the pH of intestinal luminal contents also will affect the equilibrium between NH_4^+ and NH_3; a more alkaline lumen will shift the balance in favor of NH_3, permitting increased absorption. In theory, laxatives that cause relative acidification of luminal contents (e.g., lactulose) may be more effective as agents for the treatment of hepatic encephalopathy. However, this theoretical effect on the equilibrium between NH_4^+ and NH_3 has never been convincingly demonstrated for available laxatives.

PROTEIN SYNTHESIS AND DEGRADATION The liver is an important site of protein synthesis and degradation. Although the body muscle mass produces the greatest total amount of protein, the liver has the highest rate of synthesis per gram of tissue. The liver synthesizes not only the proteins it needs, but also and perhaps more important, it produces numerous export proteins. Among the latter, albumin is the most important; *it is produced at a rate of approximately 12 g/d,* representing 25 percent of total hepatic protein synthesis and half of all exported protein. The average normal half-life of serum albumin is 17 to 20 days. The proportion of hepatocytes carrying out active albumin synthesis varies from 10 to 60 percent depending on the body's requirements. Approximately 60 percent of albumin is found in the extravascular spaces, but plasma albumin is still the most abundant circulating protein.

Albumin contributes significantly to the plasma oncotic pressure. In addition, it is the principal binding and transport protein for numerous substances, including some hormones, fatty acids, trace metals, tryptophan, bilirubin, and other organic anions of both endogenous and exogenous origin. Despite the many important functions of albumin, rare individuals with congenital analbuminemia appear to have no major physiologic derangements other than the excessive accumulation of extravascular fluid. While many of the less

hydrophobic ligands may be transported in the unbound form, this suggests that other serum proteins also may play a role in binding and transport.

Much has been learned about the mechanisms involved in the synthesis of secretory proteins, especially albumin. Polyribosomes bound to the rough endoplasmic reticulum (RER) of the hepatocyte are the principal site of translation of messenger ribonucleic acid (mRNA) coding for export proteins; in contrast, proteins destined for intracellular use, such as ferritin, are synthesized on free rather than bound polyribosomes in the cytoplasm. After a short-term fast, there is a decrease in the amount of albumin mRNA associated with the RER; instead, more mRNA is found in the cytosol and in a state dissociated from polyribosomes. Albumin, like secretory proteins produced by other organs, appears to be synthesized initially as a larger precursor, preproalbumin. This precursor molecule contains an additional 24 extra amino acid residues on the N terminus, referred to as a *signal peptide*, which undergoes two sequential cleavages (or "processing"). The "pre" portion of preproalbumin is cleaved within the RER even before protein synthesis is completed; the "pro" segment is removed within the lumen of the RER. The molecule is then transported to the Golgi apparatus prior to secretion. Once synthesis and processing are completed, albumin is transported from the Golgi vesicles to the hepatocyte surface by mechanisms which are unclear but almost certainly involve the microfilaments and microtubule apparatus of the cell. Although the hepatic lymph space of Disse provides a potential avenue for the newly released albumin, most secreted proteins enter the plasma.

Albumin synthesis is subject to a number of regulatory influences. These include the rate of transcription of specific mRNAs and the availability of the substrate tRNA (transfer RNA). At the translational level, the integrity of polyribosomes and their synthetic abilities are modified by factors affecting initiation, elongation, and release of peptides and proteins as well as by the availability of ATP, GTP, and magnesium ions. The rate of albumin synthesis is also influenced by the availability of amino acid precursors, especially tryptophan, the scarcest of the essential amino acids. Indeed, in patients with large carcinoid tumors, albumin synthesis may decrease precipitously when tryptophan is consumed by carcinoid cells in the production of 5-hydroxytryptophan (serotonin) (see Chap. 276). The rate of albumin synthesis is also affected by colloid oncotic pressure, with increased production occurring in response to falling oncotic pressure. Finally, influences of hormones such as insulin and glucagon on hepatic protein metabolism are closely integrated with the nutritional factors discussed above.

The liver also produces a wide variety of other secretory proteins, most of which have a synthetic pathway and processing procedure similar to that of albumin. The presence of a *signal peptide*, such as the "prepro" segment of albumin, which is subsequently removed during protein maturation appears to be a general mechanism for orienting proteins in the membranes of the endoplasmic reticulum and directing them for export rather than for intracellular use or degradation. Most proteins undergo even further modification in the form of sequential *glycosylation* in the RER and Golgi apparatus. The carbohydrate moieties of these glycoproteins appear to be important in determining their site of action and their rate of tissue uptake after secretion. Some of the clinically important secretory glycoproteins include ceruloplasmin, α_1-antitrypsin, and most other alpha and beta globulins. While the site of albumin catabolism is uncertain, the removal of terminal sialic acid residues after secretion and the resultant exposure of penultimate galactose or N-acetylglucosamine residues appears to result in receptor-mediated uptake of "aged" proteins by hepatocytes and Kupffer cells, followed by their subsequent degradation. Reduced amounts of the hepatic receptor for asialoglycoproteins appear to result in elevated serum concentrations of these glycoproteins in patients with severe and chronic liver disease.

One of the clinically most important derangements in protein metabolism is the development of hypoalbuminemia, which results largely from reduced synthetic activity. Decreased synthesis may be caused by a decrease in the number as well as the function of hepatocytes. A decrease in the dietary supply of amino acids also can contribute to deficient synthesis. To some extent the body attempts to compensate for decreased albumin synthesis by reducing the rate of degradation. Attempts to raise the serum albumin level by intravenous infusions are often futile because this compensatory mechanism can be blunted and the decrease in albumin degradation may not occur. The reduced degradation of albumin is not a general phenomenon in chronic liver disease because other proteins such as fibrinogen are degraded more rapidly than normal. In the patient with ascites, the degree of hypoalbuminemia is worsened by the loss of large amounts of the body's albumin into the ascitic fluid. When there is increased hepatic venous pressure (as in postsinusoidal or hepatic vein outflow block), there may be increased hepatic lymph production with extravasation into the peritoneal cavity. In contrast to intestinal lymph, the protein content of hepatic lymph appears to be relatively uninfluenced by ascitic oncotic pressure, most likely reflecting the lack of tight junctions between sinusoidal endothelial cells.

Other proteins produced by the liver include many of the blood-clotting factors: fibrinogen (factor I), prothrombin (factor II), and factors V, VII, IX, and X, as well as inhibitors of both coagulation and fibrinolysis. Factors II, VII, IX, and X are vitamin K–responsive and are dependent on normal intestinal fat absorption. Vitamin K activates an enzyme system in liver endoplasmic reticulum which catalyzes the γ carboxylation of selected glutamyl residues in clotting factor precursors. The γ carboxylation enhances the Ca^{2+} and phospholipid-binding capacity of prothrombin and permits its rapid conversion to thrombin in the presence of factors V and X (Chap. 315).

The liver is involved in the process of hemostasis by virtue of both anabolic and catabolic functions. As expected, severe liver disease leads to reduced synthesis of prothrombin, a vitamin K–dependent clotting factor. The presence of malnutrition, the use of broad-spectrum antibiotics, or concomitant impairment of fat absorption due to reduction in intestinal bile salt concentration (e.g., cholestasis) may accentuate hypoprothrombinemia by decreasing the amount of vitamin K that can be absorbed from the intestine. In these situations, prothrombin levels may be at least partially corrected by parenteral vitamin K administration. However, when the coagulopathy results from impaired hepatocellular function and not cholestasis or intestinal factors, exogenous vitamin K is unlikely to correct or improve prothrombin synthesis. The vitamin K–dependent clotting proteins have a substantially shorter serum half-life than albumin; therefore, hypoprothrombinemia usually precedes the development of hypoalbuminemia, especially in the patient with acute hepatocellular disease. In cirrhosis, coagulopathy may be further aggravated by the thrombocytopenia resulting from hypersplenism.

Since the liver is also the site of production of non–vitamin K–dependent clotting factors, severe liver disease injury may lead to decreased plasma concentrations of factor V in addition to factors II, VII, IX, and X. It is unusual for fibrinogen to be reduced significantly, unless there is an associated disseminated intravascular coagulation (DIC). For unclear reasons, the damaged liver may actually produce increased amounts of fibrinogen as well as other proteins collectively designated acute-phase reactants (C-reactive proteins, haptoglobin, ceruloplasmin, and transferrin). The latter are produced both in response to liver injury (e.g., severe chronic active hepatitis) and in association with systemic illnesses such as cancer, rheumatoid arthritis, bacterial infections, burns, and myocardial infarctions. Cytokines, including interleukins 1 and 6, appear to be major stimuli of hepatic synthesis of acute-phase reactants. However, while the diseased liver may produce normal or increased amounts of fibrinogen, the molecules themselves may be qualitatively abnormal (i.e., structurally and functionally), reflecting more subtle derangements in protein synthesis. These functionally abnormal fibrinogen molecules may contribute to the altered hemostasis frequently found in patients with chronic liver disease.

DETOXIFICATION MECHANISMS Water-soluble drugs and endogenous substances usually are excreted unchanged in the urine or bile. However, lipid-soluble compounds tend to accumulate in the body and affect cellular processes, unless they are converted to less active compounds or to more water-soluble metabolites which are more easily excreted. Hepatic blood flow, protein binding, and the intrinsic capacity of the liver to eliminate a drug are all primary determinants of hepatic drug clearance. The liver has an important role in the metabolism of many exogenous drugs and endogenous hormones by virtue of several enzyme systems involved in biochemical transformation as well as the "first-pass effect" of blood flow from virtually the entire gastrointestinal tract through the liver via the portal circulation. The relative importance of these various factors differs depending on how well a drug is extracted by the liver. There are two major types of reactions. The first, *phase I reactions*, result in chemical modification of reactive groups by oxidation, reduction, hydroxylation, sulfoxidation, deamination, dealkylation, or methylation. Such modifications usually involve one of several enzymatic systems, including the mixed-function oxidases, cytochromes b_5 and P-450 (microsomal), and the glutathione S-acyltransferases (cytoplasmic). These biochemical reactions usually lead to *inactivation* of drugs such as barbiturates and benzodiazepines. However, *activation* also may occur. For example, cortisone is activated to cortisol and prednisone to prednisolone (both products being more potent than the parent compounds); imipramine, a depressant, is converted to desmethylimipramine, an antidepressant. In the same manner, phase I reactions may even convert a nontoxic compound to a toxic one, as in the metabolism of isoniazid and acetaminophen. Similarly, some carcinogens may be activated by formation of highly reactive epoxide intermediates in the liver, while other carcinogens may be detoxified.

The enzymes responsible for phase I reactions, especially those involving the cytochrome P-450 system, can be induced by drugs such as ethanol, barbiturates, haloperidol, and glutethimide. Conversely, hepatic microsomal enzymes may be inhibited by agents such as chloramphenicol, cimetidine, disulfiram, dextropropoxyphene, allopurinol, and, paradoxically, ethanol. The concomitant administration of two drugs metabolized by the same microsomal enzyme may result in modification, potentiation, or diminution of the pharmacologic efficacy of either or both drugs. Activity of phase I reactions also may change with aging.

Phase II reactions may follow phase I reactions or proceed independently; these involve the conversion of substances to their glucuronide, sulfate, acetyl, taurine, or glycine derivatives, thereby converting lipophilic substances to water-soluble derivatives and permitting their excretion in bile or urine. Conjugation catalyzed by microsomal UDP (uridine diphosphate)-glucuronyltransferases to form glucuronide derivatives is one of the most common phase II reactions. In general, the conjugates are more soluble than the parent compound and are pharmacologically inactive.

An awareness that there may be varying degrees of impairment in the hepatic uptake, detoxification, and excretion of certain drugs is important in the clinical management of patients with chronic liver disease. Portal-systemic shunting of blood may decrease the "first-pass effect" of drugs absorbed from the gut. In cirrhosis, altered intrahepatic hemodynamics due to a disordered liver architecture also may reduce the rates of hepatic drug clearance. Hypoalbuminemia will permit drugs usually bound to albumin to be present in increased concentrations of their unbound form in the circulation and extracellular spaces; this may result in an increased activity of such drugs. Most important, a decrease in the amount of function of microsomal enzymes responsible for phase I and phase II reactions will result in slower rates of drug inactivation and elimination. Drugs for which there may be a decreased clearance in patients with liver disease include anticonvulsants (e.g., phenytoin, phenobarbital), anti-inflammatory agents (e.g., acetaminophen, phenylbutazone, glucocorticoids), minor tranquilizers, cardioactive drugs (e.g., lidocaine, quinidine, propranolol), and antibiotics (e.g., nafcillin, chloramphenicol, tetracyclines, clindamycin, trimethoprim, rifampin, pyrazinamide). This will lead to decreased dosage requirements and a narrowing of the range between therapeutic and toxic drug levels. Finally, the patient with chronic liver disease may demonstrate alterations in the pharmacologic effects of drugs in addition to or independent of changes in their pharmacokinetics, such as an increased central nervous system sensitivity to opiates and other sedatives.

The difficulties in safely administering pharmacologic agents to patients with both acute and chronic liver disease are underscored by the frequency with which administration of benzodiazepines is cited as precipitating hepatic coma. It may be very difficult clinically to determine whether agitation, confusion, and irrational behavior are due to early hepatic encephalopathy or are related to the concurrent use of benzodiazepines, opiates, barbiturates, and other depressants. It should be recognized that there is great variation of drug clearance in patients with liver disease; although data on average clearances may provide a reasonable estimate for initial dosages, subsequent adjustments in dose need to be individualized in order to attain the desired plasma drug concentration.

The mechanism by which some agents exert a hepatotoxic effect may involve the same metabolic pathways responsible for normal drug detoxification. The mechanism of acetaminophen toxicity is particularly illustrative. Acetaminophen is metabolized and detoxified by the hepatic mixed-function oxygenase system, but one of the intermediate products is a potent free radical (postulated metabolite N-acetylimidoquinone) which can inactivate many enzymes and proteins by binding irreversibly to their sulfhydryl groups. Normally, this interaction can be prevented by reduced glutathione. In the presence of excessive amounts of the acetaminophen free radical (e.g., from overdosage or underlying liver disease), the glutathione levels of the hepatocytes are readily exhausted, and the excess free radicals can lead to inactivation of cellular proteins and produce widespread hepatocellular necrosis. In the case of acetaminophen overdosage, the very early administration of sulfhydryl groups in the form of N-acetylcysteine can often prevent this drug-induced liver injury.

HORMONE METABOLISM In addition to its role in the metabolism of diverse pharmacologic agents, the liver is also responsible for inactivation or modification of several endogenous hormones; therefore, chronic liver disease may be accompanied by signs of apparent hormonal imbalance. Some hormones (e.g., insulin and glucagon) are inactivated in the liver by proteolysis or deamination. Thyroxine and triiodothyronine are metabolized in the liver by reactions involving deiodination. Steroid hormones, such as glucocorticoids and aldosterone, are first inactivated to their tetrahydro derivative (by reduction of the Δ^4 double bond and the 3-keto group), followed by conjugation, mostly with glucuronic acid. Testosterone is metabolized to the isomeric 17-ketosteroids androsterone and etiocholanolone and excreted in the urine mostly as sulfate conjugates. Estrogens, such as estradiol, may be converted to estriol and estrone and then conjugated with glucuronic acid or sulfate. Abnormalities in estrogen (and testosterone) metabolism are believed to be involved in the development of the spider angiomas, loss of axillary or pubic hair, and testicular atrophy frequently seen in patients with chronic liver disease. In addition, increased portal-systemic shunting of testosterone and androstenedione secondary to portal hypertension may lead to the development of gynecomastia in cirrhotic males due to increased peripheral conversion to estradiol and estrone, especially in patients with alcoholic cirrhosis. In patients with alcoholic liver disease, feminization also may be related to the direct toxic effects of alcohol on the gonadal-pituitary-hypothalamic axis which lead to the overall reduction in serum testosterone found in patients with cirrhosis. Similar effects are also seen in patients with hemochromatosis due to deposition of iron in these sites. However, gynecomastia is often lacking in the latter, apparently due to a coincident reduction in plasma concentration of androstenedione, a major precursor for estrogen synthesis.

Estrogens also act directly on the liver to impair hepatic secretory activity. Estradiol and related estrogens, such as those present in

contraceptive pills, interfere with sodium sulfobromophthalein and bile salt excretion and worsen the preexisting defect in secretion of conjugated bilirubin in patients with Dubin-Johnson syndrome; they also may elevate plasma alkaline phosphatase levels (see Chap. 263). Related steroids such as etiocholanolone and pregnanediol have been shown to stimulate δ-aminolevulinic acid (ALA) synthetase activity, leading to increased porphobilinogen excretion. Since these steroids exert these effects only in their unconjugated form, the increased hepatic levels of δ-aminolevulinic acid synthetase in patients with alcoholic cirrhosis may be secondary to the action of gonadal steroids.

LIPID METABOLISM: FATTY ACIDS AND TRIGLYCERIDES Under normal conditions, most of the fatty acids taken up by the liver and esterified to triglyceride are derived from adipose tissue or the diet. Some fatty acids (especially saturated ones) are synthesized in the liver from acetate. The fatty acids may then be converted enzymatically to triglyceride, esterified with cholesterol, incorporated into phospholipids, or oxidized to CO_2 or ketone bodies. Most of the triglyceride is produced for export, but in order to be secreted it must be converted to lipoproteins by combining with relatively specific apoprotein moieties. This emphasizes the importance of protein synthesis for the release and secretion of triglyceride from the liver. It should be noted that the liver plays a major role in regulating lipoprotein levels by virtue of both its degradative and synthetic functions. Thus the liver is quantitatively the major site of low-density lipoprotein (LDL) catabolism, with dual high- and low-affinity receptor-mediated pathways playing a role. In addition, chylomicron remnants are removed and degraded by the liver, where their constituents have a number of metabolic effects. The liver is not only the primary site of very low density lipoprotein (VLDL) secretion but also accounts for a major portion of its subsequent degradation by mechanisms similar to that of chylomicron remnant degradation and conversion to LDL via the action of hepatic lipase. The liver also may play a role in high-density lipoprotein (HDL) catabolism. It is noteworthy that with the exception of cholestatic disease (see below), clinically significant alterations in lipoprotein and cholesterol metabolism are usually not found in patients with chronic liver disease.

Studies on the production of fatty liver have shown that singly or in combination, one or more of the steps depicted in Fig. 264-3 may be involved. An increased influx of fatty acids mobilized from adipose tissue due to drugs (e.g., ethanol or glucocorticoids) or secondary to diabetic ketosis may lead to a fatty liver. Similarly, increased levels of fatty acids in the liver, either from enhanced fatty acid synthesis or from decreased fatty acid oxidation, may lead to increased triglyceride formation. In some instances (e.g., ethanol excess) there also may be increases in the carbohydrate backbone, α-glycerophosphate, involved in fatty acid esterification to triglyceride. Since release of triglyceride involves the formation of lipoproteins, lipid accumulation may occur because of decreased apoprotein synthesis. This appears to be the case in fatty livers seen in patients with protein-calorie malnutrition (kwashiorkor) and due to toxins such as carbon tetrachloride, phosphorus, or ethionine, as well as following excessive doses of antibiotics such as tetracycline that can inhibit protein synthesis. Finally, there may be impaired lipoprotein secretion from the liver. Different alterations disrupting hepatic fat metabolism may lead to different patterns of fat accumulation designated *macrovesicular* (most common) and *microvesicular*; these are reviewed in Chap. 270. Alcohol is perhaps the most common agent leading to a fatty liver, but the mechanism(s) whereby alcohol leads to increased liver triglyceride is not clear. Depending on factors such as dose or duration, alcohol ingestion may affect any of the seven steps shown in Fig. 264-3; however, the primary factor for the production of the alcohol-induced fatty liver remains to be determined. The alterations in the redox state due to excessive accumulation of NADH resulting from oxidation of alcohol also may contribute.

In addition to the changes leading to fatty liver, there are many metabolic alterations which may be found in the blood of patients following the ingestion of large amounts of alcohol. These include, among others, *increased* plasma levels of lactate, proline, urate, and

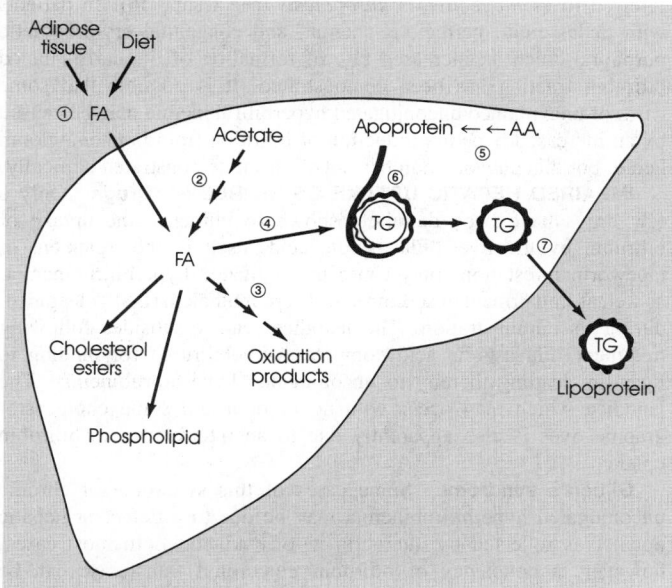

FIGURE 264-3 Factors in the uptake and esterification of fatty acids to triglyceride by the liver, including the formation and release of triglyceride as lipoprotein. The numbers refer to steps, which, if altered, may result in increased liver triglyceride (i.e., fatty liver).

triglycerides and *decreased* plasma levels of glucose, magnesium, phosphate, and triiodothyronine (T_3).

CHOLESTEROL Cholesterol and bile acid synthesis is carried out primarily by the liver. Cholesterol synthesis is subject to a number of metabolic controls, most of them mediated via the rate-limiting biosynthetic enzyme 3-hydroxy-3-methylglutaryl coenzyme A reductase (HMG-CoA reductase). Cholesterol exists either free or combined with fatty acids in the form of cholesterol esters; in the plasma, both are found primarily in association with β-lipoproteins. The plasma and liver also contain lecithin–cholesterol acyltransferase (LCAT), an enzyme involved in the conversion of free cholesterol to its esterified form. Since there is exchange of free cholesterol between tissues, changes in plasma cholesterol levels reflect changes in total body cholesterol. However, decreases in plasma cholesterol esters may reflect hepatic damage and impaired hepatic cholesterol esterification.

Severe liver injury often leads to a decrease in *total* serum cholesterol levels, including both free and esterified fractions. This may be due to decreased synthesis of cholesterol and cholesterol esters, decreased apoprotein synthesis, or both. In cholestasis (either intra- or extrahepatic), total serum cholesterol often increases strikingly. Disorders of cholestasis are associated with marked abnormalities of lipoprotein metabolism. In primary biliary cirrhosis there are pronounced elevations in serum free cholesterol and LDL; conversely, serum HDL is reduced and may disappear from the serum in patients with long-standing disease. Similar but less marked changes are seen in other cholestatic conditions.

The increase in serum free cholesterol (and phospholipid) and the concomitant decrease in esterified cholesterol in cholestasis may be related to a decrease in the hepatic production of LCAT. Reduced levels of LCAT are also correlated with the appearance of an abnormal LDL, referred to as *lipoprotein X* (LP-X). Although LP-X, which has a high content of free cholesterol and triglyceride, was originally thought to be a specific indicator of biliary tract obstruction, it is evident that it appears in any cholestatic condition. While the depressed hepatic production of LCAT may be responsible for altered lipid content and composition of lipoproteins, the factors leading to the overall increase in total serum cholesterol are not clear. In experimental animals, bile duct ligation results in a net increase in hepatic cholesterol synthesis, and in "regurgitation" of bile salts, cholesterol, and LP-X into venous radicals. However, it is difficult

to translate these experimental findings to the patient with primary biliary cirrhosis unless any insult to cells lining the biliary canaliculi and ductules can impair the delicate balance of lipid synthesis and removal.

The alterations in cholesterol and related substances resulting from liver disease may lead to significant changes in the composition of erythrocyte membranes. Such changes in composition lead to altered morphology with the development of spur and burr cell forms. The presence of these altered erythrocytes is usually an ominous sign of advanced liver disease.

Most of the derangements of hepatic metabolism discussed above are evident only in patients with severe or long-standing liver disease. Indeed, in all but the most severe cases of acute viral hepatitis, hepatic metabolic functions are remarkably well preserved, and in most cases of mild to moderate acute viral hepatitis, it is uncommon to observe clinically important alterations in carbohydrate, protein, and lipid metabolism. However, in the patients with severe or fulminant hepatitis, whether from a viral or toxic agent, the metabolic derangements may be similar to those seen in more chronic disease. For example, in fulminant hepatitis there may be pronounced hypoprothrombinemia and impaired coagulation, hypoalbuminemia, and the relatively acute development of ascites, as well as hyperammonemia and encephalopathy. However, in contrast to patients with cirrhosis, abnormalities in carbohydrate metabolism are more likely to lead to profound hypoglycemia than to hyperglycemia. This hypoglycemia appears to reflect both a marked decrease in hepatic glycogen stores and a diminished glucagon responsiveness. There also may be poor oral intake due to nausea and anorexia together with increased glucose utilization secondary to hyperinsulinemia (due to portal-systemic shunting and decreased insulin degradation).

REFERENCES

ARIAS IM et al: *The Liver: Biology and Pathophysiology*, 2d ed. New York, Raven, 1988

BUTTERWORTH RF: Pathogenesis and treatment of portal-systemic encephalopathy: An update. Dig Dis Sci 37:321, 1992

CAVALLO-PERIN P et al: Mechanism of insulin resistance in human liver cirrhosis. Evidence of a combined receptor and post-receptor defect. J Clin Invest 75:1659, 1985

COOPER AD: Role of the liver in the degradation of lipoproteins. Gastroenterology 88:192, 1984

FLANNERY DB et al: Current status of hyperammonemic syndromes. Hepatology 2:495, 1982

HOYUMPA AM et al: Hepatic encephalopathy. Gastroenterology 77:803, 1979

KLEG HK et al: Conversion of androgens to estrogens in idiopathic hemochromatosis: Comparison with alcoholic liver disease. J Clin Endocrin Metab 61:1, 1985

MILLWARD-SADLER GH et al: *Wright's Liver and Biliary Disease*, 3d ed. London, Saunders, 1992

OWEN OE et al: Hepatic, gut and renal substrate flux rates in patients with hepatic cirrhosis. J Clin Invest 68:240, 1981

ROTHSCHILD MA et al: Serum albumin. Hepatology 8:355, 1988

SHERLOCK S, DOOLEY J: *Diseases of the Liver and Biliary System*, 9th ed. Oxford, Blackwell, 1993

SMITH AR et al: Alteration in plasma and CSF amino acids, amines and metabolites in hepatic coma. Ann Surg 187:343, 1978

WILLIAMS RC: Drug administration in hepatic disease. N Engl J Med 309:1616, 1983

ZAKIM D, BOYER TD: *Hepatology, A Textbook of Liver Disease*, 2d ed. Philadelphia, Saunders, 1990

265 BILIRUBIN METABOLISM AND HYPERBILIRUBINEMIA

KURT J. ISSELBACHER

The normal metabolism of bilirubin and the approach to the patient with jaundice have been presented in Chap. 42. With a consideration of these pathways, the disorders of bilirubin metabolism can be divided into four major categories, namely, those due to (1) increased pigment production, (2) reduced hepatic uptake of bilirubin, (3) impaired hepatic conjugation, and (4) decreased excretion of the conjugated pigment from the liver into bile. The first three of these disorders are associated with predominantly unconjugated hyperbilirubinemia. The fourth group, defective excretion, is associated with predominantly conjugated hyperbilirubinemia and bilirubinuria.

DISORDERS CAUSING PREDOMINANTLY UNCONJUGATED HYPERBILIRUBINEMIA

The plasma concentration of unconjugated bilirubin is determined by (1) the rate at which newly synthesized bilirubin enters the plasma (bilirubin turnover) and (2) the rate of removal of bilirubin by the liver (hepatic bilirubin clearance). Disturbances of the latter can result from derangements of hepatic bilirubin uptake, conjugation, or both. Measurements of these variables, although not routinely available, permit a classification of patients into those with *increased bilirubin turnover* (e.g., hemolysis), those with *decreased bilirubin clearance* (e.g., Gilbert's syndrome), and those in whom both mechanisms operate.

OVERPRODUCTION OF BILIRUBIN (INCREASED TURNOVER) Increased destruction of circulating erythrocytes (intravascular and extravascular hemolysis)
In disorders associated with hemolysis, most commonly the hemolytic anemias, the rate of bilirubin production is increased and may even exceed the amount that can be removed by a normal liver. The resulting jaundice is primarily an unconjugated hyperbilirubinemia. There is often also a small increase in the serum conjugated bilirubin. If significant anemia or other adverse factors are present (e.g., fever, sepsis, hypoxemia, or vascular collapse), the ability of the liver to handle the pigment load will be compromised, and the degree of jaundice will be greater.

The clinical and diagnostic features of the various hemolytic anemias are described in Chap. 307. The presence of reticulocytosis, shortened red blood cell survival, and increased fecal urobilinogen, in the absence of clinical and laboratory evidence of liver disease, strongly suggest hemolysis and overproduction of bilirubin as the cause of the jaundice. It is obvious, however, that in some cases (e.g., cirrhosis, tumors, and sepsis), hemolysis *plus* deranged liver function may be present. In most cases of uncomplicated hemolytic states, the mean serum bilirubin level will be in the range of 51 to 68 μmol/L (3 to 4 mg/dL); rarely, higher levels may be seen.

Jaundice due to increased pigment production also may be seen as a consequence of *tissue infarction* (e.g., pulmonary infarcts) and large *collections of blood in tissues* (e.g., leakage from blood vessels after catheterization studies, rupture of an aortic aneurysm). If hypotension and hypoxemia also supervene, jaundice is usually more pronounced, and the resulting impairment of liver function also may lead to a significant increase in the serum conjugated bilirubin level (see "Postoperative Jaundice," below).

Except in early infancy, elevations of serum unconjugated bilirubin levels are not harmful per se, and the prognosis is that of the hemolytic process itself. However, in the neonatal state and infancy, unconjugated bilirubin levels above 340 μmol/L (20 mg/dL) may lead to *kernicterus* due to bilirubin deposition in the lipid-rich basal ganglia (see Chap. 378). Chronic overproduction of bilirubin may result in the formation of gallstones composed predominantly of bilirubin ("pigment stones"). In this situation, all the potential complications of calculus disease of the biliary tract (Chap. 272) may be superimposed on the chronic hemolytic state which produced it.

Increased production of bilirubin from sources other than circulating erythrocytes
About 15 to 20 percent of the circulating bilirubin is normally derived from sources other than the destruction of circulating red blood cells. This represents the so-called early-labeled fraction; it includes the synthesis of bilirubin from nonhemoglobin heme in the liver and from hemoglobin heme in the marrow.

In some conditions, jaundice results from an increased destruction of red blood cells or their precursors in the marrow—a process referred to as *ineffective erythropoiesis* (see Chap. 56). In patients with thalassemia, pernicious anemia, and congenital erythropoietic porphyria, such an increased rate of formation of the early-labeled bilirubin fraction has been demonstrated. It is possible that some cases of unexplained unconjugated hyperbilirubinemia may be caused by an increased hepatic production of bilirubin from nonhemoglobin heme, but this phenomenon has not yet been demonstrated clinically.

IMPAIRED HEPATIC UPTAKE OF BILIRUBIN   Drugs
Only a few drugs have been definitely shown to influence the uptake of bilirubin by the liver. Flavaspidic acid, used in the treatment of tapeworm infestation, may cause unconjugated hyperbilirubinemia, as well as impairment of sodium sulfobromophthalein (BSP) clearance, during its administration. The jaundice readily subsides following treatment. Flavaspidic acid competes with bilirubin for binding to ligandin, leading thereby to unconjugated hyperbilirubinemia. The jaundice which may occur with novobiocin and some cholecystographic dyes is also apparently due to an interference in bilirubin uptake.

Gilbert's syndrome
Some cases of this syndrome of chronic unconjugated hyperbilirubinemia may be due to a defect in hepatic uptake (as reflected by alteration in BSP kinetics). In most cases, however, a deficiency of bilirubin glucuronyl transferase can be demonstrated. Hence this syndrome is best considered as a defect in bilirubin conjugation (see below).

IMPAIRED BILIRUBIN CONJUGATION (DECREASED ACTIVITY OF BILIRUBIN GLUCURONOSYL TRANSFERASE)   Neonatal jaundice (physiologic jaundice of the newborn)
Almost every infant exhibits some transient unconjugated hyperbilirubinemia between the second and fifth days of life. While during gestation the placenta serves to clear bilirubin from the fetus, after birth infants must detoxify the pigments themselves. However, at this stage the hepatic enzyme glucuronosyl transferase is still "immature" and inadequate for the task. As a result, unconjugated bilirubinemia develops, usually not exceeding 86 μmol/L (5 mg/dL). The activity of glucuronosyl transferase increases within several days to 2 weeks after birth, and concomitantly, the serum bilirubin level returns to normal. In the premature infant, the glucuronosyl transferase activity is less, and the neonatal jaundice may be more pronounced. The "maturation" of the fetal and neonatal liver may be enhanced by treatment of the pregnant mother or the newborn infant with phenobarbital or related drugs. This results in a clear-cut reduction of the degree and duration of unconjugated hyperbilirubinemia in the newborn. In infants with a superimposed hemolytic process (e.g., erythroblastosis), the excessive pigment load leads to more pronounced jaundice, and bilirubin levels may exceed 340 μmol/L (20 mg/dL). It should be emphasized that neonatal jaundice is not present at the time of delivery; if jaundice is present at birth, other causes must be considered.

The cytoplasmic liver cell protein ligandin (glutathione-S-transferase B) binds bilirubin in the hepatocyte and may assist in the transfer of bilirubin to the endoplasmic reticulum for conjugation (Chap. 42). Deficiency of ligandin may contribute to neonatal jaundice.

An additional facet of the "immature" liver is a concomitant defect in the excretion of *conjugated* bilirubin. Rarely this defect persists beyond the time needed for the development of adequate glucuronide conjugation and may explain the occasional presence of conjugated hyperbilirubinemia in infants with erythroblastosis (*inspissated bile syndrome*).

When in the neonatal state unconjugated bilirubin levels approach or exceed 340 μmol/L (20 mg/dL), the infants may develop and die of *kernicterus* (bilirubin encephalopathy). This condition results from unconjugated bilirubin deposition in the lipid-rich basal ganglia. In the past, treatment consisted of exchange transfusions, and albumin infusions were used to increase binding of bilirubin in the circulation and diminish its entry into the brain. The current approach is *phototherapy;* intense illumination of these patients with strong white or blue light leads to the *photoisomerization* of bilirubin to water-soluble isomers that are rapidly excreted in the bile without the prior

TABLE 265-1 Hereditary unconjugated hyperbilirubinemias with deficiency of glucuronosyl transferase

Features	Mild (Gilbert's syndrome)	Moderate (Crigler-Najjar syndrome type II)	Severe (Crigler-Najjar syndrome type I)
Inheritance	Unclear*	Dominant†	Recessive
Serum bilirubin, μmol/L (mg/dL)	17–102 (1–6)	102–340 (6–20)	340–770 (20–45)
Kernicterus	No	Rare	Yes
Conjugated bilirubin in bile	Yes (↑ monoconjugates)	Yes (↑ ↑ monoconjugates)	No
Response to phenobarbital	Yes	Yes	No
Bilirubin conjugation	↓ ‡	↓ ↓	Absent

* Many cases have no familial incidence.
† Variable expressivity.
‡ Other defects such as occult hemolysis and decreased bilirubin uptake may coexist.

need of conjugation. Another novel approach involves decreasing bilirubin production from heme by inhibitors of the enzyme heme oxygenase. Synthetic protoporphyrins, such as tin protoporphyrin, have been administered successfully to patients with neonatal hyperbilirubinemia with marked reduction in the serum bilirubin and with no major side effects.

Hereditary glucuronosyl transferase deficiency   There are currently three syndromes that fall into this category. As indicated in Table 265-1, they reflect progressive decreases in the activity of glucuronosyl transferase and thus may be part of a spectrum, i.e., from minimal deficiency to complete absence of bilirubin glucuronosyl transferase.

GILBERT'S SYNDROME   Since the original report by Gilbert in 1907, there has been an increased recognition of this benign but chronic disorder characterized by mild, persistent, unconjugated hyperbilirubinemia. The patient usually does not manifest this disorder until after the second decade and is often unaware of the jaundice until it is detected by physical examination or routine laboratory testing. The total serum bilirubin level usually ranges and fluctuates from 21 to 51 μmol/L (1.2 to 3 mg/dL) and rarely exceeds 86 μmol/L (5 mg/dL). With the van den Bergh diazo reaction, less than 20 percent of bilirubin gives a direct reaction; however, studies using more accurate methods (such as high-pressure liquid chromatography) show that the serum bilirubin in patients with Gilbert's syndrome is almost all unconjugated. Typically, the jaundice fluctuates and is exacerbated following prolonged fasting (see below), surgery, fever or infection, and excessive exertion or alcohol ingestion. Liver function tests are normal, and the liver cells usually appear normal by light microscopy.

With the exception of hemolytic anemias, Gilbert's syndrome is probably the most common cause of mild unconjugated hyperbilirubinemia. Detailed studies show these patients to have a partial deficiency of bilirubin glucuronosyl transferase. Some patients also manifest decreased bilirubin uptake and increased hemolysis. Decreased glucuronosyl transferase alone or together with a decrease in bilirubin uptake appears to account for the observed *decrease in hepatic bilirubin clearance*. A decreased clearance and hepatic uptake of bile salts also have been shown.

Previously, Gilbert's syndrome was traditionally defined as mild, chronic, unconjugated hyperbilirubinemia occurring in the absence of hemolysis. However, with the use of radiobilirubin kinetics and erythrocyte half-life studies, at least two forms of Gilbert's syndrome have been described. One group includes patients with decreased bilirubin clearance and *no hemolysis*. A second group includes those who also have *evidence of hemolysis* (often occult) and hence increased bilirubin turnover. The simultaneous presence of both derangements appears to be a chance occurrence of two not uncommon disorders

in the same patient and does not imply a causal relationship. There is additional evidence of the heterogeneity of patients with Gilbert's syndrome. Thus, some patients have an increase in hepatocyte lipofuscin and an increase in the smooth endoplasmic reticulum (SER); others show an increase in hepatic lysosomal enzymes.

A feature of Gilbert's syndrome which can be useful diagnostically is the increase in serum bilirubin following prolonged fasting or calorie deprivation. Patients with this disorder, when placed on 1255 kJ (300 kcal) per day for 2 days, will increase their serum bilirubin by 25 μmol/L (1.5 mg/dL) or more, the major increase being in the unconjugated fraction. A decrease in glucuronosyl transferase activity is needed to obtain this effect. Patients with hemolysis do not show an increase in serum bilirubin with fasting. As a reflection of the mild decrease in glucuronosyl transferase in Gilbert's syndrome, (1) serum bilirubin levels will decrease when the enzyme activity is enhanced following phenobarbital administration, and (2) the bile shows a modest increase in monoconjugates of bilirubin (see Table 265-1).

In general, the diagnosis of this benign but not uncommon disorder is made by exclusion. The syndrome is suspected in a patient with low-grade unconjugated hyperbilirubinemia with (1) no systemic symptoms, (2) *no overt* or clinically recognizable hemolysis, (3) normal tests of routine liver function, and (4) a liver biopsy (although usually not necessary) that is normal by light microscopy.

CRIGLER-NAJJAR SYNDROME (TYPES I AND II)   This disorder is known to exist in two forms. Type I is the clinically *severe* form (originally described by Crigler and Najjar) and is due to *absence of glucuronosyl transferase* (or lack of function of one or more isoenzymes of the transferase). Type II has more *moderate* clinical findings due to *partial deficiency of glucuronosyl transferase*. The major differences are summarized in Table 265-1.

Type I (Crigler-Najjar) is a rare disorder. Infants develop high unconjugated bilirubin levels in the serum [340 to 770 μmol/L (20 to 45 mg/dL)]. Absence of the enzyme can be demonstrated in the liver by enzymatic or molecular genetic techniques. Routine liver function tests are normal, as is liver histology. Because of the lack of glucuronosyl transferase activity, no conjugated bilirubin is formed by the liver; hence no bilirubin is secreted into the bile and liver, and the bile is colorless.

Phototherapy may temporarily and transiently reduce the unconjugated bilirubin level. Phenobarbital has no effect, since the enzyme defect is complete and no drug "induction" is therefore possible. Affected infants usually die within the first year of life, although some patients have survived to the second or third decade of life. Death is usually from kernicterus. A strain of rats (Gunn rat) with the type I defect exists and is widely used as an animal model of the Crigler-Najjar syndrome (type I).

Type II patients have a *partial deficiency* of glucuronosyl transferase (due to a mutation of the enzyme) and their disorder is less severe. Serum unconjugated bilirubin levels are lower [103 to 340 μmol/L (6 to 20 mg/dL)], jaundice may not appear until adolescence, and neurologic complications are uncommon. The bile contains variable amounts of conjugated bilirubin with a significant increase in monoconjugates. Phenobarbital is effective in lowering the serum bilirubin level in type II patients. However, the disorder is relatively benign in those patients whose bilirubin level is less than 308 to 340 μmol/L (18 to 20 mg/dL).

Acquired deficiency of glucuronosyl transferase   As with any enzyme, glucuronosyl transferase is susceptible to inhibition by a variety of agents, and because of the decreased activity of the enzyme in the neonatal state, such inhibition may be more evident at that time. Neonatal jaundice may be aggravated or prolonged in infants treated with *drugs* such as chloramphenicol or novobiocin or with *vitamin K*. In some breast-fed infants, jaundice has been ascribed to the presence in *breast milk* of pregnane-3β,20α-diol, an inhibitor of glucuronosyl transferase. When the infant is removed from the breast, the "breast-milk jaundice" subsides.

Hypothyroidism delays the normal "maturation" of glucuronosyl transferase. In cretins, neonatal jaundice may be prolonged for weeks or months. In fact, the presence of prolonged unconjugated hyperbilirubinemia after birth may be a clue to an underlying hypothyroidism.

In the infant, as well as in the adult, *liver cell damage* leads to impairment in glucuronide conjugation as a result of decreased transferase activity. However, since excretion is probably the rate-limiting step in bilirubin metabolism, and since this step appears to be interfered with to a greater extent than conjugation in parenchymal liver disease, the pigment which accumulates in the blood is predominantly conjugated bilirubin.

DISORDERS CAUSING COMBINED CONJUGATED AND UNCONJUGATED HYPERBILIRUBINEMIA

In jaundice due to primary liver disease, the plasma usually exhibits elevated levels of both conjugated and unconjugated bilirubin, and *urine contains bilirubin.* The relative proportions of the two pigments are highly variable. In many familial hepatic abnormalities (described below) and in some forms of liver injury, the jaundice is largely due to increases in conjugated bilirubin. Such a serum pigment pattern is also seen with extrahepatic biliary obstruction. One *cannot differentiate* intrahepatic and extrahepatic causes of jaundice from either the levels or proportions of unconjugated and conjugated bilirubin in serum. Thus the main purpose of the initial fractionation of the serum bilirubin is to distinguish hepatic parenchymal and biliary obstructive disease from the disorders associated with predominantly unconjugated hyperbilirubinemia.

FAMILIAL DEFECTS IN HEPATIC EXCRETORY FUNCTION
Dubin-Johnson syndrome   This disorder, also called *chronic idiopathic jaundice*, is a benign, autosomally inherited hyperbilirubinemia characterized by the presence of a dark pigment in the centrilobular region of the liver cells. Functionally, there exists a *defect in biliary excretion* of bilirubin, cholephilic dyes, and porphyrins. Using the diazo method for measuring bilirubin, the serum pigment in these patients typically is in the range of 51 to 257 μmol/L (3 to 15 mg/dL) and predominantly of the conjugated type. However, with the newer and more accurate method (alkaline methanolysis and high-pressure liquid chromatography), homozygous patients with the Dubin-Johnson syndrome have been shown to have significant levels of serum *unconjugated bilirubin.* This finding may in part reflect pigment which, after conjugation by the liver, is deconjugated in the hepatobiliary system and refluxed into the plasma. Moreover, the serum contains more diconjugated than monoconjugated bilirubin, just the reverse of what is seen in acquired hepatobiliary disease and Rotor syndrome. This reversed ratio is believed to be characteristic and diagnostic for homozygous patients.

Patients with Dubin-Johnson syndrome may be asymptomatic or have vague constitutional or gastrointestinal symptoms. Not infrequently the liver is slightly enlarged; in about one-fourth of cases there is mild hepatic tenderness. Oral and intravenous cholangiography fails to visualize the biliary tract. There is typically and characteristically a late rise in the plasma BSP elimination curve at *90 min*. This is caused by the reflux from the liver of the conjugated dye and reflects the defect in the hepatic excretory transport maximum (T_m). It is noteworthy that there is no such secondary rise in plasma when dyes that are not conjugated by the liver are given, such as indocyanine green. When bile salts such as ursodeoxycholic acid are given, these patients show a decreased hepatic uptake and clearance. In the liver the striking feature is the presence of a *brown or black pigment in the hepatocytes.* Some findings suggest that this unique pigment is "melanin-like"; others indicate it to be a polymer of epinephrine metabolites.

These patients also show an abnormality in coproporphyrin excretion. Normal urine contains mostly coproporphyrin III and small amounts of coproporphyrin I; Dubin-Johnson patients show a reversal of this pattern; i.e., they excrete predominantly coproporphyrin I. Heterozygotes show an intermediate excretory pattern.

There is impaired excretion of many metabolites, including conjugated bilirubin, BSP, and iodinated dyes. Excretion of bile acids, however, is normal. Oral contraceptive agents may accentuate hyperbilirubinemia or may produce jaundice for the first time. Features of cholestasis such as pruritus or steatorrhea are usually lacking, and specifically, serum alkaline phosphatase levels are *not* elevated. The overall prognosis of the disorder is excellent.

Rotor syndrome   This is similar in many respects to the Dubin-Johnson syndrome. However, *there is no pigment in the liver cells*, and the serum conjugated bilirubin has more monoconjugates than diglucuronide conjugates. The gallbladder is usually visualized on cholecystography, and there is an increase in the *total* urinary coproporphyrins but *not* an increased percentage in excretion of coproporphyrin I. The BSP excretion pattern does *not* show a secondary rise at 90 min. The impairment in excretion which is typical of Dubin-Johnson syndrome is not present; instead, in most cases of the Rotor syndrome there is impairment of *hepatic storage capacity (S)*. This rare syndrome is inherited as an autosomal recessive trait and is genetically distinct from Dubin-Johnson syndrome.

Benign familial recurrent cholestasis   This is a relatively rare syndrome characterized by recurrent attacks of pruritus and jaundice. During an attack, the serum alkaline phosphatase and bile acid levels are markedly elevated, and liver biopsy shows the morphologic features of cholestasis. However, there is no mechanical biliary obstruction, with cholangiography revealing a patent biliary tree. Remissions are the rule, and at such times hepatic function tests and liver morphologic features are usually normal. The cause of the disorder is unknown; cirrhosis does not develop, and the disorder is benign. A congenital origin has been postulated on the basis of the early age of onset and familial incidence.

Recurrent jaundice of pregnancy   This form of jaundice is also known as *intrahepatic cholestasis of pregnancy.* During a normal pregnancy, some derangements in liver function occur, especially during the last trimester. Usually these consist of slight increases in BSP retention and in serum alkaline phosphatase. This mild increase in alkaline phosphatase during pregnancy is normally of placental rather than of hepatic origin. With a normal pregnancy, elevations of serum bilirubin level either do not occur or are less than 34 μmol/L (2 mg/dL).

In a small number of pregnant women an intrahepatic cholestasis may appear. This usually occurs in the third trimester but may develop any time after the seventh week of gestation. The clinical features consist primarily of pruritus and jaundice. Serum bilirubin levels are usually less than 103 μmol/L (6 mg/dL). The serum alkaline phosphatase and cholesterol levels are elevated significantly, while other liver function tests are only mildly deranged. Histologically, the liver shows varying degrees of cholestasis but only a few parenchymal cell changes. The clinical and laboratory abnormalities subside promptly after delivery and are usually normal within 7 to 14 days.

This condition has been seen more frequently in Scandinavia and Europe than in the United States. Since steroid hormones and specifically estrogens can induce changes in hepatic excretory function in normal individuals (see Chap. 264), these patients probably have an increased susceptibility or sensitivity to the hepatic effects of estrogenic and progestational hormones. The intrahepatic cholestasis is usually termed *recurrent*, since the syndrome often (but not always) reappears in subsequent pregnancies. The process is benign and self-limited, and treatment is usually not needed, but cholestyramine administration will diminish the pruritus. This disorder must be distinguished from the many other causes of jaundice not unique to pregnancy, such as viral hepatitis. It also must be distinguished from the idiopathic *acute fatty liver of pregnancy* and the *tetracycline-induced fatty liver.* The latter two conditions are rare, occur in the last trimester, and have a high fatality rate; however, in these disorders there is evidence of diffuse parenchymal damage and not only cholestasis.

TABLE 265-2 Conditions causing or contributing to postoperative jaundice

Increased pigment load
  A Hemolytic anemia
  B Transfusions (especially of stored blood)
  C Resorption of hematomas, blood in extravascular spaces
Impaired hepatocellular function
  A Hepatitis-like picture
    1 Halothane anesthesia
    2 Drugs
    3 Shock
    4 Infection with hepatitis viruses
  B Cholestatic picture
    1 Hypotension, hypoxemia
    2 Drugs
    3 Sepsis
Extrahepatic obstruction
  A Bile duct injury
  B Choledocholithiasis

ACQUIRED DEFECTS OF HEPATIC EXCRETORY FUNCTION

Drug-induced cholestasis A condition entirely analogous to the intrahepatic cholestasis of pregnancy may occur in some women following the use of oral contraceptive agents. In some, mild cholestatic jaundice may occur, liver function returns to normal when the drugs are withdrawn, and chronic liver disease does not result. It is relevant that one-third of the reported patients with jaundice due to oral contraceptives also have a history of recurrent intrahepatic cholestasis of pregnancy.

The nature of these changes produced by the natural and synthetic female sex hormones is very similar to those resulting from the administration of certain testosterone analogues, especially those with α substitutions at the 17 position of the steroid nucleus. These agents (such as methyltestosterone and norethandrolone) commonly cause BSP retention and less commonly cause jaundice or significant changes in other liver functions. However, unlike the female hormones, these agents have been implicated as a cause of chronic liver disease, especially biliary cirrhosis.

Because of these phenomena, synthetic steroid sex hormones should not be used in patients with liver disease. Conversely, in individuals using these agents, the appearance of jaundice or elevations in serum aminotransferase (transaminase) or alkaline phosphatase levels contraindicates their further use. However, mild to moderate increases in BSP retention alone are probably not of clinical significance, although liver function tests should be carried out periodically.

As is discussed in detail in Chap. 266, there are many drugs which may produce not only cholestasis but liver injury resembling acute hepatitis or cholestatic hepatitis. In contrast to the jaundice produced by the steroid hormones, the clinical features are those of fever, rash, arthralgia, and sometimes eosinophilia, with the liver showing a pronounced inflammatory reaction. These features suggest that such

TABLE 265-3 Laboratory features in icteric states

Bilirubin disorder	Serum bilirubin Unconjugated	Conjugated	Urine bilirubin	Comments
OVERPRODUCTION				
A Hemolysis (intra- and extravascular)	↑	N	0	↑ Bilirubin turnover; serum bilirubin rarely exceeds 68 μmol/L (4 mg/dL)
B Ineffective erythropoiesis	↑	N	0	Splenomegaly; normal RBC survival; normoblasts in marrow
DEFECTIVE HEPATIC UPTAKE				
A Some drugs (e.g., flavaspidic acid, novobiocin)				
B Gilbert's syndrome (some cases)	↑	N	0	Normal liver biopsy
DEFECTIVE CONJUGATION				
A Neonatal jaundice	↑	Low	0	↓ Glucuronosyl transferase; ? ↓ ligandin
B Gilbert's syndrome	↑	Low	0	↓ Glucuronosyl transferase and ↓ bilirubin uptake; some may have ↑ hemolysis; bile contains ↑ monoconjugates
C Crigler-Najjar syndrome (types I and II)	↑	Low	0	Type I = absence of transferase Type II = deficiency of transferase; bile contains ↑↑ monoconjugates
DEFECTIVE EXCRETION				
A Intrahepatic obstruction				
1 Familial syndromes				
a Dubin-Johnson	↑	↑	+	Abnormal BSP curve, hepatic lipochrome pigment; ↑ urinary coproporphyrin type I
b Rotor	↑	↑	+	No liver pigment; ↑ total urinary coproporphyrin
2 Drugs (e.g., chloramphenicol, methyltestosterone)	↑	↑	+	↑ Alkaline phosphatase but other function tests usually normal
3 Benign recurrent cholestasis	↑	↑	+	↑ Alkaline phosphatase
4 Recurrent jaundice of pregnancy (third trimester)	↑	↑	+	↑ Alkaline phosphatase; may be reproduced in afflicted subjects by estrogens or progesterone
B Extrahepatic obstruction (tumors, stone, stricture of bile duct)				↑↑ Alkaline phosphatase (often > fourfold)
1 Partial	↑	↑	+	
2 Complete	↑	↑	+	
HEPATOCELLULAR DISEASE*				
A Hepatitis	↑	↑	+	Conjugated/total serum bilirubin >50–70%; liver biopsy important for diagnosis
B Cirrhosis: Same as hepatitis	↑	↑		

* Note that in hepatocellular disease there is generally an interference in all pathways of bilirubin metabolism (i.e., impaired uptake, conjugation, and excretion).

reactions are *allergic* or *toxic* in nature and therefore differ from the effects caused by the steroid hormones, which probably represent an exaggerated response by the liver to the normal action of these hormones.

Postoperative jaundice   The occurrence of postoperative jaundice is a problem of increasing importance. It is perhaps seen more frequently now than in earlier years because patients are able to undergo more major surgical procedures (i.e., cardiac surgery, repair of ruptured aneurysms) and survive. In approaching this problem, the possible pathogenic mechanisms listed in Table 265-2 need to be considered. The patient may have *pigment overload*, especially from blood transfusions (with hemolysis of stored blood), from resorption of blood in extravascular spaces, and less commonly, from hemolytic anemia. *Hepatocellular damage* and decreased liver cell function may occur due to concurrent use of hepatotoxic drugs (Chap. 266) or anesthetics such as halothane. Hepatocellular necrosis may follow profound shock; with lesser degrees of hypotension or hypoxemia, morphologic damage may be slight, but significant impairment of function may occur. Hence prior shock or hypotension plus pigment overload may produce significant jaundice. Extensive sepsis also can produce jaundice, often of a cholestatic type. Concurrent renal impairment due to hypotension and hypoxemia may enhance the degree of jaundice because the renal excretion of conjugated bilirubin is decreased. *Extrahepatic obstruction* due to surgical damage or stones needs to be considered and may be excluded by sonography.

A form of jaundice referred to as *benign postoperative intrahepatic cholestasis* may be seen. In the typical case, the patient has had major and prolonged surgery for a catastrophic event such as a ruptured aortic aneurysm complicated by hypotension and hypoxemia, extensive blood loss into tissues, and massive blood replacement. Jaundice may be noted on the second or third postoperative day, and the serum bilirubin, predominantly conjugated, may reach 340 to 680 µmol/L (20 to 40 mg/dL) by the eighth to tenth day. Serum alkaline phosphatase levels may be elevated three- to tenfold. Typically, the serum aspartate aminotransferase (AST, SGOT) is only mildly elevated. The liver morphology is striking in that necrosis is not seen, only cholestasis and erythrophagocytosis.

The cause of this type of postoperative cholestatic jaundice is uncertain. However, it probably reflects (1) increased pigment load, (2) decreased liver function due to hypoxemia and hypotension, and (3) decreased renal bilirubin excretion due to varying degrees of tubular necrosis as a result of shock. This diagnostic possibility must be considered in the postoperative patient with marked cholestatic jaundice. The course of the jaundice is self-limited and will subside if the other systemic complications do not predominate and lead to death.

Hepatitis and cirrhosis   These disorders, discussed in detail in Chaps. 266 to 268, constitute the *most common disorders associated with jaundice*. As has been stated previously, when the liver cell is damaged, as in viral hepatitis, there is often impairment in all three major hepatic phases of bilirubin metabolism, namely, uptake, conjugation, and excretion. Since the excretory step is the one which is rate-limiting and most readily affected by injury, significant amounts of conjugated bilirubin reenter the systemic circulation. There are also lesser increases in the serum unconjugated bilirubin. This phenomenon is probably a reflection of the impaired uptake and conjugation and is due in part to the shortened life span of red blood cells often found in liver disease. In most patients with hepatitis and cirrhosis, the total serum bilirubin levels tend not to exceed 860 µmol/L (50 mg/dL). (For a summary of laboratory features in icteric states, see Table 265-3.)

EXTRAHEPATIC BILIARY OBSTRUCTION   Anatomic or mechanical obstruction of the bile ducts is most commonly due to stones, tumors, or strictures. The clinical picture is quite similar to that of intrahepatic cholestasis, with pronounced elevations of the serum conjugated bilirubin and alkaline phosphatase levels. Usually, but not always, fever, pain, and chills may be present. In contrast to hepatitis and cirrhosis, the serum bilirubin level often tends to plateau and

rarely exceeds levels of 600 µmol/L (35 mg/dL). The reason for this plateau is not clear but may be related to renal excretion of conjugated bilirubin or alternative pathways of bilirubin catabolism in obstructive jaundice.

REFERENCES

Benign familial recurrent cholestasis

DePagter AGF et al: Familial benign intrahepatic cholestasis. Gastroenterology 71:202, 1976

Endo T et al: Bile acid metabolism in benign recurrent intrahepatic cholestasis. Gastroenterology 76:1002, 1979

Dubin-Johnson and Rotor syndromes

Rosenthal P et al: Homozygous Dubin-Johnson syndrome exhibits a characteristic serum bilirubin pattern. Hepatology 1:540, 1981

Swartz HM et al: On the nature and excretion of the hepatic pigment in the Dubin-Johnson syndrome. Gastroenterology 76:958, 1979

Wolkoff AW et al: Hereditary jaundice and disorders of bilirubin metabolism, in *The Metabolic Basis of Inherited Disease*, 6th ed. CR Scriver et al (eds). New York, McGraw, 1989, pp 1367–1408

Wolpert E et al: Abnormal sulfobromophthalein metabolism in Rotor's syndrome and obligate heterozygotes. N Engl J Med 206:1099, 1977

Glucuronosyl transferase deficiency states

Berthelot P, Dhumeaus D: New insights into the classification and mechanisms of hereditary, chronic, non-hemolytic hyperbilirubinemia. Gut 19:474, 1978

Bosma PJ et al: Mechanism of inherited deficiencies of multiple UDP-glucuronosyl transferase isoforms in two patients with Crigler-Najjar syndrome type I. FASEB J 6:2859, 1992

Chowdury JR, Chowdury NR: Unveiling the mysteries of inherited disorders of bilirubin glucuronidation. Gastroenterology 105:288, 1993

Dawson J et al: Gilbert's syndrome: Evidence of morphologic heterogeneity. Gut 20:848, 1979

Fevery J et al: Unconjugated bilirubin and an increased proportion of bilirubin monoconjugates in the bile of patients with Gilbert's syndrome and Crigler-Najjar disease. J Clin Invest 60:970, 1977

Ohkubo H et al: Ursodeoxycholic acid oral tolerance test in patients with constitutional hyperbilirubinemias and effect of phenobarbital. Gastroenterology 81:126, 1981

Olsson R et al: Gilbert's syndrome: does it exist? A study of the prevalence of symptoms in Gilbert's syndrome. Acta Med Scand 224:485, 1988

Ritter JK et al: Identification of a genetic alteration in the code for bilirubin UDP-glucuronosyl transferase in the UGT1 gene complex of a Crigler-Najjar type I patient. J Clin Invest 90:150, 1992

van ES HG et al: Immunochemical analysis of uridine diphosphate glucuronosyl transferase in four patients with the Crigler-Najjar syndrome type I. J Clin Invest 85:1199, 1990

Postoperative jaundice

Hootegem PV et al: Serum bilirubins in hepatobiliary disease: Comparison with other liver function tests and changes in the postobstructive period. Hepatology 5:112, 1985

LaMont JT, Isselbacher KJ: Postoperative jaundice. in *Wright's Liver and Biliary Disease*, 3d ed, GH Millward-Sadler et al (eds). Philadelphia. Saunders, 1992

266   ACUTE HEPATITIS

JULES L. DIENSTAG / KURT J. ISSELBACHER

ACUTE VIRAL HEPATITIS

Acute viral hepatitis is a systemic infection affecting the liver predominantly. Five categories of viral agents have been implicated: hepatitis A virus (HAV), hepatitis B virus (HBV), hepatitis C virus (HCV), the HBV-associated delta agent or hepatitis D virus (HDV), and hepatitis E virus (HEV). Although these agents can be distinguished by their antigenic properties, all five types produce clinically similar illnesses. These range from asymptomatic and inapparent to fulminant and fatal acute infections common to all five types, on the one hand, and from subclinical persistent infections to rapidly progressive chronic liver disease with cirrhosis and even hepatocellular carcinoma, common to the bloodborne types (HBV, HCV, and HDV), on the other.

FIGURE 266-1 *A*. Electron micrograph of 27-nm hepatitis A virus particles purified from stool of a patient with acute hepatitis A virus infection and aggregated by hepatitis A antibody. *B*. Electron micrograph of concentrated serum from a patient with acute hepatitis B infection, demonstrating the 42-nm virions, tubular forms, and spherical 22-nm particles of hepatitis B surface antigen. 132,000×. (Hepatitis D resembles 42-nm virions of hepatitis B but is smaller, 35 to 37 nm; hepatitis E resembles hepatitis A virus but is slightly larger, 32 to 34 nm; hepatitis C has not been visualized.)

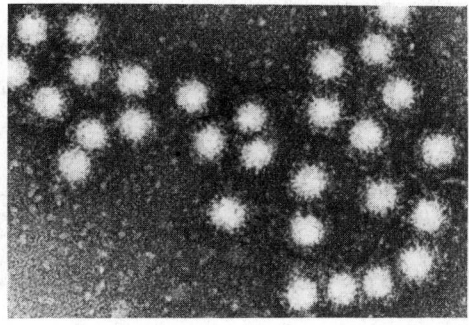

A

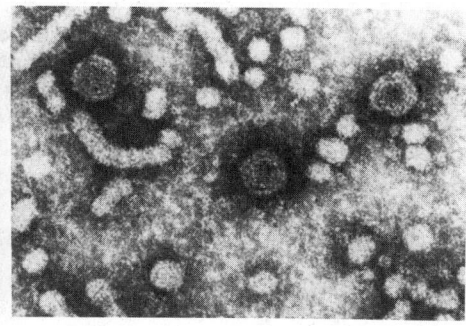

B

VIROLOGY AND ETIOLOGY **Hepatitis A** Hepatitis A virus (HAV) is a nonenveloped 27-nm, heat-, acid-, and ether-resistant RNA virus in the picornavirus family; classified initially as enterovirus type 72, it is now classified within the heparnavirus genus of the picornavirus family (Fig. 266-1). Its virion contains four capsid polypeptides designated VP1 to VP4, which are cleaved posttranslationally from the polyprotein product of a 7500-nucleotide genome. Inactivation of viral activity can be achieved by boiling for 1 min, by contact with formaldehyde and chlorine, or by ultraviolet irradiation. Despite nucleotide sequence variation of up to 20 percent among isolates of HAV, all strains of this virus identified to date are immunologically indistinguishable and belong to one serotype. Hepatitis A has an incubation period of approximately 4 weeks. Its replication limited to the liver, the virus is present in the liver, bile, stools, and blood during the late incubation period and acute preicteric phase of illness. Despite persistence of virus in the liver, viral shedding in feces, viremia, and infectivity diminish rapidly once jaundice becomes apparent. Unlike other hepatitis viruses, hepatitis A virus will replicate in tissue culture but replicates poorly compared with other picornaviruses.

Antibodies to HAV (anti-HAV) can be detected during acute illness when serum aminotransferase activity is elevated and fecal HAV shedding is still occurring. This early antibody response is predominantly of the IgM class and persists for several months, only rarely for 6 to 12 months. During convalescence, however, anti-HAV of the IgG class becomes the predominant antibody (Fig. 266-2). Therefore, the diagnosis of hepatitis A is made during acute illness by demonstrating high-titer anti-HAV of the IgM class. Following acute illness, anti-HAV of the IgG class remains detectable indefinitely, and patients with serum anti-HAV are immune to reinfection. Indeed, neutralizing antibody activity parallels the appearance of anti-HAV, and the IgG anti-HAV present in immune globulin accounts for the protection it affords against HAV infection.

FIGURE 266-2 Scheme of typical clinical and laboratory features of viral hepatitis type A.

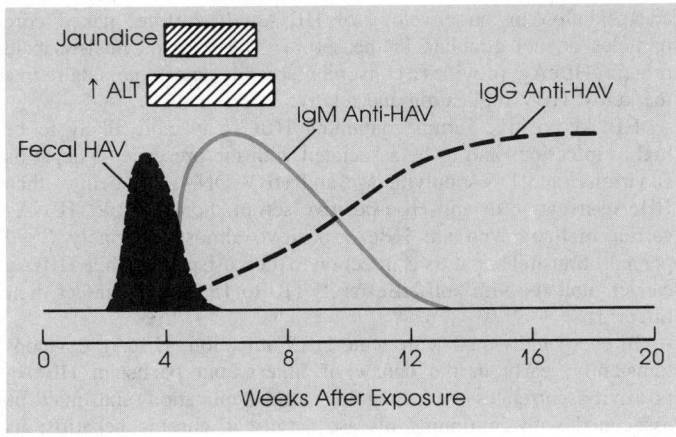

Jaundice
↑ ALT
Fecal HAV
IgM Anti-HAV
IgG Anti-HAV

Weeks After Exposure
0   4   8   12   16   20

Hepatitis B Hepatitis B virus is a DNA virus with a remarkably compact genomic structure; despite its small, circular, 3200-base-pair size, HBV DNA codes for four sets of viral products and has a complex, multiparticle structure. HBV achieves its genomic economy by relying on an efficient strategy of encoding proteins from four overlapping genes: S, C, P, and X, as detailed below. Once thought to be unique among viruses, HBV is now recognized as one of a family of animal viruses, hepadnaviruses (hepatotropic DNA viruses), and is classified as hepadnavirus type 1. Similar viruses infect certain species of woodchucks, ground and tree squirrels, and Pekin ducks, to mention the most carefully characterized. Like HBV, all have the same distinctive three morphologic forms, have counterparts to the envelope and nucleocapsid virus antigens of HBV, replicate within the liver but exist in extrahepatic sites, contain their own endogenous DNA polymerase, have partially double-stranded, partially single-stranded genomes, are associated with acute and chronic hepatitis and hepatocellular carcinoma, and rely on a replicative strategy unique among DNA viruses but typical of retroviruses. Instead of DNA replication directly from a DNA template, hepadnaviruses rely on reverse transcription (effected by the DNA polymerase) of minus-strand DNA from a "pregenomic" RNA intermediate. Then plus-strand DNA is transcribed from the minus-strand DNA template by the DNA-dependent DNA polymerase. Viral proteins are translated by the pregenomic RNA, and the proteins and genome are packaged into virions and secreted from the hepatocyte. Although HBV is difficult to cultivate in vitro in the conventional sense from clinical material, several cell lines have been transfected with HBV DNA. Such transfected cells support in vitro replication of the intact virus and its component proteins.

Three particulate forms of HBV (Table 266-1) can be demonstrated by electron microscopy (see Fig. 266-1). The most numerous are the 22-nm particles, which appear as spherical or long filamentous forms; these are antigenically indistinguishable from the outer surface or coat of HBV, and they are thought to represent excess viral coat protein. Outnumbered in serum by a factor of 100 or 1000 to 1 compared with the spheres and tubules are large, 42-nm, double-shelled spherical particles which represent the intact hepatitis B virion. The protein expressed on the outer surface of the virion and on the smaller spherical and tubular structures is referred to as *hepatitis B surface antigen* (HBsAg). Infection with HBV is unique in that the concentration of HBsAg and virus particles in the blood may reach 500 μg/mL and 10 trillion particles per milliliter, respectively. The envelope protein, HBsAg, is the product of the S gene of HBV.

HBsAg consists primarily of two major polypeptides, one of 24,000 mol wt and its glycosylated counterpart of 28,000 mol wt. A number of different HBsAg subdeterminants have been identified. There is a common group-reactive antigen, *a*, shared by all HBsAg isolates. In addition, HBsAg may contain one of several subtype-specific antigens, namely, *d* or *y*, *w* or *r*, as well as other more recently characterized specificities. These HBsAg subtypes provide additional epidemiologic markers in evaluating the transmission of hepatitis B infection in that subtypes "breed true." For example, studies of hepatitis outbreaks have shown that index cases and their

TABLE 266-1 Nomenclature and features of hepatitis viruses

Hepatitis type	Virus particle	Morphology	Genome*	Classification	Antigen(s)	Antibodies	Remarks
HAV	27 nm	Icosahedral nonenveloped	7.5-kb RNA, linear, ss, +	Heparnavirus	HAV	anti-HAV	Early fecal shedding Diagnosis: IgM anti-HAV Previous infection: IgG anti-HAV
HBV	42 nm	Double-shelled virion (surface and core) spherical	3.2-kb DNA, circular, ss/ds	Hepadnavirus	HBsAg HBcAg HBeAg	anti-HBs anti-HBc anti-HBe	Bloodborne virus; carrier state Acute diagnosis: HBsAg, IgM anti-HBc Chronic diagnosis: IgG anti-HBc, HBsAg Markers of replication: HBeAg, HBV DNA Liver, lymphocytes, other organs.
	27 nm	Nucleocapsid core			HBcAg HBeAg	anti-HBc anti-HBe	Nucleocapsid contains DNA and DNA polymerase; present in hepatocyte nucleus; HBcAg does not circulate; HBeAg (soluble, nonparticulate) and HBV DNA circulate—correlate with infectivity and complete virions.
	22 nm	Spherical and filamentous; represents excess virus coat material			HBsAg	anti-HBs	HBsAg detectable in >95% of patients with acute hepatitis B; found in serum, body fluids, hepatocyte cytoplasm; anti-HBs appears following infection—protective antibody.
HCV	Not visualized; approx. 30–60 nm	Enveloped	9.4-kb RNA, linear, ss, +	Flavivirus-like	HCV C100-3 C33c C22-3	anti-HCV	Bloodborne agent, formerly labeled non-A, non-B hepatitis Acute diagnosis: anti-HCV (C33c, C22-3), HCV RNA Chronic diagnosis: anti-HCV (C100-3, C33c, C22-3) and HCV RNA; cytoplasmic location in hepatocytes
HDV	35–37 nm	Enveloped hybrid particle with HBsAg coat and HDV core	1.7-kb RNA, circular, ss, −	Resembles viroids and plant satellite viruses	HBsAg HDVAg	anti-HBs anti-HDV	Defective RNA virus, requires helper function of HBV (hepadnaviruses); HDVAg present in hepatocyte nucleus Diagnosis: IgM/IgG anti-HDV, HDV RNA; HBV/HDV coinfection—IgM anti-HBc and anti-HDV; HDV superinfection—IgG anti-HBc and anti-HDV.
HEV	32–34 nm	Nonenveloped icosahedral	7.6-kb RNA, linear, ss, +	Alphavirus-like	HEVAg	anti-HEV	Agent of enterically transmitted non-A, non-B hepatitis; rare in USA; occurs in Asia, Mediterranean countries, Central America Diagnosis: IgM/IgG anti-HEV (assays being developed); virus in stool, bile, hepatocyte cytoplasm

* ss = single-stranded; ss/ds = partially single-stranded, partially double-stranded; − = minus-stranded; + = plus-stranded.

contacts have identical HBsAg subtypes. Clinical course and outcome, however, are independent of subtype.

Upstream of the S gene are the pre-S genes, which code for pre-S gene products, including receptors on the HBV surface of polymerized human serum albumin and for hepatocyte receptors. The pre-S region actually consists of both pre-S1 and pre-S2. Depending on where translation is initiated, three potential HBsAg gene products are synthesized. The protein product of the S gene is HBsAg (*major protein*), the product of the S region plus the adjacent pre-S2 region is the *middle protein*, and the product of the pre-S1 plus pre-S2 plus S regions is the *large protein*. Compared with the smaller spherical and tubular particles of HBV, complete 42-nm virions are enriched in the large protein. Both pre-S proteins and their respective antibodies can be detected during HBV infection, and the period of pre-S antigenemia appears to coincide with other markers of virus replication, as detailed below.

The intact 42-nm virion can be disrupted by mild detergents and the 27-nm nucleocapsid core particle isolated. Nucleocapsid proteins are coded for by the C gene. The antigen expressed on the surface of the nucleocapsid core is referred to as *hepatitis B core antigen* (HBcAg), and its corresponding antibody is anti-HBc. A third HBV antigen is *hepatitis B e antigen* (HBeAg), a soluble, nonparticulate, nucleocapsid protein that is immunologically distinct from intact HBcAg but is a product of the same C gene. The C gene has two initiation codons, a precore and a core region. If translation is initiated at the precore region, the protein product is HBeAg, which has a signal peptide that binds it to the smooth endoplasmic reticulum and leads to its secretion into the circulation. If translation begins with

the core region, HBcAg is the protein product; it has no signal peptide, it is not secreted, but it assembles into nucleocapsid particles which bind to and incorporate RNA and which, ultimately, contain HBV DNA. Also packaged within the nucleocapsid core is a DNA polymerase, which directs replication and repair of HBV DNA. In vitro, the polymerase can repair the single-stranded gap and render it double-stranded; it directs the synthesis of plus-strand DNA from a minus-strand template. When packaging within viral proteins is complete, synthesis of the incomplete plus strand stops; this accounts for the single-stranded gap and for differences in the size of the gap. HBcAg particles remain in the hepatocyte, where they are readily detectable by immunohistochemical staining, and are exported after encapsidation by an envelope of HBsAg. Therefore, naked core particles do not circulate in the serum. The secreted nucleocapsid protein, HBeAg, provides a convenient, readily detectable, qualitative marker of HBV replication and relative infectivity.

HBsAg-positive serum containing HBeAg is more likely to be highly infectious and to be associated with the presence of hepatitis B virions (and DNA polymerase and HBV DNA, see below) than HBeAg-negative or anti-HBe-positive serum. For example, HBsAg carrier mothers who are HBeAg-positive almost invariably (>90 percent) transmit hepatitis B infection to their offspring, while HBsAg carrier mothers with anti-HBe rarely (10 to 15 percent) infect their offspring.

In every individual with acute HBV infection, HBeAg develops transiently, early in the course of illness, but persistent HBeAg positivity correlates with ongoing viral replication and may be associated with continuing disease actvity in chronic hepatitis; its disappearance may be a harbinger of biochemical improvement and potential resolution of infection. Unfortunately, HBeAg is not a sufficiently discriminating marker to support prognostic predictions or to substitute for morphologic evaluation of severity in patients with chronic hepatitis.

The third of the HBV genes is the largest, the P gene, which codes for the DNA polymerase; as noted above, this enzyme has both DNA-dependent DNA polymerase and RNA-dependent reverse transcriptase activities. The fourth gene, X, codes for a small, nonparticulate protein which has been shown to be capable of transactivating the transcription of both viral and cellular genes. Such transactivation may enhance the replication of HBV, leading to the clinical association observed between the expression of the product of the X gene, hepatitis B x antigen (HBxAg), and antibodies to it in patients with severe chronic active hepatitis and hepatocellular carcinoma. The transactivating activity can enhance the transcription of other viruses besides HBV, such as HIV. Therefore, HBV may be responsible for enhanced replication of other viruses. Cellular processes transactivated by X include the human interferon-β gene and class I major histocompatibility genes; potentially, these effects could contribute to enhanced susceptibility of HBV-infected hepatocytes to cytolytic T cells. The X gene and its protein product, however, are absent in nonmammalian hepadnaviruses; therefore, X is not essential for hepadnavirus replication.

After infection with HBV, the first virologic marker detectable in serum is HBsAg (Fig. 266-3). Circulating HBsAg precedes elevations of serum aminotransferase activity and clinical symptoms and remains detectable during the entire icteric or symptomatic phase of acute hepatitis B and beyond. In typical cases, HBsAg becomes undetectable 1 to 2 months following the onset of jaundice and rarely persists beyond 6 months. After HBsAg disappears, antibody to HBsAg (anti-HBs) becomes detectable in serum and remains detectable indefinitely thereafter. Because HBcAg is sequestered within an HBsAg coat, HBcAg is not detectable routinely in the serum of patients with HBV infection. On the other hand, antibody to HBcAg (anti-HBc) is readily demonstrable in serum, beginning within the first 1 to 2 weeks after the appearance of HBsAg and preceding detectable levels of anti-HBs by weeks to months. Because variability exists in the time of appearance of anti-HBs following HBV infection, occasionally a gap of several weeks or longer may separate the disappearance of HBsAg and the appearance of anti-HBs. During this "gap" or "window" period, anti-HBc may represent serologic evidence of current or recent HBV infection, and blood containing anti-HBc in the absence of HBsAg and anti-HBs has been implicated in the development of transfusion-associated hepatitis B. In part because the sensitivity of immunoassays for HBsAg and anti-HBs has increased, however, this

window period is rarely encountered. In some persons, years after HBV infection, anti-HBc may persist in the circulation longer than anti-HBs. Therefore, isolated anti-HBc does not necessarily indicate active virus replication; most instances of isolated anti-HBc represent hepatitis B infection in the remote past. Rarely, however, isolated anti-HBc represents low-level hepatitis B viremia, with HBsAg below the detection threshold; occasionally, isolated anti-HBc represents a cross-reacting or false-positive immunologic specificity. Distinction between recent and remote HBV infection can be accomplished by determination of the immunoglobulin class of anti-HBc. Anti-HBc of the IgM class (IgM anti-HBc) predominates during the first approximately 6 months after acute infection, whereas IgG anti-HBc is the predominant class of anti-HBc beyond 6 months. Therefore, patients with current or recent acute hepatitis B, including those in the anti-HBc window, have IgM anti-HBc in their serum. In patients who have recovered from hepatitis B in the remote past as well as those with chronic HBV infection, anti-HBc is predominantly of the IgG class. Infrequently, in no more than 1 to 5 percent of patients with acute HBV infection, levels of HBsAg are too low to be detected; in such cases, the presence of IgM anti-HBc establishes the diagnosis of acute hepatitis B. When isolated anti-HBc occurs in the rare patient with chronic hepatitis B whose HBsAg level is below the sensitivity threshold of contemporary immunoassays (a low-level carrier), the anti-HBc is of the IgG class. Generally, in persons who have recovered from hepatitis B, anti-HBs and anti-HBc persist indefinitely.

The temporal association between the appearance of anti-HBs and resolution of HBV infection as well as the observation that persons with anti-HBs in serum are protected against reinfection with HBV suggest that *anti-HBs is the protective antibody*. Therefore, strategies for prevention of HBV infection are based on providing susceptible persons with circulating anti-HBs (see below). Occasionally, in 10 to 20 percent of patients with chronic hepatitis B, low-level, low-affinity anti-HBs can be detected. This antibody is directed against a subtype determinant different from that represented by the patient's HBsAg; its presence is thought to reflect the stimulation of a related clone of antibody-forming cells, but it has no clinical relevance and does not signal imminent clearance of hepatitis B.

The other readily detectable serologic marker of HBV infection, HBeAg, appears concurrently with or shortly after HBsAg. Its appearance coincides temporally with high levels of virus replication and reflects the presence of circulating intact virions, DNA polymerase, and HBV DNA. Pre-S1 and pre-S2 proteins are also expressed during periods of peak replication, but assays for these gene products are not routinely available. In self-limited HBV infections, HBeAg becomes undetectable shortly after peak elevations in aminotransferase activity, before the disappearance of HBsAg, and anti-HBe then becomes detectable, coinciding with a period of relatively lower infectivity (see Fig. 266-3). Because markers of HBV replication appear transiently during acute infection, testing for such markers is of little clinical utility in typical cases of acute HBV infection. In contrast, markers of HBV replication provide valuable information in patients with protracted infections. Departing from the pattern typical of acute HBV infections, in chronic HBV infection, HBsAg remains detectable beyond 6 months, anti-HBc is primarily of the IgG class, and anti-HBs is either undetectable or detectable at low levels (see "Laboratory Features," below) (Fig. 266-4). During early chronic HBV infection, HBV DNA can be detected both in serum and in hepatocyte nuclei, where it is present in free or episomal form. This *replicative stage* of HBV infection is the time of maximal infectivity and liver injury; HBeAg is a qualitative marker and HBV DNA a quantitative marker of this replicative phase, during which all three forms of HBV circulate, including intact virions. Over time, the replicative phase of chronic HBV infection gives way to a relatively *nonreplicative phase*. This occurs at a rate of approximately 10 percent per year and is accompanied by seroconversion from HBeAg-positive to anti-HBe-positive. In most cases, this seroconversion coincides with a transient, acute hepatitis–like elevation in aminotransferase activity, believed to reflect cell-mediated clearance

FIGURE 266-3   Scheme of typical clinical and laboratory features of acute viral hepatitis type B.

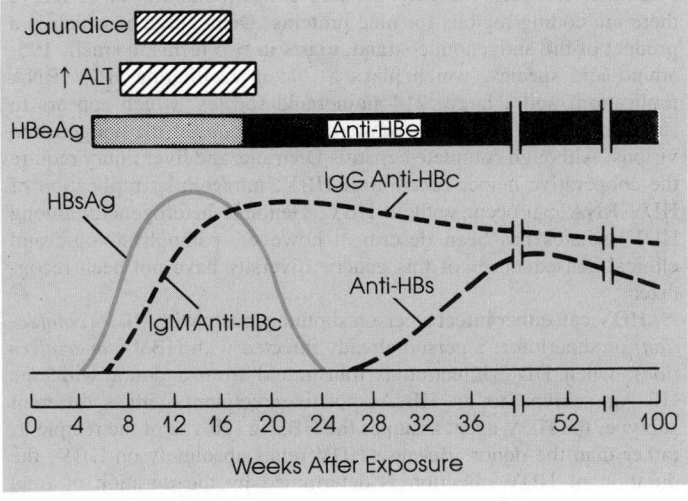

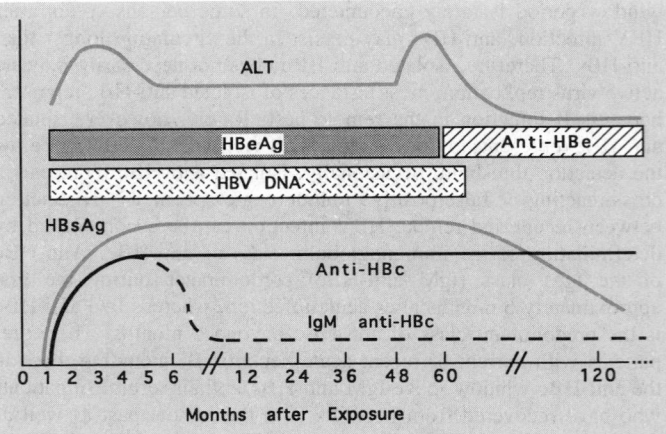

FIGURE 266-4   Scheme of typical laboratory features of chronic viral hepatitis type B. HBeAg and HBV DNA can be detected in serum during the *replicative phase* of chronic infection, which is associated with infectivity and liver injury. Seroconversion from the replicative phase to the *nonreplicative phase* occurs at a rate of approximately 10 to 15 percent per year and is heralded by an acute hepatitis–like elevation of ALT activity; during the nonreplicative phase, infectivity and liver injury are limited.

of virus-infected hepatocytes. In the nonreplicative phase of chronic infection, when HBV DNA is demonstrable in hepatocyte nuclei, it tends to be integrated into the host genome. In this phase, only spherical and tubular forms of HBV, *not intact virions*, circulate, and liver injury tends to subside. Most such patients would be characterized as asymptomatic HBV *carriers*. In reality, the designations *replicative* and *nonreplicative* are only relative; even in the so-called nonreplicative phase, HBV replication can be detected with highly sensitive amplification probes such as the polymerase chain reaction. Still, the distinctions are pathophysiologically and clinically meaningful. Occasionally, nonreplicative HBV infection converts back to replicative infection. Such spontaneous reactivations are accompanied by reexpression of HBeAg and HBV DNA as well as by exacerbations of liver injury.

Recently, attention has focused on molecular variants of HBV. Variation occurs throughout the HBV genome, and clinical isolates of HBV that do not express viral proteins have been attributed to mutations in individual or even multiple gene locations. For example, variants have been described which lack nucleocapsid proteins, envelope proteins, or both. Two categories of HBV have attracted the most attention. One of these was identified initially in Mediterranean countries among patients with an unusual serologic-clinical profile. They have severe chronic HBV infection and detectable HBV DNA but with anti-HBe instead of HBeAg. These patients were found to be infected with an HBV mutant that contained an alteration in the precore region rendering the virus incapable of encoding HBeAg. Although several potential mutation sites exist in the pre-C region, the region of the C gene necessary for the expression of HBeAg (see "Virology and Etiology," above), the most commonly encountered in such patients is a single base substitution, from G to A, which occurs in the second to last codon of the pre-C gene at nucleotide 1896. This substitution results in the replacement of the TGG tryptophan codon by a stop codon (TAG), which prevents the translation of HBeAg. Patients with such precore mutants that are unable to secrete HBeAg tend to have severe liver disease that progresses rapidly to cirrhosis and that does not respond readily to antiviral therapy. Both "wild-type" HBV and precore mutant HBV can coexist in the same patient, or mutant HBV may arise during wild-type HBV infection. In addition, clusters of fulminant hepatitis B in Israel and Japan have been attributed to common-source infection with a precore mutant. Fulminant hepatitis B in North America and western Europe, however, occurs in patients infected with wild-type

HBV, in the absence of precore mutants, and both precore mutants and other mutations throughout the HBV genome occur commonly even in patients with typical, self-limited, milder forms of HBV infection. Therefore, additional investigation will be necessary to define the effect of precore mutants on the pathogenicity and natural history of HBV infection.

The second important category of HBV mutants consists of *escape mutants*, in which a single amino acid substitution, from glycine to arginine, occurs at position 145 of the immunodominant *a* determinant common to all subtypes of HBsAg. This change in HBsAg leads to a critical conformational change that results in a loss of neutralizing activity by anti-HBs. This specific HBV/*a* mutant has been observed in two situations, active and passive immunization, in which humoral immunologic pressure may favor evolutionary change ("escape") in the virus—in a small number of hepatitis B vaccine recipients who acquired HBV infection despite the prior appearance of neutralizing anti-HBs and in liver transplant recipients who underwent the procedure for hepatitis B and who were treated with a high-potency human monoclonal anti-HBs preparation. Although such mutants have not been appreciated frequently, their existence raises a concern that may complicate vaccination strategies and serologic diagnosis.

Hepatitis B antigens and HBV DNA have been identified in extrahepatic sites, including lymph nodes, bone marrow, circulating lymphocytes, spleen, and pancreas. Although the virus does not appear to be associated with tissue injury in any of these extrahepatic sites, its presence in these "remote" reservoirs has been invoked to explain the recurrence of HBV infection after orthotopic liver transplantation. A more complete understanding of the clinical relevance of extrahepatic HBV remains to be defined.

Hepatitis D   The delta hepatitis agent, or hepatitis D virus (HDV), is a defective RNA virus which coinfects with and requires the helper function of HBV (or other hepadnaviruses) for its replication and expression. Slightly smaller than HBV, delta is a formalin-sensitive, 35- to 37-nm virus with a hybrid structure. Its nucleocapsid expresses delta antigen, which bears no antigenic homology with any of the HBV antigens, and contains the virus genome. The delta core is "encapsidated" by an outer envelope of HBsAg, indistinguishable from that of HBV except in its relative compositions of major, middle, and large HBsAg component proteins. The genome is a small, 1700-nucleotide, circular, single-stranded RNA (minus strand) that is nonhomologous with HBV DNA (except for a small area of the polymerase gene) but that has features and the rolling circle model of replication common to genomes of plant satellite viruses or viroids. HDV RNA contains many areas of internal complementarity; therefore, it can fold on itself by internal base pairing to form an unusual, very stable, rodlike structure. HDV RNA replicates via RNA-directed RNA synthesis by transcription of genomic RNA to a complementary antigenomic (plus strand) RNA; the antigenomic RNA, in turn, serves as a template for subsequent genomic RNA synthesis. Between the genomic and antigenomic RNAs of HDV, there are coding regions for nine proteins. Delta antigen, which is a product of the antigenomic strand, exists in two forms, a small, 195-amino-acid species, which plays a role in facilitating HDV RNA replication, and a large, 214-amino-acid species, which appears to suppress replication but is required for assembly of the antigen into virions. Although complete hepatitis D virions and liver injury require the cooperative helper function of HBV, intracellular replication of HDV RNA can occur without HBV. Genomic heterogeneity among HDV isolates has been described; however, pathophysiologic and clinical consequences of this genetic diversity have not been recognized.

HDV can either infect a person simultaneously with HBV (*coinfection*) or superinfect a person already infected with HBV (*superinfection*); when HDV infection is transmitted from a donor with one HBsAg subtype to an HBsAg-positive recipient with a different subtype, the HDV agent assumes the HBsAg subtype of the recipient, rather than the donor. Because HDV relies absolutely on HBV, the duration of HDV infection is determined by the duration of (and cannot outlast) HBV infection. HDV antigen is expressed primarily in hepatocyte nuclei and is occasionally detectable in serum. During acute HDV infection, anti-HDV of the IgM class predominates, and 30 to 40 days may elapse after symptoms appear before anti-HDV can be detected. In self-limited infection, anti-HDV is low titer and transient, rarely remaining detectable beyond the clearance of HBsAg and HDV antigen. In chronic HDV infection, anti-HDV circulates in high titer, and both IgM and IgG anti-HDV can be detected. HDV antigen in the liver and HDV RNA in serum and liver can be detected during HDV replication.

Hepatitis C (formerly called non-A, non-B hepatitis)   Sensitive serologic tests for identifying both types A and B hepatitis have led to the identification of hepatitis cases with incubation periods and modes of transmission consistent with an infectious disease but without serologic evidence of hepatitis A or B infection. Identified initially among recipients of transfused blood, these cases of so-called non-A, non-B hepatitis have not been associated serologically with Epstein-Barr virus or cytomegalovirus (except in rare instances) or with other viruses known to involve the liver.

An almost 15-year quest to identify an agent of non-A, non-B viral hepatitis ended in 1988 with the identification of an RNA virus with immunologic specificity for transfusion-associated non-A, non-B hepatitis. Among complementary DNA (cDNA) fragments cloned in *Escherichia coli* from the pellet of a chimpanzee plasma with unusually high infectivity, one clone, designated 5-1-1, expressed a protein that reacted with antibody in convalescent serum but not preillness serum from chimpanzees with experimentally induced non-A, non-B hepatitis. This viral clone hybridizes with the livers of infected, but not uninfected-control, chimpanzees. A protein product of this virus-specific clone was expressed in yeast, and this protein, designated C100-3, was used as an antigen in the first immunoassay to detect antibody in serum. Validation of the relationship between this agent and non-A, non-B hepatitis came most convincingly from the ability of the antibody immunoassay to distinguish, in panels of coded serum samples, between pedigreed non-A, non-B hepatitis cases and pedigreed negative, noninfectious samples as well as other-disease controls. Analysis of overlapping clones permitted identification of the entire genome, and the agent has been labeled *hepatitis C virus* (HCV). HCV is a linear, single-stranded, positive-polarity, 9400-nucleotide RNA virus with a single open reading frame (gene) that codes for a virus polyprotein of approximately 3000 amino acids. Five distinct genotypes have been identified by nucleotide mapping, although they all appear to be antigenically similar. The 5' end of the genome consists of an untranslated region adjacent to the genes for structural proteins, the nucleocapsid core and the viral envelope. The 5' untranslated and core genes are highly conserved among genotypes, but the envelope proteins are coded for by the hypervariable region, which varies from isolate to isolate and even within the same agent isolated over time from the same patient. This allows the virus to evade host immunologic mechanisms directed at virus-envelope proteins. The 3' end of the genome contains the genes for nonstructural (NS) proteins 1 through 5. The original clone, 5-1-1, and the nucleotide sequence coding for C100-3 reside within the NS4 gene, and the RNA-dependent RNA polymerase through which HCV replicates is coded for by the NS5 region (Fig. 266-5). The genome of HCV has no homology with HBV, retroviruses, or other hepatitis viruses, and because it does not replicate via a DNA intermediate, HCV does not integrate into the host genome. Studies of its gene structure suggest that HCV is a distant relative of flaviviruses, animal pestiviruses, and plant potyviruses. Like other flaviviruses and pestiviruses, HCV will probable be included in the family Flaviviridae but will comprise a new genus. HCV tends to circulate in very low titer (100 to 1000 virions per milliliter); therefore, no virus particles have been visualized. Although in vitro HCV replication is difficult to accomplish convincingly, the chimpanzee has proven to be an invaluable animal model. Neutralizing antibodies have not been identified.

As noted above, the first assay introduced detected antibodies to C100-3, a recombinant polypeptide derived from the NS4 region of the genome. In most patients with transfusion-associated hepatitis C, antibody detected with this assay appears between 1 to 3 months after the onset of acute hepatitis but sometimes not for a year or longer. Second-generation assays incorporate recombinant proteins from the nucleocapsid core region, C22-3, and the NS3 region, C33c (expressed in combination with C100-3 as C200); these assays are more sensitive (by approximately 20 percent) and detect anti-HCV 30 to 90 days earlier, during the period of acute hepatitis. Because nonspecificity has been encountered in clinical samples tested for anti-HCV, a supplementary recombinant immunoblot assay (RIBA) was introduced. Reactivity in an immunoassay is "confirmed" by incubation with a nitrocellulose strip which contains individual bands for the proteins of the first-generation (the product of recombinant bacterial clone 5-1-1 and recombinant yeast polypeptide C100-3, both nonstructural proteins) and second-generation immunoassays (nonstructural polypeptide C33c and core polypeptide C22-3) as well as a superoxide dismutase (SOD, a fusion protein with which recombinant HCV proteins are expressed in yeast and to which some false-positive reactivity is directed) band. This approach allows the demonstration of individual antibodies to nonstructural and structural viral proteins and identifies false-positive reactivity associated with bacterial, yeast, or SOD immunologic specificities. Still, detection of anti-HCV is insufficient to identify all persons infected with HCV. The most sensitive indicator is the presence of HCV RNA, which requires molecular amplification by polymerase chain reaction (Fig. 266-6). HCV RNA can be detected within a few days of exposure to HCV, well before the appearance of anti-HCV, and tends to persist for the duration of HCV infection; however, in patients with chronic HCV infection, occasionally, HCV RNA may be detectable only intermit-

FIGURE 266-5   Organization of the hepatitis C virus genome and its associated proteins. Structural genes at the 5' end include the nucleocapsid region, C, and the envelope regions, E1 and E2. The 5' untranslated region and the C region are highly conserved among isolates, while the envelope domain E2/NS1 contains the hypervariable region. At the 3' end are five nonstructural (NS) regions. Viral proteins included in the first-generation (c100-3) and second-generation (c200, a fusion protein of c100-3 and c33c, and c22-3) immunoassays and in the recombinant immunoblot assay (5-1-1, c100-3, c33c, c22-3) are presented below their corresponding genes (AA = amino acid).

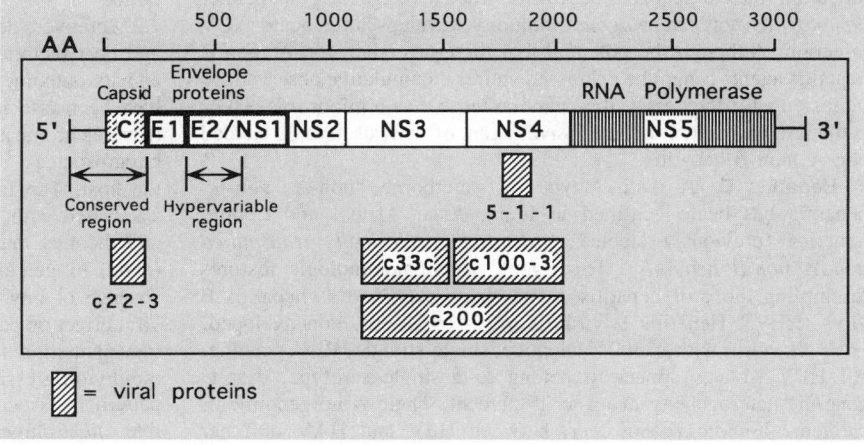

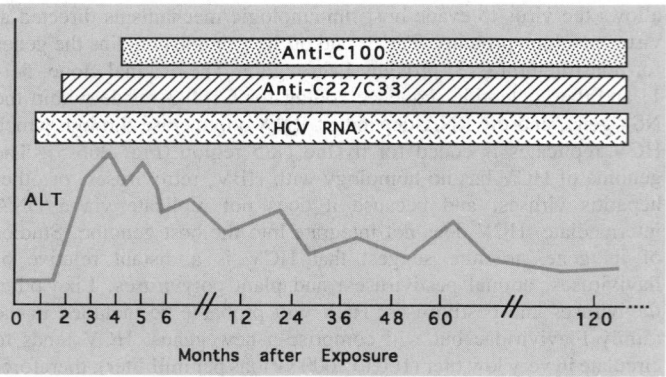

FIGURE 266-6 Scheme of typical laboratory features during acute hepatitis type C progressing to chronicity. HCV RNA is the first detectable event, preceding ALT elevation and the appearance of anti-HCV. The appearance of antibody to C100, detectable with first-generation assays, is delayed from 1 to 3 months after the appearance of antibody to C22 and C33, antibodies which are included in second-generation immunoassays. Anti-HCV detectable with second-generation assays appears during acute hepatitis C.

tently. Application of sensitive molecular probes for HCV RNA has revealed the presence of replicative HCV in peripheral blood lymphocytes of infected persons; however, as is the case for HBV in lymphocytes, the clinical relevance of HCV lymphocyte infection is not known.

Long before HCV was identified as an agent of non-A, non-B hepatitis, cross-challenge studies in chimpanzees suggested that there are at least two bloodborne non-A, non-B hepatitis agents. One, isolated from clotting factor VIII concentrates and the agent of most cases of transfusion-associated hepatitis, is chloroform-sensitive and induces ultrastructural cytoplasmic tubular changes in hepatocytes. This agent is HCV. The other, isolated from clotting factor IX concentrates, is chloroform-resistant and does not induce cytoplasmic tubular changes in hepatocytes. Theoretically, the chloroform-resistant agent could be a "non-A, non-B, non-C" hepatitis agent. The fact that all serologic and molecular markers of HCV are absent in a substantial proportion of sporadic cases of non-A, non-B hepatitis, a small proportion of cases of transfusion-associated hepatitis and "cryptogenic" cirrhosis, and almost all cases of non-A, non-B fulminant hepatitis also lends support to the existence of another agent. On the other hand, exhaustive attempts to identify another such viral agent have failed, and reinterpretation of the original cross-challenge studies in chimpanzees with serologic and molecular assays for HCV infection indicates that what were thought to be new infections with a distinct agent actually represented infection with a different genotype of HCV or reinfection with the *same* HCV agent. Whether rechallenge was with the same inoculum or a different inoculum, the chimpanzees became reinfected, suggesting that neither *homologous* nor *heterologous* immunity develops after acute HCV infection. Although the potential that there are other non-A, non-B hepatitis agents cannot be dismissed entirely, cumulative observations indicate that if they exist, they play no more than a minor role. HCV is the predominant, if not exclusive, agent of what used to be labeled non-A, non-B hepatitis.

Hepatitis E A distinct type of waterborne "non-A, non-B" hepatitis has been identified in India, Asia, Africa, and Central America (previously labeled *epidemic* or *enterically transmitted non-A, non-B hepatitis*). This agent, with epidemiologic features resembling those of hepatitis A, has been classified as hepatitis E virus (HEV). Hepatitis E virus is a 32- to 34-nm, nonenveloped, HAV-like virus with a 7600-nucleotide, single-stranded RNA genome. All HEV isolates appear to belong to a single serotype, despite genomic heterogeneity of up to 25 percent. There is no genomic or antigenic homology, however, between HEV and HAV or other

picornaviruses, and HEV, although resembling calciviruses, appears to be sufficiently distinct from any known agent to merit a new classification of its own within the alphavirus group. The virus has been detected in stool, bile, and liver from infected patients, as well from experimentally infected nonhuman primates, chimpanzees, and cynomolgus macaques. The entire virus genome has been characterized by molecular cloning of complementary DNA constructed from virus RNA extracted from bile obtained from an infected macaque. Studies in humans and experimental animals have shown that HEV is excreted in the stool during the late incubation period and that immune responses to viral antigens occur very early during the course of acute infection. Both IgM anti-HEV and IgG anti-HEV can be detected, but both fall rapidly after acute infection, reaching low levels within 9 to 12 months. Currently, serologic testing for HEV infection remains in the domain of research laboratories, but the availability of tests for routine clinical purposes is anticipated.

PATHOGENESIS Under ordinary circumstances, none of the hepatitis viruses is known to be directly cytopathic to hepatocytes. Evidence suggests that the clinical manifestations and outcomes following acute liver injury associated with viral hepatitis are determined by the immunologic responses of the host. Studies of the pathogenesis of hepatitis A, C, D, and E have been limited, but the immunopathogenesis of hepatitis B has been studied extensively. Certainly for this agent, the existence of asymptomatic hepatitis B carriers with normal liver histology and function suggests that the virus is not directly cytopathic. The facts that lymphoid cells are juxtaposed with necrotic hepatocytes in the livers of patients with liver injury and that patients with defects in cellular immune competence are more likely to remain chronically infected rather than to clear the virus are cited to support the role of cellular immune responses in the pathogenesis of hepatitis B–related liver injury. To date, however, because adequate animal and laboratory models are lacking, support for this hypothesis remains circumstantial. Still, the model that has the most experimental support involves cytolytic T cells sensitized specifically to recognize host and hepatitis B viral antigens on the liver cell surface. Although HBsAg was initially thought to be the most likely viral target antigen on the hepatocyte surface, recent laboratory observations suggest that nucleocapsid proteins (HBcAg and possibly HBeAg), present on the cell membrane in minute quantities, are the viral target antigens that, with host antigens, invite cytolytic T cells to destroy HBV-infected hepatocytes. Still, this hypothesis is insufficient to explain differences in outcomes between those who recover after acute hepatitis and those who progress to chronic hepatitis or between those with mild and severe (fulminant) acute HBV infection. As convincing as are the cumulative data supporting nucleocapsid proteins as the target of cell-mediated immunologic injury, attention has been refocused on the envelope protein, HBsAg, by the demonstration that in transgenic mice with the gene for HBsAg inserted into their genomes, cytolytic T cells directed against HBsAg can be shown to destroy hepatocytes. Therefore, HBsAg cannot be dismissed as a potential immunologic target.

Moreover, debate continues over the relative importance of viral and host factors in the pathogenesis of HBV-associated liver injury and its outcome. As noted above, precore genetic mutants of HBV have been associated with the more severe outcomes of HBV infection (severe chronic and fulminant hepatitis), suggesting that, under certain circumstances, relative pathogenicity is a property of the virus, not the host. The fact that concomitant HDV and HBV infections are associated with more severe liver injury than HBV infection alone and the fact that cells transfected in vitro with the gene for HDV (delta) antigen express HDV antigen and then become necrotic in the absence of any immunologic influences are also consistent with a viral effect on pathogenicity. Similarly, in patients who undergo liver transplantation for end-stage chronic HBV infection, occasionally, rapidly progressive liver injury appears in the new liver. This clinical pattern is associated with an unusual histologic pattern in the new liver, *fibrosing cholestatic hepatitis*, which, ultrastructurally, appears to represent a choking of the cell with overwhelming quantities of HBsAg. This observation suggests that under the influence of the potent immunosuppressive agents required to prevent allograft rejection, HBV may have a direct cytopathic effect on liver cells, independent of the immune system.

Although the precise mechanism of liver injury in HBV infection remains elusive, studies of nucleocapsid proteins have shed light on the profound immunologic tolerance to HBV of babies born to mothers with highly replicative (HBeAg-positive), chronic HBV infection. In HBeAg-expressing transgenic mice, in utero exposure to HBeAg, which is sufficiently small to traverse the placenta, induces T cell tolerance to both nucleocapsid proteins. This, in turn, may explain why, when infection occurs so early in life, immunologic clearance does not occur, and protracted, lifelong infection ensues.

Although the mechanism of HBV-induced liver injury remains uncertain, immune complex–mediated tissue damage appears to play a major pathogenetic role in the extrahepatic manifestations of acute hepatitis B. The occasional prodromal serum sickness–like syndrome observed in acute hepatitis B appears to be related to the deposition in tissue blood vessel walls of circulating immune complexes leading to activation of the complement system. The clinical consequences are urticarial rash, angioedema, fever, and arthritis. During the early prodrome of HBV infection in these patients, HBsAg in high titer in association with small amounts of anti-HBs leads to the formation of soluble, circulating immune complexes (in antigen excess). Complement components in the serum are depressed during the arthritic phase of the illness and are also detectable in the circulating immune complexes. In addition to complement components, these complexes contain HBsAg, anti-HBs, IgG, IgM, IgA, and fibrin. After the patient recovers from the serum sickness–like syndrome, these immune complexes disappear.

In patients who become carriers of HBsAg following acute hepatitis, other types of immune-complex disease may be seen. Glomerulonephritis with the nephrotic syndrome is occasionally observed; HBsAg, immunoglobulin, and C3 deposition has been found in the glomerular basement membrane. While polyarteritis nodosa develops in considerably fewer than 1 percent of patients with HBV infection, 20 to 30 percent of patients with polyarteritis nodosa have HBsAg in serum. In these patients, the affected small and medium-sized arterioles have been shown to contain HBsAg, immunoglobulins, and complement components. Another extrahepatic manifestation of viral hepatitis, essential mixed cryoglobulinemia (EMC), was reported initially to be associated with hepatitis B. The disorder is characterized clinically by arthritis and cutaneous vasculitis (palpable purpura) and serologically by the presence of circulating cryoprecipitable immune complexes of more than one immunoglobulin class. Many patients with this syndrome have chronic liver disease, but the association with HBV infection has always been controversial. Recent reevaluation of patients with EMC suggests instead that a substantial proportion have chronic HCV infection. Their circulating immune complexes contain HCV RNA at a concentration that exceeds its serum concentration; this observation argues against secondary trapping of HCV in the immune complexes and favors a primary role for the virus in the pathogenesis of EMC.

PATHOLOGY   The typical morphologic lesions of hepatitis A, B, C, D, and E are often similar and consist of panlobular infiltration with mononuclear cells, hepatic cell necrosis, hyperplasia of Kupffer cells, and variable degrees of cholestasis. Hepatic cell regeneration is present, as evidenced by numerous mitotic figures, multinucleated cells, and "rosette" or "pseudoacinar" formation. The mononuclear infiltration consists primarily of small lymphocytes, although plasma cells and eosinophils are occasionally seen. Liver cell damage consists of hepatic cell degeneration and necrosis, cell dropout, ballooning of cells, and acidophilic degeneration of hepatocytes (forming so-called Councilman-like bodies). Large hepatocytes with a ground glass appearance of the cytoplasm may be seen in chronic but not in acute HBV infection; these cells have been shown to contain HBsAg and can be identified histochemically with orcein or aldehyde

fuchsin. In uncomplicated viral hepatitis, the reticulin framework is preserved.

In hepatitis C, the histologic lesion is often remarkable for a relative paucity of inflammation, a marked increase in activation of sinusoidal lining cells, the presence of fat, and occasionally, bile duct lesions in which biliary epithelial cells appear to be piled up without interruption of the basement membrane. Occasionally microvesicular steatosis occurs in hepatitis D. In hepatitis E, a common histologic feature is marked cholestasis. A cholestatic variant of slowly resolving acute hepatitis A also has been described.

A more severe histologic lesion, *bridging hepatic necrosis*, also termed *subacute* or *confluent necrosis*, is occasionally observed in some patients with acute hepatitis. "Bridging" between lobules results from large areas of hepatic cell dropout, with collapse of the reticulin framework. Characteristically, the bridge consists of condensed reticulum, inflammatory debris, and degenerating liver cells that span adjacent portal areas, portal to central veins, or central vein to central vein. This lesion has been thought to have prognostic significance; in many of the originally described patients with this lesion, a subacute course terminated in death within several weeks to months, or chronic active hepatitis and postnecrotic cirrhosis developed. More recent investigations have failed to uphold the association between bridging necrosis and such a poor prognosis in patients with acute hepatitis. Although the frequency of bridging may be higher among hospitalized patients with severe acute hepatitis, and although cirrhosis, chronic hepatitis, and even death have been observed in this group, the frequency of bridging necrosis in uncomplicated acute viral hepatitis is probably on the order of 1 to 5 percent. Prospective studies have failed to demonstrate a difference in prognosis between patients with acute hepatitis who have bridging necrosis and those who do not. Therefore, although demonstration of this lesion in patients with chronic hepatitis has prognostic significance (see Chap. 267), its demonstration during acute hepatitis is less meaningful, and liver biopsies to identify this lesion are no longer undertaken routinely in patients with acute hepatitis. In *massive hepatic necrosis* (fulminant hepatitis, acute yellow atrophy), the striking feature at postmortem examination is the finding of a small, shrunken, and soft liver. Histologic examination reveals massive necrosis and dropout of liver cells of most lobules with extensive collapse and condensation of the reticulin framework.

Immunofluorescence and immunoperoxidase antibody studies have been instrumental in localizing HBsAg to the cytoplasm and plasma membrane of infected liver cells. In contrast, HBcAg predominates in the nucleus, but occasionally, scant amounts are also seen in the cytoplasm and on the cell membrane. Electron-microscopic studies of liver biopsy material have demonstrated the presence of HBsAg particles in the cytoplasm and HBcAg particles in the nucleus of liver cells during hepatitis B infection. These morphologic observations suggest that DNA is synthesized and packaged within core particles in the nucleus, while the surface coat is assembled in the cytoplasm, resulting in the formation of intact hepatitis B virus. HDV antigen is localized to the hepatocyte nucleus, while HAV, HCV, and HEV antigens are localized to the cytoplasm.

EPIDEMIOLOGY   Prior to the availability of serologic tests for hepatitis viruses, all viral hepatitis cases were labeled either as "infectious" or "serum" hepatitis. Modes of transmission overlap, however, and *a clear distinction among the different types of viral hepatitis cannot be made solely on the basis of clinical or epidemiologic features* (Table 266-2). The most accurate means to distinguish the various types of viral hepatitis involves specific serologic testing.

Hepatitis A   *This agent is transmitted almost exclusively by the fecal-oral route.* Person-to-person spread of HAV is enhanced by poor personal hygiene and overcrowding, and large outbreaks as well as sporadic cases have been traced to contaminated food, water, milk, and shellfish. Intrafamily and intrainstitutional spread are also common. Early epidemiologic observations suggested that there is a predilection for hepatitis A to occur in late fall and early winter. In

TABLE 266-2 Clinical and epidemiologic features of viral hepatitis

Feature	HAV	HBV	HCV	HDV	HEV
Incubation (days)	15–45, mean 30	30–180, mean 60–90	15–160, mean 50	30–180, mean 60–90	14–60, mean 40
Onset	Acute	Insidious or acute	Insidious	Insidious or acute	Acute
Age preference	Children, young adults	Young adults (sexual and percutaneous), babies, toddlers	Any age, but more common in adults	Any age (similar to HBV)	Young adults (20–40 years)
Transmission:					
Fecal-oral	+ + +	−	−	−	+ + +
Percutaneous	Unusual	+ + +	+ + +	+ + +	−
Perinatal	−	+ + +	±[a]	+	−
Sexual	±	+ +	±[a]	+ +	−
Clinical:					
Severity	Mild	Occasionally severe	Moderate	Occasionally severe	Mild
Fulminant	0.1%	0.1–1%	0.1%	5–20%[b]	1–2%[f]
Progression to chronicity	None	Occasional (1–10%) (90% of neonates)	Common (50%)	Common[d]	None
Carrier	None	0.1–30%[c]	0.5–1.0%	Variable[e]	None
Cancer	None	+ (neonatal infection)	+	±	None
Prognosis	Excellent	Worse with age, debility	Moderate	Acute, good Chronic, poor	Good
Prophylaxis	IG Inactivated vaccine	HBIG Recombinant vaccine	None	HBV vaccine (none for HBV carriers)	Unknown
Therapy	None	Interferon 40% effective	Interferon 50% effective	Unknown	None

[a] Primarily with HIV coinfection.
[b] Up to 5% in acute HBV/HDV coinfection; up to 20% in HDV superinfection of chronic HBV infection.
[c] Varies considerably throughout the world and in subpopulations within countries; see text.
[d] In acute HBV/HDV coinfection, the frequency of chronicity is the same as that for HBV; in HDV superinfection, chronicity is invariable.
[e] 10–20% in pregnant women.
[f] Common in Mediterranean countries, rare in North America and western Europe.

temperate zones, epidemic waves have been recorded every 5 to 20 years as new segments of nonimmune population appeared; however, in developed countries, the incidence of type A hepatitis has been declining, presumably as a function of improved sanitation, and these cyclic patterns are no longer being observed. No HAV carrier state has been identified after acute type A hepatitis; perpetuation of the virus in nature depends presumably on nonepidemic, inapparent subclinical infection.

In the general population, anti-HAV, an excellent marker for previous HAV infection, increases in prevalence as a function of increasing age and of decreasing socioeconomic status. In the 1970s, serologic evidence of prior hepatitis A infection occurred in about 40 percent of urban populations in the United States, most of whom never recalled having had a symptomatic case of hepatitis. In subsequent decades, however, the prevalence of anti-HAV has been declining in the United States. In developing countries, exposure, infection, and subsequent immunity are almost universal in childhood. As the frequency of subclinical childhood infections declines in developed countries, a susceptible cohort of adults emerges. Hepatitis A tends to be more symptomatic in adults; therefore, paradoxically, as the frequency of HAV infection declines, the likelihood of clinically apparent, even severe, HAV illnesses increases in the susceptible adult population. Travel to endemic areas is a common source of infection for adults from nonendemic areas. More recently recognized epidemiologic foci of HAV infection include child-care centers, neonatal intensive care units, promiscuous homosexual men, and intravenous drug users.

Hepatitis B It has long been recognized that a major route of hepatitis B transmission is percutaneous, but the outmoded designation "serum hepatitis" is an inaccurate label for the epidemiologic spectrum of HBV infection recognized today. As detailed below, most of the hepatitis transmitted by blood transfusion is not caused by HBV; moreover, in approximately half of patients with acute type B hepatitis, there is no history of an identifiable percutaneous exposure. We now recognize that many cases of type B hepatitis result from less obvious modes of nonpercutaneous or covert percutaneous transmission. HBsAg has been identified in almost every body fluid from infected persons—saliva, tears, seminal fluid, cerebrospinal

fluid, ascites, breast milk, synovial fluid, gastric juice, pleural fluid, and urine, and even rarely in feces. Although there is abundant evidence to suggest that feces are not infectious, at least some of these body fluids—most notably semen and saliva—have been shown to be infectious, albeit less so than serum, when administered percutaneously or nonpercutaneously to experimental animals. Among the nonpercutaneous modes of HBV transmission, oral ingestion has been documented as a potential route of exposure but one whose efficiency is quite low. On the other hand, the two nonpercutaneous routes considered to have the greatest impact are intimate (especially sexual) contact and perinatal transmission.

In sub-Saharan Africa, intimate contact among toddlers is considered instrumental in contributing to the maintenance of the high frequency of HBsAg in the population. Perinatal transmission occurs primarily in infants born to HBsAg carrier mothers or mothers with acute hepatitis B during the third trimester of pregnancy or during the early postpartum period. Perinatal transmission is uncommon in North America and western Europe but occurs with great frequency and is the most important mode of HBV perpetuation in the Far East and developing countries. Although the precise mode of perinatal transmission is unknown, and although approximately 10 percent of infections may be acquired in utero, epidemiologic evidence suggests that most infections occur approximately at the time of delivery and are not related to breast feeding. Likelihood of perinatal transmission of HBV correlates with the presence of HBeAg; 90 percent of HBeAg-positive mothers but only 10 to 15 percent of anti-HBe-positive mothers transmit HBV infection to their offspring. In most cases, acute infection in the neonate is clinically asymptomatic, but the child is very likely to become an HBsAg carrier.

The more than 200 million HBsAg carriers in the world constitute the main reservoir of hepatitis B in human beings. Serum HBsAg is infrequent (0.1 to 0.5 percent) in normal populations in the United States and western Europe; however, a prevalence of up to 5 to 20 percent has been found in the Far East and in some tropical countries and as high as 30 percent in persons with Down's syndrome, lepromatous leprosy, leukemia, Hodgkin's disease, polyarteritis nodosa, patients with chronic renal disease on hemodialysis, and needle-using drug addicts.

Other groups with high rates of HBV infection include spouses of acutely infected persons, sexually promiscuous persons (especially promiscuous homosexual men), health care workers exposed to blood, persons who require repeated transfusions especially with pooled blood product concentrates (e.g., hemophiliacs), residents and staff of custodial institutions for the mentally retarded, prisoners, and, to a lesser extent, family members of chronically infected patients. In volunteer blood donors, the prevalence of anti-HBs, a reflection of previous HBV infection, ranges from 5 to 10 percent, but the prevalence is higher in lower socioeconomic strata, older age groups, and persons—including those mentioned above—exposed to blood products.

Prevalence of infection, modes of transmission, and human behavior conspire to mold geographically different epidemiologic patterns of HBV infection. In the Far East and Africa, hepatitis B, a disease of the newborn and young children, is perpetuated by a cycle of maternal-neonatal spread. In North America and western Europe, hepatitis B is primarily a disease of adolescence and early adulthood, the time of life when intimate sexual contact as well as recreational and occupational percutaneous exposures tend to occur.

Hepatitis D   Infection with HDV has a worldwide distribution, but two epidemiologic patterns exist. In Mediterranean countries (northern Africa, southern Europe, the Middle East), HDV infection is endemic among those with hepatitis B, and the disease is transmitted predominantly by nonpercutaneous means, especially close personal contact. In nonendemic areas, such as the United States and northern Europe, HDV infection is confined to persons exposed frequently to blood and blood products, primarily drug addicts and hemophiliacs. HDV infection can be introduced into a population through drug addicts or by migration of persons from endemic to nonendemic areas. Thus patterns of population migration and human behavior facilitating percutaneous contact play important roles in the introduction and amplification of HDV infection. Occasionally, the migrating epidemiology of hepatitis D is expressed in explosive outbreaks of severe hepatitis, such as those which have occurred in remote South American villages as well as in urban centers in the United States. Ultimately, such outbreaks of hepatitis D—either of coinfections with acute hepatitis B or of superinfections in those already infected with HBV—may blur the distinctions between endemic and nonendemic areas.

Hepatitis C (non-A, non-B hepatitis)   Routine screening of blood donors for HBsAg and the elimination of commercial blood sources in the early 1970s reduced the frequency of, but did not eliminate, transfusion-associated hepatitis. During the 1970s, the likelihood of acquiring hepatitis after transfusion of voluntarily donated, HBsAg-screened blood was approximately 10 percent per patient (up to 0.9 percent per unit transfused). Although hepatitis B accounted for up to 5 to 10 percent of these cases, the remaining 90 to 95 percent were classified, based on serologic exclusion, as "non-A, non-B" hepatitis. For patients requiring transfusion of pooled products, such as clotting factor concentrates, the risk was even higher, up to 20 to 30 percent, while for those receiving such products as albumin and immune globulin, because of prior treatment of these materials by heating to 60°C or cold ethanol fractionation, there was then, and there remains now, no risk of hepatitis.

During the 1980s, voluntary self-exclusion of blood donors with risk factors for AIDS and, then, the introduction of donor screening for anti-HIV reduced further the likelihood of transfusion-associated hepatitis to under 5 percent. During the late 1980s and early 1990s, the introduction first of "surrogate" screening tests for non-A, non-B hepatitis [alanine aminotransferase (ALT) and anti-HBc, both shown to identify blood donors with a higher likelihood of transmitting non-A, non-B hepatitis to recipients] and, subsequently, after the discovery of HCV, first-generation immunoassays for anti-HCV reduced the frequency of transfusion-associated hepatitis even further. A prospective analysis of transfusion-associated hepatitis conducted between 1986 and 1990 showed that the incidence of transfusion-associated hepatitis at one urban university hospital fell from a baseline of 3.8 percent per patient (0.45 percent per unit transfused) to 1.5 percent per patient (0.19 percent per unit) after the introduction of surrogate testing to 0.6 percent per patient (0.03 percent per unit) after the introduction of first-generation anti-HCV assays. The introduction of second-generation anti-HCV assays will reduce the frequency of transfusion-associated hepatitis C even further, potentially to almost imperceptible levels.

In addition to being transmitted by transfusion, hepatitis C can be transmitted by other percutaneous routes, such as self-injection with intravenous drugs. In addition, this virus can be transmitted by occupational exposure to blood, and the likelihood of infection is increased in hemodialysis units. Although the frequency of transfusion-associated hepatitis C has fallen as a result of blood donor screening, the overall frequency of hepatitis C has remained the same, primarily because of increases in other modes of transmission, especially intravenous drug use.

Serologic evidence for HCV infection occurs in >90 percent of patients with transfusion-associated non-A, non-B hepatitis, hemophiliacs, and intravenous drug users; 60 to 70 percent of patients with sporadic non-A, non-B hepatitis (in the absence of a known risk factor); and 0.5 percent of volunteer blood donors (i.e., a carrier rate of 0.5 percent in the general population). The vast majority of asymptomatic blood donors found to have circulating, reproducible anti-HCV do not belong to high-risk groups. How they become infected remains a mystery. The potential exists that such infections of undefined source represent sexually transmitted infection or infection acquired by perinatal transmission; however, although these routes of infection can occur (especially when the source of infection is also infected with HIV), both sexual and perinatal transmission of HCV are rare. In all likelihood, the inefficiency of these less than direct routes of transmission is a reflection of the relatively low infectivity titer of HCV. Infections of household contacts are rare as well. Among patients with reported cases of acute hepatitis C, 40 percent have no readily identifiable risk factor.

The risk of HCV infection is increased in organ transplant recipients and in patients with AIDS; in all immunosuppressed groups, levels of anti-HCV may be undetectable, and a diagnosis may require testing for HCV RNA. Chronic hepatitis C occurs in as many as 20 percent of renal transplant recipients. In the early years after transplantation, the death rate in these patients with hepatitis is increased not as a result of liver failure but of severe infections outside the hepatobiliary tree. This effect has been attributed to the immunosuppressive impact of HCV infection on the host. Five to 10 years after transplantation, however, complications of chronic liver disease account for increased morbidity and mortality. The impact of HCV infection on liver transplant recipients is controversial, associated with severe liver disease in some series but with trivial morbidity in others.

Hepatitis E   The enteric form of non-A, non-B hepatitis identified in India, Asia, Africa, and Central America resembles hepatitis A in its primarily enteric mode of spread. The commonly recognized cases occur after contamination of water supplies such as after monsoon flooding, but sporadic, isolated cases occur. An epidemiologic feature that distinguishes HEV from other enteric agents is the rarity of secondary person-to-person spread from infected persons to their close contacts. Infections arise in populations that are immune to HAV and favor young adults. It is not known if hepatitis E occurs outside of recognized endemic areas, for example, in the United States, but preliminary studies suggest that HEV does not account for any of the sporadic "non-A, non-B" cases in nonendemic areas. Cases imported from endemic areas have been found in the United States.

CLINICAL AND LABORATORY FEATURES   Symptoms and signs   Acute viral hepatitis occurs after an incubation period that varies according to the responsible agent. Generally, incubation periods for hepatitis A range from 15 to 45 days (mean 4 weeks), for hepatitis B and D from 30 to 180 days (mean 4 to 12 weeks), for hepatitis C from 15 to 160 days (mean 7 weeks), and for hepatitis E from 14 to 60 days (mean 5 to 6 weeks). The *prodromal symptoms* of acute viral hepatitis are systemic and quite variable. Constitutional symptoms of anorexia, nausea and vomiting, fatigue, malaise, arthralgias, myalgias, headache, photophobia, pharyngitis, cough, and coryza may precede the onset of jaundice by 1 to 2 weeks. The nausea, vomiting, and anorexia are frequently associated wth alterations in olfaction and taste. A low-grade fever between 38 and 39°C (100 to 102°F) is more often present in hepatitis A and E than in hepatitis B or C, except when hepatitis B is heralded by a serum sickness–like syndrome; rarely, a fever of 39.5 to 40°C (103 to 104°F) may accompany the constitutional symptoms. Dark urine and clay-colored stools may be noticed by the patient from 1 to 5 days prior to the onset of clinical jaundice.

With the onset of *clinical jaundice*, the constitutional prodromal symptoms usually diminish, but in some patients mild weight loss (2.5 to 5 kg) is common and may continue during the entire icteric phase. The liver becomes enlarged and tender and may be associated with right upper quadrant pain and discomfort. Infrequently, patients present with a cholestatic picture, suggesting extrahepatic biliary obstruction. Splenomegaly and cervical adenopathy are present in 10 to 20 percent of patients with acute hepatitis. Rarely, a few spider angiomas appear during the icteric phase and disappear during convalescence. During the *recovery phase*, constitutional symptoms disappear, but usually some liver enlargement and abnormalities in biochemical tests of hepatic function are still evident. The duration of the posticteric phase is variable, ranging from 2 to 12 weeks, and usually is more prolonged in acute hepatitis B and C. Complete clinical and biochemical recovery is to be expected 1 to 2 months after all cases of hepatitis A and E and 3 to 4 months after the onset of jaundice in three-quarters of uncomplicated cases of hepatitis B and C. In the remainder, biochemical recovery may be delayed. A substantial proportion of patients with viral hepatitis never become icteric.

Infection with HDV can occur in the presence of acute or chronic HBV infection; the duration of HBV infection determines the duration of HDV infection. When acute HDV and HBV infection occur simultaneously, clinical and biochemical features may be indistinguishable from those of HBV infection alone, although occasionally they are more severe. As opposed to patients with *acute* HBV infection, patients with *chronic* HBV infection can support HDV replication indefinitely. This can happen when acute HDV infection occurs in the presence of a nonresolving acute HBV infection. More commonly, acute HDV infection becomes chronic when it is superimposed on an underlying chronic HBV infection. In such cases, the HDV superinfection appears as a clinical exacerbation or an episode resembling acute viral hepatitis in someone already chronically infected with HBV. In the past, events resembling acute hepatitis in an HBV carrier or a patient with chronic hepatitis B were attributed to superimposed "non-A, non-B" hepatitis or to the natural history of the disease. A proportion of such episodes, however, represent acute superinfection with HDV. Superinfection with HDV in a patient with chronic hepatitis B often leads to clinical deterioration (see below).

In addition to superinfections with other hepatitis agents, acute hepatitis-like clinical events in persons with chronic hepatitis B may accompany spontaneous HBeAg–to–anti-HBe seroconversion or spontaneous reactivation, i.e., reversion from nonreplicative to replicative infection. Such reactivations can occur as well in therapeutically immunosuppressed patients with chronic HBV infection when cytotoxic-immunosuppressive drugs are withdrawn; in these cases, restoration of immune competence is thought to allow resumption of previously checked cell-mediated cytolysis of HBV-infected hepatocytes.

Laboratory features　　The serum aminotransferases AST and ALT (previously designated SGOT and SGPT) show a variable increase during the prodromal phase of acute viral hepatitis and precede the rise in bilirubin level (see Figs. 266-2 and 266-3). The acute level of these enzymes, however, does not correlate well with the degree of liver cell damage. Peak levels vary from 400 to 4000 IU or more; these levels are usually reached at the time the patient is clinically

icteric and diminish progressively during the recovery phase of acute hepatitis. The diagnosis of anicteric hepatitis is difficult and requires a high index of suspicion; it is based on clinical features and on aminotransferase elevations, although mild increases in conjugated bilirubin also may be found.

Jaundice is usually visible in the sclera or skin when the serum bilirubin value exceeds 43 µmol/L (2.5 mg/dL). When jaundice appears, the serum bilirubin typically rises to levels ranging from 85 to 340 µmol/L (5 to 20 mg/dL). The serum bilirubin may continue to rise despite falling serum aminotransferase levels. In most instances, the total bilirubin is equally divided between the conjugated and unconjugated fractions. Bilirubin levels above 340 µmol/L (20 mg/dL) extending and persisting late into the course of viral hepatitis are more likely to be associated with severe disease. In certain patients with underlying hemolytic anemia, however, such as glucose-6-phosphate dehydrogenase deficiency and sickle cell anemia, a high serum bilirubin level is common, resulting from superimposed hemolysis. In such patients, bilirubin levels greater than 513 µmol/L (30 mg/dL) have been observed and are not necessarily associated with a poor prognosis.

Neutropenia and lymphopenia are transient and are followed by a relative lymphocytosis. Atypical lymphocytes (varying between 2 and 20 percent) are common during the acute phase. These atypical lymphocytes are indistinguishable from those seen in infectious mononucleosis. Measurement of the prothrombin time (PT) is important in patients with acute viral hepatitis, for a prolonged value may reflect a severe synthetic defect, signify extensive hepatocellular necrosis, and indicate a worse prognosis. Occasionally, a prolonged PT may occur with only mild increases in the serum bilirubin and aminotransferase levels. Prolonged nausea and vomiting, inadequate carbohydrate intake, and poor hepatic glycogen reserves may contribute to hypoglycemia noted occasionally in patients with severe viral hepatitis. Serum alkaline phosphatase may be normal or only mildly elevated, while a fall in serum albumin is uncommon in uncomplicated acute viral hepatitis. In some patients, mild and transient steatorrhea has been noted as well as slight microscopic hematuria and minimal proteinuria.

A diffuse but mild elevation of the gamma globulin fraction is common during acute viral hepatitis. Serum IgG and IgM are elevated in about one-third of patients during the acute phase of viral hepatitis, but serum IgM elevation is seen more characteristically during acute hepatitis A. During the acute phase of viral hepatitis, antibodies to smooth muscle and other cell constituents may be present, and low titers of rheumatoid factor, antinuclear antibody, and heterophil antibody also can be found occasionally. In hepatitis C and D, antibodies to liver-kidney microsomes (LKM) occur; however, the species of LKM antibodies in the two types of hepatitis are different from each other as well as from the LKM antibody species characteristic of autoimmune chronic active hepatitis type 2 (see Chap. 267). The autoantibodies in viral hepatitis are nonspecific and also can be associated with other viral and systemic diseases. In contrast, virus-specific antibodies, which appear during and after hepatitis virus infection, are serologic markers of diagnostic importance.

As described above, serologic tests are available with which to establish a diagnosis of hepatitis A, B, D, and C. Tests for fecal or serum HAV are not routinely available. Therefore, a diagnosis of type A hepatitis is based on detection of IgM anti-HAV during acute illness (see Fig. 266-2). Rheumatoid factor can give rise to false-positive results in this test.

A diagnosis of HBV infection can usually be made by detection of HBsAg in serum. Infrequently, levels of HBsAg are too low to be detected during acute HBV infection even with the current generation of highly sensitive immunoassays. In such cases, the diagnosis can be established by the presence of IgM anti-HBc. Alternatively, de novo appearance of anti-HBc and anti-HBs during illness and convalescence may support the diagnostic impression.

The titer of HBsAg bears little relation to the severity of clinical disease. Indeed, there may be an inverse correlation between the serum concentration of HBsAg and the degree of liver cell damage. For example, titers are highest in immunosuppressed patients, lower in chronic liver disease (but higher in chronic persistent than in chronic active hepatitis), and very low in acute fulminant hepatitis. These observations suggest that in hepatitis B the degree of liver cell damage and the clinical course are probably related to variations in the patient's immune response to HBV rather than to the amount of circulating HBsAg. In immunocompetent persons, however, there is a correlation between markers of HBV *replication* and liver injury (see below).

Another serologic marker that may be of value in patients with hepatitis B is HBeAg. Its principal clinical usefulness is as an indicator of relative infectivity. Because HBeAg is invariably present during early acute hepatitis B, HBeAg testing is indicated primarily during follow-up of chronic infection.

In patients with hepatitis B surface antigenemia of unknown duration, e.g., blood donors whose blood is found to be HBsAg-positive and who are referred to a physician for evaluation, testing for IgM anti-HBc may be useful to distinguish between acute or recent infection (IgM anti-HBc-positive) and chronic HBV infection (IgM anti-HBc-negative, IgG anti-HBc-positive). A false-positive test for IgM anti-HBc may be encountered in patients with high-titer rheumatoid factor.

Anti-HBs is rarely detectable in the presence of HBsAg in patients with *acute* hepatitis B, but 10 to 20 percent of persons with *chronic* HBV infection may harbor low-level anti-HBs. This antibody is directed not against the common group determinant, *a*, but against the heterotypic subtype determinant (e.g., HBsAg of subtype *ad* with anti-HBs of subtype *y*). In most cases, this serologic pattern cannot be attributed to infection with two different HBV subtypes, and the presence of this antibody is not a harbinger of imminent HBsAg clearance. When such antibody is detected, its presence is of no recognized clinical significance.

After immunization with hepatitis B vaccine, which consists of HBsAg alone, anti-HBs is the only serologic marker to appear. A summary of the commonly encountered serologic patterns of hepatitis B and their interpretations appears in Table 266-3. Tests for the detection of HBV DNA in liver and serum are now available. Like HBeAg, serum HBV DNA is an indicator of HBV replication, but tests for HBV DNA are more sensitive and quantitative. These markers are useful in following the course of HBV replication in patients with chronic hepatitis B receiving antiviral chemotherapy, e.g., with interferon (see Chap. 267). In immunocompetent persons, a general correlation does appear to exist between the level of HBV replication, as reflected by the level of HBV DNA in serum, and the degree of liver injury. High serum HBV DNA levels, increased

expression of viral antigens, and necroinflammatory activity in the liver go hand in hand unless immunosuppression interferes with cytolytic T cell responses to virus-infected cells; reduction of HBV replication with antiviral drugs, such as interferon, tends to be accompanied by an improvement in liver histology.

Before the availability of reliable serologic tests for hepatitis C, a diagnosis of non-A, non-B hepatitis was made by serologic exclusion of HAV and HBV infection in the setting of a compatible history. A helpful clinical clue is the episodic pattern of aminotransferase elevation seen frequently in non-A, non-B hepatitis. Currently, a specific serologic diagnosis of hepatitis C can be made by demonstrating the presence in serum of anti-HCV. When a second-generation immunoassay (that detects antibodies to nonstructural and nucleocapsid proteins) is used, anti-HCV can be detected in acute hepatitis C during the initial phase of elevated aminotransferase activity. This antibody may never become detectable in 20 to 30 percent of patients with acute hepatitis C, and levels of anti-HCV may become undetectable after recovery from acute hepatitis C. In patients with chronic hepatitis C, anti-HCV is detectable in >90 percent of cases. Because nonspecificity can confound immunoassays for anti-HCV, a supplementary recombinant immunoblot assay should be done to establish the specific viral proteins to which anti-HCV is directed (see "Virology and Etiology," above). Still a research tool, a polymerase chain reaction assay for HCV RNA is the most sensitive test for HCV infection. This test can detect HCV RNA even before acute elevation of aminotransferase activity and before the appearance of anti-HCV in patients with acute hepatitis C. In addition, HCV RNA remains detectable indefinitely, continuously in most but intermittently in some, in patients with chronic hepatitis C (even detectable in some persons with normal liver tests, i.e., asymptomatic carriers). Thus a diagnosis of hepatitis C can be supported by detection of anti-HCV and by exclusion of false-positive reactivity. In the small minority of patients with hepatitis C who lack anti-HCV, a diagnosis can be supported by detection of HCV RNA, if available. If all these tests are negative and the patient has a well-characterized case of hepatitis following percutaneous exposure to blood or blood products, a diagnosis of "non-A, non-B," perhaps caused by another agent, can be entertained. A proportion of patients with hepatitis C have isolated anti-HBc in their blood, a reflection of a common risk in certain populations to multiple bloodborne hepatitis agents. The anti-HBc in such cases is almost invariably of the IgG class and represents either HBV infection in the remote past or current HBV infection with low-level virus carriage.

The presence of HDV infection can be identified by demonstrating intrahepatic HDV antigen or, more practically, an anti-HDV seroconversion (a rise in titer of anti-HDV or de novo appearance of IgM

TABLE 266-3 Commonly encountered serologic patterns of hepatitis B infection

HBsAg	Anti-HBs	Anti-HBc	HBeAg	Anti-HBe	Interpretation
+	−	IgM	+	−	Acute HBV infection, high infectivity
+	−	IgG	+	−	Chronic HBV infection, high infectivity
+	−	IgG	−	+	Late-acute or chronic HBV infection, low infectivity
+	+	+	+/−	+/−	*1* HBsAg of one subtype and heterotypic anti-HBs (common) *2* Process of seroconversion from HBsAg to anti-HBs (rare)
−	−	IgM	+/−	+/−	*1* Acute HBV infection *2* Anti-HBc window
−	−	IgG	−	+/−	*1* Low-level HBsAg carrier *2* Remote past infection
−	+	IgG	−	+/−	Recovery from HBV infection
−	+	−	−	−	*1* Immunization with HBsAg (after vaccination) *2* Remote past infection (?) *3* False-positive

TABLE 266-4 Simplified diagnostic approach in patients presenting with acute hepatitis

	Serologic tests of patient's serum			
HBsAg	IgM anti-HAV	IgM anti-HBc	anti-HCV	Diagnostic interpretation
+	−	+	−	Acute hepatitis B
+	−	−	−	Chronic hepatitis B
+	+	−	−	Acute hepatitis A superimposed on chronic hepatitis B
+	+	+	−	Acute hepatitis A and B
−	+	−	−	Acute hepatitis A
−	+	+	−	Acute hepatitis A and B (HBsAg below detection threshold)
−	−	+	−	Acute hepatitis B (HBsAg below detection threshold)
−	−	−	+	Acute hepatitis C

anti-HDV). Circulating HDVAg, also diagnostic of acute infection, is detectable only briefly, if at all. Because IgM anti-HDV is transient and IgG anti-HDV is often undetectable once HBsAg disappears, retrospective serodiagnosis of acute self-limited, simultaneous HBV and HDV infection is difficult. Early diagnosis of acute infection may be hampered by a delay of up to 30 to 40 days in the appearance of anti-HDV.

When a patient presents with acute hepatitis and has HBsAg and anti-HDV in the serum, determination of the class of anti-HBc is helpful in establishing the relationship between infection with HBV and HDV. Although IgM anti-HBc does not distinguish *absolutely* between acute and chronic HBV infection, its presence is a reliable indicator of recent infection and its absence a reliable indicator of infection in the remote past. In simultaneous acute HBV and HDV infections, IgM anti-HBc will be detectable, while in acute HDV infection superimposed on chronic HBV infection, anti-HBc will be of the IgG class.

In the future, tests for the presence of HDV RNA will be useful for determining the presence of ongoing HDV replication and relative infectivity. Currently, probes for this marker are restricted to a limited number of research laboratories. Similarly, diagnostic tests for hepatitis E are cumbersome and remain limited to a small number of research laboratories. Routine diagnostic tests are being developed, however.

Liver biopsy is rarely necessary or indicated in acute viral hepatitis, except when there is a question about the diagnosis or when there is clinical evidence suggesting a diagnosis of chronic active hepatitis.

A diagnostic algorithm can be applied in the evaluation of cases of acute viral hepatitis. A patient with acute hepatitis should undergo four serologic tests, HBsAg, IgM anti-HAV, IgM anti-HBc, and anti-HCV (Table 266-4). The presence of HBsAg, with or without IgM anti-HBc, represents HBV infection. If IgM anti-HBc is present, the HBV infection is considered acute; if IgM anti-HBc is absent, the HBV infection is considered chronic. A diagnosis of acute hepatitis B can be made in the absence of HBsAg when IgM anti-HBc is detectable. A diagnosis of acute hepatitis A is based on the presence of IgM anti-HAV. If IgM anti-HAV coexists with HBsAg, a diagnosis of simultaneous HAV and HBV infections can be made; if IgM anti-HBc (with or without HBsAg) is detectable, the patient has simultaneous acute hepatitis A and B, and if IgM anti-HBc is undetectable, the patient has acute hepatitis A superimposed on chronic HBV infection. The presence of anti-HCV, if confirmable, supports a diagnosis of acute hepatitis C. Occasionally, repeat anti-HCV testing later during the illness is necessary to establish the diagnosis. Absence of all serologic markers is consistent with a diagnosis of "non-A, non-B" hepatitis, if the epidemiologic setting is appropriate.

In patients with chronic hepatitis, initial testing should consist of HBsAg and anti-HCV. Anti-HCV supports the diagnosis of chronic hepatitis C. If a serologic diagnosis of chronic hepatitis B is made, testing for HBeAg and anti-HBe is indicated to evaluate relative infectivity. Testing for HBV DNA in such patients provides a more quantitative and sensitive test for the level of virus replication and, therefore, is very helpful during antiviral therapy (see Chap. 267). In patients with hepatitis B, testing for anti-HDV is useful under the following circumstances: severe and fulminant cases, severe chronic cases, cases of acute hepatitis-like exacerbations in patients with chronic hepatitis B, persons with frequent percutaneous exposures, and persons from areas where HDV infection is endemic.

PROGNOSIS Virtually all previously healthy patients with hepatitis A recover completely from their illness with no clinical sequelae. Similarly, in acute hepatitis B, 95 percent of patients have a favorable course and recover completely. There are, however, certain clinical and laboratory features which suggest a more complicated and protracted course. Patients of advanced age and with serious underlying medical disorders may have a prolonged course and are more likely to experience severe hepatitis. Initial presenting features such as ascites, peripheral edema, and symptoms of hepatic encephalopathy suggest a poorer prognosis. In addition, a prolonged prothrombin time, low serum albumin level, hypoglycemia, and very high serum bilirubin values suggest severe hepatocellular disease. Patients with these clinical and laboratory features deserve prompt hospital admission. The case-fatality rate in hepatitis A and B is very low (approximately 0.1 percent) but is increased by advanced age and underlying debilitating disorders. Among patients ill enough to be hospitalized for acute hepatitis B, the fatality rate is 1 percent. Hepatitis C occurring after transfusion is less severe during the acute phase than type B hepatitis and is more likely to be anicteric; fatalities are rare, but the precise case-fatality rate is not known. In outbreaks of waterborne hepatitis E in India and Asia, the case-fatality rate is 1 to 2 percent and up to 10 to 20 percent in pregnant women. Patients with simultaneous acute hepatitis B and hepatitis D do not necessarily experience a higher mortality rate than do patients with acute hepatitis B alone; however, in several recent outbreaks of acute simultaneous HBV and HDV infection among drug addicts, the case fatality rate has been approximately 5 percent. In the case of HDV superinfection of a person with chronic hepatitis B, the likelihood of fulminant hepatitis and death is increased substantially. Although the case-fatality rate for hepatitis D has not been defined adequately, in outbreaks of severe HDV superinfection in isolated populations with a high hepatitis B carrier rate, the mortality rate has been recorded in excess of 20 percent.

COMPLICATIONS AND SEQUELAE A small proportion of patients with hepatitis A experience *relapsing hepatitis* weeks to months after apparent recovery from acute hepatitis. Relapses are characterized by recurrence of symptoms, aminotransferase elevations, occasionally jaundice, and fecal excretion of HAV. Another unusual variant of acute hepatitis A is *cholestatic hepatitis*, characterized by protracted cholestatic jaundice and pruritus. Rarely, liver test abnormalities persist for many months, even up to a year. Even when these complications occur, hepatitis A remains self-limited and does not progress to chronic liver disease. During the prodromal phase of acute hepatitis B, a serum sickness–like syndrome characterized by arthralgia or arthritis, rash, angioedema, and rarely hematuria and proteinuria may develop in some patients. This syndrome occurs prior to the onset of clinical jaundice, and these patients are often erroneously diagnosed as having rheumatoid arthritis or other rheumatologic diseases such as systemic lupus erythematosus. This syndrome occurs in about 5 to 10 percent of patients with acute hepatitis B. The diagnosis can be established by measuring serum aminotransferase levels, which are almost invariably elevated, and serum HBsAg.

The most feared complication of viral hepatitis is *fulminant hepatitis* (massive hepatic necrosis); fortunately, this is a rare event. This is primarily seen in hepatitis B and D, as well as hepatitis E, but rare fulminant cases of hepatitis A occur primarily in older adults and in persons with underlying chronic liver disease. Hepatitis B accounts for more than 50 percent of fulminant hepatitis cases, a sizable proportion of which are associated with HDV infection. Participation of HDV can be documented in approximately one-third of patients with acute fulminant hepatitis B and two-thirds of patients with fulminant hepatitis superimposed on chronic hepatitis B. Fulminant hepatitis is seen rarely in hepatitis C, but hepatitis E, as noted above, can be complicated by fatal fulminant hepatitis in 1 to 2 percent of all cases and in up to 20 percent of cases occurring in pregnant women. Patients usually present with signs and symptoms of encephalopathy that may evolve to deep coma. The liver is usually small and the prothrombin time excessively prolonged. The combination of rapidly shrinking liver size, rapidly rising bilirubin level, and marked prolongation of the prothrombin time, together with clinical signs of confusion, disorientation, somnolence, ascites, and edema, indicates that the patient has hepatic failure with encephalopathy. Cerebral edema is common; brainstem compression, gastrointestinal bleeding, sepsis, respiratory failure, cardiovascular collapse, and renal failure are terminal events. The mortality is exceedingly high (greater than 80 percent in patients with deep coma), but patients who survive may have a complete biochemical and histologic recovery.

It is particularly important to document the disappearance of HBsAg following apparent clinical recovery from acute hepatitis B. Before laboratory methods were available to distinguish between acute and acute hepatitis–like exacerbations (*spontaneous reactivations*) of chronic hepatitis B, observations suggested that approximately 10 percent of patients remained HBsAg-positive for longer than 6 months after the onset of clinically apparent acute hepatitis B. Half these persons were found to clear the antigen from their circulations during the next several years, but the other 5 percent remained chronically HBsAg-positive. More recent observations suggest that the true rate of chronic infection after clinically apparent acute hepatitis B is as low as 1 to 2 percent in normal, immunocompetent, young adults. Earlier, higher estimates may have been biased by inadvertent inclusion of acute exacerbations in chronically infected patients; these patients, chronically HBsAg-positive before exacerbation, were unlikely to seroconvert to HBsAg-negative thereafter. Whether the rate of chronicity is 10 or 1 percent, such patients have anti-HBc in serum; anti-HBs is either undetected or detected at low titer against the opposite subtype specificity of the antigen (see "Laboratory Features," above). These patients may (1) be asymptomatic carriers, (2) have low-grade chronic persistent hepatitis, or (3) have chronic active hepatitis with or without cirrhosis. The likelihood of becoming an HBsAg carrier after acute HBV infection is especially high among neonates, persons with Down's syndrome, chronically hemodialyzed patients, and immunosuppressed patients, including persons with human immunodeficiency virus infection.

Chronic active hepatitis is a major late complication of acute hepatitis B occurring in a small proportion of acute cases but more common in those who present with chronic infection without having experienced an acute illness (see Chap. 267). Certain clinical and laboratory features suggest progression of acute hepatitis to chronic active hepatitis: (1) lack of complete resolution of clinical symptoms of anorexia, weight loss, and fatigue and the persistence of hepatomegaly; (2) the presence of bridging or multilobular hepatic necrosis on liver biopsy during protracted, severe acute viral hepatitis; (3) failure of the serum aminotransferase, bilirubin, and globulin levels to return to normal within 6 to 12 months following the acute illness; and (4) the continued presence of HBsAg and HBeAg 6 months or more after acute hepatitis, suggesting chronic, replicative viral infection of the liver.

Although acute hepatitis D infection does not increase the likelihood of chronicity of simultaneous acute hepatitis B, hepatitis D has the potential for contributing to the severity of chronic hepatitis B. Hepatitis D superinfection can transform asymptomatic or mild chronic hepatitis B into severe, progressive chronic active hepatitis and cirrhosis; it also can accelerate the course of chronic active

hepatitis B. Some HDV superinfections in patients with chronic hepatitis B lead to fulminant hepatitis. Although HDV and HBV infections are associated with severe liver disease, mild hepatitis and even asymptomatic carriage have been identified in some patients. After transfusion-associated acute hepatitis C, as many as 50 percent of patients have abnormal biochemical liver tests for more than a year. In a majority of such patients, liver histology is consistent with chronic active hepatitis. Although many of these patients have no symptoms and a nonprogressive course, ultimately, cirrhosis develops in as many as 20 percent of those with *chronic* posttransfusion hepatitis C within 10 years of acute illness. The likelihood of chronic hepatitis is also approximately 50 percent after sporadic hepatitis C occurring in the absence of identifiable percutaneous inoculation with blood products or contaminated needles. In contrast, neither HAV nor HEV causes chronic liver disease.

Rare complications of viral hepatitis include pancreatitis, myocarditis, atypical pneumonia, aplastic anemia, transverse myelitis, and peripheral neuropathy. *Carriers* of HBsAg, particularly those infected in infancy or early childhood, have an enhanced risk of hepatocellular carcinoma. The risk of hepatocellular carcinoma is increased as well in patients with cirrhosis associated with chronic hepatitis C (see Chap. 269). In children, hepatitis B may present rarely with anicteric hepatitis, a nonpruritic papular rash of the face, buttocks, and limbs, and lymphadenopathy (papular acrodermatitis of childhood or Gianotti-Crosti syndrome).

DIFFERENTIAL DIAGNOSIS   Viral diseases such as infectious mononucleosis; those due to cytomegalovirus, herpes simplex, and coxsackieviruses; and toxoplasmosis may share certain clinical features with viral hepatitis and cause elevation in serum aminotransferase and less commonly in serum bilirubin levels. Tests such as the differential heterophil and serologic tests for these agents may be helpful in the differential diagnosis if HBsAg, anti-HBc, IgM anti-HAV, and anti-HCV determinations are negative. A complete drug history is particularly important, for many drugs and certain anesthetic agents can produce a picture of either acute hepatitis or cholestasis (see below). Equally important is a past history of unexplained "repeated episodes" of acute hepatitis. This should alert the physician to the possibility that the underlying disorder is chronic active hepatitis. Alcoholic hepatitis also must be considered, but usually the serum aminotransferase levels are not as markedly elevated and other stigmata of alcoholism may be present. The finding on liver biopsy of fatty infiltration, a neutrophilic inflammatory reaction, and "alcoholic hyaline" would be consistent with alcohol-induced rather than viral liver injury. Because acute hepatitis may present with right upper quadrant abdominal pain, nausea and vomiting, fever, and icterus, it is often confused with acute cholecystitis, common duct stone, or ascending cholangitis. Patients with acute viral hepatitis may tolerate surgery poorly; therefore, it is important to exclude this diagnosis, and in confusing cases, a percutaneous liver biopsy may be necessary prior to laparotomy. Viral hepatitis in the elderly is often misdiagnosed as obstructive jaundice resulting from a common duct stone or carcinoma of the pancreas. Because acute hepatitis in the elderly may be quite severe and the operative mortality high, a thorough evaluation including biochemical tests, radiographic studies of the biliary tree, and even liver biopsy may be necessary to exclude primary parenchymal liver disease. Another clinical constellation that may mimic acute hepatitis is right ventricular failure with passive hepatic congestion or hypoperfusion syndromes, such as those associated with shock, severe hypotension, and severe left ventricular failure. Clinical features are usually sufficient to distinguish between the two entities. Very rarely, malignancies metastatic to the liver can mimic acute or even fulminant viral hepatitis. Occasionally, genetic or metabolic liver disorders (e.g., Wilson's disease, α_1-antitrypsin deficiency) are confused with viral hepatitis.

MANAGEMENT   Treatment of acute attack   There is no specific treatment for *typical acute viral hepatitis*. Although hospitalization may be required for clinically severe illness, most patients do not require hospital care. Forced and prolonged bed rest is not essential for full recovery, but many patients will feel better with restricted physical activity. A high-calorie diet is desirable, and because many patients may experience nausea late in the day, the major caloric intake is best tolerated in the morning. Intravenous feeding is necessary in the acute stage if the patient has persistent vomiting and cannot maintain oral intake. Drugs capable of producing adverse reactions such as cholestasis and drugs metabolized by the liver should be avoided. If severe pruritus is present, the use of the bile salt–sequestering resin cholestyramine will usually alleviate this symptom. Glucocorticoid therapy has no value in acute viral hepatitis. Even in severe cases associated with *bridging necrosis*, controlled trials have failed to demonstrate the efficacy of steroids. In fact, such therapy may be hazardous.

Physical isolation of patients with hepatitis to a single room and bathroom is rarely necessary except in the case of fecal incontinence for hepatitis A and E or uncontrolled, voluminous bleeding for hepatitis types B (with or without concomitant hepatitis D) and hepatitis C. Because most patients hospitalized with hepatitis A excrete little if any HAV, the likelihood of HAV transmission from these patients during their hospitalization is low. Therefore, burdensome *enteric precautions are no longer recommended*. Although gloves should be worn when the bedpans or fecal material of patients with hepatitis A are handled, these precautions do not represent a departure from sensible procedure for all hospitalized patients. For patients with hepatitis types B and C, emphasis should be placed on blood precautions, i.e., avoiding direct, ungloved hand contact with blood and other body fluids. Enteric precautions are unnecessary. The importance of simple hygienic precautions, such as hand washing, cannot be overemphasized.

Hospitalized patients may be discharged when there is substantial symptomatic improvement, a significant downward trend in the serum aminotransferase and bilirubin values, and a return to normal of the prothrombin time. Mild aminotransferase elevations should not be considered contraindications to the gradual resumption of normal activity.

In *fulminant hepatitis*, the goal of therapy is to support the patient by maintenance of fluid balance, support of circulation and respiration, control of bleeding, correction of hypoglycemia, and treatment of other complications of the comatose state in anticipation of liver regeneration and repair. Protein intake should be restricted and oral lactulose or neomycin administered. Massive doses of glucocorticoids have been administered, but such therapy has been shown in controlled trials to be ineffective. Likewise, exchange transfusion, plasmapheresis, human cross-circulation, porcine liver cross-perfusion, and hemoperfusion have not been proven to enhance survival. Meticulous intensive care is the one factor that does appear to improve survival. Orthotopic liver transplantation is resorted to with increasing frequency, with excellent results, in patients with fulminant hepatitis (see Chap. 271).

HAZARDS TO MEDICAL AND PARAMEDICAL PERSONNEL Health care workers exposed frequently to blood, body tissues, and fluids have an increased risk of viral hepatitis, primarily hepatitis B. Approximately 15 percent of health workers have one or more serologic markers of HBV infection, and 1 percent are HBsAg-positive. The risk is higher in surgeons, pathologists, laboratory technologists who process blood specimens, technologists who draw blood and insert intravenous cannulas, hemodialysis staff, and others who perform invasive procedures. Transmission of HBV infection in health care settings, however, appears to be unidirectional, from patients to staff. With rare exceptions, HBsAg-positive health personnel do not increase the risk of HBV infection for their patients. Asymptomatic HBsAg carriers represent the greater risk to health personnel, because there are no readily identifiable clinical features that allow their recognition. Approximately 1 percent of all patients admitted to large metropolitan hospitals are HBsAg-positive, but 90 percent of these are not identified routinely. Patients with a past history of hepatitis or multiple transfusions, patients from countries where hepatitis B is endemic, sexually active homosexual men,

intravenous drug abusers, and patients with chronic liver disease, chronic renal failure, polyarteritis nodosa, and Down's syndrome should have routine HBsAg determinations because of the high frequency of HBsAg positivity in these groups. If positive, they are potentially infectious, and appropriate precautions should be taken during operative or other acute care procedures. In hemodialysis units, introduction of patient and staff education, routine periodic screening for HBsAg and aminotransferase elevations, and segregation of HBsAg-positive patients from susceptible patients have reduced dramatically the incidence of new HBV infections in both patients and medical personnel. Immunization with hepatitis B vaccine is another important measure in limiting the spread of hepatitis B to health workers (see below). Despite the fact that hepatitis B and C are transmitted by comparable routes, the risk of HCV infection in health workers is substantially lower than that for HBV infection. This may result from the very-low-level viremia associated with hepatitis C. Occupational exposure to HAV is very rare, but outbreaks have been reported among health workers in neonatal intensive care units. Transfusion-associated hepatitis A, rare as it is, has been implicated in the introduction of the virus into these units, but transmission to other babies and to hospital workers appears to have been enteric.

PROPHYLAXIS Because there is no therapy for acute viral hepatitis, and because antiviral therapy for chronic viral hepatitis is effective in only a proportion of patients (see Chap. 267), emphasis is placed on prevention through immunization. The prophylactic approach differs for each of the types of viral hepatitis. In the past, immunoprophylaxis relied exclusively on passive immunization with antibody-containing globulin preparations purified by cold ethanol fractionation from the plasma of hundreds of normal donors. Currently, for hepatitis B, active immunization with a vaccine is available as well, and development of hepatitis A vaccines is nearing completion.

Hepatitis A All preparations of immune globulin (IG) contain anti-HAV. Although the titers may vary, all IG preparations appear to have an antibody concentration sufficient to be protective. When administered before exposure or during the early incubation period, IG is effective in preventing clinically apparent type A hepatitis. In some cases, IG does not abort infection but, by attenuating it, renders it inapparent. As a result, long-lasting "passive-active" immunity occurs; however, this is now considered to be the exception rather than the rule. For intimate contacts (household, institutional) of persons with hepatitis A, administration of 0.02 mL/kg is recommended as early after exposure as possible; it may be effective even when administered as late as 2 weeks after exposure. Prophylaxis is not necessary for casual contacts (office, factory, school, or hospital), for most elderly persons, who are very likely to be immune, or for those known to have anti-HAV in their serum. In day-care centers, recognition of hepatitis A cases in children or staff should provide a stimulus for immunoprophylaxis in the center and in the children's family members. By the time most common-source outbreaks of type A hepatitis are recognized, it is usually too late in the incubation period for IG to be effective; however, prophylaxis may limit the frequency of secondary cases. For travelers to tropical countries, developing countries, and other areas outside standard tourist routes, IG prophylaxis is recommended. When such travel lasts less than 3 months, 0.02 mL/kg is given; for longer travel or residence in these areas, a dose of 0.06 mL/kg every 4 to 6 months is recommended. The high-dose, repeated approach is recommended as well for certain primate handlers and laboratory personnel who work with HAV or fecal specimens. Administration of plasma-derived globulin is safe; it has not been associated with transmission of AIDS to recipients, and the AIDS virus (human immunodeficiency virus, HIV) is inactivated by 25% alcohol, to which plasma is subjected during the cold ethanol fractionation process. Formalin-inactivated vaccines made from HAV strains attenuated in tissue culture have been shown to be immunogenic, safe, and highly effective in preventing hepatitis A. Ultimately, they will supplant IG for preexposure prophylaxis.

Although protection is achieved after a single dose, three injections will be recommended.

Hepatitis B Until 1982, prevention of hepatitis B was based on *passive* immunoprophylaxis either with standard IG, containing modest levels of anti-HBs, or hepatitis B immune globulin (HBIG), containing high-titer anti-HBs. The efficacy of standard IG has never been established and remains questionable; even the efficacy of HBIG, demonstrated in several clinical trials, has been challenged, and its contribution appears to be in reducing the frequency of clinical *illness*, not in preventing *infection*. Although HBV cannot be cultivated in vitro in the classical sense, a vaccine for *active* immunization was prepared from purified, noninfectious 22-nm spherical forms of HBsAg derived from the plasma of healthy HBsAg carriers. The vaccine was subjected to three different chemical inactivation steps which, cumulatively, destroy the infectivity of every known virus, including HIV. In controlled clinical trials among high-risk persons, this plasma-derived vaccine was shown to be immunogenic, highly effective in preventing HBV infection, and, despite its unconventional source, very safe. In 1987, the plasma-derived vaccine was supplanted by a genetically engineered vaccine derived from recombinant yeast. The latter vaccine consists of HBsAg particles that are nonglycosylated but are otherwise indistinguishable from natural HBsAg; this second-generation vaccine is comparable in immunogenicity, protective efficacy, and safety to the first-generation, plasma-derived vaccine. Current recommendations can be divided into those for preexposure and postexposure prophylaxis.

For *preexposure* prophylaxis against hepatitis B in settings of frequent exposure (health workers exposed to blood, hemodialysis patients and staff, residents and staff of custodial institutions for the developmentally handicapped, intravenous drug abusers, inmates of long-term correctional facilities, promiscuous homosexual men as well as promiscuous heterosexuals, persons such as hemophiliacs who require long-term, high-volume therapy with blood derivatives, household and sexual contacts of HBsAg carriers, and persons living in or traveling extensively in endemic areas), three intramuscular (deltoid, not gluteal) injections of hepatitis B vaccine are recommended at 0, 1, and 6 months. Pregnancy is *not* a contraindication to vaccination. In areas of low HBV endemicity such as the United States, despite the availability of safe and effective hepatitis B vaccines, a strategy of vaccinating persons in high-risk groups has not been effective. The incidence of new hepatitis B cases has continued to increase in the United States after introduction of vaccines, fewer than 10 percent of all targeted persons in high-risk groups have actually been vaccinated, and approximately 30 percent of persons with sporadic acute hepatitis B do not fall into any high-risk-group category. Therefore, to have an impact on the frequency of HBV infection in an area of low endemicity such as the United States, universal hepatitis B vaccination in childhood has been recommended.

Plasma-derived hepatitis B vaccine is no longer routinely available in the United States. There are two comparable recombinant hepatitis B vaccines available, one containing 10 μg HBsAg (Recombivax-HB) and the other containing 20 μg HBsAg (Engerix-B), and recommended doses for each injection vary between the two preparations. For Recombivax-HB, 2.5 μg is recommended for children <11 years of age of HBsAg-negative mothers, 5 μg for infants of HBsAg-positive mothers (see below) and for children and adolescents 11 to 19 years of age, 10 μg for immunocompetent adults, and 40 μg for dialysis patients and other immunosuppressed persons. For Engerix-B, 10 μg is recommended for children aged 10 and under, 20 μg for immunocompetent children older than 10 years of age and adults, and 40 μg for dialysis patients and other immunocompromised persons.

For unvaccinated persons sustaining an exposure to HBV, *postexposure* prophylaxis with a combination of HBIG (for rapid achievement of high-titer circulating anti-HBs) and hepatitis B vaccine (for achievement of long-lasting immunity as well as its apparent efficacy in attenuating clinical illness after exposure) is recommended. For

perinatal exposure of infants born to HBsAg-positive mothers, a single dose of HBIG, 0.5 mL, should be administered intramuscularly in the thigh *immediately after birth*, followed by a complete course of three injections of recombinant hepatitis B vaccine (see doses above) to be started within the first 12 h of life. For those experiencing a direct percutaneous inoculation or transmucosal exposure to HBsAg-positive blood or body fluids (e.g., accidental *needle stick*, other mucosal penetration, or ingestion), a single intramuscular dose of HBIG, 0.06 mL/kg, administered as soon after exposure as possible, is followed by a complete course of hepatitis B vaccine to begin within the first week. For those exposed by *sexual* contact to a patient with acute hepatitis B, a single intramuscular dose of HBIG, 0.06 mL/kg, should be given within 14 days of exposure, to be followed by a complete course of hepatitis B vaccine. When both HBIG and hepatitis B vaccine are recommended, they may be given at the same time but at separate sites.

The precise duration of protection afforded by hepatitis B vaccine is unknown; however, approximately 80 to 90 percent of immunocompetent vaccinees retain protective levels of anti-HBs for at least 5 years. Thereafter and even after anti-HBs becomes undetectable, protection persists against clinical hepatitis B, hepatitis B surface antigenemia, and chronic HBV infection. Currently, *booster* immunizations are not recommended routinely, except in immunosuppressed persons who have lost detectable anti-HBs or immunocompetent persons who sustain percutaneous HBsAg-positive inoculations after losing detectable antibody. Specifically, for hemodialysis patients, annual anti-HBs testing is recommended after vaccination; booster doses are recommended when anti-HBs levels fall below 10 mIU/mL.

Hepatitis D Infection with the hepatitis D can be prevented by vaccinating susceptible persons with hepatitis B vaccine. No product is available for immunoprophylaxis to prevent HDV superinfection in HBsAg carriers; for them, avoidance of percutaneous exposures and limitation of intimate contact with persons who have HDV infection are recommended.

Hepatitis C For transfusion-associated hepatitis C, the effectiveness of IG prophylaxis has not been demonstrated consistently and is not recommended. The most effective measure for reducing the frequency of posttransfusion hepatitis C is the elimination of commercially obtained donor blood and reliance exclusively on volunteer blood donors. The presence of elevated ALT and/or anti-HBc in donor blood was found to correlate with the risk of hepatitis C (non-A, non-B hepatitis) in recipients. Both these markers appear to identify segments of the blood donor population with an increased risk of bloodborne viral infections. In the late 1980s, screening of donor blood for these surrogate markers was introduced. At the same time, exclusion of blood donors in high-risk groups for AIDS and screening of blood donors for anti-HIV were introduced. These measures, introduced to limit transfusion-associated AIDS, lowered the risk of infection with other bloodborne agents, like HCV, as well. Finally, the recent introduction of blood donor screening for anti-HCV reduced further the risk of hepatitis C after transfusion to less than 1 percent per patient and 0.03 percent per unit of blood. Another approach, chemical treatment of blood products and concentrates to inactivate hepatitis virus infectivity, is also being pursued. Studies to test the efficacy of standard IG after needle stick, sexual, or perinatal exposure to hepatitis C have not been done. Because the inoculum is considerably smaller in these settings than that associated with transfusion, and because of its safety and low cost, some authorities do recommend postexposure prophylaxis with a single dose of IG, 0.06 mL/kg (or 0.5 mL for neonatal exposure), in these situations. The efficacy of IG for prevention of hepatitis E remains to be evaluated.

TOXIC AND DRUG-INDUCED HEPATITIS

Liver injury may follow the inhalation, ingestion, or parenteral administration of a number of pharmacologic and chemical agents.

TABLE 266-5 Some features of toxic and drug-induced hepatic injury

Features	Direct toxic effect		Idiosyncratic			Other
	(Carbon tetrachloride, e.g.)	(Acetaminophen, e.g.)	(Halothane, e.g.)	(Isoniazid, e.g.)	(Chlorpromazine, e.g.)	(Oral contraceptive agents, e.g.)
Predictable and dose-related toxicity	+	+	0	0	0	+
Latent period	Short	Short	Variable	Variable	Variable	Variable
Arthralgia, fever, rash, eosinophilia	0	0	+	0	+	0
Liver morphology	Necrosis, fatty infiltration	Centrilobular necrosis	Similar to viral hepatitis	Similar to viral hepatitis	Cholestasis *with* portal inflammation	Cholestasis *without* portal inflammation, vascular lesions

These include industrial toxins (e.g., carbon tetrachloride, trichloroethylene, and yellow phosphorus), the heat-stable toxic bicyclic octapeptides of certain species of *Amanita* and *Galerina* (hepatotoxic mushroom poisoning), and more commonly, pharmacologic agents used in medical therapy. It is essential that any patient presenting with jaundice or impaired liver function be questioned carefully about exposure to chemicals used in work or at home and drugs taken by prescription or bought "over the counter." In general, two major types of chemical hepatotoxicity have been recognized: (1) direct toxic type and (2) idiosyncratic type.

As shown in Table 266-5, direct toxic hepatitis occurs with predictable regularity in individuals exposed to the offending agent and is dose-dependent. The latent period between exposure and liver injury is usually short (often several hours), although clinical manifestations may be delayed for 24 to 48 h. Agents producing toxic hepatitis are generally systemic poisons or are converted in the liver to toxic metabolites. The direct hepatotoxins result in morphologic abnormalities which are reasonably characteristic and reproducible for each toxin. For example, carbon tetrachloride and trichloroethylene characteristically produce a centrilobular zonal necrosis, whereas yellow phosphorus poisoning typically results in periportal injury. The hepatotoxic octapeptides of *Amanita phalloides* usually produce massive hepatic necrosis. The lethal dose of the toxin is about 10 mg, the amount found in a single deathcap mushroom. Tetracycline, when administered in intravenous doses greater than 1.5 g daily, leads to microvesicular fat deposits in the liver. Liver injury, which is often only one facet of the toxicity produced by the direct hepatotoxins, may go unrecognized until jaundice appears.

In idiosyncratic drug reactions the occurrence of hepatitis is usually infrequent and unpredictable, the response is not dose-dependent, and it may occur at any time during or shortly after exposure to the drug. Extrahepatic manifestations of hypersensitivity, such as rash, arthralgias, fever, leukocytosis, and eosinophilia occur in about one-quarter of patients with idiosyncratic hepatotoxic drug reactions; this observation and the unpredictability of idiosyncratic drug hepatotoxicity contributed to the hypothesis that this category of drug reactions is immunologically mediated. More recent evidence, however, suggests that, in most cases, even idiosyncratic reactions represent direct hepatotoxity but are caused by drug metabolites rather than by the intact compound. Even the prototype of idiosyncratic hepatoxicity reactions, halothane hepatitis, and isoniazid hepatotoxicity, associated frequently with hypersensitivity manifestations, are now recognized to be mediated by toxic metabolites which damage liver cells directly. Currently, most idiosyncratic reactions are thought to result from differences in metabolic reactivity to specific agents; host susceptibility is mediated by the kinetics of toxic metabolite generation, which differs among individuals. Occasionally, however, the clinical features of an allergic reaction (e.g., prominent tissue eosinophilia, autoantibodies, etc.) are difficult to ignore. In vitro models have been described in which lymphocyte cytotoxicity can be demonstrated against rabbit hepatocytes altered by incubation with the potential offending drug. Similarly, in selected cases, a drug or its metabolite

has been shown to bind to a host cellular component forming a hapten; the immune response to this "neoantigen" is postulated to play a role in the pathogenesis of liver injury. Therefore, some authorities subdivide idiosyncratic drug hepatotoxicity into hypersensitivity (allergic) and "metabolic" categories. Several unusual exceptions notwithstanding, true drug allergy is difficult to support in most cases of idiosyncratic drug-induced liver injury.

Idiosyncratic reactions lead to a morphologic pattern that is more variable than those produced by direct toxins; a single agent is often capable of causing a variety of lesions, although certain patterns tend to predominate. Depending on the agent involved, idiosyncratic hepatitis may result in a clinical and morphologic picture indistinguishable from viral hepatitis (e.g., halothane) or may simulate extrahepatic bile duct obstruction clinically with morphologic evidence of cholestasis and minimal hepatocellular damage (e.g., chlorpromazine). Morphologic alterations also may include bridging hepatic necrosis (e.g., methyldopa), or, infrequently, hepatic granulomas (e.g., sulfonamides).

Not all adverse hepatic drug reactions can be classified as either toxic or idiosyncratic in type. For example, oral contraceptives, which combine estrogenic and progestational compounds, may result in impairment of hepatic function and occasionally in jaundice. However, they do not produce necrosis or fatty change, manifestations of hypersensitivity are generally absent, and susceptibility to the development of oral contraceptive–induced cholestasis appears to be genetically determined.

Because drug-induced hepatitis is often a presumptive diagnosis and many other disorders produce a similar clinicopathologic picture, evidence of a causal relationship between the use of a drug and subsequent liver injury may be difficult to establish. The relationship is most convincing for the direct hepatotoxins, which lead to a high frequency of hepatic impairment after a short latent period. Idiosyncratic reactions may be reproduced, in some instances, when rechallenge, after an asymptomatic period, results in a recurrence of signs, symptoms, and morphologic and biochemical abnormalities. Rechallenge, however, is often ethically unfeasible, because severe reactions may occur.

Treatment of toxic and drug-induced hepatic disease is largely supportive, as in acute viral hepatitis. Withdrawal of the suspected agent is indicated at the first sign of an adverse reaction. In the case of the direct toxins, liver involvement should not divert attention from renal or other organ involvement which also may threaten survival.

In Table 266-6, several classes of chemical agents are listed, together with examples of the pattern of liver injury produced by them. Certain drugs appear to be responsible for the development of chronic as well as acute hepatic injury. For example, oxphenisatin, alpha methyldopa, and isoniazid have been associated with chronic active hepatitis, and halothane and methotrexate have been implicated in the development of cirrhosis. A syndrome resembling primary biliary cirrhosis has been described following treatment with chlorpromazine, methyl testosterone, tolbutamide, and other drugs. Portal

TABLE 266-6 Principal alterations of hepatic morphology produced by some commonly used drugs and chemicals*

Principal morphologic change	Class of agent	Example
Cholestasis	Anabolic steroid	Methyl testosterone†
	Antithyroid	Methimazole
	Antibiotic	Erythromycin estolate, nitrofurantoin
	Oral contraceptive	Norethynodrel with mestranol
	Oral hypoglycemic	Chlorpropamide
	Tranquilizer	Chlorpromazine†
	Oncotherapeutic	Anabolic steroids, busulfan, tamoxifen
	Immunosuppressive	Cyclosporine
	Anticonvulsant	Carbamazine
	Calcium channel blocker	Nifedipine, verapamil
Fatty liver	Antibiotic	Tetracycline
	Anticonvulsant	Sodium valproate
	Antiarrhythmic	Amiodarone
	Oncotherapeutic	Asparaginase, methotrexate
Hepatitis	Anesthetic	Halothane‡
	Anticonvulsant	Phenytoin, carbamazine
	Antihypertensive	Methyldopa,‡ captopril, enalapril
	Antibiotic	Isoniazid,‡ rifampicin, nitrofurantoin
	Diuretic	Chlorothiazide
	Laxative	Oxyphenisatin‡
	Antidepressant	Iproniazid, amitriptyline, imipramine
	Anti-inflammatory	Ibuprofen, indomethacin
	Antifungal	Ketoconazole, fluconazole
	Antiviral	Zidovudine, dideoxyinosine
	Calcium-channel blocker	Nifedipine, verapamil, diltiazem
Mixed hepatitis/cholestatic	Immunosuppressive	Azathioprine
	Lipid-lowering	Nicotinic acid, lovastatin
Toxic (necrosis)	Hydrocarbon	Carbon tetrachloride
	Metal	Yellow phosphorus
	Mushroom	*Amanita phalloides*
	Analgesic	Acetaminophen
	Solvent	Dimethylformamide
Granulomas	Anti-inflammatory	Phenylbutazone
	Antibiotic	Sulfanomides
	Xanthine oxidase inhibitor	Allopurinol
	Antiarrhythmic	Quinidine
	Anticonvulsant	Carbamazine

* Several agents cause more than one type of liver lesion and appear under more than one category.
† Rarely associated with primary biliary cirrhosis–like lesion.
‡ Occasionally associated with chronic active hepatitis or bridging hepatic necrosis or cirrhosis.

hypertension in the absence of cirrhosis may result from alterations in hepatic architecture produced by vitamin A or arsenic intoxication, industrial exposure to vinyl chloride, or administration of thorium dioxide. The latter three agents also have been associated with angiosarcoma of the liver. Oral contraceptives have been implicated in the development of hepatic adenoma and, rarely, hepatocellular carcinoma and occlusion of the hepatic vein (Budd-Chiari syndrome). Another unusual lesion, peliosis hepatis (blood cysts of the liver), has been observed in some patients treated with anabolic steroids. The existence of these hepatic disorders expands the spectrum of liver injury induced by chemical agents and emphasizes the need for a thorough drug history in all patients with liver dysfunction.

The following are the patterns of adverse hepatic reactions for some prototypic agents.

ACETAMINOPHEN HEPATOTOXICITY (DIRECT TOXIN) Acetaminophen has caused severe centrolobular hepatic necrosis when ingested in large amounts in suicide attempts or accidentally by children. A single dose of 10 to 15 g, occasionally less, may produce clinical evidence of liver injury. Fatal fulminant disease is usually (although not invariably) associated with ingestion of 25 g or more. Blood levels of acetaminophen correlate with the severity of hepatic injury (levels above 300 μg/mL 4 h after ingestion are predictive of the development of severe damage, while levels below 150 μg/mL suggest that hepatic injury is highly unlikely). Nausea, vomiting, diarrhea, abdominal pain, and shock are early manifestations occurring 4 to 12 h after ingestion. Then 24 to 48 h later, when these features are abating, hepatic injury becomes apparent. Maximal abnormalities and hepatic failure may not be evident until 4 to 6 days after ingestion. Renal failure and myocardial injury may be present.

Acetaminophen hepatotoxicity is mediated by a toxic reactive metabolite formed from the parent compound by the cytochrome P450 mixed-function oxidase system of the hepatocyte. This metabolite is detoxified by binding to glutathione. When excessive amounts of the metabolite are formed, glutathione levels in the liver fall, and the metabolite is covalently bound to nucleophilic hepatocyte macromolecules. This process is believed to lead to hepatocyte necrosis; the precise sequence and mechanism are unknown. Hepatic injury may be potentiated by prior administration of alcohol or other drugs, by conditions which stimulate the mixed-function oxidase system, or by conditions such as starvation which reduce hepatic glutathione levels. In chronic alcoholics, the toxic dose of acetaminophen may be as low as 2 g.

Treatment of acetaminophen overdosage includes gastric lavage, supportive measures, and oral administration of activated charcoal or cholestyramine to prevent absorption of residual drug. Neither of the latter agents appears to be effective if given more than 30 min after acetaminophen ingestion; if they are used, the stomach lavage should be done before other agents are administered orally. In patients with high acetaminophen blood levels (>200 μg/mL measured at 4 h or >100 μg/mL at 8 h after ingestion), the administration of sulfhydryl compounds (e.g., cysteamine, cysteine, or N-acetylcysteine) appears to reduce the severity of hepatic necrosis. These agents appear to act by providing a reservoir of sulfhydryl groups to bind the toxic metabolites or by stimulating synthesis and repletion of hepatic glutathione. Therapy should be begun within 8 h of ingestion but may be effective even if given as late as 24 to 36 h after overdose. Later administration of sulfhydryl compounds is of uncertain value.

Survivors of acute acetaminophen overdose usually have no evidence of hepatic sequelae. In a few patients, prolonged or repeated administration of acetaminophen in therapeutic doses appears to have led to the development of chronic active hepatitis and cirrhosis.

HALOTHANE HEPATOTOXICITY (IDIOSYNCRATIC REACTION) Halothane, a nonexplosive fluorinated hydrocarbon anesthetic agent that is structurally similar to chloroform, has been reported to result in severe hepatic necrosis in a small number of individuals, many of whom have previously been exposed to this agent. The failure to produce similar hepatic lesions reliably in animals, the rarity of hepatic impairment in human beings, and the delayed appearance of hepatic injury suggest that halothane is not a direct hepatotoxin but may be a sensitizing agent. However, manifestations of hypersensitivity are seen in fewer than 25 percent of cases. A genetic predisposition leading to an idiosyncratic metabolic reactivity has been postulated and appears to be the most likely mechanism of halothane hepatotoxicity. Supporting this postulate is the demonstration in patients with halothane hepatitis and their family members of increased lymphocyte susceptibility to damage in vitro by electrophilic drug metabolites. Adults (rather than children), obese people, and women appear to be particularly susceptible. Fever, moderate leukocytosis, and eosinophilia may occur in the first week following halothane administration. Jaundice usually is noted 7 to 10 days after exposure but may occur earlier in previously exposed patients. Nausea and vomiting may precede the onset of jaundice. Hepatomegaly is often mild, but liver tenderness is common. The serum aminotransferase levels are elevated. The pathologic changes at autopsy are indistinguishable from massive hepatic necrosis resulting from viral hepatitis. The case-fatality rate of halothane hepatitis is not known but may vary from

20 to 40 percent in cases with severe liver involvement. In rare instances, cirrhosis has been observed following repeated bouts of halothane hepatitis; however, in most patients who recover, the liver returns to normal. It is strongly suggested that patients in whom unexplained spiking fever, especially delayed fever, or jaundice develops after halothane anesthesia not receive this agent again. Because cross-reactions between halothane and methoxyfluorane have been reported, the latter agent should not be used after halothane reactions. Later-generation halogenated hydrocarbon anesthetics are felt to be associated with a lower risk of hepatotoxicity; however, rare cases have been observed.

METHYLDOPA HEPATOTOXICITY (TOXIC AND IDIOSYNCRATIC REACTION)   Minor alterations in liver tests are reported in about 5 percent of patients treated with this antihypertensive agent. These trivial abnormalities typically resolve despite continued drug administration. In less than 1 percent of patients, acute liver injury resembling viral hepatitis, or chronic active hepatitis, or rarely a cholestatic reaction is seen 1 to 20 weeks after methyldopa is started. In 50 percent of cases the interval is shorter than 4 weeks. A prodrome of fever, anorexia, and malaise may be noted for a few days before the onset of jaundice. Rash, lymphadenopathy, arthralgia, and eosinophilia are rare. Serologic markers of autoimmunity are infrequently detected, and fewer than 5 percent of patients have a Coombs-positive hemolytic anemia. In about 15 percent of patients with methyldopa hepatotoxicity, the clinical, biochemical, and histologic features are those of chronic active hepatitis with or without bridging necrosis and macronodular cirrhosis. With discontinuation of the drug, the disorder usually resolves, although progression has been seen in a few patients.

ISONIAZID HEPATOTOXICITY (TOXIC AND IDIOSYNCRATIC REACTION)   In approximately 10 percent of adults treated with the antituberculosis agent isoniazid, elevated serum aminotransferase levels develop during the first few weeks of therapy; this appears to represent an adaptive response to a toxic metabolite of the drug. Whether or not isoniazid is continued, these values (usually below 200 units) return to normal in a few weeks. In about 1 percent of treated patients, an illness develops which is indistinguishable from viral hepatitis; approximately half of these cases occur within the first 2 months of treatment, while in the remainder, clinical disease may be delayed for many months. Liver biopsy reveals morphologic changes similar to those of viral hepatitis or bridging hepatic necrosis. The disease may be severe, with a case-fatality rate of 10 percent. Important liver injury appears to be age-related, increasing substantially in frequency after age 35; the highest frequency is in patients over age 50, the lowest under the age of 20. Isoniazid hepatotoxicity is enhanced by alcohol and rifampicin. Fever, rash, eosinophilia, and other manifestations of drug allergy are distinctly unusual. A reactive metabolite of acetylhydrazine, a metabolite of isoniazid, may be responsible for liver injury. A picture resembling chronic active hepatitis has been observed in a few patients.

SODIUM VALPROATE HEPATOTOXICITY (TOXIC AND IDIOSYNCRATIC REACTION)   Sodium valproate, an anticonvulsant useful in the treatment of petit mal and other seizure disorders, has been associated with the development of severe hepatic toxicity and, rarely, fatalities in both children and adults. Asymptomatic elevations of serum aminotransferase levels have been recognized in as many as 45 percent of treated patients. These ''adaptive'' changes, however, appear to have no clinical importance, for major hepatotoxicity is not seen in the majority of patients despite continuation of drug therapy. In those rare patients in whom jaundice, encephalopathy, and evidence of hepatic failure are found, examination of liver tissue reveals microvesicular fat and bridging hepatic necrosis predominantly in the centrolobular zone. Bile duct injury also may be apparent. It seems likely that sodium valproate is not directly hepatotoxic but that its metabolite, 4-pentenoic acid, may be responsible for hepatic injury.

PHENYTOIN HEPATOTOXICITY (IDIOSYNCRATIC REACTION)   Phenytoin, formerly diphenylhydantoin, a mainstay in the treatment of seizure disorders, has been associated in rare instances with the development of severe hepatitis-like liver injury leading to fulminant hepatic failure in some instances. In many patients the hepatitis is associated with striking fever, lymphadenopathy, rash (Stevens-Johnson syndrome or exfoliative dermatitis), leukocytosis, and eosinophilia, suggesting an immunologically mediated hypersensitivity mechanism. Despite these observations, there is also evidence that metabolic idiosyncrasy may be responsible for hepatic injury. In the liver, phenytoin is converted by the cytochrome P450 system to metabolites which include the highly reactive electrophilic arene oxides. These metabolites are normally metabolized further by epoxide hydrolases. A defect (genetic or acquired) in epoxide hydrolase activity could permit covalent binding of arene oxides to hepatic macromolecules, thereby leading to hepatic injury. Regardless of the mechanism, hepatic injury is usually manifest within the first 2 months after beginning phenytoin therapy. With the exception of an abundance of eosinophils in the liver, the clinical, biochemical, and histologic picture resembles that of viral hepatitis. In rare instances, bile duct injury may be the salient feature of phenytoin hepatotoxicity with striking features of intrahepatic cholestasis. Asymptomatic elevations of aminotransferase and alkaline phosphatase levels have been observed in a sizable proportion of patients receiving long-term phenytoin therapy. These liver changes are believed by some authorities to represent the potent hepatic enzyme–inducing properties of phenytoin and are accompanied histologically by swelling of hepatocytes in the absence of necroinflammatory activity or evidence of chronic liver disease.

CHLORPROMAZINE HEPATOTOXICITY (CHOLESTATIC IDIOSYNCRATIC REACTION)   In about 1 percent of patients receiving chlorpromazine, intrahepatic cholestasis with jaundice develops after 1 to 4 weeks of treatment. In rare instances, jaundice has been reported after a single exposure. Anicteric reactions are frequent. The onset may be abrupt, with fever, rash, arthralgias, lymphadenopathy, nausea, vomiting, and epigastric or right upper quadrant pain. Pruritus may precede the appearance of jaundice, dark urine, and light stools. Eosinophilia with or without mild leukocytosis may be present, and conjugated hyperbilirubinemia, moderately elevated serum alkaline phosphatase, and mildly elevated serum aminotransferase levels (100 to 200 units) are noted. Liver biopsy reveals cholestasis, bile plugs in dilated bile canaliculi, and a dense portal infiltrate of polymorphonuclear, eosinophilic, and mononuclear leukocytes. Occasionally, scattered foci of hepatic parenchymal necrosis may be evident. Jaundice and pruritus usually subside within 4 to 8 weeks following cessation of therapy, without sequelae, and fatalities are rare. Cholestyramine may be of value in relieving severe pruritus. In a small number of patients, jaundice is prolonged for several months to years; rarely, a disorder resembling but distinct from primary biliary cirrhosis may develop.

AMIODARONE HEPATOTOXICITY (TOXIC AND IDIOSYNCRATIC REACTION)   Therapy with this potent antiarrhythmic drug is accompanied in 15 to 50 percent of patients by modest elevation of serum aminotransferase levels that may remain stable or diminish despite continuation of the drug. Such abnormalities may appear days to many months after beginning therapy. A proportion of those with elevated aminotransferase levels have detectable hepatomegaly, and clinically important liver disease develops in fewer than 5 percent of patients. Features that represent a direct effect of the drug on the liver and that are common to the majority of long-term recipients are ultrastructural phospholipidosis, unaccompanied by clinical liver disease, and interference with hepatic mixed-function oxidase metabolism of other drugs. The relatively common elevations in aminotransferase levels are also considered a predictable, dose-dependent, direct hepatotoxic effect. On the other hand, in the rare patient with clinically apparent, symptomatic liver disease, liver injury resembling that seen in alcoholic liver disease is observed. The so-called pseudoalcoholic liver injury can range from steatosis, to alcoholic hepatitis–like neutrophilic infiltration and Mallory's hyaline, to cirrhosis. Electron-microscopic demonstration of phospholipid-laden lysosomal lamellar bodies can help to distinguish amiodarone hepatotoxicity from typical alcoholic hepatitis. This category of liver injury appears to be a metabolic idiosyncracy which allows hepatotoxic metabolites to be generated. Rarely, an acute idiosyncratic hepatocellular injury resembling viral hepatitis or cholestatic hepatitis occurs. Hepatic granulomas have occasionally been observed. Because amiodarone has a long half-life, liver injury may persist for months after the drug is stopped.

ERYTHROMYCIN HEPATOTOXICITY (CHOLESTATIC IDIOSYN-CRATIC REACTION) The most important adverse effect associated with erythromycin is the infrequent occurrence of a cholestatic reaction. Although most of these reactions have been associated with erythromycin estolate, other erythromycins also may be responsible. The reaction usually begins during the first 2 or 3 weeks of therapy and includes nausea, vomiting, fever, right upper quadrant abdominal pain, jaundice, leukocytosis, and moderately elevated aminotransferase levels. The clinical picture can resemble acute cholecystitis or bacterial cholangitis. Liver biopsy reveals variable cholestasis, portal inflammation comprising lymphocytes, polymorphonuclear leukocytes, and eosinophils, and scattered foci of hepatocyte necrosis. Symptoms and laboratory findings usually subside within a few days of drug withdrawal, and evidence of chronic liver disease has not been found on follow-up. The precise mechanism remains ill-defined.

ORAL CONTRACEPTIVE HEPATOTOXICITY (CHOLESTATIC RE-ACTION) The administration of oral contraceptive combinations of estrogenic and progestational steroids results in significant bromsulphthalein (BSP) retention in a high proportion of patients and, to a far lesser extent, elevation of serum alkaline phosphatase. Weeks to months after taking these agents, intrahepatic cholestasis with pruritus and jaundice is noted in a small number of patients. Especially susceptible seem to be patients with recurrent idiopathic jaundice of pregnancy, severe pruritus of pregnancy, or a family history of these disorders. Laboratory studies, with the exception of liver biochemical tests, are normal, and extrahepatic manifestations of hypersensitivity are absent. Liver biopsy reveals cholestasis with bile plugs in dilated canaliculi and striking bilirubin staining of liver cells. In contrast to chlorpromazine-induced cholestasis, portal inflammation is absent. The lesion is reversible on withdrawal of the agent, and sequelae have not been reported. The two steroid components appear to act synergistically on hepatic function, although the estrogen may be primarily responsible. Oral contraceptives are contraindicated in patients with a history of recurrent jaundice of pregnancy. Primarily benign but, rarely, malignant neoplasms of the liver, hepatic vein occlusion, and peripheral sinusoidal dilatation have also been associated with oral contraceptive therapy.

17,α-ALKYL-SUBSTITUTED ANABOLIC STEROIDS (CHOLE-STATIC REACTION) In the majority of patients receiving these agents, used therapeutically mainly in the treatment of bone marrow failure but used surreptitiously and without medical indication by athletes to improve their performance, mild hepatic dysfunction develops. Impaired excretory function is the predominant defect, but the precise mechanism is uncertain. Jaundice, which appears to be dose-related, develops in only a minority of patients and may be the sole clinical manifestation of hepatotoxicity, although anorexia, nausea, and malaise are described in some patients. Pruritus is not a prominent feature. Serum aminotransferase levels are usually under 100 units, and serum alkaline phosphatase levels are normal, mildly elevated, or, in less than 5 percent of patients, three or more times the upper limit of normal. Examination of liver tissue reveals cholestasis without inflammation or necrosis. Hepatic sinusoidal dilatation and peliosis hepatis have been found in a few patients. The cholestatic disorder is usually reversible on cessation of treatment, although fatalities have been linked to peliosis. An association with hepatic adenoma and hepatocellular carcinoma has been reported.

TRIMETHOPRIM-SULFAMETHOXAZOLE HEPATOTOXICITY (ID-IOSYNCRATIC REACTION) This antibiotic is used routinely for urinary tract infections in immunocompetent persons and for prophylaxis against and therapy of *Pneumocystis carinii* pneumonia in immunosuppressed persons (transplant recipients, patients with

AIDS). With its increasing use, its occasional hepatotoxicity is being recognized with growing frequency. Its likelihood is unpredictable, but when it occurs, trimethoprim-sulfamethoxazole hepatotoxicity follows a relatively uniform latency period of several weeks and is often accompanied by eosinophilia, rash, and other features of a hypersensitivity reaction. Biochemically and histologically, acute hepatocellular necrosis predominates, but cholestatic features are quite frequent. Occasionally, cholestasis without necrosis occurs, and very rarely, a severe cholangiolytic pattern of liver injury is observed. In most cases, liver injury is self-limited, but rare fatalities have been recorded. The hepatotoxicity is attributable to the sulfamethoxazole component of the drug and is similar in features to that seen with other sulfonamides; tissue eosinophilia and granulomas may be seen.

REFERENCES

Viral hepatitis

AACH RD et al: Hepatitis C virus infection in post-transfusion hepatitis: An analysis with first- and second-generation assays. N Engl J Med 325:1325, 1991

ALTER HJ et al: Detection of antibody to hepatitis C virus in prospectively followed transfusion recipients with acute and chronic non-A, non-B hepatitis. N Engl J Med 321:1494, 1989

BROWN JL et al: The clinical significance of molecular variation within the hepatitis B virus genome. Hepatology 15:144, 1992

CARMAN WF, THOMAS HC: Genetic variation in hepatitis B virus. Gastroenterology 102:711, 1992

CENTERS FOR DISEASE CONTROL: Protection against viral hepatitis: Recommendations of the Immunization Practices Advisory Committee (ACIP). Morb Mort Week Rep 39 (no. RR-2):1, 1990

CHOO Q-L et al: Isolation of a cDNA clone derived from a blood-borne non-A, non-B viral hepatitis genome. Science 244:359, 1989

COHEN JI: Hepatitis A virus: Insights from molecular biology. Hepatology 9:889, 1989

DEFRANCHIS R et al: The natural history of asymptomatic hepatitis B surface antigen carriers. Ann Intern Med 118:191, 1993

DI BISCEGLIE AM et al: Long-term clinical and histologic follow-up of chronic posttransfusion hepatitis. Hepatology 14:969, 1991

DIENSTAG JL: Non-A, non-B hepatitis: I. Recognition, epidemiology, and clinical features. II. Experimental transmission, putative virus agents and markers, and prevention. Gastroenterology 85:439, 743, 1983

——— (ed): Viral hepatitis. Semin Liver Dis 11:73, 1991

DONAHUE JG et al: The declining risk of post-transfusion hepatitis C virus infection. N Engl J Med 327:369, 1992

ESTEBAN JI et al: High rate of infectivity and liver disease in blood donors with antibodies to hepatitis C virus. Ann Intern Med 115:443, 1991

FARCI P et al: A long-term study of hepatitis C virus replication in non-A, non-B hepatitis. N Engl J Med 325:98, 1991

HOLLINGER FB et al (eds): *Viral Hepatitis and Liver Disease.* Baltimore, Williams & Wilkins, 1991

HOOFNAGLE JH: Type D (delta) hepatitis. JAMA 261:1321, 1989

HOUGHTON M et al: Molecular biology of the hepatitis C viruses: Implications for diagnosis, development and control of viral disease. Hepatology 14:381, 1991

KATKOV WN, DIENSTAG JL: Prevention and therapy of viral hepatitis. Semin Liver Dis 11:165, 1991

LEMON SM: Type A viral hepatitis: New developments in an old disease. N Engl J Med 313:1059, 1985

MILLER RH et al: Compact organization of the hepatitis B virus genome. Hepatology 9:322, 1989

REYES GR et al: Isolation of a cDNA from the virus responsible for enterically transmitted non-A, non-B hepatitis. Science 247:1335, 1990

RIZZETTO M: The delta agent. Hepatology 3:729, 1983

SEEFF LB et al: A serologic follow-up of the 1942 epidemic of post-vaccination hepatitis in the United States Army. N Engl J Med 316:965, 1987

VYAS GN et al (eds): *Viral Hepatitis and Liver Disease.* Orlando, Grune & Stratton, 1984

WERZBERGER A et al: A controlled trial of formalin-inactivated hepatitis A vaccine in healthy children. N Engl J Med 327:453, 1992

ZUCKERMAN AJ (ed): *Viral Hepatitis and Liver Disease.* New York, Liss, 1988

Drug-induced hepatitis

BLACK M et al: Isoniazid-associated hepatitis in 114 patients. Gastroenterology 69:389, 1975

———: Acetaminophen hepatotoxicity. Annu Rev Med 35:577, 1984

DIEHL AM et al: Cholestatic hepatitis from erythromycin ethylsuccinate. Am J Med 76:931, 1984

HARRISON PM et al: Improved outcome of paracetamol-induced fulminant hepatic failure by late administration of acetylcysteine. Lancet 335:1572, 1990

ISHAK KG, IREY NS: Hepatic injury associated with the phenothiazines: Clinicopathologic and follow-up study of 36 patients. Arch Pathol 93:283, 1972

KAPLOWITZ N (ed): Recent advances in drug metabolism and hepatotoxicity. Semin Liver Dis 10:233, 1990

——— et al: Drug-induced hepatotoxicity. Ann Intern Med 104:826, 1986

LEWIS JH et al: Amiodarone hepatotoxicity: Prevalence and clinicopathologic correlations among 104 patients. Hepatology 9:679, 1989

LUDWIG J, AXELSEN R: Drug effects on the liver: An updated tabular compilation of drugs and drug-related hepatic diseases. Dig Dis Sci 28:651, 1983

MITCHELL JR, JOLLOW DJ: Metabolic activation of drugs to toxic substances. Gastroenterology 68:392, 1975

SMILKSTEIN MJ et al: Efficacy of N-acetylcysteine in the treatment of acetaminophen overdose. N Engl J Med 319:1557, 1988

ZIMMERMAN HJ: *Hepatotoxicity.* New York, Appleton-Century-Crofts, 1978

———, ISHAK KG: Valproate-induced hepatic injury: Analysis of 23 fatal cases. Hepatology 2:591, 1982

267   CHRONIC HEPATITIS

JULES L. DIENSTAG / KURT J. ISSELBACHER*

Chronic hepatitis represents a series of liver disorders of varying causes and severity in which hepatic inflammation and necrosis continue for at least 6 months. Milder forms are nonprogressive or only slowly progressive, while more severe forms may be associated with scarring and architectural organization, which, when advanced, lead ultimately to cirrhosis. Several categories of chronic hepatitis have been recognized. These include chronic viral hepatitis, drug-induced chronic hepatitis (see Chap. 266), and autoimmune chronic hepatitis. In many cases, clinical and laboratory features are insufficient to allow assignment into one of these three categories; these "idiopathic" cases are also believed to represent autoimmune chronic hepatitis. Finally, clinical and laboratory features of chronic hepatitis are observed occasionally in patients with such hereditary/metabolic disorders as Wilson's disease (copper overload) and even occasionally in patients with alcoholic liver injury. Although all types of chronic hepatitis share certain clinical, laboratory, and histopathologic features, chronic viral and chronic autoimmune hepatitis are sufficiently distinct to merit separate discussions.

PATHOLOGIC CLASSIFICATION OF CHRONIC HEPATITIS Common to all forms of chronic hepatitis are histopathologic distinctions based on localization and extent of liver injury. These vary from the milder forms, chronic persistent hepatitis and chronic lobular hepatitis, to the more severe form, chronic active hepatitis. When first defined, these designations were felt to have prognostic implications, which have been challenged by more recent observations. Still, these histopathologic categories remain useful. Clinical features alone are insufficient—liver biopsy is necessary—to distinguish among the histopathologic categories of chronic hepatitis.

Chronic persistent hepatitis In chronic persistent hepatitis, a mononuclear inflammatory infiltrate expands, but is localized to and contained within, portal tracts. The "limiting plate" of periportal hepatocytes is intact, and there is no extension of the necroinflammatory process into the liver lobule. A "cobblestone" arrangement of liver cells, indicative of hepatic regenerative activity, is a common feature, and although minimal periportal fibrosis may be present, *cirrhosis is absent.* As a general rule, patients with chronic persistent hepatitis are asymptomatic or have relatively mild constitutional symptoms (e.g., fatigue, anorexia, nausea); have normal physical findings, except, perhaps for liver enlargement, without the usual stigmata of chronic liver disease (see below); and have modest elevations of aminotransferase activities. Progression to more severe lesions (chronic active hepatitis and cirrhosis) is very unlikely, especially in patients with autoimmune or idiopathic chronic persistent hepatitis; however, progressive disease has been recognized in patients with chronic persistent *viral* hepatitis and in those with chronic persistent hepatitis following spontaneous or therapeutic remission of autoimmune chronic active hepatitis.

Chronic lobular hepatitis In patients with chronic lobular hepatitis, in addition to portal inflammation, histologic examination of the liver reveals foci of necrosis and inflammation in the liver lobule. Morphologically, chronic lobular hepatitis resembles slowly resolving acute hepatitis. The limiting plate remains intact, periportal fibrosis is absent or limited, lobular architecture is preserved, and progression to chronic active hepatitis and cirrhosis is felt to be rare. Thus chronic lobular hepatitis can be considered a variant of chronic persistent hepatitis with a lobular component, and clinical/laboratory features are comparable. Occasionally, the clinical activity of chronic lobular hepatitis may increase spontaneously; elevation of aminotransferase activity may resemble that seen in acute hepatitis, and transient histologic deterioration can be documented. The same qualifications in prognostic import mentioned above for chronic persistent hepatitis apply to chronic lobular hepatitis.

Chronic active hepatitis Chronic active hepatitis is characterized clinically by continuing hepatic necrosis, portal/periportal and, to a lesser extent, lobular inflammation, and fibrosis. Varying in severity from mild to severe, chronic active hepatitis is recognized to be a progressive disorder that can lead to cirrhosis, liver failure, and death. Morphologic characteristics of chronic active hepatitis include (1) a dense mononuclear infiltrate of the portal tracts, which are substantially expanded into the liver lobule (in the autoimmune type, plasma cells represent a component of the infiltrate), (2) destruction of the hepatocytes at the periphery of the lobule, with erosion of the limiting plate of hepatocytes surrounding the portal triads (so-called piecemeal necrosis), (3) connective tissue septa surrounding portal tracts and extending from the portal zones into the lobule, isolating parenchymal cells into clusters and enveloping bile ducts, and (4) evidence of hepatocellular regeneration—"rosette" formation, thickened liver cell plates, and regenerative "pseudolobules." This process may be patchy, with individual liver lobules spared, or it may be diffuse. Histologic evidence of single-cell coagulative necrosis, Councilman or acidophilic bodies, appear in the periportal areas. Piecemeal necrosis is the minimal histologic requirement to establish a diagnosis of chronic active hepatitis, but this change is seen even in mild, relatively nonprogressive forms of chronic active hepatitis. A more severe lesion, *bridging hepatic necrosis* (originally termed *subacute hepatic necrosis*), characterizes a more severe and progressive form of chronic active hepatitis. Although bridging necrosis can be seen occasionally in patients with acute hepatitis, in whom it carries no prognostic importance, in chronic active hepatitis this lesion is associated with progression to cirrhosis. Bridging necrosis is characterized by hepatocellular dropout that spans lobules (i.e., between portal tracts—the periphery of the lobule—or between portal tracts and central veins—the centrizonal part of the lobule). Collapse of the reticulin network is a hallmark of bridging necrosis, and bridging fibrosis follows, leading ultimately to architectural reorganization by nodular regeneration, i.e., cirrhosis. A more extensive and ominous variant of bridging necrosis is multilobular collapse, in which ridging necrosis is widespread throughout the liver and which is associated clinically with rapid deterioration and even acute liver failure.

Although progression to cirrhosis is difficult to demonstrate in patients with chronic active hepatitis who have isolated piecemeal necrosis, in more severe forms of chronic active hepatitis, progression to cirrhosis is common. Among patients with chronic active hepatitis on liver biopsy, 20 to 50 percent also have cirrhosis, even early during the course of the disease. In fact, many cases of "cryptogenic" cirrhosis are believed to have resulted from chronic active hepatitis. Generally, chronic active hepatitis is more severe clinically than chronic persistent and lobular hepatitis. Although a sizable proportion of patients with chronic active hepatitis are asymptomatic, the majority tend to have mild to severe constitutional symptoms, especially fatigue. Specific clinical and laboratory features vary depending on the cause of the chronic active hepatitis; these will be discussed below. Generally, physical findings associated with chronic liver disease and portal hypertension are more common, aminotransferase

* The authors acknowledge the contribution of Jack Wands in the 12th edition.

levels tend to be higher, and jaundice and hyperbilirubinemia are more frequent in this form of chronic hepatitis.

CHRONIC VIRAL HEPATITIS Both the enterically transmitted forms of viral hepatitis, hepatitis A and E, are self-limited and do not cause chronic hepatitis (rare reports notwithstanding in which acute hepatitis A serves as a trigger for the onset of autoimmune chronic active hepatitis in genetically susceptible patients). In contrast, the entire clinicopathologic spectrum of chronic hepatitis occurs in patients with chronic viral hepatitis B and C as well as in patients with chronic hepatitis D superimposed on chronic hepatitis B.

Chronic hepatitis B The likelihood of chronicity after acute hepatitis B varies as a function of age. Infection at birth is associated with a clinically silent acute infection but a 90 percent chance of chronic infection, while infection in young adulthood is associated typically with clinically apparent acute hepatitis but a risk of chronicity of only 1 to 2 percent. Most cases of chronic hepatitis B among adults, however, occur in patients who never had a recognized episode of clinically apparent acute viral hepatitis. The degree of liver injury in patients with chronic hepatitis B is variable, ranging from none in asymptomatic carriers, to mild in chronic persistent hepatitis, to severe in chronic active hepatitis. Among adults with chronic hepatitis B, histologic features are of prognostic importance. In one long-term study of patients with chronic hepatitis B, investigators found a 5-year survival of 97 percent for patients with chronic persistent hepatitis, of 86 percent for patients with chronic active hepatitis, and of only 55 percent for patients with chronic active hepatitis and postnecrotic cirrhosis. On the other hand, more recent observations do not allow us to be so sanguine about the prognosis in patients with chronic persistent hepatitis; among patients with chronic persistent hepatitis followed for 1 to 13 years, progression to chronic active hepatitis and cirrhosis has been observed in more than a quarter of cases.

Probably more important to consider than histology alone in patients with chronic hepatitis B is the degree of hepatitis B virus (HBV) replication. As reviewed in Chap. 266, chronic hepatitis B can be divided into two phases based on the relative level of HBV replication. The relatively *replicative phase* is characterized by the presence in the serum of markers of HBV replication (HBeAg, HBV DNA), by the presence in the liver of detectable intrahepatocyte nucleocapsid antigens (primarily HBcAg), by high infectivity, and by accompanying liver injury; HBV DNA can be detected in the liver but is extrachromosomal. In contrast, the relatively *nonreplicative phase* is characterized by the absence of conventional markers of HBV replication (HBeAg and HBV DNA detectable by hybridization) but associated with anti-HBe, the absence of intrahepatocytic HBcAg, limited infectivity, and minimal liver injury; HBV DNA can be detected in the liver integrated into the host genome. Those in the replicative phase tend to have more severe chronic hepatitis (e.g., chronic active hepatitis), while those in the nonreplicative phase tend to have mild chronic hepatitis (chronic persistent hepatitis) or to be asymptomatic hepatitis B carriers; however, distinctions in HBV replication and in histologic category do not always coincide. The likelihood of converting spontaneously from relatively replicative to

nonreplicative chronic HBV infection is approximately 10 to 15 percent per year. As noted in Chap. 266, the conversion from replicative to nonreplicative chronic hepatitis B is associated with a transient elevation in aminotransferase activity resembling acute hepatitis; occasionally, spontaneous resumptions of replicative activity occur in nonreplicative infection; and rarely, HBV variants occur in which serologic markers of replication (HBeAg) are absent, despite the presence of replicative infection. As reviewed in Chap. 269, chronic HBV infection, especially when acquired at birth or in early childhood, is associated with an increased risk of hepatocellular carcinoma. A discussion of the pathogenesis of liver injury in patients with chronic hepatitis B appears in Chap. 266.

The spectrum of *clinical features* of chronic hepatitis B is broad, ranging from asymptomatic infection to debilitating disease or even end-stage, fatal hepatic failure. As noted above, the onset of the disease tends to be insidious in most patients, with the exception of the very few in whom chronic disease follows failure of resolution of clinically apparent acute hepatitis B. The clinical and laboratory features associated with progression from acute to chronic hepatitis B are discussed in Chap. 266. *Fatigue* is a common symptom, and persistent or intermittent *jaundice* is a common feature in severe or advanced cases. Intermittent deepening of jaundice and recurrence of malaise and anorexia, as well as worsening fatigue, are reminiscent of acute hepatitis; such exacerbations may occur spontaneously, often coinciding with evidence of virologic reactivation, may lead to progressive liver injury, and when superimposed on well-established cirrhosis, may cause hepatic decompensation. Complications of cirrhosis occur in end-stage chronic active hepatitis and include ascites, edema, bleeding gastroesophageal varices, hepatic encephalopathy, coagulopathy, or hypersplenism. Occasionally, these complications bring the patient to initial clinical attention. Extrahepatic complications of chronic hepatitis B, similar to those seen during the prodromal phase of acute hepatitis B, are associated with deposition of circulating hepatitis B antigen-antibody immune complexes. As reviewed in Chap. 266, these include arthralgias and arthritis, which are common, and the more rare purpuric cutaneous lesions (leukocytoclastic vasculitis), immune-complex glomerulonephritis, and generalized vasculitis (polyarteritis nodosa).

Laboratory features of chronic hepatitis B do not distinguish adequately between histologically mild and severe hepatitis. Aminotransferase elevations tend to be modest for chronic hepatitis B but may fluctuate in the range of 100 to 1000 units. As is true for acute viral hepatitis B, alanine aminotransferase (ALT or SGPT) tends to be more elevated than aspartate aminotransferase (AST or SGOT); however, once cirrhosis is established, AST tends to exceed ALT. Levels of alkaline phosphatase activity tend to be normal or only marginally elevated. In severe cases, moderate elevations in serum bilirubin (3 to 10 mg/dL or 51.3 to 171 μmol/L) occur. Hypoalbuminemia and prolongation of the prothrombin time occur in severe or end-stage cases. Hyperglobulinemia and detectable circulating autoantibodies are distinctly absent in chronic hepatitis B (in contrast to autoimmune chronic active hepatitis). Viral markers of chronic HBV infection are discussed in Chap. 266.

TABLE 267-1 Clinical and laboratory features of chronic hepatitis

Type of hepatitis	Diagnostic test(s)	Autoantibodies	Therapy
Chronic hepatitis B	HBsAg, IgG anti-HBc, HBeAg, HBV DNA	Uncommon	Interferon-α
Chronic hepatitis C	Anti-HCV (EIA* and RIBA‡), HCV RNA	Anti-LKM1†	Interferon-α
Chronic hepatitis D	Anti-HDV, HDV RNA, HBsAg, IgG anti-HBc	Anti-LKM3	Interferon-α (?)
Autoimmune chronic active hepatitis	ANA (homogeneous), anti-LKM1(±), hyperglobulinemia	ANA, anti-LKM1	Prednisone, azathioprine

* Enzyme immunoassay.
† Antibodies to liver-kidney microsomes type 1.
‡ Recombinant immunoblot assay.

Management of chronic hepatitis B depends on the level of virus replication. Although progression to cirrhosis is more likely in chronic active than in chronic persistent or lobular hepatitis B, all three forms of chronic viral hepatitis can be progressive. Randomized, prospective, controlled trials have established that patients with well-compensated chronic replicative hepatitis B, selected to have chronic hepatitis on liver biopsy and aminotransferase elevations, regardless of histologic features, respond to antiviral therapy with interferon-α. A 4-month (16-week) course of subcutaneous injections, daily at a dose of 5 million units or three times a week at a dose of 10 million units, is associated with an approximately 40 percent seroconversion from replicative (HBeAg and HBV DNA detectable in serum) to nonreplicative (anti-HBe detectable) HBV infection, with a concomitant improvement in liver histologic features and an approximately 10 percent chance of losing detectable HBsAg. In most cases, successful interferon therapy and seroconversion is accompanied by an acute hepatitis–like elevation in aminotransferase activity, which is believed to represent an immunostimulatory effect of interferon on the interaction between the cellular immune system and virus-infected hepatocytes. Relapse after successful therapy is rare indeed (1 to 2 percent). The likelihood of responding to interferon is higher in patients with moderate to low levels of HBV DNA (<200 pg/mL) and in patients with substantial elevations of aminotransferase activities (e.g., >100 to 200 units). The likelihood of losing HBsAg *during therapy* is increased in patients with brief-duration disease (mean duration 1½ years); followed sufficiently long after successful interferon-induced loss of replicative markers, approximately 70 percent of such patients have been observed to lose HBsAg, i.e., all serologic markers of infection, over a 5-year period. Immunosuppressed patients with chronic hepatitis B do not appear to be responsive to interferon therapy.

Complications of interferon therapy include systemic "flulike" symptoms, marrow suppression, emotional lability (irritability commonly, depression rarely), autoimmune reactions (especially autoimmune thyroiditis), and miscellaneous side effects such as alopecia, rashes, diarrhea, and numbness and tingling of the extremities. With the possible exception of autoimmune thyroiditis, all these side effects are reversible upon dose lowering or cessation of therapy.

In patients with chronic active hepatitis B, long-term therapy with glucocorticoids is not only ineffective but also detrimental. Under certain circumstances, however, the predicted impact of glucocorticoids on HBV and the immune system can be exploited for the patient's benefit. Glucocorticoids increase HBV replication and expression in hepatocytes and depress the activity of cytolytic T cells. Theoretically, then, if steroids are administered for a brief time and then withdrawn, cytolytic T cells, suppressed while HBV replication was being steroid-induced, could resume their presteroid function and be capable of attacking and destroying the new crop of HBV antigen–expressing hepatocytes. Such appears to be the case; an acute hepatitis–like elevation of aminotransferase activity follows and may be accompanied by a dramatic drop in, or even a loss of, HBV replication. A preliminary 6-week period of glucocorticoid therapy (prednisone at doses of 60 mg for 2 weeks, 40 mg for 2 weeks, and 20 mg for 2 weeks), followed by its abrupt withdrawal, has been shown to be of benefit in conjunction with interferon therapy (5 million units subcutaneously daily for 4 months) in patients with chronic hepatitis B, primarily those with near-normal or only modest elevations in aminotransferase levels.

No treatment is indicated or available for asymptomatic, nonreplicative hepatitis B carriers, and antiviral therapy should be withheld from patients with decompensated hepatitis B, in whom treatment may be associated with hepatic decompensation. Such patients should be referred to research centers involved in clinical trials. Other interferons and several nucleoside analogues active against HBV are being evaluated in experimental trials.

For patients with end-stage chronic hepatitis B, liver transplantation is the only potential lifesaving intervention. Reinfection of the new liver is almost universal; however, the likelihood of liver injury associated with hepatitis B in the new liver is variable. The majority of patients become high-level viremic carriers with minimal liver injury. Unfortunately, an unpredictable proportion experience severe hepatitis B–related liver injury, sometimes a fulminant-like hepatitis, sometimes a rapid recapitulation of the original severe chronic hepatitis B (see Chap. 271).

Chronic hepatitis D (delta hepatitis) The clinical and laboratory features of chronic HDV infection are summarized in Chap. 266. Chronic hepatitis D may follow acute coinfection with HBV but at a rate no higher than the rate of chronicity of hepatitis B. That is, although HDV coinfection can increase the severity of acute hepatitis B, HDV does not increase the likelihood of progression to chronic hepatitis B. When, however, HDV superinfection occurs in a person who is already chronically infected with HBV, long-term HDV infection is the rule and a worsening of the liver disease the expected consequence. Except for severity, chronic hepatitis B plus D has similar clinical and laboratory features to those seen in chronic hepatitis B alone. Chronic active hepatitis, with or without cirrhosis, is the rule and chronic persistent hepatitis the exception. A distinguishing serologic feature of chronic hepatitis D is the presence in the circulation of antibodies to liver-kidney microsomes (anti-LKM); however, the anti-LKM seen in hepatitis D are designated anti-LKM3 and are distinct from anti-LKM1 seen in patients with autoimmune chronic active hepatitis and in a subset of patients with chronic hepatitis C.

Management is not well defined. Glucocorticoids are ineffective and are not used. Preliminary experimental trials of interferon-α suggested that conventional doses and durations of therapy lower levels of HDV RNA and aminotransferase activity only transiently during treatment but have no impact on the natural history of the disease. A more recent trial suggests that high-dose interferon-α (9 million units) three times a week for 12 months may be associated with a sustained loss of HDV replication and clinical improvement in up to 50 percent of patients. Antiviral therapy for chronic hepatitis D remains the subject of experimental trials. In patients with end-stage liver disease secondary to chronic hepatitis D, liver transplantation has been effective. If hepatitis D recurs in the new liver without the expression of hepatitis B (an unusual serologic profile in immunocompetent persons, but common in transplant patients), liver injury is limited. In fact, the outcome of transplantation for chronic hepatitis D is superior to that for chronic hepatitis B (see Chap. 271).

Chronic hepatitis C (non-A, non-B hepatitis) Regardless of the epidemiologic mode of acquisition of HCV infection, chronicity follows acute hepatitis C in approximately 50 percent of cases. What is more, in patients with chronic transfusion-associated hepatitis followed for 10 years, progression to cirrhosis has been recorded in 20 percent. Such is the case even for patients with relatively clinically mild chronic hepatitis, including those without symptoms, with only modest elevations of aminotransferase activity, and with chronic persistent hepatitis on liver biopsy. Even in cohorts of well-compensated patients with chronic hepatitis C (no complications of chronic liver disease and with normal hepatic synthetic function), the prevalance of cirrhosis may be as high as 50 percent. Many cases of hepatitis C are identified in asymptomatic patients who have no history of acute hepatitis C, e.g., those discovered while attempting to donate blood or as a result of routine laboratory screening tests. The source of HCV infection in most of these cases remains a mystery, and the natural history of chronic hepatitis C identified under these circumstances is unknown. Among asymptomatic persons with anti-HCV, even when aminotransferase levels are normal, between a third and a half have been reported to have chronic hepatitis on liver biopsy. In these asymptomatic persons with normal aminotransferase levels, the presence of detectable circulating HCV RNA appears to distinguish those with chronic hepatitis on biopsy from those with normal liver histology.

Despite this substantial rate of progression of chronic hepatitis C, and despite the fact that liver failure can result from end-stage chronic hepatitis C, the long-term prognosis for chronic hepatitis C in a majority of patients is relatively benign. Mortality over 10 to 20 years among patients with transfusion-associated chronic hepatitis C (non-A, non-B hepatitis) has been shown not to differ from mortality in a matched population of transfused patients in whom non-A, non-B hepatitis did not develop. Although death in the hepatitis group is more likely to result from liver failure, and although hepatic decompensation may occur in approximately 15 percent of such patients over the course of a decade, the majority (almost 60 percent) of patients remain asymptomatic and well compensated, with no clinical sequelae of chronic liver disease. Overall, then, chronic hepatitis C tends to be very slowly and insidiously progressive. The impact of relative levels of HCV replication or of HCV genotype on long-term prognosis in patients with chronic hepatitis C has not been studied. On the other hand, severity of chronic hepatitis is greater and progression of chronic liver disease is more accelerated in patients who have chronic hepatitis C as well as other liver processes, including alcoholic liver disease, chronic hepatitis B, and α_1-antitrypsin deficiency. No other epidemiologic or clinical features of chronic hepatitis C (e.g., severity of acute hepatitis, level of aminotransferase activity, presence or absence of jaundice) are predictive of eventual outcome. Despite its relative benignity over time, cirrhosis following chronic hepatitis C has been associated with the late development, after several decades, of hepatocellular carcinoma (see Chap. 269).

Clinical features of chronic hepatitis C are similar to those described above for chronic hepatitis B. Generally, *fatigue* is the most common symptom; jaundice is rare. Extrahepatic complications of chronic hepatitis C are less common than they are in chronic hepatitis B, with the exception of essential mixed cryoglobulinemia (see Chap. 266). *Laboratory features* of chronic hepatitis C are similar to those in patients with chronic hepatitis B, but aminotransferase levels tend to fluctuate more (the characteristic episodic pattern of aminotransferase activity) and to be lower, especially in patients with long-standing disease. An interesting and occasionally confusing finding in patients with chronic hepatitis C is the presence of autoantibodies. Rarely, patients with autoimmune chronic active hepatitis (see below) and hyperglobulinemia have false-positive enzyme immunoassays for anti-HCV. On the other hand, a proportion of patients with serologically confirmable chronic hepatitis C have circulating autoantibodies to liver-kidney microsomes (anti-LKM). These antibodies are anti-KLM1, as seen in patients with autoimmune chronic active hepatitis *type 2* (see below), and are directed against a 33-amino-acid sequence of P450 IID6. The occurrence of anti-KLM1 in some patients with chronic hepatitis C may result from the partial sequence homology between the epitope recognized by anti-LKM1 and two segments of the HCV polyprotein. In addition, the finding of this autoantibody in some patients with chronic hepatitis C suggests that autoimmunity may be playing a role in the pathogenesis of chronic hepatitis C. Histopathologic features of chronic hepatitis C, especially those which distinguish hepatitis C from hepatitis B, are described in Chap. 266.

In the *management* of chronic hepatitis C, glucocorticoids are ineffective. Based on the outcome of prospective, randomized, controlled clinical trials, interferon-α has been approved for the treatment of chronic hepatitis C. Doses ranging from 2 to 5 million units three times a week have been shown to be effective in these trials, but the officially approved dose recommendation is 3 million units by subcutaneous injection three times a week for 6 months (24 weeks). This regimen is associated with a likelihood of biochemical response (return of ALT to normal or a 50 percent reduction of ALT to within 1.5 times the upper limit of normal) in approximately 50 percent of patients. Unlike hepatitis B, in chronic hepatitis C a successful response to interferon is not accompanied by an acute hepatitis-like elevation in aminotransferase activity; instead, ALT levels fall precipitously. Between 85 and 90 percent of responses occur within the first 3 months of therapy; responses thereafter are rare. In addition, histologic improvement in periportal and lobular inflammation has been demonstrated, primarily in biochemically responding patients, but also in biochemical nonresponders. After completion of 6 months of therapy, at least 50 percent of responding patients experience a biochemical relapse. Thus the likelihood of a sustained response is no greater than 25 percent. In those who relapse after responding, however, retreatment with interferon leads invariably to response again. Neither longer initial therapy, e.g., for 12 months, nor higher-dose therapy lowers the frequency of relapse. Whether sustained, long-term even indefinite therapy will be necessary or effective in those who relapse remains to be determined. Similarly, the impact of short-term therapy on the long-term natural history of chronic hepatitis C continues to be studied.

Levels of HCV RNA fall in tandem with ALT levels during interferon therapy, but loss of detectable HCV RNA does not preclude relapse. In fact, no single clinical or laboratory feature of chronic hepatitis C has been found which is predictive of responsiveness to interferon. Responses occur in patients with established cirrhosis, although, some observers report, at a frequency lower than that seen in patients with chronic active hepatitis without cirrhosis. Some observers report that responsiveness in chronic persistent hepatitis exceeds that in chronic active hepatitis.

Although a consensus exists that patients with symptomatic chronic active hepatitis should be treated with interferon, treatment of asymptomatic patients and those with mild chronic persistent hepatitis remains controversial. Because progression to cirrhosis can occur in an unpredictable proportion of such cases, the potential benefit of therapy should not be dismissed out of hand in these patients. Additional study is needed. Currently, no authorities advocate treating asymptomatic hepatitis C "carriers" with normal aminotransferase levels or patients with decompensated cirrhosis secondary to chronic hepatitis C. For those with decompensated, end-stage disease, liver transplantation is an option. Although the likelihood of reexpressing detectable anti-HCV after transplantation is low, the likelihood of reinfection of the new liver is almost universal. Nevertheless, and the occasional exception notwithstanding, most patients who undergo liver transplantation for chronic hepatitis C experience little, if any, morbidity, allograft loss, or mortality associated with recurrent hepatitis C infection (see Chap. 271).

AUTOIMMUNE CHRONIC ACTIVE HEPATITIS **Definition** Autoimmune chronic active hepatitis is a chronic disorder characterized by continuing hepatocellular necrosis and inflammation, usually with fibrosis, which tends to progress to cirrhosis and liver failure. When fulfilling criteria of severity, this type of chronic active hepatitis may have a 6-month mortality of as high as 40 percent. The prominence of extrahepatic features of autoimmunity as well as seroimmunologic abnormalities in this disorder supports an autoimmune process in its pathogenesis, and this concept is reflected in the labels "lupoid," plasma cell, or autoimmune chronic active hepatitis. Because autoantibodies and other typical features of autoimmunity do not occur in all cases, however, a broader, more appropriate designation for this type of chronic active hepatitis is "idiopathic" or cryptogenic. Cases in which hepatotropic viruses, metabolic/genetic derangements, and hepatotoxic drugs have been excluded merit this designation and probably include a spectrum of heterogeneous liver disorders of unknown cause, a proportion of which have characteristic autoimmune features.

Immunopathogenesis The weight of evidence suggests that the progressive liver injury in patients with idiopathic/autoimmune chronic active hepatitis is the result of a cell-mediated immunologic attack directed against liver cells; in all likelihood, predisposition to autoimmunity is inherited, while the liver specificity of this injury is triggered by environmental (e.g., chemical or viral) factors. For example, patients have been described in whom apparently self-limited cases of acute hepatitis A or B led to autoimmune chronic active hepatitis, presumably because of genetic susceptibility or predisposition. Evidence to support an autoimmune pathogenesis in chronic active hepatitis includes the following: (1) In the liver, the histopathologic lesions are composed predominantly of cytotoxic T cells and plasma cells; (2) circulating autoantibodies (nuclear, smooth muscle, thyroid, etc.; see below), rheumatoid factor, and hyperglobulinemia are common; (3) other autoimmune disorders—such as thyroiditis, rheumatoid arthritis, autoimmune hemolytic anemia, ulcerative colitis, proliferative glomerulonephritis, juvenile diabetes mellitus, and Sjögren's syndrome—occur with increased frequency in patients who have chronic active hepatitis and in their relatives; (4) histocompatibility haplotypes associated with autoimmune diseases, such as HLA-B1, -B8, -DRw3, and -DRw4, are common in patients with autoimmune chronic active hepatitis; and (5) this type of chronic active hepatitis is responsive to glucocorticoid/immunosuppressive therapy, effective in a variety of autoimmune disorders.

Cellular immune mechanisms appear to be important in the pathogenesis of autoimmune chronic active hepatitis. In vitro studies have suggested that in patients with this disorder, lymphocytes are capable of becoming sensitized to hepatocyte membrane proteins and of destroying liver cells. Abnormalities of immunoregulatory control over cytotoxic lymphocytes (impaired suppressor cell influences) may play a role as well. Studies of genetic predisposition to autoimmune chronic active hepatitis demonstrate that certain haplotypes are associated with the disorder. These include HLA-B8, -DR3, -Dw3 and certain complement alleles, C2 and C4. The precise triggering factors, genetic influences, and cytotoxic and immunoregulatory mechanisms involved in this type of liver injury remain poorly defined.

Intriguing clues into the pathogenesis of chronic active hepatitis come from the observation that circulating autoantibodies are prevalent in patients with this disorder. Among the autoantibodies described in these patients are antibodies to nuclei (so-called antinuclear antibodies, ANA, primarily in a homogeneous pattern), smooth muscle (so-called anti-smooth-muscle antibodies, ASMA, directed at actin), antibodies to liver-kidney microsomes (anti-LKM; see below), antibodies to "soluble liver antigen" (anti-SLA, directed at cytokeratins), as well as antibodies to the liver-specific asialoglycoprotein receptor (or "hepatic lectin") and other hepatocyte membrane proteins. Although some of these provide helpful diagnostic markers, their involvement in the pathogenesis of autoimmune chronic active hepatitis has not been established.

Humoral immune mechanisms have been shown to play a role in the extrahepatic manifestations of chronic active hepatitis. Arthralgias, arthritis, cutaneous vasculitis, and glomerulonephritis occurring in patients with autoimmune (and viral) chronic active hepatitis appear to be mediated by the deposition in affected tissue vessels of circulating immune complexes, followed by complement activation, inflammation, and tissue injury. While specific viral antigen-antibody complexes can be identified in acute and chronic viral hepatitis, the nature of the immune complexes in autoimmune chronic active hepatitis has not been defined.

Many of the *clinical features* of autoimmune chronic active hepatitis are similar to those described for chronic viral hepatitis. The onset of disease may be insidious or abrupt; the disease may present initially like, and be confused with, acute viral hepatitis; and a history of recurrent bouts of what had been labeled acute hepatitis is not uncommon. A subset of patients with autoimmune chronic active hepatitis has distinct features. Such patients are predominantly young to middle-aged women with marked hyperglobulinemia and high-titer circulating ANA. This is the group with positive LE preparations (initially labeled "lupoid" hepatitis) in whom other autoimmune features are common. Fatigue, malaise, anorexia, amenorrhea, acne, arthralgias, and jaundice are common. Occasionally, arthritis, maculopapular eruptions (including cutaneous vasculitis), erythema nodosum, colitis, pleurisy, pericarditis, anemia, azotemia, and sicca syndrome (keratoconjunctivitis, xerostomia) occur. In some patients, complications of cirrhosis, such as ascites and edema (associated with hypoalbuminemia), encephalopathy, hypersplenism, coagulopathy, or variceal bleeding, may bring the patient to initial medical attention.

The course of chronic active hepatitis may be variable. In those with mild disease or limited histologic lesions (e.g., piecemeal necrosis without bridging), progression to cirrhosis is limited. In those with severe symptomatic chronic active hepatitis (aminotransfer-ase levels >10 times normal, marked hyperglobulinemia, "aggressive" histologic lesions—bridging necrosis or multilobular collapse, cirrhosis), the 6-month mortality without therapy may be as high as 40 percent. Such severe disease accounts for only 20 percent of cases; the natural history of milder disease is variable, often accentuated by spontaneous remissions and exacerbations. Especially poor prognostic signs include multilobular collapse at the time of initial presentation and failure of the bilirubin to improve after 2 weeks of therapy. Death may result from hepatic failure, hepatic coma, other complications of cirrhosis (e.g., variceal hemorrhage), and intercurrent infection. In patients with established cirrhosis, hepatocellular carcinoma may be a late complication (see Chap. 269).

Laboratory features of autoimmune chronic active hepatitis are similar to those seen in chronic viral hepatitis. Liver biochemical tests are invariably abnormal but may not correlate with the clinical severity or histopathologic features in individual cases. Many patients with chronic active hepatitis have normal serum bilirubin, alkaline phosphatase, and globulin levels with only minimal aminotransferase elevations. Serum aspartate aminotransferase (AST or SGOT) and alanine aminotransferase (ALT or SGPT) levels are increased and fluctuate in the range of 100 to 1000 units. In severe cases, the serum bilirubin level is moderately elevated [51 to 171 μmol/L (3 to 10 mg/dL)]. Mild hypoalbuminemia occurs in patients with very active or advanced disease. Serum alkaline phosphatase levels may be moderately elevated or near normal. In a small proportion of patients, marked elevations of alkaline phosphatase activity occur; in such patients, clinical and laboratory features overlap with those of primary biliary cirrhosis (see Chap. 268). The prothrombin time is often prolonged, particularly late in the disease or during active phases.

Hypergammaglobulinemia (>2.5 g/dL) is common in autoimmune chronic active hepatitis. Rheumatoid factor is common as well. As noted above, circulating autoantibodies are also common. The most characteristic are antinuclear antibodies (ANA) in a homogeneous staining pattern. Smooth-muscle antibodies are less specific, seen just as frequently in chronic viral hepatitis. Because of the high levels of globulins achieved in the circulation of some patients with autoimmune chronic active hepatitis, occasionally the globulins may bind nonspecifically in solid-phase binding immunoassays for viral antibodies. This has been recognized most commonly in tests for antibodies to hepatitis C virus, as noted above. In fact, studies of autoantibodies in chronic active hepatitis have led to the recognition of new categories of autoimmune chronic active hepatitis. *Type I* autoimmune chronic active hepatitis is the classic syndrome occurring in young women, associated with marked hyperglobulinemia, lupoid features, and circulating ANA. *Type II* autoimmune chronic active hepatitis, often seen in children and more common in Mediterranean populations, is associated not with ANA but with antibodies to liver-kidney microsomal antigens (anti-LKM). Actually, anti-LKM represent a heterogeneous group of antibodies. In type II autoimmune chronic active hepatitis, the antibody is anti-LKM1, directed against P450 IID6. This is the same anti-LKM seen in some patients with chronic hepatitis C. Anti-LKM2 is seen in drug-induced hepatitis, and anti-LKM3 is seen in patients with chronic hepatitis D. Type II autoimmune chronic active hepatitis has been subdivided by some authorities into two categories, one more typically autoimmune and the other associated with viral hepatitis type C. Autoimmune chronic active hepatitis type 2a is felt to be autoimmune, is more likely to occur in young women, is associated with hyperglobulinemia, is associated with high-titer anti-LKM1, responds to glucocorticoid therapy, and is seen commonly in western Europe and the United Kingdom. Type 2b chronic active hepatitis is associated with hepatitis C virus infection, tends to occur in older men, is associated with normal globulin levels and low-titer anti-LKM1, responds to interferon, and occurs most commonly in Mediterranean countries.

The mainstay of *management* in autoimmune or idiopathic (nonviral) chronic active hepatitis is glucocorticoid therapy. Several controlled clinical trials have documented that such therapy leads to symptomatic, clinical, biochemical, and histologic improvement as well as increased survival. A therapeutic response can be expected in up to 80 percent of patients. Unfortunately, therapy has not been shown to prevent ultimate progression to cirrhosis. Although some advocate the use of prednisolone, the hepatic metabolite of prednisone, prednisone is just as effective and is favored by most authorities. Therapy may be initiated at 20 mg/d, but a popular regimen in the United States relies on an initiation dose of 60 mg/d. This high dose is tapered successively over the course of a month down to a maintenance level of 20 mg/d. An alternative, but equally effective, approach is to begin with half the prednisone dose (30 mg/d) along with azathioprine (50 mg/d). The advantage of the combination approach is a reduction, over the course of an 18-month course of therapy, in serious, life-threatening complications of steroid therapy from 66 percent down to under 20 percent. Azathioprine alone, however, is not effective in achieving remission, nor is alternate-day glucocorticoid therapy. Although therapy has been shown to be effective for severe chronic active hepatitis, therapy is not indicated for chronic persistent hepatitis or chronic lobular hepatitis, and the efficacy of therapy in mild or asymptomatic chronic active hepatitis has not been established.

Improvement of fatigue, anorexia, malaise, and jaundice tends to occur within days to several weeks; biochemical improvement occurs over the course of several weeks to months, with a fall in serum bilirubin and globulin levels and an increase in serum albumin. Serum aminotransferase levels usually drop promptly, but improvements in AST and ALT alone do not appear to be a reliable marker of recovery in individual patients; histologic improvement, characterized by a decrease in mononuclear infiltration and in hepatocellular necrosis—conversion from chronic active hepatitis to a less severe lesion, such as chronic persistent hepatitis—may be delayed for 6 to 24 months. Still, if interpreted cautiously, aminotransferase levels are valuable indicators of relative disease activity, and many authorities do *not* advocate serial liver biopsies to assess therapeutic success or to guide decisions to alter or stop therapy. Therapy must continue for at least 12 to 18 months. After tapering and cessation of therapy, the likelihood of relapse is at least 50 percent, even if posttreatment histology has improved to show chronic persistent hepatitis, and the majority of patients require therapy at maintenance doses indefinitely. Continuing azathioprine alone after cessation of prednisone therapy may reduce the frequency of relapse.

If medical therapy fails, or when chronic active hepatitis progresses to cirrhosis and is associated with life-threatening complications of liver decompensation, liver transplantation is the only recourse (see Chap. 271). Recurrence of autoimmune chronic active hepatitis in the new liver has not been documented to occur.

DIFFERENTIAL DIAGNOSIS Early during the course of chronic active hepatitis, the disease may resemble typical *acute viral hepatitis*. Without histologic assessment, chronic active hepatitis cannot be readily distinguished based on clinical or biochemical criteria from *chronic persistent hepatitis* and *chronic lobular hepatitis*. In adolescence, *Wilson's disease* may present with features of chronic active hepatitis long before neurologic manifestations become apparent and before the formation of Kayser-Fleischer rings; in this age group, serum ceruloplasmin and serum and urinary copper determinations and measurement of liver copper levels will establish the correct diagnosis. *Postnecrotic* or *cryptogenic cirrhosis* and *primary biliary cirrhosis* share clinical features with chronic active hepatitis; biochemical, serologic, and histologic assessments are usually sufficient to allow these entities to be distinguished from chronic active hepatitis. Of course, the distinction between autoimmune ("idiopathic") and viral chronic active hepatitis is not always straightforward, especially when viral antibodies occur in patients with autoimmune disease or when autoantibodies occur in patients with viral disease. Finally, the presence of extrahepatic features such as arthritis, cutaneous vasculitis, or pleuritis—not to mention the presence of circulating autoantibodies—may cause confusion with *rheumatologic disorders* such as rheumatoid arthritis and systemic lupus erythematosus. The existence of clinical and biochemical features of progressive necroinflammatory

liver disease distinguishes chronic active hepatitis from these other disorders, which are not associated with severe liver disease.

REFERENCES

CZAJA AJ et al: Laboratory assessment of severe chronic active liver disease during and after corticosteroid therapy: Correlation of serum transaminase and gamma globulin levels with histologic features. Gastroenterology 80:687, 1981

——— et al: Sustained remission after corticosteroid therapy of severe hepatitis B surface antigen-negative chronic active hepatitis. Gastroenterology 92:215, 1987

——— et al: Features reflective of early prognosis in corticosteroid-treated severe autoimmune chronic active hepatitis. Gastroenterology 95:448, 1988

——— et al: Frequency and significance of antibodies to liver/kidney microsome type 1 in adults with chronic active hepatitis. Gastroenterology 103:1290, 1992

DAVIS GL et al: Treatment of chronic hepatitis C with recombinant interferon alfa: A multicenter randomized, controlled trial. N Engl J Med 321:1501, 1989

DIENSTAG JL, ISSELBACHER KJ: Therapy for acute and chronic hepatitis. Arch Intern Med 141:1419, 1981

FATTOVICH G et al: Natural history and prognostic factors for chronic hepatitis type B. Gut 32:294, 1991

HOMBERG J-C et al: Chronic active hepatitis associated with antiliver/kidney microsome antibody type 1: A second type of "autoimmune" hepatitis. Hepatology 7:1333, 1987

KATKOV WN, DIENSTAG JL: Prevention and therapy of viral hepatitis. Semin Liver Dis 11:165, 1991

KRAWITT EL, WEISNER RH (eds): *Autoimmune Liver Diseases*. New York, Raven, 1991

LUNEL F et al: Liver/kidney microsome antibody type 1 and hepatitis C virus infection. Hepatology 16:630, 1992

MEYER ZUM BÜSCHENFELDE K-H (ed): Autoimmune hepatitis. Semin Liver Dis 11:183, 1991

PERRILLO RP et al: A randomized, controlled trial of interferon alpha-2b alone and after prednisone withdrawal for the treatment of chronic hepatitis B. N Engl J Med 323:295, 1990

SEEFF LB et al. Long-term mortality after transfusion-associated non-A, non-B hepatitis. N Engl J Med 327:1906, 1992

STELLON AJ et al: Maintenance of remission in autoimmune chronic active hepatitis with azathioprine after corticosteroid withdrawal. Hepatology 8:781, 1988

SUMMERSKILL WHJ et al: Prednisone for chronic active liver disease: Dose titration, standard dose, and combination with azathioprine compared. Gut 16:876, 1975

WEISSBERG JI et al: Survival in chronic hepatitis B: An analysis of 379 patients. Ann Intern Med 101:613, 1984

268 ALCOHOL-RELATED LIVER DISEASE AND CIRRHOSIS

DANIEL K. PODOLSKY / KURT J. ISSELBACHER

Cirrhosis is a pathologically defined entity which is associated with a spectrum of characteristic clinical manifestations. The cardinal pathologic features reflect irreversible chronic injury of the hepatic parenchyma and include extensive fibrosis in association with the formation of regenerative nodules. These features result from hepatocyte necrosis, collapse of the supporting reticulin network with subsequent connective tissue deposition, distortion of the vascular bed, and nodular regeneration of remaining liver parenchyma. The pathologic process should be viewed as a final common pathway of many types of chronic liver injury. Clinical features of cirrhosis derive from the morphologic alterations and often reflect the severity of hepatic damage rather than the etiology of the underlying liver disease. Loss of functioning hepatocellular mass may lead to jaundice, edema, coagulopathy, and a variety of metabolic abnormalities; fibrosis and distorted vasculature lead to portal hypertension and its sequelae, including gastroesophageal varices and splenomegaly. Ascites and hepatic encephalopathy result from both hepatocellular insufficiency and portal hypertension.

Classification of the various types of cirrhosis based solely on etiology or morphology is unsatisfactory. A single pathologic pattern may result from a variety of insults, while the same insult may produce several morphologic patterns. Nevertheless, most types of cirrhosis may be usefully classified by a mixture of etiologically and morphologically defined entities as follows: (1) alcoholic, (2) cryptogenic and postviral or postnecrotic, (3) biliary, (4) cardiac, (5) metabolic, inherited, and drug-related, and (6) miscellaneous. This chapter considers first the various types of cirrhosis and then the major clinical complications of chronic liver disease and cirrhosis.

ALCOHOLIC LIVER DISEASE AND CIRRHOSIS

Definition   *Alcoholic cirrhosis*, historically referred to as *Laennec's cirrhosis*, is the most common type of cirrhosis encountered in North America and many parts of western Europe and South America. It is usually characterized by diffuse fine scarring, fairly uniform loss of liver cells, and small regenerative nodules, and therefore, it is sometimes referred to as *micronodular cirrhosis*. However, micronodular cirrhosis also may result from other types of liver injury (e.g., following jejunoileal bypass), and thus *alcoholic cirrhosis* and *micronodular cirrhosis* are not necessarily synonymous. Conversely, alcoholic cirrhosis may progress to macronodular cirrhosis with time.

Alcoholic cirrhosis is only one of many consequences resulting from chronic alcohol ingestion, and it often accompanies other forms of alcohol-induced liver injury. The three principal alcohol-induced hepatic lesions are designated (1) *alcoholic fatty liver*, (2) *alcoholic hepatitis*, and (3) *alcoholic cirrhosis*. These morphologic categories are rarely found in a pure form, and features of each may be present to varying degrees in an individual patient.

Etiology   Although chronic alcoholism is the most common cause of cirrhosis, the quantity and duration of drinking necessary to cause cirrhosis remain unclear. The typical alcoholic patient with cirrhosis has had a daily consumption of a pint or more of whiskey, several quarts of wine, or an equivalent amount of beer for at least 10 years. The amount and duration of ethanol ingestion, rather than the type of alcoholic beverage or the pattern of ingestion, appear to be the important determinants of liver injury. In general, the latent period preceding the development of cirrhosis is inversely related to the level of daily alcohol intake. Rates of ethanol metabolism are under genetic control, but no metabolic defect has been identified in cirrhotic patients or their families to suggest a unique "susceptibility" to ethanol or its toxic effects. Although malnutrition per se does not appear to lead to cirrhosis, it is possible that nutritional factors may augment the detrimental effects of chronic alcohol ingestion on the liver. The finding that only 10 to 15 percent of alcoholics develop cirrhosis suggests that other factors may affect the impact of alcohol on the liver. Women, on average, appear to develop alcohol-induced liver injury at lesser levels of consumption than men, suggesting that hormonal factors may play a role in susceptibility.

Alcoholic fatty liver occurs in most heavy drinkers but is reversible on cessation of alcohol consumption and is not thought to be an inevitable precursor of alcoholic hepatitis or cirrhosis. In contrast, alcoholic hepatitis, an inflammatory lesion characterized by infiltration of the liver with leukocytes, liver cell necrosis, and alcoholic hyaline, is thought to be the major precursor of cirrhosis. Subsequent healing accompanied by fibrosis distorts the normal lobular architecture. Indeed, *deposition of collagen in perivenular spaces* may be the earliest manifestation of the process which ultimately leads to cirrhosis.

Pathology and pathogenesis   ALCOHOLIC FATTY LIVER   The liver is enlarged, yellow, greasy, and firm. Hepatocytes are distended by large macrovesicular cytoplasmic fat vacuoles which push the hepatocyte nucleus against the cell membrane. Accumulation of fat in the liver of the alcoholic results from the combination of impaired fatty acid oxidation, increased uptake and esterification of fatty acids to form triglycerides, and diminished lipoprotein biosynthesis and secretion.

ALCOHOLIC HEPATITIS   Morphologic features include hepatocyte degeneration and necrosis, often with ballooned cells, and an infiltrate of polymorphonuclear leukocytes and lymphocytes. The polymorphonuclear cells may encircle damaged hepatocytes which contain *Mallory bodies*, or *alcoholic hyaline*. These are clumps of perinuclear, deeply

eosinophilic material believed to represent aggregated intermediate filaments. Mallory bodies are highly suggestive of, but *not specific* for, alcoholic hepatitis, since morphologically similar material has been seen in association with morbid obesity, jejunoileal bypass surgery, poorly controlled diabetes mellitus, and a variety of other disorders, including Wilson's disease and Indian childhood cirrhosis. Deposition of collagen around the central vein and in perisinusoidal areas, often termed *central hyaline sclerosis*, may be associated with an increased likelihood of progression to cirrhosis.

ALCOHOLIC CIRRHOSIS   With continued alcohol intake and destruction of hepatocytes, fibroblasts (including myofibroblasts with contractile properties) appear at the site of injury and stimulate collagen formation. Weblike septa of connective tissue appear in periportal and pericentral zones and eventually connect portal triads and central veins. This fine connective tissue network surrounds small masses of remaining liver cells which regenerate and form nodules. Although regeneration occurs within the small remnants of parenchyma, cell loss generally exceeds replacement. With continuing hepatocyte destruction and collagen deposition, the liver shrinks in size, acquires a nodular appearance, and becomes hard as "end-stage" cirrhosis develops. Although alcoholic cirrhosis is usually a progressive disease, appropriate therapy and strict avoidance of alcohol may arrest the disease at most stages and permit functional improvement.

Clinical features   SIGNS AND SYMPTOMS   Clinical manifestations of *alcoholic fatty liver* are often minimal or entirely absent, and the disorder may not be recognized unless another illness (frequently alcohol-related) brings the patient to medical attention. Hepatomegaly, at times accompanied by tenderness, may be the only finding. Jaundice, ascites, and edema are only seen with more serious liver injury.

The clinical severity of *alcoholic hepatitis* varies enormously, ranging from asymptomatic or mild illness to fatal hepatic insufficiency. Typically, the clinical features of alcoholic hepatitis resemble those of viral or toxic liver injury. Patients often experience anorexia, nausea and vomiting, malaise, weight loss, abdominal distress, and jaundice. Fever sometimes as high as 39.4°C (103°F) may be seen in about half of cases. On physical examination, tender hepatomegaly is common, and splenomegaly is found in about one-third of patients. The patient may have cutaneous arterial "spider" angiomas and jaundice. More severe cases may be complicated by ascites, edema, bleeding, and encephalopathy. At the time of initial presentation, the central nervous system findings may be difficult to distinguish from manifestations of concurrent alcohol intoxication or withdrawal (see below).

Although jaundice, ascites, and encephalopathy may subside with abstinence, continued alcohol excess and poor dietary habits usually lead to repeated acute episodes of hepatic decompensation. Some patients die during these acute exacerbations, but most recover after several weeks or months. Even after complete abstinence, clinical recovery may be protracted, and histologic abnormalities can persist up to 6 months or longer. Cholestatic jaundice mimicking biliary tract obstruction also may develop in some cases of acute alcoholic hepatitis.

Alcoholic cirrhosis also may be clinically silent; in fact, 10 percent of cases are discovered incidentally at laparotomy or autopsy. In many cases symptoms are insidious in onset, occurring usually after 10 or more years of excessive alcohol use and progressing slowly over subsequent weeks and months. Anorexia and malnutrition lead to weight loss and a reduction in skeletal muscle mass. The patient may experience easy bruising, increasing weakness, and fatigue. Eventually the clinical manifestations of hepatocellular dysfunction and portal hypertension ensue, including progressive jaundice, bleeding from gastroesophageal varices, ascites, and encephalopathy. The abrupt onset of one of these complications may be the first event prompting the patient to seek medical attention. In other cases, cirrhosis first becomes evident when the patient requires treatment of symptoms related to alcoholic hepatitis.

A firm, nodular liver may be an early sign of disease; the liver may be either enlarged, normal, or decreased in size. Other frequent findings include jaundice, palmar erythema, spider angiomas, parotid and lacrimal gland enlargement, clubbing of fingers, splenomegaly, muscle wasting, and ascites with or without peripheral edema. Men may have decreased body hair and/or gynecomastia and testicular atrophy, which, like the cutaneous findings, result from disturbances in hormonal metabolism, including increased peripheral formation of estrogen due to diminished hepatic clearance of the precursor androstenedione. Testicular atrophy may reflect hormonal abnormalities or the toxic effect of alcohol on the testes. In women, signs of virilization or menstrual irregularities may occasionally be encountered. Dupuytren's contractures resulting from fibrosis of the palmar fascia with resulting flexion contracture of the digits are associated with alcoholism but are not specifically related to cirrhosis.

Over a period of 3 to 5 years, the cirrhotic patient typically becomes emaciated, weak, and chronically jaundiced. Ascites and other signs of portal hypertension become increasingly prominent. Most patients with advanced cirrhosis die in hepatic coma, commonly precipitated by hemorrhage from esophageal varices or intercurrent infection. Progressive renal dysfunction often complicates the terminal phase of the illness.

LABORATORY FINDINGS Routine hematologic and biochemical blood tests are usually normal in patients with alcoholic fatty liver, except for minimal elevations of the serum AST (aspartate aminotransferase); occasionally alkaline phosphatase and bilirubin levels are also elevated. In more advanced alcoholic liver disease, abnormalities of laboratory tests are more common. Anemia may result from acute and chronic gastrointestinal blood loss, coexistent nutritional deficiency (notably of folic acid and vitamin B_{12}), hypersplenism, and a direct suppressive effect of alcohol on the bone marrow. Hemolytic anemia, presumably due to effects of hypercholesterolemia on erythrocyte membranes resulting in unusual spurlike projections (acanthocytosis), has been described in some alcoholics with cirrhosis. Leukocytosis is often present in severe alcoholic hepatitis; however, some patients with this disorder may have leukopenia and thrombocytopenia due to hypersplenism or an inhibitory effect of alcohol on the bone marrow. Mild or pronounced hyperbilirubinemia may be found, usually in association with varying elevations of serum alkaline phosphatase levels. Levels of serum AST are frequently elevated, but levels greater than 5 μkat (300 units) are unusual and should prompt one to look for other coincident or complicating factors. In contrast to viral hepatitis, the serum AST is usually disproportionately elevated relative to ALT (alanine aminotransferase) i.e., AST/ALT ratio >2. This discrepancy may result from the proportionally greater inhibition of ALT synthesis by ethanol, which may be partially reversed by pyridoxal phosphate.

The serum prothrombin time is frequently prolonged, reflecting reduced synthesis of clotting proteins, most notably the vitamin K–dependent factors (see "Coagulopathy" below). The serum albumin level is usually depressed, while serum globulins are increased. Hypoalbuminemia reflects in part overall impairment in hepatic protein synthesis, while hyperglobulinemia is thought to result from nonspecific stimulation of the reticuloendothelial system. Elevated blood ammonia levels in patients with hepatic encephalopathy reflect diminished hepatic clearance because of impaired liver function and shunting of portal venous blood around the cirrhotic liver into the systemic circulation (see below and Chap. 264).

A variety of metabolic disturbances may be detected. Glucose intolerance due to endogenous insulin resistance may be present; however, clinical diabetes is uncommon. Central hyperventilation may lead to respiratory alkalosis in patients with cirrhosis. *Dietary deficiency* and *increased urinary losses* lead to hypomagnesemia and *hypophosphatemia*. In patients with ascites and dilutional hyponatremia, hypokalemia may occur from increased urinary potassium losses due in part to hyperaldosteronism. Prerenal azotemia is also observed in such patients.

Diagnosis *Alcoholic fatty liver* should be suspected in alcoholic patients with hepatomegaly and normal or minimally deranged liver function tests. Alcoholic fatty liver may be seen in combination with alcoholic hepatitis or established cirrhosis. *Alcoholic hepatitis* should be considered in an alcoholic who has been drinking heavily and demonstrates jaundice, fever, an enlarged, tender liver, or ascites. The clinical impression is often supported by the deranged results of tests of liver function and other laboratory abnormalities described above. Alcoholic hepatitis or fatty liver may be present in association with alcoholic cirrhosis.

Alcoholic cirrhosis should be strongly suspected in patients with a history of prolonged or excessive alcohol intake and physical signs of chronic liver disease. The clinical features and laboratory findings are usually sufficient to provide reasonable indication of the presence and extent of hepatic injury. Although a percutaneous needle biopsy of the liver is not usually necessary to confirm the typical findings of alcoholic hepatitis or cirrhosis, it may be helpful in distinguishing patients with less advanced liver disease from those with cirrhosis and in excluding other forms of liver injury such as viral hepatitis. Biopsy also may be helpful as a diagnostic tool in evaluating patients with clinical findings suggestive of alcoholic liver disease who deny alcohol intake. In patients with features of cholestasis, ultrasonography may be appropriate to exclude the presence of extrahepatic biliary obstruction. When the clinical status of an otherwise stable cirrhotic patient deteriorates without an obvious explanation, complicating conditions, such as infection, portal vein thrombosis, and hepatocellular carcinoma, should be sought.

Prognosis The patient with an alcoholic fatty liver and no complications has a good prognosis; rapid and complete resolution usually follows cessation of alcohol intake. In patients with alcoholic hepatitis, the presence of marked hyperbilirubinemia, rising serum creatinine, marked prolongation of the prothrombin time (>1.5 times control), ascites, and encephalopathy are associated with a poor short-term prognosis; the in-hospital mortality in these patients may exceed 50 percent. In milder cases, clinical recovery may be complete, but repeated bouts of alcoholic hepatitis usually lead to irreversible and progressive chronic liver injury. Abstinence from alcohol as well as early and appropriate medical care can decrease long-term morbidity and mortality and delay or prevent the appearance of further complications. Patients who have had a major complication of cirrhosis and who continue to drink have a 5-year survival of less than 50 percent. However, those patients who remain abstinent have a substantially better prognosis. In general, overall outlook in patients with advanced liver disease remains poor; most of these patients eventually die as a result of massive variceal hemorrhage and/or profound hepatic encephalopathy.

Treatment Alcoholic hepatitis and cirrhosis are serious illnesses that require long-term medical supervision and careful management. Therapy of the underlying liver disease is largely supportive. Specific treatment is directed at particular complications such as variceal bleeding and ascites (see below). Some studies suggest that administration of prednisone or prednisolone in moderately large doses may be helpful in patients with severe alcoholic hepatitis and encephalopathy. However, the use of glucocorticoids in acute alcoholic hepatitis remains controversial and should probably be reserved for those with severe disease. Although a number of studies have supported the use of propylthiouracil in the management of acute alcoholic hepatitis, the way it works is as yet undefined, and its efficacy has not been unequivocally established. More recently, maintenance therapy with colchicine (0.6 mg PO bid) has been shown to slow disease progression and increase longevity of the patient with alcoholic liver disease in one long-term study. Other agents, such as penicillamine and intravenous infusion of insulin and glucagon, have been used experimentally, but their therapeutic efficacy and safety have not been demonstrated.

In the absence of signs of impending hepatic coma, the patient should be placed on a diet containing at least 1 g protein per kilogram of body weight and 8500 to 12,500 kJ (2000 to 3000 kcal) per day. Use of diets enriched in branched-chain amino acids has been advocated in patients predisposed to hepatic encephalopathy, but the value of these diets in patients with compensated cirrhosis is unproven. Daily multivitamin supplements should be prescribed, with the addition of large parenteral doses of thiamine in patients with Wernicke-Korsakoff disease (see Chap. 377). The patient should be made to realize that there is no medication that will protect the liver against the effects of further alcohol ingestion. Therefore, alcohol should be absolutely forbidden. An important component of the complete care of such patients is encouragement to become involved in an appropriate alcohol counseling program.

All medicines must be administered with caution in the patient with cirrhosis, especially those eliminated or modified through hepatic metabolism or biliary pathways. In particular, care must be taken to avoid overzealous use of drugs that may directly or indirectly precipitate complications of cirrhosis. For example, vigorous treatment of ascites with diuretics may result in electrolyte abnormalities or hypovolemia, which can lead to coma. Similarly, even modest doses of sedative can lead to deepening encephalopathy.

POSTNECROTIC CIRRHOSIS, POSTVIRAL CIRRHOSIS

Definition Postnecrotic cirrhosis represents the final common pathway of many types of advanced liver injury. *Coarsely nodular, posthepatitic,* and *multilobular cirrhosis* are terms synonymous with *postnecrotic cirrhosis.* The term *cryptogenic cirrhosis* has been used interchangeably with *postnecrotic cirrhosis,* but this designation should be reserved for those cases in which the etiology of cirrhosis is unknown (approximately 10 percent of all patients with cirrhosis).

Postnecrotic cirrhosis is characterized morphologically by (1) extensive confluent loss of liver cells, (2) stromal collapse and fibrosis resulting in broad bands of connective tissue containing the remains of many portal triads, and (3) irregular nodules of regenerating hepatocytes, varying in size from microscopic to several centimeters in diameter.

Etiology *Postnecrotic cirrhosis* is a morphologic term referring to a defined stage of advanced chronic liver injury of both specific and unknown (cryptogenic) causes. Epidemiologic and serologic evidence suggests that viral hepatitis (hepatitis B or hepatitis C) may be an antecedent factor in from one-fourth to three-fourths of cases of apparently cryptogenic postnecrotic cirrhosis. In areas where hepatitis B virus infection is endemic (e.g., Southeast Asia, sub-Saharan Africa), up to 15 percent of the population may acquire the infection in early childhood, and cirrhosis may ultimately develop in one-fourth of these chronic carriers. Although hepatitis B infection is much less prevalent in the United States, it is relatively common among certain high-risk groups (e.g., promiscuous homosexual men, intravenous drug abusers) and contributes to an increased incidence of cirrhosis. In the United States, hepatitis C appears to account for many cases of cirrhosis following blood transfusions. Before hepatitis C screening of blood donors was introduced, hepatitis C occurred in 5 to 10 percent of blood recipients. In as many as half of those surviving 20 years or more, cirrhosis may ultimately develop. Conversely, the recent identification of hepatitis C virus and the availability of specific serologic markers have led to the demonstration that more than half of patients with cryptogenic chronic liver disease have evidence of hepatitis C infection. Postnecrotic cirrhosis also may develop in patients with chronic active hepatitis of the autoimmune type (see Chaps. 266 and 267).

Other probable causes of postnecrotic cirrhosis, including drugs and toxins, are listed in Table 268-1. In some instances, advanced alcoholic liver disease and primary biliary cirrhosis may lead to postnecrotic cirrhosis.

Pathology The postnecrotic liver is typically shrunken in size, distorted in shape, and composed of nodules of liver cells separated by dense and broad bands of fibrosis. The microscopic picture is consistent with the gross impression: Nodules are highly variable in

TABLE 268-1 Cirrhosis and/or liver disease associated with various disorders

INFECTIOUS DISEASES

Brucellosis (Chap. 121)
Echinococcus (Chap. 184)
Schistosomiasis (Chap. 183)
Toxoplasmosis (Chap. 177)
Viral hepatitis [hepatitis B, hepatitis C, hepatitis D, cytomegalovirus (Chaps. 146, 266, and 267)]

INHERITED AND METABOLIC DISORDERS (see also Chap. 270)

Alpha$_1$-antitrypsin deficiency (Chap. 270)
Fanconi's syndrome (Chap. 349)
Galactosemia (Chap. 354)
Gaucher's disease (Chap. 349)
Glycogen storage disease (Chap. 350)
Hemochromatosis (Chap. 345)
Hereditary fructose intolerance (Chap. 354)
Hereditary tyrosinemia (Chap. 352)
Wilson's disease (Chap. 348)

DRUGS AND TOXINS (Chap. 266)

Arsenicals
Isoniazid
Methotrexate
Methyldopa
Oral contraceptives (Budd-Chiari)
Oxyphenisatin
Perhexilene maleate
Pyrrolidizine alkaloids (venoocclusive disease)

OTHER OR UNPROVEN CAUSES

Chronic inflammatory bowel disease (Chap. 255)
Cystic fibrosis (Chap. 222)
Diabetes mellitus (Chap. 337)
Graft-versus-host disease (Chap. 313)
Jejunoileal bypass (Chap. 40)
Sarcoidosis (Chap. 266)

size, with large amounts of connective tissue separating the disorganized islands of regenerating parenchyma.

Clinical features In patients with cirrhosis of known etiology in whom there is progression to a postnecrotic stage, the clinical manifestations are an extension of those resulting from the initial disease process. Usually clinical symptoms are related to portal hypertension and its sequelae, such as ascites, splenomegaly, hypersplenism, encephalopathy, and bleeding esophageal varices. The hematologic and liver function abnormalities resemble those seen with other types of cirrhosis. In a few patients with postnecrotic cirrhosis the diagnosis may be made incidentally at operation, at postmortem, or by a needle biopsy of the liver performed to investigate asymptomatic hepatosplenomegaly.

Diagnosis and prognosis Postnecrotic cirrhosis should be suspected in patients with signs and symptoms of cirrhosis or portal hypertension. Needle or operative liver biopsies confirm the diagnosis, although nonuniformity of the pathologic process may result in sampling errors. The diagnosis of cryptogenic cirrhosis is reserved for those patients in whom no known etiology can be demonstrated. About 75 percent of patients have progressive disease despite supportive therapy and die within 1 to 5 years from complications, including exsanguinating variceal hemorrhage, hepatic encephalopathy, or superimposed hepatocellular carcinoma.

Treatment Management is usually limited to treatment of the complications of portal hypertension, including control of ascites, avoidance of drugs or excessive protein intake that may induce hepatic coma, and prompt treatment of infections (see below). In patients with asymptomatic cirrhosis, expectant management alone is appropriate. In those patients in whom postnecrotic cirrhosis has developed as a result of a treatable condition, therapy directed at the primary disorder may limit further progression (e.g., Wilson's disease, hemochromatosis).

BILIARY CIRRHOSIS

Biliary cirrhosis results from injury to or prolonged obstruction of either the intrahepatic or extrahepatic biliary system. It is associated with impaired biliary excretion, destruction of hepatic parenchyma, and progressive fibrosis. Primary biliary cirrhosis is characterized by chronic inflammation and fibrous obliteration of intrahepatic bile ductules. Secondary biliary cirrhosis is the result of long-standing obstruction of the larger extrahepatic ducts. Although primary and secondary biliary cirrhosis are separate pathophysiologic entities with respect to the initial insult, many clinical features are similar.

PRIMARY BILIARY CIRRHOSIS   Etiology and pathogenesis The cause of primary biliary cirrhosis remains unknown. Several observations suggest that a disordered immune response may be involved. Primary biliary cirrhosis (PBC) is frequently associated with a variety of disorders presumed to be autoimmune in nature, such as the CRST syndrome (calcinosis, Raynaud's phenomenon, sclerodactyly, telangiectasia), the sicca syndrome (dry eyes and dry mouth), autoimmune thyroiditis, and renal tubular acidosis.

Most important, a circulating IgG antimitochondrial antibody (AMA) is detected in more than 90 percent of patients with primary biliary cirrhosis and only rarely in other forms of liver disease. In recent years, it has been demonstrated that these autoantibodies recognize three to five inner mitochondrial membrane proteins identified as enzymes of the pyruvate dehydrogenase complex (PDC), the branched chain α-ketoacid dehydrogenase complex (BCKDC), and the α-ketoglutarate dehydrogenase complex (KGDC). The major autoantigen in PBC (found in 90 percent of patients) has been identified as the 74-kDa E2 component of the PDC, dihydrolipoamide acetyltransferase. The antibodies are directed to a region essential for binding of a lipoic acid cofactor and inhibit the overall enzymatic activity of PDC. Other AMA autoantibodies in PBC patients are directed to similar constituents of BCKDC and KGDC and also inhibit their enzymatic function. Despite the demonstrated ability of autoantibodies found in PBC sera to inhibit key enzymatic activities, it is unclear whether these properties have a direct pathogenetic role in the development of PBC. In addition to AMA, elevated serum levels of IgM and cryoproteins consisting of immune complexes capable of activating the alternate complement pathway are found in 80 to 90 percent of patients. Lymphocytes are prominent in the portal regions and surround damaged bile ducts. These histologic findings resemble those noted in graft-versus-host disease following liver and bone marrow transplantation and suggest that damage to bile ducts may be immunologically mediated, perhaps reflecting a defect in a suppressor cell population.

Pathology Primary biliary cirrhosis is often divided into four stages based on morphologic findings. The earliest recognizable lesion (stage I), termed *chronic nonsuppurative destructive cholangitis*, is a necrotizing inflammatory process of the portal triads. It is characterized by destruction of medium and small bile ducts, a dense infiltrate of acute and chronic inflammatory cells, mild fibrosis, and occasionally, bile stasis. At times, periductal granulomas and lymph follicles are found adjacent to affected bile ducts. Subsequently, the inflammatory infiltrate becomes less prominent, the number of bile ducts is reduced, and smaller bile ductules proliferate (stage II). Progression over a period of months to years leads to a decrease in interlobular ducts, loss of liver cells, and expansion of periportal fibrosis into a network of connective tissue scars (stage III). Ultimately, cirrhosis, which may be micronodular or macronodular, develops (stage IV).

Clinical features SIGNS AND SYMPTOMS   Many patients with primary biliary cirrhosis are asymptomatic, and the disease is initially detected on the basis of elevated serum alkaline phosphatase levels during routine screening. The majority of such patients remain asymptomatic for prolonged periods, although many may ultimately develop progressive liver injury.

Among patients with symptomatic disease, 90 percent are women aged 35 to 60. Often the earliest symptom is pruritus, which may be either generalized or limited initially to the palms and soles. In addition, fatigue is commonly a prominent early symptom. After several months or years, jaundice and gradual darkening of the exposed areas of the skin (melanosis) may ensue. Other early clinical manifestations of primary biliary cirrhosis reflect impaired bile excretion. These include steatorrhea and the malabsorption of lipid-soluble vitamins, often resulting in easy bruising (vitamin K deficiency), bone pain due to osteomalacia (vitamin D deficiency) which is typically present in conjunction with osteoporosis, occasionally night blindness (vitamin A deficiency), and dermatitis (possibly vitamin E and/or essential fatty acid deficiency). Protracted elevation of serum lipids, especially cholesterol, leads to subcutaneous lipid deposition around the eyes (xanthelasmas) and over joints and tendons (xanthomas). Over a period of months to years, the itching, jaundice, and hyperpigmentation slowly worsen. Eventually signs of hepatocellular failure and portal hypertension develop and ascites appears. Progression may be quite variable. Whereas a proportion of asymptomatic patients may show no signs of progression for a decade or longer, in others, death due to hepatic insufficiency may occur within 5 to 10 years after the first signs of the illness. Such decompensation is often precipitated by uncontrolled variceal hemorrhage or infection.

Physical examination may be entirely normal in the early phase of the disease, when patients are asymptomatic or pruritus is the sole complaint. Later, there may be jaundice of varying intensity, hyperpigmentation of the exposed skin areas, xanthelasmas and tendinous and planar xanthomas, moderate to striking hepatomegaly, splenomegaly, and clubbing of the fingers. Bone tenderness, signs of vertebral compression, ecchymoses, glossitis, and dermatitis may all be noted. Clinical evidence of the sicca syndrome can be found in as many as 75 percent of patients, and serologic evidence of autoimmune thyroid disease in 25 percent. Other conditions encountered with increased frequency include rheumatoid arthritis, CRST syndrome, scleroderma, pernicious anemia, and renal tubular acidosis. Bone disease is often a significant problem encountered over the course of the disease. While osteomalacia occurs due to diminished vitamin D absorption, accelerated osteoporosis in this patient population (the majority of whom are postmenopausal women) is even more common.

LABORATORY FINDINGS   Primary biliary cirrhosis is increasingly diagnosed at a presymptomatic stage, prompted by the finding of a two- to fivefold elevation of the serum alkaline phosphatase during routine screening. Serum 5′-nucleotidase activity is also elevated. In this setting, serum bilirubin and aminotransferase levels are usually normal, but the diagnosis is supported by a positive antimitochondrial antibody test (titer > 1:40). The latter is both *relatively* specific and sensitive; a positive test is found in over 90 percent of symptomatic patients. As the disease evolves, the serum bilirubin level rises progressively and may reach 510 μmol/L (30 mg/dL) or more in the final stages. Serum aminotransferase values rarely exceed 2.5 to 3.3 μkat (150 to 200 units). Hyperlipidemia is common, and a striking increase of the serum unesterified cholesterol is often noted. An abnormal serum lipoprotein (lipoprotein X) may be present in primary biliary cirrhosis but is not specific and appears in other cholestatic conditions. A deficiency of bile salts in the intestine leads to moderate steatorrhea and impaired absorption of the fat-soluble vitamins and hypoprothrombinemia. Patients with primary biliary cirrhosis have elevated liver copper levels, but this finding is not specific and is found in all disorders in which there is prolonged cholestasis.

Diagnosis Primary biliary cirrhosis should be considered in middle-aged women with unexplained pruritus or an elevated serum alkaline phosphatase level and in whom there may be other clinical or laboratory features of protracted impairment of biliary excretion. Although a positive serum antimitochondrial antibody determination provides important diagnostic evidence, false-positive results do occur, and therefore, liver biopsy should be performed to confirm the diagnosis. In most cases the biliary tract should be evaluated to exclude remediable extrahepatic biliary tract obstruction, especially in view of the frequent presence of coexisting cholelithiasis.

Treatment There is no specific therapy for primary biliary cirrhosis. Glucocorticoids are ineffective and may actually worsen the bone disease. D-Penicillamine has been tried because of its ability to chelate copper and because of its possible antifibrotic and immunomodulating activities. However, the drug appears to be ineffective and has a high incidence of unacceptable side effects. While some have suggested that azathioprine may be helpful in slowing the progression of disease, this has not been established. Colchicine has been shown to have some limited effectiveness in slowing the progression of disease in symptomatic patients and should be tried (0.6 mg PO bid) unless gastrointestinal intolerance is limiting. Treatment with low-dose methotrexate has been reported to halt or reverse progression of primary biliary cirrhosis. Controlled trials may eventually settle the proper role of this agent in the management of symptomatic primary biliary cirrhosis. Cyclosporine has been suggested to slow disease progression in one relatively small trial. However, the benefit needs to be weighed against the relatively frequent nephrotoxicity caused by this agent before it can be advocated for a condition which will persist for the life of the individual. Recently, ursodiol treatment (13 to 15 mg/kg per day) also has been reported to achieve both symptomatic improvement and "improvement" in serum biochemical markers in patients with clinically overt primary biliary cirrhosis. The mechanism of action of ursodeoxycholic acid in achieving this benefit remains obscure. While further confirmation is needed, this agent is generally well tolerated and safe.

Treatment is generally directed toward the relief of symptoms. Although the mechanism of the protracted pruritus is not entirely clear, cholestyramine, an oral bile salt–sequestering resin, may be helpful in doses of 8 to 12 g/d to decrease both the pruritus and the hypercholesterolemia. Steatorrhea can be reduced by a low-fat diet and substituting medium-chain triglycerides for dietary long-chain triglycerides. Fat-soluble vitamins A and K should be given by parenteral injection at regular intervals to prevent or correct night blindness and hypoprothrombinemia, respectively. Zinc supplementation may be necessary if night blindness is refractory to vitamin A therapy. Osteomalacia and osteoporosis may be ameliorated by dietary calcium supplements in conjunction with oral vitamin D. In advanced disease, $25(OH)D_3$ or $1,25(OH_2)D_3$ may be preferred to vitamin D, since poor hepatic function may limit conversion of vitamin D to the active metabolites. Progression of primary biliary cirrhosis leads to the typical complications of advanced liver disease.

The management of ascites, variceal hemorrhage, and encephalopathy is described below. Over the past several years, it has been well documented that orthotopic liver transplantation is a highly effective treatment for patients with advanced primary biliary cirrhosis. Stratified analysis of patients with a wide variety of risk levels utilizing a validated prognostic model demonstrated enhanced survival for all. Hepatic transplantation, when available, is the treatment of choice for advanced primary biliary cirrhosis.

SECONDARY BILIARY CIRRHOSIS **Etiology** Secondary biliary cirrhosis results from prolonged partial or total obstruction of the common bile duct or its major branches. In adults, obstruction is most frequently caused by postoperative strictures or gallstones, usually with superimposed infectious cholangitis. Chronic pancreatitis may lead to biliary stricture and secondary cirrhosis. Secondary biliary cirrhosis also may develop in patients with pericholangitis or idiopathic sclerosing cholangitis. Patients with malignant tumors of the common bile duct or pancreas rarely survive long enough to develop secondary biliary cirrhosis. In children, congenital biliary atresia and cystic fibrosis are common causes of secondary biliary cirrhosis. Choledochal cysts, if unrecognized, also may be a rare cause of secondary biliary cirrhosis.

Pathology and pathogenesis Unrelieved obstruction of the extrahepatic bile ducts leads to (1) bile stasis and focal areas of centrilobular necrosis followed by periportal necrosis, (2) proliferation and dilatation of the portal bile ducts and ductules, (3) sterile or infected cholangitis with accumulation of polymorphonuclear infiltrates around bile ducts, and (4) progressive expansion of portal tracts by edema and fibrosis. Extravasation of bile from ruptured interlobular bile ducts into areas of periportal necrosis leads to the formation of "bile lakes" surrounded by cholesterol-rich pseudoxanthomatous cells. As in other forms of cirrhosis, injury is accompanied by regeneration in residual parenchyma. These changes gradually lead to a finely nodular cirrhosis. In general, at least 3 to 12 months is required for biliary obstruction to result in cirrhosis. Relief of the obstruction is frequently accompanied by biochemical and morphologic improvement.

Clinical features SIGNS AND SYMPTOMS The signs and symptoms of secondary biliary cirrhosis are similar to those of primary biliary cirrhosis. Jaundice and pruritus are usually the most prominent features. In addition, fever and/or right upper quadrant pain, reflecting bouts of cholangitis or biliary colic, are typical. The manifestations of portal hypertension are found only in advanced cases.

LABORATORY TESTS Elevations in serum alkaline phosphatase and 5′-nucleotidase as well as conjugated hyperbilirubinemia are nearly always present. There is a moderate increase in serum aminotransferases. When the disease is complicated by cholangitis, elevations in aminotransferase levels and leukocytosis are more pronounced. As in primary biliary cirrhosis, there are abnormalities in serum lipids (including the presence of lipoprotein X) and laboratory findings consistent with steatorrhea. However, the antimitochondrial antibody test is usually negative.

Diagnosis Secondary biliary cirrhosis should be considered in any patient with clinical and laboratory evidence of prolonged obstruction to bile flow, especially when there is a history of previous biliary tract surgery or gallstones, bouts of ascending cholangitis, or right upper quadrant pain. Cholangiography (either percutaneous or endoscopic) usually demonstrates the underlying pathologic process. Liver biopsy, although not always necessary from a clinical standpoint, can document the development of cirrhosis.

Treatment Relief of obstruction to bile flow, by either surgical or endoscopic means, is the most important step in the prevention and therapy of secondary biliary cirrhosis. Effective decompression of the biliary tract results in a significant improvement in both symptoms and survival, even in patients with established cirrhosis. When obstruction cannot be relieved, as in sclerosing cholangitis, antibiotics may be helpful acutely in controlling superimposed infection or, when administered on a chronic basis, as prophylactic therapy in suppressing recurring episodes of ascending cholangitis. Without relief of obstruction, there is a steady progression to end-stage cirrhosis and its terminal manifestations.

CARDIAC CIRRHOSIS

Definition Prolonged, severe right-sided congestive heart failure may lead to chronic liver injury and cardiac cirrhosis. The characteristic pathologic features of fibrosis and regenerative nodules distinguish cardiac cirrhosis from both reversible passive congestion of the liver due to acute heart failure and acute hepatocellular necrosis ("ischemic hepatitis" or "shock liver") resulting from systemic hypotension and hypoperfusion of the liver.

Etiology and pathology In right-sided heart failure, retrograde transmission of elevated venous pressure via the inferior vena cava and hepatic veins leads to congestion of the liver. Hepatic sinusoids become dilated and engorged with blood, and the liver becomes tensely swollen. With prolonged passive congestion and ischemia from poor perfusion secondary to reduced cardiac output, necrosis of centrilobular hepatocytes ensues and leads to fibrosis in these central areas. Ultimately, centrilobular fibrosis develops, with collagen extending outward in a characteristic stellate pattern from the central vein. Gross examination of the liver shows alternating red (congested) and pale (fibrotic) areas, a pattern often referred to as "nutmeg liver." Improvement in management of cardiac disorders, particularly advances in surgical treatment, has reduced the frequency of cardiac cirrhosis.

Clinical features In acute passive congestion, the liver becomes enlarged and tender, and the patient may complain of severe right upper quadrant pain due to stretching of Glisson's capsule. The serum bilirubin is usually only mildly increased and may be predominantly either conjugated or unconjugated. The AST level is also typically mildly elevated but may be transiently very high following a period of marked systemic hypotension (shock liver), when the clinical picture can mimic acute viral or drug-induced hepatitis. The serum albumin and prothrombin are usually normal, but may become abnormal in shock liver or with the development of cirrhosis. In cases of tricuspid insufficiency the liver may be pulsatile, but this finding disappears as cirrhosis develops. With prolonged right-sided heart failure the liver is enlarged, firm, and usually nontender. The signs and symptoms of heart failure usually overshadow the liver disease. Bleeding from esophageal varices is rare, but chronic encephalopathy may be prominent with a waxing and waning course reflecting variations in the severity of right-sided heart failure. Ascites and peripheral edema, often primarily related to the underlying cardiac dysfunction, may be worsened by the superimposed liver disease.

Diagnosis The presence of a firm, enlarged liver with signs of chronic liver disease in a patient with valvular heart disease, constrictive pericarditis, or cor pulmonale of long duration (>10 years) should suggest cardiac cirrhosis. Liver biopsy can confirm the diagnosis but is usually contraindicated because of coagulopathy or ascites. Coexistent chronic heart and liver disease should also raise the possibility of hemochromatosis, amyloidosis, or other infiltrative diseases.

Budd-Chiari syndrome resulting from the occlusion of the hepatic veins or inferior vena cava may be confused with acute congestive hepatomegaly. In this condition the liver is grossly enlarged and tender, and severe intractable ascites is present. However, signs and symptoms of heart failure are notably absent. The most common cause is thrombosis of the hepatic veins, often in the setting of polycythemia rubra vera, myeloproliferative syndromes, paroxysmal nocturnal hemoglobinuria, oral contraceptive use, or other hypercoagulable states; it also may result from invasion of the inferior vena cava by tumor, such as renal cell or primary hepatocellular carcinoma. Idiopathic membranous obstruction of the inferior vena cava is the most common cause of this syndrome in Japan. Hepatic venography or liver biopsy showing centrilobular congestion and sinusoidal dilatation in the absence of right-sided heart failure establishes the diagnosis of Budd-Chiari syndrome. Venoocclusive disease affecting the sublobular branches of the hepatic veins and the hepatic venules may result from hepatic irradiation, treatment with some antineoplastic agents, or ingestion of pyrrolidizine alkaloids present in some herbal teas ("bush tea disease") and can mimic congestive hepatomegaly.

Treatment Prevention or treatment of cardiac cirrhosis depends on the diagnosis and therapy of the underlying cardiovascular disorder. Improvement in cardiac function frequently results in improvement of liver function and stabilization of the liver disease.

METABOLIC, HEREDITARY, DRUG-RELATED, AND OTHER TYPES OF CIRRHOSIS (See Table 268-1) Cirrhosis or hepatitis may result from a wide variety of other processes encompassing the spectrum of etiologic factors listed in Table 268-2. Although some of these disorders have distinctive clinical or morphologic features, the manifestations of cirrhosis are largely independent of the underlying pathogenic mechanism.

NONCIRRHOTIC FIBROSIS OF THE LIVER Several diseases, either congenital or acquired, may be associated with localized or generalized hepatic fibrosis. They are distinguished from cirrhosis by the absence of hepatocellular damage and the lack of nodular regenerative activity. The clinical manifestations in such cases are largely secondary to portal hypertension. The different types of

---

TABLE 268-2 Some causes of noncirrhotic hepatic fibrosis

Idiopathic portal hypertension (noncirrhotic portal fibrosis, Banti's syndrome); three variants:
   Intrahepatic phlebosclerosis and fibrosis
   Portal and splenic vein sclerosis
   Portal and splenic vein thrombosis
Schistosomiasis ("pipe-stem" fibrosis with presinusoidal portal hypertension)
Congenital hepatic fibrosis (may be associated with polycystic disease of liver and kidneys)

---

these disorders are indicated in Table 268-2; with the exception of schistosomiasis, all these conditions are relatively rare.

MAJOR SEQUELAE OF CIRRHOSIS

The clinical course of patients with advanced cirrhosis is usually complicated by a number of important sequelae which are independent of the etiology of the underlying liver disease. These include portal hypertension and its consequences (i.e., gastroesophageal varices and splenomegaly), ascites, hepatic encephalopathy, spontaneous bacterial peritonitis, hepatorenal syndrome, and hepatocellular carcinoma.

PORTAL HYPERTENSION Definition and pathogenesis Normal pressure in the portal vein is low (10 to 15 cm saline) because vascular resistance in the hepatic sinusoids is minimal. Portal hypertension (>30 cm saline) most commonly results from increased resistance to portal blood flow. Because the portal venous system lacks valves, resistance at any level between the right side of the heart and splanchnic vessels results in retrograde transmission of an elevated pressure. Increased resistance can occur at three levels relative to the hepatic sinusoids: (1) presinusoidal, (2) sinusoidal, and (3) postsinusoidal. Obstruction in the *presinusoidal* venous compartment may be anatomically outside the liver (e.g., portal vein thrombosis) or within the liver itself but at a functional level proximal to the hepatic sinusoids so that the liver parenchyma is not exposed to the elevated venous pressure (e.g., schistosomiasis). *Postsinusoidal* obstruction also may occur outside the liver at the level of the hepatic veins (e.g., Budd-Chiari syndrome), the inferior vena cava, or, less commonly, within the liver (e.g., venoocclusive disease in which the central hepatic venules are the primary site of injury). When cirrhosis is complicated by portal hypertension, the increased resistance is usually sinusoidal. While distinctions between pre-, post-, and sinusoidal processes are conceptually appealing, functional resistance to portal flow in a given patient may occur at more than one level. Portal hypertension also may arise from increased blood flow (e.g., massive splenomegaly or arteriovenous fistulas), but the low outflow resistance of the normal liver makes this a rare clinical problem.

Cirrhosis is the most common cause of portal hypertension in the United States. Clinically significant portal hypertension is present in greater than 60 percent of patients with cirrhosis. *Portal vein obstruction* is the second most common cause; it may be idiopathic or occur in association with cirrhosis, infection, pancreatitis, or abdominal trauma. *Hepatic vein thrombosis* (Budd-Chiari syndrome) and hepatic venoocclusive disease are relatively infrequent causes of portal hypertension (see above). Portal vein occlusion may result in massive hematemesis from gastroesophageal varices, but ascites is usually found only with cirrhosis. Noncirrhotic portal fibrosis accounts for only a few patients with portal hypertension.

Clinical features The major clinical manifestations of portal hypertension include hemorrhage from gastroesophageal varices, splenomegaly with hypersplenism, ascites, and acute and chronic hepatic encephalopathy. All these features are related, at least in part, to the development of portal-systemic collateral channels. The absence of valves in the portal venous system facilitates retrograde (hepatofugal) blood flow from the high-pressure portal venous system to the lower-pressure systemic venous circulation. Major sites of collateral flow involve the veins around the rectum (hemorrhoids), cardioesophageal junction (esophagogastric varices), retroperitoneal space, and the falciform ligament of the liver (periumbilical or abdominal wall collaterals). Abdominal wall collaterals appear as tortuous epigastric vessels that radiate from the umbilicus toward the xiphoid and rib margins (caput medusae).

Diagnosis In patients with known liver disease, the development of portal hypertension usually becomes evident by the appearance of splenomegaly, ascites, encephalopathy, and/or esophageal varices. Conversely, the finding of any of these features should lead one to evaluate the patient for the presence of underlying portal hypertension and liver disease. Varices are most reliably documented by fiberoptic esophagoscopy; their presence lends indirect support to the diagnosis of portal hypertension. Although rarely necessary, portal venous pressure may be measured directly by percutaneous transhepatic "skinny needle" catheterization or indirectly through transjugular cannulation of the hepatic veins. Both free and wedged hepatic vein pressure (WHVP) should be measured. While WHVP is elevated in sinusoidal and postsinusoidal portal hypertension, including cirrhosis, this measurement is usually normal in presinusoidal portal hypertension. In patients in whom additional information is necessary (e.g., preoperative evaluation before portal-systemic shunt surgery) or percutaneous catheterization is not feasible, mesenteric and hepatic angiography may be helpful. Particular attention should be directed to the venous phase to assess the patency of the portal vein and the direction of portal blood flow.

Treatment Although treatment is usually directed toward a specific complication of portal hypertension, attempts are sometimes made to reduce the pressure in the portal venous system. Surgical decompression procedures have been used for many years to lower portal pressure in patients with bleeding esophageal varices (see below). However, portal-systemic shunt surgery does not result in improved survival rates in patients with cirrhosis. Beta-adrenergic blockade with propranolol or nadolol reduces portal pressure through vasodilatory effects on both the splanchnic arterial bed and the portal venous system in combination with reduced cardiac output. Such therapy has been shown to be effective in preventing both a first variceal bleed and subsequent episodes after an initial bleed. Treatment of patients with clinically significant sequelae of portal hypertension, especially variceal bleeding, with doses of propranolol titrated to reduce the resting pulse by 25 percent is reasonable if no contraindications exist.

Vigorous treatment of patients with alcoholic hepatitis and cirrhosis, chronic active hepatitis, and other liver diseases may lead to a fall in portal pressure and to a reduction in variceal size. In general, however, portal hypertension due to cirrhosis is not reversible. In appropriately selected patients hepatic transplantation will be beneficial.

VARICEAL BLEEDING   Pathogenesis While vigorous hemorrhage may arise from any portal-systemic venous collaterals, bleeding is most common from varices in the region of the gastroesophageal junction. The factors contributing to bleeding from gastroesophageal varices are not entirely understood but include the degree of portal hypertension and the size of the varices. Esophagitis with erosion of underlying varices does not appear to play an important role.

Clinical features and diagnosis Variceal bleeding often occurs without obvious precipitating factors and usually presents with painless but massive hematemesis with or without melena. Associated signs range from mild postural tachycardia to profound shock, depending on the extent of blood loss and degree of hypovolemia. Because patients with varices may bleed from other gastrointestinal lesions (e.g., peptic ulcer, gastritis), exclusion of other bleeding sources is important even in patients with prior variceal hemorrhage. Fiberoptic endoscopy is the best choice for evaluating upper gastrointestinal hemorrhage in patients with known or suspected portal hypertension.

Treatment Variceal bleeding is a life-threatening emergency. Prompt estimation and vigorous replacement of blood losses to maintain intravascular volume are essential and take precedence over

diagnostic studies and more specific intervention to stop the bleeding. Replacement of clotting factors with fresh frozen plasma is important in patients with coagulopathy. Patients are best managed in an intensive care unit and often require close monitoring of central venous or pulmonary capillary wedge pressures, urine output, and mental status. Only when the patient is hemodynamically stable should attention be directed toward specific diagnostic studies (especially endoscopy) and other therapeutic modalities to prevent further or recurrent bleeding.

About half of all episodes of variceal hemorrhage cease without intervention, although the risk of rebleeding is very high. The medical management of acute variceal hemorrhage includes the use of vasoconstrictors (vasopressin or somatostatin), balloon tamponade, and endoscopic sclerosis of varices (sclerotherapy) or endoscopic ligation of varices and beta-adrenergic blockade. Intravenous infusion of *vasopressin* at a rate of 0.1 to 0.5 units per minute results in generalized vasoconstriction leading to diminished blood flow in the portal venous system. Intravenous infusion of vasopressin has been shown to be as effective as selective intraarterial administration. Control of bleeding can be achieved in up to 80 percent of cases, but bleeding recurs in more than half after the vasopressin is tapered and discontinued. Furthermore, a number of serious side effects, including cardiac and gastrointestinal tract ischemia, acute renal failure, and hyponatremia, may be associated with vasopressin therapy. It appears that concurrent treatment with venodilators such as nitroglycerin as an intravenous infusion or isosorbide dinitrate sublingually may enhance the effectiveness of vasopressin and reduce complications. Somatostatin is also a direct splanchnic vasoconstrictor. In some studies this peptide, given as an initial 250-μg bolus followed by constant infusion (250 μg/h), has been found to be as effective as vasopressin. If bleeding is too vigorous or endoscopy is not available, *balloon tamponade* of the bleeding varices may be accomplished with a triple-lumen (Sengstaken-Blakemore) or four-lumen (Minnesota) tube with esophageal and gastric balloons. Because of the high risk of aspiration, endotracheal intubation should be performed prior to attempts to place one of these tubes. After the tube is introduced into the stomach, the gastric balloon is inflated and pulled back into the cardia of the stomach. If bleeding does not stop, the esophageal balloon is inflated for additional tamponade. Complications are common, occurring in 15 percent or more of patients, and include aspiration pneumonitis as well as esophageal rupture.

Where available, *endoscopic* intervention should be employed as the first line of treatment to control bleeding acutely. Over the past decade, endoscopic sclerosis of varices has been extensively employed. In this procedure, the varices are injected with one of several sclerosing agents (e.g., sodium morrhuate) via a needle-tipped catheter passed through the endoscope. After initial endoscopic identification of varices as the presumed source of bleeding, such "sclerotherapy" controls acute bleeding in up to 90 percent of cases. In addition, repeated sclerotherapy can be performed until obliteration of all varices is accomplished in an effort to prevent recurrent bleeding. While available data support the efficacy of sclerotherapy in controlling bleeding acutely, repeated sclerotherapy to obliterate varices has not been documented to consistently prolong survival. Mucosal ulceration resulting from injection of the caustic sclerosant is sometimes seen and may result in further hemorrhage or stenosis. More recently, endoscopic ligation of varices has proven to be equally effective in controlling bleeding with fewer treatment-related complications. In this technique, varices are ligated and strangled with small, elastic O-rings placed endoscopically. Prophylactic sclerosis of esophageal varices in the absence of proven bleeding is not indicated.

The effectiveness of beta-adrenergic blocking agents (e.g., propranolol) in the management of acute variceal bleeding is limited due to concomitant hypotension resulting from hypovolemia. However, a number of studies suggest they may be of value in reducing the risk of recurrent upper gastrointestinal hemorrhage in the patient with portal hypertension. Moreover, prophylactic treatment with propranolol or nadolol in patients with large varices that have never bled may decrease the incidence of bleeding and prolong survival. Patients with portal hypertension without specific contraindications should be given propranolol in doses to effect a 25 percent reduction in the resting heart rate. Propranolol also may prevent recurrent bleeding from severe portal hypertensive gastropathy in patients with cirrhosis.

Surgical therapy of portal hypertension and variceal bleeding involves the creation of a portal-systemic shunt to permit decompression of the portal system. Two types of portal systemic shunts have been used: *nonselective shunts* to decompress the entire portal system and *selective shunts* intended to decompress only the varices while maintaining blood flow to the liver itself. Nonselective shunts include end-to-side or side-to-side portacaval and proximal splenorenal anastomoses; selective shunts include the distal splenorenal shunt. Nonselective shunts are more likely to be complicated by encephalopathy than selective shunts. Emergency portal-systemic nonselective shunts may control acute hemorrhage, but such surgery is usually used only as a last resort because early operative mortality is greater than 30 percent. The role of portal-systemic shunt surgery after initial control of bleeding by nonoperative means is also uncertain. Surgically created shunts effectively reduce the risk of recurrent hemorrhage, but the overall mortality of patients undergoing such surgery is comparable with that of unoperated patients. Although patients who have undergone portal-system surgery succumb to recurrent bleeding less commonly than unoperated patients, this improvement is counterbalanced by increased morbidity from encephalopathy and death from progressive liver failure. Prophylactic shunt surgery should not be performed in patients with nonbleeding varices. Increasingly, therapeutic portal-systemic shunt has been reserved for patients who experience further bleeding despite serial endoscopic sclerotherapy. Recently, techniques have been developed to create a portal-systemic shunt by a percutaneous approach. In this technique, designated *transjugular intrahepatic portosystemic shunt* (TIPS), an expandable metal stent is advanced to the hepatic veins under angiographic guidance and then through the substance of the liver to create a direct portacaval channel. Although control trials are needed, this technique may prove to be an appropriate alternative to surgery for refractory bleeding due to portal hypertension. Other surgical procedures (e.g., esophageal transection) also have been advocated for the management of acute variceal bleeding, although their efficacy remains unproven. Even though recent trials found that esophageal transection was as effective as endoscopic sclerotherapy, transection is considered a last resort by most authorities.

Portal hypertensive gastropathy Although variceal hemorrhage is the most commonly encountered bleeding complication of portal hypertension, many patients will develop a congestive gastropathy due to the venous hypertension. In this condition, identified by endoscopic examination, the mucosa appears engorged and friable. Indolent mucosal bleeding rather than the brisk hemorrhage resulting from a variceal source is typical. Beta-adrenergic blockade with propranolol (which reduces splanchnic arterial pressure as well as portal pressure) is sometimes effective in ameliorating this condition. H-2 receptor antagonists or other agents useful in the treatment of peptic disease are usually not helpful.

SPLENOMEGALY Definition and pathogenesis Congestive splenomegaly is common in patients with severe portal hypertension. Rarely, massive splenomegaly from nonhepatic disease leads to portal hypertension due to increased blood flow in the splenic vein.

Clinical features Although usually asymptomatic, splenomegaly may be massive and contribute to the thrombocytopenia or pancytopenia of cirrhosis. In the absence of cirrhosis, splenomegaly in association with variceal hemorrhage should suggest the possibility of splenic vein thrombosis.

Treatment Splenomegaly usually requires no specific treatment, although massive enlargement of the spleen may occasionally necessitate splenectomy at the time of shunt surgery. Splenectomy also may be indicated if splenomegaly is the cause rather than the result of portal hypertension. Thrombocytopenia alone is rarely severe enough to necessitate removal of the spleen.

ASCITES Definition Ascites is the accumulation of excess fluid within the peritoneal cavity. It is most frequently encountered in patients with cirrhosis and other forms of severe liver disease, but a number of other disorders may lead to either transudative or exudative ascites (see Chap. 43).

Pathogenesis The accumulation of ascitic fluid represents a state of total-body sodium and water excess, but the event that initiates this imbalance is unclear. Three theories have been proposed (see Fig. 268-1). The "underfilling" theory suggests that the primary abnormality is inappropriate sequestration of fluid within the splanchnic vascular bed due to portal hypertension and a consequent decrease in effective circulating blood volume. According to this theory, an apparent decrease in intravascular volume (underfilling) is sensed by the kidney, which responds by retaining salt and water. The "overflow" theory suggests that the primary abnormality is inappropriate renal retention of salt and water in the absence of volume depletion. A third theory, the peripheral arterial vasodilation hypothesis, has been proposed to account for the constellation of arterial hypotension and increased cardiac output in association with high levels of vasoconstrictor substances which are routinely found in patients with cirrhosis and ascites. Again, sodium retention is considered secondary to arterial vascular underfilling, but the result of a disproportionate increase of the vascular compartment due to arteriolar vasodilation rather than decreased intravascular volume. According to this theory, portal hypertension results in splanchnic arteriolar vasodilation leading to underfilling of the arterial vascular space and baroreceptor-mediated stimulation of renin-angiotensin, sympathetic output, and antidiuretic hormone release.

Regardless of the initiating event, a number of factors contribute to accumulation of fluid in the abdominal cavity (see Fig. 268-1). Elevated levels of serum epinephrine and norepinephrine have been well documented. *Increased central sympathetic outflow* is found in patients with cirrhosis and ascites but not in those with cirrhosis alone. Increased sympathetic output results in diminished natriuresis by activation of the renin-angiotensin system and diminished sensitivity to atrial natriuretic peptide. *Portal hypertension* plays an important

FIGURE 268-1 Multiple factors involved in development of ascites. Current concepts suggest that initiating factor may be primary sodium retention ("overflow"), diminished effective intravascular volume ("underfilling"), or arteriolar vasodilation.

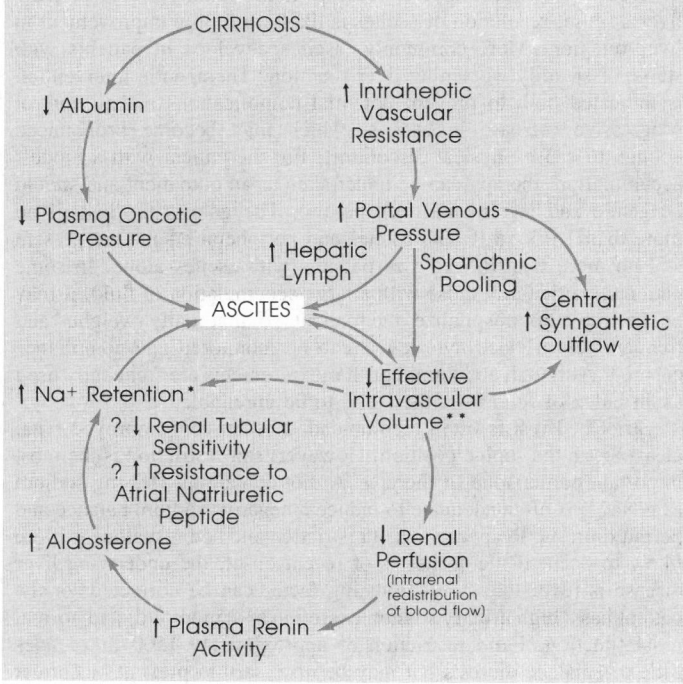

role in the formation of ascites by raising hydrostatic pressure within the splanchnic capillary bed. *Hypoalbuminemia* and *reduced plasma oncotic pressure* also favor the extravasation of fluid from plasma to the peritoneal cavity, and thus ascites is infrequent in patients with cirrhosis unless both portal hypertension and hypoalbuminemia are present. *Hepatic lymph* may weep freely from the surface of the cirrhotic liver due to distortion and obstruction of hepatic sinusoids and lymphatics and contribute to ascites formation. In contrast to the contribution of transudative fluid from the portal vascular bed, hepatic lymph may weep into the peritoneal cavity even in the absence of marked hypoproteinemia because the endothelial lining of the hepatic sinusoids is discontinuous. This mechanism may account for the high protein concentration present in the ascitic fluid of some patients with the Budd-Chiari syndrome.

Renal factors also play an important role in perpetuating ascites. Patients with ascites fail to excrete a water load in a normal fashion. They have increased renal sodium reabsorption by both proximal and distal tubules, the latter due largely to increased plasma renin activity and secondary hyperaldosteronism. Insensitivity to circulating atrial natriuretic peptide, often present in elevated concentrations in patients with cirrhosis and ascites, may be an important contributory factor in many patients. This insensitivity has been documented in those patients with the most severely impaired sodium excretion, who typically also exhibit low arterial pressure and marked overactivity of the renin-aldosterone axis. Renal vasoconstriction, perhaps resulting from increased serum prostaglandin or catecholamine levels, also may contribute to sodium retention.

Clinical features and diagnosis Usually ascites is first noticed by the patient because of increasing abdominal girth. More pronounced accumulation of fluid may cause shortness of breath because of elevation of the diaphragm. When peritoneal fluid accumulation exceeds 500 mL, ascites may be demonstrated on physical examination by the presence of shifting dullness, a fluid wave, or bulging flanks. Ultrasound examination, preferably with a Doppler study, can detect smaller quantities of ascites and should be performed when physical examination is equivocal or when the cause of the recent onset of ascites is not clear (e.g., exclude Budd-Chiari syndrome or portal vein thrombosis). Paracentesis usually should be performed with a small-gauge needle at the time of initial evaluation or at the time of any clinical deterioration of a cirrhotic patient. A small amount of fluid (<200 mL) should be obtained and examined for evidence of infection, tumor, or other possible causes and complications of ascites.

Treatment When ascites develops in the setting of severe, acute liver disease, resolution of ascites is likely to follow improvement in liver function. More commonly, ascites develops in patients with stable or steadily worsening liver function. Therapeutic intervention is indicated both to prevent potential complications and to control progressive increase in ascites, which may become pronounced enough to cause physical discomfort. For the patient with a modest accumulation, therapy can be undertaken as an outpatient and should be gentle and incremental (see below). The goal is the loss of no more than 1.0 kg/d if both ascites and peripheral edema are present and no more than 0.5 kg/d in patients with ascites alone. In some patients, particularly those with a large accumulation of fluid, it may be desirable to hospitalize the patient so that daily weights and frequent serum electrolyte levels can be monitored and compliance ensured. Although abdominal girth measurements are frequently used as an index of fluid loss, they tend to be unreliable.

Strict bed rest is often recommended because of improved renal clearance in the supine position. However, salt restriction is the most important cornerstone of therapy. A diet containing 800 mg sodium (2 g NaCl) is often adequate to induce a negative sodium balance and permit diuresis. Response to salt restriction and bed rest alone is more likely to occur if the ascites is of recent onset, the underlying liver disease is reversible, a precipitating factor can be corrected, or the patient has a high urinary sodium excretion (~25 mmol/d) and normal renal function. Fluid restriction of approximately 1500 mL/d does little to enhance diuresis but may be necessary to prevent or correct

hyponatremia. If sodium restriction alone fails to result in diuresis and weight loss, diuretic therapy should be instituted. Because of the role of hyperaldosteronism in sustaining salt retention, spironolactone or other distal tubule–acting diuretics (triamterene, amiloride) are the drugs of choice. These agents are also preferred because of their gentle action and specific potassium-sparing properties. Spironolactone is initially given in a dose of 25 mg four times a day and is increased as needed by 100 mg/d every several days up to a maximum dose, which rarely exceeds 400 mg/d. An indication of the minimum effective dose of spironolactone may be obtained by monitoring urinary electrolyte concentrations for a rise in sodium and fall in potassium levels reflecting effective competitive inhibition of aldosterone. Conversely, the development of azotemia or hyperkalemia may be dose-limiting or even warrant a reduction in the amount of this medication. In some patients, diuresis cannot be initiated despite maximal doses of distal tubule–acting agents (e.g., 400 mg spironolactone) because of avid proximal tubular sodium absorption. When this occurs, more potent and proximally acting diuretics (furosemide, thiazide, or ethacrynic acid) may be added cautiously to the regimen. Spironolactone plus furosemide, 20 or 80 mg/d, is usually sufficient to initiate a diuresis in most patients. However, such aggressive therapy must be used with great caution to avoid plasma volume depletion, azotemia, and hypokalemia, which may lead to encephalopathy.

In patients with a large accumulation of ascitic fluid, particularly those requiring hospitalization, large-volume paracentesis has proven to be an effective and less costly approach to initial management than prolonged bed rest and conventional diuretic treatment. In this approach, 4 to 6 L of fluid is removed by peritoneal cannula using strict aseptic techniques and monitoring hemodynamic and renal function. Albumin is infused intravenously, replacing that lost, to avoid depleting the intravascular space and precipitating hypotension. Paracentesis can be repeated daily or until all fluid has been removed. Maintenance diuretic therapy in conjunction with sodium restriction may then be instituted to avoid recurrent ascites.

A minority of patients with advanced cirrhosis have "refractory ascites" or rapidly reaccumulate fluid after control by paracentesis. In some patients, a side-to-side *portacaval shunt* may result in improvement in ascites, although generally these patients are extremely poor surgical risks. Intractable ascites also can be treated with the surgical implantation of a plastic *peritoneovenous shunt* which has a pressure-sensitive, one-way valve allowing ascitic fluid to flow from the abdominal cavity to the superior vena cava. However, the usefulness of this technique is limited by a high rate of such complications as infection, disseminated intravascular coagulation, and thrombosis of the shunt. Nonetheless, recent controlled studies have indicated equal effectiveness with medical therapies, although no benefit in survival could be documented.

SPONTANEOUS BACTERIAL PERITONITIS (SBP) Patients with ascites and cirrhosis may develop acute bacterial peritonitis without an obvious primary source of infection. Patients with very advanced liver disease are particularly susceptible to SBP. The ascitic fluid in these patients typically has especially low concentrations of albumin and other so-called opsonic proteins which normally may provide some protection against bacteria. Typical features include abrupt onset of fever, chills, generalized abdominal pain, and rebound abdominal tenderness accompanied by cloudy ascitic fluid with a high white cell count and usually positive bacterial cultures. However, the clinical symptoms *may be minimal*, and some patients manifest only worsening jaundice or encephalopathy in the absence of localizing abdominal complaints. The diagnosis is based on careful examination of the ascitic fluid. An ascitic fluid leukocyte count of greater than 500 cells per cubic millimeter or more than 250 polymorphonuclear leukocytes should suggest the possibility of bacterial peritonitis while results of bacterial cultures of ascitic fluid are pending. Other measurements such as fluid pH or determination of gradients between serum and fluid pH or lactate are generally not necessary.

A variant of SBP, designated *monomicrobial nonneutrocytic*

bacterascites, is sometimes seen. In these patients, culture of ascitic fluid yields bacteria, but the neutrophil count is less than 250 cells per cubic millimeter. These patients often have less severe liver disease than those found initially to have typical SBP. While many patients with this variant have cleared the bacterascites at the time of a subsequent paracentesis, nearly 40 percent will develop typical SBP; thus follow-up paracentesis is usually warranted in this setting.

Empirical therapy with cefotoxanine or ampicillin and an aminoglycoside should be initiated when the diagnosis is first suspected because enteric gram-negative bacilli are found in the majority of cases; less frequently, the infection is caused by pneumococci and other gram-positive bacteria. Cefotoxanine may be preferable due to the lower rate of renal toxicity. Specific antibiotic therapy can be selected once the specific organism is identified. Therapy is usually administered for 10 to 14 days, although one controlled study has suggested that a 5-day course of intravenous antibiotics may be as effective.

While appropriate antibiotic therapy is usually effective in the treatment of an episode of SBP, recurrent episodes are relatively common; as many as 70 percent of patients will experience at least one recurrence within a year of the first episode. The risk of recurrence likely reflects the predisposing role of the underlying advanced liver disease which contributed to the development of the first episode of SBP. Although the mechanism of SBP is still unclear, trials have suggested some benefit from prophylactic maintenance therapy with norfloxacin (400 mg/d) to prevent relapse or recurrence. This agent presumably causes selective decontamination of the intestine, eliminating many aerobic gram-negative bacilli.

HEPATORENAL SYNDROME Definition and pathogenesis Hepatorenal syndrome is a serious complication in the patient with cirrhosis and ascites and is characterized by worsening azotemia with avid sodium retention and oliguria in the absence of identifiable specific causes of renal dysfunction. The exact basis for this syndrome is not clear, but altered renal hemodynamics appear to be involved. The kidneys are structurally intact; urinalysis and pyelography are usually normal. Renal biopsy, although rarely needed, is also normal, and in fact, kidneys from such patients have been used successfully for renal transplantation. There are indications that an imbalance in certain metabolites of arachidonic acid (prostaglandins and thromboxane) may play a pathogenetic role.

Clinical features and diagnosis Worsening azotemia, hyponatremia, progressive oliguria, and hypotension are the hallmarks of the hepatorenal syndrome. This syndrome, which is distinct from prerenal azotemia, may be precipitated by severe gastrointestinal bleeding, sepsis, or overly vigorous attempts at diuresis or paracentesis; it also may occur without an obvious cause. It is essential to exclude other causes of renal impairment often seen in these patients. These include prerenal azotemia or acute tubular necrosis due to hypovolemia (e.g., secondary to gastrointestinal bleeding or diuretic therapy) or an increased nitrogen load such as that seen as a result of bleeding. Drug nephrotoxicity is also often a consideration, particularly in the patient who has received agents such as aminoglycosides or contrast dye. The diagnosis is supported by the demonstration of avid urinary sodium retention. Typically, the urine sodium concentration is less than 5 mmol/L, a concentration lower than that generally found in uncomplicated prerenal azotemia. The urinary sediment is unremarkable.

Treatment Treatment is usually unsuccessful. Although some patients with hypotension and decreased plasma volume may respond to infusions of salt-poor albumin, volume expansion must be undertaken with caution to avoid precipitating variceal bleeding. Vasodilator therapy, including intravenous infusion of dopamine, is not effective.

HEPATIC ENCEPHALOPATHY Definition Hepatic (portal-systemic) encephalopathy is a complex neuropsychiatric syndrome characterized by disturbances in consciousness and behavior, personality changes, fluctuating neurologic signs, asterixis or "flapping tremor," and distinctive electroencephalographic changes. Encephalopathy may be *acute* and reversible or *chronic* and progressive. In

severe cases, irreversible coma and death may occur. Acute episodes may recur with variable frequency.

Pathogenesis The specific cause of hepatic encephalopathy is unknown. The most important factors in the pathogenesis are severe hepatocellular dysfunction and/or intrahepatic and extrahepatic shunting of portal venous blood into the systemic circulation so that the liver is largely bypassed. As a result of these processes, various toxic substances absorbed from the intestine are not detoxified by the liver and lead to metabolic abnormalities in the central nervous system (CNS). Ammonia is the substance most often incriminated in the pathogenesis of encephalopathy. Many, but not all, patients with hepatic encephalopathy have elevated blood ammonia levels, and recovery from encephalopathy is often accompanied by declining blood ammonia levels. Other compounds and metabolites which may contribute to the development of encephalopathy include mercaptans (derived from intestinal metabolism of methionine), short-chain fatty acids, and phenol. Several observations suggest that excessive concentrations of γ-aminobutyric acid (GABA), an inhibitory neurotransmitter, in the CNS are important in the reduced levels of consciousness seen in hepatic encephalopathy. Increased CNS GABA may reflect failure of the liver to efficiently extract precursor amino acids or to remove GABA produced in the intestine. False neurochemical transmitters (e.g., octopamine), resulting in part from alterations in plasma levels of aromatic and branched-chain amino acids, also may play a role. An increase in the permeability of the blood-brain barrier to some of these substances may be an additional factor involved in the pathogenesis of hepatic encephalopathy. There is also evidence to suggest that endogenous benzodiazepines may contribute to the development of hepatic encephalopathy. This evidence includes isolation of 1,4-benzodiazepines from brain tissue of patients with fulminant hepatic failure as well as the partial response observed in some patients and experimental animals after administration of flumazenil, a benzodiazepine antagonist. The benzodiazepine receptor is closely associated with the GABA receptor and may facilitate GABA neurotransmission. However, the inconsistent effect of flumazenil in patients with encephalopathy, as well as potential methodologic pitfalls in the measurement of endogenous benzodiazepines, precludes definitive attribution of a role to these substances in the pathogenesis of hepatic encephalopathy.

In the patient with otherwise stable cirrhosis, hepatic encephalopathy often follows a clearly identifiable precipitating event (see Table 268-3). Perhaps the most common predisposing factor is *gastrointestinal bleeding*, which leads to an increase in the production

---

TABLE 268-3 Common precipitants of hepatic encephalopathy

INCREASED NITROGEN LOAD

Gastrointestinal bleeding
Excess dietary protein
Azotemia
Constipation

ELECTROLYTE IMBALANCE

Hypokalemia
Alkalosis
Hypoxia
Hypovolemia

DRUGS

Narcotics, tranquilizers, sedatives
Diuretics (see "Electrolyte imbalance")

MISCELLANEOUS

Infection
Surgery
Superimposed acute liver disease
Progressive liver disease

of ammonia and other nitrogenous substances which are then absorbed. Similarly, *increased dietary protein* may precipitate encephalopathy as a result of increased production of nitrogenous substances by colonic bacteria. *Electrolyte disturbances*, particularly hypokalemic alkalosis secondary to overzealous use of diuretics, vigorous paracentesis, or vomiting, may precipitate hepatic encephalopathy. Systemic alkalosis causes an increase in the amount of nonionic ammonia (NH_3) relative to ammonium ions (NH_4^+). Only nonionic (uncharged) ammonia readily crosses the blood-brain barrier and accumulates in the central nervous system. Hypokalemia also directly stimulates renal ammonia production. Hypoxia, injudicious use of CNS-depressing drugs (e.g., barbiturates, benzodiazepines) and acute infection may trigger or aggravate hepatic encephalopathy, although the mechanisms involved are not clear. Other potential precipitating factors include superimposed acute viral hepatitis, alcoholic hepatitis, extrahepatic bile duct obstruction, surgery, and other coincidental medical complications.

Clinical features and diagnosis Hepatic encephalopathy has protean manifestations, and any neurologic abnormality, including focal deficits, may be encountered. In patients with acute encephalopathy, neurologic deficits are completely reversible upon correction of underlying precipitating factors and/or improvement in liver function, but in patients with chronic encephalopathy, the deficits may be irreversible and progressive. Cerebral edema is frequently present and contributes to the clinical picture and overall mortality in patients with both acute and chronic encephalopathy.

The diagnosis of hepatic encephalopathy should be considered when four major factors are present: (1) acute or chronic hepatocellular disease and/or extensive portal-systemic collateral shunts (the latter may be either spontaneous, e.g., secondary to portal hypertension, or surgically created, e.g., portacaval anastomosis), (2) disturbances of awareness and mentation which may progress from forgetfulness and confusion to stupor and finally coma, (3) shifting combinations of neurologic signs, including asterixis, rigidity, hyperreflexia, extensor plantar signs, and rarely, seizures, and (4) a characteristic (but nonspecific) symmetric, high-voltage, slow-wave (2 to 5 per second) pattern on the electroencephalogram. Asterixis ("liver flap," "flapping tremor") is a nonrhythmic asymmetric lapse in voluntary sustained position of the extremities, head, and trunk. It is best demonstrated by having the patient extend the arms and dorsiflex the hands. Because elicitation of asterixis depends on sustained voluntary muscle contraction, it is not present in the comatose patient. Asterixis is nonspecific and also occurs in patients with other forms of metabolic brain disease. Alterations in personality, mood disturbances, confusion, deterioration in self-care and handwriting, and daytime somnolence are additional clinical features of encephalopathy. *Fetor hepaticus*, a unique musty odor of the breath and urine believed to be due to mercaptans, may be noted in patients with varying stages of hepatic encephalopathy. Some patients may develop spastic paraparesis or *chronic progressive hepatocerebral degeneration*, the latter a clinical variant of hepatic encephalopathy characterized by a slow decline in intellectual function, tremor, cerebellar ataxia, choreoathetosis, and psychiatric symptoms.

Grading or classifying the stages of hepatic encephalopathy is often helpful in following the course of the illness and assessing response to therapy. One useful classification is shown in Table 268-4.

The diagnosis of hepatic encephalopathy is usually one of exclusion. There are no diagnostic liver function test abnormalities, although an elevated serum ammonia level in the appropriate clinical setting is highly suggestive of the diagnosis. Examination of the cerebrospinal fluid is unremarkable, and computed tomography of the brain shows no characteristic abnormalities. A number of conditions, particularly disorders related to acute and chronic alcoholism, can mimic the clinical features of hepatic encephalopathy. These include acute alcohol intoxication, sedative overdose, delirium tremens, Wernicke's encephalopathy, and Korsakoff's psychosis (see Chap. 377). Subdural hematoma, meningitis, and hypoglycemia or other metabolic encephalopathies also must be considered, especially in

TABLE 268-4 Clinical stages of hepatic encephalopathy

Stage	Mental status	Asterixis	EEG
I	Euphoria or depression, mild confusion, slurred speech, disordered sleep	+/−	Usually normal
II	Lethargy, moderate confusion	+	Abnormal
III	Marked confusion, incoherent speech, sleeping but arousable	+	Abnormal
IV	Coma; initially responsive to noxious stimuli, later unresponsive	−	Abnormal

patients with alcoholic cirrhosis. In young patients with liver disease and neurologic abnormalities, Wilson's disease should be excluded.

Treatment Early recognition and prompt treatment of hepatic encephalopathy are essential. Patients with acute, severe hepatic encephalopathy (stage IV) require the usual supportive measures for the comatose patient. Specific treatment of hepatic encephalopathy is aimed at (1) elimination or treatment of precipitating factors and (2) lowering of blood ammonia (and other toxin) levels by decreasing the absorption of protein and nitrogenous products from the intestine. In the setting of acute gastrointestinal bleeding, blood in the bowel should be promptly evacuated with enemas and laxatives in order to reduce the nitrogen load. Protein should be excluded from the diet, and constipation should be avoided. Ammonia absorption can be decreased by the administration of lactulose, a nonabsorbable disaccharide that acts as an osmotic laxative. Metabolism of lactulose by colonic bacteria also may result in an acid pH that favors conversion of ammonia to the poorly absorbed ammonium ion. In addition, lactulose may actually diminish ammonia production through its direct effects on bacterial metabolism. Lactulose syrup can be administered in a dose of 30 to 50 mL every hour until diarrhea occurs; thereafter the dose is adjusted (usually 15 to 30 mL three times daily) so that the patient has two to four soft stools daily. Intestinal ammonia production by bacteria also can be decreased by oral administration of the antibiotic neomycin, at a dose of 0.5 to 1.0 g every 6 h. Although poorly absorbed, neomycin may reach sufficient concentrations in the bloodstream to cause renal toxicity. The use of agents such as levodopa, bromocriptine, keto analogues of essential amino acids, and intravenous amino acid formulations rich in branched-chain amino acids in the treatment of acute hepatic encephalopathy remains of unproven benefit. Flumazenil, a short-acting benzodiazepine antagonist, may have a role in management of hepatic encephalopathy precipitated by use of benzodiazepines, if there is a need for urgent therapy. Hemoperfusion to remove toxic substances and therapy directed primarily toward coincident cerebral edema in acute encephalopathy are also of unproven value.

Chronic encephalopathy may be effectively controlled by administration of lactulose. Management of patients with chronic encephalopathy should include dietary protein restriction, sometimes to levels as low as 40 g/d, in combination with low doses of lactulose or neomycin. Nephrotoxicity or ototoxicity may be limiting in prolonged usage of neomycin. There are suggestions that vegetable protein may be preferable to animal protein.

OTHER SEQUELAE OF CIRRHOSIS Coagulopathy Patients with cirrhosis often demonstrate a variety of abnormalities in both cellular and humoral clotting function. Thrombocytopenia may result from hypersplenism. In the alcoholic patient, there may be direct bone marrow suppression by ethanol. Diminished protein synthesis may lead to reduced production of fibrinogen (factor I), prothrombin (factor II), and factors V, VII, IX, and X. Reduction in levels of all factors except factor V may be worsened by the coincident malabsorption of the fat-soluble cofactor vitamin K due to cholestasis (see Chap. 254). Recent reports have documented the appearance of normal factor VIII levels following liver transplantation in patients with classical hemophilia, probably as a result of production by nonhepatocellular components of the donor organ.

Hepatocellular carcinoma See Chap. 269.

REFERENCES

Alcoholic and postnecrotic cirrhosis

ARROYO V, GINÉS P: Arteriolar vasodilation and the pathogenesis of the hyperdynamic circulation and renal sodium and water retention in cirrhosis. Gastroenterology 102:1077, 1992

BARRY RE, McGIVAN JD: Acetaldehyde alone may initiate hepatocellular damage in acute alcoholic liver disease. Gut 26:1065, 1985

BASKIN B et al: Ethanol and liver regeneration. Hepatology 8:408, 1988

BROWN J et al: Seroprevalence of hepatitis C virus nucleocapsid antibodies in patients with cryptogenic chronic liver disease. Hepatology 15:175, 1992

CARITHERS RL et al: Methylprednisolone therapy in patients with severe alcoholic hepatitis: A randomized multicenter trial. Ann Intern Med 110:685, 1989

GLUUD C et al: Prognostic indicators in alcoholic cirrhotic men. Hepatology 8:222, 1988

JEFFERS LJ et al: Prevalence of antibodies to hepatitis C virus among patients with cryptogenic chronic hepatitis and cirrhosis. Hepatology 15:187, 1992

KERSHENOBICH D et al: Colchicine in the treatment of cirrhosis of the liver. N Engl J Med 318:1709, 1988

ORREGO H et al: Long-term treatment of alcoholic liver disease with propylthiouracil. N Engl J Med 317:1421, 1987

RAMOND M-J et al: A randomized trial of prednisolone in patients with severe alcoholic hepatitis. N Engl J Med 326:507, 1992

Biliary cirrhosis

BESWICK DR et al: Asymptomatic primary biliary cirrhosis: A progress report on long-term follow-up and natural history. Gastroenterology 89:267, 1985

BODENHEIMER H JR et al: Evaluation of colchicine therapy in primary biliary cirrhosis. Gastroenterology 95:124, 1988

CHRISTENSEN E et al: Beneficial effects of azathioprine and predictor of prognosis in primary biliary cirrhosis: Final results of an international trial. Gastroenterology 89:1084, 1985

FREGEAU DR et al: Antimitochondrial antibodies of primary biliary cirrhosis recognize dihydrolipoamide acyltransferase and inhibit enzyme function of the branched chain α-ketoacid dehydrogenase complex. J Immunol 142:3815, 1989

———— et al: Inhibition of α-ketoglutarate dehydrogenase activity by a distinct population of autoantibodies recognizing dihydrolipoamide succinyltransferase in primary biliary cirrhosis. Hepatology 11:975, 1990

KAPLAN MM, KNOX TA: Treatment of primary biliary cirrhosis with low-dose weekly methotrexate. Gastroenterology 101:1332, 1991

MARKUS BH et al: Efficacy of liver transplantation in patients with primary biliary cirrhosis. N Engl J Med 320:1709, 1989

POUPON RE et al: A multicenter, controlled trial of ursodiol for the treatment of primary biliary cirrhosis. N Engl J Med 324:1548, 1991

WIESNER RH et al: A controlled trial of cyclosporine in the treatment of primary biliary cirrhosis. N Engl J Med 322:1419, 1990

YEAMAN SJ et al: Primary biliary cirrhosis: Identification of two major M2 mitochondrial autoantigens. Lancet 1:1067, 1988

Hepatic encephalopathy

BASILE AS et al: Elevated brain concentrations of 1,4-benzodiazepines in fulminant hepatic failure. N Engl J Med 325:473, 1991

BASSETT ML et al: Amelioration of hepatic encephalopathy by pharmacologic antagonism of the GABA-Benzodiazepene receptor complex in a rabbit model of fulminant hepatic failure. Gastroenterology 93:1069, 1987

BUTTERWORTH RF: Pathogenesis and treatment of portal-systemic encephalopathy: An update. Dig Dis Sci 37:321, 1992

DUDLEY FJ et al: Hepatorenal syndrome without avid sodium retention. Hepatology 6:248, 1986

FRASER CL, ARIEFF AI: Hepatic encephalopathy. N Engl J Med 313:865, 1985

JONES EA et al: The neurobiology of hepatic encephalopathy. Hepatology 4:1235, 1984

MORGAN MY, HAWLEY KE: Lactitol vs. lactulose in the treatment of acute hepatic encephalopathy in cirrhotic patients: A double blind randomized study. Hepatology 7:1278, 1987

SKOLNICK P: The γ-aminobutyric acid A (GABA$_A$)-benzodiazepine receptor complex, pp 534–536, in: Jones EA, moderator. The γ-aminobutyric A (GABA$_A$) receptor complex and hepatic encephalopathy: Some recent advances. Ann Intern Med 110:532, 1989

Portal hypertension and ascites

BURROUGHS AK et al: Randomized, double-blind, placebo-controlled trial of somatostatin for variceal bleeding. Gastroenterology 22:1388, 1990

CELLO JP et al: Endoscopic sclerotherapy versus portacaval shunt in patients with severe cirrhosis and variceal hemorrhage. N Engl J Med 311:1589, 1984

EPSTEIN M: The sodium retention of cirrhosis: A reappraisal. Hepatology 6:312, 1986

FLORAS JS et al: Increased sympathetic outflow in cirrhosis and ascites: Direct evidence from intraneural recordings. Ann Intern Med 114:373, 1991

GINÉS P et al: Comparison of paracentesis and diuretics in the treatment of cirrhotics with tense ascites: Results of a randomized study. Gastroenterology 93:234, 1987

———— et al: Paracentesis with intravenous infusion of albumin as compared with peritoneovenous shunting in cirrhosis with refractory ascites. N Engl J Med 325:829, 1991

MILLIKAN WJ et al: The Emory prospective randomized trial: Selective versus nonselective shunt to control variceal bleeding. Ann Surg 201:712, 1985

NICHOLLS KM et al: Sodium excretion in advanced cirrhosis: Effect of expansion of central blood volume and suppression of plasma aldosterone. Hepatology 6:235, 1986

PAGLIARO L et al: Prevention of first bleeding in cirrhosis: A meta-analysis of randomized trials of nonsurgical treatment. Ann Intern Med 117:59, 1992

PASTA L et al: Propranolol for prophylaxis of bleeding in cirrhotic patients with large varices: A multicenter randomized clinical trial. Hepatology 8:1, 1988

PINTO PC et al: Large-volume paracentesis in nonedematous patients with tense ascites: Its affect on intravascular volume. Hepatology 8: 207, 1988

PINZANI M et al: Altered furosemide pharmacokinetics in chronic alcoholic liver disease with ascites contributes to diuretic resistance. Gastroenterology 92:294, 1987

PYNARD T et al: Beta-adrenergic-antagonist drugs in the prevention of gastrointestinal bleeding in patients with cirrhosis and esophageal varices. N Engl J Med 324:1532, 1991

RING EJ et al: Using transjugular intrahepatic portosystemic shunts to control variceal bleeding before liver transplantation. Ann Intern Med 116:304, 1992

STIEGMANN GV et al: Endoscopic sclerotherapy as compared with endoscopic ligation for bleeding esophageal varices. N Engl J Med 326:1527, 1992

TERBLANCHE J et al: Controversies in the management of bleeding esophageal varices. N Engl J Med 320:1394, 1469, 1989

Spontaneous bacterial peritonitis

CROSSLEY JR, WILLIAMS R: Spontaneous bacterial peritonitis. Gut 26:325, 1985

DEPARTMENT OF MEDICINE, UNIVERSITY OF NEW MEXICO SCHOOL OF MEDICINE et al: Monomicrobial nonneutrocytic bacterascites: A variant of spontaneous bacterial peritonitis. Hepatology 12:710, 1990

GINÉS P et al: Norfloxacin prevents spontaneous bacterial peritonitis recurrence in cirrhosis: Results of a double-blind, placebo-controlled trial. Hepatology 12:716, 1990

RUNYON BA et al: Short-course versus long-course antibiotic treatment of spontaneous bacterial peritonitis: A randomized controlled study of 100 patients. Gastroenterology 100: 1737, 1991

TITÓ L et al: Recurrence of spontaneous bacterial peritonitis in cirrhosis: Frequency and predictive factors. Hepatology 8:27, 1988

---

269 TUMORS OF THE LIVER

KURT J. ISSELBACHER / JULES L. DIENSTAG*

BENIGN LIVER TUMORS

HEPATOCELLULAR ADENOMAS Hepatocellular adenomas are benign tumors of the liver found predominantly in women in their third and fourth decades. Their preponderance in women suggests a hormonal influence in their pathogenesis, and oral contraceptives have been implicated. There has been a striking increase in these adenomas since oral contraceptives were introduced, and the majority of patients in whom the tumors are found have been on these hormonal agents. Multiple hepatic adenomas have been associated with glycogen storage disease type I.

Hepatic adenomas occur predominantly in the right lobe of the liver, may be multiple, and are often quite large (i.e., >10 cm). Microscopically, they consist of normal or slightly atypical hepatocytes. They have an increase in glycogen, making them appear paler and larger than normal. Clinical features include pain and the presence of a palpable mass or features of intratumor hemorrhage (pain and circulatory collapse). The diagnosis is usually made by a combination of techniques: sonography, computed tomographic (CT) scan, selective hepatic arteriography, and radionuclide scans. The angiographic appearance is typically hypervascular but often also with hypovascular regions. Technetium 99m scans usually show a defect because phagocytosing Kupffer cells are absent. There is a risk of malignant change in the range of 10 percent; the risk is increased in large (>10 cm) and multiple adenomas.

As far as management is concerned, a patient taking oral contraceptives should stop doing so. If the lesion is large (i.e., 8 to 10 cm),

* The authors acknowledge Jack Wands' contribution to this chapter in the 12th edition.

near the surface, and resectable, surgery is appropriate. Because of the risk of rupture, pregnancy should be avoided.

FOCAL NODULAR HYPERPLASIA Focal nodular hyperplasia is a benign tumor often picked up accidentally on CT scans or at laparoscopy done for other reasons. It also occurs predominantly in women, but in contrast to hepatic adenomas, oral contraceptives do not appear to be implicated, and hemorrhage and necrosis are rare. The risk of hemorrhage, however, appears to be increased in women taking oral contraceptives. Typically, it is a solid tumor, often in the right lobe, with a fibrous core and stellate projections. In the fibrous projections, one may find atypical hepatocytes, biliary epithelium, Kupffer cells, and inflammatory cells. A radionuclide technetium scan will usually show a hot spot because of the presence of Kupffer cells. The lesion appears vascular on angiography, and septations may be detectable. If the lesion is asymptomatic, surgery is not indicated.

HEMANGIOMA AND OTHER BENIGN TUMORS *Hemangiomas* are probably the most common benign liver tumors, occurring predominantly in women and usually detected when abdominal imaging is done for unrelated symptoms or unexpectedly at surgery. The prevalence in the general population is in the range of 0.5 to 7.0 percent. These vascular lesions are usually asymptomatic and can be identified by magnetic resonance imaging (MRI), contrast-enhanced CT, labeled red blood cell nuclide scans, or hepatic angiography. They do not need to be removed unless they are large and are producing a mass effect. Hemorrhage is rare, and malignant change does not occur.

Nodular regenerative hyperplasia consists of multiple hepatic nodules resulting from periportal hepatocyte regeneration with surrounding atrophy. It may be associated with underlying conditions such as malignancy or connective tissue disease. Portal hypertension (in the absence of cirrhosis) is the most common clinical manifestation. Other less common benign hepatic lesions include *bile duct adenomas* and *cystadenomas. Juvenile hemangioendotheliomas* occur in children together with congestive heart failure and cutaneous hemangiomas.

CARCINOMAS OF THE LIVER

HEPATOCELLULAR CARCINOMA **Epidemiology and etiology** Primary hepatocellular carcinoma is one of the most common tumors in the world. It is especially prevalent in regions of Asia and sub-Saharan Africa, where the annual incidence is up to 500 cases per 100,000 population. In the United States and western Europe, it is much less common, accounting for only 1 to 2 percent of malignant tumors at autopsy. Hepatocellular carcinoma is up to four times more common in men than in women and usually arises in a cirrhotic liver. The peak incidence occurs in the fifth to sixth decades of life in western countries but one to two decades earlier in regions of Asia and Africa with a high prevalence of liver carcinoma.

The principal reason for the high incidence of hepatocellular carcinoma in parts of Asia and Africa is the frequency of chronic infection with *hepatitis B virus* (HBV) and *hepatitis C virus* (HCV). These chronic infections frequently lead to cirrhosis, which itself is an important risk factor for hepatocellular carcinoma; 60 to 90 percent of these tumors occur in patients with macronodular cirrhosis. The role of HBV as a factor is fairly convincing. Studies in regions of Asia where hepatocellular carcinoma and HBV infection are prevalent have shown that the incidence over time of this cancer is about 100-fold higher in individuals with evidence of HBV infection than in noninfected controls. In patients with HBV infection and hepatocellular carcinoma, HBV DNA may be integrated into host genomic DNA, both in the tumor cells and in adjacent, uninvolved hepatocytes. In addition, there can be modifications of cellular gene expression by insertional mutagenesis, chromosomal rearrangements, or the transcriptional transactivating activity of the X and the pre-52/S regions of the HBV genome. These alterations probably occur during the process of liver cell injury and repair.

Since the discovery in 1989 of hepatitis C viruses as the agent responsible for most cases of non-A, non-B hepatitis, an increasing body of evidence has implicated HCV in hepatocellular carcinoma. In fact, studies of patients in Europe and Japan have shown HCV to be substantially more prevalent than HBV in cases of hepatocellular carcinoma. In some patients, both HBV and HCV can be demonstrated, but the clinical course of the liver malignancy does not appear to differ between patients with both infections and those in whom only one of the two viruses is implicated. One distinction in high-prevalence areas between hepatocellular carcinoma associated with HBV infection and that associated with HCV infection is in the timing of onset. In Asia, hepatitis B is acquired at birth via perinatal transmission, while HCV infection is acquired primarily during adulthood from transfused blood. As a reflection of this distinction in time of infection, the onset of liver carcinoma occurs one to two decades earlier in those with lifelong hepatitis B than it does in adult-acquired hepatitis C.

Any agent or factor that contributes to chronic, low-grade liver cell damage and mitosis makes hepatocyte DNA more susceptible to genetic alterations. Thus, as indicated above, *chronic liver disease* of any type is a risk factor and predisposes to the development of liver cell carcinoma. This includes alcoholic liver disease, α_1-antitrypsin deficiency, hemochromatosis, and tyrosinemia. In Africa and southern China, *aflatoxin B$_1$* is an important public health hazard. This mycotoxin appears to induce a very specific mutation at codon 249 in the tumor suppressor gene p53.

The loss, inactivation, or mutation of the p53 gene has been implicated in tumorigenesis and is the most common genetic derangement present in human cancers. Thus HBV and aflatoxin B$_1$ have been implicated in the pathogenesis of hepatocellular carcinoma in regions of Africa and southern China where both agents are prevalent.

In view of the male predominance in liver cancer, hormonal factors also may play a role. Hepatocellular tumors may occur with long-term androgenic steroid administration, with exposure to thorium dioxide or vinyl chloride (see below), and possibly with exposure to estrogens in the form of oral contraceptives.

Clinical and laboratory features Cancers of the liver initially may escape clinical recognition because they often occur in patients with underlying cirrhosis, and the symptoms and signs may suggest progression of the underlying disease. The most common presenting features are abdominal *pain* with detection of an abdominal mass in the right upper quadrant. There may be a *friction rub* or *bruit* over the liver. Blood-tinged ascites occurs in about 20 percent of cases. Jaundice is rare, unless there is significant deterioration of liver function or mechanical obstruction of the bile ducts. Serum elevations of alkaline phosphatase and alpha fetoprotein (AFP) are common (see below). An abnormal type of prothrombin, des-γ-carboxy prothrombin, is also detectable and in general correlates with AFP elevations.

A small percentage of patients with hepatocellular carcinoma may have evidence of *paraneoplastic syndrome;* erythrocytosis may result from erythropoietin-like activity produced by the tumor, or hypercalcemia may result from secretion of a parathyroid-like hormone. Other manifestations may include hypercholesterolemia, hypoglycemia, acquired porphyria, dysfibrinogenemia, and cryofibrinogenemia.

Imaging procedures used to detect liver tumors include ultrasound, CT, MRI, hepatic artery angiography (see Chap. 248), and radionuclide scans with technetium 99m. Ultrasound is frequently used to screen high-risk populations and should be the first procedure if hepatocellular carcinoma is suspected; it is less costly than scanning procedures, is relatively sensitive, and can detect most tumors greater than 3 cm. MRI, however, is being used with increasing frequency.

Alpha fetoprotein (AFP) levels greater than 500 μg/L are found in about 70 to 80 percent of patients with hepatocellular carcinoma. Lower levels may be found in patients with large metastases from gastric or colonic tumors and in some patients with acute or chronic hepatitis. The presence and persistence of high levels of serum AFP (over 500 to 1000 μg/L) in an adult with liver disease and without an obvious gastrointestinal tumor strongly suggest hepatocellular carcinoma. Increasing levels with time suggest progression of the tumor or recurrence after hepatic resection or therapeutic approaches such as chemotherapy or chemoembolization (see below).

Percutaneous *liver biopsy* can be diagnostic if taken in an area localized by ultrasound or CT. The risk that tumor cells will migrate along the biopsy track exists, but it is small; because these tumors tend to be vascular, percutaneous biopsies should be done with caution. Cytologic examination of ascitic fluid is invariably negative for tumor cells. Occasionally, *laparoscopy* or *minilaparotomy* may be required, permitting liver cell biopsy under direct vision. This approach has the additional advantage of identifying the occasional patient with localized resectable tumor suitable for partial hepatectomy.

Course and management   The course of the disease is rapid; if untreated, most patients die within 3 to 6 months of diagnosis. In selected cases, therapy may prolong life. *Surgical resection* offers the only chance for cure; however, few patients have a resectable tumor at the time of presentation because of underlying cirrhosis, involvement of both hepatic lobes, or distant metastases (common sites are lung, brain, bone, and adrenal), and the 5-year survival is low. In patients at high risk for the development of hepatocellular carcinoma, such as HBsAG-positive patients and patients with cirrhosis, including that caused by chronic hepatitis C, screening programs have been initiated to identify small tumors when they are still resectable. Because 20 to 30 percent of patients with hepatocellular carcinoma do not have elevated levels of circulating AFP, ultrasonographic screening is recommended as well. In a study in the Far East, HBsAg-positive persons, with or without liver disease, were screened serially; a number of patients with small, subclinical tumors were identified and surgical resection undertaken. Follow-up observation revealed a 5-year survival rate in this group of 70 percent and a 10-year survival rate of 50 percent. These Asian patients, however, were unusual in that they had minimal or no liver disease and their tumors tended to be unifocal or encapsulated. The findings of this Asian study stand in contrast to a study in a large population of Italian patients with cirrhosis associated in most cases with chronic HBV and HCV infections; screening every 3 to 12 months permitted the detection of a 3 percent annual incidence of cancer in this cohort but in most cases failed to achieve the goal of early detection of surgically treatable disease.

Liver transplantation may be considered as a therapeutic option, but recurrence of tumor or metastases after transplantation have limited its usefulness (see Chap. 271). Other experimental approaches that are being evaluated include (1) hepatic artery embolization with chemotherapy (chemoembolization), (2) alcohol ablation via ultrasound-guided percutaneous injection, (3) ultrasound-guided cryoablation, (4) immunotherapy with monoclonal antibodies tagged with cytotoxic agents, and (5) gene therapy with retroviral vectors containing genes expressing cytotoxic agents.

OTHER MALIGNANT TUMORS

Fibrolamellar carcinoma differs from the typical hepatocellular carcinoma in that it tends to occur in young adults without underlying cirrhosis. This tumor is nonencapsulated but well circumscribed and contains fibrous lamellae; it grows slowly and is associated with a longer survival if treated. Surgical resection has resulted in 5-year survivals exceeding 50 percent; if the lesion is nonresectable, liver transplantation is an option, and the outcome far exceeds that observed in the nonfibrolamellar variety of liver cancer. *Hepatoblastoma* is a tumor of infancy typically with very high serum AFP levels. The lesions are usually solitary, may be resectable, and have a better 5-year survival than hepatocellular carcinoma. *Cholangiocarcinoma* is uncommon but has been associated with primary sclerosing cholangitis and in the Far East with clonorchiasis or opisthorchiasis. Often, the lesion occurs at the bifurcation of the common bile duct ("Klatskin

tumor"). These lesions are almost never resectable, and they invariably recur if liver transplantation is attempted. Biliary diversion, originally achieved surgically and nowadays accomplished by the insertion of stents, either percutaneously or endoscopically, can relieve biliary obstruction, but the prognosis remains poor. *Angiosarcoma* consists of vascular spaces lined by malignant endothelial cells. Etiologic factors include prior exposure to thorium dioxide (Thorotrast), polyvinyl chloride, arsenic, and androgenic anabolic steroids. *Epithelioid hemangioendothelioma* is of borderline malignancy; most are benign, but metastases occur. This tumor occurs in early adulthood, presents with right upper quadrant pain, is heterogeneous on sonography, hypodense on CT, and without neovascularity on angiography. Immunohistochemical staining reveals expression of factor VIII antigen. In the absence of extrahepatic metastases, these lesions can be treated by surgical resection or liver transplantation.

METASTATIC TUMORS   Metastatic malignant tumors of the liver are common in clinical practice, ranking second only to cirrhosis as a cause of fatal liver disease. In the United States, the incidence of clinically significant metastatic carcinoma is at least 20 times greater than that of primary carcinoma. Hepatic metastases have been reported at autopsy in 30 to 50 percent of patients dying from malignant disease.

Pathogenesis   The liver is uniquely vulnerable to invasion by tumor cells. Its size, high rate of blood flow, double perfusion by hepatic artery and portal vein, and its Kupffer cell filtration function combine to make it the most common site of metastases, except for the lymph nodes. In addition, local tissue factors or endothelial membrane characteristics appear to enhance metastatic implants. Virtually all types of neoplasms except those primary in the brain may metastasize to the liver. The most common primary tumors are those of the gastrointestinal tract, lung, breast, and melanomas. Less common are metastases from tumors of the thyroid, prostate, and skin.

Clinical features   Most patients with metastatic malignancy of the liver present with (1) symptoms usually referable only to the primary tumor, with asymptomatic hepatic involvement discovered in the course of clinical evaluation; (2) nonspecific symptoms of weakness, weight loss, fever, sweating, and loss of appetite, or rarely, (3) features indicating active hepatic disease, especially abdominal pain, hepatomegaly, or ascites.

Patients with widespread metastatic liver involvement usually have suggestive clinical signs of cancer and hepatic enlargement. Some have localized induration or tenderness, and occasionally, a friction rub may be found over tender areas of the liver.

Abdominal liver biochemical tests are frequent but often mildly elevated and nonspecific. They reflect the effects of fever and wasting, as well as those of the infiltrating neoplastic process itself. An increase in serum alkaline phosphatase is the most common and frequently the only abnormality noted. Hypoalbuminemia, anemia, and occasional mild elevation of aminotransferase levels also may be found with more widespread disease. Greatly elevated serum levels of carcinoembryonic antigen (CEA) are usually found when the metastases are from primary malignancies in the gastrointestinal tract, breast, or lung.

Diagnosis   Evidence of metastatic invasion of the liver should be sought actively in any patient with a primary malignancy, especially of the lung, gastrointestinal tract, or breast, before resection of the primary lesion is undertaken. Abnormal liver biochemical tests, particularly an elevated alkaline phosphatase, or demonstration of a mass by liver ultrasound, CT, or MRI may provide a presumptive diagnosis. Blind percutaneous needle biopsy of the liver will result in a positive diagnosis of metastatic disease in only 60 to 80 percent of cases with hepatomegaly and elevated alkaline phosphatase levels. Serial sectioning of specimens, two or three repeat biopsies, or cytologic examination of biopsy smears may increase the diagnostic yield by 10 to 15 percent. The yield is greatly increased when biopsies are directed by ultrasound or CT or obtained at laparoscopy.

Treatment   Most metastatic carcinomas respond poorly to all forms of treatment, which is usually only palliative. Surgical removal of a single, large metastasis is rarely feasible. Systemic chemotherapy with combinations of different chemotherapeutic agents may slow tumor growth briefly and reduce symptoms in some patients but does not significantly alter the prognosis. Chemoembolization, intrahepatic chemotherapy, and alcohol ablation may provide palliation. It remains to be determined whether newer drugs, combination chemotherapy, or novel strategies (including immunologic targeting) will eventually prove to be more effective.

REFERENCES

COLOMBO M et al: Hepatocellular carcinoma in Italian patients with cirrhosis. N Engl J Med 325:675, 1991

DiBISCEGLIE AM: Hepatocellular carcinoma. Ann Intern Med 108:390, 1988

KERLIN P et al: Hepatic adenoma and focal nodular hyperplasia: Clinical pathologic and radiologic features. Gastroenterology 84:994, 1983

KEW MC: Hepatic tumors. Semin Liver Dis 4:89, 1984

OKUDA K: Hepatocellular carcinoma: Recent progress. Hepatology 15:948, 1992

OZTURK M: p53 mutation in hepatocellular carcinoma after aflatoxin exposure. Lancet 338:1356, 1991

SAITO I et al: Hepatitis C virus infection is associated with the development of hepatocellular carcinoma. Proc Natl Acad Sci USA 87:6547, 1990

TABOR E et al: *Etiology, Pathology, and Treatment of Hepatocellular Carcinoma in North America.* Houston, Gulf Publishing, 1991

TAO LC: Oral contraceptive–associated liver cell adenoma and hepatocellular carcinoma: Cytomorphology and malignant transformation. Cancer 68:341, 1991

VENOOK AP et al: Chemoembolization for hepatocellular carcinoma. J Clin Oncol 8:1108, 1990

270   INFILTRATIVE AND METABOLIC DISEASES AFFECTING THE LIVER

KURT J. ISSELBACHER / DANIEL K. PODOLSKY

Many disseminated, systemic, or metabolic diseases involve the liver in a diffuse manner by the infiltration of abnormal cells or the accumulation of chemical substances or metabolites. Chemical accumulation may be extracellular or intracellular and may involve hepatocytes, Kupffer cells, or other elements of the reticuloendothelial system. Although infiltrative diseases may vary widely in cause and extrahepatic manifestations, the findings in the liver may be quite similar. Generalized enlargement and firmness of the liver, gradual and nonspecific deterioration of liver function, and, less often, signs of portal hypertension or ascites are typical features of this group of diseases. Differential diagnosis by clinical means may be difficult on occasion, but in patients in whom ancillary clinical findings do not establish the diagnosis, the diffusely infiltrated liver provides an excellent source of tissue for diagnostic purposes.

FATTY LIVER (See also Chap. 264)

Slight to moderate enlargement of the liver due to a diffuse accumulation of neutral fat (triglycerides) in hepatocytes is an important clinical and pathologic finding. Imaging procedures such as computed tomography (CT), ultrasound, and magnetic resonance imaging (MRI) may each yield alterations suggesting increased fat in the liver. As discussed in Chap. 264, fatty liver can be due to increased amounts of fat reaching the liver via the bloodstream or lymphatics, increased synthesis or decreased oxidation of lipids in the liver, and/or decreased export of very low density lipoproteins (VLDL) from the liver. Fatty liver can be separated into two categories based on whether the fat droplets in the hepatocytes are macrovesicular or macrovesicular fat (Table 270-1).

TABLE 270-1   Causes of fatty liver

Macrovesicular (large fat droplets in hepatocytes)
  A Alcohol, alcoholic liver disease
  B Diabetes mellitus
  C Obesity
  D Protein-calorie malnutrition
  E Glucocorticoid therapy
  F Total parenteral nutrition
  G Drugs, e.g., methotrexate
Microvesicular (small fat droplets in hepatocytes)
  A Reye's syndrome
  B Acute fatty liver of pregnancy
  C Jamaican vomiting sickness
  D Valproic acid, tetracycline toxicity

MACROVESICULAR FATTY LIVER   This is the most common type of fatty liver and is seen most frequently in alcoholism or alcoholic liver disease, diabetes mellitus, obesity, and prolonged parenteral nutrition. Hematoxylin and eosin–stained liver sections show hepatocytes with large, empty vacuoles with the nucleus "pushed" to the periphery of the cell. In general, fat in the liver is not damaging per se, and the fat will disappear with improvement or elimination of the predisposing condition.

Etiology   The major causes of fatty liver with macrovesicular fat depend on the age, geographic location, and metabolic-nutritional status of the patient population. *Chronic alcoholism* is the most common cause of fatty liver in this country and in other countries with a high alcohol intake. The severity of fatty involvement is roughly proportional to the duration and degree of alcoholic excess. *Protein malnutrition*, especially in infancy and early childhood, accounts for most cases of severe fatty liver in the tropical zones of Africa, South America, and Asia. The hepatic changes may be associated with other clinical and pathologic features of kwashiorkor. Patients with adult-onset *diabetes mellitus*, especially those who are overweight and are poorly controlled, often have fatty livers. *Obesity* is commonly associated with fatty infiltration of the liver; this recedes as weight reduction occurs. However, *jejunoileal bypass* for surgical treatment of morbid obesity is sometimes associated with severe fatty liver and hepatic failure that may be fatal. In patients with Cushing's syndrome and in those receiving large doses of glucocorticoids, fatty infiltration of the liver may occur. In many *chronic illnesses*, especially those complicated by impaired nutrition or malabsorption, increased fat is found in liver cells. For example, patients with severe ulcerative colitis, chronic pancreatitis, or protracted heart failure frequently have moderately fatty livers at the time of death. Patients maintained on prolonged *total parenteral nutrition* also may develop fatty livers.

Acute fatty liver is caused by a number of hepatotoxins and is frequently accompanied by signs and symptoms of liver failure. Carbon tetrachloride intoxication, DDT poisoning, and ingestion of substances containing yellow phosphorus result in severe fatty liver. Acute and prolonged alcohol ingestion also may be considered in this category and may be associated with a rapidly enlarging and fat-laden liver.

Clinical features   The signs and symptoms of fatty liver are related to the degree of fat infiltration, the time course of its accumulation, and the underlying cause. The obese or diabetic patient with chronic fatty liver is usually asymptomatic and has only mild tenderness over the enlarged liver. The liver function tests are normal or show mild elevations of alkaline phosphatase, transaminases, or aminotransferases. In contrast, the rapid accumulation of fat seen in the setting of hyperalimentation may lead to marked tenderness, presumably resulting from stretching of Glisson's capsule. Similarly, alcoholic patients with acute fatty liver following a bout of heavy drinking may have right upper quadrant pain and tenderness often with laboratory evidence of cholestasis. The clinical presentation of acute fatty liver of pregnancy or fatty liver from hepatotoxins is similar to that of fulminant hepatic failure arising from any cause, with evidence of hepatic encephalopathy, marked elevations of prothrombin time and transaminases, and variable degrees of jaundice.

Diagnosis The findings of a firm, nontender, and generally enlarged liver with minimal hepatic dysfunction in a patient with chronic alcoholism, malnutrition, poorly controlled diabetes mellitus, or obesity should suggest a fatty liver. This can usually be detected by CT scans, MRI, or ultrasound. When diagnostic uncertainty exists, needle biopsy of the liver will demonstrate the increased fatty content and possibly the underlying primary disorder.

Treatment Adequate nutritional intake, removal of alcohol or offending toxins, and correction of any associated metabolic disorders usually result in recovery. There is no clinical rationale for the use of lipotropic agents such as choline. When indicated, attention should be directed to abstinence from alcohol, careful control of diabetes, weight loss, or correction of intestinal absorptive defects. In the alcoholic fatty liver there is gradual disappearance of fat from the liver after 4 to 8 weeks of adequate diet and abstinence from alcohol. Similarly, fatty infiltration usually resolves within 2 weeks after discontinuation of parenteral hyperalimentation. However, patients with jejunoileal bypass may develop progressive liver inflammation and fibrosis in addition to fatty liver; hence restitution of intestinal continuity may not prevent progression of disease.

MICROVESICULAR FATTY LIVER This is the less common form of fatty liver. On microscopic examination, the fat is present in many small vacuoles. Although the droplets consist of triglycerides in both the macrovesicular and microvescicular forms, the reason for this difference in morphologic appearance is not clear.

REYE'S SYNDROME (FATTY LIVER WITH ENCEPHALOPATHY) This acute illness is encountered exclusively in children below 15 years of age. It is characterized clinically by vomiting and signs of progressive central nervous system damage, signs of hepatic injury, and hypoglycemia. Morphologically, there is extensive fatty vacuolization of the liver and renal tubules. There is mitochondrial dysfunction with decreased activity of hepatic mitochondrial enzymes. The cause is unknown, although viral and toxic agents, especially salicylates, have been implicated. Increased aspirin use and much higher serum salicylate levels in children with this illness than in the general population have been described during outbreaks of Reye's syndrome. However, it seems clear that this illness also may occur in the absence of exposure to salicylates. In fatal cases, the liver is enlarged and yellow with striking diffuse fatty microvacuolization of cells. Peripheral zonal hepatic necrosis also has been present in some cases. Fatty changes of the renal tubular cells, cerebral edema, and neuronal degeneration of the brain are the major extrahepatic changes. Electron-microscopic studies show structural alterations of mitochondria in liver, brain, and muscle.

The onset usually follows an upper respiratory tract infection, especially influenza or chickenpox. Within 1 to 3 days, persistent vomiting occurs, together with stupor, which usually progresses rapidly to generalized convulsions and coma. The liver is enlarged, but *jaundice is characteristically absent or minimal*. Elevations in serum aminotransferases and prothrombin time, hypoglycemia, metabolic acidosis, and elevated serum ammonia levels are the major laboratory findings. The mortality rate in Reye's syndrome is approximately 50 percent. Therapy consists of infusions of glucose and fresh frozen plasma, as well as intravenous mannitol to reduce the cerebral edema. Chronic liver disease has not been reported in survivors.

Acute fatty liver of pregnancy is a syndrome that occurs late in pregnancy and is often associated with jaundice and hepatic failure. In half the cases it is associated with preeclampsia. If diagnosed in time, the disease usually resolves with termination of the pregnancy.

Microvesicular fat accumulation also may be seen as a toxic reaction to *valproic acid* and with excessive doses of *tetracycline*. It is a typical finding in *Jamaican vomiting sickness*, which is caused by hypoglycin A present in unripened ackee fruit.

STORAGE DISEASES

Lipid storage diseases include the hereditary disorders of Gaucher's and Niemann-Pick disease. Other rare disorders associated with increased fat in the liver include abetalipoproteinemia, Tangier disease, Fabry's disease, and types I and V hyperlipoproteinemia (see Chap. 344 for details). Hepatic enlargement caused by distention of liver cells with glycogen is present in some poorly controlled diabetics and frequently in juvenile diabetes. More often, however, hepatomegaly is due to fatty infiltration. Ketoacidosis and vigorous insulin therapy may further enhance hepatic enlargement. In the absence of cirrhosis, hepatomegaly usually decreases with control of the diabetes.

HEPATIC MINERAL ACCUMULATION

WILSON'S DISEASE (See Chap. 348) This rare disease, predominantly of young people, is characterized by cirrhosis, softening and degeneration of the basal ganglia, and pigmentation of the cornea (Kayser-Fleischer rings). Increased copper deposition in the tissues seems to be responsible for the liver and basal ganglia changes. Liver cells are ballooned and show increased glycogen with glycogen vacuolization in the nuclei. The liver shows all grades of changes, from minimal to severe periportal or macronodular cirrhosis.

HEMOCHROMATOSIS (See Chap. 345) This relatively common genetically determined disorder involves accumulation of abnormal amounts of iron due to inappropriate absorption in the intestine. The liver, as a primary site of iron storage, is affected most directly. There is diffuse deposition of excess iron in hepatocytes, in contrast to the characteristic accumulation of iron in the reticuloendothelial compartment typical of secondary iron overload and hemosiderosis. Hepatic iron overload commonly results in hepatomegaly. Although liver function is initially well preserved, if the disease is untreated, progressive impairment is followed by the development of cirrhosis.

OTHER INFILTRATIVE DISEASES

HURLER'S SYNDROME (See Chap. 349) This is an uncommon hereditary disease that is characterized by the widespread tissue deposition of mucopolysaccharide (chondroitin sulfate B and heparan sulfate) in many tissues. The liver is frequently enlarged and firm. Microscopically, Kupffer cells and other macrophages are enlarged and filled with metachromatic granular material. Cirrhosis may be a late complication.

α₁-ANTITRYPSIN DEFICIENCY (See also Chap. 223) Patients with homozygous deficiency of serum α_1-antitrypsin (α1AT) are prone to develop emphysema in adult life. The disease is suggested by the absence of alpha₁ globulin on serum electrophoresis (α1AT makes up 90 percent of this fraction normally) and confirmed by direct measurement of α1AT. The exact phenotype can then be determined by starch electrophoresis. Although there are 16 recognized alleles, only PiZ and PiS are associated with clinical disease. The molecular bases of these altered products have been related to single nucleic acid substitutions, e.g., PiZ is caused by a G (guanine) to A (adenine) transposition, which results in a substitution of a glutamic acid for lysine at residue 292 in the α1AT protein. Hepatocytes of some patients with this deficiency contain globules positive to the periodic acid Schiff (PAS) reaction. Approximately 10 percent of children with homozygous deficiency (PiZZ phenotype) of α1AT will develop significant liver disease, including neonatal hepatitis and progressive cirrhosis. It has been suggested that 15 to 20 percent of all chronic liver disease in infancy may be attributed to α1AT deficiency. In adults, the most common manifestation of α1AT deficiency is asymptomatic cirrhosis, which may progress from a micronodular to a macronodular state and may be complicated by the development of hepatocellular carcinoma. The occurrence of liver disease in these patients is not dependent on the development of lung disease.

RETICULOENDOTHELIAL DISORDERS (See also Chaps. 58 and 311)

Moderate to massive hepatomegaly and splenomegaly occur frequently in the various types of *leukemia* and *lymphoma*. Jaundice, when present, is usually slight and results from hemolysis. Deep and protracted jaundice is distinctly rare and is caused by obstruction of the intrahepatic or extrahepatic bile ducts by tumor. Liver biopsy specimens reveal portal and sinusoidal infiltrates in most cases of leukemia, but the cellular pattern may be mixed and nonspecific. Liver biopsy is diagnostic in only 5 percent of patients with *Hodgkin's disease*. This percentage is increased in those with advanced disease or splenomegaly. Directed biopsy at laparoscopy or laparotomy is more likely to be positive than "blind" needle biopsy. Nonspecific histologic changes in the liver have been described in patients with lymphoma and may contribute to the abnormal liver function tests.

Myeloid metaplasia and other myeloproliferative disorders associated with extramedullary hematopoiesis produce hepatomegaly which may reach huge proportions, especially following splenectomy. Serum alkaline phosphatase elevations are often found. Ascites and portal hypertension, resulting from diffuse involvement of portal venules and lymphatics, are rare complications.

GRANULOMATOUS INFILTRATIONS

Perhaps as a result of the large population of mononuclear phagocytes, a number of systemic granulomatous diseases involve the liver, including sarcoidosis, miliary tuberculosis, histoplasmosis, brucellosis, schistosomiasis, berylliosis, and drug reactions (Table 270-2). In addition, isolated granulomas of no diagnostic importance may be found occasionally in patients with various forms of cirrhosis and hepatitis. The liver infiltrated by granulomas may be slightly enlarged and firm, but hepatic dysfunction is usually limited and manifested only by mild increases in serum alkaline phosphatase and occasionally aminotransferase levels. In a few patients with sarcoidosis or brucellosis, portal hypertension may develop, and extensive postnecrotic scarring or postnecrotic cirrhosis may follow healing of the granulomatous lesions, as in schistosomiasis.

In AIDS, evidence of liver disease is quite common but is usually mild with minimal morbidity. In these patients, hepatic granulomatous disease is often present and may be caused by opportunistic infections, with *Mycobacterium avium-intracellulare* being the most frequent pathogen. Cytomegalovirus hepatitis and hepatic mycoses are less common. These patients are frequently being treated for *Pneumocystis carinii* infections with sulfonamides, which also may cause hepatic granulomatous disease. AIDS cholangiopathy has been described with features of primary sclerosing cholangitis and infiltration of the biliary tree with cryptosporidia.

Needle biopsy of the liver often provides the first definite evidence of a systemic or disseminated granulomatous disease. In patients with sarcoidosis who have neither clinical nor laboratory evidence of hepatic involvement, needle biopsy is positive in about 80 percent of cases. In cases of suspected miliary tuberculosis, a portion of the biopsy should be cultured and stained for mycobacteria. The organism can be detected in the majority of cases, particularly when caseating granulomas are present. Serial sections of the biopsy specimen should be examined if granulomas are not apparent. Individual granulomas are rarely specific in their microscopic appearance, and final diagnosis usually requires other clinical, laboratory, or histologic data.

In approximately 20 percent of patients it is not possible to identify a cause for the granulomatous infiltration. When these infiltrates are accompanied by fever of unknown origin, the diagnosis of granulomatous hepatitis should be considered. This is an uncommon disorder of unknown cause and is diagnosed by exclusion. While granulomatous hepatitis invariably responds to moderate doses of corticosteroids, relapses are frequent, and such therapy should never be undertaken unless tuberculous disease or other causes of granulomatous infiltration have been excluded. This may include an initial empiric trial of antituberculous therapy.

AMYLOIDOSIS (See also Chap. 281)

Systemic amyloidosis, whether primary and idiopathic, familial, or secondary to chronic inflammatory or neoplastic diseases, often involves the liver. Grossly, the liver infiltrated with amyloid is enlarged and pale and rubbery in consistency. Microscopically, the birefringent amyloid deposits appear as homogeneous waxy material within the space of Disse, often being concentrated in the periportal areas and associated with atrophy of adjacent liver cell plates. Selective involvement of the walls of blood vessels, especially of the hepatic arterioles, may be a striking feature of primary amyloidosis. With this possible exception, however, the hepatic lesions are the same in all forms of amyloidosis and are present in 60 to 90 percent of cases.

An enlarged and firm liver is found in about 60 percent of patients, and ascites occurs in advanced stages of the disease in about 20 percent. Jaundice, portal hypertension, and other signs of chronic liver disease are usually absent. Liver function changes, although frequent, correlate poorly with the extent of liver infiltration. Hypoalbuminemia and elevated serum alkaline phosphatase are common. Hypoalbuminemia, however, may be related to the nephrotic syndrome owing to renal involvement; the prothrombin time is usually normal. The diagnosis is established by biopsy of rectum, skin, liver, or other involved organs and demonstration of the characteristic Congo red–staining deposits by polarizing microscopy.

TABLE 270-2　Some causes of hepatic granulomas

Systemic disease
  A　Sarcoidosis
  B　Hodgkin's and non-Hodgkin's lymphoma
  C　Primary biliary cirrhosis
  D　Berylliosis
  E　Crohn's disease
  F　Wegener's granulomatosis
  G　Granulomatous hepatitis, idiopathic
Infections
  A　Bacterial
    1　Tuberculosis
    2　Mycobacterium avium intracellulare
    3　Brucellosis
    4　Leprosy
  B　Viral
    1　Epstein-Barr virus
    2　Cytomegalovirus
    3　Chicken pox
  C　Parasitic
    1　Schistosomiasis
  D　Rickettsial
    1　Q fever
  E　Spirochetes
    1　Syphilis
  F　Drugs
    1　Sulfonamides
    2　Isoniazid
    3　Allopurinol

REFERENCES

CRYSTAL RG: Alpha 1-antitrypsin deficiency, emphysema and liver disease: Genetic basis and strategy for therapy. J Clin Invest 85:1343, 1990

GISHAN FK, GREENE HL: Liver disease in children with PIZZ α₁-antitrypsin deficiency. Hepatology 8:307, 1988

HOFFMAN MS et al: Hepatic amyloidosis presenting as severe intrahepatic cholestasis: A case report and review of the literature. Am J Gastroenterol 83:783, 1988

HURWITZ ES et al: Public Health Service Study on Reye's syndrome and medications. N Engl J Med 313:842, 1985

HUTCHISON DC: Natural history of alpha 1-protease inhibitor deficiency. Am J Med 84:3, 1988

MINAKAMI H et al: Pre-eclampsia: A microvesicular fat disease of the liver. Am J Obstet Gynecol 159:1043, 1988

PERLMUTTER DH: The cellular basis for liver injury in alpha 1-antitrypsin deficiency. Hepatology 13:172, 1991

RILEY C et al: Acute fatty liver of pregnancy: A reassessment based on observations in nine patients. Ann Intern Med 106:703, 1987

RUSTGI VK: Liver disease in pregnancy. Med Clin North Am 73:1041, 1989

SCRIVER CR et al (eds): *The Metabolic Basis of Inherited Disease*, 6th ed. New York, McGraw-Hill, 1989

SHERLOCK S, DOOLEY J: *Diseases of the Liver and Biliary System*, 9th ed. Oxford, Blackwell, 1993

STERNLIEB I: Perspectives on Wilson's disease. Hepatology 12:1234, 1990

VAN COSTA RN et al: Adult Reye's syndrome: A review with new evidence for a generalized defect in intramitochondrial enzyme processing. Neurology 41:1815, 1991

271 LIVER TRANSPLANTATION

JULES DIENSTAG

Liver transplantation, the replacement of the native, diseased liver by a normal organ (allograft) recovered from a brain-dead donor, has matured from an experimental procedure reserved for desperately ill patients to an accepted, lifesaving operation applied much earlier in the natural history of end-stage liver disease. The preferred and technically most advanced approach is *orthotopic transplantation,* in which the native organ is removed and the donor organ is inserted in the same anatomic location. Pioneered in the 1960s by Starzl at the University of Colorado and, later, at the University of Pittsburgh and by Calne in Cambridge, England, liver transplantation is now performed routinely by dozens of centers throughout North America and western Europe. Success and survival have improved from approximately 30 percent in the 1970s to almost 60 percent today. These improved prospects for prolonged survival; dating back to the early 1980s, resulted from refinements in operative technique (including the introduction of venovenous bypass to allow venous return from the extremities and visceral circulation during clamping of the inferior vena cava), improvements in organ procurement and preservation, advances in immunosuppressive therapy, and, perhaps most influentially, more enlightened patient selection and timing. Despite the perioperative morbidity and mortality, the technical and management challenges of the procedure, and its costs, liver transplantation has become the approach of choice for selected patients whose chronic or acute liver disease is progressive, life-threatening, and unresponsive to medical therapy. Based on the current level of success, the number of liver transplants has continued to grow each year; in 1990, over 2500 patients received liver allografts in the United States

INDICATIONS Potential candidates for liver transplantation are children and adults who, in the absence of contraindications (see below), suffer from severe, irreversible liver disease for which alternative medical or surgical treatments have been exhausted or are unavailable. *Timing of the operation is of critical importance.* Indeed, improved timing and better patient selection are felt to have contributed more to the increased success of liver transplantation in the 1980s and beyond than all the impressive technical and immunologic advances combined. Although the disease should be advanced, and although opportunities for spontaneous or medically induced stabilization or recovery should be allowed, the procedure should be done sufficiently early to give the surgical procedure a fair chance for success. Ideally, transplantation should be considered in patients with end-stage liver disease who are experiencing or have experienced a life-threatening complication of hepatic decompensation, whose quality of life has deteriorated to unacceptable levels, or whose liver disease will result predictably in irreversible damage to the central nervous system (CNS). If this is done sufficiently early, the patient will not have developed any contraindications or extrahepatic systemic deterioration. Although patients with well-compensated cirrhosis can survive for many years, many patients with quasi-stable chronic liver disease have much more advanced disease than may be apparent. As discussed below, the better the status of the patient prior to transplantation, the higher will be the anticipated success rate of transplantation. The decision about *when* to transplant is complex and requires the combined judgment of an experienced team of hepatologists, transplant surgeons, anesthesiologists, and specialists in support services, not to mention the well-informed consent of the patient and the patient's family.

Transplantation in children Indications for transplantation in children are listed in Table 271-1. The most common is *biliary atresia. Inherited or genetic disorders of metabolism* associated with liver failure constitute another major indication for transplantation in children and adolescents. In Crigler-Najjar disease type I and in certain hereditary disorders of the urea cycle and of amino acid or lactate-pyruvate metabolism, transplantation may be the only way to prevent impending deterioration of CNS function, despite the fact that the native liver is structurally normal. Combined heart and liver transplantation has yielded dramatic improvement in cardiac function and in cholesterol levels in children with homozygous familial hypercholesterolemia; combined liver and kidney transplantation has been successful in patients with hereditary oxalosis. In hemophiliacs with transfusion-associated hepatitis and liver failure, liver transplantation has been associated with recovery of normal factor VIII synthesis.

Transplantation in adults Liver transplantation is indicated for end-stage *cirrhosis* of all causes (see Table 271-1). In sclerosing cholangitis and *Caroli's disease* (multiple cystic dilatations of the intrahepatic biliary tree), recurrent infections and sepsis associated with inflammatory and fibrotic obstruction of the biliary tree may be an indication for transplantation. Because prior biliary surgery complicates, and is a relative contraindication for, liver transplantation, surgical diversion of the biliary tree has been all but abandoned for patients with sclerosing cholangitis. In patients who undergo transplantation for *hepatic vein thrombosis (Budd-Chiari syndrome),* postoperative anticoagulation is essential; underlying myeloproliferative disorders may have to be treated but are not a contraindication to liver transplantation. If a donor organ can be located quickly, before life-threatening complications—including cerebral edema—set in, patients with *fulminant hepatitis* are candidates for liver

---

TABLE 271-1 Indications for liver transplantation

Children	Adults
Biliary atresia	Primary biliary cirrhosis
Neonatal hepatitis	Secondary biliary cirrhosis
Congenital hepatic fibrosis	Primary sclerosing cholangitis
Alagille's disease*	Caroli's disease‡
Byler's disease†	Cryptogenic cirrhosis
α₁-Antitrypsin deficiency	Chronic active hepatitis with cirrhosis
Inherited disorders of metabolism	Hepatic vein thrombosis
Wilson's disease	Fulminant hepatitis
Tyrosinemia	Alcoholic cirrhosis§
Glycogen storage diseases	Chronic viral hepatitis§
Lysosomal storage diseases	Primary hepatocellular malignancies§
Protoporphyria	Hepatic adenomas
Crigler-Najjar disease type I	
Familial hypercholesterolemia	
Hereditary oxalosis	
Hemophilia	

* Arteriohepatic dysplasia, with paucity of bile ducts, and congenital malformations, including pulmonary stenosis.
† Intrahepatic cholestasis, progressive liver failure, mental and growth retardation.
‡ Multiple cystic dilatations of the intrahepatic biliary tree.
§ Controversial indications (see text).

transplantation. More controversial as candidates for liver transplantation are patients with *alcoholic cirrhosis, chronic viral hepatitis,* and *primary hepatocellular malignancies.* Although all three of these categories are considered to be high risk, liver transplantation can be offered to carefully selected patients. Patients with alcoholic cirrhosis can be considered as candidates for transplantation if they meet strict criteria for abstinence and reform. Patients with chronic hepatitis C have done as well as any other subset of patients after transplantation, despite the fact that recurrent infection in the donor organ is the rule. In patients with chronic hepatitis B, the success of transplantation is reduced by approximately 10 to 20 percent; however, the majority of patients do well for at least several years. Issues of disease recurrence are discussed in more detail below. Patients with nonmetastatic primary hepatobiliary tumors—primary hepatocellular carcinoma, cholangiocarcinoma, hepatoblastoma, angiosarcoma, epithelioid hemangioendothelioma, and multiple or massive hepatic adenomata—have undergone liver transplantation; however, for hepatobiliary malignancies, overall survival is significantly lower than that for other categories of liver disease. To minimize the very high likelihood of recurrent tumor after transplantation, some centers are evaluating experimental adjuvant chemotherapy protocols. Because the likelihood of recurrent cholangiocarcinoma is almost universal, this tumor is no longer considered an indication for transplantation.

CONTRAINDICATIONS   *Absolute contraindications* for transplantation include life-threatening systemic diseases, uncontrolled extrahepatic bacterial or fungal infections, preexisting advanced cardiovascular or pulmonary disease, multiple uncorrectable life-threatening congenital anomalies, metastatic malignancy, active drug or alcohol abuse, and human immunodeficiency virus (HIV) infection. Because carefully selected patients in their sixties and even seventies have undergone transplantation successfully, advanced age per se is no longer considered an absolute contraindication; however, in older patients, a more thorough preoperative evaluation should be undertaken to exclude ischemic cardiac disease. Advanced age (>60 years), however, may be considered a *relative contraindication,* that is, a factor to be taken into account with other relative contraindications. Other relative contraindications include highly replicative hepatitis B, portal vein thrombosis, preexisting renal disease not associated with liver disease, intrahepatic or biliary sepsis, severe hypoxemia resulting from right-to-left intrapulmonary shunts, previous extensive hepatobiliary surgery, and any uncontrolled serious psychiatric disorder. Any one of these relative contraindications is insufficient in and of itself to preclude transplantation. For example, the problem of portal vein thrombosis can be overcome by constructing a graft from the donor liver portal vein to the recipient's superior mesenteric vein.

TECHNICAL CONSIDERATIONS   Donor selection   Donor livers for transplantation are procured primarily from victims of head trauma. Organs from brain-dead donors up to age 60 are acceptable if the following criteria are met: hemodynamic stability, adequate oxygenation, absence of bacterial or fungal infection, serologic exclusion of hepatitis B and C viruses and HIV, absence of abdominal trauma, and absence of hepatic dysfunction. Cardiovascular and respiratory functions are maintained artificially until the liver can be removed. Compatibility in ABO blood group and organ size between donor and recipient are important considerations in donor selection; however, ABO-incompatible or reduced-donor-organ transplants can be performed in emergency or marked donor-scarcity situations. Tissue typing for HLA matching is not required, and preformed cytotoxic HLA antibodies do not preclude liver transplantation. Following perfusion with cold electrolyte solution, the donor liver is removed and packed in ice. The use of University of Wisconsin (UW) solution, rich in lactobionate and raffinose, has permitted the extension of cold ischemic time up to 20 h; however, 12 h may be a more reasonable limit. Improved techniques for harvesting multiple organs from the same donor have increased the availability of donor livers, but the availability of donor livers is far outstripped by the demand. Currently, in the United States, all donor livers are distributed through a nationwide organ-sharing network (United Network of Organ Sharing) designed to allocate available organs based on regional considerations and recipient acuity. Recipients who require the highest level of care (intensive care) have the highest priority.

Surgical technique   Removal of the recipient's native liver is technically difficult, particularly in the presence of portal hypertension with its associated collateral circulation and extensive varices, and even more so in the presence of scarring from previous abdominal operations. The combination of portal hypertension and coagulopathy (elevated prothrombin time and thrombocytopenia) translates into large blood product transfusion requirements. After the portal vein and infrahepatic and suprahepatic inferior vena cavae are dissected, a pump-driven venovenous bypass system is applied to reroute blood from the portal vein and inferior vena cava, preventing congestion of visceral organs. After the hepatic artery and common bile duct are dissected, the native liver is removed and the donor organ inserted. During the anhepatic phase, coagulopathy, hypoglycemia, hypocalcemia, and hypothermia are encountered and must be managed by the anesthesiology team. Caval, portal vein, hepatic artery, and bile duct anastomoses are performed in succession, the last by end-to-end suturing of the donor and recipient common bile ducts or by choledochojejunostomy to a Roux en Y loop if the recipient common bile duct cannot be used for reconstruction (e.g., in sclerosing cholangitis). A typical transplant operation lasts 8 h, with a range of 6 to 18 h. Because of excessive bleeding, large volumes of blood, blood products, and volume expanders may be required during surgery.

POSTOPERATIVE COURSE AND MANAGEMENT   Immunosuppressive therapy   The introduction in 1980 of cyclosporine as an immunosuppressive agent contributed substantially to the improvement in survival after liver transplantation. Cyclosporine depresses both humoral and cell-mediated immunity via inhibition of interleukin 2 production. This process occurs without affecting rapidly dividing cells in the bone marrow, which may account for the reduced frequency of posttransplantation systemic infections. The most common and important side effect of cyclosporine therapy is nephrotoxicity. Cyclosporine causes dose-dependent renal tubular injury and direct renal artery vasospasm. Following renal function, therefore, is important in monitoring cyclosporine therapy, perhaps even a more reliable indicator than blood levels of the drug. Nephrotoxicity is reversible and can be managed by dose reduction. Other adverse effects of cyclosporine therapy include hypertension, hyperkalemia, tremor, hirsutism, and gum hyperplasia. Like azathioprine, cyclosporine appears to be associated with a risk of lymphoproliferative malignancies (see below), which may occur earlier after cyclosporine than after azathioprine therapy. Because of these side effects, combinations of cyclosporine, prednisone, and azathioprine—all at reduced doses—are preferable regimens for immunosuppressive therapy.

In patients with pretransplant renal dysfunction or renal deterioration that occurs intraoperatively or immediately postoperatively, cyclosporine therapy may not be practical; under these circumstances, induction or maintenance of immunosuppression with monoclonal antibodies to T cells, OKT3, may be appropriate. Therapy with OKT3 has been especially effective in reversing acute rejection in the posttransplant period and is the standard treatment for acute rejection that fails to respond to methylprednisolone boluses. Intravenous infusions of OKT3 may be complicated by transient fever, chills, and diarrhea. When this drug is used to induce immunosuppression initially or to provide "rescue" in those who reject despite "conventional" therapy, the incidence of bacterial, fungal, and especially cytomegalovirus infections is increased during and after such therapy. In some centers, ganciclovir antiviral therapy is initiated prophylactically as a routine along with OKT3. A new, experimental drug, FK-506, is being introduced and is being tested primarily for "rescue" therapy in patients who fail to respond to other immunosuppressive agents. This drug is a macrolide antibiotic isolated from a Japanese soil fungus, *Streptomyces tsukubaensis,* with similar immunosuppressive effects and mechanisms to those of cyclosporine but with substantially higher potency. The use of FK-506 is still limited to research trials; unfortunately, it has similar nephrotoxicity to that of cyclosporine, and the nephrotoxicity is especially profound when the two drugs are used together. The important principle about immunosuppression is that the ideal approach strikes a balance between immunosuppression and immunological competence. Given sufficient immunosuppression, acute liver allograft rejection is always reversible; however, if the cumulative dose of immunosuppressive therapy is too large, the patient will succumb to opportunistic infection. Therefore, immunosuppressive drugs must be used judiciously, with strict attention to the infectious consequences of such therapy.

Postoperative complications Complications of liver transplantation can be divided into hepatic and nonhepatic categories. In addition, both immediately postoperative and late complications are encountered. Patients who undergo liver transplantation as a rule have been chronically ill for protracted periods and may be malnourished and wasted. The impact of such chronic illness and the multisystem failure that accompanies liver failure continues to require attention in the postoperative period. Because of the massive fluid losses and fluid shifts that occur during the operation, patients may remain fluid overloaded during the immediate postoperative period, straining cardiovascular reserve; this effect can be amplified in the face of transient renal dysfunction and pulmonary capillary vascular permeability. Continuous monitoring of cardiovascular and pulmonary function, measures to maintain the integrity of the intravascular compartment and to treat extravascular volume overload, and scrupulous attention to potential sources of and sites of infection are of paramount importance. Cardiovascular instability may result as well from the electrolyte imbalance that may accompany reperfusion of the donor liver. Pulmonary function may be compromised further by paralysis of the right hemidiaphragm associated with phrenic nerve injury. The hyperdynamic state with increased cardiac output that is characteristic of patients with liver failure reverses rapidly after successful liver transplantation.

Other immediate management issues include renal dysfunction; prerenal azotemia, acute kidney injury associate with hypoperfusion (acute tubular necrosis), and renal toxicity caused by antibiotics or cyclosporine are frequently encountered in the postoperative period, sometimes necessitating dialysis. Occasionally, postoperative intraperitoneal bleeding may be sufficient to increase intraabdominal pressure, which, in turn, may reduce renal blood flow—this effect is rapidly reversible when abdominal distention is relieved by exploratory laparotomy to identify and ligate the bleeding site and to remove intraperitoneal clot. Anemia also may result from acute upper gastrointestinal bleeding or from transient hemolytic anemia, which may be autoimmune, especially when blood group O livers are transplanted into blood group A or B recipients. This autoimmune hemolytic anemia is mediated by donor intrahepatic lymphocytes that recognize red blood cell A or B antigens on recipient erythrocytes. Transient in nature, this process resolves once the donor liver is repopulated by recipient bone marrow–derived lymphocytes; the hemolysis can be treated by transfusing blood group O red blood cells and/or by administering higher doses of glucocorticoids. Transient thrombocytopenia is encountered commonly as well. Aplastic anemia, a late occurrence, is rare but has been reported in almost 30 percent of patients who underwent liver transplantation for acute, severe hepatitis of unknown cause.

Bacterial, fungal, or viral infections are common and may be life-threatening postoperatively. Early after transplant surgery, common postoperative infections predominate—pneumonia, wound infections, infected intraabdominal collections, urinary tract infections, and intravenous line infections—rather than opportunistic infections; these infections may involve the biliary tree and liver as well. Beyond the first postoperative month, the toll of immunosuppression becomes evident, and opportunistic infections—cytomegalovirus, herpes viruses, fungal infections (*Aspergillus, Nocardia, Candida,* cryptococcal disease), mycobacterial infections, parasitic infections (*Pneumo-*

cystis, Toxoplasma), *Legionella,* and *Listeria*—predominate. Rarely, early infections represent those transmitted with the donor liver, either infections present in the donor or infections acquired during procurement processing. De novo viral hepatitis infections acquired from the donor organ or from transfused blood products occur after typical incubation periods for these agents (well beyond the first month). Obviously, infections in an immunosuppressed host demand early recognition and prompt management; prophylactic antibiotic therapy is administered routinely in the immediate postoperative period. Use of sulfamethoxazole with trimethoprim reduces the incidence of postoperative *Pneumocystis carinii* pneumonia.

Neuropsychiatric complications include seizures, commonly associated with cyclosporine toxicity, encephalopathy, depression, and difficult psychosocial adjustment. Rarely, diseases are transmitted by the allograft from the donor to the recipient. In addition to viral and bacterial infections, malignancies of donor origin have occurred. Lymphoproliferative malignancies, especially B cell lymphoma, are a recognized complication associated with immunosuppressive drugs such as azathioprine and cyclosporine (see above). Epstein-Barr virus has been shown to play a contributory role in some of these tumors, which may regress when immunosuppressive therapy is reduced.

Hepatic complications Hepatic dysfunction after liver transplantation is similar to the hepatic complications encountered after major abdominal and cardiothoracic surgery; however, in addition, there may be complications such as primary graft failure, vascular compromise, failure or obstruction of the biliary anastomoses, and rejection. As in nontransplant surgery, postoperative jaundice may result from prehepatic, intrahepatic, and posthepatic sources. *Prehepatic* sources represent the massive hemoglobin pigment load from transfusions, hemolysis, hematomas, ecchymoses, and other collections of blood. *Early intrahepatic* liver injury includes effects of hepatotoxic drugs and anesthesia; hypoperfusion injury associated with hypotension, sepsis, and shock; and benign postoperative cholestasis. *Late intrahepatic* sources of liver injury include posttransfusion hepatitis and recurrent primary disease (see below). *Posthepatic* sources of hepatic dysfunction include biliary obstruction and reduced renal clearance of conjugated bilirubin. Hepatic complications unique to liver transplantation include primary graft failure associated with ischemic injury to the organ during harvesting; vascular compromise associated with thrombosis or stenosis of the portal vein or hepatic artery anastomoses; stenosis, obstruction, or leakage of the anastomosed common bile duct; and rejection.

Transplant rejection Despite the use of immunosuppressive drugs, rejection of the transplanted liver still occurs in a majority of patients, beginning 1 to 2 weeks after surgery. Clinical signs suggesting rejection are fever, right upper quadrant pain, and reduced bile pigment and volume. Leukocytosis may occur, but the most reliable indicators are increases in serum bilirubin and aminotransferase levels. Because these tests lack specificity, it may be difficult to distinguish among rejection and biliary obstruction, primary graft nonfunction, vascular compromise, viral hepatitis, cytomegalovirus infection, drug hepatotoxicity, and recurrent primary disease. Radiographic visualization of the biliary tree and/or percutaneous liver biopsy often help to establish the correct diagnosis. Morphologic features of acute rejection include portal infiltration, bile duct injury, and/or endothelial inflammation ("endothelialitis"); some of these findings are reminiscent of graft-versus-host disease and primary biliary cirrhosis. As soon as transplant rejection is suspected, treatment consists of intravenous methylprednisolone in repeated boluses; if this fails to abort rejection, many centers use antibodies to lymphocytes, such as OKT3, or polyclonal antilymphocyte globulin.

Chronic rejection is a relatively rare outcome that may follow repeated bouts of acute rejection or that occurs unrelated to preceding rejection episodes. Morphologically, chronic rejection is characterized by progressive cholestasis, focal parenchymal necrosis, mononuclear infiltration, vascular lesions (intimal fibrosis, subintimal foam cells, fibrinoid necrosis), and fibrosis. This process may be reflected as ductopenia—the vanishing bile duct syndrome. Some of the histologic hallmarks of chronic rejection may be so similar to those of chronic viral hepatitis that differentiation between the two may be difficult. Reversibility of chronic rejection is limited; in patients with therapy-resistant chronic rejection, retransplantation has yielded encouraging results.

OUTCOME **Survival** The survival rate for patients undergoing liver transplantation has improved steadily since 1983. One-year survival rates have increased from approximately 70 percent in the early 1980s to 80 to 85 percent at the end of the decade. Currently, the 5-year survival rate approaches 60 percent. An important observation is the relation between clinical status before transplantation and outcome. For patients who undergo liver transplantation when their level of compensation is high (e.g., still working or only partially disabled), a 1-year survival rate of 85 percent is the rule. For those whose level of decompensation mandates continuous in-hospital care prior to transplantation, the 1-year survival rate is about 70 percent, while for those who are so decompensated that they require life support in an intensive care unit, the 1-year survival rate is approximately 50 percent. Indeed, the trend toward transplantation earlier in the natural history of end-stage liver disease is a major factor in the increased success of liver transplantation during the 1980s. Another important distinction in survival has been drawn between high-risk and low-risk patient categories. For patients who do not fit any "high risk" designations, 1-year and 4-year survival rates of 85 and 80 percent, respectively, have been recorded. In contrast, among patients in "high risk" categories—cancer, fulminant hepatitis, hepatitis B, age >60, concurrent renal failure, respirator dependence, portal vein thrombosis, and history of a portacaval shunt or multiple right upper quadrant operations—survival statistics fall into the range of 65 percent at 1 year and just above 50 percent at 4 years. Survival after retransplantation for primary graft nonfunction is approximately 50 percent. Causes of failure of liver transplantation vary with time. Failures within the first 3 months result primarily from technical complications, postoperative infections, and hemorrhage. Transplant failures after the first 3 months are more likely to result from infection, rejection, or recurrent disease (such as malignancy or viral hepatitis).

Recurrence of primary disease The recurrence of autoimmune chronic active hepatitis or primary sclerosing cholangitis has not been reported. There have been reports of recurrent primary biliary cirrhosis after liver transplantation; however, the histologic features of primary biliary cirrhosis and acute rejection are virtually indistinguishable and occur as frequently in patients with primary biliary cirrhosis as in patients undergoing transplantation for other reasons. Hereditary disorders such as Wilson's disease and α_1-antitrypsin deficiency have not recurred after liver transplantation; however, recurrence of disordered iron metabolism has been observed in some patients with hemochromatosis. Hepatic vein thrombosis (Budd-Chiari syndrome) may recur; this can be minimized by treating underlying lymphoproliferative disorders and by anticoagulation. Cholangiocarcinoma recurs almost invariably; therefore, few centers now transplant such patients. In patients with hepatocellular carcinoma, tumor recurrence in the liver is common after approximately 1 year. Trials are underway to assess the benefit of adjuvant chemotherapy.

Hepatitis A can recur after transplantation for fulminant hepatitis A, but such acute reinfection has no serious clinical sequelae. In fulminant hepatitis B, recurrence is not the rule; however, hepatitis B recurs almost invariably after transplantation for end-stage chronic hepatitis B. With sufficient immunosuppressive therapy to prevent allograft rejection, levels of hepatitis B viremia increase markedly, regardless of pretransplantation values. A majority of patients undergoing transplantation for chronic hepatitis B become high-level HBV carriers without liver injury; however, some patients experience a rapid recapitulation of severe injury—chronic active hepatitis or even fulminant hepatitis—after transplantation. *Fibrosing cholestatic hepatitis* is a histologic feature linked to rapidly progressive liver injury in approximately 10 percent of patients transplanted for hepatitis B. These patients experience marked hyperbilirubinemia, substantial prolongation of the prothrombin time (both out of proportion to

relatively modest elevations of aminotransferase activity), and rapidly progressive liver failure. This lesion has been suggested to represent a "choking off" of the hepatocyte by an overwhelming density of HBV proteins. Complications such as sepsis and pancreatitis also have been observed more frequently in patients undergoing liver transplantation for hepatitis B. Thus the outcome of transplantation for hepatitis B is unpredictable. Some centers have relied on continuing infusions of hepatitis B immune globulin to prevent recurrent hepatitis B, but trials demonstrating an advantage over no therapy have not been done. Patients who undergo liver transplantation for chronic hepatitis B plus D have a better survival rate than patients transplanted for hepatitis B alone. Recurrence of hepatitis C virus (HCV) after liver transplantation can be documented in almost every patient, if sufficiently sensitive virus markers are used. Although, occasionally, patients have succumbed to HCV-associated liver injury, in the vast majority of patients the impact of recurrent hepatitis C on graft and patient survival appears to be negligible.

Posttransplantation quality of life Full rehabilitation is achieved in the majority of patients who survive the early postoperative months and escape chronic rejection or unmanageable infection. Psychosocial maladjustment interferes with medical compliance in a small number of patients, but most manage to adhere to immunosuppressive regimens, which must be continued indefinitely. In one study, 85 percent of patients who survived their transplants returned to gainful activities. In fact, some women have conceived and carried pregnancies to term after transplantation without demonstrable injury to their infants.

REFERENCES

DAVIES SE et al: Hepatic histological findings after transplantation for chronic hepatitis B virus infection, including a unique pattern of fibrosing cholestatic hepatitis. Hepatology 13:150, 1991

FERAY C et al: Reinfection of liver graft by hepatitis C virus after liver transplantation. J Clin Invest 89:1361, 1992

LAU JYN et al: High-level expression of hepatitis B viral antigens in fibrosing cholestatic hepatitis. Gastroenterology 102:956, 1992

LUCEY MR et al: Selection for and outcome of liver transplantation in alcoholic liver disease. Gastroenterology 102:1736, 1992

MADDREY WC (ed): *Transplantation of the Liver*. New York, Elsevier, 1988

———, VAN THIEL DH: Liver transplantation: An overview. Hepatology 8:948, 1988

MARTIN P et al: Liver transplantation for viral hepatitis: Current status. Am J Gastroenterol 87:409, 1992

MUNOZ SJ, FRIEDMAN LS: Liver transplantation. Med Clin North Am 73:1011, 1989

SORRELL MF, SHAW BW JR (guest eds): A primer of liver transplantation for the referring physician. Semin Liver Dis 9:159, 1989

STARZL TE et al: Liver transplantation. N Engl J Med 321:1014, 1092, 1989

WEISNER RH (guest ed): Hepatic allograft rejection. Semin Liver Dis 12:1, 1992

———, et al: Hepatic allograft rejection: New developments in terminology, diagnosis, prevention, and treatment. Mayo Clin Proc 68:69, 1992

WRIGHT TL et al: Recurrent and acquired hepatitis C viral infection in liver transplant recipients. Gastroenterology 103:317, 1992

272 DISEASES OF THE GALLBLADDER AND BILE DUCTS

NORTON J. GREENBERGER / KURT J. ISSELBACHER

PHYSIOLOGY OF BILE PRODUCTION AND FLOW **Bile secretion and composition** Bile formed in the hepatic lobules is secreted into a complex network of canaliculi, small bile ductules, and larger bile ducts which run with lymphatics and branches of the portal vein and hepatic artery in portal tracts situated between hepatic lobules. These interlobular bile ducts coalesce to form larger septal bile ducts that join to form the right and left hepatic ducts, which in turn unite to form the common hepatic duct. The common hepatic duct is joined by the cystic duct of the gallbladder to form the common bile duct which enters the duodenum (often after joining the main pancreatic duct) through the ampulla of Vater.

Hepatic bile is a pigmented isotonic fluid with an electrolyte composition resembling blood plasma. The electrolyte composition of gallbladder bile differs from that of hepatic bile because most of the inorganic anions, chloride and bicarbonate, have been removed by reabsorption across the basement membrane.

Major components of bile by weight include water (82 percent), bile acids (12 percent), lecithin and other phospholipids (4 percent), and unesterified cholesterol (0.7 percent). Other constituents include conjugated bilirubin, proteins (IgA, by-products of hormones, and other proteins metabolized in the liver), electrolytes, mucus, and, often, drugs and their metabolic by-products.

The total daily basal secretion of hepatic bile is approximately 500 to 600 mL. The metabolic products of hepatocyte uptake and synthesis are secreted into the bile canaliculi, which are lined by microvillus membrane components associated with microfilaments of actin, microtubules, and other contractile elements. Within the hepatocyte, conjugation of many of the bile constituents may occur, while other components of bile, such as primary bile acids, lecithin, and some cholesterol, are synthesized de novo. Three mechanisms are important in regulating bile flow: (1) active transport of bile acids from hepatocytes into the canaliculi, (2) bile acid–independent ATPase-mediated transport of sodium, and (3) ductular secretion. The last is a secretin-mediated and cyclic AMP–dependent phenomenon which appears to result from the active transport of sodium and bicarbonate into the ductule with resulting passive movement of water across the cell membrane.

The bile acids   The primary bile acids, cholic and chenodeoxycholic acids, are synthesized from cholesterol in the liver, conjugated with glycine or taurine, and excreted into the bile. Secondary bile acids, including deoxycholate and lithocholate, are formed in the colon as bacterial metabolites of the primary bile acids. However, lithocholic acid is much less efficiently absorbed from the colon than deoxycholic acid. Other secondary bile acids, found in trace amounts, which include ursodeoxycholic acid (a stereoisomer of chenodeoxycholate) and a variety of other unusual or "aberrant" bile acids, may be produced in increased amounts in patients with chronic cholestatic syndromes. In normal bile, the ratio of glycine to taurine conjugates is about 3:1, while in patients with cholestasis, increased concentrations of sulfate and glucuronide conjugates of bile acids are often found.

Bile acids are detergents which in aqueous solutions and above a critical concentration of about 2 mM form molecular aggregates called *micelles*. Cholesterol alone is poorly soluble in aqueous environments, and its solubility in bile depends on both the lipid concentration and the relative molar percentages of bile acids and lecithin. Normal ratios of these constituents favor the formation of solubilizing *mixed micelles*, while abnormal ratios promote the precipitation of cholesterol crystals in bile.

In addition to facilitating the biliary excretion of cholesterol, bile acids are necessary for the normal intestinal absorption of dietary fats via a micellar transport mechanism (see Chap. 254). Bile acids also serve as a major physiologic driving force for hepatic bile flow and aid in water and electrolyte transport in the small bowel and colon.

Enterohepatic circulation   Bile acids are efficiently conserved under normal conditions. Conjugated and unconjugated bile acids are absorbed by *passive diffusion* along the entire gut. Quantitatively much more important for bile salt recirculation, however, is the *active transport* mechanism for conjugated bile acids in the distal ileum (see Chap. 254). The reabsorbed bile acids enter the portal bloodstream and are taken up rapidly by hepatocytes, reconjugated, and resecreted into bile (enterohepatic circulation).

The normal bile acid pool size is approximately 2 to 4 g. During digestion of a meal, the bile acid pool undergoes at least one or more enterohepatic cycles depending on the size and composition of the meal. Normally, the bile acid pool circulates approximately 5 to 10 times daily. Intestinal absorption of the pool is about 95 percent

efficient, so fecal loss of bile acids is in the range of 0.3 to 0.6 g/d. This fecal loss is compensated by an equal daily synthesis of bile acids by the liver, and thus the size of the bile salt pool is maintained. Bile acids returning to the liver suppress de novo hepatic synthesis of primary bile acids from cholesterol by inhibiting the rate-limiting enzyme 7α-hydroxylase. While the loss of bile salts in stool is usually matched by increased hepatic synthesis, the maximum rate of synthesis is approximately 5 g/d, which may be insufficient to replete the bile acid pool size when there is pronounced impairment of intestinal bile salt reabsorption.

Gallbladder and sphincteric functions   In the fasting state, the sphincter of Oddi offers a high-pressure zone of resistance to bile flow from the common bile duct into the duodenum. This tonic contraction serves to (1) prevent reflux of duodenal contents into the pancreatic and bile ducts and (2) promote bile filling of the gallbladder. The major factor controlling the evacuation of the gallbladder is the peptide hormone cholecystokinin, which is released from the duodenal mucosa in response to the ingestion of fats and amino acids. Cholecystokinin produces (1) powerful contraction of the gallbladder, (2) decreased resistance of the sphincter of Oddi, (3) increased hepatic secretion of bile, and thus (4) enhanced flow of biliary contents into the duodenum.

Hepatic bile is "concentrated" within the gallbladder by energy-dependent transmucosal absorption of water and electrolytes. Almost the entire bile acid pool may be sequestered in the gallbladder following an overnight fast for delivery into the duodenum with the first meal of the day. The normal capacity of the gallbladder is 30 to 75 mL of bile.

DISEASES OF THE GALLBLADDER

CONGENITAL ANOMALIES   Anomalies of the biliary tract may be found in 10 to 20 percent of the population, including abnormalities in number, size, and shape (e.g., agenesis of the gallbladder, duplications, rudimentary or oversized "giant" gallbladders, and diverticula). Phrygian cap is a clinically innocuous entity in which a partial or complete septum (or fold) separates the fundus from the body. Anomalies of position or suspension are not uncommon and include left-sided gallbladder, intrahepatic gallbladder, retrodisplacement of the gallbladder, and "floating" gallbladder. The latter condition predisposes to acute torsion, volvulus, or herniation of the gallbladder.

GALLSTONES   Pathogenesis of gallstones   Gallstones are quite prevalent in most western countries. In the United States, autopsy series have shown gallstones in at least 20 percent of women and in 8 percent of men over the age of 40. It is estimated that 16 to 20 million persons in the United States have gallstones and that approximately 1 million new cases of cholelithiasis develop each year.

Gallstones are crystalline structures formed by concretion or accretion of normal or abnormal bile constituents. These stones are divided into three major types; cholesterol and mixed stones account for 80 percent of the total, with pigment stones comprising the remaining 20 percent. Mixed and cholesterol gallstones usually contain more than 70 percent cholesterol monohydrate plus an admixture of calcium salts, bile acids and bile pigments, proteins, fatty acids, and phospholipids. Pigment stones are composed primarily of calcium bilirubinate; they contain less than 10 percent cholesterol.

CHOLESTEROL AND MIXED STONES AND BILIARY SLUDGE   Cholesterol is relatively water insoluble and requires aqueous dispersion into either micelles or vesicles, both of which require the presence of a second lipid to "liquify" the cholesterol. When the cholesterol content of bile exceeds the amount which can be solubilized by bile salt and bile salt–lecithin micelles, the excess is dispersed in larger lipid vesicles (Fig. 272-1). Vesicles are spherical particles composed of lecithin and cholesterol and contain only traces of bile salts. Vesicles

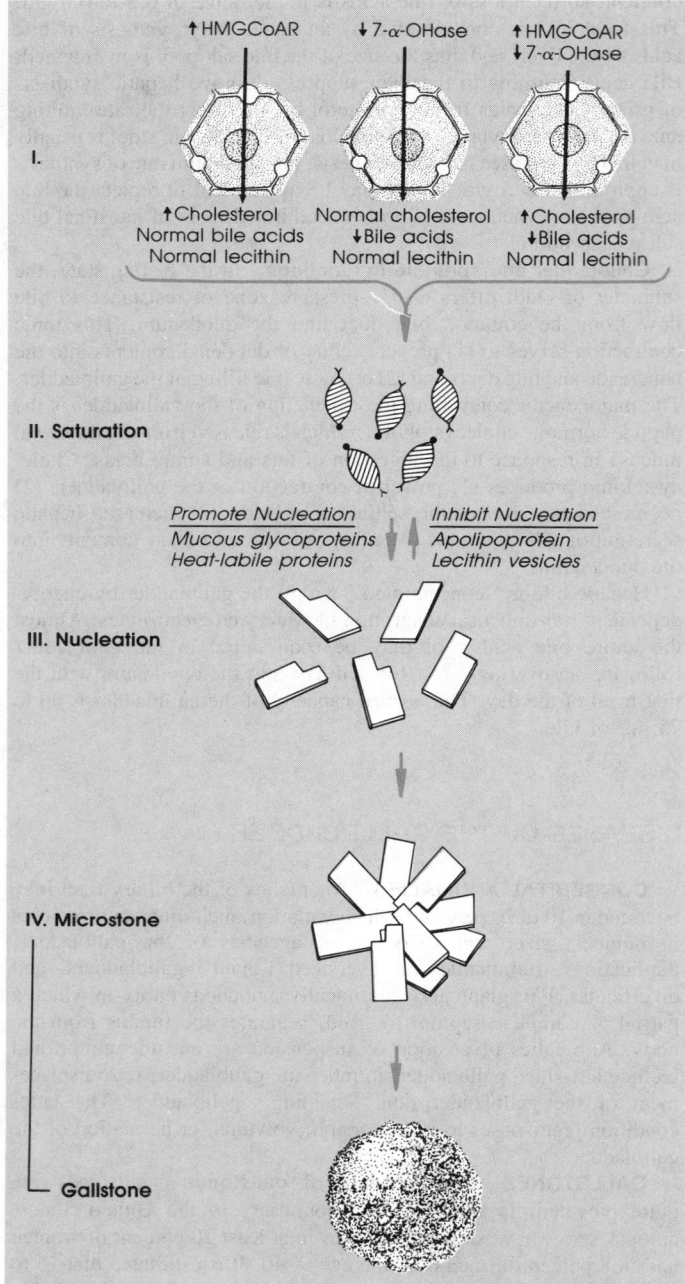

FIGURE 272-1 Scheme showing pathogenesis of gallstone formation. Conditions or factors that increase the ratio of cholesterol to bile acids and lecithin favor gallstone formation (HMG-CoAR = hydroxymethylglutaryl–coenzyme A reductase; 7-α-OHase = 7α-hydroxylase).

and micelles are important cholesterol-solubilizing and -transport agents in bile supersaturated with cholesterol.

There are several important mechanisms in the formation of lithogenic (stone-forming) bile. The most important is increased biliary secretion of cholesterol. This may occur in association with obesity, high-caloric diets, or drugs (e.g., clofibrate) and may result from increased activity of hydroxymethylglutaryl–coenzyme A (HMG-CoA) reductase, the rate-limiting enzyme of hepatic cholesterol synthesis. In some patients, impaired hepatic conversion of cholesterol to bile acids also may occur, resulting in an increase of the lithogenic cholesterol/bile acid ratio. Lithogenic bile also results from decreased hepatic secretion of bile salts and phospholipids which may follow impaired hepatic synthesis (e.g., rare inborn errors of metabolism such as cerebrotendinous xanthomatosis) or conditions affecting

the enterohepatic circulation of these constituents (e.g., prolonged parenteral alimentation or ileal disease or resection). In addition, most patients with gallstones appear to have reduced activity of hepatic cholesterol 7α-hydroxylase, the rate-limiting enzyme for primary bile acid synthesis.

Thus an excess of biliary cholesterol in relation to bile acids and phospholipids may be due to hypersecretion of cholesterol, hyposecretion of bile acids, or both. While cholesterol saturation of bile is an important prerequisite for gallstone formation, it is not sufficient by itself to produce cholesterol precipitation in vivo. Most people with supersaturated bile do not develop stones because the time required for cholesterol crystals to nucleate and grow is longer than the time bile spends in the gallbladder. Two additional disturbances of bile acid metabolism which are likely to contribute to supersaturation of bile with cholesterol are (1) reduction of the bile acid pool and (2) enhanced conversion of cholic acid to deoxycholic acid with replacement of the cholic acid pool by an expanded deoxycholic acid pool. The first disorder may be caused by more rapid loss of primary bile acid from the small intestine into the colon. The second disturbance may result from enhanced dehydroxylation of cholic acid and increased absorption of newly formed deoxycholic acid.

A second important abnormality is defective vesicle formation. Ordinarily, cholesterol and phospholipid are secreted into bile as unilamellar bilayered vesicles which are unstable and are converted, along with bile acids, into other lipid aggregates such as micelles. During micellation of vesicles, more phospholipid than cholesterol is transferred to mixed micelles, leading to unstable cholesterol-rich vesicles which aggregate into larger multilamellar vesicles from which cholesterol crystals aggregate.

A third important mechanism is *nucleation* of cholesterol monohydrate crystals, which is greatly accelerated in human lithogenic bile; it is this feature rather than the degree of cholesterol supersaturation that distinguishes lithogenic from normal gallbladder bile. Accelerated nucleation of cholesterol monohydrate in bile may be due to either an *excess of pronucleating factors* or a *deficiency of antinucleating factors*. Nonmucin and mucin glycoproteins and lysine phosphatidylcholine appear to be pronucleating factors, while apolipoproteins AI and AII and other glycoproteins appear to be antinucleating factors. However, the characterization of additional pronucleating and antinucleating factors remains incomplete. Cholesterol monohydrate crystal nucleation and crystal growth probably occur within the mucin gel layer. Vesicle fusion leads to liquid crystals, which, in turn, nucleate into solid cholesterol monohydrate crystals. Continued growth of the crystals occurs by direct nucleation of cholesterol molecules from supersaturated unilamellar or multilamellar biliary vesicles.

A fourth important mechanism in cholesterol gallstone formation concerns *biliary sludge*. Biliary sludge is a thick mucous material which upon microscopic examination reveals lecithin-cholesterol crystals, cholesterol monohydrate crystals, calcium bilirubinate, and mucin thread or mucous gels. Biliary sludge typically forms a crescent-like layer in the most dependent portion of the gallbladder and is recognized by characteristic echoes on ultrasonography (see below). In vitro, cholesterol monohydrate crystals (>50 μm) mixed with mucus produce echoes that are indistinguishable from gallbladder sludge observed in patients. The presence of biliary sludge implies two abnormalities: (1) the normal balance between gallbladder mucin secretion and elimination has become deranged; and (2) nucleation from biliary solutes has occurred. That biliary sludge is a precursor form of gallstone disease is evident from several observations. In one study, 96 patients with gallbladder sludge were followed prospectively by serial ultrasound studies. In 17 patients (18 percent), biliary sludge disappeared and did not recur for at least 2 years. In 58 patients (60 percent), biliary sludge disappeared and reappeared. Importantly, gallstones developed in 14 patients, in 8 of whom the gallstones were "silent." In 12 patients, cholecystectomies were performed, 6 for gallstone-associated biliary pain and 3 in symptomatic patients with sludge but without gallstones who had prior attacks of pancreatitis;

the latter did not recur after cholecystectomy. It should be emphasized that biliary sludge can develop with disorders that cause gallbladder hypomotility, i.e., surgery, burns, total parenteral nutrition, pregnancy, and oral contraceptives—all of which are associated with gallstone formation. Finally, biliary sludge can account for the observation that most cholesterol gallstones have a pigmented center.

To summarize, cholesterol gallstone disease occurs because of several defects, which include (1) bile supersaturation with cholesterol, (2) nucleation of cholesterol monohydrate with subsequent crystal retention and stone growth, and (3) abnormal gallbladder motor function with delayed emptying and stasis. Other important factors known to predispose to cholesterol stone formation are summarized in Table 272-1.

PIGMENT STONES   Gallstones composed largely of calcium bilirubinate are much more common in the orient than in western countries. The presence of increased amounts of unconjugated, insoluble bilirubin in bile results in the precipitation of bilirubin which may aggregate to form pigment stones or may fuse to form the nidus for growth of mixed cholesterol gallstones. In western countries, chronic hemolytic states (with increased conjugated bilirubin in bile) or alcoholic liver disease are associated with an increased incidence of pigment stones. Deconjugation of soluble bilirubin mono- and diglucuronide may be mediated by the enzyme β-glucuronidase, which is sometimes produced when bile is chronically infected by bacteria. Pigment stone formation is especially prominent in Asians and is often associated with infections in the biliary tree (see Table 272-1).

Diagnosis of gallstones   Procedures of potential use in the diagnosis of cholelithiasis and other diseases of the gallbladder are detailed in Table 272-2. The plain abdominal film may detect gallstones containing sufficient calcium to be radiopaque (10 to 15

percent of cholesterol and mixed stones and approximately 50 percent of pigment stones). Plain radiography also may be of use in the diagnosis of emphysematous cholecystitis, porcelain gallbladder, limey bile, and gallstone ileus.

Ultrasonography of the gallbladder is very accurate in the identification of cholelithiasis and has several advantages over oral cholecystography (see Fig. 272-2A). The gallbladder is easily visualized with the technique, and in fact, failure to image the gallbladder successfully in a fasting patient correlates well with the presence of underlying gallbladder disease. Stones as small as 2 mm in diameter may be confidently identified provided that firm criteria are used [e.g., acoustic "shadowing" of opacities that are within the gallbladder lumen and that change with the patient's position (by gravity)]. In major medical centers, the false-negative and false-positive rates for ultrasound in gallstone patients are about 2 to 4 percent. Biliary sludge is material of low echogenic activity that typically forms a layer in the most dependent position of the gallbladder. This layer shifts with postural changes but fails to produce acoustic shadowing; these two characteristics distinguish sludges from gallstones.

Oral cholecystography (OCG) is a useful procedure for the diagnosis of gallstones but has been largely replaced by ultrasound. False-positive results are rare, but the oral cholecystogram may be falsely negative (when good opacification is achieved) in approximately 5 to 10 percent of patients with gallstones. Factors which may produce nonvisualization of the OCG are summarized in Table 272-2. When these can be excluded, nonvisualization of the gallbladder following a second dose of oral contrast agent is highly correlated with underlying cystic duct obstruction or chronic inflammation of the gallbladder.

Radiopharmaceuticals such as ^{99m}Tc-labeled N-substituted iminodiacetic acids (HIDA, DIDA, DISIDA, etc.) are rapidly extracted from the blood and are excreted into the biliary tree in high concentration even in the presence of mild to moderate serum bilirubin elevations. Failure to image the gallbladder in the presence of biliary ductal visualization may indicate cystic duct obstruction, acute or chronic cholecystitis, or surgical absence of the organ. Such scans have their greatest application in the diagnosis of acute cholecystitis.

Symptoms of gallstone disease   Gallstones usually produce symptoms by causing inflammation or obstruction following their migration into the cystic duct or common bile duct. The most specific and characteristic symptom of gallstone disease is biliary colic. Obstruction of the cystic duct or common bile duct by a stone produces increased intraluminal pressure and distention of the viscus which cannot be relieved by repetitive biliary contractions. The resultant visceral pain is characteristically a severe, steady ache or pressure in the epigastrium or right upper quadrant of the abdomen with frequent radiation to the interscapular area, right scapula, or shoulder.

Biliary colic begins quite suddenly and may persist with severe intensity for 1 to 4 h, subsiding gradually or rapidly. An episode of biliary pain is sometimes followed by a residual mild ache or soreness in the right upper quadrant which may persist for 24 h or so. Nausea and vomiting frequently accompany episodes of biliary colic, and mild elevations of serum bilirubin [not exceeding 85.5 μmol/L (5 mg/dL)] occur in 25 percent of patients. Persistence of a high serum bilirubin level suggests common duct stones. Fever or chills (rigors) with biliary colic usually imply an underlying complication, i.e., cholecystitis, pancreatitis, or cholangitis. Complaints of vague epigastric fullness, dyspepsia, eructation, or flatulence, especially following a fatty meal, should not be confused with biliary colic. Such symptoms are frequently elicited from patients with gallstone disease but are not specific for biliary calculi. Biliary colic may be precipitated by eating a fatty meal, by consumption of a large meal following a period of prolonged fasting, or by eating a normal meal.

Natural history of gallstones   Gallstone disease discovered in an asymptomatic patient or in a patient whose symptoms are not referable to cholelithiasis is a common clinical problem. The natural history of "silent" or asymptomatic gallstones has occasioned much debate. In contrast to previous reports, a study of predominantly male silent

---

TABLE 272-1   Predisposing factors for cholesterol and pigment gallstone formation

CHOLESTEROL AND MIXED STONES

A Demography
  1 Northern Europe and North and South America greater than Asia, probable familial, hereditary aspects
B Obesity
  1 Normal bile acid pool and secretion but increased biliary secretion of cholesterol
C Weight loss
  1 Mobilization of tissue cholesterol leads to increased biliary cholesterol secretion while enterohepatic secretion of bile salt is decreased
D Female sex hormones
  1 Estrogens stimulate hepatic lipoprotein receptors, increase uptake of dietary cholesterol, and increase biliary cholesterol secretion
  2 Natural estrogens, other estrogens, and oral contraceptives lead to decreased bile salt secretion
E Ileal disease or resection
  1 Malabsorption of bile acids leads to decreased bile acid pool and decreased biliary secretion of bile salts
F Increasing age
  1 Increased biliary secretion of cholesterol, decreased size of bile acid pool, decreased biliary secretion of bile salts
G Gallbladder hypomotility leading to stasis and formation sludge/stools
  1 Prolonged parenteral nutrition
  2 Fasting
  3 Pregnancy
  4 Drugs such as octreotide
H Clofibrate therapy
  1 Increased biliary secretion of cholesterol
I Miscellaneous
  1 ? Diabetes mellitus
  2 High-calorie, high-fat diet

PIGMENT STONES

A Demographic/genetic factors: Asia, rural setting
B Chronic hemolysis
C Alcoholic cirrhosis
D Chronic biliary tract infection, parasite infestation
E Increasing age

TABLE 272-2   Diagnostic evaluation of the gallbladder

Diagnostic advantages	Diagnostic limitations	Comment
PLAIN ABDOMINAL X-RAY		

Low cost
Readily available
	Relatively low yield
	?Contraindicated in pregnancy
		Pathognomonic findings in:
		  Calcified gallstones
		  Limey bile, porcelain GB
		  Emphysematous cholecystitis
		  Gallstone ileus

ORAL CHOLECYSTOGRAM (OCG)		

Low cost
Readily available
Accurate identification of gallstones (90–95%)
Identification of GB anomalies, hyperplastic cholecystoses
Identification of chronic GB disease after nonvisualization on double dose
	?Contraindicated in pregnancy
	?Contraindicated with history of reaction to iodinated contrast
	Nonvisualization with:
	  Serum bilirubin >34–68 μmol/L (2–4 mg/dL)
	  Failure to ingest or absorb tablets
	  Impaired hepatic excretion
	Very small stones may be undetected
	More time-consuming than GBUS
		A useful procedure in identification of gallstones if diagnostic limitations prevent GBUS; largely superseded by GBUS

GALLBLADDER ULTRASOUND (GBUS)		
Rapid Accurate identification of gallstones (>95%) Simultaneous scanning of GB, liver, bile ducts, pancreas "Real-time" scanning allows assessment of GB volume, contractility Not limited by jaundice, pregnancy May detect very small stones	Bowel gas Massive obesity Ascites Recent barium study	Procedure of choice for detection of stones
RADIOISOTOPE SCANS (HIDA, DIDA, ETC.)		
Accurate identification of cystic duct obstruction Simultaneous assessment of bile ducts	?Contraindicated in pregnancy Serum bilirubin >103–205 μmol/L (6–12 mg/dL) Cholecystogram of low resolution	Indicated for confirmation of suspected cholecystitis; useful in diagnosis of acalculous cholecystopathy, especially if given with CCK to assess gallbladder emptying

FIGURE 272-2 Examples of ultrasound and radiologic studies of the biliary tract. *A*. An ultrasound study showing a distended gallbladder containing a single large stone (*arrow*) which casts an acoustic shadow. *B*. Endoscopic retrograde cholangiopancreatogram (ERCP) showing normal biliary tract anatomy. In addition to the endoscope and large vertical gallbladder filled with contrast dye, the common hepatic duct (chd), common bile duct (cbd), and pancreatic duct (pd) are shown. The arrow points to the ampulla of Vater. *C*. Percutaneous transhepatic cholangiogram (PTHC) showing choledocholithiasis. The biliary tract is dilatated and contains multiple radiolucent calculi (*small arrows*). The dilatation is due to obstruction by a large stone in the distal portion of the duct (*large arrow*). *D*. ERCP showing sclerosing cholangitis. The common bile duct is to the right of the endoscope. Following retrograde cholangiography, the common bile duct shows thickening of the wall with a narrow, beaded lumen typical of sclerosing cholangitis.

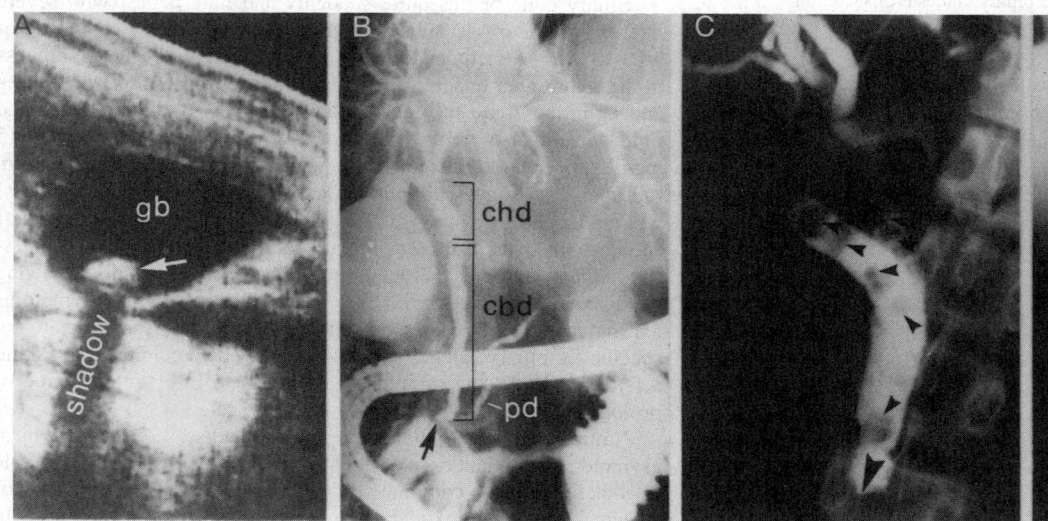

gallstone patients suggests that the cumulative risk for the development of symptoms or complications requiring surgery is relatively low— 10 percent at 5 years, 15 percent at 10 years, and 18 percent at 15 years. Patients remaining asymptomatic for 15 years were found to be unlikely to develop symptoms during further follow-up, and most patients who did develop complications from their gallstones experienced *prior* warning symptoms. Similar conclusions apply to diabetics with silent gallstones. Decision analysis has suggested that (1) the cumulative risk of death due to gallstone disease while on expectant management is small, and (2) prophylactic cholecystectomy is not warranted.

Complications requiring cholecystectomy appear to be much more common in gallstone patients who have developed symptoms of biliary colic. Patients found to have gallstones at a young age are more likely to develop symptoms from cholelithiasis than are patients older than 60 years at the time of initial diagnosis. Patients with diabetes mellitus and gallstones may be somewhat more susceptible to septic complications, but the magnitude of risk of septic biliary complications in diabetic patients is incompletely defined. In addition, asymptomatic gallstone patients with nonvisualization of the gallbladder on OCG appear to have an increased tendency to develop symptoms and complications.

Treatment of gallstones SURGICAL THERAPY Although the management of silent gallstones remains controversial, the risk of developing symptoms or complications requiring surgery is quite small (in the range of 1 to 2 percent per year) in most asymptomatic gallstone patients. Thus a recommendation for prophylactic cholecystectomy in a patient with gallstones should probably be based on assessment of three factors: (1) the presence of symptoms which are frequent enough or severe enough to interfere with the patient's general routine, (2) the presence of a prior complication of gallstone disease, i.e., history of acute cholecystitis, pancreatitis, gallstone fistula, etc., or (3) the presence of an underlying condition predisposing the patient to increased risk of gallstone complications (e.g., calcified or porcelain gallbladder, cholesterolosis, adenomyomatosis, nonvisualizing gallbladder on OCG, and/or a previous attack of acute cholecystitis regardless of current symptomatic status). Patients with very large gallstones (over 2 cm in diameter) and patients having gallstones in a congenitally anomalous gallbladder also might be considered for prophylactic cholecystectomy. Although age under 50 years is a worrisome factor in asymptomatic gallstone patients, few authorities would now recommend routine cholecystectomy in all young patients with silent stones. Laparoscopic cholecystectomy is a minimal-access approach for the removal of the gallbladder together with its stones. Because of a markedly shortened hospital stay as well as decreased cost and a mortality rate of less than 1 percent, it is the procedure of choice for most patients referred for elective cholecystectomy; in only 4 to 5 percent of patients are surgeons compelled to convert to open cholecystectomy.

MEDICAL THERAPY—GALLSTONE DISSOLUTION Oral bile acid therapy is essentially ineffective in dissolving (1) pigment gallstones, which represent approximately 20 percent of radiolucent stones, (2) radiopaque or calcified gallstones, (3) gallstones greater than approximately 1.5 cm in diameter, and (4) gallstones in gallbladders poorly opacified following oral cholecystography. Treatment with oral chenodeoxycholic acid (CDCA, chenic acid) or its 7β-epimer ursodeoxycholic acid (UDCA) to dissolve cholesterol or mixed gallstones has resulted in complete or partial dissolution of such stones in approximately 50 to 60 percent of *selected* patients with radiolucent gallstones. The major therapeutic effect of CDCA is thought to be secondary to a decrease in HMG-CoA reductase activity, which, in turn, results in decreased hepatic cholesterol synthesis. UDCA administration appears to produce a lamellar liquid crystalline phase in bile which allows a dispersion of cholesterol from stones by physicochemical means. Ursodeoxycholic acid also may retard cholesterol crystal nucleation. UDCA is therapeutically more effective at lower doses (5 to 10 mg/kg per day) than CDCA and has not been

associated with the relatively high incidence of diarrhea and serum aminotransferase elevations seen in CDCA-treated patients.

In *carefully selected* patients with radiolucent stones less than 15 mm in a functioning gallbladder, complete dissolution can be achieved within 2 years with UDCA or a combination of UDCA with CDCA in approximately 50 to 60 percent. The highest success rate, i.e., approximately 70 to 80 percent, occurs in patients with small (<5 mm), floating, radiolucent gallstones. If bile acid therapy is limited to patients with small, floating, radiolucent stones, probably no more than 10 percent of patients with symptomatic cholelithiasis are candidates for such treatment. However, in addition to the vexing problem of recurrence, there is also the factor of taking a costly drug for an indefinite period of time.

After complete dissolution of gallstones by either CDCA or UDCA and withdrawal of such treatment, there is a recurrence rate of 30 to 55 percent over 3 to 12 years of follow-up. There appears to be an approximately linear increase in gallstone recurrence of 10 to 15 percent per annum over the first 3 to 5 years, after which there may be a plateau with no further recurrence. The recurrence rate is lower in patients who had a single gallstone compared with those with multiple stones. In clinical trials designed to prevent recurrences, UDCA in doses of 3 mg/kg or 200 to 300 mg/d may delay and/or reduce recurrence.

Direct dissolution of gallstones within a period of hours using methyl tertiary butyl ether or other solvents through percutaneously placed biliary catheters also has been reported. Such solvent dissolution of gallbladder or ductal stones by continuous perfusion appears promising.

GALLSTONE LITHOTRIPSY Gallbladder stones may be fragmented by extracorporeal shock waves generated by the use of electrohydraulic, piezoceramic, or electromagnetic devices. Such shock-wave lithotripsy combined with medical litholytic therapy is a safe and effective treatment in carefully selected patients with gallbladder calculi. The usual criteria for selection of patients include (1) a history of biliary colic, (2) radiolucent stones, (3) a functioning gallbladder with opacification by oral cholecystography or normal emptying by cholecystokinin scintigraphy, (4) up to a maximum of three stones but preferably solitary stones ≤20 mm, and (5) absence of acute cholecystitis, cholangitis, biliary obstruction, acute pancreatitis, and pregnancy. The best results have been obtained in patients with solitary stones ≤20 mm; 60 to 70 percent of such patients remain stone- and fragment-free at 8 to 12 months. Results are less satisfactory for stones larger than 20 mm or for two or three stones. Side effects, caused mostly by passage of fragments after lithotripsy, include biliary colic (35 percent), pancreatitis (2 percent), and cholecystitis (1 percent). Approximately 5 percent of lithotripsy-treated patients have required cholecystectomy or urgent endoscopic sphincterotomy. If lithotripsy of gallstones is restricted to patients with symptomatic solitary gallstones ≤20 mm, only 10 to 15 percent of all patients with symptomatic gallstones will be eligible. There are still two problematic areas: (1) *recurrence* of gallstones in 10 to 15 percent of patients 2 years after lithotripsy combined with medical litholytic therapy, and (2) the *cost* of taking UDCA or UDCA plus CDCA for an indefinite period. Importantly, while the utilization of gallstone lithotripsy has decreased considerably since the emergence of laparoscopic cholecystectomy, lithotripsy does remain an option for carefully selected patients who wish to avoid surgery.

ACUTE AND CHRONIC CHOLECYSTITIS **Acute cholecystitis** Acute inflammation of the gallbladder wall usually follows obstruction of the cystic duct by a stone. Inflammatory response can be evoked by three factors: (1) *mechanical inflammation* produced by increased intraluminal pressure and distention with resulting ischemia of the gallbladder mucosa and wall, (2) *chemical inflammation* caused by the release of lysolecithin (due to the action of phospholipase on lecithin in bile) and other local tissue factors, and (3) *bacterial inflammation*, which may play a role in 50 to 85 percent of patients with acute cholecystitis. The organisms most frequently isolated by culture of gallbladder bile in these patients include *Escherichia coli,* *Klebsiella* species, group D *Streptococcus, Staphylococcus* species, and *Clostridium* species.

Acute cholecystitis often begins as an attack of biliary colic which progressively worsens. Approximately 60 to 70 percent of patients report having experienced prior attacks which resolved spontaneously. As the episode progresses, however, the pain of acute cholecystitis becomes more generalized in the right upper abdomen. As with biliary colic, the pain of cholecystitis may radiate to the interscapular area, right scapula, or shoulder. Peritoneal signs of inflammation such as increased pain with jarring or on deep respiration may be apparent. The patient is anorectic and often nauseated. Vomiting is relatively common and may produce symptoms and signs of vascular and extracellular volume depletion. Jaundice is unusual early in the course of acute cholecystitis but may occur when edematous inflammatory changes involve the bile ducts and surrounding lymph nodes.

A low-grade fever is characteristically present, but shaking chills or rigors are not uncommon. The right upper quadrant of the abdomen is almost invariably tender to palpation. An enlarged, tense gallbladder is palpable in one-quarter to one-half of patients. Deep inspiration or cough during subcostal palpation of the right upper quadrant usually produces increased pain and inspiratory arrest (Murphy's sign). A light blow delivered to the right subcostal area may elicit a marked increase in pain. Localized rebound tenderness in the right upper quadrant is common, as are abdominal distention and hypoactive bowel sounds from paralytic ileus, but generalized peritoneal signs and abdominal rigidity are usually lacking, absent perforation.

The diagnosis of acute cholecystitis is usually made on the basis of a characteristic history and physical examination. The triad of sudden onset of right upper quadrant tenderness, fever, and leukocytosis is highly suggestive. Typically, leukocytosis in the range of 10,000 to 15,000 cells per microliter with a left shift on differential count is found. The serum bilirubin is mildly elevated [less than 85.5 μmol/L (5 mg/dL)] in 45 percent of patients, while 25 percent have modest elevations in serum aminotransferases (usually less than a fivefold elevation). The radionuclide (e.g., HIDA) biliary scan may be confirmatory if bile duct imaging is seen without visualization of the gallbladder. Ultrasound will demonstrate calculi in 90 to 95 percent of cases.

Approximately 75 percent of patients treated medically have remission of acute symptoms within 2 to 7 days following hospitalization. In 25 percent, however, a complication of acute cholecystitis will occur despite conservative treatment (see below). In this setting, prompt surgical intervention is required. Of the 75 percent of patients with acute cholecystitis who undergo remission of symptoms, approximately one-quarter will experience a recurrence of cholecystitis within 1 year, and 60 percent will have at least one recurrent bout within 6 years. In view of the natural history of the disease, acute cholecystitis is best treated by early surgery whenever possible.

ACALCULOUS CHOLECYSTITIS   In 5 to 10 percent of patients with acute cholecystitis, calculi obstructing the cystic duct are not found at surgery. In over 50 percent of such cases an underlying explanation for acalculous inflammation is not found. An increased risk for the development of acalculous cholecystitis is especially associated with serious trauma or burns, with the postpartum period following prolonged labor, and with orthopedic and other nonbiliary major surgical operations in the postoperative period. Other precipitating factors include vasculitis, obstructing adenocarcinoma of the gallbladder, diabetes mellitus, torsion of the gallbladder, "unusual" bacterial infections of the gallbladder (e.g., *Leptospira, Streptococcus, Salmonella,* or *Vibrio cholerae*), and parasitic infestation of the gallbladder. Acalculous cholecystitis also may be seen with a variety of other systemic disease processes (sarcoidosis, cardiovascular disease, tuberculosis, syphilis, actinomycosis, etc.) and may possibly complicate periods of prolonged parenteral hyperalimentation.

Although the clinical manifestations of acalculous cholecystitis are indistinguishable from those of calculous cholecystitis, the setting of acute gallbladder inflammation complicating severe underlying illness is characteristic of acalculous disease. Ultrasound, CT scanning, or radionuclide examinations demonstrating a large, tense, static gallbladder without stones and with evidence of poor emptying over a prolonged period may be diagnostically useful in some cases. The complication rate for acalculous cholecystitis exceeds that for calculous cholecystitis. Successful management of acute acalculous cholecystitis appears to depend primarily on early diagnosis and surgical intervention with meticulous attention to postoperative care.

ACALCULOUS CHOLECYSTOPATHY   Disordered motility of the gallbladder can produce recurrent biliary pain in patients without gallstones. Infusion of an octapeptide of cholecystokinin (CCK) can be used to measure the gallbladder ejection fraction during cholescintigraphy. In a representative study, CCK cholescintigraphy using ^{99mm}Tc-diisopropyl iminodiacetic acid (DIDA) identified 21 patients with an abnormal gallbladder ejection fraction (<40 percent at 45 min); 10 of 11 patients who underwent surgery became asymptomatic, whereas all 10 who did not undergo surgery showed abnormalities, i.e., chronic cholecystitis, gallbladder muscle hypertrophy, and/or a markedly narrowed cystic duct. From this and other similar studies, the following criteria can be used to identify patients with acalculous cholecystopathy: (1) recurrent episodes of typical right upper quadrant (RUQ) pain characteristic of biliary tract pain, (2) abnormal CCK cholescintigraphy demonstrating a gallbladder ejection fraction of less than 40 percent, (3) infusion of CCK reproduces the patient's pain, and (4) prior history of transient abnormalities in liver tests that accompanied episodes of RUQ pain. An additional clue would be the identification of a large gallbladder on ultrasound examination. Finally, it should be noted that sphincter of Oddi dysfunction also can give rise to recurrent RUQ pain and CCK-scintigraphic abnormalities.

EMPHYSEMATOUS CHOLECYSTITIS   So-called emphysematous cholecystitis is thought to begin with acute cholecystitis (calculous or acalculous) followed by ischemia or gangrene of the gallbladder wall and infection by gas-producing organisms. Bacteria most frequently cultured in this setting include anaerobes such as *Clostridium welchii,* or *perfringens,* and aerobes such as *E. coli.* This condition occurs most frequently in elderly men and in patients with diabetes mellitus. The clinical manifestations are essentially indistinguishable from those of nongaseous cholecystitis. The diagnosis is usually made on plain abdominal film by the finding of gas within the gallbladder lumen, dissecting within the gallbladder wall to form a gaseous ring, or in the pericholecystic tissues. The morbidity and mortality rates with emphysematous cholecystitis are considerable. Prompt surgical intervention coupled with appropriate antibiotics is mandatory.

Chronic cholecystitis   Chronic inflammation of the gallbladder wall is almost always associated with the presence of gallstones and is thought to result from repeated bouts of subacute or acute cholecystitis or from persistent mechanical irritation of the gallbladder wall. The presence of bacteria in the bile occurs in more than one-quarter of patients with chronic cholecystitis. Although the presence of infected bile in a patient with *chronic* cholecystitis undergoing elective cholecystectomy probably adds little to the operative risk, intraoperative Gram's staining and routine culturing of bile have been advocated to identify those patients whose gallbladder is colonized with *Clostridium* species. Appropriate antibiotics intra- and postoperatively are recommended in such patients because colonization with these organisms may be associated with devastating septic complications following surgery. Chronic cholecystitis may be asymptomatic for years, may progress to symptomatic gallbladder disease or to acute cholecystitis, or may present with complications (see below).

Complications of cholecystitis   EMPYEMA AND HYDROPS   Empyema of the gallbladder usually results from progression of acute cholecystitis with persistent cystic duct obstruction to superinfection of the stagnant bile with a pus-forming bacterial organism. The clinical picture resembles that of cholangitis with high fever, severe RUQ pain, marked leukocytosis, and often, prostration. Empyema of the gallbladder carries a high risk of gram-negative sepsis and/or perforation. Emergency surgical intervention with proper antibiotic coverage is required as soon as the diagnosis is suspected.

Hydrops or mucocele of the gallbladder also may result from prolonged obstruction of the cystic duct, usually by a large solitary calculus. In this instance, the obstructed gallbladder lumen is progressively distended, over a period of time, by mucus (mucocele) or by a clear transudate (hydrops) produced by mucosal epithelial cells. A visible, easily palpable, nontender mass often extending from the right upper quadrant into the right iliac fossa may be found on physical examination. The patient with hydrops of the gallbladder frequently remains asymptomatic, although chronic RUQ pain also may occur. Cholecystectomy is indicated, since empyema, perforation, or gangrene may complicate the condition.

GANGRENE AND PERFORATION Gangrene of the gallbladder results from ischemia of the wall and patchy or complete tissue necrosis. Underlying conditions often include marked distention of the gallbladder, vasculitis, diabetes mellitus, empyema, or torsion resulting in arterial occlusion. Gangrene usually predisposes to perforation of the gallbladder, but perforation also may occur in chronic cholecystitis without premonitory warning symptoms. *Localized perforations* are usually contained by the omentum or by adhesions produced by recurrent inflammation of the gallbladder. Bacterial superinfection of the walled-off gallbladder contents results in abscess formation. Most patients are best treated with cholecystectomy, but some seriously ill patients may be managed with cholecystostomy and drainage of the abscess. *Free perforation* is less common but is associated with a mortality rate of approximately 30 percent. Such patients may experience a sudden transient relief of RUQ pain as the distended gallbladder decompresses; this is followed by signs of generalized peritonitis.

FISTULA FORMATION AND GALLSTONE ILEUS *Fistulization* into an adjacent organ adherent to the gallbladder wall may result from inflammation and adhesion formation. Fistulas into the duodenum are most common, followed in frequency by those involving the hepatic flexure of the colon, stomach or jejunum, abdominal wall, and renal pelvis. Clinically "silent" biliary-enteric fistulas occurring as a complication of chronic cholecystitis have been found in up to 5 percent of patients undergoing cholecystectomy. Asymptomatic cholecystoenteric fistulas may sometimes be diagnosed by finding gas in the biliary tree on plain abdominal films. Barium contrast studies or endoscopy of the upper gastrointestinal tract or colon may demonstrate the fistula, but oral cholecystography will almost never result in opacification of either the gallbladder or the fistulous tract. Treatment in the symptomatic patient usually consists of cholecystectomy, common bile duct exploration, and closure of the fistulous tract.

Gallstone ileus refers to mechanical intestinal obstruction resulting from the passage of a large gallstone into the bowel lumen. The stone customarily enters the duodenum through a cholecystoenteric fistula at that level. The site of obstruction by the impacted gallstone is usually at the ileocecal valve, provided that the more proximal small bowel is of normal caliber. The majority of patients do not give a history of either prior biliary tract symptoms or complaints suggestive of acute cholecystitis or fistulization. Large stones over 2.5 cm in diameter are thought to predispose to fistula formation by gradual erosion through the gallbladder fundus. Diagnostic confirmation may occasionally be found on the plain abdominal film (e.g., small-intestinal obstruction with gas in the biliary tree and a calcified, ectopic gallstone) or following an upper gastrointestinal series (cholecystoduodenal fistula with small bowel obstruction at the ileocecal valve). Early laparotomy is indicated with enterolithotomy and careful palpation of the more proximal small bowel and gallbladder to exclude other stones.

LIMEY (MILK OF CALCIUM) BILE AND PORCELAIN GALLBLADDER Calcium salts may be secreted into the lumen of the gallbladder in sufficient concentration to produce calcium precipitation and diffuse, hazy opacification of bile or a layering effect on plain abdominal roentgenography. This so-called limey bile or milk of calcium bile is usually clinically innocuous, but cholecystectomy is recommended because limey bile most often occurs in an hydropic gallbladder. In the entity called *porcelain gallbladder*, calcium salt deposition within the wall of a chronically inflamed gallbladder may be detected on the plain abdominal film. Cholecystectomy is advised in all patients with porcelain gallbladder because in a high percentage of cases this finding appears to be associated with the development of carcinoma of the gallbladder.

Treatment of cholecystitis MEDICAL THERAPY Although surgical intervention remains the mainstay of therapy for acute cholecystitis and its complications, a period of in-hospital stabilization may be required before cholecystectomy. Oral intake is eliminated, nasogastric suction is initiated, and extracellular volume depletion and electrolyte abnormalities are repaired. Meperidine or pentazocine are usually employed for analgesia because they may produce less spasm of the sphincter of Oddi than drugs such as morphine. Intravenous antibiotic therapy is usually indicated in patients with severe acute cholecystitis even though bacterial superinfection of bile may not have occurred in the early stages of the inflammatory process. Postoperative complications of wound infection, abscess formation, or sepsis are reduced in antibiotic-treated patients. Effective single-agent antibiotics include ampicillin, cephalosporins, ureidopenicillins, or aminoglycosides, but in diabetic or debilitated patients and in those with signs of gram-negative sepsis, combination antibiotic treatment may be preferable (see also Chap. 98).

SURGICAL THERAPY The optimal timing of surgical intervention in patients with acute cholecystitis remains controversial. Urgent (emergency) cholecystectomy or cholecystostomy is probably appropriate in most patients in whom a complication of acute cholecystitis such as empyema, emphysematous cholecystitis, or perforation is suspected or confirmed. In uncomplicated cases of acute cholecystitis, up to 30 percent of patients fail to resolve their symptoms on appropriate medical therapy, and progression of the attack or a supervening complication leads to the performance of early operation (within 24 to 72 h). The technical complications of surgery are not increased in patients undergoing early as opposed to delayed cholecystectomy. Delayed surgical intervention is probably best reserved for (1) patients in whom the overall medical condition imposes an unacceptable risk for early surgery and (2) patients in whom the diagnosis of acute cholecystitis is in doubt. Early cholecystectomy is the treatment of choice for most patients with acute cholecystitis. Mortality figures for emergency cholecystectomy in most centers approach 3 percent, while the mortality risk for elective or early cholecystectomy approximates 0.5 percent in patients under age 60. Of course, the operative risks increase with age-related diseases of other organ systems and with the presence of long- or short-term complications of gallbladder disease. Seriously ill or debilitated patients with cholecystitis may be managed with cholecystostomy and tube drainage of the gallbladder. Elective cholecystectomy may then be done at a later date.

Postcholecystectomy complications Early complications following cholecystectomy include atelectasis and other pulmonary disorders, abscess formation (often subphrenic), external or internal hemorrhage, biliary-enteric fistula, and bile leaks. Jaundice may indicate absorption of bile from an intraabdominal collection following a biliary leak or mechanical obstruction of the common bile duct by retained calculi, intraductal blood clots, or extrinsic compression. Routine performance of intraoperative cholangiography during cholecystectomy has helped to reduce the incidence of these early complications.

Overall, cholecystectomy is a very successful operation which provides total or near-total relief of preoperative symptoms in 75 to 90 percent of patients. The most common cause of persistent postcholecystectomy symptoms is an overlooked extrabiliary disorder (e.g., reflux esophagitis, peptic ulceration, postgastrectomy syndrome, pancreatitis, or irritable bowel syndrome). In a small percentage of patients, however, a disorder of the extrahepatic bile ducts may result in persistent symptomatology. These so-called postcholecystectomy syndromes may be due to (1) biliary strictures, (2) retained biliary calculi, (3) cystic duct stump syndrome, (4) stenosis or dyskinesia of the sphincter of Oddi, or (5) bile salt–induced diarrhea or gastritis.

CYSTIC DUCT STUMP SYNDROME   In the absence of cholangiographically demonstrable retained stones, symptoms resembling biliary colic or cholecystitis in the postcholecystectomy patient have frequently been attributed to disease in a long (>1 cm) cystic duct remnant (cystic duct stump syndrome). Careful analysis, however, reveals that postcholecystectomy complaints are attributable to other causes in almost all patients in whom the symptom complex was originally thought to result from the existence of a long cystic duct stump. Accordingly, considerable care should be taken to investigate the possible role of other factors in the production of postcholecystectomy symptoms before attributing them to cystic duct stump syndrome.

PAPILLARY DYSFUNCTION, PAPILLARY STENOSIS, SPASM OF THE SPHINCTER OF ODDI, AND BILIARY DYSKINESIA   Symptoms of biliary colic accompanied by signs of recurrent, intermittent biliary obstruction may be produced by papillary stenosis, papillary dysfunction, spasm of the sphincter of Oddi, and biliary dyskinesia. Papillary stenosis is thought to result from acute or chronic inflammation of the papilla of Vater or from glandular hyperplasia of the papillary segment. Five criteria have been used to define papillary stenosis: (1) upper abdominal pain, usually right upper quadrant or epigastric, (2) abnormal liver tests, (3) dilatation of the common bile duct upon endoscopic retrograde cholangiopancreatogram (ERCP) examination, (4) delayed (longer than 45 min) drainage of contrast material from the duct, and (5) increased basal pressure of the sphincter of Oddi, a finding that may be of only minor significance. A useful alternative to ERCP is hepatobiliary scintigraphy using ^{99m}Tc-diisopropyl iminodiacetic acid (DIDA), especially if ERCP and/or biliary manometry are either unavailable or not feasible. In patients with papillary stenosis, quantitative hepatobiliary scintigraphy has revealed delayed transit from the common bile duct to the bowel, ductal dilatation, and abnormal time-activity dynamics. This technique also can be used before and after sphincterotomy to document improvement in biliary emptying. Treatment consists of endoscopic or surgical sphincteroplasty to ensure wide patency of the distal portions of both the bile and pancreatic ducts. The greater the number of the preceding criteria present, the greater the likelihood that a patient does have a degree of papillary stenosis sufficient to justify correction. The factors usually considered as indications for sphincterotomy include (1) prolonged duration of symptoms, (2) lack of response to symptomatic treatment, (3) presence of severe disability, and (4) the patient's choice of sphincterotomy over surgery (given a clear understanding on his or her part of the risks involved in both procedures).

Criteria for diagnosing dyskinesia of the sphincter of Oddi are even more controversial than those for papillary stenosis. Proposed mechanisms include spasm of the sphincter, denervation sensitivity resulting in hypertonicity, and abnormalities of the sequencing or frequency rates of sphincteric contraction waves. When thorough evaluation has failed to demonstrate another cause for the pain, and when cholangiographic and manometric criteria suggest a diagnosis of biliary dyskinesia, medical treatment with nitrites or anticholinergics to attempt pharmacologic relaxation of the sphincter has been proposed. Endoscopic sphincterotomy or surgical sphincteroplasty may be indicated in patients who fail to respond to a 2- to 3-month trial of medical therapy, especially if basal sphincter of Oddi pressures are elevated.

BILE SALT–INDUCED CATHARSIS AND GASTRITIS   Postcholecystectomy patients may develop symptoms and signs of gastritis, which has been attributed to duodenogastric reflux of bile. However, firm data linking an increased incidence of bile gastritis with surgical removal of the gallbladder are lacking. Similarly, the occurrence of cholestyramine-responsive diarrhea in a small number of patients following cholecystectomy has been attributed to an alteration of the enterohepatic circulation of bile acids induced or unmasked by removal of the gallbladder.

THE HYPERPLASTIC CHOLECYSTOSES   The term *hyperplastic cholecystoses* is used to denote a group of disorders of the gallbladder characterized by excessive proliferation of normal tissue components.

Adenomyomatosis is characterized by a benign proliferation of gallbladder surface epithelium with glandlike formations, extramural sinuses, transverse strictures, and/or fundal nodule (''adenoma'' or ''adenomyoma'') formation. Outpouchings of mucosa termed *Rokitansky-Aschoff sinuses* may be seen on oral cholecystography in conjunction with hyperconcentration of contrast medium. Characteristic dimpled filling defects also may be seen.

Cholesterolosis is characterized by abnormal deposition of lipid, especially cholesterol esters, in the lamina propria of the gallbladder wall. In its diffuse form (''strawberry gallbladder''), the gallbladder mucosa is brick red and speckled with bright yellow flecks of lipid. The localized form shows solitary or multiple ''cholesterol polyps'' studding the gallbladder wall. Cholesterol stones of the gallbladder are found in nearly half the cases. Cholecystectomy is indicated in both adenomyomatosis and cholesterolosis when symptomatic or when cholelithiasis is present.

CANCER OF THE GALLBLADDER   Most cancers of the gallbladder develop in conjunction with stones rather than polyps. In patients with gallstones, the risk for developing gallbladder cancer, while increased, is still quite low. In one study, gallbladder cancer developed in only 5 of 2583 patients with gallstones followed for a median of 13 years. In the United States, adenocarcinomas comprise the vast majority of the estimated 6500 new cases of gallbladder cancer diagnosed each year. The female/male ratio is 4:1, and the mean age at diagnosis is approximately 70 years. The clinical presentation is most often one of unremitting right upper quadrant pain associated with weight loss, jaundice, and a palpable right upper quadrant mass. Cholangitis may supervene. The preoperative diagnosis of the condition is difficult. Once symptoms have appeared, spread of the tumor outside the gallbladder by direct extension or by lymphatic or hematogenous routes is almost invariable. Over 75 percent of gallbladder carcinomas are unresectable at the time of surgery, the exceptions being tumors discovered incidentally at laparotomy. The 1-year mortality rate for unresectable disease is approximately 95 percent, and only 5 percent of patients survive 5 years or more from the time of diagnosis. Radical operative resection does not appear to improve survival. Results of trials with radiation and chemotherapy of primary gallbladder cancer also have been disappointing.

DISEASES OF THE BILE DUCTS

CONGENITAL ANOMALIES   Biliary atresia and hypoplasia Atretic and hypoplastic lesions of the extrahepatic and major intrahepatic bile ducts are the most common biliary anomalies of clinical relevance encountered in infancy. The clinical picture is one of severe obstructive jaundice during the first month of life, with pale stools. The diagnosis is confirmed by surgical exploration with operative cholangiography. Approximately 10 percent of cases of biliary atresia are treatable with roux-en-Y choledochojejunostomy, with the Kasai procedure (hepatic portoenterostomy) being attempted in the remainder in an effort to restore some bile flow. Most patients, even those having successful biliary-enteric anastomoses, eventually develop chronic cholangitis, extensive hepatic fibrosis, and portal hypertension.

Choledochal cysts   Cystic dilatation may involve the free portion of the common bile duct, i.e., choledochal cyst, or may present as diverticulum formation in the intraduodenal segment. In the latter situation, chronic reflux of pancreatic juice into the biliary tree can produce inflammation and stenosis of the extrahepatic bile ducts leading to cholangitis or biliary obstruction. Because the process may be gradual, approximately 50 percent of patients present with onset of symptoms after age 10. The diagnosis may be made by ultrasound, abdominal CT, or cholangiography. Surgical treatment involves excision of the "cyst" and biliary-enteric anastomosis. Patients with choledochal cysts are at increased risk for the subsequent development of cholangiocarcinoma.

Congenital biliary ectasia Cystic dilatation of the intrahepatic bile ducts may involve either the major intrahepatic radicles (Caroli's disease) or the inter- and intralobular ducts (congenital hepatic fibrosis) or both. In Caroli's disease, clinical manifestations include recurrent cholangitis, abscess formation in and around the affected ducts, and sometimes, gallstone formation within portions of ectatic intrahepatic biliary radicles. The CT scan and cholangiographic patterns are usually diagnostic, and treatment with ongoing antibiotic therapy is usually undertaken in an effort to limit the frequency and severity of recurrent bouts of cholangitis. Progression to secondary biliary cirrhosis with portal hypertension, amyloidosis, extrahepatic biliary obstruction, cholangiocarcinoma, or recurrent episodes of sepsis with hepatic abscess formation is common.

CHOLEDOCHOLITHIASIS Pathophysiology and clinical manifestations Passage of gallstones into the common bile duct occurs in approximately 10 to 15 percent of patients with cholelithiasis. The incidence of common duct stones increases with increasing age of the patient so that up to 25 percent of elderly patients may have calculi in the common duct at the time of cholecystectomy. Undetected duct stones are left behind in approximately 1 to 5 percent of cholecystectomy patients. The overwhelming majority of bile duct stones are cholesterol or mixed stones formed in the gallbladder which then migrate into the extrahepatic biliary tree through the cystic duct. Primary calculi arising de novo in the ducts are usually pigment stones developing in patients with (1) chronic hemolytic diseases, (2) hepatobiliary parasitism or chronic, recurrent cholangitis, (3) congenital anomalies of the bile ducts (especially Caroli's disease), or (4) dilated, sclerosed, or strictured ducts. Common duct stones may remain asymptomatic for years, may pass spontaneously into the duodenum, or (most often) may present with biliary colic or a complication.

Complications CHOLANGITIS Cholangitis may be acute or chronic, and symptoms result from inflammation, which usually requires at least partial obstruction to the flow of bile. Bacteria are present on bile culture in approximately 75 percent of patients with acute cholangitis early in the symptomatic course. The characteristic presentation of acute cholangitis involves biliary colic, jaundice, and spiking fevers with chills (Charcot's triad). Blood cultures are frequently positive, and leukocytosis is typical. *Nonsuppurative* acute cholangitis is most common and may respond relatively rapidly to supportive measures and to treatment with antibiotics (see Chap. 98). In *suppurative* acute cholangitis, however, the presence of pus under pressure in a completely obstructed ductal system leads to symptoms of severe toxicity—mental confusion, bacteremia, and septic shock. Response to antibiotics alone in this setting is relatively poor, multiple hepatic abscesses are often present, and the mortality rate approaches 100 percent unless prompt surgical correction of the obstructing lesion and drainage of infected bile is carried out.

OBSTRUCTIVE JAUNDICE Gradual obstruction of the common bile duct over a period of weeks or months usually leads to initial manifestations of jaundice or pruritus without associated symptoms of biliary colic or cholangitis. Painless jaundice may occur in patients with choledocholithiasis, but this manifestation is much more characteristic of biliary obstruction secondary to malignancy of the head of pancreas, bile ducts, or ampulla of Vater.

In patients whose obstruction is secondary to choledocholithiasis, associated chronic calculous cholecystitis is very common, and the gallbladder in this setting may be relatively indistensible. The absence of a palpable gallbladder in most patients with biliary obstruction from duct stones is the basis for *Courvoisier's law*, i.e., that the presence of a palpably enlarged gallbladder suggests that the biliary obstruction is secondary to an underlying malignancy rather than to calculous disease. Biliary obstruction causes progressive dilatation of the intrahepatic bile ducts as intrabiliary pressures rise. Hepatic bile flow is suppressed, and regurgitation of conjugated bilirubin into the bloodstream leads to jaundice accompanied by dark urine (bilirubinuria) and light-colored (acholic) stools.

Common bile duct stones should be suspected in any patient with cholecystitis whose serum bilirubin level exceeds 85.5 μmol/L (5 mg/dL). The maximum bilirubin level is seldom over 256.5 μmol/L (15.0 mg/dL) in patients with choledocholithiasis unless concomitant hepatic disease or another factor leading to marked hyperbilirubinemia exists. Serum bilirubin levels of 342.0 μmol/L (20mg/dL) or more should suggest the possibility of neoplastic obstruction. The serum alkaline phosphatase level is almost always elevated in biliary obstruction. A rise in alkaline phosphatase often precedes clinical jaundice and may be the only abnormality in routine liver function tests. There may be a two- to tenfold elevation of serum aminotransferases, especially in association with acute obstruction. Following relief of the obstructing process, serum aminotransferase elevations usually return rapidly to normal, while the serum bilirubin level may take 1 to 2 weeks to return to normal. The alkaline phosphatase level usually falls slowly, lagging behind the decrease in serum bilirubin.

PANCREATITIS The most common associated entity discovered in patients with nonalcoholic acute pancreatitis is biliary tract disease. Biochemical evidence of pancreatic inflammation complicates acute cholecystitis in 15 percent of cases and choledocholithiasis in over 30 percent, and the common factor appears to be the passage of gallstones through the common duct. Coexisting pancreatitis should be suspected in patients with symptoms of cholecystitis who develop (1) back pain or pain to the left of the abdominal midline, (2) prolonged vomiting with paralytic ileus, or (3) a pleural effusion, especially on the left side. Surgical treatment of gallstone disease is usually associated with resolution of the pancreatitis.

SECONDARY BILIARY CIRRHOSIS Secondary biliary cirrhosis may complicate prolonged or intermittent duct obstruction with or without recurrent cholangitis. Although this complication may be seen in patients with choledocholithiasis, it is more common in cases of prolonged obstruction from stricture or neoplasm. Once established, secondary biliary cirrhosis may be progressive even after correction of the obstructing process, and increasingly severe hepatic cirrhosis may lead to portal hypertension or to hepatic failure and death. Prolonged biliary obstruction also may be associated with clinically relevant deficiencies of the fat-soluble vitamins A, D, and K.

Diagnosis and treatment The diagnosis of choledocholithiasis is usually made by cholangiography (Table 272-3), either preoperatively or intraoperatively at the time of cholecystectomy. The incidence of coexisting common duct stones in patients with cholelithiasis is relatively high. Operative cholangiography should be performed routinely during surgical procedures on the biliary tract. Preoperative indications for common duct exploration include (1) cholangiographic demonstration of ductal stones, (2) jaundice or cholangitis preceding operation, (3) a history of gallstone-related pancreatitis, and (4) cholangiographic evidence of a markedly enlarged common bile duct. Operative indications for exploration of the duct include (1) manual palpation of stones in the common bile duct, (2) positive intraoperative cholangiogram, (3) enlargement of the common bile duct or cystic duct at operation, (4) multiple small stones or "sand" in the gallbladder, and (5) a gallbladder empty of stones at surgery in a patient with previously documented gallstones.

In most cases of choledocholithiasis, the treatment of choice is cholecystectomy with choledocholithotomy and T-tube drainage of the bile ducts. A T-tube cholangiogram is usually performed prior to T-tube removal on or before the tenth postoperative day. Retained calculi seen on T-tube cholangiography may be removed percutaneously by placement of a steerable basket catheter under radiographic guidance through the matured T-tube sinus tract. Endoscopic sphincterotomy followed by spontaneous or basket stone extraction is an additional nonoperative alternative in the management of patients with common duct stones, especially in elderly or poor-risk patients.

TRAUMA, STRICTURES, AND HEMOBILIA Benign strictures of the extrahepatic bile ducts result from surgical trauma in approximately 95 percent of cases and occur in about 1 in 500 cholecystectomies.

TABLE 272-3 Diagnostic evaluation of the bile ducts

Diagnostic advantages	Diagnostic limitations	Contraindications	Complications	Comment
HEPATOBILIARY ULTRASOUND (HBUS)				
Rapid Simultaneous scanning of GB, liver, bile ducts, pancreas Accurate identification of dilated bile ducts Not limited by jaundice, pregnancy Guidance for fine-needle biopsy	Bowel gas Massive obesity Ascites Barium Partial bile duct obstruction Poor visualization of distal CBD	None	None	Initial procedure of choice in investigating possible biliary obstruction
COMPUTED TOMOGRAPHY (CT)				
Simultaneous scanning of GB, liver, bile ducts, pancreas Accurate identification of dilated bile ducts, masses Not limited by jaundice, gas, obesity, ascites High-resolution image Guidance for fine-needle biopsy	Extreme cachexia Movement artifact Ileus Partial bile duct obstruction High cost May not be readily available	Pregnancy	Reaction to iodinated contrast, if used	Indicated for evaluation of hepatic or pancreatic masses Procedure of choice in investigating possible biliary obstruction if diagnostic limitations prevent HBUS
PERCUTANEOUS TRANSHEPATIC CHOLANGIOGRAM (PTHC)				
Extremely successful when bile ducts dilated Best visualization of proximal biliary tract Possible separate visualization of obstructed left ductal system Bile cytology/culture Percutaneous transhepatic drainage	Nondilated or sclerosed ducts	Pregnancy Uncorrectable coagulopathy Massive ascites ? Hepatic abscess	Bleeding Hemobilia Bile peritonitis Bacteremia, sepsis	Usually, initial cholangiogram of choice when bile ducts are dilated
ENDOSCOPIC RETROGRADE CHOLANGIOPANCREATOGRAM (ERCP)				

Simultaneous pancreatography
Visualization/biopsy of ampulla and duodenum
Best visualization of distal biliary tract
Bile or pancreatic cytology
Endoscopic sphincterotomy and stone removal
Biliary manometry
Not limited by ascites, coagulopathy, abscess
	Gastroduodenal obstruction
	? Roux en Y biliary-enteric anastomosis
		Pregnancy
		? Acute pancreatitis
		? Severe cardiopulmonary disease
			Pancreatitis
			Cholangitis, sepsis
			Infected pancreatic pseudocyst
			Perforation (rare)
			Hypoxemia, aspiration
				Cholangiogram of choice in:
				  Absence of dilated ducts
				  ? Pancreatic, ampullary or gastroduodenal disease
				  Prior biliary surgery
				  PTHC contraindicated or failed
				  Endoscopic sphincterotomy a treatment possibility

NOTE: Intravenous cholangiography (IVC) is an obsolete technique because 40 percent of common duct stones are missed and there is poor resolution even with tomography. There are few indications for its use especially since other cholangiographic techniques are usually available.

Strictures may present with bile leak or abscess formation in the immediate postoperative period or with biliary obstruction or cholangitis as long as 2 years or more following the inciting trauma. The diagnosis is established by percutaneous or endoscopic cholangiography. Successful operative correction by a skillful surgeon with duct-to-bowel anastomosis is usually possible, although mortality rates from surgical complications, recurrent cholangitis, or secondary biliary cirrhosis are high.

Hemobilia may follow traumatic or operative injury to the liver or bile ducts, intraductal rupture of a hepatic abscess or aneurysm of the hepatic artery, biliary or hepatic tumor hemorrhage, or mechanical complications of choledocholithiasis or hepatobiliary parasitism. Diagnostic procedures such as liver biopsy, percutaneous transhepatic cholangiography (PTHC), and transhepatic biliary drainage catheter placement also may be complicated by hemobilia. Patients often present with a classic triad of biliary colic, obstructive jaundice, and melena or occult blood in the stools. The diagnosis is sometimes made by cholangiographic evidence of blood clot in the biliary tree, but selective angiographic verification may be required. Although minor episodes of hemobilia may resolve without operative intervention, surgical ligation of the bleeding vessel is frequently required.

EXTRINSIC COMPRESSION OF THE BILE DUCTS Partial or complete biliary obstruction may sometimes be produced by extrinsic compression of the ducts. The most common cause of this form of obstructive jaundice is carcinoma of the head of the pancreas. Biliary obstruction also may occur as a complication of either acute or chronic pancreatitis or involvement of lymph nodes in the porta hepatis by lymphoma or metastatic carcinoma. The latter should be distinguished from cholestasis resulting from massive replacement of the liver by tumor.

HEPATOBILIARY PARASITISM Infestation of the biliary tract by adult helminths or their ova may produce a chronic, recurrent pyogenic cholangitis with or without multiple hepatic abscesses, ductal stones, or biliary obstruction. This condition is relatively rare but does occur in inhabitants of southern China and elsewhere in Southeast Asia. The organisms most commonly involved are trematodes or flukes, including *Clonorchis sinensis, Opisthorchis viverrini* or *felineus*, and *Fasciola hepatica*. The biliary tract also may be involved by intraductal migration of adult *Ascaris lumbricoides* from the duodenum or by intrabiliary rupture of hydatid cysts of the liver produced by *Echinococcus* species. The diagnosis is made by cholangiography and the presence of characteristic ova on stool examination. When obstruction is present, the treatment of choice is laparotomy under antibiotic coverage, with common duct exploration and a biliary drainage procedure. It should be emphasized that in the Orient, one also sees cholangiohepatitis associated with pigment lithiasis, which may, in fact, be more common than cholangitis due to parasites.

SCLEROSING CHOLANGITIS Primary or idiopathic sclerosing cholangitis is a disorder characterized by a progressive, inflammatory, sclerosing, and obliterative process affecting the extrahepatic and, often, the intrahepatic bile ducts. The lesion may appear as an isolated entity or may occur in association with inflammatory bowel disease, especially ulcerative colitis, or with multifocal fibrosclerosis syndromes such as retroperitoneal, mediastinal, and/or periureteral fibrosis, Riedel's struma, or pseudotumor of the orbit. Papillary stenosis and sclerosing cholangitis are also important complications of AIDS; cytomegalovirus and cryptosporidia infections have been observed frequently in such patients, raising the question whether these microbes may be a pathogenetic factor in primary sclerosing cholangitis. Secondary sclerosing cholangitis may occur as a long-term complication of choledocholithiasis, cholangiocarcinoma, operative or traumatic biliary injury, or contiguous inflammatory processes.

Patients with sclerosing cholangitis often present with signs and symptoms of chronic or intermittent biliary obstruction: jaundice, pruritus, right upper quadrant abdominal pain, or acute cholangitis. Late in the course, complete biliary obstruction, secondary biliary cirrhosis, hepatic failure, or portal hypertension with bleeding varices may occur. The diagnosis is usually established by finding thickened ducts with narrow, beaded lumina on cholangiography (see Fig. 272-2D). The cholangiographic technique of choice in suspected cases is probably ERCP, since intrahepatic ductal involvement may make PTHC difficult. When a diagnosis of sclerosing cholangitis has been established, a search for associated diseases, especially for chronic inflammatory bowel disease, should be carried out.

Therapy with cholestyramine may help control symptoms of pruritus, and antibiotics are useful when cholangitis complicates the clinical picture. Vitamin D and calcium supplementation may help prevent the loss of bone mass frequently seen in patients with chronic cholestasis. Glucocorticoids have not been shown to be efficacious. Preliminary studies have identified three promising drugs that appear to be of benefit, i.e., urodeoxycholic acid, methotrexate, and cyclosporine. In cases where complete or high-grade biliary obstruction has occurred, balloon dilatation or surgical intervention may be appropriate. Efforts at biliary-enteric anastomosis or stent placement may, however, be complicated by recurrent cholangitis and further progression of the stenosing process. The role of colectomy in patients with sclerosing cholangitis complicating chronic ulcerative colitis is uncertain. The prognosis is unfavorable, with a mean survival of 4 to 10 years following the diagnosis, regardless of therapy. Primary sclerosing cholangitis is one of the most common indications for liver transplantation. In one study, the mean follow-up time from the diagnosis of primary sclerosing cholangitis to the time of liver transplantation was 5.8 years.

CHOLANGIOCARCINOMA Benign tumors of the extrahepatic bile ducts are extremely rare causes of mechanical biliary obstruction. The majority of these are papillomas, adenomas, or cystadenomas which present with obstructive jaundice or hemobilia. Adenocarcinoma of the extrahepatic ducts is relatively more common. There is a slight male preponderance (60 percent), and the peak age incidence is in the fifth to seventh decades. Apparent predisposing factors include (1) some chronic hepatobiliary parasitic infestations, (2) congenital anomalies with ectactic ducts, (3) sclerosing cholangitis and chronic ulcerative colitis, and (4) occupational exposure to possible biliary tract carcinogens (workers in rubber or automotive plants). Cholelithiasis is not clearly associated with cholangiocarci-

noma as a predisposing factor. The lesions may be diffuse or nodular; the latter often arise at the confluence of the hepatic ducts (Klatskin tumors). This tumor is usually associated with a *collapsed* gallbladder, and such a finding mandates that the proximal hepatic ducts be optimally visualized by cholangiography.

Patients with cholangiocarcinoma usually present with biliary obstruction, painless jaundice, pruritus, weight loss, and acholic stools. A deep-seated, vaguely localized RUQ pain may be an associated complaint. Hepatomegaly and a palpable, distended gallbladder are frequent accompanying signs. Fever is unusual unless associated with ascending cholangitis. Because the obstructing process is gradual, the cholangiocarcinoma is often far advanced by the time it presents clinically. The diagnosis is most frequently made by cholangiography following ultrasound demonstration of dilated intrahepatic bile ducts. Any focal strictures of the bile ducts should probably be considered malignant until proved otherwise. Long-term palliation of the tumor is possible in some cases when radiation and/or chemotherapy are combined with palliative drainage of the biliary tree.

CARCINOMA OF THE PAPILLA OF VATER The ampulla of Vater may be involved by extension of tumor arising elsewhere in the duodenum or may itself be the primary site of origin of sarcomas, carcinoid tumors, or adenocarcinomas. Papillary adenocarcinomas are associated with slow growth and a more favorable clinical prognosis than diffuse, infiltrative cancers of the ampulla, which are more frequently widely invasive. The presenting clinical manifestation is usually obstructive jaundice. ERCP is probably the preferred diagnostic technique when ampullary carcinoma is suspected, because it allows for direct endoscopic inspection and biopsy of the ampulla as well as for performance of pancreatography to exclude a diagnosis of pancreatic malignancy. Cancer of the papilla is usually treated by wide, often radical, surgical excision. Lymph node or other metastases are present at the time of surgery in approximately 20 percent of cases, and the 5-year survival rate following surgical therapy in this group is only 5 to 10 percent. In the absence of metastases, however, radical pancreaticoduodenectomy (Whipple procedure) is associated with 5-year survival rates as high as 40 percent, and several long-term survivors have been reported.

REFERENCES

BARKUN JS et al: Randomised controlled trial of laparoscopic versus mini cholecystectomy. Lancet 340:1116, 1992

BARR F et al: Disorders of bile acid metabolism in cholesterol gallstone disease. J Clin Invest 90:589, 1992

CAREY MC et al: Whither biliary sludge? Gastroenterology 95:508, 1988

CELLO JP: Acquired immunodeficiency syndrome cholangiopathy: Spectrum of disease. Am J Med 86:539, 1989

DOWLING RH et al: Gallstone recurrence and post dissolution management, in *Enterohepatic Circulation of Bile Acids and Sterol Metabolism*, G Paumgartren, A Stichl, W Gersk (eds). Lancaster, PA, MTP Press, 1985, pp 361–369

GEENEN JE et al: The efficacy of endoscopic sphincterotomy after cholecystectomy in patients with sphincter-of-Oddi dysfunction. N Engl J Med 320:82, 1989

GRACIE WA, RANSOHOFF DF: The natural history of silent gallstones. The innocent gallstone is not a myth. N Engl J Med 307:798, 1982

HOLZBACH RT et al: Biliary proteins: Unique inhibitors of cholesterol crystal nucleation in human gallbladder bile. J Clin Invest 72:35, 1984

JOHNSTON DE, KAPLAN MM: Medical progress: Pathogenesis and treatment of gallstones. N Engl J Med 328:412, 1993

LEE SP et al: Origin and fate of biliary sludge. Gastroenterology 94:170, 1988

LEVY PF et al: Human gallbladder mucin accelerates nucleation of cholesterol in artifical bile. Gastroenterology 87:270, 1984

MARINGHINI A et al: Gallstones, gallbladder cancer, and other gastrointestinal malignancies: An epidemiologic study in Rochester, Minnesota. Ann Intern Med 107:30, 1987

MEYERS WC: A prospective analysis of 1518 laparoscopic cholecystectomies. N Engl J Med 324:1073, 1991

PAUMGARTNER G et al: Gallstones: Pathogenesis. Lancet 338:1117, 1991

PODDA M et al: Efficacy and safety of a combination of dienodeoxycholic acid and ursodeoxycholic acid for gallstone dissolution. Gastroenterology 96:222, 1989

PORAYKO MK et al: Patients with asymptomatic primary sclerosing cholangitis frequently have progressive disease. Gastroenterology 98:1594, 1990

RANSOHOFF DF: Assessment of prophylactic cholecystectomy and medical therapy for diabetics with silent gallstones. Gastroenterology 92:1588, 1987

SACKMAN M et al: The Munich gallbladder lithotripsy study: Results of the first five years with 711 patients. Ann Intern Med 114:290, 1991

SAUERBRUCH T et al: Fragmentation of bile duct stones by extracorporeal shock waves. Gastroenterology 96:222, 1989
———— et al: Gallbladder stones: Management. Lancet 338:1121, 1991
SHAFFER EA et al: Cholescintigraphic detection of functional obstruction of the sphincter of Oddi: Effect of papillotomy. Gastroenterology 90:728, 1986
SILVIS SE et al: What is the post-cholecystectomy pain syndrome? Gastrointestinal Endoscopy 31:401, 1985
SMITH BF, LAMONT JT: The central issue of cholesterol gallstones. Hepatology 6:529, 1986

THISTLE JL et al: Dissolution of cholesterol gallbladder stones by methyl-tert-butyl ether administered by percutaneous transhepatic catheter. N Engl J Med 320:633, 1989
WIESNER RH et al: Comparison of clinicopathologic features of primary sclerosing cholangitis and primary biliary cirrhosis. Gastroenterology 88:108, 1985
YAP L et al: Acalculous biliary pain: Cholecystectomy alleviates symptoms in patients with abnormal cholescintigraphy. Gastroenterology 101:786, 1991

section 3   Disorders of the pancreas

273   APPROACH TO THE PATIENT WITH PANCREATIC DISEASE

PHILLIP P. TOSKES / NORTON J. GREENBERGER

GENERAL CONSIDERATIONS

Inflammatory disease of the pancreas may be acute or chronic. Although good data exist concerning the frequency of acute pancreatitis (about 5000 new cases per year in the United States with a mortality rate of about 10 percent), the number of patients who suffer with recurrent acute pancreatitis or chronic pancreatitis is largely undefined. Only one prospective study on the incidence of chronic pancreatitis is available; this showed an incidence of 8.2 new cases per 100,000 per year and a prevalence of 26.4 cases per 100,000. These numbers probably underestimate considerably the true incidence and prevalence, since non-alcohol-induced pancreatitis was largely ignored. At autopsy, the prevalence of chronic pancreatitis ranges from 0.04 to 5 percent. The relative inaccessibility of the pancreas to direct examination and the nonspecificity of the abdominal pain associated with pancreatitis make the diagnosis of pancreatitis difficult and usually dependent on elevation of blood amylase levels. Many patients with chronic pancreatitis do not have elevated blood amylase levels. Some patients with chronic pancreatitis develop signs and symptoms of pancreatic exocrine insufficiency, and thus objective evidence for pancreatic disease can be demonstrated. However, there is a very large reservoir of pancreatic exocrine function. Greater than 90 percent of the pancreas must be damaged before maldigestion of fat and protein is manifested. Even the secretin stimulation test, which is the most sensitive method of assessing pancreatic exocrine function, is probably abnormal only when greater than 60 percent of exocrine function has been lost. Noninvasive, indirect tests of pancreatic exocrine function (bentiromide, serum trypsinogen) are much more likely to be abnormal in patients with obvious pancreatic disease, i.e., pancreatic calcification, steatorrhea, or diabetes mellitus, than in patients with occult disease. Thus the number of patients who have subclinical exocrine dysfunction (i.e., less than 90 percent loss of function) is unknown.

The clinical manifestations of acute and chronic pancreatitis and pancreatic insufficiency are protean. Thus patients may present with hypertriglyceridemia, vitamin B_{12} malabsorption, hypercalcemia, hypocalcemia, hyperglycemia, ascites, pleural effusions, and chronic abdominal pain with normal amylase levels. Indeed, if the clinician considers pancreatitis as a possible diagnosis only when presented with a patient having classic symptoms (i.e., severe, constant epigastric pain that radiates through to the back, along with an elevated blood amylase level), only a minority of the patients with pancreatitis will be diagnosed correctly.

As emphasized in Chap. 274, the etiologies as well as the clinical manifestations are quite varied. Although it is well appreciated that *pancreatitis* is frequently secondary to alcohol abuse and biliary tract disease, pancreatitis is also caused by drugs, trauma, and viral infections and is associated with metabolic and connective tissue disorders. In addition, in approximately 20 percent of patients with acute pancreatitis and 25 to 40 percent of patients with chronic pancreatitis, the etiology is obscure.

TESTS USEFUL IN THE DIAGNOSIS OF PANCREATIC DISEASE

Several tests have proved of value in the evaluation of pancreatic exocrine function. Examples of specific tests and usefulness in the diagnosis of acute and chronic pancreatitis are summarized in Table 273-1. At most institutions, pancreatic function tests are performed if the diagnosis of pancreatic disease remains a possibility after noninvasive tests (ultrasound, computed tomographic scan) and invasive tests (ERCP) are normal or inconclusive. In this regard, tests employing *direct* stimulation of the pancreas are the most sensitive.

PANCREATIC ENZYMES IN BODY FLUIDS   The serum amylase level is widely used as a screening test for acute pancreatitis in the patient with acute abdominal pain or back pain. A value greater than 150 Somogyi units per deciliter should raise the question of acute pancreatitis. Levels greater than 300 units make the diagnosis more likely, and values greater than three times normal virtually clinch the diagnosis if gut perforation or infarction is excluded. In acute pancreatitis the serum amylase is usually elevated within 24 h and remains so for 1 to 3 days. Levels return to normal within 3 to 5 days unless there is extensive pancreatic necrosis, incomplete ductal obstruction, or pseudocyst formation. Approximately 85 percent of patients with acute pancreatitis will have an elevated serum amylase. Normal values, however, may occur if (1) there is a delay (2 to 5 days) in obtaining blood samples, (2) the underlying disorder is chronic pancreatitis rather than acute pancreatitis, and (3) hypertriglyceridemia is present. Patients with hypertriglyceridemia and proven pancreatitis have been found to have spuriously low levels of amylase and lipase activity.

The serum amylase is often elevated in other conditions (Table 273-2), in part because the enzyme is found in many organs in addition to the pancreas (salivary glands, liver, small intestine, kidney, fallopian tube) and can be produced by various tumors (carcinoma of the lung, esophagus, breast, and ovary). Isoenzymes of amylase fall into two general categories, those arising from the pancreas (P isoamylases) and those from nonpancreatic sources (S isoamylases). The measurement of serum isoamylases is of clinical importance. Isoamylase analysis of normal serum shows that about

TABLE 273-1 Tests useful in the diagnosis of acute and chronic pancreatitis and pancreatic tumors

Test	Principle	Comment
PANCREATIC ENZYMES IN BODY FLUIDS		
Amylase		
1 Serum	Pancreatic inflammation leads to increased enzyme levels	Simple; 20–40% false-negatives and -positives; reliable if test results are three times the upper limit of normal
2 Urine	Renal clearance of amylase is increased in acute pancreatitis	May be abnormal when serum levels normal; false-negatives and -positives
3 Amylase/creatinine clearance ratio (C_{am}/C_{cr})	Renal clearance of amylase greater than clearance of creatinine	No more sensitive than the serum amylase; many false-positives
4 Ascitic fluid	Disruption of gland or main pancreatic duct leads to increased amylase concentration	Can establish diagnosis of pancreatitis; false-positives with intestinal obstruction and perforated ulcer
5 Pleural fluid	Exudative pleural effusion with pancreatitis	False-positives with carcinoma of the lung and esophageal perforation
6 Isoenzymes	P isoamylases arise from the pancreas; S isoamylases are from other sources	More sensitive than total serum amylase in diagnosis of acute pancreatitis; useful in identifying nonpancreatic causes of hyperamylasemia
Serum lipase	Pancreatic inflammation leads to increased enzyme levels	New methods of determination greatly simplified; positive in 70–85% of cases.
Serum trypsin-like immunoreactivity (TLI)	Pancreatic inflammation leads to increased levels	*Elevated* in acute pancreatitis; *decreased* in chronic pancreatitis *with* steatorrhea; normal in chronic pancreatitis *without* steatorrhea and steatorrhea with normal pancreatic function
Pancreatic polypeptide (PP)	PP confined almost totally to the pancreas; release stimulated by nutrients and hormones; such release parallels pancreatic enzyme secretion	Basal, meal-simulated, and hormone (secretin CCK)-stimulated PP levels *decreased* in chronic pancreatitis; fasting PP levels >125 pg/mL argues against chronic pancreatitis and pancreatic cancer
STUDIES PERTAINING TO PANCREATIC STRUCTURE		
Radiologic and radionuclide tests		
1 Plain film of the abdomen	Abnormal in acute and chronic pancreatitis	Simple; normal in >50% of both acute and chronic pancreatitis
2 Upper gastrointestinal x-rays	Abnormally thickened duodenal folds; displacement of stomach or widening of duodenal loop suggests a pancreatic mass (inflammatory, neoplastic, cystic)	Simple; frequently normal; largely superseded by US and CT scanning
3 Ultrasonography (US)	Can provide information on edema, inflammation, calcification, pseudocysts, and mass lesions	Simple, noninvasive; sequential studies quite feasible; useful in diagnosis of pseudocyst
4 CT scan	Permits detailed visualization of pancreas and surrounding structures	Useful in the diagnosis of pancreatic calcification, dilated pancreatic ducts, and pancreatic tumors; may not be able to distinguish between inflammatory and neoplastic mass lesions
5 Selective angiography	Can identify pancreatic neoplasms (1) by sheathing of celiac or superior mesenteric branches by tumor or (2) by tumor staining; displacement of vessels by tumor	Indicated (1) in suspected islet cell tumors and (2) prior to pancreatic or duodenal resection; most reliable features reflect nonresectable pancreatic cancer
6 Endoscopic retrograde cholangiopancreatography (ERCP)	Cannulation of pancreatic and common bile duct permits visualization of pancreatic-biliary ductal system	Provides diagnostic data in 60–85% of cases; differentiation of chronic pancreatitis from pancreatic carcinoma may be difficult
Pancreatic biopsy with US or CT guidance	Percutaneous biopsy with skinny needle and localization of lesion by US	High diagnostic yield; laparotomy avoided; requires special technical skills
TESTS OF EXOCRINE PANCREATIC FUNCTION		
Direct stimulation of the pancreas with analysis of duodenal contents		
1 Secretin-pancreozymin (CCK) test	Secretin leads to increased output of pancreatic juice and HCO_3^-; CCK leads to increased output of pancreatic enzymes; pancreatic secretory response related to functional mass of pancreatic tissue	Sensitive enough to detect occult disease; involves duodenal intubation and fluoroscopy; poorly defined normal enzyme response; overlap in chronic pancreatitis; large secretory reserve capacity of the pancreas
Indirect stimulation of pancreas with measurement of pancreatic enzymes		
1 Lundh test meal	Test meal (fat, carbohydrate, and protein) causes increased release of CCK, which causes increased enzyme output; trypsin concentration measured	Useful in pancreatic exocrine insufficiency; false-negatives with delayed gastric emptying; false-positives in primary mucosal disease of the gut and choledocholithiasis; does not measure secretory capacity
2 Benzoyl-tyrosyl-*p*-aminobenzoic (Bz-Ty-PABA, bentiromide) test	Synthetic peptide (Bz-Ty-PABA) specifically cleaved by chymotrypsin, liberating PABA which is absorbed and PABA metabolite excreted in the urine	Simple and reliable test of pancreatic exocrine function. Measurement of blood PABA level increases sensitivity.
3 Pancreolauryl test	Fluorescein dilaurate is hydrolyzed by pancreatic elastase which is absorbed and fluorescein measured in urine	Sensitivity and specificity similar to Bentiromide test

TABLE 273-1   Tests useful in the diagnosis of acute and chronic pancreatitis and pancreatic tumors *(continued)*

Test	Principle	Comment
Measurement of intraluminal digestion products		
1 Microscopic examination of stool for undigested meat fibers and fat	Lack of proteolytic and lipolytic enzymes causes decreased digestion of meat fibers and triglycerides	Simple, reliable; not sensitive enough to detect milder cases of pancreatic insufficiency
2 Quantitative stool fat determination	Lack of lipolytic enzymes brings about impaired fat digestion	Reliable, reference standard for defining severity of malabsorption; does not distinguish between maldigestion and malabsorption
3 Fecal nitrogen	Lack of proteolytic enzymes leads to impaired protein digestion, increase in stool nitrogen	Does not distinguish between maldigestion and malabsorption; low sensitivity
Measurement of pancreatic enzymes in feces		
1 Chymotrypsin	Pancreatic secretion of proteolytic enzymes	May be useful in cystic fibrosis; tedious; 10% false-positive and false-negative results
Miscellaneous tests		
1 Dual-labeled Schilling test	Intrinsic factor [^{57}Co]cobalamin and Hog R protein [^{58}Co]cobalamin are given together. Since proteases are necessary to cleave R protein, the ratio of labeled cobalamin excreted in urine is an index of exocrine dysfunction.	Time-consuming and expensive

35 to 45 percent of the amylase is of pancreatic origin. For example, in patients with acute pancreatitis, the total serum amylase level returns to normal more rapidly than pancreatic isoamylase. Thus, in patients seen after the first day, the pancreatic isoamylase level is a more sensitive indicator of pancreatitis than the total serum amylase level. In addition, in certain conditions, such as the postoperative

state, acute alcohol intoxication, and diabetic ketoacidosis, it had been assumed that elevations in serum amylase indicated acute pancreatitis. However, the elevation of serum amylase in such conditions has been shown to actually be of the S type. Simple tests to distinguish pancreatic amylase from nonpancreatic amylase are no longer readily available, and such tests are often not reliable when the total amylase is minimally to moderately elevated. The serum trypsinogen (performed by several commercial laboratories) is quite helpful in this regard. Since this enzyme is secreted specifically by the pancreas, a normal serum trypsinogen level in a patient with minimal elevation of serum amylase essentially rules out acute pancreatitis. Urinary amylase measurements, including the amylase/creatinine clearance ratio, offer no increased sensitivity or specificity over blood amylase levels.

Elevation of ascitic fluid amylase occurs in acute pancreatitis as well as (1) in pancreatogenous ascites due to disruption of the main pancreatic duct of a leaking pseudocyst and (2) in other abdominal disorders which simulate pancreatitis (e.g., intestinal obstruction, intestinal infarction, and perforated peptic ulcer). Elevation of pleural fluid amylase occurs in acute pancreatitis, chronic pancreatitis, carcinoma of the lung, and esophageal perforation.

Lipase may now be the single best enzyme to measure for the diagnosis of acute pancreatitis. Improvements in substrates and technology offer clinicians improved options, especially when a turbidometric assay is used. The newer lipase assays have colipase as a cofactor and are fully automated. Nevertheless, a word of caution is in order. Many hospital laboratories are now using the Ektachem technique because it is rapid and contains the appropriate substrates. However, at least two reports have demonstrated poor specificity with this technique, i.e., patients with nonpancreatic disorders having elevated lipase levels.

Assay for trypsinogen (or trypsin-like immunoreactivity) has a theoretical advantage over amylase and lipase determinations in that the pancreas is the only organ that contains this enzyme. The test appears to be useful in the diagnosis of both acute and chronic pancreatitis. Sensitivity and specificity are comparable to amylase and lipase determinations. Since trypsinogen is also excreted by the kidney, elevated values are found in renal failure, as is the case with serum amylase and lipase levels. No single blood test is reliable for the diagnosis of acute pancreatitis in patients with renal failure. Whether a patient with renal failure and abdominal pain has pancreatitis remains a difficult clinical problem. A recent study found that in patients with renal dysfunction, serum amylase levels were elevated only when creatinine clearance was less than 50 mL/min. In such patients, the serum amylase level was invariably less than 500 IU/L in the absence of objective evidence of acute pancreatitis. In that

TABLE 273-2   Causes of hyperamylasemia and hyperamylasuria

PANCREATIC DISEASE

A Pancreatitis
  1 Acute
  2 Chronic: ductal obstruction
  3 Complications of pancreatitis
    a Pancreatic pseudocyst
    b Pancreatogenous ascites
    c Pancreatic abscess
B Pancreatic trauma
C Pancreatic carcinoma

NONPANCREATIC DISORDERS

A Renal insufficiency
B Salivary gland lesions
  1 Mumps
  2 Calculus
  3 Irradiation sialadenitis
  4 Maxillofacial surgery
C "Tumor" hyperamylasemia
  1 Carcinoma of the lung
  2 Carcinoma of the esophagus
  3 Breast carcinoma, ovarian carcinoma
D Macroamylasemia
E Burns
F Diabetic ketoacidosis
G Pregnancy
H Renal transplantation
I Cerebral trauma
J Drugs: morphine

OTHER ABDOMINAL DISORDERS

A Biliary tract disease: cholecystitis, choledocholithiasis
B Intraabdominal disease
  1 Perforated or penetrating peptic ulcer
  2 Intestinal obstruction or infarction
  3 Ruptured ectopic pregnancy
  4 Peritonitis
  5 Aortic aneurysm
  6 Chronic liver disease
  7 Postoperative hyperamylasemia

SOURCE: After WB Salt II, S Schenker, Medicine 55:269, 1976.

study, serum lipase and trypsin levels paralleled serum amylase values.

A recent study evaluated the sensitivity and specificity of five assays used to diagnose acute pancreatitis: two amylase assays, one lipase, one trypsin-like immunoreactivity (TLI), and one pancreatic isoamylase. The data obtained show that (1) if the best cutoff level is used, all assays have similar specificities and suggest that (2) total serum amylase is as good an indicator of acute pancreatitis as any of the others. However, inherent in many such studies is the problem that the recognition and diagnosis of acute pancreatitis hinge on the finding of an elevated serum amylase level. The question arises as to whether any diagnostic test result can be proved superior to the total serum amylase level if hyperamylasemia is required for the diagnosis. In other studies, when "objective" confirmation of the clinical diagnosis of pancreatitis was required (ultrasonography, computed tomography, laparotomy), the sensitivity of the serum amylase has been as low as 68 percent. With these limitations in mind, the recommended screening tests for acute pancreatitis are *total serum amylase* and *serum lipase activities*. Serum amylase values greater than three times normal are highly specific.

STUDIES PERTAINING TO PANCREATIC STRUCTURE   Radiologic tests   Plain films of the abdomen provide useful information in 30 to 50 percent of patients with acute pancreatitis. The most frequent abnormalities include (1) a localized ileus usually involving the jejunum ("sentinel loop"), (2) a generalized ileus with air-fluid levels, (3) the "colon cutoff sign," which results from isolated distention of the transverse colon, (4) duodenal distention with air-fluid levels, and (5) a mass, which is frequently a pseudocyst. In chronic pancreatitis, an important radiographic finding is pancreatic calcification, which characteristically is localized adjacent to and superimposed on the second lumbar vertebra (see Fig. 274-3A).

Upper gastrointestinal x-rays may reveal displacement of the stomach by the retroperitoneal mass (see Fig. 274-2A) or widening and effacement of the duodenal C loop, which also suggest the presence of a pancreatic mass that could be an inflammatory, cystic, or neoplastic process. However, their use has been largely superseded by ultrasound.

Ultrasonography (echography) can provide important information in patients with acute pancreatitis, chronic pancreatitis, pancreatic calcification, pseudocyst, and pancreatic carcinoma. It is a useful procedure in the evaluation of the patient with acute pancreatitis. Echographic appearances can indicate the presence of edema, inflammation, and calcification (not obvious on plain films of the abdomen), as well as pseudocysts, mass lesions, and gallstones (see Figs. 274-2B and 274-3B). In acute pancreatitis, the pancreas is characteristically enlarged. In pancreatic pseudocyst, the usual appearance is that of an echo-free, smooth, round fluid collection. Pancreatic carcinoma distorts the usual landmarks, and mass lesions greater than 3.0 cm are usually detected as localized, echo-free solid lesions. Ultrasound is often the initial investigation for most patients with suspected pancreatic disease. However, obesity, excess small- and large-bowel gas, and recently performed barium contrast examinations can interfere with ultrasound studies, which are often technically unsatisfactory.

Computed tomography (CT) is the best imaging study for initial evaluation of a suspected chronic pancreatic disorder and for the complications of acute and chronic pancreatitis. It is especially useful in the detection of pancreatic tumors, fluid-containing lesions such as pseudocysts and abscesses, and calcium deposits (see Figs. 274-3C and 274-4A). Most lesions are characterized by (1) enlargement of the pancreatic outline, (2) distortion of the pancreatic contour, or (3) fluid-containing lesions that have different attenuation coefficients than normal pancreas. However, it is occasionally difficult to distinguish between inflammatory and neoplastic lesions. Oral water-soluble contrast agents may be used to opacify the stomach and duodenum during CT scans; this permits more precise delineation of various organs as well as mass lesions. Dynamic (rapid intravenously administered contrast) CT scans are useful in estimating the degree of pancreatic necrosis and in predicting morbidity and mortality.

Selective catheterization of the celiac and superior mesenteric arteries combined with superselective catheterization of others such as the hepatic, splenic, and gastroduodenal arteries permits visualization of the pancreas and detection of pancreatic neoplasms and pseudocysts. Pancreatic neoplasms can be identified by the sheathing of blood vessels by a mass lesion (see Fig. 274-1D). Hormone-producing pancreatic tumors are especially likely to exhibit increased vascularity and tumor staining. Angiographic abnormalities are noted in many patients with pancreatic carcinoma but are uncommon in patients without pancreatic disease. Angiography complements ultrasonography and endoscopic retrograde cholangiopancreatography (ERCP) in the study of a patient with a suspected pancreatic lesion and may be carried out if ERCP is either unsuccessful or nondiagnostic.

Endoscopic retrograde cholangiopancreatography   ERCP may provide useful information on the status of the pancreatic ductal system and thus aid in the differential diagnosis of pancreatic disease (see Figs. 274-1C, 274-3D, and 274-4B). Pancreatic carcinoma is characterized by stenosis or obstruction of either the pancreatic duct or the common bile duct; both ductal systems are often abnormal. In chronic pancreatitis, ERCP abnormalities include (1) luminal narrowing, (2) irregularities in the ductal system with stenosis, dilatation, sacculation, and ectasia, and (3) blockage of the pancreatic duct by calcium deposits. Differentiation from carcinoma may be difficult because of similar overlapping features, i.e., ductal stenosis and irregularity. Elevated serum and/or urine amylase levels following ERCP have been reported in 25 to 75 percent of patients, but clinical pancreatitis is uncommon. In a series of 300 patients, pancreatitis occurred in only 5 patients following ERCP. If no lesion is found within the biliary and/or pancreatic ducts in a patient with repeated attacks of acute pancreatitis, manometric studies of the sphincter of Oddi may be indicated. Such studies, however, do increase the risk of post-ERCP/manometry acute pancreatitis. Such pancreatitis appears to be more common in patients with a nondilated pancreatic duct.

Pancreatic biopsy with radiologic guidance   Percutaneous aspiration biopsy of a pancreatic mass often distinguishes a pancreatic inflammatory mass from a pancreatic neoplasm.

TESTS OF EXOCRINE PANCREATIC FUNCTION

Pancreatic function tests (see Table 273-1) can be divided into the following:

1 *Direct stimulation of the pancreas* by intravenous infusion of secretin or secretin plus cholecystokinin (CCK) followed by collection and measurement of duodenal contents
2 *Indirect stimulation of the pancreas* utilizing nutrients or amino acids, fatty acids, and synthetic peptides followed by assay of proteolytic, lipolytic, and amylolytic enzymes
3 Study of *intraluminal digestion products* such as undigested meat fibers, stool fat, and fecal nitrogen
4 *Measurement of fecal pancreatic enzymes* such as chymotrypsin

The secretin test, used to detect diffuse pancreatic disease, is based on the physiologic principle that the pancreatic secretory response is directly related to the functional mass of pancreatic tissue. In the standard assay, secretin is given intravenously in a dose of 1 clinical unit (CU) per kilogram, either as a bolus or continuous infusion. Obviously, results will vary with the secretin preparation used, dose, mode of administration, and completeness of collection of duodenal contents. Normal values for the standard secretin test are (1) volume output >2.0 mL/kg per hour, (2) bicarbonate (HCO_3^-) concentration >80 mmol/L, and (3) HCO_3^- output >10 mmol in 1 h. The most reproducible measurement having the highest level of discrimination between normal subjects and patients with chronic pancreatitis appears to be the maximal bicarbonate concentration.

The *combined secretin-CCK test* permits measurement of pancreatic amylase, lipase, trypsin, and chymotrypsin. Although there is overlap in the distribution of enzyme output in normal subjects and patients with pancreatitis, markedly decreased enzyme outputs suggest advanced damage and destruction of acinar cells. With frank exocrine pancreatic insufficiency there is usually an overall reduction in both HCO_3^- concentration and output of several enzymes. However, with lesser degrees of pancreatic damage there may be a dissociation between HCO_3^- concentration and enzyme output. There also may be a dissociation between the results of the secretin test and other tests of absorptive function. For example, patients with chronic pancreatitis often have abnormally low outputs of HCO_3^- after secretin but have normal fecal fat excretion. Thus the secretin test measures the secretory capacity of ductular epithelium, while fecal fat excretion indirectly reflects intraluminal lipolytic activity. Steatorrhea does not occur until intraluminal levels of lipase are markedly reduced, underscoring the fact that only small amounts of enzymes are necessary for intraluminal digestive activities. An abnormal secretin test should suggest only that chronic pancreatic damage is present; it will not consistently distinguish between chronic pancreatitis and pancreatic carcinoma.

Another test of exocrine pancreatic function, which indirectly reflects intraluminal chymotrypsin activity, has been evaluated in patients with pancreatic disease. This test (the *tripeptide hydrolysis* or *bentiromide test*) utilizes a synthetic peptide, N-benzoyl-L-tyrosyl-p-aminobenzoic acid (Bz-Ty-PABA), that is specifically cleaved by chymotrypsin to Bz-Ty and PABA. Normally, after oral administration, the peptide reaches the small intestine, where it is hydrolyzed by chymotrypsin with the liberation of PABA, which is rapidly absorbed and excreted in the urine. Results in several hundred patients with chronic pancreatitis and other disorders indicate that PABA excretion is significantly lower in chronic pancreatitis compared with controls. Depending on the severity of pancreatic exocrine impairment, the overall sensitivity is 60 percent (range 46 to 74 percent), and the specificity if coupled with a D-xylose test approximates 90 percent. Measurement of blood PABA levels increases sensitivity.

Measurement of *intraluminal digestion products*, i.e., undigested muscle fibers, stool fat, and fecal nitrogen, is discussed in Chap. 254. Measurement of chymotrypsin in stool reflects pancreatic output of this proteolytic enzyme. Decreased chymotrypsin activity in stool has been reported in patients with chronic pancreatitis and cystic fibrosis. However, normal values may occur in patients with pancreatic insufficiency, and false-positive results have been reported in up to 10 percent of normal individuals.

Tests useful in the diagnosis of exocrine pancreatic insufficiency and the differential diagnosis of malabsorption are also discussed in Chaps. 254 and 274.

274   ACUTE AND CHRONIC PANCREATITIS

NORTON J. GREENBERGER / PHILLIP P. TOSKES / KURT J. ISSELBACHER

BIOCHEMISTRY AND PHYSIOLOGY OF PANCREATIC EXOCRINE SECRETION

GENERAL CONSIDERATIONS   The pancreas secretes 1500 to 3000 mL isosmotic alkaline (pH >8.0) fluid per day containing about 20 enzymes and zymogens. The pancreatic secretions provide the enzymes needed to effect the major digestive activity of the gastrointestinal tract and provide an optimal pH for the function of these enzymes.

REGULATION OF PANCREATIC SECRETION   Hormonal and

neural mechanisms   The exocrine pancreas is under both hormonal and neural control, with hormonal control being of primary importance. *Gastric acid* is the stimulus for the release of secretin, a peptide with 27 amino acids. Sensitive radioimmunoassay studies for secretin suggest that the pH threshold for the release of secretin from the duodenum and jejunum is 4.5. Secretin stimulates the secretion of pancreatic juice rich in *water and electrolytes*. Release of cholecystokinin (CCK) from the duodenum and jejunum is largely produced by long-chain fatty acids, certain essential amino acids (tryptophan, phenylalanine, valine, methionine), and gastric acid itself. CCK evokes an *enzyme-rich secretion from the pancreas*. Gastrin, although it shares an identical terminal tetrapeptide with CCK, is a weak stimulus for pancreatic enzyme output. The *parasympathetic nervous system* (via the vagus) exerts some control over pancreatic secretion. Part of this is mediated by the release of gastrin, and part is secondary to a direct effect of acetylcholine on the pancreatic acinar cell. Also, vagal stimulation effects release of vasoactive intestinal peptide (VIP), a secretin agonist. Vagal control of pancreatic secretion seems to be most important following a truncal vagotomy, but even in such patients severe maldigestion does not ensue. Bile salts also stimulate pancreatic secretion, thereby integrating the functions of the biliary tract, pancreas, and small intestine.

Pancreatic secretion at the cellular level   There appear to be two functionally distinct pathways by which secretagogues can stimulate pancreatic secretion. Studies with isolated pancreatic acinar cells indicate that secretin, VIP, and cholera toxin interact with receptors on the acinar cell, leading to an increase in cellular cyclic adenosine monophosphate (cyclic AMP). CCK, acetylcholine, gastrin, and various other peptides (e.g., bombesin, caerulein) react with other receptors on the acinar cell to cause an increased turnover of phosphatidylinositol and the release of membrane calcium and induce changes in the electrical properties of the pancreatic acinar cell surface and junctional membranes. When a secretagogue that increases cyclic AMP is added to a secretagogue that increases calcium outflux, potentiation of enzyme secretion occurs.

WATER AND ELECTROLYTE SECRETION   Although sodium, potassium, chloride, calcium, zinc, phosphate, and sulfate are found within pancreatic secretion, *bicarbonate is the ion of primary physiologic importance*. In the acini and in the ducts, secretin causes the cells to add water and bicarbonate to the fluid. In the ducts, an exchange occurs between bicarbonate and chloride. There is a good correlation between the maximal bicarbonate output after stimulation with secretin and the pancreatic mass. The bicarbonate output of 120 to 300 mmol/d helps neutralize gastric acid production and creates the appropriate pH for the activity of the pancreatic enzymes.

ENZYME SECRETION   The pancreas secretes amylolytic, lipolytic, and proteolytic enzymes. Amylolytic enzymes such as amylase hydrolyze starch to oligosaccharides and to the disaccharide maltose. The *lipolytic enzymes* include lipase, phospholipase A, and cholesterol esterase. Bile salts *inhibit* lipase, but colipase, another constituent of pancreatic secretion, binds to lipase and prevents this inhibition. Bile salts *activate* phospholipase A and cholesterol esterase. *Proteolytic enzymes* include *endopeptidases* (trypsin, chymotrypsin), which act on the internal peptide bonds of proteins and polypeptides; exopeptidases (carboxypeptidases, aminopeptidases), which act on the free carboxyl-terminal end and free amino-terminal end of peptides, respectively; and elastase. The proteolytic enzymes are secreted as inactive precursors (zymogens). Ribonucleases (deoxyribonucleases, ribonuclease) are also secreted. While parallel secretion of pancreatic enzymes usually occurs, nonparallel secretion can occur as a result of exocytosis from heterogeneous sources within the pancreas. *Enterokinase*, an enzyme found within the duodenal mucosa, cleaves the lysine-isoleucine bond of trypsinogen to form trypsin. Trypsin then activates the other proteolytic zymogens in a cascade phenomenon. All pancreatic enzymes have pH optima in the alkaline range.

AUTOPROTECTION OF THE PANCREAS   Autodigestion of the pancreas is prevented by the packaging of proteases in precursor form and by the synthesis of protease inhibitors. These protease inhibitors are found within the acinar cell, the pancreatic secretions, and the alpha$_1$- and alpha$_2$-globulin fractions of plasma.

EXOCRINE-ENDOCRINE RELATIONSHIPS Pancreatic glucagon (29 amino acid residues) has a high degree of structural similarity to secretin. It decreases volume and enzyme secretion by the pancreas but not bicarbonate secretion. Glucose, in large concentrations, also may inhibit pancreatic exocrine secretion. The choleretic and insulinotropic effects of secretin are shared by glucagon.

ENTEROPANCREATIC AXIS AND FEEDBACK INHIBITION Pancreatic enzyme secretion in human beings is controlled, at least in part, by a negative feedback mechanism induced by the presence of active serine proteases in the duodenum. To illustrate, intraduodenal perfusion with phenylalanine causes a prompt increase in plasma CCK levels as well as increased secretion of chymotrypsin. However, simultaneous perfusion with trypsin blunts both responses. Conversely, duodenal perfusion with protease inhibitors actually leads to enzyme hypersecretion. It appears that serine proteases inhibit pancreatic secretion by acting on a CCK-releasing peptide found within the lumen of the small intestine.

ACUTE PANCREATITIS

GENERAL CONSIDERATIONS Pancreatic inflammatory disease may be classified as (1) acute pancreatitis and (2) chronic pancreatitis by primarily clinical criteria, the obvious difference between them being restoration of normal function in the former and permanent residual damage in the latter. The pathologic spectrum of acute pancreatitis varies from *edematous pancreatitis*, which is usually a mild and self-limited disorder, to *necrotizing pancreatitis*, in which the degree of pancreatic necrosis correlates with the severity of the attack and its systemic manifestations. The term *hemorrhagic pancreatitis* is less meaningful in a clinical sense because variable amounts of interstitial hemorrhage can be found in pancreatitis as well as in other disorders such as pancreatic trauma, pancreatic carcinoma, and severe congestive heart failure.

The incidence of pancreatitis varies in different countries and depends on cause, e.g., alcohol, gallstones, metabolic factors, and drugs (Table 274-1). In the United States, for example, acute pancreatitis is related to alcohol ingestion more commonly than to gallstones; in England, the opposite obtains. Epidemiologic data based on autopsy data indicate that in the United States the overall prevalence of acute pancreatitis is approximately 0.5 percent. An upward trend has been noted in the crude death rate.

ETIOLOGY AND PATHOGENESIS There are many causes of acute pancreatitis (see Table 274-1), but the mechanisms by which these conditions trigger pancreatic inflammation have not been identified. Alcoholic patients with pancreatitis may represent a special subset, since most alcoholics do not develop pancreatitis. The list of identifiable causes is growing, and it is likely that pancreatitis related to viral infections, drugs, and as yet undefined factors is more common than heretofore recognized.

Approximately 5 percent of cases of acute pancreatitis are drug related (see Table 274-1). The pancreatitis can be mild or severe; over 85 drugs have been implicated, but many of these reports involve single cases. Drugs cause pancreatitis either by a hypersensitivity reaction or generation of a toxic metabolite, although in some cases this differentiation is not clear. Conventional criteria for establishing that a drug definitely causes pancreatitis are as follows: (1) no other drugs are involved, (2) other causes are excluded, and (3) there is a positive rechallenge. However, in some instances in which a drug has been implicated in several dozen cases, the latter criterion has not been met.

Autodigestion is one pathogenetic theory which proposes that proteolytic enzymes (e.g., trypsinogen, chymotrypsinogen, proelastase, and phospholipase A) are activated within the pancreas rather than in the intestinal lumen. A number of factors (e.g., endotoxins, exotoxins, viral infections, ischemia, anoxia, and direct trauma) are

TABLE 274-1 Causes of acute pancreatitis

Alcohol ingestion (acute and chronic alcoholism)
Biliary tract disease (gallstones)
Postoperative (abdominal, nonabdominal)
Postendoscopic retrograde cholangiopancreatography (ERCP)
Trauma (especially blunt abdominal type)
Metabolic
  A Hypertriglyceridemia
  B Apolipoprotein CII deficiency syndrome
  C Hypercalcemia (e.g., hyperparathyroidism), drug-induced
  D Renal failure
  E After renal transplantation*
  F Acute fatty liver of pregnancy†
Hereditary pancreatitis
Infections
  A Mumps
  B Viral hepatitis
  C Other viral infections (coxsackievirus, echovirus)
  D Ascariasis
  E Mycoplasma
Drug-associated
  A Definite association
    1 Azathioprine, 6-mercaptopurine
    2 Sulfonamides
    3 Thiazide diuretics
    4 Furosemide
    5 Estrogens (oral contraceptives)
    6 Tetracycline
    7 Valproic acid
    8 Pentamidine
    9 Dideoxyinosine (ddI)
  B Probable association
    1 Acetaminophen
    2 Chlorthalidone
    3 Ethacrynic acid
    4 Procainamide
    5 Erythromycin
    6 L-Asparaginase
    7 Metronidazole
    8 Nonsteroidal anti-inflammatory drugs (NSAIDs)
    9 Angiotensin-converting enzyme (ACE) inhibitors
Connective tissue disorders with vasculitis
  A Systemic lupus erythematosus
  B Necrotizing angiitis
  C Thrombotic thrombocytopenic purpura
Penetrating peptic ulcer
Obstruction of the ampulla of Vater
  A Regional enteritis
  B Duodenal diverticulum
Pancreas divisum
Recurrent bouts of acute pancreatitis without obvious cause
  A Consider
    1 Occult disease of the biliary tree or pancreatic ducts, especially occult gallstones (microlithiasis, sludge)
    2 Drugs
    3 Hypertriglyceridemia
    4 Pancreas divisum
    5 Pancreatic cancer
    6 Sphincter of Oddi dysfunction
    7 Cystic fibrosis
    8 Truly idiopathic

---

* Pancreatitis occurs in 3 percent of renal transplant patients and is due to many factors including surgery, hypercalcemia, drugs (glucocorticoids, azathioprine, L-asparaginase, diuretics), and viral infections.
† Pancreatitis also occurs in otherwise uncomplicated pregnancy and is most often associated with cholelithiasis.

believed to activate these proenzymes. Activated proteolytic enzymes, especially trypsin, not only digest pancreatic and peripancreatic tissues but also can activate other enzymes such as elastase and phospholipase. The active enzymes then digest cellular membranes and cause proteolysis, edema, interstitial hemorrhage, vascular damage, coagulation necrosis, fat necrosis, and parenchymal cell necrosis. Cellular injury and death result in the liberation of activated enzymes. In addition, activation and release of bradykinin peptides and vasoactive substances (e.g., histamine) are believed to produce vasodilatation, increased vascular permeability, and edema. There is thus a cascade of events culminating in the development of acute necrotizing pancreatitis.

The autodigestion theory has largely eclipsed two older theories.

First, the "common channel" theory holds that such an anatomic arrangement facilitates reflux of bile into the pancreatic duct, and this results in activation of pancreatic enzymes. (Actually, a common channel with free communication between the common bile duct and main pancreatic duct is infrequently encountered.) The second theory is that obstruction and hypersecretion are pivotal in the development of pancreatitis. Obstruction of the main pancreatic duct, however, produces pancreatic edema but not pancreatitis.

A recent hypothesis to explain the intrapancreatic activation of zymogens is that they become activated by *lysosomal hydrolases* within the pancreatic acinar cell itself. In two different types of experimental pancreatitis, it has been demonstrated that digestive enzymes and lysosomal hydrolases become admixed; as a result, the former can be activated within the acinar cell by the latter. In vitro, lysosomal enzymes such as cathepsin B can activate trypsinogen, and trypsin can activate the other protease precursors. It is still not clear, however, whether the appropriate pH (i.e., about 3.0) occurs within the human acinar cell to allow activation of trypsinogen by lysosomal hydrolases.

CLINICAL FEATURES *Abdominal pain* is the major symptom of acute pancreatitis. Pain may vary from a mild and tolerable discomfort to severe, constant, and incapacitating distress. Characteristically, the pain, which is steady and boring in character, is located in the epigastrium and periumbilical region and often radiates to the back as well as to the chest, flanks, and lower abdomen. The pain is frequently more intense when the patient is supine, and patients often obtain relief by sitting with the trunk flexed and knees drawn up. Nausea, vomiting, and abdominal distention due to gastric and intestinal hypomotility and chemical peritonitis are also frequent complaints.

Physical examination frequently reveals a distressed and anxious patient. Low-grade fever, tachycardia, and hypotension are fairly common. Shock is not unusual and may result from (1) hypovolemia secondary to exudation of blood and plasma proteins into the retroperitoneal space (i.e., a "retroperitoneal burn"), (2) increased formation and release of kinin peptides which cause vasodilatation and increased vascular permeability, and (3) systemic effects of proteolytic and lipolytic enzymes released into the circulation. Jaundice occurs infrequently; when present, it usually is due to edema of the head of the pancreas with compression of the intrapancreatic portion of the common bile duct. Erythematous skin nodules due to subcutaneous fat necrosis may occur. In 10 to 20 percent of patients there are pulmonary findings, including basilar rales, atelectasis, and pleural effusion, the latter most frequently left-sided. Abdominal tenderness and muscle rigidity are present to a variable degree, but compared with the intense pain, these signs may be unimpressive. Bowel sounds are usually diminished or absent. A pancreatic pseudocyst may be palpable in the upper abdomen. A faint blue discoloration around the umbilicus (Cullen's sign) may occur as the result of hemoperitoneum, and a blue-red-purple or green-brown discoloration of the flanks (Turner's sign) reflects tissue catabolism of hemoglobin. The latter two findings, which are uncommon, indicate the presence of a severe necrotizing pancreatitis.

LABORATORY DATA The diagnosis of acute pancreatitis is usually established by the presence of an increased serum amylase. Values elevated threefold above normal virtually clinch the diagnosis if overt salivary gland disease and gut perforation or infarction are excluded. However, there appears to be no definite correlation between the severity of pancreatitis and the degree of serum amylase elevation. After 48 to 72 h, even with continuing evidence of pancreatitis, total serum amylase values tend to return to normal. However, pancreatic isoamylase and lipase levels may remain elevated for 7 to 14 days. It will be recalled that amylase elevations in serum and urine occur in many conditions other than pancreatitis (see Table 273-2). Importantly, patients with *acidemia* (arterial pH ≤7.32) may have spurious elevations in serum amylase. In one study, 12 of 33 acidemic patients had an elevated serum amylase, but only 1 had an elevated lipase value; 9 had salivary-type amylase as the predominant

serum isoamylase. This explains why patients with diabetic ketoacidosis may have marked elevations in serum amylase without any other evidence to support a diagnosis of acute pancreatitis. The urine amylase C_{am}/C_{cr} ratio is usually elevated in patients with severe pancreatitis; this ratio usually is not increased in patients with normal serum amylase. Serum lipase activity increases in parallel with amylase activity, and measurement of both enzymes increases the diagnostic yield. An elevated serum lipase or trypsin value is usually diagnostic of acute pancreatitis; these tests are especially helpful in patients with nonpancreatic causes of hyperamylasemia (see Table 273-4). Markedly increased levels of peritoneal or pleural fluid amylase [>1500 nmol/L (>5000 units per deciliter)] are also helpful, if present, in establishing the diagnosis.

Leukocytosis (15,000 to 20,000 leukocytes per microliter) occurs frequently. More severe cases may show hemoconcentration with hematocrit values exceeding 50 percent because of loss of plasma into the retroperitoneal space and peritoneal cavity. *Hyperglycemia* is common and is due to multiple factors that include decreased insulin release, increased glucagon release, and increased output of adrenal glucocorticoids and catecholamines. *Hypocalcemia* occurs in approximately 25 percent of cases, and its pathogenesis is incompletely understood. While earlier studies suggested that the parathyroid gland response to a decrease in serum calcium is impaired, subsequent observations have failed to confirm this. Intraperitoneal saponification of calcium by fatty acids in areas of fat necrosis occurs occasionally with large amounts (up to 6.0 g) dissolved or suspended in ascitic fluid. Such "soap formation" also may be significant in patients with pancreatitis, mild hypocalcemia, and little or no obvious ascites. *Hyperbilirubinemia* [serum bilirubin >68 μmol/L (>4.0 mg/dL)] occurs in approximately 10 percent of patients. However, jaundice is transient, and serum bilirubin levels return to normal in 4 to 7 days. Serum alkaline phosphatase and aspartate aminotransferase (AST) levels are also transiently elevated and parallel serum bilirubin values. When markedly elevated [i.e., >8.5 μmol/L (>500 units per deciliter)], serum lactic dehydrogenase (LDH) levels suggest a poor prognosis. Serum albumin is decreased to ≤30 g/L (≤3.0 g/dL) in about 10 percent of cases and is associated with more severe pancreatitis and an increased mortality rate (Table 274-2). *Hypertriglyceridemia* occurs in 15 to 20 percent of cases, and serum amylase levels in such patients are often spuriously normal (see Chap. 273). Most patients with hypertriglyceridemia and pancreatitis, when subsequently examined, show evidence of an underlying derangement in lipid metabolism which probably antedated the pancreatitis, and this is discussed below. Approximately 25 percent of patients have *hypoxemia* (arterial $P_{O_2} \leq 60$ mmHg), which may herald the onset of

---

TABLE 274-2   Factors adversely affecting survival in acute pancreatitis

Ranson/Imrie criteria
  A At admission or diagnosis
    1 Age >55 years
    2 Leukocytosis >16,000 per cubic millimeter
    3 Hyperglycemia >11 mmol/L (>200 mg/dL)
    4 Serum LDH >400 IU/L
    5 Serum AST >250 IU/L
  B During initial 48 h
    1 Hematocrit fall >10 percent
    2 Fluid sequestration >4000 mL
    3 Hypocalcemia <1.9 mmol/L (<8.0 mg/dL)
    4 Hypoxemia (P_{O_2} <60 mmHg)
    5 BUN rise >1.8 mmol/L (>5 mg/dL) after IV fluids
    6 Hypoalbuminemia <32 g/L (<3.2 g/dL)
Acute physiology and chronic health evaluation (APACHE II) score > 12
Hemorrhagic peritoneal fluid
Key indicators
  A Hypotension (BP <90 mmHg) or tachycardia >130 beats per minute
  B P_{O_2} <60 mmHg
  C Oliguria (<50 mL/h) or increasing BUN, creatinine
  D Metabolic [serum calcium <1.9 mmol/L (<8.0 mg/dL) or serum albumin <32 g/L (<3.2 g/dL)]

adult respiratory distress syndrome. Finally, the electrocardiogram is occasionally abnormal in acute pancreatitis with ST-segment and T-wave abnormalities simulating myocardial ischemia.

Radiologic studies useful in the diagnosis of acute pancreatitis are listed in Table 273-1 and discussed in Chap. 273. Although one or more of the abnormalities are found in over 50 percent of patients, the findings are inconstant and nonspecific. The chief value of conventional x-rays [chest; kidney, ureter, and bladder (KUB)] in acute pancreatitis is to help exclude other diagnoses, especially a perforated viscus. Upper gastrointestinal tract x-rays have been superseded by ultrasonography and computed tomographic scanning. A CT scan may confirm the clinical impression of acute pancreatitis even in the face of normal serum amylase levels. Importantly, CT is quite helpful in indicating the severity of acute pancreatitis and its expected morbidity and mortality (see below). Sonography and radionuclide scanning (PIPIDA, HIDA) are useful in acute pancreatitis to evaluate the gallbladder and biliary tree.

DIAGNOSIS Any severe acute pain in the abdomen or back should suggest acute pancreatitis. The diagnosis is usually entertained when a patient with a possible predisposition to pancreatitis presents with severe and constant abdominal pain, nausea, emesis, fever, tachycardia, and abnormal findings on abdominal examination. Laboratory studies frequently reveal leukocytosis, abnormal x-rays of the abdomen and chest, hypocalcemia, and hyperglycemia. The diagnosis is usually confirmed by finding an elevated serum amylase and/or lipase. Obviously, not all the above features have to be present for the diagnosis to be established.

The *differential diagnosis* should include consideration of the following disorders: (1) perforated viscus, especially peptic ulcer, (2) acute cholecystitis and biliary colic, (3) acute intestinal obstruction, (4) mesenteric vascular occlusion, (5) renal colic, (6) myocardial infarction, (7) dissecting aortic aneurysm, (8) connective tissue disorders with vasculitis, (9) pneumonia, and (10) diabetic ketoacidosis. A penetrating duodenal ulcer usually can be identified by upper gastrointestinal x-rays and/or endoscopy. A perforated duodenal ulcer is readily diagnosed by the presence of free intraperitoneal air. It may be difficult to differentiate acute cholecystitis from acute pancreatitis, since an elevated serum amylase may be found in both disorders. Pain of biliary tract origin is more right-sided and gradual in onset, and ileus is usually absent; sonography and radionuclide scanning are helpful in establishing the diagnosis of cholelithiasis and cholecystitis. Intestinal obstruction due to mechanical factors can be differentiated from pancreatitis by the history of colicky pain, findings on abdominal examination, and x-rays of the abdomen showing characteristic changes of mechanical obstruction. Acute mesenteric vascular occlusion is usually evident in elderly debilitated patients with brisk leukocytosis, abdominal distention, and bloody diarrhea, in whom paracentesis shows sanguineous fluid and arteriography shows vascular occlusion. Serum as well as peritoneal fluid amylase levels are increased, however, in patients with intestinal infarction. Systemic lupus erythematosus and polyarteritis nodosa may be confused with pancreatitis, especially since pancreatitis may develop as a complication of these diseases. Diabetic ketoacidosis is often accompanied by abdominal pain and elevated total serum amylase levels, thus closely mimicking acute pancreatitis. However, the serum lipase and pancreatic isoamylase are not elevated in diabetic ketoacidosis.

COURSE OF THE DISEASE AND COMPLICATIONS It is important to identify those patients with acute pancreatitis who have an increased risk of dying. Ranson and Imrie have utilized multiple prognostic criteria and have demonstrated that there is an increased mortality rate with three or more risk factors identifiable either at the time of admission to the hospital or during the initial 48 h of hospitalization (see Table 274-2). The acute physiology and chronic health evaluation scoring system (APACHE II) utilizes the worst values of 12 physiologic measurements, age, and previous health status and provides a good description of illness severity for a wide range of common diseases; this score also correlates with outcome. Prospective studies have compared APACHE II with multiple prognos-

tic criteria, i.e., Ranson and Imrie scores, in predicting the severity of acute pancreatitis. On admission, APACHE II identified approximately two-thirds of severe attacks, and after 48 h, the prognostic accuracy of APACHE II is comparable with Ranson and Imrie's scoring system. The drawbacks of APACHE II are (1) complexity, (2) requirement of a computer for scoring, and (3) standardization regarding peak values and cutoff scores. McMahon and colleagues have shown that the presence of a "toxic broth" or dark (hemorrhagic) fluid in abdominal pancreatitis is also an important prognostic indicator in acute pancreatitis. These multiple-factor scoring systems are difficult to use and have not been embraced consistently by clinicians. There is a great need for a reliable simple biochemical test consistently capable of predicting outcome in patients with acute pancreatitis. Two candidate markers which show great promise are serum granulocyte elastase and urinary trypsinogen activation peptide (TAP). The key indicators of a severe attack of acute pancreatitis are also listed in Table 274-2. Importantly, the presence of any one of these factors is associated with an increased risk of complications and any two criteria with a 20 to 30 percent mortality rate. The high mortality rate of such severely ill patients is due in large part to infection and warrants intensive radiologic intervention and monitoring and/or a combination of radiologic and surgical means as discussed in detail below.

The local and systemic complications of acute pancreatitis are listed in Table 274-3. Patients frequently develop an inflammatory mass in the first 2 to 3 weeks after pancreatitis. These may be phlegmons, abscesses, or pseudocysts (see below). Systemic complications include pulmonary, cardiovascular, hematologic, renal, metabolic, and central nervous system abnormalities. Pancreatitis, hypertriglyceridemia, and alcoholism constitute a triad in which cause and effect remain incompletely understood. However, several reasonable conclusions can be drawn. First, hypertriglyceridemia can precede and apparently cause the development of pancreatitis. Second, the vast majority (>80 percent) of patients with acute pancreatitis do not have hypertriglyceridemia. Third, almost all patients with pancreatitis and hypertriglyceridemia are *either* alcoholics who have been drinking shortly before the onset of pancreatitis *or* patients with preexisting hypertriglyceridemia. Fourth, many of the patients with this triad have persistent hypertriglyceridemia after recovery from pancreatitis and abstention from alcohol and are prone to recurrent episodes of pancreatitis. Fifth, any factor (e.g., drugs, alcohol) that causes an abrupt increase in serum triglycerides to levels greater than 11 mmol/L (1000 mg/dL) can precipitate a bout of pancreatitis that can be associated with significant complications and even become fulminant. Finally, patients with a deficiency of apolipoprotein CII have an increased incidence of pancreatitis; apolipoprotein CII activates lipoprotein lipase, which is important in clearing chylomicrons from the bloodstream.

Purtscher's retinopathy, a relatively unusual complication, refers to the sudden and severe loss of vision in patients with acute pancreatitis. It is characterized by a peculiar funduscopic appearance with cotton-wool spots and hemorrhages confined to an area limited by the optic disk and macula; it is believed to be due to posterior retinal artery occlusion with aggregated granulocytes.

The two most common causes of acute pancreatitis are alcoholism and biliary tract disease; other causes are listed in Table 274-1. However, after a conventional workup, a specific cause will not be identified actually in 10 to 20 percent of patients. It is important to note that ultrasound examinations will not detect gallstones, especially microlithiasis and/or sludge, in 4 to 7 percent of patients. In one series of 31 patients initially diagnosed as having idiopathic acute pancreatitis, 23 were found to have occult gallstone disease. Thus approximately two-thirds of patients with recurrent acute pancreatitis without an obvious cause actually have occult gallstone disease. Other diseases of the biliary tree and pancreatic ducts that can cause acute pancreatitis include choledochocele, ampullary tumors, pancreas divisum, and pancreatic duct stones, stricture, and tumor. Approximately 2 percent of patients with pancreatic carcinoma present with acute pancreatitis.

TABLE 274-3 Complications of acute pancreatitis

LOCAL

A Pancreatic phlegmon
B Pancreatic abscess
C Pancreatic pseudocyst
  1 Pain
  2 Rupture
  3 Hemorrhage
  4 Infection
  5 Obstruction of gastrointestinal tract (stomach, duodenum, colon)
D Pancreatic ascites
  1 Disruption of main pancreatic duct
  2 Leaking pseudocyst
E Involvement of contiguous organs by necrotizing pancreatitis
  1 Massive intraperitoneal hemorrhage
  2 Thrombosis of blood vessels
  3 Bowel infarction
F Obstructive jaundice

SYSTEMIC

A Pulmonary
  1 Pleural effusion
  2 Atelectasis
  3 Mediastinal abscess
  4 Pneumonitis
  5 Adult respiratory distress syndrome
B Cardiovascular
  1 Hypotension
    a Hypovolemia
    b Hypoalbuminemia
  2 Sudden death
  3 Nonspecific ST-T changes in electrocardiogram simulating myocardial infarction
  4 Pericardial effusion
C Hematologic
  1 Disseminated intravascular coagulation (DIC)
D Gastrointestinal hemorrhage*
  1 Peptic ulcer disease
  2 Erosive gastritis
  3 Hemorrhagic pancreatic necrosis with erosion into major blood vessels
  4 Portal vein thrombosis, variceal hemorrhage
E Renal
  1 Oliguria
  2 Azotemia
  3 Renal artery and/or renal vein thrombosis
F Metabolic
  1 Hyperglycemia
  2 Hypertriglyceridemia
  3 Hypocalcemia
  4 Encephalopathy
  5 Sudden blindness (Purtscher's retinopathy)
G Central nervous system
  1 Psychosis
  2 Fat emboli
H Fat necrosis
  1 Subcutaneous tissues (erythematous nodules)
  2 Bone
  3 Miscellaneous (mediastinum, pleura, nervous system)

* Aggravated by coagulation abnormalities (DIC).

TREATMENT In most patients (approximately 85 to 90 percent) with acute pancreatitis, the disease is self-limited and subsides spontaneously, usually within 3 to 7 days after treatment is instituted. Medical therapy is aimed at reducing pancreatic secretion and, in essence, "putting the pancreas at rest." Conventional measures include (1) analgesics for pain, (2) intravenous fluids and colloids to maintain normal intravascular volume, (3) no oral alimentation, and (4) nasogastric suction to decrease gastrin release from the stomach and prevent gastric contents from entering the duodenum. Recent controlled trials, however, have shown that nasogastric suction offers no clear-cut advantages in the treatment of mild to moderately severe acute pancreatitis. Its use, therefore, must be considered elective rather than mandatory.

It has been demonstrated that CCK-stimulated pancreatic secretion is almost abolished in four different experimental models of acute pancreatitis. This probably explains why drugs to block pancreatic secretion in acute pancreatitis have failed to have any therapeutic benefit. For this and other reasons, anticholinergic drugs are not indicated in acute pancreatitis. Although antibiotics have been used in the treatment of acute pancreatitis, three recent randomized, prospective trials have shown no benefit from the use of antibiotics in acute pancreatitis of mild to moderate severity. However, because secondary infection of necrotic pancreatic tissue (phlegmon, abscess, pseudocyst) or obstructed biliary passages (ascending cholangitis, complicating choledocholithiasis) contributes to much of the late mortality, appropriate *antibiotic therapy of established infection* is obviously quite important. Several other drugs have been evaluated by prospective, controlled trials and found *ineffective* in the treatment of acute pancreatitis. The list, by no means complete, includes glucagon, H-2 blockers, protease inhibitors such as aprotinin, glucocorticoids, calcitonin, somatostatin analogues such as octreotide, and nonsteroidal anti-inflammatory drugs (NSAIDs).

A CT scan, especially a contrast-enhanced dynamic CT (CECT) scan, provides valuable information on the severity and prognosis of acute pancreatitis (Fig. 274-1 and Table 274-4). In particular, the CECT allows estimation of the presence and extent of pancreatic necrosis. Recent studies suggest that the likelihood of prolonged pancreatitis or a serious complication is negligible when the CT severity index is 1 or 2 and unlikely with scores of 3 to 6. However, patients with CT severity index scores of 7 to 10 had a 92 percent morbidity and 17 percent mortality. A CECT is indicated in patients with three or more of Ranson's signs, in all seriously ill patients, and in patients who show evidence of clinical deterioration. The patient with mild to moderate pancreatitis usually requires treatment with intravenous fluids, fasting, and possibly nasogastric suction for 2 to 4 days. A clear liquid diet is frequently started on the third to sixth day and a regular diet by the fifth to seventh day. The patient with unremitting *fulminant pancreatitis* usually requires inordinate amounts of fluid and close attention to complications such as cardiovascular collapse, respiratory insufficiency, and pancreatic infection. The latter should be managed by a combination of radiologic and surgical means (see below). While earlier uncontrolled studies suggested that *peritoneal lavage* via a percutaneous dialysis catheter is helpful in severe pancreatitis, recent studies indicate that such treatment does not influence the outcome of such attacks. Laparotomy with adequate drainage and removal of necrotic tissue should be considered if conventional therapy does not halt the patient's deterioration. The use of parenteral nutrition makes it possible to give nutritional support to patients with severe, acute, or protracted pancreatitis who are unable to eat normally. Patients with severe gallstone-induced pancreatitis may improve dramatically if papillotomy is carried out within the first 36 to 72 h of the attack. Recent studies indicate that only those patients with gallstone pancreatitis who are in the very severe group should be considered for urgent endoscopic retrograde cholangiopoanancreatography (ERCP). Finally, the treatment for patients with hypertriglyceridemia-associated pancreatitis include (1) weight loss to ideal weight, (2) lipid-restricted diet, (3) exercise, (4) avoidance of alcohol and drugs that can elevate serum triglycerides (i.e., estrogens, vitamin A, thiazides, and beta-blockers), and (5) control of diabetes.

PANCREATIC PHLEGMON, ABSCESS, AND PSEUDOCYST

The *phlegmon* is a solid mass of swollen, inflamed pancreas often containing patchy areas of necrosis; it may be present for 1 to 2 weeks. This prolonged inflammatory process should not be confused with a pseudocyst, a differentiation which is usually accomplished by sonography. A phlegmon should be suspected if abdominal pain, fever, leukocytosis, and hyperamylasemia persist for more than 5 days and especially if an abdominal mass is also present. Differentiation from an abscess may be difficult even with a CT scan. Occasionally, extensive areas of pancreatic necrosis develop in phlegmons and require incision and drainage, especially if infected. Phlegmons also may be secondarily infected, resulting in abscess formation. The latter occurs in 10 percent of patients with acute pancreatitis. The early diagnosis of pancreatic infection can be

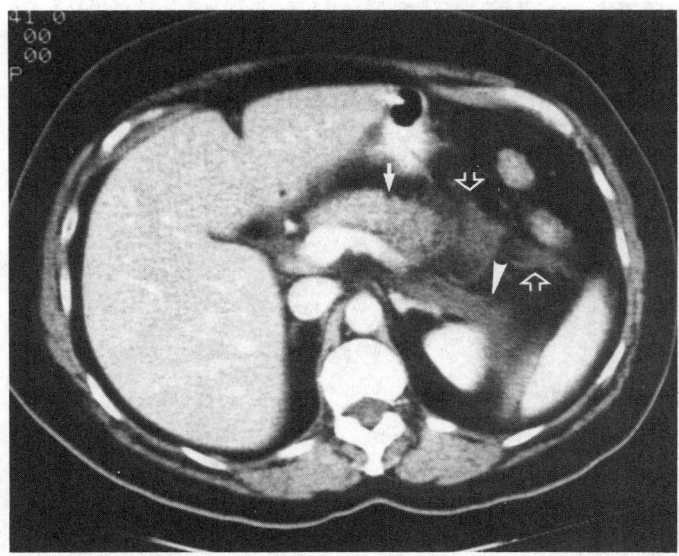

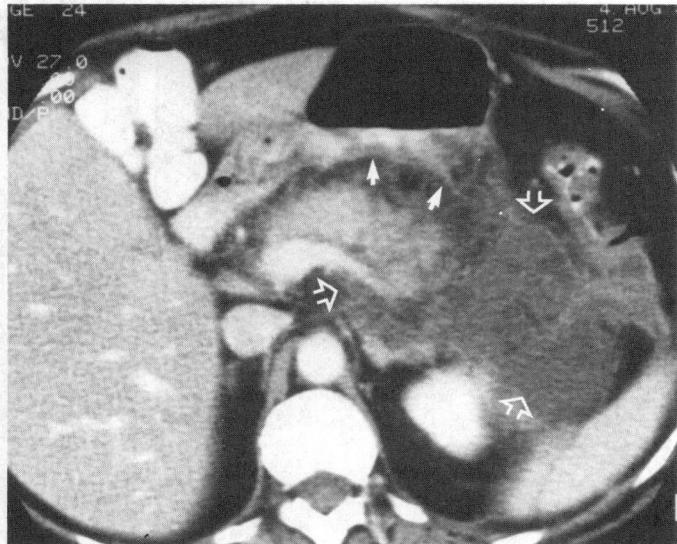

A

B

FIGURE 274-1   Acute pancreatitis: CT evolution. *A.* Contrast-enhanced CT scan of the abdomen performed on admission of a patient with clinical evidence of acute pancreatitis. Note the mildly decreased density of the body of the pancreas to the left of the midline (*arrow*). There are a few linear strands in the peripancreatic fat, suggesting inflammation (*open arrows*). A small amount of fluid is seen in the anterior pararenal space (*arrowhead*). *B.* Nine days after admission, there is a marked worsening with severe inflammation of the pancreas evidenced by anterior displacement of the posterior gastric wall (*arrows*), increased inflammation of the peripancreatic fat, and increased pancreatic effusion in the anterior perirenal space and around the splenic vein (*open arrows*). (*Courtesy of Dr. P.R. Ros, University of Florida College of Medicine.*)

accomplished by CT-guided needle aspiration. In one study, 60 patients, representing 5 percent of all admissions for acute pancreatitis, were suspected of harboring a pancreatic infection on the basis of fever, leukocytosis, and an abnormal CT scan (phlegmon, pseudocyst, or extrapancreatic fluid collection). Importantly, 36 of 60 patients (60 percent) had a pancreatic infection, with 20 of the 36 (55 percent) developing infection within the first 2 weeks. This study suggests that only guided aspiration can reliably distinguish sterile from infected pancreatic necrosis. The following are guidelines for patients meeting the above selection criteria: (1) pseudocysts and phlegmons should be aspirated promptly because more than half could be infected; (2) extrapancreatic fluid collections need not be aspirated promptly because most are sterile; (3) if a phlegmon is found initially to be sterile but fever and leukocytosis persist, allow several days of observation before considering reaspiration, since clinical improvement frequently occurs; and (4) if fever and leukocytosis recur after an interval of well-being, consider reaspiration.

Severe pancreatitis with the presence of three or more risk factors, postoperative pancreatitis, early oral feeding, early laparotomy, and perhaps injudicious use of antibiotics predispose to the development of pancreatic abscess, which occurs in 3 to 4 percent of patients with acute pancreatitis. Pancreatic abscess also may develop because of communication of a pseudocyst with the colon, after inadequate surgical drainage of a pseudocyst, or after needling of a pseudocyst. The characteristic signs of abscess are fever, leukocytosis, ileus, and rapid deterioration in a patient initially recovering from pancreatitis. However, the only manifestations may be persistent fever and signs of continuing pancreatic inflammation. Drainage of pancreatic abscesses by nonsurgical percutaneous catheter techniques, using CT guidance, has been only moderately successful (resolution in 50 to 60 percent of patients). Accordingly, laparotomy with radical sump drainage and possibly resection of necrotic tissue is usually required because the mortality rate for undrained pancreatic abscess approaches 100 percent. Multiple abscesses are common and reoperation is frequently required.

Pseudocysts of the pancreas are collections of tissue, fluid, debris, pancreatic enzymes, and blood which develop over a period of 1 to 4 weeks after the onset of acute pancreatitis in approximately 15 percent of patients. In contrast to true cysts, pseudocysts do not have epithelial lining, and the walls consist of necrotic tissue, granulation tissue, and fibrous tissue. Disruption of the pancreatic ductal system is common. However, the subsequent course of this disruption varies widely, namely, from spontaneous healing to continuous leakage of pancreatic juice, causing tense ascites. Pseudocysts are preceded by pancreatitis in 90 percent of cases and by trauma in 10 percent. Approximately 85 percent are located in the body or tail of the pancreas and 15 percent in the head. Some patients have two or more pseudocysts. Abdominal pain, with or without radiation to the back, is the usual presenting complaint. A palpable, tender mass may be found in the middle or left upper abdomen. The serum amylase level is elevated in 75 percent of patients some time during their illness and may fluctuate markedly.

Pseudocysts often displace some portion of the gastrointestinal tract on x-ray examination in 75 percent of cases (Fig. 274-2). Sonography, however, is reliable in detecting pseudocysts. Sonography also permits differentiation between an edematous and an inflamed pancreas (pancreatic phlegmon), which can give rise to a palpable mass and an actual pseudocyst. Furthermore, serial ultrasound studies

TABLE 274-4   Severity index in acute pancreatitis

	Points
GRADE OF ACUTE PANCREATITIS	
A Normal pancreas	0
B Pancreatic enlargement alone	1
C Inflammation compared with pancreas and peripancreatic fat	2
D One peripancreatic fluid collection	3
E Two or more fluid collections	4
DEGREE OF PANCREATIC NECROSIS	
A No necrosis	0
B Necrosis of one-third of pancreas	2
C Necrosis of one-half of pancreas	4
D Necrosis of more than one-half of pancreas	6

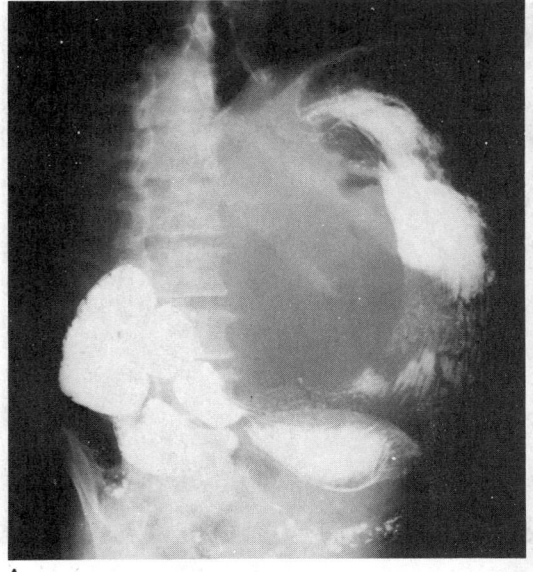

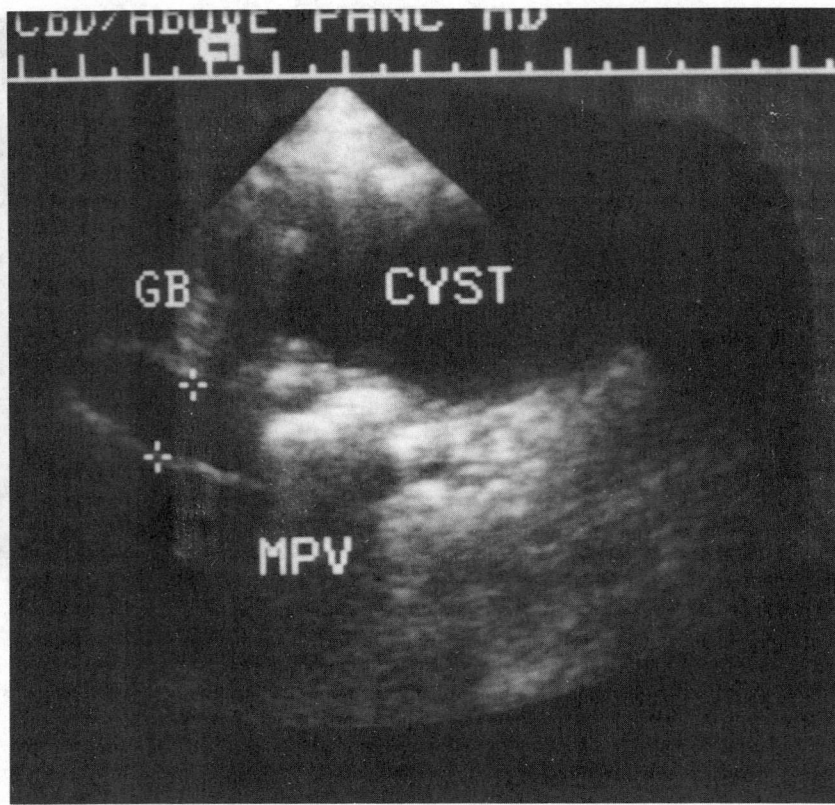

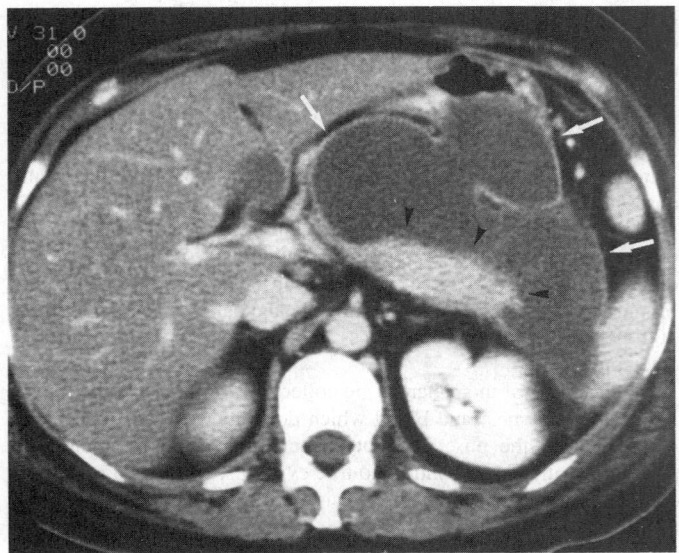

FIGURE 274-2 Pseudocyst of pancreas. *A.* Upper gastrointestinal x-ray showing displacement of stomach by pseudocyst. *B.* Sonogram showing pseudocyst (*cyst*). GB = gallbladder; MVP = portal vein. Behind the large pseudocyst is seen the calcified head of the pancreas. A dilated common bile duct (*asterisk*) is noted. (*Courtesy of Dr. C. E. Forsmark, University of Florida College of Medicine.*) *C.* CT scan showing pseudocyst. Note the large lobulated fluid collection (*arrows*) surrounding the tail of the pancreas (*arrowheads*). Note the dense, thin rim in the periphery representing the fibrous capsule of the pseudocyst. (*Courtesy of Dr. P. R. Ros, University of Florida College of Medicine.*)

will indicate whether a pseudocyst has resolved. CT scanning complements the use of ultrasound in the diagnosis of pancreatic pseudocyst (see Fig. 274-2), especially when it is infected.

In studies utilizing sonography, pseudocysts resolved in 25 to 40 percent of patients. However, pseudocysts that are greater than 5 cm and that persist for longer than 6 weeks rarely disappear. In others, serious complications may occur such as (1) pain caused by expansion of the lesion and pressure on other viscera, (2) rupture, (3) hemorrhage, and (4) abscess. Rupture of a pancreatic pseudocyst is a particularly serious complication. Shock almost always supervenes, and mortality rates range from 14 percent if the rupture is not associated with hemorrhage to over 60 percent if hemorrhage has occurred. Rupture and hemorrhage are the prime causes of mortality in pancreatic

pseudocyst. A triad of findings, i.e., increase in size of the mass, localized bruit over the mass, and a sudden decrease in hemoglobin and hematocrit levels without obvious signs of external blood loss, should alert one to the diagnosis of hemorrhage from a pseudocyst. Thus, in pseudocyst patients who are stable and uncomplicated and in whom serial ultrasound studies show a decreasing pseudocyst, conservative therapy is indicated. Conversely, patients with a pseudocyst which is expanding and which is complicated by rupture, hemorrhage, and abscess should be operated on. Using ultrasound or CT guidance, sterile chronic pseudocysts can be treated safely with single or repeated needle aspiration or more prolonged catheter drainage with an expected success rate of 45 to 75 percent. The success rate with infected pseudocysts is considerably less, i.e., 40 to 50 percent. Patients not responding to drainage require surgical therapy. Therapy consists of internal or external drainage of the cyst. Prolonged observation of a nonresolving pancreatic pseudocyst exposes the patient to increased risks which exceed those of elective surgery.

Pseudoaneurysms develop in up to 10 percent of patients with acute pancreatitis at sites reflecting the distribution of pseudocysts and fluid collections. The splenic artery is most frequently involved, followed by the inferior and superior pancreatic duodenal arteries. The diagnosis should be suspected in patients with pancreatitis who develop either upper gastrointestinal bleeding without an obvious cause or in whom a contrast-enhanced lesion is demonstrated within or adjacent to a suspected pseudocyst as determined by thin-cut CT examination. Arteriography is necessary to confirm the diagnosis.

PANCREATIC ASCITES AND PANCREATIC PLEURAL EFFU-SIONS Pancreatic ascites is usually due to disruption of the main pancreatic duct, often associated with an internal fistula between the duct and the peritoneal cavity or a leaking pseudocyst (see also Chap. 43). The diagnosis of pancreatic ascites is suggested in a patient with an elevated serum amylase level who also has increased levels of albumin [>30 g/L (>3.0 g/dL)] and amylase in the ascitic fluid. In addition, ERCP will often demonstrate passage of contrast material from a major pancreatic duct or a pseudocyst into the peritoneal cavity. As many as 15 percent of patients with pseudocysts have concurrent pancreatic ascites. The differential diagnosis should include intraperitoneal carcinomatosis, tuberculous peritonitis, constrictive pericarditis, and Budd-Chiari syndrome.

If the pancreatic duct disruption is posterior, an internal fistula may develop between the pancreatic duct and pleural space producing a pleural effusion, which is usually left-sided and often massive. This often requires thoracentesis or chest tube drainage.

Treatment usually involves placing the patient on nasogastric suction and parenteral alimentation to decrease pancreatic secretion. In addition, paracentesis is performed to keep the peritoneal cavity free of fluid and, it is hoped, effect sealing of the leak. The long-acting somatostatin analogue (octreotide) which inhibits pancreatic secretion is also useful in pancreatic ascites and pleural effusion. If ascites continues to recur after 2 to 3 weeks of medical management, the patient should be operated on following pancreatography to define the anatomy of the abnormal duct. Two or more sites of extravasation on ERCP identify patients unlikely to respond to conservative management.

CHRONIC PANCREATITIS AND PANCREATIC EXOCRINE INSUFFICIENCY

GENERAL AND ETIOLOGIC CONSIDERATIONS Chronic inflammatory disease of the pancreas may present as episodes of acute inflammation superimposed on a previously injured pancreas or as chronic damage with persistent pain or malabsorption. The causes of relapsing chronic pancreatitis are similar to those of acute pancreatitis (see Table 274-1), except that frequently there is an appreciable incidence of cases of undetermined origin. In addition, the pancreatitis associated with gallstones is predominantly acute or relapsing acute in nature. A cholecystectomy is almost always performed in patients after the first or second attack of gallstone-associated pancreatitis. Patients with chronic pancreatitis may present with persistent abdominal pain, with or without steatorrhea, and some may present with steatorrhea and no pain.

Patients with chronic pancreatitis who develop extensive destruction of the pancreas (i.e., less than 10 percent of exocrine function remaining) will demonstrate steatorrhea and azotorrhea. In the adult in the United States, alcoholism is the most common cause of clinically apparent pancreatic exocrine insufficiency, while cystic fibrosis is the most frequent cause in children. In up to 25 percent of adults in the United States with chronic pancreatitis, the cause is not known; i.e., they have idiopathic chronic pancreatitis. In other parts of the world, severe protein-calorie malnutrition is a common cause. Table 274-5 lists other causes of pancreatic exocrine insufficiency, but they are relatively uncommon.

PATHOPHYSIOLOGY Unfortunately, the events that initiate an inflammatory process within the pancreas are still not well understood, and the many hypotheses will not be reviewed. In the case of alcohol-induced pancreatitis, however, it has been suggested that the primary defect may be the precipitation of protein (inspissated enzymes) within the ducts. The resulting ductal obstruction can lead to duct dilatation, diffuse atrophy of the acinar cells, fibrosis, and eventual calcification of some of the protein plugs. However, that some alcoholic patients with recurrent acute pancreatitis show no evidence of chronic pancreatitis does not support the intraductal protein precipitation hypothesis. In fact, experimental and clinical observations have shown the direct toxic effects of alcohol on the pancreas. While patients with alcohol-induced pancreatitis generally consume large amounts of alcohol, some consume very little (i.e., 50 g/d or less). Thus prolonged consumption of "socially acceptable" amounts of alcohol is compatible with the development of pancreatitis. In addition, the finding of extensive pancreatic fibrosis in patients who have expired during their first attack of clinical acute alcohol-induced pancreatitis supports the concept that such patients already have chronic pancreatitis.

CLINICAL FEATURES Patients with relapsing chronic pancreatitis may present with symptoms identical to those found in acute pancreatitis, but their pain may be continuous or intermittent, or pain may be absent. The pathogenesis of this pain is poorly understood. Although the classic description is that of epigastric pain radiating through the back, the pain pattern is often atypical. The pain may be maximal in the right or left upper quadrants in the back or diffuse throughout the upper abdomen; it may even be referred to the anterior chest or flank. Characteristically, the pain is persistent, deep-seated, and unresponsive to antacids. It often is increased by alcohol and ingestion of heavy meals (especially foods rich in fat). Often the pain is so severe as to require the frequent use of narcotics.

Weight loss, abnormal stools, and other signs or symptoms suggestive of malabsorption (see Table 254-5) are common in chronic pancreatitis. However, clinically apparent deficiencies of fat-soluble vitamins are surprisingly rare. The physical findings in these patients are usually not impressive, such that there is a disparity between the severity of the abdominal pain and the paucity of physical signs (save some abdominal tenderness and mild temperature elevation).

DIAGNOSTIC EVALUATION (See Chap. 273) In contrast to patients with relapsing acute pancreatitis, the serum amylase and lipase levels are usually not elevated. Elevations of the serum bilirubin and alkaline phosphatase may indicate cholestasis secondary to chronic inflammation around the common bile duct (Fig. 274-3). Many

---

TABLE 274-5 Causes of pancreatic exocrine insufficiency

Alcohol, chronic alcoholism
Cystic fibrosis
Severe protein-calorie malnutrition with hypoalbuminemia
Pancreatic and duodenal neoplasms
Pancreatic resection
Gastric surgery
  A Subtotal gastrectomy with Billroth I anastomosis
  B Subtotal gastrectomy with Billroth II anastomosis
  C Truncal vagotomy and pyloroplasty
Gastrinoma (Zollinger-Ellison syndrome)
Hereditary pancreatitis
Traumatic pancreatitis
Hemochromatosis
Shwachman's syndrome (pancreatic insufficiency and bone marrow dysfunction)
Trypsinogen deficiency
Enterokinase deficiency
Isolated deficiencies of amylase, lipase, or proteases
α_1-Antitrypsin deficiency
Idiopathic pancreatitis

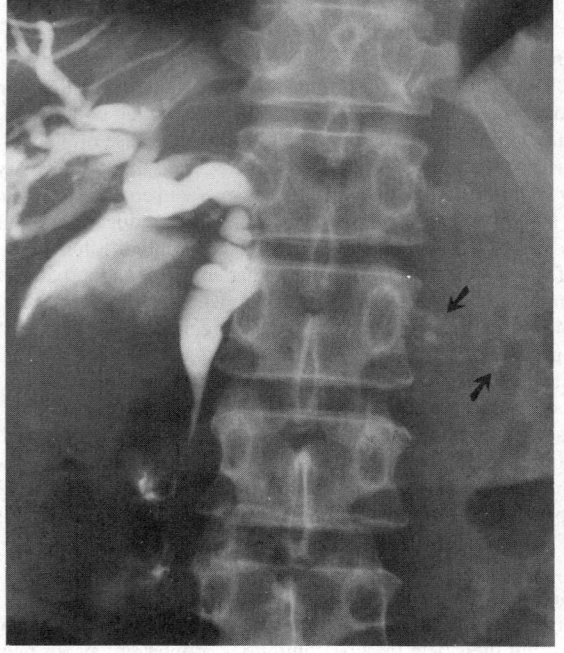

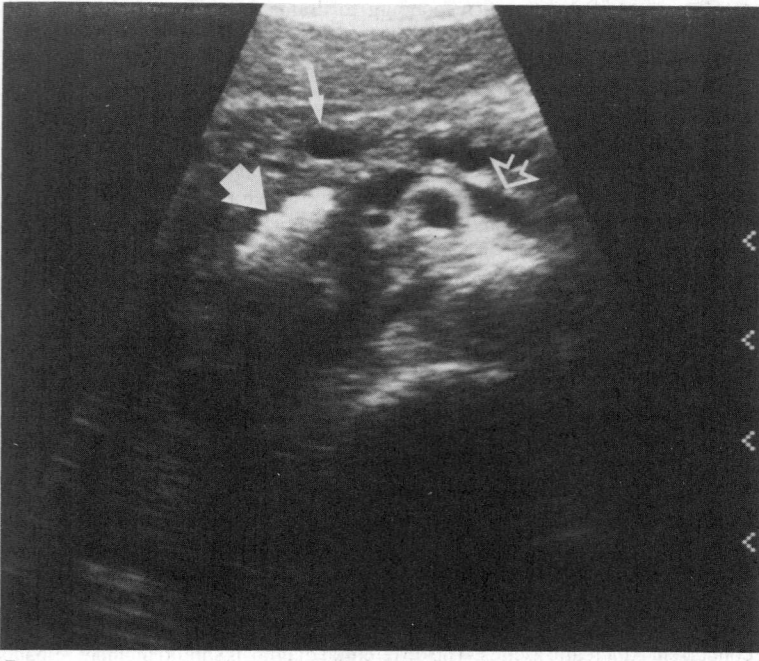

A   B

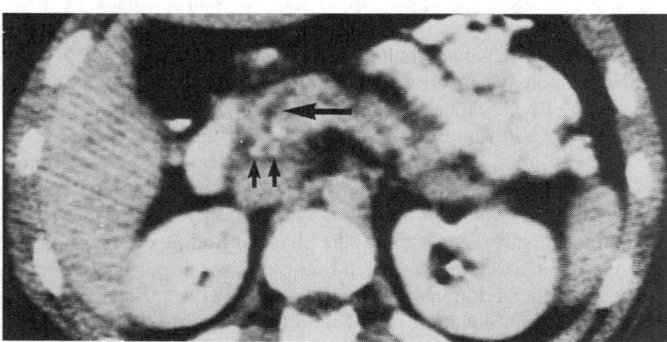

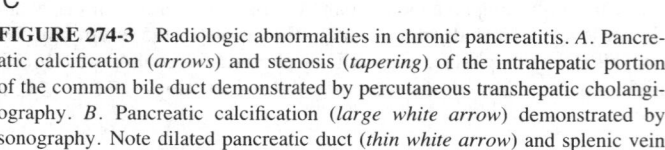

C   D

FIGURE 274-3   Radiologic abnormalities in chronic pancreatitis. *A*. Pancreatic calcification (*arrows*) and stenosis (*tapering*) of the intrahepatic portion of the common bile duct demonstrated by percutaneous transhepatic cholangiography. *B*. Pancreatic calcification (*large white arrow*) demonstrated by sonography. Note dilated pancreatic duct (*thin white arrow*) and splenic vein (*clear arrow*). *C*. Pancreatic calcification (*vertical arrows*) and dilated pancreatic duct (*horizontal arrow*) demonstrated by CT scan. *D*. Endoscopic retrograde cholangiogram shows grossly dilated pancreatic ducts (*arrows*) in a patient with long-standing pancreatitis.

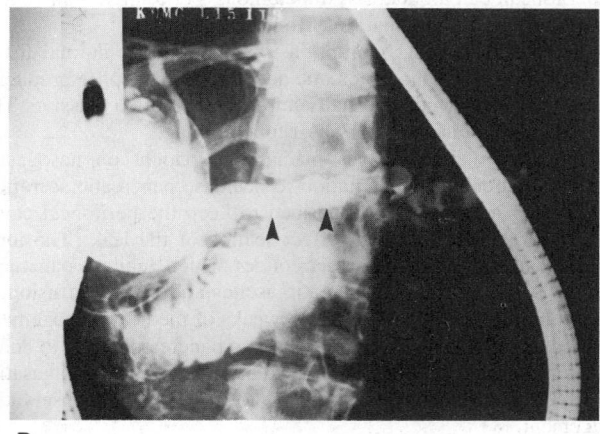

patients demonstrate impaired glucose tolerance, and some may have an elevated fasting blood glucose level.

The classic triad of pancreatic calcification, steatorrhea, and diabetes mellitus usually establishes the diagnosis of chronic pancreatitis and exocrine pancreatic insufficiency but is found in less than one-third of chronic pancreatitis patients. Accordingly, it is often necessary to perform an intubation test such as the *secretin stimulation test*, which usually becomes abnormal when 60 percent or more of pancreatic exocrine function has been lost. Approximately 40 percent of patients with chronic pancreatitis have *cobalamin (vitamin B₁₂) malabsorption* which is corrected by the administration of oral pancreatic enzymes. There is usually a marked excretion of fecal fat (see Chap. 254), which can be reduced with the administration of oral pancreatic enzymes. The bentiromide test (Chap. 273) and D-xylose urinary excretion test are useful in patients with "pancreatic steatorrhea," since the bentiromide test will be abnormal and the D-xylose excretion usually normal. A decreased serum trypsinogen level strongly suggests pancreatic exocrine insufficiency.

The radiographic hallmark of chronic pancreatitis is the presence of scattered calcification throughout the pancreas (see Fig. 274-3). Diffuse pancreatic calcification indicates that significant damage has occurred and obviates the need for a secretin test. Alcohol is by far the most common cause of pancreatic calcification, but it also may be seen in severe protein-calorie malnutrition, hereditary pancreatitis, posttraumatic pancreatitis, hyperparathyroidism, islet cell tumors, and idiopathic chronic pancreatitis. An ongoing prospective study of 107 patients has shown convincingly that pancreatic calcification may decrease or even disappear either following ductal decompression or spontaneously in one-third of patients with severe chronic pancreatitis. Pancreatic calcification is a dynamic process that is incompletely understood.

Special techniques such as sonography, CT scanning, and ERCP have added new dimensions to the diagnosis of pancreatic disease. In addition to excluding pseudocysts and pancreatic cancer, sonography may show calcification or dilated ducts associated with chronic pancreatitis (Fig. 274-4). Similar benefits can be derived from CT

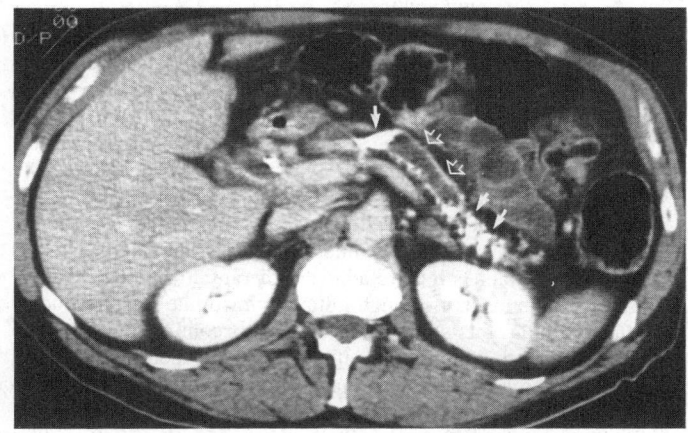

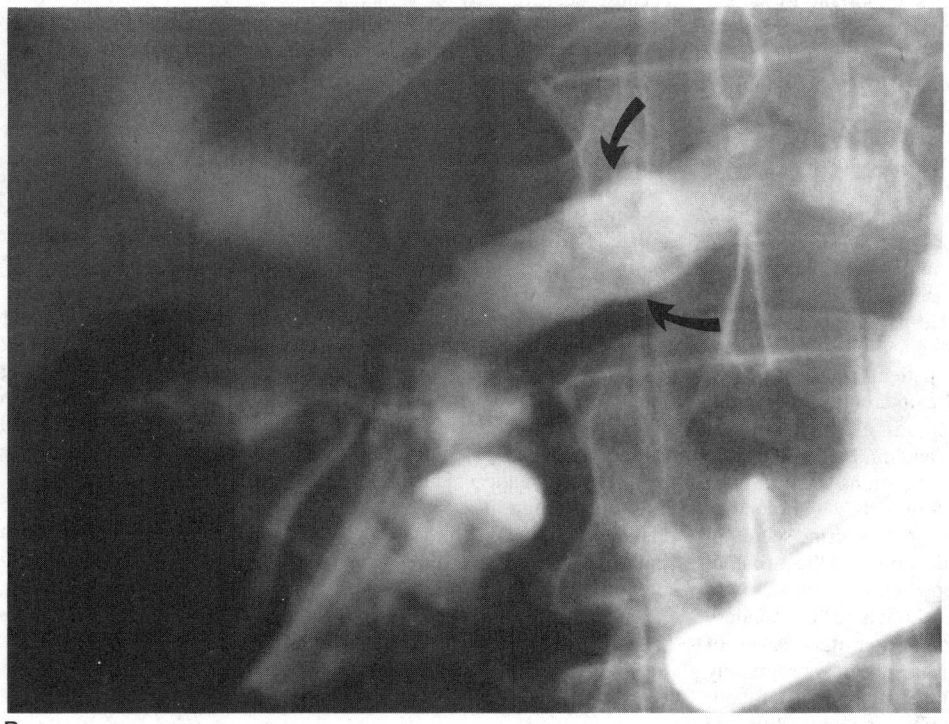

FIGURE 274-4 Chronic pancreatitis and pancreatic calculi: CT scan and ERCP appearance. *A.* In this contrast-enhanced CT scan of the abdomen, there is evidence of an atrophic pancreas with multiple calcifications (*arrows*). Note a markedly dilated pancreatic duct seen in this section through the body and tail (*open arrows*). *B.* ERCP in the same patient demonstrates the dilated pancreatic duct as well as an intrapancreatic duct calculus (*arrows*). These findings correlate nicely with the CT scan appearance.

scans. ERCP is the only nonoperative technique which provides a direct view of the pancreatic duct. In patients with alcohol-induced pancreatitis, ERCP may reveal a pseudocyst missed by sonography or CT scan.

COMPLICATIONS OF CHRONIC PANCREATITIS The complications of chronic pancreatitis are protean. *Cobalamin (vitamin B₁₂) malabsorption* occurs in 40 percent of patients with alcohol-induced chronic pancreatitis and in virtually all with cystic fibrosis. The cobalamin malabsorption is consistently corrected by the administration of pancreatic enzymes (containing proteases). The cobalamin malabsorption may be due to excessive binding of cobalamin by nonintrinsic factor cobalamin-binding proteins. The latter are ordinarily destroyed by pancreatic proteases, but with pancreatic insufficiency the nonspecific binding proteins escape degradation and compete with intrinsic factor for cobalamin binding. Although the majority of patients show *impaired glucose tolerance*, the development of diabetic ketoacidosis and coma is uncommon. Similarly, end organ damage (retinopathy, neuropathy, nephropathy) is also uncommon, and the appearance of these complications should raise the question of concomitant genetic diabetes mellitus. A nondiabetic retinopathy, peripheral in location and secondary to vitamin A and/or zinc

deficiency, is common in these patients. High-amylase-containing *effusions* occur within the pleura, pericardium, or peritoneum. *Gastrointestinal bleeding* may occur from a peptic ulcer, gastritis, a pseudocyst eroding into the duodenum, or ruptured varices secondary to splenic vein thrombosis due to inflammation of the tail of the pancreas. *Icterus* may occur, owing to either edema of the head of the pancreas compressing the common bile duct or chronic cholestasis secondary to chronic inflammatory reaction around the intrapancreatic portion of the common bile duct (see Fig. 274-3). This chronic obstruction may lead to cholangitis and ultimately biliary cirrhosis. *Subcutaneous fat necrosis* may appear as tender red nodules on the lower extremities. *Bone pain* may be secondary to intramedullary fat necrosis. Inflammation of the large and small joints of the upper and lower extremities may occur. The incidence of pancreatic carcinoma is probably increased in patients with diffuse calcification. Perhaps the most common and troublesome complication is addiction to narcotics.

TREATMENT AND APPROACH TO MANAGEMENT Therapy for patients with chronic pancreatitis is directed toward two major problems, namely, pain and malabsorption. Patients with intermittent attacks of pain are essentially treated like those with acute pancreatitis (see above). Patients with severe and persistent pain should avoid alcohol completely and avoid large meals rich in fat. Since the pain is often severe enough to require frequent use of narcotics (and hence addiction), a number of surgical procedures have been developed for pain relief. ERCP allows the surgeon to plan the operative approach. If there is a stricture of the pancreatic duct, then a *local resection* may ameliorate the pain. Unfortunately, isolated localized strictures are not common. In most patients with alcohol-induced disease, the pancreas is diffusely involved, and surgically correctible localized ductal disease is rare. When there is primary ductal obstruction and dilatation, ductal decompression may provide effective pain palliation. Short-term pain relief may be achieved in up to 80 percent of patients, while long-term pain relief occurs in approximately 50 percent. In some of these patients, however, pain relief can be achieved only by resecting 50 to 95 percent of the gland. Although pain relief is achieved in three-quarters of these patients, they tend to develop pancreatic endocrine and exocrine insufficiency and must be on pancreatic enzyme replacement therapy. It is important to screen patients carefully, for such radical surgery is contraindicated in those who are severely depressed or suicidal or continue to drink. Procedures such as sphincteroplasty, splanchnicectomy and celiac ganglionectomy, and nerve blocks usually bring only temporary relief and are not recommended. Although there is current enthusiasm for treating the pain of chronic pancreatitis by endoscopic placement of stents into the pancreatic duct, adequate control studies have not been carried out. In addition, significant complications, i.e., acute pancreatitis, pancreatic abscess, damage to the pancreatic duct, and death, have occurred in up to 36 percent of patients following stent placement.

Three double-blind trials have demonstrated that pancreatic enzymes decrease the abdominal pain in selected patients with chronic pancreatitis. In these trials, pain relief was obtained in approximately 75 percent of the patients evaluated. The patients most likely to respond to such therapy with amelioration of pain are those with mild to moderate exocrine pancreatic dysfunction, as evidenced by an abnormal secretin test, normal fat absorption, and minimal abnormalities on ERCP examination. These clinical observations seem to fit in with data in human beings and experimental animals which demonstrate a negative feedback regulation for pancreatic exocrine secretion controlled by the amount of proteases within the lumen of the proximal small intestine. It seems reasonable to approach the patient with severe persistent or continuous abdominal pain thought to be secondary to chronic pancreatitis in the following manner: After other causes of abdominal pain (peptic ulcer, gallstones, etc.) have been appropriately excluded, a pancreatic *sonogram* should be done. If no mass is found, a *secretin test* may be performed, since with chronic pancreatitis and pain this test usually will be abnormal. If the secretin test is abnormal (i.e., decreased bicarbonate concentration or volume output), a 3- to 4-week *trial of pancreatic enzymes* is appropriate. Eight conventional tablets or three enteric-coated capsules are taken at meals and at bedtime. If no relief is obtained, and especially if the volume secreted during the secretin test is very low, ERCP should be performed. If a pseudocyst or a localized ductal obstruction is found, surgery should be considered. A provocative study from South Africa questions the significance of the relationship of dilated ducts and/or strictures to pain. The finding of an appreciable obstruction or stricture in 65 percent of the patients who were pain-free more than 1 year, compared with 79 percent of the group with pain, suggests that factors other than duct obstruction or narrowing may be important in the pathogenesis of pain. It may be that the most important factors in the relief of pain are abstinence from alcohol and progressive pancreatic dysfunction rather than the surgical procedure per se. If no surgically remedial lesion is found and severe pain continues despite abstinence from alcohol, subtotal pancreatic resection may be necessary.

The treatment of malabsorption rests on the use of pancreatic enzyme replacement therapy. Although diarrhea and steatorrhea are usually improved, the results are frequently less than satisfactory. The major problem is delivery of enough active enzyme into the duodenum. Steatorrhea can be abolished if 10 percent of the normal amount of lipase could be delivered into the duodenum at the proper time. This concentration of lipase cannot be achieved with the presently available preparations of pancreatic enzymes, even if the latter are given in large doses. These poor results may be due to inactivation of lipase by gastric acid, food emptying from the stomach more rapidly than the exogenously administered pancreatic enzymes, and variation in the enzyme activity of various batches of commercially available pancreatic extracts.

For the usual patient, three to eight tablets or capsules of a potent enzyme preparation should be administered with meals. Some patients on conventional tablets require adjuvant therapy to improve enzyme replacement treatment. Although initially cimetidine was considered an effective adjuvant, studies have failed to confirm this. Sodium bicarbonate (1.3 g with meals) is effective and inexpensive. Antacids containing calcium carbonate or magnesium hydroxide are not effective and may actually result in increased steatorrhea. Adjuvant therapy should not be given with enteric-coated microsphere preparations because such therapy may increase the gastric pH such that these preparations would release their enzymes into the stomach rather than the small intestine.

Patients with severe exocrine pancreatic insufficiency secondary to alcohol who continue to drink have a high mortality (in one series 50 percent were dead when followed for 5 to 12 years) and significant morbidity (weight loss, lassitude, vitamin deficiency, and narcotic addiction). Pain may abate if progressive severe exocrine insufficiency continues. If abstinence is pursued and vigorous replacement therapy is utilized for the maldigestion-malabsorption, the patients do reasonably well.

HEREDITARY PANCREATITIS   Hereditary pancreatitis is a rare disease similar to chronic pancreatitis except for an early age of onset and evidence of hereditary factors (involving an autosomal dominant gene with incomplete penetrance). These patients have recurring attacks of severe abdominal pain which may last from a few days to a few weeks. The serum amylase and lipase levels may be elevated during acute attacks but are usually normal. Patients frequently develop pancreatic calcification, diabetes mellitus, and steatorrhea, and in addition, they have an increased incidence of pancreatic carcinoma. Such patients often require ductal decompression to obtain pain relief. Abdominal complaints in relatives of patients with hereditary pancreatitis should raise the question of pancreatic disease.

PANCREATIC ENDOCRINE TUMORS

Pancreatic endocrine tumors are summarized in Table 274-6 and are discussed in Chap. 276.

OTHER CONDITIONS

ANNULAR PANCREAS   When there is a failure in communication of the ventral and dorsal anlage of the pancreas, a ring of pancreatic tissue encircles the duodenum. Such an annular pancreas may cause intestinal obstruction in the neonate or the adult. Symptoms of postprandial fullness, epigastric pain, nausea, and vomiting may be present for years before the diagnosis is entertained. The radiographic findings are symmetric dilatation of the proximal duodenum with bulging of the recesses on either side of the annular band, effacement of the duodenal mucosa without destruction of the mucosa, accentuation of the findings in the right anterior oblique position, and lack of change on repeated examinations. The differential diagnosis should include duodenal webs, tumors of the pancreas or duodenum, postbulbar peptic ulcer, regional enteritis, and adhesions. Patients with annular pancreas have an increased incidence of pancreatitis and peptic ulcer. Because of these and other potential complications, the treatment is surgical even though the condition has been present for years. Retrocolic duodenojejunostomy is the procedure of choice,

TABLE 274-6   Pancreatic endocrine tumors

Syndrome	Hormone(s) produced	Primary hormone effects	Pathologic features	Clinical features
Zollinger-Ellison	Gastrin	Gastric acid hypersecretion with basal acid outputs usually >15 mmol/h (>15 meq/h)	Delta cell islet tumors; 10% aberrant (duodenal); 60% malignant	Severe peptic ulcer disease often refractory to therapy; ectopic ulcers; diarrhea; multiple endocrine adenomas (parathyroid, pituitary, adrenal, thyroid)
Insulinoma	Insulin	Hypoglycemia with inappropriately increased serum insulin levels	Beta cell islet tumors; 80–90% benign	Hypoglycemic symptoms
Glucagonoma	Glucagon; pancreatic polypeptide	Hyperglucagonemia →glucose intolerance	Alpha cell islet tumors; 60% malignant	Slow-growing pancreatic tumor; hyperglycemia; bullous and eczematoid dermatitis, weight loss; anemia; gastric and intestinal motor abnormalities
Somatostatinoma	Somatostatin; pancreatic polypeptide	Somatostatin inhibits insulin, gastrin and pancreatic enzyme secretion; decreased bile flow	Delta cell islet tumor	Pancreatic tumor; diarrhea; steatorrhea; gallstones; diabetes mellitus; anemia
Pancreatic cholera	Vasoactive intestinal peptide (VIP) ? Gastric inhibitory polypeptide ? Prostaglandin E ? Pancreatic peptide	Net secretion of salt and water by gut	? Delta cell tumor; >50% malignant	Pancreatic tumor with severe watery diarrhea; flushing; weight loss; hypokalemia; hypercalcemia; hypochlorhydria; hyperglycemia; inordinate fecal water and electrolyte losses
Carcinoid	Serotonin; prostaglandins	Altered gut motility; diarrhea	Enterochromaffin cells; non-beta cell islet tumors	Carcinoid syndrome with flushing; wheezing; diarrhea; alcohol intolerance; hepatomegaly

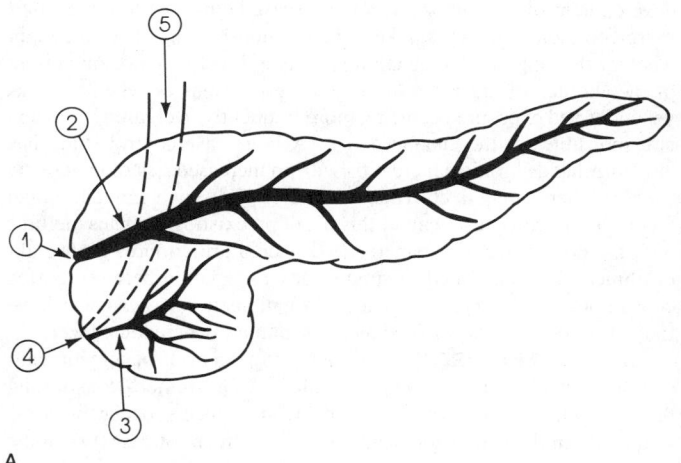

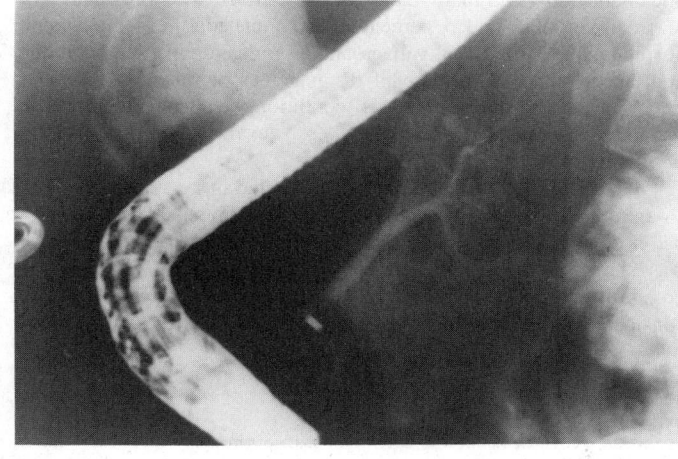

B

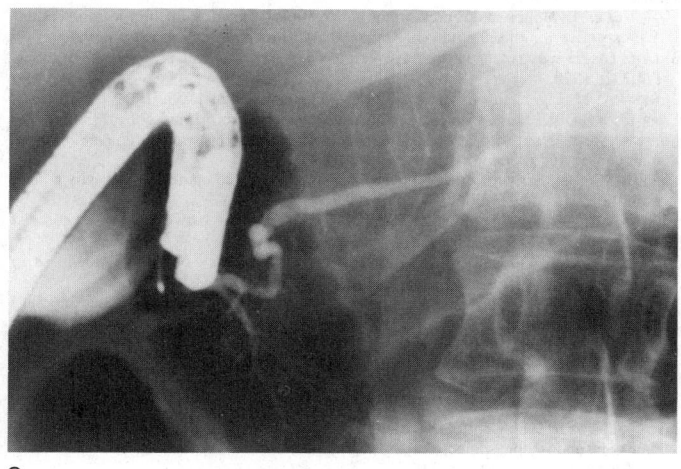

C

FIGURE 274-5 Illustration of the pancreatic ducts and typical ERCP of pancreas divisum. *A.* Diagram of the ventral and dorsal structures of the pancreas: (1) duct of Santorini, (2) pancreatic duct from the dorsal anlage, (3) pancreatic duct from the ventral anlage, (4) duct of Wirsung, and (5) common bile duct. *B.* ERCP, through the major papilla, demonstrating the ventral duct which does not communicate with the dorsal duct. *C.* ERCP demonstrating that the dorsal duct cannulated through the minor papilla does not communicate with the major papilla. (*Courtesy of Dr. C. E. Forsmark, University of Florida College of Medicine.*)

A

although some surgeons advocate Billroth II gastrectomy, gastroenterostomy, and vagotomy.

PANCREAS DIVISUM   Pancreas divisum occurs when the embryologic ventral and dorsal parts of the pancreas fail to fuse so that pancreatic drainage is accomplished mainly through the accessory papilla. Pancreas divisum is the most common congenital anatomic variant of the human pancreas. Current evidence indicates that this anomaly is not a predisposing factor to the development of pancreatitis in the great majority of patients with the anomaly. However, the combination of pancreas divisum and a small accessory orifice could result in dorsal duct obstruction. The challenge is to identify this subset of patients with dorsal duct pathology. Cannulation of the dorsal duct by ERCP is not as easily done as is cannulation of the ventral duct (Fig. 274-5). Patients with pancreatitis and pancreas divisum demonstrated by ERCP should be treated with conservative measures, including pancreatic enzyme therapy. Many of these patients have idiopathic pancreatitis unrelated to the pancreas divisum and will respond well to pancreatic enzyme therapy. Endoscopic or surgical intervention is indicated only when the above methods fail. If marked dilation of the dorsal duct can be demonstrated, surgical ductal decompression should be performed. The appropriate therapy for those patients without dilation of the dorsal duct is not yet defined. It should be stressed that the ERCP appearance of pancreas divisum, i.e., a small-caliber ventral duct with an arborizing pattern, may be confused with an obstructed main pancreatic duct secondary to a mass lesion.

MACROAMYLASEMIA   In macroamylasemia amylase circulates in the blood in a polymer form too large to be easily excreted by the kidney. The patient with this condition will demonstrate an elevated serum amylase value, a low urinary amylase value, and a C_{am}/C_{cr} ratio of less than 1 percent. The presence of macroamylase can be documented by chromatography of the serum. The prevalence of macroamylasemia is 1.5 percent of the nonalcoholic general adult hospital population. Usually macroamylasemia is an incidental finding and is not related to disease of the pancreas or other organs. It is important to be aware of this condition so that patients with macroamylasemia will not be needlessly evaluated and treated for pancreatic disease.

Macrolipasemia has now been documented in a patient with non-Hodgkin's lymphoma and in a patient with cirrhosis. These patients had normal ultrasound and CT examinations of the pancreas. Lipase was shown to be complexed with immunoglobulin A. Thus the possibility of *both* macroamylasemia and macrolipasemia should be considered in patients with elevated blood levels of these enzymes.

REFERENCES

AGARWAL N et al: Assessment of severity in acute pancreatitis. Am J Gastroenterol 86:1385, 1991

AMMANN RW: A critical appraisal of interventional therapy in chronic pancreatitis. Endoscopy 23:191, 1991

———— et al: Evolution and regression of pancreatic calcification in chronic pancreatitis: A prospective long-term study of 10 patients. Gastroenterology 95:1018, 1988

BALTHAZAR EJ et al: Acute pancreatitis: Value of CT in establishing prognosis. Radiology 174:331, 1990

BANKS PA: Management of pancreatic pain. Pancreas 6(suppl 1):52, 1991

CARR-LOCKE DL: Pancreas divisum: The controversy goes on. Endoscopy 23:88, 1991

COPENHAGEN PANCREATIC STUDY: An interim report from a prospective epidemiological multicenter study. Scand J Gastroenterol 16:305, 1981

GERZOF SG et al: Early diagnosis of pancreatic infection by computed tomography guided aspiration. Gastroenterology 93:1315, 1987

JOHNSON CD et al: CT of acute pancreatitis: Correlation between lack of contrast enhancement and pancreatic necrosis. AJR 156:92, 1991

KOLARS JC et al: Comparison of serum amylase, pancreatic isoamylase and lipase in patients with hyperamylasemia. Dig Dis Sci 29:289, 1984

LEE SP et al: Biliary sludge as a cause of acute pancreatitis. N Engl J Med 326:589, 1992

MCMAHON MJ et al: A comparative study of methods for reproduction of severity of attacks of acute pancreatitis. Br J Surg 67:22, 1985

MOOSSA AR: Surgical treatment of chronic pancreatitis: An overview. Br J Surg 74:661, 1987

NEOPTOLEMOS JP et al: Control trial of urgent endoscopic retrograde cholangiopancreatography and endoscopic sphincterotomy versus conservative treatment for acute pancreatitis due to gallstones. Lancet 2:979, 1988

NIEDERAU C, GRENDELL JH: Diagnosis of chronic pancreatitis. Gastroenterology 88:1973, 1985

SARLES H: Definitions and classifications of pancreatitis. Pancreas 6:470, 1991

SLAFF J et al: Protease specific suppression of pancreatic exocrine secretion. Gastroenterology 87:44, 1984

STEINBERG WM et al: Diagnostic assays in acute pancreatitis: A study of sensitivity and specificity. Ann Intern Med 102:576, 1985

TOSKES PP: Biochemical tests in pancreatic disease. Curr Opin Gastroenterol 8:814, 1992

————: Medical therapy of chronic pancreatitis. Semin Gastrointest Dis 2:188, 1991

————: Hyperlipidemic pancreatitis. Gastroenterol Clin North Am 19:783, 1990

WILSON C et al: Prediction of outcome in acute pancreatitis: A comparative study of APACHE II, clinical assessment, and multiple screening systems. Br J Surg 77:1260, 1990

275   PANCREATIC CANCER

ROBERT J. MAYER

INCIDENCE AND ETIOLOGY   The incidence of pancreatic carcinoma in the United States has increased significantly as the median life expectancy of the American population has been prolonged. The tumor results in the death of more than 95 percent of afflicted patients. Approximately 25,000 individuals died of pancreatic cancer in 1993, making it the fifth most common cause of cancer-related mortality. The disease appears to occur somewhat more frequently in males than in females and in blacks than in whites. It rarely develops prior to the age of 50.

Little is known about the causes of pancreatic cancer. Cigarette smoking represents the most consistently observed risk factor for the development of the tumor, with the disease being two to three times more common in heavy smokers than in nonsmokers. It is uncertain whether this apparent association reflects a direct carcinogenic effect of metabolites of cigarette smoke on the pancreas or whether an as yet undefined exposure occurring more frequently in cigarette smokers is responsible for the enhanced risk. A large case control study has also correlated chronic pancreatitis with an increased risk of pancreatic cancer. There are no convincing data to link such epidemiologic factors as alcohol abuse, cholelithiasis, or preexisting diabetes mellitus with the development of pancreatic cancer. Furthermore, the weight of clinical data has failed to support any association between coffee consumption and pancreatic cancer. Mutations in c-K-*ras* genes have frequently been found in specimens of human pancreatic cancer.

CLINICAL FEATURES   More than 90 percent of pancreatic cancers are ductal adenocarcinomas, with islet cell tumors constituting the remaining 5 to 10 percent. Pancreatic cancers occur twice as frequently in the pancreatic head (about 70 percent of cases) as in the body (about 20 percent) or tail (about 10 percent) of the gland.

With the exception of jaundice, the initial symptoms associated with pancreatic cancer are often insidious in nature and are usually present for longer than 2 months prior to the time the cancer is diagnosed (Table 275-1). Pain and weight loss are present in more than 75 percent of patients. The pain typically has a gnawing, visceral

---

TABLE 275-1   Presenting signs and symptoms of pancreatic carcinoma

Frequent
   Abdominal pain
   Weight loss
   Jaundice (lesions of pancreatic head only)
Infrequent
   Glucose intolerance
   Palpable gallbladder
   Migratory thrombophlebitis
   Gastrointestinal hemorrhage
   Splenomegaly

quality, occasionally radiating from the epigastrium to the back, and generally representing a more severe problem in lesions arising in the body or tail since such tumors may become quite large prior to being detected. Characteristically, the pain improves somewhat on bending forward. The development of significant pain is suggestive of retroperitoneal invasion and infiltration of the splanchnic nerves, indicating the primary lesion to be far advanced and surgically unresectable. Rarely, such pain may be transient and associated with hyperamylasemia, indicative of acute pancreatitis caused by ductal obstruction by tumor. The weight loss observed in the majority of patients having pancreatic carcinoma is primarily the result of anorexia, although in the initial period of the disease, subclinical malabsorption may also be a contributing factor.

Jaundice due to biliary obstruction is found in more than 80 percent of patients having tumors in the pancreatic head and is typically accompanied by darkening of urine, a claylike appearance of stool, and pruritus. In contrast to the "painless jaundice" sometimes observed in patients having carcinomas of the bile ducts, duodenum, or periampullary regions, the majority of icteric individuals having ductal carcinomas of the pancreatic head will complain of significant abdominal discomfort. Although the gallbladder is usually enlarged in patients with carcinoma of the head of the pancreas, it is palpable in less than 50 percent of cases (Courvoisier's sign). The presence, however, of an enlarged gallbladder in a jaundiced patient without biliary colic should suggest malignant obstruction of the extrahepatic biliary tree.

The vast majority of patients with pancreatic cancer do not develop clinical diabetes mellitus; in one study, glucose intolerance was found in only 6 percent of a group of 924 patients whose presenting symptoms were carefully analyzed. Other uncommon initial manifestations include venous thrombosis and migratory thrombophlebitis, gastrointestinal hemorrhage resulting from varices due to tumor compression of the portal venous system, and splenomegaly caused by cancerous encasement of the splenic vein.

DIAGNOSTIC PROCEDURES (Fig. 275-1) Despite the availability of serologic tests for tumor-associated antigens such as the carcinoembryonic antigen (CEA) and CA 19-9 and noninvasive imaging techniques such as CT scanning and ultrasonography, the early diagnosis of a potentially resectable pancreatic carcinoma remains extremely difficult. The nonspecificity of the initial symptoms and the poor sensitivity of both serologic assays and noninvasive techniques have frustrated the development of effective screening procedures. When the disease is clinically suspected in a patient having vague, persistent abdominal complaints, ultrasound should be performed to visualize the gallbladder and the pancreas, as well as upper GI contrast radiographs to rule out a hiatal hernia or a peptic ulcer. If these studies fail to provide an explanation for the symptoms, a CT scan should be considered. It should encompass not only the pancreas but also the liver, retroperitoneal lymph nodes, and pelvis, since pancreatic cancer frequently spreads within the abdomen. While more costly than ultrasonography, CT is technically simpler, more reproducible, provides better definition of the body and tail of the pancreas, and requires less interpretive skill. CT generally detects a malignant pancreatic lesion in over 80 percent of cases; in 5 to 15 percent of patients with proven pancreatic carcinoma, the CT scan shows only generalized pancreatic enlargment suggestive of pancreatitis rather than malignancy. False-positive results have also been reported in about 5 to 10 percent of cases where no tumor was found on laparotomy. At present, magnetic resonance imaging (MRI) has not been shown superior to CT in the evaluation of pancreatic lesions.

In selected situations where clinical circumstances dictate additional diagnostic evaluation, endoscopic retrograde cholangiopancreatography (ERCP) may clarify the cause of ambiguous CT or ultrasound findings. The characteristic findings are stenosis or obstruction of either the pancreatic or the common bile duct; both duct systems are abnormal in over half the cases. The differentiation between carcinoma and chronic pancreatitis by ERCP can be quite difficult, particularly if both diseases are present. False-negative results with ERCP are

quite infrequent (less than 5 percent) and usually occur in the setting of islet cell, rather than ductal, carcinomas.

Selective and superselective angiography may be of value in some patients. Angiography is an effective means of detecting carcinomas in the body and tail of the pancreas by demonstrating vascular narrowing, displacement, or occlusion by tumor. Angiography is also useful in assessing whether encasement of peripancreatic vessels is present; this is of importance in determining the potential for surgical resection.

Regardless of the results of the above diagnostic studies, a histologic confirmation of a presumed pancreatic cancer is mandatory to be absolutely certain that malignancy exists and to rule out the presence of such other neoplasms as an islet cell tumor or a lymphoma, for which the therapeutic approach and prognosis differ significantly from those for the usual ductal carcinoma. Such tissue confirmation may often be obtained through a percutaneous needle aspiration biopsy of the pancreas with CT or ultrasonographic guidance, thereby obviating surgical exploration.

It should be emphasized that patients with carcinoma of the pancreas may undergo several months of investigation before a diagnosis is established. In the past, this period of diagnostic delay and accompanying emotional uncertainty erroneously led to an impression that the pain and weight loss might not have had an organic cause, resulting in an association of pancreatic cancer and depression. The availability of CT scans has resulted in a prompter diagnosis and dispelled this incorrect notion. Unfortunately, however, even laparotomy may not provide a definitive diagnosis, because chronic pancreatitis may also produce a hard mass in the head of the pancreas, making it indistinguishable from carcinoma by palpation. Furthermore, a superficial biopsy of such a mass may not show neoplastic tissue, revealing only evidence of pancreatitis since the cancer itself is often surrounded by edematous, inflamed, and fibrotic tissue (i.e., changes associated with chronic pancreatitis).

TREATMENT Complete surgical resection of pancreatic tumors offers the only effective treatment for this disease. Unfortunately, such "curative" operations are only possible in 10 to 15 percent of patients with pancreatic cancer and are limited, for all practical purposes, to those individuals having tumors in the pancreatic head in whom jaundice was the initial symptom. Patients considered for such a procedure should have no evidence of metastatic spread on a chest radiogram and abdominal-pelvic CT scan, should undergo preoperative celiac angiography (to exclude evidence of surgical unresectability such as vascular invasion by tumor), and should receive their care from an experienced surgeon, since mortality rates of greater than 15 percent have been associated with this procedure. Although the potential for cure in patients with pancreatic cancer is restricted to those few who are able to undergo a complete surgical resection, the 5-year survival rate following such operations is only 10 percent. Nonetheless, an attempt at the procedure merits strong consideration, particularly for lesions in the pancreatic head, since ductal carcinomas often cannot be distinguished preoperatively from ampullary, duodenal, and distal bile duct tumors or pancreatic cyst adenocarcinomas, all of which have far higher resectability and cure rates. Furthermore, survival is prolonged three- to fourfold in patients who eventually experience disease recurrence following resection over those whose tumor is not excised, indicating that such operations have a palliative as well as curative potential. The risk for tumor recurrence is unaffected by the type of operative procedure [i.e., total pancreatectomy versus pancreaticoduodenectomy ("Whipple resection")] but is increased by the presence of lymph node metastases or tumor invasion into adjacent viscera. As a rule, pancreaticoduodenectomy or distal pancreatectomy seems preferable to total pancreatectomy because of the retention of exocrine function and avoidance of brittle diabetes.

The median survival for patients whose pancreatic cancers are surgically unresectable is approximately 5 months. Management of such individuals should be directed at symptomatic palliation. Ambulatory patients having tumors in the pancreatic head should be

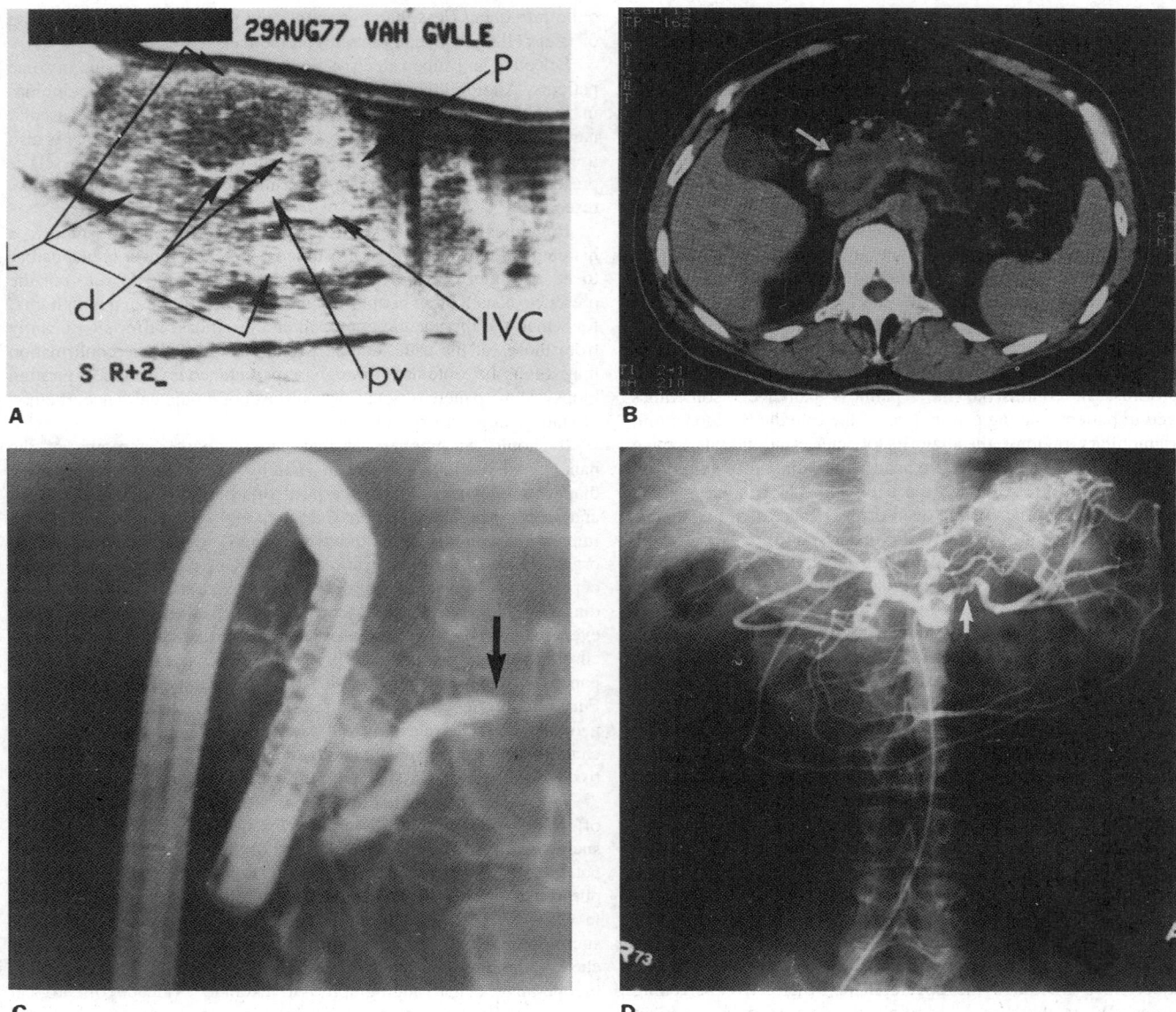

FIGURE 275-1   Carcinoma of the pancreas. *A.* Sonogram showing pancreatic carcinoma (P), dilated intrahepatic bile ducts (d), dilated portal vein (pv), and inferior vena cava (IVC). *B.* CT scan showing pancreatic carcinoma (arrow). *C.* ERCP showing abrupt cut off of the duct of Wirsung (arrow). *D.* Arteriogram showing sheathing of splenic artery by tumor encasement (arrow).

considered for surgical diversion of the biliary system. If jaundice has already developed, therapeutic options include either nonoperative biliary decompression by endoscopic or percutaneous, transhepatic biliary drainage or surgical biliary bypass. External beam radiation in patients with unresectable tumors which have not spread beyond the pancreas does not appear to prolong survival, although a sufficient reduction in tumor size may lead to palliation of pain. However, the addition of 5-fluorouracil (5-FU) chemotherapy to external beam irradiation has increased the survival time for these patients, perhaps by acting as a radiosensitizing agent. A similar combination of radiation therapy and 5-FU appears to have prolonged the survival and increased the cure rate when compared to a prospectively randomized nontreatment control group of patients who had a complete surgical resection of their pancreatic cancer. This observation has been made in a small patient population and thus demands confirmation prior to the general acceptance of the efficacy of postoperative ("adjuvant") treatment. The application of such chemoradiation therapy at diagnosis prior to surgery ("neoadjuvant") treatment as a means of increasing the potential for resectability is under investigation.

The experience utilizing chemotherapy in the management of patients with widely metastatic pancreatic cancer has been disappointing. No presently available drug regimen can be considered as being "standard." Newer forms of therapy must be developed and should constitute the initial treatment for consenting, ambulatory patients.

Pancreatic endocrine tumors are discussed in Chap. 276.

REFERENCES

Berg RJ, Connelly RR: Updating the epidemiologic data on pancreatic cancer. Semin Oncol 6:275, 1979

Cancer of the Pancreas Task Force: Staging of cancer of the pancreas. Cancer 47:1631, 1981

Connolly MM et al: Survival in 1001 patients with carcinoma of the pancreas. Ann Surg 206:366, 1987

Gastrointestinal Tumor Study Group: Pancreatic cancer. Adjuvant combined radiation and chemotherapy following curative resection. Arch Surg 120:899, 1985

Gudjonsson B et al: Cancer of the pancreas. Diagnostic accuracy and survival statistics. Cancer 42:2494, 1978

Lin A, Feller ER: Pancreatic carcinoma as a cause of unexplained pancreatitis: Report of ten cases. Ann Intern Med 113:166, 1990

Lowenfels AB et al: Pancreatitis and the risk of pancreatic cancer. N Engl J Med 328:1433, 1993

MOERTEL CT et al: Therapy of locally unresectable pancreatic adenocarcinoma: A randomized comparison of high dose (6,000 rads) radiation alone, moderate dose radiation (4,000 rads) + 5-fluorouracil, and high dose radiation + 5-fluorouracil. The Gastrointestinal Tumor Study Group. Cancer 48:1705, 1981

MOOSA AR, LEVIN B: The diagnosis of "early" pancreatic cancer: The University of Chicago experience. Cancer 47:1688, 1981

O'CONNELL MJ: Current status of chemotherapy for advanced pancreatic and gastric cancer. J Clin Oncol 3:1031, 1985

SPEER AG et al: Randomized trial of endoscopic versus percutaneous stent insertion in malignant obstructive jaundice. Lancet 2:57, 1987

STEINBERG WM et al: Comparison of the sensitivity and specificity of the CA 19-9 and carcinoembryonic antigen assays in detecting cancer of the pancreas. Gastroenterology 90:343, 1986

WARSHAW AL, FERNANDO-DEL CASTILLO C: Pancreatic carcinoma. N Engl J Med 326:455, 1992

TABLE 276-1   Distribution of APUD tumors

Origin	Tumors
Gastrointestinal tract	Carcinoid tumor
Pancreas	Islet cell carcinoma
Central nervous system	Ganglioneuroblastoma, neuroblastoma, chemodactoma, paraganglionoma
Thyroid	Medullary thyroid carcinoma
Skin	Melanoma
Adrenal medulla	Pheochromocytoma
Lung	Carcinoid tumor, small cell carcinoma

276   ENDOCRINE TUMORS OF THE GASTROINTESTINAL TRACT AND PANCREAS

LEE M. KAPLAN

Tumors arising from neuroendocrine cells of the gastrointestinal tract and pancreas present special challenges in diagnosis and therapy. Unlike other gastrointestinal neoplasms, these tumors often cause symptoms from excess hormone secretion rather than from growth, invasion, or local anatomic effects. Frequently slow growing, they may nonetheless be life-threatening because of uncontrolled release of specific hormones and neurotransmitters. These neoplasms arise from within the gastrointestinal mucosa and pancreatic islets in cells that normally secrete regulatory monoamines and peptide hormones. For example, gastrin-secreting G cells within the gastric and duodenal mucosa regulate gastric acid secretion, and insulin-secreting β cells within the pancreatic islets have a crucial role in the homeostatic control of glucose metabolism. Overall, more than 30 distinct secretory products have been identified within neuroendocrine cells of the gut.

BIOLOGIC CONSIDERATIONS

A striking feature of neuroendocrine tumors is the preservation of highly differentiated cell function. Tumor cells contain secretory granules and maintain the capacity for *a*mine *p*recursor *u*ptake and *d*ecarboxylation (APUD), a process essential for the production of monoamine neurotransmitters such as serotonin, dopamine, and histamine. This characteristic has fostered the term *APUDomas* for neoplasms derived from these cells, which can be located in the thyroid (C cells), adrenal medulla, lung (neuroendocrine cells), skin (melanocytes), and nervous system (glial cells and neuroblasts), as well as the gastrointestinal tract and pancreas. These cells also synthesize and secrete *peptide* hormones by a separate mechanism. Several of the known APUDomas are listed in Table 276-1. It was postulated that this specialized capability implies a common embryologic origin for these diverse cells, but in fact, cells of *varied* heritage can acquire the APUD phenotype during differentiation.

Studies of neuroendocrine cell physiology have revealed several important characteristics of secretory cells and the clinical syndromes caused by their humoral products:

1 Cellular phenotype does not predict the nature of the secreted product. Thus neurons may secrete peptide "hormones" into the synaptic cleft, and endocrine cells may secrete monoamines previously classified as "neurotransmitters." Individual cells have the capacity to synthesize and secrete both peptide and monoamine

transmitters, which may coexist in individual secretory granules. Many symptoms of enterochromaffin cell tumors (carcinoid tumors) appear to arise from the combined actions of monoamine and peptide products.

2 Transmitter secretion by neuroendocrine cells is frequently episodic or pulsatile. Although the regulation of secretion is incompletely understood, the temporal pattern of hormone release may vary depending on the hormonal milieu, physiologic state, or stage of development. Thus symptoms produced by abnormal secretion of hormones from neuroendocrine tumors may be intermittent, especially in early stages when tumor cells may behave more like their normal counterparts.

3 Individual cells have the *potential* to secrete a wide array of transmitters. This feature is particularly evident for the peptide hormones. Depending on the stage of development, cellular environment, and other as yet unidentified factors, neuroendocrine cells can change secretory profiles dramatically. For example, in cell culture, clonal populations may suddenly change from the secretion of insulin to cholecystokinin, gastrin, or even glucagon. Endocrine tumors may contain heterogeneous populations of cells so that within individual tumors a single cell type may predominate, or there may be multiple cell types in varying proportions. In addition, the secretory profile of a tumor may vary with time, producing a dramatic alteration of symptoms. Individual metastatic implants also can display different phenotypes from the primary tumor and from each other.

4 Individual hormones and transmitters secreted by neuroendocrine cells may regulate physiologic activity (e.g., secretion, absorption, or contractility), stimulate or inhibit growth, or affect the development of target cells. Thus the humoral activity of gut neuroendocrine tumors can cause a wide variety of effects, including gastric acid hypersecretion, abnormal intestinal motility, gastric epithelial hyperplasia, gallstone formation, mesenteric and cardiac fibrosis, and necrosis of the skin.

5 Hormone production by neuroendocrine cells is tightly regulated at many levels, including RNA transcription, precursor peptide processing, and secretion. These cells, in addition, may be subject to control by neighboring secretory cells *(paracrine regulation)*. Thus multiple cell types may act in concert to control the growth, secretory characteristics, and thus the clinical manifestations of individual tumors. Abnormal secretion by the tumors themselves may disrupt the normal regulated function of neighboring neuroendocrine cells, and neoplastic transformation may disturb hormone secretion by these cells. Cells may secrete partially processed hormone precursors, leading to unpredictable effects, or display altered susceptibility to regulation by exogenous stimuli. Occasionally, such characteristics can be exploited to permit specific diagnostic tests for individual tumors.

Neuroendocrine tumors of the gastrointestinal tract can be classified by cell type, major hormone secreted, and site of origin. These characteristics, alone or in combination, correlate well with the observed clinical syndromes. Table 276-2 lists the important tumors in this category, along with their clinical presentations, major secreted products, cells of origin, and biologic behavior.

TABLE 276-2   Gastrointestinal endocrine tumor syndromes

Syndrome	Cell type	Clinical features	Percentage malignant	Major products
Carcinoid syndrome	Enterochromaffin, enterochromaffin-like	Flushing, diarrhea, wheezing, hypotension	~100	Serotonin, histamine, miscellaneous peptides
Zollinger-Ellison, gastrinoma	Non-ß islet cell, duodenal G cell	Peptic ulcers, diarrhea	~70	Gastrin
Insulinoma	Islet ß cell	Hypoglycemia	~10	Insulin
VIPoma (Verner-Morrison, WDHA)	Islet D_1 cell	Diarrhea, hypokalemia, hypochlorhydria	~60	Vasoactive intestinal peptide
Glucagonoma	Islet A cell	Mild diabetes mellitus, erythema necrolytica migrans, glossitis	>75	Glucagon
Somatostatinoma	Islet D cell	Diabetes mellitus, diarrhea, steatorrhea, gallstones	~70	Somatostatin
GRFoma	Non-ß islet cell	Acromegaly	–	Growth hormone-releasing hormone (GRF)
CRFoma	Non-ß islet cell	Cushing's syndrome	–	Corticotropin-releasing hormone (CRF)
PPoma	Islet PP cell	Rare necrolytic erythema	–	Pancreatic polypeptide (PP)
Neurotensinoma	Non-ß islet cell	None	–	Neurotensin
Miscellaneous tumors	Non-ß islet cell	Hypercalcemia, inappropriate ADH, hyperpigmentation	–	Parathyroid hormone, vasopressin, melanocyte-stimulating hormone

DIAGNOSTIC CONSIDERATIONS

Several distinct syndromes of hormone excess have been described in which symptoms may suggest the presence of an endocrine tumor of the gastrointestinal tract or pancreas. Moreover, these tumors may present as part of the type 1 multiple endocrine neoplasia (MEN 1) syndrome (see Chap. 343). MEN 1 patients frequently develop parathyroid and pituitary adenomas that may produce symptoms of hypercalcemia, hyperprolactinemia, hyperthyroidism, or growth hormone excess. Diagnosis is suggested by history, physical findings, elevated blood levels of the relevant peptide hormone(s), or elevated urinary levels of the major metabolites of monoamine transmitters. Further confirmation of hormone-producing tumors may be provided by provocative tests that reveal abnormalities in the regulation of hormone secretion. For example, tolbutamide may enhance somatostatin secretion from somatostatinoma cells. Normal somatostatin-secreting D cells do not show this effect. Other examples of *abnormal* regulation in tumor cells include enhancement by secretin of gastrin secretion in gastrinomas and pentagastrin stimulation of calcitonin secretion in medullary thyroid (C cell) tumors.

Anatomic definition for pancreatic tumors should be sought by computed tomography (CT), and endoscopic visualization or barium contrast studies should be obtained for suspected mucosal and submucosal tumors. In cases where tumors are too small to be visualized by these noninvasive methods, angiography or selective venous sampling for hormone determination may provide anatomic localization. CT and magnetic resonance imaging (MRI) are the preferred means of assessing metastatic spread, since the liver and lymph nodes are the initial sites of tumor metastasis.

THERAPEUTIC CONSIDERATIONS

Therapy of endocrine tumors has two goals: (1) to decrease or reverse the growth and spread of the tumor and (2) to relieve the symptoms of hormone overproduction. When the tumor is localized, both goals may be accomplished by surgical excision. However, most of these tumors are malignant and have spread by the time of diagnosis, and control of growth in such malignant tumors has proven difficult. Thus far, the greatest benefit has been seen with chemotherapeutic regimens that include streptozocin, alone or in combination with fluorouracil or doxorubicin. Control of hepatic metastases has been achieved with hepatic artery embolization or direct injection with cytotoxic agents (e.g., ethanol), although these approaches are palliative rather than curative.

Several approaches are used to control the effects of excess hormone production by these tumors. The most common is to block the function of the target tissue. For example, gastric acid hypersecretion induced by gastrin-producing tumors may be reversed by medications that inhibit acid secretion (e.g., H-2 receptor blockers or proton pump blockers) or by surgical resection of the stomach. Diazoxide is used to help reverse the effects of hyperinsulinemia, and hypomotility agents may ameliorate the diarrhea caused by hypersecretion of vasoactive intestinal peptide (VIP), gastrin, somatostatin, neurotensin, or serotonin.

A second approach is to block release of the transmitter from the tumor cells. The success of this approach depends on the continued ability of the tumor cells to respond to such physiologic or pharmacologic stimuli. Initial trials used somatostatin, a peptide hormone that inhibits the release of numerous hormones and amine transmitters. While somatostatin controls the symptoms of many of these tumors, it has a short half-life and must be given intravenously. These limitations have been largely overcome by the use of octreotide, a longer-acting analogue of somatostatin with similar actions that can be administered subcutaneously. The chemical structures of somatostatin and octreotide are shown in Fig. 276-1 (see also Chap.

FIGURE 276-1 Structures of somatostatin-14 and octreotide. The double circle denotes the substitution of D-tryptophan for the naturally occurring L-tryptophan. This substitution inhibits peptide degradation and prolongs serum half-life.

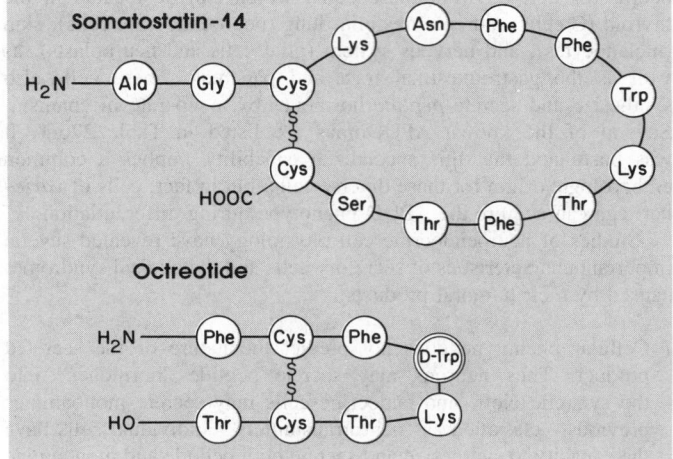

TABLE 276-3 Clinical uses of octreotide in gastrointestinal disease

Hormone-secreting tumors

Carcinoid tumor	Inhibits cutaneous flushing, controls diarrhea, reverses hypotension, aids perioperative management, ?inhibits growth
VIPoma	Controls diarrhea
Insulinoma	Controls hypoglycemia acutely, aids perioperative management
Gastrinoma	Perioperative management, ?controls diarrhea
Glucagonoma	Controls necrolytic erythema
Dumping syndrome	Controls diarrhea, vasomotor symptoms
Diarrhea	Inhibits intestinal secretion, motility
Short-bowel syndrome	
Ileostomy	
Diabetic neuropathy	
AIDS	
Fistulas	Inhibits fluid and enzyme secretion, promotes healing
Pancreatic	
Enteric	
Crohn's disease	
Gastrointestinal bleeding	
Portal hypertensive gastropathy	Reduces portal pressure, splanchnic blood flow
Esophageal and gastric varices	Reduces portal pressure, splanchnic blood flow

331). Octreotide frequently relieves the symptoms of several endocrine tumors that are inadequately controlled by tumor resection or ablation. In addition, tumor regression has occurred in occasional patients, suggesting that the hormone agonist may have some growth-inhibiting effects. The major known side effects of octreotide are dose-dependent and are similar to symptoms of somatostatin excess, including steatorrhea, mild hyperglycemia, nausea, and abdominal pain. Patients on long-term therapy with this agent have an increased tendency to develop gallstones. The clinical disorders that respond to therapy with octreotide are summarized in Table 276-3.

CARCINOID TUMORS

Carcinoid tumors are the most protean and the most common gastrointestinal endocrine tumors, accounting for approximately 55 percent of such neoplasms. The incidence of carcinoid tumors in the United States is approximately 15 per 1 million population per year. They may present with gastrointestinal bleeding, abdominal pain, obstruction from tumor growth or tumor-induced mesenteric fibrosis, or symptoms arising from tumor-secreted hormones. The name *carcinoid* was applied to these tumors because slow growth and the homogeneous appearance of tumor cells led early investigators to underestimate their malignant potential. They pursue an indolent course, and the interval between onset of symptoms and diagnosis averages 4.5 years. Carcinoid tumors arise from neuroendocrine cells throughout the body but are most prevalent in the gastrointestinal tract, pancreas, and pulmonary bronchi. Ninety percent of these tumors arise in the enterochromaffin, or Kulchitsky, cells within the gastrointestinal tract. The tumors can be found anywhere from the stomach to the rectum and are most common in the appendix, ileum, and rectum. Gastrointestinal carcinoids frequently cause abdominal pain, bleeding, or intestinal obstruction. Although they are rarely large, the tumors may become the leading point for intussusception. In addition, mesenteric spread stimulates a local fibrous reaction, causing intestinal kinking, obstruction, and vascular compromise. Rare sites of carcinoid tumors include the thymus, esophagus, biliary duct, Meckel's diverticulum, breast, and ovary. No risk factors have been clearly defined for these tumors, although the incidence of gastric carcinoids may be increased in patients with pernicious anemia, achlorhydria, and Hashimoto's thyroiditis. Carcinoids of the bronchus, stomach, and duodenum may occur in association with MEN 1. Thymic carcinoids may be associated with hyperparathyroidism or Cushing's syndrome.

Appendiceal tumors comprise nearly half of all carcinoid tumors and are incidental findings in 0.3 to 0.7 percent of routine appendectomy specimens. They are usually small, solitary, and benign. Local invasion is common but metastatic spread is rare, and the presence of tumor does not appear to confer appreciable morbidity or mortality. Colorectal carcinoids have a similarly benign course and are usually asymptomatic. In contrast, small-bowel and bronchial carcinoids have a more malignant course. Local transmural invasion, early metastasis to lymph nodes and liver, and symptoms from hormone secretion are common. Other sites of metastatic spread include bone and, less commonly, heart, breast, and eye. The risk of metastatic spread is dependent on tumor size. Metastases are found in fewer than 2 percent of tumors less than 1 cm in diameter but in nearly 100 percent of tumors greater than 2 cm. Additional primary tumor implants within the gastrointestinal tract are found in 40 percent of patients.

CARCINOID SYNDROME Enterochromaffin cells secrete a variety of hormones and are embryologically related to thyroid C cells, adrenal medullary cells, and melanocytes. Tumors of each of these cell types may produce syndromes of hormone excess. Hormone secretion by carcinoid cells can cause distinctive and debilitating effects (carcinoid syndrome) long before local growth or metastatic spread is otherwise apparent. Manifestations of the carcinoid syndrome include the "classic" triad of cutaneous flushing, diarrhea, and valvular heart disease and, less commonly, telangiectasias, wheezing, and paroxysmal *hypo*tension. Flushing, which is present in approximately 85 percent of patients with carcinoid syndrome, is also seen with many other conditions, including menopause, autonomic nervous system dysfunction, ethanol ingestion, disulfiram treatment, drug withdrawal, and a variety of hormone-secreting tumors, including pheochromocytoma, medullary thyroid carcinoma, VIPoma, and mastocytosis. It is estimated that approximately 5 percent of individuals presenting with the new onset of flushing will be found to have the carcinoid syndrome. Early in the course, symptoms are usually episodic and may be provoked by stress, catecholamines, and ingestion of food or alcohol. During acute paroxysms, systolic blood pressure typically falls 20 to 30 mmHg. Diarrhea may result from several mechanisms. The most common type is mixed secretory and hypermotility-induced, producing watery stools unresponsive to fasting. Other causes include partial mechanical obstruction from tumor or fibrosis and mesenteric vascular insufficiency from local fibrosis. Endocardial fibrosis can cause valvular heart disease, usually affecting the proximal side of the tricuspid and pulmonary valves and leading to tricuspid insufficiency, pulmonary stenosis, and secondary right-sided heart failure. Left-sided valvular disease may occur in association with bronchial carcinoids, presumably because venous effluent from these tumors passes directly into the pulmonary veins, avoiding inactivation of the hormone mediators in the lung.

Approximately 5 percent of all patients with carcinoid tumors experience one or more symptoms of the carcinoid syndrome. The likelihood of developing symptoms is strongly dependent on the origin and behavior of the tumor. While 30 to 60 percent of small-bowel carcinoids are associated with systemic manifestations, only 3.5 percent of lung, 1 percent of appendix, and virtually no rectal carcinoids produce the syndrome. In patients with intestinal carcinoids, the humoral symptoms only develop in the setting of metastatic disease to the liver. Bronchial and other extraintestinal carcinoids, whose hormone products are not immediately cleared by the liver, may produce the carcinoid syndrome in the absence of metastasis.

Carcinoid tumors may be classified on the basis of embryonic origin (Table 276-4). Clinical features, secreted hormones, diagnostic evaluation, and prognosis vary according to whether a carcinoid arises in foregut, midgut, or hindgut structures. For example, carcinoid syndrome is less common in patients with foregut carcinoids than midgut tumors, but the syndrome, when it occurs, is more likely to include wheezing. Patients with foregut carcinoid syndrome more often have dramatic cutaneous flushing involving the whole body than those with tumors of midgut or hindgut organs. The flush of bronchial carcinoids may be prolonged (lasting hours to days); associated with

TABLE 276-4   Characteristics of carcinoid tumors

Embryonic origin	Site of primary tumor	Carcinoid syndrome		
		Frequency, %	Characteristics	Monoamines
Foregut	Bronchus	3.5	Intense flush, lasting up to several hours; associated lacrimation, salivation, facial edema; wheezing; diarrhea; left- and right-sided cardiac lesions	5-HT, ± histamine
	Stomach	~5	Intense, patchy, whole body flush, with defined borders, wheals, usually lasting several minutes; pruritus; wheezing; diarrhea	5-HTP, histamine, ± 5-HT
	Duodenum, jejunum	~40	Diarrhea	5-HT
	Pancreas, gallbladder	Rare	Occasional necrolytic erythema	
		~40	Facial flush, usually lasting seconds to minutes; telangiectasias; cardiac lesions; peritoneal fibrosis; diarrhea	5-HT, ± histamine
	Illeum	~1		
Midgut	Appendix			
	Colon	Rare	Mild facial flush	5-HT
Hindgut	Rectum	0	Diarrhea	

NOTE: 5-HT = 5-hydroxytryptamine (serotonin); 5-HTP = 5-hydroxytryptophan.

excessive lacrimation, salivation, and facial edema; and occasionally producing significant hypotension. The cutaneous manifestations of gastric carcinoids, though lasting only minutes, are frequently well-circumscribed and associated with wheals, pruritus, and high levels of histamine secretion. Midgut carcinoids commonly cause the carcinoid syndrome. Acute episodes of flushing tend to be less severe than those associated with foregut tumors, but facial telangiectasias may develop late in the course. Midgut tumors are more frequently associated with cardiac manifestations and peritoneal fibrosis. Hindgut tumors rarely cause the carcinoid syndrome. A rare variant syndrome associated with ovarian carcinoids causes severe peritoneal fibrosis.

Serotonin (5-hydroxytryptamine, 5-HT) is the most common secretory product of carcinoid tumors. As shown in Fig. 276-2, carcinoid tumors synthesize serotonin by enzymatic modification of circulating tryptophan. Up to 50 percent of the dietary intake of tryptophan can be converted to serotonin by these cells, which may leave inadequate substrate for incorporation into proteins and conversion to niacin. As a result, patients with widely metastatic carcinoid tumors may suffer symptoms of protein malnutrition (see Chap. 72) or mild pellagra (see Chap. 77). Serotonin induces intestinal secretion, inhibits intestinal absorption, and stimulates intestinal motility. High serotonin levels are likely the cause of diarrhea in most cases of carcinoid syndrome. Serotonin also stimulates fibroblast growth and fibrogenesis and thus may mediate or accelerate the peritoneal and cardiac valvular fibrosis in this disease. Excess serotonin secretion alone does not account for cutaneous flushing. Multiple monoamine and peptide factors contribute to the vasomotor changes; the relative contributions of each mediator may vary from patient to patient.

Carcinoid tumors elaborate multiple monoamines and peptide hormones, including histamine, catecholamines, bradykinins, tachykinins, enkephalins and endorphins, vasopressin, gastrin, adrenocorticotrophin, and prostaglandins (Table 276-5). Many secrete somatostatin, neurotensin, substance P, neurokinin A, and motilin. The elevated circulating levels of these substances mediate many of the pathophysiologic changes of carcinoid syndrome, although the relative contributions of each remain to be identified.

DIAGNOSIS   The diagnosis of carcinoid tumors is influenced by the presenting features of the tumor. Patients with nonfunctional tumors (i.e., without the carcinoid syndrome) usually present with symptoms due to the direct effects of the tumor in the gastrointestinal tract, including abdominal pain or tenderness, nausea, malaise, weight loss, intestinal or biliary obstruction, or gastrointestinal bleeding. Depending on the location of the tumor and whether metastases are present, endoscopy, barium studies, or CT may allow anatomic localization. Radiographic studies should include small-bowel follow-through or direct instillation of radiographic contrast material into the small bowel (enteroclysis) to identify tumors in the jejunum and ileum. Despite the improved detection of tumors, however, their

pathologic identity is usually not suspected before resection or liver biopsy.

Evaluation of patients with clinical features of carcinoid syndrome is based on the observation that serotonin is secreted by the large majority of functional carcinoid tumors. As shown in Fig. 276-2, serotonin is metabolized in the blood to 5-hydroxyindoleacetic acid (5-HIAA), which is cleared by the kidneys. Plasma and platelet serotonin and urinary 5-HIAA levels are usually elevated in the setting of carcinoid syndrome. Measurement of urinary 5-HIAA excretion is the most useful diagnostic test, and approximately 75 percent of patients excrete more than 80 μmol/d (15 mg/d). Specificity of this test approaches 100 percent after exclusion of ingested substances

FIGURE 276-2   Metabolic pathway of serotonin in the carcinoid syndrome.

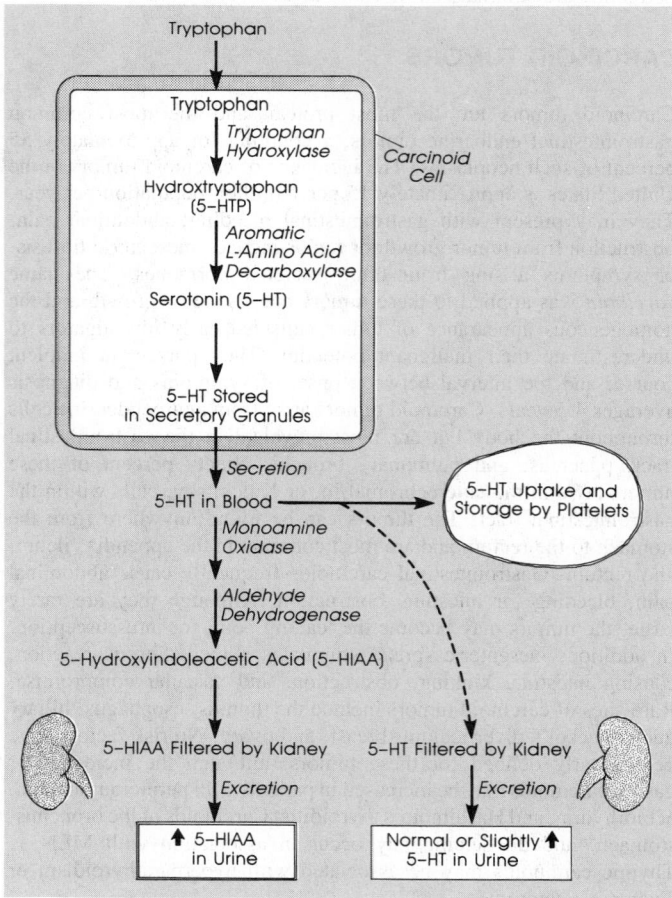

TABLE 276-5 Hormone mediators of carcinoid syndrome

Clinical feature	Frequency, %	Candidate mediators
Diarrhea	78	5-HT, histamine, prostaglandins, VIP, glucagon, gastrin, calcitonin
Cutaneous flushing	94	5-HT, 5-HTP, kallikrein, NKA, histamine, SK, SP, prostaglandins
Telangiectasia	25	Unknown
Wheezing	18	5-HT, histamine
Abdominal pain	51	Tumor, hepatic enlargment, bowel ischemia (fibrosis)
Heart disease		5-HT
Right-sided	40	
Left-sided	13	
Pellagra dermatosis	7	Tryptophan depletion (5-HT synthesis)

NOTE: 5-HT = 5-hydroxytryptamine (serotonin); 5-HTP = 5-hydroxytryptophan; NKA = neurokinin A; SK = substance K; SP = substance P; VIP = vasoactive intestinal peptide.
SOURCE: After W Creutzfeldt and F Stockmann, Am J Med 82:4, 1987.

known to elevate 5-HIAA levels; these include bananas, plantain, pineapple, kiwi fruit, walnuts, plums, pecans, avocados, guaifenesin, and acetaminophen. Conversely, aspirin and levodopa ingestion can cause a falsely depressed 5-HIAA level. In some patients with carcinoid syndrome and normal urinary 5-HIAA, documentation of elevated plasma or platelet serotonin concentrations may establish the diagnosis. However, many gastric carcinoid tumors lack the aromatic L-amino acid decarboxylase and convert 5-hydroxytryptophan (5-HTP) to serotonin with low efficiency. Since 5-HTP is not metabolized to 5-HIAA, urinary studies may be misleading. These patients may have elevated urinary serotonin levels, since renal cells contain aromatic L-amino acid decarboxylase. Diagnosis in these cases may be confirmed by demonstrating elevated plasma 5-HTP, histamine, or peptide hormone levels, although it frequently rests on the anatomic detection of the tumor itself. Attempts to provoke cutaneous flushing are helpful for documenting flushing in cases when the clinical history is equivocal. Ethanol, pentagastrin, or *micro*gram quantities of epinephrine can be used for this purpose. Abdominal ultrasonography, CT, and selective angiography are the most sensitive tests for detecting metastatic disease in the liver. Since most patients with the humoral syndrome have metastases, liver biopsy is the most common access to histologic diagnosis. Additional information about bone metastases and cardiac sequelae may be obtained with bone scans and echocardiography, respectively. In patients in whom a tumor cannot be detected, imaging with radiolabeled metaiodobenzyl guanidine (MIBG) or octreotide may be helpful. MIBG is concentrated by neuroendocrine cells and accumulates in many carcinoid tumors, and octreotide binds to somatostatin receptors, which are expressed in large numbers by many such tumors.

TREATMENT Effective treatment of the carcinoid syndrome may require more than one approach. Therapy should be selected according to the severity of symptoms. Since nearly all patients with carcinoid syndrome have metastatic disease, resection is rarely curative. Mild diarrhea may be controlled with hypomotility agents such as loperamide or diphenoxylate/atropine. In patients who have undergone ileal resection, diarrhea can be exacerbated by bile salt malabsorption and frequently responds to cholestyramine. Flushing, if rare and mild, may not require therapy. Combination therapy with histamine H-1 and H-2 receptor antagonists (e.g., diphenhydramine and ranitidine) can inhibit the cutaneous flush associated with foregut carcinoids. Phenoxybenzamine may provide additional benefit by inhibiting the release of bradykinin. Methylxanthine bronchodilators and glucocorticoids are helpful in relieving the dyspnea and wheezing associated with bronchial carcinoids. Beta-adrenergic agonists should be avoided because they may provoke acute exacerbations. Serotonin antagonists, including cyproheptadine and methysergide, have been used to provide

relief of diarrhea. Unfortunately, these agents have little effect on flushing and other vasomotor symptoms, and methysergide can induce fibrosis similar to that caused by the carcinoid itself.

Octreotide is a potent inhibitor of hormone secretion by carcinoid cells. Indeed, this agent provides effective control of diarrhea, flushing, and wheezing in more than 75 percent of cases. Octreotide is effective in the management of acute manifestations of the carcinoid syndrome such as hypotension or resulting angina, as well as the transient exacerbation caused by hepatic artery embolization or the induction of general anesthesia. However, octreotide must be administered in two or three subcutaneous injections each day. It is not yet known whether octreotide can prevent the observed cardiac (or mesenteric) fibrosis. Established valvular heart disease is not reversed by any form of medical therapy.

Surgery, hepatic artery embolization, and chemotherapy have been used to reduce the burden of tumor tissue. Surgery is the treatment of choice for small (<2 cm diameter) carcinoid tumors of the appendix or large bowel. Patients with carcinoid syndrome from isolated bronchial or other extraintestinal carcinoids also may be amenable to curative resection. Most patients with carcinoid syndrome, however, have gross metastatic disease. Hepatic resection generally provides only transient amelioration of symptoms and no improvement in survival. In isolated cases, however, long-term palliation has been achieved by resection of a *single* hepatic metastasis after removal of the primary tumor. Several less invasive approaches have been tried to limit the hepatic tumor burden and control humoral symptoms, including local irradiation, selective hepatic artery infusion of chemotherapy, CT-guided instillation of ethanol into metastatic implants, and hepatic arterial occlusion combined with chemoembolization. Unfortunately, carcinoid tumors are generally radioresistant and respond weakly to chemotherapy. Arterial occlusion by Gelfoam embolization provides transient relief of symptoms in approximately 90 percent of patients. Its success derives in part from the fact that the hepatic artery supplies less than half the blood supply of normal liver tissue but nearly all the blood supply of the tumor. Side effects of therapy include pain, fever, and occasional synthetic liver dysfunction. Effectiveness of therapy can be monitored with serum transaminase levels, which should rise substantially over the first 24 to 48 h after embolization. Patients undergoing embolization may experience acute exacerbation of carcinoid symptoms provoked by the sudden release of hormones from the tumor. Although such effects are rarely life-threatening, prophylactic treatment with histamine-receptor blockers and octreotide is recommended.

Several systemic chemotherapeutic protocols have been evaluated. Various combinations of streptozocin, fluorouracil, cyclophosphamide, and doxorubicin induce objective responses in approximately one-third of patients with metastatic disease, although the effect on survival is minimal. Leukocyte interferon decreases tumor size in approximately 20 percent and decreases urinary 5-HIAA excretion in about half of patients. Although octreotide has induced objective responses in a few cases, controlled trials have not yet demonstrated a significant effect.

The prognosis is highly dependent on the site and stage of the disease at diagnosis. As noted above, appendiceal and rectal carcinoids rarely affect survival. For other gastrointestinal carcinoids, 5-year survival is approximately 95 percent with local disease, 65 percent with lymph node involvement, and 18 percent with liver metastases. Median survival is $2\frac{1}{2}$ years after the first episode of flushing. Prognosis is inversely correlated with the degree of urinary 5-HIAA elevation. Despite attempts at therapy, patients excreting >800 μmol/d (>150 mg/d) have a median survival of only 1 year.

PANCREATIC ISLET-CELL TUMORS

GASTRINOMA (ZOLLINGER-ELLISON SYNDROME) (See also Chap. 252) In 1955, Zollinger and Ellison reported the association of severe peptic ulcer disease and gastrin-secreting tumors of the pancreas. These gastrinomas generate high serum gastrin levels, leading to hypersecretion of gastric acid and consequent duodenal and jejunal ulcers. Gastrinomas are the most common of the hormone-secreting tumors of the pancreatic islets, comprising nearly one-tenth of gastroenteropancreatic endocrine tumors and occurring with a frequency of approximately 4×10^{-7} in an unselected population in Ireland. Zollinger-Ellison syndrome may account for up to 0.1 percent of patients with duodenal ulcer disease in the United States. Ulcer disease develops in almost all patients with gastrinoma and is the presenting problem in approximately 70 percent. More than half of patients experience diarrhea (either watery stools or steatorrhea), and approximately 30 percent present with diarrhea alone. Radiologic and endoscopic examinations frequently reveal increased gastric fluid and thickened rugal folds. The age distribution of patients with gastrinoma is similar to that in ordinary acid peptic disease, with a broad peak in the fifth to eighth decades. Gastrinoma should be considered in all patients with recurrent or refractory ulcer disease, ulcers associated with gastric hypertrophy, ulcers in the distal duodenum or jejunum, ulcers in patients with diarrhea, kidney stones, hypercalcemia, or pituitary disease, or a strong family history of duodenal ulcer disease or endocrine tumors.

Between one-fourth and one-half of gastrinomas occur in association with the MEN 1 syndrome (see Chap. 343). Hyperparathyroidism is the most common component of MEN 1 and occurs in about 80 percent of patients with this form of Zollinger-Ellison syndrome. All gastrinoma patients should be screened for possible MEN 1 by measurement of serum calcium, phosphorus, cortisol, and prolactin levels and imaging of the sella turcica. First-degree relatives of patients with MEN 1 also should be similarly screened.

Approximately 80 percent of gastrin-secreting tumors arise in pancreatic islets, including nearly all those associated with MEN 1, and most are located in the pancreatic head. Another 10 to 15 percent arise from G cells in the duodenum, and the remainder are scattered in the distal small bowel, stomach, spleen, liver, lymph nodes, and ovary (mucinous cystadenoma). The tumors are usually small and are frequently multifocal, especially when associated with MEN 1. The biologic behavior may be variable. In most reported series, one-half to two-thirds of these tumors are malignant, with metastases in lymph nodes and liver and less frequently in bone. However, the prevalence of metastatic disease at the time of diagnosis appears to have decreased, perhaps owing to the more widespread consideration and earlier detection of these tumors. Such observations have important therapeutic implications, since isolated tumors are more likely to be cured by resection. Gastrinomas, like most other islet cell tumors, are generally slow-growing, but growth patterns vary widely and metastases may be more aggressive than the primary tumor itself.

Treatment of Zollinger-Ellison syndrome is directed at the sequelae of excess gastrin secretion and at the tumor itself. The availability of potent inhibitors of gastric acid secretion, including H-2 receptor blockers and the H^+,K^+-ATPase inhibitor omeprazole, has reduced the need for gastric surgery in these patients. The rare patient who fails to respond to medical therapy should be treated surgically. However, patients with coexistent hyperparathyroidism should undergo parathyroid resection before a decision is made about gastric surgery, since resolution of hypercalcemia may permit better medical control of gastric acid secretion.

Because of the effective control of hormone-mediated symptoms, morbidity and mortality from gastrinoma are increasingly related to the growth and spread of tumor itself. Curative resection of the gastrinoma is possible in 15 to 20 percent of cases and is favored by an extrapancreatic location and an inability to detect the tumor mass preoperatively. Gastrinomas in association with MEN 1 syndrome are not amenable to surgical cure, although these tumors generally have a benign natural history. Preoperative evaluation with CT and selective angiography is used to exclude multiple primary tumors and metastases. Treatment of unresectable gastrinoma includes chemotherapy, hormonal therapy, and hepatic artery embolization. Chemotherapeutic regimens including streptozocin and fluorouracil, with or without doxorubicin, commonly induce partial responses. Leukocyte interferon also may cause objective response, but octreotide does not appear to be effective. Hepatic artery embolization may decrease hepatic tumor burden and ameliorate pain. Unfortunately, none of these approaches prolongs survival of patients with metastatic disease, which approximates 25 percent at 10 years. For more information about the diagnosis and therapy of Zollinger-Ellison syndrome, refer to Chap. 252.

INSULINOMA (β CELL TUMOR) The hallmark of pancreatic β cell tumors is the development of symptomatic hypoglycemia from unregulated insulin hypersecretion (see also Chap. 338). Insulinomas are the second most common functioning islet cell tumors and have a reported prevalence of approximately 8×10^{-7} in an unselected Irish population. They arise most frequently in the fifth to seventh decades, although cases have been reported at all ages. In infants and children, insulinoma must be distinguished from diffuse β cell adenomatosis and nesidioblastosis. Whipple's triad describes the classic presentation of insulinoma and includes fasting hypoglycemia, *symptoms* of hypoglycemia, and immediate relief after intravenous glucose administration. Weight gain may result from increased food ingested to combat symptoms of hypoglycemia. In the current era, the diagnosis of insulinoma is made by demonstrating fasting hypoglycemia in the presence of normal or elevated plasma insulin levels. Symptoms related to the hypoglycemia include headache, slurred speech, psychological alterations, visual disturbances, confusion, and, ultimately, coma and death. Hypoglycemia also induces the secondary release of catecholamines, leading to tremulousness, diaphoresis, pallor, palpitations, cardiac arrhythmias, and behavioral irritability. Because of the episodic release of insulin, symptoms early in the course may be intermittent or occur only after somewhat prolonged periods of fasting. However, symptoms do develop early so that tumors are usually small and solitary at the time of diagnosis. Multiple primary tumors are found in approximately 10 percent of patients. An additional 10 percent are malignant, with spread to the local lymph nodes and the liver. As with gastrinomas, insulinomas are frequently associated with MEN 1 (see Chaps. 338 and 343), and such tumors are more likely to be multifocal. Extrapancreatic insulin-secreting tumors are rare and usually arise in ectopic pancreatic tissue.

Diagnosis is made by demonstrating fasting hypoglycemia and an inadequate response of insulin to the hypoglycemia (see Chap. 338 for details). Patients are fasted under close supervision for up to 72 h, followed, if necessary, by an exercise tolerance test. The majority of patients with insulinoma develop hypoglycemia within 24 h, as evidenced by a serum glucose less than 2.8 mmol/L (50 mg/dL) in men or 2.5 mmol/L (45 mg/dL) in women. However, there is no absolute glucose level which defines hypoglycemia, so the diagnosis of insulinoma depends on demonstrating inadequate insulin suppression in the face of falling glucose levels. Documentation of rising cortisol levels excludes hypoglycemia secondary to hypothalamic-pituitary-adrenal dysfunction. It is also necessary to exclude other causes of fasting hypoglycemia, including administration of exogenous insulin, sulfonylurea ingestion, severe liver failure, and tumors that secrete insulinlike growth factors (e.g., fibrosarcoma, mesothelioma, and hemangiopericytoma). Exogenous insulin administration can be excluded by measuring levels of the C peptide of proinsulin, which normally vary in parallel with the plasma insulin concentrations. Since insulin administration suppresses endogenous insulin secretion, detection of normal or elevated C-peptide levels is inconsistent with insulin abuse. In addition, because insulinoma cells often process proinsulin incompletely, the serum often has an increased ratio of proinsulin to insulin. A ratio greater than 20 percent in the appropriate clinical setting is suggestive of insulinoma. Serum levels of sulfonyl-ureas should be elevated if hyperinsulinemic hypoglycemia is caused by these agents. Normal glucose/insulin ratios exclude liver failure and tumors which secrete insulin-like growth factors. (Refer to Chap. 338 for a more complete discussion of hypoglycemia syndromes.)

Once a diagnosis of insulinemia is established, acute treatment is supportive with intravenous glucose infusion as required to maintain plasma levels within the normal range. Hyperglycemic agents, including diazoxide, beta-adrenergic receptor blockers, and phenytoin can be used to support serum glucose levels, but their effects are variable and may last only a short time. Octreotide frequently inhibits insulin secretion by these tumors and may be an effective agent for acute management. Definitive therapy is accomplished by surgical resection. Because insulinomas are usually small (most are <2 cm in diameter), only half are detected by CT. Angiography with selective venous sampling for insulin levels is about 80 percent sensitive, and palpation at laparotomy detects 80 to 90 percent of tumors. At surgery, detectable tumors should be resected. The effectiveness of intervention is monitored by determination of intraoperative blood glucose levels. If no detectable tumors are found, stepwise distal pancreatectomy is performed until frozen sections of resected specimens and/or blood glucose measurements indicate that all tumor has been removed. If no tumor is found, or if multiple tumors are present, pancreatectomy is limited to 70 to 80 percent to preserve digestive and endocrine pancreatic function.

Patients with metastatic disease and those whose insulinomas are not removed by partial pancreatectomy can frequently be managed with hyperglycemic agents such as diazoxide or octreotide. In one study, all seven patients with metastatic insulinoma showed a response to octreotide, although the degree of response was variable. However, hypoglycemia may be worsened by octreotide administration, perhaps owing to inhibition of glucagon or growth hormone by this agent. Diazoxide, though frequently effective, can cause troubling side effects, including salt and fluid retention, hypertrichosis, and gastrointestinal upset. The combination of streptozocin and doxorubicin is the mainstay of chemotherapy for metastatic disease; it is superior to streptozocin-fluorouracil. These agents induce objective remission in approximately half of patients and are associated with a modest but significant increase in survival. Patients with residual tumor should be followed carefully for changes in secretory profile which may affect therapy. Such changes may include development of hyperglycemia as a result of glucagon-secreting metastases.

VIPOMA [VERNER-MORRISON SYNDROME; WATERY DIARRHEA, HYPOKALEMIA, ACHLORHYDRIA (WDHA) SYNDROME

Verner and Morrison described a syndrome of watery diarrhea, hypokalemia, and renal failure in association with non-β cell tumors of the pancreatic islets. The clinical features of this syndrome are caused by the high levels of vasoactive intestinal peptide (VIP) secreted by the tumors. VIPomas comprise approximately 2 percent of gastroenteropancreatic tumors and have a prevalence of approximately 1×10^{-7} in the Irish population studied. The manifestations of VIPoma include secretory diarrhea, profound weakness, hypokalemia, and hypochlorhydria. Stool volume is greater than 3 L/d in the majority of patients, and non-anion-gap acidosis usually occurs as a result of bicarbonate losses in the stool. Other electrolyte abnormalities include hypercalcemia in approximately two-thirds of patients and hypophosphatemia. Approximately half of patients develop hyperglycemia, which results from hypokalemia- and VIP-induced glycogenolysis in the liver, and a fifth of patients experience cutaneous flushing. Although most symptoms can be reproduced by infusion of exogenous VIP, these tumors also contain other peptide hormones, including the VIP-related peptide histidine-methionine (PHM), somatostatin, helodermin, and neurotensin, each of which may contribute to clinical features exhibited by individual patients. Diagnosis rests on the demonstration of high plasma VIP levels in the setting of a stool volume of at least 1 L/d. Lesser increases in VIP levels occur in patients with hepatic failure and intestinal ischemia.

VIPomas are most commonly pancreatic tumors. Unlike gastrinomas and insulinomas, however, VIPomas frequently grow to a large size before becoming clinically apparent. On average, the size of these tumors at the time of diagnosis is second only to that of nonfunctioning pancreatic islet cell tumors. Although they are slow-growing, these tumors are usually malignant. Approximately three-fifths are metastatic at the time of diagnosis. Most VIPomas are located in the body or tail of the pancreas. A few cases have been seen in association with MEN 1. However, there is no constant relation between the two syndromes. Between 10 and 15 percent of VIP-secreting tumors arise from neuroendocrine cells in the intestinal mucosa, and a few are ganglioneuroblastomas, mastocytomas, pheochromocytomas, or small cell carcinomas of the lung.

Treatment is surgical extirpation whenever possible. However, metastases may preclude this approach. Preoperative evaluation should include CT to localize the tumor and any metastases that may be present. In addition to supportive therapy with fluids and electrolytes, prednisone is frequently effective in reducing the volume of diarrhea, despite its inability to alter serum VIP levels. Octreotide inhibits the secretion of VIP and ameliorates symptoms in most patients. VIPomas often produce symptoms related to the large size of the tumor itself. Surgery may be indicated to relieve local effects or to remove a single large primary tumor. For patients with symptomatic metastatic disease, chemotherapy and hepatic artery embolization have the greatest benefit on tumor burden. Regimens combining streptozocin and doxorubicin or streptozocin-fluorouracil are the most effective chemotherapy, inducing objective partial remission in up to 90 percent of cases.

GLUCAGONOMA In 1966, McGovern described a rare syndrome of diabetes mellitus and necrolytic migratory erythema in association with a pancreatic islet cell tumor. The observation that these tumors secrete high levels of glucagon suggested a cause for the diabetes and that the peptide may have a role in the other clinical features. Although these tumors frequently synthesize and secrete additional peptides, including pancreatic polypeptide, somatostatin, insulin, and gastrin, the common link is hyperglucagonemia. Glucagonomas are characteristically single, large, and slow-growing. More than 75 percent have metastasized at the time of diagnosis, most commonly to the liver and bones. Glucagonoma has been reported in association with MEN 1 (see Chap. 343). A fasting plasma glucagon of >1000 ng/L (>1000 pg/mL) establishes the diagnosis. More modest elevations of plasma glucagon levels may occur in diabetic ketoacidosis, renal failure, hepatic failure, sepsis, prolonged fasting, and gluten-sensitive enteropathy. Hypocholesterolemia and hypoaminoacidemia are common, with alanine, glycine, and serine levels usually less than 25 percent of normal. Glucagonoma may be distinguished from other hyperglucagonemic syndromes by the failure of glucose to suppress and the failure of arginine to enhance serum glucagon concentrations.

The characteristic glucagonoma skin rash is erythematous, raised, scaly, sometimes bullous, sometimes psoriatic, and ultimately crusted. It is located primarily on the face, abdomen, perineum, and distal extremities. After resolution, the regions of the acute eruption usually remain indurated and hyperpigmented. Patients also may experience glossitis, stomatitis, angular cheilitis, dystrophic nails, and hair thinning. The diabetes is usually mild or asymptomatic and may manifest only as an abnormality on an oral glucose tolerance test. Ketoacidosis has not been reported. Weight loss, hypoaminoacidemia, anemia, and thromboembolic disease also occur in association with this syndrome. A causal association between hyperglucagonemia and skin disease has been difficult to prove, leading to speculation that the rash may result from nutritional deficiency. In some patients, the rash responds to oral zinc or intravenous amino acid therapy. Octreotide therapy also has yielded good results. However, dermatologic symptoms frequently recur after each of these therapies.

Because the tumor is usually large and found only in the pancreas, it is easily identified by CT, ultrasound, or angiography. Surgical therapy is curative in approximately 30 percent of patients. Resection is more frequently aimed at decreasing tumor burden. Despite occasional objective responses, attempts at chemotherapy with combinations of streptozocin, fluorouracil, doxorubicin, and dacarbazine have little impact. Fortunately, the slow-growing nature of the tumor allows for prolonged survival even in many cases of metastatic disease.

SOMATOSTATINOMA Somatostatin-secreting tumors are the most recent group to be identified with a defined clinical syndrome. The classic triad of somatostatinoma comprises diabetes mellitus, steatorrhea, and cholelithiasis. These symptoms derive from the widespread inhibitory actions of somatostatin, including inhibition of insulin release, pancreatic enzyme and bicarbonate secretion, and gallbladder motility, respectively. The diabetes is usually mild, and in a few cases, *hypo*glycemia has been seen, perhaps from the cosecretion of other peptides. Individual somatostatinomas have been shown to secrete insulin, calcitonin, gastrin, VIP, adrenocorticotrophin, prostaglandins, substance P, motilin, and glucagon. Patients with somatostatinomas also may develop hypochlorhydria, weight loss, and paroxysmal hypertension.

Approximately 60 percent of reported somatostatinomas are located in the pancreas. The second most common site is in the small intestine, although intestinal tumors are associated with lower plasma somatostatin levels and are more commonly asymptomatic. Like glucagonomas and VIPomas, these tumors are usually single, large, and metastatic at the time of diagnosis. Somatostatinomas have not been reported in association with MEN 1. Curiously, the occasional coincidence of pheochromocytoma, café au lait spots, and neurofibromatosis suggests a possible association with MEN type 2b (see Chap. 343). Small cell lung carcinomas, medullary thyroid carcinomas, pheochromocytomas, and paragangliomas that secrete somatostatin also have been described.

MISCELLANEOUS FUNCTIONAL ISLET CELL TUMORS   In addition to the diseases described above, islet cell tumors have been associated with several other syndromes of hormone excess, including acromegaly (growth hormone or growth hormone–releasing hormone), hypercalcemia (parathormone-like peptide), diarrhea and diabetes mellitus (neurotensin), and Cushing's syndrome (corticotropin-releasing factor or adrenocorticotropin).

NONFUNCTIONING ISLET CELL TUMORS (See also Chap. 275) More than 15 percent of pancreatic islet cell tumors are not associated with any definable hormone-mediated syndrome. Nonetheless, many of these nonfunctioning islet cell tumors synthesize and secrete one or more regulatory peptides, including pancreatic polypeptide, substance P, and motilin. With increasing availability of radioimmunoassay and immunohistochemical reagents, protein products will probably be defined for more and more of these tumors. Nonetheless, most of these tumors behave in a similar fashion. They arise most commonly in the head and tail of the pancreas and are frequently large (5 to 10 cm in diameter) at the time of diagnosis. The most common clinical manifestations are abdominal pain, jaundice, a palpable mass, malaise, and bleeding esophageal or gastric varices (from splenic vein compression). Though slow-growing, at least half of these tumors present with metastases to the liver or lymph nodes. Surgical cure is achieved in approximately 20 percent. The remainder

are poorly responsive to chemotherapy. Streptozocin with or without fluorouracil induces objective responses in approximately 60 percent of patients. Five-year survival for patients with these tumors is approximately 40 percent, with many long-term survivors despite known metastatic disease.

REFERENCES

Carcinoid tumors and syndrome

ERICKSSON B, OBERG K: Peptide hormones as tumor markers in neuroendocrine gastrointestinal tumors. Acta Oncol 30:477, 1991

FELDMAN JM: Carcinoid tumors and syndrome. Semin Oncol 14:237, 1987

GODWIN JD: Carcinoid tumors: An analysis of 2837 cases. Cancer 36:560, 1975

JOENSUU H et al: Treatment of metastatic carcinoid tumor with recombinant interferon-alpha. Eur J Cancer 28A:1650, 1992

KVOLS LK et al: Treatment of the malignant carcinoid syndrome: Evaluation of a long-acting somatostatin analogue. N Engl J Med 315:663, 1986

MOERTEL CG et al: Carcinoid tumor of the appendix: Treatment and prognosis. N Engl J Med 317:1699, 1987

NORHEIM I et al: Malignant carcinoid tumors: An analysis of 103 patients with regard to tumor localization, hormone production, and survival. Ann Surg 206:115, 1987

OBERG K: The action of interferon-alpha on human carcinoid tumors. Semin Cancer Biol 3:35, 1992

SAINI A, WAXMAN J: Management of carcinoid syndrome. Postgrad Med 67:506, 1991

THORSON A et al: Malignant carcinoid of the small intestine with metastases to the liver, valvular disease of the right side of the heart, peripheral vasomotor symptoms, bronchoconstriction, and an unusual type of cyanosis: A clinical and pathologic syndrome. Am Heart J 47:795, 1954

Islet cell tumors

BIESMA B et al: Recombinant interferon alpha-2b in patients with metastatic apudomas: Effect on tumors and tumor markers. Br J Cancer 66:850, 1992

BLOOM SR, POLAK JM: Glucagonoma syndrome. Am J Med 82 (Suppl 5B):25, 1987

BOSTWICK DG et al: Expression of opioid peptides in tumors. N Engl J Med 317:1439, 1987

GORDEN P et al: Somatostatin and somatostatin analogue (SMS 201-995) in treatment of hormone-secreting tumors of the pituitary and gastrointestinal tract and non-neoplastic diseases of the gut. Ann Intern Med 110:35, 1989

JONES DV JR et al: Metastatic glucagonoma: A clinical response to a combination of 5-fluorouracil and alpha-interferon. Am J Med 93:348, 1992

KLEIN S et al: In vivo assessment of the metabolic alterations in glucagonoma syndrome. Metabolism 41:1171, 1992

KREJS GJ: VIPoma syndrome. Am J Med 82 (Suppl 5B):37, 1987

KVOLS LK et al: Treatment of metastatic islet cell carcinomas with a somatostatin analogue (SMS 201-995). Ann Intern Med 107:162, 1987

MOERTEL CG et al: Streptozocin-doxorubicin, streptozocin-fluorouracil or chlorozocin in the treatment of advanced islet cell carcinoma. N Engl J Med 326:519, 1992

ROSCH T et al: Localization of pancreatic islet cell tumors by endoscopic ultrasonography. N Engl J Med 326:1721, 1992

VINIK AI et al: Somatostatinomas, PPomas, neurotensinomas. Semin Oncol 14:263, 1987

WYNICK D et al: Symptomatic secondary hormone syndromes in patients with established malignant pancreatic endocrine tumors. N Engl J Med 319:605, 1988

section 1 Disorders of the immune system

277 CELLULAR AND MOLECULAR BASIS OF IMMUNITY

BARTON F. HAYNES / ANTHONY S. FAUCI

Basic research in immunology has resulted in advances in a wide range of clinical disciplines, from allergy and rheumatology to neurology and cardiology. Monoclonal antibody technology has revolutionized the study of cell surface molecules of effector and regulatory immune cells and has provided specific reagents for essentially any target molecule. The isolation, cloning, and sequencing of genes for antigen receptors and their associated molecules on B cells and T cells, as well as the delineation of the structures of major histocompatibility complex (MHC) class I and class II molecules (see Chap. 64), have provided the information necessary to understand immune cell recognition and effector function. Thus, in recent years, breakthroughs in new technology have explained diversification of the T and B cell receptor for antigen repertoires, induction of self-tolerance (self-antigen nonreactivity), and regulation of immune cell growth and differentiation.

The normal function of the immune system is essential for health, and dysfunction of the immune system leads to myriad diseases (Table 277-1). Deficiency of immune cell production or defective immune cell function can lead to a wide spectrum of immunodeficiency diseases (see Chap. 278). Overactivity of various components of the immune system leads to the development of allergic or autoimmune diseases. Leukemias and lymphomas are the result of malignant transformation in cells of the immune system (see Chaps. 310 and 311). With these new insights into immune system function have come new and specific modes of therapy for autoimmune, immunodeficiency, and malignant immune system diseases. The aim of this chapter is to provide the essentials of the cellular and molecular basis of immunity, with emphasis on those principles relevant to understanding at a basic level the protean clinical and laboratory manifestations of disordered immunity.

THE CD CLASSIFICATION OF HUMAN LYMPHOCYTE DIFFERENTIATION ANTIGENS The development of monoclonal antibody technology led to the discovery of a large number of new leukocyte surface molecules. In 1982, the First International Workshop on Leukocyte Differentiation Antigens was held to establish a nomenclature for cell surface molecules of human leukocytes. From this and subsequent leukocyte differentiation workshops has come the cluster of differentiation (CD) classification of leukocyte antigens (Table 277-2). The data presented in Table 277-2 establish a context to facilitate study of the extraordinary complex series of events that transpire during normal and aberrant human immune system function.

PHENOTYPE AND FUNCTION OF IMMUNE CELLS

The dual limbs of the immune system are the thymus-derived (T) lymphocyte and the bone marrow–derived or bursa-equivalent (B) lymphocyte, both of which derive from a common stem cell. The principal effector and regulator cells of the immune system are T, B, and large granular lymphocytes and monocytes-macrophages. Nonlymphoid cells such as neutrophils, eosinophils, basophils, and tissue mast cells play non-antigen-specific roles in inflammatory responses that result from immune-mediated reactions and, as such, must be considered in the scheme of immune cell function (Fig. 277-1).

Cytokines are soluble proteins produced by a wide variety of hematopoietic and nonhematopoietic cell types. Activation of immune system cells is in large part regulated by the ordered production of myriad cytokines that control gene activation and functional cell surface molecule expression. Many cytokines have similar functions, and considerable redundancy in cytokine capabilities is important for normal immune system function. In addition, many different cell types have receptors for the same cytokine, giving rise to the concept of "cytokine networks" wherein many cell types secrete a variety of cytokines capable of binding and stimulating multiple cell types. In this chapter the cytokines that affect various cell types are discussed in the context of each type of immune cell.

The proportion and distribution of immunocompetent cells in various tissues reflect cell traffic, homing patterns, and functional capabilities. Bone marrow is the major site of maturation of B cells, monocytes-macrophages, and granulocytes and contains pluripotent stem cells which under the influence of various colony stimulating factors (CSF) are capable of giving rise to all hematopoietic cell types (Table 277-3). Granulocyte (G)–CSF stimulates the production of neutrophils and stem cell division; granulocyte/macrophage (GM)–CSF stimulates neutrophil, monocyte, eosinophil, and erythroid and megakaryocytoid cell growth and synergizes with interleukin 3 (IL-3), interleukin 11 (IL-11), and stem cell factor (SCF) for stem cell activation. Macrophage (M)–CSF drives monocyte differentiation, while IL-3 drives neutrophil, monocyte, eosinophil, basophil, and erythroid and megakaryocytoid cell differentiation and promotes hematopoietic stem cell survival. T cell precursors also arise from hematopoietic stem cells but leave the yolk sac, fetal liver, or bone marrow while immature and home to the thymus for completion of maturation. Mature T lymphocytes, B lymphocytes, and monocytes enter the circulation and home to peripheral lymphoid organs (lymph nodes, spleen) and the gut-associated lymphoid tissue (tonsil, Peyer's patches, and appendix) and await activation by foreign antigen.

T CELLS T lymphocytes differ from other immune effector cell types in that the pool of effector T cells is established in the thymus early in life and is maintained throughout life by antigen-driven

TABLE 277-1   Disorders of the immune system

IMMUNODEFICIENCIES

Primary immunodeficiencies
  Combined immunodeficiencies
    Severe combined immunodeficiency
      X-linked
      Autosomal recessive
    Adenosine deaminase (ADA) deficiency
    Purine nucleoside phosphorylase (PNP) deficiency
    MHC class II deficiency
    MHC class I deficiency (bare leukocyte syndrome)
    Reticular dysgenesis
  Predominantly antibody deficiencies
    X-linked agammaglobulinemia
    X-linked hypogammaglobulinemia with growth hormone deficiency
    Ig deficiency with increased IgM (hyper-IgM syndrome)
    Ig heavy chain gene deletions
    κ chain deficiency
    IgA deficiency
    Selective deficiency of IgG subclasses
    Common variable immunodeficiency (CVID)
    Transient hypogammaglobulinemia of infancy
    Secretory component deficiency
  Other well-defined immunodeficiency syndromes
    Wiskott-Aldrich syndrome
    Ataxia-telangiectasia
    Third and fourth pouch/arch syndrome (Di George)
  Syndromes associated with immunodeficiency
    Chromosome abnormalities
      Bloom syndrome
      Fanconi syndrome
      Down syndrome
    Multiple organ system abnormalities
      Partial albinism
      Short-limbed dwarfism
      Cartilage hair hypoplasia
      Agenesis of corpus callosum
    Hereditary metabolic defects
      Transcobalamin II deficiency
      Acrodermatitis enteropathica (zinc deficiency)
      Type I orotic aciduria
      Biotin dependent carboxylase deficiency
    Hypercatabolism of Ig
      Familial hypercatabolism of Ig
      Myotonic dystrophy
      Intestinal lymphangiectasia
    Other
      Hyper-IgE syndrome
      Chronic mucocutaneous candidiasis
      Thymoma
      Immunodeficiency following hereditarily determined
        susceptibility to Epstein-Barr virus (Duncan's syndrome)
Acquired immunodeficiencies
  Acquired immunodeficiency syndrome (AIDS)
  Iatrogenic
  Idiopathic CD4+ T lymphocytopenia

ALLERGIC DISEASES

Generalized
  Anaphylaxis
  Serum sickness
  Generalized drug reactions
  Food allergy
  Insect venom allergy
  Mastocytosis
Airways
  Allergic rhinitis
  Asthma
  Hypersensitivity pneumonitis
Skin
  Urticaria
  Angioedema
  Eczema
  Atopic dermatitis
  Allergic contact dermatitis
  Erythema multiforme and Stevens-Johnson syndrome
Ocular allergy
  Allergic conjunctivitis
  Atopic keratoconjunctivitis
  Venereal keratoconjunctivitis
  Giant papillary conjunctivitis
  Contact allergy

AUTOIMMUNITY

Organ specific
  Endocrine system
    Thyroid gland
      Hashimoto's thyroiditis
      Graves' disease
      Thyroiditis with hyperthyroidism
    Type I autoimmune polyglandular syndrome
    Type II autoimmune polyglandular syndrome
    Insulin-dependent diabetes mellitus
    Immune-mediated infertility
    Autoimmune Addison's disease
  Skin
    Pemphigus vulgaris
    Pemphigus foliaceus
    Bullus pemphigoid
    Dermatitis herpetiformis
    Linear IgA dermatosis
    Epidermolysis bullosa acquisita
    Autoimmune alopecia
    Erythema nodosa
    Contact dermatitis
    Herpes gestationis
    Cicatricial pemphigoid
    Chronic bullous disease of childhood
  Hematologic system
    Autoimmune hemolytic anemia
    Autoimmune thrombocytopenic purpura
      Idiopathic
      Drug-related
    Autoimmune neutropenia
  Neuromuscular system
    Myasthenia gravis
    Acute disseminated encephalomyelitis
    Multiple sclerosis
    Guillain-Barré syndrome
    Chronic inflammatory demyelinating polyradiculoneuropathy
  Hepatobiliary system
    Autoimmune chronic active hepatitis
    Primary biliary sclerosis
    Sclerosing cholangitis
  Gastrointestinal tract
    Gluten-sensitive enteropathy
    Pernicious anemia
    Inflammatory bowel disease
Organ nonspecific
  Connective tissue diseases
    Systemic lupus erythematosus
    Rheumatoid arthritis
    Systemic sclerosis (scleroderma)
    Ankylosing spondylitis
    Reactive arthritides
    Polymyositis/dermatomyositis
    Sjögren's syndrome
    Mixed connective tissue disease
    Behçet's syndrome
    Psoriasis
  Vasculitic syndromes
    Systemic necrotizing vasculitides
      Classic polyarteritis nodosa
      Allergic angiitis and granulomatosis (Churg-Strauss disease)
      Polyangiitis overlap syndrome
    Hypersensitivity vasculitis
    Wegener's granulomatosis
    Temporal arteritis
    Takayasu's arteritis
    Kawasaki's disease
    Isolated vasculitis of the central nervous system
    Thromboangiitis obliterans
    Miscellaneous vasculitides
  Sarcoidosis
  Graft-versus-host disease
  Cryopathies

TABLE 277-1 Disorders of the immune system (*continued*)

NEOPLASMS

T cell neoplasms
  Adult T cell leukemia/lymphoma
  Acute lymphocytic leukemia
  Cutaneous T cell lymphoma
  Non-Hodgkin's lymphoma
  Hairy cell leukemia
  Acute lymphoblastic leukemia
  Chronic lymphocytic leukemia (rare)
B cell neoplasms
  Chronic lymphocytic leukemia
  Multiple myeloma
  Burkitt's lymphoma
  Hairy cell leukemia
  Acute lymphoblastic leukemia
  Non-Hodgkin's lymphoma
  Waldenström's macroglobulinemia
  Primary amyloidosis
  Heavy chain diseases
    gamma (Franklin's disease)
    alpha (Seligmann's disease)
    mu
Monocyte neoplasms
  Acute monocytic leukemia
  Hodgkin's disease
  Histiocytic lymphoma
  Histiocytosis X
    Eosinophilic granuloma
    Letterer-Siwe disease
    Hand-Schüller-Christian disease
  Malignant histiocytosis (histiocytic medullary reticulosis)
Other
  Proliferation of large granular lymphocytes

expansion of virgin peripheral T cells into "memory" T cells that reside primarily in peripheral lymphoid organs. Mature T lymphocytes contribute 70 to 80 percent of normal peripheral blood lymphocytes, 90 percent of thoracic duct lymphocytes, 30 to 40 percent of lymph node cells, and 20 to 30 percent of spleen lymphoid cells. In lymph nodes, T cells occupy deep paracortical areas around B cell germinal centers, and in the spleen, they are in periarteriolar areas of white pulp (see Chap. 58). T cells are the primary effectors of cell-mediated

immunity, with subsets of T cells maturing into cytotoxic cells capable of lysis of virus-infected or foreign cells. T cells are also the primary regulatory cells of T and B lymphocyte and monocyte function by the production of lymphokines and by direct cell contact. In addition, T cells regulate erythroid cell maturation in bone marrow.

Human T cells express cell surface proteins that mark stages of intrathymic T cell maturation; many of these molecules mediate or augment specific T cell function (Table 277-2, Fig. 277-2).

A number of cytokines regulate the process of T cell proliferation and differentiation (Table 277-4). The earliest identifiable cells of T lineage are CD34+ pro-T cells (i.e., cells in which T cell receptor genes are neither rearranged nor expressed); they are found in fetal liver, yolk sac, and postnatal bone marrow. In the thymus, CD7+ T cell precursors begin cytoplasmic (c) synthesis of components of the CD3 complex of T cell receptor–associated molecules (see Fig. 277-2). Within CD7+, CD2+, and cCD3+ T cell precursors, T cell receptor (TCR) gene rearrangement begins and eventuates in two T cell lineages, expressing either TCRαβ chains or TCRγδ chains (see Chap. 278). T cells expressing the TCRαβ chains comprise the majority of peripheral T cells in blood, lymph node, and spleen and terminally differentiate into either CD4+ or CD8+ cells. Cells expressing TCRγδ chains circulate as a minor population in blood; their functions, although not fully known, have been postulated as immune surveillance at epithelial surfaces and in cellular defenses against mycobacterial organisms. CD1, CD4, and CD8 are expressed on immature cortical thymocytes; however, upon functional maturity, T cell expression of CD1 ceases and T cell subset antigens CD4 and CD8 are reciprocally expressed. Mature CD4+ TCRαβ+ cells induce B cell differentiation, induce CD8+ cytotoxic T cell proliferation, produce various lymphokines, and regulate certain stages of erythropoiesis. A subset of CD4+ cells also may function as cytotoxic effector cells, recognizing foreign peptide antigen fragments that are physically associated with MHC class II molecules on antigen-presenting cells. CD8+ TCRαβ+ cells function as suppressors of B cell antibody synthesis or as cytotoxic effector T cells, recognizing foreign peptide antigen fragments associated with MHC class I molecules (see Chap. 64).

T cell maturation stages are clinically relevant in that T cell acute lymphoblastic leukemia and lymphomas are malignancies of pro-T, pre-T, or immature T cells, while forms of cutaneous T cell lymphoma

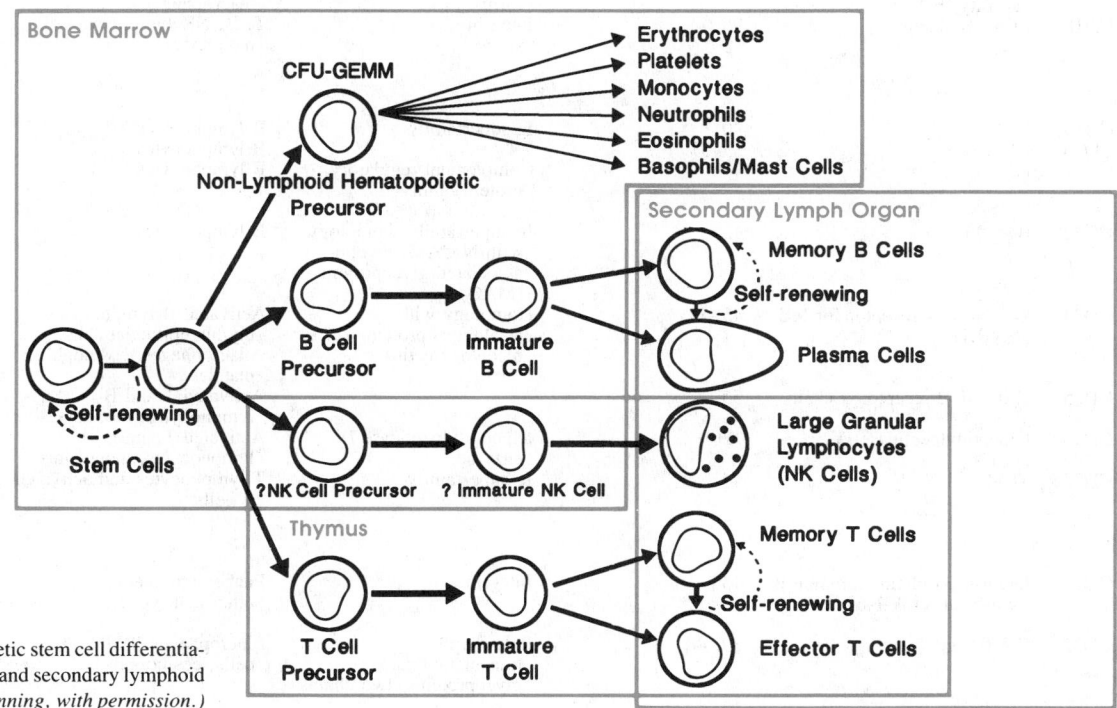

FIGURE 277-1 Hematopoietic stem cell differentiation in bone marrow, thymus, and secondary lymphoid organs. (*After Haynes and Denning, with permission.*)

TABLE 277-2   CD classification of human lymphocyte surface molecule

CD	Other names	Molecular mass, kDa	Molecular structure	Tissue/lineage	Function
CD1	T6	49,000	Ig superfamily associated with β2M	Cortical thymocytes, Langerhans cells, interdigitating cells	Antigen presentation to TCRγδ cells
CD2	T11, LFA-3 receptor, E-rosette receptor	50,000	Ig superfamily	T lymphocytes	Binds LFA-3 (CD58) on RBC, monocytes, thymic epithelial cells; alternative pathway of T cell activation
CD3	T3, CD3 complex, Leu4	CD3γ—26 CD3δ—20 CD3ε—20 CD3ζ—16 CD3η—28	CD3γ,δ,ε Ig superfamily; CD3 η, ζ; homologous to each other and with FcRε ζ chain comprise α family of signal transducers	CD3γ,δ,ε,ζ,η, T lymphocytes, cytoplasmic CD3ε, NK cells	T cell–associated molecules; transduce signals from T cell receptors
CD4	T4, Leu3a	59	Ig superfamily	T lymphocytes, monocytes, tissue macrophages, microglial cells, EBV-transformed B lymphocytes	Receptor for HIV env gp120; binds to HLA class II; associated with p56-lck tyrosine kinase
CD5	T1	67	Ig superfamily	T lymphocytes, B lymphocyte subset	Comitogenic for T lymphocytes; ligand for CD72
CD6	T12	100	Scavenger receptor type I superfamily	Subset of T and B lymphocytes	?
CD7	3A1, Leu9	40	Ig superfamily	T lymphocytes, NK cells; on subsets of T, B, and myeloid precursors	Comitogenic for T lymphocytes; Ca^{2+} inducible gene
CD8	T8, Leu2a	CD8α—38 CD8β—38	CD8 α, β, Ig superfamily	T cell subset	Receptor for MHC class I; associated with p56-lck tyrosine kinase
CD10	J5, CALLA, neutral endopeptidase	100	Endopeptidase enzyme	B lymphoid progenitor cells	Peptide cleavage
CD11a	LFA-1α chain	180	Integrin	T, B, NK lymphocytes, monocytes	With β2 integrin, ligand for ICAM-1 (CD54), ICAM-2, and ICAM-3; mediates leukocyte adhesion and leukocyte-endothelial adherence
CD11b	MAC-1, MO-1α chain, CR3	165	Integrin	NK cells, PMNs, monocytes	With β2 integrin, receptor for C3bi, fibrinogen, factor X
CD11c	gp150/95 α chain, CR4	150	Integrin	NK cells, PMNs, monocytes	With β2 integrin, mediates cell binding to C3bi
CD14	LeuM3, MO-2	55	Phosphoinositol-linked transmembrane glycoprotein	Monocytes	Endotoxin binding protein
CD15	Sialyl Lewis X (sLe^x)	Carbohydrate	Neu Acα 2–3 Gal β1–4 (Fucα1–3) GlcNac	Granulocytes; cryptic form of CD15 is on T cells [Cutaneous lymphocyte antigen (CLA)]	Ligand for ELAM-1 on endothelial cells; CLA mediates T cell homing to skin
CD16	Fc receptor for IgG (low affinity) FcγRIII	50–65	Ig superfamily, PI and TM forms	NK cells, PMN, macrophages	FcR for IgG
CD18	LFA-1β chain	95	Integrin	T, B, NK lymphocytes, monocytes	Ligand for ICAM-1 (CD54), ICAM-2, and ICAM-3; mediates leukocyte-endothelial interactions
CD19	B4	90	Ig superfamily	B lymphocytes	Regulates B cell activation
CD20	B1, Bp35	35–37	—	B lymphocytes	Mediates B cell activation
CD21	B2	140	Complement regulatory protein family	B lymphocytes	C3d/EBV receptor, complement receptor 2 (CR2), ligand for CD23
CD22	Bgp135	135	Ig superfamily, homology with N-CAM, myelin-associated glycoprotein (MAG)	B lymphocytes	Comitogenic for B cell activation, interacts with CD45RO on T cells and CD75 on B cells
CD23	Low-affinity receptor for IgE FcεRII	45–50	Homology with asialoglycoprotein receptor (lectin)	Activated B lymphocytes, thymic epithelial cells, macrophages, eosinophils, platelets	FcεRII, soluble CD23 activates immature T cells, ligand for CD21
CD25	TAC, IL-2 receptor α chain	55	—	Activated T and B lymphocytes, monocytes	Low-affinity receptor for IL-2
CD26	Dipeptidylpeptidase IV, gp120	120	Dipeptidylpeptidase IV enzyme	Activated T and B lymphocytes, monocytes	Serine exopeptidase; binds collagen
CD28	Tp44	44	Ig superfamily	T lymphocytes and activated B cells	Comitogenic for T lymphocytes, regulates T cell cytokine stability, Ligand for B7/BB1 molecules
CD29	Integrin β1 chain; common β subset of VLA-1-6	130	Integrin	Panhematopoietic, many other cell types	Ligand for many extracellular matrix molecules
CD32	FcδRII, gp40	39, 48	Polymorphic transmembrane glycoproteins, two chains	Macrophages, PMNs, B cells, eosinophils	Fc receptor for aggregated IgG, ligation leads to cell activation

TABLE 277-2   CD classification of human lymphocyte surface molecule (*continued*)

CD	Other names	Molecular mass, kDa	Molecular structure	Tissue/lineage	Function
CD34	MY10	105–120	Sialomucin with unique protein sequence	T lymphocyte, other hematopoietic precursors	?
CD35	CR1, C3b receptor	160–250	—	B cells, subset NK cells, PMNs, monocytes, RBC	Binds immune complexes
CD38	OKT10, T10	45	Single-chain glycoprotein	Activated lymphocytes, immature B cells	?
CD39	gp80	70–100	—	Activated B lymphocytes, T lymphocytes, and NK cells	Mediates homotypic adhesion of B cells
CD40	gp50	44–48	Homology with nerve growth factor receptor, fas(APO-1), and TNF receptor	B cells, follicular dendritic cells, macrophages	B cell activation, homotypic adhesion; binds to a TNF-like molecule, gp39, that is defective in X-linked hyper-IgM syndrome
CD43	Leukosialin, sialophorin, leukocyte sialoglycoprotein	95	Cell surface sialomucin	T, B, NK cells, monocytes	Involved in leukocyte activation, deficient in Wiskott-Aldrich syndrome, ligand for ICAM-1
CD44	Pgp-1, In(Lu)-related p80, Hermes, extracellular matrix receptor III	80–120	Cartilage link protein, core proteoglycan homology; multiple isoforms generated by alternative splicing	T, B, NK cells, monocytes, RBC	Transmembrane hyaluronate receptor, promotes leukocyte adhesion; comitogenic for T cells, mediates leukocyte-endothelial binding; promotes carcinoma metastasis
CD45	Leukocyte common antigen, T200	CD45RO—180 CD45RA—220 CD45RB—220, 205, 190	Multiple isoforms generated by alternative splicing	Leukocytes	Cytoplasmic domain is a tyrosine phosphatase, regulates lymphocyte activation, CD45RO in T cells is a ligand for CD22 on B cells
CD49b	VLA-2α chain	170	Integrin	Activated T cells, platelets	With β1 integrin, binds collagen
CD49d	VLA-4α chain	150	Integrin	T and B lymphocytes, monocytes	With β integrin, is the receptor for endothelial VCAM-1; mediates leukocyte–endothelial cell binding in Peyer's patches
CD54	ICAM-1	40	Ig superfamily	Endothelial cells, activated lymphocytes	Ligand for LFA-1, rhinoviruses, falciparum malaria, CD43
CD56	N-CAM, NKH-1	140	Ig superfamily, homology with N-CAM	NK cells	Mediates NK cell homotypic adhesion
CD57	HNK1, Leu7	110		NK cells, subset of T cells	?
CD58	LFA-3	40–65	Ig superfamily	Widespread, activated lymphocytes	Ligand for CD2
CD64	FcgRI, high-affinity receptor for IgG	75	Transmembrane glycoprotein	Monocytes, tissue macrophages	Binds monomeric IgG with high affinity, ligation leads to cell activation
CD69	Activation inducer molecule, EA-1, gp34/28	28, 34	Homodimer; type II membrane protein related to NK cell activation protein family	Activated B, T, NK cells, monocytes	Ligand binding to CD69 triggers cytolytic activity of NK and TCRγδ T cells
CD71	T9, transferrin receptor	95	Heterodimer	Activated T and B lymphocytes, monocytes, proliferating cells of many types	Binds transferrin
CD72	—	39, 43	Heterodimer	B cells	Ligand for CD5 molecule
CD73	Ecto-5′ nucleotidase	69	Nucleotidase enzyme	Subsets of B and T lymphocytes	Regulates uptake of nucleotides

(mycosis fungoides, Sézary syndrome) and the syndrome of adult T cell leukemia (associated with HTLV-I infection) share the phenotype of mature (usually CD4+) T cells.

Molecular basis of T cell recognition of antigen The T cell antigen receptor is a complex of molecules consisting of an antigen-binding heterodimer of either αβ or γδ chains noncovalently linked with five CD3 subunits (γ, δ, ε, ζ, and η) (Fig. 277-3). The CD3 ζ chains are either disulfide-linked homodimers (CD3-ζ₂) or disulfide-linked heterodimers composed of one ζ chain and one η chain. TCRαβ or TCRγδ molecules must be associated with CD3 molecules to be inserted into the T cell surface membrane, TCRα being paired with TCRβ and TCRγ being paired with TCRδ. Molecules of the

CD3 complex mediate transduction of T cell activation signals via T cell receptors, while TCRα and β or γ and δ molecules combine to form the TCR antigen-binding site.

The α, β, γ, and δ T cell antigen receptor molecules have amino acid sequence homology and structural similarities to immunoglobulin heavy and light chains, and like many functionally relevant molecules of immune cells (e.g., MHC class I or II, CD2, CD4, CD8), they are therefore members of the *immunoglobulin gene superfamily* of molecules. The TCRβ and δ chains contain four separately encoded regions, namely, the V (variable), D (diversity), J (joining), and C (constant) regions, and the TCRα and γ chains consist of V, J, and C regions. Thus molecules of the T cell antigen receptor have constant

TABLE 277-3 Cytokines that regulate multipotent or pluripotent hematopoietic stem cell (HSC) proliferation and differentiation

Cytokine	Other names/abbreviation	Effect on stem cells
Interleukin 1α,β	IL-1αβ	Indirectly stimulates HSC by inducing IL-6 production from BM stromal cells
Interleukin 3	IL-3	Promotes survival of HSC; synergizes with IL-11, LIF, and SCF for entry of HSC into cell cycle
Interleukin 4	IL-4, B cell differentiating factor (BCDF)	Synergizes with IL-11 for entry of HSC into cell cycle
Interleukin 6	IL-6	Synergizes with IL-3 for HSC differentiation into myeloid lineages
Interleukin 11	IL-11	Synergizes with IL-3 and SCF for entry of HSC into cell cycle
Stem cell factor	SCF, c-kit ligand, steel factor (SLF), mast cell differentiating factor	Synergizes with IL-3, IL-6, IL-11, G-CSF, and GM-CSF for HSC proliferation
Basic fibroblast growth Factor	BFGF	Synergizes with IL-3 and GM-CSF for HSC activation
Granulocyte colony stimulating factor	G-CSF	Stimulates HSC entry into cell cycle
Granulocyte/monocyte-macrophage colony stimulating factor	GM-CSF	Synergizes with SCF, IL-11, and IL-3 for HSC activation
Leukemia inhibitory factor	LIF, HILDA, DIA	Inhibits proliferation of HSC
Macrophage inflammatory protein 1α	MIP1α, stem cell inhibitor 1 (SCI-1)	Inhibits proliferation of embryonic stem cells but synergizes with SCF entry of HSC into cell cycle
Transforming growth factor β	TGF-β	Inhibits proliferation of HSC

SOURCE: Adapted with permission from Haynes and Denning.

and variable regions, and the genes encoding the α, β, γ, and δ chains of these molecules undergo rearrangement during T cell maturation, culminating in synthesis of the completed molecule.

The variable region elements of α, β, γ, and δ genes, which are separate in the germ line, are brought together by DNA rearrangement and deletion during intrathymic differentiation of the T lymphocyte.

Thus TCR diversity is due to the large numbers of V-J or V-D-J combinations formed during TCR gene rearrangement. As T cells mature in the thymus, the repertoire of antigen-reactive T cells is generated by selection processes that eliminate many autoreactive T cells, enhance the proliferation of needed antigen-reactive T cells, and allow T cells with nonuseful TCR to die (see below).

FIGURE 277-2 Human T cell maturation. sCD3 = surface CD3 expression, cCD3 = cytoplasmic CD3 expression.

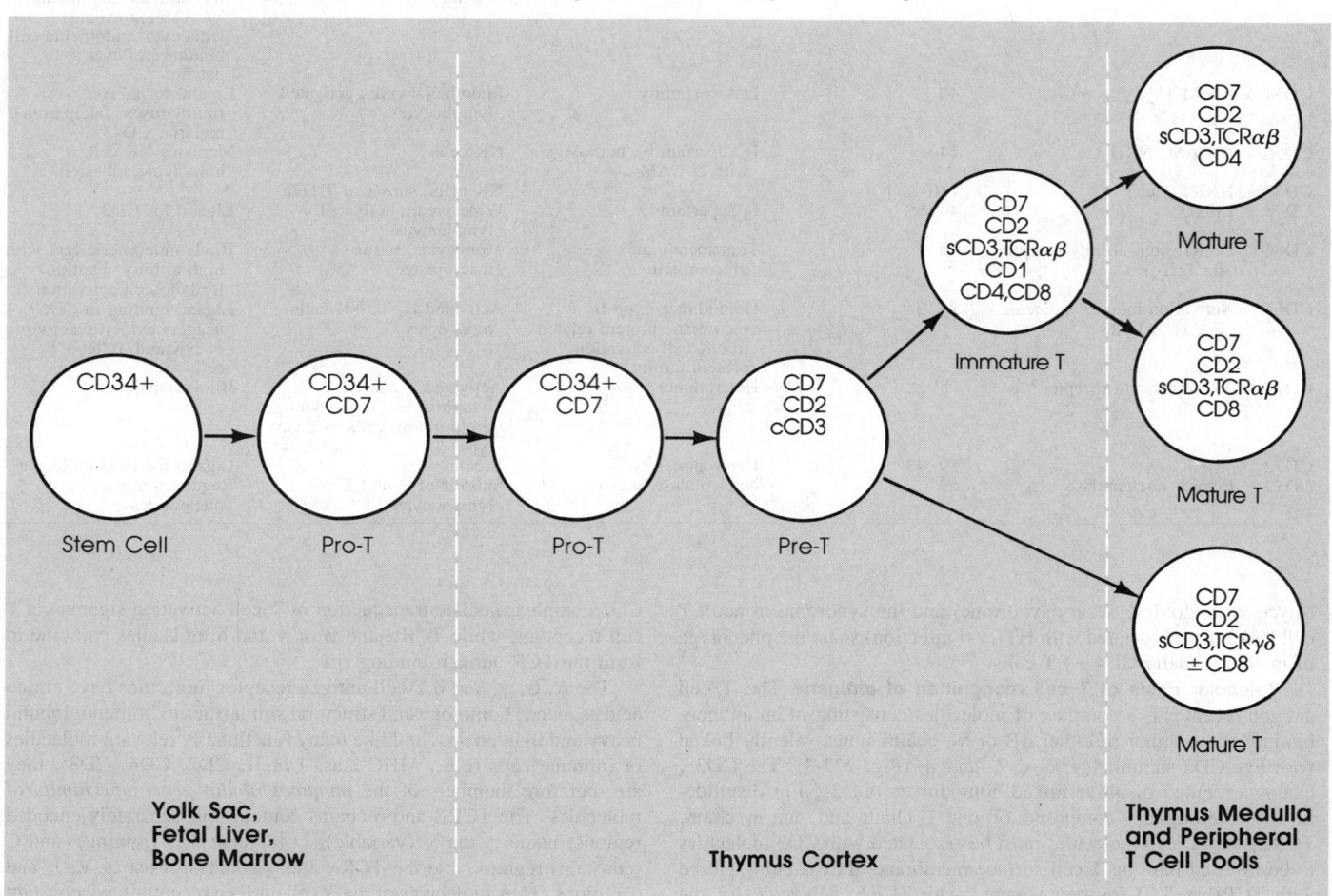

TABLE 277-4 Roles of cytokines in T cell proliferation and differentiation

Cytokine	Source within thymus	Function
IL-1α,β	Macrophages, TE cells, fibroblasts, endothelial cells, dendritic cells	Induces proliferation of thymocytes; induces production of other cytokines (i.e., IL-6, GM-CSF); with sCD23, induces TCRαβ maturation in T cell precursors
IL-2	Activated T cells	Induces proliferation of mature and immature thymocytes
IL-4	T cells	Induces proliferation of thymocytes; inhibits growth of TE cells
IL-5	Activated T cells	Induces cytotoxic T cell differentiation
IL-6	Activated T and B cells, macrophages, fibroblasts, TE cells, endothelial cells	Synergizes with mitogen or IL-1 for T cell/thymocyte proliferation
IL-7	Fibroblasts, BM stromal cell line	Comitogenic factor for thymocytes and T cells
IL-8	Monocytes-macrophages	Chemotactic for T cells
IL-10	Fetal and postnatal thymocytes, B cells	Costimulant for immature and mature thymocyte proliferation and maturation; inhibits cytokine production by mature T cells
Soluble CD23 (FcεRII)	TE cells, B cells	With IL-1, induces TCRαβ maturation in T cell precursors
GM-CSF	Activated T cells, fibroblasts, endothelial cells, T cells	Promotes growth of early T cell leukemias; promotes proliferation of immature thymocytes
G-CSF	TE cells, macrophages, fibroblasts	?Mitogenic for immature thymocytes
M-CSF	TE cells, monocytes, fibroblasts, endothelial cells	Supports differentiation of progenitors committed to the monocyte-macrophage lineages; ?mitogenic for immature thymocytes
LIF	TE cells, activated cells	?Prevents multilineage differentiation of intrathymic stem cells prior to signal to become T cell precursors
IFN-γ	Activated T cells, thymocytes	Up-regulates expression of TE, fibroblast, and macrophage CD54 (ICAM-1) and MHC class II; antiproliferative effect on thymocytes via adenylate cyclase pathway
TNF-α	Macrophages, activated T and B cells, thymocytes	IL-1–like effects
TGF-α	Activated macrophages, TE cells	Regulates production of other cytokines (IL-1 and IL-6) by TE cells; drives TE cell proliferation and/or differentiation via EGF receptor
TGF-β	?TE cells, T cells	Regulates expression of several oncogenes; suppresses lymphocyte responses to other cytokines; ?inhibits TE cell proliferation
EGF	?Monocytes-macrophages, ?fibroblasts, ?TE cells	Drives TE cell proliferation

NOTE: Unless otherwise stated, effect reported or postulated is in humans. TE = thymic epithelial; BM = bone marrow; EGF = epidermal growth factor; LIF = leukemia inhibitory factor; IFN-γ = γ-interferon; TNF = tumor necrosis factor; TGF = transforming growth factor; FcεRII = Fc receptor for IgE type II; IL = interleukin.
SOURCE: After Haynes et al.

T cells do not recognize native protein, carbohydrate or lipid antigens. Instead, T cells recognize only short (approximately 9 to 13 amino acids) peptide fragments that are derived from protein antigens taken up or produced in antigen-presenting cells. Foreign antigen is either taken up by endocytosis (exogenous antigen-presentation pathway) or arises exogenously (i.e., from an infectious agent) in antigen-presenting cells such as macrophages or dendritic cells (exogenous antigen-presentation pathway). Antigen-presenting cells proteolytically degrade foreign proteins and display peptide fragments embedded in the MHC class I or II antigen recognition site on the MHC molecule surface, where foreign peptide fragments bind to TCRαβ or TCRγδ chains of reactive T cells. CD4 molecules act as an adhesive and, by direct binding to MHC class II (DR, DQ, or DP) molecules, stabilize the interaction of TCR with peptide antigen (see Fig. 277-3). Similarly, CD8 molecules stabilize the TCR-antigen interaction by direct binding to MHC class I (A, B, or C) molecules.

Whereas it is generally agreed that the TCRαβ receptor recognizes peptide antigens in MHC class I or class II molecules, recent data suggest that the TCRγδ receptor may bind to other non-MHC molecules such as CD1.

Just as foreign antigens are degraded and their peptide fragments presented in the context of MHC class I or class II molecules on antigen-presenting cells, endogenous self-proteins are also degraded and self-peptide fragments are presented to T cells in the context of MHC class I or class II molecules on antigen-presenting cells. In peripheral lymphoid organs, T cells are present that are capable of recognizing self-protein fragments but normally are *anergic* and are nonresponsive to self-antigenic stimulation.

The specificity of reactivity of mature T cells is largely determined within the thymus during fetal and early postnatal development. In the thymus, the recognition of self-peptides on thymic epithelial cells and thymic macrophages is thought to play an important role in shaping the T cell repertoire to recognize foreign antigen *(positive selection)* and in eliminating highly autoreactive T cells *(negative selection)*. As immature cortical thymocytes begin to express surface TCR, autoreactive thymocytes are destroyed *(negative selection)*, thymocytes with TCR capable of interacting with foreign antigen peptides in the context of self MHC antigens are activated and develop to maturity *(positive selection)*, and thymocytes with TCR that are incapable of binding to self MHC antigens die of attrition *(no selection)*. Mature thymocytes that are positively selected are either CD4 + helper T cells or MHC class II–restricted cytotoxic (killer) T cells, or they are CD8 + T cells destined to become MHC class I–restricted cytotoxic T cells. For T cells to be *MHC class I–* or *class II–restricted* means that T cells recognize antigen peptide fragments as immunogenic only when they are presented in the antigen recognition site of the same MHC antigens expressed by the thymic microenvironment during the time of T cell selection.

Once ligation of mature T cell TCR by foreign peptide occurs in the context of self MHC class I or class II molecules (see Fig. 277-3), binding of non-antigen-specific adhesion ligand pairs such as CD54-CD11/CD18 and CD58/CD2 is up-regulated to stabilize MHC peptide–TCR binding (see Fig. 277-3). Once TCR-MHC binding is stabilized, activation signals are transmitted to the T cell via tyrosine kinases associated with CD4 or CD8 molecules (p56-lck) and CD3 molecules (pp59-fyn), and ligation of CD28 by B7/BB1 molecules on antigen-presenting cells leads to T cell cytokine (IL-2, IL-4) mRNA stabilization. All these events lead to enhanced T cell activation. For control of T cell activation, the cytoplasmic tyrosine phosphatase domain of the CD45 family of molecules modulates the activation status of the triggered T cells by modifying the activity of intracellular tyrosine kinases p56-lck and pp59-fyn. Thus a concert of molecular and biochemical events is required for normal T cell recognition of antigen and subsequent T cell activation.

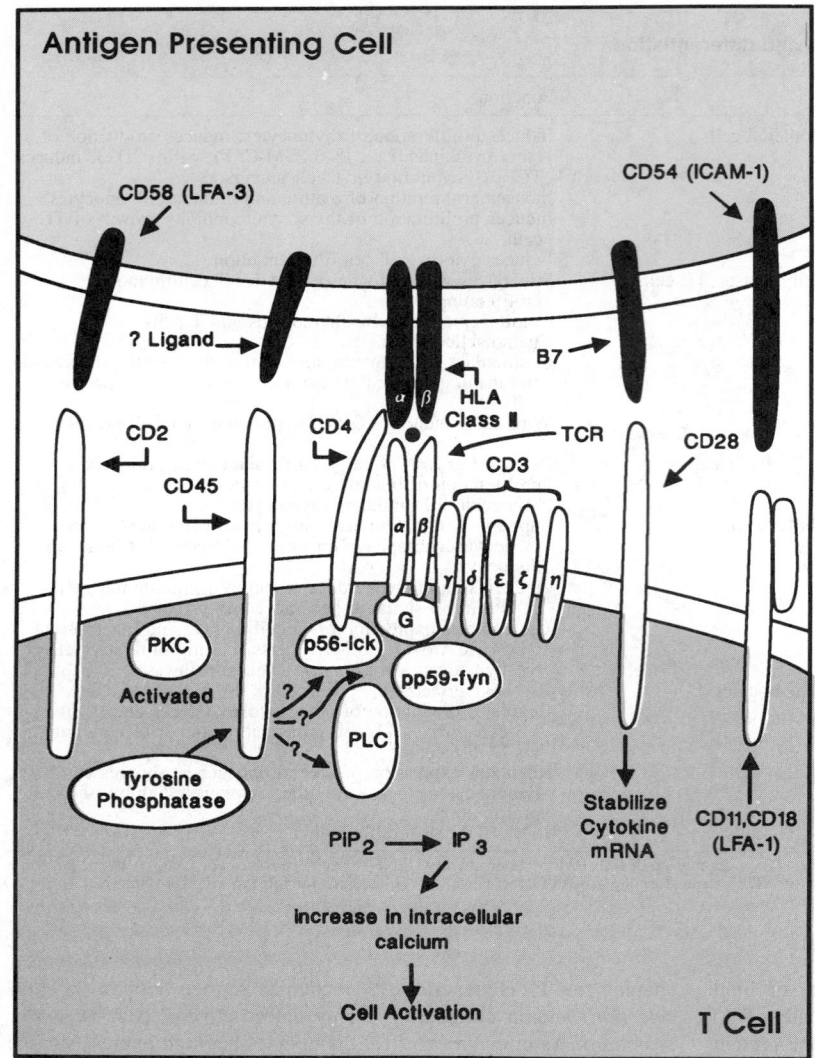

FIGURE 277-3   Molecules involved in human T cell recognition of antigen and in human T cell activation. The black circle at the tip of the αβ chains of HLA class II molecules represents a peptide fragment of "processed" protein antigen. TCRαβ and HLA (MHC) class II αβ + peptide interactions are stabilized by adhesion-ligand pairs such as LFA-1/ICAM-1 and CD2/LFA-3. Ligand binding to T cell CD28 induces stabilization of T cell–activating cytokines such as IL-2 and promotes T cell activation. Intracellular signals for T cell activation are mediated by the CD3 TCR-associated molecules and involve the activation of protein kinase C (PKC), the production of phospholipase C (PLC), and phosphorylation of proteins by the tyrosine kinases p56-lck and pp59-fyn. These events lead to production of phosphoinositol molecules (PIP2 and IP3) that mediate rises in intracellular calcium and eventually cell activation.

Superantigens in T cell development   *Superantigens* are protein molecules capable of activating up to 20 percent of the peripheral T cell pool, whereas conventional antigens activate fewer than 1 in 10,000 T cells. T cell superantigens include staphylococcal enterotoxins, other bacterial products, and retroviral proteins. Conventional antigens bind to MHC class I or II molecules in the groove of the αβ heterodimer and bind to T cells via V regions of both TCRα and β chains. In contrast, superantigens bind directly to TCRβ chains and MHC class II β chains at sites that differ from conventional antigen peptides and stimulate T cells based solely on the Vβ gene utilized regardless of the D, J, and Vα chain present (Fig. 277-4). Superantigen stimulation of human peripheral T cells occurs in the clinical setting of the *staphylococcal toxic shock syndrome* leading to massive overproduction of T cell cytokines (see Chap. 102).

B CELLS   Mature B cells comprise 10 to 15 percent of human peripheral blood lymphocytes, 50 percent of splenic lymphocytes, and approximately 10 percent of bone marrow lymphocytes. B cells express on their surface intramembrane immunoglobulin (Ig) molecules that function as B cell antigen receptors in a complex of Ig-associated α and β signaling molecules with intracellular signaling events similar to those in T cells (Fig. 277-5). B cells also express surface receptors for the Fc region of IgG molecules (CD32) as well as receptors for activated complement components (C3d or CD21, C3b or CD35). The primary function of B cells is to produce antibodies. Mature B cells are derived from bone marrow precursor cells that arise continuously throughout life (see Fig. 277-1).

B lymphocyte development can be separated into two phases: antigen-independent and antigen-dependent B cell development. Antigen-independent B cell development occurs in primary lymphoid organs, including fetal liver and bone marrow, and includes all stages of B cell maturation up to the surface (s) Ig + mature B cell. Antigen-dependent B cell maturation is driven by the interaction of antigen with B cell sIg leading to memory B cell induction and plasma cell formation. Antigen-dependent stages of B cell maturation occur in secondary lymphoid organs, including lymph node, spleen, and gut Peyer's patches. In contrast to the T cell repertoire that is generated intrathymically before contact with foreign antigen, the repertoire of B cells expressing diverse antigen-reactive sites is generated by further recombination of immunoglobulin genes after contact with antigen— a process called *somatic mutation*.

During B cell development, diversity of the antigen-binding variable region of Ig is generated by an ordered set of Ig gene rearrangements. First, the process brings diversity (D) segments to joining (J) segments and then brings a variable (V) gene segment and constant (C) segments to yield a functional Ig heavy chain gene (V-D-J-C). During later stages, a functional κ or λ light chain gene is generated by rearrangement of a V segment to a J segment, ultimately yielding an intact Ig molecule composed of heavy and light chains. The most immature B cell precursors (pro-B cells) express surface CD10 and CD34, lack B lineage–specific antigens CD19 and CD22, and also lack cytoplasmic (c) and surface (s) Ig (Fig. 277-6).

The next stage in B cell development, the pre-pre-B cell, is marked

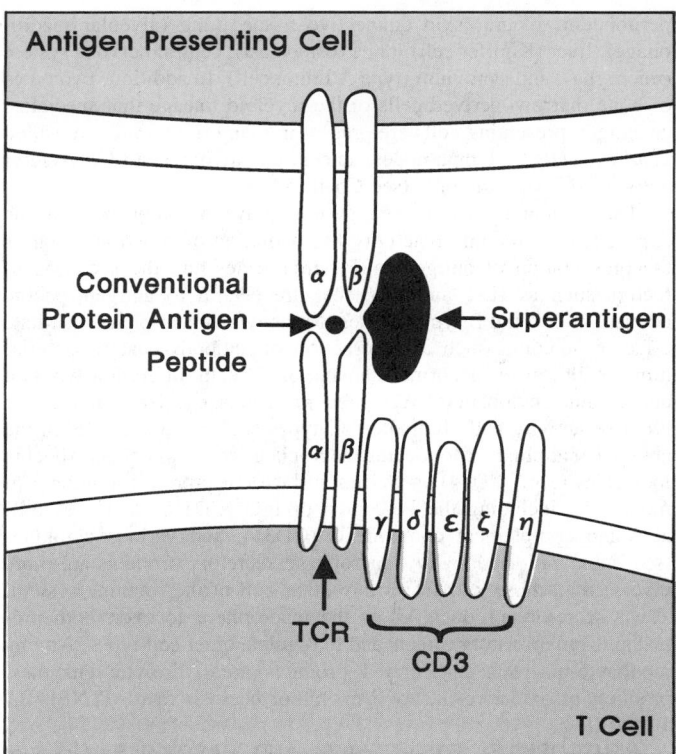

FIGURE 277-4 Comparison of site of superantigen binding to T cell receptor with the site of binding to T cell receptor of processed conventional antigen.

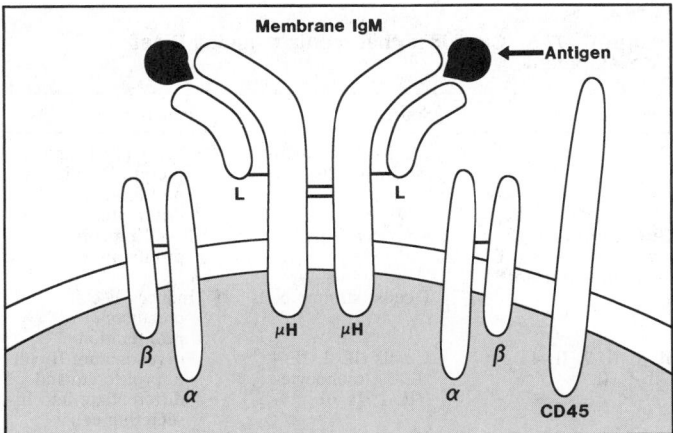

FIGURE 277-5 B cell antigen receptor for antigen-associated molecules. Immunoglobulin (Ig) associated α and β chains are disulfide-linked molecules that mediate the delivery of intracellular activation signals to B cells following interaction of membrane Ig with antigen. CD45 modulates the activation state of B cells by the tyrosine phosphatase activity of the cytoplasmic domain of CD45 molecules.

by the acquisition of CD19 and CD22 B cell antigens. Ig genes undergo rearrangement in pre-pre-B cells, but Ig heavy chain protein is not expressed. The hallmark of the next maturation stage, the pre-B cell, is expression of cμ heavy chain in association with expression of CD73 and CD21 surface proteins. Immature B cells have rearranged Ig light chain genes and express sIgM. As immature B cells develop into mature B cells, sIgD is expressed as well as sIgM and CD23. At this point, B lineage development in bone marrow is complete,

and B cells exit into the peripheral circulation and migrate to secondary lymphoid organs. There are approximately 300 VK genes and 5 JK genes, resulting in the pairing of VK and JK genes to create 1500 different light chain combinations. The number of distinct κ light chains that can be generated is increased by somatic mutations within the VK and JK genes, thus creating a large number of specificities from a limited amount of germ-line genetic information.

In heavy chain immunoglobulin gene rearrangement, the VH domain is created by the joining of three types of germ-line genes called VH, DH, and JH, thus allowing for even greater diversity in the variable region of heavy chains than for light chains (see Chap. 278).

A number of cytokines synergize to drive sequential stages of B cell maturation (Table 277-5). Bone marrow stromal cell– and T cell–derived IL-3 and IL-7 drive the earliest stages of B cell differentiation. Low-molecular-weight B cell growth factor (BCGF) binds to high-

FIGURE 277-6 Antigen-independent human B lymphocyte maturation. (*After Haynes and Denning, with permission.*)

	Stem Cell	Pro-B	Pre-Pre-B	Pre-Pre-B	Pre-B	Immature B	Mature B
	CD34	CD34	CD34	CD34	-	-	-
		CD10	CD10	CD10	-	-	-
			CD19	CD19	CD19	CD19	CD19
			CD40	CD40	CD40	CD40	CD40
				CD73	CD73	CD73	CD73
				CD22	CD22	CD22	CD22
				CD38	CD38	-	-
					CD21	CD21	CD21
							CD23
IL-7 Receptor	-	+	+	-	-	-	-
IL-3 Receptor	-	+	+	+	+	-	-
IL-4 Receptor	-	-	-	-	+	+	+
Immunoglobulin Gene Rearrangement	-	-	+	+	+	+	+
IgM Expression	-	-	-	-	cytoplasm	surface	surface
IgD Expression	-	-	-	-	-	-	surface

TABLE 277-5 Cytokines that regulate human B cell development

Cytokine	Source	Function
IL-7	T cells, bone marrow stromal cells	Drives pro-B and pre-pre-B cells to proliferate and differentiate
BCG-F (low-molecular-weight B cell growth factor)	Activated T cells	B cell precursor proliferation
IL-3	T cells, stromal cells	Induces B cell precursor proliferation
IL-1, IL-2, IL-4, IL-5, IL-6	T cells (IL-2, IL-4, IL-5), monocytes (IL-1, IL-6)	Drives mature B cells to proliferate and differentiate into Ig-secreting cells

affinity receptors expressed on all B cell precursors except pro-B cells and also triggers B cell differentiation. IL-1, IL-2, IL-4, IL-5, and IL-6 synergize to drive mature B cells to proliferate and differentiate into Ig-secreting cells.

LARGE GRANULAR LYMPHOCYTES Large granular lymphocytes (LGL) (previously called "null cells") constitute approximately 5 to 10 percent of peripheral blood lymphocytes and are nonadherent, nonphagocytic cells with large azurophilic cytoplasmic granules. LGL express surface receptors for the Fc portion of IgG (CD16), and many LGL express some T lineage markers and proliferate in response to IL-2. LGL arise in both bone marrow and thymic microenvironments (see Fig. 277-1).

Functionally, LGL share features with both monocytes-macrophages and neutrophils in that subsets of LGL mediate antibody-dependent cellular cytotoxicity (ADCC) and natural killer (NK) activity. ADCC is the binding of an opsonized (antibody-coated) target cell to an Fc receptor–bearing effector cell via the Fc region of antibody resulting in lysis of the target by the effector cell. Natural killer (NK) cell activity is the nonimmune (i.e., effector cell never having had previous contact with the target), non-antibody-mediated killing of target cells, which are usually malignant cell types or transplanted foreign cells. Thus LGL that mediate NK activity may play an important role in immune surveillance and destruction of cells that spontaneously undergo malignant transformation in vivo. Lymphokine-activated killer, or LAK, cells are NK lymphocytes that proliferate in vitro to high levels of IL-2 and develop the ability to kill tumor cells efficiently. LAK cells generated with IL-2 in vitro or in vivo from patients with solid tumors such as renal cell carcinomas have shown promising antitumor activity. Rare patients with complete absence of NK cells have been described who lack both NK activity and CD56+, CD16+ lymphocytes but have normal T and B cell function. NK cell hyporesponsiveness is also observed in patients with the *Chédiak-Higashi syndrome,* an autosomal recessive disease associated with fusion of cytoplasmic granules and defective degranulation of neutrophil lysosomes. Recently, a series of studies has suggested that NK cells can specifically recognize normal allogeneic cells in a clonal fashion. Studies of allogeneic target cells suggest that the genetic locus controlling NK alloantigen lysis is different from conventional MHC products, is inherited as an autosomal recessive trait, and is located on chromosome 6 in the same region as MHC class I genes.

MONOCYTES-MACROPHAGES Monocytes arise from precursor cells within bone marrow (see Fig. 277-1) and circulate with a half-life ranging from 1 to 3 days. Monocytes leave the peripheral circulation by marginating in capillaries and then migrating into a vast extravascular pool. Tissue macrophages arise by migration of monocytes from the circulation and by proliferation of macrophage precursors in tissue. Common locations of tissue macrophages (and some of their specialized names) are lymph node, spleen, bone marrow, perivascular connective tissue, serous cavities such as the peritoneum, pleura, skin connective tissue, lung (alveolar macrophage), liver (Kupffer cell), bone (osteoclast), central nervous system (microglia), and synovium (type A lining cell). In addition, two types of bone marrow–derived cells of the myeloid lineage that specialize as antigen-presenting cells are present in many tissues and are called *dendritic cells* (in lymph nodes, spleen, and thymus) and *Langerhans cells* (in skin and thymus) (see Chap. 58).

The monocyte-macrophage system plays a major role in the expression of immune reactivity by mediation of functions such as the presentation of antigen to T lymphocytes and the secretion of factors such as IL-1 and IL-6 that are central to antigen-specific activation of T and B lymphocytes. Monocytes-macrophages mediate effector functions such as destruction of antibody-coated bacteria, tumor cells, or even normal hematopoietic cells in certain types of autoimmune cytopenias. Activated macrophages also can mediate NK-like activity and eliminate cell types such as tumor cells in the absence of antibody. Monocytes-macrophages express lineage-specific molecules (e.g., CD14) as well as surface receptors for a number of molecules, including the Fc region of IgG (CD16, CD32, CD64), activated complement components (CD35), and various cytokines (see Table 277-2). Finally, macrophage secretory products are more diverse than those known for any other cell of the immune system. These secretory products allow the macrophage to exert both pro- and anti-inflammatory effects and to regulate other cell types. Among monocyte-macrophage–secreted products are hydrolytic enzymes, products of oxidative metabolism, tumor necrosis factor (TNF), IL-1, and IL-6.

NEUTROPHILS, EOSINOPHILS, AND BASOPHILS Granulocytes are present in nearly all forms of inflammation and are nonspecific amplifiers and effectors of specific immune responses. Unchecked accumulation and activation of granulocytes can lead to host tissue damage, as seen in neutrophil- and eosinophil-mediated *systemic necrotizing vasculitis.* Granulocytes are derived from stem cells in bone marrow (see Fig. 277-1). Each type of granulocyte (neutrophil, eosinophil, or basophil) is derived from a different subclass of progenitor cell which is stimulated to proliferate by colony stimulating factors. During terminal maturation of granulocytes, class-specific nuclear morphology and cytoplasmic granules appear that allow for histologic identification of granulocyte type.

Neutrophils express Fc receptors for IgG (CD16) and receptors for activated complement components (C3b or CD35) (see Table 277-2). Upon interaction of neutrophils with immune complexes, azurophilic granules (containing myeloperoxidase, lysozyme, elastase, and other enzymes) and specific granules (containing lactoferrin, lysozyme, collagenase, and other enzymes) are released, and microbicidal superoxide radicals (O_2) are generated at the neutrophil surface. The generation of superoxide leads to inflammation by direct injury to tissue and by alteration of macromolecules such as collagen and DNA.

Eosinophils express Fc receptors for IgG (CD32) and are potent cytotoxic effector cells for various parasitic organisms. Intracytoplasmic contents of eosinophils, such as major basic protein, eosinophil cationic protein, and eosinophil-derived neurotoxin, are capable of directly damaging tissues and may be responsible in part for the organ system dysfunction in the *hypereosinophilic syndromes* (see Chap. 59). Since the eosinophil granule contains anti-inflammatory types of enzymes (histaminase, arylsulfatase, phospholipase D), eosinophils may down-regulate or terminate ongoing inflammatory responses in normal inflammation homeostasis.

The normal functions of basophils and tissue mast cells are not completely understood; the capacity of basophil mediators to increase local delivery of antibodies and complement by increasing vascular permeability is hypothetical. Thus the basophil is identified principally with allergic reactions and some delayed cutaneous hypersensitivity states. Certainly the promotion of increased vascular permeability by basophils is important in the genesis of inflammatory lesions in some vasculitis syndromes (see Chap. 291). Basophils express surface receptors for IgE (CD23) and, upon cross-linking of basophil-bound

TABLE 277-6 Mediators released from human mast cells and basophils

Mediator	Actions
Histamine	Smooth-muscle contraction, increased vascular permeability
Slow reacting substance of anaphylaxis (SRSA) (leukotriene C_4, D_4, E_4)	Smooth-muscle contraction
Eosinophil chemotactic factor of anaphylaxis (ECF-A)	Chemotactic attraction of eosinophils
Platelet-activating factor	Activates platelets to secrete serotonin and other mediators; smooth-muscle contraction; induces vascular permeability
Neutrophil chemotactic factor (NCF)	Chemotactic attraction of neutrophils
Leukotactic activity (leukotriene B_4)	Chemotactic attraction of neutrophils
Heparin	Anticoagulant
Basophil kallikrein of anaphylaxis (BK-A)	Cleaves kininogen to form bradykinin

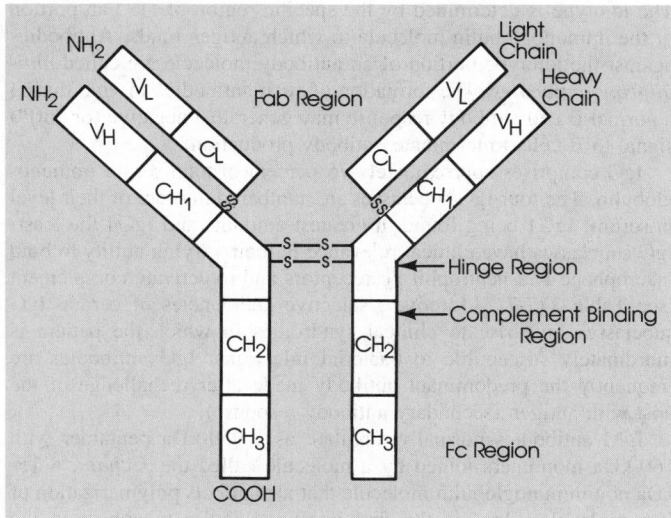

FIGURE 277-7 Schematic structure of the immunoglobulin G (IgG) molecule.

IgE by antigen, release histamine, eosinophil chemotactic factor of anaphylaxis, and neutral protease—all mediators of immediate (anaphylaxis) hypersensitivity responses (Table 277-6). In addition, basophils express surface receptors for activated complement components (C3a, C5a), through which mediator release can be directly effected (see Chap. 282 for a discussion of tissue mast cells).

HUMORAL MEDIATORS OF SPECIFIC IMMUNITY: IMMUNOGLOBULINS

Immunoglobulins are the products of differentiated B cells and mediate the humoral arm of the immune response. The primary functions of antibodies are to bind specifically to antigen and bring about the inactivation or removal of the offending toxin, microbe, parasite, or other foreign substance from the body. The structural basis of immunoglobulin molecule function and immunoglobulin gene organization has provided insight into the role of antibodies in normal protective immunity and in pathologic immune-mediated damage by immune complexes and autoantibody formation against host determinants.

All immunoglobulins have the basic structure of two heavy and two light chains (Fig. 277-7). Immunoglobulin isotype (i.e., G, M, A, D, E) is determined by the type of Ig heavy chain present. IgG and IgA isotypes can be divided further into subclasses (G1, G2, G3,

G4, and A1, A2) based on specific antigenic determinants on Ig heavy chains. The characteristics of human immunoglobulins are outlined in Table 277-7. The four chains are covalently linked by disulfide bonds. Each chain is made up of a variable (V) region and constant (C) regions (also called *domains*), themselves made up of units of approximately 110 amino acids. Light chains have one variable (VL) and one constant (CL) unit; heavy chains have one variable unit (VH) and three or four constant (CH) units, depending on isotype. As the name suggests, the constant regions of immunoglobulin molecules are made up of homologous sequences and share the same primary structure as all other immunoglobulin chains of the same isotype and subclass. Constant regions are involved in biologic functions of immunoglobulin molecules. The CH2 domain of IgG and the CH4 units of IgM are involved with the binding of the C1q portion of C1. The CH region at the carboxy-terminal end of the IgG molecule, the Fc region (see Fig. 277-7), binds to surface Fc receptors (CD16, CD32, CD64) of macrophages, large granular lymphocytes, B cells, neutrophils, and eosinophils.

Variable regions (VL and VH) constitute the antibody-binding (Fab) region of the molecule. Within the VL and VH regions are hypervariable regions (extreme sequence variability) that constitute the antigen-binding site unique to each immunoglobulin molecule.

TABLE 277-7 Characteristics of human immunoglobulins

	IgG	IgM	IgA	IgD	IgE
Molecular mass, kDa	150	190 (950)*	160 (385)†	175	190
Heavy chain	$\gamma1$, $\gamma2$, $\gamma3$, $\gamma4$	μ	$\alpha1$, $\alpha2$	δ	ϵ
Light chain	κ or λ	κ or λ	κ or λ	κ or λ	κ or λ
Adult average serum level, mg/dL	1250 ± 300	125 ± 50	210 ± 50	4	0.03
Half-life, d	23.0	5.1	5.8	2.8	2.5
Classic pathway	IgG1, IgG2, IgG3 yes; IgG4 no	Yes	No	No	No
Alternative pathway	IgG1, IgG2, IgG3 no; IgG4 yes	No	Yes	Yes	Yes
Binding cells via Fc	Macrophages, neutrophils, eosinophils, large granular lymphocytes	Lymphocytes	Lymphocytes	None	Mast cells, basophils, B cells
Other biologic properties	Placental transfer	Primary antibody response, rheumatoid factor	Antibody in mucous secretions	Primary lymphocyte surface molecules	Mediates anaphylaxis, allergy

* IgM circulates as a pentameric molecule.
† Secretory IgA is a dimer.
SOURCE: Adapted with permission from CA Haseman and JD Capra, in *Fundamental Immunology*, WE Paul (ed), 2d ed. New York, Raven, 1989.

The idiotype is determined by the specific region of the Fab portion of the immunoglobulin molecule to which antigen binds. Antibodies against the idiotype portion of an antibody molecule are called *anti-idiotype antibodies*. The formation of such antibodies in vivo during a normal B cell antibody response may generate a negative (or "off") signal to B cells to terminate antibody production.

IgG comprises approximately 75 percent of total serum immunoglobulin. The four IgG subclasses are numbered in order of their level in serum, IgG1 being found in greatest amounts and IgG4 the least. IgG subclasses have clinical relevance in their varying ability to bind macrophage and neutrophil Fc receptors and to activate complement (see Table 277-7). Moreover, selective deficiencies of certain IgG subclasses give rise to clinical syndromes in which the patient is inordinately susceptible to bacterial infections. IgG antibodies are frequently the predominant antibody made after rechallenge of the host with antigen (secondary antibody response).

IgM antibodies normally circulate as a 950-kDa pentamer with 160-kDa monomers joined by a molecule called the *J chain,* a 15-kDa nonimmunoglobulin molecule that also effects polymerization of IgA molecules. IgM is the first immunoglobulin to appear in the immune response (primary antibody response) and is the initial type of antibody made by neonates. Membrane IgM in the monomeric form also functions as a major antigen receptor on the surface of mature B cells (see Fig. 277-5). IgM is an important component of immune complexes in autoimmune diseases. For instance, IgM antibodies against IgG molecules (rheumatoid factors) are present in high titers in *rheumatoid arthritis,* other collagen diseases, and some infectious diseases *(subacute bacterial endocarditis).* IgM antibody binds the C1 component of complement via the CH4 domain and thus is a potent activator of complement.

IgA comprises only 10 to 15 percent of total serum immunoglobulin but is the predominant class of immunoglobulin in secretions. IgA in secretions (tears, saliva, nasal secretions, gastrointestinal tract fluid, and human milk) is in the form of secretory IgA (sIgA), a polymer consisting of two IgA monomers, a joining molecule called the *J chain,* and a glycoprotein called the *secretory protein.* Of the two IgA subclasses, IgA1 is primarily found in serum, whereas IgA2 is more prevalent in secretions. IgA fixes complement via the alternative complement pathway and has potent antiviral activity in humans by prevention of virus binding to respiratory and gastrointestinal epithelial cells.

IgD is found in minute quantities in serum (see Table 277-7) and along with IgM is a major receptor for antigen on the B cell surface. Present in serum is very low concentrations (see Table 277-7), IgE is the major class of immunoglobulin involved in arming mast cells and basophils by binding to these cells via the Fc region. Antigen cross-linking of IgE molecules on basophil and mast cell surfaces results in release of mediators of the immediate hypersensitivity response (see Table 277-6).

CELLULAR INTERACTIONS IN REGULATION OF THE NORMAL IMMUNE RESPONSE

The net result of activation of the humoral (B cell) and cellular (T cell) arms of the immune system by foreign antigen is the elimination of antigen directly by immune effector cells or in concert with specific antibody. In addition, a series of regulatory cells is activated which modulate T effector cell activation and B cell antibody production. Figure 277-8 is a simplified schematic diagram of the immune system outlining some of these cellular interactions.

T CELL–T CELL AND T CELL–B CELL INTERACTIONS The expression of immune cell function is the result of a complex series of immunoregulatory events that occur in phases. Both T and B lymphocytes mediate immune functions, and each of these cell types, when given appropriate signals, passes through stages, from activation and induction through proliferation, differentiation, and ultimately effector functions. The effector function expressed may be at the end point of a response, such as secretion of antibody by a differentiated plasma cell, or it might serve a regulatory function that modulates other functions, such as is seen with CD4+ inducer or CD8+ regulatory T lymphocytes, which modulate both differentiation of B cells and activation of CD8+ or CD4+ cytotoxic T cells.

CD4 inducer (or helper) T cells can be subdivided on the basis of cytokines produced. Activated TH1-type inducer T cells secrete interferon-γ (IFN-γ) and IL-2, while activated TH2-type inducer T cells secrete IL-4, IL-5, IL-6, and IL-10. TH1 CD4+ T cells provide T cell help for generation of cytotoxic T cells and generally respond to antigens that lead to delayed hypersensitivity types of immune responses (such as *Mycobacterium tuberculosis*). In contrast, TH2 cells regulate the intensity of immune responses by the secretion of a cytokine, IL-10, that inhibits the production of other cytokines (see Table 277-4). In addition, TH2 CD4+ T cells provide help to B cells for specific Ig production and respond to antigens that require high antibody levels for foreign antigen elimination (such as in certain parasite infections).

As shown in Fig. 277-8, upon activation by antigen-presenting cells, regulatory T cell subsets that produce IL-2, IL-3, IFN-γ, and/or IL-4, IL-5, IL-6, and IL-10 are generated that exert positive and negative forces on effector T and B cells. For B cells, trophic effects are mediated by a variety of cytokines, particularly T cell–derived IL-3, IL-4, and IL-5, which act at sequential stages of B cell maturation, resulting in B cell proliferation, differentiation, and ultimately antibody secretion (see Table 277-5). For cytotoxic T cells, trophic factors include inducer T cell secretion of IL-2 and IFN-γ (see Table 277-4). In addition, B cells themselves are capable of serving as antigen-presenting cells, processing and presenting antigens to T cells, and secreting TNF-α and IL-6.

MONOCYTE–T CELL INTERACTIONS Many of the activation and regulatory effects of lymphocytes and monocytes occur via soluble mediators that regulate T and B cell maturation (see Tables 277-3, 277-4, and 277-5). Monocytes-macrophages are required for optimal activation of T cells by antigens or by mitogens (nonspecific activators of lymphocytes). A soluble macrophage product, IL-1, can substitute in some cases for intact macrophages for activation of lymphocytes. Upon contact with antigens or mitogens, macrophages secrete IL-1, IL-6, and TNF, two effects of which are (1) the induction of receptors for IL-2 on T cells and (2) the induction of T cell IL-2, IL-4, and other cytokine secretion. IL-2, IL-4, and other cytokines, in turn, activate other T cells, resulting in expansion of effector and regulatory T cells that also have been induced to express IL-2, IL-4, and IL-7 receptors (see Fig. 277-8). Effector T cells mediate a variety of functions, including the killing of virus-infected cells, graft rejection, graft-versus-host reaction, delayed-type hypersensitivity, and the release of a wide spectrum of immunoregulatory cytokines (see Tables 277-3, 277-4, and 277-5).

THE COMPLEMENT SYSTEM

The complement system is a cascading series of plasma enzymes, regulatory proteins, and proteins capable of cell lysis whose principal site of synthesis is the liver. There are two arms of the complement system (Fig. 277-9). Activation of the classic complement pathway via C1, C4, and C2 and activation of the alternative complement pathway via factor D, C3, and factor B both lead to cleavage and activation of C3. C3 is a protein whose activation fragments, when bound to target surfaces such as bacteria and other foreign antigens, are critical for opsonization (coating by antibody and complement) in preparation for phagocytosis.

The protein fragment C3b, split from C3, is necessary for activation of the terminal complement components C5–9. These form the membrane attack complex which, when inserted into cell membranes, brings about osmotic lysis of the cell.

C3b also joins with a cleavage product of factor B (called Bb) to form C3bBb, also known as the *alternative pathway C3 convertase.*

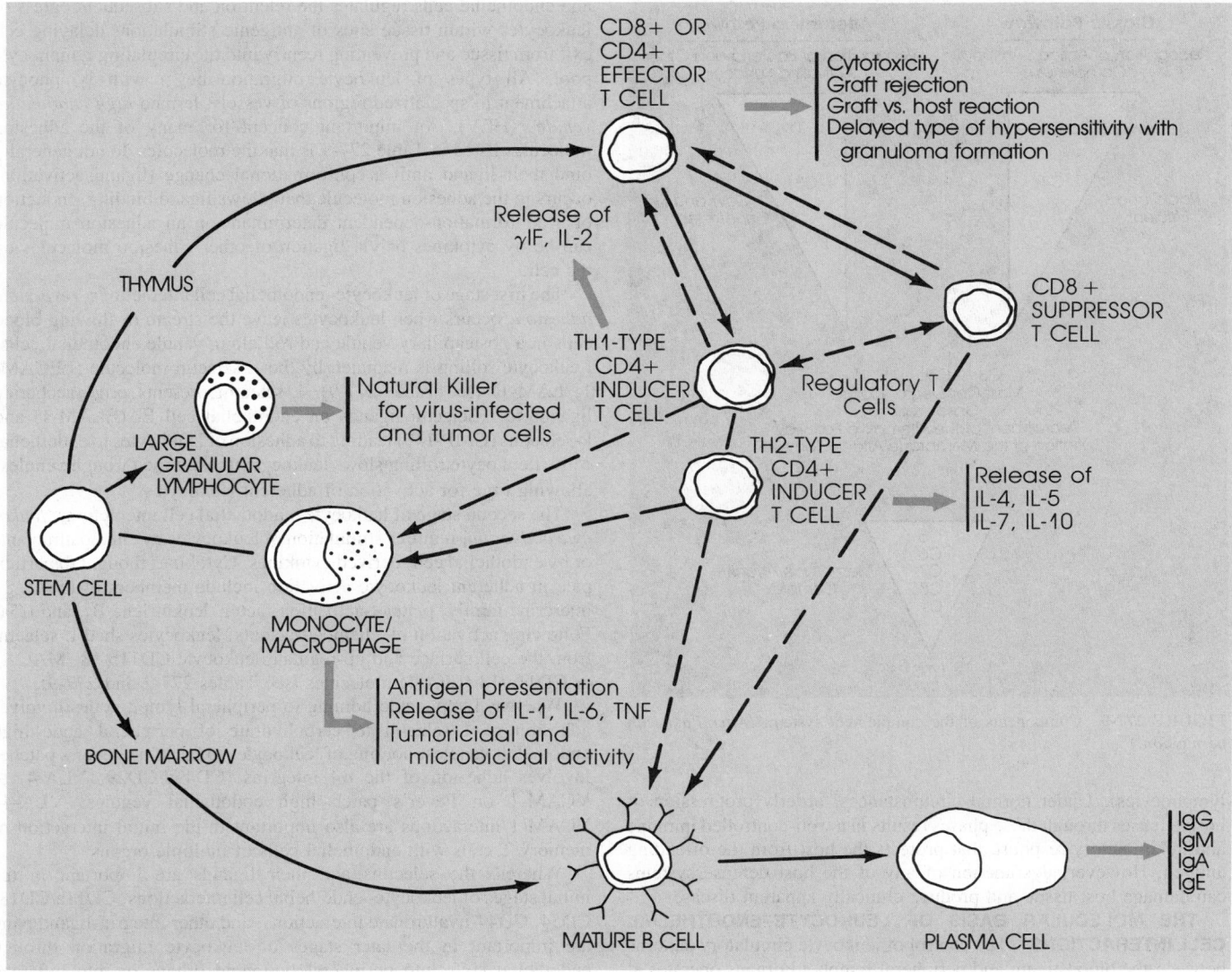

FIGURE 277-8 Schematic model of intercellular interactions of immune cells during the ontogeny and activation stages of immune responses.

Activation of the classic complement pathway results in cleavage of C4 and C2 with a resulting complex of fragments, C4b2a, also called the *classic pathway C3 convertase*. Both the classic pathway C3 convertase (C4b2a) and the alternative pathway C3 convertase (C3bBb) function to cleave C3 to form active C3b, thus driving activation of the C5–9 membrane attack complex. The fact that C3b can combine with Bb to form the alternative pathway C3 convertase gives rise to a potent positive feedback loop for production of C3b and thus continued activation of terminal complement components.

Activation of the classic complement pathway is by interaction of antigen and antibody to form immune complexes that bind C1q, a subunit of C1. Immunoglobulin isotypes that bind C1q and activate the classic pathway are IgM, IgG1, IgG2, and IgG3. In contrast, IgA1, IgA2, and IgD activate complement via the alternative pathway. Activation of the complement cascade via the classic pathway by IgG- or IgM-containing immune complexes is a rapid and efficient pathway to activation of terminal complement components. In contrast, activation of the alternative complement pathway via IgA-containing immune complexes or by bacterial endotoxin is a slower and less efficient pathway to terminal component activation. Thus the immunoglobulin isotype composition of immune complexes is a critical factor in determining complement activation and the efficiency of clearance of immune complexes by C3 receptor–bearing cells.

In addition to the role of complement in opsonization of bacteria and cell lysis, several complement component fragments are potent mediators of immune cell activation. C3a and C5a bind to receptors on mast cells and basophils, resulting in release of histamine and other mediators of anaphylaxis. C5a is also a potent chemoattractant for neutrophils and monocytes-macrophages (Table 277-8).

MECHANISMS OF IMMUNE DAMAGE

Several responses by the host to foreign antigen culminate in the rapid and efficient elimination of nonself substances. In these scenarios, the classic weapons of the immune system (T cells, B cells, macrophages) interface with cells and soluble products that are mediators of inflammatory responses (neutrophils, eosinophils, basophils, kinin and coagulation systems, and complement cascade).

There are four general phases of host defenses: (1) migration of leukocytes to sites of antigen localization; (2) specific and nonspecific recognition of foreign antigens mediated by T and B lymphocytes, macrophages, and the alternative complement pathway; (3) amplification of the inflammatory response with recruitment of specific and nonspecific effector cells by complement components, lymphokines and monokines, kinins, arachidonic acid metabolites, and mast cell–basophil products; and (4) macrophage, neutrophil, and lymphocyte participation in antigen destruction with ultimate removal of antigen particles by phagocytosis (by macrophages or neutrophils) or by direct cytotoxic mechanisms (involving macrophages, neutrophils, and

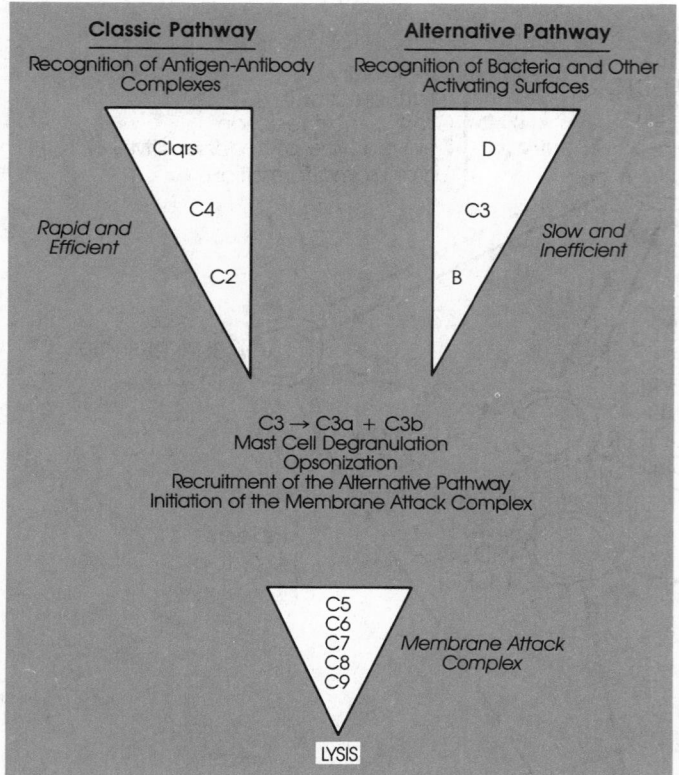

FIGURE 277-9   Components of the complement system. *(After Paul with permission.)*

lymphocytes). Under normal circumstances, orderly progression of host defenses through these phases results in a well-controlled immune and inflammatory response that protects the host from the offending antigen. However, dysfunction of any of the host defense systems can damage host tissue and produce clinically apparent disease.

THE MOLECULAR BASIS OF LEUKOCYTE–ENDOTHELIAL CELL INTERACTIONS   The control of leukocyte circulatory patterns between the bloodstream and peripheral lymphoid organs operates at the level of lymphocyte–endothelial cell interactions to control the specificity of lymphocyte subset entry into organs. Similarly, leukocyte–endothelial cell interactions regulate the entry of leukocytes into inflamed tissue. Adhesion molecule expression on leukocytes

TABLE 277-8   Biologic activities of some complement components

Component	Activity
C4a weak anaphylatoxin	Evokes histamine release from basophils and mast cells
C3a	Anaphylatoxin; evokes histamine release from basophils and mast cells
C5a	Anaphylatoxin; evokes histamine release from basophils and mast cells; potent chemoattractant for monocytes and neutrophils
C3b, C3bi	Enhancement of phagocytosis by neutrophils and monocytes; promotes immune complex binding to cells within monocyte-macrophage system, as well as neutrophils; C3b with Bb forms alternative pathway C3 convertase and amplifies alternative pathway; promotes solubilization of immune complexes
C5–9	Membrane attack complex; forms transmembrane channels leading to cell destruction

SOURCE: Adapted with permission from S Ruddy, in Kelley et al.

and endothelial cells regulates the retention and subsequent egress of leukocytes within tissue sites of antigenic stimulation, delaying cell exit from tissue and preventing reentry into the circulating lymphocyte pool. All types of leukocyte migration begin with lymphocyte attachment to specialized regions of vessels, termed *high endothelial venules* (HEV). An important concept for many of the adhesion molecules listed in Table 277-9 is that the molecules do not generally bind their ligand until a conformational change (ligand activation) occurs in the adhesion molecule that allows ligand binding. Induction of a conformation-dependent determinant on an adhesion molecule can be by cytokines or via ligation of other adhesion molecules on the cell.

The first stage of leukocyte–endothelial cell interactions, *reversible adhesion*, occurs when leukocytes leave the stream of flowing blood cells in a postcapillary venule and roll along venule endothelial cells. Leukocyte rolling is mediated by the L-selectin molecule (LECAM-1, LAM-1) (see Table 277-9). L-selectin presents oligosaccharide ligands to L-selectin ligands on endothelial cell E- (ELAM-1) and P-selectins (GMP-140) leading to adhesion of leukocytes to endothelial cells. Leukocyte rolling slows leukocyte transit time through venules, allowing time for activation of adherent leukocytes.

The second stage of leukocyte–endothelial cell interactions, *leukocyte activation*, requires stimulation of leukocytes by chemoattractants or by endothelial cell–derived cytokines. Cytokines thought to participate in adherent leukocyte activation include members of the IL-8–intercrine family, platelet-activation factor, leukotriene B_4, and C5a. Following activation by chemoattractants, leukocytes shed L-selectin from the cell surface and up-regulate leukocyte CD11b/18 (MAC-1) or CD11a/18 (LFA 1) molecules (see Tables 277-2 and 277-9).

Whereas lymphocyte homing to peripheral lymph nodes involves adhesion of L-selectin to carbohydrate of peripheral node high endothelial venules, homing of leukocytes to intestine Peyer's patches involves adhesion of the α4 integrins (CD49d/CD29, VLA-4) to VCAM-1 on Peyer's patch high endothelial venules. VLA-4–VCAM-1 interactions are also important in the initial interaction of memory T cells with endothelial cells of multiple organs.

Whereas the selectins and their ligands are important in the initial stages of leukocyte–endothelial cell interactions, CD11a/CD18, CD54, CD44-hyaluronate interactions, and other integrin-ligand pairs are important in the later stages of leukocyte migration through endothelial cells into peripheral lymphoid organs or into inflamed tissue.

IMMUNE-COMPLEX FORMATION   Clearance of antigen by immune-complex formation between antigen and antibody is a highly effective mechanism of host defense. However, depending on the level of immune complexes formed and their physicochemical properties, immune complexes may or may not result in host and foreign cell damage. After antigen exposure, certain types of soluble antigen-antibody complexes freely circulate and, if not cleared by the reticuloendothelial system, can be deposited in blood vessel walls and in other tissues such as renal glomeruli. The precise mechanisms whereby immune complexes damage tissues, particularly blood vessels, are discussed in Chaps. 283 and 291.

IgE-MEDIATED ALLERGIC REACTIONS—ANAPHYLAXIS   T helper cells that drive antiallergen IgE responses are usually TH2-type inducer T cells that secrete IL-4, IL-5, IL-6, and IL-10. Mast cells and basophils have receptors for the Fc portion of IgE (CD23), and cell-bound antiallergen IgE effectively "arms" basophils and mast cells. Mediator release is triggered by antigen (allergen) interaction with Fc receptor–bound IgE; the mediators released are responsible for the pathophysiologic changes of allergic diseases (see Table 277-6). Mediators released from mast cells and basophils can be divided into three broad categories of action: (1) those which increase vascular permeability and contract smooth muscle (histamine, platelet-activating factor, SRS-A, BK-A); (2) those which are chemotactic for or activate other inflammatory cells (ECF-A, NCF, leukotriene B_4); and (3) those which modulate the release of other mediators (BK-A, platelet-activating factor) (see Chap. 282).

TABLE 277-9 Leukocyte–endothelial cell adhesion molecules

Molecule	Distribution	Ligand	Functions
SELECTIN FAMILY			
L-selectin (LECAM-1, LAM-1)	Leukocyte	Lymph node addressin, sialylated oligosaccharides	Regulates leukocyte binding to inflamed endothelium; lymph node homing receptor
P-selectin (GMP-140)	Endothelial cells, alpha granules of platelets	Sialylated derivatives of Lewis X oligosaccharides	Involved in initial leukocyte–endothelial cell interactions
E-selectin (ELAM-1)	Endothelial cells	Sialylated derivatives of Lewis X oligosaccharides	Involved in initial leukocyte–endothelial cell interactions
INTEGRIN FAMILY			
$\alpha 1\beta 1$ (VLA-1, CD49a)	Activated T cells, monocytes, endothelial cells	Laminin, collagen	Activation-dependent adhesion receptor; marker for memory T cells
$\alpha 2\beta 1$ (VLA-2, CD49b)	Lymphocytes, endothelial cells, widespread	Collagen, laminin	Activation-dependen adhesion receptor
$\alpha 3\beta 1$ (VLA-3, CD49c)	Lymphocytes, endothelial cells, widespread	Fibronectin, collagen, laminin	Activation-dependent adhesion receptor
$\alpha 4\beta 1$ (VLA-4, CD49d)	Lymphocytes	VCAM-1, fibronectin fragment, vascular addressin	Involved in organ-specific homing; activation up-regulates adhesion
$\alpha 5\beta 1$ (VLA-5, CD49e)	Lymphocytes, endothelial cells, widespread	Fibronectin	Activation-dependent adhesion receptor; marker for memory T cells
$\alpha 6\beta 1$ (VLA-6, CD49f)	Widespread	Laminin	Adhesion to endothelial cells
$\alpha L\beta 2$ (LFA-1, CD11a)	Leukocytes	ICAM-1, ICAM-2, ICAM-3	Activation-dependent adhesion receptor
$\alpha M\beta 2$ (MAC-1, CD11b)	Myeloid, NK cells	ICAM-1, C3bi, factor X	Activation-dependent adhesion receptor; mediates adhesion of myeloid cells to endothelial cells
$\alpha X\beta 1$ (p150, 95, CD11c)	Myeloid cells, subset of lymphocyte	?	Activation-dependent adhesion receptor; mediates binding of myeloid cells to ligands derived from complement cascade
IMMUNOGLOBULIN GENE SUPERFAMILY			
CD2	T cells, NK cells	CD58 (LFA-3)	Activation-dependent adhesion receptor; can transmit proliferation signal
CD54 (ICAM-1)	Activated lymphocytes, thymic epithelium, cytokine (IL-1, TNF-α, IFN-γ)–stimulated endothelial cells	LFA-1, rhinoviruses, *P. falciparum*	Up-regulated expression on many tissues; mediates endothelial-leukocyte adherence
ICAM-2	Endothelial cells	LFA-1	Mediates leukocyte-endothelial adherence
ICAM-3	All resting leukocytes	LFA-1	Leukocyte-leukocyte interactions prior to leukocyte activation
CD58 (LFA-3)	Most tissue cell types	CD2	Up-regulated expression in lymphoid tissues; involved in CTL–target cell interactions
VCAM-1 (InCAM-110)	TNF-α– and IL-1–stimulated endothelial cells, follicular dendritic cells	VLA-4 ($\alpha 4\beta 1$)	Mediates homing of VLA-4 + leukocytes to Peyer's patches; mediates binding of B cells to germinal centers
CARTILAGE LINK PROTEIN FAMILY			
CD44 (Hermes, Pgp1, EcMRIII)	Leukocytes, widespread	Hyaluronan (hyaluronic acid)	Mediates leukocyte adhesion to endothelial cells, probably by activation-dependent adhesion; binds to various cytokines

SOURCE: Adapted with permission from Haynes and Denning.

CYTOTOXIC REACTIONS OF ANTIBODY In this type of immunologic injury, complement-fixing (C1-binding) antibodies against normal or foreign cells or tissues (IgM, IgG1, IgG2, IgG3) bind complement via the classic pathway and initiate a sequence of events similar to that initiated by immune-complex deposition, resulting in cell lysis or tissue injury. Examples of antibody-mediated cytotoxic reactions include red cell lysis in *transfusion reactions, Goodpasture's syndrome* with anti-glomerular basement membrane antibody formation, and *pemiphigus vulgaris* with antiepidermal antibodies inducing blistering skin disease.

CLASSIC DELAYED-TYPE HYPERSENSITIVITY REACTIONS Inflammatory reactions initiated by mononuclear leukocytes and not by antibody alone have been termed *delayed-type hypersensitivity reactions*. The term *delayed* has been used to contrast a secondary cellular response which appears 48 to 72 h after antigen exposure with an *immediate* hypersensitivity response generally seen within 12 h of antigen challenge and initiated by basophil mediator release or preformed antibody. For example, in an individual previously infected with *M. tuberculosis* (TB) organisms, intradermal placement of TB purified-protein derivative (PPD) as a skin test challenge results in an indurated area of skin at 48 to 72 h, indicating previous exposure to TB.

The cellular events that result in classic delayed-type hypersensitivity responses are centered around T cells (predominantly IFN-γ, IL-2, and lymphotoxin-secreting TH1-type helper T cells) and macrophages. First, local immune and inflammatory responses at the site of foreign antigen up-regulate endothelial cell adhesion molecule expression, promoting the accumulation of leukocytes at the tissue site. In the general scheme outlined in Fig. 277-8, antigen is processed by monocytes-macrophages and presented to T cells expressing a T cell receptor specific for the antigen. Macrophage-secreting IL-1 and IL-6 amplify the clonal expansion of antigen-specific T cells, and lymphokines (primarily IL-2, IFN-γ, and lymphotoxin) are secreted to recruit other T cells and macrophages to participate in the cellular inflammatory response. In particular, cytotoxic T cells are activated to become active killer cells by IL-2. Once recruited, macrophages frequently undergo epithelioid cell transformation and form giant cells in response to IL-4 and IFN-γ. This type of mononuclear cell infiltrate is termed *granulomatous inflammation*. Examples of diseases in which delayed-type hypersensitivity plays a major role are fungal infections *(histoplasmosis)*, mycobacterial infections *(TB, leprosy)*, chlamydial infections *(lymphogranuloma venereum)*, helminth infections *(schistosomiasis)*, reactions to toxins *(berylliosis)*, and hypersensitivity reactions to organic dusts *(hypersensitivity pneumonitis)*. In addition, delayed-type hypersensitivity responses may play a role in tissue damage in autoimmune diseases such as *rheumatoid arthritis* and *Wegener's granulomatosis* (see Chaps. 285 and 291).

AUTOIMMUNE DISEASE   Autoimmune disease is characterized by production of either antibodies that react with host tissue or immune effector T cells that are autoreactive to endogenous self peptides. Since B cell responses in humans generally require inducer T cells, a B cell autoantibody response directly implies disordered T cell immunoregulatory control. In some instances, autoantibodies may arise by a normal T and B cell response activated by foreign organisms or substances that contain antigens, particularly polysaccharides, that cross-react with similar self antigens in body tissues. This phenomenon is called *molecular mimicry*. Examples of clinically relevant autoantibodies are antibodies against acetylcholine receptors in *myasthenia gravis* and anti-DNA, antierythrocyte, and antiplatelet antibodies in *systemic lupus erythematosus*.

As mentioned above in the description of immunoglobulins, the unique portion of the variable region of the immunoglobulin molecule where antigen binds is called the *idiotype*, and an antibody that reacts specifically with that region is called an *anti-idiotype antibody*. Anti-idiotype antibodies may arise during the course of the normal immune response. For example, anti-idiotypes against antitetanus antibodies develop during normal immunization of humans to tetanus toxoid and serve to deliver "off" signals to B cells secreting antitetanus antibodies. Antibodies may be an important component of the normal immunoregulatory network. Anti-idiotype antibodies also may be relevant to two types of autoimmunity: (1) dysfunction of the idiotype–anti-idiotype antibody system could lead to B cell hyperreactivity by failure to generate "off" signals for B cell differentiation, and (2) some antireceptor antibodies produced in autoimmune diseases (anti-acetylcholine receptor antibodies in myasthenia gravis, anti-insulin receptor antibodies in forms of type I diabetes mellitus, and anti-thyrotropin receptor antibodies in autoimmune thyroid disease) may be anti-idiotype antibodies made against the antibody-combining site (idiotype) of an autoantibody.

Genetic factors likely play a role in the genesis of autoimmune disease, either by selecting for inherent B cell hyperreactivity and tendency toward autoantibody formation or, in the case of MHC antigen association with autoimmune diseases, via presentation of self or foreign peptides that stimulate an inappropriate antiself response. Myasthenia gravis, autoimmune thyroid disease, and pernicious anemia are all associated with HLA-B8 (MHC class I) and -DR3 (MHC class II) expression (see Chap. 64) and are also associated with certain immunoglobulin heavy chain markers. There is also a strong association of certain DR types with the development of rheumatoid arthritis.

Whereas organ-specific autoimmune diseases are likely the result of the combined effects of several factors that lead to inappropriate targeting of a particular organ or system to immune damage, generalized autoimmune diseases such as systemic lupus erythematosus can be thought of as diseases in which there is episodic breakdown of immunologic tolerance to self molecules. Recent studies have demonstrated that in a mouse model of autoimmunity (the MRL mouse), the cause of autoimmune disease is a defect in a cell surface molecule (fas/APO-1) on T cells that is required for the intrathymic death of autoreactive T lymphocytes. The defective fas/APO-1 molecule prevents negative selection of autoreactive T cells, leading to seeding of peripheral lymphoid organs with excessive numbers of autoreactive T cells. It is thought that rare serious multisystem lupus erythematosus–like syndromes in children may be the human homologues of murine MRL autoimmune disease. Instead of a defect in central (thymic) tolerance, adult acquired systemic lupus erythematosus is more likely to be a generalized defect in maintenance of peripheral tolerance in which the peripheral immune system lacks the ability to maintain anergy to self antigens. While the molecules involved in maintenance of peripheral tolerance/anergy to self antigens are not fully known, recent data suggest that T cell CD28 and B cell B7/BB1 molecules are involved in regulating this process.

CLINICAL EVALUATION OF IMMUNE FUNCTION

Clinical assessment of immunity requires investigation of the four major components of the immune system that participate in host defense and in pathogenesis of autoimmune diseases: (1) humoral immunity (B cells), (2) cell-mediated immunity (T cells, monocytes), (3) phagocytic cells of the reticuloendothelial system (macrophages), as well as polymorphonuclear leukocytes, and (4) complement. Clinical problems that require an evaluation of immunity include chronic infections, recurrent infection, unusual infecting agents, and certain autoimmune syndromes. The type of clinical syndrome under evaluation can provide information regarding possible immune defects (see Chap. 278). Defects in cellular immunity generally result in viral, mycobacterial, and fungal infections. An extreme example of deficiency in cellular immunity is the acquired immunodeficiency syndrome (AIDS) (see Chap. 279). Antibody deficiencies result in recurrent bacterial infections, frequently with organisms such as *Streptococcus pneumoniae* and *Haemophilus influenzae* (see Chap. 278). Disorders of phagocyte function frequently are manifested by recurrent skin infections, often due to *Staphylococcus aureus* (see Chap. 59). Finally, deficiencies of early and late complement components are associated with autoimmune phenomena and recurrent *Neisseria* infections (Table 277-10). Chapter 278 summarizes useful initial screening tests of immune function.

INTERVENTIONAL IMMUNOTHERAPY

Most current therapies for autoimmune and inflammatory diseases involve the use of nonspecific immune-modulating or immunosuppressive agents such as glucocorticoids or cytotoxic drugs. The goal of development of new treatments for immune-mediated diseases is to design ways to specifically interrupt pathologic immune responses, leaving nonpathologic immune responses intact. Novel ways to interrupt pathologic immune responses that are under investigation include the use of monoclonal antibodies against T lymphocytes as therapeutic agents, the use of toxin-labeled cytokines and/or specific cytokine inhibitors as anti-inflammatory agents, and the use of soluble adhesion molecules to interrupt inflammatory reactions associated with up-regulated adhesion molecule expression. For some animal models of organ-specific autoimmune disease, the TCR types of pathogenic T cells have been oligoclonal or monoclonal, giving hope

TABLE 277-10 Complement deficiencies and associated diseases

Component	Associated diseases
CLASSIC PATHWAY	
C1q, C1r, C1s, C4	Immune-complex syndromes,* pyogenic infections
C2	Immune-complex syndromes,* few with pyogenic infections
C1 inhibitor	Rare immune-complex disease, few with pyogenic infections
C3 AND ALTERNATIVE PATHWAY C3	
C3	Immune-complex syndromes,* pyogenic infections
D	Pyogenic infections
Properdin	*Neisseria* infections
I	Pyogenic infections
H	Hemolytic uremic syndrome
MEMBRANE ATTACK COMPLEX	
C5, C6, C7, C8	Recurrent *Neisseria* infections, immune-complex disease
C9	Rare *Neisseria* infections

* Immune-complex syndromes include SLE and SLE-like syndromes, glomerulonephritis, and vasculitis syndromes.
SOURCE: Adapted with permission from JA Schifferli and DK Peters, Lancet 88:957, 1983.

that anti-TCR therapy (TCR peptides, inducing anti-TCR antibodies or anti-TCR regulatory T cells) may be feasible. However, to date, pathologic T cells in human autoimmune disease have remained difficult to define, and specific TCR-directed therapy of T cell–mediated autoimmune diseases remains only a theoretical possibility.

REFERENCES

CLARK SC, KAMEN R: The human hematopoietic colony-stimulating factors. Science 236:1229, 1987

DAVIS MM: Molecular genetics of T cell antigen receptors. Hosp Pract 23:157, 1988

FINKEL TH et al: T-cell development and transmembrane signaling: Changing biological responses through an unchanging receptor. Immunol Today 12:79, 1991

FRANK MM: Complement in the pathophysiology of human disease. N Engl J Med 316:1525, 1987

GLEICH GJ: Eosinophils, basophils and mast cells. J Allergy Clin Immunol 84:1024, 1989

HAYNES BF, DENNING SM: Lymphopoiesis, in *The Molecular Basis of Blood Diseases*, 2d ed, G Stamatoyannopoulos et al (eds). Philadelphia, Saunders, 1993

—— et al: Intrathymic T cell maturation. Semin Immunol 2:67, 1990

HERMAN A et al: Superantigens: Mechanism of T-cell stimulation and the role in immune responses. Annu Rev Immunol 9:745, 1991

KELLEY WN et al (eds): *Textbook of Rheumatology*, 4th ed. Philadelphia, Saunders, 1993, chaps. 6, 7, 10, 13, 15, 16

PAUL WE (ed): *Fundamental Immunology*, 2d ed. New York, Raven, 1989

RETH M et al: The B-cell antigen receptor complex. Immunol Today 12:196, 1991

SPRINGER TA: Adhesion receptors of the immune system. Nature 346:425, 1990

278 PRIMARY IMMUNE DEFICIENCY DISEASES

MAX D. COOPER / ALEXANDER R. LAWTON III

Immunologic functions are mediated by two developmentally independent, but functionally interacting, families of lymphocytes. The activities of B and T lymphocytes and their products in host defense are closely integrated with the functions of other cells of the reticuloendothelial system. Macrophages, dendritic cells, and the Langerhans' cells in the skin play an important role in the trapping and presentation of antigens to T and B cells to initiate the immune response. Macrophages also become effector cells, especially when activated by cytokine products of lymphocytes. The scavenger activity of polymorphonuclear leukocytes is directed and made specific by antibodies in concert with cytokines and the complement system. Natural killer (NK) cells, a population of granular lymphocytes, may spontaneously kill tumor and virus-infected cells, activities that are enhanced by the cytokine products of immune and inflammatory cells. Killing by NK cells also can be targeted by IgG antibodies for which NK cells have cell-surface receptors. The interaction of basophils and tissue mast cells with IgE antibodies in causation of immediate-type hypersensitivity is discussed in Chap. 282. Consideration of these interrelationships is an important part of the analysis of patients with suspected immune deficiency.

CLINICAL DISEASE FEATURES COMMON TO IMMUNE DEFICIENCY Immunodeficiency syndromes, whether congenital, spontaneously acquired, or iatrogenic, are characterized by unusual susceptibility to infection and not infrequently to autoimmune disease and lymphoreticular malignancies. The types of infection often provide the first clue to the nature of the immunologic defect.

Patients with *defects in humoral immunity* have recurrent or chronic sinopulmonary infection, meningitis, and bacteremia, most commonly caused by pyogenic bacteria such as *Haemophilus influenzae, Streptococcus pneumoniae*, and staphylococci. These and other pyogenic organisms also cause frequent infections in individuals who have either neutropenia or a deficiency of the pivotal third component of complement (C3). The tripartite collaboration of antibody, complement, and phagocytes in host defense against pyogenic organisms makes it important to assess all three systems in individuals with unusual susceptibility to bacterial infections.

Antibody-deficient patients in whom cell-mediated immunity is intact have an interesting response to viral infections. The clinical course of primary infection with viruses such as varicella-zoster or rubeola, unless complicated by bacterial infection, does not differ significantly from that of the normal host. However, long-lasting immunity may not develop, and as a result, multiple bouts of chickenpox and measles may occur. Such observations suggest that intact T cells may be sufficient for control of established viral infections, while antibodies play an important role in limiting the initial dissemination of virus and in providing long-lasting protection. Exceptions to this generalization are becoming more widely recognized. Agammaglobulinemic patients fail to clear hepatitis B virus from their circulation and have a progressive, and often fatal, course. Poliomyelitis has occurred following live-virus vaccination in some patients. Chronic encephalitis, which may progress over a period of months to years, is a particular threat in congenitally agammaglobulinemic boys. Echoviruses and adenoviruses have been isolated from brain, spinal fluid, or other sites in such patients; in others no agent has been detected.

The occurrence of an unusually serious infection, for example, *H. influenzae* meningitis in an older child or adult, warrants consideration of humoral immune deficiency. Bacterial infections in certain sites also may suggest this possibility. Chronic otitis media occurs frequently in patients with hypogammaglobulinemia and is significant because of its relative rarity in normal adults. Pansinusitis, although almost invariably present in immunoglobulin deficiency, is a less helpful finding because it is not rare in apparently normal people. Bacterial infections of the skin or urinary tract are less frequent problems in hypogammaglobulinemic patients.

Infestation with the intestinal parasite *Giardia lamblia* is a frequent enough cause of diarrhea in antibody-deficient patients to warrant diagnostic duodenal aspiration and intestinal biopsy when the organism cannot be demonstrated in the stool.

Abnormalities of cell-mediated immunity predispose to disseminated virus infections, particularly with latent viruses such as herpes simplex (see Chap. 143), varicella zoster (see Chap. 144), and cytomegalovirus (see Chap. 146). In addition, patients so affected

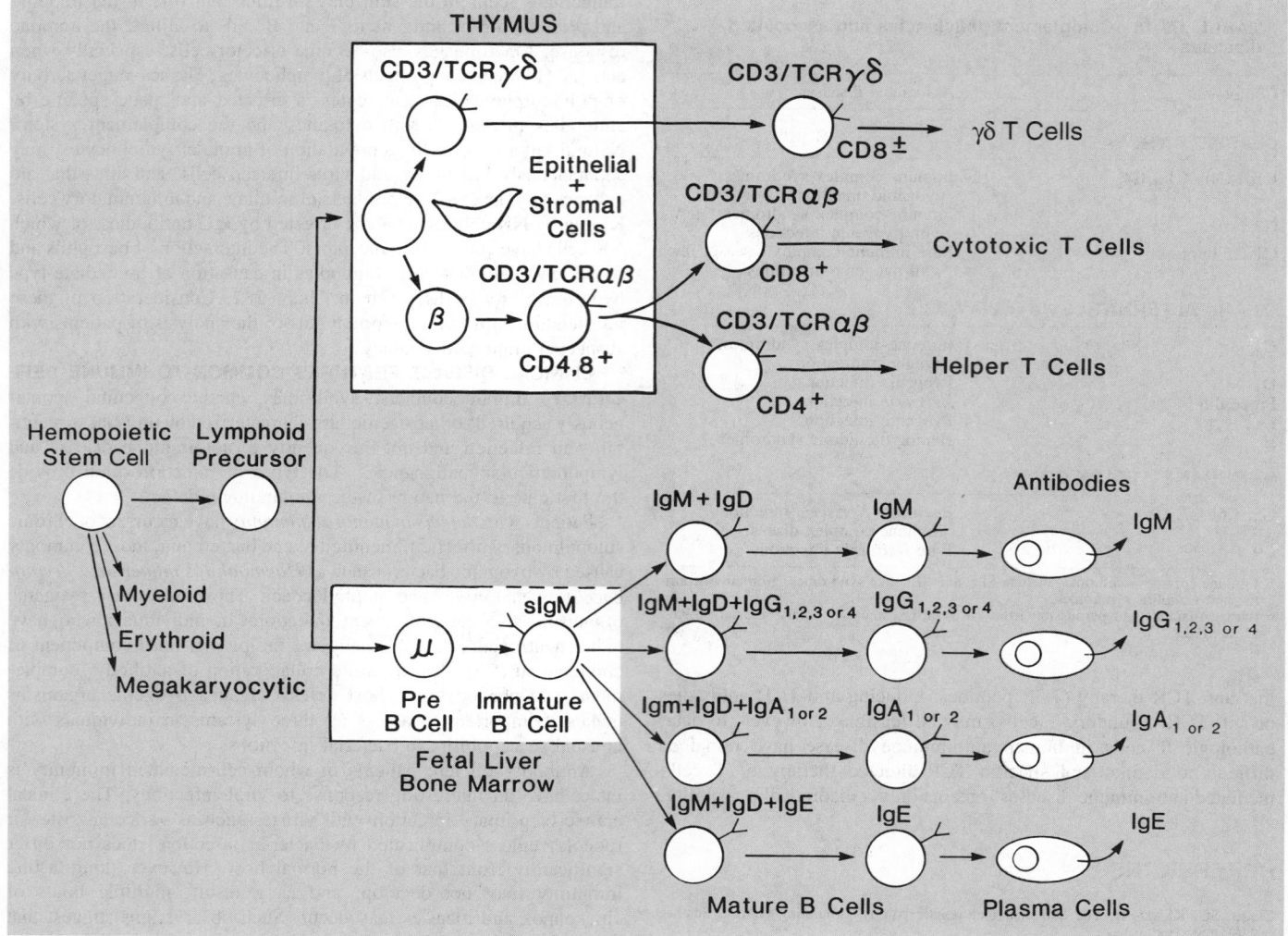

FIGURE 278-1 Hypothetical model outlining the differentiation of hemopoietic stem cells along T and B cell lineages. Failure to develop T and B cells may result from defective stem cells or from inborn metabolic errors affecting both cell types. Rarely, other hematopoietic cell lines are also absent. Absence of either T or B cells suggests malfunction of central lymphoid tissues, including the thymus and the fetal liver–bone marrow complex. B cell deficiency may result from failure to generate pre-B cells from their stem cell precursors or from failure of pre-B cells to give rise to their B lymphocyte progeny. Similarly, differentiation may be arrested at several levels within the T cell lineage; arrests at the thymocyte level and failure to develop the helper subset have been observed in immunodeficient patients. Agammaglobulinemia and deficiencies of some T cell functions may occur despite the presence of normal numbers of B or T cells in the circulation. Failure of B lymphocytes to differentiate to plasma cells can be due to intrinsic cellular abnormalities or to faulty T cell regulation.

almost invariably develop mucocutaneous candidiasis and frequently acquire systemic fungal infections. Pneumonia caused by *Pneumocystis carinii* is also common (see Chap. 178).

T cell deficiency is always accompanied by some abnormality of antibody responses (see Fig. 278-1), although this may not be reflected by hypogammaglobulinemia. This explains in part why patients with primary T cell defects are also subject to overwhelming bacterial infection.

The most severe form of immune deficiency occurs in individuals, often infants, who lack both cell-mediated and humoral immune functions. Individuals with severe combined immunodeficiency are susceptible to the whole range of infectious agents including organisms not ordinarily considered pathogenic. Multiple infections with viruses, bacteria, and fungi occur, often simultaneously. Because donor lymphocytes cannot be rejected by these recipients, blood transfusions can produce fatal graft-versus-host disease.

DIFFERENTIATION OF T AND B CELLS The functional deficits which occur in both congenital and acquired immunodeficiencies are usefully viewed as being caused by defects at various points along the differentiation pathways of immunocompetent cells. For this reason, certain features of the development and differentiation of T and B cells that are especially relevant to the analysis of immunodeficiency are briefly presented here; Chap. 277 provides a general account of their roles in cellular and humoral immunity.

A subpopulation of hematopoietic stem cells may become restricted to lymphoid differentiation prior to migration to the thymus, where T cells are generated, or to the fetal liver and adult bone marrow, where B cell development begins (see Fig. 278-1). A major function of these central lymphoid tissues is to generate the clonal diversity characteristic of the immune system. Each T or B lymphocyte is induced to express surface receptor molecules of a unique specificity for antigen. The receptors of B lymphocytes are immunoglobulin molecules which are formed by paired heavy and light chains of either κ or λ type. The heavy chain gene loci are on the long arm of chromosome 14; the 5'-3' order of these is V_H (variable), D (diversity), and J_H (joining) minigene families followed by the C_H (constant region) genes, C_μ, C_δ, $C_{\gamma3}$, $C_{\gamma1}$, $C_{\alpha1}$, $C_{\gamma2}$, $C_{\gamma4}$, C_ϵ, and $C_{\alpha2}$. The κ gene family, consisting of V_κ, J_κ, and C_κ genes, is located on chromosome 2 and the homologous λ gene loci on chromosome 22.

The T cell receptors are related cell surface molecules with antigen-binding specificity. The receptor on most T cells is composed of two polypeptide chains, called α and β. The β-chain family is located on chromosome 7 and consists of V_β, D_β, J_β, and C_β minigene loci. The α-chain family on chromosome 14 similarly consists of a series of V_α, D_α, J_α, and C_α genes. A smaller subpopulation of T cells express a T cell receptor composed of γ and δ polypeptide chains. The γ-chain gene family is located on chromosome 7, and the δ-chain family is located in the midst of the α gene locus on chromosome 14.

The genetic strategy for creating functional gene complexes encoding antigen receptors is similar for T and B cells. For example, a functional V region gene of the immunoglobulin heavy chain is formed by productive rearrangement of one each of the V_H, D, and J_H genes and deletion of the intervening DNA to generate a contiguous coding structure which is then transcribed together with the nearest C_H gene. Functional light chain genes are formed by a V-J rearrangement in either the κ or λ gene loci. The V_β gene is similarly composed of a rearranged set of V_β, D_β, and J_β genes forming a contiguous coding structure, which the T cell then transcribes along with the nearest C_β gene. Because there are many different V, D, and J genes, they can be put together in various combinations to encode a large number of receptor molecules having different antigen-binding specificities.

Generation of clonal diversity requires cellular proliferation, such that each of the different receptor specificities encoded in the genome comes to be uniquely expressed by individual cells. A clone consists of all cells that express the identical antigen-binding receptors. Estimates for the total number of B cell clones usually vary between 10 and 100 million. T cell clonal diversity may be equally extensive. The initial step in clonal development is independent of antigen and reflects a genetically programmed sequence of differentiation analogous to that of primary erythropoiesis or myelopoiesis. This phase, termed *primary differentiation*, begins early in human fetal development and may continue into adult life.

The most primitive morphologically identifiable cell in the B lineage is called a *pro-B cell*. These cells are marked by the cell surface CD19 antigen and the nuclear expression of terminal deoxynucleotidyl transferase (Tdt). Pro-B cells undergo productive $V_H DJ_H$ rearrangement to express cytoplasmic μ chains (the heavy chain of IgM) and become pre-B cells. Since light chain gene rearrangement usually occurs later, pre-B cells lack the characteristic membrane-bound immunoglobulin receptors which characterize B lymphocytes but may express μ-chain/surrogate light chain receptors encoded by the nonrearranged V pre-B and 14.1 genes in the λ light chain gene locus. Pre-B cells are generated in the fetal liver and in bone marrow throughout life, dividing in response to growth factors made by neighboring stromal cells. After undergoing a productive rearrangement of light chain VJ genes, pre-B cells become immature B lymphocytes that express surface IgM receptors. These B lymphocytes differ from their more mature counterparts in an important physiologic characteristic; they are highly susceptible to inactivation when their receptors bind antigen. Consequently, immature B cells encountering self-antigens may be eliminated or rendered anergic. The antigen receptors on B cells are multichain units. In order for membrane-bound immunoglobulins to reach the B cell surface, they require association with Ig-α and Ig-β chains, which serve as signal transduction elements for the antigen receptor complex.

The developmental sequence for expression of diverse immunoglobulin classes by human B lymphocytes begins with expression of IgM. The expression of IgD- on IgM-bearing cells occurs later. Lymphocytes committed to synthesis of IgG, IgA, and IgE are derived from IgM-bearing precursors through a genetic switch mechanism. Each of the heavy chain constant region genes except C_δ is preceded by a switch region composed of repetitive nucleotide sequences. The heavy chain class switch is initiated by splicing of the switch region of μ with the switch region in front of the downstream heavy chain gene to be expressed next and is completed by the terminal differentiation of plasma cells producing the new heavy chain class. Completion of the switch process thus involves antigenic stimulation

and the help of T cells which produce soluble switch factors, such as interleukin 4 and tumor growth factor β for IgA responses.

T lineage cells also undergo sequential rearrangements of the minigene families encoding their antigen receptors. On entering the epithelial thymus, lymphoid precursor cells may follow one of two T cell pathways. The first involves rearrangement of V_γ and J_γ genes to express γ chains and rearrangement of V_δ, D_δ, and J_δ genes to express δ chains. These associate with the CD3 proteins to form the CD3/γδ T cell receptor (TCR) complex of γδ T cells. Pre-T cells beginning development along the second differentiation pathway in the thymus rearrange one each of the V_β, D_β, and J_β genes prior to the expression of a complete β chain. At a later differentiation stage, similar rearrangements of V_α and J_α genes occur in the α-chain family, and then the completed antigen receptor molecule of one α chain and one β chain is expressed together with the CD3 protein complex on the cell surface of an immature αβ T cell. Initially, the αβ T cells express both the CD4 and CD8 accessory molecules on their surface. As these cells mature under the influence of a self-antigen selection process, they either down-regulate the CD8 molecule to become CD4 + T cells with helper cell potential or they cease to express the CD4 molecule to become CD8 + T cells with cytotoxic potential. The CD4 + αβ T cells leaving the thymus have been selected to recognize peptide fragments presented in the groove of class II major histocompatibility (MHC) molecules of antigen-presenting cells. The CD8 + αβ T cells migrating from the thymus have been selected to recognize peptide fragments in the cleft of class I MHC molecules expressed by virtually all types of nucleated cells. The CD4 and CD8 molecules are called *accessory receptors* because they have binding affinity for class II or class I MHC molecules, respectively, and are coupled to tyrosine kinase molecules that are active in signal transduction. While the γδ T cells express neither CD4 nor CD8 molecules during their intrathymic development, they may express CD8 molecules as mature T cells in the periphery. Expression of these and other cell surface molecules can be defined by specific monoclonal antibodies, thus providing a powerful tool for elucidating the developmental status of both T and B lymphocytes (see Fig. 278-1).

The αβ T cells bearing the CD4 markers constitute approximately 70 percent of circulating T cells and function as helper-inducer cells, necessary for expression of effector functions of both T and B cells. The αβ T cells expressing CD8 molecules constitute 20 to 30 percent of circulating T cells, mediate cytotoxic reactions, and may be responsible for suppression of immune responses. The γδ T cells constitute a minor population of T cells. While their function is still unclear, they may serve a protective role along epithelial surfaces and to eliminate damaged cells. Developmental arrests or failure of function of one or more of these T cell subsets may be responsible for immunodeficiency or autoimmune diseases.

The events designated *secondary differentiation* follow stimulation of specific clones of lymphocytes by antigen. These processes are synonymous with the immune response (see Chap. 277). Particularly important in consideration of immunodeficiencies are the collaborative interactions among macrophages, T cells, and B cells. While B lymphocytes may differentiate to IgM-secreting plasma cells when stimulated by thymus-independent antigens, such as lipopolysaccharides, most antibody responses, particularly those of the IgA and IgG classes, require intimate collaboration between T and B cells. Antigens bound to the antibody receptors on B cells are internalized, partially digested, and recycled to the cell surface, where they are presented on class II molecules to the T cell. The activated T cell in turn produces soluble factors that promote growth and differentiation of the B cell or inflammatory responses. These factors, which include interleukins IL-2, IL-4, IL-5, IL-6, and IL-10 and interferon-γ, may be differentially produced by individual T cells depending on their prior mode of activation.

Differentiation of T or B cells may be arrested at either the primary or secondary stages. Reflecting the complex cellular interactions involved in immune responses and the pivotal role played by T lymphocytes, immune deficiencies primarily involving T cells are usually also associated with abnormal B cell function. Conversely, immunodeficiencies manifested primarily by inability to produce antibodies may be caused by T cell defects not associated with abnormal cell-mediated immunity.

EVALUATION OF IMMUNODEFICIENT PATIENTS   A careful history and physical examination will usually indicate whether the major problem involves the antibody-complement-phagocyte system or cell-mediated immunity. A history of a normal response to smallpox vaccination or of contact dermatitis due to poison ivy suggests intact cellular immunity. Persistent mucocutaneous candidiasis suggests deficient cell-mediated immunity. Lymphopenia and the absence of palpable lymph nodes may be important findings. However, patients with profound immunodeficiency may have diffuse lymphoid hyperplasia. Most immunodeficiencies may be diagnosed by thoughtful use of tests available in local or regional clinical laboratories. More precise evaluation of immunologic functions and treatment may require referral to specialized centers. Table 278-1 presents a résumé of widely available laboratory investigations.

Humoral immunity   With rare exceptions, deficiency of humoral immunity is accompanied by diminished serum concentration of one or more classes of immunoglobulin. Normal values vary with age, and adult concentrations of IgM (1.0 g/L) are reached at about 1 year, of IgG (8.0 g/L) at 5 to 6 years, and of IgA (2.0 g/L) at puberty (see Chap. 277). Also, the wide range of values among normal adults creates difficulty in defining the lower limits of normal. Reasonable estimates for low normal values are 0.4 g/L for IgM, 5 g/L for IgG, and 0.5 g/L for IgA. In the presence of borderline hypogammaglobulinemia, assessing the patient's capacity to produce specific antibodies becomes particularly important. Isohemagglutinins, anti-streptolysin O, and "febrile agglutinins" are valuable standard assays, and measurements of pre- and postimmunization titers to tetanus toxoid, diphtheria toxoid, *H. influenzae* capsular polysaccharide, and *S.*

pneumoniae serotypes provide a comprehensive assessment of humoral responsiveness.

Estimation of numbers of circulating B lymphocytes is of value in determining the pathogenesis of certain types of immune deficiency. B lymphocytes are identified by the presence of membrane-bound immunoglobulins, their associated α- and β-chain units, and other lineage-specific molecules on the B cell surface (Table 278-1), which can be identified and enumerated by specific monoclonal antibodies.

Since antibody deficiency may be mimicked clinically by deficiency of complement components, measurement of total hemolytic complement (CH_{50}) should be a part of the evaluation of host defense. Measurement of C3 alone is inadequate for screening, since deficiencies of both early and late complement components may predispose to bacterial infection (see Chap. 277).

Cellular immunity   Human T lymphocytes may be enumerated by their expression of the TCR/CD3 complex of surface molecules. The CD2 antigenic molecule is also expressed by almost all the T cells and a few non-T lineage lymphocytes. The CD4 molecule serves as a marker for helper T cells, but macrophages also express this molecule in relatively low levels. Conversely, the CD8 molecule is expressed by cytotoxic T cells. This cell surface molecule also may be expressed by γδ T cells and by natural killer cells.

Normal levels of serum immunoglobulins and antibody responsiveness are reliable indices of intact helper T cell function. T lymphocyte function can be measured directly by delayed hypersensitivity skin testing using a variety of antigens to which the majority of older children and adults have been sensitized. The most generally useful skin test antigen is a 1:5 dilution of tetanus toxoid injected intradermally, since almost all individuals will have been sensitized. Purified protein derivative (PPD), histoplasmin, mumps antigen, and extracts of *Candida* or *Trichophyton* also may be used.

T lymphocyte function may be estimated in vitro by the capacity of cells to proliferate in response to antigens to which the patient has been sensitized, to lymphocytes from an unrelated donor, to antibodies that cross-link the CD3/TCR complex, or to the T cell mitogens, which include phytohemagglutinin, concanavalin A, and pokeweed mitogen. The response is usually quantified by measurement of incorporation of radioactive thymidine into newly synthesized DNA. It is also possible to measure the production of cytokines (or interleukins) by activated T cells. Finally, the ability of T cells activated in mixed lymphocyte culture to lyse target cells can be measured.

CLASSIFICATION   Primary immunodeficiencies may be either congenital or acquired and are currently classified according to mode of inheritance and whether the defect involves T cells, B cells, or both (Table 278-2). The following discussion emphasizes three related concepts: (1) that immunodeficiencies are most logically viewed as defects of cellular differentiation, (2) that these defects may involve either primary development of T or B cells or the antigen-dependent phase of their differentiation, and (3) that defects of secondary B cell differentiation may in some instances reflect faulty T-B collaboration.

Secondary immunodeficiencies are those not caused by intrinsic abnormalities in development or function of T and B cells. The best known of these is AIDS, which may follow infection with the human immunodeficiency virus (see Chap. 279). Other examples are immune deficiency associated with malnutrition, protein-losing enteropathy, and intestinal lymphangiectasia. Also considered secondary are immunodeficiencies resulting from hypercatabolic states such as occur in myotonic dystrophy, immunodeficiency associated with lymphoreticular malignancy, and immunodeficiency resulting from treatment with x-rays, antilymphocyte serum, or cytotoxic drugs.

Incidence   As a group, the primary immunodeficiencies are relatively common. The most frequent, isolated IgA deficiency, occurs in approximately 1 in 600 individuals in North America.

The more severe forms of primary immunodeficiency have their onset early in life and all too frequently result in death during childhood. Immunodeficiencies may become apparent at any age, however, and patients with congenital hypogammaglobulinemia may

---

TABLE 278-1   Laboratory evaluation of host defense status

INITIAL SCREENING ASSAYS*

Complete blood count with differential smear
Serum immunoglobulin levels: IgM, IgG, IgA, IgD, IgE

OTHER READILY AVAILABLE ASSAYS

Quantification of blood mononuclear cell populations by immunofluorescence assays employing monoclonal antibody markers[†]
 T cells: CD3, CD4, CD8, TCRαβ, TCRγδ
 B cells: CD19, CD20, CD21, Ig(μ, δ, γ, α, κ, λ), Ig-associated molecules
   (α, β)
 NK cells: CD16
 Monocytes: CD15
 Activation markers: HLA-DR, CD25, B7/BB1 antigen (B cells)
T cell functional evaluation
 1 Delayed hypersensitivity skin tests (PPD, *Candida* histoplasmin, tetanus toxoid)
 2 Proliferative response to mitogens (anti-CD3 antibody, phytohemagglutinin, concanavalin A) and allogeneic cells (mixed lymphocyte response)
 3 Cytokine production
B cell functional evaluation
 1 Natural or commonly acquired antibodies: isohemagglutinins; antibodies to common viruses (influenza, rubella, rubeola) and bacterial toxins (diphtheria, tetanus)
 2 Response to immunization with protein (tetanus toxoid) and carbohydrate (pneumococcal vaccine, *H. influenza B* vaccine) antigens
 3 Quantitative IgG subclass determinations
Complement
 1 CH_{50}
 2 C3, C4
Phagocyte function
 1 Reduction of nitroblue tetrazolium
 2 Chemotaxis assays
 3 Bactericidal activity

* Together with a history and physical examination, these tests will identify more than 95 percent of patients with primary immunodeficiencies.
† The menu of monoclonal antibody markers may be expanded or contracted to focus on particular clinical questions.

TABLE 278-2 WHO classification of primary immunodeficiencies

COMBINED IMMUNODEFICIENCIES

Severe combined immunodeficiency (SCID):
1 X-linked
2 Autosomal recessive ("Swiss-type agammaglobulinemia")
Adenosine deaminase (ADA) deficiency
Purine nucleoside phosphorylase (PNP) deficiency
MHC class II deficiency
Reticular dysgenesis

PREDOMINANTLY ANTIBODY DEFICIENCIES

X-linked agammaglobulinemia
X-linked hypogammaglobulinemia with growth hormone deficiency
Ig deficiency with increased IgM ("hyper-IgM syndrome")
Ig heavy chain–gene deletions
κ-Chain deficiency
IgA deficiency
Selective deficiency of IgG subclasses (with or without IgA deficiency)
Common variable immunodeficiency (CVID)
Transient hypogammaglobulinemia of infancy

OTHER WELL-DEFINED IMMUNODEFICIENCY SYNDROMES

Wiskott-Aldrich syndrome
Ataxia telangiectasia
3d and 4th pouch/arch syndrome (DiGeorge)

SYNDROMES ASSOCIATED WITH IMMUNODEFICIENCY

Chromosome abnormalities:
1 Bloom syndrome
2 Fanconi anemia
3 Down syndrome
Multiple organ system abnormalities:
1 Partial albinism
2 Short-limbed dwarfism
3 Cartilage hair hypoplasia
4 Agenesis of the corpus callosum
Hereditary metabolic defects:
1 Transcobalamin II deficiency
2 Acrodermatitis enteropathica (zinc deficiency)
3 Type I orotic aciduria
4 Biotin-dependent carboxylase deficiency
Hypercatabolism of Ig:
1 Familial hypercatabolism of Ig
2 Myotonic dystrophy
3 Intestinal lymphagiectasia
Other:
1 Hyper-IgE syndrome
2 Chronic mucocutaneous candidiasis
3 Thymoma
4 Immunodeficiency following hereditarily determined susceptibility to Epstein-Barr virus

---

survive to middle age or beyond. In a referral center for patients with immunodeficiency diseases, approximately two-thirds of the immunodeficient patients will be adults. Improved methods of diagnosis and treatment may increase this ratio in the future.

Severe combined immunodeficiency (SCID) This syndrome is characterized by gross functional impairment of both humoral and cell-mediated immunity and by susceptibility to devastating fungal, bacterial, and viral infections. It is usually congenital, may be inherited either as an X-linked or autosomal recessive defect, or may occur sporadically. Affected infants rarely survive beyond 1 year without treatment. This syndrome has been associated with a diversity of defects in development of immunocompetent cells, some of which may be related to specific enzymatic abnormalities.

The classic example of SCID, *Swiss-type agammaglobulinemia*, is characterized by severe lymphopenia and is inherited with an autosomal recessive pattern. A genetic defect in the Ig and TCR recombination mechanism may underlie this failure in both T and B cell development. Rarely, other hematopoietic cell lines fail to develop in a variant form of SCID called *reticular dysgenesia*. About half of patients with autosomal recessive SCID are deficient in an enzyme involved in purine metabolism, adenosine deaminase (ADA), due to

deletions or point mutations in the ADA gene. Studies of the pathophysiologic relationship of ADA deficiency to abortive lymphoid differentiation suggest that intracellular accumulation of adenosine and deoxyadenosine nucleotides interferes with critical metabolic functions, including DNA synthesis. Improvement of both clinical status and immunologic function occurs in some patients treated with exogenous ADA conjugated to polyethylene glycol to prolong its half-life. The cellular defect in the lymphopenic forms of SCID logically rests with the precursor cells for both T and B lineages. The immunologic defects in all these types of SCID patients have been repaired following transplantation of bone marrow or fetal liver as a source of stem cells, confirming the hypothesis that the stromal microenvironments of the thymus and bone marrow of these patients are capable of supporting T and B cell differentiation of normal stem cells.

SCID also may occur with an X-linked inheritance pattern. Affected boys have normal numbers of B lymphocytes with few or no circulating T lymphocytes. This developmental disorder also can be repaired by transplantation of bone marrow stem cells from a histocompatible sibling. Transplants of haploidentical bone marrow, depleted of donor T cells to prevent graft-versus-host disease, also may correct the T cell deficit, but antibody deficiency requiring immunoglobulin therapy may persist for years in this instance.

Treatment of SCID patients should be performed in centers with a strong research interest in this problem. It is crucial that these patients be recognized early and not be given live viral vaccines or blood transfusions, which may cause fatal graft-versus-host disease.

T cell immunodeficiency Reflecting the diversity of T cell functions, abnormalities of T cell development may be responsible for a wide spectrum of immune deficiencies, including severe combined immunodeficiency, selective defects in cell-mediated immunity, and syndromes presenting as antibody deficiency with apparently normal cell-mediated immunity. These defects may be acquired (see Chap. 279) as well as congenital. Until recently, laboratory assays of T lymphocyte function were limited to correlates of cell-mediated immunity; no means were available for studying T cell regulatory functions. Improved assays of T cell subsets and their functional integrity are expanding the spectrum of immunodeficiencies primarily related to T cell abnormalities.

DI GEORGE'S SYNDROME This is the classic example of isolated T cell deficiency which results from maldevelopment of thymic epithelial elements derived from the third and fourth pharyngeal pouches. Defective development of organs dependent on cells of embryonic neural crest origin includes congenital cardiac defects, particularly those involving the great vessels; hypocalcemic tetany, due to failure of parathyroid development; and absence of a normal thymus. Associated abnormalities may include abnormal ears, shortened philtrum, micrognathia, and hypertelorism. Serum immunoglobulin concentrations are frequently normal, but antibody responses, particularly of IgG and IgA isotypes, are usually impaired. Lymphocyte levels are reduced, and most of the circulating lymphocytes are B cells. Affected individuals usually have a tiny, histologically normal thymus located near the base of the tongue or in the neck. With time, most patients develop functional T cells.

Children lacking the congenital anomalies associated with Di George's syndrome may present with severe impairment of cell-mediated immunity. Some patients have normal or even increased immunoglobulin levels, while others have selective deficiencies of one or more immunoglobulin classes. Specific antibody responses are usually impaired even in patients with normal concentrations of immunoglobulins. This ill-defined entity has been called the *Nezelof's syndrome*.

Inherited deficiency of the enzyme purine nucleoside phosphorylase (PNP) is associated with an often severe and selective deficiency of T lymphocyte function. This enzyme functions in the same purine salvage pathway as ADA; toxic effects of the *PNP deficiency* may be related to intracellular accumulation of deoxyguanosine triphosphate (GTP).

ATAXIA-TELANGIECTASIA   This is an autosomal recessive genetic disorder characterized by cerebellar ataxia, oculocutaneous telangiectasia, and immunodeficiency. The responsible gene has been mapped to the q22–23 region on chromosome 11. Onset of truncal ataxia usually occurs in infancy and is progressive. Immunodeficiency may be clinically manifest by recurrent and chronic sinopulmonary infection leading to bronchiectasis. However, not all patients have immunodeficiency. The two most frequent causes of death are chronic pulmonary disease and malignancy. Lymphomas are most common, although carcinomas also have occurred.

The immunologic abnormalities seem to be related to maldevelopment of the thymus. The thymus is markedly hypoplastic and similar in appearance to an embryonic thymus. The peripheral T cell pool is frequently reduced in size, especially in lymphoid tissue compartments. Cutaneous anergy and delayed rejection of skin grafts are common. Although the number and class distribution of B lymphocytes are usually normal, most patients are deficient in serum IgE and IgA, and a smaller number have reduced serum levels of IgG, particularly of the IgG2, IgG4 subclasses. IgM and IgD are usually normal.

There is circumstantial evidence that ataxia-telangiectasia may involve a generalized defect in cellular differentiation related to the defects in DNA repair mechanisms which have been identified in these patients. Cultured cells from these patients are highly susceptible to radiation-induced chromosomal damage. Defective DNA repair mechanisms may account for the high incidence of malignancies in these patients. Ovarian agenesis also occurs frequently. Persistence of very high serum levels of oncofetal proteins, including alpha fetoprotein and carcinoembryonic antigen, may be of diagnostic value.

Only symptomatic treatment is available. Unless a severe IgG deficiency is present, therapy with immunoglobulin is not indicated. Unusual sensitivity to x-irradiation should be kept in mind in planning therapy for patients who develop cancer.

Immunoglobulin deficiency syndromes X-LINKED AGAMMAGLOBULINEMIA   Males with this syndrome often begin to have recurrent bacterial infections late in the first year of life, when maternally derived immunoglobulins have disappeared. Affected individuals have very few immunoglobulin-bearing B lymphocytes in their circulation and lack primary and secondary lymphoid follicles. However, B cell precursors are found in normal frequency in the bone marrow. This developmental block at the pre-B cell level contrasts with earlier and later arrests in B cell differentiation characterizing other immunodeficiencies (see below and Fig. 278-1). The defective kinase gene is located in the Xq 22 region. B cells from obligate carriers utilize the normal X chromosome exclusively, while T cells and myeloid cells express either X chromosome. *X-linked agammaglobulinemia with growth hormone deficiency* is a rare variant disorder that maps to the same region of the X chromosome.

Agammaglobulinemia is a misnomer, since most patients with this and other forms of severe panhypogammaglobulinemia synthesize some immunoglobulins. Within the same family, some affected males have had substantial levels of IgM, IgG, and IgA, while others have been nearly agammaglobulinemic. All these patients were markedly deficient in circulating B lymphocytes. This observation indicates that the few B lymphocytes that escape the block in differentiation are capable of plasma cell maturation and immunoglobulin synthesis. However, antibody replacement therapy is needed in all these patients because of the limited number of B cell clones that are generated.

Sinopulmonary infections constitute the most frequent clinical problem. A form of arthritis with some of the features of rheumatoid disease occurs in some of these patients. *Mycoplasma* organisms are sometimes the cause of the arthritis. Chronic encephalitis of viral etiology can be a fatal complication. Some of these patients have an associated dermatomyositis. The frequency with which these complications occur is reduced by adequate treatment with intravenous immunoglobulin.

TRANSIENT HYPOGAMMAGLOBULINEMIA OF INFANCY   This is a reversible syndrome in which normal physiologic hypogammaglobulinemia of infancy is unusually prolonged and severe. IgG levels normally drop to 3.0 to 4.0 g/L between 3 and 6 months of age as maternally derived IgG is catabolized. The IgG levels subsequently rise, reflecting the infants' increased synthetic capacity. Periodic immunologic assessment is needed to differentiate transient hypogammaglobulinemia from other forms of antibody deficiency. Antibody replacement therapy is recommended only in rare instances of severe or recurrent infections.

ISOLATED DEFICIENCY OF IGA   This immunodeficiency occurs with a frequency of approximately 1 in 600 individuals of European origin. IgA deficiency is much less common in people of Asian and African origin. In Japan, for example, the incidence is approximately 1 in 18,500. While the precise genetic basis for this difference in incidence is unknown, IgA deficiency is frequently associated with certain MHC haplotypes in Caucasians.

With rare exceptions, IgA1 and IgA2 subclasses are both deficient in serum and in mucous secretions. While most individuals with isolated IgA deficiency appear healthy, others have an increased number of respiratory infections of varying severity, and a few have severe pulmonary disease such as bronchiectasis. Chronic diarrheal disease also occurs. The incidence of asthma and other atopic diseases among IgA-deficient patients is high, and conversely, the incidence of IgA deficiency among atopic children has been found to be 20 to 40 times that in the normal population. IgA deficiency is also significantly associated with autoimmune diseases such as rheumatoid arthritis and systemic lupus erythematosus. Selective reductions in the IgG2 and IgG4 subclasses have been associated with the increased infections seen in some IgA-deficient individuals. Finally, IgA-deficient patients may develop significant levels of antibodies to IgA. These patients may have severe anaphylactic reactions when transfused with normal blood or blood products.

IgA deficiency is often familial. It also can occur in association with congenital intrauterine infections, such as toxoplasmosis, rubella, and cytomegalovirus infection, or following treatment with phenytoin, penicillamine, or other medications in genetically susceptible individuals.

The pathogenesis of IgA deficiency, whether genetic or induced by environmental insult, involves a block in terminal differentiation of B lymphocytes. The IgA-bearing lymphocytes in these patients also bear surface IgM. This immature phenotype, also prevalent in normal neonates, may reflect a primary defect in essential regulatory interactions between T and B cells.

Treatment of IgA deficiency is essentially symptomatic. IgA cannot be effectively replaced by exogenous immunoglobulin or plasma, and use of either can increase the risk of development of antibodies to IgA. IgA-deficient patients in need of transfusion should be screened for the presence of antibodies to IgA and ideally should be given blood only from IgA-deficient donors. Treatment with immunoglobulin may benefit the exceptional IgA-deficient person in whom IgG2 and IgG4 subclass deficiencies are associated with severe infections. The risk of anaphylactic reactions to contaminating IgA must always be considered in treating IgA-deficient patients.

IGG SUBCLASS DEFICIENCIES   Selective deficiencies in one or more of the four IgG subclasses are seen in some patients with repeated infections. The IgG subclass deficiency may easily go undetected when the total serum IgG level is measured, because IgG2, IgG3, and IgG4 together account for only 30 to 40 percent of the IgG antibodies. Even a deficiency in IgG1 may be masked by increases in the remaining IgG isotypes. However, the availability of subclass-specific monoclonal antibodies allows precise measurement of IgG subclass levels.

Homozygous deletions of genes encoding the constant region of the different γ chains is the basis for the IgG subclass deficiency in some individuals. For example, deletion of the $C_{\alpha 1}$, $C_{\gamma 2}$, $C_{\gamma 4}$, and C_{ϵ} genes on both chromosomes 14 was responsible for one individual's inability to make IgA1, IgG2, IgG4, and IgE. Interestingly, individuals with this and other patterns of C_H-gene deletions may not have unusual infections.

Most of the IgG subclass–deficient individuals with repeated infections appear to have regulatory defects which prevent normal B cell differentiation. The defect may extend to other isotypes. IgA deficiency may accompany IgG2 and IgG4 subclass deficiencies (see "Isolated Deficiency of IgA," above), and an inability to produce IgM antibodies to polysaccharide antigens often reflects a broader defect in antibody responsiveness. While patients with IgG subclass deficiency may benefit from administration of immunoglobulin, a thorough immunologic assessment is needed to identify the relatively few who need this therapy.

COMMON VARIABLE IMMUNODEFICIENCY This diagnostic category includes a heterogeneous group of males and females, mostly adults, who have in common the clinical manifestations of deficient production of all major immunoglobulin classes. The majority of these panhypogammaglobulinemic patients have normal numbers of B lymphocytes which are clonally diverse but phenotypically immature. B lymphocytes in these patients are able to recognize antigens and can proliferate in response but fail to differentiate to become plasma cells. This abortive differentiation pattern leads to the frequent occurrence of nodular lymphoid hyperplasia, including splenomegaly and intestinal lymphoid hyperplasia. Three types of defects in B lymphocyte differentiation have been tentatively identified. First, an intrinsic abnormality of B lymphocytes may prevent their differentiation into immunoglobulin-secreting plasma cells even when provided with differentiation factors from normal T cells. Second, in some patients the T cells, or their products, may actively suppress the terminal differentiation of normal B lymphocytes. Third, the defective B cell response may reflect a deficiency of helper T cell function which may be associated with reduced numbers of CD+ T cells.

Common variable immunodeficiency and IgA deficiency may represent polar ends of a clinical spectrum due to the same underlying gene defect in a large subset of these patients. The two disorders feature similar B cell differentiation arrests, differing only in the numbers of immune globulin classes involved. Both disorders occur frequently within the same family, and the same MHC haplotypes are associated with both immunodeficiency patterns. The data suggest an underlying susceptibility gene in both disorders.

It is important to consider the diagnosis of common variable immunodeficiency in adults with chronic pulmonary infections, some of whom will present with unexplained bronchiectasis. Intestinal diseases, including chronic giardiasis, intestinal malabsorption, and atrophic gastritis with pernicious anemia, are common in this group of patients. Patients with common variable immunodeficiency also may present with signs and symptoms highly suggestive of lymphoid malignancy, including fever, weight loss, splenomegaly, generalized lymphadenopathy, and lymphocytosis. Routine histologic examination of lymphoid tissues usually reveals germinal center hyperplasia which may be difficult to distinguish from nodular lymphoma (see Chap. 311). Demonstration of a normal distribution of immunoglobulin isotypes and light chain classes on circulating and tissue B lymphocytes can serve to distinguish these patients from those having a monoclonal B cell malignancy with secondary hypogammaglobulinemia. The monthly administration of intravenous immunoglobulin in adequate doses (see below) is an essential part of the prevention and treatment of all these complications.

X-LINKED IMMUNODEFICIENCY WITH INCREASED LEVELS OF IGM In this syndrome, IgG and IgA levels are very low or undetectable, while IgD levels may be high. The normal development of B lymphocytes bearing IgM and IgD and the absence of IgG and IgA B lymphocytes indicate a defect in isotype switching. The defective gene in these patients may encode a transmembrane molecule on T cells that is the ligand for the CD40 molecule on B cells. The failure to express this CD40 ligand prevents normal T and B cell cooperation and isotype switching. The clinical patterns of infection are similar to those occurring with other hypogammaglobulinemic states. Lymphoid hyperplasia may be severe. Neutropenia often occurs in affected males and can increase their vulnerability to infections. Adequate antibody replacement by immunoglobulin administration may reverse the neutropenia and reduce the frequency of infections requiring antibiotic therapy.

ISOLATED DEFICIENCY OF IGM This syndrome has been reported rarely in the United States but was detected frequently in a British population. Approximately 60 percent of these patients had severe recurrent infections, often with bacteremia. Pneumococcal pneumonia and meningococcal meningitis have been noted in IgM-deficient patients. Other associated conditions included gastrointestinal disease, atopy, splenomegaly, and development of malignancy. The condition was frequently familial and was four times more common in males than in females. The number of circulating B lymphocytes has varied from very low to normal.

Miscellaneous immunodeficiency syndromes Infection with *Candida albicans* is the almost universal accompaniment of severe deficiencies in cell-mediated immunity. The syndrome of *chronic mucocutaneous candidiasis* is different because superficial candidiasis is usually the only major manifestation of immunodeficiency. These patients rarely develop systemic infection with *Candida* or other fungal agents and are not unusually susceptible to virus or bacterial disease. The syndrome is often congenital and may be associated with single or multiple endocrinopathies as well as iron deficiency. Treatment of associated conditions may lead to improvement or even cure of *Candida* infection.

No uniformity of immunologic defects has been identified in these patients, although defects of antibody formation have been detected occasionally. Humoral immunity, including ability to make specific anti-*Candida* antibodies, is usually normal. Many patients are anergic, some to a variety of antigens and some only to *Candida;* anergy in some patients has been related to inability of their lymphocytes to produce the cytokine called *migration inhibition factor.*

Results of treatment with antifungal agents, such as amphotericin B, have been variable. In some patients, intensive treatment with amphotericin B coupled with surgical removal of infected nails has led to sustained improvement. Ketoconazole, an oral antifungal agent, also may be effective, but long-term remissions are rarely achieved with therapeutic means that are presently available.

IMMUNODEFICIENCY WITH THYMOMA The association of hypogammaglobulinemia with spindle cell thymoma usually occurs relatively late in adult life. Bacterial infections and severe diarrhea often reflect the antibody deficiency, whereas fungal and viral infections are infrequent complications. T cell numbers and cell-mediated immunity are usually intact, but these patients are very deficient in circulating B lymphocytes and pre-B cells in the bone marrow. They also frequently have eosinopenia and may develop erythroid aplasia. Complete bone marrow failure has occurred in a few immunodeficient patients with thymoma. The relationship between the thymoma and apparent abnormalities of hematopoietic stem cells remains conjectural.

WISKOTT-ALDRICH SYNDROME This is an X-linked genetic disease characterized by eczema, thrombocytopenia, and repeated infections. The platelets are small and have a shortened half-life. Affected male infants often present with bleeding, and most do not survive childhood, dying of complications of bleeding, infection, or lymphoreticular malignancy. The immunologic defects are well characterized phenotypically but are poorly understood. Serum concentrations of IgM are usually decreased, while IgA and IgG are normal and IgE is frequently increased. Synthetic rates for all three classes may be elevated, indicating a significant element of hypercatabolism. The number and class distribution of B lymphocytes are usually normal. Functionally, these boys are consistently unable to make antibodies to polysaccharide antigens normally; responses to protein antigens are often impaired late in the course of the disease. While most patients acquire T cell deficiencies, serial appraisal suggests that the T cell defects are secondary. Affected boys frequently become anergic, and their T cells do not respond normally to challenge with ubiquitous antigens. The nature of the primary defect is still unknown.

Transplantation of histocompatible bone marrow from a sibling donor has corrected both hematologic and immunologic abnormalities in several patients. In patients lacking a suitable donor, splenectomy may improve platelet counts and reduce the risk of serious hemorrhage. Because of the increased risk of pneumococcal bacteremia, splenectomized patients should probably receive prophylactic penicillin.

X-LINKED LYMPHOPROLIFERATIVE SYNDROME   This is an X-linked recessive disease in which there appears to be a selective impairment in immune elimination of Epstein-Barr virus (EBV). Infectious mononucleosis in affected males may have a fulminant and fatal outcome, may be associated with development of B cell malignancies, or may result in acquired hypogammaglobulinemia, aplastic anemia, or agranulocytosis. Antibodies to EBV have been detected in some patients but are often absent in the face of infection. Generation of cytotoxic T cells appears to be the primary mechanism of control of EBV infection in normal persons, and natural killer cells also may play a role in eliminating EBV-infected B cells. While the gene defect has been mapped to the Xq 24–27 region, the nature of the cellular defect which prevents a normal response to EBV in patients with the X-linked lymphoproliferative syndrome has not been defined.

HYPER-IGE SYNDROME   The *hyper IgE syndrome* (see Chap. 54) is characterized by recurrent abscesses involving skin, lungs, and other organs and very high IgE levels. Staphylococcal infection is common to all patients, but most have infections with other pyogenic organisms as well. Males and females of all races are affected in an inheritance pattern suggesting an autosomal dominant defect with variable penetrance. A specific immunologic defect has not been identified. Abnormal neutrophil chemotaxis is an inconsistent finding, and diminished antibody responses to secondary immunization have been noted in some patients. Prophylaxis with penicillinase-resistant penicillins or cephalosporins is highly recommended to prevent staphylococcal infections. Pneumatocoeles, a frequent complication of penumonias, may require surgical excision.

Metabolic abnormalities associated with immunodeficiency The relation of deficiencies of the purine salvage enzymes adenosine deaminase and purine nucleoside phosphorylase to immunodeficiency was discussed earlier. The syndrome of *acrodermatitis enteropathica* includes severe desquamating skin lesions, intractable diarrhea, bizarre neurologic symptoms, variable combined immunodeficiency, and an often fatal outcome. This disease is apparently caused by an inborn error of metabolism resulting in malabsorption of dietary zinc and can be treated effectively by parenteral or large oral doses of zinc. Zinc deficiency might in part account for the immunodeficiency which accompanies severe malnutrition. Inherited *deficiency of transcobalamin II*, the serum carrier molecule responsible for transport of vitamin B_{12} to tissues, is associated with failure of immunoglobulin production as well as megaloblastic anemia, leukopenia, thrombocytopenia, and severe malabsorption. All abnormalities of this rare disorder are reversed by administration of vitamin B_{12}.

TREATMENT OF IMMUNODEFICIENCIES   Immunodeficiency diseases involving severe abnormalities of T cell function, with or without hypogammaglobulinemia, are often treatable with bone marrow transplants (see Fig. 278-1). Histocompatible marrow from a sibling donor is preferred, but haploidentical marrow may be used after removal of T cells. This therapy is complex and is best done by experienced research teams.

Replacement therapy with human immunoglobulin currently should be used in patients who have recurrent bacterial infections and are deficient in IgG. Maintenance of serum IgG levels above 5.0 g/L is sufficient to prevent most systemic infections and, together with antibiotic therapy, enhances reversal of chronic sinopulmonary infection. These serum levels usually can be achieved by intravenous administration of IgG, 400 mg/kg, at monthly intervals.

The advantage of intravenous immunoglobulin over intramuscular preparations is that higher amounts of antibodies can be given with less discomfort. Since higher levels of serum antibodies afford better protection from infections, intravenous antibody replacement is currently considered the treatment of choice for hypogammaglobulinemia. In patients with mild to moderate IgG deficiency (3.0 to 4.0

g/L), the decision to treat should be based on clinical symptoms and response to antigenic challenge.

Immunoglobulin treatment is of no value in patients with deficiencies of immunoglobulins other than IgG. This form of treatment is not benign. Some patients develop symptoms of diaphoresis, tachycardia, flank pain, and hypotension during or immediately following injections. This reaction may be mediated by aggregates of IgG or other biologically active substances, but it also may occur as a consequence of antibodies produced by the patient against donor immunoglobulins, particularly IgA (see Chap. 312).

Use of plasma or immunoglobulin selected on the basis of a high titer of antibodies to a particular agent may be indicated in certain situations. For example, antibodies to the causative virus may dramatically improve the chronic enteroviral encephalitis which occurs in some agammaglobulinemic patients.

Therapy with exogenous IgG may not suffice to eliminate the chronic sinopulmonary inflammation and its progression to pulmonary fibrosis and bronchiectasis. Therefore, maintenance of good pulmonary toilet with regular postural drainage can be an especially important part of patient management. The principles of antibiotic therapy are not different in these than in other patients, except that the index of suspicion of bacterial infection should remain very high.

The availability of purified interferon-γ and other biologically active cytokines promises to be important in the therapy of certain immunologic disorders. Gene therapy also holds great promise for therapy of defined genetic defects of the immune system.

REFERENCES

ARNAIR-VILLENA A et al: Human T cell activation deficiencies. Immunol Today 13:259, 1992

BLAESE RM, CULVER KW: Gene therapy for primary immunodeficiency disease. Immunodeficiency Rev 3:329, 1992

BUCKLEY RH, SHIFF RI: The use of intravenous immune globulin in immunodeficiency diseases. N Engl J Med 325:110, 1991

COOPER MD: B lymphocytes: Normal development and function. N Engl J Med 317:1452, 1987

FISCHER A: Severe combined immunodeficiencies. Immunodeficiency Rev 3:83, 1992

GOOD RA: Bone marrow transplantation for immunodeficiency diseases. Am J Med Sci 294:68, 1987

PAUL WE: *Fundamental Immunology*, 2d ed. New York, Raven, 1989

PREUD'HOMME JL, HANSON LA: IgG subclass deficiency. Immunodeficiency Rev 2:83, 1990

ROIFMAN CM, GELFAND EW: Replacement therapy with high dose intravenous gammaglobulin improves sinopulmonary disease in patients with hypogammaglobulinemia. Pediatr Infect Dis J 7:S92, 1988

ROSEN FS et al: Primary immunodeficiency diseases—Report of a WHO Scientific Group. Immunodeficiency Rev 3:195, 1992

ROYER HD, REINHERZ EL: T lymphocytes: Ontogeny, function, and relevance to clinical disorders. N Engl J Med 274:1171, 1987

SCHAFFER FM et al: IgA deficiency. Immunodeficiency Rev 3:15, 1991

279   HUMAN IMMUNODEFICIENCY VIRUS (HIV) DISEASE: AIDS AND RELATED DISORDERS

ANTHONY S. FAUCI / H. CLIFFORD LANE

The 1990s mark the second decade of the HIV/AIDS pandemic. The disease was first recognized in the United States in the summer of 1981 when the Centers for Disease Control (CDC) reported the unexplained occurrence of *Pneumocystis carinii* pneumonia in 5 previously healthy homosexual men in Los Angeles and Kaposi's sarcoma in 26 previously healthy homosexual men in New York and Los Angeles. Within months, the disease became recognized in male and female injection drug users (IDUs) and soon thereafter in recipients of blood transfusions and hemophiliacs who received plasma-derived coagulation factors. Early on in the epidemic, because of the disproportionate number of cases in Haitians, this group was incorrectly designated as a "risk" group. It soon because clear that the disease in Haitians was following a pattern of sexual transmission, both homosexual and heterosexual, the latter of which was virtually identical to the predominant mode of transmission in certain developing countries in Africa and elsewhere in the world (see below). As the epidemiologic pattern of the disease unfolded, it became clear that a microbe transmissible by sexual contact and blood or blood products was the most likely etiologic agent of the epidemic.

In 1983, HIV was isolated from a patient with lymphadenopathy and by 1984 it was clearly demonstrated to be the causative agent of AIDS. This retrovirus of the lentivirus family (see below) was formerly called *lymphadenopathy associated virus (LAV), human T lymphotropic virus III (HTLV-III)*, and *AIDS-associated retrovirus (ARV)*. In 1985, a sensitive enzyme-linked immunosorbent assay (ELISA) blood test was developed which has led to an appreciation of the scope of HIV infection among cohorts of individuals who admittedly practice high-risk behavior (see below) as well as among selected populations which have been screened such as blood donors, military recruits and active duty military personnel, Job Corps applicants, and patients in various sentinel hospitals (see below). This surveillance approach together with monitoring of levels of CD4+ T cell counts as a parameter of immunosuppression has led to the clear appreciation that there is a broad spectrum of HIV disease ranging from the asymptomatic infected individual up to advanced clinical disease which has been referred to as *AIDS*.

In the 1980s, the care of AIDS patients in the United States was with few exceptions confined to relatively restricted groups of physicians and hospitals, mostly in urban areas particularly on the northeastern and western seaboards. Toward the end of the 1980s and certainly in the 1990s it has become evident that virtually every practicing physician in the country will be required to have some degree of familiarity with the workup, diagnosis, and treatment of HIV-infected individuals. HIV-infected patients are now and in increasing numbers will be presenting to their family practice physicians, internists, obstetrician/gynecologists, pediatricians, and surgeons with clinical problems that may be directly or indirectly related, or totally unrelated, to their HIV infection.

Scientific advances are occurring at an extremely rapid pace in the areas of molecular virology of HIV, pathogenesis (both virologic and immunopathogenic) and treatment of HIV, as well as the opportunistic diseases associated with HIV infection, prophylaxis of opportunistic infections, and vaccine development. Despite such advances the HIV pandemic is growing in magnitude worldwide and the cost in human life and suffering is staggering. Physicians and other health care providers are in the unusual position of caring for HIV-infected individuals within the framework of a rapidly evolving scientific and clinical discipline. The purpose of this chapter is to present the most current information available on the scope of the epidemic, on its pathogenesis, treatment, and prevention, and on prospects for vaccine development. Above all the aim is to provide the reader with a solid scientific basis and practical guidelines for a state of the art approach to the HIV-infected patient.

DEFINITION AIDS was originally defined for surveillance purposes by the CDC prior to the identification of HIV as the etiologic agent as the presence of a reliably diagnosed "opportunistic" disease that is at least moderately indicative of an underlying defect in cell-mediated immunity in the absence of known causes of underlying immune defects such as iatrogenic immunosuppression or malignant neoplasms. Upon the availability of sensitive and specific diagnostic tests for HIV, the case definition of AIDS has undergone several revisions with regard to inclusion and exclusion criteria. The current

---

TABLE 279-1 CDC surveillance case definition for AIDS (1993)

A Indicator diseases diagnosed definitively in the absence of other causes of immunodeficiency and without laboratory evidence of HIV infection
  1 Candidiasis of the esophagus, trachea, bronchi, or lungs
  2 Cryptococcosis, extrapulmonary
  3 Cryptosporidiosis with diarrhea persisting >1 month
  4 Cytomegalovirus disease of any organ excluding liver, spleen, and lymph nodes in a patient >1 month of age
  5 Herpes simplex virus infection causing a mucocutaneous ulcer persisting >1 month; or bronchitis, pneumonia, or esophagitis in a patient >1 month of age
  6 Kaposi's sarcoma in a patient <60 years old
  7 Lymphoma of the brain (primary) in a patient <60 years of age
  8 Lymphoid interstitial pneumonia and/or pulmonary lymphoid hyperplasia in a child <13 years of age.
  9 *Mycobacterium avium* complex or *M. kansasii* disease (disseminated)
  10 *Pneumocystis carinii* pneumonia
  11 Toxoplasmosis of the brain in a patient >1 month of age
B Indicator diseases diagnosed definitively regardless of the presence of other causes of immunodeficiency and in the presence of laboratory evidence of HIV infection
  1 Any disease listed in section A
  2 Bacterial infections (multiple or recurrent) in children <13 years of age caused by *Haemophilus, Streptococcus*, or other pyogenic bacteria.
  3 Coccidioidomycosis, disseminated
  4 HIV encephalopathy
  5 Histoplasmosis, disseminated
  6 Isosporiasis with diarrhea persisting >1 month
  7 Kaposi's sarcoma at any age
  8 Non-Hodgkin's lymphoma of B cell or unknown phenotype and having the histologic type of small noncleaved lymphoma or immunoblastic sarcoma
  9 Any mycobacterial disease, disseminated, excluding *M. tuberculosis*
  10 *M. tuberculosis*, extrapulmonary
  11 *Salmonella* (nontyphoid) septicemia, recurrent
  12 HIV wasting syndrome
C Indicator diseases diagnosed presumptively in the presence of laboratory evidence of HIV infection
  1 Candidiasis of the esophagus
  2 Cytomegalovirus retinitis with loss of vision
  3 Kaposi's sarcoma
  4 Lymphoid interstitial pneumonia and/or pulmonary lymphoid hyperplasia in a child <13 years of age
  5 Mycobacterial disease, disseminated
  6 *Pneumocystis carinii* pneumonia
  7 Toxoplasmosis of the brain in a patient >1 month of age
D Indicator diseases diagnosed definitively in the absence of other causes of immunodeficiency and in the presence of negative results for HIV infection
  1 *Pneumocystis carinii* pneumonia
  2 Other indicator diseases listed in section A and CD4+ T lymphocyte count <400 per microliter
E The 1993 expanded definition includes:
  1 All HIV-infected persons who have <200 CD4+ T lymphocyte counts per microliter, or a CD4+ T lymphocyte percentage of total lymphocytes of <14.
  2 Pulmonary tuberculosis
  3 Recurrent pneumonia
  4 Invasive cervical cancer

From: Morb Mort Week Rep (Suppl 1):1, 1987; Morb Mort Week Rep 41, no. RR-17, 1993.

---

surveillance case definition is shown in Table 279-1. In 1993, the case definition was further expanded to include any HIV-infected individual with a CD4+ T cell count less than 200 per microliter, even without symptoms, as well as HIV-infected individuals with pulmonary tuberculosis (TB), recurrent episodes of pneumonia, or invasive cervical carcinoma. This definition is complex and comprehensive; however, the clinician should view HIV disease simply as a broad spectrum ranging from the primary infection, with or without the acute HIV syndrome, to the asymptomatic infected state to advanced disease (see below), rather than focusing on the presence or absence of AIDS, a strict definition that was established not for the practical care of patients but for surveillance.

TABLE 279-2 The human retroviruses

Virus	Culture characteristics	Diseases
HTLV-I	Transforming	Leukemias/lymphomas of CD4+ T lymphocytes; tropical spastic paraparesis (TSP); HTLV-1–associated myelopathy (HAM)
HTLV-II	Transforming	None recognized
HIV-1	Cytopathic	HIV disease/AIDS
HIV-2	Cytopathic	HIV disease/AIDS; may be less virulent than HIV-1

ETIOLOGY

The etiologic agent of AIDS is HIV, which belongs to the family of human retroviruses and the subfamily of lentiviruses. Nononcogenic lentiviruses cause disease in other animal species including sheep, horses, goats, cattle, cats, and monkeys. The four recognized human retroviruses belong to two distinct groups: the human T lymphotropic viruses, HTLV-I and II, and the human immunodeficiency viruses, HIV-1 and -2 (Table 279-2). The reader is referred to Chap. 151 for a detailed description of the biology of the human retroviruses. The most common cause of HIV disease throughout the world and certainly in the United States is HIV-1. HIV-2 was first identified in 1986 in West African patients and was originally confined to West Africa. However, a number of cases of HIV-2 have been reported in Europe, South America, Canada, and the United States. Although HIV-2 has approximately 40 percent nucleotide sequence homology with HIV-1 it is much more closely related phylogenetically to the simian immunodeficiency virus (SIV) found in sooty mangabees. HIV-1 is more closely related to an SIV isolated from chimpanzees in 1990. The taxonomic relationship among primate lentiviruses is shown in Fig. 279-1.

MORPHOLOGY Electron microscopy illustrates that the HIV-1 virion is an icosahedral structure (Fig. 279-2A) containing numerous external spikes formed by the two major viral envelope proteins, the external gp120 and the transmembrane gp41. The virion buds from the surface of the infected cell and incorporates a variety of host proteins including major histocompatibility complex (MHC) class I and II antigens (see Chap. 64) into its lipid bilayer. The structure of HIV-1 is schematically diagrammed in Fig. 279-2B (see also Chap. 151).

FIGURE 279-1 Taxonomy of primate lentiviruses. Figure illustrates the various percents of nucleotide sequence homologies among the different viruses. (*From RC Desrosiers, A finger on the missing link. Nature 345:288, 1990.*)

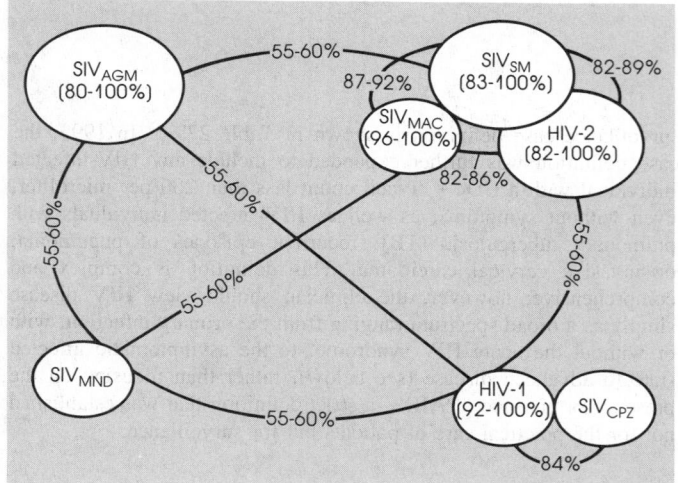

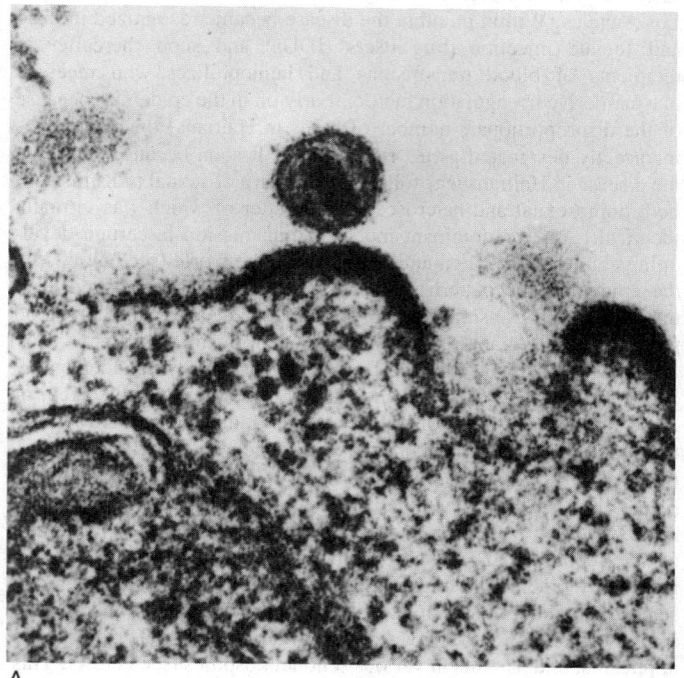

A

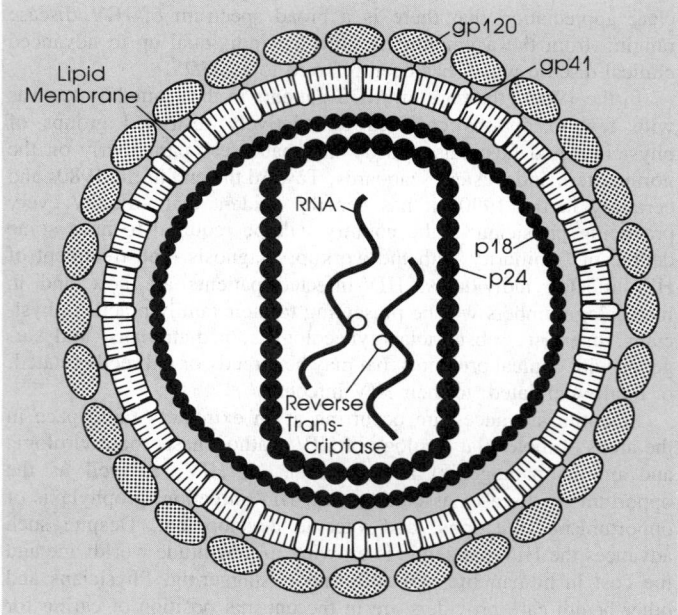

B

FIGURE 279-2 *A.* Electron micrograph of HIV. Figure illustrates a typical virion following budding from the surface of a CD4+ T lymphocyte together with two additional incomplete virions in the process of budding from the cell membrane. *B.* Structure of HIV-1, including the gp120 outer membrane, gp41 transmembrane components of the envelope, genomic RNA, enzyme reverse transcriptase, p18(17) inner membrane, and p24 core protein. (*Adapted from RC Gallo, The human immunodeficiency virus (HIV), Scientific American, January, 1987.*)

LIFE CYCLE The hallmark of the life cycle of HIV infection is the reverse transcription of genomic RNA to DNA by the enzyme called *reverse transcriptase*. The HIV life cycle begins with the high-affinity binding of the gp120 protein via a portion of its V1 region near the *N*-terminus to its receptor on the host cell surface, the CD4 molecule (Fig. 279-3). The CD4 molecule is a 55-kDa protein found

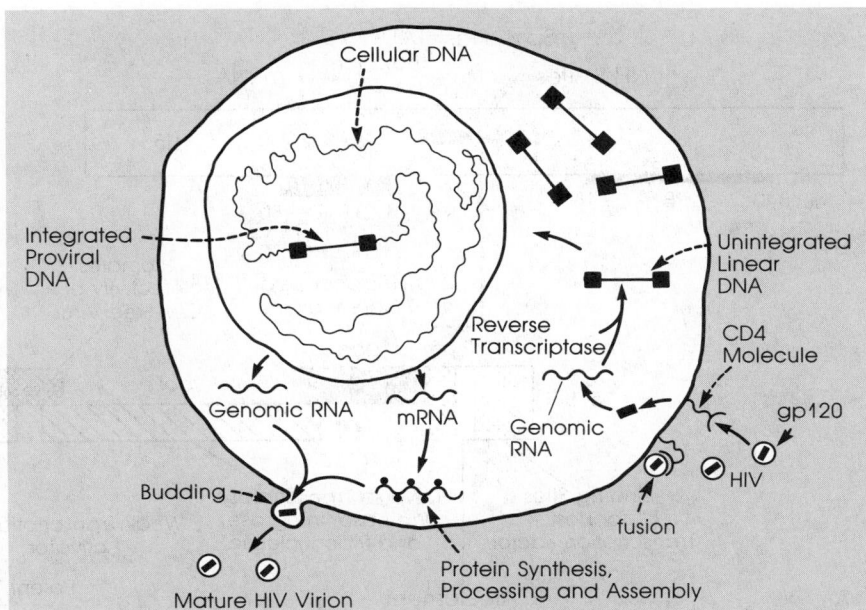

FIGURE 279-3 The life cycle of HIV. See text for description. *(From AS Fauci, The human immunodeficiency virus: Infectivity and mechanisms of pathogenesis. Science 239:617, 1988.)*

predominantly on a subset of T lymphocytes responsible for helper or inducer function in the immune response (see Chap. 277). It is also expressed on the surface of cells of the monocyte/macrophage lineage. Following binding, fusion with the host cell membrane occurs via the gp41 molecule, and the HIV genomic RNA is un-coated and internalized. The reverse transcriptase enzyme which was contained in the virion then catalyzes the reverse transcription of the genomic RNA into double-stranded DNA. The DNA migrates to the nucleus where it is integrated into the host cell chromosomes through the action of another virally encoded enzyme, *integrase*. The incorporation of this "provirus" into the cell genome is permanent. This provirus may remain transcriptionally inactive (latent) or manifest high levels of gene expression with active production of virus.

Cellular activation plays an important role in the life cycle of HIV. The activation of HIV expression from the latent state depends upon the interaction of a number of cellular and viral factors (see below). Incompletely reverse-transcribed DNA intermediates are labile in quiescent cells and will not be efficiently integrated into the host cell genome unless cellular activation occurs shortly after infection. Furthermore, activation of the host cell is required for the initiation of transcription of the integrated proviral DNA into either genomic or messenger RNA. Following transcription, HIV mRNA is translated into proteins which undergo modification through cleavage, glycosylation, myristilation, and phosphorylation. The viral core is formed by the assembly of HIV proteins, enzymes, and genomic RNA at the plamsa membrane of the cells. Budding of the progeny virion occurs through the host cell membrane, where the core acquires its external envelope.

HIV GENOME A schematic diagram of the HIV-1 genome is shown in Fig. 279-4. Similar to other retroviruses, HIV-1 comprises genes which encode the structural proteins of the virus: *gag* encodes the proteins that form the virion core (including p24 antigen); *pol* encodes the enzymes responsible for reverse transcription and integration; and *env* encodes the envelope glycoproteins. However, HIV-1 is more complex than other retroviruses in that it also contains at least six other genes (*tat, rev, nef, vif, vpr,* and *vpu*) that encode for proteins which are involved in the regulation of HIV expression (see Chap. 151). Flanking these genes are the long terminal repeats (LTRs) which contain regulatory elements involved in gene expression (see below), such as the polyadenylation signal sequence, the TATA promoter sequence, the NF-κB and SP1 enhancer binding sites, the transactivating response (TAR) sequences where the *tat* protein binds,

and the negative regulatory element (NRE) whose deletion increases the level of gene expression (Fig. 279-4). The major difference in the genomes of HIV-1 and HIV-2 is the fact that HIV-2 lacks the *vpu* gene and HIV-2 has a *vpx* gene not contained in HIV-1.

TRANSMISSION

HIV is transmitted by sexual contact, homosexual and heterosexual; by blood or blood products; and by infected mother to infant intrapartum, perinatally, or via breast milk. Well into the second decade of the epidemic, there is absolutely no evidence that HIV is transmitted by casual contact or that the virus can be spread by insects such as by a mosquito bite.

SEXUAL TRANSMISSION Sexual contact is the major mode of transmission worldwide. Although transmission through homosexual contact has been the most common form of sexual transmission in the United States (see below), heterosexual transmission is the most common modality of transmission worldwide, particularly in developing countries; in addition, it is being seen with increasing frequency in the United States. HIV virus has been demonstrated in the semen both within infected mononuclear cells and in the cell-free seminal fluid. The virus appears to concentrate in the seminal fluid particularly in situations in which there are increased numbers of lymphocytes in the fluid, as in genital inflammatory states such as urethritis and epididymitis, conditions closely associated with other sexually transmitted diseases. The virus has also been demonstrated in cervical smears and vaginal fluid. There is a strong association of transmission of HIV with receptive anal intercourse, likely due to the fact that there is only a thin and fragile rectal mucosal membrane separating the deposited semen from potentially susceptible cells within and beneath the mucosa as well as the fact that there may be trauma associated with anal intercourse. The trauma associated with anal douching and receptive insertion of a clenched fist into the rectum ("fisting") also increases the likelihood of infection during receptive anal intercourse. Although the vaginal mucosa is several layers thicker than the rectal mucosa and less likely to be traumatized during intercourse, it is clear that the virus can be transmitted to either partner through vaginal intercourse. There is approximately a twenty times greater chance of transmission of HIV from a man to a women than from a woman to a man through vaginal intercourse. This may be in part due to the prolonged exposure of the vaginal and cervical

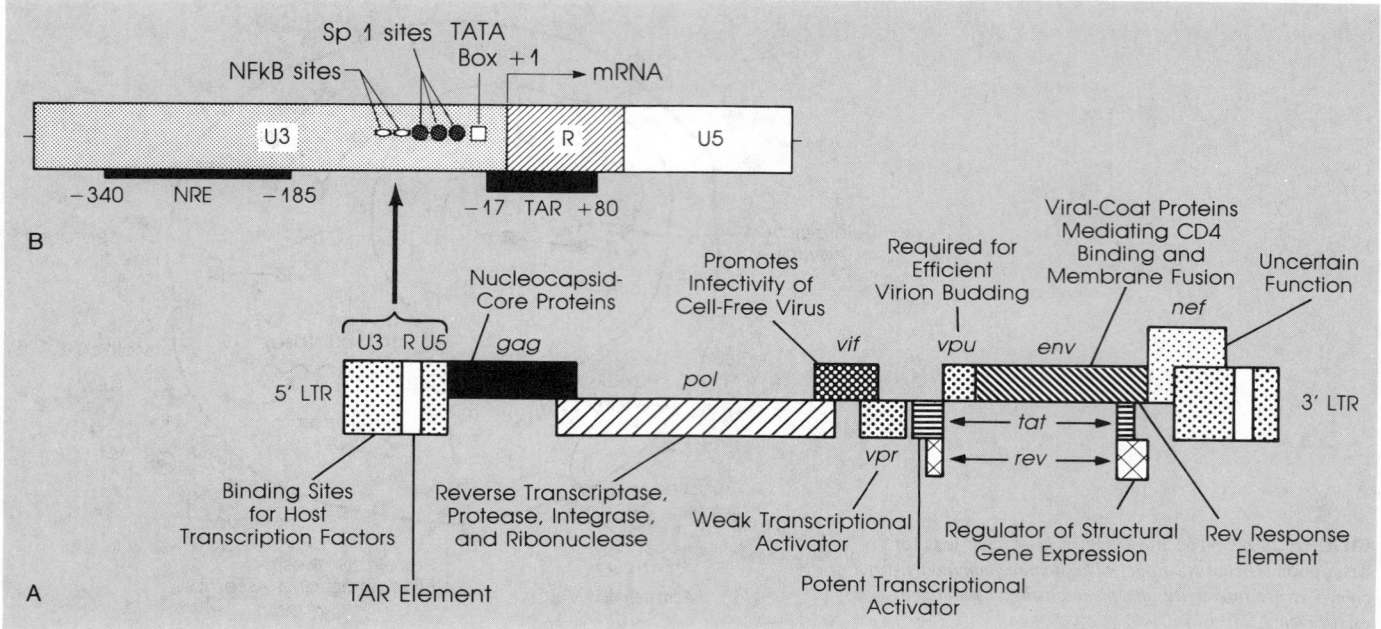

FIGURE 279-4 *A.* The genome of HIV. *(From WC Greene, N Engl J Med, 324:308, 1991.) B.* The long terminal repeat of HIV. *(From ZF Rosenberg and AS Fauci, Immunol Today 11:176, 1990.)*

mucosa as well as the endometrium (which semen enters through the cervical os) to the infected semen. This is in comparison to the relatively brief period that the penis and urethral orifice are exposed to infected vaginal fluid. There is a close association of genital ulcerations and transmission, both from the standpoint of susceptibility to infection and infectivity. Infections with microorganisms such as *Treponema pallidum* (see Chap. 133), *Haemophilus ducreyi* (see Chap. 112), and herpes simplex virus (see Chap. 143) are important causes of genital ulcerations linked to transmission of HIV. Further-more, there have been individual reports of associations of cervical ectopy as well as cervical erosions resulting from infection due to *Chlamydia trachomatis* (see Chap. 140) and *Neisseria gonorrhoeae* (see Chap. 110) with transmission of HIV infection. Thus, these phenomena in certain cases can be considered as *cofactors* for HIV transmission.

Oral sex appears to be a much less efficient mode of transmission of HIV; however, there have been rare individual reports of HIV transmission resulting from receptive fellatio and insertive cunni-lingus.

BLOOD AND BLOOD PRODUCTS   The virus can be transmitted by blood and blood products both in individuals who share contami-nated needles for intravenous drug use and in those who receive transfusions of blood or blood products. HIV infection and AIDS among IDUs continues to increase in the United States (see below). Infection occurs through the intravenous exposure to infected blood via contaminated needles and other drug paraphernalia. The risk of infection increases with the duration of injection drug use, the frequency of needle sharing, participation in the ''shooting gallery'' drug culture where several individuals share the same needle, and using injection drugs in a geographic area with a high prevalence of HIV infection such as in certain inner city areas particularly on the eastern seaboard.

From the late 1970s until the Spring of 1985 when mandatory testing of donated blood for HIV-1 was initiated, it has been estimated that over 10,000 individuals in the United States were infected through transfusions of blood or blood products (see Chap. 312). Approximately 5000 individuals who survived their primary illness for which the transfusion was administered have developed AIDS. It is estimated that 90 to 100 percent of those who were transfused with

HIV-infected blood became infected. Transfusion of whole blood, packed red blood cells, platelets, leukocytes, and plasma are all capable of transmitting HIV infection, while hyperimmune gamma-globulin, hepatitis B immune globulin, plasma-derived hepatitis B vaccine, and Rh_0 (O) immune globulin have not been associated with transmission of HIV infection. The procedures involved in processing these products either inactivate or remove the virus.

In addition to the above, several thousand hemophiliacs were infected with HIV by receipt of HIV-infected fresh frozen plasma or concentrates of clotting factors. Approximately 2000 have developed AIDS. Currently, in the United States and in most developed countries, the combination of screening all blood for HIV antibody by ELISA and confirmatory western blot where applicable; the self-deferral of donors on the basis of risk behavior; the screening out of HIV-negative individuals with positive surrogate laboratory parameters for HIV infection such as hepatitis B and C; and serologic test for syphilis has made the risk of transmission of HIV infection by transfused blood or blood products extremely small. One study estmated that the risk of HIV-1 infection via transfused blood from an HIV-infected, but seronegative, donor ranged from 1 in 40,000 to 1 in 250,000, while in another study the estimate was 1 in 61,000. There have been no reported cases of transmission of HIV-2 in the United States via donated blood, and currently donated blood is screened for both HIV-1 and HIV-2 antibodies. The chance of infection of a hemophiliac via clotting factor concentrates has essentially been eliminated because of the added layer of safety resulting form heat treatment of the concentrates.

A small number of cases of transmission of HIV via semen used in artificial insemination and tissues used in organ transplantation have been well documented. Therefore, donors of such tissues are now screened for HIV infection prior to transplantation.

OCCUPATIONAL TRANSMISSION OF HIV: HEALTH CARE AND LABORATORY WORKERS   There is a small but definite occupa-tional risk of HIV transmission among health care workers, laboratory personnel, and potentially others who work with HIV-infected speci-mens, particularly when sharp objects are involved. Large multi-institutional studies have indicated that the risk of HIV transmission following skin puncture from a needle or other sharp object that was contaminated with blood from a person with documented HIV infection is approximately 0.3 percent. The risk of a similar type of exposure to hepatitis B infection is 20 to 30 percent. There have been reports of health care workers who have become infected by exposure of mucous membranes or abraded skin to HIV-infected material.

However, the risk is much smaller than that for exposure via actual skin puncture with a contaminated object such as a needle (see "HIV and the Health Care Worker" below).

In 1990, the CDC reported that an HIV-infected dentist, by then deceased, had transmitted HIV infection to five of his patients on whom he had performed invasive dental procedures. Although the mechanisms of the transmission were never fully delineated, it was surmised that the infections occurred through instruments contaminated with HIV; the dentist supposedly used the same instruments on himself that he used in his practice and a breakdown in sterile procedures was suspected, but never proven. Subsequently, a number of epidemiologic studies were performed tracing the patients of several HIV-infected dentists, physicians, and surgeons and not a single case of HIV infection that could be linked to them was identified. Thus, the risk of transmission from an infected health care worker to his/ her patient is extremely low and at this point too low to be measured. The very occurrence of HIV transmission as well as hepatitis B and C to and from health care workers underscores the importance of the use of universal precautions when caring for all patients (see below and Chap. 98).

MATERNAL-FETAL/INFANT TRANSMISSION HIV can be transmitted from an infected mother to her fetus during pregnancy or to her infant during delivery. Virologic analysis of aborted fetuses indicate that the fetus can be infected during pregnancy, as early as the first and second trimester. However, it is felt that maternal transmissions to the fetus/infant occur most commonly in the perinatal period. This is based on the time frame of identification of infection by culture or polymerase chain reaction (PCR) techniques in the infant following delivery (negative at birth and positive several months later) as well as the demonstration that the first born twin of an infected mother is more commonly infected than is the second born twin.

The rate of transmission of HIV from mother to fetus/infant averages approximately 30 percent with a low of 12.9 percent in a European collaborative study and a high of 45 percent in Nairobi, Kenya. These differences may relate to adequacy of prenatal care of the mother as well as to the stage of disease in the mother during pregnancy. Higher rates of transmission have been associated with a symptomatic mother and low maternal CD4+ T cell counts. In addition, it has been speculated that if the mother gets infected during pregnancy there is a higher rate of transmission to the fetus due to the high levels of viremia following primary infection.

Postnatal mother-to-infant transmission of HIV has been clearly documented, strongly implicating colostrum and breast milk as the vehicles of infection. Virus can be isolated from both. In rare cases, mothers have been infected by transfusions following delivery and have transmitted the infection to their infants with the only risk factor being breast feeding. Where possible, breast feeding by an infected mother should be avoided; however, this becomes problematic in certain developing countries where the only consistent source of adequate nutrition as well as immunity against potentially serious infections for the infant is breast milk.

OTHER BODY FLUIDS There is no convincing evidence that saliva can transmit HIV infection either by kissing or by other exposures such as occupationally to health care workers. Although HIV has been isolated from saliva, this has been successful in only a small percentage of infected individuals. Furthermore, saliva has been demonstrated to contain inhibitory activity to HIV. However, a most unusual form of HIV transmission from infected children to mothers in the former Soviet Union has been identified. In those cases, the children (infected through transfusion) were said to have bleeding sores in the mouth and the mothers were said to have lacerations and abrasions on and around the nipples of the breast resulting from trauma from the children's teeth. Breast feeding had been continued until the children were older than is usual in the United States and other developed countries.

There have been conflicting reports of the isolation of HIV from other body fluids such as tears, sweat, and urine. However, there is no evidence that HIV transmission can occur as a result of exposure to these fluids. Nonetheless, bodily wastes of patients should be handled according to universal precautions (see below).

EPIDEMIOLOGY

AIDS IN THE UNITED STATES By June 1, 1993, there were 302,000 cumulative cases of AIDS reported in adults and adolescents in the United States (Table 279-3) and approximately 60 percent of these have died thus far. The majority of these cases are among men who have had sex with men (56 percent), and there will continue to be large numbers of new cases of AIDS within this group in the future. However, over the past few years, the numbers of newly reported cases of AIDS among IDUs has surpassed those of men who have had sex with men in certain cities with a high IV drug usage.

TABLE 279-3   AIDS cases in adults/adolescents in the United States as of June 1, 1993

Exposure category	White, not Hispanic No. (%)	Black, not Hispanic No. (%)	Hispanic No. (%)	Asian/ Pacific Islander No. (%)	American Indian/ Alaskan Native No. (%)	Total* No. (%)
Men who have sex with men	115,988 (74)	30,786 (33)	19,406 (39)	1,395 (71)	329 (54)	168,249 (56)
Injecting drug use (IDU) (female and heterosexual male)	15,031 (10)	36,007 (39)	19,665 (39)	96 (5)	104 (17)	71,053 (24)
Men who have sex with men and inject drugs	10,864 (7)	5,297 (6)	2,743 (6)	49 (2)	85 (14)	19,054 (6)
Hemophilia/ coagulation disorder	2,206 (1)	237 (0)	206 (0)	33 (2)	11 (2)	2,699 (1)
Heterosexual contact	4,472 (3)	12,201 (13)	4,068 (8)	105 (5)	32 (5)	20,909 (7)
Receipt of transfusion of blood, blood components, or tissue	3,743 (2)	1,056 (1)	681 (1)	122 (6)	11 (2)	5,621 (2)
Other/undetermined	4,880 (3)	6,320 (7)	3,095 (6)	171 (9)	32 (5)	14,580 (5)
Adult/adolescent subtotal	157,184	91,904	49,864	1,971	604	302,165
Percent of total adult/ adolescent AIDS cases	(52)	(30)	(17)	(<1)	(<1)	(100)

* Includes 638 persons of unknown race/ethnicity.
SOURCE: Centers for Disease Control and Prevention, USPHS.

TABLE 279-4   Pediatric (<13 years) AIDS cases in the United States as of June 1, 1993

Exposure category	White, not Hispanic No. (%)	Black, not Hispanic No. (%)	Hispanic No. (%)	Asian/ Pacific Islander No. (%)	American Indian/ Alaskan Native No. (%)	Total* No. (%)
Hemophilia/coagulation disorder	134 (14)	27 (1)	34 (3)	3 (14)	1 (7)	199 (4)
Mother with/at risk for AIDS/ HIV infection:	616 (66)	2,378 (95)	1,005 (89)	11 (52)	14 (93)	4,034 (87)
IV drug related	369	1,426	754	6	8	2,596
Sex with bisexual male	37	27	18	1	—	83
Sex with person with hemophilia	12	5	3	—	—	20
Receipt of blood transfusion, blood components, or tissue	28	40	25	—	—	93
Other	143	880	205	4	6	1,242
Receipt of transfusion of blood, blood components, or tissue	164 (18)	72 (3)	75 (7)	7 (33)	—	319 (7)
Undetermined	15 (2)	37 (1)	11 (1)	—	—	63 (1)
Pediatric subtotal	929	2,514	1,125	21	15	4,615
Percent of total pediatric AIDS cases	(20)	(54)	(24)	(<1)	(<1)	(100)

* Includes 11 children of unknown race/ethnicity.
SOURCE: Centers for Disease Control and Prevention, USPHS.

In addition, the relative number of cases among heterosexuals, women, and children have been increasing, reflecting directly and indirectly the increase in numbers of cases among IDUs (see below). By June 1, 1993, there were 4615 cumulative cases of AIDS among children less than 13 years of age and greater than 50 percent have died (Table 279-4). Greater than 80 percent of these were born to infected mothers and in approximately 70 percent of those cases the mother was either an IDU or the heterosexual partner of an IDU. The increasing prevalence of HIV infection and AIDS over the past decade among infants and children directly reflects the increase in prevalence of HIV infection among women who are IDUs or who have heterosexual partners who are IDUs. The majority of these cases are among minorities (African-Americans and Hispanics), especially those who live in inner cities in the Northeast and Southeast regions of the country. In this regard, HIV infection and AIDS has disproportionately affected minority populations in the United States. African-Americans and Hispanics comprise only 12 percent and 9 percent of the population, respectively, yet they account for 30 percent and 17 percent of adult/adolescent AIDS cases, respectively, and 54 percent and 24 percent of AIDS cases in children, respectively. The majority of IDUs in these inner cities are African-Americans and Hispanics and the above statistics reflect the high prevalence of HIV infection among IDUs in such areas. The relationship of geographic area of the country to the demography of HIV infection and AIDS, particularly the interconnection among geography, IDU, heterosexual transmission, and HIV infection in women and consequently in children is illustrated by the rate of reported cases of AIDS per 100,000 population by state comparing adolescent/adult men and adolescent/adult women (Fig. 279-5). The more diffuse distribution of cases among men throughout the various states reflects the wider distribution of cases representing men who have had sex with men. The concentrations on the East and West Coasts as well as in Texas and Nevada further reflect the higher densities of men who have had sex with men and to a lesser extent IDUs in those states. In contrast, the disproportionately high rate of AIDS cases among women in the Northeast and Florida, which have the highest rates of IV drug use and a relatively lower rate of AIDS, and in women on the West Coast and Texas compellingly link IDU to heterosexual transmission and infection in women in the United States at the present time. Forty-nine percent of women with AIDS have become infected through IDU compared to 20 percent of men with AIDS; 36 percent of women with AIDS have become infected by heterosexual contact compared to 3 percent of men with AIDS (Table 279-3). Only 1 percent of

AIDS cases are among hemophiliacs and 2 percent are among recipients of blood transfusions, blood products, or transplanted tissue. This relative percent will gradually decrease despite the fact that individuals previously infected through this mode of transmission

FIGURE 279-5   Rate of reported AIDS cases per 100,000 adolescents and adults, by sex and state of residence, in the United States in 1990. *[From Morb Mort Week Rep 40 (22) 1990.]*

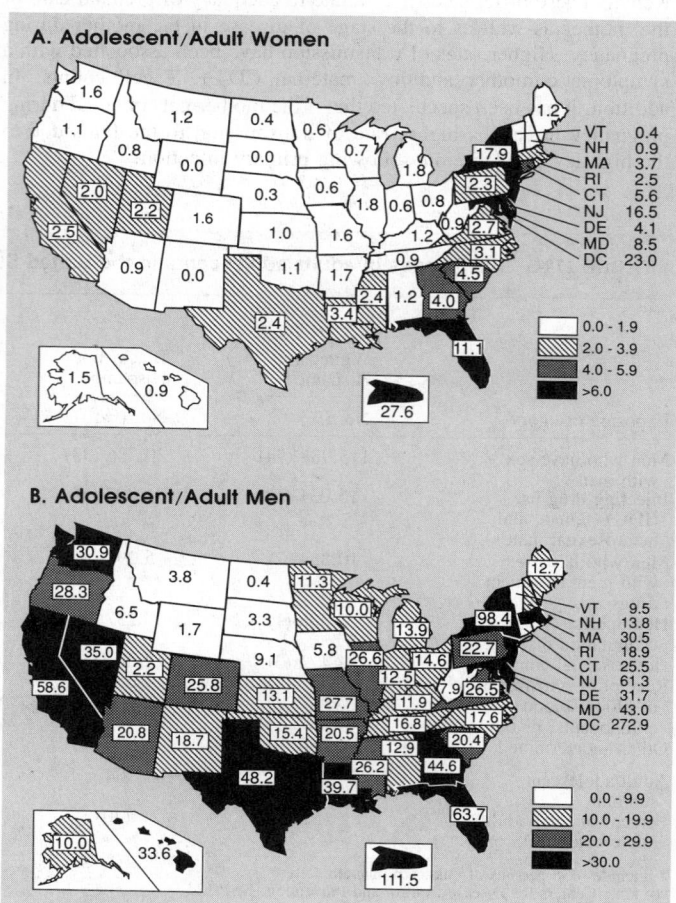

TABLE 279-5   Projected number of persons diagnosed with AIDS and projected number of deaths in the United States, 1989–1994

Year	Cases	Deaths
1989	48,000	32,000
1990	52,000	36,000
1991	58,000	44,000
1992	47,000–77,000	45,000–57,000
1993	47,000–85,000	46,000–67,000
1994	43,000–93,000	45,000–76,000
Total	415,000–535,000	320,000–385,000

SOURCE: Centers for Disease Control and Prevention, USPHS.

will continue to develop AIDS. The risk of additional infections via this mode of transmission in the United States is extremely small (see above).

The actual number of cases of AIDS and deaths due to AIDS in the United States per year from 1989 through 1991 and the projected range of cases from 1992 through 1994 are shown in Table 279-5. By 1994, there will have been a cumulative number of 415,000 to 535,000 cases with 320,000 to 385,000 deaths. The National Center for Health Statistics report of January, 1992, indicated that for 1989 (the latest analyzed data available) HIV infection was the third leading cause of death in the United States for all races aged 25 to 44 years and the sixth leading cause of death in African-American men of any age. In 1990, AIDS was the leading cause of death for men and women aged 25 to 44 in several cities in the United States (Fig. 279-6).

HIV PREVALENCE IN THE UNITED STATES   The U.S. Public Health Service estimates that there are approximately 1 million HIV-infected people in the United States. These estimates are made on the basis of a combination of HIV seroprevalence data, statistical modeling, and evolving information on the natural history of HIV infection. Short of universal testing, there are problems inherent in any attempt to estimate the true prevalence of HIV infection. Considerable data exist on the seroprevalence of HIV among groups practicing high-risk behavior such as men who have sex with men and who have attended sexually transmitted (STD) clinics; IDUs; and prostitutes. These studies obviously indicate an extremely high prevalence rate of HIV infection and do not reflect the true national prevalence. On the other hand, national surveillance data collected from first-time blood donors and military recruits reflect a falsely low prevalence rate because IDUs and men who have sex with men are discouraged from applying to the military and from donating blood. Other serosurveys have included Job Corps applicants and newborn infants. The aggregate results of these studies indicate that the prevalence of HIV infection nationwide is low (approximately 0.5 percent). However, there is a great deal of variability related to geography, race, economic status, age, sex, and, of course, behavior.

A series of unlinked serosurveys of HIV prevalence were conducted by the CDC in a variety of settings in a number of metropolitan areas throughout the country from 1988 through 1990. Men who have sex with men and who were attendees of over 100 STD clinics in 46 metropolitan areas showed high prevalence rates throughout the entire country. However, there was considerable variability, ranging from approximately 10 to over 60 percent; rates were somewhat higher in the eastern half of the country. Rates of new infection among this population have shown several trends over the past 10 years. The rate of new infection among homosexual men attending STD clinics in San Francisco in 1982 and 1983 was approximately 19 percent per year. By the mid and late 1980s, the rate had dropped to less than 1 percent per year, likely due to a combination of a saturational effect and significant behavioral modification. However, in the early 1990s, there has been a disturbing trend in the annual rate of new infection, up to 3 percent among young homosexual men who are "coming out"; they have not likely witnessed firsthand the devastation of the epidemic to the degree that their older counterparts have and apparently

are engaging in a greater degree of high-risk behavior. The range of HIV seroprevalence among IDUs in 61 treatment programs in 29 metropolitan areas was 0 percent to 49 percent. The rates varied considerably depending on the geographic location, with the highest rates observed on the eastern seaboard and much lower rates in the West and Southwest. In this regard, in other studies HIV prevalence rates among female prostitutes also varied greatly, from 0 to approximately 50 percent, with the rates directly reflecting the degree of IDU among the groups surveyed as well as the prevalence of HIV in the IDUs in that geographic location at the time of the survey. The seroprevalence rates among 35 tuberculosis clinics in 18 metropolitan areas ranged from 0 to 58 percent with the highest rates on the East Coast. The overall range of HIV seroprevalence by state in childbearing women was 0 to 0.66 percent. Much higher rates were found in women from large metropolitan areas, with states along the Atlantic coast manifesting higher rates than other regions of the country. The HIV national prevalence for childbearing women in 1990 was 0.15 percent or over 1 in every 700 mothers of newborns. This translates to approximately 6000 infected mothers giving birth in 1990, resulting in approximately 2000 infected newborns.

On the other end of the spectrum, screening of blood donors gives a different picture of national prevalence because of the confounding issue of self-deferral among individuals practicing high-risk behavior (see above). In 1985, 4 million blood donors were screened at 50 American Red Cross blood banks; the overall seroprevalence was 0.0245 percent with a prevalence of 0.0859 percent for first-time donors. A comparable survey was repeated in 1989; the overall seroprevalence was 0.0084 percent with a prevalence of 0.0415

FIGURE 279-6   AIDS as a leading cause of death for New York City men and women ages 20 to 39, 1983–1990. *(From New York State Department of Health—1991.)*

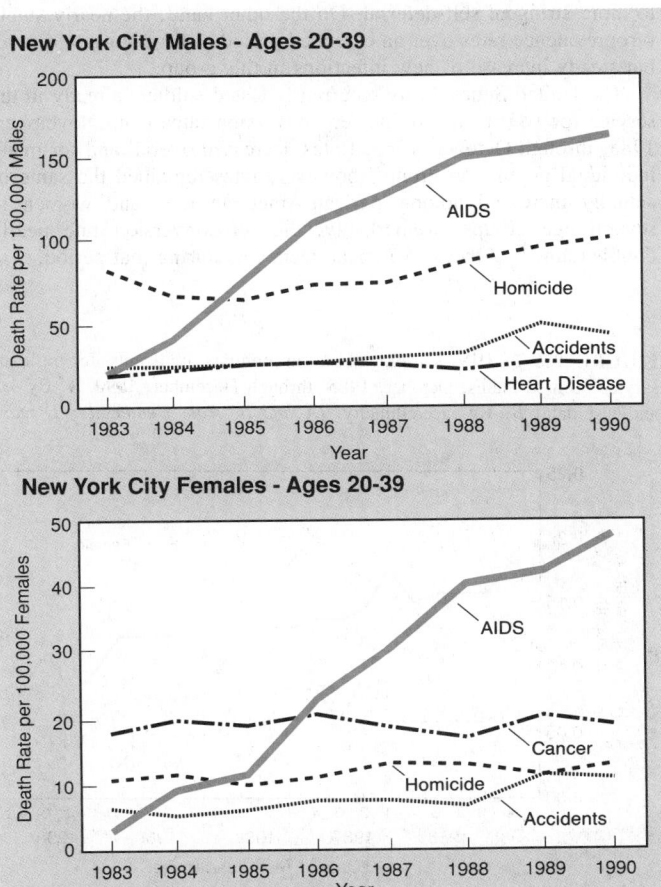

percent for first-time donors. It is likely that the decrease over the 4-year period reflects at least in part a greater adherence to self-deferral associated with a greater general awareness of what constitutes high-risk behavior.

Other national surveys directed towards the "general" population, but unavoidably encompassing a more restricted population, have also lent insight into the scope and trend of HIV infection, particularly among individuals who might not perceive that they are at risk and so may not self-defer. HIV seroprevalence studies of civilian applicants for military service conducted by the Department of Defense have provided extremely useful information regarding HIV prevalence in young sexually active persons in this country (Fig. 279-8A). Nearly 3 million applicants were screened from October, 1985, through December, 1990; the cumulative HIV seroprevalence was 0.12 percent with rates more than twice as high for males as for females and much higher for African-Americans and Hispanics than for other subgroups (Fig. 279-7B). The geographic distribution of HIV-positive male applicants paralleled the incidence of AIDS cases in males in those areas of the country; the highest rates were seen in the Middle Atlantic states and Puerto Rico, with the lowest rates seen in the central Midwest and Mountain states. The geographic distribution of HIV-positive female applicants indicated that the highest rates were in the northeast and southeast seaboard states, as well as Puerto Rico, reflecting a pattern similar to that for AIDS cases in women and children and for HIV prevalence in IDUs and in childbearing women in those areas. Additional important information was gathered by observing the seroprevalence of new applicants over the 50-month period covered by the survey (Fig. 279-7A). HIV seroprevalence decreased slightly in men and remained nearly stable in women, indicating that the incidence of new HIV infection apparently is not increasing in those groups of people that apply for military service. However, as mentioned above for blood donors over time, it is likely that the downward trend in males is due at least in part to an increased appreciation over time of what constitutes high-risk behavior, leading to more stringent self-deferral. On the other hand, the nearly stable seroprevalence rates over an extended period of time suggest a small but steady increase of new infections in this group.

The United States Army recurrently tested soldiers already in the service for HIV to determine seroconversion rates from November, 1985, through October, 1989. Rates decreased overall and for many individual population groups; however, rates remained the same or actually increased among African-American men and women in several age groups. Remarkably, the seroconversion rate nearly doubled among African-American teenagers during that period.

Another window into the HIV seroprevalence of a certain segment of sexually active young people in the United States comes from the serosurvey of Job Corps applicants. The Job Corps is a federal training program for socially and educationally disadvantaged young persons (16 to 21 years) in the United States. Data from 1988 through 1990 indicate a higher rate of seroprevalence (0.36 percent) than that of military recruits of the same age. Rates were especially high among African-Americans and Hispanics, and seroprevalence was similar in males and females. The study underscores the seriousness of the problem of HIV infection in disadvantaged adolescents, particularly young women and minorities.

Still another perspective of HIV seroprevalence among sexually active young people comes from a serosurvey conducted at 19 universities throughout the United States between April, 1988, and February, 1989, in which 30 of 16,863 specimens (0.2 percent) were positive for HIV antibodies. Positive specimens were found in 9 of the 19 schools. Of note is the fact that all but 2 of the 30 infected students were men, likely primarily reflecting infection of men who have sex with men, giving a seroprevalence rate for men of 0.5 percent, while the rate for women was 0.02 percent, a figure in sharp contrast to that of the largely socially and educationally disadvantaged young women in the Job Corps survey (0.32 percent).

Finally, serosurveys conducted at 38 sentinel hospitals throughout the United States from 1988 through 1990 underscore the wide variation in seroprevalence based largely on geographic location. Specimens were taken from patients hospitalized for diseases unlikely to be associated with HIV infection. The median seroprevalence was 0.9 percent, with a nearly 80-fold variation among hospitals (0.1 to 7.6 percent). In a 1992 report, a serosurvey of a District of Columbia sentinel hospital revealed that 11.3 percent of white and 16.9 percent of African-American men were HIV infected.

Thus, HIV infection and AIDS is widespread in the United States and is spreading rapidly among certain populations and stabilizing and even decreasing among others. Similar to other STDs, it is highly unlikely that HIV infection will spread homogeneously throughout the population of the United States. However, it is clear that anyone who practices high-risk behavior is at risk for HIV infection. In addition, the alarming increase in infections and AIDS cases among IDUs, their heterosexual partners, women, infants born of infected children, and adolescents, as well as the spread within certain inner city areas particularly among underserved minority populations with inadequate access to health care delivery testifies to the fact that the epidemic of HIV infection in the United States is a public health problem of major proportion.

FIGURE 279-7 HIV seroprevalence in civilian applicants for military service, United States, October, 1985, through December, 1990. A. By sex and test date. B. By race/ethnicity. *(A and B, from Centers for Disease Control, National HIV Serosurveillance Summary, Results through 1990, June, 1992.)*

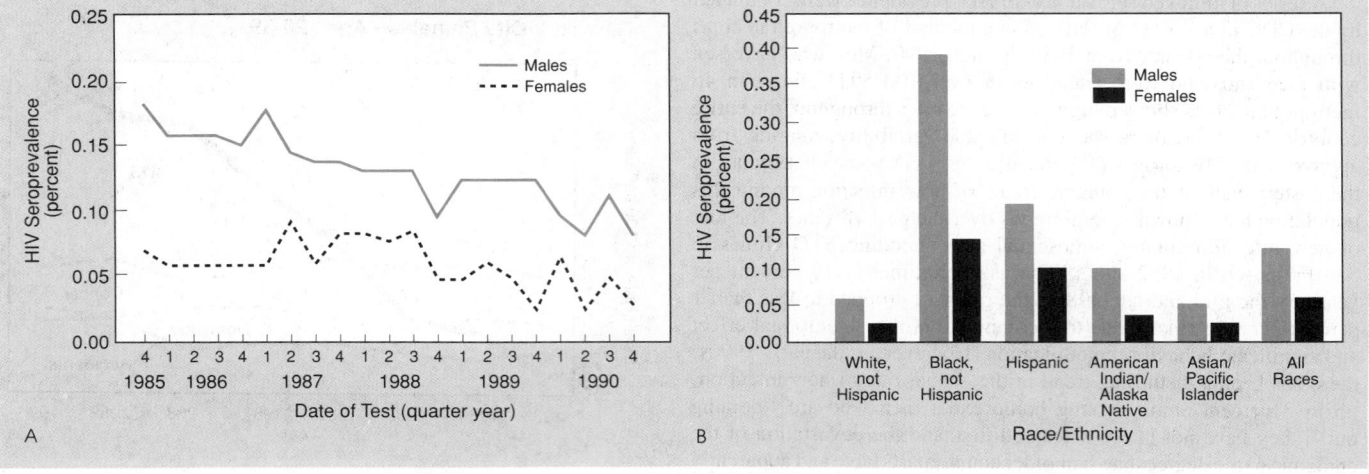

TABLE 279-6   Cumulative worldwide cases of AIDS reported to the World Health Organization as of July 1, 1993

Country/Region	Cases
Africa	247,577
Americas	371,086
Canada	7,770
Caribbean/Bahamas	9,250
Central America	4,436
Mexico	13,259
South America	47,051
United States of America	289,320
Asia	3,561
Europe	92,482
Oceania	4,188
Total	718,894

SOURCE: WHO, *Weekly Epidemiological Record*, No. 27, July 2, 1993.

HIV INFECTION AND AIDS WORLDWIDE HIV infection/AIDS is truly a global pandemic with cases reported from every continent. The reported cases of AIDS worldwide are a gross underestimate of the true incidence, mostly because of the incomplete reporting mechanisms available in certain developing countries. The reported cumulative cases of AIDS as of July 1, 1993, are shown in Table 279-6 and the estimated global distribution of adult HIV infections for the same time period is illustrated in Fig. 279-8. There is not and most likely will not be a uniform pandemic of AIDS worldwide. What is being witnessed are waves of epidemics with somewhat different characteristics in different regions of the world depending upon the demographics of the country or region in question and the timing of the introduction of HIV into the population. Considerable devastation has already been experienced in certain developing countries, particularly in sub-Saharan Africa, with respect to AIDS cases and deaths. This reflects the extensive spread of HIV which apparently began in the late 1970s and early 1980s. The major mode of transmission in this region is that of WHO Pattern II, which is heterosexual sex where the number of infected males and females are approximately equal. This is in contrast to North America and most of South America, Western Europe, Scandinavia, Australia, and New Zealand (Pattern I) where approximately 90 percent of cases are among men who have sex with men or among IDUs. Of note is the fact that the annual incidence of HIV infections in sub-Saharan Africa is believed still to be on the increase, signaling even worse devastation through the 1990s. In South America and the Caribbean, the annual incidence of infection is also believed to be increasing, but at lower levels than sub-Saharan Africa. WHO estimates that 1 million HIV-infected children have been born since the start of the HIV pandemic and more than half of these have developed AIDS and have died. In addition, approximately 2 million uninfected children are currently or will become AIDS orphans; approximately 90 percent of children born to HIV-infected women are in sub-Saharan Africa. In certain sub-Saharan African countries such at Zaire and Uganda, available seroprevalence data indicate that 3 to 6% of the entire population may be infected.

Other Pattern II regions are the Caribbean and certain areas of South America. During the early phases of the epidemic in Haiti, the primary mode of transmission was via men who had sex with men but who were predominantly bisexual males. These infected bisexual men then began infecting their heterosexual partners and by the mid-1980s heterosexual spread emerged as the major mode of transmission, with increasing number of women becoming infected; accompanying this trend was an increase in infection rate among infants.

In certain developing countries, transmission of HIV by contaminated blood or blood products remains a major problem because of lack of facilities and/or resources for screening of blood donors and inadequare blood banking facilities. Significant outbreaks of HIV infection have occurred in Romania and the former Soviet Union by a breakdown or lack of sterile techniques involving needles and syringes as well as an inappropriate use of blood transfusions.

HIV-2 was first described in asymptomatic West Africans (see above) and remains a major cause of HIV disease in West Africa. However, a number of cases have now been reported in other regions of Africa, Western Europe, South America (particularly Brazil), Canada, and the United States. Infection is felt to cause a more indolent disease than HIV-1 with advanced disease evolving over a longer period of time than with HIV-1.

Substantial transmission of HIV was documented in only a few countries in South Asia and Southeast Asia in the late 1980s. However, the spread in certain countries in this region, particularly Thailand and India, has been rapid since then. The situation in Thailand is of particular note in that the epidemic began in earnest in 1988 and has subsequently emerged rapidly. During the early and mid 1980s,

FIGURE 279-8 Estimated distribution of adult HIV infections for late 1993. *(From WHO.)*

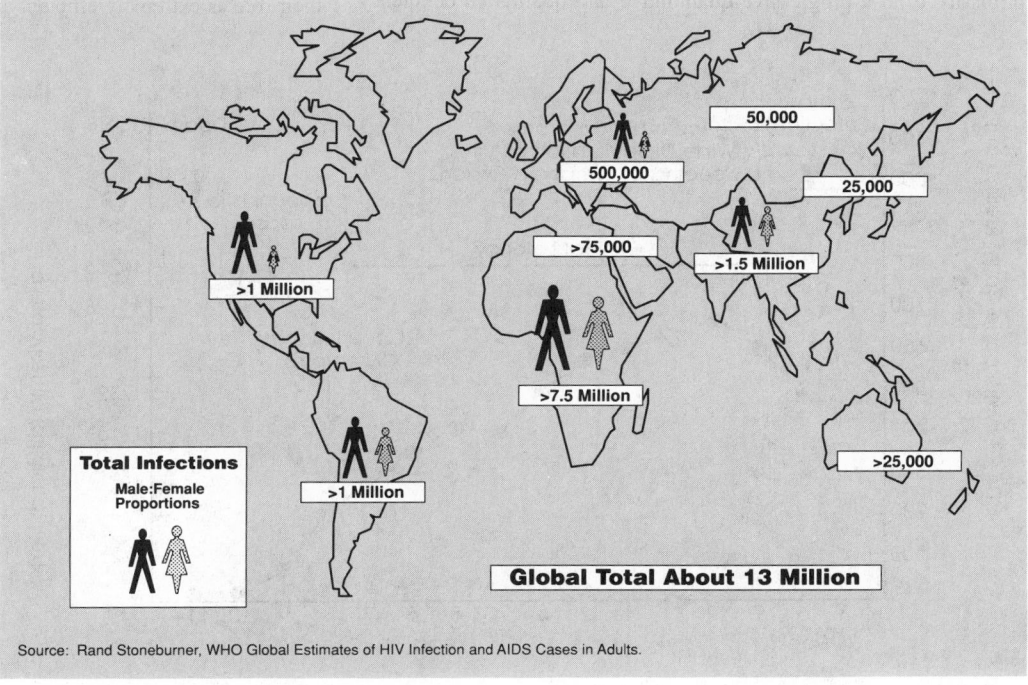

Source: Rand Stoneburner, WHO Global Estimates of HIV Infection and AIDS Cases in Adults.

Thailand was considered a Pattern III country, along with countries in Eastern Europe, North Africa, the Middle East, other Asian countries, and certain countries in the Pacific. Pattern III countries have relatively few cases of HIV infection/AIDS and most of these individuals have had contact with Pattern I and II countries. However, this paradigm was broken in Thailand. A single HIV-positive person was identified in Thailand among 101 male prostitutes in Bangkok in 1985, and it was expected that gay men would experience the first wave of rapid transmission. From 1985 through 1987 serosurveys among IDUs in Thailand revealed a prevalence of 0 to 1 percent, and similar surveys conducted among female prostitutes from 1985 through 1989 reported rates of less than 1 percent. There was not a wide appreciation of the potential for the epidemic to emerge into the general population. It was anticipated that it would remain confined to men who have sex with men and possibly to IDUs and would not substantially involve people who are generally considered to be at low risk. However, a remarkable pattern began to emerge in 1988. There was an extraordinary explosion of HIV prevalence among IDUs, from 1 percent at the beginning of 1988 to 32 to 43 percent by August-September of 1988. Thus unexpectedly, the first wave of HIV infection spread rapidly among IDUs. This was followed by successive waves of transmission to female prostitutes, then to their non-IDU male clients, and then ultimately into the low-risk, non-prostitute wives and girlfriends of these men in the general population. An indication of the extent of the HIV epidemic in Thailand is the prevalence among military recruits. Military service is mandatory for Thais at age 21. Serosurveys of conscripts indicate that in the northern provinces, including Chang Mai, the overall HIV prevalence among 21-year-old men is 10.3 percent. It is feared that such explosive patterns will also be seen in other Asian countries, particularly developing countries, such as India, which will equal and surpass sub-Saharan Africa as the most severely afflicted region in the remainder of the 20th century and into the 21st century.

WHO estimates that by the year 2000 there will be at least 40 million people worldwide infected with HIV. Other estimates are even higher ranging from 60 to 120 million. It is clear that the global impact of HIV infection and disease into the 21st century will be immense.

PATHOPHYSIOLOGY AND IMMUNOPATHOGENESIS

The hallmark of HIV disease is a profound immunodeficiency resulting primarily from a progressive quantitative and qualitative deficiency of the CD4+ subset of T lymphocytes referred to as the helper or inducer T cells. This subset of T cells is defined phenotypically by the presence on its surface of a CD4 molecule (see Chap. 277), which is the cellular receptor for HIV. Although the CD4+ T cell is the predominant cell type that is actually infected with HIV, virtually any human cell which expresses a CD4 molecule (written as CD4+) is capable of binding to and becoming infected with HIV. Although a number of mechanisms responsible for cytopathicity and immune dysfunction of CD4+ T cells have been demonstrated in vitro (see below), it is still unclear which mechanism or combination of mechanisms is primarily responsible for the progressive depletion and functional impairment of these cells in vivo. Nonetheless, when the CD4+ T cells decline beneath a certain level (see below) the patient is at high risk of developing a variety of opportunistic diseases, particularly infections and certain neoplasms which are AIDS-defining illnesses. Other features of AIDS such as Kaposi's sarcoma and neurologic abnormalities cannot be explained completely by the immunosuppressive effect of HIV since these complications may occur prior to the development of severe immunologic impairment.

The combination of viral pathogenic and immunopathogenic events which occur during the course of HIV disease from the moment of initial infection through the development of advanced disease are complex and heterogeneous. Although the precise sequence of events has not been fully delineated, there are reproducible in vivo and in vitro observations that have clarified certain of these real and potential mechanisms. It is highly likely that these mechanisms are quantitatively and qualitatively different at different stages of disease and so it is essential to consider the typical course of an HIV-infected individual in order to more fully appreciate these pathogenic events (Fig. 279-9).

PRIMARY INFECTION It is likely that the initial infection of susceptible cells varies somewhat with the route of infection. Virus that enters directly into the bloodstream via infected blood or blood products (i.e., transfusions, use of contaminated needles for IDU, sharp object injury, maternal to fetal transmission either intrapartum or perinatally, or in certain cases via sexual intercourse where there is trauma sufficient to cause bleeding) is likely cleared from the circulation to the lymphoid organs where it replicates to a critical level and then leads to a burst of viremia. It is uncertain which cell in the blood or lymphoid tissue is the first to actually become infected. It has been assumed that the CD4+ T cell or monocyte was the initial target. However, dendritic cells have been demonstrated to be efficient transporters or presenters of HIV to CD4+ T cells consistent with their role as extremely efficient antigen-presenting cells in the course

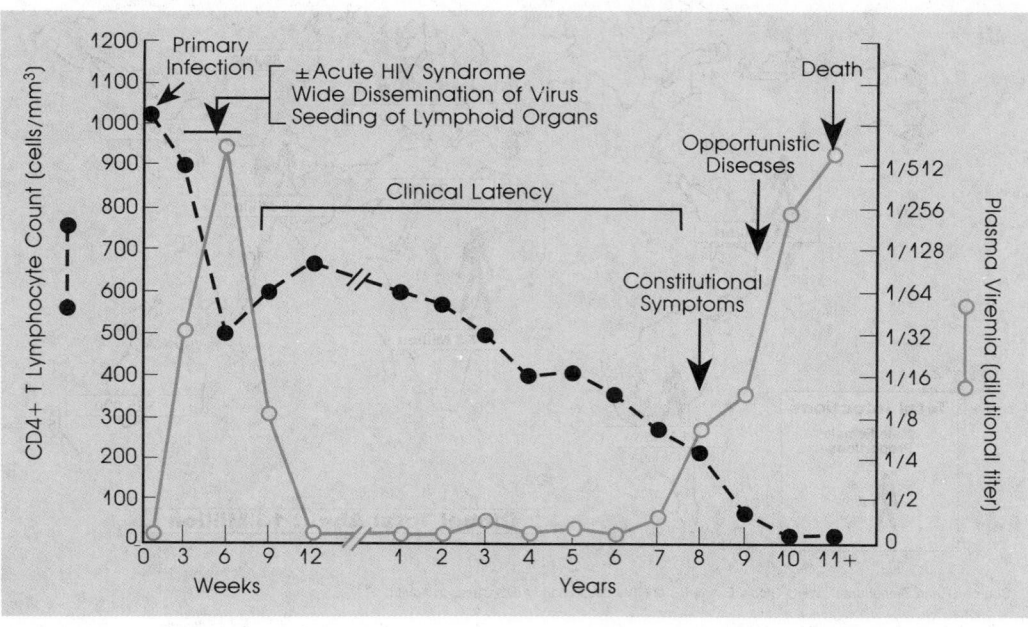

FIGURE 279-9 Typical course of an HIV-infected individual. See text for detailed description. *(From G Pantaleo et al, N Engl J Med 328:327, 1993.)*

of the normal immune response to antigen (see Chap. 277). One likely scenario is that dendritic cells carry virus to tissues, particularly lymph nodes, where they put the virus in contact with susceptible CD4+ T cells; this is somewhat different from the role of the follicular dendritic cells (FDC) residing in the germinal centers of the lymph nodes; these FDCs serve as traps or filters for the virus (see below). Dendritic cells have been reported to express low levels of CD4. However, there are conflicting reports as to whether the dendritic cells themselves can actually become infected with HIV. In circumstances where the virus enters "locally," such as via the rectum and the vagina in intercourse; the upper gastrointestinal tract via swallowed infected semen or vaginal fluid; or infected breast milk, it is likewise unclear which is the initial cell to becomer infected. Although infection of various mucosal cells of the gastrointestinal and genitourinary tract have been reported, it remains unclear whether they play a role in initial infection or whether CD4+ tissue macrophages and/or resident CD4+ T cells are the initial targets. Cells of dendritic cell lineage in the tissues could serve the same role as mentioned above by binding virus and "presenting" it to T cells. The common denominator of local infection would be a drainage to the regional lymph nodes with replication of virus and subsequent viremia which would then lead to more widespread infection of lymph nodes. A more detailed description of the role of lymphoid tissue in the immunopathogenesis of HIV infection is given below.

INITIAL VIREMIA AND DISSEMINATION OF VIRUS   It has been well documented that patients who experience the "acute HIV syndrome" following primary infection have high levels of viremia which last for several weeks (see below). The acute mononucleosis-like symptoms are well correlated with the presence of viremia. It is highly likely that most patients develop some degree of viremia which contributes to virus dissemination even though they remain asymptomatic or do not recall experiencing symptoms. It is these early events which likely play a major role in the subsequent course of infection in that the degree of initial virus replication and seeding of organs such as lymph nodes establishes the magnitude of virus burden which the immune system will be required to contain and which will expose susceptible cells to infection. A combination of the development of an HIV-specific immune response (both humoral and cell-mediated) (see below) and the efficient trapping of virions in the FDC of the lymph node germinal centers leads to the curtailment of viremia, disappearance of symptoms, and the beginning of so-called clinical latency, which lasts for variable periods, with a median duration of approximately 10 years (Fig. 279-9).

IMMUNOPATHOGENIC EVENTS DURING CLINICAL LATENCY It has been the consistent observation of clinicians caring for AIDS patients that, with few exceptions, there is a gradual and progressive diminution over time of the level of CD4+ T cells. The slope of the decline is highly predictive of the pattern of the clinical course and the development of advanced disease. Most patients are entirely asymptomatic during this progressive decline of CD4+ T cells (see below), which has led to the term *clinical latency*. Culturable viremia and p24 antigenemia are uncommon during this period, and there are very few cells (usually 1:1000 to 1:10,000) which contain HIV provirus and at least 1 log less cells which are actively expressing HIV mRNA during this period. In most patients, it is extremely difficult to detect active virus replication in the peripheral blood mononuclear cells during this period. However, the progressive decline of CD4+ T cells belies true viral latency since both cytopathic effects and qualitative dysfunction of T cells that cannot be explained by mere lymphocyte depletion occur. It has been demonstrated that even during this prolonged clinically latent period, there is copious virus contained in the lymph nodes and active virus replication in the lymph nodes (see below). Therefore, it is essential to distinguish between clinical latency and true microbiologic latency.

ADVANCED HIV DISEASE   After variable periods of time, usually measured in years, the CD4+ T cell count falls below a critical level (less than 200 cells per microliter) and the patient becomes highly susceptible to opportunistic disease. The patient may experience constitutional signs and symptoms or may develop an opportunistic disease without any prior symptoms. Even within this severely immunosuppressed state, the defect is progressive and unrelenting. It is not uncommon for CD4+ T cell counts to drop as low as 10 per microliter or even to zero, yet the patient may survive for months to more than 1 year. This is more common now that patients are more aggressively treated as well as given prophylaxis against the common life-threatening opportunistic infections such as *Pneumocystis carinii* pneumonia (see below). Ultimately, patients who progress to this severest form of immunosuppression will succumb to opportunistic diseases.

ROLE OF LYMPHOID ORGANS   The lymph nodes are the major anatomic sites for the establishment as well as the acute and chronic propagation of HIV infection. Out of logistic necessity, most studies on the pathogenesis of HIV infection have focused on the peripheral blood mononuclear cells. However, the fact remains that lymphocytes in the peripheral blood at any given time represent only approximately 2 percent of the total body lymphocyte pool and so may not always accurately reflect the status of the entire immune system; the bulk of the body's lymphocytes reside in the lymphoid organs such as the lymph nodes, spleen, and gut-associated lymphoid tissue. Since HIV disease is an infectious disease of the immune system, it is critical to appreciate the pathogenic events that occur in the lymphoid tissue in HIV infection.

Certain patients will experience progressive generalized lymphadenopathy (see below) relatively early in the course of infection; others may experience varying degrees of transient lymphadenopathy. It has been suggested that progressive generalized lymphadenopathy represents an exaggerated immune response to HIV and carries a more favorable prognosis (see below); however, lymph node involvement is a common denominator of virtually all patients with HIV infection, even those without easily detectable lymphadenopathy. Simultaneous examination of lymph node and peripheral blood mononuclear cells in the same patients during various stages of HIV disease including the early asymptomatic stage (when CD4+ T cell levels generally are greater than 500 per microliter), the intermediate stage (when these levels are 200 to 500 per microliter), and the advanced stage of disease (when they are 0 to 200 per microliter) has led to substantial insight into the pathogenesis of HIV infection. By a combination of polymerase chain reaction (PCR) techniques for HIV DNA and RNA, in situ hybridization for HIV RNA, and electron microscopy, the following picture has emerged. In most patients, early in the course of infection prior to significant immunosuppression (CD4+ T cell levels of greater than 500 per microliter) culturable viremia or p24 antigenemia is uncommon, the viral burden in the peripheral blood mononuclear cells is extremely low, and expression of HIV in these cells in minimal or undetectable. Remarkably, at this time there are copious amounts of extracellular virions trapped within the germinal centers of the lymph nodes (Fig. 279-10A) and in situ hybridization reveals expression of virus in individual cells of the paracortical area and to a lesser extent the germinal center (Fig. 279-10B). The architecture of the germinal centers is preserved and may even be hyperplastic due to in situ proliferation of cells and recruitment of cells to the lymph nodes. Electron microscopy demonstrates a fine network of FDCs with interdigitating processes that envelop virtually every lymphocyte in the germinal center (Fig. 279-10C). Extracellular virions can be seen attached to the processes, yet the FDCs appear to be relatively healthy. It is difficult to demonstrate infection of the FDC at this point or even in advanced disease; however, rare examples of virus budding off FDCs have been reported. As the disease progresses, the architecture of the germinal centers begins to show disruption, and the trapping efficiency of the node diminishes. Electron microscopy reveals swollen organelles in the FDC and cell death. At this time, the relative burden of HIV as well as the expression of HIV in the peripheral blood mononuclear cells increase and begin to equilibrate with the relative viral burden per given number of cells in the lymph node. As the disease progresses to the advanced stage, there is complete disruption of the architecture of the germinal center.

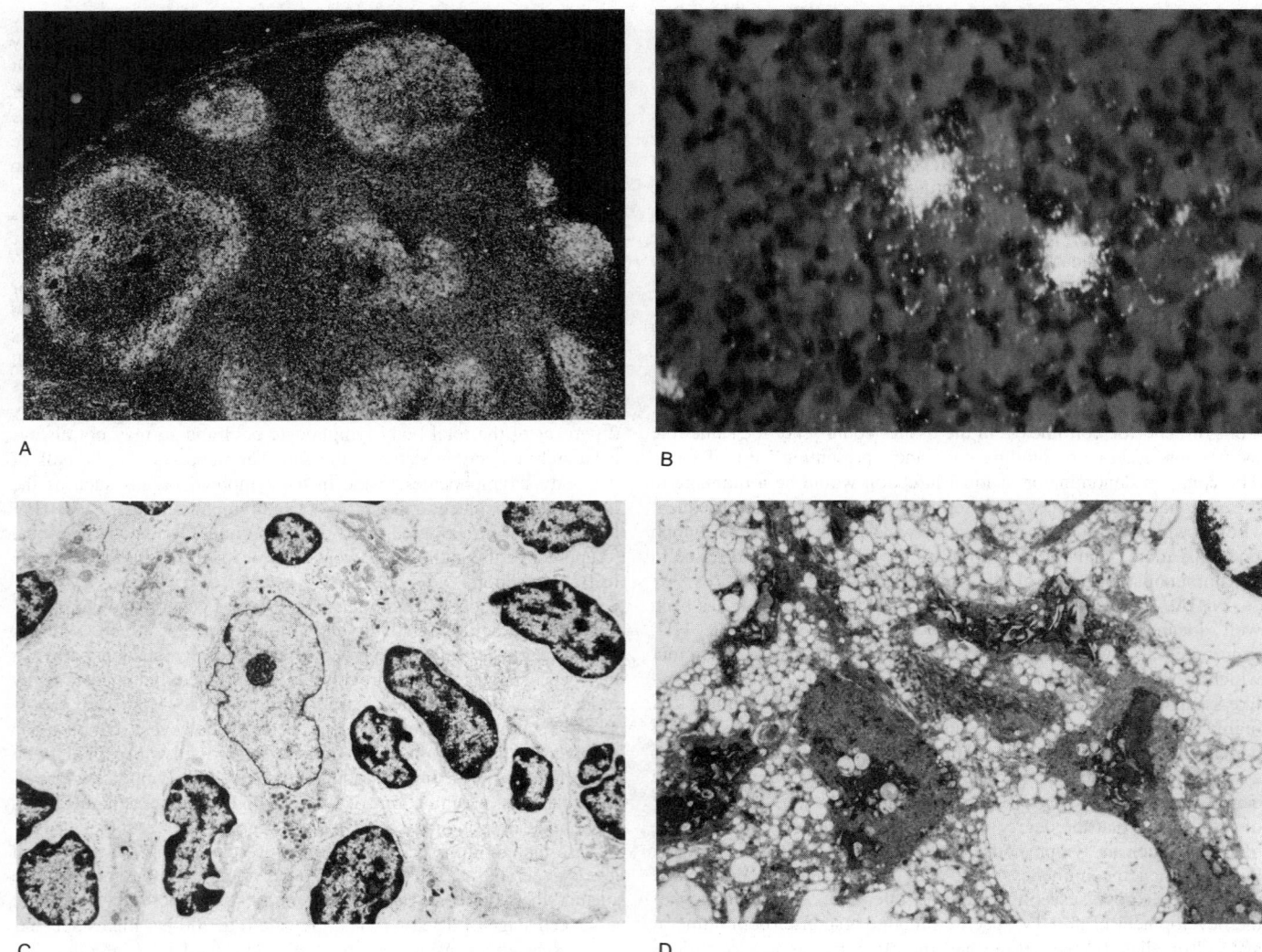

FIGURE 279-10 HIV in the lymph nodes of HIV-infected individuals. *A.* Cervical lymph node from an asymptomatic individual with no culturable viremia or p24 antigenemia. In situ hybridization using a molecular probe for HIV RNA reveals copious virus demarcating the numerous germinal centers (bright areas) of the node. The virus was extracellular and bound to the processes of the follicular dendritic cells which interdigitate within the confines of the germinal centers. Original ×25. *(Courtesy of Dr. Cecil Fox.) B.* Individual cells infected with HIV. Two cells in the paracortical area of the lymph node are shown expressing HIV RNA by in situ hybridization using a radiolabeled molecular probe. Original × 250 *(Courtesy of Dr. Cecil Fox.) C.* Follicular dendritic cell in cervical lymph node of an asymptomatic HIV- infected individual. Electron microscopy reveals a follicular dendritic cell with a prominent nucleolus surrounded by several lymphocytes within the germinal center of the node. Higher magnification of several fields indicates that multiple processes of the follicular dendritic cell surround and are in contact with several lymphocytes. Original × 1920 *(Courtesy of Dr. Jan Orenstein.) D.* Dissolution of follicular dendritic cells in the germinal center of a cervical lymph node from a patient with advanced HIV disease. Widespread death of follicular dendritic cells is associated with a loss of ability of the lymph node to trap virus late in the course of HIV disease. Original × 3744. *(Courtesy of Dr. Jan Orenstein. Adapted from G Pantaleo et al, N Engl J Med 328:327, 1993.)*

This is accompanied by dissolution of the FDC network and massive dropout of FDCs (Fig. 279-10*D*). The trapping function of the lymph node is completely lost and virus freely spills over into the circulation. Simultaneous PCR analysis of lymph node and peripheral blood mononuclear cells indicates that the relative viral burden and expression of HIV in the blood versus the lymph node approach equilibrium at this stage. This advanced stage is accompanied by a burst of viremia which may represent a true increase in virus replication due in part to an escape from the immune system curtailment (see below) as well as a mechanical escape from the lymph node trapping function. At this point, the lymph nodes are characterized as "burnt out." It is unclear what the mechanism of FDC death is; there is no indication by electron microscopy of copious virus replication or budding of virions off the cell in great quantities. Thus, the lymphoid tissues play a major role in the pathogenesis of HIV disease. They serve as an important reservoir of the virus, a filter or trapping apparatus of free virions, and a prominent milieu for the exposure of susceptible cells to large amounts of virus trapped among the processes of the FDC, which activate adjacent cells as well as present virus to these cells. Active virus replication occurs in individual cells within the lymph node throughout the entire course of HIV disease, even during the time of clinical latency when little, if any, virus or virus replication can be demonstrated in peripheral blood mononuclear cells. Understanding the pathogenic events that occur within the lymph node throughout the course of HIV disease adds considerably to our appreciation of how and why CD4 + T cells continue to progressively diminish in number during the time that the disease appears to be latent and so little viral burden and activity can be detected in peripheral blood. A schematic diagram of the role of lymphoid tissue in the pathogenesis of HIV disease is shown in Fig. 279-11.

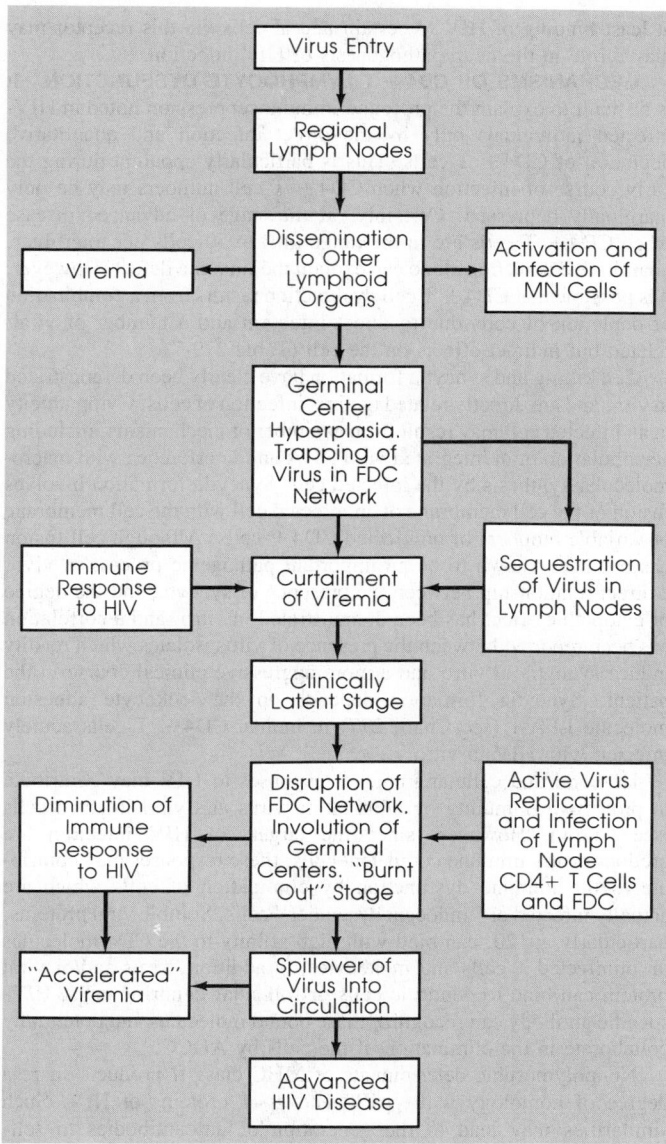

FIGURE 279-11 The role of lymphoid organs in the pathogenesis of HIV infection. *(Adapted from G Pantaleo et al, N Engl J Med 328:327, 1993.)*

T LYMPHOCYTE ABNORMALITIES The range of T cell abnormalities in advanced HIV infection is broad. The defects are both quantitative and qualitative and impact every limb of the immune system (see below), bespeaking the critical dependence of the integrity of the immune system on the inducer/helper function of the CD4 + T cell. Virtually all the immune defects in advanced HIV disease can be explained by the quantitative depletion of CD4 + T cells. However, T cell dysfunction can be demonstrated in patients early in the course of infection even when the CD4 + T cell count is within the low-normal range. The degree of these dysfunctions increases as the disease progresses. One of the first abnormalities to be detected is a defect in response to soluble antigen at a time when mononuclear cells can still respond normally to mitogen stimulation. The mechanisms for this selective defect are unclear, but may involve abnormal antigen recognition as well as aberrant cell triggering (see below). In addition, the memory subset of T cells appears to be affected earlier and more profoundly than the naive subset. Essentially every T cell function has been reported to be abnormal at some stage of HIV infection. Certain of these abnormalities include defective T cell cloning and colony forming efficiencies, impaired expression of interleukin 2 receptors, defective IL-2 production, decreased interferon-gamma

(IFN-γ) production in response to antigens, depressed HLA class I–restricted cytotoxic T lymphocyte responses against a number of viruses, decreased allogeneic responses, and decreased ability to help B cells to produce immunoglobulin.

HIV-specific CD8 + cytolytic T cells have been demonstrated in HIV-infected individuals early in the course of disease (see below). As the disease progresses, this functional capability is lost. The cause of this loss of cytolytic activity is unclear. However, it has been demonstrated that, as the disease progresses, CD8 + T cells assume an abnormal phenotype characterized by expression of activation markers such as HLA-DR with an absence of expression of the IL-2 receptor (CD25) and a loss of clonogenic potential. The levels of CD8 + T cells varies throughout the course of disease and may be normal, elevated, or decreased. It has been demonstrated in vitro that CD8 + T cells can suppress the induction of HIV expression, likely by secretion of a soluble factor.

B LYMPHOCYTE ABNORMALITIES B cells from HIV-infected individuals manifest abnormal activation reflected by increased spontaneous proliferation and immunoglobulin secretion, and by increased spontaneous secretion of tumor necrosis factor alpha (TNF-α) and IL-6. The enhanced spontaneous in vitro transformation of B cells with Epstein-Barr virus (EBV) is probably due to defective T cell immune surveillance and has as its in vivo counterpart an increase in incidence of EBV-related B cell lymphomas. Untransformed B cells cannot be infected with HIV. However, HIV or its products (particularly gp120) can directly activate B cells to secrete TNF-α and IL-6. It is likely that the in vivo activation of B cells by virus products accounts at least in part for the spontaneous activation of these cells noted in vitro. In vivo, this activated state manifests itself by hypergammaglobulinemia and by the presence of circulating immune complexes and autoantibodies. The B cells are also defective in that they respond poorly to in vitro stimulation with antigens and mitogens. HIV-infected individuals respond poorly to primary and secondary immunization with protein and polysaccharide antigens. These B cell defects are likely responsible in part for the increase in bacterial infections seen in advanced HIV disease in adults, as well as for the important role of bacterial infections in HIV-infected children who cannot mount an adequate humoral response to common bacterial pathogens.

MONOCYTE/MACROPHAGE ABNORMALITIES Circulating monocytes are normal in number in HIV-infected individuals. Monocytes express the CD4 molecule on their surface and thus are targets for HIV infection. Certain strains of HIV have been demonstrated to have a selective tropism for CD4 + monocytes versus CD4 + T cells. Of note is the fact that the degree of cytopathicity of HIV for cells of the monocyte lineage is low and HIV can replicate extensively in cells of the monocyte lineage under certain circumstances with little cytopathic effect. Hence, monocyte lineage cells can serve as reservoirs of HIV infection and may play a role in the dissemination of HIV in the body. Infection of circulating monocytes occurs infrequently; however, infection of tissue macrophages and macrophage lineage cells in the brain and lung (pulmonary alveolar macrophages) can be easily demonstrated. Infection of monocyte precursors in the bone marrow may directly or indirectly be responsible for certain of the hematologic abnormalities in HIV-infected individuals. The predominant cells in the brain that are infected with HIV are cells of the monocyte lineage, infiltrating either macrophages or resident microglial cells (see below). A number of abnormalities of circulating monocytes have been reported in HIV-infected individuals, including defects in chemotaxis, secretion of IL-1, certain cytotoxic functions, and the ability to present antigen to T cells. The reported functional abnormalities of circulating monocytes are likely related in part to abnormal activation of these cells in vivo by cytokines.

NATURAL KILLER (NK) CELL ABNORMALITIES The presumed role of NK cells is to provide immunosurveillance against virus-infected cells, certain tumor cells, and allogeneic cells (see Chap. 277). HIV-infected individuals manifest functionally defective NK cell activity despite the fact that NK cells have been normal in numbers and phenotype in most studies. The abnormality in NK cell function is thought to result from a defect in postbinding lysis. However, the lytic machinery does not appear to be impaired since NK cells from HIV-infected individuals mediate antibody dependent cellular cytotoxicity (ADCC) normally. It has been demonstrated that the addition of IL-2 enhanced the depressed NK cell activity in vitro. The in vivo mechanism for defective NK cell activity is unknown; however, it may be related to the lack of normal inductive signals from CD4 + T lymphocytes.

AUTOIMMUNE PHENOMENA Autoimmune phenomena are commonly noted in HIV-infected individuals. This usually occurs in the absence of autoimmune disease (see below). Autoimmune phenomena include antibodies to lymphocytes and less commonly to platelets and neutrophils. Antiplatelet antibodies have some clinical relevance in that they may contribute to the thrombocytopenia of HIV infection (see below). Antibodies to nuclear and cytoplasmic components of cells have been reported as have antibodies to cardiolipin. In addition, autoantibodies to a range of serum proteins including albumin, immunoglobulin, and thyroglobulin have been reported. Antibodies to MHC class II molecules may interfere with the antigen-presenting capabilities of certain cells or may contribute to their depletion via ADCC mechanisms.

OTHER CELL TYPES Although the CD4 + T lymphocyte and CD4 + cells of the monocyte lineage are the principal targets of HIV, virtually any cell that expresses the CD4 molecule can potentially be infected with the virus. Circulating dendritic cells have been reported to express low levels of CD4, and there have been conflicting reports of whether these cells can be infected with the virus. Epidermal Langerhans cells express CD4 and have been demonstrated to be infected in vivo with HIV. A variety of other cell types which express low levels of CD4, no detectable CD4, or only CD4 mRNA have been reported to be infected with HIV. These include megakaryocytes, astrocytes and oligodendrocytes, follicular dendritic cells, microglial cells, CD8 + T cells (under certain conditions), enterochromaffin cells, retinal cells, renal epithelial cells, cervical cells, rectal and colonic mucosal cells, trophoblastic cells, and cardiac myocytes. In certain of those studies in which in situ hybridization of tissue specimens was performed, it was not entirely clear whether monocytes in these tissues were the cells actually infected with HIV. In addition, a large number of established cell lines have been shown to be infected with HIV. However, the significance of these observations with regard to pathogenesis of HIV infection, including dysfunction of respective organs which contain such cells, is unclear. At present, the only cells that have unequivocally been shown to harbor HIV in vivo are CD4 + T lymphocytes and cells of monocyte/macrophage lineage.

Of potentially important clinical relevance is the demonstration that thymic precursor cells which were assumed to be negative for CD3, CD4, and CD8 molecules actually do express low levels of CD4 and can be infected with HIV in vitro. In addition, human thymic epithelial cells when transplanted into an immunodeficient mouse can be infected with HIV by direct inoculation of virus into the thymus. Since these cells likely play a role in the normal replenishment of CD4 + T cells, it is possible that their infection and depletion interferes with the replenishment of the CD4 + T cell pool in infected individuals, including those in whom antiretroviral therapy has at least temporarily suppressed virus replication (see below). In addition, CD34 + monocyte precursor cells residing in bone marrow are capable of being infected in vitro with HIV, and these cells may serve as a reservoir of HIV as well as play a role in the suppression of hematopoiesis. Furthermore, CD34 + bone marrow precursor cells have been shown to be infected in vivo in patients with advanced HIV disease. It is likely that these cells express low levels of CD4 and therefore it is not essential to invoke CD4-independent mechanisms to explain the infection. Other studies have demonstrated that the galactosyl ceramide molecule can serve as an alternative receptor for HIV in CD4-negative neural and colonic epithelial cells (see "Neuropathogenesis" below). CD4-independent infection of or

at least binding of HIV to certain neural cells via this receptor may play a role in the neuropathogenesis of HIV infection.

MECHANISMS OF CD4 + T LYMPHOCYTE DYSFUNCTION It is difficult to explain the profound immunosuppression noted in HIV-infected individuals only by the direct infection and quantitative depletion of CD4 + T cells. This is particularly apparent during the early course of infection when CD4 + T cell numbers may be only marginally depressed. Certainly, at the stage of advanced disease when CD4 + T cells are in the range of 0 to 50 cells per microliter, quantitative depletion alone can explain the immune defect. However, it is possible that CD4 + T cell dysfunction results from a combination of depletion of cells due to direct infection and a number of viral-related but indirect effects on the cell (Table 279-7).

Cell killing and syncytia formation have clearly been demonstrated in vitro and are directly related to virus infection of cells. Cytopathicity in an infected cell may result from a number of mechanisms, including accumulation of unintegrated viral DNA and interference with macro-molecular synthesis by the infected cell. Syncytia formation involves fusion of the cell membrane of an infected cell with the cell membrane of variable numbers of uninfected CD4 + cells. Although cell fusion has not been shown to be an important pathogenic process in vivo, a direct relationship between the presence of syncytia and the degree of cytopathic effect has been demonstrated in vitro, and a correlation has been reported between the presence of virus isolates which readily induce syncytia in vitro and a more aggressive clinical course in the patient. Syncytia formation depends on the leukocyte adhesion molecule LFA-1 (see Chap. 277) in human CD4 + T cells acutely infected with HIV in vitro.

Humoral and cellular immune responses to HIV may contribute to protective immunity by eliminating virus and viral infected cells (see below). However, since the targets of HIV infection are predominantly immune competent cells, these responses may contribute to the immune dysfunction by elimination of cells which are actually infected or "innocent bystander" cells. Soluble viral proteins, particularly gp120, can bind with high affinity to the CD4 molecules on uninfected T cells and monocytes; in addition, virus and/or viral protein can bind to dendritic cells or follicular dendritic cells. HIV-specific antibody can recognize these bound molecules and potentially collaborate in the elimination of the cells by ADCC.

Nonpolymorphic determinants of MHC class II products share a degree of homology with gp120 and gp41 proteins of HIV. Such similarities may lead to the generation of autoantibodies to self-MHC determinants. In fact, anti-HLA-DR antibodies have been demonstrated in the sera of HIV-infected individuals. These antibodies could contribute to the elimination of HLA-DR expressing cells by ADCC; in addition, it has been suggested that these antibodies may inhibit certain T cell functions which involve HLA-DR molecules.

Following binding of gp120/anti-gp120 complexes to the CD4 molecule, CD4 + T cells become refractory to further stimulation in vitro via the CD3 molecule. In addition, peripheral blood mononuclear cells acutely infected with HIV in vitro no longer respond to stimulation with anti-CD3 antibodies. Thus it has been hypothesized

---

TABLE 279-7 Potential mechanisms of CD4 + T lymphocyte dysfunction/depletion in HIV infection

HIV-mediated direct cytopathicity (single-cell killing)
HIV-mediated syncytia formation
Virus-specific immune responses:
  HIV specific cytolytic T lymphocytes
  Antibody dependent cellular cytotoxicity
  Natural killer cells
Autoimmune mechanisms
Anergy caused by inappropriate cell signalling via gp120/CD4 interaction
Superantigen-mediated pertubation of T cell subsets
Programmed cell death (apoptosis)

* From G Pantaleo et al., N Engl J Med 328:327, 1993.

that a negative or anergic signal is delivered to the cell upon interaction with gp120 or gp120/anti-gp120 complexes. Antibodies directed against gp120 have been detected on CD4+ T cells in HIV-infected individuals.

Conventional antigens bind in the groove of the MHC molecule of the antigen-presenting cell (see Chap. 277) and interact with the variable components of the T cell receptor alpha and beta chains in order to activate the T cell. Thus any given conventional antigenic peptide can stimulate only a very small fraction ($<1/100,000$) of total T cells. In contrast, certain microbial antigens are capable of binding to and activating entire subsets of T cells, not through true antigen receptor binding but by binding to another site on the variable (V) region of the beta (β) chain of the T cell receptor. This binding, to all members of a particular Vβ subset (1 to 10 percent of all T cells) can induce massive stimulation and expansion of T cells and/or, depending upon the state of activation of the T cell, result in deletion or anergy of the T cells bearing the specific Vβs. For this reason, these antigens have been referred to as *superantigens*. It has been hypothesized that superantigen(s), either retrovirally encoded or unrelated to HIV, may contribute to the immunopathogenesis of HIV infection. This hypothesis stems from the observations that endogenous or exogenous retroviral-encoded superantigens react with CD4+ T cells in the developing immune system of certain strains of mice, leading to anergy or deletion of the CD4+ T cells bearing specific Vβs. Certain studies have demonstrated that there are quantitative perturbations of certain Vβ subsets of CD4+ T cells in HIV-infected individuals, lending credence to the possibility that one or more superantigens may be involved in the nonrandom and preferential depletion of certain subsets of CD4+ T cells over others. It is unclear whether this process of direct superantigen-driven depletion actually occurs in vivo. However, it is certain that superantigens can activate CD4+ T cells, and so by simply increasing the susceptibility of certain T cell subsets to HIV infection they may contribute indirectly to their ultimate depletion.

Cells may die through one of two main mechanisms. The first of these, necrosis, is generally triggered by an exogenous injury. It is, for the most part random and accompanied by inflammation as cells spill their cytoplasmic contents into surrounding tissues. The other, programmed cell death, or apoptosis, is a more controlled process that serves a normal physiologic function in a variety of organ systems. It is part of the ontogeny of the immune system and is a mechanism for the clonal deletion of autoreactive T cells in the thymus. It depends on the process of cellular activation. It has been hypothesized that in HIV infection, sequential activation signals delivered to CD4+ T cells induce programmed cell death. Cross-linking of the CD4 molecule by gp120 or gp120/anti-gp120 complexes (see above) delivers the first of two signals to the cell which is required for apoptosis. The second signal, leading to cell death, is delivered via the T cell receptor upon activation by a conventional antigen or a superantigen. The latter would link the apoptosis and superantigen hypotheses of the depletion and/or functional impairment of CD4+ T cells in the absence of direct infection by HIV. Alternatively, HIV-induced alterations in tyrosine kinase activity may also trigger the cell to undergo programmed death.

INDUCTION OF HIV EXPRESSION   Although HIV can initially infect both resting and activated CD4+ T cells in vitro with approximately the same efficiency, the ability of the virus to effectively reverse transcribe its genomic RNA and integrate its provirus into the cellular genome is heavily dependent on the state of activation of the cell. In addition, the process of expression of HIV in an infected cell followed by virion production and spread to other susceptible cells relies on a variety of inductive or activation signals. These inductive signals can derive from a wide range of sources and can be considered as cofactors for the spread of virus within a host. Coinfection or simultaneous cotransfection of cells with HIV and other heterologous viruses or viral genes has demonstrated that certain viruses such as cytomegalovirus (CMV), herpes simplex virus, human herpes virus

6, hepatitis B virus, and HTLV-I can up-regulate HIV expression. Furthermore, other microbes such as mycoplasma have been reported to contribute to the induction of HIV expression.

The immune system is homeostatically regulated by a complex network of immunoregulatory cytokines which are pleiotropic, redundant, and operate in a paracrine and autocrine manner. They are continuously being expressed even during periods of apparent quiescence of the immune system. Upon perturbation of the immune system by antigenic challenge, these cytokines are further expressed to varying degrees. Cytokines which are important components of this immunoregulatory network have been demonstrated to play a major role in the regulation of HIV expression in vitro. IL-1, IL-2, IL-3, IL-6, TNF-α and β, IFN-γ, GM-CSF, and M-CSF may induce expression of HIV in chronically infected cells in vitro. IFN-α and -β suppress whereas transforming growth factor (TGF)-β and IL-4 both induce and suppress HIV expression. Several of these cytokines synergize in their inductive capabilities and others function in an autocrine and paracrine manner in the induction of HIV expression similar to their physiologic function in the regulation of the immune system. Molecular mechanisms of induction of virus expression range from stimulating new transcription via transcription-activating factors such as NF-κB, as is true with TNF-α, to predominantly posttranscriptional induction of virus as with IL-6 and GM-CSF. TGF-β interferes with both transcriptional and posttranscriptional induction of virus expression. Elevated levels of TNF-α and IL-6 have been reported in the plasma and cerebrospinal fluid of HIV-infected individuals, and increased expression of certain cytokines such as IFN-γ have been demonstrated in certain tissues such as lymph nodes of HIV-infected individuals. Thus, this complex network of immunoregulatory cytokines which is operable even during apparent immunologic quiescence likely contributes to the baseline induction of HIV expression, particularly in the lymph nodes.

NEUROPATHOGENESIS   HIV infection can lead to a variety of neurologic abnormalities due to opportunistic infections and neoplasms as well as to direct effects of HIV or its products (see below). With regard to the latter, HIV has been demonstrated in the brains of infected individuals with neuropsychiatric abnormalities. In addition, the virus can be isolated from the cerebrospinal fluid of a high percentage of infected individuals without detectable neuropsychiatric findings. The predominant cells within the brain that are infected with HIV are of the monocyte/macrophage lineage such as microglial cells. It has been reported that virus isolates from brain are preferentially monocyte tropic as opposed to T cell tropic when cultured in vitro. There is no convincing evidence that neurons can be infected with HIV in vivo. However, galactosyl ceramide has been demonstrated to be an essential component of the neural receptor for HIV gp120 and antibodies to galactosyl ceramide inhibit enttry of HIV into neural cell lines in vitro.

HIV-infected individuals may manifest both white matter lesions as well as neuronal loss. The HIV-mediated effects on brain tissue are felt to be due to a combination of direct toxic or functional inhibitory influences of gp120 on neuronal cells as well as the toxic effects of a variety of cytokines released from infiltrating macrophages, resident microglial cells, and astrocytes. Neurotoxicity due to gp120 can be blocked in vitro in certain types of neurons by antagonists of L-type voltage-dependent calcium channels or by antagonists of N-methyl-D-aspartate (NMDA), which is a type of glutamate receptor. Factors which might be toxic or inhibitory to neurons include TNF-α, IL-1, IL-6, TGF-β, and endothelin. Reactive gliosis has been demonstrated in the brains of HIV-infected individuals and TNF-α and IL-6 have been shown to induce astrocyte proliferation. Elevated TNF-α levels have been demonstrated in the cerebrospinal fluid of HIV-infected individuals. In addition, astrocyte-derived IL-6 can induce HIV expression in infected cells in vitro. The likelihood that HIV or its products are involved directly or indirectly in neuropathogenesis is supported by the observation that neuropsychiatric abnormalities may undergo remarkable and rapid improvement upon the initiation of zidovudine therapy, particularly in HIV-infected children.

PATHOGENESIS OF KAPOSI'S SARCOMA Kaposi's sarcoma does not result from a neoplastic transformation of cells and so is not truly a sarcoma. It is a manifestation of excessive proliferation of spindle cells which are believed to be of vascular origin with features in common with endothelial and smooth muscle cells. No chromosomal abnormalities nor evidence of viral infection have been identified in Kaposi's sarcoma cells cultured from HIV-infected individuals. It is a cytokine-mediated disease in which a number of factors including oncostatin M, basic fibroblast growth factor, IL-1ß, IL-6, and GM-CSF function in an autocrine and paracrine manner to sustain the growth and chemotaxis of the sarcoma cells (see Chap. 151). The pathogenic link between HIV infection and Kaposi's sarcoma is the fact that these inflammatory and angiogenic cytokines cooperate with the HIV-derived *tat* protein, which itself serves as a growth factor in the induction and progression of Kaposi's sarcoma in HIV-infected individuals. It remains unclear why there is a much greater incidence of Kaposi's sarcoma among HIV-infected homosexual men than among individuals with other risks for HIV infection. Theories which have been proposed include the presence in homosexual men of a chronically immune activated state and the possibility that another virus may be involved; neither of these have been substantiated by firm evidence (see below).

IMMUNE RESPONSE TO HIV

As detailed below, following an initial bout of viremia, individuals infected with HIV mount an immune response that appears to contribute to slowing the progression of infection and to delaying the ultimate development of clinically apparent disease for a median of 10 years. This immune response contains elements of both humoral and cell-mediated immunity (Table 279-8) and is directed toward multiple antigenic determinants of the HIV virion, as well as toward viral proteins produced within infected cells. Paradoxically, those CD4 + elements of the immune system with antigen receptors specific for HIV are theoretically those most likely to bind to infected cells and themselves become infected and destroyed. Thus, relatively early in the course of HIV infection there is destruction of the specific cellular components of host defense that are most important for the control of HIV infection.

Although a great deal of investigation has been directed toward attempting to dissect and understand the individual elements of this immune response, it remains unclear which of these phenomena are most important in delaying progression of infection and which, if any, may actually be playing a role in the pathogenic process.

THE HUMORAL IMMUNE RESPONSE As discussed below, antibodies to HIV usually appear within 2 weeks of the onset of the

acute syndrome following primary infection and almost invariably within 8 weeks following initial infection (Fig. 279-12). It is the detection of these antibodies that forms the basis of most screening tests for HIV infection. Despite earlier claims to the contrary, there is currently no evidence to suggest that, apart from extremely rare exceptions, the period between initial infection and development of an antibody response is any longer than 3 months. The first antibodies detected are those directed toward the structural or *gag* proteins of HIV, p24 and p17 and the *gag* precursor, p55. The development of antibodies to p24 is associated with a decrease in the serum levels of free p24 antigen. Antibodies to the *gag* proteins are followed by the appearance of antibodies to the envelope proteins (gp160, gp120, p88, and gp41) and to the products of the *pol* gene (p31, p51, and p66). Additionally, one may see antibodies to low-molecular-weight proteins from HIV-infected cells corresponding to antibodies to the regulatory proteins produced by the HIV genes *vpr, vpu, vif, rev, tat,* and *nef.*

While antibodies are made to multiple antigens of HIV, the precise functional significance of these different antibodies is unclear. The best studied have been the antibodies directed toward the envelope proteins of the virus. As noted above, the envelope of HIV consists of an outer envelope glycoprotein, with a molecular weight of 120 kDa, and a transmembrane glycoprotein, with a molecular weight of 41kDa. These are initially synthesized as a 160 kDa precursor. The majority of the antienvelope antibodies are directed toward an epitope that lies within the gp41 region, from amino acid 579 to amino acid 613.

Antibodies directed toward the envelope proteins of HIV have been characterized as both protective and possibly contributing to the overall pathogenesis. Among the protective antibodies are those that function to directly neutralize HIV and prevent the infection of additional cells, as well as those that participate in ADCC. Neutralizing antibodies appear to be of two forms, type specific and group specific. Type-specific neutralizing antibodies are generally directed to a hypervariable region of the gp120 molecule known as the *V3 loop* (amino acids 303 to 338). These antibodies only neutralize viruses of a given strain and are present in low titer in most infected individuals. Group-specific antibodies, on the other hand, are capable of neutralizing a wide variety of HIV isolates. At least two forms of group-specific antibodies have been identified, those binding to amino acids 423 to 437 of gp120 and those binding to amino acids 728 to 745 of gp41. The other major class of protective antibodies are those that participate in ADCC. This is actually a form of cell-mediated immunity (see Chap. 277) in which Fc receptor–bearing natural killer cells, armed with specific anti-HIV antibodies via binding of the Fc portion of the antibodies to the cellular Fc receptors bind to and

FIGURE 279-12 Relationship between antigenemia and the development of antibodies to HIV. Antibodies to HIV proteins are generally seen 6 to 12 weeks following infection and to 3 to 6 weeks after the development of plasma viremia. Late in the course of illness, antibody levels to p24 decline, generally in association with a rising titer of p24 antigen.

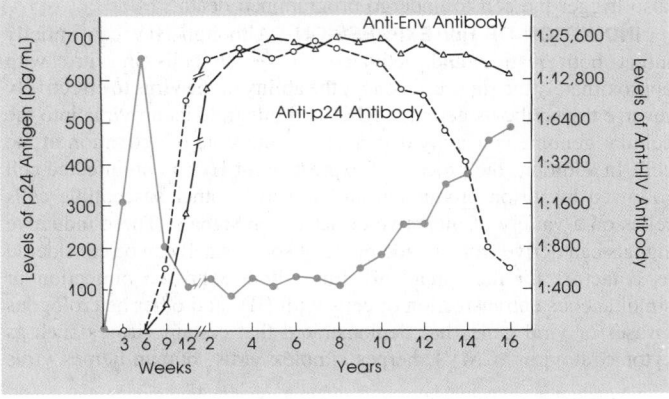

TABLE 279-8 Elements of the immune response to HIV

HUMORAL IMMUNITY

A Binding antibodies
B Neutralizing antibodies
   1 Type specific
   2 Group specific
C Antibodies participating in ADCC
   1 Protective
   2 Pathogenic (bystander killing)
D Enhancing antibodies

CELL MEDIATED IMMUNITY

A Helper CD4 + T lymphocytes
B Class I MHC-restricted cytotoxic CD8 + T lymphocytes
C CD8 + T cell-mediated inhibition (noncytolytic)
D Antibody-dependent cellular cytotoxicity
E Natural killer cell

destroy cells expressing HIV antigens (Fig. 279-13). Antibodies to both gp120 and gp41 have been shown to participate in ADCC-mediated killing of HIV infected cells. Levels of antienvelope antibodies capable of mediating ADCC are highest in patients at the earlier stages of HIV infection. ADCC-mediated killing can be augmented in vitro IL-2.

In addition to playing a role in host defense, HIV-specific antibodies also have been implicated in the pathogenesis of the disease. Antibodies directed to gp41, in low titer, have been shown

FIGURE 279-13 Schematic of the different immunologic effector mechanisms felt to be active in the setting of HIV infection. Detailed descriptions are given in the text.

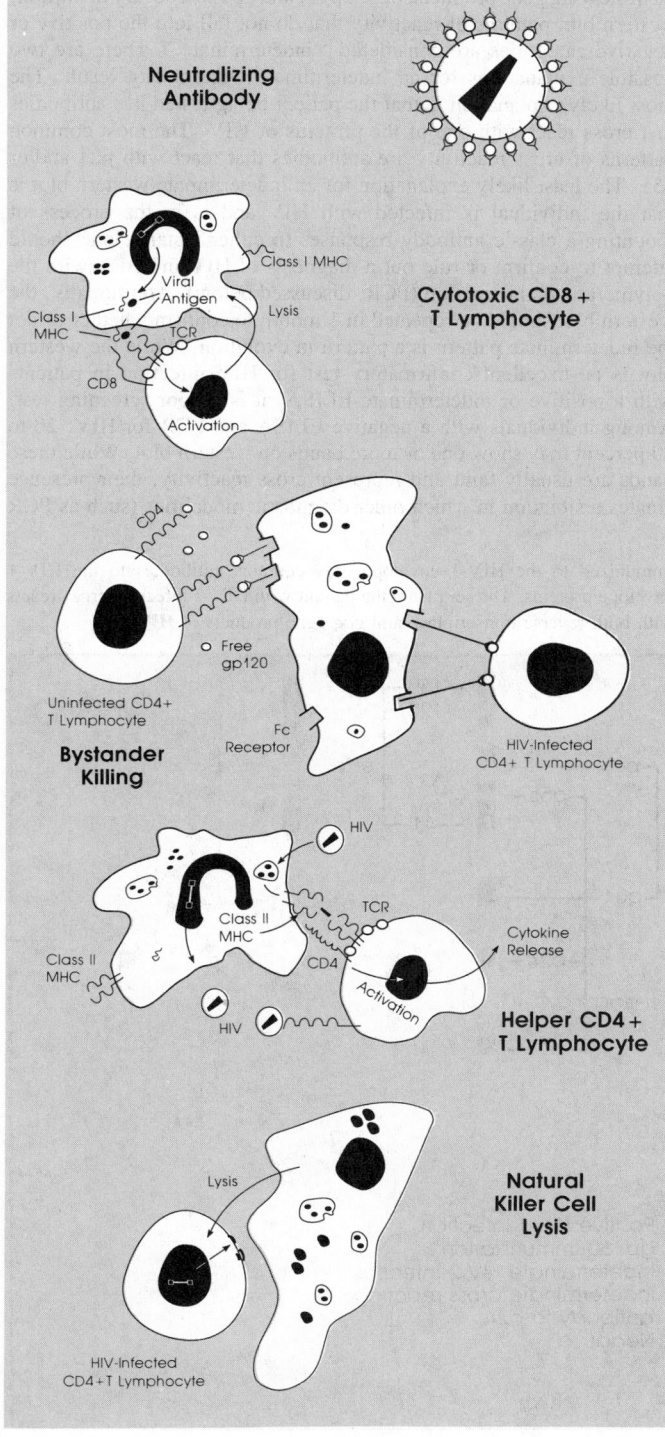

to be capable of facilitating infection of cells through an Fc receptor–mediated mechanism known as *antibody enhancement*. The same regions of the envelope protein of HIV that give rise to antibodies capable of mediating ADCC also elicit the production of antibodies that are capable of facilitating infection of uninfected cells. Additionally, it has been postulated that anti-gp120 antibodies participating in the ADCC killing of HIV-infected cells might also kill uninfected CD4 + T cells if the uninfected cells had bound free gp120 from the circulation, a phenomenon referred to as *bystander killing* (see above) (Fig. 279-13).

THE CELLULAR IMMUNE RESPONSE Given the fact that T cell–mediated immunity is known to play a major role in host defense against most viral infections (see Chap. 277), it is generally felt that this is an important component of the host immune response to HIV. T cell immunity can be divided into two major categories, that of the helper/inducer or CD4 + T cell and that of the cytotoxic/suppressor or CD8 + T cell. It has been very difficult to directly demonstrate the presence of HIV-specific CD4 + T cells in HIV-infected patients. This may be related to the fact that these cells, with their high affinity for binding to HIV-infected cells, may be among the first cells that are infected and destroyed during HIV infection. Nonetheless, through the use of computer modeling several regions of the HIV-1 envelope molecule have been identified that are structurally analogous to other known T cell epitopes by virtue of possessing structures known as *amphipathic helices*. Peptides from these envelope regions have been used to demonstrate the presence of T cells that are specific for these regions in the peripheral blood of HIV-infected individuals. Other studies have demonstrated that healthy, HIV-negative volunteers also possess T cells in their peripheral blood that react to the envelope proteins of HIV.

Classic, MHC class I–restricted, CD8 + cytotoxic T lymphocytes specific for HIV have been identified in the peripheral blood of HIV-infected patients. In this form of immunologic surveillance, CD8 + T lymphocytes, through their HIV-specific antigen receptors, bind to and cause the lytic destruction of HLA-identical cells expressing HIV antigens complexed with class I MHC molecules on the surface of the cell (Fig. 279-13). These cytotoxic T cells have been identified in the peripheral blood of HIV-infected individuals predominantly in the early stages of HIV infection with a relatively high precursor frequency of approximately 10 to 20 cytotoxic T cells per 10,000 peripheral blood mononuclear cells. Longitudinal studies have demonstrated that over time, paralleling the loss of CD4 + T lymphocytes, this element of specific host defense is lost, reenforcing the concept that the CD4 + T lymphocyte is an important element in maintaining antigen-specific cytotoxic T cell responses. Multiple HIV antigens appear capable of eliciting HIV-specific cytotoxic T cell responses and class I–restricted cytotoxic lymphocytes directed toward at least four of the HIV gene products, namely gag, envelope, polymerase, and nef have been identified.

In addition to classic, MHC-restricted cytotoxic T lymphocytes and the helper/inducer CD4 + T lymphocyte, at least three other forms of cell-mediated immunity to HIV have been described. These are CD8 + T cell–mediated inhibition, ADCC, and natural killer cell activity. CD8 + T cell–mediated inhibition refers to the ability of CD8 + T cells from an HIV-infected patient to inhibit the replication of HIV in tissue culture. This phenomenon requires that the T cells be from an HIV-infected individual; however, there is no requirement for HLA compatibility between the CD8 + T cells and the infected cells. It is likely that this effector mechanism is mediated by soluble factors expressed by activated CD8 + T lymphocytes. ADCC, as described above under humoral immunity, involves the killing of HIV-expressing cells by natural killer cells armed with specific antibody directed toward HIV antigens. Finally, natural killer cells alone have been shown capable of killing HIV-infected target cells in tissue culture systems. This primitive element of cytotoxic host defense, geared toward nonspecific surveillance of neoplastic transformation and viral infection, can also be enhanced by IL-2, similar to ADCC.

DIAGNOSIS AND LABORATORY MONITORING OF HIV INFECTION

Prior to the identification of HIV-1 as the causative agent of AIDS, a diagnosis of AIDS was made solely on clinical grounds. The establishment of HIV as the causative agent of AIDS and related syndromes early in 1984 was followed by the rapid development of sensitive screening tests for HIV infection and by March, 1985, blood donors in the United States were routinely being screened for antibodies to HIV (see above). At present a wide array of laboratory tests are available for both diagnosing and monitoring patients with HIV infection.

DIAGNOSIS OF HIV INFECTION The diagnosis of HIV infection is dependent upon the demonstration of antibodies to HIV and/or the direct detection of HIV or one of its components. As noted above, antibodies to HIV generally appear in the circulation 4 to 8 weeks following infection.

The standard screening test for HIV is the *enzyme-linked immuno-sorbent assay (ELISA)*. This solid-phase assay is an extremely good screening test, with a sensitivity of over 99.5 percent. Of note is the fact that the majority of diagnostic laboratories use a commercial ELISA kit that contains both HIV-1 and HIV-2 and thus either will be detected on routine screening. ELISA tests are generally scored as positive (highly reactive), negative (nonreactive), or indeterminate (partially reactive). While the ELISA is an extremely sensitive assay, it is not optimal with regard to specificity. In fact, in studies of low-risk individuals, such as volunteer blood donors, only 13 percent of ELISA-positive individuals actually had HIV infection. For this reason, anyone suspected of having HIV infection on the basis of an inconclusive or positive ELISA test must have that test result confirmed with a more specific assay.

The most commonly used confirmatory test is the *western blot* (Fig. 279-14). It takes advantage of the fact that multiple antigens of HIV, of different well-characterized molecular weights, elicit the production of specific antibodies. These antigens can be separated on the basis of molecular weight, and antibodies to each individual component can be detected as discrete bands on the western blot. A negative western blot is one in which no bands are present at molecular weights corresponding to HIV gene products. In a patient with a positive or indeterminate ELISA and a negative western blot, one can conclude with certainty that the ELISA reactivity was a false positive. On the other hand, a positive western blot, defined as one demonstrating antibodies to members of all three of the major gene products of HIV (*gag, pol,* and envelope proteins) is conclusive evidence of infection with HIV. In fact, according to most experts, as well as the criteria established by the Association of State and Territorial Public Health Laboratory Directors, a western blot can be considered positive for HIV-1 if it contains bands to at least two of the following gene products: p24, gp41, and gp120/160. By definition, western blot patterns of reactivity that do not fall into the positive or negative categories are considered "indeterminate." There are two possible explanations for an indeterminate western blot result. The most likely explanation is that the patient being tested has antibodies that cross react with one of the proteins of HIV. The most common patterns of cross reactivity are antibodies that react with p24 and/or p55. The least likely explanation for an indeterminate western blot is that the individual is infected with HIV and is in the process of mounting a classic antibody response. In either instance one should attempt to confirm or rule out a diagnosis of HIV infection with the polymerase chain reaction (PCR, discussed below). Additionally, the western blot should be repeated in 1 month to confirm whether or not the indeterminate pattern is a pattern in evolution. While the western blot is an excellent confirmatory test for HIV infection in patients with a positive or indeterminate ELISA, it is a poor screening test. Among individuals with a negative ELISA and PCR for HIV, 20 to 30 percent may show one or more bands on western blot. While these bands are usually faint and represent cross reactivity, their presence creates a situation in which other diagnostic modalities (such as PCR

FIGURE 279-14 *A.* Schematic representation of how a western blot is performed. *B.* Examples of patterns of western blot reactivity. In each instance the western blot strip contains antigens to HIV-1. The sera from the patient immunized to the HIV-1 envelope only contains antibodies to the HIV-1 envelope proteins. The sera from the patient with HIV-2 infection cross-reacts with both reverse transcriptase and *gag* gene products of HIV-1.

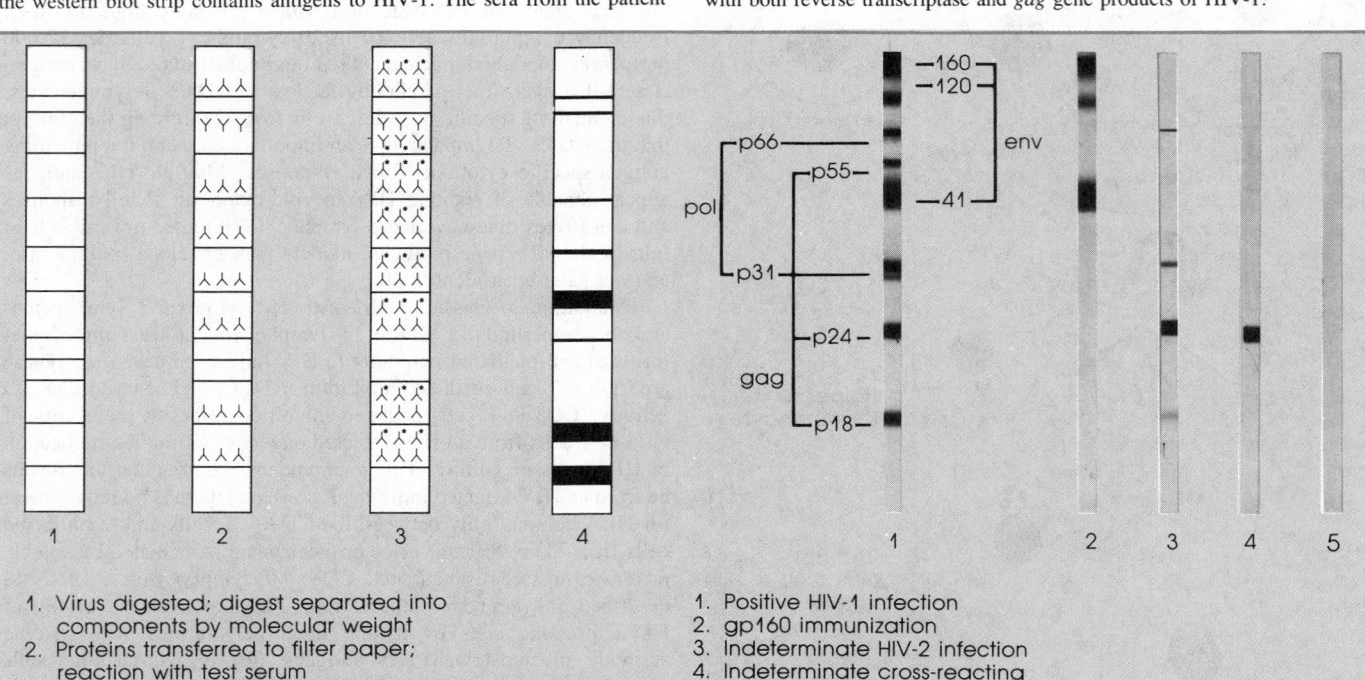

A
1. Virus digested; digest separated into components by molecular weight
2. Proteins transferred to filter paper; reaction with test serum
3. Enzyme-conjugated antihuman antibody added
4. Substrate added and color noted

B
1. Positive HIV-1 infection
2. gp160 immunization
3. Indeterminate HIV-2 infection
4. Indeterminate cross-reacting antibody to p24
5. Negative

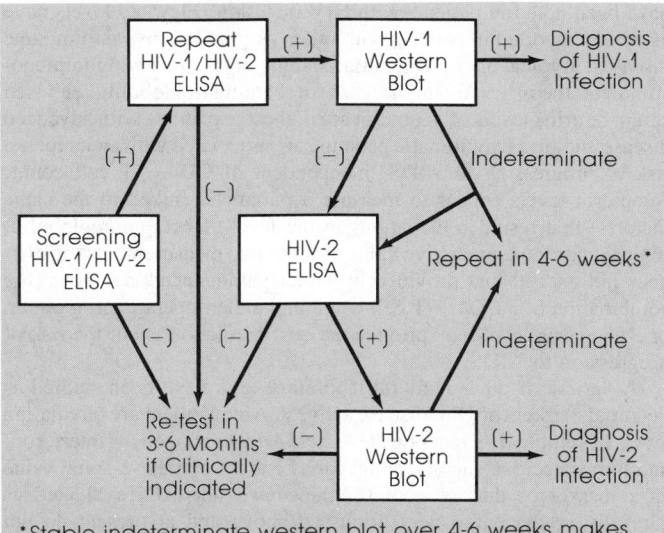

FIGURE 279-15 Algorithm for the use of serologic tests in the diagnosis of HIV-1 or HIV-2 infection.

or p24 antigen capture) must be employed to insure that the bands are not indicative of early HIV infection.

A guideline for the use of these serologic tests in attempting to make a diagnosis of HIV infection is depicted in Fig. 279-15. In a patient in whom HIV infection is suspected, the appropriate initial test is ELISA. If this is negative, unless one has a high suspicion of early HIV infection, such as an exposure within the previous 3 months, this result is sufficient to rule out the diagnosis and retesting should be performed only as clinically indicated. If the ELISA is indeterminate or positive, the test should be repeated. If the repeat is negative on two occasions, one can assume that the initial positive reading was due to a technical error in the performance of the assay and that the patient is negative. If the repeat is indeterminate or positive one should proceed to the western blot. If the western blot is positive, one has a diagnosis of HIV infection. If the western blot is negative, the ELISA can be assumed to have been a false positive and the diagnosis of HIV infection is ruled out. If the western blot is indeterminate one should proceed to the PCR with a repeat western blot in 1 month. If the PCR is negative and there is no progression in the western blot, a diagnosis of HIV is ruled out. If the PCR is positive and/or the western blot shows progression a diagnosis of HIV infection can be made.

A variety of other laboratory tests are available for the direct detection of HIV or its components. Although at present the ELISA and the western blot are the only licensed tests for making a diagnosis of HIV infection, many of these other tests are in common use in the research laboratory and are of considerable help when the western blot results are indeterminate. In addition, several of these direct measurements of HIV are currently being used to assess the antiviral activity of experimental therapies for HIV. The simplest of these is the *p24 antigen capture assay*. This is an ELISA-type assay in which the solid phase consists of antibodies to the p24 antigen of HIV. The viral protein p24 can be detected in the peripheral blood of HIV-infected individuals where it exists either as free antigen or complexed to anti-p24 antibodies. Overall, approximately 30 percent of individuals with HIV infection have detectable levels of free p24 antigen. This percentage increases to about 50 percent when samples are treated with a weak acid to dissociate antigen-antibody complexes prior to assay. Throughout the course of HIV infection an equilibrium appears to exist between p24 antigen and anti-p24 antibodies. During the first few weeks of infection, prior to the development of an

immune response, there is a brisk rise in p24 antigen levels. Following the development of anti-p24 antibodies these levels decline. Late in the course of infection, when circulating levels of free virus are high, p24 antigen levels also increase, particularly when detected by the use of techniques to dissociate antigen-antibody complexes. While the precise pathophysiologic significance of p24 antigenemia is unclear, it has been shown that for a group of asymptomatic patients with HIV infection and similar CD4+ T cell counts, those with detectable levels of p24 antigen are, on the average, three times more likely to show progression to AIDS than those in whom p24 antigen levels cannot be detected. Additionally, multiple clinical trials have demonstrated that patients receiving antiretroviral therapy will show a decline in their circulating levels of p24 antigen, and some have advocated the use of this assay for monitoring the effectiveness of such treatment. However, the validity of this recommendation has yet to be established. At present the p24 antigen capture assay seems to have its greatest utility as a screening test for HIV infection in patients suspected of having the acute HIV syndrome, and in whom high levels of p24 antigen are present prior to the development of antibodies.

The *direct cultivation of HIV* from plasma or peripheral blood mononuclear cells is a technique employed in many research laboratories and has proven very useful for monitoring the effects of experimental antiretroviral agents and generating isolates of HIV for studies of antiviral resistance and analysis of genomic drift. Most of the techniques employed involve cocultivation of patient material with an indicator cell line capable of supporting HIV replication, most commonly peripheral blood mononuclear cells that have been activated with phytohemagglutinin. When used as a clinical monitoring tool, the sample being studied (either cells or plasma) is serially diluted and an endpoint titration is determined. Cultures generally need to be maintained for up to 28 days, during which time they are periodically observed for the formation of syncytia or giant cells, and supernatants are sampled for the presence of HIV p24, using the antigen capture assays mentioned above. There is no role at present for HIV culture in the routine management of patients with HIV infection; however, such tests may become more common as one attempts to tailor antiretroviral therapy according to the sensitivities of patient-derived viral isolates.

The *polymerase chain reaction* is a diagnostic technique that has gained acceptance in many areas of clinical microbiology. Although the extreme sensitivity of this technique leads in many cases to false positives, in a well-controlled setting PCR has been of extraordinary value in furthering our understanding of the pathogenesis of HIV and has provided a true gold standard for the diagnosis of HIV infection. This is particularly true for the diagnosis of HIV infection in at-risk neonates. Two forms of PCR are used in the study of HIV infection, DNA PCR and RNA PCR. The DNA PCR is used for making a diagnosis of HIV infection by amplifying proviral DNA. In performing a DNA PCR test for HIV, peripheral blood mononuclear cells are lysed and the DNA region of interest is amplified utilizing primer pairs from relatively constant regions of the HIV genome. Primer pairs from both the *gag* and LTR regions are usually employed. The amplified DNA is then characterized utilizing nucleic acid hybridization techniques and, with the proper controls to check for contamination and success of amplification, it is possible to determine whether or not HIV proviral DNA is present at a frequency of one copy per 10,000 cells. Studies of this type have clearly documented that the interval between HIV infection and antibody positivity is on the order of 1 to 3 months.

In addition to being a diagnostic tool, DNA PCR is also useful for amplifying defined areas of proviral DNA for sequence analysis, and in this regard has become an important technique for studies of sequence diversity and microbial resistance to antiretroviral agents. RNA PCR has been used most frequently for monitoring changes in the level of the HIV genome present in plasma. In this technique, following DNAase treatment, a cDNA copy is made of all RNA species present in plasma. Insofar as HIV is an RNA virus (see above and Chap. 151), this will result in the production of DNA copies of HIV proportional to the amount of HIV present in plasma. This proviral cDNA is then amplified and characterized using the PCR technique employing primer pairs that can distinguish genomic cDNA from messenger cDNA. In the patient with a positive or indeterminate ELISA test and an indeterminate western blot and in the patient in whom serologic testing may be unreliable (such as in a patient with hypogammaglobulinemia), PCR is a valuable diagnostic tool for making a diagnosis of HIV infection. Given the cost and problems with contamination that can occur with PCR, however, its use as a diagnostic tool should be reserved for these instances where standard serologic testing has failed to give a definitive result.

LABORATORY MONITORING OF PATIENTS WITH HIV INFECTION The epidemic of HIV infection and AIDS has provided the clinician with new challenges in the integration of clinical and laboratory data. The close relationship between clinical manifestations of HIV infection and CD4+ T cell count has made this immunologic test an essential part of routine evaluation of HIV-infected individuals. In addition, other tests such as the p24 antigen capture assay (described above), serum neopterin, and serum beta$_2$microglobulin levels may also provide information of value to the clinician.

At present, the CD4+ T cell count is the only laboratory test generally accepted as a reliable indicator of the progression of HIV infection. This measurement, which is the product of the percent of CD4+ T cells (determined by flow cytometry) and the total lymphocyte count (determined by the WBC and differential) has been shown to correlate very well with clinical progression. Patients with CD4+ T counts under 200 per microliter are at high risk of infection with *Pneumocystis carinii* while patients with CD4+ T cell counts under 100 per microliter are at high risk of infection with CMV and *Mycobacterium avium-intracellulare* (MAI). Patients with an initial diagnosis of HIV infection should have CD4+ T cell measurements performed approximately every 6 months and more frequently if a declining trend is noted. Antiretroviral therapy is indicated when the CD4+ T cell count falls below 500 per microliter, and a declining CD4 count may provide an indication for changing therapy. Once the CD4 count is under 200 per microliter patients should be placed on a regimen for *Pneumocystis carinii* pneumonia (PCP) prophylaxis. All effective forms of antiretroviral therapy to date have been associated with causing at least a transient increase in either CD4+ T cell count or CD4 percent.

Beta$_2$ microglobulin is an 11kDa protein that is expressed on the surface of most nucleated cells. It forms a heterodimer with the class I MHC molecules and exhibits amino acid homology with the constant region of immunoglobulin. Free beta$_2$microglobulin can be measured in both serum and urine. Levels of beta$_2$microglobulin are elevated in a variety of conditions characterized by lymphocyte activation and/or lymphocyte destruction, among them lymphoproliferative syndromes, autoimmune disease, and viral infections, including HIV infection. In addition, beta$_2$microglobulin is excreted by the renal tubule, and levels may be elevated in patients with renal disease. Levels of beta$_2$microglobulin correlate with the degree of disease progression in patients with HIV infection. The highest levels are seen in patients with AIDS, the lowest levels in patients with asymptomatic HIV infection. Levels of beta$_2$microglobulin have a predictive value for progression to AIDS that is independent of their inverse relationship to CD4+ T cell counts. In one large study the level of serum beta$_2$microglobulin was the single most important predictor of development of AIDS. In another study, 34 percent of patients with a beta$_2$microglobulin level over 3.8 µg/mL went on to develop AIDS over a 3-year period compared to only 7 percent of patients with a beta$_2$microglobulin level under 2.9 µg/mL. Levels of beta$_2$microglobulin have been shown to decrease in a dose-dependent fashion in patients treated with zidovudine (AZT).

Neopterin (6-D-erythro-trihydroxypropylpterin) is a low-molecular-weight compound derived from an intermediate product of the de novo biosynthesis of tetrahydrobiopterin from guanosine triphosphate (GTP). It is produced by activated monocytes and increased levels have been noted in patients with HIV infection. Elevated levels have also been reported in patients with other viral infections, autoimmune diseases, atypical phenylketonuria, and in patients receiving immunostimulant therapy. As in the case of beta$_2$microglobulin, elevated serum or urine levels of neopterin are highest in patients with advanced disease and, in asymptomatic patients, are associated with an increased risk of progressing to AIDS, independent of CD4+ T cell count. Neopterin levels appear to measure a parameter linked to the same factor(s) that result in elevations in the level of beta$_2$microglobulin. In this regard, the predictive value of these two measurements together does not exceed that provided by either parameter alone. Thus, the combination of a CD4+ T cell count and either a beta$_2$microglobulin or a neopterin level may provide the best prediction about the risk of progression to AIDS.

A variety of other nonviral laboratory tests have been studied as potential markers of HIV disease activity. Among them are circulating levels of soluble IL-2 receptor, IgA, acid-labile endogenous interferon, and tumor necrosis factor. While each of these may have some value as a marker of disease activity, they have not been evaluated as carefully as the parameters discussed above and at present do not play a major role in the laboratory monitoring of patients with HIV-1 infection.

CLINICAL MANIFESTATIONS

The clinical consequences of HIV infection encompass a spectrum ranging from an acute syndrome associated with primary infection to a prolonged asymptomatic state to advanced disease. It is preferable to adopt the concept that HIV disease is manifested in various stages. As mentioned above, active virus replication and progressive immunologic impairment occur throughout the course of HIV infection, and so HIV disease actually progressses even during the clinically latent stage. HIV disease can be empirically divided on the basis of the degree of immunosuppression into an early stage (CD4+ T cell count greater than 500 per microliter), an intermediate stage (CD4+ T cell count between 200 and 500 per microliter), and an advanced stage (CD4+ T cell count less than 200 per microliter). Most AIDS-defining opportunistic infections and true malignancies occur within the advanced stage, while neurologic disease and Kaposi's sarcoma are not as strictly related to the level of immunosuppression. There are no recognized HLA associations with HIV infection or with the development of any particular manifestation of HIV disease. However, it has been reported that HLA-B35 is associated with an accelerated progression to AIDS (see Chap. 64). The two major classification systems for staging HIV infection are the CDC system (Table 279-9) and the Walter Reed Medical Center system (Table 279-10). Each has its own advantages and disadvantages, with the CDC system relying more on clinical condition for classification and the Walter Reed system relying more on immunologic status such as level of CD4+ T cell count and presence or absence of delayed cutaneous hypersensitivity. For the purposes of describing the clinical syndromes seen in patients with HIV infection, separate sections

---

TABLE 279-9   Centers for Disease Control classification system for HIV disease

Group I	Acute HIV syndrome
Group II	Asymptomatic infection
Group III	Persistent generalized lymphadenopathy
Group IV	Other diseases:
Subgroup A	Constitutional disease
Subgroup B	Neurologic disease
Subgroup C	Secondary infectious diseases
Subgroup D	Secondary neoplasms
Subgroup E	Other conditions

SOURCE: Modified from the Centers for Disease Control and Prevention, USPHS, 1986 and 1987.

TABLE 279-10 Walter Reed staging classification of HIV infection

Stage	HIV Antibody	Chronic lymphadenopathy	CD4 cells/mm³	DTH skin testing	Thrush	Opportunistic infections
WR0	−	−	>400	Normal (reactive to ≥2 skin test antigens)	−	−
WR1	+	−	>400	Normal	−	−
WR2	+	+	>400	Normal	−	−
WR3	+	+/−	<400	Normal	−	−
WR4	+	+/−	<400	Partial defect (reactive to 1 skin test antigen)	−	−
WR5	+	+/−	<400	Anergy and/or thrush (reactive to 0 skin test antigens)	−	
WR6	+	+/−	<400	Normal, partial defect or anergy	+/−	+

☐ absolute criteria required to be fulfilled for stage assignment

Abbreviations: + = present; − = absent; DTH = delayed type hypersensitivity
SOURCE: Modified from Redfield et al: The Walter Reed staging classification for HTLV-III/LAV infection. N Engl J Med 314:131, 1986.

will deal with the acute syndrome, the asymptomatic stage, early symptomatic disease, neurologic disease, secondary infections, neoplasms and organ-specific syndromes.

THE ACUTE HIV SYNDROME   It is estimated that approximately 50 to 70 percent of individuals with HIV infection experience an acute syndrome approximately 3 to 6 weeks following primary infection (Fig. 279-16). Varying degrees of clinical severity have been reported, and it has been suggested that symptomatic seroconversion may be prognostic of an increased risk for a more accelerated course. The typical clinical findings are listed in Table 279-11 and are accompanied by a burst of plasma viremia and p24 antigenemia. The syndrome is typical of an acute viral infection and has been likened to acute mononucleosis. Symptoms usually persist for 1 to 2 weeks and gradually subside as an immune response to HIV develops. Opportunistic infections have been reported during this stage of infection, presumably as a result of the transient immunosuppression. In this regard, a number of immunologic abnormalities accompany the acute HIV syndrome including multiphasic perturbations of the numbers of circulating lymphocyte subsets. Total lymphocyte and T cell subsets (CD4 and CD8) are initially reduced. An inversion of the

CD4+ to CD8+ T cell ratio occurs later because of a rise in the number of CD8+ T cells. The CD8+ T cell levels return to normal, but the CD4+ T cell levels remain somewhat depressed, resulting in the persistence of an abnormal ratio. Lymphadenopathy occurs in approximately 70 percent of people with symptomatic primary HIV infection. Lymph node biopsies show a reduction of extrafollicular B cells, CD8+ T cell follicular infiltration, and relatively little activation and proliferation of the germinal center cells. From 1 week to 3 months following the onset of symptoms, humoral and cellular immune responses are detected and coincide with the disappearance of symptoms and the decrease and/or disappearance of plasma viremia and p24 antigenemia. As mentioned above, the decrease in viremia is likely due to a combination of an immune clearance of virus and the sequestration of virus in the lymph nodes. Most patients recover spontaneously from this syndrome and are left with mild degrees of decrease in CD4+ T lymphocyte counts that may still remain within the normal range. However, an occasional patient will manifest a fulminant course of immunologic deterioration following primary infection even after disappearance of symptoms. In the vast majority of patients, primary infection, with or without the acute syndrome, is followed by a prolonged period of clinical latency.

THE ASYMPTOMATIC STAGE—CLINICAL LATENCY   Although the length of time from initial infection to the development of clinical disease (Table 279-9; Group IV) varies greatly from individual to

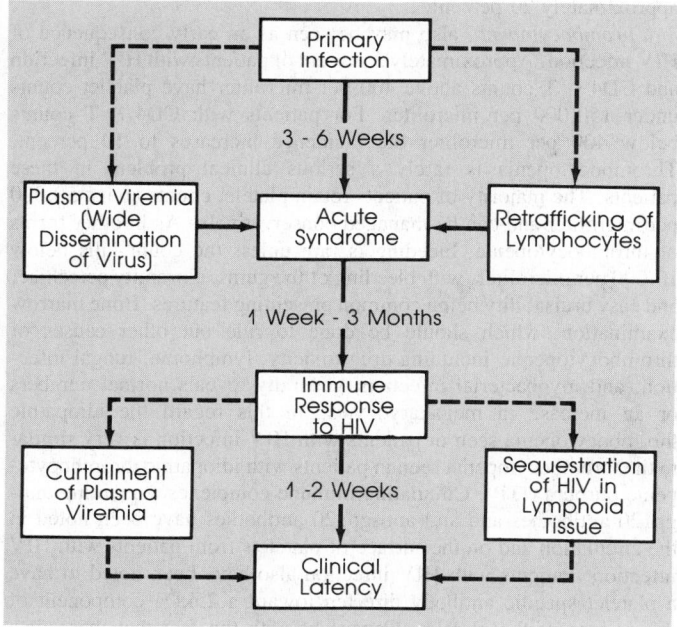

FIGURE 279-16   The acute HIV syndrome. See text for detailed description. (*From G Pantaleo et al, N Engl J Med 328:327, 1993.*)

TABLE 279-11 Clinical findings in the acute HIV syndrome*

GENERAL

Fever
Pharyngitis
Lymphadenopathy
Headache/retro-orbital pain
Arthralgias/myalgias
Lethargy/malaise
Anorexia/weight loss
Nausea/vomiting/diarrhea

NEUROPATHIC

Meningitis
Encephalitis
Peripheral neuropathy
Myelopathy

DERMATOLOGIC

Erythematous maculopapular rash
Mucocutaneous ulceration

* From B Tindal and DA Cooper.

individual, the median time is approximately 10 years for homosexual or bisexual men. This median time varies somewhat with the mode of infection, with IDUs generally having a more aggressive course than homosexual men and hemophiliacs. As emphasized above, HIV disease with active virus replication progresses during this asymptomatic period. Certain patients will remain entirely asymptomatic despite the fact that their CD4 + T cell counts fall to extremely low levels. Initial symptoms may be associated with the first manifestations of an opportunistic disease. Other patients experience varying degrees of intermittent symptoms such as malaise, lethargy, weakness, and anorexia which are not persistent enough to be categorized as constitutional disease (Table 279-9; Group IVA). Certain patients, otherwise asymptomatic, develop persistent generalized lymphadenopathy (Table 279-9; Group III) (see below). With few exceptions, there is a progressive diminution of CD4 + T cell counts during this asymptomatic period which ultimately leads to a state of immunosuppression that is severe enough (CD4 + T cell count <200 per microliter) to place the patient at high risk for opportunistic, and hence clinically apparent, disease.

EARLY SYMPTOMATIC DISEASE As noted above, viral replication continues and the immunologic function of the HIV-infected individual declines during the period of clinical latency. At some point in that decline, usually after the CD4 + T cell count has fallen below 500 cells per microliter, patients begin to develop signs and symptoms of clinical illness (Table 279-12). Many of these problems can be traced to minor opportunistic infections, not sufficiently indicative of a defect in cell mediated immunity to be considered an AIDS-defining illness, while some of them appear to be a direct effect of long-standing HIV infection. This stage of HIV infection has been given a variety of names in the past, among them *pre-AIDS* and *AIDS-related complex (ARC)*. These clinical findings, while indicative of a decline in immune function, are generally less predictive of the patient's overall status than are the data obtained from serial measurement of CD4 + T cell counts. At present antiretroviral therapy is indicated for patients in this group, particularly if their CD4 + T cell count is under 500 cells per microliter.

Generalized lymphadenopathy, defined as the presence of enlarged lymph nodes (>1 cm) in two or more extrainguinal sites for more than 3 months without an obvious cause, is often the earliest symptom of HIV infection following the acute syndrome. It is due to a marked follicular hyperplasia in response to HIV infection. In this condition the nodes are generally discrete and freely moveable. This feature of HIV disease, which may be seen at any point along the immunologic spectrum, is not associated with any increased likelihood of developing AIDS. Paradoxically, a loss in lymphadenopathy or a decrease in lymph node size may be a poor prognostic marker and indicative of disease progression. In the early and intermediate stages of HIV infection, as defined by CD4 + T cell counts above 200 per microliter, the main differential diagnosis is an adenopathic form of Kaposi's sarcoma. Late in the course of disease, one must extend the differential diagnosis to include mycobacterial infection, lymphoma, and bacillary angiomatosis. Lymph node biopsy is not indicated in early patients unless there are accompanying signs and symptoms of systemic illness such as fever and weight loss or if the nodes begin to enlarge, become fixed, or coalesce.

Oral lesions are particularly common during this phase of HIV infection. Among them are thrush, hairy leukoplakia, and aphthous

ulcers. Thrush, due to *Candida* infection, and oral hairy leukoplakia, presumed due to Epstein-Barr virus, are usually indicative of fairly advanced immunologic decline, generally occurring in patients with less than 300 CD4 + T cells per microliter. In one study, 59 percent of patients with oral candidiasis went on to develop AIDS over the next year. Thrush appears as a white, cheesy exudate, often on an erythematous mucosa (see Fig. A1-41). While most commonly seen on the soft palate, early lesions may be found along the gingival border. The diagnosis is made by direct examination of a scraping for pseudohyphal elements. Culturing is of no value insofar as the majority of patients with HIV infection will have a positive throat culture for *Candida* even in the absence of thrush. Oral hairy leukoplakia presents as a filamentous white lesion, generally along the lateral borders of the tongue (see Fig. A1-40). While usually more a sign of HIV-induced immunodeficiency than a clinical problem, severe cases have been noted to respond to therapy with acyclovir. Aphthous ulcers of the posterior oropharynx are also seen with regularity in patients with HIV infection. These lesions are of unknown etiology and can be quite painful and interfere with swallowing. Topical anesthetics are usually the best symptomatic treatment although the relief provided is of short duration. Recent reports that thalidomide may be of some help in this situation suggest that the pathophysiology may involve the action of tissue-destructive cytokines.

Reactivation herpes zoster or shingles (see Fig. A1-37) is seen in 10 to 20 percent of patients with HIV infection. This reactivation syndrome of varicella-zoster virus is an indication of modest decline in immune function and is often the first clnical indication of immunodeficiency. In one series, patients who developed shingles were noted to do so on the average of 5 years following HIV infection. In a cohort of patients with HIV infection, AIDS was noted to develop in 1 percent of the cohort per month following the diagnosis of localized zoster. In that study, AIDS was more likely to develop in those patients with severe pain, extensive disease, or disease involving cranial or cervical dermatomes. In patients who developed both shingles and oral hairy leukoplakia or thrush, shingles was noted to devleop approximately 1 year earlier. The clinical manifestations of reactivation zoster in HIV-infected patients, although indicative of immunologic compromise, are not as severe as that seen in other immunodeficient conditions. Thus, while lesions may extend over several dermatomes and frank cutaneous dissemination may be seen, visceral involvement has not been reported. In contrast to patients without a known underlying immunodeficiency, patients with HIV infection tend to have recurrences of zoster, with a relapse rate of approximately 20 percent.

Thrombocytopenia also may be seen as an early consequence of HIV infection. Approximately 3 percent of patients with HIV infection and CD4 + T counts above 400 per microliter have platelet counts under 150,000 per microliter. For patients with CD4 + T counts below 400 per microliter the incidence increases to 10 percent. Thrombocytopenia is rarely a serious clinical problem in these patients. The majority of patients retain platelet counts above 50,000 per microliter and can be managed conservatively. As in other forms of thrombocytopenia, bleeding is rare unless the count falls below 10,000 per microliter, with bleeding of the gums, extremity petechiae, and easy bruisability being common presenting features. Bone marrow examination, which should be done to rule out other causes of thrombocytopenia, including drug toxicity, lymphoma, fungal infection, and myobacterial infection, generally reveals normal numbers or an increase in megakaryocytes. In this regard the idiopathic thrombocytopenia seen in patients with HIV infection is very similar to the thrombocytopenia seen in patients with idiopathic thrombocytopenic purpura (ITP). Circulating immune complexes containing anti-gp120 antibodies and anti-anti-gp120 antibodies have been noted in the circulation and on the surface of platelets from patients with HIV infection. Patients with HIV infection also have been noted to have a platelet specific antibody directed toward a 25kDa component of the surface of the platelet. Consistent with the fact that these data

---

TABLE 279-12   Clinical characteristics of early symptomatic disease

Generalized lymphadenopathy
Thrush
Oral hairy leukoplakia
Shingles
Thrombocytopenia
Molluscum contagiosum

point to an immunologic basis for the thrombocytopenia seen in patients with AIDS, most of the therapeutic interventions that have been employed have been immune based. Either high dose intravenous immunoglobulin (IVIG) or glucocorticoids are capable of inducing transient increases in platelet counts; however, they do not generally provide long-term solutions. It has also been suggested that the thrombocytopenia in patients with HIV infection may be due to the direct effects of HIV on megakaryocytes, as evidenced by a decrease in platelet production. Consistent with this is the fact that the most effective medical approach to this problem has been the use of zidovudine. Even in patients without thrombocytopenia, therapy with zidovudine has been associated with a significant increase in platelet count and should be considered the treatment of choice for HIV-associated thrombocytopenia. Approximately 70 percent of patients with HIV-associated thrombocytopenia will have a satisfactory response to zidovudine. For patients with platelet counts below 20,000 per microliter the approach to therapy should be to initiate treatment with IVIG or glucocorticoids for an immediate response coupled with zidovudine for a more lasting response. Splenectomy is a viable option in patients refractory to medical management. The majority of patients with HIV-associated thrombocytopenia will respond to this surgical treatment. Because of the propensity to develop serious infections with encapsulated organisms, physicians should ensure that all patients with HIV infection, especially those about to undergo splenectomy, are immunized with pneumococcal polysaccharide. It should be noted that in addition to causing an increase in platelet count, removal of the spleen will result in an increase in total lymphocyte count, making determinations of total CD4+ T counts unreliable. In this situation one should rely on the CD4 percent for making diagnostic decisions with respect to the likelihood of opportunistic infections in the HIV-infected patient. Thrombocytopenia has also been reported in early HIV-infected patients as a consequence of classic thrombotic thrombocytopenic purpura (see Chap. 307). This clinical syndrome, consisting of fever, thrombocytopenia, hemolytic anemia, and neurologic and renal dysfunction is a rare complication of early HIV infection. As in other settings, the appropriate management is the use of salicylates and plasma exchange.

Miscellaneous clinical conditions frequently seen in patients with early stages of HIV infection include molluscum contagiosum, basal cell carcinomas of the skin, headache, condyloma acuminata, and recurrent bouts of oral or genital herpes simplex. In the past, unexplained fever, weight loss and diarrhea were included under the general heading of ARC. Many of these cases are now being diagnosed as specific opportunistic infections. In addition, this syndrome has been classified as an AIDS-defining illness in patients in whom no other diagnosis can be found, and is discussed below under generalized wasting.

NEUROLOGIC DISEASE Clinical disease of the nervous system accounts for a significant degere of morbidity in a high percentage of patients with HIV infection (Table 279-13). The neurologic problems that occur in the HIV-infected population may be primary to the overall pathogenic processes of HIV infection or may be secondary to opportunistic infections or neoplasms. Among the opportunistic infections and neoplasms that involve the central nervous system (CNS) are toxoplasmosis, cryptococcosis, progressive multifocal leukoencephalopathy, CMV, HTLV-I, mycobacterium tuberculosis, syphilis, and primary CNS lymphoma. These occur in about one-third of patients with AIDS and are discussed in more detail below under the various opportunistic infections and neoplasms. Primary processes related to HIV infection of the nervous system are somewhat similar to those seen with other lentiviruses such as the Visna-Maedi virus of sheep. Neurologic problems occur throughout the course of disease and may be inflammatory, demyelinating, or degenerative in nature. While only one of these, the AIDS dementia complex, is considered an AIDS-defining illness, most HIV-infected patients will have some neurologic problem during the course of their disease. As noted in the section on pathogenesis, damage to the CNS may be a direct result of viral infection of CNS macrophages or glial cells or

TABLE 279-13 Neurologic diseases in patients with HIV infection

OPPORTUNISTIC INFECTIONS

Toxoplasmosis
Cryptococcosis
Progressive multifocal leukoencephalopathy
Cytomegalovirus
Syphilis
Mycobacterium tuberculosis
HTLV-I

NEOPLASMS

Primary CNS lymphoma
Kaposi's sarcoma

PRIMARY HIV-1 INFECTION

Aseptic meningitis
AIDS dementia complex
Myelopathy
    Vacuolar myelopathy
    Pure sensory ataxia
    Paresthesia/dysesthesia
Peripheral neuropathy
    Acute demyelinating polyneuropathy
    Mononeuritis multiplex
    Distal symmetric polyneuropathy
Myopathy

secondary to the release of potentially toxic cytokines such as TNF and TGF-β. Virtually all patients with HIV infection have some degree of involvement of the nervous system with HIV. This is evidenced by the fact that cerebrospinal fluid (CSF) findings are abnormal in approximately 90 percent of patients, even at the asymptomatic stage of HIV infection. Included in these abnormalities are pleocytosis in 50 to 65 percent, isolation of virus in approximately 50 percent, elevated CSF protein in 35 percent, and evidence of intrathecal synthesis of anti-HIV antibodies in 89 percent. It should be pointed out, however, that evidence of CNS infection with HIV does not imply the presence of impairment of cognitive function, and while neurologic problems related to HIV infection can be seen at all stages of the illness, the mere presence of HIV infection in the CNS does not necessarily mean that the patient has a clinically relevant neurologic problem. In this regard the neurologic function of an HIV-infected individual should be considered normal unless clinical signs and symptoms suggest otherwise.

Aseptic meningitis may be seen throughout all but the very late stages of HIV infection. As noted above, in the setting of acute seroconversion patients may experience a syndrome of headache, photophobia, and, in some instances, frank encephalitis. CSF findings include a lymphocytic pleocytosis, elevated protein, and normal glucose. Cranial nerve involvement may be seen, predominantly cranial nerve VII, occasionally V, and/or VIII. This syndrome usually resolves spontaneously within 2 to 4 weeks; however, in some patients signs and symptoms may persist as a chronic problem. Such episodes may occur any time throughout the course of HIV infection; however, they become increasingly rare following the development of AIDS. This suggests that aseptic meningitis seen in the context of HIV infection is an immunologically mediated disease.

The AIDS dementia complex refers to a constellation of signs and symptoms of CNS disease that generally occurs late in the course of HIV infection (Table 279-14). As suggested by its name, a major feature of this entity is the development of dementia, which is defined as a decline in cognitive ability from a previously attained level. This may present as impaired ability to concentrate, increased forgetfulness, or increased difficulty performing complex tasks. Initially these symptoms may be indistinguishable from findings of situational depression or fatigue. In addition to dementia, patients with the AIDS dementia complex also may have motor and behavioral abnormalities.

TABLE 279-14   Clinical Staging of the AIDS Dementia Complex

Stage O (normal)	Normal mental and motor function.
Stage 0.5 (equivocal/subclinical)	Absent, minimal, or equivocal symptoms without impairment of work or capacity to perform activities of daily living (ADL). Mild signs (snout response, slowed ocular or extremity movements) may be present. Gait and strength are normal.
Stage 1 (mild)	Able to perform all but the more demanding aspects of work or ADL but with unequivocal evidence (signs or symptoms that may include performance on neuropsychological testing) of functional intellectual or motor impairment. Can walk without assistance.
Stage 2 (moderate)	Able to perform basic activities of self-care but cannot work or maintain the more demanding aspects of daily life. Ambulatory, but may require a single prop.
Stage 3 (severe)	Major intellectual incapacity (cannot follow news or personal events, cannot sustain complex conversation, considerable slowing of all output) or motor disability (cannot walk unassisted, usually with slowing and clumsiness of arms as well).
Stage 4 (end stage)	Nearly vegetative. Intellectual and social comprehension and output are at a rudimentary level. Nearly or absolutely mute. Paraparetic or paraplegic with urinary and fecal incontinence.

Adapted from JJ Sidtis and RW Price: Early HIV infection and the AIDS dementia complex. Neurology 40:197, 1990.

Among the motor problems are unsteady gait, poor balance, and difficulty with rapid alternating movements. Findings of increased tone and deep tendon reflexes may be present in patients with spinal cord involvement (see below). Late stages may be complicated by bowel and/or bladder incontinence. Behavioral problems include apathy and lack of initiative with progression to a vegetative state in some instances. In most instances these changes occur without significant changes in level of alertness, in contrast to the findings in patients with dementia due to toxic/metabolic encephalopathies.

The AIDS dementia complex is the initial AIDS-defining illness in approximately 10 percent of patients with HIV infection and thus rarely occurs prior to clinical evidence of immunodeficiency.

Clinically significant AIDS dementia complex eventually develops in approximately two-thirds of patients with HIV infection. As immunologic function declines, the risk and severity of the AIDS dementia complex increases. Autopsy series suggest that 80 to 90 percent of patients with HIV infection have histologic evidence of CNS involvement. Several classification schemes have been developed for grading AIDS dementia complex. The most commonly used clinical staging system is outlined in Table 279-14.

The precise cause of the AIDS dementia complex remains unclear although it is felt to represent the end result of the direct effects of HIV on the CNS. HIV has been demonstrated to be present in the brains of patients with AIDS dementia complex by Southern blot, in situ hybridization, and electron microscopy. Multinucleated giant cells, macrophages, and microglial cells appear to be the main cell types harboring virus in the CNS. Histologically, the major changes are seen in the subcortical areas of the brain and thus fit under the general category of subcortical dementia. In this regard AIDS dementia complex is similar to the dementia seen in patients with Parkinson's disease (see Chap. 371) and Huntington's chorea (see Chap. 370) and distinct from that seen in patients with Alzheimer's disease (see Chap. 370). Among the histopathologic changes are white matter pallor and gliosis, multinucleated giant cell encephalitis and vacuolar myelopathy. Less commonly, diffuse or focal spongiform changes in the white matter occur.

There are no specific criteria upon which a diagnosis of AIDS dementia complex rests, and thus this syndrome must be distinguished from a number of other diseases which affect the CNS of HIV-infected patients (Table 279-15). The diagnosis of dementia depends upon demonstrating a decline in cognitive function. This can be accomplished objectively with the use of the Mini-Mental Status Examination (Table 279-16) in patients for whom prior scores are available. For this reason it is advisable for all patients with a diagnosis of HIV infection to have a baseline Mini-Mental Status Examination. Imaging studies of the CNS, either computerized tomography (CT) or magnetic reasonance imaging (MRI), often demonstrate evidence of cerebral atrophy (Fig. 279-17). MRI also may reveal small areas of increased density of T2-weighted images, often referred to as "unidentified bright objects." While a lumbar puncture is an important element of the evaluation of patients with HIV infection and neurologic abnormalities, it is generally most helpful in the diagnosis of opportunistic infections. In AIDS dementia complex, patients may have an increase in CSF cells and protein; however, these findings are nonspecific, and the diagnosis is truly one that can be made only after opportunistic pathogens and neoplasms have been ruled out. While HIV is often able to be isolated from the

TABLE 279-15   Characterization of the most common central nervous system diseases in patients with HIV infection

Disease	Approximate incidence, %	Clinical features	Characteristic CSF findings	Characteristic radiologic findings
AIDS dementia complex	67	Personality changes, dementia, unsteady gait, seizures	Nonspecific	Cortical atrophy, ventricular dilatation, bright spots on T2-weighted MRI
Toxoplasmosis	15	Fever, headache, focal neurologic deficits, seizure + antibodies in 85%	Nonspecific	Multiple ring-enhancing lesions in multiple locations
Cryptococcal meningitis	6–12	Fever, nausea, vomiting, confusion, headache	Elevated protein, low glucose, positive crypto Ag/culture	Nonspecific
Progressive multifocal leukoencephalopathy virus	4	Multiple focal deficits without changes in level of consciousness	Nonspecific	Multiple white matter lesions on T2-weighted images
Neurosyphilis	1	Meningitis, neuroretinitis, deafness, focal neurologic deficits	VDRL	Nonspecific
Central nervous system	1	Seizure, focal neurologic deficits, headache	Nonspecific in 1°CNS lymphoma; malignant cells in systemic lymphoma	Single or few ring-enhancing lesions
Tuberculous meningitis	1	Fever, headache, confusion, meningitis, cough	Elevated protein, low glucose, pleocytosis, positive AFB smear/culture	Mass lesions in approximately 50%, abnormal chest x-ray

TABLE 279-16   The Folstein Mini-Mental Status Examination

Question	Scoring	Maximum Score
1 Where are (state, county, city, hospital, clinic)?	1 point for each	5
2 What are the (day, date, month, season, year, time)?	1 point for each	5
3 "Say these three words after me: (yellow, apple, Ohio)"	1 point for each	3
4 Ask patient to begin with 100 and count backwards by 7's. Or, if patient refuses, ask to spell "world" backwards.	Stop after 5, score no. correct. Or, 1 point for each correct letter	5
5 Recall the three words given in question no. 3.	1 point for each	3
6 Ask the patient to name "watch" then "pencil."	1 point for each	2
7 Ask the patients to repeat "No ifs, ands, or buts."	1 point if correct	1
8 Three-stage command: Take this paper in your right hand, fold it in half, and put it on the floor.	1 point for each correct	3
9 Ask the patient to read silently and obey the command (print in block letters): CLOSE YOUR EYES.	1 point if correct	1
10 Ask the patient to write a sentence.	1 point if it contains a subject and verb and makes sense (ignore spelling and grammar)	1
11 "Draw a clock with numbers and hands showing the time to be 8:20"	2 points if correct	2
12 Have the patient copy this design:	1 point if all sides and angles are preserved and if intersecting sides form a quadrangle.	1

CSF of these patients, this finding is not specific for AIDS dementia complex and, in fact, there appears to be no correlation between the presence of HIV in the CSF and the presence of AIDS dementia complex. Elevated levels of beta$_2$microglobulin, neopterin, and quinolinic acid (a metabolite of tryptophan reported to cause CNS injury) have been noted in the CSF of patients with AIDS dementia complex. These findings suggest that cytokines may be involved in the pathogenesis of this syndrome; however, at this time definitive evidence is still lacking.

While there is no specific treatment for the AIDS dementia complex, multiple reports suggest that treatment with antiretroviral agents may be of benefit. Improvement in neuropsychiatric tests have been noted for both adult and pediatric patients treated with either zidovudine or didanosine. In fact, the rapid symptomatic improvement in cognitive function noted with the initiation of antiretroviral therapy suggests that at least some component of this problem is quickly

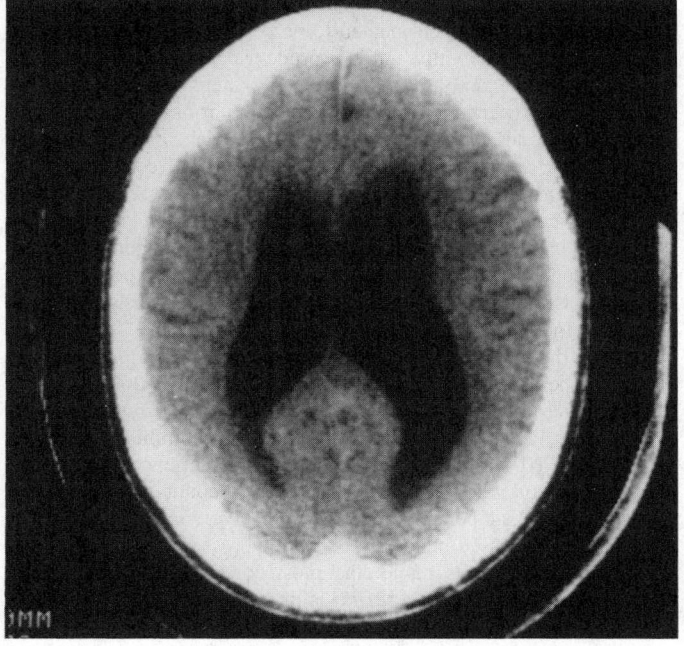

FIGURE 279-17   Computed tomogram of the central nervous system of a patient with AIDS dementia complex. CT demonstrates cortical thinning and dilatation of the ventricles.

reversible, again supporting at least a partial role of soluble mediators in the pathogenesis.

It should also be noted that these patients have an increased sensitivity to the side effects of neuroleptic drugs. The use of these drugs for symptomatic treatment is associated with an increased risk of extrapyramidal side effects, thus requiring that patients with AIDS dementia complex who receive these agents be monitored carefully.

Seizures are a relatively frequent complication of HIV infection and may be seen as a consequence of opportunistic infections, neoplasms, or AIDS dementia complex (Table 279-17). Seizures are seen in 15 to 40 percent of patients with cerebral toxoplasmosis, 15 to 35 percent of patients with primary CNS lymphoma, 8 percent of patients with cryptococcal meningitis, and 7 to 50 percent of patients with AIDS dementia complex. Seizures may also be seen in patients with CNS tuberculosis, aseptic meningitis, and progressive multifocal leukoencephalopathy. Seizures may be the presenting clinical symptom of HIV disease. In one study of 100 patients with HIV infection presenting with a first seizure, cerebral mass lesions were the most common cause, responsible for 32 of 100 new onset seizures. Of these 32, 28 were due to toxoplasmosis and 4 to lymphoma. AIDS dementia complex accounted for an additional 24 new-onset seizures. Cryptococcal meningitis was the third most common diagnosis, responsible for 13 of the 100 seizures. In 23 cases, no cause could be found and it is possible that these represent a subcategory of the AIDS dementia complex. Thus, the AIDS dementia complex may be the single leading cause of seizures in patients with HIV infection. Of these 23 cases, 16 (70 percent) had two or more seizures, suggesting that anticonvulsant therapy is indicated in all patients with HIV infection and seizure unless a rapidly correctable cause is noted. In this regard, while phenytoin remains the initial treatment of choice, hypersensitivity reactions to this drug have been reported in over 10 percent of patients with AIDS, and therefore the use of phenobarbital or valproic acid must be considered as alternatives.

TABLE 279-17   Leading causes of seizures in patients with HIV infections

Disease	Overall contribution to seizures
AIDS dementia complex	24–47%
Cerebral toxoplasmosis	28%
Cryptococcal meningitis	13%
Primary central nervous system lymphoma	4%
Progressive multifocal leukoencephalopathy	1%

From DM Holtzman et al.

Spinal cord disease is present in approximately 20 percent of patients with AIDS, often as part of the AIDS dementia complex. In fact, 90 percent of the patients with HIV-associated myelopathy have some evidence of dementia, suggesting that similar pathologic processes may be responsible for both conditions. Three main types of spinal cord disease, or myelopathy, are seen in patients with AIDS. The first of these is a vacuolar myelopathy as discussed above under AIDS dementia complex. This is pathologically similar to subacute combined degeneration of the cord such as occurs with pernicious anemia. Although B_{12} deficiency is common in patients with AIDS, it does not appear to be responsible for the cord disease seen in these patients, given the fact that there is no response to treatment with parenteral B_{12}. Vacuolar myelopathy is characterized by a subacute onset and often presents with gait disturbances, predominantly ataxia and spasticity. This may progress to include bladder and bowel dysfunction. Physical findings include evidence of increased deep tendon reflexes and extensor plantar responses. The second form of spinal cord disease involves the dorsal columns and presents as a pure sensory ataxia. The third form is also sensory in nature and presents with paresthesias and dysesthesias of the lower extremities. In contrast to the cognitive problems seen in patients with the AIDS dementia complex these spinal cord syndromes do not generally respond to therapy with antivirals and therapy is mainly supportive. Other diseases involving the spinal cord in patients with HIV infection include HTLV-I–associated myelopathy (HAM) (see Chap. 151), neurosyphilis (see Chap. 133), herpesvirus infections (varicella-zoster, simplex, and CMV) (see Chaps. 143 and 144), tuberculosis (see Chap. 130), and lymphoma (see Chap. 311).

Peripheral neuropathies are common in patients with HIV infection; they occur at all stages of illness and take a variety of forms. Early in the course of HIV infection, an acute inflammatory demyelinating polyneuropathy resembling Guillain-Barré syndrome may occur (see Chap. 373). Patients commonly present with progressive weakness, areflexia, and minimal sensory changes. CSF examination reveals a pleocytosis, and peripheral nerve biopsy demonstrating a perivascular infiltrate suggesting an autoimmune etiology. Although generally a self-limited disease, in severe cases plasma exchange, intravenous immunoglobulin, or systemic glucocorticoids have been tried and have been reported to have variable degrees of success. Because of the immunosuppressive effect of glucocorticoids, they should be reserved for severe cases refractory to other measures. Another autoimmune peripheral neuropathy seen in patients with AIDS is mononeuritis multiplex (see Chap. 291). This necrotizing arteritis generally occurs in patients with moderate degrees of immunosuppression and may be managed as outlined above. However, the most common peripheral neuropathy in patients with HIV infection is a distal, symmetric, painful polyneuropathy generally seen only in patients with advanced HIV infection and AIDS. Although it is present clinically in only 30 to 40 percent of patients, two-thirds of patients with AIDS may be shown by electrophysiologic studies to have some evidence of peripheral nerve disease. This polyneuropathy, which is felt to be due to HIV-mediated axonal degeneration, most often presents as bilateral painful burning sensations in the feet and lower extremities. Antiretrovirals have been of little benefit in the management of this problem. Therapy is predominantly symptomatic through the use of tricyclics and analgesics. There are two important entities in the differential diagnosis of peripheral neuropathy in the HIV-infected patient. The first is CMV-associated progressive polyradiculopathy. This entity is generally fulminant in onset, with lower extremity and sacral paresthesias, difficulty in walking, areflexia, ascending sensory loss, and urinary retention. CSF examination reveals a predominantly neutrophilic pleocytosis. Therapy with ganciclovir or foscarnet can lead to rapid improvement. The second entity is dideoxynucleoside-associated peripheral neuropathy. This painful complication of either didanosine, zalcitabine, or stavudine therapy is most commonly seen at high doses and usually resolves following discontinuation of therapy. It is discussed in more detail below.

Myopathy may also complicate the course of HIV infection.

Among the causes of myopathy in the setting of HIV infection are HIV itself, zidovudine, and the generalized wasting syndrome (see below). HIV-associated myopathy may range in severity from asymptomatic elevation in creatine kinase to a subacute syndrome characterized by proximal muscle weakness and myalgias. Quite pronounced elevations in creatine kinase may occur in asymptomatic patients, particularly following exercise. The clinical significance of this finding is unclear. A variety of both inflammatory and non-inflammatory pathologic processes have been noted in patients with more severe myopathy including myofiber necrosis with inflammatory cells, nemaline rod bodies, cytoplasmic bodies and mitochondrial abnormalities. Profound muscle wasting may be seen after prolonged zidovudine therapy. This toxic side effect of the drug appears to be related to its ability to interfere with the function of mitochondrial polymerases and is reversible following discontinuation of treatment.

SECONDARY INFECTIONS   Secondary infections are a late complication of HIV infection, for the most part occurring in patients with less than 200 CD4 cells per microliter. While characteristically caused by opportunistic organisms, such as *Pneumocystis carinii,* CMV, and other organisms that do not ordinarily cause disease in the absence of a compromised immune system, the spectrum of serious secondary infections that may be seen in patients with HIV infection also includes common bacterial and mycobacterial pathogens. Secondary infections are the leading cause of morbidity and mortality in patients with HIV infection. Approximately 80 percent of AIDS patients die as a direct result of an infection other than HIV, with infections due to opportunistic organisms heading the list. The clinical spectrum of diseases caused by secondary infections is constantly changing as patients live longer, and as new and better approaches to treatment and prophylaxis are developed.

Protozoal infections   *Pneumocystis carinii* (see Chap. 178) is one of the most common infections in patients with HIV infection; however, with the development of effective prophylactic regimens its incidence and relative contribution to morbidity and mortality have been decreasing. Approximately 70 to 80 percent of patients with HIV infection will experience at least one bout of *Pneumocystis carinii* pneumonia (PCP) at some time during the course of their disease and PCP is listed as the immediate cause of death in 15 to 20 percent of patients dying with AIDS. Depending upon the severity, the probability of death from a single episode of PCP varies from 10 to 50 percent. As a result of the AIDS epidemic PCP has become an increasing cause of community-acquired pneumonia. While the mode of transmission is unclear, infections with PCP probably represent reactivation of latent infection or failure of host defense mechanisms to combat a ubiquitous inhabitant of the environment. Nonetheless, in the hospital environment person-to-person spread of infection has been suggested anecdotally and it is prudent not to place a patient at risk for PCP (for example an HIV-infected patient with less than 200 CD4 + T cells per microliter) in the same room with someone suffering from an acute episode of PCP. The risk of infection with *Pneumocystis carinii* increases as the CD4 + T cell count declines. In this regard, in the patient with HIV infection, PCP is most commonly seen in patients who have experienced a previous bout of PCP and in patients who have under 200 CD4 + T cells per microliter. In the absence of PCP prophylaxis, following a primary bout of PCP, 31 percent will experience a second bout within 6 months, 66 percent within 12 months. For patients with over 200 CD4 + T cells per microliter, the attack rate for PCP is approximately 0.5 percent over a 6-month period. In contrast, for patients with under 200 CD4 + T cells per microliter the attack rate is 8 percent over 6 months and 18 percent over 12 months. For this reason, it is recommended that all patients with HIV infection who have either experienced a previous bout of PCP or who have a CD4 + T cell count under 200 per microliter (or CD4 percent under 15), receive some form of PCP prophylaxis (discussed below).

As suggested by its name, the most common manifestation of infection with *Pneumocystis carinii* is pneumonia. Patients generally present with fever and a cough that is usually nonproductive or productive of only scant amounts of white sputum. They may complain of a characteristic retrosternal chest pain that is usually worse on inspiration and described as either sharp or burning. In more severe cases, patients usually note dyspnea on exertion, fatigue, and weight loss. In stark contrast to PCP in the non-HIV setting, which is often a fulminant disease with patients usually presenting within 5 days of the onset of symptoms, HIV-associated PCP may have an indolent course characterized by weeks of vague symptoms prior to presentation or diagnosis. PCP should be included in the differential diagnosis of fever, pulmonary symptoms, or unexplained weight loss in any patient with HIV infection and less than 200 CD4 + T cells per microliter. Findings on physical examination are minimal. The usual findings for pneumonia are not present. Breath sounds are usually clear; however, they may be slightly diminished. While occasional rhonchi or wheezes may be heard, especially in patients with some other underlying pulmonary disease, findings of consolidation are usually absent. Chest x-ray may reveal a variety of patterns; however the most common finding is either a normal film, if the disease is suspected early, or a faint bilateral interstitial infiltrate. The classic finding of a dense, perihilar infiltrate described in patients with non-HIV–associated PCP is rarely seen in patients with AIDS. In patients with PCP who have been receiving aerosolized pentamidine for prophylaxis one may see a chest x-ray pattern with upper lobe cavitary disease, reminiscent of tuberculosis. Other less common findings on chest film include lobar infiltrates and pleural effusions.

PCP is complicated by pneumothorax in approximately 2 percent of cases. Pneumothorax is more common in patients with prior episodes of PCP and in patients who have received aerosolized pentamidine for prophylaxis, presumably due to the increased propensity for these patients to have apical cavitary disease. The mortality for patients with PCP-associated pneumothorax is approximately 10 percent and aggressive medical (sclerotherapy) and/or surgical intervention may be required.

The laboratory evaluation is usually of little help in the differential diagnosis of PCP. A mild leukocytosis is common; however, given the fact that HIV-infected patients generally have leukopenia with baseline WBC values in the range of 1500 to 3000 cells per microliter, a WBC on the order of 4000 to 6000 per microliter may represent an elevation. The serum LDH is often elevated, and arterial blood gases may indicate hypoxemia with a decline in Pa_{O_2} and an increase in the arterial-alveolar (a–A) gradient. Indeed, arterial blood gases not only aid in making the diagnosis of PCP but also provide important information for staging the severity of the disease and directing treatment (see below and Chap. 178).

A definitive diagnosis of PCP requires demonstration of the trophozoite or cyst forms of the organisms in samples obtained from induced sputum, bronchoalveolar lavage, transbronchial biopsy, or open lung biopsy (see Chap. 178). The diagnosis may be somewhat more difficult in patients who have been receiving aerosolized pentamidine for PCP prophylaxis insofar as the burden of organisms may be reduced. In this setting, the diagnostic yield from induced sputum decreases from 92 percent to 64 percent while the yield from bronchoalveolar lavage drops from 95 percent to 80 percent. More recently, PCR has been used in an attempt to identify specific DNA sequences for *Pneumocystis carinii* in clinical specimens. This technique may provide somewhat better sensitivity that that obtained through histologic staining. The differential diagnosis of PCP in patients with HIV infection includes CMV pneumonia, fungal pneumonia, nonspecific interstitial pneumonitis, tuberculosis and Kaposi's sarcoma (see below).

In addition to pneumonia, a number of other clinical problems have been reported in the HIV-infected patient as a result of infection with *Pneumocystis carinii*. Most of these reports, with the exception of otic disease, involve patients receiving aerosolized pentamidine as prophylaxis for PCP. This form of prophylaxis, while quite effective in preventing PCP, is ineffective in preventing disease outside the lung. *Pneumocystis carinii* appears capable of hematogenous spread and of seeding a variety of organ systems as well as causing a primary infection of the ear (Table 279-18). These "extrapulmonary" manifestations of *Pneumocystis carinii* occur in approximately 2.5 to 5.0 percent of patients with HIV infection.

Otic involvement with *Pneumocystis carinii* is most commonly seen as a primary infection, i.e., in patients with no evidence of pulmonary disease. It usually presents as a unilateral polypoid mass that involves the external auditory canal. It may also involve the middle ear and may extend to the mastoid, resulting in radiographic abnormalities on plain films of the skull. Patients often complain of ear pain and decreased hearing. Perforation of the tympanic membrane has been reported in over half of the cases. In contrast, most of the other extrapulmonary forms of pneumocystis are seen in patients with a history of PCP. Most common in this group are ophthalmic lesions of the choroid that are usually noted on routine examination or in the context of evaluation for CMV retinitis. Multiple, bilateral lesions 0.5 to 2 disc diameters in size that appear as slightly elevated yellow-white plaques are generally seen. They are usually asymptomatic and are often confused with the cotton wool spots of the retina that are associated with HIV infection. *Pneumocystis carinii* has been reported to cause a necrotizing vasculitis that resembles Buerger's disease, bone marrow hypoplasia, and intestinal obstruction. Among the other organ systems involved have been the lymph nodes, spleen, liver, kidney, pancreas, pericardium, heart and adrenals. Of note has been the presentation of disease in either liver, kidney, or spleen which is generally asymptomatic; however, it can be associated with cystic lesions that appear calcified on CT or ultrasound.

A variety of therapeutic options are available for the patient with PCP or disseminated pneumocystis (Table 279-19) (see Chap. 178). The gold standard for therapy at present is trimethoprim/sulfamethoxazole which is effective in approximately 90 percent of patients. Trimethoprim/sulfamethoxazole is available in both intravenous and oral forms. The major disadvantage to this therapy is the relatively high incidence of side effects. In contrast to the non-HIV population where a 10 percent incidence of side effects is seen, there is a 50 to 65 percent incidence of side effects in the HIV-infected population. These include rash, fever, leukopenia, thrombocytopenia, and hepatitis, and although therapy need not be stopped when these occur, it is important to remain vigilant for more serious hypersensitivity reactions such as Stevens-Johnson syndrome. In addition, it may be advisable to withhold other myelotoxic drugs such as zidovudine and ganciclovir during therapy with trimethoprim/sulfamethoxazole. In patients with mild disease, side effects may be minimized by slightly reducing dosage. Ideally, treatment with trimethoprim/sulfamethoxazole or the other agents mentioned below should be continued for 21 days. It should be noted that in contrast to many other infections in which one expects a stabilization, if not improvement, in clinical course wiithin 24 to 48 hours of initiation of appropriate antimicrobial therapy, patients with PCP often do not begin to improve until the end of the first week. In fact, during the first 5 days of treatment, particularly in moderate to severe cases, there is often a worsening of the patient's condition, presumably secondary to the inflammatory response resulting from the death of large numbers of organisms in the lung. This inflammatory response and its adverse clinical consequences can be markedly reduced by the adjunct use of

TABLE 279-18 Extrapulmonary manifestations of *Pneumocystis carinii* infection in patients with HIV infection

Acute otitis
Retinitis
Visceral cystic calcifications
Necrotizing vasculitis
Intestinal obstruction
Lymphadenopathy
Bone marrow involvement
Ascites
Thyroiditis

TABLE 279-19   Manifestations and treatment of secondary infections in patients with HIV disease

Infecting Agent	Manifestations	Treatment	Prophylaxis	Drug Toxicities	Comment
Pneumocystis carinii			TMP/SMX 1 DS daily Aerosolized pentamidine 300 mg/month	Rash, fever, neutropenia Bronchospasm	Begin once CD4+ T cell count <200/μL or CD4% <15
	Mild to moderate pneumonia [Pa$_{O_2}$≥70 mm Hg and (A-a)dO$_2$≤35] mmHg	TMP/SMX 15–20 mg/kg/d PO		Rash, fever, neutropenia	Treat for 21 d if possible, no less than 14 d
		TMP 20 mg/kg/d PO + dapsone 100 mg PO qd		Methemoglobinemia	Contraindicated in patients with G6PD deficiency
		Clindamycin 600 mg PO q6h + primaquine 15 mg PO qd		C. difficile colitis Rash, neutropenia	Contraindicated in patients with G6PD deficiency
		Intravenous pentamidine 3–4 mg/kg/d		Nephritis, pancreatitis, hypoglycemia, diabetes	
		Aerosolized pentamidine 300 mg/d		Bronchospasm	Provides no systemic effects. Not recommended but an option for multidrug allergic pt with mild pneumonia
	Severe pneumonia [Pa$_{O_2}$≤70mmHg or (A-a)dO$_2$≤35mmHg]	TMP/SMX 15–20 mg/kg/d IV initially (total course 14–21 d)		Rash, fever, leukopenia, thrombocytopenia, hepatitis	Prednisone, 40 mg bid for 2 d, then 40 mg/d for 5 d, then 20 mg/d to the end of therapy (21 d total) added to specific antimicrobial ASAP and no later than 36 h after diagnosis
		Pentamidine 3–4 mg/kg/d IV for 14–21 d		Nephritis, pancreatitis, hypoglycemia, diabetes	
		Clindamycin 900 mg IV q8h then 450 mg PO q6h + primaquine 30 mg PO qd for total of 14–21 d		C. difficile colitis Rash, neutropenia	Contraindicated in patients with G6PD deficiency
		Atovoquone 250 mg PO q6h for 14–21 d		Skin rash, neutropenia	For patients intolerant of other regimes. Less effective than standard therapy.
		Trimetrexate (dose from manufacturer)		Skin rash, neutropenia	Available only through treatment IND: call 1-800-TRIALSA. Bone marrow suppressive effects blunted by use of leucovorin
		Eflornithine (DFMO) 100 mg/kg IV q6h for 14 d followed by 75 mg/kg PO q6h for 4–6 weeks		Thrombocytopenia	1-800-TRAILSA for information
	Disseminated disease	Any of the systemic therapies outlined above			
Toxoplasma gondii			TMP/SMX 1 DS qd	Rash, fever neutropenia	More specific regimens under study
	Encephalitis, brain abscess, chorioretinitis, myocarditis	Sulfadiazine 1–2 g PO qid + pyrimethamine 25–100 mg qd		Crystalluria, rash Rash, fever, neutropenia	Treatment is generally for life. Leucovorin to minimize bone marrow suppression
		Clindamycin initially 200–400 mg IV q6h + pyrimethamine 25–100 mg qd followed by clindamycin 300–900 mg PO q8h + pyrimethamine 25–100 mg qd		C. difficile colitis Rash, fever, neutropenia	Leucovorin to minimize bone marrow suppression
		Atovoquone 250 mg PO q6h + pyrimethamine 25–100 mg qd		Rash, fever, neutropenia	Leucovorin to minimize bone marrow suppression
		Macrolides (clarithromycin or azithromycin)			Early results disappointing
Isospora belli	Diarrhea	TMP/SMX 10 mg/kg/d PO for 10 d then 1/2 dose for 3 months		Rash, fever, neutropenia	
Cryptosporidia/ Microsporidia	Diarrhea	No known specific therapy, supportive measures include somatostatin, parenteral nutrition			

TABLE 279-19   Manifestations and treatment of secondary infections in patients with HIV disease (Continued)

Infecting Agent	Manifestations	Treatment	Prophylaxis	Drug Toxicities	Comment
M. avium intracellulare			Rifabutin 100 mg PO qd		Begin prophylaxis once CD4+ T cell count <100/µL
	Disseminated disease that may involve lung, bone marrow, liver	Ethambutol 15 mg/kg qd + clofazimine 100 mg PO qd + ciprofloxicin 750 mg PO qd + macrolide (azithromycin or clarithromycin)		Hepatitis, neuropathy (peripheral/optic) Darkening of skin, hepatitis	Treatment is generally for life
Mycobacterium tuberculosis	Asymptomatic, PPD+	Isoniazid, 15 mg/kg up to 900 mg PO twice a week or 300 mg, PO daily for 1 y		Hepatitis	
	Active disease	Isoniazid, 300 mg PO × 1 y + rifampin 600 mg PO qd × 1 y + pyrazinamide 30 mg/kg/d in 2 doses		Hepatitis Hepatitis Hepatitis	Treat with 3 drugs for 2 months. If isolate is sensitive to isoniazid and rifampin then switch to those 2 drugs. Treat 9 months and at least 6 months after third negative culture.
	Active disease in a setting when there is a possibility of multidrug resistance	Add ethambutol 15–25 mg/kg/d and streptomycin or amikacin for active disease		Neuropathy (peripheral/optic) Nephrotoxicity, hearing loss	Quinolones may also be considered as a fifth drug
Candida albicans			Fluconazole 200 mg PO qd	Hepatotoxicity	Begin once CD4+ cell count <100/µL
	Thrush, vaginitis	Clotrimiazole troches, nystatin Fluconazole 200 mg PO qd		Hepatotoxicity	Treatment is generally prn (as needed)
	Esophagitis	Fluconazole 200 mg PO qd for 7–14 days Amphotericin B 0.25 mg/kg/d IV for 7–10 days		Hepatotoxicity Nephrotoxicity, fever/chills	
Crytoptococcus neoformans			Fluconazole 100–200 mg PO qd	Hepatotoxicity	Begin prophylaxis if CD4+ T cell count < 100/µL
	Meningitis, brain abscess, penumonia, disseminated disease	Amphotericin B 0.3 mg/kg/d IV + flucytosine 150 mg/kg/d PO for 6 weeks followed by fluconazole 100–200 mg PO qd indefinitely		Nephrotoxicity, fever/chills Bone marrow suppression Hepatotoxicity	Approximately 50% will need to have flucytosine held during therapy due to neutropenia. An alternative is amphotericin B alone at a dose of 0.8 mg/kg/d.
Histoplasma encapsulatum	Disseminated disease, pneumonia	Amphotericin B 0.6–1 mg/kg/d to a total 1 g then itraconazole 200 mg qd indefinitely		Nephrotoxicity, fever/chills Hepatitis	
Cytomegalovirus	Retinitis, esophagitis, colitis and pneumonia	Ganciclovir 5 mg/kg q12h for 14 d followed by 5 mg/kg qd IV indefinitely Foscarnet 60 mg/kg q8h for 14 d followed by 90–120 mg/kg qd IV indefinitely		Neutropenia Interstitial nephritis, seizure, hypocalcemia	Neutropenia may be ameliorated by colony stimulating factors Should be preceded by saline infusion
Herpes simplex	Recurrent perioral, perirectal, or genital ulcers	Acyclovir 200–400 mg PO 5id as needed			Foscarnet 60 mg/kg q8h × 14 d for patients with acyclovir-resistant herpes simplex or zoster
	Esophagitis; acute retinal necrosis	Acyclovir 5 mg/kg IV q8h for 10–14 days			
Herpes zoster	Cutaneous (local or disseminated); retinal necrosis	Acyclovir 800 mg PO 5id or 10 mg/kg IV q8h for 10–14 days or longer			
Treponema pallidum	Early syphilis	Benzathine penicillin G 2.4 million units IM weekly for 3 weeks			Approx 20% relapse, need retreatment. Immunologic abnormalities may cause inaccurate serology.
	Late or neurosyphilis	Aqueous penicillin G 2.4 million units IV daily for 10–14 d Procaine penicillin G, 1.2 million units IM daily for 10–14 d Ceftriaxone 1–2 g IM or IV qd 10–14 d			May be given with probnecid 500 mg PO qid

glucocorticoids. Glucocorticoids are now indicated for use in the treatment of any patient with HIV infection and PCP in whom the Pa_{O_2} is under 70 mmHg or in whom the a-A gradient is over 35 mmHg. In this setting, several clinical trials have shown clear benefit from glucocorticoids with approximately a 50 percent decrease in mortality (from 40 to 20 percent), and a 50 percent decrease in the number of patients requiring mechanical ventilatory support. The only significant side effect has been an increased incidence of thrush. Adjunct glucocorticoid therapy should begin as soon as possible after the diagnosis is made, perferably no later than 36 to 72 h. In fact, glucocorticoids added later in the course of disease have not been shown to confer any clinical benefit and have been associated with an increased risk of other opportunistic infections. The recommended course of glucocorticoid therapy is 21 days (Table 279-19), although some prefer to stop steroids 48 to 72 h prior to stopping antimicrobial therapy in order to allow one to assess the baseline status of the patient no longer receiving steroids yet still receiving antimicrobials.

In patients unable to tolerate trimethoprim/sulfamethoxazole several options are available. Pentamidine isethionate is also licensed for treatment of PCP. This drug must be administered parenterally. The development of sterile abscess following intramuscular administration makes intravenous administration the route of choice. In addition, it has been proposed that for mild cases the drug may be administered as an aerosol. Although some therapeutic successes have been noted by this route of administration, it is ineffective for extrapulmonary disease, and aerosolized pentamidine is best reserved for prophylaxis of PCP in patients unable to tolerate systemic prophylaxis (see below). When given by the intravenous route, pentamidine must be introduced slowly to prevent cardiovascular effects. Although comparable in efficacy to trimethoprim/sulfamethoxazole, therapy with pentamidine is associated with a greater number of serious side effects. Among the side effects are nephrotoxicity, often necessitating dose reduction of 20 to 50 percent; pancreatitis, necessitating discontinuation; thrombocytopenia and dysregulation of glucose metabolism resulting in either hyper- or hypoglycemia. The latter side effect is seen in 14 percent of patients receiving pentamidine and is probably secondary to pancreatic injury during therapy. Fatal hypoglycemia as well as the development of insulin-requiring diabetes mellitus have been noted. These disorders of glucose metabolism are seen with increased frequency in patients who develop renal damage during therapy, are generally noted later in the course of therapy, and are more common in patients receiving total doses above 4 g and in patients who have received pentamidine in the past. Pentamidine-associated hypoglycemia has been reported as late as 2 weeks following the discontinuation of drug and thus, patients must be alerted to be vigilant for this side effect.

Among the alternatives to trimethoprim/sulfamethoxazole and intravenous pentamidine are trimethoprim/dapsone (oral only), clindamycin/primaquine (oral and parenteral), atovoquone (oral only), trimetrexate/leucovorin (oral and parenteral), and eflornithine (DFMO, oral and parenteral). The combination of trimethoprim and dapsone has been shown to be similar in efficacy to trimethoprim/sulfamethoxazole and to be associated with fewer toxicities. Some clinicians choose this combination as first-line treatment in patients with mild disease. One side effect of dapsone therapy is the development of methemoglobinemia, and its use is contraindicated in patients with G6PD deficiency. Dapsone as a single agent is not effective therapy. Similarly, while neither clindamycin alone nor primaquine alone are effective for the treatment of pneumocystosis, in combination response rates are as high as 86 percent. The main side effects are rash and methemoglobinemia. Atovoquone (BW566C80) is a hydroxynapthoquinone that interferes with electron transport in mitochondria and as such interferes with pyrimidine synthesis in protozoa. In a series of clinical trials, this drug has been shown to have activity against *Pneumocystis carinii*; however, despite a lower incidence of side effects, overall response rates are somewhat less than that of trimethoprim/sulfamethoxazole and relapses are more common, thus placing this agent as second-line therapy. Trimetrexate, an inhibitor

of dihydrofolate reductase, is another agent shown to be effective in the treatment of patients with PCP. This drug, whose bone marrow suppressive side effects can be greatly minimized by the concomitant use of folinic acid (leucovorin), is associated with response rates of approximately 70 percent. While not appropriate as initial therapy, trimetrexate may be of use in the patient unable to tolerate or failing other forms of treatment. Eflornithine (DFMO) is an irreversible inhibitor of decarboxylase and thus interferes with the synthesis of polyamines. Its main side effect is thrombocytopenia. As in the case of trimetrexate this drug has been shown to have some efficacy as a salvage treatment; however, lower overall response rates when compared to trimethoprim/sulfamethoxazole suggest that this drug not be used for initial therapy. While neither trimetrexate not DFMO are licensed, both are available on a compassionate use basis for treatment of PCP or disseminated pneumocystosis.

Once one has made a diagnosis of, or suspects, infection with *Pneumocystis carinii,* appropriate systemic therapy is initiated with one of the agents or combinations of agents noted above. For patients with moderate to severe disease, glucocorticoids are included as part of the treatment regimen and specific antimicrobial therapy should be administered parenterally (see above). After 7 to 14 days of therapy, clearcut clinical improvement should be noted. If it is not, a change in therapy must be considered, with the general practice being to switch treatment regimens, rather than add new drugs and, if the situation is worsening, to consider a repeat bronchoscopy to confirm that the initial diagnosis was correct and to rule out the possibility of a second infection. For patients who develop respiratory failure, intubation and mechanical ventilation remain an option, and given the current range of therapeutic options available for treatment, patients have been successfully treated and extubated.

Pneumocystis prophylaxis is one of the cornerstones in management of the HIV-infected patient. As mentioned above, prophylaxis is indicated for any HIV-infected individual who has experienced a previous bout of PCP, who has fewer than 200 CD4+ T cells per microliter, or who has a CD4 percentage of 15 or lower. As in treatment, the preferred medication for prophylaxis is trimethoprim/sulfamethoxazole given as a single double-strength tablet anywhere from three times a week to twice a day. In studies of the twice a day regimen, no cases of PCP were noted in the treatment group as opposed to 16 cases in the untreated control group. In addition, in this study, which had a minimum follow-up of 24 months, the median survival for the treatment group was 22.9 months compared to 12.6 months for the control group. In more recent trials, examining a once a day regimen of trimethoprim/sulfamethoxazole and comparing it to aerosolized pentamidine at a dose of 300 mg every 4 weeks, 1-year and 18-month recurrence rates of 4.5 percent and 11.4 percent, respectively, were noted for the trimethoprim/sulfamethoxazole group compared to 18.5 percent and 27.6 percent, respectively, for the aerosolized pentamidine group. These data, coupled with the increased incidence of pneumothorax and disseminated pneumocystosis seen with aerosolized pentamidine, point to systemic therapy with trimethoprim/sulfamethoxazole as the preferred regimen for prophylaxis. Unfortunately, however, many patients are unable to tolerate trimethoprim/sulfamethoxazole and there is a great need for alternative regimens. In this regard many regimens, most of them variations on the themes outlined above have been proposed. A recent study of dapsone was prematurely stopped when it was observed that there was a higher incidence of death due to bacterial infections in the dapsone group than in the trimethoprim/sulfamethoxazole group. This may have been due to the broad-spectrum antibacterial activity of the combination regimen or due to some adverse effect of dapsone on neutrophil function. Aerosolized pentamidine, 300 mg every 4 weeks delivered by a Respirgard II or equivalent nebulizer, remains an option for patients unable to tolerate systemic therapy. Among the alternative systemic regimens currently under study, however, no clear recommendations emerge at the present time.

Toxoplasma gondii, the etiologic agent of toxoplasmosis (see Chap. 177), is the most common secondary CNS infection in patients with AIDS, accounting for 38 percent of all secondary CNS infections. It accounts for 50 to 60 percent of all mass lesions in the CNS of patients with HIV infection and is responsible for 28 percent of first seizures. Overall, toxoplasmosis is seen in approximately 15 percent of patients with AIDS and is most common in patients from the Caribbean. Toxoplasmosis is generally a late complication of HIV infection and usually occurs in patients with less than 100 CD4+ T cells per microliter. It is felt to represent a reactivation syndrome and is 10 times more common in patients with antibodies to the organism, an indicator of prior infection, than in patients who are seronegative. However, due to the abnormalities of B cell function seen in patients with HIV infection (see above), serologic testing cannot be used to eliminate a diagnosis of toxoplasmosis and 5 to 10 percent of cases occur in HIV-infected patients who are seronegative for *Toxoplasma gondii*. Approximately 30 percent of AIDS patients with antibodies to *Toxoplasma gondii* will go on to develop CNS infection at some time during the course of their disease.

Primary infection is usually asymptomatic, occurring early in life although some may experience a chorioretinitis such as is seen following congenital infection. While primary infection in an immuno-compromised host may result in a disseminated lethal infection involving lung, myocardium and brain, this syndrome is rarely seen in patients with HIV infection. The most common clinical presentation in patients with HIV infection is one of fever, headache, and focal neurologic deficits with the last occurring in approximately 90 percent of patients. Patients may present with seizure, hemiparesis, or aphasia as a manifestation of focal neurologic defects or with a picture more related to accompanying cerebral edema consisting of confusion, dementia, lethargy, and progression to coma. The latter are obviously similar to problems encountered in patients with the AIDS dementia complex. In this clinical setting the diagnosis is suspected based upon radiologic findings. MRI or double-dose contrast CT are the preferable techniques with the MRI clearly the most sensitive. Findings generally include multiple lesions in multiple locations, although in some cases only a single lesion may be seen. Pathologically these lesions generally exhibit central necrosis and as a result are ring enhancing on contrast CT or MRI (Fig. 279-18). There is usually evidence of surrounding edema. While the definitive diagnostic procedure is a brain biopsy, given the morbidity frequently associated with this procedure, it is usually more appropriate in the patient in whom one suspects toxoplasmosis (multiple ring-enhancing lesions on CT, seropositive) to initiate specific therapy (see below) and only proceed to biopsy in those patients who do not show a therapeutic response within 2 to 4 weeks. In addition to the classic presentation as a CNS mass lesion a variety of other clinical problems have been encountered and reported in the HIV-infected patient as a consequence of infection with *Toxoplasma gondii*. Among them are a CNS presentation more characteristic of herpes simplex with a negative CT scan, chorioretinitis, pneumonia, peritonitis with ascites, and orchitis.

The standard treatment is combination therapy with pyrimethamine and sulfadiazine (Table 279-19), which has a response rate of approximately 90 percent. Given the fact that the relapse rate is over 50 percent at 6 months, the requirement for therapy is generally lifelong. Leukopenia, the main side effect of this combination, may be ameliorated with the concomitant use of folinic acid (leucovorin). If the patient is receiving other myelosuppressive agents, such as zidovudine or ganciclovir, the dosages of these medications may require modifications. Other complications of therapy include fever, rash, thrombocytopenia, and renal failure due to sulfadiazine crystalluria. Crystalluria can be managed by administering fluids and alkalinizing the urine without discontinuing the medications. Overall, 45 to 70 percent of patients will develop side effects from treatment, with approximately 33 percent of patients requiring a change in therapy. At present there are two main options for alternative therapy. The first of these is the combination of clindamycin and pyrimethamine. Clindamycin appears to be almost as good as sulfadiazine in combination with pyrimethamine and is an alternative for the sulfa-allergic patient. The other option is atovoquone. As mentioned above, this

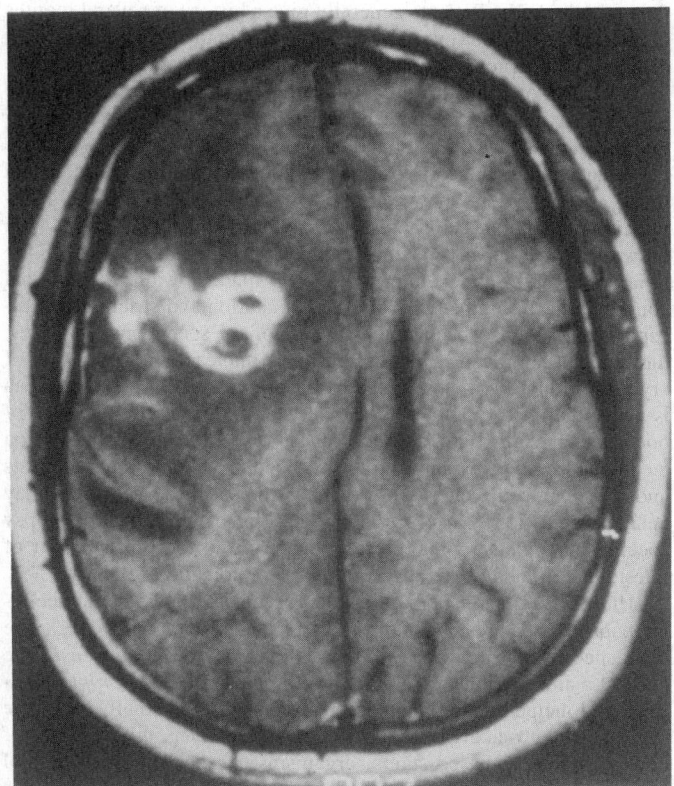

FIGURE 279-18 Contrast-enhanced MRI of the central nervous system of a patient with central nervous system toxoplasmosis. Several ring-enhancing lesions can be noted in the temporoparietal area.

inhibitor of mitochondrial electron transport has activity against a wide range of protozoa. It has been shown both as a single agent and in combination with pyrimethamine to be a viable alternative for treatment of toxoplasmosis in patients who have failed or who have developed adverse reactions to standard therapy. In the patients for whom the sulfa component of treatment appears to cause side effects, the use of pyrimethamine alone as a maintenance regimen has been advocated. Although not as effective as the combination it does appear to provide some protection from relapse. While animal model data suggest that the macrolide antibiotics, clarithromycin and azithromycin, might be of benefit for treatment of toxoplasmosis, clinical trial results thus far have been disappointing. Glucocorticoids are recommended for the management of the patient with cerebral edema.

Given the frequency of toxoplasmosis in the HIV-infected population (overall incidence of approximately 15 percent), there is a great need to develop an effective strategy for prophylaxis. Unfortunately, aside from atovoquone, most of the agents or combination of agents with activity have sufficient side effects to question their role in primary prophylaxis. Patients receiving trimethoprim/sulfamethoxazole for prophylaxis of PCP have a decreased incidence of toxoplasmosis, again underscoring the potential importance of this particular regimen for antimicrobial propylaxis.

Cryptosporidia, Microsporidia, and Isospora belli (see Chap. 179) are the most common opportunistic protozoa that infect the gastrointestinal tract and cause diarrhea in patients with HIV infection. *Cryptosporidium* is a well-known cause of diarrhea in animals and may cause a self-limited diarrheal infection in the immunocompetent host. It is spread through fecal-oral contact and nosocomial outbreaks have been noted. In the HIV-infected individual, cryptosporidial infection may present in a variety of ways from a self-limited or intermittent diarrheal illness in the relatively early stages of HIV infection to a severe, life-threatening diarrhea in severely immunodeficient individuals. Patients generally give a history of several months of intermittent diarrhea evolving to a several-month history of persistent diarrhea with copious watery stools, often up to several liters per day. In 75 percent of cases this is accompanied by crampy abdominal pain with approximately 25 percent of patients noting nausea and/or vomiting. This intestinal infection may be complicated by lactose intolerance and malabsorption. In addition to involving the intestinal tract, cryptosporidia may cause biliary tract disease in the HIV-infected population. Biliary disease may present as cholecystitis with or without accompanying cholangitis. Radiographic studies of the biliary tree reveal thickening of the gall bladder wall with luminal abnormalities accompanying bile duct dilatation and stricture. Cryptosporidia have also been noted in pulmonary specimens; however, the clinical significance in this setting is unclear. The diagnosis of cryptosporidial diarrhea is made by stool examination. The diarrhea is non-inflammatory and the characteristic finding is the presence of oocysts that stain with acid-fast dyes. Use of a sucrose flotation technique followed by concentration procedures to enrich for the cysts and to separate the cysts from other particles in the specimen may enhance detection. On electron microscopy of small bowel biopsy specimens, organisms may be seen adhering to the brush border of intestinal epithelial. Therapy is purely symptomatic at present.

Microsporidia are small unicellular organisms, obligate intracellular parasites that reside within the cytoplasm of enteric cells. The main species causing disease in man is *Enterocytozoon bieneusi*. The clinical manifestations are similar to those described for *Cryptosporidium* and include abdominal pain and diarrhea. The small size of the organism may make it difficult to detect; however, with the use of new chromotrope-based stains, organisms can be identified in stool samples by light microscopy. Definitive diagnosis generally depends upon electron microscopic examination of stool specimen, intestinal aspirate, or intestinal biopsy. In contrast to cryptosporidia, Microsporidia have been noted in a variety of extraintestinal locations, including the eye, muscle, and liver and have been associated with conjunctivitis and hepatitis. As in the case of *Cryptosporidium*, no effective therapies have been identified and treatment is purely symptomatic.

Isospora belli is a coccidian parasite, most commonly found as a cause of diarrhea in patients from the Caribbean and Africa. Its cysts appear in the stool as large acid-fast structures that can be differentiated from cryptosporidia by virtue of differences in size, shape, and number of sporocysts. Clinical syndromes caused by this organism appear identical to those caused by cryptosporidia; however, one important difference is that this infection can be treated with trimethoprim/sulfamethoxazole. While relapses are common, a three-times-a-week regimen, similar to that used to provide prophylaxis against PCP, appears adequate to prevent recurrence.

Entamoeba histolytica (see Chap. 173) and *Giardia lamblia* (see Chap. 179), although not opportunistic pathogens in that they can also cause disease in immunocompetent individuals, are seen with an increased frequency in patients with HIV infection. These treatable protozoa should be carefully looked for in any patient with HIV infection and persistent diarrhea. Other strains of *Entamoeba* and *Blastocystis hominis* are also seen with an increased frequency in homosexual men with HIV infection; however, these organisms are felt to be of little if any clinical significance.

Miscellaneous protozoal infections are being reported with increased frequency as the AIDS epidemic spreads in other regions of the world. In this regard visceral leishmaniasis (Chap. 175) is recognized with increasing frequency in patients who live in or travel to endemic areas. The clinical presentation is one of hepatosplenomegaly, fever, and hematologic abnormalities. Lymphadenopathy and other constitutional symptoms may be present. Organisms can be isolated from cultures of bone marrow aspirates, while histologic stains are often negative and antibody titers are of little help in diagnosis. Patients usually respond well initially to standard therapy although, as with most infections in HIV-infected individuals, eradication of the organisms is difficult and relapses are common. Among other protozoal infections that have been reported are severe and

recurrent babesiosis (Chap. 179), Chagas disease (Chap. 176) presenting as a CNS mass lesion, and meningoencephalitis due to *Acanthamoeba* or *Naegleria* (Chap. 173). No significant changes have been noted in the clinical manifestations of malaria in patients with HIV infection.

Bacterial infections Atypical mycobacteria (see Chap. 132) account for a large number of opportunistic infections in patients with HIV infection although their overall contribution to mortality remains small. In the United States, disseminated infection with atypical mycobacteria, particularly *Mycobacterium avium* complex (MAC) is diagnosed in approximately 40 percent of HIV-infected patients antemortem and is seen in 80 percent of patients at autopsy. MAC accounts for 95 percent of the atypical mycobacterial infections seen in patients with AIDS in the United States; however, infections with at least 12 different mycobacteria, including *M. bovis* and representatives of all four Runyon groups, have been reported. Infections with MAC, which consists of *M. avium* and *M. intracellulare*, are predominantly seen in U.S. patients and are rare in Africa.

MAC infection probably represents an acute infection with organisms that are ubiquitous in the environment in both soil and water. The presumed portals of entry are the gastrointestinal and respiratory tract. MAC infection is a late complication of HIV infection, occurring in patients with CD4+ T cell counts under 100 cells per microliter. In one study the median CD4+ T cell count for patients with MAC was 60 cells per microliter. HIV-infected patients presenting with MAC infection have been reported to have a median survival of approximately 6 to 10 months, which likely reflects the late stage of HIV infection. While a variety of clinical syndromes have been attributed to MAC infections, the most common presentation is fever, weight loss, and night sweats, presumably due to disseminated disease. At least 85 percent of HIV-infected patients with MAC infection are mycobacteremic, and enormous numbers of organisms can often be demonstrated on bone marrow biopsy. Liver involvement is common and MAC infection should be suspected in any HIV-infected individual with a low CD4+ T cell count, unexplained fever, and an elevated alkaline phosphatase. The chest x-ray is abnormal in approximately 25 percent of patients. The most common radiographic pattern is a bilateral lower lobe interstitial infiltrate, suggestive of miliary spread. In addition, alveolar or nodular infiltrates and hilar and/or mediastinal adenopathy occur. Endobronchial lesions have also been reported. Other clinical findings include lymphadenopathy, abdominal pain, and diarrhea. Diagnosis is suspected by demonstration of long, slender acid-fast bacilli on bone marrow, lymph node, or liver biopsy or upon examination of stool specimens and confirmed by culture of blood or involved tissue. The finding of two consecutive sputum samples positive for MAC is highly suggestive of pulmonary infection. Cultures generally turn positive within 2 weeks. In earlier studies, treatment with various combination regimens that usually included ethambutol, clofazamine, and rifabutin, with or without an aminoglycoside, where shown to have little effect on mycobacteremia and to increase only marginally the median survival of patients with MAC infection from 6 months to 8 months. Given these data and the considerable toxicity encountered with these treatment regimens many clinicians chose not to treat MAC infection unless there was clear evidence of disease. However, both the macrolide and the fluoroquinolone classes of antibiotics now show considerable promise. Clarithromycin and azithromycin are two macrolide antibiotics that are licensed for the treatment of common respiratory tract infections. They are both characterized by broad spectrum antimicrobial activity, good tissue penetration, and good activity in vitro against MAC. Clarithromycin has been shown in a controlled trial to cause significant decreases in the titer of MAC organisms in the blood and to improve the patients' sense of well being. Similar encouraging data have been generated for azithromycin in open trials. Ciprofloxacin, ofloxacin, and sparfloxacin are fluorinated members of the quinoline family. While ciprofloxacin is the only one currently licensed, all three have shown activity against MAC in vitro, and clinical trials are currently underway to assess their efficacy in vivo. Given these data many physicians now choose to treat patients with MAC infection with a combination regimen consisting of ethambutol, clofazamine, ciprofloxacin, and a macrolide. As with all of the potentially life-threatening infections seen in patients with AIDS, prophylactic regimens when available should be employed. In this regard, the use of rifabutin in patients with advanced HIV infection has been shown to delay the onset of bacteremia and is now a recommend prophylaxis regimen for patients with under 100 CD4+ T cells per microliter.

A number of other atypical mycobacteria have been reported to cause infections in patients with HIV infection. Infection with *M. kansasii* generally presents as a pulmonary infection with 20 to 30 percent of patients showing evidence of disseminated disease. Patients usually present with fever, cough, and night sweats. Chest x-ray reveals upper lobe cavitation in approximately half of the patients, while a lower lobe interstitial pattern consistent with hematogenous spread may be seen in other patients. Organisms are usually identified easily in pulmonary secretions; evidence of disease is found in over 75 percent of the patients with a positive culture. *M. kansasii* infection is a particularly important diagnosis to make since it is relatively easy to treat with a combination regimen of isoniazid, rifampin, and ethambutol. *M. fortuitus, M. chelonia, M. marinum,* and *M. hemophilum* have all been reported to cause cutaneous lesions in patients with HIV infection; *M. hemophilum* is also reported to cause disseminated disease and septic arthritis. *M. gordonae*, generally a nonpathogen in humans, and *M. xenopi*, a colonizer of water storage tanks, have both been reported to cause disseminated disease. Therapy of these latter organisms is extremely difficult.

M. tuberculosis, while once thought to be on its way to extinction in the United States, has experienced a major resurgence in the context of the HIV epidemic (see Chap. 130). A 20-year decline in the number of new cases in the United States ended in 1986, and the number of new cases per year has since been on a steady increase. Approximately 5 percent of the patients with AIDS are reported to have active tuberculosis. While the prevalence and incidence of infection with *M. tuberculosis* as determined by Purified Protein Derivative (PPD) skin testing appears quite comparable among members of the same risk group regardless of HIV status, HIV infection increases the risk of developing active tuberculosis by a factor of 15 to 30. For the patient with HIV infection and a positive PPD skin test, the rate of reactivation is approximately 8 percent per year. Although the majority of tuberculosis cases in the HIV-infected population are felt to represent reactivation, acute infection and reinfection are being seen with an alarming frequency, especially in the context of the new outbreaks of multidrug resistant (MDR) tuberculosis. Active tuberculosis appears to be most common in patients of ages 25 to 44, in African-Americans and Hispanics, in patients in New York City and Miami, and in patients in developing countries. In these areas, 20 to 70 percent of the new cases of active tuberculosis are in patients with HIV infection. Given the fact that, in contrast to HIV infection, infection with *M. tuberculosis* can be spread through casual contact and respiratory droplets, this emerging second epidemic probably represents the greatest health risk to the general public and the health care profession to emerge from the HIV crisis. In contrast to infection with MAC, active tuberculosis often develops relatively early in the course of HIV infection and may be among the earliest clinical signs of HIV infection. In one study, the median CD4+ T cell count at presentation was 326 cells per microliter. The clinical manifestations of tuberculosis in the HIV-infected patients are quite varied and generally show different patterns as a function of the patient's CD4+ T cell count. In patients with relatively high CD4+ T cell counts, a typical pattern of pulmonary reactivation occurs in which patients present with fever, cough, dyspnea on exertion, weight loss, night sweats, and a chest x-ray revealing cavitary apical disease of the upper lobes. Disseminated disease is more common in patients with low CD4 counts. The chest x-ray in patients with disseminated disease may also reveal diffuse or lower lobe bilateral reticulonodular infiltrates consistent with miliary spread, pleural effusions, and hilar and/or mediastinal adenop-

athy. Infection may be present in bone, brain, meninges, gastrointestinal tract, lymph node (particularly cervical nodes), and viscera. Cases of visceral abscesses of the liver and prostate have been reported. Approximately 60 to 80 percent of patients will have pulmonary disease and 30 to 40 percent will have extrapulmonary disease.

Respiratory isolation and a negative-pressure room should be employed with patients in whom a diagnosis of pulmonary tuberculosis is being considered. This approach is critical in order to limit nosocomial and community spread of infection. A definitive diagnosis is made by culture of the organism from an involved site. Blood cultures are positive in 15 percent of cases. However, given the importance of making an early diagnosis and initiating treatment, especially given the emergence of MDR tuberculosis (see below), a presumptive diagnosis should be made based upon a positive acid fast stain and consistent clinical presentation while awaiting culture results. A positive PPD in a HIV-infected person is defined as any area of induration $\geq$ 5 mm. While this can be used to support the diagnosis and identify candidates for isoniazid prophylaxis, up to 50 percent of patients with HIV infection and active tuberculosis may be anergic, and thus a negative skin test does not rule out a diagnosis.

Standard therapy for tuberculosis is generally as successful in the HIV-infected patient as it is in the HIV-negative patient. In most cases, one initiates therapy with three drugs for a total course of at least 9 months and no less than 6 months beyond a third negative culture. Patients with HIV infection have a slightly higher incidence of adverse drug reactions. In one series, 18 percent of patients experienced a drug reaction, predominantly rash and hepatitis related to rifampin.

A major, emerging problem has been the increasing identification of strains of *M. tuberculosis* resistant to two or more first-line drugs, usually isoniazid and rifampin, so-called MDR tuberculosis (see Chap. 130). Outbreaks of MDR-tuberculosis have been reported from New York, Florida, Michigan, and Missouri. Of the initial 87 cases reported, 83 occurred in patients with HIV infection. Due to delays in obtaining antimicrobial sensitivities patients often received inadequate treatment regimens, and the initial mortality from MDR-tuberculosis has been as high as 72 to 89 percent. Thus therapy should be initiated with a five-drug regimen while awaiting formal sensitivity results for anyone contracting tuberculosis in an area where MDR-tuberculosis has become a problem.

Prevention of active tuberculosis can be a reality if the health care profession is aggressive in looking for evidence of latent tuberculosis by making sure that all patients at risk for tuberculosis and all patients with HIV infection receive a PPD skin test. As mentioned above, in the setting of HIV infection, an induration of $\geq$ 5 mm should be considered positive, and such patients should be treated for 1 year with isoniazid. Given the fact that 50 percent of patients will be anergic, some experts also recommend that any patient with HIV infection who is anergic and at high risk for TB be given a 1-year course of isoniazid.

Nonmycobacterial bacteria account for a high number of infections in patients with AIDS and are the second leading cause of death following opportunistic infections. Bacterial infections most frequently present clinically as respiratory tract infections, sepsis, and/or gastroenteritis. In addition, syphilis and bacillary angiomatosis may present with atypical features. Patients with HIV infection appear to be particularly prone tio infections with encapsulated organisms, perhaps as a consequence of altered B cell activation and/or defects in neutrophil function that may be secondary to disease or drugs. *Streptococcus pneumonia* (see Chap. 101) and *Haemophilus influenzae* (see Chap. 112) are among the two most common bacterial infections seen in patients with HIV infection. These two organisms are responsible for the majority of cases of bacterial pneumonia in patients with AIDS and also contribute to the increased incidence of sinusitis that has been reported in this patient population. Patients with HIV infection have a 6-fold increase in the incidence of pneumoccal pneumonia and a 100-fold increase in the incidence of pneumococcal bacteremia. For these reasons, all patients with HIV infections should be receive immunization with pneumococcal polysaccharide. *Staphylococcus aureus* infections (see Chap. 102) are also seen with increased frequency in the setting of HIV infection. Carriage of staphylococcal organisms in HIV infected patients is approximately twice that seen in the general population. Staphylococcal infections are usually responsible for catheter-related sepsis with the risk increasing as the CD4 + T cell count declines. Pyomyositis is another complication of staphylococcal infection and is seen with increased frequency in the HIV-infected patient group. This disease, which was formerly rare in the United States, is generally seen in association with muscle injury; it has been postulated that the myopathy of HIV infection may be a predisposing factor.

Infections with enteric pathogens such as salmonella, shigella, and campylobacter are more common in homosexual men and are often more severe and more prone to relapse in patients with HIV infection. The latter patients have approximately a 20-fold increased risk of infection with *Salmonella typhimurium* (see Chap. 117). They may present with a variety of nonspecific symptoms, including fever, anorexia, fatigue, and malaise of several weeks' duration. Diarrhea, although common, may be absent. Diagnosis is made by culture of blood and stool. Although treatment is generally not indicated for salmonella gastroenteritis, because of the protracted course and high rate of recurrence in the HIV-infected population, long-term therapy is usually prescribed for them; the greatest degree of success has been reported with oral ciprofloxacin. Patients with HIV infection have an increased incidence of infection with *Salmonella typhi* in areas of the world where typhoid is a problem (see Chap. 117).

Shigella infections (see Chap. 118) cause particularly severe gastrointestinal disease in HIV-infected individuals, characterized by diarrhea and fever. *Shigella flexneri* is the most common species isolated, and up to 50 percent of patients with HIV infection and shigellosis are bacteremic in contrast to otherwise healthy hosts, where bacteremia is rare.

Campylobacter infections (see Chap. 119) occur with an increased frequency in HIV-infected patients. While *C. fetus* and *jejuni* are the strains most frequently isolated, infections with many other strains have been reported. Patients usually present with crampy abdominal pain, fever, and bloody diarrhea; infection may also present as proctitis. Stool examination reveals the presence of fecal leukocytes. Systemic infection may be seen with up to 10 percent of infected patients exhibiting bateremias. As in the case of the other enteric pathogens, infections with *Campylobacter* species are often persistent or recurrent, and prolonged therapy is usually needed. Most strains are sensitive to erythromycin; however, resistant strains have been reported.

Infections with *Treponema pallidum*, the etiologic agent of syphilis, play an important role in the HIV epidemic (see Chap. 133). In the HIV-negative individual, genital syphilitic ulcers rank with the ulcers of chancroid as major predisposing factors for heterosexual transmission of HIV (see above). While most HIV-infected individuals with syphilis will have a typical presentation, a variety of formerly rare clinical problems may be encountered. Among them are lues maligna, an ulcerating lesion of the skin due to a necrotizing vasculitis; unexplained fever; nephrotic syndrome; and neurosyphilis. Neurosyphilis may be asymptomatic or may present as acute meningitis, neuroretinitis, deafness, or stroke. In one series, 44 percent of all cases of neurosyphilis were found to occur in patients with HIV infection; the rate of neurosyphilis in this population may be as high as 1.5 percent. Given the immunologic abnormalities seen in patients with HIV infection, diagnosis through standard serologic testing may be challenging. On the one hand, a significant number of patients may have a false positive VDRL due to a polyclonal B cell activation. On the other hand, the development of a positive VDRL may be delayed in the patient with new infection and the anti-FTA antibody test may be negative due to immunodeficiency. Darkfield examination of appropriate specimens should be performed in any patient in whom a diagnosis of syphilis is suspected, even if the patient has a negative VDRL. Similarly, given the spinal fluid abnormalities seen with HIV

infection alone, a diagnosis of neurosyphilis may be difficult to make. Any patient with a positive serum VDRL with neurologic findings who has an abnormal spinal fluid examination, with or without a positive CSF VDRL, should be considered a possible case of neurosyphilis. In the HIV infected patient with syphilis, treatment should follow standard guidelines. However, standard treatment may be inadequate and may need to be repeated in patients who fail to respond or who show evidene of relapse. In these patients, one also needs to have a high index of suspicion for neurosyphilis and treat accordingly with high-dose IV penicillin if this diagnosis is suspected.

Bacillary angiomatosis, a vascular proliferative disease felt to be due to the rickettsia-like organism *Rochalimaea henselae*, is seen with an increased frequency in patients with HIV infection (see Chap. 124). This disease usually presents with cutaneous erythematous papules that may appear similar to Kaposi's sarcoma. While 93 percent of patients have cutaneous manifestations, the disease may also involve lymph node, bone, and viscera. Fever, weight loss, and malaise are seen in the majority of patients. Mass lesions with abscess-like characteristics in spleen, liver, and CNS have been described. The disease may be associated with peliosis hepatica, a condition in which the liver contains multiple, cystic, blood-filled spaces resulting in hepatomegaly and abdominal pain. The diagnosis is made by demonstration of bacillary organisms on Warthin-Starry stain of appropriate clinical specimens. Patients usually respond well to treatment with erythromycin or tetracycline, although relapses occur in approximately 15 percent of cases.

Fungal infections *Candida* infections are the most common fungal infections occurring in patients with HIV infection; virtually all patients experience some candida infection over the course of their illness (see Chap. 166). Infections are often seen early in the course of HIV infection, heralding the onset of clinically apparent immunodeficiency. Although they are a significant cause of morbidity, *Candida* infections are generally easy to control and usually involve only the mucosal surfaces. Invasive disease is extremely rare and occurs predominantly as a consequence of iatrogenic measures such as indwelling catheters, broad spectrum antibiotics, and/or drug induced neutropenia.

Superficial infection of the oral cavity with *Candida* (thrush) generally presents as a white, cheesy exudative on the posterior oropharynx (Fig A1-41). Early lesions also may be detected along the gingival-labial margins. The exudate is easy to scrape, and branching pseudohyphae are readily detectable on wet-mount KOH preparations. In women with HIV infection, vaginal yeast infections are seen as an early sign of immunodeficiency.

Later in the course of HIV infection, generally in association with CD4 + T cell counts under 100 cells per microliter, candida infections of the esophagus, trachea, bronchi, or lungs may occur. These infections are felt to be indicative of a serious defect in cell-mediated immunity and are among the AIDS-defining conditions (Table 279-1). Perhaps the most common of these is esophagitis. While generally a late manifestation of HIV infection, *Candida* esophagitis has also been reported during the acute HIV syndrome. Esophagitis generally presents as odynophagia and retrosternal pain or burning. Oral thrush is often present as well, although it may be absent in patients who have been receiving topical oral medications. A definitive diagnosis is made through upper endoscopy and observation of characteristic white plaques shown by wet mount to contain pseudohyphae. However, a high index of suspicion based upon history and/or a barium swallow demonstrating a grossly irregular mucosa (Fig. 279-19) is sufficient to justify an empiric trial of antifungal therapy. If improvement does not occur within 4 to 6 days of therapy, upper endoscopy is needed to eliminate the other possible causes of esophagitis, namely CMV, herpes simplex virus, Kaposi's sarcoma, and lymphoma.

Oral and vaginal *Candida* infections may be treated with topical nystatin or clotrimazole troches; the frequency of administration should match the severity of disease. Nonetheless, many find it more convenient to use systemic therapy with either ketoconazole or

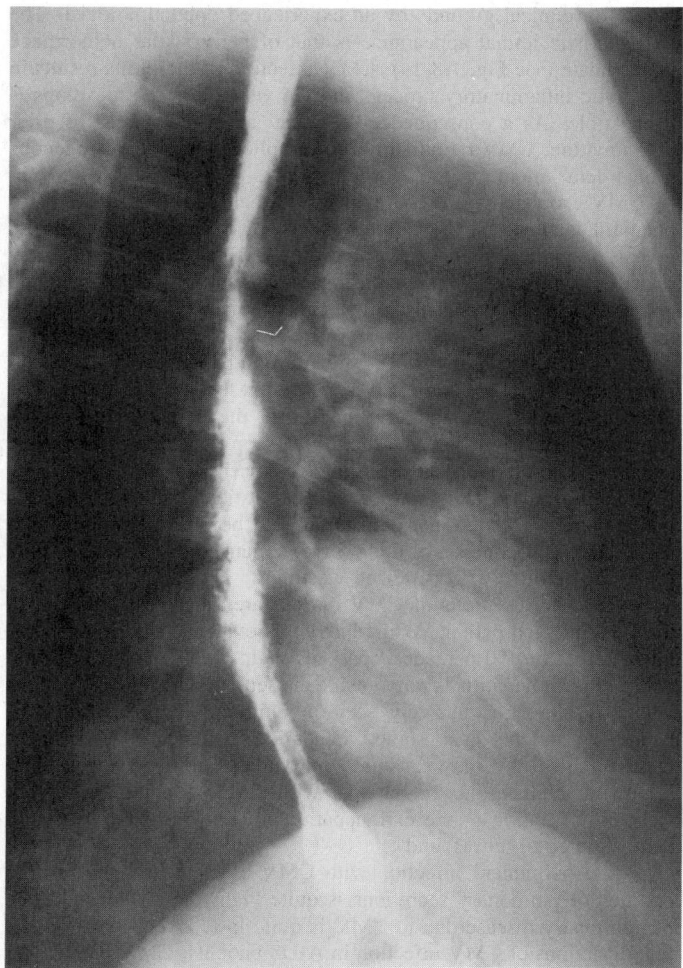

FIGURE 279-19 Barium swallow of a patient with *Candida* esophagitis. The flow of barium along the mucosal surface is grossly irregular.

fluconazole, both of which are effective in the majority of cases. Although fluconazole is more expensive, somewhat better results have been achieved, which may, at least in part, reflect the poor absorption of ketoconazole in patients with high gastric pH. A short course of intravenous therapy with amphotericin B followed by oral therapy with fluconazole may be indicated in particularly severe cases of candida infection.

Cryptococcus neoformans is the leading cause of meningitis in patients with AIDS (see Chap. 165). This ubiquitous, yeast-like fungus with a polysaccharide capsule causes serious, life-threatening infection in 6 to 12 percent of patients with AIDS. It is the initial AIDS-defining condition in 1.5 percent of patients, generally occurring in fairly advanced patients as defined by a CD4 + T cell count under 100 cells per microliter. The median survival of a patient with HIV infection following a diagnosis of cryptococcal infection is 9 months. Cryptococcal meningitis is particularly common in patients with AIDS in Africa, occurring in approximately 20 percent of individuals; it was the initial illness suggesting that a new epidemic of immunodeficiency was occurring in Africa. Although initial exposure is felt to occur via the respiratory route, the most common site of infection is the brain and meninges. CNS infection is seen in 67 to 85 percent of AIDS patients with cryptococcal disease; the majority of patients present with a picture of subacute meningoencephalitis. In addition to meningitis, patients may develop cryptoccomas which appear on MRI as multiple ring-enhancing lesions. Patients with CNS cryptococcal disease often display symptoms for weeks to months prior to diagnosis and, as is the case with many AIDS-associated

opportunistic infections, a high index of suspicion is essential in order to make an early diagnosis. Among the symptoms commonly seen are fever in virtually 100 percent of patients, nausea and vomiting in 40 percent, and altered mental status, headache, and meningeal signs in 25 percent. The incidence of seizures and focal neurologic defects is low. Pulmonary disease is seen in 40 percent of patients, 90 percent of whom will also have CNS infection. Patients with pulmonary disease present with fever, cough, dyspnea and, in some cases, hemoptysis. A focal or diffuse interstitial infiltrate is seen on chest x-ray in over 90 percent of patients. Chest x-ray may also reveal lobar disease, cavitary disease, pleural effusions, and hilar or mediastinal adenopathy. Over half the patients will be fungemic. In patients with fungemia fever, malaise and fatigue are common. While the majority of patients with cryptococcal disease present with CNS infection, 4 to 10 percent may present with pulmonary disease in the absence of other manifestations and 4 to 8 percent may present with fungemia as the only manifestation of infection. Uncommon manifestations of cryptoccocal infection in patients with HIV infection include skin lesions resembling molluscum contagiosum, lymphadenopathy, palatal and glossal ulcers, arthritis, gastroenteritis, myocarditis, and prostatitis. In fact, the prostate gland may serve as a reservoir for smoldering infection.

A presumptive diagnosis of cryptococcal infection can be made upon identification of organisms in spinal fluid on India ink examination, by measuring the presence of cryptococcal antigen in blood or spinal fluid, or by histologic evidence of cryptococcal infection in a biopsy specimen. A definitive diagnosis is made by culturing the organism from spinal fluid, blood, bone marrow, sputum, or tissue. A positive culture for *Cryptococcus neoformans*, regardless of site, should be considered significant and an indication for treatment. Cryptococcal antigen is present in the CSF of virtually all cases of cryptococcal meningitis, although in 15 percent of cases all other findings may be normal. In cryptococcal meningitis, the CSF WBC is over 20 cells per microliter in less than 50 percent of patients, the protein is elevated in 35 to 70 percent, and the glucose is low in about 50 percent. In patients with CNS cryptoccomas, both CSF antigen and culture may be negative and biopsy may be required to make the diagnosis.

Therapy with amphotericin B should be started immediately in any patient with evidence of cryptococcal infection, either by antigen or culture. Standard therapy in the HIV-infected patient consists of 6 weeks of amphotericin B at a daily dose of 0.3 mg/kg in combination with 150 mg/kg of flucytosine. Approximately 50 percent of patients will require that the flucytosine be omitted for at least part of the course of therapy due to neutropenia. Given the fact that with this therapy alone over 50 percent of patients will relapse, it is recommended that at the termination of amphotericin therapy patients be placed on fluconazole, 100 to 200 mg daily, indefinitely. Many physicians choose to place all patients with HIV infection on fluconazole, 100 to 200 mg daily, once the CD4 + T cell count falls below 100 cells per microliter as prophylaxis against both candida and cryptococcal infections.

Histoplasmosis is an opportunistic infection that is seen most frequently in patients in the Mississippi and Ohio River valleys, Puerto Rico, Dominican Republic, and South America; all of these are areas in which infection with *Histoplasma encapsulatum* is endemic (see Chap. 162). Because of this limited geographic distribution, the percentage of AIDS cases in the United States with histoplasmosis is only approximately 0.5 percent. In endemic areas, however, the incidence is much higher. The organism exists in the mycelial phase in soil, and large numbers of organisms are found in soil that contains droppings from birds or bats. The organism exists in the yeast phase at body temperature. Histoplasmosis is generally a late manifestation of HIV infection; however, it may be the initial AIDS-defining condition. The median CD4 + T cell count for patients with histoplasmosis was 33 cells per microliter in one study. While disease due to *H. encapsulatum* may present as a primary infection of the lung, disseminated disease, presumably due to reactivation, is the most common presentation in the HIV-infected patients. These patients usually present with a 4- to 8-week history of fever and weight loss. Hepatosplenomegaly and lymphadenopathy are each seen in about 25 percent of patients. CNS disease, either meningitis or a mass lesion, is seen in 15 percent of patients. Bone marrow involvement is common, with thrombocytopenia, neutropenia, and anemia occurring in 33 percent of patients. Approximately 7 percent of patients have mucocutaneous lesions, consisting of a maculopapular rash, skin, or oral ulcers. Although respiratory symptoms are usually minimal, with cough and dyspnea seen in 10 to 30 percent of patients, the chest x-ray is abnormal in about 50 percent of patients, revealing either a diffuse interstitial infiltrate or diffuse small nodules. Diagnosis is made by culturing the organism from blood, bone marrow, or tissue. Levels of fungal polysaccharide antigen may be detected in the blood and can be used to follow the course of therapy; however, this test may not be readily available commercially. Treatment consists of an initial course of amphotericin B, 0.6 mg/kg daily to a total dose of 1 g, followed by an indefinite maintenance regimen of either amphotericin, 1 mg/kg biweekly or oral itraconazole.

Coccidioides immitis is a mold that resides in the soil and causes a predominantly pulmonary infection in both immunologically intact hosts and patients with HIV infection (see Chap. 163). As in the case of histoplasmosis, infection with *C. immitis* is limited to certain geographic areas; it is endemic in the southwest United States. In these endemic areas, the annual rate of infection is approximately 3 percent and most of the disease seen in patients with HIV infection is felt to be a result of reactivation. Coccidioidal infection may develop relatively early in the course of HIV infection; however, most patients have CD4 + T cell counts under 250 cells per microliter. Patients generally present with fever, weight loss, and cough and fairly extensive abnormalities on chest x-ray. Diffuse reticulonodular infiltrates are the most common finding on chest x-ray, although nodules, cavities, pleural effusions, and hilar adenopathy also occur. While pulmonary disease is the most common manifestation of infection, seen on close to 70 percent of patients, 12 percent develop meningitis, 9 percent have lymphadenopathy, 9 percent have hepatic involvement, and 5 percent develop cutaneous disease. Abdominal infection and peritonitis have also been reported. Diagnosis is made by culture. While serologic testing is usually helpful in the immunocompetent host, serologies may be negative in 25 percent of HIV-infected individuals with coccidioidal infection. Treatment is amphotericin B, 1 mg/kg daily to a total dose of 1 g followed by indefinite maintenance with either fluconazole or itraconazole.

Viral infections   Human herpesvirus infections present substantial problems throughout the clinical course of HIV infection. In addition to causing clinical disease in their own right, predominantly in the form of reactivation syndromes, these DNA viruses are also felt to act as cofactors, enhancing the replication of HIV. Among the members of this group that are particularly disabling for patients with HIV infection are CMV (see Chap. 146), herpes simplex viruses (see Chap. 143), herpes zoster viruses (see Chap. 144), and Epstein-Barr virus (see Chap. 145).

CMV causes an acute infection, generally early in life, after which it exists in a latent state (see Chap. 146). Over 95 percent of patients with HIV infection are seropositive for CMV and at autopsy 90 percent of patients have some evidence of reactivated CMV disease. Clinical manifestations of CMV generally occur late in the course of HIV infection, for the most part in patients with less than 100 CD4 + T cells per microliter; however, evidence of active CMV replication such as excretion of CMV in throat washing or urine can be detected quite early in HIV-infected individuals. Retinitis, esophagitis, and colitis are the most common manifestations of CMV infection in patients with AIDS.

Perhaps the most devastating manifestion of CMV is retinitis, occurring in 25 to 30 percent of patients. CMV retinitis usually presents as a painless, progressive loss of vision; patients may complain of floaters. The disease is usually bilateral, affecting one eye more than the other, and the diagnosis is generally made

purely on clinical grounds by an experienced ophthalmologist. The characteristic retinal appearance is that of perivascular hemorrhage and exudate (see Fig. A8-14). CMV infection of the retina results in a necrotic inflammatory process and the visual loss that develops is irreversible. As a consequence of retinal atrophy in areas of prior inflammation, CMV retinitis may be complicated by rhegmatogenous retinal detachment.

CMV esophagitis presents with substernal chest pain and odynophagia. Diagnosis usually requires endoscopy which characteristically reveals a single, large shallow ulcer in the distal esophagus. Biopsy reveals characteristic intranuclear and intracytoplasmic inclusion bodies. While CMV may also involve the stomach and small intestine, the most frequent gastrointestinal manifestation of CMV infection is colitis, which is seen in 5 to 10 percent of all patients with AIDS and presents as diarrhea, abdominal pain, weight loss, and anorexia. The diarrhea is usually nonbloody and, as in the case of esophagitis, diagnosis is usually achieved through endoscopy and biopsy; characteristically, multiple mucosal ulcerations are seen. Barium enema is of little value and, in fact, may be normal. Patients with CMV colitis may experience abdominal perforation and become bacteremic as a result. One consequence of CMV involvement of the gastrointestinal tract may be diffuse, generalized wasting.

Other manifestations of CMV disease are much less common in the HIV-infected patient. While histologic evidence of hepatitis may be seen in 33 to 50 percent of patients with CMV elsewhere, in the body, clinical hepatitis is rare outside the setting of primary infection, which is almost exclusively seen in children. Approximately 33 percent of patients show some biochemical evidence of biliary tract disease, and CMV may cause a syndrome of papillary stenosis and sclerosing cholangitis. In patients with CMV-associated papillary stenosis, dilatation of the extrahepatic common bile duct is usually demonstrated on ultrasound.

While pulmonary infection with CMV as evidenced by positive cultures of pulmonary secretions is quite high, the actual incidence of pulmonary disease due to CMV is quite low. In contrast to other manifestations of CMV infection in AIDS patients, CMV pneumonia responds quite poorly to therapy, as is the case with individuals without HIV infection.

CMV can cause an ascending myelitis and subacute polyneuropathy that may respond well to treatment. Other manifestations of CMV infection include adrenalitis, epididymitis, cervicitis, and pancreatitis.

The diagnosis of clinically significant CMV infection can be difficult. Given the fact that most patients with advanced HIV infection actively excrete CMV, positive throat, urine, blood, and/or tissue cultures are quite common and of little diagnostic significance. Aside from CMV retinitis, where the diagnosis is made on clinical grounds, a diagnosis of CMV infection requires the histologic demonstration of large intranuclear bodies and cytoplasmic inclusions in the suspect tissue, in the absence of other possible pathologic processes.

Two drugs, ganciclovir and foscarnet, are currently licensed for treatment of CMV infection. Initial response rates for retinitis with either agent are approximately 80 to 90 percent; however, relapse rates are extremely high and patients must receive long-term maintenance therapy. Ganciclovir is somewhat easier to administer for initial therapy; it is given as a short infusion twice a day for 14 days. However, it is associated with a high incidence of bone marrow suppression and usually cannot be given in combination with zidovudine or trimethoprim/sulfamethoxazole. Foscarnet therapy is associated with a high incidence of renal and electrolyte disorders and for initial therapy must be given as three 2-h infusions daily for 14 days. Maintenance therapy for both drugs consists of a single daily infusion. While both drugs were shown to have similar degrees of efficacy in a randomized controlled trial, patients without renal insufficiency treated with forscarnet had a slightly longer survival than patients treated with ganciclovir. The reason for this finding is unclear; however, it may be related to the fact that in addition to being a potent anti-CMV agent, foscarnet also has activity against HIV. Hence, some clinicians recommend that patients with CMV retinitis

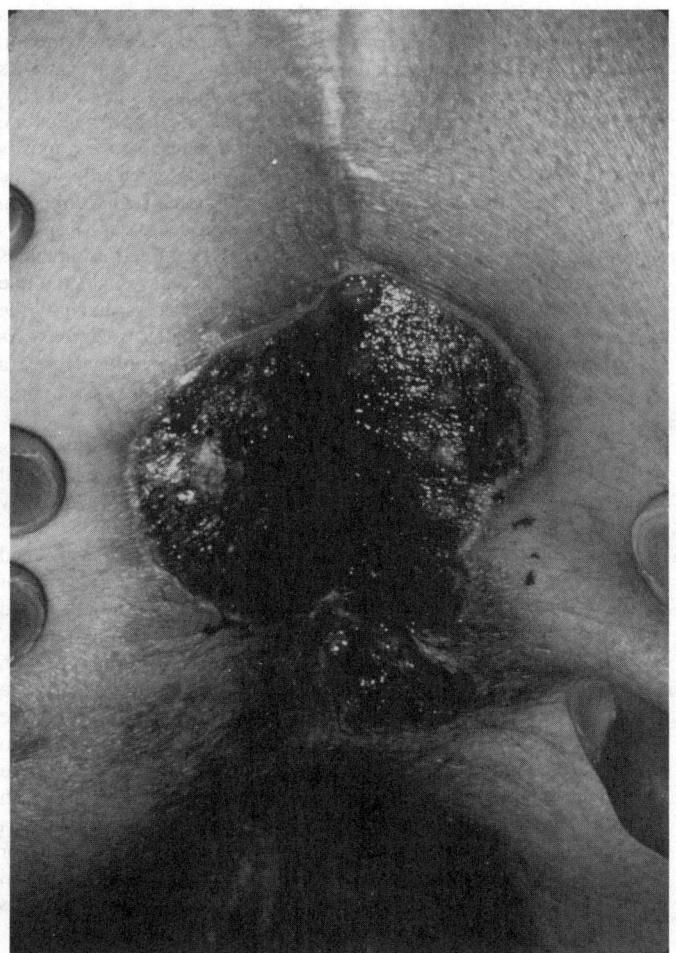

FIGURE 279-20   Severe, erosive perirectal herpes simplex in a patient with AIDS.

be treated with an initial course of the more convenient drug, ganciclovir, followed by maintenance with foscarnet. Strains of CMV that are resistant to ganciclovir have been identified; foscarnet is clearly the agent of choice in this situation. While CMV infections remain a major cause of morbidity in patients with HIV infection, the lack of any relatively benign form of therapy has precluded the development of an effective prophylactic strategy. Studies are currently underway evaluating the role of CMV hyperimmune Ig as a means of preventing CMV disease in HIV-infected patients. For the small percentage of HIV-infected individuals who are antibody negative for CMV and who require blood products, they should be obtained from CMV negative donors, if at all possible.

Infection with *herpes simplex virus* (HSV) in HIV-infected individuals is associated with recurrent orolabial, genital and perianal lesions (see Chap. 143). As HIV infections progress and as the CD4+ T cell count declines, these infections become more frequent and severe. Lesions often appear beefy red, are exquisitely painful, and have a predilection to occur high in the gluteal cleft (Fig. 279-20). Perirectal HSV may be associated with proctitis and anal fissures. HSV should be high on the differential diagnosis in any HIV-infected patients with a poorly healing, painful perirectal lesion. As in the case of CMV, HSV may cause esophagitis. HSV esophagitis often occurs together with active orolabial lesions. In contrast to CMV, where esophagitis is usually associated with a single, large ulcer, HSV esophagitis generally occurs as multiple small ulcers. Recurrent herpetic whitlow is another problem in patients with HIV infection. It may present with painful vesicles or extensive cutaneous erosion and is a more severe version of the form seen in the immunologically

intact host. Both herpes simplex and herpes zoster (see below) may rarely cause a widespread, bilateral necrotizing retinitis referred to as the *acute retinal necrosis syndrome*. This syndrome, in contrast to CMV retinitis, is associated with pain, keratitis, and iritis. It is often associated with orolabial HSV or trigeminal zoster. Ophthalmologic examination reveals widespread, pale gray, peripheral lesions; this condition is often complicated by retinal detachment. Herpetic encephalitis is extremely rare in HIV-infected patients despite its association with other immunosuppressed conditions.

Treatment of severe or recurrent HSV infection is acyclovir, 200 mg orally five times per day, for most cases and intravenously at higher doses for more serious conditions. The development of microbial resistance due to alterations in the viral thymidine kinase enzyme is becoming an increasing problem in the HIV-infected population. These resistant strains are also resistant to ganciclovir; however, they are usually sensitive to foscarnet. The development of acyclovir resistance should be considered in patients with herpetic lesions refractory to acyclovir therapy.

Varicella zoster virus (VZ), the etiologic agent of chickenpox, assumes a latent form in dorsal root ganglia following primary infection (see Chap. 144). Later in life, reactivation is associated with shingles; the appearance of shingles in any patient under 50 should be an indication for workup of an underlying immunodeficiency, particularly HIV. Shingles is an early manifestation of HIV-induced immunodeficiency and in one African study, 91 percent of the patients developing shingles had underlying HIV infection. VZ infection in a patient with HIV infection is almost exclusively confined to the skin, although the skin eruptions may be extensive, over several dermatomes, and extremely painful (see Fig. A1-37). A recurrence rate of 23 percent was noted in one report. A disseminated cutaneous form of zoster that very much resembles a mild form of chickenpox may be seen in patients with advanced HIV disease. As noted above, a small number of patients may develop the acute retinal necrosis syndrome, often in association with trigeminal shingles. Visceral involvement is extremely rare as a reactivation syndrome in an HIV-infected patient, in contrast to many other severe immunodeficiency states. Hence, patients need not be hospitalized and placed in strict isolation. Primary infection, on the other hand, can be lethal and should be treated aggressively with acyclovir and hyperimmune immunoglobulin. While treatment for shingles is not required, it can often result in a reduction in the time to resolution of the lesions, and most physicians choose to treat with high-dose oral or intravenous acyclovir. Acyclovir-resistant strains have been noted and characteristically present as hyperkeratotic lesions; under these circumstances forscarnet is a useful alternative.

Epstein-Barr virus (EBV), one of the causative agent of infectious mononucleosis, is also a very common infection in patients with HIV infection (see Chap. 145). Many patients with HIV actively shed EBV throughout the course of their illness. Aside from the association with lymphoma (discussed below), EBV is felt to play a causative role in oral hairy leukoplakia (OHL). OHL presents as white, frond-like lesions on the lateral aspect of the tongue, and is sometimes seen on the adjacent buccal mucosa (see Fig. A1-40). These lesions are sometimes confused with candida; however, they are quite distinct and, in contrast to candida lesions, cannot be scraped. EBV genome has been demonstrated in these lesions by in situ hybridization. This observation coupled with the fact that there are reports that these lesions regress following therapy with high-dose oral acyclovir have supported the concept that there is a cause and effect relationship between EBV and OHL. Despite this therapeutic option, these lesions are rarely of sufficient clinical consequence to require therapy; they have a relatively high spontaneous remission rate (25 to 50 percent), and are more important for what they represent, namely the presence of immunodeficiency.

JC virus, a human papovavirus that is the etiologic agent of progressive multifocal leukoencephalopathy (PML), is an important opportunistic infection in patients with AIDS (see Chap. 375). While approximately 70 percent of the general adult population has antibodies to JC virus, indicative of prior infection, less than 10 percent show any evidence of ongoing viral replications. In contrast, close to 33 percent of HIV-infected individuals have evidence of active replication of JC virus. PML, the only known clinical manifestation of JC virus infection is seen in 4 percent of HIV-infected individuals and is a late manifestation of AIDS. PML is a demyelinating disease that begins as small foci in subcortical white matter that eventually coalesce. The cerebral hemispheres, cerebellum, and brainstem may all be involved. Histologically, swollen oligodendritic nuclei with inclusions due to the nucleocapsid proteins of JC are seen. Death of the oligodendrocyte leads to demyelination without inflammation. Patients have a protracted clinical course, often developing multiple focal deficits without changes in mental status. Patients with PML may exhibit ataxia, hemiparesis, visual field cuts, aphasia, and sensory defects. The diagnosis is usually made by MRI, which reveals multiple white matter lesions on T2-weighted images. The clinical picture is generally much more impressive than the findings on MRI. Death usually occurs within 3 to 6 months of the onset of symptoms. Intrathecal cytosine arabinoside leads to improvement in some cases; however, no consistently effective therapy is currently available.

Evidence of infection with *human papilloma virus* is approximately twice as common in HIV-infected individuals (81 percent of patients in one series) as in the general population. The association of this virus with epidermal dysplasia suggests that both anal and cervical carcinomas will be seen in the HIV-infected population with increased frequency as survival is prolonged through the use of better antiretroviral regimens (see below).

Over 95 percent of HIV-infected patients have evidence of infection with *hepatitis B*: coinfection with *hepatitis C* and *hepatitis D* is also quite common. HIV infection has several effects on hepatitis virus infection. It is associated with approximately a threefold increase in the development of persistent hepatitis B surface antigenemia. However, patients with hepatitis B infection in the presence of HIV infection have decreased evidence of inflammatory liver disease, presumably due to the effects of HIV on the immune system. Hepatitis D is a defective RNA virus that requires concomitant infection with hepatitis B in order to replicate, and thus infection is only seen together with hepatitis B infection. Hepatitis D infection is more common in patients with HIV infection, is associated with higher levels of hepatitis B virus replication, and seems to be associated with slightly worse hepatic disease as evidenced by slightly higher levels of hepatic transaminases.

NEOPLASTIC DISEASES   A variety of neoplastic and premalignant diseases occur with increased frequency in HIV-infected individuals. Among them are Kaposi's sarcoma, lymphoma, and intraepithelial dysplasia of the cervix and anus. These diseases are significant contributors to the morbidity and mortality of patients with HIV infection. The clinical manifestations of these complications as well as their epidemiologic profiles have undergone considerable change as new approaches to treatment develop and as the epidemic involves different demographic groups.

Kaposi's sarcoma is a multicentric neoplasm consisting of multiple vascular nodules appearing in the skin, mucous membranes, and viscera. The course ranges from indolent, with only minor skin or lymph node involvement, to fulminant, with extensive cutaneous and visceral involvement. In the initial period of the AIDS epidemic Kaposi's sarcoma was a prominent clinical feature of the first cases of AIDS, occurring in 79 percent of the patients diagnosed in 1981. By 1989 it was seen in only 25 percent of cases and by 1992 this number had decreased to 9 percent. Part of this decrease is a reflection of the fact that AIDS-related Kaposi's sarcoma, in contrast to classical or endemic forms, is a disease that occurs predominantly in homosexual men, with 96 percent of all cases occurring in that risk group. As the percentage of AIDS cases in other risk groups increases, the percentage of cases complicated by Kaposi's sarcoma decreases. This, however, is only a partial explanation for the observed decreased incidence in Kaposi's sarcoma in patients with AIDS. A growing body of epidemiologic data points to the possibility that a sexually transmitted cofactor may play a role in the development of Kaposi's sarcoma. In this regard, Kaposi's sarcoma is four times more common in women who have had sexual contact with bisexual men, Kaposi's sarcoma has been seen in homosexual men without evidence of HIV infection, and homosexual men in New York and Los Angeles are more likely than homosexual men in the central states to have Kaposi's sarcoma. As safer sex practices are employed, especially in the homosexual community, the risk of transmission of this unknown cofactor and thus the risk of Kaposi's sarcoma decreases. Kaposi's sarcoma has been an early manifestation of HIV infection, at times occurring in patients with normal CD4+ T cell counts. Thus the rate of new cases of Kaposi's sarcoma may be influenced as much by the rate of new HIV infections as the total number of HIV infections. As the rate of new HIV infections among homosexual men decreases, a decrease in the overall incidence of new cases of Kaposi's sarcoma would be expected.

From a pathophysiologic perspective, Kaposi's sarcoma appears more like a consequence of disordered cytokine regulation of cell growth than a true cancer (see above and Chap. 151). Generally speaking, the tumor respects tissue planes and is rarely invasive.

Clinically, Kaposi's sarcoma may present in a variety of ways and may be seen at any stage of HIV infection, even in the presence of normal CD4+ T cell counts. The initial lesion may be a small, raised reddish purple nodule on the skin, a discoloration on the oral mucosa, or a swollen lymph node (see Fig. A1-22). Lesions often appear in sun-exposed areas, particularly the tip of the nose, and have a propensity to occur in areas of trauma (Kebner phenomenon). Because of the vascular nature of the tumors and the presence of extravasated red blood cells in the lesions, their color ranges from reddish to purple to brown and may often take on the appearance of a bruise with yellowish discoloration and tattooing. Lesions range in size from a few millimeters to several centimeters and may be either discrete or confluent. Kaposi's sarcoma lesions most commonly appear as raised macules; however, they also appear papular, particularly in patients with higher CD4 counts. Confluent lesions may give rise to surrounding lymphedema and may be quite disfiguring when they involve the face and disabling when they involve the lower extremities or the surfaces of joints. Lymph nodes, gastrointestinal tract, and lung are the organ systems most commonly affected by Kaposi's sarcoma; however, lesions have been reported in virtually every organ system including the heart and the CNS. In contrast to most malignancies where lymph node involvement implies metastatic spread and a poor prognosis, lymph node involvement may be seen very early in Kaposi's sarcoma and is of no special clinical significance. In fact, some patients may present with disease limited to the lymph nodes. These are generally patients with relatively intact immune function and thus have the best prognosis. Pulmonary involvement generally presents as shortness of breath. The chest x-ray characteristically shows bilateral lower lobe infiltrates that obscure the margins of the mediastinum and diaphragm (Fig. 279-21). Pleural effusions are seen in 70 percent of cases of pulmonary Kaposi's sarcoma, a fact that is often helpful in the differential diagnosis. Gastrointestinal involvement usually takes one of two forms. The first is mucosal involvement that may lead to bleeding that can be severe. These patients on occasion may also develop symptoms of gastrointestinal obstruction if large lesions develop. The second gastrointestinal manifestation is biliary tract involvement. Kaposi's sarcoma lesions may infiltrate the gallbladder and biliary tree leading to a clinical picture of obstructive jaundice similar to that seen with sclerosing cholangitis. In an effort to create a set of uniform parameters upon which to stage the extent of Kaposi's sarcoma, several systems have been proposed. Given the unique nature of this disorder, standard oncologic staging systems have not been useful. An excellent staging system has been developed by the National Institute of Allergy and Infectious Diseases AIDS Clinical Trials Group; it distinguishes patients on the basis of tumor extent, immunologic function, and presence or absence of systemic disease (Table 279-20).

A diagnosis of Kaposi's sarcoma is based upon biopsy of a

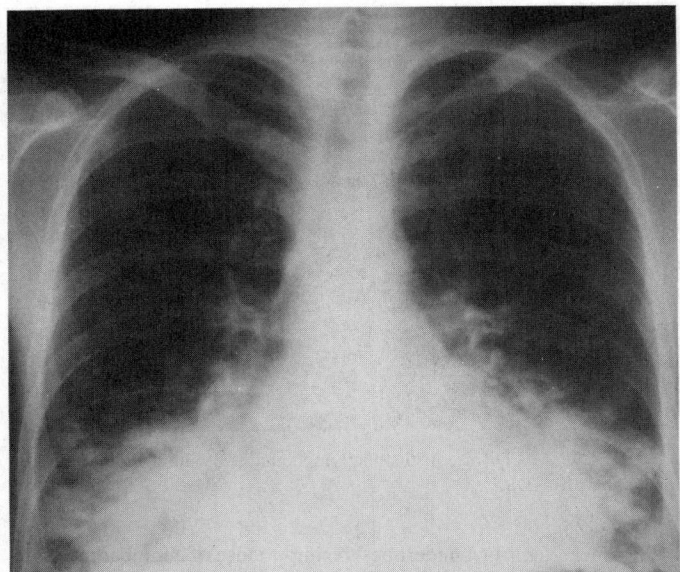

FIGURE 279-21 Chest x-ray of a patient with AIDS and pulmonary Kaposi's sarcoma. The characteristic findings include dense bilateral lower lobe infiltrates obscuring the heart borders and a pleural effusion.

suspicious lesion. Histologically one sees a proliferation of spindle cells, a proliferation of endothelial cells, and extravasation of red blood cells. Hemosiderin laden macrophages and, in early cases, an inflammatory cell infiltrate may be present. Included in the differential diagnoses are lymphoma (oral lesions), bacillary angiomatosis, and cutaneous mycobacterial infections.

Management of Kaposi's sarcoma (Table 279-21) should be carried out in consultation with an expert since definitive guidelines do not exist. In some cases lesions remain quite indolent and many patients can be managed with no specific treatment. Given the fact that less than 10 percent of AIDS patients with Kaposi's sarcoma die as a consequence of their malignancy and that death from opportunistic infections is much more common, whenever possible one should avoid treatment regimens that may further suppress the immune system and render the patients more susceptible to opportunistic infections. Treatment is indicated under two main circumstances. The first is when a single lesion or a limited number of lesions are causing significant discomfort or cosmetic problems. Examples of this would be prominent facial lesions, lesions overlying a joint, or lesions in the posterior oropharynx that interfere with swallowing. Under these circumstances treatment with localized radiation, intralesional vinblastine, or cryotherapy may be indicated. Patients with HIV infection are particularly sensitive to the side effects of radiation therapy. This is especially true with respect to the development of radiation-induced mucositis; doses of radiation directed at mucosal

surfaces, particularly in the head and neck region should be adjusted accordingly. The use of systemic single-agent chemotherapy should be considered in patients with a large number of lesions. Response rates varying from 26 to 80 percent have been seen with etoposide, vinblastine, doxorubicin, bleomycin, or IFN-α. The single most important determinant of response appears to be the CD4 + T cell count. It is ironic that the patients most likely to respond to therapy are those who need it the least and who generally should not be treated aggressively for fear of further compromising immune function. This relationship between response rate and baseline CD4 + T cell count is particularly true for IFN-α, where the response rate for patients with over 600 CD4 + T cells per microliter is approximately 80 percent, while for patients with under 150 CD4 + T cells it is under 10 percent. In contrast to the other single therapy agents, IFN-α provides an added advantage of having antiretroviral activity and thus may be considered an appropriate first choice for single-agent systemic therapy for the early patient with disseminated disease. Combination chemotherapy offers the best overall response rate for patients with life-threatening disease, with close to 90 percent of all patients responding to a low-dose combination regimen of doxorubicin, bleomycin, and vinblastine. As noted above, Kaposi's sarcoma is a radiation-sensitive tumor, and for patients with severe pulmonary involvement, one may also consider radiation therapy.

Lymphomas occur with an increased incidence in patients with either congenital or acquired T cell immunodeficiencies (see Chap. 278). AIDS is no exception to this general observation, with at least 3 percent of all patients developing lymphoma at some time during the course of their illness. This represents a 60-fold increased incidence compared to the general population. Lymphoma is seen in all risk groups, with the highest incidence (5.2 percent) in patients with hemophilia, and the lowest (1 percent), in patients from the Caribbean or Africa with heterosexually acquired infection. Lymphoma is a late manifestation of HIV infection, generally occurring in patients with under 200 CD4 + T cells per microliter. As HIV disease progresses, the risk of lymphoma increases. In contrast to Kaposi's sarcoma, which occurs at a relatively constant rate (2.4 percent per year) throughout the course of illness, the attack rate for lymphoma rises exponentially with increasing duration of HIV infection and decreasing level of immunologic function. At 3 years following infection, the risk of lymphoma is 0.8 percent per year. By 8 years following infection it has increased to 2.6 percent per year.

Three main categories of lymphoma are seen in patients with HIV infection. These are grade III or IV immunoblastic lymphoma, Burkitt's lymphoma, and primary CNS lymphoma (see Chap. 311). Approximately 90 percent of these lymphomas are B cell in phenotype and half contain Epstein-Barr virus DNA. These tumors may be either monoclonal or oligoclonal in origin and are probably in some way related to the pronounced polyclonal B cell activation seen in patients with AIDS (see "Pathophysiology and Immunopathogenesis" above).

Immunoblastic lymphomas account for approximately 60 percent of the cases of lymphoma in patients with AIDS. These are generally

TABLE 279-20 National Institute of Allergy and Infectious Diseases AIDS Clinical Trials Group TIS Staging System for Kaposi's sarcoma

Parameter	Good risk (stage 0): All of the following	Poor risk (stage 1): Any of the following
Tumor (T)	Confined to skin and/or lymph nodes and/or minimal oral disease	Tumor-associated edema or ulceration Extensive oral lesions Gastrointestinal lesions Nonnodal visceral lesions
Immune system (I) Systemic illness (S)	CD4 + T cell count ≥200 cells/μL No B symptoms* Karnofsky performance status >70 No history of opportunistic infection neurologic disease, lymphoma, or thrush	CD4 + T cell count < 200 cells/μL B symptoms* present Karnofsky performance status < 70 History of opportunistic infection neurologic disease, lymphoma, or thrush

* Defined as unexplained fever, night sweats, >10% involuntary weight loss, or diarrhea persisting for more than 2 weeks.

TABLE 279-21   Management of AIDS-associated Kaposi's sarcoma

Observation
Single or limited number of lesions
  Radiation
  Intralesional vinblastine
  Cryotherapy
Extensive, non-life-threatening disease
  Single-agent chemotherapy (etoposide; vinblastine; advanycin, or
  bleomycin)
  Interferon-α (if CD4+ T cell >150/μL)
Life-threatening disease
  Combination chemotherapy with low-dose, doxorubicin, bleomycin
  and vinblastine (ABV)
  Radiation

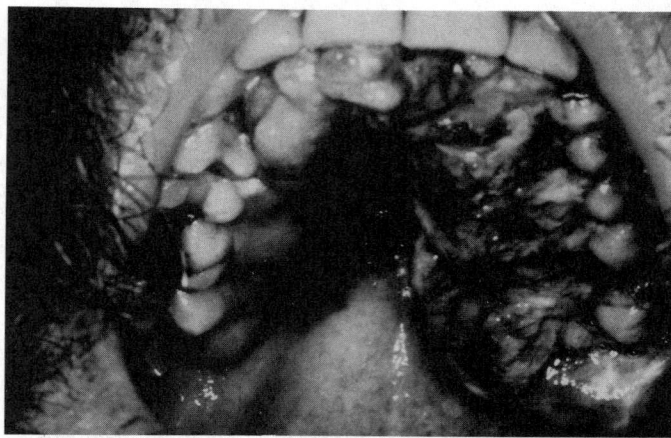

FIGURE 279-22   Diffuse histiocytic lymphoma involving the hard palate of a patient with AIDS.

high-grade and would have been classified as diffuse histiocytic lymphomas in earlier classification schemes. This tumor is more common in older patients, increasing from an incidence of 0 percent in HIV-infected individuals less than 1 year of age to over 3 percent in those over 50 years of age.

Small noncleaved cell or *Burkitt's lymphoma* accounts for approximately 20 percent of the cases of lymphoma in patients with AIDS. These are most frequent in patients 10 to 19 years of age and usually demonstrate characteristic *c-myc* translocations from chromosome 8 to chromosomes 14 or 22. Burkitt's lymphoma is not commonly seen in the setting of immunosuppression, and the incidence of this tumor in the setting of HIV infection is over 1000-fold higher than that seen in the general population. In contrast to African Burkitt's lymphoma, where 97 percent of cases contain an Epstein-Barr virus genome, less than 50 percent of HIV-associated Burkitt's lymphoma are Epstein-Barr positive.

Primary CNS lymphoma accounts for approximately 20 percent of the cases of lymphoma in patients with HIV infection. In contrast to the HIV-associated Burkitt's lymphoma, primary CNS lymphomas are more commonly Epstein-Barr virus positive; in one study, the incidence was 100 percent and the lymphomas did not appear to have a predilection for any particular age group. The median CD4+ T cell count at time of diagnosis for patients with primary CNS lymphoma is approximately 40 cells per microliter, compared to a mean of approximately 190 cells per microliter for patients with systemic lymphoma. This highlights the fact that CNS lymphoma generally presents at a later stage of HIV infection than does systemic lymphoma, and this may at least in part explain the poorer prognosis for this particular subset of patients (discussed below).

The clinical presentation of lymphoma in the patient with HIV infection is quite varied, ranging from focal seizures to rapidly growing mass lesions in the oral mucosa (Fig. 279-22) to persistent unexplained fever. At least 80 percent of patients will present with extranodal disease and a similar percentage will have B type symptoms of fever, night sweats, or weight loss. Virtually any site in the body may be involved. The most common extranodal site is the CNS, involved in approximately one-third of all patients with lymphoma; approximately 60 percent of these will be primary CNS lymphoma. Primary CNS lymphoma generally presents with focal neurologic deficits including cranial nerve findings, headaches, and/or seizures. MRI or CT generally reveals a limited number (one to three) of 3 to 5-cm lesions. The lesions are often ring enhancing with contrast and may occur in any location. The main differential diagnosis is cerebral toxoplasmosis, although cerebral Chagas disease may manifest a similar clinical picture. Prognosis is poor; the median survival following diagnosis is 2 to 3 months.

In addition to the 20 percent of all lymphomas in HIV-infected individuals that are primary CNS lymphomas, CNS disease unrelated to lymphoma is also seen in HIV-infected patients with systemic lymphoma, and approximately 20 percent of patients with systemic lymphoma will have CNS disease in the form of leptomeningeal

involvement. This fact underlines the importance of a lumbar puncture in the staging evaluation of patients with systemic lymphoma.

The second most common extranodal site is the GI tract, with involvement noted in 25 percent of patients. Any site in the GI tract may be involved, and patients may complain of difficulty swallowing or abdominal pain. The diagnosis is usually suspected based upon CT or MRI of the abdomen. Bone marrow involvement occurs in approximately 20 percent of patients and may be associated with a pancytopenia. Liver and lung involvement are each seen in approximately 10 percent of patients. Pulmonary disease may present as either a mass lesion, multiple nodules, or an interstitial infiltrate.

Both conventional and nonconventional approaches have been employed in an effort to treat HIV-related lymphomas. Initial attempts using standard intensive therapeutic regimens have largely been abandoned due to low response rate (20 to 30 percent) and a high incidence of fatal opportunistic infections. The median survival for patients treated with intensive regimens is approximately 4 to 6 months. These figures predominantly reflect results in patients with fairly advanced HIV infection and low CD4+ T cell counts. Patients with higher CD4+ T cell counts do better with intensive chemotherapy, and in these earlier-stage patients, response rates as high as 72 percent and disease-free intervals exceeding 15 months have been reported. Clinical trials are currently underway comparing standard chemotherapeutic approaches with low-dose modified regimens. At present, the median survival for patients with HIV-related systemic lymphoma is 10 months. Treatment of primary CNS lymphoma is almost uniformly unsuccessful. Palliative measures such as radiation therapy and/or glucocorticoids aimed at reducing the size of the lesion(s) and the accompanying cerebral edema may provide some symptomatic relief. The prognosis is poor for patients with primary CNS lymphoma; median survival is 2 to 4 months.

Intraepithelial dysplasia of either the cervix or the anus has been increasingly recognized as a complication of long-standing HIV infection. This human papilloma virus–associated condition correlates with the subsequent development of intraepithelial neoplasia and eventually invasive cancer. In two separate studies, HIV-infected men without anorectal symptoms were studied for evidence of dysplasia, and Papanicolaou smears were found to be abnormal in about 40 percent. These changes were persistent at 1-year follow-up, raising the possibility of a subsequent transition to a more malignant condition. While the incidence of an abnormal Papanicolaou smear of the cervix is approximately 5 percent in the otherwise healthy population, the incidence of abnormal smears in women with HIV infection is 60 percent, and invasive cervical carcinoma has been added to the list of AIDS-defining conditions. Thus far only small increases in the incidence of cervical or anal cancer have been seen as a consequence of HIV infection. However, given these findings, as patients with HIV infection live longer through the use of improved treatment strategies, it is likely that such conditions will begin to appear more frequently. For these reasons, all patients with HIV infection should have periodic rectal and/or pelvic examinations with Papanicolaou smears to look for evidence of cellular dysplasia.

A variety of other neoplastic conditions have been described in patients with HIV infection. While none of these other conditions have been reported to occur at a higher rate than that seen in the general population, these cancers may be more fulminant and difficult to treat in an HIV-infected patient. In this regard, Hodgkin's disease in the setting of HIV infection often presents as extensive disease with mixed cellular or lymphocyte depletion pathologic types. In contrast to the excellent results and high cure rates for Hodgkin's disease in the general population, the patient with HIV infection and Hodgkin's disease has a median survival of only 12 to 15 months. As the epidemic of HIV infection continues, additional neoplastic complications are to be expected.

ORGAN-SPECIFIC SYNDROMES Virtually every organ system in the body is vulnerable to disease either as a direct consequence of HIV infection or secondary to other infectious or neoplastic conditions. While the majority of these diseases are due to opportunistic infections or neoplasms (see above), there are also a variety of clinical problems for which no specific pathogens are clearly identified.

Pulmonary disease is seen in virtually every patient with HIV infection. Its evaluation is one of the most important components in management, given the importance of early diagnosis and initiation of specific therapy. The most common manifestation of pulmonary disease is pneumonia and the most common cause of pneumonia is *Pneumocystis carinii*. Other major causes of pneumonia include nonspecific interstitial pneumonitis, Kaposi's sarcoma, mycobacterial infections, and fungal infections. Although there are some distinguishing clinical and radiographic characteristics (Table 279-22), in most cases an accurate diagnosis is based upon histologic or microbiologic identification of the causative organism. Specimens for examination are derived from induced sputum, bronchoalveolar lavage, transbronchial biopsy, or open lung biopsy. In most of the conditions seen in HIV-infected patients, the chest x-ray reveals bilateral diffuse interstitial infiltrates. In patients with mycobacterial or fungal infections, hilar or mediastinal adenopathy may also be seen. In Kaposi's sarcoma the infiltrates are dense and often obliterate the borders of the heart and diaphragm; there is usually an accompanying pleural effusion. Upper-lobe cavitary disease is suggestive of reactivation TB or *Pneumocystis carinii* pneumonia in a patient receiving aerosolized pentamidine. The presence of a pneumothorax is most consistent with this latter condition. With the exception of bacterial pneumonias, sputum production is usually scant. Hemoptysis may be seen in the setting of cryptococcal pneumonia, tuberculosis, or Kaposi's sarcoma.

Two forms of idiopathic interstitial pneumonia have been described in patients with HIV infection; these are lymphoid interstitial pneumonitis (LIP) and nonspecific interstitial pneumonitis (NIP). LIP, while a common finding in children, is quite rate in adults, occurring in approximately 1 percent of patients. This disorder is characterized by a benign lymphocytic infiltrate of the lung and is felt to be part of the systemic polyclonal activation of lymphocytes seen in the context of HIV and EBV infections. Transbronchial biopsy is diagnostic in 50 percent of cases; an open lung biopsy is required for diagnosis in the remainder. This condition is generally self-limited and no specific treatment is necessary. Severe cases have been managed with a brief course of glucocorticoids. NIP is seen in up to half of all patients with AIDS and in some series is responsible for up to one-third of all pulmonary disease. Interstitial infiltrates with lymphocytes and plasma cells in a perivascular and peribronchial distribution are seen on histologic examination. Symptoms include fever and nonproductive cough occasionally accompanied by mild chest discomfort. Chest x-ray, which is normal in 50 percent of cases, may demonstrate a faint interstitial pattern. Similar to LIP, this is a self-limited process for which no therapy is indicated.

In addition to pneumonia, *sinusitis* is a common respiratory tract complication of HIV infection and is seen at all stages of infection. More severe cases are seen in patients with lower CD4+ T cell counts. Sinusitis presents as fever, nasal congestion, and headache; the diagnosis is best made by CT or MRI. Maxillary sinuses are most commonly involved; however, disease is frequently seen in ethmoid, sphenoid, and frontal sinuses as well. Although over 80 percent of patients show clinical improvement regardless of whether or not antibiotics are given, radiographic improvement is quicker and more pronounced in patients who have received antimicrobial therapy. It is postulated that this high incidence of sinusitis results from the increased frequency of infections with encapsulated organisms such as *Haemophilus influenzae* and *Streptococcus pneumoniae*, although this has not been formally proven.

Gastrointestinal disease is a common feature of HIV infection and is most frequently due to a secondary infection. The oral mucosa, in addition to being involved with thrush, oral hairy leukoplakia, and Kaposi's sarcoma also may be affected by large, shallow, painful aphthous ulcers. These lesions, which may be painful enough to result in a decrease in oral intake, are of unknown cause. While no specific therapy exists, some reports suggest that brief courses of high-dose glucocorticoids or thalidomide may be of help. Esophagitis (Fig. 279-19) generally presents with odynophagia and retrosternal pain and may be due to *Candida*, CMV, or HSV. In addition, the esophagus may be involved with Kaposi's sarcoma and lymphoma. The esophageal mucosa, similar to the oral mucosa, may have large, painful ulcers of unclear etiology. These lesions are somewhat similar in appearance to the ulcers of CMV esophagitis but do not respond to antiviral therapy and can pose a significant problem with regard to nutrition. Achlorhydria is a common problem in patients with HIV infection; however, gastric problems are otherwise rare. Kaposi's sarcoma as well as lymphoma may involve the stomach. Infections of the small and large intestine are among the most significant gastrointestinal problems in the HIV-infected patient. They usually present with diarrhea, abdominal pain, occasionally fever and, in severe cases, weight loss. In addition to specific secondary infections, patients with HIV infection may also experience a chronic diarrheal syndrome for which no etiologic agent other than HIV can be identified and which is generally referred to as *AIDS* or *HIV enteropathy*. This is a clinical condition resembling chronic gastroenteritis with diarrhea of more than 1 month duration for which no cause can be found. This condition is most likely a direct result of HIV infection within the gastrointestinal tract. Histologic examination of the small bowel in these patients reveals low-grade mucosal atrophy with a decrease in mitotic figures suggesting a hyporegenerative state. Patients often have decreased or absent small bowel lactase and malabsorption with accompanying weight loss.

TABLE 279-22 Characteristics of pneumonia in patients with HIV infection

Etiology	Sputum	Chest x-ray
Pneumocystis carinii	Scant	Normal/interstitial infiltrate
Pneumocystis carinii in setting of aerosolized pentamidine	Scant	Upper lobe cavitary lesions; pneumothorax
Bacterial	Neutrophils, organisms	Consolidation
Atypical mycobacteria	Scant	Interstitial infiltrate; hilar adenopathy
Reactivation *Mycobacterium tuberculosis*	White blood cells, organisms, occasional hemoptysis	Cavitary or miliary infiltrates; hilar adenopathy
Nonspecific interstitial pneumonitis (NIP)	Scant	Normal/interstitial infiltrate
Kaposi's sarcoma	Scant, occasional hemoptysis	Dense, bilateral lower lobe infiltrates; pleural effusions

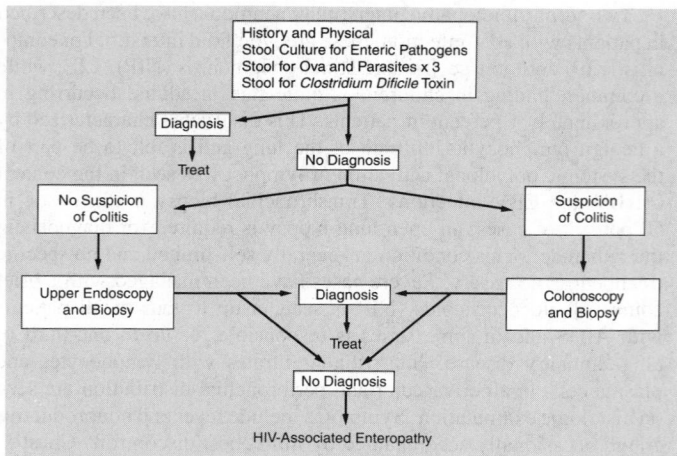

TABLE 279-23   **Causes of bone marrow suppression in patients with HIV infection**
HIV infection
Mycobacterial infection
Fungal infections
B19 Parvovirus infection
Lymphoma
Medications
Zidovudine
Dapsone
Trimethoprim/sulfamethoxazole
Pyrimethamine
5-Flucytosine
Ganciclovir
Interferon-α
Trimetrexate
Foscarnet

FIGURE 279-23   Algorithm for the evaluation of diarrhea in a patient with HIV infection. HIV-associated enteropathy is a diagnosis of exclusion and can be made only after other, generally treatable, forms of diarrheal illness have been ruled out.

In working up a patient with HIV infection and gastrointestinal problems, a set of stool examinations, including culture, examination for ova and parasites, and examination for *Clostridium difficile* toxin should form the initial part of the evaluation. Approximately 50 percent of the time this work-up will demonstrate infection with pathogenic bacteria such as salmonella, shigella, campylobacter; mycobacteria (both atypical and *Mycobacterium tuberculosis*); protozoa such as giardia, *E. histolytica*, cryptosporidia, or *Isospora*; or *Clostridium difficile*. If these stool examinations are negative, additional evaluation, including upper and/or lower endoscopy with biopsy may establish a diagnosis of microsporidial or mycobacterial infection of the small intestine or CMV colitis in over half the patients. In patients for whom this diagnostic evaluation is nonrevealing and, if diarrhea has persisted for over 1 month, a presumptive diagnosis of HIV enteropathy can be made. An algorithm for the evaluation of diarrhea in patients with HIV infection is given in Fig. 279-23.

Rectal lesions are common in HIV-infected patients, particularly the perirectal ulcers and erosions due to the reactivation of HSV (Fig. 279-21). These may appear quite atypical, without vesicles, and respond well to treatment with acyclovir. Other rectal lesions more commonly seen in HIV-infected patients include condyloma acuminatum, Kaposi's sarcoma, and intraepithelial neoplasia.

Several different forms of hepatobiliary disease occur in patients with HIV infection. Biliary tract disease in the form of papillary stenosis or sclerosing cholangitis has been reported in the context of cryptosporidiosis, CMV infection, and Kaposi's sarcoma. Hepatic disease may take the form of hepatocellular injury due to hepatitis viruses, granulomatous hepatitis due to mycobacterial or fungal infections, or hepatic masses secondary to tuberculous abscess or peliosis hepatis. Fatty infiltration has also been reported, and it has been suggested that this may be related in some patients to nucleoside therapy.

Pancreatic injury is most commonly due to drug toxicity, notably that secondary to pentamidine or dideoxynucleosides. While up to 50 percent of patients with HIV infection may have biochemical evidence of pancreatic injury, and there is often evidence of pancreatic infection with CMV and MAC at autopsy, fewer than 5 percent of patients show any clinical evidence of pancreatitis that is not linked to a drug toxicity.

Hematologic problems are common throughout the course of HIV infection and occur as a direct consequence of HIV, as a manifestation of secondary infections and neoplasms, and as a side effect of therapy (Table 279-23). HIV has been shown to be present in the bone marrow, and there is evidence that it is capable of infecting early hematopoietic precursor cells. Bone marrow suppression may also be associated with disseminated mycobacterial infections, fungal infections, and lymphoma. Direct histologic examination and culture of bone marrow in patients with HIV infection and unexplained hematologic abnormalities are often diagnostic. A significant percentage of bone marrow aspirates have been reported to contain lymphoid aggregates, the precise significance of which is unknown.

Anemia is the most common hematologic abnormality seen with HIV infection and is present in 18 percent of asymptomatic seropositive individuals, 50 percent of patients with early symptoms, and 75 percent of patients with AIDS. While generally mild, anemia can be quite severe and may require chronic blood transfusion. Among the specific reversible causes of anemia in HIV-infected individuals are drug toxicity, systemic fungal and mycobacterial infections, nutritional deficiences, and parvovirus B19 infections.

Zidovudine is a major contributor to the anemia seen in patients with advanced HIV infection. This nucleoside analogue (discussed below), has a somewhat selective ability to block erythroid maturation, an effect that is seen prior to effects on other marrow elements. A characteristic feature of zidovudine therapy is an elevated MCV. Another drug with selective effects on the erythroid series is dapsone. This agent can cause a serious hemolytic anemia in patients who are G6PD-deficient as well as create a functional anemia in others through induction of methemoglobemia.

Folate levels are usually normal in HIV-infected individuals; however, B_{12} levels may be depressed in patients with AIDS, presumably as a consequence of long-standing achlorhydria and malabsorption. Replacement therapy with B_{12} seems to have a minimal effect on HIV-associated anemia. True autoimmune hemolytic anemia is rare, although approximately 20 percent of patients with HIV infection may have a positive direct antiglobulin test, presumably as a consequence of polyclonal B cell activation. Some patients do develop a syndrome of increased peeripheral destruction or splenic sequestration of erythrocytes that in some instances has been reported in association with zidovudine treatment.

In addition to the more common secondary infections described above, patients with HIV infection have been reported to develop anemia secondary to infection with parvovirus B19. This is an important cause of anemia to be aware of, since it responds to treatment with intravenous immunoglobulin. Baseline erythropoietin levels in patients with HIV infection and anemia are generally less than expected, given the degree of anemia. The exception is zidovudine-associated anemia, where levels may be quite high. In fact, in patients with zidovudine-associated anemia and low erythropoietin levels, treatment with erythropoietin at a dose of 100 μg/kg three times a week may result in an increase in hemoglobulin levels. Erythropoietin seems to be of less benefit in patients with elevated erythropoietin levels and in patients with anemia due to causes other than zidovudine toxicity.

Neutropenia is seen in approximately half the patients with HIV infection. It is mild in most instances; however, it can be severe and place patients at risk of spontaneous bacterial infections. This is usually seen in patients receiving any of a number of myelosuppressive therapies used in the treatment of HIV infection and its complications. Zidovudine, ganciclovir, pyrimethamine, and trimethoprim/sulfa-methoxazole are among the drugs that most commonly cause severe neutropenia in patients with HIV infection. Neutropenia is most severe in patients with more advanced disease. Folinic acid (leucovorin) may ameliorate the neutropenia induced by pyrimethamine. The role of colony stimulating factors in the management of patients with HIV infection and neutropenia has undergone extensive evaluation. Both G-CSF and GM-CSF have been shown to increase neutrophil counts in patients with HIV infection. These effects have been seen in both drug-induced and nondrug-induced neutropenias. While G-CSF is theoretically more attractive as a colony stimulating agent due to the fact that HIV replication is enhanced in vitro by GM-CSF, additional studies need to be performed to determine precisely the role of either of these factors in the management of patients with HIV infection and neutropenia.

Thrombocytopenia occurs in approximately 40 percent of patients with HIV infection and, in contrast to neutropenia and anemia, is often an early, primary manifestation of HIV infection (see above). The thrombocytopenia seen as direct result of HIV infection resembles that of idiopathic thrombocytopenic purpura (ITP) and responds not only to conventional strategies but, in a large number of cases, to therapy with antiretrovirals. Thrombocytopenia may also be seen as a side effect of medications; however, it is rarely a dose-limiting side effect. Other causes for thrombocytopenia in patients with HIV infection include bone marrow involvement with lymphoma, myco-bacterial infection, or fungal infections.

Lymphadenopathy is also a common finding in patients with HIV infection, ranging from the generalized follicular hyperplasia seen early in disease to involvement secondary to opportunistic infections and neoplasms. Lymph node biopsy is not indicated in the lymphade-nopathy seen early in disease unless it is associated with rapid enlargement, unusual consistency, or coalescence. While Kaposi's sarcoma may present in a lymphadenopathic form early in disease there are no data to suggest that early treatment is indicated. In contrast, new-onset lymphadenopathy in the setting of more advanced HIV infection, for example CD4+ T cell counts under 200 cells per microliter may be the first sign of a secondary infection or neoplasm and should be examined both histologically and with culture. Among the secondary infections commonly associated with lymphadenopathy are mycobacterial infections, fungal infections, and bacillary angio-matosis. In addition to Kaposi's sarcoma, lymphoma may also present as lymphadenopathy.

Renal disease may be associated with HIV infection (see Chaps. 241 and 242). Although renal disease is often the result of a drug-induced injury, a significant portion of patients with AIDS (up to 10 percent in some series) may develop renal disease as a direct consequence of HIV infection; this is designated as *AIDS-* or *HIV-associated nephropathy*. Secondary infections rarely result in significant renal impairment; however, one may see nephrocalcinosis as a result of infection with mycobacteria or *Pneumocystis carinii*.

Among the drugs commonly associated with renal damage in patients with AIDS are pentamidine, amphotericin, and foscarnet. In addition, trimethoprim/sulfamethoxazole may compete for tubular secretion of creatinine and cause an increase in the serum creatinine level, while sulfadiazine may crystallize in the kidney and result in an easily reversible form of renal shutdown.

HIV-associated nephropathy closely resembles heroin-associated nephropathy seen in IVDUs and initially was thought to be that condition in patients with HIV infection; however, it is now recognized as a true direct complication of HIV infection. HIV-associated nephropathy can be an early manifestation of HIV infection and is also seen in children. The severity of renal disease and propensity to develop end-stage renal failure appear to be a function of race and much more of a problem among blacks than whites, perhaps more so than any other manifestation of HIV infection. Given the fact that ir

most series over 50 percent of patients with HIV-associated nephropa-thy were IVDUs, it was originally thought that this racial predilection was merely reflective of the increased portion of blacks in the IVDU group rather than a true race-related phenomenon. However, the incidence by race of HIV-associated end-stage renal failure in non-IVDU homosexual men suggests that race does play a major role and that end-stage renal failure occurs disproportionately among blacks.

The prototypic lesion of HIV-associated nephropathy is a focal segmental glomerulosclerosis, and is seen in approximately 80 percent of patients with this complication. Patients present with heavy proteinuria without edema or hypertension. Ultrasound examination usually reveals enlarged, hyperechogenic kidneys; a definitive diagno-sis is obtained through renal biopsy. Progression to end-stage renal failure usually occurs within 1 year. The remainder of patients (approximately 20 percent) with HIV-associated nephropathy present with a mesangial hyperplasia with minimal glomerulosclerosis. It is believed that this may be the precursor lesion to focal segmental glomerulosclerosis.

There is no successful management for HIV-associated nephropa-thy. There seems to be little overall benefit of zidovudine on this complication of HIV infection, although temporary improvement following initiation of therapy has been noted by some investigators. In patients in whom renal disease is detected relatively early, at the stage of mesangial hyperplasia with minimal glomerulosclerosis, it has been proposed that a short course of glucocorticoids may be of value. While this seems a reasonable option it must be done with awareness of the potentially devastating effects of long-term glucocorticoid use in patients with HIV infection.

Dermatologic problems are common in patients with HIV infection (see Chap. 54). From the macular, roseola-like rash seen with the acute seroconversion syndrome to extensive end-stage Kaposi's sarcoma, cutaneous manifestations are present throughout the course of HIV infection. While many of these manifestations are covered elsewhere in this chapter under their respective causes and under the heading of early symptomatic disease, there are some additional dermatologic problems seen in the context of HIV infection that have not yet been discussed (see Chaps. 51, 52, and 54). Among these are seborrheic dermatitis, eosinophilic pustular folliculitis, and several minor cutaneous infections.

Seborrheic dermatitis occurs in 3 percent of the general population; however, it is seen in up to 50 percent of patients with HIV infection and is among the most common noninfectious manifestations of HIV infection. In fact, in the early days of the AIDS epidemic, patients with a community-acquired pneumonia and seborrheic dermatitis were often given a presumptive diagnosis of PCP. Seborrheic dermatitis increases in prevalence and severity as the CD4 count declines. Several reports have noted that in HIV-infected patients, seborrheic dermatitis may be aggravated by concomitant infection with *Pityro-sporon*, a yeast-like fungus, and have recommended that topical antifungals may be of help in cases refractory to standard topical treatment.

Eosinophilic pustular folliculitis is a rare dermatologic condition seen with increased frequency in patients with HIV infection. It presents as multiple urticarial perifollicular papules that may coalesce to plaque-like lesions. Skin biopsy reveals an eosinophilic infiltrate of the hair follicle that in certain cases has been associated with the presence of a mite. Patients typically have an elevated IgE level and may respond to treatment with topical antihelminthics. There is at least one report of a patient with AIDS developing a severe form of Norwegian scabies with hyperkeratotic, psoriasiform skin lesions.

Although they are not reported to be increased in frequency, both psoriasis and icthyosis may be particularly severe when they occur in patients with HIV infection. Preexisting psoriasis may become guttae in appearance and more refractory to treatment.

As mentioned above there are a variety of secondary infections that present with cutaneous manifestations. Among them are HSV that causes severe erosive orolabial, genital, perirectal (Fig. 279-20), and whitlow lesions and VZ that causes both shingles and a forme fruste of chickenpox secondary to cutaneous dissemination. Similarly, molluscum contagiosum and condyloma acuminatum may be significantly more serious in HIV-infected individuals. Atypical mycobacterial infections may present as erythematous cutaneous nodules, as may certain fungal infections. Extrapulmonary pneumocystosis may result in necrotizing vasculitis.

The skin of patients with HIV infection is often a target organ for drug reactions (see Chap. 52). Although most skin reactions will be mild and not necessarily an indication to discontinue treatment, patients may have particularly severe cutaneous eruptions, including erythroderma and Stevens-Johnson syndrome as a reaction to drugs, particularly sulfa drugs. Similarly, patients with HIV infection are often very photosensitive and burn easily following exposure to sunlight or as a side effect of radiation therapy (see Chap. 55).

Certain of the cosmetic changes that accompany HIV infection and treatment may be less clinically important, but nonetheless troubling to patients. Both yellowing of the nails and straightening of the hair, particularly in black patients, have been reported as a consequence of infection. Zidovudine therapy has been associated with elongation of the eyelashes and the development of a bluish discoloration to the nails, again more commonly seen in black patients. Therapy with clofazamine may cause a yellow-orange discoloration to the skin.

Heart disease, while relatively common at postmortem examination (25 to 75 percent in autopsy series), is rarely a clinical problem in patients with AIDS or HIV infection. The most common clinically significant finding is a dilated cardiomyopathy associated with congestive heart failure (see Chap. 205); this generally occurs as a late complication of HIV infection and, histologically, most closely resembles a myocarditis. HIV has been detected in cardiac tissue and there is debate over whether it plays a direct role in this condition. Patients present with the classic findings of congestive heart failure, namely edema and shortness of breath. Treatment is no different from that of any other patient with congestive heart failure although one must be certain that drug toxicity is not the cause. In this regard, both IFN-α and nucleoside analogues have been reported to cause a cardiomyopathy in patients with HIV infection that reverses once therapy is discontinued. Similarly, Kaposi's sarcoma, cryptococcosis, and toxoplasmosis can involve the myocardium, resulting in cardiomyopathy. In one series, the majority of patients with a treatable myocarditis were found to have myocarditis associated with toxoplasmosis. Most of these patients also had evidence of CNS toxoplasmosis. Thus, an MRI or double-dose contrast CT scan of the brain should be included in the work-up of any patient with advanced HIV infection and an unexplained cardiomyopathy.

A variety of other cardiovascular problems have been noted in the setting of HIV infection. Pericardial disease may be due to Kaposi's sarcoma, mycobacterial infections, cryptococcal disease, or lymphoma. Tamponade and death have been noted in association with pericardial Kaposi's sarcoma, presumably secondary to acute hemorrhage. Clinically significant ischemic heart disease is not seen to an increased degree in HIV-infected individuals, despite the fact that a high percentage of patients are noted to have hypertriglyceridemia and coronary artery disease has been a relatively frequent finding at autopsy. Nonbacterial thrombotic endocarditis has been reported and should be considered in patients with unexplained embolic phenomena. As mentioned above, nucleoside analogues and IFN-α have been associated with cardiac toxicity in HIV-infected patients. In addition, intravenous pentamidine, when given rapidly, can result in hypotension as a consequence of cardiovascular collapse.

Immunologic and rheumatologic disorders are common in patients with HIV infection and range from excessive immediate hypersensitivity–type reactions to an increase in the incidence of reactive arthritis to conditions characterized by a diffuse infiltrative lymphocytosis. These phenomena occur in an apparent paradox to the profound immunodeficiency that characterizes this infection. Drug allergies are the most significant allergic reactions occurring in HIV-infected patients and seem to be more common as the disease progresses; they

occur in 65 percent of patients who receive therapy with trimethoprim/sulfamethoxazole for PCP. In general, these drug reactions are characterized by an erythematous, morbilliform eruption that is pruritic, tends to coalesce, and is often associated with fever. Nonetheless, approximately 33 percent of patients can successfully be maintained on the offending therapy, and thus these reactions are not an immediate indication to stop the drug. Anaphylaxis is extremely rare in patients with HIV infection, and patients with a cutaneous eruption during a single course of therapy can still be considered candidates for future treatment or prophylaxis with the same agent. In addition, desensitization regimens are moderately successful in HIV-infected patients. While the mechanisms underlying these allergic-type phenomena remain unknown, patients with HIV infection have been noted to have elevated IgE levels that increase as the CD4+ T cell count declines, and there are numerous examples of patients with multiple drug reactions suggesting some common pathway. It is anticipated that allergic drug reactions will become an increasingly difficult aspect of managing patients with HIV infection, especially with the expanding need for multidrug regimens for the treatment of tuberculosis.

HIV infection shares many similarities with a variety of autoimmune diseases. A substantial polyclonal B cell activation that is associated with a high incidence of antiphospholipid antibodies, including anticardiolipin antibodies, VDRL antibodies, and lupus-like anticoagulants is common to both settings. Some reports indicate that patients with HIV infection have an increased incidence of positive antinuclear antibodies. However, there is no evidence that patients with HIV infection have an increase in two of the more common autoimmune diseases, namely systemic lupus erythematosus and rheumatoid arthritis. In fact, it has been observed that these diseases may be somewhat ameliorated by the concomitant presence of HIV infection, suggesting that an intact CD4 limb of the immune response plays an integral part in their pathogenesis. Similarly, one patient with common variable immunodeficiency, characterized by hypogammaglobulinemia, was noted to have a restoration of Ig levels following the development of HIV infection, suggesting a possible role for overactive CD4 immunity in some forms of that disease. The one autoimmune disease that may occur with an increased frequency in patients with HIV infection is a variant of primary Sjögren's syndrome (see Chap. 288). Patients with HIV infection can develop a syndrome consisting of parotid gland enlargement, dry eyes, and dry mouth that is characterized by lymphocytic infiltrates of the salivary gland and lung. In contrast to Sjögren's syndrome where these infiltrates are composed predominantly of CD4+ T cells, in patients with HIV infection the infiltrates are composed predominantly of CD8+ T cells. In addition, while patients with Sjögren's syndrome are predominantly women who have autoantibodies to Ro and La and are frequently HLA-DR3 or -B8, patients with this syndrome in the setting of HIV infection are often African-American men who do not have anti-Ro or anti-La and are predominantly HLA-DR5. In at least one case the syndrome improved following zidovudine therapy. The term *diffuse infiltrative lymphocytosis syndrome* (DILS) has been proposed to describe this entity and distinguish it from Sjögren's syndrome.

Approximately 33 percent of patients with HIV infection experience arthralgias. Furthermore, 5 to 10 percent of patients with HIV infection are diagnosed as having some form of reactive arthritis such as Reiter's syndrome or psoriatic arthritis. These syndromes occur with increasing frequency as the immune system declines and may be related to an increase in the number of infections with organisms that may act as a trigger for a reactive arthritis. These arthritides generally respond adequately to standard treatment; however, therapy with methotrexate has been associated with an increase in the incidence of opportunistic infections and should be used with caution and only in severe cases.

Patients with HIV infection also experience a variety of joint problems with no obvious cause that are generically referred to as *HIV-* or *AIDS-associated arthropathy*. This syndrome is a subacute obligoarticular arthritis developing over a period of 1 to 6 weeks and lasting 6 weeks to 6 months. It generally involves the large joints, predominantly knees and ankles, and is nonerosive with only a mild inflammatory response. Joint films are nonrevealing. Nonsteroidal antiinflammatory drugs are marginally helpful; however, prompt relief has been noted with the use of intraarticular steroids. A second form of arthritis also felt to be secondary to HIV infection is called "painful articular syndrome." This condition, described in as many as 10 percent of a cohort of AIDS patients, present as acute, severe, sharp pain in the joint. It predominantly affects the knees, elbows, and shoulders, lasts 2 to 24 h and may be severe enough to require narcotic analgesics. The cause of this arthropathy is unclear; however, it is felt that it results from a direct effect of HIV on the joint. This is a reasonable assumption, given the fact that other lentiviruses, in particular the caprine arthritis-encephalitis virus, are capable of causing arthritis.

A variety of other immunologic or rheumatologic diseases have been reported in patients with HIV infection, either de novo or in association with opportunistic infections or drugs. Using the criteria of widespread musculoskeletal pain of at least 3 months' duration and at least 11 of 18 possible tender points by digital palpation, 11 percent of an HIV-infected cohort consisting of 55 percent IVDUs could be diagnosed as having fibromyalgia. While the incidence of frank arthritis was less in this population than in other studies that predominantly consisted of homosexual men, these data support the concept that there are musculoskeletal problems that occur as a direct result of HIV infection. In addition, there have been reports of leukocytoclastic vasculitis in the setting of zidovudine therapy, CNS angiitis, and polymyositis in HIV-infected individuals. Septic arthritis is surprisingly rare, especially given the increased incidence of staphylococcal bacteremias seen in this population. When septic arthritis has been reported it has usually been due to systemic fungal infections with *Sporothrix schencki*, *Cryptococcus neoformans*, or *Histoplasma capsulatum*, or systemic mycobacterial infection with *M. hemophilum*.

Ophthalmologic problems are seen in over 50 percent of patients with HIV infection, generally as a late mainfestation of disease. The most common abnormal findings on funduscopic examination are cotton-wool spots. These hard white spots that appear on the surface of the retina and often have an irregular edge, represent areas of retinal ischemia, secondary to microvascular disease. At times they are associated with small areas of hemorrhage and thus are difficult to distinguish from CMV retinitis. In contrast to CMV retinitis, however, these spots are not associated with visual loss and tend to remain stable or improve over time.

Second to cotton-wool spots, the most common disease of the eye in patients with HIV infection is CMV retinitis. This is almost invariably a late manifestation of HIV disease, occurring in patients with less than 100 CD4 + T cells per microliter. CMV causes a progressive necrotizing retinitis that results in permanent visual loss. Fundoscopically one sees perivascular hemorrhage and exudate that is usually bilateral and progressive over time (see Fig. A8-14). Retinal detachment may occur in areas of retinal scarring secondary to burned-out infection. The treatment is detailed above and at present is limited to either ganciclovir or foscarnet.

Several other secondary infections may cause ocular problems in the HIV-infected patient. among them are *Pneumocystis carinii*, toxoplasmosis, and herpesviruses. *Pneumocystis carinii* causes a severe choroiditis that is most commonly seen in the absence of pulmonary disease. Lesions appear as slightly raised yellow-white plaques and may be confused with cotton-wool spots. Toxoplasmic retinitis is usually an accompaniment of CNS toxoplasmosis. It may be very difficult to distinguish from CMV retinitis and should be considered in anyone with a diagnosis of CMV retinitis who is not responding well to initial therapy. In contrast, the infections of the retina caused by HSV and HZV, referred to as *acute retinal necrosis syndrome*, are quite distinct, causing a painful inflammation of the eye that may be associated with keratitis or iritis. Fundoscopic

examination reveals multiple, usually bilateral pale gray lesions. This entity is often seen in association with trigeminal zoster or orolabial HSV and is associated with an increased risk of retinal detachment.

Endocrinologic and *metabolic* abnormalities are frequently seen in patients with HIV infection. The most common abnormality is hyponatremia, seen in up to 30 percent of all patients. This is generally related to the syndrome of inappropriate antidiuretic hormone (vasopressin) secretion (SIADH) as a consequence of increased free water intake and decreased free water excretion (see Chap. 45). SIADH is generally seen in the context of pulmonary or CNS disease; however, the presence of a low serum sodium in the presence of a high serum potassium should alert one to the possibility of adrenal insufficiency. Although the majority of patients with HIV infection studied at autopsy had involvement of the adrenal gland, less than 10 percent had prior evidence of adrenal insufficiency. CMV is the most common cause of adrenal gland disease in HIV infection. Other causes include mycobacterial infections, Kaposi's sarcoma, cryptococcal disease, histoplasmosis, and ketoconazole toxicity.

Hypogonadism is seen in approximately 50 percent of patients with HIV infection and is generally a complication of the underlying illness; however, testicular dysfunction may also be induced by ganciclovir therapy. In several surveys, 67 percent of patients with HIV infection noted decreased libido and 33 percent complained of impotence. Twenty-five percent of women with HIV infection in African studies were noted to be amenorrheic. Thyroid function is generally normal, despite histologic evidence of thyroid gland involvement with several pathologic processes, including CMV, *Cryptococcus neoformans*, *Pneumocystis carinii*, and Kaposi's sarcoma.

As noted above, pancreatitis leading to abnormalities of glucose metabolism may be seen in patients with HIV infection; however, this is most often due to complications of therapy with either pentamidine or dideoxynucleosides.

Generalized wasting defined as involuntary weight loss of greater than 10 percent associated with intermittent or constant fever and chronic diarrhea or fatigue for more than 30 days in the absence of a defined cause other than HIV infection, is a AIDS-defining condition (Table 279-9). It is the primary AIDS-defining illness in Africa and is the sixth leading AIDS diagnosis in New York City. A constant feature is major muscle wasting with scattered myofiber degeneration and occasional evidence of myositis. Glucocorticoids may be of some benefit; however, this approach must be carefully weighed against the potential risk of added immunosuppression. While similar findings may be seen with CMV disease or MAC bacteremia in the setting of advanced HIV infection, the generalized wasting syndrome appears to be a true direct effect of HIV.

IDIOPATHIC CD4 + T LYMPHOCYTOPENIA (ICL)

A syndrome was reported in 1992–93 characterized by an absolute CD4 + T cell count of less than 300 cells per microliter or less than 20 percent of total T cells on more than one occasion, no evidence of HIV-1, HIV-2, HTLV-I or HTLV-II on testing, and the absence of any defined immunodeficiency or therapy associated with decreased levels of CD4 + T cells. By mid-1993, approximately 100 patients had been described. After extensive multicenter investigation, a series of reports were published in early 1993 which cumulatively allowed the following conclusions: ICL is a very rare syndrome, as determined by studies of blood donors and cohorts of HIV-seronegative homosexual men. The syndrome is almost certainly not new or just emerging. Cases were clearly identified as early as 1983, and cases remarkably similar to ICL were identified decades ago. The recent definition of ICL based on CD4 + T cell counts coincided with the ready availability of testing for CD4 + T cells in patients suspected of being immunosuppressed. Although as a result of immunosuppression, certain patients with ICL develop some of the opportunistic diseases seen with HIV-infected patients, the syndrome is demographically, clinically, and immunologically dissimilar to HIV infection and AIDS. Less than half of the ICL patients had risk factors for HIV infection, and there were wide geographic and age distributions. The fact that a significant proportion of patients did have risk factors is probably a reflection of selection bias in that physicians who take care of HIV-infected patients are more likely to monitor CD4+ T cells. Approximately one-third of the patients are women compared to 11 percent of women among HIV-infected individuals in the United States. Many patients with ICL remained clinically stable and their condition did not progressively deteriorate as is so commonly seen with seriously immunosuppressed HIV-infected patients. Certain patients with ICL even experienced spontaneous reversal of the CD4+ T lymphocytopenia. Immunologic abnormalities in ICL are somewhat different from those in HIV infection. ICL patients often have decreases in CD8+ T cells as well as B cells. Furthermore, immunoglobulin levels were either normal or, more commonly, decreased in ICL compared to the usually observed hypergammaglobulinemia of HIV-infected individuals. Finally, virologic studies revealed no evidence of HIV-1, HIV-2, HTLV-I, or HTLV-II or of any other mononuclear cell-tropic virus. Furthermore, there was no epidemiologic evidence to suggest that a transmissible microbe was involved. The cases of ICL were widely dispersed with no clustering. Close contacts and sexual partners who were studied were clinically well with negative serologic, immunologic, and virologic studies for HIV. ICL is a heterogeneous syndrome and it is highly likely that there is no common cause; however, there may be certain common causes among subgroups of patients that are currently unrecognized.

Patients who present with the laboratory data consistent with ICL should be worked up for underlying diseases which may be responsible for the immunosuppression. If no underlying cause is detected, no specific therapy should be initiated. However, if opportunistic disease occur, they should be treated appropriately (see below). Depending on the level of the CD4+ T cell count, patients should receive prophylaxis for the appropriate commonly encountered opportunistic infections.

TREATMENT OF HIV INFECTION AND ITS COMPLICATIONS

GENERAL PRINCIPLES OF PATIENT MANAGEMENT The treatment of patients with HIV infection requires not only a comprehensive knowledge of the disease processes to be experienced but also the ability to deal with the problems of a chronic, life-threatening illness. Specific antiretroviral therapy and antimicrobial treatment and prophylaxis are critical measures in prolonging an acceptable quality of life; however, counseling and education are also of paramount importance in providing patients with optimal overall care. Patients must be educated about the infectious potential of their condition, with frank discussions about sexual practices and sharing of intravenous needles. The treating physician must not only be aware of the latest medications available for HIV infection and its complications but must also take the time to educate patients concerning the natural history of the illness and to listen to and be sensitive to their fears and concerns. As with other diseases, decisions about therapeutic maneuvers should be done in consultation with the patient when possible and with the patient's proxy if the patient is no longer capable of making decisions. In this regard, it is recommended that all patients with HIV infection and in particular those with under 200 CD4+ T cells per microliter give someone they trust durable power of attorney to make medical decisions on their behalf, if necessary.

No matter how well prepared patients may feel they are for adversity, initial awareness of a diagnosis of HIV infection is an invariably devastating event. For this reason it is recommend that anyone about to undergo testing have "pretest counseling" to at least partially prepare them should the results come back positive. Following a diagnosis of HIV infection the physician should be ready with immediate support systems for the newly diagnosed patient; these should include an experienced social worker or nurse who can spend time talking to the person and insuring that he/she is emotionally stable. Most communities have HIV crisis centers that can be of great help in these difficult situations.

Following an initial diagnosis of HIV infection there are several examinations and laboratory studies that should be performed to help stage the extent of disease and provide baseline standards for future reference. In addition to routine chemistry, hematology screening panels, and chest x-ray, one should also obtain a CD4+ T cell count and a VDRL. A PPD skin test should be done and a Mini-Mental Status Examination performed and recorded (Table 279-16). In addition, patients should be counseled with regard to sex practices and needle sharing, and counseling should be offered to others whom the patient knows or suspects may also be infected. Once these baseline activities are performed, short-term and long-term medical management strategies should be developed based on the information below.

ANTIRETROVIRAL THERAPY The cornerstone of medical management of HIV infection is antiretroviral therapy. Suppression of HIV replication is an important component in prolonging life as well as improving the quality of life of patients with HIV infection. Many questions such as "When is the best time to start antiretroviral therapy?," "What is the best regimen to start with?," "When should therapy be changed?," and "What regimen should one change to?" currently lack definitive answers. Nonetheless, the physician and patient must come to a mutually agreeable plan based upon the best available data. At present an extensive clinical trials network involving both clinical investigators and patient advocates is in place attempting to develop improved approaches to therapy. As a result, new therapies and new therapeutic strategies are emerging and new drugs are often available through expanded access programs prior to official licensure. For these reasons, management of patients with HIV infection is best accomplished with the input of someone who is an expert in the field.

Zidovudine (AZT, 3'-azido-2',3'-dideoxythymidine) was the first approved drug for the treatment of HIV infection and is the prototype drug for the general class of compounds referred to as nucleoside analogues (Table 279-24). These compounds, in which the hydroxyl group in the 3' position of the ribose moiety is substituted with a hydrogen or other chemical group, act as DNA chain terminators due to their inability to form a 3'-5' phosphodiester linkage with another nucleoside. They bind much more avidly to the active site of the RNA-dependent DNA polymerase of HIV (reverse transcriptase) than they bind to the active site of mammalian cell DNA polymerases. This may, at least in part, explain their selective effect on HIV replication. Zidovudine also has a relatively high avidity for the DNA polymerase gamma of human mitochondria. This may contribute to the development of the myopathy sometimes seen in patients receiving zidovudine. The active form of zidovudine is the triphosphate, and the rate of phosphorylation, a thymidine kinase–dependent pathway, may be different in different cells. This may explain why zidovudine protects some cell types from HIV better than others. Zidovudine is well-absorbed orally, with a serum half-life of approximately 1 h. Hence, most recommended dosing regimens employ an every-4-h or five-times-a-day schedule. Given the fact that, as in the case of didanosine (see below), the intracellular half-life may be much longer, the rationale for this dosing schedule is unsubstantiated and a variety of more convenient schedules are often employed, particularly when zidovudine is given as part of a combination regimen.

The clinical efficacy of zidovudine was clearly established in a phase II, placebo-controlled trial in which 282 patients who had either experienced a single bout of PCP or who had a variety of AIDS-associated symptoms were randomized to receive either placebo or zidovudine at a dose of 200 mg every 4 h. The trial was stopped prematurely when it became clear that there were far fewer deaths and far fewer new opportunistic infections occurring in the patients receiving zidovudine (Fig. 279-24). In addition to this clinical benefit, patients treated with zidovudine were noted to have increases in total lymphocyte counts, including CD4+ T cell counts, declines in

TABLE 279-24 Currently licensed antiretroviral drugs

Drug	Structure	Standard dose	Other regimens	Toxicities	Special considerations
AZT, Zidovudine 3′ Azido-2′, 3′-dideoxythymidine		100 mg, 5 id	200 mg tid, 300 mg bid	Anemia, leukopenia, myopathy	
ddl, Didanosine 2′,3′ dideoxyinosine		200 mg bid, > 60 kg 100 mg bid, < 60 kg		Peripheral neuropathy, pancreatitis	Need at least 2 tablets dose
ddc, Zalcitabine 2′,3′ dideoxycytidine		0.75 mg tid		Peripheral neuropathy, pancreatitis	Only licensed in combination with AZT, 200 mg tid
d4T, Stavudine 2′,3′-didehydro-3′-deoxythymidine		10–40 mg bid		Peripheral neuropathy, hepatitis	

circulating levels of p24 antigen, and weight gain. In subsequent trials a beneficial effect was also noted in patients with neurologic disease and in earlier disease with higher CD4+ T cell counts. At the present time, zidovudine is indicated therapy for anyone with HIV infection and less than 500 CD4+ T cells per microliter. This recommendation is based upon the U.S. Food and Drug Administration approval and licensure process, which in turn is based solely upon the results of controlled clinical trials. Thus, the eventual indications

FIGURE 279-24 Comparison of number of events (deaths or new opportunistic infections) occurring in patients randomized to receive either oral palcebo or AZT (zidovudine). Following 6 weeks of therapy, fewer events were seen in the patients randomized to AZT. (*Courtesy of Burroughs Wellcome Co.*)

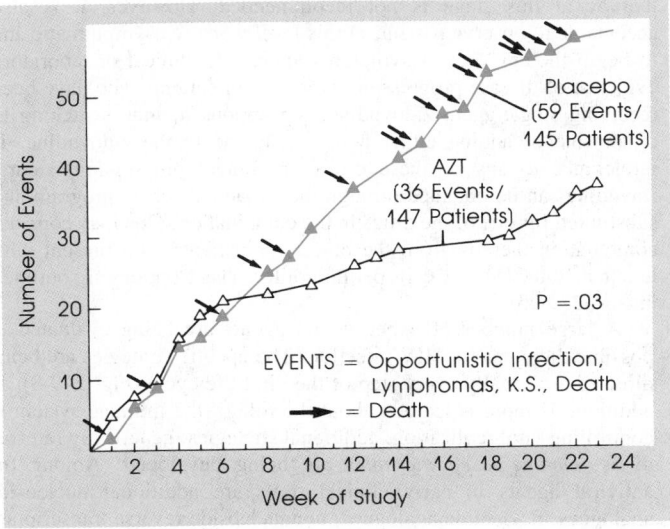

for zidovudine therapy may be even broader than those currently in place. Only controlled clinical trials will provide definitive guidelines whether to initiate antiretroviral therapy earlier than the currently recommended decision point.

Similarly, a great deal of effort has been directed toward defining the optimal dose of zidovudine. While the earliest trials, employing doses of 1200 mg/d showed benefit, there was also substantial toxicity. Subsequent trials have demonstrated that doses as low as 400 to 600 mg/d are equivalent in efficacy to higher-dose regimens and are significantly less toxic. At present the dose most frequently employed is 100 mg five times a day, although in patients taking other medications on a twice a day schedule or three times a day schedule, zidovudine regimens of 200 mg twice or three times a day may be used (Table 279-24).

While many patients experience fatigue, malaise, nausea, and headache upon the initiation of zidovudine therapy these side effects often subside overtime. The major toxicities of zidovudine are on the bone marrow. Patients often develop a macrocytic anemia which, when seen in association with low serum erythropoietin levels, may be ameliorated somewhat with injections of recombinant erythropoietin beginning at a dose of 100 μ/kg three times a week. Although zidovudine-induced anemia is macrocytic, there is no evidence that deficiencies in B_{12} or folate play a role; exogenous administration of these vitamins is of no help. In addition to anemia, patients receiving zidovudine, especially advanced patients, may experience neutropenia and in some cases thrombocytopenia. Other common toxicities of zidovudine include a proximal myopathy characterized by weakness, muscle wasting, and in some patients an elevation in creatine kinase; and a bluish discoloration of the nails that is particulary noticeable in black patients. It has been suggested that some forms of HIV-associated cardiomyopathy may actually be a side effect of nucleosides; this is also true of some cases of fatty infiltration of the liver. Although an increased incidence of tumors of the vaginal epithelium has been noted in rodents treated with extremely high doses of zidovudine, no increases in cancers in AIDS patients have thus far been attributed to zidovudine therapy. However, lymphomas are being seen with increased frequency as patients with AIDS live longer. Given these potential side effects, it is recommended that patients starting therapy with zidovudine be monitored for toxicity at least every other week for the first month and then monthly.

Considerable concern has been raised over the observation that strains of HIV resistant to zidovudine have been identified. This is usually seen in patients receiving zidovudine for periods of 6 months or longer, however, it has also been reported in isolates obtained at the time of seroconversion. Resistance is seen more quickly in late-stage patients where there is presumably a greater degree of viral replication and thus more chance for mutation. This resistance is secondary to mutations in the HIV reverse transcriptase and at least five different mutations have been identified that are associated with zidovudine resistance (codons 41, 67, 70, 215, and 219). Zidovudine resistance is not associated with resistance to either didanosine or zalcitabine. While the clinical significance of this observation has not been precisely defined, it does appear that this may be one factor limiting the long-term usefulness of zidovudine as monotherapy and provides a strong rationale for the early use of combination regimens.

Didanosine (ddI, 2′,3′-dideoxyinosine) was the second drug licensed for the treatment of HIV infection. In a series of open trials, didanosine was shown to be capable of causing increases in CD4+ T cell counts and declines in p24 antigen levels. Licensure was based upon the demonstration in a controlled, randomized trial that patients who had received zidovudine for a minimum of 16 weeks and were switched to didanosine experienced increases in CD4+ T cell counts and fewer new opportunistic infections. Data are still being generated in a randomized trial comparing zidovudine to didanosine as initial therapy. At present, didanosine is an FDA-approved therapy for any patient with HIV infection who has received prolonged zidovudine therapy. Didanosine therapy is usually reserved for patients who have begun to show evidence of clinical or laboratory decline while receiving zidovudine. In this event, rather than switching patients to didanosine one may chose to merely add it to the zidovudine regimen. As in the case of zidovudine, patients receiving didanosine develop strains of HIV that are resistant to didanosine. At least some of these isolates, occurring in patients who had originally developed zidovudine-resistant isolates as a consequence of prior zidovudine therapy, have regained some degree of sensitivity to zidovudine. Strains of HIV resistant to didanosine are generally also resistant to zalcitabine.

The standard dose of didanosine is 200 mg twice a day for patients over 60 kg and 100 mg twice a day for patients under 60 kg. Didanosine is best absorbed on an empty stomach at a neutral pH. For this reason the current formulations of didanosine contain a buffer and each dose must be administered in no less than two tablets. Thus, a patient who requires 100 mg twice a day, should take two 50-mg tablets twice a day rather than one 100-mg tablet twice a day.

The toxicity profile of didanosine is quite different from that of zidovudine. The most frequent toxicity of didanosine is a painful sensory peripheral neuropathy that occurs in approximately 30 percent of patients receiving doses above 200 mg twice a day. This generally resolves with discontinuation of drug and may not recur when patients are retreated at a reduced dose. The other major toxicity is pancreatitis; it was reported to occur in 9 percent of patients in the early clinical trials, although the frequency was somewhat less in later studies using lower doses. Pancreatitis can be fatal, and for this reason all patients receiving didanosine should be monitored carefully. Didanosine should be discontinued if a patient experiences abdominal pain consistent with pancreatitis or elevated amylase and/or lipase and edematous pancreas on ultrasound. These patients should not be retreated and, as a general rule, didanosine is contraindicated for a patient with a prior history of pancreatitis, regardless of etiology. Didanosine has minimal effects on the bone marrow and can be given in combination with bone marrow toxic drugs such as zidovudine, ganciclovir, or trimethoprim/sulfamethoxazole.

Zalcitabine (ddC, 2′,3′-dideoxycytidine) is the third drug currently licensed for treatment of HIV infection. In contrast to zidovudine and didanosine, zalcitabine is not licensed for use as monotherapy and is only licensed as part of a combination regimen with zidovudine. This is a reflection of the results of the initial clinical trials designed to assess the efficacy of zalcitabine in the therapy of HIV infection. A direct comparison of zalcitabine to zidovudine was stopped prematurely when it was noted that there were significantly more deaths occurring in the zalcitabine-treated group (59 vs. 33). In a separate trial, however, the combination of zalcitabine with zidovudine was shown to cause greater and more sustained elevations in CD4+ T cell counts than zidovudine alone. Based upon these results, zalcitabine (0.75 mg/kg three times a day) was licensed as part of a combination regimen with zidovudine (200 mg three times a day) for patients with advanced HIV infection. Similar to didanosine, the main toxicity is a reversible peripheral neuropathy. While cases of pancreatitis have been reported in patients receiving zalcitabine, it has not been seen to the same degree as that reported with didanosine. Nonetheless, zalcitabine is also contraindicated in patients with a prior history of pancreatitis. The precise role of the zidovudine/zalcitabine combination regimen in the treatment of HIV infection has yet to be established, although some experts choose this regimen as initial therapy for patients with HIV infection who present with less than 200 CD4+ T cells per microliter, while others add zalcitabine to zidovudine monotherapy in patients showing an immunologic or clinical decline.

Stavudine (d4T,2′,3′-didehydro-3′-deoxythymidine) is another nucleoside analogue. This agent is currently available for use under an expanded access program and thus formal approval is anticipated. Stavudine has an activity profile comparable to that of zidovudine in preclinical studies. Thus far, clinical trials have demonstrated that stavudine therapy is associated with increases in CD4+ T cell counts, declines in p24 antigen levels, and an improved sense of well being. In contrast to zidovudine, stavudine appears to have minimal myelosuppressive toxicity. Peripheral neuropathy and elevations in SGPT have been the primary toxicities observed to date. At present, stavudine is available only directly from the manufacturer (1-800-842-8036), and its use is limited to patients who are unable to take either zidovudine or didanosine because of intolerance or clinical failure.

One strategy for the institution of antiretroviral therapy is as follows: withhold therapy and follow patients with CD+ T cell counts greater than 500 per microliter. As mentioned, active virus replication occurs throughout HIV infection, and theoretically it would be justifiable to begin therapy as soon as the diagnosis is made, as some clinicians do. However, given the toxicity of the available retroviral agents and the potential for the development of resistance to antivirals, therapy at this stage is not recommended. However, it is also acceptable to observe patients at this level who are asymptomatic and to begin therapy only if symptoms appear. If clinical or laboratory evidence of disease progression is present in patients who have been receiving single-agent zidovudine, the options include switching to didanosine or adding either it or zalcitabine to the zidovudine. If intolerance to any of these drugs or clinical progression occurs, stavudine can be obtained through the expanded access program and substituted for one of the drugs in the combination. One may consider combination therapy from the outset for patients who present with less than 200 CD4+ T cells per microliter. These options are outlined in Fig. 279-25.

A large number of experimental agents are being evaluated as possible therapies for HIV infection. Therapeutic strategies are being directed at virtually every step of the viral life cycle (Fig. 279-3). In addition, as more is learned about the role of the immune system in controlling viral replication, additional strategies, generically referred to as *immune-based therapies* are being developed. Among the antiviral agents in early clinical trials are additional nucleoside analogues, nucleotide analogues, nonnucleoside reverse transcriptase

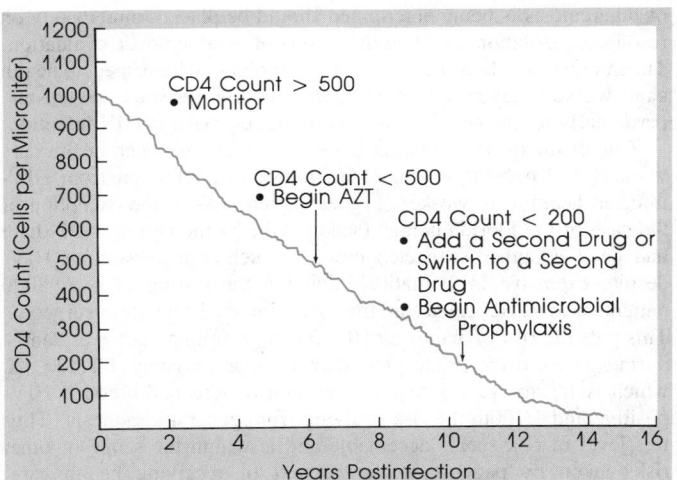

FIGURE 279-25 One possible strategy for the management of patients with HIV infection. In the early stages of illness, as long as the CD4 count is above 500 cells per cubic millimeter observation is the rule. Once the count falls below that level, therapy is initiated with a single agent, usually AZT. However, observation alone is acceptable if patients remain asymptomatic at this level of CD4 count. Combination therapy is given to the patient with more advanced disease, or the patient showing progression while on AZT alone.

inhibitors, *tat* inhibitors, protease inhibitors, and antisense nucleic acids. Among the immune-based therapies being tried are IFN-α, bone marrow transplantation with adoptive transfer of lymphocytes, active immunotherapy with subunit envelope vaccines or autologous cells genetically engineered to express viral proteins, passive immunotherapy with inactivated anti-HIV antisera or monoclonal antibodies, and IL-2. In addition, clinical trials are planned employing the techniques of molecular biology to combat HIV infection through the infusion of cells genetically modified to resist infection with HIV.

TREATMENT OF SECONDARY INFECTIONS, KAPOSI'S SARCOMA, AND LYMPHOMAS Treatment guidelines are outlined in Tables 279-19 and 279-21 and discussed in detail in the sections dealing with the secondary infections and neoplastic complications of HIV infection.

PROPHYLAXIS AGAINST SECONDARY INFECTIONS Enhanced survival and improved quality of life for patients with HIV infection can be traced not only to the introduction of zidovudine and related compounds but also to improved regimens for preventing secondary infections. As a result, the clinical profile of HIV-infected patients is continually evolving as immunodeficient patients live longer and at less risk of formerly inevitable problems such as PCP. Because certain secondary infections occur with predictability only when the competence of the immune system, as measured by the CD4+ T cell count, declines below a certain level, this knowledge can be used to help devise effective strategies for minimizing these risks.

PCP rarely occurs before the CD4+ T cell count drops below 200 cells per microliter or before the CD4 percent declines below 15 percent. At this point, patients should be started on a regimen of PCP prophylaxis. The preferred regimen, for patients able to tolerate it, is trimethoprim/sulfamethoxazole at a dose of 1 double-strength tablet twice a day. Another benefit of trimethoprim/sulfamethoxazole as a prophylaxis regimen is that it also provides protection against toxoplasmosis as well as certain bacterial infections. Alternate strategies for pneumocystis prophylaxis including atovoquone and clindamycin/pyrimethamine are currently being evaluated for patients who are sulfa intolerant. Aerosolized pentamidine remains an option for those unable to tolerate any systemic therapy.

Another opportunistic infection for which primary prophylaxis is clearly indicated is MAC. This infection is extremely common among

patients in the United States but is rarely seen with CD4+ T cell counts above 100 cells per microliter. Rifabutin, 100 mg/d, was effective in a clinical trial in delaying the onset of MAC bacteremia by an average of 6 months. Based upon these data, rifabutin has been licensed for use as a primary prophylaxis for MAC infection in patients with HIV infection and less than 100 CD4+ T cells per microliter.

Given the resurgence of tuberculosis in the HIV-infected population, any patient with HIV infection and at least 5 mm of induration on PPD skin testing should receive a 1-year course of isoniazid. In addition, any patient with HIV infection who is anergic and at high risk of tuberculosis should be given a year of isoniazid. These measures could be quite effective not only in helping the individual patient but also in curtailing the spread of tuberculosis in the community.

Patients with HIV infection are at increased risk for infection with encapsulated bacteria, particularly *H. influenzae* and *S. pneumoniae*. For this reason patients with HIV infection and especially patients in whom splenectomy is being considered should be vaccinated with the pneumococcal polysaccharide and *H. influenzae* type b vaccines.

While no generally accepted guidelines exist, many physicians recommend primary prophylaxis against cryptococcal and candidal infections with fluconazole; clinical trials of a candidate cryptococcal vaccine are underway. In addition, clinical trials are being conducted to evaluate the role of intermittent clindamycin/pyrimethamine as primary prophylaxis for toxoplasmosis in patients unable to tolerate trimethoprim/sulfamethoxazole and to evaluate the role of CMV IgG to prevent CMV reactivation syndromes.

Secondary prophylaxis, the prevention of second or subsequent episodes of a given infection, is indicated for virtually every opportunistic infection experienced by the patient with AIDS. These infections are usually impossible to eradicate and, with the exception of tuberculosis, life-long therapy or secondary prophylaxis is the rule (see Table 279-19). It is obvious that as the number of medications given to an individual patient increases, the chance for untoward drug reactions and interactions to occur increases. Thus, patients must be monitored carefully for such reactions. However, with the judicious use of prophylactic regimens a significant improvement in the quality of life for the patient with HIV infection and advanced immunodeficiency is clearly possible.

HIV AND THE HEALTH CARE WORKER

There is a small but definite risk that a health care worker, especially one who deals with large numbers of HIV-infected patients, may become infected with HIV in the course of his/her work (see "Occupational Transmission of HIV" above). By 1991, there had been a total of 27 well-documented seroconversions in health care workers that occurred as a direct result of exposure to contaminated blood or bloody body fluids. Twenty of these were due to a needle stick injury, two were due to cuts with contaminated objects, two were large mucous membrane exposures, two were felt to be the result of exposure of known open wounds to contaminated blood, and one was the the result of repeated and extensive cutaneous exposure to blood and body fluids. Twenty-four of these accidents involved blood, one involved bloody pleural fluid, and two involved concentrated virus stocks. In addition, another 109 HIV-infected health care workers had been identified with no identifiable risk for HIV infection other than occupational exposure. Taken together, the data from several large studies suggest that the risk of HIV infection following a percutaneous injury with an HIV-contaminated hollow-bore needle (in contrast to a solid bore, i.e., suture, needle) is approximately 0.3 percent. A seroprevalence survey conducted in May, 1991, of 3420 orthopedic surgeons, 75 percent of whom practiced in an area with a relatively high HIV infection rate and 39 percent of whom reported percutaneous exposure to patient blood, failed to reveal any cases of possible occupational infection, suggesting that the risk of infection with a suture needle may be considerably less than that with a blood-drawing needle.

The majority of cases of health care worker seroconversions occur as a result of needle stick injuries. When one considers the circumstances that result in needle stick injuries, it is immediately obvious that adhering to the standard guidelines for dealing with sharp objects would result in a significant decrease in this sort of accident. In this regard, in one study, 27 percent of needlestick injuries were the result of improper disposal of the needle (over half of these were due to recapping the needle), 23 percent occurred while attempting to start an intravenous line, 22 percent occurred during blood drawing, 16 percent were associated with an intramuscular or subcutaneous injection, and 12 percent were associated with giving an intravenous infusion.

The best management for a percutaneous injury with a needle contaminated with blood from a patient with HIV infection is a debated subject. While all agree that the wound should be immediately cleansed and antiseptic applied, the role of zidovudine prophylaxis is unclear. Among the arguments against the use of zidovudine are the fact that three separate SIV primate studies have failed to show any evidence of protection, that protection has been seen in the feline leukemia virus model only when the drug is given prior to exposure, that there are multiple anecdotes of health care workers who have serconverted despite immediately beginning zidovudine prophylaxis, and that the side effects of zidovudine are considerable. In one study, 70 percent of health care workers taking zidovudine for postexposure prophylaxis reported one or more side effects, particularly nausea, malaise, and headache. Arguments in favor of zidovudine prophylaxis are that the risk of a serious side effect is minimal while the potential benefit is great, and that if infection were to occur the patient would have started therapy at the earliest possible point in time. The ultimate decision must be individualized and reached after careful discussion between the injured health care worker and his/her physician. Since zidovudine prophylaxis, if it is going to be given, should probably be started as soon as possible (within 2 to 4 h) after the injury, health care workers at potential risk should think beforehand about what they would do if they were to be in this position.

There are several things health care workers can do to minimize their risk of an occupational HIV infection. These are listed in the July, 1991, CDC guidelines and include: adherence to universal precautions; refraining from direct patient care if one has exudative lesions or weeping dermatitis; and disinfecting and sterilizing reusable devices employed in invasive procedures. The premise of universal precautions is that each and every specimen should be handled as if it came from someone infected with a blood-borne pathogen. In this regard, all samples should be double bagged, gloves should be worn when drawing blood, and spills should be immediately disinfected with bleach.

In attempting to put this small but definite risk to the health care worker in perspective, it is important to point out that approximately 200 health care workers die each year as a result of occupationally acquired hepatitis B infection. The tragedy in this instance is that these infections and deaths due to hepatitis B could be greatly decreased by more extended use of the hepatitis B vaccine. The risk of hepatitis B infection following a needle stick injury from an antigen-positive patient is much higher than the risk of HIV infection (see "Transmission," above). There are multiple examples of needle stick injuries where the patient was positive for both hepatitis B and HIV and the health care worker became infected only with hepatitis B. For these reasons it is advisable, given the high prevalence of hepatitis B infection in patients with HIV infection, that all health care workers dealing with HIV-infected patients be immunized with the hepatitis B vaccine.

Tuberculosis is another infection common to patients with HIV infection that can be transmitted to the health care worker. For this reason, all health care workers should know their PPD status, have it checked yearly, and receive a year of isoniazid (INH) should their skin test become positive. In addition, all patients in whom a diagnosis of tuberculosis is being entertained should be placed immediately on respiratory isolation, pending the results of the diagnostic evaluation. Tuberculosis will become an increasing problem with respect to health care workers given the emergence of drug-resistant organisms, particularly for the health care worker with preexisting HIV infection.

One of the most charged issues ever to come between health care workers and patients is that of tranmission of infection from HIV-infected health care workers to their patients. With the exception of the case of the Florida dentist (see above), by the end of 1992 there had been no other suspected cases of such transmission of HIV, despite extensive investigation inlcuding the testing of over 8000 patients who had received care from HIV-infected dentists or surgeons. This puts the risk of acquiring HIV infection from a doctor or dentist during an exposure-prone procedure at approximately 1/1,000,000 which is 1/10th the risk that a given unit of screened blood is HIV-positive and 1/100th the risk of dying from general anesthesia. Thus this level of risk seems acceptable and is within the scope of other risks taken by patients in the context of receiving health care. Theoretically, the same universal precautions that are being used to protect the health care worker from the patient with HIV infection will also protect the patient from the HIV-infected health care worker.

VACCINES

Given the fact that human behavior, especially human sexual behavior, is extremely difficult to change, the best hope for preventing the spread of HIV infection rests with the development of a safe and effective vaccine. This task is extremely problematic for a number of reasons, including the high degree of mutability of the virus, the fact that the infection can be transmitted by cell-free or cell-associated virus, and the likely need for the development of effective mucosal immunity. However, studies using animal models have been encouraging (see below). It should be pointed out that while the ideal goal of a vaccine for HIV is to prevent infection, a vaccine that does not necessarily prevent infection but significantly alters the course of disease after a person gets infected also may have a major impact on public health.

Preclinical work in the area of vaccine development has been greatly facilitated through the use of animal models of lentivirus infections. Perhaps the most useful model to date has been the simian immunodeficiency virus (SIV) infection of rhesus monkeys. SIV, a lentivirus that is closely related to HIV-2 and differs from HIV-1 in that it lacks the *vpu* gene and contains the *vpx* gene, causes an acute infection that leads to immunodeficiency, secondary injection, and death when administered to susceptible animals. Studies by several groups have clearly demonstrated that infection can be prevented by prior immunization of animals with either inactivated virus, recombinant vaccinia virus expressing the SIV envelope followed by a booster immunization with recombinant protein, or attenuated virus lacking the *nef* gene. Even in other studies using antigens that did not confer protection from infection, the clinical course following infection appeared to be delayed. Of note is the fact that in those studies demonstrating protection it has not always been obvious what components of the immune response were conferring the protection. In fact, in the studies of inactivated virus it has been shown that the protective elements of the immune response were not directed toward components of the virus at all but toward components of the cells used in growing up the viral stocks. These data suggest that antibodies to certain cell surface proteins that participate in SIV binding may provide excellent protection against infection, a hypothesis that have been supported in studies of CD4-immunized monkeys. While the protection studies carried out with envelope-expressing recombinant vaccinia virus and recombinant envelope boosting point to an immune response to the envelope as potentially protective there is still much to be learned with respect to the correlates of immunity involved in protection against infection and/or disease.

The only suitable animal model for HIV infection is the chimpanzee. However, this model has significant drawbacks in that chimpanzees are expensive, they are an endangered species, and although they can be infected with HIV, they do not develop disease. Thus unless a candidate vaccine prevents infection in this model, its overall impact on disease progression cannot be assessed. Most recently, however, immunization of chimps with either whole inactivated virus followed by protein or peptide boosting or with recombinant envelope proteins has been shown to confer protection against infection with HIV-1. These data from animal models suggest the feasibility of inducing at least partial protection against HIV infection in man by vaccination.

While awaiting clear signals from the preclinical animal work, clinical trials of candidate vaccines have nonetheless begun in man. In this regard both recombinant envelope proteins and recombinant vaccinia viruses expressing HIV envelope have been demonstrated to be safe and immunogenic in healthy uninfected volunteers. Certain of these vaccines are also being tested as forms of active immunotherapy in patients who are already infected. At present, one can state with a fair degree of certainty that humans can safely be immunized to several of the antigens of HIV and it is only a matter of time until one or more of these vaccine candidates will be tested in a vaccine efficacy trial. It is clear, however, that it will take several years of clinical trials to establish the efficacy or lack thereof of a candidate vaccine for HIV.

PREVENTION

Education, counseling, and behavior modification are the cornerstones of prevention of HIV infection. Widespread voluntary testing of individuals in whom there is any possibility that they had been or are in a high-risk behavior situation, together with counseling of infected individuals, should prove helpful in behavioral modification programs for infected individuals who might otherwise have been unaware of their HIV status and who could infect their sexual partners. In uninfected and infected individuals, the practice of safe sex is the most effective way to avoid contracting and spreading HIV infection. Abstinence from sexual relations is the only absolute way to prevent sexual transmission. However, this may not be feasible, and so there are a number of relatively safe practices that can markedly decrease the chances of transmission of HIV infection. Partners engaged in monogamous sexual relationships who wish to be assured of safety should both be tested for HIV antibody. It must be understood that any divergence from the monogamous nature of the relationship by either party puts both parties at risk; therefore, open discussions regarding the importance of honesty in such relationships should be encouraged by counseling parties. Where the HIV status of either of the partners is not known, there are a number of options. Use of condoms preferably together with the HIV-inhibiting spermatacide nonoxynol-9 can markedly decrease the chance of transmission of HIV. It should be remembered that condoms are not 100 percent effective in preventing transmission of HIV infection, and there is an approximately 10 percent failure rate of condoms used for contraceptive purposes. Most condom failures result from breakage or improper usage. Latex condoms are preferable as virus has been shown to leak through natural skin condoms. Petroleum-based gels should never be used for lubrication of the condom as they increase the likelihood of condom rupture. Nontraumatic mutual masturbation is considered safe provided there is no ingestion of semen, vaginal secretions, or other potentially infected body fluids. Kissing is considered safe although there remains the theoretical possibility of transmission via virus contained in saliva if saliva is exchanged.

The most effective way to prevent transmission of HIV infection among IVDUs is to stop the use of injecting drugs. Unfortunately, since addiction to injecting drugs is an illness, it is extremely difficult to accomplish this without entering the addict into a treatment program. For those who will not or cannot do so and who will continue to inject drugs, the avoidance of sharing of needles and other paraphernalia (''works'') is the next best way to avoid transmission of infection. The cultural and social factors that contribute to the sharing

of paraphernalia are complex and difficult to overcome. In addition, needles and syringes may be in short supply, adding to the imperative to share. Under these curcumstances, works should be cleaned after each usage with a virucidal solution such as undiluted sodium hypochlorite (household bleach). Certain countries in Western Europe as well as certain communities in the United States have adopted programs of providing free needles and syringes in exchange for used paraphernalia. It is important for IVDUs to be tested for HIV infection and counseled in order to avoid transmission of HIV to their sexual partners. This form of transmission has increased greatly in the United States (see above).

Prevention of HIV transmission through tranfused blood or blood products has been dramatically decreased by a combination of screening of all blood donors for HIV infection as well as self-deferral of individuals who may be at risk for HIV infection. In addition, clotting factor concentrates are heat treated. Autologous tranfusions are preferable to transfusions from another individual. However, logistic contraints as well as the unpredictability of the need for most transfusions lessen the feasibility of this approach.

HIV can be transmitted via breast milk and colostrum. The avoidance of breast feeding may not be practical in developing countries where nutritional concerns override the risk of HIV transmission. However, in countries such as the United States where there is an option to breast feeding, bottled formula and milk should be used when a mother is HIV positive.

REFERENCES

AIDS in New York State. New York State Department of Health, 1991

ANDERSON RE et al: Use of ß2-microglobulin level and CD4 lymphocyte count to predict development of acquired immunodeficiency syndrome in persons with human immunodeficiency virus infection. Arch Intern Med 150:73, 1990

BERAL V et al: Kaposi's sarcoma among persons with AIDS: A sexually transmitted infection? Lancet 2:123, 1990

BHAT S et al: Galactosyl ceramide or a derivative is an essential component of the neural receptor for human immunodeficiency virus type 1 envelope glycoprotein gp120. Proc Natl Acad Sci USA 88:7131, 1991

BUSCH MP et al: Evaluation of screened blood donations for human immunodeficiency virus type I infection by culture and DNA amplification of pooled cells. N Engl J Med 325:1, 1991

CAMERON PU et al: Dendritic cells exposed to human immunodeficiency virus type-1 transmit a vigorous cytopathic effect to CD4 + T cells. Science 257:383, 1992

CEASE KB et al: Helper T cell antigenic site identification in the acquired immunodeficiency syndrome virus gp120 envelope protein and induction of immunity in mice to the native protein using a 16-residue synthetic peptide. Proc Natl Acad Sci USA 84:4249, 1987

CENTERS FOR DISEASE CONTROL: *National HIV Seroprevalence Surveys—Summary of Results: Data from seroprevalence activities through 1989.* DHHS publication # HIV/CID/9-90-006

————: *National HIV Serosurveillance Summary, vol. 2. Results through 1990.* DHHS publication # HIV/NCID/11-91/011

CHIN J: Global estimates of HIV infection and AIDS cases: 1991. AIDS 5 (suppl 2): S57, 1991

CIESIELSKI C et al: Transmission of human immunodeficiency virus in a dental practice. Ann Intern Med 116:798, 1992

CLERICI M et al: Interleukin-2 production used to detect antigenic peptide recognition by T-helper lymphocytes from asymptomatic HIV-seropositive individuals. Nature 339:383, 1989

COLLIER AC et al: Central nervous system manifestations in human immunodeficiency virus infection without AIDS. J Acquir Immune Defic Synd 5:229, 1992

COOMBS RW et al: Plasma viremia in human immunodeficiency virus infection. N Engl J Med 321:1626, 1989

DAGLEISH AG et al: Neutralization of diverse HIV-1 strains by monoclonal antibodies raised against a gp41 synthetic peptide. Virology 165:209, 1988

DAVEY RT, HC LANE: Laboratory methods in the diagnosis and prognostic staging of infection with human immunodeficiency virus type 1. Rev Inf Dis 12:912, 1990

ENSOLI B et al: Cytokines and growth factors in the pathogenesis of AIDS-associated Kaposi's sarcoma. Immunol Rev 127:147, 1992

EPSTEIN LG, GENDELMAN HE: Human immunodeficiency virus type 1 infection of the nervous system: Pathogenic mechanisms. Ann Neurol 33:429, 1993

EUROPEAN COLLABORATIVE STUDY: Children born to women with HIV-1 infection: Natural history and risk of infection. Lancet 337:253, 1991

FAUCI AS: CD4 + T lymphocytopenia without HIV infection—no lights, no camera, just facts. N Engl J Med 328:429, 1993

FISCHL MA et al: Safety and efficacy of sulfamethoxazole and trimethoprim chemoprophylaxis for *Pneumocystis carinii* pneumonia in AIDS. JAMA 259:1185, 1988

GAYLE HD et al: Prevalence of the human immunodeficiency virus among university students. N Engl J Med 323:1538, 1990

GELDERBLOM HR: Assembly and morphology of HIV: potential effect of structure on viral function. AIDS 5:617, 1991

GREENE WC: The molecular biology of human immunodeficiency virus type I infection. N Engl J Med 324:308, 1991

GREENSPAN D et al: Relation of oral hairy leukoplakia to infection with the human immunodeficiency virus and risk of developing AIDS. J Infect Dis 155:475, 1987

HAYNES BF: Scientific and social issues of human immunodeficiency virus vaccine development. Science 260:1279, 1993

HIRSCH MS, D'AQUILA RT: Therapy for human immunodeficiency virus infection. N Engl J Med 328:1686, 1993

HOLLANDER H, STRINGARI S: Human immunodeficiency virus associated meningitis. Am J Med 83:813, 1987

ITESCU S et al: A sicca syndrome in HIV infection: Association with HLA-DR5 and CD8 lymphocytosis. Lancet 466, 1989

JOHNSTON MI, HOTH DF: Present status and future prospects for HIV therapies. Science 260:1286, 1993

KARON JM et al: Projections of the number of persons diagnosed with AIDS and the number of immunosuppressed HIV-infected persons—United States. Morb Mort Wk Rep 41:1, 1993

KARZON DT et al: Development of a vaccine for the prevention of AIDS. A critical appraisal. Vaccine 10:1039, 1992

KAYE BR: Rheumatologic manifestations of infection with human immunodeficiency virus (HIV). Ann Intern Med 111:158, 1989

KLEIN RS et al: Oral candidiasis in high-risk patients as the initial manifestation of the acquired immunodeficiency syndrome. N Engl J Med 311:354, 1984

KRAMER A et al: Neopterin: A predictive marker of acquired immune deficiency syndrome in human immunodeficiency virus infection. J Acquir Immune Defic Synd 2:291, 1989

KROWN SE et al: Kaposi's sarcoma in the acquired immunodeficiency syndrome: A proposal for a uniform evaluation, response and staging criteria. J Clin Oncol 7:1201, 1989

LINDGREN S et al: HIV and child-bearing: Clinical outcome and aspects of mother-to-infant transmission. AIDS 5:1111, 1991

MASUR H et al: CD4 counts as predictors of opportunistic pneumonias in human immunodeficiency virus (HIV) infection. Ann Intern Med 111:223, 1989

MATSUSHITA S et al: Characterization of a human immunodeficiency virus neutralizing monoclonal antibody and mapping of the neutralizing epitope. J Virol 62:2107, 1988

MCARTHUR JC: Neurologic manifestations of AIDS. Medicine 66:407, 1987

MCNEIL JG et al: Trends of HIV seroconversion among young adults in the US Army, 1985 to 1989. JAMA 265:1709, 1991

MELBYE M et al: Risk of AIDS after herpes zoster. Lancet I:728, 1987

MILES SA et al: AIDS Kaposi sarcoma-derived cells produce and respond to interleukin 6. Proc Natl Acad Sci USA 87:4068, 1990

Monthly vital statistics report. Final data from the National Center for Health Statistics 40:1, 1992. DHHS publication # (PHS) 92-1120

MOSS AR et al: Seropositivity for HIV and the development of AIDS or AIDS related conditions: Three year follow-up of the San Francisco General cohort. Br Med J 296:745, 1988

MUSHER DM et al: Syphilis, the response to penicillin therapy, neurosyphilis and the effect of human immunodeficiency virus infection. Ann Intern Med 113:872, 1990

NAVI BA et al: Cerebral toxoplasmosis complicating the acquired immunodeficiency syndrome: Clinical and neuropathological findings in 27 patients. Ann Neurol 19:224, 1986

PADIAN NS et al: Female-to-male transmission of human immunodeficiency virus. JAMA 266:1664, 1991

PANTALEO G et al: HIV infection is active and progressive in lymphoid tissue during the clinically latent stage of disease. Nature 362:355, 1993

———: The immunopathogenesis of human immunodeficiency virus infection. N Engl J Med 328:327, 1993

PIZZO PA, BUTLER KM: In the vertical transmission of AIDS, timing is everything. N Engl J Med 325:652, 1991

PLATANIAS LC et al: Thrombotic thrombocytopenic purpura as the first manifestation of human immunodeficiency virus infection. Am J Med 87:699, 1989

POLI G, FAUCI AS: The effect of cytokines and pharmacologic agents on chronic HIV infection. AIDS Res Hum Retrovirus 8:191, 1992

POLK BF et al: Predictors of the acquired immunodeficiency syndrome developing in a cohort of seropositive homosexual men. N Engl J Med 316:61, 1987

RATNER L: Human immunodeficiency virus-associated autoimmune thrombocytopenic purpura: A review. Am J Med 86:194, 1989

RAVIGLIONE MC: Extrapulmonary pneumocystosis: The first 50 cases. Rev Inf Dis 12:1127, 1990

ROBINSON WE et al: Two immunodominant domains of gp41 bind antibodies which enhance human immunodeficiency virus type I infection in vitro. J Virol 65:4169, 1991

ROOK AH et al: Interleukin-2 enhances the depressed natural killer and cytomegalovirus specific activities of lymphocytes from patients with the acquired immune deficiency syndrome. J Clin Invest 72:398, 1982

ROSENBERG PS et al: Population-based monitoring of an urban HIV/AIDS epidemic. Magnitude and trends in the District of Columbia. JAMA 268:495, 1992

ROSENBERG ZF, FAUCI AS: Immunopathogenesis of human immunodeficiency virus infection. Adv Immunol 47:377, 1989

———, ———: Immunology of HIV infection, in Immunology, 2d ed, WE Paul (ed). New York, Raven, in press

SAFAI B et al: Spectrum of Kaposi's sarcoma in the epidemic of AIDS. Cancer Res 45:466s, 1985

SATTLER FR, FEINBERG J: New developments in the treatment of Pneumocystis carinii pneumonia. Chest 101:451, 1992

SCHRIER RD et al: B and T lymphocyte responses to an immunodominant epitope of human immunodeficiency virus. J Virol 62:2531, 1988

SCHWARTZ JS et al: Human immunodeficiency virus test: Evaluation, performance and use. JAMA 259:2574, 1988

SELIK RM et al: HIV infection as leading cause of death among young adults in US cities and states. JAMA 269:2991, 1993

SIMMS RW et al: Fibromyalgia syndrome in patients infected with human immunodeficiency virus. Am J Med 92:368, 1992

STEIN M et al: Causes of death in patients with human immunodeficiency virus infection. Am J Med 93:387, 1992

STEINMAN RM: The dendritic cell system and its role in immunogenicity. Ann Rev Immunol 9:271, 1991

ST. LOUIS ME et al: Human immunodeficiency virus infection in disadvantaged adolescents. Findings from the US Job Corps. JAMA 266:2387, 1991

TINDAL B, COOPER DA: Primary HIV infection: Host responses and intervention strategies. AIDS 5:1, 1991

WAKEFIELD AE et al: DNA amplification on induced sputum samples for diagnosis of Pneumocystis carinii pneumonia. Lancet 337:1378, 1991

WALKER BD et al: HIV specific cytotoxic T lymphocytes in seropositive individuals. Nature 328:345, 1987

WALKER CM et al: CD8 + lymphocytes can control HIV infection in vitro by suppressing virus replication. Science 234:1563, 1986

WEINHOLD KJ et al: Cellular anti-gp120 cytolytic reactivities in HIV-1 seropositive individuals. Lancet 1:902, 1988

WEISS RA: How does HIV cause AIDS? Science 260:1273, 1993

WENIGER BG et al: The epidemiology of HIV infection and AIDS in Thailand. AIDS 5 (suppl 2): S71, 1991

280   PLASMA CELL DISORDERS

DAN L. LONGO

GENERAL PRINCIPLES   The *plasma cell disorders* are monoclonal neoplasms related to each other by virtue of their development from common progenitors in the B lymphocyte lineage. Multiple myeloma, Waldenström's macroglobulinemia, primary amyloidosis (see Chap. 281), and the heavy chain diseases comprise this group and may be designated by a variety of synonyms such as *monoclonal gammopathies*, *paraproteinemias*, *plasma cell dyscrasias*, and *dysproteinemias*. A schema for the normal development of B lymphocytes is depicted in Fig. 280-1. Mature B lymphocytes destined to produce IgG bear surface immunoglobulin molecules of both M and G heavy chain isotypes with both isotypes having identical idiotypes (variable regions). Under normal circumstances, maturation to antibody-secreting plasma cells is stimulated by exposure to the antigen for which the surface immunoglobulin is specific; however, in the plasma cell disorders the control over this process is lost. The clinical manifestations of all the plasma cell disorders relate to the expansion of the neoplastic cells, to the secretion of cell products (immunoglobulin molecules or subunits, lymphokines), and to some extent to the host's response to the tumor.

There are three categories of structural variation among immunoglobulin molecules that form antigenic determinants, and these are used to classify immunoglobulins (Chap. 277). *Isotypes* are those determinants that distinguish among the main classes of antibodies of a given species and are the same in all normal individuals of that species. Therefore, isotypic determinants are, by definition, recognized by antibodies from a distinct species (heterologous sera) but not by antibodies from the same species (homologous sera). There are five heavy chain isotypes (M, G, A, D, E) and two light chain isotypes (kappa, lambda). *Allotypes* are distinct determinants that reflect regular small differences between individuals of the same species in the amino acid sequences of otherwise similar immunoglobulins. These differences are determined by allelic genes, and by definition, they are detected by antibodies made in the same species. *Idiotypes* are the third category of antigenic determinants. They are unique to the molecules produced by a given clone of antibody-producing cells. Idiotypes are formed by the unique structure of the antigen-binding portion of the molecule.

Antibody molecules (see Fig. 280-2) are composed of two heavy chains (mol wt ~50,000) and two light chains (mol wt ~25,000). Each chain has a constant portion (limited amino acid sequence variability) and a variable region (extensive sequence variability).

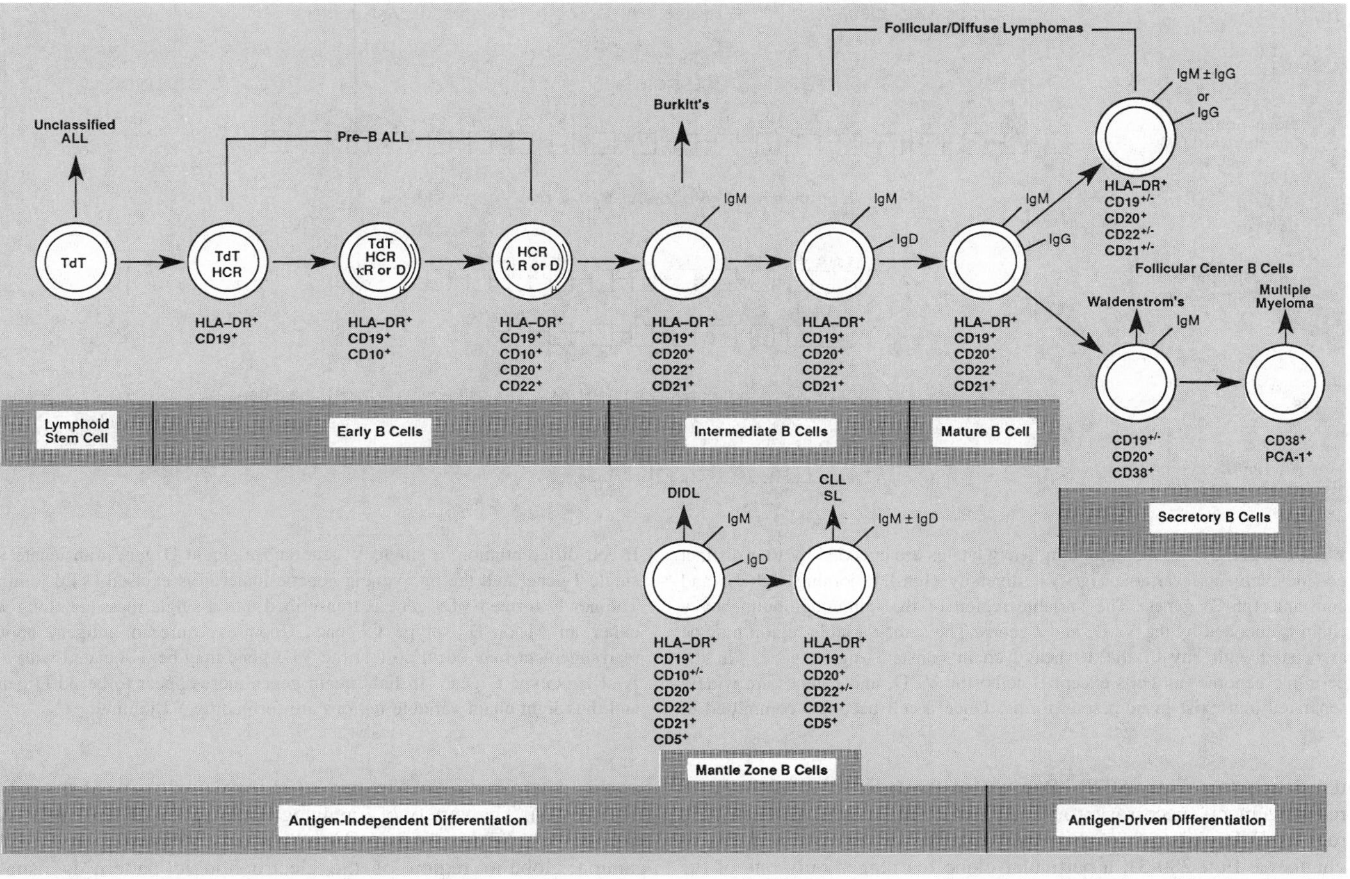

FIGURE 280-1 Schematic representation of the pathway of differentiation of normal B cells. HLA-DR, CD10, CD19, CD20, CD21, CD22, CD5, and CD38 are cell markers used to distinguish stages of development. Terminal transferase (TdT) is a cellular enzyme. Immunoglobulin heavy chain gene rearrangement (HCR) and light chain gene rearrangement or deletion (kappa R or D, lambda R or D) occur early in B cell development. The approximate stage of differentiation arrest for each B cell lymphoproliferative disorder is shown. The following abbreviations are used: ALL, acute lymphoblastic leukemia; CLL, chronic lymphocytic leukemia; DIDL, diffuse intermediately differentiated lymphocytic lymphoma; SLL, small lymphocytic lymphoma. The mantle zone B cells give rise to CLL and DIDL, but the relationship between this lineage and follicular center B cells is not yet clear.

The light and heavy chains are linked by disulfide bonds and are aligned so that their variable regions are adjacent to one another. This variable region forms the antigen recognition site of the antibody molecule; its unique structural features form a particular set of determinants, or idiotypes, that are reliable markers for a particular clone of cells because each antibody is formed and secreted by a single clone. Each chain is specified by distinct genes, synthesized separately, and assembled into an intact antibody molecule after

FIGURE 280-2 Schematic depiction of an IgG molecule. Each molecule consists of two heavy and two light chains linked by disulfide bonds. There are two types of light chains, kappa (genes on chromosome 2) and lambda (chromosome 22), each containing two domains. There are 10 types of heavy chains: 4 types of G (G1 to G4), 2 of A (A1, A2), 2 of M (M1, M2), and 1 each of D and E (all on chromosome 14), each with four domains. A domain is 100 to 110 amino acids in length. Within each domain is an intrachain disulfide bond that produces a loop. V_H (variable domain of the heavy chain) and V_L (variable domain of the light chain) form an antigen binding site whose unique determinants form an idiotype. Immunoglobulins of the same isotype (e.g., IgG1κ) differ between individuals. The determinants that distinguish them are called allotypic determinants and are located on C_L (constant domain of the light chain) and C_{H2} (second constant domain of the heavy chain). C_{H2} is also the main site of glycosylation (CHO) and complement binding. Papain cleaves the molecule into antigen-binding (Fab) and crystallizable (Fc) components. The portion of the heavy chain in an Fab fragment is called the Fd piece. Fc receptors on cells bind to the C_{H3} domain. IgM and IgA occur as polymers and each unit of two heavy and two light chains is connected by a J (joining) chain. The heavy chain isotypes determine the function of the antibody.

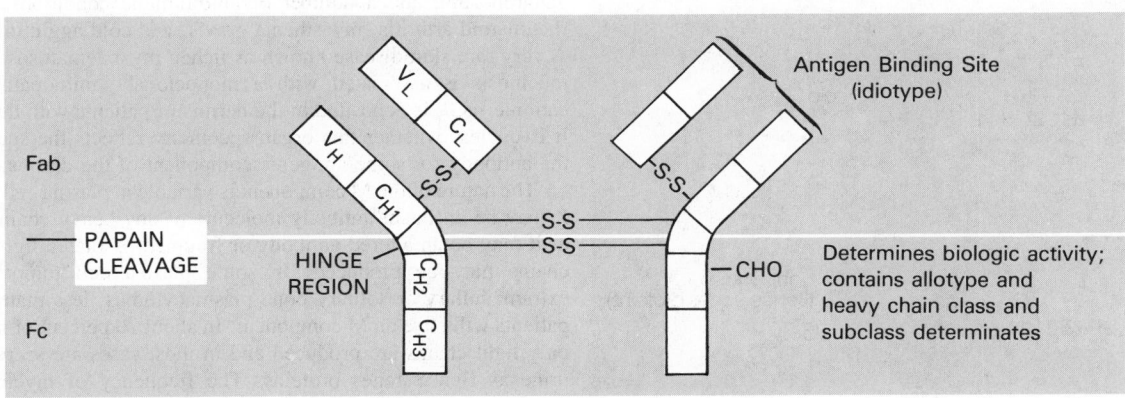

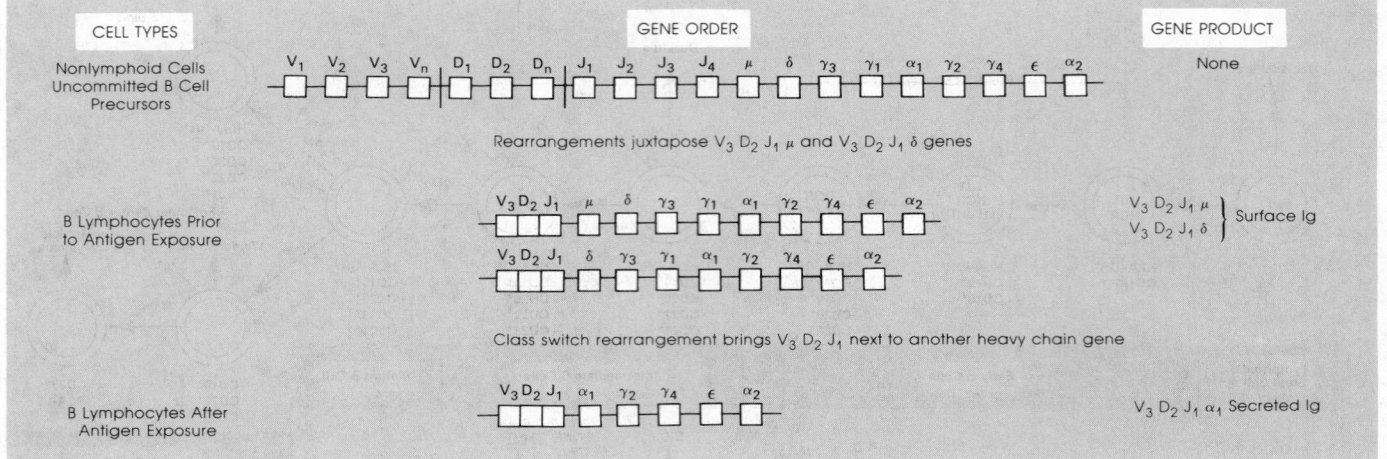

FIGURE 280-3   Immunoglobulin heavy chains are encoded by four distinct genetic elements, variable (Igh-V), diversity (Igh-D), joining (Igh-J), and constant (Igh-C) genes. The variable region of the immunoglobulin heavy chain is encoded by the V, D, and J genes. The same variable region may be associated with any of the 10 heavy chain constant region genes. In the germline genome (all cells except B cells) the V, D, and J genes are widely separated and exist in numerous forms. Once a cell becomes committed to B cell differentiation, a single V gene and a single D gene translocate to a single J gene, and the intervening genetic material is excised (VDJ joining). The newly formed VDJ gene is transcribed into a single message along with either an M or D isotype C gene. Upon exposure to antigen, another rearrangement may occur so that the VDJ gene may be associated with a G, A or E isotype C gene. In light chain genes there appear to be no D genes, and thus light chain variable regions are formed by VJ joining.

translation (see Fig. 280-3). Because of the mechanics of the gene rearrangements necessary to specify the immunoglobulin variable regions (VDJ joining for the heavy chain, VJ joining for the light chain; see Fig. 280-3), a particular clone rearranges only one of the two chromosomes to produce an immunoglobulin molecule of only one light chain isotype and only one allotype (allelic exclusion). After exposure to antigen, the variable region may become associated with a new heavy chain isotype (class switch). Each clone of cells performs these sequential gene arrangements in a unique way. This results in each clone producing a unique immunoglobulin molecule. In most cells, light chains are synthesized in slight excess, are secreted as free light chains by plasma cells, and are cleared by the kidney, but less than 10 mg of such light chains is excreted per day.

Electrophoretic analysis of components of the serum proteins

FIGURE 280-4   Representative electrophoretic patterns of serum and urine. The upper panel illustrates the normal pattern of serum and urine protein on electrophoresis. Since there are many different immunoglobulins in the serum, their differing mobilities in an electric field produce a broad peak. The lower panel illustrates the patterns of serum and urine proteins in a patient with myeloma. The predominance of a product of a single cell is reflected by a "church spire" sharp peak. The presence of free light chains in the urine is reflected in a peak, as well.

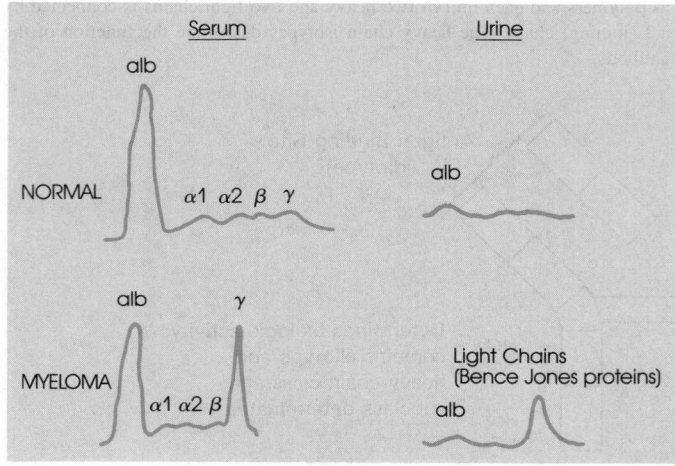

permits determination of the amount of immunoglobulin in the serum (Fig. 280-4). The variety of immunoglobulins move heterogeneously in an electric field and form a broad peak in the gamma region. The gamma globulin region of the electrophoretic pattern is usually increased in the sera of patients and animals with plasma cell tumors. There is a sharp spike in this region called an *M component* (M for monoclonal). Less commonly, the M component may appear in the beta$_2$ or alpha$_2$ globulin region. The antibody must be present at a concentration of at least 5 g/L (0.5 g/dL) to be detectable by this method. This corresponds to approximately 10^9 cells producing the antibody. Confirmation that such an M component is truly monoclonal relies on the use of immunoelectrophoresis that shows a single light and heavy chain type. Hence immunoelectrophoresis and electrophoresis provide qualitative and quantitative assessment of the M component, respectively. Once the presence of an M component has been confirmed, electrophoresis provides the more practical information for managing patients with monoclonal gammopathies. In a given patient, the amount of M component in the serum is a reliable measure of the tumor burden. This makes the M component an excellent tumor marker, yet it is not specific enough to be used to screen asymptomatic patients. In addition to the plasma cell disorders, M components may be detected in other lymphoid neoplasms such as chronic lymphocytic leukemia and lymphomas of B or T cell origin; nonlymphoid neoplasms such as chronic myelogenous leukemia, breast and colon cancer; a variety of nonneoplastic conditions such as cirrhosis, sarcoidosis, parasitic diseases, Gaucher's disease, and pyoderma gangrenosum; and a number of autoimmune conditions, including rheumatoid arthritis, myasthenia gravis, and cold agglutinin disease. A very rare skin disease known as lichen myxedematosus or papular mucinosis is associated with a monoclonal gammopathy. Highly cationic IgGλ is deposited in the dermis of patients with this disease. It is unclear whether this organ specificity reflects the specificity of the antibody for some antigenic component of the dermis.

The nature of the M component is variable in plasma cell disorders. It may be an intact antibody molecule of any heavy chain subclass, or it may be an altered antibody or fragment. Isolated light or heavy chains may be produced. In some plasma cell tumors such as extramedullary or solitary bone plasmacytomas, less than a third of patients will have an M component. In about 20 percent of myelomas, only light chains are produced and in most cases are secreted in the urine as Bence Jones proteins. The frequency of myelomas of a particular heavy chain class is roughly proportional to the serum concentration, and therefore IgG myelomas are more common than IgA and IgD myelomas.

MULTIPLE MYELOMA Definition Multiple myeloma represents a malignant proliferation of plasma cells. The terms *multiple myeloma* and *myeloma* may be used interchangeably. The disease results from the uncontrolled proliferation of plasma cells derived from a single clone. The tumor, its products, and the host response to it result in a number of organ dysfunctions and symptoms of bone pain or fracture, renal failure, susceptibility to infection, anemia, hypercalcemia, and occasionally clotting abnormalities, neurologic symptoms, and vascular manifestations of hyperviscosity.

Etiology The cause of myeloma is not known. Myeloma was found to occur with increased frequency in those exposed to the radiation of nuclear warheads in World War II after a 20-year latency. There is no direct evidence implicating oncogenes in human myeloma. In contrast to most other B cell tumors, consistent chromosomal alterations have not been found in patients with myeloma. Overexpression of *myc* or *ras* genes has been noted in some cases. The murine plasmacytoma models suggest that the induction of plasmacytomas (e.g., with mineral oil injection) may require exposure to foreign antigens as well as a cellular event. Thus chronic antigenic stimulation may play a role in the transformation of a particular B cell clone. There is also some evidence for a genetic predisposition to myeloma in humans. Myeloma has been seen more commonly than expected among farmers, wood workers, leather workers, and those exposed to petroleum products. The neoplastic event in myeloma may involve cells earlier in B cell differentiation than the plasma cell. Circulating B cells bearing surface immunoglobulin that share the idiotype of the M component are present in myeloma patients. It is possible that the malignant clone escapes normal control mechanisms at a pre-plasma cell stage of differentiation and the chronic exposure to a particular antigenic stimulus drives the cell to terminal differentiation. It remains difficult to distinguish benign from malignant plasma cells on the basis of morphologic criteria in all but a few cases.

Incidence and prevalence Myeloma increases in incidence with age. The median age at diagnosis is 68 years. It is rare under age 40. The yearly incidence is around 4 per 100,000 and remarkably similar in countries throughout the world. Males are slightly more commonly affected than females, and blacks have nearly twice the incidence of whites. In the age group over 25 the incidence is 30 per 100,000. Myeloma accounts for about 1 percent of all malignancies in whites and 2 percent in blacks; 13 percent of all hematologic cancers in whites and 33 percent in blacks.

Pathogenesis and clinical manifestations (Table 280-1) Bone pain is the most common symptom in myeloma, affecting nearly 70 percent of patients. The pain usually involves the back and ribs, and unlike the pain of metastatic carcinoma, which often is worse at night, the pain of myeloma is precipitated by movement. Persistent localized pain in a patient with myeloma usually signifies a pathologic fracture. The bone lesions of myeloma are caused by the proliferation of the tumor cells and the activation of osteoclasts which destroy the bone. The osteoclasts respond to osteoclast activating factors (OAF) made by the myeloma cells (OAF activity can be mediated by several cytokines, including interleukin 1, lymphotoxin, and tumor necrosis factor). However, production of these factors stops following administration of corticosteroids or interferon-γ. The bone lesions are lytic in nature and are rarely associated with osteoblastic new bone formation; therefore, radioisotopic bone scanning is less useful in diagnosis than plain radiography. The bony lysis results in substantial mobilization of calcium from bone, and serious acute and chronic complications of hypercalcemia may dominate the clinical picture (see below). Localized bone lesions may expand to the point that mass lesions may be palpated, especially on the skull (Fig. 280-5), clavicles, and sternum, and the collapse of vertebrae may lead to symptoms of spinal cord compression.

The next most common clinical problem in patients with myeloma is susceptibility to bacterial infections. The most common infections

TABLE 280-1 Pathogenesis and clinical manifestations of multiple myeloma

Clinical finding	Underlying cause	Pathogenic mechanism
Hypercalcemia, pathologic fractures, cord compression, lytic bone lesions, osteoporosis, bone pain	Skeletal destruction	Tumor expansion; production of osteoclast activating factors (OAF) by tumor cells
Renal failure	Light chain proteinuria, hypercalcemia, urate nephropathy, amyloid glomerulopathy (rare)	Toxic effects of tumor products, light chains, OAF, DNA breakdown products
	Pyelonephritis	Hypogammaglobulinemia
Anemia	Myelophthisis, decreased production, increased destruction	Tumor expansion; production of inhibitory factors and autoantibodies by tumor cells
Infection	Hypogammaglobulinemia, decreased neutrophil migration	Decreased production due to tumor-induced suppression; increased IgG catabolism
Neurologic symptoms	Hyperviscosity, cryoglobulins, amyloid deposits	Products of tumor; properties of M component; light chains
	Hypercalcemia, cord compression	OAF
Bleeding	Interference with clotting factors, amyloid damage of endothelium, platelet dysfunction	Products of tumor; antibodies to clotting factors; light chains; antibody coating of platelets
Mass lesions		Tumor expansion

are pneumonias and pyelonephritis, and the most frequent pathogens are *Streptococcus pneumoniae*, *Staphylococcus aureus*, and *Klebsiella pneumoniae* in the lungs and *Escherichia coli* and other gram-negative organisms in the urinary tract (Chap. 81). In about 25 percent of patients, recurrent infections are the presenting features, and over 75 percent of patients will have a serious infection at some time in their course. The susceptibility to infection has several contributing causes. First, patients with myeloma have diffuse hypogammaglobulinemia

FIGURE 280-5 Bony lesions in multiple myeloma. The skull demonstrates the typical "punched out" lesions characteristic of multiple myeloma. The lesion represents a purely osteolytic lesion with little or no osteoblastic activity. *(Courtesy of Dr. Geraldine Schechter.)*

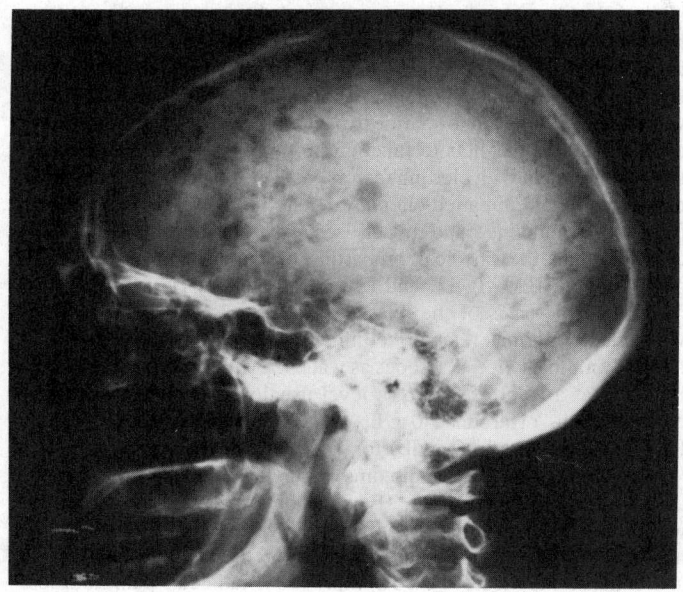

if the M component is excluded. The hypogammaglobulinemia is related to both decreased production and increased destruction of normal antibodies. Moreover, some patients generate a population of circulating regulatory cells in response to their myeloma that can suppress normal antibody synthesis. In the case of IgG myeloma, normal IgG antibodies are broken down more rapidly than normal because the catabolic rate for IgG antibodies varies directly with the serum concentration. The large M component results in fractional catabolic rates of 8 to 16 percent instead of the normal 2 percent. These patients have very poor antibody responses, especially to polysaccharide antigens such as those on bacterial cell walls. Such responses are normally T cell–independent. Most measures of T cell function in myeloma are normal, but a subset of CD4+ cells may be decreased. Granulocyte lysozyme content is low, and granulocyte migration is not as rapid as normal in patients with myeloma, probably the result of a product of the tumor. There are also a variety of abnormalities in complement functions in myeloma patients. All these factors contribute to the immune deficiency of these patients.

Renal failure occurs in nearly 25 percent of myeloma patients, and some renal pathology is noted in over half. There are many contributing factors. Hypercalcemia is the most common cause of renal failure. Glomerular deposits of amyloid, hyperuricemia, recurrent infections, and occasional infiltration of the kidney by myeloma cells all may contribute to renal dysfunction. However, tubular damage associated with the excretion of light chains is almost always present. Normally, light chains are filtered, reabsorbed in the tubules, and catabolized. With the increase in amount of light chains presented to the tubule, the tubular cells become overloaded with these proteins, and tubular damage results either directly from light chain toxic effects or indirectly from the release of intracellular lysosomal enzymes. The earliest manifestation of this tubular damage is the adult Fanconi syndrome (a type 2 proximal renal tubular acidosis) with increased loss of glucose, amino acids, and defects in the ability of the kidney to acidify and concentrate the urine. The proteinuria is not accompanied by hypertension, and the protein is nearly all light chains. Generally, there is very little albumin in the urine because glomerular function is usually normal. When the glomeruli are involved, the proteinuria is nonselective. Patients with myeloma also have a decreased anion gap [i.e., sodium minus (chloride plus bicarbonate)] because the M component is cationic, resulting in retention of chloride. This is often accompanied by hyponatremia that is felt to be artificial (pseudohyponatremia) because each volume of serum has less water as a result of the increased protein.

Anemia occurs in about 80 percent of myeloma patients. It is usually normocytic and normochromic and related both to the replacement of normal marrow by expanding tumor cells and to the inhibition of hematopoiesis by factors made by the tumor. In addition, mild hemolysis may contribute to the anemia. A larger than expected fraction of patients may have megaloblastic anemia due to either folate or vitamin B_{12} deficiency. Granulocytopenia and thrombocytopenia are very rare. Clotting abnormalities may be seen due to the failure of antibody-coated platelets to function properly or to the interaction of the M component with clotting factors I, II, V, VII, or VIII. Raynaud's phenomenon and impaired circulation may result if the M component forms cryoglobulins, and hyperviscosity syndromes may develop depending on the physical properties of the M component (most common with IgM, IgG3, and IgA paraproteins). Hyperviscosity is defined on the basis of the relative viscosity of serum as compared with water. Normal relative serum viscosity is 1.8 (i.e., serum is normally almost twice as viscous as water). Symptoms of hyperviscosity occur at a level of 5 to 6, a level usually reached at paraprotein concentrations of around 40 g/L (4 g/dL) for IgM, 50 g/L (5 g/dL) for IgG3, and 70 g/L (7 g/dL) for IgA.

Although neurologic symptoms occur in a minority of patients, they may have many causes. Hypercalcemia may produce lethargy, weakness, depression, and confusion. Hyperviscosity may lead to headache, fatigue, visual disturbances, and retinopathy. Bony damage and collapse may lead to cord compression, radicular pain, and loss of bowel and bladder control. Infiltration of peripheral nerves by amyloid can be a cause of carpal tunnel syndrome and other sensorimotor mono- and polyneuropathies.

Many of the clinical features of myeloma, e.g., cord compression, pathologic fractures, hyperviscosity, sepsis, and hypercalcemia, can present as medical emergencies. Despite the widespread distribution of plasma cells in the body, tumor expansion is dominantly within bone and bone marrow and, for reasons unknown, rarely causes enlargement of spleen, lymph nodes, or gut-associated lymphatic tissue.

Diagnosis and staging   The classic triad of myeloma is marrow plasmacytosis (>10 percent), lytic bone lesions, and a serum and/or urine M component. The diagnosis may be made in the absence of bone lesions if the plasmacytosis is associated with a progressive increase in the M component over time or if extramedullary mass lesions develop. There are two important variants of myeloma, solitary bone plasmacytoma and extramedullary plasmacytoma. These lesions are associated with an M component in less than 30 percent of the cases, they may affect younger individuals, and both are associated with median survivals of 10 or more years. Solitary bone plasmacytoma is a single lytic bone lesion without marrow plasmacytosis. Extramedullary plasmacytomas usually involve the submucosal lymphoid tissue of the nasopharynx or paranasal sinuses without marrow plasmacytosis. Both tumors are highly responsive to local radiation therapy. If an M component is present, it should disappear after treatment. Solitary bone plasmacytomas may recur in other bony sites or evolve into myeloma. Extramedullary plasmacytomas rarely recur or progress.

The most difficult differential diagnosis in patients with myeloma involves their separation from people with benign monoclonal gammopathies or monoclonal gammopathies of uncertain significance (MGUS). MGUS are vastly more common than myeloma, occurring in 1 percent of the population over age 50 and in up to 10 percent over age 75. Patients with MGUS usually have fewer than 20 g/L (2 g/dL) of M components, no urinary Bence Jones protein, less than 5 percent marrow plasmacytosis, and no anemia, renal failure, lytic bone lesions, or hypercalcemia. When bone marrow cells are exposed to radioactive thymidine in order to quantitate dividing cells, patients with MGUS always have a labeling index of less than 1 percent and patients with myeloma always have a labeling index of greater than 1 percent. Other discriminators include plasma cell acid phosphatase and β-glucuronidase, both of which are low in MGUS patients, and the salmon calcitonin stimulation test, which is positive only in patients with active ongoing bone destruction. Only about 11 percent of patients with MGUS go on to develop myeloma. Typically, patients with MGUS require no therapy.

The clinical evaluation of patients with myeloma includes a careful physical examination searching for tender bones and masses. It is paradoxic that only a small minority of patients have an enlargement of the spleen and lymph nodes, the physiologic sites of antibody production. Chest and bone radiographs may reveal lytic lesions or diffuse osteopenia. A complete blood count with differential may reveal anemia. Erythrocyte sedimentation rate is elevated. Very rare patients (~2 percent) may have plasma cell leukemia with more than 2000 plasma cells per microliter. This may be seen in disproportionate frequency in IgD (~12 percent) and IgE (~25 percent) myelomas. Serum calcium, urea nitrogen, creatinine, and uric acid may be elevated. Protein electrophoresis and measurement of serum immunoglobulins are useful for detecting and characterizing M spikes, supplemented by immunoelectrophoresis, which is especially sensitive for identifying low concentrations of M components not detectable by protein electrophoresis. A 24-h urine specimen is necessary to quantitate protein excretion, and a concentrated aliquot is used for electrophoresis and immunologic typing of any M component. Serum alkaline phosphatase is usually normal even with extensive bone involvement because of the absence of osteoblastic activity. It is also important to quantitate serum beta$_2$ microglobulin (see below).

The serum M component will be IgG in 53 percent of patients, IgA in 25 percent, and IgD in 1 percent, and 20 percent of patients will have only light chains in serum and urine. Dipsticks for detecting proteinuria are not reliable at identifying light chains, and the heat test for detecting Bence Jones protein is falsely negative in about 50 percent of patients with light chain myeloma. Fewer than 1 percent of patients have no identifiable M component, and these are usually light chain myelomas in which renal catabolism has made them undetectable in the urine. About two-thirds of patients with serum M components also have urinary light chains. The light chain isotype may have an impact on survival. Patients secreting lambda light chains have a significantly shorter overall survival than those secreting kappa light chains. It is not clear whether this is due to some genetically important determinant of cell proliferation or because lambda light chains are more likely to cause renal damage and form amyloid than are kappa light chains. The heavy chain isotype may have an impact on patient management as well. About half of patients with IgM paraproteins develop hyperviscosity compared with only 2 to 4 percent of patients with IgA and IgG M components. Among IgG myelomas, it is the IgG3 subclass that has the highest tendency to form both concentration- and temperature-dependent aggregates, leading to hyperviscosity and cold agglutination at lower serum concentrations.

The staging system for patients with myeloma is a functional system for predicting survival and is based on a variety of clinical and laboratory tests, unlike the anatomic staging systems for solid tumors. Details of the staging system are given in Table 280-2. Based on the hemoglobin, calcium, M component, and degree of skeletal involvement, the total-body tumor burden is estimated to be low (stage I, $<0.6 \times 10^{12}$ cells per square meter), intermediate (stage II, 0.6 to 1.2×10^{12} cells per square meter), or high (stage III, $>1.2 \times 10^{12}$ cells per square meter), and the stages are further subdivided on the basis of renal function (A if serum creatinine < 2 mg/dL, B if > 2). Patients in stage IA have a median survival of more than 5 years and those in stage IIIB about 15 months. Beta$_2$ microglobulin is a protein of 11,000 mol wt with homologies with the constant region of immunoglobulins that is the light chain of the class I major histocompatibility antigens (HLA-A, -B, -C) on the surface of every cell. Serum beta$_2$ microglobulin is the single most powerful predictor of survival and can substitute for staging. Patients with beta$_2$ microglobulin levels less than 0.004 g/L have a median survival of 43 months and those with levels higher than 0.004 g/L only 12 months. It is also felt that once the diagnosis of myeloma is firm, histologic features of atypia may also exert an influence on prognosis. Interleukin 6 may be an autocrine and/or paracrine growth factor for myeloma cells; elevated levels are associated with more aggressive disease. High labeling index and high levels of lactate dehydrogenase and thymidine kinase are also associated with poor prognosis.

Treatment and course About 10 percent of patients with myeloma will have an indolent course demonstrating only very slow progression of disease over many years. Such patients only require antitumor therapy when the serum myeloma protein rises above 50 g/L (5 g/dL) or progressive bone lesions develop. Patients with solitary bone plasmacytomas and extramedullary plasmacytomas may be expected to enjoy prolonged disease-free survival after local radiation therapy to a dose of around 40 Gy. There is a low incidence of occult marrow involvement in patients with solitary bone plasmacytoma. Such patients are usually detected because their serum M component falls slowly or disappears initially only to return after a few months. These patients respond well to systemic chemotherapy.

The vast majority of patients with myeloma require therapeutic intervention. In general, such therapy is of two sorts: systemic chemotherapy to control the progression of myeloma and symptomatic supportive care to prevent serious morbidity from the complications of the disease. All patients with stage II or III disease and stage I patients exhibiting Bence Jones proteinuria, progressive lytic bone lesions, vertebral compression fractures, recurrent infections, or rising serum M component should be treated with systemic combination chemotherapy. Therapy can prolong and improve the quality of life for myeloma patients.

TABLE 280-2   Myeloma staging system

Stage	Criteria	Estimated tumor burden ($\times 10^{12}$ cells/m^2)
I	All the following:	
	1 Hemoglobin >100 g/L (10 g/dL)	<0.6 (low)
	2 Serum calcium <12 mg/dL	
	3 Normal bone x-ray or solitary lesion	
	4 Low M-component production	
	a IgG level <50 g/L (<5 g/dL)	
	b IgA level <30 g/L (<3 g/dL)	
	c Urine light chain <4 g/24 h	
II	Fitting neither I nor III	0.6–1.20 (intermediate)
III	One or more of the following:	
	1 Hemoglobin <85 g/L (<8.5 g/dL)	>1.20 (high)
	2 Serum calcium (>12 mg/dL)	
	3 Advanced lytic bone lesions	
	4 High M-component production	
	a IgG level >70 g/L (>7 g/dL)	
	b IgA level >50 g/L (>5 g/dL)	
	c Urine light chains >12 g/24 h	

SUBCLASSIFICATION BASED ON SERUM CREATININE LEVELS

Level	Stage	Median survival, months
A < 2 mg/dL	IA	61
B > 2 mg/dL	IIA,B	55
	IIIA	30
	IIIB	15

STAGING BASED ON SERUM BETA$_2$ MICROGLOBULIN LEVELS

Level	Stage	Median survival, months
<4 μg/mL	I	43
>4 μg/mL	II	12

The standard treatment has consisted of intermittent pulses of an alkylating agent [L-phenylalanine mustard (L-PAM, melphalan), cyclophosphamide, or chlorambucil] and prednisone administered for 4 to 7 days every 4 to 6 weeks. The alkylating agents appear to be roughly equally active, but resistance to one agent is often accompanied by resistance to the others. The usual doses are as follows: melphalan, 8 mg/m^2 of body surface area per day; cyclophosphamide, 200 mg/m^2 per day; chlorambucil, 8 mg/m^2 per day; prednisone, 25 to 60 mg/m^2 per day. Because of their near equivalence in antitumor efficacy, we favor cyclophosphamide as the alkylating agent because it is less toxic to the marrow stem cell compartment and results in a lower incidence of acute myelodysplastic syndromes than do the other alkylating agents. Doses may need adjustment based on marrow tolerance. However, there are few constraints on the dose of the steroid pulse, and it appears that more is better. Recent evidence suggests that higher dose-intensity (i.e., mg/m^2 per week) of the steroid is associated with significantly longer survival. Patients responding to therapy generally have a prompt and gratifying reduction in bone pain, hypercalcemia, and anemia and often have fewer infections. The serum M component lags substantially behind the symptomatic improvement, often taking 4 to 6 weeks to fall. This fall depends on the rate of tumor kill and the fractional catabolic rate of immunoglobulin, which in turn depends on the serum concentration (for IgG). Light chain excretion, with a functional half-life of approximately 6 h, may fall within the first week of treatment. However, since urine light chain levels may relate to renal tubular function, they are not a reliable measure of tumor cell kill. Calculations of tumor cell kill are made by extrapolation of the serum M component level and rely heavily on the assumption that every tumor cell produces immunoglobulin at a constant rate. About 60 percent of patients will achieve at least a 75 percent reduction in serum M component level and tumor cell mass in response to an alkylating agent and prednisone.

Although this is a tumor reduction of less than one log, clinical responses may last many months. Efforts to improve the fraction of patients responding and the degree of response have involved adding other active chemotherapeutic agents to the treatment program. Patients with more advanced disease may benefit most from such an approach, but three- to five-drug therapy is experimental at this time. High-dose therapy with hematopoietic support is also being tested in younger patients.

The ideal duration of therapy has not been determined. Most physicians treat every 4 to 6 weeks for 1 or 2 years. Cessation of therapy is followed by relapse, usually within a year. Retreatment may be associated with a second response in up to 80 percent of patients. Maintenance therapy (e.g., with interferon-α) may prolong the duration of response, but no study has demonstrated this to result in prolonged survival. The regrowth rate of the tumor during relapse accelerates with each relapse. Patients primarily resistant to initial therapy have a median survival of less than a year. High-dose pulsed steroids used alone (200 mg prednisone every other day or 1 g/m^2 per day methylprednisolone for 5 days) or VAD combination chemotherapy (vincristine, 0.4 mg/d in a 4-day continuous infusion; doxorubicin, 9 mg/m^2 per day in a 4-day continuous infusion; dexamethasone, 40 mg/d for 4 days per week for 3 weeks) may offer useful palliation in patients resistant to primary therapy.

About 15 percent of patients die within the first 3 months after diagnosis, and subsequently, the death rate is about 15 percent per year. The disease usually follows a chronic course for 2 to 5 years before developing an acute terminal phase, usually marked by the development of pancytopenia with a cellular marrow that is refractory to treatment. Widespread organ infiltration by myeloma cells occurs, and survival is less than 6 months. About 46 percent of patients die in the chronic phase of disease from progressive myeloma (16 percent) and renal failure (10 percent), sepsis (14 percent), or both (6 percent). Death in the acute terminal phase (26 percent) is chiefly from progressive myeloma (13 percent) and sepsis (9 percent). Five percent of patients die of acute leukemia, myeloblastic or monocytic, and although it has been debated that this is related to the primary disease, it appears more likely to be the result of chronic therapy with alkylating agents. Nearly 23 percent of patients die of myocardial infarction, chronic lung disease, diabetes, or stroke, all intercurrent illnesses related more to the age of the patient group than to the tumor.

Supportive care directed at the anticipated complications of the disease may be as important as primary antitumor therapy. The hypercalcemia generally responds well to corticosteroid therapy, hydration, and natriuresis. Calcitonin may add to the inhibitory effects of steroids on bone resorption. Diphosphonates have also been shown to reduce osteoclastic bone resorption. Treatments aimed at strengthening the skeleton, such as fluorides, calcium, and vitamin D with or without androgens, have been suggested but are not of proven efficacy. Iatrogenic worsening of renal function may be prevented by the use of allopurinol during chemotherapy to avoid urate nephropathy and by maintaining a high fluid intake to help excrete light chains and calcium. In the event of acute renal failure, plasmapheresis is approximately 10 times more effective at clearing light chains than peritoneal dialysis, and acutely reducing the protein load may result in functional improvement. Urinary tract infections should be watched for and treated early. Chronic dialysis probably should not be initiated in patients who have failed to respond to antitumor therapy. Plasmapheresis may be the treatment of choice for hyperviscosity syndromes. Although the pneumococcus is a dreaded pathogen in myeloma patients, they do not respond to pneumococcal polysaccharide vaccines. The advent of intravenous gamma globulin preparations raises some hope that prophylactic administration may prevent some serious infections, but this has not been tested. Chronic oral antibiotic prophylaxis is probably not warranted. Patients developing neurologic symptoms in the lower extremities, severe localized back pain, or problems with bowel and bladder control may need emergency myelography and radiation therapy for palliation.

Most bone lesions respond to analgesics and chemotherapy, but certain painful lesions may respond most promptly to localized radiation. The chronic anemia may respond to hematinics (iron, folate, cobalamin), and some have responded to androgens. The pathogenesis of the anemia should be established and specific therapy instituted, where possible.

WALDENSTRÖM'S MACROGLOBULINEMIA In 1948, Waldenström described a malignancy of lymphoplasmacytoid cells that secreted IgM. In contrast to myeloma, the disease was associated with lymphadenopathy and hepatosplenomegaly, but the major clinical manifestation was the hyperviscosity syndrome. The disease resembles the related diseases chronic lymphocytic leukemia, myeloma, and lymphocytic lymphoma. Waldenström's macroglobulinemia and IgM myeloma both follow a similar clinical course. The diagnosis of IgM myeloma is usually reserved for patients with lytic bone lesions and is important only because of the hazard of pathologic fractures.

The cause of macroglobulinemia is unknown. The disease is similar to myeloma in being slightly more common in men and occurring with increased incidence with age (median 64 years). There have been reports that the IgM in some patients with macroglobulinemia may have specificity for myelin-associated glycoprotein (MAG), a protein that has been associated with demyelinating disease of the peripheral nervous system and may be lost earlier and to a greater extent than the better known myelin basic protein in patients with multiple sclerosis. There is a surface antigen on natural killer cells that is cross-reactive with the MAG, and coincidentally, natural killer cells are decreased in multiple sclerosis. Sometimes patients with macroglobulinemia develop a peripheral neuropathy before the appearance of the neoplasm. There is speculation that the whole process begins with a viral infection that may elicit an antibody response that cross-reacts with a normal tissue component.

Like myeloma, the disease involves the bone marrow, but unlike myeloma, it does not cause bone lesions or hypercalcemia. Like myeloma, a serum M component is present in the serum in excess of 30 g/L (3 g/dL), but unlike myeloma, the size of the IgM paraprotein results in little renal excretion and only around 20 percent of patients excrete light chains. Therefore, renal disease is not common. The light chain isotype is kappa in 80 percent of the cases. Patients present with weakness, fatigue, and recurrent infections, similar to myeloma patients, but epistaxis, visual disturbances, and neurologic symptoms such as peripheral neuropathy, dizziness, headache, and transient paresis are much more common in macroglobulinemia. Physical examination reveals adenopathy and hepatosplenomegaly, and ophthalmoscopic examination may reveal vascular segmentation and dilatation of the retinal veins characteristic of hyperviscosity states. Patients may have a normocytic, normochromic anemia, but rouleaux formation and a positive Coombs' test are much more common than in myeloma. Malignant lymphocytes are usually present in the peripheral blood. About 10 percent of macroglobulins are cryoglobulins. These are pure M components and are not the mixed cryoglobulins seen in rheumatoid arthritis and other autoimmune diseases. Mixed cryoglobulins are composed of IgM or IgA complexed with IgG, for which they are specific. In both cases, Raynaud's phenomenon and serious vascular symptoms precipitated by the cold may occur, but mixed cryoglobulins are not commonly associated with malignancy. Patients suspected of having a cryoglobulin based on history and physical examination should have their blood drawn into a warm syringe and delivered to the laboratory in a container of warm water to avoid errors in quantitating the cryoglobulin.

Control of serious hyperviscosity symptoms such as an altered state of consciousness or paresis can be achieved acutely by plasmapheresis because 80 percent of the IgM paraprotein is intravascular. Aside from this, management is identical to that of myeloma. About 80 percent of patients respond to chemotherapy, and their median survival is over 3 years. The absence of other serious organ toxicities results in a longer life span of patients with macroglobulinemia compared with those with myeloma.

HEAVY CHAIN DISEASES The heavy chain diseases are rare

lymphoplasmacytic malignancies. Their clinical manifestations vary with the heavy chain isotype. Patients secrete a defective heavy chain that usually has an intact Fc fragment and a deletion in the Fd region. Gamma, alpha, and mu heavy chain diseases have been described, but no reports of delta or epsilon heavy chain diseases have appeared. Molecular biologic analysis of these tumors has revealed structural genetic defects that may account for the aberrant chain secreted.

Gamma heavy chain disease (Franklin's disease) This disease affects people of widely different age groups and countries of origin. It is characterized by lymphadenopathy, fever, anemia, malaise, hepatosplenomegaly, and weakness. Its most distinctive symptom is palatal edema, resulting from node involvement of Waldeyer's ring, and this may progress to produce respiratory compromise. The diagnosis depends on the demonstration of an anomalous serum M component [often <20 g/L (<2 g/dL)] that reacts with anti-IgG but not anti-light chain reagents. The M component is typically present in *both serum* and *urine*. Most of the paraproteins have been of the gamma₁ subclass, but other subclasses have been seen. The patients may have thrombocytopenia, eosinophilia, and nondiagnostic bone marrow. Patients usually have a rapid downhill course and die of infection; however, some patients have survived 5 years with chemotherapy.

Alpha heavy chain disease (Seligmann's disease) This is the most common of the heavy chain diseases. It is closely related to a malignancy known as *Mediterranean lymphoma*, a disease that affects young people in parts of the world such as the Mediterranean, Asia, and South America in which intestinal parasites are common. The disease is characterized by an infiltration of the lamina propria of the small intestine with lymphoplasmacytoid cells that secrete truncated alpha chains. Demonstrating alpha heavy chains is difficult because the alpha chains tend to polymerize and appear as a smear instead of a sharp peak on electrophoretic profiles. Despite the polymerization, hyperviscosity is not a common problem in alpha heavy chain disease. Without J chain–facilitated dimerization, viscosity does not increase dramatically. Light chains are absent from serum and urine. The patients present with chronic diarrhea, weight loss, and malabsorption and have extensive mesenteric and paraaortic adenopathy. Respiratory tract involvement occurs rarely. Patients may vary widely in their clinical course. Some may develop diffuse aggressive histologies of malignant lymphoma. Chemotherapy may produce long-term remissions. Rare patients appear to have responded to antibiotic therapy, raising the question of the etiologic role of antigenic stimulation perhaps by some chronic intestinal infection.

Mu heavy chain disease The secretion of isolated mu heavy chains into the serum appears to occur in a very rare subset of patients with chronic lymphocytic leukemia. The only features that may distinguish patients with mu heavy chain disease are the presence of vacuoles in the malignant lymphocytes and the excretion of kappa light chains in the urine. The diagnosis requires ultracentrifugation or gel filtration to confirm the nonreactivity of the paraprotein with the light chain reagents because some intact macroglobulins fail to interact with these serums. The tumor cells seem to have a defect in the assembly of light and heavy chains because they appear to contain both in their cytoplasm. There is no evidence that such patients should be treated differently from other patients with chronic lymphocytic leukemia.

REFERENCES

ALEXANIAN R et al: Prognosis of asymptomatic multiple myeloma. Arch Intern Med 148: 1963, 1988

BARLOGIE B et al: Plasma cell myeloma—New biological insights and advances in therapy. Blood 73:865, 1989

————, ALEXANIAN R: Second International Workshop on Myeloma: Advances in biology and therapy of multiple myeloma. Cancer Res 49:7172, 1989

BATAILLE R et al: Serum levels of interleukin 6, a potent myeloma cell growth factor, as a reflection of disease severity in plasma cell dyscrasias. J Clin Invest 84:2008, 1989

CHAK LY et al: Solitary plasmacytoma of bone: Treatment, progression and survival. J Clin Oncol 5:1811, 1987

GREGORY WM et al: Combination chemotherapy versus melphalan and prednisone in the treatment of multiple myeloma: An overview of published trials. J Clin Oncol 10:334, 1992

GRIEPP PR et al: Value of beta-2-microglobulin level and plasma cell labeling indices as prognostic factors in patients with newly diagnosed myeloma. Blood 72:219, 1988

KYLE RA (ed): Myeloma and related disorders, in *Neoplastic Diseases of the Blood*. New York, Churchill Livingstone, 1991, pp 325–571

LOKHORST HM, DEKKER AW: Advances in the treatment of multiple myeloma. Cancer Treat Rev 19:113, 1993

MANDELLI F et al: Maintenance treatment with recombinant interferon-alpha-2b in patients with multiple myeloma responding to conventional induction chemotherapy. N Engl J Med 322:1430, 1990

PALMER M et al: Dose-intensity analysis of melphalan and prednisone in multiple myeloma. J Natl Cancer Inst 80:414, 1988

281 AMYLOIDOSIS

ALAN S. COHEN

DEFINITION AND CLASSIFICATION *Amyloidosis* may be defined as the extracellular deposition of the fibrous protein amyloid in one or more sites of the body. It was named by Virchow in 1854 on the basis of its color after staining with iodine and sulfuric acid. This protein has unique ultrastructural, x-ray diffraction, and biochemical characteristics. It can be deposited locally, where it has no clinical consequences, or it may involve virtually any organ system of the body, leading to severe pathophysiologic changes, or the disease may fall between these two extremes. The natural history of amyloidosis is poorly understood, and the clinical diagnosis is often not made until the disease is far advanced. It is now clear that there are multiple clinically and biochemically different forms of amyloid that are so classified because of the unique fibrous structure they all possess. The following classification is clinically the most useful: (1) primary (AL type) amyloidosis (no evidence for preexisting or coexisting disease), (2) amyloid associated with multiple myeloma (also AL type), (3) secondary or reactive (AA type) amyloidosis associated with chronic infectious diseases (e.g., osteomyelitis, tuberculosis, leprosy) or chronic inflammatory diseases (e.g., rheumatoid arthritis), (4) heredofamilial amyloidosis, a variety of neuropathic [AF transthyretin (prealbumin) type], renal, cardiovascular, and other syndromes, plus the amyloidosis associated with familial Mediterranean fever (AA type), (5) local amyloidosis (focal, often tumor-like, deposits which occur in isolated organs, often endocrine, without evidence of systemic involvement), (6) amyloidosis associated with aging, especially in the heart and in the brain, and (7) amyloid associated with long-term hemodialysis. These clinical forms and their current biochemical classification are listed in Table 281-1.

PATHOLOGY AND STRUCTURE Amyloid is amorphous, eosinophilic, extracellular, and ubiquitous in distribution. The involved organs may have a rubbery consistency and a waxy, pink or gray appearance. Organ enlargement, especially of the liver, kidney, spleen, and heart, may be prominent.

Microscopically, amyloid stains pink with the hematoxylin-eosin stain and shows metachromasia with crystal violet. The Congo red stain imparts a unique green birefringence when sections are viewed in the polarizing microscope. This is the single most useful procedure for establishing the presence of amyloid. Amyloid deposits may be focal in almost any area of the body but are most often perivascular.

The heart may show focal or diffuse interstitial deposits in the myocardium, endocardium, or pericardium. In the aged heart, the atrium is usually focally involved, or there may occur more diffuse lesions of the atria and ventricles. In the kidney, the glomerulus is primarily affected, although interstitial, peritubular, and vascular amyloid occur. In early lesions, small nodular or diffuse deposits appear near the basement membrane, and as the disease progresses, the glomerulus may be massively laden with amyloid and its capillary

TABLE 281-1   The 1990 guidelines for nomenclature and classification of amyloid and amyloidosis

Amyloid protein[a]	Protein precursor	Protein type of variant	Clinical
AA[b]	apoSSA		Reactive (secondary) Familial Mediterranean fever Familial amyloid nephropathy with urticaria and deafness (Muckle-Wells syndrome)
AL	kappa, lambda (e.g., k III)	Ak, A, (e.g., A k III)	Idiopathic (primary), myeloma or macroglobulinemia-associated
AH	IgG 1(γ1)	Aγ1	
ATTR	Transthyretin	e.g., Met 30[c]	Familial amyloid polyneuropathy (Portuguese)
		e.g., Met 111	Familial amyloid cariomyopathy (Danish)
		TTR or Ile 122	Systemic senile amyloidosis
AApoAI	apoAI	Arg 26	Familial amyloid polyneuropathy (Iowa)
AGel	Gelsolin	Asn 187[d] (15)	Familial amyloidosis (Finnish)
ACys	Cystatin C	Gln 68	Hereditary cerebral hemorrhage with amyloidosis (Icelandic)
AB	B protein precursor (e.g., BPP_{695})[e]	Gln 618 (22)	Alzheimer's disease Down's syndrome Hereditary cerebral hemorrhage amyloidosis (Dutch)
AB_2M	$Beta_2$ microglobulin		Associated with chronic dialysis
AScr	Scrapie protein, precursor 33–35 kDa cellular form	Scrapie protein 27–30 kDa	Creutzfeldt-Jakob disease, etc.
		e.g., Leu 102	Gerstmann-Straussler-Scheinker syndrome
ACal	(Pro)calcitonin	(Pro)calcitonin	Medullary carcinoma of thyroid
AANF	Atrial natriuretic factor		Isolated atrial amyloid
AIAPP	Islet amyloid polypeptide		Islets of Langerhans Diabetes type II, Insulinoma

[a]Nonfibrillar proteins, e.g., protein AP (amyloid P component) excluded
[b]Abbreviation not explained in table: AA = amyloid A protein, SAA = serum amyloid A protein, apo = apolipoprotein, L = immunoglobulin light chain, H = immunoglobulin heavy chain
[c]ATTR Met 30 when used in text
[d]Amino acid positions in the mature precursor protein. The position in the amyloid fibril protein is given in parentheses
[e]Number of amino acid residues
SOURCE: Cohen, 1991.

bed occluded. In the gastrointestinal tract, there may be perivascular deposits only, or irregular or diffuse deposits may be found in the submucosa, the muscularis mucosa, or subserosa. The amyloid may appear at any level or portion of the gastrointestinal tract, including the gallbladder and pancreas. In the nervous system, amyloid has been described along peripheral nerves, in autonomic ganglia, and in senile plaques, neurofibrillary tangles, and blood vessels ("congophilic angiopathy") of the central nervous system. It may be found in any portion of the orbit, including the vitreous humor and cornea. In summary, there is virtually no area of the body that is spared. This ubiquitous distribution elicits a wide variety of clinical symptoms and signs.

All types of human amyloid consist of fine, nonbranching, rigid fibrils that in tissue sections measure approximately 10×10^{-9} m (100 Å) in diameter. Isolated amyloid fibrils have a delicate, thin, nonbranching fibrous character. The individual fibril (or filament) has a diameter of about 7×10^{-9} m (70 Å) and tends to aggregate laterally. Each fibril (filament) has subunit protofibrils of 3 to 3.5 × 10^{-9} m (30 to 35 Å) diameter. X-ray diffraction of isolated amyloid fibrils reveals a cross beta pattern, the "pleated sheet" of Pauling and Corey, indicating that the polypeptide chain runs transversely to the long axis of the fibril specimen.

A second component, the plasma component or pentagonal unit (P component or AP) with a different ultrastructure, x-ray diffraction pattern, and chemical characteristics, also has been isolated from amyloid and is identical with a serum alpha globulin (SAP). It has many similarities to C-reactive protein, but it does not behave in

humans as a classic acute-phase protein. It is not responsible for the characteristic tinctorial properties or ultrastructure of amyloid.

BIOCHEMISTRY OF AMYLOID FIBRILS The bulk of amyloid deposits consists of fibrils. Purified amyloid derived from the fibril is a protein. The chemical composition of the different clinical forms of amyloid are distinct and allow for more precise diagnosis (Table 281-1). The homology of the fibril of primary and myeloma amyloid to the N-terminal region of the variable fragment of an immunoglobulin light chain, and subsequently, in a limited number of cases, to a homogeneous light polypeptide chain, has been demonstrated. These light chain–related proteins range in size from about 5000 to 25,000 Da and are now termed amyloid light chain (AL) or AL_κ or AL_λ (Table 281-1). Amino acid sequence analysis indicates that most primary amyloid proteins contain the N-terminal amino acid residue identical to the variable regions of the light chain. Lambda chain class predominates over kappa in AL by a 2:1 ratio, whereas in multiple myeloma the reverse is true. Indeed, almost all lambda VI chains have been associated with amyloid. One heavy chain–related amyloid (AH) has been described recently.

Another protein, amyloid A (AA), unrelated to any known immunoglobulin, has been described in the secondary amyloid deposits. This protein can be isolated from the amyloid of patients with secondary amyloidosis and from that associated with familial Mediterranean fever. It is a unique protein with a molecular weight of about 8400 Da made up of approximately 76 amino acid residues arranged in a single chain. Some heterogeneity has been demonstrated (i.e., AAs of different molecular weights). AA is derived from serum

TABLE 281-2 **Hereditary amyloid syndromes—1990**

Clinical aspects*	Geographic or ethnic association	Protein and mutation
FAP—Distal limb peripheral neuropathy (sensory/motor); autonomic neuropathy with alternate constipation and diarrhea; nephropathy; cardiopathy with congestive failure (CHF) and arrhythmias; pupillary abnormalities in late disease (scalloped pupil); occasional vitreous opacities	Portuguese, Japanese, Swedish, Greek, Italian, Turkish	Transthyretin Met 30 (ATTR Met 30)
FAP—Peripheral neuropathy; autonomic neuropathy; cadiopathy, no renal (yet)	USA/German	ATTR Ala 30
FAP—Similar; few details known (neuropathy, diarrhea, vitreous opacities)	Israeli (Polish extraction)	ATTR Ile 33
FAP—Cardiomyopathy, vitreous opacities, mild neuropathy, renal (early report)	USA/Greek	ATTR Pro 36
FAP—Peripheral neuropathy; gastrointestinal (early report)	Japanese (Osaka)	ATTR Gly 42
FAP—Peripheral neuropathy; liver (early report)	Japanese	ATTR Arg 50
FAP—Cardiopathy; vitreous opacities	USA/Maryland/German extraction	ATTR His 58
FAP—Severe cardiopathy (often late in life); less peripheral neuropathy; occasional carpal tunnel syndrome	USA/West Virginia/ Appalachia (English-Irish-German extraction	ATTR Ala 60
FAP—Neuropathy, diarrhea, nephropathy, cardiomyopathy	USA/Illinois/Texas (German extraction)	ATTR Tyr 77
FAP—Marked carpal tunnel syndrome; marked vitreous opacities, gastrointestinal symptoms	USA/Indiana (Swiss extraction)	ATTR Ser 84
FAC—Late-onset cardiopathy; vitreous opacities; no neuropathy as yet (early report)	USA/Italian	ATTR Asn 84
FAP—Severe cardiomyopathy; mild sensory neuropathy; vitreous opacities	USA/Italian	ATTR Asn 90
FAC—Primarily heart disease with congestive failure and arrhythmias	Danish	ATTR Met 111
FAP—Peripheral neuropathy; vitreous opacities; gastrointestinal; kidney (heart probable, early report)	Japanese (Osaka)	ATTR Cys 114
FAP—Lower limb neuropathy; nephropathy	USA/Iowa (Scottish-Irish-English)	Apolipoprotein AI Arg 26 (AApoAI Arg 26)
FAP—Cranial nerve neuropathy; skin changes; lattice corneal dystrophy; nephropathy	Finnish	Gelsolin Asn 187 (15) (AGel Asn 187 (15))
Hereditary cerebral hemorrhage with amyloidosis: cerebral angiopathy with spontaneous bleeds	Icelandic	Cystatin C Glh 68 (ACys Gln 68)
	Dutch	Beta protein
Familial(?) amyloid (senile, systemic) cardiopathy; heart disease in elderly patients; diagnosis at autopsy	Black	ATTR Ile 122
Familial Mediterranean fever—Fever; joint pain; polyserositis; skin rash; mostly autosomal recessive	Sephardic Jews, Armenians, Kurds	AA
Familial nephropathy with urticaria and deafness (Muckle-Wells syndrome)		AA

* FAP = familial amyloid polyneuropathy; FAC = familial amyloid cardiomyopathy.
SOURCE: Cohen, 1991.

amyloid A (SAA) by proteolysis. SAA is synthesized in the liver, migrates as an HDL complex, and is known as apoSAA. SAA is a polymorphic protein, expressed as SAA_1 and SAA_2, the former of which is the major component of tissue-extracted AA protein. To date, four human SAA genes have been described. Data from the mouse indicate that in that species only SAA_2 contributes to tissue amyloid deposits. These collective data suggest that minimal amino acid differences can affect amyloidogenicity, a concept supported by studies in other (i.e., hereditary) amyloidoses.

SAA behaves as an acute-phase reactant and is elevated in infection and inflammation. In addition, SAA is elevated in amyloid-resistant animals, suggesting that the appearance of amyloid is not solely determined by the level of SAA. An SAA inducing factor (now known to be interleukin 1) is released from stimulated macrophages and causes the release of SAA from hepatocytes, the site of SAA synthesis. The precise regulation of the conversion of SAA to the insoluble AA protein of amyloidosis is not understood.

Familial amyloid polyneuropathy (FAP) is a dominant hereditary disease affecting kinships originating in Portugal, Japan, Sweden,

and elsewhere. A 14,000-Da protein has been isolated from the tissues of patients from each of the above-noted geographically distributed kinships. Immunologic and amino acid sequence analyses have identified it as transthyretin (prealbumin), the first association of this molecule with a disease. It also has been shown that in many kinships there is a single amino acid substitution, methionine for valine at position 30, in the transthyretin isolated from the amyloid. Multiple other variants also have been shown to exist (Table 281-2).

A number of other amyloid proteins have been isolated and characterized. These include several from focal endocrine-related amyloid lesions such as precalcitonin from the amyloid of medullary carcinoma of the thyroid and insulinoma amyloid polypeptide (IAPP) of the pancreas found not only in association with insulinomas but with adult-onset diabetes mellitus as well. Transthyretin also has been isolated from senile cardiac amyloid, and atrial natriuretic peptide has been isolated as a distinct and separate protein from these lesions. $Beta_2$ microglobulin has been identified as the protein from the amyloid associated with chronic hemodialysis.

Of great interest is confirmation that the lesions known as senile plaques (which contain amyloid) and the meningeal vascular amyloid of Alzheimer's disease consist of a newly described protein, beta protein (or A4 protein), a 39 to 43 amino acid fragment of the large molecule known as beta protein precursor.

P component of amyloid   In addition to the characteristic fibrils described above, a second component, the P component, has been noted in most amyloid deposits. P component (AP) has been recognized by electron microscopy as a pentagonal-shaped structured unit having an outside diameter of about 9×10^{-9} m (90 Å) and an inside diameter of about 4×10^{-9} m (40 Å). On immunoelectrophoresis it migrates as an alpha globulin, and it possesses antigenic identity with a constituent of normal human plasma (SAP). The amino acid sequence is distinct from that of the amyloid fibrils. Its pentagonal ultrastructure is similar to C-reactive protein (CRP), but the latter is one-half the molecular weight of AP and has other well-defined differences despite a 50 to 60 percent homology on amino acid sequence. AP binds to amyloid fibrils in a calcium-dependent fashion almost universally and has been used as a marker of amyloid.

IMMUNOBIOLOGY OF AMYLOID   The precise etiology and pathogenesis of amyloidosis are unknown. Experimentally, the induction of AA amyloidosis has been shown to be a multifactorial process that is contributed to by the type of inflammatory stimulation, the nature of the SAA isotype, and the genetic background of the host. During inflammation, the mediator, interleukin 1, stimulates hepatic cells to produce increased SAA. SAA is partially degraded by monocyte or leukocyte surface enzymes to form AA. It is likely that macrophages play a role in the SAA degradation. Related abnormalities such as altered connective tissue glycosaminoglycans, altered macrophage enzymes, or enzyme inhibitors have all been postulated.

In AL amyloid, a monoclonal population of bone marrow plasma cells appears to be present and either consistently produces small lambda or kappa fragments or clones of immunoglobulins that are processed (cleaved) in an abnormal fashion by macrophage enzymes to produce the partially degraded light chains responsible for AL amyloidosis.

The formation of amyloid also may be determined in part by the intrinsic beta configuration of at least a portion of the polypeptide chain such as in transthyretin, beta$_2$ microglobulin, and other amyloidogenic proteins. Clearly, in the hereditary amyloidoses the substitution of a single amino acid variant contributes to the overall pathogenesis.

It also has been demonstrated that a substance known as amyloid enhancing factor (AEF), possibly a cytokine, contributes at least to the accelerated formation of secondary and probably other forms of amyloid.

CLINICAL MANIFESTATIONS   The clinical manifestations of amyloidosis are varied and depend entirely on the area of the body which is involved.

Kidney   Renal involvement may consist of mild proteinuria or frank nephrosis. In some cases, the urinary sediment may show only a few red blood cells. The renal lesion is usually not reversible and in time leads to progressive azotemia and death. The prognosis does not appear to be related to the degree of the proteinuria; when azotemia finally develops, the prognosis is grave. In one series, the mean survival of patients with renal amyloid from the time of biopsy was 29 months, but in a few cases there was presumptive evidence of regression of the renal amyloid. The utilization of chronic hemodialysis and of kidney transplantation has clearly improved the prognosis of renal amyloid. Hypertension is rare, except in long-standing amyloidosis. Renal tubular acidosis or renal vein thrombosis may occur. Localized accumulation of amyloid may be noted in the ureter, bladder, or other parts of the genitourinary tract. Renal pathology occurs in AA, AL, and many forms of heredofamilial disease and does not enable one to distinguish among the various types.

Liver   While hepatic involvement is common, liver function abnormalities are minimal and occur late in the disease. The two tests most useful in indicating hepatic amyloid are the Bromsulphalein (BSP) extraction and serum alkaline phosphatase activity; however, no liver function tests are truly specific or sensitive for amyloid. Liver scans produce variable and nonspecific results. Portal hypertension occurs but is uncommon. Intrahepatic cholestasis has been noted in about 5 percent of patients with AL (primary) amyloidosis. In a series of 38 patients in whom liver tissue was available for examination, all 38 had some amyloid present, irrespective of the type of amyloidosis (primary or secondary), and contrary to previous notions, parenchymal amyloid was more extensive in the AL cases. Hepatomegaly is common, and AL hepatic amyloid is usually accompanied by the nephrotic syndrome and congestive heart failure. Prognosis is poor, and one group of 80 patients with proven AL hepatic amyloid had a median survival of 9 months. Amyloidosis of the spleen characteristically is not associated with leukopenia and anemia. Hepatic amyloid is uncommon and rarely of clinical importance in heredofamilial amyloidosis.

Heart   Cardiac manifestations consist primarily of congestive failure and cardiomegaly (with or without murmurs) and a variety of arrhythmias. Cardiac amyloidosis is common in primary (AL) and heredofamilial amyloidosis and very rare in the secondary (AA) form. Although the cardiac manifestations predominantly reflect diffuse myocardial amyloid, the endocardium, valves, and pericardium may be involved as well. Pericarditis with effusion is rare, although the differential diagnosis of constrictive pericarditis versus restrictive cardiomyopathy frequently arises. Echocardiography has demonstrated symmetric thickening of the left ventricular wall, hypokinesia and decreased systolic contraction and thickening of the interventricular septum and left ventricular posterior wall, and left ventricular cavities of small to normal size. Two-dimensional echocardiography produces the characteristic findings of thickened right and left ventricles, a normal left ventricular cavity, and especially a diffuse hyperrefractile "granular sparkling" appearance. Hearts which are heavily infiltrated with amyloid may or may not show an enlarged silhouette. Fluoroscopy usually shows decreased mobility of the ventricular wall; angiographic studies usually demonstrate thickened ventricular wall, decreased ventricular mobility, and absence of rapid ventricular filling in early diastole. Cardiac amyloidosis can present as intractable heart failure. Electrocardiographic abnormalities include a low-voltage QRS complex and abnormalities in atrioventricular and intraventricular conduction, often resulting in varying degrees of heart block. Owing to their propensity to develop conduction defects and arrhythmias, patients with cardiac amyloidosis appear to be especially sensitive to digitalis, and this drug should be used with caution. Radionuclide techniques utilizing technetium 99m pyrophosphate for cardiac scanning are often positive, especially in patients with amyloid-related congestive heart failure.

Skin   Involvement of the skin is one of the most characteristic manifestations of primary (AL) amyloidosis. The lesions may consist of slightly raised, waxy papules or plaques which usually are clustered in the folds of the axillae, anal, or inguinal regions, the face and neck, or mucosal areas such as ear or tongue. Periorbital ecchymoses ("black eye syndrome") have been reported. The lesions are seldom pruritic. Involvement of the skin or mucosa may not be apparent clinically but may be demonstrated by biopsy. Gentle rubbing of the skin may induce bleeding into the skin, leading to purpura. Cutaneous involvement also can occur in secondary amyloidosis; in one series it was found in 42 percent of such patients, in 55 percent of a group of patients with primary disease, and in all 11 patients with hereditary amyloid neuropathy.

Gastrointestinal tract   Gastrointestinal symptoms are common in all systemic types of amyloidosis. They may result from direct involvement of the gastrointestinal tract at any level or from infiltration of the autonomic nervous system with amyloid. The symptoms include those of obstruction, ulceration, malabsorption, hemorrhage, protein loss, and diarrhea. Infiltration of the tongue occasionally leads to macroglossia. When not enlarged, the tongue may become stiffened and firm to palpation. While infiltration of the tongue is characteristic of primary amyloidosis (AL) or amyloidosis accompanying multiple myeloma, it is occasionally seen in the secondary (AA) form of the disease.

Gastrointestinal bleeding may occur from any of a number of sites, notably the esophagus, stomach, or large intestine, and may be severe. Amyloid infiltration of the esophagus may lead to an incompetent or nonrelaxing lower esophageal sphincter, nonspecific motility disorders of the esophageal body, or rarely achalasia. Small bowel lesions may lead to clinical and x-ray changes of obstruction. A malabsorption syndrome is seen at times. Amyloidosis may develop in association with other entities involving the gastrointestinal tract, especially tuberculosis, granulomatous enteritis, lymphoma, and Whipple's disease; differentiation of these conditions, which give rise to secondary amyloidosis, from diffuse primary amyloidosis of the small bowel may be difficult. Similarly, amyloidosis of the stomach may closely mimic gastric carcinoma, with obstruction, achlorhydria, and the radiologic appearance of tumor masses.

Nervous system   Neurologic manifestations may include peripheral neuropathy, postural hypotension, inability to sweat, Adie's pupil, hoarseness, and sphincter incompetence. These manifestations are especially prominent in the heredofamilial amyloidoses. The cranial nerves are generally spared, except for those involving the pupillary reflexes. Carpal tunnel syndrome may be caused by several amyloidoses, especially primary (AL) and chronic hemodialysis (B_2M) amyloid. Peripheral neuropathy is frequent in the former type. Amyloid occurs in the central nervous system as a component of senile plaques, neurofibrillary tangles, and in blood vessels ("congophilic angiopathy"). The protein concentration in the cerebral spinal fluid may be increased. Infiltrates of the cornea or vitreous body may be present in hereditary amyloid syndromes. Certain of these syndromes are characterized by a bilateral scalloping appearance of the pupil.

Endocrine   Amyloid may infiltrate the thyroid or other endocrine glands but rarely causes endocrine dysfunction. Local amyloid deposits almost invariably accompany medullary carcinoma of the thyroid. Amyloid is often found in the adrenal gland, pituitary gland, and pancreas. Little if any clinical dysfunction is present unless there is massive replacement of the gland by amyloid.

Joints   Amyloid can directly involve articular structures by its presence in the synovial membrane and synovial fluid or in the articular cartilage. Amyloid arthritis can mimic a number of rheumatic diseases because it can present as a symmetric arthritis of small joints with nodules, morning stiffness, and fatigue. Most patients with amyloid arthropathy eventually are found to have multiple myeloma. The synovial fluid usually has a low white blood cell count, a good to fair mucin clot, a predominance of mononuclear cells, and no crystals. Studies of surgical specimens suggest a significant incidence of amyloid in cartilage, capsule, and synovium in osteoarthritis. Amyloid infiltration of muscle may lead to a pseudomyopathy.

Respiratory system   The nasal sinuses, larynx, and trachea may be involved by accumulations of AL amyloid which block the ducts, in the case of the sinuses, or the air passages. Amyloidosis of the lung involves the bronchi and alveolar septa diffusely. The lower respiratory tract is affected most frequently in primary (AL) amyloidosis and in the disease associated with dysproteinemia. Pulmonary symptoms attributable to amyloid are present in about 30 percent of these patients and in some are the most serious manifestations of the disease. In secondary (AA) amyloidosis, pulmonary disease is a frequent histopathologic accompaniment but seldom gives rise to clinically significant symptoms. Amyloid also may be localized in the bronchi or pulmonary parenchyma and may resemble a neoplasm. In these cases, local excision should be attempted and, when successful, may be followed by prolonged remissions.

Hematopoietic system   Hematologic changes may include fibrinogenopenia, increased fibrinolysis, and selective deficiency of clotting factors. Deficient factor X seems to be due to nonspecific calcium-dependent binding to the polyanionic amyloid fibrils. Splenectomy in the patient with such a factor X deficiency can relieve the deficiency and the associated bleeding disorder, since factor X has been shown to bind to the large masses of splenic amyloid.

HEREDOFAMILIAL AMYLOIDOSIS   Until recently, there was no generally accepted nosology for the heredofamilial amyloid syndromes. Some reports emphasized the site of predominant organ involvement as neuropathic, nephropathic, or cardiopathic amyloidosis, while others stressed the genetic aspects. To date, virtually all analyses of pedigrees have shown that, with one major exception, the mode of inheritance is autosomal dominant. The exception is amyloidosis of familial Mediterranean fever (FMF), which is inherited as an autosomal recessive disorder and is an AA type of amyloid. Even in FMF amyloid, however, several kinships with autosomal dominant inheritance have been reported. While the recognizable clinical patterns can be used as the basis for classification, classification according to the specific point mutation is preferable (Table 281-2).

The heredofamilial amyloidoses include a group primarily involving the nervous system. The prototype is the lower limb neuropathy [familial amyloid polyneuropathy (FAP)], first described in Portugal, which has a poor prognosis and is characterized by progressively severe neuropathy, including marked autonomic nervous system involvement. This variety also has been described in Japan, Sweden, and in families of Greek, Swedish, and Italian origin. In some of these individuals, bilateral "scalloped" pupils are pathognomonic of the disease. The second type of neuropathy has been found in families of Swiss origin in Indiana and of German origin in Maryland. It is a milder disease and is often associated with a carpal tunnel syndrome and vitreous opacities. A more severe variety of generalized neuropathy associated with renal amyloidosis has been described in Iowa in a family of English-Irish-Scottish ancestry.

Several types of severe familial renal disease in association with amyloid have been described. Possibly the most remarkable is FMF, a disorder subdivided into phenotype I, with irregularly occurring fever and abdominal, chest, or joint pain, preceding or accompanying renal amyloid, and phenotype II, in which renal amyloidosis is the first or only manifestation of the disease. Colchicine treatment prevents attacks of FMF and appears to prevent subsequent deposition of amyloid as well. Sporadically, other hereditary forms of renal amyloidosis have been described, including the curious association of urticaria, deafness, and renal amyloid.

Severe familial amyloid heart disease has been described in a Danish family and familial persistent atrial standstill with amyloid in a family of Mexican-American origin. Hereditary cerebral amyloid with hemorrhage in an Icelandic family appears to be due to gamma trace protein (cystatin C) deposits and is associated with a decrease of these proteins in the cerebrospinal fluid. A similar disorder (but caused by beta protein) has been reported from the Netherlands. Miscellaneous hereditary amyloid syndromes include hereditary multiple endocrine neoplasms type II (including medullary carcinoma of the thyroid with amyloid) as well as others listed in Table 281-1.

DIAGNOSIS   The specific diagnosis of amyloidosis depends on obtaining a tissue specimen by biopsy and the demonstration of amyloid with appropriate stains. First, of course, the disease must be suspected. When a patient with a chronic disorder predisposing to amyloid such as rheumatoid arthritis, tuberculosis, paraplegia, multiple myeloma, bronchiectasis, or leprosy develops hepatomegaly, splenomegaly, malabsorption, cardiac disease, or, most important, proteinuria, secondary (AA) amyloid should come to mind. In addition, in any heredofamilial syndromes, especially those which have a dominant autosomal mode of inheritance and are characterized by peripheral neuropathy, nephropathy, or cardiopathy, the diagnosis of amyloid should be considered. Finally, primary systemic (AL) amyloid should be considered in any individual with a diffuse noninflammatory infiltrative disease involving either mesenchymal tissues—blood vessels, heart, gastrointestinal tract—or parenchymal tissues—kidney, liver, spleen, adrenal.

When the diagnosis is suspected, it is good practice to perform an abdominal subcutaneous fat pad aspirate or rectal biopsy. If there is a specific reason for not carrying out these procedures, such other sites as skin, gums, or the suspected organ—kidney, liver—may be biopsied. All tissues obtained must be stained with Congo red and examined in the polarizing microscope for green birefringence. A modified potassium permanganate stain will allow reasonably accurate differentiation of the AA type from AL amyloid. In the former, pretreatment with permanganate, followed by the standard Congo red stain, abolishes the green birefringence (i.e., the tissue is permanganate-sensitive). Beta$_2$ microglobulin amyloid is also permanganate-sensitive. The AL and hereditary types are permanganate-resistant.

In order to establish the relationship of immunoglobulin-related amyloid to multiple myeloma, electrophoretic and immunoelectrophoretic studies on serum and urine should be performed when the biopsy reveals amyloid deposition. Most of these patients will have only relatively small paraprotein components, and only a few will have frank multiple myeloma.

PROGNOSIS AND TREATMENT The course of amyloidosis is difficult to document, since dating the time of origin of the disease is rarely possible. When amyloidosis develops in patients with rheumatoid arthritis, it seldom becomes evident when the arthritis is less than 2 years in duration. The mean duration of arthritis before amyloidosis was detected was 16 years in one series. When amyloidosis develops in patients with multiple myeloma, manifestations leading to initial hospitalization are more apt to be related to amyloid disease than to myeloma. In these cases, prognosis is very poor, and life expectancy is usually less than 6 months.

Instances have been reported of amyloidosis accompanying treatable infections, such as osteomyelitis, in which at least partial remission has occurred following treatment of the primary disease. There have been similar experiences following successful treatment of tuberculosis or drainage of chronic empyema. However, many such reports are not substantiated by biopsy proof of resorption.

Generalized amyloidosis is usually a slowly progressive disease that leads to death in several years, but it may have a better prognosis than was suspected in the past. The average survival in most large series is 1 to 4 years, but a number of individuals with amyloid have been followed 5 to 10 years and longer.

The major causes of death are heart disease and renal failure. Sudden death, presumably due to arrhythmias, is common. Occasionally, gastrointestinal hemorrhage, respiratory failure, intractable heart failure, and superimposed infections are the terminal events.

There is no specific therapy for any variety of amyloidosis. Rational therapy should be directed at (1) decreasing chronic antigenic stimuli that produce amyloid, (2) inhibition of the synthesis and extracellular deposition of amyloid fibrils, and (3) promoting lysis or mobilization of existing amyloid deposits.

A variety of agents have been used to treat amyloidosis. Proof of their efficacy is not available. The finding that a portion of the immunoglobulin light chain is incorporated in the amyloid of patients with primary amyloidosis and its presumed synthesis by plasma cells has led to the use of alkylating agents. However, these agents cause bone marrow depression, and there are reports of acute leukemia developing in amyloidosis patients receiving melphalan. Recent trials have indicated that a prednisone/melphalan regimen or a prednisone/melphalan/colchicine program prolongs life. Studies in several centers are underway to compare these programs with each other and with colchicine alone (see below).

Patients with severe renal amyloidosis and azotemia have been treated by dialysis or kidney transplantation with very good outcomes. This has significantly improved the prognosis in patients whose major manifestations are renal. Heart transplantation also has been successful in a small number of carefully selected cases.

Colchicine has been shown to be effective in preventing acute attacks in patients with FMF, and two groups of investigators independently have reported the inhibition of amyloid deposition in the mouse model by colchicine. It is conceivable, therefore, that colchicine is effective in blocking amyloid deposition. One large study has shown it to be effective in prolonging life in primary (AL) amyloidosis using a life-table survivorship analysis. However, the exact mechanism of its action is unknown. The use of dimethylsulfoxide (DMSO) in the treatment of amyloid has had variable results.

REFERENCES

COHEN AS: Amyloidosis. N Engl J Med 277:522, 1967

———, JONES LA: Advances in amyloidosis. Curr Opin Rheumatol 5:62, 1993

———, SKINNER M: Diagnosis of amyloidosis, in *Laboratory Diagnostic Procedures in the Rheumatic Diseases*, 3d ed, AS Cohen (ed). Orlando, Fla, Grune & Stratton, 1985, pp 377–399

GLENNER GG et al: Amyloid fibril proteins: Proof of homology with immunoglobulin light chains by sequence analyses. Science 172:1150, 1971

HUSBY G et al: The 1990 guidelines for nomenclature and classification of amyloid and amyloidosis, in *Amyloid and Amyloidosis*, JB Natvig et al (eds). Dordrecht, Netherlands, Kluwer, 1990, pp 813–816

KYLE RA, GREIPP PR: Amyloidosis (AL): Clinical and laboratory features in 229 cases. Mayo Clin Proc 58:665, 1983

NATVIG JB et al (eds): *Amyloid and Amyloidosis*. Dordrecht, Netherlands, Kluwer, 1990

section 2 Disorders of immune-mediated injury

282 DISEASES OF IMMEDIATE TYPE HYPERSENSITIVITY

K. FRANK AUSTEN

The term *atopic allergy* implies a familial tendency to manifest alone or in combination such conditions as asthma, rhinitis, urticaria, and eczematous dermatitis (atopic dermatitis). However, individuals without an atopic background also may develop hypersensitivity reactions, particularly urticaria and anaphylaxis, associated with the same class of antibody, IgE, found in atopic individuals. The designation *diseases of immediate type hypersensitivity* presents a more suitable framework than the broad term *allergy* or the restrictive definition of atopy.

The fixation of IgE to human basophils has been demonstrated by radioautography and electron microscopy and to intraepithelial and perivenular mast cells in tonsils, adenoids, and nasal polyps of humans by immunofluorescence. IgE-dependent mediator generation and release also occur in the mast cells of human lung slices, nasal polyps, or skin and have been observed in those tissues most involved in diseases of immediate type hypersensitivity.

The high-affinity receptor for IgE, designated $Fc_\epsilon RI$, is composed of one α, one β, and two disulfide-linked γ chains, which together cross the plasma membrane seven times. The α chain is solely responsible for IgE binding, and the γ chains are responsible for signal transduction that results from the aggregation of the tetrameric receptors by polymeric antigen. The stereospecific receptor perturbation activates a polyphosphatidyl inositol–selective phospholipase C to elaborate 1,2-diacylglycerols (1,2-DAG) and inositol-1,4,5-*tris*-phosphate (IP_3), which in turn activate protein kinase C and mobilize intracellular calcium ions, respectively. These events may be augmented by the formation of calcium ion channels and attenuated by the activation of adenylate cyclase with formation of cyclic 3′,5′-adenosine monophosphate (cyclic AMP) and activation of cyclic AMP–dependent protein kinase. The calcium ion–dependent activation of phospholipases cleaves membrane phospholipids to generate lysophospholipids, which, like 1,2-DAG, are fusogenic and may facilitate the fusion of the secretory granule perigranular membrane with the cell membrane, a step that releases the membrane-free granule containing the preformed or primary mediators of mast cell effects. The arachidonic acid cleaved directly from phospholipids by phospholipase A_2 and secondarily from intermediates generated from phospholipase C– and D–activated pathways is processed to bioactive lipid mediators (Fig. 282-1). The lysophospholipid formed from release of arachidonic acid from 1-*O*-alkyl-2-acyl-*sn*-glyceryl-3-phosphorylcholine can be acetylated in the second position to form platelet-activating factor (PAF). The secretory granule of the human mast cell has a crystalline structure, unlike mast cells of lower species, and IgE-dependent cell activation can be characterized morphologically by solubilization and swelling of the granule contents within the first minute of receptor perturbation; this reaction is followed by the ordering of intermediate filaments about the swollen granule, movement toward the cell surface, and fusion of the perigranular membrane with that of other granules and with the plasmalemma to form extracellular channels for mediator release while maintaining cell viability.

Important insight into the diversity of mast cells within a species has been gained from studies of serosal mast cells considered to be connective tissue mast cell (CTMC) and mucosal mast cell (MMC)

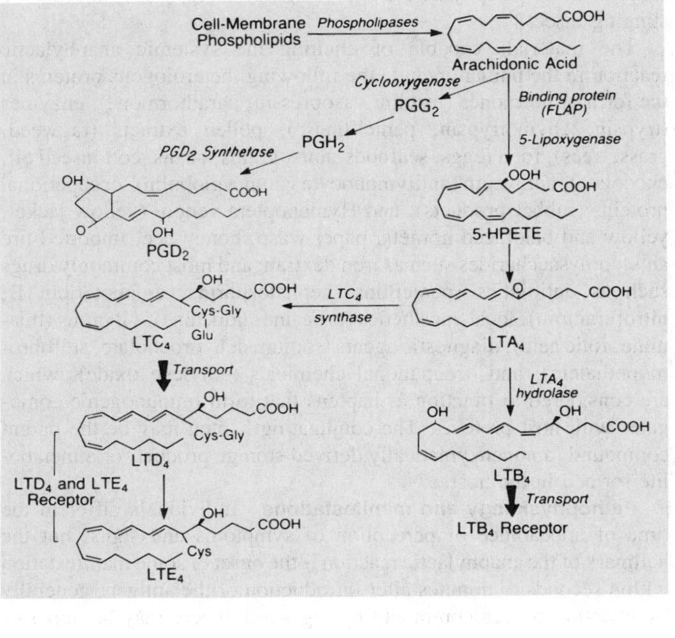

populations from rats infected with *Nippostrongylus brasiliensis*. The CTMC secretory granules stain with alcian blue and counterstain with safranin; contain large amounts of histamine, heparin proteoglycan, chymotryptic protease termed *neutral protease I*, and carboxypeptidase A; generate prostaglandin D_2 upon IgE-Fc–dependent activation; and remain viable ex vivo in coculture with fibroblasts in the absence of added T cell factors. The MMC secretory granules stain with alcian blue but not safranin, synthesize chondroitin sulfate diB and E proteoglycan rather than heparin proteoglycan, contain small amounts of histamine and a distinct chymotryptic protease termed *neutral protease II*, generate leukotriene C_4 in preference to prostaglandin D_2 (PGD_2) during activation-secretion, and are T cell factor–dependent for appearance in vivo or generation from progenitors in vitro. The cloning of the cDNA and corresponding genes for four chymotryptic serine proteases of the mouse mast cell secretory granule has allowed demonstration of early expressed genes in the interleukin 3–dependent bone marrow–derived precursor population and subclass-specific, late expressed genes for CTMC and MMC, respectively.

The evidence for diversity of mast cells within the human is more subtle than in the rat but nonetheless is sufficient to suggest possible functional implications. Mast cells of human lung, intestine, and skin each stain with alcian blue but not safranin and have a similar histamine content. Dispersed partially purified human lung and intestinal mast cells respond to activation by IgE-Fc–dependent mechanisms with generation of LTC_4 and PGD_2, are not activated by various peptide agonists, are enriched for the secretory granule neutral protease tryptase but lack chymase and carboxypeptidase A, and exhibit secretory granules with a scroll and crystalline ultrastructure. In the lung they synthesize heparin proteoglycan in a 2:1 ratio to chondroitin sulfate E proteoglycan, and in the intestine they are T cell–dependent, as revealed by their absence from mucosal sites in patients with T cell deficiencies. The skin mast cells are readily stimulated for exocytosis by diverse peptides such as C5a anaphylatoxin, substance P, and f-Met-Leu-Phe; they elaborate PGD_2 with IgE-Fc receptor–dependent activation; they are much enriched for the secretory granule neutral proteases—tryptase, chymase, and carboxypeptidase A—and for heparin proteoglycan; they exhibit secretory granules with a lattice and crystalline ultrastructure; and they are present in the intestinal submucosa of patients with T cell deficiencies. Although there are, at least, two genes for human secretory granule mast cell tryptases, the homology of their expressed proteins is so great that they are not distinguished by immunohistochemical studies with monoclonal antibodies; hence it is likely that lung and mucosal mast cells contain a tryptase different from that in skin and submucosal mast cells. Whether mast cell diversity is determined entirely by the microenvironment or is dictated in part by different progenitors derived from a common marrow precursor is not established.

Mast cells bearing specific recognition units are distributed at cutaneous and mucosal surfaces and in deeper tissues about venules, are an expansile population during T cell stimulation, and could regulate the entry of foreign substances by their rapid response capability. Upon stimulus-specific activation in vitro, histamine and selected secretory granule–associated acid hydrolases are solubilized, whereas the neutral proteases, which are cationic, remain largely complexed to the anionic proteoglycans. It is speculated that the macromolecular complex serves to deliver the neutral proteases so that the endo- and exoproteases can function in concert at the substrate site to clear damaged tissue and facilitate repair. In addition to these preformed mediators, after activation, mast cells generate lipid mediators from membrane phospholipids and transcribe and translate a range of cytokines (Fig. 282-2). Histamine and the various lipid mediators alter venular permeability, thereby allowing influx of plasma proteins such as complement and immunoglobulins, and the cysteinyl leukotrienes constrict both vascular and nonvascular smooth muscle. Leukotrienes C_4 and D_4 (LTC_4 and LTD_4) are logs more potent than histamine in constricting human airway smooth muscle

FIGURE 282-1 Pathways for biosynthesis and release of membrane-derived lipid mediators from mast cells. In the 5-lipoxygenase pathway leukotriene A_4 (LTA_4) is the intermediate from which the terminal-pathway enzymes generate the distinct final products, leukotriene C_4 (LTC_4) and leukotriene B_4 (LTB_4), which leave the cell by separate saturable transport systems. Gamma glutamyl transpeptidase and a dipeptidase then cleave glutamic acid and glycine from LTC_4 to form LTD_4 and LTE_4, respectively, for which there appears to be a common receptor. The only mast cell product of the cyclooxygenase system is PGD_2.

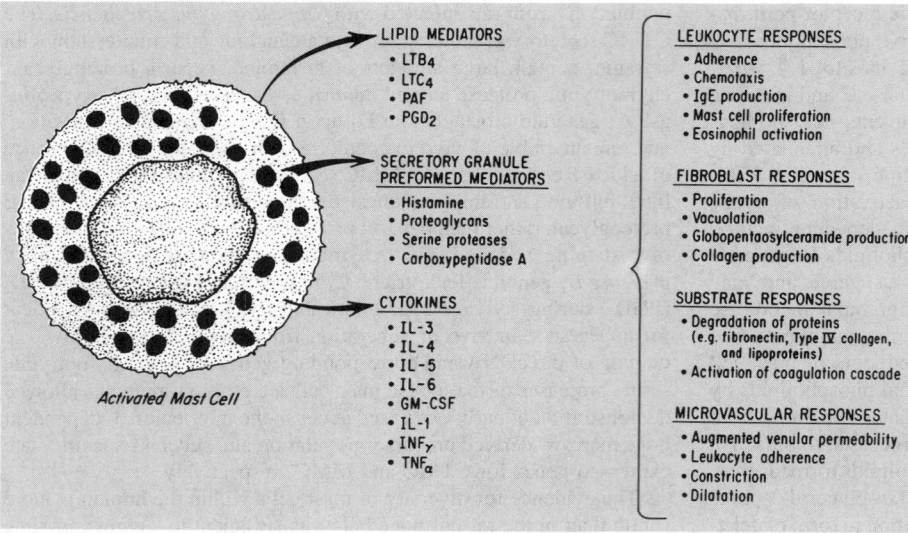

LIPID MEDIATORS
- LTB$_4$
- LTC$_4$
- PAF
- PGD$_2$

SECRETORY GRANULE PREFORMED MEDIATORS
- Histamine
- Proteoglycans
- Serine proteases
- Carboxypeptidase A

CYTOKINES
- IL-3
- IL-4
- IL-5
- IL-6
- GM-CSF
- IL-1
- INF$_\gamma$
- TNF$_\alpha$

Activated Mast Cell

LEUKOCYTE RESPONSES
- Adherence
- Chemotaxis
- IgE production
- Mast cell proliferation
- Eosinophil activation

FIBROBLAST RESPONSES
- Proliferation
- Vacuolation
- Globopentaosylceramide production
- Collagen production

SUBSTRATE RESPONSES
- Degradation of proteins (e.g. fibronectin, Type IV collagen, and lipoproteins)
- Activation of coagulation cascade

MICROVASCULAR RESPONSES
- Augmented venular permeability
- Leukocyte adherence
- Constriction
- Dilatation

FIGURE 282-2 Bioactive mediators of three categories generated by IgE-dependent activation of murine mast cells can elicit common but sequential target cell effects leading to acute and sustained inflammatory responses. *(Modified from Stevens and Austen.)*

when administered by aerosol, and leukotriene E$_4$ (LTE$_4$), the most stable member of the family, is also somewhat more potent than histamine. The 5-lipoxygenation of arachidonic acid to 5S-hydroperoxy-6-*trans*-8,11,14-*cis*-eicosatetraenoic acid (5-HPETE) and then to 5,6-*trans*-oxido-7,9-*trans*-11,14-*cis*-eicosatetraenoic acid (LTA$_4$) is followed by the adduction of glutathione via a microsomal LTC$_4$ synthase to yield 5S-hydroxy-6R-S-glutathionyl-7,9-*trans*-11,14-*cis*-eicosatetraenoic acid (LTC$_4$); upon transport across the membrane to the extracellular environment, LTC$_4$ undergoes sequential cleavage of the glutathione portion to yield the cysteinylglycyl (LTD$_4$) and cysteinyl (LTE$_4$) derivatives. Alternatively, a cytosolic LTA$_4$ epoxide hydrolase converts LTA$_4$ into 5S-12R-dihydroxy-6,14-*cis*-8,10-*trans*-eicosatetraenoic acid (LTB$_4$), which mediates leukocyte margination and directed (chemotactic) migration in human sites. This proinflammatory response would be sustained by a cytokine such as tumor necrosis factor alpha (TNF-α). Interleukin 4 is critical to the B cell switch for IgE biosynthesis, and IL-3 and IL-4 cause the proliferation of immature mast cells from bone marrow progenitors for tissue-directed differentiation. Thus there is the possibility of an autocrine mechanism for IgE/mast cell–mediated disease. There is even evolving evidence that mast cells, via their constituents, can regulate fibroblast proliferation and/or angiogenesis. Local and subclinical regulation of the tissue microenvironment would represent an initial and homeostatic physiologic response, whereas an intense or continuous stimulus would result in inflammation and tissue injury that could be either beneficial or detrimental (hypersensitivity) depending on the appropriateness of the immunologic specificity.

Consideration of the mechanism of immediate type hypersensitivity diseases in the human has focused largely on the IgE-dependent recognition of otherwise nontoxic substances. Support for this thesis has come from the finding that clinical atopic allergy is associated with elevated total levels of IgE and in some instances with an immune response that is specifically linked to the histocompatibility locus. Populations of allergic whites have a significantly higher total serum level of IgE than nonallergic individuals, and highly atopic persons with asthma have significantly higher serum levels of IgE than those with fewer allergic manifestations. IgE distribution in normal families is consistent with the dominant inheritance of the low-IgE phenotype. As a result of the action of a single IgE regulator gene, the majority of family members would have elevated IgE levels as a possible basis for their atopic state. The association between HLA histocompatibility type and the immediate hypersensitivity response has been noted in persons of the low-IgE phenotype who were studied with highly purified allergens, generally of small size. Such presumptive evidence of immune-response (Ir) genes by linkage disequilibrium, i.e., the association of the hypersensitivity response

with a particular histocompatibility haplotype, represents an additional element in the polygenic atopic allergic state. Nonetheless, all the studies taken together, both of families and of populations, seem to indicate that the genetically determined elevated IgE levels found in about three-fourths of atopic allergic subjects exert the predominant influence on most specific IgE responses. It is also likely that diseases of immediate type hypersensitivity may occur because of deficient intracellular controls of mediator generation or release, or both, or that the extracellular controls directed against mediator inactivation may be impaired.

ANAPHYLAXIS **Definition** The life-threatening anaphylactic response of a sensitized human appears within minutes after administration of specific antigen and is manifested by respiratory distress often followed by vascular collapse or by shock without antecedent respiratory difficulty. Cutaneous manifestations exemplified by pruritus and urticaria with or without angioedema are characteristic of such systemic anaphylactic reactions. Gastrointestinal manifestations include nausea, vomiting, crampy abdominal pain, and diarrhea.

Predisposing factors and etiology There is no convincing evidence that age, sex, race, occupation, or geographic location predisposes a human to anaphylaxis except through exposure to some immunogen. According to most studies, atopy does not predispose individuals to anaphylaxis from penicillin therapy or venom of a stinging insect.

The materials capable of eliciting the systemic anaphylactic reaction in the human include the following: heterologous proteins in the form of hormones (insulin, vasopressin, parathormone), enzymes (trypsin, chymotrypsin, penicillinase), pollen extracts (ragweed, grass, trees), food (eggs, seafoods, nuts, grains, beans, cottonseed oil, chocolate), antiserum (antilymphocyte gamma globulin), occupational proteins (rubber products), and Hymenoptera venom (yellow jacket, yellow and baldfaced hornets, paper wasp, honey bee, imported fire ants); polysaccharides such as iron dextran; and most commonly drugs such as antibiotics (penicillins, cephalosporins, amphotericin B, nitrofurantoin), local anesthetics (procaine, lidocaine), vitamins (thiamine, folic acid), diagnostic agents (sodium dehydrocholate, sulfobromophthalein), and occupational chemicals (ethylene oxide), which are considered to function as haptens that form immunogenic conjugates with host proteins. The conjugating hapten may be the parent compound, a nonenzymatically derived storage product, or a metabolite formed in the host.

Pathophysiology and manifestations Individuals differ in the time of appearance of perception of symptoms and signs, but the hallmark of the anaphylactic reaction is the onset of some manifestation within seconds to minutes after introduction of the antigen, generally by injection or less commonly by ingestion. There may be upper or lower airway obstruction or both. Laryngeal edema may be experienced as a "lump" in the throat, hoarseness, or stridor, while bronchial obstruction is associated with a feeling of tightness in the chest or audible wheezing. A particularly characteristic feature is the eruption of well-circumscribed, discrete cutaneous wheals with erythematous, raised, serpiginous borders and blanched centers. These urticarial eruptions are intensely pruritic and may be localized or distributed. They may coalesce to form giant hives, and they seldom persist beyond 48 h. A localized, nonpitting, deeper edematous cutaneous process, angioedema, also may be present. It may be asymptomatic or cause a burning or stinging sensation.

In fatal cases with clinical bronchial obstruction, the lungs show marked hyperinflation on gross and microscopic examination. The microscopic findings in the bronchi, however, are limited to luminal secretions, peribronchial congestion, submucosal edema, and eosinophilic infiltration, and the acute emphysema is attributed to intractable bronchospasm that subsides with death. The angioedema resulting in death by mechanical obstruction occurs in the epiglottis and larynx, but the process is also evident in the hypopharynx and to some extent the trachea; on microscopic examination there is wide separation of the collagen fibers and the glandular elements; vascular congestion and eosinophilic infiltration are also present. Patients dying of vascular collapse without antecedent hypoxia from respiratory insufficiency have visceral congestion with a presumptive loss of intravascular blood volume. The associated electrocardiographic abnormalities, with or without infarction, noted in some patients could reflect a primary cardiac event or be secondary to a critical reduction in plasma volume.

The angioedematous and urticarial manifestations of the anaphylactic syndrome have been attributed to release of endogenous histamine. A role for the cysteinyl leukotrienes in altering pulmonary mechanics by causing marked bronchiolar constriction seems likely. Vascular collapse without respiratory distress in response to experimental challenge with the sting of a hymenopteran was associated not only with marked and prolonged elevations in blood histamine but also with evidence of intravascular coagulation and kinin generation. Based on the findings that patients with systemic mastocytosis and episodic hypotension proceeding to vascular collapse excrete large amounts of PGD_2 in addition to histamine and are controlled by administration of a nonsteroidal agent but not by antihistamines alone, it may be that PGD_2 is also of importance in the hypotensive anaphylactic reactions. Because of the marked coronary arterial constrictor action of the cysteinyl leukotrienes upon administration to experimental animals, these substances may be involved in the disease process of patients with myocardial ischemia without or with infarction.

Diagnosis The diagnosis of an anaphylactic reaction depends largely on an accurate history revealing the onset of the appropriate symptoms and signs within minutes after the responsible material is encountered. When only a portion of the full syndrome is present, such as isolated urticaria, sudden bronchospasm in an asthmatic patient, or vascular collapse after intravenous administration of an agent, it is difficult to exclude a nonimmunologic, toxicologic, or idiosyncratic response. For example, intravenous administration of a chemical mast cell–degranulating agent may elicit generalized urticaria, angioedema, and a sensation of retrosternal oppression with or without clinically detectable bronchoconstriction or hypotension. Furthermore, nonsteroidal anti-inflammatory agents such as indomethacin, aminopyrine, mefenamic acid, and aspirin may precipitate a life-threatening episode of obstruction of upper or lower airways in asthmatic subjects that is clinically reminiscent of anaphylaxis but is not associated with a detectable IgE response. This syndrome may reflect a unique reactivity to an imbalance in the ratio of prostaglandin to leukotriene biosynthesis when cyclooxygenase is inhibited.

The presence of a labile reagin (IgE) in the heart blood of a patient dying of systemic anaphylaxis has been demonstrated at postmortem by passive transfer of the serum intradermally into a normal recipient, followed in 24 h by antigen challenge into the same site, with

subsequent development of a wheal and flare, the Prausnitz-Küstner reaction. Indeed, such a reagin can be transiently identified in the serum of most patients who develop systemic anaphylaxis to a variety of different agents. In order to avoid the hazards of transferring hepatitis to the recipient in the Prausnitz-Küstner reaction, it is preferable to employ the less sensitive monkey recipient or a human leukocyte suspension enriched with basophils for subsequent antigen challenge. It is presumed that the activity responsible for most cases of systemic anaphylaxis resides with the IgE class, since the Prausnitz-Küstner activity in the sera of patients with systemic reactions to Hymenoptera venom or human seminal plasma protein can be removed by IgE immunosorbent columns. Furthermore, radioimmunoassays have demonstrated specific IgE antibodies in patients with anaphylactic reactions to insulin and to parathormone, but such approaches require purified antigens. In the transfusion anaphylactic reaction that occurs in patients with IgA deficiency, the responsible specificity resides in IgG anti-IgA rather than in IgE; the mechanism of the reaction is presumed to be complement activation with secondary mast cell participation.

Treatment and prevention Early recognition of an anaphylactic reaction is mandatory, since death occurs within minutes to hours after the first symptoms. Mild symptoms such as pruritus and urticaria can be controlled by administration of 0.2 to 0.5 mL of 1:1000 epinephrine subcutaneously, with repeated doses as required at 20-min intervals for a severe reaction. If the antigenic material was injected into an extremity, the rate of absorption may be reduced by prompt application of a tourniquet proximal to the reaction site, administration of 0.2 mL of 1:1000 epinephrine into the site, and removal without compression of an insect stinger, if present. An intravenous infusion should be initiated to provide a route for administration of 5.0 mL epinephrine, diluted 1:10,000, at 5- to 10-min intervals, volume expanders, and vasopressor agents such as dopamine if intractable hypotension occurs. Epinephrine provides both alpha- and beta-adrenergic effects, resulting in vasoconstriction, bronchial smooth-muscle relaxation, and attenuation of enhanced venular permeability. Beta blockers are relatively contraindicated in persons at risk for anaphylactic reactions, especially those sensitive to Hymenoptera venom or those undergoing immunotherapy for respiratory system allergy. When epinephrine fails to control the situation, hypoxia due to airway obstruction or related to a cardiac arrhythmia, or both, must be considered. Oxygen via a nasal catheter or intermittent positive-pressure breathing of oxygen with 0.5 mL isoproterenol diluted 1:200 in saline may be helpful, but either endotracheal intubation or a tracheostomy is mandatory for oxygen delivery if progressive hypoxia exists. Ancillary agents such as the antihistamine diphenhydramine, 50 to 80 mg intramuscularly or intravenously, and aminophylline, 0.25 to 0.5 g intravenously, are appropriate for urticaria-angioedema and bronchospasm, respectively. Intravenous corticosteroids are not effective for the acute event but may be considered for persistent bronchospasm and hypotension.

Prevention of anaphylaxis must take into account the sensitivity of the recipient, the dose and character of the diagnostic or therapeutic agent, and the effect of the route of administration on the rate of absorption. If there is a definite history of a past anaphylactic reaction, even though mild, it is advisable to select another agent or procedure. A knowledge of cross-reactivity among agents is critical since, for example, cephalosporins share a common β-lactam ring with the penicillins. A skin test should be performed before the administration of certain materials producing a high incidence of anaphylactic reactions, such as horse serum or allergenic extracts, or when the nature of the past adverse reaction is unknown. Since even a skin or conjunctival test can produce a serious reaction, a scratch test should precede these tests in a high-risk situation. With regard to penicillin, two-thirds of patients with a positive reaction history and positive intradermal skin tests to benzylpenicilloyl-polylysine (BPL) and/or the minor determinant mixture (MDM) of benzylpenicillin products experience allergic reactions with treatment, and these are almost uniformly of the anaphylactic type in those patients with minor determinant reactivity. Even patients without a history of previous clinical reactions have a 6 percent incidence of positive skin tests to the two test materials, and about 3 per 1000 with a negative history experience anaphylaxis with therapy, with a mortality of about 1 per 100,000. The value of skin testing is both to permit therapy with the agent in question when the risk does not exist and to emphasize the hazards where the sensitivity is confirmed. In the event that an agent must be used despite a positive history, a positive skin test, or both, the following precautionary measures should be taken: An intravenous infusion should be started, with intubation equipment and a tracheostomy set at hand; the material should be given intradermally, then subcutaneously, and then intramuscularly in increasing doses at 20- to 30-min intervals so that the initial dose by the next route does not exceed the final dose by the previous route. It is difficult to be certain that the mediator-containing cells have been exhausted, and therapeutic use of the agent may be accompanied by untoward consequences. It may be critical to give the therapeutic agent at regular intervals to prevent the reestablishment of a sensitized cell pool of large size.

A different form of protection involves the development of blocking antibody of the IgG class which is protective against Hymenoptera venom–induced anaphylaxis by interacting with antigen so that less reaches the sensitized tissue mast cells; to be effective, this immunotherapy requires the use of specific or cross-reacting Hymenoptera venom rather than whole-insect-body extracts.

Because sensitization can be transient, the maximal risk for systemic anaphylactic reactions in persons with Hymenoptera sensitivity occurs in association with a currently positive skin test. Although there is only low-grade cross-reactivity between honey bee and yellow jacket venoms, there is a high degree of cross-reactivity between yellow jacket venom and the rest of the vespid venoms (yellow or baldfaced hornets and wasps). Prevention involves modification of outside activities to exclude bare feet, wearing perfumed toiletries, eating in certain areas, clipping hedges or grass, and hauling away trash or fallen fruit. As with each anaphylactic sensitivity, the individual should wear an informational bracelet and have immediate access to an unexpired epinephrine kit located within the home, the vehicle, and/or carried. The limitations of lifestyle and the psychological duress can be addressed by venom immunotherapy to achieve a venom-specific IgG titer above 3.0 μg/mL of serum. Present knowledge favors indefinite continuation of venom therapy with a maintenance schedule or until the skin test becomes negative, with confirmation by immunochemical measurement of specific IgE in serum. For children with a systemic reaction limited to skin, the likelihood of progression to more serious respiratory or vascular manifestations is low, and thus immunotherapy is not recommended.

URTICARIA AND ANGIOEDEMA Definition Urticaria and angioedema may appear separately or together as cutaneous manifestations of localized nonpitting edema; a similar process may occur at mucosal surfaces of the upper respiratory or gastrointestinal tract. *Urticaria* involves only the superficial portion of the dermis, presenting as well-circumscribed wheals with erythematous raised serpiginous borders with blanched centers that may coalesce to become giant wheals. *Angioedema* is a well-demarcated localized edema involving the deeper layers of the skin, including the subcutaneous tissue. Recurrent episodes of urticaria and/or angioedema of less than 6 weeks' duration are considered acute, whereas attacks persisting beyond this period are designated chronic.

Predisposing factors and etiology The occurrence of urticaria and angioedema is probably more frequent than usually described because of the evanescent, self-limited nature of such eruptions, which seldom require medical attention when limited to the skin. Although persons in any age group may experience acute or chronic urticaria and/or angioedema, these lesions increase in frequency after adolescence, with the highest incidence occurring in persons in the third decade of life; indeed, one survey of college students indicated that some 15 to 20 percent had experienced a pruritic wheal reaction.

The classification of urticaria-angioedema presented in Table 282-1 focuses on the different mechanisms for eliciting clinical disease.

TABLE 282-1 Classification of urticaria with angioedema

IgE-dependent
  A Atopic diathesis
  B Specific antigen sensitivity (pollens, foods, drugs, fungi, molds, Hymenoptera venom, helminths)
  C Physical: dermographism, cold, light, cholinergic, vibratory, exercise-related

Complement-mediated
  A Hereditary angioedema: type 1, type 2
  B Acquired angioedema: type 1, type 2
  C Necrotizing vasculitis
  D Serum sickness
  E Reactions to blood products

Nonimmunologic
  A Direct mast cell–releasing agents: opiates, antibiotics, curare, D-tubocurarine, radiocontrast media
  B Agents which presumably alter arachidonic acid metabolism: aspirin and nonsteroidal anti-inflammatory agents, azo dyes, and benzoates

Idiopathic

Only the IgE-dependent and the IgG-mediated reactions in IgA-deficient persons should be considered immediate hypersensitivity. However, the other mechanisms are important for differential diagnosis, and most cases of chronic urticaria are idiopathic. The appearance of urticaria and angioedema in atopic persons in the absence of a specific exposure is attributed to the atopic diathesis and implies an IgE mechanism. Urticaria and/or angioedema occurring during the appropriate season in patients with seasonal respiratory allergy or as a result of exposure to animals or molds is attributed to inhalation of pollens, animal dander, and mold spores, respectively. However, urticaria and angioedema secondary to inhalation are relatively uncommon compared with ingestion of fresh fruits, shellfish, chocolate, nuts, tomatoes, and various drugs, including penicillin-contaminated milk products, that may elicit not only the anaphylactic syndrome with prominent gastrointestinal complaints but also chronic urticaria.

Additional etiologies include physical stimuli such as cold, solar rays, exercise, and mechanical irritation. The physical urticarias can be distinguished by the precipitating event and other aspects of the clinical presentation. *Dermographism*, which occurs in 1 to 4 percent of the population, is defined by the appearance of a linear wheal at the site of a brisk stroke with a firm object or by any configuration appropriate to the eliciting event. Dermographism has a prevalence that peaks in the second to third decades. It is not influenced by an atopic diathesis and has a duration generally of less than 5 years. *Pressure urticaria*, which often accompanies dermographism or chronic idiopathic urticaria, presents in response to a sustained stimulus such as a shoulder strap or belt, running (feet), or manual labor (hands). *Cholinergic urticaria* is distinctive in that the pruritic wheals are of small size (1–2 mm) and are surrounded by a large area of erythema; attacks are precipitated by fever, a hot bath or shower, or exercise and are presumptively attributed to a rise in core body temperature. *Exercise-related anaphylaxis* begins with erythema and pruritic urticaria but progresses to angioedema of the face, oropharynx, larynx, or intestine or to vascular collapse; it is distinguished from cholinergic urticaria by presenting with wheals of conventional size and by not occurring with fever or a hot bath. *Cold urticaria*, either acquired or hereditary, is local at the exposed site (ice cube) or exposed body areas (ambient temperature) but can progress to vascular collapse with immersion in cold water (swimming). *Solar urticaria* is subdivided into three groups by the response to specific portions of the light spectrum. *Vibratory angioedema* may occur after years of occupational exposure or can be idiopathic; it may be accompanied by cholinergic urticaria. Other rare forms of physical allergy, always defined by stimulus-specific elicitation, include *local heat urticaria*, *aquagenic urticaria* from contact with water of any temperature, and *contact urticaria* from direct interaction with some chemical substance.

Angioedema without urticaria occurs with C$\overline{1}$ inhibitor (C$\overline{1}$INH) deficiency that can be inborn as an autosomal dominant characteristic or can be acquired. The urticaria and angioedema associated with classical serum sickness or with idiopathic cutaneous necrotizing angiitis are believed to be an immune-complex disease when hypocomplementemia is a concomitant. The idiosyncratic drug reactions to mast cell granule–releasing agents and to nonsteroidal antiinflammatory drugs can be systemic, resembling anaphylaxis, or limited to cutaneous sites.

Pathophysiology and manifestations Urticarial eruptions are distinctly pruritic, involve any area of the body from the scalp to the soles of the feet, and appear in crops of 24- to 72-h duration, with old lesions fading as new ones appear. The most common sites are the extremities, external genitalia, and face, particularly the region of the eyes and lips. Although self-limited in duration, angioedema of the upper respiratory tract may be life-threatening due to laryngeal obstruction, while gastrointestinal involvement may present with abdominal colic, with or without nausea and vomiting, and may precipitate unnecessary surgical intervention. No residual discoloration occurs with either urticaria or angioedema unless there is an underlying process leading to superimposed extravasation of erythrocytes.

The pathology of urticaria and angioedema is usually characterized by massive edema of the dermis in urticaria and of the subcutaneous tissue as well as the dermis in angioedema. Collagen bundles in affected areas are widely separated, and the venules are sometimes dilated. The perivenular infiltrate may consist of lymphocytes, eosinophils, and neutrophils that are present in varying combination and number throughout the dermis. Allergen-induced wheal-and-flare reactions are characterized by mast cell degranulation and an accumulation of eosinophils over hours to days. The elicitation of a wheal-and-flare response upon injection of the relevant allergen into a patient with urticaria and/or angioedema or into a site in a normal recipient prepared with serum from the patient, the Prausnitz-Küstner reaction, indicates an IgE-dependent mast cell–mediated reaction.

Perhaps the best-studied example of mast cell–mediated urticaria and angioedema is *cold urticaria*. Cryoglobulins, cryofibrinogens, cold agglutinins, or hemolysins may be recognized, but not in the majority of patients. The finding in a number of patients of a serum factor, characterized as being of the IgE class, that is capable of transferring the cold urticaria reaction to a skin site of a normal recipient has focused attention on the mast cell in this condition. Immersion of an extremity in an ice bath precipitates angioedema of the distal portion with urticaria at the air interface within minutes of the challenge. Histologic studies reveal marked mast cell degranulation with associated edema of the dermis and subcutaneous tissues. The venous effluent of the cold-challenged and angioedematous extremity reveals a marked rise in plasma content of histamine, low-molecular-weight eosinophilotactic activity, and high-molecular-weight neutrophil chemotactic activity, which are presumably of mast cell origin, whereas the venous effluent of the contralateral normal extremity contains none of these mediators. Elevated levels of histamine have been found in the plasma content of venous effluent and in the fluid of suction blisters at experimentally induced lesional sites in patients with dermographism, pressure urticaria, vibratory angioedema, light urticaria, and heat urticaria. By ultrastructal analysis, the pattern of mast cell degranulation in cold urticaria resembles an IgE-mediated response with solubilization of granule contents, fusion of the perigranular and cell membranes, and discharge of granule contents, whereas in a dermographic lesion there is an additional superimposed zonal (piecemeal) degranulation. Elevations of plasma histamine with biopsy-proven mast cell degranulation also have been demonstrated with systemic attacks of *cholinergic urticaria* and *exercise-induced erythema-angioedema* precipitated experimentally by exercise on a treadmill while wearing a wet suit; however, only in cholinergic urticaria is there a concomitant decrease in pulmonary function.

Diagnosis The rapid onset and self-limited nature of urticarial and angioedematous eruptions are distinguishing features. Additional characteristics are the occurrence of the urticarial crops in various stages of evolution and the asymmetric distribution of the angioedema. Urticaria and/or angioedema involving IgE-dependent mechanisms are often appreciated by historical considerations implicating specific allergens or physical stimuli, by seasonal incidence, and by exposure to certain environments. Direct reproduction of the lesion with physical stimuli is particularly valuable because it so often establishes the cause of the lesion. The diagnosis of an environmental allergen can be sought by careful skin testing with the putative substance to determine if a local wheal and flare results. Passive transfer by the injection of serum from an affected individual of such a reaction into a skin site of a normal recipient followed by allergen challenge, the Prausnitz-Küstner phenomenon, is not appropriate because of the risks associated with any injection of donor serum. Passive transfer to the skin of a nonhuman primate or in vitro to human basophils may be attempted. IgE-mediated urticaria and/or angioedema may or may not be associated with an elevation of total IgE or with peripheral eosinophilia. Fever, leukocytosis, or an elevated sedimentation rate are characteristically absent.

The classification of urticarial and angioedematous states noted in Table 282-1 in terms of possible mechanisms necessarily includes some differential diagnostic points. Hypocomplementemia is not observed in IgE-mediated mast cell disease and can reflect either an acquired abnormality generally attributed to the formation of immune complexes or a genetic deficiency of C$\overline{1}$INH. Chronic recurrent urticaria, generally in females, associated with arthralgias, an elevated sedimentation rate, and normo- or hypocomplementemia suggests an underlying cutaneous necrotizing angiitis. Confirmation depends on a biopsy that reveals cellular infiltration, nuclear debris, and fibrinoid necrosis of the venules. The same pathobiologic process accounts for the urticaria in association with such diseases as systemic lupus erythematosus, Sjögren's syndrome, or viral hepatitis with or without an associated arteritis. Serum sickness per se or a similar clinical entity due to drugs includes not only urticaria but also pyrexia, lymphadenopathy, myalgia, and arthralgia or arthritis. Urticarial reactions to blood products or IgG treatment are defined by the event and generally are not progressive unless the recipient is IgA deficient in the former case or the reagent is aggregated in the latter.

Hereditary angioedema is an autosomal dominant state associated with the absence of functional C$\overline{1}$INH. The diagnosis is suggested not only by family history but also by the lack of urticarial lesions, the prominence of recurrent gastrointestinal attacks of colic, and episodes of laryngeal edema. Laboratory diagnosis depends on demonstrating the antigenic lack of C$\overline{1}$INH (type 1) in most kindreds, but some kindreds have an antigenically intact nonfunctional protein (type 2) and require a functional assay to establish the diagnosis. The natural substrates of uninhibited C$\overline{1}$, C4, and C2 are chronically depleted but fall further during attacks due to the activation of additional C1 to C$\overline{1}$. Because the C$\overline{1}$INH protein also regulates the Hageman factor–initiated activation of kallikrein and of plasmin, the vasoactive peptides responsible for the angioedema are likely some combination of bradykinin and a plasmin-derived fragment of C$\overline{1}$-cleaved C2. An acquired form of C$\overline{1}$INH deficiency, associated with lymphoproliferative disorders, has the same clinical manifestations and differs in the lack of a familial element; in the reduction of C1/C$\overline{1}$ as well as C$\overline{1}$INH, C4, and C2; and in the presence of an antiidiotypic antibody to the monoclonal immunoglobulin expressed on the B cells (type 1). In a second acquired form of C$\overline{1}$INH deficiency with angioedema due to appearance of IgG anti-C$\overline{1}$INH (type 2) B cell malignancy has not been prominent.

Urticaria and angioedema must be differentiated from contact sensitivity, an acute vesicular eruption that progresses to chronic thickening of the skin with continued allergenic exposure. They must also be differentiated from atopic dermatitis, a condition that may present as erythema, edema, papules, vesiculation, and oozing proceeding to a subacute and chronic stage in which vesiculation is less marked or absent and scaling, fissuring, and lichenification predominate in a distribution that characteristically involves the flexor surfaces. In cutaneous mastocytosis, the reddish brown macules and papules, characteristic of urticaria pigmentosa, urticate with pruritus upon trauma; and in systemic mastocytosis, without or with urticaria pigmentosa, there is an episodic systemic flushing with or without urticaria but no angioedema.

Prevention and treatment Identification of the etiologic factor(s) and their elimination provide the most satisfactory therapeutic program; this approach is feasible to varying degrees with IgE-mediated reactions to allergens or physical stimuli. Topically applied steroids are of no benefit in the management of urticaria and/or angioedema; and while systemic steroids have no general value, they are helpful in an occasional patient with necrotizing cutaneous angiitis, pressure urticaria, or even ordinary urticaria and angioedema. Antihistamines of the H1 class and sympathomimetic agents often provide symptomatic relief; cyproheptadine, hydroxyzine, and a combination of H1 and H2 antihistamines are held to be even more beneficial. The therapy of inborn C$\overline{1}$INH deficiency has been simplified by the finding that attenuated androgens correct the biochemical defect and afford prophylactic protection. Since the affected individuals are heterozygous, with the depletion of C$\overline{1}$INH being due to a combination of deficient synthesis and excessive utilization of the normal gene product, the efficacy of the attenuated androgens is attributed to production by the normal gene of an amount of functional C$\overline{1}$INH sufficient to control the spontaneous activation of C1 to C$\overline{1}$. Since the use of such agents for children and pregnant women is not yet accepted, the antifibrinolytic agent ε-aminocaproic acid may be used occasionally to control spontaneous attacks or for preoperative prophylaxis in some patients.

SYSTEMIC MASTOCYTOSIS **Definition** *Systemic mastocytosis* is defined by mast cell hyperplasia that in most instances is indolent and nonneoplastic. Since human mast cells originate from pluripotent bone marrow cells (CD34 +) and disseminate as unrecognized progenitors for tissue-specific proliferation and maturation, the hyperplasia is generally recognized in bone marrow and such peripheral sites as skin, gastrointestinal mucosa, liver, and spleen. Mastocytosis occurs at any age and has a slight preponderance in males. The prevalence of systemic mastocytosis is not known, and a familial occurrence has not been established.

Classification, pathophysiology, and clinical manifestations A recent consensus classification for systemic mastocytosis recognizes four forms (Table 282-2). The form designated as *indolent* accounts for the majority of patients and is not known to alter life expectancy. When a patient is classified as having indolent systemic mastocytosis, the concomitant clinical findings must be carefully noted, since they define the complications and directions for management. In systemic mastocytosis *associated with hematologic disorders*, the prognosis is determined by the nature of that disorder, which can range from dysmyelopoiesis to frank leukemia. In *aggressive* systemic mastocytosis, mast cell proliferation in parenchymal organs such as liver, spleen, and lymph nodes is marked and in a subset of patients is associated with prominent eosinophilia; the prognosis is limited. *Mast cell leukemia* is the rarest form of the disease and is invariably fatal at present.

With the recognition from studies with mouse bone marrow–derived mast cells that some nine recombinant cytokines can regulate

proliferation and/or cellular phenotype, systemic mastocytosis of the human is viewed as a disorder of regulation in which the clinical manifestations are largely due to the chemical mediators provided by mast cells, with some contribution from the space occupancy of the mast cell load itself. The pharmacologically induced manifestations are pruritus, flushing, palpitations and vascular collapse, gastric distress, lower abdominal crampy pain, and recurrent headache. The increase in cell burden is evidenced by the small, reddish brown macules or papules, termed *urticaria pigmentosa*, at skin sites but also contributes to bone pain and malabsorption. The mast cell–mediated fibrotic changes are limited to liver, spleen, and bone marrow and presumably relate to the functional characteristics of mast cells developing at those sites, as opposed to those prominent at sites without fibrosis, such as the gastrointestinal tissue or skin. Immunofluorescent analysis of bone marrow and skin lesions in mastocytosis reveals only one mast cell phenotype with the epitopes of tryptase, chymase, and carboxypeptidase A.

The cutaneous lesions of urticaria pigmentosa respond to trauma with urtication and erythema (Darier's sign). Because of the difficulty in diagnosing systemic mastocytosis in the absence of skin lesions to biopsy, the apparent incidence of these lesions of 90 percent or greater in patients with indolent systemic mastocytosis may be an overestimation. Approximately 1 percent of patients with indolent mastocytosis have skin lesions that appear as tan-brown macules with striking patchy erythema and associated telangiectasia (telangiectasia macularis eruptiva perstans). In the gastrointestinal tract, histamine-mediated hypersecretion is the most common problem, with resultant gastritis and peptic ulcer. The diarrhea and abdominal pain attributed to disease of the small intestine can be aggravated by malabsorption with nutritional insufficiency and osteomalacia. The periportal fibrosis associated with mast cell infiltration and a prominence of eosinophils can, on occasion, lead to portal hypertension and ascites. In some patients, flushing and recurrent vascular collapse are markedly aggravated by an idiosyncratic response to minimal dosage of nonsteroidal anti-inflammatory agents. The neuropsychiatric disturbances are clinically most evident as impaired recent memory and "migraine-like" headaches. Patients in every category of systemic mastocytosis can experience exacerbation of a specific clinical sign or symptom with alcohol ingestion, use of mast cell–interactive narcotics, and ingestion of nonsteroidal anti-inflammatory agents, to which the response is idiosyncratic.

Diagnosis Although the diagnosis is generally suspected on the basis of the clinical history and physical findings, the contention can be strengthened by certain laboratory procedures and established only by a tissue diagnosis. A 24-h urine collection for measurement of histamine, histamine metabolites, or metabolites of PGD_2 is currently the most common noninvasive approach. A convenient alternative, but with a lesser incidence of positivity, is to measure blood levels of histamine or the mast cell–derived neutral protease tryptase. Additional studies directed by the presentation include a bone scan or skeletal survey; contrast studies of the upper gastrointestinal tract with small bowel follow-through, CT scan, or endoscopy; and a neuropsychiatric evaluation, including an EEC. The tissue diagnosis is straightforward if there are lesions of urticaria pigmentosa, but the diagnosis of systemic mastocytosis requires involvement of other organs and is most frequently established by bone marrow biopsy and aspiration. The bone marrow lesions consist of focal and paratrabecular aggregates of mast cells, often mixed with eosinophils, lymphocytes, and, on occasion, plasma cells, histiocytes, and fibroblasts.

The differential diagnosis requires the exclusion of other flushing disorders. The 24-h urine assessment of 5-hydroxy-indoleacetic acid and metanephrines should exclude a carcinoid tumor or a pheochromocytoma. Most patients with recurrent anaphylaxis, including the idiopathic group, present with angioedema, which is not a manifestation of systemic mastocytosis.

Treatment The management of systemic mastocytosis uses a stepwise and symptom-sign–directed approach that includes an H1 antihistamine for flushing and pruritus, an H2 antihistamine or proton

---

TABLE 282-2 Classification of systemic mastocytosis

Type	Description
I	*Indolent* with cutaneous manifestations, vascular collapse, ulcer disease, malabsorption, skeletal disease, hepatosplenomegaly, or lymphadenopathy
II	*Concomitant hematologic disorder*, either myelodysplastic or myeloproliferative
III	*Aggressive* per se or lymphadenopathic mastocytosis with eosinophilia
IV	*Mastocytic leukemia*

pump inhibitor for gastric acid hypersecretion, oral cromolyn sodium for diarrhea and abdominal pain, and a nonsteroidal anti-inflammatory agent for severe flushing associated with vascular collapse despite use of H1 and H2 antihistamines to block biosynthesis of PGD$_2$. Although systemic glucocorticoids appear to alleviate the malabsorption, their use is complicated by disease of the upper gastrointestinal tract or bone. Chemotherapy is not appropriate for patients with indolent mastocytosis and apparently does not prolong survival in patients with mast cell leukemia. It is appropriate for associated hematologic disorders of other cell types and for the aggressive form of systemic mastocytosis.

ALLERGIC RHINITIS Definition Allergic rhinitis is characterized by sneezing; rhinorrhea; obstruction of the nasal passages; conjunctival, nasal, and pharyngeal itching; and lacrimation, all occurring in a temporal relationship to allergen exposure. Although commonly seasonal due to elicitation by airborne pollens, it can be perennial in an environment of chronic exposure. The incidence of allergic rhinitis in North America is about 7 percent, with the peak occurring in childhood and adolescence.

Predisposing factors and etiology Allergic rhinitis generally presents in atopic individuals, i.e., in persons with a family history of a similar or related symptom complex and a personal history of collateral allergy expressed as eczematous dermatitis, urticaria, and/or asthma (see Chap. 217). Symptoms generally appear before the fourth decade of life and tend to diminish gradually with aging, although complete spontaneous remissions are uncommon. A relatively small number of weeds that depend on wind rather than insects for cross-pollination, as well as certain grasses and trees, produce sufficient quantities of pollen suitable for wide distribution by air currents to elicit seasonal allergic rhinitis. The dates of pollination of these species generally vary little from year to year in a particular locale but may be quite different in another climate. Molds, which are widespread in nature because they occur in soil or decaying organic matter, may propagate spores in a pattern dependent on climatic conditions. Perennial allergic rhinitis occurs in response to allergens that are present throughout the year such as in desquamating epithelium in animal dander, the processed materials or chemicals utilized in an industrial setting, or the dust accumulating at work or at home. Dust has a diverse content including mites, and many patients with perennial rhinitis are sensitive only to house dust. Moreover, in many patients with perennial rhinitis, no clear-cut allergen can be demonstrated. The ability of allergens to cause rhinitis rather than lower respiratory symptoms may be attributed to their size, 10 to 100 μm, and retention within the nose. However, even when the allergen penetrates to the lower respiratory tract, whether it elicits a bronchoconstrictor response resulting from mediator release depends on the presence of chronically hyperirritable airways.

Pathophysiology and manifestations Episodic rhinorrhea, sneezing, and obstruction of the nasal passages with lacrimation and pruritus of the conjunctiva, nasal mucosa, and oropharynx are the hallmarks of allergic rhinitis. The nasal mucosa is pale and boggy, but the nares are not reddened or excoriated. The conjunctiva may be congested and edematous; the pharynx is generally unremarkable but may appear injected. Swelling of the turbinates and mucous membranes with obstruction of the sinus ostia and eustachian tubes precipitates secondary infections of the sinuses and middle ear, respectively, commonly in perennial but rarely in seasonal disease. Nasal polyps often arise concurrently with edema and/or infection within the sinuses and increase obstructive symptoms.

The nose presents a large mucosal surface area through the folds of the turbinates and serves to adjust the temperature and moisture content of inhaled air and to filter out particulate materials. The convoluted nasal passages readily filter out particles above 10 μm in size by impingement in a mucous blanket at bends in their course; ciliary action then moves the entrapped particles toward the pharynx. Entrapment of pollen and digestion of the outer coat by mucosal enzymes such as lysozymes release protein allergens generally of 10,000 to 40,000 molecular weight. Although the initial interaction

occurs between the allergen and intraepithelial mast cells sensitized with specific IgE, the bulk of the mast cells are located beneath the mucosal surface and are recruited secondarily. During the symptomatic season when the mucosa are already swollen and hyperemic, there is enhanced adverse reactivity to the seasonal pollen as well as to antigenically unrelated pollens for which there is underlying hypersensitivity. This priming effect is attributed to improved penetration of the allergens to the deeper perivenular mast cells. Biopsy specimens of nasal mucosa during an episodic allergic reaction show profound submucosal edema with infiltration predominantly by eosinophils, although some neutrophil polymorphonuclear leukocytes are present. Polyps, a feature in perennial rhinitis, are mucosal protrusions containing chiefly edema fluid with variable degrees of eosinophilic infiltration.

The mucosal surface fluid contains not only IgA that is present preferentially because of its secretory piece but also IgE, which apparently arrives by diffusion from plasma cells distributed in proximity to mucosal surfaces. IgE fixes to mucosal and submucosal mast cells, and the intensity of the clinical response to inhaled allergens is quantitatively related to the naturally occurring or experimentally defined pollen dose. Specific IgE is distributed not only to tissue mast cells but also to circulating basophilic leukocytes; patients with more severe clinical disease have basophils that release histamine in response to lesser concentrations of allergen in vitro than do cells from patients with milder disease. Human nasal polyps from ragweed-sensitive patients release histamine, eosinophilotactic peptides, and spasmogenic leukotrienes upon challenge with ragweed allergen in vitro. In sensitive individuals, the introduction of allergen into the nose is associated with sneezing, "stuffiness," and discharge, and the fluid contains histamine, PGD$_2$, and leukotrienes. Thus the mast cells of nasal polyp tissue, and of the nasal mucosa and submucosa, generate and release mediators through IgE-dependent reactions which are capable of producing tissue edema and eosinophilic infiltration.

Diagnosis The diagnosis of seasonal allergic rhinitis depends largely on an accurate history of occurrence coincident with the pollination of the offending weeds, grasses, or trees. The continuous character of perennial allergic rhinitis due to contamination of the home or place of work makes historical analysis difficult, but there may be a variability in symptoms that can be related to animal exposure or work habits. Patients with perennial rhinitis commonly develop the problem in adult life, are more often women than men, and manifest nasal polyps and thickening of the sinus membranes by x-ray. The term *vasomotor rhinitis* designates a symptom complex resembling perennial allergic rhinitis without an established allergic basis. Other entities to be excluded are exposure to irritants, upper respiratory infection, pregnancy with prominent nasal mucosal edema, prolonged topical use of alpha-adrenergic agents in the form of nose drops, and the use of certain therapeutic agents such as rauwolfia. Nasal polyps are a characteristic of perennial allergic rhinitis and are often associated with sinus infection.

The nasal secretions of allergic patients are rich in eosinophils, and peripheral eosinophilia with elevations in relation to clinical exacerbations is a common feature. Local or systemic neutrophilia implies infection. Total serum IgE is frequently elevated, but the demonstration of immunologic specificity for IgE is critical to an etiologic diagnosis. Some normal individuals will exhibit a wheal-and-flare skin response to intracutaneous inoculation of high concentrations of common airborne allergens. The diagnosis rests not only on the skin test alone but also on the correlation of the clinical history with skin reactivity to concentrations of allergen selected by controlled testing. This provides the best balance of selectivity with specificity. Scratch tests with food allergens are unreliable, while intracutaneous testing may be dangerous, and elimination diets are the best approach to the diagnosis. Regardless of method of testing, food allergy is uncommon as a significant cause of allergic rhinitis.

Although standard radioimmunodiffusion techniques can be used to screen for patients with markedly elevated levels of IgE, their sensitivity of less than 1000 ng/mL is insufficient to detect the elevations in most atopic allergic patients. A commonly employed technique, sensitive to about 50 ng/mL, is known as the *competitive radioimmunosorbent test* (RIST). In this procedure, the IgE of the serum competes with radiolabeled IgE for solid-phase–bound anti-IgE; the displacement of radiolabeled IgE is compared with a standard curve to yield the IgE concentration of the serum. Other assays, such as the noncompetitive RIST, in which the anti-IgE immunosorbent is exposed to a series of standard IgE preparations before introducing the unknown, and double-antibody radioimmunoprecipitin test (RIP), have greater sensitivity and reproducibility, respectively, and, like the competitive RIST, establish a normal geometric mean serum IgE for nonallergic whites of less than 120 ng/mL. Even more useful is the measurement of specific anti-IgE in serum by its binding to a solid-phase allergen and quantitation by the subsequent uptake of radiolabeled anti-IgE. This radioallergosorbent technique (RAST) correlates satisfactorily with the bioassay of specific IgE by skin test or histamine release from peripheral blood leukocytes and is convenient for the patients; however, it requires defined allergens and full standardization. Further, neither the immunochemical nor bioassay detection of a previous immune response to a foreign material mandates a therapeutic intervention, unless there is relevant concomitant evidence of a significant clinical problem.

Prevention and treatment   Avoidance of exposure to the offending allergen is the most effective means of controlling allergic diseases; removal of pets from the home to avoid animal danders, utilization of air filtration devices to minimize the concentrations of airborne pollens, travel to nonpollinating areas during the critical periods, and even a change of domicile to eliminate a mold spore problem may be necessary.

Management with pharmacologic agents represents the standard approach to seasonal or perennial allergic rhinitis. Antihistamines of the H1 class are effective for nasopharyngeal itching, sneezing, and watery rhinorrhea and for such ocular manifestations as itching, tearing, and erythema, but they are not efficacious for the nasal congestion. The older antihistamines are sedating, and their anticholinergic (muscarinic) effects include visual disturbance, urinary retention, and even arrhythmias. Because the newer H1 antihistaminics such as terfenadine or astemizole are less lipophilic, their ability to cross the blood-brain barrier is reduced, and therefore, their sedating and anticholinergic side effects are minimized. Alpha-adrenergic agents are generally used topically to alleviate nasal congestion and obstruction, but the duration of efficacy is limited because of rebound rhinitis and such systemic responses as insomnia, irritability, and hypertension. The latter are more frequent with use of oral alpha-adrenergic agonists. Cromolyn sodium, a liquid nasal metered-dose spray, is essentially without side effects and is the only intervention of a prophylactic nature; thus it is used to attenuate episodic allergen activation of nasal mast cells. Intranasal high-potency glucocorticoids such as beclamethasone or flunisolide are the most potent drugs available for the relief of established rhinitis, seasonal or perennial, and even vasomotor rhinitis; they provide efficacy with substantially reduced side effects as compared with this same class of agent administered orally. Their most frequent side effect is local irritation, with *Candida* overgrowth being a rare occurrence. Thus, for patients who do not benefit adequately from a full dosage of nonsedating H1 antihistamine and a maintenance dosage of cromolyn sodium, an alpha-adrenergic agent for short-term relief should be replaced by high-potency topical glucocorticoids.

Immunotherapy, often termed *hyposensitization*, consists of repeated subcutaneous injections of gradually increasing concentrations of the allergen(s) considered to be specifically responsible for the symptom complex. Controlled studies in ragweed and grass allergic rhinitis have established that patients are partially relieved of their symptoms by such treatments applied over a period of years. Improvement appears to be dose-related, and the end point is based either on severe adverse local or systemic reactions to the allergen injection or on satisfactory relief of symptoms. The immunologic

characteristics of a response include a rise in antibodies of the IgG class, a small increase in specific IgE early in the treatment course followed by a plateau or decline, and a decline in the percentage of histamine released from peripheral blood basophilic leukocytes challenged with a fixed concentration of the allergen. The antibodies of the IgG class might well reduce or neutralize the quantity of allergen available for interaction with the tissue mast cells but, more important, could modify the seasonal booster response in specific IgE synthesis. None of the individual parameters of the response to immunotherapy correlates well with the assessments of clinical efficacy, suggesting that benefit is derived from a complex of effects. Immunotherapy should be reserved for clearly documented seasonal diseases that cannot be managed with drugs because of their side effects.

REFERENCES

Austen KF: The anaphylactic syndrome, in *Immunological Diseases*, 4th ed, M Samter et al (eds). Boston, Little, Brown, 1988

Craig SS et al: Ultrastructural analysis of human T and TC mast cells identified by immunoelectron microscopy. Lab Invest 58:682, 1988

Gordon JR et al: Mast cells as a source of multifunctional cytokines. Immunol Today 11:458, 1990

Lewis RA et al: Leukotrienes and other products of the 5-lipoxygenase pathway: Biochemistry and relation to pathobiology in human diseases. N Engl J Med 323:645, 1990

Metcalfe DD (ed): Clinical advances in mastocytosis: An interdisciplinary roundtable discussion. J Invest Dermatol 96:1S, 1991

Naclerio RM: Allergic rhinitis. N Engl J Med 325:860, 1991

Ravetch JV, Kinet J-P: Fc receptors. Annu Rev Immunol 9:457, 1991

Soter NA: Urticaria and angioedema, in *Dermatology In General Medicine*, 4th ed, TB Fitzpatrick et al (eds). New York, McGraw-Hill, 1993

Stevens RL, Austen KF: Recent advances in the cellular and molecular biology of mast cells. Immunol Today 10:381, 1989

Valentine MD, Golden DBK: Insect venom allergy, in *Immunological Diseases*, 4th ed, M Samter et al (eds). Boston, Little, Brown, 1988

283   IMMUNE-COMPLEX DISEASES

MICHAEL M. FRANK / THOMAS J. LAWLEY

DEFINITION   The term *immune-complex disease* refers to a group of diseases thought to be mediated by the deposition of immune complexes in specific organ or tissue sites including the glomerulus of the kidney and blood vessel walls. In general, these immune deposits are thought to arise from antigen-antibody complexes formed in the circulation. In some cases the antigens appear to be self- or autoantigens. In many cases these antigens are components of or are stimulated by infectious agents. Once deposited in tissues, the complexes activate a variety of potent soluble mediators of inflammation, such as the complement proteins, causing an influx of polymorphonuclear neutrophils and monocytes. They activate a variety of cells with surface membrane receptors for immunoglobulins, often directly inducing the release of cytokines. These activated cells release toxic products of oxygen and arginine metabolism as well as various proteases and other enzymes, ultimately causing tissue damage. While the specific etiology of these diseases is variable, they share a common pathophysiology. The clinical features of these diseases are quite diverse, ranging from mild cutaneous eruptions to severe organ involvement with pericarditis, glomerulonephritis, and vasculitis.

PATHOPHYSIOLOGY   The introduction of foreign or noxious substances into an individual is often followed by an immune response. Specific antibody produced in the course of this response binds to antigen, forming immune complexes. In general, these complexes are phagocytosed and destroyed by neutrophils and macrophages locally in tissue sites. If formed or released into the circulation, they are cleared from the circulation by phagocytic cells of the reticuloendothelial system. However, at times these complexes are deposited in tissues, causing inflammation and tissue damage. In recent years there has been a concerted effort to understand the mechanisms underlying this damage.

The biologic activity of the complexes has been studied in detail. It has been shown that the isotype of antibody affects biologic activity. Thus IgG- and IgM-containing complexes activate the classic complement pathway, and IgA-containing complexes often activate the alternative complement pathway. In contrast, cell surface IgE complexes are capable of mediating the degranulation of mast cells by a noncytotoxic, complement-independent mechanism.

The size of the immune complexes in the circulation is an important parameter of toxicity. In general, the larger (>19 S) complexes cause more tissue damage than the smaller complexes. The size is related to the concentration and molar ratio of antibody and antigen, as well as to the avidity of the antibody for the antigen. The ratio of antigen to antibody may range from antibody excess through antigen-antibody equivalence to antigen excess. In marked antibody excess, antigen valences are saturated, and in general, the complexes are small. Under conditions of marked antigen excess, antibody-combining sites are saturated, chances for lattice formation are limited, and, again, the complexes are small. At equivalence or mild antigen excess, lattice formation is facilitated, and large complexes can form. Immune complexes formed at moderate antigen excess are thought to be most pathogenic, perhaps because they are most efficient at activating the various mediator systems such as the complement cascade.

Net charge of antigen and antibody also appears to be important in determining the pathophysiologic effect of the complexes. It has been shown that positively charged immune complexes or immune complexes containing antigens with patches of positive charged groups tend to deposit in renal glomeruli, while complexes containing similar antigen with neutral charge tend to penetrate glomeruli slowly. This is presumably due to the fact that the glomerulus presents a negatively charged surface to the circulation. Similarly, there is a relationship between the degree of binding of immune complexes to the basement membrane of skin, which is also negatively charged, and the degree of positive charge of the complexes.

The first human disease in which circulating immune complexes were thought to play a pathogenic role was serum sickness. In their classic monograph, "Die Serumkrankheit," Clemens von Pirquet and Bela Schick described in great detail their experiences with the use of horse antidiphtheria toxin in children. They found that a reproducible reaction pattern occurred 8 to 13 days following the subcutaneous injection of horse serum protein. The patients developed fever, malaise, cutaneous eruptions, arthralgias, leukopenia, lymphadenopathy, and albuminuria. The authors suggested that this reaction pattern was caused by the interaction of host antibody, formed in the 8 days following the injection of the horse serum, with horse serum protein circulating in the recipient. They believed that this interaction led to the deposition of antigen-antibody complexes in tissue with resulting tissue damage, but the technology necessary to pursue this hypothesis was not available.

Numerous large retrospective studies of human serum sickness confirmed the observations of von Pirquet and Schick, but it was not until the studies of Germuth and Dixon that evidence for the role of circulating immune complexes in serum sickness was obtained. These investigators utilized rabbit models of serum sickness.

In the acute serum sickness model, the injection of antigen is followed by a period of intravascular equilibration, then by intravascular-extravascular equilibration lasting several days, and then by a progressive decline in the level of antigen in the circulation, representing the normal degradation of the injected serum protein. Following this period of decay, there is a sudden acceleration in the clearance of the antigen from the circulation, usually beginning at about 7 to 8 days. The period of rapid decline in the level of antigen in the circulation is due to the development of an immune response in the recipient animal. This results in the formation of antigen-antibody

complexes and subsequent clearance of the complexes from the circulation by phagocytes of the reticuloendothelial system (RES) (Fig. 283-1). During the period in which the complexes are being formed in the circulation, there is a fall in the animal's serum complement levels. At this time, pathologic changes occur in large arteries, renal glomeruli, joints, and cardiac vessels. The glomerulonephritis noted during this period has been studied extensively. It is characterized by swelling of the endothelial cells and marked proteinuria with little hematuria; an infiltrate of monocytes but very few granulocytes is found in the renal glomeruli. Immunofluorescence studies have shown that antigen, host immunoglobulin, and C3 are deposited along the glomerular basement membrane in a typical granular pattern. On electron-microscopic examination of kidney sections, few abnormalities are seen except swelling of endothelial cells. Late in the reaction, subepithelial deposits of electron-dense material are noted in some animals; however, at this time fluorescent antibody examination is negative for immunoglobulin and complement in the glomeruli. The deposits may represent immunologically altered immunoglobulin or complement.

There is also a very high incidence of arteritis in the coronary artery outflow tract and at branching points of the aorta in the acute serum sickness model. The arteritis is characterized by marked intimal proliferation of endothelium. This is followed by degradation of the internal elastic lamina and adventitia with resulting fibrinoid necrosis of the vessel. On immunofluorescence microscopy, host immunoglobulin, antigen, and C3 are found roughly in the region of the internal elastic lamina, but these immunoreactive materials are rapidly removed and are gone in several days. It has been suggested that the polymorphonuclear neutrophils present in the lesions phagocytize these complexes. In contrast to the findings in glomerulonephritis, materials which decrease complement activity or inhibit the polymorphonuclear leukocytic response diminish or block the development of arteritis.

FIGURE 283-1 The rabbit model of acute serum sickness. Radiolabeled antigen is injected at day 0. After a period of equilibration of antigen between the intravascular and extravascular space, there is progressive elimination of antigen from the circulation. With the onset of the animal's immune response there is rapid elimination of antigen from the circulation. Coincident with the phase of rapid elimination is the appearance of antigen-antibody complexes in the circulation and a fall in serum complement. Complete antigen clearance is associated with the appearance of free antibody in the circulation. At the time when antigen-antibody complexes are seen in the circulation, immunopathologic findings are maximal.

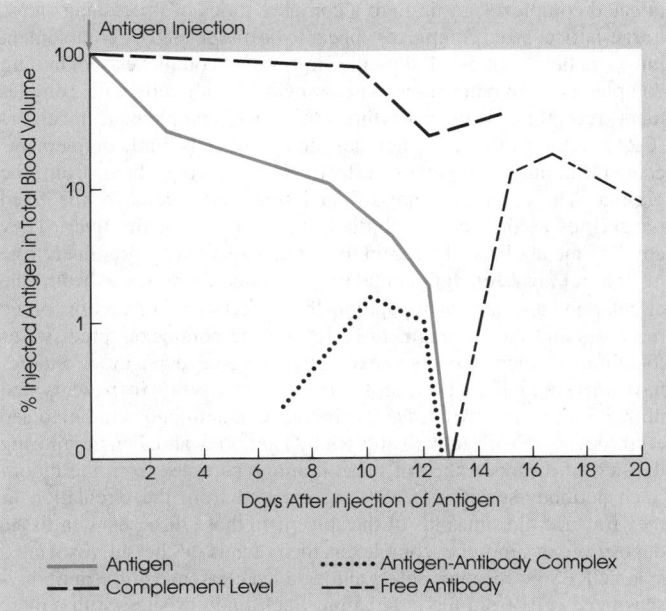

At the time of the development of serum sickness in this animal model, there are high-molecular-weight immune complexes in the circulation; the animals that become sick regularly have complexes that are greater than 19 S in their sedimentation characteristics. Acute serum sickness is present only as long as these circulating immune complexes persist and resolves rapidly once the antigen is cleared from the circulation and the immune complexes are gone.

It is possible to induce chronic glomerulonephritis in animals by the repeated intravenous injection of the antigen. The dose of antigen injected is critical to the development of the disease. Antigen excess must be produced after each antigen administration, and immune complexes must circulate in the animals. These animals develop glomerulonephritis but not the arteritis characteristic of acute serum sickness.

Other animal models of immune-complex disease closely resemble systemic lupus erythematosus. The most widely studied and best characterized is the disease that occurs spontaneously in the F_1 hybrid of New Zealand Black (NZB) and New Zealand White (NZW) mice. These animals develop antibodies to nucleic acids including double-stranded DNA and have decreased numbers of suppressor T cells. They also develop circulating immune complexes and an immune-complex–mediated glomerulonephritis that eventuates in renal insufficiency and death. Direct immunofluorescence microscopy of the kidneys in these animals reveals deposits of DNA, antibodies to DNA, and C3 in the glomerular basement membrane. The female NZB-NZW mice develop these changes before the males, and this sex difference may be related to a switch in the class of antibodies to DNA from IgM to IgG that occurs much earlier in the females than in the males.

Over the years, a great deal of attention has been paid in animal models to the fate of immune complexes in an attempt to understand exactly why they are deposited in tissues in autoimmune diseases. Injection of antigens into immunized animals is followed by the deposition of the antigen in the liver, spleen, and lung, all elements of the RES. Detailed studies have examined the fate of preformed immune complexes of carefully determined size in a variety of animals. In general, the findings of these studies have paralleled those reported in the animal models of serum sickness. The very large insoluble complexes are rapidly removed from the circulation. Soluble complexes that are greater than 19 S in their sedimentation characteristics are removed by the liver and persist in the circulation for only a matter of minutes. The major factor appearing to govern the rate of clearance of these large, preformed complexes from the circulation is the rate of hepatic blood flow. In some studies, complement activation by complexes is also important in their metabolism, and injected complexes go through a complex series of processing steps. Large-lattice–sized complexes appear to be dissociated by complement into smaller entities. Following injection, complexes containing complement components become associated with cells with complement receptors. Human erythrocytes have complement receptors (CR1) on their surface membranes, and these cells bind complement-coated immune complexes, effectively removing them from the plasma. The complexes are stripped from these cells by the fixed phagocytes as they course through the sinusoids of the liver. They are then metabolized. Fc receptors for IgG also play a prominent role in the removal of IgG-containing immune complexes from the circulation, and any manipulation that affects the interaction of Fc receptors and the Fc fragment of IgG in the complexes predisposes to failure to clear the complexes and to tissue deposition. Studies have measured RES Fc-receptor functional activity in patients and normal individuals by intravenously injecting autologous radiolabeled erythrocytes sensitized with anti-Rh IgG antibody and then monitoring the rate of disappearance of these immune particles from the blood. Such antibody-sensitized cells are removed from the circulation as they traverse the sinusoids of the spleen. In those diseases with tissue deposition of immune complexes there tends to be an associated splenic RES Fc-receptor defect and delayed clearance of the antibody-sensitized cells from the circulation. Such findings suggest that there

may be a failure in adequate removal of the complexes from the circulation, allowing for their tissue deposition. Studies in animals support these conclusions and suggest that failure of normal clearance mechanisms precedes the development of immune-complex deposition. Recent work suggests that mechanisms that promote the degranulation of mast cells with histamine release (e.g., the formation of IgE antibody) facilitate immune-complex deposition by decreasing vascular endothelial cell contact.

Another form of immune-complex–mediated tissue damage follows local formation of immune complexes in tissues such as the kidney. Glomerular subepithelial immune-complex deposits are thought to form at times on an in situ basis. This may occur as a result of antibody binding to fixed glomerular antigens or antibody binding to "planted" nonglomerular antigens. In the latter instance it is believed that certain cationic antigens can bind to the laminae rarae of the capillary wall in a glomerulus through charge-dependent mechanisms. This "planted" antigen is then recognized by antibody, and local tissue damage results. The pathophysiologic events leading to tissue damage in immunologically mediated inflammation are under intense study. In order for circulating leukocytes to exit from blood vessels into tissue at sites of inflammation, they must first bind to the endothelial cells that line the postcapillary venules. This is accomplished by proteins or glycoproteins, known as *cell adhesion molecules*, on the surface of the leukocytes interacting with other cell adhesion molecules on the endothelial cells. The interaction of one cell adhesion molecule with another appears to be quite specific. The expression and/or affinity of many cell adhesion molecules can be induced or upregulated by exposure of endothelial cells to cytokines such as interleukin 1 or tumor necrosis factor-α. Thus an endothelial cell in a postcapillary venule, when exposed to tumor necrosis factor-α, will rapidly begin to express the cell adhesion molecule P-selectin and will begin to upregulate the expression of ICAM-1 on its surface. P-selectin will bind to sialyl Lewis X on leukocytes, and ICAM-1 will bind to leukocyte LFA-1. This cell-cell interaction will lead to binding of the leukocytes to the endothelium with subsequent transmigration to areas of immune-complex deposition.

DETECTION OF CIRCULATING IMMUNE COMPLEXES Many different assays are available for the detection of soluble immune complexes in various biologic fluids. Although these assays vary in their sensitivity and reproducibility, they have expanded our understanding of circulating immune complexes and their role in various disease states. In general, early tests for the detection of circulating immune complexes relied on physical characteristics of the immune complexes, such as their high molecular weight or cold insolubility. These rather insensitive techniques have been replaced by assays for immunologic components or biologic activities of immune complexes. Although there are now sensitive radioimmunoassays for the detection of circulating immune complexes containing IgG, IgM, and IgA, these tests are not antigen-specific. In fact, in most cases in which circulating immune complexes are demonstrable, the component antigen(s) is (are) unknown. As with most laboratory tests, immune-complex assays may be influenced by other factors. Anticoagulants, endotoxin, and free DNA as well as immunoglobulin aggregates formed after the sample is obtained may result in false-positive results. The impact of these factors can be reduced by the selection of immune-complex assays that are unaffected by these variables and by the use of two or more different assays in situations in which critical evaluation of circulating immune complexes is desired. Several of the most sensitive and commonly used immune-complex assays will be described briefly: (1) C1q binding, or solid-phase radioassays, (2) Raji cell assays, and (3) conglutinin assays. *C1q* is a subcomponent of the first component of complement and will bind to immune complexes containing IgG subclasses 1 to 3 or IgM via noncovalent attachment to a specific site on the Fc portion of immunoglobulin. *Raji cells* are a lymphoblastoid cell line with cell surface receptors for complement, especially C3. The assays are based on the ability of circulating immune complexes that contain bound complement components in their lattices to bind to the surface of the Raji cells via the complement receptors. The bound complexes are easily detected. *Conglutinin* is a 750-kDa nonimmunoglobulin protein found in certain bovine sera that will bind to a cleavage fragment of human C3 known as iC3b. Immune complexes containing iC3b will bind to conglutinin attached to a solid-phase substrate and can be detected.

SERUM SICKNESS Drug hypersensitivity reactions are the most common cause of serum sickness today. It is hypothesized that the drug acting as a hapten binds to a plasma protein. The drug-protein complex induces an immune response which in turn causes typical serum sickness. Commonly occurring signs and symptoms of serum sickness include fever, cutaneous eruptions (morbilliform and/or urticarial), arthralgias, lymphadenopathy, and albuminuria. Less common manifestations are arthritis, nephritis, neuropathy, and vasculitis. The time required for primary sensitization to an offending agent is approximately 1 to 3 weeks. However, clinical manifestations may develop within 12 to 36 h if there is a history of a previous immunizing exposure. Drug-induced serum sickness usually abates within days after withdrawal of the causative agent. Reactions may persist for longer intervals, particularly if repository or long-acting agents are responsible for the problem. Drugs responsible for serum sickness include penicillin, sulfonamides, thiouracils, hydantoins, *p*-aminosalicylic acid, phenylbutazone, thiazides, and streptomycin. Foreign antisera and blood products also may induce serum sickness reactions.

Studies of patients receiving intravenous infusions of horse antithymocyte globulin (ATG) as therapy for bone marrow failure have confirmed and expanded the immunologic findings in animal models of serum sickness in humans. The patients develop signs and symptoms of serum sickness 8 to 13 days after beginning therapy with ATG (Fig. 283-2). These include fever; malaise; cutaneous eruptions; arthralgias and arthritis, mainly of the large joints; gastrointestinal distress with nausea, vomiting, and melena; lymphadenopathy; and proteinuria. Clinical disease coincides with the development of very high levels of circulating immune complexes as measured by the ^{125}I-labeled C1q binding assay and marked decreases in serum C3, C4, and CH$_{50}$ levels. The first cutaneous manifestation of serum sickness is a serpiginous band of erythema occurring along the sides of the hands, feet, fingers, and toes at the junction of palmar or plantar skin with the dorsolateral surface. Direct immunofluorescence of involved skin during serum sickness reveals deposits of immunoglobulins and C3 in the walls of small cutaneous blood vessels in most patients.

These studies provide strong support for a pathogenic role for circulating immune complexes in the pathophysiology of human serum sickness.

SYSTEMIC LUPUS ERYTHEMATOSUS Systemic lupus erythematosus (SLE) is a multisystem disease associated with a number of immunologic abnormalities, including the production of autoantibodies, hypergammaglobulinemia, suppressor T cell abnormalities, decreased levels of serum complement, and increased levels of circulating immune complexes (see Chap. 284). Immune complexes are thought to play a critical role in the pathophysiology of SLE. Early evidence for the role of circulating immune complexes in SLE included the finding by direct immunofluorescence of glomerular deposits of immunoglobulin, complement, and DNA in kidney biopsies. Mixed IgM-IgG cryoglobulins were found in the sera of a substantial number of SLE patients, and when the antibody specificity of these cryoprecipitates was examined, reactivity was found against single- and double-stranded DNA as well as ribonucleoprotein. Utilizing the newer, more sensitive assays, circulating immune complexes have been found in a high percentage of patients with SLE. Studies demonstrating a defect in the clearance by the spleen of autologous red cells sensitized with anti-Rh antibody have led to the suggestion that these patients have impaired function of RES Fc-IgG receptors. Such impaired function might allow complexes to circulate until they deposited in tissues. The prolonged RES clearance in patients with active SLE was found to be correlated with increased levels of circulating immune complexes as measured by the C1q binding assay and with clinical disease activity. Studies in the same patients after their disease improved with treatment revealed a significant correlation between clinical improvement, improvement of Fc-mediated clearance, and decreased levels of circulating immune complexes. Individuals with SLE also have decreased numbers of C3b receptors on their erythrocytes, which also may contribute to abnormalities in immune-complex clearance. Whether the decreased number of receptors is primary or secondary remains to be established. Nonetheless, abnormalities of both Fc-IgG and C3b receptors which are responsible for phagocytosis of circulating immune complexes are present in patients with SLE.

VASCULITIS There is strong circumstantial evidence for the role of circulating immune complexes in the various forms of hypersensitivity or necrotizing vasculitis (see Chap. 291). Features of the classic "palpable purpura" of cutaneous necrotizing vasculitis closely resemble the clinical, histopathologic, and immunopathologic

FIGURE 283-2 Serum sickness in human beings. Horse antithymocyte globulin was injected into patients with aplastic anemia daily for 10 days. After the fifth day of injection, C1q binding activity begins to rise (*A*). At the same time there is a dramatic fall in plasma levels of C3 and C4 and onset of clinical symptoms (*B*).

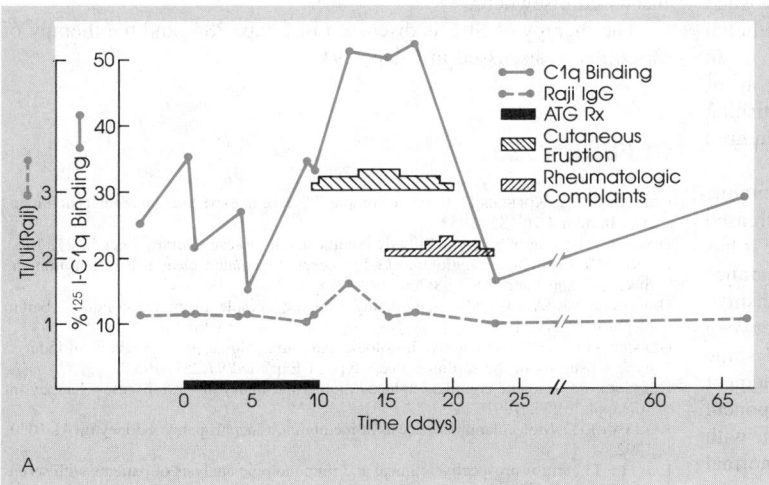

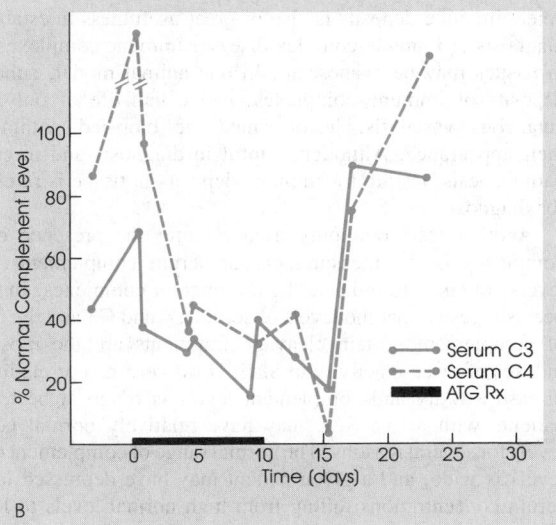

features of the Arthus reaction. The Arthus reaction is a model for immune-complex–mediated vascular damage in which antigen is injected intradermally into an animal which possesses circulating antibody against that antigen. In both vasculitis and the Arthus reaction, deposits of immunoglobulin and complement are found in the walls of blood vessels in early lesions. The histopathology of both consists of infiltrates of polymorphonuclear neutrophils, leukocytoclasis, endothelial cell damage and necrosis, hemorrhage, and perivascular deposits of fibrin. Electron microscopy of lesions of cutaneous necrotizing vasculitis reveals subendothelial electron-dense deposits compatible with immune complexes. The available evidence indicates the presence of immune complexes at the site of tissue damage in necrotizing vasculitis. In accord with these findings is the demonstration of circulating immune complexes in a high percentage of patients with this disease.

LABORATORY FINDINGS   In theory, the essential feature of immune-complex disease would be the finding of circulating immune complexes. In practice, there is great variability from disease to disease in the frequency of positive immune-complex assays. In some diseases, such as SLE, there is a high frequency of positive immune-complex assays. In others, such as membranoproliferative glomerulonephritis, the frequency of positive assays is much lower. Part of the reason for this has to do with the stage of disease under study. In some cases immunologic phenomena are responsible for the initiation of the disease and the initial tissue insult. However, subsequent injury is caused by scarring, inflammation, and repair mechanisms that result in more extensive tissue damage. Thus progression of disease may occur at a time when immunologic injury is no longer occurring. A second reason for the failure to detect circulating immune complexes in diseases thought to be mediated by them has to do with technical difficulties in the measurement of such complexes. There are many types of assays for immune complexes. Most are indirect and rely on a biologic or biochemical property of the complexes such as the binding of complement components. The pattern of positive reaction clearly varies from disease to disease. Clearly, each assay recognizes a different type of complex with maximal efficiency. Since multiple assays are rarely performed on one specimen, complexes, although present, may not be detected. Finally, although a disease is classified as immune-complex–related because of the finding of immune deposits in affected tissues or because of the similarity of its pathologic findings to those of animal models of immune-complex disease, the disease may not be actually caused by circulating immune complexes. For example, antibody may be formed to a tissue component, bind to it in a tissue site, and induce damage. Such is thought to be the case in Goodpasture's disease. For all these reasons, assays for the detection of circulating immune complex, while often useful, are rarely critical for diagnosis or patient management.

Examination of tissues using immunofluorescence techniques to detect immune deposits is also of great usefulness in establishing the diagnosis of immune-complex disease. Immune complexes deposited in tissues may be evanescent. In one animal model, subendothelial deposits of immune complexes, had a half-life of only 3.9 h. In cutaneous vasculitis, lesions must be biopsied within 12 h of their appearance. Although helpful in diagnosis and in establishing pathogenesis, testing for immune deposits in tissue is rarely required for diagnosis.

Another test commonly used to infer the presence of immune complexes is the measurement of serum complement. Decreased levels are taken to indicate the presence of complexes. In fact, it has been suggested that the levels of serum C4 and C3 and the appearance of complement protein cleavage fragments are the most sensitive indexes of disease activity in SLE. However, the correlation between disease activity and complement levels is rough at best, and some patients with active SLE may have relatively normal complement levels for several reasons. The normal range of complement component levels is wide, and a given patient may have depressed levels, with serum concentrations falling from high-normal levels to low-normal levels. In general, complement components act as acute-phase re-

actants, and the lowering of serum complement may be masked by increased synthesis. Moreover, activation of complement may mediate profound pathophysiologic effects, although relatively few molecules of complement are actually involved. For example, complement binding to red cells may be responsible for much of the red cell destruction that occurs with ABO-mismatched transfusions, yet serum complement levels may be unchanged because too few molecules are used in erythyrocyte destruction to detect a fall in titer. Finally, all types of complexes do not activate complement in the same way. Massive antigen release from red cells occurring during the course of vivax malaria infection leads to the rapid formation of antigen-antibody complexes in the circulation. For unknown reasons, these complexes only interact with the early components of the classic complement pathway, while C3 and the later complement components are not recruited. Thus, if one measures levels of C3, no fall in titer is noted, although complexes are present and massive complement activation has taken place. The complexes formed in SLE activate optimally the classic pathway; presumably those involved in IgA glomerulonephritis activate the alternative pathway. Therefore, the complement test chosen for examination may be important.

Other tests may suggest indirectly the presence of immune-complex disease. For example, a finding of mixed IgG-IgM cryoprecipitates suggests the presence of immune complexes. The presence of antinuclear antibodies suggests autoimmunity, as does the presence of a number of tissue component–specific antibodies. Similarly, the presence of specific antigen such as hepatitis B surface antigen in the circulation together with appropriate clinical symptoms may suggest an immune-complex disease. Most patients with active immune-complex–mediated disease have an elevated erythrocyte sedimentation rate, although this is not invariably the case. Patients with Takayasu's arteritis may have a normal erythrocyte sedimentation rate during the later phases of the evolution of lesions, when most pathology is caused by scarring, fibrosis, and repair within vessel walls. Finally, specific laboratory test findings such as red cell casts in the urine in glomerulonephritis or mild cerebrospinal fluid pleocytosis in the presence of cerebritis are discussed in the chapters concerning those diseases.

TREATMENT   The therapy of immune-complex–mediated disease relies on removal of the offending antigen and interruption of the inflammatory response. In general, serum sickness is a self-limited disease that is seldom life-threatening. In the case of drug-induced serum sickness, it is most important to discontinue the offending agent. In recent years, plasmapheresis (particularly in concert with cytotoxic agents) has been used to blunt the manifestations of acute immune-complex tissue injury. In many instances, supportive care combined with antihistamines for urticaria and acetaminophen for fever, myalgias, and arthralgias is adequate. If serious renal, vascular, or central nervous system involvement occurs, the use of systemic glucocorticoid therapy is indicated. These approaches to therapy are discussed elsewhere.

The therapy of SLE is discussed in Chap. 284, and the therapy of vasculitis is discussed in Chap. 291.

REFERENCES

COCHRANE CB, KOFFLER D: Immune complex disease in experimental animals and man. Adv Immunol 16:185, 1963

DIXON F: The role of antigen-antibody complexes in disease. Harvey Lect 52:21, 1963

FRANK MM et al: Immunoglobulin G–Fc receptor mediated clearance in autoimmune diseases. Ann Intern Med 98:206, 1983

GAUTHIER VJ, ABRASS CK: Circulating immune complexes in renal injury. Semin Nephrol 12:379, 1992

GERMUTH FC JR.: A comparative histologic and immunologic study in rabbits of induced hypersensitivity of the serum sickness type. J Exp Med 97:257, 1953

GLASSOCK RJ: Immune complex–induced glomerular injury in viral diseases. Kidney Int 40(suppl 35):55, 1991

KERJASCHKI D: Molecular pathogenesis of membranous nephropathy. Kidney Int 41:1090, 1992

LAWLEY TJ et al: A prospective clinical and immunologic analysis of patients with serum sickness. N Engl J Med 311:1407, 1984

MANNIK M, AREND WP: Fate of preformed immune complexes in rabbits and rhesus monkeys. J Exp Med 134:19s, 1971

MULLIGAN ME et al: Tissue injury caused by deposition of immune complexes is L-arginine–dependent. Proc Natl Acad Sci USA 88:6338, 1991

VON PIRQUET C, SCHICK B: *Serum Sickness.* Baltimore, Williams & Wilkins, 1951

THEOFILOPOULOS AN, DIXON FJ: The biology and detection of immune complexes. Adv Immunol 28:89, 1979

284 SYSTEMIC LUPUS ERYTHEMATOSUS

BEVRA HANNAHS HAHN

DEFINITION AND PREVALENCE Systemic lupus erythematosus (SLE) is a disease of unknown cause in which tissues and cells are damaged by pathogenic autoantibodies and immune complexes. Ninety percent of cases are in women, usually of childbearing age, but children, men, and the elderly can be affected. In the United States, the prevalence of SLE in urban areas varies from 15 to 50 per 100,000 population; it is more common in blacks than in whites. Hispanic and Asian populations are also susceptible.

PATHOGENESIS AND ETIOLOGY SLE probably results from interactions between susceptibility genes and the environment. This interaction results in abnormal immune responses with T and B lymphocyte hyperactivity which is not suppressed by the usual immunoregulatory circuits. Evidence for genetic predisposition includes increased concordance for disease in monozygotic compared with dizygotic twins, a 10 percent frequency of patients with more than one affected family member, and correlations of certain genes (especially MHC classes II and III) with disease and autoantibodies. C4AQO, a defective class III allele which fails to encode a functional C4A protein, is the most common genetic marker associated with SLE in many ethnic groups (found in 40 to 50 percent of patients compared with 15 percent of healthy controls). Certain extended haplotypes, such as B8.DR3.DQw2.C4AQO, predispose to SLE in some populations. The strongest single gene associations occur between HLA class II (especially DQ_{beta}) and autoantibodies which define clinical subsets of lupus. For example, high titers of IgG anti-DNA are associated with lupus nephritis and with DQB1*0201, *0602, and *0302 inherited with either DR2 or DR3. Antibodies to Ro/La (SS-A/SS-B) are associated with the dermatitis of subacute cutaneous lupus and with certain DQA and DQB genes inherited with DR3 (occasionally DR2). The lupus anticoagulant, correlated clinically with clotting, is associated with DQB*0301, *0302, *0303, and *0602 inherited with DR4 or DR7. The DQA or DQB susceptibility genes in each group share amino acid sequences that may determine the ability to make a particular autoantibody. Family studies suggest that genes unlinked to HLA also participate in susceptibility and that females are more likely than males to express the autoimmune manifestations of their genotypes. The more susceptibility genes one has, the higher is the relative risk for SLE; three or four different genes are probably required.

Environmental factors that flare SLE are largely unknown, with the exception of UV-B (and sometimes UV-A) light. As many as 70 percent of patients are photosensitive. Other factors such as ingested alfalfa sprouts and chemicals such as hydrazines and hair dye have been implicated. Searches for viral/retroviral disease inducers, currently in progress, are inconclusive. Although some drugs can induce lupus-like disease, there are notable clinical and autoantibody differences between drug-induced and spontaneous lupus. Femaleness is clearly a susceptibility factor, since the prevalence in women of childbearing years is seven to nine times higher than in men, whereas the female-to-male ratio is 3:1 in pre- and postmenopausal years. Metabolism of estrogenic and androgenic hormones may be abnormal in lupus patients. Sex hormones also influence immune tolerance.

Abnormal immune responses include sustained production of pathogenic subsets of autoantibodies and immune complexes (ICs). No immunoglobulin genes have been identified that exclusively encode harmful autoantibodies, although certain V-region genes (especially V_H) seem to be preferentially used, and there is probably clonal selection of B cells secreting high-avidity antibodies to autoantigens. In most murine lupus models, T cell help is critical to development of full-blown disease; there is active investigation of T cell suppression as a therapeutic intervention in patients. The abnormalities that permit hyperactivated self-reactive B and T cells to dominate immune repertoires in SLE are unclear. These cells escape normal tolerizing mechanisms; they are neither deleted nor anergized. Recent evidence in mice suggests that defective apoptosis, genetically encoded, may prevent elimination of self-reactive cells. There is some evidence that bone marrow stem cell precursors of B and, perhaps, of T lymphocytes are intrinsically abnormal. Alternatively, the microenvironment in which these stem cells develop may be abnormal. Perhaps genes, sex hormones, and exogenous antigens influence tolerance and cell activation. Alternatively, these cells could be altered by antilymphocyte antibodies. The structure of antigens that stimulate autoantibodies is under investigation. Some are clearly derived from self (histones, RNP, erythrocyte surface antigens); others may be from the external environment and mimic self (e.g., components of vesicular stomatitis virus mimic peptides in Ro antigen). Some autoantibodies induce disease by direct reaction with their antigens, such as those directed against surface antigens on erythrocytes or platelets. Others may attach to cell membranes (such as glomerular basement membrane, GBM) via cationic charge or because they cross-react with tissue constituents (e.g., some anti-DNA antibodies react with laminin in GBM). If these antibodies, when complexed with antigen, can fix complement, tissue damage occurs. Alteration of cell function after antibodies bind to membranes also occurs independent of complement activation. Autoantibodies characteristic of SLE are listed in Table 284-1.

Abnormalities of immune regulation are required to develop SLE. Immune complexes are cleared inadequately. CR1 receptors on erythrocytes are low in number (usually because they are stripped by high levels of IC, occasionally because of genetic control) so that many ICs are not transported to the mononuclear phagocyte system (MPS). The MPS is unable to process ICs normally. Idiotype–anti-idiotype networks fail to suppress hyperactivated T and B cells. T lymphocytes are heavily skewed toward help: CD4 + CD8 −, CD4 − CD8 +, CD4 − CD8 −, alpha/beta, and gamma/delta T cells have all been shown to help B cell production of autoantibodies in SLE. Therefore, the usual suppressor functions attributed to CD4 − CD8 + cells and to the NK cells with which T cells interact are absent. Finally, normal tolerance mechanisms that eliminate or inactivate strongly autoreactive T and B lymphocytes are impaired.

In summary, some individuals are genetically predisposed to SLE. Under the influence of multiple genes, often triggered by environmental challenges and highly influenced by sex, they may develop a number of different clinical syndromes which fulfill diagnostic criteria for SLE. The cause of these syndromes is complex and probably differs between patients.

CLINICAL MANIFESTATIONS At onset, SLE may involve only one organ system (additional manifestations occur later) or may be multisystemic. Clinical manifestations are listed in Table 284-2; those which fulfill American Rheumatism Association criteria for a diagnosis of SLE are listed in Table 284-3. Autoantibodies are detectable at disease onset. Severity varies from mild and intermittent to persistent and fulminant. Most patients experience exacerbations interspersed with periods of relative quiescence. True remissions with no symptoms and requiring no therapy occur in less than 10 percent. Systemic symptoms are usually prominent and include fatigue, malaise, fever, anorexia, and weight loss.

Musculoskeletal Almost all patients experience arthralgias and myalgias; most develop intermittent arthritis. Pain is often out of proportion to physical findings of symmetric fusiform swelling in

TABLE 284-1 Autoantibodies in patients with SLE

	Incidence, %	Antigen detected	Clinical importance
Antinuclear antibodies	95	Multiple nuclear and cytoplasmic antigens	Human cell line substrates are more sensitive than standard murine tissues. A repeatedly negative test on both makes SLE diagnosis unlikely. Multiple antibodies are detected.
Anti-DNA	70	DNA	Anti-dsDNA is relatively disease specific; anti-ssDNA is not. Associated with nephritis and clinical activity.
Anti-Sm	30	Protein complexed to 6 species of small nuclear RNA	Specific for SLE.
Anti-RNP	40	Protein complexed to U1RNA	High titer seen in syndromes with features of polymyositis, scleroderma, lupus, and mixed connective tissue disease. If present in SLE without anti-DNA, risk for nephritis is low.
Anti-Ro (SSA)	30	Protein complexed to Y_1–Y_5 RNA	Associated with Sjögren's syndrome, DR3 haplotype, subacute cutaneous lupus, inherited complement deficiencies, ANA-negative lupus, lupus in the elderly, neonatal lupus, congenital heart block in infants. Can cause nephritis.
Anti-La (SSB)	10	Phosphoprotein complexed with RNA pol III transcripts	Always associated with anti-Ro; risk for nephritis is low if present in SLE. Associated with Sjögren's syndrome.
Antihistone	70	Histones	More frequent in drug-induced LE (95%) than in spontaneous SLE.
Anticardiolipin	50	Phospholipid	Increases risk for venous or arterial thrombosis, thrombocytopenia, valvular heart disease, and spontaneous abortion. Associated with prolonged PTT (lupus anticoagulant) and false-positive VDRL.
Antierythrocyte	60	Erythrocyte surface antigens	A small proportion of these patients develop overt hemolysis.
Antiplatelet	—	Platelet surface	Associated with thrombocytopenia.
Antilymphocyte	70	Lymphocyte surface antigens	Probably associated with leukopenia and abnormal T cell function.
Antineuronal	60	Neuronal and lymphocyte surface antigens	In CSF, high IgG titers correlate with diffuse CNS lupus.

joints [most frequently proximal interphalangeal (PIP) and metacarpophalangeal (MCP) joints of the hands, wrists, and knees], diffuse puffiness of hands and feet, and tenosynovitis. Joint deformities are unusual, with 10 percent of patients developing swan-neck deformities of fingers and ulnar drift at MCP joints. Erosions are rare; subcutaneous nodules occur. Myopathy can be inflammatory (during periods of active disease) or secondary to treatment (hypokalemia, glucocorticoid myopathy, hydroxychloroquine myopathy). Ischemic necrosis of bone is a common cause of hip, knee, or shoulder pain in patients receiving glucocorticoids.

Cutaneous　The malar ("butterfly") rash is a fixed erythematous rash, flat or raised, over the cheeks and bridge of the nose, often involving the chin and ears. It is photosensitive. Scarring is absent; telangiectasias may develop. A more diffuse maculopapular rash, predominant in sun-exposed areas, is also common and usually indicates disease flare. Loss of scalp hair is usually patchy but can be extensive; hair often regrows in SLE lesions but not in discoid lupus lesions (DLE). DLE occurs in about 20 percent of patients with SLE and can be disfiguring, since the lesions have central atrophy and scarring, with permanent loss of appendages. DLE lesions are circular and characterized by an erythematous raised rim, scaliness, follicular plugging, and telangiectasia. They occur over the scalp, ears, face, and sun-exposed areas of the arms, back, and chest. Only 5 percent of patients with DLE subsequently develop SLE. Less frequent SLE skin lesions include urticaria, bullae, erythema multiforme, lichen planus–like lesions, and panniculitis ("lupus profundus").

Patients with subacute cutaneous lupus (SCLE) are a distinct subset with recurring extensive dermatitis. Arthritis and fatigue are frequent; central nervous system and renal involvement are not.

Some patients are antinuclear antibody (ANA)–negative. Most have antibodies to Ro (SS-A) or to single-stranded (ss) DNA and are HLA-DR3, -DQw1, or -DQw2. Skin lesions are photosensitive and may be annular or papulosquamous psoriasiform lesions over the arms, trunk and face; they become hypopigmented but do not scar.

Patients with SLE, DLE, or SCLE can develop vasculitic skin lesions. These include purpura, subcutaneous nodules, nail fold infarcts, ulcers, vasculitic urticaria, and gangrene of digits. Shallow, slightly painful ulcers in the mouth and nose are frequent in patients with SLE.

Renal　Most patients with SLE have immunoglobulins deposited in glomeruli, but only one-half have clinical nephritis, defined by proteinuria. Early in the disease most are asymptomatic, although some develop the edema of nephrotic syndrome. Urinalysis shows hematuria, cylindruria, and proteinuria. Most patients with mesangial or mild focal proliferative nephritis (see discussion under "Pathology" below) maintain good renal function. Patients with diffuse proliferative nephritis develop renal failure if untreated. Since severe nephritis requires aggressive immunosuppression with high-dose glucocorticoids and cytotoxic drugs and mild lesions do not, renal biopsy may provide information that affects therapy. Patients with rapidly deteriorating renal function and active urine sediment require prompt, aggressive therapy; biopsy is not necessary unless such patients fail to respond to therapy. However, patients with a slow rise in creatinine to levels > 265 μmol/L (>3 mg/dL) may show a high proportion of sclerotic glomeruli on biopsy; they are unlikely to respond to immunosuppressive therapies and are candidates for dialysis or transplantation. Patients with persistently abnormal urinalyses, high titers of anti-dsDNA, and/or hypocomplementemia are at risk for severe nephritis; kidney biopsy may guide therapy.

TABLE 284-2 Clinical manifestations of SLE

	Percent of patients positive during course of disease
Systemic	95
Fatigue, malaise, fever, anorexia, nausea, weight loss	
Musculoskeletal	95
Arthralgias/myalgias	95
Nonerosive polyarthritis	60
Hand deformities	10
Myopathy/myositis	40/5
Ischemic necrosis of bone	15
Cutaneous	80
Malar rash	50
Discoid rash	15
Photosensitivity	70
Oral ulcers	40
Other rashes—maculopapular, urticarial, bullous, subacute cutaneous lupus	40
Alopecia	40
Vasculitis	20
Panniculitis	5
Hematologic	85
Anemia (of chronic disease)	70
Hemolytic anemia	10
Leukopenia ($<4000/mm^3$)	65
Lymphopenia ($<1500/mm^3$)	50
Thrombocytopenia ($<100,000/mm^3$)	15
Circulating anticoagulant	10–20
Splenomegaly	15
Lymphadenopathy	20
Neurologic	60
Cognitive dysfunction	50
Organic brain syndromes	35
Psychosis	10
Seizures	20
Other CNS (see text)	15
Peripheral neuropathy	15
Cardiopulmonary	60
Pleurisy	50
Pericarditis	30
Myocarditis	10
Endocarditis (Libman-Sachs)	10
Pleural effusions	30
Lupus pneumonitis	10
Interstitial fibrosis	5
Pulmonary hypertension	<5
ARDS/hemorrhage	<5
Renal	50
Proteinuria >500 mg/24 h	50
Cellular casts	50
Nephrotic syndrome	25
Renal failure	5–10
Gastrointestinal	45
Nonspecific (anorexia, nausea, mild pain, diarrhea)	30
Vasculitis with bleeding or perforation	5
Ascites	<5
Abnormal liver enzymes	40
Thrombosis	15
Venous	10
Arterial	5
Fetal loss	30 (of pregnancies)
Ocular	15
Retinal vasculitis	5
Conjunctivitis/episcleritis	10
Sicca syndrome	15

Nervous system Any region of the brain can be involved in SLE, as can the meninges, spinal cord, and cranial and peripheral nerves. Central nervous system (CNS) events may be single or multiple and often occur when SLE is active in other organ systems. Mild cognitive dysfunction is the most frequent manifestation. Seizures of any type may occur. Less frequent manifestations include

TABLE 284-3 The 1982 criteria for classification of systemic lupus erythematosus

1	Malar rash	Fixed erythema, flat or raised, over the malar eminences
2	Discoid rash	Erythematous raised patches with adherent keratotic scaling and follicular plugging; atrophic scarring may occur
3	Photosensitivity	
4	Oral ulcers	Includes oral and nasopharyngeal, observed by physician
5	Arthritis	Nonerosive arthritis involving two or more peripheral joints, characterized by tenderness, swelling, or effusion
6	Serositis	Pleuritis or pericarditis documented by ECG or rub or evidence of pericardial effusion
7	Renal disorder	Proteinuria greater than 0.5 g/d or greater than 3+, or cellular casts
8	Neurologic disorder	Seizures without other cause or psychosis without other cause
9	Hematologic disorder	Hemolytic anemia or leukopenia (less than $4000/mm^3$) or lymphopenia (less than $1500/mm^3$) or thrombocytopenia (less than $100,000/mm^3$) in the absence of offending drugs
10	Immunologic disorder	Positive LE cell preparation or anti-dsDNA or anti-Sm antibodies or false-positive VDRL
11	Antinuclear antibodies	An abnormal titer of ANAs by immunofluorescence or an equivalent assay at any point in time in the absence of drugs known to induce ANAs

If four of these criteria are present at any time during the course of disease, a diagnosis of systemic lupus can be made with 98 percent specificity and 97 percent sensitivity.

SOURCE: Criteria published by Tan EM et al: The 1982 revised criteria for the classification of systemic lupus erythematosus. Arthritis Rheum 25:1271, 1982.

psychosis, organic brain syndromes, headache (including migraine), focal infarcts, extrapyramidal disorders, cerebellar dysfunction, hypothalamic dysfunction with inappropriate antidiuretic hormone (ADH) secretion, pseudotumor cerebri, subarachnoid hemorrhage, aseptic meningitis, transverse myelitis, optic neuritis, cranial nerve palsies, and peripheral sensorimotor neuropathy. Depression and anxiety are frequent.

Laboratory diagnosis of CNS lupus can be difficult. Abnormal electroencephalograms occur in about 70 percent of patients and usually show diffuse slowing or focal abnormalities. Cerebrospinal fluid (CSF) shows elevated protein levels in 50 percent and increased mononuclear cells in 30 percent of patients; oligoclonal bands, increased Ig synthesis and antineuronal antibodies may be found. Lumbar puncture should be performed whenever CNS symptoms could result from infection, especially in immunosuppressed patients. CT scans and angiograms are most likely to be positive when focal neurologic deficits are present and are less helpful in cases with diffuse manifestations. Magnetic resonance imaging is the most sensitive radiographic technique to detect changes of SLE; changes are often nonspecific. Laboratory measures of disease activity (Table 284-4) often do not correlate with neurologic manifestations. Neurologic problems (with the exception of deficits resulting from large infarcts) usually improve with immunosuppressive therapy and/or time; recurrences are common.

Vascular Thrombosis in vessels of any size can be a major problem. Although vasculitis may underlie thrombosis, there is increasing evidence that antibodies against phospholipids (lupus anticoagulant, anticardiolipin) are associated with clotting without inflammation. In addition, degenerative vascular changes after years of exposure of blood vessels to circulating immune complexes and hyperlipidemia from glucocorticoid therapy predispose to degenerative coronary artery disease in lupus patients. Therefore, anticoagulation is more appropriate than immunosuppression in some patients.

Hematologic Anemia of chronic disease occurs in most patients

TABLE 284-4 Laboratory manifestations of SLE

Tests that help *confirm the clinical diagnosis and predict severity*	Tests that may be helpful in *following the clinical course**
Relatively specific for SLE:	Titer of anti-dsDNA
Anti-dsDNA	Serum complement levels
Anti-Sm	Westergren erythrocyte sedimentation rate
Not specific:	Hematocrit
ANA (most sensitive)	Leukocyte count
THC, C3, C4	Platelet count
Anti-Ro	Urinalysis
Direct Coombs' test	Serum creatinine
VDRL	
PTT	
Anticardiolipin	
Hematocrit	
Leukocyte count	
Platelet count	
Urinalysis	
Serum creatinine	

* For each patient, the pattern of laboratory abnormalities (if any) associated with a disease flare should be established and only those tests used subsequently as adjuncts to clinical assessment.

when lupus is active. Hemolysis occurs in a small proportion of those with positive Coombs' tests; it is usually responsive to high-dose glucocorticoids; resistant cases may respond to splenectomy. Leukopenia (usually lymphopenia) is common but is rarely associated with recurrent infections and does not require treatment. Mild thrombocytopenia is common; severe thrombocytopenia with bleeding and purpura occurs in 5 percent of patients and should be treated with high-dose glucocorticoids. Short-term improvement can be achieved by administration of intravenous gamma globulin. If the platelet count fails to reach acceptable levels in 2 weeks, splenectomy should be considered.

The lupus anticoagulant (LA) belongs to a family of antiphospholipid antibodies. It is recognized by prolongation of the partial thromboplastin time and failure of added normal plasma to correct the prolongation. More sensitive tests include the Russell viper venom time and the rabbit brain neutral phospholipid test. Antibodies to cardiolipin (aCL) are detected in ELISA assays. Clinical manifestations of LA and aCL include thrombocytopenia, recurrent venous or arterial clotting, recurrent fetal loss, and valvular heart disease. If the LA is associated with hypoprothrombinemia or thrombocytopenia, bleeding may occur. Less commonly, antibodies to clotting factors (VIII, IX) arise; they cause bleeding. Bleeding syndromes usually respond to glucocorticoids; clotting syndromes do not.

Cardiopulmonary Pericarditis is the most frequent manifestation of cardiac lupus; effusions can occur and occasionally lead to tamponade; constrictive pericarditis is rare. Myocarditis can cause arrhythmias, sudden death, and/or heart failure. Valvular insufficiency (usually arotic or mitral) is an uncommon sequel of Libman Sachs endocarditis; it may be associated with antiphospholipids. Myocardial infarcts usually result from degenerative disease, although they can result from vasculitis.

Pleurisy and pleural effusions are common manifestations of SLE. Lupus pneumonitis causes fever, dyspnea, and cough; x-rays show fleeting infiltrates and/or areas of platelike atelectasis; this syndrome respond to glucocorticoids. However, *the most common cause of pulmonary infiltrates in patients with SLE is infection.* Interstitial pneumonitis leading to fibrosis occurs occasionally; the inflammatory phase may respond to treatment; the fibrosis does not. Pulmonary hypertension is an uncommon, grave manifestation of SLE. Infrequent pulmonary manifestations with high mortality include adult respiratory distress syndrome and massive intraalveolar hemorrhage.

Gastrointestinal Common gastrointestinal (GI) symptoms include nausea, diarrhea, and vague discomfort. Symptoms may result from lupus peritonitis. Vasculitis of the intestine is the most dangerous manifestation, presenting with acute crampy abdominal pain, vomiting, and diarrhea. Intestinal perforation can occur and usually requires immediate surgery. Patients with pseudoobstruction have abdominal pain; x-rays show dilated loops of small bowel which may be edematous; surgery should be avoided unless frank obstruction is present. Glucocorticoid therapy is useful for all these GI syndromes. Some patients have GI motility disorders similar to those in scleroderma; they are not benefited by steroids. Acute pancreatitis occurs and can be severe, resulting from active SLE or from therapy with glucocorticoids or azathioprine. Elevated amylase levels may reflect pancreatitis, salivary gland inflammation, or macroamylasemia. Elevated serum transaminases are common in patients with active SLE but are not associated with significant hepatic damage; they return to normal as the disease is treated.

Ocular Retinal vasculitis is a serious manifestation; blindness can develop over a few days, and aggressive immunosuppression should be instituted. Examination shows areas of sheathed, narrow retinal arterioles and cytoid bodies (white exudates) adjacent to vessels. Other ocular abnormalities include conjunctivitis, episcleritis, optic neuritis, and the sicca syndrome.

PATHOLOGY **Cutaneous lesions** Lesions of acute SLE, discoid lupus (DLE), and subacute cutaneous LE (SCLE) show similar histopathology, with degeneration of the basal layer of the epidermis, disruption of the dermal-epidermal junction (DEJ), and mononuclear infiltrates around vessels and appendages in the upper dermis. In DLE, follicular plugging and hyperkeratosis are prominent. Deposits of immunoglobulins (Ig) and C′ are seen in the DEJ in 80 to 100 percent of lesional and 50 percent of nonlesional skin in active SLE; the proportions are lower during remissions. Only 50 percent of SCLE lesions are positive for Ig and C′ deposits. Ig deposition in the DEJ is not specific for LE. Vasculitis skin lesions usually show leukocytoclastic angiitis.

Renal lesions Glomerulonephritis (GN) is caused by deposition of circulating immune complexes or in situ complex formation in mesangium and glomerular basement membranes (GBM). Renal biopsy should be considered when results would affect therapy. Information regarding location of immune deposits, histologic pattern of renal damage, and activity and chronicity of lesions is all useful in predicting prognosis and selecting appropriate treatment. In mild GN unlikely to lead to renal failure, Ig deposits are confined to the mesangium, and histology shows no changes or mesangial proliferation. If Ig and C′ are deposited outside the mesangium in capillary GBM, prognosis worsens. Histologic changes that should be treated with aggressive immunosuppression include focal proliferative, membranoproliferative, and diffuse proliferative GN (see Chap 241). Progression from focal to diffuse lesions can occur. Membranous changes without proliferation are uncommon but have a better prognosis than proliferative GN. Activity and chronicity scores indicate severity and reversibility of lesions. *Reversible "active" lesions* associated with high risk of progression to renal failure are glomerular necrosis, cellular epithelial crescents, hyaline thrombi, interstitial inflammatory infiltrates, and necrotizing vasculitis. *Irreversible changes unlikely to respond to immunosuppression* and highly associated with renal failure include glomerular sclerosis, fibrous crescents, interstitial fibrosis, and tubular atrophy. In patients with high chronicity scores, treatment of lupus should be determined by extrarenal disease.

LABORATORY MANIFESTATIONS The presence of characteristic antibodies (see Table 284-1) confirms the diagnosis of SLE. Antinuclear antibodies (ANAs) are the best screening test. If the test substrate contains human nuclei (WIL-2 or HEP-2 cells), more than 95 percent of lupus patients will be positive. A positive ANA test is not specific for SLE; ANAs occur in some normal individuals (usually in low titer); the frequency increases with aging. Other autoimmune diseases, viral infections, chronic inflammatory processes, and several drugs induce ANAs. Therefore, a positive ANA test supports the diagnosis of SLE but is not specific; a negative ANA test makes the diagnosis unlikely but not impossible. Antibodies to double-stranded

DNA (dsDNA) and to Sm are relatively specific for SLE; other autoantibodies listed in Table 284-1 are not. However, determining the complete autoantibody profile of each patient helps predict clinical subsets. High serum levels of ANAs and anti-dsDNA antibodies and low levels of complement usually reflect disease activity, especially in patients with nephritis. Total functional hemolytic complement (CH_{50}) levels are the most sensitive measure of complement activation but are also most subject to laboratory error. Quantitative levels of C2 and C4 are widely available. Very low levels of CH_{50} with normal levels of C3 suggest inherited deficiency of a complement component, which is highly associated with SLE and with ANA negativity.

Hematologic abnormalities include anemia (usually normochromic normocytic but occasionally hemolytic), leukopenia, lymphopenia, and thrombocytopenia. The Westergren erythrocyte sedimentation rate correlates with disease activity in some patients.

Urinalysis and serum creatinine determinations should be done periodically in patients with SLE. With active nephritis, the urinalysis usually shows proteinuria, hematuria, and cellular or granular casts. Urinary protein excretion measured over 24 h increases during periods of activity. See the discussion under "Pathology" for a description of renal biopsy.

PREGNANCY Fertility rates are normal in patients with SLE, but spontaneous abortion and stillbirths are frequent (30 to 50 percent), especially in women with lupus anticoagulant and/or antibodies to cardiolipin. Treatment of women with prior fetal loss and antiphospholipid antibodies is controversial. Options are no intervention, daily low-dose aspirin until the last month of pregnancy, low-dose aspirin plus daily high-dose glucocorticoids, and twice-daily subcutaneous heparin in full anticoagulating doses; there are data to support each approach.

Pregnancy has varied effects on SLE activity. Disease flares in a small proportion, especially during the 6 weeks postpartum. If severe renal or cardiac disease is absent and SLE activity is controlled, most patients complete pregnancy safely and deliver normal infants. Glucocorticoids (except dexamethasone and betamethasone) are inactivated by placental enzymes and do not cause fetal abnormalities; they should be used to suppress disease activity. Neonatal lupus, caused by transmission of maternal anti-Ro antibodies across the placenta, consists of transient skin rash and (rarely) permanent heart block. Transient thrombocytopenia from maternal antiplatelet antibodies also occurs.

DIFFERENTIAL DIAGNOSIS The American Rheumatism Association published diagnostic criteria for SLE (see Table 284-3). Any four of the manifestations listed establish a diagnosis of SLE. Early disease confined to a few systems is more difficult to classify; it may take several years for a patient to fulfill criteria. Disorders with which SLE can be confused include rheumatoid arthritis; various forms of dermatitis; neurologic disorders such as epilepsy, multiple sclerosis, and psychiatric disorders; and hematologic diseases such as idiopathic thrombocytopenic purpura. Many autoimmune disorders have overlapping features, so exact classification may be difficult. Mixed connective tissue disease has features of SLE, rheumatoid arthritis, polymyositis, and scleroderma, accompanied by high titers of anti-RNP antibodies (Chap 287); patients have a low incidence of nephritis and CNS disease and a high incidence of pulmonary manifestations and evolution into scleroderma. Therapy should be directed toward the dominant manifestations in each patient. The possibility of drug-induced lupus should always be considered.

DRUG-INDUCED LUPUS Several drugs can cause a syndrome resembling SLE, including procainamide, hydralazine, isoniazid, chlorpromazine, D-penicillamine, practolol, methyldopa, quinidine, alpha interferon, and possibly hydantoins, ethosuximide, and oral contraceptives. The syndrome is rare with all but procainamide, the most frequent offender, and hydralazine. There is genetic predisposition to drug-induced lupus, partly determined by drug acetylation rates. Procainamide induces ANAs in 50 to 75 percent of individuals within a few months; hydralazine induces ANAs in 25 to 30 percent. Ten to 20 percent of ANA-positive individuals develop lupus-like symptoms. Most common are systemic complaints and arthralgias; polyarthritis and pleuropericarditis occur in 25 to 50 percent. Renal and CNS diseases are rare. All patients have ANAs, and most have antibodies to histones. Antibodies to dsDNA and hypocomplementemia are rare—a helpful point in distinguishing drug-induced from idiopathic lupus. Anemia, leukopenia, lupus anticoagulant, anticardiolipin antibodies, thrombocytopenia, cryoglobulins, rheumatoid factors, and false-positive VDRL and positive direct Coombs' tests can occur. The initial therapeutic approach is withdrawal of the offending drug; most patients improve in a few weeks. If symptoms are severe, a short course (2 to 10 weeks) of glucocorticoids is indicated. Symptoms rarely persist more than 6 months; ANAs may persist for years. Most lupus-inducing drugs can be used safely in patients with idiopathic SLE.

PROGNOSIS Survival in patients with SLE is approximately 70 percent over 10 years. Survival is lowest in nonwhite patients, low socioeconomic groups, and patients with severe involvement of kidneys, brain, lungs, or heart. Disability is common. Infection and renal failure are the leading causes of death.

TREATMENT There is no cure for SLE. Complete remissions are rare. Therefore, patient and physician should plan (1) to control acute, severe flares and (2) to develop maintenance strategies in which symptoms are suppressed to an acceptable level, usually at the cost of some drug side effects. Approximately 25 percent of LE patients have mild disease with no life-threatening manifestations, although pain and fatigue may be disabling. These patients should be managed without glucocorticoids. Arthralgias, arthritis, myalgias, fever, and mild serositis may improve on nonsteroidal anti-inflammatory drugs (NSAIDS) including salicylates. However, NSAID toxicities such as elevated liver enzymes, aseptic meningitis, and renal impairment are especially frequent in SLE. The dermatitides of SLE and, occasionally, lupus arthritis may respond to antimalarials. Doses of 400 mg hydroxychloroquine daily may improve skin lesions in a few weeks. Side effects are uncommon and include retinal toxicity, rash, myopathy, and neuropathy. Regular ophthalmologic examinations should be performed at least annually, since retinal toxicity is related to cumulative dose. Other therapies for rash include sunscreens (an SPF rating of 15 or higher is recommended), topical or intralesional glucocorticoids, quinacrine, retinoids, and dapsone. Systemic glucocorticoids should be reserved for patients with severe lesions unresponsive to other measures.

Life-threatening, severely disabling manifestations of SLE that are responsive to immunosuppression should be treated with high doses of *glucocorticoids* (1 to 2 mg/kg per day). When disease is active, glucocorticoids should be given in divided doses every 8 to 12 h. After the disease is controlled, therapy should be consolidated to one morning dose; thereafter, the daily dose should be tapered as rapidly as clinical disease permits. Ideally, patients should be slowly converted to alternate-day therapy with a single morning dose of short-acting glucocorticoid (prednisone, prednisolone, methylprednisolone) to minimize side effects. However, the disease may flare on the day off steroids, in which case the lowest single daily dose that suppresses disease should be used. Undesirable effects of chronic glucocorticoid therapy include cushingoid habitus, weight gain, hypertension, infection, capillary fragility, acne, hirsutism, accelerated osteoporosis, ischemic necrosis of bone, cataracts, glaucoma, diabetes mellitus, myopathy, hypokalemia, irregular menses, irritability, insomnia, and psychosis. Prednisone doses of 15 mg daily (or less) given before noon usually do not suppress the hypothalamic pituitary axis. Some side effects can be minimized; hyperglycemia, hypertension, edema, and hypokalemia should be treated; infections should be identified and treated early; immunizations with influenza and pneumococcal vaccines are safe and should be given if disease is stable. To minimize osteoporosis, supplemental calcium (1000 mg daily) should be added in most patients; in those with 24-h urinary calcium excretion < 120 mg, vitamin D 50,000 units one to three times weekly can be added (monitor for hypercalcemia), and estrogen replacement therapy should be considered at menopause. Calcitonin and bisphosphonates also may be useful. Acutely ill lupus patients, including those with proliferative GN, can be treated with 3 to 5 days of 1000-mg intravenous "pulses" of methylprednisolone, followed by maintenance daily or alternate-day glucocorticoids. Disease is probably controlled more rapidly by this approach, but it is unclear whether long-term outcome is changed.

The use of *cytotoxic agents* (azathioprine, chlorambucil, cyclophosphamide) in SLE is probably beneficial in controlling active disease, reducing the rate of disease flares, and reducing steroid requirements. Patients with lupus nephritis have significantly less renal failure if treated with combinations of glucocorticoids plus cyclophosphamide; azathioprine as the second drug is less beneficial but is also effective. However, overall survival is not different, probably because renal failure usually leads to dialysis or transplantation rather than to death. Undesirable side effects of cytotoxic drugs include bone marrow suppression, increased infection with opportunistic organisms such as herpes zoster, irreversible ovarian failure, hepatotoxicity (azathioprine), bladder toxicity (cyclophoshamide), alopecia, and increased risk for malignancy. Azathioprine is the least toxic; recommended doses are 2 to 3 mg/kg per day orally. Cyclophosphamide is the most effective and the most toxic. Intravenous pulse doses (10 to 15 mg/kg) once every 4 weeks have less urinary bladder toxicity than daily oral doses, but bone marrow suppression can be severe. Cyclophosphamide also can be used in daily oral doses (1.5 to 2.5 mg/kg per day of each). After disease activity has been controlled for a few months, tapering of cytotoxic agents and attempts to discontinue them are appropriate.

Some manifestations of SLE do not respond to immunosuppression, including clotting disorders, some behavioral abnormalities, and end-stage GN. Anticoagulation is the therapy of choice for prevention of clotting; chronic warfarin therapy is effective in preventing venous clotting and possibly in reducing arterial clotting; the effects of aspirin and heparin on arterial thrombosis are unclear. Psychoactive drugs should be used when appropriate. "Pure" membranous GN may not respond to immunosuppression; several weeks of therapy can be tried but should be abandoned if improvement is not obvious. The survival of lupus patients on dialysis or after transplantation is similar to that of patients with other forms of GN in most series.

Several experimental therapies are being studied, including plasma-pheresis accompanied by intravenous cyclophosphamide, cyclosporine, intravenous gamma globulin, total lymph node irradiation, fish oil, and antibodies to T lymphocytes.

REFERENCES

ARNETT FC: The genetic basis of lupus erythematosus, in *Dubois' Lupus Erythematosus*, 4th ed, D Wallace, BH Hahn (eds). Philadelphia, Lea & Febiger, 1992

AUSTIN HA III et al: Prognostic factors in lupus nephritis. Am J Med 75:382, 1983

BALOW JE et al: NIH Conference: Lupus nephritis (includes treatment). Ann Intern Med 106:79, 1987

CALLEN JP: Treatment of cutaneous lesions in patients with lupus erythematosus. Dermatol Clin 8:355, 1990

EBLING FM, HAHN BH: Pathogenic subsets of antibodies to DNA. Int Rev Immunol 5:79, 1989

GINZLER E, SCHORN AK: Outcome and prognosis in systemic lupus erythematosus. Rheum Dis Clin North Am 14:67, 1988

KIMBERLY RP: Treatment: Corticosteroids and anti-inflammatory drugs. Rheum Dis Clin North Am 14:2, 1988

NAKAMURA RM, TAN EM: Update on autoantibodies to intracellular antigens in systemic rheumatic diseases. Clin Lab Med 12:1, 1992

NOSSENT HC et al: Systemic lupus erythematosus after renal transplantation: Patient and graft survival and disease activity. Ann Intern Med 114:183, 1991

SAMMARITANO LR, GHARAVI AE: Antiphospholipid antibody syndrome. Clin Lab Med 12:41, 1992

STEINBERG AD et al: Systemic lupus erythematosus: NIH Conference (pathogenesis). Ann Intern Med 115:548, 1991

285 RHEUMATOID ARTHRITIS

PETER E. LIPSKY

Rheumatoid arthritis (RA) is a chronic multisystem disease of unknown cause. Although there are a variety of systemic manifestations, the characteristic feature of RA is persistent inflammatory synovitis, usually involving peripheral joints in a symmetric distribution. The potential of the synovial inflammation to cause cartilage destruction and bone erosions and subsequently joint deformities is the hallmark of the disease. Despite its destructive potential, the course of RA can be quite variable. Some patients may experience only a mild oligoarticular illness of brief duration with minimal joint damage, while others will have a relentless progressive polyarthritis with marked joint deformity. Most patients will experience an intermediate course.

EPIDEMIOLOGY AND GENETICS The prevalence of RA is approximately 1 percent of the population (range 0.3 to 2.1 percent); women are affected approximately three times more often than men. The prevalence increases with age, and sex differences diminish in the older age group. RA is seen throughout the world and affects all races. However, the incidence and severity seem to be less in rural sub-Saharan Africa. The onset is most frequent during the fourth and fifth decades of life, with 80 percent of all patients developing the disease between the ages of 35 and 50. The incidence of RA is more than six times as great in 60- to 64-year-old women compared to 18- to 29-year-old women.

Family studies indicate a genetic predisposition. For example, severe RA is found at approximately four times the expected rate in first-degree relatives of individuals with seropositive disease; approximately 10 percent of patients with RA will have an affected first-degree relative. Moreover, monozygotic twins are at least four times more likely to be concordant for RA than dizygotic twins, who have a similar risk of developing RA as nontwin siblings. The role of genetic influences in the etiology of RA was established by the demonstration of an association with the class II major histocompatibility complex gene product HLA-DR4. As many as 70 percent of patients with classic or definite RA express HLA-DR4 compared with 28 percent of control individuals. An association with HLA-DR4 has been noted in many populations, including North American and European whites, African-Americans, Chippewa Indians, Japanese, and native populations in India, Mexico, South America, and southern China. In a number of groups, including Israeli Jews, Asian Indians, and Yakima Indians of North America, however, there is no association between the development of RA and HLA-DR4. In these individuals, there is an association between RA and HLA-DR1 in the former two groups and HLA-Dw16 in the latter. Molecular analysis of HLA-DR antigens has provided insight into these apparently disparate findings. The HLA-DR molecule is composed of two chains, a nonpolymorphic α chain and a highly polymorphic β chain. Allelic variations in the HLA-DR molecule reflect differences in the amino acids of the β chain, with the major amino acid changes occurring in the three hypervariable regions of the molecule. Each of the HLA-DR molecules that is associated with RA has the same or a very similar sequence of amino acids in the third hypervariable region of the β chain of the molecule (Table 285-1). Thus the β chains of the HLA-DR molecules associated with RA, including HLA-Dw4 (DRβ1*0401), HLA-Dw14 (DRβ1*0404), HLA-Dw15 (DRβ1*0405), HLA-DR1 (DRβ1*0101), and HLA-Dw16 (DRβ1*1402), contain the same amino acids at positions 67 through 74, with the exception of a single change of one basic amino acid for another (arginine → lysine) in position 71 of HLA-Dw4. All other HLA-DR β chains have amino acid changes in this region that alter either their charge or hydrophobicity. These results indicate that a particular amino acid sequence in the third hypervariable region of the HLA-DR molecule is a major genetic element conveying

TABLE 285-1 Amino acid sequence of the third hypervariable region of the β chains of HLA-DR alleles associated with rheumatoid arthritis

HLA-DR	β chain	Amino acid*								Associated with rheumatoid arthritis
		67	68	69	70	71	72	73	74	
DR4/Dw4	β1*0401	L	L	E	Q	K	R	A	A	+
DR4/Dw14	β1*0404	–	–	–	–	R	–	–	–	+
DR4/Dw15	β1*0405	–	–	–	–	R	–	–	–	+
DR1	β1*0101	–	–	–	–	R	–	–	–	+
Dw16	β1*1402	–	–	–	–	R	–	–	–	+
DR4/Dw10	β1*0402	I	–	–	D	E	–	–	–	–
DR4/Dw13	β1*0403	–	–	–	–	R	–	–	E	–

* Single-letter amino acid code

susceptibility to RA, regardless of whether it occurs in HLA-DR4, HLA-Dw16, or HLA-DR1. Since this region of the HLA-DR molecule is involved in selection of the CD4+ T cell repertoire during development in the thymus and also in the presentation of antigenic peptides to CD4+ T cells in the periphery, it is possible that the association between particular HLA-DR molecules and RA may be explained by the capacity of CD4+ T cells of individuals expressing these HLA-DR determinants to recognize an antigen that initiates the disease process. The lack of association of HLA-DR4 and RA in certain populations is explained by the major member of the DR4 family found in that population. HLA-DR4 is a family of closely related, serologically defined molecules, including HLA-Dw4, -Dw10, -Dw13, and -Dw15. Different members of the HLA-DR family of molecules are found to predominate in different ethnic groups. Thus, in HLA-DR4–positive North American whites, HLA-Dw4 and -Dw14 are the most frequent, whereas HLA-Dw15 is most frequent in Japanese and southern Chinese. Each of these is associated with RA. By contrast, HLA-Dw10, which is not associated with RA and contains nonconservative amino acid changes in positions 70 and 71 of the β chain, is most common is Israeli Jews. Therefore, HLA-DR4 is not associated with RA in this population.

Additional genes in the HLA-D complex also may convey susceptibility to RA. The haplotype HLA-DR4, DQw7 may be associated with more severe manifestations of RA, including Felty's syndrome, although this could reflect linkage disequilibrium with the HLA-Dw4 subtype of DR4, whereas pulmonary involvement in RA is associated with HLA-DR4. It has been estimated, however, that HLA genes contribute only a portion of the genetic susceptibility to RA. Thus genes outside the HLA complex also contribute. These include genes controlling the expression of the antigen receptor on T cells and both immunoglobulin heavy and light chains.

Genetic risk factors do not fully account for the incidence of RA, suggesting that environmental factors also play a role in the etiology of the disease. This is emphasized by epidemiologic studies in Africa that have indicated that climate and urbanization have a major impact on the incidence and severity of RA in groups of similar genetic background.

Besides an association between the development of RA and genes of the major histocompatibility complex, there appears to be a genetic predisposition for the development of certain toxic reactions induced by drugs used to treat RA. For example, the presence of the HLA-DR3 allele is highly associated with the development of side effects to gold therapy, including proteinuria, thrombocytopenia, and perhaps skin rash. Similarly, the presence of this allele appears to predispose to the development of proteinuria following therapy with D-penicillamine. In general, no association has been noted between HLA type and the response to therapy.

ETIOLOGY The cause of RA remains unknown. It has been suggested that RA might be a manifestation of the response to an infectious agent in a genetically susceptible host. Because of the worldwide distribution of RA, it has been hypothesized that the infectious organism is ubiquitous. A number of possible causative agents have been suggested, including *Mycoplasma*, Epstein-Barr virus, cytomegalovirus, parvovirus, and rubella virus, but convincing evidence that these or other infectious agents cause RA has not emerged. The process by which an infectious agent might cause chronic inflammatory arthritis also remains a matter of controversy. One possibility is that there is persistent infection of articular structures or retention of microbial products in the synovial tissues which generates a chronic inflammatory response. Alternatively, the microorganism or response to the microorganism might induce an immune response to components of the joint by altering its integrity and revealing antigenic peptides. In this regard, reactivity to type II collagen and heat shock proteins has been demonstrated. Another possibility is that the infecting microorganism might prime the host to cross-reactive determinants expressed on joint structures as a result of "molecular mimicry." Finally, products of infecting microorganisms might induce the disease. Recent work has focused on the possible role of "superantigens" produced by a number of microorganisms, including staphylococci, streptococci and *Mycoplasma arthritidis*. Superantigens are proteins with the capacity to bind to HLA-DR molecules and particular Vβ segments of the heterodimeric T cell receptor and stimulate specific T cells expressing the Vβ gene products (see Chap. 277). The role of superantigens in the etiology of RA remains speculative.

Other potential etiologic mechanisms in RA include a breakdown in normal self-tolerance leading to reactivity to self-antigens in the joint, such as type II collagen, or loss of immunoregulatory control mechanisms resulting in polyclonal T cell activation.

PATHOLOGY AND PATHOGENESIS Microvascular injury and an increase in the number of synovial lining cells appear to be the earliest lesions in rheumatoid synovitis. The nature of the insult causing this response is not known. Subsequently, an increased number of synovial lining cells is seen along with perivascular infiltration with mononuclear cells. As the process continues, the synovium becomes edematous and protrudes into the joint cavity as villous projections.

Light-microscopic examination discloses a characteristic constellation of features which include hyperplasia and hypertrophy of the synovial lining cells; focal or segmental vascular changes, including microvascular injury, thrombosis, and neovascularization; edema; and infiltration with mononuclear cells, often collected into aggregates around small blood vessels. The endothelial cells of the rheumatoid synovium have the appearance of high endothelial venules (HEV) of lymphoid organs and have been altered by cytokine exposure to facilitate entry of cells into tissue. Rheumatoid synovial endothelial cells express increased amounts of various adhesion molecules involved in this process. Although this pathologic picture is typical of RA, it also can be seen in a variety of other chronic inflammatory arthritides. The mononuclear cell collections are variable in composition and size. The predominant infiltrating cell is the T lymphocyte. CD4+ T cells (helper-inducer) predominate over CD8+ T cells (suppressor-cytotoxic) and are frequently found in close proximity to HLA-DR+ macrophages and dendritic cells. An increased number of a separate population of T cells expressing the γδ form of the T cell receptor also has been found in the synovium, but their role in RA has not been delineated. Analysis of T cells in synovial fluid has documented an enrichment in CD29, CD45RO-expressing memory CD4+ T cells and a marked reduction in the number of CD45RA-expressing naive CD4+ T cells. In addition, the CD8+ T cells are largely of the cytotoxic and not the suppressive phenotype. Besides the accumulation of T cells, rheumatoid synovitis is also characterized by the infiltration of large numbers of B cells that differentiate locally into antibody-producing plasma cells. These cells produce both polyclonal immunoglobulin and the autoantibody rheumatoid factor that results in the local formation of immune complexes.

Although the etiologic stimuli have not been identified, established rheumatoid synovitis is characterized by persistent immunologic activity. The infiltrating T cells appear to be activated, since they express activation antigens such as HLA-DR. In addition, they express an increased density of molecules, such as leukocyte function associated antigen 1 (LFA-1, CD11a/CD18), that have been implicated in a variety of cell-to-cell interactions, including binding of circulating cells to postcapillary venules just prior to entry into sites of tissue inflammation. Finally, the T cells appear to have proliferated locally in the synovial tissue, perhaps in response to sequestered antigen, since they express determinants such as very late antigen-1 (VLA-1) that appears on T cells only after prolonged proliferation. Evidence of B cell activation also can be found in the inflamed synovium, and plasma cells producing immunoglobulin and rheumatoid factor are characteristic features of rheumatoid synovitis. Large numbers of macrophages with an activated phenotype are also found in rheumatoid synovium.

The rheumatoid synovium is characterized by the presence of a number of secreted products of activated lymphocytes, macrophages, and other cell types. The local production of these cytokines appears to account for many of the pathologic and clinical manifestations of RA. Table 285-2 lists cytokines that have been identified in rheumatoid synovial fluid and indicates their putative role in the rheumatoid inflammatory process. These cytokines include those that are derived from T lymphocytes such as interleukin 2 (IL-2), IL-6, granulocyte-macrophage colony stimulating factor (GM-CSF), tumor necrosis factor α, and transforming growth factor β; those originating from activated macrophages, including IL-1, tumor necrosis factor α, IL-6, IL-8, GM-CSF, macrophage CSF, platelet-derived growth factor, insulin-like growth factor, and transforming growth factor β; as well as those secreted by other cell types in the synovium, such as fibroblasts and endothelial cells, including IL-1, IL-6, IL-8, GM-CSF, and macrophage CSF. The activity of these cytokines appears to account for many of the features of rheumatoid synovitis, including the synovial tissue inflammation, synovial fluid inflammation, synovial proliferation, and cartilage and bone damage, as well as the systemic manifestations of RA. In addition to the production of cytokines that propagate the inflammatory process, local factors are produced that tend to slow the inflammation, including specific inhibitors of cytokine action and additional cytokines, such as transforming growth factor β, which inhibits many of the features of rheumatoid synovitis including T cell activation and proliferation, B cell differentiation, and migration of cells into the inflammatory site.

These findings have suggested that the propagation of RA is an immunologically mediated event, although the original initiating stimulus has not been characterized. One view is that the inflammatory process in the tissue is driven by the CD4+ helper-inducer T cells infiltrating the synovium. Evidence for this includes (1) the predominance of CD4+ T cells in the synovium, (2) the increase in soluble IL-2 receptors, a product of activated T cells, in blood and synovial fluid of patients with active RA, and (3) amelioration of the disease by removal of T cells by thoracic duct drainage or peripheral lymphapheresis or suppression of their function by total lymphoid irradiation. In addition, administration of monoclonal antibodies directed at T cells or the CD4+ T cell subset has been shown to suppress rheumatoid inflammation in some patients. Finally, patients with established RA who become infected with the human immunodeficiency virus (HIV) also have been noted to improve. T lymphocytes produce a number of cytokines, including interferon-γ and GM-CSF, that can lead to activation of macrophages and also increased expression of HLA molecules. Moreover, T lymphocytes produce a variety of cytokines that promote B cell proliferation and differentiation into antibody-forming cells and therefore also may promote local B cell stimulation. The resultant production of immunoglobulin and rheumatoid factor can lead to immune-complex formation with consequent complement activation and exacerbation of the inflammatory process by the production of the anaphylatoxins, C3a and C5a, and the chemotactic factor C5a. The tissue inflammation is reminiscent of delayed-type hypersensitivity reactions occurring in response to soluble antigens or microorganisms. It is, however, unclear whether this represents a response to a persistent exogenous antigen or to altered autoantigens such as collagen, immunoglobulin, or one of the heat shock proteins. Alternatively, it could represent persistent responsiveness to activated autologous cells such as might occur as a result of Epstein-Barr virus infection or persistent response to a foreign antigen or superantigen in the synovial tissue. Finally, rheumatoid inflammation could reflect persistent stimulation of T cells by synovial-derived antigens that cross-react with determinants introduced during antecedent exposure to foreign antigens or infectious microorganisms.

Overriding the chronic inflammation in the synovial tissue is an acute inflammatory process in the synovial fluid. The exudative synovial fluid contains more polymorphonuclear leukocytes than mononuclear cells. A number of mechanisms play a role in stimulating the exudation of synovial fluid. Locally produced immune complexes can activate complement and generate anaphylatoxins and chemotactic factors. Local production by mononuclear phagocytes of factors such as IL-1, tumor necrosis factor α (TNF-α), and leukotriene B$_4$, as well as products of complement activation, can stimulate the endothelial cells of postcapillary venules to become more efficient at binding circulating cells, whereas TNF-α, IL-8, C5a, and leukotriene B$_4$ stimulate the migration of polymorphonuclear leukocytes into the synovial site. In addition, vasoactive mediators such as histamine produced by the mast cells that infiltrate the rheumatoid synovium also may facilitate the exudation of inflammatory cells into the synovial fluid. Finally, the vasodilatory effects of locally produced prostaglandin E$_2$ also may facilitate entry of inflammatory cells into the inflammatory site. Once in the synovial fluid, the polymorphonuclear leukocytes can ingest immune complexes, with the resultant production of reactive oxygen metabolites and other inflammatory mediators, further adding to the inflammatory milieu. Locally produced cytokines such as TNF-α, IL-8, and GM-CSF can additionally stimulate polymorphonuclear leukocytes. The production of large amounts of cyclooxygenase and lipoxygenase pathway products of arachidonic acid metabolism by cells in the synovial fluid and tissue further accentuates the signs and symptoms of inflammation.

TABLE 285-2 Cytokines in rheumatoid inflammation

Manifestation	Cytokine involved
1 Synovial tissue inflammation	
a Increased adherence of postcapillary venules	IL-1, TNF-α, IFN-γ
b Chemotaxis of T cells	IL-8
c T cell activation and proliferation	IL-1, TNF-α, IL-6, IL-2
d B cell differentiation and antibody formation	IL-1, TNF-α, IL-6, IL-2, IFN-γ
e Increased expression of HLA antigens	IFN-γ, TNF-α, GM-CSF
f Macrophage activation	IFN-γ, GM-CSF, M-CSF, IL-2
2 Synovial fluid inflammation	
a Increased adherence of postcapillary venules	IL-1, TNF-α, IFN-γ
b Chemotactic for PMN	TNF-α, IL-8
c Activation of PMN	TNF-α, GM-CSF, IL-8
3 Synovial proliferation	
a Fibroblast growth	PDGF, IL-1, IGF, FGF, TGF-β, EGF
b Neovascularization	TNF-α, FGF, TGF-β
4 Cartilage and bone damage	
a Activation of chondrocytes	IL-1, TNF-α
b Activation of fibroblasts	IL-1, TNF-α
c Activation of osteoblasts-osteoclasts	IL-1, TNF-α
5 Systemic manifestations	
a Fever, constitutional symptoms	IL-1, TNF-α
b Acute phase reactants	IL-1, TNF-α, IL-6

NOTE: IL-1, interleukin 1; IL-2, interleukin 2; IL-6, interleukin 6; TNF-α, tumor necrosis factor α; IFN-γ, interferon-γ; GM-CSF, granulocyte-macrophage colony stimulating factor; M-CSF, macrophage colony stimulating factor; PDGF, platelet-derived growth factor; PMN, polymorphonuclear cells; IGF, insulin-like growth factor; FGF, fibroblast growth factor; TGF-β, transforming growth factor β; EGF, epidermal growth factor.

The precise mechanism by which bone and cartilage destruction occurs has not been completely resolved. Although the synovial fluid contains a number of enzymes potentially able to degrade cartilage, the majority of destruction occurs in juxtaposition to the inflamed synovium, or pannus, that spreads to cover the articular cartilage. This vascular granulation tissue is composed of proliferating fibroblasts, small blood vessels, and a variable number of mononuclear cells and produces a large amount of degradative enzymes, including collagenase and stromelysin, that may facilitate tissue damage. The cytokines IL-1 and tumor necrosis factor α play an important role by stimulating the cells of the pannus to produce collagenase and other neutral proteases. These same two cytokines also activate chondrocytes in situ, stimulating them to produce proteolytic enzymes that can degrade cartilage locally. Finally, these two cytokines may contribute to the local demineralization of bone by activating osteoclasts. Prostaglandin E_2 produced by fibroblasts and macrophages also may contribute to bone demineralization. Systemic manifestations of RA can be accounted for by release of inflammatory effector molecules from the synovium. These include IL-1, TNF-α, and IL-6, which account for many of the manifestations of active RA, including malaise, fatigue, and elevation of serum acute phase reactants. In addition, immune complexes produced within the synovium and entering the circulation may account for other features of the disease, such as systemic vasculitis.

CLINICAL MANIFESTATIONS   Onset   Characteristically, RA is a chronic polyarthritis. In approximately two-thirds of patients, it begins insidiously with fatigue, anorexia, generalized weakness, and vague musculoskeletal symptoms until the appearance of synovitis becomes apparent. This prodrome may persist for weeks or months and defy diagnosis. Specific symptoms usually appear gradually as several joints, especially those of the hands, wrists, knees, and feet, become affected in a symmetric fashion. In approximately 10 percent of individuals, the onset is more acute, with a rapid development of polyarthritis, often accompanied by constitutional symptoms, including fever, lymphadenopathy, and splenomegaly. In approximately one-third of patients, symptoms may initially be confined to one or a few joints. Although the pattern of joint involvement may remain asymmetric in a few patients, a symmetric pattern is more typical.

Signs and symptoms of articular disease   Pain, swelling, and tenderness may initially be poorly localized to the joints. Pain in affected joints, aggravated by movement, is the most common manifestation of established RA. It corresponds in pattern to the joint involvement but does not always correlate with the degree of apparent inflammation. Generalized stiffness is frequent and is usually greatest after periods of inactivity. Morning stiffness of greater than 1-h duration is an almost invariable feature of inflammatory arthritis and serves to distinguish it from various noninflammatory joint disorders. The length and intensity of the stiffness can be used as a crude assessment of disease activity. The majority of patients will experience constitutional symptoms such as weakness, easy fatigability, anorexia, and weight loss. Although fever to 40°C occurs on occasion, temperature elevation in excess of 38°C is unusual and suggests the presence of an intercurrent problem such as infection.

Clinically, synovial inflammation causes swelling, tenderness, and limitation of motion. Warmth is usually evident on examination, especially of large joints such as the knee, but erythema is infrequent. Pain originates predominantly from the joint capsule, which is abundantly supplied with pain fibers and is markedly sensitive to stretching or distention. Joint swelling results from accumulation of synovial fluid, hypertrophy of the synovium, and thickening of the joint capsule. Initially, motion is limited by pain. The inflamed joint is usually held in flexion to maximize joint volume and minimize distention of the capsule. Later, fibrous or bony ankylosis or soft tissue contractures lead to fixed deformities.

Although inflammation can affect any diarthrodial joint, RA most often causes symmetric arthritis with characteristic involvement of certain specific joints such as the proximal interphalangeal and metacarpophalangeal joints. The distal interphalangeal joints are rarely involved. Synovitis of the wrist joints is a nearly uniform feature of RA and may lead to limitation of motion, deformity, and median nerve entrapment (carpal tunnel syndrome). Synovitis of the elbow joint often leads to flexion contractures that may develop early in the disease. The knee joint is commonly involved with synovial hypertrophy, chronic effusion, and frequently ligamentous laxity. Pain and swelling behind the knee may be caused by extension of inflamed synovium into the popliteal space (Baker's cyst). Arthritis in the forefoot, ankles, and subtalar joints can produce severe pain with ambulation as well as a number of deformities. Axial involvement is usually limited to the upper cervical spine. Involvement of the lumbar spine is not seen, and lower back pain cannot be ascribed to rheumatoid inflammation. On occasion, inflammation from the synovial joints and bursae of the upper cervical spine leads to atlantoaxial subluxation. This usually presents as pain in the occiput but on rare occasions may lead to compression of the spinal cord.

With persistent inflammation, a variety of characteristic deformities develop. These can be attributed to a number of pathologic events, including laxity of supporting soft tissue structures; destruction or weakening of ligaments, tendons, and the joint capsule; cartilage destruction; muscle imbalance; and unopposed physical forces associated with the use of affected joints. Characteristic deformities of the hand include (1) radial deviation at the wrist with ulnar deviation of the digits often with palmar subluxation of the proximal phalanges (''Z'' deformity), (2) hyperextension of the proximal interphalangeal joints, with compensatory flexion of the distal interphalangeal joints (swan-neck deformity), (3) flexion deformity of the proximal interphalangeal joints and extension of the distal interphalangeal joints (boutonnière deformity), and (4) hyperextension of the first interphalangeal joint and flexion of the first metacarpophalangeal joint with a consequent loss of thumb mobility and pinch. Typical deformities also may develop in the feet, including eversion at the hindfoot (subtalar joint), plantar subluxation of the metatarsal heads, widening of the forefoot, hallux valgus, and lateral deviation and dorsal subluxation of the toes.

Extraarticular manifestations   RA is a systemic disease with a variety of extraarticular manifestations. Although these occur frequently, not all of them have clinical significance. However, on occasion, they may be the major evidence of disease activity and source of morbidity and require management per se. As a rule, these manifestations occur in individuals with high titers of autoantibodies to the Fc component of immunoglobulin G (rheumatoid factors).

Rheumatoid nodules develop in 20 to 30 percent of persons with RA. They are usually found on periarticular structures, extensor surfaces, or other areas subjected to mechanical pressure, but they can develop elsewhere, including the pleura and meninges. Common locations include the olecranon bursa, the proximal ulna, the Achilles tendon, and the occiput. Nodules vary in size and consistency and are rarely symptomatic, but on occasion they break down as a result of trauma or become infected. They are found almost invariably in individuals with circulating rheumatoid factor. Histologically, rheumatoid nodules consist of a central zone of necrotic material including collagen fibrils, noncollagenous filaments, and cellular debris, a midzone of palisading macrophages that express HLA-DR antigens, and an outer zone of granulation tissue. Examination of early nodules has suggested that the initial event may be a focal vasculitis.

Clinical weakness and atrophy of skeletal muscle are common. Muscle atrophy may be evident within weeks of the onset of RA and usually is most apparent in musculature approximating affected joints. Muscle biopsy may show type II fiber atrophy and muscle fiber necrosis with or without a mononuclear cell infiltrate.

Rheumatoid vasculitis (see Chap. 291) which can affect nearly any organ system is seen in patients with severe RA and high titers of circulating rheumatoid factor. Rheumatoid vasculitis is very uncommon in African Americans. In its most aggressive form, rheumatoid vasculitis can cause polyneuropathy and mononeuritis multiplex, cutaneous ulceration and dermal necrosis, digital gangrene, and visceral infarction. While such widespread vasculitis is very rare, more limited forms are not uncommon, especially in white patients with high titers of rheumatoid factor. Neurovascular disease presenting either as a mild distal sensory neuropathy or as mononeuritis multiplex may be the only sign of vasculitis. Cutaneous vasculitis usually presents as crops of small brown spots in the nail beds, nail folds, and digital pulp. Larger ischemic ulcers, especially in the lower extremity, also may develop. Myocardial infarction secondary to rheumatoid vasculitis has been reported, as has vasculitic involvement of lungs, bowel, liver, spleen, pancreas, lymph nodes, and testes. Renal vasculitis is rare.

Pleuropulmonary manifestations, which are more commonly observed in men, include pleural disease, interstitial fibrosis, pleuropulmonary nodules, pneumonitis, and arteritis. Evidence of pleuritis is found commonly at autopsy, but symptomatic disease during life is infrequent. Typically, the pleural fluid contains very low levels of glucose in the absence of infection. Pleural fluid complement is also low compared with the serum level when these are related to the total protein concentration. Pulmonary fibrosis can produce impairment of the diffusing capacity of the lung. Pulmonary nodules may appear singly or in clusters. When they appear in individuals with pneumoconiosis, a diffuse nodular fibrotic process (Caplan's syndrome) may develop. On occasion, pulmonary nodules may cavitate and produce a pneumothorax or bronchopleural fistula. Rarely, pulmonary hypertension secondary to obliteration of the pulmonary vasculature occurs. In addition to pleuropulmonary disease, upper airway obstruction from cricoarytenoid arthritis or laryngeal nodules may develop.

Clinically apparent heart disease attributed to the rheumatoid process is rare, but evidence of asymptomatic pericarditis is found at autopsy in 50 percent of cases. Pericardial fluid has a low glucose level and is frequently associated with the occurrence of pleural effusion. Although pericarditis is usually asymptomatic, on rare occasions death has occurred from tamponade. Chronic constrictive pericarditis also may occur.

RA tends to spare the central nervous system directly, although vasculitis can cause peripheral neuropathy. *Neurologic manifestations* also may result from atlantoaxial or midcervical spine subluxations. Nerve entrapment secondary to proliferative synovitis or joint deformities may produce neuropathies of median, ulnar, radial (interosseous branch), or anterior tibial nerves.

The rheumatoid process involves the *eye* in less than 1 percent of patients. Affected individuals usually have long-standing disease and nodules. The two principal manifestations are episcleritis, which is usually mild and transient, and scleritis, which involves the deeper layers of the eye and is a more serious inflammatory condition. Histologically, the lesion is similar to a rheumatoid nodule and may result in thinning and perforation of the globe (scleromalacia perforans). Fifteen to twenty percent of persons with RA may develop Sjögren's syndrome with attendant keratoconjunctivitis sicca.

Felty's syndrome consists of chronic RA, splenomegaly, neutropenia, and on occasion anemia and thrombocytopenia. It is most common in individuals with long-standing disease. These patients frequently have high titers of rheumatoid factor, subcutaneous nodules, and other manifestations of systemic rheumatoid disease. Felty's syndrome is very uncommon in African Americans. It may develop after joint inflammation has regressed. Circulating immune complexes are often present, and evidence of complement consumption may be seen. The leukopenia is a selective neutropenia with polymorphonuclear leukocyte counts of less than 1500 cells per microliter and sometimes less than 1000 cells per microliter. Bone marrow examination usually reveals moderate hypercellularity with a paucity of mature neutrophils. However, the bone marrow may be normal, hyperactive, or hypoactive; maturation arrest may be seen. Hypersplenism has been proposed as one of the causes of leukopenia, but splenomegaly is not invariably found and splenectomy does not always correct the abnormality. Excessive margination of granulocytes caused by antibodies to these cells, complement activation, or binding of immune

complexes may contribute to granulocytopenia. Patients with Felty's syndrome have increased frequency of infections usually associated with neutropenia. The cause of the increased susceptibility to infection is related to the defective function of polymorphonuclear leukocytes as well as the decreased number of cells.

Osteoporosis secondary to rheumatoid involvement is common and may be aggravated by corticosteroid therapy. Corticosteroid treatment may cause significant loss of bone mass, especially early in the course of therapy, even when low doses are employed. Osteopenia involves both juxtaarticular bone and long bones distant from involved joints. RA is associated with a modest decrease in mean bone mass and a moderate increase in the risk of fracture. Bone mass appears to be adversely affected by functional impairment and active inflammation, especially early in the course of the disease.

LABORATORY FINDINGS   No tests are specific for diagnosing RA. However, rheumatoid factors, which are autoantibodies reactive with the Fc portion of IgG, are found in more than two-thirds of adults with the disease. Widely utilized tests largely detect IgM rheumatoid factors. The presence of rheumatoid factor is not specific for RA. Rheumatoid factor is found in 5 percent of healthy persons. The frequency of rheumatoid factor in the general population increases with age, and 10 to 20 percent of individuals over 65 years old have a positive test. In addition, a number of conditions besides RA are associated with the presence of rheumatoid factor. These include systemic lupus erythematosus, Sjögren's syndrome, chronic liver disease, sarcoidosis, interstitial pulmonary fibrosis, infectious mononucleosis, hepatitis B, tuberculosis, leprosy, syphilis, subacute bacterial endocarditis, visceral leishmaniasis, schistosomiasis, and malaria. In addition, rheumatoid factor may appear transiently in normal individuals after vaccination or transfusion and also may be found in relatives of individuals with RA.

The presence of rheumatoid factor does not establish the diagnosis of RA but can be of prognostic significance because patients with high titers tend to have more severe and progressive disease with extraarticular manifestations. Rheumatoid factor is uniformly found in patients with nodules or vasculitis. The predictive value of the presence of rheumatoid factor in determining a diagnosis of RA is poor. Thus less than one-third of unselected patients with a positive test for rheumatoid factor will be found to have RA. The test is not useful as a screening procedure but can be employed to confirm a diagnosis in individuals with a suggestive clinical presentation and, if present in high titer, to designate patients at risk for severe systemic disease.

Normochromic, normocytic anemia is frequently present in active RA. It is thought to reflect ineffective erythropoiesis; large stores of iron are found in the bone marrow. In general, anemia and thrombocytosis correlate with disease activity. The white blood cell count is usually normal, but a mild leukocytosis may be present. Leukopenia also may exist without the full-blown picture of Felty's syndrome. Eosinophilia, when present, usually reflects severe systemic disease.

The erythrocyte sedimentation rate is increased in nearly all patients with active RA. A variety of other acute phase reactants including ceruloplasmin and C-reactive protein are also elevated, and generally such elevations correlate with disease activity and the likelihood of progressive joint damage.

Synovial fluid analysis confirms the presence of inflammatory arthritis, although none of the findings is specific. The fluid is usually turbid, with reduced viscosity, increased protein content, and a slightly decreased or normal glucose concentration. The white cell count varies between 5 and 50,000 cells per microliter; polymorphonuclear leukocytes predominate. Total hemolytic complement, C3, and C4 are markedly diminished in synovial fluid relative to total protein concentration as a result of activation of the classic complement pathway by locally produced immune complexes.

When monoclonal antibodies specific for T lymphocyte subsets are used to examine peripheral blood mononuclear cells of patients with RA, no specific changes in the numbers of circulating CD4 +

(helper-inducer) or CD8+ (suppressor-cytotoxic) T cells are noted. However, an increased number of circulating T cells expressing HLA-DR, an indication of T cell activation, can be observed. This finding is most frequent in patients with active joint disease.

RADIOGRAPHIC EVALUATION Early in the disease, roentgenograms of the affected joints are usually not helpful in establishing a diagnosis. They reveal only that which is apparent from physical examination, namely, evidence of soft tissue swelling and joint effusion. As the disease progresses, abnormalities become more pronounced, but none of the radiographic findings is diagnostic of RA. The diagnosis, however, is supported by a characteristic pattern of abnormalities, including the tendency toward symmetric involvement. Juxtaarticular osteopenia may become apparent within weeks of onset. Loss of articular cartilage and bone erosions develop after months of sustained activity. The primary value of radiography is to determine the extent of cartilage destruction and bone erosion produced by the disease, particularly when one is considering therapy with disease-modifying drugs or surgical intervention. Other means of imaging bones and joints, including ^{99m}Tc bisphosphonate bone scanning and magnetic resonance imaging, may be capable of detecting early inflammatory changes but are rarely necessary in the routine evaluation of patients with RA.

CLINICAL COURSE AND PROGNOSIS The course of RA is quite variable and difficult to predict in an individual patient. Most patients experience persistent but fluctuating disease activity, accompanied by a variable degree of joint deformity. After 10 to 12 years, fewer than 20 percent of patients will have no evidence of disability or deformity. Features of patients that predict the development of disability include older age, female sex, more severe radiographic involvement, and the presence of rheumatoid nodules or elevated titers of rheumatoid factor. The pattern of disease onset does not appear to predict the development of disabilities. Approximately 15 percent of patients with RA will have a short-lived inflammatory process that remits without major deformity.

Several features of patients with RA appear to have prognostic significance. Remissions of disease activity are most likely to occur during the first year. White females tend to have more persistent synovitis and more progressively erosive disease than males. Persons who present with high titers of rheumatoid factor, C-reactive protein, and haptoglobin also have a worse prognosis, as do individuals with subcutaneous nodules or radiographic evidence of erosions at the time of initial evaluation. Although sustained disease activity of more than 1 year's duration portends a poor outcome, the rate of progression of joint abnormalities is not constant; the greatest progression takes place during the first 6 years of disease and at a much slower rate thereafter. Indeed, the rate of progression of joint damage is greater during the first year of observation compared with the second and third years. Within 3 years of disease, as many as 70 percent of patients will have some radiographic evidence of damage to joints. Foot joints are affected more frequently than hand joints. Despite the decrease in the rate of progressive joint damage with time, functional disability, which develops early in the course of the disease, continues to worsen at the same rate.

The median life expectancy of persons with RA is shortened by 3 to 7 years. Of the 2.5-fold increase in mortality rate, RA itself is a contributing feature in 15 to 30 percent. The increased mortality rate seems to be limited to patients with more severe articular disease and can be attributed largely to infection and gastrointestinal bleeding. Drug therapy also may play a role in the increased mortality rate seen in these individuals. Factors correlated with early death include disability, disease duration or severity, corticosteroid use, age, and male sex.

DIAGNOSIS The diagnosis of RA is easily made in persons with typical established disease. In a majority of patients, the disease assumes its characteristic clinical features within 1 to 2 years of onset. The typical picture of bilateral symmetric inflammatory polyarthritis involving small and large joints in both the upper and lower extremities with sparing of the axial skeleton except the cervical spine suggests the diagnosis. Constitutional features indicative of the inflammatory nature of the disease, such as morning stiffness, support the diagnosis. Demonstration of subcutaneous nodules is a helpful diagnostic feature. Additionally, the presence of rheumatoid factor, inflammatory synovial fluid with increased numbers of polymorphonuclear leukocytes, and radiographic findings of juxtaarticular bone demineralization and erosions of the affected joints substantiate the diagnosis.

The diagnosis is somewhat more difficult early in the course when only constitutional symptoms or intermittent arthralgias or arthritis in an asymmetric distribution may be present. A period of observation may be necessary before the diagnosis can be established. A definitive diagnosis of RA depends predominantly on characteristic clinical features and the exclusion of other inflammatory processes. The isolated finding of a positive test for rheumatoid factor or an elevated erythrocyte sedimentation rate, especially in an older person with joint pains, should not itself be used as evidence of RA.

Recently, the American College of Rheumatology has developed revised criteria for the classification of rheumatoid arthritis (Table 285-3). The newer criteria are simpler to apply than the previous ones and demonstrate a sensitivity of 91 to 94 percent and a specificity of 89 percent when used to classify patients with RA compared with control subjects with rheumatic diseases other than RA. The major differences between the new and old criteria are that results of invasive procedures such as biopsies are not included, the classifications of probable, definite, and classic RA have been eliminated, and patients with more than a single diagnosis are not eliminated by exclusion criteria. Although these criteria were developed as a means of disease classification for epidemiologic purposes, they are useful as guidelines for establishing the diagnosis. Failure to meet these criteria, however, especially during the early stages of the disease, does not exclude the diagnosis.

TREATMENT General principles The goals of therapy of RA are (1) relief of pain, (2) reduction of inflammation, (3) preservation of functional capacity, (4) resolution of the etiopathogenic process, and (5) facilitation of healing. Currently available medications are capable of providing pain relief and some reduction in inflammation. Since the etiology of RA is unknown, the pathogenesis is speculative, and the mechanisms of action of many of the therapeutic agents employed are uncertain, therapy remain empirical. None of the therapeutic interventions are curative, and therefore, all must be viewed as palliative, aimed at relieving the signs and symptoms of

---

TABLE 285-3 The 1987 revised criteria for the classification of rheumatoid arthritis

1 Guidelines for classification

   a Four of seven criteria are required to classify a patient as having rheumatoid arthritis.

   b Patients with two or more clinical diagnoses are not excluded.

2 Criteria*

   a Morning stiffness: Stiffness in and around the joints lasting 1 h before maximal improvement.

   b Arthritis of three or more joint areas: At least three joint areas, observed by a physician simultaneously, have soft tissue swelling or joint effusions, not just bony overgrowth. The 14 possible joint areas involved are right or left proximal interphalangeal, metacarpophalangeal, wrist, elbow, knee, ankle, and metatarsophalangeal joints.

   c Arthritis of hand joints: Arthritis of wrist, metacarpophalangeal joint, or proximal interphalangeal joint.

   d Symmetric arthritis: Simultaneous involvement of the same joint areas on both sides of the body.

   e Rheumatoid nodules: Subcutaneous nodules over bony prominences, extensor surfaces, or juxtaarticular regions observed by a physician.

   f Serum rheumatoid factor: Demonstration of abnormal amounts of serum rheumatoid factor by any method for which the result has been positive in less than 5 percent of normal control subjects.

   g Radiographic changes: Typical changes of RA on posteroanterior hand and wrist radiographs which must include erosions or unequivocal bony decalcification localized in or most marked adjacent to the involved joints.

* Criteria *a–d* must be present for at least 6 weeks. Criteria *b–e* must be observed by a physician.

the disease. The various therapies employed are directed at nonspecific suppression of the inflammatory or immunologic process in the hope of ameliorating symptoms and preventing progressive damage to articular structures.

Management of patients with RA involves an interdisciplinary approach which attempts to deal with the various problems that these individuals encounter with functional as well as psychosocial interactions. A variety of physical therapy modalities may be useful in decreasing the symptoms of RA. Rest ameliorates symptoms and can be an important component of the total therapeutic program. In addition, splinting to reduce unwanted motion of inflamed joints may be useful. Exercise directed at maintaining muscle strength and joint mobility without exacerbating joint inflammation is also an important aspect of the therapeutic regimen. A variety of orthotic devices can be helpful in supporting and aligning deformed joints to reduce pain and improve function.

Medical management of RA involves three general approaches. The first is the use of aspirin and other nonsteroidal anti-inflammatory drugs, simple analgesics, and, if necessary, low-dose glucocorticoids to control the symptoms and signs of the local inflammatory process. These agents are rapidly effective at mitigating signs and symptoms, but they appear to exert minimal effect on the progression of the disease. The second line of therapy includes a variety of agents that have been classified as the disease-modifying or slow-acting antirheumatic drugs. These agents appear to have the capacity to decrease elevated levels of acute phase reactants in treated patients and, therefore, are thought to modify the destructive capacity of the disease. Other second-line agents are the immunosuppressive and cytotoxic drugs that have been shown to ameliorate the disease process in some patients. The third approach involves the use of a number of experimental modalities, such as total-lymphoid irradiation, lymphoplasmapheresis, the administration of the immunosuppressive agent cyclosporine, and the administration of monoclonal antibodies to T cells and T cell subsets. Although some show potential for ameliorating disease, none has been shown to be a safe and cost-effective way to treat patients on a long-term basis. Recently, substitution of dietary omega-6 essential fatty acids with omega-3 fatty acids such as eicosapentaenoic acid found in certain fish oils also has been shown to provide symptomatic improvement in patients with RA. A variety of nontraditional approaches also have been claimed to be effective in treating RA, including diets, plant and animal extracts, vaccines, hormones, and topical preparations of various sorts. Many of these are costly, and none has been shown to be effective. However, belief in their efficacy ensures their continued use by some patients.

Nonsteroidal anti-inflammatory drugs   Besides aspirin, there are now several additional nonsteroidal anti-inflammatory drugs (NSAIDs) available to treat RA. These include etodolac, fenoprofen, ibuprofen, indomethacin, ketoprofen, nabumetone, naproxen, meclofenamate, piroxicam, sulindac, tolmetin, diclofenac, oxaprozin, and flurbiprofen. As a result of the capacity of these agents to block the activity of the enzyme cyclooxygenase and therefore the production of prostaglandins, prostacyclin, and thromboxanes, they have analgesic, anti-inflammatory, and antipyretic properties. In addition, the agents may exert other anti-inflammatory effects. These agents are all associated with a wide spectrum of toxic side effects. Some, such as gastric irritation, azotemia, platelet dysfunction, and exacerbation of allergic rhinitis and asthma, are related to the inhibition of cyclooxygenase activity, while a variety of others, such as rash, liver function abnormalities, and bone marrow depression, may not be. Elderly patients on diuretics may be at higher risk for certain toxic effects. None of the NSAIDs has been shown to be more effective than aspirin in the treatment of RA. However, these nonaspirin drugs are associated with a lower incidence of gastrointestinal intolerance. None of the newer NSAIDs appears to show significant therapeutic advantages over the other available agents. In addition, there is no consistent advantage of any of these newer agents over the others with respect to the incidence or severity of toxic manifestations.

Disease-modifying antirheumatic drugs (DMARDs)   Clinical ex-

perience has delineated a number of agents that appear to have the capacity to alter the course of RA. This group of agents includes gold compounds, D-penicillamine, the antimalarials, and sulfasalazine. Despite having no chemical or pharmacologic similarities, in practice, these agents share a number of characteristics. They exert minimal direct nonspecific anti-inflammatory or analgesic effects, and therefore, NSAIDs must be continued during their administration, except in a few cases when true remissions are induced with them. The appearance of benefit from DMARD therapy is usually delayed for weeks or months. As many as two-thirds of patients develop some clinical improvement as a result of therapy with any of these agents, although the induction of true remissions is unusual. In addition to clinical improvement, there is frequently an improvement in serologic evidence of disease activity, and titers of rheumatoid factor and C-reactive protein and the erythrocyte sedimentation rate frequently decline. Despite this, there is minimal evidence that DMARDs actually retard the development of bone erosions or facilitate their healing.

Each of these drugs is associated with considerable toxicity, and therefore, careful patient monitoring is necessary. Which DMARD should be the drug of first choice remains controversial, and trials have failed to demonstrate a consistent advantage of one over the other. Toxicity of the various agents thus becomes important in determining the drug of first choice. Failure to respond or development of toxicity to one agent does not preclude responsiveness to another. For example, a similar percentage of RA patients who have failed to respond to gold will respond to D-pencillamine when it is given as the second disease-modifying drug.

No characteristic features of patients have emerged that predict responsiveness to a DMARD. Moreover, the indications for the initiation of therapy with one of these agents are not well defined, although recently the trend has been to begin DMARD therapy early in the course of the disease. There is no convincing evidence that therapy with multiple DMARDs is more effective than treatment with a single agent.

Glucocorticoid therapy   Although systemic glucocorticoid therapy can provide effective symptomatic therapy in patients with RA, these drugs should be avoided if possible because they do not alter the course of the disease and the potential toxicity of long-term therapy is substantial. Low-dose (less than 7.5 mg/d) prednisone has been advocated as useful additive therapy to control symptoms, but trials have not provided convincing evidence of efficacy. Monthly pulses with high-dose corticosteroids may be useful in some patients and may hasten the response when therapy with a DMARD is initiated.

Immunosuppressive therapy   The immunosuppressive drugs azathioprine and cyclophosphamide have been shown to be effective in the treatment of RA and to exert therapeutic effects similar to those of the DMARDs. However, these agents appear to be no more effective than the DMARDs. Moreover, they cause a variety of toxic side effects, and cyclophosphamide appears to predispose the patient to the development of malignant neoplasms. Therefore, these drugs have been reserved for patients who have clearly failed therapy with DMARDs. On occasion, extraarticular disease such as rheumatoid vasculitis may require cytotoxic immunosuppressive therapy.

The folic acid antagonist methotrexate, given in an intermittent low dose (7.5 to 15 mg once weekly), also may be useful in the treatment of RA. Recent trials have documented the efficacy of methotrexate and have indicated that its onset of action is more rapid than other DMARDs, and patients tend to remain on therapy with methotrexate longer than they remain on other DMARDs because of better clinical responses and less toxicity. Long-term trials have indicated that methotrexate does not induce remission, but rather suppresses symptoms while it is being administered. Maximal improvement is observed after 6 months of therapy, with little additional improvement thereafter. Major toxicity includes gastrointestinal upset, oral ulceration, and liver function abnormalities that appear to be dose-related and reversible and hepatic fibrosis that can be quite insidious, requiring liver biopsy for detection in its early stages. Drug-induced pneumonitis also has been reported. Because of its therapeutic benefit and toxicity profile, methotrexate is used before other second-line drugs by many rheumatologists.

Recent trials have suggested that cyclosporine also may be effective in the treatment of RA. Although high-dose therapy may induce rapid improvement, it is associated with frequent renal and gastrointestinal toxicity. Lower doses of cyclosporine (<5 mg/kg per day), however, appear to cause slower but nonetheless significant improvement in disease activity with fewer toxic side effects that are reversed upon lowering the dose. Currently, cyclosporine has not been approved for use in RA.

Surgery Surgery plays a role in the management of patients with severely damaged joints. Although arthroplasties and total joint replacements can be done on a number of joints, the most successful procedures are carried out on hips and knees. Realistic goals of these procedures are relief of pain, correction of deformity, and modest functional improvement. Reconstructive hand surgery may lead to cosmetic improvement and some functional benefit. Open or arthroscopic synovectomy may be useful in some patients with persistent monarthritis, especially of the knee. Although synovectomy may offer short-term relief of symptoms, there is no evidence that it retards bone destruction or the natural history of the disease. In addition, early tenosynovectomy of the wrist may prevent tendon rupture.

Approach to the patient with RA At the onset of disease it is difficult to predict the natural history of an individual patient's illness. Therefore, the usual approach is to attempt to alleviate the patient's symptoms with NSAIDs. Some patients may have mild disease that requires no additional therapy. Since the DMARDs are potentially toxic and not universally effective, their use is usually delayed until it is apparent that symptoms cannot be controlled adequately with NSAIDs.

At some time during most patients' course, the possibility of initiating second-line therapy is entertained. With aggressive disease this might occur sooner, often within 1 to 3 months of diagnosis, whereas in patients with more indolent disease, smoldering activity may not require such therapy for many years. The development of bone erosions or radiographic evidence of cartilage loss is clear-cut evidence of the destructive potential of the inflammatory process and indicates the need for second-line drug therapy. The other indications, such as persistent pain, joint swelling, or functional impairment, are much more subjective, however. The decision to begin use of a second-line drug requires careful monitoring of joint swelling and functional activity, as well as an understanding of the patient's pain tolerance and expectation of therapy. In this setting, the fully informed patient must play an active role in the decision to begin second-line drug therapy, after careful review of the therapeutic and toxic potential of the various drugs.

If a patient responds to a second-line drug, therapy is continued with careful monitoring to avoid toxicity. All second-line drugs provide a suppressive effect and therefore require prolonged administration. Even with successful therapy, local injection of glucocorticoids may be necessary to diminish inflammation that may persist in a limited number of joints. In addition, NSAIDs may be necessary to mitigate symptoms. Even after inflammation has totally resolved, symptoms from loss of cartilage and supervening degenerative joint disease or deformities may require additional treatment. Surgery also may be necessary to relieve pain or diminish the functional impairment secondary to deformity. Only when patients have persistent inflammatory disease or severe extraarticular manifestations is the use of cytotoxic immunosuppressive drugs or experimental procedures justified. Recently an alternative approach to treat patients with RA has been suggested. This involves the initiation of therapy with multiple agents early in the course of disease in an attempt to control inflammation, followed by maintenance on one or more agents as necessary to control disease activity. The effectiveness of this therapeutic alternative has not been proven.

REFERENCES

ARNETT FC et al: The American Rheumatism Association 1987 revised criteria for the classification of rheumatoid arthritis. Arthritis Rheum 31:315, 1988

BOERS M, RAMSDEN M: Long-acting drug combinations in rheumatoid arthritis: A formal overview. J Rheumatol 18:316, 1991

BROOKS PM, DAY RO: Nonsteroidal anti-inflammatory drugs: Differences and similarities. N Engl J Med 324:1716, 1991

CUSH J, LIPSKY PE: Cellular basis for rheumatoid inflammation. Clin Orthop 265:9, 1991

FELSON DT et al: The comparative efficacy and toxicity of second-line drugs in rheumatoid arthritis. Arthritis Rheum 33:1449, 1990

GREGERSEN PK et al: The shared epitope hypothesis. Arthritis Rheum 30:1205, 1987

HARRIS ED JR: Rheumatoid arthritis: Pathophysiology and implications for therapy. N Engl J Med 322:1277, 1990

KAVANAUGH AF, LIPSKY PE: Gold, penicillamine, antimalarials and sulfasulazine, in Inflammation: Basic Principles and Clinical Correlates, 2d ed, JI Gallin et al (eds). New York, Raven, 1992, pp 1083–1101

KREMER JM, PHELPS CT: Long-term prospective study of the use of methotrexate in the treatment of rheumatoid arthritis. Arthritis Rheum 35:138, 1992

LAAN RFJM: Bone mass in patients with rheumatoid arthritis. Ann Rheum Dis 51:826, 1992

LEIGH JP, FRIES JF: Mortality predictors among 263 patients with rheumatoid arthritis. J Rheumatol 18:1307, 1991

NEPOM GT et al: The molecular basis for HLA class II associations with rheumatoid arthritis. J Clin Immunol 7:1, 1987

OCHI T et al: Effect of early synovectomy on the course of rheumatoid arthritis. J Rheumatol 18:1794, 1991

TUGWELL P et al: Low-dose cyclosporine versus placebo in patients with rheumatoid arthritis. Lancet 335:1051, 1990

VAN DER HEIJDE DMFM et al: Biannual radiographic assessments of hands and feet in a three-year prospective followup of patients with early rheumatoid arthritis. Arthritis Rheum 35:26, 1992

WEINBLATT ME et al: Long-term prospective study of methotrexate in the treatment of rheumatoid arthritis: 84-month update. Arthritis Rheum 35:129, 1992

WOLFE F, CATHEY MA: The assessment and prediction of functional disability in rheumatoid arthritis. J Rheumatol 18:1298, 1991

WORDSWORTH P, BELL J: Polygenic susceptibility in rheumatoid arthritis. Ann Rheum Dis 50:343, 1991

286 SYSTEMIC SCLEROSIS (SCLERODERMA)

BRUCE C. GILLILAND

DEFINITION Systemic sclerosis (SSc) is a multisystem disorder of unknown cause characterized by fibrosis of the skin, blood vessels, and visceral organs, including the gastrointestinal tract, lungs, heart, and kidneys. The degree and rate of skin and internal organ involvement vary among patients. Two subsets, however, can be identified, even though there is some overlap. One subset is referred to as *diffuse cutaneous scleroderma* and is characterized by the rapid development of symmetric skin thickening of proximal and distal extremity, face, and trunk. These patients are at greater risk for developing kidney and other visceral disease early in their course. The other subset is *limited cutaneous scleroderma*, which is defined by symmetric skin thickening limited to distal extremities and face. This subset frequently has features of CREST syndrome, an acronym standing for calcinosis, Raynaud's phenomenon, esophageal dysmotility, sclerodactyly, and telangiectasia. The prognosis in limited cutaneous scleroderma is better except for the occasional patient who, after many years, develops pulmonary arterial hypertension or biliary cirrhosis. Systemic sclerosis of visceral organs also may occur in the absence of any skin involvement, which is referred to as *systemic sclerosis without scleroderma*. Survival is determined by the severity of visceral disease, especially involving the heart, lungs, and/or kidneys.

Scleroderma also can occur in a localized form limited to the skin, subcutaneous tissue, and muscle and without systemic involvement. The two localized forms are morphea, which occurs as single or multiple plaques of skin induration, and linear scleroderma, which involves an extremity or face.

SSc also occurs in association with features of other connective tissue diseases. The term *overlap syndrome* has been used to describe such patients. *Undifferentiated connective tissue disease* has been suggested as a designation for patients who do not have diagnostic criteria for any one connective tissue disease. *Mixed connective tissue disease* is a syndrome involving features of systemic lupus erythematosus, systemic sclerosis, polymyositis, and rheumatoid arthritis and very high titers of circulating antibody to nuclear ribonucleoprotein antigen (see Chap. 287). *Eosinophilic fasciitis* and the *eosinophilia-myalgia syndrome* associated with L-tryptophan ingestion are scleroderma-like illnesses and will be discussed in this chapter.

EPIDEMIOLOGY SSc has a worldwide distribution and affects all races. The onset of disease is usually in the third to fifth decade, and the incidence increases with age. Women are affected approximately three times as often as men, and even more often during the childbearing years. The onset of scleroderma in childhood is unusual. The annual incidence has been estimated to be 14.1 cases per million population based on a 20-year study performed in Allegheny County, Pennsylvania. The role of heredity has not been clarified. Several examples of familial SSc have been reported, and the finding of other connective tissue diseases and autoantibodies in relatives of involved patients suggests a hereditary predisposition. Some studies have shown an association of SSc with DR1, DR3, and DR5.

Several environmental factors have been associated with the development of SSc and scleroderma-like illnesses. SSc appears to be more common in coal and gold miners, especially in those with more extensive exposure, suggesting that silica dust may be a predisposing factor. Workers exposed to polyvinyl chloride may develop Raynaud's phenomenon, acroosteolysis, scleroderma-like skin lesions, and nailfold capillary abnormalities similar to those observed in SSc. These workers also may develop hepatic fibrosis and angiosarcoma. The development of scleroderma has been associated with exposure to vinyl chloride, epoxy resins, and aromatic hydrocarbons such as benzine and toluene. In 1981, in Spain, a multisystem disease resembling scleroderma occurred following the ingestion of adulterated cooking oil (rapeseed oil). Approximately 20,000 people were affected. The patients initially develop interstitial pneumonitis, eosinophilia, arthralgias, arthritis, and myositis, followed subsequently by joint contractures, skin thickening, Raynaud's phenomenon, pulmonary hypertension, sicca syndrome, and resorption of the distal fingertips. Extensive sclerosis of the dermis and subcutaneous tissue has been noted in patients receiving pentazocine, a nonnarcotic analgesic agent. Bleomycin, an anticancer agent, produces fibrotic skin nodules, linear hyperpigmentation, alopecia, gangrene of fingers, and pulmonary fibrosis affecting mainly the lower lobes. Scleroderma and other connective tissue diseases have been reported in women who have had silicone breast implants. At present, the evidence is not conclusive that women with these implants carry an increased risk for developing scleroderma or other connective tissue diseases. Localized fibrosis, however, can occur around the implant. The development of a scleroderma-like illness has been associated with the ingestion of products containing L-tryptophan and is referred to as the *eosinophilia-myalgia syndrome* (see Chap. 384).

PATHOGENESIS The outstanding feature of SSc is overproduction and accumulation of collagen and other extracellular matrix proteins in skin and other organs. While the pathogenesis of SSc remains to be further elucidated, the disease process involves immunologic mechanisms, vascular damage, and activation of fibroblasts.

An early event in SSc that precedes fibrosis is vascular damage involving small arteries, arterioles, and capillaries in the skin, gastrointestinal tract, kidneys, heart, and lungs. Raynaud's phenomenon, the initial symptom of SSc in the majority of patients, is a clinical expression of this damage. Endothelial cell injury occurs early and is followed by thickening of the intima, narrowing of the lumen, and eventual obliteration of the vessel. As vascular damage progresses, the microvascular bed in the skin and other sites is diminished, producing a state of chronic ischemia. Vascular damage can be observed in the nailfolds by wide-field microscopy, which shows drop-out of capillaries with dilatation and tortuosity of remaining ones. In the skin, remaining capillaries may proliferate and dilate to become visible telangiectasia.

Several mechanisms for endothelial injury in SSc patients have been proposed. In the sera of some patients an endothelial cytotoxic factor has been found and identified as a serine protease present in granules of activated T cells. The sera of some patients mediate antibody-dependent cellular cytotoxicity directed against human endothelial cells. Circulating antiendothelial antibodies, present in some patients, may be yet another mechanism for cell injury. Tumor necrosis factor also can induce endothelial injury as well as stimulate fibrosis. Endothelial cell damage is reflected by elevated levels of factor VIII/von Willebrand factor in the sera of many but not all patients with SSc. The binding of von Willebrand factor to subendothelium mediates platelet activation with release of factors that alter vascular permeability, leading to edema. Activated platelets also release platelet-derived growth factor (PDGF), which is chemotactic and mitogenic for both smooth-muscle cells and fibroblasts, and transforming growth factor β (TGF-β), which stimulates fibroblast collagen synthesis. These and other cytokines stimulate intimal fibrosis and with their passage through the injured endothelium also could account for adventitial and perivascular fibrosis. Endothelial damage along with a deficiency of tissue plasminogen activator factor enhances intravascular coagulation and, when extensive, can lead to microangiopathic hemolytic anemia observed in those patients at risk for developing acute renal failure.

Existing evidence indicates that cell-mediated immunity plays an important role in the development of fibrosis. Perivascular and diffuse mononuclear infiltrates consisting predominantly of T cells and monocytes are found in macroscopically normal appearing skin adjacent to areas of skin fibrosis. The T cells in these infiltrates are mostly helper T cells (CD4). Elevated levels of circulating interleukin 2 (IL-2), IL-2 receptors, and CD4 antigens are found in SSc patients, indicating activation of helper T cells. In early SSc, elevated levels of circulating IL-2 and IL-2 receptors have been shown to be associated with disease progression. The CD4+/CD8+ T cell ratio is increased in peripheral blood of SSc patients due usually to an increase number of CD4+ T cells and a decrease number of CD8+ T cells. Laminin and type IV collagen, components of the endothelial basement membrane, induce in vitro transformation of lymphocytes from SSc patients, suggesting that the target of cell-mediated immunity might be endothelium. Increased levels of circulating IL-1 and tumor necrosis factor in SSc patients indicate in vivo activation of monocytes. These two cytokines have been shown to stimulate fibroblasts. Additional support for involvement of cell-mediated immunity in the pathogenesis of SSc is the appearance of scleroderma-like lesions in patients with graft-versus-host disease (GVHD) after bone marrow transplantation and in a murine model of chronic GVHD, conditions known to be associated with activated T cells. Mast cells also may be involved in the development of fibrosis. Increased numbers of mast cells are found in the dermis in both involved and uninvolved skin. Mast cell degranulation has been noted in skin that subsequently became fibrosed. Interaction with T cells may be one mechanism for mast cell degranulation resulting in release of products that stimulate fibroblast collagen synthesis. Release of histamine from mast cells also may contribute to edema observed in early disease.

Humoral immune abnormalities are also present in patients with SSc. Antinuclear antibodies are found in approximately 95 percent of patients (see "Laboratory Findings," below), and antibodies to type IV collagen and laminin may be present. The role of these antibodies in the pathogenesis of SSc is not presently understood.

Regulatory mechanisms control fibroblast growth and synthesis of collagen, fibronectin, and glycosaminoglycans. Compared with fibroblasts from normal persons, the fibroblasts from SSc appear to have aberrant regulation of growth. When fibroblasts from affected SSc skin are removed and cultured in vitro, they continue to produce excessive quantities of collagen. The collagen is biochemically normal, and the proportion of type I to type III is the same as in normal skin. Fibroblasts from SSc patients appear to be in a state of permanent activation most likely as a result of stimulation by cytokines. These activated cells are thought to represent an expanded subpopulation of fibroblasts that inherently express increased matrix genes. Studies have revealed a subpopulation of SSc fibroblasts that produces two to three times more collagen than other cells from the same tissue. Fibroblasts expressing elevated levels of messenger RNA for types I and III collagen have been demonstrated by in situ hybridization particularly around dermal blood vessels in affected SSc skin. A small number of fibroblasts expressed increased levels of mRNA for type VI collagen. Platelet-derived growth factor receptors are expressed on SSc fibroblasts on cells not only from affected areas but also from macroscopically normal appearing skin. Fibroblasts from normal persons lack expression of these receptors. TGF-β has been shown to upregulate the expression of these receptors in SSc fibroblasts but not in normal cells and, in conjunction with PDGF, stimulates SSc fibroblast proliferation. Macrophages and fibroblasts are capable of secreting PDGF and TGF-β, and activated T cells release TGF-β.

Fibroblasts may activate T cells to release cytokines that stimulate fibrosis. Fibroblasts in SSc patients have been shown to have increased expression of an adhesion molecule which facilitates binding of T cells. This binding allows interaction between T cell antigen receptor and class II molecules and antigen on fibroblasts resulting in T cell activation and cytokine release. T cells also may be activated by their interaction with extracellular matrix molecules.

Chromosomal abnormalities have been noted in greater than 90 percent of SSc patients. These acquired abnormalities include chromatid breaks, acentric fragments, and ring chromosomes and are found in approximately 30 percent of mitotic cells. A chromosomal breakage factor has been found in the serum of SSc patients and their first-degree relatives. A recent study has shown that chromosome breaks are associated with the HLA haplotype A1, B8, and DR3. The significance of these chromosomal abnormalities is unknown.

PATHOLOGY Skin In the skin, a thin epidermis overlies compact bundles of collagen which lie parallel to the epidermis. Finger-like projections of collagen extend from the dermis into the subcutaneous tissue and bind the skin to the underlying tissue. Dermal appendages are atrophied, and rete pegs are lost. In early stages of disease, increased numbers of T cells, monocytes, plasma cells, and mast cells are found, particularly in the lower dermis of involved skin.

Gastrointestinal tract In the lower two-thirds of the esophagus, the histologic findings consist of a thin mucosa and increased collagen in the lamina propria, submucosa, and serosa. The degree of fibrosis is less than in the skin. Atrophy of the muscularis in the esophagus and throughout the involved portions of the gastrointestinal tract is more prominent than the amount of fibrotic replacement of muscle. Ulceration of the mucosa is often present and may be due to either SSc or superimposed peptic esophagitis. Striated muscles in the upper third of the esophagus are relatively spared. Similar changes may be found throughout the gastrointestinal tract, especially in the second and third portions of the duodenum, in the jejunum, and large intestine. Atrophy of the muscularis of the large intestine may lead to the development of large-mouth diverticula. In the later stages of the disease, the involved portions of the gastrointestinal tract become dilated. Infiltration of lymphocytes and plasma cells in the lamina propria is also present.

Lung With pulmonary involvement, diffuse interstitial fibrosis, thickening of the alveolar membrane, and peribronchial fibrosis are observed. Bronchiolar epithelial proliferation accompanies the pulmonary fibrosis. Rupture of septa produces small cysts and areas of bullous emphysema. Small pulmonary arteries and arterioles show intimal thickening, fragmentation of the elastica, and muscular hypertrophy; this may occur without interstitial pulmonary fibrosis and produce pulmonary hypertension.

Musculoskeletal system The synovium in patients with arthritis is similar to that seen in early rheumatoid arthritis and shows edema with infiltration of lymphocytes and plasma cells. A characteristic finding is a thick layer of fibrin overlying and within the synovium. Later in the disease the synovium may become fibrotic. Fibrinous deposits appear on the surfaces of tendon sheaths and in the overlying fascia and may lead to audible creaking over moving tendons.

Histologic features of primary myopathy consist of interstitial and perivascular lymphocytic infiltrations, degeneration of muscle fibers, and interstitial fibrosis. Arterioles may be thickened, and capillaries may be decreased in number. Pathologic and electrophysiologic findings of polymyositis in proximal muscles are present in the few patients who are considered to have the overlap syndrome of SSc and polymyositis.

Heart Cardiac involvement consists of degeneration of myocardial fibers and irregular areas of interstitial fibrosis that are most prominent around blood vessels. Fibrosis also involves the conduction system, leading to atrioventricular conduction defects and arrhythmias. The wall of smaller coronary arteries may be thickened. Fibrinous pericarditis and pericardial effusions are found in some patients.

Kidney Renal involvement is found in over half the patients and consists of intimal hyperplasia of the interlobular arteries, fibrinoid necrosis of the afferent arterioles, including the glomerular tuft, and thickening of the glomerular basement membrane. Small cortical infarctions and glomerulosclerosis may be present. The renal pathologic change is often indistinguishable from that observed in malignant hypertension. Renal vascular lesions, however, may be present in the absence of hypertension. Immunofluorescence studies of kidney have shown IgM, complement components, and fibrinogen in the walls of affected vessels. Angiographic renal studies in patients with SSc may show constriction of the intralobular arteries, a finding that simulates the vasospasm of the digital arteries observed in Raynaud's phenomenon. Cold-induced Raynaud's phenomenon has been shown to decrease renal blood flow.

Other organs Primary liver involvement is not common. Primary biliary cirrhosis occurs in some patients, particularly in those with the limited cutaneous form of SSc. Fibrosis of the thyroid gland may develop in the presence or absence of autoimmune thyroiditis.

Thickening of the periodontal membrane with replacement of the lamina dura is demonstrated radiographically as widening of the periodontal space and rarely causes loosening of the teeth.

CLINICAL MANIFESTATIONS Raynaud's phenomenon Systemic sclerosis usually begins insidiously; the first symptoms are frequently Raynaud's phenomenon and puffy fingers. Ninety-five percent of patients will experience Raynaud's phenomenon, which is defined as episodic vasoconstriction of small arteries and arterioles of fingers, toes, and sometimes the tip of the nose and earlobes. Episodes are brought on by cold exposure, vibration, or emotional stress. Patients experience pallor and/or cyanosis followed by rubor on rewarming. Pallor and/or cyanosis is usually associated with coldness and numbness of fingers and/or toes, and rubor with pain and tingling. Not all patients appreciate the three color phases. A history of digit pallor appears to be the most reliable symptom for the presence of Raynaud's phenomenon. Raynaud's phenomenon may precede skin changes by several months or even years in those patients who subsequently develop the limited cutaneous form of SSc. After 2 or more years of Raynaud's phenomenon, few patients who have this as their only symptom will subsequently develop SSc.

Skin features In early disease, fingers and hands are swollen. Swelling also may involve forearms, feet, lower legs, and face. However, lower extremities are relatively spared. This edematous phase may last for a few weeks, months, or even longer. The edema may be pitting or nonpitting. The skin gradually becomes firm, thickened, and eventually tightly bound to underlying subcutaneous tissue (indurative phase). In patients with diffuse cutaneous scleroderma, skin changes will become generalized and involve the extremities, face, and trunk. Rapid progression of these changes over a 2- to 3-year period is associated with a greater risk of visceral disease, particularly of the lungs, heart, or kidneys. On the other hand, patients with limited cutaneous scleroderma will usually have a more gradual progression of skin changes which are restricted to fingers or distal extremity and face. After many years of disease, the skin may soften and return to normal thickness or become thin and atrophic.

In the extremities, the taut skin over fingers gradually limits full extension, and flexion contractures develop. Ulcers may appear on the volar pads of the fingertips and over bony prominences such as elbows, malleoli, and the extensor surface of the proximal interphalangeal joints of the hands. These ulcers may become secondarily infected. The volar pads of the fingertips develop pitting scars and lose soft tissue. In some instances, resorption of the terminal phalanges occurs. Skin over the extremities, face, and trunk may become darkly pigmented, even without exposure to the sun. Pigmentation of the skin may occur over superficial blood vessels and tendons. The skin loses hair, oil, and sweat glands and so becomes dry and coarse. Vaginal dryness occurs and may cause dyspareunia.

In some patients, particularly those with the limited cutaneous form of disease, calcific deposits develop in intracutaneous and subcutaneous tissue. The sites commonly involved are periarticular tissue, digital pads, olecranon and prepatellar bursae, and skin along the extensor surface of the forearms. The overlying skin may break down, with drainage of calcific material. Involvement of the face results in loss of skin wrinkles and facial expression, as well as microstomia, which may make eating and dental hygiene difficult. The capillary beds of nailfolds of the fingers may show enlargement of capillaries with little or no capillary loss, usually indicative of limited cutaneous scleroderma. In diffuse cutaneous scleroderma, there is disorganization of the capillary beds with dilated capillaries interspersed with areas where capillaries have disappeared. These capillary changes, which are observed by wide-angle microscopy or with an ophthalmoscope used as a magnifier, are not found in patients who have only Raynaud's phenomenon.

Musculoskeletal features   More than half the patients with SSc complain of pain, swelling, and stiffness of the fingers and knees. Symptoms of carpal tunnel syndrome may occur. A symmetric polyarthritis resembling rheumatoid arthritis may be seen. In more advanced stages of the disease, leathery crepitation can be palpated over moving joints, especially the knee. Extensive fibrotic thickening of the tendon sheaths in the wrist can produce a carpal tunnel syndrome. Muscle weakness usually is present in patients with severe skin involvement and, in most cases, is due to disuse atrophy. There is a distinctive histologic myopathy that accompanies SSc which is not associated with muscle enzyme abnormalities. A few patients develop a myositis characterized by proximal muscle weakness and muscle enzyme elevations that are identical to polymyositis (overlap syndrome). In addition to terminal phalanges, resorption of bone may involve ribs, clavicle, and angle of mandible.

Gastrointestinal features   Symptoms attributable to esophageal involvement are present in more than 50 percent of patients and include epigastric fullness, burning pain in the epigastric or retrosternal regions, and regurgitation of gastric contents. These symptoms, most noticeable when the patient is lying flat or bending over, are due to the reduced tone of the gastroesophageal sphincter and to dilatation of the distal esophagus. Peptic esophagitis frequently occurs and may lead to strictures and narrowing of the lower esophagus. However, it seldom results in bleeding. Dysphagia, particularly of solid foods, may occur independent of other esophageal symptoms and is caused by loss of esophageal motility due to neuromuscular dysfunction. Manometry or cineradiography reveals decreased amplitude or disappearance of peristaltic waves in the lower two-thirds of the esophagus.

Raynaud's phenomenon in the absence of a connective tissue disease is also associated with esophageal dysmotility. Later in the course of the illness, dilatation and atony of the lower portion of the esophagus as well as reflux are seen. With gastric involvement, barium studies show dilatation, atony, and delayed gastric emptying.

Hypomotility of the small intestine produces symptoms of bloating and abdominal pain and may suggest an intestinal obstruction or paralytic ileus (pseudoobstruction). Malabsorption syndrome with weight loss, diarrhea, and anemia is due to bacterial overgrowth in the atonic intestine or possibly to obliteration of lymphatics by fibrosis. Roentgenographic features of the second and third portions of the duodenum and of the jejunum include dilatation, loss of the usual feathery pattern, and delayed disappearance of barium. Pneumatosis intestinalis occasionally occurs and appears as radiolucent cysts or linear streaks within the wall of the small intestine. Benign pneumoperitoneum may result from the rupture of these cysts. Involvement of the large intestine may cause chronic constipation and fecal impaction with episodes of bowel obstruction. A segment of atonic bowel may act as a fulcrum for intussuception to occur. Barium studies of the large intestine may show dilatation, atony, and large-mouth diverticula. Some patients may have gastrointestinal features of SSc with little or no cutaneous or other organ involvement.

Pulmonary features   The lungs are affected in SSc in at least two-thirds of the patients. The most common symptom is exertional dyspnea, often accompanied by a dry, nonproductive cough. Symptoms may occur in the absence of pulmonary fibrosis, and patients with pulmonary fibrosis can be relatively asymptomatic. Bilateral basilar rales may be present. Restriction of chest movement caused by extensive skin involvement of the thorax rarely occurs. Aspiration pneumonia may result from gastric reflux due to lower esophageal atony. Superimposed bacterial or viral pneumonia can be a serious complication in patients with pulmonary fibrosis. There is an increased frequency of alveolar cell and bronchogenic carcinoma in patients with pulmonary fibrosis. Pulmonary function tests are frequently abnormal and show a reduction in vital capacity and decreased lung compliance. Impairment of gas exchange is reflected by a low diffusing capacity and low P_{O_2} with exercise. These abnormalities may be present even when the chest radiograph is normal. Chest film may show a pattern of linear densities, mottling, and honeycombing involving most prominently the lower two-thirds of the lung. Early pulmonary disease can be detected by high-resolution computed tomography (HRCT) and bronchoalveolar lavage (BAL). The recovery by BAL of increased number of cells, mostly alveolar macrophages accompanied by neutrophils and eosinophils, is evidence for alveolitis. Treatment of alveolitis with drugs such as cyclophosphamide conceivably may be more effective when alveolitis is detected early, although this is not proven. In the absence of significant interstitial fibrosis, a severe form of pulmonary arterial hypertension develops after many years of disease in patients with limited cutaneous scleroderma. Less than 10 percent of patients will develop this complication, which is caused by narrowing and obliteration of pulmonary arteries and arterioles by intimal fibrosis and medial hypertrophy. Pulmonary hypertension is manifested by progressive worsening of dyspnea and eventually by the appearance of right-sided heart failure. Electrocardiographic evidence of pulmonary hypertension is usually present. The prognosis is extremely poor with the development of pulmonary hypertension; the mean duration of survival is approximately 2 years.

Cardiac features   Primary cardiac involvement in SSc includes pericarditis with or without effusions, heart failure, and varying degrees of heart block or arrhythmias. The majority of patients with diffuse cutaneous SSc have cardiac abnormalities. Cardiomyopathy attributable to myocardial fibrosis appears in fewer than 10 percent of patients and involves primarily those patients with diffuse cutaneous scleroderma. Radionuclide studies have shown abnormalities of left ventricular function due to myocardial fibrosis. Cold-induced vasospasm of the hands produces defects in myocardial thallium perfusion. The characteristic pathologic feature of contraction band necrosis results from cardiac muscle damage caused by intermittent vasospasm of coronary vessels. Patients may experience angina pectoris even though coronary angiograms are normal. Patients also can develop left ventricular failure secondary to systemic hypertension or cor pulmonale secondary to pulmonary arterial hypertension.

Renal features Renal failure is the leading cause of death in SSc, accounting for almost half the deaths. Significant renal disease occurs mostly in those patients with diffuse cutaneous scleroderma. A high risk of renal crisis is present in those patients who have rapidly progressive widespread skin thickening in their first 2 to 3 years of disease. Renal crisis is characterized by malignant hypertension, which can rapidly progress to renal failure. These patients manifest hypertensive encephalopathy, severe headache, retinopathy, seizures, and left ventricular failure. Hematuria and proteinuria are followed by oliguria and renal failure. The mechanism for the hypertensive crisis is activation of the renin-angiotensin system. Before the advent of effective antihypertensive drugs, the majority of these patients died within 6 months. A small number of patients may develop renal crises in the absence of hypertension. Renal failure also can develop insidiously later in the course of disease in the setting of mild to moderate hypertension and proteinuria. In these patients or those with clinically unrecognized renal disease, reduction of renal plasma flow secondary to heart failure or volume depletion resulting from overdiuresis may precipitate renal crisis. An indicator of impending renal failure is microangiopathic anemia, which may occur in a normotensive patient. The presence of a chronic pericardial effusion may also herald subsequent renal failure.

Other features Symptoms of dry eyes and/or dry mouth are frequently present in patients with SSc. Lip biopsy may show lymphocytic infiltration of minor salivary glands characteristic of Sjögren's syndrome or intraglandular or periglandular fibrosis. Antibodies to SS-A (Ro) and/or SS-B (La) are found in those patients with lip biopsies consistent with Sjögren's syndrome and not in those with salivary gland fibrosis.

Hypothyroidism occurs in a significant number of patients and may be associated with high levels of antithyroid antibodies. Fibrosis of the thyroid gland may be present but also occurs in the absence of autoimmune thyroiditis. Other manifestations of SSc include trigeminal neuralgia and male impotence secondary to decreased penile tumescence. These men have normal serum levels of testosterone and gonadotropins. Pathogenesis of this abnormality has been considered to be vascular and/or autonomic nervous system abnormalities.

LABORATORY FINDINGS The erythrocyte sedimentation rate may be elevated. Hypoproliferative anemia related to chronic inflammation is the most common cause of anemia in SSc. Anemia also may be caused by iron deficiency secondary to gastrointestinal bleeding. Bacterial overgrowth due to atony of the small bowel may lead to vitamin B_{12} and/or folic acid–deficiency anemia. Microangiopathic hemolytic anemia is most often associated with renal involvement and is caused by the presence of intravascular fibrin in renal arterioles. Hypergammaglobulinemia, consisting mostly of IgG, is found in approximately half the patients. Rheumatoid factor, in low titer, is present in 25 percent of patients. Antinuclear antibodies detected by using a cultured human laryngeal carcinoma cell line (HEp-2) substrate are present in 95 percent of patients. Antinuclear antibodies that have a high specificity for SSc are antitopoisomerase 1 (Scl-70), antinucleolar, and anticentromere. Antitopoisomerase 1, originally called anti-Scl-70, recognizes the nuclear enzyme DNA topoisomerase 1. These antibodies are found in about 20 percent of patients and are associated with diffuse cutaneous involvement and interstitial pulmonary disease. They are seldom present in other disorders or in conjunction with anticentromere antibodies. Antinucleolar antibodies are relatively specific for SSc and are present in approximately 20 to 30 percent of patients. Anticentromere antibodies react with protein antigens located in the kinetochore region of chromosomes and are strongly associated with limited cutaneous scleroderma or CREST syndrome. Anticentromere antibodies are found in only about 10 percent of patients with diffuse cutaneous

scleroderma and rarely in other connective tissue diseases. They are found occasionally in patients with only Raynaud's phenomenon and may indicate subsequent development of limited cutaneous disease. Several antinucleolar antibodies have been associated with SSc: Anti-RNA polymerase 1 is found in patients with diffuse cutaneous SSc who have a higher prevalence of renal and cardiac involvement, anti-Th has been found in patients with limited cutaneous SSc, and anti-PM-Scl, formerly referred to as anti-PM1, may be found in SSc patients with polymyositis and renal involvement. *Anti-U3 nucleolar RNP is also highly specific for SSc, is more frequent in African Americans, and is associated with skeletal muscle disease and pulmonary arterial hypertension*. High titers of anti-RNP are present in those patients with features of mixed connective tissue disease. Anti-SS-A and/or anti-SS-B are present in those patients with overlap syndrome of SSc and Sjögren's syndrome.

DIAGNOSIS The diagnosis of SSc presents no difficulty in the presence of Raynaud's phenomenon, with typical skin lesions and visceral involvement. Although Raynaud's phenomenon may be the first symptom of SSc, most patients with Raynaud's phenomenon alone do not develop a connective tissue disease. Other causes of Raynaud's phenomenon include thoracic outlet (scalenus anticus and cervical rib) syndromes, shoulder-hand syndrome, trauma (jackhammer or vibratory machine operators), previous cold injury, vinyl chloride exposure, and circulating cryoglobulins or cold agglutinins. Linear scleroderma and morphea are localized forms of scleroderma that can usually be distinguished clinically. In early disease, SSc may initially be confused with rheumatoid arthritis, systemic lupus erythematosus, or polymyositis when articular or muscle involvement is prominent. SSc without cutaneous involvement should be considered in patients with unexplained pulmonary fibrosis, pulmonary hypertension, cardiomyopathies, heart block, dysphagia, or malabsorption syndrome. Several conditions have scleroderma-like features but lack the visceral involvement. Scleredema (scleredema adultorum of Buschke) occurs predominantly in children and is characterized by painless edematous induration involving the face, scalp, neck, trunk, and proximal portions of the extremities. Involvement of the hands and feet usually does not occur. Scleredema may be associated with previous streptococcal infection and is usually self-limited, resolving in 6 to 12 months. Histology reveals accumulation of mucopolysaccharides in the dermis and skeletal muscle. A rare entity, scleromyxedema (lichen myxedematosus), is manifested by yellowish or pale red papules in association with diffuse skin thickening which may involve the face and hands. Acid mucopolysaccharide deposits are found in the dermis. Monoclonal IgG may be detected in some of these patients. Primary amyloidosis may involve the skin of the extremities and face diffusely to give the appearance of scleroderma. Biopsy will clearly differentiate these entities.

COURSE AND PROGNOSIS The course of SSc is quite variable. Until disease differentiates into recognizable subsets, prognosis in early disease is difficult to predict. Patients with limited cutaneous scleroderma, especially those with anticentromere antibodies, have a good prognosis, with the notable exception of those few patients, less than 10 percent, who after 10 to 20 years or longer develop pulmonary arterial hypertension. Malabsorption syndrome and primary biliary cirrhosis are the causes of morbidity and mortality in some patients with limited cutaneous disease. On the other hand, the prognosis is generally worse in patients with diffuse cutaneous disease, particularly when the onset occurs at an older age. In addition, males have a worse prognosis. Renal and other visceral organ disease may develop early in the course of those patients with rapidly progressive generalized skin thickening. Death occurs most often from cardiac, renal, or pulmonary involvement. In one study the 10-year cumulative survival of patients with only renal involvement was 30 percent, and of patients with only lung involvement, 50 percent. In patients without heart, lung, or kidney involvement, survival was 71 percent.

Skin may spontaneously soften after years of disease. Softening occurs in the reverse order of original skin involvement, beginning with the trunk and followed by the proximal and then the distal extremities. Sclerodactyly may persist. Skin thickness may eventually approach normal.

TREATMENT Even though SSc cannot be cured, treatment of involved organ systems can relieve symptoms and improve function. The doctor-patient relationship is extremely important in caring for patients with this chronic debilitating illness. Once the diagnosis of SSc has been made, the patient and family should be instructed about this disorder. The patient will need repeated explanations and reassurances throughout his or her illness. Depending on the severity of illness, the patient will require monitoring of blood pressure, blood counts, urinalysis, and renal and pulmonary function on a regular basis.

Effectiveness of drug therapy in SSc is difficult to evaluate because of the variable course and severity of the disease. Many drugs have been used in the treatment of SSc without any consistent or prolonged benefit. In uncontrolled studies D-penicillamine has been reported to reduce skin thickening and prevent development of significant organ involvement. This drug interferes with inter- and intramolecular cross-linking of collagen and is also immunosuppressive. Its immunosuppressive activity also may lead to decreased collagen production. Penicillamine is better tolerated when started at a low dose, usually 250 mg/d, and then increased at 1- to 3-month intervals up to 1.5 g/d as tolerated. Although a few patients can tolerate higher doses, most patients are maintained on a dose between 0.5 and 1 g/d. For optimal absorption, it is important to give this drug 1 h before or 2 h after a meal. This drug can be quite toxic; its more serious complications include glomerulonephritis with nephrotic syndrome, aplastic anemia, leukopenia, thrombocytopenia, and myasthenia gravis. Other side effects are fever, rash, anorexia, nausea, and loss of taste. Patients should have monthly complete blood counts (including platelet count) and urinalyses. Azathioprine and other immunosuppressives also have been used in SSc and should be reserved for those patients with rapidly progressive and life-threatening disease. Control studies are lacking. Trials of treatment with recombinant interferon γ, 5-fluorouracil, and *extracorporeal photochemotherapy* have shown improvement in some disease parameters. No therapy, however, has been clearly demonstrated in a controlled, prospective study to suppress or reverse the disease process of SSc.

Antiplatelet therapy may play a role in the treatment of SSc, since the biologic products of platelets affect blood vessels. Low doses of aspirin block the formation of thromboxane A_2, a powerful vasoconstrictor and platelet aggregator. In addition, dipyridamole, 200 to 400 mg in divided daily doses, also decreases platelet adhesion to damaged vessel walls. While these drugs have a reasonable therapeutic rationale, a 2-year double-blind study did not show any benefit from their use. Reports of beneficial effects of colchicine or chlorambucil have not been documented in controlled studies.

Glucocorticoids are indicated in those patients with inflammatory myositis or pericarditis. The initial dose is 40 to 60 mg/d and is tapered based on clinical improvement. Prednisone 10 mg/d or less may be beneficial in treating arthritis refractory to nonsteroidal anti-inflammatory drugs and in reducing edema associated with the edematous phase of early skin involvement. Glucocorticoids are not otherwise indicated in the long-term treatment of SSc. High doses of glucocorticoids may play a role in precipitating acute renal failure. However, this association remains unclear.

The management of Raynaud's phenomenon is directed at control of vasospasm. Patients should be advised to dress warmly and wear mittens and socks, not to smoke, to remove causes of external stress, and to avoid drugs such as amphetamine and ergotamine. Beta blocking drugs may make Raynaud's phenomenon worse. Warmth of the central body induces peripheral vasodilatation. Drugs that block sympathetic vasoconstriction, such as reserpine, α-methyldopa, phenoxybenzamine, and prazosin, may be useful in the treatment of Raynaud's phenomenon, but their side effects often curtail extended use. The calcium channel blockers nifedipine and diltiazem can be effective in alleviating Raynaud's phenomenon, but side effects of light-headedness and palpitations may limit their use. The dose of nifedipine is 10 to 20 mg tid. Ketanserin, an oral serotonin antagonist, also has been shown to be effective. Studies with iloprost, a prostacyclin analogue, have shown a decrease in frequency and severity of Raynaud's phenomenon and healing of digital ulcers in some patients. Techniques of biofeedback also have been used with variable success for teaching patients to control the temperature of their hands. Surgical sympathectomy usually provides only temporary improvement, and it, along with other forms of therapy, does not prevent progression of the vascular lesion. The response to any therapy for Raynaud's phenomenon is limited by the degree of existing structural narrowing of digital arteries. Gangrene of distal digits may occur and require surgical amputation.

Numerous drugs have been claimed to soften the hidebound skin, but documentation in controlled studies is lacking. These drugs include D-penicillamine, colchicine, p-aminobenzoic acid, and vitamin E. Dryness of the skin may be reduced by avoiding frequent use of detergent soaps and by regularly applying hydrophilic ointments and bath oils. Regular exercise helps to maintain flexibility of extremities and pliability of skin. Massaging the skin several times a day also may be beneficial. Fingertip ulcerations can be protected by applying a guard or cage over the end of the finger. The use of an occlusive dressing over a noninfected ulcer may promote healing and protect the finger. Skin ulcers should be kept clean by soaking or by surgical or chemical debridement. Sympatholytic drugs or local nitroglycerine paste applied to the ulcer may be beneficial in promoting healing. Infected ulcers can usually be treated with topical antibiotics but may require systemic antibiotics, especially when there is a question of underlying osteomyelitis.

Patients with reflux esophagitis are treated with small, frequent meals, antacids between meals, and elevation of the head of the bed. Patients should be advised not to lie down for a few hours after a meal and to avoid coffee, tea, and chocolate, which reduce the pressure of the lower esophageal sphincter. Cimetidine or ranitidine may be beneficial. Omeprazole has been effective in treating erosive esophagitis in some patients. Metoclopramide, which increases esophageal motility and increases lower esophageal sphincter tone, also can be of help in some patients. Patients with dysphagia should be instructed to chew their food thoroughly and wash it down with fluids. Malabsorption syndrome due to duodenal hypomotility and bacterial overgrowth may improve with intermittent use of appropriate antibiotics. Patients with severe debilitating malabsorption may benefit from parenteral hyperalimentation. Stool softeners and mild laxatives are usually adequate for treating constipation caused by hypomotility of the colon.

Acute myositis is usually responsive to glucocorticoids; these drugs should not be used for the indolent primary form of muscle disease of SSc. Articular symptoms are treated with aspirin or other nonsteroidal anti-inflammatory agents.

Pulmonary fibrosis is not reversible, and therefore treatment is directed at symptoms or complications. Pulmonary infection requires prompt treatment with antibiotics. Hypoxia necessitates giving low concentrations of oxygen. The role of glucocorticoids in preventing progression of interstitial lung disease is not clear. Patients should receive Pneumovax and yearly influenza immunizations.

Recognition of early renal failure is important in order to preserve remaining function. Renal involvement is often accompanied by hypertension and mild to moderate proteinuria. An occasional patient may be normotensive. Antihypertensive agents are often effective in lowering blood pressure and stabilizing or reversing renal failure. These drugs include propranolol, clonidine, and minoxidil. Particularly effective are the angiotensin-converting enzyme inhibitors, which include captopril, enalapril, and lisinopril. Dialysis may be required in patients with progressive renal failure. Some patients, however, have a slow return of renal function after several months and may no longer require dialysis.

Patients with cardiac failure require careful monitoring of digitalis and diuretic administration. Pericardial effusions also may improve with diuretics. Care should be taken to avoid overdiuresis, which may lead to decreased renal blood flow, decreased cardiac output, and renal failure.

EOSINOPHILIC FASCIITIS Eosinophilic fasciitis is a scleroderma-like syndrome of unknown cause characterized by inflammation followed later by sclerosis of the dermis, subcutis, and deep fascia. The disease affects adults and often occurs after strenuous physical activity. Patients do not have Raynaud's phenomenon or internal organ involvement. Several immunologic abnormalities have been associated with eosinophilic fasciitis and include aplastic anemia, myelodysplastic syndrome, and thrombocytopenia. Patients usually have the abrupt onset of symmetric tenderness and swelling of the extremities which is rapidly followed by induration of the skin and subcutaneous tissue. The skin takes on a cobblestone or puckered appearance. Carpal tunnel syndrome appears early in the course, and flexion contractures develop later. A low-grade myositis is often present, but creatinine kinase levels are usually normal. A marked eosinophilia is found in the early stage of disease and subsequently decreases. Increased levels of polyclonal IgG and immune complexes are often present in the serum. A full-thickness biopsy consisting of skin, fascia, and superficial muscle shows perivascular infiltration of histiocytes, eosinophils, lymphocytes, and plasma cells. Biopsies later in the course show sclerosis. Spontaneous improvement and occasionally complete remission may occur after 2 to 5 years of disease. Some patients have persistent disease, while others are left with flexion contractures. Administration of glucocorticoids may provide symptomatic improvement and will decrease the eosinophilia. Improvement has been reported with the use of the H-2 blocker cimetidine.

EOSINOPHILIA-MYALGIA SYNDROME In 1989, reports of patients with scleroderma-like skin changes, myalgias, and eosinophilia dramatically increased. Most, but not all, of these cases were associated with ingestion of L-tryptophan manufactured by a single Japanese company. Batches of L-tryptophan implicated in eosinophilia-myalgia syndrome (EMS) were found to contain trace amounts of a contaminant identified as a dimer of L-tryptophan which appeared in 1988 after changes were made in the method of manufacturing this drug. It is not clear whether this chemical contaminant is the etiologic agent or another unidentified substance is responsible. L-*Tryptophan products were taken off the market in 1990*. The onset of EMS can be either abrupt or insidious. In the early phases of the disease, clinical manifestations include low-grade fever, fatigue, dyspnea, cough, arthralgias/arthritis, evanescent erythematous rashes, muscle cramping, and severe myalgias. Pulmonary infiltrates may be present. Over the next 2 to 3 months, scleroderma-like skin changes appear. Some patients develop a peripheral neuropathy which may persist. An ascending polyneuropathy may lead to paralysis and respiratory failure requiring ventilatory assistance. Cognitive dysfunction with impairment of memory and concentration has been recognized in this syndrome. Myocarditis and cardiac arrhythmias occur in some patients, and a few patients develop pulmonary hypertension. Approximately a third of patients have features of eosinophilic fasciitis. EMS most closely resembles toxic oil syndrome; however, Raynaud's phenomenon does not occur, and there is a lower prevalence of pulmonary hypertension and thromboembolic disease. The peripheral eosinophil count is greater than 1000 cells per cubic millimeter in most patients. The histologic findings on biopsy of skin, fascia, and superficial muscle are similar to that found in eosinophilic fasciitis. The clinical features of EMS may persist after L-tryptophan has been discontinued. EMS may run a chronic course, and response to therapy has been variable. Treatment has included glucocorticoids, antimalarial drugs, immunosuppressive drugs, and plasmapheresis. The pathogenesis and natural course of this disease are not yet known (see also Chap. 384).

REFERENCES

ABRAHAM D et al: Expression and function of surface antigens on scleroderma fibroblasts. Arthritis Rheum 34:1164, 1991

ALTMAN RD et al: Predictors of survival in systemic sclerosis (scleroderma). Arthritis Rheum 34:403, 1991

CARPENTIER PH, MARICQ HR: Microvasculature in systemic sclerosis. Rheum Dis Clin North Am 16:75, 1990

DEGIANNIS D et al: Soluble interleukin-2 receptors in patients with systemic sclerosis: Clinical and laboratory correlations. Arthritis Rheum 33:375, 1990

KAHALEH MB: Soluble immunologic products in scleroderma sera. Clin Immunol Immunopathol 58:139, 1991

———: Vascular disease in scleroderma: Endothelial T lymphocyte-fibroblast interactions. Rheum Dis Clin North Am 16:53, 1990

KAUFMAN LD: The eosinophilia-myalgia syndrome: Current concepts and future directions. Clin Exp Rheumatol 10:87, 1992

LAKHANPAL S et al: Eosinophilic fasciitis: Clinical spectrum and therapeutic response in 52 cases. Semin Arthritis Rheum 17:221, 1988

LEROY EC et al: Scleroderma (systemic sclerosis): Classification, subsets and pathogenesis. J Rheumatol 15:202, 1988

MEDSGER TA J: Systemic Sclerosis (Scleroderma), Localized forms of Scleroderma, and Calcinosis, in *Arthritis and Allied Conditions*, 12th ed, DJ McCarty (ed). Philadelphia, Lea & Febiger, 1993, p 1253

NEEDLEMAN BW et al: In vitro identification of subpopulation of fibroblasts that produces high levels of collagen in scleroderma patients. Arthritis Rheum 33:842, 1990

SEIBOLD J: Scleroderma, in *Textbook of Rheumatology*, 4th ed, WN Kelly et al (eds). Philadelphia, Saunders, Chap. 66, 1993

——— et al: Dermal mast cell degranulation in systemic sclerosis. Arthritis Rheum 33:1702, 1990

STEEN VD et al: Outcome of renal crisis in systemic sclerosis: Relation to availability of angiotensin converting enzyme (ACE) inhibitors. Ann Intern Med 113:352, 1990

YAMAKAGE A et al: Selective upregulation of platelet-derived growth factor α receptors by transforming growth factor β in scleroderma fibroblasts. J Exp Med 175:1227, 1992

287 MIXED CONNECTIVE TISSUE DISEASE

GORDON C. SHARP

DEFINITION Mixed connective tissue disease (MCTD) is an overlap syndrome characterized by a combination of clinical features similar to those of systemic lupus erythematosus (SLE) (see Chap. 284), scleroderma (see Chap. 286), polymyositis (see Chap. 384), and rheumatoid arthritis (see Chap. 285) and unusually high titers of circulating antibody to a nuclear ribonucleoprotein (RNP) antigen.

ETIOLOGY, PATHOGENESIS, AND PATHOLOGY The etiologic and pathogenic mechanisms of MCTD remain unknown, but characteristic immune findings include (1) immunoregulatory abnormalities with persistence of extremely high titers of antibody to nuclear RNP and a marked polyclonal hypergammaglobulinemia indicative of B cell hyperactivity, (2) circulating immune complexes during active disease but with normal clearance by the reticuloendothelial system in most patients, in contrast to SLE, (3) deposition of IgG, IgM, and complement within vascular walls and along sarcolemmal and glomerular basement membranes, and (4) widespread lymphocytic and plasma cell infiltration of numerous tissues. One of the chief underlying pathologic findings in some patients with MCTD is a vascular lesion with intimal proliferation and medial hypertrophy, resulting in narrowing of the lumen of large vessels (e.g., pulmonary, renal, and coronary arteries) and of small arterioles of many organs. Such lesions in the lungs in the absence of significant pulmonary fibrosis, in contrast to scleroderma, may contribute to pulmonary hypertension and abnormalities of pulmonary function.

CLINICAL MANIFESTATIONS The age range in published reports of MCTD is from 4 to 80 years, with a mean of 37 years. Approximately 80 percent of patients have been female. Typical clinical features include Raynaud phenomenon, polyarthritis, swollen hands or sclerodactyly, esophageal dysfunction, pulmonary involvement, and inflammatory myopathy. Malar rash, alopecia, lymphadenopathy, and cardiac and renal disease are less frequent.

Cutaneous features of MCTD include a swollen, sausage-like appearance of the fingers, nonscarring alopecia, lupus-like rashes, heliotrope eyelids, erythematous patches over the knuckles, periungual telangiectasia, and "squared" telangiectasia over the hands and face. Scleroderma-like changes may be present but rarely become extensive.

Musculoskeletal abnormalities occur in most patients. Arthritis is usually nondeforming but may resemble rheumatoid arthritis. Proximal muscle weakness is frequent and may be severe. Serum levels of creatine kinase and aldolase are often markedly elevated, electromyograms are typical of inflammatory myopathy, and biopsies show degeneration of muscle fibers and interstitial and perivascular infiltrates of lymphocytes and plasma cells.

Esophageal dysfunction has been demonstrated in 80 percent, including 70 percent who are asymptomatic. Abnormalities include reduced upper and lower esophageal sphincter pressures and decreased amplitude of peristalsis in the distal two-thirds of the esophagus.

Pulmonary involvement occurred in 85 percent of one series of MCTD patients and often was clinically silent until far advanced. Clinical findings include exertional dyspnea, pleuritic pain, and bibasilar rales. Reduced diffusing capacity for carbon monoxide is the most frequent functional abnormality. Pulmonary hypertension is the most frequent serious complication in MCTD.

Cardiac disease is less common than pulmonary involvement in adults but may be more frequent in children. Pericarditis is the most common finding; other findings have included mitral valve prolapse, myocarditis, congestive heart failure, and aortic insufficiency.

Renal disease in children and adults with MCTD has a combined prevalence of about 28 percent. Progressive renal failure is unusual; clinical and histologic findings suggest that vascular lesions may represent a more serious problem than immune-complex nephritis in MCTD.

Less frequent clinical manifestations include fever, lymphadenopathy, neurologic abnormalities, Sjögren's syndrome (see Chap. 288), hepatosplenomegaly, and intestinal involvement similar to that seen in scleroderma.

LABORATORY FINDINGS   Almost all patients have positive fluorescent antinuclear antibody tests at high titers with a speckled pattern and very high titers of antibodies directed against the ribonuclease-sensitive nuclear RNP component of extractable nuclear antigen (ENA). Elevated anti–native DNA antibody titers and antibodies to the ribonuclease-resistant Sm component of ENA are uncommon in MCTD; their presence is usually associated with a severe flare-up of lupus-like features. High titers of circulating RNP antibodies usually persist for years, but antibody levels may decline significantly or become undetectable in patients in prolonged remission.

Recent studies have further elucidated the nature of the RNP and Sm antigens. Antibodies to RNP immunoprecipitate U1 snRNA-protein complexes and react with proteins designated 70K, A, and C, whereas Sm antibodies immunoprecipitate complexes containing U1, U2, U4, U5, and U6 snRNAs and react with proteins designated B/B' and D. Furthermore, these antigenic complexes have been shown to have important biologic roles in the processing of messenger RNA. Several reports indicate that antibodies to the 70K protein are associated with anti-U1 RNP antibodies in MCTD but rarely occur in SLE. Immunogenetic studies have revealed that U1 70K-positive MCTD patients have disease associated with the presence of either HLA-DR4 or HLA-DR2 but not with HLA-DR3, as is found in patients with SLE. A sequence of shared amino acids or a "shared epitope" within HLA-DR, which is common to both HLA-DR4 and HLA-DR2, may be the basis for this association.

Rheumatoid factor is found, often at very high titers, in half the patients. Less frequent findings include hypocomplementemia, leukopenia, anemia, and thrombocytopenia (mainly in children).

DIAGNOSIS   The diagnosis of MCTD is based on a combination of typical overlapping clinical findings and high titers of circulating antibody to nuclear U1 RNP. In some, all the clinical manifestations may be present on initial evaluation. However, MCTD is now being recognized in an earlier phase in patients with minimal symptoms (e.g., Raynaud phenomenon, arthralgias, myalgias, and swollen hands). In some this mild "undifferentiated connective tissue disease"

syndrome may persist for years, but a prospective, long-term study showed that the majority of patients with high titers of U1 RNP antibodies and limited clinical manifestations ultimately developed signs and symptoms consistent with a diagnosis of MCTD.

TREATMENT AND PROGNOSIS   Lacking controlled studies, specific treatment recommendations for MCTD are based on anecdotal information. Salicylates, other nonsteroidal anti-inflammatory agents, hydroxychloroquine, vasodilators, and/or low doses of glucocorticoids are used to treat mild disease. If the disease is more severe and significantly involves major organ systems, higher doses of glucocorticoids (e.g., 1 mg/kg per day of prednisone) are usually required. As with SLE, a cytotoxic agent may be added in steroid-resistant or -dependent cases. However, the efficacy of this latter therapeutic regimen has not been substantiated by controlled clinical trials. The prognosis for MCTD is generally similar to that of SLE and somewhat better than for scleroderma.

REFERENCES

KANEOKA H et al: Molecular genetic analysis of HLA-DR and HLA-DQ genes among anti-U1-70kD autoantibody-positive connective tissue disease patients. Arthritis Rheum 35:83, 1992

PETTERSSON I ET AL: The use of immunoblotting and immunoprecipitation of (U) small nuclear ribonucleoproteins in the analysis of sera of patients with mixed connective tissue disease and systemic lupus erythematosus. Arthritis Rheum 29:986, 1986

SHARP GC, SINGSEN BH: Mixed connective tissue disease, in Arthritis and Allied Conditions, 12th ed, DJ McCarty, W Koopman (eds). Philadelphia, Lea & Febiger, 1992, p 1213

TAKEDA Y ET AL: Enzyme-linked immunosorbent assay using isolated (U) small nuclear ribonucleoprotein polypeptides as antigens to investigate the clinical significance of autoantibodies to these polypeptides. Clin Immunol Immunopathol 50:213, 1989

288   SJÖGREN'S SYNDROME

HARALAMPOS M. MOUTSOPOULOS

DEFINITION   Sjögren's syndrome is a chronic, slowly progressive autoimmune disease characterized by lymphocytic infiltration of the exocrine glands resulting in xerostomia and dry eyes. Approximately one-third of patients present with extraglandular (systemic) manifestations. A small but significant number of the patients may develop malignant lymphoma. The disease can be seen alone (primary Sjögren's syndrome) or in association with other autoimmune rheumatic diseases such as rheumatoid arthritis, systemic lupus erythematosus, or scleroderma (secondary Sjögren's syndrome).

INCIDENCE AND PREVALENCE   The disease affects predominantly middle-aged women (female-to-male ratio 9:1), although it can be seen in all ages, including childhood. The incidence of the disease is still unknown, but it is considered to be very common since, in addition to the primary syndrome, 30 percent of patients with rheumatoid arthritis, systemic lupus erythematosus, and scleroderma suffer from secondary Sjögren's syndrome.

PATHOGENESIS   The two main autoimmune phenomena observed in Sjögren's syndrome are lymphocytic infiltration of the exocrine glands and B lymphocyte hyperreactivity, as illustrated by circulating autoantibodies. The latter is accompanied by an oligomonoclonal B cell process, which is characterized by serum and urine monoclonal light chains and cryoprecipitable monoclonal immunoglobulins.

Sera of patients with Sjögren's syndrome often contain a number of autoantibodies directed against non-organ-specific antigens such as immunoglobulins (rheumatoid factors) and extractable nuclear and cytoplasmic antigens (Ro/SSA, La/SSB) (Table 288-1). Molecular characterization and cloning have shown that Ro/SSA autoantigen consists of three polypeptide chains (52,000, 54,000, and 60,000 Da) in conjunction with HY_1, HY_3, HY_4, and HY_5 RNAs, whereas La/SSB protein of 48,000 Da is bound to RNA III polymerase transcripts. Autoantibodies to organ-specific antigens such as salivary duct cells, thyroid gland cells, and gastric mucosa also have been described. The presence of autoantibodies to Ro/SSA and La/SSB antigens in Sjögren's syndrome is associated with earlier disease onset, longer disease duration, salivary gland enlargement, severity of lymphocytic infiltration of minor salivary glands, and certain extraglandular manifestations such as lymphadenopathy, purpura, and vasculitis.

Phenotypic and functional studies have shown that the predominant cell infiltrating the affected exocrine glands is the helper/inducer T cell with characteristics of memory cells. Both B and T infiltrating lymphocytes are activated, as illustrated by production of immunoglobulins with autoantibody activity, spontaneous release of interleukin 2, as well as expression on the T cell surface of activation markers such as class II HLA molecules and LFA-1. Macrophages and NK cells are rarely detected in infiltrates, while epithelial cells of the affected glands inappropriately express class II molecules and possess messages for c-*myc* protooncogene and tranforming growth factor beta. All these phenomena suggest that the epithelial cell of the exocrine glands in Sjögren's syndrome may act as an antigen presenting cell, and recent studies indicate that a retrovirus may be the initiator of the autoimmune process.

Immunogenetic studies have demonstrated that HLA-B8, -DR3, and -DRw52 are prevalent in primary Sjögren's syndrome patients as compared with the normal control population. Further analysis of HLA class II genes by molecular techniques revealed that Sjögren's syndrome patients with anti-Ro/SSA and/or anti-La/SSB antibodies possess DQA_1/DQB_1 chains containing specific amino acid residues in their second hypervariable region.

CLINICAL MANIFESTATIONS The majority of the patients with Sjögren's syndrome have symptoms related to diminished lacrimal and salivary gland function. In most patients, the primary syndrome runs a slow and benign course. The initial manifestations can be nonspecific (such as arthralgias, fatigue, Raynaud's phenomenon), and usually 8 to 10 years elapse from the initial symptoms to full-blown development of the disease.

The principal oral symptom of Sjögren's syndrome is dryness (xerostomia). This is described as difficulty in swallowing dry food, inability to speak continuously, a burning sensation, increase in dental caries, and problems in wearing complete dentures. Physical examination shows a dry, erythematous, sticky oral mucosa. There is atrophy of the filiform papillae on the dorsum of the tongue, and saliva from the major glands is either not expressible or is cloudy. Enlargement of the parotid or other major salivary glands occurs in two-thirds of patients with primary Sjögren's syndrome but is uncommon in those with the secondary syndrome. Diagnostic tests include sialometry, sialography, and scintigraphy. All these techniques exhibit high sensitivity but not well established disease specificity. In contrast, the labial minor salivary gland biopsy exhibits higher specificity, permitting histopathologic confirmation of the focal lymphocytic infiltrates.

Ocular involvement is the other major manifestation of Sjögren's syndrome. Patients usually complain of dry eyes, with a sandy or gritty feeling under the eyelids. Other symptoms include burning, accumulation of thick strands at the inner canthi, decreased tearing, redness, itching, eye fatigue, and increased photosensitivity. These symptoms are attributed to the destruction of corneal and bulbar conjunctival epithelium defined as keratoconjunctivitis sicca. Diagnostic evaluation of keratoconjunctivitis sicca includes measurement of tear flow by Schirmer's I test and tear composition as assessed by the tear breakup time or tear lysozyme content. The most specific diagnostic procedure, however, is slit-lamp examination of the cornea and conjunctiva after rose Bengal staining. This test reveals punctate corneal ulcerations and attached filaments of corneal epithelium.

Involvement of other exocrine glands occurs less frequently and includes a decrease in mucous gland secretions of the upper and lower respiratory tree resulting in dry nose, throat, and trachea (xerotrachea) and diminished secretion of the exocrine glands of the gastrointestinal tract leading to esophageal mucosal atrophy, atrophic gastritis, and subclinical pancreatitis. Dyspareunia due to dryness of the external genitalia and dry skin also may occur.

Extraglandular (systemic) manifestations are seen in one-third of patients with Sjögren's syndrome (Table 288-2), while they are very rare in patients with Sjögren's syndrome associated with rheumatoid arthritis. These patients complain more often of easy fatigability, low-grade fever, myalgias, and arthralgias. Most patients with primary Sjögren's syndrome experience at least one episode of nonerosive arthritis during the course of their disease. Manifestations of pulmonary involvement are frequent but rarely important clinically, with subclinical diffuse interstitial lung disease being the most common. Renal involvement includes interstitial nephritis, clinically manifested by hypostenuria and renal tubular dysfunction with or without acidosis and Fanconi's syndrome. Untreated acidosis may lead to nephrocalcinosis. Glomerulonephritis is a rare finding that occurs in patients with systemic vasculitis, cryoglobulinemia, or systemic lupus erythematosus overlapping with Sjögren's syndrome. Renal biopsy reveals either membranous or membranoproliferative glomerulonephritis. Vasculitis affects small and medium-sized vessels. The most common clinical features are purpura, recurrent urticaria, skin ulcerations, and mononeuritis multiplex. Histologically, leukocytoclastic, lymphocytic, acute necrotizing angiitis, and endarteritis obliterans are seen.

It has been suggested that primary Sjögren's syndrome with vasculitis also may present with multifocal, recurrent, and progressive nervous system disease, such as hemiparesis, transverse myelopathy, hemisensory deficits, seizures, and movement disorders. Aseptic meningitis and multiple sclerosis also have been reported in these patients.

Lymphoma and Waldenström's macroglobulinemia are well-known manifestations of Sjögren's syndrome. Most lymphomas are of B cell origin. Pseudolymphoma or frank lymphoma should always be suspected when persistent major salivary gland enlargement, lymphadenopathy, lung nodules, or hilar or mediastinal lymphadenopathy is observed. Parenchymal organs, such as lungs and gastrointestinal tract can be affected. Lymphomas may appear in Sjögren's

TABLE 288-1 Incidence of non-organ-specific autoantibodies in Sjögren's syndrome (SS) compared with systemic lupus erythematosus (SLE)

	SS (% positive)	SLE (% positive)
Rheumatoid factor	80	25–30
Antibodies to double-stranded DNA	Absent	70–80
Antibodies to Ro/SSA	60	10–25
Antibodies to La/SSB	50	10

TABLE 288-2 Incidence of extraglandular manifestations in primary Sjögren's syndrome

Clinical manifestation	Percent
Arthralgias/arthritis	60
Raynaud's phenomenon	37
Lymphadenopathy	14
Lung involvement	14
Vasculitis	11
Kidney involvement	9
Liver involvement	6
Lymphoma	6
Splenomegaly	3
Peripheral neuropathy	2
Myositis	1

TABLE 288-3   Differential diagnosis of sicca symptoms

Xerostomia	Dry eye	Bilateral parotid gland enlargement
Viral infections	Inflammation	Viral infections
Drugs	Stevens-Johnson	Mumps
Psychotherapeutic	syndrome	Influenza
Parasympatholytic	Pemphigoid	Epstein-Barr
Antihypertensives	Chronic conjunctivitis	Coxsackievirus A
Psychogenic	Chronic blepharitis	Cytomegalovirus
Irradiation	Sjögren's syndrome	Human immunodefi-
Diabetes mellitus	Toxicity	ciency virus
Trauma	Burns	Sarcoidosis
Sjögren's	Drugs	Amyloidosis
syndrome	Neurologic conditions	Sjögren's syndrome
	Impaired lacrimal gland	Metabolic
	function	Diabetes mellitus
	Impaired eyelid function	Hyperlipoproteinemias
	Miscellaneous	Chronic pancreatitis
	Trauma	Hepatic cirrhosis
	Hypovitaminosis A	Endocrine
	Blink abnormality	Acromegaly
	Lid scarring	Gonadal hypofunction
	Anesthetic cornea	
	Epithelial irregularity	

syndrome patients after several years of an apparently benign course and are observed more often in patients with systemic disease.

Routine laboratory tests reveal mild normochromic, normocytic anemia. An elevated erythrocyte sedimentation rate is found in approximately 70 percent of patients.

DIAGNOSIS AND DIFFERENTIAL DIAGNOSIS   Diagnosis of Sjögren's syndrome is based on the presence of two of three of the following manifestations: keratoconjunctivitis sicca, xerostomia, and rheumatoid arthritis or another connective tissue syndrome. Salivary or lacrimal gland enlargement may or may not be present.

The differential diagnosis of Sjögren's syndrome includes other conditions which may cause dry mouth or eyes or parotid salivary gland enlargement (Table 288-3). HIV infection (see Chap. 279) also appears to produce a clinical picture indistinguishable from Sjögren's syndrome in certain patients (Table 288-4). Infiltrative processes such as sarcoidosis may cause parotid gland enlargement. This is distinguished from Sjögren's syndrome by minor salivary gland biopsy, which usually reveals noncaseating granulomas in sarcoidosis patients. These patients also lack autoantibodies.

TREATMENT   Sjögren's syndrome remains fundamentally an incurable disease, since no therapeutic modality has been identified that can alter the course of the disease. Hence treatment of Sjögren's syndrome is aimed at symptomatic relief and limiting the damaging local effects of chronic xerostomia and keratoconjunctivitis sicca by substitution of the missing secretions.

The sicca complex is treated with fluid replacement supplied as often as necessary. To replace deficient tears, there are several readily available ophthalmic preparations (Tearisol; Liquifilm; 0.5% methylcellulose; Hypo Tears). In severe cases, it may be necessary for patients to use these as often as every 30 min. If corneal ulceration

TABLE 288-4   Differential diagnosis of Sjögren's syndrome with HIV infection

HIV infection and sicca syndrome	Sjögren's syndrome
Predominant in young males	Predominant in middle-aged women
Lack of autoantibodies to Ro/SSA and/or La/SSB	Presence of autoantibodies
Lymphoid infiltrates of salivary glands by CD8-positive lymphocytes	Lymphoid infiltrates of salivary glands by CD4-positive lymphocytes
Association with HLA-DR5	Association with HLA-DR3 and -DRw52
Positive serologic tests for HIV	Negative serologic tests for HIV

is present, eye patching and boric acid ointments are recommended. Certain drugs which may increase lacrimal and salivary hypofunction such as diuretics, antihypertensive drugs, and antidepressants should be avoided. Propionic acid gels may be used to treat vaginal dryness.

Bromhexine given orally at high doses (48 mg/d) appears to improve sicca manifestations. However, frequent ingestion of fluids, particularly with meals, is often the best solution.

Preliminary studies suggest that hydroxychloroquine 200 mg/d partially corrects hypergammaglobulinemia and decreases IgG antibodies to La/SSB antigen and erythrocyte sedimentation rate while increasing the hemoglobin levels.

Glucocorticoids (1 mg/kg per day) or other immunosuppressive agents (i.e., cyclophosphamide) are indicated for the treatment of extraglandular manifestations, particularly when renal or severe pulmonary involvement and systemic vasculitis have been documented.

REFERENCES

MOUTSOPOULOS HM et al: Sjögren's syndrome (sicca syndrome): Current issues. Ann Intern Med 92:212, 1980

———, YOUINOU P: New developments in Sjögren's syndrome. Curr Opin Rheumatol 3:815, 1991

——— et al: Immunopathogenesis of Sjögren's syndrome: "Facts and fancy." Autoimmunity 5:17, 1989

——— et al: Nephrocalcinosis in Sjögren's syndrome: A late sequela of renal tubular acidosis. J Int Med 230:187, 1991

REVEILLE JD et al: Specific amino acid residues in the second hypervariable region of HLA-DQA1 and DQB1 chain genes promote the Ro (SS-A)/La (SS-B) autoantibody responses. J Immunol 146:3871, 1991

SKOPOULI FN et al: c-*myc* mRNA expression in minor salivary glands of patients with Sjögren's syndrome. J Rheumatol 19:693, 1992

TALAL N et al: *Sjögren's syndrome: Clinical and immunological aspects.* Berlin, Springer-Verlag, 1987

289   ANKYLOSING SPONDYLITIS, REACTIVE ARTHRITIS, AND UNDIFFERENTIATED SPONDYLOARTHROPATHY

JOEL D. TAUROG / PETER E. LIPSKY

The spondyloarthropathies are a group of disorders that share certain clinical features. In addition, each of these conditions is associated with expression of the HLA-B27 gene product. The similarity in clinical manifestations and in genetic predisposition suggest that the spondyloarthropathies may have a related pathogenic mechanism. These disorders include ankylosing spondylitis, Reiter's syndrome, reactive arthritis, psoriatic arthritis and spondylitis, enteropathic arthritis and spondylitis, juvenile-onset spondyloarthropathy, and the less clearly defined undifferentiated spondyloarthropathy.

ANKYLOSING SPONDYLITIS

Ankylosing spondylitis (AS) is an inflammatory disorder of unknown cause that primarily affects the axial skeleton; peripheral joints and extraarticular structures also may be involved. The disease usually begins in the second or third decade; the prevalence in men is approximately three times that in women. It is considered the prototype of the spondyloarthropathies. In Europe, AS is often referred to as *Marie-Strümpell disease* or *Bechterew's disease*.

EPIDEMIOLOGY   Ankylosing spondylitis shows a striking correlation with the histocompatibility antigen HLA-B27 and occurs worldwide roughly in proportion to the prevalence of this antigen (see Chap. 64). In North American Caucasians, the general prevalence of HLA-B27 is 7 percent, whereas over 90 percent of patients with AS have inherited this antigen. The association with HLA-B27 is independent of disease severity.

In population surveys, 1 to 2 percent of adults inheriting HLA-B27 have been found to have AS. In contrast, in families of patients with AS, 10 to 20 percent of adult first-degree relatives inheriting HLA-B27 have been found to have the disease. The concordance rate in identical twins is estimated to be 60 percent or less. These epidemiologic findings indicate that both genetic and environmental factors play a role in the pathogenesis of the disease and that the genetic factors may include allelic genes in addition to HLA-B27.

PATHOLOGY   Sacroiliitis is usually one of the earliest manifestations of AS. The early lesion consists of subchondral granulation tissue-containing lymphocytes, plasma cells, mast cells, macrophages, and chondrocytes. Usually, the thinner iliac cartilage is eroded first, then the thicker sacral cartilage. The irregularly eroded, sclerotic margins of the joint are gradually replaced by fibrocartilage regeneration and then by ossification. Ultimately, the joint may be totally obliterated. Radiographically, this progression is evident as erosion of the cortical margins of the joint with subchondral bony sclerosis, followed by apparent widening of the joint space caused by extensive erosion of the cortical margins, bony bridging, and then fusion.

In the spine, the initial lesion consists of inflammatory granulation tissue at the junction of the annulus fibrosus of the disk cartilage and the margin of vertebral bone. The outer annular fibers are eroded and eventually replaced by bone, forming the beginning of a bony excrescence called a *syndesmophyte*, which then grows by continued enchondral ossification, ultimately bridging the adjacent vertebral bodies. Ascending progression of this process leads to the ''bamboo spine'' observed radiographically. Other lesions in the spine include diffuse osteoporosis, erosion of vertebral bodies at the disk margin (Romanus lesion), ''squaring'' of vertebrae, and inflammation and destruction of the disk-bone border. Inflammatory arthritis of the apophyseal joints is common; early, there is pannus eroding cartilage, often followed by bony ankylosis.

The pathology of peripheral joint arthritis in AS can show synovial hyperplasia, lymphoid infiltration, and pannus formation, but the process lacks the exuberant synovial villi, fibrin deposits, ulcers, and plaques of plasma cells seen in rheumatoid arthritis (see Chap. 285). Central cartilaginous erosions due to proliferation of subchondral granulation tissue are common in AS but rare in rheumatoid arthritis.

The enthesis, the site of tendinous or ligamentous attachment to bone, is another common site of pathology in AS, especially at sites localized around the spine and pelvis. Enthesitis is characterized by erosive, inflammatory lesions that may eventually undergo ossification.

Acute anterior uveitis occurs in approximately 20 percent of patients with AS. Few cases have been studied histologically, none at an early stage. After recurrent attacks, the iris shows nonspecific inflammatory changes, scarring, increased vascularity, and many macrophages laden with pigment.

Aortic insufficiency develops in a small percentage of cases. There is thickening of the aortic valve cusps and the aorta near the sinuses of Valsalva, with dense adventitial scar tissue and intimal fibrous proliferation, the scar tissue often extending into the ventricular septum with resultant heart block.

Microscopic inflammatory lesions of the colon and ileocecal valve have been found in a majority of patients with AS, even in those lacking any clinical evidence of inflammatory bowel disease. IgA nephropathy has been reported with increased frequency.

PATHOGENESIS   The pathogenesis of AS is poorly understood. A number of features of the disease implicate immune-mediated mechanisms, including elevated serum levels of IgA and acute phase reactants, inflammatory histology, and close association with HLA-B27. No specific event or exogenous agent that triggers the onset of disease has been identified, although overlapping features with reactive arthritis and inflammatory bowel disease suggest that enteric bacteria may play a role. Evidence has been obtained suggesting antigenic interrelatedness between HLA-B27 and certain enteric bacteria, but it is not yet known whether this contributes to the pathogenesis of AS. Evidence that HLA-B27 plays a direct role is provided by the finding that rats transgenic for B27 spontaneously develop spondylitis.

CLINICAL MANIFESTATIONS   The symptoms of the disease are usually first noticed in late adolescence or early adulthood; onset after age 40 is unusual. The initial symptom is usually dull pain, insidious in onset, felt deep in the lower lumbar or gluteal region, accompanied by low-back morning stiffness of up to a few hours' duration that improves with activity and returns following prolonged periods of inactivity. Within a few months of onset, the pain usually has become persistent and bilateral, and nocturnal exacerbation of the pain that forces the patient to get up and move around may be frequent.

In some patients bony tenderness may accompany back pain or stiffness, while in others it may be the predominant complaint. Common sites include the costosternal junctions, spinous processes, iliac crests, greater trochanters, ischial tuberosities, tibial tubercles, and heels. Occasionally, chest pain is the presenting complaint because of involvement of the thoracic spine and chest wall articulations. Arthritis in the hips and shoulders occurs in 25 to 35 percent of patients overall and can lead to early symptoms. Arthritis of peripheral joints other than the hips and shoulders has been reported in up to 30 percent of patients and can occur at any stage of the disease. Peripheral arthritis is usually asymmetric. Neck pain and stiffness, indicating involvement of the cervical spine, is usually a relatively late manifestation. Occasional patients, especially those with a juvenile onset, present with predominantly constitutional symptoms such as fatigue, anorexia, fever, weight loss, or night sweats.

The most common extraarticular manifestation is acute anterior uveitis, which can antedate the spondylitis. Attacks are typically unilateral and tend to recur, causing pain, photophobia, and increased lacrimation. Aortic insufficiency, sometimes producing the symptoms of congestive heart failure, occurs in a few percent of patients and occasionally occurs early in the course of the spinal disease. A high percentage of patients have inflammation in the colon or ileum, but this is usually asymptomatic.

Initially, physical findings reflect the manifestations of the inflammatory process. The most specific findings involve loss of spinal mobility, with limitation of anterior flexion, lateral flexion, and extension of the lumbar spine, and limitation of chest expansion. Limitation of motion is usually out of proportion to the degree of bony ankylosis, reflecting spasm secondary to pain and inflammation. Pain in the sacroiliac joints may be elicited either with direct pressure or with maneuvers that stress the joints. In addition, there is commonly tenderness upon palpation at the sites of symptomatic bony tenderness and paraspinous muscle spasm.

The Schober test is a useful measure of forward flexion of the lumbar spine. The patient stands erect, with heels together, and marks are made directly over the spine 5 cm below and 10 cm above the lumbosacral junction (identified by a horizontal line between the posterosuperior iliac spines.) The patient then bends forward maximally, and the distance between the two marks is measured. The distance between the two marks increases 5 cm or more in the case of normal lumbar mobility and less than 4 cm in the case of decreased lumbar mobility. Chest expansion is measured as the difference between maximal inspiration and maximal forced expiration in the fourth intercostal space in males or just below the breasts in females. Normal chest expansion is 5 cm or greater.

Limitation or pain with motion of the hips or shoulders is usually present if either of these joints is involved. Careful examination is also necessary to detect inflammatory disease of peripheral joints. It should be emphasized that early in the course of mild cases, symptoms may be mild and nonspecific, and the physical examination may be completely normal.

The course of the disease is extremely variable, ranging from the individual with mild stiffness and radiographically equivocal sacroiliitis to the patient with a totally fused spine, severe bilateral hip arthritis, and ankylosis, possibly accompanied by severe peripheral arthritis and extraarticular manifestations. Pain tends to be persistent early in the disease and then to become intermittent, with alternating exacerbations and quiescent periods. In a typical severe case with progression of the spondylitis to syndesmophyte formation, the patient's posture undergoes characteristic changes. The lumbar lordosis is obliterated with accompanying atrophy of the buttocks. The thoracic kyphosis is accentuated. If the cervical spine is involved, there may be a forward stoop of the neck. Hip involvement with ankylosis may lead to flexion contractures, compensated by flexion at the knees. The progression of the disease may be followed by measuring the patient's height, chest expansion, Schober test, and occiput-to-wall distance when the patient stands erect with the heels and back flat against the wall. Occasional individuals are encountered with advanced physical findings suggestive of long-standing AS who report having never had significant symptoms.

Onset of the disease in adolescence correlates both with a worse prognosis and more severe hip involvement. The disease in women tends to progress less frequently to total spinal ankylosis, although there is some evidence for an increased prevalence of isolated cervical ankylosis and of peripheral arthritis in women.

The most serious complication of the spinal disease is spinal fracture, which can occur with even minor trauma to the rigid, osteoporotic spine. The cervical spine is most commonly involved, and this can lead to quadriplegia. Cauda equina syndrome is another infrequent complication of long-standing spinal disease in AS. Pulmonary involvement, characterized by slowly progressive upper lobe fibrosis, is a rare complication of long-standing AS; eventually, the lesions can cavitate and become colonized by *Aspergillus*. Although cardiovascular involvement can occur early in the course of the disease, the prevalence of aortic insufficiency and of cardiac conduction disturbances, including third-degree heart block, increases with prolonged disease. Prostatitis has been reported to have an increased prevalence in men with AS. Amyloidosis is only rarely of clinical concern.

Despite the persistence of the disease, most patients with AS are able to remain gainfully employed. Only in uncommon instances does the disease appear to shorten life, these being largely the result of spinal trauma, complications of therapy such as upper gastrointestinal hemorrhage, aortic insufficiency, respiratory failure, or amyloid nephropathy. An excess mortality from leukemia was noted in patients treated with deep x-ray therapy to the spine, a common mode of therapy for AS until effective anti-inflammatory medications became available in the mid-1950s.

LABORATORY FINDINGS   There is no laboratory test that is diagnostic of AS. In most ethnic groups, the HLA-B27 gene is present in approximately 90 percent of patients with AS; American blacks appear to represent an exception, since the prevalence of B27 in this group has been reported to be only 50 percent. Most patients with active disease have an elevated erythrocyte sedimentation rate and an elevated C-reactive protein. A mild normochromic, normocytic anemia may be present. Patients with severe disease may show an elevated alkaline phosphatase. Elevated serum IgA levels are common. Rheumatoid factor and antinuclear antibodies are uniformly absent unless caused by a coexistent disease unrelated to AS. Synovial fluid from inflamed peripheral joints in AS is not distinctly different from that of other inflammatory joint diseases. In cases with restriction of chest wall motion, pulmonary function tests may demonstrate decreased vital capacity and increased functional residual capacity, but airflow measurements are normal and ventilatory function is usually well maintained.

RADIOGRAPHIC FINDINGS   Radiographically demonstrable sacroiliitis is usually present in AS. The earliest changes in the sacroiliac joints demonstrable by plain x-ray radiography show blurring of the cortical margins of the subchondral bone, followed by erosions and sclerosis. Progression of the erosions leads to "pseudowidening" of the joint space; as fibrous and then bony ankylosis supervene, the joints may become obliterated radiographically. The changes and progression of the lesions are usually symmetric.

In mild cases, years may elapse before unequivocal sacroiliac abnormalities are evident on plain radiographs. Although computed tomography and magnetic resonance imaging can detect abnormalities reliably at an earlier stage than plain radiography, these techniques are not generally used for routine diagnostic purposes.

Roentgenographic abnormalities generally appear in the sacroiliac joints before appearing elsewhere in the spine. In the lumbar spine, progression of the disease leads to straightening caused by loss of lordosis and reactive sclerosis caused by osteitis of the anterior corners of the vertebral bodies with subsequent erosion, leading to "squaring" of the vertebral bodies. Progressive ossification of the superficial layers of the annulus fibrosus leads to eventual formation of marginal syndesmophytes, visible on plain films as bony bridges connecting successive vertebral bodies on the anterior and lateral sides.

DIAGNOSIS   The diagnosis of early AS before the development of irreversible deformity can be difficult to establish. Currently, modified New York criteria (1984) are widely used for diagnosis. These consist of the following: (1) a history of inflammatory back pain (see below), (2) limitation of motion of the lumbar spine in both the sagittal and frontal planes, (3) limited chest expansion, relative to standard values for age and sex, and (4) definite radiographic sacroiliitis. Under these criteria, the presence of radiographic sacroiliitis plus any one of the other three criteria is sufficient for a diagnosis of definite AS. The increased sensitivity of these modified criteria is largely the result of the inclusion of earlier stages of radiographic sacroiliitis than are permitted under the original New York criteria.

Several studies have identified a sizable population of B27+ individuals with symptoms typical of AS who lack definite radiographic sacroiliitis. However, when followed over time, most of these patients eventually develop radiographic changes. These studies indicate that diagnostic criteria based on radiographic findings may in some cases be too insensitive for the diagnosis of early AS. The B27 test is useful only as a diagnostic adjunct, since the presence of B27 is neither necessary nor sufficient for the diagnosis, but it can be helpful in patients who have not yet developed radiographic sacroiliitis.

AS must be differentiated from numerous other causes of low-back pain. The inflammatory back pain of AS is usually distinguished by the following five features: (1) age of onset below 40, (2) insidious onset, (3) duration greater than 3 months before medical attention is sought, (4) morning stiffness, and (5) improvement with exercise or activity. The most common causes of back pain other than AS are primarily mechanical or degenerative rather than inflammatory and do not show these features. Less common metabolic, infectious, and malignant causes of back pain also must be differentiated from AS.

Marked calcification and ossification of paraspinous ligaments occur in *diffuse idiopathic skeletal hyperostosis* (DISH). Although DISH is often categorized as a variant of osteoarthritis, diarthrodial joints are not involved. Ligamentous calcification and ossification are usually most prominent in the anterior spinal ligaments and give the appearance of "flowing wax" on the anterior bodies of the vertebrae. However, a radiolucency may be seen between the newly deposited bone and the vertebral body, differentiating DISH from the marginal osteophytes in spondylosis. Intervertebral disk spaces are preserved, and sacroiliac and apophyseal joints appear normal, helping to differentiate DISH from spondylosis and from ankylosing spondylitis, respectively.

DISH occurs in the middle-aged and the elderly and is more common in men than in women. Patients are frequently asymptomatic but may have musculoskeletal stiffness. Radiographic changes are generally much more severe than might be predicted from the mild symptoms caused by DISH.

TREATMENT   There is no definitive treatment for AS. The principal goal of management is the conscientious participation by the patient in an exercise program designed to maintain functional posture and to preserve range of motion. Most patients require anti-inflammatory agents to achieve sufficient symptomatic relief to be able to remain functional and carry out the exercise program. It is not known whether drug treatment alone can alter the progression of the disease.

Worldwide, the most commonly used drug therapy for AS is indomethacin, although several other nonsteroidal anti-inflammatory drugs (NSAIDs) also have been proven to be effective in reducing pain and stiffness and are commonly used. Indomethacin is particularly effective as a 75-mg slow-release preparation taken once or twice daily. Although phenylbutazone, at doses of 200 to 400 mg/d, has been considered by several authorities to be the most effective agent in AS, because of its greater potential for serious side effects such as aplastic anemia and agranulocytosis, its use in the United States is confined to patients with severe disease whose symptoms do not respond well to other agents. Recent controlled trials suggest that sulfasalazine,* in doses of 2 to 3 g/d, may be useful in reducing peripheral joint symptoms as well as reversing laboratory evidence of inflammation. Its effects on axial arthritis and natural progression of the disease are unclear. The peripheral arthritis also may respond to the folic acid antagonist methotrexate.* No therapeutic role for gold, penicillamine, immunosuppressive drugs, or systemic glucocorticoids has been documented in AS. Occasionally, intralesional or intraarticular glucocorticoid injections may be beneficial in patients with persistent enthesopathy or synovitis unresponsive to anti-inflammatory agents.

The most common indication for surgery in patients with AS is severe hip joint arthritis, the pain and stiffness of which are often dramatically relieved by total hip arthroplasty. A small number of patients may benefit from surgical correction of extreme flexion deformities of the spine or of atlantoaxial subluxation.

Attacks of acute anterior uveitis are usually effectively managed with local glucocorticoid administration in conjunction with mydriatic agents. Coexistent cardiac disease may require pacemaker implantation or aortic valve replacement.

REACTIVE ARTHRITIS AND UNDIFFERENTIATED SPONDYLOARTHROPATHY

Reactive arthritis (ReA) refers to acute nonpurulent arthritis complicating an infection elsewhere in the body. In recent years, the term has been used primarily to refer to spondyloarthropathies following enteric or urogenital infections and occurring predominantly in individuals with the histocompatibility antigen HLA-B27. Included in this category is the constellation of clinical findings often referred to as *Reiter's syndrome*. Other forms of reactive arthritis not associated with HLA-B27 and showing a different spectrum of clinical features, such as rheumatic fever, are discussed elsewhere in this book (see Chap. 200).

HISTORICAL BACKGROUND In 1916, Reiter described a patient who, following an episode of bloody diarrhea, developed a systemic illness with polyarthritis, conjunctivitis, and nongonococcal urethritis. Although similar cases had been described previously, this report served to focus attention on the triad of arthritis, urethritis, and conjunctivitis, which subsequently was referred to as *Reiter's syndrome*. Additional clinical features, particularly mucocutaneous lesions, were later recognized to be frequent accompaniments of the syndrome.

The identification of bacterial species capable of triggering the clinical syndrome and the finding that three-fourths of the patients possess the HLA-B27 antigen have led to the unifying concept of reactive arthritis as a clinical syndrome triggered by a specific etiologic agent in a genetically susceptible host. A similar spectrum of clinical manifestations can be triggered by enteric infection with any of several

Shigella, Salmonella, Yersinia, and *Campylobacter* species, by genital infection with *Chlamydia trachomatis,* and possibly by other agents as well. Although Reiter's syndrome can be said to represent one part of the spectrum of the clinical manifestations of ReA, it can be reasonably argued that the term is now largely of historical interest. Undifferentiated spondyloarthropathy is a diagnosis given to patients with clinical findings suggestive of a spondyloarthropathy but whose disease does meet criteria for other diagnoses.

EPIDEMIOLOGY Like AS, ReA occurs predominantly in individuals who have inherited the HLA-B27 gene; in most series, 60 to 85 percent of patients are B27+. In epidemics of arthritogenic bacterial infection, e.g., *S. flexneri,* it has been estimated that ReA develops in ~20 percent of exposed B27+ individuals. Some studies of families with multiple cases of AS or ReA have suggested that the two conditions tend to "breed true"; i.e., the two conditions are uncommonly found together within an individual family. Whether this is caused by genetic or environmental factors is not known. The disease is most common in individuals 18 to 40 years of age, but it is well recognized both in children over 5 years of age and in older adults.

The sex ratio in ReA following enteric infection is nearly 1:1, whereas venereally acquired ReA is predominantly a male disease. The overall prevalence and incidence of ReA are difficult to assess because of the variable prevalence of the triggering infections and genetic susceptibility factors in different populations. Certain populations, such as the Navajo Indians of the southwestern United States and the Inuit Eskimos of Greenland, show a very high occurrence of ReA, whereas the disease is quite uncommon in certain other populations such as the Haida Indians, with an equally high prevalence of HLA-B27. The reasons for these differences are not clear.

A particularly severe form of peripheral spondyloarthropathy has been described in patients with AIDS (see Chap. 279). Most of these patients are HLA-B27+. Whether B27+ individuals with HIV infection develop this syndrome at a higher than expected frequency is controversial.

PATHOLOGY Synovial histology is similar to that of other inflammatory arthropathies. Enthesitis is a common clinical finding in ReA; the histology of this lesion resembles that of AS. Microscopic histopathologic evidence of inflammation has been noted in the colon and ileum of patients with postvenereal as well as postenteric ReA. The skin lesions of keratoderma blenorrhagica are histologically indistinguishable from psoriatic lesions.

ETIOLOGY AND PATHOGENESIS The first bacterial infection to be causally related to ReA was *S. flexneri.* An outbreak of shigellosis among Finnish troops in 1944 resulted in numerous cases of ReA. Of the four species of *Shigella, sonnei, boydii, flexneri,* and *dysenteriae, S. flexneri* has most often been implicated in cases of ReA, both sporadic and epidemic. *S. sonnei,* although responsible for the majority of cases of shigellosis in the United States, has only rarely been implicated in cases of ReA.

Other bacteria that have been definitively identified as triggers of ReA include several *Salmonella* species, *Y. enterocolitica, C. jejuni,* and *C. trachomatis.* There is suggestive evidence implicating several other microorganisms, including *Y. pseudotuberculosis, Clostridium difficile, Neisseria gonorrhoeae, Ureaplasma urealyticum,* and *Streptococcus pyogenes.* There are also numerous isolated reports of acute arthritis preceded by other bacterial, viral, or parasitic infections, but whether the microorganisms involved are actual triggers of ReA remains to be determined.

It has not been determined whether ReA occurs by the same pathogenic mechanism following infection with each of these microorganisms, nor has the mechanism been fully elucidated in the case of any one of the known bacterial triggers. Most, if not all, of the triggering organisms share a capacity to invade host cells and survive intracellularly. Antigens from *Chlamydia, Yersinia,* and *Salmonella* have been shown to persist in the synovium of patients with ReA for long periods following the acute attack. CD4+ T cells that specifically

*This drug has not been approved for this purpose by the Food and Drug Administration at the time of publication.

respond to antigens of the inciting organism are typically found in inflamed synovium but not in peripheral blood of patients with ReA. Their role in disease pathogenesis is not known.

Additional evidence for an unusual persistence of the immune response to the infecting organism in those individuals in whom ReA develops comes from studies of *Yersinia*-induced ReA. In comparison with individuals who fail to develop ReA following enteric infection with *Yersinia*, patients with ReA show fewer gastrointestinal symptoms attributable to the infection, a smaller initial IgM response, stronger and more persistent IgA and IgG responses, higher levels of IgA anti-*Yersinia* antibodies with a secretory component, and reduced T cell proliferative responses to *Yersinia* antigens. Similarly, patients with *Chlamydia*-induced ReA have more persistent IgA anti-*Chlamydia* titers than individuals with *Chlamydia* infection and no arthritis.

The role of HLA-B27 in ReA and undifferentiated spondyloarthropathy remains to be determined. Transgenic rats with high expression of B27 spontaneously develop a multiple organ system inflammatory disease affecting the gut, peripheral and axial joints, male genital tract, and skin that clinically and histologically strikingly resembles these human conditions. The role of bacteria in the rat disease is not yet clear. In both the rat and human diseases, it remains to be determined whether the primary process is an autoimmune response against host tissues or an immune response against antigens of the triggering organism that have disseminated to the target tissues, and the specific role of B27 itself remains to be determined. Antigenic cross-reactivity between the B27 molecule and envelope glycoproteins of arthritogenic bacteria, including *S. flexneri* and *Y. pseudotuberculosis*, has been well documented, but the pathogenic significance of this is not known. Many but not all B27— individuals with ReA possess HLA-B alleles that are antigenically cross-reactive with HLA-B27, notably HLA-B7.

CLINICAL FEATURES   The clinical manifestations of ReA constitute a spectrum that ranges from an isolated, transient monarthritis to a more severe multisystem disease. In the majority of cases, a careful history will elicit some evidence of an antecedent infection 1 to 4 weeks before the onset of symptoms of the reactive disease. However, in a sizable minority, particularly in cases of relapse, no clinical or laboratory evidence of an antecedent infection can be found. In many cases of presumed venereally acquired reactive disease, there is a history of a recent new sexual partner, even in the absence of laboratory evidence of infection.

Constitutional symptoms are common, including fatigue, malaise, fever, and weight loss. The musculoskeletal symptoms are usually acute in onset. Arthritis is usually asymmetric and additive, with involvement of new joints occurring over a period of a few days to 1 to 2 weeks. The joints of the lower extremities, especially the knee, ankle, and subtalar, metatarsophalangeal, and toe interphalangeal joints, are the most common sites of involvement, but the wrist and fingers can be involved as well. The arthritis is usually quite painful, and tense joint effusions are not uncommon, especially in the knee. Dactylitis, or "sausage digit," a diffuse swelling of a solitary finger or toe, is a distinctive feature of both ReA and psoriatic arthritis. Tendinitis and fasciitis are particularly characteristic lesions, producing pain at multiple insertion sites, especially the Achilles insertion, the plantar fascia, and sites along the axial skeleton. Spinal and low-back pain are quite common and may be caused by insertional inflammation, muscle spasm, acute sacroiliitis, or, presumably, arthritis in intervertebral articulations.

Urogenital lesions may occur throughout the course of the disease. In males, urethritis may be marked or relatively asymptomatic and may be either an accompaniment of the triggering infection or a result of the reactive phase of the disease. Prostatitis is also common. Similarly, in females, cervicitis or salpingitis may be caused either by the infectious trigger or by the sterile reactive process.

Ocular disease is common, ranging from transient, asymptomatic conjunctivitis to an aggressive anterior uveitis that occasionally proves refractory to treatment and may result in blindness.

Mucocutaneous lesions are frequent. Oral ulcers tend to be superficial, transient, and often asymptomatic. The characteristic skin lesions, keratoderma blenorrhagica, consists of vesicles that become hyperkeratotic, ultimately forming a crust before disappearing. It is most common on the palms and soles but may occur elsewhere as well. In patients with HIV infection, these lesions are often extremely severe and extensive, to the point of dominating the clinical picture. Lesions on the glans penis, termed *circinate balanitis*, are common; these consist of vesicles that quickly rupture to form painless superficial erosions, which in circumcised individuals can form crusts similar to those of keratoderma blenorrhagica. Nail changes are common and consist of onycholysis, distal yellowish discoloration, and/or heaped-up hyperkeratosis.

Less frequent or rare manifestations of ReA include cardiac conduction defects, aortic insufficiency, central or peripheral nervous system lesions, and pleuropulmonary infiltrates.

Long-term follow-up studies suggest that some joint symptoms persist in many, if not most, patients with ReA. Recurrences of the acute syndrome are common, and as many as 25 percent of patients either become unable to work or are forced to change occupations because of persistent joint symptoms. Chronic heel pain is often a particularly distressing symptom. Ankylosing spondylitis is also a common sequela. In most studies, HLA-B27 + patients have a worse outcome than B27— patients. The extent to which the long-term prognosis varies with different inciting agents is not known. However, patients with *Yersinia*-induced arthritis appear to have less chronic disease than those whose initial episode follows epidemic shigellosis. The course of undifferentiated spondyloarthropathy remains to be studied.

LABORATORY AND RADIOGRAPHIC FINDINGS   The erythrocyte sedimentation rate is elevated during the acute phase of the disease. Mild anemia may be present, and acute phase reactants tend to be increased. Synovial fluid is nonspecifically inflammatory, showing an elevated white cell count with a predominance of neutrophils. In most ethnic groups, three-fourths of the patients are B27 + . Although it is unusual for the triggering infection to persist through the time of onset of the reactive disease, it may occasionally be possible to culture the organism, e.g., in the case of *Shigella*- or *Chlamydia*-induced disease. Serologic evidence of a recent infection may be present, such as a marked elevation of antibodies to *Yersinia* or *Chlamydia*.

In early or mild disease, radiographic changes may be absent or confined to juxtaarticular osteoporosis. With long-standing persistent disease, marginal erosions and loss of joint space can be seen in affected joints. Periostitis with reactive new bone formation is characteristic of the disease, as it is with all the spondyloarthropathies. Spurs at the insertion of the plantar fascia are common.

Sacroiliitis and spondylitis similar to those described for AS may be seen as late sequelae. However, sacroiliitis is more commonly asymmetric than in AS, and the spondylitis, rather than ascending symmetrically from the lower lumbar segments, can begin anywhere along the lumbar spine. The syndesmophytes may be coarse and nonmarginal, arising from the middle of a vertebral body, a pattern rarely seen in primary AS.

DIAGNOSIS   ReA is a clinical diagnosis, there being no definitively diagnostic laboratory test or radiographic finding. The diagnosis should be entertained in any patient with an acute inflammatory, asymmetric, additive arthritis or tendinitis. The evaluation of such a patient should include careful questioning regarding possible antecedent triggering events such as an episode of diarrhea or dysuria. On physical examination, careful attention must be paid to the distribution of the joint and tendon involvement and to possible sites of extraarticular involvement, such as the eyes, mucous membranes, skin, nails, and genitalia. Synovial fluid aspiration and analysis may be helpful in excluding septic or crystal-induced arthritis.

Although typing for B27 is not needed to secure the diagnosis in clear-cut cases, it has prognostic significance in terms of severity, chronicity, and the propensity for spondylitis and uveitis. Furthermore, it can be helpful diagnostically in atypical cases, a positive test increasing and a negative test decreasing the probability that the diagnosis of ReA is correct.

It is particularly important to differentiate ReA from disseminated gonococcal disease, both of which can be venereally acquired and associated with urethritis (see Chap. 110). Gonococcal arthritis and tenosynovitis tend to involve both upper and lower extremities equally, whereas in ReA the symptoms usually predominate in the lower extremities. Back pain is common in ReA but is not a feature of gonococcal disease, whereas the vesicular skin lesions characteristic of disseminated gonococcal disease are not found in ReA. A positive gonococcal culture from the urethra or cervix does not exclude a diagnosis of ReA; however, culturing gonococci from blood, skin lesion, or synovium establishes the diagnosis of disseminated gonococcal disease. Occasionally, the only definitive way to distinguish the two is through a therapeutic trial of antibiotics.

ReA shares many features in common with psoriatic arthropathy, including the asymmetry of the arthritis, a propensity for "sausage digits" and nail involvement, an association with uveitis, and skin lesions of similar histology (see Chap. 298). However, psoriatic arthritis is usually gradual in onset, the arthritis tends to affect primarily the upper extremities, and there is far less associated periarthritis. Psoriatic arthritis is not associated with mouth ulcers, urethritis, or bowel symptoms. Although psoriatic arthropathy shows some distinctive radiographic features that are not found in ReA, these occur only late in the disease and are of little help diagnostically. Only psoriatic spondylitis, not the peripheral arthritis, is associated with HLA-B27, about 50 percent of patients being positive. Occasional patients, usually B27+, following what appears to be a typical episode of ReA, will develop typical psoriasis and persistent arthritis such that the two entities become indistinguishable. Undifferentiated spondyloarthropathy is diagnosed in patients who lack evidence of an antecedent infection that might incriminate ReA and who do not meet criteria for AS but who show clinical features of these disorders.

TREATMENT   Most patients with ReA are benefitted to some degree by NSAIDs, although rarely are symptoms of the acute arthritis completely ameliorated, and some patients fail to respond at all. Indomethacin, 75 to 150 mg/d in divided doses, is the initial treatment of choice. Other NSAIDs may be tried, with phenylbutazone, 100 mg tid or qid, being the NSAID of last resort because of its potentially serious side effects.

Recent controlled data suggest that prolonged administration of a long-acting tetracycline may ameliorate *Chlamydia*-induced ReA. Previously, the prevailing dogma held that antibiotics were of no benefit. Whether other antibiotic regimens may be effective for ReA triggered by other agents is under investigation.

Patients with debilitating symptoms refractory to NSAID therapy may respond to immunosuppressive agents such as azathioprine, 1 to 2 mg/kg per day, or methotrexate, 7.5 to 15 mg per week. Recent studies have suggested that sulfasalazine, up to 3 g/d in divided doses, also may be beneficial to patients with persistent ReA.* Systemic glucocorticoids are not routinely used but may occasionally be helpful in mobilizing a severely affected bedridden patient. Antimalarials, gold, and penicillamine are not useful in the treatment of ReA.

Tendinitis and other enthesitic lesions occasionally may benefit from intralesional glucocorticoids. Uveitis may require aggressive treatment with glucocorticoids to prevent serious sequelae. Skin lesions ordinarily require only symptomatic treatment. In patients with HIV infection and ReA, many of whom have severe skin lesions, the skin lesions in particular appear to respond to systemic treatment with zidovudine. Cardiac complications are managed conventionally; management of neurologic complications is symptomatic.

Patients need to be educated about the nature of the disease and the factors that predispose to its recurrence. Comprehensive management includes counseling of patients in the use of condoms and avoidance of sexual promiscuity and exposure to enteropathogens.

Appropriate use of physical therapy, vocational counseling, and continued surveillance for long-term complications such as ankylosing spondylitis are also part of comprehensive care.

REFERENCES

CALIN A (ed): *Spondylarthropathies*. Orlando, Grune & Stratton, 1984

DOUGADOS M et al: The European Spondylarthropathy Study Group preliminary criteria for the classification of spondylarthropathy. Arthritis Rheum 34:1218, 1991

GRANFORS K et al: *Salmonella* liposaccharide in synovial cells from patients with reactive arthritis. Lancet 335:685, 1990

HAMMER RE et al: Spontaneous inflammatory disease in transgenic rats expressing HLA-B27 and human β2-m: An animal model of HLA-B27-associated human disorders. Cell 63:1099, 1990

LAUHIO A et al: Double-blind, placebo-controlled study of three-month treatment with lymecycline in reactive arthritis, with special reference to *Chlamydia* arthritis. Arthritis Rheum 34:6, 1991

LIPSKY PE, TAUROG JD (eds): *B27+ Spondyloarthropathies*. New York, Elsevier, 1991

LEIRISALO-REPO M et al: Ten-year follow-up study of patients with *Yersinia* arthritis. Arthritis Rheum 31:533, 1988

MIELANTS H et al: Gut inflammation in the spondyloarthropathies: Clinical, radiologic, biologic and genetic features in relation to the type of histology. A prospective study. J Rheumatol 18:1542, 1991

WINCHESTER R: AIDS and the rheumatic diseases. Bull Rheum Dis 39(5):1, 1990

ZEIDLER H et al: Unidifferentiated spondyloarthopathies. Rheum Dis Clin North Am 18:187, 1992

290   BEHÇET'S SYNDROME

HARALAMPOS M. MOUTSOPOULOS

DEFINITION   Behçet's syndrome is a multisystem disorder presenting with recurrent oral and genital ulcerations as well as ocular involvement. Recently, internationally agreed diagnostic criteria have been proposed (Table 290-1).

PREVALENCE, PATHOGENESIS, AND PATHOLOGY   The disease has a worldwide distribution. The prevalence of Behçet's syndrome ranges from 1:10,000 in Japan to 1:500,000 in North America and Europe. It affects mainly young adults, with men having more severe disease than females.

The etiology and pathogenesis of this syndrome remain obscure; it is considered an autoimmune disease since vasculitis is the main pathologic lesion and circulating autoantibodies to human oral mucous membrane are found in approximately 50 percent of the cases. Familial occurrence has been reported, and in patients from eastern Mediterranean countries and Japan, the disease appears to be linked to HLA-B5 and HLA-DR5 alloantigens.

CLINICAL FEATURES   The recurrent aphthous ulcerations are a sine qua non for the diagnosis. The ulcers are usually painful, 2 to 10 mm in diameter, shallow or deep with a central yellowish necrotic base, appear singly or in crops, and are located anywhere in the oral cavity. The ulcers persist for 1 to 2 weeks and subside without leaving scars. The genital ulcers resemble the oral ones. Vaginal ulcers are usually painless, while ulcers on the external genitalia may be painful.

Skin involvement includes folliculitis, erythema nodosum, an acne-like exanthem, and infrequently vasculitis. Nonspecific skin

TABLE 290-1   Diagnostic criteria of Behçet's disease

Recurrent oral ulceration plus 2 of:

Recurrent genital ulceration
Eye lesions
Skin lesions
Pathergy test

---

*Azathioprine, methotrexate, and sulfasalazine have not been approved for this purpose by the Food and Drug Administration at the time of publication.

inflammatory reactivity to any scratches or intradermal saline injection (pathergy test) is a common and specific manifestation in Japanese and eastern Mediterranean patients.

Eye involvement is the most dreaded complication, since it occasionally progresses rapidly to blindness. The eye disease is usually present at the onset but also may develop within the first few years. In addition to iritis, posterior uveitis, retinal vessel occlusions, and optic neuritis can be seen in some cases of the syndrome. Hypopyon uveitis, which is considered the hallmark of Behçet's syndrome, is in fact a rare manifestation.

The arthritis of Behçet's syndrome is not deforming and affects the knees and ankles.

Superficial or deep peripheral vein thrombosis is seen in one-fourth of the patients. Pulmonary emboli is a rare complication. The superior vena cava is obstructed occasionally, producing a dramatic clinical picture. Arterial involvement occurs infrequently and presents with aortitis or peripheral arterial aneurysm and arterial thrombosis. Pulmonary artery vasculitis presenting with dyspnea, cough, chest pain, hemoptysis, and infiltrates on chest roentgenograms has been reported recently in 5 percent of patients.

Central nervous system involvement is found more frequently in northern Europe and the United States. The most common lesions are benign intracranial hypertension, a multiple sclerosis–like picture, pyramidal involvement and psychiatric disturbances.

Gastrointestinal involvement is reported in patients from Japan and includes mucosal ulcerations of the gut.

Laboratory findings are mainly nonspecific indices of inflammation such as leukocytosis and elevated erythrocyte sedimentation rate as well as C-reactive protein levels; antibodies to human oral mucosa are also found.

PROGNOSIS AND TREATMENT   The severity of the syndrome usually abates with time. Apart from the cases with neurologic complications, the life expectancy seems to be normal, and the only serious complication is blindness.

Treatment of Behçet's syndrome is symptomatic and empirical. Mucous membrane involvement may respond to topical corticosteroids in the form of mouthwash or paste. The arthritis responds to rest and analgesics. Thrombophlebitis is treated with aspirin, 500 mg/d, and dipyridamole, 150 mg/d. Colchicine can be beneficial in the mild forms of the syndrome. Uveitis and central nervous system involvement require systemic corticosteroid therapy (prednisone, 1 mg/kg per day) and azathioprine, 2 to 3 mg/kg per day or cyclosporin A, 5 to 10 mg/kg per day.

REFERENCES

INTERNATIONAL STUDY GROUP FOR BEHÇET'S DISEASE: Criteria of diagnosis of Behçet's disease. Lancet 335:1078, 1990

NUSSENBLATT RB et al: Effectiveness of cyclosporin therapy for Behçet's disease. Arthritis Rheum 28:671, 1985

PLOTKIN GR et al: *Behçet's Disease: A Contemporary Synopsis*. New York, Futura, 1988

RAZ I et al: Pulmonary manifestations in Behçet's syndrome. Chest 95:585, 1989

YAZICI H, MOUTSOPOULOS HM: Behçet's disease, in *Current Therapy in Allergy and Immunology*, LM Lichtenstein, AS Fauci (eds). Philadelphia, Decker, 1985

——— et al: A controlled trial of azathioprine in Behçet's syndrome. N Engl J Med 322:281, 1990

291   THE VASCULITIS SYNDROMES

ANTHONY S. FAUCI

DEFINITION   *Vasculitis* is a clinicopathologic process characterized by inflammation of and damage to blood vessels. The vessel lumen is usually compromised, and this is associated with ischemia of the tissues supplied by the involved vessel. A broad and heterogeneous group of syndromes may result from this process, since any type, size, and location of blood vessel may be involved. Vasculitis and its consequences may be the primary or sole manifestation of a disease; alternatively, vasculitis may be a secondary component of another primary disease. Vasculitis may be confined to a single organ such as the skin, or it may simultaneously involve several organ systems.

PATHOPHYSIOLOGY AND PATHOGENESIS   Generally, most of the vasculitic syndromes are assumed to be mediated at least in part by immunopathogenic mechanisms (see Table 291-1). However, evidence to this effect is for the most part indirect and may reflect epiphenomena as opposed to true causality. Deposition of immune complexes in tissues (see Chap. 283) is the most widely accepted pathogenic mechanism of vasculitis. Nonetheless, the causal role of immune complexes has not been clearly established in most of the vasculitic syndromes. Circulating immune complexes need not result in deposition of the complexes in blood vessels with ensuing vasculitis, and many patients with active vasculitis do not have demonstrable circulating or deposited immune complexes. The actual antigen contained in the immune complex has only rarely been identified in vasculitic syndromes. In this regard, hepatitis B antigen has been identified in both the circulating and deposited immune complexes in a subset of patients with systemic vasculitis, most notably within the polyarteritis nodosa group (see below).

The mechanisms of tissue damage in immune-complex–mediated vasculitis resemble those described for serum sickness (Chap. 283). In this model, antigen-antibody complexes are formed in antigen excess and are deposited in vessel walls whose permeability has been increased by vasoactive amines such as histamine, bradykinin, and leukotrienes released from platelets or from mast cells as a result of IgE-triggered mechanisms. The deposition of complexes results in activation of complement components, particularly C5a, which is strongly chemotactic for neutrophils. These cells then infiltrate the vessel wall, phagocytose the immune complexes, and release their intracytoplasmic enzymes, which damage the vessel wall. As the process becomes subacute or chronic, mononuclear cells infiltrate the vessel wall. The common denominator of the resulting syndrome is compromise of the vessel lumen with ischemic changes in the tissues supplied by the involved vessel.

TABLE 291-1   Potential pathogenic mechanisms of blood vessel damage in the vasculitis syndromes

IMMUNOPATHOGENIC MECHANISMS

In situ formation or deposition of immune complexes in blood vessel wall
Direct antibody-mediated damage via antibodies directed at endothelial cells or other tissue components
Antibody-dependent cellular cytotoxicity directed against blood vessel tissue
Cytotoxic T lymphocytes directed at blood vessel components
Granuloma formation in blood vessel wall or adjacent to blood vessel
Cytokine-induced (i.e., interleukin 1, TNF-α), expression of adhesion molecules for leukocytes on endothelial cells

NONIMMUNOPATHOGENIC MECHANISMS

Infiltration of blood vessel wall or surrounding tissue by microbial agents
Direct invasion of blood vessel wall by neoplastic cells
Unidentified mechanisms

In addition to the classic immune-complex–mediated mechanisms of vasculitis, other immunopathogenic mechanisms may be involved in damage to vessels. The most prominent of these are delayed hypersensitivity and cell-mediated immune injury as reflected in the histopathologic feature of granulomatous vasculitis. However, immune complexes themselves may induce granulomatous responses. Vascular endothelial cells can express HLA class II molecules following activation by cytokines such as interferon-γ. This allows these cells to participate in immunologic reactions such as interaction with CD4+ T lymphocytes in a manner similar to antigen-presenting macrophages. Endothelial cells can secrete interleukin 1 (IL-1), which may activate T lymphocytes and initiate or propagate in situ immunologic processes within the blood vessel. In addition, IL-1 and tumor necrosis factor alpha are potent inducers of endothelial-leukocyte adhesion molecule 1 (ELAM-1) and vascular cell adhesion molecule 1 (VCAM-1), which may enhance the adhesion of leukocytes to endothelial cells in the blood vessel wall. Other mechanisms such as direct cellular cytotoxicity or antibody directed against vessel components or antibody-dependent cellular cytotoxicity have been suggested in certain types of vessel damage. However, there is no convincing evidence to support their causal contribution to the pathogenesis of any of the recognized vasculitic syndromes. Finally, antibodies to neutrophil cytoplasmic components have been described for certain of the vasculitis syndromes, particularly Wegener's granulomatosis (see below), but their pathogenic significance, if any, is unclear.

It is unknown why certain individuals develop vasculitis in response to certain antigenic stimuli, whereas others do not. However, it is likely that a number of factors are involved in the ultimate expression of a vasculitic syndrome. These include the genetic predisposition, the regulatory mechanisms associated with immune response to certain antigens, and the ability of the reticuloendothelial system to clear circulating complexes from the blood. The size and physicochemical properties of immune complexes, the relative degree of turbulence of blood flow, the intravascular hydrostatic pressure in different vessels, and the preexisting integrity of the vessel endothelium likely explain why only certain types of immune complexes cause vasculitis and why the vasculitic process is selective for only certain vessels in individual patients.

CLASSIFICATION OF VASCULITIC SYNDROMES A major feature of the vasculitic syndromes as a group is the fact that there is a great deal of heterogeneity at the same time as there is considerable overlap among them. This has led to both difficulty and confusion with regard to the categorization of these diseases. The classification scheme listed in Table 291-2 takes into account this heterogeneity and overlap and will serve as a matrix to emphasize the fact that certain syndromes are predominantly systemic in nature and almost invariably lead to irreversible organ system dysfunction and even death if untreated, while others are usually localized to the skin and rarely result in irreversible dysfunction of vital organs. The distinguishing and overlapping features of the diseases listed in Table 291-2, which justify this classification scheme, will be discussed below.

SYSTEMIC NECROTIZING VASCULITIS

CLASSIC POLYARTERITIS NODOSA **Definition** *Polyarteritis nodosa* (PAN) in its classic form was described in 1866 by Kussmaul and Maier. It is a multisystem, necrotizing vasculitis of small and medium-sized muscular arteries in which involvement of the renal and visceral arteries is characteristic. Classic PAN does not involve pulmonary arteries, although bronchial vessels may be involved; granulomas, significant eosinophilia, and an allergic diathesis are not part of the classic syndrome.

Incidence and prevalence It is difficult to establish an accurate incidence of this disease because of the fact that many reports of PAN actually have included diseases other than the classic syndrome.

TABLE 291-2 Classification of the vasculitic syndromes

Systemic necrotizing vasculitis
  Classic polyarteritis nodosa
  Allergic angiitis and granulomatosis of Churg-Strauss
  Polyangiitis overlap syndrome
Hypersensitivity vasculitis
  Exogenous stimuli proved or suspected
    Henoch-Schönlein purpura
    Serum sickness and serum sickness–like reactions
    Other drug-induced vasculitides
    Vasculitis associated with infectious diseases
  Endogenous antigens likely involved
    Vasculitis associated with neoplasms (particularly lymphoid malignacies)
    Vasculitis associated with connective-tissue diseases
    Vasculitis associated with other underlying diseases
    Vasculitis associated with congenital deficiencies of the complement system
Wegener's granulomatosis
Giant cell arteritis
  Temporal arteritis
  Takayasu's arteritis
Other vasculitic syndromes
  Kawasaki disease
  Isolated central nervous system vasculitis
  Thromboangiitis obliterans (Buerger's disease)
  Behçet's syndrome
  Miscellaneous vasculitides

It is clearly an uncommon, but not a rare, disease. The mean age at onset is 48 years, and the male-to-female ratio is 1.6:1.

Pathophysiology and pathogenesis The vascular lesion in classic PAN is a necrotizing inflammation of small and medium-sized muscular arteries. The lesions are segmental and tend to involve bifurcations and branchings of arteries. They may spread circumferentially to involve adjacent veins. However, involvement of venules is not seen in classic PAN and, if present, suggests the polyangiitis overlap syndrome (see below). In the acute stages of disease, polymorphonuclear neutrophils infiltrate all layers of the vessel wall and perivascular areas, which results in intimal proliferation and degeneration of the vessel wall. Mononuclear cells infiltrate the area as the lesions progress to the subacute and chronic stages. Fibrinoid necrosis of the vessels ensues with compromise of the lumen, thrombosis, infarction of the tissues supplied by the involved vessel, and, in some cases, hemorrhage. As the lesions heal, there is collagen deposition, which may lead to further occlusion of the vessel lumen. Aneurysmal dilatations up to 1 cm in size along the involved arteries are characteristic of classic PAN. Granulomas and substantial eosinophilia with eosinophilic tissue infiltrations are not characteristically found and suggest allergic angiitis and granulomatosis (see below).

Multiple organ systems are involved, and the clinicopathologic findings reflect the degree and location of vessel involvement and the resulting ischemic changes (Table 291-3). As mentioned above, pulmonary arteries are not involved in classic PAN, and bronchial artery involvement is uncommon. The pathology in the kidney is predominantly that of arteritis; however, glomerulitis occurs in up to 30 percent of patients. In patients with significant hypertension, typical pathologic features of glomerulosclerosis may be seen alone or superimposed on lesions of glomerulonephritis. In addition, pathologic sequelae of hypertension may be found elsewhere in the body.

The presence of hepatitis B antigenemia in approximately 20 to 30 percent of patients with systemic vasculitis, particularly of the classic PAN type, together with the isolation of circulating immune complexes composed of hepatitis B antigen and immunoglobulin, and the demonstration by immunofluorescence of hepatitis B antigen, IgM, and complement in the blood vessel walls, strongly suggest the role of immunologic phenomena in the pathogenesis of this disease. Hairy cell leukemia can be associated with classic PAN; the pathogenic mechanisms of this association are unclear.

TABLE 291-3   Classic PAN: Organ system involvement at autopsy

Organ system	Percent
Kidney	85
Heart	76
Liver	62
Gastrointestinal tract:	51
Jejunum	37
Ileum	27
Mesentery	24
Colon	20
Duodenum	10
Gallbladder	10
Rectosigmoid	10
Appendix	7
Muscle	39
Pancreas	35
Testes	33
Peripheral nerves	32
Central nervous system	27
Skin	20

SOURCE: Cupps and Fauci, 1981, p 32.

TABLE 291-4   Clinical manifestations related to organ system involvement in classic PAN

Organ system	Percent incidence	Clinical manifestations
Renal	60	Renal failure, hypertension
Musculoskeletal	64	Arthritis, arthralgia, myalgia
Peripheral nervous system	51	Peripheral neuropathy, mononeuritis multiplex
Gastrointestinal tract	44	Abdominal pain, nausea and vomiting, bleeding, bowel infarction and perforation, cholecystitis, hepatic infarction, pancreatic infarction
Skin	43	Rash, purpura, nodules, cutaneous infarcts, livedo reticularis, Raynaud's phenomenon
Cardiac	36	Congestive heart failure, myocardial infarction, pericarditis
Genitourinary	25	Testicular, ovarian, or epididymal pain
Central nervous system	23	Cerebral vascular accident, altered mental status, seizure

SOURCE: Cupps and Fauci, 1981, p 29.

Clinical and laboratory manifestations   Nonspecific signs and symptoms are the hallmarks of classic PAN. Fever, weight loss, and malaise are present in over one-half of cases. Patients usually present with vague symptoms such as weakness, malaise, headache, abdominal pain, and myalgias. Specific complaints related to the vascular involvement within a particular organ system also may dominate the presenting clinical picture as well as the entire course of the illness (Table 291-4). Renal involvement most commonly manifests as ischemic changes in the glomeruli; however, glomerulonephritis is seen in approximately 30 percent of patients. Hypertension may be related to both the renal polyarteritis and the glomerulitis and may dominate the clinical picture. Classic PAN may involve any organ system; the clinical manifestations related to specific organ system involvement are listed in Table 291-4. No clinical features have been identified that discriminate PAN patients with or without hepatitis B antigenemia.

There are no diagnostic serologic tests for classic PAN. In over 75 percent of patients, the leukocyte count is elevated with a predominance of neutrophils. Eosinophilia is seen only rarely and, when present at high levels, suggests the diagnosis of allergic angiitis and granulomatosis. The anemia of chronic disease may be seen, and an elevated erythrocyte sedimentation rate (ESR) is almost always present. Other common laboratory findings reflect the particular organ involved. Hypergammaglobulinemia may be present, and up to 30 percent of patients have a positive test for hepatitis B surface antigen. Arteriograms may demonstrate characteristic abnormalities such as aneurysms in the small and medium-sized muscular arteries of the kidneys and abdominal viscera.

Diagnosis   The diagnosis of classic PAN is based on the demonstration of characteristic findings of vasculitis on biopsy material of involved organs. In the absence of easily accessible tissue for biopsy, the angiographic demonstration of involved vessels, particularly in the form of aneurysms of small and medium-sized arteries in the renal, hepatic, and visceral vasculature, is sufficient to make the diagnosis. Aneurysms of vessels are not pathognomonic of classic PAN; furthermore, aneurysms need not always be present, and angiographic findings may be limited to stenotic segments and obliteration of vessels. Biopsy of symptomatic organs such as nodular skin lesions, painful testes, and muscle groups provides the highest diagnostic yields, while blind biopsy of asymptomatic organs is frequently negative.

Treatment and prognosis   The prognosis of untreated classic PAN is extremely poor. The usual clinical course is characterized either by fulminant deterioration or by relentless progression associated with intermittent acute flare-ups. Death usually results from renal failure; from gastrointestinal complications, particularly bowel infarcts and perforation; and from cardiovascular causes. Intractable hypertension often compounds dysfunction in other organ systems, such as the kidneys, heart, and central nervous system, leading to additional late morbidity and mortality. The 5-year survival rate of untreated patients has been reported to be 13 percent, while glucocorticoid treatment may increase this figure to over 40 percent. Extremely favorable therapeutic results have been reported in classic PAN with the combination of prednisone, 1 mg/kg per day, and cyclophosphamide, 2 mg/kg per day (see section on "Wegener's Granulomatosis" for a detailed description of this therapeutic regimen). This regimen has been reported to result in up to a 90 percent long-term remission rate even following the discontinuation of therapy. In addition, long-term remissions have been reported in PAN associated with hepatitis B virus antigenemia using the antiviral agent vidarabine in combination with plasma exchange with and without glucocorticoids. Careful attention to the treatment of hypertension can lessen the acute and late morbidity and mortality associated with renal, cardiac, and central nervous system complications of PAN.

ALLERGIC ANGIITIS AND GRANULOMATOSIS (CHURG-STRAUSS DISEASE)   Definition   *Allergic angiitis and granulomatosis* was described in 1951 by Churg and Strauss and is a disease characterized by granulomatous vasculitis of multiple organ systems, particularly the lung. It is similar in many respects to classic PAN, except that the former has a high frequency of lung involvement, vasculitis of blood vessels of various types or sizes (including veins and venules), intra- and extravascular granuloma formation together with eosinophilic tissue infiltration, and a strong association with severe asthma and peripheral eosinophilia.

Incidence and prevalence   Allergic angiitis and granulomatosis is an uncommon disease whose exact incidence, similar to classic PAN, is difficult to determine due to the grouping of multiple types of vasculitic syndromes in many reported series. The disease can occur at any age with the possible exception of infants. The mean age of onset is 44 years, with a male-to-female ratio of 1.3:1.

Pathophysiology and pathogenesis   The vasculitis which is characteristic of allergic angiitis and granulomatosis is similar to that of classic PAN (see above) with certain notable exceptions. In addition to small and medium-sized muscular arteries, capillaries, veins, and venules can be involved in the former disease. The characteristic histopathologic features of allergic angiitis and granulomatosis are granulomatous reactions that may be present in the tissues or even within the walls of the vessels themselves. These are usually associated with infiltration of the tissues with eosinophils. This process can occur in any organ in the body; however, in sharp contrast to classic PAN, lung involvement is predominant, with skin, cardiovascular system, kidney, peripheral nervous system, and gastrointestinal tract also commonly involved. Although the precise pathogenesis of this disease is uncertain, its strong association with asthma, its clinicopathologic manifestations which strongly suggest hypersensitivity phenomena, and its close similarity to classic PAN point to aberrant immunologic phenomena.

Clinical and laboratory manifestations Patients with allergic angiitis and granulomatosis exhibit nonspecific manifestations such as fever, malaise, anorexia, and weight loss similar to patients with classic PAN. In contrast to the latter disease, the pulmonary findings in allergic angiitis and granulomatosis clearly dominate the clinical picture with severe asthmatic attacks and the presence of pulmonary infiltrates. Skin lesions occur in approximately 70 percent of patients and include purpura in addition to cutaneous and subcutaneous nodules. Apart from the characteristic pulmonary findings, the multisystem involvement in this disease is quite similar to that of classic PAN (see above); an important exception is the fact that the renal disease in allergic angiitis and granulomatosis is less common and generally less severe than that of classic PAN.

The characteristic laboratory finding in virtually all patients with allergic angiitis and granulomatosis is a striking eosinophilia which reaches levels greater than 1000 cells per microliter in more than 80 percent of patients. The other laboratory findings are similar to those of classic PAN and reflect the organ systems involved.

Diagnosis Similar to classic PAN, the diagnosis of allergic angiitis and granulomatosis is made by biopsy, demonstrating vasculitis in a patient with the characteristic clinical manifestations. The biopsy findings are distinctive in the latter disease in that granulomatous vasculitis with eosinophilic tissue involvement together with peripheral eosinophilia are typical. Furthermore, pulmonary involvement is extremely common and is usually manifested by severe asthma associated with pulmonary infiltrates that may be fleeting in nature.

Treatment and prognosis The prognosis of untreated allergic angiitis and granulomatosis is poor, with a reported 5-year survival of 25 percent. Unlike classic PAN, the cause of death is more likely to be related to pulmonary and cardiac disease as opposed to renal or gastrointestinal involvement. Glucocorticoid therapy has been reported to increase the 5-year survival to more than 50 percent. In certain patients, the disease may be quite mild and may remit spontaneously or with short courses of glucocorticoids. In glucocorticoid failures or in patients who present with fulminant multisystem disease, the treatment of choice is a combined regimen of cyclophosphamide and alternate-day prednisone, which has resulted in a high rate of complete remission similar to the experience with classic PAN (see above).

POLYANGIITIS OVERLAP SYNDROME Many patients with systemic vasculitis manifest clinicopathologic characteristics which do not fit precisely into any classification but which have overlapping features of classic PAN, allergic angiitis and granulomatosis, Wegener's granulomatosis, Takayasu's arteritis, and the hypersensitivity group of vasculitides. This subgroup has been referred to as the *polyangiitis overlap syndrome* and is part of the major grouping of systemic necrotizing vasculitis. This entity has been designated with a distinct classification in order to avoid confusion in attempting to fit such overlap syndromes into one or other of the more classic vasculitic syndromes. This subgroup is truly a systemic vasculitis with the same potential for resulting in irreversible organ system dysfunction as the other systemic necrotizing vasculitides. The diagnostic and therapeutic considerations as well as the prognosis for this subgroup are the same as those for classic PAN and allergic angiitis and granulomatosis.

HYPERSENSITIVITY VASCULITIS

DEFINITION The term *hypersensitivity vasculitis* has been used to designate a heterogeneous group of disorders which are characterized by a vasculitic syndrome presumed to be associated with a hypersensitivity reaction following exposure to an antigen such as an infectious agent, a drug, or other foreign or endogenous substances. The terminology assigned to this particular group of vasculitis syndromes may be somewhat misleading, since most of the other groups of vasculitis syndromes are probably also associated with some form of hypersensitivity or aberrant immunologic reaction to as yet unidentified antigens.

The common denominator of this group of diseases is the involvement of small vessels. Although any organ can be involved with this type of vasculitis, skin involvement generally dominates the clinical picture, and the extracutaneous involvement is usually much less severe than that of the systemic vasculitides. There are multiple subgroups within the larger category of hypersensitivity vasculitis.

INCIDENCE AND PREVALENCE Although the exact incidence of this group of vasculitic syndromes is uncertain, it is clearly more common than the systemic necrotizing vasculitis group. The disease can occur at any age and in both sexes; however, different subgroups have a higher incidence in certain age groups, and some are more common in males than females, or vice versa.

PATHOPHYSIOLOGY AND PATHOGENESIS The typical histopathologic feature of the hypersensitivity vasculitides is the presence of vasculitis of small vessels. Postcapillary venules are the most commonly involved vessels; capillaries and arterioles may be involved less frequently. This vasculitis is characterized by a leukocytoclasis which refers to the nuclear debris remaining from the neutrophils that have infiltrated in and around the vessels during the acute stages. In the subacute or chronic stages, mononuclear cells predominate; in certain subgroups, eosinophilic infiltration is seen. Erythrocytes often extravasate from the involved vessels, leading to palpable purpura.

Immune-complex deposition is generally considered to be the immunopathogenic mechanism of this type of vasculitis; however, formal proof that this is the case has not been established for all subgroups (see above). The hypersensitivity vasculitides can be broken down empirically into two major categories depending on the type of putative antigen involved in the hypersensitivity reaction. In the originally described group, the antigen was foreign to the host, i.e., a drug, microbe, or foreign protein. In the second category, the antigen is felt to be endogenous to the host. Examples of these are the "self" proteins such as DNA or immunoglobulin which form immune complexes with their respective antibodies and lead to vasculitic complications in systemic lupus erythematosus and rheumatoid arthritis, respectively; other examples are the recognized and putative tumor antigens which form immune complexes with antibody and lead to vasculitis associated with certain neoplasms. Certain lymphoid malignancies also may secrete cytokines which contribute to the pathogenic process (see Table 291-1).

CLINICAL AND LABORATORY MANIFESTATIONS The hallmark of the broad group of hypersensitivity vasculitides is the predominance of skin involvement. Skin lesions may appear typically as palpable purpura; however, other cutaneous manifestations of the vasculitis may occur, including macules, papules, vesicles, bullae, subcutaneous nodules, ulcers, and recurrent or chronic urticaria. Despite the fact that skin lesions predominate, other organ systems may be involved to varying degrees, and the extent to which this occurs may define a relatively distinct subgroup. Even in patients with isolated cutaneous involvement, the disease may be characterized by systemic signs and symptoms such as fever, malaise, myalgia, and anorexia. The skin lesions may be pruritic or even quite painful, with a burning or stinging sensation. Lesions most commonly occur in the lower extremities in ambulatory patients or in the sacral area in bedridden patients due to the effects of hydrostatic forces on the postcapillary venules. Edema may accompany certain lesions, and hyperpigmentation often occurs in areas of recurrent or chronic lesions.

There are no specific laboratory tests which are diagnostic of hypersensitivity vasculitis. A mild leukocytosis with or without eosinophilia is characteristic, as is an elevated ESR. Cryoglobulins and rheumatoid factor may be seen in certain cases, and serum complement levels follow no definite pattern. Laboratory abnormalities related to specific organ dysfunction reflect the involvement of these organs in the particular syndrome in question.

Henoch-Schönlein purpura The most distinctive subgroup of the hypersensitivity vasculitides is *Henoch-Schönlein purpura*, also referred to as *anaphylactoid purpura*, which is characterized by palpable purpura (most commonly distributed over the buttocks and lower extremities), arthralgias, gastrointestinal signs and symptoms, and glomerulonephritis. The disease is usually seen in children; however, individuals of any age may be affected. It has a remarkable tendency to resolve and recur several times over a period of weeks or months, usually ending in spontaneous resolution. A small percentage of patients progress to chronic disease. A number of antigens have been implicated in the immunopathogenesis of this disease, including infectious agents, drugs, certain foods, insect bites, and immunizations. IgA is the antibody class most often seen in the immune complexes of these patients. The typical palpable purpura is seen in virtually all patients; most patients develop polyarthralgias in the absence of frank arthritis. Gastrointestinal involvement, which is seen in almost 70 percent of pediatric patients, is characterized by colicky abdominal pain usually associated with nausea, vomiting, diarrhea, or constipation and which is frequently accompanied by the passage of blood and mucus per rectum; bowel intussusception may occur rarely. The renal involvement is usually characterized by a mild glomerulitis leading to hematuria with red blood cell casts (see also Chap. 241). Most patients recover completely, and some do not require therapy. When glucocorticoid therapy is required, it is usually administered as 1 mg/kg per day of prednisone and tapered according to the clinical response.

Serum sickness and serum sickness–like reactions These reactions are characterized by the occurrence of fever, urticaria, polyarthralgias, and lymphadenopathy 7 to 10 days after primary exposure and 2 to 4 days after secondary exposure to a heterologous protein (classic serum sickness) or a nonprotein drug such as penicillin or sulfa (serum sickness–like reaction). Most of the manifestations are not due to a vasculitis; however, occasional patients will have typical cutaneous venulitis which may progress rarely to a systemic vasculitis. This disorder is discussed in detail in Chap. 283.

Vasculitis associated with other underlying primary diseases A number of diseases have vasculitis as a secondary manifestation of the underlying primary process. Foremost among these are the connective tissue diseases, particularly *systemic lupus erythematosus* (Chap. 284), *rheumatoid arthritis* (Chap. 285), and *Sjögren's syndrome* (Chap. 288). The most common form of vasculitis in these conditions is the small-vessel venulitis isolated to the skin and clinically indistinguishable from the hypersensitivity vasculitides noted in response to an exogenous antigen. However, certain patients may develop a fulminant systemic necrotizing vasculitis indistinguishable from the PAN group.

Cryoglobulinemia may be seen in a number of the diverse vasculitic syndromes. *Essential mixed cryoglobulinemia* (see Chap. 241) may present as a typical hypersensitivity vasculitis confined to the skin. However, typically, it is associated with glomerulonephritis, arthralgias, hepatosplenomegaly, and lymphadenopathy in addition to skin involvement. The cryoglobulins usually consist of cryoprecipitable IgM rheumatoid factor directed against normal endogenous IgG.

Vasculitis can be associated with certain *malignancies*, particularly lymphoid or reticuloendothelial neoplasms. Leukocytoclastic venulitis confined to the skin is the most common finding; however, widespread systemic vasculitis may occur. Of particular note is the association of *hairy cell leukemia* (Chap. 310) with classic PAN.

A leukocytoclastic vasculitis predominantly involving the skin with occasional involvement of other organ systems may be a minor component of many other diseases. These include *subacute bacterial endocarditis*, *Epstein-Barr virus infection*, *chronic active hepatitis*, *ulcerative colitis*, *congenital deficiencies of various complement components*, *retroperitoneal fibrosis*, and *primary biliary cirrhosis*. Association of hypersensitivity vasculitis with *alpha₁-antitrypsin*

deficiency, *intestinal bypass surgery*, and *relapsing polychondritis* has been reported.

DIAGNOSIS The diagnosis of hypersensitivity vasculitis is made by the demonstration of vasculitis on biopsy. Given the predominance of cutaneous involvement, biopsy material is generally readily available. Patients who present with what appears to be isolated cutaneous vasculitis should undergo a systemic (usually noninvasive) workup of other organ systems, since skin involvement is often the presenting feature of systemic vasculitis.

TREATMENT AND PROGNOSIS Most cases of hypersensitivity vasculitis resolve spontaneously, and others, such as Henoch-Schönlein purpura, remit and relapse before finally remitting completely. In those patients in whom persistent cutaneous disease evolves or in whom extracutaneous organ system involvement occurs, a variety of therapeutic regimens have been tried with variable results. In general, the treatment of this type of vasculitis has not been satisfactory. This is in contrast to the systemic necrotizing vasculitis group (see above) and Wegener's granulomatosis (see below), which generally are much more serious diseases than hypersensitivity vasculitis but usually respond dramatically to the combination of prednisone and cyclophosphamide. Fortunately, since the disease is generally limited to the skin, this lack of consistent response to therapy usually does not lead to a life-threatening situation. When an antigenic stimulus is recognized as the precipitating factor in the vasculitis, it should be removed; if this is a microbe, appropriate antimicrobial therapy should be instituted. If the vasculitis is associated with another underlying disease, treatment of the latter often results in resolution of the former. In situations where disease is apparently self-limited, no therapy, except possibly symptomatic therapy, is indicated. When disease persists or results in progressive organ system dysfunction, such as renal failure in Henoch-Schönlein purpura, glucocorticoid therapy should be instituted, usually as prednisone, 1 mg/kg per day, in a regimen aimed at rapid tapering where possible, either directly to discontinuation or by conversion to an alternate-day regimen followed by ultimate discontinuation. In cases that prove refractory to glucocorticoids in which irreversible organ system dysfunction is likely, a trial of a cytotoxic agent such as cyclophosphamide in the regimen described above for systemic vasculitis is warranted. Patients with chronic vasculitis isolated to cutaneous venules rarely respond dramatically to any therapeutic regimen, and cytotoxic agents should be used only as a last resort in these patients. Plasmapheresis has been used with some success in fulminant cases. Dapsone has been tried in a number of patients with isolated cutaneous vasculitis with rare anecdotal reports of success. However, this drug has been consistently beneficial as therapy for cutaneous vasculitis only in patients with erythema elevatum diutinum (see below).

WEGENER'S GRANULOMATOSIS

DEFINITION *Wegener's granulomatosis* is a distinct clinicopathologic entity characterized by granulomatous vasculitis of the upper and lower respiratory tracts together with glomerulonephritis. In addition, variable degrees of disseminated vasculitis involving both small arteries and veins may occur.

INCIDENCE AND PREVALENCE Wegener's granulomatosis is an uncommon disease whose true incidence is difficult to determine. It is extremely rare in blacks compared with whites; the male-to-female ratio is 1:1. The disease can be seen at any age; approximately 15 percent of patients are less than 19 years of age, and only rarely does the disease occur before adolescence; the mean age of onset is approximately 40 years.

PATHOPHYSIOLOGY AND PATHOGENESIS The histopathologic hallmarks of Wegener's granulomatosis are necrotizing vasculitis of small arteries and veins together with granuloma formation which may be either intravascular or extravascular. Lung involvement typically appears as multiple, bilateral, nodular cavitary infiltrates

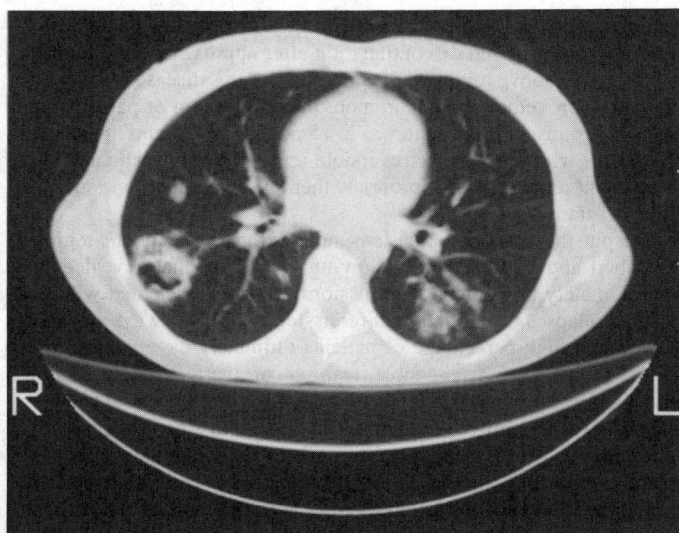

FIGURE 291-1 CT scan of a patient with Wegener's granulomatosis. Patient developed multiple, bilateral, nodular, and cavitary infiltrates.

(Fig. 291-1) which on biopsy almost invariably reveal the typical necrotizing granulomatous vasculitis. Endobronchial disease, either in its active form or as a result of fibrous scarring, may lead to obstruction with atelectasis. Upper airway lesions, particularly those in the sinuses and nasopharynx, typically reveal inflammation, necrosis, and granuloma formation with or without vasculitis.

In its earliest form, renal involvement is characterized by a focal and segmental glomerulitis which may evolve into a rapidly progressive crescentic glomerulonephritis. Granuloma formation is only rarely seen on renal biopsy. In addition to the classic triad of upper and lower respiratory tracts and kidney disease, virtually any organ can be involved with vasculitis, granuloma, or both.

The immunopathogenesis of this disease is unclear, although the involvement of upper airways and lungs suggests an aberrant hypersensitivity response to an exogenous or even endogenous antigen that enters through or resides in the upper airway.

Although circulating and deposited immune complexes have been demonstrated in certain patients with Wegener's granulomatosis, there is no convincing evidence that immune complexes play a causal pathogenic role in this disease. The presence of granulomas with copious, well-defined multinucleated giant cells, particularly in involved pulmonary tissue, suggests delayed hypersensitivity and/or foreign-body reactions. However, direct evidence for either of these mechanisms is lacking.

A high percentage of patients with Wegener's granulomatosis develop antineutrophil cytoplasmic antibodies (ANCAs). The terminology of *cytoplasmic* or *c-ANCAs* refers to the coarse, granular pattern observed by immunofluorescence microscopy when serum antibodies bind to certain cytoplasmic components on indicator neutrophils. Proteinase-3, the 29-kDa neutral serine proteinase present in neutrophil azurophil granules, has been identified as the major c-ANCA antigen. Although ANCAs, particularly perinuclear or p-ANCAs (usually directed against myeloperoxidase or elastase), have been described in other vasculitic syndromes, c-ANCAs are a sensitive (88 percent) and specific (95 percent) marker for active Wegener's granulomatosis. There is no clear evidence that ANCAs plays a primary role in the pathogenesis of Wegener's granulomatosis.

The bronchoalveolar lavage fluid of patients with active Wegener's granulomatosis contains a high percentage of neutrophils compared with that of other granulomatous lung diseases such as sarcoidosis, in which increased numbers of lymphocytes are noted (see Chap. 292). The pathogenic significance of this difference is unclear.

CLINICAL AND LABORATORY MANIFESTATIONS A typical patient presents with severe upper respiratory tract findings such as paranasal sinus pain and drainage and purulent or bloody nasal discharge with or without nasal mucosal ulceration (Table 291-5). Nasal septal perforation may follow, leading to saddle nose deformity. Serous otitis media may occur as a result of eustachian tube blockage.

Pulmonary involvement may be manifested as asymptomatic infiltrates or may be clinically expressed as cough, hemoptysis, dyspnea, and chest discomfort. It is present in 85 to 90 percent of patients. Subglottic stenosis resulting from active disease or scarring occurs in approximately 15 percent of patients and may result in severe airway obstruction.

Eye involvement (52 percent of patients) may range from a mild conjunctivitis to dacryocystitis, episcleritis, scleritis, granulomatous sclerouveitis, ciliary vessel vasculitis, and retroorbital mass lesions leading to proptosis.

Skin lesions (46 percent of patients) appear as papules, vesicles, palpable purpura, ulcers, or subcutaneous nodules; biopsy reveals vasculitis, granuloma, or both. Cardiac involvement (8 percent of patients) manifests as pericarditis, coronary vasculitis, or, rarely, cardiomyopathy. Nervous system manifestations (23 percent of patients) include cranial neuritis, mononeuritis multiplex, or, rarely, cerebral vasculitis and/or granuloma.

Renal disease (77 percent of patients) generally dominates the clinical picture and, if left untreated, accounts directly or indirectly for most of the mortality in this disease. Although it may smolder in some cases as a mild glomerulitis with proteinuria, hematuria, and

TABLE 291-5 Wegener's granulomatosis: Frequency of clinical manifestations in 158 patients studied at the National Institutes of Health

Manifestation	Percent at disease onset	Percent throughout course of disease
Kidney		
Glomerulonephritis	18	77
Ear/nose/throat	73	92
Sinusitis	51	85
Nasal disease	36	68
Otitis media	25	44
Hearing loss	14	42
Subglottic stenosis	1	16
Ear pain	9	14
Oral lesions	3	10
Lung	45	85
Pulmonary infiltrates	25	66
Pulmonary nodules	24	58
Hemoptysis	12	30
Pleuritis	10	28
Eyes		
Conjunctivitis	5	18
Dacryocystitis	1	18
Scleritis	6	16
Proptosis	2	15
Eye pain	3	11
Visual loss	0	8
Retinal lesions	0	4
Corneal lesions	0	1
Iritis	0	2
Other*		
Arthralgias/arthritis	32	67
Fever	23	50
Cough	19	46
Skin abnormalities	13	46
Weight loss (greater than 10 percent body weight)	15	35
Peripheral neuropathy	1	15
Central nervous system disease	1	8
Pericarditis	2	6
Hyperthyroidism	1	3

*Less than 1 percent had parotid, pulmonary artery, breast, or lower genitourinary (urethra, cervix, vagina, testicular) involvement.
SOURCE: Hoffman et al, 1992.

red blood cell casts, it is clear that once clinically detectable renal functional impairment occurs, rapidly progressive renal failure usually ensues unless appropriate treatment is instituted.

While the disease is active, most patients have nonspecific symptoms and signs such as malaise, weakness, arthralgias, anorexia, and weight loss. Fever may indicate activity of the underlying disease but more often reflects secondary infection, usually of the upper airway.

Characteristic laboratory findings include a markedly elevated ESR, mild anemia and leukocytosis, mild hypergammaglobulinemia (particularly of the IgA class), and mildly elevated rheumatoid factor. Thrombocytosis may be seen as an acute-phase reactant; hypocomplementemia is not seen despite the presence of circulating immune complexes in some patients. Eighty-eight percent of patients with active disease and 43 percent of patients in remission are positive for c-ANCAs (see above).

DIAGNOSIS The diagnosis of Wegener's granulomatosis is a clinicopathologic one made by the demonstration of necrotizing granulomatous vasculitis on biopsy of appropriate tissue in a patient with the clinical findings of upper and lower respiratory tract disease together with evidence of glomerulonephritis. Pulmonary tissue, preferably obtained by open thoracotomy, offers the highest diagnostic yield, almost invariably revealing granulomatous vasculitis. Biopsy of upper airway tissue usually reveals granulomatous inflammation with necrosis but may not show vasculitis. Renal biopsy confirms the presence of glomerulonephritis. The finding of elevated titers of c-ANCAs further supports the diagnosis.

In its typical presentation, the classic clinicopathologic complex of Wegener's granulomatosis usually provides ready differentiation from other disorders. However, if all the typical features are not present at once, it needs to be differentiated from the other vasculitides, particularly allergic angiitis and granulomatosis, Goodpasture's syndrome (see Chap. 241), tumors of the upper airway or lung, and infectious or noninfectious granulomatous diseases. Of particular note is the differentiation from idiopathic midline destructive disease (idiopathic midline granuloma; see Chap. 294) and upper airway neoplasms which may erode through the skin of the face, a feature very rarely seen in Wegener's granulomatosis.

Of particular importance in the differential diagnosis is a disease called *lymphomatoid granulomatosis*. It is characterized by lung, skin, central nervous system, and kidney involvement in which atypical lymphocytoid and plasmacytoid cells infiltrate tissue in an angioinvasive manner. In this regard, it clearly differs from Wegener's granulomatosis in that it is not an inflammatory vasculitis in the classic sense but an infiltration of vessels with atypical mononuclear cells; granuloma may be present in involved tissues. Approximately 50 percent of patients develop a true malignant lymphoma. The presence of c-ANCAs proves extremely helpful in the differentiation from all the preceding diseases.

TREATMENT AND PROGNOSIS Wegener's granulomatosis was formerly universally fatal, usually within a few months after the onset of clinically apparent renal disease. Glucocorticoids alone led to some symptomatic improvement, with little effect on the ultimate course of the disease. It has been well established that the treatment of choice in this disease is cyclophosphamide given in doses of 2 mg/kg per day orally. The leukocyte count should be monitored closely during therapy, and the dosage should be adjusted in order to maintain the count above 3000 per cubic millimeter, which generally maintains the neutrophil count at approximately 1500 per microliter. With this approach, clinical remission can usually be induced and maintained without causing severe leukopenia with its associated risk of infection. Cyclophosphamide should be continued for 1 year following the induction of complete remission and gradually tapered and discontinued thereafter.

At the initiation of therapy, glucocorticoids should be administered together with cyclophosphamide. This can be given as prednisone, 1 mg/kg per day initially (for the first month of therapy) as a daily regimen, with gradual conversion to an alternate-day schedule followed by tapering and discontinuation after approximately 6 months.

Using the above regimen, the prognosis of this disease is excellent; marked improvement is seen in more than 90 percent of patients, and complete remissions are achieved in 75 percent of patients. A number of patients who developed irreversible renal failure but who achieved subsequent remission on appropriate therapy have undergone successful renal transplantation.

Despite the dramatic remissions induced by the therapeutic regimen described above, long-term follow-up of patients has revealed that approximately 50 percent of remissions are later associated with one or more relapses. Reinduction of remission is almost always achieved; however, a high percentage of patients ultimately have some degree of morbidity from irreversible features of their disease, such as varying degrees of renal insufficiency, hearing loss, tracheal stenosis, saddle nose deformity, and chronically impaired sinus function.

Certain types of morbidity are related to toxic side effects of treatment. Since the preceding therapeutic regimen calls for conversion to alternate-day glucocorticoid therapy within 3 months and ultimate discontinuation within 6 to 12 months, glucocorticoid-related side effects such as diabetes mellitus, cataracts, life-threatening infectious disease complications, serious osteoporosis, and severe cushingoid features are infrequently encountered except in those patients requiring prolonged courses of daily glucocorticoids. However, cyclophosphamide-related toxicities are more frequent and severe. Cystitis to varying degrees occurs in 43 percent of patients, bladder cancer in 4 percent, and myelodysplasia in 2 percent.

Despite its life-saving effects in patients with Wegener's granulomatosis, cyclophosphamide cannot be tolerated by certain patients, such as those who develop severe neutropenia at low doses of drug or those who develop severe cystitis or bladder cancer. In these patients, alternative treatment regimens should be initiated. Azathioprine, in doses of 1 to 2 mg/kg per day, has proven effective in some patients, particularly in maintaining remission in those in whom remission was induced by cyclophosphamide. The drug should be administered together with the glucocorticoid regimen described above. Anecdotal reports have indicated therapeutic success with less frequent and severe toxic side effects using intermittent boluses of intravenous cyclophosphamide (1 g/m² per month) in place of daily drug administered orally. However, we have found that although 6 months of such a regimen induced improvement in approximately 90 percent of patients with remissions in 50 percent, 72 percent of patients were unable to maintain remission despite further treatment over 6 to 24 months. Although certain reports have indicated that trimethoprim-sulfamethoxazole may be of benefit in the treatment of Wegener's granulomatosis, there are no firm data to substantiate this, particularly in patients with serious renal and pulmonary disease. A regimen of methotrexate in doses up to 25 mg per week with alternate-day glucocorticoids has shown some promise in treatment of patients with moderate disease. Further studies over extended periods of time are needed to substantiate these early results.

TEMPORAL ARTERITIS

DEFINITION *Temporal arteritis*, also referred to as *cranial* or *giant cell arteritis*, is an inflammation of medium- and large-sized arteries. It characteristically involves one or more branches of the carotid artery, particularly the temporal artery, hence the name *cranial* or *temporal arteritis*. However, it is a systemic disease that can involve arteries in multiple locations.

INCIDENCE AND PREVALENCE Temporal arteritis is an uncommon disease, estimated to occur in 24 per 100,000 people. It is a disease of the elderly, occurring almost exclusively in individuals older than 55 years; however, well-documented cases have occurred in patients 40 years old or younger. It is more common in women than in men and is rare in blacks. Familial aggregation of this disease has been reported.

PATHOPHYSIOLOGY AND PATHOGENESIS Although the temporal artery is most frequently involved in this disease, patients often have a systemic vasculitis of multiple medium- and large-sized arteries which may go undetected. Histopathologically, the disease is a panarteritis with inflammatory mononuclear cell infiltrates within the vessel wall with frequent giant cell formation. There is proliferation of the intima and fragmentation of the internal elastic lamina. Pathophysiologic findings in organs result from the ischemia related to the involved vessels. Immunopathogenic mechanisms, particularly cell-mediated immunity, are felt to be involved in this disease, although the etiology is entirely unknown.

CLINICAL AND LABORATORY MANIFESTATIONS The disease is characterized clinically by the classic complex of fever, anemia, high ESR, and headaches in an elderly patient. Other manifestations include malaise, fatigue, anorexia, weight loss, sweats, and arthralgias. Temporal arteritis is closely associated with the polymyalgia rheumatica syndrome, which is characterized by stiffness, aching, and pain in the muscles of the neck, shoulders, lower back, hips, and thighs.

In patients with involvement of the temporal artery, headache is the predominant symptom and may be associated with a tender, thickened, or nodular artery which may pulsate early in the disease but may become occluded later. Scalp pain and claudication of the jaw and tongue may occur. A well-recognized and dreaded complication of temporal arteritis, particularly in untreated patients, is ocular involvement due primarily to ischemic optic neuritis, which may lead to serious visual symptoms, even sudden blindness in some patients. However, most patients have complaints relating to the head or eyes for months before objective eye involvement. Attention to such symptoms with institution of appropriate therapy (see below) will usually avoid this complication. Claudication of the extremities, strokes, myocardial infarctions, aortic aneurysms and dissections, and infarctions of visceral organs have been reported.

Characteristic laboratory findings in addition to the elevated ESR include a normochromic or slightly hypochromic anemia. Liver function abnormalities are common, particularly increased alkaline phosphatase levels. Increased levels of IgG and complement have been reported, as have increased levels of circulating immune complexes.

DIAGNOSIS The diagnosis of temporal arteritis and its associated clinicopathologic syndrome often can be made clinically by the demonstration of the classic picture of fever, anemia, and high ESR with or without symptoms of polymyalgia rheumatica in an elderly patient. The diagnosis is confirmed by biopsy of the temporal artery. Since involvement of the vessel may be segmental, the diagnosis may be missed on routine biopsy; serial sectioning of biopsy specimens is recommended. Dramatic response to a trial of glucocorticoid therapy can confirm the diagnosis.

TREATMENT AND PROGNOSIS Temporal arteritis and its associated symptoms are exquisitely sensitive to glucocorticoid therapy. Treatment should begin with prednisone, 40 to 60 mg per day, followed by a gradual tapering to a maintenance dose of 7.5 to 10 mg per day. In order to lessen glucocorticoid side effects in elderly individuals, conversion to alternate-day therapy may be attempted, but only after the disease has been put into remission with daily therapy. When ocular signs and symptoms occur, it is important that therapy be initiated or adjusted to control them. Because of the possibility of relapse, therapy should be continued for at least 1 to 2 years. The prognosis is generally good, and most patients achieve complete remission that is often maintained after withdrawal of therapy.

TAKAYASU'S ARTERITIS

DEFINITION *Takayasu's arteritis* is an inflammatory and stenotic disease of medium- and large-sized arteries characterized by a strong predilection for the aortic arch and its branches. For this reason, it is often referred to as the *aortic arch syndrome*.

INCIDENCE AND PREVALENCE Takayasu's arteritis is an uncommon disease, much less common than temporal arteritis. It is most prevalent in adolescent girls and young women. Although it is more common in the Orient, it is neither racially nor geographically restricted. An association of the disease has been described with HLA-DR2, MB1 in Japan and HLA-DR4, MB3 in the United States.

PATHOPHYSIOLOGY AND PATHOGENESIS The disease involves medium- and large-sized arteries, with a strong predilection for the aortic arch and its branches; the pulmonary artery also may be involved. The most commonly affected arteries seen by angiography are the subclavians, followed by the aortic arch, ascending aorta, carotids, and femorals. The involvement of the major branches of the aorta is much more marked at their origin than distally. Partial renal artery occlusion with resulting hypertension is common. The disease is a panarteritis with inflammatory mononuclear cell infiltrates and occasionally giant cells. There is marked intimal proliferation and fibrosis, scarring and vascularization of the media, and disruption and degeneration of the elastic lamina. Narrowing of the lumen occurs with or without thrombosis. The vasa vasorum are frequently involved. Pathologic changes in various organs reflect the compromise of blood flow through the involved vessels.

Immunopathogenic mechanisms, the precise nature of which is uncertain, are suspected in this disease. As with several of the vasculitis syndromes, circulating immune complexes have been demonstrated, but their pathogenic significance is unclear.

CLINICAL AND LABORATORY MANIFESTATIONS Takayasu's arteritis is a systemic disease with generalized as well as local symptoms. The generalized symptoms include malaise, fever, night sweats, arthralgias, anorexia, and weight loss which may occur months before vessel involvement is apparent. These symptoms may merge into those related to pain over the involved vessels followed by symptoms of ischemia in organs supplied by the compromised vessels. Pulses are commonly absent in the involved vessels, particularly the subclavian artery. Aortic regurgitation may occur; hypertension is seen in almost 50 percent of patients. Cardiomegaly and cardiac failure secondary to aortic or pulmonary hypertension occur commonly; the coronary arteries are uncommonly involved. Carotid artery involvement leads to a variety of central nervous system signs and symptoms with over half of patients experiencing syncopal episodes; stroke, which occurs in 15 percent of patients, may represent the first sign of disease; ocular signs and symptoms are present in 60 percent of patients.

The clinical course may be fulminant, may progress gradually, or may stabilize. Complications are related to the distribution of the involved vessels. Death usually occurs from congestive heart failure or cerebrovascular accidents.

Characteristic laboratory findings include an elevated ESR, mild anemia, and elevated immunoglobulin levels.

DIAGNOSIS The diagnosis of Takayasu's arteritis should be suspected strongly in a young woman who develops a decrease or absence of peripheral pulses, discrepancies in blood pressure, and arterial bruits. The diagnosis is confirmed by the characteristic pattern on arteriography which includes irregular vessel walls, stenosis, poststenotic dilatation, aneurysm formation, occlusion, and evidence of increased collateral circulation. Histopathologic demonstration of inflamed vessels adds confirmatory data; however, tissue is rarely readily available for examination.

TREATMENT AND PROGNOSIS The course of the disease is variable, and spontaneous remissions may occur. Reported mortality statistics range from less than 10 percent to 75 percent. Although glucocorticoid therapy in doses of 40 to 60 mg prednisone per day alleviates symptoms, there are no convincing studies which indicate that they alone increase survival. The combination of glucocorticoid therapy for acute signs and symptoms and an aggressive surgical and/or angioplastic approach to stenosed vessels has markedly improved survival and decreased morbidity by lessening the risk of stroke, correcting hypertension due to renal artery stenosis, and improving blood flow to ischemic viscera and limbs. Most recent mortality figures using this therapeutic approach are less than 10 percent. In individuals who are refractory to glucocorticoids, methotrexate in doses up to 25 mg per week has yielded encouraging results; however, long-term studies will be needed to confirm this.

KAWASAKI DISEASE

Kawasaki disease (mucocutaneous lymph node syndrome) is an acute, febrile, multisystem disease of children. It is characterized by unresponsiveness to antibiotics, nonsuppurative cervical adenitis, and changes in the skin and mucous membranes such as edema, congested conjunctivae, erythema of the oral cavity, lips, and palms, and desquamation of the skin of the fingertips. Although the disease is generally benign and self-limited, it is associated with coronary artery aneurysms in approximately 25 percent of cases, with an overall case fatality rate of 0.5 to 2.8 percent. These complications usually occur between the third and fourth weeks of illness during the convalescent stage. Vasculitis of the coronary arteries is seen in almost all the fatal cases which have been autopsied. There is typical intimal proliferation and infiltration of the vessel wall with mononuclear cells. Beadlike aneurysms and thromboses may be seen along the artery. Most investigators agree that many of the cases of PAN formerly reported in children were actually arteritic complications of unrecognized mucocutaneous lymph node syndrome. Other manifestations include pericarditis, myocarditis, myocardial ischemia and infarction, and cardiomegaly.

It is likely that immune-mediated injury to blood vessel endothelium is involved in the pathogenesis of this disease. Patients with Kawasaki disease have been demonstrated to have evidence of increased immune activation characterized by increased activated helper T cells and monocytes, elevated serum-soluble interleukin 2 receptor levels, elevated levels of spontaneous interleukin 1 production by peripheral blood mononuclear cells, anti-endothelial cell antibodies, and increased cytokine-inducible activation antigens on their vascular endothelium.

Apart from the up to 2.8 percent of patients who develop fatal complications, the prognosis of this disease for uneventful recovery is excellent. High-dose intravenous gamma globulin (2 g/kg as a single infusion over 10 h) together with aspirin (100 mg/kg per day for 14 days followed by 3 to 5 mg/kg per day for several weeks) have been shown to be effective in reducing the prevalence of coronary artery abnormalities when administered early in the course of the disease.

ISOLATED VASCULITIS OF THE CENTRAL NERVOUS SYSTEM

Isolated vasculitis of the central nervous system is an uncommon clinicopathologic entity characterized by vasculitis restricted to the vessels of the central nervous system without other apparent systemic vasculitis. Although the arteriole is most commonly affected, vessels of any size can be involved. The inflammatory process is usually composed of mononuclear cell infiltrates with or without granuloma formation. Cases have been associated with cytomegalovirus, syphilis, pyogenic bacterial, and varicella-zoster infections, as well as with Hodgkin's disease and amphetamine abuse; however, in most cases no underlying disease process has been identified.

Patients may present with severe headaches, altered mental function, and focal neurologic defects. Systemic symptoms are generally absent. Devastating neurologic abnormalities may occur depending on the extent of vessel involvement. The diagnosis is generally made by demonstration of characteristic vessel abnormalities on arteriography and confirmed by biopsy of the brain parenchyma

and leptomeninges. The prognosis of this disease is poor; however, in certain patients the disease may remit spontaneously, and some reports indicate that glucocorticoid therapy alone or together with cyclophosphamide in steroid-resistant patients administered as described above for the systemic vasculitides has induced sustained clinical remissions in a small number of patients.

THROMBOANGIITIS OBLITERANS (BUERGER'S DISEASE)

Thromboangiitis obliterans is an inflammatory occlusive peripheral vascular disease of unknown etiology which affects arteries and veins. Thrombosis of the vessels is likely the primary event, and so this disease is not a classic vasculitis. However, it is considered among the vasculitides because of the intense inflammatory response within the thrombus and the fact that there is often a vasculitis of the vasa vasorum in the arterial wall. The disease is discussed in detail in Chap. 211.

BEHÇET'S SYNDROME

Behçet's syndrome is a clinicopathologic entity characterized by recurrent episodes of oral and genital ulcers, iritis, and cutaneous lesions. The underlying pathologic process is a leukocytoclastic venulitis, although vessels of any size and in any organ can be involved. This disorder is described in detail in Chap. 290.

MISCELLANEOUS VASCULITIDES

A variety of disorders, many of which are uncommon, are characterized by varying degrees of inflammatory responses involving blood vessels. *Cogan's syndrome* is a disease characterized by nonsyphilitic interstitial keratitis together with vestibuloauditory symptoms. It may be associated with a systemic vasculitis involving vessels of different sizes as well as the aortic valve.

Erythema nodosum is a common disease which is recognized as a hypersensitivity manifestation of a number of other disorders. It is a painful nodular process of the dermis and subcutaneous tissues. However, histopathologically, there is a vasculitis of small venules (see Chap. 51).

Erythema elevatum diutinum is a rare chronic skin disorder of unknown etiology characterized by persistent red, purple, and yellowish papules, plaques, and nodules usually distributed symmetrically over the extensor surface of the limbs which on biopsy demonstrate a leukocytoclastic venulitis together with a marked dermal inflammatory infiltrate. The disease responds dramatically to dapsone therapy.

Certain *infections* may be associated with an inflammatory vasculitic process. For example, rickettsias can invade and proliferate in the endothelial cells of small blood vessels causing a vasculitis (see Chap. 138). In addition, the inflammatory response around blood vessels associated with certain systemic fungal diseases such as histoplasmosis (see Chap. 162) may mimic a primary vasculitic process.

Eales' disease is a retinal vasculitis which predominantly affects males in the second and third decades of life and which produces a syndrome of recurrent hemorrhages into the retina and vitreous.

APPROACH TO THE PATIENT WITH VASCULITIS

When a physician is presented with a patient in whom the diagnosis of vasculitis has been established clinically or pathologically, there are certain guidelines that may prove helpful to follow (Table 291-6). Each patient is unique and will require individual decision making; however, this framework should serve as a matrix. Expansion of each of the points in Table 291-6 is found in the text above.

1 Properly categorize the syndrome. Is it a specific syndrome (i.e., Wegener's granulomatosis, temporal arteritis, etc.)?
2 If syndrome is associated with an underlying disease or an offending antigen, treat underlying disease or remove offending antigen where possible.
3 Determine the extent of disease activity.
4 Institute therapy with appropriate agents in diseases in which therapy is essential and of proven benefit, such as with glucocorticoids in temporal arteritis and glucocorticoids and cyclophosphamide in Wegener's granulomatosis.
5 When feasible, avoid immunosuppressive therapy (glucocorticoids or cytotoxic agents) in diseases which rarely result in irreversible organ system dysfunction and which usually do not respond to such agents (i.e. chronic isolated cutaneous vasculitis).
6 Institute glucocorticoid therapy in patients with systemic vasculitis. Add a cytotoxic agent such as cyclophosphamide if an adequate response does not result or if a disease will historically respond only to cytotoxic agents, such as with Wegener's granulomatosis (see 4).
7 Be aware of the toxic side effects of therapeutic agents employed.
8 Continually attempt to taper glucocorticoids to an alternate-day regimen and discontinuation when possible. When using cytotoxic agents, taper and discontinue drug as soon as is feasible upon induction of remission according to established protocols.
9 Use alternative agents where the clinical situation dictates, such as with lack of responsiveness to or unacceptable toxic side effects with recommended agents.

REFERENCES

CUPPS TR, FAUCI AS: *The Vasculitides*. Philadelphia, Saunders, 1981
———— et al: Isolated angiitis of the central nervous system. Prospective diagnostic and therapeutic experience. Am J Med 74:97, 1983
FAUCI AS et al: The spectrum of vasculitis: Clinical, pathologic, immunologic, and therapeutic considerations. Ann Intern Med 89:660, 1978
———— et al: Wegener's granulomatosis: Prospective clinical and therapeutic experience with 85 patients for 21 years. Ann Intern Med 98:76, 1983
GIORDANO JM et al: Experience with surgical treatment of Takayasu's disease. Surgery 109:252, 1991
GROSS WL et al: ANCA and associated diseases: Immunodiagnostic and pathogenetic aspects. Clin Exp Immunol 91:1, 1993
HOFFMAN GS et al: Bronchoalveolar lavage analyses in Wegener's granulomatosis: A method to study disease pathogenesis. Am Rev Respir Dis 143:401, 1991
———— et al: Wegener's granulomatosis: An analysis of 158 patients. Ann Intern Med 116:488, 1992
KADISON P, HAYNES BF: Mechanisms of vessel damage, in *Inflammation: Basic Principles and Clinical Correlates*, JI Gallin et al (eds). New York, Raven Press, 1988, pp 703–717
KATZ P, FAUCI AS: Systemic vasculitis, in *Immunological Diseases*, M Sampter et al (eds). Boston, Little, Brown, 1988, pp 1417–1435
LEAVITT RY, FAUCI AS: Wegener's granulomatosis. Curr Opin Rheumatol 3:8, 1991
LEUNG DYM: New developments in Kawasaki disease. Curr Opin Rheumatol 3:46, 1990
NEWBURGER JW et al: A single intravenous infusion of gamma globulin as compared with four infusions in the treatment of acute Kawasaki disease. N Engl J Med 324:1633, 1991
SHELHAMER JH et al: Takayasu's arteritis and its therapy. Ann Intern Med 103:121, 1985
TREPO C et al: Superiority of a new curative etiopathogenic treatment of hepatitis B–related polyarteritis, using a short corticosteroid course, vidarabine, and plasma exchanges. Presse Med 17:1527, 1988

292 SARCOIDOSIS

RONALD G. CRYSTAL

DEFINITION Sarcoidosis is a chronic, multisystem disorder of unknown cause characterized in affected organs by an accumulation of T lymphocytes and mononuclear phagocytes, noncaseating epithelioid granulomas, and derangements of the normal tissue architecture. Although there are usually skin anergy and depressed cellular immune processes in the blood, sarcoidosis is characterized at the sites of disease by exaggerated T helper lymphocyte immune processes. All parts of the body can be affected, but the organ most frequently affected is the lung. Involvement of the skin, eye, and lymph nodes

is also common. The disease is often acute or subacute and self-limiting, but in many individuals it is chronic, waxing and waning over many years.

ETIOLOGY The cause of sarcoidosis is unknown. A variety of infectious and noninfectious agents have been implicated, but there is no proof that any specific agent is responsible. However, all available evidence is consistent with the concept that the disease results from an exaggerated cellular immune response (acquired, inherited, or both) to a limited class of antigens or self-antigens.

INCIDENCE AND PREVALENCE Sarcoidosis is a relatively common disease affecting individuals of both sexes and almost all ages, races, and geographic locations. Females appear to be slightly more susceptible than males. Cases of sarcoid have been described in all of the major races, and the disease is found throughout the world. It has been suggested that sarcoid is more common in certain geographic areas such as the southeastern part of the United States, but when case-matched controls have been used, these geographic differences are less convincing. There is a remarkable diversity of the prevalence of sarcoidosis among certain ethnic and racial groups. The prevalence of sarcoidosis is from 10 to 40 per 100,000 in the United States and Europe. In the United States, the majority of patients are black, with a ratio of blacks to whites ranging from 10:1 to 17:1. In Europe, however, the disease affects mostly whites. Furthermore, while the prevalence per 100,000 in Sweden is 64, in France it is 10, in Poland 3, yet for Irish females living in London it is 200. In contrast, the disease is very rare among Eskimos, Canadian Indians, New Zealand Maoris, and Southeast Asians.

Most patients present with sarcoidosis between the ages of 20 and 40, but it can occur in children and in the elderly. Several hundred kindred groups with familial sarcoidosis have been described, and the disease has been observed in twins, more commonly in monozygotic than in dizygotic pairs. There also have been several instances of husband-wife pairs identified, and geographic foci of sarcoid among unrelated individuals living closely within a community, arguing for some environmental factors in the pathogenesis of the disease. Although the disease is believed to result from exaggerated cellular immune responses to a limited class of antigens, no clear patterns in any HLA locus have emerged. Unlike many diseases in which the lung is involved, sarcoidosis favors nonsmokers.

PATHOPHYSIOLOGY AND IMMUNOPATHOGENESIS The first manifestation of the disease is an accumulation of mononuclear inflammatory cells, mostly T helper lymphocytes and mononuclear phagocytes, in affected organs. This inflammatory process is followed by the formation of granulomas, aggregates of macrophages and their progeny, epithelioid cells, and multinucleated giant cells. The typical sarcoid granuloma is a compact structure composed of an aggregate of mononuclear phagocytes surrounded by a rim of T helper-inducer lymphocytes and, to a far lesser extent, B lymphocytes. The overall structure is relatively discrete and is interspersed with fine collagen fibrils, presumably remnants of the underlying connective tissue matrix. The giant cells within the granuloma can be of the Langhans' or foreign-body variety and often contain inclusions such as Schaumann bodies (conchlike structures), asteroid bodies (stellate-like structures), and residual bodies (refractile calcium-containing inclusions).

Together the accumulated T cells, mononuclear phagocytes, and granulomas represent the active disease. Other than the fact that they take up space and thus their bulk modifies the local architecture, there is no evidence that the mononuclear inflammatory cells dispersed in the tissue or in the granuloma injure the affected organ by releasing mediators that damage the normal parenchymal cells or the extracellular matrix. Rather, organ dysfunction in sarcoid results mostly from the accumulated inflammatory cells distorting the architecture of the affected tissue; if a sufficient number of structures vital to the function of the tissue are involved, the disease becomes clinically apparent in that organ. Thus, while autopsy series show that, to some extent, sarcoidosis involves most organs in the majority of patients, the disease manifests clinically only in organs where it affects function (such as the lung and eye) or in organs where it is readily observed

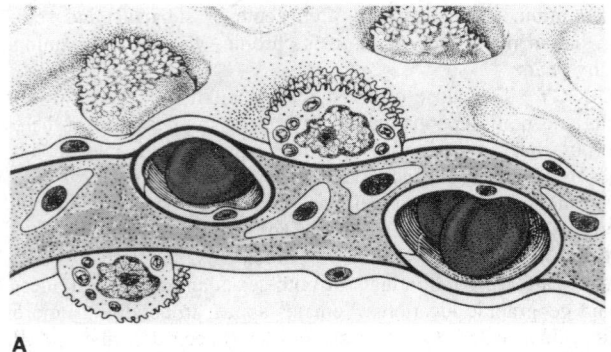

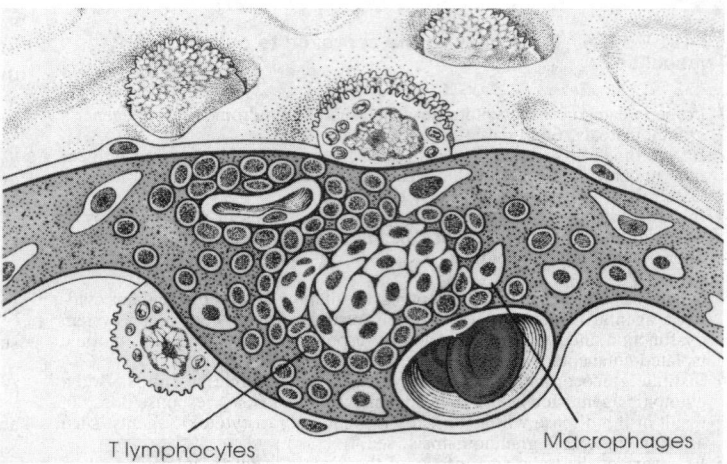

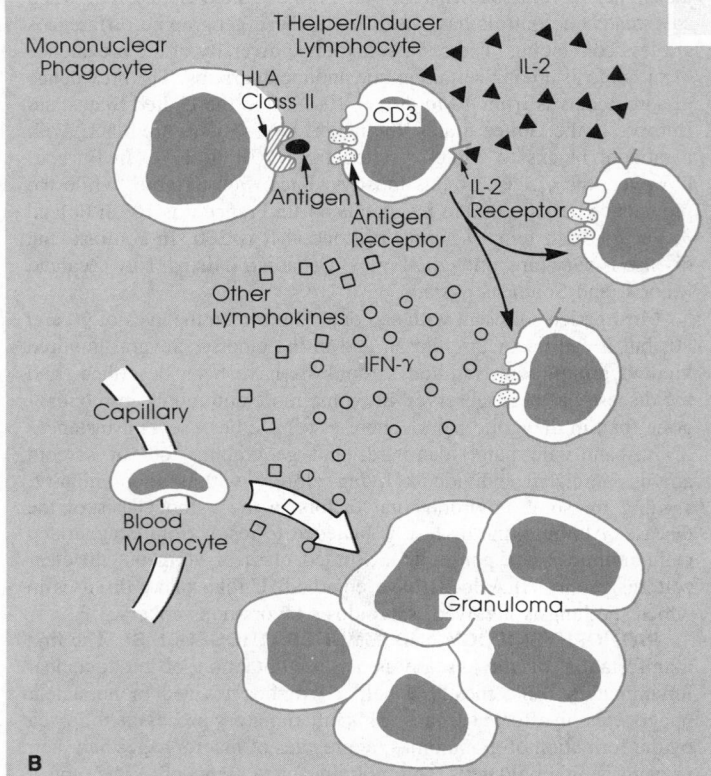

FIGURE 292-1 Pathogenesis of sarcoidosis. *A*. Histologic abnormalities. Normal alveoli *(left)* and alveoli in active sarcoidosis *(right)*. The latter are distorted by the accumulated T helper-inducer lymphocytes, alveolar macrophages, and macrophages aggregated into granulomas. There is mild damage to alveolar epithelial and endothelial cells. *B*. The exaggerated processes of T helper-inducer lymphocytes in affected organs result in the accumulation of these cells along with macrophages and macrophages aggregated into granulomas. The trigger for the T helper-inducer cells is unknown. It may be a limited class of antigens or self-antigens presented in the context of class II HLA surface molecules by mononuclear phagocytes to the T helper-inducer lymphocyte. The antigen class II HLA complex is identified by the T-cell antigen receptor, the CD3 signal transducing complex is triggered, and the T cell is activated. Consequent to this process the immune response is exaggerated and skewed to produce activated T helper-inducer cells that release interleukin 2, which drives the accumulation of more T helper cells. The activated T helper-inducer cells also release interferon-γ (IFN-γ) and other lymphokines, mediators that contribute to the recruitment and activation of blood monocytes and hence to granuloma formation.

(such as the skin or, by x-ray, the hilar nodes). For example, in the lung, the inflammatory cells and granulomas distort the walls of the alveoli, bronchi, and blood vessels (Fig. 292-1*A*), thus altering the intimate relationships between air and blood necessary for normal gas exchange. When a sufficient amount of pulmonary tissue is involved, it is sensed by the individual as dyspnea. In contrast, most individuals with sarcoidosis have granulomatous mononuclear cell inflammation in the liver but usually do not have symptoms or functional derangements referable to that organ, likely because the disease process does not modify the local structures sufficiently to affect function.

If the disease is suppressed, either spontaneously or with therapy, the mononuclear inflammation is reduced in intensity and the number of granulomas is reduced. The granulomas resolve either by dispersion of the cells or by centripetal proliferation of fibroblasts from the periphery of the granuloma inward, to form a small scar. In chronic cases, the mononuclear cell inflammation persists for years. If the intensity of the inflammation is sufficiently high for a sufficiently long period, the derangements to the affected tissues result in extensive damage, the development of fibrosis, and permanent loss of organ function.

All available evidence suggests that active sarcoidosis results from

an exaggerated cellular immune response to a variety of antigens or self-antigens, in which the process of T lymphocyte triggering, proliferation, and activation is skewed in the direction of helper-inducer T lymphocyte processes (Fig. 292-1*B*). The result is an exaggerated helper-inducer T cell response and thus the accumulation of large numbers of activated T cells in the affected organs. Since the activated helper-inducer T lymphocyte releases mediators that attract and activate mononuclear phagocytes, it is likely that the process of granuloma formation is a secondary phenomenon which is a consequence of the exaggerated helper-inducer T cell process. In this context, the current hypotheses of the cause of sarcoidosis, not mutually exclusive, include (1) the disease is caused by a class of antigens, nonself or self, that trigger only the helper-inducer T cell arm of the immune response, (2) the disease results from an inadequate suppressor arm of the immune response, such that helper-inducer T cell processes cannot be shut down in a normal fashion, or (3) the disease results from inherited (and/or acquired) differences in immune response genes, such that the response to a variety of antigens is an exaggerated, helper-inducer T cell process.

Independent of the inciting agent(s) or the reason why there is an exaggerated helper-inducer T cell response, there is a general understanding of the processes responsible for the maintenance of the inflammation and the development of the granuloma. The T helper-inducer lymphocytes accumulate at the sites of disease, at least in part, because they proliferate in these sites at an exaggerated rate. This T cell proliferation is maintained by the spontaneous release of interleukin 2 (IL-2), the T cell growth factor, by activated T helper-inducer cells in the local milieu. In this regard, sarcoidosis is a remarkable example of compartmentalization of the immune system and a dramatic illustration of why disease activity of sarcoidosis cannot be assessed by evaluating the immune system only in the blood. Whereas the T helper-inducer cells in the involved organs are releasing IL-2 and proliferating at an enhanced rate, the T cells in other sites, such as blood, are quiescent. Furthermore, while there is a marked enhancement of the number of T helper-inducer cells at the sites of disease, the numbers of T helper-inducer cells in the blood are normal or slightly reduced. In the involved organs, the ratio of helper-inducer to suppressor-cytotoxic T cells may be as high as 10:1 compared to the ratio of 2:1 found in normal tissues or in the blood of affected individuals.

In addition to driving other T helper-inducer cells in the affected organs to proliferate, the T helper-inducer cells at the sites of disease are activated and release mediators that both recruit and activate mononuclear phagocytes. The T helper-inducer cells accomplish this by releasing a variety of mediators (lymphokines) including proteins capable of recruiting blood monocytes to the local milieu of the activated T cells and interferon-γ, a protein that, among its many actions, activates mononuclear phagocytes. Together these mediators recruit blood monocytes to the affected organs and activate them, providing the building blocks for the formation of the granuloma.

In addition to these exaggerated cellular immune processes, active sarcoid is also characterized by hyperglobulinemia. Included among the immunoglobulins are antibodies against a variety of infectious agents as well as IgM anti-T cell antibodies. However, there is no evidence that any of these antibodies plays a role in the pathogenesis of the disease, and they are thought to result from the nonspecific polyclonal stimulation of B cells by the activated T cells at the site of disease.

If the damage in the affected organs is sufficiently extensive that the remaining parenchymal cells cannot reestablish the normal tissue architecture, the usual result is fibrosis, the proliferation of mesenchymal cells, and deposition of their connective tissue products. There is convincing evidence that the fibroblast proliferation is directed by tissue macrophages spontaneously releasing growth signals for fibroblasts, including platelet-derived growth factor, fibronectin, and insulin-like growth factor 1. It is not known, however, why this fibrotic process occurs only in a relatively small proportion of individuals with sarcoidosis.

CLINICAL MANIFESTATIONS Sarcoidosis is a systemic disease, and thus the clinical manifestations may be generalized or focused on one or more organs. However, because the lung is almost always involved, most patients have symptoms referable to the respiratory system. Independent of the site, the clinical manifestations of the disease relate directly to the exaggerated helper-inducer T cell–mononuclear phagocyte granulomatous inflammatory process itself or to the sequelae resulting from the permanent damage caused by this process.

Sarcoidosis is occasionally discovered in a completely asymptomatic individual, but more commonly it presents abruptly over 1 to 2 weeks or the affected individual develops symptoms insidiously over several months. Independent of the mode of presentation, about 75 percent of all cases present when the individual is less than 40 years of age.

The asymptomatic form is usually detected by a routine examination, such as a chest film. In the United States, this represents about 10 to 20 percent of all cases, but in countries where chest films are mandatory in preemployment screening programs, the proportion of asymptomatic patients is higher.

So-called acute or subacute sarcoidosis develops abruptly over a period of a few weeks and represents 20 to 40 percent of all cases. These individuals usually have constitutional symptoms such as fever, fatigue, malaise, anorexia, or weight loss. These symptoms are usually mild, but in approximately 25 percent of the acute cases the constitutional complaints are extensive. Many patients have respiratory symptoms, including cough, dyspnea, or a vague retrosternal chest discomfort. Two syndromes have been identified in the acute group. Löfgren's syndrome, frequent in Scandinavian, Irish, and Puerto Rican females, includes the complex of erythema nodosum and x-ray findings of bilateral hilar adenopathy, often accompanied by joint

symptoms. The Heerfordt-Waldenstrom syndrome describes individuals with fever, parotid enlargement, anterior uveitis, and facial nerve palsy.

The insidious form of sarcoidosis develops over months and is associated usually with respiratory complaints without constitutional symptoms. In the United States, 40 to 70 percent of all sarcoid patients are in this category. About 10 percent of these individuals have symptoms referable to organs other than the lung. It is the individuals who present with the insidious form of sarcoidosis who most commonly go on to develop chronic sarcoidosis, with permanent damage to the lung and other organs.

Despite the fact that sarcoidosis is a systemic disease and some evidence of inflammation can be detected in most organs in the majority of patients, sarcoidosis is important clinically because of the pulmonary abnormalities and, to a lesser extent, lymph node, skin, and eye involvement. Far less commonly, other organs are involved significantly.

Lung Of individuals with sarcoidosis, 90 percent have an abnormal chest x-ray at some time during their course. Overall, approximately 50 percent develop permanent pulmonary abnormalities and 5 to 15 percent have progressive fibrosis of the lung parenchyma. Sarcoidosis of the lung is primarily an interstitial lung disease (see Chap. 224) in which the inflammatory process involves the alveoli, small bronchi, and small blood vessels. These individuals typically have symptoms of dyspnea, particularly with exercise, and a dry cough. In acute and subacute cases, physical examination usually reveals dry rales. Hemoptysis is rare, as is production of sputum. Occasionally, the large airways are involved to a degree sufficient to cause dysfunction. Distal atelectasis can result from endobronchial sarcoidosis or from external compression from enlarged intrathoracic nodes. Rarely, wheezing is heard, incorrectly suggesting asthma. Large-vessel pulmonary granulomatous arteritis is common, but it rarely causes major problems. If it dominates the pulmonary lesions, it is sometimes called *necrotizing sarcoidal granulomatosis*. The pleura is involved in 1 to 5 percent of cases, almost always manifesting as a unilateral pleural effusion with characteristics of an exudate containing lymphocytes. The effusions usually clear within a few weeks, but chronic pleural thickening can result. Pneumothorax is very rare.

Lymph nodes Lymphadenopathy is very common in sarcoidosis. Intrathoracic nodes are enlarged in 75 to 90 percent of all patients; usually this involves the hilar nodes, but the paratracheal nodes are commonly involved (Fig. 292-2A). Less frequently, there is enlargement of subcarinal, anterior mediastinal, or posterior mediastinal nodes. Peripheral lymphadenopathy is very common, particularly involving the cervical, axillary, epitrochlear, and inguinal nodes. The nodes in the retroperitoneal area and in the mesenteric chain also can enlarge. All these nodes are nonadherent, with a firm, rubbery texture. Palpation causes no pain. Unlike nodes in tuberculosis, the nodes do not ulcerate. The lymphadenopathy rarely causes a problem for the affected individual; however, if it is massive, it can be disfiguring and can impinge on other organs and lead to functional impairment.

Skin Sarcoidosis involves the skin in about 25 percent of cases. The most common lesions are erythema nodosum, plaques, maculopapular eruptions, subcutaneous nodules, and lupus pernio. Erythema nodosum, comprising bilateral, tender red nodules on the anterior surface of the legs, is not specific for sarcoidosis but is common, particularly in acute sarcoidosis, in combination with systemic symptoms and polyarthralgias. Treatment is not required, since the lesions resolve spontaneously in 2 to 4 weeks. Erythema nodosum is much more common among sarcoid patients in Europe than in the United States. Skin plaques associated with sarcoid are purple, indolent lesions, often raised, and usually occur on the face, buttocks, and extremities. The maculopapular eruptions occur on the face around the eyes and nose, on the back, and on the extremities. These are elevated lesions less than 1 cm in diameter with a flat, waxy top. Subcutaneous nodules are most common on the trunk and extremities. Lupus pernio is characterized by indurated blue-purple,

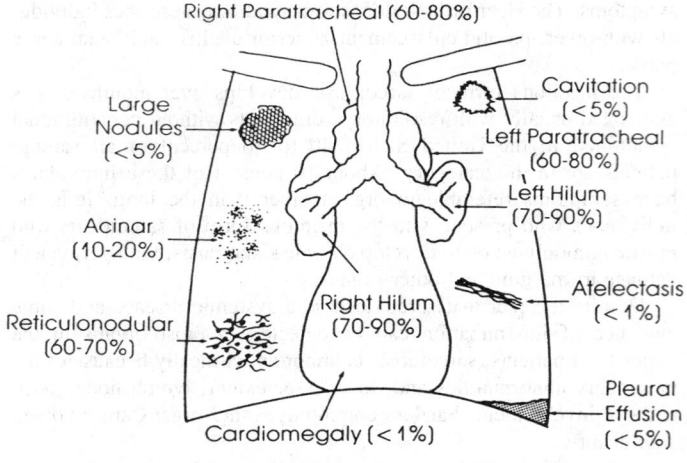

A

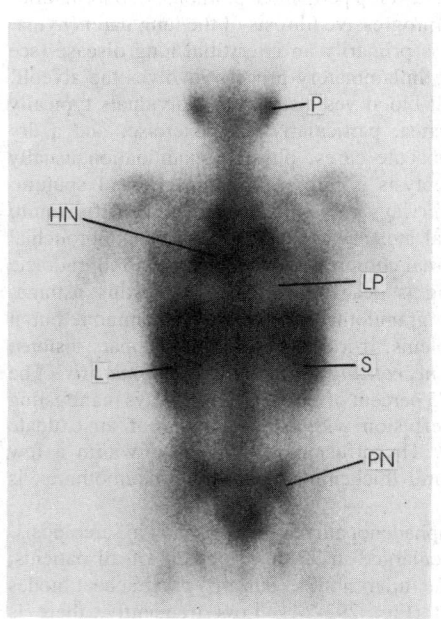

B

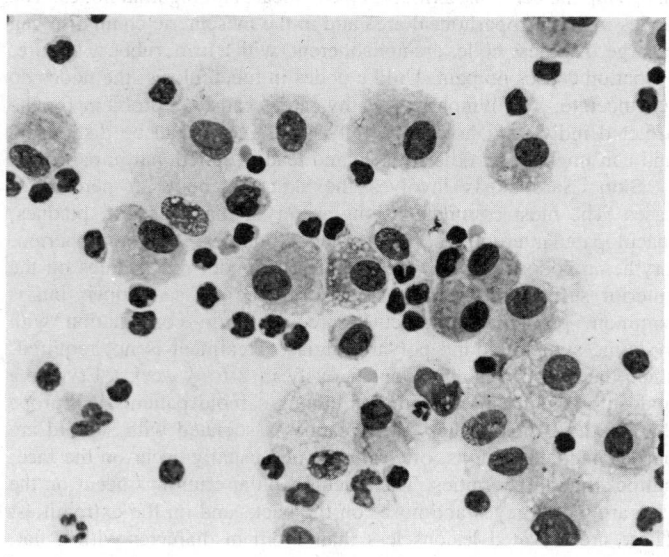

C

swollen, shiny lesions on the nose, cheeks, lips, ears, fingers, and knees. The lesions on the tip of the nose cause a bulbous appearance, sometimes associated with varicosities. The nasal mucosa is usually involved, and underlying bone can be destroyed. Sarcoidosis also can involve old surgical scars and tattoos. Although it may be disfiguring, cutaneous sarcoidosis rarely causes major problems. Clubbing of the fingers is occasionally observed in sarcoidosis, usually in association with extensive pulmonary fibrosis.

Eye   Eye involvement occurs in approximately 25 percent of patients with sarcoidosis, and it can cause blindness. The usual lesions involve the uveal tract, iris, ciliary body, and choroid. Of those cases with eye involvement, approximately 75 percent have anterior uveitis and 25 to 35 percent have posterior uveitis. There is blurred vision, tearing, and photophobia. The uveitis can develop rapidly and may clear spontaneously over a 6- to 12-month period. It also can develop insidiously and be chronic. Conjunctival involvement is also common, usually with small, yellow nodules. When the lacrimal gland is involved, a keratoconjunctivitis sicca syndrome, with dry, sore eyes, can result.

Upper respiratory tract   The nasal mucosa is involved in up to 20 percent of patients, usually presenting with nasal stuffiness. Any of the structures of the mouth can be involved, particularly the tonsils. Sarcoidosis involves the larynx in about 5 percent of cases. The epiglottis and areas around the true vocal cords are usually involved, but the cords themselves are not. These individuals are usually hoarse, and they have dyspnea, wheezing, and stridor; complete obstruction can occur.

Bone marrow and spleen   Sarcoidosis of the marrow is reported in 15 to 40 percent of cases, but it rarely causes hematologic abnormalities other than a mild anemia, neutropenia, eosinophilia, and occasionally, thrombocytopenia. Although splenomegaly occurs in only 5 to 10 percent of patients, celiac angiography or splenic biopsy reveals involvement in 50 to 60 percent of cases. The presentation and complications of splenomegaly in sarcoidosis are similar to those of splenomegaly in general.

Liver   Although liver biopsy reveals liver involvement in 60 to 90 percent of cases, liver dysfunction is usually not important clinically. Sarcoidosis involves generally the periportal areas. Approximately 20 to 30 percent have hepatomegaly and/or biochemical evidence of liver involvement. Usually these changes reflect a cholestatic pattern and include an elevated alkaline phosphatase level; the bilirubin and aminotransferases are only mildly elevated, and jaundice is rare. Rarely, portal hypertension can occur, as can intrahepatic cholestasis with cirrhosis.

Kidney   Clinically apparent primary renal involvement in sarcoidosis is rare, although tubular, glomerular, and renal artery diseases have been reported. More commonly, but still in only 1 to 2 percent of all cases, there is a disorder of calcium metabolism with hypercalciuria, with or without hypercalcemia. If chronic, nephrocalcinosis and nephrolithiasis can result. It is believed that the calcium abnormalities are associated with enhanced calcium absorption in the gut, which is related to an abnormally high level of circulating 1,25-dihydroxyvitamin D produced by mononuclear phagocytes in the granulomas.

FIGURE 292-2   Common laboratory findings of sarcoidosis. *A.* Schematic view of the abnormal findings on the chest x-ray. Shown are changes observed with the average frequency of occurrence. *B.* Typical gallium 67 scan of an individual with active sarcoidosis. The isotope has accumulated in the lung parenchyma (LP), liver (L), spleen (S), parotid (P), hilar nodes (HN), and pelvic nodes (PN). *C.* Cells recovered by bronchoalveolar lavage of an individual with active pulmonary sarcoidosis. The lavage analysis reflects the inflammation in the tissue. Shown are alveolar macrophages (*large cells*) and lymphocytes (*small cells*). The cell population is dominated by lymphocytes, in contrast to normals, in whom lymphocytes represent <20 percent of the cell population.

Nervous system All components of the nervous system can be involved in sarcoidosis. Neurologic findings are observed in about 5 percent of patients. Seventh nerve involvement with unilateral facial paralysis is most common. It occurs suddenly and is usually transient. Other common manifestations of neurosarcoid include optic nerve dysfunction, papilledema, palate dysfunction, hearing abnormalities, hypothalamic and pituitary abnormalities, chronic meningitis, and occasionally, space-occupying lesions. Psychiatric disturbances have been described, and seizures can occur. Rarely, multiple lesions occur which mimic multiple sclerosis, spinal cord abnormalities, and peripheral neuropathy.

Musculoskeletal system The bones, joints, and/or muscles can be involved in sarcoidosis. Bone lesions are observed in 5 percent of patients and include variable-sized cysts in areas of expanded bone, well-defined, round, punched-out lesions, or lattice-like changes. Hand and foot bones are the common sites, but most bones can be involved. Occasionally, the bone lesions are tender and painful. Joint involvement is more common, with an incidence of 25 to 50 percent in known cases of sarcoidosis. Arthralgias and frank arthritis occur mostly in large joints; they can be migratory and are usually transient, but they can be chronic and result in deformities. Although muscle biopsy frequently demonstrates granulomatous inflammation, muscle dysfunction is rare. However, nodules, polymyositis, and chronic myopathy have been described.

Heart Approximately 5 percent of patients have significant heart involvement, with clinical evidence of cardiac dysfunction. Left ventricular wall involvement is common. Arrhythmias are frequent, and serious conduction disturbances, including complete heart block, can occur. Papillary muscle dysfunction, pericarditis, and congestive heart failure are also observed. Cor pulmonale secondary to chronic pulmonary fibrosis may occur but is uncommon.

Endocrine and reproductive system The hypothalamic-pituitary axis is the part of the endocrine system most commonly involved; this usually presents as diabetes insipidus. Anterior pituitary dysfunction is also seen, manifesting as a deficiency in one or more pituitary hormones. Complete hypopituitarism is rare. Much less frequently, sarcoidosis can cause primary dysfunction of other endocrine glands. Adrenal cortical involvement resulting in Addison's syndrome has been described. Involvement of the reproductive organs occurs, but infertility is rare. Pregnancy is not affected by sarcoidosis, and patients with sarcoidosis who become pregnant usually improve during pregnancy. However, the disease may flare post partum; presumably this variation results from fluctuations in endogenous glucocorticoid production.

Exocrine glands Parotid enlargement is a classic feature of sarcoidosis, but clinically apparent parotid involvement occurs in less than 10 percent of patients. Bilateral involvement is the rule. The gland is usually nontender, firm, and smooth. Xerostomia can occur; other exocrine glands are affected only rarely.

Gastrointestinal tract Although sarcoidosis involvement of the gastrointestinal tract is found occasionally at autopsy, it rarely has clinical importance. Occasionally, patients have esophageal or gastric symptoms.

COMPLICATIONS The respiratory tract abnormalities cause most of the morbidity and mortality associated with sarcoidosis. The major problems are those characteristic of interstitial lung disease (see Chap. 224), particularly dyspnea and insufficient oxygen delivery to vital organs. Respiratory failure with carbon dioxide retention is rare. In some patients, lung destruction results in formation of bullae that may harbor mycetomas, which are usually aspergillomas; erosion into the parenchyma can result in massive bleeding. The most common complications apart from the lung are associated with the eye; however, with therapy blindness is rare. Complications of other organs include a gamut of abnormalities. The most serious are CNS lesions or cardiac involvement leading to congestive heart failure or sudden death.

LABORATORY ABNORMALITIES Common abnormalities in the blood include lymphocytopenia, an occasional mild eosinophilia, an increased erythrocyte sedimentation rate, hyperglobulinemia, and an elevated level of angiotensin-converting enzyme. Hypercalcemia is rare. Other serum abnormalities relate to involvement of specific organs such as liver, kidney, or endocrine glands.

Because the lung is involved so commonly, the routine chest film is almost always abnormal (Fig. 292-2A). The three classic x-ray patterns of pulmonary sarcoidosis are type I—bilateral hilar adenopathy with no parenchymal abnormalities; type II—bilateral hilar adenopathy with diffuse parenchymal changes; and type III—diffuse parenchymal changes without hilar adenopathy. The type III pattern is sometimes split into two categories, with films that show fibrosis and upper lobe retraction classified separately. Although patients with type I x-rays tend to have the acute or subacute, reversible form of the disease while those with types II and III often have the chronic, progressive disease, these patterns do not represent consecutive "stages" of sarcoidosis. Thus, except for epidemiologic purposes, this x-ray categorization is mostly of historic interest. The hilar adenopathy is almost always bilateral, but unilateral node enlargement can be seen. Nodes are also common in the paratracheal region. The diffuse parenchymal changes are typically reticulonodular infiltrates, but an acinar pattern is observed occasionally. Large nodules, similar to those of metastatic disease, are unusual but can occur. When there is massive fibrosis, the hila are pulled upward and there are conglomerate masses in the midlung zones. Some of the unusual chest x-ray findings in sarcoidosis include "egg shell" calcification of hilar nodes, pleural effusions, cavitation, atelectasis, pulmonary hypertension, pneumothorax, and cardiomegaly.

The lung function abnormalities of sarcoidosis are typical for interstitial lung disease (see Chap. 224) and include decreased lung volumes and diffusing capacity with a normal or supernormal ratio of the forced expiratory volume in 1 s to the forced vital capacity. Occasionally there is evidence of airflow limitation. There is usually mild hypoxemia and a mild, compensated hypocarbia.

The gallium 67 lung scan is usually abnormal, showing a pattern of diffuse uptake. If present, enlarged nodes are detected in these scans, as is inflammation in a variety of extrathoracic sites that usually have no clinical importance (Fig. 292-2B). Bronchoalveolar lavage demonstrates typically an increased proportion of lymphocytes, most of which are activated helper-inducer T lymphocytes (Fig. 292-2C). The remainder of the cells are mostly alveolar macrophages. In patients with significant fibrosis, a small number of neutrophils are also found. Eosinophils are rare.

The other laboratory features of sarcoidosis depend on the specific organ involved.

DIAGNOSIS For a typical case, the diagnosis of sarcoidosis is made by a combination of clinical, radiographic, and histologic findings. In a young adult with constitutional complaints, respiratory symptoms, erythema nodosum, blurred vision, and bilateral hilar adenopathy, the diagnosis is almost always sarcoidosis. Commonly, however, the findings are more subtle. Furthermore, because sarcoidosis can occur in almost any place in the body, like tuberculosis or syphilis, it can be confused with many other disorders. In this context, the differential diagnosis of sarcoidosis must cover a wide range. However, it is confused most commonly with neoplastic diseases such as lymphoma or with disorders characterized also by a mononuclear cell granulomatous inflammatory process, such as the mycobacterial and fungal disorders.

The presence of skin anergy is typical but not diagnostic of sarcoidosis. The Kveim-Siltzbach skin test, the intradermal injection of a heat-treated suspension of a sarcoidosis spleen extract which is biopsied 4 to 6 weeks later, yields sarcoidosis-like lesions in 70 to 80 percent of individuals with sarcoidosis with less than 5 percent false-positive results. However, the material is not widely available, and with the use of the transbronchial biopsy to obtain lung parenchyma for diagnostic purposes, the Kveim-Siltzbach test is not in general use.

No blood findings are diagnostic of the disease. Angiotensin-converting enzyme is elevated in the serum in approximately two-thirds of patients with sarcoidosis, but false-positive and false-negative results are common. An elevated 24-h urine calcium level is consistent with the diagnosis but is not specific.

The chest x-ray cannot be used as the sole criterion for the diagnosis of sarcoidosis. While the finding of bilateral hilar adenopathy is the hallmark of this disease, a similar pattern is occasionally observed in lymphoma, tuberculosis, coccidioidomycosis, brucellosis, and bronchogenic carcinoma.

The pattern of the gallium 67 scan is not diagnostic for sarcoidosis, nor is the finding of an increased proportion of lymphocytes among the cells recovered by bronchoalveolar lavage. However, the typical patterns of these tests (Fig. 292-2B and C) put the diagnosis in the general category of granulomatous lung disorders.

Whether or not the presentation is "classic," biopsy evidence of a mononuclear cell granulomatous inflammatory process is mandatory in order to make a definitive diagnosis of sarcoidosis. Because the lung is involved so frequently, it is the most common site to be biopsied, usually through a fiberoptic bronchoscope. Less common, but acceptable, sites for biopsy are the hilar nodes (by mediastinoscopy), the skin, conjunctiva, or lip. Rarely, the spleen, intraabdominal nodes, muscle, parotid or other salivary glands, upper respiratory tract, or the heart is biopsied for diagnostic purposes. At any of these sites, the findings must include the typical noncaseating granulomas. However, although histologic evidence is mandatory for a definitive diagnosis of sarcoidosis, the histologic findings are not sufficiently specific to make the diagnosis by themselves, since noncaseating granulomas are found in a number of other diseases, including infections and malignancy. Furthermore, although the liver or scalene nodes often reveal "positive" biopsies in cases of sarcoidosis, noncaseating granulomas from other causes are so frequent in these sites that they are not considered acceptable sites for establishing the diagnosis. Thus the definitive diagnosis of sarcoidosis is based on the biopsy in the context of the history, physical examination, blood tests, x-ray, lung function, and, if available, gallium 67 scan and bronchoalveolar lavage. Patients with immunodeficiency virus (HIV) infection commonly have lymphocytopenia, chest x-ray abnormalities, positive gallium 67 chest scans, and increased proportions of lavage lymphocytes (early in the course of the disease), and they can have lung granulomas, and thus serologic testing for HIV infection should always be done in individuals suspected of having sarcoidosis.

PROGNOSIS Overall, the prognosis in sarcoidosis is good. Most individuals who present with the acute disease are left with no significant sequelae. Approximately half of all patients have some permanent organ dysfunction, but for most this is mild, stable, and progresses rarely. In approximately 15 to 20 percent of cases, the disease remains active or recurs intermittently. Death is attributable directly to the disease in about 10 percent of all those affected.

TREATMENT The therapy of choice for sarcoidosis is glucocorticoids. A variety of other drugs have been tried, including indomethacin, oxyphenbutazone, chloroquine, methotrexate, p-aminobenzoate, allopurinol, levamisole, and cyclophosphamide, but there is no evidence, apart from anecdotal, uncontrolled reports, to support their efficacy. Cyclosporine is ineffective for the pulmonary manifestations of the disease; anecdotal reports suggest that it may be useful in extrathoracic sarcoid not responding to glucocorticoids.

The major problem in treating sarcoidosis is in deciding when to treat. Because the disease clears spontaneously in about 50 percent of patients, and because the permanent organ derangements often do not improve with glucocorticoids, there is controversy among clinicians as to the criteria for treatment. However, there is no question that glucocorticoids suppress effectively the activated T helper-inducer cell processes occurring at the sites of disease. Thus the major problem in making decisions concerning therapy in sarcoidosis is to determine the extent and activity of the inflammatory process in the organs at greatest risk, such as the lung, eye, heart, and central nervous system.

For the lung, this is based on a combination of history, physical findings, chest x-ray, and pulmonary function tests. Centers that see large numbers of these individuals also use criteria based on gallium 67 lung scans and bronchoalveolar lavage findings. The serum level of the angiotensin-converting enzyme has been suggested as a criterion for disease activity, but it is not specific for the lung. Unless the respiratory impairment is devastating, active pulmonary sarcoidosis is observed usually without therapy for 2 to 3 months; if the inflammation does not subside spontaneously, therapy is instituted. For the eye, decisions concerning therapy are based on slit-lamp examination and tests for visual acuity. For the heart and central nervous system, decisions are based on an estimate of the severity of the involvement; patients with minor dysfunction are usually observed, while patients with significant cardiac or neurologic abnormalities are treated. Usually, it is not necessary to treat the systemic symptoms, but occasionally the extent of the fevers, fatigue, and/or weight loss will necessitate therapy.

The usual therapy for sarcoidosis is prednisone, 1 mg/kg, for 4 to 6 weeks, followed by a slow taper over 2 to 3 months. This is repeated if the disease again becomes active. Alternate-day therapy is used by some clinicians, but there is no evidence that it is as effective. High-dose bolus intravenous glucocorticoids are used occasionally but are probably not as effective as oral therapy. Inhaled glucocorticoids are not efficacious. Mild ocular disease responds usually to local therapy, but suppression of the uveitis often requires systemic glucocorticoids.

REFERENCES

CRYSTAL RG Interstitial lung disease of unknown etiology: Disorders characterized by chronic inflammation of the lower respiratory tract. N Engl J Med 310:154, 235, 1984

FANBURG BL, PITT EA: Sarcoidosis, in *Textbook of Respiratory Medicine*, JF Murray, JA Nadel (eds). Philadelphia, Saunders, 1988, pp 1486–1500

GRASSI C et al: *Sarcoidosis and Other Granulomatous Disorders, Proceedings of the XI World Congress*. Amsterdam, Excerpta Medica, 1988

DUBOIS R et al: Granulomatous processes, in *The Lung: Scientific Foundations*, RG Crystal, JB West (eds). New York, Raven, 1991, pp 1925–1938

JOHNS CJ: Sarcoidosis, in *Pulmonary Diseases and Disorders*, AP Fishman (ed). New York, McGraw-Hill, 1988, pp 645–666

MOLLER DR et al: Bias toward use of a specific T-cell receptor β-chain variable region in a subgroup of individuals with sarcoidosis. J Clin Invest 82:1183, 1988

PINKSTON P et al: Spontaneous release of interleukin-2 by lung T-lymphocytes in active pulmonary sarcoidosis. N Engl J Med 208:793, 1983

ROBINSON BWS et al: Gamma interferon is spontaneously released by alveolar macrophages and lung T-lymphocytes in patients with pulmonary sarcoidosis. J Clin Invest 75:1488, 1985

SALTINI C et al: Spontaneous release of interleukin-2 by lung T-lymphocytes in active pulmonary sarcoidosis is primarily from the Leu3 + DR + T-cell subset. J Clin Invest 77:1962, 1986

SHARMA OP: Pulmonary sarcoidosis and corticosteroids. Am Rev Resp Dis 147:1598, 1993

VENET A et al: Enhanced alveolar macrophage-mediated antigen-induced T-lymphocyte proliferation in sarcoidosis. J Clin Invest 75:293, 1985

293 FAMILIAL MEDITERRANEAN FEVER (FAMILIAL PAROXYSMAL POLYSEROSITIS)

SHELDON M. WOLFF

DEFINITION Familial Mediterranean fever (FMF) is an inherited disorder of unknown etiology, characterized by recurrent episodes of fever, peritonitis, and/or pleuritis. Arthritis, skin lesions, and amyloidosis are seen in some patients.

TERMINOLOGY The variety of names given to FMF has led to confusion concerning its clinical features. None of the names, including FMF, is completely satisfactory. *Benign paroxysmal peritonitis* is inappropriate because many of the patients have involvement of serosal surfaces other than the peritoneum, and some die of amyloidosis. *Familial paroxysmal polyserositis* is an acceptable alternative for the term *familial Mediterranean fever.*

ETHNOLOGY AND GENETICS FMF occurs predominantly in patients of non-Ashkenazi (Sephardic) Jewish, Armenian, and Arabic ancestry. However, the disease is not restricted to these groups, and has been seen in patients of Italian, Ashkenazi Jewish, and Anglo-Saxon descent as well as others.

The earliest studies of the genetics of FMF were done in Israel, where the disease appears to be inherited as an autosomal recessive. Nevertheless, approximately 50 percent of patients give no family history of the disease. Consanguinity among the parents of FMF patients is as high as 20 percent, a figure which may be an underestimate. Approximately 60 percent of patients are male.

A recent paper in which 27 non-Ashkenasi Jewish families were studied reported that the gene that most likely causes FMF is located in the short arm of chromosome 16. Of great importance should be data derived from similar studies on FMF patients from other ethnic groups.

ETIOLOGY Although numerous pathogenetic mechanisms have been suggested, the cause of FMF is unknown. Fever and inflammation are such prominent signs that frequent attempts have been made to implicate infectious agents and/or their products. However, extensive studies have failed to implicate these or any other specific infectious agents. Others have suggested a deficiency in an inhibitor of C5a, thus implicating alterations in the immune system. Substantiation of such potential pathogenic mechanisms is awaited.

Because many FMF patients note that certain emotional or environmental changes may have profound effects on the frequency with which episodes of their disease occur, a psychosomatic basis has been suggested for the illness. There is no question that most patients eventually have transient or even permanent psychological alterations, which probably reflect their reaction to a chronic recurring illness that is forever threatening their social, economic, and personal well-being, but there is no evidence for a functional etiology for FMF.

The demonstration that FMF is inherited as an autosomal recessive disorder has led to the thesis that it is another inborn error of metabolism. Despite extensive studies, no such error has been found. Reported instances of excessive urinary excretion of porphyrins in FMF are probably examples of true porphyria and not FMF.

PATHOLOGY Despite the striking clinical manifestations during an acute attack of FMF, no specific pathologic alterations have been found. At laparotomy, only acute peritoneal inflammation in which the exudate contains a predominance of polymorphonuclear leukocytes is found to be present. A disproportionately large number of male patients develop gallbladder disease with and without cholelithiasis, but extensive histopathologic examination has failed to reveal any specific pathologic changes. Pleural and joint inflammation are also nonspecific.

In the amyloidosis which accompanies FMF, amyloid is deposited in the intima and media of the arterioles, the subendothelial region of venules, the glomeruli, and the spleen. Aside from their vessels, the heart and liver are uninvolved.

MANIFESTATIONS In the majority of patients, the symptoms of FMF begin between the ages of 5 and 15, although attacks sometimes commence during infancy, and onset has occurred as late as age 52. The duration and frequency of attacks vary greatly in the same patient, and there is no set rhythm or periodicity to their occurrence. The usual acute episode lasts 24 to 48 h, but some may be prolonged for 7 to 10 days. The attacks range in frequency from twice weekly to once a year, but 2 to 4 weeks is the commonest interval. Spontaneous remissions lasting years have been seen. In the majority of cases, pregnancy is associated with an absence of acute episodes, and many patients note less frequent attacks in the summer than in the winter. There may be a decrease in the severity and frequency of the attacks with age or with development of amyloidosis.

Fever Fever is a cardinal manifestation of FMF and is present during most but not all attacks. Rarely, fever may be present without serositis. The temperature may be preceded by a chill and will peak in 12 to 24 h. Defervescence is often accompanied by diaphoresis. The fever ranges from 38.5 to 40°C but is quite variable.

Abdominal pain Abdominal pain occurs in more than 95 percent of patients, and may vary in severity in the same patient. Minor premonitory discomfort may precede an acute episode by 24 to 48 h. The pain usually starts in one quadrant and then spreads to involve the whole abdomen. The initial site is usually very tender. Tenderness may remain localized with referred pain in other areas, and there may be radiation to the back. There may be splinting of the chest and pain in one or both shoulders, typical of diaphragmatic irritation. Nausea and vomiting sometimes occur. The abdomen is usually distended, and may become rigid with decreased or absent bowel sounds. On x-ray, the wall of the small intestine may appear edematous, transit of barium is slowed, and fluid levels may be seen. An abdominal operation may precipitate an acute attack of FMF which may be confused with other postoperative complications.

Chest pain Most patients with abdominal attacks have referred chest pain at one time or another, and 75 percent also develop acute pleuritic pain with or without abdominal symptoms. In 30 percent, the attacks of pleuritis precede the onset of abdominal attacks by varying periods of time, and a small number of patients never develop abdominal attacks. Chest pain is usually unilateral and is associated with diminished breath sounds, a friction rub, or a transient pleural effusion.

Joint pain In Israel, 75 percent of patients report at least one episode of acute arthritis. Arthritis can be distinct from abdominal or pleural attacks, can be acute or, rarely, chronic, and may involve one or several joints. Effusions are common and the large joints are involved most frequently. Radiologic findings are nonspecific. Despite careful search, frank arthritis rarely has been seen in the United States. Some patients have a history of rheumatic fever–like illness in childhood, but in a large series of patients, including 30 from the Middle East, acute arthritis was not observed. Mild arthralgia is common during acute attacks but is nonspecific.

Skin manifestations Skin involvement is reported by 25 to 35 percent of patients. These lesions consist of painful, erythematous areas of swelling from 5 to 20 cm in diameter, usually located on the lower legs, the medial malleolus, or the dorsum of the foot. They may occur without abdominal or pleural pain and subside within 24 to 48 h.

Other signs and symptoms Involvement of other serosal membranes has been reported, but pericarditis and meningitis are rare. Hematuria, splenomegaly, and small white dots called *colloid bodies* in the ocular fundus are among the findings of questionable significance. Rarely migraine-like headaches accompany acute abdominal attacks, and some patients have become somewhat irrational or show extreme emotional lability during attacks. Whether these are primary manifestations of FMF or secondary effects of pain and fever is not known.

Complications A serious, but increasingly rare, complication of FMF is drug addiction or habituation. Obviously, efforts should be made to avoid use of narcotics. Depression and lack of motivation are common, and patients with FMF require considerable encouragement and support. A striking number of patients in one American series have developed gallbladder disease.

Amyloidosis has been reported in Israel, North Africa, and elsewhere in the Middle East, but there have been only rare reported instances of amyloidosis complicating FMF in the United States. These findings are even more striking because there are probably as many known FMF patients in the United States as in Israel. These differences are unexplained and suggest that environmental or nutritional, as well as genetic, factors may play a role in the development of amyloidosis in FMF.

LABORATORY FINDINGS Polymorphonuclear leukocytosis ranging from 10,000 to 30,000 cells per microliter is almost invariable during acute attacks. The erythrocyte sedimentation rate is elevated during attacks but returns to normal between attacks. Plasma fibrinogen, serum haptoglobin, ceruloplasmin, and C-reactive protein increase during the episodes. Plasma lipids are normal, and there are no consistent abnormalities of hepatic or renal function. When amyloidosis is present, laboratory findings are typical of a nephrotic syndrome followed by renal insufficiency. Electrocardiographic and electroencephalographic changes are inconstant and nonspecific.

DIAGNOSIS   When the typical acute attacks of FMF occur in an individual of appropriate ethnic background who has a family history of FMF, the diagnosis is easy. When a patient is seen for the first time, a variety of other febrile illnesses must be excluded by appropriate study or observation. These include acute appendicitis, acute pancreatitis, porphyria, cholecystitis, intestinal obstruction, and other major abdominal catastrophes.

Some of the inherited forms of the hyperlipidemias may mimic the clinical picture of FMF, but lipid analysis will eliminate them from consideration. The patient with FMF is not immune to other diseases, and when an attack differs from the usual pattern or is more prolonged, consideration should be given to other diagnostic possibilities. The pleural form of the disease is sometimes difficult to differentiate from acute pulmonary infection or infarction, but the rapid disappearance of signs and symptoms resolves the problem. The joint manifestations may be more prolonged than other forms of FMF, and differentiation from septic arthritis, gout, and acute rheumatoid disease may be necessary. The erythema is sometimes difficult to differentiate from superficial thrombophlebitis or cellulitis.

Whether or not the patient is of the appropriate ethnic group, the most difficult diagnostic problem in FMF is the patient who presents with fever alone. In this situation, an extensive diagnostic workup for fever of unknown origin may be required. Fortunately, such patients are rare, and all eventually develop serosal involvement. Until specific diagnostic tests for FMF are available, patients with recurrent fever but without signs of inflammation of one of the serosal membranes should not be categorized as having FMF.

It has been reported that FMF patients have increased levels of plasma dopamine beta-hydroxylase (RHP) activity and that these levels returned to normal during colchicine treatment. Others have not confirmed these findings.

PROGNOSIS   Despite the severity of the symptoms during some acute attacks, most patients are remarkably free of any debilitation during the intervals between attacks. With encouragement and an understanding of their disease, most FMF patients lead fairly normal lives. The greatest hazard to patients is prolonged periods of hospitalization due to erroneous diagnoses or failure to understand the disease. In the United States, the prognosis of patients with FMF does not seem to be different from that of patients with other chronic nonfatal illnesses. Death usually results from causes unrelated to the underlying disease.

In the past, the complication of amyloidosis in Israel, parts of North Africa, Turkey, and other parts of the Middle East made the prognosis quite different from that in America. In the past, approximately 25 percent of FMF patients in Israel were known to have amyloidosis, and this complication usually led to death. However, the widespread use of colchicine has resulted in dramatically decreasing the incidence of amyloidosis.

TREATMENT   Among the therapies tried have been antibiotics, hormones (including estrogens and adrenal corticosteroids), antipyretic drugs, immunotherapy, psychotherapy, elimination and low-fat diets, chloroquine, and phenylbutazone. When carefully studied and followed up, none of these therapies proved effective.

During the past 20 years, the outlook of patients with FMF has been altered dramatically. Goldfinger reported in 1972 that the prophylactic use of colchicine in five patients dramatically reduced the number of attacks. Subsequently, controlled trials in the United States and Israel have shown that chronic administration of colchicine will greatly reduce the number of acute attacks of FMF. It is recommended that 0.6 mg colchicine be taken by mouth three times a day. Patients often develop gastrointestinal side effects with this dose, however, in which case the dose should be reduced to 0.6 mg

taken twice a day. Although an occasional patient will respond to 0.6 mg taken only once a day, this amount is less likely to be beneficial. Most FMF patients will respond favorably to colchicine prophylaxis.

REFERENCES

DINARELLO CA et al: Colchicine therapy for familial Mediterranean fever. A double-blind trial. N Engl J Med 291:934, 1974

MATZNER Y et al: C5a-Inhibitor deficiency in peritoneal fluids from patients with familial Mediterranean Fever. N Engl J Med 314:1001, 1986

MEYERHOFF J: Familial Mediterranean fever: Report of a large family, review of the literature, and discussion of the frequency of amyloidosis. Medicine 59:66, 1980

PRAS E et al: Mapping of a gene causing familial Mediterranean fever to the short arm of chromosome 16. N Engl J Med 326:1509, 1992

ZEMER D et al: Colchicine in the prevention and treatment of the amyloidosis of familial Mediterranean fever. N Engl J Med 314:1001, 1986

294   MIDLINE GRANULOMA

SHELDON M. WOLFF

DEFINITION   Midline granuloma is an uncommon disease characterized by localized inflammation, destruction, and often mutilation of the tissues of the upper respiratory tract and face. This condition has also been referred to as *lethal midline granuloma, malignant granuloma*, and *granuloma gangrenescens*, none of which is an appropriate term.

ETIOLOGY   The etiology of midline granuloma is unknown. In view of the intense granulomatous inflammation, the disease is thought to represent a localized hypersensitivity reaction which leads to tissue destruction and mutilation. However, the responsible antigen(s) is unknown, and there is no immunologic evidence supporting this hypothesis. A variety of microorganisms have been considered as possible causative agents, but detailed microbiologic investigations have failed to detect the consistent presence of pathogenic organisms. In view of the clinical and pathologic features of the illness as well as the fact that some tumors, in particular, lymphomas, can elicit a similar intense inflammatory response, some authors have suggested a neoplastic basis for midline granuloma. However, when malignant tissue is found in the lesions, the diagnosis of midline granuloma is no longer tenable.

It is possible that midline granuloma is part of the spectrum of what has been recently termed *angiocentric immunoproliferative lesions*. The latter are considered to represent a spectrum of postthymic T cell proliferative lesions. In fact, the association of malignant reticulosis and also of lymphomatoid granulomatosis with this group seems justified. Whether "idiopathic" midline granuloma is an early or arrested form of angiocentric immunoproliferative lesions awaits the kind of sophisticated immunocytologic studies that have been performed in patients with T cell lymphoproliferative diseases.

PATHOLOGY   The most characteristic pathologic finding is acute or chronic inflammation with necrosis. Superimposed pyogenic infection of the involved tissues, including the sinuses, may contribute to nonspecific histologic findings. The pathologic hallmark, noncaseating granulomas, with or without giant cells, may be obscured by the inflammatory reaction, but when present this is strong evidence in favor of the diagnosis. Primary vasculitis is seen rarely; when it occurs, a search for other causes, most notably Wegener's granulomatosis, should be made (see Chap. 291). The presence of malignant cells makes the diagnosis of midline granuloma unacceptable. Until a cause is established, the diagnosis of midline granuloma will rest on the characteristic clinical features outlined below.

CLINICAL FEATURES   The disease may occur at any age, but the majority of patients are in the fifth and sixth decades. It is more common in women than men and has been reported in all races. Many patients report recurrent "sinus" problems, and some have histories of allergic rhinitis, although the significance of these features is unknown.

The major symptoms are usually related to the nose. Patients frequently complain of nasal stuffiness and occasionally of discharge. The first symptom in a smaller percentage of patients relates to ulceration of the mucosa of the nose, the buccal mucosa, or the gums. This has led to loosening of the teeth, and dentists are often consulted first by these patients. Rarely, patients will present first with eye findings related to conjunctival inflammation or even ulceration. Although the progression of symptoms in some patients may be slow, all too often the disease steadily, and sometimes rapidly, progresses. The characteristic symptoms of nasal discharge, difficulty in breathing through the nose, and pain over the sinuses, nose, or eye become more prominent with time. Once ulceration begins, the disease often progresses rapidly. The ulcers frequently involve the nasal septum and will lead to the characteristic septal perforation and a saddlenose deformity. The majority of patients develop ulceration and eventually perforations of the soft and hard palates. Untreated, the disease can lead to massive destruction and mutilation of the tissues involved, including the skin of the face and the eyes. Frequently, the necrotic tissue becomes infected, and systemic symptoms such as fever and anorexia appear. The destructive lesions can become very malodorous. The disease extends to involve local tissues and does not progress below the neck; if this happens, other diseases should be considered. As the necrotic process progresses and involves vital organs, patients may lose sight in the affected eye, experience dysphagia, and have difficulty in speech. Although spontaneous temporary remissions have been reported, untreated midline granuloma is fatal. The progression of the disease can be rapidly accelerated by surgical procedures in the affected areas. The patient usually dies from secondary infection, although erosion by the process into a major blood vessel or penetration into the central nervous system with superimposed meningitis can also cause death.

Aside from the granulomatous inflammation, necrosis, and destruction, no other specific clinical or pathologic findings are associated with midline granuloma. Occasionally, with superimposed infection, local lymphadenopathy may be noted, but it is not characteristic of the disease per se.

LABORATORY FINDINGS With progression of the disease, a variety of nonspecific abnormalities may be noted. These changes are characteristic of inflammatory processes in general or of secondary infections. For example, mild anemia, leukocytosis, elevated sedimentation rate, and hyperglobulinemia are common in these patients. Radiographic examination reveals pansinusitis, and as the disease advances, destruction of bone in the involved areas is characteristic.

DIFFERENTIAL DIAGNOSIS The diagnosis of midline granuloma is made by finding the characteristic histologic lesions in biopsies of the affected tissues. When the specimens show only inflammatory tissue, a presumptive diagnosis of midline granuloma can be made only when the characteristic clinical picture is present and other diseases with similar presentation have been excluded. The diagnosis of Wegener's granulomatosis is ruled out by the absence of vasculitis in the biopsy specimens and the localized nature of midline granuloma (i.e., no pulmonary or renal involvement). In addition, Wegener's granulomatosis rarely, if ever, causes erosion through facial tissues. It is often difficult to differentiate true midline granuloma from neoplasms of the upper airways such as malignant reticulosis and certain lymphomas. These may be clinically similar to midline granuloma and are often associated with granulomatous inflammation. Careful examination of generous biopsy material as well as concomitant workup for disseminated neoplasm often provides the clinicopathologic distinction. Other diseases to be excluded by appropriate laboratory techniques are histoplasmosis, blastomycosis, coccidioidomycosis, leprosy, tuberculosis, syphilis, mucocutaneous leishmaniasis, rhinoscleroma, and pseudotumor of the orbit. Occasional patients who inhale cocaine develop septal perforations with inflammation that may be difficult to differentiate from midline granuloma (if the patients deny cocaine abuse).

TREATMENT The complications of midline granuloma such as superimposed infections can be treated specifically. Although adrenal glucocorticoids are often used in the therapy of midline granuloma, they are of no value and probably are contraindicated if infection is present. Sporadic reports of therapy with cytotoxic agents are difficult to interpret, since some of the patients reported clearly had lymphoma or Wegener's granulomatosis, diseases where such agents are of definite value. However, some patients appear to respond to cytotoxic chemotherapy. Surgical removal of the involved tissue has been attempted but is useless and may, in fact, cause rapid progression of the disease.

The treatment of choice is radiotherapy to the local lesion. Although low dosages [1000 cGy (1000 rad) and below] have been reported to be effective, many patients relapse after such therapy. Radiotherapy should be given in a dose of 5000 cGy (5000 rad) to the involved areas. Where such a regimen is employed, long-lasting remissions (more than 20 years) and probable cures have been achieved. Following irradiation and after an appropriate period to allow for tissue healing (usually 1 year), reconstructive and plastic surgery, which may be of enormous cosmetic and functional value, can be undertaken.

REFERENCES

FAUCI AS et al: Radiation therapy of midline granuloma. Ann Intern Med 84:140, 1976
FECHNER RE, LAMPPIN DW: Midline malignant reticulosis. Arch Otolaryngol 95:467, 1972
GRANGE C et al: Centrofacial malignant granulomas. Medicine 71:179, 1992
LIPFORD EH JR: Angiocentric immunoproliferative lesions: A clinicopathologic spectrum of post-thymic T-cell proliferation. Blood 72:1674, 1988

section 3   Disorders of the joints

295   APPROACH TO ARTICULAR AND MUSCULOSKELETAL DISORDERS

JOHN J. CUSH / PETER E. LIPSKY

Musculoskeletal complaints account for more than 10 percent of all outpatient evaluations in general medical practice. Many of the musculoskeletal complaints that cause patients to seek medical attention are related to self-limited conditions requiring minimal evaluation and only symptomatic therapy and reassurance. However, some patients with similar symptoms may have a more serious condition that requires additional laboratory testing to confirm the suspected diagnosis or document the extent and nature of the pathologic process. The initial goal of the clinician is to diagnose accurately and provide timely therapy while avoiding excessive diagnostic testing and unnecessary treatment.

Individuals with musculoskeletal complaints should be evaluated in a uniform, logical manner with a thorough history, a comprehensive physical examination, and appropriate laboratory testing. With such an approach and an understanding of the pathophysiologic processes underlying musculoskeletal complaints, an adequate diagnosis can be made in the vast majority of individuals. However, some patients will not fit immediately into an established diagnostic category. Many musculoskeletal disorders resemble each other at the outset and may take months or even years to evolve fully into a specific, recognizable syndrome. Such knowledge should temper the desire to establish a definitive diagnosis at the first encounter. A logical approach to the evaluation of patients with musculoskeletal complaints is shown in Fig. 295-1.

A paramount objective during the initial encounter is to determine whether the condition requires additional evaluation or immediate therapy. To make this decision, a knowledge of the particular anatomic site(s) of involvement (articular, periarticular, or extraarticular) and the nature of the pathologic process (inflammatory or noninflammatory) is important (Table 295-1). In addition to the four cardinal signs of inflammation (erythema, warmth, pain, and swelling), inflammatory disorders may manifest morning stiffness, fever, systemic symptoms, and/or laboratory evidence of inflammation (i.e., elevated erythrocyte sedimentation rate, thrombocytosis, etc.). Information derived from the patient's symptoms and signs allows the clinician to narrow the diagnostic considerations and assess the need for immediate diagnostic testing, therapeutic intervention, or continued observation over a period of time.

CLINICAL HISTORY   Historic features of the disorder are important in establishing the nature and extent of the pathologic process and also may provide important clues to the diagnosis. Aspects of the patient profile, including age, sex, race, and family history, can provide important information. Certain diagnoses are more frequent in different *age* groups. Systemic lupus erythematosus, rheumatic fever, and Reiter's syndrome occur more frequently in the young, whereas fibrositis is most frequent in middle age and osteoarthritis and polymyalgia rheumatica are more prevalent among the elderly. Diagnostic clustering is also evident when *sex* and *race* are considered. Gout and the spondyloarthropathies are more common in men, whereas rheumatoid arthritis and fibrositis are more frequent in

women. Racial predilections are noted with disorders such as polymyalgia rheumatica and giant cell arteritis (whites) and sarcoidosis (blacks). *Familial aggregation* may be seen in disorders such as ankylosing spondylitis, gout, rheumatoid arthritis, and Heberden's nodes of osteoarthritis.

The type of clinical presentation also provides important diagnostic clues. The *mode of onset* is characteristically acute in septic arthritis or gout, whereas osteoarthritis, rheumatoid arthritis, and fibrositis may have more indolent presentations.

Precipitating events such as trauma, drug administration, or antecedent illnesses should be sought. The *number and pattern* of involved structures often provide useful information. Complaints secondary to trauma and gout are typically focal, whereas others, such as polymyositis, rheumatoid arthritis, and fibrositis, are more diffuse. Rheumatoid arthritis tends to be symmetric, whereas the spondyloarthropathies are asymmetric. The upper extremities are frequently involved in rheumatoid arthritis, whereas lower extremity arthritis is characteristic of Reiter's syndrome and gout at their onsets. Involvement of the axial skeleton is common in ankylosing spondylitis but is infrequent in rheumatoid arthritis, with the notable exception of the cervical spine. The *chronology and evolution* of the patient's complaints also may be useful in suggesting diagnostic possibilities. Chronic (osteoarthritis), intermittent (gout), migratory (rheumatic fever), and additive (Reiter's syndrome) patterns are suggestive of certain disease processes. The duration of signs and symptoms alters the diagnostic considerations. Thus the musculoskeletal signs and symptoms of hepatitis B virus infection may be identical with those of early rheumatoid arthritis, but they rarely persist beyond 2 to 3 weeks.

Associated features outside the musculoskeletal system also may provide useful diagnostic information. A variety of musculoskeletal disorders may be associated with systemic features such as fever (systemic lupus erythematosus, infection), rash (systemic lupus erythematosus, Reiter's syndrome, dermatomyositis), or morning stiffness (inflammatory arthritis). In addition, some are associated with involvement of other organs, including the eyes (Behçet's disease, sarcoid, Reiter's syndrome), the organs of the gastrointestinal tract (scleroderma, inflammatory bowel disease), the genitourinary tract (Reiter's syndrome, gonococcemia), or the nervous system (Lyme disease, vasculitis).

PHYSICAL EXAMINATION   The goal of the physical examination is to ascertain the structures involved, the nature of the disorder, the extent and functional consequences of the process, and the presence of systemic manifestations. A knowledge of topographic anatomy is necessary to identify the primary site(s) of involvement and differentiate between articular, periarticular, and extraarticular disease. The musculoskeletal evaluation is largely dependent on careful inspection, palpation, and a variety of specific physical maneuvers to elicit diagnostic signs.

Examination of involved and uninvolved joints will determine the absence or presence of *warmth, erythema,* or *swelling.* The examination should distinguish true articular swelling caused by synovial effusion or synovial proliferation from periarticular involvement which usually extends beyond the normal joint margins. Synovial effusion can be distinguished from synovial hypertrophy or bony hypertrophy by palpation. Bursal effusions (i.e., olecranon, prepatellar) overlie bony prominences and are fluctuant with sharply defined borders. Joint *stability* can be assessed by palpation and by the

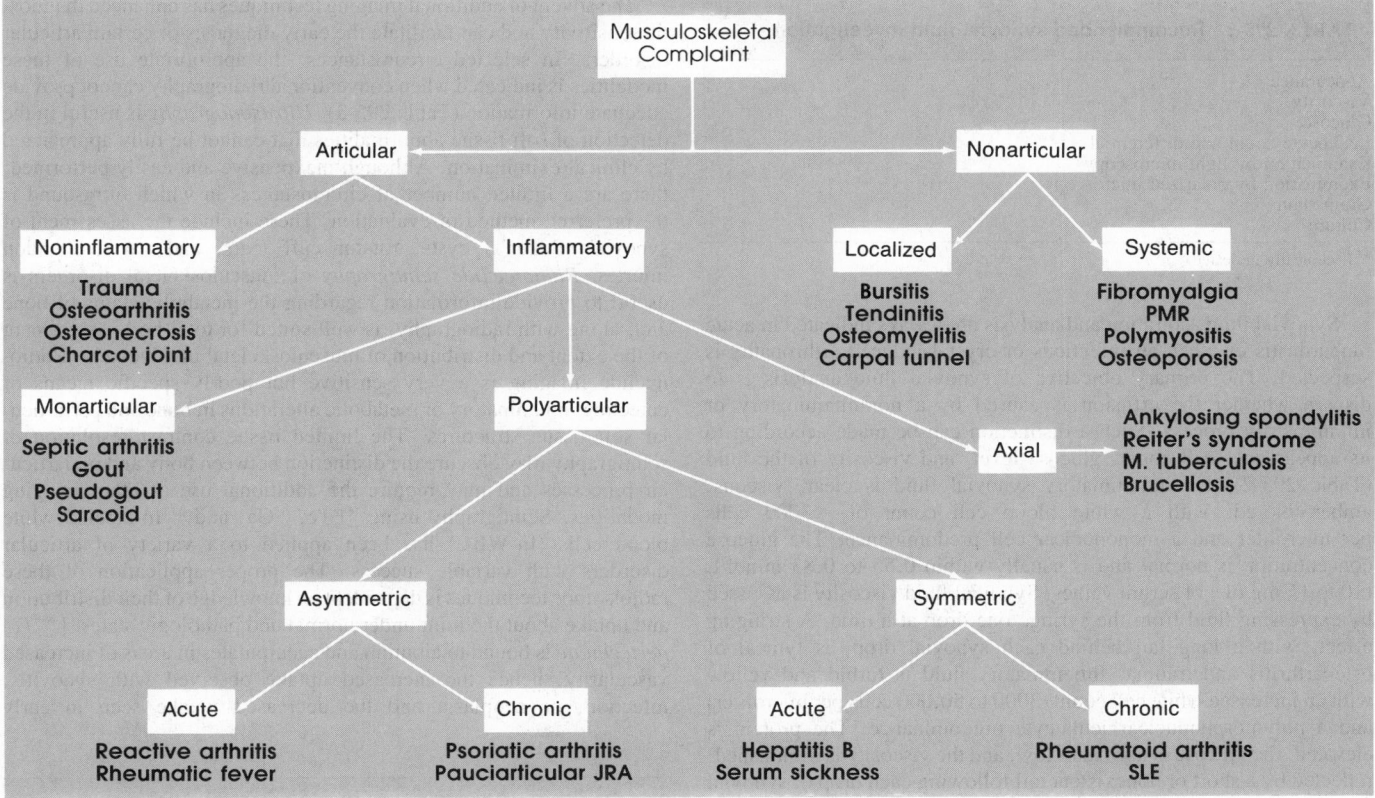

FIGURE 295-1   Approach to musculoskeletal disorders. An algorithm based on several rheumatologic symptoms and signs enables the physician to formulate a differential diagnosis (shown in italics) (PMR, polymyalgia rheumatica; SLE, systemic lupus erythematosus; JRA, juvenile rheumatoid arthritis).

application of manual stress. Subluxation or dislocation, which may be secondary to traumatic, mechanical, or inflammatory causes, can be assessed by inspection and palpation. Joint *volume* can be assessed by palpation. Distention of the articular capsule by various processes causes pain. The patient will attempt to minimize the pain by maintaining the joint in the position of greatest volume and least intraarticular pressure, usually partial flexion. Clinically, this may be reflected as obvious swelling, voluntary or eventually fixed flexion deformities, or diminished range of motion, especially on extension when joint volumes are decreased. Active and passive *range of motion* should be assessed in all planes and is best quantified by a goniometer with contralateral comparison. Joint *crepitus* may be felt during these maneuvers and may be prominent in degenerative disorders. Limitation of motion is frequently caused by effusion, pain, deformity, or

contracture. Contractures may be an indication of antecedent synovial inflammation or trauma. Joint *deformity* usually indicates a long-standing pathologic process. Deformities may result from ligament destruction, soft tissue contracture, bony enlargement, ankylosis, erosive disease, or subluxation. Examination of the musculature will document strength and the presence of atrophy and also will elicit pain or spasm. The examiner should assess carefully for periarticular involvement, especially when articular complaints are not supported by objective findings referable to the joint capsule. The identification of musculoskeletal pain of soft tissue origin (periarticular or extraarticular) will prevent unwarranted and often expensive further evaluations.

ADDITIONAL INVESTIGATIONS   The vast majority of musculoskeletal disorders can be easily diagnosed by a complete history and physical examination. However, in a number of circumstances, additional investigations may be required to establish the diagnosis or confirm a suspected etiology. A number of features indicate the need for additional evaluation. Patients with *acute monarticular* conditions require additional evaluation, as do those who present with *traumatic* or *inflammatory* conditions or those with *neurologic changes* or *systemic manifestations* of serious disease. Finally, individuals with *chronic (>6 weeks)* symptoms, even of minor severity, are candidates for additional evaluation. The extent and nature of the additional investigation should be dictated by the pattern of the involvement and suspected pathologic process. Broad batteries of diagnostic tests and radiographic procedures are rarely a useful or cost-effective means to establish a diagnosis.

Besides a complete blood count, including a white blood cell and differential count, the routine evaluation should include a determination of the erythrocyte sedimentation rate or C-reactive protein, which can be useful in discriminating inflammatory from noninflammatory musculoskeletal disorders. Serum uric acid determinations are only useful when clinically indicated.

TABLE 295-1   Characterizing musculoskeletal disorders

Anatomic sites of involvement	Pathologic processes
Articular	**Inflammatory**
Synovium	Infectious
Articular cartilage	Crystal-induced
Juxtaarticular bone	Immunologic
Other—menisci, capsule	Reactive
Periarticular	Idiopathic
Tendon	**Noninflammatory**
Bursa	Traumatic
Ligament	Mechanical or degenerative
Extraarticular	Functional
Bone	Neoplastic
Muscle	Other
Nerve	
Fascia	
Skin and subcutaneous tissue	

TABLE 295-2 Recommended synovial fluid investigation

Appearance
Viscosity
Glucose
Leukocyte count and differential
Examination by light microscopy
Examination by polarized microscopy
Gram stain*
Culture*

---

* If clinically indicated.

Synovial fluid aspiration and analysis are always indicated in acute monarthritis or when an infectious or crystal-induced arthropathy is suspected. The primary objective of synovial fluid analysis is to discern whether the effusion is caused by a noninflammatory or inflammatory process. Such a distinction can be made according to its appearance, cell count, glucose level, and viscosity of the fluid (Table 295-2). Noninflammatory synovial fluid is clear, viscous, amber-colored, with a white blood cell count of <3000 cells per microliter and a mononuclear cell predominance. The glucose concentration is normal and is usually within 0.55 to 0.83 mmol/L (10 to 15 mg/dL) of serum values. Synovial fluid viscosity is assessed by expressing fluid from the syringe one drop at a time. A stringing effect, with a long tail behind each synovial drop, is typical of osteoarthritis and trauma. Inflammatory fluid is turbid and yellow with an increased white cell count (3000 to 50,000 cells per microliter) and a polymorphonuclear leukocyte predominance. The protein is elevated, the glucose is normal or low, and the viscosity is diminished, reflected by a short or nonexistent tail following each drop of synovial fluid. Such effusions are found in rheumatoid arthritis, gout, other inflammatory arthritides, and occasionally septic arthritis. Infectious fluid is turbid and opaque, with a white cell count >50,000 cells per microliter and a polymorphonuclear leukocyte predominance. The protein is elevated, the glucose is often low, and viscosity is poor. Such effusions are typical of septic arthritis but may rarely occur with sterile inflammatory arthritides such as rheumatoid arthritis or gout. Additionally, hemorrhagic synovial fluid may be seen with hemarthrosis or trauma. Synovial fluid should be analyzed immediately for cellularity and crystals using a polarizing microscope. Monosodium urate, seen in gouty effusions, appears as long, needle-shaped, negatively birefringent, usually intracellular crystals, whereas calcium pyrophosphate dihydrate, found in chondrocalcinosis and pseudogout, is usually seen as short, rhomboid-shaped, positively birefringent crystals. Whenever infection is a possibility, synovial fluid should be Gram-stained and cultured appropriately. If gonococcal arthritis is suspected, immediate plating of the fluid on appropriate culture medium is indicated. It should be noted that on occasion both crystal-induced arthritis and infection may occur in the same joint.

Serologic tests for rheumatoid factor (antibodies to IgG), antinuclear antibodies, complement levels, or antistreptolysin O titers should be carried out only when there is clinical evidence to suggest a specific diagnosis, since these have poor predictive value as screening tests.

DIAGNOSTIC IMAGING IN JOINT DISEASES Historically, *conventional radiography* has played an integral part in the diagnosis and staging of articular disorders. Plain films are most appropriate when there is a history of prior trauma, suspected chronic infection, progressive disability, or monarticular involvement; when therapeutic alterations are considered; or when they are useful as a baseline assessment for what appears to be a chronic process. However, in most inflammatory disorders, early radiography is rarely helpful in establishing a diagnosis and often reveals only soft tissue swelling and juxtaarticular demineralization. As the disease progresses, calcification (soft tissue, cartilage, or bone), joint space narrowing, erosions, bony ankylosis, new bone formation (sclerosis, osteophytes, or periostitis), or subchondral cysts may develop and provide diagnostic information. The use of high-quality films and proper positioning can eliminate the need for further studies.

The advent of additional imaging techniques has enhanced diagnostic sensitivity and can facilitate the early diagnosis of certain articular disorders. In selected circumstances, the appropriate use of these modalities is indicated when conventional radiography cannot provide adequate information (Table 295-3). *Ultrasonography* is useful in the detection of soft tissue abnormalities that cannot be fully appreciated by clinical eximination. Although inexpensive and easily performed, there are a limited number of circumstances in which ultrasound is the preferred method of evaluation. These include the assessment of synovial (Baker's) cysts, rotator cuff tears, and various tendon injuries. *Radionuclide scintigraphy* of musculoskeletal disorders is useful to provide information regarding the metabolic status of bone and, along with radiography, is well suited for total-body assessment of the extent and distribution of musculoskeletal involvement. Radionuclide imaging is a very sensitive but poorly specific means of detecting inflammatory or metabolic alterations in bone and periarticular soft tissue structures. The limited tissue contrast resolution of scintigraphy may obscure the distinction between bony and periarticular processes and may require the additional use of other imaging modalities. Scintigraphy using ^{99m}Tc, ^{67}Ga, and ^{111}In-labeled white blood cells (In-WBC) has been applied to a variety of articular disorders with variable success. The proper application of these radioisotope techniques is dependent on knowledge of their distribution and uptake about the joint under normal and pathologic states. [^{99m}Tc] *pertechnate* is bound to albumin and accumulates in areas of increased vascularity, hence the increased uptake observed with synovitis, infection, or neoplasia and the decreased uptake seen in early

TABLE 295-3 Diagnostic imaging techniques for musculoskeletal disorders

	Imaging time (h)	Cost*	Imaging capacity	Indications
ULTRASOUND†				
	<1	+	Focal	Synovial cysts, rotator cuff tears, tendon injury
RADIONUCLIDE SCINTIGRAPHY				
^{99m}Tc	1–4	+ +	Diffuse	Metastatic bone survey, evaluation of Paget's disease, quantitative joint assessment, acute infection, acute and chronic osteomyelitis
^{111}In-WBC	24	+ + +	Diffuse	Acute infection, prosthetic infection, acute osteomyelitis
^{67}Ga	24–48	+ + + +	Diffuse	Acute and chronic infection, acute osteomyelitis
COMPUTED TOMOGRAPHY				
	<1	+ + +	Focal	Herniated intervertebral disk, sacroiliitis, spinal stenosis, spinal trauma, osteoid osteoma, tarsal coalition
MAGNETIC RESONANCE IMAGING				
	1/2–2	+ + + + +	Focal	Avascular necrosis, osteomyelitis, intraarticular derangement and soft tissue injury, derangments of axial skeleton and spinal cord, pigmented villonodular synovitis, inflammatory and metabolic muscle pathology

* Relative imaging cost.
† Operator dependent.

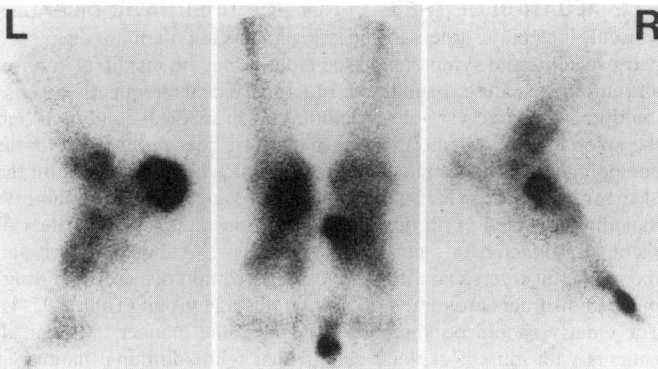

FIGURE 295-2 [^{99m}Tc] diphosphonate scintigraphy of the feet of a 33-year-old black male with Reiter's syndrome, manifested by sacroiliitis, urethritis, uveitis, asymmetric oligoarthritis, and enthesitis. This bone scan demonstrates increased uptake indicative of enthesitis involving the insertions of the left Achilles tendon, plantar aponeurosis, and the right tibialis posterior tendon and arthritis of the right first interphalangeal joint.

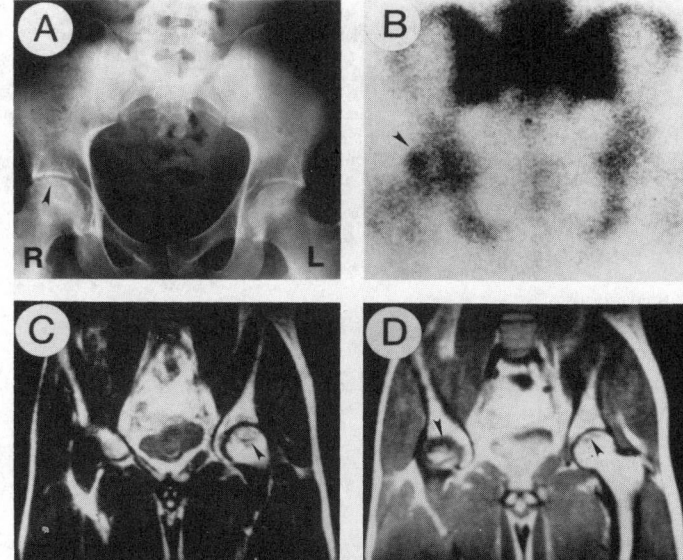

FIGURE 295-3 Superior sensitivity of magnetic resonance imaging in the diagnosis of osteonecrosis of the femoral head. A 25-year-old white male taking high-dose glucocorticoids for idiopathic thrombocytopenic purpura developed bilateral hip pain. Conventional x-ray films (*A*) demonstrated abnormalities only in the right hip consistent with stage II osteonecrosis (arrow). A bone scan (*B*) revealed increased uptake in the right hip only (arrow). MRI using spin-echo proton density images (*C* and *D*) demonstrated low-density signals from both femoral heads (arrows), indicative of bilateral osteonecrosis.

osteonecrosis. By contrast, [^{99m}Tc] *diphosphonate* is utilized as a bone-seeking radionuclide, whose distribution is dependent on blood flow and uptake during new bone formation. Increased uptake is seen with inflammation, increased blood flow, bone remodeling, and heterotopic bone formation (Fig. 295-2). The poor specificity of ^{99m}Tc scanning has limited its use to investigational and serial assessments of joint/bone involvement, inflammatory or infectious processes, and metastatic bone surveys. ^{67}Ga binds to serum and cellular transferrin and lactoferrin and is preferentially taken up by neutrophils, macrophages, bacteria, and tumor tissue (i.e., lymphoma) and is thus useful in the identification of infection and malignancies. Scanning with ^{111}In-WBC has been used to detect both infectious and inflammatory arthritis. Although both have been used with success, ^{111}In-WBC scanning is superior to ^{67}Ga in the early diagnosis of osteomyelitis and infected prosthetic joints. Prior treatment with antibiotics reduces the diagnostic sensitivities of both ^{67}Ga and ^{111}In-WBC scintigraphy. Other radionuclide conjugates (i.e., [^{111}In]chloride, ^{111}In- and ^{125}I-labeled polyclonal IgG, [^{99m}Tc]liposomes, and [^{99m}Tc]hexamethylpropyleneamine oxine) have been developed and used with variable success in the detection of infectious or inflammatory musculoskeletal disorders. Further comparative studies are needed to define the diagnostic indications for these modalities.

Computed tomography (CT) provides rapid reconstruction of sagittal, coronal, and axial images and spatial relationships among anatomic structures. It has proved to be most useful in the assessment of the axial skeleton because of its ability to visualize in the axial plane. Articulations previously considered difficult to visualize using conventional radiography, such as the zygoapophyseal, sacroiliac, sternoclavicular, and hip joints, can be evaluated effectively using CT. CT has been demonstrated to be useful in the diagnosis of low-back pain syndromes, sacroiliitis, avascular necrosis, osteoid osteoma, tarsal coalition, osteomyelitis, and intraarticular osteochondral fragments.

Magnetic resonance imaging (MRI) has emerged as a significant

advancement in musculoskeletal imaging. MRI has the advantages of providing multiplanar images with fine anatomic detail and contrast resolution (Figs. 295-3 and 295-4). Moreover, the lack of ionizing radiation and adverse effects and the superior ability to visualize bone marrow and soft tissue periarticular structures have led to increased use of this modality. The advantages of MRI are counterbalanced by high costs and long procedural time, factors that have limited its use in the evaluation of musculoskeletal disorders. Therefore, it is recommended that MRI only be employed when less expensive and noninvasive modalities fail to provide necessary information that will affect the patient's clinical management.

MRI is capable of imaging fascia, vessels, nerve, muscle, cartilage, ligaments, tendons, pannus, synovial effusions, cortical bone, and bone marrow. Visualization of these structures can be enhanced by altering enumerable pulse sequences. In musculoskeletal imaging, the most frequently utilized techniques include T1-weighted and T2-weighted spin-echo, gradient-echo, and inversion recovery (including STIR) images. T1-weighted images usually demonstrate superior anatomic detail, whereas T2-weighted images enhance the visualization of soft tissues enriched in water molecules, thereby facilitating the visualization of fluid, edema, inflammation, and tumors. Structures containing few mobile hydrogen protons (cortical bone, fibrocartilage, tendons, and ligaments) will appear dark or black on T1- and T2-

FIGURE 295-4 Coronal magnetic resonance images of the wrist in a 54-year-old female with rheumatoid arthritis. *A*. T1-weighted image demonstrates an erosion of the triquetrum (arrow). *B*. Gadopentetate dimeglumine enhanced T1-weighted image demonstrates enhancement of the same erosion (arrow), indicating the presence of vascularized pannus. *C*. Inversion recovery (STIR) image demonstrates a fluid-dense, high-intensity signal near the triquetrum (arrow) and in the intercarpal spaces, suggesting widespread intercarpal inflammation.

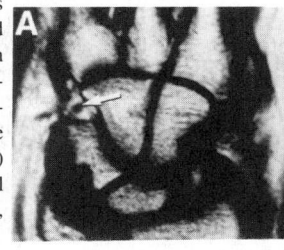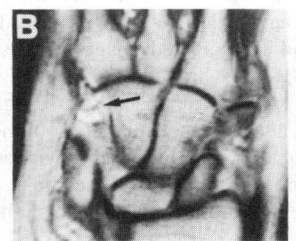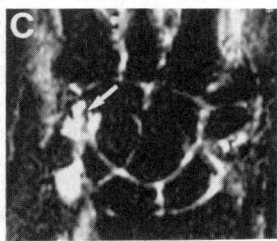

TABLE 295-4   Musculoskeletal disorders in the elderly

INFLAMMATORY

Polymyalgia rheumatica/giant cell arteritis
Vasculitis (polyarteritis, cholesterol emboli syndrome)
Crystal arthropathies (gout, pseudogout)
Septic arthritis
Older-onset lupus

MECHANICAL

Osteoarthritis
Spinal stenosis
Low back pain
Trauma
Heel spurs

METABOLIC/ENDOCRINE

Osteoporosis
Paget's disease
Hypothyroidism/myxedema
Amyloid
Diabetes

NEOPLASIA-RELATED

Secondary gout
Carcinomatous arthropathy or neuromyopathy
Dermatomyositis
Sjögren's syndrome
Vasculitis (lymphoma, hairy cell leukemia)
Cryoglobulinemia
Panniculitis (pancreatic cancer, lymphoproliferative disorders)
Hypertrophic osteoarthropathy
Metastasis to bone
Atrial myxoma

DRUG-INDUCED

Gout (diuretics, low-dose salicylates, cytotoxics, alcohol)
Drug-induced lupus (procainamide, hydralazine, methyldopa, phenytoin, isoniazid, quinidine)
Myopathy (glucocorticoids, lovastatin, clofibrate, taxol, colchicine, penicillamine, hydroxychloroquine)
Osteonecrosis (glucocorticoids, ethanol, radiation, hip surgery)
Osteopenia (glucocorticoids, heparin, phenytoin)
Toxicity (salicylates, NSAIDs, narcotics)

EVALUATION OF THE ELDERLY FOR RHEUMATIC DISEASES

Musculoskeletal disorders in geriatric patients are often not diagnosed because signs and symptoms in the elderly may be insidious in onset and chronic in nature. In addition, older individuals frequently possess multiple interactive variables, including other medical conditions and therapies that may obscure the nature of the problem. This is compounded by the diminished reliability of laboratory testing in the elderly owing to the wider range of nonpathologic serologic variability, including elevated erythrocyte sedimentation rates and low titers of rheumatoid factor or antinuclear antibodies. Although nearly all rheumatic disorders can afflict the elderly, certain diseases and drug-induced disorders are more common in this age group (Table 295-4). The elderly should be approached in the same manner used for all patients with musculoskeletal complaints, with additional inquiry to exclude common geriatric musculoskeletal disorders. An emphasis on identifying the rheumatic consequences of intercurrent medical conditions and therapies is extremely important. Drug-induced lupus erythematosus, polymyalgia rheumatica, gout, and chronic salicylate toxicity are all more common in the elderly. The physical examination should emphasize coexistent disease that may influence subsequent diagnosis and treatment.

REFERENCES

BROWER AC: Imaging techniques and modalities, in *Arthritis in Black and White*, AC Brower (ed). Philadelphia, Saunders, 1988, p 1

CALINS E: Arthritis in the elderly. Bull Rheum Dis 40(3):1, 1991

FRIES JF: Assessment of the patient with rheumatic disease, in *Textbook of Rheumatology*, 4th ed, WN Kelley et al (eds). Philadelphia, Saunders, 1993

HASSELBACHER P: Arthrocentesis and synovial fluid analysis, in *Primer on the Rheumatic Diseases*, HR Schumacher Jr et al (eds). Atlanta, Arthritis Foundation, 1988, pp 55–60

MICHET CJ, HUNDER GG: Examination of the joints, in *Textbook of Rheumatology* 4th ed, WN Kelley et al (eds). Philadelphia, Saunders, 1993

MURAKAMI DM et al: Advances in imaging of rheumatoid arthritis. Clin Orthop 265:83, 1991

SHMERLING RH, DELBANCO TL: The rheumatoid factor: An analysis of clinical utility. Am J Med 91:528, 1991

——— et al: Synovial fluid tests: What should be ordered? JAMA 264:1009, 1990

STOLLER DW, GENANT JK: Magnetic resonance imaging of the knee and hip. Arthritis Rheum 33:441, 1990

TUMEH SS, TOHMEH AG: Nuclear medicine techniques in septic arthritis and osteomyelitis. Rheum Dis Clin North Am 17:559, 1991

WERNICK R: Avoiding laboratory test misinterpretation in geriatric rheumatology. Geriatrics 44:61, 1989

weighted images. The high fat content in bone marrow produces a bright signal on T1- and T2-weighted images and is nullified on STIR images. Whereas static fluid and fluid-dense structures appear dark to intermediate on T1-weighted images and bright on T2-weighted and STIR images, flowing blood does not generate a signal. As a result, vessels appear dark or black on most standard spin-echo sequences. Muscle, nerve, articular cartilage, and proliferative synovium demonstrate an intermediate signal on T1-weighted images and decreases on T2-weighted sequences.

Because of its sensitivity to changes in marrow fat, MRI has been shown to be a sensitive but nonspecific means of detecting osteonecrosis and osteomyelitis. The enhanced soft tissue contrast resolution of MRI is superior to arthrography and CT in the diagnosis of soft tissue injuries (i.e., meniscal and rotator cuff tears), intraarticular derangements, and spinal cord damage following vertebral injury, subluxation, and synovitis. MRI is also useful in the diagnosis of pigmented villonodular synovitis. In this condition, the synovial tissues are enriched in hemosiderin-laden macrophages, leading to a low signal intensity on T1- and T2-weighted images because of the paramagnetic effects of iron.

Newer imaging techniques such as gadopentetate dimeglumine–enhanced MRI, single-photon-emission computed tomography (SPECT), positron-emission tomography (PET), and magnetic resonance spectroscopy offer enhanced resolution and metabolic imaging of affected tissues. These modalities are currently investigational, and their clinical applicability remains to be determined.

296   OSTEOARTHRITIS

KENNETH D. BRANDT*

Osteoarthritis (OA), also termed *degenerative joint disease*, represents failure of the diarthrodial (movable, synovial-lined) joint. In idiopathic (primary) OA, the most common form of the disease, no predisposing factor is apparent. Secondary OA is pathologically indistinguishable from idiopathic OA but is attributable to an underlying cause (Table 296-1).

EPIDEMIOLOGY/RISK FACTORS   OA is the most common joint disease of mankind. Knee OA is the leading cause of chronic disability in developed countries; some 100,000 people in the United States are unable to walk independently from bed to the bathroom because of OA of the knee or hip.

Under the age of 55 years, the joint distribution of OA in men and women is similar; in older individuals, hip OA is more common in men, while OA of interphalangeal joints and the thumb base is

* The author acknowledges the contribution of Karen Kovalov-St. John to this chapter in the 12th edition.

TABLE 296-1 Classification of OA

IDIOPATHIC

Localized
 Hands: Heberden's and Bouchard's nodes (nodal), erosive interphalangeal arthritis (nonnodal), carpal-1st metacarpal
 Feet: hallux valgus, hallux rigidus, contracted toes (hammer/cock-up toes), talonavicular
 Knee:
  Medial compartment
  Lateral compartment
  Patellofemoral compartment
 Hip:
  Eccentric (superior)
  Concentric (axial, medial)
  Diffuse (coxae senilis)
 Spine:
  Apophyseal joints
  Intervertebral joints (disk)
  Spondylosis (osteophytes)
  Ligamentous (hyperostosis, Forestier's disease, diffuse idiopathic skeletal hyperoslosis)
 Other single sites, e.g., glenohumoral, acromioclavicular, tibiotalar, sacroiliac, temporomandibular
Generalized (GOA): Includes three or more areas listed above (Kellgren-Moore)

SECONDARY

Trauma
 Acute
 Chronic (occupational, sports)
Congenital or developmental
 Localized diseases: Legg-Calvé-Perthes, congenital hip dislocation, slipped epiphysis
 Mechanical factors: unequal lower extremity length, valgus/varus deformity, hypermobility syndromes
 Bone dysplasias: epiphyseal dysplasia, spondyloapophyseal dysplasia, osteonychondystrophy
Metabolic
 Ochronosis (alkaptonuria)
 Hemochromatosis
 Wilson's disease
 Gaucher's disease
Endocrine
 Acromegaly
 Hyperparathyroidism
 Diabetes mellitus
 Obesity
 Hypothyroidism
Calcium deposition diseases
 Calcium pyrophosphate dihydrate deposition
 Apatite arthropathy
Other bone and joint diseases
 Localized: fracture, avascular necrosis, infection, gout
 Diffuse: rheumatoid (inflammatory) arthritis, Paget's disease, osteopetrosis, osteochondritis
Neuropathic (Charcot joints)
Endemic
 Kashin-Beck
 Mseleni
Miscellaneous
 Frostbite
 Caisson's disease
 Hemoglobinopathies

SOURCE: From Mankin et al.

TABLE 296-2 Risk factors for OA

Age
Female sex
Race
Genetic factors
Major joint trauma*
Repetitive stress, e.g., vocational*
Obesity*
Congenital/developmental defects*
Prior inflammatory joint disease
Metabolic/endocrine disorders

* Potentially modifiable
SOURCE: After Hochberg M, J Rheumatol 18:1438, 1991.

Thus the mother of a woman with distal interphalangeal joint OA (Heberden's nodes) is twice as likely to exhibit OA in these joints—and the proband's sister three times as likely—as the mother and sister of an unaffected woman. A point mutation in the cDNA coding for type II collagen was identified recently in several generations of a family with chondrodysplasia and polyarticular secondary OA. The prevalence of genetic abnormalities in matrix molecules will be a major focus of OA research in the coming years.

The most powerful risk factor for OA is age. A progressive increase in prevalence of OA is seen with increasing age. In a radiographic survey of women less than 45 years of age, only 2 percent had OA; between the ages of 45 to 64 years, however, the prevalence was 30 percent, while for those older than 65 years it was 68 percent. In males, the figures were similar but somewhat lower in the older age groups.

Major trauma and repetitive joint use both are risk factors for OA. In both humans and animal models, anterior cruciate ligament insufficiency and meniscus damage (and removal) lead to knee OA. Damage to the articular cartilage may occur at the time of injury or subsequently (during use of the affected joint), but even normal cartilage will degenerate when the joint is unstable.

The pattern of joint involvement is influenced by prior vocational or avocational overload. Thus ankle OA is common in ballet dancers and metacarpophalangeal joint OA in prize fighters, while OA is not common at either of these sites in the general population. The person with a trimalleolar fracture will almost certainly develop ankle OA.

In view of the growing participation of the population of this country in sports in general and in running in particular, it is important to note that there are no convincing data to support an association between specific athletic activities and arthritis if major trauma is excluded. This may, however, be due to the lack of good long-term studies and the difficulty of retrospective assessment of activities. Thus long-distance running and jogging have not been noted to cause OA, although selection bias, i.e., early discontinuation of the activity by those incurring joint damage, cannot be excluded.

In contrast, activities such as those performed by jackhammer operators, cotton mill workers, shipyard workers, coal miners, and others have been shown to lead to OA in those joints exposed to repetitive occupational use. In a study of three groups of textile workers, each of whom performed a different repetitive manual task, OA was more common in joints involved in repetitive usage than in other joints of the hand. Men whose jobs required knee bending and at least medium physical demand had higher rates of radiographic evidence of knee OA, and the radiographic changes were more likely to be more severe than those in men whose jobs required neither.

While the association between obesity and knee OA has been well documented, only recently has a causal relationship between the two been clearly shown. For those in the highest quintile for body mass index at baseline examination, the relative risk for developing knee OA in the ensuing 36 years was 1.5 for men and 2.1 for women. For *severe* knee OA, the relative risk rose to 1.9 for men and 3.2 for women, suggesting that obesity plays an even larger role in the etiology of the most serious cases of knee OA.

more common in women. Similarly, radiographic evidence of knee OA, especially *symptomatic* knee OA, appears to be more common in women than in men (Table 296-2).

Racial differences exist in both the prevalence of OA and the pattern of joint involvement. The Chinese in Hong Kong have a lower incidence of hip OA than whites; OA is more frequent in Native Americans than in whites. Interphalangeal joint OA and, especially, hip OA are much less common in South African blacks than in whites in the same population. Whether these differences are genetic or due to differences in joint usage related to life-style or occupation is unknown.

In other cases, the relationship of heredity to OA is less ambiguous.

While joint pain is the major feature leading the patient with OA to seek medical attention, the correlation between the pathologic severity of OA and symptoms is poor. Thus many individuals with radiographic changes of advanced OA are asymptomatic. The risk factors for *pain and disability* in affected individuals are poorly understood. Notably, for the same degree of pathologic severity, women are more likely to be symptomatic than men, those on welfare are more likely than those who are working, and divorced individuals are more likely than those who are married. In addition, for individuals with OA who had poor social support, a biweekly telephone call from a trained lay interviewer was as effective as a nonsteroidal anti-inflammatory drug (NSAID) in reducing joint pain, emphasizing the importance of psychosocial factors as determinants of pain in patients with OA.

PATHOLOGY   The most striking changes in OA are usually seen in load-bearing areas of the articular cartilage. In the early stages the cartilage is thicker than normal, but with progression of OA the joint surface thins, the cartilage softens, the integrity of the surface is breached, and vertical clefts develop (fibrillation) (Fig. 296-1). Deep cartilage ulcers, extending to bone, may appear. Areas of fibrocartilaginous repair may develop, but the repair tissue is inferior to pristine hyaline articular cartilage in its ability to withstand mechanical stress. All the cartilage is metabolically active, and the chondrocytes replicate, forming clusters (clones). Later, however, the cartilage becomes hypocellular.

Remodeling and hypertrophy of bone are also major features. Appositional bone growth occurs in the subchondral region, leading to the "sclerosis" seen radiographically. The abraded bone under a cartilage ulcer may take on the appearance of ivory (eburnation). Growth of cartilage and bone at the joint margins leads to osteophytes (spurs), which alter the contour of the joint and may restrict movement. Soft tissue changes include a patchy chronic synovitis and thickening of the joint capsule, which may further restrict movement. Periarticular muscle wasting is common. These changes may play a major role in symptoms and disability.

PATHOGENESIS   Articular cartilage, the major target organ in OA, serves two essential functions within the joint, both of which are mechanical. First, it provides a remarkably smooth bearing surface so that with joint movement one bone glides effortlessly over the other. (With synovial fluid as lubricant, the coefficient of friction for cartilage rubbed against cartilage, even with physiologic loading, is 15 times lower than that of two ice cubes passed across each other.) Second, articular cartilage prevents the concentration of stresses so that the bones do not shatter when the joint is loaded.

OA develops in either of two settings: (1) The biomaterial properties of the articular cartilage and subchondral bone are normal, but excessive loads applied to the joint cause the tissues to fail; or (2) the applied load is physiologically reasonable, but the material properties of the cartilage or bone are inferior.

Although articular cartilage is highly resistant to wear under conditions of repeated oscillation, repetitive impact loading soon leads to joint failure. This accounts for the high prevalence of OA at specific sites related to vocational or avocational overload (e.g., shoulders and elbows of baseball pitchers, ankles of ballet dancers, metacarpophalangeal joints of boxers, knees of basketball players). In general, the earliest progressive degenerative changes in OA occur at those sites within the joint which are subject to the greatest compressive loads. More than 80 percent of all cases of "idiopathic" OA of the hip may be due to subtle congenital or developmental defects, such as congenital subluxation/dislocation, acetabular dysplasia, Legg-Calvé-Perthes disease, or slipped capital femoral epiphysis, which increase joint congruity and concentrate dynamic loads. Notably, the institution in the 1940s of screening of newborns and infants for congenital hip disease has led to a marked decrease in the prevalence of hip OA in adults in Brittany.

Clinical conditions that reduce the ability of the cartilage or subchondral bone to deform are associated with development of OA. In ochronosis, for example, accumulation of homogentisic acid polymers leads to stiffening of the cartilage; in osteopetrosis, stiffness of the subchondral trabeculae occurs. In both conditions, severe

FIGURE 296-1   *A.* Normal articular cartilage. Note the intact surface and even distribution of chondrocytes. Mitotic figures are not present in normal adult articular cartilage. *B.* Osteoarthritic cartilage. Note the disruption of surface integrity, with vertical fissures (fibrillation) and irregular distribution of cells. Many of the chondrocytes have replicated and exist in clusters. Stained with safranin-O, which binds to the sulfated glycosaminoglycan chains of proteoglycans. Note patchy areas of diminished staining (pale extracellular matrix) due to proteoglycan depletion.

A

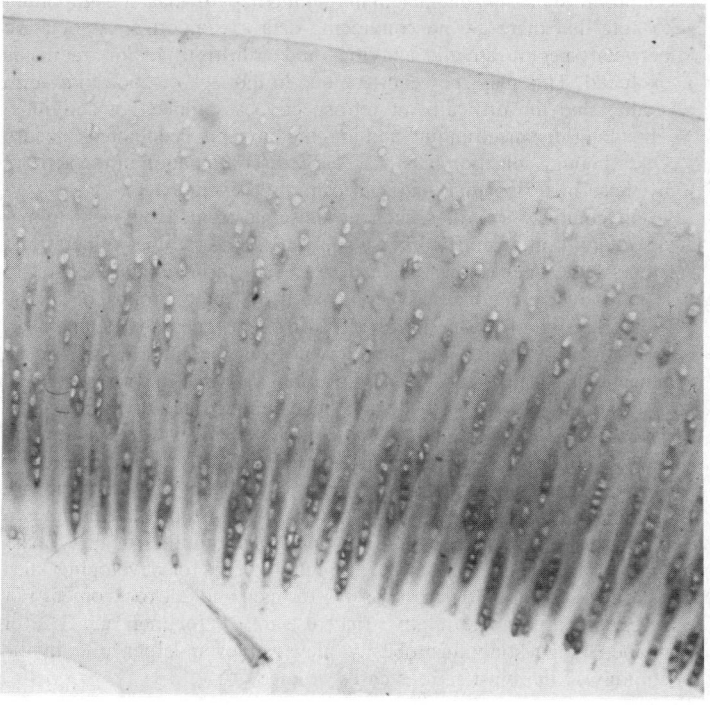

B

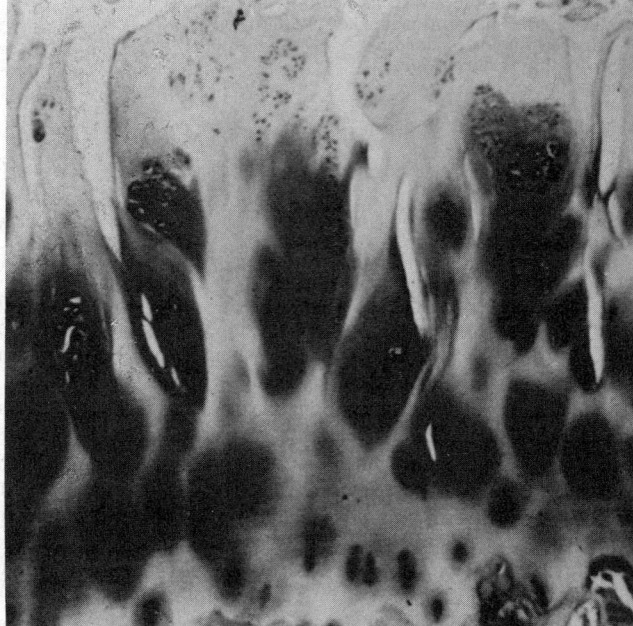

generalized OA is usually apparent by age 40. In the laboratory, if the subchondral bone is stiffened experimentally, repetitive impact loading leads rapidly to degeneration of the overlying cartilage. Conversely, osteoporosis, in which the bone is abnormally soft, may protect against OA. The elderly patient with a hip fracture rarely has hip OA.

The extracellular matrix of articular cartilage: Normal turnover
Articular cartilage is composed of two major macromolecular species: proteoglycans (PGs), which are responsible for the stiffness of the tissue and its ability to withstand load, and collagen, which provides tensile strength and resistance to shear. Although lysomal proteases (cathepsins) have been demonstrated within the cells and matrix of normal articular cartilage, their low pH optimum makes it likely that the proteoglycanase activity of these enzymes will be confined to intracellular sites or to the immediate pericellular area. However, cartilage also contains a family of metalloproteinases, including stromelysin, collagenase, and gelatinase, which can degrade all the components of the extracellular matrix at neutral pH. Each is secreted by the chondrocyte as a proenzyme that must be activated by proteolytic cleavage of its *N*-terminal sequence. Net expression of neutral metalloproteinase activity represents the balance between activation of the latent forms and inhibition of the activity by tissue inhibitors.

The turnover of normal cartilage is effected through a degradative cascade, for which many investigators consider the driving force to be interleukin 1 (IL-1), a cytokine produced by mononuclear cells (including synovial lining cells) and synthesized by chondrocytes. IL-1 stimulates the synthesis and secretion of latent collagenase, latent stromelysin, latent gelatinase, and tissue plasminogen activator. Plasminogen, the substrate for the latter enzyme, may be synthesized by the chondrocyte or may enter the cartilage by diffusion from the synovial fluid. In addition to its catabolic effects, at concentrations even lower than those needed to stimulate cartilage degradation, IL-1 suppresses PG synthesis by the chondrocyte, inhibiting matrix repair (see below).

It is obvious that the preceding materials are potentially very destructive to cartilage. The balance of the system lies with at least two inhibitors: tissue inhibitor of metalloproteinase (TIMP) and plasminogen activator inhibitor 1 (PAI-1), both of which are synthesized by the chondrocyte and limit the degradative activity of active neutral metalloproteinases and plasminogen activator, respectively. If TIMP or PAI-1 are destroyed or present in insufficient concentrations relative to the active enzymes, stromelysin and plasmin are free to act on matrix substrates. Stromelysin can degrade the protein core of the PG and can activate latent collagenase. Conversion of latent stromelysin to an active, highly destructive protease by plasmin provides a second mechanism for matrix degradation.

Polypeptide mediators, e.g., insulin-like growth factor 1 (IGF-1) and transforming growth factor β (TGF-β), stimulate biosynthesis of PGs. They regulate matrix metabolism in normal cartilage and may play a role in matrix repair in OA. Notably, these growth factors modulate catabolic as well as anabolic pathways of chondrocyte metabolism; not only do they increase PG synthesis but, by downregulating chondrocyte receptors for IL-1, they also decrease PG degradation. Whether age-related changes occur in matrix concentrations of IGF-1 or TGF-β or in the responsiveness of the OA chondrocyte to these mediators is unknown.

In addition to its responsiveness to cytokines and a variety of other biologic mediators, chondrocyte metabolism in normal cartilage can be modulated directly by mechanical loading. Whereas static loading and prolonged cyclic loading inhibit synthesis of PGs and protein, loads of relatively brief duration may stimulate matrix biosynthesis.

Pathophysiology of cartilage changes in OA Most investigators feel that the primary changes in OA begin in the cartilage. Even though no alteration in collagen content occurs in OA, a change in the arrangement and size of the collagen fibers is apparent. The biochemical data are consistent with a defect in the collagen network of the cartilage, perhaps due to disruption of the "glue" that binds adjacent collagen fibers together in the matrix. This is among the earliest matrix changes observed and appears to be irreversible.

Although "wear" may be a factor in the loss of cartilage, strong evidence supports the concept that lysosomal and neutral metalloproteinases account for much of the loss of cartilage matrix in OA. Whether their synthesis and secretion are stimulated by IL-1 or by other factors (e.g., mechanical stimuli), neutral metalloproteinases, plasmin, and cathepsins all appear to be involved in the breakdown of articular cartilage in OA. TIMP and PAI-1 may work to stabilize the system, at least temporarily, and growth factors, such as IGF-1, TGF-β, and basic fibroblast growth factor (FGF), are implicated in repair processes that may heal the lesion or, at least, stabilize the process. A stoichiometric imbalance appears to exist between the levels of active enzyme, which may be several-fold higher than those in normal cartilage, and the level of TIMP, which may be only modestly increased.

The chondrocytes in OA cartilage undergo active cell division and are very active metabolically, producing increased quantities of collagen and PGs. Prior to the loss of cartilage and PG depletion, this marked biosynthetic activity may lead to an increase in PG concentration, which may be associated with thickening of the cartilage and "compensated," stabilized OA. (It is inaccurate to call OA "degenerative" joint disease.) These homeostatic mechanisms may maintain the joint in a reasonable functional state for years. The repair tissue, however, often does not hold up as well under mechanical stresses as normal hyaline cartilage. Eventually, at least in some cases, the rate of PG synthesis falls off and "end-stage" OA develops, with full-thickness loss of cartilage.

Is OA a focal joint disease or a systemic disorder? Several observations suggest that OA may be the result of a systemic abnormality of articular cartilage: First, although it may present in only a single joint, OA usually does not remain monarticular; in knees, hips, and small joints of the hand in particular, OA tends to become bilateral. Furthermore, knee OA is strongly associated with hand OA. The "monarthritis multiplex" pattern of OA, however, could as well be due to local mechanical factors as to a systemic cartilage abnormality.

CLINICAL FEATURES The joint pain of OA is often described as a deep ache, localized to the involved joint. Typically, the pain of OA is aggravated by joint use and relieved by rest, but as the disease progresses it may become persistent. Nocturnal pain, interfering with sleep, is seen particularly in advanced OA of the hip and may be enervating. Stiffness of the involved joint upon arising in the morning or after a period of inactivity (e.g., an automobile ride or an evening in a theater seat) may be prominent but usually lasts less than 20 minutes. Systemic manifestations are not a feature of primary OA.

Since articular cartilage is aneural, the joint pain in OA must arise from other structures (Table 296-3). In some patients it may be due to stretching of nerve endings in the periosteum covering osteophytes. In others it may arise from microfractures in subchondral bone or medullary hypertension caused by distortion of blood flow by thickened subchondral trabeculae. Muscle spasm and joint instability leading to stretching of the joint capsule also may be sources of pain.

In some patients with OA, joint pain may be due to synovitis. In advanced OA, histologic evidence of synovial inflammation may be as marked as that in the synovium of a patient with rheumatoid

---

TABLE 296-3 Causes of joint pain in patients with OA

Source	Mechanism
Synovium	Inflammation
Subchondral bone	Medullary hypertension, microfractures
Osteophyte	Stretching of periosteal nerve endings
Ligaments	Stretch
Capsule	Inflammation, distention
Muscle	Spasm

arthritis. Synovitis in OA may be due to phagocytosis of shards of cartilage and bone from the abraded joint surface (wear particles), release from the cartilage of soluble matrix macromolecules, (e.g., glycosaminoglycans or PGs), or the presence of crystals of calcium pyrophosphate or calcium hydroxyapatite. In other cases, immune complexes containing antigens derived from cartilage matrix may be sequestered in collagenous tissue of the joint, leading to low-grade chronic synovitis. In contrast, in the earlier stages of OA, even in the patient with chronic joint pain, synovial inflammation may be absent, suggesting that the pain is due to one of the other factors mentioned above. Notably, even in the absence of synovitis, joint pain in OA may be relieved by a nonsteroidal anti-inflammatory drug (NSAID), consistent with the fact that these drugs have analgesic actions independent of their anti-inflammatory effects.

Physical examination of the OA joint may reveal localized tenderness and bony or soft tissue swelling. Bony crepitus (the sensation of bone rubbing against bone, evoked by joint movement) is characteristic. Synovial effusions, when present, are usually not large. Palpation may reveal some warmth over the joint. Periarticular muscle atrophy may be due to disuse or to reflex inhibition of muscle contraction. In advanced stages of OA, gross deformity, bony hypertrophy, subluxation, and marked loss of joint motion may be striking. The notion that OA is inexorably progressive is incorrect. In many patients the disease stabilizes; in some, regression of joint pain, and even of radiographic changes, occurs.

LABORATORY AND RADIOGRAPHIC FEATURES The diagnosis of OA is usually based on clinical and radiographic features. In the early stages, radiographs may be normal, but joint space narrowing becomes evident as articular cartilage is lost. Other characteristic radiographic findings include subchondral bone sclerosis, subchondral cysts, and marginal osteophytes. A change in the contour of the joint, due to bony remodeling, and subluxation may be seen. Although tibiofemoral joint space narrowing has been considered to be a radiographic surrogate for articular cartilage thinning, in patients with early OA who do not have radiographic evidence of bony changes (e.g., subchondral sclerosis or cysts, osteophytes), joint space narrowing alone does not accurately predict the status of the articular cartilage. Similarly, osteophytosis alone, in the absence of other radiographic features of OA, may be due to aging rather than to OA.

As indicated above, great disparity often exists between the severity of radiographic findings, severity of symptoms, and functional ability in OA. Thus, while more than 90 percent of people over age 40 have some radiographic changes of OA in weight-bearing joints, only 30 percent of these will have symptoms.

No laboratory studies are diagnostic of OA, but specific laboratory testing may help in identifying one of the underlying causes of secondary OA (see Table 296-1). Since primary OA is not systemic, the erythrocyte sedimentation rate, serum chemistry determinations, blood counts, and urinalysis are normal. Analysis of synovial fluid reveals mild leukocytosis (<2000 white blood cells per microliter), with a predominance of mononuclear cells.

Prior to the appearance of radiographic changes, the ability to clinically diagnose OA without an invasive procedure (e.g., arthroscopy) is limited. Approaches such as magnetic resonance imaging (MRI) and ultrasonography are expensive and not widely available, and the limits of resolution do not justify their routine clinical use for diagnosis of OA or for monitoring disease progression. Much effort is currently being devoted to evaluation of serologic tests for these purposes. The approach depends on detection in synovial fluid and/or serum of macromolecules (e.g., PGs, glycosaminoglycans) released from degenerating cartilage or bone. None of these tests has yet proved suitable for clinical use.

The Osteoarthritis Criteria Subcommittee of the American College of Rheumatology has recently developed sets of criteria that permit a diagnosis of OA of the hip, knee, or hand based on algorithms that utilize clinical data with or without radiographic and routine clinical laboratory data (e.g., synovial fluid analysis, erythrocyte sedimenta-

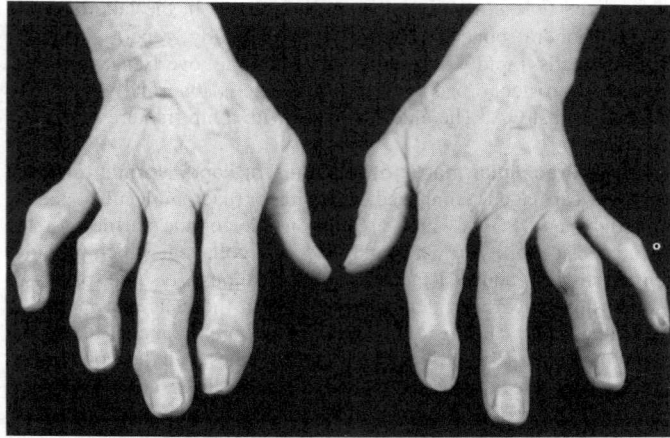

FIGURE 296-2 Nodal osteoarthritis. Note bony enlargement of distal and proximal interphalangeal joints (Heberden's nodes and Bouchard's nodes, respectively). *(From American College of Rheumatology.)*

tion rate). The sensitivity and specificity of these criteria for OA at each of the preceding sites are approximately 90 percent.

OA AT SPECIFIC JOINT SITES   Interphalangeal joints Heberden's nodes, bony enlargements of the distal interphalangeal joints, represent the most common form of idiopathic OA (Fig. 296-2). A similar process at the proximal interphalangeal joints leads to Bouchard's nodes. Often, Heberden's nodes develop gradually, with little or no discomfort. However, they may present acutely with pain, redness, and swelling, sometimes triggered by minor trauma. Gelatinous dorsal cysts, filled with hyaluronic acid, may develop at the insertion of the digital extensor tendon into the base of the distal phalanx.

EROSIVE OA   In erosive OA (EOA), distal and/or proximal interphalangeal joints of the hands are most prominently affected. EOA tends to be more destructive than typical nodal OA. Radiographic evidence of collapse of the subchondral plate is characteristic, and bony ankylosis may occur. Joint deformity and functional impairment may be severe. Pain and tenderness are commonly episodic. The synovium is much more extensively infiltrated with mononuclear cells than in other forms of OA.

GENERALIZED OA   Generalized OA (GOA) is characterized by involvement of three or more joints or groups of joints (distal interphalangeal and proximal interphalangeal joints are counted as one group each). Heberden's and Bouchard's nodes are prominent. Symptoms may be episodic, with "flare-ups" of inflammation marked by soft tissue swelling, redness, and warmth. The erythrocyte sedimentation rate may be elevated, but serum rheumatoid factor tests are negative.

Thumb base The second most frequent area of involvement in OA is the thumb base. Swelling, tenderness, and marked crepitus on movement of the joint are typical. Osteophytes may lead to a "squared" appearance of the thumb base (Fig. 296-3). In contrast to Heberden's nodes, which usually do not interfere significantly with function, OA at the base of the thumb frequently impairs function because of loss of motion and strength. Pain with pinch leads to adduction of the thumb and contracture of the first web space, often resulting in compensatory hyperextension of the first metacarpophalangeal joint and swan-neck deformity of the thumb.

The hip Congenital or developmental defects (e.g., acetabular dysplasia, Legg-Calvé-Perthes disease, slipped capital epiphysis) may be implicated in as many as 80 percent of cases of hip OA. Twenty percent of patients will develop bilateral involvement. Pain from hip OA is generally referred to the inguinal area but may be referred to the buttock or proximal thigh. Less commonly, hip OA presents as knee pain. Pain can be evoked by putting the involved hip through

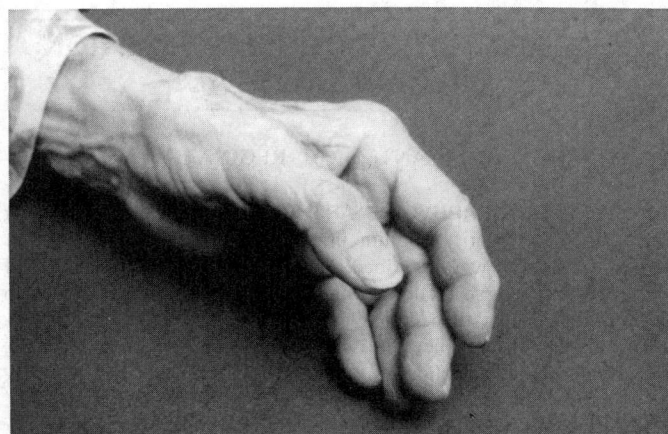

FIGURE 296-3 Osteoarthritis of the first carpometacarpal joint. Note the squared appearance of the thumb base due to bony enlargement and remodeling of the joint.

its range of motion initially; flexion may be painless, but internal rotation will exacerbate pain. Loss of internal rotation occurs early, followed by loss of extension, adduction, and flexion due to capsular fibrosis and/or buttressing osteophytes.

The knee OA of the knee may involve medial or lateral femorotibial compartments and/or the patellofemoral compartment. Palpation may reveal bony hypertrophy (osteophytes) and tenderness. Effusions, if present, are generally small. Joint movement commonly elicits bony crepitus. OA in the medial compartment may result in a varus (bow-legged) deformity; in the lateral compartment it produces a valgus (knock-knee) deformity. A positive ''shrug'' sign (pain when the patella is compressed manually against the femur during quadriceps contraction) may be a sign of OA in the patellofemoral joint.

Chondromalacia patellae, which also is characterized by knee pain and a positive shrug sign, is a syndrome of patellofemoral pain, often bilateral, occurring in teenagers and young adults. It is more common in females than in males. It may be caused by a variety of factors (e.g., abnormal quadriceps angle, patella alta, trauma). Although exploration of the knee may reveal softening and fibrillation of cartilage on the posterior aspect of the patella, this is usually not progressive, and in most cases, chondromalacia patellae is not a precursor of OA. Analgesics or NSAIDs and physical therapy are usually effective; in some, pain may be relieved by surgical correction of patellar malalignment.

The spine Degenerative disease of the spine can involve the apophyseal joint, intervertebral disks, and/or paraspinous ligaments. *Spondylosis* refers to degenerative *disk* disease. The term *OA of the spine* should be reserved for degeneration of the apophyseal joints (true diarthrodial joints). Symptoms of spinal OA include localized pain and stiffness. Nerve root compression by an osteophyte blocking a neural foramen, prolapse of a degenerated disk, or subluxation of an apophyseal joint may cause radicular pain and motor weakness. OA of the spine must be differentiated from diffuse idiopathic skeletal hyperostosis (DISH), which is characterized by marked calcification and ossification of the paraspinous ligaments (see Chap. 289).

TREATMENT No cure exists for OA. Treatment is aimed at reducing pain, maintaining mobility, and minimizing disability. The vigor of the therapeutic intervention should be dictated by the condition of the individual patient. For those with only mild disease, reassurance, instruction in joint protection, and an occasional analgesic may be all that is required.

Drug therapy Drug therapy in OA is symptomatic. Often the joint pain can be controlled with just a simple analgesic (e.g., acetaminophen). For more severe pain, dextrapropoxyphene hydrochloride may be used. Narcotics are rarely indicated in OA.

NSAIDs often decrease pain and improve mobility in OA. However, it is unclear whether this is due to their anti-inflammatory effect or to an analgesic action independent of their effect on inflammation. As indicated above, patients with OA may obtain symptomatic benefit from an NSAID even when evidence of synovitis is lacking. In a recent double-blind, controlled trial, an anti-inflammatory dose of ibuprofen (2400 mg/d) was no more effective than a chiefly analgesic dose of ibuprofen (1200 mg/d) or than acetaminophen in patients with symptomatic knee OA. Furthermore, the presence of clinical signs of inflammation (i.e., synovial swelling, tenderness) did not accurately predict that the response to anti-inflammatory therapy would be better than that to acetaminophen. Nonetheless, if simple analgesics are inadequate, it is reasonable to prescribe an NSAID for the patient with OA.

Claims have been made that some agents, such as polysulfated glycosaminoglycans, retard the progression of OA in human beings; it has been suggested that some NSAIDs also may have a ''chondroprotective'' effect. However, adequately controlled long-term clinical trials in human beings to support such claims are lacking.

Systemic glucocorticoids have no place in the treatment of OA. However, intra- or periarticular injection of a depot glucocorticoid preparation may provide marked symptomatic relief. The injection should not be repeated in a given joint more often than every 4 to 6 months, since too frequent injections may accelerate cartilage breakdown.

Capsaicin cream, which depletes local sensory nerve endings of substance P, a neuropeptide mediator of pain, may reduce joint pain and tenderness when applied topically by patients with hand or knee OA.

Reduction of joint loading OA may be caused or aggravated by poor body mechanics. Correction of poor posture and a support for excessive lumbar lordosis can be helpful. Excessive loading of the involved joint should be avoided. Overloading of the knee due to pronated feet or varus or valgus knee deformities may be corrected by orthotics or osteotomy. A wedged insole may decrease joint pain in patients with early medial OA of the knee. Running shoes also may be helpful in cushioning load.

Patients with OA of the knee or hip should avoid prolonged standing, kneeling, and squatting. Obese patients should be counseled to lose weight. In a strain of guinea pigs that develops spontaneous knee OA, dietary restrictions sufficient to result in a 28 percent decrease in body weight resulted in a 40 percent reduction in the severity of OA lesions. Moreover, while there are no data to show that it will decrease the prevalence of OA in obese humans, weight loss did reduce the risk of knee *symptoms* in obese women with radiographic evidence of knee OA.

Rest periods during the day also may be of benefit, but complete immobilization of the painful joint is rarely indicated. In patients with unilateral OA of the hip or knee, a cane, held in the contralateral hand, may reduce joint pain by reducing the joint contact force. Bilateral disease may necessitate the use of crutches or a walker.

Physical therapy Application of heat to the OA joint may reduce pain and stiffness. A variety of modalities are available. Often, the least expensive and most convenient is a hot shower or bath. Occasionally, better analgesia may be obtained with ice than with heat. Transcutaneous electrical nerve stimulation (TENS) may be helpful, especially for back pain due to OA of the lumbar spine.

Disuse of the OA joint and reflex inhibition of muscle contraction because of pain leads to muscle atrophy. Since they play a major role in protecting articular cartilage from stress, strengthening periarticular muscles is important. The atrophy of joint cartilage and bone which develops with disuse of a limb is due chiefly to reduction in loading of the joint by contraction of periarticular muscles (e.g., hamstrings and quadriceps for the knee). Exercises should be designed to maintain range of motion and strengthen muscles surrounding the joint. Isometric exercises are generally preferable to isotonic exercises, since they minimize joint stress. In a randomized trial in patients with moderately severe knee OA (judged radiographically), strengthening of quadriceps and hamstring muscles by an isometric exercise program significantly decreased joint pain. In contrast, in the control group, which performed range-of-motion exercise, no gains in muscle strength occurred, and knee pain worsened during the period of observation. The decrease in pain in the isometric exercise group was comparable with that which can be achieved with NSAIDs.

Orthopedic surgery   Total joint arthroplasty (joint replacement surgery) should be reserved for patients with advanced OA in whom aggressive medical management has failed. In such cases it may be remarkably effective in relieving pain and increasing mobility. Osteotomy, which is surgically more conservative, can eliminate concentrations of peak dynamic loading and may provide effective pain relief in patients with hip or knee OA. It is of greatest benefit when the disease is only moderately advanced. Arthroscopic removal of loose cartilage fragments can prevent locking and relieve pain. Lavage of the joint with large quantities of saline or Ringer's lactate to flush out fibrin, cartilage shards, and other debris may provide months of comfort for patients whose joint pain has been refractory to analgesics, NSAIDs, and intraarticular steroid injections. However, invasive procedures such as this may produce a large placebo effect, and studies that include a sham lavage control group have not been performed.

Chondroplasty (abrasion arthroplasty) also has gained some popularity as treatment for OA. Well-controlled studies of its efficacy are lacking, however, and the fibrocartilage which resurfaces the abraded bone is inferior to normal hyaline cartilage in its ability to withstand mechanical loads. Interestingly, in patients who had undergone tibial osteotomy for medial compartment knee OA, knee pain and function were not related to the degree of cartilage regeneration seen at arthroscopy 2 years later.

Note: This work was supported in part by grants AR 20582 and 39250 from the National Institute of Arthritis and Musculoskeletal and Skin Diseases.

REFERENCES

ALTMAN R et al: Criteria for classification and reporting of osteoarthritis of the hip. Arthritis Rheum 34:505, 1991

——— et al: Criteria for classification and reporting of osteoarthritis of the hand. Arthritis Rheum 33:1601, 1990

——— et al: Development of criteria for the classification and reporting of osteoarthritis: Classification of osteoarthritis of the knee. Arthritis Rheum 29:1039, 1986

ANDERSON JJ, FELSON DT: Factors associated with osteoarthritis of the knee in the first national health and nutrition examination survey (HANES I): Evidence for an association with overweight, race, and physical demands of work. Am J Epidemiol 128:179, 1988

BRADLEY JD et al: Comparison of an anti-inflammatory dose of ibuprofen, an analgesic dose of ibuprofen, and acetaminophen in the treatment of patients with osteoarthritis of the knee. N Engl J Med 325:87, 1991

BRANDT KD: Management of osteoarthritis, in *Textbook of Rheumatology*, 4th ed. WN Kelley et al (eds). Philadelphia, Saunders, 1993

———, FLUSSER D: Osteoarthritis, in *Prognosis in the Rheumatic Diseases*, N Bellamy (ed). Lancaster, UK, Kluwer Academic, 1991, pp 11–35

———, MANKIN HJ: Pathogenesis of osteoarthritis, in *Textbook of Rheumatology*, 4th ed, WN Kelley et al (eds). Philadelphia, Saunders, 1993

———, RADIN E: The physiology of articular stress: Osteoarthrosis. Hosp Pract 103, 1987

MANKIN HJ: Clinical features of osteoarthritis, in *Textbook of Rheumatology*, 4th ed, WN Kelley et al (eds). Philadelphia, Saunders, 1993

——— et al: Workshop on etiopathogenesis of osteoarthritis. J Rheumatol 13:1127, 1986

297   ARTHRITIS DUE TO DEPOSITION OF CALCIUM CRYSTALS

GARY S. HOFFMAN / ANTONIO J. REGINATO

CRYSTALLOGRAPHY AND ARTHRITIS   The use of polarizing microscopy to identify sodium urate crystals in synovial fluid of patients with gout was described in 1961. Since then, application of this relatively simple technique and research tools such as electron microscopy, energy-dispersive elemental analysis, and x-ray diffraction have established the role of additional types of microcrystals, including calcium pyrophosphate dihydrate (CPPD), calcium hydroxyapatite (HA), and calcium oxalate (CaOx), in other forms of arthritis. Each of these crystals may cause acute or chronic arthritis or periarthritis. In spite of differences in crystal morphology, chemistry, and physical properties, the clinical events that result from deposition and release of sodium urate, CPPD, HA, and CaOx may be indistinguishable. Prior to the use of crystallographic techniques in rheumatology, much of what was considered to be gouty arthritis, in fact, was not. The great frequency (at least 60 percent) with which either HA or CPPD is found in chronic effusions from osteoarthritic joints has raised many questions about their role in causing or enhancing arthritis in the elderly. Patients with the most severe osteoarthritis appear to have the highest incidence of concurrent HA and/or CPPD synovitis, implying an additive or synergistic relationship. The occasional coexistence of sodium urate, CPPD, HA, or CaOx in the same joint further emphasizes the importance of crystallographic analysis for these potentially difficult diagnostic problems. In the setting of acute articular or periarticular inflammation, aspiration and analysis of effusions are most important to assess the possibility of infection. Polarization microscopy alone may identify most typical crystals and allow diagnosis. HA, however, represents an exception. Because these crystals are not birefringent and are extremely small, more sophisticated techniques would be required to confirm their presence. Apart from the identification of specific microcrystalline materials or organisms, synovial fluid characteristics are not pathognomonic. Chronic monarticular or pauciarticular effusions of uncertain etiology should be approached with an inquisitiveness similar to that given to the acute effusion. Although chronicity makes septic arthritis far less likely, it remains part of the differential diagnosis, as does microcrystalline arthropathy.

CPPD DEPOSITION DISEASE   Pathogenesis   CPPD crystal deposition in articular cartilage, synovium, and periarticular ligaments and tendons is most common in the elderly, affecting 10 to 15 percent of persons 65 to 75 years old and 30 to 60 percent of those more than 85 years old. In most cases this process is asymptomatic, and the cause of CPPD deposition is uncertain. Because over 80 percent of patients are more than 60 years old and 70 percent have preexisting joint damage from other conditions, it is likely that physical and chemical changes in aging cartilage favor crystal nucleation. Examples of such chemical alterations include the following: (1) Increased production of inorganic pyrophosphate and decreased levels of pyrophosphatases in cartilage extracts from patients with CPPD arthritis. The increase in pyrophosphate appears related to enhanced activity of ATP pyrophosphohydrolase and 5'-nucleotidase, which catalyze the reaction of ATP to adenosine and pyrophosphate, which could combine with calcium to form CPPD crystals within matrix vesicles. (2) Diminution of cartilage glycoproteins that normally inhibit and regulate crystal nucleation. Inhibitor deficiencies may thus lead to increased crystal deposition. (3) In vitro studies have demonstrated that transforming growth factor β1 and epidermal growth factor both stimulate pyrophosphate elaboration by articular cartilage and thus may contribute to deposition of CPPD crystals. The release of CPPD crystals in the joint space is followed by neutrophil phagocytosis of crystals and the release of inflammatory substances. In addition, neutrophils release a glycopeptide that is

TABLE 297-1   Conditions associated with CPPD disease

Aging
Disease-associated
  Primary hyperparathyroidism
  Hemochromatosis
  Hypophosphatasia
  Hypomagnesemia
  Chronic tophaceous gout
  Post-meniscectomy
Hereditary: Slovakian-Hungarian, Chilean-Spanish, French, Swedish,
  Dutch, Canadian, Mexican-American, Italian-American, German-
  American, Japanese, Tunisian, Jewish, English

chemotactic for other neutrophils, thus augmenting inflammatory events. The same substance is present in gout. In both gout and CPPD arthritis, production of this glycopeptide can be suppressed by colchicine.

A minority of patients with CPPD arthropathy have an increased incidence of metabolic abnormalities or hereditary CPPD disease (Table 297-1). These associations suggest that a variety of different metabolic products may enhance CPPD deposition. Included among these conditions are hyperparathyroidism, hemochromatosis, gout, hypophosphatasia, hypomagnesemia, and ochronosis. Hemochromatosis and hyperparathyroidism are good examples. Ferrous ions and hypercalcemia may either directly alter cartilage or inhibit inorganic pyrophosphatases, leading to enhanced susceptibility to CPPD deposition. The presence of CPPD arthritis in individuals less than 50 years old should lead to consideration of these metabolic disorders and inherited forms of disease, including those identified in a variety of ethnic groups (Table 297-2). Investigation should include inquiry for evidence of familial aggregation and evaluation of serum calcium, phosphorus, alkaline phosphatase, magnesium, serum ferritin, and transferritin saturation.

Clinical manifestations   CPPD arthropathy may be asymptomatic, acute, subacute, or chronic or cause acute synovitis superimposed on chronically involved joints. Acute CPPD arthritis was originally termed "pseudogout" by McCarty and coworkers because of its striking similarity to gout. He and others have since recognized that the clinical sequelae of CPPD deposition include (1) induction or enhancement of some forms of osteoarthritis, (2) induction of severe resorptive disease that may radiographically mimic neuropathic arthritis, (3) production of symmetric proliferative synovitis, clinically similar to rheumatoid arthritis, and (4) calcification of intervertebral disks and restriction of spine mobility mimicking ankylosing spondylitis.

The knee is the most frequently affected joint in CPPD arthropathy. Other sites include the wrist, shoulder, ankle, elbow, and hands. Rarely, the temporomandibular joint and ligamentum flavum of the

spinal canal may be involved. Clinical and radiographic evidence indicates that CPPD deposition is polyarticular in at least two-thirds of patients. When acute synovitis occurs, diagnosis is made by identification of rod- or rhomboid-shaped weakly positively birefringent crystals (Fig. 297-1) in synovial fluid. When the clinical picture resembles that of slowly progressive osteoarthritis, diagnosis may be more difficult. Joint distribution may provide important clues, suggesting CPPD disease. For example, primary osteoarthritis almost never involves the metacarpophalangeal, wrist, elbow, shoulder, or ankle joint. If radiographs reveal punctate and/or linear radiodense deposits in fibrocartilaginous joint menisci or articular hyaline cartilage (chondrocalcinosis), the diagnostic certainty of CPPD is further enhanced. *Definitive diagnosis* requires demonstration of typical crystals in synovial fluid or articular tissue. In the absence of joint effusion or indications to obtain a synovial biopsy, chondrocalcinosis is presumptive of CPPD deposition. One exception is chondrocalcinosis due to CaOx in some patients with chronic renal failure.

Acute attacks of CPPD arthritis may be precipitated by trauma, such as physical injury to an extremity, joint surgery, a sprain, or even a long walk. These events are believed to cause cartilaginous abrasion and microcrystal shedding into the joint space. Rapid diminution of serum calcium concentration, as may occur in severe medical illness or after surgery (especially parathyroidectomy), also can lead to pseudogout. How transient calcium disequilibrium may facilitate CPPD release is unclear.

In as many as 50 percent of cases, CPPD pseudogout may be associated with low-grade fever and on occasion temperature as high as 40°C. Whether or not radiographic proof of chondrocalcinosis is evident in the involved joint(s), synovial analysis with microbial stains and cultures is essential to rule out the possibility of infection. In fact, infection in a joint with any microcrystalline deposition process can lead to crystal shedding and subsequent synovitis from both crystals and microorganisms. Synovial fluid in uncomplicated pseudogout has inflammatory qualities. The WBC count can range from several thousand cells to 100,000 cells per milliliter, the mean being about 24,000 cells per milliliter and the predominant cell being the neutrophil. Polarization microscopy usually reveals weakly positively birefringent crystals in the extracellular fluid and within neutrophils.

Untreated, acute attacks may last a few days to as long as a month. *Treatment* by joint aspiration (to decrease intraarticular pressure) and nonsteroidal anti-inflammatory agents or intraarticular glucocorticoid injection may result in return to prior status within 10 days or less. For patients with frequent recurrent attacks of pseudogout, daily

FIGURE 297-1   Calcium pyrophosphate dihydrate crystals, as seen in a fresh preparation of synovial fluid, illustrate rod- and rhomboid-shaped weakly birefringent crystals (compensated polarized light microscopy; × 400).

TABLE 297-2   Conditions associated with HA deposition disease

Aging
Osteoarthritis
Hemorrhagic effusions in the elderly
Destructive arthropathy
Tendinitis, bursitis
Tumoral calcinosis (sporadic cases)
Disease-associated
  Hyperparathyroidism
  Milk alkali syndrome
  Renal failure/long-term dialysis
  Connective tissue diseases (e.g., progressive systemic sclerosis,
    CREST syndrome, idiopathic myositis)
  Heterotopic calcification following neurologic catastrophes (e.g.,
    stroke, spinal cord injury)
Hereditary
  Bursitis, arthritis
  Tumoral calcinosis

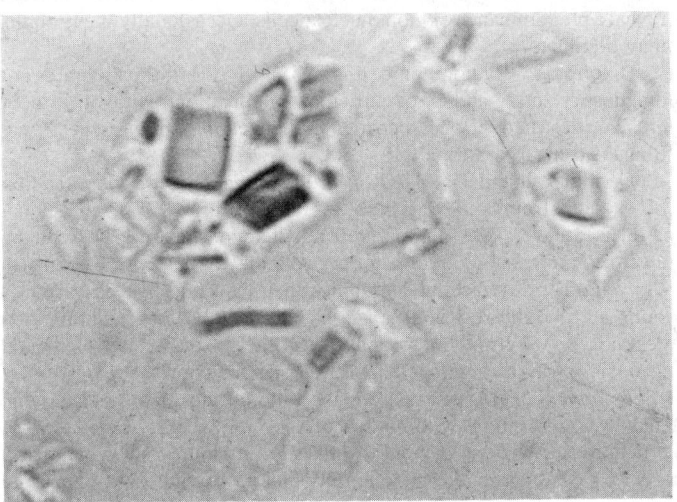

prophylactic treatment with low doses of colchicine may be helpful. Unfortunately, effective treatment does not exist to remove CPPD deposits from cartilage and the joint capsule. As a result, CPPD tends to cause progressive forms of arthritis.

CALCIUM HA DEPOSITION DISEASE **Pathogenesis** Calcium hydroxyapatite is the primary mineral of bone and teeth. Abnormal accumulation can occur in areas of tissue damage (dystrophic calcification), in hypercalcemic or hyperparathyroid states (metastatic calcification), and in certain conditions of unknown cause (Table 297-2). In chronic renal failure, hyperphosphatemia enhances HA deposits within as well as around joints. It was not until 1976 that HA was clearly established as a cause of arthritis.

HA and other basic calcium phosphates may be released from exposed bone and cause the acute synovitis occasionally seen in chronic stable osteoarthritis (e.g., the "hot" Heberden's node). HA deposition is also an important factor in an extremely destructive chronic arthropathy of the elderly that occurs most often in knees and shoulders. Joint destruction is associated with attenuation or rupture of supporting structures, leading to instability and deformity. Progression tends to be indolent, and synovial fluid WBC counts are usually less than 1000 cells per milliliter. Symptoms range from minimal to severe pain and disability that may lead to joint replacement surgery. Whether severely affected patients merely represent an extreme synovial tissue response to HA crystals that are so common in osteoarthritis is uncertain. Observations that favor articular HA deposition and joint destruction being a unique entity rather than just a sequel of osteoarthritis include the following: (1) Primary osteoarthritis of the shoulders is infrequent. (2) High levels of activated collagenase and neutral protease, as well as fragments of collagen, have been found in the noninflammatory synovial fluids of patients with severe HA arthropathy; the concentration of these enzymes exceeded those for rheumatoid arthritis and uncomplicated osteoarthritis. (3) Synovial membrane tissue cultures exposed to HA crystals (or CPPD) markedly increased release of these enzymes, underscoring the destructive potential of abnormally stimulated synovial lining cells.

Clinical manifestations Periarticular and articular deposits may coexist and be associated with acute and/or chronic damage to the joint capsule, tendons, bursa, or articular surfaces. The most common sites of HA deposition include those in and/or around the knees, shoulders, hips, and fingers. Clinical manifestations include asymptomatic radiographic abnormalities, acute synovitis or tendinitis, and chronic destructive arthropathy. Most patients with HA arthropathy are elderly. Although the true incidence of HA arthritis is not known, 30 to 50 percent of patients with osteoarthritis have HA microcrystals in their synovial fluid. Such crystals can frequently be identified in clinically stable osteoarthritic joints but are more likely to come to attention in persons experiencing acute or subacute worsening of joint pain and swelling. The synovial fluid WBC count in HA arthritis is usually low (<2000 cells per milliliter) but may at times have as many as 50,000 cells per milliliter. Most synovial fluid analyses reveal a predominance of mononuclear cells. Occasionally, neutrophils may dominate.

Diagnosis Radiographic findings in HA arthropathy are not diagnostic. Intra- and/or periarticular calcifications with or without erosive, destructive, or hypertrophic changes may be present. X-ray films also may be normal.

Definitive diagnosis of HA arthropathy depends on identification of crystals from synovial fluid or tissue (Fig. 297-2). Individual crystals are very small, nonbirefringent, and can only be seen by electron microscopy. Clumps of crystals may appear as 1- to 20-μm shiny intra- or extracellular globules that stain purplish on Wright's stain and bright red with alizarin red S. Absolute identification depends on electron microscopy with energy dispersive elemental analysis, x-ray diffraction, or infrared spectroscopy.

Treatment of HA arthritis is nonspecific. Acute attacks of synovitis may be selflimiting within days to several weeks. Aspiration of effusions and the use of nonsteroidal anti-inflammatory agents for 2 weeks or intraarticular injection of glucocorticoid salts appear to

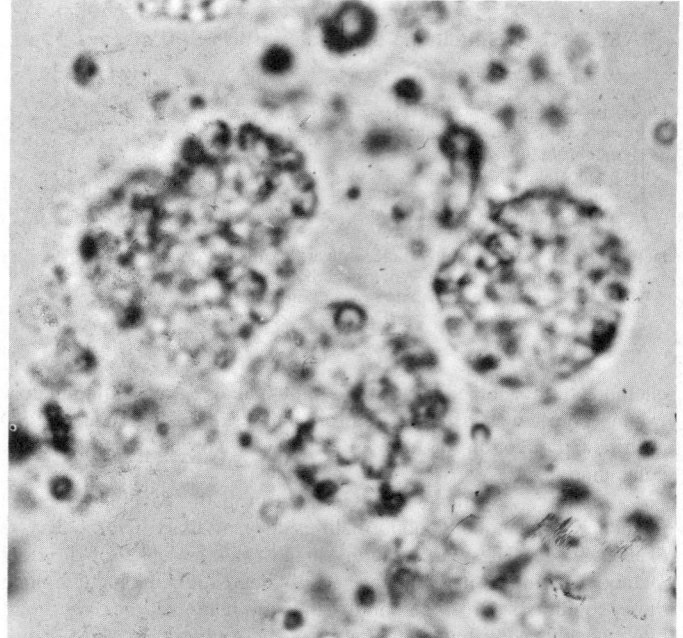

A

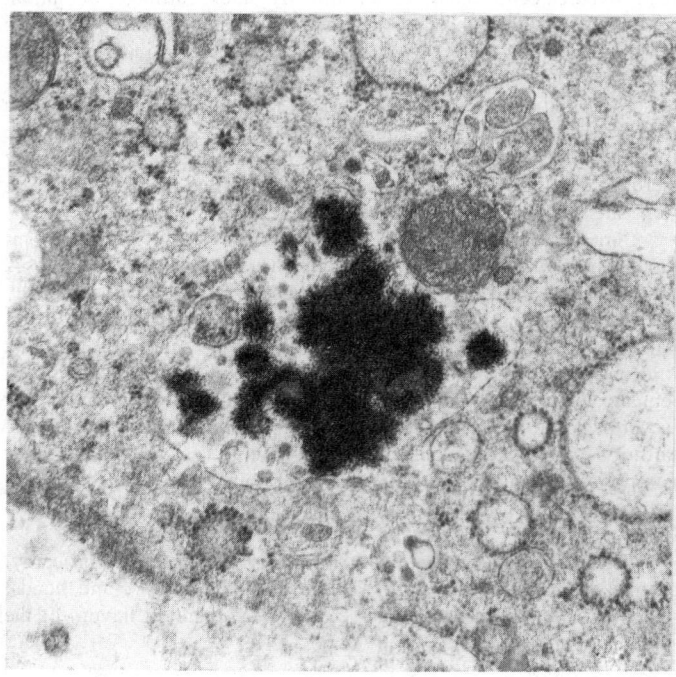

B

FIGURE 297-2 *A*. Cytoplasmic round inclusions inside synovial fluid cells represent aggregates of apatite crystals (fresh preparation, ordinary light microscopy; × 400). *B*. An electron micrograph demonstrates a cluster of dark apatite crystals within a synovial fluid mononuclear cell (× 30,000).

shorten the duration and intensity of symptoms. In patients with underlying severe destructive articular changes, response to medical therapy is usually less rewarding.

CaOx DEPOSITION DISEASE **Pathogenesis** *Primary oxalosis* is a rare hereditary metabolic disorder (Chap. 352). Enhanced production of oxalic acid may result from at least two different enzyme defects, leading to hyperoxalemia and deposition of calcium oxalate crystals in tissues. Nephrocalcinosis, renal failure, and death usually occur prior to 20 years of age. Acute and/or chronic CaOx arthritis and periarthritis may complicate primary oxalosis during later years of illness.

Secondary oxalosis is more common than the primary disorder. It is one of the many metabolic abnormalities that complicate end-stage renal disease (ESRD). In ESRD, calcium oxalate deposits have long been recognized in visceral organs, blood vessels, bones, and even cartilage. However, it was not until 1982 that such deposits were demonstrated to be one of the causes of arthritis in chronic renal failure. Thus far, reported patients have been dependent on long-term hemodialysis or peritoneal dialysis (see also Chap. 238), and many had received vitamin C (ascorbic acid) supplements. Ascorbic acid is metabolized to oxalate, which is inadequately cleared in uremia and by dialysis. Such supplements are now usually avoided in dialysis programs because of the risk of enhancing hyperoxalosis and its sequelae.

Clinical manifestations and diagnosis As was noted for the other calcium salts, CaOx aggregates can be found in bone, articular cartilage, synovium, and periarticular tissues. From these sites, crystals may be shed, causing acute synovitis. Persistent aggregates of CaOx may, like HA and CPPD, stimulate synovial proliferation and enzyme release, resulting in progressive articular destruction. Few well-studied cases have been reported. Deposits have been documented in fingers, wrists, elbows, knees, ankles, and feet. Any articular site could potentially be involved.

Each of the known microcrystalline arthropathies may be a complication of ESRD, and rare patients may have more than one type of crystal present in a joint effusion. The advent of crystallographic techniques has made it clear that most arthritic problems in ESRD are not, as was once believed, due to gout. Clinical features of acute CaOx arthritis may not be distinguishable from those due to sodium urate, CPPD, or HA. Radiographs may reveal chondrocalcinosis, a feature of either CPPD or CaOx deposition. CaOx-induced synovial effusions are usually noninflammatory, with less than 2000 leukocytes per milliliter. Predominant cell types have varied from being either neutrophils or mononuclear cells. In most instances, crystals are extracellular, although CaOx has been identified within neutrophils. Synovial membranes show modest signs of inflammation. CaOx has a variable shape and variable birefringence to polarized light. The most easily recognized forms are bipyramidal and strongly positively birefringent (Fig. 297-3).

Treatment of CaOx arthropathy with nonsteroidal anti-inflammatory agents, colchicine, intraarticular glucocorticoids, and increased frequency of dialysis has produced only slight improvement.

FIGURE 297-3 Bipyramidal and small polymorphic calcium oxalate crystals (ordinary light microscopy; × 400).

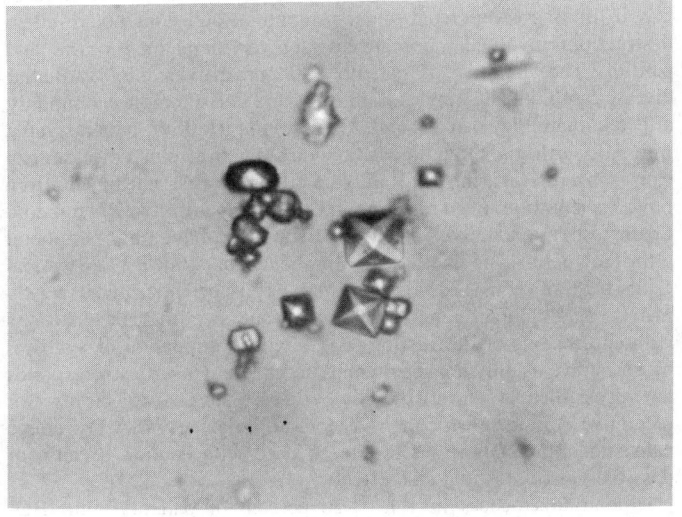

REFERENCES

ALVARELLOS A, SPILBERG I: Colchicine prophylaxis in pseudogout. J Rheumatol 13:804, 1986

BETH A et al: Articular cartilage vesicles generate calcium pyrophosphate dihydrate-like crystals in vitro. Arthritis Rheum 35:231, 1992

DIEPPE PA et al: Apatite deposition disease: A new arthropathy. Lancet 1:266, 1976

DOHERTY M et al: Inorganic pyrophosphate in metabolic diseases predisposing to calcium pyrophosphate dihydrate crystal deposition. Arthritis Rheum 34:1297, 1991

———— et al: Familial chondrocalcinosis due to calcium pyrophosphate dihydrate crystal deposition in English families. Br J Rheumatol 30:10, 1991

HALVERSON P, MCCARTY DJ: Basic calcium phosphate (apatite, octacalcium phosphate, tricalcium phosphate crystal deposition diseases), in *Arthritis and Allied Conditions*, 11th ed, DJ McCarty (ed). Philadelphia, Lea & Febiger, 1989

HOFFMAN GS et al: Calcium oxalate microcrystalline-associated arthritis in end-stage renal disease. Ann Intern Med 97:36, 1982

MCCARTY DJ et al: The significance of calcium phosphate crystals in the synovial fluid of arthritic patients: The "pseudogout syndrome." Ann Intern Med 56:711, 1962

REGINATO AJ, KURNIK B: Calcium oxalate and other crystals associated with kidney diseases and arthritis. Semin Arthritis Rheum 18:198, 1989

————, SCHUMACHER HR: Crystal associated arthropathies. Clin Geriatr Med 4:295, 1988

ROSENTHAL AK et al: Transforming growth factor beta 1 stimulates inorganic pyrophosphate elaboration by porcine cartilage. Arthritis Rheum 34:904, 1991

SCHUMACHER HR, REGINATO AJ: *Atlas of Synovial Fluid Analysis and Crystal Identification*. Philadelphia, Lea & Febiger, 1991, chaps 8, 9, and 10

298 PSORIATIC ARTHRITIS AND ARTHRITIS ASSOCIATED WITH GASTROINTESTINAL DISEASE

PETER H. SCHUR

PSORIATIC ARTHRITIS

Psoriatic arthritis is a chronic inflammatory arthritis that affects 5 to 8 percent of people with psoriasis.

ETIOLOGY AND PATHOGENESIS To date, the cause and pathogenesis are unknown. Indirect evidence has suggested that (viral) infections, trauma, increased cellular immunity to streptococci, decreased suppressor cell activation, immune complexes, and abnormal polymorphonuclear leukocyte (PMN) function may each play a role. Widespread severe psoriasis with rapidly progressive arthritis should make one suspect HIV infection (see Chap. 279). Familial aggregation suggests the influence of genetic factors. Although HLA-B13, B17, and CW6 are increased in frequency in patients with psoriasis, most studies have observed an increased frequency of HLA-B17, CW6, and/or B27 in patients with psoriatic spondylitis, while B27, B38, B39, and DR7a have been noted in association with peripheral arthritis in different studies.

CLINICAL MANIFESTATIONS Three major types of psoriatic arthritis have been identified: asymmetric inflammatory arthritis, symmetric arthritis, and psoriatic spondylitis. A mean of 47 percent of patients (range 16 to 70 percent) have an asymmetric inflammatory arthritis. Disease appears equally in men and women. Psoriasis tends to precede the arthritis by many years, although many complain of morning stiffness. The proximal and distal interphalangeal (PIP, DIP) joints are most frequently involved [with characteristic sausage-shaped digits (dactylitis)], while knees, hips, ankles, and wrists are less frequently involved. Most patients have onychodystrophy (onycholysis, ridging, pitting of nails), whose course does not parallel that of the synovitis. The prognosis is good, with only one-fourth of the patients developing progressive destructive disease; one-third develop inflammatory ocular complications (conjunctivitis, iritis, episcleritis).

A mean of 25 percent of patients (range 15 to 39 percent) develop symmetric arthritis resembling rheumatoid arthritis (see Chap. 285).

The disease occurs twice as frequently in women. Psoriasis and inflammatory arthritis usually develop simultaneously; again, most patients experience morning stiffness. The DIP, PIP, MCP, MTP, and, in particular, large peripheral joints are involved. Practically all have onychodystrophy, which helps distinguish these patients from those with rheumatoid arthritis. Over half this group goes on to develop destructive arthritis, including arthritis mutilans. Eye complications are uncommon. None have subcutaneous nodules, but one-fourth have rheumatoid factors.

A mean of 23 percent of the patients (range 5 to 33 percent) have psoriatic "spondylitis," with or without peripheral joint involvement. Psoriasis tends to precede the arthritis by a few years, and low-back pain with morning stiffness is common. Psoriatic spondylitis is more common in men. About half this group has spondylitis and the other sacroilitis. The back disease is usually slowly progressive with little clinical deterioration as compared with ankylosing spondylitis; the peripheral disease also tends not to be destructive except for the occasional patient with arthritis mutilans. Enthesopathy, i.e., inflammation of tendons and ligamentous attachments to bone, is characteristic, viz., tendo Achillis, plantar fascia causing heel pain. Many have onychodystrophy, while few have inflammatory ocular complications.

Some authors have described additional subsets of psoriatic arthritis: predominant DIP joint involvement (6 percent of cases), arthritis mutilans (5 percent), juvenile psoriatic arthritis (2 percent), and SAPHO (sternoclavicular hyperostosis, chronic sterile multifocal osteomyelitis, hyperostosis of the spine, and a peripheral arthritis).

The pathology is similar to that seen in rheumatoid arthritis: synoviocytic hyperplasia, early PMN infiltration and later mononuclear cell infiltration, cartilage erosion, and pannus formation. Fibrosis of the joint capsule and marrow is prominent in many patients.

LABORATORY FINDINGS   There are a few laboratory abnormalities. Elevated erythrocyte sedimentation rates, C-reactive proteins, and complement levels reflect inflammation. Rheumatoid factors are uncommon and are more likely to be observed in those with symmetric arthritis. Immunoglobulin levels are normal. Uric acid levels may be elevated; sodium urate crystals in joint fluids suggest gout.

Radiologic investigation reveals findings quite similar to those of rheumatoid arthritis: soft tissue swelling, loss of the cartilage space, erosions, bony ankylosis, subluxations, subchondral cysts, but less demineralization. More unique and suggestive of psoriatic arthritis are erosions at DIP joints, expansion of the base of the terminal phalanx, tapering of the proximal phalanx and cuplike erosions of and bony proliferation of the distal terminal phalanx ("pencil-in-cup" appearance), proliferation of bone near osseous erosions, terminal phalangeal osteolysis, bone proliferation and periostitis (especially of phalanges), and telescoping of one bone into its neighbor, leading to the "opera-glass" deformity. The axial skeleton shows asymmetric or unilateral sacroiliitis and large asymmetric nonmarginal syndesmophytes.

DIAGNOSIS   The diagnosis of psoriatic arthritis should be considered in individuals with arthritis and psoriasis. Psoriasis should be distinguished from seborrheic dermatitis and eczema. Psoriatic lesions may be quite small peripherally or often hidden in the scalp, umbilicus, and gluteal folds. Fungal infection of nails can be distinguished from psoriasis, for the latter will demonstrate pitting and onycholysis. Furthermore, onychodystrophy is uncommon (20 percent) in uncomplicated psoriasis. Patients with ankylosing spondylitis (see Chap. 289) have more back symptoms and less (and less severe) peripheral arthritis than those with psoriatic arthritis. It is often difficult to distinguish Reiter's syndrome (see Chap. 289) from psoriatic arthritis, since both manifest dactylitis. Reiter's syndrome usually presents in younger individuals, especially males, is less frequently progressive or destructive, and more likely is associated with characteristic skin lesions (keratoderma blenorrhagica), urethritis, and conjunctivitis. Gout can be distinguished by the presence of intraarticular sodium urate crystals (see Chap. 347). Psoriasis in association with Heberden's nodes or Bouchard's nodes of the DIP and PIP joints, respectively, rather suggests osteoarthritis (see Chap. 296). Psoriatic arthritis differs

from rheumatoid arthritis by the relative lack of rheumatoid factors; the tendency to asymmetry, dactylitis, iritis, enthesopathy, onychodystrophy; the high frequency of HLA-B27, especially in patients with axial skeletal involvement; and characteristic radiologic features.

TREATMENT   The treatment of psoriatic arthritis begins with patient education and physical and occupational therapy to maintain muscle strength and joint and muscle function. Orthotics and occasional intraarticular glucocorticoids for isolated acutely and severely inflamed joints may be added as needed. The mainstay, however, is the use of nonsteroidal anti-inflammatory drugs (NSAIDs), including salicylates, which reduce inflammation and alleviate pain for the majority of patients. Oral colchicine has been reported to be beneficial. For patients with more severe involvement, a disease-modifying antirheumatic drug should be utilized. While hydroxychloroquine is often successful in creating either amelioration or remission, it carries a significant risk of exacerbation of psoriasis. Sulfasalazine has been reported to be of benefit. Intramuscular gold salts have created remission in over 50 percent of patients, with few side effects. For more severe cases, especially with extensive skin involvement, methotrexate is recommended. A total of three doses of 2.5 to 5 mg given 12 h apart once a week is recommended. Most patients respond well with respect to both skin lesions and arthritis. Patients who are resistant to oral therapy may respond to intravenous therapy. Renal and liver function tests and a complete blood count should be monitored frequently, and any abnormalities should suggest withholding of the drug until tests normalize. Liver biopsies are recommended after a total of 1.5 g methotrexate and then every 2 years to identify patients with fibrosis and cirrhosis, which necessitate withdrawal of the drug. This occurrence is rare. However, patients are advised to avoid nephrotoxic and hepatotoxic (e.g., ethanol) drugs. If methotrexate cannot be tolerated, 6-mercaptopurine and azathioprine have proven successful. The arthritis of few patients responds to the psoriasis therapy known as PUVA (psoralen with UV-A radiation). Advanced forms of therapy such as cyclosporine should be provided only in consultation with or by persons expert in their use.

ARTHRITIS ASSOCIATED WITH GASTROINTESTINAL DISEASE

INFLAMMATORY BOWEL DISEASE (IBD)   Peripheral arthritis occurs in 9 to 20 percent of patients with IBD (e.g., ulcerative colitis, Crohn's disease; see Chap. 255). Arthritis is somewhat more likely to occur in patients with large bowel disease and in those patients with complications such as abscesses, pseudomembranous polyposis, perianal disease, massive hemorrhage, erythema nodosum, stomatitis, uveitis, and pyoderma gangrenosum. Males and females are affected equally. The arthritis tends to be acute, is associated with flares of the bowel disease, occurs early in the course of the bowel disease, is self-limiting (90 percent under 6 months), and does not result in destruction. Involved joints are swollen, erythematous, warm, and painful. The majority of patients (90 percent) have polyarticular disease with knees, ankles, elbows, and wrists more commonly affected than PIP, MCP, and MTP joints. Half of patients have migratory arthritis. Granulomas, associated with Crohn's disease, can cause an erosive arthritis. Rarely, a psoas abscess can result from bowel perforation, even resulting in (septic) hip arthritis. Rheumatoid factor tests are negative. In those persons who have only peripheral arthritis, there is no increase in frequency in HLA-B27. Synovial fluids have 5000 to 12,000 white blood cells per microliter, mostly PMNs. Radiographs demonstrate soft-tissue swelling and effusions without erosions or destruction. Pathologic examination of synovial biopsies reveals only nonspecific inflammation. The arthritis responds to successful treatment of the bowel disease such as colectomy (for ulcerative colitis), glucocorticoids, or sulfasalazine. NSAIDs relieve pain and inflammation but should be used with caution because of possible gastrointestinal side effects.

Spondylitis occurs in 1.1 to 26 percent of patients with IBD.

Males are somewhat more frequently affected. Patients will typically complain of stiffness in the back and/or buttocks in the morning or after rest. Stiffness and associated pain are often relieved by exercise. Back symptoms are unrelated to those of the gastrointestinal disease. Physical examination reveals limited spinal flexion and reduced chest expansion. Some patients may have peripheral arthritis, especially of the hips and/or shoulders. Iritis is a frequent complication. Radiographs of the back show the typical findings of ankylosing spondylitis and bilateral sacroiliitis. HLA-B27 is found in 53 to 75 percent of these patients. Treatment includes NSAIDs, gluococorticoids for the bowel disease, and physical therapy. The axial disease progresses in a slow manner akin to ankylosing spondylitis.

Asymptomatic sacroiliitis detected by radiography occurs in 4 to 25 percent of patients with IBD. By contrast, 52 percent of patients with IBD have abnormal technetium pyrophosphate bone scans of the sacroiliac joint. There is no increased frequency of HLA-B27. This "disease" does not necessarily progress to spondylitis.

Other complications of chronic IBD include (1) finger clubbing (observed in 4 to 13 percent of patients with Crohn's disease, especially those with small bowel involvement) which may regress after surgery, (2) development of amyloid, especially in association with Crohn's disease, and (3) osteoporosis resulting from inactivity, malabsorption, and/or treatment with glucocorticoids. Osteomalacia can result from malabsorption. In this setting, with acutely increased back pain, one should suspect compression fracture.

INTESTINAL BYPASS ARTHRITIS   Intestinal bypass surgery was developed for the treatment of obesity in 1952; 11 years later arthritis was recognized as a postoperative complication. Polyarthralgia and sometimes arthritis may occur weeks, even years, following surgery in 8 to 36 percent of patients. Pain and tenderness exceed objective findings in most cases; others have noted episodes of abrupt onset of pain and inflammation. Tenosynovitis is common, with episodes possibly lasting for days and even months; it tends to affect the knee, wrist, ankle, shoulder, and finger joints and cause pain in the neck and back. This syndrome occurs more likely after jejunocolic than after jejunoileal surgery and more in females than in males. There is often an associated urticarial, vesicular, pustular, macular, or nodular eruption. Raynaud's symptoms appear in one-third of patients. X-rays generally show no joint damage, except marginal erosions in patients with persistent arthritis. Synovial fluids generally have white blood cell counts of 500 to 27,000 cells per microliter, mostly PMNs. Synovial biopsies show chronic synovitis with lymphocytes but without lymphoid follicles. Tests for rheumatoid factors, antinuclear antibodies, and HLA-B27 are usually negative, while immune complexes (and cryoglobulins) are often present. They contain bacterial antigens, their antibodies, IgA secretory component, and various complement components. These observations suggest that the syndrome has the following pathogenesis: Bacteria proliferate in intestinal blind loops, bacterial antigens are absorbed, and antibodies to these antigens develop and combine with them to form immune complexes which deposit in synovial tissue to cause arthritis. NSAIDs and glucocorticoids can relieve the joint symptoms, but more lasting results can be achieved by tetracycline therapy to decrease bacteria; even better is reanastomosis of the bowel.

WHIPPLE'S DISEASE (INTESTINAL LIPODYSTROPHY)   Whipple's disease is rare and occurs mostly in middle-aged Caucasian males who develop arthritis, prolonged diarrhea, malabsorption, and weight loss. Up to 90 percent of patients develop arthritis, usually prior to other symptoms. Knees and ankles and, to a lesser extent, fingers, hips, shoulders, elbows, and wrists are involved. The arthritis is acute in onset and is characterized by tender, red, swollen joints. Symptoms are migratory, usually lasting just a few days, and are rarely chronic or cause permanent joint damage. Associated symptoms may include fever (54 percent), edema, serositis (pleurisy, pericarditis, endocarditis), pneumonia, hypotension, lymphadenopathy (54 percent), hyperpigmentation (54 percent), subcutaneous nodules, clubbing, and uveitis. Central nervous system involvement (43 percent) may develop, with loss of memory, confusion, depression, headache,

diplopia, and papilledema, and may be appreciated by abnormalities in magnetic resonance images of the brain. Laboratory abnormalities include anemia (75 percent), low serum carotene (95 percent) and albumin levels (93 percent), and HLA-B27 (8 to 30 percent) in those patients with axial arthritis. Synovial fluids have been reported to contain 450 to 36,000 white blood cells per microliter (30 to 95 percent neutrophils) or a mild monocytosis. Joint x-rays rarely show erosions but may show a sacroiliitis in those occasional patients who have axial skeletal symptoms; abdominal x-rays, computed tomographic scans, or ultrasound may reveal lymphadenopathy. The diagnosis is generally established by the detection of PAS-staining bacilliform structures in the lamina propria and/or in foamy macrophages in small intestine. These inclusion-containing foamy macrophages also have been detected in the synovium, synovial fluid, abdominal and peripheral lymph nodes, pericardium, myocardium, liver, spleen, kidney, brain, and other tissues. Electron microscopy reveals rod-shaped organisms in the lamina propria of the small intestine. Although bacteria have not been isolated or cultured from these patients, the syndrome responds well to long-term antibiotic therapy, e.g., penicillin, tetracyline, or erythromycin, 0.5 g qid for 1 year. Some have recommended an initial 2-week course of penicillin and streptomycin. Trimethoprim-sulfamethoxazole is beneficial in the event of central nervous system involvement.

REACTIVE ARTHRITIS   A Reiter's-like syndrome of arthritis 2 to 3 weeks following diarrhea caused by either *Shigella*, *Salmonella*, *Yersinia*, *Chlamydia trachomatis*, or *Campylobacter* organisms is described elsewhere (see Chap. 289).

REFERENCES

FLEMING JL et al: Whipple's disease: Clinical, biochemical and histopathologic features and assessment of treatment in 29 patients. Mayo Clin Proc 63:539, 1988

GLADMAN DD et al: Longitudinal study of clinical and radiological progression in psoriatic arthritis. J Rheumatol 17:809, 1990

GRAVELLESE EM, KANTROWITZ GF: Arthritic manifestations of inflammatory bowel disease. Am J Gastroenterol 83:703, 1988

HELLIWELL P et al: A re-evaluation of the osteoarticular manifestations of psoriasis. Br J Rheumatol 30:339, 1991

KAMMER GM et al: Psoriatic arthritis: A clinical, immunologic and HLA study of 100 patients. Semin Arthritis Rheum 9:75, 1979

KERR R, RESNICK D: Radiology of the seronegative spondyloarthropathies. Clin Rheum Dis 11:113, 1985

KHAN MA, VAN DER LINDEN SM: Ankylosing spondylitis and other spondyloarthropathies. Rheumatol Clin North Am 16:551, 1990

WOLHEIM FA: Enteropathic arthritis, in *Textbook of Rheumatology*, 4th ed, WN Kelley et al (eds). Philadelphia, Saunders, 1993

WOODROW JC: Genetic aspects of the spondyloarthropathies. Clin Rheum Dis 11:1, 1985

299 RELAPSING POLYCHONDRITIS AND MISCELLANEOUS ARTHRITIDES

BRUCE C. GILLILAND

RELAPSING POLYCHONDRITIS

Relapsing polychondritis is an episodic and often progressive inflammatory disorder of unknown cause affecting predominately the cartilage of the ears, nose, and tracheobronchial tree, as well as internal structures of the eyes and ears. Other manifestations include polyarthritis, vasculitis, cardiac abnormalities, skin lesions, and glomerulonephritis. It is most common between the ages of 40 to 60 years but may affect children and the elderly. Relapsing polychondritis is an uncommon disorder which has been found in all races. Both sexes are equally affected, and no familial tendency is apparent. Approximately 30 percent of patients with relapsing polychondritis will have another rheumatologic disorder, the most frequent being systemic vasculitis, rheumatoid arthritis, systemic lupus erythematosus, or Sjögren's syndrome.

PATHOLOGY AND PATHOPHYSIOLOGY The earliest abnormality of cartilage noted histologically is a focal or diffuse loss of basophilic staining indicating depletion of proteoglycan from the cartilage matrix. Inflammatory infiltrates are found adjacent to involved cartilage and consist predominantly of mononuclear cells and occasional plasma cells. In acute disease, polymorphonuclear white cells also may be present. Destruction of cartilage begins at the outer edges and advances centrally. There is lacunar breakdown and loss of chondrocytes. Degenerating cartilage is replaced by granulation tissue and later by fibrosis and focal areas of calcification. Small loci of cartilage regeneration may be present. Immunofluorescence studies have shown immunoglobulins and complement at sites of involvement. Fine granular material observed in the degenerating cartilage matrix by electron microscopy has been interpreted to be enzymes or immunoglobulins.

Immunologic mechanisms play a role in the pathogenesis of relapsing polychondritis. Immunoglobulin and complement deposits are found at sites of inflammation. In addition, antibodies to type II collagen and immune complexes are detected in the sera of some patients. The possibility that an immune response to type II collagen may be important in the pathogenesis is supported experimentally by the occurrence of auricular chondritis in rats immunized with type II collagen. Antibodies to type II collagen are found in the sera of these animals, and immune deposits are detected at sites of ear inflammation. Cell-mediated immunity also may be operative in causing tissue injury, since lymphocyte transformation can be demonstrated when lymphocytes of patients are exposed to cartilage extracts.

Dissolution of cartilage matrix can be induced by the intravenous injection of crude papain, a proteolytic enzyme, into young rabbits, which results in collapse of their normally rigid ears within 4 h. Reconstitution of the matrix occurs in about 7 days. In relapsing polychondritis, loss of cartilage matrix also most likely results from action of proteolytic enzymes released from chondrocytes, polymorphonuclear white cells, and monocytes that have been activated by inflammatory mediators.

CLINICAL MANIFESTATIONS Auricular chondritis is the most frequent presenting manifestation of relapsing polychondritis and eventually affects about 90 percent of patients. Usually both ears are involved. Patients experience the sudden onset of pain, tenderness, and swelling of the cartilaginous portion of the ear. Earlobes are spared because they do not contain cartilage. The overlying skin has a beefy red or violaceous color. Prolonged or recurrent episodes result in a flabby or droopy ear. Swelling may close off the eustachian tube to cause otitis media or the external auditory meatus, either of which can impair hearing. Inflammation of the internal auditory artery or its cochlear branch produces hearing loss, vertigo, ataxia, nausea, and vomiting. The cartilage of the nose becomes inflamed during the first or subsequent attacks. Approximately 80 percent of patients will eventually have nose involvement. Patients may experience nasal stuffiness, rhinorrhea, and epistaxis. The bridge of the nose becomes red, swollen, and tender and may collapse, producing a saddle deformity. In some patients, the saddle deformity develops insidiously without overt inflammation.

Arthritis is the presenting manifestation in relapsing polychondritis in approximately one-third of patients and may be present for several months before other features appear. Eventually, more than half the patients will have arthritis. The arthritis is usually asymmetric, oligo- or polyarticular, and involves both large and small peripheral joints. An episode of arthritis lasts from a few days to several weeks and resolves spontaneously without residual joint deformity. Attacks of arthritis may not be temporally related to other manifestations of relapsing polychondritis. The joints are warm, tender, and swollen.

Joint fluid has been reported to be noninflammatory. In addition to peripheral joints, inflammation may involve the costochondral, sternomanubrial, and sternoclavicular cartilages. Destruction of these cartilages may result in a flail anterior chest wall. Relapsing polychondritis may occur in patients with preexisting rheumatoid arthritis, Reiter's syndrome, psoriatic arthritis, or ankylosing spondylitis.

Eye manifestations occur in greater than half of patients and include conjunctivitis, episcleritis, iritis, and keratitis. Ulceration and perforation of the cornea may occur and cause blindness. Other manifestations include cataracts, proptosis, optic neuritis, extraocular muscle palsies, retinal vasculitis, and renal vein occlusion.

Laryngotracheal involvement occurs in approximately 70 percent of patients. Symptoms include hoarseness, a nonproductive cough, and tenderness over the larynx and proximal trachea. Mucosal edema, strictures, and/or collapse of laryngeal or tracheal cartilage may cause stridor and life-threatening airway obstruction necessitating tracheostomy. Collapse of cartilage in bronchi leads to pneumonia and, when extensive, to respiratory insufficiency.

Aortic regurgitation occurs in about 15 percent of patients and is due to progressive dilatation of the aortic ring or to destruction of the valve cusps. Other heart values can be affected. Other cardiac manifestations include pericarditis, myocarditis, and conduction abnormalities. Aneurysms of the proximal, thoracic, or abdominal aorta may occur and occasionally rupture.

Vasculitis in relapsing polychondritis ranges from small to large vessel disease and can result in thrombosis of intracerebral, mesentery, and peripheral arteries. Manifestations of small vessel vasculitis include cutaneous lesions and peripheral and cranial nerve neuropathy. Cranial nerves VI and VII are most often involved. Segmental necrotizing glomerulonephritis with crescent formation has been noted in some patients. Approximately 25 percent of patients have skin lesions, none of which is characteristic for this disease. Skin lesions include cutaneous lesions of leukocytoclastic vasculitis, erythema nodosum, erythema multiforme, angioedema/urticaria, livedo reticularis, and panniculitis.

The course of disease is highly variable, with episodes lasting from a few days to several weeks and then subsiding spontaneously. In other patients, disease may have a chronic, smoldering course. In one study, the 5-year estimated survival rate was 74 percent and the 10-year survival rate 55 percent. In contrast to earlier series, only about half the deaths could be attributed to relapsing polychondritis or complications of treatment. Pulmonary complications accounted for only 10 percent of all fatalities. In general, patients with more widespread disease have a worse prognosis.

LABORATORY FINDINGS Mild leukocytosis and normocytic, normochromic anemia are often present. The erythrocyte sedimentation rate is usually elevated. Rheumatoid factor and antinuclear antibody tests are occasionally positive in low titer. Circulating immune complexes may be detected, especially in patients with early active disease. Elevated levels of gamma globulin may be present. Tracheal stenosis can be demonstrated by regular tomograms or computed tomography of the neck. Bronchography is performed for demonstrating bronchial narrowing. Intrathoracic airway obstruction also can be evaluated by inspiratory-expiratory flow studies. On a chest film, narrowing of main bronchi and, when aortic insufficiency is present, cardiomegaly can be observed. Radiographs may show calcification at previous sites of cartilage damage involving ear, nose, larynx, or trachea.

DIAGNOSIS Diagnosis is based on recognition of the typical clinical features. Biopsies of the involved cartilage from the ear, nose, or respiratory tract will confirm the diagnosis but are only necessary when clinical features are not typical. Patients with Wegener's granulomatosis may have a saddle nose and pulmonary involvement but can be distinguished by the absence of auricular involvement and the presence of granulomatous lesions in the tracheobronchial tree. Patients with Cogan's syndrome have interstitial keratitis and vestibular and auditory abnormalities, but this syndrome does not involve the respiratory tract or ears. Reiter's syndrome may initially resemble relapsing polychondritis because of oligoarticular arthritis and eye involvement, but it is distinguished in time by the appearance of urethritis and typical mucocutaneous lesions and the absence of nose or ear cartilage involvement. Rheumatoid arthritis may initially suggest relapsing polychondritis because of arthritis and eye inflammation. The arthritis in rheumatoid arthritis, however, is erosive and symmetric. In addition, rheumatoid factor titers are usually high compared with relapsing polychondritis. Bacterial infection of the pinna may be mistaken for relapsing polychondritis but differs by usually involving only one ear, including the earlobe. Auricular cartilage also may be damaged by trauma or frostbite.

Relapsing polychondritis may develop in patients with a variety of autoimmune disorders, including systemic lupus erythematosus, rheumatoid arthritis, Sjögren's syndrome, and vasculitis. In most cases, these disorders antedate the appearance of polychondritis usually by months or years. It is likely that these patients have an immunologic abnormality that predisposes them to development of this group of autoimmune disorders.

TREATMENT Prednisone, 40 to 60 mg/d, is often effective in suppressing disease activity and is tapered gradually once disease is controlled. In some patients prednisone can be stopped, while in others low doses in the range of 10 to 15 mg/d are required for continued suppression of disease. Immunosuppressive drugs such as cyclophosphamide or azathioprine should be reserved for patients who fail to respond to prednisone. Heart valve replacement or repair of an aortic aneurysm may be necessary.

MISCELLANEOUS ARTHRITIDES

NEUROPATHIC JOINT DISEASE Neuropathic joint disease (Charcot's joint) is a severe form of osteoarthritis associated with loss of pain sensation, proprioception, or both. In addition, normal muscular reflexes that modulate joint movement are decreased. Without these protective mechanisms, joints are subjected to repeated trauma, resulting in progressive cartilage damage. The distribution of joint involvement depends on the underlying neurologic disorder. In tabes dorsalis, knees, hips, and ankles are most commonly affected; in syringomyelia, the glenohumeral joint, elbow, and wrist; and in diabetes mellitus, the tarsal and tarsometatarsal joints. Resorption of metatarsals and phalanges is also seen in diabetic patients. In children, neuropathic joint disease is caused by congenital indifference to pain or meningomyelocele. Neuropathic joint disease is also observed in patients with amyloidosis and leprosy or following frequent repeated intraarticular glucocorticoid injections. The mechanism of injury in the latter situation is thought to be an analgesic effect of steroids leading to overuse of a previously damaged joint which results in accelerated cartilage deterioration.

Neuropathic joint disease usually begins in a single joint and then progresses to involve other joints, depending on the underlying neurologic disorder. The involved joint progressively becomes enlarged from bony overgrowth and synovial effusion. Loose bodies may be palpated in the joint cavity. Joint instability, subluxation, and crepitus occur as the disease progresses. Charcot's joints may develop rapidly, and a totally disorganized joint with multiple bony fragments may evolve in a patient within weeks or months. The amount of pain experienced by the patient is less than would be anticipated based on the degree of joint involvement. Patients may experience sudden joint pain from intraarticular fractures of osteophytes or condyles. Initially, radiographs show early features of osteoarthritis followed subsequently by marked destructive and hypertrophic changes. Large, bizarre-shaped osteophytes and intraarticular bone fragments are observed. The radiographic findings of the diabetic Charcot's foot may be difficult to distinguish from those of osteomyelitis. Osteomyelitis is often suspected when the diabetic patient has an infected cutaneous ulcer on the foot. The Charcot's joint radiographically shows osteopenia, sharp cortical margins, and severe disruption and disorganization of the midtarsal and tarsometatarsal joints. In osteomyelitis, the bone margins are indistinct. The synovial fluid from a neuropathic joint is usually noninflammatory, may be bloody or xanthochromic, and may contain fragments of synovium, cartilage, and/or bone.

The primary focus of treatment is to provide stabilization of the joint. Treatment of the underlying disorder, even if successful, usually does not alter the joint disease. Braces and splints are helpful. Their use requires close surveillance, since patients may be unable to appreciate pressure from a poorly adjusted brace. In the diabetic patient, early recognition and treatment of a Charcot's foot by prohibiting weight bearing of the foot for at least 8 weeks may possibly prevent severe disease from developing. Fusion of a very unstable joint may improve function, but nonunion is frequent, especially when immobilization of the joint is inadequate.

HYPERTROPHIC OSTEOARTHROPATHY Hypertrophic osteoarthropathy (HOA) is characterized by clubbing of digits, periosteal new bone formation, and arthritis. HOA occurs in a primary or familial form beginning usually in childhood. The secondary form of HOA is associated with intrathoracic malignancies, suppurative lung disease, congenital heart disease, and a variety of other disorders and is more common in adults. Clubbing is almost always a feature of HOA but can occur as an isolated manifestation. It is unclear whether clubbing alone represents a partial expression of HOA or is a separate entity. The presence of only clubbing in a patient usually has the same clinical significance as HOA.

Pathology and pathophysiology In HOA, the periosteum becomes elevated, and new bone is deposited beneath the periosteum while endosteal bone is resorbed. These changes occur primarily at the distal ends of metacarpals, metatarsals, and long bones of the extremities. Occasionally, scapulae, clavicles, ribs, and pelvic bones are also affected. Mononuclear cell infiltration may be present in the adjacent soft tissue. Proliferation of connective tissue occurs in the nail bed and volar pad of digits, giving the distal phalanges a clubbed appearance. Small blood vessels in the clubbed digits are dilated and have thickened walls. In addition, the number of arteriovenous anastomoses is increased. The synovium of involved joints is edematous and may have an infiltration of lymphocytes and plasma cells.

The pathogenesis of HOA is not known. Both neurogenic and humoral theories have been proposed. In support of a neurogenic mechanism is the observation that the disorders most often associated with HOA involve sites innervated by the vagus nerve. Also, vagotomy may result in resolution of symptoms. A neural reflex initiated by vagal stimulation from the site of disease is thought to lead to vasodilatation and other features of HOA. The humoral theory postulates that a substance produced by the underlying disease and normally inactivated or removed by its passage through the lung reaches the systemic circulation in an active form and induces the changes of HOA. Several humoral substances, including immunoreactive growth hormone, estrogens, prostaglandins, bradykinin, ferritin, and platelet-derived growth factor have been suggested but not proven to be mediators of HOA.

Clinical manifestations Primary HOA, also referred to as *pachydermoperiostitis* or *Touraine-Solente-Golé syndrome*, usually begins insidiously at puberty. It is inherited as an autosomal dominant trait with variable expression and is more common in boys than in girls. The skin of the face and scalp thickens, producing deep nasolabial folds, furrowed forehead, and corrugated scalp, which give the face a leonine appearance. The skin of the face and scalp is usually greasy, and there is excessive sweating, particularly of the palms and soles. The distal extremities are thickened due to proliferation of new bone and soft tissue, and when the process is extensive, they may resemble elephant feet. Marked clubbing of hands and feet produces a spade-like deformity and clumsiness. Acrolysis of the terminal phalanges of the feet and hands may occur. Symptoms of bone and joint pain are usually seen only in those who have had the disease for two decades or longer.

HOA secondary to an underlying disease occurs more frequently than primary HOA. It accompanies a variety of disorders and may precede clinical features of the associated disorder by months. The progression of HOA tends to be more rapid when associated with malignancies, most notably bronchogenic carcinoma. Patients experience a burning or deep-seated aching pain in the distal extremities due to periostitis. The pain can be quite incapacitating and is aggravated by dependency and relieved by elevation of the affected limbs. Joint manifestations vary from arthralgias to very painful arthritis, most often affecting the metacarpophalangeal and metatarsophalangeal joints, wrists, ankles, and knees. The involved joints are warm, tender, and swollen. Joint effusions are usually small, and the fluid is noninflammatory, containing only a few white cells. The distal extremities may be swollen and the overlying skin warm and erythematous. Pressure applied over the distal end of the forearms and lower legs may be quite painful. Clubbing is usually asymptomatic, except for occasional warmth or burning of the fingertips. Clubbing usually evolves over months and often is first noted by the physician and not the patient. Patients, especially those with lung tumor, may experience severe skeletal pain prior to the appearance of clubbing. Clubbing is characterized by widening of the fingertips, enlargement of the distal volar pad, convexity of the nail contour, and the loss of the normal 15° angle between the proximal nail and cuticle. The thickness of the digit at the base of the nail is greater than the thickness at the distal interphalangeal joint. The base of the nail feels spongy when compressed, and the nail can be easily rocked on its bed. Marked periungual erythema is usually present. When clubbing is advanced, the finger may have a drumstick appearance. Excessive sweating, oiliness of the skin, and thickening of the facial skin are uncommon in secondary HOA.

HOA occurs in 5 to 10 percent of patients with intrathoracic malignancies, the most common being bronchogenic carcinoma and pleural tumors. Lung metastases infrequently cause HOA. HOA is also seen in patients with intrathoracic infections, including lung abscesses, empyema, bronchiectasis, chronic obstructive lung disease, and pulmonary tuberculosis. HOA also may accompany chronic interstitial pneumonitis, sarcoidosis, and cystic fibrosis. In the latter, clubbing is more common than the full syndrome of HOA. Other causes of clubbing include congenital heart disease with right-to-left shunts, Crohn's disease, ulcerative colitis, sprue, and neoplasms of the esophagus, liver, and small and large bowel. In patients with congenital heart disease with right-to-left shunts, clubbing alone occurs more often than the full syndrome of HOA.

Unilateral clubbing has been found in association with aneurysms of the aorta, subclavian, or innominate artery and with arteriovenous fistula of brachial vessels. Clubbing of the toes but not fingers has been associated with an infected abdominal aortic aneurysm. Clubbing of a single digit may follow trauma and has been reported in tophaceous gout and sarcoidosis.

Hyperthyroidism (Graves' disease), treated or untreated, may occasionally be associated with clubbing and periostitis of the bones of the hands and feet. This condition is referred to as *thyroid acropachy*. Periostitis is asymptomatic and occurs in the midshaft and diaphyseal portion of the metacarpal and phalangeal bones. The long bones of the extremities are seldom affected. Elevated levels of long-acting thyroid stimulator (LATS) are found in the serum of these patients.

Laboratory findings The laboratory abnormalities reflect the underlying disorder. The synovial fluid of involved joints has less than 500 white cells per microliter, and they are predominantly mononuclear. Radiographs show a faint radiolucent line beneath the new periosteal bone along the shaft of long bones at their distal end. These changes are observed most frequently at the ankles, wrists, and knees. The ends of the distal phalanges may show osseous resorption. Radionuclide studies show pericortical linear uptake along the cortical margins of long bones that may be present before any radiographic changes.

Treatment The treatment of hypertrophic osteoarthropathy is to identify the associated disorder and treat it appropriately. The symptoms and signs of hypertrophic osteoarthropathy may disappear completely with removal or effective chemotherapy of a tumor or with antibiotic therapy and drainage of a chronic pulmonary infection. Vagotomy or percutaneous block may lead to symptomatic relief in some patients. Aspirin, other nonsteroidal anti-inflammatory drugs, or analgesics may help control symptoms of hypertrophic osteoarthropathy.

FIBROMYALGIA Fibromyalgia, also termed *fibrositis*, is a commonly encountered disorder characterized by diffuse musculoskeletal pain, stiffness, paresthesia, nonrestorative sleep, and easy fatigability which affects predominantly women between the ages of 25 and 45 years. The term *fibrositis* is a misnomer, since this is not an inflammatory disorder of connective tissue; therefore, the term *fibromyalgia* is now preferred. Several causative mechanisms for fibromyalgia have been postulated. A disturbance of normal stage 4 (non-REM) sleep has been suggested as playing a role in its development. Symptoms of fibromyalgia were produced in normal subjects by disturbing stage 4 sleep with a buzzer without wakening them. Sleep studies in patients with fibromyalgia have shown more alpha-wave intrusion and less REM sleep, indicating disturbed and unrefreshed sleep; however, patients with chronic pain from other causes may have similar sleep patterns. Psychological factors, muscle abnormalities, and autonomic nervous system dysfunction also have been proposed to play a role in this disorder. Emotional stress, medical illness, surgery, thyroid disease, and trauma have been implicated in triggering fibromyalgia. Fibromyalgia has appeared in some patients with HIV infection, parvovirus B19 infection, or Lyme disease. In the last, fibromyalgia continued despite adequate antibiotic treatment for Lyme disease. A better understanding of fibromyalgia awaits further studies.

Symptoms are generalized aching and stiffness of the trunk, hip, and shoulder girdles. Other patients complain of generalized aching and muscle weakness. Patients perceive that their joints are swollen; however, joint examination is normal. Stiffness is usually present on arising in the morning and improves during the day but may last all day in some patients. Patients complain of exhaustion and wake up tired. They also awake frequently at night and have trouble falling back asleep. Symptoms are made worse by stress or anxiety, cold, damp weather, and overexertion. Patients often feel better during warmer weather and vacations. Disorders commonly associated with fibromyalgia include irritable bowel syndrome, irritable bladder, headaches (including migraine headaches), and dysmenorrhea. Symptoms of fibromyalgia also occur in patients who carry the diagnosis of chronic fatigue syndrome.

The characteristic physical feature is the demonstration of specific tender sites which are exquisitely more tender than adjacent areas. Tender sites should be distinguished from the trigger points found in myofascial pain syndromes. Pressure over trigger points causes pain to be referred to a nearby site, while pressure over tender sites causes pain only at that site. The patient may suddenly jump or withdraw when the tender site is palpated. The sites of tenderness are remarkably constant in location. Common sites of tenderness are bilaterally over the suboccipital muscle insertion at the base of the skull, the anterior aspect of the intertransverse process spaces at C5–C7, the midpoint of the upper border of the trapezius muscle, above the scapular spine near the medial border of the scapula, the second costochondral junction, the lateral epicondyle, the upper outer quadrant of the buttock, the posterior aspect of the trochanteric prominence, and the medial fat pad of the knee. Skinfold tenderness may be present, particularly over the upper scapular region. Subcutaneous nodules may be felt at sites of tenderness. Nodules in similar locations are present in normal persons but are not tender.

The diagnosis of fibromyalgia is made by recognizing the clinical manifestations. The joint and muscle examination is normal, and there are no laboratory abnormalities. The American College of Rheumatology in 1990 published uniform diagnostic criteria for fibromyalgia that required patients to have widespread pain in combination with 11 of the 18 tender sites described above. These criteria serve a useful purpose for enrolling patients in clinical studies; however, not all patients with fibromyalgia meet these criteria. Fibromyalgia may occur in patients with rheumatoid arthritis or other connective tissue diseases. A distinction is no longer made between primary and secondary fibromyalgia (concomitant with other disease).

Patients should be informed that they have a treatable condition which is not a crippling, deforming, or degenerative process. Salicylates or other nonsteroidal anti-inflammatory drugs only partially improve symptoms. Glucocorticoids have been of little benefit and should not be used in these patients. Local measures such as heat, massage, injection of tender sites with steroids or lidocaine, and acupuncture provide only temporary relief of symptoms. The use of tricyclics such as amitriptyline, 10 to 25 mg, doxepin, 10 to 25 mg, and cyclobenzaprine, 10 to 20 mg, at bedtime will give the patient restorative sleep resulting in clinical improvement. Higher doses of these medications may be necessary. A combination of alprazolam, 0.5 to 3 mg/d, and ibuprofen, 2.4 g/d, has been shown in a controlled study to be more effective than either drug alone. Patients also may benefit by regular aerobic exercises and by reducing the stress in their lives. While treatment of fibromyalgia may be effective in some patients, others continue to have chronic disease which may be only partially relieved, if at all.

PSYCHOGENIC RHEUMATISM   Patients may experience severe joint pain involving a few to several joints without physical findings of arthritis. These patients are often convinced that they have rheumatoid arthritis, systemic lupus erythematosus, or another connective tissue disease. This disorder is recognized by the inconsistencies, exaggerations, and emotional lability of the patient during the history and physical examination. Laboratory studies are normal. Organic disease needs to be excluded, which requires seeing the patient at regular intervals. This condition also needs to be distinguished from fibromyalgia. Anti-inflammatory or other drugs are not helpful.

CARPAL TUNNEL SYNDROME   Carpal tunnel syndrome is an entrapment neuropathy of the median nerve at the wrist producing paresthesias and weakness of the hands. The syndrome is caused by pressure on the median nerve where it passes in company with the flexor tendons of the fingers through the tunnel formed by carpal bones and the transverse carpal ligament.

Compression of the median nerve is produced by any process that encroaches on the carpal tunnel. Localized tenosynovitis of the flexor tendons of the fingers is a frequent cause of carpal tunnel syndrome, particularly in middle-aged women. Premenstrual edema or edema occurring in pregnancy also may cause these symptoms. Symptoms can be precipitated by activities which require repeated flexion, pronation, and supination of the wrist, e.g., sewing, driving, operating computers and cash registers, and playing squash or golf. Other causes of carpal tunnel syndrome, often bilateral, are rheumatoid arthritis, acromegaly, hypothyroidism, and amyloidosis. Unilateral carpal tunnel syndrome is more likely due to trauma, physical activities involving one wrist, tuberculosis, gout, or calcium pyrophosphate deposition disease.

Patients experience numbness or paresthesias of the palmar surface of the thumb, index and middle fingers, and radial half of the ring finger. Numbness or paresthesias of the whole hand may occur. Pain may be referred to the forearm and less commonly to the shoulder and neck regions. Pain or tingling of the fingers often occurs at night and is relieved by shaking or exercising the hand. Weakness and atrophy of the thenar muscles usually appear later and can occur without significant sensory symptoms.

Thenar muscle weakness is manifested by decreased strength of abduction, opposition, and flexion of the thumb. On examination, symptoms of paresthesia or pain in the fingers may be reproduced by percussion over the volar surface of the wrist (Tinel's sign) or by full flexion of the wrist for 1 min (Phalen's maneuver). A more sensitive and specific diagnostic maneuver to elicit symptoms of carpal tunnel syndrome is compressing the carpal tunnel with a modified sphygmomanometer set at 150 mmHg for up to 60 s. Decreased touch or hyperpathia to pinprick and widening of two-point discrimination may be demonstrated over the sensory distribution of the median nerve. Nerve conduction studies of the median nerve show delayed latency across the wrist, confirming the diagnosis.

Treatment of patients with only sensory symptoms and minor nerve conduction abnormalities consists of a wrist splint to be worn mainly at night, anti-inflammatory drugs, and local injection with steroids. If symptoms persist or motor abnormalities are present, surgical decompression of the carpal tunnel with release of the transverse carpal ligament and debridement is indicated.

TARSAL TUNNEL SYNDROME   Tarsal tunnel syndrome is an entrapment neuropathy of the posterior tibial nerve at the ankle producing aching, burning, tingling, and numbness of the plantar surface of the foot and toes. The syndrome is caused by compression of the posterior tibial nerve and its branches as they pass through the tunnel beneath the flexor retinaculum on the medial side of the ankle inferior and posterior to the medial malleolus. Also passing through this tunnel are the flexor tendons of the toes, vascular bundle, and the medial and lateral plantar branches of the posterior tibial nerve. Compression of the nerve in the tunnel may be caused by tenosynovitis or ganglia resulting from overuse or trauma and by inflammatory arthritis such as rheumatoid arthritis. A bony prominence from a talocalcaneal coalition also may compress the tunnel. Other causes include pregnancy, myxedema, and amyloidosis.

Patients experience paresthesias of the plantar surface of the foot and toes which may radiate up the calf. Symptoms often occur at night and after standing and may be relieved by movement of the foot and ankle. On examination, there may be loss of sensation over the plantar surface of the foot, but this is variable. Symptoms may be reproduced by percussion over the flexor retinaculum (Tinel's sign) or by applying firm pressure to this area. Diagnosis is confirmed by nerve conduction studies that show prolonged latency across the tunnel. Treatment consists of anti-inflammatory drugs and local injection of steroids. If symptoms persist, surgical decompression is indicated.

REFLEX SYMPATHETIC DYSTROPHY SYNDROME   The reflex sympathetic dystrophy syndrome (RSDS) is characterized by pain and tenderness usually of a distal extremity accompanied by signs and symptoms of vasomotor instability, trophic skin changes, and the rapid development of bony demineralization. A precipitating event can be identified in two-thirds of cases. These include local trauma, myocardial infarction, strokes, peripheral nerve injuries, antituberculosis drugs, barbiturates, and recently, cylosporin A in patients undergoing renal transplantation. RSDS is observed most often in individuals over the age of 50, reflecting the frequency of the accompanying disorder. The sex distribution is equal. An entire hand or foot is usually affected. Occasionally, RSDS will involve an isolated site such as the patella, hip, or one or two rays of a foot or hand. The contralateral side may be affected in up to 50 percent of patients, and subclinical disease may be present in virtually all patients. The pathogenesis of RSDS is poorly understood. The vasomotor manifestations are thought to be caused by abnormal stimulation of the sympathetic nervous system.

RSDS evolves through three clinical phases. The clinical manifestations of the first phase are pain and swelling of a distal extremity, which develop weeks to months following the precipitating event. The pain has an intense, burning quality. The involved extremity is warm, edematous, and tender especially around joints. Increased sweating and hair growth occur. In 3 to 6 months, the skin gradually becomes thin, shiny, and cool (second phase). Clinical features of the first two phases overlap. In another 3 to 6 months, the skin and subcutaneous tissue become atrophic, and irreversible flexion contractures of the hand or foot develop (third phase). Motion of the shoulder on the affected side is frequently painful and greatly restricted, a condition referred to as *shoulder-hand syndrome* (see "Adhesive Capsulitis," below).

The laboratory abnormalities are those of the associated disorder.

Radiographs of the involved distal extremity demonstrate mottled osteopenia referred to as *Sudeck's atrophy*. Later in the course, diffuse osteopenia develops. Similar changes, however, are observed in an immobilized limb following a fracture or paralysis. Bone scan in the early phase shows asymmetric and increased blood flow followed subsequently by increased radionuclide uptake in the periarticular bone of the involved side. Uptake also may be increased on the contralateral side indicating subclinical involvement.

Early recognition and treatment are important to prevent permanent disability. RSDS may be reversible in its early phases. Appropriate mobilization of the patient following a myocardial infarction, stroke, or injury may help to prevent this syndrome. Pain should be properly controlled. Application of heat or cold packs and active range-of-motion exercises under the surveillance of a physical therapist can be effective. A short course of high-dose prednisone has been beneficial in some patients when given early in phase 1 and occasionally may need to be repeated. Prednisone is started at 60 mg/d for 4 days and then is gradually tapered over a 3-week period. Sympathetic nerve block may be effective in reducing pain by blocking the pain cycle. A long-acting local anesthetic is injected into the stellate ganglion for the upper extremity and into the lumbar paravertebral region for the lower extremity. A sustained response may not be achieved, in which case the block can be repeated three to four times. Patients who have a good response with a sympathetic nerve block usually have good results with surgical sympathectomy. Another method of treatment is a postganglionic regional block, which is done by injecting intravenously guanethidine (investigational use only) or bretylium. In some patients, an intravenous regional block with a local anesthetic agent (Bier's block) or intravenous injection of glucocorticoids into the affected extremity may be beneficial. While the disease can be reversed in stage 1, and sometimes in stage 2, once the patient is in stage 3, treatment is mainly symptomatic. Tendon releases can be done to relieve flexion contractures.

TIETZE'S SYNDROME AND COSTOCHONDRITIS   Tietze's syndrome is manifested by painful swelling of one or more costochondral articulations. Age of onset is usually before 40, and both sexes are equally affected. Most patients have only one joint involved, usually the second or third costochondral joint. The onset of anterior chest pain may be sudden or gradual. The pain may radiate to the arms or shoulder and is aggravated by sneezing, coughing, deep inspirations, or twisting motions of the chest. The term *costochondritis* is often used interchangeably with Tietze's syndrome, but some restrict the former term to pain of the costochondral articulations without swelling. Costochondritis is observed in patients over age 40, tends to affect the third, fourth, and fifth costochondral joints, and occurs more often in women. Both syndromes may mimic cardiac or upper abdominal causes of pain. Rheumatoid arthritis, ankylosing spondylitis, and Reiter's syndrome may involve costochondral joints but are distinguished easily by their other clinical features. Other skeletal causes of anterior chest wall pain are xiphoidalgia and the slipping rib syndrome, which usually involves the tenth rib. Malignancies such as breast cancer, prostate cancer, plasma cell cytoma, and sarcoma can invade ribs, thoracic spine, or chest wall and produce symptoms suggesting Tietze's syndrome and should be easily distinguishable by radiographs and biopsy. Analgesics, anti-inflammatory drugs, and local steroid injections usually relieve symptoms.

MUSCULOSKELETAL DISORDERS ASSOCIATED WITH HYPER-LIPIDEMIA   Musculoskeletal manifestations may be the first indication of a hereditary disorder of lipoprotein metabolism. Patients with type II hyperlipoproteinemia may have recurrent migratory polyarthritis involving knees and other large peripheral joints and, to a lesser degree, peripheral small joints. The involved joints can be warm, erythematous, and swollen. Arthritis usually has a sudden onset, lasts from a few days to 2 weeks, and does not cause joint damage. Several attacks occur a year. Synovial fluid from involved joints is not inflammatory and contains few white cells and no crystals. Joint involvement may actually represent inflammatory periarthritis

or peritendinitis and not intraarticular disease. The recurrent transient nature of the arthritis may suggest rheumatic fever, especially since patients with lipoproteinemia have an elevated erythrocyte sedimentation rate and a falsely elevated antistreptolysin O titer. Furthermore, patients may have aortic valvular disease secondary to atherosclerosis. Patients with type II hyperlipoproteinemia also have tendinous xanthomas in the Achilles, patellar, and extensor tendons of the hands and feet. These are located within tendon fibers and appear in childhood in homozygous patients and after the age of 30 in heterozygous patients. Tuberous xanthomas appear only in patients homozygous for type II hyperlipoproteinemia. They are located over the extensor surfaces of the elbows, knees, and hands, as well as on the buttocks. Patients with type IV hyperlipoproteinemia also may have a mild inflammatory arthritis affecting large and small peripheral joints, usually in an asymmetric pattern with only a few joints involved at a time. Arthritis may be persistent or recurrent with episodes lasting a few days. Joint fluid is noninflammatory. Periarticular hyperesthesia may be present. Large juxtaarticular bone cysts have been noted in a few patients. The pathogenesis of arthritis in both types of hyperlipoproteinemia is not well understood. Salicylates, other NSAIDs, or analgesics usually provide relief of symptoms.

PERIARTICULAR DISORDERS   Bursitis   Bursitis is inflammation of a bursa, which is a thin-walled sac lined with synovial tissue. The function of the bursa is to facilitate movement of tendons and muscles over bony prominences. Excessive frictional forces, trauma, systemic disease (e.g., rheumatoid arthritis, gout), or infection may cause bursitis. Subacromial bursitis (subdeltoid bursitis) is the most common form of bursitis. Another is trochanteric bursitis, which involves the bursa around the insertion of the gluteus medius to the greater trochanter of the femur. Patients experience pain over the lateral aspect of the hip and upper thigh and are tender over the posterior aspect of the greater trochanter. External rotation and resisted abduction of the hip elicit pain. Olecranon bursitis occurs over the posterior elbow, and when the area is acutely inflamed, infection should be excluded by aspirating and culturing fluid from the bursa. Achilles bursitis involves the bursa located above the insertion of the tendon to the calcaneus and results from overuse and wearing tight shoes. Retrocalcaneal bursitis involves the bursa which is located between the calcaneus and posterior surface of the Achilles tendon. The pain is experienced at the back of the heel, and swelling appears on the medial and/or lateral side of the tendon. It occurs in association with spondyloarthropathies, rheumatoid arthritis, gout, and trauma. Ischial bursitis (weaver's bottom) affects the bursa separating the gluteus medius from the ischial tuberosity and develops from prolonged sitting on hard surfaces. Iliopsoas bursitis affects the bursa that lies between the iliopsoas muscle and hip joint and is lateral to the femoral vessels. Pain is experienced over this area and is made worse by hip extension and flexion. Bursitis results from trauma or overuse but can also be seen in patients with rheumatoid arthritis. Anserine bursitis is an inflammation of the sartorius bursa located over the medial side of the tibia just below the knee and is manifested by pain on climbing stairs. Tenderness is present over the insertion of the conjoint tendon of the sartorius, gracilis, and semitendinosus. Prepatellar bursitis (housemaid's knee) occurs in the bursa situated between the patella and overlying skin and is caused by kneeling on hard surfaces. Treatment of bursitis consists of prevention of the aggravating condition, rest of the involved part, a nonsteroidal anti-inflammatory drug, and local steroid injection.

Rotator cuff tendinitis and impingement syndrome   Tendinitis of the rotator cuff is the major cause of a painful shoulder and is currently thought to be caused by impingement of the tendon(s). Of the tendons forming the rotator cuff, the supraspinatus tendon is most often affected, probably because of its repeated impingement between the humeral head and the undersurface of the anterior third of the acromium and coracoacromial ligament above as well as its reduced blood supply occurring with abduction of the arm (Fig. 299-1). The tendon of the infraspinatus or the long head of the biceps is

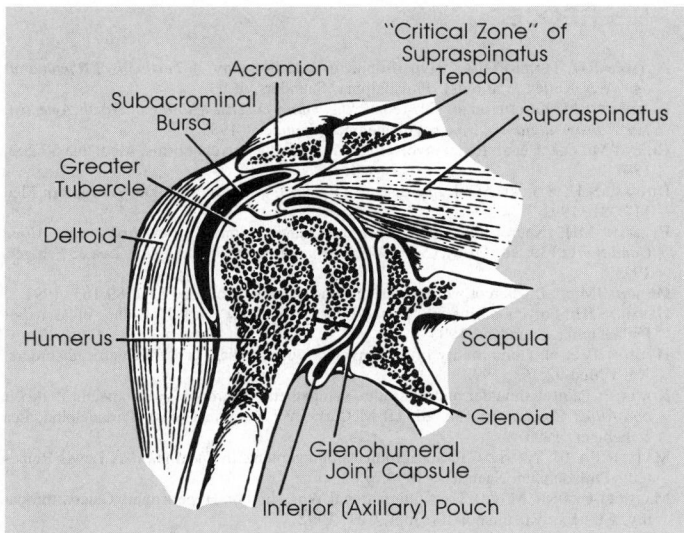

FIGURE 299-1 Coronal section of the shoulder illustrating the relationships of the glenohumeral joint, the joint capsule, the subacromial bursa, and the rotator cuff (supraspinatus tendon). *(From Kozin.)*

less commonly involved. The process evolves through edema and hemorrhage of the rotator cuff, followed by fibrotic thickening and eventually rotator cuff degeneration with tendon tears and bone spurs. Subacromial bursitis also accompanies this syndrome. Symptoms usually appear after injury or overuse, especially with activities involving elevation of the arm with some degree of forward flexion. Impingement syndrome occurs in persons participating in baseball, tennis, swimming, or occupations that require repeated elevation of the arm. Those over age 40 are particularly susceptible. Patients complain of a dull aching in the shoulder that may interfere with sleep. Severe pain is experienced when the arm is actively abducted into an overhead position. The arc between 60 and 120° is especially painful. Tenderness is present over the lateral aspect of the humeral head just below the acromion. Nonsteroidal anti-inflammatory drugs, local steroid injection, and physical therapy may relieve symptoms.

Patients may tear the supraspinatus tendon acutely by falling on an outstretched arm or lifting a heavy object. Symptoms are pain, along with weakness of abduction and external rotation of the shoulder. Atrophy of the supraspinatus muscles develops. The diagnosis is established by arthrogram or ultrasound. Surgical repair may be necessary in patients who fail to respond to conservative measures. In patients with moderate to severe tears and functional loss, surgery is indicated.

Calcific tendinitis   This is characterized by deposition of calcium salts, primarily hydroxyapatite, within a tendon. The exact mechanism for calcification is not known but may be due to ischemia or degeneration of the tendon. The supraspinatus tendon is most often affected because of its frequent impingement and reduced blood supply when the arm is abducted. It usually develops after age 40. Calcification within the tendon may evoke acute inflammation, producing sudden and severe pain in the shoulder. Tendon calcification, however, may be asymptomatic or not related to the patient's symptoms.

Bicipital tendinitis and rupture   Bicipital tendinitis, or tenosynovitis, is produced by friction on the tendon of the long head of the biceps as it passes through the bicipital groove. When the inflammation is acute, patients experience anterior shoulder pain which radiates down the biceps into the forearm. Abduction and external rotation of the arm are painful and limited. The bicipital groove is very tender to palpation. Pain may be elicited along the course of the tendon by resisting supination of the forearm with the elbow at 90° (Yergason's

supination sign). Acute rupture of the tendon may occur with vigorous exercise of the arm and is often painful. In a young patient, it should be repaired surgically. Rupture of the tendon in an older person may be associated with little or no pain and is recognized by the presence of persistent swelling of the biceps ("Popeye" muscle) produced by the retraction of the long head of the biceps. Surgery is usually not necessary in this setting.

Adhesive capsulitis   Often referred to as "frozen shoulder," adhesive capsulitis is characterized by pain and restricted movement of the shoulder usually in the absence of intrinsic shoulder disease. Adhesive capsulitis, however, may follow bursitis or tendinitis of the shoulder or be associated with systemic disorders such as chronic pulmonary disease, myocardial infarction, and diabetes mellitus. Prolonged immobility of the arm contributes to the development of adhesive capsulitis, and reflex sympathetic dystrophy is thought to be a pathogenic factor. The capsule of the shoulder is thickened, and a mild chronic inflammatory infiltrate and fibrosis may be present.

Adhesive capsulitis occurs more commonly in women after age 50. Pain and stiffness usually develop gradually over several months to a year but may progress rapidly in some patients. Pain may interfere with sleep. The shoulder is tender to palpation, and both active and passive movement are restricted. Radiograph of the shoulder shows osteopenia. The diagnosis is confirmed by arthrogram, in that only a limited amount of contrast material, usually less than 15 mL, can be injected under pressure into the shoulder joint.

The majority of patients improve spontaneously 12 to 18 months after the onset of disease, but some may have permanent restriction of movement. Early mobilization of the arm following an injury to the shoulder may prevent the development of this disease. Slow but forceful injection of contrast material into the joint may lyse adhesions and stretch the capsule, resulting in improvement of shoulder motion. Manipulation under anesthesia may be helpful in some patients. Once the disease is established, therapy may have little effect on its natural course. Local injections of glucocorticoids, nonsteroidal anti-inflammatory drugs, and physical therapy may provide relief of symptoms.

TUMORS OF JOINTS   Primary tumors and tumor-like disorders of synovium are uncommon but should be considered in the differential diagnosis of monarticular joint disease. In addition, metastases to bone and primary bone tumors adjacent to a joint may produce joint symptoms.

Pigmented villonodular synovitis is characterized by exuberant proliferation of synovial cells usually involving a single joint. It occurs most often in young adults and affects both sexes equally. The cause of this disorder is unknown.

The synovium is a brownish color and has numerous large, finger-like villi which fuse to form pedunculated nodules. There is marked hyperplasia of synovial cells within the stroma of the villi. Hemosiderin granules and lipids are found in the cytoplasm of macrophages and in the interstitial tissue. Multinucleated giant cells may be present. The proliferative synovium grows into the subsynovial tissue and invades adjacent cartilage and bone.

The clinical picture of pigmented villonodular synovitis is characterized by the insidious onset of swelling and pain in one joint, most commonly the knee. Other joints affected include the hips, ankles, calcaneocuboid joints, elbows, and small joints of the fingers or toes. The disease also may involve the common flexor sheath of the hand. Symptoms may be mild, intermittent, and present for years before the patient seeks medical attention. Radiographs may show joint space narrowing, erosions, and subchondral cysts. The joint fluid contains blood and is dark red or almost black in color. Lipid containing macrophages may be present in the fluid. The joint fluid may be clear if hemorrhages have not occurred.

The treatment of pigmented villonodular synovitis is complete synovectomy. With incomplete synovectomy, the villonodular synovitis recurs, and the rate of tissue growth may be faster than occurred originally. Irradiation of the involved joint has been successful in some patients.

Synovial chondromatosis is a disorder characterized by multiple focal metaplastic growths of normal-appearing cartilage in the synovium or tendon sheath. Segments of cartilage break loose and continue to grow as loose bodies. When calcification and ossification of loose bodies occur, the disorder is referred to as *synovial osteochondromatosis*. The disorder is usually monarticular and affects young to middle-aged individuals. The knee is most often involved, followed by hip, elbow, and shoulder. Symptoms are pain, swelling, and decreased motion of the joint. Radiographs may show several rounded calcifications within the joint cavity. Treatment is synovectomy; however, the tumor may recur.

Hemangiomas occur in synovium and in tendon sheaths. The knee is affected most commonly. Recurrent episodes of joint swelling and pain usually begin in childhood. The joint fluid is bloody. Treatment is excision of the lesion. *Lipomas* occur most often in the knee, originating in the subsynovial fat on either side of the patellar tendon. Lipomas also appear in tendon sheaths of the hands, wrists, feet, and ankles. In some instances, surgical removal is necessary.

Synovial sarcoma (malignant synovioma) is a neoplasm of connective origin arising from tissue adjacent to large joints and seldom from the joint itself. It occurs most often in young adults and is more common in men. The tumor presents as a slowly growing mass near a joint, without much pain. The tumor spreads along tissue planes. The most common site of visceral metastasis is lung. The diagnosis is made by biopsy. Treatment is wide resection of the tumor including adjacent muscle and regional lymph nodes. Amputation of the involved distal extremity may be required. Chemotherapy may be beneficial in some patients with metastatic disease.

Synovial chondrosarcoma may arise in the synovium, tendon sheath, or bursa and is very rare. Treatment is radical excision or amputation.

REFERENCES

ALTMAN RD, TENENBAUM J: Hypertrophic osteoarthropathy, in *Textbook of Rheumatology*, WN Kelley et al (eds). Philadelphia, Saunders, 1993

BENNETT RM, GOLDENBERG DL (eds): *Rheumatic Disease Clinics of North America: The Fibromyalgia Syndrome*. Philadelphia, Saunders, 1989

CHANG-MILLER A et al: Renal involvement in relapsing polychondritis. Medicine 66:202, 1987

DINERMAN H, STEERE AC: Lyme disease associated with fibromyalgia. Ann Intern Med 117:281, 1992

ELLMAN MH: Neuropathic joint disease (Charcot joints), in *Arthritis and Allied Conditions*, 13th ed, DJ McCarty, WJ Koopman (eds). Philadelphia, Lea & Febiger, 1993

GIURINI JM et al: Charcot's disease in diabetic patients. Postgrad Med 89:163, 1991

HERMAN JH: Polychondritis, in *Textbook of Rheumatology*, WN Kelley et al (eds). Philadelphia, Saunders, 1993

HUDSON JI et al: Comorbidity of fibromyalgia with medical and psychiatric disorders. Am J Med 92:363, 1992

KOZIN F: Painful shoulder and the reflex sympathetic dystrophy syndrome, in *Arthritis and Allied Conditions*, 13th ed, DJ McCarty, WJ Koopman (eds). Philadelphia, Lea & Febiger, 1993

MATSEN FA III, ARNTZ CT: Subacromial impingement, in *The Shoulder*, Lewis Reines (ed). Philadelphia, Saunders, 1990, p 623

MATUCCI-CERINIC M (ed): First International Workshop on Hypertrophic Osteoarthropathy. Clin Exp Rheumatol 10(suppl. 7):1, 1992

MICHET CJ: Vasculitis and relapsing polychondritis. Rheum Dis Clin North Am 16:441, 1990

MUÑOZ-GOMEZ J et al: Reflex sympathetic dystrophy syndrome of the lower limbs in renal transplant patients treated with Cyclosporin A. Arthritis Rheum 34:625, 1991

NEER CS II: Impingement lesions. Clin Orthop 173:70, 1983

PINEDA C et al: The spectrum of soft tissue and skeletal abnormalities of hypertrophic osteoarthropathy. J Rheumatol 17:626, 1990

SCHILLER AL: Tumors and tumor-like lesions involving joints, in *Textbook of Rheumatology*, WN Kelley et al (eds). Philadelphia, Saunders, 1993

UHTHOFF HK, SARKAR K: An algorithm for shoulder pain caused by soft-tissue disorders. Clin Orthop 254:121, 1990

WEISMAN MH: Arthritis associated with hematologic disorders, storage diseases, disorders of lipid metabolism, and dysproteinemias, in *Arthritis and Allied Conditions*, 13th ed, DJ McCarty, WJ Koopman (eds). Philadelphia, Lea & Febiger, 1993

WOLFE F et al: The American College of Rheumatology 1990 criteria for the classification of fibromyalgia: Report of the multicenter criteria committee. Arthritis Rheum 33:160, 1990

PART TWELVE

HEMATOLOGY AND ONCOLOGY

300 IMPACT OF MOLECULAR BIOLOGY ON HEMATOLOGY

STUART H. ORKIN

Phenotypic variation is the essence of genetics, whether reflected in normal polymorphism or inherited disease. Differences between individuals are encoded in cellular DNA (the *genome*), the reservoir of genetic information for the individual as well as the species. Until recently the precise relationship between a given phenotype (a trait or a disease) and a specific alteration in cellular DNA could only be inferred. For example, where a specific protein was known to be structurally abnormal in a clinical condition, demonstration of an amino acid replacement in the mutant product allowed one to predict a substitution in the DNA on the basis of the genetic code. Thus, the substitution of glutamic acid by valine at the sixth amino acid of the beta chain of sickle hemoglobin could be accounted for by a change in a single nucleotide in cellular DNA (Chap. 60).

During the past 15 years a revolution has occurred in the biomedical sciences with the introduction of the powerful methods of recombinant DNA that permit isolation of genes in pure form and their precise characterization. In many spheres of medicine recombinant DNA technology offers great promise, only one tangible consequence of which is the commercial production of new proteins such as growth factors, hormones, and enzymes. Nowhere has the impact of recombinant DNA been more immediate than in the understanding, diagnosis, and potential treatment of hematologic diseases.

IMMEDIATE IMPACT ON HEMATOLOGIC DISEASE

The application of recombinant DNA technology to the analysis of disease has expanded greatly since its introduction in about 1978; therefore discussion of its impact on hematologic disease must of necessity be selective. Consideration of the hemoglobinopathies, particularly thalassemia syndromes, is particularly instructive.

DETERMINING THE MOLECULAR BASIS OF DISEASE For nearly three decades it has been appreciated that thalassemia syndromes result from unbalanced synthesis of globin chains (Chap. 306). Prior to recombinant DNA methods, reduced (or absent) synthesis of specific globin polypeptides in various thalassemia syndromes was established, as was deficiency of specific messenger RNAs. Whether deficiency was secondary to mutations in globin genes per se or in genes that regulate their expression, and how specific mutations led to reduced mRNA synthesis or function, were largely unknown. This changed with the advent of procedures that permitted isolation of globin genes from patients with thalassemias, determination of their nucleotide sequences, and analysis of expression of the cloned genes upon their reintroduction into cells. It became possible to elucidate the precise molecular basis of these syndromes. Rather than representing a single type of mutation, thalassemia syndromes reflect the entire spectrum of molecular defects that might be predicted to interfere with gene expression. Lesions include gross gene deletions, but more commonly consist of *single base substitutions* in globin genes that adversely affect gene transcription, proper removal of intervening sequences during RNA splicing, mRNA polyadenylation, translatability, or stability.

The thalassemia syndromes were the first genetic disorders to be described in detail at the molecular level. The comprehensive dissection of the thalassemia syndromes relied on combining gene cloning with RFLP haplotype analysis. The latter method takes advantage of RFLPs, or *restriction fragment length polymorphisms,* to characterize the chromosome vicinity of the globin genes. In a given chromosomal region, the pattern of restriction site differences constitutes a RFLP haplotype, much as differences at histocompatibility loci form a haplotype. It was reasoned that haplotype differences surrounding the human β-globin gene might provide a signature for different chromosomal backgrounds upon which mutations in the β-globin gene producing thalassemia might have arisen. It thus became possible to group potentially identical mutant alleles together and focus attention on those among them that differ from the others. Therefore, examination of cloned β-globin genes (representing different chromosome haplotypes) revealed a comprehensive picture of mutations in thalassemia with high efficiency and speed.

IMPACT ON DIAGNOSIS At the clinical level, the new genetic methods have had their greatest impact on diagnosis. This has resulted from the development of techniques for the detection of specific gene defects in uncloned DNA samples. The feasibility of identifying specific defects in small DNA samples permits examination of the distribution of mutations in populations, carrier detection in families at risk (or those possibly at risk), and prenatal diagnosis as early as the first trimester by chorionic villus biopsy sampling and later by amniocentesis.

Although extensive DNA deletion, insertion, or rearrangement may often be the molecular basis of an inherited disorder, most gene mutations in inherited disorders are single nucleotide changes that cannot be detected by gross examination of gene structure. To diagnose such defects, highly sensitive assays are required that distinguish mutant from normal DNA sequences in a specific region of a gene. With a catalogue of clinically relevant gene mutations for which individuals may be surveyed (as is available for the thalassemia syndromes), these procedures may be applied with great precision. The detection of the sickle cell mutation is already a classic demonstration of the application of recombinant DNA methods to diagnosis. A substitution of T for A in the sixth codon of the β-globin gene, which directs the replacement of valine for glutamic acid, is the underlying basis for sickle cell anemia. Quite fortuitously, this single change abolishes a recognition site in the gene for a restriction enzyme (Mst II) and, thereby, alters the fragments of the gene generated upon digestion of total DNA by this enzyme. With the procedure of Southern, in which DNA fragments are electrophoretically separated in gels and then probed for specific sequences by molecular hybridization (see Chap. 61), the relevant β-globin gene fragments may be visualized. In this manner a molecular diagnosis of normal, sickle trait, or sickle cell anemia can be achieved accurately and reliably with a small DNA sample from blood cells or fetal material. This approach has been used in the prenatal diagnosis of sickle cell anemia with considerable success (Chap. 306).

APPLICATIONS OF POLYMERASE CHAIN REACTION (PCR) The newer and simpler PCR method was also first applied in the analysis of the sickle cell mutation. With synthetic DNA primers flanking the sickle mutation, the critical DNA segment can be amplified in vitro more than a millionfold to provide material sufficient for analysis by restriction enzyme digestion, molecular hybridization, or even direct DNA sequencing. Since the method requires only minute samples, takes hours rather than days, and can be automated, PCR has rapidly found its way into clinical as well as research laboratories.

The extraordinary power of PCR methodology is perhaps best exemplified by its application to the analysis of minimal residual disease in hematologic malignancies. In many forms of cancer very specific cytogenetic alterations occur (Chap. 317). Often these involve breakage and union of ordinarily separate chromosomal regions; typical examples are the translocations found in chronic myelogenous leukemia (Chap. 310). To the extent that such translocations are found within a limited target region, these chromosomal abnormalities may be detected with PCR primers flanking the breakpoints. An especially informative example is follicular lymphoma, in which there is frequently a chromosome 14;18 translocation. The 14;18 breakpoints connect one of six immunoglobulin heavy chain joining (J_h) regions on chromosome 14 to a small breakpoint region on the *BCL2* gene on chromosome 18. With PCR (using primers flanking the junctures), a single abnormal cell is detectable among more than 10^6 normal cells. Therefore, PCR presents the means to identify the subclinical presence of residual neoplastic cells. Although the precise clinical significance of small numbers of residual leukemic cells in patients in apparent remission remains to be determined, it is highly likely that correlations of the residual neoplastic cell burden with clinical outcome and treatment will be important for management of hematologic malignancies.

DETECTION OF CLONALITY IN CELL POPULATIONS   A related application of recombinant DNA methods to hematologic malignancies is the detection of *clonality in cell populations*. The clonal expansion of lymphoid cells is generally taken to reflect proliferation of malignant cells, whereas polyclonal expansion is not. Rearrangements of immunoglobulin genes and T cell receptor loci normally accompany differentiation of B and T cells, respectively. In light of this, Southern blot analysis of lymphoid cell DNA with appropriate molecular probes can provide evidence regarding the clonality of cell populations. Taken together with other findings, such information can make clinical diagnoses more precise.

Using DNA probes that detect RFLPs, the cellular DNAs of virtually any two (or more) individuals can be distinguished, particularly if highly polymorphic probes (called *fingerprinting probes*) are employed. The capability of distinguishing the genotypes of cells has also found an application in the management of patients following bone marrow transplantation. Analysis of RFLPs following allogeneic transplantation enables assessment of the relative contribution of host and donor hematopoietic cells. Engraftment of donor marrow, reemergence of host elements, and mixed cell chimerism can be evaluated with RFLP analysis.

Selected applications of recombinant DNA methods in clinical diagnosis are summarized in Table 300-1.

IMPACT ON THE UNDERSTANDING OF DISEASE AND NORMAL BIOLOGY

Some diseases reflect a disturbance of normal cellular physiology. An understanding of their biochemical basis can often provide novel insights into normal biology. Until recently, the analysis of inherited human disorders required identification and characterization of specific proteins and their corresponding genes.

Many conditions, however, including those affecting the hematopoietic system, display phenotypes for which adequate biochemical explanations are lacking. In general, animal models that faithfully mimic human disorders are not available. However, using an approach that combines classic genetics and recombinant DNA methods, the gene affected in a disorder can now be identified without specific

TABLE 300-1   Recombinant DNA analysis in clinical diagnosis

Application	Examples
Detection of specific mutations in populations and families at risk	Carrier detection of sickle cell anemia
	Estimation of specific β-thalassemia mutations in populations
Prenatal diagnosis of disease	β Thalassemia, sickle cell anemia
Detection of minimal residual disease in malignancy	Chromosome 14;18 translocation in follicular lymphoma
Detection of clonality in cell populations	Rearrangement of Ig and T cell receptor gene loci in lymphomas
Distinguishing genotypes of hematopoietic cells	Assessment of host/donor cell contributions following allogeneic bone marrow transplantation

knowledge of the protein product. With DNA probes that recognize RFLPs within families at risk for an inherited condition, markers that are very closely linked to a particular disease locus may be identified. By a variety of methods, the region of the relevant gene may be further delimited by additional linkage mapping or by use of patient samples bearing DNA deletions or chromosomal translocations. Ultimately, a region of DNA that gives rise to an mRNA that is structurally or quantitatively deranged in the disease defines the gene itself. This approach to the identification and characterization of the affected gene and its product is now referred to as *positional cloning*.

IMPACT OF POSITIONAL CLONING OF DISEASE GENES   Examples of the impact of this approach to disease are rapidly emerging. One of the first involved the analysis of an inherited hematologic disorder, the X-linked variety of chronic granulomatous disease (X-CGD). In this disease activated phagocytic white blood cells of affected males fail to produce superoxide anion, an important chemical component of the host defense system against microorganisms (Chap. 79). The cellular biochemistry of superoxide generation and its derangement in X-CGD has been actively studied since the first description of this rare disorder more than 30 years ago. Nonetheless, considerable controversy existed regarding the nature of the essential cellular proteins and the X-chromosome-encoded locus in the disease. Although the details are beyond the scope of this chapter, the molecular cloning of the gene involved in X-CGD rapidly demonstrated the requirement for an unusual cytochrome molecule in white blood cell superoxide production. In addition, further work has provided useful biochemical and molecular reagents with which to pursue dissection of superoxide production in greater depth. Positional cloning has also elucidated the genetic defects in Duchenne muscular dystrophy and in retinoblastoma, neurofibromatosis, and fragile-X syndrome, among others.

The great promise of positional cloning to the understanding of inherited disorders relates to the power of recombinant DNA methods, where in rapid succession (1) the protein product of a gene can be determined from a DNA sequence; (2) specific reagents to that protein can be generated either by immunization with synthetic peptides deduced from the sequence or with material manufactured in bacteria; and (3) the normal versions of the involved genes can be introduced into mammalian cells to analyze protein function. This approach will facilitate understanding of normal cellular physiology as well as efforts to correct disease phenotypes.

NEW MODELS OF HEMATOLOGIC DISEASE   In addition to providing the relevant genes and the tools with which to study their encoded proteins and expression, recombinant DNA methods applied to mice allow for the generation of animal models of disease. For example, introduction of genes found at the sites of chromosomal translocations in various leukemias or lymphomas into the germline of mice ultimately leads to transgenic lines that develop malignancies which closely mimic those seen in humans. Furthermore, targeted gene mutation by homologous recombination provides the means to create mice with specific genetic deficiencies. In the coming years it is highly likely that mouse models for most of the inherited and acquired hematologic disorders will be developed.

IMPACT OF THE NEW GENETICS ON TREATMENT OF HEMATOLOGIC DISORDERS

In at least four areas recombinant DNA technology has had a major impact on clinical hematology (Tables 300-1 and 300-2). First, as noted above, identification of the specific gene mutations leading to thalassemia syndromes has led to effective and efficient prenatal diagnosis of disease. In geographic areas where these conditions are prevalent, programs for prenatal diagnosis, coupled with routine hematologic screening and genetic counseling, have dramatically reduced the incidence of births of newly affected individuals. This is a monumental achievement in public health management of a genetic disorder.

Second, as also noted above, the development of new methods for the detection of specific DNA abnormalities in only a few cells among many allows better assessment of residual disease in hematologic malignancies. Correlation of clinical outcome with residual disease status and treatment is likely to lead to improved therapy.

Third, the availability of new hematopoietic growth factors through molecular cloning and gene expression is beginning to change the clinical management of several conditions. For example, the introduction of erythropoietin into the clinic constitutes a major new approach to the treatment of the anemia of chronic renal disease. Abnormalities of white blood cell production, particularly the transient neutropenia accompanying cancer chemotherapy, is now more effectively managed by administration of growth factors (colony stimulating factors) for myelomonocytic cells.

Fourth, production of blood clotting factors by recombinant DNA methods provides a promising approach to the treatment of hemophilias.

Other applications of recombinant DNA technology in clinical hematology are more speculative, but two warrant discussion.

DRUG MANIPULATION OF GENE EXPRESSION Since the production of fetal hemoglobin generally reduces the consequences of sickle cell anemia or thalassemia, studies have focused on the pharmacologic stimulation of fetal hemoglobin production in adults. Based on the observation that the modification of cellular DNA by methylation is often associated with gene inactivity, 5-azacytidine, a drug that causes widespread demethylation, has been tested for its effects on fetal hemoglobin production in patients with thalassemia or sickle cell anemia. While an augmentation in production was observed, the molecular basis for the effect has remained controversial. Nonetheless, this research has led to the testing of a variety of cytotoxic agents (such as hydroxyurea) and a variety of butyrate derivatives that appear to exert a similar effect on fetal hemoglobin production. Although the precise mechanisms by which such drugs exert their effect is unclear, increases in fetal hemoglobin production are often in the range predicted to be of clinical benefit. Hence, it is apparent that knowledge of the molecular biology of specific gene systems should generate novel therapies for the management of severe inherited hematologic disorders.

SOMATIC GENE THERAPY A potential application of recombinant DNA technology to clinical hematology now being explored is *somatic gene therapy*. The ability to clone genes and reintroduce them into cells offers prospects for correcting inherited disease by genetic means. The intent of such an approach would be to treat only somatic cells of the affected individual (somatic gene therapy), rather than attempting to correct the germline. At present, somatic gene therapy is envisioned only for severe, life-threatening disorders for which conventional medical management is unsatisfactory. Many methods for the introduction of the normal version of a gene into a cell bearing defective versions have been considered. At present, the most promising avenue would appear to be the use of modified, recombinant RNA viruses (retroviruses) to achieve efficient transfer of new genetic material into hematopoietic stem cells. Recent attention has focused on modified adenoviruses as an alternative delivery vehicle.

In principle, the hematopoietic system is an attractive target for gene therapy because pluripotent stem cells self-renew and also give rise to cell progenitors and mature blood cells. Furthermore, extensive experience in bone marrow transplantation provides a strong base for management of the host, the handling of marrow cells, and the reconstitution of the hematopoietic system by infusion of donor cells. In somatic therapy, genetically modified cells of the affected patient, rather than stem cells from another individual, would be used for cellular reconstitution. The inherited disorders that seem most appropriate for this approach include immunodeficiencies, such as severe combined immunodeficiency due to lack of adenosine deaminase (Chap. 278), hemoglobinopathies (thalassemia and sickle cell anemia), storage disorders (such as Gaucher's disease), and coagulation factor deficiencies (such as hemophilia A). Although considerable progress in the methodologies required for somatic gene therapy has been made, efficient infection of sufficient numbers of stem cells by recombinant retroviruses and adequate expression of the introduced gene in hematopoietic stem cells and their progeny remain formidable problems retarding clinical use. Nonetheless, numerous research protocols are under study in many laboratories and should form the basis for attempts to cure various disorders by gene therapy. Preliminary attempts to manage adenosine deaminase deficiency by retroviral infection of host T cells and subsequent expansion of the cells in vitro appear promising. Because correction of a mutant gene in the chromosome (rather than introduction of a normal gene copy randomly into the host cell genome) would be preferable, since regulated expression would be guaranteed, attention is also being directed to the use of targeted gene insertion.

Current and potential applications of recombinant DNA methods in the management of hematologic disease are summarized in Table 300-2.

Disorders of the hematopoietic system have proved to be a fruitful arena for the application of recombinant DNA methods to clinical medicine. Progressively greater impact of these methods on diagnosis and on the understanding of pathophysiology is virtually assured. Sensitive diagnostic approaches to clonality and minimal residual disease are likely to guide future management of malignant disease. Finally, we can be cautiously optimistic about the potential of recombinant DNA technology to provide novel approaches to treatment, including pharmacologic manipulation of gene expression and somatic genetic therapy.

TABLE 300-2 Recombinant DNA and management of hematologic disease

Application	Examples
Current	
Prenatal diagnosis of inherited disorders	β Thalassemia and sickle cell anemia
Detection of minimal residual disease in malignancy	Translocation in follicular lymphoma
	Ig or T cell receptor gene rearrangements
Administration of hematopoietic growth factors	Erythropoietin for anemia of chronic renal disease
Administration of clotting factors	Factor VIII for hemophilia A
Under study	
Modulation of gene expression to ameliorate severity of clinical disease	Stimulation of fetal hemoglobin production in sickle cell anemia
	Use of γ-interferon in chronic granulomatous disease
Possible for future	
Somatic therapy for the correction of inherited disease	Candidates
	Hemoglobinopathies
	Adenosine deaminase deficiency
	Storage disorders
	Coagulation deficiencies

REFERENCES

ANDERSON WF: Human gene therapy. Science 256:808, 1992

COLLINS FS: Positional cloning: Let's not call it reverse anymore. Nature Genet 1:3, 1992

ERLICH HA (ed): *PCR Technology: Principles and Applications for DNA Amplification.* New York, Stockton Press, 1989

MULLIGAN RC: The basic science of gene therapy. Science 260:926, 1993

ORKIN SH: Molecular genetics and inherited human disease, in *The Metabolic Basis of Inherited Disease,* 6th ed, CR Scriver et al (eds). New York, McGraw-Hill, 1989

———, KAZAZIAN HH JR: Mutation and polymorphism of the human beta-globin gene and its surrounding DNA. Annu Rev Genet 18:131, 1984

ANDERSON WF: Human gene therapy. Science 256:808, 1992

COLLINS FS: Positional cloning: Let's not call it reverse anymore. Nature Genet 1:3, 1992

section 1 Disorders of the hematopoietic system

301 MOLECULAR AND CELLULAR HEMATOPOIESIS

MARK A. GOLDBERG / H. FRANKLIN BUNN

The understanding of blood cell formation, or hematopoiesis, has been greatly enhanced by recent advances in cell culture techniques and the application of recombinant DNA technology. The cloning and characterization of an array of hematopoietic growth factors have provided new insights into the regulation of production and the biologic function of hematopoietic cells. Several of these recombinant proteins have now been produced on a large scale and have made the transition from the laboratory bench to the bedside, where clinical applications are being investigated extensively.

HEMATOPOIETIC STEM CELLS All the cells circulating in the blood are descendents of a very small number of pluripotent stem cells. These ancestral cells, which comprise less than 0.01 percent of the nucleated cells in the bone marrow, are capable of restoring normal hematopoiesis in irradiated animals and in patients with bone marrow aplasia. The pluripotent stem cell has the unique capacity for self-renewal and the potential for growth and differentiation along granulocytic, monocytic, erythroid, megakaryocytic, and lymphoid lineages. Some stem cells divide and give rise to progeny that lose their ability to differentiate along multiple pathways and become committed to a specific hematopoietic lineage. These committed progenitor cells continue to proliferate and differentiate into morphologically identifiable precursor cells which then undergo terminal maturation, thereby developing highly specialized functions and losing their ability to proliferate. Techniques have been developed which support the growth and differentiation of hematopoietic progenitor cells in vitro. Using these techniques, hematopoietic colonies of mixed and single lineages have been identified and characterized with respect to the factors required for their growth. These hematopoietic colonies are termed *colony forming units* (CFU) or *burst forming units* (BFU), with the specific type of colony designated by suffixes indicating the constituent cell types. Figure 301-1 depicts an outline of hematopoietic differentiation from the pluripotent stem cell to the highly specialized terminally matured blood cells.

CLONAL ORIGIN OF HEMATOPOIETIC MALIGNANCIES Hematologic malignancies arise as a clonal proliferation of one of the progenitor cells depicted in Fig. 301-1. The clinical manifestations of a particular malignancy depend on the stage of differentiation and lineage of the affected cell as well as on the specific nature of the initial mutation and of subsequent mutations that may appear during clonal evolution. In order for the abnormal clone of cells to attain sufficient tumor mass to produce clinical symptoms and signs, it must possess a growth advantage over the normal cells.

Molecular techniques can be used to establish the clonal origin of known and suspected tumor cells. A monoclonal proliferation of cells

in the blood, bone marrow, or lymph nodes can be distinguished from a polyclonal proliferation by morphologic examination of chromosomes in search of clonal karyotypic abnormalities. Alternatively, analysis of DNA by Southern blot hybridization or the polymerase chain reaction can be used to identify (1) clonal immunoglobulin gene rearrangements in suspected B lymphocyte malignancies, (2) clonal T cell receptor gene rearrangements in T lymphocyte malignancies, and (3) diagnostic gene translocations such as the *bcr-abl* translocation seen in chronic myelogenous leukemia. In females with the appropriate polymorphic loci on the X chromosome, clonality can be established by glucose-6-phosphate dehydrogenase isoenzyme patterns or analysis of DNA restriction fragments. This information is useful for several purposes: It may allow one to establish a definitive diagnosis of a malignancy; it may provide insight into the cell of origin and the steps in tumor progression; and it also may provide a sensitive tool for assessing remission or early relapse.

Clonal analysis of mature blood cells indicates that the myeloproliferative disorders generally arise in the pluripotent stem cell. Similarly, many of the myelodysplastic syndromes appear to be clonal stem cell disorders. The cell of origin in the acute leukemias and its effect on response to therapy and prognosis are currently being studied. Understanding the cell of origin in the various lymphoid malignancies has facilitated the classification of this complex group of disorders.

HEMATOPOIETIC GROWTH FACTORS Also depicted in Fig. 301-1 are many of the known hematopoietic growth factors and cytokines necessary for growth and differentiation of cells in the various lineages. The biologic activities of most of these hematopoietic cytokines have been determined largely by in vitro cell culture experiments. Their in vivo regulation and physiologic roles are currently the object of intense study. As depicted in the diagram, some of the growth factors, such as stem cell factor (SCF; also known as *steel factor* or *c-kit ligand*), interleukin 3 (IL-3), and granulocyte-macrophage colony stimulating factor (GM-CSF), have the potential to influence the proliferation and differentiation of several hematopoietic lineages; in addition, they have overlapping and synergistic activities. Other growth factors, such as erythropoietin, granulocyte colony stimulating factor (G-CSF), and macrophage colony stimulating factor (M-CSF) act primarily on later progenitor cells committed to a single lineage. G-CSF also has been shown recently to play a synergistic role in stimulating early multilineage progenitors in hematopoietic cell culture experiments, though the in vivo importance of this observation is unknown. Furthermore, G-CSF, M-CSF, GM-CSF, and IL-3 have been shown not only to stimulate proliferation and differentiation of hematopoietic cells but also to modulate the function of mature granulocytes and mononuclear phagocytes.

The hematopoietic growth factors act by binding to specific receptors present on the surface of target cells. An increasing number of these growth factor receptors have been cloned; they share limited homologies with one another and appear to constitute a superfamily of growth factor receptor genes. The expression of a specific receptor

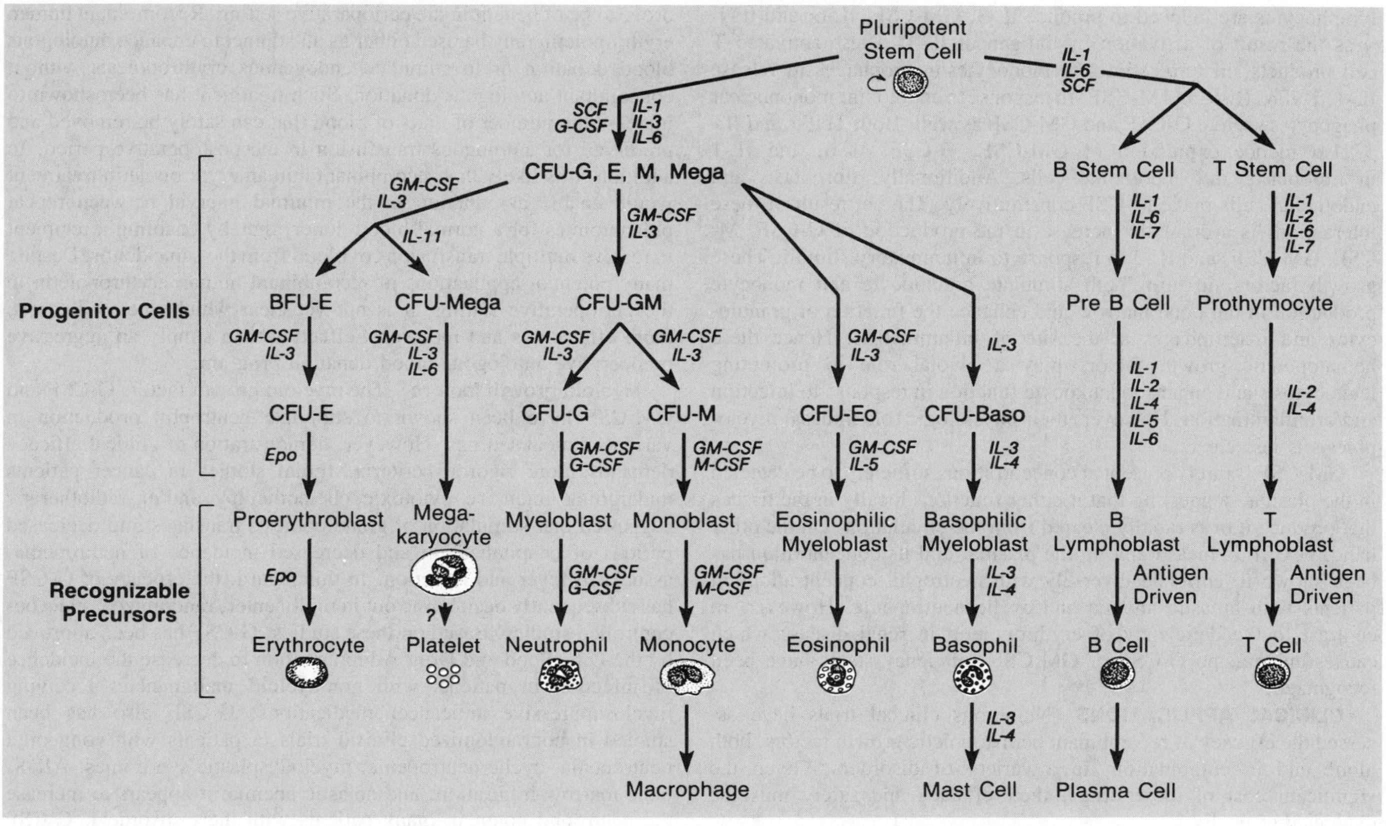

FIGURE 301-1 A depiction of the stem cell model of hematopoiesis. Growth factors and cytokines influencing particular steps in the differentiation pathway are shown. Abbreviations not in the text: G, granulocyte; E, erythrocyte; M, monocyte; Mega, megakaryocyte; Eo, eosinophil; Baso, basophil; Epo, erythropoietin.

or combination of receptors on the cell surface may determine the cell's ultimate path of differentiation.

Erythropoietin   This 30-kDa glycoprotein hormone is crucial to the regulation of erythropoiesis. The primary site of erythropoietin production after birth is the kidney, probably in peritubular interstitial cells located in the inner cortex and outer medulla. In the fetus, the liver is the major site of erythropoietin production. In response to the sensing of hypoxia in the kidney and liver, erythropoietin gene transcription increases, leading to increased erythropoietin mRNA and increased production and secretion of erythropoietin protein. The hormone travels to hematopoietic tissues, where it binds to its receptor on erythroid progenitor cells, stimulating proliferation and differentiation. This results in an increase in the oxygen-carrying capacity of the blood, thereby alleviating the hypoxic stimulus and providing a negative feedback loop. In patients with normal renal function, serum erythropoietin levels are inversely proportional to the hemoglobin concentration.

Myeloid growth factors   G-CSF, M-CSF, GM-CSF, and IL-3 work together to stimulate granulocyte and monocyte/macrophage proliferation, differentiation, and function in vitro. Furthermore, GM-CSF and IL-3 contribute to in vitro stimulation of megakaryopoiesis and erythropoiesis (Fig. 301-1). Like erythropoietin, the myeloid cytokines are all relatively small glycoproteins. However, unlike erythropoietin, the recombinant proteins do not appear to require glycosylation for in vivo biologic activity. Many cell types can produce G-CSF, M-CSF, and GM-CSF in the setting of inflammation (Fig. 301-2), while IL-3 production appears to be limited to T lymphocytes and mast cells. The regulation of their production involves a complex network of signaling and feedback loops which are in large part influenced by inflammatory cytokines, including interleukin 1 (IL-1), tumor necrosis factor α (TNFα), interleukin 6 (IL-6), and interferon-γ (IFN-γ), as well as by foreign antigens. T

FIGURE 301-2 Network of signaling and feedback loops and sites of production of the hematopoietic growth factors and cytokines involved in the regulation of the inflammatory response.

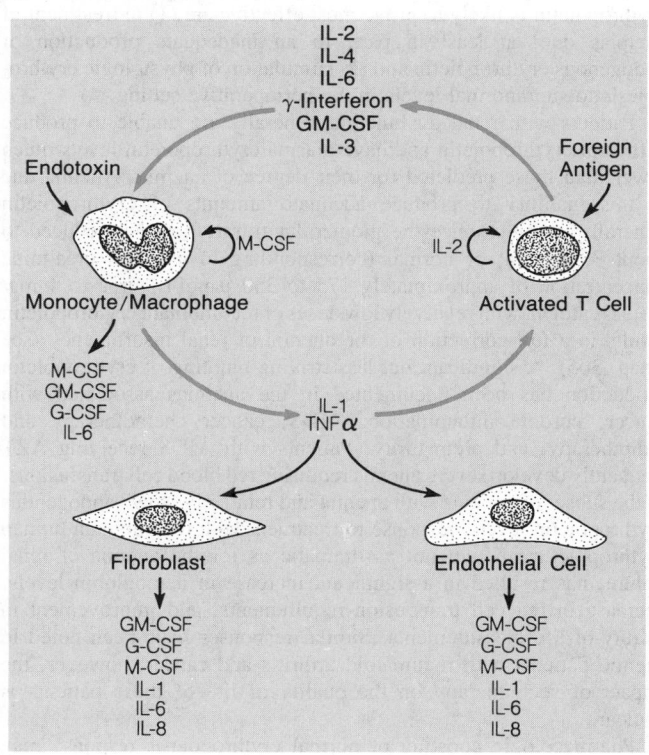

lymphocytes are induced to produce IL-3, GM-CSF, IL-6, and IFN-γ as the result of activation by antigen or IL-1. These activated T cell products, in turn, stimulate monocytes/macrophages to release IL-1, TNFα, IL-6, and M-CSF. In response to endotoxin, mononuclear phagocytes secrete G-CSF and GM-CSF as well. Both TNFα and IL-1 also induce expression of GM-CSF, G-CSF, IL-6, and IL-1 in fibroblasts and endothelial cells. Additionally, fibroblasts and endothelial cells make M-CSF constitutively. The net result of these interactions is a dramatic increase in the production of G-CSF, M-CSF, GM-CSF, and IL-3 in response to inflammatory stimuli. These growth factors, in turn, both stimulate granulocyte and monocyte production in the bone marrow and enhance the function of granulocytes and macrophages at the site of inflammation. Hence these hematopoietic growth factors play a pivotal role in promoting leukocytosis and enhanced leukocyte function in response to infection and/or inflammation. However, their physiologic role in basal myelopoiesis is less clear.

GM-CSF is rarely present at concentrations sufficient to be detected in the plasma, suggesting that it either functions locally in the tissues that produce it or is rapidly cleared from the circulation. On the other hand, G-CSF is measurable in the plasma, and its concentration has been shown to correlate inversely with neutrophil concentrations in patients with aplastic anemia and cyclic neutropenia. However, in contrast to the deficiency of erythropoietin in renal disease which causes anemia, no G-CSF or GM-CSF deficiency states have been recognized.

CLINICAL APPLICATIONS   Numerous clinical trials have assessed the efficacy of recombinant hematopoietic growth factors, both alone and in combination, in a variety of disorders. Given the significant cost of these drugs, their efficacy and safety must be evaluated critically.

Erythropoietin   In patients with any type of anemia, intervention is generally warranted only to treat symptoms. Hence there is little need to correct a relatively mild anemia with few associated symptoms. Although it has been clearly demonstrated that recombinant human erythropoietin can increase the red cell mass in various patient groups as well as in normal individuals, the true utility of recombinant human erythropoietin depends on demonstrating that it can be used to decrease the need for homologous red blood cell transfusions and/or to improve the quality of life. The two general areas in which recombinant human erythropoietin is likely to prove most effective are (1) in treatment of anemias due, at least in part, to an inadequate production of endogenous erythropoietin and (2) stimulation of physiologic erythropoiesis to supranormal levels in the perioperative setting.

Patients with renal dysfunction generally are unable to produce sufficient erythropoietin and have plasma erythropoietin levels much lower than those predicted for their degree of anemia. Anemia due to this inability to produce adequate amounts of erythropoietin generally develops once the glomerular filtration rate is reduced to about 30 percent of normal (corresponding to a serum creatinine concentration of approximately 175 to 350 μmol/L, or 2 to 4 mg/dL). Treatment with relatively low doses of recombinant erythropoietin results in a full correction of the anemia of renal insufficiency (see Chap. 305). A significant but less striking blunting of erythropoietin production has been documented in the anemias associated with cancer, chronic inflammation, AIDS, cancer chemotherapy and radiotherapy, and prematurity. Patients with AIDS receiving AZT frequently develop severe anemia requiring red blood cell transfusions. In the subset of patients with anemia and relatively "low" endogenous erythropoietin levels, response to treatment with recombinant human erythropoietin, though not as dramatic as for the anemia of renal failure, has resulted in a significant increase in hemoglobin levels, decrease in red cell transfusion requirements, and improvement in quality-of-life measurements. Similar responses have been noted in anemic patients with rheumatoid arthritis and cancer; however, the impact of such therapy on the quality of life of these patients is unclear.

Pharmacologic boosting of normal erythropoiesis response may prove to be of benefit in the perioperative setting. Recombinant human erythropoietin may be used either as an adjunct to enhance autologous blood donation or to stimulate endogenous erythropoiesis without concomitant autologous donation. Such treatment has been shown to increase the number of units of blood that can safely be removed and preserved for autologous transfusion in the postoperative period. In addition, it is likely that recombinant human erythropoietin treatment would enable a reduction in the minimal interval between repeat phlebotomies for a normal blood donor, thereby enabling a recipient to receive multiple transfusions of blood from the same donor. Despite many potential applications of recombinant human erythropoietin in the perioperative setting, it is not yet clear which ones will prove more efficacious and more cost-effective than simply an aggressive preoperative autologous blood donation program.

Myeloid growth factors   The myeloid growth factors G-CSF and GM-CSF have been shown to stimulate neutrophil production in various clinical settings. However, demonstration of clinical efficacy demands more rigorous criteria. Initial studies in cancer patients undergoing intensive cytotoxic chemotherapy and/or radiotherapy suggested that stimulation of granulopoiesis translates into decreased periods of hospitalization and decreased incidence of neutropenia-associated fever and infection. In this regard, the efficacy of G-CSF has subsequently been borne out in multicenter, randomized, placebo-controlled studies. Based on these studies, G-CSF has been approved by the U.S. Food and Drug Administration to decrease the incidence of infection in patients with nonmyeloid malignancies receiving myelosuppressive anticancer medications. G-CSF also has been studied in nonrandomized clinical trials in patients with congenital neutropenia, cyclic neutropenia, myelodysplastic syndromes, AIDS, bone marrow infiltration, and aplastic anemia; it appears to increase the neutrophil count in many patients with these disorders. G-CSF often increases the neutrophil count sufficiently in patients with congenital and cyclic neutropenia and so decreases the frequency and severity of infection. In myelodysplastic syndromes, G-CSF also generally increases the neutrophil count. However, effects on the frequency of infection, progression to acute myelogenous leukemia, and survival are uncertain. G-CSF has been generally well tolerated with no apparent dose-limiting toxicity. The most frequent toxicity has been bone pain, which is usually responsive to mild analgesics.

GM-CSF has been used in settings similar to those in which G-CSF has been studied. Although GM-CSF has proliferative effects on a broader range of hematopoietic progenitors in vitro (see Fig. 301-1), its primary clinical benefit in vivo has been on granulopoiesis. On the basis of well-controlled clinical trials, it has been approved by the U.S. Food and Drug Administration for the acceleration of myeloid recovery following autologous bone marrow transplantation for lymphoid malignancies as well as for use in patients who have undergone allogeneic or autologous bone marrow transplantation in whom engraftment has failed or is delayed. The potential efficacy of GM-CSF in other settings is unclear. Unlike G-CSF, GM-CSF does not appear to be very effective in stimulating neutrophil production in patients with congenital and cyclic neutropenia. In myelodysplastic syndromes, GM-CSF frequently increases the neutrophil and eosinophil counts and occasionally may stimulate other hematopoietic lineages. However, as with G-CSF, its effects on the frequency of infection, progression to acute myelogenous leukemia, and survival in patients with myelodysplastic syndromes are uncertain. Likewise, neither G-CSF nor GM-CSF appears to be generally efficacious in treating severe aplastic anemia. In AIDS patients with neutropenia, the results of studies with GM-CSF have been similar to those with G-CSF. GM-CSF appears to be more toxic than G-CSF. In addition to bone pain, GM-CSF has been noted to cause rash, fevers, myalgias, fatigue, anorexia, phlebitis, thrombosis, eosinophilia, and, at high doses, capillary leak syndrome with pleural and pericardial effusions and edema. The side effects of GM-CSF, especially fever, can complicate the management of critically ill patients with severe neutropenia.

The use of G-CSF or GM-CSF in myeloid malignancies is still

experimental. The potential benefits of these growth factors in these conditions, including stimulating cells to differentiate or chemotherapy sensitization by putting resting cells into cycle, must be weighed against the possibility of enhancing proliferation of a malignant clone, thereby accelerating the pace of the disease.

Based on current information, definitive indications as to when to use G-CSF versus GM-CSF are unclear. Nonetheless, it is becoming evident that if stimulation of neutrophil production is the primary goal, this can be done more specifically, and with fewer potential side effects, with G-CSF. However, because of differences in the spectrum of activity of these cytokines, in situations other than the treatment of neutropenia, the relative utility of G-CSF versus GM-CSF remains to be determined.

Future applications Clinical trials are underway investigating the safety and efficacy of IL-3 and IL-6 in various clinical settings. Studies of many of the other hematopoietic growth factors and cytokines are sure to follow in short order. Many will focus on the potential synergy of combinations of these factors. A particularly exciting property shared by several of these growth factors, including G-CSF, GM-CSF, and IL-3, is the ability to increase markedly the concentration of progenitor cells and stem cells in the peripheral blood. These circulating progenitor cells can be collected by leukapheresis and reinfused along with hematopoietic growth factors following intensive myelosuppressive chemotherapy. In this setting, the combination of peripheral blood progenitor cells and growth factor has been shown to stimulate not only granulopoiesis but also megakaryopoiesis and erythropoiesis. Using combinations of peripheral blood progenitor cells and hematopoietic growth factors may allow further dose intensification of anticancer therapy with the hope of increasing response rates and survival. It also may allow peripheral blood stem cell transplantation to play an increasing role in clinical practice and, in selected patients, may supplant autologous bone marrow transplantation.

REFERENCES

BAGBY GC, SEGAL GM: Growth factors and the control of hematopoiesis, in *Hematology: Basic Principles and Practice*, R Hoffman et al (eds). New York, Churchill Livingstone, 1991, pp 97–121

CRAWFORD J et al: Reduction by granulocyte colony-stimulating factor of fever and neutropenia induced by chemotherapy in patients with small-cell lung cancer. N Engl J Med 325:164, 1991

EMERSON SG: The stem cell model of hematopoiesis, in *Hematology: Basic Principles and Practice*, R Hoffman et al (eds). New York, Churchill Livingstone, 1991, pp 72–81

ESCHBACH JW et al: Correction of the anemia of end-stage renal disease with recombinant human erythropoietin: Results of a combined phase I and II clinical trial. N Engl J Med 316:73, 1987

FLEISCHMAN RA: Southwestern Internal Medicine Conference: Clinical use of hematopoietic growth factors. Am J Med Sci 305:248, 1993

GARNICK MB (ed): *Erythropoietin in Clinical Applications: An International Perspective.* New York, Marcel Dekker, 1990

LIESCHKE GJ, BURGESS AW: Granulocyte colony stimulating factor and granulocyte-macrophage colony stimulating factor. N Engl J Med 327:28, 1992

OGAWA M: Differentiation and proliferation of hematopoietic stem cells. Blood 81:2844, 1993

SINGER JW: Use of recombinant hematopoietic growth factors in bone marrow transplantation. Am J Pediatr Hematol Oncol 15:175, 1993

302 PATHOPHYSIOLOGY OF THE ANEMIAS

H. FRANKLIN BUNN

There is a large and coherent body of information on the birth, life, and death of red cells. Familiarity with erythropoiesis and erythrocyte structure and function is necessary to understand the pathogenesis of the various anemias as well as to develop an orderly approach to diagnosis and management. Conversely, investigation of specific red cell disorders has provided unique insights into normal erythroid physiology.

RED CELL PRODUCTION Red cells are derived from an undifferentiated progenitor cell in the bone marrow called the *pluripotent stem cell* (Fig. 302-1). As explained in more detail in Chap. 301, a stem cell is one which is capable of both self-renewal and differentiation. Erythrocytes, as well as granulocytes, monocytes, platelets, and lymphocytes evolve from this ancestor cell. As Fig. 302-1 shows, the most primitive erythroid progenitor which has been cultured from both bone marrow and peripheral blood is called the *erythroid burst-forming unit* (BFU$_e$). After 10 to 15 days in tissue culture, it produces a large colony of recognizable red cell precursors. The BFU$_e$ is responsive to high doses of the erythroid-promoting hormone erythropoietin, which acts synergistically with other hematopoietic growth factors (see Chap. 301). A more mature progenitor cell, the *erythroid colony forming unit* (CFU$_e$), is very sensitive to erythropoietin, producing a smaller clone of erythroid cells after 4 to 7 days in culture.

Erythropoietin is a glycoprotein hormone having a molecular weight of 30,400. Erythropoietin is produced, primarily by the kidneys, in response to hypoxia and is secreted into the plasma. Accordingly, anemic patients have increased plasma levels of this hormone, inversely proportional to their hemoglobin level. In contrast, patients with uremia usually have a marked impairment of erythropoietin production and therefore relatively low plasma levels.

Erythropoietin interacts with a specific receptor on the surface of committed erythroid stem cells, inducing them to differentiate into proerythroblasts, the earliest red cell precursor that can be recognized on examination of the bone marrow. Normally, the transition from the proerythroblast to the most mature normoblast involves three or four cell divisions over a 4-day period (see Fig. 302-1). During this time, the nucleus becomes smaller, and an increasing amount of hemoglobin is produced in the cytoplasm. Following the last division, the pyknotic nucleus is removed from the normoblast. What remains is the reticulocyte, which stays in the bone marrow for 2.5 to 3 days. The reticulocyte is then released into the general circulation, where it remains for another 24 h before it loses its mitochondria and ribosomes and assumes the morphologic appearance of a mature red cell.

Erythroid precursor cells ranging from the pronormoblast to the reticulocyte possess a specific surface receptor for the iron-transferrin complex, enabling them to incorporate sufficient iron for hemoglobin production (Fig. 302-2). The use of a radioactive iron label such as ^{59}Fe permits a quantitative assessment of erythropoiesis. From the rate at which injected ^{59}Fe-labeled transferrin disappears from the plasma, plasma iron turnover can be calculated. This parameter is generally proportional to the total developing erythroid cell mass. Normally, about 80 percent of ^{59}Fe bound to plasma transferrin goes to erythroid cells in the marrow. After 4 to 6 days, the labeled iron reappears in circulating erythrocytes. The extent to which circulating red cells acquire the label provides an index of the efficiency or effectiveness of erythropoiesis.

The normal marrow is capable of increasing its red cell production to about three to five times the normal rate within a week or two following stimulation by high levels of erythropoietin. In chronic hemolytic anemias, erythropoiesis may increase five- to sevenfold. As the erythroid marrow expands, fat is replaced by erythroid cells, and formerly inactive or "yellow" marrow becomes active or "red."

HEMOGLOBIN BIOSYNTHESIS Erythroid cell development involves the production of hemoglobin-containing cells. Hemoglobin is a tetramer composed of two pairs of polypeptides, e.g., $\alpha_2\beta_2$. The globin subunits, α, β, γ, and δ, are each covalently linked to a heme group. The synthesis of a particular globin subunit is directed by a corresponding gene inherited from each parent. As shown in Fig. 302-1, there is a marked amplification in the transcription of globin mRNA during the development of proerythroblasts. About 98 percent of the protein in the cytoplasm of circulating red cells is hemoglobin.

In the red cells of normal adults, hemoglobin A ($\alpha_2\beta_2$) constitutes

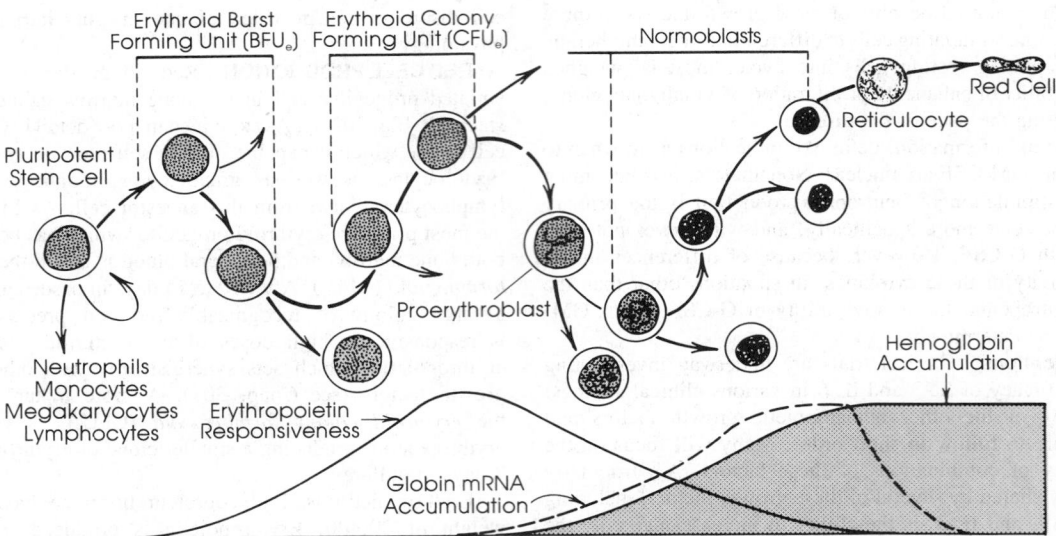

FIGURE 302-1 Differentiation and morphologic maturation of erythroid cells. Erythroid cells are derived from pluripotent stem cells (shown on left) which are also capable of differentiating into neutrophils, monocytes (macrophages), megakaryocytes, and lymphocytes. Under the influence of erythropoietin, erythroid progenitor cells (BFU$_e$ → CFU$_e$) differentiate into proerythroblasts, the earliest recognizable erythroid cells in the bone marrow. During further maturation, globin mRNA accumulates, directing the cell to synthesize hemoglobin.

about 97 percent of the total hemoglobin. The remaining 3 percent is primarily hemoglobin A$_2$ ($\alpha_2\delta_2$). As discussed in Chap. 306, this minor component is increased in patients with β thalassemia. Fetal hemoglobin (HbF or $\alpha_2\gamma_2$) usually accounts for less than 1 percent of total hemoglobin in normal adult red cells. HbF is localized to 1 to 7 percent of red cells. In contrast, it is the main hemoglobin component of fetal red cells. During the last 3 months of gestation, γ-chain synthesis switches to β-chain synthesis. However, in certain types of congenital hemolytic anemias such as the β thalassemias and sickle cell anemia, the production of γ chains (and therefore of HbF) persists. In addition, increased levels of HbF also may be encountered in certain acquired anemias in which there is disordered red cell proliferation.

Normally α- and β-chain synthesis in erythroid precursors is evenly balanced. In contrast, the thalassemias (Chap. 306) are characterized by imbalance in globin chain synthesis.

The synthesis of *heme* in red cell precursors is closely matched to globin chain production. As shown in Fig. 302-3, the initial and rate-limiting step is the condensation of succinyl coenzyme A (CoA) and glycine to form δ-aminolevulinic acid. This reaction, which takes place in mitochondria, requires that glycine be activated by pyridoxal phosphate. Accordingly, patients with sideroblastic anemia, in whom heme synthesis is usually defective, may sometimes respond to pyridoxine therapy (Chap. 303). The next steps of heme synthesis take place in the cytosol. Two molecules of δ-aminolevulinic acid condense to form a ring structure, porphobilinogen. This colorless pyrrole is elevated in acute intermittent porphyria and can be detected in urine by the Watson-Schwartz test. The subsequent steps in prophyrin synthesis are also shown in Fig. 302-3. The last three reactions take place in mitochondria. Iron is inserted into protoporphyrin IX to form heme. In iron deficiency, as well as in lead poisoning, increased levels of protoporphyrin can be detected in red cells.

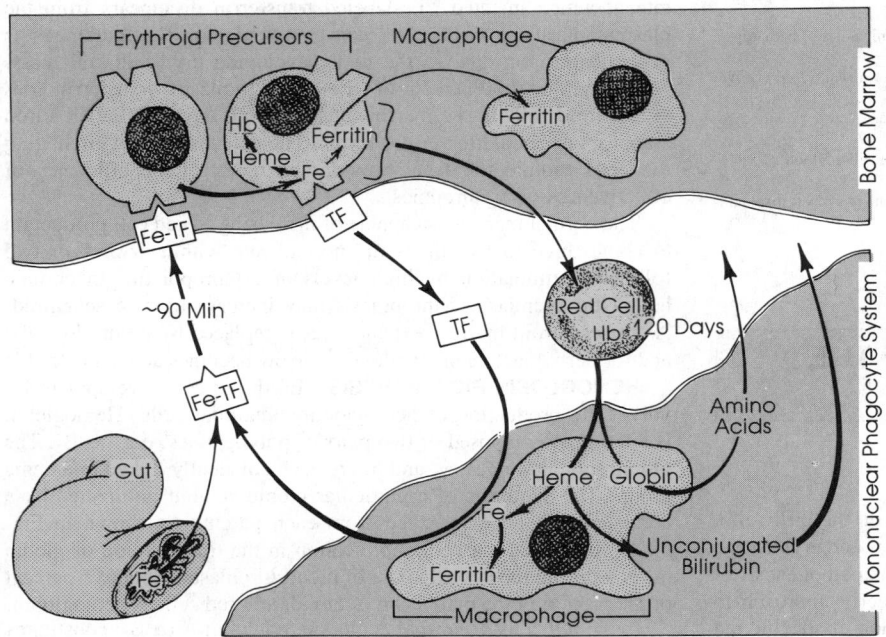

FIGURE 302-2 Erythrocyte production, circulation, and destruction. Circulating iron-bound transferrin (TF) is bound to specific receptors on the surface of erythroid progenitors and precursors in the marrow. Most of this iron is incorporated into hemoglobin; the remainder is stored as ferritin. Following maturation of the erythroid precursor, the nucleus is shed and the red blood cell emerges from the marrow into the plasma where it circulates for approximately 120 days. The senescent red blood cell is taken up by the mononuclear phagocyte system and is destroyed. The heme iron is initially incorporated into ferritin. This storage iron is available for transport to the marrow via transferrin.

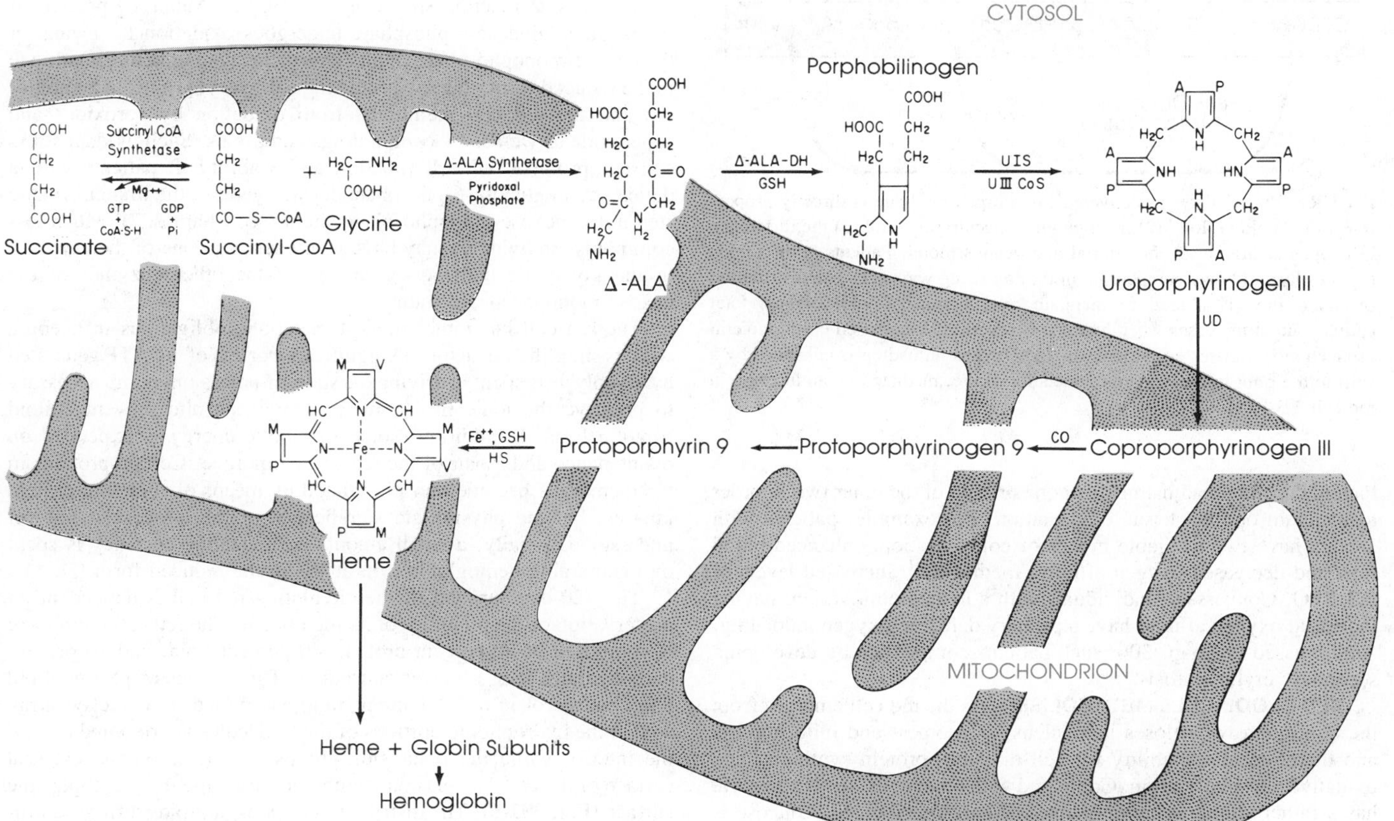

CYTOSOL

Porphobilinogen

Uroporphyrinogen III

Protoporphyrin 9 ← Protoporphyrinogen 9 ← Coproporphyrinogen III

Heme

Heme + Globin Subunits

↓

Hemoglobin

MITOCHONDRION

FIGURE 302-3 The biosynthesis of heme. Enzymatic steps that occur in mitochondria are shown. The following abbreviations are used: CoA, coenzyme A; GTP, guanosine triphosphate; GDP, guanosine diphosphate; Pi, inorganic phosphorus; GSH, glutathione; δ-ALA-DH, δ-aminolevulinate dehydrase; UIS, uroporphyrinogen I synthetase; UIII CoS, uroporphyrinogen III cosynthetase; UD, uroporphyrinogen decarboxylase; CO, coproporphyrinogen oxidase; HS, heme synthetase; A, acetate; P, proprionate; M, methyl; V, vinyl.

Disorders of porphyrin synthesis and metabolism are discussed in Chap. 346.

HEMOGLOBIN STRUCTURE AND FUNCTION The primary role of red cells is to transport oxygen from lungs to tissues and to transport carbon dioxide in the reverse direction. Both functions are assumed by hemoglobin. The three-dimensional structure of human hemoglobin has been determined from x-ray crystallographic analysis. The important functional properties of hemoglobin such as subunit cooperativity, the pH dependency of oxygen affinity (the Bohr effect), and the interaction with 2,3-bisphosphoglycerate can now be understood in stereochemical terms. This structural information also has been useful in explaining the abnormal functional properties of a number of human hemoglobin variants which are associated with clinical and hematologic manifestations (see Chap. 306).

During circulation through the lungs, hemoglobin becomes almost fully saturated with oxygen (1.34 mL O_2 per gram of hemoglobin). As red cells perfuse the capillary beds, oxygen is extracted. Efficient unloading of oxygen at relatively high oxygen tensions is possible because of the sigmoid shape of the oxygen dissociation curve (subunit cooperativity) (see Fig. 302-4). The affinity of hemoglobin for oxygen is modified by three intracellular cofactors: hydrogen ion, carbon dioxide, and 2,3-bisphosphoglycerate (2,3-BPG). Increasing the concentrations of each of these three effectors results in a ''shift to the right'' in the oxygen dissociation curve. In human red cells, 2,3-BPG is an important regulator of hemoglobin function. One molecule of 2,3-BPG binds to the β chains of deoxyhemoglobin, thereby decreasing oxygen affinity. Elevated levels of 2,3-BPG have been noted in various states of hypoxia. The resulting decrease in oxygen affinity permits enhanced oxygen release. The oxygenation of a particular organ or tissue depends on three main factors (depicted in

Fig. 302-5): blood flow, oxygen-carrying capacity of the blood (hemoglobin concentration), and the affinity of the hemoglobin for oxygen. Patients with a primary abnormality of one of these three

FIGURE 302-4 The oxyhemoglobin dissociation curve of normal blood. The major factors influencing the position of the curve are pH, temperature, and the intracellular concentration of 2,3-BPG. An increase in plasma pH or a decrease in temperature and 2,3-BPG causes an increase in oxygen affinity (shift to the left) and a relative decrease in oxygen unloading when going from an arterial P_{O_2} of 12.7 kPa (95 mmHg) to a venous P_{O_2} of 5.3 kPa (40 mmHg). Conversely, a decrease in pH or an increase in either temperature or 2,3-BPG causes a decrease in oxygen affinity (shift to the right) and a relative increase in oxygen unloading.

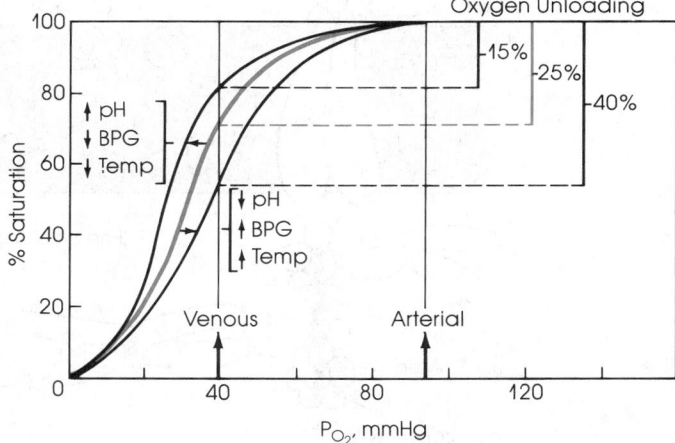

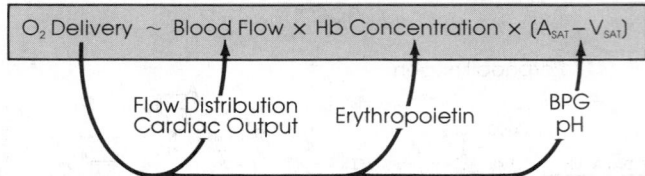

$$O_2 \text{ Delivery} \sim \text{Blood Flow} \times \text{Hb Concentration} \times (A_{SAT} - V_{SAT})$$

Flow Distribution
Cardiac Output   Erythropoietin   BPG
                                    pH

FIGURE 302-5 Oxygen delivered to an organ or tissue is directly proportional to (1) blood flow, (2) hemoglobin concentration, and (3) the difference in oxygen saturation of the arterial and venous blood. Patients with various types of hypoxia may compensate in the following ways: (1) The distribution of blood flow is altered to maintain oxygenation of vital organs; total cardiac output increases when hypoxia is severe. (2) Increased erythropoietin production stimulates erythropoiesis. (3) Oxygen unloading is enhanced by a shift to the right in the oxygen dissociation curve, mediated by an increase in red cell 2,3-BPG.

factors depend on adjustments in one or both of the other two in order to maintain optimal tissue oxygenation. For example, patients with anemia have two available modes of compensation: enhanced blood flow and decreased oxygen affinity, mediated by increased levels of 2,3-BPG. Conversely, individuals with a hemoglobin variant having increased oxygen affinity have a primary defect in oxygen unloading. As discussed in Chap. 306, such patients compensate by developing secondary erythrocytosis.

RED BLOOD CELL METABOLISM As the red cell emerges from the bone marrow, it loses its nucleus, ribosomes, and mitochondria and therefore all capability for cell division, protein synthesis, and oxidative phosphorylation. Compared with other cells, the erythrocyte has a rather simple scheme of intermediary metabolism. Glucose is virtually the only fuel utilized by the red cell. It readily enters the red cell by facilitated diffusion and is then converted to glucose-6-phosphate. There are two major pathways available for glucose-6-phosphate (see Fig. 307-2). About 80 to 90 percent of this intermediate is converted to lactate by means of the glycolytic (or Embden-Meyerhof) pathway. Two moles of adenosine triphosphate (ATP) are generated for every mole of glucose metabolized. The intracellular mediator of hemoglobin function, 2,3-bisphosphoglycerate, is synthe-

sized in a side reaction shown in Fig. 307-2. About 10 percent of intracellular glucose-6-phosphate undergoes oxidation by means of the hexose-monophosphate shunt. This pathway maintains glutathione in the reduced form, thereby protecting sulfhydryl groups in hemoglobin and the red cell membrane from oxidation by peroxides and superoxide as well as by certain drugs and toxins. Such oxidant stress can compromise red cell function and viability in patients with a deficiency in glucose-6-phosphate dehydrogenase, the first enzymatic step in the hexose-monophosphate shunt (see Chap. 307). Much less commonly, individuals may have a deficiency in one of the enzymes of the glycolytic pathway or in one of the other enzymes of the hexose-monophosphate shunt.

The red cell has rather modest metabolic obligations in keeping with its simplified structure. A significant portion of the ATP generated by glycolysis is spent in driving the sodium-potassium pump necessary to preserve the ionic milieu in the cytoplasm and prevent colloid osmotic lysis. In addition, some metabolic energy is expended on maintenance and repair of the red cell membrane. Certain proteins in the membrane become phosphorylated by means of ATP and protein kinases, but the physiologic significance of this process is not yet understood. Finally, a small amount of metabolic currency is spent on maintaining hemoglobin iron atoms in the reduced form (Fe^{2+}).

The 120-day survival of the circulating red cell is dependent on preservation of the pliability of its membrane. The red cell membrane is composed of 50 percent protein, 40 percent lipid, and 10 percent carbohydrate. It is a bilayer consisting of molecules of phospholipid and cholesterol in a 1.2:1 molar ratio assembled in a stacked array so that the hydrophobic portions of the molecules are oriented toward the interior while the polar side groups are either on the external surface of the cell (the plasma membrane) or on the inner cytoplasmic surface (Fig. 302-6). The distribution of phospholipids differs significantly in the two portions of the bilayer. The outer surface is relatively rich in lecithin and sphingomyelin, while the inner surface has relatively more phosphatidyl serine and phosphatidyl ethanolamine. The lipids on the outer surface exchange freely with plasma lipids.

The red cell membrane contains a limited number of major proteins depicted in Fig. 302-6 and a large number of minor components. These proteins can be divided into two groups. Among those that span the lipid bilayer are glycophorin, which contains a number of

FIGURE 302-6 Diagram of a cross section of the red blood cell membrane. Spectrin, actin, tropomyosin, and protein 4.1 form a meshwork which laminates the inner surface of the membrane. In contrast, other proteins such as the glycophorins (GP) and protein 3 (the anion transport channel) traverse the lipid bilayer. Long polysaccharide chains are covalently attached to these proteins on the outer surface of the cell and also to glycolipid. Ankyrin and

protein 4.2 form a bridge between spectrin and a fraction of the anion transport proteins. Protein 4.1 binds to GP. Phospholipids in the lipid bilayer include phosphatidylcholine (PC) and sphingomyelin (SM), which are located primarily on the outer surface of the membrane, and phosphatidyl serine (PS) and phosphatidyl ethanolamine (PE), which are located primarily on the inner surface of the membrane.

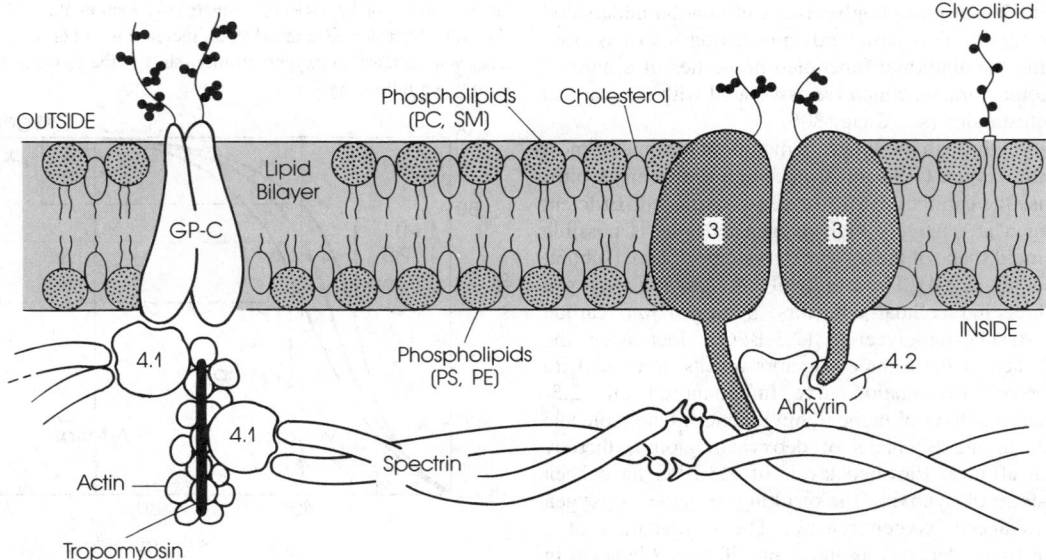

polysaccharide blood group antigens, and band 3, which serves as a channel for the passage of anions in and out of the red cell. Other proteins bind only to the inner surface of the red cell membrane. These include structural proteins such as spectrin and actin, which interact to form a meshwork that laminates the cytoplasmic surface of the membrane.

It is likely that the physiologic demise of 120-day-old red cells is due to a loss of membrane flexibility, preventing them from negotiating the narrow-bore channels of the microcirculation, including the sinusoids of the spleen. The factors responsible for red cell senescence are poorly understood. Experimental evidence indicates that deterioration of the red cell's metabolic machinery sufficient to deplete it of ATP can cause the cell to become spiculated (echinocytic) and lose its normal pliability. Depletion of ATP disrupts the spectrin and actin meshwork lining the inner membrane surface, resulting in aggregation of these proteins. Other factors such as coating with immunoglobulin also may contribute to the recognition of the senescent red cell by the mononuclear phagocyte system. In contrast to normal red cells, there is a large and well-documented body of information on the mechanisms responsible for red cell destruction in various hemolytic anemias. These are discussed in Chap. 307.

Once the senescent red cell is sequestered (see Fig. 302-2), hemoglobin is readily catabolized. Amino acids are released by proteolytic digestion and subsequently reutilized or metabolized. The heme group is catabolized by a microsomal oxidizing system. The porphyrin ring is converted to bile pigments which are excreted almost quantitatively by the liver. One mole of carbon monoxide is formed per mole of heme broken down. Endogenous carbon monoxide production correlates directly with erythroid cell destruction. As Fig. 302-2 shows, the iron released during heme catabolism is initially incorporated into the storage protein ferritin, but it is eventually transported to marrow erythroid precursors by transferrin, the plasma iron–binding protein.

If red cell production is disordered, there may be significant destruction of erythroid cells within the bone marrow. A number of anemias are characterized by *ineffective erythropoiesis*, particularly those in which erythroid maturation is morphologically abnormal and the circulating red cells are abnormal in size. Examples discussed in detail elsewhere include megaloblastic anemias, sideroblastic anemias, and β thalassemia major. Such disorders are characterized by erythroid hyperplasia in the bone marrow and rapid uptake of labeled iron into the marrow but a low recovery of the labeled iron in circulating red cells. Endogenous carbon monoxide production and plasma levels of unconjugated bilirubin are generally elevated in ineffective erythropoiesis.

REFERENCES

BABIOR BM, STOSSEL TP: *Hematology: A Pathophysiological Approach*, 2d ed. New York, Churchill Livingston, 1990

BECK WS (ed): *Hematology*, 5th ed. Boston, MIT Press, 1991

BUNN HF, FORGET BG: *Hemoglobin: Molecular, Genetic and Clinical Aspects*. Philadelphia, Saunders, 1986

JANDL JH: *Blood Pathophysiology*. Boston, Blackwell, 1991

JELKMANN W: Erythropoietin: Structure, control of production and function. Physiol Rev 72:449, 1992

PALEK J (ed): Cellular and molecular biology of the red cell membrane proteins in health and disease. Semin Hematol 29:229-239, 1992

303   ANEMIAS WITH DISTURBED IRON METABOLISM

KENNETH R. BRIDGES / H. FRANKLIN BUNN

Iron is involved in a broad repertoire of biochemical reactions, making it essential to all life. When complexed with porphyrin, iron forms heme, the prosthetic group for many proteins such as hemoglobin, where it binds oxygen reversibly, and cytochromes, where it is vital to oxidation-reduction reactions. Since the inorganic form of the element is highly toxic, specific processes have evolved for the assimilation, transport, and storage of iron. Under normal circumstances, iron homeostasis is precisely maintained, but it can go awry in a variety of clinical settings, leading either to iron deficiency or iron overload.

PHYSIOLOGY OF IRON

IRON ABSORPTION   Iron absorption occurs predominantly in the duodenum and upper jejunum. Inorganic iron salts exist in either of two valence states, Fe^{2+} (ferrous) or Fe^{3+} (ferric). Most dietary iron consists of ferric salts, which form insoluble ferric oxyhydroxide complexes that precipitate at physiologic pH. Absorption is aided by gastric acidity, which maintains ferric iron in a soluble form. Normally, about 10 percent of the 10 to 20 mg of iron ingested per day in an average diet is absorbed by a poorly characterized mechanism. Heme is much more readily absorbed than inorganic iron. Unfortunately, a dearth of meat in the diets of many people throughout the world limits the availability of this excellent iron source.

The absorption of inorganic iron is greatly influenced by dietary compounds that may chelate the element. Citrate and ascorbate, for example, increase iron absorption by forming soluble complexes which readily enter the epithelial cells lining the upper gastrointestinal tract. Other compounds such as tannins, which are found in teas, plant phytates, and phosphates, form very tight complexes with iron and significantly inhibit absorption. The metabolic machinery involved in iron absorption is shared with several heavy metals, including lead, cadmium, and strontium. Increased iron absorption, as occurs, for instance, in iron deficiency, enhances the uptake of these elements.

TRANSPORT AND STORAGE   Despite intense scrutiny, the precise mechanism by which iron is translocated across the epithelial barrier in the intestine is unknown. Once this task is accomplished, however, the element is coupled to transferrin, an 80-kDa serum glycoprotein that can bind two iron atoms and delivers iron to tissues throughout the body (Fig. 303-1). The aggregate binding sites of all the transferrin in the circulation comprise the total iron binding capacity (TIBC) of plasma. Normally, 20 to 45 percent of the iron binding sites of transferrin are filled. Specific receptors on the plasma membranes of cells recognize transferrin, leading to the internalization of the protein and the release of iron into the cell cytoplasm. As might be expected, erythroid precursor cells in the bone marrow, which have a high requirement for iron, have a correspondingly high density of transferrin receptors.

Excess iron is stored in the body as ferritin or hemosiderin. The iron in ferritin is enclosed within a protein shell, apoferritin, which can take up Fe^{2+} and oxidize it to Fe^{3+} that is deposited within the iron core. Iron stimulates the synthesis of apoferritin. With time, ferritin is engulfed by lysosomes and catabolized to hemosiderin, a nonspecific mixture of partially degraded protein, lipid, and iron. Iron enters and leaves the ferritin molecule in a metabolically controlled fashion, making it available for the normal physiologic functions of the cell. In contrast, the iron trapped in the hemosiderin meshwork returns to the metabolic mainstream of the cell in a slow and unregulated fashion. Small quantities of ferritin appear in serum.

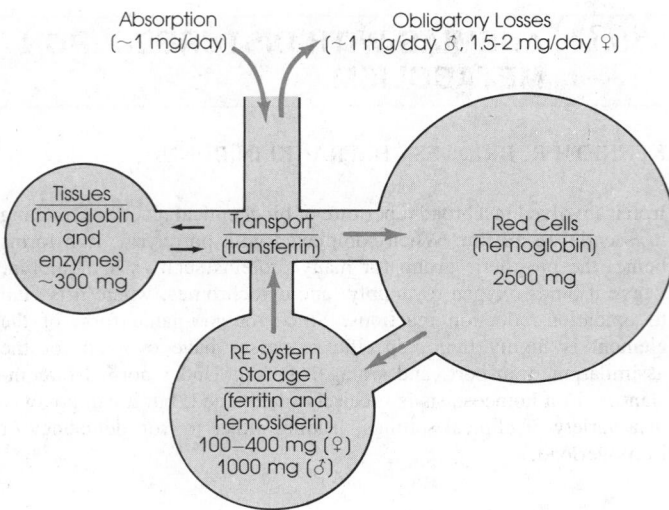

FIGURE 303-1 The distribution of iron in normal adults and internal iron kinetics. Bold arrows indicate major pathways of iron movement; RE = reticuloendothelial.

Normally, a close correlation exists between the serum ferritin concentration and body iron stores, with 1 μg/L serum ferritin equivalent to approximately 10 mg storage iron.

Body iron stores are assiduously conserved. In fact, no physiologic pathway of iron removal exists. About 1 mg of the element is lost daily from the shedding of senescent cells along the gastrointestinal and genitourinary tracts and from desquamation of skin (see Fig. 303-1). Menstruation results in the additional loss of about 1 mg/day of iron in women. Normally, these losses are closely balanced by daily absorption of about 10 percent of ingested iron. An increase in the demand for iron due to growth spurts, pregnancy, or pathologic hemorrhage can boost iron absorption to about 20 percent. Frank iron deficiency can increase the absorption of the element to between 30 and 40 percent of the amount ingested. With iron overload, absorption decreases.

Iron kinetics   Between 80 and 90 percent of absorbed iron is delivered to the bone marrow for erythropoiesis. The dynamics of iron utilization by the peripheral tissues can be monitored by loading plasma transferrin with the radioisotope ^{59}Fe and injecting the labeled protein back into the circulation. Such ferrokinetic studies reveal an exponential loss of label from the plasma, with a half-life of about 75 min. The plasma iron turnover (PIT) is the absolute amount of iron released from transferrin per unit of time and is determined largely by the rate of erythropoiesis. Effective erythropoiesis results in the incorporation of 80 to 90 percent of iron into hemoglobin in circulating erythrocytes. A small fraction of developing normoblasts are destroyed by marrow macrophages in a process termed *ineffective erythropoiesis*. The normoblasts are ineffective at the task of producing mature circulating erythrocytes. With some anemias, such as the thalassemias, the megaloblastic anemias, and sideroblastic anemia, this medullary destruction is markedly exaggerated. The result is a high PIT, reflecting the increase in erythropoietic activity, but a diminished incorporation of the labeled iron into circulating erythrocytes. When erythropoiesis is diminished because of marrow hypoplasia, the PIT is correspondingly reduced.

LABORATORY INVESTIGATION OF IRON STORES   **Direct assay**   This requires biopsy specimens. Most storage iron is found in the reticuloendothelial cells of the bone marrow, liver, and spleen or in hepatic parenchymal cells. The liver is a homogeneous tissue and therefore an excellent source by which to gauge iron stores. Prussian blue staining of liver biopsies, a commonly used technique, provides only a semiquantitative estimation of iron stores, whereas atomic absorption spectroscopy furnishes accurate quantitative data.

Formalin-fixed samples can be evaluated by this technique, allowing for transport and later testing. Liver biopsy with atomic absorption spectroscopic measurements is the touchstone for quantitative evaluation of iron overload. Bone marrow specimens are not reliable in the estimation of iron excess but are useful in the evaluation of iron deficiency. Because of the cellular heterogeneity of the marrow, histologic evaluation of iron deposits must focus on storage in macrophages. An absence of Prussian blue staining reliably indicates a deficiency in iron stores.

Indirect assay   The simplest indirect assay is the ratio of serum iron to TIBC (Fig. 303-2). Iron deficiency depresses serum iron levels and boosts the TIBC. Therefore, the transferrin is generally less than 10 percent saturated. Iron loading increases the serum iron with little effect on the TIBC, leading to greater than 70 percent saturation of transferrin. The iron-to-TIBC ratio must be viewed with the patient's total clinical picture in mind. For example, serum iron and transferrin levels are depressed by conditions such as inflammation, cancer, and liver disease, leading at times to skewed ratios. These variables are particularly difficult to interpret in the elderly and in hospitalized patients. For these individuals the plasma ferritin reflects body iron stores most reliably.

Ferritin in the circulation is a secretory form of the protein which is glycosylated and differs in subunit composition from the storage form found in cells. The physiologic function of serum ferritin is presently unknown. The protein normally contains very little iron. The concentration of serum ferritin rises with iron loading and declines with depletion of tissue iron stores. The serum ferritin level also increases with inflammation, cancer, and liver disease. In addition, the normal ranges for serum ferritin vary with age and sex. Therefore, corrections for these factors should be made when values on a specific patient are interpreted. Using bone marrow biopsy as an absolute measure of iron stores, patients with values below about 14 μg/L are almost invariably iron deficient.

In patients with iron deficiency, protoporphyrin IX accumulates in the red cell because there is insufficient iron to convert it to heme (Fig. 302-3, p. 1719). The fluorometric assay of free erythrocyte protoporphyrin (FEP) is a reliable and cost-effective way of screening large groups of individuals such as school children for iron deficiency. Elevation of FEP occurs in other conditions that disrupt porphyrin metabolism, such as lead poisoning, therapy with isoniazid, and sideroblastic anemia. Exclusion of these conditions markedly enhances the specificity for iron deficiency of a high FEP.

Computed tomography (CT) of the liver provides an excellent assessment of body iron stores, particularly in patients with iron overload. The iron content of liver biopsy samples correlates well with determination by dual-energy CT scanning. Another sensitive

FIGURE 303-2 Serum iron and total iron binding capacity in various disorders.

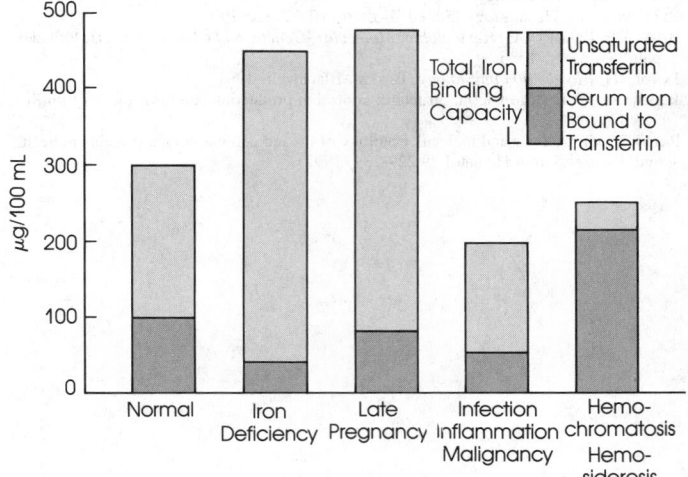

noninvasive technique for evaluating liver iron deposition is magnetic resonance imaging (MRI). Both instruments permit longitudinal evaluation and are valuable adjuncts in monitoring and treating patients with iron overload.

IRON-DEFICIENCY ANEMIA

ETIOLOGY Iron deficiency occurs when the rate of loss or utilization of the element exceeds its rate of assimilation. The stages of iron deficiency are shown in Table 303-1. Utilization is greatest during the rapid growth spurts of infancy and adolescence (Table 303-2). Depleted iron stores, if not frank anemia, are commonly seen in children in these two age groups. Neonates born to iron-deficient women are rarely anemic but do have low body iron stores. These infants lack the reserves needed for the swift growth that occurs after birth. Breast milk is a marginally adequate source of iron, whereas cow's milk has an even lower iron content. Iron deficiency during childhood has a number of deleterious consequences, including impaired cognition. Therefore, infants should receive iron supplementation.

In western countries, the increased demand for iron during adolescence is often accompanied by voluntary consumption of foods with low iron content. Among the elderly and the poor, financial constraints often produce a similar pattern of inadequate iron intake. Large numbers of people throughout the world have become inured to diets consisting of grains or cereals, which provide inadequate quantities of iron. The added burden of blood loss due to parasites such as hookworm makes iron deficiency a problem of staggering proportions.

Decreased absorption of iron This can occur in many clinical settings. After partial or total gastrectomy, the assimilation of dietary iron is impaired, owing primarily to increased motility and bypass of the proximal intestine, which is the primary site of iron absorption. Achlorhydria also contributes to decreased iron absorption. Patients with chronic diarrhea or intestinal malabsorption also can develop iron deficiency, particularly when the duodenum and proximal jejunum are involved. Sometimes iron-deficiency anemia is a harbinger of nontropical (celiac) sprue.

Iron loss This can be physiologic or pathologic. Examples of physiologic iron loss include menstruation and pregnancy. Menstrual blood loss doubles the daily iron requirement. With a term pregnancy, about 900 mg iron is lost by the mother to the fetus, the placenta, and to parturitional hemorrhage. Increased gastrointestinal absorption of the element by the mother compensates partially for these losses. In the absence of supplemental iron, however, the mother's stores will be depleted to meet the needs of the fetus. Currently, the vast majority of pregnant women who seek medical attention routinely receive prophylactic treatment with iron salts. Pregnant women who do not receive adequate antenatal care have a high incidence of clinically significant iron deficiency.

The gastrointestinal tract is most often responsible for pathologic blood loss and subsequent iron-deficiency anemia. The process is often insidious; the patient's presenting symptoms may be due solely

TABLE 303-2 Causes of iron deficiency

Increased iron utilization
  Postnatal growth spurt
  Adolescent growth spurt

Physiologic iron loss
  Menstruation
  Pregnancy

Pathologic iron loss
  Gastrointestinal bleeding
  Genitourinary bleeding
  Pulmonary hemosiderosis
  Intravascular hemolysis

Decreased iron intake
  Cereal-rich, meat-poor diets
  Pica
  Elderly and indigent
  Food faddists
  Malabsorption

to anemia. Common causes of chronic gastrointestinal blood loss include peptic ulcer disease, gastritis, hemorrhoids, angiodysplasia of the colon, and colonic adenocarcinoma. Salicylate ingestion often produces occult blood in the stool and occasionally causes significant blood loss. Gastrointestinal cancer is a specter haunting all patients with iron-deficiency anemia. Therefore, a complete gastrointestinal workup is necessary in men and postmenopausal women who are iron deficient. Stool guaiacs should be performed on six different occasions along with a digital rectal examination. Radiologic examination of the gastrointestinal tract, endoscopic procedures, or both are obligatory.

In about 15 percent of patients with documented gastrointestinal bleeding, no source is found, even after extensive radiologic and endoscopic investigation. In tropical areas, parasitic infestations, particularly hookworm, are a major cause of blood loss. Occasionally, as in patients with hereditary telangiectasia or in those with a bleeding diathesis, gastrointestinal bleeding arises from multiple sites. Thrombocytopenia, qualitative platelet disorders, and von Willebrand's disease are more apt to cause gastrointestinal bleeding than are deficiencies of the soluble coagulation factors.

Blood loss from other sources rarely produces iron-deficiency anemia. Bleeding in the genitourinary tract usually is sufficiently alarming that medical attention is sought early in the process. Intravascular hemolysis with hemoglobin loss in the urine, e.g., paroxysmal nocturnal hemoglobinuria, is very unusual. Pulmonary hemorrhage, secondary to bronchiectasis or idiopathic pulmonary hemosiderosis, also may cause iron-deficiency anemia.

CLINICAL CONSEQUENCES Iron deficiency impairs cell growth and proliferation. The production of red blood cells is in particular jeopardy owing to their high requirement for iron. Many symptoms of iron-deficiency anemia, including weakness, lassitude, palpitations, and sometimes exertional dyspnea, are common to all forms of chronic anemia. No definite link between these symptoms and tissue depletion of iron-dependent enzymes and cofactors has been established.

After the cells of the bone marrow, those of the gastrointestinal tract proliferate most actively. Consequently, many of the signs and symptoms of iron deficiency are localized to this organ system. Glossitis characterized by a reddened, swollen, smooth, shiny, and tender tongue occurs sporadically. Angular stomatitis involves erosion, tenderness, and swelling at the corners of the mouth. Gastric atrophy with achlorhydria occurs occasionally. A postcricoid web (Plummer-Vinson syndrome) may develop with long-standing iron deficiency. Koilonychia, or spoon-shaped nails, result from slowing in the rate of growth of the nail plate.

Menorrhagia is a common symptom in iron-deficient women. Both menorrhagia and gastric atrophy (mentioned above) may be a consequence as well as a cause of iron deficiency. In one study of

TABLE 303-1 Stages in the development of iron deficiency

	Normal	Mild	Moderate	Severe
Hemoglobin:	150 g/L	130 g/L	100 g/L	50 g/L
MCV	N	↓	↓	↓↓
MCHC	N	N	↓	↓↓
Marrow Fe stores	Present	Absent	Absent	Absent
Serum Fe/TIBC, μg/L	1000/3000	~750/3000	~500/4500	~250/6000

NOTE: MCV = mean corpuscular volume; MCHC = mean corpuscular hemoglobin concentration; TIBC = total iron-binding capacity; N = normal; ↓ = decreased.

600 female American blood donors, 13 percent were found to be iron deficient by FEP determinations. A recent evaluation of several thousand unselected women in Iceland revealed iron deficiency in 20 percent and iron-deficiency anemia in about 3 percent.

One peculiar symptom that is quite characteristic of iron deficiency is pica. Patients develop cravings for substances such as starch (amylophagia), ice (pagophagia), and clay (geophagia). Some of these materials, such as starch and clay, bind iron in the gastrointestinal tract, worsening the deficiency. The basis of this bizarre behavior is unknown.

A particularly invidious consequence of iron deficiency is increased intestinal absorption of lead. Children from impoverished families, who often have both iron deficiency and pica, are at greatest risk of developing lead poisoning. The toxicity of lead is due at least in part to a disruption of heme synthesis in neural tissues, a process abetted by iron deficiency. These unfortunate children are thereby placed in double jeopardy.

LABORATORY FINDINGS The development of iron deficiency progresses in stages (see Table 303-1), each of which correlates with clinical laboratory abnormalities. *Storage iron depletion* occurs first, during which iron reserves are lost without compromise of the iron supply for erythropoiesis. At this stage, a bone marrow aspirate stained with Prussian blue shows markedly reduced or absent deposits of iron in macrophages. This condition is accompanied by a decrease in the level of serum ferritin. The next stage is *iron-deficient erythropoiesis*, during which the erythroid iron supply is reduced without the development of anemia. The iron binding capacity of the serum (TIBC) first rises, followed by a drop in serum iron. As a result, the fractional saturation of transferrin falls markedly. The level of transferrin saturation that is necessary to support erythropoiesis is about 15 percent. Iron-deficient erythropoiesis is inevitable below this value. The circulating red cells become microcytic and hypochromic. This is accompanied by an increase in FEP. The final stage is the development of frank *iron-deficiency anemia*, wherein the red cells become more severely hypochromic and microcytic (Plate A9-4). Often only a thin rim of cytoplasm appears at the periphery of the red cell. Small fragments and bizarre poikilocytes are also seen. The membranes of these iron-deficient erythrocytes are stiff, and these misshapen red cells have shortened survival in the circulation. Although the percentage of reticulocytes is usually normal, the absolute reticulocyte count, usually about 50,000 cells per cubic milliliter, is low. The white count is usually normal, while the platelet count is normal or increased. The bone marrow displays moderate erythroid hyperplasia. Many of the late normoblasts have scanty cytoplasm.

Transferrin receptors are shed from the plasma membranes of cells and can be detected in the plasma. The major source of plasma transferrin receptors is the hematopoietic cells of the bone marrow. The quantity of transferrin receptors in the plasma rises in patients with iron deficiency, providing another possible diagnostic test for this condition.

DIFFERENTIAL DIAGNOSIS In a patient with hypochromic, microcytic anemia, the major diagnostic possibilities are iron deficiency, thalassemia, anemia of chronic inflammation, lead poisoning, and sideroblastic anemia. Several laboratory tests (Table 303-3) are useful in the differential diagnosis. Mild iron deficiency may be readily confused with β thalassemia trait or with the two-deletion forms of α thalassemia (α-/α- or --/$\alpha\alpha$) (see Chap. 322). In these mild forms of thalassemia, microcytosis is much more marked than hypochromia; accordingly, the mean corpuscular hemoglobin concentration (MCHC) is usually normal. The red cell size distribution is more uniform than that in iron deficiency. Target cells and basophilic stippling are usually more prominent in thalassemia than in iron deficiency. Hemoglobin A_2 is elevated in β thalassemia trait and decreased in iron deficiency and α thalassemia. If a patient with β thalassemia trait develops iron deficiency, the level of hemoglobin A_2 may fall to normal. The serum iron is normal or elevated in the thalassemias and decreased in both iron deficiency and the anemia of

TABLE 303-3 Differential diagnosis of microcytic, hypochromic anemia

	Iron-deficiency anemia	β Thalassemia trait	Anemia of chronic disease	Sideroblastic anemia
Serum iron	↓	N	↓	↑
TIBC	↑	N	↓	N
Serum ferritin	↓	N	↑	↑
Red cell protoprophyrin	↑	N	↑	↑ or N
Hb A₂	↓	↑	N	↓

NOTE: ↑ = increased; ↓ = decreased, N = normal; TIBC = total iron-binding capacity.

chronic disease. However, as Fig. 303-2 shows, the transferrin level is also decreased in the latter condition. The laboratory tests shown in Table 303-3 are not very helpful in determining whether a patient with a chronic inflammatory disease, such as rheumatoid arthritis, has become iron deficient. The finding of a low serum ferritin level or absent iron stores in a bone marrow aspirate would be diagnostic of iron deficiency in such patients. A trial of iron therapy may be necessary to settle the issue. The diagnosis of sideroblastic anemia rests on the demonstration of ringed sideroblasts in the bone marrow. These patients often have a population of hypochromic, microcytic red cells, even though the MCHC is usually normal.

THERAPY Iron deficiency responds very well to the administration of oral agents such as iron salts (e.g., ferrous sulfate) or iron polysaccharide preparations (e.g., ferric polymaltose). Ferrous sulfate, which contains 50 mg elemental iron per 325-mg tablet, should be administered three times daily. Iron is best absorbed when taken between meals. Unfortunately, abdominal discomfort, characterized by bloating, fullness, and occasional pain, occurs commonly with this iron preparation. Ferrous gluconate and ferrous lactate often are better tolerated, particularly when taken at mealtime. Polysaccharide iron complex frequently fares better than any iron salt, despite the fact that each tablet contains 150 mg elemental iron. Iron-containing vitamin cocktails generally should be avoided, since these preparations are costly and contain suboptimal amounts of iron.

A reticulocytosis commences 3 to 4 days after the initiation of iron therapy, with a peak at about 10 days. Patients may not respond to iron replacement as a result of (1) an incorrect diagnosis, (2) noncompliance, (3) blood loss exceeding the rate of replacement, (4) bone marrow suppression by tumor, chronic inflammation, etc., or (5) malabsorption. Malabsorption of iron is an infrequent problem, but when it occurs, it requires parenteral iron replacement. Iron-dextran complex may be administered as intramuscular injections following a 25-mg dose to test for allergic reactions. A total of 100 mg iron-dextran per treatment session can be given in this fashion. Administration is repeated weekly until iron stores are replete. A Z-tract should be used for the injections to prevent oozing of the compound into the dermis, which can produce intractable skin discoloration. Iron-dextran can be given intravenously to patients who cannot tolerate the intramuscular injections or who require more rapid correction of iron deficiency. The most convenient approach is to dilute 500 mg of the compound into 100 mL sterile saline and to infuse a test dose of 1 mL. If no adverse reaction is noted, the remainder of the solution can be delivered over 2 h. The intravenous administration of up to 4 g iron at a single sitting allows the correction of iron deficiency at a single session. About 20 percent of patients experience arthralgias, chills, and fever which are dose-dependent and may persist for several days after the infusion. Iron-dextran should be used sparingly, if at all, in patients with rheumatoid arthritis since these symptoms are markedly enhanced with this disease. Nonsteroidal anti-inflammatory agents usually control these symptoms. Anaphylaxis, a serious complication of the administration of iron-dextran, occurs rarely. Intravenous administration of iron-dextran allows better control of this problem, since symptoms occur immediately with the beginning of the test dose. The infusion can be stopped, and correction of the condition with benadryl and epinephrine can be started. The 25-mg test dose used for the intramuscular injection cannot be retrieved should anaphylaxis develop, however. The amount of iron required for replacement can be calculated from the deficit in the red cell mass, with an additional 1000 mg to replace the body stores. Blood transfusions are rarely necessary except for patients in whom severe iron-deficiency anemia threatens cardiovascular or cerebrovascular function.

ANEMIAS WITH SECONDARY IRON LOADING

Iron overload in individuals with chronic anemias may result either from multiple transfusions or increased gastrointestinal absorption of the element owing to ineffective erythropoiesis.

SIDEROBLASTIC ANEMIAS These comprise a group of disorders of diverse causes (Table 303-4) characterized by ringed sideroblasts in the nucleated erythroid precursors in the bone marrow. Greater than 10 percent of the normoblasts contain iron-laden mitochondria that surround the nucleus and appear as pathognomonic ''rings'' with Prussian blue staining. A number of metabolic abnormalities have been noted in the sideroblastic anemias, including defects in one or more of the steps in heme synthesis. Since the initial and final steps of heme synthesis are located in the mitochondrion (see Fig. 302-3), it is difficult to know whether such abnormalities are the cause or the result of iron loading. In addition to the presence of ringed sideroblasts, these disorders share certain other features: bone marrow erythroid hyperplasia with decreased red cell production (ineffective erythropoiesis); a population of hypochromic, microcytic red cells reflecting defective heme synthesis; and a marked increase in serum iron and transferrin saturation, sometimes accompanied by generalized iron overload.

Hereditary sideroblastic anemia is a rare X-linked disorder. Some cases have been associated with defective activity of δ-aminolevulinic acid synthetase, the initial and rate-limiting enzyme in heme biosynthesis. Affected males have anemia of variable severity that occasionally responds to treatment with large doses of pyridoxine.

Acquired sideroblastic anemias may be caused by a variety of insults, including ethanol and isoniazid, which disrupt heme metabolism, and lead, which inhibits several steps in the heme synthetic pathway (Table 303-4). Ringed sideroblasts are found in about 30 percent of patients hospitalized for alcohol abuse, particularly in the setting of coexistent folate deficiency and malnutrition. This morphologic abnormality disappears within several days following cessation of alcohol ingestion. Secondary sideroblastic anemia also has been observed in a variety of inflammatory and neoplastic states. A particularly intractable form of the disorder sometimes occurs following treatment of malignancy, especially multiple myeloma, with alkylating chemotherapeutic agents.

Most commonly, however, acquired sideroblastic anemia is idiopathic, appearing spontaneously in older individuals. Disturbed growth and maturation occur in all the lines that emanate from the hematopoietic stem cells. Chromosomal abnormalities involving bone marrow cells occur commonly. Neutropenia develops in a significant

---

TABLE 303-4 The sideroblastic anemias

Hereditary or congenital sideroblastic anemias
Acquired sideroblastic anemias
 Associated with drugs and toxins (e.g., alcohol, lead, isoniazid, chloramphenicol)
 Associated with neoplastic and inflammatory disease (e.g., carcinoma, leukemia, lymphoma, rheumatoid arthritis)
 Alkylating agent chemotherapy (e.g., cyclophosphamide)

---

number of patients, as does thrombocytopenia. Some individuals have normal numbers of platelets that are, however, dysfunctional. A bleeding diathesis often results. About 10 percent of individuals with sideroblastic anemia will develop a particularly intractable form of acute myelogenous leukemia. This proportion appears to be higher in cases arising from therapy with alkylating agents.

The treatment of secondary sideroblastic anemia focuses primarily on withdrawal of the offending agent. No specific treatment is presently available for idiopathic cases. Since pyridoxine is innocuous and inexpensive, all patients should receive a trial of the vitamin at 200 mg/d for 2 to 3 months, despite the low probability of response in the acquired disorder. Occasionally, an improvement in hematocrit occurs with androgen therapy. This therapy should be used cautiously in patients with liver disease, diabetes, or benign prostatic hypertrophy. Ongoing clinical trials are attempting to define the role of cytokines such as granulocyte-monocyte colony stimulating factor (GM-CSF), interleukin 3, and erythropoietin in the treatment of sideroblastic anemia. Supportive therapy, including blood transfusions, is indicated in all patients.

TRANSFUSIONAL HEMOCHROMATOSIS Repeated blood transfusion is the most common cause of iron overload in patients with anemia. One unit of blood contains 200 to 250 mg iron. Therefore, a patient who requires 3 units of blood per month will accumulate about 8 g iron over the course of a year, enough to cause early clinical sequelae of iron loading. In order for the consequences of iron loading to play a major clinical role, a requirement for chronic transfusions must be coupled with a relatively long survival. The disorders that fulfill these criteria at present include (1) thalassemia major, (2) myeloproliferative and myelodysplastic syndromes (including sideroblastic anemia), (3) pure red cell aplasia, and (4) aplastic anemia of moderate severity. Patients with chronic renal failure on dialysis once fell into this category. The recent introduction of cloned erythropoietin has largely obviated this problem for these individuals.

Transfusional iron overload produces a spectrum of problems similar to those seen with idiopathic hemochromatosis. Of these, the most serious result from myocardial and hepatic iron deposition. Cardiac siderosis leads to arrhythmias, conduction defects, and a restrictive cardiomyopathy. Echocardiography (Chap. 190) is useful in detecting early myocardial dysfunction. Iron deposition in the liver injures hepatocytes, leading to necrosis, fibrosis, and ultimately cirrhosis. Since hepatic iron deposition produces very little inflammation as fibrosis progresses, serum transaminase levels are usually only modestly elevated. Disturbed glucose metabolism occurs commonly, although an oral glucose tolerance test is sometimes needed to demonstrate the defect. Gonadal dysfunction and ACTH deficiency are much less frequent. Hyperpigmentation reflects increased melanin production due to dermal iron deposition. Fair-skinned patients whose melanocytes are incapable of boosting melanin production (and who tan poorly) show little or no hyperpigmentation. In the assessment of these patients, liver biopsy provides the greatest yield of information, since iron content as well as the pathologic state of the organ can be determined. Liver CT scanning and MRI are the most reliable noninvasive methods of estimating iron deposition. The iron/TIBC ratio and serum ferritin level are both elevated with transfusional hemochromatosis but do not accurately establish the degree of iron overload.

The only treatment presently available for transfusional hemochromatosis is chelation. Desferrioxamine is the only agent that has been extensively evaluated and shown to prevent or reverse the complications of iron overload. The drug must be given parenterally over a period of 12 to 16 h by subcutaneous infusion with a portable syringe pump. No safe and effective oral iron chelating agent has been devised. Oral ascorbic acid supplementation markedly enhances iron excretion in patients on desferrioxamine therapy. The vitamin increases the availability of storage iron to the chelator by slowing the degradation of ferritin to hemosiderin. Cardiac toxicity has occurred in patients with hemochromatosis who consumed excessive amounts of ascorbic acid, however. The generation of injurious free radicals by iron released from storage sites is the probable mechanism of this effect. Further investigation into the basis of cellular injury in patients with hemochromatosis treated with ascorbic acid is needed to clarify the possible therapeutic utility of this vitamin.

REFERENCES

BRIDGES KR: Transfusion hemochromatosis, in *Transfusion Medicine*, WH Churchill, S Kurtz (eds). Cambridge, Mass, Blackwell, 1988, p 129

BURNS ER et al: Clinical utility of serum tests for iron deficiency in hospitalized patients. Am J Clin Pathol 93:240, 1990

JANSEN BM et al: Screening with zinc protoporphyrin for iron deficiency in non-anemic female blood donors. Clin Chem 36:846, 1990

LANZKOWSKY P: Problems in diagnosis of iron deficiency anemia. Pediatr Ann 14:618, 1985

NATHAN DG (ed): Oral iron chelators. Semin Hematol 27:83, 1990

PIOMELLI S et al: Lead-induced abnormalities of porphyrin metabolism: The relationship with iron deficiency. Ann NY Acad Sci 514:278, 1987

SKIKNE BS et al: Serum transferrin receptor: A quantitative measure of tissue iron deficiency. Blood 75:1870, 1990

VANDERMOLEN L et al: Ringed sideroblasts in primary myelodysplasia: Leukemic propensity and prognostic factors. Arch Intern Med 148:653, 1988

YIP R, DALLMAN PR: Developmental changes in erythrocyte protoporphyrins: Roles of iron deficiency and lead toxicity. J Pediatr 104:710, 1984

304   MEGALOBLASTIC ANEMIAS

BERNARD M. BABIOR / H. FRANKLIN BUNN

The megaloblastic anemias are disorders caused by impaired DNA synthesis. Cells primarily affected are those having relatively rapid turnover, especially hematopoietic precursors and gastrointestinal epithelial cells. Cell division is sluggish, but cytoplasmic development progresses normally, so megaloblastic cells tend to be large, with an increased ratio of RNA to DNA. Megaloblastic erythroid cells tend to be destroyed in the marrow in excessive numbers, an abnormality termed *ineffective erythropoiesis* (Chaps. 56 and 302).

Most megaloblastic anemias are due to a deficiency of cobalamin (vitamin B_{12}) and/or folic acid. The various clinical entities associated with megaloblastic anemia are listed in Table 304-1. This classification is easier to comprehend if the physiologic and biochemical principles discussed below are kept in mind.

PHYSIOLOGIC CONSIDERATIONS

FOLIC ACID   Folic acid is the common name for pteroylmonoglutamic acid. It is synthesized by many different plants and bacteria. Fruits and vegetables constitute the primary dietary source of the vitamin. Some forms of dietary folic acid are labile and may be destroyed by cooking. The minimum daily requirement is normally about 50 μg, but this may be increased severalfold during periods of enhanced metabolic demand such as pregnancy.

The assimilation of adequate amounts of folic acid is dependent on the nature of the diet and its means of preparation. Folates in various foodstuffs are largely conjugated to polyglutamic acid. This highly polar side chain impairs the intestinal absorption of the vitamin. However, conjugases (γ-glutamyl carboxypeptidases) in the lumen of the gut convert polyglutamates to mono- and diglutamates, which are readily absorbed in the proximal jejunum.

There are binding proteins in plasma for folates, but their physiologic significance is unclear. Plasma folate is primarily in the form of N^5-methyltetrahydrofolate, a monoglutamate. N^5-Methyltetrahydrofolate is transported into cells by a carrier which is specific for the tetrahydro forms of the vitamin. Once in the cell, the N^5-

TABLE 304-1   Classification of the megaloblastic anemias

COBALAMIN DEFICIENCY

A Inadequate intake: vegetarians (rare)
B Malabsorption
  1 Inadequate production of intrinsic factor (IF)
    a Pernicious anemia
    b Gastrectomy
    c Congenital absence or functional abnormality of IF (rare)
  2 Disorders of terminal ileum
    a Tropical sprue
    b Nontropical sprue
    c Regional enteritis
    d Intestinal resection
    e Neoplasms and granulomatous disorders (rare)
    f Selective cobalamin malabsorption (Imerslund's syndrome) (rare)
  3 Competition for cobalamin
    a Fish tapeworm
    b Bacteria: blind loop syndrome
  4 Drugs: *p*-aminosalicylic acid, colchicine, neomycin
C Other
  1 Nitrous oxide
  2 Transcobalamin II deficiency (rare)

FOLIC ACID DEFICIENCY

A Inadequate intake: unbalanced diet (common in alcoholics, teenagers, some infants)
B Increased requirements
  1 Pregnancy
  2 Infancy
  3 Malignancy
  4 Increased hematopoiesis (chronic hemolytic anemias)
  5 Chronic exfoliative skin disorders
  6 Hemodialysis
C Malabsorption
  1 Tropical sprue
  2 Nontropical sprue
  3 Drugs: Phenytoin, barbiturates, (?) ethanol
D Impaired metabolism
  1 Inhibitors of dihydrofolate reductase: methotrexate, pyrimethamine, triamterene, pentamidine, etc.
  2 Alcohol
  3 Rare enzyme deficiencies: dihydrofolate reductase, others

OTHER CAUSES

A Drugs which impair DNA metabolism
  1 Purine antagonists: 6-mercaptopurine, azathioprine, etc.
  2 Pyrimidine antagonists: 5-fluorouracil, cytosine arabinoside, etc.
  3 Others: procarbazine, hydroxyurea, acyclovir, zidovudine
B Metabolic disorders (rare)
  1 Hereditary orotic aciduria
  2 Others
C Megaloblastic anemia of unknown etiology
  1 Refractory megaloblastic anemia
  2 Di Guglielmo's syndrome*
  3 Congenital dyserythropoietic anemia

* A form of acute nonlymphocytic leukemia with atypical, dysplastic changes in erythroid series.

methyl group is removed in a cobalamin-requiring reaction (see below), and the folate is then reconverted to the polyglutamate form. The polyglutamate form may be useful for retention of folate by the cell.

Normal individuals have about 5 to 20 mg folic acid in various body stores, half in the liver. In light of the minimum daily requirement, it is not surprising that a deficiency will occur within months if dietary intake or intestinal absorption is curtailed.

COBALAMIN   This vitamin is a complex organometallic compound in which a cobalt atom is situated within a corrin ring, a structure similar to the porphyrin from which heme is formed (see Fig. 302-3). Unlike heme, however, cobalamin cannot be synthesized in the human body and must be supplied in the diet. The only dietary source of cobalamin is animal products: meat and dairy foods. The minimum daily requirement for cobalamin is about 2.5 μg.

During gastric digestion, cobalamin in food is released and forms a stable complex with gastric R binder, one of a group of closely related glycoproteins of unknown function which are found in secretions (e.g., saliva, milk, gastric juice, bile), phagocytes, and plasma. On entering the duodenum, the cobalamin–R binder complex is digested, releasing the cobalamin, which then binds to intrinsic factor (IF). This glycoprotein of molecular weight 50,000 is produced by the parietal cells of the stomach. The secretion of intrinsic factor generally parallels that of hydrochloric acid. The cobalamin-IF complex is resistant to proteolytic digestion and travels to the distal ileum, where specific receptors on the mucosal brush border bind the cobalamin-IF complex, thereby enabling the vitamin to be absorbed. Thus intrinsic factor, like transferrin (see Chap. 303), serves as a cell-directed carrier protein. The receptor-bound cobalamin-IF complex is taken into the ileal mucosal cell, where over the course of several hours the IF is destroyed and the cobalamin is transferred to another transport protein, transcobalamin II (TC II). The cobalamin–TC II complex is then secreted into the circulation, from which it is rapidly taken up by the liver, bone marrow, and other cells. The pathway of cobalamin absorption is shown in Fig. 304-1. Normally, about 2 mg cobalamin is stored in the liver, and another 2 mg is stored elsewhere in the body. In view of the minimum daily requirement, about 3 to 6 years would be required for a normal individual to become deficient in cobalamin if absorption were to cease abruptly.

Although TC II is the acceptor for newly absorbed cobalamin,

FIGURE 304-1 The assimilation of cobalamin. On entering the stomach, dietary cobalamin (Cbl) forms a complex with R binding protein. As this protein is digested, cobalamin is transferred to intrinsic factor (IF). This complex passes through the intestine until it reaches specific receptors on the mucosa of the distal ileum. The internalized Cbl is then transferred to transcobalamin II (TC II), which circulates in the plasma until it binds to receptors on cells throughout the body and is internalized.

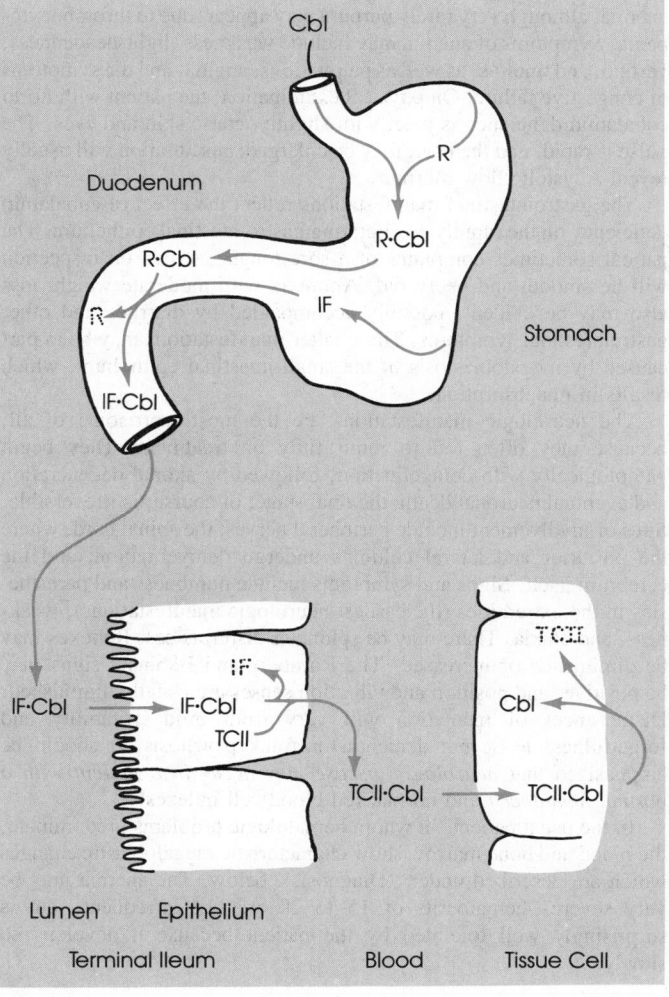

most circulating cobalamin is bound to transcobalamin I (TC I), a glycoprotein closely related to gastric R binder. TC I appears to be derived in part from leukocytes. The paradox that most circulating cobalamin is bound to TC I rather than TC II, even though TC II initially carries all the cobalamin that is absorbed by the intestine, is explained by the fact that cobalamin bound to TC II is rapidly cleared from the blood ($t_{1/2}$ about 1 h), while clearance of cobalamin bound to TC I requires many days. The function of TC I is unknown.

BIOCHEMICAL CONSIDERATIONS

FOLATE The *prime function* of this vitamin is to transfer 1-carbon moieties such as methyl and formyl groups to various organic compounds (see Fig. 304-2). The source of these 1-carbon moieties is usually serine, which reacts with tetrahydrofolate to produce glycine and $N^{5,10}$-methylenetetrahydrofolate. An alternative source is formiminoglutamic acid, an intermediate in histidine catabolism, which gives up its formimino group to tetrahydrofolate to yield N^5-formiminotetrahydrofolate and glutamic acid. These derivatives provide entry into an interconvertible donor pool consisting of tetrahydrofolate derivatives carrying various 1-carbon moieties (see Fig. 304-2). The constituents of this pool can donate their 1-carbon moieties to appropriate acceptor compounds to form metabolic intermediates which are ultimately converted to building blocks used in the synthesis of biologic macromolecules. The most important building blocks are (1) purines, in which the C-2 and C-8 atoms are introduced in folate-dependent reactions, (2) deoxythymidylate monophosphate (dTMP), synthesized from $N^{5,10}$-methylenetetrahydrofolate and deoxyuridylate monophosphate (dUMP), and (3) methionine, formed by the transfer of a methyl group from N^5-methyltetrahydrofolate to homocysteine. Cobalamin is also required for the formation of methionine from homocysteine (see below).

In all but one of the 1-carbon transfer reactions, tetrahydrofolate is produced. It can immediately accept a 1-carbon moiety and reenter the donor pool. The single exception is the thymidylate synthetase reaction (dUMP → dTMP), in which dihydrofolate is the product (Fig. 304-2). This must be reduced to tetrahydrofolate by the enzyme dihydrofolate reductase before it can reenter the donor pool. A number of drugs are able to inhibit dihydrofolate reductase, thereby diverting folate from the donor pool and producing what amounts to a state of folate deficiency in the face of normal tissue folate concentrations.

COBALAMIN In humans there are two metabolically active forms of cobalamin, identified by the alkyl group attached to the sixth coordination position of the cobalt atom: methylcobalamin and adenosylcobalamin. The vitamin preparation which is used therapeutically is cyanocobalamin (also called vitamin B_{12}). Cyanocobalamin

FIGURE 304-2 Scheme of folate metabolism.

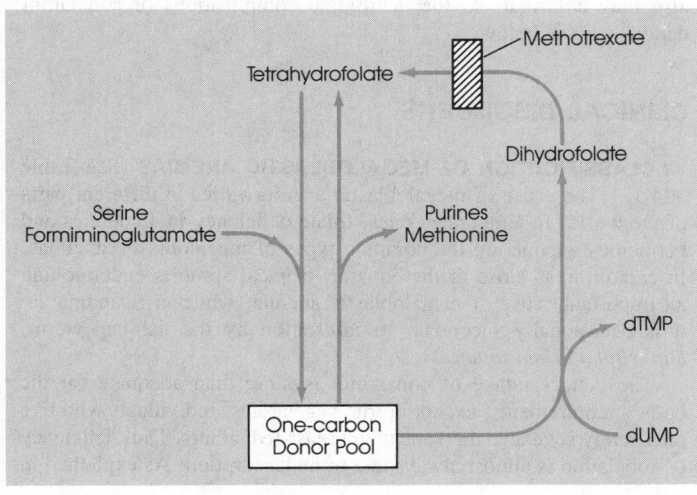

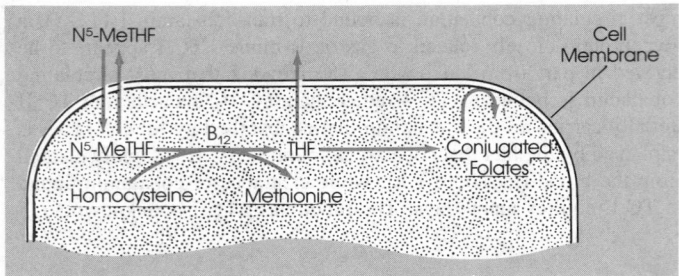

FIGURE 304-3 Diagram showing the interrelationship between cobalamin (methylcobalamin, B_{12}) and folate metabolism within the cell. N^5-MeTHF = N^5 methyltetrahydrofolate; THF = tetrahydrofolate.

has no known physiologic role and must be converted to a biologically active form before it can be used by tissues.

Methylcobalamin is an essential cofactor in the conversion of homocysteine to methionine (Fig. 304-3). When this reaction is impaired, folate metabolism is deranged, and it is this derangement which is thought to underlie the defect in DNA synthesis and the megaloblastic maturation pattern in patients who are deficient in cobalamin (see Fig. 304-3). In cobalamin deficiency, the unconjugated N^5-methyltetrahydrofolate newly taken from the bloodstream cannot be converted to other forms of tetrahydrofolate by methyl transfer. This is the so-called folate trap hypothesis. Since N^5-methyltetrahydrofolate is a poor substrate for the conjugating enzyme (this has been shown in rats and pigs but has not yet been demonstrated in humans), it largely remains in the unconjugated form and slowly leaks from the cell. Tissue folate deficiency therefore develops, and this results in megaloblastic hematopoiesis. This hypothesis explains why tissue folate stores in cobalamin deficiency are substantially reduced, with a disproportionate reduction in conjugated as compared with unconjugated folates, despite normal or supranormal serum folate levels. It also explains why large doses of folate can produce a partial hematologic remission in patients with cobalamin deficiency.

Impairment in the conversion of homocysteine to methionine also may be partly responsible for the neurologic complications of cobalamin deficiency (see below). The methionine formed in this reaction is needed for the production of choline and choline-containing phospholipids. Nervous system damage is postulated to result at least in part from interference with these processes due to decreased methionine production in cobalamin deficiency.

Adenosylcobalamin is required for the conversion of methylmalonyl coenzyme A (CoA) to succinyl CoA. Lack of this cofactor leads to large increases in the tissue levels of methylmalonyl CoA and its precursor, propionyl CoA. As a consequence, nonphysiologic fatty acids containing an odd number of carbon atoms are synthesized and incorporated into neuronal lipids. This biochemical abnormality also may contribute to the neurologic complications of cobalamin deficiency (see below).

CLINICAL DISORDERS

CLASSIFICATION OF MEGALOBLASTIC ANEMIAS (See Table 304-1) The cause of megaloblastic anemia varies in different parts of the world. In temperate zones, folate deficiency in alcoholics and pernicious anemia are the common types of megaloblastic anemias. In certain areas close to the equator, tropical sprue is endemic and an important cause of megaloblastic anemia, while in Scandinavia, it is occasionally secondary to infestation by the fish tapeworm, *Diphyllobothrium latum*.

The dietary intake of cobalamin is more than adequate for the body's requirements, except in true vegetarians (individuals who live on a purely vegetable diet) and their breast-fed infants. Thus deficiency of cobalamin is almost always due to malabsorption. As explained in

the section above, the absorption of cobalamin depends on a specific binding protein produced in the stomach and uptake by a specific receptor in the mucosa of the distal ileum. Accordingly, several steps in this process can go awry and lead to malabsorption. In contrast, the dietary intake of folic acid is marginal in many parts of the world. Furthermore, since the body's stores of folate are relatively low, folic acid deficiency can arise rather suddenly during periods of decreased dietary intake or increased metabolic demand. Finally, folic acid deficiency may be due to malabsorption. Often two or more of these factors coexist in a given patient.

Combined deficiencies of cobalamin and folic acid are not uncommon. Patients with tropical sprue are often deficient in both vitamins. The biochemical lesion that results in megaloblastic maturation of bone marrow cells also causes structural and functional abnormalities of the rapidly proliferating epithelial cells of the intestinal mucosa. Thus severe deficiency of one vitamin can lead to malabsorption of the other. Furthermore, as discussed above, a deficiency of cobalamin causes a secondary reduction in cellular folic acid.

Finally, megaloblastic anemias may occasionally be induced by factors unrelated to a vitamin deficiency. Most such cases are caused by one or more of the many drugs which interfere with DNA synthesis. Less commonly, megaloblastic maturation is encountered in certain acquired defects of hematopoietic stem cells. Rarest of all are specific congenital enzyme deficiencies in which megaloblastic anemia is characteristically encountered.

COBALAMIN DEFICIENCY There are many conditions in which cobalamin deficiency may develop. Although each has its own characteristic manifestations, certain clinical features are common to all. These clinical features involve the blood, the gastrointestinal tract, and the nervous system.

The hematologic manifestations are almost entirely the result of anemia, although very rarely purpura may appear, due to thrombocytopenia. Symptoms of anemia may include weakness, light-headedness, vertigo, and tinnitus, as well as palpitations, angina, and the symptoms of congestive failure. On physical examination, the patient with florid cobalamin deficiency is pale, with slightly icteric skin and eyes. The pulse is rapid, and the heart may be enlarged; auscultation will usually reveal a systolic flow murmur.

The gastrointestinal manifestations reflect the effect of cobalamin deficiency on the rapidly proliferating gastrointestinal epithelium. The patient sometimes complains of a sore tongue, which on inspection will be smooth and beefy red. Anorexia with moderate weight loss also may be evident, possibly accompanied by diarrhea and other gastrointestinal symptoms. These latter manifestations may be in part caused by megaloblastosis of the small-intestinal epithelium, which results in malabsorption.

The neurologic manifestations are the most worrisome of all, because they often fail to remit fully on treatment. They begin pathologically with demyelination, followed by axonal degeneration and eventual neuronal death; the final stage, of course, is irreversible. Sites of involvement include peripheral nerves; the spinal cord, where the posterior and lateral columns undergo demyelination; and the cerebrum itself. Signs and symptoms include numbness and paresthesias in the extremities (the earliest neurologic manifestations), weakness, and ataxia. There may be sphincter disturbances. Reflexes may be diminished or increased. The Romberg and Babinski signs may be positive, and position and vibration senses are usually diminished. Disturbances of mentation will vary from mild irritability and forgetfulness to severe dementia or frank psychosis. It should be emphasized that *neurologic disease may occur in a patient with a normal hematocrit* and normal red blood cell indexes.

In the usual patient, in whom hematologic problems predominate, the blood and bone marrow show characteristic megaloblastic changes which are described under "Diagnosis" below. The anemia may be very severe—hematocrits of 15 to 20 are not infrequent—but is surprisingly well tolerated by the patient because it develops so slowly.

Pernicious anemia The most common cause of cobalamin deficiency in temperate climates is pernicious anemia, in which intrinsic factor secretion ceases owing to atrophy of the gastric mucosa. It is most frequently seen in individuals of northern European descent and African-Americans and is much less common in southern Europeans and Asians. Men and women are equally affected. It is a disease of the elderly, the average patient presenting near age 60; it is rare under age 30, although typical pernicious anemia can be seen in children under age 10 (juvenile pernicious anemia). Inherited conditions in which a histologically normal stomach secretes either an abnormal intrinsic factor or none at all will induce cobalamin deficiency in infancy or early childhood.

There is considerable evidence for immunologic abnormalities in pernicious anemia. The incidence of pernicious anemia is substantially increased in patients with other diseases thought to be of immunologic origin, including Graves' disease, myxedema, thyroiditis, idiopathic adrenocortical insufficiency, vitiligo, and hypoparathyroidism. Patients with pernicious anemia also have abnormal circulating antibodies related to their disease: 90 percent have antiparietal cell antibody, while 60 percent have anti-intrinsic factor antibody. Antiparietal cell antibody is also found in 50 percent of patients with gastric atrophy without pernicious anemia, as well as in 10 to 15 percent of an unselected patient population, but anti-intrinsic factor antibody is usually absent from these patients. Relatives of patients with pernicious anemia have an increased incidence of the disease, and even clinically unaffected relatives may have anti-intrinsic factor antibody in their serum. Finally, treatment with corticosteroids has been reported to reverse the disease both pathologically and clinically.

The destruction of parietal cells in pernicious anemia is thought to be mediated by complement-fixing antibodies against the parietal cell surface. The observation that pernicious anemia is unusually common in patients with agammaglobulinemia, however, suggests that the cellular immune system also may play a role in its pathogenesis.

Pathologically, the most characteristic finding in pernicious anemia is gastric atrophy affecting the acid- and pepsin-secreting portion of the stomach; the antrum is spared. Other pathologic changes are secondary to the deficiency of cobalamin; these include megaloblastoid alterations in the gastric and intestinal epithelium and the neurologic changes described above. The abnormalities in the gastric epithelium appear as cellular atypia in gastric cytology specimens, a finding which must be carefully distinguished from the cytologic abnormalities seen in gastric malignancy.

The *clinical manifestations* are primarily those of cobalamin deficiency, as described above. The disease is of insidious onset and progresses slowly. Laboratory examination will reveal hypergastrinemia and pentagastrin-fast achlorhydria as well as the hematologic and other laboratory abnormalities discussed below under "Diagnosis."

Through appropriate replacement therapy, patients with pernicious anemia should experience complete and lifelong correction of all abnormalities which are due to cobalamin deficiency, except to the extent that irreversible changes in the nervous system may have occurred prior to treatment. These patients, however, are unusually subject to gastric polyps and have about twice the normal incidence of cancer of the stomach. In view of the latter complication, patients should be followed with frequent stool guaiac examinations together with further diagnostic studies when indicated.

Postgastrectomy Following total gastrectomy or extensive damage to gastric mucosa as, for example, by ingestion of corrosive agents, megaloblastic anemia may develop because the source of intrinsic factor has been removed. In such patients, the absorption of orally administered cobalamin is impaired. Megaloblastic anemia also may follow partial gastrectomy, but the incidence is lower than after total gastrectomy, in which cobalamin malabsorption occurs in 100 percent of patients. The cause of cobalamin deficiency after partial gastrectomy may be intestinal overgrowth of bacteria, but it does not always respond to antibiotics.

Intestinal organisms Megaloblastic anemia may occur with intestinal stasis due to anatomic lesions (strictures, diverticula, anastomoses, "blind loops") or pseudoobstruction (diabetes mellitus, scleroderma, amyloid). This anemia is caused by colonization of the small intestine by large masses of bacteria which divert cobalamin from the host. Steatorrhea also may be seen under these circumstances, because bile salt metabolism is disturbed when the intestine is heavily colonized with bacteria. Hematologic responses have been observed after administration of oral antibiotics such as tetracycline and ampicillin.

Megaloblastic anemia is seen, in Scandinavia especially, in persons harboring the fish tapeworm, *D. latum*. The anemia has been attributed to competition by the worm for cobalamin. Destruction of the worm eliminates the problem.

Ileal abnormalities Cobalamin deficiency is commonly found in tropical sprue, while it is an unusual complication of nontropical sprue (gluten-sensitive enteropathy; see Chap. 254). Virtually any disorder which compromises the absorptive capacity of the distal ileum can result in cobalamin deficiency. Specific entities include regional enteritis, Whipple's disease, and tuberculosis. Segmental involvement of the distal ileum by disease can cause megaloblastic anemia without any other manifestations of intestinal malabsorption such as steatorrhea. Cobalamin malabsorption is also seen after ileal resection. The Zollinger-Ellison syndrome (intense gastric hyperacidity due to a gastrin-secreting tumor) may cause cobalamin malabsorption by acidifying the small intestine. This will retard the transfer of the vitamin from R binder to intrinsic factor and will impair the binding of the cobalamin-IF complex to the ileal receptors. Chronic pancreatitis also may cause cobalamin malabsorption by impairing the transfer of the vitamin from R binder to intrinsic factor. This abnormality can be detected by tests of cobalamin absorption (see below, Schilling test), but it is invariably mild and never causes clinical cobalamin deficiency. Finally, there is a rare congenital disorder, Imerslund-Gräsbeck disease, in which a selective defect in cobalamin absorption is accompanied by proteinuria.

FOLIC ACID DEFICIENCY Patients with folic acid deficiency are more apt to be malnourished than those with cobalamin deficiency. Accordingly, they are likely to appear wasted. The gastrointestinal manifestations are similar to but may be more widespread and more severe than those of pernicious anemia. Diarrhea is often present, and cheilosis and glossitis are also encountered. However, in contrast to cobalamin deficiency, neurologic abnormalities do not occur.

The hematologic manifestations of folic acid deficiency are the same as those of cobalamin deficiency. Folic acid deficiency can generally be attributed to one or more of the following factors: inadequate intake, increased demand, and malabsorption.

Inadequate intake Folic acid malnutrition is commonly encountered among a number of groups. Alcoholics frequently become folate deficient because their main source of caloric intake is alcoholic beverages. Distilled spirits are virtually devoid of folic acid, while beer and wine do not contain enough of the vitamin to satisfy the daily requirement. In addition, alcohol may interfere with folate metabolism. Narcotic addicts are also prone to become folate deficient because of malnutrition. Many indigent and elderly individuals who subsist primarily on canned foods or "tea and toast" and occasional teenagers whose diet consists of "junk food" develop folate deficiency.

Increased demand Tissues with a relatively high rate of cell division such as the bone marrow or gut mucosa have a large requirement for folate. Therefore, patients with chronic hemolytic anemias or other causes of very active erythropoiesis may become deficient if their high folate requirement is not met by dietary intake. Likewise, a pregnant woman may become deficient in folic acid because of the high demand of the developing fetus. Deficiency in pregnancy can cause neural tube defects in newborns. Folate deficiency also may occur during the growth spurts of infancy and adolescence. Patients on chronic hemodialysis may require supplementary folate to replace that lost in the dialysate.

Malabsorption Folic acid deficiency is a common accompaniment of tropical sprue. Both the gastrointestinal symptoms and malabsorption are improved by the administration of either folic acid or antibiotics by mouth. Patients with nontropical sprue (gluten-sensitive enteropathy) also may develop significant folic acid deficiency which parallels other parameters of malabsorption. Similarly, folate deficiency in alcoholics may be due in part to malabsorption. In addition, other primary small-bowel disorders are sometimes associated with vitamin deficiency. These entities are all discussed in Chap. 254.

DRUGS Next to deficiency of folate or cobalamin, the most common cause of megaloblastic anemia is drug ingestion. Drugs which cause megaloblastic anemia do so by interfering with DNA synthesis, either directly or by antagonizing the action of folate. They can be classified as follows:

1 *Direct inhibitors of DNA synthesis.* The drugs in this category are used in the treatment of malignancy. Their efficacy depends on their ability to impair DNA synthesis. They include purine analogues (6-thioguanine, azathioprine, 6-mercaptopurine), pyrimidine analogues (5-fluorouracil, cytosine arabinoside), and other drugs which interfere with DNA synthesis by a variety of mechanisms (hydroxyurea, procarbazine).

   The antiviral agent zidovudine (AZT), used for treating the human immunodeficiency virus (HIV), often causes severe megaloblastic anemia, a problem also seen with acyclovir, which is used to treat herpes infections.
2 *Folate antagonists.* The most toxic of these is methotrexate, an exceedingly powerful inhibitor of dihydrofolate reductase which is used in the treatment of certain malignancies. Much less toxic but still capable of inducing a megaloblastic anemia are several weak dihydrofolate reductase inhibitors that are used to treat a variety of nonmalignant conditions. These include pentamidine, trimethoprim, triamterene, and pyrimethamine.

   The megaloblastic changes in methotrexate poisoning appear to result from a buildup of dUMP owing to impaired methylation to dTMP. The excess dUMP is partially phosphorylated to dUTP, which accumulates in the cell and is incorporated into newly synthesized DNA. As a result, defective strands of DNA are produced in which T is partly replaced by U.
3 *Nitrous oxide.* Nitrous oxide inhalation causes the destruction of endogenous cobalamin. As ordinarily used, this anesthetic does not destroy enough cobalamin to cause clinical manifestations. Repeated or protracted exposure, however, may lead to a megaloblastic anemia. Fatal megaloblastic anemia has been reported in patients with tetanus who were given nitrous oxide continuously for weeks.
4 *Others.* A number of drugs antagonize folate by mechanisms which are poorly understood but are thought to involve an effect on absorption of the vitamin by the intestine. In this category are the anticonvulsants phenytoin (Dilantin) and primidone (Mysoline) and phenobarbital (Luminal). Megaloblastic anemia induced by these agents is mild.

ACUTE MEGALOBLASTIC ANEMIA Occasionally, a full-blown megaloblastic state can develop over the course of just a few days. This is usually seen following nitrous oxide anesthesia but may occur in any patient with a serious illness requiring intensive care, especially a patient receiving multiple transfusions, dialysis, or total parenteral nutrition. An acute megaloblastic state also can be precipitated by the administration of a weak antifolate (e.g., trimethoprim) to a patient with marginal tissue folate stores.

The condition resembles an immune cytopenia, with a rapidly developing thrombocytopenia and/or leukopenia in the absence of anemia. The blood smear may be completely normal, but the marrow is always floridly megaloblastic. Acute megaloblastic anemia responds rapidly to treatment with folate plus cobalamin in the usual therapeutic doses.

OTHER Hereditary Megaloblastic anemia may be seen in several hereditary disorders. It is a regular feature of orotic aciduria, a deficiency of orotidylic decarboxylase and phosphorylase, leading to a defect in pyrimidine metabolism and characterized by retarded growth and development as well as by the excretion of large amounts of orotic acid. Megaloblastic anemia has been reported in a single case of the Lesch-Nyhan syndrome, a condition resulting from a deficiency of hypoxanthine-guanine phosphoribosyltransferase whose clinical manifestations include gout, mental retardation, and self-mutilation. It also has been described in methylmalonic aciduria due to a combined defect in the biosynthesis of methyl and adenosyl cobalamins, although it is not seen in methylmalonic aciduria due to methylmalonyl CoA mutase deficiency. Congenital folate malabsorption causes megaloblastic anemia, accompanied by ataxia and mental retardation. Megaloblastic anemia has been reported to accompany the congenital deficiency of two other folate-metabolizing enzymes: dihydrofolate reductase and N^5-methyltetrahydrofolate:homocysteine methyltransferase. These deficiencies are less well documented than is congenital folate malabsorption. A thiamine-responsive megaloblastic anemia accompanied by nerve deafness and diabetes mellitus has been reported in several children. Megaloblastic changes as well as multinuclearity of red blood cell precursors are seen in the marrow of certain patients with congenital dyserythropoietic anemia, a group of inherited disorders characterized by mild to moderate anemia presenting at any age and pursuing a benign course.

Transcobalamin II deficiency, like the congenital abnormalities in cobalamin absorption described previously, causes pronounced deficiency in cobalamin in infancy or early childhood, with all the accompanying manifestations. Megaloblastic anemia is not seen in hereditary transcobalamin I deficiency.

Refractory megaloblastic anemia This is a form of myelodysplasia in which megaloblastic erythropoiesis may sometimes be seen. Megaloblastic changes are restricted to the red blood cell series; large granulocyte precursors and giant metamyelocytes are not seen (see below). Like other forms of myelodysplasia, acquired sideroblastic anemia is associated with an increased incidence of acute leukemia.

Megaloblastic changes are seen in erythremic myelosis and acute erythroleukemia (di Guglielmo), where red blood cell precursors are prominently involved. Here, the marrow is characterized by bizarre erythroid maturation, with multinuclearity and multipolar mitotic figures in the red blood cell precursors. Erythremic myelosis is discussed further in Chap. 310.

DIAGNOSIS The finding of significant macrocytosis [mean corpuscular volume (MCV) > 100 fL] suggests the presence of a megaloblastic anemia. Other causes of macrocytosis include hemolysis, liver disease, alcoholism, hypothyroidism, and aplastic anemia. If the macrocytosis is marked (MCV > 110 fL), the patient is much more likely to have a megaloblastic anemia. Macrocytosis is less marked with concurrent iron deficiency or thalassemia. The reticulocyte count is low, and the leukocyte and platelet count also may be decreased, particularly in severely anemic patients. The blood smear (Fig. A9-2) demonstrates marked anisocytosis and poikilocytosis, together with macroovalocytes, which are large, oval, fully hemoglobinized erythrocytes typical of megaloblastic anemias. There is some basophilic stippling, and an occasional nucleated red blood cell may be seen. In the white blood cell series, the neutrophils show hypersegmentation of the nucleus. This is such a characteristic finding that a single cell with a nucleus of six lobes or more should raise the immediate suspicion of a megaloblastic anemia. A rare myelocyte also may be seen. Bizarre, misshapen platelets are also observed. The bone marrow examination is very helpful in the diagnosis of megaloblastic anemia. The marrow is hypercellular with a decreased myeloid/erythroid ratio and abundant stainable iron. Red blood cell precursors are abnormally large and have nuclei that appear much less mature than would be expected from the development of the cytoplasm (nuclear-cytoplasmic asynchrony). The nuclear chromatin is more dispersed than it should be and consequently stains less intensely than normal. To the extent that it is aggregated, it condenses in a peculiar fenestrated pattern which is very characteristic of megaloblastic erythropoiesis. Abnormal mitoses may be seen. Granulocyte precursors are also affected, many being larger than normal, including giant bands and metamyelocytes. Megakaryocytes are decreased and show abnormal morphology.

Megaloblastic anemias are characterized by ineffective erythropoiesis (Chap. 302). In a severely megaloblastic patient, as many as 90 percent of the red blood cell precursors may be destroyed before they are released into the bloodstream, compared with 10 to 15 percent in the normal subject. Enhanced intramedullary destruction of erythroblasts results in an increase in unconjugated bilirubin and lactic acid dehydrogenase (isoenzyme 1) in plasma. Abnormalities in iron kinetics also attest to the presence of ineffective erythropoiesis, with increased iron turnover but low incorporation of labeled iron into circulating red blood cells.

In evaluating a patient with megaloblastic anemia, it is important to determine whether there is a specific vitamin deficiency by measuring serum cobalamin and folate levels. The normal range of cobalamin in serum is 200 to 900 pg/mL; values less than 100 pg/mL indicate clinically significant deficiency. The normal serum concentration of folic acid ranges from 6 to 20 ng/mL; values of 4 ng/mL or less are generally considered to be diagnostic of folate deficiency. Unlike serum cobalamin, serum folate levels may reflect recent alterations in dietary intake. Measurement of red blood cell folate level occasionally provides useful information, since it is not subject to short-term fluctuations in folate intake and is, therefore, a better index of tissue folate stores than serum folate.

Once cobalamin deficiency has been established, its pathogenesis can be delineated by means of a Schilling test. A patient is given radioactive cobalamin by mouth, followed shortly thereafter by an intramuscular injection of unlabeled cobalamin. The proportion of the administered radioactivity excreted in the urine during the next 24 h provides an accurate measure of absorption of cobalamin, assuming that a complete urine sample has been collected. Since cobalamin deficiency is almost always due to malabsorption (see Table 304-1), this first stage of the Schilling test should be abnormal. The patient is then given labeled cobalamin bound to intrinsic factor. Absorption of the vitamin will now approach normal if the patient has pernicious anemia or some other type of intrinsic factor deficiency. If cobalamin absorption is still decreased, the patient may have bacterial overgrowth ("blind loop" syndrome) or ileal disease (including an ileal absorptive defect secondary to the cobalamin deficiency itself). Cobalamin malabsorption due to bacterial overgrowth can frequently be corrected by the administration of antibiotics. The Schilling test can provide equally reliable information after the patient has had adequate therapy with parenteral cobalamin.

Low serum cobalamin levels occur in some patients who are hematologically normal and have normal Schilling tests. Many of these patients absorb cobalamin poorly when the vitamin is mixed with food. Other patients show normal serum cobalamin levels but elevated levels of serum methylmalonic acid, a metabolic marker of cobalamin deficiency. Both these groups of patients are generally considered to have mild or "subtle" cobalamin deficiency. Poorly defined neuropsychiatric abnormalities occur in many of these patients, and it has been suggested that these abnormalities may be due to the patients' cobalamin-deficient state. Whether this is so remains to be conclusively demonstrated, but until the question is settled, the safest course is to treat these patients with cobalamin.

TREATMENT

COBALAMIN DEFICIENCY Apart from specific therapy related to the underlying disorder (e.g., antibiotics for intestinal overgrowth with bacteria), the mainstay of treatment for cobalamin deficiency is replacement therapy. Since the defect is one of absorption, replacement should be administered parenterally, specifically in the form of intramuscular cyanocobalamin. (If intramuscular administration is contraindicated or refused, cobalamin deficiency can be managed by oral replacement therapy, but at doses of 300 to 1000 μg daily, it is an expensive mode of treatment which requires very close medical supervision to avoid relapse.) Treatment should be started with 100 μg cobalamin per day for a week. The frequency of administration of the vitamin may then be decreased, the goal being to give a total of 2000 μg during the first 6 weeks. The patient may then be placed on 100 μg cyanocobalamin intramuscularly every month, a regimen that must be maintained for the rest of the patient's life. If necessary, larger doses may be given at less frequent intervals (e.g., 1 mg every 2 to 4 months), but the risk of relapse is substantially greater than if the vitamin is given monthly.

The response to treatment is gratifying. Shortly after treatment is begun, and several days before a hematologic response is evident in the peripheral blood, the patient will experience an increase in strength and an improved sense of well-being. Marrow morphology begins to revert toward normal within a few hours after treatment is initiated. Reticulocytosis begins 4 to 5 days after therapy is started and peaks at about day 7 (Fig. 304-4), with subsequent remission of the anemia over the next several weeks. If a reticulocytosis does not occur, or if it is less brisk than expected from the level of the hematocrit, a search should be made for other factors contributing to the anemia (e.g., infection, coexisting folate deficiency, or hypothyroidism). Hypokalemia and salt retention may occur early in the course of therapy.

In most cases, replacement therapy is all that is needed for the treatment of cobalamin deficiency. Occasionally, however, a patient with a severe anemia will have such a precarious cardiovascular status that emergency transfusion is necessary. This must be done with great care, since it is very easy to precipitate florid congestive failure in such patients by fluid overload. Blood must be administered slowly in the form of packed cells, with very close observation, giving as an initial dose no more than 100 mL. This small volume will frequently be enough to ameliorate the cardiovascular problems sufficiently that further therapy can be restricted to cobalamin replacement. If necessary, blood may be administered by exchanging patient blood (mostly plasma) for packed cells.

With lifelong treatment, patients should experience no further manifestations of cobalamin deficiency. As previously stated, neurologic symptoms may not be fully corrected even by optimal therapy. The potential for late development of gastric carcinoma in pernicious anemia necessitates careful follow-up of the patient.

FOLATE DEFICIENCY Like cobalamin deficiency, folate deficiency is treated by replacement therapy. The usual dose of folate is 1 mg/d, by mouth, but higher doses (up to 5 mg/d) may be required

FIGURE 304-4 Hematologic response of a patient with pernicious anemia to an intramuscular injection of 100 μg cobalamin on day 0. (*From A Erslev, TG Gabuzda, Pathophysiology of Blood, Philadelphia, Saunders, 1975.*)

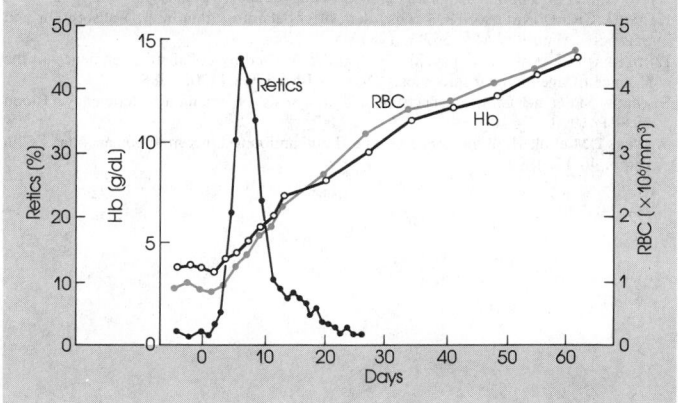

for folate deficiency due to malabsorption. Parenteral folate is rarely necessary. The hematologic response is similar to that seen after replacement therapy for cobalamin deficiency—that is, a brisk reticulocytosis after about 4 days, followed by correction of the anemia over the next 1 to 2 months. The duration of therapy depends on the basis of the deficiency state. Patients with a continuously increased requirement (such as patients with hemolytic anemia) or those with malabsorption or chronic malnutrition should continue to receive oral folic acid indefinitely. In addition, the patient should be encouraged to maintain an optimal diet containing adequate amounts of folate.

Folate, particularly in large doses, can correct the megaloblastic anemia of cobalamin deficiency without altering the neurologic abnormalities. The neurologic manifestations may even be aggravated by folate therapy. Cobalamin deficiency can thus be masked in patients who for one reason or another are taking large doses of folate. For this reason, a hematologic response to folate must never be used to rule out cobalamin deficiency in a given patient; cobalamin deficiency can be excluded only by appropriate laboratory evaluation.

OTHER CAUSES OF MEGALOBLASTIC ANEMIA   Megaloblastic anemia due to drugs can be treated, if necessary, by reducing the dose of the drug or eliminating it altogether. The effects of folate antagonists which inhibit dihydrofolate reductase can be counteracted by folinic acid (citrovorum factor) in a dose of 100 to 200 mg/d. Since folinic acid is a derivative of tetrahydrofolate, it circumvents the block in folate metabolism imposed by dihydrofolate reductase inhibitors, replenishing the tissues with a form of folate which can directly enter the 1-carbon donor pool. Certain of the congenital megaloblastic anemia–producing enzyme deficiencies can be treated by appropriate specific therapeutic regimens. For the megaloblastic forms of sideroblastic anemia, pyridoxine in pharmacologic doses (as high as 300 mg/d) should be tried. A few patients will respond to this therapy. Simple supportive measures are all that appear to be in order for treatment of refractory megaloblastic anemia. Acute erythroleukemia (di Guglielmo's disease) is usually treated like other types of acute nonlymphocytic leukemia (see Chap. 310).

REFERENCES

BABIOR BM: The megaloblastic anemias, in *Hematology*, 4th ed, WJ Williams et al (eds). New York, McGraw-Hill, 1990

BECK WS: Diagnosis of megaloblastic anemia, in *Annual Review of Medicine, 1991*, WP Creger (ed). Stanford, Calif, Annual Reviews, Inc., 1991

———: Neuropsychiatric consequences of cobalamin deficiency. Adv Intern Med 36:33, 1991

BORCH K: Epidemiologic, clinicopathologic, and economic aspects of gastroscopic screening of patients with pernicious anemia. Scand J Gastroenterol 21:21, 1986

CHANARIN I et al: Cobalamin and folate: Recent developments. J Clin Pathol 45:227, 1992

COOPER BA, ROSENBLATT DS: Inherited defects of vitamin B_{12} metabolism. Annu Rev Nutr 7:291, 1987

HERBERT V: Don't ignore low serum cobalamin (vitamin B_{12}) levels. Arch Intern Med 148:1705, 1988

———: Nutritional anemias in the elderly, in *Nutrition and Aging*, DM Prinsley et al (eds). New York, Alan R. Liss, 1990

HSING AW et al: Pernicious anemia and subsequent cancer. Cancer 71:745, 1993

KAPADIA CR, DONALDSON RM: Disorders of cobalamin (vitamin B_{12}) absorption and transport. Annu Rev Med 36:93, 1985

LINDENBAUM J et al: Neuropsychiatric disorders caused by cobalamin deficiency in the absence of anemia or macrocytosis. N Engl J Med 318:1720, 1988

STABLER SP et al: Clinical spectrum and diagnosis of cobalamin deficiency. Blood 75:871, 1990

WATERS HM et al: High incidence of type II autoantibodies in pernicious anemia. J Clin Pathol 46:45, 1993

305   ANEMIA ASSOCIATED WITH CHRONIC DISORDERS

H. FRANKLIN BUNN

Among the most commonly encountered anemias are those which accompany a variety of chronic underlying diseases. They can be corrected only if the primary condition is reversible. As shown in Table 305-1, these anemias can be subdivided into several groups.

ANEMIA OF CHRONIC INFLAMMATION

CLINICAL FEATURES   Patients who have a chronic systemic inflammatory disorder persisting more than a month usually develop a mild or moderate anemia. The extent of the anemia is roughly proportional to the duration and severity of the inflammatory process. These disorders include chronic infections such as subacute infective endocarditis, osteomyelitis, lung abscess, tuberculosis, and pyelonephritis. Noninfectious inflammatory disorders often associated with chronic anemia include rheumatoid arthritis, systemic lupus erythematosus, vasculitides (such as temporal arteritis), sarcoidosis, regional enteritis, and tissue injury such as fracture.

This kind of anemia is also commonly encountered in neoplastic disorders, including Hodgkin's disease and a variety of solid tumors such as carcinoma of the lung and breast. Other factors may contribute to the development of more severe anemia in cancer patients. In those with gastrointestinal or uterine cancer, blood loss can be the predominant factor. Chronic bleeding will lead to iron deficiency. Furthermore, cancer patients may develop progressive anemia if the bone marrow is invaded with tumor cells. Myelophthisic anemia is discussed in Chap. 308. Cancer patients are often malnourished and may be deficient in folate. Rarely, patients with disseminated malignancy develop severe traumatic hemolytic anemia (Chap. 307). Finally, suppression of hematopoiesis by chemotherapeutic agents or radiation therapy may aggravate anemia.

HEMATOLOGIC FEATURES   Hemoglobin values generally range between 90 and 110 g/L. A hemoglobin level less than 80 g/L indicates the presence of one or more of the aggravating factors mentioned above. Although this group of anemias is generally classified as normocytic, normochromic, red blood cells are often slightly microcytic. The mean corpuscular hemoglobin concentration is about 320 g/L (normal $\cong$ 340 g/L). Examination of the bone marrow reveals normal erythroid maturation. However, the red blood cell precursors have less stainable iron than normal (i.e., fewer sideroblasts), while the macrophages in the marrow usually contain increased amounts of iron. Myeloid hyperplasia and an increase in plasma cells are often seen in chronic infections.

The corrected reticulocyte count is low. Careful measurement of red blood cell survival generally reveals moderately shortened erythrocyte life span. Cross-transfusion studies point to an extracorpuscular mechanism, probably hyperplasia of the mononuclear phagocyte system. There is seldom any other evidence of significant hemolysis. However, in certain chronic infections such as subacute

TABLE 305-1   Anemias secondary to chronic systemic diseases

1 Anemia of chronic inflammation
  a Infection
  b Connective tissue disorders, etc.
  c Malignancy
2 Anemia of uremia
3 Anemia due to endocrine failure
4 Anemia of liver disease

infective endocarditis and miliary tuberculosis, splenomegaly can contribute to further shortening of the red blood cell life span, thereby increasing the severity of the anemia. In this setting, spherocytes are often seen on the blood smear.

Serum iron is characteristically subnormal in this group of anemias, but in contrast to iron deficiency, the total transferrin level is also reduced (see Fig. 303-2). The fractional saturation of transferrin is lower than normal. The serum iron level falls within hours or days following the onset of the inflammation, whereas several weeks elapse before the transferrin level falls. Serum ferritin is increased in patients with inflammatory disorders. Certain other plasma proteins are characteristically elevated in chronic inflammation, probably under the stimulus of interleukin 1 (IL-1) and tumor necrosis factor, cytokines released by activated macrophages. These "phase reactants" include gamma globulin, the third component of complement, haptoglobin, α_1-antitrypsin, orosomucoid, and fibrinogen. The latter is usually not measured, since protein electrophoresis is routinely done on serum rather than plasma. Elevation of these proteins is responsible for the increased rate of red blood cell sedimentation which is so commonly observed.

It is often difficult to detect iron deficiency in a patient with chronic inflammation. The serum iron level is low, and red blood cell protoporphyrin is increased in both conditions. When iron deficiency is superimposed on a chronic inflammatory state, the serum ferritin level falls to less than 60 μg/L. The serum transferrin level rises, usually to within normal limits. Under such circumstances, the amount of storage iron in the bone marrow is unpredictable. This problem is commonly encountered in patients with rheumatoid arthritis who may have developed iron deficiency owing to gastrointestinal blood loss. Because of this diagnostic uncertainty, it is often prudent to give such a patient a trial of iron and ascertain whether the hemoglobin level increases. However, it is important to avoid prolonged administration of iron unless a true deficiency state persists.

PATHOGENESIS The anemia of chronic inflammation is primarily due to defective red blood cell production and failure to compensate for the slightly decreased red blood cell life span. The subnormal amounts of iron in erythroblasts, despite an abundance of storage iron, suggest a defect in the transfer of iron to the developing erythroid cells. It is likely that inflammatory cytokines, such as IL-1, induce increased translation of ferritin in macrophages, thereby trapping iron and hindering release to transferrin. The cells that are formed are somewhat "iron deficient" and therefore tend to be small and pale. As in true iron deficiency, increased red blood cell protoporphyrin reflects the reduced availability of iron for heme synthesis. This block in iron utilization can be measured by iron kinetic studies. If radioactive iron bound to transferrin is administered, there is normal uptake into erythroblasts and incorporation into circulating red cells. In contrast, if hemoglobin labeled with radioactive iron is injected, the incorporation of label into circulating red cells is only half normal. The hyperplastic mononuclear phagocyte system which is responsible for decreased survival of circulating red cells probably traps the hemoglobin iron and prevents its transfer to the bone marrow. The macrophages' increased avidity for iron may be due to one of the actions of IL-1, i.e., release of lactoferrin from neutrophils. The iron binding protein lactoferrin captures free iron and rapidly transfers it to macrophages.

The modest suppression of red blood cell production is caused in part by decreased availability of iron. In addition, erythropoietin levels tend to be lower than expected for the degree of anemia. However, erythropoietin levels are not as low as in the anemia of renal failure (see below) and probably do not play a significant role in the pathogenesis of the anemia.

MANAGEMENT The anemia of chronic inflammation is not responsive to hematinic agents such as iron, folic acid, or vitamin B_{12}. Since the anemia is seldom severe, blood transfusion is rarely indicated. Efforts should be directed toward correcting the underlying disorder. In addition, if the anemia is more severe than expected, it is essential to search for other factors such as blood loss or drug-induced myelosuppression that could contribute to the reduction of red blood cell mass. While erythropoietin therapy can increase the hematocrit, the improvement is modest and by itself does little to improve the patient's functional state.

ANEMIA OF UREMIA

Anemia almost always accompanies the uremic syndrome (Chap. 237). Although the hemoglobin level is highly variable among uremic patients, the severity of the anemia is roughly proportional to the degree of azotemia. The cause of the renal failure usually has little bearing on the extent of anemia. However, for any level of serum creatinine, patients with polycystic disease tend to be less anemic than those with other types of renal disease. In contrast to anemias associated with other chronic disorders discussed in this chapter, the anemia of uremia can be very severe, with hemoglobin levels as low as 40 g/L. However, patients often tolerate such marked anemia fairly well. This is largely due to compensatory adjustments such as redistribution of blood flow and a decrease in the oxygen affinity of the blood (see Chap. 302).

The anemia of uremia is normochromic and normocytic. Examination of the bone marrow seldom reveals any abnormalities. Red blood cell morphology is usually normal. In about one-third of patients, so-called burr cells are seen in the peripheral blood smear. These red blood cells have a characteristic evenly scalloped border (see Fig. A9-9). Neither the degree of anemia nor the red blood cell life span is influenced by the presence of burr cells. In most patients the corrected reticulocyte count is low, and the red blood cell survival is only modestly decreased. Thus the low red blood cell mass is due to decreased red blood cell production. The primary basis for this defect is that the diseased kidneys are unable to secrete adequate amounts of erythropoietin. Plasma erythropoietin levels are much lower than those of nonuremic patients with a comparable degree of anemia. Erythropoietin production is further impaired but not abolished in patients who have undergone bilateral nephrectomy. In addition, erythropoiesis may be somewhat suppressed by the accumulation of substances that are normally cleared by the kidneys. Iron kinetic measurements reveal impaired incorporation of iron into circulating red blood cells. Thus it is likely that the anemia is due in part to ineffective erythropoiesis (see Chap. 302). Improvement in the rate of utilization of iron by the bone marrow has been noted following hemodialysis.

A small minority of uremic patients, particularly those with advanced disease, have brisk hemolysis. Red blood cell survival studies indicate that the hemolysis is extracorpuscular. Either metabolic or mechanical factors may contribute to the hemolysis. Some patients may acquire a defect in the hexose monophosphate shunt which renders the red blood cell vulnerable to the formation of Heinz bodies (see Chap. 307). The hemolysis can be aggravated by oxidant drugs or oxidant compounds such as chloramine in the dialysis bath. If the renal failure is due to thrombotic thrombocytopenic purpura or hemolytic-uremic syndrome, patients will have a severe form of microangiopathic hemolytic anemia, with characteristic abnormalities of red blood cell morphology (see Chap. 307).

In some patients, aluminum salts that contaminate the tap water used in hemodialysis cause a worsening of anemia and the emergence of microcytosis and hypochromia.

Treatment of the anemia of uremia should focus on an attempt to reverse the renal failure. Red cell production may be modestly improved following hemodialysis. A prompt and dramatic correction of the anemia follows successful renal transplantation. Occasionally, polycythemia may be encountered following the renal engraftment and may be a harbinger of impending rejection.

The development of recombinant human erythropoietin has enabled definitive treatment of the anemia of uremia. Administration of this genetically engineered product either by intravenous infusion or by subcutaneous injection results in correction of anemia and gratifying symptomatic improvement. The agent is identical in structure to native erythropoietin and therefore safe and virtually free of side effects. However, overtreatment should be avoided, since it can aggravate hypertension and increase the likelihood of thromboses. Accordingly, sufficient recombinant erythropoietin should be given to maintain the patient's hematocrit between 0.32 and 0.37.

It is important to be aware of other factors that may aggravate the anemia of renal disease. Uremic patients have a propensity to hemorrhage, owing to a qualitative defect in platelet function. Thus gastrointestinal blood loss is commonly encountered. Furthermore, a small but significant amount of blood loss occurs during hemodialysis. For these reasons, some uremic patients become iron deficient. Folic acid deficiency also may occur owing to the poor nutrition of many patients or to the loss of this vitamin during dialysis.

ANEMIA SECONDARY TO ENDOCRINE FAILURE

A number of hormones, including thyroxine, glucocorticoids, testosterone, and growth hormone, are known to affect proliferation of human erythroid cells in vitro. Therefore, it is not surprising that a mild to moderate normochromic, normocytic anemia generally accompanies a number of endocrine deficiency states, including hypothyroidism, Addison's disease, hypogonadism, and panhypopituitarism. It is possible that the anemias associated with hypothyroidism and hypopituitarism are related to the decreased need for oxygen transport, since oxygen consumption is reduced when thyroid hormone or growth hormone is lacking.

The anemia of *myxedema* is usually normocytic. Red blood cell life span is normal, and erythropoiesis is effective. A minority of patients have macrocytic red blood cells which can usually be attributed to either folic acid or B_{12} deficiency. Patients with myxedema have an increased incidence of pernicious anemia. Hypothyroid patients, particularly females with menorrhagia, often develop iron deficiency and a microcytic anemia. Because the plasma volume may be reduced along with the red blood cell mass, the anemia of hypothyroidism may be masked. Since the signs and symptoms of myxedema are sometimes elusive, this diagnosis should be considered in the evaluation of any patient with unexplained anemia.

The anemia of *Addison's disease* is also masked by a decrease in plasma volume. Untreated patients have an average hemoglobin level of about 130 g/L. Upon hormone replacement, the plasma volume is rapidly reconstituted, and the hemoglobin level falls to 80 percent of its pretreatment value. With continued therapy, the red blood cell mass returns to normal.

Testosterone has a physiologic influence on red blood cell mass. During passage through adolescence, the mean hemoglobin level of males increases from 130 to 150 g/L. Eunuchoid males generally have a mean hemoglobin level averaging 130 g/L. Pituitary dysfunction or ablation is associated with a mild normochromic, normocytic anemia as well as occasional leukopenia.

The anemias secondary to endocrine failure are all readily corrected when adequate hormone replacement is given.

ANEMIA OF LIVER DISEASE

Patients with chronic liver disease, regardless of etiology, usually have a mild to moderate anemia which is normocytic or slightly macrocytic. An increased plasma volume may artificially lower the hematocrit and make the anemia seem worse than it is. Red blood cell morphology is normal, except for the presence of target cells (see Fig. A9-3) and occasional stomatocytes, which have increased membrane surface area owing to increased deposits of cholesterol and phospholipid. The bone marrow is usually normal. Erythropoiesis fails to compensate for a moderate shortening of red blood cell life span. The anemia persists as long as hepatic function is defective, but it may be corrected if normal hepatic function can be restored.

The situation is much more complex in patients with *alcoholic liver disease*. Many factors can contribute to the development of anemia. Alcohol is a direct suppressor of erythropoiesis. In alcoholics who have continued to drink up to the time of clinical evaluation, the bone marrow often reveals vacuoles in the cytoplasm of red and white blood cell precursors. In addition, ringed sideroblasts may be observed, particularly in patients who are malnourished. In alcoholics there is often suboptimal intake of dietary folic acid and impairment of folate utilization. Furthermore, anemia in alcoholics is commonly compounded by significant hemorrhage from gastritis, esophageal varices, or duodenal ulcer. The risk of gastrointestinal blood loss is further increased by the presence of thrombocytopenia or deficiencies in soluble clotting factors. Although alcoholics usually have increased iron stores, they may become iron deficient after prolonged gastrointestinal bleeding. Rarely, patients with alcoholic cirrhosis develop a severe hemolytic anemia accompanied by the appearance of rigid red blood cells with irregular borders called *acanthocytes*, or "spur" cells (see Fig. A9-8) (Chap. 307). In addition, alcoholics may acquire a defect in the erythrocyte hexose monophosphate shunt, similar to that encountered in patients with uremia.

REFERENCES

BUDMAN DR, STEINBERG AD: Hematologic aspects of systemic lupus erythematosus. Ann Intern Med 86:220, 1977
ESCHBACH JW, ADAMSON J: Anemia of end-stage renal disease. Kidney Int 28:1, 1985
——— et al: Correction of the anemia of end-stage renal disease with recombinant human erythropoietin. N Engl J Med 316:73, 1987
MEANS RT, KRANTZ SB: Progress in understanding the pathogenesis of the anemia of chronic disease. Blood 80:1639, 1992
MOWAT AG: Hematologic abnormalities in rheumatoid arthritis. Semin Arthritis Rheum 1:195, 1972
SAVAGE D, LINDENBAUM J: Anemia in alcoholics. Medicine 65:322, 1986
SEARS DA: Anemia of chronic disease. Med Clin North Am 76:567, 1992

306   DISORDERS OF HEMOGLOBIN

H. FRANKLIN BUNN

In 1910, Herrick wrote of a medical student from Jamaica who had a hemolytic anemia in conjunction with elongated, "sickled" red blood cells. Subsequently, sickle cell disease was shown to associate with an electrophoretically abnormal hemoglobin (designated Hb S) which differed from normal Hb A by the substitution of valine for glutamic acid at the sixth position of the β chain. Since then, over 500 structurally different human hemoglobin variants have been discovered in widely scattered parts of the world. Generally, a new hemoglobin is named after the place where it is first encountered. No more than a third of these mutant hemoglobins are associated with significant clinical manifestations. The remainder have been discovered by serendipity or as a result of large population surveys.

This chapter focuses on the clinically significant hemoglobin variants. In addition, disorders of the biosynthesis of globin (the thalassemias) and methemoglobinemia are discussed.

GENETIC CONSIDERATIONS The synthesis of each of the subunits of hemoglobin (α, β, γ, δ, ε, ζ) is governed by separate genes. The ε and ζ subunits are found only in embryonic hemoglobin. Normal individuals inherit two β-chain genes (one from each parent), four α-chain genes, and four γ-chain genes. The ε-, γ-, δ-, and β-chain genes occupy adjacent loci on chromosome 11 (see Fig. 306-1). The ζ and α genes are located on chromosome 16. The structure and function of normal hemoglobin ($\alpha_2\beta_2$) are discussed in Chap. 302. The inheritance of abnormal hemoglobins follows classic mendelian genetics. If both parents are heterozygous for a hemoglobin variant

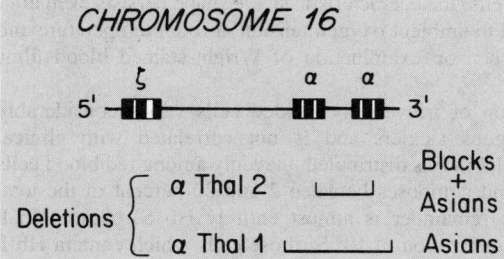

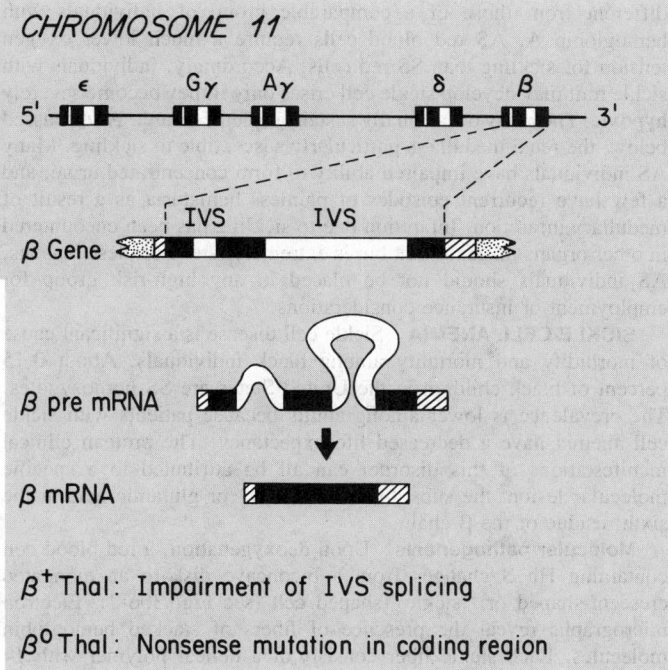

FIGURE 306-1 Diagram of human globin genes. (*Left*) The α-globin gene complex includes the embryonic ζ gene as well as two α genes. In the vast majority of individuals with α thalassemia 2 (α−) one α gene is deleted owing to a nonhomologous crossover between adjacent α genes. In α thalassemia 1 (− −) both α genes are deleted. (*Right*) The β-globin gene complex includes the embryonic ε gene, two fetal genes (^Gγ and ^Aγ), the δ gene, and the β gene. Below is a diagram of the β gene showing the coding regions (■), the intervening segments (IVS), (□), and the flanking regions (▨) that are transcribed into mRNA below. Most cases of β⁺ thalassemia in Mediterranean individuals involve a base substitution causing partial impairment of splicing of an IVS. Most cases of β⁰ thalassemia in Mediterraneans involve a base substitution that creates either a stop codon or a frame shift.

such as Hb S, statistically one-quarter of their offspring will be SS homozygotes, another quarter will be normal (AA genotype), and half will have sickle trait (AS). The commonly encountered hemoglobinopathies such as S, C, and E are β-chain variants. Occasionally, an individual inherits two different β-chain variants, one from each parent. Hemoglobin SC disease is an example of such a compound heterozygous state. Genes for β thalassemia are located on the β-chain structural gene. Accordingly, an individual can inherit from one parent (and pass on to a child) either β thalassemia or a β-chain variant, but not both. Among the hemoglobinopathies associated with sickling (described below), only the homozygous state (Hb SS) or double heterozygous state (Sβ thalassemia or SC) has important clinical manifestations. In contrast, the unstable variants and those having abnormal oxygen-binding properties are encountered only in heterozygotes. In some cases, the homozygous state would be incompatible with life.

About 90 percent of these abnormal hemoglobins are single amino acid replacements due to a single base substitution in the corresponding triplet codon. The structural information accumulated on human mutant hemoglobins has provided ample verification of the fidelity of the genetic code. Other genetic mechanisms must be invoked to explain the structure of a few interesting hemoglobin variants. The Lepore hemoglobins have arisen because of nonhomologous crossover between the adjacent δ- and β-chain genes, giving rise to a fusion subunit in which the *N*-terminal end has the amino acid sequence of the δ chain and the *C*-terminal end has the sequence of the β chain (see Fig. 306-1). Some of the unstable hemoglobins have deletions

of one or more residues in sequence within a subunit. Finally, there are a few variants which have elongated subunits (e.g., Hb Constant Spring). These have arisen either because of a base substitution in the termination codon or because of a frame shift which puts the termination codon out of phase.

CLINICAL CLASSIFICATION The clinically significant hemoglobin variants are classified in Table 306-1. By far the most important and prevalent type of hemoglobinopathy is due to the presence of sickle hemoglobin, either in the homozygous state or in conjunction with another type of hemoglobin abnormality. The inheritance of an unstable hemoglobin variant may give rise to congenital hemolytic anemia associated with the presence of inclusions of precipitated hemoglobin within the red blood cells (Heinz bodies). Finally, hemoglobin variants may have abnormal functional or spectral properties, resulting in familial erythrocytosis or familial cyanosis.

SICKLE SYNDROMES

SICKLE CELL TRAIT About 8 percent of black Americans are heterozygous for Hb S. The gene frequency is highest in central Africa, particularly in regions where malaria is endemic. In some parts of Nigeria, over 30 percent of the population has sickle trait. The gene has persisted because heterozygotes gain slight protection against falciparum malaria. This is an example of balanced polymorphism.

The diagnosis of sickle trait or any of the other sickle syndromes depends on the demonstration of sickling under reduced oxygen tension. In the widely used sickle preparation, sickled cells can be visualized microscopically after the addition of an oxygen-consuming reagent such as metabisulfite. Many clinical laboratories prefer a solubility test which depends on the fact that deoxyhemoglobin S has a low solubility at high ionic strength. These tests are reasonably specific for Hb S, although some of the unstable variants may give a false-positive solubility test. Therefore, if one of these screening tests is positive, hemoglobin electrophoresis should be performed. Individuals with sickle trait usually have about 35 to 40 percent Hb S and 55 to 60 percent Hb A.

Hemoglobin S heterozygotes have minimal clinical problems. Their overall life expectancy and frequency of hospitalization are no

---

TABLE 306-1 Clinically important hemoglobin variants

I **Sickle syndromes**
  A Sickle cell trait (AS)
  B Sickle cell anemia (SS)
  C Compound heterozygous states: sickle β thalassemia, sickle C disease (SC), sickle D disease (SD)
II **Unstable hemoglobin variants: congenital Heinz body hemolytic anemia**
III **Variants with high oxygen affinity: familial erythrocytosis**
IV **M hemoglobins: familial cyanosis (see Table 306-3)**

different from those of a comparable group of individuals with hemoglobin A. AS red blood cells require a much lower oxygen tension for sickling than SS red cells. Accordingly, individuals with sickle trait may develop sickle cell crises only if they become severely hypoxic. They may occasionally sustain a splenic infarct. As discussed below, the renal medulla is particularly susceptible to sickling. Many AS individuals have impaired ability to form concentrated urine, and a few have recurrent episodes of painless hematuria as a result of medullary infarction. Infarction due to sickling has been encountered in other organs in sickle trait but is extremely rare. For these reasons, AS individuals should not be placed in any high-risk group for employment or insurance considerations.

SICKLE CELL ANEMIA   Sickle cell disease is a significant cause of morbidity and mortality among black individuals. About 0.15 percent of black children in the United States are SS homozygotes. The prevalence is lower among adults because patients with sickle cell anemia have a decreased life expectancy. The protean clinical manifestations of this disorder can all be attributed to a specific molecular lesion: the substitution of valine for glutamic acid at the sixth residue of the β chain.

Molecular pathogenesis   Upon deoxygenation, a red blood cell containing Hb S changes from a biconcave disk to an elongated crescent-shaped or ''sickle''-shaped cell (see Fig. 306-2). Electron micrographs reveal the presence of fibers of stacked hemoglobin molecules. Each sickle fiber consists of a helical polymer with 14 strands. The polymer is stabilized by hydrophobic bonding between β6 valine and a complementary site on another portion of the β chain on an adjacent strand (Fig. 306-2). In addition, there are many other interactions between neighboring molecules. Sickling, both within the intact red blood cell and in free solution, is greatly affected by the presence of non-S hemoglobin. Hb A participates more readily than Hb F in copolymerization with Hb S.

Cellular pathogenesis   As discussed in Chap. 302, the ability of red blood cells to traverse the microcirculation depends in large part on their pliability. As sickle polymers are formed during deoxygenation, the red blood cell becomes rigid and, as a result, may obstruct capillary blood flow. The rate at which polymerization occurs depends primarily on the intracellular concentration of Hb S and the extent of deoxygenation. If polymerization occurs before the red cell escapes the narrow-bore capillary, obstruction may occur, resulting in local tissue hypoxia, further deoxygenation, and further sickling. This vicious cycle may result in the amplification of microscopic obstruction into a larger area of infarction. The oxygen-dependent sickle cycle is ordinarily reversible. However, the membrane of SS red blood cells may become sufficiently damaged that the cells lose potassium and water, leading to the formation of irreversibly sickled

forms. In these cells, the characteristic sickle shape persists even after they are exposed to ambient oxygen tension at room temperature and can readily be seen on examination of Wright-stained blood films (see Fig. A9-6).

The proportion of irreversibly sickled cells varies considerably among homozygous sicklers and is not correlated with clinical severity. Hemoglobin F is distributed unevenly among red blood cells of SS patients and composes between 2 and 20 percent of the total hemoglobin (the remainder is almost entirely Hb S). Since Hb F inhibits the polymerization of Hb S, those cells which contain Hb F are protected from sickling, whereas those cells which lack Hb F are at risk of becoming irreversibly sickled. It is not surprising that these rigid cells are readily culled from the circulation and destroyed. The continuous formation and destruction of irreversibly sickled cells contributes significantly to the severe hemolytic anemia shared by all patients with sickle cell anemia. Furthermore, these rigid cells may initiate small-vessel occlusions even if they lack sickle fibers.

Factors such as acidosis or increased erythrocyte 2,3-biphospho-glycerate, both of which lower the oxygen affinity of red blood cells, will enhance the formation of deoxyhemoglobin and, therefore, will promote intracellular polymerization and eventual sickling. In addition, sickling is highly dependent on hemoglobin concentration. Any pathophysiologic process which tends to pull water out of sickle red blood cells will greatly increase their tendency to sickle. Thus the hypertonic environment of the renal medulla can cause local sickling and the formation of papillary infarcts, even in individuals with sickle trait.

SS red blood cells have increased adherence to capillary endothelial cells. This interaction is likely to delay the transit time in the microcirculation, thereby increasing the extent of polymer formation.

Clinical manifestations   Patients with homozygous sickle cell anemia have a variety of clinical problems broadly outlined in Table 306-2. Signs and symptoms usually do not appear until after the sixth month of life, at which time most of the Hb F has been replaced by Hb S. Among the *constitutional* manifestations of sickle cell anemia are delay of growth and development. In addition, these patients have an increased tendency to develop serious infections, particularly due to pneumococcus. SS patients have marked impairment of splenic function, preventing effective clearance of circulating bacteria. With the passage of time, the organ sustains recurrent infarcts and eventually becomes a remnant of fibrous tissue.

ANEMIA   SS homozygotes have a severe hemolytic anemia with hematocrit values between 18 and 30 percent. The mean red blood cell survival is about 10 to 15 days. Those cells having relatively low levels of Hb F have a shorter life span, in part due to a greater chance of becoming irreversibly sickled. As a result of accelerated red blood

FIGURE 306-2   Polymerization of sickle hemoglobin. When the red cell (A) is deoxygenated, deoxyhemoglobin S aggregates to form domains of elongated rodlike polymers (B). In most cells these fibers align and distort the cell into the classic sickle shape (C). The individual Hb S molecules form a closely packed polymer consisting of 14 strands having a helical configuration (D). A close-up of the contacts between a pair of aligned strands (E) shows the abnormal β6 valine forming a hydrophobic contact with an acceptor site on the β chain of a molecule on the adjacent strand.

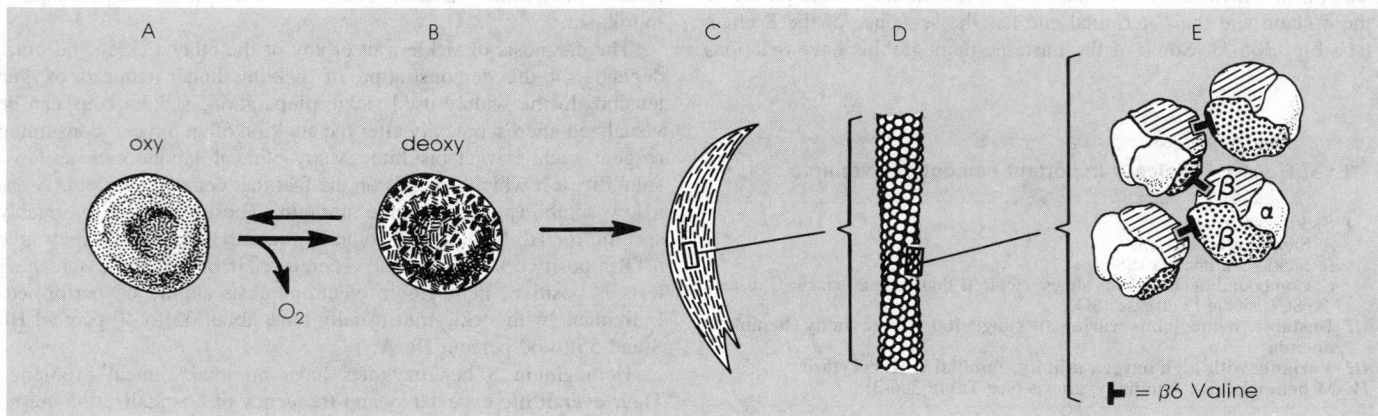

TABLE 306-2 Clinical manifestations of sickle cell anemia

I Constitutional
  A Impaired growth and development
  B Increased susceptibility to infection

II Vasoocclusive
  A Microinfarcts → Painful crises
  B Macroinfarcts
                    Organ damage

III Anemia
  A Severe hemolysis
  B Aplastic crises

---

cell breakdown, patients with sickle cell disease have characteristic clinical and laboratory findings as discussed in Chap. 302. Even though hemolysis is primarily extravascular, plasma haptoglobin is generally low or absent, and plasma hemoglobin levels are moderately elevated.

The anemia becomes increasingly severe if erythropoiesis is suppressed. There are two main causes of "aplastic crises"—infection and folic acid deficiency. As discussed in Chap. 305, infection brings about a transient reduction in red blood cell production. In particular, parvovirus infection causes an abrupt suppression of erythropoiesis. In SS patients with severe ongoing hemolysis, this usually results in a rapid drop in hematocrit (see Table 306-2).

ACUTE PAIN CRISIS The morbidity and mortality of sickle cell disease are due primarily to recurrent vasoocclusive phenomena. As shown in Table 306-2, these can be divided into two groups. Throughout their lives, SS patients are plagued by recurrent *painful crises*. These episodes may appear with explosive suddenness and attack various parts of the body, particularly the abdomen, chest, back, and joints. About one quarter of painful crises are preceded by a viral or bacterial infection. The frequency of painful crises is highly variable. A given patient may have months or even years without a crisis and then have a cluster of frequent, severe attacks. In some individuals, crises occur more frequently in cold weather, perhaps precipitated by reflex vasospasm. In others, crises come more often in warm weather, during times when patients are likely to become dehydrated. It is often difficult to distinguish between painful sickle crisis and some other type of acute process such as biliary colic, appendicitis, or a perforated viscus. Many patients have been subjected to abdominal exploration because they were considered to have an acute surgical problem. Patients having abdominal sickle crises usually have normal bowel sounds and no rebound tenderness. If the abdominal pain is due to sickling, the surgeon usually finds no gross evidence of infarction or ischemia.

SS homozygotes frequently develop attacks of acute pleuritic chest pain with fever. Although the initial chest x-ray is often unremarkable, an infiltrate may evolve. The important differential diagnosis is between pneumonitis and pulmonary infarction. Culture and Gram's stain of the sputum will be helpful in establishing the presence of pneumonia. In these patients, pulmonary infarctions are much more likely due to thrombosis in situ than to emboli. Occasionally, pulmonary infarcts become secondarily infected.

When a sickle crisis is localized in the extremities, it may induce acute synovitis and joint effusion. Examination of the joint fluid is helpful in distinguishing sickle crisis from other causes of acute arthritis, such as sepsis, gout, or rheumatoid disease. If the effusion is due to sickling, the fluid will be clear and yellow, with a low white blood cell count (100 to 1000 mononuclear cells per cubic millimeter) and an absence of crystals or bacteria.

Sickle crises may occasionally involve the central nervous system. Patients can present with a seizure, stroke, or coma. Although such crises are frequently reversible, they may be fatal.

CHRONIC ORGAN DAMAGE By the time that patients reach adulthood, there is often objective evidence of anatomic or functional damage to various tissues due to the cumulative effects of recurrent vasoocclusive episodes. Almost any organ may be involved, but the most common are the lungs, kidneys, liver, skeleton, and skin.

Cardiopulmonary Impairment of pulmonary function is a common complication of sickle cell disease. Resting arterial P_{O_2} is usually reduced in part because of intrapulmonary arterial-venous shunting. Since SS red blood cells have decreased oxygen affinity, arterial blood will be significantly undersaturated, leading to an increased tendency for red cells to sickle when they reach the peripheral circulation. SS homozygotes frequently develop congestive heart failure. The chronic severe anemia and hypoxemia impose a sustained burden on the heart. Most patients have a systolic ejection murmur as a result of their hyperdynamic circulation. Even though more oxygen is extracted by the myocardium than any other tissue, SS patients rarely develop vasoocclusive sickling in the myocardium, probably because of rapid transit through the microcirculation.

Genitourinary (See also Chaps. 241 and 243) The hypertonic and acidic environment of the renal medulla promotes sickling, resulting in microinfarcts. Virtually all patients have isosthenuria. The inability to form concentrated urine increases the risk of significant dehydration. In addition, like those with sickle trait, Sβ thalassemia, or SC disease, SS homozygotes may develop significant and prolonged painless hematuria as a result of papillary infarcts. Hematuria may be so extensive that iron deficiency develops. ε-Aminocaproic acid has proved to be effective in severe cases but must be used with caution because it may prevent the lysis of clots in the renal pelvis.

Mild nitrogen retention is commonly encountered, accompanied by moderate hyperuricemia. However, patients rarely have uric acid nephropathy or gout. As SS patients survive into the fourth and fifth decades, a substantial proportion develop progressive renal failure. The pathogenesis of the glomerular dysfunction is unclear. Male patients with sickle cell anemia occasionally develop priapism (spontaneous and painful engorgement of the penis). This distressing complication occurs with about equal frequency in prepubertal and postpubertal patients, although the latter are more difficult to treat and may develop impotence following the acute episode. Patients should be treated conservatively with sedation, analgesia, and intravenous fluids. The administration of packed red blood cells also may be effective. Surgical intervention is rarely indicated.

Hepatobiliary Like other patients with congenital hemolytic anemia, those with sickle cell anemia are icteric, owing to elevated nonconjugated bilirubin in the plasma, and have an increased tendency to form gallstones. As a rule, cholecystectomy is not recommended unless gallstones cause symptoms. It is often difficult to distinguish between the abdominal pain of acute cholecystitis and that due to a sickle crisis. Jaundice deepens markedly if a patient develops choledocholithiasis, and bilirubin levels as high as 855 μmol/L (50 mg/dL) have been reported. In addition, patients with sickle cell anemia may develop hepatic infarcts which occasionally become infected, resulting in abscess formation. If a significant portion of hepatic parenchyma becomes infarcted, fibrosis and deterioration of liver function may result, with deepening of jaundice.

Skeletal Like other patients with congenital hemolytic anemia, patients with sickle cell anemia demonstrate radiologic abnormalities due to the expansion of red marrow. However, the development of bony infarcts results in more characteristic x-ray abnormalities. The biconcave or "fishmouth" vertebrae are virtually pathognomonic of sickle cell disease. Skeletal infarction generally leads to increased bony trabeculation and sclerosis. Aseptic necrosis of the head of the femur is particularly common in patients with sickle cell disease and can lead to considerable disability. Selected patients benefit from surgical intervention, ranging from core decompression to total hip replacement. Like infarcts in other organs, bony infarctions are more likely to become infected. In patients who develop osteomyelitis, salmonella is a frequent pathogen.

Skin Chronic skin ulcers often occur in the distal lower extremities. The lesions appear to be more common in patients with more severe anemia. Ankle ulcers also have been encountered in rare patients with other types of congenital hemolytic anemia. This complication is seen more commonly in tropical areas. Ankle ulcers generally respond to conservative management, such as elevation of the leg, maintenance of strict cleanliness, and application of a mild chemical debriding agent. In patients with refractory ulcers, a hypertransfusion regimen is probably indicated. Skin grafting should be undertaken only after all other measures have failed.

Ocular   A variety of ocular abnormalities are encountered in patients with SS and SC disease. These include retinal infarcts, peripheral vessel disease, arteriovenous anomalies, vitreous hemorrhage, retinitis proliferans, and retinal detachment. In addition, when viewed with a strong magnifying lens, angulated and "corkscrew" vessels can be seen in the bulbar conjunctiva. The major ocular complications are more commonly encountered in SC and sickle β thalassemia patients than in SS patients. The early diagnosis of retinal lesions in sickle disease is important because retinal detachment may be prevented by appropriate therapy.

Neurologic   A variety of central nervous system manifestations may be encountered in sickle cell anemia. Although cerebral thrombosis is the principal neurologic complication, these patients also have an increased incidence of subarachnoid hemorrhage. An SS patient has about a 25 percent lifelong chance of developing some type of neurologic complication. Hemiplegia is encountered more frequently than coma, convulsions, or visual disturbances. Patients generally make a full recovery, particularly from their first cerebral vascular accident. A hypertransfusion program is beneficial to children who have sustained a major neurologic complication.

Diagnosis   The diagnosis of sickle cell anemia should be considered in any black patient with a hemolytic anemia. The history of painful crises, arthropathy, ankle ulcers, etc. can be very helpful. If a patient has a relatively mild form of the disease, the diagnosis may not have been made during childhood. A number of laboratory tests are useful in distinguishing sickle cell anemia from other hemoglobinopathies. Examination of the peripheral blood smear reveals normochromic normocytic red blood cells, many of which appear as targets. The presence of irreversibly sickled forms is very helpful (see Fig. A9-6). In addition, the presence of Howell-Jolly bodies, siderocytes, and occasional normoblasts attests to the absence of effective splenic function. A positive test for sickling, such as the metabisulfite preparation or the solubility test, indicates the presence of Hb S but does not distinguish between SS, AS, and compound heterozygotes (SβThal, SC). Hemoglobin electrophoresis is necessary to establish the diagnosis. Patients with homozygous sickle cell anemia have about 2 to 20 percent Hb F and 2 to 4 percent Hb A_2. The remainder is Hb S. No Hb A is detected unless the patient has been transfused within the past 4 months. Patients with sickle β thalassemia will have hypochromic microcytic red blood cells, fewer irreversibly sickled forms, and a variable proportion of Hb A (0 to 30 percent). SC diseases can be readily diagnosed by hemoglobin electrophoresis. In hemoglobin SD disease, the two hemoglobin variants comigrate during conventional electrophoresis at pH 8.6 but can be separated by agar gel electrophoresis at pH 6.0.

Treatment   Understanding the molecular pathogenesis of sickling is beginning to lead to the development of rational and effective therapy. A large array of antisickling regimens are effective in vitro but have unacceptable toxicity. Hydroxyurea therapy significantly increases Hb F levels and reduces hemolysis. Its effect on pain crises and other vasoocclusive manifestations is under study. Additional investigation is focusing on stimulating the production of Hb F by other agents such as butyrate and recombinant erythropoietin.

Currently accepted management of sickle cell anemia is primarily supportive and conservative. Since patients with sickle cell anemia are at increased risk of developing infections, many of which trigger painful and aplastic crises, it is very important to detect infection early and give appropriate antibiotics promptly. Malaria prophylaxis should be administered in endemic areas. The development of pneumococcal sepsis in children may be prevented by the administration of the polyvalent vaccine and prophylactic penicillin.

The anemia of sickle cell disease increases markedly if the patient becomes deficient in folic acid. Since these patients have a continuously increased requirement for folic acid, it is reasonable to maintain them on a daily oral supplement.

Painful crises should be treated promptly with adequate analgesia and hydration. Some patients feel that their crises can be aborted if treated early. Therefore, it is expedient to give these patients a supply of an analgesic such as codeine which can be taken at home. However, these patients are at risk of becoming addicted to opiates. Oxygen should be administered during acute pain crisis if the patient has arterial hypoxemia.

Blood transfusions play a limited role in the management of sickle cell anemia. Between crises, patients tolerate anemia quite well and do not derive much subjective benefit from transfusions. However, partial replacement of the patients' red blood cells by transfused red cells (hypertransfusion) may be an effective way of preventing vasoocclusive crises. In order to lower the viscosity of the patient's blood significantly, it is necessary that over 50 percent of the patient's red blood cells be of donor origin. Hypertransfusion is a reasonable approach to getting a patient through a limited period of risk such as surgery. However, the problems of isoimmunization, iron overload, and transmission of infection dictate against its widespread use.

Prevention   Genetic counseling can play an important role in the prevention of sickle cell anemia. Parents who are both AS heterozygotes should be informed that there is a 25 percent chance that their offspring will be homozygous. The antenatal diagnosis of sickle cell anemia can be made in the first trimester of pregnancy by obtaining fetal cells from a chorionic villus and analyzing the DNA following digestion with a restriction endonuclease that recognizes the codon involved in the β6 valine mutation. If it is established that the fetus is an SS homozygote, the parents may decide to terminate the pregnancy.

Prognosis   The clinical course of patients with sickle cell anemia is highly variable. Many assessments of prognosis that have appeared in the literature have been unduly pessimistic. During the past 30 years there has been considerable improvement in the care of patients with sickle cell anemia. An increasing number of patients are surviving into adulthood and bearing offspring. There also has been a decline in the mortality of SS mothers during pregnancy and childbirth. However, in underdeveloped nations, the mortality in sickle cell anemia remains very high.

No single clinical or laboratory finding is a consistent predictor of prognosis in sickle cell disease. Although those patients who have relatively high amounts of Hb F tend to have milder clinical manifestations, this relationship is of no prognostic value in any given patient. Considerable variation in the severity of sickle cell disease has been reported among different ethnic and geographic groups. A group of Shi Arabs from Saudi Arabia has been found to have a less severe form of sickle cell anemia with very high levels of Hb F (15 to 30 percent). A relatively mild type of sickle cell anemia also has been encountered in central India. SS patients with coexisting α thalassemia have less severe hemolysis but do not have a significant reduction in vasoocclusive phenomena.

SICKLE β THALASSEMIA   This disease is highly variable in its clinical severity and complications. It is commonly encountered in people from the Mediterranean countries as well as those from central Africa. Sickle β thalassemia tends to be milder in blacks, just as homozygous β thalassemia is much less severe in blacks than in the Mediterranean populations. Patients have a congenital hemolytic anemia of variable severity, accompanied by splenomegaly in about 70 percent of cases. Individuals who produce no normal β chains (sickle $β^0$ thalassemia) have vasoocclusive manifestations comparable with those encountered in homozygous SS disease. In contrast, patients who are able to produce some normal β chains (sickle $β^+$ thalassemia) have less severe anemia, fewer pain crises, and less organ damage.

Examination of the blood film reveals hypochromic microcytic red blood cells with polychromatophilia, target cells, stippling, and rare fixed sickle forms. The electrophoretic pattern shows from 60 to 90 percent Hb S and 10 to 30 percent Hb F. Hemoglobin A will be about 10 to 30 percent if the β-thalassemia gene is capable of producing some β^A chains (β$^+$ thalassemia, see below). In patients who have sickle β^0 thalassemia, no Hb A will be present, and therefore the disorder may be difficult to distinguish from homozygous sickle cell anemia. Hemoglobin A$_2$ is moderately elevated in sickle β thalassemia, but it is difficult to measure this minor component accurately in the presence of Hb S. Occasional patients may derive benefit from splenectomy if the spleen is sequestering a significant amount of red blood cells.

SICKLE C DISEASE   Although the gene frequency among blacks in the United States for Hb C (β6 Glu→Lys) is only one-fourth that for Hb S, the prevalence of SC disease among adults is almost as high as SS disease, since the former group of patients has a nearly normal life expectancy. These individuals have a mild to moderate hemolytic anemia, usually accompanied by splenomegaly. On peripheral blood smears, target cells and occasional plump sickled forms are seen. Hemoglobin electrophoresis reveals 50 percent Hb S and 50 percent Hb C. Hemoglobin S copolymerizes with Hb C to the same extent as with Hb A. The increased tendency of SC red blood cells to sickle, compared with sickle-trait cells, can be explained by two phenomena: increased intracellular hemoglobin concentration and significantly higher percent Hb S. Patients with SC disease may occasionally have painful crises or organ infarcts. They are at particular risk of developing ocular complications described above, including proliferative retinopathy and retinal detachment. In addition, patients with SC disease are at relatively high risk of developing hematuria from renal medullary infarcts and avascular necrosis of the femoral head. Women with SC disease have a higher rate of complications during pregnancy. Individuals with an electrophoretic pattern suggestive of Hb SC disease but with more severe clinical manifestations may be double heterozygotes for Hb S and Hb O Arab (β121 Glu→Lys).

SICKLE D DISEASE   A number of hemoglobins comigrate with Hb S on routine electrophoresis. The most commonly encountered variant is Hb D Los Angeles (β121 Glu→Gln). Hemoglobins S and D can be separated by special electrophoretic methods. The diagnosis of Hb SD disease is suggested by the demonstration of a positive sickle cell preparation in only one of the patient's two parents. SD double heterozygotes have moderately severe anemia and vasoocclusive complications.

HOMOZYGOUS Hb C DISEASE   Patients have a mild congenital hemolytic anemia accompanied by splenomegaly. Hemoglobin C (β6 Glu→Lys) has a tendency to form intracellular crystals, particularly if red blood cells are suspended in a hypertonic medium. The intracellular hemoglobin concentration is markedly increased owing to loss of potassium and water from the cytoplasm. As a result, the blood film reveals striking target cells. Red blood cell osmotic fragility is decreased. Patients rarely develop significant complications. No specific therapy is indicated.

HEMOGLOBIN E   The second most common hemoglobin variant worldwide is Hb E (β26 Glu→Lys). It has very high prevalence in Southeast Asia, with gene frequencies in Thailand, Laos, and Cambodia approaching 0.1. Because of the recent emigration of refugees from Southeast Asia, Hb E is now encountered quite commonly in the United States. Hb E has nearly normal O$_2$ binding properties and stability, but its synthetic rate is impaired owing to the fact that the base substitution at codon 26 creates a new splicing sequence that causes abnormal mRNA processing and decreased production of mature β^E message. As a result, individuals with Hb E have a thalassemic phenotype (see below). Heterozygotes (AE) have slightly microcytic red cells. Homozygotes have more marked microcytosis (MCV of 65 to 70 fL) and prominent target cells. Hb E is not associated with anemia or any other clinical manifestations unless inherited along with a β-thalassemia gene. These compound heterozygotes (E/β thalassemia) have severe anemia and most of the other findings encountered in β thalassemia major (see below).

UNSTABLE HEMOGLOBIN VARIANTS

Hemolytic anemia is sometimes due to a mutant hemoglobin that precipitates within red blood cells, forming solid inclusions. Currently, over 100 different unstable and poorly soluble hemoglobin variants have been identified. The great majority are single amino acid substitutions in the β chain. A few are due to deletion of one or more amino acids within the β chain. Patients present with a hemolytic anemia of variable degree. Severe cases are usually detected in late infancy or early childhood and have jaundice, splenomegaly, and dark-colored urine. An autosomal dominant mode of inheritance can usually be established, although about a fifth of the cases appear to be spontaneous mutants.

Pathogenesis   These hemoglobin variants have structural alterations at sites in the molecule that drastically affect its stability and solubility. As a result, the abnormal hemoglobin forms an intracellular precipitate (Heinz body). Red blood cells which contain this type of inclusion are recognized by the mononuclear phagocyte system and are either cleansed of their intracellular debris (pitting) or destroyed. The degree of instability of these hemoglobin variants and, therefore, the extent of hemolysis vary considerably. In some, an additional oxidant stress, such as the ingestion of certain drugs, is required for significant hemolysis. The degree of anemia is influenced not only by the severity of the hemolysis but also by the ability of the blood to unload oxygen. Thus patients having unstable variants with increased oxygen affinity may have compensated hemolysis with a near-normal hemoglobin level.

Diagnosis   The red blood cell morphology is somewhat variable. Often, patients with a functioning spleen have normal-appearing red blood cells. Slight hypochromia and basophilic stippling are not uncommon. The blood may have to be incubated in order to bring out Heinz bodies. In some cases, red blood cells appear as if a bite had been taken from a margin. It is tempting to speculate that at this site a Heinz body had been pitted. Following splenectomy, red blood cells appear much more abnormal, and Heinz bodies are larger and more numerous.

The diagnosis of a congenital Heinz body hemolytic anemia is established by the following laboratory tests and results:

1 *Hemoglobin electrophoresis* will often reveal an abnormal component, usually composing less than 30 percent of the total.
2 *Heinz bodies* can be demonstrated by incubating a freshly drawn sample of blood with a supravital stain.
3 A significant *precipitate* is formed when the hemolysate is incubated at 50°C or in the presence of 17% isopropanol.
4 The *oxygen dissociation curve* is often abnormal.

If these tests are negative in a patient with congenital nonspherocytic hemolytic anemia, a defect of the membrane or of one of the red blood cell enzymes is likely (Chap. 307).

Treatment   The treatment of congenital Heinz body hemolytic anemia is primarily supportive. Anemia is rarely severe enough to warrant blood transfusion. Oxidant drugs should be avoided. Those with severe hemolysis often benefit from prophylactic folate therapy. Although patients with severe hemolysis may benefit from splenectomy, this operation is not curative. Because of the risk of bacterial sepsis in infants and young children who have been splenectomized, this treatment should be postponed until the child is over 4 years old. The diagnostic tests cited above become more abnormal following splenectomy. For this reason, in some cases the diagnosis may not be definitely established until after the operation.

STABLE VARIANTS HAVING ABNORMAL OXYGEN AFFINITY

More than 50 hemoglobin variants with high oxygen affinity have been encountered in families with erythrocytosis. Their structural alterations tend to be at sites which influence hemoglobin's functional

TABLE 306-3   Differential diagnosis of cyanosis

I **Decreased oxygenation of hemoglobin (↑ deoxyhemoglobin)**
  A Reduced arterial oxygen tension (common)
    1 Pulmonary disease
    2 Cardiac right-to-left shunt
  B Hemoglobin variant having decreased oxygen affinity (rare)
II **Methemoglobinemia (rare)**
  A Hereditary
    1 M hemoglobins
    2 Cytochrome b_5 reductase deficiency
  B Acquired
    1 Nitrites and nitrates: sodium nitrite, amyl nitrite, nitroglycerin, nitroprusside, silver nitrate
    2 Aniline dyes
    3 Acetanilid and phenacetin
    4 Sulfonamides
    5 Other: lidocaine, chlorate, phenazopyridine

behavior. As a result of the hemoglobin's increased oxygen affinity, oxygen unloading to tissues is decreased, and there is an erythropoietin-mediated stimulus to erythropoiesis. This disorder is manifested in the heterozygous state and follows an autosomal codominant pattern of inheritance. Hematocrit levels are rarely high enough to cause a significant increase in blood viscosity. Thus affected individuals are generally asymptomatic and lack any pertinent physical findings other than a ruddy complexion. The diagnosis should be suspected in all patients with unexplained erythrocytosis, particularly when other family members are similarly affected, and can be established by the demonstration of increased oxygen affinity of the whole blood. About two-thirds of the high-affinity variants can be readily separated from Hb A by electrophoresis. No treatment is indicated. The patient should be reassured that the disorder is benign.

Hemoglobin variants having a marked decrease in oxygen affinity cause one form of familial cyanosis (Table 306-3). Because of the abnormality of hemoglobin function, arterial blood is partially unsaturated despite normal oxygen tension. Thus the cyanosis is due to increased levels of deoxyhemoglobin in the blood. Except for this cosmetic problem, affected individuals have no other clinical manifestations. Blood values are otherwise normal.

METHEMOGLOBINEMIA

Oxygen transport depends on the maintenance of intracellular hemoglobin in the reduced (Fe^{2+}) state. When hemoglobin is oxidized to methemoglobin, the heme iron becomes Fe^{3+} and is now incapable of binding oxygen. Normal red cells contain less than 1 percent methemoglobin. A small amount of hemoglobin autooxidizes as red cells circulate. This process probably occurs by the dissociation of the superoxide anion from oxyhemoglobin:

$$Hb^{2+}O_2 \rightarrow Hb^{3+} + O_2^-$$

Normally, the methemoglobin that is formed is reduced by the following reaction:

$$Hb^{3+} + RedCyt\ b_5 \rightarrow Hb^{2+} + OxCyt\ b_5$$

Reduced cytochrome b_5 (RedCyt b_5) is regenerated by the enzyme cytochrome b_5 reductase (methemoglobin reductase):

$$OxCyt\ b_5 + NADH \xrightarrow[\text{reductase}]{\text{Cytochrome }b_5} RedCyt\ b_5 + NAD$$

Hereditary methemoglobinemia is due either to the presence of one of the M hemoglobins (see below) or to the deficiency of the enzyme cytochrome b_5 reductase (Table 306-3). These inherited disorders are clinically mild, while the induction of methemoglobinemia by drugs or toxins can be life-threatening.

If methemoglobin exceeds 15 g/L (1.5 g/dL) (10 percent of the total hemoglobin), affected individuals will have clinically obvious cyanosis. The color of the skin is indistinguishable from the much more common cyanosis due to impairment of oxygen saturation that may occur in pulmonary and cardiac disorders (see Table 306-3). With higher amounts of methemoglobin, patients become symptomatic. At a methemoglobin level of about 35 percent, the affected individual experiences headache, weakness, and breathlessness. Levels in excess of 80 percent are usually incompatible with life.

The toxicity of methemoglobinemia can be readily explained in terms of hemoglobin function. The fact that a certain proportion of the heme moieties is no longer able to bind oxygen is not a serious physiologic handicap per se. A proportion of 30 percent methemoglobin is much more deleterious than a 30 percent decrement in red cell mass, because the oxidized hemes have a marked effect on the remaining functional hemes in the hemoglobin tetramer. The conformation of methemoglobin (like that of carboxyhemoglobin) is very similar to that of oxyhemoglobin. Thus a partially oxidized hemoglobin tetramer has the same tertiary and quaternary structures as a molecule that is comparably oxygenated. In each case, the affinity of the remaining hemes for oxygen is increased. For this reason, methemoglobinemia [as well as carbon monoxide (Chap. 395)] causes a "shift to the left" of the oxyhemoglobin dissociation curve and, consequently, impaired unloading of oxygen to tissues.

CYTOCHROME b_5 REDUCTASE (METHEMOGLOBIN REDUCTASE) DEFICIENCY   This condition is inherited in an autosomal recessive pattern. The enzyme is a flavoprotein having properties similar to those of liver microsomal cytochrome b_5 reductase. The soluble erythrocyte enzyme is formed by cleavage of a hydrophobic tail from the microsomal enzyme.

Individuals with cytochrome b_5 reductase deficiency have lifelong cyanosis of variable degree, depending on the level of methemoglobin, but usually have no associated symptoms or other physical findings. Some may have mild polycythemia owing to increased oxygen affinity. Others have been noted to be mentally retarded. Untreated individuals usually have 15 to 30 percent methemoglobin. Methemoglobin levels are higher in the older population of red cells because the activity of the abnormal enzyme declines markedly with red cell age. There appears to be considerable heterogeneity in the variant enzymes from different families, as shown by differences in their electrophoretic mobility and kinetic parameters. In these ways, cytochrome b_5 reductase deficiency resembles glucose-6-phosphate dehydrogenase deficiency (Chap. 307).

ACQUIRED METHEMOGLOBINEMIA   This disorder is generally due to exposure to certain drugs or toxins. Compounds which can cause clinically significant methemoglobinemia are listed in Table 306-3. Some agents such as nitrite and chlorate oxidize the heme iron directly. Others such as sulfa drugs and aniline must undergo biochemical transformation before they cause methemoglobinemia. Few drugs currently in use cause significant methemoglobinemia, unless the individual is unusually susceptible. Exposure to local anesthetics such as procaine and to nitroprusside occasionally causes severe methemoglobinemia. As might be expected, individuals heterozygous for methemoglobin reductase deficiency are much more likely than normal individuals to develop clinically apparent methemoglobinemia after exposure to an oxidant stress. Thus the extent of methemoglobinemia depends not only on the dose of the toxic agent but also on the susceptibility of the exposed individual.

M HEMOGLOBINS   Five hemoglobin variants have abnormal absorbance spectra, owing to the oxidation of the heme iron in the affected subunit. They involve substitutions of amino acid residues responsible for the binding of the heme iron to the globin. These so-called M hemoglobins (Table 306-3) result in a rare form of congenital and familial cyanosis. Individuals with the α-chain variants Hb M Boston and Hb M Iwate are cyanotic at birth, while cyanosis does not appear in those with the β-chain variants (Hb M Saskatoon, Hb M Hyde Park, and Hb M Milwaukee) until about 4 to 6 months of age, when fetal hemoglobin has been replaced by adult hemoglobin. As with the unstable and high-affinity variants, an autosomal codominant inheritance pattern is found. Except for cyanosis, patients are asymptomatic.

DIAGNOSIS Methemoglobinemia should be considered in any cyanotic patient with no evidence of heart or lung disease. If the cyanosis is due to decreased oxygen saturation, a blood specimen will change from a purple to a red color upon mixing with air. In contrast, a blood specimen from a methemoglobinemic individual remains a chocolate brown color irrespective of exposure to air. Methemoglobinemia can be documented by spectroscopic examination of the hemolysate. Individuals with hereditary methemoglobinemia will have lower levels than patients symptomatic from acquired methemoglobinemia. Patients who have ingested an oxidant drug may have an additional hemoglobin derivative called *sulfhemoglobin* in which the protoporphyrin has been chemically modified. Sulfhemoglobinemia tends to cause cyanosis even more readily than methemoglobinemia. Unlike methemoglobin, the absorbance of sulfhemoglobin at 620 to 630 nm is not decreased by the addition of cyanide. The M hemoglobins have characteristic spectral abnormalities which differ from those obtained when normal Hb A is partially oxidized. Furthermore, these hemoglobin variants can be detected by hemoglobin electrophoresis.

TREATMENT In individuals with methemoglobin reductase deficiency, the oral administration of methylene blue (100 to 300 mg/d) or ascorbic acid (300 to 500 mg/d) will result in a marked reduction in the level of methemoglobin. The purpose of treatment is primarily cosmetic. Severe toxic methemoglobinemia is treated by the intravenous administration of methylene blue (2 mg/kg; repeat if needed). Within an hour, the methemoglobin level is usually reduced by at least 50 percent. Treatment is neither possible nor necessary in individuals having Hb M.

THALASSEMIAS

The thalassemias are a diverse group of congenital disorders in which there is a defect in the synthesis of one (or more) of the subunits of hemoglobin. As a result of decreased production of hemoglobin, the red blood cells are microcytic and hypochromic (see Table 56-2). The thalassemias involve a spectrum ranging from subtle morphologic abnormalities to life-threatening disease. In contrast to the qualitative hemoglobin abnormalities listed in Table 306-1, the thalassemias are quantitative abnormalities of subunit synthesis. Thus the β chains of patients with β thalassemia have normal structure but are produced in reduced and sometimes undetectable amounts. Conversely, patients with α thalassemia have impaired production of α chains. The reduction in globin chain synthesis can be demonstrated in vitro by incubating reticulocytes with labeled amino acids and determining the incorporation of radioactivity into globin subunits (Table 306-4). Most forms of thalassemia can be identified from the information summarized in Table 306-4. Establishing a definitive diagnosis requires analysis of globin gene structure.

α THALASSEMIA As mentioned at the beginning of this chapter, normal individuals inherit two α-chain genes from each parent. The great majority of cases of α thalassemia can be explained by deletions of α-chain genes owing to nonhomologous crossover (see Fig. 306-1). Specific gene deletions can be identified by analysis of patients' DNA following digestion by restriction endonucleases. The clinical manifestations of α thalassemia depend on the number of genes deleted (see Table 306-4). In the silent carrier state, heterozygous α thalassemia 2 (α−/αα), one of the four genes is deleted. Affected individuals have no hematologic abnormalities. Individuals with deletion of two of the four α-chain genes (α-thalassemia trait) have either homozygous α thalassemia 2 (α−/α−) or heterozygous α thalassemia 1 (−−/αα). They have microcytic and slightly hypochromic red blood cells but no significant hemolysis or anemia. Hemoglobin electrophoresis is normal except for a decreased amount of Hb A₂. Deletion of three α-chain genes (−−/α−) produces a well-compensated hemolytic state with microcytic hypochromic red blood cells including many target cells. Intracellular inclusions or Heinz bodies are formed by the precipitation of Hb H, a tetramer composed of β chains which accumulates because of the marked impairment of α-chain synthesis. The most severe form of α thalassemia, hydrops fetalis, is usually due to deletion of all four α-chain genes. The affected fetus has red blood cells containing only Hb Barts, a tetramer composed of γ chains. This condition is incompatible with life, since oxygen transport depends on the presence of heterotetramers such as $\alpha_2\beta_2$ and $\alpha_2\gamma_2$. In Southeast Asians, both the α− and the −− haplotypes are relatively common; thus both Hb H disease and hydrops fetalis are frequently encountered. In contrast, blacks and individuals from the Mediterranean and the Middle East commonly have the α− haplotype (gene frequency in blacks ≅ 0.15) but rarely have the −− haplotype. Therefore, Hb H disease is uncommon among them, and hydrops fetalis is extremely rare. Homozygous α thalassemia 2 is encountered in about 2 percent of blacks and is therefore a relatively common cause of microcytosis in an individual who is otherwise healthy and not iron-deficient.

The elongated α-chain variant Hb Constant Spring, often encountered among Southeast Asians, also has an α-thalassemia phenotype and, when inherited with the −− haplotype, can cause Hb H disease.

β THALASSEMIA Since individuals inherit only one β-chain gene from each parent, affected individuals are either heterozygotes, homozygotes, or compound heterozygotes. The gene frequency for β thalassemia approaches 0.1 in southern Italy and certain Mediterranean islands. β Thalassemia is also encountered quite commonly in central Africa, the Middle East, Southeast Asia, including certain parts of India, and the south Pacific. Statistically, one-quarter of the offspring of two heterozygotes (β-thalassemia trait) will have the homozygous state: β thalassemia major or Cooley's anemia. An individual may inherit a β-thalassemia gene from one parent and a β-chain structural variant from the other. Sickle β

TABLE 306-4 Classification of the thalassemias

Diagnosis	Globin chain synthesis in reticulocytes	RBC morphology	Hb electrophoresis	Clinical severity
α Thalassemia:	α/β*			
Silent carrier (α−/αα)	0.9	Normal	Normal, ↓ Hb A₂	0
α-thalassemia trait [(α−/α−) or (−−/αα)]	0.7	↓ MCV† ↓ MCV	Normal, ↓ Hb A₂	0
Hb H disease (−−/α−)	0.3	Heinz bodies, targets	↑ Hb H (β₄) (10–15%)	2+
Hydrops fetalis (−−/−−)	0	↑↑ Nucleated RBC	↑↑ Hb Barts (γ₄)	4+
β Thalassemia:	β/α*			
Heterozygous	0.5	↓ MCV, stippling ↓ MCV, hypochromic	↑ Hb A₂ (± ↑ Hb F)	0 to +
Homozygous (or compound heterozygous)	0–0.3	Nucleated RBC, targets bizarre shapes	↑↑ Hb F	4+ (major) 2−3+ (intermedia)

* Normal = 1.
† MCV = mean corpuscular volume.

thalassemia (discussed above) is a commonly encountered example of such a compound heterozygous state.

The molecular pathogenesis of the β thalassemias is more complex and heterogeneous than that of α thalassemia. In contrast to α thalassemia, gene deletion is an uncommon cause of β thalassemia. Among the recognized types of β-gene deletion, an entity known as "hereditary persistence of fetal hemoglobin" has minimal clinical manifestations owing to efficient synthesis of γ chains on the chromosome in which the β and δ genes are deleted. In the great majority of cases of β thalassemia, restriction endonuclease maps reveal no gross abnormalities of the β-globin gene complex. Nevertheless, there are several steps in β-globin synthesis that could go awry and lead to a thalassemic phenotype. A number of cases involve mutations in or near one of the intervening sequences of the β-globin gene, leading to errors in the splicing of mRNA. Often β^A chains are made but in reduced amounts (β^+ thalassemia) (see Fig. 306-1). Other cases have nonsense mutations in the coding region, causing premature termination of β-globin chains. This is the most common cause of β^0 thalassemia (Fig. 306-1).

Cellular pathogenesis   As a result of imbalance in globin chain synthesis, the β thalassemias have varying degrees of ineffective erythropoiesis (see Chap. 302) and hemolysis. In β thalassemia major there is a marked relative excess of α-chain production. Free α chains have decreased solubility and will form insoluble aggregates or inclusions within red blood cell precursors in the bone marrow. Like congenital Heinz body hemolytic anemia due to unstable hemoglobin variants, the inclusion bodies in thalassemia bring about abnormalities in membrane permeability as well as entrapment and destruction of red blood cells by the macrophages in the mononuclear phagoycte system. As a result, β thalassemia is characterized by both intramedullary erythroid destruction and a shortening of the life span of circulating red blood cells that emerge from the bone marrow. Thus these patients have the characteristic parameters of both ineffective erythropoiesis (increased plasma iron turnover, decreased incorporation of iron into red blood cells) and peripheral hemolysis. Because these red blood cells are under double jeopardy, there is an enormous compensatory stimulus to erythropoiesis, resulting both in expansion of the red marrow and in extramedullary hematopoiesis in the liver and spleen. Chain imbalance in β thalassemia is attenuated to a variable degree by the "compensatory" synthesis of γ chains which are able to combine with excess free α chains and form a stable tetramer (Hb F). Patients with β thalassemia major who have a relatively high rate of γ-chain production have a less severe clinical course. Individuals with β thalassemia minor have absent or very mild ineffective erythropoiesis and hemolysis, detectable in some patients by a slight elevation in fecal urobilinogen and a modest shortening of the red blood cell life span.

β Thalassemia minor   This common entity, also referred to as β-*thalassemia trait*, is rarely associated with significant clinical manifestations. The diagnosis is generally made in patients being evaluated for mild anemia or in follow-up of abnormalities found on routine blood studies. Most individuals with β-thalassemia trait escape diagnosis. About one-fifth of affected individuals have modest splenomegaly. Icterus is occasionally noted, particularly in those individuals who also have Gilbert's disease, another common and benign congenital disorder (see Chap. 265).

In otherwise healthy individuals with β-thalassemia trait, the mean hemoglobin level is about 15 percent lower than in normal persons of the same age and sex; the red blood cell count is usually elevated, and the cells are microcytic. Indeed, at any level of hematocrit, patients with β thalassemia minor have more marked microcytosis than those with iron deficiency. In contrast, the mean corpuscular hemoglobin concentration is normal. In addition to microcytosis, examination of the blood film reveals occasional target cells, cigar-shaped cells, and a moderate amount of basophilic stippling; the reticulocyte count is normal. Special isotope techniques are required to demonstrate a slightly reduced red blood cell life span. The red blood cells have decreased osmotic fragility. Serum iron is normal

unless the patient also happens to be iron deficient. Hemoglobin electrophoresis is very useful in establishing the diagnosis of β thalassemia minor. Most affected individuals will have a twofold increase in Hb A_2 ($\alpha_2\delta_2$), i.e., 5 percent versus normal of 2.5 percent. In contrast, Hb A_2 is subnormal in α thalassemia, iron deficiency, and sideroblastic anemias. Patients with β-thalassemia trait who become iron deficient usually have a "normal" level of Hb A_2 which increases to above normal after correction of the deficiency. Approximately half of individuals with β thalassemia minor also have a modest elevation of Hb F ($\alpha_2\gamma_2$), i.e., 2 to 3 percent. In the less common state, δβ thalassemia, in which there is a deletion of the adjacent δ- and β-chain genes, Hb A_2 levels will be normal or decreased, but Hb F is increased (5 to 15 percent).

No treatment is indicated for individuals with β-thalassemia trait. They should be reassured that they do not have a serious hematologic problem. The genetic implications of thalassemia should be explained, particularly to those of childbearing age. Many individuals have been given long-term iron treatment on the mistaken impression that they had iron-deficiency anemia. These patients may gradually develop clinically significant siderosis. Establishing the diagnosis of β thalassemia minor should prevent such inappropriate therapy.

β Thalassemia major   Also termed *Cooley's anemia*, this is probably the most severe form of congenital hemolytic anemia. Clinical manifestations generally appear after the first 4 to 6 months of life when the switch from γ-chain to β-chain production normally occurs. Patients develop a severe anemia with a hematocrit of less than 20 percent unless they are supported by transfusions. Accordingly, patients have all the signs and symptoms associated with severe anemia. In addition, they have findings related to severe intramedullary and peripheral hemolysis as well as to iron overload. Inadequately treated patients often have marked wasting and appear malnourished. Children have slow rates of growth and development. In adolescents, the onset and development of secondary sex characteristics are delayed. Patients have a peculiar skin color owing to a combination of icterus, pallor, and increased melanin deposition. They usually have skeletal abnormalities, secondary to expansion of the erythroid marrow. Enlargement of the malar bones may give the characteristic "chipmunk" facies or cause malocclusion of the jaw. Patients invariably have cardiomegaly, which may be accompanied by signs of congestive heart failure. Marked hepatomegaly and splenomegaly are always found in these patients.

The *diagnosis* of β thalassemia major should be considered in any patient with a severe hemolytic anemia and hypochromic microcytic red blood cells. Examination of the peripheral blood smear reveals marked variations in the size and shape of red blood cells, including many target and stippled cells as well as teardrop- and cigar-shaped cells (see Fig. A9-5). Normoblasts are usually seen, particularly if the patient has undergone splenectomy. Hemoglobin electrophoresis shows the presence of increased amounts of Hb F and variable amounts of Hb A. In patients who are homozygous for β^0 thalassemia, no Hb A can be detected. Hemoglobin A_2 is usually increased about twofold, although it can be normal in β thalassemia major.

Patients with β thalassemia major have a short life expectancy. It is unusual for a patient with the most severe form of the disease to survive into adulthood. Most patients have such severe anemia that they are dependent on transfusions. The chronic administration of large amounts of blood along with an inappropriate increase in iron absorption from the gastrointestinal tract inevitably leads to clinically significant hemosiderosis. As a result of iron overload, these patients develop abnormalities in cardiac, endocrine, and hepatic function. The combination of chronic hypoxia and myocardial siderosis leads to cardiac arrhythmias, congestive failure, and ultimately death.

Homozygotes who survive into adulthood are likely to have a less severe form of the disease, designated as β *thalassemia intermedia*. There are several genetic subtypes which are associated with less severe clinical manifestations: (1) β thalassemia with unusually high levels of Hb F synthesis, (2) δβ thalassemia in which there is absence of δ-chain as well as β-chain synthesis, and (3) the presence of α thalassemia in combination with homozygous β thalassemia, leading to more balanced subunit synthesis. A milder clinical course is also seen in individuals who are doubly heterozygous for β thalassemia and hereditary persistence of Hb F. Patients with the preceding genotypes usually have moderately severe anemia but do not require transfusions.

Treatment of β thalassemia major includes supportive measures and, when feasible, bone marrow transplantation. The obvious benefits of transfusion therapy are partially offset by the risk of iron overload, alloimmunization, and transmission of infection. Despite these problems, children with Cooley's anemia fare better if their hemoglobin is maintained at greater than 90 g/L (9 g/dL). In view of the increased demands of the hyperplastic marrow, it is reasonable to maintain these patients on a daily supplement of folic acid. Since splenic sequestration contributes to shortened red blood cell survival, many patients derive some benefit from splenectomy. The prevention and treatment of iron overload are a continuing concern in these patients. Continuous subcutaneous injection of desferrioxamine permits the mobilization and excretion of significant amounts of iron and, when administered over a prolonged period, can prevent or retard the development of chronic iron toxicity.

Bone marrow transplantation provides definitive therapy in patients who have a histocompatible donor and access to a transplant facility. If the procedure is performed before the onset of iron-induced organ damage, about 80 percent of patients have disease-free long-term survival and can be considered cured.

Considerations of genetic counseling and antenatal diagnosis are as relevant in the *prevention* of β thalassemia major as they are for sickle cell anemia (see above). Prenatal diagnosis can usually be made by DNA analysis of amniotic fluid cells. However, in some cases it is necessary to take the risk of obtaining fetal red blood cells for globin chain synthesis measurements.

REFERENCES

ADAMS JG, HONIG GR: *Human Hemoglobin Genetics.* New York, Springer Verlag, 1986

BUNN HF, FORGET BG: *Hemoglobin: Molecular, Genetic and Clinical Aspects.* Philadelphia, Saunders, 1986

————: Sickle hemoglobin and other hemoglobin mutants, in *The Molecular Basis of Blood Diseases,* Stamatoyannopoulos G et al (eds). Philadelphia, Saunders, 1993

DABROW MB, WILKINS JC: Hematologic emergencies. Management of transfusion reactions and crises in sickle cell disease. Postgrad Med 93:183, 1993

EMBURY S: The clinical pathophysiology of sickle cell disease. Annu Rev Med 37:36, 1986

FORGET BG: The pathophysiology and molecular genetic of beta thalassemia. Mt Sinai J Med 60:95, 1993

HEBBEL RP: Beyond hemoglobin polymerization: The red blood cell membrane and sickle disease pathophysiology. Blood 77:214, 1991

KAZAZIAN HH: The thalassemia syndromes: Molecular basis and prenatal diagnosis in 1990 (review). Semin Hematol 27:209, 1990

LUCARELLI G et al: Bone marrow transplantation in patients with thalassemia. N Engl J Med 322:417, 1990

MANSOURI A, LURIE AA: Consise review: Methemoglobinemia. Am J Hematol 42:7, 1993

NAGEL RL, RANNEY HM: Genetic epidemiology of structural mutations of the β-globin gene. Semin Hematol 27:342, 1990

————, ROTH EF: Malaria and red cell genetic defects. Blood 74:1213, 1989

ROBINSON A: Sickle cell disease, the thalassemias, Tay-Sachs disease: Protein to gene. Can Med Assoc J 148:1481, 1993

WAYNE AS et al: Transfusion management of sickle cell disease. Blood 81:1109, 1993

307 HEMOLYTIC ANEMIAS

WENDELL ROSSE / H. FRANKLIN BUNN

Red blood cells normally survive 90 to 120 days in the circulation. Red cell life span may be shortened in a number of disorders, often resulting in anemia as the bone marrow is not able to adequately replenish the prematurely destroyed red cells. Hemolytic anemias are generally identified by the abnormality that brings about the premature destruction of the red cells. In this chapter we will describe the general attributes of this important group of anemias, the diagnostic procedures useful in identifying the causes of the accelerated red cell breakdown, and the pathogenesis and management of specific hemolytic disorders.

In many patients with hemolytic anemia, the diagnosis can be deduced from a careful history and physical examination. The patient often complains of fatigue and other symptoms of anemia (see Chap. 56). Less commonly, jaundice and even red-brown urine (hemoglobinuria) are reported. A complete drug history is often critical. The family history is especially helpful in the diagnosis of an inherited hemolytic anemia. The patient's physical examination provides equally useful information. Icterus and splenomegaly are encountered in a variety of hemolytic anemias. As discussed in detail in this chapter, a wide array of other historical and physical findings is associated with specific hemolytic anemias.

Laboratory tests may be used initially to demonstrate the presence of hemolysis (Table 307-1) and then to demonstrate the cause of hemolysis. Elevation of the reticulocyte count in the anemic patient is the single most useful indicator of hemolysis, reflecting erythroid hyperplasia of the bone marrow. Accordingly, biopsy of the bone marrow is often unnecessary. Reticulocytes are also elevated in patients with active blood loss, those with myelophthisis, and those who are recovering from suppression of erythropoiesis (see Chap. 56).

The morphology of the red cells as seen on the peripheral blood film is often abnormal and may provide evidence both of hemolysis and of its cause; the characteristic abnormalities and their associated causes and syndromes are listed in Table 307-2. While in no case can the peripheral blood smear be totally diagnostic by itself, in many cases it is a low-cost, important clue to the presence of hemolysis and to diagnosis.

Red blood cells may be lysed by their removal from the circulation by macrophages, particularly those of the spleen and liver (extravascular lysis), or less commonly by disruption of the membrane during their circulation (intravascular hemolysis). In intravascular hemolysis, the release of hemoglobin may result in hemoglobinuria. Both mechanisms result in increased heme catabolism and enhanced formation of the tetrapyrrole unconjugated bilirubin, which is normally metabolized by the liver by conjugation and subsequent excretion. As mentioned above, the plasma level of unconjugated bilirubin may be high enough to produce readily apparent jaundice. The unconjugated (indirect) bilirubin level can be further elevated by a commonly encountered defect in transport of bilirubin (Gilbert's

TABLE 307-1 Laboratory evaluation of hemolysis

	Moderate hemolysis (RBC life span 20–40 days)	Severe hemolysis (RBC life span 5–20 days)
HEMATOLOGIC		
Routine blood film	Polychromatophilia	Polychromatophilia
Reticulocyte count	↑	↑ ↑
Bone marrow examination	Erythroid hyperplasia	Erythroid hyperplasia
PLASMA OR SERUM		
Bilirubin	↑ Unconjugated	↑ Unconjugated
Haptoglobin	↓ , absent	Absent
Plasma hemoglobin	↑	↑ ↑
Lactate dehydrogenase	↑ (variable)	↑ ↑ (variable)
URINE		
Bilirubin	0	0
Hemosiderin	0, +	+
Hemoglobin	0	+ *

* Intravascular hemolysis.

TABLE 307-2 The value of red blood cell morphology in diagnosis of hemolytic anemia

Morphology	Cause	Syndromes
Spherocytes	Loss of membrane	Hereditary spherocytosis, autoimmune hemolytic anemia
Target cells	Increased ratio of red blood cell surface area to volume	Hemoglobin disorders: thalassemias, HbS, C, etc.; liver disease
Schistocytes	Traumatic disruption of membrane	Microangiopathic conditions, intravascular prostheses
Sickled cells	Polymerization of HbS	Sickle cell disease syndromes
Acanthocytes	?Abnormal membrane lipids	Severe liver disease (spur cell anemias)
Agglutinated cells	Presence of IgM antibody	Cold agglutinin disease
Heinz bodies	Precipitated hemoglobin	Unstable hemoglobin, oxidant stress

TABLE 307-3 Classifications of hemolytic anemias

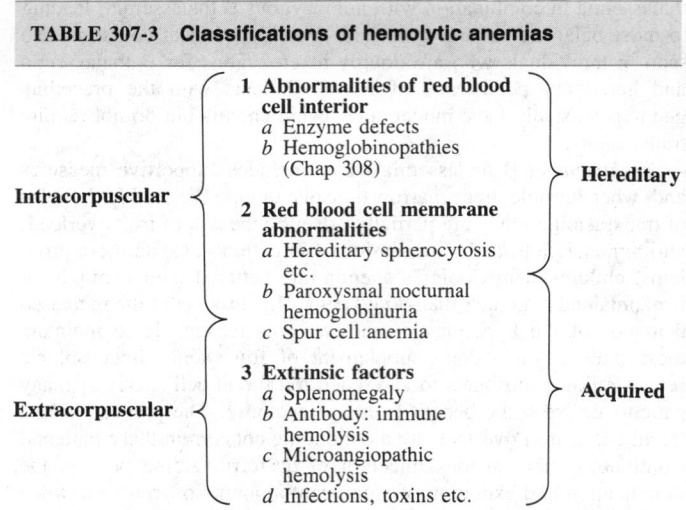

syndrome) (see Chap. 263). In patients with hemolysis, the level of unconjugated bilirubin never exceeds 70 to 85 μmol/L (4 to 5 mg/dL), unless liver function is impaired.

Other serum tests are also useful in the assessment of hemolysis. *Haptoglobin* is an alpha globulin which is present in high concentration (~1.0 g/L) in the plasma (and serum). It binds specifically and tightly to the protein (globin) in hemoglobin. The hemoglobin-haptoglobin complex is cleared within minutes by the mononuclear phagocyte system. Thus patients with significant hemolysis, either intravascular or extravascular, have low or absent levels of serum haptoglobin. Haptoglobin synthesis is decreased in patients with hepatocellular disease. Conversely, synthesis is enhanced in inflammatory states. These facts must be considered in the interpretation of serum haptoglobin. Plasma hemoglobin is increased in proportion to the degree of hemolysis but may be falsely elevated owing to lysis of red cells in vitro. Once the haptoglobin binding capacity of the plasma is exceeded, free hemoglobin permeates renal glomeruli. This filtered hemoglobin is reabsorbed by the proximal tubule, where it is catabolized in situ, and the heme iron is incorporated into storage proteins (ferritin and hemosiderin). The presence of hemosiderin in the urine, detected by staining the sediment with Prussian blue, indicates that a significant amount of circulating free hemoglobin has been filtered by the kidneys. When the absorptive capacity of the tubular cells is exceeded, hemoglobinuria ensues. The presence of hemoglobinuria indicates severe intravascular hemolysis. Sometimes the clinician is faced with the dilemma of whether benzidine-positive heme pigment in the urine is hemoglobin or myoglobin. The easiest way to distinguish between these alternatives is to examine an anticoagulated blood specimen after centrifugation. The plasma of patients with hemoglobinuria has a reddish brown color. Conversely, patients with myoglobinuria have normal-appearing plasma. Because of its higher molecular weight, hemoglobin has lower glomerular permeability than myoglobin and is less rapidly cleared by the kidneys.

CLASSIFICATION The hemolytic anemias can be conveniently grouped in three different ways, shown in Table 307-3. From an anatomic vantage point, the cause of accelerated red cell destruction can be regarded as either (1) a molecular defect (hemoglobinopathy or enzymopathy) inside the red cell, (2) an abnormality in membrane structure and function, or (3) an environmental factor such as mechanical trauma or an autoantibody. In *intracorpuscular* types of hemolysis, the patient's red cells have an abnormally short life span in a normal recipient (with a compatible blood type), while compatible normal red cells survive normally in the patient. The opposite is true in *extracorpuscular* types of hemolysis. Finally, as exemplified in the organization of the remainder of this chapter, hemolytic disorders can be conveniently classified as either inherited or acquired.

INHERITED HEMOLYTIC ANEMIAS

RED CELL MEMBRANE DISORDERS There are four types of inherited abnormalities of the red cell membrane: hereditary spherocytosis, hereditary elliptocytosis, hereditary pyropoikilocytosis, and hereditary stomatocytosis. A large body of information has recently been amassed on the molecular mechanisms underlying these disorders.

Hereditary spherocytosis Affected individuals have congenital hemolysis arising from a defect in one of the proteins in the red cell membrane leading to a decreased ratio of surface area to volume and consequently spherocytes. This disorder has an autosomal dominant inheritance pattern and an incidence of approximately 1:4500. In 20 percent of patients, the absence of hematologic abnormalities in family members suggests either autosomal recessive inheritance or a spontaneous mutation. The disorder is sometimes clinically apparent in early infancy but often escapes detection until adult life.

CLINICAL MANIFESTATIONS The major clinical features of hereditary spherocytosis are anemia, splenomegaly, and jaundice. The prominence of the last finding accounts for its prior designation "congenital hemolytic jaundice" and is due to an increased concentration of unconjugated (indirect-reacting) bilirubin in plasma. Jaundice may be intermittent and tends to be less pronounced in early childhood. Because of the increased bile pigment production, gallstones of pigment type are common, even in childhood. Compensatory normoblastic hyperplasia of the bone marrow occurs with the extension of red marrow into the midshafts of long bones and occasionally with extramedullary erythropoiesis, at times leading to the formation of paravertebral masses visible on chest x-ray. Because the bone marrow's capacity to increase erythropoiesis by six- to eightfold exceeds the usual rate of hemolysis in this disease, anemia is usually mild or moderate and may even be absent in an otherwise healthy individual. Compensation may be temporarily interrupted by episodes of erythroid hypoplasia precipitated by infections, particularly parvovirus. Splenomegaly is a very common finding in hereditary spherocytosis. The hemolytic rate may increase transiently during systemic infections which induce further splenic enlargement. Chronic leg ulcers, similar to those observed in sickle cell anemia, occur occasionally.

The characteristic erythrocyte abnormality is the spherocyte (Fig. A9-10). The mean corpuscular volume (MCV) is usually normal or slightly decreased, and the mean corpuscular hemoglobin concentration (MCHC) is increased to 350 to 380 g/L. Spheroidicity may be quantitatively assessed in terms of osmotic fragility (Fig. 307-1). Because spherocytes have a decreased surface area per unit volume, they lyse more readily when exposed to solutions of low salt

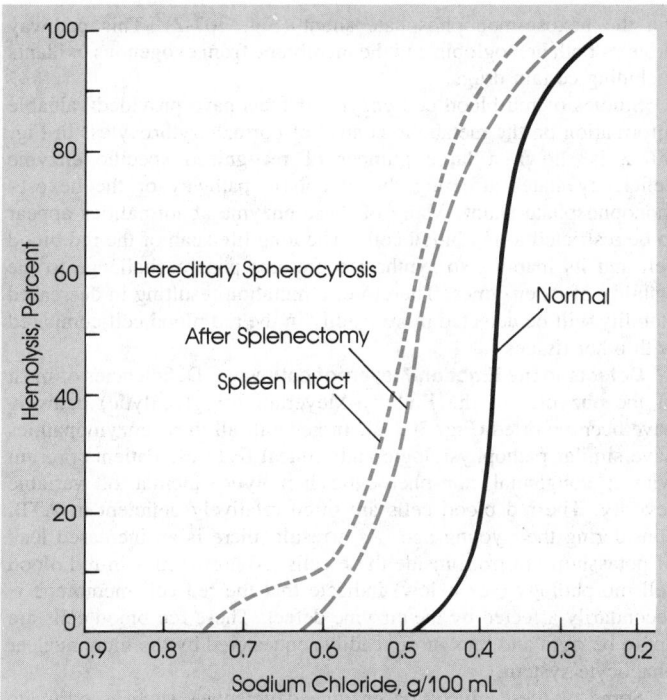

FIGURE 307-1 Osmotic fragility of red blood cells in hereditary spherocytosis. When the spleen is present, a small subpopulation of cells which are "conditioned" in the spleen form the fragile "tail" of the osmotic fragility curve. After splenectomy a single population exists which is more osmotically fragile than normal.

concentration. On microscopic examination, spherocytes are usually detected even when present in very small numbers. However, they will ordinarily not influence the osmotic fragility test unless they constitute more than 1 or 2 percent of the total cell population. A prominent increase in the osmotic fragility of red blood cells following sterile incubation of whole blood for 24 h at 37°C is also characteristic of hereditary spherocytosis. The autohemolysis test is an extension of this latter procedure and measures the amount of spontaneous hemolysis occurring after 48 h of sterile incubation. In hereditary spherocytosis, about 10 to 50 percent of the red blood cells are lysed (versus less than 4 percent of normal red blood cells). Autohemolysis of these red blood cells is largely prevented by the addition of glucose prior to incubation.

PATHOGENESIS   The molecular abnormality in hereditary spherocytosis involves the proteins of the cytoskeleton. Nearly all patients have a significant deficiency of spectrin which is often secondary to the inherited molecular defect and correlates with the severity of the anemia. Many patients have a decrease and/or a structural abnormality in ankyrin, the protein that links spectrin to protein 3 (see Fig. 302-6). Other molecular defects include decreased production of spectrin and impaired assembly of spectrin with protein 4.1. The spheroidal contour and rigid structure of the red blood cells impede their passage through the spleen. There, the red blood cells are exposed to an environment in which their increased metabolic rate cannot be sustained. The first injury imposed on them by the spleen is a further loss of surface membrane. This "conditioning" produces a subpopulation of hyperspheroidal red blood cells in the peripheral blood. These are subsequently destroyed in the spleen.

DIAGNOSIS   Hereditary spherocytosis must be distinguished from the spherocytic hemolytic anemias associated with red blood cell antibodies. The family history is helpful, when present. The diagnosis of immune spherocytosis is usually readily established by a positive direct Coombs test. Spherocytes, often in considerable numbers, are seen in association with hemolysis induced by splenomegaly in

patients with cirrhosis or chronic infections, and a few spherocytes are seen in the course of a wide variety of hemolytic disorders, particularly glucose-6-phosphate dehydrogenase (G6PD) deficiency.

TREATMENT AND PROGNOSIS   Splenectomy reliably corrects the anemia, although the red blood cell defect persists. The operative risk is low. Red blood cell survival after splenectomy is normal or nearly so. Rare relapses have been reported and are probably attributable to postoperative growth of splenic autotransplants or to hyperplasia of secondary spleens which were overlooked at operation. Because of the potential for gallstones and for episodes of bone marrow hypoplasia or hemolytic crises, splenectomy should be performed in individuals in whom the disease causes symptoms. Splenectomy in children should be postponed until age 4, if possible. Beyond age 3, severe infections following splenectomy in hereditary spherocytosis are rare. Nonetheless, polyvalent pneumococcal vaccine should be administered to all patients who are to undergo splenectomy. Because of the increased requirement for folic acid in patients with hemolysis, they sometimes become deficient in this vitamin. Therapy with folic acid may result in an increased hemoglobin level.

Hereditary elliptocytosis and hereditary pyropoikilocytosis
Red blood cells of oval or elliptic shape are normally found in birds, reptiles, camels, and llamas; however, they occur in appreciable numbers in humans only in *hereditary elliptocytosis*, a disorder which is transmitted as an autosomal dominant and affects 1 per 4000 to 5000 of the population, a frequency similar to that of hereditary spherocytosis. In most affected individuals, a structural abnormality of erythrocyte spectrin leads to impaired assembly. Others often have a deficiency of erythrocyte membrane protein 4.1, which is important in stabilizing the interaction of spectrin and actin in the cytoskeleton (see Fig. 302-6). Homozygotes with total absence of this protein have more marked hemolysis. In Southeast Asia there is a high incidence of hereditary ovalocytosis, in which a partial deletion of protein 3 confers resistance against malaria.

The great majority of patients manifest only mild hemolysis, with hemoglobin levels above 120 g/L, reticulocytes less than 4 percent, depressed haptoglobin levels, and red blood cell survivals just under the normal range. In 10 to 15 percent of patients, the rate of hemolysis is substantially increased, with chromium half-survival times of red blood cells as short as 5 days and reticulocytes ranging to 20 percent. Hemoglobin levels rarely fall below 90 to 100 g/L. Red blood cell destruction occurs predominantly in the spleen, which is enlarged in patients with overt hemolysis, and hemolysis is corrected by splenectomy.

In both the anemic and nonanemic varieties of this disorder the red blood cells are normochromic and normocytic. At least 25 percent and, more commonly, greater than 75 percent of red blood cells are elliptic, with an axial ratio (width/length) of less than 0.78. Patients with hemolysis frequently have microovalocytes, bizarre-shaped red blood cells, and red cell fragments, all of which increase in number following splenectomy. The degree of hemolysis does not correlate with the percentage of elliptocytes. Osmotic fragility is usually normal but may be increased in patients with overt hemolysis.

Hereditary pyropoikilocytosis (HPP) is related to hereditary elliptocytosis, since both have been encountered in the same family. HPP is a rare disorder characterized by bizarre-shaped, microcytic red cells which undergo disruption at temperatures of 44 to 45°C (in contrast to the normal thermal instability at 49°C). This results from an abnormality of spectrin self-assembly. Hemolysis, which is usually severe, is recognized in childhood and is partially responsive to splenectomy.

Hereditary stomatocytosis   Stomatocytes are red blood cells having a slitlike central zone of pallor on dried smears. The syndrome of hereditary hemolytic anemia and stomatocytic red blood cells is inherited in an autosomal dominant pattern. Two major red blood cell defects have been delineated in this syndrome. First, the red blood cells have an increased permeability to sodium and potassium, which is compensated for by an increased active transport of these cations. Second, red cells have an increased surface area associated with an

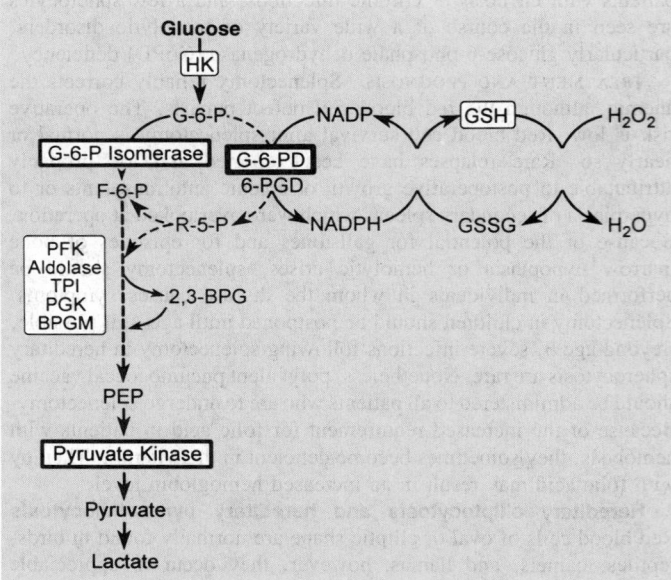

FIGURE 307-2 Metabolic pathways in the red blood cell. The glycolytic pathway from glucose to lactate is outlined vertically on the left. The pentose phosphate pathway is shown on the upper right. Dashed arrows indicate multiple reaction steps. Enzyme deficiency states in order of prevalence: glucose-6-phosphate dehydrogenase (G6PD) >>> pyruvate kinase > glucose-6-phosphate (G-6-P) isomerase > rare deficiency states reported in occasional families and enclosed here in lightly outlined boxes. These include deficiencies in hexokinase (HK), phosphofructokinase (PFK), aldolase, triose phosphate isomerase (TPI), phosphoglycerate kinase (PGK), and 2,3-BPG mutase (BPGM), and in the enzymes involved in the synthesis of glutathione. Other abbreviations: H_2O_2, hydrogen peroxide; GSH and GSSG, reduced and oxidized glutathione, respectively; NADP and NADPH, oxidized and reduced pyridine nucleotide, respectively; 6-PGD, 6-phosphogluconate dehydrogenase; R-5-P, ribose-5-phosphate; F-6-P, fructose-6-phosphate; 2,3-BPG, 2,3-bisphosphoglycerate; PEP, phosphoenol pyruvate. (*Courtesy of Donald Paglia.*)

increase in membrane lipid content, particularly phosphatidylcholine. In some patients, the red blood cell is swollen with an excess of ions and water and a decreased mean corpuscular hemoglobin concentration (overhydrated stomatocytes, "hydrocytosis"); in other patients, the red cell is shrunken with a decreased ion and water content and an increased mean corpuscular hemoglobin concentration (dehydrated stomatocytes, "desiccytosis"). Those patients in whom the red blood cells are overhydrated have true stomatocytes on dried smears. Dehydrated stomatocytes assume the morphology of target cells on dried smears. In both instances, red blood cells are cup- or bowl-shaped when examined in wet preparation. Osmotic fragility is increased in overhydrated stomatocytes and decreased in underhydrated stomatocytes. Autohemolysis is increased and is corrected by glucose.

Most patients have splenomegaly and mild anemia. Splenectomy decreases but does not totally correct the hemolytic process. Its indications are similar to those for hereditary spherocytosis.

RED CELL ENZYME DEFECTS During its maturation, the red blood cell loses its nucleus, ribosomes, and mitochondria and thus its capability for protein synthesis and oxidative phosphorylation. The mature circulating red blood cell has a relatively simple pattern of intermediary metabolism (Fig. 307-2) in keeping with its modest metabolic obligations. As discussed in Chap. 302, some ATP must be generated from the Embden-Meyerhof pathway to drive the cation pump which maintains the ionic milieu within the red blood cell. Smaller amounts of energy are needed for the preservation of hemoglobin iron in the ferrous (Fe^{2+}) state, and perhaps for the renewal of the lipids in the red blood cell membrane. About 10 percent of the glucose consumed by the red blood cell is metabolized

via the hexose-monophosphate shunt (Fig. 307-2). This pathway protects both hemoglobin and the membrane from exogenous oxidants including certain drugs.

Studies of red blood cell enzyme defects have provided valuable information on the metabolic control of normal erythrocytes. In Fig. 307-2 is shown a large number of recognized specific enzyme deficiency states affecting the glycolytic pathway or the hexose-monophosphate shunt. Many of these enzyme abnormalities appear to be restricted to red blood cells. The long life span of the red blood cell and its inability to synthesize proteins pose a challenge to the stability of its enzymes. Therefore, a mutation resulting in decreased stability will be detected more readily in the red blood cell compared with other tissues.

Defects in the Embden-Meyerhof pathway Deficiencies of most of the enzymes of the Embden-Meyerhof (or glycolytic) pathway have been reported (Fig. 307-2). In general, all these enzymopathies have similar pathophysiologic and clinical features. Patients present with a congenital nonspherocytic hemolytic anemia of variable severity. The red blood cells are often relatively deficient in ATP, considering their young age. As a result, there is an increased leak of potassium ion from inside these cells. Abnormalities in red blood cell morphology (see below) indicate that the red cell membrane is secondarily affected by the enzyme defect. These red blood cells are apt to be rigid and thus more readily sequestered by the mononuclear phagocyte system.

Some of these glycolytic enzyme deficiencies such as pyruvate kinase (PK) deficiency and hexokinase deficiency are localized to the red blood cell, with no apparent metabolic abnormality in leukocytes or other cells that have been studied. In other disorders, the enzyme deficiency is more widespread. Glucose phosphate isomerase deficiency and phosphoglycerate kinase deficiency also involve leukocytes, although affected individuals have no apparent abnormalities of white blood cell function. Individuals with deficiency of triose phosphate isomerase have decreased levels of enzyme in leukocytes, muscle cells, and central nervous system fluid. Furthermore, they have a progressive neurologic disorder. Some patients with phosphofructokinase deficiency have a myopathy.

Among the reported defects of glycolytic enzymes, about 95 percent are due to PK deficiency and about 4 percent are due to glucose phosphate isomerase deficiency. The remainder, shown in Fig. 307-2, are extremely rare. Most have been encountered in isolated families. There is considerable variability in the clinical manifestations and laboratory findings among reported cases of PK deficiency. This is probably due to the fact that a number of different PK variants have been reported. This heterogeneity probably also applies to the other less common glycolytic enzyme defects. Accordingly, the clinical manifestations of these disorders are quite variable.

GENETICS Most of the glycolytic enzyme defects are inherited in an autosomal recessive pattern. Thus the parents of affected patients are heterozygotes. Heterozygotes generally possess half-normal levels of enzyme activity which are more than adequate for normal metabolic function. Thus these individuals are entirely asymptomatic. Since the gene frequency for this group of enzymopathies is low, it is not surprising that true homozygotes are often the offspring of a consanguineous mating. Alternatively, affected individuals may be compound heterozygotes, inheriting an abnormal allele from each parent. Phosphoglycerate kinase deficiency is inherited as a sex-linked disorder. Affected males have a severe hemolytic anemia, while female carriers may have a mild hemolytic process.

CLINICAL MANIFESTATIONS Patients with severe hemolysis usually present during early childhood with anemia, icterus, and splenomegaly. Other stigmata of chronic hemolysis are occasionally seen. Occasionally, siblings are similarly affected.

LABORATORY FINDINGS Patients have a normocytic (or slightly macrocytic), normochromic anemia with reticulocytosis. In those with PK deficiency, bizarre erythrocytes are noted on the peripheral smear with large numbers of spiculated red blood cells. Spherocytes are usually infrequent or absent. Hence the term *congenital nonsphero-*

cytic hemolytic anemia has been applied to these disorders. Unlike hereditary spherocytosis, the osmotic fragility of freshly drawn blood is usually normal. Incubation brings out an osmotically fragile population of red blood cells.

The diagnosis of this group of anemias depends on specific enzymatic assays. An abnormality in enzyme kinetics may be demonstrated. In addition, differences in electrophoretic mobility, pH optimum, or heat stability may be noted. This information is useful in documenting heterogeneity among enzyme variants. The molecular defects of some PK variants have been identified at the DNA level.

TREATMENT   Most patients do not require therapy. Those with severe hemolysis should be given a daily supplement of folic acid (1 mg/d). Blood transfusions may be necessary during a hypoplastic crisis. Patients with PK deficiency may benefit from splenectomy. Because of their enzymatic defect, the younger cells (reticulocytes) depend on mitochondrial respiration rather than glycolysis for maintenance of ATP. However, in the hypoxic environment of the spleen, aerobic metabolism is curtailed and the ATP-depleted cells are destroyed in situ. Following splenectomy, patients with PK deficiency often have a marked increase in circulating reticulocytes. Patients with deficiency of glucose phosphate isomerase also may improve by splenectomy. There is not sufficient information to indicate whether this operation would help individuals with other glycolytic enzymopathies.

Defects in the hexose-monophosphate shunt   The normal red blood cell is well endowed to protect itself against oxidant stress. Upon exposure to an offending drug or toxin, the amount of glucose that is metabolized via the hexose-monophosphate shunt is increased severalfold. In this way reduced glutathione is regenerated, protecting the sulfhydryl groups of hemoglobin and the red blood cell membrane from oxidation. Individuals with an inherited defect in the hexose-monophosphate shunt are unable to maintain an adequate level of reduced glutathione in their red blood cells. As a result, hemoglobin sulfhydryl groups become oxidized, and the hemoglobin tends to precipitate within the red blood cell forming Heinz bodies.

Among the congenital shunt defects, by far the most common is *G6PD deficiency*. It affects more than 200 million people throughout the world. Like the glycolytic enzymopathies, there is considerable genetic heterogeneity among affected individuals. Indeed, over 400 variants of G6PD have been described. Abnormalities in primary DNA or protein sequence have been established in about 30 of the G6PD variants. The remainder are presumed to have abnormal structure because of differences in electrophoretic mobility, enzyme kinetics, pH optimum, and heat stability. Like many of the hemoglobin variants, some G6PD mutants were discovered by chance and are not associated with any significant functional abnormalities. The normal G6PD is designated as type B. About 20 percent of blacks have a G6PD (designated A+) which differs electrophoretically but is functionally normal. Among the clinically significant G6PD variants, the most common is the so-called A− type encountered primarily in blacks who originated from central Africa. The A− G6PD has the same electrophoretic mobility as the A+ type, but it is unstable and has abnormal kinetic properties. Like the HbS gene, the A− type of G6PD may confer protection against malaria. This variant is found in about 11 percent of black males in the United States. A second relatively common G6PD variant is encountered among peoples of the eastern Mediterranean area, particularly Sephardic Jews. A third relatively common variant occurs in the Chinese.

The G6PD gene is located on the X chromosome. Thus the deficiency state is a sex-linked trait. Affected males (hemizygotes) inherit the abnormal gene from their mothers who are usually carriers (heterozygotes). Because of inactivation of one of the two X chromosomes (Lyon hypothesis; see Chap. 60), the heterozygote has two populations of red blood cells: normal and deficient in G6PD. Most female carriers are asymptomatic. Those who happen to have a high proportion of deficient cells resemble the male hemizygotes.

G6PD activity normally declines about 50 percent during the 120-day life span of the red blood cell. This decay is moderately accelerated

TABLE 307-4   Drugs causing hemolysis in subjects deficient in G6PD

Antimalarials: Primaquine, pamaquine, dapsone
Sulfonamides: Sulfamethoxazole
Nitrofurantoin
Analgesics: Acetanilid
Miscellaneous: Vitamin K (water-soluble form), doxorubicin, methylene blue, nalidixic acid, furazolidone, niridazole, phenazopyridine

in A− red blood cells and markedly so in red blood cells containing the Mediterranean variant. Individuals with the A− variant may have a slightly shortened red blood cell survival, but they are not anemic. Clinical problems arise only when the affected individual is subjected to some type of environmental stress. Most often, hemolytic episodes are triggered by viral and bacterial infections. The mechanism for this is unknown. In addition, drugs or toxins which pose an oxidant threat to the red blood cell cause hemolysis in individuals deficient in G6PD (Table 307-4). Of these, sulfa drugs, antimalarials, and nitrofurantoin are most commonly incriminated. Although aspirin is frequently mentioned as a likely offender, it has no deleterious effect in A− individuals. Accidental ingestion of toxic compounds such as naphthalene (found in moth balls) may cause severe hemolysis. Finally, metabolic acidosis can precipitate an episode of hemolysis in subjects deficient in G6PD.

CLINICAL AND LABORATORY FEATURES   The patient may experience an acute hemolytic crisis within hours of exposure to the oxidant stress. In severe cases, hemoglobinuria and peripheral vascular collapse can develop. Since only the older population of red blood cells is rapidly destroyed, the hemolytic crisis is usually self-limited, even if the exposure to the oxidant continues. Among black males with the A− variant, the red cell mass decreases by a maximum of 25 to 30 percent. During the period of acute hemolysis, a rapid drop in hematocrit is accompanied by a rise in plasma hemoglobin and unconjugated bilirubin and a decrease in plasma haptoglobin. The oxidation of hemoglobin leads to the formation of Heinz bodies, visualized by means of a supravital stain such as crystal violet. However, Heinz bodies are usually not seen after the first day or so, since these inclusions are readily removed by the spleen. Their removal leads to the formation of "bite cells," red cells which have lost a peripheral portion of the cell. Multiple bites cause the formation of fragments. Small numbers of spherocytes also may be present.

Individuals with the *Mediterranean type G6PD* have a more unstable enzyme and, therefore, a much lower overall enzyme activity than blacks with the A− variant. As a result, they have more severe clinical manifestations. Some have a chronic hemolytic anemia, even in the absence of any exposure to oxidants. A minority of patients are exquisitely sensitive to fava beans and will develop a fulminant hemolytic crisis following exposure. Sensitivity to *Vicia fava* is a poorly understood phenomenon that appears to be determined by a separate gene. Favism is not encountered in blacks with the A− variant. Individuals with the Mediterranean variant sometimes have a temporary episode of hemolysis during the newborn period.

The *diagnosis* of G6PD deficiency should be considered in any individual, particularly a black male, who experiences an acute hemolytic episode. The patient should be thoroughly questioned about possible exposure to oxidant agents. A number of screening tests are available to establish the diagnosis. However, since the deficiency occurs primarily in older red blood cells, a false-negative test may be seen during a hemolytic episode when there is a high proportion of young red blood cells. It may be necessary to repeat these diagnostic tests after the patient has recovered. Unusual features in the case should prompt further investigation, including a more complete and specific characterization of the enzyme.

TREATMENT   Since hemolysis in patients deficient in A− G6PD is usually self-limited, no specific treatment is necessary. Splenectomy does not appear to be of benefit to Mediterranean patients with chronic hemolysis. Blood transfusions are rarely indicated. If a patient develops a severe hemolytic episode with hemoglobinuria, maintaining adequate urine output is important.

Attention should be directed toward the *prevention* of hemolytic episodes. Infections ought to be treated promptly. Subjects deficient in G6PD should be warned about risks posed by oxidant drugs and fava beans. Any black patient about to be given an oxidant drug should be screened for G6PD deficiency.

OTHER DEFECTS OF THE HEXOSE-MONOPHOSPHATE SHUNT   A few kindreds have been found to have congenital deficiency in red blood cell glutathione due to a defect in either of the two enzymes responsible for the synthesis of this tripeptide. Affected individuals have a hemolytic anemia with Heinz bodies that is aggravated by oxidant drugs. Deficiency of glutathione reductase has been reported, but its relationship to clinically significant hemolysis is not well established. Sometimes the deficiency state can be corrected by the administration of riboflavin (5 mg/d). There are also isolated reports of deficiencies of glutathione peroxidase and 6-phosphogluconate dehydrogenase, but again, their association with hemolysis is uncertain.

Other enzyme defects   Hemolytic anemia may sometimes be caused by abnormalities in enzymes of nucleotide metabolism. A growing number of individuals with pyrimidine 5'-nucleotidase deficiency have been encountered. Their red cells have marked basophilic stippling. Hemolytic anemia also has been noted in individuals whose red blood cells have supranormal levels of adenosine deaminase and relatively low levels of ATP.

HEMOGLOBINOPATHIES   The sickling disorders constitute an important form of congenital hemolytic anemia. Less commonly, hemolysis may be due to the inheritance of an unstable hemoglobin variant. These disorders of hemoglobin are discussed in Chap. 306.

ACQUIRED HEMOLYTIC ANEMIAS

In patients with acquired hemolytic anemia, red cells are made normally but are prematurely destroyed because of damage acquired in the circulation; the single exception is rare disorders characterized by acquired dysplasia of the cells of the bone marrow and the production of structurally and functionally abnormal red cells. The damage that occurs may be mediated by antibodies or toxins that mark the cell for premature death or may be due to vicissitudes encountered during the circulation, including an overactive reticuloendothelial system or traumatic lysis by natural or artificial impediments to smooth circulation.

SPLENOMEGALY AND HYPERSPLENISM   The spleen is particularly efficient in trapping and destroying red blood cells which have minimal defects, often so mild as to be undetectable by in vitro techniques. This unique ability of the spleen to filter mildly damaged red blood cells results from its unusual vascular anatomy. Almost all the blood circulating through the spleen flows rapidly from arterioles in the white pulp to sinuses in the spleen's red pulp and then into the venous system. In contrast, a small portion of splenic blood flow (normally 1 to 2 percent) leaves the arterioles of the white pulp to enter a nonendothelial portion of the spleen. In this sense, it is extravascular, although the entire spleen may be considered as a specialized part of the vascular system. This blood passes into the "marginal zone" of the lymphatic white pulp. Although the cells which occupy this zone are not phagocytic, they serve as a mechanical filter that hinders the progress of severely damaged blood cells. As red blood cells leave this zone and enter the red pulp, they flow into narrow cords which end blindly but which communicate with sinuses through small openings between the lining cells of the sinuses. These openings, averaging 3 μm in diameter, test the ability of red blood cells to undergo a deformation of shape. Red blood cells which do not pass the stringent test imposed on them by the spleen filter are engulfed by phagocytic cells and destroyed.

The normal spleen poses no threat to normal red blood cells until they become senescent. However, splenomegaly exaggerates the adverse conditions to which red blood cells are exposed. Splenic enlargement may be considered in three broad categories. In the first are infiltrative diseases (such as myeloproliferative disorders; Chap. 309), lymphomas (Chap. 311), and storage diseases such as Gaucher's disease; (Chap. 349). In the second are systemic inflammatory diseases leading to splenic hypertrophy. In the third are diseases which cause congestive splenomegaly, particularly cirrhosis of the liver and thrombosis of the splenic, portal, or hepatic veins. Hemolysis may occur whenever the spleen is enlarged. Its occurrence is least predictable in infiltrative diseases of the spleen, where substantial splenomegaly may exist with no apparent hemolysis. Inflammatory and congestive splenomegaly is commonly associated with mild to moderate shortening of red blood cell survival, along with granulocytopenia and thrombocytopenia (hypersplenism). Patients with cytopenia(s) sufficient to produce symptoms generally benefit from splenectomy.

IMMUNOLOGIC CAUSES OF HEMOLYSIS   Immune hemolysis in the adult may be induced by three general types of antibodies:

1 Alloantibodies acquired by blood transfusions or pregnancies and directed against transfused red blood cells (Chap. 312).
2 Antibodies (usually IgG) reactive at body temperature and directed against the patient's own red blood cells (Table 307-5).
3 Antibodies (usually IgM) reactive in cold and directed against the patient's own red blood cells (Table 307-5).

The Coombs antiglobulin test is the major tool for diagnosing these disorders. This test relies on the ability of antibodies prepared in animals or by hybridomas and directed against specific human serum proteins to agglutinate red blood cells if these human serum proteins are present on the red blood cell surface. The serum proteins of particular interest are IgG and C3. The ability of anti-IgG or anti-C3 antisera to agglutinate the patient's red blood cells is referred to as the *direct Coombs test*. The presence or absence of IgG or C3 may give important information about the origin of the immune hemolytic anemia (see Table 307-5). Rarely, neither IgG nor complement may be found on the red cells of the patient (Coombs-negative immune hemolytic anemia).

At times, it may be important to demonstrate antibody in the serum of the patient by reacting the serum with normal red cells. IgM antibodies (usually cold-reacting) may be detected by agglutination of normal or fetal red cells. IgG antibodies may be directed by the *indirect Coombs test*, in which the serum of the patient is incubated with normal red cells and antibody is detected with anti-IgG as in the direct Coombs test.

"Warm" antibodies   Antibodies that react with protein antigens usually are IgG and react at body temperature; occasionally, they are IgA. This acquired syndrome is frequently designated *autoimmune hemolytic anemia, warm antibody type*. In recent years, as a number of drugs which induce this clinical syndrome have become recognized, attention has focused on the exogenous factors which may underlie the formation of these red blood cell antibodies, and the expression *immunohemolytic anemia* is preferred.

Clinical manifestations   Immunohemolytic anemia induced by warm-reacting IgG antibody occurs at all ages but is more common

---

TABLE 307-5   Use of the direct Coombs test in diagnosing the cause of autoimmune hemolytic anemia

Reaction with:

Anti-IgG	Anti-C3	Causes
Yes	No	Antibodies to Rh protein, hemolysis caused by α-methyldopa or penicillin; not seen in SLE
Yes	No	Antibodies to glycoprotein antigens, SLE
No	Yes	Cold-reacting antibodies (agglutinins or Donath-Landsteiner antibody), most drug-related antibodies, IgM antibodies, IgG antibodies of low affinity, activation of complement by immune complexes

in adults, particularly women and older individuals. In approximately one-fourth of patients this disorder occurs as a complication of an underlying disease affecting the immune system, especially chronic lymphocytic leukemia, non-Hodgkin's lymphoma, and systemic lupus erythematosus (SLE) (Table 307-6). Occasionally, immunohemolytic anemia is seen in patients with advanced, active Hodgkin's disease. Case reports link it to a variety of nonlymphoid neoplasms.

The presentation and course of IgG immunohemolytic anemia are quite variable. In its mildest form, the only manifestation is a positive direct Coombs test. In this instance, insufficient antibody is present on the red blood cell surface to permit the reticuloendothelial system to recognize the cell as abnormal. This is particularly common in SLE. A large fraction of patients with immunohemolytic anemia have a chronic mild anemia and splenomegaly. In other cases this disorder may be more severe, with hemoglobin levels less than 70 g/L and reticulocyte counts of 30 percent and higher. Spherocytosis is usually marked (Fig. A9-11). Both the direct and indirect Coombs tests may be positive. In its most severe form, immunohemolytic anemia presents with fulminant, overwhelming hemolysis associated with hemoglobinemia, hemoglobinuria, and shock, a syndrome which may be fatal.

Associated findings include hyperbilirubinemia, decreased or absent haptoglobin levels, splenomegaly, and occasionally hepatomegaly. Thrombocytopenia also may be present. The coexistence of immune destruction of red blood cells and platelets is referred to as *Evans' syndrome*, a disorder in which separate antibodies are directed against platelets and red blood cells. Occasionally, venous thrombosis occurs.

Pathogenesis   IgG antibodies bring about the destruction of the cells by two mechanisms: (1) immune adherence of red cells to destructive cells of the immune system mediated by the antibody itself and by complement components that become fixed to the membrane and (2) completion of the complement sequence, resulting in rupture of the membrane. In IgG-mediated immune adherence, the affixed antibody reacts with Fc receptors on macrophages; this binds the target to the destroyer and activates phagocytic processes that internalize the target, destroying it. Complement-mediated immune adherence is mediated by C3b and C4b interacting with a series of receptors on the macrophage; this is much less likely to lead to destruction of the target by itself but markedly increases the immune adherence due to IgG. Immune adherence is also enhanced by the peculiar circulation of the spleen, which brings cells into intimate contact with phagocytic cells. If internalization is only partial, membrane is preferentially removed; this results in the formation of spherocytes. These spherocytes are not able to pass through the fenestrations in the wall of the splenic sinus and thus accumulate in the spleen, where they are destroyed.

TABLE 307-6   Hemolysis due to antibodies

WARM-ANTIBODY IMMUNOHEMOLYTIC ANEMIA

A Idiopathic
B Lymphomas: Chronic lymphocytic leukemia, non-Hodgkin's lymphomas, Hodgkin's disease (infrequent)
C Systemic lupus erythematosus and other collagen-vascular diseases
D Drugs
   1 α-Methyldopa type
   2 Penicillin type (stable hapten)
   3 Quinidine type (unstable hapten)
E Post-viral infections
F Other tumors (rare)

COLD-ANTIBODY IMMUNOHEMOLYTIC ANEMIA

A Cold agglutinin disease
   1 Acute: *Mycoplasma* infection, infectious mononucleosis
   2 Chronic: Idiopathic, lymphoma
B Paroxysmal cold hemoglobinuria

Lysis by the direct lytic action of complement does not commonly occur because the mechanisms for the down-regulation of its activation are so effective that insufficient sequences are completed to breach the cell membrane.

Therapy and prognosis   In the initial evaluation of the patient, it is important to be sure that drugs which are known to cause immunohemolytic anemia are not involved. This topic is discussed below.

Patients having a mild degree of hemolysis usually do not require therapy. In those with clinically significant hemolysis, initial therapy consists of glucocorticoids (e.g., prednisone, 1.0 mg/kg per day). A rise in hemoglobin is frequently noted within 3 or 4 days and occurs in most patients within 1 week. Prednisone is continued until the hemoglobin level has risen to normal values, and thereafter it is tapered slowly over the course of several months. More than 75 percent of patients will achieve an initial significant and sustained reduction in hemolysis; however, in half these patients the disease will relapse either during the period of steroid tapering or following the cessation of steroid therapy. Steroids appear to have two modes of action: an immediate effect due to inhibition of the clearance of IgG-coated red blood cells by the mononuclear phagocyte system and a later effect due to steroid-induced inhibition of antibody synthesis.

Patients with severe anemia may require blood transfusions. Because the antibody in this disease is a "panagglutinin," reacting with nearly all normal donor cells, the usual cross matching is impossible. The goal in selecting blood for transfusion is to avoid administering red cells with antigens to which patients have previously been sensitized and which are known to be associated with complement lysis and intravascular hemolysis. In addition to A and B, Kell, Kidd (Jk^a), and Duffy (Fy) account for almost all examples of this type of hemolysis. A common procedure is to adsorb the panagglutinin present in patient's serum using the patient's own red cells from which antibody has been eluted previously. Serum freed of autoantibody in this way can then be tested for the presence of alloantibody to specific donor blood groups. ABO-compatible red cells matched in this fashion are administered slowly, with attention paid to the possibility of an immediate-type transfusion reaction.

Splenectomy is the second line of therapy in immune hemolytic anemia due to IgG. It is recommended for patients who cannot tolerate or fail to respond to steroid therapy. To provide prophylaxis against pneumococcal infection, a risk in splenectomized individuals, patients should be immunized with polyvalent pneumococcal antiserum.

Patients who have been refractory to steroid therapy and to splenectomy have been treated with immunosuppressive drugs. The greatest experience is with azathioprine and cyclophosphamide. A variable success rate has been reported with each. Intravenous gamma globulin may be used when rapid cessation of hemolysis is required. However, it is not nearly as effective in this disorder as it is in immune thrombocytopenia.

In the majority of patients, this disease is controlled by steroid therapy alone, by splenectomy, or by a combination. In most of the remaining patients, a partial degree of control is achieved. Fatalities occur among three categories: (1) rare patients with overwhelming hemolysis in whom death is directly attributable to anemia, (2) those with major thrombotic events coincident with active hemolysis, and (3) those whose host defenses are impaired by glucocorticoids, splenectomy, and/or immunosuppressives. In patients in whom immunohemolysis develops as a complication of an underlying disorder, the prognosis is dominated by that of the primary disease.

Immunohemolytic anemia secondary to drugs   Drugs which have been directly implicated in immunohemolytic anemia are of two kinds, as distinguished by their mechanisms of action: (1) drugs, such as α-methyldopa, an antihypertensive (Chap. 209), that induce a disorder identical almost in every respect to the warm-antibody immunohemolytic anemia described above, and (2) drugs that can become associated with the red blood cell surface and induce the formation of an antibody directed against the red blood cell–drug complex. The association of drug and glycoprotein may be relatively tight, as in the case of penicillin, or relatively loose, as in the case of quinidine.

A positive direct Coombs test is observed in up to 10 percent of patients receiving α-methyldopa therapy in a dose of 2.0 g/d. A small minority of these patients develop spherocytosis and hemolysis, often of severe degree. This "autoimmune" disorder is probably due to the fact that α-methyldopa alters the protein(s) bearing the Rh antigens so that the drug becomes immunogenic; the resulting antibodies cross-react with the normal Rh protein. Thus the antibody does not react with the drug, and the indirect Coombs test is positive even when the drug is not added to the test. Two distinctive features are that the indirect Coombs test is positive in almost all patients with hemolysis and that the red cells are coated with IgG but not C3. Hemolysis decreases over the course of several weeks after cessation of drug therapy, although the direct Coombs test may remain positive for more than 1 year.

In most other cases when a drug induces an immune hemolytic reaction, the antibody is directed against the combination of the drug and the membrane glycoprotein to which it is attached. Therefore, the indirect Coombs test is not positive unless the drug is added to reaction mixture. Further, the hemolytic reaction in vivo is also dependent on the presence of the drug and usually ceases shortly after the drug has been discontinued. Penicillin and its congeners may cause this type of reaction if the drug is given in very high doses (10 million units per day or more). The drug adheres relatively firmly to the glycoprotein of the red cell membrane. The hemolysis in vivo is usually not severe. Since the antibody is usually IgG, spherocytosis and splenic destruction may occur. Most other drugs do not adhere as tightly to their glycoprotein, and they and the antibodies that they have generated are removed during the washing steps of the Coombs reaction. Most of these antibodies are able to fix complement (especially those which are IgM), and these components remain on the red cell surface; thus the direct Coombs test is positive with anti-C3 but not anti-IgG. Again, the antibody is detected in the *indirect* Coombs test only when the drug is added to the incubation mixture. Hemolysis may be quite severe, sometimes resulting in signs of intravascular hemolysis; resolution is usually prompt after the drug is discontinued. In addition to quinine and quinidine, a number of drugs, including sulfonamides, sulfonureas, phenacetin, stibophen, and dipyrone, have been shown to cause this reaction.

Immune hemolysis due to cold-reactive antibodies   Antibodies that react with polysaccharide antigens are usually IgM and react better at lower temperatures, hence the name *cold-reactive antibodies*. The clinical manifestations associated with IgM antibodies (the more common cold agglutinins) differ from those associated with IgG antibodies, the relatively uncommon Donath-Landsteiner antibody of paroxysmal cold hemoglobinuria.

Cold agglutinins arise in two clinical settings: (1) monoclonal antibodies as the product of lymphocytic neoplasia and (2) polyclonal antibodies in a response to infection. In many elderly patients, the "neoplasm" is benign monoclonal gammopathy, and although chronic, it does not progress and the protein product remains its only manifestation. In a few patients, the lymphoma may be aggressive. Occasionally, cold agglutinins are found in patients with nonlymphocytic neoplasms.

Transient cold agglutinins occur commonly in two infections: *Mycoplasma pneumoniae* infection and infectious mononucleosis. In both, the titer of antibody is usually too low to cause clinical symptoms, but its presence is of diagnostic value; only occasionally is hemolysis present. Cold agglutinins are less frequently encountered in a number of other viral infections. Their manifestations are usually benign.

The specificity of the antibody may be of diagnostic value. Cold agglutinins reacting more strongly with adult cells than fetal (cord) cells are called *anti-I*; these antibodies are seen in benign lymphoproliferation (chronic cold agglutinin monoclonal gammopathy) and in *Mycoplasma* infections. Those reacting more strongly with cord cells are called *anti-i*; these antibodies are seen in aggressive lymphomas

and in infectious mononucleosis. Rarely, the antibody may react with other antigens that are equally expressed on adult and cord cells.

The clinical manifestations elicited by the antibody are of two sorts: acrocyanosis and hemolysis. Acrocyanosis is the marked purpling of the extremities, ears, and nose when the blood becomes cold enough to agglutinate in the veins; it clears on warming and does not have the vasospastic characteristics of Raynaud's phenomenon (see Chap. 211).

The hemolysis is usually not severe and is manifest by a mild reticulocytosis, agglutination on the blood film, and agglutination during analysis of the blood by particle analysis (giving rise to a falsely high mean corpuscular volume). The degree of hemolysis depends on several variables.

1 Antibody titer. In general, the titer in symptomatic patients is above 1:2000 dilution of serum and may range to as high as 1:50,000. When collecting samples for testing the titer, great care must be taken that the serum is separated from the cells while maintaining the sample at 37°C so that the antibody will not adsorb onto the patient's own cells.
2 Thermal amplitude of the antibody (the highest temperature at which the antibody will react with the red cell). For most antibodies, this is 23 to 30°C. Those with a higher thermal amplitude (up to 37°C) will be more hemolytic, since it is more likely that these temperatures will be reached during the circulation of the cells.
3 Environmental temperature. Since the reaction can only occur at temperatures below body temperature, frequency and degree of exposure to cold are major determinants of the rate of hemolysis.

The hemolysis that occurs is due primarily to the hemolytic action of complement, since there are no functional Fc receptors for the IgM antibody. Complement is readily fixed, since a single molecule of antibody is enough to effect binding of C1 and initiate the sequence of reactions. However, the normal human red cell is remarkably resistant to the hemolytic action of complement because of several defense mechanisms. Therefore, severe hemolysis with hemoglobinuria will occur only with massive activation of the antibody, such as by sudden chilling. The activation of complement is always marked by the accumulation of a degradation product of C3, C3dg, on the surface; this is what is detected with appropriate antisera in the direct Coombs test in all patients with significant cold agglutinin disease.

THERAPY   The cutaneous manifestations of this disorder are best treated by maintaining the patient in a warm environment. Because transfusion of normal blood presents to the patient a large number of red blood cells which have not been exposed previously to the cold agglutinin and are therefore not "protected," transfusion may be associated with an acceleration of the hemolytic process. Splenectomy is usually not of value in this disorder. Glucocorticoids are of limited value, although patients with the panthermal variety of cold agglutinin disease may respond favorably to this therapy. Chlorambucil and cyclophosphamide are the most commonly employed agents in those patients in whom therapy is indicated. Although some patients have experienced a dramatic improvement, the effectiveness of this therapy is usually marginal.

Cold agglutinin disease tends to be chronic and unremitting. The overall prognosis is dominated by the underlying lymphoproliferative disease, if present. In those patients in whom cold agglutinin disease appears to arise spontaneously, lymphoproliferative disease may become apparent after several years.

Paroxysmal cold hemoglobinuria (PCH)   Now a rare disorder, PCH was more frequent at a time when tertiary syphilis was more prevalent. It results from the formation of the Donath-Landsteiner antibody, an IgG antibody which is directed against the P antigen complex and which can induce complement-mediated lysis. Attacks are precipitated by exposure to cold and are associated with hemoglobinemia and hemoglobinuria; chills and fever; back, leg, and abdominal pain; headache; and malaise. Recovery from the acute episode is prompt, and between episodes patients are asymptomatic. When this syndrome accompanies acute viral infections (e.g., measles and

TABLE 307-7   Disturbances of the formed elements of blood secondary to intravascular trauma

Etiology	Fragments	Hemolysis	Thrombo-cytopenia
Impact: march hemoglo-binuria, etc.	0	+	0
Cardiac (turbulence):			
Aortic valve prosthesis	+ + + +	+ + + +	0
Mitral valve prosthesis	+ +	+ +	0
Calcific aortic stenoses	+	±	0
Vessel disease*	+ + +	+	+
Thrombotic thrombo-cytopenic purpura	+ + + +	+ + + +	+ + + +
Hemolytic uremic syndrome	+ + + +	+ + + +	+ + + +
Adenocarcinoma	+ + + +	+ + + +	+ + + +
Disseminated intravas-cular coagulation	+ +	±	+ + + +

* Malignant hypertension, eclampsia, renal graft rejection, hemangiomas, immune disease (scleroderma).

mumps), it is self-limited. Although the direct Coombs test may show complement to be present (seldom IgG), this test may be completely negative. The diagnosis is made by demonstrating cold-reacting IgG antibodies either by lytic tests (when the titer is very high) or by special antiglobulin tests. When PCH is secondary to syphilis, it responds favorably to specific therapy for this disorder. Chronic autoimmune PCH may respond to prednisone or cytotoxic therapy (azathioprine or cyclophosphamide) but does not respond to splenectomy. Despite the severity of individual episodes, the natural history of this disease extends over many years.

TRAUMA IN THE CIRCULATION   Mechanical trauma can cause hemolysis in three ways: (1) when red blood cells flow through small vessels over the surface of bony prominences and are subject to external impact during various physical activities, (2) when they flow across a pressure gradient created by an abnormal heart valve or valve prosthesis and are disrupted by a shear stress, and (3) when the deposition of fibrin in the microvasculature exposes them to a physical impediment that fragments them (Table 307-7).

External impact   Hemoglobinemia and hemoglobinuria have been observed in individuals who have undergone a prolonged march or a prolonged jog, most typically on a hard surface and while wearing thin-soled shoes. The role of direct external trauma in this process has been demonstrated by the fact that hemolysis can be prevented by the insertion of a soft inner sole in the runner's shoes. Similar types of hemolysis have been described following karate and the playing of bongo drums. No abnormality of red blood cell morphology has been demonstrated, even during the acute episode, and no underlying red blood cell abnormality has been uncovered. A large percentage of individuals will develop hemoglobinemia and hemoglobinuria when exposed to the conditions described above. As a result of muscle damage during some of these activities, myoglobinuria also may occur, but renal function is preserved. No specific therapy is required.

Cardiac hemolysis   Hemolysis associated with fragmented red blood cells (Fig. A9-7) occurs in approximately 10 percent of patients with artificial aortic valve prostheses. This incidence is somewhat greater with valves having stellite rather than Silastic occluders, greater with small valves as compared with larger valves, and greater when valves are cloth-covered or when there is a paravalvular leak. Traumatic hemolysis is much less common in recipients of porcine valves. Severe hemolysis may occur after repair of ostium primum or endocardial cushion defects with a prosthetic patch. Mitral valve prostheses also have been associated with hemolysis, but since the pressure gradient across these values is lower than across aortic prostheses, the incidence is lower. A moderately shortened red blood cell survival with little or no anemia occurs in some patients with severe calcific aortic stenosis. Indeed, almost any intracardiac lesion that alters hemodynamics may lead to some shortening of red blood

cell survival. In addition, traumatic hemolysis has been observed in patients who have undergone aortofemoral bypass.

CLINICAL MANIFESTATIONS   In severe cases, hemoglobin levels fall to 50 to 70 g/L with reticulocytosis, fragmented red blood cells in the peripheral blood, depressed haptoglobin, elevated serum lactate dehydrogenase (LDH), and hemoglobinemia and hemoglobinuria. Iron loss (as hemoglobin or hemosiderin) in the urine may lead to iron deficiency. The direct Coombs test may rarely become positive.

PATHOGENESIS   A number of factors combine to cause the fragmentation and destruction of red blood cells in this disorder. Direct mechanical trauma of red blood cells at the time of seating of the occluder of the prosthetic valve, the deposition of fibrin across disrupted attachment points, and, probably most important, the shear stress resulting from turbulent blood flow may all result in the fragmentation of red blood cells. The turbulence explains the higher incidence of hemolysis in patients who have a paravalvular leak and therefore greater velocity of blood flow across the aortic orifice during systole.

THERAPY AND PROGNOSIS   Iron deficiency should be corrected by the administration of oral iron. The elevated hemoglobin which results may permit a decrease in the cardiac output and a slowing of the hemolytic rate. Limitation in physical activity also lessens the hemolytic rate. When these measures fail, any paravalvular leak must be repaired or the prosthetic valve replaced.

Deposition of fibrin in the microvasculature   Fibrin deposition in the microvasculature fragments red blood cells and traps platelets under three general conditions: (1) abnormalities of the vessel wall in recognized disorders, such as malignant hypertension, eclampsia, rejection of a renal allograft, disseminated cancer, and hemangiomas, (2) two potentially fatal syndromes of unknown etiology, thrombotic thrombocytopenic purpura and the hemolytic uremic syndrome, and (3) disseminated intravascular coagulation.

ABNORMALITIES OF THE VESSEL WALL   The degree of hemolysis induced by this family of disorders is usually quite mild, although the number of fragments in the peripheral blood may be striking. In some patients, thrombocytopenia may be severe. In each case, therapy is best directed at the primary disease. Thus reversal of renal graft rejection, treatment of malignant hypertension and eclampsia, control of cancer, etc. lead to a cessation of the hemolytic process. The relative importance of the primary vascular abnormality and of the deposition of fibrin in causing hemolysis is unclear.

Thrombotic thrombocytopenic purpura (TTP)   This disease of unknown etiology affects individuals of all ages but primarily young adults, more often women.

CLINICAL MANIFESTATIONS   Hemolysis is a striking feature of this disease. Anemia occurs in association with fragmented red blood cells, nucleated red cells in the peripheral blood, an elevated reticulocyte count, and thrombocytopenia of varying degree. Platelet counts range from 5000 to 100,000 per cubic millimeter. Mild jaundice can occur, and petechiae may be present, although usually to a less striking degree than in idiopathic thrombocytopenic purpura (ITP). Typically, the LDH level is very elevated, indicating the intravascular hemolysis. Tests of coagulation, such as the prothrombin time, partial thromboplastin time, fibrinogen concentration, and the level of fibrinogen split products, are usually normal or only mildly abnormal. If the coagulation tests indicate a major consumption of procoagulants, the diagnosis of TTP is doubtful. Erythroid hyperplasia and an increased number of megakaryocytes are present in the bone marrow. A positive antinuclear antibody (ANA) determination is obtained in approximately 20 percent of patients. Some patients experience significant, although not severe, bleeding of uterine, gastrointestinal, or other origin. Fever is present in many patients, and many experience nonspecific constitutional symptoms such as nausea, abdominal pain, and arthralgias. The spleen and liver usually are not palpable.

The course of TTP spans days to weeks in most patients but occasionally continues for months. As the disease progresses, the brain and kidneys can become involved, and their dysfunction is the ultimate cause of death in the majority of patients. Proteinuria and a moderate elevation of blood urea nitrogen may be found on initial presentation, and there can be a continued rise in blood urea nitrogen and a fall in urine output if the patient develops renal failure. Neurologic symptoms develop in more than 90 percent of patients whose disease terminates in death. Initially, there may be changes in mental status such as confusion, delirium, or altered states of consciousness. Focal findings include seizures, hemiparesis, aphasia, and visual field defects. These neurologic symptoms may fluctuate and terminate in coma. Involvement of myocardial blood vessels may be a cause of sudden death in some patients.

PATHOGENESIS The cause of TTP is unknown, but the manifestations can be explained by *localized* platelet thrombi and fibrin deposition. Arterioles are filled with hyalin material, presumably fibrin and platelets, and similar material may be seen beneath the endothelium of otherwise uninvolved vessels. Immunofluorescence studies have shown the presence of immunoglobulin and complement in arterioles. Microaneurysms of arterioles are often present. Controversy exists concerning the specificity of these changes, some authorities noting them in the hemolytic uremic syndrome (particularly in the kidney) and in disseminated intravascular coagulation. An association with SLE, scleroderma, and Sjögren's syndrome suggests an immunologic origin. A high-molecular-weight form of von Willebrand's protein, as well as a platelet-aggregating protein, has been identified in the plasma of TTP patients and may contribute significantly to the pathogenesis of the microvascular defect.

DIAGNOSIS The combination of hemolytic anemia with fragmented and nucleated red blood cells, thrombocytopenia, fever, neurologic disorders, and renal dysfunction is virtually pathognomonic of TTP. The diagnosis is further supported by the finding of normal coagulation tests, although occasional patients have an isolated abnormality of coagulation. Although they are not usually required for diagnosis, biopsies of skin and muscle, gingiva, lymph node, or bone marrow may demonstrate the pathologic abnormalities described above. TTP should be considered in every patient in whom the diagnosis of ITP or Evans' syndrome (ITP plus immunohemolytic anemia) is made. The finding of fragmented red blood cells in the peripheral blood is particularly helpful in this regard. Because the clinical course can fluctuate widely, therapy is difficult to evaluate.

THERAPY AND PROGNOSIS Until recently, this disease was almost universally fatal. A large number of therapeutic modalities have been attempted with variable success. These include glucocorticoids, splenectomy, and antiplatelet drugs. Patients are initially treated with high doses of glucocorticoids (60 to 100 mg prednisone per day). However, additional therapy is indicated. The definitive treatment which produces a 60 to 80 percent complete response rate occurs with plasmapheresis. Because large volumes are required (2 to 4 L/d), plasmapheresis is preferred over exchange transfusion. Splenectomy may be effective, but with a lower frequency of response and with additional risk in these critically ill patients. The benefit of antiplatelet drugs (dipyridamole, sulfinpyrazone, dextran, aspirin) is unclear, but they are commonly used together with the therapeutic measures described above. Aspirin may increase the risk of bleeding and should be employed with caution. Vincristine may be effective in otherwise refractory patients. Because of the ever-present risk of sudden death, therapy should be instituted promptly. Even deep coma is not a contraindication to therapy, since full neurologic recovery is the rule in patients responding to therapy. If treatment is instituted early in the disease, remission occurs in approximately two-thirds of patients. Relapses have been noted in approximately 10 percent of patients but are usually responsive to therapeutic intervention. Platelet transfusions should not be given because they can precipitate thrombotic events.

Hemolytic uremic syndrome This disorder is usually encountered in young children and has laboratory features similar to those of TTP. Often the patient has a prodrome of a gastroenteritis, which may consist of bloody diarrhea. Many of these children have gastroenteritis caused by *Escherichia coli* 0157:H7. Very rarely, the disorder appears to be familial. Patients present with acute hemolytic anemia, thrombocytopenic purpura, and acute oliguric renal failure. Most patients have either hemoglobinuria or anuria. Unlike TTP, neurologic manifestations are uncommon. The peripheral blood findings and coagulation tests are usually indistinguishable from those of TTP. Pathologic changes are similar but restricted to the kidney. Patients are treated with dialysis and transfusions. The efficacy of glucocorticoids, dextran, and heparin is uncertain. The mortality in children ranges from 5 to 20 percent but is considerably higher in adults. A disorder resembling the hemolytic uremic syndrome has recently been described in adults treated with the antineoplastic drug mitomycin C, usually in combination with other drugs.

Disseminated intravascular coagulation (DIC) Red blood cell fragmentation in the microvasculature (microangiopathic hemolytic anemia) is seen in about one-fourth of patients with DIC (Chap. 316). The degree of hemolysis is much less in DIC than in either TTP or the hemolytic uremic syndrome, and anemia with reticulocytosis and nucleated red blood cells is distinctly rare.

DIRECT TOXIC EFFECTS A variety of infections may be associated with severe hemolysis. The microorganisms in bartonellosis (Chap. 124), malaria (Chap. 174), and babesiosis (Chap. 179) directly parasitize red blood cells. Other infectious organisms exert their damaging effects on red blood cells indirectly. The most striking is that resulting from septicemia with *Clostridium welchii* (Chap. 108). The phospholipase produced by this organism is capable of cleaving the phosphoryl bond of lecithin, thereby lysing human red blood cells. A mild, transient hemolysis frequently accompanies bacteremia with diverse organisms such as pneumococci, staphylococci, and *E. coli*.

Hemolysis may result from the direct action of snake and spider venoms on the red blood cell. Although cobra venom is directly lytic in vitro, the clinical disease induced by the bite of the cobra is one of moderate hemolysis associated with spherocytosis. Spider bites are known to induce acute intravascular hemolysis associated with spherocytosis. It is thought that the brown recluse spider which inhabits the central and southern portions of the United States and portions of South America is responsible. The hemolytic disease continues for several days up to 1 week.

Copper has a direct hemolytic effect on red blood cells. Hemolysis has been observed following exposure of individuals to copper salts (such as during hemodialysis). In addition, the transient episodes of hemolysis observed in patients with Wilson's disease are probably due to copper toxicity.

The red blood cell membrane is unstable at temperatures above 49°C due to denaturation of the cytoskeletal protein spectrin. When studied in vitro, the red blood cell undergoes a process of budding, cleavage, and resealing above this temperature. The same process is observed in individuals who have suffered extensive burns. These patients have prominent spherocytosis as well as hemoglobinemia and sometimes hemoglobinuria.

ACQUIRED RED CELL MEMBRANE DISORDERS

SPUR CELL ANEMIA Hemolytic anemia with bizarre-shaped red blood cells occurs in some patients with severe hepatocellular disease. Most patients with spur cell anemia have advanced Laennec's cirrhosis. This hemolytic disorder is observed in approximately 5 percent of patients with manifestations of severe cirrhosis, such as ascites, jaundice, and hepatic encephalopathy. Spur cell anemia has also been reported in neonatal hepatitis.

Clinical manifestations Anemia is moderate to severe, with hematocrit levels ranging from 0.16 to 0.30. Thus the anemia is more severe than is observed in otherwise uncomplicated cirrhosis, in which hematocrit levels are rarely below 0.28, unless there is accompanying folic acid deficiency, blood loss, iron deficiency, etc. (Chap. 305). Splenomegaly is a constant feature, and the spleen is generally more prominent than in patients who have cirrhosis but who do not have spur cell anemia. Jaundice is also a constant feature, and hepatic encephalopathy is common. Other tests of liver function are similar to values obtained in most patients with severe cirrhosis, although there is a tendency to longer prothrombin times. Chromium half-survival times of red blood cells are decreased to as short as 6 days (normal being 26 to 32 days), and red cell destruction is localized to the spleen. Normal transfused red blood cells have a survival similar to that of the patient's own red blood cells. Red blood cells are irregularly shaped with multiple spicules, and a small number of bizarre-shaped fragments are commonly seen on peripheral blood smears (see Fig. A9-8). Reticulocytes range from 5 to 15 percent.

Pathogenesis The surface membrane of spur cells contains 50 to 70 percent excess cholesterol, but its total phospholipid content is normal. In this way, spur cells are distinct from the more usual target red blood cells in liver disease, which possess an excess of both cholesterol and phospholipid. Cholesterol out of proportion to phospholipid decreases the fluidity of the spur cell membrane, and cell deformability is also decreased. Normal red blood cells acquire the spur abnormality when incubated in serum from affected patients. This results from the presence in serum of an abnormal low-density lipoprotein with an increased mole ratio of free (unesterified) cholesterol to phospholipid. These rigid, cholesterol-laden red blood cells are detected by the filtering system of the spleen, aided by congestive splenomegaly in cirrhosis. In contrast to circulating spur cells, normal red blood cells which have acquired cholesterol in vitro have an increased surface area and a decreased osmotic fragility, and they have a regular pattern of spicule deformity. This is also true in vivo for normal red blood cells during their initial 24 h in the patient's circulation. However, during continued circulation in vivo in the presence of the spleen, cholesterol-rich spur cells lose surface area and transform to the irregular pattern of spiculation associated with acanthocytes (see "Red Blood Cell Morphology" above). This process of membrane "conditioning" by the spleen continues, and the cell is destroyed in the spleen.

Diagnosis Increasing anemia in a patient with chronic cirrhosis most commonly results from blood loss, folic acid deficiency, or iron deficiency. The hemolytic rate may increase transiently during periods of acute fatty liver. The combination of an elevated reticulocyte count and elevated bilirubin level in the presence of the characteristic morphologic abnormality on peripheral blood smear is diagnostic. Red blood cells of similar morphologic appearance are seen in patients with abetalipoproteinemia. However, these individuals have a minimal amount of hemolysis.

Spur cells and acanthocytes must be distinguished from regularly scalloped, crenated red blood cells (echinocytes). These are a frequent artifact on blood smears, and they are present in some patients with uremia ("burr cells") (Fig. A9-9). Small, dense crenated spheres (spheroechinocytes) are sometimes seen in congenital nonspherocytic hemolytic anemia due to enzyme deficiencies in the Embden-Meyerhof pathway (see below).

Treatment Since normal red blood cells acquire the spur abnormality when transfused into patients with this form of anemia, transfusion therapy is of limited benefit. Attempts to influence red blood cell cholesterol by the use of various lipid-lowering agents have been unsuccessful. Splenectomy has been reported to prevent both the conditioning of red blood cells in the spleen and their premature destruction. However, splenectomy carries a high risk in patients with severe liver disease complicated by portal hypertension and coagulation defects, and it must be reserved for selected patients in whom hemolysis is a major clinical problem and who appear to be relatively good surgical risks.

Prognosis In most patients, spur cell anemia occurs during the late stages of cirrhosis, and more than 90 percent of patients succumb to their underlying liver disease within 1 year of the diagnosis of spur cell anemia.

PAROXYSMAL NOCTURNAL HEMOGLOBINURIA (PNH) This condition is distinctive among hemolytic disorders in humans because it is an intracorpuscular defect acquired at the stem cell level. It occurs primarily in young adults.

Clinical manifestations Anemia is of exceedingly variable degree with hematocrit values of 0.20 and lower in occasional patients and normal values in others. Mild granulocytopenia and thrombocytopenia are commonly present. Although regarded as a classic feature of this disease, gross hemoglobinuria is present only intermittently in most patients and never occurs in some. Hemosiderinuria is usually present. Other features of diagnostic significance are a low leukocyte alkaline phosphatase and a low red blood cell acetylcholinesterase. Red blood cells are normochromic and normocytic unless iron deficiency has occurred from the chronic loss of iron in the urine. The diagnosis is established by a positive acid hemolysis test or sucrose lysis test, both of which demonstrate the enhanced sensitivity of PNH red blood cells to complement (see below).

The demonstration of a deficiency of the membrane proteins decay accelerating factor (DAF) and CD59 by flow cytometry on red cells, platelets, or granulocytes is likely to become the definitive test for the disorder.

Venous thrombosis is a common complication of this disorder and has been reported in peripheral veins as well as in mesenteric, hepatic, portal, and cerebral veins. Thrombosis is a common cause of death in patients severely affected with PNH. A second manifestation, possibly related to thromboses in small veins, is the occurrence of acute back and abdominal pain similar in character to that which occurs in sickle cell anemia. Headache also has been reported.

Pathogenesis PNH is an acquired clonal disease, probably arising from a single abnormal stem cell. It may be seen in association with other stem cell disorders, including aplastic anemia (frequently), myelofibrosis, and (rarely) other myelodysplastic or myeloproliferative disorders. The normal clone of stem cells and its descendants does not completely disappear, and the proportion of cells that are abnormal varies from patient to patient and from time to time in a single patient.

The fundamental defect in PNH is the partial or complete inability of a clone of hematopoietic cells to construct a glycosyl-phosphatidylinositol anchor for the attachment of a variety of membrane proteins to the bilayer. Two of these proteins [(DAF, CD55) and membrane inhibitor of reactive lysis (MIRL, CD59)] make the cells more sensitive to the effect of complement. In the red cells, this is manifest as the marked sensitivity of the cells to the hemolytic action of complement. DAF normally disrupts the enzyme complexes from either the classical (antibody-driven) pathway or the alternative pathway that activate C3 and C5; CD59 modulates the conversion of C9 by the membrane attack complex C5B-8 to a polymeric complex capable of penetrating the membrane.

The platelets also lack these proteins; however, the life span of the platelet is normal. On the other hand, the activation of complement indirectly stimulates platelet aggregation and hypercoagulability; this is probably responsible for the tendency to thrombosis seen in PNH.

The third major manifestation of PNH, relative marrow hypoplasia, is present in almost all patients to a greater or lesser degree. It is not known how this may be related to the lack of GPI-linked proteins.

Diagnosis PNH should be suspected in anyone with otherwise unexplained hemolytic anemia, especially with leukopenia and/or thrombocytopenia and with evidence of intravascular hemolysis (hemoglobinemia, hemoglobinuria, hemosiderinuria, elevated LDH of the erythrocyte type). The diagnosis is often delayed because (1) it is not considered, (2) hemoglobinuria is confused with hematuria, and (3) elevation of the LDH is confused with that seen in liver disease.

The most specific diagnostic test commonly available is the acidified serum lysis (Ham) test, which is performed by incubating the patient's red blood cells with normal serum acidified to a pH of 6.2. Complement is activated under these conditions, and the defective PNH cells are lysed but not normal cells (including the normal cells of the patient). The sensitivity of the test is increased by optimizing the Mg^{2+} concentration and by using sera of normal donors known to be potent in this test. The test may miss small populations of abnormal cells but is falsely positive only in a rare form of congenital dyserythropoietic anemia which can be readily distinguished on clinical grounds. The sucrose lysis test, in which complement is activated by reduction of the ionic strength of the incubation medium, is more sensitive but less specific. The most sensitive and specific test is determination of the absence of the GPI-linked proteins on granulocytes and platelets by flow cytometry; this test is not generally available.

Treatment   Transfusion therapy is useful in PNH not only for raising the hemoglobin level but also for suppressing the marrow production of red blood cells during episodes of sustained hemoglobinuria or of sustained painful crisis. Whole blood transfusions infrequently cause an exacerbation of the hemolytic process. This can be prevented by using washed red blood cells rather than whole blood.

Therapy with androgens frequently results in a rise in hemoglobin level. Adrenocortical steroids also may be effective in reducing the rate of hemolysis but should be given in moderate doses (25 to 30 mg prednisone) only on alternate days.

Because of iron loss in the urine, iron deficiency is common. An exacerbation of hemolysis often follows the administration of iron because of the formation of a large number of young red blood cells, many of which are sensitive to complement. This may be minimized by giving prednisone (60 mg/d) or by suppressing the bone marrow with transfusions.

Acute thrombosis in PNH, particularly the Budd-Chiari syndrome and cerebral thrombosis, should be treated aggressively with thrombolytic agents. Heparin therapy should be instituted rapidly and maintained for several days before changing to coumadin therapy.

Antithymocyte globulin (ATG) is often of use in treating marrow hypoplasia, as it is in the related disease, aplastic anemia. A total dose of 150 mg/kg is given over 4 to 10 days; large doses of prednisone are usually needed to counteract the immune-complex disease that results from the administration of this foreign protein.

In patients, especially the younger ones, with either hypoplasia or thrombosis who have an appropriate sibling donor, marrow transplantation should be considered early in the course of the disease. The usual conditioning programs are sufficient to eradicate the aberrant clone.

REFERENCES

AMIDON TM et al: Mitral and aortic paravalvular leaks with hemolytic anemia. Am Heart J 125:266, 1993

BECKER PS, LUX SE: Disorders of the red cell membrane, in *Hematology of Infancy and Childhood*, DG Nathan, FA Oski (eds). Philadelphia, Saunders, 1992

BEUTLER E: Study of glucose-6-phosphate dehydrogenase: History and molecular biology. Am J Hematol 42:53, 1993

BEUTLER E: Glucose-6-phosphate deficiency. N Engl J Med 329:169, 1991

COOPER RA: Hemolytic syndromes and red cell membrane abnormalities in liver disease. Semin Hematol 17:103, 1980

HIRONO A et al: Enzymatic diagnosis in non-spherocytic hemolytic anemia. Medicine 67:110, 1988

KELTON JG et al: The platelet aggregating factors of thrombotic thrombocytopenic purpura. Prog Clin Biol Rev 337:141, 1990

MOAKE JL: The role of von Willebrand factor (vWF) in thrombotic thrombocytopenic purpura. Prog Clin Biol Rev 337:135, 1990

PALEK J, SAHR SE: Mutations of the red blood cell membrane proteins: From clinical evaluation to detection of the underlying genetic defect. Blood 80:308, 1992

ROSSE WF: Autoimmune hemolytic anemia. Hosp Prac 20:105, 1985

———: *Clinical Immunohematology*. Cambridge, Blackwell Scientific, 1989

ROBSON WL et al: Hemolytic-uremic syndrome. Curr Probl Pediatr 23:16, 1993

THOMPSON CE: Thrombotic microangiopathies in the 1980s: Clinical features. Blood 80:1890, 1992

308   BONE MARROW FAILURE: APLASTIC ANEMIA AND OTHER PRIMARY BONE MARROW DISORDERS

JOEL M. RAPPEPORT / H. FRANKLIN BUNN

An important group of anemias is caused by primary disorders of the bone marrow in which the formation of erythropoietic precursors is impaired. The term *aplastic anemia* should be restricted to conditions in which a markedly hypocellular bone marrow results in pancytopenia (anemia, neutropenia, and thrombocytopenia). Rare patients develop selective aplasia of only erythroid cells (*pure red cell aplasia*). Alternatively, in *myelophthisic anemia*, erythropoiesis is suppressed because the marrow is infiltrated with tumor, granulomas, or fibrosis. The dysmyelopoietic or myelodysplastic anemias are associated with variable neutropenia and thrombocytopenia resulting from an acquired disorder of the hematopoietic pluripotent stem cell.

APLASTIC ANEMIA

ETIOLOGY   Aplastic anemia is thought to be due to injury or destruction of a common pluripotential stem cell affecting all subsequent cell populations. Table 308-1 classifies aplastic anemia by cause. In approximately half the cases of aplastic anemia in the United States, no cause can be identified. In areas of the world where a larger percentage of the population may be exposed to toxins such as insecticides and benzenes in uncontrolled dose, the percentage of idiopathic cases is smaller. In some cases, disordered hematopoiesis results from an abnormal stem cell clone. In others, a damaged marrow microenvironment may contribute to marrow failure. In a substantial subset of patients, immune mechanisms appear to contribute to the pathogenesis of aplasia.

Congenital causes   Fanconi's anemia, the most common type of constitutional aplastic anemia, is an autosomal recessively inherited disease usually appearing in childhood. This disorder is often associated with multiple congenital anomalies, including short stature, renal malformations, hyperpigmentation of the skin, and bony abnormalities, particularly hypoplastic or absent thumbs or radii. Most patients

---

TABLE 308-1   Causes of pancytopenia

Aplastic anemia
  A Idiopathic anemias
  B Constitutional anemias (Fanconi's anemia)
  C Chemical and physical agents
    1 Dose-related: benzene, ionizing irradiation, alkylating agents, antimetabolites (folic acid antagonists, purine and pyrimidine analogues), mitotic inhibitors, anthracyclines, inorganic arsenicals
    2 Idiosyncratic: chloramphenicol, phenylbutazone, sulfa drugs, methylphenylethylhydantoin, gold compounds, organic arsenicals, insecticides
  D Immunologically mediated aplasia
  E Other associations: hepatitis, other viral infections, systemic lupus erythematosus, diffuse eosinophilic fasciitis, transfusion-associated graft-versus-host disease, pregnancy

Pancytopenia with normal or increased bone marrow cellularity
  A Myelodysplastic syndromes
  B Hypersplenism (Chap. 58)
  C Vitamin B_{12} and folate deficiencies (Chap. 304)
  D AIDS (Chap. 279)

Paroxysmal nocturnal hemoglobinuria (Chap. 307)

Bone marrow replacement
  A Hematologic malignancies (Chaps. 151, 310, 311)
  B Nonhematologic metastatic tumor
  C Storage cell disorders (Chap. 349)
  D Osteopetrosis (Chap. 362)
  E Myelofibrosis (Chap. 309)

have chromosomal abnormalities owing to defective DNA repair. Patients who survive the complications of progressive marrow failure are at high risk of developing leukemia or other malignancies. Other congenital disorders have been associated with bone marrow failure, including dyskeratosis congenita.

Immune causes   A number of clinical observations have led to the concept that a significant proportion of cases of aplastic anemia may be mediated by immunologic mechanisms. These include recovery following immunosuppressive preparation for autologous marrow grafting and, in some patients, the necessity of immunosuppression for hematopoietic reconstitution following marrow transplantation from identical twin donors. A variety of in vitro culture techniques also have supported a humoral or cellular immune process in some patients with aplasia. However, in any given case, the identification of an immune mechanism may be difficult.

Drugs and toxins   Multiple and seemingly unrelated drugs and chemical agents have been incriminated as causes of aplastic anemia. The association varies from a predictable dose-related aplasia to idiosyncratic reactions unrelated to dose.

Agents which in an adequate dose will predictably produce bone marrow depression include the antineoplastic and immunosuppressive drugs along with ionizing radiation. These drugs include folic acid antagonists, alkylating agents, the anthracyclines, and the nitrosoureas, as well as purine and pyrimidine analogues. The degree of aplasia is dose related but may vary from individual to individual. The effects of combination chemotherapy may be additive. Withdrawal of the drug usually permits recovery of the marrow elements, although aplasia is occasionally irreversible. Marrow aplasia also may be induced by x-ray therapy, by chronic low-dose x-ray exposure, or, less commonly, by acute exposure from a laboratory or industrial accident. The severity of aplasia is dependent on the dose and rate of the exposure as well as the extent of marrow irradiated.

Benzene derivatives and other hydrocarbons have been associated with multiple hematologic abnormalities, including aplastic anemia. Benzene-induced aplasia may result from both industrial and domestic use of benzene-containing products. This aplasia may be reversible, although mild abnormalities such as macrocytosis may persist.

Chloramphenicol, a broad-spectrum antibiotic, is associated with two forms of bone marrow toxicity. The more common effect on the bone marrow is a reversible dose-related suppression of erythroid and, on occasion, granulocytic and megakaryocytic precursors. This condition is characterized by a transient anemia, associated with a drop in reticulocytes and elevation of serum iron. This bone marrow suppression is related to the dose and duration of administration of chloramphenicol. The bone marrow reveals vacuoles in the cytoplasm of early erythroid and granulocytic precursors. Similar morphologic features are seen much more commonly in patients who have ingested large amounts of alcohol.

The more serious form of bone marrow failure associated with chloramphenicol is an "idiosyncratic" reaction. This nitrobenzene compound has been the single most commonly incriminated drug in cases of aplastic anemia. These patients develop severe pancytopenia and often irreversible, fatal marrow aplasia. This complication is estimated to occur in approximately 1 in 50,000 patients who take the drug. The development of aplastic anemia seems to be unrelated to dose or duration of administration. Marrow aplasia cannot be anticipated or prevented by hematologic monitoring, since it may appear after cessation of the drug. Unfortunately, many cases of fatal aplastic anemia have occurred in patients who received chloramphenicol for trivial or dubious reasons. Therefore, this antibiotic should not be used when there are reasonable alternatives.

Other unrelated chemicals and drugs may be responsible for the development of aplastic anemia. These agents can be placed into two classes: those in which a number of associations have been reported and, therefore, a definite toxic potential has been established, and those in which only a few reported cases exist and, therefore, only a possibility of toxic potential exists at present. The establishment of these relationships is often confounded by the fact that many of the patients have taken multiple drugs. Agents in which a definite potential toxicity exists are shown in Table 308-1.

Infections   A number of cases of aplastic anemia have been reported following infectious hepatitis. The antecedent hepatitis is not distinguished by its severity, and the aplastic anemia commonly appears as the hepatitis resolves. Aplasia has usually followed non-A, non-B hepatitis, including hepatitis C, but on occasion has been associated with types A and B. The aplasia tends to be severe and frequently has a fatal outcome. Other viruses, including Epstein-Barr virus, have been implicated in aplastic anemia. Many cases of so-called idiopathic aplastic anemia are preceded by a benign-appearing viral respiratory illness. Parvovirus selectively infects erythroblasts and therefore acutely aggravates anemia in patients with hemolysis (Chap. 307).

Some patients infected with human immunodeficiency virus will develop pancytopenia and a hypoplastic bone marrow. Contributing factors include direct suppression of hematopoietic cells by the virus, opportunistic infections such as cytomegalovirus or *Mycobacterium avium intracellulare*, and myelotoxic drugs such as trimethoprim-sulfamethoxazole and azidothymidine.

Aplastic anemia also has been reported in association with a number of other illnesses (see Table 308-1). The clinical and laboratory findings associated with paroxysmal nocturnal hemoglobinuria may accompany or precede the development of aplasia. Aplastic anemia that develops during pregnancy may remit following delivery of the fetus.

CLINICAL MANIFESTATIONS   The onset of aplastic anemia is usually insidious. Initial presenting symptoms include mild progressive weakness and fatigue attributable to the anemia and/or hemorrhage from the skin, nose, gums, vagina, or gastrointestinal tract due to the thrombocytopenia. The bleeding is usually mild, but occasionally retinal or central nervous system hemorrhage may be the initial mode of presentation. Although the patient may be severely neutropenic, it is less common for the initial presentation to be a bacterial infection.

Physical examination generally reveals pallor. Petechiae or ecchymoses may be noted in the skin, mucous membranes, conjunctivae, and fundi. Lymphadenopathy and hepatosplenomegaly are notably absent. Fever may be present, but despite the presence of an infection, the usual signs of inflammation may be absent because of neutropenia.

The *course* of the disease is generally determined by the severity of the aplasia, rather than by the etiology. Mild disease can progress to a more severe disorder. Conversely, complete recovery or partial recovery of one or more cell lines may develop. It is important to obtain an accurate assessment of the degree of aplasia. *Severe aplasia* is defined as marked pancytopenia with at least two of the following criteria: granulocytes fewer than 500 per microliter, platelets fewer than 20,000 per microliter, or anemia with corrected reticulocyte count less than 1 percent. The bone marrow is markedly hypoplastic and depleted of hematopoietic cells. Patients with severe disease have a high risk of dying from bleeding and/or infections in a matter of months, while patients with a milder form of the disease may live for years. The clinical course of the disease is affected primarily by infections and by the nature and location of bleeding. Although infections may not dominate the clinical picture initially, they assume greater importance with the passage of time. Because of the need for multiple red blood cell and platelet transfusions, over a period of time one may encounter the sequelae of hemosiderosis and/or hepatitis. Even those patients who recover may have mild thrombocytopenia and persistent macrocytosis for many years. Long-term survivors are at increased risk of developing acute leukemia, the myelodysplastic syndrome, or paroxysmal nocturnal hemoglobinuria.

LABORATORY DIAGNOSIS   The diagnosis of aplastic anemia and the assessment of its relative severity depend on a thorough laboratory evaluation. The peripheral blood usually shows pancytopenia. The absolute granulocyte count is low or becomes progressively depressed during the illness. The red blood cells are normochromic and usually somewhat macrocytic, reflecting stress erythropoiesis, and the corrected reticulocyte count is inappropriately low. Since serious bleeding and/or infection correlates with the degree of thrombocytopenia or neutropenia, these values must be determined initially and followed serially. A bone marrow aspirate may yield a "dry tap," but a bone marrow biopsy will reveal a severely hypocellular or aplastic marrow with replacement by fat. There is usually a severe depression of megakaryocytes and myeloid cells and a marked but relatively less severe depression of the erythroid precursors.

Elevated serum iron level coupled with a normal level of transferrin results in elevated transferrin saturation. Because of the reduction in erythroid precursors, plasma iron clearance is prolonged, and incorporation of iron into red blood cells is markedly decreased. There is no evidence of increased red blood cell destruction.

DIFFERENTIAL DIAGNOSIS   The diagnosis of aplastic anemia implies the exclusion of the other causes of pancytopenia that are listed in Table 308-1. Splenomegaly and/or lymphadenopathy argue strongly against aplastic anemia. Malignant and nonmalignant invasion of the bone marrow must be excluded by microscopic examination of the marrow. Paroxysmal nocturnal hemoglobinuria and systemic lupus erythematosus should be ruled out by appropriate tests, including the sugar water and acid hemolysis tests. Vitamin B_{12} and folate deficiencies can be excluded by serum assays and morphologic changes. Pancytopenia rarely may be secondary to various infections, including AIDS. Before aplastic anemia can be classified as idiopathic, a careful history must exclude exposure to all known and suspected agents. In our complex society, all patients are exposed to potentially toxic agents in the environment. Nevertheless, this difficulty should not discourage a careful and extensive search for a cause.

TREATMENT   The management of aplastic anemia has become one of the most challenging aspects of modern medicine, requiring a diligent multidisciplinary team of caregivers in a well-equipped tertiary care center. For patients with mild aplasia, every effort should be made to do as little as possible except to remove possible etiologic agents in expectation of spontaneous recovery. As noted below, androgens may be of value in mild aplasia. Patients with severe aplasia should be considered for an immediate bone marrow transplantation, if a suitable donor is available. As discussed in detail in Chap. 313, the great majority of patients who undergo marrow transplantation have complete correction of the hematopoietic defect.

Supportive care   Regardless of the therapy chosen, the mainstay of treatment is good supportive care. The first and most immediate step is the removal of any suspected cause. If the disease is mild at presentation, no further supportive care need be instituted, unless there is subsequent deterioration. If a severe neutropenia exists (polymorphonuclear leukocytes fewer than 500 per microliter), the patient should be shielded from potential infections. Prophylactic systemic antibiotics should not be utilized. Intramuscular injections should be avoided. Established infections should be treated vigorously with specific antibiotics, and fever of undetermined etiology may, after appropriate bacteriologic evaluation, call for broad-spectrum antibiotic coverage until a specific diagnosis is established. Menstruating females should be placed on suppressive doses of birth control pills.

Transfusions   Blood products should be used *judiciously* and restricted to appropriate component therapy, since future therapy and ultimate survival may be affected by transfusions. Red blood cells should be administered to maintain the well-being of the patient rather than to establish a certain hemoglobin level. Transfusions pose significant risks, such as development of hepatitis or hemosiderosis, as well as sensitization to both red blood cell antigens and transplantation antigens. Platelet transfusions should be administered in the face of serious hemorrhage. Some groups employ prophylactic transfusions when the platelet count is lower than 20,000 per microliter. Others, fearful of the development of resistance to future transfusions, administer platelets only when faced with hemorrhage. Responses to platelet transfusions may be blunted by the presence of infection. If a patient develops immune resistance to platelet transfusions, HLA-compatible platelet transfusions may be useful (Chap. 312). Should

a bone marrow transplant be considered, family members should be avoided as a source of blood products, since the patient may develop antibodies to minor transplantation antigens. Leukocyte transfusions are not administered prophylactically. However, white blood cell infusions may be of value in patients with documented gram-negative infections and severe neutropenia who have failed to respond to antimicrobial therapy.

Marrow-stimulating agents   Although patients with mild aplasia sometimes respond to androgens, and a few appear to be androgen-dependent, those with severe aplasia are usually unresponsive. Patients with mild aplasia should be treated with adequate doses of androgens as the initial mode of therapy. The most widely used drugs at present are oxymetholone, fluoxymesterone, and nandrolone decanoate. Responses may occur as long as 3 to 6 months after the initiation of therapy. The administration of recombinant hematopoietic growth factors, either alone or in combination, is under active investigation. To date, granulocyte-macrophage colony stimulating factor is somewhat effective in boosting neutrophil, eosinophil, and monocyte counts but has little effect on platelets or red cell production.

Immunosuppressive agents   Increasing clinical and laboratory evidence suggests that 40 to 50 percent of patients will have a complete or, more likely, partial response to a variety of immunosuppressive agents. The specificity and mechanism of this therapy are as yet undefined. The most commonly administered therapy is animal antisera directed against human lymphocytes and thymocytes. The effectiveness, as well as the dose and duration of administration, of these heterogeneous sera is variable from batch to batch. Serious side effects may accompany the administration of these heteroantisera. Very high doses of glucocorticoids or the immunosuppressive agent cyclosporine may yield similar responses.

In general, splenectomy has no role in the management of aplastic anemia.

Bone marrow transplantation   (See Chap. 313)

OTHER PRIMARY BONE MARROW DISORDERS

PURE RED CELL APLASIA   Pure red cell aplasia involves a selective failure in the production of erythroid elements in the bone marrow. Granulopoiesis and megakaryocytopoiesis remain normal. Patients have a normochromic, normocytic anemia with normal granulocyte count and platelet count. Severe reticulocytopenia exists, and the bone marrow is characterized by a virtual absence of any erythroid precursors in the face of otherwise normal cellular elements. An increase in lymphocytes may be seen in the marrow.

Constitutional red cell aplasia   Blackfan-Diamond syndrome, a rare chronic constitutional red blood cell aplasia, may appear in infants from the time of birth to the age of 2 years. Twenty-five percent of patients have minor congenital anomalies. The disorder is of unknown etiology but has been corrected by both glucocorticoids and marrow transplantation.

Acquired red cell aplasia   The rare acquired form of pure red cell aplasia is seen predominantly in middle-aged adults. About one-third of patients have thymomas. Five percent of all patients with thymomas have pure red cell aplasia. The association between thymoma and myasthenia gravis is somewhat stronger. In many patients, both with and without thymomas, erythropoiesis is inhibited by a complement-fixing IgG immunoglobulin which has selective cytotoxicity for marrow erythroblasts. A much smaller group of patients has been noted to have an inhibitor against erythropoietin. Occasionally, pure red cell aplasia is encountered in patients with T cell chronic lymphatic leukemia. The circulating T cells are distinguished by the presence of receptors for the Fc portion of IgG. Other disorders sometimes associated with pure red cell aplasia include acquired hypogammaglobulinemia, systemic lupus erythematosus, T-gamma lymphocytosis, and AIDS.

TREATMENT   Since these patients have virtually no endogenous red blood cell production, they are totally dependent on red blood cell transfusion. If thymic enlargement is noted, a thymectomy may induce a remission in approximately 50 percent of patients. If the thymus is normal, thymectomy is of no benefit. Patients without thymoma or those with an unsuccessful thymectomy should receive glucocorticoids, alone or in combination with immunosuppressive agents such as cyclophosphamide, azathioprine, cyclosporine, or antithymocyte globulin. Treatment often results in both prolonged clinical remission and disappearance of the inhibitor.

MYELODYSPLASTIC SYNDROMES   Also known as the *refractory dysmyelopoietic anemias*, these anemias are a heterogeneous group of normocytic anemias often associated with neutropenia, thrombocytopenia, and/or monocytosis. The bone marrow varies in cellularity and usually reveals disordered maturation of erythroid, myeloid, and megakaryocytic cells. In some patients, bilobed neutrophils (Pelger-Huet cells) can be detected on blood films. In others, erythroid cells accumulate large amounts of iron in mitochondria (ringed sideroblasts) (Chap. 303). The FAB (French, American, British) classification of the myelodysplastic syndrome includes five categories: refractory anemia (RA), refractory anemia with ringed sideroblasts (RARS), refractory anemia with excess of blasts (RAEB), chronic myelomonocytic leukemia (CMML), and refractory anemia with excess of blasts in transformation (RAEB-T). This intrinsic disorder of the hematopoietic pluripotential stem cell is most frequently noted in older people. Although the etiology of these disorders is unclear, some patients appear to develop the syndrome secondary to chemotherapy, particularly alkylating agents with or without accompanying radiation therapy. The most common cytogenetic abnormalities noted include the deletion of the long arm of chromosome 5 (5q−), deletion of chromosome 7 or 5 (−7, −5), or trisomy 8. Over time, a variety of additional cytogenetic changes may be observed. Survival is variable among the subtypes, with longer median survivals of 76 months noted in RARS and short median survivals of 3 to 6 months noted in RAEB-T. Patients frequently succumb to infections and hemorrhage because of the associated neutropenia and thrombocytopenia. These clonal disorders are frequently preleukemic, with subsequent conversion to frank leukemia in 5 to 20 percent of patients with RARS and greater than 50 percent of patients with RAEB-T.

The mainstay of treatment is supportive: appropriate transfusion therapy and antibiotics for febrile episodes. Occasional long-term survivors may require therapy for iron overload. Rarely, patients with sideroblastic anemia will respond to pyridoxine or pyridoxal phosphate. Although differentiation agents such as vitamin D, retinoic acid, and low-dose cytosine arabinoside are effective in vitro, their therapeutic efficacy has been disappointing. Bone marrow transplantation in the appropriate setting has been curative for the myelodysplastic syndromes, as it has for de novo leukemias. Stimulation of the bone marrow by a variety of agents has been studied. Androgen therapy has in some cases resulted in moderate improvement. Recombinant human hematopoietic growth factors, including GM-CSF (granulocyte-macrophage colony stimulating factor), G-CSF (granulocyte colony stimulating factor), IL-3 (interleukin 3), erythropoietin, and combinations thereof, are currently under investigation and offer the potential for stimulating blood cell production. Both their long-term therapeutic effect and the possibility of accelerating the development of leukemia are still to be determined. The treatment of leukemia evolving from the myelodysplastic syndrome is discussed in Chap. 310.

MYELOPHTHISIC ANEMIA   Infiltration of the bone marrow with tumor, fibrosis, or granulomas can result in the development of a severe anemia. Tumor may be derived from cell lines indigenous to the bone marrow, as in leukemia, lymphoma, or myeloma, or the marrow may be invaded by metastatic deposits of solid tumor, usually carcinoma. Among the solid tumors most frequently associated with myelophthisic anemia are carcinoma of the breast, stomach, prostate, lung, and thyroid. Hepatomegaly and splenomegaly may develop in this setting, along with marrow fibrosis.

Fibrosis in the bone marrow, usually in association with myeloid metaplasia (see Chap. 309), can cause myelophthisic anemia. Granulomatous involvement of the bone marrow is usually due to advanced tuberculosis. Primary lipid storage disorders, such as Gaucher's disease and Niemann-Pick disease, occasionally produce a myelophthisic anemia, and the rare disorder osteopetrosis, or marble bone disease, also may give a similar hematologic picture.

The invasion of the bone marrow by tumor or granulomas impairs both erythropoiesis and thrombopoiesis. In contrast, neutrophil production is generally normal or increased. It is unlikely that the anemia and thrombocytopenia are due merely to "crowding" of the bone marrow space by extrinsic cells. Myelophthisis also causes a distortion of the microcirculation of the marrow, with premature release of immature cells.

Myelophthisis usually results in a severe normochromic, normocytic anemia. A variety of misshapen erythrocytes are noted, particularly teardrop cells and fragmented cells with some basophilic stippling. In addition, normoblasts are usually seen in the peripheral blood. The reticulocyte percentage is often slightly increased (3 to 6 percent). However, when corrected for the anemia and the premature release from the bone marrow, the absolute reticulocyte count is actually reduced and reflects a decrease in red blood cell production. While thrombocytopenia is usually present, the white blood cell count is often elevated, with a marked shift to the left in the differential count. The combination of immature myeloid cells and normoblasts in the peripheral blood constitutes the "leukoerythroblastic" morphology so characteristic of myelophthisic anemia. Striking abnormalities are usually seen on examination of the bone marrow. Often an aspirate yields a "dry tap" owing to the infiltration of the marrow with abnormal tissue, although, on occasion, tumor cells will be identified. Marrow biopsy is more likely to be diagnostic, revealing leukemia, lymphoma, or foci of metastatic tumor or granuloma. However, marrow involvement is often segmental, so the primary pathologic process may be missed on a single biopsy.

Treatment   Treatment consists of attempts to reverse the primary pathologic process. It is particularly important to search for the presence of tuberculosis, since this disease is readily treatable. More often, however, the underlying disease is not amenable to therapy and requires supportive measures, such as blood transfusions.

REFERENCES

BACIGALUPO A et al: Bone marrow transplantation (BMT) versus immunosuppression for the treatment of severe aplastic amenia (SAA): A report of the EBMT SAA writing party. Br J Haematol 70:177, 1988

ESTEY EH: Prognosis and therapy of myelodysplastic syndromes. Cancer Treat Res 64:233, 1993

GORDON-SMITH EC: Fanconi anemia: Constitutional aplastic anemia. Semin Hematol 28(2):104, 1992

HAMBLIN T: Recent advances in the management of myelodysplastic syndromes. Hematol Oncol 11 (suppl I):27, 1993

NISSEN C: The pathophysiology of aplastic anemia. Semin Hematol 28(4):313, 1991

ROBINSON BE, QUESENBERY PJ: Hematopoietic growth factors: Overview and clinical applications. Am J Med Sci 300:163, 1990

ROSSE WF: Evolution of clinical understanding: Paroxysmal nocturnal hemoglobinuria as a paradigm. Am J Hematol 42:122, 1993

SPIVAK J: Pure red cell aplasia. Curr Issues Anemia 4(1): 2, 1992

STEWART FM: Hypoplastic/aplastic anemia: Role of bone marrow transplantation. Med Clin North Am 76(3):683, 1992

YOUNG N: The problem of clonality in aplastic anemia. Blood 79:1385, 1992

---

309 THE MYELOPROLIFERATIVE DISEASES

DAVID W. GOLDE / SUBHASH C. GULATI

DEFINITION   The myeloproliferative diseases are a family of disorders characterized by increased blood cell production which arise in a clonal manner from abnormalities at the level of the hematopoietic stem cell. Specific syndromes in this family include chronic myelogenous leukemia (CML), polycythemia vera (PV), agnogenic myeloid metaplasia with myelofibrosis (MF, also called *idiopathic myelofibrosis*), and essential thrombocytosis (ET). While there is commonality in the pathologic and clinical manifestations, distinct transitions from one disease to another are unusual. The myeloproliferative disorders usually have a chronic course but also may transform to an aggressive phase or acute leukemia.

CHRONIC MYELOGENOUS LEUKEMIA (CML)

DEFINITION AND ETIOLOGY   CML is a clonal stem cell disorder characterized by markedly increased myelopoiesis and the presence of the Philadelphia (Ph) chromosome. The Philadelphia chromosome involves a translocation of the Abelson (*abl*) proto-oncogene on chromosome 9 to the breakpoint cluster region (*bcr*) of chromosome 22 with formation of a fusion gene called *bcr-abl*. CML is an acquired disorder. Although no specific etiologic agent has been identified, an increased incidence of CML was observed in survivors of the atomic bomb in Japan. The peak incidence of CML was seen 5 to 12 years after radiation exposure and appeared to be dose related.

PATHOPHYSIOLOGY   The Ph chromosome results from an exchange of DNA on the long arms of chromosomes 9 and 22 forming the translocation (9;22) (q34;q11). This rearrangement creates the *bcr-abl* fusion gene and leads to expression of a novel bcr-abl protein product (Fig. 309-1). The common translocations result in bcr-abl proteins of 210 (p210) and 190 (p190) kDa which differ in the amount of bcr amino acid residues included. The p190 protein is mainly associated with Ph-positive acute lymphoblastic leukemia (ALL), whereas p210 is found both in Ph-positive ALL and in CML. Retroviral constructs incorporating the p210 and p190 *bcr-abl* genes have been introduced into mouse bone marrow cells and transplanted into lethally irradiated mice. A variety of hematopoietic malignancies developed, including a CML-like disorder, lymphoblastic leukemia, histiocytosis, and erythroleukemia. Transgenic mice have been created

where every cell had a p190 *bcr-abl* gene and the leukemias that developed were mainly of B lymphoblasts.

Transcription of the *bcr-abl* fusion gene results in a hybrid messenger RNA that is subsequently translated into a 210- or 190-kDa protein. The tyrosine kinase activity of the 190-kDa protein is greater than that of the 210-kDa protein, which, in turn, is greater than that of the normal 145-kDa c-*abl* gene product. It is likely that the bcr-abl protein provides a growth advantage to the CML cells by virtue of increased protein kinase activity which may amplify normal proliferative signals. Thus in CML there is expansion of committed myeloid precursor compartments associated with overproduction of mature myeloid elements. Genetic instability in the CML clone apparently leads to subsequent transformation into an acute leukemic phase with further chromosomal abnormalities, including a double Ph chromosome.

Using the polymerase chain reaction (PCR), minimal residual disease can be detected in CML by amplifying *bcr-abl* fusion RNA. Use of this technique also can confirm the diagnosis in patients who do not have a visible Ph chromosome. Rare patients with the CML syndrome have no Ph chromosome or evidence for the *bcr-abl* rearrangement. Even though Ph chromosome–containing cells predominate in the bone marrow in CML, normal stem cells remain but are suppressed by the Ph-positive clone. These normal diploid cells may be observed after long-term bone marrow culture in vitro and following treatment with interferon or high-dose chemotherapy.

SYMPTOMS AND SIGNS   The usual course of CML involves a chronic phase of variable duration, followed by blastic transformation, with some patients experiencing a distinct intermediate accelerated phase. Most patients are diagnosed in the chronic phase when an elevated white blood cell count is found in association with splenomegaly. At diagnosis, the white blood cell count can exceed 200,000 cells per microliter. Patients may present without symptoms after the incidental finding of an elevated white blood cell count or may complain of left upper quadrant discomfort from splenomegaly.

FIGURE 309-1   Formation of the Ph chromosome.

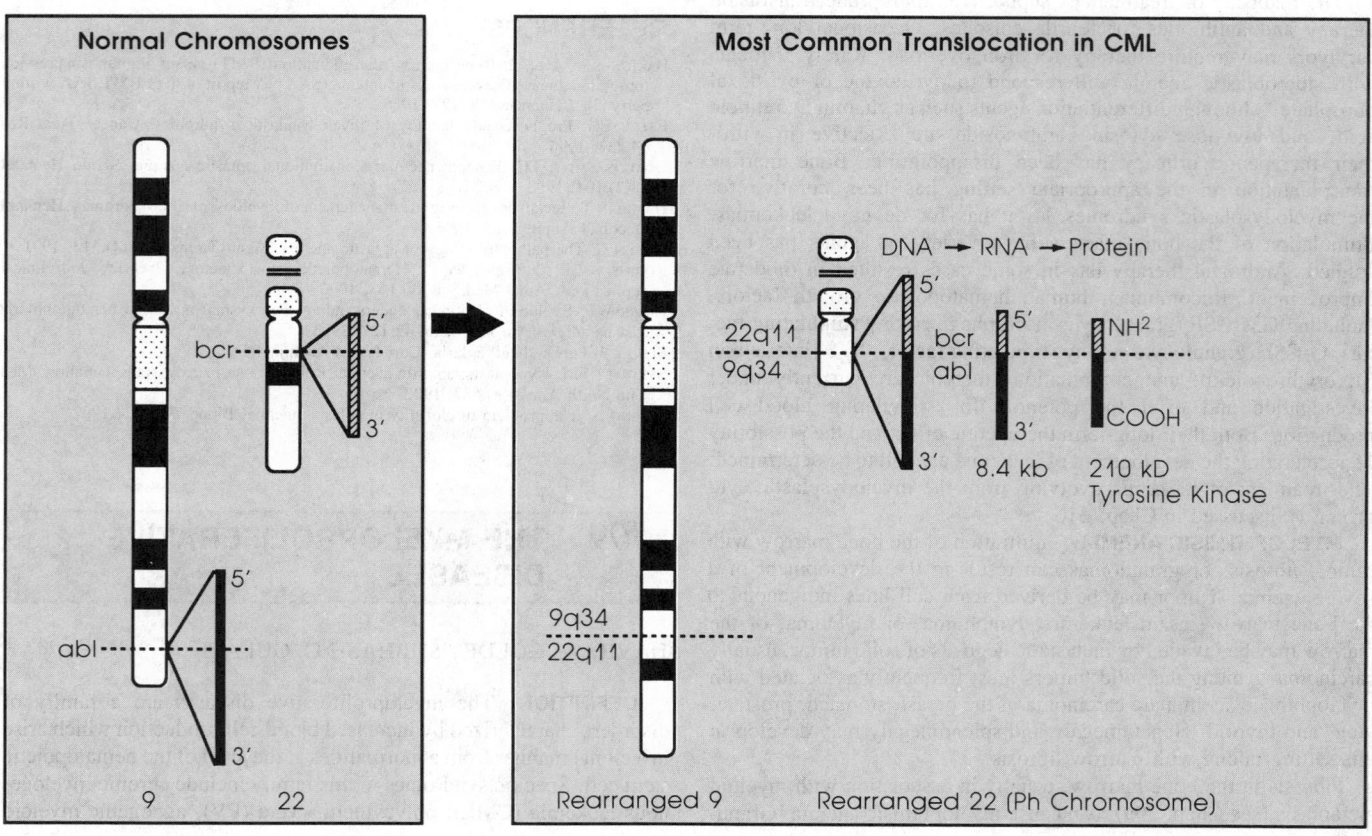

| Normal Chromosomes | Most Common Translocation in CML |

Other presenting symptoms relate to anemia or hypermetabolism with consequent weight loss, fatigue, fever, and elevated uric acid levels. The most consistent physical sign in CML is splenomegaly. An enlarged spleen is found in more than 90 percent of the patients. Hepatomegaly or, in rare instances, lymphadenopathy is observed and may suggest the transition to acute leukemia.

Bone pain and pain from splenic infarction are uncommon in the early stages of CML but are observed with disease progression. The accelerated phase is characterized by increasing resistance to therapy, progressive organomegaly, worsening anemia, thrombocytosis or thrombocytopenia, myelofibrosis, and fever. Blast crisis is associated with signs and symptoms of acute leukemia, often with extramedullary disease.

LABORATORY FINDINGS   Table 309-1 summarizes the distinguishing laboratory features of the myeloproliferative disorders. A white blood cell count over 100,000 cells per microliter is common at presentation in patients with CML, but with the increased use of laboratory screening, CML may be discovered at an early stage. The peripheral blood smear shows a marked increase in granulocytes with a left shift in differentiation, including increase in promyelocytes, myelocytes, and metamyelocytes. Eosinophilia and basophilia may be prominent. The neutrophil (leukocyte) alkaline phosphatase score is low or zero, in contrast to the high score seen in leukemoid reactions. Platelet function and morphology are usually normal in CML. A prominent elevation of serum vitamin B_{12} level, as well as an increased serum vitamin B_{12}–binding capacity, is noted because of increased granulocyte production of transcobalamin I.

A hemoglobin concentration of less than 11 g/dL is observed in one-third of the patients, and half of patients have a platelet count over 450,000 cells per microliter. The bone marrow is hypercellular with a marked increase in the myeloid-to-erythroid ratio. Occasionally, increased reticulin or collagen fibrosis is observed. In CML the marrow as well as the spleen may contain glycolipid-laden phagocytes, which resemble Gaucher cells or sea-blue histiocytes, due to the increased turnover of glucocerebrosides and sphingolipids. Hyperuricemia is often observed due to increased cell turnover in CML and can be exacerbated by cytotoxic treatment. The granulocytes in CML have near-normal phagocytic and bactericidal activity.

Features indicative of progression into blastic phase include bone lesions, pancytopenia, enlarging liver and spleen, and increase in the percentage of blasts in the bone marrow and blood. Blast crisis is usually of the myeloid type. About 30 percent of patients have lymphoblastic transformation, which needs to be distinguished from the myeloid blast crisis, since it is treated differently. Lymphoid characteristics include lymphoblast morphology, presence of the enzyme terminal deoxynucleotidyl transferase (TdT), and expression of the common acute lymphoblastic leukemia antigen (CALLA). Lymphoid transformation is associated with a lower-molecular-weight p190 *bcr-abl* translocation product. Blast crisis of erythroid, basophilic, and megakaryoblastic type is also seen.

DIAGNOSIS   The diagnosis of CML depends on the association of markedly increased myelopoiesis, splenomegaly, and the presence of the Ph chromosome. Examination of the peripheral blood smear and bone marrow usually leads to accurate diagnosis in the proper clinical setting. Cytogenetic studies are confirmatory. In some patients with the CML syndrome, the Ph chromosome is not observed. In 50 percent of such patients the *bcr-abl* abnormality can be detected by polymerase chain reaction, thus confirming the diagnosis of CML. A few patients with otherwise characteristic disease have no detectable *bcr-abl* translocation (Ph-negative CML). A rare form of myeloproliferative disease, called *juvenile CML*, is seen in patients less than 4 years of age. It is distinguished from adult-type CML by the absence of the Ph chromosome, elevated fetal hemoglobin, thrombocytopenia, and prominent monocytosis. Usually, moderate leukocytosis and a normal cytogenetic karyotype are observed. Patients with juvenile CML rarely undergo blastic transformation and usually die of infection or organ failure from monocyte and macrophage infiltration. Typically, CML can be differentiated from a leukemoid reaction associated with infection or neoplasm by the presence of the Ph chromosome, eosinophilia, basophilia, and a low neutrophil alkaline phosphatase score. Agnogenic myeloid metaplasia usually presents with marked myelofibrosis and splenomegaly with absence of the Ph chromosome.

THERAPY AND PROGNOSIS   Allogeneic bone marrow transplantation is the only curative treatment presently available for patients with CML. Early identification of possible histocompatible bone marrow donors is important, and all siblings should be HLA typed. Long-term disease-free survival is obtained in 50 to 70 percent of patients in the chronic phase who are treated by HLA-matched sibling bone marrow transplantation. Patients transplanted in an accelerated phase have a poorer prognosis, and transplantation in the blastic phase is curative in less than 10 percent of patients. After transplantation, patients may have reappearance of some cells containing the Ph chromosome or *bcr-abl* positivity by PCR. The long-term clinical significance of this mixed chimeric state in the early stages after bone marrow transplantation is not known.

Young patients who do not have an HLA-compatible sibling donor should be considered for HLA-matched unrelated bone marrow transplantation if a trial of interferon-α (IFN-α) therapy has not resulted in a major cytogenetic response. The search for a potential donor should be initiated at diagnosis. Unrelated, allogeneic bone marrow transplantation presents special hazard and should be performed in centers with sophisticated programs in the prevention and management of graft-versus-host disease. Patients who relapse after bone marrow transplantation often benefit from IFN-α therapy. The timing of bone marrow transplantation in patients with sibling histocompatible donors is controversial. Some clinicians prefer a trial of IFN-α prior to accepting the immediate risk of morbidity and mortality associated with bone marrow transplantation. Most centers, however, recommend bone marrow transplantation within the first year of diagnosis. Unfortunately, two-thirds of patients with CML do not have HLA-compatible siblings or are too old to tolerate the transplant conditioning regimen.

Emergency treatment of CML is usually not necessary unless the patient has evidence of leukostasis, painful splenomegaly, or a dangerously high white blood cell count. Hyperuricemia is common at presentation and can be managed with allopurinol and hydration. Patients with white blood cell counts in the 30,000 cells per microliter range with no symptoms can be observed until a definitive plan of therapy is determined.

The general goal of treatment for patients in chronic phase CML is to decrease myelopoiesis, thereby controlling the disease and its symptoms. Many chemotherapeutic drugs can accomplish this aim, but none are selective for the Ph-positive clone or are capable of delaying the development of blast crisis. IFN-α, which has not yet been approved for the treatment of CML in the United States, appears to be partially selective in inhibiting the neoplastic clone and therefore is often the first therapeutic option. The chemotherapeutic drug of choice for managing chronic-phase CML is hydroxyurea, which is

TABLE 309-1 **The myeloproliferative diseases**				
	CML	PV	MF	ET
Hematocrit	Normal or ↓	↑↑	↓	Normal
White blood cell count	↑↑↑	↑	↑ to ↓	Normal
Platelet count	↑ to ↓	↑	↑ to ↓	↑↑↑
Splenomegaly	+ + +	+	+ + +	+
Ph chromosome or *bcr/abl*	+	0	0	0
Marrow fibrosis	±	± or ↓	+ + +	±
Neutrophil alkaline phosphatase	↓ to 0	↑↑	↑ or normal	↑ or normal

preferred over busulfan because of ease of use and lower incidence of side effects. Hydroxyurea is usually given in doses of 1 to 3 g/d orally, with adjustments to keep the white blood cell count between 10,000 and 20,000 cells per microliter. Hydroxyurea can cause diarrhea, mucositis, or rash but is usually well tolerated. Serious side effects of busulfan include sterility, amenorrhea after prolonged use, pulmonary and retroperitoneal fibrosis, marrow fibrosis and aplasia, and hyperpigmentation of the skin. Busulfan can be given intermittently by mouth, but the dosage may be difficult to regulate. Other alkylating agents, such as cyclophosphamide, can control excess myelopoiesis and may be used if hydroxyurea is not tolerated or becomes ineffective in controlling blood counts.

Although still experimental in the treatment of CML, IFN-α is an effective agent in reducing the white blood cell and platelet counts. IFN-α appears to have preferential antiproliferative effects on CML progenitor cells. Durable complete cytogenetic responses may occur but are rare. Responding patients, however, show reemergence of normal hematopoietic precursors and a relative decrease in Ph-positive cells. It is not yet clear whether the development of blast crisis is delayed in these patients, although the observation of long-term disease control in cytogenetically responding patients supports the concept. IFN-α is usually started at 3 to 5 million units daily, intramuscularly or subcutaneously, and the dosage is adjusted to maintain the white blood cell count above 5000 cells per microliter. Patients can be maintained on a' 3- to 5-day per week treatment schedule. Some clinicians use IFN-α in conjunction with hydroxyurea or low-dose cytosine arabinoside. Liver function tests and blood counts should be monitored during interferon therapy, and cytogenetic analyses are needed to assess response. During interferon therapy, patients often experience a flulike syndrome associated with fever and myalgias. These side effects may be severe and lead to discontinuation of interferon, but symptoms usually respond to acetaminophen and interferon dose adjustment. Leukopenia and thrombocytopenia also may occur. IFN-α is relatively contraindicated in patients with depression or preexisting psychiatric disorders and should be used with caution in patients with liver, thyroid, or cardiac disease.

Age, spleen size, high platelet count, presence of circulating blasts, marked basophilia or eosinophilia, and the presence of additional chromosomal abnormalities (double Ph, 8 + , 17q +) are all associated with poor prognosis. Death seldom occurs during the chronic phase of CML. The risk of transformation from the chronic to the blastic phase is approximately 20 percent per year after the first year. Eighty-five percent of patients die while in the blastic phase. The overall median survival of patients in chronic phase of CML is 4 to 5 years. Patients in the accelerated phase have a median survival of 85 weeks, whereas patients in the blastic phase of CML have a median survival of only 15 to 20 weeks.

The optimal treatment strategy for chronic phase CML has not been determined. Young patients with HLA-matched sibling or unrelated donors should be offered bone marrow transplantation as the only known curative option. For older patients and those without a matched sibling bone marrow donor, an initial trial of IFN-α is warranted. Hydroxyurea is the chemotherapeutic drug of choice for controlling the excessive myelopoiesis in chronic phase disease.

Myeloid blast crisis is difficult to treat. A course of induction therapy for acute myeloblastic leukemia is usually warranted and can lead to reversion to chronic-phase disease or, rarely, cytogenetic remission. It is important to diagnose the lymphoid type of blast crisis accurately, since it may be treated effectively with aggressive acute lymphoblastic leukemia regimens that include vincristine and prednisone. Once remission is attained with the induction regimen, allogeneic bone marrow transplantation is an option for a few patients with HLA-matched siblings. Splenectomy or irradiation of the spleen is rarely used today, although elderly patients or those with splenic infarcts may be palliated by these procedures.

POLYCYTHEMIA VERA

DEFINITION AND ETIOLOGY   Polycythemia vera (PV) is a myeloproliferative disorder resulting from clonal expansion of a transformed hematopoietic stem cell associated with prominent overproduction of erythrocytes and, to a lesser extent, expansion of granulocytic and megakaryocytic elements. PV is gradual in onset and has a slowly progressive course. The disease generally begins in late middle life, and there is a slight male predominance. PV is relatively uncommon in blacks and occurs with increased frequency in Jews of European ancestry. Rare cases of PV in monozygotic twins and a minimal increased incidence in first-degree relatives of affected patients suggest a genetic role in rare cases. The cause of PV is unknown, and there is no known link to radiation exposure. A PV-like disease is seen in mice infected with certain strains of Friend erythroleukemia virus, but no viral relationship has been found for the human disease.

PATHOPHYSIOLOGY AND SYMPTOMATOLOGY   Polycythemia vera is a neoplastic stem cell disorder associated with excessive proliferation of erythroid, granulocytic, and megakaryocytic precursors. Since erythrocytosis is the primary manifestation of PV, it must be differentiated from secondary causes of erythrocytosis which usually are associated with syndromes of increased elaboration of erythropoietin (Table 309-2). The serum concentration of erythropoietin is low in PV but is not absent. While initially it was believed that PV erythropoiesis was autonomous, it is now known that the erythroid precursors in PV patients respond to erythropoietin and may be hypersensitive to its action. Bone marrow cells from patients with PV form colonies of erythroid precursors in culture in the absence of added erythropoietin. This phenomenon is rarely seen in other conditions. Much of this "endogenous" erythroid colony formation in PV is abrogated by the addition of antibodies to erythropoietin, suggesting increased sensitivity to erythropoietin. Some red cell

---

TABLE 309-2   Classification of polycythemia

PRIMARY (AUTONOMOUS)

Polycythemia vera
"Pure" erythrocytosis ("erythremia")
   Familial
   Sporadic

SECONDARY

Physiologically appropriate (decreased tissue oxygenation)
  High altitude
  Chronic lung disease
  Alveolar hypoventilation
  Cardiovascular right-to-left shunt
  High-oxygen-affinity hemoglobinopathy
  Carboxyhemoglobinemia ("smoker's erythrocytosis")
  Congenitally decreased erythrocyte 2,3,-DPG
Physiologically inappropriate (normal tissue oxygenation)
  Tumors producing erythropoietin or other erythropoietic stimuli
    Renal cell carcinoma
    Hepatocellular carcinoma
    Cerebellar hemangioblastoma
    Uterine leiomyoma
    Ovarian carcinoma
    Pheochromocytoma
  Renal diseases
    Cysts
    Hydronephrosis
    Diffuse parenchymal disease
    Bartter's syndrome
    Renal transplantation
    Nephrotic syndrome
    Long-term hemodialysis
  Adrenal cortical hypersecretion
  Exogenous androgens, erythropoietin, cobalt
  Unexplained ("essential")

RELATIVE POLYCYTHEMIA (SPURIOUS OR STRESS ERYTHRO-CYTOSIS, GAISBÖCK'S SYNDROME)

SOURCE: Hocking and Golde.

production in PV, however, may be autonomous with respect to erythropoietin. As with chronic myelogenous leukemia, there are increased myeloid and megakaryocytic progenitors in the bone marrow, indicating that the panmyelosis in PV is characterized by expansion of the committed precursor cell pools.

Patients with PV usually present with symptoms referable to an expanded blood volume. They may complain of headaches, vertigo, tinnitus, or blurred vision. Occasionally, patients present with thrombotic complications or hemostatic defects manifested by easy bruisability, epistaxis, or gastrointestinal hemorrhage. Other symptoms include weight loss, sweating, pain in the feet, peptic ulceration, or severe pruritus, which is often aggravated by bathing in warm water. These symptoms relate to hypermetabolism, hyperhistaminemia, hypervolemia, and abnormal platelet function. Approximately one-third of the patients have hypertension. An occasional patient will present with symptoms referable to splenomegaly or hyperuricemia. Asymptomatic patients are often identified by routine blood count determinations.

Physical examination typically shows plethora and, occasionally, dusky cyanosis. There is often venous prominence with engorgement of the retinal veins, and splenomegaly is present in approximately 75 percent of patients. Splenomegaly is a key physical finding in terms of differentiating PV from secondary polycythemia.

LABORATORY FINDINGS The diagnostic criteria of the Polycythemia Study Group are presented in Table 309-3. These criteria were developed to help ensure uniformity with regard to the diagnosis of PV, but they are stringent and may exclude early stages of the disease. Typically, patients present with an elevated hemoglobin concentration and hematocrit associated with thrombocytosis, leukocytosis, and splenomegaly. In these cases, diagnosis is straightforward. Patients presenting only with erythrocytosis need a systematic evaluation to establish a firm diagnosis. The confirmation of true polycythemia requires determination of a chromium 51 red cell mass and a plasma volume study. If the red cell mass is normal and the plasma volume low-normal or reduced, the patient does not have true polycythemia but, rather, a relative increase in hemoglobin concentration. This circumstance can be seen in patients receiving diuretic therapy or in those who fall in a heterogeneous group of patients previously referred to as having *Gaisböck's syndrome*, now known as *spurious* or *stress erythrocytosis*. If true polycythemia is documented by an increased red cell mass, PV needs to be distinguished from secondary causes of erythrocytosis (see Table 309-2). Signs of panmyelosis, including leukocytosis, basophilia, thrombocytosis, and splenomegaly, strongly point to the diagnosis of PV. In obvious cases, no elaborate testing is required. Bone marrow examination is usually not needed, but iron deposits may be absent and mild reticulin fibrosis may be present at the time of diagnosis. Cytogenetic studies in PV may show clonal markers ($+1$, $+8$, $+9$, 20q-) in up to 30 percent of the patients.

In the absence of clear-cut signs of PV, additional laboratory testing is necessary. Determination of the serum erythropoietin concentration is important in distinguishing primary from secondary causes of polycythemia. An elevated erythropoietin concentration suggests secondary erythrocytosis, while a low level is compatible with PV. An oxygen saturation of less than 92 percent suggests hypoxemia as the cause for erythrocytosis. Direct measurement of carboxyhemoglobin and arterial oxygen saturation can be helpful. Measurement of the P_{50} of the oxyhemoglobin dissociation curve is useful in detecting high-oxygen-affinity hemoglobins. Radiographic evaluation of the kidneys may be necessary to rule out a renal lesion secreting erythropoietin. In some patients, examination of the liver or the posterior fossa of the brain may be indicated to exclude hepatic lesions or cerebellar hemangioblastoma associated with abnormal erythropoietin production.

In PV, the neutrophil alkaline phosphatase score is frequently increased, as is the serum vitamin B_{12} level and serum vitamin B_{12}-binding capacity. Although they are included as part of the Polycythemia Vera Study Group criteria, these laboratory findings are seldom helpful in differential diagnosis.

COURSE AND PROGNOSIS The use of ^{32}P and myelosuppressive therapy with alkylating agents, while providing disease control, has led to an increased incidence of acute leukemia, and these therapies are rarely used today. The so-called spent or burnt-out phase of PV is characterized by marked splenomegaly and anemia associated with bone marrow fibrosis. Modern therapy may lead to an altered disease course, and survival in excess of 12 years is now common. The majority of patients in the past have died of vascular complications of the disease. Acute leukemia may occur in 2 percent of patients who have not been exposed to alkylating agents or radiotherapy.

TREATMENT While treatment for the patient with polycythemia vera needs to be individualized, phlebotomy is indicated initially in all patients to reduce the hematocrit to less than 46 percent. In young patients with normal cardiac function, a 1-unit phlebotomy can often be performed on alternating days or every third day until a safe hematocrit is achieved. Patients with cardiovascular disease and older patients should have smaller-volume phlebotomies performed twice weekly. Therapy should be directed toward maintaining the hematocrit between 42 and 44 percent. With continued phlebotomy, there is the inevitable development of iron deficiency, which will impair red cell production and permit phlebotomy at widely spaced intervals. Iron deficiency itself, however, may cause unwanted side effects, and secondary microcytosis may increase whole blood viscosity. Some iron supplementation may be required and necessitate phlebotomy at more frequent intervals. Patients who are managed by phlebotomy alone have a measurably high risk of thrombotic complications over a 5- to 7-year period after diagnosis. Thrombosis in patients treated with phlebotomy alone is more common in older patients, but hematocrit and platelet count do not have a significant impact on the risk of thrombosis.

The results of the Polycythemia Vera Study Group experience indicated that patients treated with ^{32}P or chlorambucil had a greater than 10 percent incidence of acute leukemia. Therefore, chlorambucil is now contraindicated in the treatment of PV. ^{32}P can only be recommended for the very elderly or for unusual circumstances where the patient cannot have regular medical supervision. Hydroxyurea has been shown to be highly effective in controlling the polycythemic syndrome, and approximately three-quarters of patients can achieve long-term disease control with this drug. While the lack of mutagenicity of hydroxyurea has been called into question, it appears to be one of the safest myelosuppressants available. Other alkylating agents are also effective in controlling the disease but appear to have leukemogenic potential equivalent to that of chlorambucil. IFN-α, an experimental agent in the treatment of PV that decreases panmyelosis and can control the erythrocytosis, has considerable promise. While the role of IFN-α in the treatment of PV is not yet determined, it is an active and useful agent without apparent leukemogenic potential. It also may be combined with intermittent phlebotomy or with hydroxyurea in difficult to manage patients. At present, it is not known if interferon has a selective effect on the neoplastic clone in PV as it does in CML.

TABLE 309-3 Diagnostic criteria for polycythemia vera

Category A
  1 Significantly elevated red cell mass
  2 Arterial blood oxygen saturation $\geq 92\%$
  3 Splenomegaly
Category B
  1 Thrombocytosis >400,000 per microliter
  2 Leukocytosis >12,000 per microliter
  3 Increased leukocyte alkaline phosphatase score in absence of fever or infection
  4 Serum vitamin B_{12} level greater than 900 pg/mL or vitamin B_{12}-binding capacity greater than 2200 pg/mL

Diagnosis of polycythemia vera if: A1 + A2 + A3 or A1 + A2 + any two factors from category B

SOURCE: Adapted from the Polycythemia Vera Study Group criteria.

Special problems arise in the management of patients with PV. Elective surgery should not be performed in uncontrolled PV, since hemorrhagic and thrombotic complications lead to a markedly increased perioperative mortality. Generally, such surgery should be postponed until the disease has been under control for 2 months. In emergency situations, isovolemic phlebotomy should be performed prior to surgery.

Severe pruritus may be an important problem, and attempts to treat it with agents such as hydroxyzine, cyproheptadine, or cimetadine are warranted, but inhibition of hematopoiesis with hydroxyurea or IFN-α may be required for symptom control. The use of antiplatelet agents in PV is controversial, particularly since they may increase the risk of hemorrhage. Small doses of aspirin (baby aspirin) may be indicated in patients with a thrombotic tendency. Where the platelet count cannot be controlled with hydroxyurea, IFN-α or anagrelide can be used. Hyperuricemia should be treated with allopurinol, and hemorrhagic complications may rarely require platelet transfusion.

AGNOGENIC MYELOID METAPLASIA WITH MYELOFIBROSIS (MF)

DEFINITION AND ETIOLOGY Agnogenic myeloid metaplasia with myelofibrosis (MF), also called *idiopathic myelofibrosis*, is a clonal disorder of the hematopoietic stem cell characterized by bone marrow fibrosis and extramedullary hematopoiesis. Gradual fibrosis of the bone marrow and hyperplasia of myeloid elements result in progressive anemia and variable changes in granulocyte and platelet counts associated with increasing splenomegaly. The disease begins in late middle life and is gradual in onset, chronic, and progressive. Males and females are equally affected, and there is a rare reported familial occurrence.

PATHOPHYSIOLOGY AND SYMPTOMATOLOGY Idiopathic MF is a clonal hematopoietic disorder in which fibroblastic proliferation is thought to be due to release of growth factors such as platelet-derived growth factor or tumor growth factor from platelets and megakaryocytes. Type III collagen is usually the cause of myelofibrosis. Bone marrow fibroblasts have been demonstrated not to be part of the neoplastic clone. MF commonly presents with symptoms related to anemia and splenomegaly. Splenomegaly is present in all patients, and in some, splenic enlargement may be massive. The splenomegaly may be present for years prior to diagnosis and can cause pain, abdominal fullness, and early satiety. Hepatomegaly is seen in approximately 50 to 75 percent of patients but is not observed in the absence of splenomegaly. As the disease progresses, patients may experience weight loss, skin and mucous membrane bleeding, and, less commonly, bone pain, jaundice, and lymphadenopathy.

LABORATORY FINDINGS Anemia is observed in over half of patients at diagnosis and ultimately develops in all patients. Initially, the anemia is due to ineffective erythropoiesis, but subsequently, there is increased pooling of red blood cells in the spleen and decreased red cell survival. Folate deficiency and, rarely, autoimmune hemolytic anemia or acquired hemoglobin H disease may develop. Examination of the peripheral blood smear reveals poikilocytosis with prominent teardrop forms. Fragmented red cells and nucleated red blood cells are commonly observed. An increase in platelet count is seen in half of patients, and giant platelets or megakaryocytes may be seen in the peripheral blood. A moderate elevation in neutrophil count is observed in most patients, but neutropenia is seen in up to 25 percent of the cases. Often there is a left shift toward early granulocytic forms, and occasionally, circulating blasts may be found. Some patients have an increase in absolute basophil count. The neutrophil alkaline phosphatase score is elevated in about half of patients, but others have a lower than normal value. Platelet function studies often show defective platelet adhesiveness and impaired secondary release of ADP in response to epinephrine.

Radiographically demonstrable bone sclerosis is seen in about 50 percent of patients, particularly in the proximal long bones and the vertebral bodies. Rarely, osteolytic lesions are demonstrable. Routine radiographic studies usually show splenomegaly and dense bones.

Bone marrow aspiration is almost always unsuccessful in patients with MF and results in a "dry tap." Bone marrow biopsy should be performed and reveals fibrosis of marrow spaces and often osteosclerosis. MF may be extensive or focal, and megakaryocytic hyperplasia is usually observed. Pathologically, the spleen shows features of extramedullary hematopoiesis in the red pulp.

DIAGNOSIS The diagnosis of idiopathic MF is usually not difficult, nor is it hard to distinguish it from other myeloproliferative disorders. The presence of the Ph chromosome and a low neutrophil alkaline phosphatase score distinguish CML from idiopathic MF. While MF and PV can present with a similar pathologic picture, the history of PV is usually distinctive. Rarely, myelodysplasia with MF may create confusion. Megakaryoblastic leukemia (acute MF) normally presents with fever and pancytopenia and should be differentiated from idiopathic MF.

THERAPY There is no definitive therapy for idiopathic MF. Bone marrow transplantation offers the only potential curative therapeutic option. Marrow fibrosis may be reversible after bone marrow transplantation, but few patients are of an appropriate age or have an HLA-matched sibling donor. Normally when therapy is required for idiopathic MF, it is because of anemia. Since the anemia may be multifactorial, a search for folate or iron deficiency and/or autoimmune hemolytic anemia is indicated, since specific therapy in these circumstances is effective. Treatment with androgens will lead to responses in approximately 30 to 40 percent of anemic patients. Danazol, 200 mg three times daily, orally, or testosterone enanthate, 400 mg weekly, intramuscularly, in men has been employed with some success, although the precise mechanism of androgen action is unknown. Androgen side effects may be serious, particularly in older men with occult prostate cancer. Measurement of the serum erythropoietin level can be helpful in guiding potential therapy with erythropoietin, although there are little controlled data regarding the utility of erythropoietin in this disease. Transfusions are necessary for unresponsive anemia.

In the face of marked splenomegaly, the issue of splenectomy must be addressed. Splenectomy performed under appropriate conditions offers an important opportunity to enhance the quality of life for patients with idiopathic MF. In the older literature, however, splenectomy was associated with unacceptable perioperative morbidity and mortality. While splenectomy does not affect the overall survival of patients with idiopathic MF, it can be a useful therapeutic approach to manage hemolytic anemia, thrombocytopenia, and painful splenic infarction, as well as portal hypertension. Splenectomy, however, is contraindicated in the face of increased platelet counts, and it is important to achieve optimal disease control beforehand.

Chemotherapy can be useful in the management of symptomatic patients with idiopathic MF. The drug of choice in these situations is hydroxyurea, which can reduce the leukocytosis and constitutional symptoms associated with the disease and may reduce spleen size and splenic discomfort. Hydroxyurea should be initiated at doses of approximately 0.5 to 1.0 g/d, but higher doses may be required to reduce platelet counts. The effect of hydroxyurea on marrow fibrosis is uncertain. Alkylating agents are now contraindicated, but IFN-α may be useful in selective patients with marked thrombocytosis. Overall experience with IFN-α is currently too limited to decide on its role. Glucocorticoids may be useful if autoimmune hemolytic anemia is associated with the MF and to reduce constitutional symptoms, but side effects limit its chronic use. Radiation therapy for massive splenomegaly has limited application in the palliation of debilitated and elderly patients.

ESSENTIAL THROMBOCYTOSIS

DEFINITION AND ETIOLOGY Essential thrombocytosis (ET) is a myeloproliferative disorder characterized by markedly elevated platelet production, with blood platelet counts above 600,000 cells

TABLE 309-4   Differential diagnosis of thrombocytosis

MYELOPROLIFERATIVE DISORDERS

Essential thrombocythemia
Polycythemia vera
Chronic myelogenous leukemia
Myelofibrosis

SECONDARY THROMBOCYTOSIS

Recovery from acute infection
Malignant disease
   Carcinoma
   Hodgkin's disease
   Lymphoma
Hemolytic anemia
Postoperative
   Splenectomy
   Other surgical procedures
Acute hemorrhage
Iron deficiency
Response to drugs
   Epinephrine
   Vincristine
Chronic inflammatory disorders
   Rheumatoid arthritis
   Ulcerative colitis
   Hepatic cirrhosis
   Sarcoidosis
Response to exercise, stress
Recovery from myelosuppresive drugs
Therapy of vitamin B_{12} deficiency
Others: Osteoporosis, 5q− syndrome

per microliter. Clinical involvement of hematopoietic lineages other than the megakaryocytic line is unusual. The disease must be distinguished from secondary thrombocytosis in response to inflammation, acute bleeding, iron deficiency, or neoplasia (Table 309-4). The cause of ET is unknown.

PATHOPHYSIOLOGY AND SYMPTOMATOLOGY   ET is likely a disorder of the pluripotent hematopoietic stem cell, based on the demonstration of monoclonality in the bone marrow in about 90 percent of females determined using X chromosome–linked gene probes. "Autonomous" in vitro megakaryocytic colony formation is observed in this disease, and "autonomous" erythroid colony formation also has been reported. Clinically, however, evidence of polycythemia or granulocytosis is rare.

The symptoms of ET are related to the increased platelet count and platelet dysfunction. Two-thirds of patients are asymptomatic at diagnosis, and younger patients can remain asymptomatic for long periods. Vascular occlusion may be found in 20 to 50 percent of patients at diagnosis and involves both arteries and veins. Platelet emboli or local platelet aggregation can lead to microvascular occlusion associated with transient cerebral ischemic symptoms, stroke, or digital ischemia. Occlusion of the coronary or mesenteric vessels also may occur. Erythromelalgia is a syndrome of redness and burning in the extremities, which is probably due to arteriolar occlusion. Venous thrombosis is also observed in ET and may involve the portal, hepatic, or splenic veins. Hemorrhagic manifestations are found in up to 50 percent of patients, usually involving the mucous membranes or skin, but occasionally severe gastrointestinal hemorrhage can occur. Patients may complain of easy bruisability or prolonged bleeding after minor surgery or dental procedures. Usually there is a correlation between the platelet count and symptoms, but younger patients, especially women, may have high platelet counts and may be asymptomatic for prolonged periods.

LABORATORY FINDINGS   An elevated platelet count is the most prominent abnormality in ET. The peripheral blood smear shows platelets of different size and shape, often with giant forms and hypogranularity. Functional abnormalities include impaired platelet aggregation in response to epinephrine, collagen, or adenosine diphosphate (ADP). The epinephrine defect is most characteristic.

No correlation is observed between bleeding and in vitro platelet aggregation abnormalities. Splenic enlargement is seen in two-thirds of patients and is usually modest. Anemia or granulocytosis is uncommon. Bone marrow examination reveals increased numbers of megakaryocytes which may show morphologic abnormalities, and modest reticulin fibrosis is seen in patients with advanced disease.

DIAGNOSIS   A markedly elevated platelet count in the absence of an identifiable cause of secondary thrombocytosis is usually sufficient for a diagnosis of ET. Support for the diagnosis may be obtained by in vitro platelet aggregation studies and the documentation of splenomegaly. Cytogenetic abnormalities are uncommon. Secondary thrombocytosis is usually associated with increased numbers of megakaryocytes of small diameter and low ploidy. In ET, the megakaryocytes are large and hyperploid.

The Polycythemia Vera Study Group has proposed the following diagnostic criteria for ET: (1) platelet count persistently greater than 1 million per microliter in the absence of any identifiable cause, (2) normal red cell volume or hemoglobin less than 13 g/dL, (3) presence of iron in the bone marrow, (4) absence of collagen fibrosis in the bone marrow biopsy, and (5) absence of the Philadelphia chromosome.

COURSE AND PROGNOSIS   Survival in older patients is similar to that of patients with PV. Patients usually die of hemorrhagic or thrombotic complications. ET can progress into MF in perhaps a quarter of patients and in about 5 percent transforms into an acute leukemia. The disease seems to follow a much more benign course in some young patients in whom there may not be an associated high risk of hemorrhage or thrombosis.

THERAPY   Asymptomatic younger patients often can simply be observed, even if their platelet counts are over 1 million per microliter. Such asymptomatic patients may have stable disease for many years. All patients with thrombocytosis should be strongly encouraged not to smoke. Symptomatic disease should be treated, and older patients with platelet counts approaching 1 million per microliter also should receive therapy. Radioactive phosphorus and busulfan are no longer used because of significant toxicity and mutagenicity. Hydroxyurea is generally considered to be the initial treatment of choice to lower the platelet count to 500,000 per microliter or less. Hydroxyurea is usually given in doses of 500 to 2000 mg/d orally, with few side effects. IFN-α is an experimental agent with distinct activity in ET. The dose of IFN-α must be adjusted with respect to acute toxicity and the development of neutropenia. The tolerance for IFN-α varies considerably from patient to patient, but a frequent starting point is 3 million units subcutaneously daily. IFN-α is effective in controlling the platelet count and may partially reverse platelet function defects. Little is known of the possible long-term advantages or disadvantages of IFN-α as compared with hydroxyurea. Anagrelide is a novel compound with powerful antiaggregating effects on platelets which also significantly inhibits platelet production. Anagrelide has a specific effect on thrombopoiesis and does not appear to influence other hematopoietic lineages. Control of the platelet count with anagrelide is seen in over 90 percent of patients. The major side effects are neurologic, gastrointestinal, and cardiac and lead to discontinuation of the treatment in about 15 percent of patients. Fluid retention and peripheral edema are common.

The use of antiplatelet function agents such as aspirin or dipyridole is controversial. These agents can lead to serious hemorrhage, yet they may protect against thrombosis in other patients. Control of the platelet count seems to be of primary importance, but in those rare patients in whom good control cannot be achieved or who develop thrombotic complications despite adequate lowering of the platelet count, the addition of low-dose aspirin seems warranted. Patients who hemorrhage despite control of the platelet count may rarely require platelet transfusion as a lifesaving measure.

REFERENCES

ANAGRELIDE STUDY GROUP: Anagrelide, a therapy for thrombocythemic states: Experience in 577 patients. Am J Med 69:76, 1992

BIGGS JC et al: Treatment of chronic myeloid leukemia with allogeneic bone marrow transplantation after preparation with Bu-Cy 2. Blood 5:1352, 1992

CUNNINGHAM I: Bone marrow transplantation for chronic myelogenous leukemia. Oncology 4:101, 1990

DALEY GQ et al: Induction of chronic myelogenous leukemia in mice by the P210[bcr/abl] gene of the Philadelphia chromosome. Science 247:824, 1990

DHINGRA K et al: Minimal residual disease in interferon-treated chronic myelogenous leukemia: Results and pitfalls of analysis based on polymerase chain reaction. Leukemia 6:754, 1992

GUILHOT F et al: Cytogenetic remissions in chronic myelogenous leukemia using interferon alpha-2a and hydroxyurea with or without low-dose cytosine arabinoside. Leuk Lymph 4:49, 1991

HEHLMANN R et al: Chronic myelogenous leukemia: Recent developments in prognostic evaluation and chemotherapy. Leukemia 6(suppl 3):110S, 1992

HOCKING WG, GOLDE DW: Polycythemia: Evaluation and management. Blood Rev 3:59, 1989

KOLB HJ et al: Donor leukocyte transfusions for treatment of recurrent chronic myelogenous leukemia in marrow transplant patients. Blood 76:2462, 1990

PEARSON TC: Primary thrombocythaemia: Diagnosis and management. Br J Haematol 78:145, 1991

SILVER RT: A new treatment for polycythemia vera: Recombinant interferon alpha. Blood 76:664, 1990

————: Chronic myeloid leukemia. Curr Opin Oncol 4:66, 1992

TALPAZ M et al: Interferon-alpha produces sustained cytogenetic responses in chronic myelogenous leukemia: Philadelphia chromosome-positive patients. Ann Intern Med 114:532, 1991

———— et al: Recombinant interferon-alpha therapy of Philadelphia chromosome-negative myeloproliferative disorders with thrombocytosis. Am J Med 86:554, 1989

WEINSTEIN IM: Idiopathic myelofibrosis: Historical review, diagnosis and management. Blood Rev 5:98, 1991

310   THE LEUKEMIAS

DAVID A. SCHEINBERG / DAVID W. GOLDE

Leukemias are neoplasms derived from hematopoietic cells that proliferate initially in the bone marrow before disseminating to the peripheral blood, spleen, lymph nodes, and ultimately, other tissues. As such, they are distinguished from the lymphomas, which arise primarily in the lymph nodes but also may spread (in "leukemic phase") to the blood and marrow. Classification of leukemia is broadly related to the cell of origin (e.g., lymphoid or myeloid) as well as to the rapidity of the clinical course (e.g., acute or chronic), but modern categorizations have identified specific leukemias on the basis of biologic, antigenic, and molecular characteristics of these diseases. This chapter reviews acute myelogenous leukemia (AML), the acute and chronic lymphocytic leukemias (ALL and CLL), and hairy cell leukemia. Chronic myelogenous leukemia (CML) is covered in Chap. 309.

ETIOLOGY The cause of leukemia is not known in most patients, although both genetic and environmental factors are important. There is a high concordance rate among identical twins if acute leukemia develops in the first year of life, and families with an excessive incidence of leukemia have been identified. Acute leukemia occurs with an increased frequency in a variety of congenital disorders, including the Down, Bloom, Klinefelter, Fanconi, and Wiskott-Aldrich syndromes.

Environmental factors are also known to play a role in the etiology of leukemia. Ionizing radiation causes leukemia in experimental animals, and there is a clear relationship between such exposure and the development of leukemia in humans. For example, individuals with occupational radiation exposure, patients receiving radiation therapy, and Japanese survivors of the atomic bomb explosions have a predictable and dose-related increased incidence of leukemia. Radiation exposure increases the risk of developing CML, AML, and possibly ALL, but there is no known relationship to CLL or to hairy cell leukemia. Exposure to chemicals such as benzene and other aromatic hydrocarbons or treatment with alkylating agents and other chemotherapeutic drugs also leads to an increased incidence of AML. The combination of radiation and chemotherapeutic agents, such

as in patients treated for Hodgkin's disease, results in additive leukemogenic effects. A role for electromagnetic energy in leukemogenesis remains unproven.

Although RNA-based retroviruses cause a number of leukemias in animals, a viral cause for a human leukemia has been established only for adult T cell leukemia (ATL), which is caused by the human T cell leukemia virus type I (HTLV-I). This virus can be transmitted horizontally by sexual contact or blood products as well as from mother to child (see Chap. 151). ATL is endemic in southwestern Japan and parts of the Caribbean and central Africa. The other known human leukemia virus, HTLV-II, has not yet been firmly linked to a specific leukemia. Epstein-Barr virus (EBV) has been associated with a form of ALL (L3 subtype) as well as certain aggressive lymphomas. The common forms of acute and chronic leukemia, however, are not contagious, and the incidence of leukemia is not increased among close contacts such as marital partners or in the offspring of women who develop leukemia during pregnancy.

INCIDENCE AND PREVALENCE The incidence of all leukemias is approximately 13 per 100,000 people per year, and the age-related incidence of both acute and chronic leukemias is somewhat higher in men than in women. ALL is primarily a disease of children and young adults, whereas AML, CLL, and hairy cell leukemia increase in incidence with increasing age, peaking in the sixth and seventh decades.

PATHOPHYSIOLOGY Acute leukemia is characterized by the clonal proliferation of immature hematopoietic cells. The leukemia arises following malignant transformation of a single hematopoietic progenitor, followed by cellular replication and expansion of the transformed clone. The most prominent characteristic of the neoplastic cells in acute leukemia is a defect in maturation beyond the myeloblast or promyelocyte level in AML and the lymphoblast level in ALL. The proliferating leukemia cells accumulate in the bone marrow, suppressing normal hematopoiesis and ultimately resulting in the replacement of normal elements. The consequent paucity of normal progenitors leads to the anemia, infections, and bleeding complications that characterize the disease. Leukemic cells proliferate primarily in the bone marrow, circulate in the blood, and may infiltrate into other tissues such as lymph nodes, liver, spleen, skin, gums, viscera, and the central nervous system (CNS). Although the diagnosis of leukemia is often first made by observation of large numbers of blasts in the blood, the majority of the leukemic cells are found in the marrow.

The cellular blood elements are derived from pluripotent and committed hematopoietic stem cells which reside in the bone marrow (Chap. 301). Leukemic transformation may occur in cells at several levels of differentiation. In some patients with AML who are heterozygous for glucose-6-phosphate dehydrogenase (G6PD) isoenzymes, the granulocytes, macrophages, erythrocytes, and megakaryocytes all contain the single G6PD isoenzyme present in the leukemic cells, suggesting that these cells are derived from the malignant clone and that leukemic transformation involved a multipotent stem cell. In other AML patients, only granulocytes and/or macrophages appear clonal, and in these patients, transformation may have occurred at the level of the committed granulocytic-macrophage progenitor. Clonality in different lineages also has been confirmed by fluorescence in situ hybridization studies.

The mechanism of neoplastic transformation producing leukemia is poorly understood but involves a fundamental alteration of DNA conferring hereditable malignant characteristics to the transformed cell and its progeny. In animals, leukemias can be induced by retroviruses which either carry a transforming gene (viral oncogene) or integrate into specific sites in DNA causing activation of cellular proto-oncogenes (insertional mutagenesis). The role of oncogenes in the pathogenesis of neoplasia is discussed in Chap. 63. With sensitive techniques, clonal cytogenetic abnormalities can be detected in most patients with acute and chronic leukemias. A wide range of cytogenetic abnormalities is associated with the various forms of leukemias, and distinctive nonrandom chromosomal abnormalities are found, as shown in Table 310-1. Chromosomal rearrangement in leukemic cells

TABLE 310-1 Common chromosomal abnormalities associated with leukemias

Abnormality	Associated disease	Comment
MYELOGENOUS LEUKEMIA		
t(8;21)	AML—M2	Better prognosis
t(15;17)	AML—M3	Retinoic acid receptor gene rearranged; better prognosis
inv (16); del (16q)	AML—M4 with eosinophils	Better prognosis
+8	AML—all subtypes	Poor prognosis
+21	AML—M1, M7	
+13	AML—biphenotypic	
5q−, −5, −7	AML—especially secondary AML	Poor prognosis
t(9;11)	AML—M5A	Poor prognosis
t(9;22)	CML	Poor prognosis; tyrosine kinase *bcr-abl* oncogene product created
t(4;11)	Biphenotypic leukemia	Poor prognosis
ACUTE LYMPHOCYTIC LEUKEMIA		
t(4;11)	ALL—L2	Poor prognosis
t(1;19)	ALL—L1; with clg expression	DNA binding fusion protein created
t(8;14)	ALL—L3	Poor prognosis; *myc* oncogene upregulated
Hyperdiploidy	ALL—L1, L2	Better prognosis
t(9;22)	ALL	Poor prognosis
t(10;14)	ALL—T cell	T cell receptor gene rearranged
9p−, 6q−, or 12p−	ALL	Most frequent abnormalities seen; up to 10% each in ALL
CHRONIC LYMPHOCYTIC LEUKEMIA		
+12	CLL	
14q + Abnormalities	Any B lineage leukemias	

may alter the structure or regulation of cellular oncogenes, producing quantitative or qualitative changes in their gene products that may play a role in initiating or maintaining the leukemic state. For example, the t(15;17) translocation of acute promyelocytic leukemia (APL) results in the production of a new oncogenic protein that has retinoic acid–binding properties. Treatment of patients with APL with large doses of retinoic acid results in maturation of the cells and the induction of remission. The t(9;22) translocation results in an aberrant tyrosine kinase protein; the t(8;14) translocation yields an overexpression of the growth regulatory protein myc; and the t(1;19) translocation forms a new DNA-binding protein. Most data suggest that the development of leukemia is a multistep process, and in many cases, acute leukemia develops in patients with a preexisting myelodysplastic or myeloproliferative disorder.

The pathophysiology of bone marrow failure in leukemia is complex. Pancytopenia is typically present and results at least in part from physical replacement of the normal precursor cells by leukemic cells. Some patients with acute leukemia and pancytopenia have a hypocellular bone marrow, indicating that the marrow failure is not simply due to overcrowding by leukemic cells. Leukemic cells may directly inhibit normal hematopoiesis via cell-mediated or humoral mechanisms. Normal hematopoietic stem cells do remain in the bone marrow and are capable of proliferating and restoring hematopoiesis following effective antileukemic treatment.

Some patients develop AML after a preleukemic or myelodysplastic syndrome. The myelodysplastic syndromes are a heterogeneous group of disorders typically found in middle-aged or older patients and have been subclassified into the categories of refractory anemia (RA),

refractory anemia with ringed sideroblasts (RARS), refractory anemia with excess blasts (RAEB), refractory anemia with excess blasts in transformation (RAEB-T), and chronic myelomonocytic leukemia (CMMOL) (see Chap. 308). The term *preleukemia* should be reserved for a recognizable syndrome of hematopoietic dysfunction that typically precedes the classic findings of AML. This syndrome is usually characterized by a picture of ineffective hematopoiesis with anemia, thrombocytopenia, and sometimes granulocytopenia associated with a hypercellular, dysplastic bone marrow. In preleukemia, the leukemic clone is already established, and usually there is progressive impairment of hematopoiesis and accumulation of blasts. Megaloblastic hematopoiesis is common, and folate or vitamin B_{12} deficiency must be ruled out. Cytogenetic abnormalities are frequent; the most common chromosomal abnormalities are 5q−, −5, −7, and trisomy 8. When 5q− exists as the sole abnormality, the patient usually presents with refractory anemia associated with mild thrombocytosis. This disorder, referred to as the *5q − syndrome*, only progresses to acute leukemia in a minority of patients. Many patients with preleukemic or myelodysplastic syndromes never develop overt AML but die from complications of bone marrow failure. *Smoldering AML* refers to a syndrome in which the diagnostic features of acute leukemia are present, but the disease follows an indolent or subacute course. This disorder also tends to occur in elderly patients.

ACUTE LEUKEMIAS: ALL AND AML

PATHOLOGY AND CLASSIFICATION The diagnosis of acute leukemia requires the demonstration of leukemic cells in the bone marrow, peripheral blood, or extramedullary tissues. The bone marrow is typically hypercellular with a monomorphic infiltration of leukemic blasts and a marked reduction in normal bone marrow elements. The diagnosis of the type of leukemia is currently based on a combination of morphologic, immunophenotypic, and cytochemical characteristics, as well as evidence of specific genetic translocations, when present. It is critical to distinguish ALL from AML, since these two diseases differ in natural history, prognosis, and response to various therapeutic agents. As many as one-third of adult ALL cases bear the t(9;22) translocation, with incidence increasing with age. It is important to identify these patients because prognosis is much poorer.

Acute lymphocytic leukemia can be identified and classified on the basis of morphology and immunologic phenotype related to the stage of lymphoid differentiation. The leukemic lymphoblasts in ALL are generally smaller (10 to 15 μm in diameter) than myeloblasts and typically have only a thin rim of agranular cytoplasm. The nucleus may be round or convoluted (see Fig. A9-24). Three morphologic subtypes are included in the French-American-British (FAB) classification: L1 cells are small and homogeneous with a regular nuclear membrane and a small nucleolus. L2 cells are larger, have a lower nucleus-to-cytoplasm ratio with more pleomorphism and typically have one or more prominent nucleoli. The L3 form of ALL is uncommon, occurring in less than 5 percent of cases; the leukemic cells in this variant contain large vesicular nuclei with basophilic, often vacuolated cytoplasm. L3 cells have a high mitotic index and represent the leukemic form of Burkitt's lymphoma.

Leukemic lymphoblasts in more than 90 percent of patients with ALL contain a nuclear enzyme terminal, deoxynucleotidyl transferase (Tdt), which is less commonly present in AML cells (about 20 percent). L3 ALL, a more mature subtype, is typically negative for Tdt, as are mature hematopoietic cells, CLL, and hairy cell leukemias. The leukemic cells from approximately half of patients with ALL react with the periodic acid Schiff stain, showing blocklike inclusions of glycogen. Lymphoblasts do not contain granulocytic or monocytic lysosomal enzymes and therefore do not react with cytochemical stains for peroxidase, Sudan black, and nonspecific esterase.

A large number of cell surface protein antigens on leukemia cells have now been identified by monoclonal antibodies. These antigens and antibodies are grouped according to cluster of differentiation

TABLE 310-2   Morphologic subtypes of acute leukemias

Subtype	Percent of cases	Morphology	Reactivity with special stains or markers			
			Peroxidase or Sudan black	Nonspecific esterase	Periodic acid shift	Typical protein markers
M0, undifferentiated	3	Primitive cells; absence of cytochemical stains	−	−	−	CD34, 33, 13
M1, AML without maturation	20	Few if any azurophilic granules	+/−	+/−	−	CD34, 33, 13
M2, AML with maturation	25	Blasts with promyelocytic granules, Auer rods may be present	+++	+/−	−	CD34, 33, 15, 13
M3, promyelocytic leukemia	10	Hypergranular promyelocytes often with multiple Auer rods per cell	+++	+	+/−	CD33, 13, (HLA-Dr−)
M4, acute myelomonocytic leukemia	20	Monocytoid-appearing cells in peripheral blood; M4 with eosinophilia is subtype	+/−	+++	−	CD34, 33, 15, 14, 13
M5, acute monocytic leukemia	20	Two subtypes identified: (a) undifferentiated; (b) differentiated with 80% promonocytes and monocytes	−	+++	+/−	CD33, 15, 14, 13
M6, acute erythroleukemia	5	Predominance of erythroblasts and markedly dysplastic erythroid precursors	+/−	−	+++	CD33, glycophorin
M7, acute megakaryocytic leukemia	5	Undifferentiated blasts react with antiplatelet antibodies and contain platelet peroxidase	−	+/−	++	CD33, CD41
L1 ALL	75	Small round blasts with scanty cytoplasm	−	−	+++	CD10, 19, 34, Tdt
L2 ALL	20	Pleomorphic larger blasts with more cytoplasm and prominent nucleoli	−	−	+++	CD10, 19, 34, Tdt
L3 ALL	5	Large blasts with basophilic vacuolated cytoplasm and vesicular nuclei	−	−	+++	CD19, CD20, sIg

(CD) numbers. Certain antigens are preferentially expressed on cells of specific lineage and at different stages of maturation (Tables 310-2 and 310-3). Identification of these antigens is often useful in diagnosis. Virtually all lymphocytic leukemias of B cell origin express

TABLE 310-3   Cell surface markers used in diagnosing leukemias

Marker name	Normal cell distribution	Leukemia distribution
HLA-Dr	Early myeloid, monocytoid, B lineage	ALL, AML, CLL, HCL, not APL
CD34	Stem cells	ALL, AML (early subtypes)
CD19	B Lineage	ALL (B lineage), CLL, HCL
CD20	B Lineage	ALL (B lineage), CLL, HCL
CD21	Intermediate B	CLL
Surface Ig	Intermediate and maturing B	L3-ALL, CLL, HCL
CD13	Myeloid and monocytoid	AML (all subtypes)
CD14	Myeloid and monocytoid	AML (often M4, M5)
CD15	Myeloid and monocytoid	AML (later subtypes)
CD33	Early myeloid; monocytoid	AML (all subtypes)
CD1	Early (thymic) T cells	T-ALL
CD2	T lineage	T-ALL
CD3	Mature T cells	T-CLL, ATL
CD5	T lineage	T-ALL, B-CLL
CD7	T lineage	T-ALL, 20% of AML
CD16	NK, granulocytes	NK leukemia, Tγ leukemia
CD25	Activated T and B	HCL, ATL

CD19, whereas most myeloid leukemias express CD33. acute leukemias of both lineages often express CD34, a marker of hematopoietic stem cells. T-ALL cells express markers of the T cell lineage such as CD2, CD5, or CD7. Use of an appropriate panel of antigen markers and histochemical stains allows the diagnostic classification of nearly all leukemias, even in situations where the morphology is ambiguous.

Several forms of ALL can be defined based on immunologic phenotype. Approximately 60 percent of cases are termed *common ALL*; the cells are typically Tdt+, CD34+, and CD19+ and have the common ALL antigen (CALLA) CD10. They do not express surface membrane immunoglobulin or T cell antigens. These cells are derived from precursors of the B cell lineage and have immunoglobulin gene rearrangements. About 20 percent of cases of ALL are of the *T cell type*, where the T lymphoblasts express the E-rosette receptor CD2 or other T lymphocyte–related antigens, such as CD5, CD7, or CD1. T-ALL cells are Tdt+, usually CALLA-negative, and stain positively for acid phosphatase. T cell ALL typically occurs in adolescent males and is frequently associated with a high leukocyte count and an anterior mediastinal mass. Less than 5 percent of cases of ALL are of the *B cell type* (expressing Ig). The cells in this variant produce a monoclonal immunoglobulin that is bound to the surface membrane and has L3 morphology. In B cell ALL, the cells typically contain the t(8;14) chromosomal abnormality that is also characteristic of Burkitt's lymphoma.

The leukemic cells in AML are 12 to 20 μm in diameter, larger than lymphoblasts, and have a lower nucleus-to-cytoplasm ratio. The leukemic myeloblasts usually have discrete nuclear chromatin and multiple nucleoli. Auer rods are sticklike abnormal primary granules present in the cytoplasm of leukemic cells. Such Auer rods are diagnostic of AML and are seen in 10 to 20 percent of patients with AML, particularly the M3 form (see Fig. A9-22). Dysplastic morphologic abnormalities may be prominent in granulocytic, erythroid, and megakaryocytic cells. Cytochemical stains are often helpful in classifying the pathologic subtypes of AML and in confirming the diagnosis. Myeloperoxidase, α-naphthyl-ASD-chloracetate esterase, and Sudan black are primarily present in cells undergoing granulocytic differentiation. Nonspecific esterase (α-naphthyl butyrate esterase) stains cells of the monocyte-macrophage lineage. A number of myeloid and monocytic cell surface antigens on AML cells also have been described and are useful in confirming a diagnosis in situations where the morphology and cytochemical stains are unclear (Table 310-3).

A collaborative French-American-British group divided AML into pathologic subtypes based on the degree of differentiation and maturation of the predominant cells toward granulocytes, monocytes, erythrocytes, or megakaryocytes. The characteristics of each subtype are summarized in Table 310-2. There are differences in the clinical features of some subtypes. The acute promyelocytic subtype (M3) is frequently associated with disseminated intravascular coagulation (DIC) induced by thromboplastic material released by the leukemic cells; DIC is usually present at the time of diagnosis and may be exacerbated during chemotherapy. It is important to immediately recognize the M3 APL variant because of the complications of DIC (see p. 1770) but also because remissions may be induced safely with *trans*-retinoic acid, rather than chemotherapy, as described above (p. 1765). Acute myelomonocytic leukemia (M4) and acute monocytic leukemia (M5) are more likely than other subtypes to involve extramedullary tissues, including skin, gingiva, and the nervous system. A recently defined subtype, M4EO, is characterized by increased abnormal eosinophils in the marrow, frequent CNS involvement, and an inv(16) chromosomal abnormality. There are several other specific disease syndromes associated with chromosomal abnormalities: T(4;11) is associated with a biphenotypic leukemia, splenomegaly, and poor prognosis; t(8;21) is associated with a good-prognosis AML-M2 in younger adults who often have splenomegaly or chloromas; t(9;11) is found with AML-M5; t(6;9) is seen with M2 and basophilia; and inv(3) or t(3;3) is found with increased platelets.

It may be difficult to distinguish AML without maturation (M1) from the L2 form of ALL by morphology alone. In these cases, cell surface markers and histochemistry usually define the leukemia type. Some patients have a biphenotypic or mixed-lineage acute leukemia in which the malignant cells express both myeloid and lymphoid markers. These cells may represent leukemias of primitive pluripotent stem cells, or the phenotype results from aberrant gene expression in a transformed myeloid or lymphoid progenitor.

Sensitive molecular methods for the detection of the t(9;22) translocation are now available using the polymerase chain reaction (PCR) with probes specific to the chromosomal breakpoints. These methods are capable of detecting as few as 1 leukemia cell in 1 million other cells. PCR is now available in a number of centers to document the t(15;17) translocation of APL and the immunoglobulin rearrangements seen in ALL and CLL. Less sensitive but useful fluorescence in situ hybridization (FISH) techniques also allow the identification of individual leukemia cells.

CLINICAL AND LABORATORY FEATURES ALL and AML share many clinical features. In the majority of patients, the initial symptoms of acute leukemia are present for less than 3 months. A preleukemic syndrome can be identified in approximately 25 percent of patients with AML; in these patients, anemia and other cytopenias are usually present for months to years preceding the development of overt leukemia. Patients with ALL and AML may present with pancytopenia without circulating blasts, with a normal leukocyte count, or with marked leukocytosis. Leukostasis due to occlusion of the microcirculation by leukemic blast cells can lead to hypoperfusion of vital tissues, most commonly lung and brain. Leukostasis becomes increasingly common when the number of circulating blasts exceeds 100×10^9 per liter and is seen more often with the larger blast cells in AML than in ALL. Patients may complain of manifestations of anemia such as pallor, easy fatigability, and dyspnea on mild exertion.

Bleeding is a major problem in patients with acute leukemia and is primarily related to thrombocytopenia. In some patients, megakaryocytes are derived from the leukemic clone and produce platelets with abnormal functions. Petechiae and easy bruisability are common. Hemorrhage becomes increasingly common when the platelet count is less than 20×10^9 per liter, particularly in the setting of infection or coagulapathy, typically occurring from oral (particularly gingiva) and gastrointestinal mucous membranes. Spontaneous bleeding involving the CNS, lungs, or other viscera also may occur. Patients with APL, but also with other subtypes of AML, whose cells contain granules with procoagulant activity, often present with DIC with elevated prothrombin and partial thromboplastin times, low fibrinogen levels, and plasma fibrinogen split products.

Infection is a nearly universal complication of acute leukemia. The incidence of infection is inversely related to the number of circulating neutrophils and becomes a major risk in patients with neutrophil counts less than 0.5×10^9 per liter. Neutrophils derived from leukemic progenitors also may function abnormally, further compromising host defense. The leukemia and its treatment cause a breakdown of mucosal barriers, and systemic infections usually develop from organisms colonizing the skin, throat, and gastrointestinal tract. Common sites of infections in patients with acute leukemia include the blood, skin, gingiva, perirectal tissues, lung, and urinary tract. Septicemia often occurs without an apparent source. Gram-negative bacteria, gram-positive cocci, and *Candida* species are frequent pathogens, but often no positive cultures are obtained. Patients with ALL being treated with prednisone may harbor infection despite a lack of fever.

Hepatomegaly and splenomegaly due to leukemic infiltration are present in a majority of patients with ALL and a minority of patients with AML. Visceral involvement can produce symptoms of nausea, abdominal fullness, or early satiety. Lymphadenopathy is usually found in ALL and not commonly in AML. An anterior mediastinal mass is often present in patients with the T cell variant of ALL. Acute leukemia may infiltrate into extramedullary tissues such as the skin, lung, eye, gums, nasopharynx, kidneys, or nervous system, particularly with AML-M5 or ALL but in any patient at end stage. Testicular involvement at diagnosis or relapse is seen in males with ALL. Soft tissue masses of leukemic cells (*chloromas*) can develop in any location. Occasionally, extramedullary leukemia can precede detectable involvement in the bone marrow.

Symptoms related to the expanding malignant cell mass, such as bone pain and sternal tenderness, occur in approximately half of patients with acute leukemia; osteolytic lesions are rare. Renal abnormalities can develop as a result of leukemic infiltration, ureteral obstruction by uric acid stones or enlarged lymph nodes, urate nephropathy, or from infectious or hemorrhagic complications. Because of the rapid turnover of cells, especially during treatment, allopurinol and vigorous hydration with diuresis are usually instituted as soon as possible after diagnosis to prevent urate nephropathy and other manifestations of the "tumor lysis" syndrome. Alkalinization of the urine and careful monitoring for hyperphosphatemia, hypocalcemia, and hyperkalemia are indicated. The risk of metabolic complications with rapid tumor lysis after chemotherapy increases with the size of the tumor burden as well as in particular types of leukemia such as the ALL-L3, Burkitt's type.

The neoplastic cells may infiltrate into the subarachnoid space, causing leukemic meningitis or direct involvement of the brain or spinal cord parenchyma. Neurologic involvement is unusual at the time of diagnosis, but the CNS is a frequent site of relapse, particularly in patients with ALL. The first symptoms of leukemic meningitis may be headache, nausea, or cranial nerve palsies (especially cranial nerves III through VII). Papilledema, seizures, and altered mentation develop with disease progression. Cytocentrifuge preparations of cerebrospinal fluid (CSF) characteristically reveal leukemic blast cells; elevated CSF protein and reduced CSF glucose concentrations are seen.

Patients with acute leukemia often develop metabolic abnormalities. Hyponatremia and hypokalemia are possible due to renal tubular abnormalities induced by lysozyme or other products of the leukemic cells. The serum lactate dehydrogenase (LDH) level may be increased. The metabolic activity of large numbers of blasts can lead to artifactual reductions in results of laboratory tests, especially glucose and potassium concentrations and arterial blood oxygen levels. Hyperuricemia may be present due to accelerated turnover of cells with increased purine release; lactic acidosis occurs rarely in patients with a large burden of leukemic cells.

TREATMENT OF ACUTE LEUKEMIA   General considerations
The expansion of leukemic cells follows a Gompertzian growth curve with near exponential growth at a lower cell mass and progressive slowing of the growth rate at higher leukemic cell burdens. The leukemic mass is usually near 10^{12} cells at the time of diagnosis. Chemotherapeutic agents produce a fractional cell kill; that is, a percentage of tumor cells (not an absolute number) is killed with each course of treatment. Most chemotherapeutic regimens employed for acute leukemias are probably capable of a 3 to 5 log cell kill, resulting in the elimination of 99.9 to 99.999 percent of the leukemia cells.

The treatment of acute leukemia is classically divided into phases. *Remission induction chemotherapy* involving intensive systemic chemotherapy is administered with the goal of reducing the leukemic cell mass below the level of clinical detection. When the leukemia cell mass is reduced below approximately 10^9 to 10^{10} cells, leukemia can no longer be detected in the blood or bone marrow, and the patient appears to be in complete remission. The clinical criteria for complete remission include (1) less than 5 percent blasts in the bone marrow and absence of leukemic cells in the peripheral blood, (2) the restoration of normal peripheral blood counts, and (3) the absence of physical findings attributable to extramedullary involvement of the leukemia. If no further treatment is given, however, the residual leukemic cells will expand, leading to relapse. After remission is achieved, additional systemic chemotherapy must be given to further reduce the leukemic cell mass and, ideally, eradicate the leukemia. Intensive chemotherapy administered immediately following remission induction has been referred to as *consolidation* or *early intensification treatment*. Lower-dose chemotherapy that is generally continued over several years is referred to *maintenance treatment*. Local chemotherapy or radiation may be necessary to sites of frequent relapse (''sanctuary'' sites), such as the CNS, since systemic treatment may fail to eradicate disease in these areas.

Supportive care   The supportive care of patients with pancytopenia is a critical aspect of the treatment of acute leukemia, and this primarily involves the appropriate administration of blood products and management of infections. Newer approaches to supportive care involve the use of hematopoietic growth factors and hematopoietic stem cell support.

Adequate levels of hemoglobin can usually be maintained with transfusions of packed red blood cells. An adequate number of circulating platelets can initially be attained by transfusions of platelets from unselected donors, but many transfused patients eventually develop antiplatelet antibodies which shorten platelet survival and render the patient unresponsive to further platelet transfusions. Patients who fail to respond to transfusions of platelets from unselected donors may respond to platelets from an HLA-identical donor. The risk of spontaneous hemorrhage is directly related to the degree of thrombocytopenia. It is generally advisable to transfuse platelets to maintain the platelet count above 20×10^9 per liter, especially in the setting of fever, infections, or coagulapathy. Uterine bleeding should be minimized in menstruating women with thrombocytopenia by administering an anovulatory agent.

Previous data have indicated that survival is not improved by granulocyte transfusions either to prevent infections or to treat documented infections because of technical difficulty in collecting sufficient numbers of granulocytes from normal donors and the adverse effects associated with their transfusion, such as fever, leukoagglutination, pulmonary infiltrates, and transmission of cytomegalovirus (CMV) and other infections. Newer techniques for obtaining large numbers of granulocytes will allow a reexamination of their role in infection control in leukemia. Blood products given to patients with leukemia should be irradiated with 3000 cGy to prevent potential donor stem cell engraftment and graft-versus-host effects of live lymphocytes contaminating the transfusions. White cell filtering of platelet and red cell transfusions may reduce alloimmunization as well.

The prevention and treatment of infections are of critical importance in the management of patients with acute leukemia. Since most infections are caused by organisms colonizing the skin and gastrointestinal tract, a variety of approaches have been evaluated to suppress the endogenous flora in these sites. Most centers recommend the use of face masks, careful hand washing, and isolation for visitors of granulocytopenic patients. Oral absorbable and nonabsorbable antibiotics are widely used prophylactically. They have proven useful in the reduction of febrile episodes, but it has been argued that the marginal advantage is overbalanced by the development of resistant strains. The development of bacterial and fungal infections may be delayed or avoided by these measures.

Granulocytopenic patients who develop fever or other signs of infection require prompt evaluation and immediate treatment. Fever is usually due to a bacterial, fungal, or viral infection. Gram-negative sepsis is common in this setting and may be rapidly fatal. Granulocytopenic patients with unexplained fever or overt infections should receive empirical treatment for a presumed bacterial infection until a definitive diagnosis can be established. A combination of broad-spectrum antibiotics, such as an aminoglycoside or a third-generation cephalosporin, and a semisynthetic antipseudomonal penicillin should be employed and the antibiotic program modified when the results of bacterial and fungal cultures are available. Systemic fungal infections are also common in granulocytopenic patients with leukemia and should be suspected in patients after several days of fever or in those who fail to respond to antibiotics or who respond and develop recurrent fever. Definitive diagnosis of fungal infections may be difficult, and a therapeutic trial of amphotericin B is often indicated. The problem of infections in the immunocompromised host is discussed in Chap. 81.

TREATMENT OF ACUTE LYMPHOBLASTIC LEUKEMIA   Forty-five years ago ALL was uniformly fatal, and patients had a median survival of only 2 months. Therapy developed in the 1950s through the 1970s enabled more than 50 percent of children with ALL to achieve long-term remissions and probable cure. Adults and certain high-risk subgroups of children with ALL have a poorer prognosis, and long-term remissions are still only achieved in a minority of patients. Therapy for ALL consists of four parts: (1) remission induction chemotherapy, (2) CNS prophylaxis, (3) consolidation, and (4) maintenance therapy.

The combination of vincristine and prednisone with either L-asparaginase or daunorubicin induces complete remissions in over 90 percent of children with ALL within 4 weeks. Some patients with persistent leukemia may achieve remission with 2 to 4 additional weeks of treatment with the same or alternate drugs. Failure to achieve remission can be attributed primarily to the development of drug resistance, severe infections, or CNS leukemia.

In patients who achieve remission, prophylactic treatment to the CNS is required to prevent leukemic meningitis. Since the drugs used in remission induction in ALL generally penetrate poorly into the CSF, circulating leukemic cells that infiltrated into the CNS and CSF early in the course of the disease are sheltered from the effects of systemic chemotherapy. Over the ensuing months, these cells may proliferate, producing overt leukemic meningitis. Leukemic meningitis is the initial site of relapse in up to two-thirds of patients with ALL who do not receive prophylactic therapy. Prophylactic treatment to the CNS, instituted during or immediately after remission induction, has been successful in dramatically reducing the incidence of CNS relapse. Some centers employ 18- to 24-Gy whole-brain radiation in combination with intrathecal methotrexate. Cranial irradiation does produce subtle abnormalities in neurologic function and sometimes subacute necrotizing leukoencephalopathy, particularly in the youngest children, and there is considerable interest in evaluating chemotherapy-only regimens as alternative methods of CNS treatment. Preliminary data suggest that the combination of intrathecal and high-dose systemic methotrexate may provide adequate prophylactic treatment to the CNS.

Since patients in remission still harbor leukemia cells, further systemic treatment is required to prevent or delay leukemic relapse. The optimal approach to continuation therapy involves the administration of combination chemotherapy given in doses approaching maximal tolerance using 6-thioguanine, mercaptopurine, cytarabine, methotrexate, cyclophosphamide, doxorubicin, or etoposide. The combination of 6-mercaptopurine and methotrexate is the most frequently employed maintenance regimen, but more intensive consolidation and maintenance regimens with anthracyclines and cytosine arabinoside are used for adult patients and children with poor prognostic features.

The optimal duration of maintenance chemotherapy is unknown. Many patients can discontinue chemotherapy after 2 to 3 years and remain in long-term remission. Up to one-quarter of patients will relapse, however, after maintenance therapy is discontinued. It is not known whether maintenance therapy given for more than 3 years will further reduce the likelihood of relapse. Until widespread use of methods, such as PCR, to reliably detect small numbers of residual leukemic cells is available, there is no objective means to determine when therapy can be discontinued safely.

Complications of therapy for ALL Chemotherapy-induced myelosuppression and immunosuppression are inevitable immediate side effects of the treatment of ALL. The chemotherapy directed toward the leukemic lymphoblasts also affects normal T and B lymphocytes, resulting in lymphocytopenia and immunodeficiency. Peripheral blood B cells generally recover to normal levels within several months after treatment is discontinued, but T cell numbers and function may remain depressed for up to 1 year. *Pneumocystis carinii* pneumonia can occur while patients are in remission, and trimethoprim-sulfamethoxazole prophylaxis is effective in preventing this complication. Viral infections such as herpes simplex and zoster, measles, and cytomegalovirus are common. Growth in children is somewhat retarded during the administration of chemotherapy. Catch-up growth generally occurs once therapy is discontinued, and most children ultimately attain near-normal height and weight. Sterility may result from treatment with most chemotherapeutic agents and irradiation. Gonadal function may recover after a prolonged interval. The gonads in prepubertal patients are relatively resistant to the effects of chemotherapy, and most patients undergo normal puberty after therapy is discontinued. Late complications also include CNS and neuroendocrinologic disorders that can result from cranial irradiation, secondary cancers and myeloid luekemias that may occur after both irradiation and chemotherapy, and cardiac problems from toxic drugs.

Prognosis in ALL A number of characteristics of ALL have been identified as having a prognostic impact; as therapies are tailored to specific subgroups of patients, though, these characteristics may lose their importance. The factors most affecting prognosis are age, leukemic cell DNA content (ploidy), immunophenotype, the leukocyte count at the time of diagnosis, and specific cytogenetic abnormalities. Children between the ages of 3 and 9 years with white blood counts less than 10×10^9 per liter have the best prognosis; 50 to 70 percent achieve long-term survival and probable cure with current treatment. Older patients and those with higher leukocyte counts have a poorer prognosis. Fewer than 30 percent of adults with ALL are long-term survivors in most series, and it is uncertain whether the maintenance therapy that is effective in children is of benefit in adults. Males have a worse prognosis than females; L1 subtype, which is less often seen

in adults, gives a better prognosis than the L2 form. With regard to immunophenotype, patients with cells marking for CD10 (CALLA-positive) have the best prognosis; the T cell phenotype is a better prognostic indicator in adults but not children, whereas the B cell (L3) variant of ALL has the worst prognosis.

Chromosomal abnormalities provide independent prognostic information. Approximately one-half the patients with ALL have detectable cytogenetic abnormalities, including hypodiploidy, pseudodiploidy, or hyperdiploidy. A number of nonrandom chromosomal abnormalities are associated with ALL. Between 10 and 40 percent of patients with ALL have the Philadelphia (Ph) chromosome t(9;22), with the incidence rising with age. Patients with certain translocations, such as t(8;14), t(4;11), and t(9;22) have a poor prognosis; patients with hyperdiploidy have a better prognosis.

Remission and survival rates in adult patients with ALL (those over 15 years of age) are significantly lower than for children with the same disease. Remission induction rates in adults and high-risk children are generally between 50 and 70 percent following treatment with vincristine, prednisone, and daunorubicin; the median duration of remission is 10 to 20 months, and the 5-year survival rate is 20 to 30 percent with standard chemotherapy. Several centers have reported improved results in high-risk children and in adults with more intensive, multiple-drug consolidation and maintenance programs and allogeneic bone marrow transplant, but the optimal therapy for high-risk forms of ALL is uncertain.

Treatment of recurrent ALL Leukemia may recur either in the bone marrow or in extramedullary sites. Patients who relapse while receiving maintenance therapy have a very poor prognosis with little possibility of a long-term second remission. Combination chemotherapy with a three- or four-drug regimen including vincristine, prednisone, L-asparaginase, and/or daunorubicin results in a second remission in 50 to 70 percent of these patients, and these patients should be considered for bone marrow transplantation. Remission duration, however, is usually brief, and subsequent relapse is inevitable. Patients who relapse after discontinuation of maintenance therapy have a better prognosis. Second remissions can be induced in about 90 percent of these patients. Although most will relapse again, some have achieved long-term survival. These patients should probably have chemotherapeutic CNS prophylaxis repeated to prevent recurrent disease in this extramedullary site.

Meningeal leukemia is the most common site of extramedullary relapse in patients with ALL. Cranial irradiation plus intrathecal methotrexate alone or in combination with cytarabine is the standard therapy for CNS leukemia. Ommaya reservoirs to deliver chemotherapy into ventricular CSF are usually placed surgically in patients with ALL. Testicular relapse is common in male patients with ALL and may occur during or after cessation of maintenance therapy. The treatment of choice is irradiation of the affected testicle. Patients with extramedullary relapse involving the CNS, testes, or other tissues are at very high risk for subsequent relapse in the bone marrow. Systemic reinduction therapy is indicated and may prevent generalized relapse of ALL.

TREATMENT OF ACUTE MYELOGENOUS LEUKEMIA AML cells derive from early hematopoietic progenitors, and the drugs active in AML have marginal selectivity for leukemic cells over their normal bone marrow counterparts. Induction of severe myelosuppression is necessary in order to achieve a complete remission. The combination of cytarabine with anthracyclines such as daunorubicin or demethoxy-daunorubicin results in a complete remission rate of 60 to 80 percent in patients under 60 years of age who have not had a myelodysplastic preleukemic state. Mitoxantrone or amsacrine may be substituted for the anthracycline. If residual leukemia is present 2 to 4 weeks after chemotherapy, the same treatment is often repeated. Patients who fail to enter remission with this approach have a poor prognosis.

Patients with AML who achieve complete remission still have substantial residual leukemia. Further therapy is required therefore to treat the occult disease. The benefits of available forms of consolidation and maintenance treatment are controversial. The best results have been achieved in patients receiving two to three intensive cycles of consolidation chemotherapy similar to the induction regimen. Median remission duration varies from 9 months to 2 years in most series. Between 10 and 30 percent of patients survive over 5 years free of disease, and most of these patients are probably cured. Somewhat better results have been reported in preliminary studies using very intensive consolidation regimens, including high-dose cytarabine alone or in combination with other drugs. Prospective, controlled studies have reported no benefit for patients receiving maintenance treatments. Current data suggest that the major benefit in therapy is achieved with intensive induction and consolidation treatment.

Most patients who achieve complete remission will ultimately relapse, usually in the first 2 years. At that point, the disease is less responsive to therapy, and median survival is 3 to 6 months.

CNS leukemia in AML occurs in 10 to 20 percent of patients at some point in their disease and most commonly develops in patients with monocytic (M5) or myelomonocytic (M4) subtypes or at terminal stages. Unlike ALL, the CNS is rarely an isolated site of relapse in AML. CNS involvement usually occurs in the setting of systemic relapse, and prophylactic treatment to the CNS has not improved remission duration or survival. Patients who develop meningeal leukemia are treated with cranial irradiation and/or intrathecal chemotherapy with cytarabine and/or methotrexate.

Prognostic factors in AML   Chromosomal abnormalities in AML are of prognostic value; patients with abnormalities such as t(8;21), t(15;17), or inv(16) tend to have a better prognosis than average, while −5, −7, t(9;22), and complex chromosomal abnormalities are associated with a poor prognosis.

Age is a major prognostic factor in many series; unfortunately, half of patients with AML are over 60 years of age. Patients over 60 years of age are less likely to achieve complete remission or to tolerate intensive therapy well and may be more difficult to support through the complications of pancytopenia. In addition, elderly patients are more likely to have leukemic cells with poor-risk chromosomal abnormalities such as −7 and −5 and often have a prior myelodysplastic or preleukemic syndrome. Elderly patients who do achieve remission, however, have a similar remission duration and survival as younger patients. Since the major factor influencing survival is the achievement of complete remission, intensive chemotherapy should be administered to most elderly patients, with careful attention to supportive care.

The AML leukemic subtype is of modest prognostic significance. Acute promyelocytic leukemia (M3) is typically associated with DIC; fatal CNS hemorrhage may complicate remission induction chemotherapy for this type of leukemia. *trans*-Retinoic acid differentiation therapy can induce complete remissions in this subtype and is rapidly replacing chemotherapy as the initial induction treatment. DIC is best treated with frequent platelet transfusions, as many as 6 to 12 units per day, and 2 to 4 units of fresh plasma daily, to replace lost coagulation factors and inhibitors until the fibrinogen is normalized and the white blood cell count reduced. Heparin and ε-amino caproic acid therapy remain controversial, but heparin is often used in conjunction with the preceding supportive measures. Patients with promyelocytic leukemia who do achieve remission appear to have a greater chance of long-term survival than other subgroups. Patients with erythroleukemia or monocytic or myelomonocytic leukemia, with the exception of the M4 eosinophilic variant associated with inv(16), may have a poorer prognosis than the M1 to M3 subgroups.

Patients with preleukemia or myelodysplastic syndromes evolving into AML or therapy-related leukemias respond poorly to chemotherapy; less than half of these patients achieve complete remission. Such patients also tend to have prolonged bone marrow aplasia following treatment and often succumb to complications of pancytopenia. Patients who do achieve remission have a remission duration similar to patients with de novo AML, and intensive induction therapy is usually indicated. No treatment has been consistently effective during the preleukemic phase, and intensive chemotherapy should be withheld until progressive overt leukemia develops. Efforts to treat preleuke-

mias with low doses of cytarabine, 5-azacytidine, and differentiating agents such as hexamethylene bisacetamide or retinoic acid occasionally lead to clinical improvement, but improvement in survival has not yet been documented. Studies with hematopoietic hormones such as granulocyte-macrophage or granulocyte colony stimulating factor (G-CSF, GM-CSF) suggest utility for this class of agents to improve granulopoiesis in myelodysplastic syndromes, and high-dose erythropoietin may stimulate increased red cell production. Patients who develop acute leukemia after a preexisting myeloproliferative disorder or paroxysmal nocturnal hemoglobinuria usually have a poor prognosis.

Patients who receive cytotoxic chemotherapy with or without concomitant radiation therapy have an increased risk of developing AML. Secondary or treatment-related leukemia is most commonly associated with prolonged therapy with alkylating agents, nitrosoureas, or procarbazine and has been seen primarily in patients with Hodgkin's disease, myeloma, and ovarian carcinoma. Almost all patients with treatment-related AML have chromosomal abnormalities, usually hypodiploidy with −5 and/or −7. These patients typically develop a preleukemic syndrome with pancytopenia several months before overt AML is recognized. They respond poorly to chemotherapy, and despite treatment, few survive more than 1 year.

BONE MARROW TRANSPLANTATION FOR ACUTE LEUKEMIA
Bone marrow transplantation from an identical twin or an HLA-identical sibling donor after intensive therapy is effective treatment for both ALL and AML. The objective of this approach is to administer very high doses of chemotherapy alone or with total-body irradiation and then to rescue the patient from severe myelosuppression by the transplantation of bone marrow from a normal donor. In addition, the transplantation of allogeneic bone marrow may confer an immune-mediated graft-versus-leukemia effect. Hence syngeneic (twin-donated) and T cell–depleted allogeneic marrow transplants generally result in a higher rate of relapse. The current results with bone marrow transplantation are summarized in Table 310-4. The principles of bone marrow transplantation are discussed in detail in Chap. 313.

Allogeneic bone marrow transplantation is associated with substantial risks. Approximately one-third of patients conventionally transplanted for leukemia will die from transplant-related complications, including graft-versus-host disease (GVHD), interstitial pneumonitis, and opportunistic infections. By depleting T cells from the donor marrow graft, these complications can be markedly reduced, but the relapse and graft failure rates climb so that long-term survival is largely unchanged. Most centers limit the use of bone marrow transplantation to patients under 60 years of age, since older patients generally have a poor outcome largely due to complications of GVHD and infection. Reports from several centers indicate that up to 30 percent of otherwise end-stage patients with refractory acute leukemia or patients with secondary leukemias have achieved long-term disease-

TABLE 310-4 Representative results of bone marrow transplantation (BMT) compared with conventional chemotherapy for AML and ALL

	Survival >3 years, %		
	Allo-BMT	Auto-BMT	Chemotherapy
ACUTE MYELOGENOUS LEUKEMIA			
First remission	30–70	30–60	20–50
Second remission or early relapse	30–50	20–40	<10
Third remission or relapse	10–30	20	0
ACUTE LYMPHOCYTIC LEUKEMIA			
First remission	40–60	20–40	10–50
Second remission or early relapse	20–40	20–30	<10
Third remission or relapse	10–20		0

free survival and probable cure following bone marrow transplantation. Although only a small proportion of patients in this category benefit, the results compare favorably with those obtained with other forms of treatment.

Survival figures are improved substantially when bone marrow transplantation is performed during remission, the burden of leukemic cells is low, and the patients are in relatively good general condition (see Table 310-4). In young patients with AML, transplantation in first remission is often recommended, but overall results are not consistently superior to intensive chemotherapy. Transplantation in *early first relapse* or *second remission* may be equally effective, but patients may be in poorer overall condition. Because many children with ALL can achieve a prolonged initial remission with chemotherapy, bone marrow transplantation has generally been reserved for patients in *second remission*; in this group, 30 to 60 percent have achieved prolonged survival with marrow transplantation. It is not clear that transplantation of most adults in *first remission* of ALL is more advantageous than intensive chemotherapy. Discussions regarding the time of bone marrow transplant in ALL relate to the likelihood of relapse.

Approximately 30 percent of patients with AML transplanted in *early relapse* or *second remission* have achieved long-term survival. There is controversy, though, as to whether patients with AML should receive allogeneic bone marrow transplantation or postremission chemotherapy while in *first* complete remission. Patients at high risk for relapse after chemotherapy, such as those with certain poor-risk karyotypes or with secondary leukemias, should probably be transplanted. For other patients, it is clear that the risk of recurrent leukemia is lower following bone marrow transplantation than with postremission chemotherapy; however, the transplanted patients usually represent a highly selected group. In addition, bone marrow transplantation is more likely to be associated with fatal treatment complications. In all patients, 3- or 5-year survival is 40 to 60 percent with bone marrow transplantation compared with 10 to 50 percent survival achieved with optimal chemotherapy. Patient age is a major prognostic factor with bone marrow transplantation, and the better results have been reported in children and young adults. Although young patients have better results with allogeneic bone marrow transplantation than with chemotherapy, this is less true for patients over 30 years of age. Of note is that the median age of patients with AML is 60. One major limitation of bone marrow transplantation as a general therapeutic approach is that only a minority of patients are eligible; most patients are either too old to be considered or lack an HLA-identical related donor. Recently, several large registries of potential unrelated donors have been formed, and bone marrow transplants from unrelated histocompatible donors are under active evaluation.

Autologous bone marrow transplantation also has been evaluated in patients with acute leukemia. With this approach, remission bone marrow is collected and cryopreserved. The patient may then receive intensive chemoradiotherapy followed by reinfusion of the cryopreserved bone marrow. Since remission bone marrow is likely to contain small numbers of residual leukemic cells, many centers have treated the collected marrow with antileukemic monoclonal antibodies or chemotherapy prior to cryopreservation in an attempt to "purge" residual leukemic cells. Autologous transplantation has the advantage of not requiring a matched donor and the lack of GVHD complications; thus a much larger group of patients is eligible for treatment by this approach. A disadvantage is the far higher rate of relapse. Selected patients with AML transplanted in first or second remission have achieved prolonged survival, but further studies are required to critically assess the efficacy of autologous versus allogeneic marrow transplantation for acute leukemia. Furthermore, neither the efficacy nor best methods of ex vivo treatment of the collected bone marrow to eradicate contaminating malignant cells have been demonstrated conclusively.

Because of the pace of advances in supportive care, methods of manipulating or modifying the graft-versus-leukemia effect and GVHD, newer purging methods in autologous transplantation, as well as more intensive nontransplant approaches with growth factor rescue, recommendations for the optimal therapy of acute leukemia are changing.

IMMUNOTHERAPY FOR ACUTE LEUKEMIAS Immunotherapy for acute leukemia has included the use of monoclonal antibodies that react with cell surface antigens on leukemia blasts, cytokine activation of cellular immunity, and nonspecific immunostimulatory agents. Clinical trials with nonspecific immune potentiating agents such as bacillus Calmette-Guerin (BCG), *Corynebacterium parvum*, or levamisole have not shown a benefit in prolonging the duration of remission. Interleukin 2–activated natural killer cells (LAK cells) have shown activity in reducing residual disease but not large leukemia burdens. Monoclonal antibodies to myeloid antigens have been apparently as effective at purging AML cells from autologous marrow ex vivo before reinfusion as ex vivo chemotherapy. Similar approaches to ALL therapy using antibodies to B cell antigens are also under investigation. Radiolabeled monoclonal antibodies to AML also have shown considerable antileukemic activity in vivo. At this time, the value of specific immunotherapy for acute leukemia remains to be proven in large trials.

SUMMARY AND FUTURE DIRECTIONS IN ACUTE LEUKEMIA Effective induction chemotherapy capable of inducing remission in most patients with ALL and AML is now available, but long-term survival is still achieved in only a minority of patients owing to the presence of residual leukemia. In the next decade, a focus of clinical research will be directed toward measures to prolong the duration of remission by use of innovative methods of consolidation treatment. This may include intensive chemotherapy or high-dose chemoradiotherapy with growth factor rescue, stem cell support, or bone marrow transplantation. It also will be important to develop effective, selective immunologic approaches that are capable of eliminating residual leukemic cells, such as antibody-based strategies, or vaccines against leukemia-associated oncogenic proteins, which may promote long-term active immunosuppression of relapse. For the success of these newer approaches, sensitive methods to detect and follow the presence of residual leukemia are needed in order to guide therapy. Already such PCR methods are available for the translocations causing CML and APL and for the immunoglobulin rearrangements seen in certain cases of ALL. Another aim of research will be the use of specific treatments tailored to individual types of leukemias stratified according to their genotype and immunophenotype.

CHRONIC LYMPHOCYTIC LEUKEMIA

Chronic lymphocytic leukemia (CLL) is a neoplasm of activated B lymphocytes. The CLL cells, which morphologically resemble mature, small lymphocytes of the peripheral blood, accumulate in the bone marrow, blood, lymph nodes, and spleen in large numbers. The disease is usually seen in patients over 50 years of age, but improved diagnosis has identified many younger patients. CLL is the most common form of leukemia in the United States and is more frequent in males than females. The CLL cells commonly have trisomy 12 alone or with additional chromosomal abnormalities. Clonality also can be demonstrated by expression of a single light chain (κ or λ) or immunoglobulin idiotype specificity. Rarely, cells that appear to be chronic lymphoid leukemias may be of T cell or NK cell origin. These less common varieties include diseases formerly known as T-CLL but are actually large granular lymphocytic leukemias, T suppressor leukemia, adult T cell leukemia, and T prolymphocytic leukemias. An unusual type of T cell CLL is seen in patients with ataxia-telangiectasia and is often associated with a translocation of genetic material between the number 14 chromosomes (t14;14).

The diagnosis of CLL usually can be made on the basis of physical examination and a review of the peripheral blood smear. Lymphocytosis is usually present, and the malignant cells characteristically appear as morphologically normal small lymphocytes (see Fig.

A9-23). The dual expression of B cell antigens (CD19, CD20, CD21, CD24) with a T cell antigen (CD5) on the cells is usually diagnostic of CLL. In most cases, a monoclonal immunoglobulin can be demonstrated on the cell surface, although immunofluorescent staining is relatively weak. Monoclonal surface IgM with or without IgD and occasionally IgG is characteristically present, and a small amount of this IgM paraprotein can often be detected in the serum with sensitive techniques. CLL cells have Fc receptors and the second complement receptor (CD21). Most patients develop some degree of hypogammaglobulinemia. Approximately 3 percent of patients with lymphoproliferative disorders have a T cell or, rarely, NK cell neoplasm. The neoplastic T cells form rosettes with sheep erythrocytes, in contrast to the mouse red cell rosettes formed by the more common B cell CLL. T cell CLL usually cannot be distinguished from B cell CLL morphologically, but expression of T cell markers is easily detected by flow cytometry. NK cell leukemias stain for CD16, and the neoplastic lymphocytes are usually granular.

DIFFERENTIAL DIAGNOSIS   It is important to distinguish early CLL from reactive lymphocytosis in asymptomatic patients. In reactive lymphocytosis, the cells are polyclonal and predominantly T lymphocytes, whereas in CLL they are always B cells. The demonstration of monoclonal surface membrane immunoglobulin unambiguously defines a B cell lymphocytosis as neoplastic. Chronic T cell leukemias must be distinguished from Sézary syndrome, where the cells have a characteristic lobulated nucleus and there usually is extensive skin involvement. Chronic T cell leukemias also must be distinguished from adult T cell leukemia (ATL) associated with HTLV-I. Prolymphocytic and prolymphocytoid leukemias are CLL variants seen in older people and are characterized by massive splenomegaly, often in the absence of lymphadenopathy. The neoplastic cell in these prolymphocytic leukemias is also usually of B cell origin, and it is larger than that seen in CLL, with prominent nucleolus. Prolymphocytic leukemia is typically associated with very high white blood cell counts (in excess of 200×10^9 per liter) and a poor response to therapy. Occasionally, diffuse or follicular lymphomas involving the marrow or spleen can spill out into the blood and mimic CLL morphologically. However, the cells often have a clefted nucleus, brightly staining cell surface monoclonal immunoglobulin, and the absence of CD5 staining. Lymphomas at this stage are typically far more aggressive. Splenic villous lymphomas typically cause splenomegaly, a plasma protein monoclonal band, and lower white blood cell counts than CLL. The cells have a small nucleolus and short villi. Unlike hairy cell leukemia, these cells are negative for tartrate-resistant acid phosphatase (TRAP) and CD25. Hairy cell leukemia is distinguished from CLL on the basis of the typical cellular morphology, markers such as CD25, and the presence of tartrate-resistant acid phosphatase in the hairy cells. Waldenström's macroglobulinemia is differentiated from CLL on the basis of bone marrow morphology and lower white blood cell counts, CD38 positivity, cytoplasmic Ig, and the secretion of a large amount of a monoclonal IgM paraprotein. Small lymphocytic lymphomas (diffuse well-differentiated lymphomas) are morphologically and immunophenotypically the same as CLL and appear to represent a different clinical variant of the same neoplasm.

CLINICAL FEATURES   The diagnosis of B-CLL is usually made when there is a minimum of 5×10^9 mature-appearing lymphocytes per liter of blood and 30 percent infiltration of the marrow with B cell phenotype cells bearing CD5. In more than 25 percent of patients with CLL, the disorder is discovered as an incidental finding. The common practice of ordering routine complete blood counts in adults has led to an earlier diagnosis of CLL in asymptomatic patients. The signs and symptoms of CLL usually relate to tissue infiltration, peripheral blood cytopenias, or immunosuppression. Patients may present with symptoms of anemia, lymph node enlargement, or intercurrent infection. Splenomegaly seldom leads to symptoms, and the liver is minimally enlarged in only about half of patients. The clinical course is quite variable, and prognosis is correlated directly with stage (see Table 310-4).

In CLL, the white blood cell count ranges between 5×10^9 and 200×10^9 per liter, with a preponderance of mature-appearing lymphocytes. There is little correlation between the leukocyte count and symptoms except at very high tumor burdens. Patients with advanced disease may present with anemia, granulocytopenia, and thrombocytopenia resulting from bone marrow infiltration by the leukemic cells. About 20 percent of patients develop a Coombs-positive autoimmune hemolytic anemia during the course of their disease. Occasionally, autoimmune thrombocytopenia or pure red cell aplasia occurs. CLL may evolve into an aggressive lymphocytic lymphoma (diffuse large cell lymphoma) referred to as *Richter's syndrome*, which may be due to a clonal evolution of the original leukemia.

TREATMENT   Because of the indolent nature of CLL, few attempts have been made at curative therapy. Typically, agents are given for disease control, although a number of centers are exploring strategies with curative intent. Experimental regimens have not yet prolonged survival significantly. Among a number of prognostic classifications of CLL that have been employed, the international classification is quite useful (Table 310-5). Patients with early-stage disease, limited to lymphocytosis alone or lymphocytosis plus limited lymphadenopathy, have a good prognosis. Patients with A(0) disease, characterized only by lymphocytosis without other poor prognostic signs, are unlikely to need therapy or die of CLL. Median survival exceeds 10 years; these patients usually require no treatment, and treatment may even be detrimental. Patients with more substantial lymphadenopathy and hepatosplenomegaly have an intermediate prognosis with a median survival of approximately 5 years. Patients with anemia or thrombocytopenia have a worse prognosis, with a median survival of less than 3 years. The value of these prognostic groups is changing as better therapies are used increasingly. In addition to the clinical staging classification, several other features have been proposed as prognostic indicators. Poorer prognosis is associated with an initial blood lymphocyte count of 50,000 per microliter or more, a lymphocyte count doubling time of under 12 months, complex chromosomal abnormalities, and a diffuse marrow infiltration pattern.

The indications for therapy in CLL include hemolytic anemia, important cytopenias, disfiguring lymphadenopathy, symptomatic organomegaly, or marked systemic symptoms. When treatment is required, the cornerstone of therapy is usually an alkylating agent. Chlorambucil is the most frequently prescribed drug for CLL, utilizing either small daily doses or a larger pulse every 3 to 6 weeks. Daily or pulse cyclophosphamide appears to be as effective as chlorambucil in the treatment of CLL. Maintenance therapy has no definite value, and continuing alkylating agent therapy may increase the risk of

TABLE 310-5   International workshop on CLL staging classification*

Stage	Description	Median survival, years
A	Lymphocytosis with clinical involvement of fewer than 3 lymph node groups[†]; no anemia or thrombocytopenia	8–10 or more
	A(0) No nodes enlarged	
	A(I) Nodes enlarged	
	A(II) Hepatomegaly or splenomegaly	
B	More than 3 lymph node groups[†] involved. No anemia or thrombocytopenia	5–6
	B(I) Nodes enlarged	
	B(II) Hepatomegaly or splenomegaly	
C	Anemia or thrombocytopenia regardless of number of lymph node groups involved	2.5
	C(III) Anemia	
	C(IV) Thrombocytopenia	

* This represents a combination of the Binet classification (A,B,C) with the Rai classification (0,I,II,III,IV).
† Lymph node groups—cervical, axillary, inguinal, liver, spleen.

future development of AML. Three newer drugs useful in the treatment of CLL include deoxycoformycin, 2-chlorodeoxyadenosine, and fludarabine monophosphate. These agents have considerable antileukemia activity, even in prior-treated patients. Fludarabine is now approved for therapy of CLL and is as effective as alkylating agent therapy in both treated and untreated patients, with response rates of 50 to 80 percent. Similarly, 2-chlorodeoxyadenosine is sometimes effective in fludarabine-resistant disease.

Glucocorticoids are useful for CLL in special circumstances, such as in the treatment of associated Coombs-positive hemolytic anemia or immune thrombocytopenia, and may be transiently effective in treating patients with pancytopenia and the "packed marrow" syndrome. Glucocorticoids have important side effects, including a predisposition to opportunistic infection, and should not routinely be used in CLL. In advanced CLL unresponsive to fludarabine and 2-chlorodeoxyadenosine, combination chemotherapy as used in lymphoma may be useful. Regimens that include an alkylating agent, vincristine, doxorubicin, and prednisone are often employed. Splenectomy may be indicated in patients with hypersplenism, refractory hemolytic anemia, or thrombocytopenia. Radiation therapy occasionally may be useful for palliating localized disease or hypersplenism in the aged. Experimental therapies such as allogeneic bone marrow transplantation, interferon α, interleukin 2, and monoclonal antibodies to cell surface antigens such as CD5, CD19, CD20, CD52, and CD25 used alone or conjugated to isotopes or toxins are currently under study with occasionally encouraging results. Hypogammaglobulinemia is common in patients with CLL, and life-threatening infectious complications may occur. Intravenous Ig preparations are effective in prophylaxis against recurrent infections, but the cost is high.

HAIRY CELL LEUKEMIA

Hairy cell leukemia is a rare lymphoid neoplasm characterized by peripheral blood cytopenias, splenomegaly, and morphologically typical malignant cells in the blood and bone marrow. Hairy cell leukemia is usually seen in male patients over 40 years of age. The disease is now recognized with increased frequency, and many large series have been reported. Hairy cell leukemia has been reported to occur worldwide.

Although originally referred to as *leukemic reticuloendotheliosis*, the term *hairy cell leukemia* is now widely accepted because it is descriptive of the characteristic cytoplasmic projections seen on the leukemic cell. The disorder is nearly always due to expansion of neoplastic B lymphocytes which express and often produce monoclonal immunoglobulin. Rare T cell variants which may represent a related disorder, including one case associated with the human retrovirus HTLV-II, have been described.

CLINICAL FEATURES AND PATHOLOGY   Patients with hairy cell leukemia usually present with symptoms due to splenomegaly, pancytopenia, infection caused by impaired host defense, or vasculitis. Many asymptomatic patients are detected on routine complete blood counts. More than three-quarters of patients will have palpable splenomegaly, and in some cases splenic involvement is massive. Lymphadenopathy is rare, and substantial hepatomegaly is uncommon at the time of diagnosis, although infiltration of the portal triads by hairy cells is often seen microscopically. Occasionally, bone lesions may cause hip pain. Approximately 30 percent of patients with hairy cell leukemia have an associated vasculitis-like disorder. Common manifestations include erythema nodosum and cutaneous nodules due to perivasculitis. Visceral involvement similar to polyarteritis nodosa may occur.

Moderate pancytopenia is usually present at diagnosis. The leukocyte count is normal or low, and characteristic hairy cells are seen in the peripheral blood. These cells are about 15 to 20 μm in diameter and have an eccentrically placed nucleus with foamy cytoplasm. Cytoplasmic projections (hairs) may be seen on smear, but they are best appreciated by phase microscopy. These cells are

TRAP-positive. The cells stain with antibodies to B cell antigens and often CD25, the interleukin 2 receptor, an activation antigen. Bone marrow aspiration is often unsuccessful because of reticulin fibrosis. The biopsy typically shows replacement of the normal architecture by mononuclear cells that are not packed together but maintain spaces between the intercellular contacts. Splenic histology is typical, consisting of mononuclear cell infiltration of the red pulp and engorgement of the sinuses.

Hairy cell leukemia must be distinguished from chronic lymphocytic leukemia, prolymphocytic leukemia, splenic villous lymphoma, and Waldenström's macroglobulinemia. Some patients with hairy cell leukemia present with a hypocellular bone marrow which may be misdiagnosed as aplastic anemia or with an inaspirable marrow leading to confusion with primary myelofibrosis. The diagnosis depends on identifying the characteristic cells in the bone marrow and peripheral blood.

TREATMENT OF HAIRY CELL LEUKEMIA   The course of hairy cell leukemia can be quite indolent; however, there is a wide spectrum of severity and rate of progression of the disease among patients. Approximately one-quarter of patients present without significant symptoms or complications of the disease; these patients require no immediate treatment. They should be followed at intervals and observed closely for infections. Infection is the primary cause of death in patients with hairy cell leukemia. Common infections include *Legionella* pneumonitis, toxoplasmosis, tuberculosis, and atypical mycobacterial disease, nocardiosis, and pyogenic infections. Patients probably benefit from pneumonococcal vaccination. Any significant fever should be evaluated thoroughly and treated aggressively with antibiotics. Since *Legionella* pneumonitis is relatively common in these patients, high-dose erythromycin should be administered to patients with pulmonary infiltrates.

Therapy directed at the leukemia is indicated in patients with pancytopenia, recurrent infections, symptomatic splenomegaly, autoimmune complications, or disease progression. Formerly, the cornerstone of therapy was splenectomy, which appeared to ameliorate the disease in a majority of patients. Splenectomy is now rarely performed except in situations where life-threatening cytopenias must be corrected immediately. Three drugs that are highly active in inducing remissions are now available: interferon α, deoxycoformycin (Pentostatin), and 2-chlorodeoxyadenosine (2CDA). Virtually all treated patients respond to interferon α, with about 70 percent achieving major hematologic benefit. Complete remissions are rare, but retreatment of recurrent disease is often successful. Pentostatin is also highly active in hairy cell leukemia, even in patients who have failed interferon-α, and often induces complete remissions. The most important new agent is 2CDA. 2CDA has an extremely high complete response rate of over 80 percent and a very low rate of relapse. Although additional follow-up is needed, this latter agent may be curative in some patients after a single course of therapy. When approved for use by the U.S. Food and Drug Administration, 2CDA will probably be the treatment of choice.

Short courses of glucocorticoids may be useful in controlling the vasculitis or autoimmune manifestations that are often associated with the disease but are not indicated as primary therapy. G-CSF may be useful during neutropenic periods. The prognosis in hairy cell leukemia is excellent, and prognosis-based published series are outdated because of the rapid recent improvements in treatment, including the application of interferon, deoxycoformycin, and 2CDA and better supportive care.

REFERENCES

General

Clarkson B: New pharmacologic approaches to treatment of leukemia. Semin Oncol 28:99, 1991

Foon K, Todd R: Immunologic classification of leukemia and lymphoma. Blood 68:1, 1986

Golde DW: The stem cell. Sci Am 265:86, 1991

MANDELLI F (ed): Therapy of actue leukemias. Leukemia 6(suppl 2):1 1992

SCHEINBERG DA: Current applications of monoclonal antibodies for the therapy of hematopoietic cancers. Curr Opin Immunol 3:679, 1991

SCHIFFER CA: Interferon studies in the treatment of patients with leukemia. Semin Oncol 18:1, 1991

ALL

CHAMPLIN R, GALE RP: Acute lymphoblastic leukemia: Recent advances in biology and therapy. Blood 73:2051, 1989

HOELZER D et al: Prognostic factors in a multicenter study for treatment of acute lymphoblastic leukemia in adults. Blood 71:123, 1988

HOROWITZ MM et al: Chemotherapy compared with bone marrow transplantation for adults with acute lymphoblastic leukemia in first remission. Ann Intern Med 115:13, 1991

LIPSHULTZ SE et al: Late cardiac effects of doxorubicin therapy for acute lymphoblastic leukemia in childhood. N Engl J Med 325:808, 1991

NEGLIA JP et al: Second neoplasms after acute lymphoblastic leukemia in childhood. N Engl J Med 325:1330, 1991

PUI C-H: Acute myeloid leukemia in children treated with epipodophyllotoxins for acute lymphoblastic leukemia. N Engl J Med 325:1682, 1991

——— et al: Biology and clinical significance of cytogenetic abnormalities in childhood acute lymphoblastic leukemia. Blood 76:1449, 1990

RIVERA GK, MAUER AM: Controversies in the management of childhood acute lymphoblastic leukemia: Treatment intensification, CNS leukemia, and prognostic factors. Semin Hematol 24:12, 1987

VAN DER PLAS DC et al: Prognostic significancer of karyotype at diagnosis in childhood acute lymphoblastic anemia. Leukemia 6:176, 1992

AML

APPELBAUM FR et al: Chemotherapy versus marrow transplantation for adults with acute nonlymphocytic leukemia: A five-year follow-up. Blood 72:179, 1988

BAGBY GC: The preleukemic syndrome (hematopoietic dysplasia). Blood Rev 2:194, 1988

BENNETT JM et al: Proposal for a recognition of minimally differentiated acute myeloid leukaemia (AML-MO). Br J Hematol 78:325, 1991

FOON KA, GALE RP: Therapy of acute myelogenous leukemia. Blood Rev 6:15, 1992

RODEGHIERO F et al: Early deaths and anti-hemorrhagic treatments in acute promyelocytic leukemia: A GIMEMA retrospective study in 286 consecutive patients. Blood 75:2112, 1990

WARRELL RP JR et al: Differentiation therapy of acute promyelocytic leukemia with tretinoin (all-*trans* retinoic acid). N Engl J Med 324:1385, 1991

CLL

BENNETT JM et al: Proposals for the classification of chronic (mature) B and T lymphoid leukaemias. J Clin Pathol 42:567, 1989

CHUN HG et al: Fludarabine phosphate: A synthetic purine antimetabolite with significant activity against lymphoid malignancies. J Clin Oncol 9:175, 1991

DIGHIERO G et al: B-cell chronic lymphocytic leukemia: Present status and future directions. Blood 78:1901, 1991

KEATING MJ et al: Fludarabine: A new agent with marked cytoreductive activity in untreated chronic lymphocytic leukemia. J Clin Oncol 9:44, 1991

TEFFERI A, PHYLIKY RL: A clinical update on chronic lymphocytic leukemia. II. Critical analysis of current chemotherapeutic modalities. Mayo Clin Proc 67:457, 1992

Hairy cell leukemia

DURRELMAN S et al: 2'-Deoxycoformycin after failure of alpha-interferon in hairy cell leukemia. Eur J Haematol 43:297, 1989

GOLOMB HM, ELLIS E: Treatment options for hairy-cell leukemia. Semin Oncol 18:7, 1991

LILL McC, GOLDE DW: Treatment of hairy cell leukemia. Blood Rev 4:238, 1990

O'DWYER PJ et al: 2'-Deoxycoformycin (Pentostatin) for lymphoid malignancies. Ann Intern Med 108:733, 1988

PIRO LD et al: Lasting remissions in hairy-cell leukemia induced by a single infusion of 2-chlorodeoxyadenosine. N Engl J Med 322:1117, 1990

SAVEN A, PIRO LD: Treatment of hairy cell leukemia. Blood 79:1111, 1992

311   MALIGNANT LYMPHOMAS

ARNOLD S. FREEDMAN / LEE M. NADLER

DEFINITION The malignant lymphomas, in contrast to leukemias, are neoplastic transformations of cells which reside predominantly in lymphoid tissues. The two major variants of malignant lymphoma are non-Hodgkin's lymphoma and Hodgkin's disease. Although both these tumors infiltrate reticuloendothelial organs, they are biologically and clinically distinct. Table 311-1 compares non-Hodgkin's and Hodgkin's lymphomas with regard to cellular deriva-

TABLE 311-1   The malignant lymphomas

	Non-Hodgkin's	Hodgkin's
Cellular derivation	90% B cell 10% T cell	Unresolved
Sites of disease:		
Localized	Uncommon	Common
Nodal spread	Discontiguous	Contiguous
Extranodal	Common	Uncommon
Mediastinal	Uncommon	Common
Abdominal	Common	Uncommon
Bone marrow	Common	Uncommon
B symptoms	Uncommon	Common
Chromosomal translocation	Common	Yet to be described
Curability	30–40%	>75%

tion, sites of disease, presence of systemic symptoms, chromosomal translocations, and curability. This comparison supports the notion that they are fundamentally different diseases.

CELLULAR AND DEVELOPMENTAL ASPECTS OF NON-HODGKIN'S AND HODGKIN'S LYMPHOMAS To date, biologic studies have provided no clear-cut explanations for the differences demonstrated in Table 311-1. A large number of studies have examined the cellular origins of these tumors in an attempt to relate the neoplastic

TABLE 311-2   Histologic classification of non-Hodgkin's lymphoma

Working formulation, malignant lymphoma	Rappaport terminology	Cellular lineage, %		Chromosomal abnormalities
		B	T	
LOW GRADE				
A Small lymphocytic cell	Diffuse-well-differentiated lymphocytic (DWDL)	98	2	Trisomy 12 t(11;14) t(14;19)
B Follicular, predominantly small cleaved cell	Nodular poorly differentiated lymphocytic (NPDL)	100	0	t(14;18) del(6)
C Follicular mixed, small cleaved and large cell	Nodular mixed lymphocytic histiocytic (NM)	100	0	t(14;18) Trisomy, 3, 7, 8
INTERMEDIATE GRADE				
D Follicular, predominantly large cell	Nodular histiocytic (NH)	100	0	Trisomy 7, 10, 12, 21 t(14;18)
E Diffuse small cleaved cell	Diffuse poorly differentiated lymphocytic (DPDL)	80	20	del(6)(q) t(3;9), t(14;18)
F Diffuse mixed, small and large cell	Diffuse mixed lymphocytic-histiocytic (DM)	90	10	Trisomy 3 t(14;18)
G Diffuse large cell	Diffuse histiocytic (DH)	80	20	Trisomy 7, 12 t(14;18), t(3;22) del(6)(q21)
HIGH GRADE				
H Large cell immunoblastic	Diffuse histiocytic (DH)	80	20	t(14;18) del(6)(q21)
I Lymphoblastic	Diffuse lymphoblastic (LL)	10	90	
J Small noncleaved cell; Burkitt's	Diffuse undifferentiated (DUL)	95	5	t(8;14), t(2;8), t(8;22)

cell to its normal cellular counterpart. By understanding the lineage and corresponding normal stage of differentiation, it should be eventually possible to further subgroup these tumors biologically according to cellular origin, ability to localize within specific microenvironments, propensity to further differentiate in vivo, production of cytokines, and response to therapy.

Non-Hodgkin's and Hodgkin's lymphomas are morphologically classified (as shown in Tables 311-2 and 311-6). In an attempt to understand the lineage derivation of these histologically defined subtypes, it is necessary to examine the normal populations of cells which reside in lymphoid tissues. To this end, B and T cell ontogeny will be reviewed. It will be within this context that the neoplastic lymphoma cell will be related to its normal cellular counterpart.

Lymphocytes can be functionally subdivided into distinct populations by their expression of unique cell surface and molecular markers. In the past, human B cells were identified by their expression of cell surface or cytoplasmic immunoglobulin and their capacity to secrete immunoglobulin. In contrast, human T lymphocytes were classically defined by the expression of sheep red blood cell receptors and their functional ability to regulate immune responses. The characterization of monoclonal antibodies (MAbs) directed against cell surface molecules expressed on human lymphoid cells has led to very significant advances in both the phenotypic and functional characterization of these cells. Monoclonal antibodies have been useful in assigning cellular lineage, identifying normal stages of lymphoid differentiation, and identifying the function of many of these molecules. Similarly, molecular biologic techniques demonstrating gene rearrangements have been helpful in defining lineage, clonality, and, to a lesser extent, stage of differentiation.

Normal B cell ontogeny   CELL SURFACE ANTIGENS   Normal B cell ontogeny has been operationally divided into functional stages, namely, pre-B cell, mature (resting) B cell, activated/proliferating B cell, differentiating B cell, and secretory (plasma) cell (Fig. 311-1). Several antigens have been very useful in defining B lineage derivation, since within the hematopoietic system they are uniquely expressed on B lymphocytes and their expression spans B cell ontogeny (see Fig. 311-1). Two of the most useful antigens are CD19 and CD20.

The most immature pre-B cells have been defined by their coexpression of cell surface antigens including major histocompatibility complex (MHC) class II (Ia) and CD19. Individual stages of pre-B cell ontogeny have been delineated by the sequential expression of the pre-B cell antigen CD10 (common acute lymphoblastic leukemia antigen, CALLA, enkephalinase), CD20, and finally, cytoplasmic immunoglobulin mu (cμ) heavy chains without the expression of light chains. As pre-B cells mature, they are exported to the peripheral blood and lymphoid tissues, where they reside until activated by antigen (mature B cell; see Fig. 311-1). Mature resting B cells continue to express cell surface Ia, CD19, and CD20 but no longer express CD10. These cells also express cell surface immunoglobulins IgM and IgD (the B cell antigen receptor), CD21 (which is the receptor for the C3d cleavage fragment of complement and for Epstein-Barr virus), and several lymphocyte homing and adhesion receptors including CD44, L-selectin, and CD11a/CD18 (LFA-1). These molecules are involved in lymphocyte recirculation, localization in distinct microenvironments, and cell-cell interactions.

Following triggering with antigen or other signals of activation, mature resting B cells are activated and subsequently proliferate (activated/proliferating B cell; see Fig. 311-1). From in vitro, in vivo, and in situ studies, the activation of resting B cells is accompanied by a sequence of cell surface antigenic changes. Resting B cells begin to lose cell surface IgD and CD21. As these antigens are lost, a number of B cell–associated and –restricted antigens sequentially appear (activation antigens). Activation antigens are cell surface molecules which are likely to be involved in the regulation of cellular proliferation and/or differentiation or alternatively play a role in the localization and binding of activated B cells within a microenvironment. These activation antigens include CD71 (transferrin receptor), CD54 (ICAM-1, ligand for LFA-1), CD25 (low-affinity interleukin 2 receptor), CD5, and B7 (adhesion molecule for T cells).

With further differentiation there is a sequential loss of the B cell activation antigens as well as pan-B cell antigens including Ia, CD19, and CD20. This stage is also characterized by the appearance of several other antigens (CD38 and PCA-1) which are expressed on plasma cells (secretory B cell).

FIGURE 311-1   Correlation of B cell differentiation and B cell malignancies.

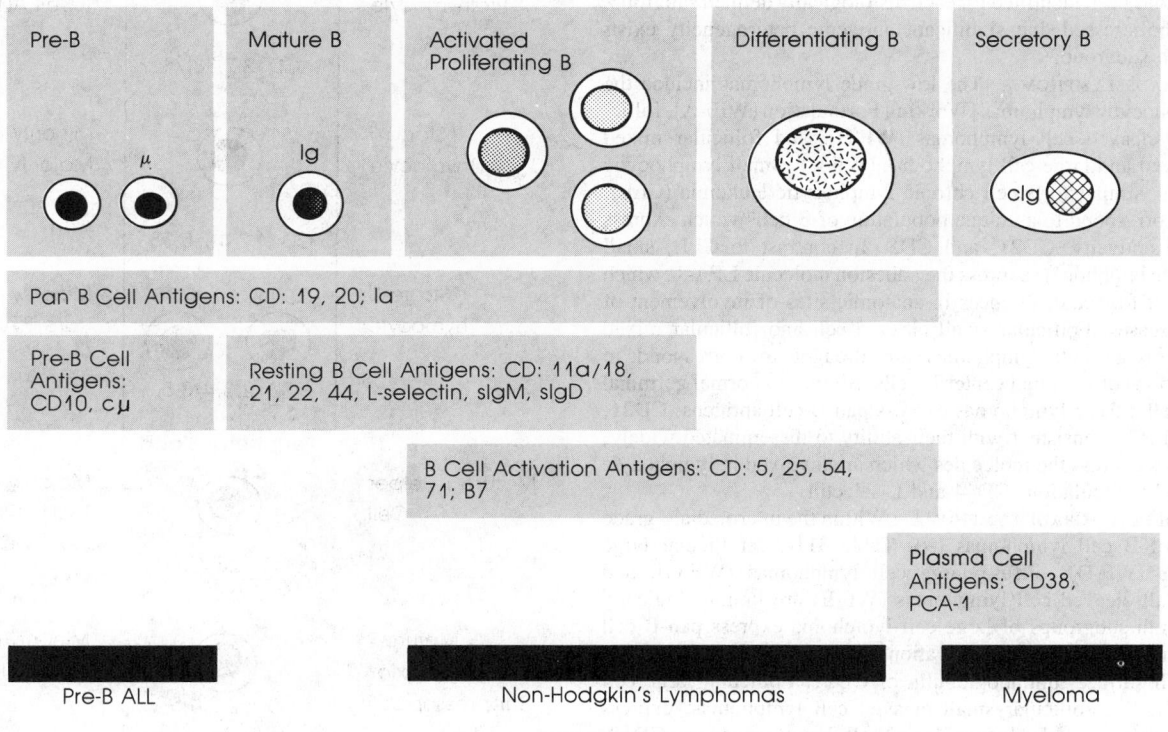

IMMUNOGLOBULIN GENE REARRANGEMENTS A vast variety and number of possible immunoglobulin molecules exist, each corresponding to a unique antigenic epitope. This diversity is the result of genetic recombination within the DNA of B lymphocytes. The germ-line DNA contains segments coding for different subunits of the immunoglobulin molecule. For the immunoglobulin heavy chain, these consist of a very large number of different variable (V) segments, a smaller number of different diversity (D) segments, a few joining (J) segments, and a constant region for each subclass of immunoglobulin.

The usual mechanism for achieving recombination of the immunoglobulin heavy chain genes involves joining together single V, D, and J segments with the appropriate constant region segment and excising the unused segments (somatic mutation). Therefore, the numbers of potential recombinants of V, D, and J segments are enormous. Light chain genes lack D segments but have a similar mechanism of rearrangement. A functional rearrangement of a heavy or light chain gene prevents rearrangements of another gene of the same chain type (allelic exclusion); however, an abnormal heavy or light chain rearrangement which cannot be transcribed will allow the other heavy chain allele or one of the other light chain alleles, respectively, to attempt rearrangement. *This functional allelic exclusion ensures that only one immunoglobulin specificity is allowed for any one B cell.* The heavy chain gene undergoes rearrangement first, followed by the kappa and then the lambda light chain genes. Clonal rearrangement of immunoglobulin genes is consistent with a B cell lineage derivation of a lymphoma.

MALIGNANT LYMPHOMAS OF B CELL ORIGIN As seen in Table 311-2, more than 90 percent of all cases of non-Hodgkin's lymphomas are of B cell derivation. *This observation is based on the expression of B lineage–restricted antigens as well as clonal rearrangements of immunoglobulin heavy and light chain genes.* Although most investigators have attempted to relate B cell lymphomas to major steps of B lymphocyte development (see Fig. 311-1), it is becoming increasing clear that these tumors correspond to major and minor subpopulations of activated B cells. It is noteworthy that no B cell neoplasm phenotypically corresponds to the resting B lymphocyte (mature B). All B cell non-Hodgkin's lymphomas express the pan-B cell antigens, including Ia, CD19, and CD20. Moreover, virtually all B cell non-Hodgkin's lymphomas express one or more B cell activation antigens and adhesion receptors. Although a common antigenic phenotype has been identified for each histologically defined subgroup, it should be stressed that significant antigenic heterogeneity exists within each subgroup.

LOW-GRADE LYMPHOMA The low-grade lymphomas include the small lymphocytic lymphomas [Working Formulation (WF)-A], follicular small cleaved cell lymphomas (WF-B), and follicular mixed small cleaved and large cell lymphomas (WF-C). Small lymphocytic lymphomas, similar to B cell chronic lymphocytic leukemia (CLL), appear to correspond to a unique population of B cells which express pan-B cell antigens, CD21, and CD5. In contrast to CLL, small lymphocytic lymphomas express the adhesion molecule LFA-1, which may account for the differences in anatomic sites of involvement of the two diseases. Follicular small cleaved cell and follicular mixed small and large cell lymphomas are thought to correspond to subpopulations of germinal center B cells. Similar to normal germinal center B cells, these lymphomas express pan-B cell antigens, CD21, CD10, and B7. Consistent with their ability to disseminated widely, these tumors express the molecules which are involved in lymphocyte homing and recirculation, CD44 and L-selectin.

INTERMEDIATE-GRADE LYMPHOMA Within the intermediate-grade subgroup of B cell lymphomas (see Table 311-2), follicular large lymphomas (WF-D), diffuse large cell lymphomas (WF-G), and diffuse small cleaved cell lymphomas (WF-E) are immunologically distinct. Both subgroups of large cell lymphoma express pan-B cell antigens and several B cell activation antigens but less frequently express cell surface immunoglobulin or CD21. Follicular large cell lymphomas, like follicular small cleaved cell lymphomas, express CD10, whereas B cell diffuse large cell lymphomas are CD10-negative. Diffuse small cleaved B cell lymphomas cytologically and phenotypically resemble follicular small cleaved cell lymphomas. They both express pan-B cell antigens and several of the B cell activation antigens. In contrast to follicular small cleaved cell lymphomas which express CD10 and frequently demonstrate a 14;18 translocation (see below), diffuse small cleaved cell lymphomas do not. A subgroup of diffuse small cleaved cell lymphomas termed *intermediate lymphocytic lymphomas,* also known as *centrocytic* or *mantle zone lymphomas,* is phenotypically similar to diffuse small cleaved cell lymphomas but also expresses surface IgD and CD5, characteristics of normal B cells which reside in the mantle zone of lymphoid follicles. These tumors have the characteristic chromosome translocation t(11;14).

HIGH-GRADE LYMPHOMA Large cell immunoblastic lymphomas (WF-H) are phenotypically identical to B cell diffuse large cell lymphomas. In contrast, the small noncleaved cell (WF-J) or Burkitt's lymphomas are related to normal germinal center B cells and follicular lymphomas in that they express pan-B cell antigens, B cell activation antigens, and CD10. The endemic (African) Burkitt's lymphoma cells which have the Epstein-Barr virus genome present in the tumor cells express the Epstein-Barr virus receptor CD21, whereas the nonendemic (American) variation does not.

Normal T cell ontogeny CELL SURFACE ANTIGENS During embryonic and early postnatal development, bone marrow precursor cells migrate to the thymus. The thymic microenvironment provides a setting for the processing and eventual development of functionally competent T cells. These cells are subsequently exported into peripheral lymphoid tissues and the circulation. A sequence of changes in cell surface antigens identified by MAbs is observed to accompany intrathymic differentiation (Fig. 311-2). The cells in the earliest stage (1) of intrathymic differentiation, which constitute 10 percent of the thymic lymphocytes, express CD2 (E rosette receptor, ligand for the LFA-3 adhesion molecule), CD71 (the transferrin receptor), CD38, and CD7.

FIGURE 311-2 Correlation of T cell differentiation and T cell malignancies.

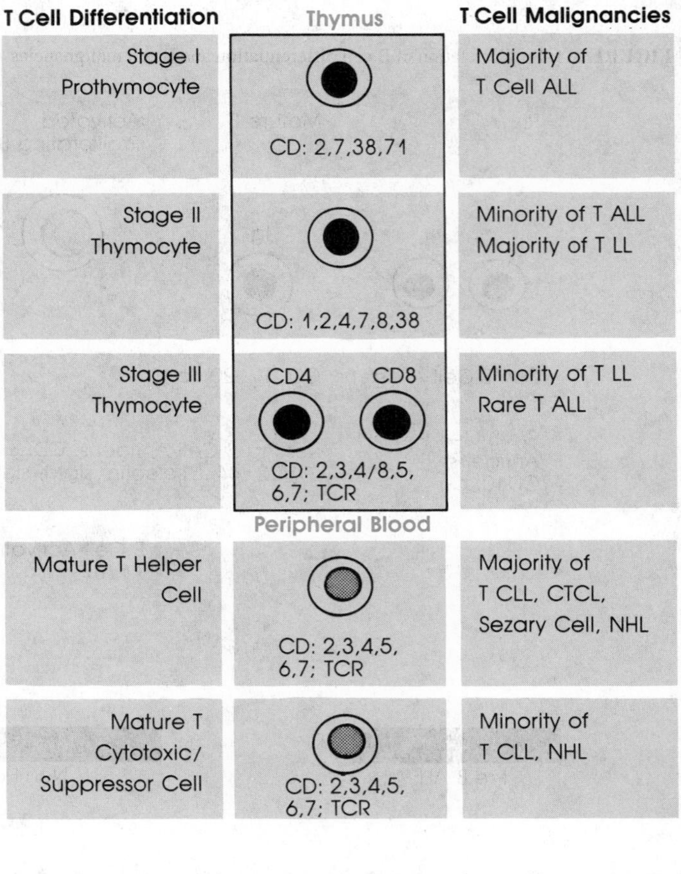

T Cell Differentiation	Thymus	T Cell Malignancies
Stage I Prothymocyte	CD: 2,7,38,71	Majority of T Cell ALL
Stage II Thymocyte	CD: 1,2,4,7,8,38	Minority of T ALL Majority of T LL
Stage III Thymocyte	CD4 CD8 CD: 2,3,4/8,5, 6,7; TCR	Minority of T LL Rare T ALL
Mature T Helper Cell	CD: 2,3,4,5, 6,7; TCR	Majority of T CLL, CTCL, Sezary Cell, NHL
Mature T Cytotoxic/ Suppressor Cell	CD: 2,3,4,5, 6,7; TCR	Minority of T CLL, NHL

Peripheral Blood

Stage II thymocytes are characterized by the loss of CD71, acquisition of CD1, and coexpression of CD4 (HIV-1 receptor) and CD8. The population coexpressing CD1, CD2, CD4, CD7, CD8, and CD38 constitutes 70 percent of thymocytes.

With further maturation, cells lose CD1 and acquire mature T cell antigens CD3, CD5, and CD6 (stage III). CD3 is a complex of chains which are noncovalently associated with the T cell antigen receptor. In parallel with the expression of CD3, cells express the T cell antigen receptor (TCR). The TCR can exist as an α/β heterodimer and recognizes antigen in the context of MHC. A second T cell receptor is also associated with CD3 and is termed γ/δ. Cells which express the γ/δ TCR appear earlier in ontogeny than α/β TCR–positive cells, are CD4- and CD8-negative, and can be associated with natural killer cell activity.

When cells leave the thymus, they are segregated into cells expressing either CD4 (helper T cell) or CD8 (cytotoxic/suppressor T cell), constituting 60 to 70 percent and 30 to 40 percent of peripheral T cells, respectively. Activated peripheral T cells undergo additional changes in cell surface antigens. They express the low-affinity interleukin 2 (IL-2) receptor (CD25), the transferrin receptor (CD71), CD9, and CD38.

T CELL RECEPTOR GENE REARRANGEMENTS   As indicated above, the T cell receptor is composed of several subunits, including a heterodimer imposed of the α and β chain in associated with the CD3 complex. The α, β, and γ chains genes undergo rearrangements in the same manner as immunoglobulin genes. V, D, and J DNA segments have been identified for the β chain gene and V and J segments for the others. There is also a temporal progression of rearrangement and gene expression, starting with γ chain gene rearrangement, followed by β chain gene rearrangement, and γ chain gene mRNA expression, then by β chain mRNA expression, and finally by α chain gene rearrangement and mRNA expression. It may be possible to utilize this progression to assign a stage within early T cell differentiation to a particular T cell lymphoma. *A neoplastic T cell population and its clonality are demonstrated by unique T cell receptor gene rearrangements.*

T CELL LYMPHOMAS   The most widely expressed T cell antigens used to define lineage are CD2 and CD7. As depicted in Fig. 311-2, T cell malignancies reflect distinct stages of T cell ontogeny. Similar to B cell neoplasms, the common cell surface phenotype for T cell neoplasms will be presented.

Lymphoblastic lymphomas correspond to stage II thymocytes, and the majority express CD1, CD2, CD4, CD7, and CD8. The remainder of the T cell lymphomas correspond to mature T cell populations, generally T helper cells. The peripheral T cell lymphomas, which histologically include diffuse small cleaved cell, diffuse mixed small and large cell, and diffuse large cell lymphomas, variably express the mature T cell antigens CD2, CD3, CD5, CD6, and CD7. Most express CD4, with a small fraction expressing CD8. Cutaneous T cell lymphomas also express a mature T helper cell phenotype: CD2, CD3, CD4, CD5, and CD7. Sézary cells generally lack CD7 and Ia antigens, whereas cells infiltrating the skin are CD7-positive and invariably express CD25 and CD71. The HTLV-1–associated adult T cell lymphomas are similar to the cutaneous T cell lymphomas in that they express CD2, CD3, CD4, CD5, CD7, and CD25.

Cellular origin of the Reed-Sternberg cell of Hodgkin's disease Reed-Sternberg cells, in the appropriate cytoarchitectural milieu, are required for the diagnosis of Hodgkin's disease. However, Reed-Sternberg cells are not only observed in Hodgkin's disease but may be seen in small numbers in several subtypes of non-Hodgkin's lymphoma. The major obstacle to determining the cellular origin of Hodgkin's disease is limited by identification and isolation of Reed-Sternberg cells. Studies to date have examined enriched populations of these cells or alternatively examined them using immunologic staining techniques in tissue sections. As discussed below, evidence exists for both lymphoid and nonlymphoid origin. Unfortunately, these studies have been complicated by contaminating normal populations admixed with Reed-Sternberg cells.

In Hodgkin's disease tissues the majority of cells are small lymphocytes with a mature T cell phenotype (CD2, CD3, CD4 or CD8, CD5) together with a variable number of presumably nonneoplastic B cells. Reed-Sternberg cells and their variants may be immunologically distinguished from the neoplastic cells of most non-Hodgkin's lymphomas by their lack of a characteristic pattern of most T and B cell–associated antigens. Reed-Sternberg cells may contain intracellular immunoglobulin, but this is polyclonal and is not thought to be produced by this cell. These cells express CD25 (low-affinity IL-2 receptor) and the transferrin receptor (CD71), which are also expressed on activated B, T, and natural killer cells. They also express MHC class II antigens, certain antigens expressed on myeloid cells (e.g., CD13), and the epithelial membrane antigen. Reed-Sternberg cells of the lymphocyte-predominant form of Hodgkin's disease express the leukocyte common antigen (CD45R), whereas all other Reed-Sternberg cells are negative, a feature of dendritic cells.

Two unique antigens are expressed on the Reed-Sternberg cell, and therefore, MAbs directed against these antigens have proven to be diagnostically useful. The first is CD15 (identified by MAb Leu M1), which is the Lewis X blood group antigen, and it functions as an adhesion receptor. CD15 is expressed on Reed-Sternberg cells in all subtypes of Hodgkin's disease except for the lymphocyte-predominant variant. The second antigen is the CD30 antigen (Ki-1), which is present on virtually all Reed-Sternberg cells. The CD30 antigen also is expressed on some activated B cells, activated T cells, dendritic cells, Epstein-Barr virus–transformed cell lines, and tumor cells isolated from some patients with large cell lymphomas (Ki-1 large cell anaplastic lymphoma).

Recent molecular studies of Reed-Sternberg–enriched populations have provided insight into the origin of Reed-Sternberg cells. Immuno-globulin gene rearrangements have been demonstrated in some specimens (usually lymphocyte-predominant Hodgkin's disease), and T cell receptor β chain rearrangements have been demonstrated in others. Clonal rearrangements have not been seen in background lymphocytes. Although rearrangements of the T cell γ chain genes have been observed, they should not be misconstrued as evidence for a clonal T cell origin, since this gene may not provide evidence for clonality. More recently, sensitive in situ hybridization studies have identified the Epstein-Barr virus (EBV) genome in Reed-Sternberg cells from about 30 percent of cases examined, supporting a role for EBV in some cases of Hodgkin's disease. Since EBV infection is restricted to B cells within the hematopoietic system, these findings support a B lineage for these Reed-Sternberg cells. Therefore, Hodgkin's disease is a heterogeneous disease derived from subpopulations of activated B cells, activated T cells, or dendritic cells. Moreover, the distinct biologic and clinical behaviors (see Table 311-1) of Hodgkin's and non-Hodgkin's lymphomas may be a reflection of their divergent cellular origins.

NON-HODGKIN'S LYMPHOMA

EPIDEMIOLOGY   About 40,000 new cases of non-Hodgkin's lymphoma occur each year in the United States, and this number appears to be increasing. Although the total number of patients is relatively small compared with some of the more common solid tumors, the malignant lymphomas are the most common neoplasm of patients between the ages of 20 and 40. Moreover, they rank fourth in the total number of person-years of life lost each year from cancer. With the increasing incidence of AIDS, the number of cases of non-Hodgkin's lymphoma has sharply increased.

ETIOLOGY   Animal studies suggest that lymphomas have a viral etiology. A herpesvirus has been isolated in avians and C-type retroviruses have been identified in rodents, cows, and subhuman primates with lymphocytic lymphomas. In contrast, in humans only endemic African Burkitt's lymphoma, some high grade B cell lymphomas, and adult T cell lymphoma have been shown to have a viral etiology. Epstein-Barr virus (EBV) has a strong association with the pathogenesis of Burkitt's lymphoma and high-grade lymphoma in immunodeficiency patients, including HIV-1 infected individuals. The human T cell leukemia virus (HTLV-1) is the causative agent in adult T cell lymphoma in endemic areas, which include southwestern Japan and the Caribbean.

Although limited progress has been made in identifying agents which might be involved in inducing non-Hodgkin's lymphomas, exciting advances have been made in identifying those genes which appear to be involved in lymphomatous transformation. Cytogenetic abnormalities have been well documented in a number of non-Hodgkin's lymphomas (see Table 311-2). DNA sequence analysis of several of these chromosomal translocations has demonstrated that genes which normally regulate heavy and light chain immunoglobulin synthesis have been juxtaposed to genes that regulate normal cellular activation and proliferation. It is postulated that these transforming genes, or *oncogenes,* have come under the control of those regulatory elements which normally control B cell proliferation and differentiation. The best-studied example is the t(8;14) or variant t(2;8) or t(8;22) translocations of Burkitt's lymphoma present in over 90 percent of Burkitt's lymphomas and a subgroup of acute lymphoblastic leukemias. In this disease, the c-*myc* oncogene on chromosome 8 is joined to either the immunoglobulin heavy chain locus on chromosome 14, the κ light chain locus on chromosome 2, or the λ light chain locus on chromosome 22, leading to activation and overexpression of the c-*myc* gene product. In contrast, the non-Burkitt's subtype lacks c-*myc* activation and expression. Another example is the t(14;18) translocation which is seen in approximately 85 percent of patients with follicular lymphomas and 35 percent of those with diffuse lymphomas. In t(14;18), the gene *bcl*-2 (chromosome 18) is juxtaposed to the immunoglobulin heavy chain locus (chromosome 14). The *bcl*-2 gene product prevents programmed cell death or apoptosis. It is hypothesized that the alteration is *bcl*-2 expression is involved in the pathogenesis of the indolent behaving low-grade lymphomas.

A number of primary diseases have an increased incidence of subsequently developing non-Hodgkin's lymphoma and to a lesser extent Hodgkin's lymphoma. As seen in Table 311-3, diseases of inherited and acquired immunodeficiency as well as autoimmune diseases are associated with an increased incidence of lymphoma. Non-Hodgkin's lymphomas which occur in the context of drug-induced immunosuppression, acquired or congenital immunodeficiency, and AIDS are frequently associated with EBV. The association between immunosuppression and induction of non-Hodgkin's lymphomas appears to be compelling, since if the immunosuppression can be reversed (e.g., discontinuing immunosuppressive agents following organ transplantation), a percentage of these lymphomas regress

spontaneously. The incidence of lymphoma in iatrogenic immune suppression, AIDS, and autoimmune disease argues strongly for immune dysregulation contributing to the development of lymphoma. Patients with certain environmental exposures have a higher incidence of lymphomas. Patients with Hodgkin's disease treated with combined-modality treatment of radiation therapy and chemotherapy exhibit an increased risk of developing secondary large cell lymphomas. Lymphoma-like syndromes also have been found in patients treated with phenytoin. Although in most cases this disease regresses when the drug is stopped, a significant number of patients still develop malignant lymphomas.

CLINICAL PRESENTATION AND DIFFERENTIAL DIAGNOSIS
More than two-thirds of patients with non-Hodgkin's lymphoma present with persistent painless peripheral lymphadenopathy. At the time of presentation, differential diagnosis includes infectious causes due to bacteria, viruses (e.g., infectious mononucleosis, cytomegalovirus, and human immunodeficiency virus), and parasites (toxoplasmosis). In young patients, Hodgkin's lymphoma must be excluded. In older patients, other neoplasms must be considered. It is generally agreed that in adults, a firm lymph node greater than 1 cm in size that is not associated with a documentable infection and that persists longer than 4 to 6 weeks should be considered for biopsy. Certain clinical features suggest the diagnosis of non-Hodgkin's lymphoma. Involvement of Waldeyer's ring, epitrochlear, and mesenteric nodes is more suggestive of non-Hodgkin's lymphoma than Hodgkin's. Unlike Hodgkin's, which can present with weight loss, fever, or night sweats (B symptoms), it is less common for patients with non-Hodgkin's lymphoma to present with systemic complaints.

Non-Hodgkin's lymphomas also present with chest, abdominal, or extranodal symptomatology. Although much less common than Hodgkin's disease, approximately 20 percent of patients with non-Hodgkin's lymphoma have mediastinal adenopathy. These patients most frequently present with persistent cough and chest discomfort or without symptoms but have an abnormal chest x-ray. Occasionally, a superior vena cava syndrome accompanies presentation, especially in patients with T cell lymphomas and to a lesser extent in those with B cell diffuse large cell lymphoma. Differential includes infectious causes (e.g., histoplasmosis, tuberculosis, or infectious mononucleosis), sarcoidosis, Hodgkin's disease, and other neoplasms. Involvement of retroperitoneal, mesenteric, and pelvic nodes is common in most histologic subtypes of non-Hodgkin's lymphoma. Unless massive or leading to obstruction, these nodes usually produce no symptoms. In contrast, patients who come to medical attention because of an abdominal mass, massive splenomegaly, or primary gastrointestinal lymphoma present with complaints similar to those associated with other abdominal space-occupying lesions. These include chronic pain, abdominal fullness, early satiety, symptoms associated with viscus obstruction, or even acute perforation and gastrointestinal hemorrhage. Symptoms due to extralymphatic disease are more common in some subtypes of diffuse non-Hodgkin's lymphoma but are uncommon in follicular lymphomas. Rarely, some patients present with symptoms of unexplained anemia and thrombocytopenia due to marrow infiltration with lymphoma or hypersplenism. Diffuse non-Hodgkin's lymphomas can present with cutaneous lesions, testicular masses, acute spinal cord compression, solitary bone lesions, and rarely, lymphomatous meningitis. Primary non-Hodgkin's lymphoma of the brain constitutes only 1 percent of all non-Hodgkin' lymphomas. However with HIV-1 infection and the increasing use of immunosuppressive therapy in organ transplant recipients, primary central nervous system (CNS) lymphoma is becoming one of the most common types of primary brain tumors.

PATHOLOGIC CLASSIFICATION   Rappaport and Working Formulation classification schemes   The pathologic classification of non-Hodgkin's lymphomas has been difficult for both pathologists and clinicians. Histologic classifications is crucial, since therapeutic options are based on histologic subtype and less frequently by stage. In 1966, Henry Rappaport presented the first clinically relevant classification scheme for non-Hodgkin's lymphomas. This classifica-

---

TABLE 311-3   Diseases or exposures associated with increase risk of development of malignant lymphoma

Inherited immunodeficiency disease
  Klinefelter's syndrome
  Chediak-Higashi syndrome
  Ataxia telangiectasia syndrome
  Wiscott-Aldrich syndrome
  Common variable immunodeficiency disease
Acquired immunodeficiency diseases
  Iatrogenic immunosuppression
  Human immunodeficiency virus-1 infection
  Acquired hypogammaglobulinemia
Autoimmune disease
  Sjögren's syndrome
  Celiac sprue
  Rheumatoid arthritis and systemic lupus erythematosus
Chemical or drug exposures
  Phenytoin
  Radiation
  Prior combination chemotherapy and radiation therapy
Viral association (other than HIV)
  Epstein-Barr virus
  Human T cell leukemia virus

tion was based on assessment of overall pattern of lymph node architecture (low-power microscopy) as well as the cytologic classification of the neoplastic cell (high-power microscopy). The Rappaport classification subdivides the non-Hodgkin's lymphomas into two major subtypes, namely, nodular (follicular) and diffuse. Nodular lymphomas retain some features of normal lymph node architecture in that the neoplastic cells appear to form "germinal centers" (nodules). In contrast, in diffuse lymphomas, the normal cortical and paracortical lymph node architecture is largely effaced. Rappaport also divided non-Hodgkin's lymphomas into subgroups according to cytologic appearance of the malignant cell: (1) well-differentiated, (2) poorly differentiated, and (3) histiocytic. This suggested that these tumors corresponded morphologically to distinct stages of lymphoid and monocytic differentiation. The importance of the Rappaport classification (see Table 311-2) was that each histologically defined subtype of non-Hodgkin's lymphoma exhibited a unique natural history and response to therapy. The nodular lymphomas generally behaved in an indolent manner, while most diffuse lymphomas had an aggressive behavior.

With the advent of modern immunology, the Rappaport classification proved to have several biologic defects. First, the term *histiocytic* was incorrect, since virtually all these tumors were of lymphoid origin. Second, certain clinical entities were not accounted for by this classification scheme. By the late 1970s, six independent pathologic schemes were in use throughout the world, and therefore, therapeutic trials could not be compared. Because of this confusion, a new classification scheme was proposed and has been termed the *Working Formulation* (see Table 311-2). The latter incorporates the best features of the various classification systems and, more important, retains clinical relevance. The Working Formulation subdivides non-Hodgkin's lymphomas into *low-*, *intermediate-*, and *high-grade* subgroups dependent on their natural history. Low-grade lymphomas are characterized by an indolent clinical course, with their natural history not significantly altered by therapy. Intermediate- and high-grade lymphomas historically were associated with very short survivals. With the advent of aggressive combination chemotherapeutic regimens, some of the patients with intermediate- and high-grade tumors demonstrate long-term disease-free survivals. It should be noted that the Working Formulation omits several important histologic subtypes, including diffuse intermediate lymphocytic lymphoma (a low-grade disease), adult T cell lymphoma associated with HTLV-1, lymphoma of mucosa associated lymphoid tissue (MALT), and cutaneous T cell lymphoma. Table 311-2 compares the Working Formulation and the Rappaport classifications. In clinical practice, these classification schemes are frequently used interchangeably.

STAGING AND DISEASE DETECTION **Conventional staging**
The Ann Arbor staging system developed for Hodgkin's disease also has been used in staging non-Hodgkin's lymphomas. This staging system focuses on the number of tumor sites (nodal and extranodal), location, and the presence or absence of systemic symptoms. Table 311-4 summaries this staging system. In stages I and II, sites of disease are on the same side of the diaphragm. Stage III disease involves both sides of the diaphragm, whereas stage IV is defined as extranodal lymphomatous involvement, most frequently of the bone marrow and liver. Systemic symptoms (fever, weight loss of more than 10 percent of body weight, and night sweats, i.e., B symptoms)

are less common in non-Hodgkin's lymphomas (about 20 percent of cases) than in Hodgkin's disease and therefore are not as useful in predicting prognosis. It must be emphasized that this classification scheme was developed specifically for Hodgkin's disease, which disseminates by contiguous lymphatic extension and to a much lesser extent hematogenously. Since non-Hodgkin's lymphomas most frequently disseminate hematogenously, this staging system has proven to be less useful in this type of lymphoma.

The concept of staging has a smaller impact on treatment strategy in patients with non-Hodgkin's lymphomas than in those with Hodgkin's disease. Only 10 percent of patients with follicular lymphoma have localized disease and are candidates for local radiation therapy. For the diffuse lymphomas, even patients with localized disease and the majority of patients with advanced stage disease now receive systemic treatment. Therefore, staging is undertaken in non-Hodgkin's lymphomas to identify those small numbers of patients who can be treated with local therapy and to stratify within histologic subtypes with the view to prognosticate and to assess the impact of therapeutic regimens.

Staging procedures after biopsy diagnosis Staging must be undertaken in the context of the Working Formulation histologic grade. A suggested staging workup for patients with non-Hodgkin's lymphoma is summarized in Table 311-5. An organized approach to staging a patient with non-Hodgkin's lymphoma is mandatory. After the initial excisional biopsy and documentation of the pathologic and, when possible, immunologic subtype of disease, blood tests should be obtained, including a complete blood count, routine chemistries, liver function tests, and serum protein electrophoresis to document the presence of circulating monoclonal paraprotein. Waldeyer's ring involvement is often associated with intestinal involvement, and

---

TABLE 311-5 Staging evaluation for non-Hodgkin's lymphoma

ESSENTIAL

1 Pathologic documentation by hematopathologist
2 Physical examination
3 Documentation of B symptoms
4 Laboratory evaluation
  a Complete blood counts
  b Liver function tests
  c Renal function tests
  d Uric acid
  e Calcium
  f Serum protein electrophoresis
5 Chest radiograph
6 CT scan of abdomen and pelvis
7 Bone marrow biopsy

ESSENTIAL UNDER CERTAIN CIRCUMSTANCES

1 Chest CT scan
2 Head CT scan
3 Lumbar puncture
4 Barium studies of GI tract
5 Endoscopic examination
6 Cytologic examination of effusion
7 Gallium scan (planar or SPECT)

USEFUL BUT NOT ESSENTIAL TESTS

1 Cell surface marker phenotypic analysis
2 Cytogenetic analysis
3 Gene rearrangement analysis
4 Polymerase chain reaction analysis of minimal residual disease
5 Flow cytometry for DNA analysis
6 Liver scan
7 Liver biopsy
8 Bone scan
9 Thallium scan
10 Lymphangiography
11 Ultrasonography
12 Magnetic resonance imaging
13 Echocardiogram
14 Laparotomy

TABLE 311-4 Ann Arbor staging system

Stage I	Involvement in single lymph node region or single extralymphatic site
Stage II	Involvement of two or more lymph node regions on the same side of diaphragm; can also include localized involvement of extralymphatic site (stage IIE)
Stage III	Involvement of lymph node regions or extralymphatic sites on both sides of diaphragm
Stage IV	Disseminated involvement of one or more extralymphatic organs with or without lymph node involvement

gastrointestinal contrast studies or endoscopy is indicated if the patient appears to have localized disease. Chest radiography is used to exclude mediastinal and hilar adenopathy, pleural effusions, and pulmonary parenchymal infiltration. Chest computed tomographic (CT) scan is used to more precisely assess the extent of disease and is strongly recommended for patients with abnormal chest radiographs. However, abdominal/pelvic CT scan is essential for accurate staging to assess lymphadenopathy in retroperitoneal, mesenteric, and retrocrural areas. Lymphangiography in less useful than in Hodgkin's disease, since common sites of disease in non-Hodgkin's lymphoma include nodes in the mesentery, hilum of liver, spleen, or kidneys as well as nodes in the deep bony pelvis, none of which is detected by this procedure. However, lymphogram may be an accurate predictor of intraabdominal lymphoma, since the majority of patients with a positive lymphogram also have disease in the liver and in abdominal nodes. The major advantage of lymphangiography over abdominal/pelvic CT scan is its ability to detect infiltrated but normal-sized retroperitoneal nodes. The major indication for lymphangiography is non-Hodgkin's lymphoma is for patients with localized inguinal disease who may be candidates for local radiotherapy, where CT scanning for intraabdominal disease may be falsely negative. Unilateral percutaneous bone marrow biopsies must be performed, since the likelihood of lymphomatous involvement of the marrow is relatively high, especially in low-grade lymphoma, where marrow involvement occurs in up to 60 percent of cases. With any indication of hepatic abnormalities on blood tests or on liver scan, a percutaneous liver biopsy may be indicated in patients who would otherwise have stage I disease. In patients with aggressive lymphomas with marrow involvement, with paranasal sinus involvement, or if clinically indicated, examination of the cerebrospinal fluid by lumbar puncture should be performed.

More invasive tests are reserved for the uncommon presentation with stage I or II non-Hodgkin's lymphoma. While staging laparotomy may be performed routinely in Hodgkin's disease, this is not so in the non-Hodgkin's lymphomas. In the diffuse non-Hodgkin's lymphomas, stages II, III, and IV can all be considered reflective of disseminated disease and are therefore usually treated with chemotherapy. In contrast, only true stage I disease or, depending on the histologic subtype, stage II disease will be considered as localized and treated with radiation alone. Therefore, for most patients with non-Hodgkin's lymphoma, it is less critical to ascertain the precise pathologic stage of disease. Moreover, it is common for these patients to exhibit disseminated disease after routine staging tests (e.g., bone marrow or liver biopsy), thus obviating the need for laparotomy to prove dissemination. For example, within follicular lymphomas, the small cleaved cell and mixed small and large cell types, following clinical staging and bone marrow biopsy, greater than 85 percent of these patients will have stage III or stage IV disease. Thus *surgical staging should never be considered a routine procedure in patients with non-Hodgkin's lymphoma.*

A number of other tests are becoming more important in both staging and advancing our knowledge of the biology of non-Hodgkin's lymphoma. Radionuclide scans, especially with gallium, appear to have clinical utility. Gallium scans are positive in virtually all intermediate- and high-grade lymphomas and in about 50 percent of low-grade lymphomas. Gallium scans, with high doses of isotope which permit delayed imaging, combined with single photon emission computed tomography (SPECT), are very sensitive in detecting tumor infiltration. These tests are also very useful in monitoring response to therapy. The role of magnetic resonance imaging (MRI) in detecting non-Hodgkin's lymphoma is under active investigation. To date, MRI appears to be most valuable for detecting occult marrow involvement. Immunologic and molecular biologic studies are proving increasingly useful in confirming diagnosis. For example, in cases with difficult histopathologic patterns, cell surface markers can distinguish between non-Hodgkin's lymphoma and carcinoma [leukocyte common antigen (CD45) is specific for lymphoma]. Similarly, MAbs directed against lineage-restricted antigens and rearrangement of immunoglobulin or

T cell receptor genes are useful in identifying lymphoid tumors. The delineation of the cell surface phenotype is becoming important because an increasing number of salvage treatment programs employ high-dose chemoradiotherapy and monoclonal antibody–purged autologous bone marrow support (see below). Definition of a specific chromosomal abnormality also may have prognostic significance.

Sensitive techniques to detect minimal residual disease The development of molecular techniques to define immunoglobulin and T cell receptor gene rearrangements has provided very sensitive tools with which to more accurately assess tumor cell infiltration. The most common and accessible tissues to be tested include peripheral blood and bone marrow. Whereas conventional histologic analysis of the bone marrow can detect 1 lymphoma cell infiltrating 20 normal cells, immunologic flow cytometric and Southern blot analysis each improve this level of detection to approximately 1 lymphoma cell in approximately 100 normal cells. Similarly, flow cytometry has been used to detect "clonal excess" in the blood of patients with B cell non-Hodgkin's lymphoma. More recently, molecular biologic techniques demonstrate that minimal disease detection can be markedly improved. For those non-Hodgkin's lymphomas with a known chromosomal translocation, it is now possible to identify a unique chromosomal "breakpoint." This has been most elegantly accomplished for the t(14;18) translocation present in the majority of follicular lymphomas and in about 30 percent of diffuse lymphomas. Based on DNA sequence, it is possible to amplify this unique stretch of DNA using specific oligonucleotide primers and the polymerase chain reaction (PCR) (see Chap. 61). With this approach, 1 tumor cell in 10^6 normal cells can be detected. Thus, while other tests may be negative, PCR may demonstrate that the blood or bone marrow is contaminated by lymphoma cells. These biologic techniques are presently being compared with more conventional staging methods. Considering their sensitivity, they may be useful in more accurately assessing complete remission and, more important, in determining whether treatment should be prolonged, truncated, or intensified.

NATURAL HISTORY BY HISTOLOGIC SUBTYPE Considering the heterogeneity of non-Hodgkin's lymphomas and the unique clinical presentation and natural history within histologically defined subtypes, it is important to briefly review these subtypes.

Low grade SMALL LYMPHOCYTIC (DIFFUSE WELL-DIFFERENTIATED LYMPHOCYTIC) This disease is the lymphomatous presentation of chronic lymphocytic leukemia (CLL) and therefore occurs in middle-aged and older patients. Patients usually present with asymptomatic generalized lymphadenopathy. Unlike CLL, the peripheral blood may be normal or reveal only a mild lymphocytosis (60 percent will have absolute lymphocytosis of >4000 per cubic millimeter at diagnosis). In contrast, the bone marrow is involved in 75 to 95 percent of cases. Serum paraprotein is found in about 20 percent of cases, and hypogammaglobulinemia is common. These patients can often be observed without treatment for 3 to 4 years, with a median survival of 8 to 10 years. A small percentage of small lymphocytic lymphomas and CLLs will undergo histologic conversion to diffuse large cell lymphoma (Richter's syndrome). These patients usually present with extensive disease, abdominal masses, and B symptoms and experience short survival.

FOLLICULAR, PREDOMINANTLY SMALL CLEAVED CELL (NODULAR POORLY DIFFERENTIATED LYMPHOCYTIC) Follicular lymphomas account for approximately 50 percent of the non-Hodgkin's lymphomas; the small cleaved cell type is the most common subtype. Patients usually present with painless peripheral adenopathy in cervical, axillary, inguinal, and femoral regions. Patients frequently note that lymph node enlargement has been present for long periods of time and these nodes have "waxed and waned." Less typically, there is enlargement of Waldeyer's ring and epitrochlear nodes. Some patients present with asymptomatic large abdominal and retroperitoneal masses with or without evidence of gastrointestinal and/or renal obstruction. Although patients may present with one or more sites of nodal disease, noninvasive workup usually demonstrates widely disseminated disease with involvement of spleen, liver, and bone marrow in over 80 percent of patients. Bone marrow involvement in follicular lymphoma reveals a unique pattern of paratrabecular infiltration. Peripheral blood involvement is seen in about 10 percent of patients, and CNS disease is rare, although epidural disease can be seen. In contrast to diffuse lymphomas, about 10 percent of patients present with extramedullary extranodal disease and less than 10 percent present with B symptoms. The course of this disease is quite variable. The conventional approach for most patients is that they can be observed with waxing and waning disease for a median of 3 years without the need for therapy. Although in patients with stage I or limited stage II disease local radiation therapy may provide long-term remissions or cure, others demonstrate more disseminated and rapid growth and require treatment because massive nodal or organ enlargement leads to pain, lymphatic obstruction, organ obstruction, or more rarely, neurologic symptoms. At the time of increasing generalized disease or rapid growth at a single site, involved nodes should be considered for rebiopsy. At that time, a significant number of patients will demonstrate a "conversion" or "transformation" to a more aggressive histologic pattern, often diffuse large cell. This conversion occurs in up 60 percent of patients with follicular small cleaved cell lymphoma. Histologic conversion can be associated with infiltration of extranodal sites, the development of systemic symptoms, and a poor prognosis, since the tumor is much less responsive to treatment. Historically, both disease-free and overall survivals of patients with follicular lymphoma have not changed despite many different therapeutic approaches. Although 40 to 70 percent of patients achieve complete remissions (noninvasively staged) with conventional single-agent or aggressive combination chemotherapy, the median duration of remission is between 2 and 3 years. Following relapse, patients can be observed or retreated; however, the median survival after first relapse is 5 years. Patients with follicular non-Hodgkin's lymphoma survive long periods of time, with median survivals for patients with stage III and IV disease approaching 7 to 9 years.

FOLLICULAR, MIXED SMALL CLEAVED AND LARGE CELL (NODULAR MIXED)   This entity has similarities with both follicular small cleaved cell and follicular large cell lymphomas. Bone marrow infiltration at presentation is less common than in small cleaved cell lymphoma, but large abdominal masses are seen more commonly. Since some studies suggest that a subset of these patients may be cured with conventional therapy, these patients are generally not observed but are treated soon after diagnosis with combination chemotherapy.

Intermediate grade   FOLLICULAR, PREDOMINANTLY LARGE CELL (NODULAR HISTIOCYTIC)   Although the follicular architecture of these tumors is preserved, this disease behaves much more like diffuse large cell lymphoma. In contrast to other follicular lymphomas, this histologic variant has less frequent infiltration of the marrow and liver and presents with large masses and frequently extranodal disease. A finite cure rate has been reported in selected series. Most follicular large cell lymphomas which are not cured by treatment eventually convert to diffuse large cell lymphoma.

DIFFUSE SMALL CLEAVED CELL (DIFFUSE POORLY DIFFERENTIATED LYMPHOCYTIC)   This disease behaves like a follicular variant. Patients are middle-aged or older. At the time of presentation, most have stage IV disease with infiltration of the spleen, liver, and bone marrow, with marrow and liver infiltration occurring in over 50 percent of patients. Later in the course of the disease, infiltration of other parenchymal organs (e.g., lungs) is observed. The overall median survival is much shorter than observed in patients with low-grade lymphomas; however, like low-grade lymphoma, aggressive combination chemotherapy has had a minimal impact on the natural history of this disease.

DIFFUSE MIXED SMALL AND LARGE CELL (DIFFUSE MIXED)   This tumor behaves most like diffuse large cell lymphoma. Some investigators consider these two tumors to be a spectrum of a single entity. In several clinical trials where patients with diffuse mixed and diffuse large cell lymphoma were treated identically, survival rates were comparable. However, in other series, a higher relapse rate was observed.

DIFFUSE LARGE CELL (DIFFUSE HISTIOCYTIC)   Patients who are generally middle-aged or older present with either nodal enlargement (especially in the neck or abdomen) or extranodal disease (in the gastrointestinal tract, testes, bone, thyroid, salivary glands, skin, and brain). During the course of the disease, the liver, kidneys, and lungs may be involved. Diffuse large cell lymphoma is highly invasive, with local compression of vessels or airways, involvement of peripheral nerves, and destruction of bone. Although bone marrow involvement initially is found in only 10 to 20 percent of patients, its detection is important because of its strong correlation with later spread to the CNS. Later in the disease, some patients demonstrate both extensive bone marrow infiltration and peripheral blood involvement. Several large studies have identified a number of clinical features considered to be associated with inability to achieve a complete remission and poor prognosis. These features include poor performance status, bulk of disease (>10-cm tumor masses), bone marrow infiltration, multiple sites of extranodal disease, markedly elevated serum lactic dehydrogenase (LDH), and systemic B symptoms. Using these prognostic variables, alternative therapies are being investigated to improve the survival for poor-prognosis patients with diffuse large cell lymphoma.

High grade   LARGE CELL IMMUNOBLASTIC (DIFFUSE HISTIOCYTIC)   This variant of diffuse large cell lymphoma demonstrates a unique pathologic appearance. This disease usually occur in adults, commonly over age 50, and often in a setting of prior immune-mediated or lymphoproliferative disease (e.g., celiac disease, Hashimoto's thyroiditis, angioimmunoblastic lymphadenopathy, Sjögren's syndrome, Mediterranean lymphoma, cold agglutinin disease, or Waldenström's macroglobulinemia). Anemia, lymphopenia, diffuse hypergammaglobulinemia, B symptoms, and advanced stage are common at presentation. Most patients present with extranodal disease, and invasion of the bone marrow and CNS is common. Although histologically distinct within the Working Formulation, with aggressive combination chemotherapy, the prognosis for these patients is similar to that for patients with diffuse large cell lymphoma.

LYMPHOBLASTIC (DIFFUSE LYMPHOBLASTIC)   Although lymphoblastic lymphomas represent a major subgroup of childhood non-Hodgkin's lymphomas, they are much less common in adults (less than 5 percent of adult non-Hodgkin's lymphomas). Patients are usually males in their twenties to thirties who present with lymphadenopathy in cervical, supraclavicular, and axillary regions (50 percent) or with a mediastinal mass (50 to 70 percent). In most patients, the mediastinal mass is anterior, >10 cm, symptomatic often with superior vena cava syndrome, and associated with pleural effusions. Less commonly, patients present with extranodal disease (e.g., skin, testicular, or bony involvement). Greater than 90 percent of patients present with stage III or IV disease, and half have B symptoms. Although the bone marrow can be normal at presentation, approximately 60 percent of patients develop bone marrow infiltration and a subsequent leukemic phase indistinguishable from T cell acute lymphoblastic leukemia. Patients with bone marrow involvement have a very high incidence of CNS infiltration. Prior to current aggressive acute leukemia–like therapy, this disease was rapidly fatal.

SMALL NONCLEAVED, BURKITT'S AND NON-BURKITT'S (DIFFUSE UNDIFFERENTIATED)   Burkitt's lymphoma is a childhood tumor which has two major clinical presentations. The endemic (African) form presents as a jaw tumor which spreads to extranodal sites, especially to the bone marrow and meninges. The nonendemic (American) form has an abdominal presentation with massive disease, ascites, and skin, bone, peripheral node involvement and, like the African form, also spreads to the bone marrow and CNS (although less than in the African form). Prior to aggressive therapeutic programs, all children died rapidly. These tumors are now treated with very aggressive chemotherapeutic programs with more gratifying results. Burkitt's lymphoma is uncommon in adults but is occasionally seen in patients up to age 35. In contrast, small noncleaved non-Burkitt's lymphomas are observed and are very aggressive and frequently present like diffuse large cell lymphoma in extranodal sites. Like Burkitt's lymphoma, these tumors have a very high propensity to invade the bone marrow and CNS.

Other subtypes AIDS-RELATED LYMPHOMAS Non-Hodgkin's lymphoma occurs in 10 to 30 percent of patients with AIDS. Most cases are grouped with high-grade tumors, including small noncleaved and large cell immunoblastic lymphomas. In these cases, extranodal involvement is common, with the CNS, bone marrow, and gastrointestinal tract the most frequent sites. Most patients present with widespread disease, rapid nodal enlargement, and B symptoms. Primary CNS lymphoma is common in AIDS patients with a short survival. AIDS lymphomas have been associated with translocations involving chromosome 8 and with EBV (in about 40 percent of cases), similar to that seen in Burkitt's lymphoma. Although treated with the most aggressive combinations of chemotherapy, results have been poor largely due the high death rate secondary to intercurrent infections.

CUTANEOUS T CELL LYMPHOMAS Cutaneous T cell lymphomas are diseases of middle-aged adults with a slight male predominance. Major variants include mycosis fungoides and the Sézary syndrome, characterized by peripheral blood involvement. Cutaneous T cell lymphomas present with an indolent course with cutaneous manifestations and lymphadenopathy. Later patients will develop hepatic, splenic, gastrointestinal tract, pulmonary, and renal involvement. Infiltration of the bone marrow and circulating leukemia (Sézary cells), usually in the presence of generalized erythroderma, are also frequent late manifestations. The median survival from diagnosis is about 10 years, with infection being the most common cause of death.

ADULT T CELL LEUKEMIA/LYMPHOMA This entity has been observed in southwestern Japan and the Caribbean, as well as in blacks in the southeastern United States, and is associated with the HTLV-1 type C retrovirus. Adult T cell leukemia/lymphoma (ATLL) presents in an aggressive manner, with generalized lymph adenopathy, hepatosplenomegaly, cutaneous infiltration, hypercalcemia, lytic bone lesions, elevated LDH, and a profound leukemia characterized by pleomorphic CD4-positive T cells. The skin lesions can vary from papules, plaques, and tumors to ulcerations. Marrow involvement is not marked, and anemia and thrombocytopenia are not common. This disease has a fulminant course, and its natural history has been minimally altered by aggressive combination chemotherapy. Although 50 to 70 percent of patients will achieve a complete remission, the median duration of remission is around 12 months. The incidence of infections, including many opportunistic infections, is very high in patients with ATLL. A chronic form also has been described with skin lesions, mild lymphocytosis without significant numbers of circulating blasts, and absence of hepatosplenomegaly or lymphadenopathy. These patients can survive for years before converting to a more aggressive form of the disease.

ANGIOIMMUNOBLASTIC LYMPHADENOPATHY (CLASSIFIED WITH LARGE CELL IMMUNOBLASTIC) This disease of older adults presents with the acute onset of generalized lymphadenopathy, rash, hepatosplenomegaly, and B symptoms. Immunologic abnormalities are common and include plasmacytosis, polyclonal hypergammaglobulinemia, and a positive Coombs' test. Although this disease is progressive and frequently fatal, it is unresolved whether it is a hyperimmune disorder or a malignant lymphoma. Limited cytogenetic and clonal T cell receptor β-chain rearrangements suggest a neoplasm akin to adult peripheral T cell lymphoma.

MONOCYTOID B CELL LYMPHOMA This disease overlaps with the lymphomas of mucosa-associated lymphoid tissue (MALT). There is no age predilection for these tumors, which are generally localized and can involve the gastrointestinal tract, respiratory tract, and lacrimal and salivary glands. Patients can present with peptic ulcer disease, abdominal pain, and sicca syndrome. The clinical behavior of this disease is similar to the indolent lymphomas.

THERAPY To decide the appropriate treatment regimen, the clinician must determine the grade and extent of disease. The next decision is whether or not to treat, and if the treatment option is selected, whether the goal is to palliate symptoms or to cure. Although some general principles are agreed on in the treatment of non-Hodgkin's lymphoma, therapeutic approaches for all histologic subtypes are actively being evaluated. Options to be chosen must consider age and the presence of comorbid diseases (cardiac, renal, pulmonary, hepatic) which might significantly affect end-organ toxicity.

Radiotherapy Radiation has a limited role in the primary treatment of non-Hodgkin's lymphoma. It should be considered only as a potential curative modality in patients who have been aggressively staged and who have stage I or II low-grade non-Hodgkin's lymphoma. Selected patients with intermediate-grade (diffuse large cell) lymphomas have been treated in the past with local radiation therapy with 60 to 90 percent long-term disease-free survival; however, several recent studies support the use of abbreviated chemotherapy (with or without local radiation) with a very high success rate (>90 percent disease-free survival). For patients with stage I disease, involved-field radiotherapy is employed, with the dose dependent on the histologic subtype. Doses of less than 3500 cGy are usually sufficient for low-grade disease, whereas high-grade disease is frequently treated with 5000 cGy or greater, which can be modified when used after combination chemotherapy. For patients with stage I follicular non-Hodgkin's lymphoma, the long-term disease-free survival ranges from 60 to 80 percent. In addition to its curative potential in stage I patients, radiotherapy is frequently used in conjunction with systemic therapy to treat sites of bulk disease. However, it remains controversial whether the addition of radiotherapy increases the overall disease-free survival. Moreover, in low-grade lymphomas, radiotherapy has been used commonly to palliate sites of symptomatic disease.

Chemotherapy This modality is used for most patients with stage II and all patients with stage III and IV non-Hodgkin's lymphoma. Chemotherapeutic options are dictated by grade and histologic subtype.

LOW-GRADE LYMPHOMA For the most part, small lymphocytic and follicular small cleaved cell lymphomas are approached similarly. Traditionally, these tumors have not been treated until they produce symptoms. This was so because single-agent chemotherapy or combinations of agents did not induce complete long-term remissions, and more important, they did not alter the overall survival of patients with these diseases. These regimens included the use of single alkylating agents such as cyclophosphamide or chlorambucil or combinations such as CVP (cyclophosphamide, vincristine, and prednisone) or CHOP (CVP plus doxorubicin). More aggressive chemotherapy regimens (see "Intermediate Grade," below) have in some studies produced more rapid and possibly higher percentages of complete remissions, but unfortunately, they have not changed the overall survival of patients with these diseases. In addition, attempts to treat patients for prolonged periods of time with single-agent therapy or the addition of long-term "maintenance" treatment also have not had an impact on survival. Following relapse, most patients can be retreated successfully; however, the ability to achieve third and subsequent remissions becomes more difficult and the duration of those remissions is shorter. Three recently developed purine analogues have shown activity in low-grade non-Hodgkin's lymphoma. Fludarabine is perhaps the most active new drug, known best for its use in chronic lymphocytic leukemia, and it will give about a 60 percent response rate in pretreated patients. Two other less widely used drugs, 2-chlorodeoxyadenosine (2-CDA), which is a highly effective agent in hairy cell leukemia, and 2′-deoxycoformycin, an inhibitor of adenosine deaminase, which is most active in T cell malignancies, have shown some activity in indolent lymphomas. A subset of patients with follicular mixed small cleaved and large cell lymphoma is reported to experience long-term remission and possible cure following treatment with combination chemotherapy (C-MOPP or CHOP); however, this remains controversial. If these diseases are to be cured, either more aggressive high-dose regimens must be evaluated or new therapeutic modalities must be employed. Recently, several approaches have been taken to treat patients with advanced-stage follicular lymphomas earlier in the course of their disease with aggressive chemotherapy combined total nodal irradiation or high-dose chemoradiotherapy and autologous bone marrow transplantation. These studies suggest that high complete response rates in the range of 80 percent or greater are possible. However, the impact of these studies on long-term disease-free survival and overall survival remains unknown due to relatively short follow-up.

INTERMEDIATE-GRADE LYMPHOMA   The regimens used to treat diffuse large cell lymphoma are also employed to treat follicular mixed, follicular large cell, and diffuse small cleaved cell lymphoma. The treatment of diffuse large cell lymphoma is one of the major success stories of modern chemotherapy. The first successful regimen for this disease was C-MOPP (cyclophosphamide, vincristine, prednisone, and procarbazine), which induced complete remissions in approximately 40 percent of patients and with long-term disease-free survival for most of the complete responders. Patients with no response or partial responses died rapidly. The inclusion of the anthracycline doxorubicin in the CHOP regimen had a significant impact on this disease, with much higher complete and durable remission and a long-term disease-free survival of 35 percent. Success with this and subsequent regimens required attention to administering full doses and adhering to schedules as strictly as possible. Over the past 15 years, attempts have been made to improve the percentage of complete remissions and overall cure rate. Additional agents have been added to CHOP, including bleomycin, methotrexate, procarbazine, nitrogen mustard, cytosine arabinoside, and etoposide (e.g., BACOD, M-BACOD, m-BACOD, ProMACE-MOPP, COP-BLAM, COMLA, MACOP-B, ProMACE/CytaBOM). In addition to the complexity of the regimen, the duration of some of these treatments has been prolonged for up to 12 months. With these approaches, the complete remission rate now approaches 80 percent for the most aggressive regimens. However, toxicities also have increased (e.g., infections as well as cardiac and pulmonary complications). Within individual institutional studies, the results with some of these third-generation regimens has been far superior to CHOP, with approximately 70 percent of patients appearing to be cured. However, a multi-institutional, randomized trial comparing CHOP with m-BACOD, ProMACE/CytaBOM, or MACOP-B found no difference in the overall survival, response rate, or time to treatment failure between the four treatment arms. Patients who survive 2 years disease-free have an excellent chance of being cured, although a continuous rate of late relapses is seen in approximately 10 percent of patients. Prolonged "maintenance" therapy has not improved overall survival. With the various treatment options and until randomized studies are completed, the selection of a treatment regimen for diffuse large cell lymphoma should be based on the therapist's experience with a particular regimen and its toxicities.

Follicular large cell lymphomas have been treated with CHOP-like regimens with high complete remission rate and controversial evidence for long-term disease-free survival. In contrast, diffuse small cleaved lymphoma has been treated with most of the preceding aggressive regimens, but while complete response rates are high, at best 25 percent of patients experience long-term disease-free survival.

HIGH-GRADE LYMPHOMA   These tumors have an extremely poor prognosis and need to be treated very aggressively. Patients with large cell immunoblastic histologies are generally treated with regimens used for diffuse large cell lymphomas. Lymphoblastic lymphoma in adults has been treated with some success, although inferior to that seen in children. A 56 percent disease-free survival at 3 years has been reported in patients treated with CHOP with high-dose methotrexate, L-asparaginase, and intrathecal methotrexate. When treated with regimens initially developed for childhood acute lymphoblastic leukemia, about 40 percent of adults are reported to survive at 5 years. CNS prophylaxis is critical in this disease, since the CNS is a frequent sanctuary site of recurrence in the absense of prophylaxis. The small noncleaved cell lymphomas (Burkitt's and non-Burkitt's) in adults have been treated with regimens designed for the pediatric population, which involve high doses of cyclophosphamide, cytosine arabinoside, and CNS prophylaxis with methotrexate. Although complete remission rates are very high, the cure rate is still much less than is observed for diffuse large cell lymphoma. Patients with good prognostic features (normal LDH, absence of CNS or marrow involvement) have better survival than those with poor prognostic characteristics.

AIDS-RELATED LYMPHOMAS   These tumors are among the most aggressive of the non-Hodgkin's lymphomas. Most are high-grade immunoblastic or small noncleaved cell types, with some intermediate-grade diffuse large cell lymphomas also observed. Initial studies with aggressive regimens yielded dismal results, with only one-third of patients achieving complete remission and a high frequency of CNS relapse and fatal opportunistic infection. Subsequent studies using modified doses of chemotherapy and CNS prophylaxis have given complete remission rates of 50 percent, with a median survival of 15 months for those patients in complete remission. Since neutropenia was a major problem even in modified-dose therapy, the addition of the hematopoietic growth factor granulocyte-macrophage colony stimulating factor (GM-CSF) has permitted tolerable escalation of chemotherapy doses. Response rates appear to be related to clinical factors, including history of AIDS and performance status. For patients who do not respond or following relapse, the results of salvage treatment are very poor, with short survival. Despite some encouraging responses, these tumors are becoming increasingly more common, and their response to therapy and prognosis is presently radically different from non-AIDS-related lymphoma of similar histologic subtype.

CUTANEOUS T CELL LYMPHOMA   Both local and systemic therapy are used in the treatment of cutaneous T cell lymphoma. Topical treatment of skin lesions with chemotherapeutic agents such as nitrogen mustard can induce remissions in up to 90 percent of patients. Similarly, local radiation induces a high remission rate; however, similar to B cell low-grade lymphomas, the vast majority of patients relapse within 3 years. Another modality with quite similar results is the use of 8-methoxypsoralen followed by ultraviolet light (PUVA). Systemic therapy with either drugs alone or combined-modality therapy can induce high response rates (up to 80 percent), but few long-term remissions are seen in advanced-stage patients. Other treatments with interferon-α, monoclonal antibodies (unconjugated and conjugated to toxins or radioisotopes), extracorporeal phototherapy, and the adenosine deaminase inhibitor 2-deoxycoformycin remain investigational.

Prognostic significance of immunophenotype in non-Hodgkin's lymphoma   A large number of studies have examined the relationship between cell surface marker expression and prognosis in non-Hodgkin's lymphoma. Although many studies have found cell surface phenotype to be an independent prognostic variable, these studies often failed to stratify patients for different histologic subtypes of non-Hodgkin's lymphoma. Despite the many attempts to determine whether immunophenotype correlates with prognosis, this still remains controversial.

The expression of non-lineage-restricted cell surface markers in relation to prognosis has been examined in several series. The expression of the transferrin receptor (CD71), which identifies proliferating normal cells, has been examined. Although early studies suggested that patients with CD71-positive tumors have decreased survival, these studies were not well controlled for histologic subtype or therapy. More recent studies which examined CD71 expression within defined histologic subtypes of both low- and intermediate/high-grade non-Hodgkin's lymphomas failed to demonstrate any correlation between antigen expression and clinical outcome. A nuclear antigen also present in proliferating cells, identified by the MAb Ki-67, also has been studied. Recently, it has been reported that in diffuse large cell lymphoma Ki-67 was an independent predictor of survival in a multivariate analysis. Patients with more than 60 percent Ki-67–positive cells had a significantly shorter median survival than patients with 60 percent or less Ki-67–positive cells.

Attempts also have been made to correlate the cellular lineage with response to treatment and survival. It remains controversial whether lineage derivation is an independent variable affecting prognosis, with some studies suggesting that non-Hodgkin's lymphomas of T cell origin have a worse prognosis than B cell–derived tumors. Within the B cell diffuse large cell lymphomas, patients with tumors with an aberrant immunophenotype (lacking HLA-DR, CD20, or CD22) had a significantly shorter survival. Expression of the homing receptor CD44 also has been associated with disseminated disease and poor survival. Although these findings are of great interest, large prospective studies will be needed to confirm these observations. Presently, the treatment of non-Hodgkin's lymphomas is not altered by immunophenotype of the tumor cells.

Salvage chemotherapy The prognosis for patients with intermediate- and high-grade non-Hodgkin's lymphoma who fail to achieve a complete remission or relapse following aggressive therapy is very poor. Salvage chemotherapy employing drugs such as cytosine arabinoside, cisplatin, etoposide, and ifosfamide, given as single agents or in combination, has been used to induce remissions. Depending on the histology and regimen, approximately 20 to 30 percent of patients attain a complete remission, with partial remissions in another 30 percent. Unfortunately, these remissions tend to be short-lived (approximately 2 to 6 months), with less than 3 percent of patients in remission beyond 2 years.

Bone marrow transplantation (BMT) Patients whose disease is resistant to conventional or salvage therapeutic regimens can still be induced into a complete remission with very high doses of chemotherapy or the combination of high-dose chemotherapy and radiotherapy. This occurs because a steep dose-response curve persists in non-Hodgkin's lymphomas even after relapse. This treatment approach is complicated by very significant and prolonged myelosuppression. To overcome the latter, bone marrow as a source of hematopoietic stem cells can be infused from an identical twin (syngeneic), an HLA-matched relative (allogeneic), or the patient (autologous). Alternatively, hematopoietic stem cells can be isolated from peripheral blood. The vast majority of transplants for patients with lymphoma employ autologous marrow. Bone marrow transplantation has become widespread in the treatment of patients with refractory or relapsed non-Hodgkin's lymphoma, and retrospective analysis clearly demonstrates that only a subgroup of patients benefits from this approach. Patients whose disease has never responded to primary therapy are presently not salvaged by this approach. Following relapse from remission, patients whose disease is resistant to all forms of salvage therapy have less than 15 percent long-term disease-free survival. In contrast, approximately 40 percent of those patients whose disease is still responsive to therapy have long-term disease-free survival with high-dose therapy and marrow transplantation. While the majority of patients undergoing BMT have intermediate- and high-grade non-Hodgkin's lymphoma, studies in patients with low-grade lymphomas suggest that some patients experience long-term disease-free survival. Early studies with BMT reported treatment-related deaths in the range of 20 to 30 percent; however, as patients with no associated comorbid disease have been treated, this mortality has significantly decreased (approximately 5 percent). The use of recombinant hematopoietic growth factors to hasten myeloid cell recovery also has significantly reduced morbidity and length of hospitalization following high-dose therapy and marrow transplantation.

Lower treatment-related mortality has led some groups to use BMT as consolidation therapy in patients with incurable non-Hodgkin's lymphomas in first remission. Selected studies have demonstrated that patients with less than a 20 percent long-term disease-free survival following conventional therapy have a disease-free survival of 80 percent following early BMT. Although this modality is capable of curing some patients with relapsed non-Hodgkin's lymphomas, many issues still remain, including optimal therapeutic regimen, timing of transplantation, source of hematopoietic stem cells, the need to purge autologous marrow, and methods to minimize morbidity and mortality.

Newer modalities A number of new therapeutic approaches have resulted from the advances in immunology and molecular biology. Over 10 years ago, MAbs directed against surface antigens expressed on non-Hodgkin's lymphoma cells were first used clinically in an attempt to specifically treat these tumors. The results of these studies suggest that MAbs by themselves do not induce significant tumor regression. Although there was initial enthusiasm about using MAbs directed against unique idiotypes expressed on B cell follicular lymphomas, few significant clinical responses have been observed. Newer trials are evaluating MAbs coupled with radionuclides or toxins to specifically produce cytotoxic effects, whereas other trials are using soluble factors (cytokines) which are potentially cytotoxic to tumor cells. The major cytokines being studied include the interferons, tumor necrosis factor, and interleukin 2. Recombinant hematopoietic growth factors which are responsible for growth of myeloid, lymphoid, and erythroid cells are also being tested. Conceptually, these growth factors will limit myelosuppression, thereby permitting higher doses and more frequent administration of chemotherapeutic drugs. Early results are encouraging, and agents such as GM-CSF and G-CSF appear to hasten recovery of myeloid cells. The role of all these agents in improving the treatment of lymphomas is being evaluated in many research centers.

HODGKIN'S DISEASE

EPIDEMIOLOGY AND ETIOLOGY Approximately 7500 new cases of Hodgkin's disease are diagnosed annually in the United States. The epidemiology of this disease has provided important information regarding the possible role of age and genetic and environmental factors associated with its development. In non-Hodgkin's lymphomas there is a linear increase in incidence with age. In contrast, in Hodgkin's disease in the United States and developed western nations, the age-specific incidence curve is characteristically bimodal, with an initial peak in young adults (15 to 35 years) and a second peak after age 50. However, in Japan, there is an absence of the early peak, and in some third-world countries, there is a shift of the first peak into childhood as well as a shift of histology from nodular sclerosis to mixed cellularity and lymphocyte predominance. Hodgkin's disease is more prevalent in males, and when the age-specific incidence curve is compared with the sex distribution of the patients, the increased male prevalence is most prominent in young adults. A disproportionate number of patients in the first modal peak exhibit nodular sclerosis histology. In childhood Hodgkin's disease, this male predominance is even more striking, with over 80 percent of patients being male. This has lead some investigators to hypothesize a sex-linked genetic or hormonally related increase in susceptibility.

Although controversial, clustering of patients with Hodgkin's has been reported. Increased risk has been associated with decreased number of siblings, single-family dwellings, decreased number of playmates, early birth order, sibling with Hodgkin's disease, tonsillectomy, and certain HLA antigens. These findings have been used to suggest that Hodgkin's disease is caused by a virus possessing an oncogenic potential which is low but increases with age from the time of infection. These observations suggest that genetic and environmental factors may be associated with the development of this disease. As in non-Hodgkin's lymphomas, there is an increased risk of Hodgkin's disease in patients with immunodeficiencies and autoimmune diseases (see Table 311-3). The major obstacle to determining the cause of Hodgkin's disease is our inability to isolate and study the neoplastic cell. Unlike non-Hodgkin's lymphomas, no chromosomal abnormalities have been consistently demonstrated.

CLINICAL FEATURES AND DIFFERENTIAL DIAGNOSIS Hodgkin's disease usually presents as a localized disease and subsequently spreads to contiguous lymphoid structures and ultimately disseminates to nonlymphoid tissues with a potentially fatal outcome. Hodgkin's disease commonly presents with a newly detected mass or group of lymph nodes which are firm, freely movable, and usually nontender. Approximately half of patients present with adenopathy in the neck or supraclavicular area, and over 70 percent of patients present with superficial lymph node enlargement. Because these are frequently not painful, detection by the patient may be delayed until the lymph nodes are quite large. Approximately 60 percent of patients present with mediastinal adenopathy. This is sometimes first detected on a routine chest x-ray. Nodes involved by Hodgkin's disease tend to be centripetal or axial in contrast to those in non-Hodgkin's lymphomas, which have a tendency to be centrifugal, involving epitrochlear, Waldeyer's ring, and abdominal nodes. In 2 to 5 percent of patients, lymph nodes or other tissues involved with Hodgkin's disease can become painful after the ingestion of alcoholic beverages. The growth of lymph nodes may be quite variable; some lesions can remain stable for long periods of time, while spontaneous and temporary regression of some nodes also may occur.

The majority of patients presenting with Hodgkin's disease have few or no symptoms related to their disease. However, 25 to 30 percent of patients have some constitutional symptoms; the most common is low-grade fever which can be associated with recurrent night sweats. For some patients, night sweats may be the sole complaint. A small number of patients may have high fluctuating fevers accompanied by drenching night sweats (Pel-Epstein fevers). These fevers can persist for several weeks, followed by afebrile intervals. Fevers and night sweats are seen more commonly in older patients and in those with more advanced stage. Some patients with extensive abdominal but limited peripheral adenopathy are first evaluated for fever and night sweats. They undergo a workup for fever of unknown origin and usually are found to have mixed cellularity or lymphocyte-depleted Hodgkin's disease. Another important presenting symptom is unexplained weight loss of greater than 10 percent over 6 months or less. Other frequent symptoms include fatigue, malaise, and weakness. Pruritus occurs in approximately 10 percent of patients at initial diagnosis; it is usually generalized and may be associated with a skin rash and rarely may be the only disease manifestation. Mediastinal, pulmonary, pleural, or pericardial involvement may be associated with cough, chest pain, shortness of breath, or hypertrophic osteoarthropathy; bone involvement may be associated with bone pain. Occasionally, a patient will present with obstruction of the superior vena cava as the first symptom. Sudden spinal cord compression can be a presenting complaint but is usually a complication of advanced progressive disease. Headache or visual disturbances may be seen in the very rare patient with intracranial Hodgkin's disease, and abdominal involvement may result in abdominal pain, bowel disturbances, and even ascites.

The differential diagnosis is similar to that described for non-Hodgkin's lymphoma. In patients with cervical adenopathy, such infections as bacterial or viral pharyngitis, infectious mononucleosis, and toxoplasmosis must be excluded. Other malignancies, such as non-Hodgkin's lymphomas, nasopharyngeal cancers, and thyroid cancers, also can present with localized cervical adenopathy. Axillary adenopathy must be differentiated from non-Hodgkin's lymphoma and breast cancer. Mediastinal adenopathy must be distinguished from infections, sarcoid, and other tumors. In older patients, the differential diagnosis includes tumors of the lung and mediastinum, specifically small cell and non-small cell carcinomas. Reactive mediastinitis and hilar adenopathy from histoplasmosis can be confused with lymphoma, since it occurs in otherwise asymptomatic people. Primary abdominal disease with hepatomegaly, splenomegaly, and massive adenopathy is uncommon, and other neoplastic diseases, especially non-Hodgkin's lymphoma, must be excluded under these circumstances.

DIAGNOSIS AND PATHOLOGIC CLASSIFICATION The diagnosis of Hodgkin's disease requires a biopsy which contains sufficient tissue to permit an accurate microscopic diagnosis. Biopsy specimens are usually from lymph nodes but may occasionally be from other tissues. Needle aspirations or needle biopsies are not adequate for the histologic diagnosis of Hodgkin's disease.

The criteria for the diagnosis and classification of Hodgkin's disease have remained unchanged since 1966 when the Rye classification was adopted (Table 311-6). As indicated above, central to the diagnosis is the presence of the *Reed-Sternberg* (RS) cell, a large cell with a bilobed or multilobulated nucleus with prominent inclusion-

TABLE 311-6 Rye classification of Hodgkin's disease

Histologic subgroup	Incidence, %	Pathology RS*	Pathology Other	Prognosis
Lymphocyte-predominant	2–10	Rare	Predominance of normal-appearing	Excellent
Nodular sclerosis	40–80	Frequent "lacunae"	Lymphoid nodules, collage bands	Very good
Mixed cellularity	20–40	Numerous	Pleomorphic infiltrate	Good
Lymphocyte-depleted	2–15	Numerous, often bizarre	Lymphocytes, pleomorphic fibrosis	Poor

* RS = Reed-Sternberg cell.

like nucleoli. There are several morphologic variants of Reed-Sternberg cells, and it is the frequency of these variants, as well as the cellular and fibrous background of the proliferation, that helps to establish the histologic subtypes of Hodgkin's disease. It is important to note that Reed-Sternberg cells may occasionally be found in other conditions such as infectious mononucleosis and non-Hodgkin's lymphomas. Thus an accurate diagnosis of Hodgkin's disease depends on additional cellular and architectural features of the tissue and optimally also with supportive immunologic studies.

In the Rye classification, Hodgkin's disease is subdivided into four types, including (1) lymphocyte predominant, (2) nodular sclerosis, (3) mixed cellularity, and (4) lymphocyte depleted. Table 311-6 summarizes the major clinical characteristics of these types associated with the Rye classification. It is very important to stress that *treatment and prognosis in Hodgkin's disease is dependent on stage of disease, whereas in non-Hodgkin's lymphoma treatment is largely based on histologic subtype.*

STAGING AND OTHER LABORATORY ABNORMALITIES   Ann Arbor classification Following biopsy and histopathologic classification of Hodgkin's disease, one must define the extent of the disease (i.e., staging), which is essential for the selection of optimal therapy. In the Ann Arbor staging classification (see Table 311-4), the patient receives both a clinical and a pathologic stage. The clinical stage is defined by the extent of disease based on physical examination and other noninvasive studies. The pathologic stage is defined by data obtained from invasive tests, including biopsy specimens obtained from different sites, usually during a staging laparotomy. The presence of localized extralymphatic disease is designated by the suffix *E*. Such extralymphatic involvement may include solitary involvement of lung, pericardium, or bone. Multifocal involvement in these organs usually is defined as disseminated disease. Bone involvement must be separated from bone marrow involvement, since bone marrow and liver involvement is always defined as stage IV disseminated disease.

The presence of systemic symptoms that are of prognostic importance is designated by the suffix *B* and their absence by the suffix *A*. The presence of both fevers and weight loss results in a less favorable prognosis, while night sweats are currently felt to be of no prognostic importance. Patients with limited disease, such as pathologic stage IA or IIA, are effectively treated with radiotherapy alone, while patients with more disseminated disease, such as pathologic stage IIIB, IVA, or IVB, are most effectively treated with chemotherapy alone or combined with radiotherapy.

Staging procedures after biopsy diagnosis The diagnostic studies recommended for complete staging are outlined in Table 311-7. There is general agreement on the studies which are considered to be essential. Detailed physical examination with attention to documentation of all sites of nodal involvement and splenomegaly is essential. The chest radiograph is usually sufficient to exclude mediastinal, hilar, pleural, and parenchymal involvement. However, in patients with demonstrable thoracic disease, chest CT scan more accurately defines extent of disease. CT scan of the abdomen and

TABLE 311-7 Staging evaluation for Hodgkin's lymphoma

ESSENTIAL

1 Pathologic documentation by hematopathologist
2 Physical examination
3 Documentation of B symptoms
4 Laboratory evaluation
  a Complete blood counts
  b Liver function tests
  c Renal function tests
  d Uric acid
  e Erythrocyte sedimentation rate
5 Chest radiograph
6 CT scan of chest, abdomen, and pelvis
7 Bone marrow biopsy

ESSENTIAL UNDER CERTAIN CIRCUMSTANCES

1 Liver biopsy
2 Bipedal lymphangiogram
3 Gallium scan
4 Staging laporotomy
5 Bone scan
6 Bone radiographs

USEFUL BUT NOT ESSENTIAL TESTS

1 Cell surface marker phenotypic analysis
2 Gene rearrangement analysis
3 Ultrasonography
4 Magnetic resonance imaging
5 Estimation of patients delayed hypersensitivity status

---

pelvis has a definite place in the staging of Hodgkin's disease for the assessment of nodal and hepatic disease, but much less for splenic disease. CT scanning can detect the exact location and extent of all enlarged nodes, including iliac, mesenteric, and retrocrural nodal areas, as compared with a lymphogram, which evaluates only the paraaortic and common internal and external iliac nodes. However, the abdominal/pelvic CT scan is limited because it requires nodal enlargement for detection and rarely can detect splenic or hepatic involvement.

A number of more invasive diagnostic tests are required if patients are clinically stage I, II, or IIIA. Lymphograms of the lower extremities are very useful to demonstrate paraaortic and iliac nodal enlargement, and they are more sensitive than abdominal/pelvic CT scans because they can detect disease in normal-sized nodes. Moreover, lymphograms are useful prior to staging laparotomy to direct the surgeon to the nodes to be biopsied. However, the safety and accuracy of this procedure are highly dependent on the experience of the radiologist. If a staging laparotomy is considered, patients should undergo a bone marrow biopsy to exclude stage IV disease. However, the frequency of a positive bone marrow biopsy in clinical stage IA or IIA disease is less than 1 percent. The role of staging laparotomy is still controversial. Staging laparotomy includes biopsy of selected lymph nodes in the retroperitoneum, splenectomy, and several needle and wedge biopsies of the liver. Traditionally, all patients without obvious stage IV disease underwent laparotomy, and nearly one-third had their initial clinical stage changed as a result of the procedure. For example, one-third of patients with normal-sized spleens had demonstrable tumor infiltration at laparotomy, whereas 35 percent of patients with clinical splenomegaly had no histologic evidence of disease. Liver involvement is more common in patients with positive lymphograms and enlarged spleens. Although very important, the routine use of staging laparotomy in all patients may not be appropriate. Laparotomy should be utilized in patients whose clinical stages make them candidates for treatment with radiation therapy alone and in whom evidence of unsuspected abdominal disease will significantly change treatment. A staging laparotomy should not be performed in patients who are to receive chemotherapy based on the presence of bulky chest disease, bulky abdominal involvement, or stage IV

disease. A staging laparotomy with splenectomy should be performed by a surgeon who is skilled in this procedure after careful review of clinical, laboratory, pathologic, and radiologic studies. Finally, a number of ancillary studies may be very useful in selected patients and are listed in Table 311-7. Gallium scintigraphy is useful in following response to treatment and in detecting early recurrences. A gallium scan is necessary at the time of initial staging to determine whether the lymphoma is gallium-avid.

Laboratory abnormalities   Routine blood counts, liver function tests, and renal function tests are all necessary parts of the medical workup but do not provide information about the extent of Hodgkin's disease or of specific organ involvement. A moderate normochromic, normocytic anemia associated with low serum iron level and low iron-binding capacity but with normal or increased iron stores in the bone marrow may be present in patients with Hodgkin's disease as well as in other neoplastic and chronic diseases. A moderate to marked leukemoid reaction is common, particularly in symptomatic patients, and usually disappears with treatment. Mild peripheral absolute eosinophilia is not uncommon, especially in patients with pruritus. Absolute monocytosis is also observed. Absolute lymphocytopenia (<1000 cells per cubic milliliter) usually occurs in patients with more advanced disease. Many tests have been evaluated as indicators of disease activity. To date, the erythrocyte sedimentation rate still is the best monitor, but it suffers from its lack of specificity and can return to normal when residual disease is still demonstrable. Other abnormal tests include increased serum levels of copper, calcium, lactic acid, alkaline phosphatase, lysozyme, globulins, C-reactive protein, and other acute phase reactants.

Immunologic abnormalities   Hodgkin's disease is associated with a well-described but poorly understood immunologic defect. Untreated patients, including those with limited disease, have defective cellular immunity characterized by anergy to routine skin tests. They also have a reversal of the CD4/CD8 ratio, suggesting that this anergy may be due to an increased number of suppressor T cells as well as a decreased number of CD4-positive cells. In several studies, decreased immune reactivity correlates both with advanced stages of disease and the presence of systemic symptoms. However, anergy to recall and neoantigens appears to have no prognostic significance. Following successful therapy, anergy reverses to recall antigens but is still present in some patients to neoantigens. In addition to anergy, other tests of T cell function, including responses to mitogens and suppressor cell function, suggest a defect in immune function prior to and following treatment. Humoral immunity with antibody production to soluble antigens is normal in untreated patients. Thus patients who undergo staging laparotomy and splenectomy will develop humoral immunity to pneumococcal antigens if immunized with the pneumococcal vaccine prior to therapy. The clinical impact of these immune defects is limited. Except for a higher than normal incidence of herpes zoster and development of warts, these patients are not plagued by opportunistic infections.

NATURAL HISTORY ACCORDING TO HISTOLOGIC SUBTYPE

Patients with lymphocyte-predominant Hodgkin's disease are usually asymptomatic at presentation and tend to have localized disease. These patients are usually young, rarely have systemic symptoms or mediastinal mass, and are predominantly males. Nodular sclerosis Hodgkin's disease is found most frequently in adolescents and young adults who usually have localized disease; a preponderance are young women who present with a large mediastinal mass. Lymphocyte-depleted Hodgkin's disease is usually disseminated at the time of diagnosis and occurs in older patients who frequently have systemic symptoms. The mixed cellularity type occurs in all age groups and stages and is only slightly more common in males. There is a tendency toward an older age peak (30 to 40 years) than with nodular sclerosis, and approximately half of these patients have advanced disease. Patients with lymphocyte-predominant and nodular sclerosis Hodgkin's disease, if untreated, have a more indolent disease associated with a longer survival and are more likely to be cured with radiotherapy.

There are several variables which adversely affect the prognosis of Hodgkin's disease. The number of involved sites and presence of bulky disease are the most important variables because extensive disease is often associated with high frequency of drug-resistant tumor cells. Large masses in the chest (greater than one-third the chest diameter) respond poorly to radiotherapy or chemotherapy alone but respond better to combined treatment. The prognosis is generally poor if a patient's disease is resistant to primary therapy or relapse occurs within 12 months. Age and systemic B symptoms are poor prognostic signs regardless of stage. Systemic B symptoms forbode a very poor prognosis, especially when both fevers and weight loss are present.

TREATMENT OF HODGKIN'S DISEASE Essentially all patients can and should be treated with curative intent. Radiotherapy may cure over 80 percent of patients with localized Hodgkin's disease and chemotherapy over 50 percent of those with disseminated disease. *The choice of treatment regimen is totally dependent on stage of disease.* As with all neoplasms, the therapy of Hodgkin's disease is constantly being reevaluated to improve disease-free survival and decrease toxicity.

Radiotherapy Radiation therapy alone has been evaluated in patients with pathologic stages IA, IIA, IB, and IIB. Although previously some patients with stage IIIA disease were treated with radiotherapy alone, more recent studies suggest that chemotherapy yields better results in patients with stage IIIA disease. While lower doses of radiation therapy will cause tumor regression, it was the recognition that 4000 cGy delivered at the rate of 1000 cGy per week could eradicate localized Hodgkin's disease that revolutionized treatment and led to substantial cure rates in patients with localized disease. With the knowledge that Hodgkin's spreads by lymphatic contiguity, three types of radiation fields were devised—namely, the mantle field, the paraaortic field, and pelvic irradiation. The *mantle field* includes the submandibular, cervical, supraclavicular, infraclavicular, axillary, mediastinal, and hilar lymph nodes. The *paraaortic field* covers the transverse processes of the abdominal vertebral bodies and the spleen, if it has not been removed. *Pelvic irradiation* includes the common iliac, hypogastric, external iliac, and inguinal nodes. When there is gross pelvic nodal involvement, the femoral nodes are also treated. Sometimes the pelvic and paraaortic fields are treated as one unit, which is then commonly called the *inverted-Y field*. The use of pelvic irradiation has recently been reduced, since stage I and II supradiaphragmatic Hodgkin's disease can be treated without pelvic irradiation and for stage III disease total nodal irradiation has only a limited role. Patients now receive mantle and paraaortic irradiation and only rarely total nodal irradiation. Patients receive doses of 3600 to 4000 cGy with an additional "cone down" dose for a total of 4000 to 4400 cGy to areas of bulk disease.

Patients with localized nodal Hodgkin's disease (pathologic stages IA and IIA) treated with mantle or paraaortic radiation therapy have nearly 80 percent long-term disease-free survival. Patients with stage IB and IIB disease have a slightly reduced disease-free survival (70 percent); however, most patients who relapse can be treated successfully with optimal combination chemotherapy. Early-stage patients with large mediastinal involvement appear to have a higher risk of relapse after radiation therapy alone (disease-free survival of 40 to 55 percent) compared with patients with minimal or no mediastinal disease and should be managed with combined-modality therapy.

Radiation therapy can lead to acute and late complications. Acute side effects of mantle irradiation include transient dry mouth, pharyngitis, fatigue, and weight loss. Approximately 15 percent of patients within several months of mantle irradiation develop paresthesias in the lower extremities upon flexion of the neck or thighs (Lhermitte's syndrome). This syndrome usually resolves spontaneously; there is no correlation between this syndrome and irreversible spinal injury. Other long-term side effects include radiation pneumonitis (severe in less than 5 percent of patients) and symptomatic pulmonary fibrosis (<1 percent). Late complications of mantle irradiation involve cardiac damage, including pericardial effusion and, very rarely, myocardial damage. Cardiac irradiation also may accelerate coronary artery disease and induce early myocardial infarctions, although recent controlled studies have reported only a borderline significant increased risk with modern techniques. Hypothyroidism may occur in up to 30 percent of patients following mantle irradiation. Paraaortic irradiation is rarely associated with significant side effects. Pelvic irradiation acutely induces transient diarrhea and bladder irritation associated with frequency. Chronic effects include potential long-term bone marrow suppression and sterility; therefore, pelvic irradiation is less frequently employed. Moreover, increasing numbers of secondary tumors are being observed. A recent study revealed a 2.8-fold observed to expected cumulative risk of development of second tumors in 15-year survivors with Hodgkin's disease treated with radiation. The most serious of these is the emergence of second malignancies, particularly acute nonlymphocytic leukemia and high-grade non-Hodgkin's lymphomas, often seen in patients who received combined-modality therapy.

Chemotherapy By 1963, five agents had been identified as effective in the treatment of Hodgkin's disease, namely, alkylating agents, vinca alkaloids, procarbazine, methotrexate, and prednisone. While disease regression occurred in 30 to 70 percent of patients, complete response occurred in only 10 percent. Based on the principles of dose, schedule, and combination chemotherapy, a four-drug combination regimen termed MOPP [mechlorethamine (nitrogen mustard), vincristine (Oncovin), procarbazine, and prednisone] was introduced. In a 14-year median follow-up of 188 patients, DeVita and colleagues found that 84 percent had achieved a complete remission and 48 percent were alive. MOPP therapy has been associated with significant toxicity. Nearly all patients experience some degree of nausea and vomiting, which can be minimized by antiemetic therapy. Bone marrow suppression with associated leukopenia and thrombocytopenia is frequently observed. Less commonly, absolute neutropenia occurs with increased susceptibility to infection. All males and nearly all females over age 35 become sterile following MOPP therapy. There is a 2 percent actuarial risk of developing secondary leukemia at 10 years following MOPP, which returns to baseline thereafter. The acute nonlymphocytic leukemia which occurs following MOPP differs from primary acute nonlymphocytic leukemia in that the former more commonly exhibits a preleukemic or myelodysplastic syndrome, a different cytogenetic profile with emphasis on partial or complete deletions of the fifth and seventh chromosomes, and a much lower response rate to antileukemia therapy. MOPP chemotherapy has not been associated with the development of second solid tumors.

Other multiple-drug regimens have been tested in the treatment of advanced Hodgkin's disease. However, none of the "MOPP-derived combinations" have been superior to the original MOPP administered at optimal dose and schedule. Regimens also have been developed to treat MOPP-resistant patients. The best known of these is ABVD (adriamycin, bleomycin, vinblastine, and dacarbazine). A series of controlled clinical trials has demonstrated that ABVD is equivalent to MOPP in the successful treatment of primary advanced Hodgkin's disease. ABVD also has led to a significant number of prolonged complete remissions in MOPP treatment failures. Although most ABVD toxicities are identical to MOPP, the ABVD regimen produces only transient germ cell toxicity in males, no drug-induced amenorrhea, and an apparent lower incidence of second tumors (although the data on this point are limited), but an increased risk of myocardial and pulmonary damage can be seen when compared with MOPP. Another regimen with similar effectiveness but less toxicity is ChlVPP (chlorambucil, vinblastine, procarbazine, and prednisone).

More recent studies have attempted to sequentially combine MOPP with ABVD to improve cure rate. In several studies, the use of MOPP alternating with ABVD appears to produce higher complete remissions and disease-free survivals compared with MOPP alone, but longer periods of observation and more patients are necessary to confirm this result.

Salvage therapy After proper restaging, further radiotherapy can be delivered (if technically feasible) to patients who have relapsed outside a radiation field or following combination chemotherapy. In patients not achieving a complete remission or relapsing after MOPP, second-line non-cross-resistant regimens are available. If patients relapse more than 12 months after the completion of MOPP therapy, they should be retreated with MOPP or an appropriate alternate regimen; if they relapse in less than 12 months, they should be treated with a salvage regimen (crossover, i.e., ABVD for MOPP and MOPP for ABVD). With ABVD as a salvage regimen, 30 to 50 percent of patients will achieve a complete remission and 10 to 30 percent will experience long-term disease-free survival. Poor prognostic variables for salvage include stage IV disease at diagnosis, B symptoms at relapse, or remission lasting <12 months. Selected chemotherapy patients who relapse in limited nodal sites, even when the first remission is less than 12 months, can be treated with salvage radiotherapy, preferably with combination chemotherapy. Finally, as with non-Hodgkin's lymphoma, autologous or allogeneic bone marrow transplantation is an effective salvage treatment for some patients. Unlike non-Hodgkin's lymphoma, total-body irradiation has minimal value, and virtually all regimens include high-dose chemotherapy. The acute lethal pulmonary and hepatic toxicity from these regimens, however, can be very high (5 to 25 percent). As with non-Hodgkin's lymphomas, patient's whose disease remains sensitive to chemotherapeutic agents are more likely to experience long-term disease-free survival in the range of 40 percent.

Therapeutic recommendations by stage STAGE IA AND IIA, NONBULKY DISEASE Following staging laparotomy in patients with supradiaphragmatic disease, subtotal nodal irradiation is the treatment of choice. Rarely, in patients with subdiaphragmatic lymphoma, radiotherapy is delivered by an inverted-Y field including the splenic pedicle in stage I disease and through total nodal irradiation in stage II disease. Some studies suggest that treatment with involved-field radiotherapy combined with chemotherapy produces comparable results, but most do not consider this accepted treatment of choice. For patients with subdiaphragmatic stage II disease of paraaortic nodes, chemotherapy is recommended.

STAGE IB AND IIB, NONBULKY DISEASE The therapy is the same as for stage IA and IIA Hodgkin's disease; however, the relapse rate is higher (30 percent). Relapse can usually be salvaged with chemotherapy. Subtotal or combination chemotherapy with involved-field irradiation remains an alternative treatment for these patients.

STAGE II, BULKY Stage II disease with bulky mediastinal/hilar adenopathy should be managed with combined-modality therapy, including chemotherapy and radiotherapy to sites of bulk disease.

STAGE IIIA Patients who present with minimal splenic disease appear to respond equally well to total lymphoid irradiation, combination chemotherapy with irradiation, or chemotherapy alone. However, randomized, prospective trials are needed to further determine the relative roles of radiation therapy and chemotherapy. For patients with enlarged paraaortic and pelvic nodes, the recommended treatment is combination chemotherapy with or without irradiation to involved sites. Alternative therapy includes combination chemotherapy alone.

STAGE IIIB, STAGE IV Combination chemotherapy is recommended. In uncontrolled studies, the addition of radiation therapy to involved sites may improved disease-free survival.

REFERENCES

ARMITAGE JO: Bone marrow transplantation in the treatment of patients with lymphoma. Blood 73:1749, 1989

————: Drug therapy: Treatment of non-Hodgkin's lymphoma. N Engl J Med 328:1023, 1993

CANELLOS GP et al.: Chemotherapy of advanced Hodgkin's disease with MOPP, ABVD, or MOPP alternating with ABVD. N Engl J Med 327:1478, 1992

CASTELLINO RA: Diagnostic imaging evaluation of Hodgkin's disease and non-Hodgkin's lymphoma. Cancer 67(suppl):1177, 1991

COLTMAN CA JR (ed): Hodgkin's disease. Semin Oncol 17:641, 1990

FREEDMAN AS, NADLER LM: Immunologic markers in non-Hodgkin's lymphomas. Hematol Oncol Clin North Am 5:871, 1991

GROSSBARD ML et al: Monoclonal antibody–based therapies of leukemia and lymphoma. Blood 80:863, 1992

KAPLAN HS: *Hodgkin's Disease*, 2d ed. Cambridge, Harvard University, 1990

LEVINE AM: Acquired immunodeficiency syndrome–related lymphomas. Blood 80:8, 1992

WILLIAMS SF, GOLUMB HM (eds.): Non-Hodgkin's lymphoma. Semin Oncol 17:1, 1990

URBA W, LONGO DL: Hodgkin's disease. N Engl J Med 326:678, 1992

312 BLOOD GROUPS AND BLOOD TRANSFUSION

HARVEY G. KLEIN

BLOOD GROUP ANTIGENS AND ANTIBODIES

Human red blood cell membranes contain hundreds of different antigenic determinants (epitopes), the molecular structure of which is determined by genes at various chromosomal loci. The term *blood group* refers to any well-defined system of red blood cell antigens controlled by a locus having a variable number of allelic genes, such as A, B, and O in the ABO system. More than 20 blood group systems are currently recognized. The term *blood type* refers to the antigen phenotype, which is the serologic expression of the inherited blood group genes.

Alloantibodies specific for the different blood group antigens may occur "naturally," in the absence of known exposure to the antigen, or in response to transfusion or pregnancy. Naturally occurring antibodies tend to be IgM molecules and probably result from a thymus-independent immune response to widely occurring carbohydrate antigens. Anti-A and anti-B are examples of such antibodies. Antibodies formed in response to transfusion initially belong to the IgM class but switch to the IgG isotype within a few weeks or months. Most alloantibodies, regardless of class, are not clinically significant. However, serologic testing detects a variety of agglutinating, hemolyzing, and coating antibodies that may affect transfusion. Serologic reactivity at 30°C or higher best predicts clinical significance.

CARBOHYDRATE BLOOD GROUP ANTIGENS **ABO system: Genes and antigens** The ABO blood group is the most important system for blood transfusion. There are four major allelic genes in this system, A1, A2, B, and O. The locus for these alleles is on the long arm of chromosome 9. The gene products of the first three genes are glycosyl transferases, which attach specific sugars by alpha linkage to oligosaccharide chains. These chains comprise the carbohydrate moiety of the glycolipids and glycoproteins on red blood cells. The A and B genes differ in a few single-base substitutions, resulting in differences in A and B transferase specificity. A single-base deletion in the O gene results in an inactive protein that cross-reacts with the A and B transferases but has no detectable enzyme activity. The A1 and A2 transferases perform the same function but have different rate constants. Red cells from subjects who inherit the A1 gene have more A-reactive sites than do those with an A2 gene.

Nearly all individuals possess naturally occurring isoagglutinins, antibodies directed against the A and B antigens not present on their own red blood cells. These isoagglutinins account for the major blood group incompatibilities. Most of the major phenotypes represent more than one genotype. In practice, the ABO type is determined by testing the red cells with anti-A and anti-B and by testing the serum against A, B, and O reagent cells. The frequencies of the major ABO phenotypes in selected populations are shown in Table 312-1.

Red blood cells of types O and A2 have large amounts of another antigen, called H, which is the immediate precursor of A and B. H specificity depends on the presence of the monosaccharide fucose, attached to the oligosaccharides by a transferase that is the product of the very common H gene. The H and ABO loci are not genetically linked. Very rare individuals who fail to inherit an H gene from either

TABLE 312-1 Percentage of ABO phenotypes in selected populations

Population*	Phenotypes					
	A$_1$	A$_2$	B	A$_1$B	A$_2$B	O
European-American	35	10	8	3	1	43
African-American	23	6	17	3	1	50
German	32.5	9.4	11	3.1	1.1	42.8
South American Indian	0	0	0	0	0	100
Australian Aborigine	55.6	0	0	0	0	44.4
Lapps	36.1	18.5	4.8	6.2	6.2	18.2

* Selected populations do not necessarily apply to racial group.

parent cannot produce this transferase. As a result, even if an A or B gene is inherited, these subjects cannot produce A, B, or H antigens, and their serum contains all three antibodies. Because patients with this rare phenotype (O$_h$, Bombay) are extremely difficult to transfuse, blood of the same type must be sought from rare-donor registries.

Antibodies in the ABO system Red blood cells of newborn infants have a decreased number of A, B, and H reactive sites, and their plasma normally contains very little anti-A or anti-B. Maternal anti-A and anti-B are primarily IgM and do not cross the placenta. However, some type O adults produce an IgG cross-reacting antibody termed anti-A,B which can cross the placenta and react with fetal cells. For this reason, ABO hemolytic disease of the newborn (HDN) usually occurs in type A or B infants of type O mothers.

Safe transfusion practice prohibits transfusing A, B, or AB blood to patients whose red cells lack the corresponding antigens, since the recipient's plasma contains incompatible antibodies. Most fatal hemolytic transfusion reactions result from patient and sample identification errors that end in such incompatible transfusions. Type A or B blood, preferably as packed red cells, may be transfused to AB recipients, since the passively infused antibody is rarely of clinical significance. Although type O red blood cells may be given to patients of type A, B, or AB when type-specific blood is not available, plasma from some type O individuals contains a potent hemolytic antibody; thus type O should not be given as whole blood except in an emergency.

Lewis system Antibodies to Lewis system antigens are the most common cause of incompatibility during pretransfusion compatibility testing. Antigens in the Lewis system are not integral components of red blood cell membranes but are glycosphingolipid molecules absorbed from the surrounding plasma. The two most common Lewis antigens, Le^a and Le^b, are carbohydrate antigens that are structurally related to the ABH antigens and result from the action of the Lewis gene product, a fucosyl transferase, on an oligosaccharide precursor.

Anti-Le^a and anti-Le^b are common, naturally occurring, complement-binding antibodies of the IgM class. Lewis antibodies rarely cross the placenta and do not result in HDN. While anti-Le^a has caused hemolytic transfusion reactions, the plasma of Le^a+ donors usually contains sufficient Lewis antigen to neutralize the patient's antibody when whole blood is transfused. Anti-Le^b rarely causes transfusion reactions.

I system The I and i antigenic determinants are heterogeneous oligosaccharides that are biochemically related to the H, A, B, Le, and P antigens. The i antigen is an unbranched oligosaccharide chain that is converted by the I gene product, a glycosyltransferase, to the I antigen branched structure. Fetal and cord red blood cells react very weakly with anti-I and strongly with anti-i, suggesting that glycosyltransferase production is developmentally regulated. Rare adult red blood cells lack I antigen.

Polyclonal anti-I is a weak, clinically unimportant cold agglutinin found in the sera of most normal adults. High-titer, monoclonal anti-I autoantibodies, on the other hand, can cause chronic red cell destruction in some patients with cold agglutinin disease and lymphoproliferative disorders. An occasional patient with mononucleosis or

Mycoplasma pneumonia will develop high-titered cold agglutinins with anti-i or anti-I specificity. These antibodies are generally monoclonal and may cause autoimmune hemolysis. The rare, genetically I-negative person may develop alloanti-I. Alloanti-i has not been reported.

When patients with anti-i autoantibodies require transfusion, compatible blood is readily available. The red blood cells of most adults lack i antigen. Because anti-I autoantibodies generally react only at low temperatures, even patients with strong cold-reacting anti-I autoantibodies can be transfused safely if the blood is kept warm during the infusion.

P system Three structurally related glycosphingolipid antigens, P, P^k, and P$_1$ are considered together under the P blood group system. As in the ABO and Lewis systems, the gene products are glycosyltransferases. P$_1$ and P, the major antigenic determinants, result from different synthetic pathways and likely represent independent genetic systems.

Anti-P$_1$ is usually a weak IgM cold agglutinin that almost never damages red blood cells. In contrast, rare individuals who lack P antigens (p phenotype) may possess potent high-titer antibodies directed against one or more of the P antigens. One such antibody, anti-P$_1$PP^k (anti-Tj^a), can cause severe hemolytic transfusion reactions and HDN and has been associated with recurrent spontaneous abortions, possibly related to the presence of P-like antigens on trophoblastic tissue. Finally, sera of patients with paroxysmal cold hemoglobinuria may contain a peculiar biphasic complement fixing autoantibody with anti-P specificity known as the *Donath-Landsteiner antibody*. Donath-Landsteiner antibodies, which bind to red blood cells in the cold and fix complement when warmed, have been reported with hemolytic syndromes associated with syphilis and different viral infections.

PROTEIN BLOOD GROUP ANTIGENS Rh system The Rhesus or Rh system is second in importance only to the ABO system in transfusion practice. The Rh locus is on chromosome 1. Rh antigenic determinants depend on poorly understood interactions between a hydrophobic 30- to 32-kDa red cell membrane protein and the posttranslational addition of phospholipid molecules. More than 40 Rh phenotypes have been defined serologically. Recent evidence identifies at least three tandem Rh loci, somewhat analogous to the HLA complex. The Rh alleles describe the structure of a set of epitope pairs, C or c, E or e, and D, the last having a postulated silent allele, d. Epitopes are inherited as haplotypes, e.g., CDe or cde.

Because Rh$_o$(D) is the most immunogenic alloantigen, donated blood is tested and labeled for the presence or absence of this antigen. Approximately 15 percent of Caucasians lack the D antigen and are classified as Rh-negative. About 80 percent of Rh-negative persons who receive a single unit of Rh-positive red blood cells will develop anti-D, an antibody that may cause severe hemolytic transfusion reactions and HDN. For this reason, Rh-negative patients are always given Rh-negative cellular blood components, except during emergency circumstances. Anti-D can be induced by as few as 0.5 mL red blood cells or 0.04 mL red blood cells when given in repeated injections. Premenopausal Rh-negative women must not receive Rh-positive blood components unless adequate amounts of Rh immunoglobulin are given to prevent primary immunization; otherwise, subsequent pregnancy with an Rh-positive child almost always stimulates a secondary immune response, resulting in HDN.

The Rh antigens C, c, E, and e are considerably less immunogenic (less than 2 percent of susceptible recipients), and matching transfusion recipients for these antigens is impractical. Of course, previously sensitized patients must receive blood lacking the corresponding specific antigen. About 20 percent of donors lack the c antigen and are therefore compatible with recipients whose plasma contains anti-c. However, only 2 percent of donors lack e antigen, so patients who have developed anti-e are difficult to match. Blood banks often maintain computerized lists of phenotyped donors for such circumstances, and autologous blood remains an option for elective surgical procedures.

MNS system   Studies of the biochemistry and molecular genetics of the MNS system have contributed more to understanding red blood cell membrane structure and function than to practical transfusion problems. Closely linked genes on chromosome 4 determine the MN and Ss antigens, which are inherited as haplotypes: MS, Ms, NS, and Ns. A transmembrane protein, glycophorin A, carries M and N specificity, while S and s are on glycophorin B. Absence of these sialoglycoproteins is associated with rare red blood cell phenotypes such as En(a-), S^u, and M^k, but there are no associated hematologic abnormalities. Anti-M and anti-N are naturally occurring IgM agglutinins directed against epitopes involving both the sugar and amino acid components of the protein. Formation of anti-S or anti-s usually requires the stimulus of transfusion or pregnancy, and unlike anti-M and anti-N, these IgG class antibodies may destroy red blood cells. A third hemolytic antibody, anti-U, is formed by sensitized black patients with the S^u phenotype. Since less than 1 percent of black patients and no white patients are U negative, compatible blood is almost impossible to find.

Kell, Duffy, and Kidd systems   The Kell blood group system contains more than 20 different antigens with multiple alleles at different loci. The Kell (K) and Cellano (k) antigens are codominant autosomal alleles, and Kell is the most potent red blood cell immunogen outside of the ABO and Rh systems. An X-linked gene determines expression of the Kell precursor antigen K_x, and rare individuals of the "McLeod phenotype" lack K_x on their red blood cells. Red blood cells of the McLeod phenotype exhibit acanthocytosis, weakened Kell antigens, and in vivo hemolysis. Furthermore, genes for K_x and for type II chronic granulomatous disease (CGD) are closely linked. Type II CGD patients may display the McLeod phenotype if the deletion affects both genes. Patients with the McLeod phenotype should avoid transfusion, since a single unit of blood may elicit antibodies that react with all Kell system red cell antigens.

The Duffy and Kidd blood group systems are composed of equally prevalent codominant alleles, Fy^a and Fy^b in the former and Jk^a and Jk^b in the latter. Both blood groups are significantly more complex at the level of the gene. Duffy blood group antigens function as receptor sites for invasion of red blood cells by at least one species of malarial parasite, *Plasmodium vivax*. More than 70 percent of native West Africans lack these red cell antigens, a rare finding among Caucasians, suggesting malaria-induced selective pressure in West Africa.

Anti-K and anti-Fy^a are commonly encountered antibodies capable of marked alloimmune red cell destruction. The Kidd antibodies, anti-Jk^a and anti-Jk^b, are notoriously transient and difficult to detect. A delayed hemolytic transfusion reaction that occurs with blood that tested compatible suggests the delayed appearance of anti-Jk^a.

BLOOD TRANSFUSION

Blood components are biologic medications licensed by the Food and Drug Administration. Responsible medical practice obliges physicians to acquire knowledge of blood to make sound transfusion judgments and to advise their patients accordingly. Physicians who use blood must understand the benefits and risks of each component.

WHOLE BLOOD AND RED BLOOD CELLS   A unit of whole blood consists of approximately 450 mL blood with about 65 g hemoglobin. When refrigerated, the red blood cells are viable for up to 6 weeks, depending on the anticoagulant-preservative solution used. Whole blood is not a reliable source of platelets or granulocytes, and the labile coagulation factors V and VIII begin to deteriorate within hours of collection. Most other plasma coagulation proteins are stable for the entire storage period.

Few clinical situations require whole blood transfusion. Whole blood should be reserved for catastrophic medical or surgical bleeding, e.g., during rapid gastrointestinal hemorrhage or with major trauma, when simultaneous restoration of oxygen carrying capacity, volume, and coagulation factors is desired. Even in hemorrhagic shock, a combination of red cells and crystalloid or colloid solution is usually effective. In emergencies, rapid volume replacement generally takes precedence over red cell replacement, and cell-free resuscitation fluids should be used while the recipient's blood type is being determined. When the red blood cell deficit is critical, uncrossmatched type-specific whole blood or type O red cells are indicated.

Fresh whole blood is a poorly defined component and is rarely advantageous. During refrigerated storage, whole blood oxygen affinity increases as red cell 2,3-diphosphoglycerate (2,3-DPG) falls. Both oxygen affinity and 2,3-DPG levels return to normal within hours of transfusion. Other storage changes include a rise in extracellular potassium and lactate concentrations and a decline in pH. The clinical importance of these observations remains controversial. Blood less than 7 days old is still recommended for neonatal exchange transfusions, and a recent study suggests that blood less than 24 h old may benefit children undergoing cardiopulmonary bypass.

Red blood cells or "packed" cells are prepared by centrifuging whole blood and expressing the plasma into a satellite bag. Red cells are concentrated to a hematocrit of 80 percent or more and to a volume of about 200 mL. The refrigerated storage period is the same as that for whole blood. Red cells permit restoration of oxygen carrying capacity with less risk of volume overload and limit the quantity of sodium, potassium, citrate, and ammonia infused. The appropriateness of red blood cell transfusion should be determined by clinical signs and symptoms and not by a preset hemoglobin level.

Red blood cells are supportive therapy for perioperative blood loss and for chronic anemia when no timely definitive therapy is available. Each unit of red cells elevates an adult's hemoglobin concentration by about 1 g/dL and the hematocrit by about 3 points. The advent of a lineage-specific growth factor, recombinant human erythropoietin (rHuEpo), has dramatically decreased the use of red cell transfusion in patients with chronic end-stage renal disease, in whom endogenous erythropoietin is deficient. rHuEpo also has replaced red blood cell transfusion for selected patients with cancer, AIDS, and transfusion-dependent myelodysplasia.

Patients with autoimmune hemolytic anemia do not ordinarily receive red blood cell transfusion. Unless the autoantibody is directed against a specific blood group antigen, the transfused red cells will be destroyed as rapidly as the patient's own cells. Serious hemolytic reactions may result from alloantibodies difficult to detect in the presence of an autoantibody. However, when anemia is severe enough to cause hypoxemia or cardiac decompensation, cautious transfusion may be lifesaving. Patients with some forms of ineffective erythropoiesis, e.g., nutritional deficiencies of vitamin B_{12}, folate, or iron, are candidates for transfusion only if they are symptomatic and only if the cause of anemia cannot be corrected expeditiously by specific replacement therapy. These conditions number among the few indications for the single-unit transfusion.

Red blood cells in a hypertonic cryoprotective glycerol solution may be stored frozen for as long as 10 years. Once thawed, the cells must be washed thoroughly, lest residual glycerol cause intravascular hemolysis. The resulting red blood cell concentrate contains almost no plasma proteins, which makes it ideal for patients who experience reactions to donor plasma proteins. The markedly reduced number of platelets and leukocytes also decreases febrile reactions, immunogenicity, and cytomegalovirus transmission. Cryopreserved red blood cells retain biochemical and posttransfusion survival characteristics similar to those present at the time of freezing. Frozen cells are generally reserved for providing blood to persons with rare phenotypes or for storing autologous units in unusual circumstances. Some institutions stockpile cryopreserved cells for inventory control, and the Department of Defense has deployed such stockpiles for military emergencies. However, the thaw and wash process is slow, logistically difficult, and expensive, and the thawed cells outdate within 24 h.

PLATELETS   Platelet concentrates are prepared either by centrifugation of platelet-rich plasma from single units of blood to yield 6×10^{10} platelets or by automated plateletpheresis to yield approximately six such units from individual donors. When stored at room temperature in gas-permeable containers to maintain aerobic metabolism and pH, platelets remain viable for up to 5 days. A unit of platelets should raise an adult's platelet count by at least 5000 cells per microliter, and platelets circulate for about a week in stable, nonimmunized, thrombocytopenic patients.

Platelet transfusions are indicated when either severe thrombocytopenia or platelet dysfunction is associated with active or imminent bleeding. Platelet transfusions usually control bleeding in thrombocytopenic patients who have suppressed platelet production, such as occurs with leukemia, chemotherapy, or radiotherapy, or who develop the dilutional thrombocytopenia observed during massive transfusion. Platelet transfusions are less effective when there is peripheral destruction, such as consumption coagulopathy or immune thrombocytopenic purpura (ITP), and are not recommended except when life-threatening hemorrhage occurs; in these situations, platelet transfusions may prevent potentially fatal hemorrhage until the cause of platelet destruction can be reversed. The use of prophylactic platelet transfusions for stable thrombocytopenic patients remains controversial. The threshold platelet count at which spontaneous bleeding occurs will vary with the cause of the thrombocytopenia and with the degree of platelet dysfunction. Most patients with platelet counts about 10,000 cells per microliter do not develop spontaneous bleeding complications. Certain complicating clinical factors such as sepsis, rapidly falling counts, medications that interfere with platelet function, and mucositis increase the risk of hemorrhage in patients receiving myelosuppressive therapy. Prophylactic platelet transfusions are often used to maintain counts above 20,000 cells per microliter in these circumstances. Patients in the immediate postoperative period and those with a second defect in hemostasis may require a platelet count of 50,000 to 100,000 cells per microliter. Platelet transfusions should be monitored with 1- or 24-h posttransfusion platelet counts.

Ideally, transfused platelets should be of the same ABO and Rh type as the patient. ABO-mismatched platelets result in lower platelet increments and may contribute to the development of platelet refractoriness. When group O donors are used for A, B, or AB recipients, donor plasma may contain sufficient antibody to destroy some of the patient's red blood cells. Incompatible plasma may be reduced for pediatric infusions or when adults require large numbers of single-donor platelets. Although platelets do not express the Rh antigen, the red blood cells present can sensitize an Rh-negative recipient of Rh-positive platelet concentrates. Rh-negative patients should receive platelets from Rh-negative donors when possible. When this is not possible, Rh immunization can be prevented by injection of Rh immune globulin. This is especially important for Rh-negative women in childbearing years.

Patients who receive platelet transfusions frequently develop alloantibodies to the HLA antigens that are expressed on lymphocytes in the platelet concentrates. Alloimmunized patients may become resistant (refractory) to further platelet transfusions unless the platelets come from HLA-compatible donors. As many as a third of alloimmunized patients fail to respond even to HLA-identical platelets. Suboptimal response to fresh histocompatible platelets suggests platelet-specific antibodies, nonimmune platelet consumption, or hypersplenism.

LEUKOCYTE-REDUCED BLOOD COMPONENTS Red blood cell and platelet components contain variable numbers of residual leukocytes, predominantly lymphocytes. Febrile reactions are common in sensitized patients who receive components containing more than 5×10^8 leukocytes, and alloimmunization to the HLA antigens of residual lymphocytes may occur when more than 10^6 lymphocytes are transfused. Certain cell-associated viruses such as cytomegalovirus (CMV) and HTLV I and II are transmitted by small numbers of lymphocytes. Recent evidence indicates that allogeneic leukocytes may activate latent viruses in the recipient. These observations have stimulated efforts to develop leukocyte-reduced cellular blood components. Cell washing procedures remove most plasma but reduce the leukocytes by only about 1 log, enough to eliminate some febrile reactions but insufficient to prevent other complications. Specially constructed filters can reduce the leukocyte content in red blood cell components or platelet concentrates by more than 3 logs to levels difficult to count with standard techniques. Blood cell separators also collect leukocyte-reduced platelets. These leukocyte-reduced components virtually eliminate febrile reactions, reduce the risk of HLA alloimmunization and cell-associated virus transmission, and may reduce reactivation of latent viruses such as CMV and HIV-1. Since transfusion-associated graft-versus-host-disease (GVHD) can result from as few as 10^4 allogeneic lymphocytes transfused to a severely immunocompromised patient, and since the outcome is frequently lethal, current leukocyte reduction techniques do not reliably protect such patients. To prevent transfusion-associated GVHD, blood components should be treated with gamma irradiation at a dose of 25 Gy.

GRANULOCYTE TRANSFUSIONS Infection has replaced bleeding as the major cause of death in severely pancytopenic patients. The frequency of infection increases as the absolute neutrophil count falls below 500 cells per microliter. Improved antibiotic regimens and recombinant myeloid growth factors (G-CSF and GM-CSF) that reduce the duration of neutropenia have improved the management of such patients. However, selected patients with fewer than 500 granulocytes per microliter and persistent fever, despite appropriate antibiotic therapy for at least 48 h, may benefit from granulocyte transfusions. Other less well documented indications include progressive fungal infections, inherited defects of granulocyte function such as CGD, and neonatal sepsis. Prophylactic transfusion of granulocytes to neutropenic patients does not appear to reduce the incidence of infections. A course of therapy consists of at least four daily transfusions of 10 to 30 $\times$ 10^9 neutrophils, probably a marginally effective number that represents only about 10 percent of normal daily neutrophil production. Transfusions are complicated by severe rigors, pulmonary injury, alloimmunization, and transmission of cell-associated viruses, particularly CMV. Leukocyte concentrates present a substantial risk of GVHD for immunosuppressed patients and premature infants. Prophylactic gamma irradiation is recommended but may adversely affect granulocyte function.

PLASMA COMPONENT THERAPY Fresh frozen plasma (FFP) and cryoprecipitate are the major plasma components used for patients with clotting disorders. (Management of inherited factor deficiencies with blood derivatives is discussed in Chap. 315.) FFP contains all coagulation factors found in fresh plasma. Each 250-mL unit infusion raises most coagulation factor levels 3 to 5 percent. FFP is used for bleeding patients with multiple coagulation factor deficiencies, such as occur in severe liver disease or dilutional coagulopathy. Warfarin-induced deficiency of vitamin K–dependent factors may be rapidly reversed with FFP, but ordinarily vitamin K administration produces a smooth reversal in 6 to 12 h. FFP is rarely indicated for prolongations of prothrombin time less than 1.5 times normal. FFP should not be used for volume expansion or prophylactically for cardiopulmonary bypass. When colloid volume expanders are indicated, human albumin fraction is equally effective and has been heat treated to inactivate viruses. Using plasma to supplement nutrition or to improve wound healing is likewise inappropriate.

Cryoprecipitate is prepared from FFP by a freeze-thaw process that concentrates about 60 percent of the fibrinogen, factor VIII, von Willebrand factor, and factor XIII into 10 percent of the original volume. Currently, the major uses are for patients with von Willebrand disease and for hypofibrinogenemia, as may occur with disseminated intravascular coagulation. Cryoprecipitate transmits the same viruses as plasma, and standard doses pooled from 12 to 20 donors carry an additive risk. Commercial clotting factor concentrates, treated to eliminate infectious agents, and recombinant clotting proteins have replaced plasma and cryoprecipitate for many uses.

HEMAPHERESIS Automated blood cell separators have made therapeutic plasmapheresis and blood cell removal rapid, safe, and easy. Two plasma volumes can be exchanged in less than 3 h, and intravascular solutes such as antibodies, immune complexes, and a variety of protein-bound toxins can be reduced by more than 50 percent with each exchange. The most established indications for plasmapheresis include symptomatic hyperviscosity syndrome, Goodpasture's syndrome, Guillain-Barré syndrome, and thrombotic thrombocytopenic purpura. For a variety of other illnesses, the efficacy and the appropriate volume, frequency, and replacement solutions have yet to be established.

Blood cells also may be efficiently exchanged or removed. Cell separators are routinely used for red cell exchange to manage acute complications of sickle cell disease such as stroke, chest syndrome, and priapism. When blast cells increase rapidly in acute leukemia, therapeutic leukapheresis can prevent associated cerebrovascular, pulmonary, and renal complications. Therapeutic plateletpheresis has been used to treat symptomatic thrombocythemia.

Recently, blood cell separators have been used to process bone marrow and to collect peripheral blood progenitor cells to support autologous bone marrow transplantation. Peripheral blood mononuclear cells also have been used for cancer and AIDS immunotherapy, as well as for somatic cell gene therapy of immune-deficient patients who lack adenosine deaminase.

CUSTOMIZED COMPONENTS Autologous transfusion The patient's own (autologous) blood may be collected and stored for future elective surgery. Other autologous techniques include intraoperative phlebotomy with crystalloid replacement (hemodilution), intraoperative collection of shed blood, and postoperative collection of blood from closed spaces such as mediastinal drainage. Autologous transfusion avoids the risks of immunologic mismatch and disease transmission. Autologous blood is recommended for patients planning elective surgical procedures that require 1 to 4 units of blood. For some patients with unstable cardiac and vascular disease, the benefits of autologous blood must be weighed against the medical risks of phlebotomy and the risks of delaying surgery. Supplemental iron with recombinant erythropoietin increases the amount of blood that can be collected, but the usefulness of this strategy has not been confirmed.

Directed donations Some patients solicit blood donations from friends and family members in order to reduce the risk of infection from routine volunteer blood. Ironically, the prevalence of laboratory markers of infectious disease in blood from these directed donors exceeds the prevalence found in unselected repeat volunteer donors. For the donor, loss of anonymity and confidentiality is a further disadvantage of directed donation. For certain medical circumstances, e.g., maternal platelets for neonates with alloimmune thrombocytopenia and rare red blood cell phenotypes from compatible family members, directed donations are the preferred therapy. In contrast, medical considerations specifically contraindicate directed donations from a prospective father to a spouse in childbearing years and from a bone marrow donor to the marrow recipient before the transplant. Finally, transfusion-associated GVHD may result if cellular components from a relative are not irradiated.

MASSIVE TRANSFUSION *Massive transfusion* is generally defined as replacement of total blood volume in less than 24 h. Dilution of platelets and, less often, of plasma coagulation factors may result when more than one blood volume is rapidly replaced with stored blood. Metabolic changes during massive transfusion are complex and interrelated. Rapid infusions of citrate anticoagulant can cause symptomatic hypocalcemia, especially in the presence of liver disease. Transient hyperkalemia and acidosis may result when the transfusion rate exceeds 100 mL/min. These changes are often followed by a metabolic alkalosis and hypokalemia as citric acid is metabolized to pyruvate and bicarbonate. Expectant use of calcium, potassium, or bicarbonate infusions is treacherous at best, and under no circumstances should these solutions be added to the blood components. When refrigerated blood infuses rapidly through large central venous lines, profound hypothermia may further complicate these metabolic changes and predispose the patient to seizures and cardiac arrhythmias. Commercial instruments are available to warm the blood during massive infusion.

COMPLICATIONS OF BLOOD TRANSFUSION Transfusion reactions are classifed as immune or nonimmune (Table 312-2).

TABLE 312-2 Complications of transfusion per unit transfused

Immune complications	Frequency*	Nonimmune complications	Frequency*
Acute hemolysis	1/6000	Hepatitis	1/3000
Delayed hemolysis	1/1000	HIV (AIDS)	1/225,000
Febrile nonhemolytic	1/200	Hypervolemia	Unknown
Allergic cutaneous	1/200	Iron overload	Unknown
Anaphylactic	1/150,000	Bacterial sepsis	Rare
Alloimmunization (RBC)	1/100	Hypothermia	Rare
Alloimmunization (HLA)	1/10		
Graft-versus-host disease	Rare		

* Estimated.

Antibody-mediated reactions are directed against red blood cells, white blood cells, platelets, and at least one class of immunoglobulin, IgA. Transfusion of viable lymphocytes can result in cell-mediated GVHD. The major nonimmune reactions are due to circulatory overload, transfusional siderosis, and transmission of infectious agents. Reports that transfusion-induced immunomodulation decreases survival of cancer patients and increases postoperative infections further emphasize the seriousness of blood transfusion.

Hemolytic transfusion reactions Red blood cell alloantibodies may lyse cells within the circulation or coat red blood cells and accelerate cell removal by the reticuloendothelial system. Approximately 1 in 100,000 units transfused will result in a fatal hemolytic reaction, usually from ABO incompatibility arising from misidentification of the patient or the blood specimen. Rapid cell destruction commonly involves the ABO system, since both anti-A and anti-B fix complement. Other antibodies reported to cause intravascular hemolysis include anti-Jk^a, anti-Fy^a, and rarely, anti-Le^a. Patients with acute hemolytic reactions may complain of flushing, pain at the infusion site, chest or back pain, restlessness, anxiety, nausea, or diarrhea. Signs include fever or chills and the typical findings of shock and renal failure. In comatose or anesthetized patients, the first indication may be hemoglobinuria or generalized bleeding resulting from disseminated intravascular coagulation.

Extravascular hemolysis is most often caused by antibodies of the Rh system, but several other antibodies, including those of Kell, Duffy, and Kidd systems, are common offenders. Malaise, jaundice, and fever are seen in about 1 in 500 patients transfused, are usually mild, and occur 5 to 10 days after transfusion. Shock and renal complications are rare. About 1 in 150 asymptomatic patients develop a new antibody about a week after transfusion, reflecting the anamnestic rise in previously undetected antibodies stimulated by the transfusion. The rare patient is found to have destroyed all the transfused cells in the absence of demonstrable antibodies.

Laboratory investigation The initial investigation of a hemolytic transfusion reaction involves a careful check of the identity of donor and recipient, since clerical errors, especially mistakes in specimen labeling, are frequently involved. The next steps involve documenting red blood cell destruction, investigating its cause, and managing the patient's clinical status.

With recent intravascular hemolysis, free hemoglobin may color both plasma and urine. The laboratory can confirm elevated free hemoglobin, presence of methemalbumin, or reduced serum haptoglobin if necessary. The best indicators of extravascular hemolysis include a rise in unconjugated bilirubin and a failure of the hematocrit to reach the expected posttransfusion level.

A pretransfusion of the patient's blood is usually retained so that determination of both donor and recipient blood types can be repeated along with the compatibility test. If antibodies are detected, the pretransfusion specimen is used to determine specificity, since alloantibodies are formed only against those antigens not present on the patient's own cells. The posttransfusion specimen may not contain the offending antibodies if they have been absorbed by the transfused incompatible red blood cells. However, the red cells can be examined to determine whether transfused cells have been removed or coated with antibody, as indicated by the direct antiglobulin (Coombs') test.

Management of patients with extravascular hemolysis should be conservative. Additional transfusions should be withheld until serology is adequately defined, unless the patient's life is otherwise threatened. Intravascular hemolysis poses a far greater hazard, but there is no specific therapy. Management of hypotension, bleeding, or renal failure is supportive.

Other immunologically related reactions In the absence of red blood cell destruction, most febrile reactions can be ascribed to immune destruction of leukocytes or platelets. Most of these are mild and can be prevented by using leukocyte-reduced components. An allergic pulmonary edema related to sequestration of antibody-coated leukocytes in the lung has been reported. These rare reactions occur when a donor's plasma contains a high-titer antibody that reacts with the recipient's leukocytes. Cutaneous allergic reactions such as urticaria can be managed by slowing the transfusion and administering antihistamines. Patients with antibodies against IgA molecules may develop hypotensive anaphylactic reactions when exposed to plasma-containing components. Such patients are best managed with IgA-deficient blood components from relatives or from rare-donor lists. When necessary, cellular components can be washed extensively to remove the offending plasma. Finally, transfusion commonly results in alloimmunization to blood cell antigens, which complicates subsequent transfusions and bone marrow or solid organ transplants.

Nonimmune transfusion reactions The most significant nonimmune transfusion reactions, aside from infectious complications, are circulatory overload and transfusional siderosis. Circulatory overload manifested by pulmonary edema is a particular risk to the elderly, the infant, the patient with cardiac or renal compromise, and the patient with chronic anemia in whom red cell mass is decreased while the plasma volume is increased. The average unit of whole blood contains about 60 mEq sodium, while the average unit of red blood cells contains between 10 and 20 mEq. Transfusion-induced iron overload is an often fatal consequence of chronic transfusion for refractory anemia. Children with thalassemia major are the single largest group affected, but a substantial number of children with congenital anemias and adults with intensely treated refractory anemia are likewise at risk. Every milliliter of red blood cells deposits 1.08 mg iron in tissues as the red blood cells age and die. Iron deposition begins to affect endocrine, hepatic, and cardiac function when the total body burden has risen to more than 20 g, the equivalent of about 100 units of red blood cells. Lethal cardiac complications occur at about 60 g, or about 300 units. Iron chelation therapy should be considered for all patients who are likely to require intensive red cell support.

Infection Numerous different viral, bacterial, and protozoal agents can be transmitted through blood transfusion. To decrease potential disease transmission, donors are screened for risk factors by medical history and tested with a battery of laboratory screening assays. Sterilization techniques have been developed for some plasma components and fractionation products, but as yet no method for sterilizing cellular blood components has been found.

Hepatitis Emphasis on voluntary blood donations, donor screening, and specific assays for hepatitis B virus (HBV) and antibody to hepatitis C have reduced the risk of posttransfusion hepatitis in the United States from rates as high as 20 percent to a current rate of about 1 percent. Hepatitis A is almost never transmitted by blood. The current incidence of transfusion-associated hepatitis B is extremely low, and an effective hepatitis B vaccine is available for susceptible patients who anticipate chronic transfusion therapy. Most transfusion-transmitted hepatitis is caused by hepatitis C virus (HCV). Hepatitis C generally presents with few signs or symptoms, but serologic and biochemical evidence of infection can be detected 2 to 26 weeks after transfusion. Despite its mild presentation and declining incidence, posttransfusion hepatitis C remains a serious health concern, since more than 50 percent of infected patients progress to chronic liver disease. Furthermore, persuasive statistical evidence links both HBV and HCV with hepatocellular carcinoma.

Retroviral infections Several human retroviruses are readily transmitted by blood transfusion. Human immunodeficiency virus type 1 (HIV-1), the agent implicated in AIDS, infects about 90 percent of patients who receive an infected blood component (see Chap. 279). Prior to routine testing of blood donors, transfusions were implicated in 2 to 3 percent of total AIDS cases. Improved donor selection criteria and specific screening tests appear to have significantly reduced this figure. The current risk of infection is estimated at about 1 case per 225,000 units transfused. A related agent, HIV-2, has been associated with AIDS, and although no transfusion-related cases have yet been reported in the United States, blood donors are being tested for this agent as well. Cellular blood components are also screened for the cell-associated retroviruses HTLV-I and II isolated from patients with tropical spastic paraparesis, T cell leukemia, and hairy cell leukemia (see Chap. 151).

Other infectious agents CMV, ordinarily a common and relatively innocuous herpesvirus, can be an important pathogen in pregnant women, premature infants, and immunosuppressed patients (see Chap. 146). These patients should receive components from seronegative donors or blood processed to remove leukocytes. Bacterial growth in refrigerated blood is unusual. However, units contaminated with *Staphylococcus aureus* or with certain gram-negative organisms such as *Yersinia enterocolitica* and *Citrobacter* species that grow well at 4°C and in citrated blood may cause shock and death. A wide variety of bacteria and spirochetes grow well in platelet concentrates stored at room temperature. Malaria and Chagas' disease are among the most important infectious causes of transfusion-related morbidity and mortality worldwide. The rare cases detected in the United States are usually found among immigrants or travelers to areas where these diseases are endemic.

REFERENCES

AGRE P, CARTRON JP: Molecular biology of the Rh antigens. Blood 78:551, 1991

ALTER HJ et al: Detection of antibody to hepatitis C virus in prospectively followed transfusion recipients with acute and chronic non-A, non-B, hepatitis. N Engl J Med 321:1494, 1989

ANDERSON KC: The role of the blood bank in hematopoietic stem cell transplantation. Transfusion 32:272, 1992

Blood, Blood Components, and Plasma Expanders (Drug Evaluations Annual 1992). Chicago, American Medical Association, 1992, chap. 94, pp 2069–2092

BLUMBERG N et al: Transfusion-induced immunomodulation and its clinical consequences. Transfusion Med Rev 4 (suppl):24, 1990

HEYMAN MR, SCHIFFER CA: Platelet transfusion therapy for the cancer patient. Semin Oncol 17:198, 1990

MOLLISON PL et al (eds): *Blood Transfusion in Clinical Medicine*, 9th ed. Oxford, Blackwell Scientific, 1993

NATIONAL BLOOD RESOURCES EDUCATION PROGRAM EXPERT PANEL: The use of autologous blood. JAMA 263:414, 1990

ROSSI EC et al (eds): *Principles of Transfusion Medicine*. Baltimore, Williams & Wilkins, 1991

WALKER R et al: *The Technical Manual*, 11th ed. Arlington, Va, American Association of Blood Banks, 1993

YAMAMOTO F et al: Molecular genetic basis of the histo-blood group ABO system. Nature 345:229, 1990

313 BONE MARROW TRANSPLANTATION

E. DONNALL THOMAS

SELECTION OF THE PATIENT Marrow transplantation is a rational therapeutic option only if the patient's disease involves the marrow or if hazard to the normal marrow is the limiting factor in aggressive treatment of a disease. A marrow transplant involves a transplant not only of the donor myeloid, erythroid, and megakaryocytic systems but also of the donor lymphoid and macrophage-monocyte systems. The rationale is illustrated by the three types of disease for which marrow transplantation has been widely utilized:

1 *Genetic disease*. For immunologic deficiency diseases, the objective is to replace the recipient's genetically defective lymphoid system with the normal lymphoid system of the donor. For genetic diseases such as thalassemia major, the abnormal marrow must be destroyed and replaced by normal marrow.

2 *Aplastic anemia*. Regardless of cause, the disease process results in loss of the marrow, and the objective is to replace the defective organ with a normal functioning organ.

3 *Malignant disease*. For leukemia and other hematologic malignancies, the objective is the complete destruction of the malignant cell population and, unavoidably, normal marrow cells by intensive chemoradiotherapy with restoration of normal marrow function by the transplanted marrow.

TYPES OF TRANSPLANTS   A *syngeneic* graft describes a graft in which donor and recipient are genetically identical, i.e., identical twins. An *allogeneic* graft is one in which donor and recipient are of different genetic origins. A *chimera* is an individual whose body contains living, proliferating cells of different genetic origin. An *autologous* marrow graft refers to the removal of a patient's marrow, administration of chemo- and/or radiotherapy, and then return of the patient's own marrow.

SELECTION OF THE DONOR   The donor must be in good health, and the donor, or an appropriate advocate, must be capable of giving informed consent. The principal risk is the anesthesia. Selection of the donor is largely determined by histocompatibility testing. Red blood cell incompatibility is not a barrier to marrow transplantation.

Histocompatibility typing (See Chap. 64)   The HLA region is composed of a series of closely linked genes on chromosome 6. The array of genes encoded on a single chromosome is known as a *haplotype*. Each individual has two haplotypes, one inherited from each parent. The antigens are encoded at loci designated HLA-A, -B, -C, -DP, -DQ, and -DR. Serologic or molecular biologic techniques are used to detect the antigens. These closely linked genetic loci, each with a large number of known alleles, make the HLA region the most complex genetic polymorphism yet described. Despite this complexity, within a family there can be only four haplotypes. Therefore, for a given patient, each sibling has one chance in four of being HLA-identical with the patient. The most widely used transplants are those between HLA-identical siblings. There is now an increasing use of other family members and volunteer unrelated donors who match the patient or differ by only one HLA antigen.

PREPARATION OF THE PATIENT   Infants with severe combined immunologic deficiency are conditioned to accept a transplant by the nature of their disease. All other patients are immunologically competent, to a greater or lesser degree, and are able to reject the marrow graft unless prepared with some form of immunosuppressive therapy. An immunosuppressive regimen commonly used for patients with aplastic anemia is large doses of cyclophosphamide. Preparation of the patient with leukemia involves high-dose chemoradiotherapy for immunosuppression and to kill leukemic cells. A commonly used regimen involves cyclophosphamide followed by total-body irradiation. Approximately 10 Gy must be used for immunosuppression sufficient to permit consistent engraftment of marrow even though only 4 to 5 Gy will cause lethal marrow injury. Patients with leukemia or with genetic disease of the marrow may be prepared with busulfan to destroy the abnormal marrow along with cyclophosphamide for immunosuppression.

Marrow aspiration and infusion   In the operating room and under general or spinal anesthesia, multiple marrow aspirations are performed on the iliac crests. For adult donors, the volume of the mixture of blood and marrow cells is from 0.5 to 1.0 L. As each aspiration is performed, the marrow is mixed with heparin and tissue culture medium. The marrow is passed through stainless steel screens to break up particles. It is then given to the recipient by intravenous infusion. The marrow stem cells pass through the lungs, and subsequent growth and reconstitution of the marrow are confined almost exclusively to the medullary cavities.

Support for the patient without marrow function   Usually 2 to 4 weeks are required before the transplanted marrow starts to produce the critical formed elements of the peripheral blood. Recently, the use of hematopoietic growth factors G-CSF or GM-CSF has shortened the period of granulocytopenia to 7 to 12 days. The patient should be cared for using the most effective available isolation facilities. Platelet transfusions are usually unnecessary at levels above 20,000 per microliter (see Chap. 314). Below that level, they should be used until values above 20,000 are sustained. If the patient becomes refractory to random donor platelets, the use of platelets from HLA-matched family members or unrelated donors may be necessary. Aspirin and other drugs that depress platelet function should be avoided. Granulocyte transfusions may be indicated for therapy of refractory infection in a granulocytopenic patient. Packed red blood cells should be given as needed to control symptoms of anemia, usually to keep the hematocrit above 25 percent. All blood products should be irradiated with at least 1.5 Gy to inactivate lymphocytes that might cause a graft-versus-host reaction.

Since infection is an ever-present danger, bacteriologic cultures should be obtained frequently. Onset of significant fever (38.5°C) should arouse a strong suspicion of infection in the granulocytopenic patient. Fever with clinical signs of bacteremia or fever sustained more than 24 h is an indication for starting systemic antibacterial therapy even if cultures are negative. Initial therapy usually includes an aminoglycoside active against *Pseudomonas* and a second agent with broad-spectrum activity against gram-negative organisms, with additional antibiotics added as indicated by culture results (see Chap. 81). Subsequently, if cultures are negative but fever persists, the addition of vancomycin and/or amphotericin may be considered. Once broad-spectrum antibiotic therapy has been initiated, it should be continued until the granulocyte count rises above 500 cells per microliter even if clinical signs of infection disappear.

Many patients coming to marrow transplantation have had inadequate nutrition because of their disease or the efforts to treat it (see Chap. 76). The preparation for marrow grafting results in nausea, vomiting, and mucositis which results in poor oral intake for at least several weeks. A Hickman modification of the Broviac catheter is installed routinely. The catheter makes it possible to administer hyperalimentation, medications, and blood products and is also used for drawing blood samples. Although some catheters are removed because of infection or suspected infection, about 90 percent of the patients have the catheter in place for approximately 3 months, the period of time when it is needed.

ENGRAFTMENT AND PROOF OF ENGRAFTMENT   Engraftment is signaled by a rise in granulocytes and platelets and the reappearance of reticulocytes. Proof of engraftment depends on use of cytogenetics, blood genetic markers, and/or restriction enzyme fragment length polymorphisms to distinguish donor from host cells. The regenerating marrow is usually entirely of donor type. Occasional patients show persistence of some host cells.

COMPLICATIONS FOLLOWING ENGRAFTMENT   The complications that may follow successful marrow engraftment are (1) graft rejection, a problem primarily occurring in patients with aplastic anemia, (2) infection, including early bacterial infections or later opportunistic infections such as cytomegalovirus (CMV) interstitial pneumonia, (3) veno-occlusive liver disease, (4) acute graft-versus-host disease (GVHD), the result of the immunologic reaction of the engrafted lymphoid elements against tissues of the recipient, (5) chronic GVHD, (6) recurrence of leukemia, and (7) miscellaneous complications such as hemorrhagic cystitis, cardiomyopathy, cataract formation, leukoencephalopathy, and sterility.

Marrow graft recipients, whether allogeneic or autologous, suffer impaired immune competence in the first few months after grafting. Hematopoietic growth factors have shortened the period of susceptibility to bacterial infections. Acyclovir and ganciclovir have reduced the complications associated with herpes simplex and CMV infection. Trimethoprim-sulfamethoxazole has removed the risk of *Pneumocystis carinii* infection.

CLINICAL RESULTS OF MARROW TRANSPLANTATION   Immunodeficiency diseases
Despite the rarity of these disorders, these patients are unique in that immunosuppressive therapy is not necessary to condition the patient to accept a graft, and because some myeloid function is usually present, rapid marrow engraftment is not essential.

Genetically determined hematologic diseases   Marrow grafts have now been reported for thalassemia major, sickle cell disease, Kostmann's syndrome, chronic granulomatous disease, Chédiak-Higashi syndrome, Blackfan-Diamond syndrome, congenital aplastic anemia, Fanconi's anemia, and several storage diseases due to enzyme deficiencies. Thalassemia major is a significant cause of death in children in many parts of the world. In developed countries, therapy with transfusions and chelating agents can prolong life for one to three decades but at great expense. Since the first transplant in 1981, more than 500 marrow transplants for thalassemia major have been done. Approximately 10 percent of the patients died of complications of marrow grafting, and 10 percent have regenerated their own marrow and again have thalassemia major. Eighty percent of the patients appear to be cured of the disease, although some 5 percent of the cured patients are under treatment for chronic GVHD. Good results are now being reported for older, multiply transfused patients.

Transplantation for severe aplastic anemia   (See Chap. 308) HLA-IDENTICAL SIBLING DONORS   Patients with severe aplastic anemia must be prepared for engraftment with immunosuppressive therapy. The most widely used regimen is cyclophosphamide (CY) 50 mg/kg on each of 4 days followed 36 h later by donor marrow. The first two successful transplants were reported in 1972, and these recipients are alive and well.

For ethical reasons, the initial marrow transplants were carried out in patients who had failed to benefit from conventional therapy after receiving multiple transfusions. One-third of the patients rejected the graft, and the long-term survival of these end-stage patients was 40 to 50 percent.

Since blood transfusions can sensitize an intended marrow transplant recipient, resulting in rejection of the marrow graft, patients with severe aplastic anemia were identified early in the course of the disease so that marrow transplantation could be carried out before blood transfusions were given. The long-term survival of these patients is more than 80 percent. Therefore, patients with severe aplastic anemia and their families should have tissue typing performed immediately upon diagnosis. If a suitable donor can be identified, marrow transplantation should be carried out promptly before transfusions become necessary.

However, many patients with severe aplastic anemia present to the physician with bleeding and/or infection, and transfusions must be given as an urgent medical necessity. Therefore, marrow transplant teams are investigating other preparative regimens designed to prevent graft rejection and to improve survival. These include regimens using various combinations of antithymocyte globulin (ATG), CY, and partial-body or total-nodal irradiation. A regimen involving the administration of 30 mg/kg of ATG between each dose of CY shows a survival of greater than 90 percent.

IDENTICAL TWIN DONORS   Aplastic anemia is not a common disease, and to find a patient with it who has an identical twin is even more uncommon. Nevertheless, a number of such transplants have been carried out. In some patients the simple intravenous infusion of marrow without any immunosuppressive treatment resulted in recovery. These results reinforce the concept that aplastic anemia is due to an acquired abnormality of the stem cell which can be corrected by transplantation of normal syngeneic stem cells. However, some patients did not recover after marrow infusion. These patients were then treated with the CY and given a second infusion of marrow from the twin, which resulted in complete hematopoietic reconstitution.

The results suggest that some cases may be due to an immune mechanism or abnormal regulators of cell growth. Whatever the mechanism, the rare patient with aplastic anemia who has a genetically identical twin has a 90 percent chance of being cured with marrow transplantation.

Transplantation for acute leukemia   Acute leukemia (see Chap. 310) has served as a prototype malignant disease of the marrow for treatment by intensive chemoradiotherapy and marrow transplantation. Until a decade ago, almost all regimens used for preparing leukemic patients for marrow transplantation employed supralethal total-body irradiation (TBI). CY, etoposide, cytosine arabinoside, or other antileukemic drugs are given with TBI to kill a greater fraction of leukemic cells. More recently, regimens using busulfan (BU) and CY (without TBI) are showing results equivalent to those with TBI.

ACUTE LEUKEMIA IN REFRACTORY RELAPSE USING HLA-IDENTICAL SIBLING DONORS   For ethical reasons, marrow transplantation was initially attempted only in patients with acute leukemia in relapse after chemotherapy. These end-stage patients presented with a heavy body burden of leukemic cells, were usually granulocytopenic and thrombocytopenic, and often were already infected with antibiotic-resistant bacteria and fungi. There were many deaths related to advanced illness, GVHD, opportunistic infections, or recurrent leukemia. Approximately 10 percent of these patients became long-term survivors with no further antileukemic therapy. The longest surviving patients are now 20 years postgrafting. Despite the use of a variety of different preparative regimens, long-term survival for these end-stage patients remains at about 5 to 15 percent.

ACUTE LEUKEMIA BEYOND FIRST REMISSION USING HLA-IDENTICAL SIBLING DONORS   Patients with acute leukemia who relapse have a high probability of dying of the disease even though additional remissions may be achieved. Transplantation in second or subsequent remission avoids the problems associated with a large body burden of leukemic cells. Marrow grafting for these patients has resulted in long-term disease-free survival of 40 to 60 percent.

Approximately one-half of patients with acute myeloid leukemia (AML) who relapse die without achieving a second remission. Transplantation in first relapse before additional chemotherapy also results in approximately 40 to 60 percent disease-free survival. Transplantation at the first sign of relapse may be the optimal timing, but relapse signaled by infection and the difficulty of quickly arranging for a transplant are obstacles.

ACUTE MYELOID LEUKEMIA IN FIRST REMISSION USING HLA-IDENTICAL DONORS   Patients with AML in first remission are known to have a poor prognosis. With combination chemotherapy, the median duration of the first remission is approximately 12 to 18 months, and only 20 to 25 percent of the patients are alive at 5 years after initial chemotherapy. Therefore, a study of marrow transplantation in those patients in first remission was considered to be ethically acceptable. Hundreds of such transplants have now been carried out, with various marrow transplant teams reporting 45 to 70 percent long-term disease-free survival.

Since about 20 percent of patients with AML in first remission already have been cured by chemotherapy, transplantation means that these patients will be exposed needlessly to the risks of this procedure. Nevertheless, five different randomized, prospective studies have demonstrated a better survival for patients given a marrow graft in first remission as compared with those treated with chemotherapy. Until methods for identifying those destined to relapse are perfected, marrow grafting is the preferred treatment.

ACUTE LYMPHOID LEUKEMIA IN FIRST REMISSION USING HLA-IDENTICAL DONORS   Patients with "good risk" characteristics of ALL at diagnosis have a 50 to 70 percent chance of being cured by chemotherapy and are not candidates for a marrow graft. Marrow grafts for patients with ALL in first remission generally have been restricted to patients who have characteristics indicating a poor prognosis with chemotherapy. Survival of such patients after marrow grafting has ranged from 10 to 60 percent, apparently depending on the criteria for selection.

CHRONIC MYELOID LEUKEMIA USING HLA-IDENTICAL DONORS
Marrow transplantation for patients with CML in blast crisis, like
other forms of advanced leukemia, has resulted in a cure rate of
approximately 15 percent.

Patients with the chronic phase of the disease are good candidates
for a marrow graft because they usually are in good condition without
infection or having had transfusions. Most CML patients have been
transplanted after preparation with CY and TBI. The disease-free
survival is approximately 60 percent, with the longest period exceeding
15 years. The absence of the Ph chromosome indicates cure of these
patients. Several more recent studies using TBI-containing regimens
or a BU-CY regimen show, on actuarial analysis, disease-free plateaus
of approximately 80 percent. The improvement in survival is probably
related to several advances in transplant technology, including the
prevention of viral infections and reduction in GVHD.

CML is a disease that can be controlled with BU or hydroxyurea
but is not cured by chemotherapy. The median survival is 30 to 50
months. Therapy with interferon-α may result in disappearance of
the Ph chromosome in some patients but, as yet, has not been
demonstrated to affect survival. Since the best results with marrow
grafting are seen when the transplant is carried out in the first 2 years
after diagnosis, all patients with CML should be considered for
marrow grafting and a donor sought.

OTHER MALIGNANT DISEASES TREATED BY MARROW GRAFTING
FROM HLA-IDENTICAL SIBLINGS Lymphomas, Hodgkin's disease,
multiple myeloma, myelodysplastic syndromes, breast cancer, ovarian
cancer, testicular cancer, and small cell lung cancer have been treated
with intensive chemoradiotherapy and a marrow graft. The results
vary widely, but in almost every category some patients have
apparently been cured of otherwise fatal disease. Particular attention
is being focused on lymphoma and Hodgkin's disease, with marrow
grafting being considered as the first form of therapy after failure of
initial standard therapy.

USE OF DONORS OTHER THAN HLA-IDENTICAL SIBLINGS Only
one-third of patients will have an HLA-identical sibling. Marrow
transplantation has been carried out between family member donor-
recipient pairs in which one of the HLA haplotypes was genetically
identical and the other haplotype phenotypically identical or differing
by only one locus. The results of these transplants are quite similar
to the results using an HLA-identical sibling donor. The outcome is
largely a function of the stage of the disease at the time of transplant.

HLA typing makes it technically possible to find a suitably matched
unrelated donor, at least for patients with the more common HLA
haplotypes. The National Marrow Donor Program has recruited more
than 600,000 donors, and more than 1400 transplants from unrelated
donors have been carried out. The recipients have more GVHD, but
disease-free survival seems almost as good as in recipients of matched
sibling grafts. The long-term results of these transplants are not yet
known.

Autologous marrow transplantation The technique for procur-
ing and cryopreserving marrow has been established for more than
20 years. The presence in the circulating blood of hematopoietic
progenitor cells (stem cells) also has been known for a long time.
Recently, it has been shown that the administration of G-CSF or GM-
CSF can markedly increase the number of stem cells in the circulating
blood and that these cells can be used for autologous grafting. Marrow
and blood stem cells can be used together to shorten significantly the
period of pancytopenia after autologous grafting. The use of autologous stem cells avoids the risk of GVHD. The following points are
pertinent in considering autologous stem cell transplantation: (1) The
stem cells should not be contaminated with malignant cells; (2)
autologous stem cells are of value only in protecting the patient
against lethal hematopoietic toxicity; (3) the tumor being treated must
show a dose-response curve such that supralethal chemoradiotherapy
can be expected to result in a significantly enhanced antitumor
response; and (4) the protocol must be designed so that the role of
autologous marrow can be demonstrated. In animals it is feasible to
administer "supralethal" therapy and to demonstrate that animals

given syngeneic marrow will survive while those not given marrow
will die. For obvious reasons, this kind of controlled experiment
cannot be done in humans. Failure to recognize these four principles
accounts for much of the current uncertainty about the value of
autologous marrow transplantation in the treatment of patients with
malignant disease.

As for allogeneic transplants, the tumors that might be expected
to show a significant improvement in response to high-dose chemoradiotherapy include the leukemias, Hodgkin's disease, non-Hodgkin's
lymphoma, multiple myeloma, small cell cancer of the lung, breast
cancer, testicular tumors, and ovarian tumors. Techniques being
explored for removal of tumor cells from the marrow include physical
separation, destruction by chemotherapeutic agents, and positive
selections of stem cells by monoclonal antibodies. The use of
cryopreserved autologous stem cells leads to successful hematopoietic
reconstitution in most patients. For hematologic malignancies, autologous transplantation after high-dose chemoradiotherapy results in
apparent cure of a significant fraction of patients; such a transplant
therefore offers an alternative to patients who do not have an HLA-
matched allogeneic donor. Autologous stem cell grafts are used
increasingly for treatment of metastatic breast cancer or breast
cancer patients with more than 10 positive nodes. The high-dose
chemotherapy includes CY, cisplatin, and carmustine. These autologous grafts are producing long-term disease-free survival of some
patients with breast cancer with an otherwise grim prognosis.

IMMUNOLOGIC ASPECTS OF MARROW TRANSPLANTATION
Marrow graft rejection *Marrow graft rejection* describes a phenomenon in which the transplanted marrow graft begins to function, but
after a few days or weeks, the peripheral blood counts suddenly drop
and marrow biopsy shows the marrow to be devoid of myeloid
elements. Immunologically mediated marrow graft rejection is usually
a consequence of sensitization by transfusions. In addition, inadequate
immunosuppressive therapy before grafting may facilitate marrow
graft rejection.

Marrow graft failure may be due to causes other than immunologic
mechanisms. With a solid organ, such as the kidney, histologic proof
of graft rejection is easily obtained, but such proof usually cannot be
obtained with a marrow graft because the myeloid marrow simply
disappears. Other possible mechanisms of graft failure include (1)
defective or inadequate numbers of stem cells in the donor marrow,
(2) defective microenvironment in the marrow recipient, (3) allogeneic
resistance not associated with HLA, and (4) susceptibility of the
donor marrow to the same etiologic mechanism(s) responsible for the
original disease process.

Acute graft-versus-host disease A "wasting disease" or "runt
disease" was described many years ago in newborn mice or in rodents
exposed to lethal TBI and given infusions of allogeneic hematopoietic
cells. The disease was recognized to be due to an immunologic
reaction of engrafted lymphoid cells, presumably T cells, against the
tissues of the host. In patients given a marrow graft from an HLA-
identical sibling and postgrafting immunosuppression, approximately
one-half develop moderate to severe GVHD.

Acute GVHD in humans usually involves the skin, gastrointestinal
tract, and/or the liver. A skin rash is usually the first sign of GVHD.
Intestinal involvement results in diarrhea and may progress to
abdominal pain and ileus. Liver disease is characterized by rises of
bilirubin, SGOT, and alkaline phosphatase. Severe immunologic
deficiency accompanies GVHD, and death from infection is frequent.

Since GVHD is immunologically mediated, efforts to prevent its
development have involved the use of immunosuppressive therapy.
Of the many agents studied, methotrexate, glucocorticoids, and
cyclosporine were found to be useful. Cyclosporine is a potent
immunosuppressive agent that does not cause mucositis, as methotrexate does, and does not suppress the marrow graft, so effective marrow
function is evident earlier. Cyclosporine is nephrotoxic, and marrow
graft recipients often receive other nephrotoxic agents such as
amphotericin. Creatinine and serum cyclosporine levels must be
monitored carefully, with prompt reduction of dosage if renal function

is threatened. A regimen using a short course of methotrexate along with cyclosporine has proved highly effective in reducing the incidence and severity of acute GVHD.

A number of studies have been carried out in an effort to treat acute GVHD once it becomes established. Recipients of HLA-identical marrow have been treated with rabbit, goat, or horse ATG, high-dose methyl prednisolone, cyclosporine, and/or anti-T cell monoclonal antibodies. About two-thirds of patients will respond to one or another of these agents. However, about one-third of the patients who develop moderate to severe GVHD will die of it or its infectious complications.

Experiments are underway designed to eliminate from the marrow inoculum the T cells believed to be responsible for GVHD while retaining hematopoietic stem cells. One approach involves treatment of the donor marrow with lectins for agglutination and separation of the T cells. Monoclonal antibodies that react with human T cells or subsets of T cells are being used in conjunction with complement or are bound to toxins, such as the A chain of ricin, to create an immunotoxin. The preliminary results of these studies indicate a reduction in the incidence and severity of GVHD. However, the incidence of graft failure and of recurrence of leukemia is significantly increased. The explanation for these problems is unknown.

Chronic GVHD   Chronic GVHD occurs in approximately one-fourth of those recipients of marrow from an HLA-identical sibling who survive beyond 100 days. The manifestations include skin disease, keratoconjunctivitis, buccal mucositis, esophageal strictures, small- and large-intestinal involvement, pulmonary insufficiency, chronic liver disease, and generalized wasting. Histologically, the disease resembles the systemic collagen vascular diseases, especially morphea and lupus erythematosus profundus. Chronic GVHD may be associated with recurrent and occasionally fatal bacterial infections.

Treatment of chronic GVHD with short courses of ATG or prolonged treatment with prednisone has been only partially effective. Twenty percent continue to have problems which may be disabling, and cyclosporine, intermittent steroids, thalidomide, or monoclonal antibodies alone or bound to a toxin are being tried for the refractory patients.

Recovery of immunologic function   Despite recovery from pancytopenia, most allogeneic recipients are susceptible to a wide variety of opportunistic infections. Historically, approximately one-fifth of patients developed an interstitial pneumonia, and cytomegalovirus was demonstrated in more than one-half of these pneumonias. The mortality rate was approximately 80 percent. Use of blood products from donors who are serologically negative for CMV for those donor-recipient pairs who also serologically negative and the use of prophylactic ganciclovir have almost eliminated CMV infection and pneumonia. Susceptibility to infection is the result of a very slow return of immunologic function, which may be made worse by GVHD and by efforts to prevent or treat GVHD. Fortunately, by the end of the first year after grafting, most patients have recovered immunologically and are able to lead normal lives without an increased incidence of infection.

Tolerance   The long-term healthy human recipients of allogeneic marrow transplants are true chimeras. Their myeloid, lymphoid, and monocyte-macrophage systems are made up of cells of donor origin. Clearly, these donor cells in the recipient are "tolerant" of the host's tissues. Studies of tolerance constitute a fascinating story in immunobiology, but a clear understanding of the state of tolerance has not emerged. At least three mechanisms may be operative, including classical central tolerance due to clonal deletion, tolerance due to clonal anergy, and tolerance related to the presence of active "suppressor" cells.

The effect of age   The success of allogeneic marrow grafting is inversely proportional to the age of the recipient. For example, for patients transplanted in first remission of AML, long-term survival for those under age 20 is approximately 75 percent, and for patients aged 30 to 50, 40 percent. The most apparent explanation for this difference is the increased incidence and severity of GVHD in older

patients. Most marrow transplant centers do not transplant patients over age 50. These age restrictions do not apply to syngeneic or autologous transplants because these patients do not have GVHD, although patients over age 50 do not tolerate intensive treatment as well as younger patients.

RECURRENT LEUKEMIA AFTER GRAFTING   Frequency   For patients with leukemia transplanted in relapse or in second remission, actuarial analysis shows a rather constant rate of recurrence of leukemia in the first year, a decreasing rate in the second year, and few recurrences thereafter. If there were no other causes of death, 30 to 70 percent would be destined to relapse. However, the risk of relapse is only 15 to 20 percent for patients with AML transplanted in first remission or CML transplanted in the chronic phase. It is evident that recurrent leukemia after grafting is a major problem for patients transplanted in relapse or in second or subsequent remission.

Nature of recurrent leukemia   Blood genetic markers, cytogenetic techniques, and restriction enzyme fragment length polymorphisms can be used to identify the donor or host origin of the leukemic cells in patients who relapse after marrow transplantation. In the vast majority of patients, the recurrent leukemia is in host-type cells, indicating that the preparative regimen and the graft did not eliminate all the leukemic cells. However, several cases have now been reported in which the recurrent leukemic cells were shown to be of donor origin. The mechanism of donor cell transformation is unknown. In more than a dozen cases a lymphoblastic lymphoma associated with Epstein-Barr virus genomes has occurred in donor cells. These highly fatal lymphomas have usually occurred in patients undergoing intensive treatment for GVHD.

Graft-versus-leukemia effect   In recipients of allogeneic marrow grafts, evidence supporting the existence of a graft-versus-leukemia effect has been difficult to obtain because of the large number of deaths from other causes among patients with severe GVHD. Statistical methods have shown that the relative relapse rate for patients transplanted in relapse or for ALL in second remission was 2.5 times greater in recipients without GVHD than in those with GVHD. Recipients of allogeneic marrow who did not develop GVHD had approximately the same relapse rate as recipients of syngeneic marrow, indicating that subclinical GVHD did not reduce the relapse rate.

GENERALIZATIONS ABOUT MARROW TRANSPLANTATION   Because of the complexity of the marrow grafting regimens, transplantation should be undertaken only by teams with all the resources needed to ensure an optimal result. The number of such teams has increased rapidly over the past few years.

Marrow transplantation is obviously an expensive undertaking, primarily because of hospital costs, but cost has been reduced appreciably by transplantation earlier in the course of the disease when the patient is in relatively good condition. The introduction of hematopoietic growth factors should further reduce cost by shortening the time in the hospital. Cost analysis studies comparing marrow transplantation with combination therapy have found marrow transplantation to be more cost-effective.

The ethical problems of exposing a patient and donor to the marrow transplant regimen and the risk of death in the first 1 to 3 months after grafting have limited the use of marrow transplantation. However, the demonstration of better long-term survival rates with marrow transplantation compared with conventional therapy for several diseases and the cure of some diseases not cured by conventional therapy should alleviate the ethical concern. Extension of this form of therapy to other malignant diseases and to a variety of genetic disorders is being reported, and the current rapid rate of progress and the availability of unrelated volunteer donors may soon make a much broader application of marrow grafting a reality.

REFERENCES

ARMITAGE JD: Drug therapy: Treatment of non-Hodgkin's lymphoma. N Engl J Med 328:1023, 1993

APPELBAUM FR et al: Chemotherapy v marrow transplantation for adults with acute nonlymphocytic leukemia: A five-year follow-up. Blood 72:179, 1988

BEATTY PG et al: Marrow transplantation from related donors other than HLA identical siblings. N Engl J Med 313:765, 1985

CLIFT RA et al: The treatment of acute non-lymphoblastic leukemia by allogeneic marrow transplantation. Bone Marrow Transplant 2:243, 1987

COPELAN JC et al: Radiation-free preparation for allogeneic bone marrow transplantation in adults with acute lymphoblastic leukemia. J Clin Oncol 10:237, 1992

GOLDMAN JM et al: Bone marrow transplantation for chronic myelogenous leukemia in chronic phase. Ann Intern Med 108:806, 1988

GOODRICH JM et al: Prevention of cytomegalovirus disease after allogeneic marrow transplant by ganciclovir prophylaxis. Ann Intern Med 118:173, 1993

KESSINGER A, ARMITAGE JO: The evolving role of autologous peripheral stem cell transplantation following high-dose therapy for malignancies. Blood 77:211, 1991

LUCARELLI G et al: Bone marrow transplantation in patients with thalassemia. N Engl J Med 322:417, 1990

MARTIN P et al: Effects of in vitro depletion of T cells in HLA-identical allogeneic marrow grafts. Blood 66:664, 1985

MEYERS JD, THOMAS ED: Infection complicating bone marrow transplantation, in *Clinical Approach to Infection in the Immunocompromised Host*, RH Rubin, LS Young (eds). New York, Plenum Press, 1981, p 507

NEMUNAITIS J et al: Recombinant granulocyte-macrophage colony-stimulating factor after autologous bone marrow transplantation for lymphoid cancer. N Engl J Med 324:1773, 1991

PHILIP T et al: High-dose therapy and autologous bone marrow transplantation after failure of conventional chemotherapy in adults with intermediate-grade or high-grade non-Hodgkin's lymphoma. N Engl J Med 316:1493, 1987

STORB R et al: Marrow transplantation for aplastic anemia. Semin Hematol 21:27, 1984

——— et al: Methotrexate and cyclosporine compared with cyclosporine alone for prophylaxis of acute graft versus host disease after marrow transplantation for leukemia. N Engl J Med 314:729, 1986

SULLIVAN KM et al: Chronic graft-versus-host disease in 52 patients: Adverse natural course and successful treatment with combination immunosuppression. Blood 57:267, 1981

THOMAS ED et al: Bone-marrow transplantation. N Engl J Med 292:832, 895, 1975

——— et al: Marrow transplantation for the treatment of chronic myelogenous leukemia. Ann Intern Med 104:155, 1986

WEIDEN PL et al: Antileukemic effect of graft-versus-host disease in human recipients of allogeneic-marrow grafts. N Engl J Med 300:1068, 1979

YEAGER AM et al: Autologous bone marrow transplantation in patients with acute nonlymphocytic leukemia, using ex vivo marrow treatment with 4-hydroperoxycyclophosphamide. N Engl J Med 315:141, 1986

ZUTTER MM et al: Epstein-Barr virus lymphoproliferation after bone marrow transplantation. Blood 72:520, 1988

---

section 2 Clotting disorders

---

314 DISORDERS OF THE PLATELET AND VESSEL WALL

ROBERT I. HANDIN

Patients with platelet or vessel wall disorders usually bleed into superficial sites such as the skin, mucous membranes, or genitourinary or gastrointestinal tract. Bleeding begins immediately after trauma and either responds to simple measures such as pressure and packing or requires systemic therapy with glucocorticoids, plasma fractions, or platelet concentrates. The most common platelet/vessel wall disorders are (1) various forms of thrombocytopenia, (2) von Willebrand's disease, and (3) drug-induced platelet dysfunction. This chapter reviews the diagnosis and treatment of quantitative and qualitative platelet disorders as well as vessel wall defects which cause bleeding. The physiology of normal hemostasis and the cardinal manifestations of bleeding arising from hemostatic disorders have been reviewed in Chap. 57.

PLATELET DISORDERS

Platelets arise from the fragmentation of megakaryocytes, which are very large, polyploid bone marrow cells produced by several cycles of chromosomal duplication without cytoplasmic division. After leaving the marrow space, approximately one-third of the platelets are sequestered in the spleen, while the other two-thirds circulate for 7 to 10 days. Normally, only a small fraction of the platelet mass is consumed in the process of hemostasis, so most platelets circulate until they become senescent and are removed by phagocytic cells. The normal blood platelet count is maintained between 150,000 and 450,000 per microliter. Although the regulatory signals are not well-defined, a decrease in platelet mass stimulates an increase in the number, size, and ploidy of megakaryocytes, releasing additional platelets into the circulation.

The platelet count varies during the menstrual cycle, rising following ovulation and falling at the onset of menses. It is also influenced by the patient's nutritional state and can be decreased in severe iron, folic acid, or vitamin B_{12} deficiency. Platelets are *acute phase reactants*, and patients with systemic inflammation, tumors, bleeding, and mild iron deficiency may have an increased platelet count, a benign condition called *secondary* or *reactive thrombocytosis*. In contrast, the increase in platelet count that is characteristic of the myeloproliferative disorders such as polycythemia vera, chronic myelogenous leukemia, myeloid metaplasia, and essential thrombocytosis can cause either severe bleeding or thrombosis.

MECHANISM OF THROMBOCYTOPENIA Thrombocytopenia is caused by one of three mechanisms—decreased bone marrow production, increased splenic sequestration, or accelerated destruction of platelets. In order to determine the etiology of thrombocytopenia, each patient should have a careful examination of the peripheral blood film, an assessment of marrow morphology by examination of an aspirate or biopsy, and an estimate of splenic size by bedside palpation supplemented, if necessary, by ultrasonography or computed tomographic (CT) scan. Occasional patients have "pseudothrombocytopenia," a benign condition in which platelets agglutinate or adhere to leukocytes when blood is collected with EDTA as anticoagulant. This is a laboratory artifact, and the actual platelet count in vivo is normal. A scheme for classifying patients with thrombocytopenia based on these clinical observations and laboratory tests is outlined in Fig. 314-1.

Impaired production Disorders that injure stem cells or prevent their proliferation in marrow frequently cause thrombocytopenia. They usually affect multiple hematopoietic cell lines so that thrombocytopenia is accompanied by varying degrees of anemia and leukopenia. Diagnosis of a platelet production defect is readily established by examination of a bone marrow aspirate or biopsy, which should show a reduced number of megakaryocytes. The most common causes of decreased platelet production are marrow aplasia, fibrosis, or infiltration with malignant cells, all of which produce highly characteristic marrow abnormalities. Occasionally, thrombocytopenia is the presenting laboratory abnormality in these disorders. Cytotoxic drugs, which are frequently used in cancer chemotherapy, impair megakaryocyte proliferation and maturation and frequently cause thrombocytopenia. There are also rare marrow disorders such as congenital amegakaryocytic hypoplasia and thrombocytopenia with absent radii

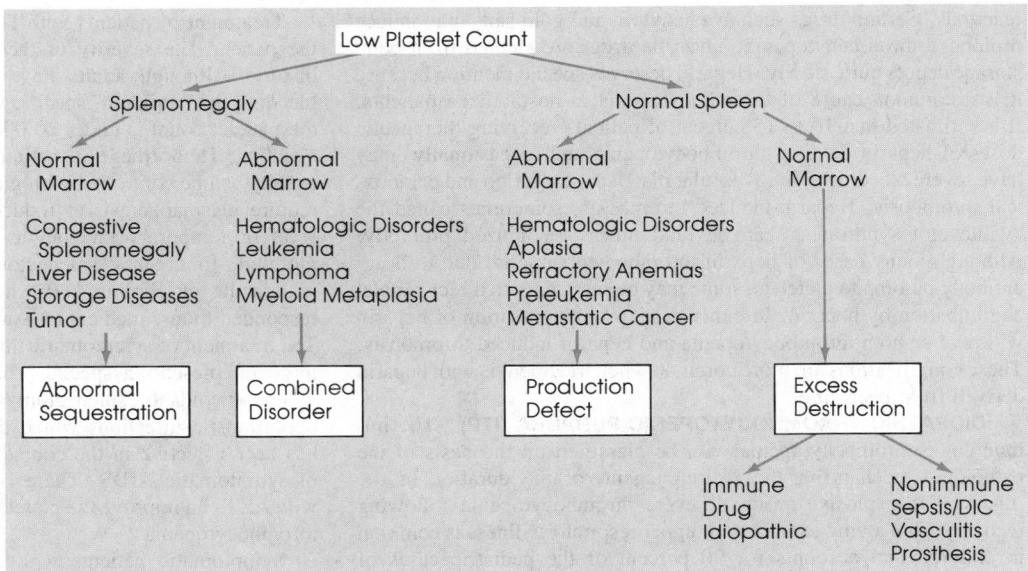

FIGURE 314-1   Clinical evaluation of patients with thrombocytopenia (*Modified from RI Handin, in W Beck (ed). Hematology, 4th ed, Cambridge, Mass, MIT Press, 1985.*)

(TAR syndrome), which selectively decrease megakaryocyte production.

Splenic sequestration   Since one-third of the platelet mass is normally sequestered in the spleen, splenectomy will increase the platelet count by 30 percent. Postsplenectomy thrombocytosis is a benign self-limited condition which does not require specific therapy. In contrast, when the spleen enlarges, the fraction of sequestered platelets increases, lowering the platelet count. The most common causes of splenomegaly are portal hypertension secondary to liver disease and splenic infiltration with tumor cells in myeloproliferative or lymphoproliferative disorders or with macrophages in storage disorders such as Gaucher's disease. Isolated splenomegaly is rare, and in most patients, splenomegaly is accompanied by other clinical manifestations of the underlying disease. Many patients with leukemia, lymphoma, or a myeloproliferative syndrome have both marrow infiltration and splenomegaly and develop thrombocytopenia from a combination of impaired marrow production and splenic sequestration of platelets.

Accelerated destruction   Abnormal vessels, fibrin thrombi, and intravascular prostheses can all shorten platelet survival and cause *nonimmunologic thrombocytopenia.* For example, thrombocytopenia is common in patients with vasculitis, the hemolytic uremic syndrome, thrombotic thrombocytopenic purpura (TTP), as one manifestation of disseminated intravascular coagulation (DIC), and in patients with prosthetic cardiac valves. In addition, platelets coated with antibody, immune complexes, or complement are rapidly cleared by mononuclear phagocytes in the spleen or other tissues inducing *immunologic thrombocytopenia.* The most common causes of immunologic thrombocytopenia are viral or bacterial infections, drugs, and a chronic autoimmune disorder referred to as *idiopathic thrombocytopenic purpura* (ITP). Patients with immunologic thrombocytopenia do not usually have splenomegaly and have an active bone marrow with an increased number of megakaryocytes.

DRUG-INDUCED THROMBOCYTOPENIA   Many common drugs can cause thrombocytopenia (Table 314-1). As previously mentioned, many chemotherapeutic agents are cytotoxic and depress megakaryocyte production. Ingestion of large quantities of alcohol has a similar marrow-depressing effect leading to transient thrombocytopenia. The syndrome is particularly common in binge drinkers. Thiazide diuretics, which are used commonly to treat hypertension or congestive heart failure, impair megakaryocyte production and can produce mild thrombocytopenia (50,000 to 100,000 per microliter), which may persist for several months after the drug is discontinued.

Most drugs induce thrombocytopenia by eliciting an immune response in which the platelet is an innocent bystander. The platelet is damaged by complement activation following the formation of drug-antibody complexes. Current laboratory tests can identify the causative agent in 10 percent of patients with clinical evidence of drug-induced thrombocytopenia. The best proof of a drug-induced etiology is a prompt rise in the platelet count when the suspected drug is discontinued. Patients with drug-induced platelet destruction also may have a secondary increase in megakaryocyte number without other marrow abnormalities.

Although most patients recover within 7 to 10 days and do not require therapy, occasional patients with platelet counts below 10,000 to 20,000 per microliter have severe hemorrhage and may require temporary support with glucocorticoids, plasmapheresis, or platelet transfusions while waiting for the platelet count to rise. A patient who has recovered from drug-induced immunologic thrombocytopenia should be instructed to avoid the offending drug in the future, since only minute amounts of drug are needed to set up subsequent immune

---

TABLE 314-1   Drugs implicated in thrombocytopenia

SUPPRESSION OF PLATELET PRODUCTION

A Myelosuppressive drugs
   1 Severe: cytosine arabinoside, daunorubicin
   2 Moderate: cyclophosphamide, busulfan, methotrexate, 6-mercaptopurine
   3 Mild: vinca alkaloids
B Thiazide diuretics
C Ethanol
D Estrogens

IMMUNOLOGIC PLATELET DESTRUCTION

A Clinical suspicion plus convincing experimental evidence
   1 Antibiotics: sulfathiazole, novobiocin, *p*-aminosalicylate
   2 Cinchona alkaloids: quinidine, quinine
   3 Foods: beans
   4 Sedatives, hypnotics, anticonvulsants: apronalide, carbamazepine
   5 Arsenical drugs used to treat syphilis
   6 Digitoxin
   7 Methyldopa
   8 Stibophen
B Clinical suspicion (major drugs implicated)
   1 Aspirin
   2 Chlorpropamide
   3 Chloroquine
   4 Chlorothiazide and hydrochlorothiazide
   5 Gold salts
   6 Insecticides
   7 Sulfadiazine, sulfisoxazole, sulfamerazine, sulfamethazine, sulfamethoxypyridazine, sulfamethoxazole, sulfatolamide

reactions. Certain drugs such as phenytoin and gold salts may induce prolonged thrombocytopenia, since the drugs are cleared from body storage depots quite slowly. Heparin deserves special mention because it is a common cause of thrombocytopenia in hospitalized patients. It is estimated that 10 to 15 percent of patients receiving therapeutic doses of heparin develop thrombocytopenia and, occasionally, may have severe bleeding or intravascular platelet aggregation and paradoxical thrombosis. Heparin-induced thrombosis, sometimes called the "white clot syndrome," can be fatal unless recognized promptly. Although many cases of heparin thrombocytopenia are due to drug-antibody binding to platelets, some may be secondary to direct platelet agglutination by heparin. In either case, prompt cessation of heparin will reverse both thrombocytopenia and heparin-induced thrombosis. These complications are more common when treatment is with heparin derived from beef lung.

IDIOPATHIC THROMBOCYTOPENIC PURPURA (ITP) The immunologic thrombocytopenias can be classified on the basis of the pathologic mechanism, the inciting agent, or the duration of the illness. The explosive onset of severe thrombocytopenia following recovery from a viral exanthem or upper respiratory illness is common in children and accounts for 90 percent of the pediatric cases of immunologic thrombocytopenia. This syndrome is usually called *acute idiopathic thrombocytopenic purpura* (acute ITP). Of these patients, 60 percent recover in 4 to 6 weeks and over 90 percent recover within 3 to 6 months. Transient immunologic thrombocytopenia also complicates some cases of infectious mononucleosis, acute toxoplasmosis, or cytomegalovirus infection and can be part of the prodromal phase of viral hepatitis. Acute ITP is rare in adults and accounts for less than 10 percent of postpubertal patients with immune thrombocytopenia. Acute ITP is caused by immune complexes containing viral antigens which bind to platelet Fc receptors or by antibodies produced against viral antigens which cross-react with the platelet. In addition to the viral disorders described above, the differential diagnosis should include atypical presentations of aplastic anemia, acute leukemias, or metastatic tumor. A bone marrow examination is essential to exclude these disorders, which can occasionally mimic acute ITP.

Most adults present with a more indolent form of thrombocytopenia which may persist for many years and is referred to as *chronic ITP*. Women aged 20 to 40 are afflicted most commonly and outnumber men by a ratio of 3:1. They may present with an abrupt fall in platelet count and bleeding similar to patients with acute ITP. More often they have a prior history of easy bruising or menometrorrhagia. These patients have an autoimmune disorder with antibodies directed against target antigens on the glycoprotein IIb-IIIa or glycoprotein Ib-IX complex (see Fig. 57-2). Although most antibodies function as opsonins and accelerate platelet clearance by phagocytic cells, occasional antibodies bind to epitopes on critical regions of these glycoproteins and impair platelet function. A number of tests have been introduced to measure platelet-associated IgG. Although the tests are quite sensitive, their specificity is a problem. First, there is a high "background" level of IgG on normal platelets. Second, an elevation in plasma immunoglobulin levels or in circulating immune complexes will nonspecifically increase platelet-associated IgG.

Since a low platelet count may be the initial manifestation of systemic lupus erythematosus (SLE) or the first sign of a primary hematologic disorder, all patients with chronic ITP should have a bone marrow examination and an antinuclear antibody determination. In addition, patients with hepatic or splenic enlargement, lymphadenopathy, or atypical lymphocytes should have serologic studies for hepatitis, cytomegalovirus, Epstein-Barr virus, toxoplasma, and HIV. HIV infection has rapidly become a common cause of immunologic thrombocytopenia and should be considered in the differential diagnosis of thrombocytopenia, especially in high-risk groups—homosexuals, hemophiliacs, intravenous drug abusers, and heterosexual individuals with multiple partners. Thrombocytopenia can be the initial symptom of HIV infection or a complication of fully developed clinical AIDS.

Treatment of patients with ITP must take into account the age of the patient, the severity of the illness, and the anticipated natural history. Although adults have a higher incidence of intracranial bleeding than children, specific therapy may not be necessary unless the platelet count is under 20,000 per microliter or there is extensive bleeding. Hemorrhage in patients with either acute or chronic ITP usually can be controlled with glucocorticoids but, in rare cases, may require plasmapheresis to reduce the antibody or immune-complex level or temporary phagocytic blockade with intravenous gamma globulin. Emergency splenectomy is usually reserved for patients with acute or chronic ITP who are desperately ill and have not responded to any medical measures designed to improve hemostasis. The treatment of symptomatic thrombocytopenia in patients with HIV infection presents a special problem because the administration of glucocorticoids or splenectomy may increase susceptibility to the opportunistic infections which threaten these patients. Splenectomy has been effective in the course of HIV infection prior to the onset of symptomatic AIDS. There is increasing evidence that treatment with AZT can improve the platelet count in patients with HIV-induced thrombocytopenia.

Symptomatic patients with chronic ITP are usually placed on glucocorticoids. In one standard regimen, 60 mg prednisone is administered for 4 to 6 weeks and then decreased over another few weeks. Approximately 50 percent of patients with chronic ITP will normalize their platelet count on high doses of prednisone. However, the majority will have a fall in platelet count following steroid withdrawal. Patients with chronic ITP who fail to maintain a normal platelet count after a course of steroids are eligible for elective splenectomy. These steroid-responsive but steroid-dependent patients are very likely to respond to splenectomy, and 70 percent will have a normal platelet count within 1 week after surgery. Some patients who do not respond to glucocorticoids may still respond to splenectomy. Occasionally, patients may fail to respond to splenectomy because of the failure to remove an accessory spleen. In other patients, a small inactive accessory spleen may grow or new splenic foci may develop from splenic cells shed at the time of surgery and cause the late onset of thrombocytopenia. In either case, the presence of splenic tissue can be diagnosed by examination of the blood smear for Howell-Jolly bodies which appear in the red cells of asplenic individuals. This can be confirmed by a radionuclide scan.

Patients who are still thrombocytopenic after steroid therapy or splenectomy or who relapse months to years after initial therapy have received a variety of immunosuppressive drugs including azathioprine, cyclophosphamiade, vincristine, and vinblastine. More recently, danazol, an impeded androgen, has been used with some success. Although each of these drugs may be beneficial, it is important to use some restraint because they have serious side effects. Intravenous gamma globulin (IVIG) has become a popular therapy, although it is only transiently effective and is quite expensive. It should be used to temporarily raise the platelet count and to support patients prior to surgery or labor and delivery. Anti-RhD therapy appears to be equally effective, although a form suitable for intravenous administration must be obtained. If a patient is not bleeding and maintains a platelet count over 20,000 per microliter, consideration should be given to withholding therapy, since there are many patients with severe chronic thrombocytopenia who have lived with their disease for two or three decades.

VON WILLEBRAND'S DISEASE Von Willebrand's disease (vWD) is the most common inherited bleeding disorder and may occur in as many as 1 in 800 to 1000 individuals. The von Willebrand factor (vWF) is a heterogeneous multimeric plasma glycoprotein with two major functions. It facilitates platelet adhesion under conditions of high shear stress by linking platelet membrane receptors to vascular subendothelium; it also serves as the plasma carrier for factor VIII, the antihemophilic factor, a critical blood coagulation protein. Discrete domains in each vWF subunit mediate each of these important functions (Fig. 314-2). The normal plasma vWF level is 10 mg/L. The vWF activity is distributed among a series of plasma multimers

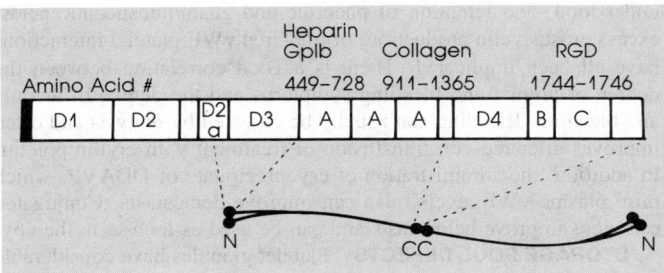

FIGURE 314-2 Domain structure of the von Willebrand protein (vWF) and its relation to the physical structure of the protein as determined by electron microscopy. The letters represent the repeated sequence elements that encode each vWF subunit. The propolypeptide, which is cleaved during multimer assembly, is encoded by the D1 and D2 repeats. The globular amino-terminal domain is encoded by the D2a and D3 repeats and the carboxy-terminal domain by the D4 repeat. The elongated filamentous region, which contains vWF binding sites for GpIb, heparin, and collagen, is encoded by the three A repeats. The amino acid residues that comprise the functional binding sites are shown at the top of the figure.

with estimated molecular weights ranging from 400,000 to over 20 million. A single large vWF precursor subunit is synthesized in endothelial cells and megakaryocytes, where it is cleaved and assembled into the disulfide-linked multimers present in plasma, platelets, and vascular subendothelium. A modest reduction in plasma vWF concentration or a selective loss in the high-molecular-weight multimers decreases platelet adhesion and causes clinical bleeding.

Although vWD is heterogeneous, there are certain clinical features which are common to all the syndromes. With one exception (type III disease), all forms are inherited as autosomal dominant traits and affected patients are heterozygous with one normal and one abnormal vWF allele. In mild cases, bleeding occurs only after surgery or trauma. More severely affected patients have spontaneous epistaxis or oral mucosal, gastrointestinal, or genitourinary bleeding. The laboratory findings are variable. The most diagnostic pattern is the combination of (1) a prolonged bleeding time, (2) a reduction in plasma vWF concentration, (3) a parallel reduction in ristocetin cofactor activity, and (4) reduced factor VIII activity. The variability in laboratory tests is related to both the heterogeneous nature of the defects in vWD and the fact that plasma levels are influenced by ABO blood group type, central nervous system disorders, systemic inflammation, and pregnancy. Since vWD is an autosomal dominant disorder, some vWF is produced by the remaining normal allele. Thus patients with mild defects may have laboratory values that fluctuate over time and may occasionally be within the normal range.

There are three major types of vWD. Patients with *type I disease*, the most common abnormality, have a mild to moderate decrease in plasma vWF. In the milder cases, although hemostasis is clearly impaired, the vWF level is just below the lower limit of normal (50 percent activity, or 5 mg/L). In type I disease, there is a parallel decrease in vWF antigen, factor VIII activity, and ristocetin cofactor activity, with a normal spectrum of multimers detected by sodium dodecyl sulfate–agarose (SDS-agarose) gel electrophoresis. Cultured endothelial cells derived from the umbilical cords of patients with vWD synthesize and secrete reduced quantities of vWF multimer and have a two- to fourfold reduction in vWF mRNA.

The variant forms of vWD (*type II disease*), which are much less common, are characterized by normal or near-normal levels of a dysfunctional protein. Patients with the *type IIa variant* of vWD have a deficiency in the high- and medium-molecular-weight forms of vWF multimer detected by SDS-agarose electrophoresis. This is due either to an inability to secrete the high-molecular-weight vWF multimers or to proteolysis of the multimers soon after they leave the endothelial cell and enter the circulation. Mutations in a localized region of the vWF A-2 domain have been identified in families with type IIa vWD. The quantity of vWF antigen and the amount of associated factor

VIII are usually normal. In the *type IIb variant*, there is also a loss in high-molecular-weight multimers. However, in type IIb disease, it is due to the inappropriate binding of vWF to platelets. This forms intravascular platelet aggregates which are rapidly cleared from the circulation, causing mild, cyclic thrombocytopenia. Mutations in a disulfide-bonded loop in the A-1 domain that binds to glycoprotein Ib-IX have been identified as the cause of the type IIb defect. A few patients have been described with a platelet membrane disorder which mimics type IIb vWD—*platelet-type vWD*. It is due to mutations in the portion of glycoprotein/IX which interacts with vWF. Levels of total vWF antigen and factor VIII are normal.

Approximately 1 in 1 million individuals have a very severe form of vWD that is phenotypically recessive (*type III disease*). Type III patients are usually the offspring of two parents with mild type I disease. However, in many cases, the parents are very mildly affected or are asymptomatic. Type III patients may inherit a different abnormality from each parent (a doubly heterozygous state) or be homozygous for a single defect. Type III patients have severe mucosal bleeding, no detectable vWF antigen or activity, and may have sufficiently low factor VIII levels to have occasional hemarthroses like mild hemophiliacs. Several type III families have been described with major deletions in the vWF gene that were detected by Southern blotting with vWF cDNA. In addition, families with nonsense mutations and a combination of a deleted and nonsense mutant allele have been described.

Appropriate therapy of vWD depends on the symptoms and the underlying type of disease. There are two therapeutic options. One involves the use of cryoprecipitate, a plasma fraction enriched in vWF, or factor VIII concentrates which retain high-molecular-weight vWF multimers (Humate-P, Koate HS). The factor VIII concentrates are highly purified and heat-treated to destroy HIV and are appropriate treatments for all the inherited forms of vWD. During surgery or after major trauma, patients should receive cryoprecipitate or factor VIII concentrate twice daily. This regimen should be continued twice daily for 48 to 72 h to ensure optimal hemostasis. Minor bleeding episodes such as prolonged epistaxis or severe menorrhagia may respond to a single transfusion. Recurrent menorrhagia, a major problem for women with severe vWD, can be treated effectively with oral contraceptive agents that suppress menses.

A second therapeutic option, which avoids the use of plasma, is the use of 1-desamino-8-D-arginine vasopressin (DDAVP), a vasopressin analogue which has minimal blood pressure-elevating and fluid-retaining properties and raises the plasma vWF level in normal individuals and patients with mild vWD. Patients with type I disease are the best candidates for DDAVP therapy. However, they must be tested for an adequate response prior to anticipated surgery, and vWF levels must be monitored closely during therapy, since the patient may develop tachyphylaxis when therapy is continued for more than 48 h. DDAVP should not be given to patients with variant forms of vWD without prior testing, since it may not improve multimer pattern or hemostasis in type IIa patients and it may actually worsen the defect by depleting high-molecular-weight multimers forming intravascular platelet aggregation and lowering the platelet count in type IIb patients. It is also ineffective therapy for most patients with the severe form (type III) of vWD.

Although most cases of vWD are inherited, there are also acquired forms of vWD caused by antibodies which inhibit vWF function or by lymphoid or other tumors which selectively adsorb vWF multimers onto their surfaces. Anti-vWF antibodies have developed in patients with severe vWD following multiple transfusions, as well as in patients with autoimmune and lymphoproliferative disorders. Adsorption of vWF to tumor surfaces has been documented in patients with Waldenström's macroglobulinemia and Wilm's tumor and inferred in other patients with lymphoma. Treatment of acquired vWD should focus on controlling the underlying disease, since plasma derivatives and DDAVP are often not effective and the disorder can be fatal.

PLATELET MEMBRANE DEFECTS   Receptors which modulate platelet adhesion and aggregation are located on the two major platelet surface glycoproteins. As previously discussed (see Chap. 57), vWF facilitates platelet adhesion by binding to glycoprotein Ib-IX, while fibrinogen links platelets into aggregates via sites on the glycoprotein IIb-IIIa complex. There are two rare but well-defined platelet defects characterized by a loss of or a defect in these glycoprotein receptors. Patients with the *Bernard-Soulier syndrome* have markedly reduced platelet adhesion and cannot bind vWF to their platelets owing to deficiency or dysfunction of the glycoprotein Ib-IX complex. They also have reduced levels of several other membrane proteins, mild thrombocytopenia, and extremely large, lymphocytoid platelets. Platelets from patients with *Glanzmann's disease* or *thrombasthenia* are deficient in or have a defect in the glycoprotein IIb-IIIa complex. Their platelets do not bind fibrinogen and cannot form aggregates, although the platelets undergo shape change and secretion and are of normal size.

Both these disorders are inherited as autosomal recessive traits and are characterized by markedly impaired hemostasis and recurrent episodes of severe mucosal hemorrhage. In keeping with the selective nature of the defects, Bernard-Soulier platelets react normally to all stimuli except ristocetin. In contrast, thrombasthenic platelets adhere normally and will agglutinate with ristocetin but will not aggregate with any of the agonists which require fibrinogen binding, such as adenosine diphosphate (ADP), thrombin, or epinephrine.

The only effective therapy for hemorrhagic episodes in these two disorders is transfusion with normal platelets. This is usually effective, although alloimmunization will eventually limit the life span of infused platelets. In addition, a few patients have developed inhibitor antibodies with specificity for the missing protein. These antibodies bind to the protein which is expressed on the transfused normal platelets and impair their function.

PLATELET RELEASE DEFECTS   The most common mild bleeding disorders arise from the ingestion of aspirin and other nonsteroidal anti-inflammatory drugs (NSAIDs) which inhibit platelet production of thromboxane A_2, an important mediator of platelet secretion and aggregation (see Figs. 57-3 and 57-4). These drugs inhibit platelet cyclooxygenase, which converts arachidonic acid to a labile endoperoxide intermediate that is critical for thromboxane formation. Aspirin is the most potent agent, since it irreversibly acetylates the platelet enzyme so that a single dose impairs hemostasis for 5 to 7 days. The other agents are competitive and reversible inhibitors with more transient effects. Blocking thromboxane A_2 synthesis partially inhibits platelet release and aggregation with weak agonists such as ADP and epinephrine and produces a mild hemostatic defect. The administration of high doses of certain antibiotics, particularly penicillin, can coat the platelet surface, block platelet release, and impair hemostasis.

Patients generally have minimal symptoms such as easy bruising, and bleeding is usually confined to the skin. Occasional patients will have prolonged oozing after surgery, particularly with procedures involving mucous membranes such as periodontal, oral, or reconstructive plastic surgery. Not surprisingly, the antiplatelet effect of drugs such as aspirin is more dramatic when they are administered to patients with underlying defects like vWD or hemophilia. Patients with drug-induced cyclooxygenase deficiency often but not always have a mildly prolonged bleeding time, and their platelets fail to aggregate when incubated with arachidonic acid, epinephrine, or low doses of ADP. Since the bleeding time is not entirely reliable, if patients have taken aspirin, they should be treated as if they have a mild hemostatic defect for the next 5 to 7 days. Platelet responses to collagen and thrombin are impaired at low doses but normal at higher doses. Symptomatic patients should be encouraged to use drugs such as acetaminophen which do not impair platelet function. Although most cases of cyclooxygenase deficiency are drug-induced, occasional patients have inherited disorders in platelet cyclooxygenase activity which impair thromboxane production or receptor level defects which prevent platelets from responding to thromboxane A_2.

Although a number of metabolic disorders can perturb hemostasis, uremic platelet dysfunction is clinically the most important. The mechanism by which uremia impairs platelet function is not well understood, and retention of phenolic and guanidinosuccinic acids, excess prostacyclin production, or impaired vWF-platelet interactions have all been implicated. There is a good correlation between the degree of uremia and bleeding symptoms and the degree of anemia and bleeding. Bleeding can usually be reversed by dialysis and often improves after red cell transfusion or treatment with erythropoietin. In addition, the administration of cryoprecipitate or DDAVP, which raise plasma vWF levels, also can improve hemostasis. Conjugated estrogens improve hemostasis and can be used as long-term therapy.

STORAGE POOL DEFECTS   Platelet granules have considerable amounts of adenine nucleotides, calcium, and adhesive glycoproteins such as thrombospondin, fibronectin, and vWF, all of which promote platelet adhesion and aggregation. Thus, it is not surprising that patients with defective platelet granules have a mild bleeding disorder. Platelet storage pool defects may be inherited as an isolated disorder or be part of systemic granule packaging defects such as oculocutaneous albinism or the Hermansky-Pudlak or Chédiak-Higashi syndromes. Clinically, these patients cannot be distinguished from those with other functional platelet disorders, since they all have easy bruising, mucosal bleeding, and a prolonged bleeding time. They can be differentiated from patients with the cyclooxygenase defects because their platelets will usually aggregate in response to arachidonic acid. In addition, their platelets have decreased levels of specific granule constituents such as ADP and serotonin and abnormalities in granule morphology that are best visualized by electron microscopy.

Occasionally, patients with acute or chronic leukemia or one of the myeloproliferative disorders develop an acquired storage pool disorder due to dysplastic megakaryocyte development. In addition, patients with liver disease and some patients with systemic lupus erythematosus or other immune-complex-mediated disorders may have circulating platelets which have degranulated prematurely. Platelet degranulation and a transient storage pool disorder also have been described following prolonged cardiopulmonary bypass. Fortunately, most patients with storage pool defects have only mildly impaired hemostasis. They can be treated with platelet transfusions. Occasional patients have responded to DDAVP.

VESSEL WALL DISORDERS

Bleeding from vascular disorders (nonthrombocytopenic purpura) is usually mild and confined to the skin and mucous membranes. The pathogenesis of bleeding is poorly defined in many of the syndromes, and classical tests of hemostasis, including the bleeding time and tests of platelet function, are usually normal. Vascular purpura arises from damage to capillary endothelium, abnormalities in the vascular subendothelial matrix or extravascular connective tissues which support blood vessels, or from the formation of abnormal blood vessels. There are also several idiopathic disorders which involve the vessel wall and which can cause more severe bleeding and organ dysfunction.

THROMBOTIC THROMBOCYTOPENIC PURPURA   Thrombotic thrombocytopenic purpura (TTP) is a fulminant, often lethal disorder that may be initiated by endothelial injury and subsequent release of vWF and other procoagulant materials from the endothelial cell. In addition, some patients with TTP may have a unique circulating protein which induces platelet aggregation. Characteristic findings include the microvascular deposition of hyaline thrombi which stain for fibrin, thrombocytopenia, microangiopathic hemolytic anemia, fever, renal failure, fluctuating levels of consciousness, and evanescent focal neurologic deficits. The presence of hyaline thrombi in arterioles, capillaries, and venules without any inflammatory changes in the vessel wall is diagnostic. Gingival biopsies are positive in 30 to 40 percent of patients, and marrow biopsies are occasionally helpful. The presence of a severe Coombs-negative hemolytic anemia with schistocytes or fragmented red blood cells in the peripheral blood smear, coupled with thrombocytopenia, and minimal activation of the coagulation system help to confirm the clinical suspicion of TTP.

This disorder should be distinguished from vasculitis and systemic lupus erythematosus, which can predispose patients to TTP. Levels of platelet-associated IgG and complement are usually normal in TTP.

The treatment of acute TTP has changed radically in the past few years. Steroids and heparin or emergency splenectomy have been abandoned, and the enthusiasm for antiplatelet therapy has diminished. Increasingly, treatment has focused on the use of exchange transfusion or intensive plasmapheresis coupled with infusion of fresh frozen plasma. With this therapeutic approach, the overall mortality has been markedly reduced, and over half the patients with TTP are recovering from this formerly fatal disorder. Most patients surviving the acute illness recover completely with no residual renal or neurologic disease. Occasional patients with a chronic, relapsing form of TTP require maintenance plasmapheresis and plasma infusion, and a few patients are only controlled with glucocorticoids.

HEMOLYTIC-UREMIC SYNDROME Hemolytic-uremic syndrome (HUS) is a disease of infancy and early childhood which closely resembles TTP. Patients present with fever, thrombocytopenia, microangiopathic hemolytic anemia, hypertension, and varying degrees of acute renal failure. In many cases, onset is preceded by a minor febrile or viral illness, and an infectious or immune-complex–mediated cause has been proposed. As in TTP, there is no evidence of disseminated intravascular coagulation. In contrast to TTP, the disorder remains localized to the kidney, where hyaline thrombi are seen in the afferent arterioles and glomerular capillaries. Such thrombi are not present in other vessels, and neurologic symptoms, other than those associated with uremia, are uncommon. There is no effective therapy; however, with dialysis for acute renal failure, the initial mortality is only 5 percent. Between 10 and 50 percent of patients are left with some chronic renal impairment.

HENOCH-SCHÖNLEIN PURPURA Henoch-Schönlein or anaphylactoid purpura is a distinct, self-limited type of vasculitis which occurs in children and young adults. Patients have an acute inflammatory reaction in capillaries, mesangial tissues, and small arterioles which leads to increased vascular permeability, exudation, and hemorrhage. Vessel lesions contain IgA and complement components. The syndrome may be preceded by an upper respiratory infection or streptococcal pharyngitis or be associated with food or drug allergies. Patients develop a purpuric or urticarial rash on the extensor surfaces of the arms and legs and on the buttocks; they also have polyarthralgias or arthritis, colicky abdominal pain, and hematuria from focal glomerulonephritis. Despite the hemorrhagic features, all coagulation tests are normal. A small number of patients may develop fatal acute renal failure, and 5 to 10 percent develop chronic nephritis. Glucocorticoids provide symptomatic relief of the joint and abdominal pains but do not alter the course of the illness.

METABOLIC AND INFLAMMATORY DISORDERS A number of acute febrile illnesses cause capillary fragility and skin bleeding. Immune complexes containing viral antigens or the viruses themselves may damage endothelial cells. In addition, certain pathogens such as the rickettsiae which cause Rocky Mountain spotted fever replicate in endothelial cells and damage them. Thrombocytopenia is also a frequent finding in acute infectious disorders and may contribute to skin bleeding. In addition, whenever the platelet count falls below 10,000 per microliter, gaps which develop between endothelial cells allow the diapedesis of red cells into the dermis leading to the formation of petechiae. Drugs such as the sulfonamides, penicillin, and allopurinol may cause vascular inflammation resulting in maculopapular or urticarial rashes. Some of these mechanisms are additive, and drug reactions in thrombocytopenic individuals cause an intensely hemorrhagic rash.

Occasionally, patients with diffuse polyclonal hyperglobulinemia will develop purpuric lesions on the lower limbs—a benign condition referred to as *hyperglobulinemic purpura*. Vascular purpura may occur in patients with various monoclonal plasma protein abnormalities, including Waldenström's macroglobulinemia, multiple myeloma, and cryoglobulinemia. These proteins markedly increase serum viscosity and may impair blood flow through capillaries. Thus retinal hemorrhage, central nervous system dysfunction, and skin necrosis have all been described in these syndromes due to the marked elevation in viscosity. In addition, the globulins may impair platelet aggregation and adhesion and interfere with fibrin polymerization. Patients with mixed cryoglobulinemia develop a more extensive maculopapular lesion due to immune-complex–mediated damage to the vessel wall. The mixed cryoglobulinemia (usually IgG and anti-IgG) may be associated with arthralgias, diffuse weakness, and unexplained nephritis. Plasmapheresis will temporarily lower the level of globulins, remove immune complexes, and improve symptoms in these patients. However, long-term management must include control of the underlying disease which produces the abnormal globulins or immune complexes.

Patients with *scurvy* (vitamin C deficiency) develop painful episodes of perifollicular skin bleeding as well as bleeding into muscles and, occasionally, into the gastrointestinal and genitourinary tracts. The diagnosis is confirmed by the presence of hyperkeratosis of skin, gum swelling, and low levels of the vitamin in leukocytes. Vitamin C–deficient patients have markedly defective collagen synthesis, since ascorbic acid is needed to synthesize hydroxyproline, an essential constituent of collagen. Patients with *Cushing's syndrome*, which is characterized by excess production of glucocorticoids, or patients on large doses of glucocorticoids develop generalized protein wasting and may show skin bleeding or easy bruising due to atrophy of the supporting connective tissue around blood vessels. Aging causes a similar atrophy of perivascular connective tissue on the extensor surfaces of the hands and arms, leading to "senile purpura." These patients develop dark purple, irregularly shaped hemorrhagic areas due to abnormal skin mobility which tears small blood vessels.

Patients with inherited disorders of the connective tissue matrix such as *Marfan's syndrome*, *Ehlers-Danlos syndrome*, and *pseudoxanthoma elasticum* also have easy bruising. In addition to having fragile skin vessels and easy bruising, patients with Ehlers-Danlos syndrome may develop aneurysms in intraabdominal vessels and apoplectic rupture and hemorrhage due to defects in the vascular collagen network. Primary vascular abnormalities also can lead to bleeding. Patients with *Osler-Weber-Rendu disease* (hereditary hemorrhagic telangiectasia), an inherited autosomal dominant disorder, have frequent episodes of nasal and gastrointestinal bleeding from abnormal telangiectatic capillaries; patients with *angiodysplasia* of the colon have increased incidence of gastrointestinal bleeding. In the *Kasabach-Merritt syndrome*, patients may have very extensive and progressively enlarging vascular malformations which may involve large portions of their extremities. Bleeding is secondary to disseminated intravascular coagulation triggered by stagnant blood flow through the tortuous abnormal vessels.

REFERENCES

HANDIN RI, WAGNER DD: Molecular and cellular biology of von Willebrand factor, in *Progress in Hemostasis and Thrombosis*, vol 9, BS Coller (ed). Philadelphia, Saunders, 1989, pp 233–259

——— et al (eds): *Blood: Principles and Practice of Hematology and Hematologic Oncology*. Philadelphia, Lippincott, 1993

MAJERUS P: Platelets, in *The Molecular Basis of Blood Diseases*, G Stamatoyanopoulis et al (eds). Philadelphia, Saunders, 1987, pp 689–722

STUART MJ, KELTON JG: The platelet: Quantitative and qualitative abnormalities, in *Hematology of Infancy and Childhood*, 4th ed, DG Nathan, FA Oski (eds). Philadelphia, Saunders, 1992, p 1343–1479

WILLIAMS WJ: et al (eds): *Hematology*, 4th ed. New York, McGraw-Hill, 1990

315　DISORDERS OF COAGULATION AND THROMBOSIS

ROBERT I. HANDIN

Patients with congenital plasma coagulation defects characteristically bleed into muscles, joints, and body cavities hours or days after an injury. Most of the *inherited* plasma coagulation disorders are due to defects in single coagulation proteins, with the two X-linked disorders, factors VIII and IX deficiency, accounting for the majority of the congenital coagulation disorders. These patients merit special attention because they may have severe bleeding and chronic disability and require specialized medical therapy. With rare exceptions, the known disorders prolong either the prothrombin time (PT), partial thromboplastin time (PTT), or both these important laboratory screening tests. If they are abnormal, quantitative assays of specific coagulation proteins are then carried out using the PT or PTT tests with plasma from congenitally deficient individuals as substrate. The corrective effect of varying concentrations of patient plasma is measured and expressed as a percentage of a normal pooled plasma standard. The interval range for most coagulation factors is from 50 to 150 percent of this average value, and the minimal level of most individual factors needed for adequate hemostasis is 25 percent.

Acquired coagulation disorders are both more frequent and more complex, arising from deficiencies of multiple coagulation proteins and simultaneously affecting both primary and secondary hemostasis. The most common acquired hemorrhagic disorders are (1) disseminated intravascular coagulation, (2) the hemorrhagic diathesis of liver disease, and (3) vitamin K deficiency and complications of anticoagulant therapy.

Although congenital and acquired bleeding disorders are relatively rare, venous and arterial thrombosis and embolism are common medical disorders which have been recognized for over a hundred years. Although risk factors such as atherosclerotic vascular disease, congestive heart failure, malignancy, and immobility predispose patients to thrombosis, specific coagulation defects have not yet been identified in most patients with thromboembolism. Several inherited coagulation abnormalities have now been described which induce a hypercoagulable or prethrombotic state and predispose patients to thrombosis. These disorders merit special attention because they affect young people, cause recurrent episodes of thromboembolism, and may involve multiple members of a single family. An understanding of the biochemical basis of thromboembolism is also important because anticoagulant and antithrombotic regimes are based on the premise that modifying critical coagulation reactions will reduce the incidence of thrombosis. This chapter will review the diagnosis, natural history, and therapy of congenital and acquired plasma coagulation disorders, as well as the inherited prethrombotic disorders. The physiology of normal hemostasis and the cardinal manifestations of the hemorrhagic and thrombotic disorders are described in Chap. 57.

FACTOR VIII DEFICIENCY—HEMOPHILIA A　Pathogenesis and clinical manifestations　The antihemophilic factor (AHF) or factor VIII coagulant protein is a large (265-kDa), single-chain protein which regulates the activation of factor X by proteases generated in the intrinsic coagulation pathway (see Figs. 57-4 and 57-6). It is synthesized in liver parenchymal cells and circulates complexed to the von Willebrand protein (vWF). Previous efforts to purify and characterize the factor VIII molecule were limited by its low concentration (10 μg/L) and susceptibility to proteolysis. However, the cloning and sequencing of complementary DNA (cDNA) encoding the factor VIII molecule and the mapping of the factor VIII gene on the X chromosome have provided a detailed picture of its structure and have led to improved methods for carrier detection and prenatal diagnosis of hemophilia A.

One in 10,000 males is born with deficiency or dysfunction of the factor VIII molecule. The resulting disorder, hemophilia A, is characterized by bleeding into soft tissues, muscles, and weight-bearing joints. Although normal hemostasis requires at least 25 percent factor VIII activity, symptomatic patients usually have factor VIII levels below 5 percent, with a close correlation between the clinical severity of hemophilia and plasma AHF level. Patients with <1 percent factor VIII activity have *severe* disease; they bleed frequently even without discernible trauma. Patients with levels between 1 and 5 percent have *moderate* disease with less frequent bleeding episodes. Those with levels over 5 percent have *mild* disease with infrequent bleeding that is usually secondary to trauma. Occasional patients with factor VIII levels as high as 25 percent are discovered when they bleed after major trauma or surgery. The majority of patients with hemophilia A have factor VIII levels below 5 percent.

Hemophilic bleeding occurs hours or days after injury, can involve any organ, and, if untreated, may continue for days or weeks. This can result in large collections of partially clotted blood putting pressure on adjacent normal tissues and can cause necrosis of muscle (compartment syndromes), venous congestion (pseudophlebitis), or ischemic damage to nerves. For example, hemophiliacs often develop femoral neuropathy due to pressure from an unsuspected retroperitoneal hematoma. They also can develop large calcified masses of blood and inflammatory tissue that are mistaken for soft tissue sarcomas (pseudotumor syndrome).

Patients with severe hemophilia are usually diagnosed shortly after birth because of an extensive cephalhematoma or profuse bleeding at circumcision. However, patients with moderate disease may not bleed until they begin to walk or crawl, and mild hemophiliacs may not be diagnosed until they are adolescents or young adults. Typically, a hemophiliac patient presents with pain followed by swelling in a weight-bearing joint, such as the hip, knee, or ankle. The presence of blood in the joint (hemarthrosis) causes synovial inflammation, and repetitive bleeding erodes articular cartilage and causes osteoarthritis, articular fibrosis, joint ankylosis, and eventually muscle atrophy. Although bleeding may occur into any joint, after a joint has been damaged, it may become a site for subsequent bleeding episodes.

Hematuria, in the absence of any genitourinary pathology, is also common. It is usually self-limited and may not require specific therapy. The most feared complications of hemophilia are oropharyngeal and central nervous system bleeding. Patients with oropharyngeal bleeding may require emergency intubation to maintain an adequate airway. Central nervous system bleeding can occur without antecedent trauma or without evidence of a specific lesion.

Patients suspected of having hemophilia should have screening tests of hemostasis, including a platelet count, bleeding time, PT, and PTT. Typically, the patient will have a prolonged PTT with all other tests normal. Because of the clinical similarity of factor VIII deficiency and factor IX deficiency, any male with an appropriate bleeding history and a prolonged PTT should have specific assays for factor VIII and factor IX.

Therapy　There are several tenets regarding the treatment of bleeding in hemophiliac patients: (1) Symptoms often precede objective evidence of bleeding. (2) Signs of bleeding may not appear until several days after well-documented trauma. Physicians caring for these patients have learned to rely on their patients to inform them of early symptoms, usually pain, and to begin treatment at that time. Early treatment is more effective, less costly, and can be lifesaving. (3) It is critical to avoid the use of aspirin or aspirin-containing drugs which impair platelet function and may cause severe hemorrhage.

Plasma products enriched in factor VIII have revolutionized the care of hemophilia patients, reduced the degree of orthopedic deformity, and permitted virtually any form of elective and emergency surgery. The widespread use of factor VIII concentrates also has produced serious complications, including viral hepatitis, chronic liver disease, and AIDS. The standard therapeutic products are cryoprecipitate and factor VIII concentrate. *Cryoprecipitate*, which contains about half the factor VIII activity of fresh frozen plasma in one-tenth the original volume, is simple to prepare and is produced in hospital or regional blood banks. It must be stored frozen and is thawed and pooled prior to administration. However, most patients utilize partially purified *factor VIII concentrate*, which is prepared from multiple donors and supplied as a lyophilized powder. It can be refrigerated and reconstituted just prior to use.

There are three recent developments which have increased the safety of factor VIII therapy. First, heating of lyophilized factor VIII concentrates under carefully controlled conditions can inactivate human immunodeficiency virus (HIV) without destroying factor VIII coagulant activity. Second, highly purified factor VIII can be produced by adsorbing and eluting factor VIII from monoclonal antibody columns. Third, recombinant factor VIII has just completed clinical trials and is being marketed. Patients with hemophilia should receive either monoclonal purified or recombinant factor VIII to minimize viral infections and exposure to irrelevant proteins.

It has been determined, empirically, that each unit of factor VIII infused, defined as the amount present in 1 mL normal plasma, will raise the plasma level of the recipient by 2 percent per kilogram of body weight. Factor VIII has a half-life of 8 to 12 h, making it necessary to infuse it continuously or at least twice daily to sustain a chosen factor VIII level. In patients with mild hemophilia, an alternative to the use of plasma products is desmopressin (DDAVP), which transiently increases the factor VIII level. DDAVP in general will increase the factor level two- to threefold. Although generally safe, it occasionally causes hyponatremia or may precipitate thrombosis in elderly patients.

An uncomplicated episode of soft tissue bleeding or an early hemarthrosis can be treated with one infusion of cryoprecipitate or factor VIII concentrate sufficient to raise the factor VIII level to 15 or 20 percent. A more extensive hemarthrosis or retroperitoneal bleeding requires twice-daily or continuous infusions in order to keep the factor VIII level between 25 and 50 percent for at least 72 h. Life-threatening bleeding into the central nervous system or major surgery may require therapy for 2 weeks with levels kept at a minimum of 50 percent of normal. In addition to the prompt infusion of factor VIII–enriched plasma products, patients need skilled orthopedic care with immobilization of inflamed joints to promote healing and to prevent contractures and physical therapy to strengthen muscles and maintain joint mobility. Prior to surgery, every patient should be screened for the presence of an inhibitor to factor VIII.

Patients with hemophilia who do not have an inhibitor should receive factor VIII infusions just prior to surgery and will require daily monitoring so that the factor VIII level is maintained above 50 percent for 10 to 14 days after surgery. When patients undergo joint replacement or other major orthopedic surgery, therapy should be continued for 3 weeks. This permits adequate wound healing and the institution of necessary joint mobilization and physical therapy.

Hemophiliacs also require treatment prior to dental procedures. Filling of a carious tooth can be managed by a single infusion of cryoprecipitate or factor VIII concentrate coupled with the administration of 4 to 6 g of ε-aminocaproic acid (EACA) four times daily for 72 to 96 h after the dental procedure. EACA is a potent antifibrinolytic agent which will inhibit plasminogen activators present in oral secretions and stabilize clot formation in oral tissue. Alternatives include tranexamic acid, a longer-acting antifibrinolytic. EACA is also effective when used as a mouthwash. For major oral and periodontal surgery and extractions of permanent teeth, patients should probably be hospitalized briefly and also treated with factor VIII concentrates. Therapy should begin just prior to surgery and be continued for a minimum of 48 to 72 h.

Many centers have organized home care programs so that patients can administer their own factor VIII infusions with the onset of symptoms. Occasional patients with very frequent bleeding receive regularly scheduled infusions. However, the expense and inconvenience usually limit the use of "prophylactic" infusions. Concern regarding transmission of AIDS has complicated therapy of hemophilia, and some patients are reluctant to treat themselves, despite the fact that current blood products carry a very low risk of transmitting HIV.

Complications Most hemophiliacs have had multiple episodes of hepatitis, and a majority have elevated hepatocellular enzyme levels and abnormalities on liver biopsy. Between 10 and 20 percent of hemophiliacs also have hepatosplenomegaly, and a small number develop chronic active or persistent hepatitis or cirrhosis. Recently, a few patients with hemophilia and end-stage liver disease have received liver transplants with cure of both diseases. Along with homosexuals and intravenous drug abusers, hemophiliacs are at high risk for AIDS because they frequently receive blood products. Hemophiliacs also can present with the full range of AIDS-related syndromes, including diffuse lymphadenopathy and immune thrombocytopenia. Although as many as 80 percent of multiply transfused hemophiliacs are HIV-positive and some have clinical AIDS, the advances in factor VIII concentrate technology discussed previously should prevent future HIV infection.

Despite frequent bleeding, severe iron-deficiency anemia is uncommon because most of the bleeding is internal and iron is effectively recycled. Mild iron deficiency from chronic epistaxis or gastrointestinal bleeding has been noted in some hemophiliacs. In addition, after receiving large doses of the older partially purified factor VIII concentrates, some patients have developed a mild Coombs-positive hemolytic anemia due to small amounts of anti-A and anti-B antibody that is present in commercial concentrates.

Following multiple transfusions, between 10 and 20 percent of patients with severe hemophilia develop inhibitors to factor VIII. Inhibitors are, generally, IgG antibodies which rapidly neutralize factor VIII activity and prevent effective transfusion therapy. There are two types of inhibitors which have different biologic characteristics and lead to different clinical presentations. Patients with type I inhibitors have a typical anamnestic response and raise their antibody titer following exposure to factor VIII. Patients with a type II inhibitor have a low antibody titer which cannot be stimulated by factor VIII infusion. Patients with the type I inhibitor should not receive factor VIII. In an emergency, control of bleeding may require intensive plasmapheresis or infusion of prothrombin complex concentrates which contain trace quantities of activated coagulation factors and can bypass the block in coagulation produced by the inhibitor. Patients with low-titer type II antibodies may respond to higher than normal doses of factor VIII.

Genetic counseling and carrier detection Until recently, carrier detection required biologic and immunologic assays which compared the ratio of factor VIII to vWF (von Willebrand factor) protein and were predictive in only 70 to 80 percent of cases. It is now possible to trace the defective allele in some families by examining the inheritance of restriction fragment length polymorphisms (RFLPs) linked to the factor VIII gene. In addition, in families in which a specific mutation has been defined in the factor VIII gene, it can be readily detected by gene amplification and allele-specific oligonucleotide hybridization. Previously, prenatal diagnosis required sampling fetal blood for coagulant activity. Now, in families with an identifiable RFLP linked to the gene or a known mutation, precise diagnosis is possible early in pregnancy from either chorionic villus biopsy or amniocentesis. The amount of material required has decreased, and the rapidity of diagnosis has increased with the introduction of the polymerase chain reaction to amplify desired segments of genomic DNA.

Female carriers of hemophilia, who are heterozygotes, usually produce sufficient factor VIII from the factor VIII allele on their normal X chromosome for normal hemostasis. However, occasional hemophilia carriers will have factor VIII levels far below 50 percent due to random inactivation of normal X chromosomes in tissue producing factor VIII. These symptomatic carriers may bleed with major surgery or bleed occasionally with menses. Rarely, true female hemophiliacs arise from consanguinity within families with hemophilia or from concomitant Turner's syndrome or XO mosaicism in a carrier female.

FACTOR IX DEFICIENCY—HEMOPHILIA B Factor IX is a single-chain, 55-kDa proenzyme which is converted to an active protease

(IXa) by factor XIa or by the tissue factor–VIIa complex. Factor IXa then activates factor X in conjunction with activated factor VIII. Factor IX is one of a group of six proteins synthesized in the liver which require vitamin K for biologic activity. As previously discussed (see Chap. 57), vitamin K is a cofactor for a unique posttranslational modification which inserts a second carboxyl group onto certain glutamic acid residues on factor IX. This modification permits calcium binding and adsorption onto phospholipid surfaces. Factor IX cDNA has been cloned, the gene mapped on the X chromosome, linked RFLPs identified, and many patients with deletions and mutations in the IX gene have now been described.

Factor IX deficiency or dysfunction (hemophilia B, Christmas disease) occurs in 1 in 100,000 male births. Accurate laboratory diagnosis is critical, since it is indistinguishable clinically from factor VIII deficiency (hemophilia A) but requires treatment with a different plasma fraction. Either fresh frozen plasma or a plasma fraction enriched in the prothrombin complex proteins is used. Monoclonally purified or recombinant factor IV preparation will soon be used in clinical trials. In addition to the expected complications of hepatitis, chronic liver disease, and AIDS, the therapy of factor IX deficiency has a special hazard. Trace quantities of activated coagulation factors in prothrombin complex concentrates may activate the coagulation system and cause thrombosis and embolism. This is particularly common in immobilized surgical patients and patients with liver disease. As a result, some centers have returned to fresh frozen plasma for factor IX–deficient surgical patients, while others have recommended the addition of small doses of heparin to the concentrate to activate antithrombin III during the infusion and reduce hypercoagulability.

FACTOR XI DEFICIENCY Factor XI is a 160-kDa dimeric protein which is activated via the intrinsic coagulation pathway. It is converted to an active protease (XIa) by factor XIIa, in conjunction with high-molecular-weight kininogen and kallikrein (see Figs. 57-4 and 57-5). Factor XI deficiency is inherited as an autosomal recessive trait and is especially common in Ashkenazi Jews. In contrast to factors VIII and IX deficiency, the correlation between factor level and propensity to bleed is not as precise, there is less spontaneous bleeding, and hemarthroses are rare. Many patients with factor XI deficiency present with posttraumatic bleeding or with bleeding in the perioperative period, and occasional factor XI–deficient women have menorrhagia. Daily infusions of fresh frozen plasma are sufficient, since the half-life of factor XI is approximately 24 h. The majority of defective factor XI alleles were accounted for by a limited number of mutations in one large study.

OTHER FACTOR DEFICIENCIES Deficiencies in factors V, VII, X, and prothrombin (factor II) are all exceedingly rare autosomal recessive disorders. Although spontaneous or posttraumatic musculoskeletal bleeding or menorrhagia can occur with these deficiencies, hemarthroses are uncommon. Fresh frozen plasma is the appropriate therapy, although prothrombin concentrates may be employed for patients with severe prothrombin or factors VII and X deficiency as long as the risks of hepatitis and thrombosis are recognized.

Defects in the contact activation pathway involving Hageman factor (factor XII), high-molecular-weight kininogen, and prekallikrein cause laboratory abnormalities but no clinical bleeding. Despite dramatic prolongation of the PTT, which is often greater than 100 s, deficient individuals have normal hemostasis and can undergo major surgery without plasma replacement therapy. It is important to recognize and diagnose these disorders because the patients should neither be treated inappropriately with plasma nor denied indicated surgery on the basis of these laboratory abnormalities. As discussed in Chap. 57, there may be as yet undefined alternative pathways to activate factor XI in vivo which bypass this apparent defect in coagulation.

AFIBRINOGENEMIA AND DYSFIBRINOGENEMIA Fibrinogen is a 340-kDa dimeric molecule made up of two sets of three covalently linked polypeptide chains. Thrombin sequentially cleaves fibrinopeptides A and B from the Aα and Bβ chains of fibrinogen to produce fibrin monomer, which then polymerizes to form a fibrin clot. Although fibrinogen is needed for platelet aggregation and fibrin formation, severe fibrinogen deficiency, paradoxically, does not usually cause serious bleeding except after surgery. Patients with afibrinogenemia, who have no detectable fibrinogen in plasma or platelets, may have infrequent, mild bleeding episodes. Preliminary genetic analyses do not show any deletion or structural changes in the genes encoding the α, β, and γ chains of fibrinogen despite the total absence of plasma fibrinogen.

Fibrinogen is an abundant plasma protein (2.5 g/L) that has been very well characterized. Mutations have been identified which alter the release of fibrinopeptides from the Aα and Bβ chains of fibrinogen, the rate of polymerization of fibrin monomers, and the sites for fibrin cross-linking. These dysfibrinogenemias are almost always inherited as autosomal dominant traits, so patients have approximately equal concentrations of normal and mutant fibrinogen in their plasma. Patients with dysfibrinogenemia have a slightly prolonged PT and PTT, a prolonged thrombin time, and a disparity between the quantity of fibrinogen measured with functional and immunologic assays. Despite these abnormalities, most patients have no symptoms, while other patients have moderate bleeding. A few dysfibrinogenemias induce a hypercoagulable state and increase the risk of thrombosis, and others have been associated with an increased incidence of abortion (see Chap. 316). Some patients with liver disease, AIDS, and lymphoproliferative disorders developed an acquired form of dysfibrinogenemia.

FACTOR XIII DEFICIENCY AND DEFECTIVE FIBRIN CROSS-LINKING Factor XIII is a transglutaminase which stabilizes fibrin clots by forming ϵ-amino–γ-glutamyl cross-links between adjacent α and γ chains of fibrin. Factor XIII deficiency is an extremely rare inherited syndrome with only a few hundred documented cases. Patients usually bleed in the neonatal period from their umbilical stump or circumcision. In addition to hemorrhage, these patients may have poor wound healing, a high incidence of infertility among males and abortion among affected females, and a high incidence of intracerebral hemorrhage. These observations suggest that the enzyme may be important in other physiologic and pathologic processes beyond hemostasis, including placental implantation, spermatogenesis, and wound healing. Several drugs, including isoniazid, may bind to cross-linking sites on fibrinogen and mimic factor XIII deficiency by blocking enzyme activity. Normal hemostasis requires only 1 percent of normal enzyme activity, which can be achieved with a single infusion of fresh frozen plasma, as factor XIII has a 14 day half-life.

VITAMIN K DEFICIENCY Vitamin K is a fat-soluble vitamin which plays a critical role in hemostasis. Dietary vitamin K is absorbed in the small intestine and stored in the liver. The vitamin is also synthesized by endogenous bacterial flora resident in the small intestine and colon; however, there is controversy regarding the quantity of endogenous vitamin K that is absorbed from the large intestine. Following absorption and transport, vitamin K is converted to an active epoxide in liver microsomes and serves as a cofactor in the enzymatic carboxylation of glutamic acid residues on prothrombin complex proteins (Fig. 315-1).

There are three major causes of vitamin K deficiency—inadequate dietary intake, intestinal malabsorption, and loss of storage sites due to hepatocellular disease. Neonatal vitamin K deficiency, which causes hemorrhagic disease of the newborn, has disappeared from western countries with the routine administration of vitamin K to all newborn infants. Although there is, theoretically, a 30-day store of vitamin K in the normal liver, acutely ill patients can become deficient within 7 to 10 days. Acute vitamin K deficiency is particularly common in patients recovering from biliary tract surgery who have no dietary intake of vitamin K, have T-tube drainage of bile, and are on broad-spectrum antibiotics. Vitamin K deficiency is also seen in chronic liver disease, particularly primary biliary cirrhosis, and in some malabsorption states (see Chaps. 254 and 268). The cephalosporin antibiotics induce vitamin K deficiency in a manner analogous to

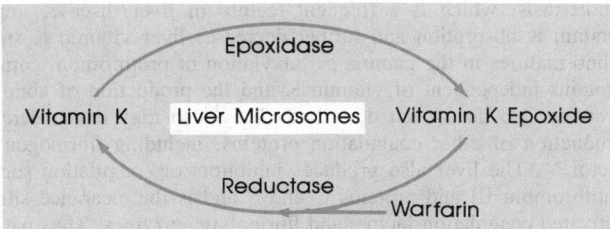

FIGURE 315-1 The mechanism of action of vitamin K, which is a cofactor in the formation of di-γ-carboxyglutamic acid residues on coagulation proteins, is depicted. Vitamin K is converted to an epoxide in liver microsomes. The epoxide is the active form and is reduced back to vitamin K by a liver membrane reductase. Warfarin blocks the action of the reductase and competitively inhibits the effects of vitamin K.

the coumarin anticoagulants—they inhibit the reduction and recycling of vitamin K.

With the onset of vitamin K deficiency, plasma levels of all the prothrombin complex proteins (factors II, VII, IX, X; protein C and protein S) decrease. Factor VII and protein C, which have the shortest half-lives, decrease first. Because of the rapid fall in factor VII, patients with mild vitamin K deficiency may have a prolonged PT and a normal PTT. Later, as the levels of the other factors fall, the PTT also will become prolonged. Parenteral administration of 10 mg vitamin K rapidly restores vitamin K levels in the liver and permits normal production of prothrombin complex proteins within 8 to 10 h. Severe hemorrhage can be treated with fresh frozen plasma, which immediately corrects the hemostatic defect. If the cause of vitamin K deficiency cannot be eliminated, patients may need monthly injections. Purified prothrombin complex concentrates should be avoided because they contain trace quantities of activated forms of the prothrombin complex proteins and can cause thrombosis in patients with liver disease. They also will expose patients to an increased risk of hepatitis.

DISSEMINATED INTRAVASCULAR COAGULATION Disseminated intravascular coagulation (DIC) can either be an explosive and life-threatening bleeding disorder or a relatively mild or subclinical disorder. Although there is a long list of diseases complicated by DIC, it is most frequently associated with obstetrical catastrophes, metastatic malignancy, massive trauma, and bacterial sepsis (Table 315-1). In each case, a tentative triggering mechanism has been identified. For example, tumors and traumatized or necrotic tissue release tissue factor into the circulation, while endotoxin from gram-negative bacteria activates several steps in the coagulation cascade. In addition to a direct effect on the activation of Hageman factor (factor XII), endotoxin induces the expression of tissue factor on the surface of monocytes and endothelial cells. These cell surfaces then accelerate coagulation reactions. This combination of potent thrombogenic stimuli causes the deposition of small thrombi and emboli throughout the microvasculature. This early thrombotic phase of DIC is then followed by a phase of procoagulant consumption and secondary fibrinolysis. Continued fibrin formation and fibrinolysis lead to hemorrhage from the depletion of coagulation proteins and platelets and the antihemostatic effects of fibrin degradation products (Fig. 315-2).

The clinical presentation varies with the stage and severity of the syndrome. Most patients have extensive skin and mucous membrane bleeding and hemorrhage from multiple sites—usually surgical incisions or venipuncture or catheter sites. Less often, patients present with peripheral acrocyanosis, thrombosis, and pregangrenous changes in digits, genitalia, and nose—areas where blood flow is markedly reduced by vasospasm or microthrombi. Some patients, particularly those with chronic DIC secondary to malignancy, have laboratory abnormalities without any evidence of thrombosis or hemorrhage.

The laboratory manifestations include thrombocytopenia and the presence of schistocytes or fragmented red blood cells which arise

TABLE 315-1 Etiologic factors and disorders causing disseminated intravascular coagulation

Liberation of tissue factors	Obstetrical syndromes—abruptio placentae, amniotic fluid embolism, retained dead fetus, second trimester abortion
	Hemolysis
	Neoplasms, particularly mucinous adenocarcinomas, acute promyelocytic leukemia
	Intravascular hemolysis
	Fat embolism
	Tissue damage—burns, frostbite, head injury, gunshot wounds
Endothelial damage	Aortic aneurysm
	Hemolytic uremic syndrome
	Acute glomerulonephritis
	Rocky Mountain spotted fever
Vascular malformation and decreased blood flow	Kasabach-Merritt syndrome
Infections	Bacterial: staphylococci, streptococci, pneumococci, meningococci, gram-negative bacilli
	Viral: arboviruses, varicella, variola, rubella
	Parasitic: malaria, kala-azar
	Rickettsial: Rocky Mountain spotted fever
	Mycotic: acute histoplasmosis

SOURCE: Modified from RI Handin, RD Rosenberg, in *Hematology*, 4th ed, WS Beck (ed), Cambridge, Mass, MIT Press, 1985.

from cell trapping and damage within fibrin thrombi; prolonged PT and PTT and thrombin time, and a reduced fibrinogen level from depletion of coagulation proteins; and elevated fibrin degradation products (FDPs) from intense secondary fibrinolysis. The cardinal manifestation of DIC, which correlates most closely with bleeding, is the plasma fibrinogen level.

Treatment DIC, although sometimes indolent, can cause life-threatening hemorrhage, and may require emergency treatment. This should include (1) an attempt to correct any reversible cause of DIC; (2) measures to control the major symptom, either bleeding or thrombosis; and (3) a prophylactic regimen to prevent recurrence in cases of chronic DIC. Treatment will vary with the clinical presentation. In patients with an obstetric complication such as abruptio placentae or acute bacterial sepsis, the underlying disorder is easy to correct, and prompt delivery of the fetus and placenta or treatment with appropriate antibiotics will reverse the DIC syndrome. In patients with metastatic tumor causing DIC, control of the primary disease may not be possible, and long-term prophylaxis may be necessary.

Patients with bleeding as a major symptom should receive fresh frozen plasma to replace depleted clotting factors and platelet concen-

FIGURE 315-2 The pathophysiology of disseminated intravascular coagulation (DIC). Shown are the interactions between coagulation and fibrinolytic pathways which result in bleeding in patients with DIC.

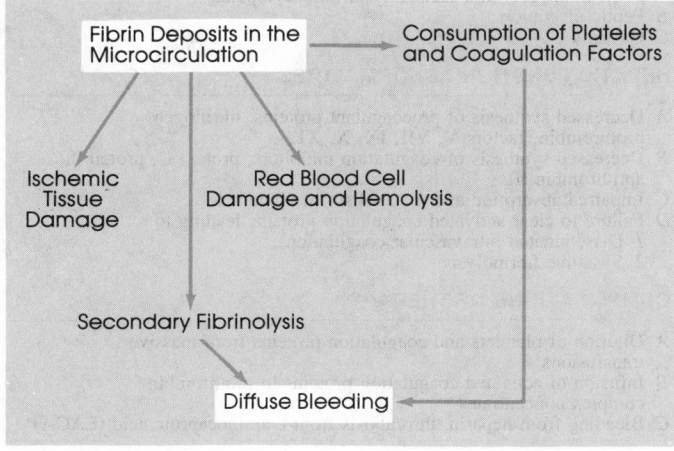

trates to correct thrombocytopenia. Those with acrocyanosis and incipient gangrene or other thrombotic problems need immediate anticoagulation with intravenous heparin. The use of heparin in the treatment of bleeding is still controversial. Although it is a logical way to reduce thrombin generation and prevent further consumption of clotting proteins, it should be reserved for patients with thrombosis or those who continue to bleed despite vigorous treatment with plasma and platelets.

Patients who initially have mild DIC and may not be symptomatic may begin to bleed following surgery or chemotherapy. For example, mild DIC, without clinical bleeding, has been documented during saline- or prostaglandin-induced midtrimester abortions. Prophylactic treatment of patients with heparin may prevent progression of a mild DIC syndrome and has been used in the treatment of patients with acute promyelocytic leukemia and in some patients with a retained dead fetus who require surgical extraction. However, most patients with low-grade DIC can be managed simply with plasma and platelet replacement and do not require heparin. Chronic DIC does not respond to oral warfarin anticoagulants, but it can be controlled with long-term heparin infusion. Occasional patients with indolent tumors and severe DIC have been maintained on heparin administered by intermittent subcutaneous injection or continuous infusion with portable pumps.

Despite our detailed understanding of the pathophysiology of DIC and a vigorous approach to therapy, there is little evidence that its treatment will change the natural history of the underlying disorder. Therapy will only stabilize the patient, prevent exsanguination or massive thrombosis, and permit institution of definitive therapy.

COAGULATION DISORDERS IN LIVER DISEASE   Since the liver plays a central role in the synthesis and metabolism of coagulation proteins, liver dysfunction is frequently accompanied by a hemostatic defect. The major causes of hemorrhage in patients with liver disease are outlined in Table 315-2. It is important to recognize that bleeding is usually due to an anatomic lesion, which can then be exacerbated by a hemostatic defect. Most patients bleed from complications of portal hypertension such as esophageal varices or from gastritis and peptic ulceration of the gastrointestinal tract. Portal hypertension also causes splenomegaly, with splenic sequestration of platelets and thrombocytopenia, which contributes to the hemostatic defect (see Chap. 268).

Patients with hepatocellular liver disease cannot store vitamin K optimally and may have some degree of vitamin K deficiency.

TABLE 315-2   Causes of bleeding in liver disease

ANATOMIC FACTORS

A Portal hypertension
　　1 Varices
　　2 Splenomegaly and secondary thrombocytopenia
B Peptic ulceration
C Gastritis

HEPATIC FUNCTION ABNORMALITIES

A Decreased synthesis of procoagulant proteins: fibrinogen, prothrombin, factors V, VII, IX, X, XI
B Decreased synthesis of coagulation inhibitors: protein C, protein S, antithrombin III
C Impaired absorption and metabolism of vitamin K
D Failure to clear activated coagulation proteins leading to
　　1 Disseminated intravascular coagulation
　　2 Systemic fibrinolysis

COMPLICATIONS OF THERAPY

A Dilution of platelets and coagulation proteins from massive transfusions
B Infusion of activated coagulation proteins in prothrombin complex concentrates
C Bleeding from heparin; thrombosis from ε-aminocaproic acid (EACA)

Cholestasis, which is a frequent feature of liver disease, impairs vitamin K absorption and further decreases liver vitamin K stores. Abnormalities in the gamma carboxylation of prothrombin complex proteins independent of vitamin K and the production of abnormal proteins also have been described. They also may have decreased production of other coagulation proteins, including fibrinogen and factor V. The liver also produces inhibitors of coagulation such as antithrombin III and proteins C and S and is the clearance site for activated coagulation factors and fibrinolytic enzymes. Thus patients with liver disease are also "hypercoagulable" and predisposed to developing DIC or systemic fibrinolysis. For these reasons, coagulation defects in advanced liver failure are often difficult to distinguish from those of DIC.

Each patient with hemorrhage and liver disease should have a PT, PTT, platelet count, and fibrinogen determination, although it is not always possible to determine the major hemostatic abnormality from a single set of laboratory values. It is helpful to have previous laboratory data available for patients with chronic liver disease who develop an acute complication. There is a good correlation between the degree of prolongation of the PT and the risk of bleeding. Most patients present with moderate prolongation of the PT and PTT, mild thrombocytopenia, and a normal fibrinogen level. However, they also may present with a more complex defect combining defective synthesis, abnormal clearance, and active consumption of coagulation proteins. Since vitamin K deficiency is so common, it is advisable to administer a single parenteral dose of vitamin K after initial laboratory studies have been obtained, even though this may only partially correct the laboratory abnormalities. The presence of severe thrombocytopenia or a low fibrinogen level suggests the additional complication of DIC and may require further studies and therapy.

The safest replacement therapy for a patient with liver disease is fresh frozen plasma, since it supplies all known coagulation factors. However, even this form of therapy has drawbacks, since large quantities of plasma may precipitate hepatic encephalopathy and cause fluid and sodium overload. Prothrombin complex concentrates should be avoided because they only replace the vitamin K–dependent factors, may be contaminated with hepatitis and AIDS virus, and contain trace quantities of activated coagulation proteins. Similarly, fibrinogen concentrates (or cryoprecipitate) which are rich in factor VIII and fibrinogen should not be used without additional fresh frozen plasma. Anticoagulation with heparin has been advocated to control DIC, but this is particularly hazardous and not recommended in cirrhosis because heparin is metabolized erratically and may thus lead to severe bleeding.

FIBRINOLYTIC DEFECTS   Bleeding also can occur from defects in the fibrinolytic system. Patients with alpha$_2$ plasmin inhibitor deficiency or plasminogen activator inhibitor-1 (PAI-1) have rapid fibrinolysis following fibrin deposition after trauma or surgery and so may experience recurrent hemorrhage. Similarly, patients with cirrhosis have an impaired clearance of tissue plasminogen activator and systemic fibrinolysis which may contribute to their hemorrhagic defect. Rarely, patients with tumors such as metastatic prostatic carcinoma may develop diffuse bleeding from primary fibrinolysis rather than DIC. Clues to the diagnosis include a disproportionately low fibrinogen level with a relatively normal PT and PTT and the presence of a normal or nearly normal platelet count. Although there are some exceptions, patients with primary fibrinolysis should have an elevated titer of fibrin degradation products (FPPs) but a normal D dimer level. However, at times it is difficult or impossible to differentiate primary fibrinolysis from the secondary fibrinolysis accompanying DIC. Patients with clearly established primary fibrinolysis should not receive heparin; they do require plasma therapy and, occasionally, fibrinolytic inhibitors such as EACA. However, EACA should not be given to patients suspected of having DIC unless they are also receiving heparin, since EACA can cause massive, often fatal, thrombosis in a patient with DIC.

CIRCULATING ANTICOAGULANTS   Circulating anticoagulants, or inhibitors, are usually IgG antibodies which interfere with coagulation reactions. Specific inhibitors inactivate individual coagulation proteins and may cause severe hemorrhage. As discussed above, they arise in 15 to 20 percent of patients with factor VIII or factor IX deficiency who have received plasma infusions. *Specific* inhibitors also occur in previously normal individuals. Although the most common target protein is factor VIII, inhibitors have been described with specificity for each of the coagulation proteins. In addition to hemophiliacs, anti-factor VIII antibodies are seen in postpartum females, in patients on various drugs, as part of the spectrum of autoantibodies in systemic lupus erythematosus patients, and in normal elderly individuals. Circulating anticoagulants also have been reported in patients with AIDS.

Nonspecific (lupus-like) inhibitors prolong coagulation tests by binding to phospholipids. They are assayed by their anticoagulant effect (LA activity) or their ability to bind to the complex phospholipid cardiolipin (ACLA activity). They do not perturb hemostasis in vivo, unless associated with thrombocytopenia or prothrombin deficiency. While they are most often encountered in patients with systemic lupus erythematosus, these nonspecific inhibitors have also been noted in patients with many other disorders and also in otherwise normal individuals.

The critical laboratory feature, which identifies the presence of either type of inhibitor, is the failure of normal plasma to correct a prolonged PT, PTT, or both. Plasma from patients with a specific inhibitor will progressively inactivate a coagulation protein and thus prolong whichever of these screening tests requires the participation of that clotting factor. This effect persists after dilution. Nonspecific inhibitors immediately prolong the PT and PTT and, at low dilution, block multiple coagulation reactions. However, these effects can be overcome by altering the quantity or type of phospholipid or by diluting the plasma.

Hemorrhage in patients with specific inhibitors may require treatment with massive plasma or concentrate infusion, the use of activated prothrombin complex concentrates to bypass the antibodies against factors VIII or IX, and plasmapheresis or exchange transfusion to lower antibody titer. Chronic immunosuppressive regimens have been sometimes employed and have been particularly useful in otherwise normal individuals with an acquired factor VIII antibody. Many patients lose their antibody and recover within 6 to 12 months, although the acute mortality rate from uncontrollable bleeding may approach 10 percent.

Patients with LA activity have normal hemostasis and will not bleed unless they have concomitant thrombocytopenia or prothrombin deficiency. Both thrombocytopenia and hypoprothrombinemia are secondary to autoantibodies which bind either to platelets or the prothrombin molecule. While these antibodies have no effect on function, they accelerate clearance of the coated platelets or the antibody-prothrombin complexes.

Although there is evidence that the presence of LA activity may predispose patients to thromboembolism and may cause midtrimester abortions, it is difficult to make firm predictions about the risk of thrombosis and the appropriate therapy for individual patients. First, tests for either LA or ACLA activity are not well standardized, and results vary among patients and can vary with serial measurements. The best predictor is a consistent prolongation of more than one coagulation test coupled with a high titer of ACLA activity. Second, the risk of thrombosis is increased in patients who have systemic lupus compared with those with idiopathic LA or ACLA activity. There is little evidence that prophylactic therapy is beneficial or that treatments aimed at reducing the titer of antibody are superior to conventional antithrombotic therapy.

Although therapy should be individualized, the following general guidelines may be helpful. They are based on personal experience and review of a rapidly expanding and changing literature. Patients with SLE and either LA or ACLA activity who have had a thrombotic episode are at high risk for a recurrence and should receive long-term anticoagulant therapy. Women who have had more than one midtrimester abortion, especially those with SLE, should have a trial

of anticoagulant therapy. Patients with a single thrombotic episode and no other risk factor except LA or ACLA activity may be treated, but the evidence for efficacy in this setting is minimal. Asymptomatic patients with laboratory abnormalities only should not be treated. Glucocorticoids should only be administered in conjunction with antithrombotic agents and are not of proven efficacy.

INHERITED PRETHROMBOTIC DISORDERS   As previously discussed (see Chap. 57), coagulation is carefully regulated by a series of inhibitors which limit thrombin generation and fibrin formation and by the fibrinolytic system which effectively removes fibrin thrombi (see Figs. 57-5 and 57-7). Inherited defects in the natural coagulation inhibitors (i.e., antithrombin, protein C, and protein S), abnormalities in the fibrinolytic system, and certain dysfibrinogenemias predispose patients to thrombosis (see Table 315-3). Although they are clearly important, defects in these proteins account for less than 10 percent of patients with recurrent thromboembolism. Antithrombin, protein C, and protein S defects are all autosomal dominant traits, so heterozygous individuals, who have a 50 percent reduction in protein concentration or a mixture of mutant and normal molecules, will have an increased risk of thrombosis. The patients all have similar clinical presentations with a strong family history of thrombosis, episodes of recurrent venous thromboembolism, and symptoms by their early twenties. Any patient with this distinctive history should be tested for the molecular abnormalities described below.

ANTITHROMBIN DEFICIENCY   Antithrombin complexes with activated coagulation proteins and blocks their biologic activity (see Fig. 57-5). The rate of this reaction is enhanced by heparin-like molecules within the vessel wall or on endothelial cells. Plasma antithrombin III content varies from 5 to 15 mg/L (50 to 150 percent), with values only slightly below normal increasing the risk of thrombosis. For optimal screening, it is important to assess both the antithrombin III concentration by immunoassay and the plasma antithrombin and heparin cofactor activity with functional assays. The most common defect is mild (heterozygous) antithrombin deficiency, which occurs in 1 in 2000 individuals. In addition, dysfunctional antithrombin molecules, with mutations affecting either the serine protease–binding site or the heparin-binding site, or activation of inhibitor by heparin have been described.

Patients with antithrombin deficiency who develop acute thrombosis or embolism can be treated with intravenous heparin, since there is usually sufficient normal antithrombin to act as a heparin cofactor. Following their first episode of thromboembolism, patients should be placed on oral anticoagulants for life to prevent recurrent thrombosis. Family studies should be conducted when an antithrombin-deficient individual is discovered, since up to half the members of a kindred may

---

TABLE 315-3   Prethrombotic disorders

INHERITED FORMS

Antithrombin III deficiency
Protein C deficiency
Protein S deficiency
Dysplasminogenemia
Dysfibrinogenemia
Defective release of plasminogen activator
Diminished venous content of plasminogen activator
Excessive release of plasminogen activator inhibitor (PAI-1)
Homocystinuria

ACQUIRED DISORDERS

Chronic congestive heart failure
Metastatic tumor
Metastatic malignancy
Extensive trauma or major surgery
Myeloproliferative disorders
Behçet's syndrome
Kawasaki's disease
Treatment with oral contraceptives or L-asparaginase GM-CSF

be affected. Asymptomatic individuals with antithrombin deficiency should receive prophylactic anticoagulation with heparin or plasma infusions to raise their antithrombin level prior to medical or surgical procedures which may increase their risk of thrombosis. Chronic oral anticoagulation is not recommended until individuals at risk have a clinical thrombotic episode.

DEFICIENCIES OF PROTEINS C AND S   Protein C is a vitamin K–dependent hepatic protein which binds to the endothelial cell surface protein thrombomodulin and is converted to an active protease by thrombin (see Fig. 57-5). Activated protein C, in conjunction with protein S, proteolyzes factors Va and VIIIa, which shuts off fibrin formation. Activated protein C also may stimulate fibrinolysis and accelerate clot lysis. Deficiencies of proteins C and S are usually autosomal dominant disorders, and deficiencies in the two proteins cause an identical syndrome of recurrent venous thrombosis and pulmonary embolism. Dysfunctional molecules also have been definitely identified in some patients with thrombosis. In addition, rare patients with homozygous protein C deficiency have fulminant neonatal intravascular coagulation and require prompt diagnosis and treatment.

The correlation between protein C and S levels and the risk of thrombosis is not as precise as for antithrombin III deficiency. In fact, as large surveys have been completed, asymptomatic individuals with protein C "deficiency" have been discovered. Protein C levels in these individuals overlap those with recurrent thromboembolism. In addition, in some well-studied protein C–deficient kindreds, asymptomatic individuals may have protein C levels as low as or lower than relatives with recurrent thrombosis. These observations raise the possibility that an as yet undiscovered comorbid condition is present in symptomatic patients. Finally, since a fraction of the available protein S is bound to C4b-binding protein and is unavailable for coagulation reactions, it may be important to measure both free and total protein S or to have a concomitant measurement of C4b-binding protein for maximum accuracy.

Heterozygous patients with protein C or S deficiencies who develop acute thrombosis should be heparinized and then placed on oral anticoagulants. There are, however, two potential problems with the use of coumarin anticoagulants in these patients. First, these vitamin K antagonists (see Fig. 315-1 and Fig. 57-5), which lower the level of the procoagulant factors II, VII, IX, and X, also may reduce the concentration of proteins C and S sufficiently to nullify the desired antithrombotic effect. In addition, there are patients with coumarin-induced skin necrosis who are protein C–deficient, suggesting that this defect may predispose patients to a rare but serious complication of oral anticoagulants. Patients with homozygous protein C deficiency require periodic plasma infusions rather than oral anticoagulants to prevent recurrent intravascular coagulation and thrombosis.

DYSFIBRINOGENEMIAS AND FIBRINOLYTIC DEFECTS   Several families have now been described with recurrent venous thrombosis and embolism due to defects in fibrinogen or plasminogen or with decreased synthesis or release of tissue plasminogen activator. While the majority of dysfibrinogenemias cause bleeding, several variants are characterized by excessively rapid release of fibrinopeptides and recurrent thromboembolism. Patients with this disorder as well as those with an abnormal plasminogen which resists activation by streptokinase and urokinase have been treated successfully with heparin and oral anticoagulants. Defects in tissue plasminogen activator content or release have not been completely characterized. One group of patients with recurrent venous thrombosis and embolism failed to increase venous blood fibrinolytic activity when challenged with local ischemia or physical exercise. The other group had impaired fibrinolytic activity in extracts prepared from biopsied veins. The cloning of cDNA for tissue plasminogen activator (tPA) coupled with the availability of immunoassays for tPA should facilitate more detailed studies of this class of defects. There is also recent evidence that young patients with acute myocardial infarction may have impaired fibrinolysis due to increased plasma levels of plasminogen

activator inhibitor (PAI), a serine protease inhibitor which binds to tPA and is derived from endothelial cells.

In addition to the inherited disorders which predispose patients to thromboembolism, many common illnesses are associated with an increased risk of thrombosis (see Table 315-3). These patients are said to have a "hypercoagulable" or "prethrombotic" state. This increased risk is seen in patients with chronic congestive heart failure and metastatic malignancy and in patients undergoing major surgery. In these patients, the generation of tissue factor activity in damaged or ischemic tissue or metastatic tumor, coupled with venous stasis and endothelial injury, induces the formation of venous and, more rarely, arterial thrombi. There are also several hematologic disorders including paroxysmal nocturnal hemoglobinuria, essential thrombocythemia, and polycythemia vera in which poorly defined abnormalities in circulating leukocytes and platelets or changes in blood flow and viscosity predispose patients to venous and arterial thrombosis. Diseases which affect the endothelial cell, such as Behçet's syndrome, Kawasaki's disease, and homocystinuria, or the administration of drugs such as the oral contraceptives, which lower antithrombin III levels, or L-asparaginase, which inhibits production of multiple coagulation factors, also may predispose patients to thrombosis. Infusion of GM-CSF has been associated with thrombosis as well.

REFERENCES

ANTONARAKIS SE: The molecular genetics of hemophilia A and B in man. Factor III and factor IX deficiency. Adv Hum Genet 17:17, 1988

FEINSTEIN DI: Lupus anticoagulant, anticardiolipin antibodies, fetal loss and systemic lupus erythematosus. Blood 80:859, 1992

GIDDINGS JC, PEAKE IR: Laboratory support in the diagnosis of coagulation disorders. Clin Haematol 14:571, 1985

GINSBURG KJ et al: Anticardiolipin antibodies and the risk for ischemic stroke and venous thrombosis. Ann Intern Med 117:997, 1992

KANE WH, DAVIE EW: Blood coagulation factors V and VIII: Structural and functional similarities and their relationship to hemorrhagic and thrombotic disorders. Blood 71:539, 1988

KASPER CK, DIETRICH SL: Comprehensive management of haemophilia. Clin Haematol 14:489, 1985

LAWN R: The molecular genetics of hemophilia. Sci Am 254:48, 1986

LUSHER JM et al: Recombinant factor VIII for the treatment of untreated patients with hemophilia A: Safety, efficacy and development of inhibitors. N Engl J Med 328:453, 1993

MAMMEN E: Congenital coagulation disorders. Semin Thromb Hemost 9:1, 1983

PIERCE GF et al: The use of purified clotting factor concentrates in hemophilia. Influence of viral safety, cost and supply on therapy. JAMA 261:3434, 1989

WHITE GC, SHOEMAKER CB: Factor VIII gene and hemophilia A. Blood 73:1, 1989

316   ANTICOAGULANT, FIBRINOLYTIC, AND ANTIPLATELET THERAPY

ROBERT I. HANDIN

ANTICOAGULANT AND FIBRINOLYTIC THERAPY

Anticoagulation with heparin, followed by treatment with oral vitamin K antagonists, is the standard treatment for acute venous thrombosis and pulmonary embolism. In addition, chronic oral anticoagulation is used to prevent cerebral arterial embolism from cardiac sources such as ventricular mural thrombi, atrial thrombi, or from an atherosclerotic, partially stenosed carotid or vertebral artery. Anticoagulants are also used, less successfully, to treat peripheral or mesenteric arterial thrombosis. These agents retard fibrin deposition on established thrombi and prevent the formation of new thrombi. The induction of a fibrinolytic state by the infusion of plasminogen activators like recombinant tissue plasminogen activator (rtPA), streptokinase (SK), or urokinase (UK) has become an accepted mode of therapy for some

TABLE 316-1 Anticoagulant therapy with heparin

Clinical indication	Dose, U.S.P. units	Route
Prophylaxis in general surgery	5000 q 12 h	SC
Prophylaxis in medical patients with congestive heart failure, cardiomyopathy, or myocardial infarction	10,000 q 12 h	SC
Venous thromboembolism (acute)	5000 (bolus) then 1000 qh	IV
Venous thromboembolism (prophylaxis in pregnancy, warfarin failures, or chronic DIC)	1000 qh	SQ pump

thromboembolic disorders. Fibrinolytic therapy has been advocated for patients with massive pulmonary embolism and systemic hypotension and to restore the patency of acutely occluded peripheral and coronary arteries. There is increasing evidence that prompt fibrinolytic therapy may reduce both myocardial damage and mortality following acute coronary occlusion (see Chap. 202).

ACUTE ANTICOAGULATION WITH HEPARIN Heparin is a naturally occurring mucopolysaccharide polymer with tetrasaccharide sequences that bind to and activate antithrombin III. It is an extremely potent anticoagulant that can dramatically reduce thrombin generation and fibrin formation in patients with acute venous and arterial thrombosis or embolism (Table 316-1). Heparin is administered to patients with acute thrombosis or embolism by continuous intravenous infusion at a rate sufficient to raise the activated partial thromboplastin time (APTT) to 1.5 to 2 times the patient's preheparin APTT. This requires infusion of approximately 1000 U.S.P. units per hour and is continued while patients are begun on oral anticoagulants and achieve appropriate prolongation of the prothrombin time. The usual duration of combined heparin-warfarin therapy is 5 to 7 days. Heparin is then discontinued, and the patient is maintained on warfarin. Alternatives to a continuous infusion include the administration of 5000 U.S.P. units of heparin four times a day either subcutaneously or intravenously. Long-term heparin administration via portable external or implantable pumps is occasionally needed for patients with recurrent thromboembolism that is refractory to oral anticoagulants, for pregnant women with thromboembolism, and for patients with chronic disseminated intravascular coagulation (DIC). Lower doses of heparin (5000 U.S.P. units every 12 h) have also been used to prevent deep venous thrombosis in high-risk surgical and medical patients. Patients with congestive heart failure, myocardial infarction, or cardiomyopathy may require 10,000 U.S.P. units every 12 h for similar protection.

The major complication of heparin therapy is bleeding—especially from surgical sites and into the retroperitoneum. Aspirin or aspirin-containing drugs impair platelet function. Thus, intramuscular injections in patients on both heparin and an antiplatelet drug may cause significant bleeding. Heparin's anticoagulant effect can be rapidly reversed by the administration of protamine sulfate. However, this is usually not necessary, since reduction or omission of heparin usually improves hemostasis and stops bleeding. Thrombocytopenia occurs in about 10 percent of heparin recipients, and is usually mild with the platelet count falling to 50,000 to 100,000 per milliliter. Thrombocytopenia is more common in patients receiving heparin derived from beef lung as opposed to porcine intestinal mucosa. Thus, porcine heparin is the preferred agent. Occasionally, thrombocytopenia can be severe and may be accompanied by intravascular platelet agglutination and arterial thrombosis. Recognition of the rare complication of thrombocytopenia and paradoxical thrombosis is critical, since discontinuing heparin can promptly reverse the syndrome and may be lifesaving. Heparin administration for longer than 2 months also carries a risk of osteoporosis.

Commercial heparin preparations are quite heterogeneous and only about 20 percent of the infused material has anticoagulant activity.

Low-molecular-weight heparin fractions, which retain anticoagulant activity, are being evaluated as an alternative to continued anticoagulation. These fractions do not interact with platelets and, thus, will not cause thrombocytopenia. However, low-molecular-weight heparin is not yet licensed for use in the United States.

CHRONIC ORAL ANTICOAGULATION The coumarin anticoagulants, which include warfarin and dicumarol (dicoumarol), prevent the reduction of vitamin K epoxides in liver microsomes and induce a state analogous to vitamin K deficiency (see Fig. 316-1). They slow thrombin generation and clot formation by impairing the biologic activity of the prothrombin complex proteins and are used to prevent the recurrence of venous thrombosis and pulmonary embolism. Although regimens employing loading doses of drug have been advocated, the simplest way to induce anticoagulation is to administer a single dose of a coumarin compound and monitor the prothrombin time (PT) until the desired prolongation is achieved. For example, treatment can be initiated with 5 to 10 mg/d of warfarin or equivalent, with the goal of prolonging the PT to 1.5 to 2 times the control value. Although the PT may reach this value after a few days of therapy, effective anticoagulation, with stable reduction of all the prothrombin complex proteins, requires at least 1 week of warfarin administration. Most patients require a daily maintenance dose of 2.5 to 7.5 mg of warfarin to remain anticoagulated. As discussed above, patients should remain on heparin until the appropriate dose of a coumarin anticoagulant, like warfarin, is established.

There is increasing concern that a more precise method is needed to assess the intensity of anticoagulation with warfarin. Commercial thromboplastins have different potencies and markedly affect the resulting PT. The International Normalized Ratio (INR) method is gradually being adopted by hospital laboratories and clinicians. In this reporting method, the ratio of the patient's PT is compared to the mean PT for a group of normal individuals. The ratio is adjusted for the sensitivity of the laboratory's thromboplastin determined by the International Sensitivity Index (ISI). Thus the INR $= (PT_{patient}/PT_{normal})^{ISI}$. Use of the INR permits physicians to obtain the appropriate level of anticoagulation independent of laboratory reagents and to follow published recommendations for intensity of anticoagulation.

Although warfarin anticoagulants reduce the recurrence of deep venous thrombosis and pulmonary or cerebral embolism, they may

FIGURE 316-1 The mechanism of action of various plasminogen activators used for thrombolytic therapy. Recombinant tissue plasminogen activator (rtPA) and pro-urokinase (proUK) preferentially activate plasminogen bound to fibrin and are called "fibrin-specific" activators. Urokinase (UK), streptokinase (SK), and acylated streptokinase-plasminogen conjugates activate both free and fibrin-bound plasminogen.

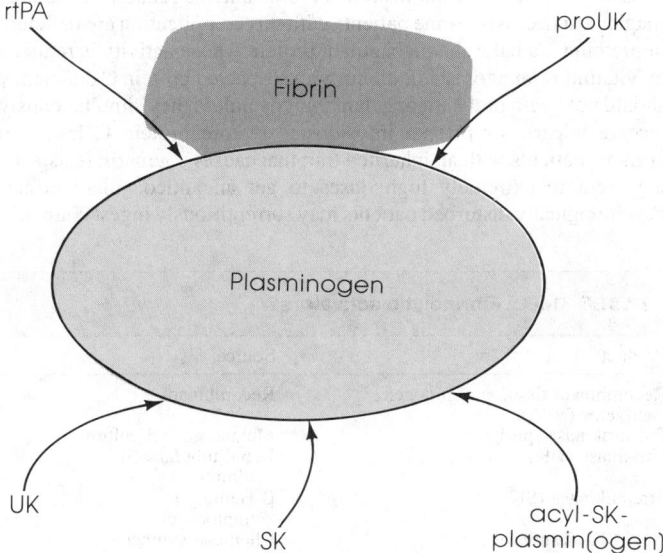

TABLE 316-2 Effect of drugs and metabolic changes on oral anticoagulant potency

Factors leading to enhanced potency and increased prothrombin time
- A Reduced coumarin clearance
  - 1 Disulfiram
  - 2 Metronidazole
  - 3 Trimethoprim-sulfamethoxazole
- B Reduced albumin binding
  - 1 Phenylbutazone
- C Additive hemostatic effect of certain drugs or disorders
  - 1 Aspirin
  - 2 Heparin
  - 3 Liver disease
  - 4 Thrombocytopenia
  - 5 Vitamin K deficiency
- D Increased turnover of vitamin K
  - 1 Clofibrate
  - 2 Hypermetabolism (e.g., hyperthyroidism)

Factors leading to diminished potency and decreased prothrombin time
- A Accelerated coumarin clearance—induction of hepatic metabolizing enzymes
  - 1 Barbiturates
  - 2 Rifampin
- B Reduced absorption
  - 1 Cholestyramine
- C Impaired metabolism
  - 1 Genetic coumarin resistance

also cause bleeding. Any patient who takes oral anticoagulants requires frequent monitoring of the PT. Despite the most careful management, fluctuations in PT can occur. Various drugs that alter liver microsomal metabolism of coumarins or compete for albumin binding sites can increase or decrease the potency of these drugs (Table 316-2).

There is a direct relation between the duration of anticoagulation and the risk of recurrent thrombosis. Although recommendations vary somewhat, most patients with a single uncomplicated thromboembolic event have maximal benefit after 3 to 6 months of anticoagulation. About 10 percent of patients on an oral anticoagulant for 1 year have a serious complication requiring medical supervision, and 0.5 to 1 percent have a fatal hemorrhagic event despite careful medical management. The anticoagulant effects of coumarins can be reversed by infusion of fresh frozen plasma or by the administration of vitamin K. In many cases, reduction or omission of several doses improves hemostasis and stops hemorrhage. Despite the risk of bleeding, patients with prosthetic heart valves, severe mitral stenosis, cardiomyopathy, chronic congestive heart failure, recurrent or persistent atrial fibrillation, or an inherited "prethrombotic" disorder may require lifelong anticoagulation.

One devastating complication of oral anticoagulation is hemorrhagic skin necrosis. Some patients with this complication are deficient in protein C, a natural anticoagulant protein whose activity is reduced by vitamin K antagonists. Patients with suspected protein C deficiency should not begin oral anticoagulant therapy unless they simultaneously receive heparin or plasma infusions to restore protein C levels to normal. Patients with an inherited trait that causes coumarin resistance may require extremely high doses to get an anticoagulant effect. Psychologically disturbed patients may surreptitiously ingest coumarin

and present with unexplained bleeding and a prolonged PT. Plasma coumarin levels can be measured to confirm such ingestion.

FIBRINOLYTIC THERAPY Fibrinolysis, an important part of the normal hemostatic process, is initiated by the release of either tPA or pro-urokinase (proUK) from endothelial cells. These agents preferentially activate plasminogen, which is adsorbed onto fibrin clots. This serves to direct and localize the lytic process to sites that contain fibrin thrombi. Although fibrinolysis begins immediately after vascular injury, clot lysis and vessel recanalization may not be complete for 7 to 10 days. As previously discussed (see Chap. 57), the fibrinolytic pathway is important in normal hemostasis, as defects can predispose patients to either hemorrhage or recurrent thrombosis (see Chap. 315). Activators of the fibrinolytic system are now being used to accelerate clot lysis in patients with thromboembolism (see Fig. 316-1, Table 316-3).

The pharmacologic agents being used to accelerate clot lysis are either derived from natural products or are chemically modified derivatives. They differ with respect to fibrin specificity and some types of complications (see Table 319-3). For example, many individuals have antistreptococcal antibodies which react with streptokinase and reduce its potency and cause febrile reactions. All fibrinolytic agents cause hemorrhage. tPA, proUK, and several other agents are relatively "fibrin-specific" and preferentially activate plasminogen in the presence of fibrin. Although this makes it theoretically possible to achieve selective clot lysis, in practice there is little difference in either the efficacy or toxicity of the "specific" and "nonspecific" fibrinolytic agents. There is, however, a substantial difference in cost, with equivalent doses of rtPA costing ten times that of SK.

It is important to remember that there is always some systemic fibrinolysis after the infusion of clinically effective doses of fibrin-specific agents. In fact, the fibrinogen level falls approximately 25 percent after infusion of lytic doses of rtPA. In addition, both the fibrin-specific and -nonspecific agents can cause hemorrhage as they cannot differentiate between vital hemostatic plugs and pathologic thrombi. To minimize the risk of bleeding, systemic lytic therapy is not recommended for patients with recent surgery or a history of neurologic lesions, gastrointestinal bleeding, or hypertension.

The current indications for fibrinolytic therapy are listed in Table 316-4. Fibrinolytic agents have been given to patients with pulmonary embolism for over 30 years. Such therapy is currently recommended for patients with massive pulmonary embolism that is complicated by hypotension, hypoxemia, and right heart strain. It is also used for selected patients with peripheral arterial embolism or occlusion and for patients with extensive iliofemoral thrombophlebitis. While lytic therapy may hasten the resolution of venous thrombi, the long-term benefit still remains unproven, and there is no firm evidence that lytic therapy reduces postphlebitic complications. In contrast, fibrinolytic therapy may be of distinct benefit in patients with axillary vein thrombosis, a condition which does not usually respond to conventional anticoagulation. Fibrinolytic agents are also used to restore the patency of occluded venous catheters and dialysis shunts. For this indication the agents are instilled locally. The extensive literature on the use of fibrinolytic agents to treat patients with coronary artery disease and myocardial infarction is reviewed in Chap. 202. When

TABLE 316-3 Fibrinolytic activators

Product	Source	MW	Fibrin	Complications
Recombinant tissue plasminogen activator (rtPA)	Recombinant	70,000	+	Bleeding
Pro-urokinase (proUK)	Melanoma cell cultures	55,000	+	Bleeding
Urokinase (UK)	Renal tubular cell cultures	33,000	+	Bleeding
Streptokinase (SK)	β-Hemolytic streptococci	47,000	−	Immune reactions—hypotension, fever Bleeding
Acyl-SK-plasmin(ogen)	Chemical synthesis	139,00	+/−	Immune reactions—hypotension, fever Bleeding

TABLE 316-4 Indications for fibrinolytic therapy

Acute coronary occlusion/infarction
Acute peripheral arterial occlusion
Massive pulmonary embolism
Axillary vein thrombosis
Massive iliofemoral vein thrombosis
Occluded A-V shunt
Arterial or venous cannulae

---

given within a few hours of infarction it appears to reduce mortality and the extent of myocardial damage.

Although the doses and mode of administration may differ slightly, the general principles and complications are the same for all the fibrinolytic agents. SK and UK are the oldest and most extensively studied fibrinolytic agents. SK is a bacterial enzyme, and UK is a product of renal tubular epithelial cells. SK is an indirect plasminogen activator that interacts with circulating plasminogen to form an equimolar complex with proteolytic activity. The SK-plasminogen complex then activates additional plasminogen molecules that initiate fibrinolysis. In contrast, UK has intrinsic proteolytic activity and can activate plasminogen directly.

In the case of SK, one usually administers a loading dose of 250,000 units irrespective of body weight. Since patients may have antistreptococcal antibodies, the loading dose may need to be repeated. In addition, patients may develop acute allergic symptoms including urticaria and, occasionally, serum sickness reactions. With UK, a loading dose of 4400 units per kg body weight is administered over 10 to 30 min. Both regimens induce an intense lytic state as evidenced by a drop in fibrinogen, prolongation of the thrombin time, and a prolongation of the euglobulin lysis time—an in vitro measure of fibrinolytic activity. After the initial loading dose, 100,000 units of SK or 4400 units of UK per kg body weight are administered hourly for 24 to 72 h. At the desired time, the lytic state is reversed by discontinuing UK or SK and by administering heparin for 7 to 10 days. Heparin can be started at the same time as the fibrinolytic agent. To enhance the likelihood of success, fibrinolytic therapy should be initiated as soon as possible after the onset of thrombosis or embolism.

Fibrin-specific agents such as rtPA or proUK are also administered intravenously. For example, systemic infusion of 100 mg rtPA over 6 h restores coronary artery patency in approximately 75 percent of patients. Patients are then maintained on heparin for several days. ProUK given in a similar manner has almost identical effects.

ANTIPLATELET DRUG THERAPY

Antiplatelet drugs have a role to play in the management of patients with arterial vascular disease and thromboembolism (see Table 316-5). Aspirin is the most widely studied of these drugs because of its unique pharmacology. A single dose of aspirin irreversibly acetylates and inactivates the enzyme cyclooxygenase and thereby inhibits platelet

TABLE 316-5 Indications for antiplatelet drug therapy

Cerebrovascular disease
 Transient ischemic attacks
 Secondary prevention of cerebrovascular accidents
Cardiovascular disease
 Unstable angina pectoris
 Primary prevention of myocardial infarction
 Secondary prevention of myocardial infarction
 Following coronary bypass grafting
 Following insertion of a prosthetic valve
Renal disease
 To maintain the patency of A-V cannulas
 ? To slow the progression of glomerular disease

---

production of thromboxane A_2. Although aspirin may also inactivate cyclooxygenase in some tissues, including endothelial cells, such cells recover rapidly by synthesizing new enzyme. Platelets, which are anucleate, cannot synthesize new enzyme and remain inactive for the rest of their life span. As little as one 160 mg tablet of aspirin daily or a 325-mg tablet every other day inhibits platelet thromboxane production and aggregation.

Patients with coronary artery disease who have unstable angina are at high risk for myocardial infarction (Chap. 202). In two large clinical trials, the prompt administration of aspirin dramatically reduced progression to myocardial infarction in this group, although aspirin had no effect on the frequency, intensity, or duration of chronic angina. Aspirin also reduces the incidence of second infarction by 25 percent when administered to men who have had a myocardial infarct. In a large study of male physicians, daily aspirin therapy also reduced the incidence of first infarcts and is now widely used for prevention of myocardial infarction. The preliminary results of large-scale clinical and epidemiologic studies carried out in women suggest that the same beneficial effects of aspirin may be expected. The combination of aspirin and dipyridamole, when begun prior to surgery, may also increase the patency of coronary bypass grafts, and the same combination reduces the incidence of cerebral emboli in patients on warfarin who have prosthetic intracardiac valves. Although dipyridamole has been a popular antithrombotic agent, it has little efficacy when given alone. There is recent evidence that aspirin is probably the only active agent in the combination aspirin-dipyridamole trials. Thus, in most cases, dipyridamole could be eliminated in favor of aspirin alone.

Aspirin also reduces the frequency of transient ischemic attacks in patients with occlusive cerebrovascular disease. It has largely supplanted anticoagulation with the coumarin compounds in patients with transient ischemia. Aspirin also reduces the incidence of a second stroke by 25 percent when administered to men following the first cerebrovascular accident. Aspirin is also effective in maintaining the patency of arteriovenous cannulas inserted into patients with renal failure who require hemodialysis. Aspirin plus dipyridamole may also slow the progression of some forms of glomerulonephritis, although these drugs are not widely used in the treatment of renal disease. However, aspirin appears not to be effective in maintaining the patency of vessels following percutaneous angioplasty.

Although aspirin is clearly the most efficacious antiplatelet agent in clinical use today, there are a large number of new drugs being tested that may soon supplement aspirin therapy. Ticlopidine, which is a potent inhibitor of platelet function, has shown some efficacy in a limited number of clinical trials. In addition, analogues of the leech anticoagulant peptide hirudin, which are potent inhibitors of thrombin, may soon be available. Finally, there are a number of agents, including monoclonal antibodies and recombinant and chemically synthesized peptides, which block either platelet adhesion or aggregation, that are undergoing animal and early clinical trials.

REFERENCES

AMERICAN COLLEGE OF CHEST PHYSICIANS: Second Conference on Antithrombotic Therapy. Chest 95(supp), 1989

COLLEN D: Towards improved thrombolytic therapy. Lancet 342:34, 1993

COLLER BS: Platelets and thrombolytic therapy. N Engl J Med 322:33, 1990

LEE TH et al: Candidates for thrombolysis among Emergency Room patients with acute chest pain: Potential true- and false-positive rates. Ann Intern Med 110:957, 1989

LEVINE MN, HIRSH J: Hemorrhagic complications of anticoagulation therapy. Semin Thromb Hemost 12L:39, 1986

LOSCALZO J, BRAUNWALD E: Tissue plasminogen activator. N Engl J Med 319:925, 1988

MARDER VJ, SHERRY S: Thrombolytic therapy: Current status (parts 1 and 2). N Engl J Med 318:1512, 1988

SAOUR JN et al: Trial of different intensities of anticoagulation in patients with prosthetic heart valves. N Engl J Med 322:428, 1990

section 3   Neoplastic diseases

317   PRINCIPLES OF NEOPLASIA

JOHN MENDELSOHN

The past few years have witnessed remarkable progress in understanding the biologic and biochemical bases for cancer. Gains in the treatment of nonresectable cancer in adults have been gradual and have focused upon those malignancies characterized by unusual sensitivity to radiation and chemotherapy. These include primarily acute leukemia, the lymphoproliferative malignancies, testicular cancer, and breast cancer. New treatment modalities involving immunotherapy and agents that promote normal cell maturation remain experimental and are under intensive investigation. Meanwhile, the search has begun for compounds which can interact with oncogene products, gene regulators, and growth factors and their receptors. Research employing modern technology in molecular genetics and immunology promises to provide a new array of anticancer agents which could move rapidly into clinical trials. This is possible because understanding cancer as a pathologic process is buttressed by new knowledge of cancer as an acquired genetic derangement.

This chapter provides an overview of the biology, etiology, and clinical sequelae of the neoplastic process, followed by a description of the general methods for diagnosing cancer and determining its stage, or extent of spread. Oncogenes and the molecular genetics of malignant transformation are discussed in Chap. 63. Cancer treatment is presented in Chap. 318, and the details of managing patients with specific types of malignant disease will be found in the chapters devoted to disorders of various specific organs.

DEFINITION   The terms cancer, neoplasia, and malignancy are usually used interchangeably in both the technical and popular literature. The disease called *cancer* is best defined by four characteristics which describe how cancer cells act differently from their normal counterparts.

1 Clonality: Cancer originates from genetic changes in a single cell, which proliferates to form a clone of malignant cells.
2 Autonomy: Growth is not properly regulated by the normal biochemical and physical influences in the environment.
3 Anaplasia: There is a lack of normal, coordinated cell differentiation.
4 Metastasis: Cancer cells develop the capacity for discontinuous growth and dissemination to other parts of the body.

Properties similar to each of these characteristics *can* be expressed by normal, nonmalignant cells at certain appropriate times—for example, during embryogenesis and wound repair—but in cancer cells the characteristic is inappropriate or excessive. Benign tumors are clonal and have some degree of autonomy but remain differentiated and do not metastasize. The process by which a normal cell is converted into one which exhibits these four characteristic traits is termed *malignant transformation.*

THE CLINICAL PROBLEM   One-third of all individuals in the United States will develop cancer. The 5-year relative survival rate for these patients (the probability of escaping death from cancer for 5 years following diagnosis) has risen to 50 percent as a result of progress in the early diagnosis and therapy of this disease. Over 6 million living Americans have a history of cancer, and about 3 million were diagnosed 5 or more years ago. Cancer remains second only to cardiovascular disease as a cause of death in this country. More than

20 percent of Americans die from cancer, and this figure has been rising steadily as the population ages and deaths from heart disease decline. In the United States, malignancy accounted for 526,000 deaths in 1992. Half of the deaths were due to the three most common types of cancer: lung, breast, and colon-rectum. Lung cancer is more prevalent in males, while breast cancer is the most common form of malignancy in females. Cancer of the colon and rectum is equally common in males and females.

Information is provided yearly by the American Cancer Society, summarizing the incidence and mortality rates for the common types of cancer. Table 317-1 and Fig. 317-1 present just a small portion of the extensive data available. Of particular importance is the clear documentation in Fig. 317-1 that deaths from lung cancer are increasing in the face of stable or falling rates for a number of other types of malignant disease.

Cancer typically presents to the physician as an abnormal growth, or tumor, which causes illness by production of biochemically active molecules, by local expansion, or by invasion into adjacent or distant tissue sites. The symptoms of the illness depend upon the specific molecular products and the location(s) of the tumor. Each type of cancer has a relatively distinctive natural history that describes the likely clinical course of the particular neoplastic process. Designing a proper treatment plan for an individual patient with malignant disease depends upon determining the extent of disease spread, together with a knowledge of the natural history and the available therapeutic alternatives for the particular type of cancer.

TUMOR CELL BIOLOGY AND BIOCHEMISTRY   Since all cells in an organism originate from a single fertilized egg (zygote), all carry the identical genetic information. The proliferation and differentiation of this cell into an embryo, and eventually into a mature organism, involve selective and coordinated expression of the genomic repertoire. Control of gene expression is accomplished through incompletely understood molecular interactions which can be modulated, in part, by chemical influences in the environment. The genomic repertoire includes information which permits cells to expand clonally, to function with varying degrees of autonomy, to differentiate, and to move from one part of the organism to another

TABLE 317-1   Estimated new cases and deaths for major sites of cancer—1992

Site or type	Number of cases	Deaths
Lung	170,000	149,000
Colon-rectum	152,000	57,000
Breast	183,000	46,000
Prostate	106,000	30,000
Urinary tract	79,000	21,000
Uterus	45,000*	10,000
Lymphoma	43,000	21,000
Oral	30,000	8,000
Pancreas	28,000	25,000
Leukemia	29,000	19,000
Melanoma	32,000[†]	7,600
Stomach	24,000	14,000
Ovary	22,000	13,000
All sites‡	1,170,000	526,000

* Includes cervix. If carcinoma in situ is included, cases total about 100,000.
† Estimated new cases of skin cancer (nonmelanoma) = about 700,000.
‡ Includes additional sites.
NOTE: Estimates by the American Cancer Society are based on rates from the N.C.I. SEER program 1987–1989.

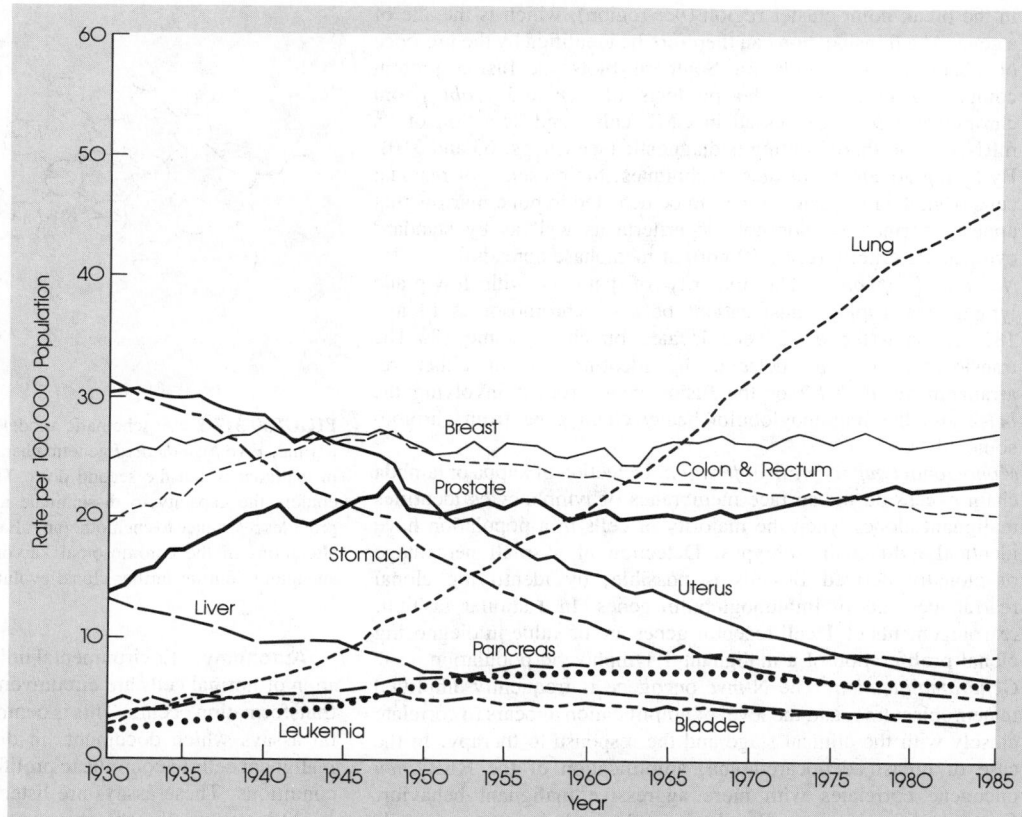

FIGURE 317-1 Cancer death rates by site in the United States, 1930 to 1985. *(Prepared by the American Cancer Society from data provided by the National Center for Health Statistics and the Bureau of the Census.)*

in a coordinated way. In the adult, the process of wound healing activates expression of these cellular characteristics in a more "embryo-like" fashion, but under well-coordinated control. In the case of malignancy, the normal control process is subverted or bypassed due to the anomalous activities of a select group of genes which have central importance to the regulation of cellular activities.

Clonality Careful cytogenetic analysis of metaphase chromosome preparations from cancer cells has yielded a wealth of information about the neoplastic process. It has become clear that virtually all solid tumors and a majority of hematopoietic malignancies display abnormalities in the chromosomal karyotype which are inherited by the population of tumor cells. These may involve translocations of chromosomal fragments into new positions, as well as additions or deletions of parts of chromosomes or whole chromosomes. A particular karyotypic alteration often occurs in a substantial fraction of all patients with a form of cancer. The first and most well known example of this is the Philadelphia chromosome (Ph) observed in 85 percent of patients with chronic myelogenous leukemia (CML), in which the long arm of chromosome 22 is translocated onto the long arm of chromosome 9. This alteration is so characteristic of CML that when analysis of some cases of acute lymphocytic leukemia demonstrated the identical translocation, it was inferred that the disease represented an unusual conversion from CML (which usually progresses to acute myelocytic leukemia). Characteristic chromosomal rearrangements have been described in a large number of other human cancers.

The observation of uniform karyotypic abnormalities in all cells within a tumor provides strong evidence for the clonal origin of the tumor. In turn, the chromosomal abnormalities serve as markers of a common malignant state in the individual cells.

A remarkable concordance between the chromosome locations of a number of human cellular oncogenes and the break points involved in chromosome translocations in human malignancies has been demonstrated. Furthermore, in many cases, these locations correlate with "fragile" sites in the chromosome. Treatment of cultured cells

with agents that inhibit the DNA repair process induces chromosomal breaks far more frequently at many of these loci. Accumulating data link these phenomena and suggest that chromosome rearrangements may result in unregulated activation of cellular oncogenes. For example, in Burkitt's lymphoma, the typical translocation between chromosomes 8 and 14 places the cellular *myc* gene adjacent to the immunoglobulin heavy chain locus, a site of gene activation in the normal lymphocyte.

The new techniques of molecular genetics permit direct assessment of genetic alterations in DNA extracts from tissues suspected of harboring malignancy, using the method of *Southern blotting*. This involves restriction endonuclease digestion, agarose gel electrophoresis, and identification of specific DNA molecular species by hybridization with labeled specific probes. Changes in gene expression can be detected by a similar technique with RNA extracts known as *northern blotting*. The new technology of molecular genetics is more powerful than cytogenetics because (1) clonal genetic abnormalities can be identified in nondividing cells, (2) genetic rearrangements are detectable even when few tumor cells exist in a population of predominantly normal cells, and (3) the sensitivity of detection is greatly enhanced by obviating assays dependent on visual identification of altered staining patterns of chromosomes. The polymerase chain reaction takes advantage of the availability of appropriate primers for certain recombinant genes to amplify abnormal genetic material present in rare cells within a population, thereby enabling detection of genetic abnormalities in these cells by Southern blotting. These approaches to the diagnosis of genetic abnormalities are presented in detail in Chap. 61.

Clonal abnormalities in the genetic makeup of cells that can be detected with molecular techniques include gene mutation, rearrangement, translocation, deletion, and amplification. Some examples will serve to demonstrate the utility of these methods.

1 CML: The Ph chromosome is formed by a translocation between chromosomes 9 and 22, with the break in chromosome 22 occurring in the break point cluster region (*bcr* region), which is the site of a gene. The translocation can therefore be identified by the presence of abnormal *bcr* bands on Southern blots. A fusion protein comprising portions of the products of *bcr* and *c-abl* (from chromosome 9) is expressed in CML cells, and detection of its mRNA by northern blotting is diagnostic (see Chaps. 63 and 310). By taking advantage of these techniques, the presence of residual cells from the malignant clone can be detected in bone marrow that appears normal by morphologic criteria as well as by standard cytogenetic criteria (e.g., 30 normal metaphase spreads).

2 *Nodular lymphoma:* The majority of patients with low-grade lymphomas display translocations between chromosomes 14 and 18, involving the *bcl*-2 gene located on chromosome 18. The translocation can be detected by identification of either re-arrangements in *bcl*-2 or the fusion gene product involving the *bcl*-2 and the immunoglobulin heavy chain gene from chromosome 14.

3 *Monoclonal lymphocyte proliferation:* Detection of kappa or lambda chain excess on the surface membranes of lymphocytes identifies malignant clones when the majority of cells in a population have identical light chain subtypes. Detection of a small percentage of clonally derived B cells is possible, by identifying clonal rearranagements of immunoglobulin genes. In a similar fashion, rearrangements of T cell receptor genes are of value in diagnosing clonal proliferation of a malignant T lymphocyte population.

4 *Gene amplification:* The N-*myc* oncogene is frequently amplified in neuroblastoma, and the level of amplification appears to correlate closely with the clinical stage and the response to therapy. In the case of breast adenocarcinoma, amplification of the HER2/*neu* oncogene correlates with more aggressive malignant behavior. Gene amplification in a clonally derived population of tumor cells is detected directly on Southern blots as increased intensity of labeling of the DNA bands derived from the amplified gene.

Studies of the selective expression of the X-linked isoenzymes of glucose-6-phosphate dehydrogenase (G6PD) in heterozygotic patients have provided further evidence for the clonal origin of cancer from a single progenitor cell. Examination of both G6PD isoenzymes and chromosomal karyotypes in CML patients has demonstrated clonal abnormalities in erythroid, myeloid, and megakaryocytic cells, as well as B lymphocytes, suggesting that this malignancy originates in a precursor cell common to all of these cell lineages.

While there is convincing evidence for the origin of cancer from genetic alterations in a single cell, further heritable alterations commonly occur, resulting in the presence of a heterogeneous mixture of subclones in a mature tumor cell population which has proliferated enough to be clinically detectable. This heterogeneity can be demonstrated by assaying a variety of characteristics in the subpopulations within a tumor; for example, further abnormalities in the chromosomal karyotype, varied drug sensitivities and metastatic capacities, difference in growth rates, and the presence or absence of hormone receptors or particular cell surface glycoproteins. With time, therefore, the progressive accumulation of heritable abnormalities in tumor subpopulations typically results in highly significant phenotypic changes which have their clinical counterpart in development of resistance to previously effective therapy or in increased metastatic spread. The appearance of new chromosomal abnormalities or other genetic alterations in patients with Ph positive CML heralds the onset of a rapidly progressive, fatal phase of the disease. A schematic model of this process of clonal progression, or clonal evolution, is shown in Fig. 317-2. It remains to be determined when in the life history of a typical malignancy the process of clonal progression occurs: genetic alterations may occur early, with later expansion of selected subpopulations from a heterogeneous mixture of cells as circumstances change; other genetic alterations may occur close to the time when they are detected by changes in the behavior of the tumor cells.

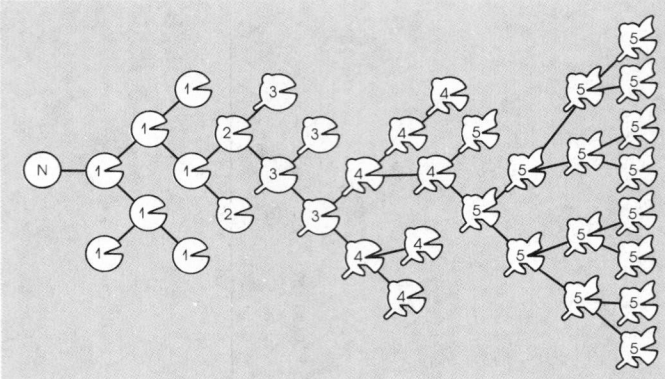

FIGURE 317-2 A schematic model of clonal progression. The N cell is normal. Five *hypothetical* genetic changes are noted. The first does not result in malignancy but the second does. The third adds invasiveness, the fourth confers the capacity to disseminate and produce metastases, and the fifth provides resistance to chemotherapy. Each may be accompanied by incremental alterations in the chromosomal karyotype, with an increasing tendency to aneuploidy during further clonal evolution.

Autonomy Environmental influences which regulate the proliferation of normal cells are circumvented when the process of malignant transformation occurs. This is demonstrable by a variety of experimental assays which document, in different ways, the capacity of the malignant cells to continue to proliferate under normally nonconducive conditions. These assays are listed in Table 317-2.

At least initially, the autonomy of human malignancies is relative rather than absolute. The well-known experiments of Huggins and associates in the 1950s led to a new form of cancer therapy which took advantage of the initial dependence of certain tumors upon the normal influences of sex hormones. The conversion of many prostatic and breast cancers from sensitivity to resistance to hormone therapy vividly demonstrates the further development of autonomy through clonal progression.

Many tumor cell lines can proliferate in culture medium without the usual requirement for serum, provided that a "cocktail" containing three to five essential growth factors and other growth-promoting agents is added. Examples of such factors are epidermal growth factor, platelet-derived growth factor, the carrier protein transferrin, and the hormone insulin. Malignant cells may find even these essential factors unnecessary. One mechanism, demonstrated experimentally and possibly of clinical significance, involves production of a growth

TABLE 317-2 Experimental detection of malignant transformation

Assay	Normal cell	Transformed cell
Capacity of single cells to form colonies in agar suspension	Unsuccessful	Successful
Density-dependent inhibition of cell proliferation in liquid culture	Yes	No
Generations obtained by continuous division in liquid culture	Limited to about 50	Unlimited
Requirements for serum or growth factors	Invariable	Reduced or absent
Capacity to grow as xenografts	Absent	Present

factor (or its analogue) by the tumor cells themselves, a process called *autocrine secretion*. In this situation a polypeptide secreted by the tumor cells may have the capacity to bind to a receptor on the surface of the cells, resulting in autostimulation (Fig. 317-3). The first growth factor to be described with the potential for autocrine stimulation of tumor cells was transforming growth factor alpha, an analogue of epidermal growth factor (EGF) which also binds to the EGF receptor.

A second mechanism by which tumor cells can reduce dependence on growth factors involves expression of increased numbers of receptors on the cell surface. Increased expression of EGF receptors is a common event in epithelial tumors, occurring in nearly all renal cell carcinomas and squamous lung carcinomas that have been examined, and in many other forms of malignancy. Tumor cells may develop a third mechanism for escaping regulation by a growth factor, by activating an internal biochemical process (e.g., the protein tyrosine kinase) ordinarily dependent upon binding of a specific growth factor to a cell surface receptor, thereby completely bypassing the need for exposure to the growth-promoting agent.

Many malignant cells also have the capacity to manipulate a key environmental element required for their growth, the development of an adequate blood supply. Angiogenesis factors produced by tumor cells, such as the fibroblast growth factors, can stimulate the entire series of events involved in the formation of capillaries and blood vessels. Recent data suggest that a high degree of tumor vascularization, observed microscopically on biopsy material, is correlated with a worse clinical prognosis. High levels of receptors for EGF or HER2 also are associated with a shorter survival in a number of malignancies.

Anaplasia   Lack of normal differentiation is a most useful characteristic in the pathologic diagnosis of malignancy. While cancer cells usually bear some of the morphologic characteristics of their normal mature counterparts, they display cellular and histologic abnormalities readily detectable with the light microscope. The cells tend to have large nuclei, with more apparent chromatin and prominent nucleoli. There are increased mitoses, as well as abnormal mitoses and giant cells containing multiple nuclei, reflecting aneuploidy and/or a failure of karyokinesis. The degree of morphologic derangement typically correlates with the extent of disease spread or the metastatic potential of the tumor. The histologic appearance of malignancy is one of disarray, with partial or complete loss of normal tissue architecture. Partial formation of structures such as glands or villi may be suggested, even in poorly differentiated malignancies.

Although the term is not used this way, the process of anaplasia

FIGURE 317-3   A diagrammatic representation of autocrine, paracrine, and endocrine secretion. Peptide growth factors are shown in latent form within the cell. The thickened, semicircular regions of the cell membrane represent receptor sites. *(From MB Sporn, GJ Todaro, N Engl J Med 303:878, 1980, by permission.)*

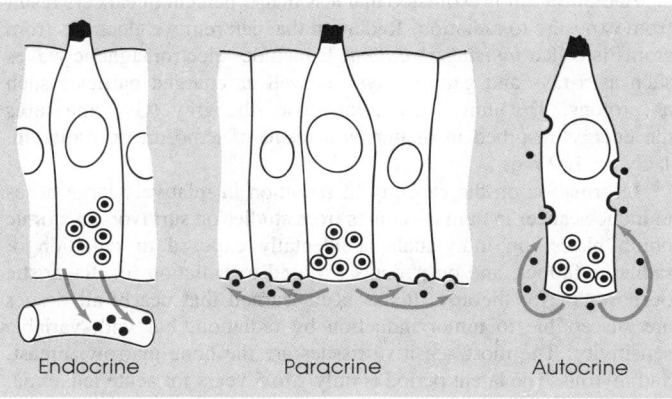

Endocrine   Paracrine   Autocrine

may be expressed at a biochemical level as production of hormones or hormone-related peptides that are either improperly regulated by normal feedback mechanisms (e.g., excessive steroid production by an adrenal carcinoma) or are not appropriate for the particular cell type if it were normally differentiated (e.g., ACTH production by a carcinoma of the lung). In such cases, the genomic repertoire of the malignant cell is expressed inappropriately. Another example is the unregulated production of immunoglobulin (partial or complete chains) by neoplastic derivatives of B lymphocytes.

Histologic features which are abnormal but do not meet the criteria of anaplasia (loss of differentiation) are designated *dysplastic*. Such changes may be seen in ''premalignant'' situations, for example, in the epithelial lining of the bronchi of cigarette smokers. These abnormalities are often reversible. Cessation of smoking can lead to normalization of the lung epithelium over a period of 5 years.

Metastasis   This term encompasses a number of phenotypic traits which together result in the clinical problem that most often leads to death from cancer. The cells lose their adherence and restrained position within an organized tissue, move into adjacent sites, develop the capacity both to invade and to egress from blood vessels, and become capable of proliferating in unnatural locations or environments. These changes in growth patterns are accompanied by an accumulation of biochemical alterations which have the capacity to promote the metastatic process. In experimental situations where tumor cells show a propensity to select a particular organ as a preferred site of metastasis, surface molecules on the metastatic cells appear to have a high affinity for endothelial cells in the vasculature of the specific target organ. The tumor cells also may be dependent upon growth factors produced in the tissues at the preferred site.

The first step in tumor cell invasion probably involves attachment to the extracellular matrix, which is mediated by receptors on the plasma membrane that bind specifically to glycoproteins such as laminin and fibronectin. The second step involves secretion of a variety of tissue-degrading enzymes including collagenases and lysosomal hydrolases. Plasminogen activators which lead to promotion of fibrinolysis are also produced. The third step, which is less well understood, involves movement of tumor cells into the degraded zone of extracellular matrix.

Many biochemical alterations appear to be involved in the progression of a tumor from a homogeneous proliferating clone to a group of heterogeneous subpopulations of cells, some of which have progressively accumulated the entire array of enzymes and surface molecules required for metastasis. It may be for this reason that the rate of metastasis is low during early tumor growth, in spite of the well-documented fact that malignant cells are often released from a tumor into the circulation continuously and in large numbers. Agents which could block critical steps in the metastatic process would be of great value in the armamentarium of antineoplastic agents.

It appears that clonal progression of a tumor generates biochemical or physiologic alterations which confer greater autonomy, greater degrees of anaplasia, and a greater capacity to metastasize. Because there is progresive selection for cells with increased tumorigenic capacity, the process has been called clonal evolution and has been compared to Darwinian evolution, in this case at a cellular level.

ETIOLOGY   Patterns of cancer incidence vary with sex, race, and geographic location. In addition, the types of tumors observed vary with age. Hereditary traits and variations in the internal environments around cells explain some of the differences in cancer incidence. It is clear from epidemiologic investigations that variations in diet and exposure to chemical and physical agents in the external environment contribute to the development of neoplasia. The environmental agents which have been linked to the incidence of cancer fall into three broad categories: radiation, a variety of chemicals, and viruses.

Genetic factors   Genetic alterations play an essential role in oncogenesis. Several lines of evidence support this conclusion: (1) There are many examples of familial aggregation for specific histologic types of tumor (e.g., retinoblastoma). (2) Chromosomal abnormalities carried in the germ line confer increased risk of developing certain types of cancer (e.g., leukemia in trisomy 21). (3) Tumors often display specific somatic rearrangement of chromosomes or genes (e.g., CML). (4) Deficiency in the capacity to repair DNA damage by mutagens is accompanied by increased risk of malignancy (e.g., xeroderma pigmentosa). (5) The capacities for agents to mutate DNA and to act as carcinogens are closely correlated. (6) Mutations or unregulated expression of particular genes can convert cells that behave normally into cells that behave in a malignant fashion.

The molecular mechanisms underlying these genetic abnormalities are beginning to be understood (see Chap. 63). They appear to fall into two major categories:

1. *Oncogenes* are genes which can cause malignant transformation when inappropriately expressed, because of mutation, amplification, or rearrangements. In most cases, they code for growth factors, receptors, or other molecules involved in signal transduction pathways, or for transcription factors that regulate gene expression. Overexpression of these genes leads to constitutive activity of key regulatory molecules that normally are modulated during the cell cycle.
2. *Suppressor genes* act by inhibiting cell growth, and a related category of genes can act by inducing programmed cell death. These genes are involved in tumorigenesis when they are lost or inactivated. Malignant transformation due to suppressor genes is recessive, in that both alleles must be altered, as in the case of the retinoblastoma gene *Rb*-1. However, the genes may appear to have a dominant inheritance pattern because one allele may be constitutionally deleted or because the abnormal gene product may inactivate the normal one, as occurs in the case of p53.

Current models in this rapidly changing field suggest that suppressor genes may act normally by binding transcription factors required for cell-cycle progression, or by serving as transcription factors that activate genes which inhibit cell-cycle progression and proliferation. Gene deletions or loss of restriction fragment length polymorphisms, which identify potential site of suppressor genes, have been described in many types of malignancy.

Data from many sources have generated an interesting model of p53 function. Normal p53 may serve as a "molecular policeman," preventing cell-cycle progression when vital cellular machinery such as the DNA has been damaged by radiation, chemotherapy, or other agents. The cell can then repair the DNA, before resuming completion of the cell cycle. If repair fails in cells that are programmed to proliferate, p53 may trigger cellular suicide by apoptosis. However, in tumor cells with mutated or inactive p53, the capacity for cell-cycle arrest may be compromised. This could provide a genetic explanation for the high incidence of mutational events in malignant cells; such events create the possibility of clonal evolution and selection for more malignant properties. Inability to arrest the cell cycle could also explain why the mutated tumor cells have a high rate of cell death and why they may be more susceptible than normal cells to the lethal effects of chemotherapy and radiotherapy.

The genetic explanation for clonal evolution has been explored by Vogelstein and his collaborators, who carefully examined the molecular changes that occur in the entire spectrum of colorectal tumors, beginning with small adenomatous polyps and ending with invasive adenocarcinoma. These tumors appear to arise as a result of mutational activation of oncogenes, combined with mutational inactivation of suppressor genes. Mutations of at least four or five genes are required for the formation of a malignant tumor. Although the genetic alterations tend to occur in a preferred sequence, it is the total accumulation of changes rather than the order of occurrence that determines the malignant behavior of the tumor cells. The genetic changes that contribute to this process in colon cancer include: (1) mutations of the *ras* oncogene; (2) loss or mutation of three suppressor genes—the familial adenomatous polyposis (*FAP*) gene, the deleted in colon carcinoma (*DCC*) gene, and p53; and (3) DNA hypomethylation (see also Chap. 256).

There have been a number of reports of potential sites of suppressor genes, identified by chromosomal deletions and/or loss of restriction fragment length polymorphism alleles. These include Wilms' tumor (11p13), lung cancer (3p), renal cell carcinoma (3p), bladder cancer (11p), colorectal carcinoma (5q), and breast cancer (13). There are intensive efforts to discover cancer-related genes encoded in the genetic loci, shown above in parentheses. The gene at 11p13, which is involved in some forms of Wilms' tumor, has been found to encode a transcription factor that is believed to regulate the differentiation of nephroblasts.

The genetic changes that play a causal role in malignancy are described in detail in Chap. 63. Somatic mutations that lead to malignant transformation are acquired during the lifetime of the individual, whereas mutations in the germ cells are inherited and form the basis for hereditary neoplasms.

For many of the common malignancies, the incidence of cancer is higher (usually up to three-fold) among patients with positive family histories than among unselected patients. However, the risk can rise to as high as twenty-five- to thirtyfold in certain groups of patients with a familial history of breast cancer or bowel cancer. In addition, there are a number of uncommon inherited disorders involving either a high risk for the occurrence of a particular neoplasm or the presence of multiple preneoplastic lesions that can progress to frank malignancy.

The hereditary neoplasms (Table 317-3) may occur as the only manifestation of a gene defect, or as part of a generalized syndrome involving multiple developmental abnormalities. The inheritance patterns in these disorders are generally autosomal dominant, with varying penetrance. Half of the children of patients with these disorders will inherit the gene defect.

The preneoplastic states are grouped into four major categories (Table 317-3). Neurofibromatosis occurs in 1 of 3000 live births. The neurofibromas undergo sarcomatous changes in about 10 percent of patients, with development of gliomas in the brain or optic nerve, meningiomas, acoustic neuromas, or pheochromocytomas. Chromosome breakage disorders are characterized by the recessive inheritance of chromosomal instability and rearrangements of karyotypes; patients have an increased incidence of acute leukemia. The immune deficiency ataxia-telangiectasia is also characterized by chromosomal fragility. Patients with hereditary or acquired immunodeficiency states have an increased incidence of neoplasia, most commonly the lymphoproliferative malignancies.

Race is a genetic factor in the incidence of cancer, but interpretation of epidemiologic data is made difficult by the concurrent effects of environmental and socioeconomic influences. Both the incidence and the death rate from cancer are higher in American blacks than in American whites, with nearly all of the difference being accounted for by the higher cancer rate in black males. It is believed that later detection and less adequate treatment may account for part, but not all, of the difference in survival. The important effect of environmental factors is made clear by documented differences in cancer incidence for Asian families that have moved to Hawaii and California.

Radiation   It is estimated that less than 3 percent of cancers result from exposure to radiation. Radiation that can remove electrons from atoms is called *ionizing radiation*. It includes electromagnetic waves such as x-rays and gamma rays, as well as charged particles such as protons. The unit of radiation dose, the gray (Gy), measures the energy absorbed in matter as a result of exposure to radiation: 1 Gy = 100 rad.

Information on the capacity of radiation in relatively large doses to induce cancer in humans comes from studies on survivors of atomic bomb blasts, on individuals accidentally exposed to radiation or radiative fallout, and on patients exposed to radiation for diagnostic purposes or for therapy. It has been learned that nearly all tissues are susceptible to tumor induction by radiation, but with variable sensitivity. The most sensitive tissues are the bone marrow, breast, and thyroid. The latent period is only 2 to 5 years for acute leukemia, and 5 to 10 years for most solid tumors. There is a higher incidence

TABLE 317-3 Hereditary neoplasms and preneoplastic conditions

Disorder	Inheritance	Features
HEREDITARY NEOPLASMS		
Retinoblastoma	AD	Often bilateral; susceptibility to second tumors, especially osteosarcoma
Familial polyposis coli	AD	Multiple adenomatous polyps and adenocarcinomas of the colon; some families have osteomas, lipomas, and fibromas (Gardner's syndrome)
Multiple endocrine neoplasia I	AD	Adenomas of the pituitary, parathyroid, and pancreatic islet cells
Multiple endocrine neoplasia II	AD	Medullary carcinoma of the thyroid, pheochromocytoma, and parathyroid tumors
HEREDITARY PRENEOPLASTIC CONDITIONS		
Phakomatoses		
Neurofibromatosis (von Reckling hausen's disease)	AD	Gliomas of the brain and optic nerve, acoustic neuroma, meningioma, and pheochromocytoma
Tuberous sclerosis	AD	Glial tumors; hamartomatous growths in several organs
von Hippel-Lindau syndrome	AD	Hemangioblastomas of cerebellum and retina; renal cell carcinoma and pheochromocytoma
DNA-chromosomal instability		
Xeroderma pigmentosum	AR	Basal and squamous cell carcinoma of skin; malignant melanomas in patients exposed to UV light
Bloom's syndrome	AR	Acute leukemias, various carcinomas
Fanconi's anemia	AR	Acute leukemias, squamous cell carcinomas, and hepatomas
Ataxia-telangiectasia	AR	Acute leukemia, lymphoma, breast cancer in females
Immune deficiency syndrome		
X-linked agammaglobulinemia	XR	Lymphomas and leukemias
Wiskott-Aldrich-syndrome	XR	Acute leukemias and lymphomas
X-linked lymphoproliferative syndrome	XR	Abnormal response to EB virus; EBV-induced B cell immunoblastic lymphomas
Cancer family syndrome	AD	Cancers of multiple organs: colon, endometrium, breast, and lung

AD = autosomal dominant; AR = autosomal recessive; XR = X-linked recessive.
SOURCE: From RS Cotran et al, p. 267.

of leukemia in patients who have received radiation therapy for neoplastic diseases and for ankylosing spondylitis, and of thyroid cancer in children irradiated for thymic enlargement.

Solar radiation, resulting from exposure to electromagnetic radiation from the sun, is the primary risk factor in skin cancer. The evidence for this linkage comes from a variety of epidemiologic and experimental observations. Skin cancer is rare in blacks and the deeply pigmented racial groups, whereas it is especially common in fair-complexioned individuals. It occurs primarily on the parts of the body exposed to sunlight and has a higher incidence in outdoor workers. Patients with genetic diseases such as xeroderma pigmentosa and albinism, which are exacerbated by sunlight, have very high risks for the development of skin cancer.

The carcinogenic effect of solar radiation is greatest in the spectral range of 290 to 320 nm (UV-B radiation), which produces delayed erythema in human skin (sunburn). This range of wavelengths correlates with the action spectrum for UV-induced damage to DNA.

Exposure to solar ultraviolet radiation is also a risk factor in melanoma. As with skin cancer, there is a higher incidence of melanoma among populations living at a latitude nearer the equator, where exposure to UV is greatest.

Tobacco Numerous epidemiologic studies have demonstrated that the principal carcinogenic agent in our environment is inhaled tobacco smoke. The incidence of lung cancer is more than tenfold higher in male smokers than in nonsmokers. Furthermore, tobacco smoking is associated with increased rates of cancer of the oral cavity, esophagus, kidney, bladder, and pancreas. Particulate matter in tobacco smoke, known as "tar," contains a long list of chemicals, primarily polycyclic hydrocarbons, which have been shown experimentally to be contact carcinogens. In addition, the metabolic activation of tobacco components, for example, the cyclic *N*-nitrosamines, can produce carcinogens with the capacity to act upon the cells of internal organs. Tobacco-related malignancies account for one-third of all cancer deaths among men in the United States and for more than 10 percent of all female cancer deaths. Unfortunately, this figure is rising in females. As a result of increased use of tobacco by women in the period since World War II, the deaths from lung cancer in females exceeded deaths from breast cancer in 1988.

Consumption of alcoholic beverages has been shown to potentiate the incidence of malignancies due to tobacco smoke. Alcohol in the absence of smoking appears to play an etiologic role in hepatocellular carcinoma.

Clearly the single most effective action which could be taken against cancer at the present time involves not an application of molecular genetic research, but cessation of smoking. Fortunately, it appears that smoking cessation results in a gradual decrease in risk, so that after 10 to 15 years, exsmokers have nearly the same risk of lung cancer as nonsmokers. Because the habit of smoking is difficult to break, the physician's role in cessation of smoking is of critical importance. Doctors should deliver a *firm* antismoking message.

Occupational exposure to carcinogens The first report of cancer related to occupational hazards was Percival Pott's observation of an unusually high frequency of scrotal cancer among London chimney sweeps in 1775. It is now known that skin cancer (including scrotal) can be induced by a variety of coal tar products, such as the materials contacted in the London chimneys. Epidemiologic studies also have related lung cancer to exposure to coal by-products. Table 317-4 provides a partial listing of industrial agents which are known to cause cancer. Chemical carcinogens, including the components of tobacco smoke, may play two roles in carcinogenesis: as mediators of genetic mutations and as promoters of proliferation of cells bearing genetic mutations.

TABLE 317-4 Examples of occupational causes of cancer

Etiology	Site of malignancy
Arsenic (inorganic)	Lung, skin, liver
Asbestos	Mesothelium, lung
Benzene	Leukemia
Benzidine	Bladder
Chromium compounds	Lung
Radiation (mining, dial painting)	Numerous locations
Mustard gas	Lung
Polycyclic hydrocarbons (coal by-products)	Lung, skin
Vinyl chloride	Angiosarcoma of liver

Air pollution   It is clear that lung cancer incidence is increased by tobacco smoking and by certain industrial and occupational exposures (primarily related to coal tar and combustion by-products). Once the risks resulting from exposure to these factors are taken into account, the epidemiologic evidence that links ambient air pollution to lung cancer remains inconclusive. Studies correlating the incidence of lung cancer with increased levels of polycyclic hydrocarbons and benzo(a)pyrene in urban air are complicated by the difficulty of eliminating the contribution of exposure to these compounds through tobacco smoking as well as occupational exposure.

Medications   Certain drugs and hormones have been shown to be carcinogenic. The synthetic nonsteroidal estrogen diethylstilbestrol (DES), which was used for a period of time to reduce fetal wastage in pregnant women, caused an increased incidence of vaginal and cervical cancer in daughters who were exposed in utero. Conjugated estrogens have been shown to increase the incidence of endometrial cancer in patients treated for menopausal symptoms. The use of progesterone concomitantly, together with decreased estrogen dose, may obviate this problem.

Alkylating agents have been shown to cause an increased incidence of acute myelocytic leukemia and probably other malignancies. They are used in therapeutic situations in which the poor prognosis of malignancy far outweighs the increased risk of an additional cancer in the future. However, because of this risk, new drug regimens which avoid the use of alkylating agents are being explored in situations where substantial long-term benefits from chemotherapy have been demonstrated, for example, in Hodgkin's disease.

The recipients of organ transplants who are treated with immunosuppressive agents, such as azathioprine and prednisone, have an increased incidence of histiocytic lymphoma as well as a variety of solid tumors. A similar increased incidence is observed in individuals with inherited and acquired immunodeficiency, for example, AIDS. This has been attributed to reduced immune surveillance, but a variety of other explanations are equally likely, such as activation of a latent oncogenic virus or chronic immunostimulation in conjunction with a compromised and malfunctioning immune system.

Diet   The role of diet and nutrition in carcinogenesis has been the subject of intensive investigation and equally intensive controversy. There are numerous nutritional hypotheses of carcinogenesis. Some of these have led to unconventional forms of cancer therapy that are based upon no scientific evidence. Unfortunately, these putative dietary therapies are propagated upon a patient population for which proven treatment modalities are often unsuccessful in achieving cure, and at a time when there is a popular emphasis on healthful nutrition.

Epidemiologic analyses of international variations in cancer incidence and comparisons of the types and frequencies of cancer in populations with different dietary habits have yielded a great deal of evidence that cancers of many major sites are influenced by diet. These studies were reviewed in an authoritative publication, *Diet, Nutrition, and Cancer*. Interim dietary guidelines are suggested which are both consistent with good nutritional practices and likely to reduce the risk of cancer: (1) Reduce the intake of fat, saturated and unsaturated, from its present average level (40 percent) to 30 percent of total energy value in the diet. (2) Include fruits (especially citrus), vegetables (especially carotene-rich and cruciferous), and whole cereal grain (fiber) in the daily diet; these provide amounts of vitamins A and C as well as fiber adequate to obviate dietary supplements. (3) Minimize consumption of salt-cured or smoked food. (4) Use alcoholic beverages in moderation, since they increase the risk of certain cancers, especially when combined with cigarette smoking.

Experimental data lend support to the inferences from epidemiologic studies, but additional research is necessary to understand how dietary factors influence carcinogenesis. For example, a number of epidemiologic studies have suggested that a high intake of fat is associated with increased risk of cancer at several sites, including breast and colon. Possible explanations for this observation include increased adiposity, leading to greater conversion of androstenedione to estrone, which could influence carcinogenesis in the breast; and stimulation of increased bile salt excretion which could alter gut flora and thereby augment the production of carcinogenic substances by the bacteria in the colon. Dietary fiber enhances the rapid transit of potential carcinogens through the colon, which could explain the low incidence of bowel cancer and rectal cancer in tropical Africa.

Vitamin C may act to prevent cancer by blocking endogenous formation of *N*-nitroso compounds in the gastrointestinal tract, but there are no data showing that taking vitamin C will prevent cancer in human beings. There is renewed interest in the possibility that increased intake of vitamins A and E may reduce the risk of malignancy. Retinoids have been shown to reduce the incidence of second malignancies, following treatment of head and neck cancers. Further clinical trials will be needed to determine the value of particular vitamins, minerals, or nutritional supplements in amounts greater than provided by a prudent diet. The physician must be alert to the scientifically unproven dietary treatments which patients with cancer may be urged to undertake. Of course the greatest tragedy occurs when patients whose malignancy could be cured by proven therapeutic modalities are misled into depending upon such dietary manipulations.

Viruses   Although there has been extensive research on viral oncogenesis with experimental murine tumors, viruses have been implicated as the direct cause of only a few human cancers. Infection with human T lymphotrophic virus I (HTLV-I) can lead to adult T cell leukemia, an aggressive malignancy of T lymphocytes, which has been reported in large series from Japan and the West Indies. The incidence of hepatocellular carcinoma in endemic regions of Asia and Africa is closely associated with previous infection with hepatitis B virus, followed by a carrier state, suggesting that a causal relationship is highly likely. Chronic hepatocyte infection by the virus might predispose to carcinogenesis in these cells. There may be a variety of contributing factors, including malaria, malnutrition, and exposure to aflatoxin. This is a serious health problem in Asia and Africa, where primary liver carcinomas represent as much as 30 percent of malignancies. There also is a strong statistical correlation between herpes simplex 2 viral infection, which is sexually transmitted, and the incidence of cervical cancer. The Epstein-Barr virus is closely associated with African Burkitt's lymphoma as well as nasopharyngeal carcinoma in Asia. Cofactors in the development of these malignancies might be holoendemic malaria in African Burkitt's lymphoma and a particular configuration of histocompatibility antigens in the case of nasopharyngeal carcinoma among Chinese. The capacity of Epstein-Barr virus to infect human B lymphocytes (infectious mononucleosis) and transform them in cell culture suggests a role for the virus in malignancy.

Risk of cancer   Knowledge of genetic and environmental factors that may contribute to cancer incidence can be utilized by the conscientious physician to identify patients who have an increased risk of malignancy. The presence of certain hereditary diseases in a patient's family may suggest procedures that can lead to early detection and prevention, for example, early surveillance by colonoscopy and prevention by prophylactic colectomy in persons who have familial polyposis of the colon. Environmental factors that increase cancer risks should be identified and avoided. It is evident, however, that changing an individual's life-style in order to avoid exposure to a carcinogen can require an extraordinary level of effort on the part of both the patient and the physician.

New methods are being discovered for detecting individuals at high risk for developing malignancies. These depend on the identification and sequencing of abnormal genes which have a causal role in cellular transformation. Polymerase chain reaction and in situ hybridization techniques can be used to identify the presence of such abnormal genes in cell specimens obtained from individuals with a positive family history. This approach will be extremely valuable in identifying high-risk individuals, who should either undergo frequent diagnostic procedures or consider prophylactic surgery, such as mastectomy. It is possible that within a decade every youngster will donate peripheral blood lymphocytes for a screening procedure that will predict susceptibility to the most common malignancies. The impact of this information on preventive versus therapeutic health care will be of major significance.

CLINICAL SEQUELAE The presence of a malignant lesion may not, in itself, cause symptoms in a patient with cancer. The primary lesion may, for a period of time, be unnoticed and unimportant for the normal maintenance of body functions, in which case its clinical significance is due to its potential for growth and spread. In addition, the presence of metastasis need not result in symptomatic illness. Patients with carcinoma of the bowel, whose disease may have spread beyond the limits of surgical curability, may live for many months or even years with easily detectable metastatic lesions in the lung or abdomen, yet remain free of symptoms until the function of a vital organ is compromised or obstructive problems appear.

Malignancies produce clinical symptoms in three general ways (Table 317-5): by direct effects resulting from invasion or compression of normal tissues; by release of cytokines, hormones, and other biologically active agents into the local and systemic environment; and by secondary psychological effects upon the patient. Each of these factors may contribute profoundly to the degree of illness experienced by the patient. Clinical symptoms resulting from released biologically active agents, as well as systemic problems caused by as yet undetermined mechanisms, are usually grouped under the category of ''paraneoplastic syndromes.''

Mass effects of malignancy In most cases tumors produce clinical problems as a result of local expansion, with obliteration of normal tissues, as the malignant cells proliferate within the confines of the involved organ: marrow replacement by leukemia results in reduced production of the normal cellular elements of the blood; lung cancer compromises oxygen exchange in involved alveoli; primary or metastatic cancer in bone causes weakened trabecular architecture, resulting in pathologic fractures; hepatomas replace normal hepatocytes and interfere with liver function. A second result of local expansion is compression of normal structures, with partial or complete obstruction of tubular organs, blood vessels, and lymphatics: colonic cancer may obstruct the gastrointestinal tract; lung cancer blocks airflow through bronchi and can obstruct pulmonary venous return; hepatic and biliary malignancies produce obstructive jaundice; a variety of intraabdominal neoplasms can encase the ureters, causing renal failure; in the extreme case, penetration of blood vessels can cause hemorrhage. A third result of local expansion is pain, due to pressure on or stretching of nerve fibers. When neoplasia causes increased pressure on nervous tissue within the confines of the skull, the symptoms include headache and vomiting as well as seizure disorders and brain dysfunction.

Paraneoplastic syndromes The malignant process is felt to develop as a result of the unregulated and/or inappropriate expression of certain genes crucial to cell proliferation and differentiation. The aggressiveness of the malignant process is increased by the subsequent uncovering of additional genetic information. In this evolutionary process, abnormal genetic information may be expressed which results in severe physiologic effects upon the patient. As noted above, there may be excessive synthesis of a gene product which is normally found in the particular cell type, or the malignant cell may produce a molecule which does not ordinarily originate from its normal counterpart.

A common type of molecule produced by malignant tumors falls into the category of polypeptide hormones. The synthesis of vasopressin or ACTH by small cell carcinoma of the lung or parathormone by some squamous cancers are examples. These can produce clinical illness by mediating normal physiologic functions to an excessive degree. Other active molecules have been detected which are homologous with or identical to known growth factors. The potential for autonomous stimulation of proliferation mediated by production of essential growth-promoting agents has been discussed.

From this brief introduction, it can be seen that biologically active agents produced by malignant cells can be clinically important for a number of reasons:

1 They may serve as markers for the presence of a type of tumor. Detection of such markers early in the course of the disease might increase chances for cure. They also may be used to follow the clinical progress of the disease and anticipate recurrence.
2 They may produce symptoms as a result of their intrinsic biologic activity. In some cases these can become the major clinical problems determining survival (e.g., hypercalcemia).
3 They may serve to promote the growth of the tumor directly. In turn, growth-promoting agents of this type may become the focus of new approaches to anticancer treatment.

The paraneoplastic sequelae of cancer which involve ectopic hormone production are described in Chap. 327, and the neurologic manifestations of neoplasia in Chap. 328. Cutaneous manifestations of internal malignancy are discussed in Chap. 54. The association of malignancy with certain metabolic disorders, hematologic abnormalities, and immunosuppression will be further described here.

Metabolic disorders One of the major and most characteristic problems seen with cancer is weight loss, usually associated with anorexia. The extensive wasting which results is known as cachexia. The cause for this commonly observed and often life-limiting disturbance remains to be determined in spite of the fact that many contributing factors have been identified. Abnormalities of taste and smell, physiologic malfunction of the gastrointestinal tract, excessive energy demands made by the tumor, and failure to adapt energy expenditure to the levels of nutrient intake have been implicated as causes of cachexia in patients with cancer. Biochemical abnormalities in energy metabolism have been well-characterized in these patients. Fatty acids are oxidized in preference to glucose, and anaerobic glucose metabolism is increased while oxidative phosphorylation is reduced. This results in an inefficient expenditure of ATP, which might lead to an energy deficit. However, none of these observations is felt to account for the magnitude of the problem.

Typically, the anorectic patient simply cannot ingest food, in spite of a clear understanding of the need for increased nourishment. The chief complaint is unpalatability. An aversion to meat has been clearly documented. While nausea may be a component of the syndrome, emesis occurs rarely. This may be because the patient feels so satiated that no food intake is tolerated.

Provision of alimentation through enteral tubes or by the intravenous route has the potential to provide total parenteral nutrition (TPN) to patients with cancer, and the techniques for performing these procedures have been well-described by investigators managing nonmalignant disease. At present there is no indication that the provision of nutritional support at this level can, by itself, affect the course of malignant disease. However, clinical trials have suggested a role for nutritional supplementation, including TPN, in preparing

---

TABLE 317-5 Symptoms caused by malignant diseases

Mass effects
  A Ablation by crowding or by invasion
  B Obstruction of vessels, tubes, and ducts
  C Rupture of blood vessels
Remote effects (paraneoplastic syndromes)
  A Ectopic hormone production
  B Neuropathies and CNS abnormalities
  C Dermatologic abnormalities
  D Metabolic disorders
    1 Anorexia, weight loss
    2 Fever
    3 Chronic inflammation
  E Hematologic disorders
  F Immunosuppression
  G Collagen vascular disorders
Psychosocial effects
  A Loss of control
  B Acceptance of personal finitude
  C Fear of pain and mutilation
  D Separation and loneliness

nutritionally deprived cancer patients for potentially beneficial surgical procedures or chemotherapy programs which otherwise might not have been tolerated due to the wasted state of the patient.

Tumor necrosis factor (TNF) is a polypeptide produced by macrophages. Administration of TNF can mimic the syndrome of cachexia in experimental animals, and it is therefore also known as cachectin. Cytokines released by inflammatory cells and tumor cells are likely candidates as etiologic agents for the debilitation and wasting that accompany aggressive malignancy.

Fever is another sign associated with malignancy, and it is usually attributable to infection. Because of the debility which often accompanies cancer, and the depression in circulating granulocytes and mononuclear cells resulting from aggressive therapeutic measures, the types of infection seen may be unusual. Infection by endogenous bacteria, fungi, viruses, and protozoa must be considered when evaluating fever of unknown etiology in patients with malignancy (see Chap. 16). There remain unusual instances when fever cannot be explained by infection and must be attributed to cytokines released by the patient's inflammatory cells or to a cause intrinsic to the neoplasm itself.

Hematologic abnormalities Anemia is found with increased incidence in advanced stages of malignant disease. The mechanisms accounting for anemia are, in nearly all cases, extrinsic to the tumor, and may be due to several causes. Increased destruction of erythrocytes can result from hypersplenism, microangiopathic hemolysis, and autoantibodies, seen especially in the lymphoproliferative malignancies. Anemia due to occult bleeding is one of the cardinal signs of malignancy in the gastrointestinal tract. Decreased production of erythrocytes may result from iron deficiency related to bleeding, vitamin B_{12} or folate deficiency, erythron depletion due to tumor crowding in the marrow, toxicity secondary to chemotherapy or radiotherapy, and the anemia associated with chronic inflammatory disease.

Granulocytopenia is commonly associated with marrow infiltration by hematologic malignancies, and also results from chemotherapy. The causes of thrombocytopenia are comparable to those associated with anemia. Depression in one or all of the circulating hematopoietic elements may result from one of the various forms of marrow failure or aplastic anemia which are known to be preleukemic.

An increase in the formed elements of the blood also may occur. Erythrocytosis resulting from inappropriate production of erythropoietin is observed not only in polycythemia vera, but also in renal cell carcinoma, hepatoma, and cerebellar hemangioma. An elevated granulocyte count may result from marrow infiltration by tumor cells or an inflammatory response to malignancy, and frank leukemoid reactions may be seen with nonhematopoietic tumors. Thrombocytosis unrelated to primary marrow disease is commonly associated with a systemic malignancy.

A hypercoagulable state is a rare clinical complication of malignancy, although it may be far more prevalent at a subclinical level. Mucin-producing tumors and adenocarcinomas, especially those of the pancreas and stomach, head the list of tumors reported to be associated with clinical disseminated intravascular coagulopathy (DIC). This may present as a migratory thrombophlebitis of unknown etiology, which can produce venous thrombosis as well as pulmonary embolism. Hypercoagulation also may be associated with marantic (nonbacterial) endocarditis and resultant thromboembolic episodes, which further complicate the clinical picture. The treatment of the primary malignancy is the only successful therapeutic attack on the problem. Anticoagulation, following the principles for treatment of DIC (Chaps. 57 and 316), may provide short-term benefits in acute situations, but with attendant risks.

Acute promyelocytic leukemia is often associated with abnormalities of hemostasis related to a hypercoagulable state. The malignant immature granulocytes can release procoagulant materials which initiate DIC.

Immunosuppression Advanced cancer is accompanied by abnormalities in immune function which can be demonstrated by skin testing against common antigens and by examination of lymphocyte responses to mitogenic stimulation in vitro. Morever, in general, the extent of malignant disease correlates well with the degree of immune dysfunction. In spite of a vast experimental literature on this subject, the two significant questions concerning immunosuppression in cancer patients continue to be unanswered: (1) What is the mechanism(s) of inhibition? (2) Is the immunosuppression merely secondary to the malignant state, or could it play an etiologic role (failure of "immune surveillance")?

Experimental data have implicated defects in both T and B cell function, as well as abnormalities of macrophages, in the etiology of the reduced immune competence in cancer patients. Primary malignancies of lymphocytes are accompanied by abnormalities in the functioning of the particular cell type involved. Some of the lymphoproliferative malignancies are characterized by an increase in autoimmune reactions, most notably in 25 percent of patients with chronic lymphocytic leukemia. In addition, both chemotherapy and radiotherapy can produce long-standing suppression of immune function.

One approach to cancer treatment involves attempts to stimulate an effective immune response with the hope that immune antitumor activity can act alone or in concert with the standard therapeutic modalities to eliminate the malignant cell population. Monoclonal antibodies against antigens present in relatively increased quantities on tumor cells may provide ways to reconstitute or hyperconstitute immune responses to malignancy. Treatment with high concentrations of cytokines such as the interferons has produced responses in a number of types of malignancy, and this is especially effective in the therapy of hairy cell leukemia and chronic myelocytic leukemia. Interleukin 2 (IL-2) is another cytokine which may produce antitumor responses in patients with renal carcinoma, when administered in pharmacologic doses alone or in combination with lymphokine-activated killer (LAK) cells.

Psychosocial effects The diagnosis of cancer immediately raises in the mind of the patient and his or her family a host of questions and fears which require the undivided attention of an empathetic, considerate, and skilled physician. This is especially true when the particular form of cancer has a poor chance for cure or when malignancy has recurred.

Of the variety of psychosocial problems experienced by patients, two which are particularly difficult to deal with are helplessness and loss of control. These involve both economic control and personal control of one's activity and one's future. Closely tied to these problems and adding to the feeling of helplessness is the difficulty of accepting personal finitude. A third major source of mental anguish is the fear of pain and mutilation. Finally, separation from loved ones, both anticipated and real, creates a void of loneliness and a fear of abandonment.

The reactions to the mental stresses which are produced by these problems can only be dealt with effectively by a professional who has become familiar with the patient's personality and his or her social and intellectual environment. Although one or another emotion may dominate at a particular time, the responses commonly observed include anger, denial, withdrawal, and depression. Added to these problems is the complexity resulting from the response of the patient's family to the illness and to the patient's own response to the illness. In spite of these stresses, some patients with incurable malignancies are able to adapt and reorient their lives in a creative and meaningful way. The intellectual and emotional challenge to the physician is obvious, and careful attention must be given to managing the patient's (and the family's) responses to malignancy in addition to providing specific treatment for the disease.

Does the patient's psychological attitude have a role in the cause or treatment of malignant disease? The question is a complex and controversial one. There is evidence, which is contested, that life stresses can predispose to systemic illness by producing anxiety or depression. One theory postulates that stress leads to a reduction in immunologic function, resulting in inadequate immune surveillance, but this explanation for the pathogenesis of cancer is not adequately supported by available clinical data. There are also reports that correction of emotional difficulties and development of positive attitudes can aid in prolonging the survival of patients with extensive malignancy. In favor of psychological support and counseling is the clear benefit to the quality of life which can be achieved by helping patients with cancer to develop positive attitudes and to gain some measure of control over *how* they are living. However, scientific evidence does not demonstrate that the patient's psyche can achieve regression or cure of the malignant process. The strongest and most responsible advocates of counseling and attitudinal approaches to cancer patient management also stress the need for concurrent treatment with standard anticancer therapies.

DIAGNOSIS AND STAGING There are a number of general goals in evaluating a patient for the presence of malignancy. The first is to detect malignancy early, since the results of therapy of cancer are far better in this situation. Second, information must be gathered leading to biopsy of a candidate lesion, which alone can establish the pathologic diagnosis of neoplasia. The third goal is to determine as precisely as possible the extent of tumor spread, both at the site of origin and as metastases. The process of obtaining this information is known as *staging*. The fourth goal is to determine the growth rate and time course of the neoplasm in the particular patient undergoing diagnostic evaluation. The dictum that "every person is different" holds for cancers as well. Each malignancy is different, although there is a natural history which broadly characterizes each type of neoplasm. The rate of tumor growth can be determined by sequential assessment, using physical examinations or radiologic techniques, occasionally aided by the measurement of serum markers of tumor activity. The physician's ingenuity and persistence often come into play; an example is determining the existence of past radiologic studies, locating them, and obtaining them for review. The fifth goal in the evaluation is to determine the effects of the malignancy upon the health and performance of the patient. The importance of this in the design of a management plan is obvious, since control of symptoms and proper modification of activity levels will improve the well-being of the patient. In addition, it has become increasingly evident that the patient's performance status provides important data in predicting prognosis as well as response to anticancer therapy. The final goal in the diagnostic evaluation is the selection of appropriate anticancer therapy. The choice will depend on the information gathered as outlined, plus a knowledge of the treatment regimens which have the highest likelihood of producing cure, durable remission, or palliation. The principles of cancer therapy are presented in Chap. 318.

There are two widely used clinical scales of performance status, the Karnofsky scale and a modification developed by the Eastern Cooperative Oncology Group. The influence of performance status upon prognosis is demonstrated by a report correlating performance and medial survival in patients with inoperable lung cancer (Table 317-6).

Clinical evaluation How does the clinician proceed to evaluate a patient for the presence of malignant disease? Early detection depends primarily on awareness of the hereditary and environmental factors contributing to the incidence of cancer, combined with thorough exploration for symptoms and signs which could lead to further diagnostic workup. The seven warning signals widely publicized by the American Cancer Society are useful to remember (Table 317-7) and are usually covered in a review of systems. A careful physical examination is especially useful in detecting early cancer of the breast, uterus, cervix, colon and rectum, prostate, mouth, skin, testes, thyroid, and lymph nodes. A number of diagnostic screening tests have proved of value in early detection: (1) the exfoliative cytology ("Pap smear") screen for cervical cancer, (2) fecal occult blood testing, accompanied by periodic sigmoidoscopy for colorectal cancer, and (3) mammograms for breast cancer. In addition, screening for elevated prostate specific antigen (PSA) is currently recommended for men over 50, although the potential benefits continue to be debated.

TABLE 317-6 Influence of pretreatment performance status on patients with inoperable lung cancer*

Performance status scale[†]			Median survival (weeks)	Patients in group (percent)
ECOG	Karnofsky	Definitions		
0	100	Asymptomatic, normal activity	34	2
1	80–90	Symptomatic, but ambulatory	24–27	32
2	60–70	Symptomatic, in bed less than 50% of day, needs minimal assistance	14–21	40
3	40–50	Symptomatic, in bed more than 50% of day, requires considerable assistance	7–9	22
4	20–30	100% bedridden, severely disabled	3–5	5

* N = 5022 males with inoperable lung cancer of all histologic types entered onto VA Lung Group protocols from 1968–1978.
† Eastern Cooperative Oncology Group (ECOG) performance status scale, and DA Karnofsky et al, Cancer 1:634, 1948.
SOURCE: Adapted from JD Minna et al, in VT DeVita, Jr et al., 1989.

The prudent guidelines for early cancer detection provided by the American Cancer Society are summarized in Tables 317-8 and 317-9.

The three most common malignancies involve bowel, lung, and breast, and it is significant that screening tests are suggested for only two of these. It has been estimated by the American Cancer Society that the 5-year survival rate for colorectal cancer could be increased from the curent level of 55 percent to as high as 85 percent, if the recommended early detection techniques were generally applied. When the recommended breast cancer detection techniques are applied, the proportion of cases found without lymph node involvement at the time of diagnosis rises from 53 percent to more than 75 percent. Unfortunately, trials of mass screening for lung cancer with chest x-rays and sputum cytology have not resulted in reduced mortality, even when subjects believed to be at high risk were followed. However, the physician who is evaluating a patient in order to attemp to detect cancer early must learn whether or not the patient smokes cigarettes and should attempt to intervene.

The approach to a patient who presents to the physician with a history of symptoms or with abnormal physical findings which could be attributed to cancer involves selection of appropriate diagnostic procedures from a wide variety of available radiologic tests and laboratory studies (Table 317-10). The choice of diagnostic procedures used in the evaluation of cancer patients is guided by the natural history of the various types of malignancy. For example, knowledge that distant spread of breast cancer most frequently occurs to the lung, liver, bone, brain, and contralateral breast leads to consideration of studies of each of these organs as part of the complete workup. The diagnostician must know the probability of spread to these various metastatic sites in the presence or absence of abnormal findings in

TABLE 317-7 Cancer's seven warning signals

Change in bowel or bladder habits
A sore that does not heal
Unusual bleeding or discharge
Thickening or lump in breast or elsewhere
Indigestion or difficulty in swallowing
Obvious change in wart or mole
Nagging cough or hoarseness

SOURCE: American Cancer Society.

TABLE 317-8   Recommended guidelines for early detection of cancer in asymptomatic average-risk women

Age	Recommendation
20–39	*Cancer-related checkup* every 3 years, to include counseling and examination of the oral cavity, thyroid, skin, lymph nodes, and ovaries, plus: – Breast self-examination, monthly – Clinical breast examination, every 3 years – Baseline mammography (35-39 years of age) – Pap test and pelvic examination every year; after 3 or more annual, consecutive satisfactory examinations, the Pap test may be performed less frequently at the discretion of the physician for women who are or have been sexually active or are age 18 or older.
40–49	*Cancer-related checkup* yearly, to include all the above plus: – Digital rectal examination, yearly – Breast self-examination, monthly – Clinical breast examination, yearly – Mammography, every 1 to 2 years – At menopause, endometrial tissue sample in high-risk women
50 and older	*Cancer-related checkup* yearly, to include all of the above, plus: – Stool blood test, yearly – Sigmoidoscopy, every 3 to 5 years – Mammography, yearly

SOURCE: From DJ Fink in Al Holleb et al, page 156.

the history, physical examination, and standard blood studies. For the asymptomatic patient with breast cancer who has no abnormal physical findings outside of a small palpable breast lesion, and normal hematologic and blood chemistry values, a chest x-ray and a mammogram are the tests typically performed to evaluate the extent of disease prior to a decision for definitive therapy. Similar considerations go into planning the diagnostic workup for patients with each of the various forms of malignancy. It is for this reason that a thorough familiarity with the natural history of malignancies of the various organs, as well as the efficacy of a wide variety of diagnostic procedures in detecting these cancers, is essential.

Pathologic diagnosis   The diagnosis of cancer is made by pathologic examination. While there are definite limitations to histologic and cytologic examination of tumor specimens, this procedure is essential in order to exclude inflammatory processes as well as hyperplasia or benign tumors. In addition, the tissue of origin of a malignancy must be known in order to select the appropriate therapy. Specimens for pathologic examination are usually obtained by biopsy of a suspicious lesion. The procedure may involve a surgical operation under general anesthesia, but in many cases tissue specimens can be obtained through local incision (e.g., breast cancer) or by removal of a piece of tissue under direct visualization (bronchoscopy, colonoscopy). When direct visualization is not possible because of the internal location of a suspected lesion, it is often possible to obtain tissue

TABLE 317-9   Recommended guidelines for early detection of cancer in asymptomatic average-risk men

Age	Recommendation
20–39	Cancer-related checkup every 3 years, to include health counseling and examination of the oral cavity, thyroid, skin, lymph nodes, testes, and prostate
40–49	Cancer-related checkup yearly, to include all of the above, plus: – Digital rectal examination with palpation of the prostate, yearly
50 and older	Cancer-related checkup yearly, to include all of the above, plus: – Stool blood test, yearly – Sigmoidoscopy, every 3 to 5 years

SOURCE: From DJ Fink in Al Holleb et al, page 155.

TABLE 317-10   Methods for diagnosis and staging

History
Physical examination, including examination of oropharynx, Pap test, and proctoscopy
Radiologic studies
  A Roentgenogram
  B Ultrasound
  C Computed tomography
  D Angiography and lymphangiography
  E Nuclear medicine
  F Magnetic resonance imaging
  G Positron emission tomography
Laboratory studies
  A Hematologic evaluation
  B Chemical tests of internal organ function
  C Tumor markers
Pathologic examination of tissue
Cytogenetics and molecular genetics

fragments or clumps of cells by fine-needle biopsy aspiration, guided by computed tomography or fluoroscopy. In addition, suitable cytologic preparations can be obtained by washing or scraping surface lesions, as is commonly done to evaluate lesions on the cervix or in bronchi. Finally, in the case of malignancy involving the hematopoietic system or growing in body cavities (e.g., ascites), needle aspiration of tumor cells in suspension can be performed.

To make the diagnosis of cancer the pathologist looks for histologic and cytologic features characteristic of the disease. These include pleomorphism of cellular and nuclear structure, a high rate of mitosis and the presence of large or multiple nuclei, disordered tissue architecture, destruction or invasion of normal tissue boundaries, and the presence of cells in inappropriate locations (metastases). Special stains are useful for identifying chemical components characteristic of particular cell types and tissues. Additional evidence can be brought to bear upon the pathologic diagnosis, using the results of immunohistochemical studies, flow cytometry data on cellular DNA content, chromosomal karyotype analysis, Southern blotting for detection of diagnostic abnormalities in rearranged or amplified genes, and electron microscopy. However, in the overwhelming majority of cases, the diagnosis is made with the light microscope, on the basis of morphologic evaluation of the cells individually and as organized into tissue structures.

After the pathologic diagnosis of malignancy is established, the description usually includes three characteristics which classify the neoplasia:

1 The tissue of origin (e.g., adenocarcinoma, epidermoid carcinoma, sarcoma, leukemia)
2 Anatomic origin (e.g., colon, lung, breast)
3 Grade, or degree of differentiation (e.g., well-differentiated or poorly differentiated)

Each of these characteristics gives the therapist information relevant to the selection of treatment and to the prognosis. Although this terminology for classification is followed in general, there are many examples of exceptions based upon customary nomenclature involving particular tissues of origin or on the use of eponyms (e.g., Hodgkin's disease, glioblastoma multiforme).

Staging of cancer   The staging of a cancer patient involves the detection of the anatomic extent of the tumor, both in its primary location and in metastatic sites. This process is of critical importance in the clinical management for a number of reasons:

1 The optimal treatment plan for an individual patient is selected on the basis of the stage of disease.
2 By determining the presence of early metastatic disease, treatment can often be designed which can increase the chance for cure, or delay the development of symptoms even if cure is not achievable.
3 Staging provides information from which the physician can better evaluate the prognosis.

4 Because half of the cases of cancer cannot be cured by the therapies available today and because rapid advances in the development of anticancer treatment are occurring, management of an individual patient often involves new drugs or experimental procedures which are in the process of being evaluated for toxicity and efficacy. Staging to determine the extent of disease accurately is essential for evaluating factors influencing the results of such new treatments.

The anatomic extent of disease is best described and communicated to other professionals by a standardized nomenclature known as the TNM system. The three elements characterized in this system are the primary *t*umor, the regional lymph *n*odes, and *m*etastases (Table 317-11). The details of classification were decided upon by the International Union against Cancer (UICC) and the American Joint Committee for Cancer Staging (AJCCS). There is a scale of subcategories with designations ranging from 0 to 4 for each of the three tumor characteristics listed in the table. These scales were chosen because they can provide useful predictions of the clinical course. The primary tumor is classified by its size and the extent of local involvement. The involvement of lymph nodes is typically stratified by the spread to locations at a varying distance from the primary lesion and by the number of involved nodes. The most relevant information regarding metastases is their presence or absence. The details of stratification within the TNM system vary for each type of malignancy and are highly individualized. They depend on the characteristic growth patterns and lymphatic drainage patterns of neoplasms of the various organs. There is not always agreement about the definitions of the TNM characteristics, which can create confusion.

The stage of the tumor is typically divided into three or four categories (e.g., I to IV). For each type of malignancy, the various T, N, and M designations are assigned to one of four stages, in order to develop separation into groupings which correlate with data on prognosis and clinical responses to therapy. This is best described by mentioning a specific example. For the neoplasm with the highest mortality rate, non-small cell carcinoma of the lung, the therapy which has the best chance for curing the patient is surgery. The staging system for lung cancer (Table 317-12) is designed in a way which stratifies patients into groups, for which different treatment protocols are indicated. For the stages I and II patients, and some stage III patients, surgery is the treatment of choice. The extent of the surgical procedure depends on the extent of disease designated by the T and N classification within these two stages. Total excision of all tumor is the therapeutic goal, with 5-year postresection survival rates of 50 percent for stage I, 30 percent for stage II, and 15 percent for stage IIIa.

Tumor markers A tumor marker is an abnormality which is specific for a particular type of malignancy. For example, the Ph chromosome abnormality in the karyotype is a marker for chronic myelogenous leukemia, and the exclusive presence of either κ or λ chains on the surface of a population of lymphocytes is a marker of the lymphoproliferative malignancies. Until recently there were no biochemical markers that were absolutely specific for and diagnostic of malignancy. However, utilization of molecular genetic technology has enabled detection of genetic alterations that are pathognomonic for particular malignancies (see discussion of ''Clonality'' above).

The term *marker* may also be used in a more restrictive sense,

referring to molecules which are produced in abnormal amounts or under abnormal circumstances and are released into the circulation. The anaplasia and autonomy of the tumor cells permit production of molecules in greater than normal amounts or at inappropriate times in the life of the organism, and in this sense the abnormalities may become specific. Assays of such markers may be of great help to the clinician in a number of ways: (1) screening of high-risk individuals for the presence of malignancy, (2) diagnosis of malignancy, (3) monitoring of the effectiveness of therapy, (4) early detection of recurrence, and (5) immunodetection of metastatic sites, using radioactive-labeled antibodies against the markers.

The tumor marker of greatest use to the clinician is human chorionic gonadotropin (hCG), which has specificity because of its nearly exclusive production by the trophoblastic epithelium of the placenta under normal circumstances. The hCG levels rise during pregnancy. The hormone also may be secreted into the blood by trophoblastic tumors, as well as germ cell neoplasms of the testes and ovaries. Other neoplasms have been reported to be associated with elevated hCG levels, but the serum concentration rarely exceeds 10,000 ng/L (10 ng/mL) whereas trophoblastic tumors can produce concentrations over 100×10^6 ng/L (100,000 ng/mL). The usefulness of the assay for hCG is markedly enhanced by clinical data which show that changes in the serum hCG concentration in patients with secreting trophoblastic malignancies accurately reflect changes in the tumor burden. Therefore, decisions on the appropriate time to discontinue therapy can be based on the time course of serum levels, and decisions to reinstate therapy for recurrent disease are made on the basis of reappearance of hCG in the serum. The clinical test for hCG utilizes a radioimmunoassay for the beta subunit, to avoid cross reactivity with luteinizing hormone.

Two clinically useful tumor markers are products of genes which are expressed during the normal differentiation of fetal tissue but are partially or completely suppressed in the adult. These markers have been termed oncofetal antigens. Carcinoembryonic antigen (CEA) was originally thought to be specific for bowel cancer, but further studies have shown it to be a nonspecific tumor-associated antigen which also may be elevated in a variety of benign conditions. In the gastrointestinal tract, the molecule, a glycoprotein with a molecular weight of 180,000, is concentrated in the glycocalyx of epithelial cells, from which it is released into the lumen of the bowel. In the presence of malignancy, CEA concentrations may be elevated in the blood and other body fluids. Serum levels of CEA above the normal concentration of 2500 ng/L (2.5 ng/mL) are found in greater than 50 percent of neoplasms involving the colon, pancreas, stomach, lung, and breast. A variety of common nonmalignant conditions are associated with elevation of CEA, but typically not over 10,000 ng/ L (10 ng/mL). These include cigarette smoking, chronic pulmonary disease, alcoholic cirrhosis, hepatitis, and inflammatory bowel dis-

TABLE 317-12 Stage Grouping of the New International Staging System for Lung Cancer*

Occult carcinoma	TX	N0	M0
Stage 0	TIS	Carcinoma in situ	
Stage I	T1	N0	M0
	T2	N0	M0
Stage II	T1	N1	M0
	T2	N1	M0
Stage IIIa	T3	N0	M0
	T3	N1	M0
	T1-3	N2	M0
Stage IIIb	Any T	N3	M0
	T4	Any N	M0
Stage IV	Any T	Any N	M1

* TX, positive cytology; TIS, carcinoma in situ; T1, less than or equal to 3 cm, no local invasion; T2, greater than 3 cm, more than 2 cm from carina; T3, direct extension to chest wall, diaphragm, pleura or pericardium; T4, invasion of mediastinum, intrathoracic organs, or vessels. N1, peribronchial or hilar nodes; N2, ipsilateral mediastinal nodes; N3, contralateral mediastinal nodes. M1, distant metastasis.
SOURCE: Mountain, CF: A new international staging system for lung cancer. Chest 89:225s–233s, 1986.

TABLE 317-11 TNM system of anatomic staging

T: Primary tumor
  T0   No evidence of primary tumor
  T1–4 Ascending degrees of increase in tumor size and involvement
N: Regional lymph nodes
  N0   No evidence of disease in lymph nodes
  N1–4 Ascending degrees of nodal involvement
M: Distant metastasis
  M0   No evidence of metastasis
  M1–4 Ascending degrees of metastatic involvement

ease. CEA is not selective for cancer, and measurements of its levels should not be used in screening for the presence of malignant disease. However, serial measurements of CEA levels in patients with secreting malignancies can provide valuable information on the efficacy of treatment and the recurrence of disease. The possibility that early elevation of serum CEA can predict recurrence of bowel cancer soon enough to allow further surgical resection for cure is under study.

The second clinically useful oncofetal antigen is alpha fetoprotein (AFP), which is produced by the liver and gastrointestinal tract epithelium during gestation and which falls to levels less than 20,000 ng/L (20 ng/mL) after birth. Serum levels are elevated in 70 percent of patients with hepatocellular cancer, the majority of patients with nonseminomatous testicular cancer, and occasional patients with neoplasms of the gastrointestinal tract. As with CEA, the serum concentration of AFP may be elevated in benign conditions, especially in inflammatory disease of the liver. Its utility is in monitoring tumor activity, especially in the case of testicular tumors.

Elevation of either AFP or hCG is found in 80 to 90 percent of all nonseminomatous germ cell tumors of the testes. However, absence or normal levels of these biochemical markers of malignancy cannot be interpreted as proof that there is no tumor. Some tumors do not produce these marker molecules. Furthermore, because of tumor heterogeneity, it is possible for marker concentrations to fall in the presence of tumor, if a nonproducing subclone begins to grow preferentially. For this reason, recurrence of disease need not be accompanied by elevation of elevated marker levels.

Other biochemical markers with clinical utility include calcitonin, with which familial medullary carcinoma of the thyroid can be detected in individuals who appear to be normal. As indicated above, elevation of serum prostate specific antigen is observed in patients with prostatic cancer, and is useful in monitoring the response to therapy.

There are many tumors which, because of increased cellular mass or loss of normal regulation, produce excessive quantities of polypeptides normally secreted into the circulation by the tissue of origin. Examples include the immunoglobulin molecules produced in multiple myeloma, and insulin or gastrin hypersecretion by islet cell tumors. In addition, tumors may secrete molecules which ordinarily are not produced in the tissue from which they are derived. This phenomenon has already been discussed in the description of the paraneoplastic syndromes, because in many cases these marker molecules have biologic activities which can produce clinical illness in the patient. In some cases of malignant disease, cultures of tumor cells have been found to secrete a variety of polypeptide hormones atypical of the tissue of origin. In addition, molecules related to normal hormones or to their precursor forms may be present in the patient's serum, in the absence of any demonstrable clinical effects. These observations provide evidence for the broad scope of genetic deregulation which may accompany the process of oncogene expression and carcinogenesis.

COST AND BENEFITS The problem of dealing with malignant disease raises many questions relevant to public health policy. It is likely that large numbers of individuals harbor genetic abnormalities which put them at high risk for developing certain types of malignancy. It is also clear that life-style issues such as smoking, dietary habits, and drinking have a major impact on cancer incidence. There will undoubtedly be increased efforts to allocate the funds and resources necessary to address cancer prevention in a more comprehensive and proactive way. However, in parallel, the expensive diagnostic equipment, procedures, and assays that are being developed, as well as the new biologic-based therapies on the horizon, make it likely that the cost of delivering care to patients with malignant disease will increase. With an increasing focus on controlling the costs of health care, it will be extremely important to carefully analyze the costs and benefits of procedures, tests, and treatment regimens, taking a critical look at the extent to which they contribute to a favorable outcome.

REFERENCES

BRUGGE J et al: *Origins of Human Cancer: A Comprehensive Review*. Cold Spring Harbor, Cold Spring Harbor Laboratory Press, 1991
COSSMAN J: *Molecular Genetics in Cancer Diagnosis*. New York, Elsevier, 1990
COTRAN RS et al: *Robbins Pathologic Basis of Disease*, 4th ed. Philadelphia, Saunders, 1989
DEVITA VT JR et al: *Cancer: Principles and Practices of Oncology*, 4th ed. Philadelphia, Lippincott, 1993
FRANKS LM et al: *Introduction to the Cellular and Molecular Biology of Cancer*. New York, Oxford University Press, 1991
GROBSTEIN C et al: *Diet, Nutrition, and Cancer*. Washington, D.C., National Academy Press, 1982
HOLLAND JF, FREI E: *Cancer Medicine*, 3d ed. Philadelphia, Lea and Febiger, 1993
HOLLEB AI et al: *American Cancer Society Textbook of Clinical Oncology*. Atlanta, American Cancer Society, Inc., 1991
VOGELSTEIN B, KINZLER KW: p53 function and dysfunction. Cell 70:523, 1992
WEINBERG RA: *Oncogenes and the Molecular Origins of Cancer*. Cold Spring Harbor, Cold Spring Harbor Laboratory Press, 1989

318 PRINCIPLES OF CANCER THERAPY

CHRISTOPHER A. SLAPAK / DONALD W. KUFE

The development of effective cancer therapy has been a major focus of biomedical research. As a direct result of fundamental and applied research efforts, some malignancies have been changed from highly lethal to often curable diseases. While progress in treating others has been frustratingly slow, advances in multiple disciplines will undoubtedly lead to improvements in these recalcitrant diseases as well.

The development of new cancer therapeutics has generated much attention and excitement. There has been a rapid increase in the discovery of biologic agents of potential clinical importance. New chemotherapeutic drugs, some of which represent novel classes of cytotoxic agents, are entering clinical trials. Differentiating agents, long a therapeutic goal, are being utilized in investigational approaches for the prevention and therapy of some malignancies.

The mainstay of cancer therapy is distributed among three interactive subspecialties. The role of the surgeon, the radiation oncologist, and the medical oncologist will continue to be reshaped as new agents become clinically available and a multimodality approach to cancer becomes the rule. The primary care physician will remain at the forefront of prevention and early detection of cancer. The further definition of cancer risk factors and the availability of more sensitive and specific screening procedures insures that the internist will influence cancer morbidity and mortality.

The approach to cancer therapy, whether it involves experimental therapeutics in a university hospital or standard state-of-the-art therapy in a community hospital, must begin with an adequate data base. Each patient requires a proper histologic diagnosis of cancer. Every patient needs adequate staging and an appropriate plan of management.

DIAGNOSIS The histologic diagnosis of cancer and the categorization of the proper tumor type is pivotal in planning further workup and in deciding on treatment options. Although a histologic diagnosis may frequently appear straightforward, the clinician must realize its limitations. Histologic subtyping with biochemical and immunologic tissue characterization has resulted in a level of distinction between diagnoses not previously possible. In addition to substantiating the diagnosis of malignancy, this subtyping provides information essential in guiding therapy. The distinction between histologically similar tumors is often critical as therapeutic options may differ. When histologic subtyping is not possible, the decision to obtain additional tissue must be made in consultation with an experienced oncologist to determine whether it will alter the approach to treatment.

STAGING The extent of malignant disease is a prime determinant in planning appropriate therapy. Staging not only guides in selecting therapeutic modalities, but provides important prognostic information and may help the clinician minimize morbid complications. There is no routine set of tests appropriate for all patients. Understanding the natural history of the primary tumor, the pattern of spread to regional lymph nodes, and the possible sites of distant metastases assists in the selection of evaluations. The risks to the patient from any study must be balanced against the benefits gained by having additional staging information.

MANAGEMENT After diagnosis and staging a plan of management must be derived. The plan must consider the biology and natural history of the tumor, the available treatment options and their appropriateness to the patient's clinical situation, and the wishes of the individual patient. The clinician must clearly establish the goals of any treatment plan and these goals should be explicitly communicated with the patient. Treatment with curative intent is clearly most desirable. The level of aggressiveness frequently required, often with attendant serious complications, requires the physician to evaluate realistically the potential for disease eradication. Treatment to improve longevity without long-term disease free survival requires the physician to consider carefully the risk-to-benefit ratios of each therapeutic option. The amount of additional time gained must be weighed against hospitalization time, potential complications, and side effects of therapy. Finally, treatment for palliation should not subject the patient to any unwarranted side effects, unnecessary complications, or other additional discomforts. The goal of palliation, relief of symptoms, prevention of complications, and maximization of quality of life, must always be kept in mind.

PRINCIPLES OF SURGICAL THERAPY

Surgery was the first modality used in the treatment of cancer dating back to the 19th century. After the development of ether anesthesia in 1840s and the principles of antisepsis in 1860s, advances in cancer surgery were pioneered by Billroth, Halsted, and others. For the first portion of this century, surgery was the only cancer treatment widely available that yielded significant disease-free survival. Surgery is still the only curative therapy in many of the most common solid tumors. However, advances in surgical techniques, as well as improved multimodality therapy, have dramatically altered the surgical approach to many cancers. More limited surgical resections that do not affect the outcome but minimize loss of normal organ function are now feasible for many tumor types. Present day surgical oncologists are an integral part of the multimodality approach to cancer therapy. Surgery has a primary role in the diagnosis, staging and treatment of many tumors.

DIAGNOSIS A significant role for surgery in the treatment of patients with cancer is in obtaining adequate tissue samples for a histological diagnosis. Accurate diagnosis is a critical first step in planning appropriate cancer therapy. Once the diagnosis of cancer is entertained, it is essential to involve a surgeon experienced in the principles of oncologic diagnosis. An improperly performed biopsy may compromise subsequent surgical management and ultimately the outcome of the patient.

Several techniques are available for obtaining tissue specimens. An *aspiration biopsy* is generally performed by inserting a fine needle into the tissue of interest and aspirating material for cytologic examination. The availability of an experienced cytologist is essential for a proper interpretation. Superficial lesions are amenable to aspiration as are internal sites under sonographic or computed tomographic guidance. A definitive diagnosis of cancer may not be possible by cytology alone. A *needle biopsy* with radiologic guidance again may permit a percutaneous approach to internal structures. With some tumors, however, particularly lymphomas and sarcomas, a larger amount of tissue is usually required for a definitive diagnosis. With either aspiration or needle biopsy, sampling errors are a significant problem. *Incisional biopsy,* removal of a section or a wedge of tissue from a larger tumor, is performed when removal of the entire tumor is impossible and is often performed prior to major surgical extirpation. An *excisional biopsy* removes the entire lesion and when possible is preferred to incisional biopsy. Excising the entire lesion ensures sufficient tissue for pathologic examination, lessens the risk of tumor dissemination, and eliminates sampling problems. The choice of the appropriate procedure is dictated by anatomic considerations, biology of the presumed tumor type, and by the requirements of the pathologist. For some tumors sufficient tissue for specialized studies such as immunophenotyping, cytogenetics, electron microscopy, or estrogen receptor status requires specialized handling and close interaction with the pathologist.

STAGING Surgery is a principal means of staging many neoplastic diseases. Exploratory laparotomy to detect intraabdominal spread of Hodgkin's disease is usually indicated when planning conservative therapy. Axillary lymph node sampling in breast carcinoma provides important prognostic information that may guide further therapy. Intraoperative staging by the sampling of celiac lymph nodes will help establish the appropriateness of an esophagectomy in a patient with esophageal carcinoma.

TREATMENT Surgery is an effective method to cure patients whose tumors are confined to particular anatomical sites. However, at presentation only about 25 percent of patients have tumors that are truly confined and amenable to surgical treatment alone. The challenge is to identify those patients who can be successfully treated by surgery alone, thus sparing unnecessary surgical morbidity for the majority of patients who will ultimately relapse. Careful clinical staging after a thorough history, physical examination, and appropriate imaging studies are often requisite to decide upon the appropriateness of surgery.

Removal of most solid tumors requires en bloc resections with adequate tumor free margins. Microscopic tumor invasion of surrounding normal tissue that is imperceptible to the surgeon may require multiple frozen biopsies to establish tumor free margins. Manipulation of the tumor should be minimized to decrease the risk of seeding distant metastases. Resection or sampling of the regional lymph node group is usually indicated; however extended resection of several involved nodal groups is generally not warranted since this has not resulted in improved survival due to the high probability of concurrent distant metastases when multiple lymph nodes are involved.

Another challenge in oncologic surgery is to identify patients for whom combined modality therapy will improve outcome and allow a decrease in the extent of surgery. The surgeon, the medical oncologist, and the radiation therapist should develop an integrated plan to deliver the most effective coordinated treatment. A dramatic example has been the impact of multimodality therapy in the treatment of early stage breast carcinoma. Radical mastectomy with extended axillary lymph node dissection has been replaced by lumpectomy with lymph node sampling together with local radiotherapy and, when indicated, systemic adjuvant chemotherapy.

Surgery has been used as means of cytoreduction when complete excision has not been possible. However, unless such surgical debulking is combined with additional therapy, such as chemotherapy for ovarian carcinoma or Burkitt's lymphoma, this approach has not yielded significant treatment benefit. A consideration of tumor cell biology demonstrates the futility of this approach: debulking a mass 10 cm in diameter containing approximately 1×10^{10} tumor cells to one 1 cm in diameter is a 1 logarithm reduction in tumor burden that will still leave the patient with 1×10^9 tumor cells.

Surgical resection of metastatic disease with intent to cure may be appropriate in special circumstances. Generally this approach is reserved for patients who have a localized metastasis occurring well after resection of the primary disease. The metastasis should be the only evidence of distant disease and it should be resectable with low morbidity. Examples include pulmonary metastases in patients with osteogenic sarcoma or solitary liver metastases in patients with colorectal carcinoma. In some patients, resection of these lesions can lead to long-term disease-free survival.

Finally, surgery is used for palliation. The selection of patients who will benefit from this approach requires considerable judgment and skill. Appropriate, judicious use of surgery in patients with metastatic disease may alleviate pain and improve the quality of life. An example is excision of an obstructing colon carcinoma in a patient with metastatic disease. However, overly aggressive surgical intervention in a palliative setting may lead to prolonged hospitalizations, unnecessary discomfort, and additional financial burden to the patient or family.

PRINCIPLES OF RADIATION THERAPY

Radiation therapy, like surgery, is a local modality used in the treatment of cancer. Its use depends to a large extent on the inherent radiosensitivity of the tumor and the adjacent normal tissues. Ideally radiation therapy should destroy cancerous tissue while causing minimal disruption to surrounding normal structures. Another consideration is the ability of the normal tissue to sustain and repair radiation-induced damage and for the patient to function adequately even if normal organ function is diminished.

PHYSICAL AND BIOLOGICAL CHARACTERISTICS Radiation therapy is dependent on the application of ionizing electromagnetic radiation to a tumor site. The term *x-ray* denotes high-energy electromagnetic radiation produced by instruments such as linear accelerators. Gamma rays are also electromagnetic radiation but are produced by radioactive isotope decay. Both are used in radiation therapy and there is no inherent difference in their physical characteristics or biologic effects.

External beam radiation therapy refers to radiation delivered from a source outside the body. High-energy, megavolt electron beams are generated from linear accelerators or from radioisotope decay of cobalt 60 and are commonly used to irradiate internal, deep-seated lesions. Linear accelerators are the more widely used and produce a more focused beam with smaller penumbra. These high-energy, penetrating beams deliver a less intense superficial dose and thus spare the skin. Lesser energy, orthovoltage beams deliver a higher dose to superficial tissues and are used to treat lesions such as skin cancers. Radiation delivered by insertion of radioactive materials within the body near or at the tumor site is called *brachytherapy*. Brachytherapy may consist of intracavitary inserts, used in the treatment of gynecologic malignancies such as cervical or vaginal carcinomas, or interstitial implants, such as those used in prostate carcinoma. Brachytherapy may be used in conjunction with external beam therapy, e.g., in head and neck carcinoma, where the implants provide a high-intensity boost to the tumor bed.

Radiation dose is defined as the unit of absorbed energy (joules) per kilogram of tissue. The rad has been replaced by the Gray (Gy). One rad equals 0.01 Gy or 1 Gy equals 100 rad. A given dose of radiation kills a constant percentage of cells, not a constant number. At high doses of radiation, cell survival decreases with first-order kinetics in proportion to increasing radiation dose. At lower radiation doses a shoulder in the curve results from a decreased rate of cell death and may represent the presence of cellular repair mechanisms.

DNA is the target for radiation-induced cell death. Ionizing radiation generates free radicals and reactive oxygen intermediates that damage local cellular substituents including DNA. Cytotoxicity produced by clinically relevant doses of radiation is dependent upon cellular division and is called *mitotic cell death*. Rapidly proliferating normal tissues such as intestinal mucosa, bone marrow, and skin are particularly susceptible to radiation-induced cytotoxicity.

Cellular repair is normally complete within 4 to 6 h after radiation exposure. The capacity and extent of cellular repair mechanisms

determine in part the radiosensitivity of a given tumor or normal tissue. Oxygen concentration is another important determinant of radiation sensitivity. Hypoxic tissues are relatively resistant to the effects of radiation. Thus, poorly vascularized central areas of larger tumor masses are likely to exhibit relative insensitivity to radiation. The presence of oxygen is important in generating and sustaining free radicals produced by radiation.

Particle beam therapy, which utilizes neutrons or charged particles such as protons, is currently available in specialized centers. Particle beams have the advantage of more precise tissue localization and are less dependent on the presence of oxygen for cytotoxicity as compared to conventional radiation therapy.

TREATMENT Radiation therapy is performed by a team of nurses, dosimetrists, physicists, and radiation oncologists. A course of radiation therapy is preceded by simulation with appropriate radiographic tumor localization. Patient positioning during simulation must be exactly reproduced for each treatment to ensure maximal tumor delivery with minimal complications.

Radiation therapy is usually delivered in fractional doses, such as 180 to 300 cGy per day, five times per week. Clinical experience has demonstrated that fractional treatment schedules markedly improve the therapeutic index (see below) and result in better tumor control. This improved outcome may be related to several factors, including cellular repair of normal tissues, repopulation of destroyed tissues, and reoxygenation of relatively hypoxic tumor sites. Additionally, radiation therapy is often delivered from multiple external sites focusing on the tumor. This approach distributes the radiotherapy and lessens toxicity to the normal tissues.

Radiation therapy with curative intent as the sole treatment modality is employed in limited stage Hodgkin's disease, some non-Hodgkin's lymphomas, certain head and neck carcinomas such as laryngeal cancer, limited stage prostate carcinoma, gynecologic tumors including vaginal and cervical carcinomas, central nervous system neoplasms, such as medulloblastoma, and some skin cancers. Radiation therapy is often an integral part of curative multimodality approaches. For example, radiation therapy combined with chemotherapy has largely replaced surgery as a curative treatment for squamous cell carcinoma of the anus. Radiation therapy is a central component of breast conservation in the multimodality treatment of early stage breast carcinoma.

Radiation therapy is also used in the palliative management of many tumors. Irradiation of bony metastases may alleviate pain and stabilize weight-bearing structures in an attempt to prevent pathologic fractures. Brain metastases are often irradiated to provide symptomatic relief and prevent further neurologic complications. Palliative radiation therapy can also be employed to treat significant bleeding, refractory visceral pain, and vital organ obstruction. In general, doses employed for palliative management are lower than those used for curative therapy and result in less acute toxicity and discomfort to the patient.

Radiation therapy may be required on an urgent basis for the treatment of complications of malignant disease. An impending spinal cord compression in a patient with metastatic carcinoma is usually best treated with radiotherapy to the involved area. Alleviation of an obstructed airway or superior vena cava is generally treated effectively by radiotherapy.

COMPLICATIONS Radiation therapy is associated with both acute toxicity and long-term sequelae. Acute reactions occur during or immediately following therapy. They are self-limited and usually do not determine the amount of radiation therapy that can be administered. Common manifestations include skin reactions with erythema and desquamation; gastrointestinal toxicity with nausea, vomiting, dysphagia, or diarrhea; and myelosuppression with leukopenia, thrombocytopenia, and anemia. If symptoms become a problem during therapy, fractional doses may need to be temporarily reduced to allow normal tissue repair.

Long-term sequelae are dose limiting and occur many months or years after the completion of therapy. Long-term complications occur rarely if known normal tissue tolerances are not exceeded. The

TABLE 318-1   Normal tissue tolerance of radiation therapy

Tissue	Dose, cGy	Complications
Brain	6000	Necrosis
Spinal cord	4500	Myelitis
Heart	4500	Pericarditis, myocardial damage
Intestine	4500	Stenosis, perforation
Liver	3000	Hepatitis, hepatic vein thrombosis
Lung	2000	Pneumonitis, fibrosis
Kidney	2000	Nephropathy, renal failure
Bone marrow	250	Aplasia

complications tend to be progressive rather than self-limited. Their occurrence does not correlate with appearance or severity of acute reactions. The mechanism behind late complications is incompletely understood but is believed to result from either the disruption of vascular endothelium or the depletion of normal tissue stem cells. Table 318-1 lists tissue tolerances of some common structures with late complications.

Radiation therapy is known to be mutagenic, carcinogenic, and teratogenic. Radiation therapy is associated with an increased risk of developing solid tumors in previously irradiated fields. The secondary tumors often appear more than 10 years after therapy is completed. The true incidence of this complication and other predisposing factors are areas of active investigation.

PRINCIPLES OF CHEMOTHERAPY

BACKGROUND   Systemic chemotherapy is the primary treatment available for disseminated malignant disease. Progress in drug therapy has resulted in the development of curative chemotherapy regimens for several tumors (Table 318-2). Chemotherapy also has a significant role in palliation, often with improved survival, in a variety of other tumors. However, in several common solid tumors chemotherapy has only minor activity.

One of the most important and still evolving roles for systemic chemotherapy is its use in the adjuvant setting. *Adjuvant* therapy is administered after a definitive surgical resection to a patient who has no clinical, radiologic, or pathologic evidence of residual malignant disease. Its purpose is to eliminate undetectable micrometastatic disease. Table 318-2 lists tumors effectively treated with adjuvant chemotherapy. The term *neoadjuvant* refers to the administration of chemotherapy prior to surgery. This approach has been utilized in the treatment of head and neck carcinoma and bladder carcinoma. A patient who responds to neoadjuvant chemotherapy may benefit from more conservative local therapy.

Chemotherapy, whether given with curative or palliative intent, usually requires multiple cycles of treatment. Assessment of therapeutic efficacy prior to completing the entire course of treatment is often desirable. Discontinuation of ineffective treatments may allow institution of other salvage regimens, or in the absence of other effective regimens, the avoidance of unnecessary toxicity. Response to therapy can be measured directly by palpating superficial tumor masses or by imaging of internal lesions. Indirect measurements are possible but generally less desirable in the evaluation of tumor response.

Uniform criteria for describing a response to therapy are widely accepted and enable comparisons of the efficacy of alternative treatments. A complete response (or complete remission) is the disappearance of all detectable malignant disease. A partial response is a 50 percent decrease in the product of the greatest perpendicular diameters of one or more lesions. There can be no increase in size of any lesion or the appearance of new lesions. Stable disease means that there is no change in measurable tumor dimensions. Progressive disease means at least a 25 percent increase in the product of the greatest perpendicular diameter of one lesion or the appearance of new lesions.

TABLE 318-2   Response of tumors to chemotherapy

CURABLE BY CHEMOTHERAPY

Acute lymphocytic leukemia
Acute myelogenous leukemia
Ewing's sarcoma
Gestational trophoblastic carcinoma
Hodgkin's disease
Non-Hodgkin's lymphoma
   Burkitt's lymphoma
   Diffuse large cell lymphoma
   Follicular mixed lymphoma
Rhabdomyosarcoma
Testicular carcinoma
Wilms' tumor

CHEMOTHERAPY HAS SIGNIFICANT ACTIVITY

Anal carcinoma
Bladder carcinoma
Breast carcinoma
Cervix carcinoma
Chronic lymphocytic leukemia
Chronic myelogenous leukemia
Endometrial carcinoma
Hairy cell leukemia
Head and neck carcinoma
Lung (small cell) carcinoma
Multiple myeloma
Non-Hodgkin's lymphoma
   Follicular lymphoma
Ovarian carcinoma

CHEMOTHERAPY HAS MINOR ACTIVITY

Brain tumors (astrocytoma)
Colorectal carcinoma
Hepatocellular carcinoma
Kaposi's sarcoma
Lung (non-small cell carcinoma)
Melanoma
Pancreatic carcinoma
Prostate carcinoma
Renal cell carcinoma
Soft tissue sarcoma

ADJUVANT CHEMOTHERAPY IS EFFECTIVE

Breast carcinoma (axillary lymph node positive)
Colorectal carcinoma (Dukes B_2 or C)
Osteogenic sarcoma
Ovarian carcinoma (stage III)
Testicular carcinoma

The modern era of chemotherapy treatment for malignant disease began after the observation in World War II that exposure to mustard gas led to bone marrow and lymph node hypoplasia. The clinical use of nitrogen mustard was pioneered by Gilman at Yale in the 1940s in the treatment of lymphoma. Farber at Harvard, also in the 1940s, first induced remissions in childhood leukemia using aminopterin, a folate antagonist. In 1955, chemotherapy was first used to cure a solid tumor, gestational trophoblastic carcinoma. The subsequent development of multidrug regimens for childhood acute leukemia and Hodgkin's disease in the 1960s demonstrated that chemotherapy could consistently cure a high percentage of patients with certain chemoresponsive diseases. To appreciate more fully the development of modern chemotherapeutic regimens and their application to treatment of neoplastic diseases, it is necessary to understand principles of cytokinetics and pharmacodynamics.

CYTOKINETICS   A primary determinant of malignant transformation is uncontrolled growth. All somatic cells, whether normal or malignant, multiply by cell division through the mitotic cell cycle (Fig. 318-1). The cell cycle is marked by two observable events; during *S-phase* (for synthesis) DNA replication occurs, and during *M-phase* (for mitosis) cellular division into two daughter cells occurs. G_1 (for gap) is the time between the end of mitosis and the start of the next S-phase; G_2 is the time between the completion of S and the

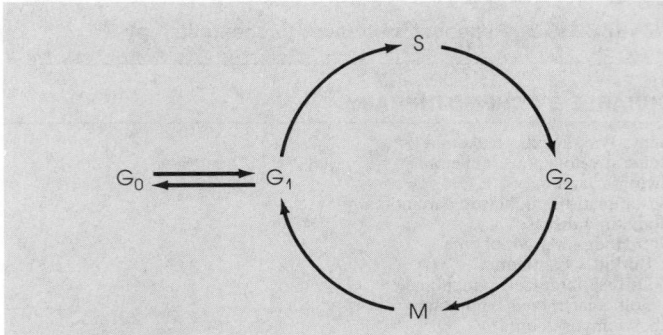

FIGURE 318-1   The cell cycle. Cellular division is marked by the events shown.

start of M. Cells that have ceased to proliferate for prolonged periods of time have entered the G_0 *phase* of the cell cycle.

Growth fraction represents the percentage of cells actively progressing through the cell cycle. *Cycle time* refers to the time required to traverse the cell cycle. Many chemotherapeutic agents, such as the antimetabolites or the alkylating agents, are cell-cycle active; i.e., they are predominantly cytotoxic to actively cycling cells. In addition, some cycle-active agents are phase specific; namely, they are cytotoxic to cells in a particular phase of the cell cycle. For example, cytarabine is a classic S-phase specific agent, while vincristine is M-phase specific. Other chemotherapeutic drugs, such as glucocorticoids, are capable of exerting cytotoxicity at any phase of the cell cycle, including G_0/G_1, and are thus not considered cycle-active.

A model elucidating the effectiveness of chemotherapy in eliminating a tumor mass was proposed by Skipper and coworkers in the 1960s. Their model of tumor cell growth and response to chemotherapy is called the *log-cell kill model* and was based on studies of the murine leukemia cell line L1210. In that model, tumor growth is exponential

with first-order kinetics and progresses at this rate regardless of tumor size until a lethal tumor burden is reached (Fig. 318-2A). The time required for a tumor to increase from a 1-μL volume of 10^6 cells to a 1-mL palpable mass of 10^9 cells (a 3-log or 1000-fold increase) is the same time for a tumor to increase from 10^9 to 10^{12} cells, a 1-L volume, and become a lethal tumor burden. In addition, a given dose of chemotherapy will result in the killing of a constant percentage of cells, not a constant number, regardless of the tumor burden at the time of treatment. Thus, if a given dose of chemotherapy kills 99.0 percent of the tumor cells, a 2-log reduction, a tumor mass of 10^{11} cells will be reduced to 10^9 cells (Fig. 318-2B). Assuming no tumor regrowth between treatments, an additional cycle of chemotherapy will reduce the tumor to 10^7 cells, whereby it would no longer be clinically detectable. Under these circumstances, the patient has achieved a complete response. However, an additional four cycles of chemotherapy would be required to reduce the tumor burden to less than one cell and therefore to achieve a cure.

While the L1210 murine leukemia models follow first-order kinetics of cell growth, most human solid tumors do not grow with a constant doubling rate. Instead, with increasing tumor size the rate of growth becomes progressively slower. This type of growth is referred to as *Gompertzian* (Fig. 318-3). In this model, as tumors enlarge the growth rate slows, the growth fraction decreases, and tumor volume begins to plateau. Patients with large tumors are likely to respond poorly to chemotherapy, primarily due to unfavorable tumor cytokinetics. Chemotherapy will be most effective with a small tumor burden when the growth fraction is the highest. Thus there is a rationale for using chemotherapy in the adjuvant setting to eliminate micrometastases when tumor burden is small and cytokinetics favor a chemotherapeutic response.

PHARMACODYNAMICS   Essentially all chemotherapeutic drugs exhibit a dose-response effect (Fig. 318-4). At sufficiently low concentrations no cytotoxicity will be observed. With increasing drug concentrations, cell kill will be proportional to drug exposure. At higher concentrations the effect will begin to plateau.

Tumor cell kill is also proportional to exposure time for many chemotherapeutic drugs. Cell-cycle–active agents in particular demonstrate increasing toxicity with prolonged exposure. With increasing time, a larger percentage of cells will enter the cell cycle, making them susceptible to the cytotoxic effects of cycle-active agents. These agents are often referred to as *schedule dependent*. Increasing the dose and exposure time of most chemotherapeutic drugs is possible only within certain limits. It is important to note that normal cells are

FIGURE 318-2   Logarithmic cell growth/kill model. *A.* Tumor cell growth proceeds with first-order kinetics from a clinically undetectable mass to a lethal tumor burden. *B.* Tumor regression in response to chemotherapy also follows first-order kinetics. A given dose of chemotherapy kills a constant

percentage of cells regardless of tumor size. As depicted here, two cycles of chemotherapy will render the tumor clinically undetectable, but six cycles will be required for total tumor eradication.

A

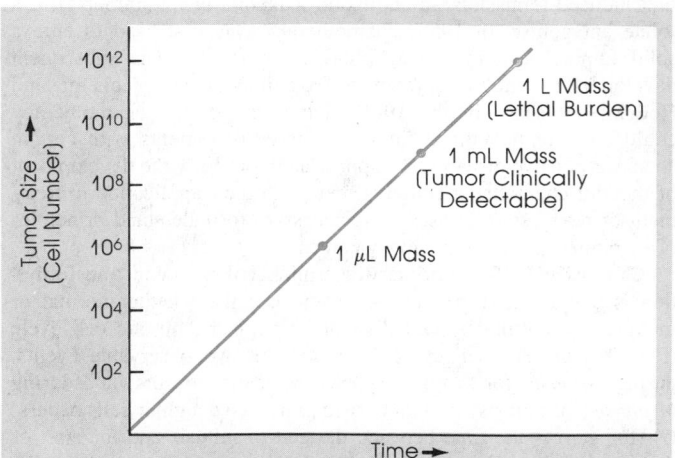

B

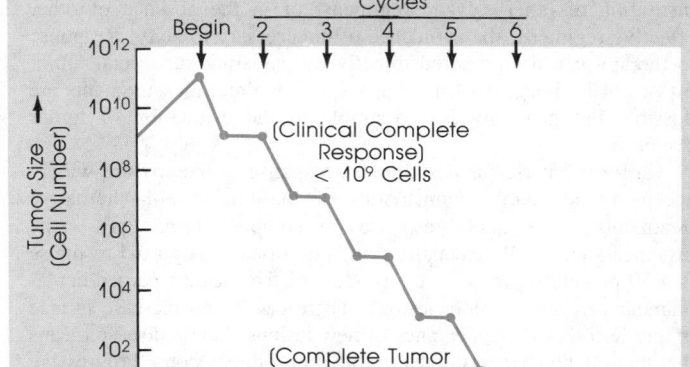

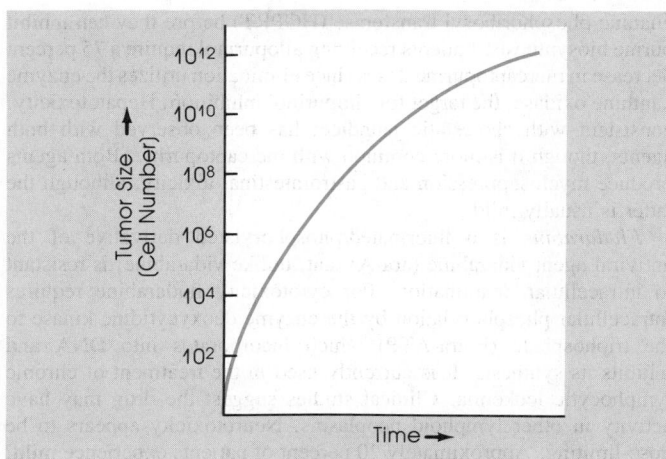

FIGURE 318-3 Gompertzian growth model. In Gompertzian growth, as the tumor size increases the growth rate slows and begins to plateau. Large tumors would exhibit chemotherapy insensitivity due primarily to unfavorable cytokinetics.

also susceptible to the cytotoxic effects of chemotherapeutic drugs and exhibit a dose-response effect. However, as seen in Fig. 318-4, the dose-response curve is shifted along the horizontal axis for tumor cells as compared to normal cells. The difference in the two dose-response curves represents the *therapeutic index.* A narrow therapeutic index limits the usefulness of many chemotherapeutic drugs. The normal tissue toxicity that limits further escalation of dose is the *dose-limiting toxicity.* The dose at which this occurs is the *maximal tolerated dose.* The most proliferative normal tissues are the bone marrow and gastrointestinal mucosa; therefore, they are generally the most susceptible to the toxicity from chemotherapy.

The ability of chemotherapy to eradicate tumor cells without causing lethal host toxicity depends on drug selectivity. The basis for anticancer drug selectivity remains incompletely understood. Although cytokinetics are important, other differences between normal and tumor cells in basic cellular processes such as metabolic pathways must also contribute. An excellent example is the ability of cytarabine to induce remissions in acute leukemia. To be effective, cytarabine must eradicate leukemic cell progenitors but spare sufficient normal bone marrow stem cells so that they can repopulate the hematopoietic system. At presentation, leukemic cells often outnumber normal bone marrow progenitors by several orders of magnitude. Leukemic cells

FIGURE 318-4 Dose-response effect. All cells, whether normal or malignant, demonstrate a dose-response effect when exposed to chemotherapeutic agents. The difference between the tumor and normal tissue response represents the therapeutic index.

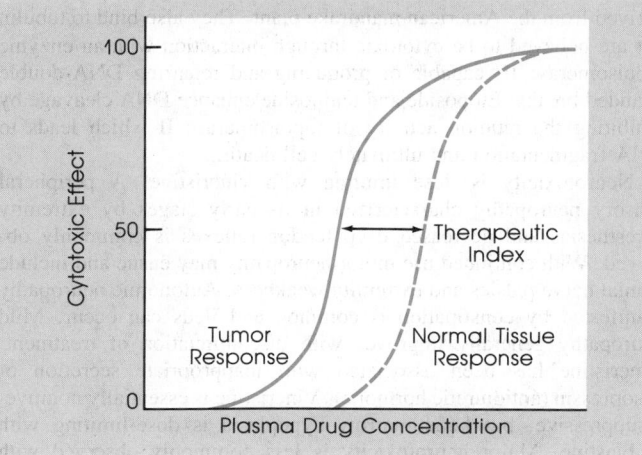

have been shown to traverse the cell cycle at rates comparable to that of normal bone marrow cells. The antileukemic effectiveness of cytarabine may relate to differences in drug uptake by cells in addition to differences in activities of intracellular kinase and deaminase pathways.

CANCER CHEMOTHERAPY Most of the commonly used cytotoxic antitumor agents are discussed below. They should be administered only by physicians experienced in their use and expert at handling potentially serious side effects. The dose of most chemotherapeutic agents is based on a patient's body surface area calculated according to a patient's height and weight. It is reported in square meters.

Antimetabolites The antimetabolites induce cytotoxicity by serving as false substrates in biochemical pathways and subsequently interfere with vital cellular processes. They are cell-cycle–active and predominantly S-phase specific drugs. Many antimetabolites are nucleoside analogues that become incorporated into DNA or RNA thereby inhibiting further nucleic acid synthesis. Other agents in this class inhibit enzymes involved in nucleotide biosynthesis.

The antifolate aminopterin, which was one of the first antitumor agents, has now been replaced by *methotrexate,* another folate analogue with more predictable clinical toxicity. Methotrexate inhibits the enzyme dihydrofolate reductase. Dihydrofolate reductase activity is necessary to maintain intracellular pools of reduced tetrahydrofolates, required for the synthesis of purine nucleotides and thymidylate. After carrier-mediated cellular uptake, methotrexate is converted to a polyglutamate derivative. Because of its increased cellular retention and enhanced inhibition of other folate-dependent enzymes, the polyglutamate compound appears to possess more antitumor activity than the parent drug. Administration of a reduced folate can overcome the cytotoxicity of methotrexate. The most commonly used agent, leucovorin, can prevent severe gastrointestinal toxicity or marked bone marrow hypoplasia if given in sufficient doses after methotrexate infusion. This so-called leucovorin rescue is generally utilized after administration of methotrexate doses >100 mg/m^2. The accumulation and subsequent prolonged release of methotrexate from third space fluids, such as pleural effusion or ascites, can markedly lengthen drug elimination and lead to unanticipated toxicities.

Use of very-high-dose methotrexate (>1000 mg/m^2) requires the monitoring of serum methotrexate levels to adjust the dose and schedule of leucovorin rescue. Methotrexate is predominantly cleared by renal excretion. Thus, patients with impaired renal function require dosage adjustments. High-dose regimens have been associated with acute renal injury, which may be prevented by vigorous hydration and alkalinization of the urine. In the absence of normal renal function, there are no satisfactory methods (including hemodialysis) to remove methotrexate from the body. Acute or chronic administration of methotrexate has been associated with hepatotoxicity. Temporary transaminase elevations have been observed in addition to portal fibrosis and even cirrhosis after chronic administration. Methotrexate is also associated with an idiosyncratic, reversible pneumonitis.

Methotrexate has activity in a wide variety of malignancies. It is currently used in the treatment of breast cancer, head and neck cancer, osteogenic sarcoma, acute lymphocytic leukemia, non-Hodgkin's lymphoma, and gestational trophoblastic carcinoma. Methotrexate is also commonly used intrathecally for leukemic or carcinomatous meningitis. Intrathecal use has been associated with chemical arachnoiditis.

Hydroxyurea inhibits the enzyme ribonucleotide reductase which prevents the conversion of ribonucleotides to deoxyribonucleotides. Its use is limited almost exclusively to myeloproliferative syndromes; it is widely used in chronic myelogenous leukemia and essential thrombocytosis. Hydroxyurea produces a predictable leukopenia which is usually reversible within days of discontinuing therapy. Gastrointestinal toxicity including nausea, vomiting, and diarrhea is usually mild. Patients who are on long term hydroxyurea therapy may develop dermatologic changes that are usually not severe enough to warrant discontinuation of therapy.

Pyrimidine-analogue antimetabolites   The fluorinated pyrimidine *5-fluorouracil* (5FU) was the result of rational drug design. For cytotoxicity, fluorouracil requires intracellular activation to one of several metabolites. Fluordeoxyuridine monophosphate (FdUMP) is a potent inhibitor of thymidylate synthase, an enzyme necessary for the synthesis of dTTP and ultimately DNA; fluorouridine triphosphate (FUTP) incorporates into RNA and interferes with its processing and function. Fluorodeoxyuridine triphosphate (FdUTP) is incorporated into DNA and eventually leads to DNA strand breakage. The importance of each of these mechanisms to fluorouracil-induced cytotoxicity has not been fully delineated. The interaction of the metabolite FdUMP with thymidylate synthase requires the presence of reduced folates. Studies suggest tumor cells may be deficient in reduced folates, so leucovorin has been administered with fluorouracil in an attempt to increase antitumor activity.

Extensive first-pass hepatic metabolism for fluorouracil has led to direct infusion into the hepatic artery for the treatment of hepatic metastases. The fluorouracil analogue *FUDR* (floxuridine), an inhibitor of thymidylate synthase with reportedly less effect on RNA synthesis than fluorouracil, is also available for intrahepatic infusion.

Like most antimetabolites, fluorouracil toxicity is schedule dependent. With bolus infusion, bone marrow suppression predominates whereas with continuous infusion therapy gastrointestinal toxicity may be more limiting. Fluorouracil has been infrequently associated with a myocardial ischemic syndrome characterized by chest pain, ECG, and isoenzyme changes. Neurologic symptoms, usually reversible, have been reported that include headaches, cerebellar ataxia, and somnolence. Dermatologic complaints are not uncommon and include dermatitis, hyperpigmentation, and skin atrophy. Fluorouracil is used predominantly in gastrointestinal malignancies including colorectal, stomach, esophageal, and pancreatic carcinomas and is widely used in combination therapy in the treatment of breast carcinoma.

Cytarabine is the 2′ epimer of cytidine. Cytarabine accumulates into cells by a carrier-mediated process using the deoxycytidine transport system. It is phosphorylated by a series of three enzymatic reactions to its active metabolite, ara-CTP. Ara-CTP incorporates into DNA and inhibits DNA replication by acting as a chain terminator. Cytarabine can be degraded intracellularly to an inactive compound (ara-U) by cytidine deaminase. The net effect of adequate cellular uptake and a balance between phosphorylation and deamination enzyme activities ultimately determines the cellular toxicity of cytarabine.

In the clinical setting cytarabine use is limited primarily to the treatment of acute myelogenous leukemia. It also has activity in acute lymphocytic leukemia and non-Hodgkin's lymphoma. Cytarabine is usually administered by a continuous 5- to 7-day infusion. High-dose cytarabine is often used in consolidation therapy or in drug refractory leukemia. When administered at low doses, cytarabine may promote myeloid cell differentiation. Intrathecal cytarabine administration is used to treat leukemic or carcinomatous meningitis but may cause chemical arachnoiditis.

When administered as a continuous infusion cytarabine causes profound myelosuppression lasting 14 to 21 days or longer. Gastrointestinal toxicity, including oral mucositis, is frequently observed. High-dose regimens are associated with a syndrome of cholestatic jaundice with elevation of liver transaminases. Cerebellar and cerebral toxicity manifested by ataxia, somnolence, and occasionally coma can be seen in patients on high-dose regimens. Patients with abnormal renal function, elevations of alkaline phosphatase (at least twofold), or age greater than 40 are at increased risk for cytarabine-induced neurotoxicity. Conjunctivitis, preventable by ophthalmic glucocorticoids, is also common with high-dose regimens.

Purine-analogue antimetabolites   The thiopurine analogues *6-mercaptopurine* (6MP) and *6-thioguanine* (6TG) have a thiol substitution for a carbonyl group in the purine base. They are used in the treatment of acute leukemia and are essentially inactive against solid tumors. Both agents require modification by the enzyme hypoxanthine-

guanine phosphoribosyl transferase (HGPRT) before they can inhibit purine biosynthesis. Patients receiving allopurinol require a 75 percent decrease in mercaptopurine doses since elimination utilizes the enzyme xanthine oxidase, the target for allopurinol inhibition. Hepatotoxicity, consistent with cholestatic jaundice, has been observed with both agents, though it is more common with mercaptopurine. Both agents produce myelosuppression and gastrointestinal toxicity, although the latter is usually mild.

Fludarabine is a fluorinated/phosphorylated derivative of the antiviral agent vidarabine (ara-A) that, unlike vidarabine, is resistant to intracellular deamination. For cytotoxicity fludarabine requires intracellular phosphorylation by the enzyme deoxycytidine kinase to the triphosphate (F-ara-ATP) which incorporates into DNA and inhibits its synthesis. It is currently used in the treatment of chronic lymphocytic leukemia. Clinical studies suggest the drug may have activity in other lymphoid neoplasms. Neurotoxicity appears to be dose-limiting. Approximately 20 percent of patients experience mild, reversible neurotoxicity, although instances of severe irreversible toxicity including coma have been reported. In addition to myelosuppression, fludarabine causes immunosuppression with episodes of serious opportunistic infections documented in some patients. Administration of fludarabine is commonly associated with fevers and chills.

Pentostatin (2′-deoxycoformycin) is a natural product that is an irreversible inhibitor of the enzyme adenosine deaminase. Inhibition of this enzyme, found in particularly high levels in lymphocytes, results in the toxic accumulation of deoxyadenosine nucleotides. Pentostatin is used in treatment of hairy cell leukemia. Its use in other lymphoid malignancies is under investigation. Pentostatin causes profound immunosuppression, especially of T cell–mediated immunity. Myelosuppression otherwise is mild. Renal function impairment has been observed which may be minimized by adequate patient hydration. CNS toxicity including somnolence and coma as well as hepatoxicity with transaminase elevations also have been seen.

Chlorodeoxyadenosine is a purine analogue that inhibits DNA replication. It is used in the treatment of hairy cell leukemia but appears to have activity in other lymphoid and myeloid malignancies. Chlorodeoxyadenosine is both myelosuppressive and immunosuppressive. Other toxicities include mild gastrointestinal toxicity and hepatotoxicity.

Plant alkaloids   The plant alkaloids currently comprise three groups: the vinca alkaloids, the taxanes, and the epipodophyllotoxins. The vinca alkaloids *vincristine* and *vinblastine* were originally isolated from the periwinkle plant *(Catharanthus roseus)*. Both are active predominately during the M-phase. They exert cytotoxicity by binding to tubulin and inhibiting microtubule assembly. Microtubule assembly and disassembly are tightly controlled cellular processes; interfering with either leads to cytotoxicity. *Paclitaxel* (Taxol), a member of the taxane family, is derived from the Pacific yew *(Taxus brevifolia)*. It functions by stabilizing microtubules and thereby preventing their disassembly. The epipodophyllotoxins *etoposide* and *teniposide* are semisynthetic derivatives of the natural product podophyllotoxin derived from the American mandrake plant. They also bind to tubulin but are believed to be cytotoxic through interaction with an enzyme topoisomerase II, capable of producing and repairing DNA-double stranded breaks. Etoposide and teniposide enhance DNA cleavage by inhibiting the reunion activity of topoisomerase II which leads to DNA fragmentation and ultimately cell death.

Neurotoxicity is dose limiting with vincristine. A peripheral sensory neuropathy characterized in its early stages by extremity paresthesias and decreased deep tendon reflexes is commonly observed. With continued use motor neuropathy may ensue and include cranial nerve palsies and extremity weakness. Autonomic neuropathy manifested by constipation is common and ileus can occur. Mild neuropathy generally improves with discontinuation of treatment. Vincristine has been associated with inappropriate secretion of vasopressin (antidiuretic hormone). Vincristine is essentially nonmyelosuppressive, but bone marrow hypoplasia is dose-limiting with vinblastine. Major neurotoxicity is less commonly observed with vinblastine. Mucositis can sometimes be severe, particularly at high doses. Vincristine is active in lymphocytic leukemia, Hodgkin's and non-Hodgkin's lymphomas, and Wilm's tumor. Vinblastine is active in testicular carcinoma, breast carcinoma, Hodgkin's and non-Hodgkin's lymphomas, and lung cancer.

Paclitaxel infusion is frequently associated with hypersensitivity reactions manifested initially by hypotension, bronchospasm, and urticaria. The vehicle in which paclitaxel is dissolved, cremophor EL (polyoxyethylated castor oil), may contribute to this high incidence. Prolonging the infusion time to 24 h and the use of extensive premedication have significantly abrogated this problem. Bradyarrhythmias, especially AV block, atypical chest pain, and rarely more severe cardiac problems have also been associated with paclitaxel infusion. Bone marrow suppression with neutropenia is the dose-limiting toxicity. Peripheral neuropathy with paresthesias in a glove-stocking distribution also is common; the ability to reverse this toxicity with cessation of therapy is unclear. Other toxicities include mucositis, myalgias, and alopecia. Paclitaxel has demonstrated activity in ovarian, breast, and head and neck carcinomas. The efficacy of paclitaxel in other malignancies is an area of intense investigation.

Leukopenia is the dose-limiting toxicity for etoposide and teniposide with white cell nadirs at approximately 14 days. Intravenous administration of either drug can be associated with fever, hypotension, bronchospasm, or rarely anaphylaxis. The incidence of these symptoms, possibly related to the drug vehicle, can be minimized by administering the drug over 1 h. A serious complication reported for both etoposide and teniposide treatment is the development of secondary leukemias. Epipodophyllotoxin-related acute myeloid leukemia appears to evolve within 3 years of receiving the drug and has been associated with cytogenetic abnormalities involving chromosome 11q23. The incidence may exceed 5 percent and appears dose and schedule dependent. The concomitant administration of cisplatin with etoposide also may increase the risk of developing secondary leukemias. Etoposide has activity in lung, testicular, and ovarian carcinomas and in refractory lymphomas and acute leukemias. Teniposide is approved for use as second-line therapy in childhood acute leukemia.

Antitumor antibiotics The antitumor antibiotics are a group of anticancer compounds isolated mainly from soil microorganisms. The anthracyclines have the widest spectrum of activity and are clinically the most important of these drugs.

The commercially available anthracyclines are *doxorubicin, daunorubicin,* and *idarubicin.* In addition, *Epirubicin* is available for clinical use outside of the United States. The anthracyclines are cell-cycle active and phase nonspecific but have pleiotropic actions upon the cell. Although they are classic DNA intercalating agents, their mechanism of cytotoxicity is likely related to interaction with the enzyme topoisomerase II with production of double-stranded DNA breaks. Other data suggest the anthracyclines undergo one- and two-electron reductions generating intracellular free radicals, particularly the hydroxyl radical, which is highly cytotoxic.

The anthracyclines are very myelosuppressive with white cell and platelet count nadirs at 10 to 14 days after treatment. The anthracyclines cause gastrointestinal toxicity including acute nausea and vomiting and mucositis later. These agents are severe vesicants. Extravasation during infusion can lead to local tissue necrosis. In extreme cases skin grafting may be required. The anthracyclines are cleared predominantly by liver metabolism; patients with elevations of serum bilirubin require dose modifications. Long-term administration is limited by cumulative dose-dependent cardiotoxicity. Irreversible cardiomyopathy with serious congestive heart failure is a significant risk in patients who have received doses in excess of 500 to 550 mg/m^2 of doxorubicin or daunorubicin. Previous chest radiotherapy or concomitant cyclophosphamide therapy may lower a patient's tolerable cumulative dose.

Doxorubicin is one of the most broadly active antitumor agents. It is used in the therapy of breast, bladder, lung, stomach, prostate, and thyroid carcinomas; Hodgkin's and non-Hodgkin's lymphomas;

and bony and soft tissue sarcomas. Daunorubicin has a much narrower range of activity and is used in the treatment of acute myeloid and lymphocytic leukemia. Idarubicin is approved for use in induction therapy for acute myeloid leukemia.

Mitoxantrone, an anthracenedione, is structurally related to the anthracyclines and was developed as a less cardiotoxic alternative to doxorubicin. The drug also appears to interact with topoisomerase II. While the incidence of cardiomyopathy is lower than for doxorubicin, it can still occur. Patients who have received lifetime doses greater than 125 mg/m^2 are at greatest risk. Complications from tissue extravasation are also less severe than with the anthracyclines. Mitoxantrone also causes marked myelosuppression. In clinical practice, mitoxantrone has not replaced the anthracyclines and is currently used as second-line therapy in breast carcinoma, acute leukemia, and non-Hodgkin's lymphomas.

Bleomycin is a mixture of cytotoxic glycopeptides. Bleomycin simultaneously interacts with the ferrous ion (Fe^{2+}) and DNA, resulting in single- and double-stranded DNA breaks through free radical generation. It is cytotoxic predominantly during the G_2–M phases of the cell cycle. Bleomycin has little myelosuppressive effect. Pulmonary toxicity manifested as a chronic interstitial pneumonitis is the most serious toxicity. Lung injury may initially present with cough, dyspnea, and infiltrates on chest radiograph, and it may ultimately progress to respiratory failure and death. Lifetime cumulative bleomycin dose is recommended not to exceed 200 U/m^2, less in patients with underlying pulmonary disease, previous chest radiotherapy, or of advanced age. Bleomycin is also associated with dermatologic toxicity characterized by hyperpigmentation and hyperkeratosis. Bleomycin infusion is associated with fever and less commonly hypotension, bronchospasm, and pulmonary edema. A test dose is often administered prior to full-dose therapy. Bleomycin is used in the treatment of Hodgkin's and non-Hodgkin's lymphoma and carcinoma of the testis and of the head and neck.

Mitomycin C is an agent used in the treatment of gastrointestinal malignancies. Mitomycin C is activated intracellularly where it is then capable of cross-linking DNA. Mitomycin C exhibits a delayed myelosuppression with leukocyte and platelet count nadirs at 4 to 6 weeks. Mitomycin C can precipitate progressive renal failure, often in association with microangiopathic anemia. The incidence of this hemolytic-uremic syndrome increases with cumulative mitomycin dose. Mitomycin C is also a severe vesicant.

Dactinomycin binds to DNA and inhibits RNA synthesis. It also appears to interact with the enzyme topoisomerase II. Its activity is limited to treatment of rhabdomyosarcoma, Ewing's sarcoma, and gestational trophoblastic carcinoma. It causes myelosuppressive and gastrointestinal toxicity.

Alkylating agents As a class, alkylating agents are among the most widely used antitumor agents. These drugs lead to inhibition of DNA synthesis by forming covalent bonds with nucleic acids. Most alkylating agents are bifunctional and are efficient at cross-linking DNA with subsequent strand breakage and ultimately cell death. These agents preferentially add alkyl groups to the N-7 of guanine in addition to other nitrogen or oxygen positions in adenine or cytidine. Although alkylation of DNA can occur at any phase of the cycle, cytotoxicity is greatest in those cells that are progressing through the cell cycle. It is most appropriate to regard these agents as cycle active, non-phase specific. The covalent alkylation of DNA is mutagenic and carcinogenic, resulting in long-term serious complications including detrimental effects on spermatogenesis and oogenesis, as well as predisposing to the development of secondary leukemias.

Azospermia resulting from alkylating agent treatment has been found in men receiving therapy for lymphoma and may persist for several years after completing therapy. The severity of gonadal injury appears to be dose dependent. In some men this complication is reversible since previously azospermic patients have subsequently fathered children. Amenorrhea and ovarian atrophy, sometimes permanent, have been associated with alkylating agent therapy in women. The possible resumption of normal menstrual cycles is inversely related to the age of the patient and the cumulative dose received.

Another serious long-term complication of alkylating agent chemotherapy is the development of secondary leukemias. In patients who have received an alkylating agent as part of combination chemotherapy for Hodgkin's or non-Hodgkin's lymphomas, the incidence of secondary acute myeloid leukemia may be as high as 5 to 10 percent. Secondary leukemias have also followed use of alkylating agent therapy for multiple myeloma and ovarian carcinoma. Not all the alkylating agents are equally leukemogenic. For example, melphalan appears to be associated with a higher incidence of secondary acute leukemia then cyclophosphamide when used in the treatment of ovarian carcinoma.

The most common dose-limiting toxicity of the alkylating agents is myelosuppression. The severity and duration varies with the individual drugs. Most of the alkyating agents are quite emetogenic and require extensive premedication. Gastrointestinal epithelial damage however is not prominent. Additional toxicities and activities of the individual agents are presented below.

Mechlorethamine (nitrogen mustard) was the first alkylating agent to receive widespread clinical use. Currently it is used almost exclusively in the therapy of Hodgkin's lymphoma. It has also been used in the treatment of malignant pleural effusions to obliterate the pleural space. Mechlorethamine is highly reactive in aqueous solution and is a severe vesicant. Administration is sometimes associated with minor cholinergic symptoms.

Cyclophosphamide is one of the most widely used broad-spectrum, antitumor agents. It is used in the treatment of carcinoma of the breast, lung, ovary, and bladder; non-Hodgkin's lymphoma; acute and chronic lymphocytic leukemias; soft tissue and bony sarcomas; and tumors of childhood including Wilms' and neuroblastoma. High doses are employed in myeloablative regimens prior to bone marrow transplantation. Cyclophosphamide is active only after microsomal liver metabolism to 4-hydroxycyclophosphamide. It is further metabolized in peripheral tissues to phosphoramide mustard and to acrolein. Cyclophosphamide therapy may be complicated by hemorrhagic cystitis, believed to be due to the metabolite acrolein, which is excreted unchanged in the urine. Adequate hydration with standard-dose therapy, and administration of the bladder protectant *mesna* with high-dose therapy, can help prevent this complication. Upon renal excretion, mesna (mercaptoethane sulfonate) is hydrolyzed to an active form which can complex with and inactivate toxic cyclophosphamide metabolites. Chronic bladder inflammation as a result of cyclophosphamide therapy has been associated with the development of malignant bladder tumors. Cyclophosphamide administration is associated with a syndrome of inappropriate antidiuresis due primarily to a distal renal tubular effect. Cyclophosphamide is also a potent immunosuppressive agent. In very high doses it has been rarely associated with acute myocardial necrosis.

Ifosfamide is a closely related analogue of cyclophosphamide that is less myelosuppressive but more urotoxic. It is usually administered with the uroprotectant agent mesna. Ifosfamide also requires hepatic metabolism for activation. A reversible neurotoxicity manifested as altered mental status can be seen in patients receiving ifosfamide. Currently ifosfamide is used in salvage therapy regimens for testicular carcinoma. Its use in other tumors including sarcoma, lymphoma, and lung carcinoma is under investigation.

Melphalan is a derivative of the amino acid phenylalanine. It has a broad antitumor activity but is used primarily in the treatment of multiple myeloma and ovarian carcinoma. Melphalan does not require hepatic activation and does not cause hemorrhagic cystitis. Melphalan appears to be one of the most leukemogenic alkylating agents. It has rarely been associated with the development of pulmonary fibrosis.

Chlorambucil is structurally related to mechlorethamine. It is available in oral form and is primarily used in the treatment of chronic lymphocytic leukemia and for indolent non-Hodgkin's lymphomas.

Busulfan is toxic to myeloid stem cells. As such it is primarily used in the treatment of myeloproliferative disorders including chronic myelogenous leukemia and in high-dose myeloablative preparative regimens prior to bone marrow transplantation. Prolonged bone marrow hypoplasia may result even after standard-dose administration. Busulfan therapy is also rarely associated with interstitial pneumonitis and progressive pulmonary fibrosis. The initial clinical symptoms of dry cough and dyspnea on exertion may progress, even with cessation of therapy, to respiratory insufficiency and death. Busulfan treatment is also associated with skin hyperpigmentation.

Thiotepa is an trivalent alkylating agent that currently has a limited clinical role. It is used as second-line therapy in breast and ovarian carcinoma. Thiotepa has a toxicity profile typical of most alkylating agents, although it is generally less emetogenic.

Alkylating agents; nitrosoureas   The nitrosoureas *carmustine* and *lomustine* are a class of alkylating agents distinguished by high lipid solubility with excellent penetration into the central nervous system and activity against CNS neoplasms. The nitrosoureas are also used in salvage regimens for Hodgkin's and non-Hodgkin's lymphoma. The nitrosoureas produce a delayed myelosuppression lasting 4 to 6 weeks and appear to have a cumulative effect on the bone marrow. Patients heavily pretreated with chemotherapy may have protracted cytopenias with a few developing bone marrow aplasia. The nitrosoureas have also been associated with development of secondary leukemias. Moderate, but reversible, elevation of hepatic enzymes is common. A pulmonary fibrosis syndrome, similar to that seen with busulfan, has been reported. Prolonged treatment with the nitrosoureas can result in progressive renal insufficiency, even after cessation of therapy.

Alkylating agents; platinum compounds   The platinum compounds *cisplatin* and *carboplatin* are the only heavy metals approved for use as antitumor agents. Although they are not true alkylating agents, they do ultimately covalently cross-link DNA. Cytotoxicity is determined by the balance between cellular enzymatic repair of damaged DNA and the extent of the DNA cross-links.

Cisplatin produces nephrotoxicity and is toxic to both the proximal and distal tubular epithelial cells. Adequate intravenous hydration with saline diuresis, accompanied by furosemide or mannitol administration, can decrease the incidence of nephrotoxicity. Nausea and vomiting may at times be severe and protracted in patients receiving cisplatin. Sensory neuropathy and high-frequency hearing loss after several cycles of therapy are not uncommon. It produces modest myelosuppression. Cisplatin has significant activity in testicular, ovarian, bladder, head and neck, and lung carcinomas. Carboplatin is a cisplatin analogue that has less nephrotoxicity, is less emetogenic, less ototoxic, but is more myelosuppressive. It has a spectrum of activity similar to cisplatin.

Other agents   *Dacarbazine* appears to exert its cytotoxicity by acting as an alkylating agent and damaging DNA after activation by hepatic microsomal enzymes. Dacarbazine is used in the treatment of melanoma, Hodgkin's disease, and soft tissue sarcomas. It produces moderate myelosuppression. Nausea and vomiting are often severe and persistent.

Procarbazine, a monoamine oxidase inhibitor, was originally developed as an antidepressant and was later discovered to have antitumor activity. It requires oxidation by hepatic enzymes after which it functions like an alkylating agent, methylating nucleic acids. Myelosuppression is moderate but dose limiting. Procarbazine produces neurotoxicity manifested by peripheral sensory neuropathy in addition to changes in mood and mental status. Nausea and vomiting may also be severe. Due to its monoamine oxidase inhibitor activity, tyramine-rich foods and medication such as sympathomimetic amines or tricyclic antidepressants may precipitate a hypertensive crisis and should be avoided. A disulfiram-like effect is also common. Procarbazine can produce gonadal atrophy and may increase the risk for development of secondary leukemias. Procarbazine is used primarily in the treatment of brain tumors and Hodgkin's disease.

L-*Asparaginase* is the only enzyme utilized as an antitumor agent. Lymphocytes have a limited ability to synthesize the amino acid L-asparagine and are dependent on circulating pools to maintain protein synthesis. Asparaginase treatment results in depletion of extracellular pools of asparagine. While this effect is associated with cytotoxicity to lymphocytes, most normal tissues are largely unaffected since they are capable of de novo asparagine synthesis. Asparaginase is used in the treatment of acute lymphocytic leukemia. Asparaginase is associated with hypersensitivity reactions including anaphylaxis or serum sickness in a significant number of patients. Anaphylaxis may occur with the first dose. The effects of inhibiting protein synthesis may lead to hypoalbuminemia, hypoinsulinemia, hyperglycemia, and mental status changes. Thrombosis due to depletion of protein C and protein S and hemorrhage due to depletion of clotting factors have been observed. Hepatotoxicity and pancreatitis are also less commonly observed.

COMBINATION CHEMOTHERAPY Most cancers are treated with multiagent combination chemotherapy. While many regimens have been derived historically by empirical means, there are a series of principles which underlie most combinations of antitumor drugs. Each of the agents within a given regimen should have demonstrated independent activity against the specific tumor. Although unanticipated synergy with other drugs in the regimen may occur, adding an agent that alone produces no responses is likely to add toxicity without benefit. Each of the agents should usually have a different mechanism of action. It is in principle advantageous to target different points along a biochemical pathway. Drugs that either inhibit the same enzyme or damage the same target are less likely to yield additive antitumor activity. Likewise, agents should be non-cross resistant. A drug-resistant tumor subpopulation selected by one agent is unlikely to be cross resistant to an agent that produces cytotoxicity through a completely different mechanism. Finally, each of the drugs should have different dose-limiting toxicities. Administering two agents with the same toxicity profile at the maximal dose of each agent can produce unacceptable toxicity. As a result of these principles, carefully chosen combination regimens should result in an improved rate of tumor cell kill. In addition, the chances of emergence of a drug-resistant clone should decrease and each agent can likely be administered at full dose.

A drug regimen commonly used in the treatment of non-Hodgkin's lymphoma illustrates these points. Treatment with the regimen of cyclophosphamide, doxorubicin, vincristine, and prednisone, often referred to as CHOP [*c*yclophosphamide, *h*ydroxydaunorubicin (doxorubicin), *o*ncovin (vincristine), *p*rednisone] can lead to long-term disease free survival in about 50 percent of patients with diffuse large cell lymphoma. Each of the four agents produces cytotoxicity by a different mechanism in the cell cycle. Cyclophosphamide and doxorubicin are cycle active non-phase specific; vincristine is cycle active M-phase specific; while prednisone is non-cycle active. Each of the agents has independent activity in the treatment of diffuse large cell lymphoma and three of the agents are capable of inducing complete responses when given alone. None of the agents would be expected to exhibit cross resistance, although in reality it does happen (see below). Finally, except with cyclophosphamide and doxorubicin, dose-limiting toxicity is nonoverlapping. In the case of cyclophosphamide and doxorubicin, dose reduction is required to prevent an unacceptable degree of myelosuppression.

While these principles can in theory be used to design new, more effective regimens, there are often great difficulties in applying them in clinical practice. For example, in many of the common solid tumors, such as colorectal carcinoma, few agents demonstrate significant single-agent activity. Furthermore, the exact mechanism of action of many antitumor drugs is not precisely understood. Moreover, agents that are known to exert cytotoxicity by different mechanisms may still be susceptible to common mechanisms of acquired drug resistance. Finally, many of the most active agents have the same dose-limiting factor, myelosuppression, rendering it impossible to use them at their maximally tolerated doses.

High-dose chemotherapy or chemoradiotherapy followed by bone marrow transplantation has been used to overcome myelosuppression. The drugs most useful for transplantation are generally the alkylating agents, such as busulfan and cyclophosphamide, which exhibit a linear response between drug dose and cell kill in vitro. Administering these drugs in myeloablative combination regimens yields improved tumor cytotoxicity. In autologous transplantation, the patient's bone marrow is harvested, cryopreserved, and then reinfused after delivery of systemic high-dose therapy. In allogeneic transplantation, bone marrow from a suitable donor, usually an HLA-compatible sibling, is used to reconstitute the patient's hematopoietic system. Substantial evidence indicates that, in addition to the high-dose preparative regimens, immune effector mechanisms contribute to control of malignant disease after allogeneic bone marrow transplantation. The precise mediators of the so-called graft-versus-tumor effect remain to be elucidated. Transplantation has been most effective in treating tumors that are initially chemoresponsive such as acute leukemia, Hodgkin's and non-Hodgkin's lymphoma, breast carcinoma, and testicular carcinoma. This approach has been ineffective, however, in treating common epithelium-derived malignancies such as non-small cell lung carcinoma and colorectal carcinoma.

COMPLICATIONS Every chemotherapeutic regimen administered in adequate doses will have some deleterious side effect on normal host tissues. Most of the complications can be anticipated and considerable expertise has been gained in treating and if possible preventing these complications. Myelosuppression, nausea and vomiting, stomatitis, and alopecia are the most frequently observed complications associated with chemotherapy administration.

Myelosuppression Chemotherapy-induced bone marrow suppression is the most important complication of therapy and is most often the dose-limiting factor. Myelosuppression, manifested as leukopenia, thrombocytopenia, and anemia, occurs with most chemotherapeutic regimens. The blood counts usually reach their nadir between 10 and 14 days of treatment, with recovery noted by day 21 and a return to normal by day 28. Thus, most chemotherapeutic regimens are administered on 21- to 28-day cycles. However, regimens that contain drugs toxic to myeloid stem cells, such as a nitrosourea, require a longer period of bone marrow recovery and are usually administered every 6 weeks.

Leukopenia, and particularly neutropenia, increases the risk of infectious complications in patients receiving chemotherapy. Fever is the hallmark of infection. Any patient with neutropenia (absolute neutrophil count $<1.0 \times 10^9$ per liter) and fever requires a prompt medical evaluation and subsequent administration of empirical, broad-spectrum parenteral antibiotics. The use of recombinant hematopoietic growth factor support, particularly granulocyte colony stimulating factor and granulocyte-macrophage colony stimulating factor, can shorten the length of neutropenia associated with chemotherapy (see "Biologic therapy," below).

Thrombocytopenia may occur in patients receiving chemotherapy but is less often dose limiting than leukopenia. An increase in a patient's bleeding time can be detected when the platelet count falls below 100×10^9 per liter, but most patients are without symptoms with platelet counts $>50 \times 10^9$ per liter. The risk for a severe hemorrhagic complication, such as spontaneous intracranial bleeding, begins to increase when the platelet count falls below 20×10^9 per liter. Thrombocytopenia to this degree is usually only observed with very intense chemotherapeutic regimens such as those used in the treatment of acute leukemia.

Anemia to some degree is to be anticipated with chemotherapy. However, except with intense chemotherapeutic regimens transfusions are usually not required. In addition, there is no hemoglobin level below which all patients should receive transfusions for chemotherapy-induced anemia. Rather, transfusions should be administered only after considering the long-term goals of therapy and weighing the risk-to-benefit ratio for each patient.

Nausea and vomiting Nausea and vomiting are major side effects of cancer chemotherapy and previously were sufficiently severe that some patients would refuse further chemotherapy treatments. However, significant progress has been made in preventing and treating chemotherapy-induced nausea and vomiting. Progress has resulted from the development of newer and more effective antiemetics, the completion of multiple clinical trials that specifically address the problem, and the education of physicians regarding its prevention and management.

Chemotherapy appears to induce nausea and vomiting through several pathways. Vomiting is controlled by two medullary centers: the vomiting center and the chemoreceptor trigger zone (see Chap. 38). The vomiting center receives input from the chemoreceptor trigger zone and coordinates the process of vomiting through multiple efferent tracts. The chemoreceptor trigger zone is directly stimulated by various toxins or drugs to release neurotransmitters, such as dopamine, which then interact with the vomiting center. The vomiting center also directly receives input from the gastrointestinal tract where appropriate stimuli can induce emesis independent of the chemoreceptor trigger zone. Finally, cerebral input, especially from visual or olfactory stimuli can trigger the vomiting center.

The chemotherapeutic agents are not all equally emetogenic. Cisplatin consistently causes the most severe side effects. Dacarbazine, doxorubicin, and mechlorethamine are also highly emetogenic agents. However several chemotherapeutic drugs, particularly the antimetabolites such as methotrexate or fluorouracil, cause only minimal nausea and vomiting.

Prevention of nausea and vomiting should be a primary goal. Antiemetic regimens always should be given on a routine schedule. Treatment only as needed is generally inappropriate. Antiemetic regimens should err on the side of being too aggressive rather than insufficient, particularly in new patients. They can subsequently be modified if required. They should be commensurate with the emetogenic potential of the particular chemotherapy program. The commonly used antiemetic agents are briefly discussed below.

The phenothiazines such as *prochlorperazine* and *chlorpromazine* are the most widely used antiemetic agents and appear to be useful drugs due to their antidopaminergic and antiserotoninergic activities. They are available in several formulations, making them useful for outpatient regimens. As single agents they are effective for only mildly emetogenic drugs such as fluorouracil.

The benzamide *metoclopramide* appears to antagonize dopamine activity peripherally and centrally. When used parenterally in high doses (1 to 2 mg/kg every 2 to 4 h) it can effectively reduce nausea and vomiting associated with even the most potently emetogenic chemotherapeutic drugs. When used in high doses extrapyramidal side effects are not uncommon, and thus it is often administered with an antihistamine such as diphenhydramine or a benzodiazepine such as lorazepam.

Serotonin antagonists such as *ondansetron* are the newest and possibly the most effective antiemetic agents. Ondansetron appears to selectively block the serotonin receptor 5-HT$_3$ which is present peripherally on the vagus nerve and centrally in the chemoreceptor trigger zone. It is effective in the treatment of nausea and vomiting due to cisplatin but is without the dystonic reactions that may accompany metoclopramide.

The cannabinoid *dronabinol* contains the principal psychoactive agent in marijuana, Δ-9-THC. It is available only in oral formulation and appears to be most effective against mild or moderately emetogenic chemotherapeutic regimens. It produces significant mood alterations including dysphoria in a substantial number of patients and is thus generally reserved for patients not responding to other therapies.

Other miscellaneous agents are frequently employed in combination antiemetic regimens. High-dose glucocorticoids such as dexamethasone are often used for brief intervals, particularly with metoclopramide. Benzodiazepines are useful as sedatives for patients with anticipatory nausea and vomiting and as amnestic agents. Antihistamines have modest antinausea properties but are most useful to prevent dystonic reactions associated with phenothiazines or metoclopramide.

Stomatitis   Stomatitis is an inflammation of the oral mucosa and a major complication of cancer chemotherapy. Early signs of stomatitis are erythema and edema which may progress to frank, painful ulcerations that persist for several days to a week or longer. The painful ulcers result in poor oral intake with subsequent dehydration and malnutrition. They also may become secondarily infected and further complicate patient management. Virtually all chemotherapeutic agents will cause stomatitis if given in sufficient dose intensity. With the antimetabolites, duration of exposure is probably a greater risk factor for developing stomatitis than peak drug level.

There currently is no known method to prevent stomatitis except for dose modification of the offending chemotherapeutic agents. Meticulous oral hygiene will help diminish pathogenic oral flora and decrease the risk of developing secondary infections. Treatment with topical oral anesthetics such as viscous xylocaine will relieve pain and help maintain adequate oral intake.

Alopecia   Chemotherapy-induced hair loss is one of the most distressing aspects of cancer treatment for some patients and is due to the direct cytotoxic effects of antineoplastic agents on the hair follicle. Hair loss tends to be patchy and most severe on the scalp, usually becoming noticeable 1 to 2 weeks after beginning therapy. After cessation of chemotherapy, hair regrowth begins and should eventually return to pretreatment levels although it may differ in texture and color. Cyclophosphamide, dactinomycin, doxorubicin, paclitaxel, and vincristine generally cause the most profound alopecia. Scalp-cooling devices that apparently decrease scalp perfusion have been employed with mixed results.

DRUG RESISTANCE   Tumor cell resistance to chemotherapeutic agents is a central problem in medical oncology. With improvements in supportive care such as a new generation of antimicrobials, multicomponent blood product and hematopoietic growth factor support, specialized oncology nursing, and high-technology intensive care units, drug resistance is probably the single most important obstacle to achieving high rates of curative cancer therapy.

The problem of drug resistance can be conveniently divided into two groups: de novo resistance and acquired resistance. In de novo resistance, tumor cells are initially unresponsive to chemotherapy. This situation unfortunately exists for many of the most common solid tumors. In acquired drug resistance, tumors are initially responsive to chemotherapy but resistance develops with continued therapy. Acquired resistance is a primary reason that only a small percentage of many responsive tumors are curable with chemotherapy.

The appearance of resistant clones within a larger population was addressed initially by Delbruck and Luria studying bacteria and later by Law and then Goldie and Coldman in tumor cells. Delbruck and Luria observed that populations of bacteria exhibited varying degrees of resistance to bacteriophage infection. They showed that resistant cells were present within the population due to spontaneous mutations that existed before exposure to the phage. Development of resistance was dependent on mutation frequency and population size.

The Delbruck-Luria principles were extended to tumor cell biology and treatment. An important property of tumor cells is genomic instability. As a tumor grows from a single transformed cell to a clinically detectable 1-mL mass of 1×10^9 cells, it undergoes spontaneous mutations and contains a heterogeneous population of cells, some of which have mutated to drug resistance purely by chance. Treatment with chemotherapy will eliminate the most sensitive cells, leaving the resistant subclones to grow. Clinically this situation occurs in patients who have responded to therapy, entered a complete remission, only later to relapse with drug-refractory tumors.

These concepts suggest some important principles to maximize chemotherapy effectiveness. Tumors are most likely to be responsive to chemotherapy when small in size prior to the development of multiple resistant subclones. Regimens that are not effective against bulky tumors may be curative when used in the adjuvant setting. Effective treatment should consist of combination chemotherapy containing non-cross resistant agents. The likelihood of two simultaneous mutations in the same cell affording resistance to two different classes of drugs is low, i.e., the product of two independent probabilities. Thus, the greater the number of truly non-cross resistant drugs administered at fully effective dose, the greater the chance of eliminating the entire tumor population.

While the combination chemotherapy concept provides useful predictions, several limitations must be understood. First, many of the antitumor agents, such as the alkylating agents, the anthracyclines, and the epipodophyllotoxins are mutagenic agents. Thus clinical drug refractoriness may result not only from prior spontaneous mutations but also from treatment with mutagenic drugs. Second, many of the antitumor drugs are cross resistant. Although the problem of multidrug resistance has gained increasing attention, much remains to be elucidated. It is clear that anticancer drug cross resistance cannot be anticipated from studies of cytotoxicity mechanisms alone.

Mechanisms of single-agent drug resistance Much of what is known about drug resistance is a result of in vitro studies. Cell lines have been made resistant to various chemotherapeutic agents by gradually selecting them in increasing concentrations of drug. By comparing resistant sublines to the parental cell lines, resistance mechanisms have been discerned. Determining the clinical importance of these in vitro mechanisms has been a slow and difficult process. Examples are given below of specific resistance mechanisms that have been determined for various agents.

DEFECTIVE TRANSPORT Several chemotherapeutic agents are transported into the cell by carrier-mediated uptake utilizing various physiologic transporters. Decreased expression or activity of a specific transporter will lead to decreased drug accumulation in the cell. For example, methotrexate resistance has been associated with loss of a folate transport protein, cytarabine resistance with loss of nucleoside transporter, and mechlorethamine resistance with loss of choline transporter.

DECREASED ACTIVATING ENZYME Some drugs require activation via intracellular biochemical pathways. A decrease in the activity of these pathways will lead to a decreased production of the cytotoxic metabolite. Decreased deoxycytidine kinase activity has been observed with cytarabine resistance, defective polyglutamylation with methotrexate resistance, and diminished HGPRT activity with thioguanine and mercaptopurine resistance.

INCREASED DRUG INACTIVATION Inactivation of cytotoxic drugs or their metabolites can also occur via intracellular biochemical pathways. Increased cytidine deaminase inactivates cytarabine, increased bleomycin hydrolase renders bleomycin inactive, and increased membrane alkaline phosphatase inactivates thioguanine and mercaptopurine.

INCREASE IN TARGET ENZYME When a chemotherapeutic drug targets a specific enzyme, increased expression of the target, often through gene amplification, can be observed. Methotrexate resistance can result from amplification of the dihydrofolate reductase gene, pentostatin resistance from amplification of the adenosine deaminase gene, and FUDR resistance from increased copy number of the thymidylate synthase gene.

ALTERATIONS IN TARGETS Rather than increasing expression of a target enzyme, the target can be structurally altered to diminish the cytotoxic effect of the drug. Tubulin alteration has been noted with vincristine resistance and paclitaxel resistance, thymidylate synthase change has been observed with decreased binding to the fluorouracil metabolite fluorodeoxyuridylate, and altered ribonucleotide reductase has been noted in resistance to hydroxyurea.

Mechanisms of multiple drug resistance The resistance mechanisms discussed above are relatively specific for a given drug. Clinical chemotherapy refractoriness, however, is often characterized by resistance to multiple drugs. The phenomenon of in vitro multidrug resistance was first described in the 1970s by Biedler and by Ling. Cells selected for resistance to one drug demonstrate cross resistance to other structurally and functionally unrelated compounds. The drugs that constitute the multidrug resistance family include the anthracyclines, the vinca alkaloids, the epipodophyllotoxins, and other agents such as dactinomycin and paclitaxel. Multidrug-resistant cells have energy-dependent decreased accumulation of cytotoxic drugs, due apparently to an outward efflux. The resistant cell lines overexpress a membrane glycoprotein of 150 to 180 kDa termed *P-glycoprotein*. The gene that codes for P-glycoprotein has been cloned

and is now recognized to belong to a family of ATP-binding cassette proteins. The human gene responsible for P-glycoprotein–mediated multidrug resistance is called *MDR1*.

P-glycoprotein–mediated efflux can be circumvented by any one of a series of ever-increasing number of reversing agents. These chemosensitizing agents, such as verapamil, quinine, and cyclosporine A, have entered clinical trials in an attempt to overcome multidrug resistance.

P-glycoprotein is expressed in normal tissues with the highest levels found on luminal surfaces such as renal tubules, small and large intestine, and bile canaliculi. The function and transport substrates of P-glycoprotein in these normal tissues remain elusive.

While P-glycoprotein expression is a well-defined mechanism of in vitro drug resistance, its role in clinical drug resistance has yet to be fully defined. Nonuniformity in assessing P-glycoprotein or *MDR1* expression in tumor specimens has led to conflicting results. Few studies compare expression in the same patients prior to therapy and after the acquisition of chemotherapeutic drug resistance. Additionally, studies that have added chemosensitizing agents to preexisting multiagent regimens have generally had marginal results or been inconclusive. In a few tumors, such as acute myeloid leukemia or childhood neuroblastoma, P-glycoprotein expression at presentation may portend a poor prognosis.

Additional mechanisms of in vitro multidrug resistance distinct from P-glycoprotein expression have been characterized. Altered activity and/or expression of the enzyme topoisomerase II has been shown to produce resistance to the anthracyclines, epipodophyllotoxins, and other drugs including dactinomycin and mitoxantrone. Altered topoisomerase activity may also exist in cells that simultaneously exhibit more than one mechanism of multidrug resistance. The clinical significance of topoisomerase II–mediated resistance is unknown.

An enhanced reducing environment with increased activity of glutathione detoxification pathways and elevated cellular pools of reduced glutathione also has been described. Resistance to alkylating agents including the nitrogen mustard derivatives and the nitrosoureas, as well as the anthracyclines, has been associated with increased glutathione detoxification. Buthionine sulfoximine, an agent that depletes cellular glutathione levels, has entered clinical trials as a chemosensitizing agent.

NEW DRUG DEVELOPMENT After the demonstration in the 1940s that some drugs have antitumor effects, the National Cancer Institute began a large-scale drug screening program. From 1955 through 1975 over 400,000 compounds were screened against murine leukemia models P388 and L1210. While many compounds were identified, the discovery of drugs with activity against rodent leukemias did not correlate well with drugs active in the treatment of the major human cancers. The drug screening protocol was then changed to include human tumors transplanted into athymic mice. It was subsequently further modified so that new compounds are now tested against a panel of about 60 human cancer cell lines representing many of the most common solid tumors. Compounds demonstrating in vitro antitumor activity are then tested against a panel of human tumor xenografts in nude mice. Compounds that are still promising then undergo further toxicology screening and formulation testing before beginning clinical trials.

Antitumor agents proceed through a series of clinical trials before they are accepted in widespread clinical use. There are currently three distinct phases of testing. From initial screening to approval by the Federal Drug Administration for a specific indication may take 10 years or longer. Table 318-3 lists some investigational anticancer agents currently in clinical trials.

Phase I trials are performed to determine drug toxicity in humans. To be eligible, patients must have a cancer not responsive to available therapies. An initial dose is chosen based on animal studies. Generally three patients are treated at a given dose before sequential dose escalation. Dose escalation proceeds until a dose-limiting toxicity is reached which defines the maximally tolerated dose. Since phase I trials are composed of relatively small numbers of often heavily

TABLE 318-3 Investigational anticancer drugs		
Drug	Category	Mechanism of action
Amifostine (WR-2721)	Aminothiol; cisplatin: toxicity protectant	Scavenges free radicals
Dexrazoxane	Anthracycline: cardioprotectant	Chelates metal ions
Edatrexate	Antifolate	Inhibits dihydrofolate reductase
Irinotecan (CPT-11)	Camptothecin derivative	Inhibits topoisomerase I
Losoxantrone	Anthrapyrazole	Inhibits topoisomerase II
Ormaplatin	Platinum analogue	Cross-links DNA
Oxaliplatin	Platinum analogue	Cross-links DNA
Pirarubicin	Anthracycline	Inhibits topoisomerase II
Piritrexim	Antifolate	Inhibits dihydrofolate reductase
Rhizoxin	Macrocyclic lactone	Inhibits microtubule assembly
Suramin	Polyanion	Modulates growth factors (?)
Taxotere	Taxane	Promotes microtubule assembly
Topotecan	Camptothecin derivative	Inhibits topoisomerase I
Tretinoin (ATRA)	Retinoid	Promotes differentiation
Trimetrexate	Antifolate	Inhibits dihydrofolate reductase
Vinorelbine	Vinca alkaloid	Inhibits microtubule assembly

pretreated patients with diverse tumor types, the lack of tumor response does not preclude an agent from ultimate clinical usefulness.

Phase II trials are designed to determine if a drug has activity in a particular tumor type. Generally small groups of patients with advanced malignancies of a particular tumor type are treated according to a dose and schedule determined from the phase I study. Patients must have measurable tumor masses to assess the efficacy of therapy. A given compound generally undergoes several phase II studies against a broad array of tumor types. After the completion of phase II trials, a decision is made based on the available data whether to proceed to phase III or to abandon further testing.

Phase III studies are designed to test an agent against the standard, existing therapy for a particular tumor. This testing usually requires a randomized, two-arm study. The malignant diseases to be tested are determined from the phase II data. Patients generally have not received prior therapy at the time of treatment. Phase III trials require large numbers of patients and frequently are multi-institutional.

ENDOCRINE THERAPY Endocrine therapy for hormone-responsive malignancies has been utilized for many years. Hormonal therapy depends on the existence of underlying cellular growth control mechanisms derived from the normal tissues from which the tumor arose. Breast carcinoma and prostate carcinoma are the solid tumors most amenable to hormonal manipulation. The presence of estrogen and progesterone receptors in breast carcinoma predicts a response to endocrine therapy. In prostate carcinoma, androgen blockade is the most effective therapy for metastatic disease.

Most of the hormonal antitumor agents are functional agonists or antagonists of the steroid family. Steroid hormones bind to specific intracellular receptors and induce a conformational receptor change. The hormone-receptor complex interacts with DNA and thereby functions as a transcription factor which regulates gene expression.

Adrenocorticosteroids The adrenal steroids have activity in the treatment of lymphocytic leukemias and lymphomas. Because of nonoverlapping toxicities with many chemotherapeutic agents, particularly lack of myelosuppression, they are frequently employed in combination regimens. They function by binding to glucocorticoid-specific receptors present in lymphoid cells and apparently cause programmed cell death or apoptosis. While several synthetic glucocor-

ticoids are available, the most commonly used agents in cancer therapy are *prednisone, methylprednisolone,* and *dexamethasone.* These agents are generally employed in relatively high doses for short periods. The most common toxicities include CNS effects with alterations in mood and personality, and metabolic derangements such as hyperglycemia, hypokalemia, and fluid retention. Suppression of the adrenocortical axis is usually not a problem with short-term administration. Likewise the development of cushingoid features, osteoporosis, and cataract formation is also less of a concern. Glucocorticoids also have been employed for palliative treatment of breast carcinoma. Dexamethasone is commonly used to alleviate intracranial edema often associated with central nervous system neoplasms.

Androgens Androgens such as *fluoxymesterone* are occasionally used in the palliative treatment of breast carcinoma. These synthetic analogues of testosterone are somewhat less virilizing than the naturally occurring hormones. However, hirsutism, weight gain, and deepening of the voice are adverse effects that may not completely reverse themselves after discontinuing therapy. Amenorrhea occurs in many women during therapy. Synthetic androgens can cause hepatotoxicity with elevations of liver function tests.

Antiandrogens The antiandrogen *flutamide* effectively blocks androgen binding to its receptor in peripheral tissues. Although serum testosterone levels may rise, levels in the target tissues are decreased. Flutamide is used in the treatment of disseminated prostate carcinoma. It is often used after orchiectomy or with leuprolide. It has predictable antiandrogen side effects in men, including gynecomastia, decreased libido, and impotence. Elevation of liver function tests also has been reported.

Estrogens Estrogen therapy was once a mainstay in the palliative treatment of disseminated prostate carcinoma. Estrogens are occasionally used in the palliative treatment of breast carcinoma. In prostate carcinoma estrogens appear to function as potent antiandrogens; their mechanism of action in breast carcinoma is not entirely understood. Two commonly used preparations are *diethylstilbestrol* (DES) and *ethinyl estradiol.* Estrogen therapy may exacerbate underlying ischemic heart disease, predispose to thromboembolic phenomena, and lead to fluid retention. Gynecomastia and impotence in men are common.

Antiestrogens The antiestrogen *tamoxifen* is widely used in the therapy of breast carcinoma. It is employed both as an adjuvant in postmenopausal women and as palliative therapy for metastatic disease in both pre- and postmenopausal women. Tamoxifen binds directly to the estrogen receptor and appears to function as a weak agonist/antagonist. It has a long plasma half-life and requires 4 weeks or longer to achieve steady-state levels. Tamoxifen can cause amenorrhea, hot flashes, and occasionally nausea and vomiting. It has been reported to modestly increase the risk of thromboembolic phenomenon. Changes in serum lipid profiles also have been noted.

Progestins Progestational agents such as *medroxyprogesterone* or *megestrol acetate* are used in the treatment of endometrial carcinoma and breast carcinoma. Their mechanism of action is unclear; however, studies suggest they may: (1) be directly cytotoxic to tumor cells; (2) disrupt the hypothalamic-pituitary-gonadal axis; (3) alter expression of estrogen receptors; and/or (4) have androgen-like effects. Progestins frequently cause menstrual irregularities. Fluid retention, hepatic enzyme elevations, and thromboembolic events all have been reported.

Aromatase inhibitor *Aminoglutethimide* inhibits several enzymes responsible for the conversion of androgens to estrogens in the peripheral tissues. It also inhibits the conversion of cholesterol to pregnenalone, a key step in steroid hormone biosynthesis. Aminoglutethimide treatment functions as a medical adrenalectomy, and patients receiving relatively high doses may need maintenance hydrocortisone to avoid adrenal insufficiency. It is used in the palliative treatment of metastatic breast carcinoma. Toxicity includes mild neurologic symptoms such as dizziness and ataxia. Lethargy is also frequent. A maculopapular skin rash, common during the first weeks of treatment, usually resolves and does not require discontinuing therapy. On rare occasions there are leukopenia and thrombocytopenia which quickly resolve with cessation of treatment.

Gonadotropin-releasing hormone agonists   The gonadotropin-releasing hormone (GnRH) agonist *leuprolide* is used in the treatment of disseminated prostate carcinoma. Continuous pituitary stimulation by GnRH, normally under pulsatile control, leads to an eventual downregulation of LH and FSH secretion with subsequent diminution of androgen levels. During the first weeks of therapy an initial LH and FSH release may precipitate a worsening of symptoms which may be avoided by instituting antiandrogen treatment. Peripheral edema with worsening of congestive heart failure also have been seen. Antiandrogen effects including gynecomastia, impotence, and hot flashes are seen to a varying degree.

Somatostatin analogues   The somatostatin analogue *octreotide* is used in the symptomatic treatment of patients with metastatic carcinoid or vasoactive intestinal peptide–secreting tumors. Somatostatin analogues suppress release of gastric and pancreatic peptides in addition to suppressing growth hormone release. Patients receiving octreotide experience a dramatic decrease in endocrine-related symptoms such as diarrhea, flushing, and hypoglycemia associated with tumor hormone secretion. The drug must be injected subcutaneously two or three times daily to maintain adequate relief of symptoms. Since somatostatin inhibits insulin secretion, patients must be monitored for hyperglycemia, particularly those with a prior history of impaired glucose tolerance. Other symptoms related to inhibition of normal gastric and pancreatic function such as indigestion, steatorrhea, abdominal pain, nausea, and vomiting also can be seen.

BIOLOGICAL THERAPY   The application of biological agents to the therapy of cancer has been eagerly anticipated by clinicians and investigators. The term *biologic response modifiers* is used to suggest that these agents function by altering the host response to cancer rather than by direct cytotoxicity. Despite much initial enthusiasm, the role of biologic agents in cancer therapy remains limited.

The availability of sufficient quantities of highly purified biologic agents has been possible only through the application of modern techniques in protein biochemistry and molecular biology. The identification and cloning of the genes coding the biologic response modifiers has allowed high-level in vitro expression of these proteins and their subsequent purification. Differences in posttranslational modification of proteins produced by nonhuman systems may result in biologic activity not identical to that of the naturally occurring products.

Assessing clinical usefulness of these agents has often been difficult since the paradigms for cytotoxic chemotherapy are generally inappropriate for biologic agents. The optimal biologic response often does not correlate with maximal tolerated dose. Biologic agents usually demonstrate peak activity within a range; concentrations higher or lower may result in suboptimal effect. Thus the optimal dose clinically is the one which produces the maximum effect, not the highest dose tolerated without unacceptable toxicity.

Monoclonal antibodies   With the development of hybridoma technology, the ability to produce monoclonal antibodies to a specific antigenic determinant led to high expectations for their widespread use in cancer therapy. While monoclonal antibodies have become important tools in cancer diagnostics, their use in cancer therapy has remained investigational. A major difficulty has been defining tumor-specific antigens serologically.

Immunophenotyping of leukemias and lymphomas utilizing monoclonal antibodies directed primarily against myeloid and lymphoid differentiation antigens has improved understanding of the natural history of these diseases and facilitated diagnostics. Immunophenotyping most often confirms the diagnosis determined by histopathology alone. Since it is impossible to determine prospectively which patients will have their diagnosis refined by immunophenotyping, however,

it is now common to immunophenotype all lymphoid and myeloid specimens.

Monoclonal antibodies do not yet have a proven role in cancer therapy, but they are being actively investigated. Antibodies directed against tumor-associated antigens have been conjugated to various drugs, radioisotopes, or toxins and administered to patients. Also, in autologous bone marrow transplantation studies, monoclonal antibodies have been used to purge harvested bone marrow of tumor cells prior to reinfusion.

Cytokines   Cytokines are a group of intercellular messenger proteins that are key immunoregulatory compounds. They comprise the largest group of biologic therapeutics in clinical trials and include the interferons, the interleukins, and the hematopoietic growth factors.

Interferons were the first biologic response modifiers to enter clinical trials. Interferons α and β share a common cellular receptor and are referred to as *type I interferons*. Interferon α is the product of a multigene family of at least 16 members, whereas interferon β is the product of a single gene. Both are produced by a variety of cell types. Type I interferons have immunoregulatory and antiproliferative effects. Recombinant interferon α is approved for use in the treatment of hairy cell leukemia and AIDS-related Kaposi's sarcoma. It also has activity in stable phase chronic myelogenous leukemia, low-grade non-Hodgkin's lymphoma, multiple myeloma, melanoma, and renal cell carcinoma. The potential clinical role of interferon β is under active investigation. Interferon γ, produced by lymphocytes, is referred to as *type II interferon* and has immunomodulatory properties distinct from type I interferons. It appears to have less single-agent antitumor activity than type I interferons. It is approved for use in chronic granulomatous disease but remains investigational as an antitumor agent. All the interferons produce a flu-like syndrome with fever, malaise, myalgias, and fatigue. Modest leukopenia is also common and hepatic transaminase elevations can also be seen.

Interleukins are cytokines that function predominantly as leukocyte messengers. Currently 12 interleukins have been identified, and several have entered clinical trials, but only recombinant interleukin 2 is an approved anticancer agent. Interleukin 2 (IL-2), previously known as T cell growth factor, is a key regulatory hormone in cell-mediated immunity. It stimulates the proliferation of T cells and natural killer (NK) cells and induces lymphokine-activated killer (LAK) cells. The latter, composed predominantly of activated NK cells, can directly lyse freshly isolated solid tumor cells. Studies at the National Cancer Institute demonstrated that infusion of high doses of IL-2 in conjunction with autologous LAK cells (expanded ex vivo) produced responses in metastatic melanoma and renal cell carcinoma. In subsequent trials, IL-2 administration produced a response in a minority of patients with metastatic renal cell carcinoma and melanoma, with a small percentage (5 to 10 percent) of patients achieving complete responses. However, cardiovascular complications were sufficient to warrant intensive care unit management. Multiple other organ system effects, generally reversible with cessation of therapy, including renal, hepatic, pulmonary, neurologic, hematopoietic and dermatologic toxicities, were noted. Subsequent studies have suggested that the use of ex vivo LAK cells may not contribute to the antitumor efficacy. The optimal dose and schedule of IL-2 administration have yet to be determined.

The other interleukins remain investigational agents for cancer therapy. Interleukin 1 activity is encoded by two proteins with minimal structural similarity, IL-1α and IL-1β. In addition a receptor antagonist, IL-1RA, has been identified. IL-1 is an important mediator of the inflammatory response and has pleiotropic biologic activities. Interleukin 3 is a hematopoietic growth factor which stimulates growth and differentiation of early myeloid progenitors and is under investigation in the treatment of myeloid malignancies. Interleukin 4 is a regulator of humoral and cell-mediated immunity, interleukin 5 is a regulator of eosinophilic growth and differentiation, and interleukin 6 has pleiotropic immunohematopoietic effects.

Tumor necrosis factor, composed of two related proteins TNF-α and TNF-β, appears to play a central role in the inflammatory response. In experimental systems, TNF administration causes direct tumor cytotoxicity, probably through the generation of free oxygen radicals. Its pronounced toxicity in humans has severely limited its clinical usefulness.

Hematopoietic growth factors Normal hematopoietic growth and differentiation is under the regulation of hematopoietic growth factors. The clinical use of these growth factors in cancer therapy has been limited mostly to ameliorating chemotherapy-induced myelosuppression. *Erythropoietin* is produced by the kidney and liver in response to hypoxia. It induces erythroid maturation in committed progenitor cells and increases the release of reticulocytes from bone marrow. The primary clinical use of recombinant erythropoietin is in treating deficiency states such as the anemia of chronic renal failure. Its role in supportive cancer therapy is limited.

Granulocyte-macrophage colony stimulating factor (GM-CSF) promotes the differentiation of the committed myeloid progenitor into mature granulocytes, monocytes, and eosinophils. It also stimulates growth of the multilineage hematopoietic stem cell. Recombinant GM-CSF hastens myeloid reconstitution after autologous bone marrow transplantation. GM-CSF administration is associated with fevers, chills, bone pain, myalgias, flushing, hypotension, anorexia, lethargy, and skin eruptions.

Granulocyte colony stimulating factor (G-CSF), stimulates the growth and differentiation of committed, neutrophilic progenitor cells. Administration to patients of recombinant G-CSF can shorten the period of neutropenia associated with chemotherapy-induced myeloid suppression. Preliminary clinical experience suggests G-CSF may be tolerated better than GM-CSF with fewer side effects. Bone pain is the most common complaint. The routine use of these agents in conjunction with chemotherapy regimens that produce significant neutropenia is under active investigation.

BIBLIOGRAPHY

CHABNER BA, COLLINS JM: *Cancer Chemotherapy: Principles and Practice.* Philadelphia, Lippincott, 1990

DEVITA VT et al (eds): *Cancer Principles and Practice of Oncology,* 4th ed. Philadelphia, Lippincott, 1993

HOLLAND JF et al (eds): *Cancer Medicine,* 3rd ed. Philadelphia, Lea and Febiger, 1993

MOOSSA AR et al (eds): *Comprehensive Textbook of Oncology,* 2d ed. Baltimore, Williams and Wilkins, 1991

PIZZO PH: Management of fever in patients with cancer and treatment-induced neutropenia. N Engl J Med 328:1323, 1993

WEISS RB (ed): New antitumor drugs in development. Semin Oncol 19(6):611, 1992

---

319 BREAST CANCER

I. CRAIG HENDERSON

Breast cancer is both one of the most common and one of the most treatable of all human malignancies. The incidence of this disease provides a poor estimate of the frequency with which breast problems are brought to the attention of physicians of all specialities. For each patient diagnosed with breast cancer, another 5 to 10 women are biopsied for suspicious symptoms, and for each patient biopsied, dozens seek consultation because of symptoms or concern. Breast cancer is one of the few tumors for which there is conclusive evidence that screening will substantially decrease mortality. In the treatment of breast cancer, radical surgical procedures have been almost entirely replaced by more limited forms of surgery, such as the modified radical mastectomy, and most breast cancer patients now have

the option of combining breast-sparing procedures (e.g., partial mastectomy or lumpectomy) with radiation therapy as an alternative to mastectomy. Medical therapies are now an important component of the treatment of almost all stages of invasive breast cancer, and medical interventions to prevent breast cancer are now being studied in randomized trials.

ETIOLOGY AND RISK FACTORS

Epidemiologic data suggest that genetic, endocrine, and environmental factors may be involved in the initiation and/or the promotion of breast cancer growth. Although the principal value of these studies is the identification of etiologic factors that may prove useful in primary prevention programs, epidemiologic data are often used to identify high-risk groups of women to be targeted for intensive surveillance or even prophylactic mastectomy. It has not been established, however, that these strategies will decrease breast cancer mortality in these high-risk groups, and an inappropriate emphasis on risk factors may obscure the fact that 70 to 80 percent of all breast cancers occur in patients without identifiable risk factors.

In the United States, the cumulative lifetime probability of developing breast cancer is 12 percent and of dying from breast cancer, 3.5 percent. Most of the risk of developing breast cancer is expressed after age 50, and the highest risk is after age 75 (Table 319-1). In counseling women regarding their risk of developing breast cancer, the use of 20- to 40-year interval probabilities may be more meaningful than the lifetime probability. For example, the probability of a woman without defined risk factors developing breast cancer between the ages of 50 and 70 is 4.67 percent; that of dying from breast cancer is 1.04 percent. A patient with a relative risk of 3 (e.g., a woman whose mother and sister have been diagnosed with breast cancer) would then have a 14 percent probability of developing breast cancer and a 3.1 percent probability of dying from breast cancer during this interval. This likely explains why no risk group with an observed cumulative incidence of breast cancer in excess of 30 to 40 percent or cumulative mortality in excess of 10 to 20 percent has been identified.

Genetic factors Although all relatives of breast cancer patients are at some increased risk of developing breast cancer, first-degree relatives (siblings, parents, children) have a two- to threefold increase in risk compared with the general population. Thus the cumulative probability that a 30-year-old woman whose sister or mother had breast cancer will herself develop breast cancer by age 70 is somewhere between 8 and 18 percent. Some investigators have observed an even higher risk when two or more relatives are affected, when the affected patient is premenopausal, or when the patient has bilateral breast cancer, but these observations have not been consistent among epidemiologic studies.

TABLE 319-1 Probability of a white female developing and dying of breast cancer in specified time intervals (1985)

Age interval, years	Risk of developing breast cancer, %	Risk of dying of breast cancer, %
Birth to 110	10.20	3.60
20–30	0.04	0.00
20–40	0.49	0.09
35–45	0.88	0.14
35–55	2.53	0.56
50–60	1.95	0.33
50–70	4.67	1.04
65–75	3.17	0.43
65–85	5.48	1.01

SOURCE: From Seidman et al, CA 35:36, 1985.

As many as 5 percent of all breast cancer patients may have inherited a specific genetic abnormality contributing to the development of their breast cancer. Point mutations of the p53 tumor suppressor gene on chromosome 17 indicate which individuals in Li-Fraumeni families will develop one or more of six different cancers, including breast cancer. Linkage studies also have demonstrated an association between loss of heterozygosity on chromosome 17q and the breast-ovarian cancer syndrome. This gene, BRCA1, is less well characterized, but penetrance may be as high as 85 percent. Possibly as many as 1 in 200 to 400 American women may be carriers. Together these two gene abnormalities account for very few breast cancers, and routine screening for these genetic abnormalities in women without evidence of a very strong family history of breast cancers diagnosed at a very young age is not warranted. However, the recent identification of these genes gives promise that more prevalent genes will eventually be identified in ongoing linkage studies.

Endocrine factors Early age of menarche, late onset of menopause, nulliparity, and late age at first pregnancy appear to be independently associated with an increased incidence of breast cancer. Since both diet and exercise may affect both age of menarche and the regularity of menses, it has been suggested that this effect of diet and exercise may explain, at least in part, variations in breast cancer incidence among women with different life-styles. Age at first full-term pregnancy is a more important determinant of risk than the number of pregnancies. Compared to women with a first pregnancy before age 18, the relative risk of breast cancer is doubled if the first pregnancy is delayed until after age 24 and about quadrupled after age 30. The risk of breast cancer is actually higher among women with their first pregnancies after age 30 than among nulliparous women, suggesting that early pregnancy is protective while late pregnancy promotes development of the disease. These observations are consistent with the hypothesis that events between menarche and the first pregnancy are critical in determining the lifetime probability of developing breast cancer.

In light of the associations between endogenous endocrine factors and breast cancer, one might anticipate that hormone administration, such as estrogen replacement therapy (ERT) for postmenopausal symptoms or oral contraceptives (OC) for birth control, would either induce or promote the growth of breast cancer. Although the results of more than 50 case-control and cohort studies performed to study possible associations have been inconsistent, recently published meta-analyses suggest that any increased risk of breast cancer from using either of these treatments for durations of 5 to 10 years is nonexistent or extremely small. However, more prolonged use of estrogens to alleviate postmenopausal symptoms may be associated with a significant increase in relative risk to the range of 1.3 to 2.2, especially if ERT is begun while the woman is still premenopausal and if stilbestrol, rather than conjugated estrogens, is used. Unopposed estrogen use increases the risk of endometrial cancer, too, but this risk can be alleviated by the concomitant or sequential use of progestins with estrogen replacement therapy. Progestins have not been shown to have a similar beneficial effect in reducing breast cancer risk and may even augment that risk. Oral contraceptive use for periods in excess of 10 years may increase the chance that a woman will develop a cancer before the age of 45, and the use of OCs for durations in excess of 4 years prior to the first full-term pregnancy has been reported to increase the relative risk of breast cancer at an early age to as high as 1.7. The increased risk from the use of ERT or OCs may be greater in women with a history of breast cancer in a first-degree relative, but interactions with other underlying risk factors have not been demonstrated. Traditionally, women with a prior history of breast cancer have not been given estrogen replacement therapy. This policy is now being reexamined, especially among women with a low probability of recurrence from their breast cancer or a high probability of developing osteoporosis. In general, the net benefit from the proper use of either ERT or OCs substantially outweighs any increased risk of dying from cancer in most groups of women.

Environmental factors Studies of atomic bomb blast victims in Hiroshima and Nagasaki demonstrate a radiation dose effect in the induction of breast cancer after a latent period of about 20 years. The highest incidence was observed among women who were aged 10 to 14 at the time of the explosion, and there was almost no increase in breast cancer incidence among women who were aged 30 to 49 at the time.

Breast cancer incidence varies widely around the world, and the highest rates occur in affluent and westernized countries. The lowest incidence is among Asians, but both immigrant and second-generation Japanese women migrating to Hawaii and southern California have an increasing risk of developing breast cancer. The search for environmental factors that might explain this phenomenon has centered on diet, and especially dietary fat. There is an excellent correlation between international variation in dietary fat intake and breast cancer incidence, and rats fed high-fat diets have a greater tendency to develop mammary tumors. However, epidemiologic studies have thus far failed to reproducibly demonstrate an association between dietary fat and the development of breast cancer. Postmenopausal women who are obese have an increased risk of breast cancer. Moderate alcohol intake has been repeatedly shown to be associated with an increased risk of 40 to 60 percent, but the explanation for this is not readily apparent. While points of circumstantial evidence linking environmental factors and breast cancer risk are numerous, none is sufficiently well established to warrant strongly urging women to change their life-style in any particular way. Of course, recommendations to reduce dietary fat content and to maintain ideal body weight may be prudent because of their beneficial effects on other organ systems even if the benefits in reducing the risk of breast cancer are minimal.

BENIGN BREAST DISEASE In general, a woman's risk of subsequently developing breast cancer after a biopsy that demonstrates benign disease is increased relative to the total population of women. The most common histologic diagnosis assigned to these biopsy specimens is "fibrocystic disease," a poorly defined term that implies the presence of macroscopic, fluid-filled cysts and a nonspecific proliferation of epithelial and mesenchymal tissue. This has led many physicians to equate all lumps and irregularities detected on physical examination or mammography with "fibrocystic disease," suggesting that the women examined are at increased risk of developing breast cancer. It has not been demonstrated that women with lumpy breasts who have *not* had a biopsy have an increased risk of breast cancer, and it is estimated that most women (probably more than 80 percent) have at least some irregular tissue densities on examination and/or mammography. For these reasons, the diagnosis of "fibrocystic disease" should not be based on nonhistologic findings, and the term probably should be abandoned by pathologists as well because of its lack of specificity.

The increased risk of breast cancer among women with benign breast disease seems to be confined entirely to that group of women who have histologic evidence of ductal or lobular cell proliferation on biopsy (about 30 percent of all patients biopsied for benign conditions), and especially those who have atypical hyperplasia (about 3 percent of biopsied patients). The relative risk for developing breast cancer in this group is 4.4 times that of an age-matched population of unselected women. In women with both atypical hyperplasia and a first-degree relative with a history of breast cancer, the risk of subsequent breast cancer is increased about ninefold. Such patients are rare (representing about 1 percent of all biopsies for benign disease), and the *observed* cumulative risk of a patient in this very high risk group developing breast cancer over a 25-year period is about 40 percent; the cumulative risk of a woman in this group dying of breast cancer is less than 10 percent. There is attenuation of this risk with time, since most women who go on to develop breast cancer do so within 10 years of a diagnosis of atypical hyperplasia.

IN SITU BREAST CANCER　There are two histologically and clinically distinct variants of carcinoma in situ (CIS): ductal and lobular. Traditionally, both were considered the earliest detectable form of malignant transformation in the breast, but increasingly, lobular CIS (or lobular neoplasia) is viewed as a risk factor akin to atypical hyperplasia. Lobular CIS does not form a palpable tumor and is usually found as an incidental finding in a premenopausal woman biopsied for some other condition. Additional biopsies will usually demonstrate additional foci of lobular CIS in the same or even the contralateral breast, and any attempt to totally excise lobular CIS by any method other than mastectomy is likely to be ineffective. Patients who have no further treatment after a diagnosis of lobular CIS have an increased lifetime risk of subsequently developing an invasive breast cancer with either a ductal or a lobular histology. Without treatment, the cumulative incidence of a subsequent breast cancer of any type (invasive or ductal in situ) is about 25 percent and the cumulative mortality somewhat less than 10 percent. Most of these cancers occur after a latent period of 5 to 20 years and occur as often in the contralateral as in the biopsied breast. For this reason, most physicians now routinely offer these patients one of two treatment options: careful observation or bilateral simple mastectomies and breast reconstruction. A patient's choice between these two disparate options is likely to depend on the anxiety generated by her perception of the risk associated with observation.

Ductal CIS (or intraductal carcinoma) may form palpable tumors. It occurs with almost equal frequency in premenopausal and postmenopausal women and is more often confined to one breast, even to one quadrant of the breast. Thus it is possible to excise this type of cancer totally by more limited surgical procedures than mastectomy. Until recently, ductal CIS was uncommon, accounting for only about 1 percent of all cancers diagnosed in the United States. However, ductal CIS is often the cause of microcalcifications seen in mammograms, and because of the increased use of routine mammography it is estimated that ductal CIS constitutes more than 10 percent of all breast cancers now diagnosed in the United States. Because these changes in incidence and mode of diagnosis are recent, it is not certain that the natural history of the ductal CIS now being diagnosed is the same as that observed in earlier eras. The diagnosis of ductal CIS may be difficult. At one extreme, it may be mistaken for atypical hyperplasia, and at the other, microscopic foci of invasion may be overlooked. Electron microscopy will reveal additional areas of invasion, and this may account for the fact that axillary lymph node metastases are seen in 1 to 2 percent of patients with a diagnosis of ductal CIS.

The natural history of ductal CIS in patients treated with less than a mastectomy has been less extensively studied than that of lobular CIS. These patients, too, are at increased risk of developing a subsequent invasive cancer throughout life, but unlike lobular CIS, this risk is more often expressed in the ipsilateral than in the contralateral breast. Until recently, the standard treatment of ductal CIS was simple mastectomy without node dissection, since only 1 to 2 percent of patients so treated die of breast cancer. Now, wide excision alone or with radiotherapy is used in a substantial percentage of patients. There are seven ongoing randomized trials comparing these two treatments; none utilizes mastectomy alone in a control group, reflecting the desire of women to decide for themselves whether they will undergo a breast-sparing procedure and the increasing acceptance by physicians of lesser surgery for this condition. The first of these randomized trials has been published with 4 years of follow-up. Among women randomized to treatment with wide excision alone, 10 percent subsequently developed a noninvasive and 11 percent an invasive cancer in the ipsilateral breast. In contrast, among women randomized to receive wide excision plus radiotherapy, only 5 percent and 3 percent, respectively, developed a noninvasive or invasive cancer. It is too early to assess the relative cancer mortality associated with these therapies, but it is unlikely that they will be significantly different in light of the long-term follow-up results from similar studies of patients with invasive cancer (see below). In addition, it is too early to determine whether these results apply equally to all the histologic subtypes of ductal CIS. Some, such as the cribriform or micropapillary variants, appear to have much less potential for subsequent recurrence than the comedo type. Until further information is available, either wide excision or wide excision plus radiotherapy may be considered for women diagnosed with ductal CIS, especially for women with small tumors who are fully informed as to the uncertainty surrounding our knowledge regarding the optimal treatment of this type of cancer at this time.

Subsequent risk for invasive cancer in the contralateral breast after mastectomy　The women with the highest risk of developing breast cancer are those who have already had one breast cancer. The risk is lifelong and occurs at a rate of 0.5 to 1.0 percent per year of follow-up. Concurrent cancers in both breasts are diagnosed in about 4 percent of patients. However, the prognosis of a patient with two breast cancers, whether concurrent or sequential, is not measurably worse than that of a patient with only one breast cancer. Since the cancer with the worst clinical and pathologic stage determines the patient's overall prognosis, patients with a good prognosis after an initial diagnosis should be monitored carefully to detect a second cancer, should it occur, as early as possible.

PREVENTION　Patients who received tamoxifen in the randomized adjuvant therapy trials (see below) were observed to have a significantly decreased incidence of contralateral breast cancer compared with that in the control groups for these studies. In addition, significant decreases in death from heart disease were observed, and data from smaller studies suggest that the incidence of osteoporosis may be decreased in postmenopausal women as well. No similar benefits were seen from the use of cytotoxic therapies. On the basis of these observations, large randomized trials evaluating the potential benefits of tamoxifen in women at high risk of developing breast cancer have begun in the United States and Europe. The primary endpoint in these studies is delay or avoidance of breast cancer onset, but the endpoints of greater importance are reduction in overall mortality, mortality from breast cancer, mortality from heart disease, and fractures from osteoporosis. Since there are not even preliminary data to suggest that overall or cause-specific mortality can be reduced by using tamoxifen in otherwise healthy women, and since there are real and potential toxicities from tamoxifen (see below), it is not recommended that this drug be used for this purpose in women not enrolled in these trials.

SCREENING ASYMPTOMATIC PATIENTS

Seven independent, randomized trials have been performed to evaluate periodic screening mammography in asymptomatic women, and these studies have demonstrated unequivocally that this strategy can reduce breast cancer mortality by 20 to 30 percent, especially in women over the age of 50. Nevertheless, substantial controversies regarding the use of screening mammography persist, including its role in women under age 50, the optimal frequency for examinations, and the amount of the benefit that could be achieved with physical examination alone.

Only one of the studies conducted thus far (the HIP trial) has demonstrated a survival advantage for screening women aged 40 to 49, and the survival benefits for this age group in this study were not seen until the second decade of follow-up. This is in marked contrast to older women, for whom the benefits were apparent within the first 5 years. There are many potential explanations for this seeming difference in efficacy among the two groups. For one, it may be an artifact of study design. Most of these trials were not meant to evaluate screening independently in younger women. Breast cancer is much less common before age 50, and a study would need to be proportionately much larger to reliably detect a benefit of 20 percent in this age group. Canadian investigators have recently published the results of a study specifically designed for women aged 40 to 49. More than 50,000 women were enrolled in the trial, but even then, no survival benefits had emerged by the seventh year of follow-up.

To obtain a definitive answer to this question, the British have recently launched a trial that will eventually enroll 200,000 women under the age of 49. The breasts of younger women are more dense than those of older women, and mammography may be less sensitive in the group aged 40 to 49. This was almost certainly true in the older studies, but in more recent studies the percentage of tumors that can be detected by mammography but not by physical examination is nearly the same in younger and older women. Breast cancers in younger women may grow more rapidly than those in older women, and if so, the lead time during which the cancer can be detected by mammography but has not spread to distant organs may be much shorter in younger women. There is substantial evidence both for and against this proposition. However, if this is the case, it certainly does not make sense to recommend mammograms less frequently in younger women, as is done by many groups now. Finally, it is unlikely that all breast cancer subtypes benefit equally from mammography, and among younger women, there may be a relatively small group with an indolent form of the disease that does benefit. If so, this could explain the delayed benefit after more than 10 years of follow-up in the HIP trial.

Even if mammography results in the same proportional reduction in risk of death among younger and older women, the absolute effects will be smaller. The chance that a woman will die of breast cancer is 0.86 percent between the ages 40 and 49 and 1.23 percent between the ages 55 and 65. With yearly mammography, the chance of dying during these age intervals may be reduced to 0.63 percent and 0.93 percent respectively. Thus the cost/benefit ratio will be less favorable among younger women. These costs include not only the expenditure for mammograms but the human suffering associated with a false-positive examination.

Although the major American trials have evaluated yearly mammography, many of the successful trials in other countries have used intervals of 2 or 3 years. It is likely that most of the benefit is achieved if mammograms are repeated every 2 years, with only a marginal increase in benefit with increased frequency, particularly among older women. No one has yet demonstrated a benefit from the use of a baseline mammogram at age 35 or 40, even though many physicians employ this as a ''halfway'' measure. The American Cancer Society dropped this from their recommendations in 1992. Most of the benefit from the earliest screening trials derived from the physical examination performed at the same time as the mammogram, but another Canadian study published in 1992 suggests that even with modern mammography techniques, much of the benefit might be achieved with physical examination alone.

Recommendations regarding the women to be screened and the frequency of screening vary widely among professional groups and between countries. However, based on the available evidence, the following guidelines appear reasonable:

1 Women aged 50 and over should undergo an annual or biennial screening examination utilizing both mammography and physical examination.
2 Mammography should generally not be used in women under age 40.
3 Women between the ages of 40 and 49 may elect to undergo periodic screening examinations, but they should be informed about the controversies regarding the use of mammography in this age group.
4 It is widely assumed that the benefits of screening are proportional to the patient's risk of developing breast cancer and that patients with a family history of breast cancer, benign breast disease, or those who are nulliparous should be screened at a younger age or more frequently. These assumptions have not been prospectively or retrospectively evaluated in any study, although in many instances such a policy seems reasonable.

Although real, the risk of radiation-induced cancers is very small and is far outweighed by the benefits in women aged 50 or over and probably in those aged 40 to 49 as well. Ultrasound will not detect microcalcifications, often the only indication of tumor and especially of very small tumors. Thermography results in unacceptably high false-positive and false-negative rates and has not even been shown to be helpful in identifying patients who should undergo mammography. Cancers appearing in patients who perform regular (e.g., monthly) breast self-examination (BSE) are, on average, smaller than those in patients who do not do BSE. The only known toxicity of BSE is the increased anxiety it causes some women. However, all published BSE studies have large length and lead-time biases. These biases occur because apparent survival advantages for patients whose cancers have been found by BSE may be due to a longer clinical observation period from diagnosis to death or to the fact that slower-growing tumors are more often detected by BSE and not due to any improved efficacy of therapy, because the tumor was diagnosed before the onset of metastasis when it is theoretically more curable. It has not yet been shown in properly controlled trials that BSE will actually decrease breast cancer mortality.

DIAGNOSIS AND INITIAL EVALUATION

More than 80 percent of cancers are diagnosed because of a suspicious mass, usually a mass found by the patient. Pain without an immediately apparent mass is a less frequent presenting symptom, and increasingly, breast cancer is being diagnosed on a routine mammogram in a totally asymptomatic patient. Nipple discharge is also an unusual presenting symptom. Most nipple discharges, whether serous or sanguineous, are caused by benign disorders, most commonly an intraductal papilloma. A nipple discharge with a negative test for hemoglobin is almost always benign, but breast cancer is the cause of a hemoglobin-positive discharge in less than 10 percent of such patients.

Physical examination should begin with a visual inspection of the breast while the patient is sitting. An underlying breast cancer may cause a protrusion, asymmetry in breast contour, or a subtle dimpling of the skin due to entrapment of Cooper's ligaments. Recent onset of nipple inversion also may be a sign of breast cancer, but both nipple inversion and asymmetry of breast size are common findings in the normal breast. Palpation of the breast is best performed when the patient is in a supine position. Breast cancers are most often described as irregularly shaped, firm or hard, painless nodules or masses, but in fact they may be of almost any shape or consistency. For this reason, any mass or thickening that is distinctly different from the surrounding tissue (i.e., any ''dominant'' lesion) should be evaluated more carefully. The most common nonmalignant finding on breast examination is a diffuse, indistinct, and somewhat elastic amalgamation of lumps often mistakenly referred to as ''fibrocystic disease'' (see above). Well-defined cysts may be quite distinct like a breast cancer, but they have a more elastic character than breast cancer. Benign fibroadenomas are often as firm as breast cancer but can be distinguished by their marble-like smoothness and slippery quality, their appearance in young women, and their recurrent nature. Fat necrosis and sclerosing adenosis, both benign conditions, usually can be distinguished from breast cancer only by biopsy. If there are signs of more locally advanced growth, mastectomy and/or radiotherapy are unlikely to substantially prolong a patient's life. These signs include fixation of the mass to the skin, the pectoralis muscle, or the chest wall; the presence of satellite skin nodules or ulcerations; the finding of matted axillary nodes; or the presence of any supraclavicular lymph nodes. Plugging of the dermal lymphatics will cause skin thickening and exaggeration of the usual skin markings, a process termed *peau d'orange*. When this is extensive and accompanied by inflammation, the patient usually has inflammatory breast cancer, a particularly virulent form of cancer best treated initially with chemotherapy and radiotherapy. Inflammatory breast cancer may be mistakenly diagnosed initially as mastitis, but infections or other inflammatory conditions of the breast are rare except in the first months postpartum or after trauma.

Further evaluation of a suspected cyst might include a repeat examination of the breast immediately following the next menstrual

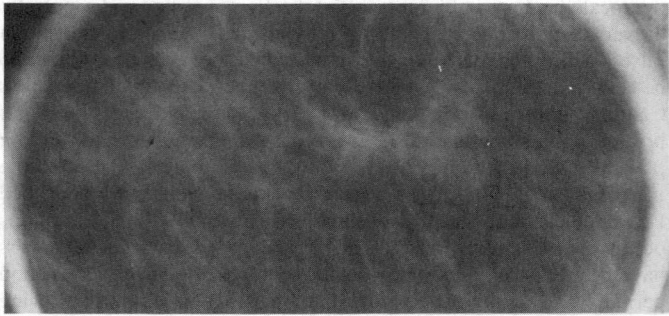

FIGURE 319-1 Focal compression mammogram shows a clinically occult 1-cm spiculated mass. Biopsy demonstrated infiltrating ductal breast cancer. *(Courtesy of Dr Paul Stomper.)*

period in a premenopausal woman, the use of ultrasound to confirm the impression that the mass is fluid-filled, or removal of the cyst fluid with a fine-gauge needle *and reexamination of the breast immediately and again some weeks later to document that the cyst has disappeared.* The latter is the preferred approach in a symptomatic patient because it will usually relieve the pain and the patient will be reassured that this is not cancer, unless the cyst fluid is grossly bloody or reaccumulates rapidly.

Mammography If breast examination leads to any suspicion that a mass is malignant, biopsy should be performed. Biopsy should be *preceded* by a mammogram, which may better define the extent of the lesion, demonstrate other suspicious masses, and serve as a baseline obtained before distortion of normal breast architecture by biopsy. Abnormalities on mammogram that suggest a breast cancer include (1) distinct, irregular, often crablike densities (Fig. 319-1), (2) *clusters* of five or more microcalcifications, each less than 1 mm in diameter and all in an area of less than 1 cm (Fig. 319-2), or (3) architectural distortion without a benign explanation such as a scar from a prior biopsy. Although more than 80 percent of suspicious microcalcifications are benign, cancers associated with such microcalcifications are usually the most curable of all breast cancers. Diagnosis can be made by radiologic placement of needles under local anesthesia

FIGURE 319-2 Mammogram shows a clinically occult 1-cm cluster of microcalcifications. Biopsy demonstrated infiltrating ductal breast cancer. *(Courtesy of Dr Paul Stomper.)*

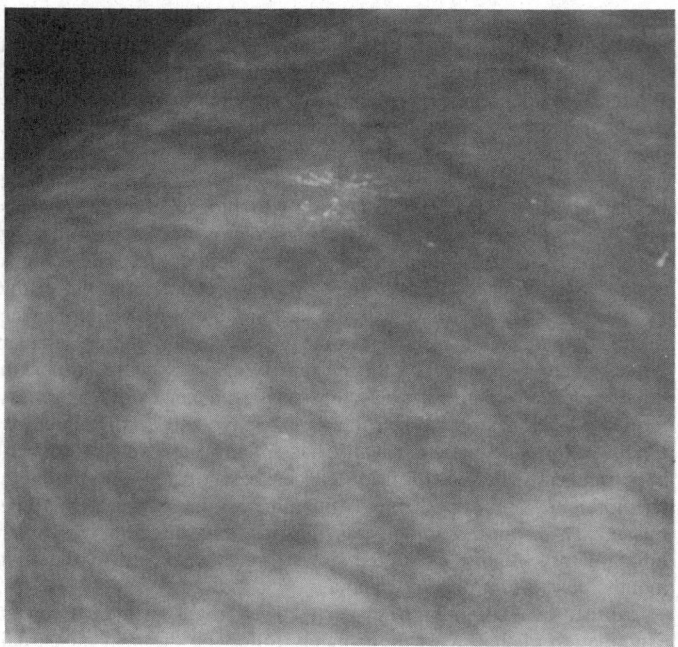

and subsequent biopsy of tissue surrounding the needle ends. The excised tissue should be x-rayed to ensure that the calcifications or other suspicious lesions have been removed, and/or the patient should have a repeat mammogram 4 to 6 weeks after biopsy when the breast is no longer tender.

In almost all instances, incisional or excisional biopsy of the breast may be performed under local anesthesia in a day surgery or an outpatient clinic, thus avoiding the additional risk of general anesthesia and permitting the patient to discuss and adjust to treatment options before undergoing definitive surgical treatment. Fine-needle aspiration and cytologic evaluation also may be diagnostic but are advisable *only* if an experienced cytologist is available and if all suspicious lesions read as negative are followed with a more definitive biopsy procedure. Tissue should be sent routinely for assay of estrogen and progesterone receptors. Additional staging procedures immediately following the diagnosis of breast cancer should include evaluation of those sites to which breast cancer most frequently metastasizes (see below).

NATURAL HISTORY AND PROGNOSTIC FACTORS

The natural history of breast cancer is characterized by long duration and marked heterogeneity. The median survival of patients who refuse all forms of treatment is between 2.5 and 3 years, but the survival of an untreated patient may exceed 20 years. Breast cancer is certainly among the more slowly growing tumors, and it has been estimated that the average tumor doubles about three times per year. If this applies to the preclinical (or prediagnostic) period of tumor growth, then the average breast cancer requires 10 years or more to grow from a single cell to 1 cm, the size at which it can be readily detected by most patients or physicians. Presumably, metastases may occur during much of this preclinical period but likely with greatest frequency during the last 3 to 4 years of preclinical growth, when the tumor mass increases from 10^6 cells to more than 10^9 cells. Microscopic or clinically undetectable micrometastases are well established by the time of diagnosis in a substantial percentage of breast cancer patients. If these patients are treated with local therapy only (i.e., surgery and/or radiotherapy), they will eventually die despite excellent local control of their disease. Because many patients' tumors metastasize late in the preclinical course, early detection with mammography will increase the survival of these patients. Because the growth rate of the disease is so variable, comparisons of treatment effects in even well-defined patient cohorts are often misleading, and large, randomized controlled trials should be used to evaluate all important treatment questions.

Clinical pathologic staging Clinical staging systems were developed by surgeons to identify *preoperatively* those patients unlikely to benefit from treatment with mastectomy. Although those with large tumor size and palpable axillary adenopathy were found to have a poorer long-term prognosis, the only patients categorically discouraged from undergoing mastectomy were those with signs of locally advanced disease (see above). About 25 to 35 percent of patients with axillary adenopathy will have no histologic evidence of tumor in lymph nodes, and the same percentage of patients without adenopathy *will* have histologic node involvement. Although information on histologic node involvement is of no value in deciding whether a patient should undergo mastectomy, this has proven to be the most accurate and reproducible prognostic factor worldwide. It is convenient to divide patients into three groups: those without node involvement, those with one to three positive nodes, or those with four or more positive nodes (Table 319-2). However, these divisions are arbitrary. A substantial number of node-negative patients will have recurrences and eventually die of breast cancer. Each additional positive node is associated with a worse prognosis, but some patients with more than 10 positive nodes will survive for 10 to 20 years or more. In general, the number of positive lymph nodes correlates with the time of recurrence as well as the probability of recurrence. For the data set

TABLE 319-2 Ten-year survival and survival without recurrence relative to histologic node status at the time of radical mastectomy (no adjuvant systemic therapy given)

Node category	Survival, % Overall	Without recurrence
All patients	60	47
Nodes negative	82	72
Nodes positive	40	25
1–3 nodes positive	54	34
4+ nodes positive	26	16

SOURCE: From Valagussa et al, CA 41:1170, 1978.

shown in Table 319-2, the median time to recurrence was 2.1 years, and the time to death was 4 years for the patients with four or more positive nodes, compared with 4.1 years and more than 10 years, respectively, for those with one to three positive nodes. The hazard of recurrence decreased in all nodal subgroups after the first 3 years but remained fairly constant thereafter. This explains why the effects of therapy on recurrence rate, especially on recurrence in patients with many positive nodes, are apparent after a short follow-up, but the effects of therapy on survival may require much longer follow-up.

Patients with a larger breast mass or a higher clinical stage are more likely to have positive nodes, but within a single-node category the size of the breast cancer has independent prognostic value. This has led to the promulgation of staging systems that combine clinical and pathologic characteristics. However, these systems have changed so frequently and are used so differently by different specialists that the categorization of patients into one of four "stages" has lost all practical meaning. For example, a 3-cm tumor mass and no histologically involved lymph nodes is considered a stage II breast cancer, as is a 1-cm mass with eight positive nodes. Both the prognosis and the likely treatment of these two patients are substantially different. Therefore, a careful description of the patient's cancer, a precise measurement of tumor size, and a simple statement of the number of histologically positive lymph nodes will provide a more accurate description of "stage" than the use of stage numbers I to IV.

Histologic subtypes More than 80 percent of breast cancers are of the invasive ductal type. The next most common variety, infiltrating lobular, constitutes almost 10 percent of all cancers and has the same prognosis as infiltrating ductal carcinoma. Medullary carcinoma, representing about 5 percent of breast cancers, is less likely to metastasize to regional lymph nodes, but the prognosis of medullary cancers with nodal metastases is the same as that of the other major histologic groups with nodal metastases. The large number of histologic types that make up the remaining 5 percent of breast cancers are generally less malignant.

Tumor grade, defined by the degree of differentiation of cytoplasmic or nuclear features, has been shown repeatedly to correlate with the probability of recurrence or death from breast cancer. Other histologic characteristics that may be important include blood vessel or intramammary lymphatic vessel invasion, mitotic frequency, lymph node sinus histiocytosis, and tumor necrosis. However, the major limitation in the use of tumor histologic features is a lack of reproducibility from one pathologist to another, especially when the pathologist has not been specifically trained and is not very experienced in the use of these grading systems. For this reason, tumor grade is not a very reliable tool for making therapeutic decisions.

Estrogen receptors Tumors with an estrogen or progesterone receptor (ER or PR) are more likely to respond to endocrine therapy used either as an adjuvant to local therapies soon after diagnosis or as a means of palliating metastatic disease symptoms later in a patient's course. Most studies have demonstrated a significantly better disease-free survival and/or overall survival during the first 10 years of follow-up for patients who have one of these receptors. However,

neither the estrogen nor the progesterone receptor identifies the 20 to 30 percent of node-negative patients likely to have recurrence, and at the end of 5 years, the difference in the recurrence rate among estrogen receptor–positive and –negative patients who are also node-negative is only about 5 percent.

Newer prognostic factors The percentage of tumor cells undergoing mitosis has been shown in a number of experimental systems to be proportional to the growth fraction (i.e., the percentage of the tumor actually growing at any one point in time) and hence to the growth rate. This growth fraction can be estimated by thymidine labeling and autoradiography to obtain a thymidine labeling index (TLI) or by flow cytometry to estimate the fraction of cells in S phase (SPF). Clinical correlations have shown that a high TLI or high SPF is associated with early relapse and earlier breast cancer death, even after correction for other prognostic factors, such as lymph node and estrogen receptor status. In general, patients with aneuploid tumors or a DNA index greater than unity will have a worse prognosis than patients with predominantly diploid tumors, but early differences in relapse rate are not large, especially among node-negative patients.

Increased levels of growth factors or receptors for growth factors also reflect increased mitotic activity, and several of these have been shown to have prognostic value. The epidermal growth factor receptor (EGFR) has been studied most extensively, and increased levels have been shown to be associated with a shorter time to relapse after initial treatment and a lower likelihood of responding to hormone therapy, even in patients whose tumors are ER-positive. Insulin-like growth factor receptor (IGF-R), somatostatin receptor (SS-R), and tumor growth factor alpha (TGFα) levels are other growth factors or growth factor receptors with prognostic value, although their value relative to other prognostic factors is not yet known.

Cathepsin D, urokinase-plasminogen activator, the products of the gene *nm23*, and adhesion molecules are all thought to be associated with invasion and/or the metastatic process. Angiogenesis is also critical to the continued growth and spread of breast cancer, and there is considerable evidence that angiogenesis factors secreted by the tumor, such as basic fibroblast growth factor (bFGF), are important in this process. Tumor levels of all theses factors have been reported to be increased in patients who relapse early or who have other poor prognostic findings, and in some centers, counts of vessels stained with factor VIII or CD31 are routinely made on newly diagnosed breast cancer.

Multiple genetic alterations have been described in breast cancers, including allelic deletions on chromosome 11 or 13 and amplification of the c-*myc* and *int*-2 genes. As described above, the tumor suppressor gene p53 is mutated in some families at high risk of developing breast cancer, but overexpression of p53 product in breast tumors has been shown to be associated with a worse prognosis as well. However, the most extensively studied is the HER-2/*neu* (or c-*erb*B-2) gene. Both amplification and overexpression of this gene on chromosome 17 are associated with a worse prognosis. This is not too suprising, however, since the HER-2/*neu* ligand and receptor are closely related to EGF and EGFR. Another possible explanation for the poor prognosis of patients with overexpression of HER-2/*neu* may be related to the observation that these patients have tumors relatively resistant to some forms of chemotherapy; ironically, they may have an increased responsiveness to others, especially regimens that include doxorubicin. These studies are the first to identify a specific factor associated with response to chemotherapy.

Before a marker is used routinely in clinical practice, the assay method(s) should be validated in more than one center, the cutoff values defining a poor or good prognostic group should be confirmed using more than one data set, the factor's value relative to other prognostic tests should be established by multivariant analyses, and the size of differences in the disease-free and overall survival of patients in poor and good prognostic categories should be determined in a prospective study with adequate sample size and appropriate patient populations. None of these newer prognostic factors, including TLI, SPF, and ploidy, fulfill all these criteria. Their inappropriate use may, in fact, result in inappropriate treatment or increased patient suffering, since a patient may erroneously conclude that her prognosis is much worse than it really is.

LOCAL THERAPY OF OPERABLE BREAST CANCER

Breast cancers are usually considered "operable" if it is technically possible to remove all cancerous tissue, if the tumor does not involve or has not become fixed to skin or structures deep to the breast, and if the tumor has not metastasized beyond the axillary or internal mammary lymph nodes. It has been demonstrated repeatedly in randomized clinical trials that more extensive surgical procedures will reduce the subsequent likelihood of tumor recurrence on the chest wall, in any remaining breast tissue, or in the nodal areas. However, these trials have failed to demonstrate that the type of surgery used will significantly affect patient survival. The evidence that local therapy has any effect on patient survival comes from the randomized trials of screening mammography (see above), in which it has been demonstrated that early mastectomy results in a lower breast cancer mortality than late mastectomy.

The most extensive surgical procedure is the *radical mastectomy,* in which the breast is removed along with the pectoralis major and minor muscles and some overlying skin (at least 4 cm on each side of the tumor biopsy site), and there is an en bloc resection of all axillary contents, including lymph nodes beyond the subclavian vein. Because of the large cosmetic defect resulting from this procedure, it is not commonly used today, and it is doubtful whether its use is ever indicated, since the same or better local control of disease can be achieved with the use of radiotherapy added to less extensive surgical procedures. Most forms of the modified radical mastectomy leave the pectoralis major muscle intact, require the removal of less skin, and usually involve a less extensive node dissection. A *simple* or *total mastectomy* is the removal of the breast and a small amount of skin. A simple mastectomy with node dissection approximates a modified radical mastectomy. Breast-conserving surgical procedures include wide excision, lumpectomy or tylectomy (Greek *tylos* = "lump"), segmental mastectomy, and quadrantectomy. These all require removal of the mass along with some normal surrounding tissue and differ only in the extent of the tissue excised. A separate incision of either a "sampling" of lymph nodes or a more complete lymph node dissection is possible with all of these procedures.

Radiotherapy   When administered after a mastectomy, radiotherapy is usually referred to as *adjuvant,* while radiotherapy given after breast-conserving surgery is often called *primary.* Adjuvant radiotherapy is used less commonly now than it once was because it was not possible to demonstrate in multiple randomized trials that its use prolonged survival. In addition, a small but statistically significant increase in mortality from second tumors and/or cardiovascular disease has been reported in patients who survived more than 10 to 15 years after receiving adjuvant radiotherapy. However, this finding was observed primarily in patients treated with now-outdated radiotherapy techniques.

When breast-conserving therapy is used, the resection margins ideally should be microscopically free of tumor before radiotherapy is given. Usually 4500 to 5000 cGy is administered in divided fractions over about 5 weeks. The same doses of radiotherapy may be administered to the axillary, supraclavicular, and internal mammary nodes, and a boost of 1600 to 1800 cGy may be added to the tumor bed. The treatment of axillary nodal areas and the use of a boost are variable and depend on the tumor characteristics of an individual patient and the treatment philosophy of the radiotherapist. When all areas are treated, primary radiotherapy is as extensive as the radical mastectomy, and local tumor control is as good or better.

The choice between breast-conserving surgery plus radiotherapy and mastectomy will depend on the patient's assessment of the relative benefits and side effects associated with each procedure. The only real advantage of breast-conserving procedures is the greater sense of body integrity and improved cosmesis that may result. This advantage may be lost if the tumor mass is large relative to the size of the breast, thus necessitating almost total removal of the breast to obtain tumor-free margins. Under the best of circumstances, the cosmetic results of limited surgery plus radiotherapy are excellent, and the treated breast may feel entirely normal and appear indistinguishable from the contralateral breast. More often the treated breast will be somewhat smaller with limited induration around the biopsy site; uncommonly (in less than 5 percent of patients) there will be marked induration, breast shrinkage, and distortion of normal breast architecture. Other complications from radiotherapy, including broken bones, brachial plexopathy, and pneumonitis, are uncommon and rarely either cause symptoms or are the source of more than transient symptomatology. There may be a subgroup of patients who have a relatively high recurrence rate (23 percent by the end of 5 years) if treated with breast-conserving surgery and radiotherapy. The histologic appearance of the tumors in these patients is characterized by extensive intraductal carcinoma in *both* the area of invasive carcinoma and adjacent tissues ostensibly free of invasive carcinoma. Although a small intraductal component in an invasive carcinoma is normal, the intraductal component comprises more than 25 percent of all tumor tissue in these patients and appears to be a marker of a tumor likely to be multifocal throughout the breast. Very limited data suggest that patients who have recurrences some years after initial surgery and radiotherapy with tumor confined entirely to the breast or breast and regional lymph nodes may be treated successfully with a secondary mastectomy and that this type of recurrence may not compromise survival.

Breast-conserving surgery *without* radiotherapy is generally not used because of the very high likelihood of local recurrence. In the only randomized trial addressing this issue, patients with tumor-free resection margins who were treated with segmental mastectomy alone had a local recurrence rate of 43 percent by the end of 9 years, compared with 12 percent for patients treated with segmental mastectomy plus radiotherapy. However, the survival of patients in these two groups is not significantly different.

Breast reconstruction   Many patients will prefer mastectomy because it requires a shorter period of initial treatment and provides the patient with an added assurance that "all the tumor has been removed." Psychological studies demonstrate that most mastectomy patients have fully recovered from the initial emotional trauma of mastectomy by the end of 1 year. Many patients feel that their lives are simplified and their sense of body integrity restored by surgical reconstruction of the breast. This may be performed at the time of mastectomy or many years later. The procedures used include simple placement of a submuscular (or less commonly, subcutaneous) saline-filled or silicone implant, the use of a tissue expander followed by saline-filled or silicone implant, the transposition of muscle and blood supply from either the back of the abdomen using the latissimus dorsi or the lower rectus abdominis muscle (TRAM flap), or the creation of a free tissue flap using the gluteus maximus muscle anastomosed to the internal mammary vessels. The choice among these procedures will depend on the extent of the patient's prior surgery and radiotherapy, the patient's willingness to undergo additional surgical procedures, and the experience and philosophy of the plastic surgeon. Under the best of circumstances, the reconstructed breast will appear to be exactly the same size and shape as the contralateral breast, but in addition to reconstruction of a nipple, this may require mammoplasty on the contralateral breast and several surgical procedures. There are anecdotal reports of collagen-vascular disease, second cancers, or failure to diagnose a cancer by mammography in an augmented breast, and because of this, the Food and Drug Administration has restricted the use of silicone implants for augmentation mammoplasty but not for reconstruction after a cancer operation. Case-control studies of breast cancer patients with silicone implants have failed to show an increased incidence of second cancers, and it is likely that such a risk, if real, is extremely small.

Node dissection The main purpose of lymph node dissection is diagnostic, not therapeutic (see above). However, the morbidity associated with the treatment of lymph nodes is greater than with any other aspect of local therapy. Even with a limited node sampling, the patient often will complain of lifelong discomfort, hyperesthesia or hypalgesia, and/or a sense of pulling and contraction. When more extensive surgery is used, when the radiotherapy field includes the upper axilla, and especially when both modalities are used, these symptoms increase in frequency and severity. Patients may experience edema of the arm and hand, and on rare occasions the patient may totally lose use of the involved extremity. For this reason, a full node dissection, as employed in the radical mastectomy, followed by radiotherapy, is usually contraindicated, and whenever possible, surgical excision should be limited to lower nodes and radiotherapy to this area avoided altogether.

Summary recommendations for local therapy All patients with invasive operable breast cancer should receive some form of local therapy. In most cases this will be either a modified radical mastectomy (simple mastectomy plus node dissection) or breast-conserving surgery and limited node dissection followed by radiotherapy to the breast. Ideally, the patient will participate in the choice between these treatment alternatives and will see both a surgeon and a radiotherapist in the process of self-education regarding the benefits and limitations of these approaches.

ADJUVANT SYSTEMIC THERAPY

Patients die from breast cancer because of metastases that could not be detected by currently available tests but that occurred months to years prior to the diagnosis and treatment of the local disease. There is no evidence that patients who die of breast cancer live any longer as a result of the local therapy. The patient is either cured or dies at about the same time she would have died without mastectomy or radiotherapy. For this reason, it makes sense that systemic therapies capable of reducing the size of these distant metastatic deposits may prolong the patient's survival. Further, some survival advantage may accrue to the patient even if she is not cured.

This hypothesis has been proven by multiple randomized trials in which thousands of women with operable breast cancer received either local treatment alone or local treatment followed by some form of systemic therapy. These systemic therapies, usually given immediately after or as an "adjuvant" to local treatment, include chemotherapy, tamoxifen, and ovarian ablation. Several meta-analyses or overviews of these trial results have been performed, providing a very accurate estimate of the benefits that might be expected from the use of these therapies in routine clinical practice. Most of the statistics that follow are taken from the overview published in 1992.

Among women aged 50 and older, 90 percent of whom were postmenopausal, the reduction in the odds of recurrence and death as a result of adjuvant tamoxifen use was 20 ± 2 percent and 19 ± 3 percent, respectively, during the first 10 years of follow-up. The benefits of tamoxifen were larger when the analysis was limited to those studies which used at least 2 years of tamoxifen. In an analysis of the chemotherapy trials using the most effective chemotherapy regimens (see below), the reduction in the odds of recurrence and death was 22 ± 3 percent and 14 ± 5 percent, respectively.

Among women less than age 50, most of whom were premenopausal, chemotherapy reduced the odds of recurrence and death by 37 ± 5 percent and 27 ± 6 percent, respectively. Adjuvant ovarian ablation reduced the odds of recurrence by 30 ± 9 percent and of death by 28 ± 9 percent. Among these younger women, adjuvant tamoxifen appeared to be less effective than either of these, with odds reductions of 27 ± 7 percent and 17 ± 10 percent, respectively.

Indirect comparison of these trial results suggests that tamoxifen is more effective than chemotherapy among older women without ovarian function. Chemotherapy suppresses ovarian function in premenopausal women, often inducing a permanent menopause. Taken together, these observations suggest that much of the benefit from adjuvant chemotherapy might be mediated through its effect on the ovary, and it would be reasonable to consider ovarian ablation as an alternative to adjuvant chemotherapy. However, a more appropriate response to these observations would be to perform a randomized trial or direct comparison of these two forms of adjuvant treatment, especially since only about 800 women were included in the ovarian ablation trials, all of which were conducted two to four decades ago. If either chemotherapy or ovarian ablation were 20 to 30 percent better than the other, it would not be possible to detect this difference using the available information.

Using trial results to make decisions about individual patients The effects of treatment may be expressed as either a proportional reduction in the odds of recurrence or death or an absolute difference in the survival of patients randomized to one or the other therapy at a single point in time. In general, the proportional effects will be constant among patients in different risk categories, while the absolute benefits of therapy will be greatest among patients with the highest risk. To better understand this, consider, for example, a trial in which 200 patients are randomized, 100 to each treatment arm of a study. At the end of 5 years of follow-up, 40 patients have died in arm A and 30 patients in arm B. The absolute difference in survival at the end of 5 years is 10 percent (70 percent in arm B minus 60 percent in arm A), but the proportional reduction in mortality is 25 percent (40 deaths expected in arm B if the therapy had no effect minus the 30 deaths actually observed divided by 40). In a second trial with 200 patients, 8 patients have died in arm A and 6 patients in arm B at the end of 5 years. In this case, the absolute difference in survival will be only 2 percent, but the proportional reduction in the odds of death will still be 25 percent.

This example correlates well with the actual results of the adjuvant therapy trials. A 25 percent reduction in the annual odds of death results in an absolute difference in survival of 10 percent at 10 years in patients with histologically positive lymph nodes. This size benefit might be expected from the use of adjuvant chemotherapy or ovarian ablation in premenopausal women or adjuvant tamoxifen in postmenopausal women. However, a 25 percent reduction in the annual odds of death from treating a patient with negative axillary lymph nodes would result in an absolute survival difference of only 6 percent if the patient were in a high-risk node-negative category (i.e., with an untreated risk of dying within 10 years of 24 percent) and 2 percent if the patient had a relatively good prognosis, node-negative breast cancer (i.e., with an untreated risk of dying of 8 percent). A less effective therapy that caused only a 12.5 percent reduction in the annual odds of death would result in a survival difference of only 5 percent at the end of 10 years. This might describe the effect of adjuvant chemotherapy in postmenopausal women.

Despite the large number of prognostic factors studied, it is not possible to identify any patient or group of patients with invasive breast cancer who will definitely not die of breast cancer. The converse is also true: Some patients will beat the odds and will survive many decades to die of causes other than breast cancer despite very bad prognostic features. For this reason, it is impossible to pick out a group of patients for whom adjuvant therapy holds no promise of benefit. Good clinical judgment in the use of adjuvant therapy requires the recognition (1) that the benefits from any therapy vary with the menopausal status of the patient, (2) that some therapies, such as chemotherapy, have substantial acute toxicity, (3) that the vast majority of patients in the good prognostic categories will derive no benefit at all because they have been cured with local therapy alone, and (4) that absolute differences in survival will be relatively small when averaged over all treated patients in the good prognostic groups.

A survival difference of 10 percent between treated and untreated patients does not mean that 10 percent of the patients have been cured and that 90 percent derived no benefit at all. Exactly the same difference might be achieved if every patient had a transient but variable prolongation of life from treatment. For example, one patient

TABLE 319-3 Dose schedules of the drug regimens and endocrine therapies most frequently used to treat early and advanced breast cancer

Drug	Dose schedule
CMF(P) (28-day cycle)	
Cyclophosphamide	100 mg/m^2 PO days 1–14
Methotrexate	60 mg/m^2 IV days 1 and 8
5-Fluorouracil	600 mg/m^2 IV days 1 and 8
Prednisone (optional)	40 mg/m^2 PO days 1–14
CAF (21-day cycle)	
Cyclophosphamide	400–500 mg/m^2 IV day 1
Doxorubicin	40–50 mg/m^2 IV day 1
5-Fluorouracil	400–500 mg/m^2 IV days 1 and 8
Tamoxifen	10 mg PO bid
Megestrol acetate	40 mg PO qid
Aminoglutethimide	250 mg PO bid
+ hydrocortisone	10 mg PO qid

might have lived 3 years from diagnosis without treatment and 4 years if treated with adjuvant systemic therapy, while another would have lived 8 years without and 11 years with treatment. Of course, it is also possible that adjuvant therapy will cure a small minority of patients and prolong the life of most of the rest. If there were a widely acceptable method for estimating the average prolongation of survival, this would be a preferable way of expressing the benefits of adjuvant treatment not only because it would better reflect the true nature of the benefit but also because the patient could then weigh the months of life to be gained against the time spent experiencing the toxicities of treatment. Possibly the closest estimate of the average prolongation of survival from treatment might be obtained by subtracting the median survival of patients randomized to the control arms of the trials included in the overview analysis from that of patients randomized to receive adjuvant therapy. For node-positive patients treated with a therapy that reduces the annual odds of death by 25 percent, this difference in medians is about 2 years. However, there is no method for even approximating the range of survival benefits around this number, and a patient also should know that her benefit could be much shorter than this or as long as several decades.

The selection of an adjuvant therapy regimen (See also Table 319-3) Combinations of drugs, such as the combination of cyclophosphamide, methotrexate, and 5-fluorouracil (CMF), are somewhat more effective than single agents, such as melphalan. While 6 months of chemotherapy is better than 1 month, durations of therapy in the range of 4 to 6 months have been shown to be as effective as more prolonged durations, such as 12 to 24 months. It has now been demonstrated in a large randomized trial that patients given full doses of chemotherapy have a significantly better survival than those treated with much lower doses. Regimens that include doxorubicin (see Table 319-3) or those given at higher doses (so that autologous bone marrow, peripheral blood stem cells, or cytokines such as G-CSF or GM-CSF are required) have not yet been shown to be more effective than CMF, even in patients with many positive lymph nodes. Adjuvant systemic therapy is usually initiated as soon as possible after the completion of local therapy, and it has been argued, largely on theoretical grounds and from uncontrolled clinical observations, that adjuvant chemotherapy should be given before definitive surgery ("neoadjuvant," "protoadjuvant," or "primary chemotherapy"). However, in a large, randomized study, chemotherapy begun 1 month after surgery was as effective as chemotherapy begun within 36 h.

Although there are theoretical reasons why longer durations of tamoxifen therapy may be more effective, there are no published data from randomized trials evaluating different durations of tamoxifen therapy. Among women aged 50 and over, the tamoxifen trials in which the drug was administered for 2 years resulted in a larger benefit than those utilizing 1 year, but no greater benefit was achieved in the trials that used more than 2 years of tamoxifen. The studies among younger women are more difficult to interpret because many

fewer women in the younger age groups were entered into those trials and most trials in younger women evaluated the effect of tamoxifen plus chemotherapy rather than the effect of tamoxifen alone. However, the available evidence suggests that much longer periods (e.g., 5 years) may be needed to demonstrate as much benefit from adjuvant tamoxifen in premenopausal women as can be achieved with 2 years of tamoxifen in postmenopausal women. Randomized trials evaluating different durations of tamoxifen therapy are ongoing. Adjuvant tamoxifen imparts a greater survival benefit to women with estrogen receptor–positive than estrogen receptor–negative tumors, but there is a small benefit in the latter group as well. In fact, the benefits from adjuvant tamoxifen in postmenopausal women with estrogen receptor–negative tumors appear to be as large as the effects of chemotherapy in this age group.

There is probably a small benefit from adding chemotherapy to tamoxifen when treating postmenopausal women and from adding tamoxifen or ovarian ablation to chemotherapy when treating premenopausal women. However, the size of these added benefits may be too small to justify the additional toxicity and cost from using chemohormonal combinations. These questions are also being evaluated in ongoing randomized trials.

Summary recommendations for adjuvant systemic therapy Premenopausal, node-positive patients should routinely receive some form of adjuvant therapy after completion of local therapy. If a formal trial is unacceptable to the patient, 6 months of therapy with CMF or 4 months of therapy with cycloplosphamide and doxorubicin (CA) or CA plus 5-fluorouracil (CAF) might be considered standard. Postmenopausal, node-positive, receptor-positive patients should routinely receive tamoxifen for 2 to 5 years. There is at present no established role for adjuvant systemic therapy in patients with in situ breast cancer or those with very small, node-negative tumors, especially those that are impalpable (e.g., found only by mammography or diagnosed with needle localization) or those that are minimally invasive. The treatment of other groups of patients should be undertaken only after full consideration of the size of the benefits and the nature of the toxicity.

TREATMENT OF DISTANT METASTASES

Breast cancer can and frequently does metastasize to almost every organ in the body but most commonly to skin, lymph nodes, lungs, liver, and bones. More than 10 percent of patients with any metastases will have central nervous system metastases at some point in the course of the disease, and new onset of frequent headaches, personality change, otherwise unexplained vomiting, or localized neurologic dysfunction should lead to a prompt evaluation that includes a head CT scan (or MRI) and cytocentrifuge examination of cerebrospinal fluid. Isolated metastases to the leptomeninges are not uncommon, and visual disturbances may be due to breast cancer metastatic to the choroid. Choroid metastases usually can be seen on funduscopic examination. Breast cancer not infrequently metastasizes to the ovary and adrenal gland, and metastases to the abdomen may mimic ovarian cancer with diffuse peritoneal studding and the development of ascites. Metastases to the skin may occur anywhere and commonly appear on the scalp. A standard evaluation for metastases might include a complete blood count, platelet count, liver function studies, chest x-ray, bone scan, and marker study such as the carcinoembryonic antigen (CEA) and CA15-3 in addition to the investigation of specific signs and symptoms.

CHOOSING AMONG THERAPIES Breast cancer recurrences, even recurrences in the skin or the chest wall or along the mastectomy scar, represent bloodborne metastases and are *never* truly isolated recurrences. Other organs will eventually manifest disease, and the time interval from the first recurrence to the second will be roughly *proportional* to the interval from primary diagnosis to the appearance of the first metastasis, usually referred to as the *disease-free interval* (DFI). Although the treatment of metastases will prolong median survival by some months and may have a profound effect on the survival of a few patients, the major value of treatment for metastatic disease is palliation of symptoms. Surgery and radiotherapy are more certain to shrink disease and palliate symptoms in a given area than systemic therapies. Systemic therapies are more likely to achieve long-term control of the disease throughout the body. Metastases to the brain and the choroid of the eye are almost always treated with radiotherapy. A local recurrence to the chest wall without evidence of distant disease might reasonably be treated with radiotherapy if the DFI is long. Malignant pleural effusions are best treated with complete chest tube drainage followed by sclerosis because the effusion may not clear even in a patient whose disease is otherwise responding to chemotherapy or endocrine therapy. The pain from bone metastases may be relieved by either systemic therapy or radiotherapy, but in a patient with multiple lesions or a short DFI, an initial course of systemic therapy is preferred, since all lesions will be affected by the systemic therapy. If the bone cortex is severely eroded, a surgical approach with placement of stabilizing rods may be preferred, since there is a long period of decreased tensile strength in a bone even after a response to radiotherapy or systemic therapy.

The median survival of all patients with metastatic breast cancer exceeds 2.5 years, and most patients will reach several, and some patients more than a dozen, decision points when treatment should or could be offered. Patients given extensive radiotherapy to bone metastases may not tolerate chemotherapy because of the effect of the radiotherapy on the bone marrow. Patients given chemotherapy may not benefit from endocrine therapy administered secondarily. There is no evidence that the treatment of asymptomatic metastases significantly prolongs survival, and a physician or patient may decide to hold therapy for some period of time both to avoid the toxicity of therapy and to better assess the pace of the disease. An asymptomatic but anxious patient who wishes to "do something" might explore the use of new or more experimental therapies first and hold therapies with known efficacy in reserve.

Endocrine therapy versus chemotherapy The patient most likely to respond to endocrine therapy is one with an estrogen and/or progesterone receptor, a long DFI, disease limited to soft tissues (e.g., lymph nodes, breast, skin) or bone as opposed to viscera, and a prior documented response to endocrine therapy. The ideal patient for chemotherapy is anyone who is symptomatic and who is deemed a poor candidate for endocrine therapy. Although only one-third of unselected patients respond to endocrine therapy, two-thirds of patients with positive receptors and/or others of the characteristics listed above will respond to endocrine therapy. About two-thirds of all patients respond to chemotherapy. There is no evidence that a response to chemotherapy will occur more rapidly. The median duration of response to endocrine therapy, about 12 to 13 months, is somewhat longer than that to chemotherapy, about 9 to 12 months, but this likely reflects differences in the responding patient populations rather than in the efficacy of the therapy. Patients on either therapy may, on occasion, continue to respond for more than a decade. The choice between these two modalities will depend on the relative probability of benefit for an individual patient based on that patient's clinical characteristics.

ENDOCRINE THERAPY Patients who respond to one endocrine therapy frequently respond to a second, often to a third, and on occasion even to a fourth or fifth sequential endocrine manipulation. Patients who fail to respond at all to one form of endocrine therapy are not likely to benefit from a different endocrine therapy. There is little difference in the efficacy of various forms of endocrine therapy, and for this reason, the least toxic therapy is usually used first. For postmenopausal women, this is tamoxifen (see Table 319-3); for premenopausal women, it might be either tamoxifen or ovarian ablation by surgery or radiation. (Studies to determine if leutenizing hormone–releasing hormone agonists are as effective as ovarian ablation are under way.) After response and progression of disease, a postmenopausal woman might be treated with either a progestin,

such as megestrol acetate or medroxyprogesterone acetate, or aminoglutethimide plus hydrocortisone (see Table 319-3).

Side effects of endocrine therapy More than 90 percent of patients treated with tamoxifen have no acute side effects at all. Others experience mild nausea that subsides after several weeks to a month, a flare reaction, menstrual disturbances if premenopausal, or hot flashes. There is an increased frequency of thrombophlebitis and thromboembolic phenomena, and about 30 percent of women on tamoxifen experience vaginal dryness. Like estrogen replacement therapy, tamoxifen treatment is associated with an increased incidence of uterine cancer. The risk appears to increase with the duration of treatment. Tamoxifen has been reported to induce hepatocellular cancer in rats, and two cases have been reported from the million-plus-patient-years of follow-up now available from patients treated with tamoxifen. Thus this seems to be a very rare event, possibly on the order of that seen from the use of oral contraceptives. Preliminary evidence suggests that tamoxifen may decrease heart disease and osteoporosis while increasing the incidence of uterine cancer. Patients usually find weight gain due to increased appetite and fluid retention the most disturbing side effect of progestin therapies.

More than 10 percent of patients with metastatic breast cancer will experience hypercalcemia at some point in the course of their disease. Often this occurs soon after the initiation of endocrine therapy as part of a "flare." In addtion to hypercalcemia, this syndrome is characterized by a sudden increase in bone pain and erythema around skin lesions, an increase in the number and intensity of lesions on bone scan, and an elevation of serum markers such as CEA and CA15-3. These signs and symptoms appear within hours to a few weeks after beginning endocrine therapy and subside by the end of a month. Unless hypercalcemia is life-threatening [calcium $\geq$ 3.5 mmol/L (14 mg/dL)], endocrine therapy should be continued and the underlying symptoms treated with pain medications, fluids, diuretics, and standard regimens for hypercalcemia (see Chap. 357).

CHEMOTHERAPY Although breast cancer responds to a long list of cytotoxic agents, three, and possibly four, appear to be especially effective and non-cross-resistant with each other: cyclophosphamide (C), doxorubicin (A), mitomycin C, and vinblastine. Phase II studies of a new drug, taxol, are also very promising, but the appropriate role for this drug, if any, has not been established. Combinations of these drugs with each other and/or with methotrexate (M) and 5-fluorouracil (F) induce higher response rates and marginally improved survival compared with serial treatment with single agents. The most popular combinations are CMF, CMF plus prednisone, and CAF (see Table 319-3). There is no evidence that survival is substantially improved by prolonged administration of these drugs, but the results of one randomized trial suggest that both response rate and quality of life are improved by some duration in excess of 3 months. A reduction of drug doses below those shown in Table 319-3 is likely to be associated with a lower response rate, but there is as yet no evidence of substantial benefit from exceeding these doses either. The use of very high dose therapy with autologous bone marrow support, peripheral blood stem cells, or cytokines such as G- or GM-CSF has not yet been proven to be beneficial in prolonging survival or improving quality of life.

Side effects of chemotherapy Although the acute side effects of chemotherapy often seem formidable, it has been repeatedly demonstrated in randomized trials that the efficacy of a regimen is a more important determinant of net quality of life than the side effects of treatment for patients with symptomatic, metastatic breast cancer. All these drugs cause dose-related myelosuppression, thrombocytopenia, and, over some months, anemia. Gastrointestinal toxicity may include everything from mild nausea to protracted vomiting, severe mucositis, and diarrhea. Both myelosuppression and gastrointestinal toxicity are mitigated by the addition of prednisone to the regimen. Alopecia may be mild and gradual in onset with the use of CMF or abrupt and total with doxorubicin combinations. Doxorubicin cardiomyopathy occurs with increasing frequency after cumulative doses in excess of 450 mg/m^2 body area have been given. All these agents, and especially the alkylating agents such as cyclophosphamide, are potential carcinogens. CMF and, to a much greater extent, melphalan have been shown to increase the incidence of leukemia and other blood dyscrasias when these drugs are used as adjuvant therapy, but the benefits far outweigh this risk in women with positive lymph nodes or other high-risk features. It is still too early to assess the danger of inducing solid tumors with these drugs, since they usually occur only after a long latent period.

SPECIAL PROBLEMS

Male breast cancer occurs with less than 1 percent of the frequency of female breast cancer. Predisposing risk factors include states of hyperestrogenism, such as Klinefelter's syndrome, schistosomiasis, a family history of breast cancer, and radiation exposure. Gynecomastia, in itself, is not an established risk factor (see Chap. 341). In other respects, male breast cancer is nearly identical to female breast cancer, with a similar prognosis, stage per stage. The primary lesion is usually treated with mastectomy, since most men are not concerned with saving the breast. There are no data from controlled trials regarding the use of adjuvant systemic therapy for men, but the treatment of metastatic disease is nearly identical.

Cystosarcoma phylloides is a rare tumor more closely related to either benign fibroadenoma, from which it apparently arises in most cases, or sarcoma. It metastasizes in less than 5 percent of cases, but the local recurrence rate may exceed 20 percent, especially if it is treated inadequately. Treatment of the benign variety of cystosarcoma phylloides consists of wide excision; for the malignant variety, wide excision or simple mastectomy. Node dissection is rarely indicated.

Paget's disease of the nipple is often mistaken initially for a simple eczema and treated with glucocorticoids. However, a crusting, eroding, or scaling nipple lesion that does not respond promptly to conservative therapy should be biopsied. Histologically, Paget's disease is characterized by noninvasive or minimally invasive tumor cells growing on the undersurface of the nipple. In some cases there will be no other tumor in the breast, and some physicians now treat apparently localized disease with wide excision. However, in over half the cases a mass will be found deep within the breast, in which case the prognosis and treatment of Paget's disease will depend on the size of the mass and the presence of involvement. The majority of the patients with Paget's disease will be treated like any other breast cancer patient.

Breast cancer is particularly difficult to diagnose and treat when it occurs *during pregnancy,* but stage per stage the prognosis approximates that of patients diagnosed in a nonpregnant state. There is no evidence that therapeutic abortion improves the prognosis. Mastectomy can be performed in the second and third trimesters, and chemotherapy has been given in the third trimester without observed damage to the fetus. *Pregnancy 2 years or more after diagnosis of breast cancer* is not associated with a higher recurrence rate or shortened survival, and counseling women regarding the advisability of pregnancy depends more on the patient's feelings regarding the possibility of not being able to see her child reach adulthood than about any potential risk to the patient from the pregnancy.

REFERENCES

General, natural history, prognostic factors, epidemiology

HARRIS JR et al: Breast cancer. N Engl J Med 327:319, 1992

HENDERSON IC: What can a woman do about her risk of dying of breast cancer? Curr Probl Cancer 14:165, 1990

——— et al: Breast Cancer, in *Cancer: Principles and Practice of Oncology*, VT De Vita Jr et al (eds). Philadelphia, Lippincott, 1989, pp 1197–1268

McGUIRE WL, CLARK GM: Prognostic factors and treatment decisions in axillary node-negative breast cancer. N Engl J Med 326:1756, 1992

Familial incidence

GARBER JE: Familial aspects of breast cancer, in *Breast Diseases*, 2d ed, JR Harris et al (eds). Philadelphia, Lippincott, 1991, p 142

Endocrine factors

DUPONT WD, PAGE DL: Menopausal estrogen replacement therapy and breast cancer. Arch Intern Med 151:67, 1991

ROMIEU I et al: Oral contraceptives and breast cancer. Review and meta-analysis. Cancer 66:2253, 1990

STEINBERG KK et al: A meta-analysis of the effect of estrogen replacement therapy on the risk of breast cancer. JAMA 265:1985, 1991

Benign breast disease, in situ carcinoma

DUPONT WD, PAGE DL: Risk factors for breast cancer in women with proliferative breast disease. N Engl J Med 312:146, 1985

FISHER B et al: Lumpectomy compared with lumpectomy and radiation therapy for the treatment of intraductal breast cancer. N Engl J Med 328:1581, 1993

SCHNITT SJ et al: Ductal carcinoma in situ (intraductal carcinoma) of the breast. N Engl J Med 318:898, 1988

Screening

CHU KC et al: Analysis of breast cancer mortality and stage distribution by age for the Health Insurance Plan clinical trial. J Natl Cancer Inst 80:1125, 1988

EDDY DM: Screening for breast cancer. Ann Intern Med 111:389, 1989

——— et al: The value of mammography screening in women under age 50 years. JAMA 259:1512, 1988

MILLER AB et al: Canadian national breast screening study: I. Breast cancer detection and death rates among women aged 40–49 years. Can Med Assoc J 147:1459, 1992

Biology

LIPPMAN ME, DICKSON RB: Mechanisms of growth control in normal and malignant breast epithelium. Rec Prog Hormone Res 45:383, 1989

Local therapy

FISHER B et al: Eight-year results of a randomized clinical trial comparing total mastectomy and lumpectomy with or without irradiation in the treatment of breast cancer. N Engl J Med 320:822, 1989

——— et al: Significance of ipsilateral breast tumor recurrence after lumpectomy. Lancet 338:327, 1991

——— et al: Lumpectomy compared with lumpectomy and radiation therapy for the treatment of intraductal breast cancer. N Eng J Med 328:1581, 1993

Adjuvant therapy

EARLY BREAST CANCER TRIALISTS' COLLABORATIVE GROUP: Systemic treatment of early breast cancer by hormonal, cytotoxic, or immune therapy: 151 randomized trials involving 32,000 recurrences and 25,000 deaths among 77,000 women. Lancet 339:1, 1992

———: *Treatment of Early Breast Cancer.* vol 1: *Worldwide Evidence 1985–1990. A Systematic Overview of All Available Randomized Trials in Early Breast Cancer of Adjuvant Endocrine and Cytotoxic Therapy.* Oxford, Oxford University press, 1990, p 207

Systemic therapy

HENDERSON IC: Endocrine therapy of metastatic breast cancer, in *Breast Diseases*, 2d ed, JR Harris et al (eds). Philadelphia, Lippincott, 1991, p 559

———: Chemotherapy for metastatic disease, in *Breast Diseases*, 2d ed, JR Harris et al (eds). Philadelphia, Lippincott, 1991, p 604

———: Window of opportunity. J Natl Cancer Inst 83:894, 1991

———, HARRIS JR: Principles in the management of metastatic disease: Intergration of local and systemic therapies, in *Breast Diseases*, 2d ed, JR Harris et al (eds). Philadelphia, Lippincott, 1991, p 547

320   MALIGNANT TUMORS OF THE HEAD AND NECK

ROBERT S. LEBOVICS

Primary malignant tumors of the head and neck arise from the multitude of tissues comprising the nasal cavity, paranasal sinuses, pharynx, larynx, salivary glands, and thyroid. Embryologic development and a complex regional anatomy contribute to the various clinical presentations of these malignancies. Tumor size, nodal status, and the presence of metastases define a tumor's classification as well as the stage of disease.

The American Joint Committee on Cancer (AJCC) has developed a standard tumor, node, and metastasis (TNM) staging system. Each anatomic site in the head and neck has its own unique clinical T-stage classification. The head and neck surgeon, for example, will be adept in the subtleties of staging laryngeal cancer involving the supraglottic larynx versus the glottic larynx. Tumors of the salivary glands are staged differently from epithelial tumors of the oropharynx. The AJCC, however, also has developed a uniform staging system for the characterization of regional lymph node (N-stage) disease in the neck (see Table 320-1).

Before definitive therapy, tumors are staged surgically, and malignancy is confirmed pathologically. Adjunctive modalities, such as computed tomography (CT) and magnetic resonance imaging (MRI), do not directly affect what is still a clinical staging system. In practice, however, treatment planning requires the incorporation of data obtained by adjunctive testing. In many institutions, cases of head and neck tumor are routinely presented to a multidisciplinary board of health professionals, including a head and neck surgeon, a radiation oncologist, a medical oncologist, a speech pathologist, and a nutritionist, as well as a diagnostic radiologist and pathologist. A frank exchange of ideas and information among these specialists will result in optimal therapy and allow each cause to be treated as unique.

NOSE AND PARANASAL SINUSES   The nose and the paranasal sinuses consist of a bony framework primarily lined with respiratory epithelium. Malignancies usually arise in either the maxillary or the ethmoid sinuses within this epithelium. Previous exposure to industrial wood products, nickel, and Thorotrast is associated with an increased incidence of malignant sinus tumors. Tumors of either the sphenoid sinus or the frontal sinus are extremely rare.

Symptoms of tumors of the maxillary sinus include facial and dental pain, localized swelling, and epistaxis. Tumors of the ethmoid sinuses may be accompanied by nasal obstruction, epistaxis, and orbital complications (proptosis and epiphora). Noninvasive tests such as CT and MRI may help to image adjacent structures—specifically, the orbit and optic nerves, prevertebral fascia, pterygopalatine fossa, cavernous sinuses, and central nervous system (CNS).

Squamous cell carcinoma is the most common tumor of the sinuses, and adenocystic carcinoma (or cylindroma) is the next most common. Uncommon tumors include adenocarcinomas and malignant melanomas. The 5-year survival rates for tumors of the maxillary and ethmoid sinuses are in the 20 percent range.

Tumors of the nose are similar to malignancies within the paranasal sinuses. Because of the abundance of minor salivary glands, both benign and malignant tumors of salivary gland origin may be manifested by nasal symptoms, including obstruction, epistaxis, foul odor, and secondary infection. Biopsy is critical for diagnosis, and follow-up imaging and staging are essential to the selection of definitive therapy.

NASOPHARYNX   The nasopharynx extends inferiorly from the posterior border of the nose at the choanae down to the junction with the oropharynx. The epithelium is primarily squamous and is richly infiltrated with lymphoid tissue. Esthesioneuroblastomas arise from olfactory epithelium connected to the cribriform plate. These tumors may either grow anteriorly and invade the nose or extend inferiorly and fill the nasopharynx. Superior extension of this tumor results in involvement of the CNS. The nasopharynx also coincides embryologically with the upper pole of the lymphoid tissue of Waldeyer's ring. This abundant tissue helps explain why nasopharyngeal masses may include lymphomas, malignant lymphoepitheliomas, and extramedullary plasmacytomas as well as squamous cell carcinomas in various degrees of differentiation. As in other head and neck tumors, histologic diagnosis of nasopharyngeal malignancies is necessary in addition to TNM staging. Electron microscopy by the surgical pathologist may be needed to confirm a histologic diagnosis. Advanced imaging techniques are usually needed for complete classification of a tumor and for the selection of optimal therapy. Since resectable tumors may invade the CNS, definitive treatment may require craniofacial resection. However, malignancies of lymphoid origins are best managed by irradiation and/or chemotherapy.

Carcinoma of the nasopharynx is infrequent in the United States, where it comprises 4 percent of head and neck malignancies. In China, however, it is more common, particularly in Kwantung Province. The incidence of nasopharyngeal carcinoma among North American–born Chinese is significantly lower than that among native-born Chinese, yet it is still higher than that among North American–born Caucasians. A possible explanation is a focus for genetic susceptibility located on the human leukocyte antigen HLA-A2 histocompatibility locus. Carcinoma of the nasopharynx also has been associated with infection by Epstein-Barr virus. Serum samples can be assayed for IgA antibodies to the viral capsid antigen (VCA) and the early antigen (EA) of this virus; titers can be predictive of prognosis.

Nearly one-half of patients with carcinoma of the nasopharynx present with regional disease in the ipsilateral neck as the only overt clinical finding. If a neck mass is found to contain squamous cell carcinoma cells and there is no known primary tumor site, occult disease within the nasopharynx must be suspected. Surgical endoscopy in addition to random biopsy of high-risk areas in the nasopharynx (including Rosenmüller's fossae) behind the eustachian tubes may help to define the primary tumor site.

Initial treatment for carcinoma of the nasopharynx is generally irradiation to the primary site and to the neck. Surgical treatment of the neck is usually reserved for persistent disease. Because of the proximity of the nasopharynx to the clivus and the base of the skull, locally invasive disease can cause isolated or multiple cranial neuropathies (especially involving cranial nerves I, III, IV, V, VI, IX, X, and XI).

ORAL CAVITY AND OROPHARYNX   The oral cavity extends from the vermilion border of the lips to the junction of the hard and soft palates superiorly and inferiorly to the circumvallate papilla. The area is divided into distinct anatomic regions, including the lips, the buccal mucosa, the alveolar ridge, the hard palate, and the anterior two-thirds of the tongue (i.e., the oral tongue). The oropharynx begins anteriorly with the oral cavity and extends inferiorly to the plane of the hyoid bone and superiorly to the plane of the hard palate. It includes the base of the tongue, the palatine tonsils, and the faucial

---

TABLE 320-1   Diagrammatic representation of TNM staging for head and neck tumors

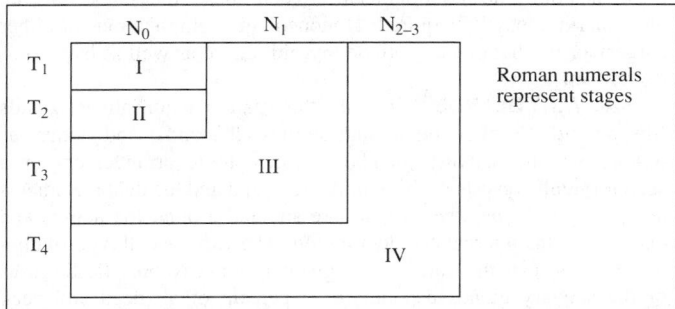

Clinical staging of the primary tumor (oral cavity, oropharynx, larynx, thyroid, salivary gland, etc.)

T stages (1–4) are separately defined for each anatomic region.

Clinical staging of neck nodes

N_0 Neck clinically negative for pathologic adenopathy.
N_1 Single ipsilateral node < 3 cm.
N_{2A} Single ipsilateral node 3-6 cm.
N_{2B} Multiple ipsilateral nodes all < 6 cm.
N_{2C} Bilateral or contralateral nodes all < 6 cm.
N_3 Single or multiple nodes, at least one > 6 cm.

Clinical staging of distant sites (brain, lung, bone, liver, etc.)

M_0 No metastatic disease.
M_1 Presence of metastasis (all M_1 tumors are stage IV).

SOURCE: AJCC, 1992.

arch encompassing the soft palate and the anterior pillar. The region inferior to the plane of the hyoid bone begins the hypopharynx, which ends at the cervical opening of the esophagus and is posterior to the true laryngeal framework. The oral cavity, oropharynx, and hypopharynx each has its own T-staging system, and in general, the larger the tumor, the higher the T stage.

Patients with squamous cell carcinoma of the oral cavity and oropharynx usually have associated medical illnesses—specifically, alcohol abuse with possible concurrent hepatic dysfunction. These patients usually also have significant smoking histories, with or without attendant pulmonary disorders. Tobacco chewing and the chewing of betel nut in India are linked to cancer of the oral cavity. Affected patients are frequently cachectic and have significant nutritional deficiencies that are difficult to correct because of odynophagia and/or alcoholism. Some of these patients have impaired cell-mediated immunity, which correlates with increased morbidity. The incidence of second primary squamous cell cancers of the oral cavity is reduced by chemoprevention with *cis*-retinoic acid. Most patients with squamous cell cancer of the oral cavity, oropharynx, and hypopharynx undergo surgery, radiation therapy, or combined-modality therapy. Chemotherapy is not used as a first-line treatment for carcinoma of the oral cavity and oropharynx. The role of chemotherapy as an adjunct or in nonresectable tumors is subject to debate. As a general rule, for a given T stage, the prognosis is best for tumors of the lips and deteriorates as the site moves toward the hypopharynx. Either stage I or stage II disease usually can be treated effectively by either surgery or irradiation; combined-modality therapy is generally preferred for patients with either stage III or stage IV disease. However, each patient should be evaluated individually by the appropriate specialists, and therapy should be based on multiple considerations, including size of tumor, side effects of planned therapy, and functional status after radical surgery. Regional disease within the neck usually requires neck dissection.

The complications of both irradiation and radical surgery are not trivial. After radiation therapy patients can suffer from xerostomia and be at increased risk for the delayed development of secondary neoplasms. Poor wound healing, fistulas, and major vessel erosion from radiation therapy are significant morbidities. Dry mouth with associated dysphagia should not be trivialized. Radical surgery can often remove a malignancy en bloc; however, both the appearance and the functional and communicative abilities of the patient may be severely compromised.

HYPOPHARYNX   The hypopharynx includes the pyriform sinus, the postcricoid region, and the inferoposterior pharyngeal wall. Approximately 5 percent of tumors of the hypopharynx are of minor salivary gland origin; the remaining 95 percent are squamous cell carcinomas. Alcohol abuse and tobacco use are the major etiologic agents for cancer of the hypopharynx. The Plummer-Vinson syndrome, iron-deficiency anemia, and dysphagia secondary to upper esophageal webs are frequently associated with carcinoma of the postcricoid region in nonsmoking women. Hypopharyngeal carcinoma most commonly originates in the pyriform sinus and usually presents in an advanced clinical stage. Symptoms, when present, generally include throat pain, otalgia, and dysphagia. Approximately 80 percent of pyriform sinus lesions are found with cervical node metastases. Because most hypopharyngeal carcinomas present as advanced lesions, therapy usually consists of a total laryngectomy with a partial pharyngectomy and complete neck dissection. Postoperative radiation therapy is usually given. Reconstructive options after radical surgery include myocutaneous flaps, gastric pull-ups, and free jejunal flaps with microvascular reanastomoses. The 5-year survival rate for carcinoma of the hypopharynx in patients undergoing both irradiation and surgery is approximately 40 percent.

LARYNX   Cancer of the larynx accounts for fewer than 2 percent of all carcinomas in the United States. The incidence of cancer of the larynx is considerably higher among men than among women (5:1). Tobacco and alcohol abuse are the prime etiologic factors. Lesions of the larynx are frequently detected earlier than those of the hypopharynx because of the associated symptoms.

Hoarseness is the most common symptom of laryngeal cancer and often motivates a patient to seek medical attention. Other associated symptoms include dyspnea, stridor, and severe pain. Dysphagia and odynophagia may be evident, and chronic cough and hemoptysis may indicate large fungating lesions. Late symptoms and signs can include weight loss, halitosis, and regional neck disease.

A clinical diagnosis is frequently made (sometimes in the doctor's office) by either mirror or fiberoptic examination of the pharynx and larynx. Once the diagnosis is suspected, appropriate adjunctive imaging should be undertaken and should be followed by formal staging endoscopy. The supraglottic larynx is embryologically different from the glottic and infraglottic larynx and consequently has a different lymphatic drainage pattern. Tumors of the true vocal cords will therefore behave differently from those originating at superior sites. Surgical endoscopy is critical for staging. Supraglottic, glottic, and infraglottic tumors are staged differently, and precise anatomic definition is a prerequisite to proper treatment. The unique anatomic characteristics of lymphatic drainage in the larynx, along with the existence of local barriers to direct extension of the tumor, theoretically make conservation laryngeal surgery an oncologically sound choice for specialized lesions. Supraglottic (horizontal) laryngectomy may be appropriate for some epiglottic lesions, while hemilaryngectomy (vertical) may be appropriate in carcinoma of the true vocal cords. T_1 and T_2 lesions of the larynx frequently can be treated successfully with irradiation or various vocal cord stripping techniques.

Total laryngectomy with or without neck dissection is reserved for advanced lesions or those which have failed to respond to radiation therapy. The morbidity (both physical and psychologic) associated with a total laryngectomy cannot be overemphasized. Patients undergo a profound change in life-style that few can appreciate preoperatively despite extensive counseling and support. Loss of the upper respiratory airway can result in anosmia and dysgeusia. Because of an open airway in the neck, patients can have a difficult time showering and cannot swim. The most profound effect, however, is loss of speech. Counseling and immediate postoperative training in the use of assistive communication devices are helpful. Some patients develop esophageal speech. Others may undergo procedures such as tracheoesophageal puncture or insertion of various prosthetic devices for the enhancement of their ability to communicate. When these measures fail, an electrolarynx may be required. Nononcologic complications of either surgery or irradiation can include thyroid failure as well as hypoparathyroidism.

SALIVARY GLANDS   There are three paired major salivary glands (the parotid, submandibular, and sublingual glands) and numerous minor exocrine salivary glands. The histologic arrangement of a secretory unit consists of the acinus at one end and the ductal elements at the other. Myoepithelial cells are situated around the acinus and extend into the intercalated duct region. The various cell types within the gland spawn the various malignant lesions. Neoplastic diseases of the salivary glands account for 5 percent of all head and neck tumors. Previous radiation therapy has been shown to be associated with the development of pleomorphic adenomas and mucoepidermoid tumors of the major salivary glands, with latencies lasting as long as several years. Persons involved in the manufacture of furniture and woodwork also run an increased risk of minor salivary gland adenocarcinoma, particularly in the sinonasal tract.

Pleomorphic adenoma is the most common tumor of the salivary glands, particularly in the parotid. While this tumor is technically benign and slow-growing, the potential for malignant degeneration exists, and surgical excision is advised in nearly all cases. In fact, nearly all tumors of the major and minor salivary glands require surgical excision because of the significant possibility of malignant degeneration. Table 320-2 lists the histologic classification of salivary tumors. As in all head and neck cancers, AJCC staging according to the TNM system is recommended during the diagnostic evaluation

TABLE 320-2 Salivary gland tumors

Benign
  Pleomorphic adenoma
  Warthin's tumor (papillary cystadenoma lymphomatosum)
  Oncocytoma
  Monomorphic adenoma
Malignant
  Malignant mixed tumor
  Mucoepidermoid carcinoma
  Adenocystic carcinoma
  Adenocarcinoma
  Acinic cell carcinoma
  Squamous cell carcinoma

and before the institution of definitive therapy. As a general rule, the larger the gland, the more likely it is that the tumor is histologically benign. While three-fourths of parotid tumors are histologically benign, the same proportion of minor salivary gland tumors are histologically malignant.

The diagnosis is based on the patient's history and physical examination along with the results of radiographic imaging studies. Paresthesias and pain may be associated with malignant tumors, particularly adenocystic carcinomas. Fine-needle aspiration is a safe method for the preoperative evaluation of salivary neoplasms, although cytologic features can be misleading in establishing a correct tissue diagnosis of malignancy. To date, there is no evidence of tumor tracking by fine-needle cytologic aspiration. The facial nerve is intricately involved with the parotid gland, and weakness in this nerve suggests the presence of a malignant tumor.

Surgical resection is the treatment of choice for salivary gland tumors. Occasionally, malignant tumors invade the facial nerve; if sacrifice of this nerve is required, immediate nerve grafting often using the sural nerve, is the treatment of choice. Reinnervation of the face may take as long as 18 months.

The prognosis of salivary gland tumors is generally a function of the stage of disease as well as tumor histology and grade at the time of initial presentation. This association is especially strong in mucoepidermoid carcinomas and acinic cell carcinomas. In adenocarcinomas and adenocystic carcinomas, the site of origin affects prognosis. Poor outcomes are frequent for tumors originating in the sinonasal tract and the laryngotracheal complex. Facial nerve involvement is especially ominous.

THYROID GLAND (See also Chap. 334) Malignant lesions of the thyroid gland arise from two functionally distinct endocrine cell lines in the thyroid gland. Follicular cells, which secrete thyroid hormone, are the cells of origin for papillary, follicular, and anaplastic carcinoma. The perifollicular cells (C cells) are neural crest derivatives and are the cells of origin for medullary carcinoma of the thyroid gland. Thyroid cancers comprise nearly 10 percent of head and neck tumors. Etiologic factors include previous irradiation to the region and, in some cases, familial syndromes associated with multiple endocrine neoplasia.

Tumors usually present as a neck mass. In some instances, extensive tracheal compression with airway compromise may be the presenting symptom, especially in aggressive neoplasms. Patients frequently complain of hoarseness, particularly in malignant neoplasms. Other risk factors for malignancy include young age, male gender, and a solid, "cold" nodule on a nuclear scan. Except in medullary carcinoma, no clinical or laboratory tests help differentiate benign from malignant thyroid nodules, although aspiration cytology is frequently helpful in defining the malignancy of a lesion.

Papillary carcinoma is the most common cancer of the thyroid; it is frequently multifocal and unencapsulated. A worse prognosis is associated with local tissue invasion and with distant lymphatic spread. Follicular carcinoma is typically solid and encapsulated; it preferentially spreads hematogenously, often involving the lungs and bones. Hürthle cell carcinoma is a variant of follicular cell cancer,

and nuclear aneuploidy is associated with a relatively poor prognosis. Anaplastic carcinoma is highly malignant and has a dismal prognosis. Diagnostic testing for patients suspected of having medullary thyroid carcinoma includes measurement of serum calcitonin. Provocative tests using calcium gluconate and pentagastrin may facilitate early diagnosis.

Surgery is the primary treatment modality for thyroid malignancies. Radioactive iodine administration, hormonal suppression by thyroid hormone supplements, external beam irradiation, and chemotherapy are useful adjuncts in some cases. Tumors whose malignancy is strongly suspected are excised, while benign tumors are generally subjected to a trial of medical management. Effective communication between the endocrinologist and the head and neck surgeon will lead to optimal therapy.

REFERENCES

Advanced techniques for management of head and neck neoplasms. Ontolaryngol Clin North Am 24:1287, 1991
HELLMAN S et al (eds): *Cancer: Principles and Practice of Oncology*, 3d ed, 1989
KOH W et al: Fast neutron radiation for inoperable and recurrent salivary gland cancers. Am J Clin Oncol 12:316, 1989
LEE NK: Molecular biology: the polymerase chain reaction. Head Neck 14:62, 1992
——: Oncogenes. Head Neck 14:235, 1992
MILLION RR: The larynx. Int J Radiat Oncol 23:691, 1992
MOISA II: Neuroendocrine tumors of the larynx. Head Neck 13:498, 1991
PAPARELLA M et al (eds): *Otolaryngology (Head and Neck)*, vol 3. Philadelphia, Saunders, 1991
PARSONS JT et al: Twice-a-day irradiation of squamous cell carcinoma. Semin Radiat Oncol 2:29, 1992
PFISTER DC et al: Current status of larynx preservation with multimodality therapy. Oncology 6:33, 1992
SESSIONS RB, DIEHL WL: Thyroid cancer and related nodularity, in *Cancer of the Head and Neck*, 2d ed, E Meyers, JY Suen (eds). New York, Churchill Livingstone, 1989, p 735
WANG CC: *Radiation Therapy for Head and Neck Neoplasms*, 2d ed. New York, Year Book Medical Publishers, 1990

321 OVARIAN CANCER

ROBERT C. BAST, JR. / ANDREW BERCHUCK

Ovarian cancer is neither common nor rare. In incidence, it ranks fifth among all malignancies of women and third among the gynecologic cancers. Ovarian cancer is, however, the most frequent cause of gynecologic cancer death because some two-thirds of cases are detected in advanced stages. Late detection reflects an absence of specific symptoms when disease is localized, as well as the lack of effective strategies for prevention or screening. The prognosis of ovarian cancer depends critically on the histologic type. More than 85 percent of ovarian cancers arise from the epithelium that covers the ovarian surface or that lines inclusion cysts, whereas less than 15 percent develop from ovarian stroma and germ cells. Although relatively rare, germ cell and stromal tumors can be cured in a majority of cases, often with preservation of reproductive function. The more common epithelial ovarian cancers respond to cytoreductive surgery and cytotoxic chemotherapy, but long-term survival is observed in only about a third of all patients with this histotype.

INCIDENCE AND EPIDEMIOLOGY In the United States, a woman's lifetime risk of developing ovarian cancer is 1 in 70. In 1992, some 21,000 cases of ovarian cancer were reported, and about 13,000 women died from the disease. Germ cell tumors generally develop within the first three decades. Stromal tumors can occur at any age. Juvenile granulosa cell and Sertoli-Leydig cell tumors are seen most frequently in younger women, whereas the peak incidence of adult granulosa cell tumors is in the perimenopausal period. The more common epithelial ovarian cancers are seldom encountered in women less than 35 years of age, but the incidence increases sharply with advancing age and peaks at ages 75 to 80. The median age of patients with epithelial ovarian cancer is 60 years. The single most important risk factor for epithelial ovarian cancer is age >40 years.

Most cases of epithelial ovarian cancer are sporadic. Less than 5 percent of ovarian cancer patients belong to families in which ovarian, breast, endometrial, or colon cancer can be tracked as an apparent autosomal dominant trait. In this setting, risk can be as high as 50 percent. Patients with two or more first-degree relatives affected by ovarian cancer are likely to belong to such families, but formal pedigree analysis is required to document risk. A single first-degree relative with ovarian cancer increases a woman's risk by at least threefold, whereas a personal history of breast or colorectal cancer increases the risk of subsequently developing ovarian cancer by twofold.

Among environmental factors, a high-fat diet has been associated with increased risk of epithelial ovarian cancer, as has the intake of lactose in subjects with relatively low tissue levels of galactose-1-phosphate uridyl transferase. Use of talc products has correlated with increased ovarian cancer risk in some studies but not in others. Endocrinologic factors are also important. Early menarche, late menopause, and nulliparity are all associated with increased risk. Conversely, pregnancy, lactation, and oral contraceptive medications decrease the risk of ovarian cancer. Use of oral contraceptives for as long as 5 years can reduce the risk of ovarian cancer by 50 percent. Thus factors that favor prolonged and persistent ovulation increase ovarian cancer risk, whereas factors that suppress ovulation decrease risk. Estrogen replacement does not appear to increase the risk of epithelial ovarian cancer in postmenopausal patients.

HISTOLOGIC CLASSIFICATION   Primary ovarian tumors can be divided into three general categories: epithelial, stromal, and germ cell tumors (Table 321-1). In addition, metastases to the ovary can occur from a variety of neoplasms, including fallopian tube, endometrial, breast, colon, gastric, and pancreatic carcinomas, as well as lymphomas and some leukemias. Krukenberg had originally described bilateral metastases to the ovarian stroma from mucin-secreting gastrointestinal cancers.

During embryologic development, the ovarian surface is derived

TABLE 321-1   Histologic classification of primary ovarian cancers

EPITHELIAL

Serous
Mucinous
Endometrioid
Clear cell "mesonephroid"
Brenner
Mixed epithelial
Undifferentiated
Unclassified

STROMAL

Granulosa cell
Thecoma, fibroma
Sertoli, Leydig cell tumors
Gynandroblastoma
Lipoid cell tumor
Sarcoma

GERM CELL

Dysgerminoma
Teratoma
Endodermal sinus tumor
Embryonal carcinoma
Polyembryoma
Choriocarcinoma
Mixed germ cell tumors
Gonadoblastoma

from the coelomic mesothelium that covers the peritoneal cavity and that also lines the müllerian duct forming the epithelial components of the fallopian tube, endometrium, and endocervix. The flattened epithelium that covers the ovarian surface is thought to retain the potential to differentiate into the cuboidal or columnar epithelia resembling müllerian duct derivatives. Serous, endometrioid, and mucinous ovarian tumors resemble epithelial components of the fallopian tube, endometrium, and endocervix, respectively. Epithelial ovarian cancers can contain a mixture of these different histotypes or can lack differentiation. Within a given histotype, benign, borderline, and frankly malignant ovarian tumors have been described. Borderline ovarian tumors contain histologically transformed cells that lack evidence of invasion. More than 75 percent of borderline lesions are found in early stage and tend to occur in younger women. Recurrence and metastasis of borderline lesions are observed, but the prognosis is dramatically better than that for most ovarian cancers. Benign and borderline ovarian tumors are not necessarily precursors of frankly malignant ovarian cancers, in contrast to cervical dysplastic lesions, which clearly give rise to invasive cervical cancer.

Granulosa, theca, Sertoli, and Leydig cell tumors resemble stromal or "sex-cord" components in the normal ovary. Similar to normal ovarian stroma, these neoplasms can produce estrogens or androgens.

In contrast to testicular lesions, germ cell tumors of the ovary are more often benign than malignant. Dermoid cysts generally contain components of all three germ layers and are most frequently benign. Calcification of bone or teeth can sometimes be detected radiographically. Among the malignant germ cell tumors, dysgerminomas, immature teratomas, endodermal sinus tumors, embryonal carcinomas, and nongestational choriocarcinomas can be differentiated histologically.

EPITHELIAL CANCERS   Biology   The ovarian surface epithelium is ordinarily quiescent with a low mitotic index. Following ovulation, surface epithelial cells proliferate to repair the defect produced when a follicle ruptures. Proliferation triggered by repeated ovulation may permit the induction or expression of genetic damage leading to malignant transformation. Invaginations of the surface epithelium can form inclusion cysts. Within the microenvironment of the stroma, proliferation of epithelial cells lining these cysts may be dysregulated.

As in the case of many other neoplasms, epithelial ovarian cancer is a clonal disease that arises from a single cell. Some four to five alterations may be required in growth factors, oncogenes, or tumor suppressor genes to dysregulate growth. Normal ovarian surface epithelial cells express transforming growth factor β that regularly inhibits their growth. A fraction of ovarian cancers appear to have lost this autocrine inhibitory loop. Conversely, a majority of ovarian cancers express both transforming growth factor α and the epidermal growth factor receptor (EGFR) to which it binds, permitting autocrine stimulation of tumor cell proliferation.

Oncogenes associated with ovarian cancers also can encode growth factors or their receptors. The HER-2/*neu* (c-*erb*B-2) gene product, a transmembrane tyrosine kinase growth factor receptor, is overexpressed in one-third of ovarian cancers. Both normal and malignant ovarian epithelia secrete macrophage colony stimulating factor (CSF-1), but only malignant cells appear to express the receptor for this growth factor encoded by the *fms* oncogene. CSF-1 is also a potent chemoattractant for macrophages. Cytokines derived from macrophages, including tumor necrosis factor α, interleukin 1, and interleukin 6, can stimulate ovarian cancer growth. Consequently, tumor-associated macrophages may provide paracrine stimulation rather than inhibition of ovarian tumor growth.

No abnormalities have been detected in the retinoblastoma (Rb) or Wilms' tumor associated suppressor genes, but approximately half of ovarian cancers have lost the normal function of p53, a DNA-binding phosphoprotein that is required for normal growth regulation. Additional suppressor loci are being sought through studies of loss of heterozygosity at different loci within tumor cells. As in many other neoplasms, genetic instability is reflected in aneuploid karyotypes for the majority of advanced ovarian cancers. Using molecular techniques, loss of heterozygosity has been observed at loci on chromosomes 1, 3, 6, 11, and 17, but there is no single karyotypic abnormality that is characteristic of ovarian cancer.

Epithelial ovarian cancer has a distinctive pattern of spread. In addition to lymphatic and hematogenous metastasis, the exfoliation, transperitoneal migration, and implantation of tumor cells can produce multiple metastatic nodules on the visceral and parietal peritoneum. Growth of these nodules and their surrounding stroma produces adhesions leading to mechanical obstruction of the intestine. Invasion of the myenteric plexus also can produce functional ileus. Early implants are found on the hemidiaphragms, particularly on the right, due to the characteristic clockwise circulation of fluid in the peritoneal cavity. Blockade of diaphragmatic lymphatics as well as exudation across tumor capillaries contributes to the intraperitoneal accumulation of ascites fluid. During embryonic development, the ovaries migrate to the pelvis from the level of the renal hilus. Consequently, ovarian lymphatic channels drain to the retroperitoneal lymph nodes at the level of the renal arteries. Retrograde metastases also can occur to femoral and inguinal lymphatics. Hematogenous metastases to the hepatic parenchyma, lung, and brain have been observed, particularly in those individuals whose intraperitoneal disease has been controlled by cytotoxic chemotherapy. Clinically significant metastases to bone are uncommon.

Clinical features and diagnosis Early-stage disease is often asymptomatic and is detected coincidentally by palpating an ovarian mass on pelvic examination. In premenopausal patients, some 95 percent of adnexal masses are benign. Even after menopause, some 70 percent of adnexal masses are benign, but detection of any ovarian enlargement in a postmenopausal patient is an indication for surgical exploration. In premenopausal patients, a mass that enlarges progressively under observation or any mass >8 cm requires exploratory surgery. In addition to primary ovarian cancers, adnexal masses can be produced by functional ovarian cysts, benign ovarian neoplasms, pedunculated uterine fibroids, hydrosalpinx, endometriosis, and inflammatory lesions of the bowel. Transvaginal sonography can aid in confirming the ovarian origin of an adnexal mass and in defining its gross morphology. Bilateral lesions and irregular, complex cysts that contain solid projections are more likely to be malignant.

In postmenopausal patients with a pelvic mass, a markedly elevated serum CA-125 level (>95 U/mL) distinguishes malignant from benign disease with a positive predictive value of 96 percent. CA-125 determinants are expressed on a high-molecular-weight glycoprotein composed of 220-kDa subunits that can be associated with cancers from a number of sites, including the ovary, endometrium, fallopian tube, endocervix, pancreas, breast, lung, and colon. Elevated levels of CA-125 in a patient with a pelvic mass should prompt her referral for initial exploration at an institution capable of proper staging of early ovarian cancer and of cytoreductive surgery for advanced disease.

Progressive enlargement of a localized ovarian cancer can produce urologic or gynecologic symptoms, including urinary frequency, dysuria, obstipation, or constipation. Rarely, torsion of an ovarian mass can produce acute abdominal symptoms. Vaginal bleeding or discharge is not frequently associated with primary ovarian cancer in postmenopausal patients, although premenopausal patients can experience heavy or irregular menstrual periods.

Approximately two-thirds of patients present with stage III or IV disease. Symptoms of more advanced disease include abdominal distention from ascites and ill-defined abdominal pain. Paracentesis usually is not required in a woman with ascites and an adnexal mass, since prompt surgical exploration is already indicated. In addition to a history, physical examination, and complete blood count, the patient's workup should include liver function studies, a serum CA-125 determination, a transvaginal sonogram, a chest film, a mammogram, and, in patients >40 years of age, a barium enema or colonoscopy. Abdominal CT and MRI have a relatively low sensitivity and specificity for diagnosing ovarian cancer and metastatic spread,

precluding their routine use in patients with a unilateral ovarian mass and normal hepatic function.

Prognostic factors Survival is directly related to stage, grade, and the amount of tumor that remains following cytoreductive surgery. Recent studies of cell growth regulation have identified relevant biologic markers. Response to treatment is also an important prognostic factor and can be assessed with serum markers and by "second look" surgical surveillance procedures.

STAGE   Stage is assessed at surgical exploration (Table 321-2). In stage I disease, tumor is limited to one or both ovaries. In stage II disease, the pelvic organs are involved without other intraperitoneal spread. In stage III disease, the tumor is limited to the abdominal cavity or retroperitoneum without invasion of the hepatic parenchyma. Stage IV disease involves hepatic parenchymal invasion or tumor spread above the diaphragm.

Careful surgical exploration is required to document early-stage disease. Although a Pfannenstiel incision is sometimes used to remove benign ovarian masses, this approach precludes exploration of the upper abdomen. A midline incision is required for adequate assessment of ovarian cancer. Surgical staging involves examination of both diaphragms, omentectomy, retroperitoneal lymph node sampling, cytologic examination of peritoneal washings, biopsy of any suspicious lesion, as well as random biopsies of apparently normal peritoneal surfaces. Reexploration following simple oophorectomy has resulted in upstaging 30 percent of patients thought to have early-stage disease.

For well-staged patients, 5-year survival in stage I can exceed 90 percent, and that in stage II, approximates 70 to 80 percent. Contemporary management produces a 20 to 30 percent long-term survival in stage III and approximately 5 percent in stage IV.

TUMOR BURDEN   With advanced disease, cytoreductive surgery is thought to be of benefit. If the bulk of tumor can be removed, leaving nodules no greater than 1.5 cm, the prognosis of patients is no worse than if only 1.5-cm disease had been present before surgery. Whether this reflects the underlying biology of the disease or the benefit from tumor removal cannot be resolved from studies presently available. Patients whose tumor can be optimally cytoreduced have a median survival of some 39 months compared with 17 months in

---

TABLE 321-2   Staging of primary ovarian cancer

Stage I	Growth limited to the ovaries
Ia	Growth limited to one ovary with an intact capsule and without ascites or tumor on the external surface
Ib	Growth limited to both ovaries with intact capsules and without ascites or tumor on the external surfaces
Ic	Growth limited to one or both ovaries with tumor on the ovarian surface(s) or with rupture of the capsule(s) or ascites present containing malignant cells or with positive peritoneal washings
Stage II	Growth involving one or both ovaries with pelvic extension
IIa	Extension and/or metastasis to the uterus and/or tubes
IIb	Extension to other pelvic tissues
IIc	Growth involving one or both ovaries with metastasis to uterus, tubes, or pelvis with tumor on the ovarian surface or with rupture of the capsule(s) or ascites present containing malignant cells or with positive peritoneal washings
Stage III	Tumor involving one or both ovaries with peritoneal implants outside the pelvis and/or positive retroperitoneal or inguinal nodes. Superficial liver metastasis indicates stage III disease. Tumor is limited to the true pelvis, but with histologically proven malignant extension to small bowel or omentum
IIIa	Tumor grossly limited to the true pelvis with negative nodes but with histologically confirmed microscopic seeding of abdominal peritoneal surfaces
IIIb	Tumor of one or both ovaries with histologically confirmed implants of abdominal peritoneal surfaces, none exceeding 2 cm in diameter. Nodes negative.
IIIc	Abdominal implants >2 cm in diameter and/or positive retroperitoneal or inguinal nodes
Stage IV	Growth involving one or both ovaries with distant metastasis. If pleural effusion is present, there must be positive cytologic test results to allot a case to stage IV. Parenchymal liver metastasis indicates stage IV.

patients with suboptimal cytoreduction in collected series. Patients with bulky disease remaining after surgery rarely experience long-term survival. Only approximately 35 percent of patients with stage III or IV ovarian cancer can be optimally cytoreduced.

HISTOLOGIC GRADE AND CELL TYPE Well-differentiated tumors are associated with a better prognosis than are moderately or poorly differentiated tumors. In some series, clear cell carcinomas are associated with a worse prognosis than are tumors of other histologic types, but among the epithelial ovarian cancers of similar stage, the tumor grade is more important than histologic subtype.

BIOLOGIC MARKERS Expression of EGFR, expression of *fms*, and overexpression of *erb*B-2 are all poor prognostic factors for ovarian cancer. Coexpression of these transmembrane tyrosine kinase growth factor receptors and their ligands may provide autocrine growth stimulation or alter resistance to cytotoxic chemotherapy. An aneuploid karyotype is also associated with a poor prognosis, particularly in borderline lesions.

SERUM MARKERS Tumor burden can be assessed during therapy in more than 80 percent of patients with the serum marker CA-125. When elevated prior to treatment, serum CA-125 levels have correlated with the clinical disease course in 90 percent of instances studied. In addition, elevations of CA-125 have preceded clinical disease recurrence by an average of 3 months, and persistently rising CA-125 values are consistently associated with progressive disease. Elevation of CA-125 (>35 U/mL) at the time of a "second look" surveillance procedure predicts persistence of disease with 96 percent accuracy. When CA-125 levels return to <35 U/mL prior to second look, small-volume residual disease can, however, still be found in 60 percent of cases. Finally, the rate at which CA-125 normalizes correlates with findings at second look procedures and survival. An apparent CA-125 half-life of <20 days is associated with a significantly better prognosis than a half-life of >20 days.

"SECOND LOOK" SURGICAL SURVEILLANCE PROCEDURES At second look laparotomy performed after 3 to 6 months of cytotoxic chemotherapy, 50 to 70 percent of patients with stage III or IV disease will be found to have persistent disease, whereas more than 90 percent of patients with stage I and II disease will be disease-free, suggesting that this procedure may not be required for patients with early-stage ovarian cancer at presentation. If gross disease is found, median survival is only approximately 12 months, whereas persistence of microscopic disease is associated with a median survival of 36 to 48 months. Although a pathologic complete response correlates with a median survival >60 months, 30 to 50 percent of patients who have a negative second look will eventually develop recurrent cancer. Whether or not reresection of disease at second look has therapeutic benefit cannot be resolved from the studies currently available.

Screening strategies Since a majority of patients with stage I and II disease can be cured using conventional therapy, earlier detection of ovarian cancer could improve survival. Pelvic examination is a relatively insensitive technique for the detection of ovarian cancer in its early stages. Cervical cytology is rarely, if ever, positive in primary ovarian cancer. Transvaginal sonography (TVS) has proven more sensitive than transabdominal sonography for detecting ovarian enlargement. Among some 8000 women screened with TVS, 11 cases of ovarian cancer were detected, with 10 in stage I. Despite high sensitivity, however, some 10 to 15 benign lesions are found at laparotomy for each case of ovarian cancer detected. Careful evaluation of morphology and Doppler flow ultrasound may reduce the number of false-positive tests.

CA-125 also may have a role in early detection of ovarian cancer in that values of the serum marker have been elevated 10 to 20 months prior to the diagnosis of the neoplasm. Sensitivity is limited in that only 60 percent of patients with early-stage ovarian cancer will have an elevated antigen level. In a premenopausal population, false-positive values are also a consideration. The first trimester of normal pregnancy, endometriosis, adenomyosis, uterine fibroids, chronic salpingitis, hepatocellular disease, pleuritis, peritonitis, and, rarely, normal menstruation can all elevate serum CA-125. Among postmeno-

pausal patients, however, only about 2 percent will have an elevation of CA-125 (>30 U/mL). In studies performed in Sweden and the United Kingdom, an abnormal CA-125 level has triggered the use of transabdominal sonography, permitting the detection of a majority of ovarian cancer cases with some in early stages of disease. Critical studies have not yet been performed to demonstrate the ability of CA-125 and TVS to improve survival of patients with ovarian cancer. At the present time neither CA-125 nor transvaginal sonography should be used routinely for screening, particularly in premenopausal populations.

Therapeutic considerations STAGES I AND II Current management of low-risk ovarian cancers (stage Ia or b and grade 1 or 2) consists of bilateral salpingo-oophorectomy (BSO), total abdominal hysterectomy (TAH), and surgical staging followed by careful observation. In selected premenopausal patients, reproductive function can be preserved by performing unilateral salpingo-oophorectomy. Patients at higher risk with grade 3 cancers or lesions of any grade that have progressed to stages Ic or II generally receive some type of adjuvant therapy following surgery. Intraperitoneal radionuclide (colloidal ^{32}P), total abdominal irradiation, single alkylating agents, or cisplatin-based combinations of cytotoxic drugs have been utilized in this setting. Although many practitioners use cisplatin-based combination chemotherapy to treat high-risk early-stage ovarian cancer, the superiority of any single approach has not been proven.

STAGES III AND IV Treatment of more advanced ovarian cancer involves TAH-BSO, omentectomy, surgical cytoreduction, and platinum-based chemotherapy for 3 to 6 months. Following cytotoxic chemotherapy, a second look laparotomy is usually performed. With current therapy, more than half of patients will have no evidence of disease by noninvasive evaluation at the completion of chemotherapy, but only about 30 to 40 percent will be free from disease when reevaluated with multiple biopsies at second look. Even in the setting of negative surveillance procedures, ovarian cancer recurs in 30 to 50 percent of patients. If residual disease is found at second look operation, investigational therapy has been attempted. This includes intraperitoneal administration of cisplatin and other compounds, use of novel agents such as taxol, and high-dose therapy with hematopoietic stem cell support.

CYTOTOXIC CHEMOTHERAPY Several different cytotoxic drugs have produced at least temporary regression of ovarian cancer (Table 321-3). Alkylating agents have proven most active, and among the alkylators, platinum-based compounds have had the greatest impact. In early studies, it was difficult to show an advantage of multiple cytotoxic drugs over single alkylating agents. With optimal cytoreduction of tumor, however, use of cyclophosphamide and cisplatin in combination has produced greater long-term survival than has cisplatin alone. Addition of doxorubicin or hexamethylmelamine to the alkylators does not appear to improve response rates or survival within individual studies, although metaanalysis suggests an advantage to the addition of doxorubicin. During the last several years, carboplatin, a cisplatin analogue, has proven less nephrotoxic, ototoxic, neuro-

---

TABLE 321-3 Cytotoxic drugs active against ovarian cancer

Alkylating agents
  Cyclophosphamide
  Ifosfamide
  Melphalan
  Chlorambucil
  Thiotepa
  Cisplatin
  Carboplatin
Antimetabolites
  5-Fluorouracil
  Hydroxyurea
Anthracyclines
  Doxorubicin
Other
  Hexamethylmelamine
  Taxol

toxic, and emetogenic but more myelotoxic than the parent compound. In two large studies, a combination of carboplatin and cyclophosphamide was as effective as, but less toxic than, a combination of cisplatin and cyclophosphamide. With carboplatin, dose can be adjusted based on renal function, which correlates effectively with myelosuppression. Current therapy for ovarian cancer includes cisplatin or carboplatin in combination with cyclophosphamide at 3- to 4-week intervals for six to eight cycles. A clinical response rate of 70 percent can be anticipated in patients with advanced epithelial ovarian cancer who have not been previously treated. Approximately 50 percent of responses will be complete judged by noninvasive techniques, and of these patients, 45 percent will have negative surgical surveillance procedures.

PERSISTENT DISEASE If persistent ovarian cancer is found at second look laparotomy or if disease subsequently recurs, options have included retreatment with platinum-based chemotherapy, intravenous administration of other drugs, intraperitoneal chemotherapy, autologous bone marrow transplantation, and immunotherapy. Retreatment with cisplatin or carboplatin has palliated patients who had previously responded to platinum-based chemotherapy and had a disease-free interval of at least 6 months. Among second-line agents, hexamethylmelamine has been used traditionally but has produced a response rate of <20 percent. Ifosfamide with the urothelial protectant mesna induced a 20 percent response rate. Recently, taxol has produced an objective response in 44 percent of patients who could still respond to cisplatin and in 30 percent of patients whose tumors had become resistant to cisplatin. Taxol is derived from the bark of the yew tree and has been in relatively short supply. New sources are being identified, and partial synthesis of the drug has been achieved. The agent has a novel mechanism of action that depends on stabilizing the polymerization of tubulin into microfilaments and mitotic spindles.

INTRAPERITONEAL THERAPY Intraperitoneal therapy produces a substantial pharmacokinetic advantage that depends on the more rapid clearance of compounds such as cisplatin from the peripheral blood than from the abdominal cavity. After intraperitoneal instillation, tumor cells within the peritoneal cavity are exposed to higher concentrations of drug than can be achieved safely by intravenous administration. Patients who have small (<5 mm) tumor nodules and who have previously responded to intravenous cisplatin are most likely to respond to IP cisplatin. As many as 40 percent of such patients have had a complete response following IP administration of cisplatin.

AUTOLOGOUS BONE MARROW TRANSPLANTATION In retrospective studies, response rates to intravenous therapy appeared to depend on the amount of cisplatin that was delivered per unit time. Substantially higher doses of alkylating agents, including platinum-based drugs, can be given with autologous bone marrow and peripheral stem cell support. Using high doses of multiple alkylating agents followed by stem cell and cytokine support, response rates of 54 to 78 percent have been achieved in patients who had failed all conventional therapy.

IMMUNOTHERAPY Different forms of immunotherapy also have been attempted for residual disease. Intraperitoneal instillation of *Corynebacterium parvum*, interferon-α, interferon-γ, or IL-2 can produce responses in approximately one-third of patients. Current trials of IP immunotherapy are evaluating combinations of interferon with standard cytotoxic drugs. Intraperitoneal administration of monoclonal antibodies linked to radionuclides also have shown activity against small volumes of disease.

STROMAL TUMORS Granulosa cell and theca cell tumors are uncommon lesions that occur most frequently in the first three decades of life. Granulosa cell tumors can produce estrogen, leading to premenarchal vaginal bleeding, menstrual irregularities, or postmenopausal bleeding. Endometrial carcinoma is associated with 5 percent of cases, possibly secondary to chronic estrogenic stimulation of the endometrium. Sertoli and Leydig cell tumors most often produce androgens with consequent virilization but can, on occasion, also produce estrogens.

Three-fourths of granulosa cell tumors present in stage I. Growth of tumors is slow, and recurrence is late, with disease-free intervals extending to 10 years. Treatment includes TAH-BSO. Cytotoxic adjuvant chemotherapy is not of proven value. Radiotherapy is of value only in the palliation of unresectable pelvic disease. For recurrent cancer, several different combinations of drugs have been used for palliative treatment, including cyclophosphamide-doxorubicin-cisplatin and actinomycin D–5-fluorouracil–cyclophosphamide.

GERM CELL TUMORS Germ cell tumors account for less than 5 percent of all ovarian cancers but comprise 75 percent of ovarian carcinomas during the first 3 decades of life. With appropriate treatment, >90 percent of patients can be cured. Histologic types include dysgerminomas, immature teratomas, endodermal sinus tumors, embryonal carcinomas, and choriocarcinomas in descending order of incidence. Endodermal sinus tumors secrete alpha fetoprotein (AFP), choriocarcinomas produce human chorionic gonadotropin (hCG), and embryonal carcinomas can express both markers. Pure dysgerminomas and immature teratomas produce neither AFP nor hCG, but elevated levels of either marker can indicate the presence of a mixed germ cell tumor that requires more aggressive treatment.

Dysgerminomas Approximately 5 percent of dysgerminomas are associated with karyotypic abnormalities of the gonads, including pure gonadal dysgenesis (46XY with bilateral streak gonads), mixed gonadal dysgenesis (45X/46XY with unilateral streak gonad and contralateral testis), or testicular feminization (46XY with bilateral testes). Tumors are bilateral in 10 to 15 percent of cases. Dysgerminomas are histologically similar to seminomas and are exquisitely sensitive to radiotherapy or chemotherapy. For disease in stage Ia, unilateral oophorectomy can be performed without additional treatment and with the expectation that radiotherapy or chemotherapy can salvage any subsequent recurrence. The retroperitoneal lymph nodes are the most frequent site of metastasis. For more advanced or recurrent disease, radiotherapy that spares the contralateral ovary or chemotherapy with bleomycin-etoposide and cisplatin (BEP) can cure the tumor and preserve reproductive function.

Nondysgerminomatous tumors Well-differentiated immature teratomas in stage Ia can be managed with surgery alone and careful follow-up. Poorly differentiated lesions or any tumor in a more advanced stage requires adjuvant chemotherapy with BEP or EP alone. In contrast to most other germ cell tumors, 75 percent of patients with endodermal sinus tumors present with pelvic pain. These aggressive tumors are rarely, if ever, bilateral and are treated with unilateral salpingo-oophorectomy, but adjuvant chemotherapy should be given in all cases. Embryonal carcinomas and the rare nongestational choriocarcinomas can be associated with precocious pseudopuberty or irregular menstrual bleeding. Conservative surgery can be undertaken to preserve reproductive function followed by adjuvant chemotherapy with BEP. Primary ovarian choriocarcinoma is less sensitive to cytotoxic chemotherapy than is gestational choriocarcinoma. Taken together, however, virtually all patients with stage I nondysgerminomatous germ cell tumors can be cured, and 50 to 80 percent of patients who present with disseminated disease also can attain long-term survival.

REFERENCES

ALBERTS DS et al: Improved therapeutic index of carboplatin plus cyclophosphamide versus cisplatin plus cyclophosphamide: Final report by the Southwest Oncology Group of a phase III randomized trial in stages III and IV ovarian cancer. J Clin Oncol 10:706, 1992

BAST RC JR et al: A radioimmunoassay using a monoclonal antibody to monitor the course of epithelial ovarian cancer. N Engl J Med 309:883, 1983

———— et al: Malignant transformation of ovarian epithelium. J Natl Cancer Inst 84:556, 1992

BERCHUCK A et al: Oncogenes in ovarian cancer. Hematol Oncol Clin North Am 6:813, 1992

BOOKMAN MA, BAST RC JR: The immunobiology and immunotherapy of ovarian cancer. Semin Oncol 18:270, 1991

CLARKE-PEARSON DL et al: Ovarian cancer, in *Comprehensive Textbook of Oncology*, 2d ed, AR Moossa et al (eds). Baltimore, William & Wilkins, 1991, pp 1006–1019

EINHORN N et al: Specificity of serum CA 125 radioimmunoassay for early detection of ovarian cancer: A prospective study. Obstet Gynecol 80:14, 1992

JACOBS I, BAST RC JR: Tumor markers for ovarian cancer, in *Manual of Clinical Laboratory Immunology*, 4th ed, NR Rose et al (eds). Washington, American Society for Microbiology, 1992, pp 811–816

JOHNSON SW et al: Mechanisms of drug resistance in ovarian cancer. Cancer 71 (2 suppl):594, 1993

LYNCH HT et al: Genetics and gynecologic cancer, in *Principles and Practice of Gynecologic Oncology*, WJ Hoskins et al (eds). Philadelphia, Lippincott, 1992, pp 27–45

MARKMAN M: Intraperitoneal chemotherapy. Semin Oncol 18:248, 1991

MCGUIRE WP, ROWINSKY EK: Old drugs revisited, new drugs, and experimental approaches in ovarian cancer therapy. Semin Oncol 18:255, 1991

OZOLS RF et al: Epithelial ovarian cancer, in *Principles and Practice of Gynecologic Oncology*, WJ Hoskins et al (eds). Philadelphia, Lippincott, 1992, pp 731–781

PIVER MS et al: Epidemiology and etiology of ovarian cancer. Semin Oncol 18:177, 1991

RUNOWICZ CD et al: Taxol in ovarian cancer. Cancer 71 (4 suppl):1591, 1993

SHPALL EJ et al: High-dose alkylating agent chemotherapy with autologous bone marrow support in patients with stage III/IV epithelial ovarian cancer. Gynecol Oncol 38:386, 1990

STANFORD JL: Oral contraceptives and neoplasia of the ovary. Contraception 43:543, 1991

SWENERTON K et al: Cisplatin-cyclophosphamide versus carboplatin-cyclophosphamide in advanced ovarian cancer: A randomized phase III study of the National Cancer Institute of Canada Clinical Trials Group. J Clin Oncol 10:718, 1992

VAN NAGELL JR JR et al: Ovarian cancer screening in asymptomatic postmenopausal women by transvaginal sonography. Cancer 68:458, 1991

WILLIAMS SD et al: Ovarian germ cell and stromal tumors, in *Principles and Practice of Gynecologic Oncology*, WJ Hoskins et al (eds). Philadelphia, Lippincott, 1992, pp 715–730

YOUNG RC et al: Adjuvant therapy in stage I and stage II epithelial ovarian cancer: Results of two prospective randomized trials. N Engl J Med 322:1021, 1990

322   TESTICULAR CANCER AND OTHER TROPHOBLASTIC DISEASES

MARC B. GARNICK

TESTICULAR CANCER

Carcinoma of the testis is a disease that serves as a model of a curable, solid neoplasm. Patients with localized forms of germinal cell cancer have a high cure rate when treated with either surgery or radiation therapy, and the advanced, metastatic forms, which in the past were almost universally fatal, are now also potentially curable. In 1977, testicular cancer was the third leading cause of cancer death in men between the ages of 15 and 34, but by 1981, the disease was no longer among the top five causes of cancer death in the same age group. The multidisciplinary principles and strategies that evolved for the management of patients with advanced testicular cancer are now being applied to other cancers.

Approximately 6600 new cases are diagnosed annually. The incidence in African-Americans is substantially lower than in whites. There is a peak frequency in early childhood and a larger peak incidence between 20 and 35 years. The disease is uncommon after age 40. A lesion suggestive of testicular neoplasm in a patient over the age of 50 should suggest a lymphoma rather than primary germinal cell carcinoma, especially with bilateral involvement of the testes.

Several factors are known to predispose to development of testicular tumor. Men with a history of cryptorchid (undescended) testes have a several-fold increased risk, intraabdominal testes being more at risk than high inguinal testes. Both the cryptorchid testis itself and the contralateral normally descended testis are at risk, suggesting that some underlying testicular defect may predispose both to maldescent and to tumor development. Although the effectiveness of orchiopexy in reducing risk is not established, it is generally agreed that a high inguinal testis should be brought into the scrotum so that it can be followed carefully. Abdominal testes that cannot be treated in this manner should probably be removed. Other predisposing factors include a history of mumps orchitis, inguinal hernia in childhood, and testicular cancer in the contralateral testis. In the majority of cases, no predisposing factor can be identified.

CLINICAL FEATURES AND DIAGNOSIS   The manifestations of testicular cancer range from an asymptomatic nodule or swelling detected while performing testicular self-examination to dyspnea secondary to massive pulmonary metastases. Most testicular cancers are diagnosed because of symptoms related to the testes, but significant delay in making a diagnosis is common and is the result of oversight by physicians and by patients. Thus high school health programs that teach testicular self-examination should be encouraged. Such programs have allowed early diagnosis, leading to more successful treatment outcomes. Most testicular cancers occur in men under age 40, and the public should be educated to the need to seek prompt medical advice for any change in previously normal testes, including the presence of a mass, a feeling of heaviness, pain, hardness, and swelling. Other causes of testicular masses include hydrocele, epididymitis, spermatocele, and orchitis, but to reduce delay in reaching a diagnosis, physicians should consider any testicular mass to be malignant until proven otherwise. Patients with testicular tumors may have pain because of associated nonneoplastic lesions, such as epididymitis.

Back or abdominal pain secondary to retroperitoneal adenopathy, weight loss, dyspnea secondary to pulmonary metastases, gynecomastia, supraclavicular lymphadenopathy, and urinary obstruction also may be present at diagnosis.

A testicular sonogram can aid in establishing the presence of a testicular parenchymal abnormality. Magnetic resonance imaging of the testis can sometimes provide useful information when the results of the physical examination and testicular ultrasound are equivocal. Once the diagnosis of a testicular neoplasm is suspected, a blood sample should be set aside, prior to orchiectomy, for subsequent determination of the tumor marker glycoproteins alpha fetoprotein (AFP) and human chorionic gonadotropin (hCG). The correct operative approach is a high radical inguinal orchiectomy. A transscrotal biopsy of the testis or a transscrotal orchiectomy should never be performed if the diagnosis of testicular cancer is likely. Because the lymphatic drainage of the testis (to the retroperitoneal lymphatics between L1 and L3) differs from that of the scrotum (to superficial and deep inguinal groin nodes), a scrotal incision in the presence of a testicular cancer may predispose to the development of local recurrences and metastases to the inguinal lymphatics. This rarely happens if a high radical inguinal orchiectomy is performed.

CLASSIFICATION AND PATHOLOGY   The most widely used classification of testicular tumors is that of Mostofi and is based on the cell type from which the tumor is derived, namely germinal or stromal (Leydig and Sertoli) cells (Table 322-1). Germinal cell tumors, the most common of these tumors and the focus of this chapter, can be subdivided into seminomas and nonseminomas. Seminomas are characterized by large cells with clear cytoplasm in a delicate fibrovascular stroma infiltrated with lymphocytes. Indeed, the granulomatous reaction around the tumor can be so intense as to

---

TABLE 322-1   Classification of testicular tumors

Germinal cell tumors (95%)
  Single cell tumors (60%)
    Seminomas
    Nonseminomas
      Embryonal cell tumors (yolk sac tumors)
      Teratomas
      Choriocarcinomas
  Combination tumors (40%)
Tumors of gonadal stroma (1–2%)
  Leydig cell
  Sertoli cell
  Primitive gonadal structures
Gonadoblastoma (germinal cell + stomal cell)

SOURCE: After FK Mostofi, Cancer 45:1735, 1980.

suggest a graft-versus-host reaction. These tumors account for about half of all testicular neoplasms and can be divided into typical, spermatocytic, and anaplastic varieties. Germinal cell tumors of the nonseminoma type can be divided into embryonal cell tumors (yolk sac tumors), teratomas, and choriocarcinomas. Embryonal carcinomas are common in children and resemble embryonal carcinomas of the ovary. Choriocarcinomas contain syncytiotrophoblastic cells. Teratomas contain at least two types of germinal cell layers and in childhood are second in frequency to embryonal tumor. Mixed tumors that contain combinations of germinal cell types account for 40 percent of germinal cell tumors; the biology of such tumors is usually determined by the least differentiated (most malignant) elements. All four types of germinal cell tumors also can originate in extragonadal sites, most commonly the mediastinum or brain. Such extragonadal tumors are presumed to arise either from aberrant migration of germinal cells during embryogenesis or, alternatively, from some common precursor stem cell line that gives rise to the germinal cells, the thymus, and the pineal.

From the clinical standpoint, the critical distinction is between _seminomas_ and _nonseminomas_ based on the histopathology of the orchiectomy specimen. The former must be in pure form; the latter may either be a mixed cancer with both seminomatous and nonseminomatous components or a pure form of a nonseminoma, such as embryonal cell carcinoma, teratoma, or choriocarcinoma. The term _teratocarcinoma_ generally refers to a mixed nonseminomatous cancer consisting of teratoma and embryonal cell cancer.

The distinction between seminoma and nonseminoma is important because the staging evaluation and subsequent management in the two differ as a consequence of the relative radioresponsiveness of seminomas compared with the radioresistance of nonseminomas. Radiation therapy to the lymphatics of the abdomen and/or chest is the mainstay of therapy in patients with pure seminoma but is rarely utilized in patients with nonseminoma. In addition, seminomas usually spread via the regional lymphatics to the retroperitoneal nodes of the abdomen and/or to the mediastinal and supraclavicular lymph nodes before gaining access to other visceral structures. Pulmonary and other hematogenous metastases (e.g., hepatic, central nervous system, osseous) are more common in patients with nonseminomas than in patients with seminomas.

BIOLOGIC AND MOLECULAR TUMOR MARKERS Germinal cell cancers of the testis often secrete biologic tumor markers that can be detected in the peripheral blood (see Chap. 327). Following orchiectomy, the presence of such markers in blood reflects the presence of metastatic disease. Such assays also can be valuable in monitoring therapy (marker levels fall with disease regression and increase with disease progression), and elevated levels in blood may predate the detection of new clinical or radiologic metastatic disease by weeks to months. The two most common markers are AFP and hCG. AFP is commonly secreted by embryonal cell cancer; its biologic half-life is approximately 6 days. AFP is not produced by pure seminoma, and its detection implies the presence of nonseminomatous elements, either in the primary lesion itself or in the metastatic site, even when the primary orchiectomy specimen is thought to be a pure seminoma. hCG is secreted by syncytiotrophoblastic giant cells, present most commonly in choriocarcinomas; such giant cells may be present in embryonal cell components and occasionally in so-called pure seminomas. The biologic half-life of hCG is approximately 24 h. hCG may be biologically active, and hCG-enhanced secretion of estrogen by the testis is the cause of gynecomastia in such patients (see Chap. 341). Several cytogenetic markers have recently been associated with germ cell cancer of the testis. Isochromosome 12p(i)(12p) is present in the majority of all forms of germ cell neoplasms and when present in multiple copies may be associated with a poorer prognosis.

STAGING EVALUATION The function of staging is to determine whether the cancer is localized to the testis or to regional lymphatics or is widely disseminated. Such information is necessary to determine if disease is amenable to local or regional therapy. If the disease is disseminated at presentation, the initial staging evaluation serves as a baseline in assessing subsequent response. Since the approach to staging and management is dictated by the pathologic diagnosis of the orchiectomy specimen, the appropriate evaluation will be outlined for each.

Pure seminoma The routine workup involves careful physical examination, an abdominal-pelvic computed tomographic (CT) scan to determine the presence of retroperitoneal adenopathy or visceral involvement, a chest x-ray with or without lung tomography, measurement of routine chemistries, and assessment of the biologic markers (AFP and hCG). In most cases, the biologic markers are undetectable. If AFP is elevated, the patient should be treated as having a nonseminoma, even though the pathologic interpretation is pure seminoma.

The portals for radiation therapy for pure seminomas were traditionally determined on the basis of bipedal lymphangiography. However, the necessity of lymphangiography for such purposes is less imperative today because CT scanning may provide similar information.

If plasma hCG is elevated in a patient with a diagnosis of pure seminoma, a search should be made for syncytiotrophoblastic giant cells. Otherwise, there may be some uncertainty as to whether occult foci of nonseminomatous components are responsible for the hCG production. Also, if the physical or radiographic examinations fail to reveal any evidence of metastatic disease and the hCG level is elevated before orchiectomy, it is necessary to follow the level of hCG sequentially. If the marker does not decline as predicted by its biologic half-life, the presence of occult metastatic cancer should be considered.

Nonseminoma The staging evaluation outlined for the seminoma is employed for the patient with a nonseminomatous germinal cell tumor of the testis. On the basis of these noninvasive staging studies, patients can be categorized as having stage I, early stage II, advanced stage II, or stage III disease. Patients with stage I disease have no clinical, radiographic, or marker evidence of tumor presence beyond the confines of the testis. Patients with early stage II have nonpalpable, small, retroperitoneal adenopathy on CT scans, usually measuring <4 to 5 cm. Advanced stage II is defined as retroperitoneal lymphadenopathy measuring >5 cm on CT scan or palpable retroperitoneal adenopathy with disease limited to lymphatics below the diaphragm. Stage III disease includes visceral involvement below the diaphragm (e.g., liver or bowel) or above the diaphragm (e.g., lung or supraclavicular lymphadenopathy). Furthermore, patients with stage III disease can be further subdivided according to anatomic location and extent of disease. Treatment decisions are often based on volume of disease in stage III patients.

Conceptually, patients with testicular cancer can be categorized pathologically as having either _seminoma_ or _nonseminoma_ and staged as having either "early" or "advanced" disease. Patients with _early_ disease would be considered to have stage I and early stage II disease, while patients with _advanced_ disease have advanced stage II or any form of stage III disease. This formulation allows rational decision making for nearly all categories of disease.

TREATMENT MODALITIES ACCORDING TO HISTOLOGY AND STAGE (Table 322-2) **Early seminoma** These patients have either a normal abdominal CT scan or retroperitoneal lymphadenopathy measuring less than 5 cm in greatest diameter. Most such patients are treated with abdominal radiotherapy, delivering 30 Gy (3000 rad) to the subdiaphragmatic lymph nodes and ipsilateral groin and a 6-Gy (600-rad) boost in areas of known disease. Although prophylactic mediastinal and supraclavicular radiation therapy was used in the past, this practice is generally not employed today. When treated with radiation following orchiectomy, patients with clinical stage I disease have a 95 to 97 percent cure rate, and patients with early stage II disease have an 85 to 90 percent survival rate.

As with stage I nonseminoma (see below), a policy of surveillance has been recommended for stage I seminoma following orchiectomy. This strategy potentially avoids the use of radiotherapy in patients cured with orchiectomy alone. In those who relapse, radiotherapy or

TABLE 322-2   Testicular cancer: General approach to management and cure rates*

	Seminoma	% Cure	Nonseminoma	% Cure
Stage I	XRT or surveillance[†]	95–97	RPLND or surveillance[†]	97
Early stage II	XRT	85–90	RPLND ± chemo[a] or Chemo[a]	85–90
Advanced stage II Stage III	Chemo[a]	80–85	Chemo[a] ± TRS ± Chemo[b]	80–85

* XRT = radiation therapy, delivered to subdiaphragmatic lymphatics; RPLND = retroperitoneal lymph node dissection; chemo[a] = combination chemotherapy (see Table 322-3); TRS = tumor-reductive surgery; chemo[b] = additional chemotherapy given if surgical specimen reveals viable cancer.
[†] Must be done in context of clinical protocol, with detailed follow-up and a compliant patient.

chemotherapy is then instituted with excellent results. Such surveillance programs must be performed within the context of a clinical trial and require highly motivated and compliant patients.

Advanced seminoma   In the past, patients with large retroperitoneal masses or mediastinal involvement were often treated with radiation therapy to fields including the subdiaphragmatic lymph nodes, whole abdomen, mediastinum, and supraclavicular nodes; however, survival rates were only 40 to 70 percent. If these patients subsequently suffered a relapse in an area outside the radiation therapy field, the ability to administer myelosuppressive combination chemotherapy was diminished and was associated with drug-related morbidity. Today, most patients with advanced forms of seminoma are treated initially with combination chemotherapy that includes cisplatin. Substantial tumor shrinkage occurs in the majority of patients. However, the proper management for partially regressed retroperitoneal masses following chemotherapy is controversial. Patients are restaged following chemotherapy, and depending on the individual treatment protocol, further treatment with chemotherapy, surgery, or radiation therapy is addressed.

Stage I nonseminoma   Patients with stage I nonseminoma are routinely treated with a retroperitoneal lymph node dissection (RPLND), using either a transabdominal or a thoracoabdominal approach. The rationale for this operation is based on the inexact data generated from the noninvasive staging evaluation of the retroperitoneal lymphatics. The false-negative rate of abdominal CT scans in patients with clinical stage I disease is 35 to 40 percent. Thus surgical removal of the retroperitoneal lymph nodes not only serves as therapy but also determines the need for possible additional therapy. If microscopic disease is detected and surgically removed, an 85 to 90 percent cure rate can be expected following RPLND.

More recently, a policy of orchiectomy followed by surveillance has been used for selected stage I nonseminoma patients. This strategy avoids a retroperitoneal lymph node dissection in a large percentage of patients. If relapse occurs, chemotherapy can then be instituted, with achievement of greater than 90 percent cure rates.

Stage II nonseminoma   The optimal management of patients with retroperitoneal lymphadenopathy measuring between 2 and 5 cm on CT scan is controversial. While RPLND may be curative, a relapse rate of 30 to 45 percent can be expected. If relapse occurs after RPLND, combination chemotherapy can be administered, or chemotherapy may sometimes be given as an adjuvant to RPLND. Alternatively, combination chemotherapy can be given prior to RPLND. If complete resolution of disease is achieved following chemotherapy, RPLND would not be performed, obviating the need for the operation in this subset of patients.

Advanced stage (bulky stage II or stage III) nonseminoma   The most common chemotherapy program includes cisplatin, bleomycin, and etoposide (BEP program). Other very active chemotherapeutic agents used in association with cisplatin include vinblastine and bleomycin (PVB program) or actinomycin D, cyclophosphamide,

TABLE 322-3   Commonly used chemotherapy programs for advanced testicular cancer

BEP	PVB	VAB-6
Etoposide	Vinblastine	Vinblastine
Bleomycin	Bleomycin	Bleomycin
Cisplatin	Cisplatin	Cisplatin
		Cyclophosphamide
		Actinomycin D

vinblastine, and bleomycin (VAB program) (Table 322-3). The use of these agents is associated with complete remission in as many as 80 to 85 percent of patients when administered cyclically over a 9- to 12-week period.

Following such therapy, patients are then restaged (with physical, radiographic, and biochemical examinations) to assess the response of areas which previously contained disease and to determine the need for additional therapy. Large abdominal masses may undergo astonishing regression. Pulmonary nodules often resolve completely, and biologic markers frequently return to normal after chemotherapy. If a residual abdominal or pulmonary mass persists despite normal levels of plasma markers, surgical removal of the mass(es) should be undertaken. Table 322-4 outlines current recommendations. Preoperatively, it is difficult to determine the nature of such residual masses. Approximately 20 percent contain residual, viable cancer; 40 percent contain fibrosis, necrosis, or hemorrhage; and an additional 40 percent demonstrate the phenomenon of "teratomatous transformation." The latter is thought to result either from chemotherapy-induced differentiation of the primary mass into a teratoma or from the selective elimination of the more malignant elements of the mass but persistence of residual teratomatous components. If either fibrosis, hemorrhage, or teratoma is found following chemotherapy, additional postoperative chemotherapy is usually not indicated. If, however, residual cancer is demonstrated, additional cisplatin combination chemotherapy is required.

If biologic markers are persistently positive following remission induction chemotherapy, additional chemotherapy is also indicated. "Tumor-reductive" surgery should not be attempted until biologic markers return to normal in most cases. Some patients experience complete resolution of physical, radiographic, and biochemical marker abnormalities after cisplatin-containing chemotherapy and may require no additional chemotherapy or surgery following their program of chemotherapy.

Testicular cancer which is refractory of BEP or other cisplatin-containing programs may sometimes respond to the addition of ifosfamide. Ifosfamide has been approved by the FDA for third-line treatment with other antineoplastics for patients with refractory germ cell tumors. The combination of cisplatin, etoposide, and ifosfamide will result in a second or third remission, which may be durable, in approximately 25 percent of patients. The use of autologous bone marrow transplantation with high-dose chemotherapy remains a

TABLE 322-4   Advanced testicular cancer, nonseminoma: Approach to management after initial chemotherapy

Biologic markers*	Radiographic abnormalities	Therapeutic choice
Positive	Present or absent	Additional chemotherapy[†]
Normal	Present	TRS[‡] ± chemotherapy[§]
Normal	Absent	Observation

* Alpha fetoprotein and human chorionic gonadotropin.
[†] Chemotherapy with a "second-line" program, with attempts to "normalize" biologic markers.
[‡] Tumor-reductive surgery.
[§] Additional chemotherapy determined by presence of "viable" cancer in surgical specimen. Chemotherapy withheld if surgical specimen contains only fibrosis or teratoma.

potential therapy for patients with refractory germ cell tumors. Although still investigational, a small percentage of patients can achieve long-term remission and even cure.

FOLLOW-UP OF PATIENTS WITH TESTICULAR CANCER All patients with testicular cancer, regardless of pathology or stage, require meticulous follow-up with monthly physical examinations, chest x-rays, and assessment of markers for 18 to 24 months. Patients with stage I disease who are treated with a surveillance policy following orchiectomy will need frequent abdominal-pelvic CT scanning in addition to the other follow-up evaluations. The frequency of these tests can be decreased in the third or fourth year following diagnosis. The goal is to detect relapse when the tumor burden is minimal. Most relapses from testicular cancer occur within the first 2 years following diagnosis, but late relapses do occur.

SIDE EFFECTS OF THERAPY   **Radiation therapy and surgery** Infertility can result both from radiation therapy and RPLND. Because these modalities are generally reserved for the management of early-stage patients, a full discussion with patients about the potential loss of fertility is appropriate. Although of questionable benefit, the possibility of sperm banking should be considered prior to the initiation of either definitive radiation therapy for early-stage seminomas or RPLND for early-stage nonseminomas. Modifications in the surgical technique of RPLND (limited nerve-sparing dissection) may decrease the incidence of fertility loss and ejaculatory disturbances.

Combination chemotherapy   When standard BEP programs are employed, the major side effects are myelosuppression, potential for nephrotoxicity, nausea and vomiting, weight loss, anemia, ileus, pulmonary toxicity, ototoxicity, peripheral neuropathy, Raynaud's phenomenon, alopecia, hypomagnesemia, and stomatitis. Neuromuscular and gastrointestinal toxicity were more frequent in vinblastine-containing programs. Infertility is usual during therapy, although fertility may return years after completion of therapy. The use of the chemotherapy programs requires skill on the part of the treating physician and should not be attempted by the occasional user. With proper expertise, these side effects can often be minimized. Hemorrhagic cystitis, which can occur with ifosfamide, can be minimized by concomitant use of the uroprotector mesna.

Bleomycin is known to cause pulmonary toxicity (see Chap. 218), and special precautions must be taken in patients who have received bleomycin and are scheduled for a surgical procedure. The acute respiratory distress syndrome has occurred in some and is thought to be related to excessive fluid overload and high inspired oxygen concentration (FI_{O_2}) during the operative procedure. Current recommendations now call for the FI_{O_2} to be maintained at ≤24 percent and for patients to be kept in a hypovolemic or euvolemic state in the perioperative period. Such measures seem to minimize the postoperative pulmonary complications. Hypercholesterolemia is found in a substantial percentage of cured patients years following completion of cisplatin-containing therapy.

THE EXTRAGONADAL GERMINAL CELL SYNDROME   Patients with extragonadal germinal cell tumors may present with a large anterior mediastinal mass, central nervous system abnormalities, or retroperitoneal disease. The response to therapy is generally lower when compared with primary testicular cancer, justifying the need for more intensive therapy. Many patients relapse years after the original diagnosis, leading to a lower cure rate compared with patients with primary testicular cancer. However, a proportion of these patients may be cured when treated with chemotherapy and tumor-reductive surgery. In addition, patients with ''undifferentiated'' cancer of the mediastinum or retroperitoneum may have an unrecognized form of extragonadal germinal cell cancer. Biologic markers and immunohistochemical staining of the biopsy material for AFP or hCG may provide useful clues. If positive, these patients should be treated as if they have potentially curable advanced testicular cancer. Extragonadal germ cell neoplasms have been associated with a spectrum of non-treatment-related hematologic abnormalities, including idiopathic thrombocytopenia, acute megakaryocytic leukemia, myelodysplasia, and malignant histiocytosis.

OTHER TROPHOBLASTIC DISEASES

Trophoblastic tumors of females encompass all proliferative trophoblastic growths that develop from pregnancy and are hence entitled *gestational trophoblastic neoplasms*. Gestational trophoblastic tumors arise most commonly from antecedent molar pregnancies but also may follow term and ectopic pregnancy and spontaneous abortions. The incidence of choriocarcinoma occurring during a term pregnancy is approximately 1 in 150,000, and approximately 75 percent of these patients demonstrate metastatic disease, the lungs being the most frequent site of metastases. The incidence of choriocarcinoma occurring with an ectopic pregnancy is approximately 1 in 5000; the incidence with spontaneous abortion is approximately 1 in 15,000.

Pathologically, the morphology of gestational trophoblastic neoplasms includes the complete and partial hydatidiform mole, invasive mole, and choriocarcinoma. The distinction between *complete* and *partial* is based on gross and microscopic appearance and karyotype. Complete moles usually demonstrate the absence of fetal or embryonic tissue; such tissue is present in a partial mole. Most complete moles have a 46,XX chromosome pattern; partial moles generally have a triploid karyotype, with the extra set of chromosomes of paternal derivation.

Based on data generated by the New England Trophoblastic Disease Center, presenting signs of patients with complete hydatidiform mole are abnormal vaginal bleeding (>90 percent), anemia (>50 percent), enlargement of the uterus (>50 percent), toxemia of pregnancy (25 percent), hyperemesis gravidarum (25 percent), and infrequently, hyperthyroidism and trophoblastic emboli to the lung. Patients with trophoblastic moles often present with the signs and symptoms of a spontaneous abortion, with vaginal bleeding being the most common feature.

Following evacuation of the molar pregnancy, approximately 15 percent of patients demonstrate localized uterine invasion, and 4 percent demonstrate metastatic disease, most often associated with choriocarcinoma.

Gestational trophoblastic neoplasms can be staged according to the FIGO staging system. Stage I is tumor localized to the uterus; stage II is tumor involving the pelvis and/or vagina; stage III is tumor involving the lung; stage IV is tumor involving other organs. The stage of the patient is generally determined after an extensive diagnostic evaluation, including a history and physical examination, measurement of hCG levels, and routine biochemical and hematologic evaluation. The metastatic workup generally includes a chest x-ray, abdominal-pelvic ultrasonography, evaluation of the liver for hepatic metastases, and, on occasion, angiography of abdominal or pelvic organs. In individuals with choriocarcinoma and documented metastases, hCG values are often measured in the cerebral spinal fluid to detect asymptomatic central nervous system involvement. Likewise, stool guaiac tests are often done to rule out lesions to the gastrointestinal tract.

The most important aspect of gestational trophoblastic neoplasms is the fact that there is a 100 percent cure rate in patients with stages I to III and approximately an 85 percent cure rate in patients with stage IV. Depending on the extent of disease and the level of hCG in the bloodstream, individuals are treated with evacuation of their pregnancy or chemotherapy. For patients having a good prognosis, single-agent methotrexate or actinomycin D are generally employed, while high-risk patients are generally treated with combination chemotherapy, including methotrexate, actinomycin D, and cyclophosphamide. More recently, for patients with evidence of metastatic disease, more intensive programs, including vinblastine, bleomycin, and cisplatin, have been used with excellent success. Treatment is continued until baselines of hCG have returned to normal.

Many patients can expect normal reproductive function following treatment. There is, however, an increased incidence of repeat episodes of moles or gestational trophoblastic neoplasms in subsequent pregnancies. The sequential determination of hCG has been extremely valuable in the monitoring of such patients.

REFERENCES

BERKOWITZ RS, GOLDSTEIN DP: Management of molar pregnancy and gestation trophoblastic disease, in *Gynecologic Oncology*, RC Knapp, RS Berkowitz (eds). New York, Macmillan, 1986

BOYLE P, ZARIDZE DG: Risk factors for prostate and testicular cancer. Eur J Cancer 29A(7):1048, 1993

EINHORN EH, DONOHUE JP: *cis*-Diamminedichloroplatinum, vinblastine, and bleomycin combination chemotherapy in disseminated testicular cancer. Ann Intern Med 87:293, 1977

FUNG CY, GARNICK MB: Clinical stage I carcinoma of the testis: A review. J Clin Oncol 6:734, 1988

GARNICK MB: Advanced testicular cancer: Treatment choices in the "land of plenty" (editorial). J Clin Oncol 3:294, 1985

GIETEMA JA et al: Long-term follow-up of cardiovascular risk factors in patients given chemotherapy for disseminated nonseminomatous testicular cancer. Ann Intern Med 116:709, 1992

NICHOLS CR et al: Hematologic neoplasia associated with primary mediastinal germ cell tumors: An update. N Engl J Med 322:1425, 1990

POTTERN LM et al: Testicular cancer risk among young men: Role of cryptorchidism and inguinal hernia. J Natl Cancer Inst 74:377, 1985

ROTH BJ, NICHOLS CR (eds): Testicular cancer. Semin Oncol 19:117, 118, 1992

STEPHENS RL, WILLIAMSON SK: Clinical stage I testicular cancer: Orchiectomy without node dissection (editorial). Ann Intern Med 109:179, 1988

WILLIAMS SD et al: Treatment of disseminated germ-cell tumors with cisplatin, bleomycin, and either vinblastine or etoposide. N Engl J Med 316:1435, 1987

—— et al: Immediate adjuvant chemotherapy versus observation with treatment at relapse in pathological stage II testicular cancer. N Engl J Med 317:1433, 1987

323 HYPERPLASIA AND CARCINOMA OF THE PROSTATE

ARTHUR I. SAGALOWSKY / JEAN D. WILSON

PROSTATIC HYPERPLASIA

Development of prostatic hyperplasia is an almost universal phenomenon in aging men. The prostate weighs only a few grams at birth; at puberty it undergoes androgen-mediated growth and reaches the adult size of about 20 g by age 20. It remains stable in size for about 25 years, and during the fifth decade a second growth spurt commences in the majority of men. Consequently, the disorder affects men over the age of 45 and increases in frequency with age so that by the eighth decade more than 90 percent of men have prostatic hyperplasia at autopsy. Because of refinements in prostatic surgery, the disorder is not a major cause of death, but it is a leading cause of morbidity in elderly men. The prostate surrounds the urethra, and prostatic hyperplasia is the most common cause of obstruction to urinary outflow in men. Overall, prostatic surgery is performed in about 10 percent of men at some time. The disorder occurs in all populations but is less common in the Orient. The mean age for development of symptomatic disease is about 65 years for whites and about 60 years for blacks. Prostatic hyperplasia does not predispose to the development of prostatic cancer.

PATHOGENESIS Unlike the pubertal growth spurt which involves the gland diffusely, prostatic hyperplasia begins in the periurethral region as a localized proliferation and progresses to compress the remaining normal gland. Histologically, the hyperplastic tissue is nodular and composed of varying amounts of glandular epithelium, stroma, and smooth muscle. The hyperplasia can compress and obstruct the urethra; rarely, the hyperplastic gland grows posteriorly to obstruct the rectum and cause constipation.

The pathogenesis is not well understood, but two necessary features for the process are aging and the presence of testes; whether the testes play a direct or permissive role is not known, but the active androgen that mediates prostatic growth at all ages is dihydrotestosterone, which is formed within the prostate from plasma testosterone (see Chap. 339). In the castrated dog, hormonal therapy that increases

dihydrotestosterone levels in the prostate causes prostatic enlargement comparable with that seen in spontaneous canine prostatic hyperplasia. Estradiol levels in men increase with age (absolutely or relative to testosterone levels), and in dogs estrogen acts synergistically with dihydrotestosterone to induce prostatic growth by enhancing the amount of androgen receptor protein in the tissue. Consequently, the role of aging in the development of prostatic hyperplasia might be explained if estradiol augments dihydrotestosterone action in humans as well.

DIAGNOSIS Urethral obstruction results from the elongation, tortuosity, and compression of the posterior urethra, but there is no straightforward relationship between obstruction and prostate size; indeed, severe obstruction can occur when the hyperplasia does not exceed the size of the normal gland. Early symptoms can be minimal because compensatory hypertrophy of the detrusor musculature of the bladder can compensate for the resistance to urine flow. With increasing obstruction, diminution in the caliber and force of the urinary stream, hesitancy in initiating voiding, postvoiding dribbling, the sensation of incomplete emptying, and on occasion urinary retention supervene. These *obstructive* symptoms must be distinguished from *irritative* symptoms such as dysuria, frequency, and urgency that also can result from inflammatory, infectious, or neoplastic causes. As the amount of residual urine increases, nocturia, overflow urinary incontinence, and a palpable bladder may be present. Eventually, the manifestations of chronic urinary retention and obstruction supervene, or acute urinary retention can be precipitated by infection, tranquilizing drugs, or alcohol. On occasion, profound obstruction can be compensated to the extent that symptoms are minimal or absent, and patients present with obstructive uropathy.

During digital rectal examination, the prostate should be characterized with regard to size, consistency, and shape. Hyperplasia commonly produces a smooth, firm, elastic enlargement, but obstruction can occur in the absence of abnormalities on rectal examination. Ultrasonography with a rectal probe or magnetic resonance imaging allows a quantitative estimate of prostate size but ordinarily provides no information beyond that provided by rectal examination. The presence of upper urinary tract obstruction and the extent of bladder emptying can be documented by an intravenous pyelogram with postvoiding film or renal sonogram with sonographic determination of bladder residual urine. Cystourethroscopy is indicated to evaluate vesicle neck obstruction. Measurement of urine flow rate and/or residual urine volume is recommended to document the degree of obstruction to outflow. More detailed urodynamic evaluation is occasionally required to rule out other causes of voiding dysfunction such as neurogenic bladder.

TREATMENT Because the majority of men above age 60 have some degree of prostatic hyperplasia, the presence of the disorder by itself is not an indication for treatment. In men who lack definite indications for intervention, it is advisable that they be examined periodically to determine the natural history of the process. Many patients who receive no therapy experience no progression in symptoms over many years. Several forms of medical or surgical treatment exist for men with more advanced symptoms. Treatment with luteinizing hormone–releasing hormone (LHRH) analogues or an inhibitor of the steroid 5α-reductase enzyme (finasteride) shrinks prostatic glandular hyperplasia by lowering tissue dihydrotestosterone levels. Therapy with alpha-adrenergic antagonists lowers bladder neck and urethral resistance but is not approved by the U.S. Food and Drug Administration for this purpose. Both finasteride and alpha-adrenergic antagonists produce moderate and durable improvements in symptoms in some patients and may be useful in symptomatic patients who do not wish to undergo surgery, but the long-term effectiveness of medical therapy is not established.

Surgery has been and is still the benchmark treatment. Indications for surgery include decrease in urine flow of sufficient magnitude to cause discomfort, persistent residual urine, acute urinary retention due to obstruction with no reversible precipitating cause, and hydronephrosis. Transurethral prostatectomy is the usual procedure of choice.

Open prostatectomy for massive glands may employ either retropubic, suprapubic, or perineal approaches. Newer surgical alternatives include simple transurethral incision prostatotomy or transurethral laser-induced prostatectomy. Nonsurgical interventional therapies receiving intense study include indwelling urethral stents and balloon dilatation of the prostate.

PROSTATIC CARCINOMA

Cancer of the prostate is the most common malignancy in men in the United States and is the second most common cause of cancer death in men above age 55 (after carcinomas of the lung and colon). In the United States there are approximately 132,000 newly diagnosed cases and more than 33,000 deaths from the disorder each year. Only about a third of cases identified at autopsy are manifest clinically. The disease is rare before age 50, and the incidence increases with age. The frequency varies in different parts of the world. The United States has 14 deaths per 100,000 men per year compared with 22 for Sweden and 2 for Japan. However, Japanese immigrants to the United States develop prostatic cancer at a frequency similar to other men in this country, suggesting that an environmental factor is the principal cause for population differences. The disease is more common among American blacks than whites; the reason for this difference is not known.

CLASSIFICATION Some carcinomas of the prostate are slow-growing and may persist for long periods without causing significant symptoms, whereas others behave aggressively. It is not known whether tumors can become more malignant with time. Insight into the natural history of a given tumor is provided by careful histopathologic grading, surgical evaluation of the pelvic lymph nodes, and measurement of the primary lesion, a size less than 1.5 mL in volume carrying a good prognosis.

Histologic grading Over 95 percent of prostatic cancers are adenocarcinomas that arise in the prostatic acini. Adenocarcinoma may begin anywhere in the prostate but has a predilection for the periphery. The tumors are frequently multifocal. Variability in cellular size, nuclear and nucleolar shape, glandular differentiation, and the content of acid phosphatase and mucin may occur within a single specimen, but the most poorly differentiated area of tumor (i.e., the area with the highest histologic grade) appears to determine its biologic behavior. In the Gleason grading scheme, the dominant and any other glandular histologic patterns are independently assigned numbers from 1 to 5 (best to least differentiated), and these numbers are summed to give a total score of 2 to 10 for each tumor. Such grading is reproducible and correlates with the course of the disease and with patient survival.

The remaining prostatic cancers are divided among squamous cell and transitional cell carcinomas that arise in the prostatic ducts, carcinoma of the prostatic utricle (a müllerian duct remnant), carcinosarcomas that arise in the mesenchymal elements of the gland, and occasional metastatic tumors (usually carcinoma of the lung, melanoma, or lymphoma). These tumors will not be considered further.

DIAGNOSIS **Symptoms and signs** Both early and advanced carcinoma of the prostate may be asymptomatic at the time of diagnosis, and more than 80 percent of patients have stage C or D disease at the time of diagnosis (see below). In symptomatic subjects, common presenting complaints (in descending order) include dysuria, difficulty in voiding, increased urinary frequency, complete urinary retention, back or hip pain, and hematuria. A high index of suspicion should be entertained in all men over age 40 with dysuria, frequency, or difficulty in voiding in the absence of mechanical urethral obstruction. Additional complications of advanced disease may include spinal cord compression for dual metastases, deep venous thrombosis and pulmonary emboli, and myelophthisis.

Digital rectal examination Palpation of the prostate is the most appropriate test for detection of all stages of disease other than stage A. Indeed, the importance of the rectal examination in the routine physical examination of men cannot be stressed too strongly. The posterior surfaces of the lateral lobes, where carcinoma begins most often, are easily palpable on digital rectal examination. Carcinoma characteristically is hard, nodular, and irregular, but induration also may be due to fibrous areas in benign prostatic hyperplasia, to focal infarcts, or to calculi as well as to tumor. The midline furrow between the lateral lobes may be obscured by either benign or malignant enlargement. Local extraprostatic extension of tumor into the seminal vesicles also can be detected by rectal examination. Scrotal and/or lower extremity lymphedema secondary to infiltration of pelvic lymph nodes indicates extensive disease.

Biochemical markers Elevation of serum prostate-specific antigen (PSA) level is the most sensitive test for the early detection of prostatic cancer. PSA level may be elevated with localized disease, whereas elevation of acid phosphatase level usually indicates extraprostatic disease. Following diagnosis and treatment, serial determinations of PSA are the best available means for assessing response. No technique of assay for either PSA or acid phosphatase (including counterimmune electrophoresis and radioimmunoassay) is sufficiently specific or sensitive for routine screening studies, and serum PSA level can be elevated in benign states, including prostatic hyperplasia, prostatitis, and prostatic infarction.

Imaging With the use of transrectal prostatic sonography, carcinoma is revealed as hypoechoic densities within the peripheral zone. The procedure is a sensitive means of identifying prostate cancer but is not specific enough for use as a screening test. Ultrasonography is also useful for directing needle biopsy and for documenting the degree of extension of the tumor into bladder and seminal vesicles. Magnetic resonance imaging (MRI) and to a lesser degree computed tomography (CT) of the prostate also may be helpful in defining the extent of tumor and locating nodes for aspiration needle biopsy. Transrectal prostatic sonography is recommended if either the digital rectal examination is positive or the PSA level is elevated. The findings on sonography, the amount of PSA elevation relative to prostate size, and the index of suspicion for carcinoma by history all affect the decision of whether or not to perform a biopsy. The combined use of these modalities allows early detection of large numbers of prostatic cancers and an increased proportion of localized and curable lesions. The biologic significance of individual lesions remains to be defined. Whether early diagnosis leads to improved survival and decreased morbidity from prostatic cancer requires further study.

Biopsy Biopsy of the prostate is essential for establishing the diagnosis and is indicated when an abnormality is detected by palpation or elevation of serum PSA level and/or by imaging or when lower urinary tract symptoms occur in men who have no known cause of obstruction. Core-needle biopsy may be performed transperineally or transrectally with less risk of bacterial contamination with the former and more precise sampling with the latter. Transrectal prostatic biopsy with a rapid-fire spring-loaded needle under sonography provides the most accurate sampling of the index lesion and the remainder of the gland and is the preferred technique. Fine-needle aspiration cytology offers immediate diagnosis with minimal patient discomfort and morbidity. Open perineal biopsy is performed infrequently because it carries the risk of at least temporary impotence and is a more extensive surgical procedure. Transurethral biopsy is also used infrequently because most early lesions are in the peripheral reigons of the gland.

Staging and assessment of metastatic disease Adenocarcinoma of the prostate may spread by three routes: direct extension, the lymphatics, and the bloodstream. The prostatic capsule is a natural boundary against growth of tumor into adjacent structures, but direct extension occurs upward into the seminal vesicles and bladder floor. Lymphatic spread can best be assessed by surgical exploration; the frequency with which it occurs correlates with the size and histologic grade of the tumor. Only about one-tenth of tumors with a grade of less than 5 have lymph node involvement, while more than 70 percent of tumors with a Gleason grade of 9 or 10 have coexisting lymphatic invasion at the time of diagnosis. The route of lymphatic spread (in decreasing order) is to obturator, internal iliac, common iliac, presacral, and paraaortic nodes. Hematogenous metastases occur to bone (pelvis > lumbar vertebrae > thoracic vertebrae > ribs) more frequently than to viscera (lung > liver > adrenal gland). Diffuse pulmonary involvement is infrequent.

The standard staging scheme is that of Whitmore. Stage A represents cancer not detectable by rectal examination but found in a surgical specimen obtained during operation for prostatic hyperplasia or at autopsy. Stage A is subdivided into two groups: stage A_1, in which well-differentiated tumor is present in only a few transurethral chips from one lobe, and stage A_2, in which involvement is more diffuse. Stage B disease is palpable but confined to the prostate. Stage B_1 disease is a single nodule involving only one lobe and surrounded by tissue that is normal to palpation; stage B_2 involves the gland more diffusely. In stage C, palpable tumor extends beyond the prostate, but there are no distant metastases. In stage D, metastatic disease is present. Stage D_1 refers to involvement of pelvic nodes only with no other metastases, whereas in the D_2 category metastatic disease is more widespread. Any of the lower stages (A, B, or C) may progress directly to stage D. Failure to include pelvic lymphadenectomy in the staging process results in marked underestimation of the frequency of lymph node metastases; for example, about one-fifth of tumors tentatively classified as A_2 solely on the basis of prostate pathology actually constitute stage D disease when appropriate surgical staging is performed. The frequency with which early hematogenous metastases are missed with the current staging procedures is uncertain.

Bony metastases from prostatic carcinoma usually contain both osteoblastic and osteolytic components. The bony pelvis and lumbar vertebrae are involved most often, and metastases also occur in thoracic vertebrae, ribs, skull, and long bones. Skeletal survey has a low sensitivity of detection because a significant portion of bone must be involved to permit detection on a routine x-ray. Bone scans using radionuclides such as technetium 99 are more sensitive, but the specificity is not high because positive scans may occur in any metabolically hyperactive bone; this includes sites of inflammation, healing fractures, osteoarthritis, and Paget's disease. Therefore, when a positive radionuclide scan is obtained during an initial survey for bone metastases, the presence of other lesions must be excluded by conventional radiography of the affected site. Radionuclide bone scans are also useful for monitoring progression and response to therapy.

Surgical staging is the common modality for assessing lymph node involvement and determining therapy. The procedure usually includes removal of the external iliac, internal iliac, and obturator lymph node chains and is either performed by open surgery or laparoscopically. Pelvic lymphadenectomy may be performed by itself or in conjunction with prostatic surgery or implantation of radioactive beads. In some centers the initial procedure is either lymphangiography or pelvic CT scan of the pelvis, followed when positive by confirmatory thin-needle biopsy of the affected lymph nodes. When the CT scan or lymphangiogram is negative, however, operative staging is mandatory.

TREATMENT   Surgery   Total prostatoseminovesiculectomy is the oldest treatment for carcinoma of the prostate. Radical perineal prostatectomy allows an easier vesicourethral anastomosis and less bleeding, while radical retropubic prostatectomy affords access to the pelvic lymph nodes. In experienced hands, both procedures have a low risk of urinary incontinence (1 percent for radical perineal and 1 to 4 percent for radical retropubic prostatectomy). Formerly, both operations caused impotence in most patients. Improvements in surgical technique for the retropubic procedure allow preservation of the neurovascular supply to the corpora cavernosa and preservation of potency in most patients below age 60 without compromising the thoroughness of the operation. Radical prostatectomy is not indicated for most stage A_1 cancer, since the disease usually is cured definitively by the simple prostatectomy at which the diagnosis is made. PSA determinations and sonographic biopsy of residual prostatic tissue aid

in identifying stage A_1 patients with additional tumor who may require further therapy. True stage A_2 disease in which pelvic nodes show no evidence of metastases may behave aggressively and be benefited by radical surgery, particularly when the neoplasm is anaplastic. Indeed, 5- and 10-year survivals equivalent to those of age-matched controls have been reported following such treatment for stage A_2 disease.

Radical prostatectomy has its clearest indication in stage B disease. Nearly all the apparent surgical cures in this stage are in men who have 1- to 2-cm nodules involving only one lobe of the prostate (e.g., stage B_1), a group historically comprising only 5 percent of prostatic carcinoma patients. Improvements in early diagnosis (see above) have increased the number of such patients diagnosed. In addition, subjects with true stage B_2 diease also may be candidates for radical prostatectomy.

The effectiveness of radical prostatectomy for locally advanced disease (stages C and D_1) is less certain. Lymphadenectomy alone has no therapeutic benefit, but diminished surgical morbidity and renewed interest in early and total androgen ablation (see below) have spurred a reassessment of a role for radical prostatectomy in locally advanced disease. Morbidity rates from local pelvic symptoms, bladder outlet obstruction, hematuria, and ureteral obstruction may be decreased by radical prostatectomy in stage C and D_1 disease, but controlled studies comparing morbidity rates after surgery with those following other therapies are lacking.

Radiation   Radiation therapy was developed as a primary treatment in prostatic carcinoma because of a desire to avoid the impotence and occasional incontinence that may follow radical prostatectomy. In most series, approximately 60 to 70 Gy (6000 to 7000 rad) is administered to the prostate over 6 weeks by a variety of delivery patterns. Pelvic nodes may or may not be radiated. Acute proctitis and urethritis are common side effects but are usually controllable by local measures and adjustments in delivery pattern. Chronic complications after full courses of external beam radiation include impotence in 30 to 60 percent, chronic proctitis in 10 to 15 percent, and occasional rectal stricture, rectal fistula, or rectal bleeding. It is not clear whether external beam radiation actually eradicates prostatic carcinoma, because many patients in whom progression of the tumor is slowed or halted have persistent tumor on rebiopsy, and the biologic potential of these persistent tumors is not clear.

The largest series on external beam radiation for prostatic cancer is that of Bagshaw; a variety of delivery techniques and doses were utilized in nearly 1300 patients, many of whom had received prior hormone manipulation. There was about 50 percent 10-year survival in stages A and B and a mean 10-year survival of 30 percent in stage C. The 5-year survival in stage D patients who received radiation to the pelvis as well was 58 percent. Several smaller studies have reported responses that in the aggregate are similar. The best results are obtained when the tumors are less than 2 cm in size at the time of therapy. There appears to be no consistent correlation between tumor grade and radiosensitivity.

Focal external beam radiation may be palliative for bone pain due to metastases. The duration of relief is variable. Radiation is less effective for alleviating ureteral obstruction secondary to metastatic tumor because the time lag for a successful response may be 6 to 8 weeks.

Interstitial radiation involves retropubic or perineal implantation of seeds of ^{125}I or ^{198}Au. This treatment avoids major extirpative surgery and provides a concentrated delivery of radiation to the target tissue. Successful seed implantation requires a well-defined primary tumor with a diameter less than 5 cm, a tumor volume less than 30 to 40 mL, and uniform distribution of seeds throughout the prostate. In the initial reports, 5-year survival following staging pelvic lymphadenectomy and retropubic implantation of ^{121}I or ^{198}Au seeds was comparable with survival rates after other forms of treatment, but the incidence of tumor progression is higher. Potency is preserved in more than 90 percent, and early complications are fewer and less severe than those after external beam radiation.

In summary, except for impotence following external beam radiation, serious morbidity is infrequent following either form of radiation therapy. Practical considerations make ^{125}I or ^{198}Au seed implantation most suited to stage B₁ disease. The long-term efficacy of either form of radiation as compared with radical prostatectomy for the treatment of localized carcinomas (stages A₂, B₁, and B₂) is not clear, but current data suggest that radiotherapy may be less curative than radical prostatectomy.

Androgen deprivation Since growth of the normal prostate is dependent on testicular androgens (see Chap. 339), it was logical to try androgen deprivation for treatment of prostatic cancer. Androgen deprivation can be achieved in four ways: (1) surgical extirpation of the glands that synthesize androgens (castration and adrenalectomy), (2) inhibition of pituitary gonadotropin (and/or adrenocorticotropin, ACTH) production (estrogen therapy, hypophysectomy, or treatment with LHRH analogues such as leuprolide or buserelin), (3) inhibition of androgen synthesis by the testes and adrenals (aminoglutethimide), and (4) inhibition of androgen binding to its receptor protein (cyproterone or flutamide). The usual means of achieving androgen deprivation are surgical castration, LHRH analogue therapy, and estrogen administration.

Since testicular secretion accounts for more than 95 percent of testosterone production, bilateral orchiectomy results in a 90 percent decline of plasma levels. Estrogens such as diethylstilbestrol are potent inhibitors of the release from the pituitary gland of luteinizing hormone (LH), the gonadotropin that regulates testosterone production, and consequently, estrogen administration also causes a fall in plasma testosterone to castration levels. Maximum depression of plasma testosterone is achieved with 3 mg/d diethylstilbestrol. Other estrogens (conjugated estrogens, ethinyl estradiol, diethylstilbestrol diphosphate) are no more effective in the lowering of plasma testosterone level than is diethylstilbestrol.

Androgen deprivation by means of bilateral orchiectomy, diethylstilbestrol therapy, or combined orchiectomy plus diethylstilbestrol was a standard form of treatment for carcinoma of the prostate for many years, based largely on comparison of treatment groups with historical controls. Subsequently, in prospective control studies, the effectiveness of high-dose diethylstilbestrol or orchiectomy, alone or in combination, in enhancing survival in any stage of prostatic cancer was not clear-cut. Furthermore, death from cardiovascular disease was more frequent in patients treated with large doses of diethylstilbestrol. LHRH analogues have largely replaced estrogen therapy because of their safer cardiovascular profile. These analogues inhibit LH secretion and lower plasma testosterone levels.

Each of the above forms of androgen ablation still leaves a small amount of circulating adrenal androgen that may be detrimental in the control of advanced prostate cancer. Androgen depletion beyond that achieved by surgical castration, LHRH analogues, or estrogen administration can be accomplished by adrenalectomy or hypophysectomy. Adrenalectomy can be accomplished either by surgical ablation or by therapy with drugs such as exogenous glucocorticoids which block the synthesis of adrenal androgen or antiandrogens such as flutamide which inhibit the binding of androgen to its cytoplasmic receptor protein. Extensive clinical trials comparing early androgen ablation alone with various forms of LHRH analogue therapy versus so-called total androgen ablation with LHRH analogues combined with nonsteroidal antiandrogens have yielded inconsistent results. In one trial, combination therapy resulted in a small but significant prolongation in both disease-free survival and overall survival; patients with the least amount of disease had the greatest degree of improvement with combination therapy. Although proof of efficacy is lacking, the current trend is for early androgen ablation and, frequently, combination androgen ablation therapy in advanced prostatic cancer.

Even when there is no beneficial effect on survival, however, androgen deprivation decreases bone pain in two-thirds of symptomatic stage D patients and hence constitutes a major adjunctive therapy in the disease. Once the decision is made to institute such therapy, the choice must be made as to which form of androgen deprivation is appropriate. When acceptable to the patient, orchiectomy is safe and inexpensive and circumvents compliance problems. Diethylstilbestrol is also inexpensive and is usually safe in dosages of 3 mg/d or less in men who do not have preexisting cardiovascular disease. In men at risk for cardiovascular complications, LHRH analogues have similar response rates and fewer cardiovascular complications than diethylstilbestrol. The role of androgen blockers such as flutamide in combination with each of the preceding means of establishing androgen deprivation remains under study.

Chemotherapy The age group at greatest risk for prostatic cancer has poor tolerance for chemotherapy. This feature, coupled with the variable course and long doubling time of the disease, makes it difficult to determine the effectiveness of such therapy. However, several comprehensive trials utilizing chemotherapy have been undertaken in stage D disease following relapse after hormonal treatment, a situation in which mean survival time is only 7 to 8 months. The agents studied most extensively are estramustine phosphate, prednimustine, and cisplatin; more limited trials have been conducted with 5-fluorouracil, melphalan, and hydroxyurea. Complete response is rare, and only one-tenth of stage D patients have an objective partial response. In other trials, combinations of chemotherapeutic agents have been tested in stage D disease, most commonly estramustine phosphate plus prednimustine and cisplatin; more limited trials have been conducted with 5-fluorouracil, melphalan, and hydroxyurea. Complete response is again rare, and only one-fourth of patients or fewer show any objective improvement. For progressive, symptomatic stage D prostatic cancer, endocrine ablation therapy should be undertaken first, but chemotherapeutic agents may provide some benefit when such patients relapse.

REFERENCES

Benign prostatic hyperplasia

GORMLEY GL et al: The effect of finasteride in men with prostatic hyperplasia. N Engl J Med 327:1185, 1992

WALSH PC: Benign prostatic hyperplasia, in *Campbell's Urology*, 6th ed, PC Walsh et al (eds). Philadelphia, Saunders, 1992, p 1007

WILSON JD: The pathogenesis of prostatic hyperplasia. Am J Med 68:745, 1980

Carcinoma of the prostate

BAGSHAW MA: External radiation therapy of carcinoma of the prostate. Cancer 45:1912, 1980

BYAR DP, CORLE DK: VACURG randomized trial of radical prostatectomy for stages I and II prostate cancer. Urology 17(suppl 4):7, 1981

CATALONA WJ, BIGG SW: Nerve-sparing radical prostatectomy: Evaluation of results after 250 patients. J Urol 143:538, 1990

——— et al: Measurement of prostate-specific antigen in serum as a screening test for prostate cancer. N Engl J Med 324:1156, 1991

COONER WH et al: Prostate cancer detection in a clinical urological practice by ultrasonography, digital rectal examination and prostate specific antigen. J Urol 143:1146, 1990

CRAWFORD ED et al: A controlled trial of leuprolide with and without flutamide in prostatic carcinoma. N Engl J Med 321:419, 1989

EISENBERGER MA et al: A critical assessment of the role of chemotherapy for endocrine resistant prostatic carcinoma. AUA Update Series Lesson 28, vol 7, 1988

GITTES RF: Carcinoma of the prostate. N Engl J Med 324:236, 1991

HENNRICKSSON P, JOHANSSON S-E: Prediction of cardiovascular complication in patients with prostatic cancer treated with estrogen. Am J Epidemiol 125:970, 1987

HERR HW: Iodine 125 implantation in the management of localized prostatic carcinoma. Urol Clin North Am 7:605, 1980

JEWETT HJ: Radical perineal prostatectomy for palpable clinically localized, non-obstructive cancer: Experience at the Johns Hopkins Hospital, 1909–1963, J Urol 124:492, 1980

JOHANSSON JE et al: High 10-year survival rate in patients with early, untreated prostatic cancer. JAMA 267:2191, 1992

NATIONAL INSTITUTES OF HEALTH CONSENSUS DEVELOPMENT CONFERENCE: The management of clinically localized prostate cancer. J Urol 138:1369, 1987

OESTERLING JE: Prostate specific antigen: A critical assessment of the most useful tumor marker for adenocarcinoma of the prostate. J Urol 145:907, 1991

STAMEY TA, MCNEAL JE: Adenocarcinoma of the prostate, in *Campbell's Urology*, PC Walsh et al (eds). Philadelphia, Saunders, 1992, p 1159

STROHMAIER WL et al: Flutamide withdrawal syndrome: Its impact on clinical trials in hormone-refractory prostate cancer. J Clin Oncol 11:1566, 1993

TYRRELL CJ et al: A multicenter randomized trial comparing the luteinizing hormone–releasing hormone analogue goserelin acetate alone and with flutamide in the treatment of advanced prostate cancer. J Urol 146:1321, 1991

324 SKIN CANCER

CARL V. WASHINGTON, JR.

Nonmelanoma skin cancer is the most common cancer in the United States, with an estimated annual incidence of more than 600,000 cases. Basal cell carcinomas (BCC) account for 70 to 80 percent of nonmelanoma skin cancers. Squamous cell carcinomas (SCC), while representing only about 20 percent of nonmelanoma skin cancers, are more significant because of their ability to metastasize. Incidence rates have risen dramatically over the past decade. While more common in men, this sexual difference has become less pronounced in recent years.

ETIOLOGY   The cause of BCC and SCC is multifactorial, with environmental and host factors being important. Recognized host factors besides age and sex include Celtic descent, fair complexion, tendency to sunburn easily, radiodermatitis, thermal burns, and certain scars and chronic ulcerations. Several heritable conditions have been associated with skin cancer (e.g., xeroderma pigmentosum). Among environmental causes, exposure to sunlight, principally the ultraviolet-B (UV-B) spectrum, appears to be the most significant. Abundant evidence exists to support the role of chronic cutaneous exposure to UV-B in skin cancer pathogenesis. The incidence of these tumors increases with decreasing latitudes. The vast majority develop on sun-exposed areas of the head and neck and are more common on the left side in the United States and the right side in England, presumably related to additional asymmetric exposure during driving. A higher incidence occurs in those with outdoor occupations. As thinning of the earth's protective ozone shield progresses, further increases in the incidence of skin cancer can be anticipated. Among chemical carcinogens, arsenic is the most important. Exposure is usually through medicinals or well water. Skin cancer in affected individuals may be seen with or without other cutaneous markers of chronic arsenism (e.g., arsenical keratoses). Drug- or disease-induced immunosuppression also predisposes to skin cancer. Transplantation patients on chronic immunosuppressive therapy are particularly prone to SCC. The frequency of skin cancer is proportional to the duration of immunosuppression and the extent of sun exposure. Human papillomaviruses (HPV) and UV-B may act as cocarcinogens. Skin cancer is not an uncommon finding in patients infected with the human immunodeficiency virus (HIV) and may be more aggressive in this setting (see Chap. 279). As the life span of HIV-infected persons increases, skin cancer may become a greater problem.

CLINICAL PRESENTATION   Basal cell carcinoma   BCC is a malignancy arising from epidermal basal cells. Several clinical types of BCC occur. The most common is the noduloulcerative BCC, which begins as a small pearly nodule, often showing small telangiectatic vessels on its surface. The nodule increases slowly in size and may undergo central ulceration. Variable amounts of melanin may be present within the tumor. BCC with heavier accumulations of pigment represent the pigmented BCC. While clinically no more aggressive than the noduloulcerative variant, it may be mistaken for malignant melanoma. The morpheaform (fibrosing) BCC manifests as a solitary, flat or slightly depressed, indurated, whitish or yellowish plaque. Borders are typically indistinct. Of BCC variants, this is the most aggressive and likely to recur. Superficial BCC consists of one or several erythematous, scaling plaques that slowly enlarge. Although more commonly found on the trunk and extremities, the head and neck are also affected. The lesions may be confused with benign inflammatory dermatoses, especially nummular eczema and psoriasis.

Squamous cell carcinoma   Primary cutaneous SCC is a malignant neoplasm of keratinizing epidermal cells. Unlike BCC, which has a very low metastatic potential, SCC can metastasize and grow rapidly. The clinical features of SCC vary widely. Commonly SCC appears as an ulcerated nodule or a superficial erosion on the skin or lower lip, but it also may present as a verrucous papule or plaque.

Unlike BCC, overlying telangiectasias are uncommon. Margins of this tumor may be ill-defined, and fixation to underlying structures may occur. Cutaneous SCC may develop anywhere on the body but usually arises on sun-damaged skin.

SCC has several premalignant forms (actinic keratosis, actinic cheilitis, and some cutaneous horns) and in situ forms (e.g., Bowen's disease) that are confined to the epidermis. Actinic keratoses (AK) and cheilitis are hyperkeratotic papules and plaques which occur on sun-exposed areas. While the potential for malignant degeneration is low in any individual lesion, the risk of SCC increases with larger numbers of lesions. Bowen's disease presents as a scaling, erythematous plaque which may occur on sun-exposed or protected sites. Individual lesions may develop into invasive SCC in up to 20 percent of cases. Controversy exists regarding the association of Bowen's disease with internal malignancy; however, recent evidence suggests no significant relationship when other predisposing factors (e.g., arsenic) are absent. Treatment of premalignant and in situ lesions reduces the subsequent risk of invasive disease.

TREATMENT   Basal cell carcinoma   Treatment modalities used with BCC include (1) electrodesiccation and curettage (ED&C), (2) excision, (3) cryosurgery, (4) radiation therapy, (5) Mohs micrographic surgery (MMS), (6) topical chemotherapy, and (7) intralesional interferon. Mode of therapy is directed by location of the tumor, histologic subtype, presence of recurrent disease, and various patient characteristics. ED&C remains the most commonly employed method by dermatologists. This method is selected for less aggressive tumors (e.g., noduloulcerative, superficial). It is best avoided in recurrent lesions, histologically aggressive tumors (e.g., morpheaform), deeply invasive or very large lesions, or in locations with high recurrence rates (e.g., nasolabial folds, medial canthus). Excision, which offers the advantage of histologic control, is usually selected for more aggressive tumors, those in high-risk locations, or in many instances for aesthetic demands. Radiation therapy, while not employed as frequently as surgical modalities, offers an excellent chance for cure in many BCC. It is useful in patients not considered surgical candidates and as a surgical adjunct in high-risk tumors. Cryosurgery utilizing liquid nitrogen may be used in certain low-risk tumors but requires specialized equipment (i.e., cryoprobes) to be used effectively for advanced neoplasms. Mohs micrographic surgery is a specialized type of surgical excision which allows for the ultimate in histologic control and preservation of uninvolved tissue. It is reserved for recurrent lesions, high-risk locations, larger and ill-defined lesions, and where maximal tissue conservation is critical (e.g., eyelids). Topical chemotherapy with 5-fluorouracil (5-FU) has limited usefulness in the management of BCC and should be used only for treating superficial BCC. Recent reports have demonstrated the effectiveness of intralesional interferon in certain primary tumors. The natural history of BCC is that of a slowly enlarging locally invasive neoplasm. The metastatic potential of BCC has been estimated to be 0.0028 to 0.1 percent.

Squamous cell carcinoma   The therapy of cutaneous SCC should be based on an analysis of risk factors influencing biologic behavior. These include size, location, degree of histologic differentiation, and age and physical condition of the patient. Surgical excision, radiation, and MMS are standard methods of treatment. Cryosurgery and ED&C have been used successfully in small primary tumors. The natural history of SCC depends on tumor and host characteristics. Tumors arising on actinically damaged skin have a lower metastatic potential than those on protected surfaces. Metastatic frequency of cutaneous SCC, reported at 0.3 to 3.7 percent, is lower than that of mucosal SCC. Tumors occurring on the lower lip have a metastatic potential approaching 11 percent. Metastases from SCC arising in burn scars, chronic ulcerations, and the genitalia have higher rates.

PREVENTION   Since the vast majority of skin cancers are related to chronic UV-B exposure, potential exists to dramatically reduce the incidence through patient and physician education. Emphasis should be placed on preventive measures beginning early in life. Patients must understand that damage from UV-B begins early, despite the fact that cancers develop years later. Regular use of sunscreens should be encouraged. Avoidance of tanning salons and sun exposure during midday (10 A.M. to 2 P.M.) is recommended. Precancerous and in situ lesions should be treated early. Chemoprophylaxis using synthetic retinoids is useful in controlling new lesions in some patients with multiple tumors.

REFERENCES

AUBRY F et al: Risk factors of squamous cell carcinoma of the skin. Cancer 55:907, 1985

FRIEDMAN RJ et al (eds): *Cancer of the Skin*. Philadelphia, Saunders, 1991, pp 27–94

GALLAGHER RP et al: Trends in basal cell carcinoma, squamous cell carcinoma, and melanoma of the skin from 1973 through 1987. J Am Acad Dermatol 23:413, 1990

KWA RE: Biology of cutaneous squamous cell carcinoma. J Am Acad Dermatol 26:1, 1992

---

325 MELANOMA AND OTHER PIGMENTED SKIN LESIONS

ARTHUR J. SOBER / HOWARD K. KOH

Pigmented skin lesions are among the most common findings on physical examination. The challenge is to distinguish cutaneous melanoma, which may be lethal, from the remainder, which with rare exception are benign.

Melanoma originates from melanocytes, pigment cells present normally in epidermis and sometimes in dermis. This tumor affects approximately 32,000 individuals per year in the United States, resulting in 6700 deaths. The incidence has increased dramatically (300 percent increase in the past 40 years); it can affect adults of all ages, even young individuals (onset from midteens); it has distinct clinical features which make it detectable at a time when cure by surgical excision is possible; and it is located on the skin surface, where it is visible. If the incidence continues to increase at the present rate, within a decade, lifetime risk of melanoma will approximate 1 percent or higher.

The reason for the increased incidence is uncertain but may stem from increased recreational sun exposure, especially early in life. Individuals of similar ethnic background who emigrate after childhood to areas of high sun exposure (Israel, Australia) have lower melanoma rates than individuals of similar age either born in these countries or who emigrated before age 10. Individuals most susceptible to development of melanoma are those with fair complexions, red or blond hair, blue eyes, and freckles and who are poor tanners and easy sunburners. In one literature survey, 9 of 11 studies linked increased melanoma risk to history of sunburn. Other factors associated with increased risk include family history of melanoma (approximately 1 in 10 melanoma patients have a family member with melanoma), presence of an atypical mole (dysplastic nevus), a giant congenital melanocytic nevus, a small to medium-sized congenital melanocytic nevus (see below), the presence of a higher than average number of ordinary melanocytic nevi, and immunosuppression (Table 325-1). A 64-fold increased risk for individuals with 50 or more moles ≥ 2 mm in size has been reported. Melanoma is relatively infrequent in heavily pigmented peoples. Dark-skinned populations (natives of India, Puerto Rico), blacks, and Orientals have rates one-seventh to one-tenth that noted for lighter-skinned Caucasians.

CLINICAL CHARACTERISTICS There are four types of cutaneous melanoma (Table 325-2). Three of these—superficial spreading melanoma, lentigo maligna melanoma, and acral lentiginous melanoma—have a period of superficial (so-called radial) growth when the lesion increases in size but does not penetrate deeply. It is during the radial growth period that melanoma is most capable of being

TABLE 325-1 Risk factors for cutaneous melanoma

High risk (>50-fold increased risk)
  Persistently changing mole
  Atypical moles in patient with two family members with melanoma
  Adulthood vs. childhood
  >50 nevi ≥ 2 mm
Intermediate risk (~10-fold)
  Family history of melanoma
  Sporadic atypical moles
  Congenital nevi (?)
  Caucasians vs. blacks or Asians
  Personal history of prior melanoma
Low risk (2- to 4-fold)
  Immunosuppression
  Sun sensitivity or excess exposure

SOURCE: Adapted from Rhodes et al.

cured by surgical excision. The fourth type, nodular melanoma, does not have a recognizable radial growth phase and usually presents as a deeply invasive lesion, fully capable of early metastasis. When tumors begin to penetrate deeply into the skin, they are in the so-called vertical growth phase. Melanomas with radial growth phases are characterized by irregular and sometimes notched borders, variation in pigment pattern, and variation in color. Increase in size or change in color is noted by the patient in 70 percent of early lesions. Bleeding, ulceration, and pain are late signs and are of little help in early recognition. Nodular melanomas are dark brown–black to blue-black nodules. Melanoma may occasionally be amelanotic, where only the biopsy of a new or changing skin nodule histologically establishes the diagnosis. Lentigo maligna melanoma usually confines itself to chronically sun-damaged, sun-exposed sites (face, neck, back of hands) in older individuals. Acral lentiginous melanoma occurs on palms, soles, nail beds, and mucous membranes. While this type occurs in whites, it is most frequent (along with nodular melanoma) in blacks and Asians. Superficial spreading melanoma is most frequent in whites. Melanomas arising in dysplastic nevi (see below) are usually of this type. The back is the most common site for melanoma in men. In women, the back and the lower leg (from knee to ankle) are frequent sites.

PROGNOSTIC FACTORS The most important prognostic factor is stage at time of presentation. (See later discussion of revised staging categories.) Five-year survival for clinical stages I and II (primary tumor; no clinical evidence of disease elsewhere) is about 85 percent. For clinical stage III (clinically palpable regional nodes that contain tumor), a 5-year survival of about 50 percent is noted when only one node is involved and about 15 to 20 percent when four or more nodes are involved. Five-year survival for clinical stage IV (disseminated disease) is less than 5 percent. Fortunately, the majority of melanomas are diagnosed in clinical stages I and II. Within stages I and II, a gradient of prognosis can be delineated based on the thickness of the primary tumor (Table 325-3). This system is based on the rationale that the likelihood of metastasis should correlate with tumor volume, with thickness the best single index of tumor volume. Melanomas less than 0.76 mm thick are usually cured by surgical removal (5-year survival rates range from 96 to 99 percent). Approximately 40 percent of primary melanomas now fall into a low-risk category (thickness < 1 mm). When low-risk patients develop metastases, the primary tumors often exhibit either extensive microscopic features of regression or a vertical growth phase. Approximately 60 percent of individuals with melanomas ≥ 3.65 mm thick will develop metastatic disease and die from their melanoma. These thick tumors are almost always raised substantially above the plane of the skin. Two intermediate categories of thickness exist (Table 325-3). Certain anatomic sites affect prognosis. The favorable sites appear to be forearm and leg (excluding feet), while unfavorable sites include scalp, hands, feet, and mucous membranes. Survival for women in stages I and II is, in general, more favorable than for men, perhaps in part because of earlier diagnosis; women frequently have melanomas

TABLE 325-2 Clinical features of malignant melanoma

Type	Site	Average age at diagnosis, years	Duration of known existence, years	Color
Lentigo maligna melanoma	Sun-exposed surfaces, particularly malar region of cheek and temple	70	5–20* or longer	In flat portions, shades of brown and tan predominant, but whitish gray occasionally present; in nodules, shades of reddish brown, bluish gray, bluish black
Superficial spreading melanoma	Any site (more common on upper back and in women on lower legs)	40–50	1–7	Shades of brown mixed with bluish red (violaceous), bluish black, reddish brown, and often whitish pink, and the border of lesion is at least in part visibly and/or palpably elevated
Nodular melanoma	Any site	40–50	Months to less than 5 years	Reddish blue (purple) or bluish black; either uniform in color or mixed with brown or black
Acral lentiginous melanoma	Palm, sole, nail bed, mucous membrane	60	1–10	In flat portions, dark brown predominantly; in raised lesions (plaques) brown-black or blue-black predominantly

* During much of this time, the precursor stage, lentigo maligna, is confined to the epidermis.
SOURCE: Adapted from AJ Sober, in *Pathophysiology of Dermatologic Diseases*, NA Soter, HP Baden (eds), New York, McGraw-Hill, 1984.

on the lower leg, where self-recognition is more likely and prognosis is better. Older individuals, in general, have poorer prognoses. This has been explained, in part, on the basis of delayed diagnosis (thicker tumors) and a higher proportion of acral melanomas (palmar-plantar), which have relatively less favorable prognoses. As in breast cancer, recurrence of melanoma may be seen after many years. About 10 to 15 percent of first-time recurrences develop after 5 years, so prolonged follow-up (at least 10 years) is warranted. The time to recurrence varies inversely with tumor thickness. Other prognostic factors for stages I and II melanoma include presence of an ulcer in the primary tumor, mitotic rate, and the presence of microscopic tumor satellites (foci of tumor ≥0.05 mm in diameter in the reticular dermis or subcutaneous fat, distinct from the main body of the tumor). The presence of microscopic satellites is also predictive of microscopic metastases to the regional lymph nodes. An alternate prognostic scheme for clinical stages I and II melanoma is based on anatomic level of invasion within the skin (Clark). Level I is intraepidermal (in situ), level II penetrates the papillary dermis, level III fills the papillary dermis, level IV penetrates the reticular dermis, and level V penetrates into the subcutaneous fat. Survival at 5 years by level of invasion averages 100, 95, 82, 71, and 49 percent, respectively.

NATURAL HISTORY Melanomas may spread by the lymphatic channels or the bloodstream. Earliest metastases are to regional lymph nodes. Clinicians attempt to predict drainage pathways using anatomic charts or by lymphoscintigraphy using technetium-99m injected around the primary tumor site. Surgical lymphadenectomy usually controls regional disease.

Liver, lung, bone, and brain are common sites of hematogenous spread, but unusual sites such as the anterior chamber of the eye also

may occur. Once widespread metastatic disease is established, likelihood of cure is low.

MANAGEMENT The entire cutaneous surface including scalp and mucous membranes should be examined in each patient. Bright room illumination is important, and a 7× to 10× hand lens is helpful for evaluating variation in pigment pattern. A history of relevant risk factors should be elicited. Any suspicious lesions should either be biopsied, evaluated by a specialist, or recorded by chart and/or photography for follow-up. Examination of the lymph nodes and palpation of the abdominal viscera are part of the staging examination for suspected melanoma. The patient should be advised to have other family members screened if either melanoma or atypical moles (dysplastic nevi) are present. The detection of early melanoma in relatives upon screening has been reported. Until causes of melanoma are more clearly understood, protection from the sun should be practiced by the patient. Routine use of a sunblock of SPF ≥ 15, use of protective clothing, and avoiding intense midday ultraviolet exposure should be recommended. The patient should be educated in the clinical features of melanoma and advised to report any new growth or other change in a pigmented lesion. Patient education brochures are available from the American Cancer Society, the American Academy of Dermatology, the National Cancer Institute, and the Skin Cancer Foundation. Self-examination at 6- to 8-week intervals may enhance the likelihood of detecting change between follow-up visits. The importance of routine follow-up visits for melanoma patients and patients with atypical moles (dysplastic nevi) should be emphasized, since this may facilitate early detection of new tumors.

PRECURSOR LESIONS Atypical moles, termed by some *dysplastic nevi*, occur in certain families affected by melanoma. In some families, melanomas occur nearly exclusively in individuals with the dysplastic nevi. These nevi appear to be transmitted as an autosomal dominant trait. In other families, the nevi may not be present in all individuals at risk of melanoma. The melanomas may arise within the atypical mole (acting as a precursor) or in normal skin (the mole acting as a marker of increased risk). An individual with atypical moles and two family members with melanoma has been reported to have a greater than 50 percent lifetime risk for developing melanoma. Table 325-4 lists the characteristic features of atypical moles and their differentiation from benign acquired nevi. The number of atypical moles may vary from one to several hundred. Atypical moles usually look different one compared with another. The borders are often hazy and indistinct, and the pigment pattern is more highly variable than

TABLE 325-3 Prognosis of localized melanoma by thickness (Breslow): 5-year survival rates for stages I and II (AJCC)

Thickness, mm	Survival, %	
	Overall	MCCG*
<0.76	96	99
0.76–1.49	87	95
1.50–2.49	75	84
2.50–3.99	66	70
≥4.00	47	44

* MCCG = Melanoma Clinical Cooperative Group.
SOURCE: From Balch et al.

TABLE 325-4 Clinical features distinguishing atypical moles from benign acquired nevi

Clinical feature	Atypical moles	Benign acquired nevi
Color	Variable mixtures of tan, brown, black, or red/pink within a single nevus; nevi may look very different from each other	Uniformly tan or brown
Shape	Irregular borders; pigment may fade off into surrounding skin; macular portion at the edge of the nevus	Round; sharp, clear-cut borders between the nevus and the surrounding skin; may be flat or elevated
Size	Usually more than 6 mm; may be more than 10 mm; occasionally smaller than 6 mm	Usually less than 6 mm in diameter
Number	Often very many (more than 100), but occasionally may be only one	In a typical adult: 10 to 40 are scattered over the body; perhaps 15% of patients have no nevi
Location	Sun-exposed areas; the back is the most common site, but dysplastic nevi may also be seen on the scalp, breasts, and buttocks	Generally on the sun-exposed surfaces of the skin above the waist; the scalp, breasts, and buttocks are rarely involved

SOURCE: Modified from Friedman et al.

that in benign acquired nevi. Since the frequency of atypical moles in melanoma-prone families is greater than 50 percent, some observers have suggested a polygenic inheritance rather than a single-gene pattern of inheritance. Of the 90 percent of melanoma patients regarded as sporadic (lacking a family history of melanoma), about 40 percent have atypical moles, as compared with an estimated 5 percent of the population at large. Further studies to determine background frequency of atypical moles are required once greater unanimity exists regarding their clinical and histopathologic features. The observation that at least 20 percent of sporadic melanomas arise in association with an atypical mole makes this nevus the most important precursor for melanoma.

Less frequent precursors include the giant congenital melanocytic nevus and the small congenital melanocytic nevus (disputed by some). Congenital melanocytic nevi are present at birth or appear in the neonatal period (tardive form). The giant melanocytic nevus, also called bathing trunk, cape, or garment nevus, is a rare malformation that affects perhaps 1 in 100,000 individuals. These nevi are usually greater than 20 cm in diameter and may cover more than half the body surface. Giant nevi often occur in association with multiple small congenital nevi. The borders are sharp, and hair may be present. The lesions are usually dark brown and may have darker and lighter areas. Pigment is haphazardly displayed. The surface is smooth to rugose to cerebriform and may vary from one portion of the lesion to another. A lifetime risk of melanoma development of 6 percent has been estimated. The greatest risk is before age 5, with the next greatest period of risk between ages 5 and 10. Early detection of melanoma is difficult in these lesions because of the deep dermal or subcutaneous origin of primary melanoma and because of the large and varied surface. Prophylactic excision early in life can be accomplished by staged removal with coverage by split-thickness skin grafts. The use of cultured keratinocytes for coverage appears promising. At present, there are no uniform management guidelines for giant congenital nevi.

The small to medium-sized congenital melanocytic nevus, affecting approximately 1 percent of people, presents usually as a raised dark to medium brown lesion with a smooth or papillomatous surface. The border is sharp, and lesions may be oriented along lines of skin cleavage. Follicular hyper- and hypopigmentation may coexist in a salt-and-pepper configuration. The lesion may have an excess of

thick, coarse hairs. The risk of developing melanoma in these lesions is at present unknown; however, melanomas can arise in these lesions. From body surface area considerations, the coincidence of melanoma and small congenital melanocytic nevi at the same site is probably higher than that calculated by chance. The remnants of a nevus with histopathologic features of a congenital nevus have been observed in 2 to 6 percent of melanomas. Management of small to medium-sized congenital melanocytic nevi remains controversial, but at many medical centers consideration is given to prophylactic removal under local anesthesia in the early teen years. Melanomas in small congenital melanocytic nevi appear to occur after this period of life.

DIFFERENTIAL DIAGNOSIS The aim of differential diagnosis is to distinguish benign pigmented lesions from melanoma and its precursors. If melanoma is a consideration, then biopsy or referral to a specialist is appropriate. It is appropriate to remove some benign look-alikes in order to decrease the chance of missing a melanoma. Table 325-5 summarizes the distinguishing features of benign lesions that may be confused with melanoma.

BIOPSY Any pigmented cutaneous lesion that has changed in size or shape or has other features suggestive of malignant melanoma is a candidate for biopsy. The recommended technique is a full-thickness excisional biopsy, since this facilitates pathologic assessment of the lesion, permits accurate measurement of thickness if the lesion is melanoma, and constitutes treatment if the lesion is benign. Shave biopsy or curettage of a suspected melanoma is contraindicated. For

TABLE 325-5 Pigmented lesions that must be distinguished from cutaneous melanoma and its precursors

Lesion	Description
Blue nevus	Gun metal or cerulean blue, blue-gray. Stable over time. One-half occur on dorsa of hand and feet. Lesions are usually single, small, 3 mm to < 1 cm. Must be distinguished from nodular melanoma.
Compound nevus	Round or oval shape, well-demarcated, smooth-bordered. May be dome-shaped or papillomatous; colors range from flesh colored to very dark brown with individual nevi being relatively homogeneous in color.
Hemangioma	Dome-shaped reddish, purple, blue nodule. Compression with a glass microscope slide may result in blanching. Must be distinguished from nodular melanoma.
Junctional nevus	Flat to barely raised brown lesion. Sharp border. Fine pigmentary stippling noted especially upon magnification.
Lentigo Juvenile Solar	Flat uniformly medium or dark brown lesion with sharp border. Solar lentigines are acquired lesions on sites of chronic solar exposure (backs of hands/face). Lesions are 2 mm to ≥1 cm. Solar lentigines have reticulate pigmentation upon magnification.
Pigmented basal cell carcinoma	Papular border. May have central ulceration. Usually solar exposed surface in older patient. Patient usually has dark brown eyes and dark brown or black hair.
Pigmented dermatofibroma	Lesion is not well demarcated visually, is firm, and dimples downward when compressed laterally. Usually on extremities. Usually < 6 mm.
Seborrheic keratosis	Rough, stuck on, waxy feeling lesions with sharp borders ranging in color from flesh to tan, to dark brown. Presence of keratin plugs in surface of help in discriminating especially dark lesions from melanoma.
Subungual hematoma	Maroon (red-brown) coloration. As lesion grows out from nailfold, a curving clear area seen.
Tattoo (medical or traumatic)	In medical tattoo lesions are small pigmentary dots often blue or green which make a regular pattern (rectangle). Traumatic tattoos are irregular, and pigmentation may appear black.

large lesions or lesions on anatomic sites where excisional biopsy may not be feasible (such as the face, hands, or feet), an incisional biopsy through the most nodular or darkest area of the lesion is acceptable; this should represent the vertical growth phase of the primary tumor. Data from prospective studies do not support the concern that an incisional biopsy might facilitate the spread of melanoma.

STAGING   Once the diagnosis of malignant melanoma has been confirmed, the tumor must be staged to determine prognosis and treatment. The history should probe for evidence of metastatic disease, such as malaise, weight loss, headaches, visual difficulty, or bone pain. The physical examination should be especially directed to the skin, regional draining lymph nodes, central nervous system, liver, and spleen. In the absence of signs or symptoms of metastasis, few laboratory or radiologic tests are indicated for staging purposes. Aside from a chest x-ray and, possibly, liver function tests, no other tests or scans are routinely indicated unless the history or physical examination suggests metastasis to a specific organ. Specifically, liver-spleen scans and computed tomography have a low yield and are not cost-effective. However, once signs of metastasis exist, favored sites of spread, such as the liver, lungs, bone, and brain, should be scanned.

Traditional staging categories have been stage I (confined to the skin), stage II (spread to regional lymph nodes), and stage III (distant metastases). Approximately 80 percent of patients with melanoma now present with stage I disease. The American Joint Commission on Cancer (AJCC) has promoted a four-stage system to divide patients more easily by risk group. This system splits the former stage I patients into low risk (new stage I: ≤1.5 mm thick) and high risk (new stage II: >1.5 mm thick).

SURGICAL MANAGEMENT   For a newly diagnosed stage I cutaneous melanoma, wide surgical excision of the lesion with a margin of normal skin is necessary to remove all malignant cells and minimize local recurrence. The outdated ''5-cm rule,'' which states that the normal skin within 5 cm of the edge of the primary cutaneous melanoma should be excised, often requires split-thickness skin grafts and is cosmetically disfiguring. Narrower margins allow for primary closure and may obviate the need for grafts or flaps without compromising overall survival rates. The appropriate width of the narrow margin is a source of controversy. A World Health Organization trial prospectively randomized between 1-cm and 3-cm margins in 612 patients with thin malignant melanomas (≤2 mm in thickness) reported that the thinner surgical margin resulted in higher rates of local recurrence but no difference in nodal metastases, distant metastases, disease-free survival, or overall survival after 7½ years of follow-up. For thicker stage I lesions, definitive data are not available, but margins up to 3 cm appear to be reasonable. Once again, for lesions on the face, hands, and feet, strict adherence to margins must give way to individual considerations about the constraints of surgery and minimization of morbidity. In all instances, however, inclusion of subcutaneous fat in the surgical specimen facilitates adequate thickness measurement and assessment of surgical margins by the pathologist.

ELECTIVE REGIONAL NODE DISSECTION   Elective regional node dissection in AJCC stage II disease (without palpable adenopathy) has been advocated, based on the hypothesis that melanoma metastasizes in an orderly fashion from the skin to regional lymph nodes and finally to distant sites. Hence surgical excision of nodal micrometastases could theoretically provide definitive treatment at a time of relatively low tumor burden and, hopefully, improve survival. The efficacy of this procedure remains controversial; while some retrospective series suggest a survival benefit, two randomized studies examining this question in patients with limb melanomas and clinical stage I disease showed no survival advantage for wide local excision followed by immediate elective regional node dissection compared with wide local excision followed by delayed dissection (only if nodes became palpable). Furthermore, the procedure has associated morbidity, and some lesions, especially those on the trunk, have

ambiguous nodal draining sites, making it difficult to decide which area to dissect. In such situations, lymphoscintigraphy can be utilized to define the nodes that serve as the primary drainage area. Certainly not all patients with clinical stage I disease require node dissections. Patients with lesions < 0.75 mm thick have excellent prognoses and need no node dissection; at the other extreme, patients with lesions > 3.50 mm have such a high risk for distant metastases that the possible benefit of an elective node dissection would be negated. A subset of patients with AJCC stage II lesions of intermediate thickness may benefit from elective regional node dissection, but there is no consensus about which patients should undergo this procedure. Ongoing randomized studies may resolve this issue.

ADJUVANT THERAPY   For patients free of disease but at high risk for metastasis, adjuvant therapy that complements surgery is needed to destroy occult micrometastases, prolong disease-free survival, and improve cure rates. Many strategies have been tried, including chemotherapy, nonspecific immunotherapy [such as immunization with bacillus Calmette-Guérin (BCG)], chemoimmunotherapy, and radiation therapy. However, such studies have been hampered by suboptimal stratification, inclusion of those at low risk, lack of randomization, small sample size, or inadequate length of follow-up. Hence no consistent evidence documents adjuvant therapy as effective in prolonging life. Current trials include studies of various melanoma vaccines to heighten the host immune response against micrometastases.

TREATMENT OF METASTATIC DISEASE   Melanoma can metastasize to any organ, the brain being a particularly favored site. Metastatic melanoma is generally incurable, and survival in patients with visceral metastases is generally less than 1 year. Thus the goal of treatment is usually palliative to improve the quality of life. Patients with soft-tissue and node metastases fare better than those with liver and brain metastases. If metastases are limited to regional nodes (AJCC stage III disease), a therapeutic lymph node dissection is indicated. Surgical excision of a single metastasis to the lung or surgically accessible brain site can be associated with prolonged survival. More often, however, patients subsequently have multiple brain metastases that require radiation and glucocorticoids. Radiation therapy can provide local palliation for recurrent tumors or metastatic sites. Chemotherapy has a response rate of only 20 to 25 percent and rarely induces complete remission. The most commonly used single agents are imidazole carboximide (dacarbazine), cisplatin, or the nitrosoureas. Combination chemotherapy does not result in consistent improvement in remission and survival rates compared with those of a single agent. Patients who have advanced regional disease isolated to a limb may benefit from hyperthermic limb perfusion with melphalan, which concentrates the chemotherapeutic agents and minimizes systemic leakage.

The lack of response to traditional treatments has spawned many trials using agents such as retinoids, high-dosage chemotherapy with autologous bone marrow transplantation, interferons, antipigmentary agents, and antibodies conjugated to isotopes, drugs, and toxins. Of all these investigational therapies, adoptive immunotherapy has received the most attention. This treatment involves exposing lymphocytes from melanoma patients to interleukin 2 (IL-2) to generate and expand lymphokine-activated killer cells (LAK cells); these LAK cells are then reinfused in conjunction with IL-2 administration. This therapy may have particular relevance to melanoma because the immune system is suspected of having a critical role in the control of melanoma metastases. However, the early response rate appears to be only about 20 percent; most of these remissions are partial, are seen in patients with skin or lung metastases, and are of short duration. In addition, treatment with IL-2 has considerable toxicity, attributable primarily to a capillary leak syndrome. Research is now focusing on improving remission rates while minimizing the toxicity; trials include high-dose IL-2, either alone or with LAK cells, with even more potent tumor-infiltrating lymphocytes, or with chemotherapeutic agents, biologic response modifiers, or other agents. The continued lack of curative treatment for metastatic disease underscores the importance of early detection and prevention of malignant melanoma to decrease avoidable mortality.

REFERENCES

ALBERT L et al: Dysplastic melanocytic nevi and cutaneous melanoma: Markers of increased melanoma risk for affected individuals and blood relatives. J Am Acad Dermatol 7:69, 1990

ARMSTRONG BK: Epidemiology of malignant melanoma: Intermittent or total accumulated exposure to the sun. J Dermatol Surg Oncol 14:835, 1988

BALCH CM et al (eds): *Cutaneous Melanoma: Clinical Management and Treatment Results Worldwide*, 2d ed. Philadelphia, Lippincott, 1992

CLARK WH JR et al: The histogenesis and biologic behavior of primary human malignant melanoma of the skin. Cancer Res 29:705, 1969

FRIEDMAN RJ et al: Malignant melanoma in the 1990s: The continued importance of early detection and the role of physician examination and self-examination of the skin. CA 41:201, 1991

HO VC, SOBER AJ: Therapy for cutaneous melanoma: An update. J Am Acad Dermatol 22:159, 1990

KOH HK et al: Adjuvant therapy of cutaneous malignant melanoma: A critical review. Med Ped Oncol 13:244, 1985

————: Cutaneous melanoma. N Engl J Med 325:171, 1991

RHODES AR: Neoplasms: Benign neoplasias, hyperplasias, and dysplasias of melanocytes, in *Dermatology in General Medicine*, TB Fitzpatrick et al (eds). New York, McGraw-Hill, 1987, pp 877–946

———— et al: Risk factors for cutaneous melanoma. JAMA 258:3146, 1987

RIGEL DS et al: Dysplastic nevi. Markers for increased risk for melanoma. Cancer 63:386, 1989

ROSENBERG SA: The immunotherapy and gene therapy of cancer. J Clin Oncol 10:180, 1992

SOBER AJ et al: Early recognition of cutaneous melanoma. JAMA 242:2795, 1979

VERONESI U et al: Delayed regional lymph node dissection in stage 1 melanoma of the skin of the lower extremities. Cancer 49:2420, 1982

————, CASCINELLI N: Narrow excision (1 cm margin), a safe procedure for thin cutaneous melanoma. Arch Surg 126:438, 1991

326 METASTATIC CANCER OF UNKNOWN PRIMARY SITE

RICHARD M. STONE

The presenting findings in up to 10 percent of cancer patients may not yield definitive identification of the site of origin of the neoplasm. Such patients with cancer of unknown primary site present difficult diagnostic and therapeutic dilemmas. First, since the number of additional studies which could be ordered may be vast, costly, and/or uncomfortable for the patient, the strategy involved in the "search for the primary" must consider what, if any, result the precise identification of the site of origin will have on the patient's treatment and length of survival. Second, while those individuals with cancer of unknown primary site fare poorly (median survival <6 months), there are subgroups of patients who are more likely to benefit from treatment and, in some cases, to enjoy long intervals without evidence of disease. The literature provides a poor guide for the care of such patients due to the largely retrospective nature of the reports, the heterogeneity of the tumors, the selection bias in small individual retrospective studies, and the variability in both the definition of the syndrome and the thoroughness of the evaluation performed to identify a primary site.

The biologic behavior of metastatic cancers of unknown primary site is unique compared with that of other nonhematopoietic neoplasms. Such cancers as breast and prostate are relatively uncommon causes of metastatic malignancy of unknown primary origin. In patients with breast cancer, for example, a breast lesion is almost always identified either prior to or simultaneously with the documentation of metastatic disease. Moreover, cancers presenting with an unknown primary site often display unusual patterns of metastatic spread (e.g., pancreatic cancer presenting with bony metastases). The predominance of tumor bulk located in distant sites rather than in the tissue of origin suggests that the genetic lesions accounting for the development of such malignancies convey a distinctly aggressive phenotype. Frequently, biopsy of an involved site will reveal a poorly differentiated histology, which represents the morphologic correlate of this biologic behavior. The relative propensity of tumor deposits in patients with metastatic cancer of unknown primary site to grow in distant locations also implies that the malignant cells may proliferate in the absence of the specific host factors (e.g., growth-promoting proteins, vascular supply) important in the development of more typical cancers. Although physiologic and genetic data which might account for the distinctive natural history of neoplasms of unknown origin are scant, cell lines derived from tumors obtained from patients with this syndrome may have abnormalities of chromosome 1, a karyotype generally associated with advanced malignancy.

DEFINITION While there is no universally accepted definition of the syndrome of metastatic cancer of unknown primary site, a helpful approach has been proposed by Ultmann and Phillip. They suggest that an occult primary neoplasm should fulfill each of the following criteria: (1) biopsy-proven malignancy, (2) history, physical examinations, chest film, complete blood counts, urinalysis, and stool test for occult blood not indicative of a primary site, (3) histologic evaluation not consistent with a primary tumor at the biopsy site, and (4) additional diagnostic studies failing to identify the primary site. Such additional diagnostic tests could include, for example, colonoscopy in a patient whose rectal examination discloses guaiac-positive stool or a meticulous otolaryngologic examination in a patient who presents with squamous cell carcinoma in a cervical node. With increased understanding of the natural history of certain tumors and with the routine use of computed tomographic (CT) scanning as well as detailed pathologic studies, there are many cases which may fulfill the definition of cancer of unknown primary site, yet where there is a reasonable suspicion that a given organ is the probable site of origin.

DIAGNOSTIC EVALUATION   History and physical examination Though usually unrevealing, a thorough history and physical examination should be carried out to elicit easily obtainable clues regarding the primary site. The patient should be questioned concerning epigastric pain, which, if present, would mandate careful exclusion of pancreatic carcinoma as well as other gastrointestinal malignancies. Symptoms referable to a given location (e.g., new cough, hematochezia, hemoptysis, change in bowel habits, unusual vaginal bleeding, nipple discharge) should prompt an aggressive, yet specific, diagnostic approach. Occupational exposure to asbestos, for example, would make the prior probability of mesothelioma much higher. The absence of prior smoking reduces the likelihood of lung cancer but, of course, does not exclude it. A history of fulguration of a skin lesion, colonic polypectomy, dilation and curettage, or prostate biopsy should prompt a review of the original histology. Other than inferences drawn from the location of the involved area (see below), the physical examination will probably be unrevealing unless a thorough pelvic and rectal examination has not been performed previously.

Additional studies In females with metastatic adenocarcinoma or poorly differentiated carcinoma, mammography should be performed. The use of abdominal/pelvic CT scans may lead to identification of the primary site in as many as 35 percent of patients and will certainly reduce the number of cases of pancreatic cancer in which the primary site is obscure before death. It is reasonable to obtain tumor markers such as an alpha fetoprotein (AFP), beta human chorionic gonadotropin (βhCG), carcinoembryonic antigen (CEA), CA-125 (associated with ovarian cancer), and prostate-specific antigen (PSA). However, since many different adenocarcinomas elaborate either CEA or CA-125, or both, the value of these markers resides in following response to therapy rather than in the identification of a primary site. Moreover, poorly differentiated colonic tumors frequently fail to elaborate CEA, and patients with benign prostate hypertrophy may have modestly elevated PSA levels, reducing the reliability of these markers in defining the primary site in a patient with metastatic cancer. Numerous studies have shown a lack of benefit of contrast studies (upper gastrointestinal series, barium enema, or intravenous pyelogram) in

TABLE 326-1 Suggested clinical evaluation of patients with metastatic cancer of unknown primary site

	Evaluate
History	Smoking history, asbestos exposure, abdominal pain

Physical examination	Lymph nodes, thyroid, skin
	  Men: prostate
	  Women: breasts, pelvic examination

Laboratory evaluation	Stool for occult blood, urinalysis, CBC, liver function tests, serum prostate specific antigen (PSA), βhCG, AFP, CEA, CA-125 (women), CXR, CT abdomen, mammography
Pathologic evaluation	See Table 326-2.

patients with metastatic cancer of unknown primary site who have no specific symptoms or no findings referable to the gastrointestinal or urinary tracts. Moreover, autopsy series reveal that the most likely primary site of origin includes epithelial tissues such as lung, stomach, colon, and kidney which give rise to tumors that respond poorly to chemotherapy, minimizing the impact of such a diagnosis. A summary of a reasonable diagnostic approach is found in Table 326-1.

Pathologic review The most important aspect in the evaluation of the patient with metastatic cancer of unknown primary site is to derive maximal information from the tissue obtained at biopsy. Vital clues pertaining to the primary site and ultimately to the patient's management can be obtained by careful review of light microscopic, immunohistochemical, ultrastructural, immunologic, and molecular biologic findings. First, if there is any question concerning the adequacy of the original biopsy sample for either confirmation of malignancy or performance of additional specialized studies, rebiopsy is mandated. The clinician must have a close working relationship with a pathologist skilled in the evaluation of tumor specimens, especially when the organ of origin is uncertain. On either the initial or subsequent biopsy, plans may be made to process the tissue for (1) routine fixation for light microscopic, histochemical, and immunohistochemical analysis, (2) freezing for DNA isolation or for additional immunologic evaluation (e.g., certain antibody-based detection methods cannot be applied to fixed, paraffin-embedded tissue), and (3) fixation, usually in glutaraldehyde, for ultrastructural analysis. Fresh tissue may be disaggregated into single-cell suspension for short-term culture for purposes of cytogenetic analysis.

If routine histologic analysis fails to suggest the tissue of origin (e.g., gland formulation in adenocarcinoma, psammoma bodies in ovarian or thyroid cancer, or spindle architecture in sarcomas), special histochemical studies may be helpful. For example, mucin positivity is helpful in recognizing poorly differentiated adenocarcinoma. Based on light microscopic review, including histochemical analysis, approximately half of those with metastatic cancer of unknown primary site are determined to have adenocarcinoma, an additional quarter have squamous cell carcinoma, usually of head and neck or lung origin, and the remainder are poorly differentiated neoplasms. In the latter group, immunohistochemical, cytogenetic, and molecular biologic studies can be extremely useful in detecting sarcoma, germ cell carcinoma, lymphoma, melanoma, or other tumors whose diagnosis would suggest a more specific therapeutic approach.

IMMUNOHISTOCHEMICAL ANALYSIS Antibodies to specific cell components and the ability to detect binding by sensitive visualization methods such as peroxidase or streptavidin-biotin permit the characterization of tumors that fail to be characterized when standard techniques are employed. Since in most situations no single antibody is of sufficient specificity to identify the primary site with certainty, a battery of such reagents must be employed. Table 326-2 provides a list of antigens that may be assessed by immunohistochemical analysis in an undifferentiated or poorly differentiated specimen. It is particularly important to exclude the diagnosis of lymphoma by employing antibodies reactive to the leukocyte common antigen (LCA, CD45). The presence of LCA suggests that the patient has a

TABLE 326-2 Possible pathologic evaluation of biopsies from patients with metastatic cancer of unknown primary site

Evaluation/findings	Suggested primary site
HISTOLOGY (HEMATOXYLIN AND EOSIN STAINING)	
Psammoma bodies, papillary configuration	Ovarian, thyroid
Signet ring cells	Stomach
IMMUNOHISTOLOGY	
Leukocyte common antigen (LCA, CD45)	Lymphoid neoplasm
Leu-M1	Hodgkin's disease
Epithelial membrane antigen	Carcinoma
Cytokeratin intermediate filaments	Carcinoma
CEA	Carcinoma
HMB 45	Melanoma
Desmin	Sarcoma
Thyroglobulin	Thyroid carcinoma
Calcitonin	Medullary carcinoma of the thyroid
Myoglobin	Rhabdomyosarcoma
PSA/prostatic acid phosphatase	Prostate
AFP	Liver, stomach, germ cell
Placental alkaline phosphatase	Germ cell
B, T cell markers	Lymphoid neoplasm
S-100	Neuroendocrine
Gross cystic fluid protein	Breast, sweat gland
FLOW CYTOMETRY	
B, T cell markers	Lymphoid neoplasm
ULTRASTRUCTURE	
Actin-myosin filaments	Rhabdomyosarcoma
Secretory granules	Neuroendocrine tumors
Desmosomes	Carcinoma
Premelanosomes	Melanoma
CYTOGENETICS	
Isochromosome 12p;12q(−)	Germ cell
t(11;22)	Ewing's sarcoma, primitive neuroectodermal tumor
t(8;14)*	Lymphoid neoplasm
3p(−)	Small cell lung carcinoma; renal cell carcinoma, mesothelioma
t(X;18)	Synovial sarcoma
t(12;16)	Myxoid liposarcoma
t(12;22)	Clear cell sarcoma (melanoma of soft parts)
t(2;13)	Alveolar rhabdomyosarcoma
RECEPTOR ANALYSIS	
Estrogen/progesterone receptor	Breast
MOLECULAR BIOLOGIC STUDIES	
Immunoglobulin, *bcl-2*, T cell receptor gene rearrangement*	Lymphoid neoplasm

* Or any other rearrangement involving an antigen-receptor gene.

lymphoid neoplasm and will respond to therapy with the same likelihood as if there was no diagnostic ambiguity. Compared with the usually poor prognosis in patients with metastatic carcinoma of unknown primary site, such a finding is indeed welcome news; long-term disease-free survival in patients with diffuse large cell lymphoma is approximately 40 percent when a regimen such as CHOP (cyclophosphamide, doxorubicin, vincristine, and prednisone) is employed. The immunohistochemical detection of specific types of filament proteins is helpful in the identification of carcinomas and sarcomas. The presence of keratin suggests carcinoma, since essentially all epithelial tumors contain this protein. However, certain sarcomas, mesotheliomas, and germ cell tumors are also keratin-positive, emphasizing the need for the judicious use of a battery of immunohistochemical markers. Sarcomas may react with antibodies to desmin. Breast, prostate, and thyroid carcinomas can each be suggested if the tissue

COLOR ATLASES

Atlas of Dermatology

1 Common Skin Diseases and Lesions
2 Cutaneous Neoplasms
3 Pigmented Lesions–Benign and Malignant
4 Infectious Disease and the Skin
5 Immunologically Mediated Skin Disease
6 Skin Manifestations of Internal Disease

7 Atlas of Endoscopic Findings
8 Atlas of Fundoscopic Examination
9 Atlas of Hematology

Atlas of Dermatology

Stephen F. Templeton
Thomas J. Lawley

1 Common Skin Diseases and Lesions

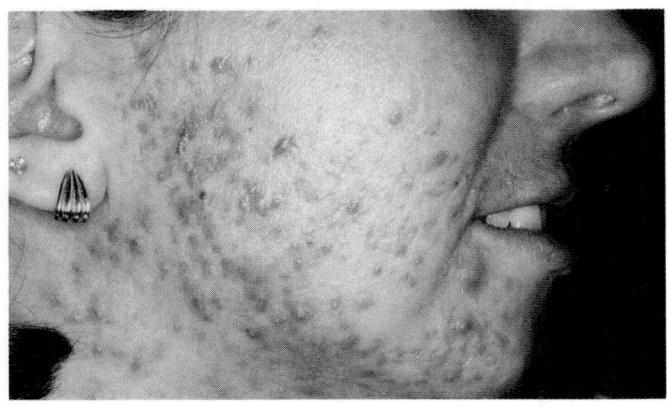

A1-1 **Acne vulgaris** with inflammatory papules, pustules, and comedones.

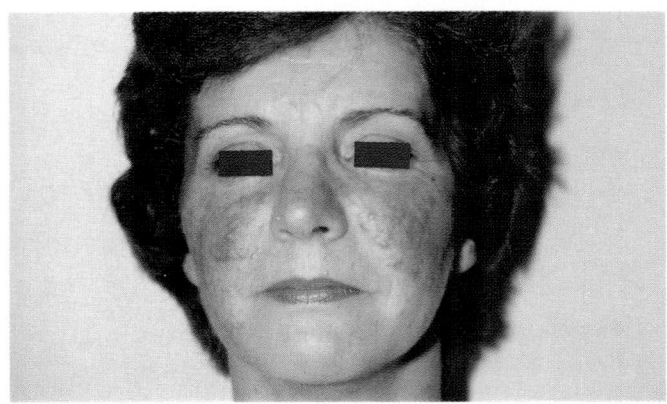

A1-2 **Acne rosacea** with prominent facial erythema, telangiectasias, scattered papules, and small pustules.

A1-4 **Atopic dermatitis** with excoriated, lichenified plaques in the popliteal fossa.

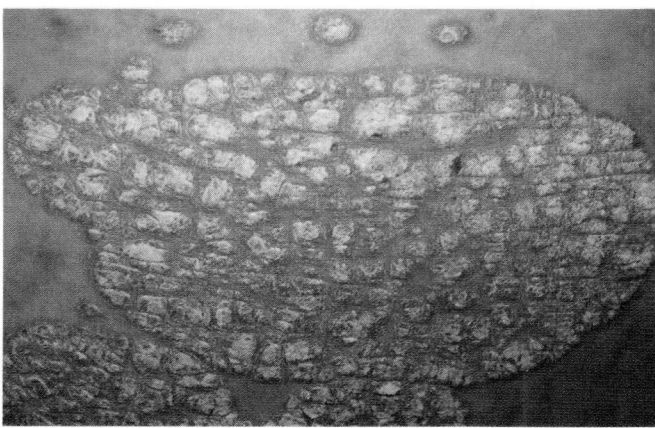

A1-3 **Psoriasis** is characterized by small and large erythematous plaques with adherent silvery scale.

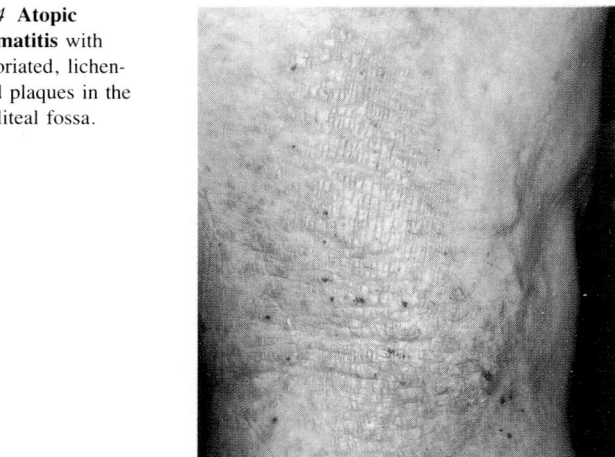

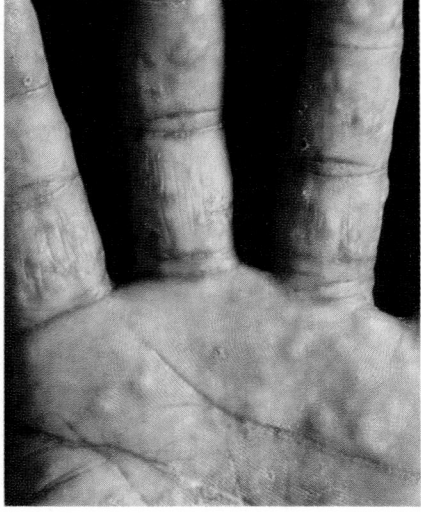

A1-5 **Dyshidrotic eczema,** characterized by deep-seated vesicles and scaling on palms and lateral fingers, is often associated with an atopic diathesis.

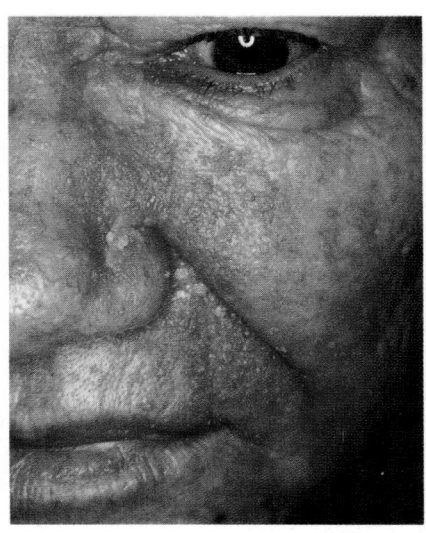

A1-6 **Seborrheic dermatitis** showing central facial erythema with overlying greasy, yellowish scale.

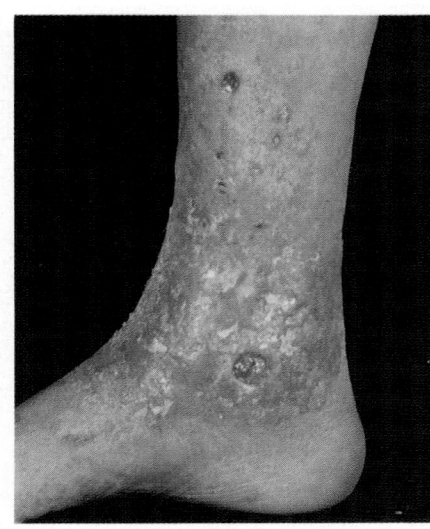

A1-7 **Stasis dermatitis** showing erythematous, scaly, and oozing patches over the lower leg. Several stasis ulcers are also seen in this patient.

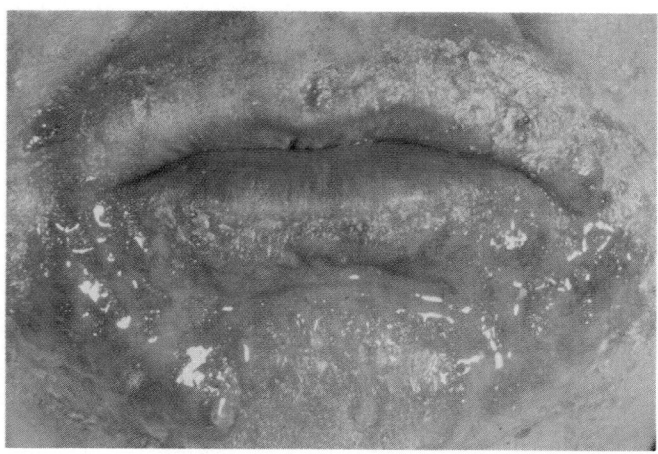

A1-8 **Allergic contact dermatitis,** acute phase, with sharply demarcated, weeping, eczematous plaques in a perioral distribution.

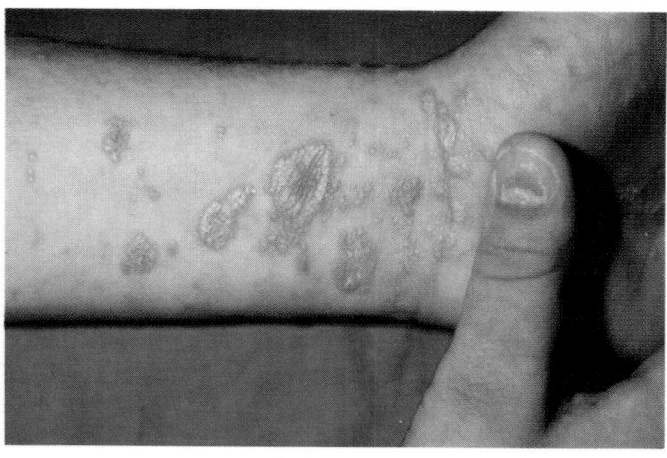

A1-9 **Lichen planus** showing multiple flat-topped, violaceous papules and plaques. Nail dystrophy as seen in this patient's thumbnail may also be a feature.

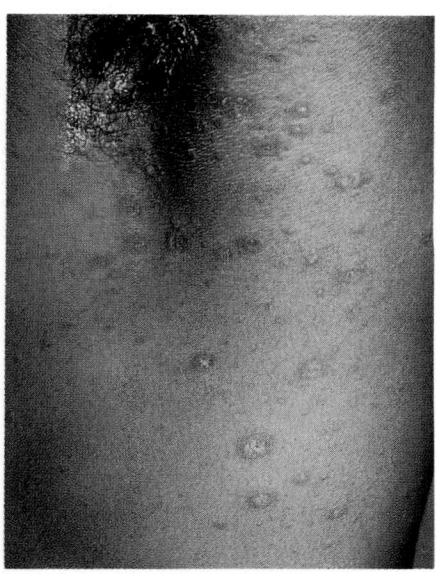

A1-10 **Pityriasis rosea.** Multiple round to oval erythematous patches with fine central scale are distributed along the skin tension lines on the trunk.

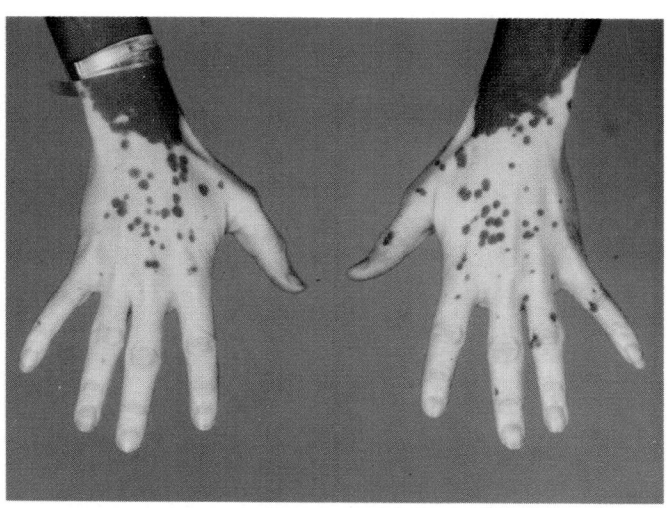

A1-11 **Vitiligo** in a typical acral distribution demonstrating striking cutaneous depigmentation, as a result of loss of melanocytes.

A1-13 **Urticaria** showing characteristic discrete and confluent, edematous, erythematous papules and plaques.

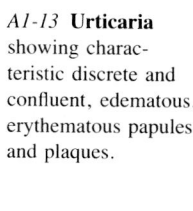

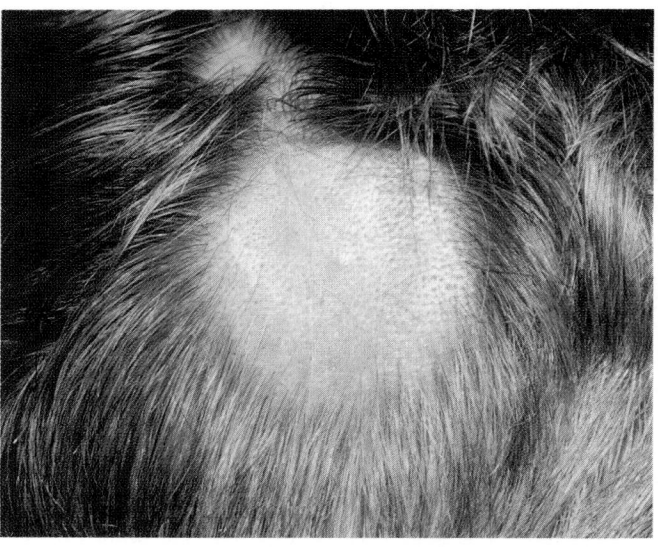

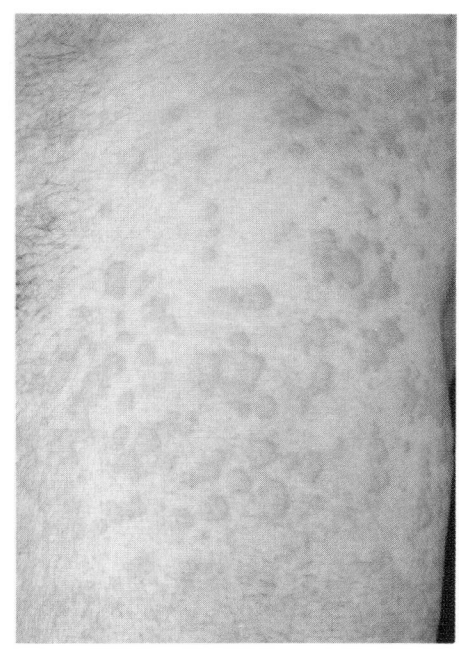

A1-12 **Alopecia areata** characterized by a sharply demarcated circular patch of scalp completely devoid of hairs. Follicular orifices are preserved, indicating a nonscarring alopecia.

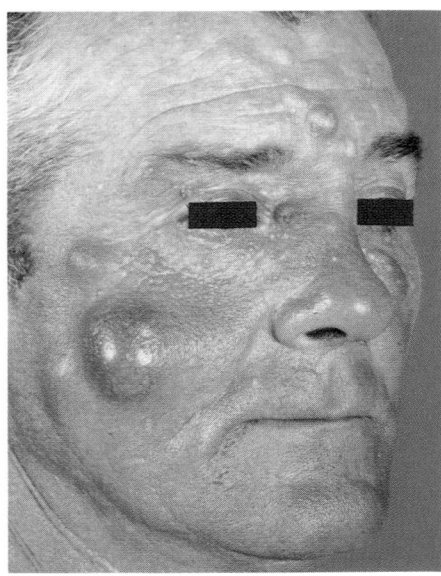

A1-14 **Epidermoid cysts.** Several inflamed and noninflamed firm, cystic nodules are seen in this patient. Often a patulous follicular punctum is observed on the overlying epidermal surface.

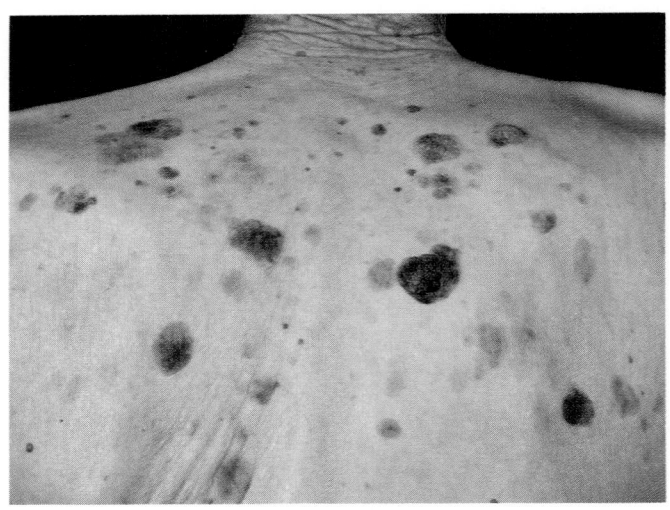

A1-15 **Seborrheic keratoses** are seen as "stuck on," waxy, verrucous papules and plaques with a variety of colors ranging from light tan to black.

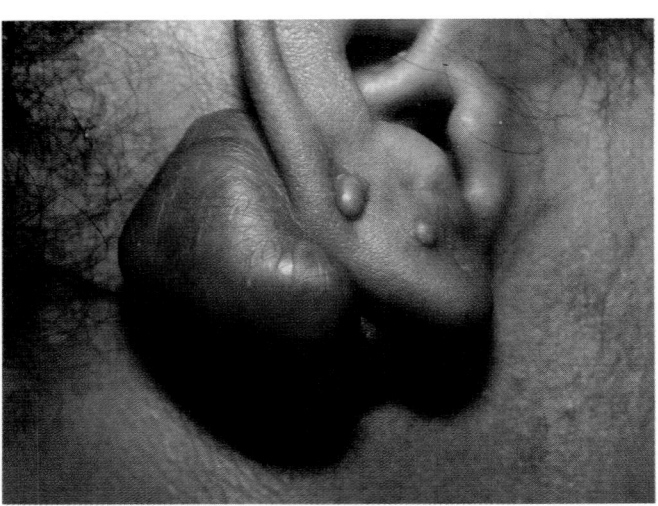

A1-16 **Keloids** resulting from ear piercing, with firm exophytic flesh-colored to erythematous nodules of scar tissue.

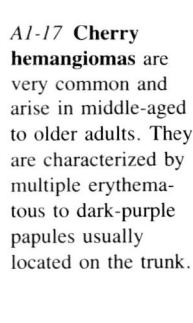

A1-17 **Cherry hemangiomas** are very common and arise in middle-aged to older adults. They are characterized by multiple erythematous to dark-purple papules usually located on the trunk.

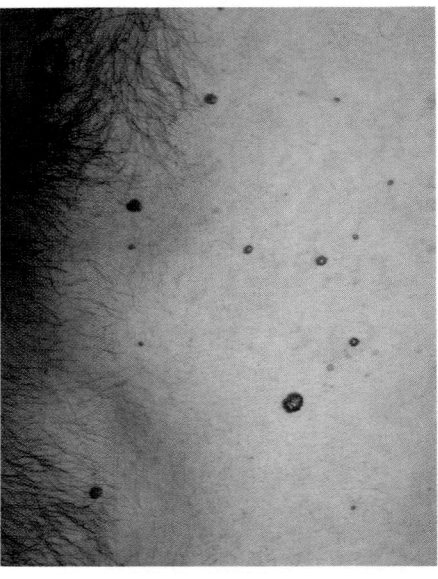

2 Cutaneous Neoplasms

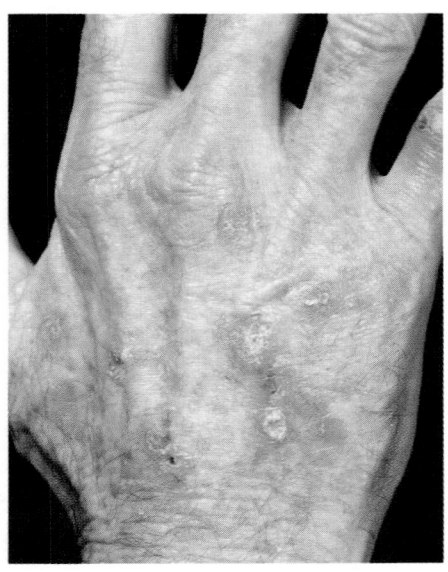

A2-18 **Actinic keratoses** consist of hyperkeratotic erythematous papules and patches on sun-exposed skin. They arise in middle-aged to older adults and have some potential for malignant transformation.

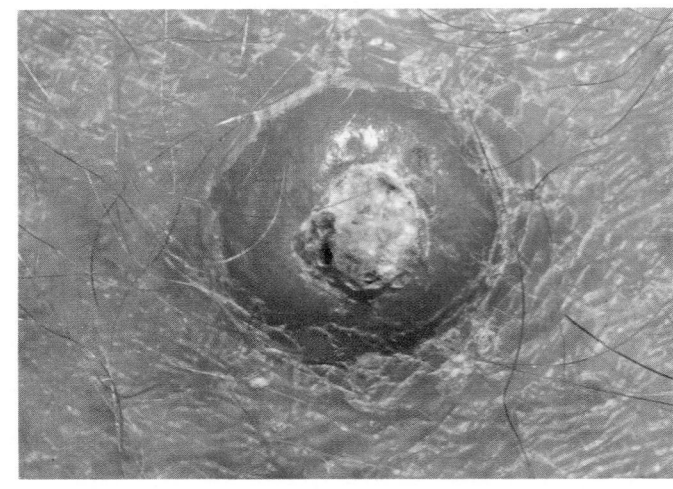

A2-19 **Keratoacanthoma** is a low-grade squamous neoplasm characterized by an exophytic nodule with central keratinous debris.

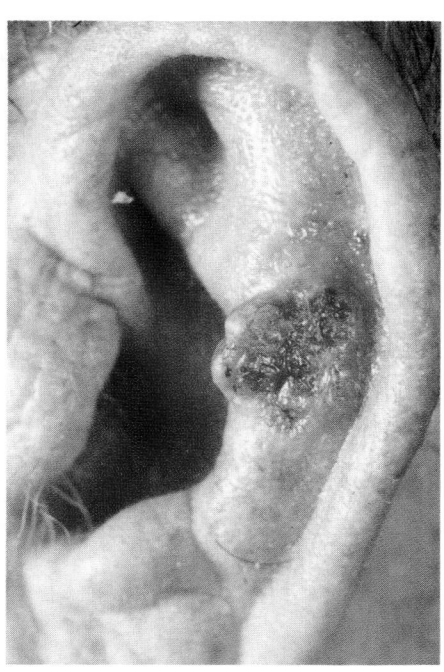

A2-20 **Basal cell carcinoma** showing central ulceration and a pearly, rolled, telangiectatic tumor border.

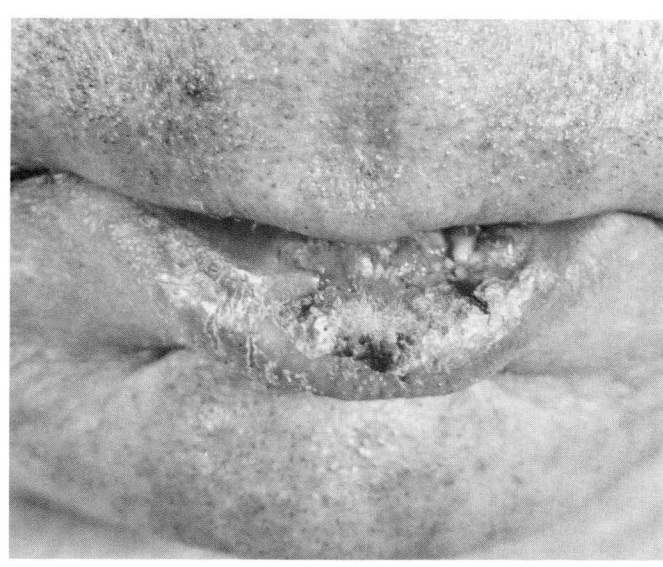

A2-21 **Squamous cell carcinoma** seen here as a hyperkeratotic crusted and somewhat eroded plaque on the lower lip. Sun-exposed skin such as the head, neck, hands, and arms are other typical sites of involvement.

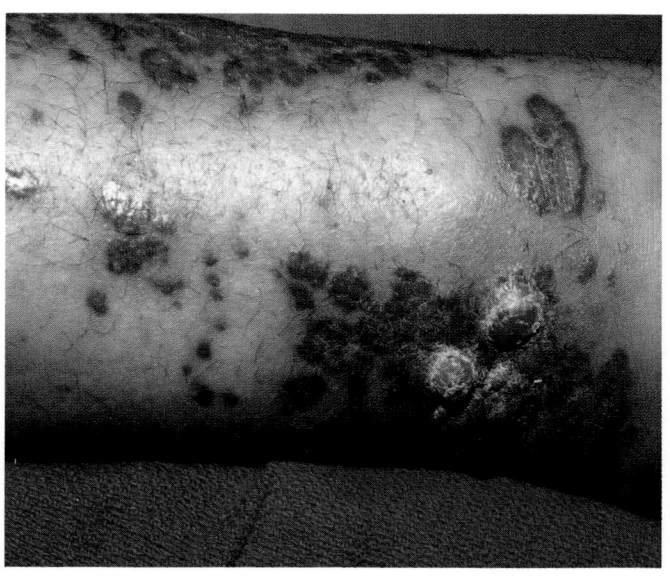

A2-22 **Kaposi's sarcoma** in a patient with AIDS demonstrating patch, plaque, and tumor stages.

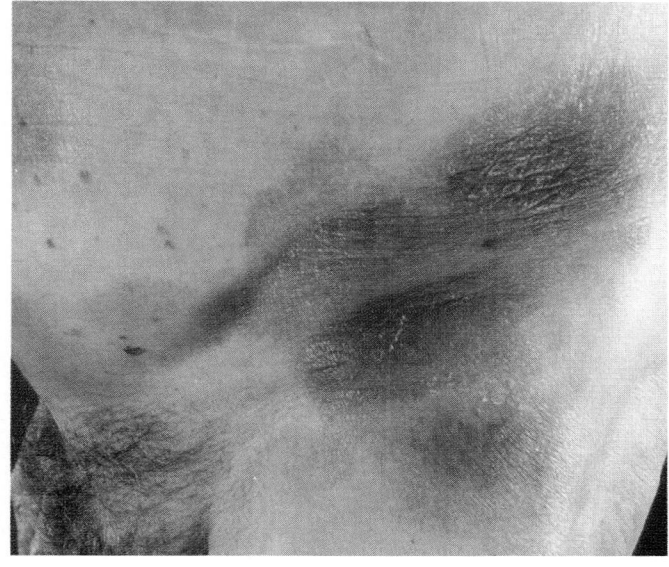

A2-23 **Mycosis fungoides** is a cutaneous T cell lymphoma, and plaque stage lesions are seen in this patient.

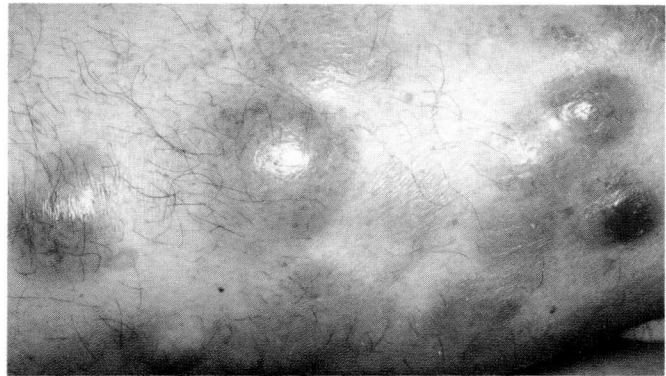

A2-24 **Non-Hodgkin's lymphoma** involving the skin with typical violaceous, "plum-colored" nodules.

A2-25 **Metastatic carcinoma** to the skin is characterized by inflammatory, often ulcerated dermal nodules.

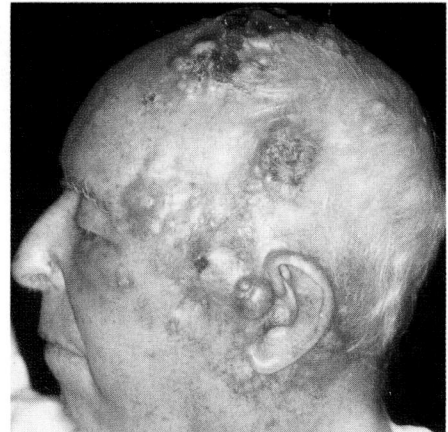

3 Pigmented Lesions—Benign and Malignant

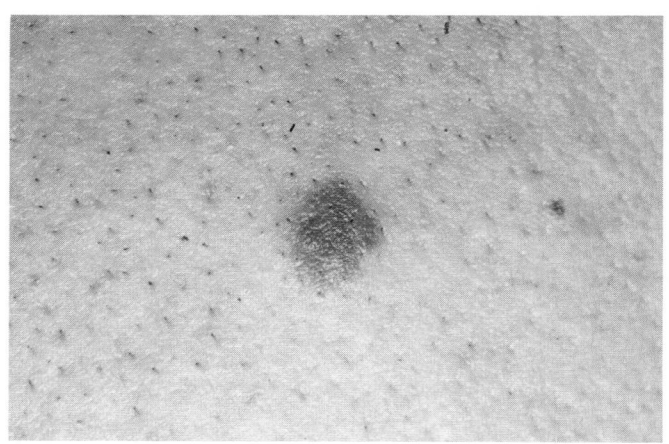

A3-26 **Nevus.** Nevi are benign proliferations of nevomelanocytes characterized by regularly shaped hyperpigmented macules or papules of a uniform color.

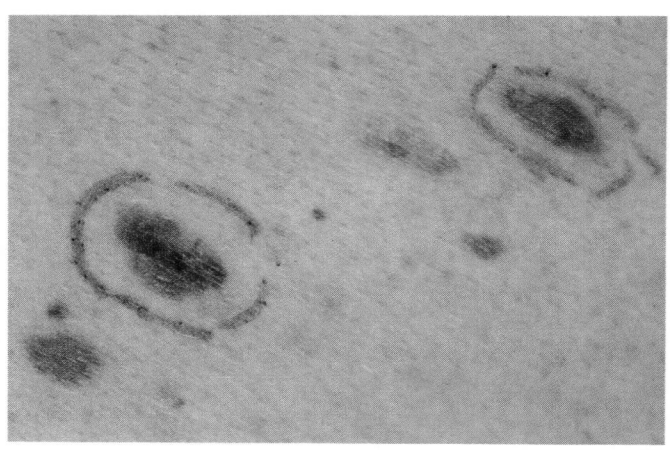

A3-27 **Dysplastic nevi** are irregularly pigmented and shaped nevomelanocytic lesions which may be associated with familial melanoma.

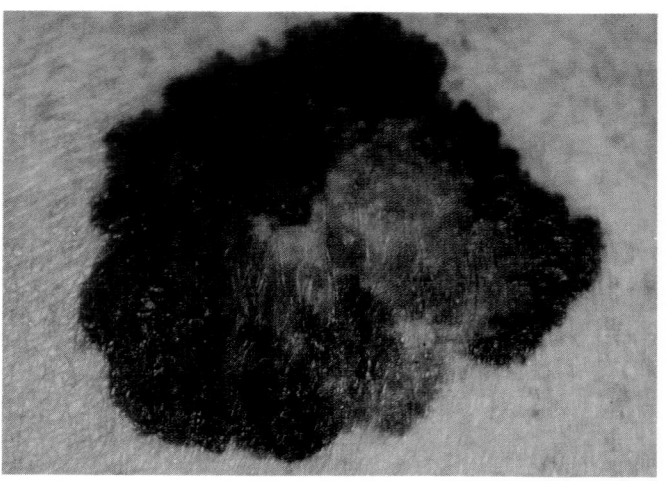

A3-28 **Superficial spreading melanoma** is the most common type of malignant melanoma and demonstrates color variegation (black, blue, brown, pink, and white) and irregular borders.

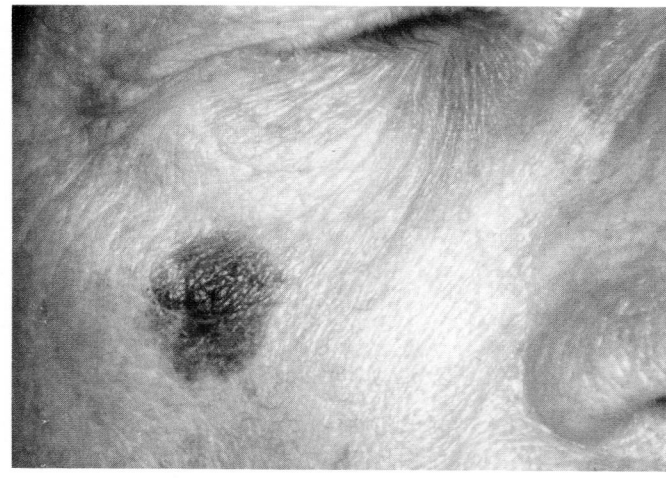

A3-29 **Lentigo maligna melanoma** occurs on sun-exposed skin as a large, hyperpigmented macule or plaque with irregular borders and variable pigmentation.

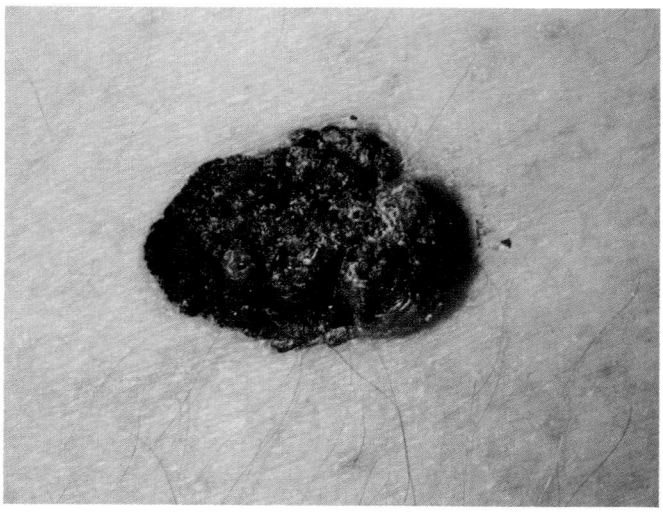

A3-30 **Nodular melanoma** most commonly manifests itself as a rapidly growing, often ulcerated or crusted black nodule.

A3-31 **Acral lentiginous melanoma** is more common in blacks, Orientals, and Hispanics and occurs as an enlarging hyperpigmented macule or plaque on the palms and soles. Lateral pigment diffusion is present.

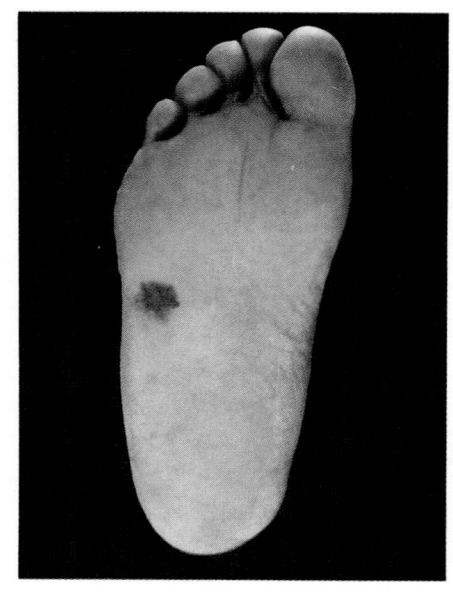

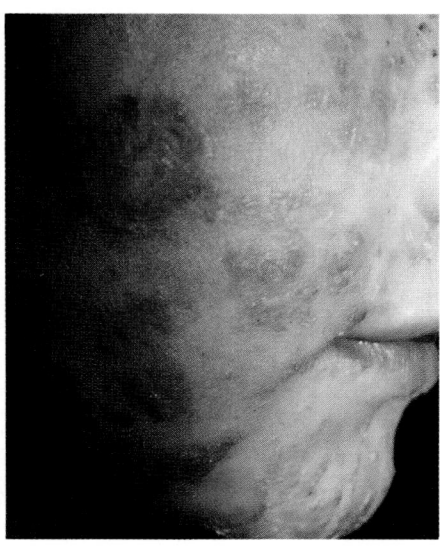

A4-32 **Impetigo contagiosa** is a superficial streptococcal or *Staph. aureus* infection consisting of honey-colored crusts and erythematous weeping erosions. Occasionally bullous lesions may be seen.

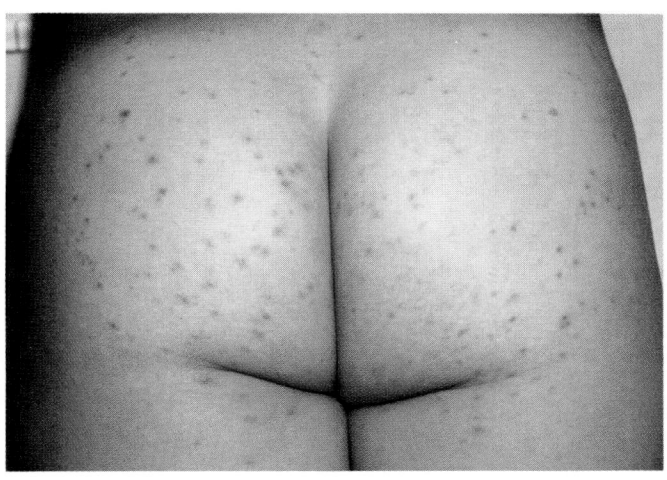

A4-33 **Folliculitis** is a bacterial infection of hair follicles and is seen as erythematous follicular papules and pustules.

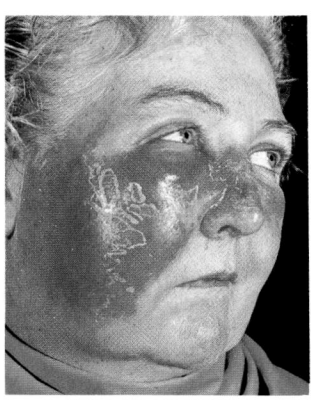

A4-34 **Erysipelas** is a streptococcal infection of the superficial dermis and consists of well-demarcated, erythematous, edematous, warm plaques.

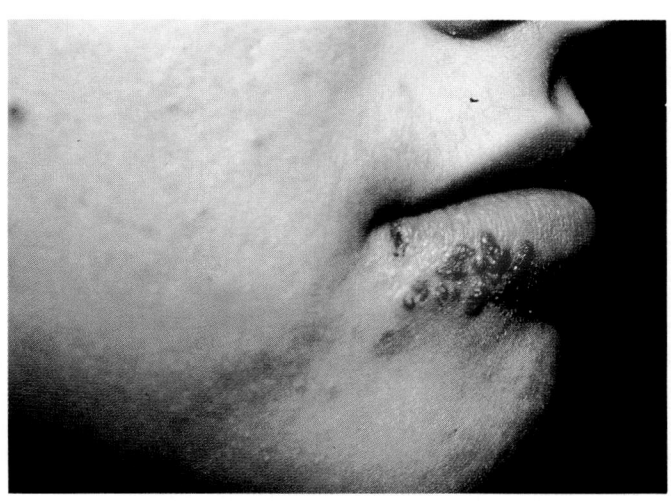

A4-35 **Herpes simplex.** Grouped vesiculopustules on an erythematous base characterize primary HSV infections.

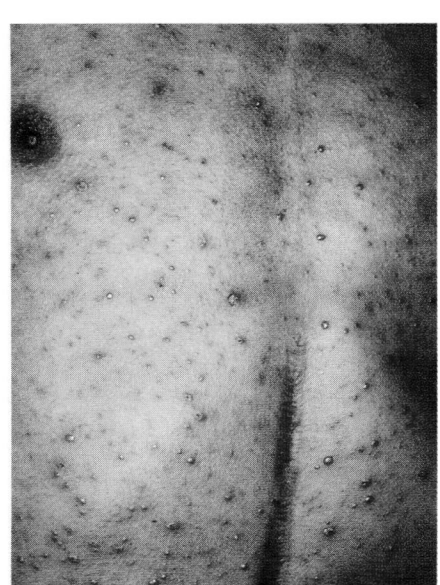

A4-36 **Varicella** showing numerous lesions in various stages of evolution: vesicles on an erythematous base, umbilicated vesicles, and crusts.

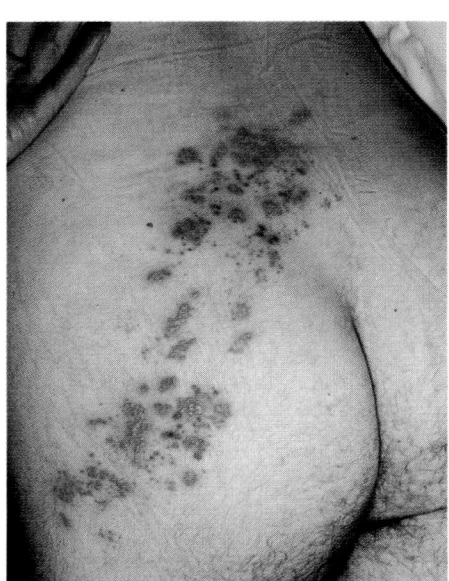

A4-37 **Herpes zoster** seen in this HIV-infected patient as hemorrhagic vesicles and pustules on an erythematous base grouped in a dermatomal distribution.

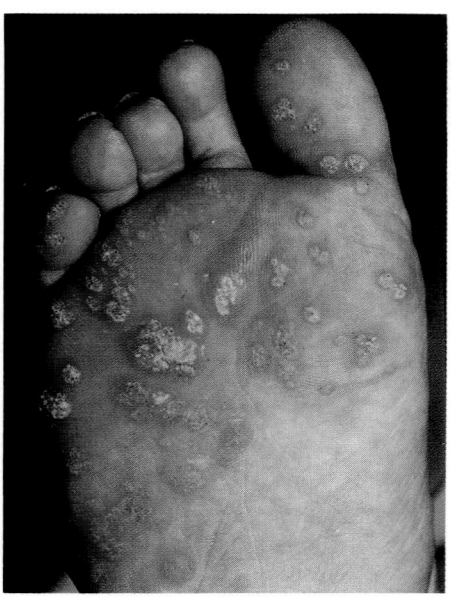

A4-38 **Verrucae** characterized as multiple hyper-keratotic, verrucous papules.

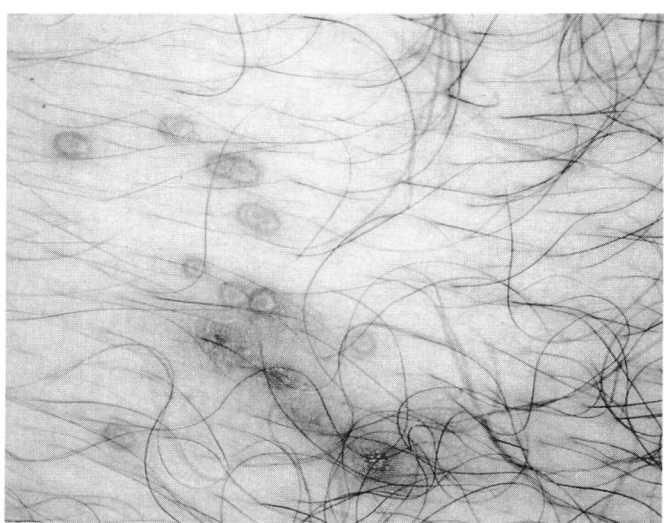

A4-39 **Molluscum contagiosum** is a cutaneous poxvirus infection characterized by multiple umbilicated flesh-colored or hypopigmented papules.

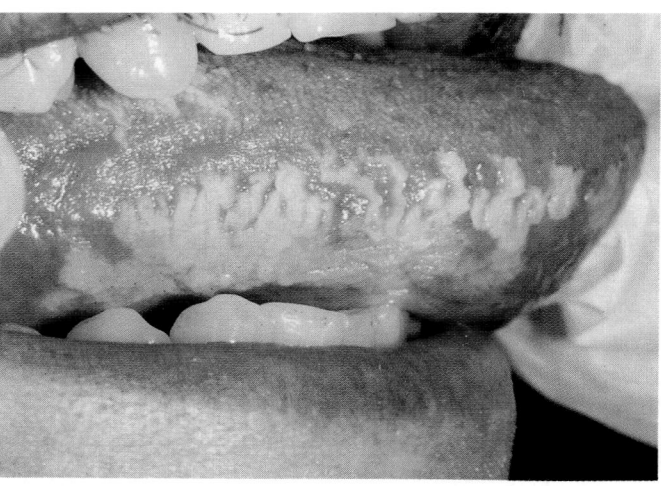

A4-40 **Oral hairy leukoplakia** often presents as white plaques on the lateral tongue and is associated with Epstein-Barr virus infection.

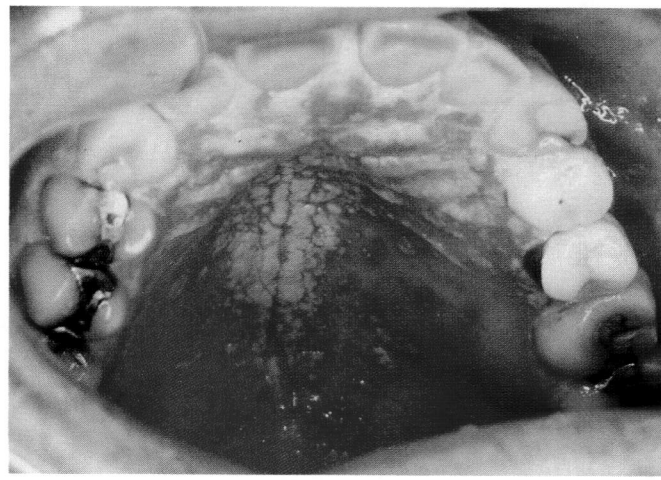

A4-41 **Pseudomembranous oral candidiasis.** Adherent white, mucoid plaques with an erythematous halo seen here on the palate often indicates an immunocompromised state.

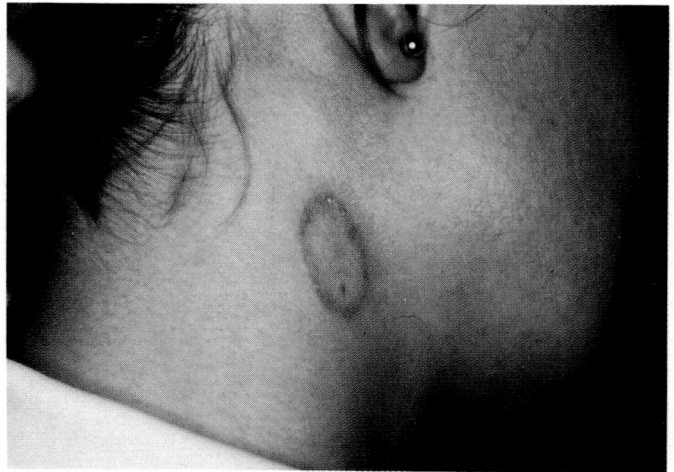

A4-42 **Tinea corporis** is a superficial fungal infection seen here as an erythematous annular scaly plaque with central clearing.

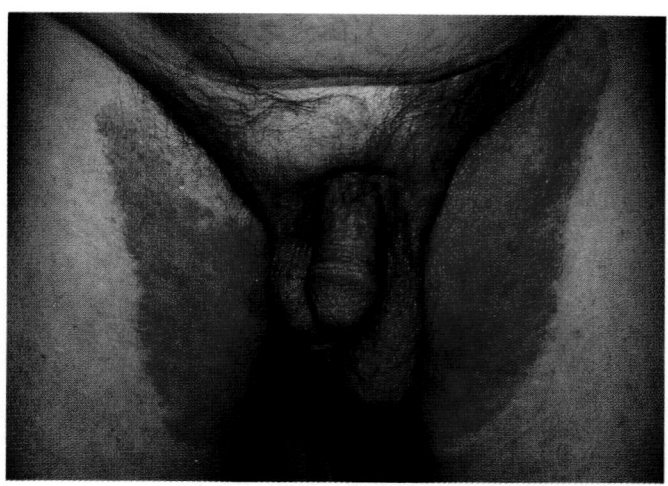

A4-43 **Tinea cruris** is a superficial dermatophyte infection with bilateral scaly, erythematous, annular plaques extending from the inguinal crease to the upper thighs.

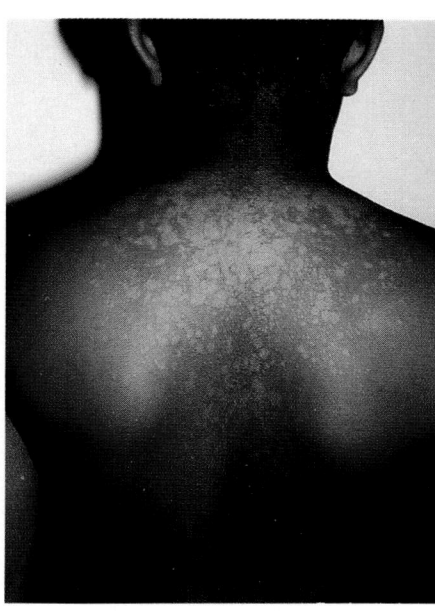

A4-44 **Tinea versicolor** is a superficial cutaneous fungal infection showing a wide variety of lesions. Finely scaling patches may be small or large, hyperpigmented or hypopigmented.

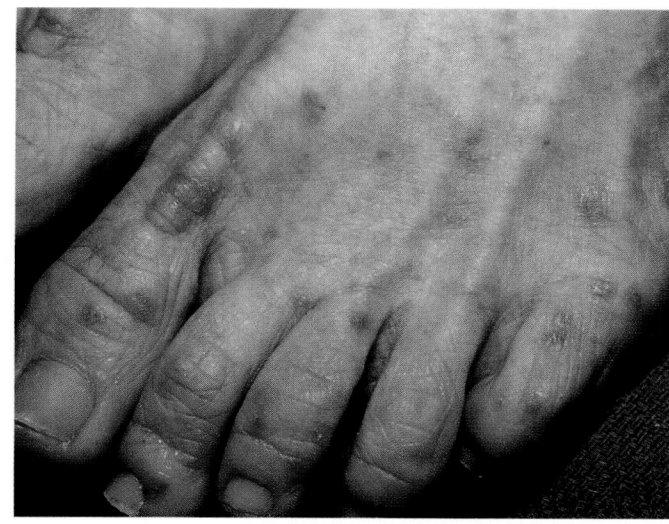

A4-45 **Scabies** showing typical scaling erythematous papules and few linear burrows.

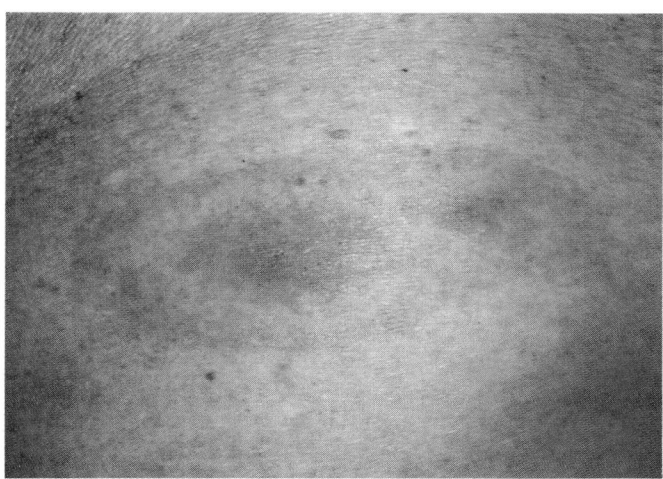

A4-46 **Erythema chronicum migrans** is the early cutaneous manifestation of Lyme disease and is characterized by erythematous annular patches, often with a central erythematous papule at the tick bite site.

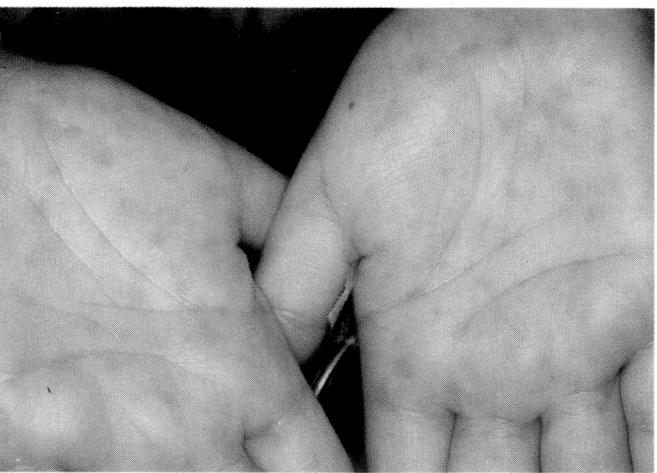

A4-47 **Rocky Mountain spotted fever** demonstrating faint erythematous palmar macules in the early phase of the disease. Lesions may become hemorrhagic (purpuric) as the disease progresses.

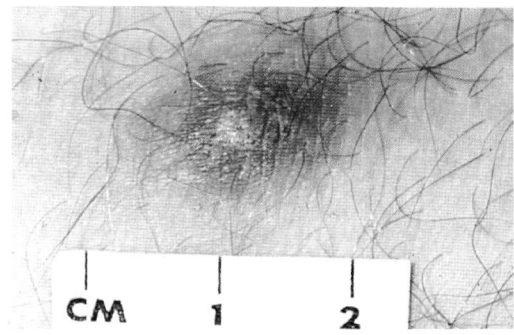

A4-48 **Disseminated gonococcemia** in the skin is seen as hemorrhagic papules and pustules with purpuric centers in an acral distribution.

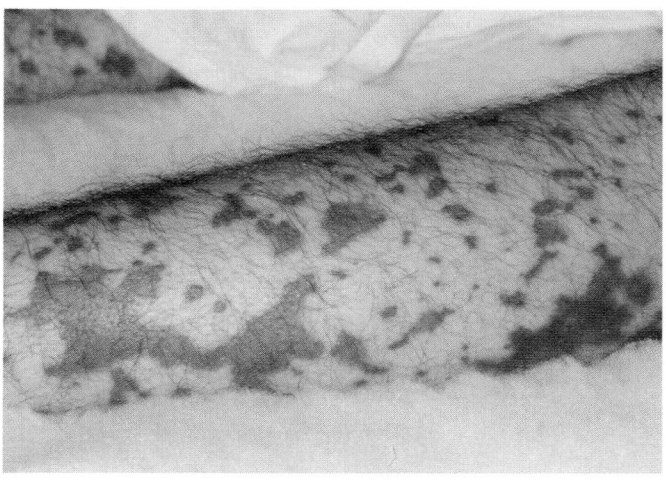

A4-49 **Fulminant meningococcemia** with extensive angular purpuric patches.

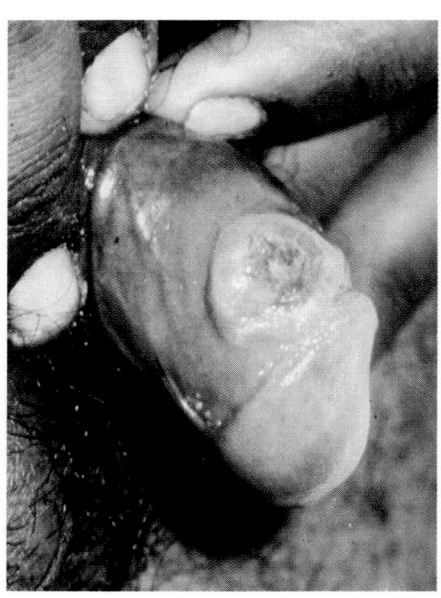

A4-50 **Primary syphilis** with a firm, nontender chancre.

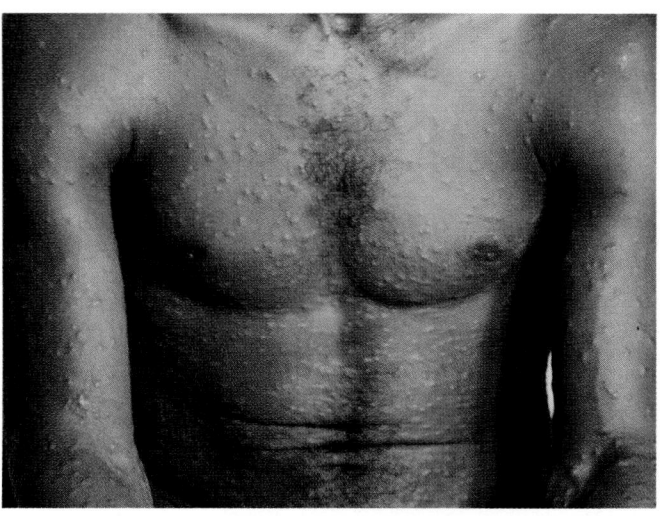

A4-51 **Secondary syphilis** demonstrating the papulosquamous truncal eruption.

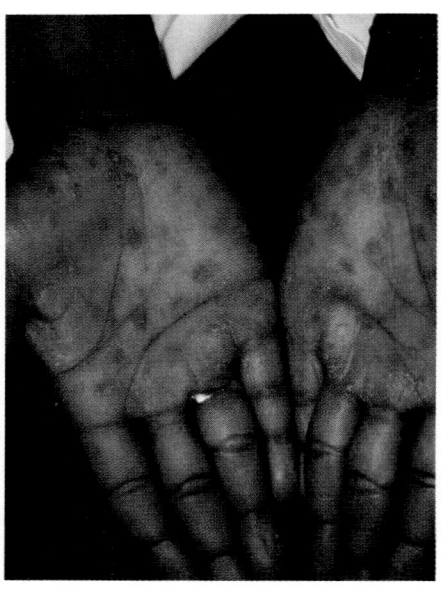

A4-52 **Secondary syphilis** commonly affects the palms and soles with scaling, firm, red-brown papules.

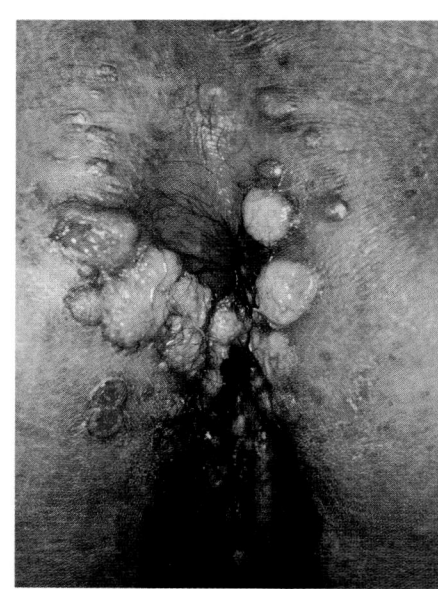

A4-53 **Condylomata lata** are moist somewhat verrucous intertriginous plaques seen in secondary syphilis.

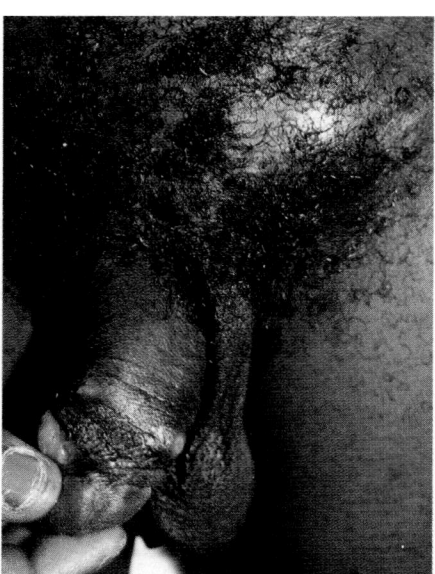

A4-54 **Chancroid** with characteristic penile ulcers and associated left inguinal adenitis (bubo).

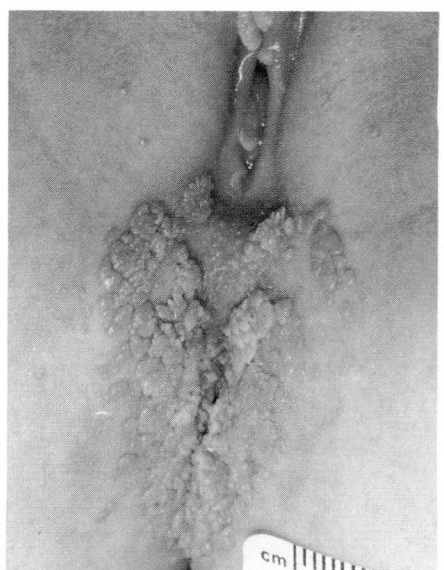

A4-55 **Condylomata acuminata** are lesions induced by human papillomavirus (HPV) and in this patient are seen as multiple verrucous papules coalescing into plaques.

5 Immunologically Mediated Skin Disease

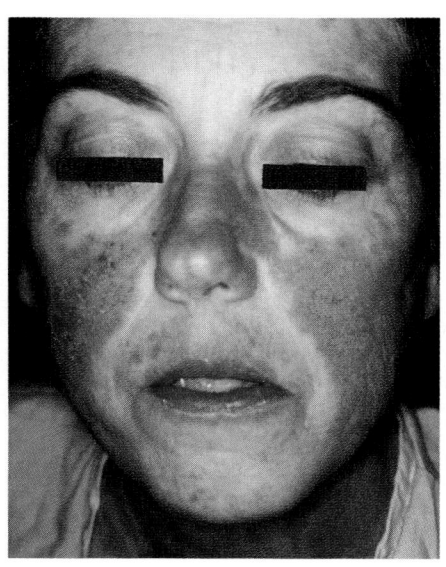

A5-56 **Systemic lupus erythematosus** showing prominent, scaly, malar erythema. Involvement of other sun-exposed sites is also common.

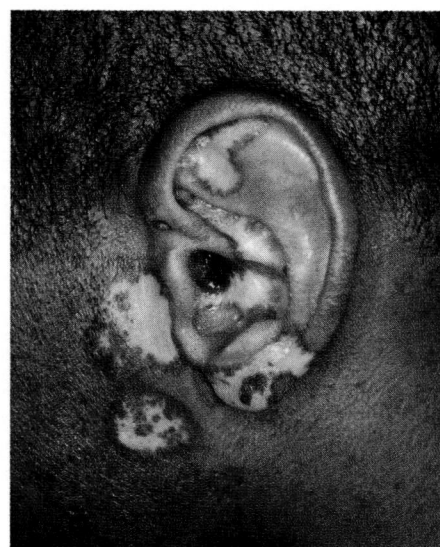

A5-57 **Discoid lupus erythematosus.** Violaceous, hyperpigmented, atrophic plaques, often with evidence of follicular plugging, which may result in scarring, are characteristic of this cutaneous form of lupus.

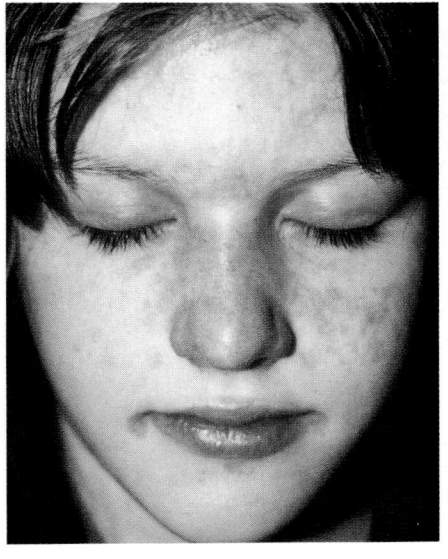

A5-58 **Dermatomyositis.** Periorbital violaceous erythema characterizes the classic heliotrope rash.

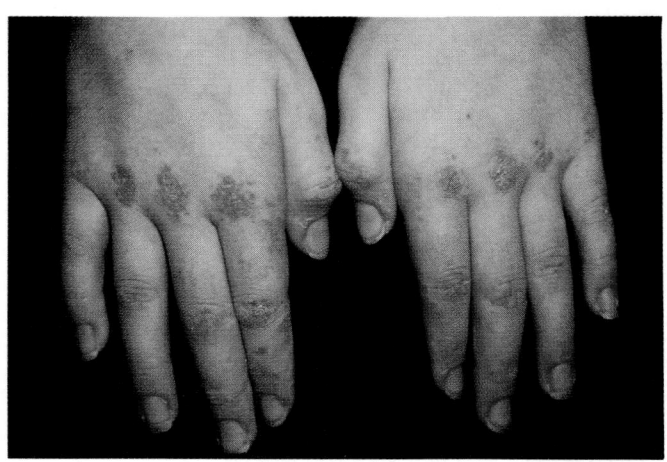

A5-59 **Dermatomyositis** often involves the hands as erythematous flat-topped papules over the knuckles (Gottron's sign) and periungal telangiectasias.

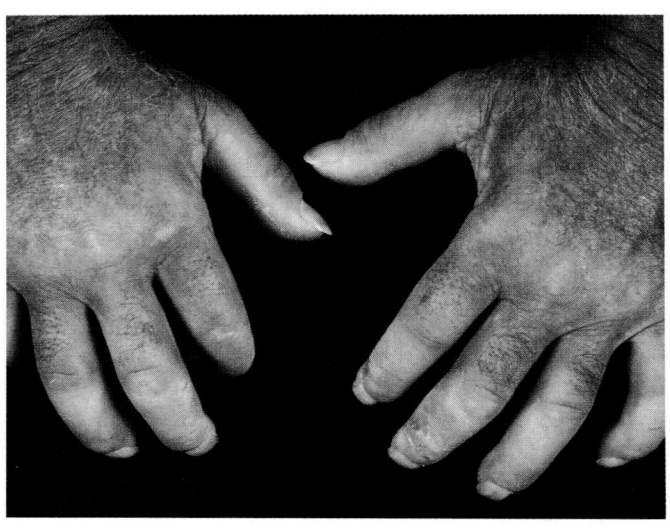

A5-60 **Scleroderma** showing acral sclerosis and focal digital ulcers.

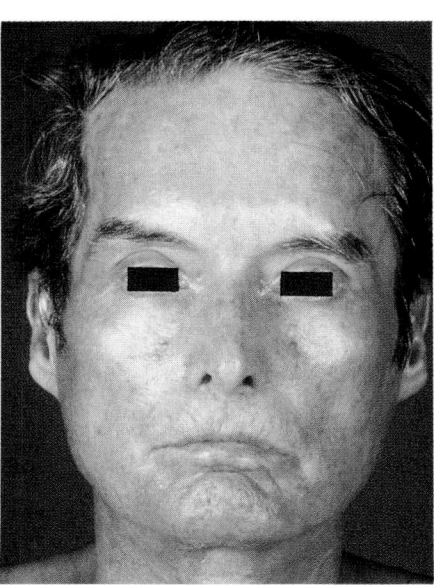

A5-61 **Scleroderma** characterized by typical expressionless, mask-like facies.

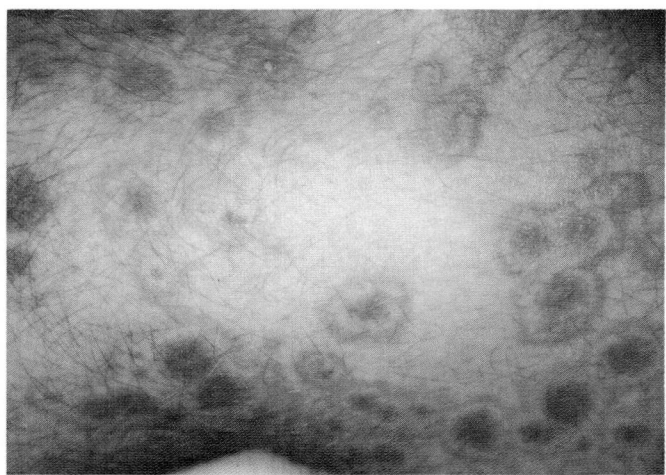

A5-62 **Erythema multiforme** is characterized by multiple erythematous plaques with a target or iris morphology and usually represents a hypersensitivity reaction to drugs or infections (especially herpes simplex virus).

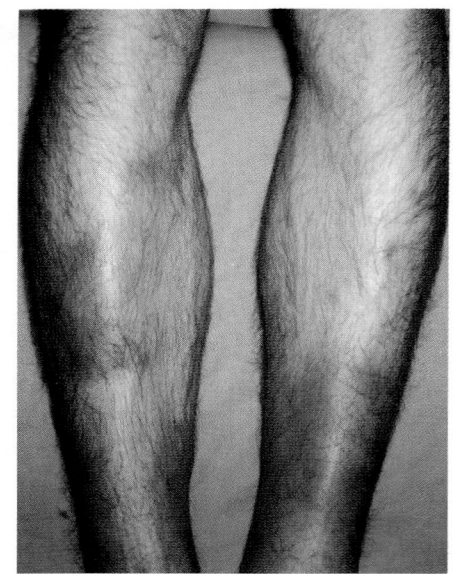

A5-63 **Erythema nodosum** is a panniculitis characterized by tender deep-seated nodules and plaques usually located on the lower extremities.

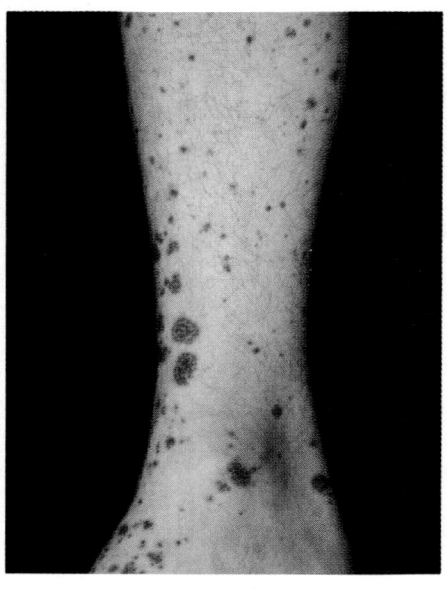

A5-64 **Vasculitis.** Palpable purpuric papules on the lower legs are seen in this patient with cutaneous small vessel vasculitis.

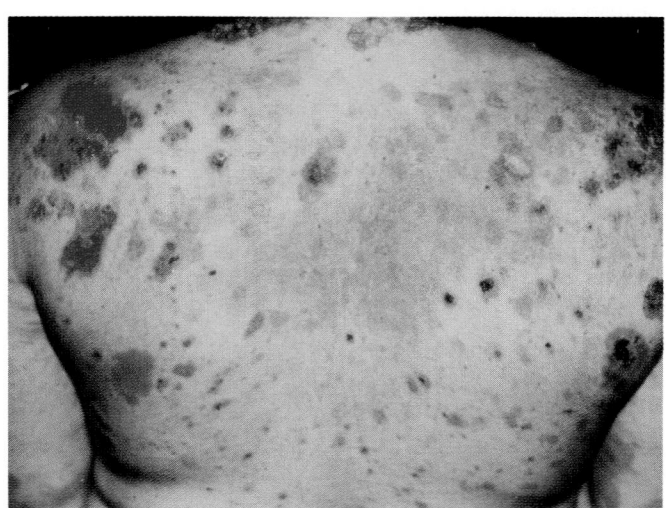

A5-65 **Pemphigus vulgaris** demonstrating flaccid bullae which are easily ruptured, resulting in multiple erosions and crusted plaques.

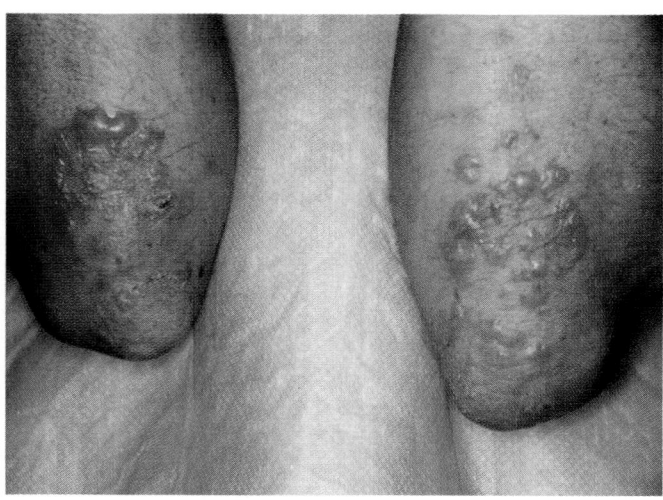

A5-66 **Dermatitis herpetiformis** manifested by pruritic, grouped vesicles in a typical location. The vesicles are often excoriated and may occur on knees, buttocks, and posterior scalp.

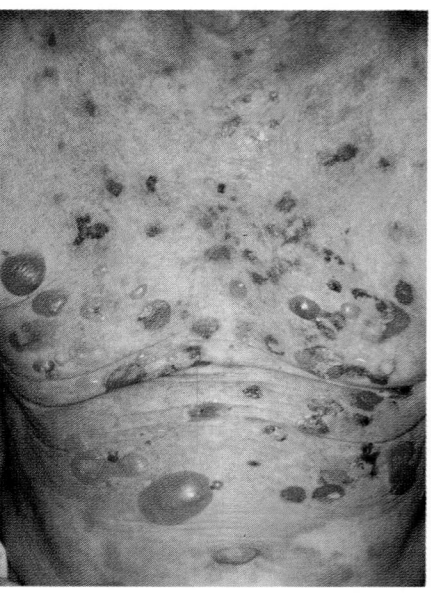

A5-67 **Bullous pemphigoid** with tense vesicles and bullae on an erythematous, urticarial base.

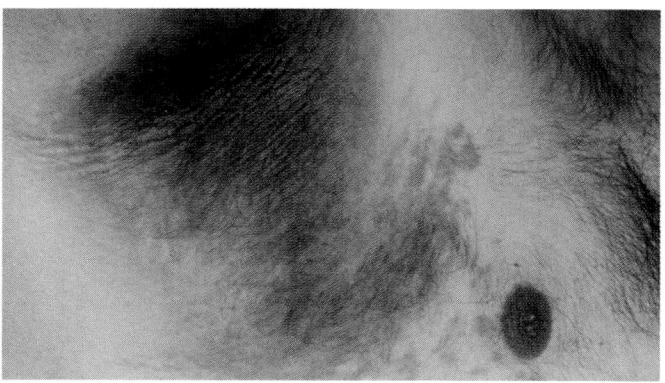

A6-68 **Acanthosis nigricans** demonstrating typical hyperpigmented axillary plaques with a velvet-like, verrucous surface.

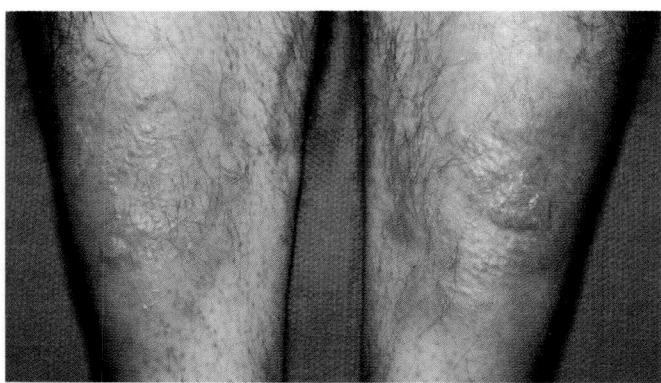

A6-69 **Pretibial myxedema** manifesting as waxy, infiltrated plaques in a patient with Graves' disease.

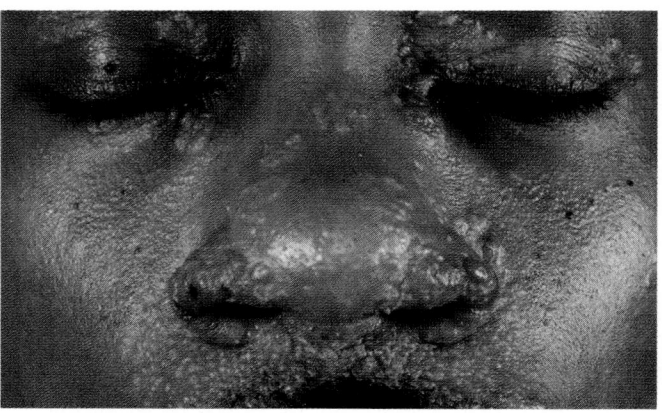

A6-70 **Sarcoid.** Infiltrated papules and plaques of variable color are seen in a typical paranasal and periorbital location.

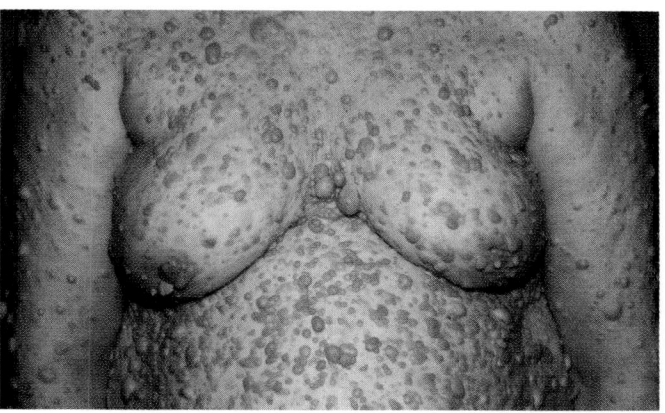

A6-71 **Neurofibromatosis** demonstrating numerous flesh-colored cutaneous neurofibromas.

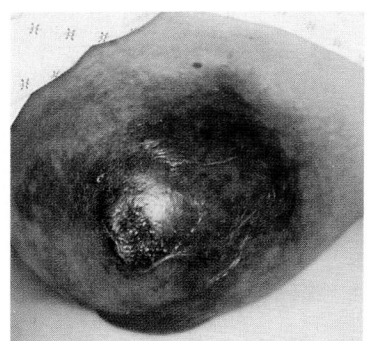

A6-72 **Coumarin necrosis** showing cutaneous and subcutaneous necrosis of a breast. Other fatty areas such as buttocks and thighs are also common sites of involvement.

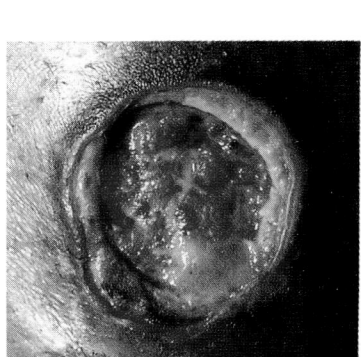

A6-73 **Pyoderma gangrenosum** showing a somewhat purulent ulcer with violaceous and undermined wound edges.

Sources of Photographs

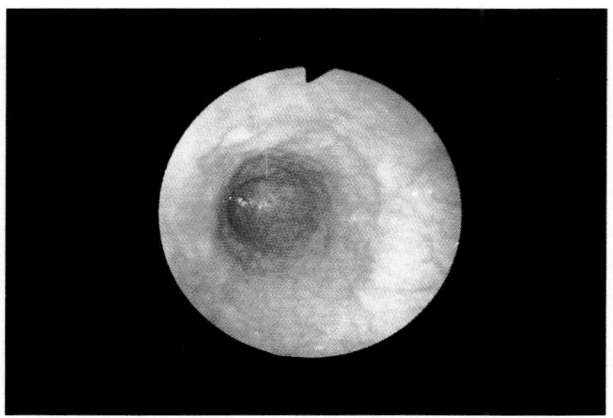

A7-1 **Normal esophagus;** fine vasculature can be seen.

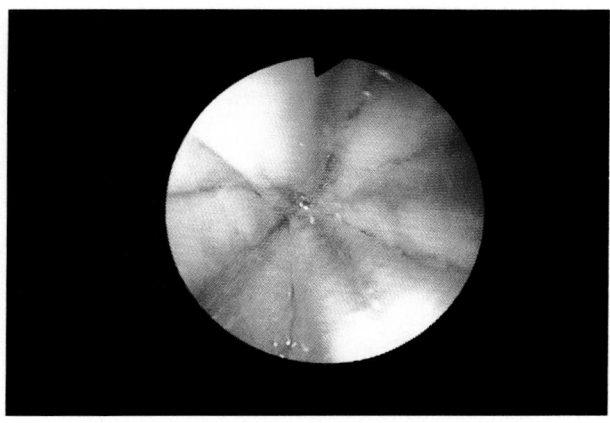

A7-2 **Peptic regurgitant esophagitis;** linear red streaks with a central white streak extend up the esophagus.

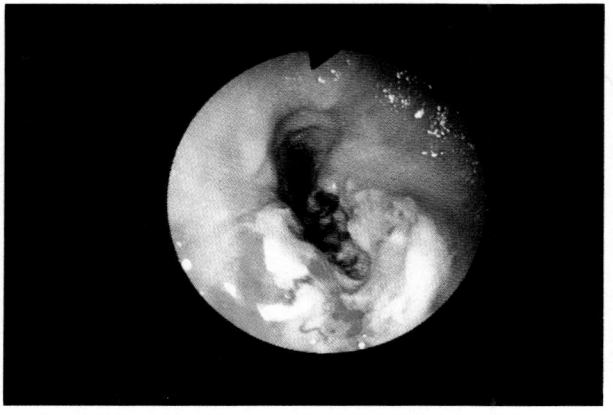

A7-3 **Ulcerated squamous cell carcinoma,** with a depressed center, involving one wall of the esophagus.

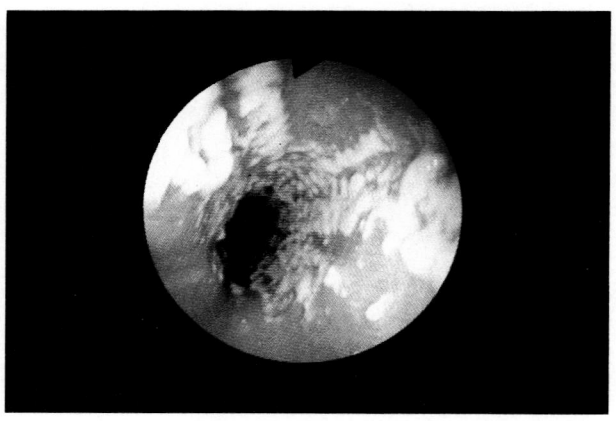

A7-4 **Moniliasis of the esophagus.** A white exudate is seen with underlying erythematous mucosa.

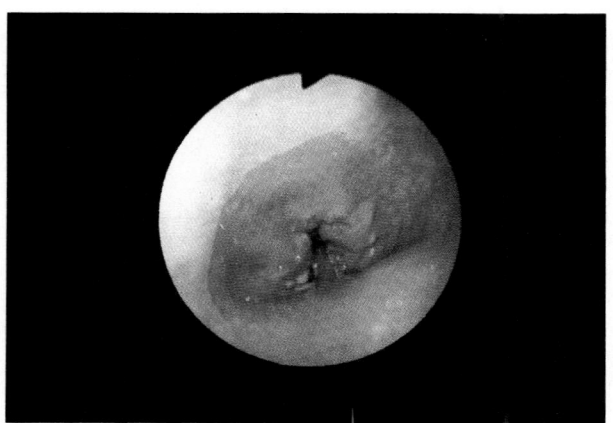

A7-5 **Barrett's metaplasia of the esophagus with an adenocarcinoma.** The squamocolumnar junction is noted in the proximal esophagus. A mucosal irregularity in the center of the photograph was an adenocarcinoma.

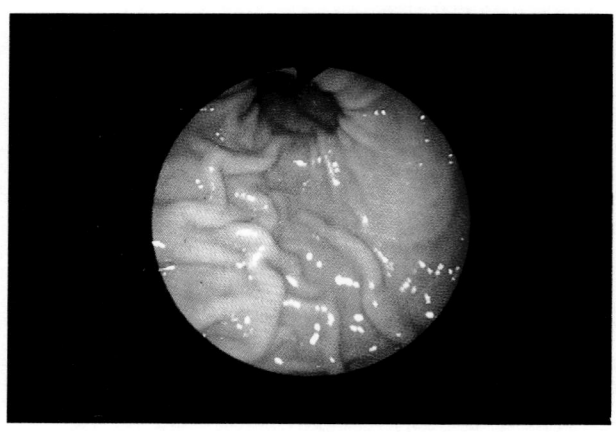

A7-6 **Normal body of the stomach with rugal folds.**

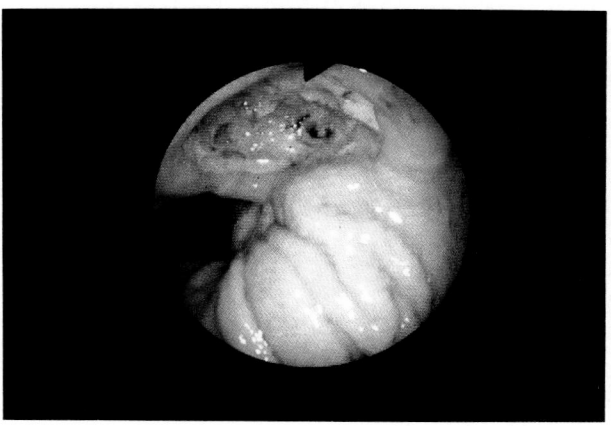

A7-7 **Large, benign, lesser curve gastric ulcer.** The folds end at the ulcer margin.

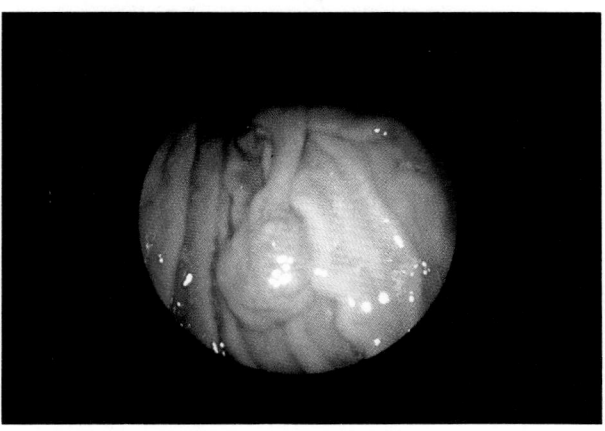

A7-8 **Gastric polyp.** The histologic type must be determined by excision and pathologic examination.

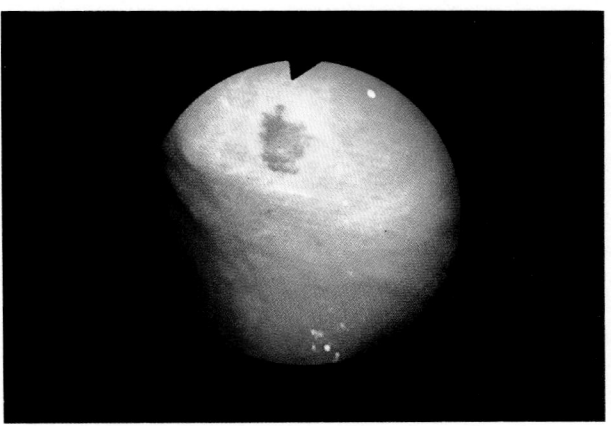

A7-9 **Arteriovenous malformation of the gastric mucosa.**

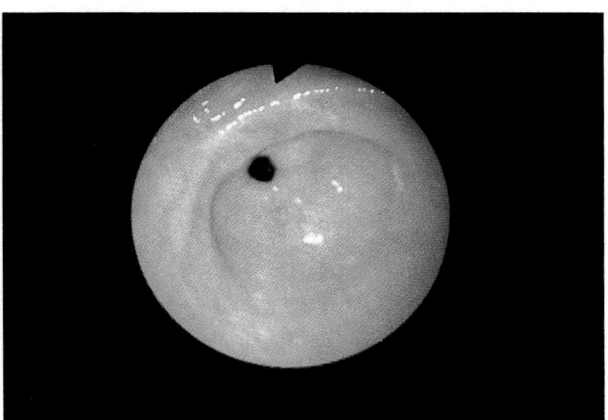

A7-10 **Normal pylorus.** Note the absence of gastric rugal folds in the antrum proximal to the pylorus.

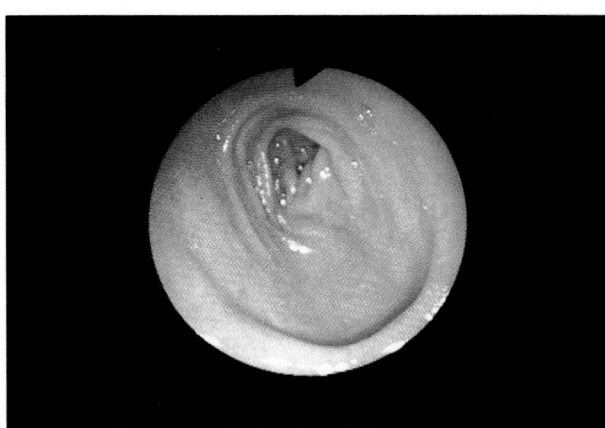

A7-11 **Normal duodenal bulb.**

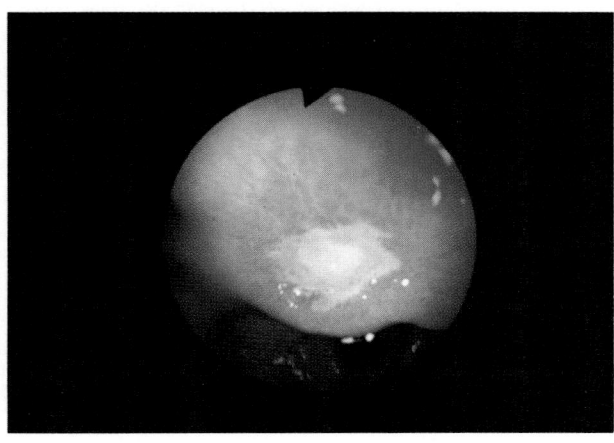

A7-12 **Duodenal ulcer.** A typical ulcer with a clean base is seen on the anterior surface of the duodenal bulb.

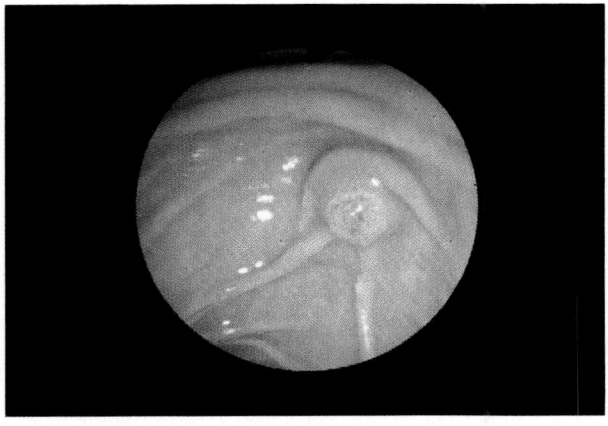

A7-13 **Normal papilla of Vater.** The fold pattern surrounding the papilla is normal; bile is seen adjacent to the papilla.

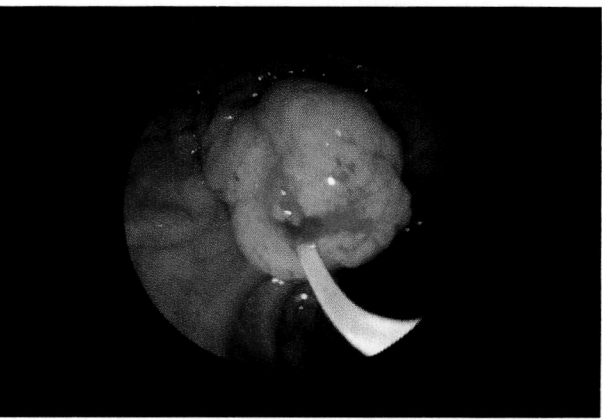

A7-14 **Periampullary carcinoma.** The mass at the papilla of Vater has been catheterized during ERCP.

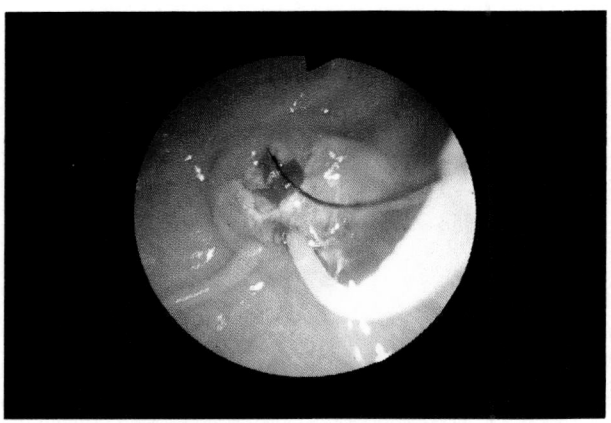

A7-15 **Endoscopic papillotomy.** A papillotome has been passed into the papilla, the wire bowed, and an incision made, with electrosurgical current, in the superior aspect of the papilla.

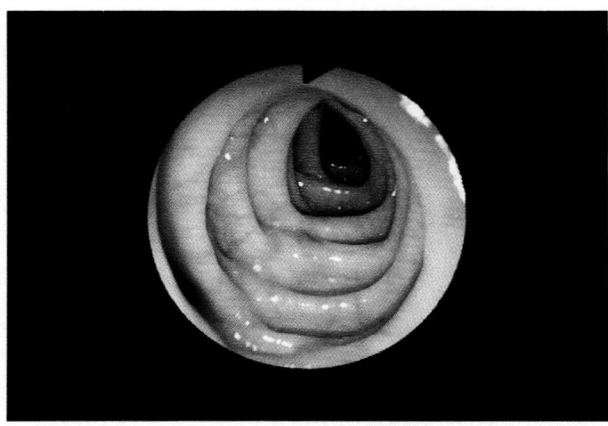

A7-16 **Normal colon;** typical folds and vascular pattern can be seen.

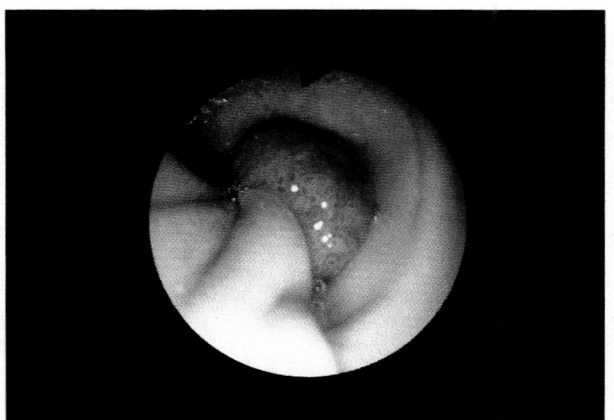

A7-17 **Colonic adenomatous polyp.** The polyp is erythematous; a stalk is seen covered with normal mucosa.

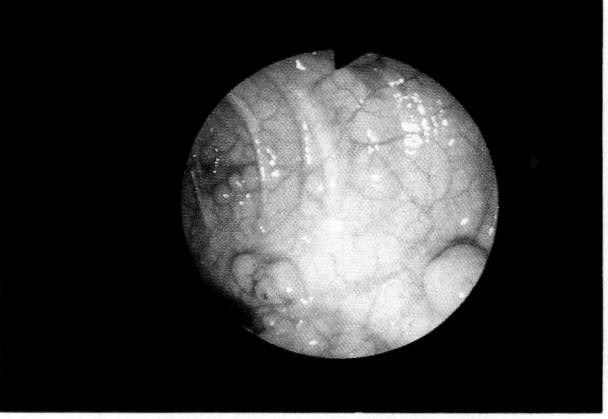

A7-18 **Multiple, small, colonic adenomatous polyps** in a case of familial polyposis coli. This colon must be removed to prevent the development of cancer.

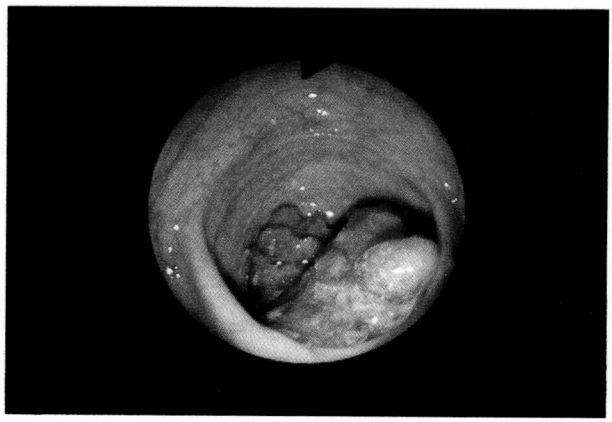

A7-19 **Colon adenocarcinoma.** The cancer is multilobed and growing into the lumen.

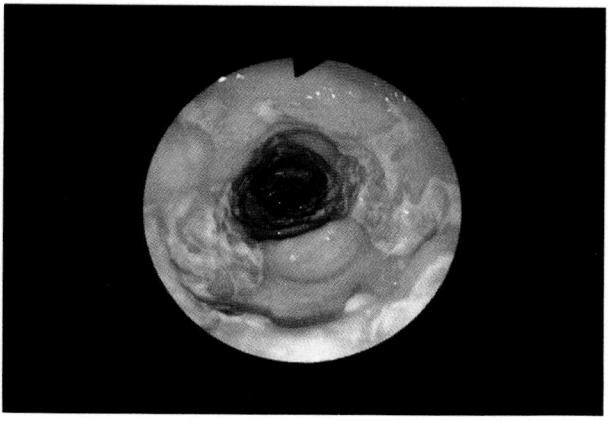

A7-20 **Crohn's colitis** with linear, serpiginous, white-based ulcers surrounded by colonic mucosa which is relatively normal.

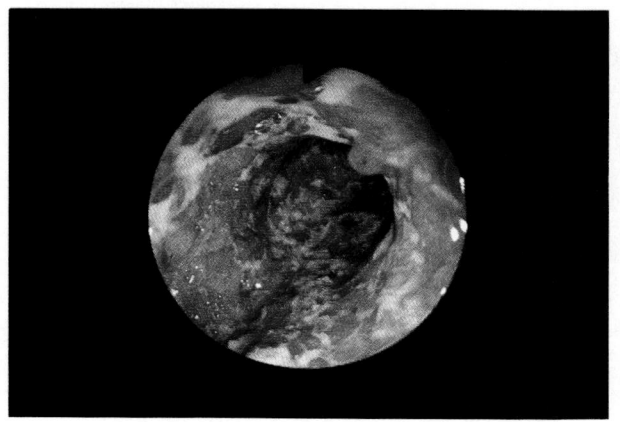

A7-21 **Severe ulcerative colitis** with diffuse ulceration, bleeding, and exudation.

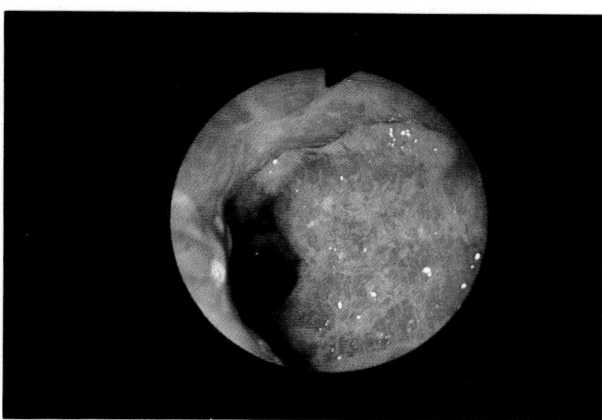

A7-22 **Kaposi's sarcoma involving the colon** in a patient with AIDS. The erythematous lesions involve most of the colonic mucosa in the photograph.

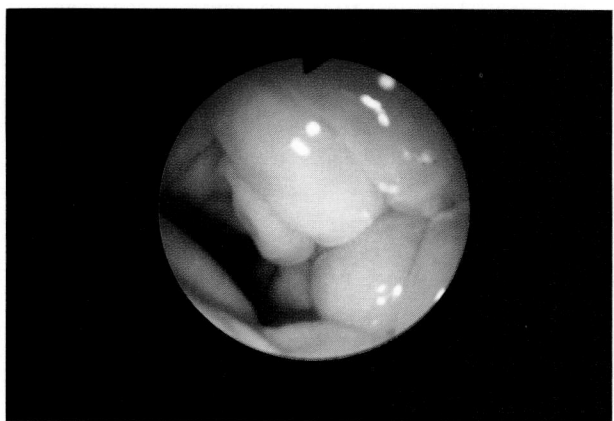

A7-23 **Colonic varices.** Multiple, serpiginous, subepithelial structures impinge on the colonic lumen.

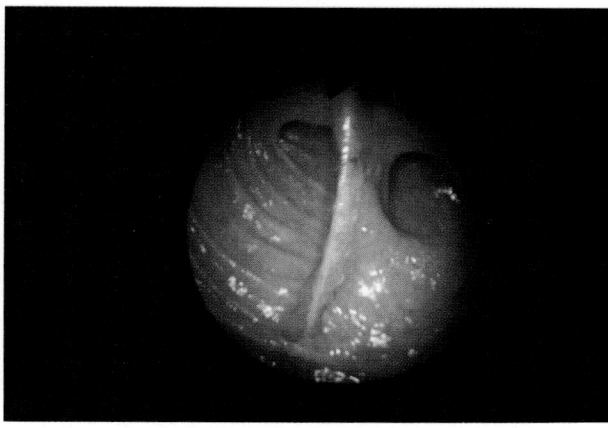

A7-24 **Ileal pouch.** The mucosa appears normal in this pouch reconstructed from ileum to provide a reservoir after total proctocolectomy and ileoanal anastomosis.

Source: All photographs except A7-12, A7-23, and A7-24 are courtesy of FE Silverstein and GN Tytgat: *Atlas of Gastrointestinal Endoscopy.* Gower Medical Publishing, New York, 1987. The three photographs listed above are courtesy of GN Tytgat.

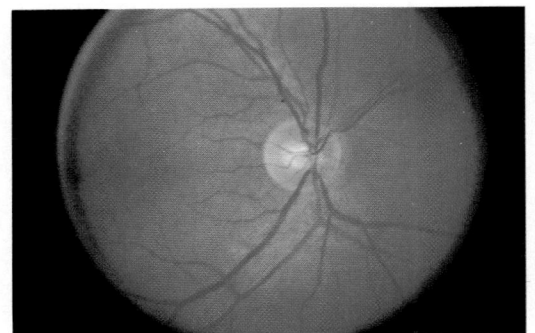

A8-1 **Normal optic nerve and retina.**

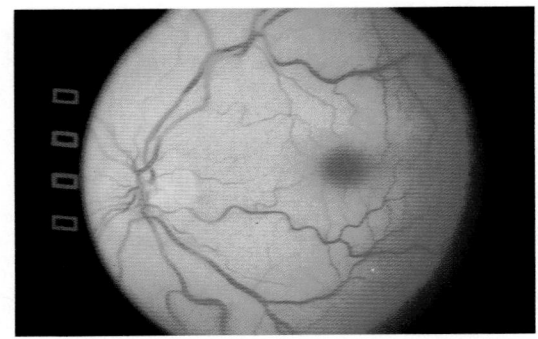

A8-2 **Central retinal artery occlusion.**

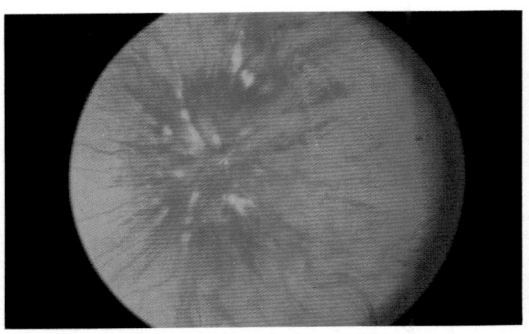

A8-3 **Central retinal vein occlusion.**

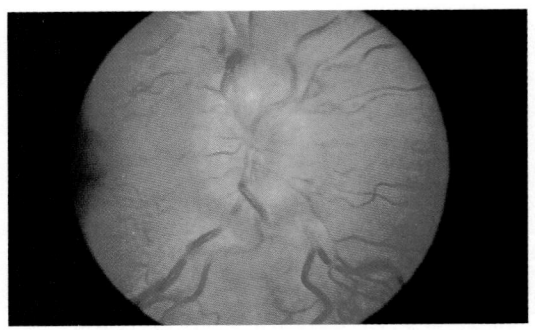

A8-4 **Early papilledema.**

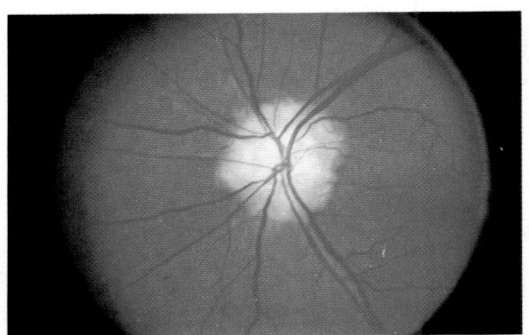

A8-5 **Drusen of the optic nerve head.**

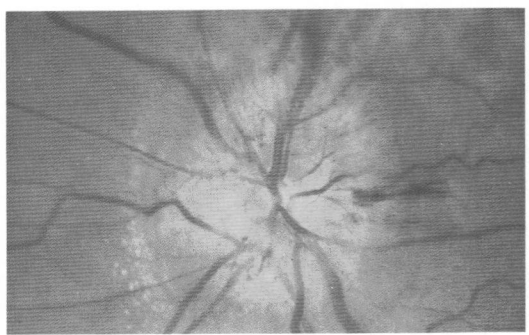

A8-6 **Anterior ischemic optic neuropathy.**

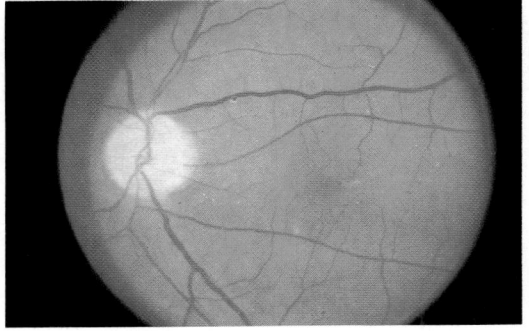

A8-7 **Primary optic atrophy.**

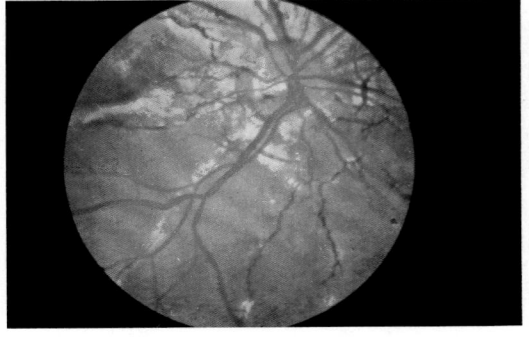

A8-8 **Angioid streaks.**

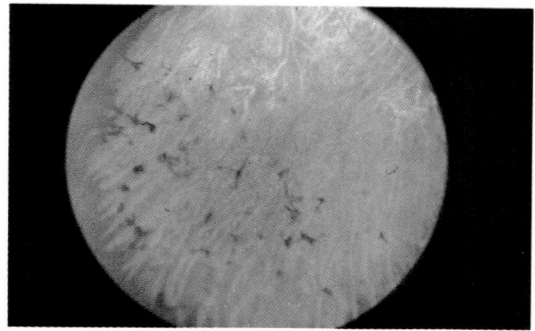

A8-9 **Retinitis pigmentosa.**

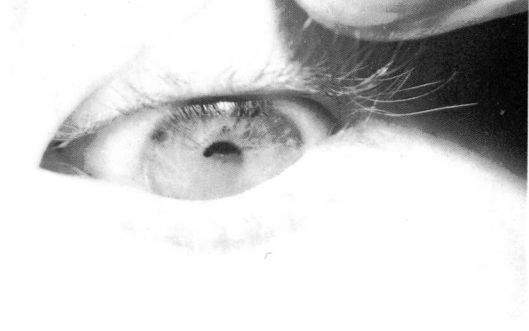

A8-10 **Band keratopathy.**

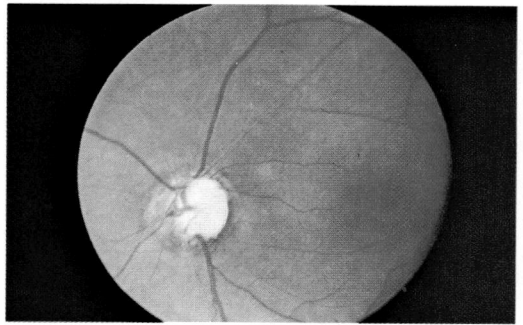

A8-11 **Glaucomatous optic disk with secondary atrophy.**

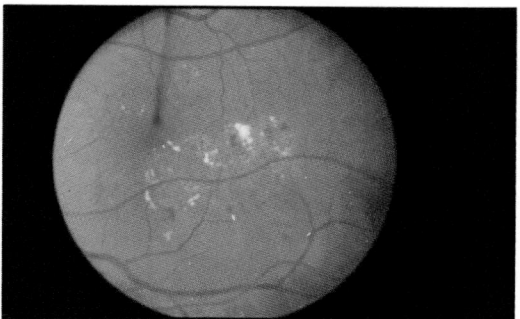

A8-12 **Diabetic retinopathy with microaneurysms.**

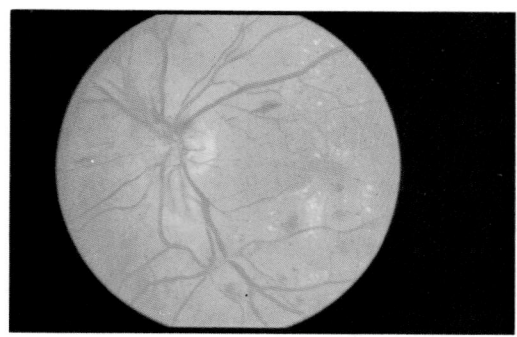

A8-13 **Proliferative diabetic retinopathy.**

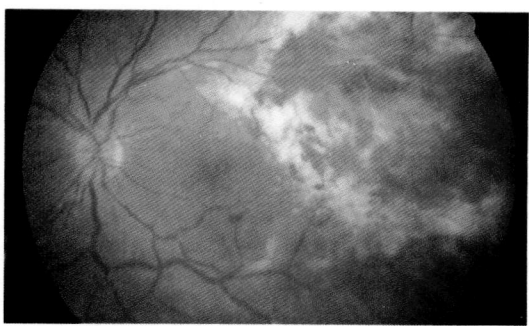

A8-14 **Cytomegalovirus retinitis in AIDS.**
(Courtesy of Donald J.D'Amico, M.D.)

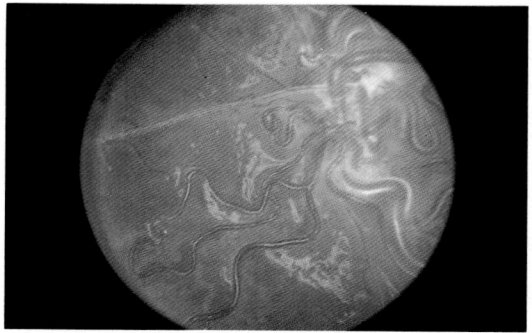

A8-15 **Retinal arteriovenous malformation in the Wyburn-Mason syndrome.**

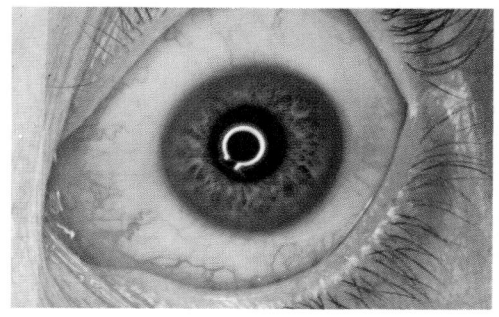

A8-16 **Kayser-Fleischer ring in Wilson's disease.**
(Note: The ring is the golden brown pigment at the periphery of the cornea and is characteristically broader superiorly and inferiorly than it is medially and laterally.)

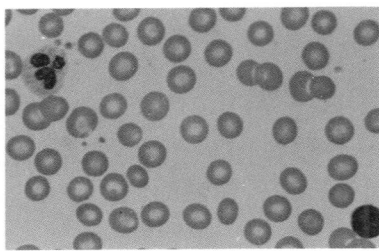

A9-1 **Normal blood smear.** Normal red blood cells are round, possess an area of central pallor, appear slightly smaller than the nucleus of a mature lymphocyte, and vary little in size (anisocytosis) or in shape (poikilocytosis).

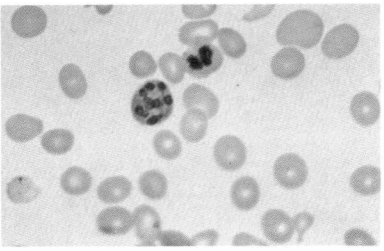

A9-2 **Megaloblastic anemia.** Oval macrocytes, well filled with hemoglobin, are admixed with lesser numbers of small teardrop-shaped red blood cells. Note also hypersegmented granulocyte.

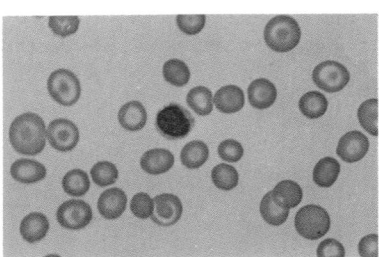

A9-3 **Liver disease.** Round macrocytes of rather uniform size are seen. Many of the macrocytes are also target cells.

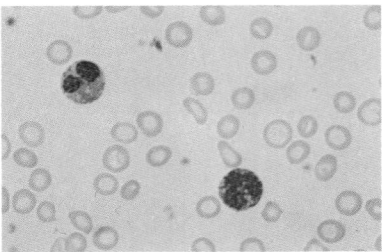

A9-4 **Iron-deficiency anemia.** In severe iron deficiency, the red blood cells are smaller than normal (microcytosis), and their central area of pallor is expanded (hypochromia) so that the cells appear to have only a thin rim of hemoglobin.

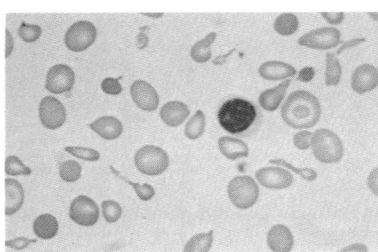

A9-5 **β Thalassemia intermedia.** Microcytic and hypochromic red blood cells are seen that resemble the red blood cells of severe iron deficiency anemia shown in Fig. A9-4. Many elliptical and teardrop-shaped red blood cells are noted.

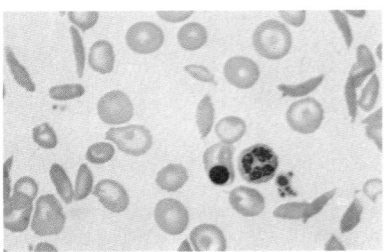

A9-6 **Sickle cell anemia.** The elongated and crescent-shaped red blood cells seen on this smear represent circulating irreversible sickled cells. Target cells and a nucleated red blood cell are also seen.

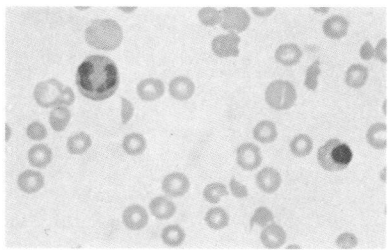

A9-7 **Traumatic hemolysis.** The helmet-shaped red blood cell and the small triangular-shaped red blood cells seen on this smear represent morphologic evidence of mechanical damage to red blood cells within the circulatory tree.

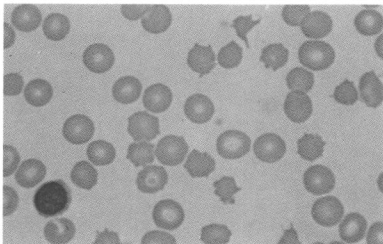

A9-8 **Spur cell anemia.** Spur cells are recognized as distorted red blood cells containing several irregularly distributed thornlike projections. Cells with this morphologic abnormality are also called acanthocytes.

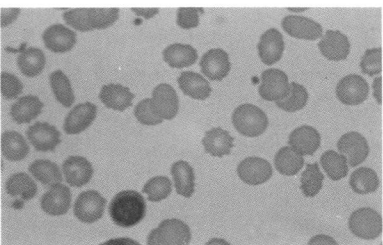

A9-9 **Uremia.** The red blood cells in uremia may acquire numerous, regularly spaced, small spiny projections. Such cells, called burr cells or echinocytes, are readily distinguishable from the irregularly spiculated acanthocytes shown in Fig. A9-8.

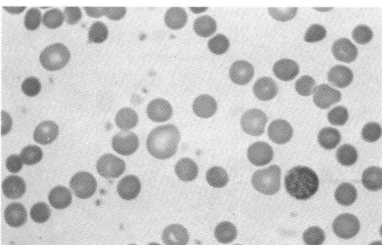

A9-10 **Hereditary spherocytosis.** Small, densely staining red blood cells are seen that have lost their central area of pallor (microspherocytes). Microspherocytes may also be found in other hemolytic disorders (Fig. A9-11).

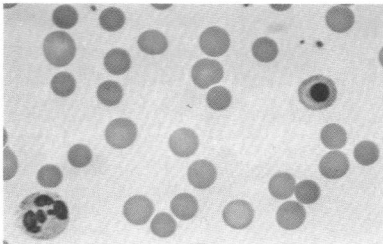

A9-11 **Immunohemolytic anemia.** Microspherocytes are seen on this blood smear along with several macrocytes with a slight purple tinge (polychromasia). The latter represent new red blood cells released early from the bone marrow. The microspherocytes seen in immunohemolytic anemia may be indistinguishable from the microspherocytes seen in hereditary spherocytosis (Fig. A9-10).

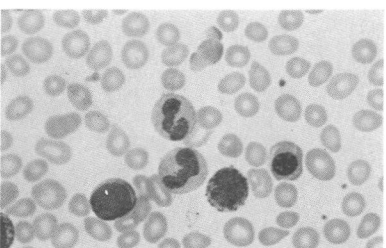

A9-12 **Myeloid metaplasia.** Teardrop-shaped red blood cells, a nucleated red blood cell, and immature myeloid cells are seen on this blood smear.

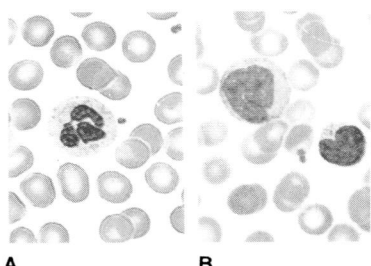

A   **B**

A9-13 A. **Normal granulocyte.** The normal granulocyte has a segmented nucleus with heavy, clumped chromatin; fine neutrophilic granules are dispersed throughout its cytoplasm. *B.* **Normal monocyte and lymphocyte.** The normal monocyte is a large cell with an indented or folded nucleus containing loose, strandlike chromatin; the cytoplasm is a blue-gray color and usually contains fine azurophilic granules. The normal lymphocyte is a smaller cell. Its nucleus is usually round but may be indented, as in the cell shown in this plate. The nuclear chromatin has a smudgy appearance; the cytoplasm is a blue color.

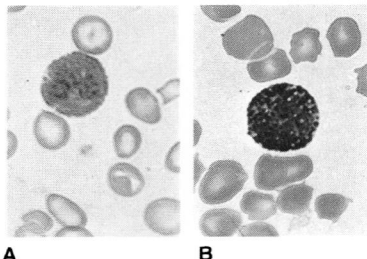

A   **B**

A9-14 A. **Normal eosinophil.** The eosinophil contains large, bright-orange granules; the nucleus is bilobed. *B.* **Basophil.** The basophil contains large purple-black granules which fill the cell and obscure the nucleus.

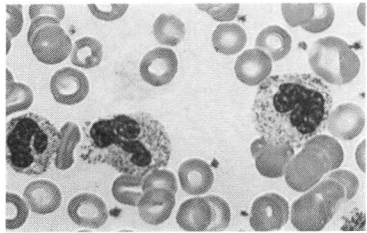

A9-16 **Neutrophils with toxic granulation.** In infection and other toxic states, azurophilic granules may become visible in mature granulocytes as coarse, dark-staining cytoplasmic granules.

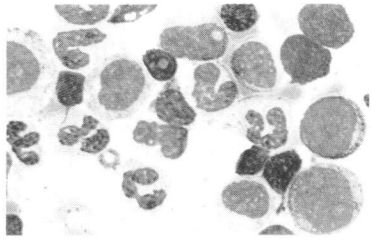

A9-15 **Normal granulocyte precursors in marrow.** The earliest granulocytic precursor (myeloblast) possesses a round nucleus with fine, punctate chromatin and one or more nucleoli; the cytoplasm is blue. As nuclear differentiation proceeds, the nucleoli disappear, the chromatin coarsens, and the nucleus becomes increasingly indented and finally segmented. As cytoplasmic differentiation proceeds, azurophilic granules appear and the cytoplasm changes color from blue to the yellow-pink-gray hue of the mature granulocyte, and as this occurs the azurophilic granules become obscured by fine neutrophilic granules.

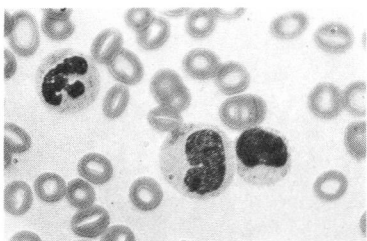

A9-17 **Band with Döhle body** (center). Döhle bodies are discrete, blue-staining nongranular areas found in the periphery of the cytoplasm of the neutrophil in infections and other toxic states. They represent aggregates of rough endoplasmic reticulum.

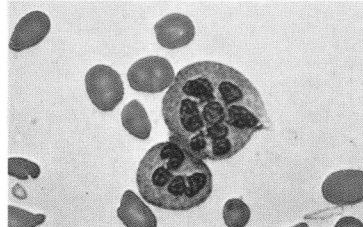

A9-18 **Hypersegmentation.** Frequent five-lobed granulocytes on a blood smear or granulocytes with more than five lobes are evidence of hypersegmentation, an important clue to the diagnosis of megaloblastic anemia.

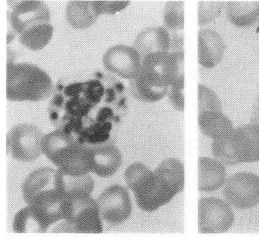

A   **B**

A9-19 A. **Chédiak-Higashi anomaly.** In this ultimately fatal disorder, the granulocytes contain huge cytoplasmic granules, formed from aggregation and fusion of azurophilic and specific granules. Large, abnormal granules are found in other granule-containing cells throughout the body. *B.* **Pelger-Hüet anomaly.** In this benign disorder, the majority of granulocytes are bilobed. The nucleus frequently has a spectacle-like or "pince-nez" configuration.

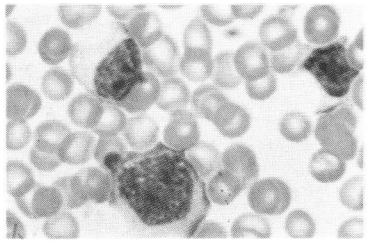

A9-20 **Reactive lymphocytes** (infectious mononucleosis). Reactive lymphocytes are usually large, cytoplasmic lymphocytes. The nucleus may be eccentrically placed and may have irregular borders and indentations (not seen on this plate). The cytoplasm contains areas that stain a darker blue due to their increased content of RNA. The cytoplasm may be indented where it abuts against a red blood cell.

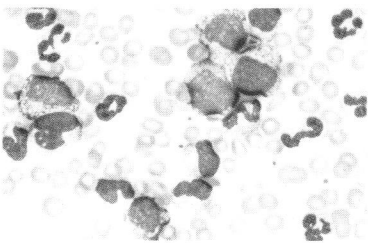

A9-21 **Chronic granulocytic leukemia.** The peripheral blood WBC count is high due to increased numbers of granulocytes and their precursors. The majority of the WBCs are segmented granulocytes or band forms, but as seen on this plate, myelocytes and promyeloblasts (not seen on this plate) may also be found on review of the blood smear.

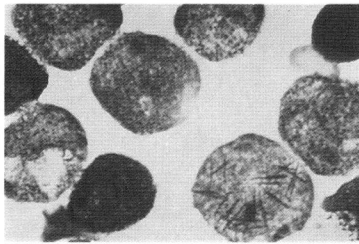

A9-22 **Leukemic cell in acute promyelocytic leukemia.** Note multiple Auer rods.

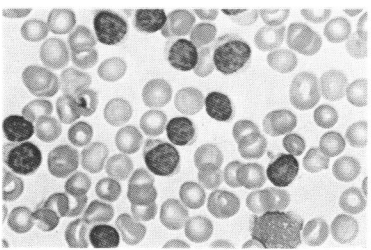

A9-23 **Chronic lymphocytic leukemia.** The peripheral blood WBC count is high due to increased numbers of small, well-differentiated lymphocytes. However, the leukemic lymphocytes are fragile, and substantial numbers of broken, smudged cells are usually also present on the blood smear.

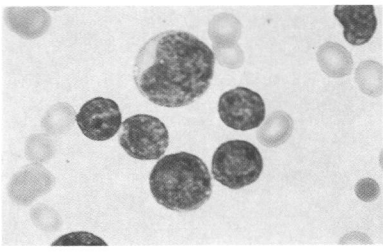

A9-24 **Leukemic cells in acute lympho-blastic leukemia** characterized by round or convoluted nuclei, high nuclear/cytoplasmic ratio and absence of cytoplasmic granules.

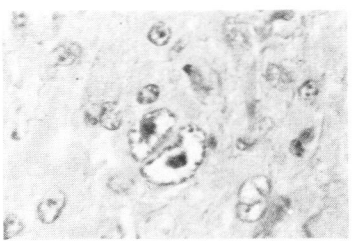

A9-25 **Hodgkin's disease:** Reed-Sternberg cell in marrow (center). The Reed-Sternberg cell is recognized by its bilobed, mirror-image nucleus, which contains in each lobe a giant, inclusion body-like nucleolus. The cytoplasmic borders of the cell cannot be identified on this plate.

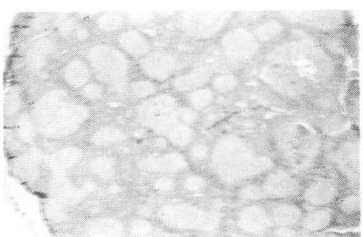

A9-26 **Non-Hodgkin's nodular lymphoma** (lymph node). This low-power view illustrates that a proliferative process has caused the normal architecture of the lymph node to be replaced by multiple nodules of varying size that extend throughout the entire lymph node.

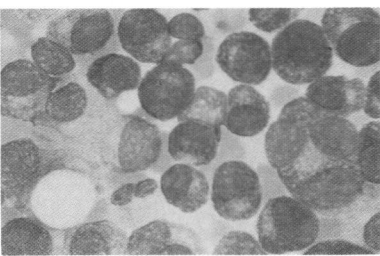

A9-27 **Multiple myeloma** (marrow). The cells bear the characteristic morphologic features of plasma cells, round or oval cells with an eccentric nucleus composed of coarsely clumped chromatin, a densely basophilic cytoplasm, and a perinuclear clear zone (hof) containing the Golgi apparatus. Binucleate and multinucleate malignant plasma cells also can be seen.

reacts with antibodies to prostate-specific antigen or prostatic alkaline phosphatase, gross cystic fluid protein, or thyroglobulin, respectively. Sarcoma subgroups including rhabdomyosarcoma (myoglobin) and angiosarcoma or Kaposi's sarcoma (factor VIII) also may be identified immunohistochemically. The finding of AFP, βhCG, or placental alkaline phosphatase staining is very helpful in assigning a germ cell origin. The S-100 protein is present in virtually all primary and metastatic melanomas, including the amelanotic variety, the latter being difficult to classify by routine techniques. However, S-100 positivity is also found in many other tumors of neuroendocrine origin (e.g., small cell lung cancer, carcinoid, neuroepithelioma); a more specific marker for melanomas is the HMB 45 (human melanoma black) antigen.

OTHER DIAGNOSTIC APPROACHES Ultrastructural analysis with electron microscopy can identify cell junctions (i.e., desmosomes, typical of epithelial cancers), neuroendocrine granules, melanosomes, and muscle filaments that can be very helpful in arriving at the tissue of origin. Though not widely utilized, cytogenetic analysis on solid tumors represents a means of classifying neoplasms associated with specific chromosomal translocations or other genetic abnormalities (see Table 326-2). Fresh tissue may be required for detection of estrogen or progesterone receptors where breast cancer is a possibility or for the determination of antigens (such as those found on certain T cells) that are not fixation-resistant. In addition to immunologic analysis, lymphomas can be diagnosed by isolating DNA from tissues and using molecular approaches to detect immunoglobulin, T cell receptor, *bcl*-2, or other lymphoid-specific gene rearrangement. Since minimal amounts of template DNA are required for amplification by polymerase chain reaction, paraffin-embedded tissue blocks may yield sufficient diagnostic material. As additional tumors are found to have specific acquired chromosomal rearrangements or mutations in genes controlling growth and differentiation, the detection of altered DNA and/or altered gene products will yield additional diagnostic capabilities.

TREATMENT Patients with cancer of unknown primary site have a median age of 62 years. However, regardless of age, the exclusion of treatable and potentially curable neoplasms is important. Patients with squamous cell carcinoma have a median survival somewhat greater (9 months) than do those with adenocarcinoma or unclassifiable neoplasms (4 to 6 months). If laboratory studies lead to a significant probability that the neoplasm is either a lymphoma, germ cell tumor, sarcoma, neuroendocrine tumor, or breast or prostate cancer, then disease-appropriate therapy should be administered. Patients who are found to have either lymphoma or germ cell neoplasm may be cured with combination chemotherapy. In other malignancies, effective palliative chemotherapy (sarcoma, breast, neuroendocrine tumor) or hormonal therapy (breast, prostate) should be strongly considered. Thus, for example, patients with neuroendocrine tumors are expected to respond to cisplatin-based chemotherapy. However, many patients, even after exhaustive pathologic review, will be left with a diagnosis of metastatic cancer (usually carcinoma or poorly differentiated malignancy) of unknown primary site. Despite these discouraging facts, patients often can be categorized as having one of several clinical features or syndromes suggesting a specific form of potentially beneficial therapy (see Table 326-3).

Unrecognized extragonadal germ cell cancer syndrome In the late 1970s, investigators identified a subset of patients with poorly differentiated carcinoma of unknown primary site who were extremely responsive to chemotherapy. These patients displayed one or more of the following features: age less than 50; tumor involving midline structures, lung parenchyma, or lymph nodes; an elevated serum AFP or βhCG level; evidence of rapid tumor growth; or tumor responsiveness to previously administered radiotherapy or chemotherapy. The administration of cisplatin-based chemotherapy has led to long-term survival in a sizable number of patients with these features, suggesting that their tumors behaved in a manner analogous to germ cell neoplasms. If all patients with poorly differentiated carcinoma are treated with a chemotherapy regimen designed for those with

TABLE 326-3 Presentations dictating specific therapy in patients with metastatic cancer of unknown primary site

Clinicopathologic features	Suspected primary site	Suggested therapy
Squamous cell carcinoma, cervical node	Head and neck cancer	Radical neck dissection; XRT
Carcinoma, axillary nodes (female)	Breast cancer	Breast XRT or mastectomy, systemic adjuvant therapy
Peritoneal carcinomatosis (female)	Ovarian cancer	Debulking surgery, cisplatin-based chemotherapy
Poorly differentiated cancer, age <50, lung or retroperitoneal or mediastinal mass or lymph nodes, elevated βhCG or AFP	Germ cell (extragonadal)	Cisplatin/VP-16–based chemotherapy
Adenocarcinoma, liver metastases, elevated CEA	Gastrointestinal malignancy	Colonoscopy, 5-FU/leucovorin

germ cell cancer (e.g., cisplatin plus etoposide or vinblastine, and often with bleomycin), about one-quarter will respond completely and a third will experience partial responses. Approximately one in six is likely to survive more than 5 years without evidence of disease. Furthermore, abnormalities of chromosome 12 similar to those described in patients with proven germ cell cancer have been detected by karyotypic analysis of clinical specimens from patients with this syndrome.

Peritoneal carcinomatosis in women Women presenting with increased abdominal girth and a pelvic mass or pain and who are found to have adenocarcinoma throughout the peritoneal cavity also may benefit from platinum-based chemotherapy. While breast cancer or a gastrointestinal malignancy also could produce these findings, peritoneal carcinomatosis is most commonly ascribed to ovarian cancer, even in those with apparently normal ovaries at the time of laparotomy. Especially if psammoma bodies or a papillary configuration is noted at the time of pathologic examination or if the CA-125 level is elevated, women with adenocarcinoma of the peritoneal cavity without a clear primary site should receive maximum surgical cytoreduction followed by cisplatin-based therapy. The stage-specific response to such therapy appears to be comparable with that observed in patients with proven ovarian cancer.

Carcinoma in an axillary lymph node in a female Women with an axillary mass proven to be adenocarcinoma or poorly differentiated carcinoma should receive treatment appropriate for stage II breast cancer whether or not a careful breast examination or mammography suggests the diagnosis of primary breast cancer and whether or not estrogen or progesterone receptors are detectable in the node. Although no lesion may be found in the breast if an immediate mastectomy is performed, patients with this syndrome who are followed and observed without local therapy have a high rate of developing primary breast tumors. Appropriate therapy would generally include either modified radical mastectomy or breast irradiation for purposes of reducing the risk of local recurrence. In addition, adjuvant systemic therapy (chemotherapy and/or tamoxifen, depending on menopausal status and whether or not estrogen receptor protein was found in the axillary tumor) to reduce the risk of developing evident metastatic breast cancer should be considered. Whether or not such systemic therapy should be administered prior to, rather than after, definitive local treatment is controversial. Women with axillary metastases without an obvious breast primary appear to have the same likelihood of prolonged disease-free survival as patients with typical stage II breast cancer.

Cervical lymph nodes It has long been recognized that patients presenting with a neck mass should be considered to have a primary tumor of the upper aerodigestive tract, usually termed *head and neck cancer,* until proven otherwise. Especially if pathologic analysis suggests squamous histology and the node is located in a high or midcervical area, a careful ear, nose, and throat examination, including direct laryngoscopy, nasopharyngoscopy, and random blind biopsies, should be undertaken. A thyroid examination and scan also must be performed to rule out a primary thyroid tumor, especially if the histology is not definitely squamous. Definitive local therapy (external beam radiation or radical neck dissection) possibly followed by platinum-based chemotherapy may lead to prolonged survival in some patients.

Adenocarcinoma and liver metastases Though not as well characterized as the unrecognized germ cell cancer syndrome and not as responsive to therapy, liver metastases proven to be adenocarcinoma have a significant likelihood of a primary stomach, biliary, or colorectal tumor. An elevated serum CEA level in this setting would provide further evidence suggesting a gastrointestinal malignancy. A flexible sigmoidoscopy or colonoscopy may be reasonable to rule out a potentially obstructive colonic lesion. Even if endoscopy fails to detect a tumor (in which case, depending on its size, resection would offer benefit), treatment with a combination of 5-fluorouracil plus leucovorin may offer palliation to some patients with presumed metastatic gastrointestinal malignancy. Given the severe and even life-threatening diarrhea that may be a consequence of this particular regimen, combined with the relative resistance of gastrointestinal tumors to chemotherapy, patients should be selected carefully prior to embarking on such therapy.

Patients not falling into one of the preceding categories should be treated palliatively. In some patients, observation is appropriate. For example, individuals without evidence of additional metastatic disease who have undergone resection of a solitary pulmonary nodule containing malignant cells may actually have undergone definitive therapy for a small primary lung tumor. Radiation therapy is indicated in patients with local disease causing bony pain or neurologic compromise. Combination chemotherapy is frequently employed in patients with an unknown primary site; however, response rates to "all purpose" regimens [e.g., FAM (5-fluorouracil, doxorubicin, mitomycin C) or FACP (5-fluorouracil, doxorubicin, cyclophosphamide, cisplatin)] are generally under 50 percent, with complete responses occurring in less than 25 percent of patients. Mitomycin C–containing regimens are associated with the risk of hemolytic-uremic syndrome. In some series, patients with a good performance status or whose disease is limited to soft tissue sites have been found more likely to respond to therapy. While patients responding to treatment have been thought to survive longer than those who do not, this seeming benefit of chemotherapy is probably related to the inherent characteristics of the tumor.

Before initiating a trial of combination chemotherapy in a patient with metastatic cancer of unknown primary site, the potential benefits must be weighed carefully against the certainty of toxicity. While some randomized studies have reported a benefit of one form of therapy over another, these reports are generally plagued by small numbers of patients and inadequate control of potential prognostic variables. Depending on motivation, eligibility, and availability, patients with metastatic cancer of unknown primary site may be candidates for evaluation of new (phase I) therapies.

REFERENCES

BELL CW et al: Unknown primary tumors: Establishment of cell lines, identification of chromosomal abnormalities, and implications for a second type of tumor progression. Cancer Res 49:4311, 1989

ELLERBROEK N et al: Treatment of patients with isolated axillary nodal metastases from an occult primary carcinoma consistent with breast origin. Cancer 66:1461, 1990

FLETCHER JA et al: Diagnostic relevance of clonal cytogenetics in malignant soft tissue tumors. N Engl J Med 324:436, 1991

HAINSWORTH JD et al: Cisplatin-based combination chemotherapy in the treatment of poorly differentiated carcinoma and poorly differentiated adenocarcinoma of unknown primary site: Results of a 12-year experience. J Clin Oncol 10:912, 1992

—— et al: Poorly differentiated carcinoma of unknown primary site: Clinical usefulness of immunoperoxidase staining. J Clin Oncol 9:1931, 1991

HORNING SJ et al: Lymphomas presenting as histologically unclassified neoplasms: Characteristics and response to treatment. J Clin Oncol 17:1281, 1989

PASTERZ R et al: Prognostic factors in metastatic carcinoma of unknown primary. J Clin Oncol 4:1652, 1986

RABER MN et al: Unknown primary tumors. Curr Opin Oncol 4:3, 1992

SPORN JR, GREENBERG BR: Empiric chemotherapy in patients with carcinoma of unknown primary site. Am J Med 88:49, 1990

STRNAD CM et al: Peritoneal carcinomatosis of unknown primary site in women. Ann Intern Med 111:213, 1989

ULTMANN JE, PHILLIPS TL: Cancer of unknown primary site, in *Principles and Practice of Oncology*, 3d ed, VT DeVita et al (eds). Philadelphia, Lippincott, 1990, chap 56

327 ENDOCRINE MANIFESTATIONS OF NEOPLASIA

LAWRENCE A. FROHMAN

Hormone secretion by tumors of nonendocrine tissue has been recognized for more than 60 years. Initially, the majority of reported cases were associated with hypoglycemia and hypercalcemia, but the term *ectopic hormone secretion* was first used in relation to Cushing's syndrome caused by adrenocorticotropin (ACTH) secretion from a variety of tumors. The spectrum of ectopic hormone secretion has expanded as a result of increased clinical awareness and the availability of sensitive assay techniques. However, the use of the term *ectopic* has been questioned with the recognition that hormones once believed to be tissue-specific may have widespread sites of production; i.e., gonadotropins are produced by the normal gonad and intestine, thyrotropin-releasing hormone (TRH) and ACTH by the pancreas, and somatostatin by the kidney and thyroid C cells. Nevertheless, the original term serves to distinguish tumor-associated hormone production from syndromes due to excess secretion of a hormone characteristically associated with a specific endocrine gland.

THEORIES OF ECTOPIC HORMONE SECRETION Several pathogenic mechanisms have been proposed to explain ectopic hormone secretion. The "sponge" theory assumed a selective uptake of the circulating hormone by tumor tissue with subsequent release on tumor cell death. This concept was abandoned, however, after the demonstration of arteriovenous differences of hormones across tumor vascular beds, the presence of hormone mRNA in tumor tissue, and hormone biosynthesis by tumors in vitro. The theory that random mutations resulted in altered DNA sequences and gene products also was discounted when it was established that the production of ectopic hormones by tumors is not random, i.e., that certain tumors are commonly associated with specific endocrinopathies. A third theory, that of gene derepression, proposed that regions of the genome not normally expressed become active and are transcribed in tumors, presumably as a result of loss of normal transcription suppressors during neoplastic transformation. Two other explanations also have been proposed: *cellular dedifferentiation*, a theory that neoplastic cells revert to a more primitive level and again produce peptide hormones that were produced normally at an earlier developmental stage, and *arrested differentiation*, whereby hormone secretion is due to persistence of a function present during development because of a failure (maturational arrest) of the developmental process. Arguments against these theories include an absence of evidence that cells can retrace their pathways of differentiation and that incompletely differentiated cells routinely secrete the hormone in question. Although the pathogenesis of ectopic hormone secretion is still unclear, the mechanism is likely the result of persistent activation of selected gene expression by an oncogene.

CRITERIA FOR DIAGNOSIS Criteria for the diagnosis of ectopic hormone secretion have changed as more precise laboratory methodology made it possible to recognize clinically inapparent cases (Table 327-1). Although many of these criteria cannot be satisfied in

TABLE 327-1 Criteria for establishing the diagnosis of ectopic hormone secretion

1 Association of a neoplasm with a syndrome attributable to excessive hormone secretion or with inappropriately elevated plasma and/or urine levels of a hormone not normally produced by the tissue from which the tumor is derived
2 Failure of plasma and/or urine hormone levels to respond to normal homeostatic suppression
3 Exclusion of other possible causal mechanisms for hormone hypersecretion
4 Reduction in hormone levels after tumor-specific therapy
5 Arteriovenous step-up gradients of hormone across tumor
6 Demonstration of hormone in tumor tissue
7 Biosynthesis and/or secretion of hormone by tumor tissue in vitro
8 Demonstration in the tumor of hormone-specific messenger RNA by cell-free translation or hybridization with cDNA

individual cases, the majority have been fulfilled in the commonly recognized syndromes.

TUMOR TYPES ASSOCIATED WITH ECTOPIC HORMONE SE-CRETION Ectopic secretion of hormones is associated with a variety of tumors. Although original reports of these syndromes described primarily lung carcinomas, carcinoids, thymomas, and fibrosarcomas, virtually all tumors have the potential of hormone secretion. Nevertheless, the frequency of occurrence of ectopic hormone secretion among various tumor types is not random. The tumors most frequently associated with clinically recognized ectopic hormone production are small cell lung carcinomas, carcinoids, and pancreatic islet tumors. Carcinoid tumors are generally found in the lung or the gastrointestinal tract. Gastrointestinal carcinoids may be present in either the foregut or the hindgut, although it is primarily foregut tumors that are hormonally active. In the lung these tumors are usually endobronchial and may remain undetected for long periods. There are many morphologic similarities between bronchial carcinoid tumors and small cell carcinoma of the lung. Indeed, the two types may have a common cell of origin, namely the Kulchitsky cell, a bronchial mucosal cell that has been called a neuroendocrine cell of the lung because of its peptide-containing granules observed on electron microscopy. A bombesin-like peptide (related to gastrin-releasing peptide) is present in Kulchitsky cells during fetal life and is the most frequent peptide produced by small cell carcinoma of the lung. Ectopic hormone secretion is also associated with other types of lung tumors, most commonly the squamous type of bronchogenic carcinomas.

In the 1960s Pearse proposed the theory that certain hormone-secreting cells are components of a "diffuse neuroendocrine system." Such cells were originally considered to be of neural crest or neuroectodermal origin and were designated APUD (amine precursor uptake and decarboxylation) cells on the basis of their ability to decarboxylate precursors of biogenic amines. Later it was discovered that many of these cells also produce the enzyme neuron-specific enolase and other neurosecretory cell markers. A corollary of the APUD theory was that tumors derived from APUD cells have the capability of hormone secretion. At present, the APUD theory appears invalid for several reasons. First, all APUD cells are not of neuroectodermal origin. Second, the APUD function of these cells is not inherently linked with peptide hormone production, and third, some ectopic hormone-secreting tumors do not possess APUD characteristics. Nevertheless, the fact that particular tumor types secrete certain hormones is useful in evaluating these syndromes.

CHARACTERIZATION OF ECTOPIC HORMONES Type of hormone secreted Of the four classes of hormones—steroids, monoamines, substituted amino acids, and peptides/proteins—only the latter are secreted ectopically. Although the explanation is not known with certainty, the ectopic production of peptide/protein hormones requires less complicated derangements in cell metabolism. For example, an oncogene serving as an inducer or enhancer of gene transcription may increase the expression of a gene coding for a peptide hormone. However, the synthesis of steroids, thyroid hormones, and monoamines requires multiple enzymatic steps and specifically

targeted translocation of the precursor molecules through various cell compartments. It is extremely unlikely that this degree of cell specialization would occur as a consequence of activation of one or several oncogenes.

Ectopic secretion of nearly all peptide hormones has been reported. These hormones may be grouped according to their usual site of origin (Table 327-2). The first group of hormones, common to the central nervous system and gastrointestinal tract, is most frequently secreted by carcinoids, small cell lung carcinomas, and pancreatic islet tumors. The second group, normally produced by the fetoplacental unit and/or the anterior pituitary, tends to be produced by gastrointestinal, hepatic, adrenal, and gonadal tumors. The third group, which includes insulin-like growth factors and parathyroid hormone–related protein, tends to be produced by mesenchymal, hepatic, genitourinary, breast, and squamous cell lung tumors. In addition to the hormones listed, other humoral factors are believed responsible for tumor-associated syndromes such as hypertrophic osteoarthropathy, polyneuropathy, hypophosphatemic osteomalacia, and anorexia.

Relation to naturally secreted hormones The primary amino acid sequences of all ectopically secreted hormones analyzed to date are identical to those of the native hormones. However, differences in structure between ectopically secreted and native hormones can occur as a result of incomplete or abnormal processing of the precursor hormone. Several abnormal forms of ectopic hormones have been defined: (1) large-molecular-weight species due to incomplete enzymatic cleavage of the precursor (proopiomelanocortin), (2) small-molecular-weight fragments due to unregulated intracellular processing (fragments of growth hormone–releasing hormone), and (3) altered glycosylation species (microheterogeneity) due either to failed cleavage of carbohydrate residues during postribosomal hormone processing (glycosylated ACTH) or failure of normal glycosylation (the alpha subunit common to the gonadotropins and TSH). The usual consequence of such altered biosynthetic processing is a hormone variant with diminished biologic activity. If modification of hormone structure is sufficient to cause loss of all biologic activity, ectopic secretion is not accompanied by clinical manifestations. Furthermore, even if a neoplastic cell can synthesize and store a biologically active hormone, a syndrome of hormone excess will not result if an effective secretory mechanism is absent. The frequency with which either an inactive hormone is synthesized or an active hormone is synthesized but not secreted is probably greater than that of classical ectopic hormone secretion, since only a small percentage of tumors that contain ectopic hormones cause clinically recognizable syndromes attributable to hormone hypersecretion.

Other considerations Hormones may be secreted by both benign and malignant tumors. Although hormone secretion normally requires a high level of cellular differentiation, an incompletely differentiated tumor may still retain secretory capability. For example, the process of granule formation and hormone storage is not generally expressed by hormone-secreting tumors; consequently, the concentration of hormone in the tumor is usually low compared with that in endocrine glands. Overall hormone secretion per unit weight is also less, and as a result, considerable tumor mass is usually present before ectopic hormone secretion is clinically apparent. One notable exception is the relatively benign, highly differentiated neoplasm, usually a carcinoid or pancreatic islet tumor, that contains and secretes hormone at a level comparable with that of normal endocrine tissue and is sufficiently small to escape detection for long periods.

Many tumors produce multiple hormones. In some this is due to the existence of a common precursor for multiple hormones; e.g., ACTH, lipotropins, melanocyte-stimulating hormones (MSHs), and endorphins are all derived from a single precursor, proopiomelanocortin (POMC), and both vasoactive intestinal peptide (VIP) and peptide histidyl-methionine (PHM) are encoded in a single precursor. In other instances, multiple hormones are produced in the absence of common precursors, e.g., production of ACTH, calcitonin, and somatostatin by medullary thyroid carcinoma and by small cell carcinoma of the lung. In some tumors separate cells secrete individual hormones,

TABLE 327-2 Spectrum of ectopic hormone production

Group/hormone	Tumor type		Group/hormone	Tumor type	
	Common	Infrequent		Common	Infrequent
NEUROENDOCRINE-GASTROINTESTINAL					
Adrenocorticotropin, β-lipotropin, endorphins, MSHs, enkephalins	Lung carcinoma (small cell), thymoma, pancreatic islet tumors, carcinoid, thyroid medullary carcinoma, pheochromocytoma, parotid tumor, prostatic carcinoma, renal carcinoma	Squamous cell, adenocarcinoma, and large cell carcinoma of the lung; breast carcinoma, colon carcinoma, gallbladder tumors, testicular carcinoma, uterine carcinoma, laryngeal carcinoma, plasmacytoma, bladder small cell carcinoma	Somatostatin	Lung carcinoma (small cell), carcinoid, pheochromocytoma	
			Calcitonin	Lung carcinoma (small cell), carcinoid	Breast carcinoma, pheochromocytoma
			Gastrin	Lung carcinoma (small cell)	Ovarian carcinoma
			Vasoactive intestinal peptide	Lung carcinoma (small cell), pancreatic islet tumors	
Vasopressin, oxytocin, neurophysin	Lung carcinoma (small cell, anaplastic, adenocarcinoma), carcinoid	Pancreatic carcinoma, duodenal carcinoma	Insulin		Gastric carcinoma, lung carcinoma, carcinoid
			Glucagon		Lung carcinoma, carcinoid, renal carcinoma
Corticotropin-releasing hormone	Lung carcinoma (small cell), carcinoid	Pituitary gangliocytoma, medullary carcinoma of thyroid	Gastrin-releasing peptide (bombesin-like)	Lung carcinoma, carcinoid	Medullary carcinoma of thyroid
Growth hormone–releasing hormone	Carcinoid, pancreatic islet adenoma, lung carcinoma, (small cell)	Adrenocortical adenoma, neurofibroma, endometrial carcinoma, pheochromocytoma, pituitary gangliocytoma			
FETOPLACENTAL AND/OR ANTERIOR PITUITARY					
Chorionic gonadotropin (and subunits)	Lung carcinoma, gastric carcinoma, ovarian carcinoma, adeno- and islet cell carcinoma of the pancreas, hepatoma, genitourinary tract tumors	Testicular carcinoma, ovarian carcinoma, adrenocortical carcinoma, breast carcinoma, melanoma, carcinoid	Growth hormone		Lung carcinoma (large cell), carcinoid, pancreatic islet tumor
			Prolactin		Lung carcinoma, renal carcinoma, gonadoblastoma, ovarian teratoma
Placental lactogen	Lung carcinoma (small cell)	Lymphoma, pheochromocytoma, hepatoma			
OTHERS					
Tissue growth factors (primary insulin-like growth factor II)	Mesenchymal tumors (i.e., fibrosarcoma), hepatoma, adrenocortical carcinoma, pancreatic/bile duct carcinoma	Lung carcinoma, ovarian carcinoma, neuroblastoma, Wilms's tumor	Parathyroid hormone–related protein	Renal carcinoma, lung carcinoma (squamous), hepatoma, pancreatic islet tumors	GI tract tumors, parotid tumors, genitourinary tract tumors, melanoma, breast carcinoma
			1,25-Dihydroxy vitamin D	Lymphoma	
Erythropoietin	Cerebellar hemangioblastoma, uterine fibroma, renal carcinoma	Adrenocortical carcinoma, hepatoma, pheochromocytoma	Parathyroid hormone		Ovarian carcinoma

whereas in others multiple hormones are produced by the same cell. Furthermore, variation may occur in cell lines cloned from such tumors, suggesting that gene expression may be unstable in succeeding generations of tumor cells both in vitro and in vivo.

FREQUENCY The frequency of ectopic hormone secretion varies with the criteria used for diagnosis. The most frequently encountered syndromes are those of ACTH hypersecretion, hypercalcemia, and organic hypoglycemia. Ectopic ACTH secretion occurs in approximately 15 to 20 percent of patients with Cushing's syndrome. Thus consideration of this diagnosis is of great importance. Similarly, nearly half of patients with hypercalcemia unrelated to volume depletion, excess ingestion of vitamin D, or sarcoidosis have a malignancy rather than hyperparathyroidism, and of these, about 70 percent secrete a hypercalcemic peptide, parathyroid hormone–related protein, that has parathyroid hormone–like biologic activity and whose amino-terminal 13 amino acids are identical to those of parathyroid hormone. In contrast, hypoglycemia due to ectopic production of insulin-like growth factor II is infrequent in patients suspected of having an

insulinoma, and ectopic growth hormone–releasing hormone (GRH) secretion is a rare (<1 percent) cause of acromegaly.

CONSEQUENCES OF ECTOPIC HORMONE SECRETION The consequences of ectopic hormone secretion may be of greater significance than the tumor itself. This is particularly true for patients with benign or slowly growing malignant ACTH- or gastrin-producing tumors in whom fulminant Cushing's syndrome or bleeding peptic ulceration may be life-threatening. In others, the hormone may cause medical problems that shorten the life span beyond that attributable to the tumor itself, i.e., severe hypercalcemia, hyponatremia, or hypoglycemia.

The symptoms of ectopic hormone secretion may be the presenting manifestations of the neoplasm or occur late in the course of the disease. The rapidity of onset of the clinical manifestations of hormone hypersecretion affects the frequency with which the syndrome is recognized. For example, excessive secretion of ACTH or vasopressin is clinically evident within weeks or months; thus a fully developed syndrome can be associated with rapidly growing malignant as well as benign tumors. In contrast, acromegaly due to ectopic GRH secretion typically requires years to become apparent and therefore is observed only when caused by benign or slowly growing malignant neoplasms. Ectopic hormone secretion, once established, does not necessarily persist for as long as the tumor is present. Hormone secretion may cease or decline to clinically insignificant levels either spontaneously or in response to radiation or chemotherapy. Hormone secretion usually, but not invariably, recurs with tumor relapse.

In addition to effects on the host, ectopic hormone secretion has numerous important biologic implications. Since tumor-secreted factors that exhibit biologic effects are not unique substances, their identification and characterization can assist in the search for the naturally occurring (eutopic) peptide. For example, tumor-secreted GRH was the source for the purification, isolation, and structural characterization of hypothalamic GRH. In addition, characterization of tumor-produced parathyroid hormone–related protein has resulted in the identification of a new hormone normally found in skin (keratinocytes), the central nervous system, lactating breast, pancreatic islets, and other tissues.

DIAGNOSIS Occasionally, the clinical manifestations of ectopic hormone secretion are so distinctive that they suggest the diagnosis before any hormones have been measured. The development of gynecomastia in the absence of associated diseases such as cirrhosis or testicular failure may suggest the presence of ectopic gonadotropin secretion, while Cushing's syndrome and increased pigmentation or severe muscle weakness (due to hypokalemia) point to ectopic ACTH secretion.

More commonly, however, clinical manifestations of hormone excess are subtle or absent. In such instances, basal serum levels of hormones, e.g., ACTH, may be elevated out of proportion to the biologic effects observed. This may be the result of the presence of ACTH precursor molecules that have little or no biologic activity. Identification of these abnormal forms can be accomplished by molecular sieve chromatography or by multiple, site-specific radioimmunoassays of serum. Similarly, disproportionate elevations of hCG may reflect the presence of the glycoprotein alpha subunit, which is biologically inactive but exhibits cross-reactivity in some radioimmunoassays. A specific alpha-subunit assay is used to confirm the diagnosis.

In other instances, the diagnosis of ectopic hormone secretion may be suggested by finding suppressed levels of hormones that are subject to feedback inhibition. Low or undetectable levels of insulin or parathyroid hormone in the presence of hypoglycemia or hypercalcemia are suggestive of tumors that secrete insulin-like growth factor II or parathyroid hormone–related protein, respectively.

Alterations in normal feedback regulation also may provide clues that elevated circulating hormone levels are derived from ectopic sources. Patients with ectopic ACTH production do not respond to suppression by glucocorticoids or to stimulation by corticotropin-releasing hormone (presumably because of the absence of appropriate receptors in the tumor tissue), an observation that helps distinguish them from patients with pituitary-dependent Cushing's disease. Apparent suppression of ACTH, which has been noted in several case reports, could be explained by intermittent secretion of ACTH by the tumor (an uncommon and poorly understood phenomenon of ectopic hormone secretion).

If the diagnosis is still in doubt, or if the source of ectopic secretion is unknown, selective venous catheterization may be an effective means of locating the tumor. As long as the tumor is actually secreting hormone at the time of study, a step-up gradient in the concentration of the hormone is of value in tumor localization and/or a search for metastases.

THERAPY Primary treatment of ectopic hormone–secreting tumors should be directed, if possible, toward removal of the tumor. Measurement of circulating hormone levels can serve as a marker for completeness of tumor excision or of the effect of radiation and chemotherapy, e.g., small cell carcinoma of the lung. In addition, recurrence of tumor may be heralded by reappearance of elevated hormone levels prior to mass effects of the tumor. However, occasional tumors may not secrete hormones at recurrence, so one cannot rely solely on hormone measurements as a marker of tumor activity.

Frequently, the tumor cannot be removed or is metastatic at the time of diagnosis. In such cases, two other approaches are available for eliminating the effects of ectopic hormone secretion. Octreotide, a long-acting somatostatin analogue, may be effective in inhibiting growth hormone–releasing hormone secretion, VIP secretion, and the clinical symptoms of the carcinoid syndrome.

The other approach involves blocking the action of the hormone when its secretion cannot be altered. Pharmacologic agents may interfere with hormone effects on target tissues. Examples include (1) demeclocycline to inhibit vasopressin action on the renal tubule in the syndrome of inappropriate antidiuretic hormone (SIADH) associated with malignancy and (2) ketoconazole and/or mitotane to inhibit adrenal steroidogenesis in the ectopic ACTH syndrome. Alternatively, surgical removal of the target tissue may avoid life-threatening complications and permit relatively symptom-free long-term survival if the tumor is benign or slowly growing. Examples include adrenalectomy for the ectopic ACTH syndrome and gastrectomy for recurrent gastrointestinal bleeding caused by gastrin-producing tumors. This form of therapy is used infrequently as more specific pharmacologic agents have become available.

ECTOPIC HORMONES AS MARKERS FOR NEOPLASIA With the initial recognition of ectopic hormone secretion, it was hoped that measurement of these hormones would provide a generally applicable means of screening for clinically silent tumors. As knowledge of the spectrum of ectopic hormone secretion has increased, however, this hope has faded. The list of ectopically secreted hormones has lengthened to the point that cost considerations preclude this form of screening. Even if the number of hormones were not as extensive, the limited correlation of tumor site and type with secretion of specific hormones necessitates an extensive workup to localize the tumor. Screening programs, when performed, have yielded few positive results. Moreover, evidence is lacking that earlier diagnosis, as a result of such procedures, reduces morbidity or mortality. Consequently, screening for ectopic hormone production is not justified in routine cancer detection programs.

REFERENCES

BURTIS WJ et al: Immunochemical characterization of circulating parathyroid hormone–related protein in patients with humoral hypercalcemia of cancer. N Engl J Med 322:1106, 1990

DOPPMAN JL: The search for occult ectopic ACTH-producing tumors. Endocrinology 2:41, 1992

——et al: Ectopic adrenocorticotropic hormone syndrome: Localization studies in 28 patients. Radiology 172:115, 1989

FROHMAN LA, DOWNS TR: Ectopic GRH syndrome, in *Acromegaly*, R Robbins et al (eds). New York, Plenum, 1987

KRENNING EP et al: Localisation of endocrine-related tumours with radioiodinated analogue of somatostatin. Lancet 1(8632):242, 1989

LEINUNG MC, et al: Diagnosis of corticotropin-producing bronchial carcinoid tumors causing Cushing's syndrome. Mayo Clin Proc 65:1314, 1990

MARTIN TJ, SUVA LJ: Parathyroid hormone–related protein in hypercalcaemia of malignancy. Clin Endocrinol (Oxf) 31:631, 1989

MUDDLE AH et al: Ectopic production of 1,25-dihydroxyvitamin D by B-cell lymphoma as a cause of hypercalcemia. Cancer 59:1543, 1987

ORTH D: Ectopic hormone production, in *Endocrinology and Metabolism*, 2d ed, P Felig et al (eds). New York, McGraw-Hill, 1987

PASS HI et al: Management of the ectopic ACTH syndrome due to thoracic carcinoids. Ann Thorac Surg 50:51, 1990

PHILIPPE J et al: Expression of peptide hormone genes in human islet cell tumors. Diabetes 37:1647, 1988

RUSSELL, PJ et al: Ectopic hormone production by small cell undifferentiated carcinomas. Mol Cell Endocrinol 71:1, 1990

SANO T et al: Growth hormone–releasing hormone–producing tumors: Clinical, biochemical, and morphological manifestations. Endocrinol Rev 9:357, 1988

STREWLER GJ, NISSENSON RA: Peptide mediators of hypercalcemia of malignancy. Annu Rev Med 41:35, 1990

TABARIN A et al: Use of ketoconazole in the treatment of Cushing's disease and ectopic ACTH syndrome. Clin Endocrinol 34:63, 1991

WYNICK D et al: Symptomatic secondary hormone syndromes in patients with established malignant pancreatic endocrine tumors. N Engl J Med 319:605, 1988

328 PARANEOPLASTIC NEUROLOGIC SYNDROMES

ROBERT H. BROWN, JR.

Neoplasia can alter neurologic function in numerous ways, as outlined in Table 328-1. Several neurologic syndromes have been delineated which are a consequence of a remotely located neoplasm but do not arise from direct involvement of the nervous system by metastasis or from a known secondary complication of cancer or its therapy (e.g., malnutrition, opportunistic infection, drug-induced neuropathy). These paraneoplastic syndromes, outlined in Table 328-2, share several characteristics. They are clinically dramatic, arising subacutely in weeks or even days to produce neurologic symptoms that may be profoundly disabling. They may precede detection of the neoplasm by months or even years; their recognition should prompt a timely search for a malignant tumor. More than one syndrome may arise with a given neoplasm. In general, as outlined in Table 328-2, certain syndromes are associated with particular types of tumors. The diagnosis of a paraneoplastic neurologic disorder depends primarily on (1) the presence of a recognized clinical syndrome, (2) careful exclusion of other cancer-related disorders (as in Table 328-1), and (3) in some instances, confirmatory laboratory studies, including serum or cerebrospinal fluid (CSF) antibodies with specific patterns of reactivity (see Table 328-3) or electromyographic studies typical of myasthenia gravis or myasthenic syndrome. CSF may show protein elevation and a mild lymphocytic pleocytosis.

INCIDENCE Studies of the incidence of these syndromes are problematic because the conditions are rare and classifications vary. In one series, these syndromes were detected in about 7 percent of nearly 1500 patients with tumors, although recent studies suggest that the incidence is somewhat lower. The paraneoplastic syndrome is encountered in up to one-sixth of all ovarian tumors, one-seventh of lung tumors, and less frequently in stomach, prostate, and breast cancers. The tumors most frequently associated with paraneoplastic syndromes are small cell lung carcinoma (47 percent), stomach (12 percent), breast (12 percent), ovary (9 percent), and colon (6 percent) tumors.

PATHOLOGIC CHANGES Pathologic features of these syndromes have been well defined. One group of paraneoplastic syndromes is characterized by *encephalomyelitis,* in which perivascular lymphocytosis, microglial proliferation, and loss of neurons occur. While these changes may be diffuse throughout the neuraxis, they often predominate in a specific anatomic location that dictates the resulting clinical abnormalities. Thus, as outlined below, the manifestations of limbic encephalitis may differ from those of brainstem encephalitis. Inflammation may be evident in dorsal root

---

TABLE 328-1 Effects of malignancy on the nervous system

Direct invasion
Metastatic invasion
  A Parenchymatous
  B Vascular (neoplastic angioendotheliosis)
  C Meningeal (meningeal carcinomatosis)
Opportunistic infections
  A Bacterial (e.g., listeria)
  B Nonbacterial
    1 Typical and atypical viral (e.g., progressive multifocal leukoencephalopathy)
    2 Fungal (e.g., cryptococcus)
Complications of antineoplastic therapy
  A Radiation (e.g., radiation necrosis)
  B Chemotherapy (e.g., vincristine neuropathy)
Metabolic complications
  A Nutritional deficiency
  B Ectopic hormone production
Paraneoplastic syndromes

---

ganglia or in gray and white matter of the spinal cord, respectively, producing ganglioradiculitis or subacute poliomyelitis. Inflammatory destruction of the sensory neuronal cell bodies (hence the term *neuronopathy*) in the dorsal root ganglia results in wallerian degeneration of axons in both peripheral nerves and corresponding ascending sensory long tracts (posterior columns of the spinal cord).

In a second pathologic form of paraneoplastic disease, severe *focal degeneration* or loss of neurons occurs without inflammation. This is exemplified by the selective but widespread loss of Purkinje neurons in the cerebellum in subacute cortical cerebellar degeneration. This disorder may occur in isolation or concurrently with findings of encephalomyelitis in other areas of the brain or spinal cord. In some cases of paraneoplastic cerebellar degeneration there may be accompanying cerebellar inflammation. In other paraneoplastic syndromes the associated pathologic changes occur in the peripheral nervous system, consisting of multifocal demyelination, myonecrosis, or abnormalities in the neuromuscular junction.

PATHOGENESIS Several mechanisms have been invoked to explain these disorders, including release by the tumor of neurotoxic substances, common viral or retroviral infections of tumor and neural tissues, and both humoral and cellular autoimmune reactivity to antigens shared between the tumor and the affected neural cells. Some paraneoplastic disorders are characterized by serum and CSF antibodies with highly specific patterns of reactivity with neural tissue or muscle. These are exemplified by the Lambert-Eaton myasthenic syndrome and myasthenia gravis, in which circulating antibodies react with pre- and postsynaptic proteins, respectively. Both syndromes have been reproduced in animals by passive administration of fractionated immunoglobulins (see Chap. 386). In some cases of paraneoplastic cerebellar degeneration, serum and CSF antibodies react specifically with cerebellar cytoplasmic antigens. In other instances, immunoglobulins from patients with a number of different paraneoplastic neurologic syndromes may produce similar patterns of reactivity with neural tissue. Thus antibodies recognizing neuronal nuclear antigens are common in patients with small cell carcinoma of the lung. Similar findings may be present in subacute sensory neuronopathy. In these cases, it appears that one or more pathogenic antibodies, possibly cross-reacting with antigens on the tumor, may provoke autoimmune neural injury in more than one region of the neuraxis. Detection of such antibodies may confirm that an evolving neurologic disorder is of paraneoplastic origin even though the antibodies are not diagnostic of a specific neurologic syndrome. Evidence suggests that some antigens may be specifically targeted by subsets of lymphocytes within affected areas of the brain.

TREATMENT Treatment of the paraneoplastic disorders is difficult and often unsuccessful. Resection of the underlying malignancy is surprisingly ineffective, although there are isolated reports of symptomatic improvement following tumor removal. Immune suppression is also of little benefit; plasmapheresis or intravenous pooled globulin may ameliorate Lambert-Eaton syndrome.

The salient features of the major paracarcinomatous neurologic syndromes are discussed below (reviewed in detail by Posner) (see Table 328-2).

BRAIN, CEREBELLUM, AND SPINAL CORD Visual paraneoplastic syndromes Patients with carcinoma of the lung (and rarely, breast, cervix, or endometrium) may develop progressive, painless loss of vision with photosensitivity due to loss of retinal photoreceptors. The electroretinogram is typically abnormal. This cancer-associated retinopathy (CAR) is commonly associated with high titers of serum antibodies to one or more CAR antigens including a 23-kDa protein.

Paraneoplastic encephalomyelitis Small cell lung carcinoma may precipitate an encephalomyelitis of variable distribution and, in consequence, variable but often overlapping clinical presentations. In addition, it is often accompanied by an inflammatory paraneoplastic sensory neuronopathy (see below). Serum and CSF from patients with paraneoplastic encephalomyelitis and neuropathy often demonstrate antibodies to neuronal nuclear antigens. This anti-Hu

TABLE 328-2 Paraneoplastic neurologic syndromes

Site	Evolution	Clinical features*	Cancer	Pathology
BRAIN AND CEREBELLUM				
Photoreceptor, retinal degeneration	Weeks to months	Painless visual loss progressing to blindness[1]	SCLC,[†] rarely cervical cancer	Loss of rods and cones, infiltration of retina with mononuclear cells
Subacute cortical cerebellar degeneration	Weeks to months	Cerebellar ataxia, dysarthria[2,3]	SCLC, ovarian and breast cancer, Hodgkin's disease	Loss of Purkinje cells
Opsoclonus-myoclonus	Weeks	Dancing eyes and feet, cerebellar ataxia, and possibly encephalopathy[2,4]	Neuroblastoma, bronchogenic carcinomas	In adults, degeneration of dentate nuclei
Paraneoplastic encephalo-myelitis				
Limbic encephalitis	Weeks to months	Agitated, confusional state, memory loss followed by dementia[2]	SCLC, ovarian and other cancers	Neuronal loss; gliosis in medial temporal lobe, amygdala and elsewhere in limbic system, perivascular and meningeal infiltration
Brainstem encephalitis	Days to weeks	Nystagmus, diplopia, vertigo, ataxia, dysarthria, dysphagia[2]	SCLC, other cancers	Neuronal loss in brainstem, inflammatory changes as above
SPINAL CORD				
Necrotizing myelopathy	Hours, days, or weeks	Para- or quadriplegia with arreflexia, sensory loss and bladder dysfunction	SCLC, lymphoma	Severe necrosis of gray and white matter
Subacute motor neuronopathy	Weeks or months	Flaccid weakness, muscle atrophy, legs affected more than arms[2]	Non-Hodgkin's lymphoma	Inflammation of ventral horns loss of anterior horn cells
PERIPHERAL NERVE				
Subacute sensory neuronopathy	Weeks to months	Severe sensory loss with arreflexia[2] and ataxia, paresthesias, pain	SCLC and other lung tumors	Inflammation and neuronal degeneration in dorsal root ganglia, secondary axon loss
Acute demyelinating neuritis (Guillain-Barré, AIDP)	Hours to days	Ascending paralysis, arreflexia, possibly ascending sensory loss, high spinal fluid protein	Hodgkin's disease	Segmental demyelination inflammation of peripheral nerves
Chronic inflammatory demyelinating polyneuropathy (CIDP)	Weeks to months	Chronic progressive or relapsing weakness with sensory loss, high spinal fluid protein	Rarely lung, breast, and gastric cancer, lymphoma, myeloma	As in AIDP
Neuropathy with paraproteinemia	Weeks to months	Chronic, may be predominantly sensory or motor[‡]	Myeloma, osteosclerotic myeloma	As in AIDP
Sensorimotor neuropathy	Weeks to months	Distal motor and sensory loss[2]	SCLC and other tumors	Axonopathy, some segmental loss of myelin
NEUROMUSCULAR JUNCTION				
Lambert-Eaton myasthenic syndrome	Weeks to months	Proximal weakness, fatiguability, dry mouth, possibly ptosis[6]	SCLC, breast, prostate, stomach tumors	Disruption of active zones on presynaptic terminals
Myasthenia gravis	Weeks to months	Weakness, fatiguability, ptosis, diplopia[7]	Thymoma	Disruption of postsynaptic junctional membrane folds
MUSCLE				
Polymyositis	Months to years	Proximal weakness, myalgias, possibly cardiomyopathy, high serum creatine kinase	Association with malignancy unclear, possibly breast, ovary, lung tumors, lymphoma	Lymphocytic inflammation of muscle interstitium, myofiber necrosis, phagocytosis
Necrotizing myopathy	Days to weeks	Rapidly progressive proximal weakness, possibly dysphagia, dyspnea	Bronchial carcinoma, SCLC	Severe myonecrosis with minimal inflammation or phagocytosis

* Superscript denotes possible association with antibody (listed Table 328-3).
† Small cell lung carcinoma.
‡ May be associated with a serum IgG or IgA M component.

antibody recognizes a 37-kDa protein specific to neuronal nuclei. The major features of paraneoplastic encephalomyelitis include the following.

LIMBIC ENCEPHALITIS In some cases, the encephalitis is limited to or most extensive within limbic structures such as the hippocampus and amygdala, producing affective changes in personality (anxiety and agitated depression), selective, early memory loss suggestive of Korsakoff psychosis, or confusion and hallucinations. In some cases the initial presentation is an amnesic syndrome. The affective disorder often prompts psychiatric evaluation. Abnormalities of the electroencephalogram or overt seizures may be present early in the syndrome. While cognition may initially be spared, dementia becomes common as the disorder progresses; symptoms referable to encephalitic involvement in other regions are often superimposed.

TABLE 328-3 Defined antibodies associated with paraneoplastic neurologic syndromes*

Antibody	Paraneoplastic syndrome	Tumor	Antigen
[1]CAR ab	Cancer-associated retinopathy	SCLC[†]	Recoverin, 25-kDa calcium-binding cone protein
[2]Anti-Hu	Encephalomyelitis, sensory neuronopathy	Predominantly SCLC[†]	37-kDa CNS nuclear protein
[3]Anti-Yo	Cerebellar degeneration	Gynecologic tumors, breast	Cerebellar leucine-zipper protein
[4]Anti-Ri	Opsoclonus-myoclonus	Breast	55- and 80-kDa CNS nuclear protein
[5]Anti-MAG IgM M protein	Demyelinating neuropathy	Myeloma	Myelin-associated glycoprotein (MAG)
[6]LEMS ab	Lambert-Eaton myasthenic syndrome	SCLC	Presynaptic calcium channel
[7]MG ab	Myasthenia gravis	Thymoma	Postsynaptic acetylcholine receptor

* Other patterns of antibody reactivity also have been described for some of these syndromes.
† Small cell lung cancer.

BRAINSTEM ENCEPHALITIS Symptoms of brainstem encephalitis relate directly to the distribution of pathologic findings. The predominant symptoms are due to medullary involvement producing nausea, vomiting, nystagmus, vertigo, and ataxia. A syndrome suggestive of progressive bulbar palsy with marked dysarthria and dysphagia may occur with pontine nuclei involvement. Mesencephalic inflammation and neuronal loss result in nuclear or internuclear eye movement abnormalities with disabling diplopia and oscillopsia. Rostral midbrain and nigral involvement may cause rigidity and in some cases stupor and coma.

CEREBELLAR ENCEPHALITIS Inflammatory changes are rare in the cerebellar cortex but may be severe in deep cerebellar nuclei such as the dentate nucleus, causing myoclonus.

MYELITIS In paraneoplastic myelitis, the gray matter of the cord is diffusely infiltrated with leukocytes leading to profound neuronal degeneration. The myelitis may be widespread through the cord or restricted to a few segmental levels. Anterior horn cell destruction typically produces muscle weakness and neurogenic atrophy which is often asymmetric. There may be selective involvement of the neck, upper extremities, or lower extremities. Corticospinal signs (hyperreflexia, weakness, Babinski signs) result from involvement of this tract in the cord or brainstem. The corticospinal tract dysfunction (and in some cases motor neuronopathy) should not be confused with motor neuron disease; typical amyotrophic lateral sclerosis does not appear to arise as a paraneoplastic complication. The appearance of sensory symptoms and signs in a patient with cancer usually denotes either dorsal root ganglioradiculitis or inflammation of the posterior horns (see below).

NECROTIZING MYELOPATHY This is a rare complication of malignancy presenting clinically as a subacute transverse myelitis, often in a thoracic location. It can be distinguished from the less fulminant encephalomyelitis described above by the evolution of an intensely necrotic, central thoracic cord lesion which tails off rostrally and caudally over several segmental levels. In some instances, there are multiple necrotic foci within the cord. Clinical findings include leg (and possibly arm) plegia, sensory loss, and urinary bladder sphincter abnormalities. The lesion is frequently initially asymmetric, mimicking the Brown-Séquard syndrome. In severe cases, the CSF protein and cell count are increased and myelography demonstrates focal cord swelling. Although not all cases are associated with tumor, cancers of the lung, lymphoma, and leukemia are known to occur in such patients.

Opsoclonus-myoclonus A syndrome of opsoclonus, myoclonus, and ataxia ("dancing eyes, dancing feet") occurs in both children and adults. About one-half of affected children have differentiated neuroblastomas, usually located in the thorax. In adults, the syndrome may be associated with solid tumors such as bronchial carcinoma. The onset is subacute, and in some patients the syndrome persists for months, to be followed by permanent encephalopathy or retardation. Pathologic findings in adults include prominent neuronal degeneration in the dentate nucleus of the cerebellum suggesting a relationship to cortical cerebellar degeneration. In some individuals, this syndrome responds to glucocorticoids or treatment of the cancer. A subgroup of women developing opsoclonus with breast cancer has been found to have an antibody (anti-Ri) directed against 55- and 80-kDa antigens on neuronal nuclei and in the tumor.

Subacute cortical cerebellar degeneration (SCCD) This is a subacute progressive cerebellar disorder characterized by profound truncal and appendicular ataxia evolving over a period of weeks in association with gynecologic tumors, oat cell carcinoma, or Hodgkin's disease. Symptoms referable to the brainstem include vertigo, dysarthria, diplopia, nystagmus, and corticospinal signs. In general, any nonfamilial ataxia arising in patients over age 45 should raise the suspicion of this entity. By contrast with paraneoplastic encephalomyelitis described above, the predominant pathologic finding in SCCD is widespread loss of cerebellar Purkinje neurons with astrogliosis and secondary loss of Purkinje cell axons. Many cases are associated with dementia for which an anatomic basis has not been well established. The CSF commonly reveals a mild pleocytosis; cerebellar atrophy may be evident on magnetic resonance imaging (MRI) or computed tomographic (CT) scan.

Several types of anti-Purkinje cell antibodies have been detected in sera of patients with SCCD. Women with cancer of the breast or ovary and SCCD demonstrate anti-antibodies (anti-Yo) recognizing cytoplasmic Purkinje cell proteins of about 34 and 62 kDa. The former is a recently cloned, novel neuronal protein expressed selectively in cerebellar Purkinje cells. A different cytoplasmic antigen is recognized by immunoglobulins from patients with SCCD and adenocarcinoma of the lung. In other patients with small cell lung carcinoma and SCCD, anti-Hu antibodies are present (see Table 328-3).

PERIPHERAL NERVES A number of clinical syndromes affecting the peripheral nerves occur in association with malignancy. *Subacute paraneoplastic sensory neuronopathy*, arguably the most clinically distinctive, is a ganglioradiculitis that may present with paraneoplastic encephalomyelitis. Other paraneoplastic neuropathies are more difficult to distinguish from noncarcinomatous neuropathies. However, their recognition is important because they are relatively common and their manifestations may precede the diagnosis of the underlying neoplasia. Neuropathy may be demonstrated in as many as 50 percent of patients with lung cancer using electrophysiologic criteria. In evaluating a paracarcinomatous neuropathy, it is helpful to ascertain whether the neuropathy (1) affects motor fibers, sensory fibers, or both, (2) predominantly involves axon or myelin, or (3) occurs with an abnormal serum paraprotein.

Subacute sensory neuronopathy This disorder primarily affects the axon, with relative sparing of myelin. The typical pathology is a ganglioradiculitis, as noted earlier. Clinically, the onset is characterized by the subacute development of paresthesias and pain (sometimes severe) in the distal limbs and associated truncal sensory ataxia. The sensory ataxia may be profoundly disabling. Although often initially restricted only to arms or legs, the symptoms eventually affect all four extremities. In a majority of cases, the underlying malignancy is oat cell cancer of the lung; the paraneoplastic neuropathy may precede the diagnosis of the tumor by more than a year. The serum of some patients contains anti-Hu antibodies.

Acute inflammatory demyelinating polyneuritis (AIDP, Guillain-Barré) This syndrome, discussed in detail in Chap. 383, may be associated with Hodgkin's disease. It is characterized by subacutely ascending paralysis, sensory loss which is often mild by comparison with the motor deficits, areflexia, and a characteristic elevation of CSF protein without pleocytosis. Histopathology reveals lymphocytic infiltration of nerves, segmental demyelination, and relative axonal sparing.

Chronic inflammatory demyelinating polyneuropathy (CIDP) Included here are a group of chronic progressive or relapsing inflammatory demyelinative peripheral neuropathies which are distinguished from acute polyneuritis by the time course, more prominent involvement of sensory nerves, lack of involvement of autonomic nerves, and responsiveness to immunotherapy. As in Guillain-Barré syndrome, the demyelinative nature of these neuropathies is defined physiologically by slowed nerve conduction velocities or dispersion of compound muscle action potentials; as in AIDP, the pathologic hallmark is segmental loss of myelin with relative preservation of axons as revealed in teased single fiber preparations. In some cases, physiologic studies may reveal only marginal slowing of conduction, whereas the biopsy demonstrates clearly selective myelin loss. Sural nerve biopsy may fail to reveal any alterations if the demyelination is proximal (and therefore detectable only with electrophysiologic methods). Elevation of CSF protein helps confirm the diagnosis.

CIDP usually occurs without any association with neoplasia. Rarely, however, it can occur in association with solid tumors of lung, breast, and stomach. It also may present in patients with Waldenström's macroglobulinemia, gamma heavy chain disease, and lymphoma. In many instances, paraneoplastic CIDP is characterized by the presence of a serum paraprotein, typically a monoclonal immunoglobulin ("M component"). As many as 20 percent of patients with monoclonal gammopathies of undetermined cause later develop hematologic disease, including malignancies.

Two chronic demyelinating neuropathies are particularly distinctive in this context. The first is associated with a monoclonal IgM that reacts with a myelin-associated glycoprotein (MAG) in peripheral nerve myelin. This pattern of reactivity occurs in about half of patients with an IgM gammopathy and neuropathy. This IgM anti-MAG neuropathy is more sensory than motor; it is slowly progressive. It remains to be established whether the anti-MAG antibody is a cause or consequence of the demyelination. The second distinctive subtype of CIDP occurs with osteosclerotic myeloma and monoclonal IgG or IgA antibodies that do not react with MAG. This polyneuropathy is predominantly motor and often quite indolent, although it may eventually produce severe limb muscle wasting. Sensory and autonomic findings are unusual. A related group of CIDP patients develop polyneuropathy, organomegaly, endocrinopathy, the M protein, and skin changes (POEMS syndrome); one-half have osteosclerotic myeloma and IgG or IgA M proteins with lambda light chains. Some patients with demyelinative neuropathies and IgM M proteins respond well to immunosuppressive therapy. Those with osteosclerotic myeloma may improve after treatment of the underlying plasmacytoma, particularly if it is solitary.

Sensorimotor neuropathy This category of mixed sensory and motor axonopathy is the most common paraneoplastic neuropathy. Symptoms depend on the severity of the neuropathy and may include muscle wasting and weakness, distal limb parasthesia, and sometimes pain. Pathologically, there is noninflammatory degeneration of axons and mild myelin loss, presumably secondary to the axonopathy. Paraneoplastic sensorimotor neuropathy has been reported with several types of tumors (lung oat cell, breast, stomach) and hematologic malignancies (Hodgkin's disease, lymphoma, multiple myeloma). In amyloidosis, itself often associated with myeloma, there may be an axonal neuropathy with intraneural deposition of amyloid fibrils derived from immunoglobulin light chains. Axonal neuropathy has been reported as a manifestation of occult insulinoma, possibly as a consequence of hypoglycemia. Infrequently, these neuropathies remit spontaneously; often they progress even with aggressive treatment of the underlying malignancy.

Subacute motor neuronopathy Another particularly striking paracarcinomatous disorder of peripheral nerves is a subacutely progressive motor neuropathy that causes slowly progressive weakness in the legs heralding an otherwise occult lymphoma. Pathologic changes include loss of motor neurons in the anterolateral gray matter of spinal cord, gliosis, loss of myelin in ventral roots, and some Schwann cell proliferation. Although there is no clearly effective treatment for this condition, many patients seem to improve following immunosuppressive therapy for the malignancy. In other patients, progression of the weakness may cease independently of the status of the lymphoma.

NEUROMUSCULAR JUNCTION Lambert-Eaton myasthenic syndrome (See also Chap. 386) This syndrome, which occurs either in association with malignancy or autoimmune disease, is characterized by weakness, myalgias, and fatigability. It is typically more severe in the lower extremities and in the proximal muscles. Ptosis may be seen. Dysautonomic features are common and may include dryness of the mouth and eyes, impotence, diminished sweating, and orthostatic symptoms. The disorder afflicts men more often than women. The incidence of associated malignancy is 70 percent in men and 25 percent in women. In most cases of either sex, the tumor is a small cell carcinoma of the lung.

The predominant clinical finding is striking reduction in strength at rest with transient improvement in power on repetitive maximal exertion. Tensilon has no effect or may slightly improve strength. Electromyography demonstrates motor unit potentials whose amplitude is low at rest but which increases with exercise or tetanic stimulation; this contrasts with the electromyographic findings in myasthenia gravis (see Chap. 386). Electron microscopy of the presynaptic motor nerve terminals at the neuromuscular junction reveals a decrease in numbers of structures believed to correspond to voltage-sensitive calcium channels. Lambert-Eaton syndrome is considered to be an autoimmune disorder associated with diminished quantal release of acetylcholine. It is associated with other autoimmune disorders and appears to be HLA-linked (B8 and DRw3 antigens). In paraneoplastic Lambert-Eaton syndrome, physiologic data incriminate antibodies directed against voltage-dependent calcium channels present both on the tumor and at distal motor nerve terminals. Treatment is directed toward the underlying neoplasm or autoimmune disease or toward augmentation of acetylcholine release with drugs that prolong presynaptic depolarization and thereby enhance calcium influx. Guanidine hydrochloride and 3,4-diaminopyridine may be beneficial either in autoimmune or paraneoplastic Lambert-Eaton myasthenic syndrome; plasma exchange and immunosuppression also may be effective.

Myasthenia gravis This disorder, discussed elsewhere in detail (Chap. 386), is characterized by exercise-induced muscle weakness caused by an antibody-mediated reduction in the numbers of acetylcholine receptors at the postsynaptic junction. About 15 percent of cases are associated with thymoma; many arise concurrently with other autoimmune or thyroid disorders.

MUSCLE Polymyositis-dermatomyositis This subject is discussed in Chap. 384. While an increased incidence of malignancy in elderly patients with dermatomyositis has long been suggested, this concept has recently been challenged by a retrospective analysis of experience with polymyositis at the Mayo Clinic.

Necrotizing myopathy Carcinoma of the bronchus may rarely be associated with a fatal subacute widespread necrotizing myopathy that involves all muscles including bulbar and diaphragmatic muscles. Intrafusal muscle fibers are also involved. Deep tendon reflexes are preserved. Muscle undergoes degeneration without phagocytosis or significant inflammatory response. The cause of the necrotizing process is unknown.

OTHER Several other neurologic syndromes have been reported to be paraneoplastic but are less well characterized. *Stiff-man syndrome,* or diffuse hypertonia due to loss of inhibitory spinal interneurons, may arise in association with carcinoma. In the nonneoplastic stiff-man syndrome, autoantibodies have been detected that react with glutamic acid decarboxylase, an enzyme essential for the synthesis of gamma aminobutyric acid, a central nervous system inhibitory neurotransmitter. Nonfamilial, subacute *chorea* and *dystonia* occur with oat cell carcinoma of the lung. *Optic neuritis* may develop as a paraneoplastic disorder, but it is difficult to exclude direct involvement of the optic nerve or chiasm by cancer cells or indirect effects of the underlying malignancy, as outlined in Table 328-1.

REFERENCES

CASCINO TL: Medical complications of systemic cancer. Med Clin North Am 77:265, 1993

DALMAU J et al: Anti-Hu–associated paraneoplastic encephalomyelitis/sensory neuronopathy: A clinical study of 71 patients. Medicine 71:59, 1992

DROPCHO EJ et al: Antineuronal (anti-Ri) antibodies in a patient with steroid-responsive opsoclonus-myoclonus. Neurology 43:207, 1993

FATHALLAH-SHAYKH H et al: Cloning of a leucine zipper protein recognized by the sera of patients with antibody-associated paraneoplastic cerebellar degeneration. Proc Natl Acad Sci USA 88:3451, 1991

FURNEAUX HM et al: Characterization of a cDNA encoding a 34-kDa Purkinje neuron protein recognized by sera from patients with paraneoplastic cerebellar degeneration. Proc Natl Acad Sci USA 86:2873, 1989

HENSON RA, URICH H: *Cancer and the Nervous System*. Oxford, Blackwell, 1982

KINSBOURNE M: Myoclonic encephalopathy of infants. J Neurol Neurosurg Psychiatry 25:271, 1964

LENNON VA, LAMBERT EH: Autoantibodies bind solubilized calcium channel–omega-conotoxin complexes from small cell lung carcinoma: A diagnostic aid for Lambert-Eaton myasthenic syndrome. Mayo Clin Proc 64:1498, 1989

LUQUE FA et al: Anti-Ri: An antibody associated with paraneoplastic opsoclonus and breast cancer. Ann Neurol 29:241, 1991

POLANS AS et al: A photoreceptor calcium-binding protein is recognized by autoantibodies obtained from patients with cancer-associated retinopathy. J Cell Biol 112:981, 1991

POSNER JB: Paraneoplastic syndromes. Neurol Clin 9:919, 1991

SAKAI K et al: Isolation of a complementary DNA clone encoding an autoantigen recognized by an anti-neuronal cell antibody from a patient with paraneoplastic cerebellar degeneration. Ann Neurol 28:692, 1990

SZABO A et al: HuD, a paraneoplastic encephalomyelitis antigen, contains RNA-binding domains and is homologous to Elav and Sex-lethal. Cell 67:325, 1991

THIRKILL CE et al: The cancer-associated retinopathy antigen is a recoverin-like protein. Invest Ophthalmol Vis Sci 33:2768, 1992

PART THIRTEEN

ENDOCRINOLOGY AND METABOLISM

section 1 Endocrinology

329 HORMONES AND HORMONE ACTION

JEAN D. WILSON

Communication between cells is largely mediated by the endocrine, nervous, and immune systems. The nervous system was originally considered distinct from the endocrine system—information was thought to be carried either by neural impulses or by chemical mediators in the blood—but it is now clear that they constitute one coordinated network. Not only may neurotransmitters such as norepinephrine circulate in blood as hormones, but neural impulses have major effects on the release of chemical mediators such as testosterone and insulin. This interlocking relationship is most apparent in the hypothalamus, which serves as the highest integrative center for the two systems. Hence, a single neuroendocrine system evolved to integrate and coordinate the metabolic activities of the organism. Endocrinology deals largely with the chemical mediators in this system, but proper understanding of the role of hormones requires knowledge of the autonomic nervous system (Chap. 68) and of the metabolic capacities of cells.

The formulation of endocrinology has been blurred in additional ways. The term *hormone* originally referred to substances that are secreted into the circulation and act as chemical effectors in other tissues. However, the capacity to form such chemical mediators is not limited to so-called endocrine organs. Some hormones, such as angiotensins II and III, are formed in the bloodstream itself. Others, such as testosterone in women and dihydrotestosterone and estradiol in men, are in part secreted and in part formed in extraglandular tissues from circulating precursors, so-called prohormones. Still other chemical mediators circulate only in restricted compartments such as the hypothalamic-pituitary portal system and do not reach the systemic circulation in appreciable quantities. Finally, certain hormones, such as insulin, dihydrotestosterone, and thyrotropin-releasing hormone (TRH), have paracrine actions in the same tissues in which they are formed and exert actions at distal sites, whereas other chemical mediators, such as müllerian-inhibiting substance, exert local actions exclusively.

BIOCHEMISTRY

SYNTHESIS The approximately 100 known mammalian hormones fall into three major categories—peptides or peptide derivatives, steroids, and amines. In the case of peptide hormones, genes code for messenger RNA, which is then translated into protein precursors. These proteins undergo posttranslational cleavage (pre-proparathyroid hormone → proparathyroid hormone → parathyroid hormone) and/or processing (thyroglobulin → thyroxine → triiodothyronine) to form the active hormone recognized by the target tissues. The distinct feature of peptide hormones is that one or a few structural genes code for the amino acid sequence of the peptide, and other genes are responsible for the alteration of the peptide to its final form. In the case of peptide hormones with subunits, the different subunits may be derived either from a single precursor (insulin) or from separate precursors ([luteinizing hormone (LH)]. Furthermore, the same peptide hormone (somatostatin) can be formed from different prohormones encoded by distinct genes, individual prohormones such as proopiomelanocortin can be metabolized to different hormones in different cells, depending on the complement of processing enzymes in the cell in question, and the primary transcripts of the calcitonin gene can be alternatively spliced in different tissues to form messenger RNA for either calcitonin or calcitonin-related peptide. Peptide hormones may also be formed ectopically in malignancies of nonendocrine origin such as carcinoma of the lung and may be formed in small amounts in normal nonendocrine tissues (see Chap. 327).

In the case of steroid hormones the fundamental precursor—cholesterol (for most steroid hormones) or 7-dehydrocholesterol (for vitamin D metabolites)—undergoes a series of enzymatic transformations to form the final products. At least six enzymes and consequently a minimum of six genes are required to transform cholesterol to estradiol. Because of the number of enzymes required, the synthesis of steroids from cholesterol is unusual in malignancies of nonendocrine tissues. However, many tissues—malignant and nonmalignant—that cannot form steroid hormones de novo from cholesterol contain enzymes that convert circulating steroids to other hormones; examples are the conversion of androgens to estrogens by trophoblastic tumors and by normal adipocytes and the conversion of progesterone to deoxycorticosterone by the kidney.

Amine hormones are synthesized by a series of reactions similar to those involved in steroid hormone synthesis except that the precursors are amino acids. For example, tyrosine is the precursor for epinephrine and norepinephrine (see Chap. 68).

STORAGE Most tissues that synthesize hormones have a limited capacity to store the completed product. For example, the normal adult testes contain only about one-sixth of the quantity of testosterone needed for daily production, and consequently the testicular pool turns over several times to provide the normal daily output of hormone. Even when tissues have special storage organelles for hormone, the amount of hormone stored is usually limited: the insulin granules in the pancreatic beta cell ordinarily contain amounts of insulin sufficient only for short-term, reserve needs. (In contrast, nerve endings may contain a several-day supply of norepinephrine.) The limited capacity to store hormones in tissues is a chemical consequence of their unsuitability for incorporation into any of the three main storage compartments of the body (lipids, glycogen, or protein). For example, most steroid hormones are too polar to be stored in large quantities in lipid compartments, and peptide and amine hormones are unsuitable for incorporation into proteins. As a consequence, the body pools of most hormones tend to be small. The major exceptions to this rule are those instances in which the precursor forms of hormone can be stored either as protein or in neutral lipid compartments; the normal thyroid gland contains the equivalent of a 2-week supply of thyroid hormones in the form of the protein thyroglobulin, and the precursor and intermediate forms of vitamin D can be stored in considerable quantity in hepatic lipid.

RELEASE   The biochemical mechanisms involved in the release process are incompletely understood. In some instances they involve conversion of insoluble to soluble derivatives (proteolysis of thyroglobulin to thyroid hormones). In others, release is due to exocytosis of storage granules (insulin, glucagon, prolactin, growth hormone). Finally, release may involve passive diffusion of newly synthesized molecules such as steroid hormones down activity gradients into plasma; under this circumstance the rate of hormone release is a function of the rate of hormone synthesis and the blood flow to the tissue.

Because of the limited capacity for storage, most hormones are released into plasma at a pace reflecting the rates of formation. The pituitary trophic hormones [LH, adrenocorticotropin (ACTH), thyrotropin (TSH)] act in their target tissues to influence rates of both hormone synthesis and release. Even when peptide hormones are stored in granules, initial release of the stored material is followed by an enhanced rate of synthesis (as, for instance, the two-phase release of insulin induced by glucose infusion). For some hormones, major diurnal, sleep-related, developmental, and neural factors influence hormone release; again, it is assumed that in most of these instances synthesis and release are tightly linked.

The rate of hormone release in many instances is periodic or rhythmic, the cycle varying in frequency from minutes to hours (ultradian), to daily (circadian), to months or years (infradian). Hormones such as LH and follicle-stimulating hormone (FSH) are released in a pulsatile fashion with bursts of secretion occurring in a repetitive pattern: ACTH (and cortisol) release varies during a 24-h cycle, and thyroid hormone release can vary on longer cycles. Whether this intermittent release is a function of alterations in synthetic rates, changes in blood flow, or other mechanisms is uncertain, but most such cycles are under neurogenic control. In many instances the physiologic significance of pulsatile release is not fully understood, but in some instances changes in frequency or amplitude of the release pattern have profound effects on hormone function; i.e., the pulsatile administration of luteinizing hormone–releasing hormone (LHRH) stimulates the release of LH by the pituitary, whereas the constant infusion of the same amount of hormone per unit time has the opposite effect. Furthermore, changes in frequency or amplitude of hormone release may characterize specific disease states; loss of the diurnal rhythm of cortisol release is characteristic of the early phase of Cushing's disease, and pulsatile release of LHRH is blunted in anorexia nervosa. Finally, understanding the rhythms by which hormones are released is essential for interpreting plasma hormone levels.

TRANSPORT   Hormones are transported via lymph, blood, and extracellular fluids from sites of release to sites of cellular action and ultimately of metabolic inactivation and degradation. The plasma is probably a passive diluent for most peptide and amine hormones, and this feature explains the short half-lives (3 to 7 min) for most nonglycosylated peptide hormones. (Glycoprotein hormones such as human chorionic gonadotropin, or hCG, have longer half-lives.) The more insoluble a hormone in water, the more important the role of transport proteins; for example, thyroid and steroid hormones are largely transported in protein-bound form. No transport protein yet characterized is exclusive; for example, testosterone can be transported both by a specific binding protein [testosterone-binding globulin (TeBG)] and by albumin; thyroxine can be transported both by prealbumin and by thyroxine-binding globulin (TBG). Protein-bound hormone (HP) cannot enter most cellular compartments and serves as a reservoir from which free hormone (H) is liberated for diffusion into intracellular compartments:

$$H + P \rightleftarrows HP$$

Distribution of bound and free hormone in plasma is determined by the amount of hormone, the amount of binding protein, and the binding affinity of hormone for the protein. However, in the intact organism the effective level of free hormone is influenced by additional factors. When the rate of dissociation of a hormone from a binding protein is rapid, the functional free fraction in vivo is also influenced by capillary transit time and membrane permeability.

The relation between free and bound hormone is complex: First, the free (dialyzable) fraction in vitro generally underestimates the actual free fraction available in vivo because hormone bound to weak binding proteins such as albumin (in contrast to that bound to specific, high-affinity binding proteins) rapidly dissociates from the albumin as the free fraction diffuses from the capillary; consequently the albumin-bound hormone can function in vivo as a free fraction. Under some conditions, measurement of the dialyzable fraction does provide a useful index of the in vivo apparent free fraction. However, in hypoalbuminemic states, the in vitro free (dialyzable) fraction may increase when the in vivo free hormone level is actually diminished. In addition, in those tissue compartments such as liver in which proteins including hormone-transport protein complexes are cleared (in contrast to peripheral tissues in which only the free hormone enters the cell) free hormone levels have lesser effects on hormone uptake by the tissue.

Second, the distribution of hormones between plasma and tissue is a function of the balance between tissue binding proteins and plasma binding proteins. Therefore, levels of true or apparent free hormone may not reflect the amounts of hormone within cells.

Third, only the free hormone interacts with receptors in target cells and participates in the regulatory feedback mechanisms that control the rates of hormone synthesis. As a consequence, changes in the amount of transport protein alone cannot cause endocrine pathology in the steady state, provided the remainder of the endocrine feedback loop is intact. For example, profound elevations or decreases in TBG (either because of genetic or other factors) are both compatible with a euthyroid state. To illustrate, an increase in TBG would lower the level of free (dialyzable) hormone and lower the amount bound to albumin; as a consequence TSH secretion would increase, and the output of thyroxine by the thyroid would increase *until* TBG is again saturated so that the level of free hormone returns to the normal range, at which time TSH levels and thyroid hormone secretion also return to normal. Likewise, a decrease in TBG would temporarily increase the level of free hormone, and TSH secretion and thyroxine output would fall until the free level returns to normal.

To summarize, a change in the amount of a specific, high-affinity binding protein can cause profound alterations in hormone levels but by itself does not cause either a steady state hormone excess or deficiency, provided the regulatory feedback mechanisms that control hormone synthesis are intact. In contrast, alteration of the amount of a binding protein may cause endocrine pathology when hormone formation is not regulated by ordinary feedback control mechanisms or when feedback control mechanisms are deranged. For example, testosterone production in women is not regulated by testosterone levels, and alterations in TeBG levels in women may alter the steady state levels of free testosterone. Likewise, changes in TBG levels in a hypothyroid patient receiving a fixed dose of levothyroxine can cause alterations in free thyroxine levels.

DEGRADATION AND TURNOVER   The plasma level (PL) of any hormone is dependent on two factors—the secretion rate (SR) of the hormone and the rates of metabolism and excretion, the so-called metabolic clearance rate (MCR):

$$PL = SR/MCR \qquad \text{or} \qquad SR = MCR \times PL$$

Metabolic clearance of hormones is accomplished by several mechanisms. Only small fractions of hormones are excreted intact in urine or bile. Degradation and inactivation of the hormone can take place in target tissues, in nontarget tissues such as liver and kidneys, or in both target and nontarget tissues. Peptide hormones are in general inactivated by proteases, largely in target tissues. Hormone metabolism frequently facilitates excretion of steroid and thyroid hormone by rendering them soluble in urine or bile. Thyroid hormones are deiodinated, deaminated, and deconjugated primarily by the liver. Steroid hormones are reduced, hydroxylated, and converted into glucuronide and sulfate conjugates. Biliary conjugates may be hydrolyzed in the gastrointestinal tract and reabsorbed into the circulation. The degradative mechanisms for different hormones have one common feature, namely, that alternative pathways exist for the catabolism of all hormones described to date.

Because of the nature of feedback control of hormone secretion, changes in rates of hormone degradation alone, like changes in plasma protein binding, do not cause endocrine pathology, provided the feedback control mechanisms that regulate synthesis are intact. For example, in severe liver disease and in myxedema, the degradation of glucocorticoids by the liver is impaired; as a consequence the turnover of cortisol slows, but the plasma level does not rise because secretion of ACTH is inhibited. Thus, a normal level of free hormone is maintained by decreasing the rate of cortisol secretion. The opposite is the case when glucocorticoid degradation is enhanced (as in thyrotoxicosis); in this situation cortisol secretion rises to keep the level of the hormone normal.

Although changes in rates of hormone degradation alone do not result in hormone deficit or excess, they may cause profound alterations in endocrine pharmacology. Thus, ordinary doses of glucocorticoids may cause the Cushing syndrome in patients with myxedema or liver disease, and consequently glucocorticoid dosage must be reduced in both conditions. Likewise, doses of glucocorticoids may have to be increased in the presence of hyperthyroidism. In addition, the development of hyperthyroidism in a patient with inadequate adrenal reserve can precipitate adrenal crisis by accelerating the rate of glucocorticoid catabolism. Thus, in circumstances in which the normal control mechanisms that regulate hormone synthesis are either circumvented or inoperative, changes in rates of hormone degradation may aggravate or cause pathology.

REGULATION OF HORMONE PRODUCTION

As stated above, fluctuations of hormone levels in the normal person are determined primarily by changes in rates of production. A unifying feature of all endocrine systems is the fact that the production of most hormones is regulated directly or indirectly by the metabolic activity of the hormone itself. This regulation is accomplished through a series of negative (and positive) feedback loops (Fig. 329-1). In some cases a fairly constant blood level of hormone is required, and some sensing device must exist to monitor either the hormone level itself or some related function such as plasma osmolality, blood glucose, plasma calcium, or body sodium content. For example, hormones produced in response to pituitary trophic hormones (cortisol, thyroxine, gonadal steroids) feed back on the hypothalamic-pituitary system to regulate their own rates of secretion. Similarly, parathyroid hormone and insulin are secreted in response to feedback signals from serum calcium and glucose levels, respectively. Feedback systems are generally more complex than this description indicates, sometimes operating indirectly by several steps; when the hormone itself acts as the direct regulator of feedback (testosterone on the hypothalamic-pituitary axis), the effect is mediated by the same receptor-effector system by which the hormone acts in other target tissues. An example of positive feedback is the stimulation of LH release by estradiol prior to ovulation. Nonhormonal and environmental factors may alter both positive and negative feedback control mechanisms or the response to such control.

A usual feature of the feedback systems is rapidity of action; indeed, most respond within minutes or hours to varying metabolic demands to maintain homeostatic control within a narrow range. The main exceptions relate to gametogenesis in the ovary and testis (see Chaps. 339 and 340). In both instances, a complex differentiative process functions in the steady state so that sperm production tends

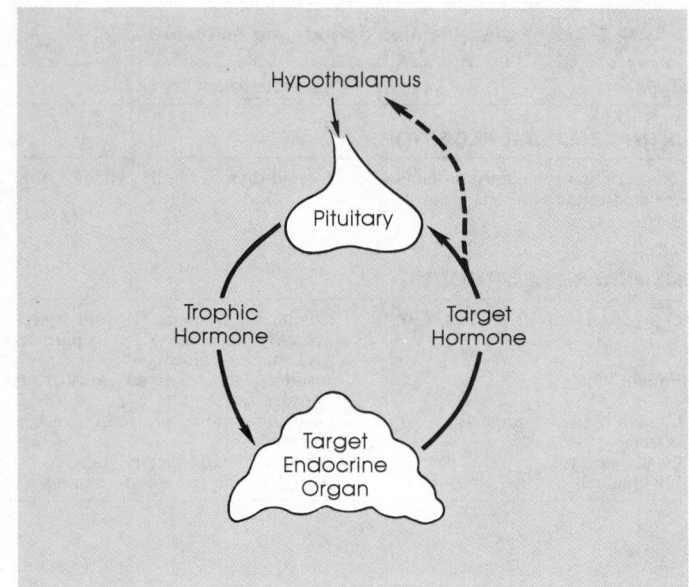

FIGURE 329-1 Feedback control of an endocrine organ such as the adrenal, thyroid, or gonads by the pituitary.

to be relatively constant from day to day whereas ovulation is cyclic. Spermatogenesis and sperm export require approximately 2 months to complete so that changes in FSH levels may not result in altered levels of sperm in the ejaculate for long periods.

The fact that the secretion of hormones is under regulatory control has several important clinical implications. First, the significance of plasma levels of hormones may be interpretable only if the appropriate regulatory factors are taken into account (Fig. 329-2). The meaning of a borderline low plasma thyroxine may become clear only when thyroid-stimulating hormone (TSH) is measured simultaneously; likewise, plasma insulin and parathyroid hormone levels may be interpretable only in conjunction with simultaneous measurements of plasma glucose and calcium, respectively. Second, the finding of simultaneous elevations of hormone pairs (or hormone regulatory factor pairs) in the absence of evidence of hormone excess suggests the presence of a hormone-resistance state. For example, simultaneous elevation of plasma glucose and insulin is characteristic of insulin resistance, and simultaneous elevation of LH and testosterone suggests androgen resistance. In contrast, simultaneous elevation of hormone pairs in the presence of signs of hormone excess suggests a trophic hormone-secreting tumor. Third, insight into the regulatory control of hormone secretion is the basis for the various dynamic tests of hormone reserve and hormone secretion (see Chap. 330).

FIGURE 329-2 Relation between target hormone level and trophic hormone level in normal and disease states (e.g., TSH and thyroid hormones, ACTH and cortisol, LH and testosterone).

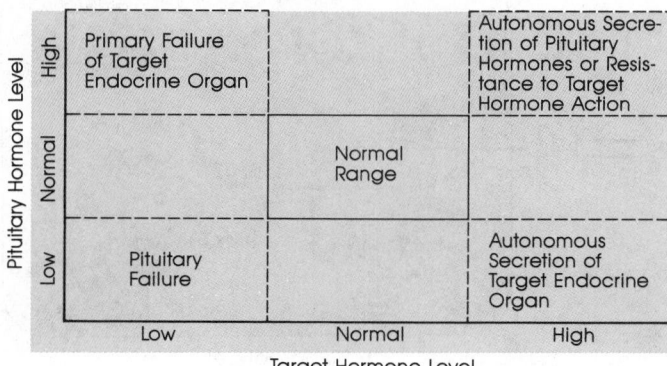

TABLE 329-1 Classification of hormone receptors

Type	Characteristic hormones	Disease states due to mutant receptor components
INTRACELLULAR RECEPTORS		
Transcription regulatory proteins related to the viral oncogene *erb*A	Steroid-thyroid family, vitamin A	Testicular feminization and related syndromes; cortisol resistance; vitamin D–dependent rickets, type II; thyroid hormone resistance; pseudohypoaldosteronism
MEMBRANE RECEPTORS		
G protein family (see Chap. 69)	Luteinizing hormone, thyroid-stimulating hormone, parathyroid hormone, epinephrine, somatostatin, vasopressin, glucagon	Pseudohypoparathyroidism, nephrogenic diabetes insipidus
Protein kinases	Insulin, platelet-derived growth factor, epidermal growth factor	Diabetes mellitus with profound insulin resistance
Growth hormone–prolactin family	Growth hormone, prolactin, cytokines, nerve growth factor	Laron dwarfism
Guanylate cyclase	Atrial natriuretic factor	
Ion channels	Acetylcholine (nicotinic), gamma-amino butyric acid	Myasthenia gravis

MECHANISMS OF HORMONE ACTION

The first step in hormone action is the binding of the hormone to specific macromolecules in the cell, so-called hormone receptors. These receptors can either be located intracellularly or in the cell membrane, and membrane-bound receptors in turn fall into several distinct classes (Table 329-1). Insight into the chemical nature of these receptors and into the mechanisms by which they participate in signal transduction has been accelerated by the cloning of the cDNAs and the genes that encode these proteins (see Chap. 61).

INTRACELLULAR RECEPTORS   Most steroid and thyroid hormones are transported in plasma bound to carrier proteins (Fig. 329-3). The protein-bound hormones (HP) are in dynamic equilibrium with small amounts of free hormones (H) that diffuse by a passive mechanism into cells. In most instances the principal form of the hormone secreted into plasma (cortisal, progesterone, aldosterone, estradiol) undergoes no further metabolism within the cell and is responsible for hormone action within the target cell. Other hormones (thyroxine, testosterone) undergo chemical conversion to more active forms (triiodothyronine and dihydrotestosterone).

H binds to specific receptor proteins (R) in the cytoplasm or nucleus to form a hormone-receptor complex (HR). The hormone-receptor complex has the capacity to bind to specific regulatory sequences in DNA (so-called hormone regulatory elements) and thus acts to control the rate of transcription. As the result of this interaction with DNA new messenger RNAs (mRNAs) are formed, and the synthesis of cytoplasmic proteins is enhanced. The cytoplasmic proteins, in turn, mediate the effects of the hormone.

The cloning of the cDNAs for the various receptors revealed that receptors of this class bear a striking homology to the viral oncogene *erb*A and to each other. The fact that members of this family of hormone-dependent transcription factors are similar in structure suggests that these receptors have evolved from a common ancestral transcription factor. Each contains a hormone-binding domain, a DNA-binding domain, and an *N*-terminal variable or immunodominant domain (Fig. 329-4). An interesting feature of this class of receptors is that more than one receptor exists for certain hormones (thyroid hormones) and that candidate receptors have been identified for which no ligand is known. Elucidation of the structures of these receptors made it possible to analyze the mutations that impair hormone action and cause several hormone-resistance syndromes (see below).

MEMBRANE-BOUND RECEPTORS   G protein family   Receptors that bind GTP (G proteins) all work by similar mechanisms but are capable of mediating a complex range of actions. In every case, binding of ligand to the receptor produces a conformational change that causes GTP to bind to the protein at a special site. The active G protein then binds to a target protein and initiates a regulatory cascade involving one (or more) intracellular mediators including adenylate cyclase, phospholipase C, and arachidonic acid. The receptors of this class are monomeric proteins with an extracellular domain that binds ligand, an intracellular G protein–binding domain, and seven transmembrane-spanning regions. Elucidation of the molecular biol-

FIGURE 329-3   Mechanism of action of hormones with intracellular receptors. H = hormone; P = plasma transport protein; R = receptor; R* = activated receptor; mRNA = messenger RNA.

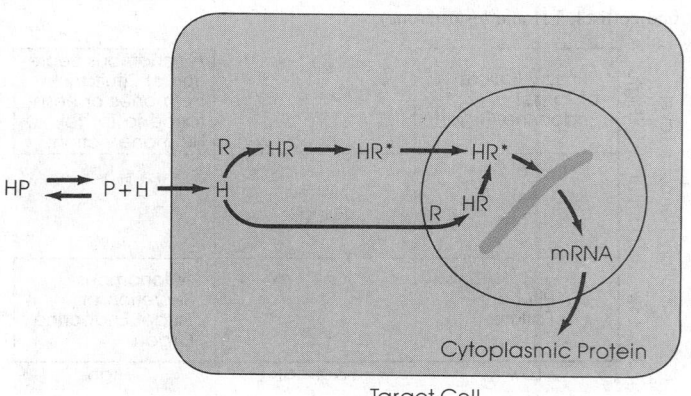

Target Cell

FIGURE 329-4   Intracellular receptors of the thyroid-steroid class. The areas of greatest homology (DNA-binding domain) are shown by the slanted bars, the areas of intermediate homology (hormone-binding domain) are shown by the stippled areas, and the areas with the least homology are shown by the open regions.

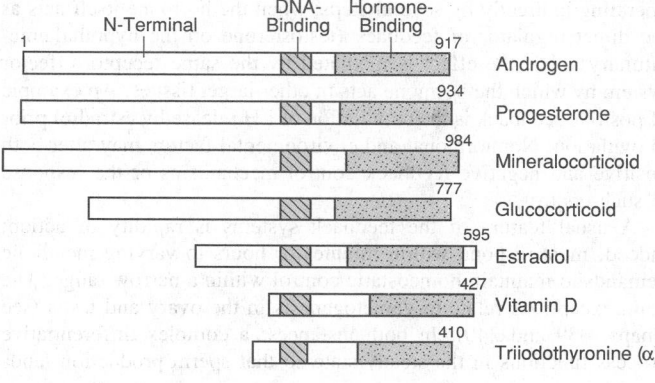

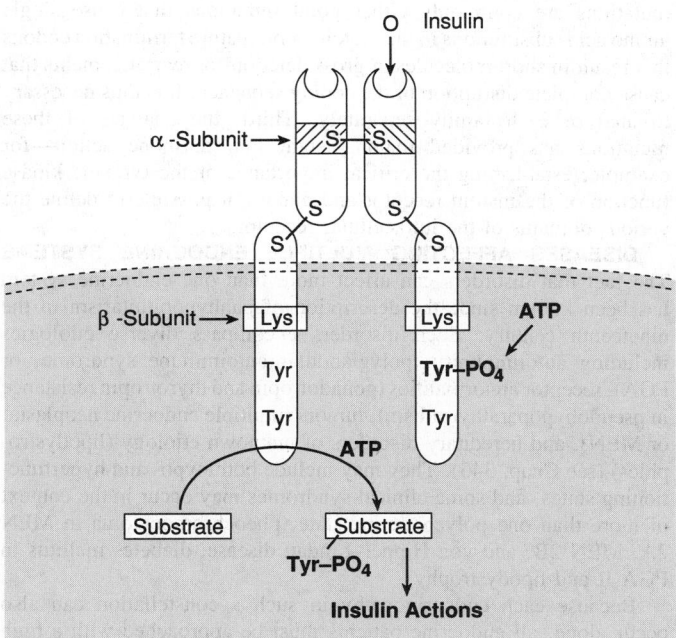

FIGURE 329-5 Schematic representation of the insulin receptor. As the result of the binding of insulin to the alpha subunit the protein kinase function of the beta receptor is activated, and both exogenous protein substrates and the beta subunit itself are phosphorylated.

ogy of the G protein has provided insight into the actions of drugs and signaling mechanisms in addition to hormones and into the pathophysiology of pseudohypoparathyroidism (see Chaps. 69 and 357 and below).

Protein kinases Receptors of this class, such as the insulin receptor and the epidermal growth factor (EGF) receptor, are glycoproteins typically composed of two alpha subunits and two beta subunits which are linked by sulfhydryl bonds (Fig. 329-5). The alpha subunits are extracellular and contain the hormone binding site, and the beta subunits are transmembrane proteins. The beta subunit of the receptor is a hormone-regulated protein kinase capable of phosphorylating itself and other substrates on tyrosine residues using ATP as the phosphate source. In the case of insulin the tyrosine activity of the receptor is essential for hormone action. Point mutations in the coding sequence of receptor genes that prevent the protein kinase activity can cause profound resistance to insulin action (see below). Exactly how receptor kinase activity is transmitted into hormone action is not entirely clear. Several endogenous substrates of the enzyme have been identified, and physiologic effects of the hormone may either be indirect or direct consequences of the phosphorylation of the substrates or of the receptor itself. The nerve growth factor receptor has an extracellular domain similar to that of the EGF and insulin receptors.

Receptors of the growth hormone/prolactin class The growth hormone receptor is a protein of approximately 600 amino acids that contains a single, centrally located transmembrane domain. Interestingly, the high-affinity growth hormone–binding protein in plasma corresponds to the extracellular hormone-binding domain of the growth hormone receptor and is believed to be cleaved from the receptor, but the role of the plasma protein in the regulation of growth is undefined. The growth hormone receptor shares approximately a 25 percent homology with the prolactin receptor [which is present in long (~ 600 amino acid) and short (~ 300 amino acid) forms] suggesting that the two receptors have evolved from a common ancestral gene. The mechanism(s) by which these receptors mediate hormone action is unclear. Mutations that impair the function of the growth hormone receptor are responsible for Laron dwarfism (see below).

Other membrane-bound receptors The receptor for atrial natriuretic factor is a guanylate cyclase that spans the plasma membrane; the extracellular portion of the receptor binds the hormone, and the intracellular portion of the protein synthesizes guanosine-3′,5′-monophosphate (cyclic GMP) which serves as the second messenger for the hormone (see Chap. 69). The nicotinic acetylcholine receptor channel is a membrane-spanning complex of proteins that forms a true ion channel containing a central pore that can be opened and closed by ligand-binding-induced conformational change to allow sodium and potassium ions to cross the membrane and hence cause depolarization of cells that contain the receptors. Autoantibodies that block the function of this receptor cause myasthenia gravis (see Chap. 380).

Receptors for gamma-aminobutyric acid and glycine, which mediate inhibitory activity in the central nervous system, show a high degree of homology with the acetylcholine receptor, suggesting that ligand-gated ion channels may be derived from a common ancestral gene.

ENDOCRINE DISORDERS

Endocrinopathy can result from hormone deficiency, hormone excess, or resistance to hormone action, and abnormalities in more than one endocrine system may coexist in the same individual.

DEFICIENCY STATES With few exceptions (calcitonin) hormone deficiency results in pathologic manifestations. The study of clinical disorders that result from hormone deficiency or absence played an important role in the evolution of endocrinology as a discipline. Such studies were followed by attempts to extract the responsible hormone from normal endocrine tissues, characterize the chemical nature (and ultimately synthesize the molecule), and administer the hormone to replace the deficit. The treatment of hypothyroidism by the administration of thyroid hormone is probably as successful as any therapeutic measure in medicine. Because clinical deficiency states can be induced in experimental animals by destruction or removal of the endocrine organ, an enormous amount is known about the pathophysiology of the deficiency states (diabetes mellitus, pituitary and adrenal insufficiency, hypothyroidism, and hypogonadism).

The nature of the destructive processes that cause failure of the endocrine organs is also understood in many instances; these include infections (adrenal insufficiency due to tuberculosis), infarction (postpartum pituitary failure) and tissue death from other causes (diabetes mellitus secondary to pancreatitis), tumors (null cell tumors of the pituitary), autoimmune processes (Hashimoto's thyroiditis), dietary inadequacy (hypothyroidism due to iodine deficiency), and hereditary defects in hormone synthesis (pituitary dwarfism). In certain forms of diabetes mellitus, the cause may be a hereditary predisposition that renders the pancreas subject to destruction by several mechanisms (see Chap. 337). In other endocrine-deficiency diseases the etiology of the defect is unidentified (congenital anorchia).

HORMONE EXCESS With few exceptions (testosterone in men, progesterone in men and women) hormone excess causes pathologic effects. Four general types of hormone excess are recognized. In one, the hormone is overproduced by the gland that is the usual site of its production (hyperthyroidism, acromegaly, Cushing's disease); such excess production results from failure of circumvention of the feedback control mechanisms that regulate production of the hormone in the normal state, but the underlying mechanism is often obscure because animal models for the diseases are rare. The second type of hormone excess results when a hormone is produced by a tissue (usually malignant) that ordinarily is not a major endocrine organ (for example, ACTH production in oat cell carcinoma of the lung, thyroid hormone secretion by struma ovarii). Such hormone-excess states have been described for many hormones (see Chap. 327). A third type of hormone-excess state involves the overproduction of hormones in peripheral tissues from circulating precursors; for example, overproduction of estrogen in liver disease because of diversion of the precursor androstenedione from its usual sites of catabolism in the liver to sites of extraglandular estrogen formation. Finally, hormone excess all too commonly results from iatrogenic causes; for example, the complications resulting from glucocorticoid therapy (see Chap. 335).

Excess of a given hormone may result from more than one cause. Thyrotoxicosis can result from overproduction of hormone by the thyroid as a result of overproduction of TSH (rare); from stimulation by extrapituitary thyroid-stimulating factors; from autonomous thyroid hyperfunction; from leakage of preformed hormone from the thyroid due to an inflammatory injury; or from excess hormone from sources other than the thyroid itself, as in thyroid hormone overdosage, accidental ingestion of meats contaminated with thyroid tissue, or secretion by struma ovarii (see Chap. 334). The unraveling of the cause of specific hormone-excess states can be one of the most challenging problems of clinical endocrinology.

PRODUCTION OF ABNORMAL HORMONES In some instances abnormal hormones can cause endocrine disease. One form of diabetes mellitus is the result of a single-gene mutation that results in the production of an abnormal insulin molecule that is ineffective because of defective binding to the insulin receptor. In other cases, hormone precursors, hormone subunits, or incompletely processed peptide hormones may be released into the circulation, as is common in so-called ectopic hormone production of neoplasia (see Chap. 327). Alternatively, immunoglobulins may bind to hormone receptors and thus exert hormonal actions, for example, the thyroid-stimulating immunoglobulins that exert TSH-like actions in hyperthyroidism (see Chap. 334) or the antibodies to the insulin receptor that have insulin-like actions (see Chap. 337).

HORMONE RESISTANCE The concept that an endocrinopathy can result because the tissues cannot respond to normal (or increased) levels of a hormone evolved from the deduction that pseudohermaphroditism is due to peripheral resistance to the action of parathyroid hormone (see Chaps. 69 and 357). This concept has had far-reaching implications. First, the concept of hormone resistance served as a major stimulus for the study of how hormones act within cells. Second, more and more forms of hormone resistance have been identified, so that diseases are now recognized to result from resistance to most hormones. Such hormone resistance is frequently due to hereditary causes. Third, hormone resistance can be due to a variety of molecular abnormalities, including defects in receptors and in postreceptor effector mechanisms for hormones, development of antibodies to hormones or hormone receptors, and the absence of target cells. Fourth, abnormalities of receptors are now implicated in the pathogenesis of diseases outside the endocrine domain, such as familial hypercholesterolemia. Hormone resistance does not necessarily involve equally all target tissues for the hormone. For example, selective resistance to thyroid hormone can be restricted to the pituitary itself, and in androgen resistance androgen action may be more severely impaired in the testis than in other target tissues.

A common feature of hormone-resistance states is the coexistence of a normal or *elevated* level of the hormone in the circulation despite deficient hormone action. This feature is a consequence of the fact that most hormones are under regulatory feedback control and failure of hormone action usually leads to increased hormone production.

The elucidation of the structures of the various receptors and the cloning of the cDNAs for these proteins has made it possible to define the molecular defects in a number of hormone-resistance states (Table 329-1). Mutations of almost every class of receptor have now been identified, and several clinical implications are now apparent. First, in the past it was only possible to identify receptor defects that caused profound hormone resistance. Now that subtle defects in receptor function can be identified, hormone resistance may prove to be a common cause of endocrinopathy. Second, at the molecular level disorders are genetically heterogeneous. Unrelated families with mutations of the insulin receptor, the growth hormone receptor, or the androgen receptor rarely have identical disorders. Furthermore, in regard to individual receptors such as the androgen receptor,

mutations are commonly either point mutations that cause single amino acid substitutions in the protein or premature termination codons that result in short molecules or gross deletions or rearrangements that cause complete disruption of the coding sequence. It is thus necessary to analyze each family separately. Third, the analysis of these mutations has provided major insight into hormone action—for example, establishing the critical importance of the tyrosine kinase function of the insulin receptor and making it possible to define the various domains of the intracellular receptors.

DISEASES AFFECTING MULTIPLE ENDOCRINE SYSTEMS
The fact that disorders can affect more than one endocrine system has been known since the description of panhypopituitarism in the nineteenth century. Such disorders encompass diverse etiologies including autoimmunity (polyglandular autoimmune syndrome, or PGA), receptor abnormalities (gonadotropin and thyrotropin resistance in pseudohypoparathyroidism), tumors (multiple endocrine neoplasia, or MEN), and hereditary disorders of unknown etiology (lipodystrophies) (see Chap. 343). They may include both hypo- and hyperfunctioning states, and some clinical syndromes may occur in the context of more than one polyendocrine state (pheochromocytoma in MEN 2A, MEN 2B, and von Hippel–Lindau disease; diabetes mellitus in PGA II and lipodystrophy).

Because each endocrinopathy in such a constellation can also occur alone, all endocrine patients must be approached with a high index of suspicion for abnormalities of multiple systems. This is of particular importance because treatment of one condition may cause worsening of another (surgical procedures such as thyroidectomy can cause worsening of unrecognized pheochromocytoma) and because in certain of the familial syndromes it is mandatory to make systematic searches for the disease in potentially affected family members.

REFERENCES

CLARK JH et al: Mechanism of action of steroid hormones, in *William's Textbook of Endocrinology*, 8th ed, JD Wilson, DW Foster (eds). Philadelphia, Saunders, 1992, pp 35–90

EVANS RM: The steroid and thyroid hormone receptor superfamily. Science 240:889, 1988

GODOWSKI PG et al: Characterization of the human growth hormone receptor gene and demonstration of a partial gene deletion in two patients with Laron-type dwarfism. Proc Natl Acad Sci USA 86:8083, 1989

HABENER JF: Genetic control of hormone formation, in *Williams' Textbook of Endocrinology*, 8th ed, JD Wilson, DW Foster (eds). Philadelphia, Saunders, 1992, pp 9–34

KAHN CR, GOLDSTEIN BJ: Molecular defects in insulin action. Science 245:13, 1989

———, WHITE MF: The insulin receptor and the molecular mechanism of insulin action J Clin Invest 82:1151, 1988

——— et al: Mechanisms of action of hormones that act at the cell surface, in *William's Textbook of Endocrinology*, 8th ed, JD Wilson, DW Foster (eds). Philadelphia, Saunders, 1992 pp 91–134

KELLY PA et al: Different forms of the prolactin receptor. Trends Endocrinol Metab 3:54, 1992

MARCELLI M et al: A single nucleotide substitution introduces a premature termination codon into the androgen receptor gene of a patient with receptor-negative androgen resistance. J Clin Invest 85:1522, 1990

MCPHAUL MJ et al: The spectrum of mutations in the androgen receptor gene that causes androgen resistance. J Clin Endocrinol Metab 76:17, 1993

PARDRIDGE WM: Serum biovailability of sex steroid hormones. Clin Endocrinol Metab 15:259,1986

TAYLOR SL et al: Mutations in the insulin receptor gene. Endocr Rev 13:566, 1992

WEISS RE, REFETOFF S: Thyroid hormone resistance. Annu Rev Med 43:363, 1992

330 ASSESSMENT OF ENDOCRINE FUNCTION

JEAN D. WILSON

Endocrine status is assessed by measuring either plasma levels of a hormone, the urinary excretion of a hormone or hormone metabolite, the rates of secretion of hormones into the circulation, hormone reserve and regulation by dynamic tests, the levels of hormone receptors, selected effects of hormone action in target tissues, or appropriate combinations of these tests. Each technique is useful in certain clinical situations.

MEASUREMENT OF PLASMA HORMONE LEVELS The plasma levels of steroid and thyroid hormones range between 1 nmol/L and 1 μmol/L, while those of peptide hormones are generally in the range of 1 pmol/L to 0.1 nmol/L. The application of modern chemical, chromatographic, bioassay, radioreceptor, radioimmunoassay, and immunometric techniques for the assessment of plasma constituents in low concentrations constitutes a significant advance in modern medicine and has made clinical endocrinology one of the most quantitative of clinical disciplines. In the case of hormones whose plasma levels are relatively constant from moment to moment and day to day (thyroxine and triiodothyronine), the measurement of isolated plasma levels alone provides a reliable assessment of the hormone status in most clinical situations.

In most instances, however, care must be exercised in assessing isolated plasma levels. For hormones with relatively simple structures (steroid and thyroid hormones) reliable assay techniques are available so that measured values usually reflect the plasma levels as of a given moment. In the case of the more complex peptide hormones, however, considerable variability may exist in the structure of physiologically active hormone molecules in the circulation, some of which may be measured poorly in some assay procedures; for example, standard radioimmunoassays for luteinizing hormone (LH) and for parathyroid hormone may on occasion either underestimate or overestimate the amount of biologically active hormone in plasma. In such situations, radioreceptor assays or in vitro bioassays may provide a better assessment of endocrine status.

Furthermore, in the case of hormones that undergo pulsatile secretion (LH, testosterone) a single value is usually not representative of mean plasma levels. In such instances it is necessary either to measure levels in several samples drawn at random or to pool aliquots of three or more samples of plasma drawn at 20- to 30-min intervals for a single determination.

When plasma levels undergo a characteristic, predictable fluctuation such as the diurnal variation of plasma cortisol, the timing of plasma sampling must be designed to provide a useful index of the hormone status. Even here, however, it is important to recognize that plasma levels may exhibit diurnal variation only during certain phases of life (plasma LH levels in early puberty). In women appropriate interpretation of plasma gonadotropins, progesterone, and estradiol during the reproductive years requires reference to the corresponding phase of the ovulatory and menstrual cycles, and it may be necessary to obtain sequential studies over many days to provide interpretable data. Seasonal variations also occur in the levels of certain hormones (such as thyroxine and testosterone), but these changes are generally so small that they do not affect the interpretation of individual values. In some situations variation in hormone levels is not the result of any obvious rhythmicity but rather the consequence of waxing and waning of disease processes; repeated measurements of cortisol or of calcium and parathyroid hormone levels over many months may be necessary to establish the diagnosis of Cushing's syndrome or of hyperparathyroidism.

In the case of steroids, thyroid hormones, and some peptide hormones such as growth hormone that are transported in plasma largely bound to proteins, measurement of total hormone concentration provides an index of endocrine status *only* to the extent that it allows a deduction of the level of the free or unbound hormone. Direct measurements of the free levels of these hormones (usually 1 percent or less of the total) can be done only in a few laboratories. Since the amount of free hormone is a function of the amount and affinity of binding of transport proteins and the amount of hormone, the total hormone level reflects the amount of free hormone only as long as the amount of binding protein(s) remains constant or fluctuates only within narrow limits. In those instances in which the level of binding protein is increased [e.g., thyroid-binding globulin (TBG) and testosterone-binding globulin (TeBG, or sex steroid–binding globulin, SHBG) in pregnancy] or decreased [hereditary decreases in TBG or cortisol-binding globulin (CBG)] it is essential to assess the amount of binding protein to allow estimation of the free hormone level (T_3 resin uptake for TBG or direct measurement of TBG, TeBG, or CBG).

Finally, the range of plasma levels of most hormones within the normal population is broad. As a consequence, the level of a hormone in an individual may be halved or doubled (and thus be abnormal for that person) but still be within the so-called normal range. For this reason it is useful to assess appropriate hormone pairs simultaneously (LH and testosterone, thyroxine and thyroid-stimulating hormone); a borderline low testosterone level in the presence of elevated plasma LH is indicative of testicular failure, whereas the same level of testosterone in the presence of a normal LH implies that the endocrine status is normal (see Fig. 329-2). Likewise, in women with increased testosterone production and secondary decrease in TeBG, plasma testosterone concentration may be normal despite increased production of the hormone.

URINARY EXCRETION Measurement of the urinary excretion of a hormone or a hormone metabolite that reflects plasma levels or secretory rates offers certain advantages over the measurement of isolated plasma levels, e.g., the urinary excretion reflects average plasma levels over the time of collection. Thus, a 24-h urine free cortisol value may provide a better estimate of the function of the adrenal cortex than isolated measurements of plasma cortisol. Again, however, certain limitations of the use of urinary measurements must be kept in mind. (1) Urinary creatinine should be measured routinely to document the adequacy of the urine collection. Women excrete on average about 1 g/d and men about 1.8 g/d. Day-to-day variation should not exceed 20 percent. (2) The excretion of individual metabolites may not reflect changes in hormone secretion under all conditions. For example, the formation of the 18-oxo derivative of aldosterone may be influenced by drugs that do not alter secretion or plasma levels of the hormone. (3) Urine values are obviously meaningless for those hormones (thyroxine, triiodothyronine) excreted into bile. Of more importance is the fact that peptide hormones such as gonadotropins may be metabolized differently in different individuals prior to excretion into the urine so that establishment of the range of normal is difficult. (4) Hormones from more than one source may be excreted as common metabolites; urinary 17-ketosteroids are derived from both adrenal and gonadal androgens, and consequently the measurement is of little value in assessing testicular androgen production in men. (5) Changes in renal function may influence rates of hormone excretion into urine. Such changes can in part be corrected by measurement of urine creatinine, but in the case of metabolites or conjugates formed in the kidney itself excretion patterns may be distorted out of proportion to the decrease in creatinine clearance.

SECRETION AND PRODUCTION RATES The measurement of the secretion rate of a hormone circumvents most problems inherent in measurement of plasma levels and urinary excretion. Such measurements involve the administration of radioactive hormone and measuring the dilution that such a hormone undergoes as a consequence of mixture with endogenously secreted, nonradioactive hormone over a given period of time. In practice the plasma hormone itself or a unique metabolite of the hormone from urine is isolated, purified to radiochemical homogeneity, and used to calculate the amount of the hormone secreted during the time of study. In the case of hormones formed principally in peripheral tissues (estradiol and dihydrotestosterone in men, triiodothyronine in both sexes) radioactive precursors can be administered, and the rates of conversion to the metabolites in question can be measured for assessment of overall production rates. Alternatively, as described above, clearance rates of hormones can be measured and, together with mean plasma levels, used to estimate secretion rates. Unfortunately, these various techniques are complex and expensive to perform, require use of radioactive isotopes, and can be done in only a few centers.

DYNAMIC TESTS OF HORMONE RESERVE AND REGULATION
When hypo- or hyperfunction is severe, measurement of the level of hormone in blood or urine may be satisfactory for making a diagnosis, particularly when the tests demonstrate appropriate feedback relationships; e.g., low plasma testosterone coupled with high plasma LH indicates primary testicular failure. In less clear-cut instances, however, stimulation tests are useful in establishing the significance of borderline low values. Likewise, suppression tests are used to document the presence of hyperfunction of endocrine systems. All such dynamic tests are designed to take advantage of the known feedback control mechanisms for various hormones (Fig. 329-1).

Two types of stimulation tests are in common use. In one, endogenous hormone production or action is blocked (cortisol production by metyrapone, estradiol action by clomiphene), and the capacity of the pituitary to respond by increasing endogenous production of the trophic hormone and/or the capacity of the target tissue to respond are then assessed; ideally such tests measure the integrity of an entire hypothalamic–pituitary–target tissue loop. In the other type of stimulation test, the trophic hormone itself is administered under some standardized regimen, and the capacity of the target tissue to respond is determined (cortisol levels before and after ACTH administration). Stimulation tests are particularly useful in four situations: (1) assessing hormone status when precise quantification of plasma levels is difficult or imperfect (ACTH), (2) assessing endocrine status when static tests are borderline low, (3) distinguishing primary from secondary (pituitary) causes of endocrine failure, and (4) assessing gonadal reserve in prepubertal subjects in whom plasma gonadotropins and gonadal steroids are difficult to interpret.

Suppression tests are useful for the diagnosis of hyperfunction because the hyperfunctioning gland by definition does not operate under normal control mechanisms. Suppression can either be quantitatively or qualitatively abnormal. For example, the feedback control of the pituitary may be reset to respond to high levels of the suppressing hormone (pituitary ACTH secretion in Cushing's disease), or secretion can be autonomous (ACTH secretion by carcinoma of the lung). In principle, the feedback regulator is administered, and the degree of inhibition of hormone secretion is assessed for the endocrine system in question (change in radioactive iodine uptake after administration of thyroid hormones, change in cortisol secretion after the administration of potent exogenous glucocorticoids, suppressibility of plasma growth hormone by glucose).

The clinical usefulness of dynamic tests of endocrine function is limited by the fact that they are altered by a multitude of secondary factors. Age, coexisting disease states, and concurrent drug regimens all interact to influence responsiveness and hence to limit the specificity of such tests. In particular, psychiatric disorders such as endogenous depression may impair endocrine dynamic tests in the absence of specific endocrine pathology.

HORMONE RECEPTORS AND ANTIBODIES   The measurement of hormone receptors in biopsy material from target tissues or in fibroblasts propagated from biopsy material is useful—for example, in the diagnosis of partial hormone-resistance states such as rickets due to vitamin D resistance, hyperglycemia and hyperinsulinemia associated with insulin resistance, and male pseudohermaphroditism due to androgen resistance (see Chap. 329). In selected laboratories the techniques of molecular biology can be applied to provide specific information about the structure of mutant receptors. Likewise, under selected conditions measurement of antibodies to hormones (such as antibodies to thyroid hormones that can cause hypothyroidism) or antibodies to target tissues (adrenal gland, gonads, thyroid) may be essential for the assessment of endocrine status. With certain exceptions (antibodies to thyroid tissue) these tests are not widely available.

TISSUE EFFECTS   Perhaps the ideal hormone test is the measurement of the peripheral end result of hormone action in the target tissues for the hormone. For example, demonstration of the capacity to concentrate urine maximally following water restriction indicates that the hypothalamic mechanisms that control the function of the posterior pituitary are intact, that the posterior pituitary has a normal capacity to secrete vasopressin, that the vasopressin receptor is intact, and that the postreceptor effector mechanisms for the hormone are operative. Optimally such a test assesses the function of the entire pathway of hormone secretion and action. In practice, many such tests are imperfect. For example, even though vasopressin secretion is normal, intrinsic renal disease can result in a fixed low urine osmolality and thus distort the interpretation of the functional test of vasopressin action. In other instances the tests are difficult to perform and subject both to artifact and to influences from diverse parameters (for example, the metabolic rate is increased by fever even when thyroid function is normal). For these reasons, the identification of additional specific tissue markers for hormone action would be very useful.

IMAGING PROCEDURES   Developments in imaging have had a profound impact in endocrinology and provide better means of identifying abnormalities in almost every endocrine system, from delineating small lesions of the pituitary and hypothalamus, to measuring bone densitometry to assess metabolic bone disease, to the noninvasive localization of functioning parathyroid tissue in patients with persistent or recurrent hyperparathyroidism. Because the rate of technologic advance in the field is so rapid, the literature evaluating the effectiveness (and limitations) of up-to-date processes inevitably lags.

A major problem in the interpretation of imaging procedures stems from the fact that small nodules of no functional significance are known from autopsy studies to occur in the pituitary, the adrenal, and, less commonly, the testes. The natural history of these nonfunctioning adenomas is not well understood; the vast majority appear to remain limited in size and nonfunctional for life, but in rare instances they may evolve into autonomous and/or hyperfunctioning tumors. In addition, malignancies—both metastatic and primary—can occur in these tissues. Now lesions of this size can be recognized in life, and the incidental discovery of adrenal and pituitary masses is a common result of CT scans or MRI performed for other reasons. Several types of criteria have been proposed for deciding which of these masses are likely to be benign and which should be removed. For example, by one guideline solid, endocrinologically silent lesions of the adrenal smaller than 3.5 cm may be followed safely with serial CT scans whereas larger lesions deserve further workup such as sonographically guided percutaneous needle biopsy or exploratory surgery. Additional experience will be required to establish the validity of these and other criteria for the assessment of such masses.

Another unresolved issue stems from the fact that it is not always clear which imaging procedure is best in a given clinical situation. In some instances evidence will be accrued that will make clear the indications for one or another procedure. In other instances definite guidelines may be harder to develop, as in the choice of MRI versus CT for delineation of the anatomy of the hypothalamic-pituitary system. In some patients small lesions are best seen with MRI whereas in others lesions in the same areas—equally small and with similar histologic features—are better delineated with CT. As a consequence, there is a tendency in the workup of complicated cases to obtain both procedures routinely. Although this practice is justified in some cases, the costs of diagnostic workups are thereby inflated.

An unexpected dividend of the developments in imaging is that it is now possible to chart the natural history of endocrine disease in a different way, as in the occasional documentation of hemorrhage into a pituitary tumor that eventuates in development of the empty sella syndrome or the uncovering of a functioning adrenal adenoma when biochemical or clinical evidence of Cushing's disease is minimal.

REFERENCES

BELLDEGRUN A et al: Incidentally discovered mass of the adrenal gland. Surg Gynecol Obstet 163:203, 1986

GORDEN P, WEINTRAUB BD: Radioreceptor and other functional hormone assays, in *Williams Textbook of Endocrinology*, 8th ed, JD Wilson, DW Foster (eds). Philadelphia, Saunders, 1992, pp 1647–1661

GRIFFIN JE: Dynamic tests of endocrine function in *Williams Textbook of Endocrinology*, 8th ed, JD Wilson, DW Foster (eds). Philadelphia, Saunders, 1992, pp 1663–1670

HAMPER UM et al: Primary adrenocortical carcinoma: Sonographic evaluation with clinical and pathologic correlation in 26 patients. Am J Roentgenog 148:915, 1987

VAITUKAITIS JL: Hormone assays, in *Endocrinology and Metabolism*, P Felig et al (eds). New York, McGraw-Hill, 1987, p 165

YALOW RS: Radioimmunoassay of hormones, in *Williams Textbook of Endocrinology*, 8th ed, JD Wilson, DW Foster (eds). Philadelphia, Saunders, 8th 1992, p 1635

331   NEUROENDOCRINE REGULATION AND DISEASES OF THE ANTERIOR PITUITARY AND HYPOTHALAMUS

GILBERT H. DANIELS / JOSEPH B. MARTIN

The pituitary, appropriately titled the master gland, produces six major hormones and stores an additional two hormones (Fig. 331-1). Growth hormone (GH) regulates growth and has important influences on intermediary metabolism (see Chap. 332). Prolactin (PRL) is necessary for lactation. Luteinizing hormone (LH) and follicle-stimulating hormone (FSH) control the gonads in men and women. Thyroid-stimulating hormone (TSH, thyrotropin) regulates thyroid

FIGURE 331-1   The relationship between the hypothalamus and pituitary. See text for details.

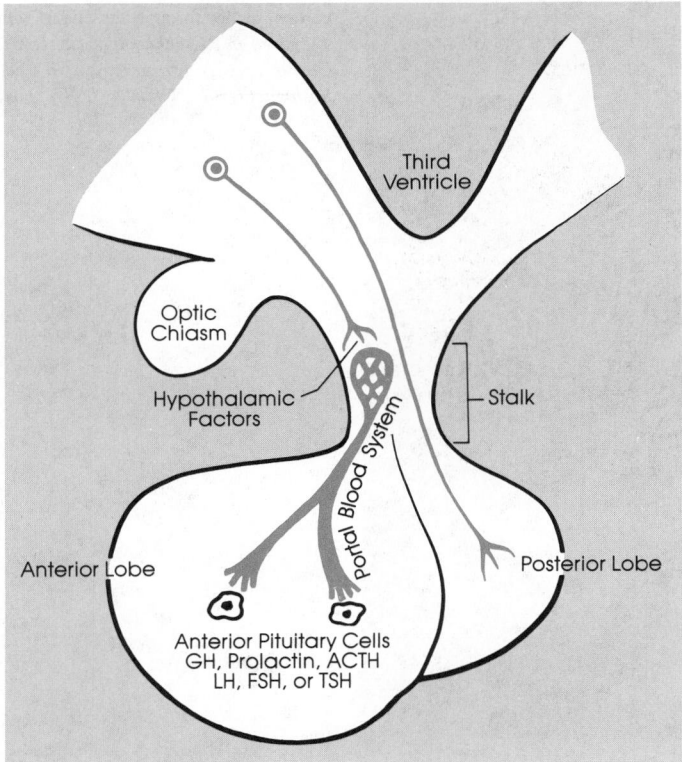

function. Adrenocorticotropin (ACTH) controls glucocorticoid function of the adrenal cortex. These hormones are all synthesized in the anterior pituitary. Vasopressin (AVP; antidiuretic hormone, ADH) and oxytocin are produced in neurons of the hypothalamus and stored in the posterior lobe of the pituitary (see Chap. 333). Vasopressin (AVP) controls water conservation by the kidneys; oxytocin is necessary for milk let-down during lactation and may aid in parturition.

A feedback relationship exists between the anterior pituitary and its three target endocrine glands—the gonads, the adrenal cortex, and the thyroid. When the gonads fail or are removed, the concentrations of LH and FSH rise, a condition known as *primary hypogonadism*. When the adrenal cortex is removed or destroyed, *primary adrenal insufficiency* (or Addison's disease) results, and the serum ACTH concentration increases. Thyroid failure results in the characteristic rise in TSH of *primary hypothyroidism*.

When the pituitary gland is removed or destroyed, loss of the trophic hormones results in secondary hypogonadism, adrenal insufficiency, or hypothyroidism. Growth hormone and prolactin function are also lost. AVP and oxytocin function are not affected by destruction of the pituitary provided their site of origin in the hypothalamus is intact.

The pituitary is, in turn, under the control of the hypothalamus, which produces a number of chemical mediators. These hormones are synthesized in the hypothalamus and enter the portal vascular system, which carries them through the pituitary stalk to the anterior lobe (see Fig. 331-1). Interruption of the pituitary stalk is followed by reduction in the release of GH, LH, FSH, TSH, and ACTH from the anterior pituitary. This implies that stimulatory influences from the hypothalamus are necessary for release of these hormones. In contrast, the level of prolactin rises after interruption of the stalk, implying a normal tonic inhibitory hypothalamic influence on prolactin secretion. The rise in prolactin secretion indicates that stalk section does not lead to pituitary destruction. If the stalk section is not at too high a level, AVP and oxytocin release continue principally from axons that terminate in the median eminence of the hypothalamus. With hypothalamic ablation, the levels of GH, LH, FSH, TSH, ACTH, AVP, and oxytocin fall, whereas prolactin levels increase (see Fig. 331-1).

Most hypothalamic factors that control secretion of the pituitary hormones are peptides (Table 331-1). Growth hormone–releasing hormone (GHRH) is the dominant influence on GH release, and

TABLE 331-1   Anterior pituitary and hypophysiotropic hormones

Pituitary hormone	Hypophysiotropic hormones	
	Name	Structure
Thyrotropin (TSH)	Thyrotropin-releasing hormone (TRH)	Tripeptide
Adrenocorticotropin (ACTH)	Corticotropin-releasing hormone (CRH) Vasopressin*	41 Amino acids
Luteinizing hormone (LH)	Luteinizing hormone–releasing hormone (LHRH)	Decapeptide
Follicle-stimulating hormone (FSH)	LHRH	Decapeptide
Growth hormone (GH)	Growth hormone–releasing hormone (GHRH)	44 Amino acids
	Growth hormone release–inhibiting hormone† (somatostatin, GIH)	14 Amino acids
Prolactin	Prolactin release–inhibiting factor (PIF)	Dopamine
	Prolactin-releasing factor (PRF)‡	Peptide

* Other peptides are also important in ACTH release.
† Somatostatin also inhibits TRH-stimulated TSH release.
‡ TRH stimulates prolactin release.

somatostatin acts as an inhibitory hormone for GH release. Although LH and FSH levels vary independently in physiologic states, one releasing hormone [luteinizing hormone–releasing hormone (LHRH), also called gonadotropin-releasing hormone (GnRH)] plays a major role in controlling their release. Thyrotropin-releasing hormone (TRH) controls TSH release and also may influence prolactin release. Corticotropin-releasing hormone (CRH) and other factors control ACTH release. In addition, dopamine acts as a prolactin inhibitory factor (PIF).

Pituitary tumors may lead to hormonal over- or underproduction or may cause mechanical problems by impinging on neighboring structures. The most common syndromes produced by pituitary tumors are due to prolactin and GH excess. Prolactin excess leads to galactorrhea and/or hypogonadism; GH excess leads to gigantism and acromegaly. ACTH-secreting tumors produce Cushing's disease; after bilateral adrenalectomy for Cushing's disease, further enlargement of ACTH-secreting tumors and hyperpigmentation (Nelson's syndrome) may develop. TSH-secreting tumors are rare causes of hyperthyroidism. Gonadotropin-secreting tumors are paradoxically most often associated with hypogonadism. Large pituitary tumors may cause partial or complete hypopituitarism by compression of the adjacent normal gland or pituitary stalk and are associated with visual field disturbances due to compression of the optic chiasm with other neurologic disturbances caused by invasion of cavernous sinuses or cranial fossae.

Hypothalamic disease may cause hypopituitarism, with the exception that secretion of prolactin may be increased. Diabetes insipidus due to AVP deficiency is virtually diagnostic of hypothalamic disease or of high interruption of the pituitary stalk. Disturbances of thirst, temperature regulation, appetite, and blood pressure may occur with hypothalamic disorders as well. Large hypothalamic masses may lead to visual field disturbances, obstruction of the third ventricle, and invasion of surrounding brain tissue.

ANATOMY AND EMBRYOLOGY

The pituitary gland (hypophysis) sits within the sella turcica ("Turkish saddle") of the sphenoid bone at the base of the skull and is composed principally of the anterior (adenohypophysis) and posterior lobes (neurohypophysis). The intermediate lobe is rudimentary in humans. The normal adult pituitary gland weighs between 0.4 and 0.8 g.

The pituitary is separated from the brain by the diaphragma sella, an extension of the dura mater, and from the sphenoid sinus anteriorly and inferiorly by a thin layer of bone. The lateral walls of the sella abut on the cavernous sinuses, which contain the internal carotid arteries and cranial nerves III, IV, V, and VI. The optic chiasm is slightly anterior to the pituitary stalk, just above the diaphragma sella. Thus tumors of the pituitary may lead to visual field defects, to cranial nerve palsies, or to invasion of the sphenoid sinus (Fig. 331-2).

The hypothalamus extends anteriorly to the margin of the optic chiasm and posteriorly to include the mammillary bodies. Superiorly, the hypothalamic sulcus of the third ventricle separates the thalamus from the hypothalamus. The rounded inferior base of the hypothalamus forms the tuber cinereum. The central portion of the base (termed the *infundibulum* or *median eminence*) is formed by the floor of the third ventricle and continues inferiorly to form the pituitary stalk. The releasing factors are synthesized in neurons situated along the margins of the third ventricle. They project fibers that terminate in the median eminence adjacent to the portal capillaries.

The cell bodies of the supraoptic and paraventricular nuclei of the hypothalamus produce vasopressin and oxytocin, which travel down nerve axons in the supraopticohypophyseal and paraventriculohypophyseal nerve tracts to reach the posterior lobe.

The communication between the hypothalamus and the anterior pituitary is chemical rather than physical. Releasing factors produced by hypothalamic neurons reach the anterior pituitary via the portal system to stimulate or inhibit hormone production. Some of the

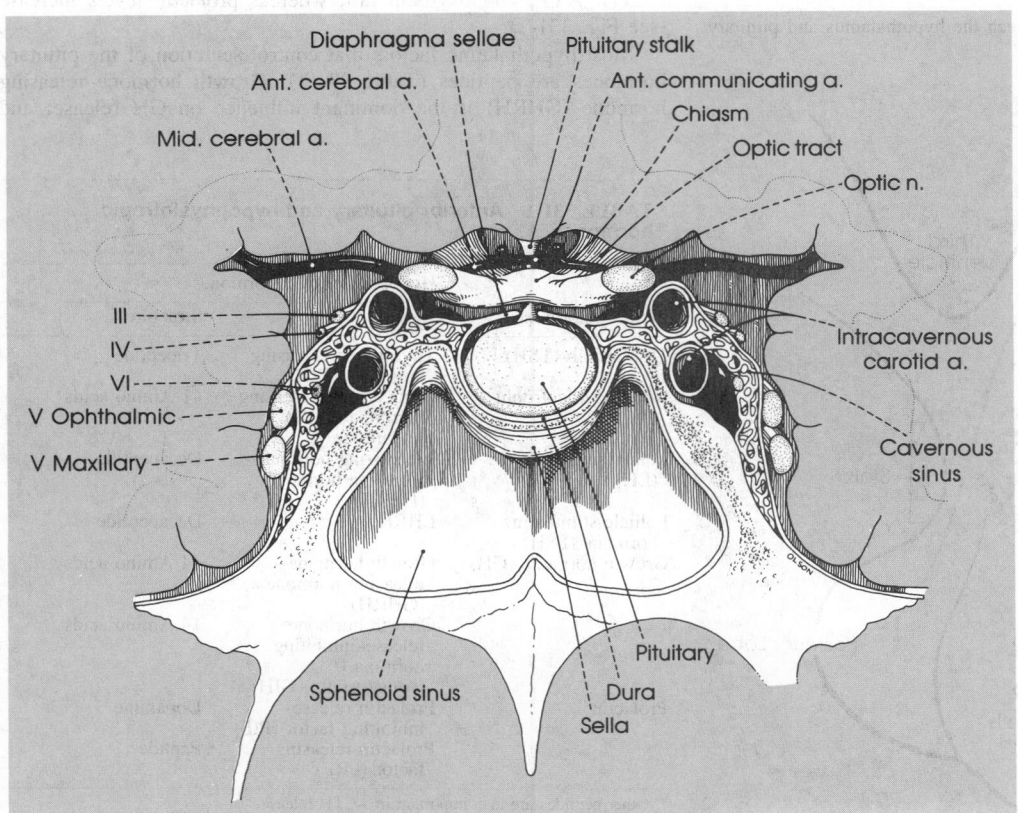

FIGURE 331-2   The relationship between the pituitary, cranial nerves, and the cavernous sinus as viewed in a coronal section through the sella. *(From JA Taren in RC Schneider et al (eds), Correlative Neurosurgery, 3d ed, Springfield, Ill., Charles C Thomas, 1982.)*

vasopressin-containing neurons also terminate in the median eminence, and vasopressin can stimulate release of ACTH and GH.

The anterior pituitary has the highest blood flow of any tissue in the body [0.8 (mL/g)/min]. The blood supply reaches the anterior pituitary by a circuitous route through the hypothalamus. Two derivatives of the internal carotid arteries, the superior hypophyseal arteries (SHA), branch in the subarachnoid space around the pituitary stalk and terminate in the capillary network of the median eminence. These capillaries have a fenestrated endothelium which allows easy access to the hypothalamic releasing hormones. Transport of substances from the capillaries to the median eminence is also facilitated because the median eminence lies outside the blood-brain barrier. The capillaries then coalesce to form 6 to 10 straight veins known as the *hypothalamic-pituitary portal circulation*. These veins constitute the main blood supply to the anterior lobe and supply it with nutrients as well as information from the hypothalamus. A direct arterial blood supply to the anterior lobe is also present, but the magnitude and importance of that circulation are uncertain. The posterior pituitary is supplied entirely by blood from the inferior hypophyseal arteries.

The anterior lobe is formed from the lateral proliferation of Rathke's pouch, an outpouching from the floor of the embryonic oral cavity. Rathke's pouch is met by a diverticulum from the floor of the third ventricle, which forms the posterior lobe.

Rathke's pouch is closed off by proliferation of the anterior and posterior lobe and forms a thin residual cleft in the gland (Rathke's cleft). This cleft may persist as a cyst lined with cuboidal or columnar epithelium. Since the pituitary rotates as it grows, these cysts usually lie in a position superior to the pituitary gland. The further growth and proliferation of these cysts can give rise to craniopharyngiomas, tumors that generally occupy a suprasellar position. Development of the sphenoid bone separates the pituitary from the oral cavity. Remnants of the pituitary, known as *pharyngeal pituitaries*, occasionally persist within or below the sphenoid bone. These remnants may produce pituitary hormones and occasionally develop into pituitary tumors.

Five distinct cell types in the anterior pituitary secrete six different hormones: lactotrophs (prolactin), somatotrophs (GH), gonadotrophs (LH and FSH), thyrotrophs (TSH), and corticotrophs (ACTH). The physiologic role of the other hormones and chemicals produced in the pituitary is uncertain.

PROLACTIN

PHYSIOLOGY   The lactotrophs constitute 15 to 20 percent of the normal pituitary and increase to 70 percent during pregnancy. The prolactin gene on chromosome 6 codes for a precursor molecule that is larger than the circulating hormone. The predominant form of the processed hormone contains 198 amino acids (23,000 mol wt) in a single polypeptide chain containing three intrachain disulfide bonds. Higher-molecular-weight forms of prolactin, up to 100,000 mol wt ("big" and "big-big" prolactin), may be present in small amounts in the circulation of normal persons and in larger amounts in patients with pituitary adenomas; these molecules react in prolactin radioimmunoassays but do not have normal biologic potency.

Prolactin is essential for lactation. Receptors for the hormone are present in human breast and gonads, whereas in other animals they are found in additional tissues. Prolactin promotes breast cancer in rodents; a similar connection has not been established in human breast cancer (see Chap. 319).

During pregnancy, increasing estrogen production stimulates the growth and replication of the pituitary lactotrophs and causes increased prolactin secretion. The pituitary doubles in size during pregnancy and returns to normal after delivery. Prolactin during pregnancy prepares the breast for postpartum lactation. High estrogen levels inhibit prolactin action at the breast so that lactation does not commence until estrogen levels decline post partum. Prolactin levels rise in the fetus beginning at about 25 weeks, probably owing to maternal estrogen transfer and stimulation of the fetal pituitary. The level falls rapidly after delivery, reaching a nadir by 2 to 4 weeks post partum. High concentrations of prolactin are present in amniotic fluid, probably of both uterine and placental origin. The functional significance of this prolactin is unknown.

Under normal circumstances, prolactin secretion by the anterior pituitary is restrained by the hypothalamus. With hypothalamic destruction or pituitary stalk section, prolactin secretion increases, and serum concentrations rise. The release of prolactin from pituitary cells after stalk section in animals requires the autocrine release of vasoactive intestinal peptide (VIP) by pituitary cells. The hypothalamic inhibitory factor for prolactin appears to be dopamine, although peptide inhibitory factors have been described. The arcuate and paraventricular nuclei of the hypothalamus produce dopamine; dopamine travels down axons to nerve terminals in the median eminence, where it is released (tuberoinfundibular dopamine system) into the portal circulation and reaches the anterior pituitary to inhibit prolactin release via interactions with pituitary D_2 receptors (adenylate cyclase–linked dopamine receptors). The intravenous administration of dopamine (2 μg/min per kilogram of body weight) or the oral administration of dopamine precursors (e.g., levodopa) or dopamine agonists (e.g., bromocriptine) inhibits prolactin release. Increased blood prolactin appears to increase hypothalamic dopamine production, which, in turn, partially inhibits prolactin release via a "short" feedback loop.

The prolactin rise during suckling appears to require a prolactin-releasing factor, which has not yet been conclusively identified. VIP may be responsible, since it is a potent stimulator of prolactin release. Suckling-induced prolactin rise is blocked by serotonin antagonists, such as methysergide, which suggests an influence of serotonin on prolactin release. TRH is also a potent stimulator of prolactin release; indeed, the lowest dose of TRH capable of stimulating TSH stimulates prolactin release as well. However, TSH and prolactin release are under independent control in most physiologic states; lactation does not lead to TSH elevation, and primary hypothyroidism is rarely associated with prolactin excess.

Prolactin concentrations rise during sleep, a phenomenon that requires the input of higher centers into the hypothalamus. Stress-related prolactin release can be blocked by opiate antagonists such as naloxone and is probably mediated by endogenous opioids. Morphine can stimulate prolactin release, which may contribute to the amenorrhea of narcotic addiction, but basal prolactin secretion is not influenced by opiate antagonists.

HYPERPROLACTINEMIA   Clinical features   Prolactin excess (hyperprolactinemia) has many causes, is associated with hypogonadism and/or galactorrhea, and may indicate the presence of a pituitary adenoma or hypothalamic disease. Of women with amenorrhea, 10 to 40 percent have hyperprolactinemia, and about 30 percent of women with amenorrhea and galactorrhea have prolactin-secreting pituitary tumors.

The hypogonadism associated with hyperprolactinemia appears to be due to inhibition of hypothalamic release of LHRH, resulting in a decrease in LH and FSH secretion. This functional hypogonadism can be regarded, in part, as a desirable physiologic mechanism whereby breast feeding causes decreased fertility and delayed resumption of menses. In general, the higher the plasma prolactin, the greater is the likelihood of amenorrhea. Milder degrees of hyperprolactinemia in women cause irregular menses or infertility due to a shortened luteal phase. Prolactin excess in men can cause impotence and infertility. In some series, 8 percent of men with impotence and 5 percent of men with infertility have hyperprolactinemia. With prolactin elevation, FSH and LH levels in men decline, and serum testosterone is often low.

Galactorrhea, defined as milk production in a patient who is not post partum, is present in 30 to 90 percent of hyperprolactinemic women (see Chap. 341). The variation in incidence reflects, in part, variation in the intensity with which clinicians search for this finding.

TABLE 331-2 Causes of hyperprolactinemia

PHYSIOLOGIC STATES

A Pregnancy
B Nursing (early)
C "Stress"
D Sleep
E Nipple stimulation
F Food ingestion

DRUGS

A Dopamine receptor antagonists
  1 Phenothiazines
  2 Butyrophenones
  3 Thioxanthenes
  4 Metoclopramide
  5 Sulpiride
B Dopamine-depleting agents
  1 Methyldopa
  2 Reserpine
C Estrogens
D Opiates

DISEASE STATES

A Pituitary tumors
  1 Prolactinomas
  2 Adenomas secreting GH and prolactin
  3 Adenomas secreting ACTH and prolactin (Nelson's syndrome and Cushing's disease)
  4 Nonfunctioning chromophobe adenomas with pituitary stalk compression
B Hypothalamic and pituitary stalk disease
  1 Granulomatous diseases especially sarcoidosis
  2 Craniopharyngiomas and other tumors
  3 Cranial irradiation
  4 Stalk section
  5 Empty sella
  6 Vascular abnormalities including aneurysm
  7 Lymphocytic hypophysitis
  8 Metastatic carcinoma
C Primary hypothyroidism
D Chronic renal failure
E Cirrhosis
F Chest wall trauma (including surgery, *herpes zoster*)
G Seizures

Galactorrhea may occur without hyperprolactinemia, particularly in parous women. However, galactorrhea is often a clue to prolactin excess; when galactorrhea is coupled with amenorrhea, hyperprolactinemia is present in 75 percent of patients. Hyperprolactinemia in men rarely causes gynecomastia or galactorrhea (see Chap. 341).

Differential diagnosis Prolactin excess has several mechanisms: (1) autonomous production (pituitary adenomas), (2) decreased dopamine or dopamine inhibitory action (e.g., due to hypothalamic disease or drugs that block dopamine synthesis, dopamine release, or dopamine action), (3) stimuli that overcome the normal dopaminergic inhibition (e.g., estrogens, possibly hypothyroidism), and (4) decreased clearance of prolactin (renal failure). No single suppression test can separate physiologic from pharmacologic or pathologic causes of hyperprolactinemia (Table 331-2).

Prolactin concentrations are slightly higher (<20 μg/L) in women than in men (<15 μg/L). During pregnancy, prolactin concentrations begin to increase during the second trimester and peak at term; maximal values are 100 to 300 μg/L, usually less than 200 μg/L. A pregnancy test is mandatory in all patients with hyperprolactinemic amenorrhea, as it is with amenorrhea alone. The mean prolactin level declines post partum but rises with each suckling episode. Over several months basal and suckling-stimulated prolactin concentrations diminish; by 4 to 6 months post partum, basal prolactin levels are normal, and the suckling-induced rise is absent despite continued nursing. Prolactin levels rise within 1 h of feeding and after seizures.

A careful drug history should be obtained in hyperprolactinemic patients. Dopamine-blocking drugs (e.g., phenothiazines, butyrophe-nones, metoclopramide) and dopamine-depleting drugs (e.g., methyldopa and reserpine) are important causes of hyperprolactinemia. Chronic cocaine use causes modest hyperprolactinemia. Prolactin concentrations are usually less than 100 μg/L with these agents, provided renal failure is not present. However, concentrations as high as 275 μg/L have been reported. Although high-dose estrogens cause hyperprolactinemia, oral contraceptives containing low doses of estrogen do not.

End-stage renal failure is associated with elevated serum prolactin in 70 to 90 percent of women and 25 to 60 percent of men. This contributes to hypogonadism in some patients with renal failure. Both decreased prolactin clearance and increased prolactin secretion may contribute to this elevation. The increased prolactin in cirrhosis of the liver has not been adequately explained.

Severe primary hypothyroidism may cause a mildly elevated serum prolactin, either due to elevated TRH or decreased dopaminergic tone. Since primary hypothyroidism also may cause enlargement of the sella turcica, mimicking a pituitary adenoma, thyroid function tests are essential in all patients with elevated serum prolactin. Rarely, primary adrenal insufficiency causes reversible serum prolactin elevation.

In 10,000 "normal" adults working at a single plant in Japan, the prevalence of hyperprolactinemia greater than 75 μg/L was 0.4 percent. Many different etiologies were found.

If a fasting hyperprolactinemic subject is not pregnant, post partum, cirrhotic, postictal, on medications, hypothyroid, or in renal failure, disease of the pituitary or hypothalamus is likely. Ectopic production of prolactin by nonpituitary tumors occurs rarely if at all. Diseases of the hypothalamus or pituitary stalk cause moderate prolactin elevation (usually less than 150 μg/L). Hyperprolactinemia occurs in 20 to 50 percent of patients with hypothalamic tumors.

Prolactin-secreting pituitary adenomas (prolactinomas) are arbitrarily divided into microadenomas (<10 mm) and macroadenomas (≥10 mm). Large, nonfunctioning pituitary adenomas also may cause modest prolactin elevation, thought to be due to stalk compression and impairment of dopamine delivery to the gland. Acromegalics (25 to 45 percent), some patients with Nelson's syndrome, and rare Cushing's patients have elevated serum prolactin levels.

Laboratory evaluation Serum prolactin levels should be measured in all people with unexplained hypogonadism or galactorrhea. If basal prolactin concentration is elevated, further evaluation is warranted after establishing that minimal prolactin elevations (e.g., less than 30 μg/L) are not due to stress or related to food intake. Blood sampling from an indwelling catheter after a 90-min rest period will exclude "needle stick" hyperprolactinemia. Levels should be assessed after fasting or more than 1 h after eating. Although there is no simple test to distinguish the various causes of hyperprolactinemia, a serum prolactin level of over 300 μg/L is diagnostic of a pituitary adenoma; a serum prolactin of over 150 μg/L in a nonpregnant patient is usually caused by a pituitary adenoma. Administration of dopamine agonists, such as bromocriptine, lowers prolactin regardless of the etiology and, therefore, is not useful as a differential test (Fig. 331-3). The majority of patients with prolactinomas have only a minimal or no rise in prolactin in response to TRH, as compared with the normal rise of 200 percent or more and the intermediate response (usually a doubling of serum prolactin) in patients with hypothalamic disease and those on dopamine-blocking agents. Unfortunately, the response to TRH is too variable to be of diagnostic value in individual patients.

In general, patients with unexplained hyperprolactinemia require magnetic resonance imaging (MRI) or contrast-enhanced computed tomography (CT) scanning of the hypothalamus and pituitary. Pituitary macroadenomas are easily visualized on these scans, but microadenomas (<10 mm) may be more difficult to delineate. Patients with amenorrhea and minimal prolactin elevations also may have hypothalamic lesions (e.g., craniopharyngiomas) or large "nonfunctioning" pituitary adenomas. When no radiologic abnormalities are found, the disorder is designated *idiopathic hyperprolactinemia*, although a

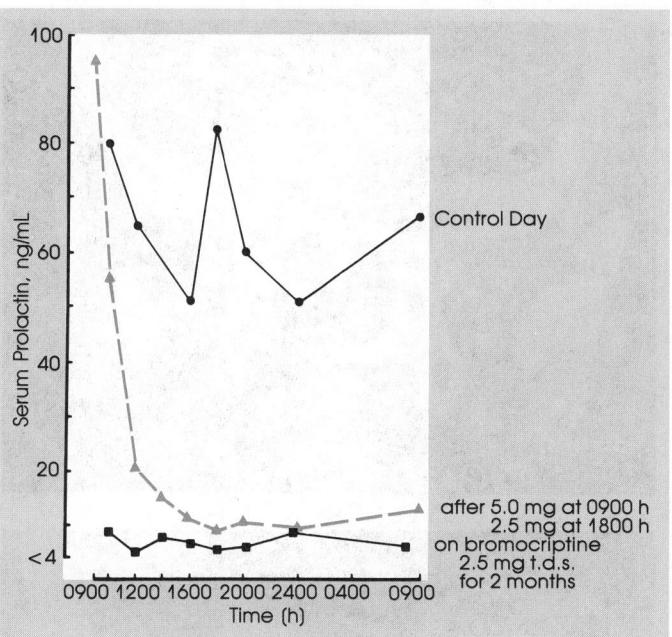

FIGURE 331-3 Changes in serum prolactin concentration in a woman with "idiopathic" hyperprolactinemia after an initial 5-mg dose of bromocriptine and when maintained on 7.5 mg daily. *(From GH Besser and MO Thorner, Postgrad Med J 52:66, 1976.)*

microadenoma may still be present. Sella tomography is not a useful screening test for small pituitary adenomas because of the high frequency of false-positive and false-negative results.

Microprolactinomas do not cause hypopituitarism (except for hypogonadism). If a small pituitary lesion is seen in a patient with hypopituitarism and hyperprolactinemia, sarcoidosis or other lesions involving the pituitary stalk should be suspected rather than a microprolactinoma. In patients with macroprolactinomas or hypothalamic lesions, evaluation of pituitary function and formal visual field examinations are essential.

Prolactinomas PATHOLOGY Prolactinomas are the most common functional pituitary adenomas. Small unsuspected microadenomas are found in 6 to 24 percent of unselected autopsies; 40 percent of these small tumors contain prolactin by immunologic staining techniques, but the fraction that actually secrete prolactin is unknown. About 70 percent of macroadenomas previously thought to be nonfunctioning are, in fact, prolactinomas. Prolactin-secreting pituitary carcinomas are rare.

Prolactinoma size correlates with hormonal output; in general, the larger the tumor, the higher are the prolactin levels. Large pituitary tumors with modest prolactin elevation (50 to 100 μg/L) are not true prolactinomas and differ in their biologic behavior. Microprolactinomas cause only hyperprolactinemia and hypogonadotropism, whereas macroprolactinomas may influence other pituitary hormones and cause headaches, visual field disturbances, and other structural problems.

CLINICAL PRESENTATION Microprolactinomas are more common than macroprolactinomas, and 90 percent of patients with microprolactinomas are women. In contrast, 60 percent of patients with macroprolactinomas are men. Irregular menses, amenorrhea, and galactorrhea are likely to result in early diagnosis, and this may partially explain the preponderance of microadenomas in women. Sexual dysfunction occurs in most men with prolactinomas, but this is the presenting complaint in 15 percent or less. Although delay in seeking medical help probably explains the larger tumors in men, more aggressive tumor behavior in men has not been excluded.

Estrogens promote the growth of lactotrophs, but an etiologic role has not been established for oral contraceptives in the pathogenesis of prolactinomas. Many women with prolactinomas first develop galactorrhea while on oral contraceptives or develop amenorrhea when the drug is discontinued. Some of these women may have been started on oral contraceptives for irregular menses that were the consequence of a prolactinoma. Although amenorrhea after discontinuing oral contraceptives is rare (about 2 percent), about a third of patients with postpill amenorrhea have prolactinomas. Development of galactorrhea in a woman on oral contraceptives mandates a prolactin determination. About 5 to 7 percent of prolactinoma patients have never menstruated (primary amenorrhea), making this an important treatable cause of primary amenorrhea. Prolactinomas may grow during pregnancy, and 15 percent of prolactinoma patients are first diagnosed in the postpartum period.

Women with prolactinomas who desire pregnancy need special consideration. Medical treatment of patients with microprolactinomas results in uneventful pregnancies 95 to 98 percent of the time; the remainder may develop headaches or visual field disturbances due to tumor enlargement that rarely requires therapy. Asymptomatic enlargement of microprolactinomas, as ascertained by radiologic studies, occurs in about 5 percent. With macroprolactinomas, the complications of tumor growth during pregnancy are more common. Symptomatic tumor enlargement occurs in about 15 percent of these patients, although prior therapy with bromocriptine may decrease this risk. The majority of patients who develop symptoms do so during the first trimester.

In prolactinoma patients, the effect of pregnancy on prolactin secretion is variable. A further rise in prolactin during pregnancy may not occur even in patients in whom tumor growth occurs. Prolactin concentrations should be measured periodically throughout pregnancy in women with prolactinomas. An increase in serum prolactin of more than 300 to 400 μg/L during pregnancy usually signals tumor growth; when this occurs, the postpartum prolactin level is usually greater than the prepartum level. Patients with stable or declining prolactin concentrations during pregnancy may have lower prolactin concentrations after pregnancy than before. In such patients, infarction or involution of the adenomas may have occurred during pregnancy. Rarely, macroprolactinomas in men grow during replacement testosterone therapy, presumably as a result of extraglandular conversion of testosterone to estrogen. The safety of oral contraceptives is uncertain, but such therapy is unlikely to cause significant tumor growth.

THERAPY The natural history of untreated hyperprolactinemia is incompletely understood. Although large pituitary adenomas must begin as small tumors, most microadenomas do not progress to macroadenomas. In general, 90 to 95 percent of untreated microprolactinomas remain stable or exhibit decreased serum prolactin concentrations over 7 years of follow-up. Serum prolactin returns to normal in a third of patients with idiopathic hyperprolactinemia (who may harbor microprolactinomas) followed for 5 years without therapy; the number increases to two-thirds if the basal prolactin is less than 40 μg/L. In 30 patients with varying degrees of hyperprolactinemia (30 to 260 μg/L) followed for a mean of 5.2 years, the prolactin level increased by more than 50 percent in a fifth, and another fifth had signs of enlargement on CT scans. The prolactin decreased by more than 50 percent in a third of the patients and returned to normal in a fifth. Abnormal x-rays returned to normal in a sixth of the patients.

Thus not all patients with microprolactinomas need therapy. Women with microprolactinomas require therapy when they desire pregnancy, have decreased libido or troublesome galactorrhea, desire regular menses, or are at risk for osteoporosis. Men with microadenomas should be treated for decreased potency or libido or when infertility is a problem. Most patients with macroprolactinomas require therapy.

Dopamine agonist drugs lower prolactin concentrations in virtually all hyperprolactinemic patients (see Fig. 331-3). Ovulatory menses and fertility are restored in more than 90 percent of premenopausal women, underscoring the direct relationship between hyperprolactinemia and amenorrhea. Bromocriptine, an ergot derivative with dopamine agonist actions, is the only effective prolactin-lowering agent licensed for this purpose in the United States. Bromocriptine should be given twice daily with food or a snack to prevent gastrointestinal irritation; some patients may be treated once a day. Therapy should begin with 1.25 mg at bedtime to minimize the side effects of nausea, vomiting, fatigue, nasal stuffiness, and postural hypotension. Gastrointestinal intolerance to oral bromocriptine may be circumvented when the drug is administered via the vagina; however, the drug is not currently licensed for vaginal administration. The dosage is gradually increased to an average of 2.5 mg twice daily. However, doses up to 15 mg/d may be required to return the prolactin concentration to normal with macroprolactinomas. Although the drug is expensive, it is effective in all forms of hyperprolactinemia and often abolishes nonhyperprolactinemic galactorrhea as well. Long-lasting parenteral and oral dopamine agonists and newer non-ergot-derived oral dopamine agonists are effective and in some cases better tolerated than bromocriptine; they are not yet licensed in the United States.

Bromocriptine is the therapy of choice for patients with microprolactinomas who have one of the indications for treatment discussed above. Prolactin concentrations return to normal in almost all who tolerate the medication, usually within days of achieving full therapeutic dosages (see Fig. 331-3). Menses usually resume within 2 months but may be delayed up to a year. Since pregnancy may occur without resumption of menses, a barrier contraceptive is recommended until menses become regular. In this way, bromocriptine can be stopped with the first missed period when pregnancy has occurred. Bromocriptine use during pregnancy is not, however, associated with an increased risk of congenital anomalies or fetal wastage. The effects of bromocriptine are usually not permanent, but a sixth of microprolactinoma patients maintain normal prolactin concentrations after stopping the drug.

In patients with macroprolactinomas, bromocriptine usually lowers the serum prolactin level and decreases tumor size (Fig. 331-4), but both effects may be incomplete. In men, testosterone concentrations usually begin to increase after 3 months of therapy but may remain subnormal. Normal sperm counts are achieved in some. Almost 90 percent of premenopausal women regain cyclic menses.

Tumor shrinkage is most rapid in the first 3 months of therapy. By 3 months, 40 percent of tumors decrease by more than 50 percent in size. Most tumors demonstrate some shrinkage; more important, abnormal visual fields improve with medical therapy in 90 percent of patients. If the visual field defect does not resolve within a short period of time (1 to 3 months), surgery should be performed. Of patients treated for 12 months without additional therapy 90 percent show tumor shrinkage of more than 50 percent. Prolactin levels fall to 20 percent of baseline in more than 90 percent and return to normal in about a third. After more than 2 years of therapy, the dosage of bromocriptine can often be reduced but rarely discontinued. In patients with persistent symptomatic hyperprolactinemia despite partial response to bromocriptine, radiation therapy or surgical debulking may be appropriate.

Although prolactin concentrations rapidly return to pretreatment levels when long-term bromocriptine is stopped, tumor regrowth may be delayed for months or years. When considering pregnancy in a patient with a macroprolactinoma, this slow regrowth should be kept in mind. Patients who conceive after prolonged bromocriptine therapy may be at less risk of tumor growth during pregnancy. In the United States, bromocriptine is generally stopped when pregnancy is confirmed; if tumor-related symptoms develop during pregnancy, bromocriptine should be reinstituted. However, many physicians outside the United States use bromocriptine throughout pregnancy in patients with macroprolactinomas. There is no evidence that bromocriptine has an adverse effect on the fetus.

Only 10 percent of large nonfunctioning pituitary adenomas with hyperprolactinemia due to stalk compression shrink with bromocriptine therapy, although prolactin concentrations usually return to normal. Alternative therapies are required. There are isolated reports

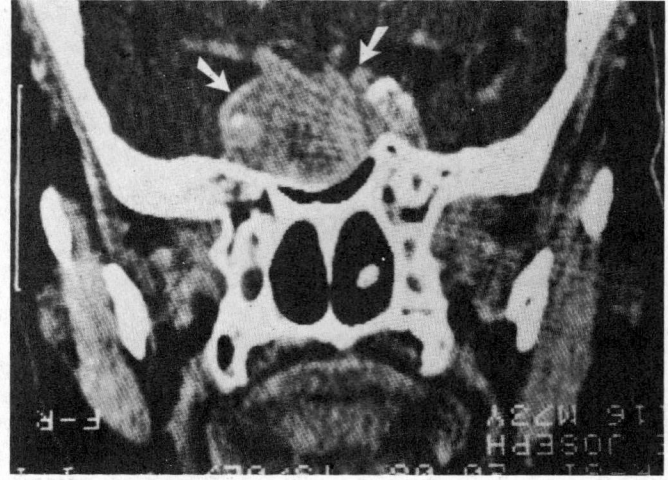

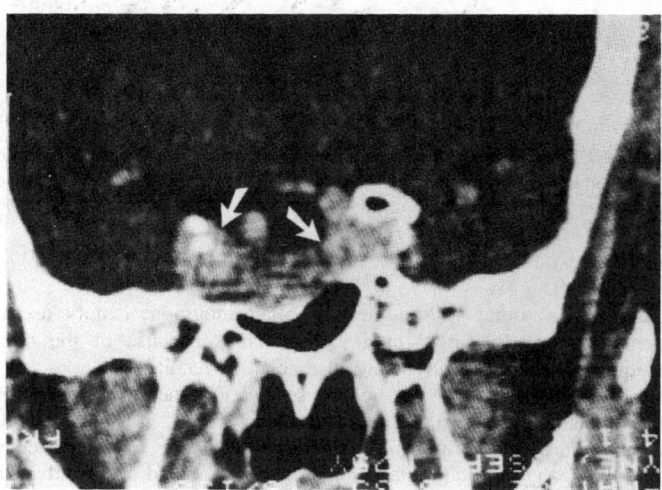

FIGURE 331-4 Frontal CT scan of a man with a large prolactin-secreting macroadenoma. (*Top*) Pretreatment scan. (*Bottom*) Scan after 1 year of treatment with bromocriptine. The upper border of the tumor is shown by arrows. (*From Molitch et al.*)

of patients with large prolactinomas refractory to bromocriptine whose tumors shrink when tamoxifen, an estrogen antagonist, is added.

Following transsphenoidal resection of microprolactinomas, serum prolactin concentration returns to normal in up to 80 to 90 percent of patients, usually within 24 h. This procedure has low morbidity and mortality. Unfortunately, recurrence rates average 17 percent after "successful" surgery and may be as high as 40 percent after 6 years of follow-up. Surgery is appropriate for women with microprolactinomas who desire pregnancy and who cannot tolerate or do not wish to take dopamine agonist drugs. Surgery may be more difficult in patients with microprolactinoma treated for more than 3 months with bromocriptine; some surgeons report increased fibrosis with a higher complication rate and lower success rate in this situation.

Surgery, whether by transsphenoidal or transcranial approach, is rarely curative for macroprolactinomas. Surgery may be necessary for patients with persistent visual field defects despite bromocriptine and for those intolerant of dopamine agonists. Tumors with large cystic or hemorrhagic components may require surgical decompression for relief of visual symptoms or headaches. Prolactin concentrations return to normal in about 30 percent of patients treated surgically, but recurrence rates may be as high as 80 percent in this subgroup. Long-term bromocriptine therapy is usually required after surgical therapy.

Radiation therapy plays a limited role in the treatment of prolactinomas. Conventional radiation therapy [4500 cGy (4500 rad) over 25 days] causes a slow decline in serum prolactin concentration. Although prolactin concentrations return to normal in about 30 percent of microprolactinomas 2 to 10 years after radiation therapy, we rarely treat microprolactinomas with radiation. The risks of hypopituitarism make this a poor fourth choice after medical, surgical, or no therapy. Radiation therapy may be necessary in macroprolactinomas with rapid or persistent tumor growth despite dopamine agonist therapy and surgery or after surgery alone in patients intolerant of dopamine agonists. The respective roles of conventional radiation, focused gamma radiation ("gamma knife"), and heavy-particle radiation (proton beam) are not established.

PROLACTIN DEFICIENCY   Prolactin deficiency is manifested as an inability to lactate. Failure of lactation is often the earliest clue to panhypopituitarism resulting from pituitary infarction during the peripartum period. The lateral wings of the pituitary have a precarious blood supply; most lactotrophs reside in this area. During pregnancy, the hypertrophied and hyperplastic lactotrophs are at risk for necrosis. If systemic hypotension develops, as with postpartum hemorrhage, the hypertrophic and hyperplastic lactotrophs may infarct (Sheehan's syndrome). Patients with diabetes mellitus are susceptible to peripartum pituitary infarction even in the absence of significant hemorrhage. Autoimmune pituitary destruction (lymphocytic hypophysitis) also may occur during late pregnancy but often is associated with elevated prolactin levels.

Many prolactin radioimmunoassays cannot distinguish normal from low concentrations; hence prolactin stimulation tests are needed to diagnose prolactin insufficiency. After administration of TRH or chlorpromazine, a rise in serum prolactin of less than 200 percent suggests prolactin deficiency. If prolactin deficiency is present, evaluation of other pituitary hormones is necessary as well to define other manifestations of hypopituitarism.

GROWTH HORMONE

PHYSIOLOGY   Growth hormone (GH, somatotropin) is secreted by somatotrophs, which make up about 50 percent of the anterior pituitary cells. The normal pituitary contains 3 to 5 mg GH and secretes 500 to 875 μg GH per day. GH shares an 85 percent structural identity with human placental lactogen (hPL, chorionic somatomammotropin). GH and hPL genes are on chromosome 17 and appear to have originated by gene duplication. Human growth hormone is a single-polypeptide chain of 191 amino acids (22,000 mol wt) and contains two intrachain disulfide bonds; it is cleaved from a larger precursor molecule (28,000 mol wt). Alternative splicing of this precursor yields a 20-kDa GH molecule of reduced biologic and immunologic activity. GH is stored in cytoplasmic granules in a high-molecular-weight polymeric form. A variant form of GH (GH-V) is found in the placenta, is the dominant form of GH circulating in the third trimester of pregnancy, and is a potent somatogen.

Multiple forms of GH exist in the circulation. The dominant form is monomeric GH (22 kDa), but larger, oligomeric forms (e.g., "big" GH, 44,000 mol wt) and smaller forms (e.g., 20 kDa) are present as well. All these variants contribute to the total circulating GH concentration. Several binding proteins for GH contribute to the heterogeneity of circulating GH. The high-affinity GH-binding protein, which is specific for the 22-kDa GH, appears to be a cleavage product of the GH receptor from the liver and possibly other tissues. A lower-affinity binding protein binds both the 22-kDa active and 20-kDa inactive GH.

Pulsatile release of GH is characteristic. Circulating levels are immeasurably low for much of the day, punctuated by four to eight bursts after meals or exercise, during slow-wave sleep, or without obvious cause. The half-life of the hormone in plasma is 20 to 30 min. GH secretion is low in infancy, slightly higher during early childhood, and dramatically increased during puberty. GH secretion is lower in adults than during puberty. After the third decade, a progressive (but individually variable) decline in GH secretion occurs.

GH is necessary for normal linear growth. GH deficiency causes short stature; GH excess (prior to epiphyseal closure) leads to gigantism. GH does not appear to be the principal direct stimulator of growth but acts indirectly by stimulating the formation of other hormones. These factors, known as *somatomedins* (SM, somatotropin-mediating hormones) or *insulin-like growth factors* (IGF), are GH-dependent and are responsible for growth stimulation (also see Chap. 332). Somatomedin C (insulin-like growth factor I, IGF-I/SM-C), the most important somatomedin for postnatal growth, is produced in the liver, chondrocytes, kidney, muscle, pituitary, and gastrointestinal tract. The liver is the main source of circulating IGF-I/SM-C. IGF-I/SM-C is a basic protein (7600 mol wt) that circulates bound to carrier proteins (IGF-binding proteins). Although the role of these carriers is under investigation, their net effect is to increase the half-life of circulating IGF-I/SM-C to 3 to 18 h as compared with the half-life of 20 to 30 min for unbound hormone. As a consequence, the concentration of IGF-I remains relatively constant throughout the day, in contrast to the fluctuating levels of GH itself. How the liver and other tissues integrate the GH pulses into IGF-I/SM-C and IGF-binding protein production is not known. Local tissue generation of IGF-I/SM-C, particularly in bone, may play an important role in growth mediation through its paracrine effects.

IGF-I is structurally similar to proinsulin and exerts some insulin-like actions. Furthermore, GH is a trophic factor for insulin release, facilitating its release in response to various secretagogues, and GH-deficient individuals have impaired insulin release to glucose challenge. Technically, one might consider insulin a somatomedin.

During the prenatal and neonatal period, growth is independent of GH, as shown by the normal birth length of GH-deficient children born to GH-deficient mothers. Nevertheless, IGF-I/SM-C levels are elevated during pregnancy; the concentration correlates with that of hPL, which may regulate IGF-I/SM-C production. IGF-I/SM-C levels at birth are lower than those of adults and rise gradually during childhood to reach the adult range by age 8 to 10 years. IGF-I/SM-C levels are dependent on nutritional status, declining in states of malnourishment. Elevated serum IGF-I/SM-C concentrations are present during the pubertal growth spurt, presumably accounting for the pubertal growth acceleration.

Although IGF-I/SM-C concentrations correlate with linear growth, the correlation is inexact, and therefore, GH may have some direct influence on growth or cause somatomedin generation in target cells.

GH exerts additional metabolic effects, including stimulation of the incorporation of amino acids into protein. Although most of this action is somatomedin-mediated, GH can directly stimulate amino acid uptake in certain systems. Some amino acids, such as arginine, are potent stimuli for GH release.

GH may have a direct effect as an insulin antagonist that inhibits glucose uptake by tissues. Patients with GH deficiency are prone to insulin-induced hypoglycemia; patients with GH excess develop insulin resistance. GH is one of the counterregulatory hormones that help restore a low blood sugar to normal (see Chap. 338). Hypoglycemia is a potent GH stimulus, and an acute rise in blood sugar inhibits GH release. Paradoxically, patients with type I diabetes mellitus have increased GH concentrations. GH increases free fatty acid release from adipocytes. The absence of this effect may be responsible for the pudgy appearance of children with GH deficiency and the higher percent body fat in adults with GH deficiency. Increased serum free fatty acid concentrations tend to blunt GH release. GH opposes the action of insulin on sugar uptake and fatty acid release and complements the anabolic action of insulin on amino acid uptake.

GH is controlled by a dual hypothalamic regulation (Table 331-3). Secretion is stimulated by growth hormone–releasing hormone (GHRH, somatocrinin) and inhibited by growth hormone release–

TABLE 331-3 Growth hormone regulation

Class of agent	Stimulation	Inhibition
Hypothalamic factors	GHRH	Somatostatin
Amines	Alpha-adrenergic stimuli (norepinephrine, clonidine)	Beta-adrenergic stimuli
	Beta-adrenergic blockers (propranolol)	Alpha-adrenergic blockers (phentolamine, dibenzyline)
	Dopaminergic stimuli (levodopa, bromocriptine, apomorphine)	Dopamine blockers (chlorpromazine)
	Serotonergic stimuli (L-tryptophan)	Serotonin blockers (methysergide, cyproheptadine)
Hormones	Decreased IGF-I/SM-C	Increased IGF-I/SM-C (obesity)
	Estrogen	Progestogens
	Vasopressin	Glucocorticoids*
	Glucagon	
Fuels	Hypoglycemia[†]	Increased blood sugar
	Decreased free fatty acids	Increased free fatty acids
	Amino acids (arginine)[†]	
Others	Exercise[†]	
	Stress[†]	
	Sleep	
	Acetylcholine	

* Acutely, glucocorticoids stimulate GH release.
[†] Probably mediated through alpha-adrenergic stimulation.

inhibitory hormone (somatostatin, somatotropin release–inhibitory factor, SRIF). GHRH appears to play the more important role, since stalk section leads to failure of GH release. Although GHRH- and somatostatin-containing neurons are separate, they have reciprocal interconnections.

Growth hormone–releasing hormone GHRH has 44 amino acids, 29 of which are necessary for full potency. GHRH belongs to a family of molecules that includes secretin, glucagon, vasoactive intestinal peptide (VIP), and gastric inhibitory peptide (GIP). The arcuate nucleus of the hypothalamus is the major site of GHRH production, although a few such neurons are in the ventromedial nucleus as well. Axons containing the peptide project to the median eminence and terminate on the portal vessels. GHRH is also present in the mucosa of the small intestine.

GHRH stimulates GH release and synthesis in vitro and in vivo, an effect that is calcium-dependent and appears to be mediated by cyclic adenosine monophosphate (cyclic AMP). GHRH enhances GH gene transcription and stimulates c-*fos*, a growth signal–transducing oncogene. Intravenous injection of GHRH (0.1 to 3.3 μg/kg body weight) produces a peak GH response at 30 to 60 min with a return to baseline by 2 to 3 h postinjection (Fig. 331-5).

Somatostatin Somatostatin, a cyclic tetradecapeptide, is the most widely distributed of the hypothalamic releasing hormones. The primary hypothalamic sources are the periventricular and medial preoptic areas of the anterior hypothalamus. Somatostatin is found in neurosecretory granules of axons that terminate in the median eminence. In addition to its function as a hormone, somatostatin is synthesized and distributed throughout the brain and serves as a neurotransmitter in many areas, including the spinal cord, brainstem, and cerebral cortex. Somatostatin is also present in the gastrointestinal tract and other organs. Somatostatin-secreting cells (D cells) of the pancreatic islets participate in the regulation of insulin and glucagon secretion, an example of paracrine regulation by this hormone (see Chap. 337).

Somatostatin is produced by processing of a larger precursor molecule and exists in both 28– and 14–amino acid forms. The 28–amino acid somatostatin has a longer half-life and is a more potent inhibitor of GH, TSH, and insulin secretion. Somatostatin 14 has a greater affinity for hypothalamic and cortical receptors and is more potent in inhibition of glucagon release, splanchnic blood flow, intestinal motility, and gastric exocrine secretion. Somatostatin analogues are effective in the therapy of acromegaly, secretory pancreatic tumors, carcinoid syndrome, and other conditions.

Somatostatin inhibits GH secretion and decreases the GH response to secretagogues without altering GH mRNA levels. Somatostatin also lowers serum TSH in normal and hypothyroid individuals and blunts TSH release in response to TRH. Somatostatin probably mediates the secondary hypothyroidism that may develop in GH-deficient children treated with GH. Somatostatin has no significant effect on the release of prolactin, gonadotropins, or ACTH in normal subjects but may lower ACTH concentrations in patients with Nelson's syndrome. Somatostatinomas are rare pancreatic islet cell or duodenal tumors that secrete somatostatin (see Chap. 276).

Growth hormone release is under complex physiologic control (see Table 331-3). The various mediators appear to act through GHRH and somatostatin. IGF-I/SM-C has an important feedback effect on GH secretion. An increased IGF-I/SM-C concentration inhibits GH release both through increased somatostatin production and by a direct

FIGURE 331-5 Response to GHRH-44 (1 μg/kg) in eight men and eight women. The shaded area shows the full range of responses at each time point and the error bars indicate the mean ± 1 SD. (*From MC Gelato et al, J Clin Endocrinol Metab 59:200, 1984.*)

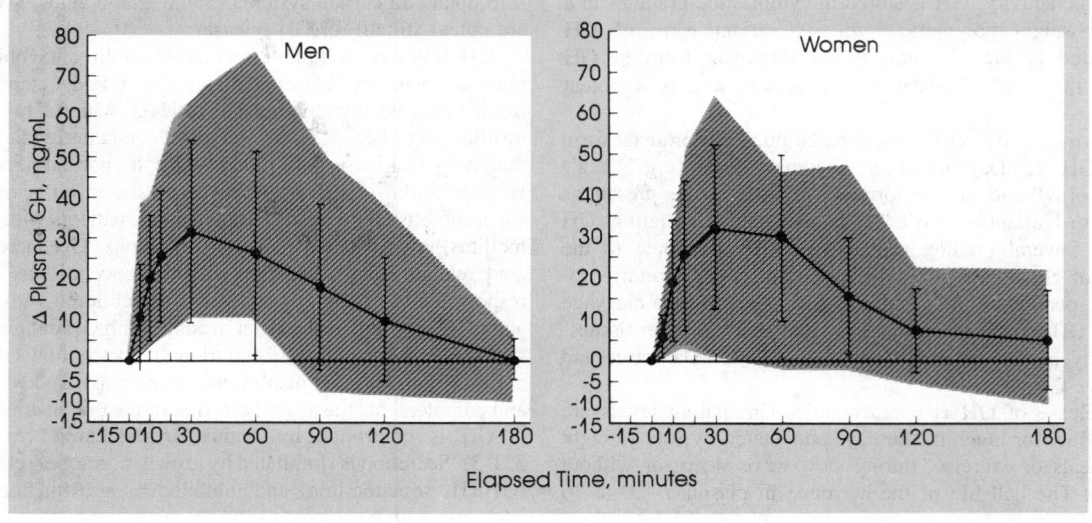

action on the pituitary. A decrease in IGF-I/SM-C, as induced by starvation, leads to a compensatory increase in GH release.

A number of neurotransmitters influence GH release:

1 Hypothalamic dopamine, the important prolactin inhibitory factor, stimulates GH through an effect on GHRH. Dopamine has a direct but weak inhibitory effect on GH release; this effect is overwhelmed by its hypothalamic stimulation of GHRH secretion. Oral administration of dopamine precursors or agonists that cross the blood-brain barrier, such as levodopa, apomorphine, or bromocriptine, causes an increase in serum GH concentration. The effects of these stimuli can be utilized to test the adequacy of GH secretion (GH reserve).

2 Alpha-adrenergic agonists, such as clonidine, stimulate GHRH and GH release, whereas phentolamine, an alpha blocker, prevents the GH rise. A number of GH stimulators, including insulin hypoglycemia, arginine, and exercise, act through alpha-adrenergic mechanisms. Beta-adrenergic blockers potentiate the GH-stimulatory effect of clonidine (and of some other agents, including levodopa), possibly by inhibiting somatostatin secretion.

3 Serotonin agonists stimulate GH release, and the nocturnal surge in GH secretion may be mediated by serotonin, since cyproheptadine (a serotonin antagonist) blocks the sleep-induced GH rise.

4 Acetylcholine increases GH release by inhibiting somatostatin. Acetylcholinesterase inhibitors increase basal GH and the GH response to GHRH.

Obesity blunts GH release in response to many stimuli, including GHRH itself. Weight reduction restores normal GH dynamics. In contrast, malnourished individuals, including women with anorexia nervosa, often have increased GH secretion and plasma concentration, partly the result of a decreased serum IGF-I/SM-C level. Oral glucose administration decreases serum GH and the GH response to GHRH. Arginine also stimulates GH release by inhibiting somatostatin release.

A number of hormones influence GH release. Most factors that stimulate GH release are more potent in women than in men, an effect mediated by estrogen. In testing GH reserve in children, estrogen priming may be necessary before adequate GH release can be demonstrated. Although estrogen increases GH concentration, it decreases its biologic effect by blocking somatomedin production. This is similar to the estrogen effect on prolactin, in which secretion is stimulated but its action in promoting lactation is inhibited. Chronic glucocorticoid administration inhibits GH release and may blunt somatomedin action as well, explaining the potent growth-inhibiting effects of these agents in children. Acute administration of glucocorticoids stimulates GH release, although the response is reduced or absent in obese individuals. ACTH and TH deficiency may be associated with reversible GH deficiency. GH-releasing peptide (GHRP) is a synthetic hexapeptide that stimulates pituitary GH release but does not interact with GHRH or opiate receptors. The therapeutic potential of this peptide is being explored.

GROWTH HORMONE EXCESS: ACROMEGALY AND GIGANTISM Clinical features GH excess results in acromegaly, an insidious, chronic debilitating disease associated with bony and soft tissue overgrowth (Table 331-4). Acromegaly occurs most frequently in middle age, with a mean age at diagnosis of 40 years in men and 45 in women. It is uncommon, with an estimated prevalence of 50 to 70 cases per million and an incidence of 3 to 4 cases per million per year. These figures may represent an underestimation due to underdiagnosis of the disorder. When GH excess develops prior to epiphyseal closure in children, increased linear growth and gigantism develop. Tumors may be more aggressive and cause more rapid onset of acromegaly in younger patients.

Most patients have soft tissue and bone enlargement which results in increased hand, foot, and hat size, prognathism, enlargement of the tongue, wide spacing of the teeth, and coarsening of facial features; these are rarely the presenting complaint. Acromegalics are said to look more like each other than like their own family members (Fig. 331-6). Laryngeal hypertrophy and sinus enlargement lead to a

TABLE 331-4 Acromegaly—Manifestations

Location	Symptoms	Signs
General	Fatigue Increased sweating Heat intolerance Weight gain	
Skin and subcutaneous tissue	Enlarging hands, feet Coarsening facial features Oily skin Hypertrichosis	Moist, warm, fleshy, doughy handshake Skin tags Acanthosis nigricans Increased heel pad
Head	Headaches	Parotid enlargement, frontal bossing
Eyes	Decreased vision	Visual field defects
Ears		Otoscope speculum cannot be inserted
Nose-throat–paranasal sinuses	Sinus congestion	Enlarged furrowed tongue
	Increased tongue size	Tooth marks on tongue
	Malocclusion Voice change	Widely spaced teeth Prognathism
Neck		Goiter Obstructive sleep apnea Enlarged sinuses
Cardiorespiratory system	Congestive heart failure	Hypertension Cardiomegaly Left ventricular hypertrophy
Genitourinary system	Decreased libido Impotence Oligomenorrhea Infertility Kidney stones	
Neurologic system	Paresthesias Hypersomnolence	Carpal tunnel syndrome
Muscles	Weakness	Proximal myopathy
Skeletal system	Joint pains (shoulders, back, knees)	Osteoarthritis

hollow-sounding voice. A moist, doughy handshake, increased skin tags, acanthosis nigricans, and oily skin are common.

Acromegaly is more than a cosmetically disfiguring disease. Patients feel weak and tired. The basal metabolic rate increases, which, in turn, causes increased sweating. Obstructive sleep apnea may be an important cause of hypersomnolence. The majority have neurologic and musculoskeletal symptoms, including headaches, paresthesias (often due to carpal tunnel syndrome), muscle weakness, and arthralgias (particularly involving the shoulders, back, and knees). The cartilage hypertrophy and osseous overgrowth often lead to degenerative arthritis, kyphoscoliosis, and on occasion spinal stenosis. Hypertension occurs in about one-third and is characterized by suppressed renin and aldosterone secretion associated with expansion of plasma volume and total-body sodium. Almost all hypertensive acromegalics and about half of nonhypertensive acromegalics have increased left ventricular mass or left ventricular wall thickness. Although it is not established whether a specific cardiomyopathy occurs, acromegalics may develop congestive heart failure in the absence of other known underlying heart disease. Amenorrhea may occur with or without hyperprolactinemia, and hirsutism is often noted. Depression may persist after successful therapy for acromegaly. Many organs, including the liver and kidneys, increase in size with no evidence of functional impairment. Goiter, which probably results from IGF-I stimulation of thyroid cell growth, is common: 3 to 7 percent of patients are hyperthyroid. Some series report abdominal pain and inguinal hernias each in about one-third of patients and nasal polyps in as many as 15 percent. Intracranial aneurysms coexist in 10 percent or less.

Patients with acromegaly probably have a shortened life expectancy with increased deaths from cardiovascular, cerebrovascular, and

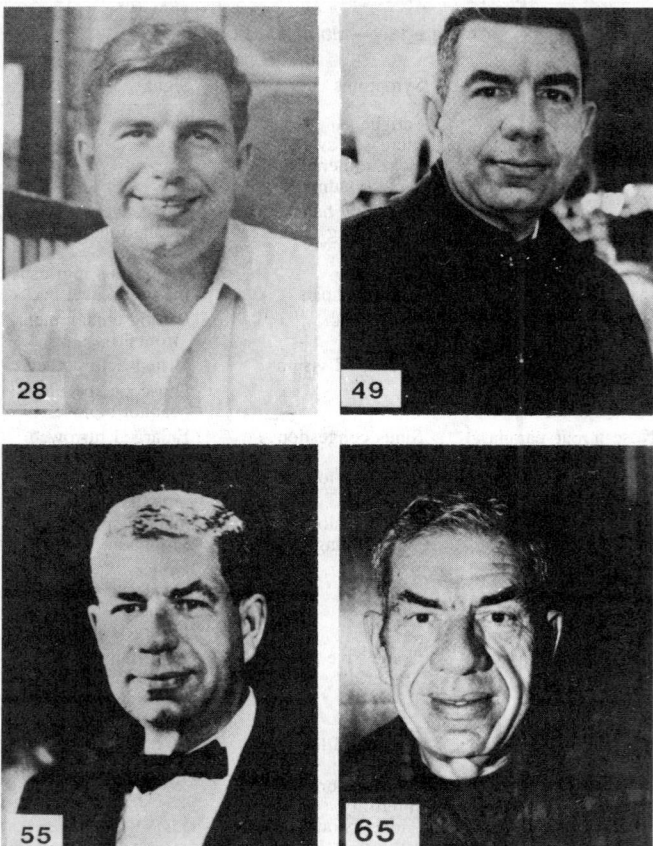

FIGURE 331-6 Serial photographs of a patient with acromegaly taken at ages 28, 49, 55, and 65 years, 6 months after removal of a GH-secreting adenoma. Note the gradual increase in the size of the nose, lips, and skin folds, particularly the nasolabial skin fold and forehead. *(From S Reichlin, Med Grand Rounds 1:9, 1982.)*

respiratory disease and, in some studies, from malignancies. In studies in which modern therapy was available, deleterious effects on life expectancy are less striking. Patients with coexisting diabetes mellitus have increased mortality. Skin tags appear to correlate with increased prevalence of colonic polyps and possibly with carcinoma of the colon. Bowel surveillance by colonoscopy has been suggested.

Laboratory investigation   Insulin resistance occurs in 80 percent, although abnormal glucose tolerance (20 to 40 percent) and clinical diabetes mellitus (13 to 20 percent) are less common. Hypercalciuria is frequent, apparently due to increased levels of circulating 1,25-dihydroxyvitamin D; renal stones occur in about one-fifth of patients. Hypercalcemia, when it occurs, is not due to acromegaly per se but suggests primary hyperparathyroidism as part of the multiple endocrine neoplasia 1 (MEN 1) syndrome (see Chap. 343). GH causes increased renal tubular reabsorption of phosphate by an undefined mechanism. Elevation of serum phosphate occurs in about one-half of patients. Hyperprolactinemia occurs in up to one-half of patients and is responsible for much of the associated galactorrhea, amenorrhea, and decreased libido.

Pathophysiology   Well-defined pituitary adenomas are found in almost all patients with acromegaly and gigantism. The tumors tend to occur in the lateral wings of the sella, where normal somatotrophs are found in abundance. Occasionally, tumors are found in ectopic locations along the lines of migration of Rathke's pouch, such as the sphenoid sinus or parapharyngeal regions.

GH levels correlate, on average, with tumor size. Tumors tend to be larger and may be more aggressive in younger patients. At the time of diagnosis, 75 percent of somatotroph adenomas are

macroadenomas; 70 percent, however, are less than 20 mm at diagnosis. Two-thirds or more of prolactinomas are microadenomas at the time of diagnosis. Aggressive screening for acromegaly on the basis of subtle clinical clues might lead to early diagnosis while tumors are still small.

Immunohistochemical staining and electron microscopy of somatotroph tumors help to predict their behavior. Densely granulated tumors have slower growth. GH-secreting carcinomas are rare and should be diagnosed only in the presence of distant metastases. Tumors that cause local invasion are called *invasive adenomas*.

Current evidence suggests a primary pituitary etiology for acromegaly. Most GH-secreting (and other pituitary) tumors are monoclonal in origin. A cellular mutation may lead to GH hypersecretion (and presumably tumor growth as well) in some patients. About 40 percent of somatotroph tumors have a mutation in the alpha subunit of a stimulatory G protein (Gs) (see Chap. 69). These G proteins normally couple surface signals to cyclic AMP production within the cells. Activation of Gs proteins is associated with GTP binding to the alpha subunit, which allows the alpha subunit to stimulate cyclic AMP production. The normal free subunit has intrinsic GTPase activity, which inactivates GTP, preventing continued cyclic AMP stimulation. The mutant alpha subunit in acromegalic patients does not possess GTPase activity; hence continued cyclic AMP stimulation results. Tumors containing these mutations tend to be smaller than those in which the mutation is absent. Further evidence for a primary etiology is the finding that peripheral concentrations of GHRH are low. Although these findings do not exclude hypothalamic GHRH excess or somatostatin deficiency as the cause in some patients, this possibility has no direct support. Abnormal GH pulsations in some surgically "cured" acromegalics could be due to an underlying hypothalamic disorder, residual tumor, or previous GH excess.

GHRH-induced acromegaly is rare (<1 percent in a one series) but is clinically indistinguishable from acromegaly caused by pituitary adenomas; prolactin excess may occur in this syndrome. This diagnosis should be considered when pituitary somatotroph hyperplasia, rather than an adenoma, is diagnosed histologically. Bronchial carcinoids and pancreatic islet cell tumors are the most likely to secrete GHRH ectopically, but small cell carcinoma of the lung, medullary thyroid carcinoma, and carcinoids of the small intestine and thymus contain GHRH as well. Many of the tumors associated with GHRH production also cause ectopic ACTH production. Hypothalamic gangliocytomas, hamartomas, and gliomas can produce GHRH (as well as somatostatin) and cause somatotroph hyperplasia and acromegaly. GHRH is not routinely measured in acromegalics unless somatotroph hyperplasia is present or an appropriate nonpituitary tumor is discovered.

Isolated ectopic production of GH has been described in a patient with a pancreatic islet cell tumor; the tumor size in this instance (420 g) suggests inefficient GH production, since GH-secreting pituitary tumors are usually small.

Diagnosis   Patients with acromegaly have symptoms for an average of 9 years and often see several physicians before the diagnosis is made. Newly consulted physicians are more likely to suspect the diagnosis than is one who has watched the insidious progress of the disease. When suggestive facial features are noted, a comparison with old pictures may be helpful (see Fig. 331-6).

Basal or random GH determinations may be elevated in normal persons, particularly in women and people with uncontrolled diabetes mellitus, renal failure, or stress; random GH determinations should not be used to screen for acromegaly. Two screening tests are available, namely, measurements of glucose-suppressed GH concentrations and IGF-I/SM-C concentrations. GH concentrations are measured 60 to 120 min after the oral administration of 100 g glucose. Although a serum GH concentration of <5 µg/L has traditionally been accepted as normal, a postsuppression value of <2 µg/L is a more rigorous criterion and should be applied. Acromegalics usually have a GH concentration after glucose administration of >10 µg/L; some suppress to values below 5 but rarely to below 2 µg/L. IGF-I/SM-C concentrations also provide an excellent screening test for acromegaly. Pitfalls include unreliable commercial assays, failure to use age-adjusted normals (especially during puberty), and possible false-negative tests with starvation. Measurements of serum IGF-I/SM-C concentration correlate with disease activity even in patients with basal GH concentrations below 10 μg/L. As GH values rise to >20 μg/L, IGF-I/SM-C concentrations plateau; this may explain why dramatic falls in GH after therapy do not cause clinical improvement. Although GH concentrations decline, IGF-I/SM-C may remain near maximal until GH falls below 20 μg/L.

GH concentrations in acromegaly may vary during the day, although they are never undetectable as in normal persons. After glucose administration to acromegalics, the GH concentrations usually are unchanged or increase, but some GH lowering may occur. GH levels increase in response to insulin-induced hypoglycemia and arginine infusion, and the response to GHRH is enhanced in most acromegalics. Somatostatin infusion lowers GH concentration but usually not to normal values. In addition, GH-secreting pituitary tumors respond to stimuli that do not affect normal somatotrophs: TRH increases GH in 80 percent, and LHRH increases GH in about 10 to 15 percent. Dopamine agonists stimulate GH release in normal persons but inhibit GH release in most acromegalics.

All patients with large pituitary adenomas should be screened with GH measurements, preferably after glucose ingestion. In rare cases patients with elevated serum GH and IGF-I/SM-C concentrations may have large pituitary tumors without clinical evidence of acromegaly. This syndrome is unexplained.

Radiologic investigation is necessary once the laboratory tests confirm the clinical suspicion of acromegaly. Although conventional skull x-rays or coned-down views of the sella turcica are abnormal in 90 percent of patients with acromegaly, MRI or CT scanning provides better definition of tumor size and is necessary for therapeutic planning. Additional clues to the diagnosis of acromegaly on conventional skull x-rays include thickening of the skull with increased bone density, enlargement of the paranasal sinuses and proliferation of the mastoid air cells, and prognathism if the jaw is included. On bone x-rays one may see enlarged vertebral bodies with anterior lipping, tufting of the distal phalanges of the hands and feet, increased thickness and lengthening of the ribs and clavicles, and bowing of the femur, tibia, and fibula. Soft tissue x-rays demonstrate increased thickness of the heel pad (>18 mm in women and 21 mm in men).

Testing for hypopituitarism and for increased prolactin should be performed. Large somatotroph adenomas commonly cause neurologic abnormalities (visual field defects or oculomotor or abducens nerve lesions). In addition, acromegaly may be associated with hyperparathyroidism and pancreatic islet cell tumors in the MEN I syndrome and rarely with pheochromocytomas or hyperaldosteronism (see Chap. 343). The alpha subunit of the glycoprotein hormones may be oversecreted in acromegaly and may serve as an additional marker of tumor regrowth.

Therapy The objectives of therapy are (1) return of GH and IGF-I/SM-C levels to normal, (2) stabilization or decrease in tumor size, and (3) preservation of normal pituitary function. The available modalities are variably successful in achieving these goals, and none is perfect. Although GH values of <5 μg/L are frequently interpreted as representing cures, a value of <2 μg/L with a normal IGF-I/SM-C level is a better criterion; patients with GH values between 2 and 5 μg/L may have persistent symptoms and increased IGF-I/SM-C concentrations.

Transsphenoidal surgery has the advantage of producing a rapid therapeutic response; it is potentially curative and is the procedure of choice. Anesthesiologists should be alerted to the potential of a difficult intubation due to anatomic changes in the jaw, tongue, epiglottis, and larynx. GH concentrations may fall to normal within hours, and soft tissue (but not bony) enlargement may melt away, even before the patient has been discharged from the hospital. The success of this procedure depends on the completeness of the resection and hence on the size of the tumor. In expert hands, apparent cure rates (GH below 5 μg/L) average 75 percent in patients with preoperative GH levels of <40 μg/L but only 35 percent in those with preoperative GH levels >40 μg/L. More stringent criteria, such as a GH level of <2 μg/L and normal IGF-I/SM-C level, are rarely used; the surgical cure rate is probably closer to 20 to 40 percent when these criteria are applied. This may explain why tumor regrowth and recurrent acromegaly are more common than previously appreciated. Persistent GH response to TRH stimulation may have predictive value in assessing risk of relapse, even in those patients with "normal" postoperative GH concentrations. Hypopituitarism may occur in 10 to 20 percent of patients with larger tumors, but up to 10 percent of patients with pituitary insufficiency prior to surgery regain normal function.

Heavy-particle pituitary radiation is successful in lowering GH concentrations in acromegaly but is slow in accomplishing this goal. Patients with suprasellar extension of the pituitary adenoma are generally excluded from this therapy. The Harvard cyclotron utilizes the Bragg peak with proton irradiation, achieving up to 12,000 cGy (12,000 rad) to the center of the pituitary adenoma. In patients with mean pretherapy GH concentration of 60 μg/L, GH concentrations are <5 μg/L in 29 percent of patients at 2 years, 40 percent at 4 years, 75 percent at 10 years, and 92 percent by 20 years. The risk of hypopituitarism is at least 20 percent.

Conventional pituitary radiation [4500 cGy (4500 rad) over 5 weeks] also has its proponents. GH generally falls 50 percent after 2 ± 1 years. GH concentrations of <5 μg/L occur in 50 percent at 5 years and in 70 percent at 10 years (after a mean pretherapy GH level of 60 μg/L). GH concentrations of <2.5 μg/L occur in 40 percent, and values <1 μg/L are seen in 20 percent at 10 to 15 years. Hypopituitarism is a common sequela, and up to 50 percent of patients require replacement therapy. The hypopituitarism is probably due to hypothalamic damage, which is possibly less common with focused heavy particles or gamma radiation. Higher doses of focused radiation [4000 to 7000 cGy (4000 to 7000 rad)] can be delivered with the cobalt 60 gamma unit ("gamma knife"), which delivers collimated radiation through multiple portals (over 200 in some units) that converge on the target in question. The radiation is delivered in a single session; radiation delivery to the tumor is the equivalent of two to three times the dosage of conventional radiation. Reports to date do not suggest an advantage (apart from convenience) over conventional radiation, either in terms of efficacy or risk of hypopituitarism; however, the data are still preliminary. We employ heavy-particle or conventional radiation in patients who have failed surgery and medical therapy or when surgery is contraindicated or is refused by the patient.

Bromocriptine is a useful adjunct to other modalities of therapy but rarely is successful alone. Clinical improvement is reported in up to 90 percent of patients with dosages of 20 to 60 mg/d. Objective decrease in hand and ring size as well as improvement in diabetes mellitus may occur in the absence of decreasing GH values. However, GH concentrations fall to <10 μg/L in only 35 percent, and values of <5 μg/L are achieved in only 21 percent; IGF-I/SM-C levels return to normal in only 8 percent. Tumor size decreases rarely.

The long-acting somatostatin analogue octreotide lowers GH to <5 μg/L and IGF-I/SM-C to normal in half of acromegalics. Modest tumor regression occurs in 30 to 50 percent of patients. The drug must be administered subcutaneously. Dosages average 100 to 200 μg every 8 h but range from 50 to 250 μg every 6 to 12 h to a maximum of 1500 μg/d. Constant subcutaneous pump therapy also has been employed. Temporary side effects are minimal and include local pain, steatorrhea, and abdominal cramps; the risk of cholelithiasis is substantial and may be due to decreased gallbladder contractility. Octreotide is 2000 times as potent as somatostatin in inhibiting GH secretion but only 1.5 to 2 times as potent an inhibitor of insulin secretion. Although impairment of glucose tolerance or worsening of diabetes mellitus may occur, the GH-lowering effects of the drug may improve glucose tolerance. Inhibition of TSH does not result in hypothyroidism. Headaches disappear quickly, possibly due to an effect on cerebral blood flow. The role of this agent as a primary treatment for acromegaly remains to be defined, but some patients have been treated successfully for over 5 years. The drug is expensive and is not licensed for this indication in the United States. It is likely that octreotide will be most useful as adjunctive therapy after unsuccessful surgery and/or radiation therapy. In preliminary studies the success rate of surgery in acromegalic patients with invasive macroadenomas has been reported to improve after octreotide pretreatment.

All acromegalic patients require long-term follow-up and evaluation for recurrent disease. Interlaboratory variation in GH levels may be considerable; whenever possible, serial GH levels should be measured by the same laboratory. False elevation of GH concentrations in some acromegalics may be due to antibodies displacing GH in the radioimmunoassays used. Surveillance for colonic polyps and/or colon cancer has been suggested for those over age 50, those with more than 10 years of acromegaly, and those with more than three skin tags; others recommend periodic colonoscopy for all acromegalics.

GH DEFICIENCY AND PITUITARY DWARFISM GH is often the first hormone to be lost in pituitary and hypothalamic disorders. In adults, GH deficiency is usually cryptic and can only be diagnosed on the basis of stimulation tests for GH release. The consequences of GH deficiency and replacement in adults are still being explored. Short-term replacement therapy in GH-deficient adults results in improved exercise tolerance, decreased body fat, and increased lean body mass. GH deficiency may contribute to the increased cardiovascular mortality in hypopituitary adults; conversely, these patients have decreased cancer mortality. Diabetics with GH deficiency show a reduction in insulin requirements and may develop hypoglycemia. In children, GH deficiency leads to impaired growth and short stature and is often a consequence of hypothalamic GHRH deficiency (see Chap. 332).

GONADOTROPINS

PHYSIOLOGY The gonadotropins, LH and FSH, are secreted by the gonadotrophs (also see Chaps. 339 and 340). These cells, which make up about 10 percent of the anterior pituitary, are dispersed throughout the anterior lobe, often situated close to the lactotrophs. Most gonadotrophs produce both LH and FSH, although a few cells produce only one hormone.

LH and FSH are glycoproteins of similar size (about 30,000 mol wt) which share a common alpha subunit [also present in TSH and human chorionic gonadotropin (hCG)] but have unique beta subunits. The alpha and beta chains are encoded by separate genes, and alpha chains are often produced in excess. The carbohydrate content of the molecules influences the biologic behavior and duration of action and may vary during the menstrual cycle. Although both FSH and LH are secreted in pulsatile fashion, the longer half-life of FSH means that FSH concentrations fluctuate less throughout the day. FSH and LH regulate ovarian and testicular function. hCG is also produced in the normal pituitary.

FSH stimulates the growth of the granulosa cells of the ovarian follicle and controls the aromatase responsible for estradiol formation within these cells. LH stimulates the ovarian theca cells to produce androgens, which diffuse to the granulosa cells, where they are converted to estrogens. Estradiol, the principal estrogen, peaks about 1 day prior to the LH surge, which, in turn, triggers ovulation. Postovulation, LH contributes to corpus luteum formation. Once conception has occurred, pituitary gonadotropin function is no longer necessary to sustain pregnancy.

In the testis, LH is primarily responsible for controlling testosterone production in the Leydig cells. FSH, in conjunction with intratesticular testosterone, stimulates the seminiferous tubules to produce sperm. Thus LH and FSH are necessary for normal spermatogenesis, whereas testosterone production requires only LH.

Luteinizing hormone–releasing hormone [LHRH, also known as *gonadotropin-releasing hormone* (GnRH)], a decapeptide produced by the arcuate nuclei of the hypothalamus, is responsible for the release of both LH and FSH. Extrahypothalamic LHRH is present in other areas of the brain as well. Noradrenergic agonists appear to facilitate, whereas endogenous opioids inhibit, LHRH release.

LHRH acts on high-affinity pituitary receptors to stimulate LH and FSH production and release. The pituitary response to LHRH varies greatly throughout life. LHRH and the gonadotropins first appear in the fetus at about 10 weeks of gestation. During the first 3 months after birth, LHRH elicits a brisk gonadotropin rise. The sensitivity to LHRH then declines until the onset of puberty. Before puberty, the FSH response to LHRH is greater than that of LH. With the onset of puberty, sensitivity to LHRH increases, and pulsatile LH secretion, first noted during sleep, ensues. Later in puberty and during the reproductive years, pulsations are present throughout the day, with LH responsiveness being greater than that of FSH. After menopause, FSH and LH concentrations rise, and postmenopausal FSH levels are higher than those of LH.

Pulsatile LHRH release results in pulsatile LH and FSH release. However, sustained infusion of LHRH and its analogues results in inhibition of LH and FSH release. This phenomenon has been utilized in the successful treatment of gonadotropin-mediated precocious puberty by the sustained administration of LHRH or its analogues. Conversely, in people with LHRH deficiency, the pulsatile administration of LHRH can restore a normal menstrual cycle or normal sperm and testosterone production.

The feedback relationship between the gonadal steroids and the hypothalamus and pituitary is detailed in Chaps. 339 and 340. Low doses of estrogens decrease the frequency of LHRH pulses and, more important, decrease the pituitary response to LHRH; this phenomenon is seen most clearly in postmenopausal women with elevated gonadotropins. However, sustained elevation of estrogens results in a positive-feedback signal that stimulates LHRH and LH release; this phenomenon is responsible, in part, for the LH surge prior to ovulation. The sensitivity of LHRH to this positive feedback by estrogen increases during middle to late puberty. Although progesterone decreases LHRH pulse frequency, the progesterone rise in the late follicular phase augments the pituitary LH response to LHRH and contributes to the LH surge. In castrated men, testosterone administration usually suppresses LH to undetectable levels and less often lowers FSH to normal (but not undetectable) concentrations. Inhibin, a peptide hormone produced by the testicular Sertoli cell and ovarian granulosa cell, is a potent inhibitor of FSH (but not LH) release. Its physiologic role is under investigation. Testosterone decreases the frequency of LH pulsations, probably by a direct effect on LHRH release, and is converted in many tissues, including the brain, to estradiol, which inhibits the pituitary response to LHRH.

Gonadotropin measurements In postmenopausal women and men with primary hypogonadism, gonadal failure results in a marked increase in FSH and LH concentrations, providing an endogenous stimulation test. Such elevated gonadotropin concentrations ensure the adequacy of pituitary gonadotroph function. On the other hand, gonadotropin measurements are rarely indicated in a woman with ovulatory menses and in men with normal sperm counts. In evaluating gonadal failure associated with low testosterone concentrations in men or low estradiol levels in women, gonadotropin measurements help separate primary from central (secondary, hypogonadotropic) hypogonadism: High gonadotropin concentrations are indicative of primary gonadal failure; low or normal gonadotropin concentrations suggest hypothalamic or pituitary disease (see Chap. 330).

HYPOGONADOTROPIC (CENTRAL, SECONDARY) HYPOGONADISM Isolated gonadotropin deficiency may be a congenital or hereditary disorder. Kallmann's syndrome is a heterogeneous genetic disorder afflicting 1 in 10,000 to 60,000 individuals; X-linked as well as autosomal inheritance has been described. Kallmann's syndrome is characterized by gonadotropin deficiency due to LHRH deficiency in association with anosmia and midline anatomic defects. LHRH-secreting neurons migrate from the olfactory placode into the brain, along with the olfactory and other nerves. The mutation in X-linked

Kallmann's syndrome results in a defect in neuronal migration. Most patients with Kallmann's syndrome secrete gonadotropins in response to LHRH administration after suitable priming. Mutations in the beta subunit of LH are another cause of hypogonadism.

Acquired defects of LHRH production are common. Hyperprolactinemia causes amenorrhea due to inhibition of LHRH release, possibly mediated by increased hypothalamic dopamine. Amenorrhea in anorexia nervosa, starvation, long-distance runners, and "stress" appears to be due to inhibition of LHRH release as well. Gonadotropin deficiency may be a relatively early defect in patients with large pituitary adenomas. Gonadotropin deficiency also occurs in patients with polyglandular endocrine deficiencies, presumably on an autoimmune basis (see Chap. 343), and in patients with hemochromatosis.

Patients with LHRH deficiency who desire fertility may respond to pulsatile therapy with LHRH or its agonists. When gonadotropin deficiency is due to pituitary disease, injections of FSH (menotropin) and chorionic gonadotropin (a hormone with LH-like activity) are necessary to achieve fertility.

ECTOPIC GONADOTROPIN SECRETION Ectopic gonadotropin production (usually hCG) can be associated with germinomas of the nonseminoma type (see Chap. 322), lung carcinomas, hepatomas, and other tumors. Children may develop precocious puberty, and men may develop gynecomastia. No distinct clinical syndrome occurs in women.

GONADOTROPIN-SECRETING PITUITARY TUMORS Gonadotropin-secreting pituitary tumors are generally large and are most commonly diagnosed in men with decreased libido, decreased serum testosterone levels, and normal or slightly elevated prolactin levels. Although 20 to 25 percent of pituitary macroadenomas are considered nonfunctioning (i.e., absence of a clinical syndrome of hormone overproduction), many of these tumors produce gonadotropin. Some produce high levels of intact gonadotropins (usually FSH or FSH in conjunction with LH, rarely LH alone), with or without a clinical syndrome. Testicular enlargement due to FSH overproduction and testosterone elevation due to LH overproduction do occur but are rare. The finding of an increased FSH concentration may be misinterpreted as primary hypogonadism if a pituitary adenoma is not suspected. Inhibin levels may be increased (as a consequence of FSH increase) in contrast to low inhibin levels in patients with primary hypogonadism. In some, the FSH has enhanced biologic activity, possibly as a result of altered glycosylation. In others, normal amounts of intact gonadotropins with unbalanced production of gonadotropin subunits, particularly alpha, FSH, or LH beta, are found. Although LH concentrations are often normal or elevated in these patients, testosterone levels are often low and respond normally to hCG administration. This suggests that the LH is biologically inactive (possible abnormal glycosylation) or that it represents immunologic cross-reactivity due to LH subunit overproduction. Some tumors secrete normal amounts of intact gonadotropins and gonadotropin subunits but demonstrate abnormal responses to TRH stimulation. FSH increase in response to TRH (e.g., 400 μg IV) occurs in 40 percent of gonadotropin-secreting tumors but not in normal individuals, hypogonadal men, or postmenopausal women; increased response of gonadotropin alpha and LH beta subunits is common as well. Some tumors express gonadotropin gene mRNA and/or hormone production in vitro but do not cause in vivo abnormalities.

In postmenopausal women with macroadenomas, it may be difficult to ascertain whether a gonadotropin elevation is due to normal menopause or to a gonadotropin-secreting adenoma. TRH testing may provide a partial answer. The majority of such tumors produce increased LH beta, FSH, or LH in response to TRH administration.

The therapy of nonfunctioning pituitary macroadenomas and gonadotropin-secreting adenomas is identical: surgery and/or radiation therapy. The response to bromocriptine, somatostatin analogue, or LHRH analogues is disappointing in terms of tumor shrinkage even when a hormonal response is achieved.

Men with primary hypogonadism (low testosterone level, elevated LH and FSH levels) are occasionally investigated for the presence of a gonadotropin-secreting tumor. There are no inexpensive ways of differentiating these two clinical situations. Primary hypogonadism is common; gonadotropin-secreting tumors are rare. The tumors are almost always large, but radiographic procedures may be necessary to exclude a tumor; whether a lateral or a posteroanterior and lateral skull x-ray will serve this purpose is uncertain. A normal testicular response to hCG administration points toward a gonadotropin-secreting adenoma but is a cumbersome, poorly standardized test.

THYROTROPIN

PHYSIOLOGY TSH is a glycoprotein hormone (28,000 mol wt) composed of an alpha subunit which it shares with LH, FSH, and hCG and a unique beta subunit that confers specificity (also see Chap. 334). TSH is produced by thyrotrophs, which constitute about 5 percent of the cells of the anterior pituitary. TSH regulates the biosynthesis, storage, and release of thyroid hormones and determines thyroid gland size. TSH first appears in the fetal pituitary at about 10 weeks of gestation. TSH levels in normal subjects average 0.5 to 5.0 mU/L, with a slight increase in the nocturnal hours.

Thyrotropin-releasing hormone (TRH), the major hypothalamic mediator of TSH release, is a tripeptide found in highest concentrations in the medial division of the hypothalamic paraventricular nuclei and in the median eminence. Extrahypothalamic TRH is found in the posterior pituitary, in other parts of the brain and spinal cord, and in the gastrointestinal tract. TRH stimulates TSH secretion by increasing cytoplasmic free calcium; phosphatidylinositol and membrane phospholipids probably participate in TRH-stimulated TSH secretion. TRH stimulation increases the glycosylation and hence the biologic activity of secreted TSH. TRH stimulates the release of prolactin as well as that of TSH. The prolactin response is enhanced in hypothyroidism and diminished in hyperthyroidism. TRH-induced GH stimulation may occur in acromegaly, renal failure, depression, in many normal children, and in occasional normal adults.

The thyroid hormones thyroxine (T_4) and triiodothyronine (T_3) inhibit TSH production directly at the pituitary level. Both T_3 and T_4 bind to receptors on pituitary nuclei, but T_3 has a 40-fold greater affinity for these receptors than does T_4. Nevertheless, exogenous T_4 is more potent than T_3 in inhibiting TSH release because circulating T_4 is a more effective means of delivering T_3 to the pituitary than is T_3 itself. Half of intrapituitary T_3 is derived from T_4 conversion within the pituitary. The effects of T_4 and T_3 on hypothalamic TRH release in humans are unknown, but in animals they cause inhibition of TRH synthesis and release. In hyperthyroidism, TSH is suppressed, and the TSH response to TRH is absent; in primary hypothyroidism, the basal TSH concentration is elevated, and the response to TRH is exaggerated.

Somatostatin decreases basal TSH release, the TSH response to TRH, and the nocturnal TSH peak. Dopamine and glucocorticoids decrease basal TSH concentration and the TSH response to TRH. Patients with untreated primary adrenal insufficiency may have slightly elevated TSH levels.

TSH concentrations can be interpreted only when serum thyroid hormone concentrations are known (see Chap. 330). In conventional hyperthyroidism, thyroid hormone levels are elevated and TSH release is inhibited. TSH-induced hyperthyroidism is rare. Only sensitive TSH assays can differentiate between low and normal concentrations. A detectable serum TSH concentration by an ultrasensitive assay excludes conventional hyperthyroidism. Low thyroid hormone and elevated serum TSH concentrations are characteristic of primary hypothyroidism. Low thyroid hormone concentrations with a "normal" or "low" TSH concentration are found in central (secondary) hypothyroidism. The TRH stimulation test (no TSH response in hyperthyroidism, exaggerated TSH response in primary hypothyroidism) has largely been supplanted by sensitive TSH measurements. The TRH stimulation test is also not useful in the diagnosis of secondary hypothyroidism or in differentiating pituitary from hypothalamic disease.

PRIMARY HYPOTHYROIDISM   Thyroid gland failure (primary hypothyroidism) leads to compensatory hypertrophy of the thyrotrophs. With thyroid failure of long duration, the pituitary gland and the sella turcica may enlarge, occasionally causing visual field defects. Although TSH-secreting tumors may develop in animals after thyroid gland removal, the increased TSH and pituitary size in human hypothyroidism is not autonomous and decreases with thyroid hormone replacement. Since hyperprolactinemia also may occur in patients with primary hypothyroidism, pituitary enlargement (hyperplasia) may be incorrectly diagnosed as a prolactinoma; however, the return to normal of prolactin concentrations with thyroid hormone therapy excludes that diagnosis. Severe primary hypothyroidism occasionally may cause impaired release of GH and ACTH after appropriate stimuli (so-called pituitary myxedema), and hypothyroid children may develop precocious puberty. These abnormalities are all corrected with thyroid hormone therapy.

SECONDARY HYPOTHYROIDISM   Hypothyroidism due to pituitary or hypothalamic disease may be difficult to diagnose. With primary hypothyroidism, serum TSH commonly rises before thyroid hormone concentrations decline below the normal range. No similar early laboratory clue exists in secondary hypothyroidism. Patients with central hypothyroidism usually do not have goiter, and many have deficiencies of other pituitary trophic hormones.

Some patients with hypothalamic hypothyroidism have mild TSH elevations, rather than normal or low concentrations, as expected. Although the TSH elevations rarely exceed 10 mU/L, they are above the expected range for hypothyroidism due to TSH deficiency. Biologically inactive but immunologically active thyrotropin is present in such cases. After TRH injection, TSH concentration rises, and the biologic potency of the TSH is increased. This suggests an additional role for TRH in controlling the biologic activity of the TSH molecule by controlling its rate of glycosylation. Although subclinical primary hypothyroidism is also characterized by mild TSH elevations, the two conditions are easily distinguished. Patients with central hypothyroidism and TSH elevations have markedly decreased T_4 concentrations; patients with subclinical hypothyroidism have normal or near-normal T_4 concentrations. TSH concentrations must not be used to guide replacement therapy in central hypothyroidism because TSH concentrations fall before full replacement is achieved; rather, peripheral levels of T_4 and free T_4 should be monitored. Severe illness may cause laboratory changes indistinguishable from central hypothyroidism, part of the so-called sick euthyroid syndrome.

PITUITARY (TSH-INDUCED) HYPERTHYROIDISM   Hyperthyroidism is not usually a disease of TSH overproduction. However, two types of TSH-mediated hyperthyroidism are recognized:

1 Pituitary tumors. These are usually macroadenomas with autonomous TSH secretion, unresponsive to thyroid hormone suppression or TRH stimulation. A hallmark of such tumors is overproduction of the glycoprotein hormone alpha subunit (TSH alpha), with a serum molar ratio of alpha to intact TSH of greater than 1:1. The free alpha subunit may be an important tumor marker and differs from the native alpha subunit in that one of its amino acids is carbohydrate-blocked and hence cannot combine with beta subunits. These tumors may produce other pituitary hormones in addition to TSH, most commonly GH. TSH and TSH alpha subunit secretion may decrease with octreotide therapy. Therapy is generally directed to the pituitary tumor, but control of hyperthyroidism may require radioactive iodine or antithyroid drugs.

2 Pituitary resistance to thyroid hormone. In this situation, thyroid hormone fails to inhibit TSH secretion appropriately in the absence of a pituitary adenoma. Since TSH secretion is not inhibited, TSH rises and stimulates thyroid hormone overproduction. The peripheral tissues are not resistant to thyroid hormone, and clinical hyperthyroidism results. The pituitary resistance to thyroid hormone is incomplete, since TSH can be suppressed with supraphysiologic levels of thyroid hormone and stimulated further with TRH; bromocriptine or octreotide may lower TSH as well. Pituitary

resistance is usually diagnosed after thyroid gland ablation, when TSH cannot be lowered to normal values with the usual therapeutic doses of thyroid hormone. However, once the hyperthyroidism has been treated, pituitary resistance is of no clinical consequence, although the TSH measurements cannot be utilized to monitor adequacy of hormone replacement.

ADRENOCORTICOTROPIN

PHYSIOLOGY   ACTH is produced by corticotrophs, which comprise about 15 percent of anterior pituitary cells, located principally in the central portion. ACTH is synthesized as part of a large precursor molecule termed *pro-opiomelanocortin* (POMC, 265 amino acids). ACTH contains 39 amino acids, with near complete biologic activity residing in the *N*-terminal 26 amino acids. In the anterior pituitary POMC is cleaved to yield ACTH, β-lipotropin, and an *N*-terminal precursor.

ACTH controls the release of cortisol from the adrenal cortex. Although aldosterone is primarily controlled by the renin-angiotensin system, ACTH also stimulates aldosterone release acutely. Other derivatives of the POMC molecule, such as γ-melanocyte-stimulating hormone (γ-MSH), also influence aldosterone production and are found in increased concentrations in the plasma of patients with idiopathic hyperaldosteronism. Patients with ACTH deficiency have near-normal aldosterone production and do not require mineralocorticoid replacement therapy.

Corticotropin-releasing hormone (CRH) is the major but not exclusive regulator of ACTH release. CRH contains 41 amino acids on a single polypeptide chain. CRH is produced primarily by neurons of the paraventricular nuclei of the hypothalamus but is also present in other areas of the brain, including the limbic system and cortex, as well as in the pancreas, gut, and adrenal medulla. Circulating CRH, which is largely of nonhypothalamic origin, is bound to a high-affinity binding protein. The placenta has the highest concentration outside the nervous system. CRH stimulates cyclic AMP production and regulates intracellular calcium and increases the concentration of POMC mRNA. Vasopressin potentiates the ACTH-releasing properties of CRH through a cyclic AMP–independent mechanism and may play a physiologic role in ACTH release. Naloxone, an opiate antagonist, releases CRH (and hence ACTH) in humans.

ACTH is released in pulses with an overriding circadian rhythm. With a normal sleeping pattern, ACTH concentration is highest in the early morning (around 4 A.M.) and lowest in late evening. The characteristic diurnal rhythm of plasma cortisol occurs in response to these ACTH changes. In primary adrenal insufficiency (Addison's disease), cortisol concentrations fall and ACTH concentrations rise. This results in hyperpigmentation owing to the melanocyte-stimulating properties of ACTH. Cortisol administration inhibits ACTH release, a phenomenon dependent on both the rate of rise of cortisol and its absolute concentration. Increased plasma cortisol inhibits CRH-induced ACTH release and also may inhibit CRH release. When supraphysiologic doses of glucocorticoids are given for prolonged periods, the hypothalamic-pituitary–adrenal cortex axis may remain suppressed for months after the drugs have been stopped, probably as the result of prolonged hypothalamic CRH suppression (see Chap. 335).

Stress, including hypoglycemia, surgery, and psychic distress, stimulates ACTH release, in part via increased CRH release. However, the magnitude of the ACTH release is greater than can be achieved during maximal stimulation with CRH. With severe illness, the requirements for cortisol may increase up to tenfold; failure to achieve these levels of cortisol during such periods may result in clinical adrenal insufficiency when adrenal reserve is impaired.

The immune system is tightly linked to the hypothalamic-pituitary-adrenal (HPA) axis. Glucocorticoids inhibit immune function, and immune mediators such as interleukin 1 are potent stimulators of ACTH secretion. These mediators may explain at least part of the link between "stress" and activation of the HPA axis, the subsequent cortisol response serving to limit the immune response.

In normal persons, ACTH circulates in low concentrations [2 to 18 pmol/L (10 to 80 pg/mL)]. It is difficult to measure ACTH in plasma and often not possible to separate low from normal values using commercial assays. Random ACTH measurements have little clinical significance. Tests for adrenal insufficiency and excess rely primarily on measurements of cortisol and its metabolites rather than on measurement of ACTH.

ACTH EXCESS (CUSHING'S DISEASE AND NELSON'S SYNDROME) Clinical features   Cortisol excess is characterized by a central distribution of adipose tissue, muscle weakness, purplish striae, hypertension, amenorrhea, osteoporosis, fatigue, and psychiatric abnormalities. This syndrome may be caused by pituitary or ectopic ACTH overproduction, adrenal tumors, or exogenous glucocorticoid administration.

The presence of cortisol excess is established by the finding of increased excretion of urine free cortisol and/or 17-hydroxycorticosteroids that fails to decrease appropriately after either overnight (1 mg at midnight) or 2-day low-dose dexamethasone administration (0.5 mg every 6 h for eight doses). Additional suppression (and occasionally stimulation) tests are required to determine whether the Cushing's syndrome is due to a pituitary lesion. In patients with pituitary ACTH hypersecretion, high-dose overnight dexamethasone administration (8 mg at midnight) results in greater than 50 percent reduction in the 8 A.M. plasma cortisol. Two-day dexamethasone administration (2 mg every 6 h for eight doses) generally results in greater than 60 percent suppression of urine 17-hydroxycorticosteroids and greater than 90 percent suppression of urine free cortisol. Urine 17-hydroxycorticosteroids increase after metyrapone administration in Cushing's disease. Plasma ACTH levels are normal or high-normal and show an exaggerated increase after CRH administration. Pituitary ACTH hypersecretion (Cushing's disease) is caused by a corticotroph microadenoma in 90 percent of patients and by a macroadenoma in most of the rest. Corticotroph hyperplasia has been documented in a few cases. The microadenomas are often small (3 to 6 mm or less) and may be difficult to find even with the use of gadolinium-enhanced MRI. Previously, pituitary surgery was often recommended on the basis of dynamic testing alone. However, bilateral inferior petrosal sinus catheterization with or without CRH administration to localize the site of ACTH production can be used to confirm the pituitary source of ACTH production and to localize adenomas when all imaging studies are negative. Nelson's syndrome (characterized by hyperpigmentation despite adequate glucocorticoid replacement therapy) is caused by growth of the residual pituitary tumor after bilateral adrenalectomy in patients with pituitary Cushing's disease. These tumors are usually easily identified on MRI or CT scanning and may exhibit aggressive growth patterns.

Treatment   Transsphenoidal microsurgery is successful in treating microadenomas in about 75 percent of patients. When surgery is successful, plasma cortisol concentrations fall almost to zero and often remain low for many months owing to delayed recovery of CRH and ACTH secretion by the hypothalamus and normal remaining pituitary. However, adrenal function eventually returns to normal in most patients. Cushing's syndrome may recur, however, even after apparently curative surgery. Previously, bilateral adrenalectomy was the therapy of choice for patients with pituitary Cushing's disease. Unfortunately, after this procedure, enlarging pituitary adenomas with increased skin pigmentation (Nelson's syndrome) develop in 10 to 30 percent of patients.

Ectopic ACTH production is a relatively common disorder and can cause great difficulty in diagnosis (see Chaps. 327 and 335). When ACTH production is caused by rapidly growing tumors such as oat cell carcinoma of the lung, symptoms of Cushing's syndrome are blunted. Rather, patients have hypokalemia, muscle weakness, weight loss, and hyperpigmentation. ACTH concentrations often exceed 66 pmol/L (300 pg/mL) and do not change with dexamethasone administration. ACTH concentrations may be lower in IRMA assays

than in radioimmunoassays; the IRMA assays do not measure larger fragments of the POMC molecule. When slow-growing tumors such as thymic carcinoids, bronchial carcinoids, medullary carcinoma of the thyroid, and pancreatic islet cell tumors produce ACTH, the typical features of Cushing's syndrome are common. In the latter group, ACTH measurements and cortisol response to dexamethasone administration may mimic those found in patients with pituitary adenomas. However, with ectopic ACTH production, ACTH concentrations generally do not change after CRH administration. When differentiation between pituitary and ectopic ACTH production is uncertain, bilateral inferior petrosal sinus catheterization is necessary. Cushing's syndrome can rarely be caused by ectopic production of CRH itself.

ACTH DEFICIENCY (SECONDARY ADRENAL INSUFFICIENCY)   ACTH deficiency may be isolated or occur in association with other anterior pituitary hormone deficiencies. Reversible isolated ACTH deficiency is common after long-term glucocorticoid administration. If glucocorticoids are withdrawn suddenly in this situation or continued in physiologic doses when severe illness is present, adrenal insufficiency may occur (see Chap. 335). Symptoms include nausea, vomiting, fatigue, joint discomfort, and dizziness, and there may be fever, hypotension, hyponatremia, and hypoglycemia. Reversible dementia may occur in the elderly. Although cortisol is necessary for free water excretion, it is not needed for potassium excretion. Hence patients with ACTH deficiency are hyponatremic but not hyperkalemic as are patients with primary adrenal insufficiency. Hyperpigmentation does not occur. These factors make diagnosis of secondary adrenal insufficiency more difficult than that of primary adrenal insufficiency. Isolated ACTH deficiency may occur without prior glucocorticoid therapy and may be of hypothalamic or pituitary origin. The diagnosis is often missed.

In general, patients undergoing pituitary surgery need to be treated with "stress" doses of glucocorticoids until normal adrenal function can be demonstrated postoperatively. All patients with pituitary macroadenomas or hypothalamic disease require testing of the pituitary-adrenal axis, but when pituitary surgery is planned, testing can be limited in focus until after surgery is completed.

THE ENDOGENOUS OPIOID PEPTIDES

The endogenous opioid peptides bind to a family of opioid receptors. The endorphins, enkephalins, and dynorphins, although chemically related, arise from different biosynthetic pathways (Fig. 331-7). In the pituitary, β-endorphin, the most abundant endorphin, is synthesized as part of a larger precursor molecule (pro-opiomelanocortin, POMC) that also contains the full sequence of ACTH, α-melanocyte-stimulating hormone (α-MSH), β-MSH, and β-lipotropin (β-LPH) (Fig. 331-8). This biosynthetic pathway represents the only pathway for pituitary ACTH synthesis. Hence ACTH and β-endorphin biosynthesis are inextricably linked in the pituitary. In adrenal insufficiency, plasma levels of both ACTH and β-endorphin are elevated; likewise, glucocorticoid administration decreases the levels of both. CRH stimulates the release of both ACTH and β-endorphin in a parallel manner; in Nelson's syndrome, the plasma levels of both ACTH and β-endorphin are elevated. Ectopic production of ACTH by tumors is also accompanied by β-endorphin excess. Although it was hoped that differential processing of POMC by tumors would allow separation of pituitary from ectopic ACTH production, analysis of metabolites is rarely helpful in individual cases. Production of "big" and "big-big" ACTH by tumors reflects the incomplete processing of the POMC precursor. Alternative processing of POMC occurs within other tissues. Therefore, although different cell types may synthesize the same primary gene product, the final profile of hormone secretion can differ completely. The hypothalamus also produces POMC in neurons and may convert POMC to smaller fragments than the anterior pituitary.

Two other opioid precursors give rise to potent endogenous

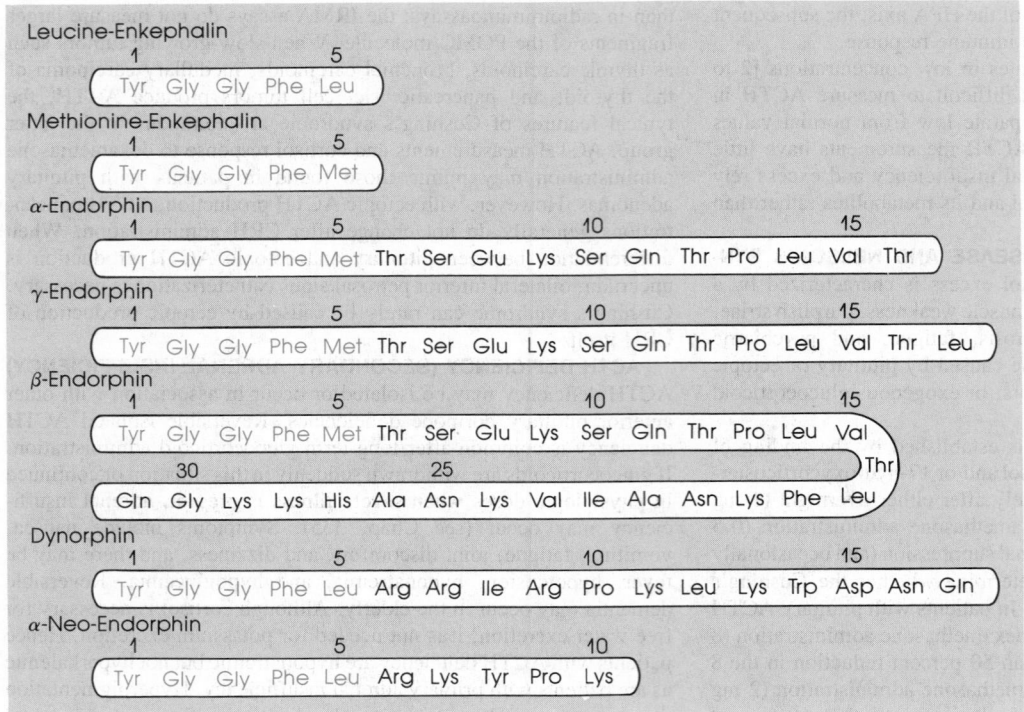

FIGURE 331-7 Structure of several endogenous opiate peptides. The amino-terminal (leftmost) four amino acids are identical in each peptide. At position 5, a methionine or leucine is found.

opioids, including the enkephalins, dynorphins, and neoendorphins. Proenkephalin A gives rise to four copies of met-enkephalin, one copy of leu-enkephalin, and several other opioid compounds; proenkephalin B (also called *prodynorphin*) includes the sequence for the potent opioid dynorphin, several neoendorphins, and other opioids. These opioid precursors are produced in many parts of the brain, including various hypothalamic nuclei. Opioids are also produced in the adrenal medulla, where they are packaged and released with epinephrine both in normal individuals and in patients with pheochromocytomas.

The pituitary is the richest site of endorphin in the body. ACTH- and endorphin-containing cells are found in the anteromedial region of the anterior lobe, at the posterior boundary of the anterior lobe, and in nerve fibers of the posterior lobe. The endorphin- and ACTH-synthesizing neurons of the hypothalamus also project to other regions of the brain. The limbic system contains substantial quantities of immunoreactive β-endorphin, suggesting a role in memory, learning, and emotion.

Neurons containing the enkephalins are even more widely distributed in the central nervous system. Levels are particularly high in the dorsal horn of the spinal cord, a region that contains opiate receptors and is involved in the transmission of pain (see Chap. 11). Enkephalins may act at this location to inhibit pain transmission by sensory nerves. Enkephalin concentrations in the myenteric plexus of the longitudinal muscles of the gastrointestinal tract are higher than in the brain. Enkephalin is released as part of the sympathetic response to stress together with epinephrine and norepinephrine; plasma enkephalin levels are high in patients with pheochromocytoma.

Two approaches have been employed to define the physiologic role of the endogenous opiates: assessment of the effects of administration of morphine or endogeneous opiate peptides and study of the effects of antagonists. Five opiate receptor types have been identified, making it difficult to draw general conclusions from the use of antagonists. Naloxone blocks the effects of endogenously secreted opiates on mu and epsilon receptors, revealing a tonic or physiologic role of opiate peptides. The opiates themselves inhibit gonadotropin release; this may explain the amenorrhea of narcotic addicts. Opiates decrease the function of the pituitary-adrenal axis in humans and stimulate GH and prolactin secretion. Naloxone causes elevations of LH and FSH levels and may prevent the stress-mediated rise in prolactin levels. ACTH and cortisol are elevated only after high doses of naloxone. Naloxone may inhibit vasopressin release in some patients with the syndrome of inappropriate vasopressin secretion (SIADH).

Physiologic actions for these hormones may include (1) morphine-like analgesic properties, (2) euphoria and other behavioral effects, and (3) neurotransmitter and neuromodulator functions. The peptides may play a role in memory, learning, response to stress, reproduction, pain transmission, and regulation of appetite, temperature, and respiration. In addition, the placebo response, acupuncture-mediated analgesia, stress-induced amenorrhea, and the pathogenesis of shock may be mediated in part by enkephalins and the endorphins. Tranquilization, irritability, agitation, violent behavior, catalepsy, narcolepsy, catatonia, the smoking habit, alcoholism, and drug addiction may all be due to biochemical abnormalities of this system.

FIGURE 331-8 Biosynthetic pathway for β-endorphin in the pituitary gland. A single precursor protein, pro-opiomelanocortin (POMC) (molecular weight of approximately 31,000), is initially synthesized from translation of a gene that encodes the structure of adrenocorticotropin (ACTH), β-lipotropin (β-LPH), and β-endorphin. Prohormone-type cleavages can generate other hormones from the same precursor, although this occurs in tissues other than the pituitary. Abbreviations: MSH = melanocyte-stimulating hormone; LPH = lipotropin; CLIP = corticotropin-like intermediate peptide; ACTH = adrenocorticotropin.

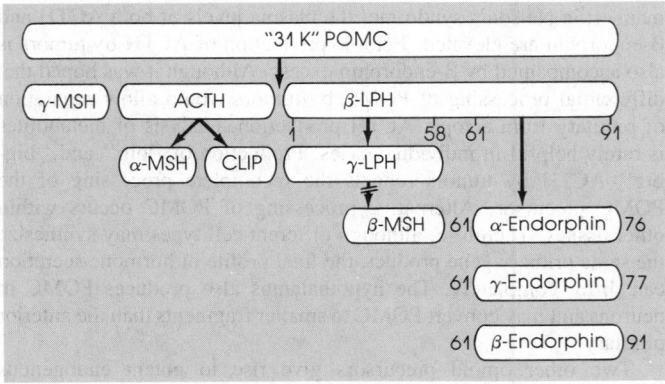

DISEASES OF THE HYPOTHALAMUS AND PITUITARY

Diseases that affect the hypothalamus and pituitary can have both endocrine and nonendocrine manifestations.

HYPOTHALAMUS The human hypothalamus weighs only about 4 g; hypothalamic dysfunction occurs only when disease is bilateral. Tumors in this region are often slow-growing and may achieve large size before symptoms appear. Signs of hydrocephalus due to third ventricle obstruction may coexist with hypopituitarism and hypothalamic dysfunction. Neurologic symptoms and signs may be caused by compression of the optic nerve, chiasm, or tract (see Chap. 19). Large tumors may affect frontal or temporal lobe function.

Nonendocrine functions of the hypothalamus include:

1 Food intake and feeding behavior. The basal hypothalamus controls maintenance of a stable weight. Several regions of the hypothalamus are implicated in hunger and satiety. The ventromedial nucleus is known to be involved in satiety, but it now appears that anterior hypothalamic regions are also concerned. Stimulation of appetite and termination of food ingestion are affected by many neuropeptides and neurotransmitters. Appetite is stimulated by γ-aminobutyric acid (GABA), dopamine, β-endorphin, enkephalin, and neuropeptide Y; appetite is inhibited by serotonin, norepinephrine, cholecystokinin, neurotensin, TRH, naloxone, somatostatin, and vasoactive intestinal peptide (VIP). Hypothalamic obesity in humans is usually associated with lesions in the vicinity of the ventromedial nucleus; this obesity appears to involve a resetting of the weight set point. With tumors in this area, aggressive behavior and marked hyperphagia (possibly related to rapid gastric emptying) occur until the new weight set point is reached. Patients often demonstrate decreased activity and finicky eating once the new set point is reached. Other factors including thyroid and adrenal hormones also influence feeding behavior. Acute hypothalamic damage often causes hyperglycemia, whereas chronic damage may rarely be associated with hypoglycemia.

2 Temperature regulation. The anterior hypothalamus contains warm- and cold-sensitive neurons that respond to local and environmental thermal gradients (see Chaps. 16 and 398). The posterior hypothalamus generates the signals necessary for heat dissipation, and serotonin stimulates heat production, which is blocked by norepinephrine and epinephrine. The temperature increase associated with infections is generated by the hypothalamus. Phagocytic cells throughout the body produce interleukin 1 (endogenous pyrogen), which stimulates the anterior hypothalamus to produce prostaglandin E_2. Prostaglandin E_2 raises the thermostat set point, leading to heat conservation (e.g., vasoconstriction) and increased heat production (e.g., muscle shivering) until blood and core temperatures match the new hypothalamic set point.

Abnormalities of temperature regulation may occur with hypothalamic disease. Hypothermia is a rare consequence of diffuse hypothalamic disease. Paroxysmal hypothermia due to sweating and vasodilatation is accompanied by fatigue, decreased alertness, hypoventilation, and arrhythmias; this syndrome is not prevented by anticonvulsants. Acute hyperthermia may accompany acute pathologic processes such as hemorrhage into the third ventricle, hypothalamic surgery, or hypothalamic infarction. Poikilothermia (a change in body temperature of greater than 1°C with change in environmental temperature) is usually a consequence of posterior hypothalamic disease. Paroxysmal hyperthermia with episodic shaking chills, spiking fevers, and autonomic phenomena is uncommon but may respond to anticonvulsants. It is important to remember that adrenal insufficiency can cause fever or hypothermia and that hypothyroidism may cause hypothermia.

3 Sleep-wake cycle. Lesions in the sleep center of the anterior hypothalamus result in insomnia and agitation, as in some patients with encephalitis. The posterior hypothalamus is important for arousal and maintenance of the waking state; posterior hypothalamic destruction due to ischemia, encephalitis, or trauma can result in a hypersomnolent state from which arousal is possible. Larger lesions extending to the reticular formation of the rostral midbrain cause coma (see Chap. 26).

4 Memory and behavior. Lesions of the ventromedial hypothalamus and premammillary region result in loss of short-term memory, often with Korsakoff's syndrome. However, dorsomedial thalamic lesions correlate best with memory loss (see Chap. 377). Longer-term memory is often intact. Large hypothalamic lesions also may cause symptoms and signs of dementia. The role of ACTH, ACTH fragments, vasopressin, and oxytocin in memory integration is under investigation. Rage reactions may result with ventromedial lesions, and lateral hypothalamic destruction may cause an apathetic state.

5 Thirst. The hypothalamus is the center for vasopressin production and for the control of thirst by serum osmolality. Impaired thirst may occur with hypothalamic lesions; rarely, primary polydipsia without diabetes insipidus is a consequence of hypothalamic lesions (see Chap. 333).

6 Autonomic nervous system function. Parasympathetic outputs are organized in the anterior hypothalamus; sympathetic pathways in the posterior hypothalamus. Diencephalic epilepsy is a rare syndrome associated with paroxysms of autonomic hyperactivity. This syndrome is not clearly epileptic in nature and does not usually respond to anticonvulsants. The clinical picture may mimic that of pheochromocytoma.

A diencephalic syndrome in children, characterized by emaciation, hyperkinesis, and inappropriate affect, often with a cheerful disposition, can be caused by invasive tumors of the anterior and basal hypothalamus. Most of these children die by the age of 2 years, but in those who survive the clinical picture changes to one of increased appetite with obesity, irritability, and rage reactions.

In general, slow-growing tumors produce dementia, disturbances of food intake (obesity or emaciation), and endocrine dysfunction. Acute destructive processes are more likely to cause coma or disturbances of the autonomic nervous system.

Diseases of the anterior hypothalamus include craniopharyngiomas, gliomas of the optic nerve, sphenoid ridge meningiomas, granulomatous disease (including sarcoidosis), germinomas, and aneurysms of the internal carotid artery. Suprasellar pituitary adenomas and tuberculum sella meningiomas may grow into the hypothalamus as well. Lesions of the posterior hypothalamus include gliomas, hamartomas, ependymomas, germinomas, and teratomas.

Precocious puberty, particularly in males, can be associated with "pinealomas." However, these pinealomas actually are germinomas, and the precocious puberty appears to result from the ectopic production of hCG by these tumors rather than from an effect on pituitary gonadotropins.

Craniopharyngiomas Craniopharyngiomas arise from remnants of Rathke's pouch and represent 3 to 5 percent of all intracranial neoplasms. Most of these tumors are suprasellar, but about 15 percent are intrasellar. The tumors are usually cystic or partially cystic, often contain calcium, and are lined with stratified squamous epithelium. Although craniopharyngiomas are usually manifested in childhood, 45 percent of patients are over age 20, and 20 percent are over age 40 at the time of diagnosis.

Children usually present with signs of increased intracranial pressure due to hydrocephalus (80 percent), including headache, vomiting, and papilledema. Visual abnormalities such as loss of vision and field cuts are found in 60 percent. Short stature is sometimes found (7 to 40 percent), but retarded bone age is more common. Delayed sexual development occurs in about 20 percent, and diabetes insipidus may be present.

About 80 percent of adults present with visual complaints, and an additional 10 percent have visual abnormalities on careful testing. Papilledema is present in about 15 percent of adults. Headaches (40 percent), mental deterioration or personality change (26 percent), and hypogonadism (35 percent) are relatively common in adults. Hyperprolactinemia is present in one-third to one-half of patients, but prolactin levels rarely exceed 100 to 150 μg/L. Diabetes insipidus (15 percent), weight gain (15 percent), and panhypopituitarism (7 percent) may occur as well. Rarely, the cyst contents spill into the cerebrospinal fluid, causing a picture of aseptic meningitis. Craniopharyngiomas may enlarge and become symptomatic during pregnancy.

Suprasellar calcification (see Fig. 331-15) in a flocculent, granular, or curvilinear pattern is present on skull x-rays in most children and in some adults with craniopharyngioma. Calcification is evident on CT scan in most of these adults, however. Hypothalamic germinomas may calcify as well. Skull x-ray abnormalities include calcification, sellar enlargement, and signs of increased intracranial pressure in 90 percent of children and 60 percent of adults.

Therapy of craniopharyngiomas is often unsatisfactory. Total removal often results in major functional deficits. We generally favor biopsy and partial resection followed by conventional radiation as a more conservative approach. Tumors less than 3 cm in diameter have a better prognosis.

Germ cell tumors   Germinomas originate in the posterior third ventricle, in the anterior third ventricle (supra- or intrasellar), or in both locations (also see Chap. 322). Germinomas (also known as *atypical teratomas*) were previously confused with parenchymal tumors of the pineal (pinealomas); when located in the anterior third ventricle, they were known as "ectopic pinealomas." Germinomas often infiltrate the hypothalamus and occasionally metastasize to the cerebrospinal fluid or distant sites.

The majority of patients have diabetes insipidus in association with variable anterior pituitary insufficiency. Precocious puberty may occur in boys, probably due to hCG production by these tumors. Diplopia, headache, vomiting, lethargy, weight loss, and hydrocephalus are common. The tumors usually begin in childhood but may be diagnosed in young adults. Because germinomas are radiosensitive, early recognition is important. Germinomas of the nonseminoma type may produce hCG and/or alpha fetoprotein, whereas pure seminomas rarely produce tumor markers (see Chap. 369). Elevated cerebrospinal fluid concentrations of hCG or alpha fetoprotein are virtually diagnostic; when elevated, a biopsy is generally unnecessary. When tumor markers are absent, a biopsy should be considered. When the tumor is located in the anterior third ventricle, biopsy by the transsphenoidal route is often possible. Tumors in the pineal region are more difficult to biopsy, leading some authors to recommend empirical radiation therapy or chemotherapy, whereas others prefer surgical biopsy or debulking followed by radiation and chemotherapy (see Chap. 369).

PITUITARY ADENOMAS   Pituitary adenomas account for about 10 to 15 percent of intracranial neoplasms. They can cause anterior pituitary hormonal imbalance, structural problems related to invasion of surrounding structures, or syndromes of hormone excess. Small pituitary tumors are present in 6 to 24 percent of adults at autopsy. Incidental pituitary tumors (pituitary "incidentalomas") are recognized with increasing frequency now that cranial MRI and CT scans are commonly performed.

Pathology   Pituitary tumors were previously classified as basophilic, acidophilic, or chromophobic on the basis of hematoxylin and eosin staining. Corticotroph adenomas are generally basophilic; the more densely granulated prolactin-secreting tumors are acidophilic; the majority of prolactinomas, sparsely granulated GH-secreting tumors, TSH-secreting and gonadotropin-secreting tumors, and nonsecreting tumors are all chromophobic. Because this classification provides little insight into hormone production, it has been abandoned. Many nonfunctioning pituitary tumors, however, are still referred to as "chromophobes." One classification is based on immunohistochemical staining: corticotroph (ACTH and POMC), somatotroph (GH), thyrotroph (TSH), gonadotroph (LH and FSH), and lactotroph (prolactin).

Pituitary tumors can also be classified by size and invasive characteristics. The following classification is used by Kovacs and Horvath. Microadenomas are <10 mm; macroadenomas are ≥10 mm in greatest diameter. Microadenomas may cause hormonal overproduction but do not cause hypopituitarism, structural problems, or sellar enlargement. Intrapituitary adenomas are within the substance of the pituitary gland; intrasellar adenomas are confined to the sella. Diffuse adenomas may fill the sella and cause focal sellar wall erosions. The distinction between intrasellar and diffuse adenomas may be difficult to make. Invasive adenomas erode through the sella into surrounding tissues, including but not limited to the sphenoid bone, cavernous sinuses, optic chiasm, third ventricle, and brain. Pituitary carcinomas are rare but can give rise to distant metastases.

Endocrine manifestations   Anterior pituitary hormone overproduction is suspected on clinical grounds and confirmed by appropriate laboratory evaluation (see Table 331-5). The most common secretory pituitary tumors are prolactinomas. They cause galactorrhea and hypogonadism, including amenorrhea, infertility, and impotence. GH-secreting tumors are the next most common secretory pituitary tumors and cause acromegaly or gigantism. Next in frequency are corticotroph (ACTH-secreting) adenomas, which cause cortisol excess (Cushing's disease). Although glycoprotein hormone–secreting pituitary adenomas are common by histologic criteria, clinical syndromes of excess LH, FSH, or TSH are rare. TSH-secreting adenomas are a rare cause of hyperthyroidism. Paradoxically, most patients with gonadotropin-secreting adenomas have hypogonadism, although testicular enlargement or testosterone excess may occur.

About 15 percent of patients with tumors that come to surgery have adenomas that secrete more than one pituitary hormone. The most common combination is GH and prolactin, and other common patterns are GH-TSH, GH-prolactin-TSH, and ACTH-prolactin. Most of these tumors have one cell secreting two hormones (unimorphous), but some tumors have two or more cell types, each of which produces a single hormone (polymorphous).

Prolactinomas in women and corticotroph adenomas in both sexes are usually diagnosed while still microadenomas. In contrast, the majority of patients with acromegaly and most men with prolactinomas have macroadenomas at the time of diagnosis. Glycoprotein hormone–secreting tumors are also usually quite large at the time of diagnosis.

About 30 to 40 percent of pituitary adenomas that come to surgery are apparently nonsecretory, although most stain immunohistochemically for pituitary hormones. These statistics are influenced by the fact that most prolactinomas do not require surgery. In some cases, particularly in the case of gonadotropin-secreting tumors, hormonal secretion is overlooked. Some of the "nonfunctioning" pituitary tumors, as well as some functional ones, secrete part of the glycoprotein hormone molecule, most commonly the alpha subunit. In general, tumors without endocrine-related symptoms are large at the time of diagnosis and often cause structural problems. Alpha subunit excess is a frequent finding in patients with TSH-secreting adenomas, and LH beta may be hypersecreted in patients with gonadotropin-secreting tumors.

Null cell tumors (no specific hormones identified by immunostaining) also are generally large when diagnosed, since no hormonal overproduction is present to provide early clues to diagnosis. Oncocytomas are nonsecretory pituitary adenomas with abundant mitochondria, commonly found in older men.

Pituitary adenomas are occasionally part of the multiple endocrine neoplasia type 1 (MEN 1) syndrome (see Chap. 343). This dominantly inherited disease causes adenomas of the pituitary gland, secretory tumors of the endocrine pancreas, and hyperparathyroidism involving multiple parathyroid glands. Pituitary adenomas may secrete GH or prolactin or may be nonfunctioning. Insulinomas and gastrinomas are the most common pancreatic tumors in MEN 1. Pancreatic GHRH-secreting tumors can cause acromegaly and pituitary hyperplasia.

Mass effects of pituitary tumors   VISUAL FIELD DEFECTS   The optic chiasm lies anterior and superior to the pituitary gland, usually 8 to 13 mm above the diaphragma sella, and in 80 percent of normal persons overlies the pituitary fossa; in about 15 percent the chiasm is anterior to the tuberculum sella (prefixed), and in 5 percent it

TABLE 331-5 Pituitary hormone evaluation

Hormone	Excess	Deficiency

Growth hormone	*1* Measurement of plasma growth hormone 1 h following glucose PO
	2 Measurement of IGF-I/SM-C
		1 Measurement of plasma growth hormone 30, 60, and 120 min after one of the following:
		  a Regular insulin 0.1 to 0.15 unit/kg IV
		  b Levodopa 10 mg/kg PO
		  c L-Arginine 0.5 mg/kg intravenously over 30 min
		2 Measurement of IGF-I/SM-C

Prolactin	*1* Measurement of basal serum prolactin, preferably fasting	*1* Measurement of serum prolactin 10 to 20 min after one of the following:
		  a TRH 200 to 500 μg IV
		  b Chlorpromazine 25 mg IM

TSH	*1* Measurement of T_4, free T_4 index, T_3, TSH, TSH alpha	*1* Measurement of T_4, free T_4, free T_4 index, TSH
Gonadotropins	*1* Measurement of FSH, LH, LH beta, testosterone, FSH beta, FSH response to TRH	*1* Measurement of basal LH, FSH in postmenopausal women; no measurements in menstruating, ovulating women *2* Testosterone, FSH, and LH in men

ACTH	*1* Measurement of urine free cortisol*
	2 Dexamethasone suppression by one of the following:
	  a Measurement of 8 A.M. plasma cortisol after administration of 1 mg dexamethasone at midnight
	  b Measurement of 8 A.M. plasma cortisol or 24-h urine 17-hydroxysteroids or free cortisol after 0.5 mg dexamethasone PO q 6 h for 8 doses†
	3 High-dose dexamethasone suppression by one of the following:
	  a Measurement of plasma cortisol after 8 mg dexamethasone PO at midnight
	  b Measurement of 8 A.M. plasma cortisol or 24-h urine 17-hydroxysteroids or free cortisol after 2 mg dexamethasone q 6 h for 8 doses
	4 Metyrapone response (same protocol as for deficiency testing)
	5 Response of plasma ACTH to ovine corticotropin releasing hormone (1 μg/kg body wt)
		1 Measurement of serum cortisol at 30 and 60 min following regular insulin 0.05 to 0.15 units per kilogram IV
		2 Metyrapone response by one of the following:
		  a Measurement of plasma 11-deoxycortisol at 8 A.M. after 30 mg/kg body wt metyrapone at midnight (maximal dose 2 g)
		  b Measurement of 24-h urinary 17-hydroxycorticoids or plasma 11-deoxycortisol day of and day after 750 mg metyrapone q 4 h for 6 doses†
		  c Measurement of 24-h urinary 17-hydroxycorticoids day of and day after 500 mg metyrapone q 2 h for 12 doses†
		3 ACTH stimulation test: Measurement of plasma cortisol and aldosterone at 0 and 60 min after IM or IV administration of 0.25 mg cosyntropin
		4 ?Response of plasma ACTH to ovine corticotropin-releasing hormone (1 μg/kg body weight)

Arginine vasopressin (AVP)	*1* Measurement of serum sodium and osmolality, urine osmolality in presence of normal renal, adrenal, thyroid function *2* Simultaneous measurement of serum osmolality and ADH levels	*1* Comparison of urine osmolality and serum osmolality under conditions of increased AVP secretion‡ *2* Simultaneous measurement of serum osmolality and AVP levels

* Tests 1 and 2 establish the diagnosis of Cushing's syndrome. Tests 3, 4, and 5 localize the Cushing's disease to the pituitary gland. Often bilateral inferior petrosal sinus catheterization will be necessary.
† Give food with metyrapone, patient hospitalized.
‡ May be achieved by water deprivation or saline administration.

overlaps the dorsum sella posteriorly (postfixed). Since 90 percent of the chiasmal axons originate in the macula, loss of central vision is an early finding. Foggy or dim vision is also described by many patients.

The most common visual field defect in patients with pituitary adenomas is a bitemporal hemianopsia, and about 8 percent of patients develop complete loss of vision in one eye with a temporal defect in the opposite eye. Alternatively, patients may demonstrate bitemporal scotomas rather than hemianopsia, particularly with a rapidly growing lesion in association with a prefixed chiasm (see Chap. 19). For this reason, visual field examinations must assess more than the lateral fields of vision. Of those patients with visual field defects, about 9 percent have a single eye defect, most commonly a superior temporal defect. Occasionally, there is a monocular field loss such as a central scotoma that mimics nonpituitary lesions. Pituitary adenomas causing visual field defects are macroadenomas with suprasellar extension; sellar enlargement is the rule.

OCULOMOTOR PALSIES Pituitary adenomas may extend laterally, invade the cavernous sinuses, and cause oculomotor palsies. When this occurs, visual field defects are usually not present. Involvement of the third cranial nerve is most common and may mimic diabetic third nerve neuropathy in that pupillary reactivity is usually preserved (see Chap. 19). Additional findings associated with lateral extension of the adenoma may include involvement of the fourth and sixth cranial nerves, pain or numbness in the distribution of the fifth cranial nerve, and compression or obstruction of the carotid artery.

Headaches are common in patients with larger tumors and are also present in the majority of patients with acromegaly. Headaches may be exacerbated by coughing. Headaches are thought to be due to stretching of the diaphragma sella but may be vascular in origin and

may be referred to several locations, including the vertex of skull and to retroorbital, frontooccipital, frontotemporal, or occipital-cervical areas.

Very large pituitary tumors may invade the hypothalamus and cause hyperphagia, abnormal temperature regulation, loss of consciousness, and loss of hormonal input from the hypothalamus. Obstructive hydrocephalus involving the third ventricle or causing diabetes insipidus is less common with pituitary adenomas than with craniopharyngiomas. Tumor invasion of the temporal lobe may cause complex partial seizures; invasion of the posterior fossa may be associated with brainstem dysfunction, and invasion into the frontal lobes causes alterations in mental state and frontal release signs.

PITUITARY APOPLEXY Acute hemorrhagic infarction of a pituitary adenoma may cause a dramatic syndrome including severe headache, nausea, vomiting, and depression of consciousness. Ophthalmoplegia, visual and pupillary disturbances, and meningismus may be present. Most of these symptoms are caused by direct pressure from the tumor, whereas meningismus results from blood in the cerebrospinal fluid. The syndrome may either evolve slowly over a period of 24 to 48 h or may lead to sudden death.

Pituitary apoplexy is found most commonly in patients with somatotroph or corticotroph adenomas, but it may be the first clinical manifestation of a pituitary tumor. Both anticoagulation and radiotherapy predispose to hemorrhagic infarction. Rarely, pituitary apoplexy produces "autohypophysectomy" with "cure" of acromegaly, Cushing's disease, or hyperprolactinemia. Hypopituitarism is a common sequela; although hormonal measurements may be normal during the acute phase, cortisol and gonadal steroid concentrations decline over the ensuing days, and thyroxine concentrations decline over weeks. Diabetes insipidus is rare.

It is important to differentiate between pituitary apoplexy and a leaking aneurysm; MRI may allow this distinction to be made, but angiography is often required. Acute pituitary apoplexy is generally considered a neurosurgical emergency and may require acute decompression of the pituitary, generally via the transsphenoidal route. Many pituitary tumors contain small hemorrhagic foci that are clinically silent.

Therapy of pituitary adenomas   Ideal therapy for pituitary adenomas would permanently correct hormonal hypersecretion without causing hypopituitarism and would shrink or remove the tumor mass without additional morbidity or mortality. Therapy for microadenomas may achieve both these goals, whereas therapy for macroadenomas is usually less successful. In considering therapy, it is critical to weigh the disability due to the tumor against any disability that may arise from the treatment. Regardless of tumor size, the therapy should not be worse than the disease. Potentially serious diseases such as Cushing's disease or acromegaly may require more aggressive treatment than do prolactinomas. (See also sections on individual pituitary hormones in this chapter.)

MEDICAL THERAPY   Bromocriptine, a dopamine agonist, is the therapy of choice in the United States for most patients with microprolactinomas who require therapy. Bromocriptine corrects hyperprolactinemia in almost all patients with microprolactinomas; however, when the drug is stopped, prolactin levels often return to pretreatment levels. More potent dopapime agonists are available outside the United States.

Bromocriptine side effects of nausea, gastric irritation, and postural hypotension can be minimized by initially giving a low dose (1.25 mg) at bedtime with a snack. Other side effects include headache, fatigue, abdominal cramps, nasal congestion, and constipation. The dosage is gradually increased to a twice-daily schedule (most commonly 2.5 mg bid). Vaginal bromocriptine is better tolerated by some patients.

Bromocriptine is also effective in large prolactin-secreting macroadenomas. (Nonfunctioning macroadenomas with minimal prolactin elevation must be excluded.) Prolactin is lowered by at least 80 percent in 90 percent and to normal values in about 37 percent of patients. Abnormal visual fields return to normal in most; the tumor shrinks by 50 percent in about 40 percent of patients within 3 months. Tumor shrinkage may be accompanied by reversal of hypopituitarism. With giant adenomas, bromocriptine-induced tumor shrinkage may rarely cause a devastating intracranial hemorrhage. Prolactin levels quickly rise when bromocriptine is stopped; however, tumor regrowth may be delayed.

Surgery is required when visual field defects do not rapidly return to normal (e.g., after 1 to 3 months of bromocriptine). Symptomatic hyperprolactinemia with inadequate response to bromocriptine requires further therapy with surgery and/or radiation. In the United States, bromocriptine is usually stopped at the onset of pregnancy and reinstituted if tumor regrowth is symptomatic; alternatively, bromocriptine can be continued throughout pregnancy, although it is not licensed for this indication in the United States.

The somatostatin analogue octreotide is the most effective adjunctive therapy in acromegaly; it also may be appropriate as temporary primary therapy or in preparation for surgery. Bromocriptine is an effective adjunct in some patients with acromegaly, particularly those with coexistent hyperprolactinemia. GH concentrations rarely return to normal, but symptomatic improvement and tumor shrinkage may occur. Bromocriptine or octreotide (though not licensed for this purpose) should be considered in acromegalic subjects whose GH or IGF-I/SM-C levels remain elevated following surgery or who are waiting for radiation therapy to be effective. Nonfunctioning and gonadotropin-secreting adenomas usually shrink 10 percent or less in response to bromocriptine, even when high doses are used. Octreotide also may be useful adjunctive therapy in patients with TSH-secreting adenomas.

SURGERY   Transsphenoidal surgery of pituitary microadenomas is safe and frequently corrects hormonal oversecretion. Hormonal overproduction is corrected within 24 h in 75 percent of patients with Cushing's disease due to corticotroph microadenomas, acromegaly with GH concentrations of <40 µg/L, and microprolactinomas associated with serum prolactin concentrations of <200 µg/L. The initial success rate for microprolactinomas varies among institutions, with reported figures ranging from 50 to 95 percent. Unfortunately, after initially successful surgery, hyperprolactinemia recurs in about 17 percent of patients followed for 3 to 5 years and possibly in 50 percent after 5 to 10 years. The recurrence rates after initially successful surgery in acromegaly and Cushing's disease are not well established but are substantial.

The mortality rate for transsphenoidal surgery of microadenomas is 0.27 percent, with a morbidity rate of about 1.7 percent, based on 2600 surgical procedures. Major complications include cerebrospinal fluid rhinorrhea, oculomotor palsy, and visual loss.

Pituitary surgery is less successful with larger secretory tumors. In patients with serum prolactin concentrations of >200 µg/L or GH concentrations of >40 µg/L, hormone concentrations return to normal in only 30 percent following surgery. Surgery is successful in about 40 to 60 percent of patients with Cushing's disease due to corticotroph macroadenomas. Recurrence rates with these secretory macroadenomas after a surgery-induced remission are uncertain; in the case of prolactin-secreting tumors, hyperprolactinemia recurs in 10 to 80 percent of patients. Whether pretreatment with octreotide in acromegalic patients with invasive macroadenomas improves the surgical success rate is under investigation.

Although visual field abnormalities are usually reversible with surgery, cure of the tumor is unlikely. The intrasellar portion of tumors invading the cavernous sinus may be debulked, but parasellar extension remains. Early series noted an 85 percent symptomatic recurrence (due to structural problems such as visual field defects) over 10 years in patients treated with surgery alone. When radiation therapy was used in combination with surgery, the 10-year recurrence was 15 percent. These series antedated modern radiologic techniques, hormone measurements, and medical therapy and may not be applicable to current practice.

Surgery for macroadenomas has a mortality rate of around 0.86 percent and a morbidity rate of about 6.3 percent. Hypopituitarism occurs in an additional 10 percent of patients. Transient diabetes insipidus occurs in about 5 percent, and permanent diabetes insipidus occurs in 1 percent. Major complications of surgery for macroadenoma include cerebrospinal fluid rhinorrhea (3.3 percent), permanent visual loss (1.5 percent), permanent oculomotor palsy (0.6 percent), and meningitis (0.5 percent).

We generally treat microprolactinomas with bromocriptine. However, we recommend surgery for those patients with microprolactinoma who require therapy and are intolerant of dopamine agonists. Surgery generally does not result in hypopituitarism in this relatively benign disease. Surgery is usually our treatment of choice in patients with acromegaly or Cushing's disease because in most instances rapid reversal of hormonal hypersecretion is essential and because cure can often be achieved. Since Cushing's disease and acromegaly are serious diseases, more extensive surgery that results in hypopituitarism may be required.

RADIATION THERAPY   Conventional radiation therapy is effective in preventing tumor growth (70 to 90 percent) but is unsatisfactory in the acute management of pituitary hyperfunction. Therapy generally consists of 4500 cGy (4500 rad) at 1.8 Gy (180 rad) per day over 5 weeks using rotational techniques. GH values of <5 µg/L are achieved in half of acromegalics after 5 years and in 70 percent after 10 years; values of <2.5 µg/L are achieved in 40 percent and <1 µg/L in only 20 percent by 10 to 15 years. Data on IGF-I/SM-C are not readily available. Conventional radiation alone is rarely successful in treating corticotroph adenomas in adults. The major complications of conventional radiation are hypopituitarism in up to 50 percent and posttherapy lassitude and fatigue lasting many months in the majority. Whether subtle cognitive defects occur is less certain. We generally use radiation as an adjunct to surgery and medical therapy for patients with continued symptomatic hormonal oversecretion (GH and prolactin) and for those with substantial residual tumor after surgery or when tumor regrowth is rapid. Slow tumor regrowth over 5 or 6 years is usually treated with repeat surgery.

The "gamma knife" delivers 4000 to 10,000 cGy (4000 to 10,000 rad) through several hundred portals in a single session, thought to be equivalent to two to three times the total dose given by conventional radiation. Preliminary results using 4000 to 7000 cGy for acromegaly are comparable with those for conventional radiation. Therapy for Cushing's disease with 7000 to 10,000 cGy is apparently successful in up to 75 percent of adults; this is comparable to heavy-particle therapy (see below) and apparently more effective than conventional radiation therapy.

Heavy-particle therapy with proton beam or alpha particles is effective in treating secretory adenomas, but response is slow. Tumors with suprasellar extension or tissue invasion are generally excluded from such series. With proton beam therapy at the Harvard cyclotron, radiation doses of up to 14,000 cGy (14,000 rad) can be given safely without damage to surrounding structures. At 2 years, 28 percent of acromegalics achieve GH values of <5 μg/L; this response increases to 56 percent at 5 years and 75 percent by 10 years. Values of IGF-I/SM-C are not reported. With Cushing's disease proton beam corrects the hypercortisolism in 55 percent at 2 years and in 80 percent by 5 years. Proton beam therapy effectively lowers ACTH and stops growth of most corticotroph adenomas in patients with Nelson's syndrome, with the exception of adenomas that are invasive at the time of therapy. Long-term results for treatment of other tumors with proton beam therapy are not available.

Complications of heavy-particle therapy include hypopituitarism in at least 20 percent of patients, although the exact long-term prevalence of this complication is uncertain. Visual field defects and oculomotor dysfunction, usually temporary, have been reported in about 1.5 percent of patients. The major drawback of all forms of radiotherapy is the length of time that must elapse before hormonal hypersecretion is corrected.

Bromocriptine (or another dopamine agonist, where available) is the therapy of choice for macroprolactinomas. Surgery and/or radiation therapy is not usually necessary but may be required for patients with persistent structural problems, symptomatic hyperprolactinemia, or intolerance to dopamine agonists. Patients with nonfunctioning macroadenomas, including "incidentalomas," require transsphenoidal surgery when the macroadenoma is symptomatic, near the optic chiasm, or growing on serial MRI or CT scans. Indications for conventional and heavy-particle radiation are discussed below. Heavy-particle therapy (or possibly the "gamma knife") is an effective alternative to surgery in patients with acromegaly, Cushing's disease, or large intrasellar nonfunctioning tumors who have contraindications to or refuse surgery. We prefer bilateral adrenalectomy in patients whose pituitary Cushing's disease is not cured by one or two transsphenoidal operations; others employ heavy-particle or "gamma knife" radiation. Persistent acromegaly is treated with medical and/or radiation therapy. Transfrontal surgery is occasionally required, particularly in patients with giant adenomas.

Pituitary adenomas may be discovered during MRI or CT scanning of the brain for other purposes (pituitary "incidentaloma"). With pituitary microadenomas, hormonal overproduction must be identified and treated; hypopituitarism and structural symptoms do not occur. A follow-up scan at 6 months, then yearly for 2 years, and subsequently every 2 to 5 years seems reasonable.

Pituitary macroadenomas, however discovered, need to be evaluated for hormonal over- and underproduction and structural effects, including visual field abnormalities. The approach to the hormonally active tumor has been described above. Should nonfunctioning tumors be treated with bromocriptine? Is prophylactic surgery or radiation therapy indicated? How often should the MRI and endocrine evaluations be repeated? The answers are unknown. We tend to recommend surgery for tumors directly abutting on the optic chiasm. For other tumors, MRI scans should be repeated at 6 and 12 months and yearly

TABLE 331-6 Causes of hypopituitarism

Isolated hormone deficiencies
 1 Congenital or acquired deficiencies
Tumors
 1 Large pituitary adenomas
 2 Pituitary apoplexy
 3 Hypothalamic tumors, e.g., craniopharyngiomas, germinomas, chordomas, meningiomas, gliomas, and others
 4 Metastatic carcinoma
Inflammatory diseases
 1 Granulomatous disease, e.g., sarcoidosis, tuberculosis, syphilis, granulomatous hypophysitis
 2 Eosinophilic granuloma
 3 Lymphocytic hypophysitis (autoimmune)
Vascular diseases
 1 Sheehan's postpartum necrosis
 2 ? Diabetic peripartum necrosis
 3 Carotid aneurysm
Destructive-traumatic events
 1 Surgery
 2 Stalk section
 3 Radiation (conventional—hypothalamus; heavy-particle—pituitary)
 4 Trauma
Developmental anomalies
 1 Pituitary aplasia
 2 Basal encephalocoele
Infiltration
 1 Hemochromatosis
 2 Amyloidosis
"Idiopathic" causes
 1 ?Autoimmune disease

thereafter. If growth occurs, surgery or radiation with conventional radiation, "gamma knife," or protons may be indicated. Ten to fifteen percent of tumors shrink with bromocriptine therapy; how many stabilize without therapy is unknown.

HYPOPITUITARISM *Hypopituitarism* refers to deficiency of one or more pituitary hormones and has many causes (Table 331-6). Pituitary hormone deficiency may be congenital or acquired (see Chap. 332). Isolated GH or gonadotropin deficiency is common. Temporary ACTH deficiency as a consequence of long-term glucocorticoid therapy is also common, but permanent isolated deficiency of ACTH or TSH is rare. Deficiency of any of the anterior pituitary hormones may occur at the level of the pituitary gland or the hypothalamus. When diabetes insipidus is present, the primary defect is almost invariably in the hypothalamus or high pituitary stalk, often in conjunction with mild hyperprolactinemia and anterior pituitary hypofunction.

Manifestations of hypopituitarism depend on the specific pituitary hormones that are lacking. Growth failure due to GH deficiency is a common presenting complaint in children. GH deficiency in adults causes more subtle manifestations such as fine wrinkling around the eyes and mouth and in subjects with diabetes mellitus increased sensitivity to insulin. The cardiovascular mortality of GH-deficient individuals is increased. Complaints related to gonadotropin deficiency include amenorrhea and infertility in women and testosterone deficiency and decreased libido, decreased beard and body hair, and preservation of a youthful scalp hairline in men. TSH deficiency causes hypothyroidism with fatigue, cold intolerance, and puffy skin in the absence of goiter. ACTH deficiency results in cortisol deficiency, manifested by fatigue; decreased appetite; weight loss; decreased skin and nipple pigmentation; abnormal response to stress characterized by fever, hypotension, and hyponatremia; and a high mortality rate. Unlike primary adrenal insufficiency (Addison's disease) ACTH deficiency does not cause hyperpigmentation, hyperkalemia, or salt loss. With combined ACTH and gonadotropin deficiency, axillary and pubic hair may be lost. Children with combined GH and cortisol deficiency often develop hypoglycemia. AVP deficiency causes diabetes insipidus with polyuria and increased thirst. When pituitary adenomas impair anterior pituitary function, GH is often the first hormone to be compromised, followed by deficiencies of gonadotropins, TSH, and ACTH. Panhypopituitarism may be accompanied by inappropriate secretion of vasopressin (see Chap. 333).

Etiology Damage to the anterior pituitary is commonly due to a pituitary adenoma (with or without infarction), pituitary surgery, heavy-particle pituitary irradiation, closed head trauma, or infarction during the postpartum period (Sheehan's syndrome). Postpartum pituitary infarction occurs in the setting of hemorrhage with systemic hypotension; vasospasm is thought to mediate the pituitary destruction that ensues. The enlarged pituitary gland of pregnancy may be more vulnerable to ischemia. Inability to lactate is the most common initial clinical clue, and other symptoms of hypopituitarism may unfold over months or years. The condition is sometimes diagnosed years after the primary event. Although clinical diabetes insipidus is rare in this setting, a decreased vasopressin response to appropriate stimuli is common. Patients with diabetes mellitus are also prone to develop hypopituitarism late in pregnancy.

Lymphocytic hypophysitis that causes hypopituitarism is primarily a disease of women either during pregnancy or in the postpartum period. In this syndrome, a mass lesion is often seen on MRI or CT scanning which, when biopsied, consists of lymphocytic infiltration. Lymphocytic hypophysitis is due to autoimmune pituitary destruction and often occurs with other autoimmune diseases such as Hashimoto's (autoimmune) thyroiditis and gastric atrophy (see Chaps. 334 and 343). Circulating antibodies to prolactin cells have been identified in some patients. It is not clear whether autoimmune hypophysitis is a common cause of "idiopathic" hypopituitarism in adults.

Hypothalamic or pituitary stalk damage has many causes (see Table 331-6). Certain lesions in this region, such as sarcoidosis, metastatic carcinoma, germinomas, histiocytosis, and craniopharyngiomas, commonly cause diabetes insipidus along with hypofunction of the anterior pituitary. Pituitary insufficiency, resulting from conventional radiation to the brain or the pituitary, is thought to be largely hypothalamic in origin, although diabetes insipidus generally does not occur.

"Functional" hypopituitarism is common. Anorexia nervosa, severe stress, and major illness are all associated with reversible LHRH deficiency. Emotional stress in children may cause GH deficiency and cessation of growth (*psychosocial dwarfism*). Severe illness may be associated with TSH and free T_4 deficiency (part of the "sick euthyroid" syndrome). ACTH deficiency occurs after long-term suppression of the hypothalamic-pituitary-adrenal axis; fortunately, ACTH deficiency is not a consequence of severe illness.

Diagnosis (See Table 331-5) To diagnose GH deficiency, the most reliable GH stimulus is insulin-induced hypoglycemia in which the blood sugar declines to less than 2.2 pmol/L (40 mg/dL) (Fig. 331-9). A GH concentration of >10 μg/L after hypoglycemia, levodopa, or arginine effectively excludes GH deficiency. Measuring the basal GH or serum IGF-I/SM-C concentration is less reliable, because GH levels are undetectable in normal persons for much of the day and because IGF-I/SM-C concentrations in patients with GH deficiency may overlap the normal range. Integrated 24-h GH secretion may be low in some short children with normal response to GH provocative stimuli.

Cortisol deficiency is potentially life-threatening. Basal cortisol function may be preserved in the face of extensive pituitary destruction; consequently, the ability of pituitary ACTH secretion to increase in response to "stress" must be assessed. Either the insulin tolerance test or the metyrapone test can be used to determine the adequacy of ACTH reserve; the ACTH stimulation test is a safer but less sensitive alternative. ACTH secretory dysfunction may occur after radiation therapy. Despite normal insulin tolerance tests, these individuals have low 24-h integrated cortisol secretion and excretion; symptomatic improvement occurs with glucocorticoid therapy.

The insulin tolerance test is safely performed on an outpatient basis in younger patients without heart disease or diseases predisposing to seizures (see Fig. 331-9 and Table 331-5). Both cortisol and GH responses are measured. If hypopituitarism is strongly suspected, a lower dose of regular insulin (0.05 to 0.1 units per kilogram of body

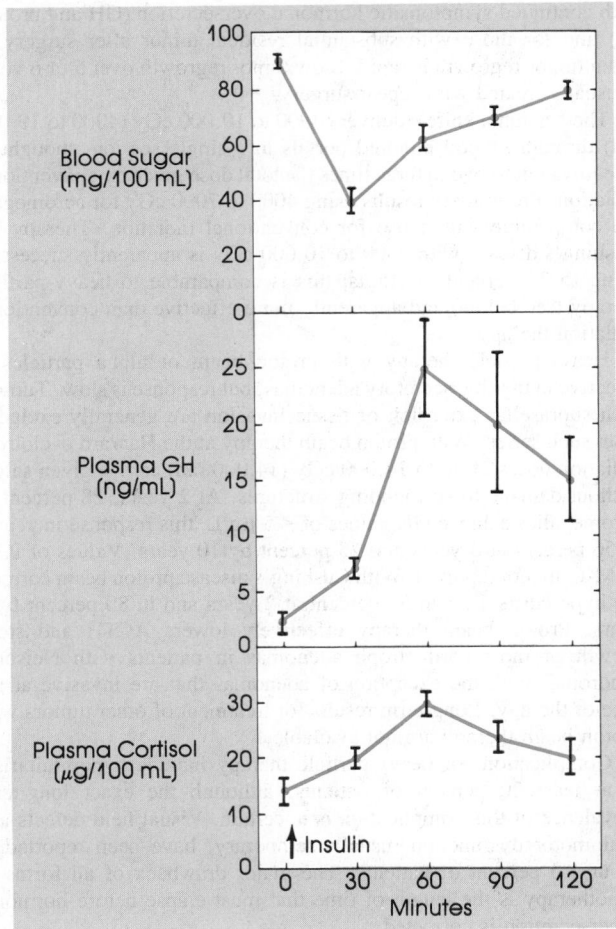

FIGURE 331-9 The insulin tolerance test. After an intravenous injection of regular insulin (0.1 unit per kilogram of body weight) a fall in blood sugar and rise in plasma GH and cortisol is expected. This test permits evaluation of both GH and ACTH in patients with pituitary disease. (*After KJ Catt, Lancet 1:933, 1970.*)

weight) should be employed. After adequate hypoglycemia, the peak plasma cortisol level should be greater than 500 nmol/L (19 μg/dL), although other criteria have been suggested. Since the metyrapone test can precipitate acute adrenal insufficiency in patients with low basal cortisol secretory rates, it should always be performed in the hospital setting when the 8 A.M. basal plasma cortisol level is less than 230 nmol/L (9 μg/dL). A normal response to metyrapone administration (see Table 331-5) has been variably defined, but one criterion is an increase of plasma 11-deoxycortisol to greater than 200 nmol/L (7.5 μg/dL) and of the urinary 17-hydroxysteroids to at least twofold over baseline, usually to a value greater than 60 μmol/d (22 mg/d). The plasma cortisol must concomitantly fall to less than 110 nmol/L (4 μg/dL) to ensure that there has been an adequate stimulus for ACTH release if these criteria have not been met. Although ACTH responses to insulin-hypoglycemia and metyrapone have not been well-standardized, a peak ACTH concentration of >40 pmol/L (200 pg/mL) is considered normal.

The rapid ACTH stimulation test (see Table 331-5) may be the safest and most convenient screening test for determining the adequacy of the pituitary-adrenal axis. Since the response of the adrenal gland to exogenous ACTH is dependent on prior endogenous ACTH exposure, it follows that patients with profound ACTH deficiency will have a deficient adrenal response to exogenous ACTH stimulation. However, the rapid ACTH stimulation test may be normal in some patients with abnormal insulin tolerance tests and therefore may not detect all who are at risk for stress-induced adrenal insufficiency.

Thus, whereas an abnormal ACTH stimulation test is indicative of an abnormal pituitary-adrenal axis, a normal response in the rapid ACTH stimulation test [cortisol >500 nmol/L (19 µg/dL)] does not always establish that the pituitary-adrenal axis is normal.

Gonadotropin function is easier to evaluate. In women with regular menses, gonadotropin secretion is normal, and gonadotropin measurements are superfluous. Likewise, a man with a normal serum testosterone level and normal spermatogenesis need not have gonadotropins measured. In postmenopausal women, gonadotropin levels are elevated (an endogenous stimulation test); "normal" levels suggest gonadotropin deficiency. Estrogen deficiency in women and testosterone deficiency in men in the absence of elevated gonadotropins imply gonadotropin deficiency.

To diagnose central hypothyroidism (thyrotropin deficiency), the serum T_4 and free T_4 (or T_3 resin uptake and free T_4 index) should first be measured. If these are in the midnormal range, TSH function is likely to be normal. If T_4 and free T_4 are low and the serum TSH level is not elevated, central hypothyroidism is present. Minimal TSH elevation (with bioinactive TSH) can occur in hypothalamic hypothyroidism, usually with low free T_4 concentrations. Mild central hypothyroidism, a consideration in patients with known pituitary disease who have low-normal T_4 and free T_4 concentrations, remains a clinical diagnosis. Before considering the diagnosis of isolated TSH deficiency in patients with the biochemical features of central hypothyroidism without evidence of other pituitary hormone deficiency, it is important to exclude the thyroxine-binding globulin (TBG) deficiency syndrome (low T_4, increased T_3 resin uptake, low to low-normal free T_4 index, normal TSH) and the "sick euthyroid" syndrome (low T_4, low free T_4 or free T_4 index, normal or low TSH) (see Chap. 334).

Several diagnostic tests utilize hypothalamic-releasing hormones to assess pituitary reserve. While these tests are *not helpful* in assessing the adequacy of anterior pituitary function, they can be useful in certain situations. In patients with isolated gonadotropin deficiency, the gonadotropin response to gonadorelin (synthetic LHRH) may be useful in predicting which patients will respond to therapy with gonadorelin. CRH testing may be useful in the differential diagnosis of Cushing's syndrome but does not indicate whether the pituitary-adrenal axis will respond appropriately to stress. TRH stimulation testing is useful in some patients in supporting the diagnosis of hyperthyroidism, recurrent acromegaly, or gonadotropin-secreting tumors and in those cases in which documentation of prolactin deficiency is necessary to support a diagnosis of more generalized anterior pituitary hormone deficiency (e.g., mild central hypothyroidism). TRH testing is not necessary in the evaluation for central hypothyroidism and is not reliable in separating pituitary from hypothalamic hypothyroidism. "Mega" tests with multiple releasing hormones have little clinical utility.

Therapy Multiple hormones must be replaced in patients with panhypopituitarism, but cortisol replacement is most important. We prefer prednisone for matters of convenience and cost, but many physicians use cortisone acetate or hydrocortisone (cortisol). Prednisone (5 to 7.5 mg) or cortisone acetate (20 to 37.5 mg) can be given to some patients as a single morning dosage, whereas others require divided doses (two-thirds at 8 A.M., one-third at 3 A.M.). Hypopituitary patients may require lower daily glucocorticoid dosages than do patients with Addison's disease and do not require mineralocorticoid replacement. In stress situations or when preparing these patients for pituitary or other surgery, higher doses of glucocorticoids should be administered (e.g., for major surgery, hydrocortisone hemisuccinate 50 to 75 mg IM/IV every 6 h or methyl prednisolone sodium succinate 15 mg IM/IV every 6 h). Levothyroxine is the therapy of choice in central hypothyroidism (0.05 to 0.15 mg/d). The free T_4 levels should be monitored rather than TSH. Since thyroxine accelerates the degradation of cortisol and can precipitate adrenal crisis in patients with limited pituitary reserve, glucocorticoid replacement should always precede levothyroxine therapy in panhypopituitarism. Hypogonadism in women is treated with estrogen-progestogen combinations

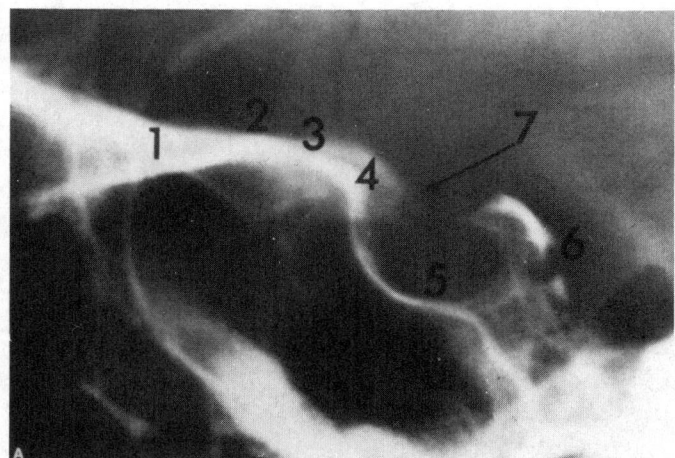

FIGURE 331-10 X-ray of the sella, lateral view. Note (1) planum sphenoidal, (2) limbus sphenoidal, (3) sulcus chiasmaticus, (4) tuberculum sellae, (5) sella floor with distinct lamina dura, (6) dorsum sellae, (7) anterior clinoid, and (8) sphenoid sinus. (*From SM Wolpert, in KD Post et al, eds, The Pituitary Adenoma, New York, Plenum, 1980.*)

and in men with testosterone esters by injection. To achieve fertility, gonadotropins must be administered by injection in patients with pituitary disease, whereas gonadorelin may be successful in those with hypothalamic disease. GH deficiency is not currently treated in adults; in children, GH administration usually is required, but GHRH injections may be effective in those with hypothalamic disease (see Chap. 332). Diabetes insipidus is treated with nasal desmopressin (usually 0.05 to 0.1 mL twice a day) (see Chap. 333).

RADIOLOGY OF THE PITUITARY Conventional posteroanterior and lateral skull x-rays define the contours of the sella turcica (Fig. 331-10). Abnormalities that may be identified on these films include enlargement, erosions, hyperostosis, and calcification in the region of the sella. However, detailed study of pituitary and hypothalamic lesions requires MRI or CT scanning (Fig. 331-11). Anterior tomograms of the sella may be required to delineate the bony anatomy before transsphenoidal surgery; however, the high radiation doses delivered by tomography and the limited information provided make routine tomography obsolete. Angiography may be required when an aneurysm or vascular malformation is suspected as a cause of an enlarged sella; MRI often obviates the need for this study.

MRI imaging (usually before and after intravenous injection of the contrast agent gadolinium DPTA; see Chap. 365) is the imaging study of choice for pituitary and hypothalamic abnormalities. Details of the optic chiasm, pituitary stalk, pituitary gland itself, intracavernous portion of the carotid artery, and relation to the cavernous sinus can be delineated on MRI scanning (Figs. 331-11 and 331-12). Advantages over CT scanning include lack of radiation, lack of iodinated contrast material, superior tissue contrast, and direct multiplanar capability. MRI is clearly superior to CT scanning in delineating microadenomas, visualizing the optic chiasm, and detecting cavernous sinus invasion. Patients with severe claustrophobia, those with ferrometallic aneurysm clips, and those with pacemakers require CT imaging. The use of sedatives and a prone position may allow patients with mild claustrophobia to tolerate the MRI. MRI is less useful when details of bony erosion or calcification are desired. Specific CT scan problems include radiation to the lens of the eye, artifacts due to bone and dental amalgam, and limited soft tissue density resolution.

The normal pituitary has an appearance similar to brain white matter on most MRI images; it has a height of 3 to 7 mm, although values up to 9 mm can be found, particularly in young women. The upper aspect is flat, concave, or, in younger patients, convex. The stalk is midline and is generally less than 2 mm in diameter. The posterior pituitary usually has a bright signal on T1-weighted images;

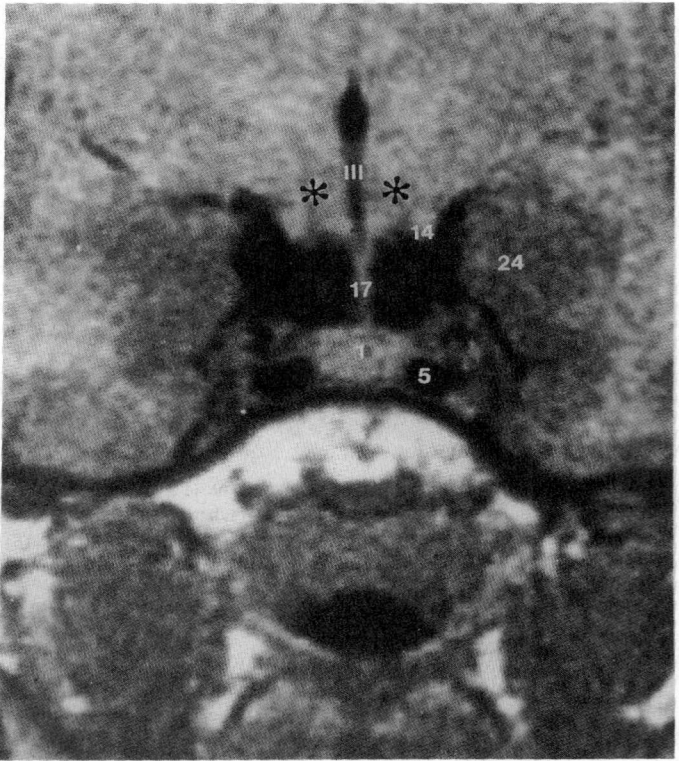

FIGURE 331-11 Coronal T1-weighted MRI scan through the posterior portion of the supraoptic hypothalamus (*). Note the anterior pituitary (1), cavernous sinus with internal carotid artery (5), proximal optic tracts (14), pituitary stalk (17), medial temporal lobes (24), and third ventricle (III). *(From Quint.)*

10 percent of normal individuals lack this intense signal. Cerebrospinal fluid appears dark on T1-weighted images and bright on T2-weighted images and is easily visualized within the sella in patients with the empty sella syndrome (Fig. 331-13). The normal pituitary gland, stalk, and cavernous sinus all show enhanced signal after intravenous gadolinium on T1-weighted images. Microadenomas do not enhance or have delayed enhancement, allowing improved resolution of these lesions (see Fig. 331-12). Five minutes after gadolinium administration, this contrast may no longer be evident. Stalk deviation and upward bulging of the pituitary suggest a microadenoma but are not specific. Up to 20 percent of normal persons show pituitary abnormalities on contrast-enhanced CT scan or MRI. In random autopsies, up to one-fourth of individuals have small pituitary abnormalities (e.g., microadenomas, cysts, metastatic tumors, pituitary infarcts), but it is unclear whether such abnormalities correspond to the focal abnormalities on CT and MRI scanning.

Localization of corticotroph adenomas in patients with Cushing's disease may be helpful in directing the surgical approach. MRI in this situation may be negative in 30 percent or more, and incidental nonfunctioning adenomas may be present in some patients with pituitary Cushing's disease. Petrosal catheterization is useful when the MRI is negative and when the question of ectopic versus pituitary Cushing's disease is unresolved. Whether it is necessary in all presumed pituitary Cushing's disease is uncertain. In patients with modest prolactin elevations, the purpose of pituitary and hypothalamic imaging is to exclude larger pathologic entities. Whether a microprolactinoma is actually visualized is less important, since this disorder is generally treated medically.

Pituitary macroadenomas causing sella enlargement with or without bony erosion may be suspected after conventional radiography. However, these findings are not specific. Additional findings on skull x-rays in acromegaly may include prognathism, enlarged paranasal sinuses, hyperostosis of the external occipital protuberance, increased density of the central bone of the sella, and an enlarged square sella

FIGURE 331-12 *A.* Coronal noncontrast T1-weighted MRI scan demonstrates pituitary gland asymmetry *(arrow)* compatible with a pituitary microadenoma. Cavernous internal carotid artery (5), optic chiasm (13), sphenoid sinus (21), and temporal lobe (24). *B.* Coronal contrast (gadolinium) enhanced T1-weighted MRI scan identifies a 4-mm right paramidline microadenoma *(arrows)*. *(From Quint.)*

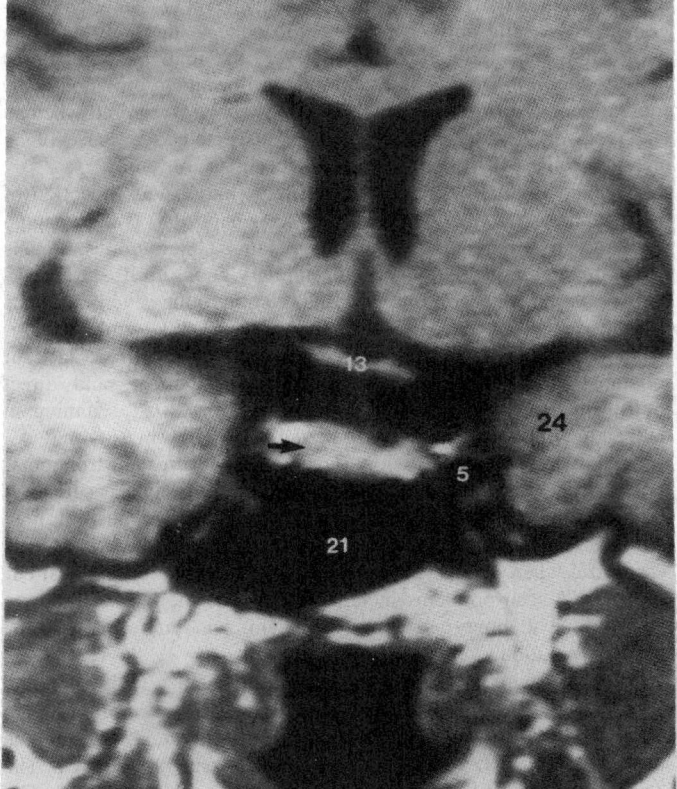

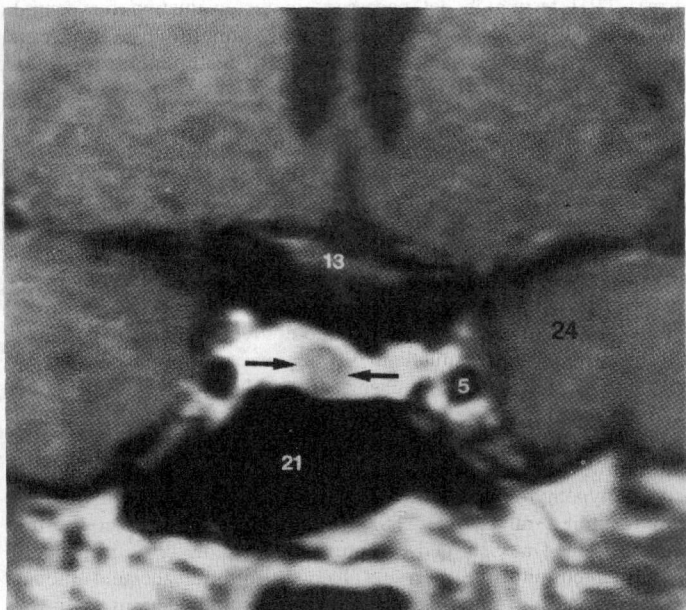

A

B

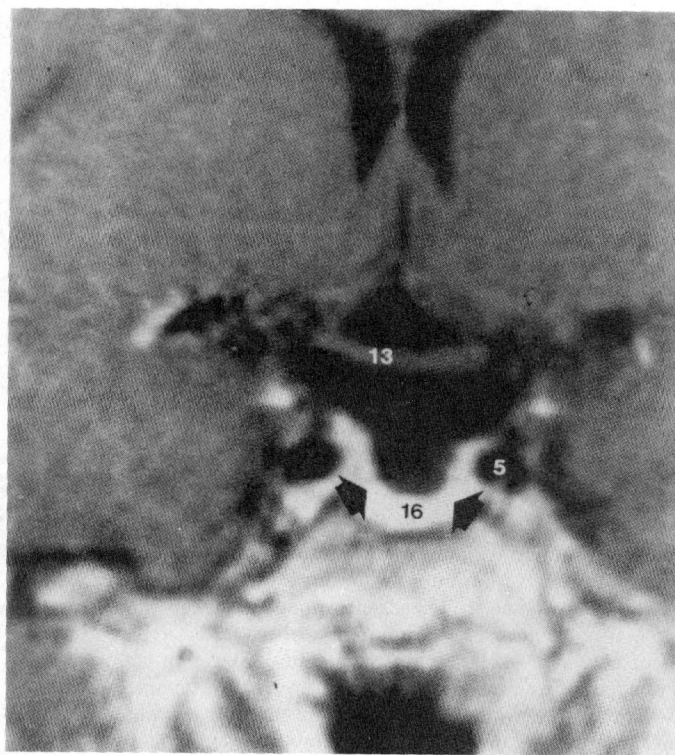

FIGURE 331-13   Empty sella. Coronal contrast-enhanced T1-weighted MRI scan through the pituitary region demonstrates an enlarged sella turcica (*arrows*) with normally enhancing pituitary tissue (16) displaced inferiorly. Note the optic chiasm (13) and intracavernous carotid artery (5). *(From Quint.)*

FIGURE 331-14   Macroadenoma. MRI scan through the pituitary region demonstrates a large sellar mass (*arrows*) elevating the optic chiasm (13) and invading the right cavernous sinus (*arrowheads*). The contrast-enhanced study differentiates the nonenhancing optic chiasm (13) from the enhancing tumor. *(From Quint.)*

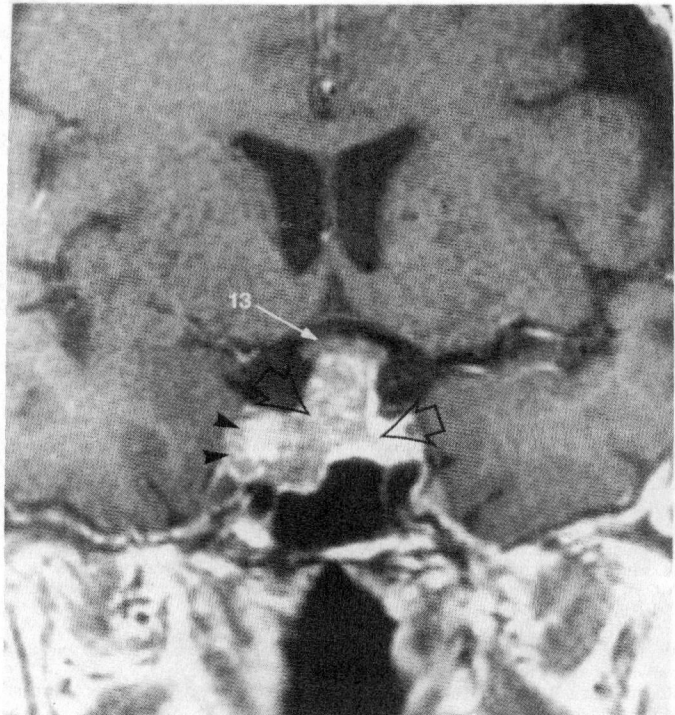

with tapered tuberculum. GH-secreting adenomas may calcify and regress to leave a calculus or stone.

Macroadenomas are well delineated on MRI. Coronal views are best (Fig. 331-14) for optic chiasm compromise, invasion of the cavernous sinus, vascular encasement, and invasion of the base of the skull. The medial wall of the cavernous sinus is thin and not directly visualized. The lateral wall of the cavernous sinus is an important landmark; the presence of tissue between the lateral wall of the cavernous sinus and the internal carotid artery is a reliable sign of invasion. Macroadenomas are hyperdense on T2-weighted images in one-third to one-half of patients; the remainder are isointense. Old hemorrhage or cyst formation results in a focally hyperintense signal and may be seen in up to 22 percent of macroadenomas (see below). (With hemorrhage, the signal is bright on T1 and T2; with fluid, the signal is of low intensity on T1 and bright on T2). Approximately one-fifth of patients with macroadenomas have a partially empty sella due to tumor degeneration or necrosis and the presence of cerebrospinal fluid density within the sella. The enlargement of the residual pituitary distinguishes this entity from the primary empty sella (see below), where the residual pituitary is normal in size. Pituitary hyperplasia (e.g., thyrotroph hyperplasia in primary hypothyroidism or lactotroph hyperplasia in pregnancy) appears as a symmetrically enlarged pituitary.

Pituitary apoplexy is caused by a sudden increase in the size of pituitary macroadenoma due to hemorrhage or infarction; enlargement of the sella is almost always evident on plain films. Acute hemorrhage (<7 days) is hypointense or isotense to brain on T1- and T2-weighted images. During the subacute stage (7 to 14 days), signal intensity is increased in the periphery of the hematoma (due to hemoglobin breakdown products such as methemoglobin), with the center remaining hypointense. After 14 days (chronic stage), the entire hematoma appears bright on T1- and T2-weighted images.

Craniopharyngiomas can often be suspected on the basis of nodular or curvilinear calcification in the suprasellar region on x-ray (Fig. 331-15). This calcification is visible in 80 to 90 percent of children and in about half of adults. On CT scanning, cystic components are present with ring or nodular calcification in most children and 80 percent of adults. The findings on MRI are variable; some cysts are cerebrospinal fluid–like in their behavior, some are not as intense as cerebrospinal fluid on T1 but brighter than cerebrospinal fluid on T2, whereas others mimic subacute hemorrhage, being hyperintense on

FIGURE 331-15   Lateral skull x-ray in a patient with a craniopharyngioma. Note dense calcification in suprasellar region (*arrow*).

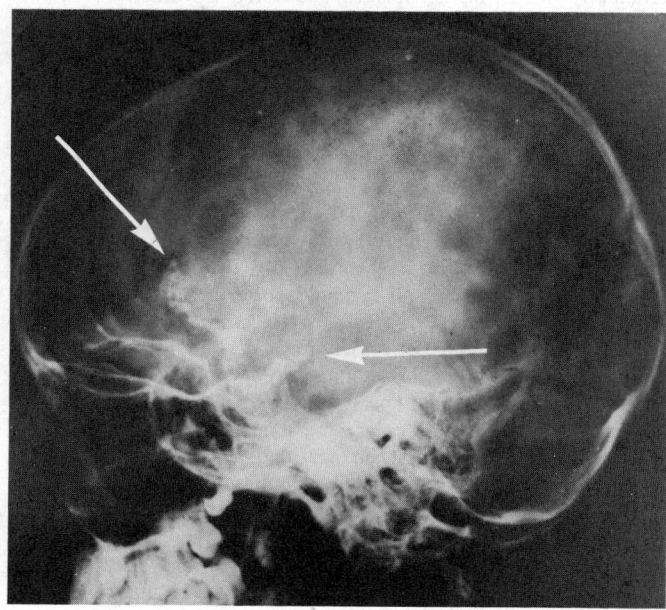

Normal

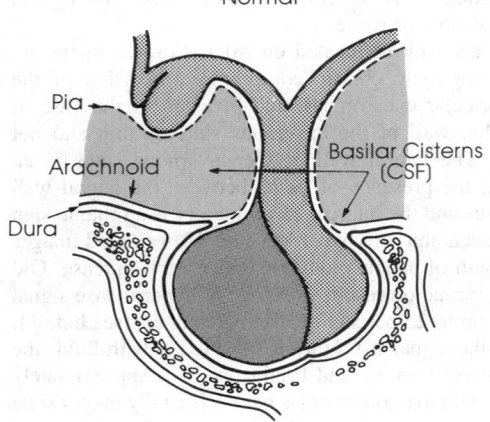

Empty Sella

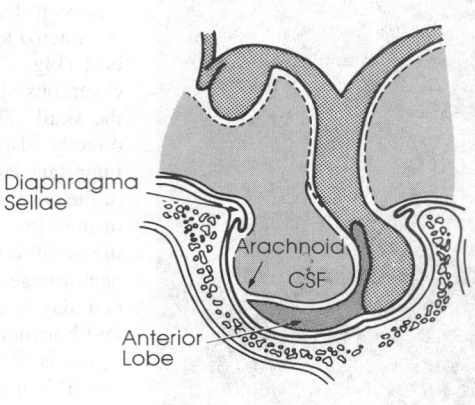

FIGURE 331-16 The findings in patients with the empty sella syndrome. (*Left panel*) The normal anatomic relationships. With the empty sella syndrome (*right panel*), ballooning of the sella results when an arachnoid diverticulum herniates through an incompetent diaphragma sellae. (*After Jordan et al.*)

T1 and T2. Calcification is usually not seen on MRI unless large amounts are present. Some craniopharyngiomas are primarily solid.

Most meningiomas of the sellar region cause abnormalities on routine skull films that include calcifications of the tumor and hyperostosis of the planum sphenoidale or of the chiasmatic sulcus. Meningiomas also may cause sella enlargement and thereby mimic pituitary adenomas. Meningiomas may be difficult to see on MRI without enhancement because they are isodense to gray matter. Almost all enhance with gadolinium, as they do with iodine contrast–enhanced CT. Delayed scanning (after 45 min) may be necessary with MRI to allow the normal enhancement of the pituitary gland and mucosal surfaces to dissipate. Vascular encasement of the carotid artery is common with meningiomas but rare with other sella region tumors.

Aneurysms in the region of the sella contain concentric calcifications demonstrable on plain skull films in about 30 percent of patients. Aneurysms can cause sella enlargement, usually with lateral depression and erosion of the sella floor. Many aneurysms are visualized on MRI with the dark appearance of a flow void as blood flows through the lumen. Multilamellated thrombi appear as a high signal on T1; adjacent brain may show a low signal on T2 due to hemosiderin deposition. In difficult cases, especially those with complete thrombosis, additional studies may be required such as digital substraction angiography, conventional angiography, and/or magnetic resonance angiography.

Other pathologic entities in the sellar region may be noted with MRI or CT scanning. In hemochromatosis, the pituitary is dark, particularly on T2-weighted images, due to iron deposition. Additional suprasellar masses include optic chiasm or hypothalamic gliomas, metastases to the hypothalamus or pituitary salk, germinomas, sarcoid granulomas, histiocytosis, dermoid tumors, epidermoid tumors, and arachnoid cysts.

THE ENLARGED SELLA–EMPTY SELLA SYNDROME Enlargement of the sella can be caused by pituitary adenomas, hypothalamic masses and cysts, aneurysms, primary hypothyroidism or hypogonadism, and increased intracranial pressure. It also can occur in patients with the primary empty sella syndrome (Fig. 331-16). In this situation, the sella tends to be symmetrically ballooned without bony erosion. The suprasellar subarachnoid space herniates through an incomplete diaphragma sella (Fig. 331-16) so that the sella is filled with cerebrospinal fluid (CSF) within an arachnoid-lined sac. An incomplete diaphragma sella is thought to be a prerequisite. It is not clear whether transient or persistent increased CSF pressure is necessary to produce sella enlargement in these patients, but CSF pressure is generally normal when measured. The pituitary is flattened and pushed to one side but tends to function normally. The fact that the CSF fills the sella can be demonstrated best with MRI scanning (see Fig. 331-13).

It is important to differentiate the primary empty sella from the enlarged partially empty sella due to a degenerated pituitary adenoma.

In the former the pituitary volume is usually normal, whereas in the latter the pituitary volume is generally increased.

Most patients with the primary empty sella syndrome are obese, multiparous women with headaches; about 30 percent have hypertension. It is of interest that multiparity, obesity, and hypertension are associated with increases in CSF pressure. Selection bias cannot be excluded in case reports, since skull x-rays may be obtained in patients with headaches, which, in turn, uncovers the enlarged sella. Endocrine abnormalities are uncommon. The report that antipituitary antibodies are present in 70 percent of these patients is therefore difficult to understand. Hyperprolactinemia occurs on occasion, possibly due to stalk stretching or coincidental microprolactinomas. GH secretory reserve is often abnormal in these patients, probably the result of obesity. Spontaneous CSF rhinorrhea and pseudotumor cerebri have each been reported in about 10 percent of the cases, but this may represent a bias of ascertainment. CSF rhinorrhea often requires surgical correction. Visual field defects have been reported and are thought to be caused by herniation of the optic chiasm into the sella turcica. Once the diagnosis of the empty sella syndrome is established by MRI or CT scan, further diagnostic studies are superfluous, and the therapy is reassurance.

REFERENCES

General

BLACK PMcL et al: *Secretory Tumors of the Pituitary Gland.* New York, Raven, 1984
BURKE CW: The pituitary megatest: Outdated. Clin Endocrinol 36:133, 1992
BURROW GN et al: Microadenomas of the pituitary and abnormal sellar tomograms in an unselected autopsy series. N Engl J Med 304:156, 1981
CROWLEY WR, ARMSTRONG WE: Neurochemical regulation of oxytocin secretion in lactation. Endocrinol Rev 13:33, 1992
HERMAN V et al: Clonal origin of pituitary adenomas. J Clin Endocrinol Metab 71:1427, 1990
HOLLENHORST RW, YOUNGE BR: Ocular manifestations produced by adenoma of the pituitary gland: Analysis of 1000 cases, in *Diagnosis and Treatment of Pituitary Tumors*, PO Kohler, GT Ross (eds). Amsterdam, Excerpta Medica, 1973, p 53
JENKINS JS, NUSSEY SS: The role of oxytocin: Present concepts. Clin Endocrinol 34:515, 1991
JONES A: Radiation oncogenesis in relation to the treatment of pituitary tumours. Clin Endocrinol 35:379, 1991
JUNEAU P et al: Malignant tumors of the pituitary gland. Arch Neurol 49:555, 1992
KLIBANSKI A: Editorial: Further evidence for a somatic mutation theory in the pathogenesis of human pituitary tumors. J Clin Endocrinol Metab 71:1415, 1990
———, ZERVAS NT: Diagnosis and management of hormone-secreting pituitary adenomas. N Engl J Med 324:822, 1991
LAMBERTS SWJ: The role of somatostatin and its analogues in the diagnosis and treatment of tumors. Endocrinol Rev 12:450, 1991
MARTIN JB, REICHLIN S: *Clinical Neuroendocrinology*, 2d ed. Philadelphia, Davis, 1987
MOLITCH ME (ed): Pituitary tumors: Diagnosis and management. Endocrinol Metab Clin North Am 16:3, 1987
———, RUSSELL EJ: The pituitary "incidentaloma." Ann Intern Med 112:925, 1990
PRYSOR-JONES RA, JENKINS J: Vasoactive intestinal peptide and anterior pituitary function. Clin Endocrinol 29:677, 1988
SCHEITHAUER BW et al: The pituitary gland in pregnancy: A clinicopathologic and immunohistochemical study of 69 cases. Mayo Clin Proc 65:461, 1990

Prolactin

BEVAN JS et al: Dopamine agonists and pituitary tumor shrinkage. Endocrinol Rev 13:220, 1992

CUNNAH D, BESSER M: Management of prolactinomas. Clin Endocrinol (Oxf) 34:231, 1991

FERRARI C et al: Functional characterization of hypothalamic hyperprolactinemia. J Clin Endocrinol Metab 55:897, 1982

KATZ E et al: Increased levels of bromocriptine following vaginal as compared to oral administration. Fertil Steril 55:882, 1991

MOLITCH ME: Pregnancy and the hyperprolactinemic woman. N Engl J Med 321:1364, 1985

———— et al: Bromocriptine as primary therapy for prolactin-secreting macroadenomas: Results of a prospective multicenter study. J Clin Endocrinol Metab 60:698, 1985

MORIONDO P et al: Bromocriptine treatment of microprolactinomas: Evidence of stable prolactin decrease after drug withdrawal. J Clin Endocrinol Metab 60:764, 1985

SCHLECTE J et al: The natural history of untreated hyperprolactinemia: A prospective analysis. J Clin Endocrinol Metab 68:412, 1989

TSAGARAKIS S et al: Megavoltage pituitary irradiation in the management of prolactinomas: Long-term follow up. Clin Endocrinol 34:399, 1991

VANCE ML et al: Bromocriptine. Ann Intern Med 100:78, 1984

———— et al: Treatment of prolactin-secreting pituitary macroadenomas with the long-acting non-ergot dopamine agonist CV 205-502. Ann Intern Med 112:668, 1990

WOOD DF et al: Dopamine, the dopamine D2 receptor and pituitary tumours. Clin Endocrinol 35:455, 1991

Growth hormone

ASA SL et al: A case for hypothalamic acromegaly: A clinicopathological study of six patients with hypothalamic gangliocytomas producing growth hormone-releasing factor. J Clin Endocrinol Metab 58:796, 1984

BARKAN AL: Acromegaly: Diagnosis and treatment. Endocrinol Metab Clin North Am 18:277, 1989

———— et al: Preoperative treatment of acromegaly with long-acting somatostatin analogue SMS 201-995: Shrinkage of invasive pituitary macroadenomas and improved surgical remission rate. J Clin Endocrinol Metab 67:1040, 1988

BAUMANN G: Growth hormone heterogeneity: Genes, isohormones, variants, and binding proteins. Endocrinol Rev 12:424, 1991

EASTMAN RC et al: Conventional supervoltage irradiation is an effective treatment for acromegaly. J Clin Endocrinol Metab 48:931, 1979

EDDY RL et al: Human growth hormone release: Comparison of provocative test procedures. Am J Med 56:179, 1974

EZZAT S, MELMED S: Are patients with acromegaly at increased risk of neoplasia? J Clin Endocrinol Metab 72:245, 1991

FROHMAN LA: Therapeutic options in acromegaly. J Clin Endocrinol Metab 72:1175, 1991

————, JANSSON J-O: Growth hormone–releasing hormone. Endocrinol Rev 7:223, 1986

HO KKY et al: Impact of octreotide, a long-acting somatostatin analogue, on glucose tolerance and insulin sensitivity in acromegaly. Clin Endocrinol 36:271, 1992

LAWRENCE JH et al: Successful treatment of acromegaly: Metabolic and clinical studies in 145 patients. J Clin Endocrinol Metab 31:180, 1970

MARCUS R et al: Effects of short-term administration of recombinant human growth hormone to elderly people. J Clin Endocrinol Metab 70:519, 1990

MELMED S: Acromegaly. N Engl J Med 322:966, 1990

———— :Etiology of pituitary acromegaly. Endocrinol Metab Clin North Am 21:539, 1992

———— et al: Pathophysiology of acromegaly. Endocrinol Rev 4:271, 1983

MOSES AC et al: Bromocriptine therapy in acromegaly: Use in patients resistant to conventional therapy and effect on serum levels of somatomedin C. J Clin Endocrinol Metab 53:752, 1981

MURUAIS C et al: Corticosteroid-induced growth hormone secretion in normal and obese subjects. Clin Endocrinol 35:485, 1991

REICHLIN S: Somatostatin. N Engl J Med 309:1495, 1983

ROSS DA, WILSON CB: Results of transsphenoidal microsurgery for growth hormone-secreting pituitary adenomas in a series of 214 patients. J Neurosurg 68:854, 1988

RUDMAN D et al: Effects of human growth hormone in men over 60 years old. N Engl J Med 323:1, 1990

SANO T et al: Growth hormone–releasing hormone–producing tumors: Clinical, biochemical and morphological manifestations. Endocrinol Rev 9:357, 1988

THORNER MO, VANCE ML: Growth hormone 1988. J Clin Invest 82:745, 1988

———— et al: Extrahypothalamic growth-hormone–releasing factor (GRF) secretion is a rare cause of acromegaly: Plasma GRF levels in 177 acromegalic patients. J Clin Endocrinol Metab 59:846, 1984

———— et al: Stereotactic radiosurgery with the cobalt-60 gamma unit in the treatment of growth hormone–producing pituitary tumors. Neurosurgery 29:663, 1991

TSH

BECK-PECCOZ P et al: Decreased receptor binding of biologically inactive thyrotropin in central hypothyroidism: Effect of treatment with thyrotropin-releasing hormone. N Engl J Med 312:1085, 1985

———— et al: Treatment of hyperthyroidism with the somatostatin analogue SMS 201-995. J Clin Endocrinol Metab 68:208, 1989

BIGOS ST et al: Spectrum of pituitary alterations with mild and severe thyroid impairment. J Clin Endocrinol Metab 46:317, 1978

FAGLIA G et al: Inappropriate secretion of thyrotropin by the pituitary. Horm Res 26:79, 1987

MAGNER JA: Thyroid-stimulating hormone: Biosynthesis, cell biology and bioactivity. Endocrinol Rev 11:354, 1990

Gonadotropins and alpha subunits

DANESHDOOST L et al: Recognition of gonadotroph adenomas in women. N Engl J Med 324:589, 1991

HESELTINE DM et al: Testicular enlargement and elevated serum inhibin concentrations occur in patients with pituitary macroadenomas secreting follicle-stimulating hormone. Clin Endocrinol 31:411, 1989

JAMESON JL et al: Glycoprotein hormone genes are expressed in clinically non-functioning pituitary adenomas. J Clin Invest 80:1472, 1987

KATZNELSON L et al: Imbalanced follicle-stimulating hormone β-subunit hormone biosynthesis in human pituitary adenomas. J Clin Endocrinol Metab 74:1343, 1992

MARSHALL JC, KELCH RP: Gonadotropin-releasing hormone: Role of pulsatile secretion in the regulation of reproduction. N Engl J Med 313:1459, 1986

MOGHISSI KS: Clinical applications of gonadotropin-releasing hormones in reproductive disorders. Endocrinol Metab Clin North Am 21:125, 1992

OPPENHEIM DS, KLIBANSKI A: Medical therapy of glycoprotein hormone–secreting pituitary tumors. Endocrinol Metab Clin North Am 18:339, 1989

———— et al: Prevalence of alpha-subunit hypersecretion in patients with pituitary tumors. J Clin Endocrinol Metab 64:1187, 1990

SNYDER PJ: Gonadotroph cell adenomas of the pituitary. Endocrinol Rev 6:552, 1985

———— et al: Secretion of uncombined subunits of luteinizing hormone by gonadotroph cell adenomas. J Clin Endocrinol Metab 59:1169, 1984

TSATSOULIS A et al: Bioactive gonadotrophin secretion in man. Clin Endocrinol 35:193, 1991

WEISS J et al: Hypogonadism caused by a single amino acid substitution in the β-subunit of luteinizing hormone. N Engl J Med 326:179, 1992

WHITCOMB RW, CROWLEY WF JR: Clinical review 4: Diagnosis and treatment of isolated gonadotropin-releasing hormone deficiency in men. J Clin Endocrinol Metab 70:3, 1990

ACTH

BATEMAN A et al: The immune-hypothalamic-pituitary-adrenal axis. Endocrinol Rev 10:92, 1989

BORST GC et al: Discordant cortisol response to exogenous ACTH and insulin-induced hypoglycemia in patients with pituitary disease. N Engl J Med 306:1462, 1982

CHROUSOS GP et al: The corticotropin-releasing factor stimulation test: An aid in the evaluation of patients with Cushing's syndrome. N Engl J Med 310:622, 1984

FLACK MR et al: Urine free cortisol in the high-dose dexamethasone suppression test for the differential diagnosis of the Cushing syndrome. Ann Intern Med 116:211, 1992

IMURA H et al: Cytokines and endocrine function: An interaction between the immune and neuroendocrine systems. Clin Endocrinol (Oxf) 35:107, 1991

LORIAUX DL, NIEMANN L: Corticotropin-releasing hormone testing in pituitary disease. Endocrinol Metab Clin North Am 20:363, 1991

ORME SM, BELCHETZ PE: Isolated ACTH deficiency. Clin Endocrinol (Oxf) 35:213, 1991

ORTH DN: Corticotropin-releasing hormone in humans. Endocrinol Rev 13:164, 1992

SCHLAGHECKE R et al: The effect of long-term glucocorticoid therapy on pituitary response to exogenous corticotropin-releasing hormone. N Engl J Med 326:226, 1992

STREETEN DHP et al: Normal and abnormal function of the hypothalamic-pituitary-adrenal system in man. Endocrinol Rev 5:371, 1984

TAHIR AH, SHEELER LR: Recurrent Cushing's disease after transsphenoidal surgery. Arch Intern Med 152:977, 1992

Endorphins

DELITALA G: Opioid peptides and pituitary function: Basic and clinical aspects, in *Brain Endocrinology*, 2d ed, M Motta (ed). New York, Raven, 1991, p 217

IMURA H et al: Endogenous opioids and related peptides: From molecular biology to clinical medicine. J Endocrinol 107:147, 1985

KROMER W: Endogenous and exogenous opioids in the control of gastrointestinal motility and secretion. Pharmacol Rev 40:121, 1989

LUNDBLAD JR, ROBERTS JL: Regulation of pro-opiomelanocortin gene expression in the pituitary. Endocrinol Rev 9:135, 1988

PFEIFFER A, HERZ A: Endocrine actions of opioids. Horm Metabol Res 16:386, 1984

Hypothalamus

BRAY GA, GALLAGHER TFJ: Manifestations of hypothalamic obesity in man: A comprehensive investigation of eight patients and a review of the literature. Medicine 54:301, 1974

DINARELLO CA: Interleukin 1 and the pathogenesis of the acute phase response. N Engl J Med 54:301, 1984

PLUM F, VAN UITERT R: Nonendocrine disease and disorders of the hypothalamus, in *The Hypothalamus*, S Reichlin et al (eds). New York, Raven, 1978, pp 415–473

Craniopharyngiomas

BANNA M: Craniopharyngiomas in adults. Surg Neurol 1:202, 1973

———— : Craniopharyngioma: Based on 160 cases. Br J Radiol 49:206, 1976

FISCHER EG et al: Treatment of craniopharyngiomas in children, 1971–1980. J Neurosurg 62:486, 1985

Hypopituitarism

ABBOUD CF: Laboratory diagnosis of hypopituitarism. Mayo Clin Proc 61:35, 1986

ARAFAH BM: Reversible hypopituitarism in patients with large nonfunctioning pituitary adenomas. J Clin Endocrinol Metab 62:1173, 1986

ASA SL et al: Lymphocytic hypophysitis of pregnancy resulting in hypopituitarism: A distinct clinicopathologic entity. Ann Intern Med 95:166, 1981

EDWARDS OM, CLARK JDA: Post-traumatic hypopituitarism. Medicine 62:281, 1986

Muir A, Maclaren NK: Autoimmune diseases of the adrenal glands, parathyroid glands, gonads and hypothalamic-pituitary axis. Endocrinol Metab Clin North Am 20:619, 1991

Oelkers W: Hyponatremia and inappropriate secretion of vasopressin (antidiuretic hormone) in patients with hypopituitarism. N Engl J Med 321:492, 1989

Rosen T, Bengtsson BA: Premature mortality due to cardiovascular disease in hypopituitarism. Lancet 336:285, 1990

Veldhuis JD, Hammond JM: Endocrine function after spontaneous infarction of the human pituitary: Report, review, and reappraisal. Endocrinol Rev 1:100, 1980

Radiology

Bruneton JN et al: Normal variants of the sella turcica. Radiology 131:99, 1979

Chakeres DW et al: Magnetic resonance imaging of pituitary and parasellar abnormalities. Radiol Clin North Am 27:265, 1989

Constine LS et al: Hypothalamo-pituitary dysfunction after radiation for brain tumors. N Engl J Med 328:87, 1993

Glick RP, Tiesi JA: Subacute pituitary apoplexy: Clinical and magnetic resonance imaging characteristics. Neurosurgery 27:214, 1990

Johnson MR et al: The evaluation of patients with a suspected pituitary microadenoma: Computed tomography compared to magnetic resonance imaging. Clin Endocrinol 36:335, 1992

Jordan RM et al: The primary empty sella syndrome: Analysis of the clinical characteristics, radiographic features, pituitary function, and cerebrospinal fluid adenohypophysial hormone concentrations. Am J Med 62:569, 1977

Quint DJ: Hypothalamic, pituitary, and pineal imaging, in *Endocrine Imaging*, MP Sandler et al (eds). Norwalk, Conn, Appleton & Lange, 1992

Wolpert SM: The radiology of pituitary adenomas. Endocrinol Metab Clin North Am 16:553, 1987

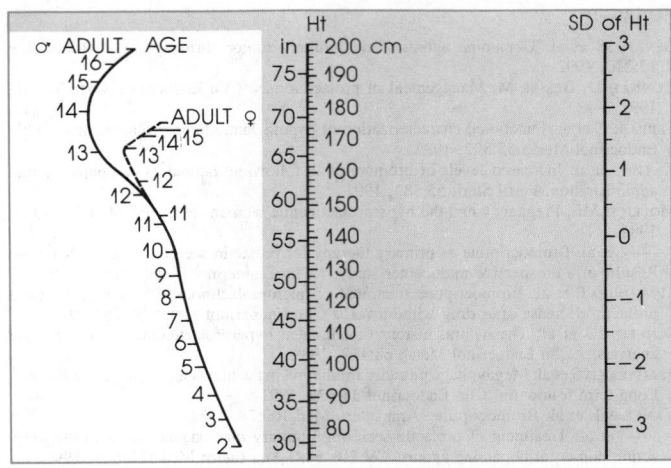

FIGURE 332-1   Nomogram for height of boys and girls.

332   DISORDERS OF GROWTH

RAYMOND L. HINTZ

NORMAL GROWTH   Children may grow rapidly over relatively short periods of time, and the physician must be aware of normal standards for growth and development as a function of age. A record of these changes can be utilized as a sensitive indicator of general health. Minimal aberrations in health may be reflected first in a deviation from the normal growth rate; conversely, an actively growing child seldom has a serious systemic disease. Thus height and growth rate provide important information.

Both longitudinal and cross-sectional studies indicate that differences exist in growth among different ethnic groups. However, normal, well-nourished children have remarkably similar growth patterns. For example, the average length of children, which at birth is about 50 cm, increases by about 25 cm in the first year of life, 12.5 cm in the second year, and 6.0 cm per year thereafter until puberty. This formula can be used to estimate average height up to about 10 years of age. Nomograms have been constructed to give a more accurate picture of average growth and the range of normal deviations from the mean (Figs. 332-1 and 332-2).

CONTROL OF GROWTH   Growth involves an increase in both the total number of cells and the synthesis of macromolecules by individual cells. The relative importance of these processes varies from organ to organ and with age. The control and integration of growth also vary among tissues and with the stage of development.

Prenatal growth   Prenatal development exemplifies the complexities of the integration and control of growth. During this time, a single cell becomes a complex organism in which billions of cells work in harmonious concert. The growth rate is astounding; the most rapid growth rate occurs during the second trimester. The control of prenatal growth is under different mechanisms from those in the postnatal period. Growth hormone and thyroid hormone have relatively minor effects on growth during prenatal life. Prenatal growth rates are dependent on uterine blood flow and other maternal influences and are less dependent on the factors that determine ultimate stature. At birth, the correlation between body length and adult height is weak ($r = 0.3$); by 2 years of age, the correlation between body length and adult height is stronger ($r = 0.7$), indicating that the factors influencing adult stature begin operating early in postnatal life.

Genetic factors   Stature is a polygenic trait (see Chap. 60), so there is no simple method of predicting on the basis of genetic factors the adult height of any given child. However, there is a correlation between the mean height of parents and the mean heights attained by their children.

Nutrition   The next most important factor affecting growth is nutrition. Severe nutritional deprivation, as in marasmus or kwashiorkor (see Chap. 72), impairs growth, as may selective deficiencies of vitamins and minerals, such as vitamin D, and subclinical deficiencies of nutrients. The trend toward increased adult stature over the last century may be due to improvement in diet, especially to an increase in protein intake during the period of rapid growth during infancy.

Hormones   GROWTH HORMONE   Growth hormone (GH or somatotropin) plays the central role in the modulation of growth of children from birth until the completion of puberty. In the total absence of GH, linear growth occurs at about half to a third the normal rate. GH also plays a role in the control of body anabolism throughout life.

GH is a member of a family of hormones that includes pituitary prolactin and human placental lactogen (hPL) (see Chap. 331). The most common form of GH in the pituitary and in the circulation is the 22,000-Da ("22K") form. This is the hormone that was purified and sequenced from human pituitary glands. The second most abundant form is a 20,000-Da ("20K") form. This variant is coded by the same gene sequence as the 22K growth hormone, but a segment of a coding exon in the growth hormone gene is not transcribed, thus resulting in a shorter hormone. Whether this variant fulfills some specific metabolic function is not clear; the 20K form seems to have

FIGURE 332-2   Nomogram for growth rate in boys and girls.

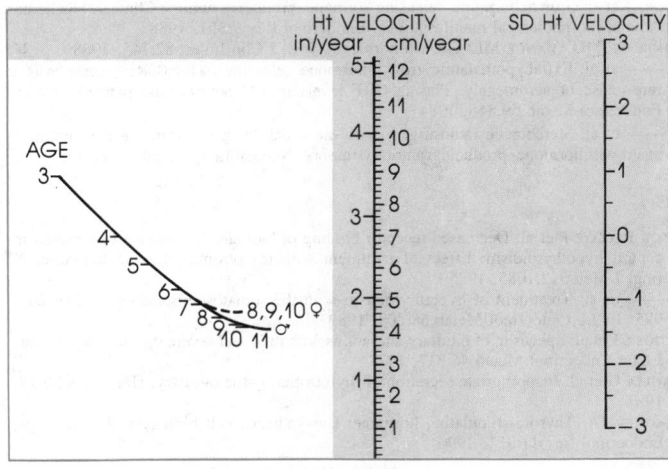

equivalent growth-promoting activity but may have less effect on carbohydrate function than the 22K form.

GH secretion is under both positive and negative hypothalamic control (see Chap. 331). The somatotropin release-inhibiting factor (somatostatin, SRIF) is a 14-amino-acid peptide that is widely distributed in tissues outside the hypothalamus and is a potent inhibitor of the secretion of many hormones, including insulin, glucagon, and gastrin.

The biologic action of GH-releasing hormone (GRH, somatocrinin) is contained in the first 29 amino acids of the 44-amino-acid peptide, and the amino-terminal amino acid is crucial for its biologic action. Patients with idiopathic GH deficiency may have a deficiency of GRH rather than an inability to make GH in the pituitary. Indeed, half or more individuals with GH deficiency respond to prolonged pulsatile administration of GRH with an increase in plasma GH and with an accelerated growth rate.

The secretion of somatostatin and GRH, and hence the release of GH, is under the influence of several factors (Fig. 332-3). Higher centers in the central nervous system have synapses that terminate on hypothalamic cells that secrete somatostatin and GRH and exert both positive and negative influences. In addition, both GH and the GH-controlled insulin-like growth factors influence the secretion or action of GRH and somatostatin. The secretion of GH is episodic, with a relatively short (10- to 15-min) half-life in plasma. A significant proportion of GH in serum is bound to a GH-binding protein GHBP that is structurally related to the GH receptor. Although small amounts of GH are secreted during waking periods, most GH secretion occurs during sleep, especially during third- and fourth-stage sleep.

THE INSULIN-LIKE GROWTH FACTORS   Although GH may exert some direct effects on growth, most of its growth-promoting actions are mediated by the insulin-like growth factor (IGF) or somatomedin peptides. Two human IGF peptides, IGF-I and IGF-II, have about 50 percent structural homology with human insulin and 70 percent homology with each other. Somatomedin C (SM-C) and IGF-I are structurally and functionally equivalent. The IGF peptides are bound tightly to six specific plasma proteins (IGFBPs) and have half-lives of hours rather than minutes. Levels of IGF-I and IGFBP-3 are dependent on GH secretion and are consequently high in acromegaly and low in hypopituitarism. Levels are also age-dependent, with low levels in early childhood, a peak during adolescence, and a decline after the age of 50 years. The plasma levels of IGF-II are also dependent on the presence of a minimal amount of GH, but supraphysiologic increases in GH do not result in a further increase in IGF-II. Thus the values of IGF-II are low in hypopituitarism but are not elevated in acromegaly. Plasma levels of IGF-II are constant from 1 year of age to beyond the eighth decade of life.

THYROID HORMONE   Unlike the pattern of growth with GH deficiency, the total absence of thyroid hormone causes an almost complete cessation of linear growth. Thus adequate thyroid hormone appears to be an absolute prerequisite for normal growth. There are several potential mechanisms for this phenomenon. Thyroid hormones exert direct effects on cell metabolism, and thyroid hormone deficiency results in diminished GH secretion in response to stimulation. In addition, the action of IGF-I on cartilage cells may be dependent on thyroid hormone.

GONADAL STEROIDS   Androgens and estrogens exert their major stimulation of growth at puberty. Much of the pubertal growth spurt is due to these hormones. Androgens have a direct stimulatory effect on the growth and maturation of bone, cartilage, and muscle. Estrogens appear to have a biphasic action, stimulating growth at low levels and inhibiting growth at high levels.

INSULIN   Insulin has strong anabolic actions separate from its effects on carbohydrate metabolism. These actions include stimulation of protein synthesis and cell division. The excessive growth of infants of diabetic mothers may be the consequence of high levels of plasma insulin in the fetus. The close structural relationship of insulin to the IGF group of growth factors and the ability of insulin to bind to the IGF-I receptor may explain some of these effects of insulin at high levels. However, insulin also has growth-stimulating actions of its own at low levels in some cell types. The role of insulin in the control of normal growth is still unclear.

OTHER FACTORS   Nerve growth factor, which is structurally related to the insulin-IGF family of peptides, has actions on the development of sympathetic neurons and possibly on the maintenance and repair of other neurons. Epidermal growth factor has potent actions on the maturation of the skin and also acts on other cell types. Platelet-derived growth factor is released from platelets upon clotting and is also a potent mitogen for many cells. The plasma levels, control mechanisms, interactions with other growth-stimulating peptides, and physiologic roles of these growth factors remain to be elucidated.

DIAGNOSIS OF GROWTH DISORDERS   Most individuals with short stature do not have a disease in the usual sense but exhibit some deviation from the normal growth pattern (Table 332-1). Thus the first step in dealing with growth disorders is to identify those individuals with a normal variation in stature who presumably do not require treatment.

Height and growth rate   An important factor in the differential diagnosis of short stature is to determine the height percentile of the patient as compared with others of the same age (see Fig. 332-1). A straightedge is placed on the patient's age and height. The intercept on the right-hand scale estimates the number of standard deviations (SD) from the mean height for age. In general, the further away the patient is from the mean height for age, the more likely that short stature is due to disease. A height above the −2-SD level indicates that the patient is likely normal. The growth rate also should be determined, if possible, either from existing growth data or by observation (see Fig. 332-2). A growth rate consistently below the mean is a cause for concern.

Because short stature is common, clinical judgment plays a large role in the approach to this problem. Individuals with severe short stature (−3 SD or greater for age) should undergo immediate evaluation, while those with less severe short stature may be serially observed so that the growth rate can be assessed. A consistently low

FIGURE 332-3   Feedback control of growth hormone secretion. GH = growth hormone; GHRH = growth hormone–releasing hormone; SM = somatomedins (insulin-like growth factors). Stimulating influences are shown by arrows in color. Inhibitory influences are shown in black.

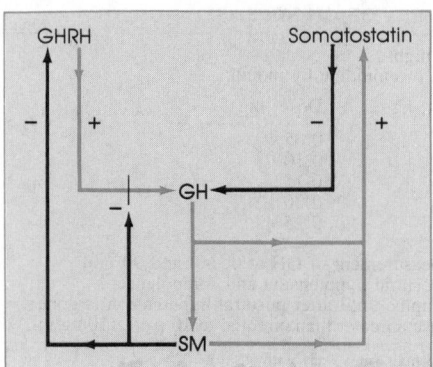

TABLE 332-1   Causes of short stature

Diagnosis	Usual practice, %	Referral center, %
Constitutional growth delay	98	80
GH deficiency	0.1	10
Hypothyroidism	0.2	4
Systemic disease	0.3	3
Chromosomal disorders	0.1	1
Bone-cartilage dysplasia	0.3	1
Psychosocial disorders	1	1

SOURCE: Modified from Horner et al, 1978.

growth rate should lead to further investigation. The diagnosis of constitutional delay is one of exclusion. In general, if hypothyroidism, GH deficiency, and the more common systemic diseases have been excluded, it is reasonable to observe the patient. However, the boundaries between "normal" and "disease" may be blurred, and the indications for treatment may change. Furthermore, continued failure to maintain a normal growth rate is an indication for reinvestigation.

History   Important features in the history include the weight and gestational age at birth, growth and development in early infancy, and presence of systemic disease. It is also crucial to assess the stature of the parents and first- and second-degree relatives and to review the growth and pubertal development patterns of parents, siblings, and other relatives. A family history of late pubertal development may be helpful diagnostically.

Physical examination   The body proportions must be evaluated. Relatively short limbs compared with the trunk suggest either long-standing hypothyroidism or one of the chondrodystrophies such as achondroplastic dwarfism; but more subtle forms of chondrodystrophy may be difficult to recognize (see also Chap. 351). It is also important to note the height-to-weight ratio. A short child who is underweight for height may have malnutrition or systemic disease. On the other hand, a child who is short but overweight is more likely to have endocrine disease. Patients with Cushing's syndrome, GH deficiency, or hypothyroidism are frequently relatively overweight for their height. Specific physical findings may suggest specific syndromes (Table 332-2).

Laboratory evaluation   Laboratory tests may either confirm the clinical impression or reveal unsuspected pathology. Assessment of bone age is useful to indicate possible pathology and to estimate final adult height. Because the manifestations of hypothyroidism may be minimal, thyroid function should be assessed routinely. IGF-I and IGFGP-3 measurements are also useful screening procedures, since most patients with GH deficiency have low values. Syndromes of GH resistance, such as Laron dwarfism, are characterized by low IGF-I levels and high GH levels. Appropriate tests may be ordered to screen for other disease states (as summarized in Table 332-3). Any girl with unexplained short stature should have a chromosomal karyotype.

TESTING OF GH SECRETION   Because GH secretion is episodic and therefore variable, random measurements of plasma GH are not adequate tests of GH deficiency. Some GH stimulation tests for screening for GH deficiency are summarized in Table 332-4 (also see Chap. 331). Because of the long half-life of IGF-I and IGFBP-3, a random measurement during the day is an accurate reflection of the mean plasma concentration. If care is taken to use age-related standards, measurements and IGF-I and IGFBP-3 provide a reasonable screen for GH deficiency. Low levels of IGF-I or IGFBP-3 should lead to more extensive evaluation. The other tests listed are indirect and largely nonphysiologic ways of provoking the release of GH. In our clinic, a GH level of 10 μg/L (10 ng/mL) after a clonidine test is considered a normal response. If that level is not achieved, more

definitive testing of GH reserve should be carried out as described in Chap. 331.

TREATMENT WITH GH   GH deficiency   The only established use of human GH is in the treatment of children who are GH-deficient. Only between 1 in 4000 and 1 in 20,000 children have a GH deficiency. About half of these cases are due to idiopathic GH deficiency, and the other half are secondary to tumor and/or radiation therapy. In approximately one-third of the latter cases, GH deficiency is isolated, and in the other two-thirds, there are multiple pituitary hormone deficiencies. If short stature is due to a systemic disease

---

TABLE 332-2   Physical findings in syndromes of short stature

Syndrome	Specific physical findings
GH deficiency	Frontal bossing, central obesity, high-pitched voice
Hypothyroidism	Dry skin, coarse hair, immature facies
Cushing's syndrome	Central obesity, striae, hypertension
Gonadal dysgenesis	Webbed neck, multiple pigmented nevi, shield chest, delayed sexual development
Pseudohypoparathyroidism	Moon facies and obesity, short metacarpals, mental retardation
Bone-cartilage dysplasia	Abnormal proportions, macrocephaly
Russell-Silver dwarfism	Small at birth, "pointed" facies, asymmetry

---

TABLE 332-3   Screening laboratory investigations in short stature

Test or x-ray	Disorder
Serum thyroxine	Hypothyroidism
IGF-I and IGFBP-3	GH deficiency
Bone age	Constitutional delay, hypothyroidism, GH deficiency
Lateral skull film	Craniopharyngioma or other central nervous system lesion
Serum calcium	Pseudohypoparathyroidism
Serum phosphate	Vitamin D–resistant rickets
Serum bicarbonate	Renal tubular acidosis
Blood urea nitrogen	Renal failure
Complete blood count	Anemia, nutritional disorder
Sedimentation rate	Inflammatory disease of bowel
Chromosomal karyotype	Gonadal dysgenesis or other abnormality

---

TABLE 332-4   Screening tests for assessing GH secretion

IGF-I RADIOIMMUNOASSAY*

Age (years)	Male Range, μg/L	Female Range, μg/L
1–2	31–160	11–206
3–4	45–230	75–320
5–6	51–288	70–320
7–8	157–385	125–396
9–10	136–308	123–330
11–12	180–440	191–462
13–14	220–616	286–660
15–16	200–836	242–660
17–18	286–627	240–506

IGFBP-3 RADIOIMMUNOASSAY*

Age	Range, mg/L	Mean, mg/L
1–12 months	0.5–1.2	1.3
1–5 years	1.4–3.0	2.1
5–7 years	1.5–3.4	2.4
7–9 years	2.1–4.2	3.0
9–11 years	2.0–4.8	3.3
11–13 years	2.1–6.2	3.8
13–15 years	2.2–5.9	4.2
15–18 years	2.5–4.8	3.8
Adults, 20–30 years	2.0–4.2	3.0

CLONIDINE TEST OF GH RELEASE

NPO after midnight
Administration of clonidine by mouth:

Body weight, kg	Dose, mg
5–15	0.05
15–25	0.10
25–35	0.15
35–50	0.20
>50	0.25

Samples for measurement of GH at 0, 60, and 90 min
Side effects: Postural hypotension and somnolence
Keep patient supine until after postural hypotension is gone
Normal response: Greater than or equal to 10 μg/L (10 ng/mL) on any sample

* Age-related normals (may vary with assay).

such as renal failure, treatment is directed toward the underlying disease state. Similarly, short stature due to hypothyroidism or cortisol excess is managed by treatment of the primary disorder. In general, the earlier the disorder is diagnosed and treated, the more successful is the growth response; if treatment of the underlying disease is delayed until after puberty, little or no improvement in stature can be expected.

Unlike the broad species specificity of peptide hormones such as insulin, GH exhibits limited species specificity. Human GH stimulates linear growth in children with GH deficiency, whereas the bovine hormone is ineffective in humans. The collection of pituitary glands from autopsy material for the preparation of human GH did not supply adequate amounts of hormone for the treatment of all children who had GH deficiency, let alone provide sufficient material for the evaluation of GH for other conditions. Furthermore, the distribution of human pituitary GH in the United States and several other countries was discontinued in 1984 because of the development of Creutzfeldt-Jakob disease in patients who had been treated with human GH. The availability since 1985 of synthetic GH has relieved the supply problem. Hormone is readily available for patients with GH deficiency, and the potentially unlimited supply has allowed exploration of other therapeutic uses of GH, including the treatment of gonadal dysgenesis.

Most children with GH deficiency respond to GH treatment with an acceleration of growth rate to normal or above normal rates. As with other hormones, there is a dose-response curve to GH. The doses that have been tested range from 0.02 to 0.2 units (0.01 to 0.1 mg) per kilogram of body weight administered as a subcutaneous injection daily. There is a wide variation in response, but the higher dosages usually result in higher average growth rates. It is possible that in selected clinical circumstances dosages of GH higher than those currently recommended should be administered. Treatment may be started at a daily dose of 0.05 or 0.1 unit/kg (0.025 or 0.050 mg/kg). The majority of GH-deficient patients have a good growth response to this dosage. If the patient fails to show an adequate growth rate, the dose can be increased until an adequate growth response is obtained or until the upper limit of 1.50 units/kg of body weight per week is achieved. As doses of GH are increased above this level, the risk of glucose intolerance increases, particularly in children who are prediabetic.

An alternative method under study for the treatment of GH deficiency is the use either of GH-releasing hormone (GHRH) or GH-releasing peptide (GHRF). Since at least half of children with GH deficiency are able to secrete GH in response to GHRH, this approach may ultimately be useful for those patients.

Short stature of other causes IDIOPATHIC SEVERE SHORT STATURE Growth hormone has been given to some patients with growth failure not due to GH deficiency. Many children with severe short stature (more than 2.5 SD below the mean for age) do not have GH deficiency. Some of these children without GH deficiency are responsive to GH treatment. Many of these patients have low IGF-I, IGFBP-3, and/or GHBP levels and may have a partial defect in the control of GH secretion. Many such children have a short-term increase in growth rate in response to GH therapy; whether the final height of these children after GH treatment is greater than their predicted height is not established. Furthermore, it is not known whether there are serious long-term side effects.

GONADAL DYSGENESIS GH also may have a role in the treatment of gonadal dysgenesis (see Chap. 62). The majority of women with gonadal dysgenesis have an average adult height between 135 and 142 cm. Androgens can cause a short-term increase in the rate of growth of girls with the disorder but do not result in an increase in final adult stature. The use of GH at modest doses is also associated with an increase in the rate of growth. Results of multicenter group studies utilizing synthetic GH either alone or in combination with androgens are encouraging in terms of both initial growth response and increases in final height.

SKELETAL DISORDERS Growth hormone also has been used to treat small numbers of subjects with a wide variety of other growth disorders, including bone-cartilage dysplasias and other genetic syndromes associated with short stature. It is not clear whether GH is of use in any of these disorders.

REFERENCES

BAUMANN G: Growth hormone heterogeneity: Genes, isohormone, variants and binding proteins. Endocr Rev 12:424, 1991

BLIZZARD R et al: Idiopathic short stature: Results of a one-year controlled study of human growth hormone treatment. J Pediatr 115:713, 1989

BLUM WF et al: A specific radioimmunoassay for the growth hormone–dependent somatomedin binding protein: Its use for diagnosis of growth hormone deficiency. J Clin Endocrinol Metab 70:1291, 1990

BROWN P: Potential epidemic Creutzfeldt-Jakob disease from human growth hormone therapy. N Engl J Med 313:728, 1985

FRASIER SD: A review of growth hormone stimulation tests in children. Pediatrics 53:929, 1974

GRUMBACH M: Growth hormone therapy and the short end of the stick. N Engl J Med 319:238, 1988

HINDMARSH PC et al: Wider indications for treatment with biosynthetic human growth hormone in children. Clin Endocrinol 34:417, 1991

HINTZ RL: Growth factors. Curr Opin Pediatr 2:786, 1990

————: Untoward events in patients treated with GH in the USA. Horm Res 38(suppl 1):44, 1992

———— et al: Efficacy of growth hormone therapy in patients without classically defined growth hormone deficiency. Growth Genet Horm 8(suppl 1):10, 1992

HORNER JM et al: Growth deceleration patterns in constitutional short stature: An aid to diagnosis. Pediatrics 62:529, 1978

LANTOS J et al: Ethical issues of growth hormone therapy. JAMA 261:1020, 1989

LEE PDK et al: Efficacy of insulin-like growth factor I levels in predicting the response to provocative growth hormone testing. Pediatr Res 27:45, 1990

ROSENFELD RG et al: Six-year results of a randomized, prospective trial of human growth hormone and oxandrolone in Turner's syndrome. J Pediatr 49:121, 1992

TANNER JM, DAVIS PSW: Clinical longitudinal standards for height and height velocity for North American children. J Pediatr 107:317, 1985

————, ISREALSOHN WJ: Parent-child correlations for body measurements of children between the ages of one month and 7 years. Ann Hum Genet 26:245, 1963

———— et al: Effect of human growth hormone treatment for 1 to 7 years on growth of 100 children with growth hormone deficiency, inherited smallness, Turner's syndrome, and other complaints. Arch Dis Child 46:317, 1985

THORNER MO et al: Growth hormone–releasing hormone and growth hormone–releasing peptide as potential therapeutic modalities. Acta Paediatr Scand (Suppl) 376:29, 1990

VIPANI OV et al: Prevalence of severe growth hormone deficiency. Br Med J 2:427, 1977

333 DISORDERS OF THE NEUROHYPOPHYSIS

ARNOLD M. MOSES / DAVID H. P. STREETEN

Axons from two largely independent hypothalamic-neurohypophyseal systems in the supraoptic and paraventricular nuclei extend through the pituitary stalk to the posterior pituitary. Hormones (vasopressin and oxytocin), formed within separate ganglion cells, migrate down the axons as part of precursor proteins. They are stored in secretory granules within the nerve terminals in the neurohypophysis and are released by exocytosis into the bloodstream in response to appropriate stimuli. Vasopressin or antidiuretic hormone (AVP or ADH) controls water conservation, and its release is coordinated with the activity of the thirst center that regulates fluid intake. Oxytocin stimulates uterine contractions and milk ejection.

VASOPRESSIN SYNTHESIS, RELEASE, AND ACTION

SYNTHESIS Vasopressin (AVP) is synthesized in the magnocellular neurons of the anterior hypothalamus. It is translated as a preprohormone which is altered in the Golgi apparatus to form a prohormone that is packaged into neurosecretory vesicles. While the prohormone is being transported to axonal terminals, enzymes generate

AVP, a 10,000 molecular weight protein called *neurophysin*, and a 39-amino-acid glycopeptide. All three products are released into the peripheral circulation.

ACTIONS   AVP conserves water by concentrating the urine. It binds to the V_2 receptor on the contraluminal surface of the distal tubular epithelium, mainly in the collecting ducts. At this site AVP enhances the hydrosmotic flow of water from the lumen to the medullary interstitium and assists in maintaining constancy of the osmolality and volume of body fluids. High concentrations of AVP acting on V_1 receptors can cause vasoconstriction, as in response to severe hypotension or to infusion of vasopressin for treatment of bleeding esophageal varices.

AVP, perhaps from axons that terminate in the cerebrum, may play a role in learning and memory, and AVP from fibers in the median eminence may influence corticotropin secretion.

NORMAL HORMONE LEVELS   AVP concentrations in plasma and urine can be measured by radioimmunoassay. The results may be expressed either as units based on pressor activity in the rat or in terms of weight of purified vasopressin. Arginine vasopressin has a biologic activity of approximately 400 units per milligram (1 mU = 2.5 ng = 2.3 pmol). The neurohypophysis under conditions of random fluid intake contains approximately 8 units, or 18 nmol (20 μg), of AVP. Under the same conditions, peripheral plasma AVP concentration ranges from 1.4 to 5.6 pmol/L (1.5 to 6 ng/L). At the latter plasma level and above, urine osmolality is maximal. The AVP concentration in blood fluctuates, with a maximum late at night and in the early morning and a minimum in the early afternoon. Under conditions of normal hydration, healthy subjects release approximately 370 to 1400 pmol (400 to 1500 ng) from the pituitary and excrete 23 to 80 pmol (25 to 90 ng) AVP in urine in 24 h. During 24 to 28 h of dehydration, the amount released increases three to five times with consequent increases in plasma and urinary levels.

METABOLISM   Inactivation of AVP occurs largely in liver and kidneys, a major mechanism being the cleavage of the terminal glycinamide to produce a biologically inactive substance. Approximately 7 to 10 percent of secreted AVP is excreted in the urine as active hormone.

CONTROL OF AVP RELEASE   The release of AVP is influenced by a number of stimuli.

Osmoregulation   Under normal conditions, AVP release is primarily regulated by osmoreceptors in the hypothalamus. Changes in the concentrations of plasma solutes to which the cellular membrane is impermeable cause alterations in the volume of the osmoreceptor cells, which in turn alter the electric activity of the neurons and control AVP release. Osmotic changes that stimulate release also enhance production of AVP. The servomechanism between effective plasma osmolality and AVP release normally maintains plasma osmolality within a very narrow range. The mean plasma osmolality of normal subjects following a water load of 20 mL/kg of body weight is 281.7 mmol/kg plasma water, and the osmolality that initiates AVP release following infusion of hypertonic saline solution into water-loaded subjects is 287.3 mmol/kg. Thus the increase in plasma osmolality from full diuresis to the initiation of antidiuresis by hypertonic saline solution is only 5.6 mmol/kg, or 2 percent.

The infusion of hypertonic saline solution into water-loaded subjects causes a linear rise in plasma osmolality with time. After an interval, there is an abrupt, progressive fall in free water clearance without a significant change in solute or creatinine excretion. We have defined the osmotic threshold for AVP release as the plasma osmolality at the onset of antidiuresis under these conditions. In 73 normal subjects, this occurred at a mean plasma osmolality of 287 mmol/kg. The osmotic threshold for AVP release also may be determined, with very similar results, by constructing a linear regression line between simultaneously obtained plasma osmolality and either plasma or urine AVP concentration during hypertonic saline infusion and extrapolating the regression line to the x-axis intercept (plasma osmolality).

Volume regulation   Decreases in plasma volume, through effects on stretch receptors in the left atrium and perhaps in the pulmonary veins, stimulate the release of AVP by reducing the tonic inhibitory impulses from the left atrium to the hypothalamus. The neural impulses travel via the vagi to the reticular formation of the midbrain and diencephalon and thence to the supraoptic and paraventricular nuclei, where they are integrated with the other stimuli that affect AVP release. Positive-pressure breathing, quiet standing, and vasodilatation may activate this mechanism, which serves to restore plasma volume, even at times overriding osmotic inhibition of AVP release. Following volume contraction, circulating AVP concentrations may reach 10 times the levels induced by hypertonicity. Increased plasma volume inhibits AVP release by the reverse mechanisms, leading to a diuresis and correction of the hypervolemia. Negative-pressure breathing, recumbency, lack of gravitational force (as in space travel), submersion in water, and exposure to cold may activate this mechanism.

Baroreceptor regulation   Activation of carotid and aortic baroreceptors in response to hypotension causes release of AVP. Hypotension due to blood loss is the most potent stimulus and may at times raise plasma levels of AVP to 560 pmol/L (600 ng/L). These concentrations of AVP may cause vasoconstriction, which probably plays a role in the restoration of blood pressure.

Neural regulation   Many neurotransmitters and neuropeptides in the hypothalamus play a role in regulating and modulating the release of AVP. Acetylcholine stimulates AVP release by its nicotinic action on supraoptic neurons. Angiotensin II, histamine, bradykinin, and neuropeptide Y probably stimulate AVP release. Norepinephrine, prostaglandins, and dopamine stimulate or inhibit AVP release, depending on the experimental conditions. Gamma aminobutyric acid appears to act as an inhibitory neurotransmitter; serotonin and substance P are also present in the supraoptic nucleus, but their influence on magnocellular neuron activity is not clear. The regulatory action of opioid peptides on AVP release is unclear, with reports indicating stimulation, inhibition, or no effect. Though the roles of these and other transmitters and peptides are still poorly defined, the antidiuretic actions of stress, emesis, and pain and the diuretic actions of hypnosis, psychological conditioning, and inhalation of carbon dioxide indicate that higher centers have an important influence on the release of AVP.

Aging   Aging is associated with enhanced AVP release in response to a rising plasma osmolality and a progressive increase in plasma AVP concentration. These changes appear to place the older individual at greater risk of developing water retention and hyponatremia, despite a concomitant decline in maximal renal concentrating capacity in response to AVP, which is usually evident beyond 60 years of age.

Pharmacologic influences   Pharmacologic agents that can stimulate AVP release include nicotine, morphine, vincristine, vinblastine, cyclophosphamide, clofibrate, chlorpropamide, and some tricyclic anticonvulsants and antidepressants. Ethanol has diuretic properties by inhibiting neurohypophyseal function under a variety of conditions. Some narcotic antagonists also inhibit AVP release. Experimentally, chlorpromazine, reserpine, and phenytoin all inhibit the loss of AVP from the pituitary and the rise in urinary excretion of AVP that result from water deprivation. In humans, phenytoin and chlorpromazine may inhibit AVP release and produce diuresis.

AVP RESPONSE TO WATER DEPRIVATION AND TO WATER LOAD   Water deprivation provides both an osmotic and a volume stimulus to vasopressin release by increasing plasma osmolality and decreasing plasma volume. The maximum urinary osmolality after water deprivation depends on renal medullary osmolality and other intrarenal factors. In response to fluid deprivation for 18 to 24 h in normal individuals, plasma osmolality rarely rises above 292 mmol/kg. The resultant stimulation of AVP release increases plasma AVP concentration to 7.4 to 14 pmol/L (8 to 15 ng/L).

The administration of water lowers plasma osmolality and expands blood volume, inhibiting the release of AVP via both osmoreceptor and atrial volume receptor mechanisms. An oral water load of 20 mL/kg in normal adults results in a fall in plasma osmolality to a mean of 281.7 mmol/kg and causes a maximum diuresis in 1 to $1\frac{1}{2}$ h with free water clearance rising to approximately 12 mL/min and urine osmolality falling to 40 to 60 mmol/kg. The delay in reaching maximal diuresis is accounted for by the time involved in absorption of water from the gut, in metabolizing previously secreted vasopressin, and in renal recovery from the action of vasopressin.

INTERACTION OF OSMOTIC AND VOLUME INFLUENCES
Under conditions of water deprivation and of water loading, volume and osmotic influences act in parallel to influence AVP release. In other circumstances, volume and osmotic influences may be competitive, and changes in plasma volume can modify the effects of hypertonic stimuli on AVP release. Osmotic factors ordinarily predominate to maintain plasma osmolality within a narrow range. Larger changes in blood volume, such as those induced by hemorrhage, may blunt and eventually overcome the osmotic influences, and hypotension can activate arterial baroreceptors to exert a powerful stimulus to the elaboration of AVP and override simultaneous inhibiting influences.

RELATION BETWEEN AVP RELEASE AND THIRST-INDUCED WATER INTAKE
Under normal conditions, there is close coordination between AVP release and thirst, both of which are regulated by small changes in plasma osmolality. The perception of thirst generally becomes apparent when plasma osmolality exceeds 292 mmol/kg. Thus water intake is not stimulated until the urine is maximally concentrated. Angiotensin II increases thirst and AVP release under conditions of extracellular volume depletion. Normally, therefore, water losses lead to slight hypernatremia which increases thirst and fluid intake to restore and maintain normal plasma osmolality. In contrast, when there is loss of thirst perception (adipsia), fluid losses are uncorrected, and hypernatremia occurs even though AVP release is adequate to concentrate the urine maximally.

EFFECTS OF GLUCOCORTICOIDS
Hormones of the adrenal cortex and the posterior pituitary have antagonistic effects on water excretion. Cortisol elevates the osmotic threshold for AVP release elicited by hypertonic saline infusion in water-loaded normal subjects, and glucocorticoids protect against water intoxication and overcome the impaired response to water loading in adrenal insufficiency.

Although the impaired ability to dilute the urine in adrenal insufficiency may be due in part to excessive circulating AVP, glucocorticoids also can act directly on the renal tubules to decrease water permeability and increase excretion of solute-free water in the absence of AVP.

CELLULAR MECHANISM OF AVP ACTIVITY
The mechanism of action of AVP in the renal tubule is shown in Fig. 333-1: (1) AVP binds to contraluminal V_2 receptor sites, (2) the receptor-hormone complex activates adenylate cyclase in the same contraluminal membrane via a guanine nucleotide binding stimulatory protein (see Chap. 69), (3) the production of cyclic AMP is increased, (4) the cyclic AMP is translocated to the luminal cell membrane where it activates a membrane-bound protein kinase, (5) the activated protein kinase causes the phosphorylation of membrane proteins, and (6) permeability of the luminal membrane to water is increased. The AVP-generated cyclic AMP may be inactivated by a phosphodiesterase. AVP also stimulates prostaglandin E_2 production, which, in turn, acts as a feedback inhibitor of adenylate cyclase activation.

The final event in the transtubular movement of water is the appearance of particle aggregates in the luminal membrane of the cell (Fig. 333-2). This aggregation relieves the rate-limiting barrier to water flow. In the presence of the aggregates, water molecules can move passively along an osmotic gradient. The transtubular movement of water depends also on the integrity of the microtubular system.

Various cations and drugs influence the action of AVP. Calcium and lithium inhibit the adenylate cyclase response to vasopressin. Lithium also interferes with a subsequent biochemical action, as does potassium deficiency. Demeclocycline inhibits adenylate cyclase

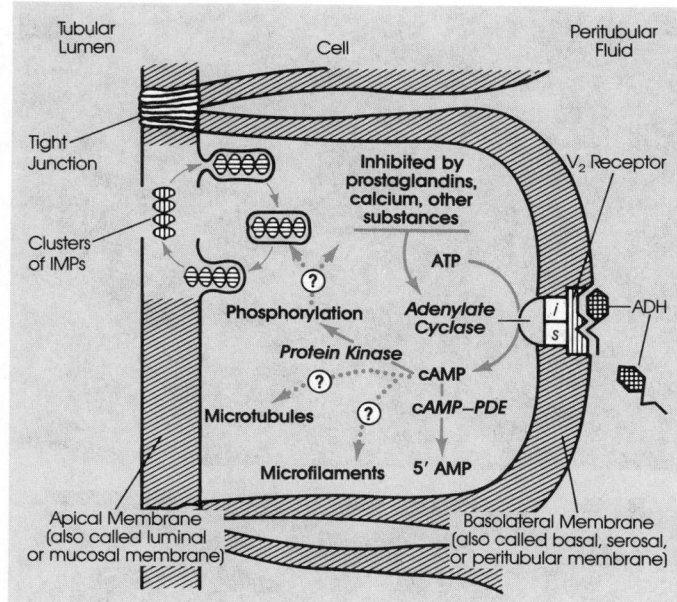

FIGURE 333-1 Schematic representation of the cellular action of vasopressin. The increased water permeability of responsive cells involves the V_2 receptor for vasopressin. Uninterrupted arrows denote steps that have been defined, interrupted arrows with question marks, postulated steps. ADH = antidiuretic hormone or vasopressin; i and s = inhibitory and stimulatory guanine nucleotide regulatory proteins; cAMP-PDE = phosphodiesterase; IMPs = intramembranous particles. (*From H Valtin, in EE Windhager, ed., Handbook of Physiology, Sect. 8: Renal Physiology, New York, Oxford, 1992.*)

stimulation by AVP and also inhibits the cyclic AMP-dependent protein kinase. In contrast, chlorpropamide increases AVP-induced activation of adenylate cyclase.

DEFICIENCY OF VASOPRESSIN: DIABETES INSIPIDUS

Diabetes insipidus refers to the passage through the body of a large quantity of dilute fluid. This state of excessive water intake and hypotonic polyuria may be due to failure of AVP release in response to normal physiologic stimuli (central or neurogenic diabetes insipidus) or failure of the kidney to respond to AVP (nephrogenic diabetes insipidus).

PATHOPHYSIOLOGY Deficiency of vasopressin release in response to the appropriate stimuli can result from lesions at several functional sites in the physiologic chain of events that regulates hormone release. Four types of central diabetes insipidus can be defined. Patients of the first type show very little rise in urine osmolality, even with a marked increase in plasma osmolality (1, Fig. 333-3) and no evidence of AVP release during hypertonic saline infusion. They are essentially devoid of releasable AVP. In the second type there is an abrupt increase in urine osmolality during dehydration (2, Fig. 333-3), but there is no evidence of an osmotic threshold during saline infusion. These patients have a defective osmoreceptor mechanism but can release AVP in response to the hypovolemia of severe dehydration. The third type of patient has some rise in urine osmolality with increasing plasma osmolality (3, Fig. 333-3) and has an elevated osmotic threshold for AVP release. These patients have a sluggish release mechanism due to a high-set osmoreceptor. In the fourth type of patient, urine and plasma osmolality coordinates are shifted to the right of normal (4, Fig. 333-3). AVP release in these patients is initiated at a normal plasma osmolality but is subnormal in amount.

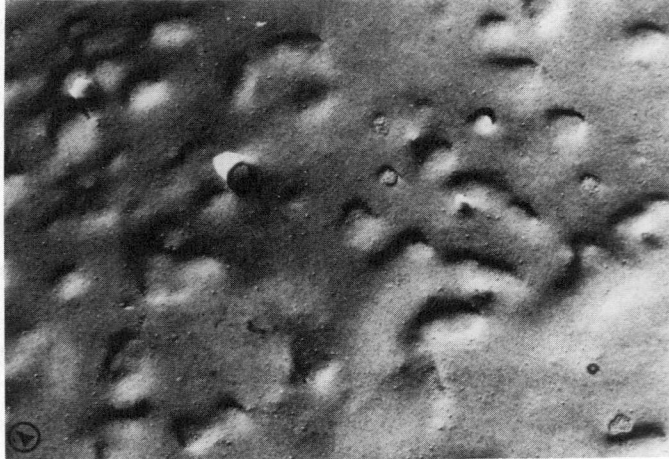

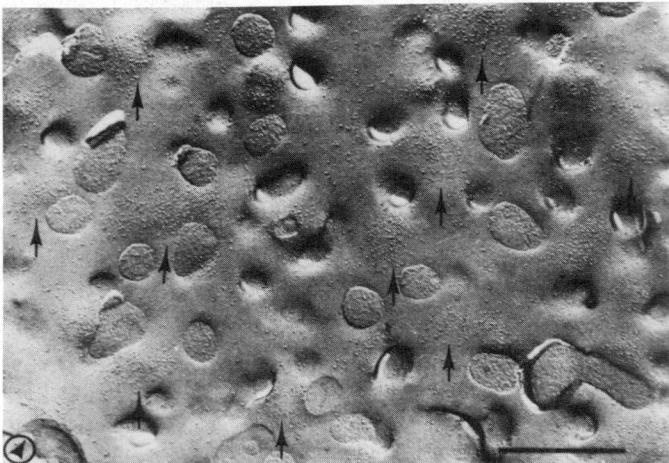

FIGURE 333-2 Virtual absence of particle clusters in renal collecting duct luminal membrane obtained from untreated Brattleboro (congenital diabetes insipidus) rat (*top*). Appearance of particle clusters (arrows) after treatment with AVP (*bottom*). (*From MC Harmanci et al, Am J Physiol 235:F440, 1978.*)

The second to fourth types of patients may develop a good antidiuresis in response to nausea, nicotine, methacholine, chlorpropamide, or clofibrate, indicating that the synthesis and storage of AVP are sufficient to allow for adequate urinary concentrating ability in the presence of an appropriate stimulus to release. In rare instances, patients of the second to fourth types may present with asymptomatic hypernatremia associated with mild or no polyuria.

ETIOLOGY The causes of central diabetes insipidus in 135 patients who satisfied the criteria described under "Diagnostic Tests" (below) and who had had the disorder for at least 6 months are shown in Table 333-1. Diabetes insipidus frequently starts in childhood or early adult life (median age of onset 24 years) and is more common in males than females. The major causes are as follows: (1) *Neoplastic or infiltrative lesions* of the hypothalamus or pituitary, including pituitary adenomas, craniopharyngiomas, germinomas, pinealomas, metastatic tumors, leukemia, histiocytosis X, and sarcoidosis, caused diabetes insipidus in 37 patients. In approximately 60 percent of these patients partial or complete loss of anterior pituitary function was present. (2) *Pituitary* or *hypothalamic surgery* caused diabetes insipidus in 32 patients and was usually associated with anterior hypopituitarism. Surgically induced diabetes insipidus usually develops between 1 and 6 days after surgery and often disappears after a few days. It may recur and become chronic after an "interphase" of 1 to 5 days. Removal of the posterior lobe of the pituitary induces permanent diabetes insipidus only if the pituitary stalk is sectioned high enough to induce retrograde degeneration of most neurons of the supraoptic nucleus. (3) *Severe head injuries*, usually associated with fractures of the skull, caused diabetes insipidus in 24 patients and were associated with anterior hypopituitarism in about one-sixth of patients. Spontaneous remissions of traumatic diabetes insipidus may occur even after 6 months, presumably because of regeneration of disrupted axons within the pituitary stalk. (4) *Idiopathic diabetes insipidus* (in 34 patients) usually starts in childhood and is seldom (<20 percent) associated with anterior pituitary dysfunction. This diagnosis can be made only after a careful search has failed to reveal evidence of a tumor, infiltrative or vascular lesion, or other presumptive cause of AVP deficiency. The presence of anterior hypopituitarism or hyperprolactinemia or radiologic evidence of lesions within or above the sella should stimulate a continuing search for a causative lesion at 3- to 12-month intervals. The diagnosis of idiopathic diabetes insipidus is made with increasing confidence as the duration of negative findings on follow-up increases. The number of neurons in

FIGURE 333-3 Relation of plasma and urinary osmolality during hydration and dehydration in normal adult subjects (shaded area) and in four types of patients with diabetes insipidus.

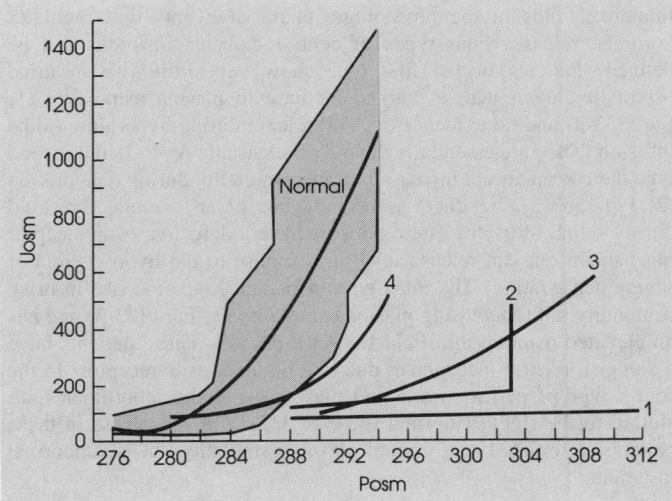

TABLE 333-1 Characteristics of 135 cases of long-standing* central diabetes insipidus diagnosed by the authors at SUNY Health Science Center, Syracuse. Categories are arranged in order of increasing median age of onset.

| Cause | Age of onset, years | | | | Percent of cases |
	Median[†]	Range	Males	Females	
Histiocytosis	2	1–30	3	2	4
Primary brain tumor —postoperative[‡]	15	6–50	9	11	15
Primary brain tumor —preoperative[§]	18	7–58	17	3	15
Idiopathic	20	<1–66	20	14	25
Head trauma	22	5–48	15	9	18
Nontraumatic encephalomalacia	43	15–73	3	4	5
Ruptured cerebral aneurysm	39		1	0	1
Post-hypophysectomy	42	24–68	4	8	9
Sarcoidosis	42		0	1	1
Metastatic cancer	56	32–72	6	5	8
			(58%)	(42%)	

* Longer than 6 months or until death.
† Median age of entire group = 24 years.
‡ 16 cases were of craniopharyngioma.
§ 5 cases were glioma, 7 germinoma, and 4 craniopharyngioma.

the supraoptic and paraventricular nuclei may be decreased in idiopathic diabetes insipidus, and circulating antibodies to hypothalamic nuclei may be present. In rare instances, diabetes insipidus may be inherited as an isolated defect or as part of an autosomal recessive syndrome (DIDMOAD) consisting of diabetes insipidus (DI), diabetes mellitus (DM), optic atrophy (OA), and deafness (D) (also called the *Wolfram syndrome*; see Chap. 343). (5) Seven patients had nontraumatic encephalomalacia from a variety of causes, including shock, cardiopulmonary arrest, hypertensive encephalopathy, poisoning, and meningitis. All the patients were brain dead and maintained on total life support systems.

Diabetes insipidus may appear during pregnancy and cease a few days after delivery, or it may commence after parturition in women with Sheehan's syndrome, especially when cortisol deficiency is treated. Mild symptoms of diabetes insipidus may either increase or improve during pregnancy. AVP-resistant diabetes insipidus also may develop during pregnancy, perhaps due to increased circulating levels of placental vasopressinase. Fortunately, such patients respond to treatment with desmopressin.

CLINICAL MANIFESTATIONS   *Polyuria, excessive thirst*, and *polydipsia* are almost invariably present in diabetes insipidus. Characteristically, these symptoms are sudden in onset, both when the disorder first presents itself and whenever the effects of administered vasopressin disappear during long-term therapy. In severe cases, the urine is pale in color, and the volume may be immense (up to 16 to 24 L/d), requiring micturition every 30 to 60 min throughout the day and night. More frequently, however, urine volume is only moderately increased (2.5 to 6 L/d), and occasionally it may be less than 2 L/d, causing no complaints on the part of the patient. Urinary concentration (less than 290 mmol/kg, specific gravity less than 1.010) is below that of the serum in severe cases but may be higher than that of serum (290 to 600 mmol/kg) in mild diabetes insipidus.

The slight rise in serum osmolality resulting from hypotonic polyuria stimulates thirst. Large volumes of fluid are imbibed, and cold drinks are preferred, patients often going to great trouble to secure cold fluids. Although thirst is probably secondary to loss of water, the administration of vasopressin may relieve or reduce thirst, even in the absence of fluid intake.

Normal function of the thirst center ensures that polydipsia closely matches polyuria, so dehydration is seldom detectable except by a mild elevation of serum sodium. However, when replenishment of excreted water is inadequate, dehydration may become severe, causing weakness, fever, psychic disturbances, prostration, and death. These features are associated with a rising serum osmolality and serum sodium concentration, the latter sometimes exceeding 175 mmol/L. Adipsia does not occur in idiopathic diabetes insipidus, but it may result from impaired function of the hypothalamic thirst center because of extension of the same abnormality that caused the diabetes insipidus. Alternatively, dehydration can occur during unconsciousness produced by surgical anesthesia, head trauma, or other causes.

Hydronephrosis and renal failure may complicate polyuria, especially in patients who fail to empty their bladders adequately because of bladder atony, urethral strictures, or other causes.

DIAGNOSTIC TESTS   The cause of hypotonic polyuria can usually be recognized by a pragmatic clinical approach. Even though stimuli such as nausea, nicotine administration, hypoglycemia, and hypotension may release AVP, the results are clinically irrelevant. It is of little consequence to the patient with symptomatic diabetes insipidus that one or more nonosmotic stimuli retains its capacity to release AVP. The following procedures, which utilize plasma and urine osmolality determinations, are readily available, reliable, and safe, and they allow the physician to establish the diagnosis and to initiate therapy rapidly. Measurements of plasma or urine AVP are expensive and time-consuming and are only occasionally needed, when osmolality measurements are inconclusive (Fig. 333-4). Diagnostic tests should not be performed in the presence of untreated thyroid or adrenocortical deficiency or when there is an osmotic diuresis (e.g., uncontrolled diabetes mellitus).

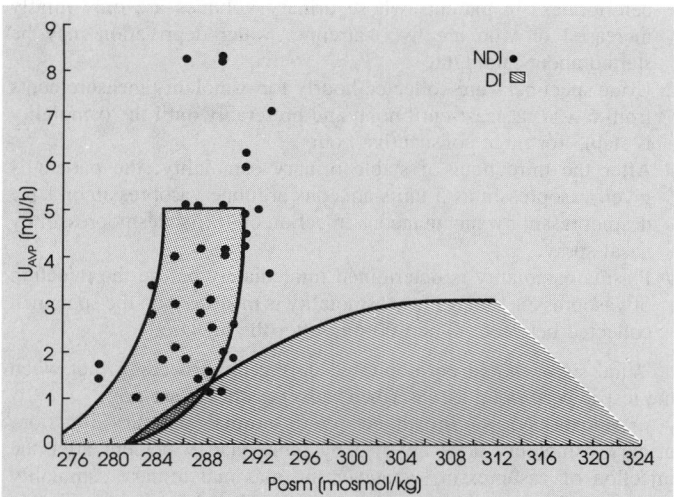

FIGURE 333-4   Relationship between plasma osmolality (Posm) and urinary AVP excretion (U_{AVP}) in normal subjects (shaded area on left), patients with central diabetes insipidus (shaded area on right), and patients with nephrogenic diabetes insipidus (individual data points). Correlates in patients with SIADH fall to the left of the normal range. [*From AM Moses, in P Czernichow and AG Robinson (eds), Frontiers of Hormone Research, vol 13: Diabetes Insipidus in Man, Basel, Karger, 1985.*]

Assessment of the relation of plasma to urine osmolality   The normal relationship between plasma osmolality (assuming no increase in blood urea or glucose) and urine osmolality is indicated in Fig. 333-3. If several simultaneously determined plasma and urine osmolalities in a patient with polyuria fall substantially to the right of the shaded area, the patient has central or nephrogenic diabetes insipidus. The latter diagnosis can be made if the response to injected vasopressin is subnormal (see "Dehydration Test," below) or if plasma or urinary AVP concentration is increased. The practice of relating plasma to urine osmolality is useful, particularly in postoperative neurosurgical cases or after head trauma, where its use can lead quickly to the differentiation of diabetes insipidus from parenteral fluid excess. If necessary, intravenous hydration can be slowed temporarily, and repeated plasma and urine osmolalities can be plotted as in Fig. 333-3, to determine whether the relationship is normal.

Dehydration test   Comparison of the urinary osmolality after dehydration with that after vasopressin administration is a simple and reliable way of diagnosing diabetes insipidus and of differentiating vasopressin deficiency from other causes of polyuria. This test should be combined with the assessment of the relationship between plasma and urine osmolality.

The maximal urinary concentrating capacity varies among individuals, and no absolute lower limits of "normal" can be defined in patients with nonspecific illnesses in whom AVP is produced in adequate amounts. It is impossible to distinguish between deficiency and sufficiency of AVP release solely by the level of the urinary osmolality attained after specified periods of water deprivation. On the other hand, if after prolonged dehydration vasopressin administration induces a further rise in urinary osmolality, there is a strong implication that vasopressin deficiency exists.

PROCEDURE

1 Fluids are withheld long enough to result in stable hourly urinary osmolalities (an hourly increase of < 30 mmol/kg for at least three successive hours). This is usually associated with a loss in body weight of at least 1 kg. In patients whose daily urinary volumes exceed 10 liters, the fluid deprivation should begin between 4 A.M. and 6 A.M. so that the patient can be carefully watched and the test terminated if weight loss exceeds 2 kg or the clinical condition deteriorates. In patients whose urinary volumes are only mildly increased or who are hyponatremic, water deprivation may be started about midnight.

2 Urine specimens are collected hourly for osmolality measurements from 6 A.M. at least until noon and preferably until the osmolality is stable for three consecutive hours.

3 After the third hour of stable urinary osmolality, the patient is given vasopressin as 5 units aqueous arginine vasopressin or 1 μg desmopressin by subcutaneous injection or 10 μg desmopressin by nasal spray.

4 Plasma osmolality is determined immediately before the injection of vasopressin, and urinary osmolality is measured on the specimen collected between 30 and 60 min after the injection.

Vital signs should be monitored during the procedure, but when the test is performed as described, adverse effects are rare.

INTERPRETATION   In subjects with normal pituitary function, urinary osmolality does not rise by more than 9 percent after the injection of vasopressin, whatever the maximal urinary osmolality achieved after dehydration alone. In central diabetes insipidus, the rise in urinary osmolality after vasopressin exceeds 9 percent. To ensure adequacy of dehydration, plasma osmolality before the vasopressin injection should be above 288 mmol/kg. Patients who have polyuria from renal diseases, potassium depletion, or nephrogenic diabetes insipidus (see below) usually show little rise in urinary osmolality with dehydration and no further rise after vasopressin injection. Patients with compulsive water drinking (primary polydipsia) often require prolonged water deprivation before plasma osmolality reaches 288 mmol/kg and before a plateau in urinary osmolality is reached; urinary osmolality rises by < 9 percent after the administration of exogenous vasopressin.

Hypertonic saline infusions   These tests are sometimes necessary to differentiate between primary polydipsia and partial central diabetes insipidus. In the former the osmotic threshold is low, normal, or slightly increased, while in the latter it is substantially increased or absent. See references for details.

DIFFERENTIAL DIAGNOSIS   Diabetes insipidus must be distinguished from other types of hypotonic polyuria (primary polydipsia and nephrogenic diabetes insipidus) and from states of osmotic diuresis (Table 333-2). Several are recognizable by the history

---

TABLE 333-2   Major polyuric syndromes

Primary disorders of water intake or output
A Excessive water intake
    1 Psychogenic polydipsia
    2 Hypothalamic disease: histiocytosis X, sarcoidosis, trauma
    3 Drug-induced polydipsia
        a Thioridazine
        b Chlorpromazine
        c Anticholinergic drugs (dry mouth)
B Inadequate tubular reabsorption of filtered water
    1 Vasopressin deficiency
        a Central diabetes insipidus
        b Drug-induced inhibition of AVP release
            (1) Narcotic antagonists
    2 Renal tubular unresponsiveness to AVP
        a Nephrogenic diabetes insipidus (congenital and familial)
        b Nephrogenic diabetes insipidus (acquired)
            (1) Several chronic renal diseases, after obstructive uropathy, unilateral renal arterial stenosis, after renal transplantation, after acute tubular necrosis
            (2) Potassium deficiencies, including primary aldosteronism
            (3) Chronic hypercalcemias, including hyperparathyroidism
            (4) Drug-induced: lithium, methoxyflurane anesthesia, demeclocycline
            (5) Various systemic disorders: multiple myeloma, amyloidosis, sickle cell anemia, Sjögren's syndrome
Primary disorders of renal absorption of solutes (osmotic diuresis)
A Glucose: diabetes mellitus
B Salts, especially sodium chloride
    1 Various chronic renal diseases, especially chronic pyelonephritis
    2 After various diuretics, including mannitol

(e.g., following lithium or mannitol administration, surgery under methoxyflurane anesthesia, or renal transplantation). In others the physical examination or simple laboratory procedures will indicate the diagnosis (evidence of glycosuria, renal disease, sickle cell anemia, hypercalcemia, or potassium depletion, including primary aldosteronism).

Congenital nephrogenic diabetes insipidus is usually inherited as an X-linked recessive trait. Affected males are totally resistant to vasopressin, while heterozygote females are asymptomatic or have mild polyuria. In several families the abnormal gene is localized to the Xq28 region of the long arm of the X chromosome. Almost all these patients have a V_2 receptor abnormality. Nephrogenic diabetes insipidus also may be inherited as an autosomal recessive trait or may occur sporadically. Females with sporadic disease appear to have a defect in the pathway of AVP action distal the V_2 receptor, and some of them respond to large doses of desmopressin. V_1 receptor–mediated functions are normal in patients with congenital nephrogenic diabetes insipidus.

When patients with nephrogenic and central diabetes insipidus cannot be differentiated by simpler means, documentation of elevated plasma or urinary AVP concentration in relation to plasma osmolality (Fig. 333-4) or of a high AVP concentration in relation to urine osmolality will allow the diagnosis of nephrogenic diabetes insipidus.

Primary polydipsia   Primary or psychogenic polydipsia may be difficult to differentiate from diabetes insipidus and occurs in two forms. Chronic overingestion of water results in hypotonic polyuria and is often confused with diabetes insipidus. The intermittent ingestion of large quantities of fluid also may lead to water intoxication and dilutional hyponatremia even though urinary diluting capacity is normal. This phenomenon is rare because normal adults can excrete between 10 and 14 mL/min of solute-free water, and it is unusual to ingest more water than this.

Polydipsia and polyuria may be erratic, even in the chronic form of primary polydipsia. This is in contrast to the sustained polydipsia and polyuria of diabetes insipidus. These patients often have no nocturnal polyuria. Of 17 patients with sustained primary polydipsia, 10 were female and 7 were male, with a median age of onset of 34 years (range 14 to 48). In three patients the onset of primary polydipsia followed head trauma, two had hypothalamic sarcoidosis, one was the sister of a patient with congenital nephrogenic diabetes insipidus, one was mentally retarded, and one had a hypothalamic lesion of unknown cause. The remaining nine patients had moderate to severe psychiatric disturbances, and some were taking psychoactive drugs with anticholinergic properties. The syndrome also has been described in patients with anorexia nervosa who drink huge quantities of water. There is a predisposition toward dilutional hyponatremia in patients who ingest excessive fluids when urinary diluting capacity is impaired by therapeutic agents such as nonsteroidal anti-inflammatory drugs or thiazide diuretics.

The diagnosis is usually evident from the combination of low plasma and urinary osmolalities. The relationship between urine and plasma osmolality during water deprivation is typically normal or supranormal (to left of normal in Fig. 333-3). There is an absent or minimal rise in urine osmolality after injection of vasopressin at the plateau of urine osmolality during dehydration. Because chronic overingestion of water may suppress release of AVP, and because chronic polyuria may cause a wash-out of the medullary osmotic gradient, urine osmolality may be subnormal in relation to plasma osmolality (to right of normal in Fig. 333-3). Therefore, it may be difficult, if not impossible, to differentiate primary polydipsia from partial central diabetes insipidus. Indeed, patients may have both problems. Treatment of these patients with vasopressin, even under close supervision, usually results in water intoxication.

A simple diagnostic approach to patients with hypotonic polyuria is shown in Fig. 333-5.

Determination of the cause of hypotonic polyuria   Once the type of the hypotonic polyuria is established, the cause must be determined (see "Etiology"). Even though treatment of the underlying

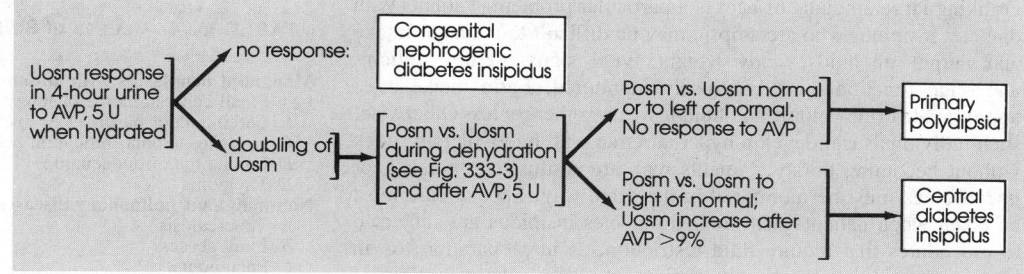

FIGURE 333-5 Approach to hypotonic polyurias.

disease only rarely causes the polyuria to regress, the underlying disease can at times be treated with success (e.g., germinoma). In this sense, the development of the polyuria can be considered a tumor marker.

The patient's history can reveal important clues such as age of onset and duration of disease, presence in other members of the family, constancy of symptoms, preference for cold or lukewarm fluids, head trauma, evidence of anterior pituitary deficiency, symptoms suggesting a space-occupying lesion, etc. Examination may reveal evidence of endocrine deficiency or excess (particularly hyperprolactinemia) or of malignant, granulomatous, or infectious disease. Routine laboratory tests and chests radiographs may provide important information.

Most patients with newly diagnosed central diabetes insipidus and primary polydipsia should have a magnetic resonance imaging study of the pituitary-hypothalamic area. In addition to providing insight into the underlying pathologic abnormality, the presence or absence of the posterior pituitary hyperintense signal with appropriate T_1-weighted imaging may confirm the diagnosis, since the signal is absent in central diabetes insipidus and present in primary polydipsia. Information obtained from lumbar puncture or even, at times, hypothalamic biopsy may diagnose lesions observed by magnetic resonance imaging. If magnetic resonance imaging is negative in patients with central diabetes insipidus, it should be repeated at increasing time intervals.

TREATMENT (See Table 333-3) Diabetes insipidus can be treated by hormone replacement. As is true of most peptides, oral administration of vasopressin is ineffective. Aqueous arginine vasopressin may be administered subcutaneously in doses of 5 to 10 units and usually has a duration of action of 3 to 6 h. The main use of this preparation is in initial management of unconscious patients with acute onset of diabetes insipidus following head trauma or a neurosurgical procedure. Its short duration of action allows recognition of the recovery of neurohypophyseal function and minimizes the development of water intoxication in patients receiving intravenous fluids.

Desmopressin has prolonged antidiuretic activity and is almost completely devoid of pressor effects. When used intranasally in amounts between 10 and 20 μg (0.1 to 0.2 mL) or by subcutaneous injection (1 to 4 μg), it has an antidiuretic action for 12 to 24 h in most patients. This analogue is the drug of choice in the treatment of most patients with diabetes insipidus. Lypressin is a nasal spray; a single application may result in an antidiuresis lasting approximately 4 to 6 h. Nasal absorption of both analogues may be decreased in the presence of an upper respiratory infection or allergic rhinitis. In such circumstances and in unconscious or uncooperative patients with diabetes insipidus, desmopressin should be given by subcutaneous injection.

Patients with diabetes insipidus who have some residual releasable AVP (types 2 to 4) may respond to oral treatment with chlorpropamide, clofibrate, or carbamazepine. Chlorpropamide stimulates AVP release and potentiates the antidiuretic action of submaximal amounts of AVP. Doses of 200 to 500 mg, usually taken once daily, are sufficient for an antidiuretic response. Its action starts within several hours of administration and usually lasts for 24 h. Chlorpropamide also may restore thirst perception and thus be useful in patients with thirst center defects. Oral hypoglycemic agents are rarely used because of hypoglycemia and other undesirable side effects.

The only way to treat most patients with nephrogenic diabetes insipidus is by solute restriction and administering thiazides or other diuretics. The resulting sodium depletion causes a fall in glomerular filtration rate with enhanced reabsorption of fluid in the proximal portion of the nephron and decreased delivery of sodium to the ascending limb of the loop of Henle and consequently reduced capacity to dilute the urine. Some women with congenital nephrogenic diabetes insipidus and some patients with lithium-induced polyuria have been treated effectively by injecting large doses of desmopressin.

When antidiuretic therapy is initiated in patients with longstanding diabetes insipidus care must be taken to avoid excessive drinking, which could result in water intoxication. Education about drinking according to thirst must be reinforced constantly in some patients.

TABLE 333-3 Agents used in treatment of diabetes insipidus

	Dose form	Usual dose	Duration of action, h
CENTRAL DIABETES INSIPIDUS			
Hormone replacement:			
Aqueous arginine vasopressin	10 or 20 units/ampul	5–10 units subcutaneously	3–6
Desmopressin	2.5 and 5.0 mL intranasal preparations, 100 μg/mL; 1- or 10-mL ampul, for injection, 4 μg/mL	10–20 μg intranasally or 1–4 μg subcutaneously	12–24
Lypressin	5-mL bottle, 50 units/mL	2–4 units intranasally	4–6
Nonhormonal agents:			
Chlorpropamide	100- and 250-mg tablets	200–500 mg daily	
Clofibrate	500-mg capsules	500 mg four times daily	
Carbamazepine	200-mg tablets	400–600 mg daily	
NEPHROGENIC DIABETES INSIPIDUS			
Hydrochlorothiazide	50-mg tablets	50–100 mg daily	
Chlorthalidone	50-mg tablets	50 mg daily	

Drinking large amounts of beer is a particular problem. Patients with diabetes insipidus who are adipsic may be difficult to manage. Intake and output of fluids, body weight, vital signs, serum sodium, and renal function must be closely monitored. Fluid intake must approximate urine volume and fluid losses by other routes. Otherwise, such individuals can develop hypernatremia with hypovolemic shock without becoming thirsty. Patients who are confused, obtunded, or unconscious must be monitored in the same way. Special care must be taken when patients with treated diabetes insipidus are subjected to procedures that require fluid restriction, as in preparation for an intravenous pyelogram, or hydration, as after administration of chemotherapy. In the former situation fluid intake must be restricted to conform to urine output. In patients receiving antidiuretic therapy fluids should not be administered beyond the amounts determined by thirst or urine output. If high urine flow rates are necessary, antidiuretic therapy can be discontinued, or furosemide may be administered while antidiuretic therapy is continued.

SYNDROMES ASSOCIATED WITH VASOPRESSIN EXCESS

Excessive blood levels or actions of vasopressin are associated with and probably cause water retention in several circumstances:

1 As a mechanism for *prevention of a rise in plasma osmolality* which would otherwise result from sodium retention in edema associated with congestive heart failure, cirrhosis with ascites, nephrosis, orthostatic edema, myxedema, and treatment with sodium-retaining drugs (fludrocortisone, nonsteroidal anti-inflammatory agents, and others)

2 As a mechanism of *defense against hypovolemia and/or hypotension* in subjects with adrenal insufficiency, excessive fluid loss (from vomiting, diarrhea, drug-induced diuresis, and excessive sweating), fluid deprivation, and probably positive-pressure respiration

3 As a consequence of *drug- or disease-induced release of vasopressin from the neurohypophysis* caused by:

  a Central nervous system disorders: head trauma, subdural hematoma, subarachnoid hemorrhage, cerebral vascular thrombosis, brain tumor, cerebral atrophy, acute encephalitis, acute psychosis, tuberculous and other meningitides

  b Drugs that release or potentiate the action of AVP: chlorpropamide, vincristine, vinblastine, cyclophosphamide, carbamazepine, general anesthetics, tricyclic antidepressants

4 In *ectopic AVP production and release:*

  a *From neoplastic tissue:* small cell carcinoma of lung, pancreatic carcinoma, lymphosarcoma, Hodgkin's disease, reticulum cell sarcoma, thymoma, carcinoma of duodenum or bladder

  b *From inflammatory lung diseases:* tuberculosis, lung abscess, pneumonias, empyema

5 *Other conditions:* Guillain-Barré syndrome, lupus erythematosus, acute intermittent porphyria, severe renovascular hypertension, and old age

SYNDROME OF INAPPROPRIATE AVP SECRETION OR SIADH
SIADH is the term applied to vasopressin excess of types 3 to 5 above, associated with hyponatremia without edema (Table 333-4). In these patients, the AVP excess is considered to be inappropriate because it occurs in the presence of plasma hypoosmolality. SIADH is analogous to abnormalities produced by administration of vasopressin and water to normal subjects. Although it may be conceptually valid to consider the AVP excess to be inappropriate in adrenal insufficiency and the edematous, hypovolemic, and hypotensive disorders listed in 1 and 2 above, their different pathogenic mechanisms and treatments make it clinically advisable not to consider these disorders as variants of the SIADH.

Pathogenesis of SIADH The ectopic origin of authentic AVP from neoplasms and pulmonary tissue of the types listed above has been documented by tissue analysis. Neoplastic cells obtained from

TABLE 333-4 Causes of SIADH

Malignant neoplasms with autonomous AVP release
  A Small cell carcinoma of lung
  B Carcinoma of pancreas
  C Lymphosarcoma, reticulum cell sarcoma, Hodgkin's disease
  D Carcinoma of duodenum
  E Thymoma
Nonmalignant pulmonary diseases
  A Tuberculosis
  B Lung abscess
  C Pneumonia
  D Viral pneumonitis
  E Empyema
  F Chronic obstructive airways disease
Central nervous system disorders
  A Skull fracture
  B Subdural hematoma
  C Subarachnoid hemorrhage
  D Cerebral vascular thrombosis
  E Cerebral atrophy
  F Acute encephalitis
  G Tuberculous meningitis
  H Purulent meningitis
  I Guillain-Barré syndrome
  J Lupus erythematosus
  K Acute intermittent porphyria
Drugs
  A Chlorpropamide
  B Vincristine
  C Vinblastine
  D Cyclophosphamide
  E Carbamazepine
  F Oxytocin
  G General anesthesia
  H Narcotics
  I Tricyclic antidepressants
Miscellaneous causes
  A Hypothyroidism
  B Positive pressure respiration

the tumors of patients with SIADH can synthesize, store, and release AVP. Both AVP and its associated neurophysin are elevated in the plasma of over 60 percent of patients with small cell carcinoma of the lung. There is excellent correlation between the increases in plasma AVP and neurophysin concentrations on the one hand and the clinical responses to treatment or the recurrences of disease on the other. Vasopressin also has been demonstrated in tuberculous lung tissue. It seems likely, but has not been established, that intracranial lesions (meningitis, encephalitis, trauma, vascular accidents) cause stimulation of AVP release from the neurohypophysis. Some drugs, such as vincristine, chlorpropamide, and carbamazepine, stimulate excessive release of AVP from the neurohypophyseal system, and others (e.g., chlorpropamide and nonsteroidal anti-inflammatory agents) potentiate the antidiuretic action of secreted AVP.

Excessive release or excessive renal tubular effect of vasopressin results in the excretion of a concentrated urine (with a urinary osmolality usually over 300 mmol/kg) despite a subnormal plasma osmolality and serum sodium concentration. Sodium excretion in the urine is maintained (usually above 20 mmol/L) by hypervolemia, suppression of the renin-angiotensin-aldosterone system, and increased plasma concentration of atrial natriuretic peptide. However, urinary sodium concentration may be below 20 mmol/L if sodium intake is low, but is higher if sodium intake is unrestricted. Blood urea nitrogen and uric acid concentrations tend to fall because of plasma dilution and increased excretion of nitrogenous compounds. Because of the hypervolemia, blood pressure shows no orthostatic fall, but in spite of hypervolemia there is no recumbent hypertension (except when plasma angiotensin II is simultaneously elevated in angiotensinogenic hypertension) and no edema (for an unknown reason). The extracellular hypotonicity leads to intracellular edema, and severe symptoms may result from cerebral edema.

Clinical manifestations of SIADH In general, the rate of fall in serum sodium concentration is more important in producing the neurologic features of SIADH than the absolute magnitude of the fall.

When SIADH is mild, with serum Na concentrations of 130 to 135 mmol/L, or develops gradually over several weeks, symptoms may be absent or limited to anorexia, nausea, and vomiting, such as occurs in other forms of hyponatremia. When hyponatremia is severe or acute in onset, body weight increases, and the symptoms of cerebral edema become predominant, including restlessness, irritability, confusion, coma, and convulsions associated with nonspecific EEG changes. Edema is almost always absent.

Diagnosis SIADH should be suspected in patients who have hyponatremia and a concentrated urine (osmolality >300 mmol/kg) associated with lethargy and in the absence of edema, orthostatic hypotension, and features of dehydration. The diagnosis of SIADH is made when other causes of enhanced AVP release are excluded. The diagnosis is supported by the finding of blood urea nitrogen, serum uric acid, creatinine, and albumin concentrations in the low-normal or subnormal range. However, it is essential in making the diagnosis to differentiate SIADH from (a) the *dilutional hyponatremias* listed in 2 above, particularly adrenocortical insufficiency, in which orthostatic hypotension with tachycardia and an elevated or high-normal BUN are characteristic, (b) the *edematous states* listed in 1 above, particularly hypothyroidism and congestive heart failure with hyponatremia, (c) *hypertensive states* associated with hyponatremia caused by renovascular stenosis or diuretic therapy, (d) *primary polydipsia* which is always associated with a dilute urine (osmolality < 150 mmol/kg), (e) *pseudohyponatremia* associated with excessive plasma glucose, triglyceride, or protein concentrations [conditions (a) through (e) are easily recognizable by the associated plasma abnormalities], and (f) the *"sick-cell"* syndrome, in which hyponatremia is due to a subnormal setting of the hypothalamic osmoreceptors, associated usually with a chronic, debilitating disease.

When the diagnosis of SIADH is not obvious after excluding other causes of hyponatremia, a positive diagnosis can usually be made with a *water-load test*. The water-load test is particularly useful in differentiating patients with a low-set osmoreceptor (who excrete the water normally) from all other hyponatremic states associated with a concentrated urine. This test should not be performed unless or until the serum sodium concentration has been elevated to a safe level (above 125 mmol/L) by restriction of water intake and/or, if necessary, by saline administration. The patient is asked to drink the water load (20 mL/kg of body weight up to 1500 mL) in 10 to 20 min, and urine is collected in hourly samples, with the patient recumbent between voidings, for 4 to 5 h in the morning. At least 65 percent of the water load should be excreted in 4 h or 80 percent in 5 h, and the lowest urinary osmolality, usually reached in the second hour, should be below 100 mmol/kg. It is essential, to prevent water intoxication in patients who fail to excrete the water load normally, to allow no further water intake for the rest of that day. Failure to excrete the water load may occur in adrenal insufficiency or renal insufficiency, as well as in SIADH. It is important to appreciate, too, that SIADH

cannot be diagnosed in the presence of severe pain, nausea, "stress," hypovolemia, hypotension, or other conditions that can stimulate AVP release even in the presence of plasma hypotonicity.

Measurements of plasma or urinary AVP (P_{AVP}, U_{AVP}) are useful adjuvants in establishing the diagnosis of SIADH. Plasma AVP is often immeasurable in hyponatremic states but is detectable, even after a water load, in SIADH. The correlates of plasma osmolality (Posm) versus P_{AVP} or U_{AVP} concentration fall to the left of the normal values in SIADH (Fig. 333-4) and in the other hyponatremic states associated with a concentrated urine. Thus, in most patients with SIADH, P_{AVP} and U_{AVP} concentrations, which may fluctuate widely, are unrelated to concomitant changes in Posm. Occasionally, this lack of correlation between Posm and P_{AVP} or U_{AVP} may be inconsistent. Rarely, for instance, the baseline, unstimulated AVP level may be inappropriately elevated and may fail to change as Posm is raised until the Posm reaches the normal range. Further increases in Posm induced by hypertonic saline infusion or water deprivation may then result in normal or subnormal increases in P_{AVP} or U_{AVP}. This unusual phenomenon may reflect uncontrolled "leakage" of AVP into the circulation.

The diagnostic approach to SIADH is depicted in Fig. 333-6.

Treatment Restriction of fluid intake to 800 to 1000 mL daily is essential. Since this intake is almost always exceeded by urinary output plus insensible fluid loss, a negative water balance ensues that results in gradual, daily reduction in weight, a progressive rise in serum Na concentration and osmolality, and symptomatic improvement. It is useful to verify the effectiveness of fluid restriction by documenting the changes in weight and serum Na concentration daily, until serum Na exceeds 135 mmol/L.

Unless and until the underlying cause of the SIADH can be corrected, fluid intake should be restricted continuously, to maintain normonatremia. In addition to restriction of fluid intake, 5% sodium chloride solution, 200 to 300 mL, should be infused intravenously over 3 to 4 h in patients with severe confusion, convulsions, or coma. It is important to avoid the possibility of inducing pontine myelinosis by not raising the serum Na concentration too rapidly. The possibility of causing congestive heart failure is remote as long as fluid is restricted but may be further reduced by the simultaneous administration of furosemide intravenously.

Attempts should be made to identify and correct the cause of the SIADH as soon as possible. The administration of water-retaining drugs should be stopped. Treatment of hypothyroidism with thyroxine should be initiated. Pulmonary tuberculosis and other pulmonary infections should be treated appropriately, and meningitis or other CNS disorders should be sought and treated, if present. When a malignant tumor is the source of autonomous AVP release and SIADH, surgery, radiation, and/or chemotherapy is often symptomatically beneficial even if the underlying neoplasm cannot be cured.

Antagonism of the release or action of AVP is not often necessary

FIGURE 333-6 Approach to diagnosis of SIADH in patients with hyponatremia.

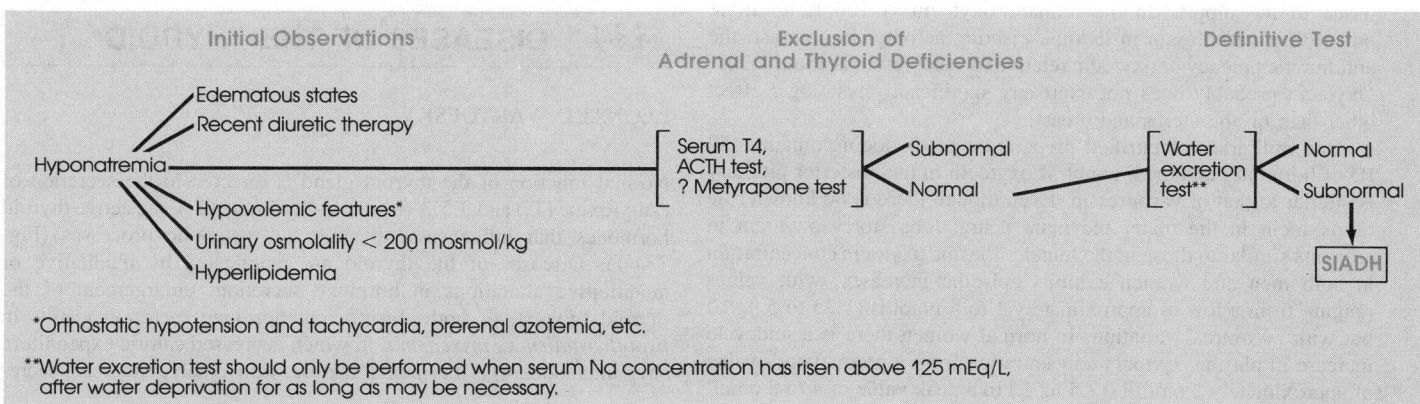

and seldom successful. Although phenytoin inhibits AVP release, it is seldom effective in SIADH. Drugs that block the effect of AVP on the renal tubule may occasionally be useful. Demeclocycline is the most potent inhibitor of AVP action available for chronic administration, in doses of 900 to 1200 mg/d. Patients receiving demeclocycline should be followed carefully to detect any evidence of renal failure, bacterial superinfection, or excessive drug-induced water loss. Lithium salts interfere with AVP action on tubular water reabsorption and can cause polyuria by this mechanism. Unfortunately, lithium can cause serious side effects in hyponatremic patients and for this reason is not recommended for treatment of SIADH.

Prognosis   The prognosis of SIADH depends on the cause. Drug-induced SIADH is rapidly and completely corrected by withdrawal of the causative agent. Similarly, the effective treatment of pulmonary or CNS infections can result in improvement and eventual cure of SIADH. Although SIADH resulting from small cell carcinoma of the lung or other malignancies can often be controlled with vigorous restriction of fluid intake, the underlying malignancy determines the prognosis in these patients.

PARAVENTRICULAR-NEUROHYPOPHYSEAL SYSTEM AND OXYTOCIN

CHEMISTRY AND PHYSIOLOGY   Oxytocin, a nonapeptide that differs by two amino acids from vasopressin, is produced in the cell bodies of the paraventricular nuclei and to a lesser extent in those of the supraoptic nuclei. It is synthesized and transported in neurosecretory granules by way of neuronal axons to the neurohypophysis, where it is stored or released, in conjunction with an oxytocin-specific neurophysin. Oxytocin release is stimulated by nerve impulses from the hypothalamus that cause depolarization of the neurosecretory terminals of the posterior pituitary and subsequent release of oxytocin through a calcium-dependent process, similar to the mechanism for vasopressin release. Estrogen stimulates release of oxytocin and its neurophysin. The secretion of oxytocin, as well as of vasopressin, is inhibited by ethanol. Some stimuli such as pain apparently release oxytocin and vasopressin simultaneously, but most stimuli release the two hormones independently. Oxytocin is liberated during suckling, whereas vasopressin is released in much greater quantities than is oxytocin after an osmotic stimulus or hemorrhage. Manipulation or distention of the female genital tract, artificially or during parturition, is a more effective stimulus to oxytocin release than suckling.

Oxytocin acts on the membranes of myometrial and myoepithelial cells to cause an increased force of contraction. Sensitivity of the myometrium to oxytocin increases with the duration of pregnancy, and a role for oxytocin in the initiation and maintenance of labor is probable but not established. Oxytocin may have survival value to the offspring, since it may hasten the final stages of birth and lessen the chances of anoxia. Oxytocin also exerts a contractile action on the myometrium postpartum and contracts the myoepithelial cells of the mammary alveoli, causing them to expel milk from the secretory tissue to the nipple. In the human, oxytocin is 100 times more potent than vasopressin in its milk-ejecting activity. In contrast, the antidiuretic potency of oxytocin relative to vasopressin is about 1:200. Oxytocin probably does not exert any significant physiologic effect other than on the uterus and breast.

One milligram of purified preparation of oxytocin contains 450 IU of hormone, and the amount of oxytocin in the posterior pituitary is similar to that of vasopressin. Even though there is no known role of oxytocin in the male, the male neural lobe stores oxytocin in amounts similar to those in the female. Plasma oxytocin concentration in both men and women exhibits episodic increases, with values ranging from a low of approximately 1 to 4 pmol/L (1.25 to 5 ng/L) but with no diurnal variation. In normal women there is a midcycle increase in plasma oxytocin concentration from a preovulatory value of approximately 2 pmol/L (2.5 ng/L) to a peak value of 4 to 8 pmol/L (5 to 10 ng/L) at the time of ovulation. During labor, plasma

oxytocin concentrations may reach high levels, with a rapid fall to prepartum levels after delivery. During suckling, plasma oxytocin levels of the mother vary but are usually about 10 to 20 pmol/L (12 to 25 ng/L). The half-life of oxytocin in plasma is about 3 to 5 min. Removal of oxytocin from the circulation is mainly by the kidneys and liver, although the uterus and mammary gland may remove some.

CLINICAL USE OF OXYTOCIN   The clinical use of oxytocin is limited to the induction of labor, control of hemorrhage following incomplete abortion and curettage, and treatment of impaired milk ejection. For discussion of the obstetric uses of oxytocin, the reader is referred to textbooks on obstetrics. Care must be taken because oxytocin may cause uterine rupture and fetal death. The antidiuretic action of oxytocin can be elicited with single intravenous doses of as little as 100 mU. Maximal antidiuresis is reached with 40 to 50 mU/min. Since 10 to 40 units of oxytocin per liter of dextrose is often used in obstetric practice, water intoxication may result. The vasodilatory action of oxytocin may cause sudden death of obstetric patients with heart disease because of hypotension, tachycardia, and arrhythmias. Anesthetics may modify the cardiovascular responses to oxytocin. For instance, in patients under cyclopropane anesthesia, oxytocin produces more hypotension but less tachycardia than in unanesthetized subjects. The vasodilatory effect of oxytocin can be blocked by vasopressin.

REFERENCES

BARTTER FC, SCHWARTZ WB: The syndrome of inappropriate secretion of antidiuretic hormone. Am J Med 42:790, 1967

BICHET DG et al: Hemodynamic and coagulation responses to 1-desamino (8-D-arginine) vasopressin in patients with congenital nephrogenic diabetes insipidus. N Engl J Med 318:881, 1988

CROSS BA, LENG G: *Progress in Brain Research*, vol 60: *The Neurohypophysis: Structure, Function and Control*. Amsterdam, Elsevier, 1983

CZERNICHOW P, ROBINSON AG: *Frontiers of Hormone Research*, vol 13: *Diabetes Insipidus in Man*. Basel, Karger, 1985

DURR JA: Diabetes insipidus in pregnancy. Am J Kidney Dis 9:276, 1987

GASH DM, BOER GJ (EDS): *Vasopressin: Principles and Properties*. New York, Plenum, 1987

MILLER M et al: Recognition of partial defects in antidiuretic hormone secretion. Ann Intern Med 73:721, 1970

MOSES AM: Osmotic thresholds for AVP release using plasma and urine AVP and free water clearance. Am J Physiol 256:R892, 1989

————, STREETEN DHP: Pathophysiologic and pharmacologic alterations in the release and action of ADH. Metabolism 25:697, 1976

———— et al: Marked hypotonic polyuria resulting from nephrogenic diabetes insipidus with partial sensitivity to vasopressin. J Clin Endocrinol Metab 59:1044, 1984

———— et al: Two distinct pathophysiological mechanisms in congenital nephrogenic diabetes insipidus. J Clin Endocrinol Metab 66:1259, 1988

———— et al: The use of T$_1$-weighted magnetic resonance imaging to differentiate between primary polydipsia and central diabetes insipidus. Am J Neuroradiol 13:1273, 1992

REICHLIN S: *The Neurohypophysis. Physiological and Clinical Aspects*. New York, Plenum, 1984

ROBERTSON GL: The regulation of vasopressin function in health and disease. Rec Progr Hormone Res 33:333, 1977

334   DISEASES OF THE THYROID*

LEONARD WARTOFSKY

Normal function of the thyroid gland is directed to the secretion of L-thyroxine (T$_4$) and 3,5,3′-triiodo-L-thyronine (T$_3$), the active thyroid hormones that influence a diversity of metabolic processes (Fig. 334-1). Diseases of the thyroid are manifested by qualitative or quantitative alterations in hormone secretion, enlargement of the thyroid (goiter), or both. Insufficient hormone secretion results in *hypothyroidism* or *myxedema*, in which decreased caloric expenditure (hypometabolism) is a principal feature. Conversely, excessive secre-

* Revision and update of work by the late Sidney Ingbar.

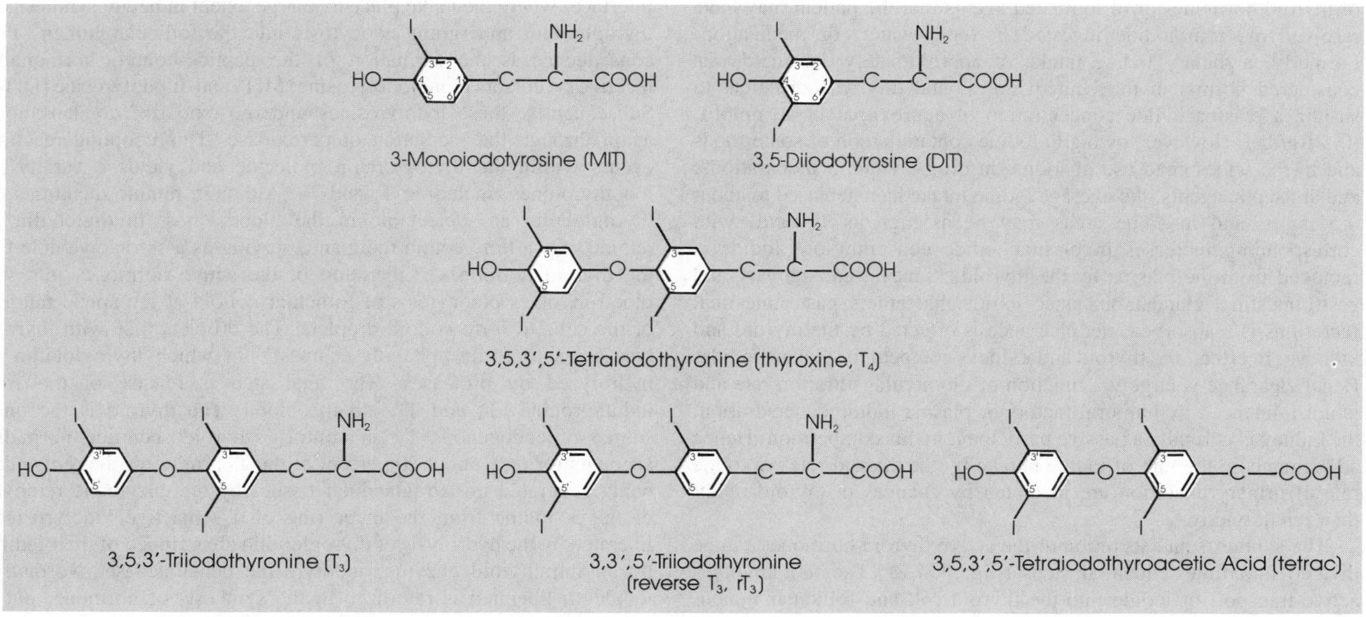

FIGURE 334-1   Structural formulas of thyroxine, its precursors, and certain of its metabolites.

tion of hormone results in hypermetabolism and other features termed *hyperthyroidism* or *thyrotoxicosis*. Enlargement of the thyroid gland (normally 15 to 20 g in adults) may be generalized or focal. Generalized enlargements may not be symmetric, the right lobe tending to enlarge more than the left. Goiters may be associated with increased, normal, or decreased hormone secretion, depending on the underlying disturbance. Focal enlargement usually reflects neoplastic disease, either benign or malignant, the former sometimes responsible for hypersecretion of hormone and hyperthyroidism, the latter rarely so. Any goiter may compress adjacent structures in the neck or mediastinum.

EMBRYOLOGY, ANATOMY, AND HISTOLOGY

The thyroid originates embryologically from an evagination of the pharyngeal epithelium with some contribution from the lateral pharyngeal pouches. Progressive descent of the midline thyroid anlage gives rise to the thyroglossal duct, which extends from the foramen cecum near the base of the tongue to the isthmus of the thyroid. Remnants of tissue may persist along the course of this tract as "lingual thyroid," thyroglossal cysts or nodules, or a structure contiguous with the thyroid isthmus called the *pyramidal lobe.* The latter is usually not discernible, except when the remainder of the gland is enlarged. Rarely, lingual thyroid may be the sole functioning thyroid tissue. In such cases, its secretion may or may not be sufficient to maintain a normal metabolic (euthyroid) state. Thyroid aplasia and functional failure of ectopic thyroid tissue are causes of sporadic neonatal hypothyroidism (1 in every 4000 or 5000 newborns), which responds to early treatment.

The fetal thyroid acquires the capacity to concentrate and organify iodine at about 10 weeks' gestation. Both T_4 and thyroid-stimulating hormone (thyrotropin, TSH) are detectable in the blood soon thereafter and increase in concentration during the second trimester. The increase in serum T_4 is due both to increasing thyroid secretion and to the appearance in plasma of thyroxine-binding globulin (TBG), and the increase in TSH is a reflection of the maturation of the fetal hypothalamus with resulting secretion of thyrotropin-releasing hormone (TRH). Maternal TRH readily crosses the placenta and may play a role in the development of the fetal pituitary-thyroid axis. Maternal TSH, by contrast, does not cross the placenta. T_3 is detectable in the blood later during the second trimester, but its concentration in blood and amniotic fluid remains low until shortly

after parturition. By contrast, the concentration of its analogue, 3,3′,5′-triiodo-L-thyronine (reverse T_3, rT_3), is increased in fetal blood and amniotic fluid relative to that in maternal blood (see Fig. 334-1). These differences are due to qualitative alterations in T_4 metabolism in the fetus. The low T_3 in fetal blood and amniotic fluid in the face of a high maternal concentration indicates that maternal-fetal transfer of T_3 is minimal, and the same is true of T_4. Hence T_4 from the fetal thyroid is the major thyroid hormone available to the fetus. Except for the possible effect of maternal TRH, therefore, the fetal pituitary-thyroid axis is a functional unit distinct from that of the mother.

The normal adult thyroid contains two lobes joined by an isthmus and lies just anterior and caudad to the cartilages of the larynx. Fibrous septa divide the gland into pseudolobules which, in turn, are composed of vesicles, called *follicles* or *acini*, surrounded by a capillary network. Normally, the follicle walls are composed of cuboidal epithelium. The lumen is filled with a proteinaceous *colloid,* which contains a unique protein, *thyroglobulin,* within the peptide sequence of which T_4 and T_3 are synthesized and stored. The thyroid contains a second smaller population of cells, the C cells. They are the source of calcitonin and give rise to medullary thyroid carcinoma when they undergo malignant transformation.

THYROID HORMONE ECONOMY: NORMAL PHYSIOLOGY

The term *thyroid hormone economy* denotes the processes involved in the synthesis of hormones within the thyroid gland, their transport in the circulation, their action and metabolism within the peripheral tissues, and the regulatory mechanisms that maintain a normal supply of thyroid hormones.

HORMONE SYNTHESIS AND SECRETION   Thyroid hormone synthesis depends on entry into the thyroid of adequate quantities of iodine, a constituent of T_4 and T_3; normal iodine metabolism within the gland; and synthesis of a receptor protein for iodine, thyroglobulin. The structure of thyroglobulin favors iodination and particularly formation of T_4 and T_3. Secretion of normal quantities of hormone, in turn, requires both a normal rate of hormone synthesis and a process for the hydrolysis of thyroglobulin and liberation of active hormones. Iodine enters the thyroid in the form of inorganic or ionic iodide, whose source is iodide derived either from the deiodination of thyroid hormones or of iodinated agents that the patient may have received or from iodide ingested in food, water, or medication. Formerly, a dietary iodine intake of approximately 0.2 mg/d was considered normal in the United States, and this was sufficient to sustain a plasma iodide concentration of approximately 40 nmol/L (0.5 μg/dL). However, owing to iodine contamination of some foods and to the widespread use of iodine in drugs, vitamin preparations, and antiseptic agents, the average iodine intake has increased to about 0.5 mg/d, and in some areas may be as high as 1 mg/d, with corresponding increases in plasma iodide concentration. Iodide is removed from the plasma by the thyroid, kidneys, and salivary and gastrointestinal glands, but since iodide that enters gastrointestinal secretions is reabsorbed, net clearance is effected by the thyroid and kidneys. In effect, the thyroid and kidneys compete for plasma iodide. Renal clearance is largely a function of glomerular filtration rate and is not influenced by humoral factors or plasma iodide concentration; the kidney is normally a passive participant in this competition. Hence adjustments in the rate of iodide uptake by the thyroid relative to the rate of urinary excretion are mediated by changes in thyroid rather than renal avidity.

The synthesis and secretion of the active thyroid hormones can be divided into four sequential steps (Fig. 334-2). The first involves active transport of iodide into the thyroid cell and follicular lumen. This occurs at a rate that exceeds passive diffusion of iodide out of the gland, with the result that the thyroid maintains concentration gradients for iodide (thyroid/plasma concentration ratios) of substantial magnitude (usually of 25 but up to 500 or more under certain conditions). Energy for iodide transport depends on oxidative metabolism within the gland. The second step in hormone biosynthesis involves oxidation of iodide to a higher valence form that is capable of iodinating tyrosyl residues in thyroglobulin, a glycoprotein of approximately 660,000 mol wt that is synthesized within the follicular cell. Oxidation of iodide is effected by a peroxidase, which utilizes hydrogen peroxide generated during the course of oxidative metabolism within the gland. Organic iodinations occur at the cell-colloid

FIGURE 334-2 Schema depicting pathways in the synthesis and secretion of thyroid hormones and mechanisms for the suprathyroidal and intrathyroidal regulation of thyroid function. Small, solid arrows indicate pathways of iodine metabolism; open arrows indicate stimulation; cross-hatched arrows indicate inhibitory influences. TRH, thyrotropin-releasing hormone; TSH, thyroid-stimulating hormone; IPO, iodide peroxidase; prot., thyroid protease; peptid., thyroid peptidase; MIT, monoiodotyrosine; DIT, diiodotyrosine; T$_4$, thyroxine; T$_3$, 3,5,3'-triiodothyronine.

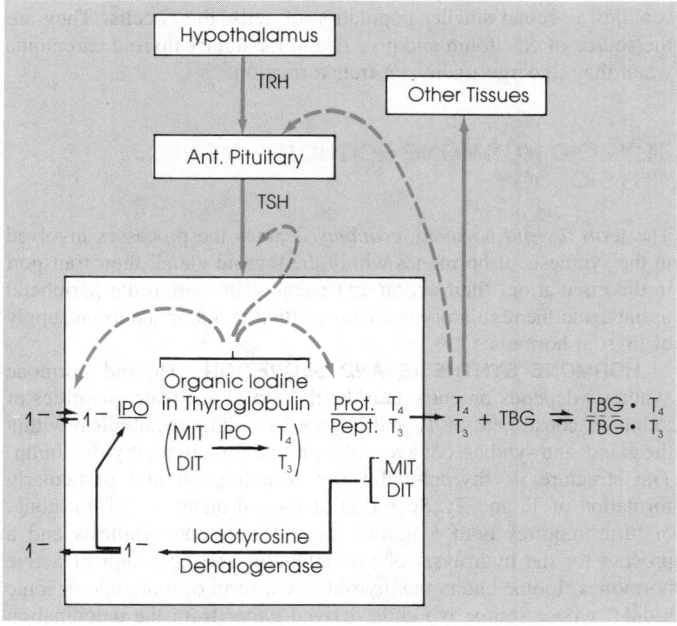

interface, where they take place to a large extent in newly synthesized thyroglobulin undergoing exocytosis into the follicular lumen. The consequence is the formation of the peptide-bound, hormonally inactive precursors monoiodotyrosine (MIT) and diiodotyrosine (DIT). Subsequently, these iodotyrosines undergo oxidative condensation, again through the mediation of peroxidase. This coupling reaction occurs within the thyroglobulin molecule and yields a variety of iodothyronines, including T$_4$ and T$_3$. Although minute quantities of thyroglobulin are detectable in the blood, most thyroglobulin is retained for a time within the gland, serving as a storage vehicle for the thyroid hormones. Liberation of the active hormones into the blood involves pinocytosis of follicular colloid at the apical margin of the cells to form colloid droplets. The droplets fuse with thyroid lysosomes to form "phagolysosomes," in which thyroglobulin is hydrolyzed by proteases. The final step is release of the free iodothyronines T$_4$ and T$_3$ into the blood. The thyroid is the only source of endogenous T$_4$; in contrast, thyroid secretion normally accounts for only about 20 percent of the T$_3$ produced, the remainder being generated in extraglandular tissues by the enzymatic removal of the 5'-iodine from the outer ring of T$_4$. Inactive iodotyrosines liberated by the hydrolysis of thyroglobulin are stripped of their iodine by an intrathyroid enzyme, iodotyrosine dehalogenase. Normally, iodide so liberated is reutilized in the synthesis of hormone, but a small proportion is lost into the blood (iodide leak); iodine leaks may become large under certain circumstances.

The thyroid also concentrates other monovalent anions such as pertechnetate, which is available as the radioactive isotope sodium [^{99m}Tc]pertechnetate. Unlike iodide, little pertechnetate is organically bound; hence its duration of stay within the thyroid is short. This property, together with its short physical half-life, makes pertechnetate a valuable radionuclide for imaging the thyroid by scintillation scanning.

The foregoing reactions are subject to inhibition by a variety of agents termed *goitrogens*, since, by virtue of their ability to inhibit hormone synthesis and indirectly stimulate TSH secretion, they induce goiter formation. Inorganic anions such as perchlorate and thiocyanate inhibit iodide transport and thereby reduce substrate for hormone formation. The goiter and hypothyroidism that follow, however, can be prevented or relieved by doses of iodide sufficiently large to enable adequate quantities to enter the gland by passive diffusion. The commonly employed antithyroid agents, such as the derivatives of thiourea and mercaptoimidazole, exert more complex actions on hormone biosynthesis. These agents inhibit the initial oxidation (organic binding) of iodide, decrease the proportion of DIT relative to MIT, and block coupling of iodotyrosines to form the hormonally active iodothyronines. The latter reaction is the most sensitive. Thus the synthesis of hormonally active iodothyronines may be decreased, although the total incorporation of iodine by the thyroid is inhibited but little. In contrast to the effect of the monovalent anions, the goitrogenic action of thioureas is not overcome by large quantities of iodine. Indeed, certain weak goitrogens, such as sulfonamides and antipyrine, are more potent when given with iodide, an effect not understood. Iodine itself, when given acutely in large doses, blocks the organic binding and coupling reactions. This action (Wolff-Chaikoff effect) is normally transient, but prolonged administration of iodide may be associated with continued inhibition of hormone synthesis and development of goiter, with or without hypothyroidism (iodide myxedema). Many patients with Graves' disease, especially after treatment with radioiodine or surgery, or with Hashimoto's disease are sensitive to the blocking effect of iodide and develop hypothyroidism when given iodides chronically. The fetal thyroid is similarly sensitive, and pregnant women should not be given iodide in large amounts because of the danger of inducing goitrous hypothyroidism in the fetus. Iodide in large doses is capable of inhibiting proteolysis of thyroglobulin and hormone release, an effect readily demonstrable in hyperfunctioning thyroids and responsible for the ameliorative action of iodides in hyperthyroidism. Excess iodide also may induce thyrotoxicosis in susceptible individuals, as discussed below. Lithium, which is administered as the carbonate salt in some patients with depression has several effects on intrathyroidal iodine metabolism, one of which is to inhibit hormone release. Glucocorticoids causes a decrease in serum thyroid hormone levels due to inhibition of TSH secretion and decreased T_4 binding to TBG. Serum T_3 is also decreased in part because of inhibition of T_4 to T_3 conversion. A direct inhibitory action of glucocorticoids on the thyroid may occur in Graves' disease, possibly by inhibition of thyroid-stimulating immunoglobulins. Dexamethasone, in conjunction with iodide, can effect a rapid reduction in the degree of thyrotoxicosis.

HORMONE TRANSPORT AND METABOLISM

HORMONE TRANSPORT In the blood, T_4 and T_3 are almost entirely bound to plasma proteins. T_4 is bound, in decreasing order of intensity, to thyroxine-binding globulin (TBG), to a T_4-binding prealbumin (transthyretin, TTR), and to albumin. High-density lipoproteins transport about 3 percent of circulating T_4 and 6 percent of T_3. By virtue of its intense affinity for T_4, TBG is the major determinant of normal binding. T_4 and its binding proteins interact in a reversible binding equilibrium in which the majority of the hormone is bound and a small proportion (normally about 0.03 percent) is free. While TTR transports only about 15 percent of circulating T_4, its contribution to free hormone is comparable to that from TBG owing to its higher dissociation constant. T_3 is not significantly bound by TTR and is bound 10 to 20 times less firmly by TBG than T_4. As a consequence, the normal proportion of free T_3 (approximately 0.3 percent) is 8 to 10 times greater than that of T_4. Only the free or unbound hormone is available to tissues; therefore, the metabolic state correlates more closely with the concentration of free than with the concentration of total hormone in plasma, and homeostatic regulation of thyroid function is directed toward maintenance of a normal concentration of free hormone. Moreover, the relatively weak binding of T_3 accounts for its more rapid onset and offset of action. Disturbances of thyroid hormone–plasma protein interaction are of two general types (see Table 334-1). In the first, the thyroid-pituitary axis is intrinsically normal, and the homeostatic control of thyroid hormone secretion is intact. Under these circumstances, disordered binding interactions result from alterations in thyroid hormone binding. For example, an increase in TBG initially lowers the concentration of free hormone and thus diminishes the quantity of hormone available to tissues. Total hormone concentration in serum then increases until the concentration of free hormone is restored to normal. The increase in total hormone concentration counterbalances the decrease in the free proportion; as a result, the absolute concentration of free hormone is normal, and the metabolic state of the patient is normal. Opposite changes occur when the concentration of TBG declines. Table 334-2 summarizes those states associated with primary alterations in

the concentration of TBG. Primary disturbances in thyroid hormone binding also occur when other binding proteins in blood are increased or when abnormal binding proteins appear. These are discussed below.

The second type of disturbance of thyroid hormone–binding interactions results from a primary alteration in the concentration of thyroid hormones in the blood, as in hypothyroidism or thyrotoxicosis. Here, normal homeostatic control of thyroid hormone secretion is lost, either because of disease within the control mechanism itself or because an intact control mechanism is incapable of overcoming the effects of disease elsewhere. Under these circumstances, the concentration of TBG is changed little, if at all, and the concentration of free hormone varies directly with the total concentration of hormone. Since homeostatic mechanisms cannot restore the concentration of free hormone to normal, primary changes in thyroid function cause persistent changes in the concentration of total and free hormone and, consequently, alterations in the metabolic state.

HORMONE METABOLISM Following penetration into the cell, T_4 and T_3 undergo reactions that lead ultimately to their excretion or inactivation. Thyroid hormones undergo sequential removal of single iodine atoms (monodeiodinations) that ultimately yields the thyronine nucleus stripped of iodine. Deiodinative pathways account for approximately 70 percent of T_4 and T_3 disposal. In the case of T_4, the most important of these is the 5′-monodeiodination that leads to the generation of T_3. Since approximately 30 percent of T_4 is converted to T_3, and since T_3 has approximately three times the metabolic potency of T_4, virtually all the metabolic action of T_4 can be ascribed to the action of the T_3 that it gives rise to. Normally, extraglandular formation accounts for about 80 percent of the T_3 in the blood and of overall T_3 production, the remainder coming from thyroid secretion. As a consequence, abnormal states and pharmacologic agents that impair T_3 formation lower the serum T_3 concentration (Table 334-3). When patients with thyroid hypofunction are treated with synthetic T_4 (levothyroxine) to sustain serum T_4 concentrations within or somewhat above the normal range, normal or nearly normal serum

TABLE 334-2 Circumstances associated with altered concentration of TBG

Increased TBG	Decreased TBG
Pregnancy	Androgens
Newborn state	Large doses of glucocorticoid
Oral contraceptives and other sources of estrogen	Chronic liver disease
Tamoxifen	Severe systemic illness
Infectious and chronic active hepatitis	Active acromegaly
Biliary cirrhosis	Nephrosis
Acute intermittent porphyria	Genetically determined
Perphenazine	Asparaginase
Genetically determined	

TABLE 334-1 Classification of the varieties of disordered thyroid hormone–plasma protein interactions

Type of abnormality	Serum T_4 and T_3	Percent FT_4 and FT_3 or RT_3U	FT_4 and FT_3 or FT_4I and FT_3I
PRIMARY ABNORMALITY IN TBG			
Increased concentration	↑	↓	N
Decreased concentration	↓	↑	N
PRIMARY DISORDER OF THYROID FUNCTION			
Hypothyroidism	↓	↓	↓
Hyperthyroidism	↑	↑	↑

NOTE: FT_4 = free T_4; FT_3 = free T_3; FT_4I = free T_4 index; FT_3I = free T_3 index; RT_3U = resin-T_3 uptake; TBG = thyroid-binding globulin.

TABLE 334-3 States associated with decreased peripheral conversion of T_4 to T_3

PHYSIOLOGIC

Fetal and early neonatal life
? Old age

PATHOLOGIC

Fasting
Malnutrition
Systemic illness
Physical trauma
Postoperative state
Drugs (propylthiouracil, dexamethasone, propranolol, amiodarone)
Radiographic contrast agents (ipodate, ipanoate)

T_3 concentrations are maintained. The generalization that the thyroid secretes relatively little T_3 does not apply to states in which the thyroid is hyperfunctioning or under increased stimulation by TSH. Under these conditions, the T_3/T_4 ratio of the secretory product and the serum concentration of T_3 relative to that of T_4 are increased. In addition, when T_4 production is decreased, as in early thyroid failure or iodine deficiency, the T_3/T_4 concentration ratio in blood is increased still further by an autoregulatory mechanism that leads to an increase in the efficiency of T_3 formation.

Approximately 40 percent of T_4 disposal is accounted for by monodeiodination at the 5 position of its inner ring to yield reverse T_3 (rT_3); this process accounts for nearly all rT_3 produced. rT_3 has little, if any, metabolic potency; therefore, the relative rates of outer- and inner-ring monodeiodination of T_4 determine the quantity of metabolically active hormone available. Factors that impair T_3 formation almost invariably increase serum rT_3 concentrations. This increase is not due to an increase in the production of rT_3 from T_4, but rather to a decrease in the 5'-monodeiodination of rT_3 to yield 3,3'-diiodothyronine (3,3'T_2); i.e., both the decreased conversion of T_4 to T_3 and the decreased degradation of rT_3 are due to a selective impairment of 5'-monodeiodination.

A second major pathway of metabolism of T_4 and T_3 and of their metabolites is conjugation in the liver, principally with glucuronate and sulfate. Conjugates either undergo deiodination locally or are secreted into the bile, but the magnitude of the enterohepatic circulation in humans is unknown. Reabsorption is incomplete at best, since the fecal excretion of T_4, T_3, and their iodine-containing metabolites accounts for approximately 20 percent of overall T_4 disposal. About 20 percent of T_4 and T_3 undergoes oxidative deamination and decarboxylation of the alanine side chain to yield tetraiodo- and triiodothyroacetic acid (tetrac and triac, respectively).

Under certain circumstances, changes in hormone synthesis and metabolism are the major determinant of the rates of metabolic clearance of T_4 and T_3. Both phenobarbital and phenytoin increase the metabolic clearance of thyroid hormones without increasing the proportion of free hormone in the blood. Indeed, in the case of phenytoin, both total and free T_4 concentrations are diminished. Nevertheless, a normal metabolic state is maintained, possibly because of an increase in T_3 formation.

HORMONE ACTION   The thyroid hormones influence the growth and maturation of tissues, cell respiration and total energy expenditure, and the turnover of essentially all substrates, vitamins, and hormones, including the thyroid hormones themselves. Some hormone actions on cell metabolism may be mediated at the level of the mitochondrion to influence oxidative metabolism and at the level of the plasma membrane and endoplasmic reticulum to influence the activity of Ca^{2+}-ATPase and transcellular flux of substrates and cations. However, the primary action of the hormone is exerted via binding to one or more intracellular receptor complexes, which, in turn, bind to specific regulatory sites in the chromosomes to influence genomic expression (see Chap. 329). There are two classes of thyroid hormone receptor (TR) which are encoded by two different genes, TRα and TRβ, located on chromosomes 17 and 3, respectively. By alternative splicing, these two genes, in turn, generate additional isoforms (e.g., α_1, α_2, β_1, β_2, etc.). The TR proteins are part of a superfamily of genes encoded by mRNAs of cellular (c-) homologues of the avian retroviral v-erb A proto-oncogene. The TR genes, c-erbA-α (TRα) and c-erb-A-β (TRβ), encode receptor proteins with a T_3-binding domain and a DNA-binding domain. The DNA-binding domain attaches to regulatory sequences in those target genes with T_3-regulated transcription (e.g., TSH, prolactin, growth hormone). In an interaction stabilized by TR auxiliary proteins (TRAPs), the activation and modulation of rates of transcription are mediated by regulatory sequences called *thyroid response elements* (TRE). Thus, in the pituitary, the binding of T_3-TR complexes to TRE serves to inhibit the expression of genes for the synthesis of the α and β subunits of TSH. While pituitary may contain the highest concentrations of TR, all tissues with high-affinity nuclear T_3 binding express TRα and

TRβ receptors. High concentrations of c-erb A-β_1 are found in brain, liver, heart, and kidney. The variable lack of T_3 responsiveness in different tissues ("resistance") is due to point mutations in the T_3-binding domain of the c-erbA-β receptor (see below).

THYROID HORMONE RESISTANCE   Generalized thyroid hormone resistance (GTHR) is a syndrome characterized by reduced responsiveness to elevated levels of thyroid hormone. The resistance to thyroid hormone action is associated with elevated circulating levels of free T_4 and free T_3, inappropriately normal or elevated (i.e., nonsuppressed) serum TSH, and intact TSH responsiveness to TRH. Kindreds have been described whose members express variable patterns of resistance, and responsiveness of target tissues may vary within the same individual. At the molecular levels, the varied phenotypes appear to be due to different gene mutations altering function of the c-erbA-β receptor. Clinical features include short stature, hyperactivity, attention deficits with mental deficiency or learning disability, and goiter. While GTRH patients are either euthyroid or hypothyroid, the differential diagnosis includes isolated pituitary resistance to thyroid hormone and a TSH-secreting pituitary tumor, disorders in which the patients usually present with hyperthyroidism. Indications for treatment of GTHR vary depending on the clinical features, but the presence of increased serum TSH reflects the need for supplemental thyroid hormone, the dosage requirement depending on parameters of tissue responses to thyroid hormone.

REGULATION OF THYROID FUNCTION   Thyroid function is regulated by two general mechanisms, one suprathyroid and one intrathyroid (Fig. 334-2). The proximate mediator of suprathyroid regulation is thyrotropin (thyroid-stimulating hormone, TSH), a glycoprotein secreted by basophilic (thyrotropic) cells in the anterior pituitary. TSH stimulates thyroid hypertrophy and hyperplasia; accelerates most aspects of intermediary metabolism in the thyroid; enhances synthesis of nucleic acid and protein, including thyroglobulin; and stimulates the synthesis and secretion of thyroid hormones. These actions result from binding of TSH to specific receptors in the surface of the follicular cell and subsequent activation of the plasma membrane enzyme adenylate cyclase. The resulting increase in the cellular cyclic 3',5'-adenosine monophosphate (cyclic AMP) concentration initiates most or all TSH responses.

Regulation of TSH secretion, in turn, is effected by two opposing influences at the level of the thyrotropic cell. Thyrotropin-releasing hormone (TRH), a tripeptide of hypothalamic origin, stimulates the secretion and synthesis of TSH, whereas thyroid hormones both inhibit the TSH secretory mechanism directly and antagonize the action of TRH. Thus homeostatic control of TSH secretion is exerted in a negative-feedback manner by thyroid hormones, and the threshold for feedback inhibition is apparently set by TRH. TRH reaches the pituitary via the hypophyseal portal blood system and binds to specific high-affinity receptors on the plasma membrane of the thyrotropic cell. Either activation of the adenylate cyclase system or a concomitant translocation of extracellular calcium into the cell initiates release of TSH. In addition to stimulating release of stored TSH, TRH enhances new synthesis of TSH via transcription and translation of the gene for the β subunit. TRH also plays a role in posttranslational processing of TSH, as indicated by the fact that TSH in patients with hypothalamic hypothyroidism has reduced biologic activity. The negative-feedback effect of the thyroid hormones appears to take place entirely at the level of the thyrotropic cell. Experimentally, thyroid hormones inhibit production of TRH mRNA and TRH prohormone as well as reduce the number of TRH receptors on the thyrotropic cell, thus impairing its responsiveness to TRH. The major negative-feedback action of the thyroid hormones is at the pituitary level, mediated by binding of the hormones to TR in the nucleus of the thyrotropic cell, resulting in reduced expression of the genes for α and β subunits of TSH. The principal arbiter of thyroid hormone action within the pituitary is T_3, both that generated locally from intrapituitary T_4 and that derived from plasma. To what extent T_4 itself is effective within the pituitary is uncertain, but other factors modify the secretion of TSH and its response to TRH. Both somatostatin and dopamine appear to be physiologic inhibitors of TRH secretion. Estrogens enhance responsiveness to TRH, whereas glucocorticoids inhibit this function. Catecholamines also play a role, with α_1-adrenergic pathways being inhibitory and α_2 pathways being stimulatory. Experimentally, tumor necrosis factor and interleukin 1 inhibit TSH secretion, possibly playing a role in the sick euthyroid syndrome.

Intrathyroid regulation of thyroid function is also important. In some manner, changes in glandular organic iodine content cause reciprocal changes in thyroid iodide transport activity and regulate growth, amino acid uptake, glucose metabolism, and nucleic acid synthesis. These influences are evident in the absence of TSH stimulation and hence may be termed *autoregulatory*, but their most important role is to modify (iodine-enrichment inhibiting and iodine-depletion enhancing) the response to TSH, probably by influencing the generation of cyclic AMP consequent to TSH stimulation. Cytokines may exert stimulatory or inhibitory effects on thyroid hormone synthesis or secretion and on interactions with TSH and in vitro, but the physiologic and pathophysiologic significance of these substances (e.g., atrial natriuretic peptide, tumor necrosis factor, transforming growth factor, epidermal growth factor, endothelin, etc.) remains to be clarified.

LABORATORY TESTS

Laboratory tests of thyroid hormone economy can be divided into five general categories: direct tests of thyroid function, tests related to the concentration and binding of thyroid hormones in blood, metabolic indexes, tests of the homeostatic control of thyroid function, and miscellaneous tests that do not fit into other categories.

DIRECT TESTS OF THYROID FUNCTION Among all tests designed to assess thyroid status, only those which involve in vivo administration of radioactive iodine test glandular function per se, and measurement of the *thyroid radioactive iodine uptake* (RAIU) is the most common. ^{131}I has been used for this purpose, but ^{123}I is preferable because of the lower radiation dose that it delivers. The administered radioiodine mixes uniformly with the endogenous iodide in the extracellular fluid and, in the steady state, can be used to assess what percentage of the iodide entering and leaving the extracellular space per unit time is accumulated by the thyroid. The RAIU is measured 24 h after administration of the isotope, since it usually reaches a plateau value at this time, but in severe thyroid hyperfunction it may peak early. The RAIU varies inversely with the plasma iodide concentration and directly with the functional state of the thyroid. At usual levels of iodine intake in the United States (up to 1 mg/d), the normal 24-h RAIU is approximately 10 to 30 percent of the administered dose. Consequently, this test discriminates poorly between normal and hypothyroid states. Values above the normal range, however, usually indicate thyroid hyperfunction and are useful in the diagnosis of hyperthyroidism. The RAIU is also a part of the thyroid suppression test (see below).

One valuable application of the RAIU is in the diagnosis of thyrotoxicosis associated with a low value of the RAIU. These include iodine-induced hyperthyroidism, thyrotoxicosis factitia, inadvertent ingestion of ground meat containing thyroid glands ("hamburger toxicosis"), and the spontaneously resolving thyrotoxicosis associated with painless chronic thyroiditis or subacute thyroiditis.

TESTS RELATED TO HORMONE CONCENTRATION AND BINDING IN BLOOD Until the evolution of highly sensitive assays for TSH, measurement of the concentration of T_4 and/or T_3 in serum, in conjunction with some assessment of hormone binding, was the traditional means of confirming a clinical diagnosis of hyperthyroidism or hypothyroidism. Highly specific and sensitive radioimmunoassays are used to measure *serum T_4* and T_3 concentrations and rarely for the measurement of *serum rT_3* concentration. The approximate normal ranges are 60 to 150 nmol/L (5 to 12 μg/dL) for T_4, 1 to 3 nmol/L (70 to 190 ng/dL) for T_3, and 0.2 to 0.6 nmol/L (10 to 40 ng/dL) for rT_3.

As mentioned above, alterations in the intensity of hormone binding by plasma proteins, as well as alterations in the rate of hormone secretion, influence the concentration of hormone in the blood. However, only alterations in hormone secretion lead to steady state alterations in the concentration of free hormone. Because they most consistently reflect the rate of hormone production, free hormone concentrations usually correlate better with the metabolic state than do total hormone concentrations. The free T_4 concentration (FT_4) can be measured directly by equilibrium dialysis of serum enriched with a tracer quantity of labeled T_4. The percent of T_4 that is dialyzable or free is thereby determined, and the product of this value and the total T_4 is the FT_4. However, since the dialysis technique is cumbersome, it has been replaced by indirect assays (see below). One traditional method, the in vitro uptake test, represents an indirect assessment of hormone binding, is simple to perform, and usually provides the same information as free T_4. Here, the serum is enriched with labeled T_4 or labeled T_3 and is then incubated with an insoluble, particulate matter, such as resin or charcoal, that binds free hormone. The percent of labeled hormone taken up by the particulate material varies inversely with both the concentration of unoccupied sites among the serum proteins and their affinity for the particular hormone being used. Labeled T_3 is usually used in preference to labeled T_4, since it is less strongly bound in the serum and hence yields higher and more accurate uptake values (resin T_3 uptake, RT_3U). In most clinical conditions, values of the RT_3U are proportionate to those of the percent of FT_4 and percent of FT_3. This proportionality reflects the fact that in normal serum, T_4 and T_3 are mainly bound by a common binding site on TBG. Therefore, alterations in binding produced by an excess or deficiency of TBG or by an excessive or insufficient supply of T_4 do not seriously disturb the relationship between the intensity of T_4 binding and that of T_3. Under these conditions, therefore, one may calculate a *free T_4 index* (FT_4I) and a *free T_3 index* (FT_3I) as the product of the RT_3U and the total T_4 and T_3 concentrations, respectively, and these are proportional to the actual FT_4 and FT_3.

Primary alterations in plasma TBG concentration (see Table 334-2) produce changes in the RT_3U that are inverse and approximately proportionate to those in the serum T_4 and serum T_3; as a result, the FT_4I and FT_3I remain normal. By contrast, alterations in T_4 secretion cause changes in the percent FT_4 and RT_3U that are in the same direction as those in serum T_4. As a result, the FT_4 and FT_4I deviate from normal values more markedly than do the percent FT_4 and RT_3U alone. Immunoradiometric (IRMA) and chemiluminescent assay methods for the direct measurement of FT_4 provide reliable results in a wide range of disorders and may replace measurement of total T_4, RT_3U, and FT_4I in the diagnosis of thyrotoxicosis and hypothyroidism.

As noted earlier, several disorders are characterized by increased plasma binding of T_4 in which, because the protein involved is not TBG, the intensity of T_4 binding relative to that of T_3 is abnormal. Most commonly, binding of T_4 is enhanced, while that of T_3 is increased little, if at all. Included among these disorders is *familial dysalbuminemic hyperthyroxinemia (FDH)*, inherited as an autosomal dominant trait, in which the plasma concentration of an albumin variant with an unusually high affinity for T_4 is increased. As a result, the serum T_4 is markedly elevated, but in keeping with the euthyroid state, FT_4 is normal. Because the RT_3U does not reflect the increase in the intensity of T_4 binding, calculated values of the FT_4I are increased, often leading to a mistaken diagnosis of thyrotoxicosis. Similar findings occur when there is *increased T_4 binding by transthyretin* (TTR, TBPA) or when the patient, usually one with autoimmune thyroid disease, develops *circulating antibodies* against T_4 itself.

In the foregoing disorders, serum T_4 is increased owing to an increase in T_4 binding, and the FT_4 and metabolic state are normal. They are therefore classified among the disorders that lead to a state of *euthyroid hyperthyroxinemia*, a term that implies the presence of hyperthyroxinemia not caused by intrinsic thyroid disease (Table 334-4). The mechanism responsible for these findings is variable and in some cases uncertain. The increases in total T_4 do not appear to

TABLE 334-4 States associated with euthyroid hyperthyroxinemia

Disorder	FT$_4$	FT$_4$I	T$_3$	TSH	Comments
Increased T$_4$ binding					
A Increased TBG	N	N	↑	N	See Tables 334-1 and 334-2
B FDH	N	↑	N,Sl ↑	N	Autosomal dominant inheritance
C Increased TBPA binding	N	↑	N	N	Increased concentration (islet-cell tumor) or affinity
D Anti-T$_4$ antibody	N	↑	N	N	Anti-T$_3$ antibody may be present
Pituitary and peripheral thyroid hormone resistance	↑	↑	↑	↑	If only pituitary resistant, patient thyrotoxic
Various disorders					
A Sick euthyroid syndrome	↑ , N	↑	↓	N, ↓	Uncommon; poorly understood
B Acute psychiatric illness	↑ , N	↑	N, ↑	N, ↑	Remits without treatment in several weeks
C Hyperemesis gravidarum	↑	↑	N	↓	Remits in several weeks
Drugs					
A Inhibitors of T$_3$-formation	↑	↑	↓	↑	Particularly ipodate and iopanoate
1 Radiographic contrast agents					
2 Propranolol	↑	↑	↓	N, ↑	Especially with large doses
3 Amiodarone	↑	↑	↓	↑	Increased TSH during first several months
B Heparin	↑	↑	N	—	Requires only small intravenous doses
C Levothyroxine therapy	↑	↑	N	↓	Hyperthyroxinemia in about 50% of cases

NOTE: FT$_4$ = free T$_4$ concentration; FT$_4$I = free T$_4$ index calculated from an in vitro T$_3$ uptake test; TSH = basal serum TSH concentration and response to TRH; N = normal; Sl = slightly.

have any impact on the metabolic state, but hyperthyroidism may be mistakenly diagnosed.

Some states are associated with an increased thyroid secretion of T$_3$, at least relative to the secretion of T$_4$. As a result, the serum T$_3$ concentration is disproportionately high relative to the serum T$_4$. This is apparently a consequence of hyperfunction of the follicular cell, since it is seen in all varieties of hyperthyroidism and in early thyroid failure, in which the gland is exposed to enhanced stimulation by TSH. Accordingly, the serum T$_3$ concentration and the derived FT$_3$I are generally superior to the corresponding values for T$_4$ in the diagnosis of hyperthyroidism. In *early* hypothyroidism, by contrast, the serum T$_3$ concentration and FT$_3$I are often normal despite subnormal values for the serum T$_4$ and FT$_4$I. Consequently, the serum T$_3$ concentration is not reliable for the diagnosis of hypothyroidism.

Measurement of the serum rT$_3$ concentration is valuable in differentiating the "low T$_3$ syndrome" (see below) from intrinsic hypothyroidism; in the former the serum rT$_3$ concentration is increased, whereas in the latter it is usually subnormal.

METABOLIC INDEXES   Tests in this category assess the metabolic impact of thyroid hormone. Though tests of this type have value in the investigative setting, none of sufficient sensitivity, specificity, and ease of performance is available for routine use. Measurements of oxygen consumption in the basal state (basal metabolic rate, BMR) were once a mainstay in the diagnosis of thyroid disease but are now of historic interest. Several blood tests may be abnormal in patients with thyroid disease, but lack of specificity limits their utility. For example, serum concentrations of creatine phosphokinase and, less frequently, lactate dehydrogenase and aspartate aminotransferase are increased in hypothyroidism and may be slightly decreased in

hyperthyroidism. The changes are nonspecific, and appreciation of them is important only in avoiding the inference that other diseases which produce similar changes are present. The concentrations in serum of testosterone-binding globulin (TeBG), the iron storage protein ferritin, and angiotensin-converting enzyme are thyroid hormone–dependent and are, therefore, increased in thyrotoxicosis, but they are of no value in the diagnosis of thyroid disease. Increases in the *serum cholesterol concentration* are common in hypothyroidism of thyroid origin, and decreases in serum cholesterol are common in thyrotoxicosis. *Systolic time indexes*, such as the preejection period and pulse-wave arrival time, are prolonged in hypothyroidism and shortened in hyperthyroidism. They may be of value in monitoring thyroid replacement therapy in elderly patients or in patients with coexisting heart disease.

TESTS OF HOMEOSTATIC CONTROL   Measurement of the basal *serum TSH concentration* is useful in the diagnosis of both advanced and subclinical hypothyroidism. The latter state represents a stage in the evolution of hypothyroidism, in which a structural or functional abnormality that impairs hormone synthesis is compensated for by hypersecretion of TSH. In thyrotoxic states, serum TSH concentration is almost always low or undetectable. While the original radioimmunoassays could not distinguish between normal and subnormal values, immunoradiometric or chemiluminescent techniques employing monoclonal antibodies provide exquisite sensitivity. Thyrotoxic patients tend to have undetectable levels (<0.1 mU/L), while values in most normal subjects range between 0.3 and 3.0 mU/L in these assays (Fig. 334-3). Thus these assays offer a significant advantage over conventional radioimmunoassays (RIA) and may be useful in confirming the diagnosis of hyperthyroidism as well as that of hypothyroidism.

FIGURE 334-3   Utility of sensitive TSH assay in evaluation of suspected thyroid dysfunction in ambulatory patients.

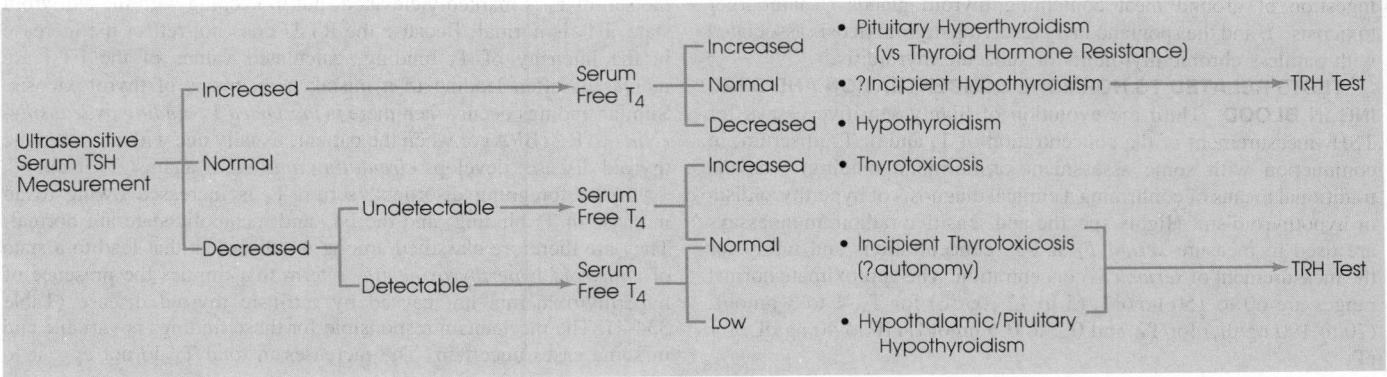

Serum TSH concentrations are absolutely or inappropriately elevated relative to serum FT_4 and FT_3 values in patients with TSH-induced hyperthyroidism. This rare syndrome results either from a TSH-secreting pituitary adenoma or resistance of the TSH secretory mechanism to feedback inhibition by T_4 and T_3. Measurement of serum TSH is the best means of distinguishing between untreated hypothyroidism of thyroid origin, in which the values are invariably increased, and pituitary or hypothalamic hypothyroidism, in which the values are usually low or within the normal range. Occasional patients with hypothyroidism of hypothalamic or pituitary origin secrete a form of TSH that is immunoactive but not bioactive. Here, serum TSH concentrations may be elevated rather than depressed.

The *thyrotropin-releasing hormone (TRH) stimulation test* assesses the functional state of the TSH-secretory mechanism and has diagnostic value in diverse circumstances. Following the intravenous injection of TRH in normal subjects, the serum TSH level begins to increase within minutes, reaches a maximum between 20 and 45 min, and then rapidly declines. The nature of the pituitary feedback mechanism is such that when hypothalamic-pituitary function is normal, one would expect an increased response to TRH when the thyrotropic cell senses a deficiency of thyroid hormone, particularly T_3, and a decreased or absent response when there is thyroid hormone excess. Thus, except in the rare instances of pituitary resistance to thyroid hormone, in which responses are usually normal, thyrotoxicosis is invariably accompanied by a blunted or absent TSH response to TRH. Owing to extreme sensitivity of the TSH-secretory mechanism to feedback inhibition, diminished responses to TRH commonly occur in apparently euthyroid patients with serum T_4 or T_3 levels within the normal range but with marginally increased T_4 or T_3 output from autonomously functioning toxic adenomas or toxic multinodular goiters. Blunted TRH responses also may be seen in some patients with euthyroid Graves' disease. In addition, responses to TRH are often decreased in elderly individuals, especially men. Despite these exceptions, a subnormal or absent response to TRH has been employed as a confirmatory test for thyrotoxicosis. With the availability of highly sensitive TSH assays, the TRH test is rarely used for this purpose. TRH tests are of even less value in the diagnosis of hypothyroidism. Responses are increased in patients with primary hypothyroidism, but the magnitude of increase is generally proportional to the extent of increase in basal serum TSH. Some patients with pituitary hypothyroidism have subnormal responses, and some with TRH deficiency due to hypothalamic disease have a near-normal response, but these responses are not seen consistently. Further, in as many as one-fourth of patients with hypothyroidism due to hypothalamic-pituitary disease, basal serum TSH levels are normal or slightly elevated, and the response to TRH is exaggerated, although some of this TSH may not be bioactive.

The *thyroid suppression test* is used to assess whether thyroid function is under normal homeostatic control. Normally, exogenous thyroid hormone suppresses pituitary TSH secretion, resulting in a decrease in the RAIU. Since liothyronine is usually employed for the test (100 μg/d for 7 to 10 days), the resulting decline in serum T_4, as well as in the RAIU, can serve as an index of suppression. A normal suppressive response is a decrease of the RAIU to less than half the control value and a decline of the serum T_4 to low normal or subnormal values. A normal suppression test is incompatible with and excludes a diagnosis of hyperthyroidism. An abnormal suppression test is always present in hyperthyroidism, irrespective of the underlying cause; this indicates either autonomy of thyroid function, the presence of an abnormal (non-TSH) thyroid stimulator, or unremitting hypersecretion of TSH. An abnormal suppression test is not pathognomonic of hyperthyroidism, however, since it may persist after treatment of hyperthyroidism in Graves' disease and is seen in about half the euthyroid patients with the ophthalmopathy of Graves' disease.

Because of the risk of adverse effects of exogenous thyroid hormone, especially liothyronine, in elderly patients and in those with cardiovascular disease, and since the TRH test is almost entirely devoid of undesirable side effects, either the latter test or highly sensitive TSH measurement has almost entirely supplanted the thyroid suppression test in the diagnosis of hyperthyroidism.

MISCELLANEOUS TESTS Various tests that do not assess thyroid function are of value in defining the nature of the thyroid disorder or in planning therapy. For example, high titers of *antithyroid peroxidase* (anti-TPO, antimicrosomal) *antibodies* or *antithyroglobulin antibodies* are found in the serum of most patients with Hashimoto's disease and in many with primary thyroprivic hypothyroidism or Graves' disease. In the latter, the serum also contains antibodies against the TSH receptor on thyroid plasma membranes. In general, these are capable of inhibiting the receptor binding of TSH (TSH-binding inhibitory immunoglobulins, TBII) and of stimulating the production of cyclic AMP therein (thyroid-stimulating antibodies or immunoglobulins, TSAb or TSI). The clinical utility of tests for TBII and TSI stems from the fact that the disappearance of the factors from the serum during a course of antithyroid therapy implies the likelihood of a long-term remission of hyperthyroidism when therapy is withdrawn. In some patients, analogous antibodies have no intrinsic stimulatory effect but block the response to endogenous TSH and produce nongoitrous hypothyroidism. Both stimulatory and blocking anti-TSH receptor antibodies have the ability to cross the placenta and, as a consequence, to produce transient hyperthyroidism (neonatal Graves' disease) or hypothyroidism, respectively, in the newborn. Measurement of these antibodies during the last months of pregnancy makes it possible to assess the likelihood of the disorders developing in the neonate.

Some patients, most commonly those with autoimmune thyroid disease, develop *circulating antibodies against T_3 or T_4*, or both. In RIAs for these hormones, because the endogenous antibody competes with the exogenous antibody for binding of the added labeled ligand, spurious high or low values for the concentration of the hormone are obtained, depending on the technique of RIA used. The true concentration of the hormone, as determined in extracts of the serum, is increased owing to the additional binding sites provided by the antibody, but antibody-bound hormone is unavailable for metabolic action. In the case of anti-T_3 antibodies, which are the more common, values of the RT_3U are low because endogenous antibody competes with the resin for binding of the added labeled T_3. Such antibodies can be detected by adding labeled hormone to serum, separating the immunoglobulins from other serum proteins, and demonstrating that they bind the labeled hormone.

Along with several other thyroid disorders, differentiated carcinomas of the thyroid release thyroglobulin into the bloodstream. As a consequence, measurements of the *serum thyroglobulin* by RIA have value not in the initial diagnosis of thyroid carcinoma but in assessing the adequacy of initial therapy and in monitoring for recurrence or dissemination of the disease. In patients with thyrotoxicosis, subnormal serum thyroglobulin concentrations together with decreased values of the RAIU suggest thyrotoxicosis factitia.

Imaging by *scintiscanning* permits localization of sites of accumulation of radioiodine or sodium [^{99m}Tc]pertechnetate. This technique is useful for defining areas of increased or decreased function within the thyroid and for detecting retrosternal goiter, ectopic thyroid tissue, hemiagenesis of the thyroid, and functioning metastases of thyroid carcinoma. Ultrasonic examination of the thyroid is also useful for differentiating cystic nodules from those which are solid. Since ultrasonic scans provide an accurate indication of size, are noninvasive, and apparently have no injurious effects, sequential scans can be employed to assess changes in the size of the thyroid as a whole or of discrete nodules over time or in response to treatment.

SICK EUTHYROID SYNDROME

Severe illness, physical trauma, or physiologic stress can induce changes in one or more aspects of thyroid hormone economy, leading to findings referred to as the *sick euthyroid syndrome* (SES). Abnormalities in SES include alterations in the peripheral transport and metabolism of the thyroid hormones, the regulation of TSH secretion, and in some cases thyroid function itself. Acting alone or together, these lead to changes in the concentrations of the circulating thyroid hormones, both total and free, that serve to define the several variants of the SES. Because of the frequency and nonspecificity of the disorders that cause it, SES is probably a more common cause of abnormalities in the concentration of thyroid hormones in the blood than intrinsic thyroid disease.

NORMAL-T_4 VARIANT OF SES Decreased production of T_3 owing to inhibition of the peripheral 5'-monodeiodination of T_4 is a consistent feature of the SES. This is reflected in a decrease in the serum total T_3 concentration that varies in severity with that of the illness. In moderately ill patients, serum total T_4 concentration is within the normal range. A decrease in the intensity of protein binding, greater for T_4 than for T_3, is an additional accompaniment. As a result, values of the RT_3U are moderately increased, and the percent FT_4 is increased to a proportionately greater extent. As a consequence, values of the free T_4 index (FT_4I) and those of the free T_4 concentrations (FT_4) are often increased. Serum rT_3 concentrations are increased, owing to a decrease in the plasma clearance of rT_3 secondary to inhibition of its 5'-monodeiodination. The plasma clearance rate of T_4 is increased, probably as a result of decreased T_4 binding, and this, in the face of normal T_4 concentrations, indicates that the overall rate of T_4 degradation and production is increased. Production rates for T_3 are decreased, and those for rT_3 are normal. Serum TSH concentration and the response of serum TSH to TRH are generally normal, although they may increase and then return to normal as recovery from the illness takes place. Despite the reduction in the serum T_3 concentration, this variant of the SES can be separated from intrinsic thyroid disease because the serum T_4 and TSH are normal and because the serum T_3 is not useful for diagnosing hypothyroidism.

LOW-T_4 VARIANT OF SES In more seriously ill patients, T_3 production rates and serum total and free T_3 concentrations decrease still further, and abnormalities in hormone binding increase in severity. As a consequence, serum T_4 concentrations decrease into the hypothyroid range. This is partly but not entirely due to decreased T_4 binding, since values of the FT_4 are frequently subnormal. These are probably the result of decreased T_4 production in the most severely ill patients and are secondary to decreased secretion of TSH. Serum TSH concentrations appear normal by conventional assay but are low with sensitive TSH assays, and TRH responses are often blunted. Hence, in this variant of the SES, there is an inappropriate hyposecretion of TSH, considering the low serum total and free T_4 and T_3 concentrations, and a diagnosis of pituitary hypothyroidism may be suggested. While the cause is unknown, low TSH in this setting may be due to effects of cytokines such as interleukin 1 and tumor necrosis factor on the pituitary. With resolution of the underlying illness, TSH levels rise, heralding recovery, and may be transiently elevated until T_4 and T_3 levels are restored to normal. Production rates for rT_3 are diminished, owing to the decreased availability of its precursor T_4; nonetheless, serum rT_3 concentrations are increased, owing to retardation of its degradation, and this provides an important means of differentiating the SES from pituitary hypothyroidism, in which serum rT_3 concentrations are low. In patients with primary hypothyroidism who have associated illness, serum TSH levels remain elevated, although generally lower than they otherwise would be.

HIGH-T_4 VARIANT OF SES An unusual variant of the SES (approximately 1 percent of sick patients) is associated with increased serum total and free T_4 concentrations during acute illness and return to normal thereafter. This variant is most often seen in elderly women, many of whom have received medications that contain iodine. The principal source of diagnostic confusion is with the syndrome of "T_4 toxicosis," i.e., true thyrotoxicosis upon which illness has been superimposed, so that serum T_4 concentrations are increased and serum T_3 concentrations are normal. In the latter, however, serum rT_3 concentrations are higher, values of the serum total T_3 and FT_3I

are higher, TSH is usually undetectable, and TRH responses are blunted to absent.

ABNORMALITIES IN HORMONE BINDING IN SES Multiple factors are responsible for the decreased binding of T_4 and, to a lesser extent, T_3 in the SES. Illness is associated with decreased synthesis of TTR and a decrease in its serum concentration, but the extent to which this contributes to decreased T_4 binding is uncertain. In chronically ill patients, serum TBG concentration is subnormal. Most often, however, the extent of decreased T_4 binding cannot be explained by decreases in serum TTR and TBG, and an inhibitor of hormone binding may be responsible. Its nature is uncertain, but it may be one or more fatty acids, which also may be responsible for diminished conversion of T_4 to T_3.

The importance of the SES is that the changes in circulating thyroid hormone concentrations should not be confused with those due to intrinsic thyroid or pituitary disease. Unresolved questions are whether the metabolic impact of thyroid hormone in peripheral tissues is decreased in the SES and whether the syndrome is a beneficial or adverse response to illness. There is no evidence that patients with low T_4 and T_3 of SES benefit from treatment with thyroid hormones.

SIMPLE (NONTOXIC) GOITER

Endemic goiter implies an etiologic factor or factors common to a particular geographic region. The term has been defined as the presence of generalized or localized thyroid enlargement in more than 10 percent of the population. *Sporadic* goiter arises in nonendemic areas as a result of factors that do not affect the population generally. Since these terms fail to define the causes of such goiters, and since thyroid enlargement of diverse etiology may exist in both endemic and nonendemic regions, it is prudent to employ a general term such as *simple* or *nontoxic goiter*. Simple or nontoxic goiter can be defined as any enlargement of the thyroid gland that does not result from an inflammatory or neoplastic process and that is not initially associated with thyrotoxicosis or myxedema.

ETIOLOGY AND PATHOGENESIS Simple goiter is sometimes due to a definable cause of impaired thyroid hormone synthesis, such as iodine deficiency, ingestion of a goitrogen, or a defect in a hormone biosynthetic pathway, but in most instances its cause is unknown. Whatever the cause, the clinical manifestations reflect the operation of a common pathophysiologic mechanism. Simple goiter occurs when one or more factors impair the capacity of the thyroid to secrete sufficient hormones to meet the needs of the peripheral tissues. Although this has been presumed to lead to increased secretion of TSH, concentrations of TSH in the serum of patients with established simple goiter are usually normal. Hence some other mechanism of goitrogenesis may be operative. A likely possibility is that depletion of glandular organic iodine accompanying impaired hormone synthesis increases the responsiveness of the thyroid to normal levels of TSH. The resulting increases in both functioning thyroid mass and cellular activity overcome mild impairment of hormone synthesis; thus the patient is metabolically normal, though goitrous. When the underlying disorder is severe, compensatory responses, now including hypersecretion of TSH, are inadequate to overcome the impairment, and the patient is both goitrous and hypothyroid. Thus simple goiter cannot be clearly separated in the pathogenic sense from goitrous hypothyroidism. Specific causes of simple goiter may exist with or without hypothyroidism (Table 334-5). Defective iodination of thyroglobulin may be an important cause in many patients. The possibility that goiter can be due to antibodies that stimulate thyroid growth but not function remains to be substantiated.

PATHOLOGY The histopathology of the thyroid in simple goiter varies with the etiology and the stage at which the examination is made. In its initial stages, the gland exhibits a uniform hypertrophy, hyperplasia, and hypervascularity. As the disorder persists or undergoes repeated exacerbations and remissions, uniformity of thyroidal

TABLE 334-5 Classification of the causes of hypothyroidism

THYROID

A Thyroprivic
1 Congenital development defect
2 Primary idiopathic
3 Postablative (radioiodine, surgery)
4 Postradiation (e.g., for lymphoma)
B Goitrous
1 Heritable biosynthetic defects
2 Maternally transmitted (iodides, antithyroid agents)
3 Iodine deficiency
4 Drug-elicited (aminosalicylic acid, iodides, phenylbutazone, iodoantipyrine, lithium)
5 Chronic thyroiditis (Hashimoto's disease)
6 Interleukin 2 and lymphokine-activated killer cells

SUPRATHYROID (TROPHOPRIVIC)

A Pituitary
1 Panhypopituitarism
2 Isolated TSH deficiency
B Hypothalamic
1 Congenital defects
2 Infection (encephalitis)
3 Neoplasm
4 Infiltrative (sarcoidosis)

SELF-LIMITED

A Following withdrawal of suppressive thyroid therapy
B Subacute thyroiditis and chronic thyroiditis with transient hypothyroidism (usually after a phase of thyrotoxicosis)

architecture is lost. Occasionally, the greater part of the gland may display a uniform involution or hyperinvolution with colloid accumulation. More often, areas of involution are interspersed with patchy areas of focal hyperplasia. Fibrosis may demarcate hyperplastic or involuted nodules. These may resemble true neoplasms (adenomas). Areas of hemorrhage and irregular calcification may be present. The evolution of the multinodular stage is almost always accompanied by the development of functional autonomy. Indeed, heterogeneity of structure and function and a degree of functional autonomy are the hallmarks of the mature stage of this disorder.

CLINICAL MANIFESTATIONS In simple goiter, the clinical manifestations arise solely from enlargement of the thyroid, since the metabolic state is normal. In goitrous hypothyroidism, symptoms caused by thyromegaly are accompanied by signs and symptoms of hormonal insufficiency. Mechanical sequelae include compression and displacement of the trachea or esophagus, occasionally with obstructive symptoms if the goiter becomes sufficiently large. Superior mediastinal obstruction may occur with large retrosternal goiters. Signs of compression can be induced in the case of large retrosternal goiters when the patient's arms are raised above the head; suffusion of the face, giddiness, or syncope may result from this maneuver (Pemberton's sign). Hoarseness due to compression of the recurrent laryngeal nerve is rare in simple goiter and suggests neoplasm. Sudden hemorrhage into a nodule may lead to an acute, painful swelling in the neck and may produce or enhance compressive symptoms. Hyperthyroidism may supervene in long-standing multinodular goiter (toxic multinodular goiter). In both endemic and sporadic multinodular goiter, the ingestion of excess iodide may result in the development of thyrotoxicosis (jodbasedow phenomenon).

In regions where iodine deficiency is severe, goitrous enlargement also may be associated with varying degrees of hypothyroidism. Cretinism, both goitrous and nongoitrous, occurs with increased frequency in the children of goitrous parents in many countries where goiter is common. Although iodine deficiency is doubtless a factor in the etiology of endemic goiter, the frequency of goiter differs greatly among persons with equally severe iodine deficiency. In such instances, dietary or waterborne goitrogens appear to be important

conditioning factors. In some areas, these goitrogens may be sufficient to cause goiter in the absence of iodine deficiency.

DIAGNOSIS The diagnosis of simple goiter requires, first, demonstration of a euthyroid state and, second, demonstration of normal serum T_4 and T_3 concentrations. The former may be difficult because manifestations of thyrotoxicosis may be subtle or atypical, especially among the elderly (see the section "Toxic Multinodular Goiter"). The latter may be problematic, since serum T_4 and especially T_3 concentrations may be near the upper limit of the normal range. In addition, the fact that serum T_3 concentrations may decrease in the euthyroid elderly complicates interpretation of this test. The RAIU is usually normal but may be increased in the presence of iodine deficiency or a biosynthetic defect. Thus a measurable TSH by a highly sensitive technique is the best index of euthyroidism. Indeed, subclinical thyrotoxicosis may be secondary to the functional autonomy of the goiter and consequently cause a decrease in both basal TSH and TSH response to TRH. Differentiation of nontoxic goiter from Hashimoto's disease is facilitated by the greater frequency of multinodularity in the former and by the presence of high titers of circulating antimicrosomal or antithyroglobulin antibodies in the latter. In some instances, emergence of a strongly dominant nodule may suggest the presence of a carcinoma. This is especially true if bleeding has caused it to increase in size rapidly and to lose the ability to accumulate iodine or pertechnetate. Appropriate radiographic studies (computed tomography, magnetic resonance imaging) and flow volume measurement should be recorded in the presence of significant substernal extension with potential for upper airway obstruction.

TREATMENT The object of treatment is to reduce the size of the goiter, either by relieving external encumbrances to hormone formation or by providing sufficient quantities of exogenous hormone to inhibit TSH secretion and thereby put the thyroid gland at rest. In disorders characterized by decreased thyroid iodide stores, such as iodine deficiency or impairment of the thyroid iodide-concentrating mechanism, small doses of iodide may prove effective. Occasionally, a known extrinsic goitrogen can be withdrawn. Most commonly, however, no specific etiologic factor can be detected, and thyroid hormone therapy is required. For this purpose, levothyroxine (L-thyroxine) is the agent of choice. In the younger patient with the early diffuse stage of simple goiter, treatment is instituted with 100 µg levothyroxine daily, and the dose is increased over the next month or so to a maximum of 150 or 200 µg/d (average dose of 1.7 µg/kg body weight per day). Complete suppression would imply reduction of serum TSH to levels less than 0.1 mU/L by an ultrasensitive assay. Until uncertainties about the association of long-term excess thyroid hormone therapy and loss of bone mineral (osteopenia) are resolved, patients should be titrated to slightly less than a fully suppressive dose. Adequacy of suppression also may be assessed by measuring the RAIU, which should decrease to less than 5 percent of the administered dose at 24 h. Lesser decreases indicate only partial suppression, which may reflect the presence of autonomous foci demonstrable by scanning techniques. In the elderly or the patient with long-standing multinodular goiter, an ultrasensitive TSH measurement or a TRH stimulation test should be undertaken before initiating treatment with levothyroxine to determine whether significant functional autonomy is present. If such is indicated by an undetectable basal TSH or a diminished or absent TSH responsiveness to TRH, suppressive therapy with levothyroxine is contraindicated, since such patients are or will eventually become thyrotoxic. Rather, consideration should be given to radioiodine ablation of the autonomous foci (see later section "Toxic Multinodular Goiter"). On the other hand, if the basal TSH or the TSH response to TRH is normal, excluding significant functional autonomy, treatment with levothyroxine can be initiated. In the elderly patient, the initial dose should not exceed 50 µg/d, and the dosage should be gradually increased, partial rather than complete suppression of the value for basal TSH and/or the RAIU being the end point. It is the practice to obtain a thyroid scan as part of the initial evaluation of all patients with multinodular goiter. In those patients in whom full suppressive doses of thyroxine are indicated, it is desirable to repeat the RAIU and scan (suppression scan), when practical, to ascertain the efficacy of suppression and/or the presence of autonomous foci.

Results of therapy vary widely. The early diffuse, hyperplastic goiter responds well, with regression or disappearance in 3 to 6 months. In the author's experience, the later, nodular stage responds less favorably, and significant reduction in gland size is achieved only in about one-third of cases; however, in the remainder, suppressive treatment may forestall further glandular growth. Internodular tissue regresses more often than do nodules themselves. The latter may therefore appear to become more prominent during treatment. After maximum regression of the goiter, suppressive medication may be maintained for prolonged periods, reduced to minimal levels, or at times withdrawn. In an unpredictable manner, goiter may remain relieved or recur. In the latter instances, if appropriate studies rule out malignancy, suppressive therapy should be reinstituted and continued indefinitely. In areas of endemic iodine deficiency, the size and prevalence of goiter and the frequency of cretinism can be reduced by the provision of iodized salt or water or the periodic injection of iodized oil.

Surgical therapy of simple goiter is physiologically unsound, but it may occasionally be necessary to relieve obstructive symptoms, especially those that persist after a trial of medical therapy. Large substernal goiters with partial upper airway obstruction also have been treated by radioactive iodine with moderate success. Surgical exploration of nodular goiter also may be indicated in some individuals when evidence suggests carcinoma. However, the concept that subtotal resection of multinodular nontoxic goiter affords effective prophylaxis against the development of thyroid carcinoma is unsound. If for some reason subtotal thyroidectomy has been performed, levothyroxine in a usual dose of about 1.7 μg/kg body weight daily is recommended to inhibit regenerative hyperplasia and further goitrogenesis.

HYPOTHYROIDISM

Hypothyroidism can result from any of a variety of abnormalities that lead to insufficient synthesis of thyroid hormone. Hypothyroidism dating from birth and resulting in developmental abnormalities is termed *cretinism*. The term *myxedema* connotes severe hypothyroidism in which there is accumulation of hydrophilic mucopolysaccharides in the ground substance of the dermis and other tissues, leading to thickening of the facial features and doughy induration of the skin.

ETIOLOGY AND PATHOGENESIS A classification of hypothyroidism is presented in Table 334-5. Overall, the primary thyroid varieties account for approximately 95 percent of cases, only 5 percent or less being suprathyroid in origin. In thyroprivic hypothyroidism, loss of thyroid tissue leads to inadequate synthesis of thyroid hormone, despite maximum stimulation of any thyroid remnant by TSH. The most common cause of thyroprivic hypothyroidism is surgical or radioiodine ablation of the thyroid gland in the treatment of Graves' disease. Thyroprivic hypothyroidism also may occur as a primary idiopathic disorder. The most common cause of primary hypothyroidism is autoimmunity and is associated with circulating antithyroid antibodies and in some cases may result from the action of antibodies that block the TSH receptor. It may coexist with diabetes mellitus and other diseases in which circulating autoantibodies are found, such as pernicious anemia, systemic lupus erythematosus, rheumatoid arthritis, Sjögren's syndrome, and chronic hepatitis. In addition, hypothyroidism can be one manifestation of a polyglandular endocrine deficiency state in which autoantibodies cause variable insufficiency of thyroid, adrenal, parathyroid, and gonadal function (see Chap. 343). All these diseases, including isolated primary hypothyroidism, are associated with an increased frequency of specific HLA haplotypes. Finally, a developmental defect may result in failure of the gland to function adequately, leading to sporadic nongoitrous cretinism or

juvenile hypothyroidism. A self-limited period of hypothyroidism is common in the course of subacute thyroiditis and in the syndrome of "painless thyroiditis," including the postpartum variant and usually after a temporary period of thyrotoxicosis. Owing to a persisting lack of TSH stimulation, intrinsically euthyroid subjects from whom chronic suppressive therapy is abruptly withdrawn experience a several-week period of thyroid hypofunction.

Inability to synthesize adequate quantities of thyroid hormone leads to hypersecretion of TSH and hence goiter. If this compensatory response is inadequate, goitrous hypothyroidism ensues. The most common cause of goitrous hypothyroidism in North America is Hashimoto's disease, in which defective organic binding of iodide and abnormal secretion of iodoproteins are frequent. Iodide-induced goiter with or without hypothyroidism appears to arise from an intrinsic defect in the organic binding mechanism, which permits a persistent Wolff-Chaikoff effect. Euthyroid patients with Graves' disease, especially after surgery or radioiodine treatment, those with Hashimoto's disease, and the normal fetus are particularly susceptible to iodide-induced goiter. In view of the susceptibility of the fetal thyroid to iodide, with resulting goiter and hypothyroidism, iodine in large doses should not be given during pregnancy. Less common causes of goitrous hypothyroidism are hereditary defects in hormone biosynthesis and ingestion of drugs that induce defects in hormone biosynthesis, such as aminosalicylic acid and lithium. Finally, in areas of environmental iodine deficiency, goitrous cretinism and hypothyroidism can occur on an endemic basis. Diminished thyroid reserve occurs as a stage in the evolution of both thyroprivic and goitrous hypothyroidism.

Rarely, long-standing hypothyroidism may lead to diffuse, nodular, or adenomatous thyrotroph hyperplasia. These patients may present with headache, visual field defects, abnormal pubertal development, galactorrhea, and pituitary enlargement, all of which disappear with levothyroxine therapy. Such patients have marked elevations in serum TSH, whereas in hypothyroidism of suprathyroid origin, the thyroid is intrinsically normal but is deprived of stimulation by TSH. Deprivation of TSH, most commonly the result of postpartum pituitary necrosis or a tumor of the pituitary or adjacent regions, results in pituitary hypothyroidism. Hypothalamic hypothyroidism is less common and results from inadequate secretion of TRH.

CLINICAL PICTURE The appearance of children with hypothyroidism depends on the age at which the deficiency began and the promptness with which replacement therapy was instituted. Cretinism may be manifested at birth but usually becomes evident within the first several months, depending on the extent of thyroid failure. Hypothyroidism is present in approximately 1 in every 5000 neonates and manifests itself in persistence of physiologic jaundice, hoarse cry, constipation, somnolence, and feeding problems; since clinical diagnosis is difficult and early treatment is crucial for normal intellectual development, all neonates should be screened for hypothyroidism with measurements of the serum T₄ or TSH. In later months, delay in reaching the normal milestones of development becomes evident, and the physical characteristics of the cretin appear. These include short stature, coarse features with protruding tongue, broad flat nose, widely set eyes, sparse hair, dry skin, protuberant abdomen with an umbilical hernia, impaired mental development, retarded bone age, epiphyseal dysgenesis, and delayed dentition.

In the older child, the clinical manifestations of hypothyroidism are intermediate between those of infantile and adult hypothyroidism. Retardation of linear growth is manifested by shortness of stature, and retardation of sexual maturation results in delayed puberty. Poor performance at school may call attention to the diagnosis. Variable manifestations of adult hypothyroidism are present. X-ray examination reveals delayed union of the epiphyses.

In the adult, early symptoms of hypothyroidism are nonspecific and of insidious onset. In the elderly patient, symptoms may be erroneously attributed to aging or other disorders such as Parkinson's disease, depression, or Alzheimer's disease. They may include fatigue, lethargy, constipation, cold intolerance, stiffness and cramping of the muscles, the carpal tunnel syndrome, and menorrhagia. Over the succeeding months, intellectual and motor activity slows, appetite declines, and weight increases. The hair becomes dry and tends to fall out, and the skin becomes dry. The voice becomes deeper and hoarse, and auditory acuity may deteriorate. Obstructive sleep apnea may occur. Ultimately, the clinical picture of florid myxedema appears, with dull expressionless face, sparse hair, periorbital puffiness, large tongue, and pale, cool skin that feels rough and doughy. Thyroid tissue is not readily palpable, except in the goitrous variety of hypothyroidism. The heart is enlarged owing to both dilation and pericardial effusion; if the heart is small, pituitary hypothyroidism (with secondary adrenal insufficiency) or coincident primary adrenal insufficiency (Schmidt's syndrome) should be considered. Adynamic ileus may cause megacolon or intestinal obstruction. Rarely, psychiatric symptoms or cerebellar ataxia may dominate the clinical picture. The relaxation phase of the deep tendon reflexes is characteristically prolonged, the so-called hung-up reflex. If left untreated, the patient with severe long-standing hypothyroidism may pass into a hypothermic, stuporous state (*myxedema coma*) that may be fatal. Respiratory depression is an important component of this state, and hence arterial P_{CO_2} may be increased. Factors that predispose to myxedema coma include cold exposure, trauma, infection, and administration of central nervous system depressants. Hyponatremia may result from impaired water excretion and from disordered regulation of vasopressin secretion.

LABORATORY TESTS The single most useful measurement is the serum TSH, which is increased in the thyroprivic and goitrous varieties and is usually normal or undetectable in pituitary or hypothalamic hypothyroidism (see Fig. 334-3). In the latter instances, hyposecretion of TSH is usually accompanied by hyposecretion of other pituitary hormones (see Chap. 331). A decrease in serum T_4 and in the FT_4I is common to all varieties of hypothyroidism. In the primary thyroid varieties, the serum T_3 may be decreased to a lesser extent than the serum T_4, presumably because the compensatory hypersecretion of TSH leads to a relative preponderance of T_3 secretion. In thyroprivic hypothyroidism, the decreased RAIU is of limited diagnostic utility because of the low value for the lower limit of the normal range. In goitrous hypothyroidism, the RAIU may be increased or display an abnormal pattern of accumulation or retention.

Manifestations of the hypothyroid state include an increased serum cholesterol level in hypothyroidism of thyroid (but not pituitary) origin and increased concentrations of serum creatine phosphokinase, aspartate transaminase, and lactate dehydrogenase. Systolic time intervals are altered in that the preejection period is prolonged and the ratio of the preejection period to left ventricular ejection time is increased. Electrocardiographic changes include bradycardia, low-amplitude QRS complexes, and flattened or inverted T waves. In primary thyroprivic hypothyroidism, pernicious anemia occurs in about 12 percent of patients; histamine-fast achlorhydria and circulating antigastric parietal cell antibodies are more common.

Some patients who appear clinically euthyroid display laboratory evidence of early thyroid failure (subclinical hypothyroidism). In mild cases, serum TSH and its response to TRH administration are increased, while serum T_4 and T_3 concentrations are normal. When thyroid failure is more advanced, serum T_4 concentration is decreased, but the serum T_3 concentration is normal or nearly so owing to TSH-induced hypersecretion of T_3 relative to T_4 and perhaps to more efficient conversion of T_4 to T_3. Subclinical hypothyroidism is most often seen in patients with Hashimoto's disease or those with Graves' disease who have been treated with ^{131}I or surgery and are usually in the evolution of frank hypothyroidism.

DIFFERENTIAL DIAGNOSIS Little difficulty is experienced in diagnosing the classic picture of cretinism or juvenile and adult hypothyroidism. Occasionally, an infant with Down's syndrome may be confused with a cretin. However, the characteristic eye changes, Brushfield's spots in the iris, hyperextensibility of the joints, and normal skin and hair texture distinguish Down's syndrome from cretinism. Chronic nephritis and the nephrotic syndrome may simulate

TABLE 334-6 Approximate therapeutic equivalence of various thyroid hormone preparations

Preparation	Average daily oral maintenance dose	Serum T_4	Undesirable lability in serum T_3
Levothyroxine	125 μg	Slightly increased	−
Liothyronine	50 μg	Decreased	+ +
Liotrix (T_4/T_3 = 4:1)	2 units	Normal	+
Thyroid extract, USP	120–180 mg	Normal	+

myxedema, particularly because of the facial puffiness and pallor. The nephrotic patient may have anemia, hypercholesterolemia, and anasarca, and the serum T_4 may be decreased if TBG is lost into the urine. However, the FT_4I is normal or increased, the serum T_3 concentration is often subnormal, as in any severe systemic illness owing to impaired peripheral generation from T_4, and the serum TSH concentration is normal.

TREATMENT Hormones available for the treatment of hypothyroidism (Table 334-6) include the synthetic hormones levothyroxine (L-thyroxine), liothyronine (L-triiodothyronine), and liotrix (a combination of the two). A preparation of natural origin still occasionally used is thyroid extract, USP. Because of their uniform potency, the author prefers the synthetic preparations and specifically levothyroxine. Unlike liothyronine, liotrix, and even thyroid extract, ingestion of levothyroxine does not lead to abrupt increases in serum T_3 concentration, which can be dangerous in the older patient or in the patient with coexisting heart disease. Rather, a stable T_3 concentration is attained through continuous generation from administered levothyroxine.

In most instances, a normal metabolic state should be restored gradually, especially in the elderly or the patient with heart disease, since sudden increases in metabolic rate may tax cardiac or coronary reserve. In adults, an initial daily dose of 25 μg levothyroxine can be increased by 25- to 50-μg increments at 4-week intervals until a normal metabolic state is attained. The dose necessary to sustain a normal metabolic state is usually about 1.7 μg/kg body weight per day, and this dose usually results in a serum T_4 at or somewhat above the upper limit of the normal range. The serum T_3 is superior to the serum T_4 as an indicator of the metabolic state in the patient receiving levothyroxine. Because of its long half-life, levothyroxine is administered as a single daily dose. The optimal dose is determined by clinical criteria and measurements of serum TSH by an ultrasensitive assay. In the patient with pituitary or hypothalamic disease, serum T_3 is the most useful parameter to follow. Elevations of the former indicate that treatment is insufficient and of the latter that it is excessive.

In neonatal, infantile, and juvenile hypothyroidism, full replacement therapy should be begun as soon as possible; otherwise, the chances of normal intellectual development and growth are poor. Infants and children require doses of levothyroxine that are disproportionately large in relation to body size. *In known or strongly suspected pituitary and hypothalamic hypothyroidism, thyroid replacement should not be instituted until treatment with hydrocortisone has been initiated*, since acute adrenocortical insufficiency may be precipitated by an increase in metabolic rate.

In some adults, hypothyroidism should be treated rapidly. This includes patients with myxedema coma and, because of the extreme sensitivity to central nervous system depressants, hypothyroid patients being prepared for emergency surgery. Here, intravenous administration of levothyroxine, in conjunction with the use of hydrocortisone, is indicated.

THYROTOXICOSIS

The term *thyrotoxicosis* denotes the clinical, physiologic, and biochemical findings that result when the tissues are exposed to, and

TABLE 334-7   Varieties of thyrotoxicosis

ASSOCIATED WITH THYROID HYPERFUNCTION*

A Excess production of TSH (rare)
B Abnormal thyroid stimulator
   1 Graves' disease
   2 Trophoblastic tumor
C Intrinsic thyroid autonomy
   1 Hyperfunctioning adenoma
   2 Toxic multinodular goiter

NOT ASSOCIATED WITH THYROID HYPERFUNCTION†

A Disorders of hormone storage
   1 Subacute thyroiditis
   2 Chronic thyroiditis with transient thyrotoxicosis
B Extrathyroid source of hormone
   1 Thyrotoxicosis factitia
   2 "Hamburger toxicosis"
   3 Ectopic thyroid tissue
      a Struma ovarii
      b Functioning follicular cacinoma

---

* Associated with increased RAIU unless body iodine burden is excessive.
† Associated with decreased RAIU.

respond to, excess thyroid hormone. Rather than a specific disease, thyrotoxicosis can originate in a variety of ways (Table 334-7). The first, and most important, encompasses those diseases that lead to sustained overproduction of hormone by the thyroid gland itself. Here, hyperfunction of the gland variously results from excessive secretion of TSH, a rare cause associated with pituitary tumor or with resistance to thyroid hormone in the pituitary but not in peripheral tissues; the action of an abnormal, homeostatically unregulated thyroid stimulator of extrapituitary origin, as in Graves' disease or hyperthyroidism in association with Hashimoto's disease or trophoblastic tumors; or the development of one or more areas of autonomous hyperfunction within the gland itself. The second category encompasses the thyrotoxic states associated with subacute thyroiditis and the syndrome termed *chronic thyroiditis with spontaneously resolving thyrotoxicosis;* an excess of preformed hormone leaks from the gland owing to the presence of inflammatory disease. New hormone formation is decreased, however, owing to the suppression of TSH secretion by the hormone excess and in some cases to the inflammatory injury itself. Since the inflammatory disorders are transitory, and since stores of preformed hormone are ultimately depleted, the thyrotoxicosis in these disorders is self-limited and is often followed by a transient period of thyroid hormone insufficiency. The third category of thyrotoxicosis is one in which the source of excess hormone is outside of the thyroid gland itself, as in thyrotoxicosis factitia, the ingestion of meat contaminated with animal thyroids ("hamburger toxicosis"), the rare functioning metastatic thyroid carcinoma, or struma ovarii.

Although the foregoing disorders are associated with thyrotoxicosis, not all are associated with *hyperthyroidism*, a term which should be used to denote only those conditions in which sustained hyperfunction of the thyroid leads to thyrotoxicosis. Thus thyrotoxic states can be classified according to whether or not they are associated with hyperthyroidism. This distinction has implications for diagnosis and for treatment. In hyperthyroidism, hyperfunction of the thyroid is reflected in an increased RAIU, whereas in the nonhyperthyroid thyrotoxic states, thyroid function (as reflected in the RAIU) is subnormal. Further, treatment of thyrotoxicosis by means intended to decrease hormone synthesis (antithyroid agents, surgery, or radioiodine) is appropriate in hyperthyroidism but is inappropriate and ineffective in other forms of thyrotoxicosis.

Though the specific diseases that cause thyrotoxicosis each make their own imprint on the clinical picture, the manifestations of the thyrotoxic state are largely the same. Since the first considered and most common is Graves' disease, the common manifestations of thyrotoxicosis are described in relation to Graves' disease.

GRAVES' DISEASE

Graves' disease, also known as Parry's or Basedow's disease, is a disorder with three major manifestations: hyperthyroidism with diffuse goiter, ophthalmopathy, and dermopathy. The three major manifestations need not appear together. Indeed, one or two need never appear, and moreover, the three may run courses that are largely independent of one another.

PREVALENCE   Graves' disease is a relatively common disorder that occurs at any age but is especially common in the third and fourth decades. The disease is more frequent in women. In nongoitrous areas, the ratio of predominance in women may be as high as 7:1. In areas of endemic goiter, the ratio is lower. Genetic factors play an important role; there is an increased frequency of haplotypes HLA-B8 and -DRw3 in Caucasian, HLA-Bw36 in Japanese, and HLA-Bw46 in Chinese patients with the disease. Not surprisingly, there is a distinct familial predisposition to Graves' disease. In addition, among family members, a clinical and immunologic overlap exists with respect to Hashimoto's disease, primary thyroprivic hypothyroidism, and pernicious anemia and probably with respect to other diseases with prominent autoimmune features. In occasional patients, the picture may change from Graves' disease to Hashimoto's disease, or vice versa, and rarely, patients with primary myxedema later become hyperthyroid. Thus it is proper to consider Graves' disease, Hashimoto's disease, and primary myxedema as closely related autoimmune thyroid diseases.

ETIOLOGY AND PATHOGENESIS   The cause is unknown. In view of the varied manifestations and their differing courses, it is possible that no single factor is responsible for the entire syndrome. With respect to hyperthyroidism, the central disorder is a disruption of homeostatic mechanisms that normally adjust hormone secretion to meet the needs of peripheral tissues. This homeostatic disruption results from the presence in plasma of an abnormal thyroid stimulator, first recognized when it was shown that the serum of patients with Graves' disease releases radioiodine from the prelabeled guinea pig or mouse thyroid. In view of its prolonged duration of action relative to that of TSH in this bioassay system, this material was designated the *long-acting thyroid stimulator* (LATS). LATS activity in the mouse assay is due to thyroid-stimulating immunoglobulins (TSI) of the IgG class elaborated by lymphocytes of patients with Graves' disease. When human thyroid tissue is used as the assay system, the measured end points are stimulation of colloid droplet or cyclic AMP generation in thyroid cells, slices, or membranes (thyroid-stimulating antibodies, TSAb) and inhibition of the binding of TSH to its receptors in human thyroid tissue (TSH-binding inhibitory immunoglobulins, TBII). These factors represent antibodies against the thyroid TSH receptor (TRAb). Activities of this type are also found in serum of some patients with euthyroid ophthalmic Graves' disease, occasional patients with Hashimoto's disease, and some euthyroid relatives of patients with Graves' disease. Presumably, the absence of thyrotoxicosis in such instances reflects predominance of blocking versus stimulatory TRAbs or intrinsic thyroid disease that prevents a hyperthyroid response. Disappearance of stimulatory factors from the serum during antithyroid treatment augurs well for long-term remission after treatment is withdrawn. Thus, while the basic cause of Graves' disease is not understood, an immunoglobulin or family of immunoglobulins directed against the TSH receptor mediates the thyroid stimulation. A heritable abnormality in immune surveillance may permit particular lymphocytes to survive, proliferate, and secrete the stimulatory immunoglobulins in response to precipitating factors.

The pathogenesis of the ophthalmic component is more enigmatic. One proposed mechanism is the development of antibodies against specific antigens in the extraocular muscles. Nothing is known of the pathogenesis of the dermopathy.

PATHOLOGY   In Graves' disease, the *thyroid gland* is diffusely enlarged, soft, and vascular. The pathology is that of parenchymatous hypertrophy and hyperplasia, characterized by increased height of the epithelium and redundancy of the follicular wall, giving the picture of papillary infoldings and cytologic evidence of increased activity. Such hyperplasia is usually accompanied by lymphocytic infiltration that reflects the immune aspect of the disease and correlates with levels of antithyroid antibodies in the blood. Following iodine medication, there is colloid storage, which sometimes causes enlargement and increased firmness of the gland. Graves' disease is associated with generalized lymphoid hyperplasia and infiltration and occasionally with enlargement of the spleen or thymus. Thyrotoxicosis may lead to degeneration of skeletal muscle fibers, enlargement of the heart, fatty infiltration or diffuse fibrosis of the liver, decalcification of the skeleton, and loss of body tissue (including fat deposits, osteoid, and muscle).

The *ophthalmopathy* is characterized by an inflammatory infiltrate of the orbital contents, exclusive of the globe, with lymphocytes, mast cells, and plasma cells. The orbital musculature is often enlarged due to infiltration with lymphocytes, mucopolysaccharides, and edema, which with fat largely accounts for the increased volume of the orbital contents that causes the globe to protrude. Muscle fibers show degeneration and loss of striations, with ultimate fibrosis.

The *dermopathy* of Graves' disease is characterized by thickening of the dermis, which is infiltrated with lymphocytes and with hydrophilic, metachromatically staining mucopolysaccharides.

CLINICAL MANIFESTATIONS The manifestations comprise those that reflect the associated thyrotoxicosis and those specifically related to Graves' disease. The former vary in intensity with the severity of the thyrotoxicosis, the age of the patient, duration of the illness, and the presence of disease in other organs, such as the heart.

Manifestations of thyrotoxicosis Common manifestations include nervousness, emotional lability, inability to sleep, tremors, frequent bowel movements, excessive sweating, and heat intolerance. Weight loss is usual despite a well-maintained or increased appetite. Proximal muscle weakness is present, with loss of strength often manifested by difficulty in climbing stairs. In premenopausal women, oligomenorrhea and amenorrhea tend to occur. Dyspnea, palpitations, and, in older patients, enhancement of angina pectoris or cardiac failure may occur. In general, nervous symptoms dominate the clinical picture in younger individuals, whereas cardiovascular and myopathic symptoms predominate in older subjects.

Usually, the patient appears anxious, restless, and fidgety. The skin is warm and moist with a velvety texture, and palmar erythema is present. Separation of the fingernail from the nailbed (Plummer's nail) is common, especially on the ring finger. The hair is fine and silky. A fine tremor of the fingers and tongue, together with hyperreflexia, is characteristic. *Ocular signs* include a characteristic stare with widened palpebral fissures, infrequent blinking, lid lag, and failure to wrinkle the brow on upward gaze. These signs result from sympathetic overstimulation and usually subside when the thyrotoxicosis is corrected. They are to be distinguished from the *infiltrative ophthalmopathy* characteristic of Graves' disease, discussed below.

Cardiovascular findings include a wide pulse pressure, sinus tachycardia, atrial arrhythmias (especially atrial fibrillation), systolic murmurs, increased intensity of the apical first sound, cardiac enlargement, and, at times, overt heart failure. A to-and-fro, high-pitched sound may be audible in the pulmonic area and may simulate a pericardial friction rub (Means-Lerman scratch).

Manifestations of Graves' disease The distinctive manifestations of Graves' disease, diffuse hyperfunctioning goiter, ophthalmopathy, and dermopathy, appear in varying combinations and in varying frequency, goiter being the most common. Premature graying of the hair and patchy vitiligo are not specific to Graves' disease and are common in other autoimmune disorders.

The *diffuse toxic goiter* may be asymmetric and lobular. The presence of a bruit over the gland usually signifies that the patient is thyrotoxic, but it may rarely be present in other disorders in which the thyroid is hyperplastic. Venous hums and carotid souffles should be distinguished from true thyroid bruits. An enlarged pyramidal lobe of the thyroid may be palpable.

The clinical signs associated with the *ophthalmopathy* of Graves' disease may be divided into two components: the spastic and the mechanical. The former includes the stare, lid lag, and lid retraction that accompany thyrotoxicosis and account for the "frightened" facies and eye signs previously described. These findings need not be associated with proptosis, may be ameliorated by adrenergic antagonists, and usually return to normal after correction of thyrotoxicosis. The mechanical component includes proptosis of varying degrees with ophthalmoplegia and congestive oculopathy characterized by chemosis, conjunctivitis, periorbital swelling, and the potential complications of corneal ulceration, optic neuritis, and optic atrophy. When exophthalmos progresses rapidly and becomes the major concern in Graves' disease, it is termed *progressive* and, if severe, *malignant exophthalmos*. The term *exophthalmic ophthalmoplegia* refers to the ocular muscle weakness that results in impaired upward gaze and convergence and strabismus with varying degrees of diplopia. Exophthalmos may be unilateral early but usually progresses to bilateral involvement.

The *dermopathy* usually occurs over the dorsum of the legs or feet and is termed *localized* or *pretibial myxedema*. It occurs in patients with past or present Graves' disease and is not a manifestation of hypothyroidism. About half of cases occur during the active stage of thyrotoxicosis. The affected area is usually demarcated from normal skin by the fact that it is raised, thickened, has a *peau d'orange* appearance and may be pruritic and hyperpigmented. The lesions are usually discrete, assuming a plaquelike or nodular configuration but in some instances are confluent. Clubbing of the fingers and toes with characteristic bony changes that differ from those of hypertrophic pulmonary osteoarthropathy may accompany the dermal changes (*thyroid acropachy*).

DIAGNOSIS When severe, Graves' disease presents little difficulty in diagnosis. Florid thyrotoxicosis is manifested by weakness, weight loss despite good appetite, nervous instability, tremor, intolerance to heat, sweating, palpitations, and hyperdefecation. When associated with diffuse thyroid enlargement, often accompanied by a bruit, and particularly when associated with ophthalmopathy, the clinical picture is virtually unique. In such instances, laboratory tests documenting undetectable TSH and increased RAIU, serum T_4 and T_3, RT_3U, and FT_4I serve as baselines for evaluation of therapy rather than necessary diagnostic aids. Occasionally, laboratory tests reveal a normal RAIU, normal serum T_4 and RT_3U, and elevated serum T_3 and FT_3I (T_3 toxicosis).

In less severe cases, particularly when ophthalmopathy is lacking, the diagnosis may be more difficult, since the symptoms of mild thyrotoxicosis are similar to those of other disorders (see "Differential Diagnosis" below). Presence of a goiter makes the diagnosis of hyperthyroidism likely, but careful palpation is necessary to determine whether toxic multinodular goiter, toxic adenoma, or subacute thyroiditis is present, since treatment of these disorders may differ from that of diffuse toxic goiter. Absence of thyroid enlargement makes the diagnosis of Graves' disease less likely but does not exclude it. In mild cases, confirmatory laboratory tests assume great importance. Unfortunately, mild thyrotoxicosis is often associated with marginal abnormalities in laboratory tests or values within the upper limit of the normal range. In such instances, an ultrasensitive TSH assay or the TRH stimulation test assumes crucial importance.

In a few (usually older) patients, the clinical picture may be one of apathy rather than hyperactivity, and evidence of hypermetabolism may be slight (*apathetic thyrotoxicosis*). In such patients, myopathic features may be pronounced. More often, cardiovascular manifestations predominate, since mild hyperthyroidism may produce severe disability in patients with underlying heart disease. Hence *all patients with unexplained cardiac failure or atrial arrhythmias should be examined for thyrotoxicosis.*

DIFFERENTIAL DIAGNOSIS Signs and symptoms of several nonthyroid disorders may simulate certain aspects of the thyrotoxic syndrome. Anxiety is a prominent feature of thyrotoxicosis, and there is thus some overlap in the symptomatology of thyrotoxicosis with that of anxiety states. Tachycardia, tremulousness, irritability, weakness, and fatigue are common to both disorders. In anxiety, however, the peripheral manifestations of excessive thyroid hormones are absent; the skin is usually cold and clammy rather than warm and moist. Weight loss, when present in emotional anxiety, is characteristically accompanied by anorexia, whereas in thyrotoxicosis the appetite is generally increased. Thyrotoxicosis can occasionally be confused with such disorders as metastatic carcinoma, cirrhosis of the liver, hyperparathyroidism, sprue, myasthenia gravis, and muscular dystrophy. Hypokalemic periodic paralysis is more common in thyrotoxic patients, especially in Oriental and Latin American men. Signs and symptoms of thyrotoxicosis may overlap with those of pheochromocytoma, which can cause heat intolerance, sweating, tachycardia with palpitations, and a hypermetabolic state. In the preceding disorders and in other conditions considered in the differential diagnosis, laboratory tests usually make it possible to differentiate them from thyrotoxicosis.

When bilateral ophthalmopathy is accompanied by goiter and thyrotoxicosis, the origin of the ophthalmopathy in Graves' disease is virtually certain. The presence of unilateral ophthalmopathy, even when associated with thyrotoxicosis, raises the possibility of some other intraorbital or intracranial disease. In the euthyroid patient with either unilateral or bilateral ophthalmopathy, other causes that must be excluded are cavernous sinus thrombosis, sphenoidal ridge meningioma, retrobulbar tumors, including leukemic deposits, and the rare granulomatous disorder pseudotumor oculi. Exophthalmos also may be seen in certain systemic disorders, such as uremia, accelerated hypertension, chronic alcoholism, chronic obstructive pulmonary disease, superior mediastinal obstruction, and Cushing's syndrome. Ophthalmoplegia in the absence of infiltrative manifestations can be confused with that which occurs in diabetes mellitus, myasthenia gravis, and myopathies. When doubt exists about the cause of ophthalmopathy, the demonstration of significant titers of TSI or TBII or of an abnormal TRH stimulation or thyroid suppression test suggests that the cause is Graves' disease, though not all patients with "euthyroid Graves' disease" demonstrate abnormal responses. In such cases, ultrasonography, magnetic resonance imaging, or computed tomography of the orbits is valuable in demonstrating characteristic thickening of the extraocular muscles.

When a thyrotoxic state occurs in a patient lacking the characteristic ophthalmopathy of Graves' disease, other causes of thyrotoxicosis must be considered. Careful palpation of the thyroid and studies with radioactive iodine are important in this regard. A symmetric, diffuse goiter of moderate or large size suggests the diagnosis of Graves' disease, especially if a bruit is present. However, the uncommon patient whose hyperthyroidism is secondary to an excess of TSH (associated with a *pituitary tumor* or resistance to feedback suppression of TSH secretion) or an abnormal stimulator of trophoblastic origin (*hydatidiform mole* or *choriocarcinoma of uterus* or *testis;* see Chap. 327) may present in this way. A single, prominent thyroid nodule or multiple nodules suggest *toxic adenoma* or *toxic multinodular goiter*, respectively. Tenderness of the thyroid associated with firm nodularity suggests *subacute thyroiditis*, while a small, firm, nontender goiter is consistent with chronic thyroiditis with spontaneously resolving thyrotoxicosis. The foregoing disorders are discussed in later sections. Absence of a palpable thyroid gland suggests an extrathyroid source of hormone, such as ectopic thyroid tissue *(struma ovarii)* or, more commonly, self-administration of hormone *(thyrotoxicosis factitia)*. Studies with radioactive iodine are also helpful. Except when hormone overproduction is secondary to increased iodine intake, values of the RAIU are increased in all disorders producing hyperthyroidism. Conversely, thyrotoxicosis that is not the result of hyperthyroidism is characterized by subnormal values of the RAIU. Subacute thyroiditis and chronic thyroiditis with spontaneously resolving thyrotoxicosis are the most common. Ectopic thyroid tissue producing thyrotoxicosis is rare. Here, the RAIU, as measured over the thyroid, is low, since TSH secretion is suppressed, but urinary excretion of radioactive iodine is slowed, owing to accumulation by the ectopic tissue.

Functioning ectopic tissue can be located by scintillation scanning. Thyrotoxicosis factitia most frequently occurs in medical or paramedical personnel or in those who have easy access to thyroid hormone. The disorder resembles thyrotoxicosis caused by ectopic thyroid tissue in that the patient's thyroid is suppressed. Consequently, the RAIU is very low, and most of administered radioactive iodine is excreted promptly in the urine. When the disorder is caused by ingestion of preparations containing T_4, such as levothyroxine or thyroid extract, the serum T_4 is increased. On the other hand, when caused by liothyronine, the serum T_4 is subnormal. Irrespective of the preparation, the serum T_3 is increased, but more so when liothyronine is the offending agent. Measurement of serum thyroglobulin is useful to confirm thyrotoxicosis factitia. Levels are elevated in Graves' disease and thyroiditis but are subnormal with exogenous thyroid hormone suppression. The demonstration of elevated titers of TRAbs in the blood also provides strong evidence that Graves' disease is the cause of thyrotoxicosis.

TREATMENT   Hyperthyroidism   Hyperthyroidism is often characterized by cyclic phases of exacerbation and remission, each of unpredictable onset and duration. Moreover, long-standing disease may be associated with progressive thyroid failure, probably consequent to chronic thyroiditis, with the supervention of hypothyroidism or decreased thyroid reserve. These characteristics have important implications in the choice of and response to therapy.

The major treatments are directed to limiting the quantity of thyroid hormones the gland can produce. Antithyroid agents interpose a chemical blockade to hormone synthesis, the effect of which is operative only as long as the drug is administered. Thus the agents can control active thyrotoxicity but probably do not prevent exacerbation at some subsequent period. The second major approach is ablation of thyroid tissue, thereby limiting hormone production. This may be achieved either by surgery or by radioactive iodine. Since these procedures induce permanent anatomic alterations of the thyroid, they can control the active phase and are more likely to prevent later exacerbation or recurrence. On the other hand, surgery or radiation is more likely to lead to hypothyroidism, either shortly after treatment or with the passage of years.

Each therapy has advantages and disadvantages, indications and contraindications. The latter are more often relative than absolute. In general, a trial of long-term antithyroid therapy is desirable in children, adolescents, young adults, and pregnant women but also may be employed in older patients. Indications for ablative procedures include relapse or recurrence following drug therapy, a large goiter, drug toxicity, failure to follow a medical regimen, or failure to return for periodic examinations. Subtotal thyroidectomy may be elected for patients under the age of 30 in whom ablative therapy is required; however, opinions differ, and some authorities employ radioactive iodine in the treatment of patients in the second or third decades. Surgery is also preferable in patients with very large goiters or with a coincident nonfunctioning nodule, especially if there is a history of radiation to the head and neck. Radioactive iodine is the ablative procedure of choice in older patients, in patients who have had previous thyroid surgery, and in those in whom systemic disease contraindicates elective surgery.

In patients selected for *long-term antithyroid therapy*, satisfactory control can almost always be achieved if sufficient drug is administered. Most patients can be managed with propylthiouracil, 100 to 150 mg every 6 or 8 h. Larger doses may be required for initial control. Methimazole is at least as effective as propylthiouracil when administered in one-tenth the dosage. However, propylthiouracil has the advantage of inhibiting the peripheral conversion of T_4 to T_3, thereby bringing about more rapid symptomatic improvement. Once euthyroidism is achieved, the daily dosage may be reduced to the smallest amount that controls the thyrotoxicosis. In some clinics the initial dose is continued and is supplemented with levothyroxine. By this latter regimen, hypothyroidism from overdosage of antithyroid drugs can be prevented. The undesirable consequences of hypothyroidism, such as enhancement of ophthalmopathy and enlargement of the goiter, may thereby be forestalled. In one study, combined therapy was associated with lower titers of TRAbs and a reduced risk of recurrence at the termination of therapy. The duration of antithyroid drug therapy is difficult to predict in the individual patient and may be a function of the natural course of the disease. The longer the course of therapy, the more likely it is that the patient will remain well when the drug is discontinued. In general a 12- to 24-month course is employed, following which one-third to one-half of patients remain well for a prolonged period or indefinitely. The likelihood of a prolonged remission is increased by a decrease in goiter size, reversion of the thyroid suppression test and TRH stimulation test to normal, or disappearance of TRAbs from the serum during treatment.

Leukopenia is the principal undesirable side effect of antithyroid drugs. A complete blood count should be obtained prior to initiating therapy to identify those patients with leukopenia related to Graves' disease. Mild transient leukopenia may occur with antithyroid drugs in approximately an additional 10 percent of patients and is not necessarily an indication for discontinuing therapy. When the absolute number of polymorphonuclear leukocytes reaches 1500 per cubic millimeter or less, antithyroid medication should be discontinued. Allergic rashes and drug sensitivity occur on occasion. These may disappear with antihistamine therapy at the same or reduced dosage of antithyroid agent, but it is probably preferable when sensitivity reactions occur to change to another drug. On rare occasions (in less than 0.2 percent), agranulocytosis occurs. This may be sudden in onset. Hepatitis, drug fever, and arthralgias occur on occasion. In the author's view, severe sensitivity reactions, including agranulocytosis, dictate the abandonment of antithyroid therapy rather than recourse to an alternate drug.

Iodide inhibits the release of hormones from the hyperfunctioning thyroid gland, and its ameliorative effects occur more rapidly than those of agents that inhibit hormone synthesis. Hence its main use is in patients with actual or impending thyrotoxic crisis and in patients with severe cardiac disease. The response to iodide alone is often incomplete and transient. Furthermore, by expanding the thyroid store of hormone, iodide may prolong the latency of response to antithyroid therapy. Therefore, iodide is safely used only in conjunction with the antithyroid agents. If the clinical course is sufficiently severe to require iodide administration, antithyroid drugs are usually the primary therapeutic agents and should be given in large doses prior to iodide. Iodide is also useful in controlling thyrotoxicosis following ^{131}I administration, during the period in which the therapeutic effect of radioiodine has not yet taken place. Large doses of *glucocorticoids* (2 mg dexamethasone every 6 h) reduce the serum T_4 concentration when relief of thyrotoxicosis is urgent. The iodinated x-ray contrast agent sodium ipodate has a similar effect. Iodine liberated from this agent inhibits thyroid secretion of T_4 and T_3, and serum T_3 is further reduced by the inhibition by ipodate of peripheral T_3 formation. Daily doses of 1 g orally are effective, but the same precautions concerning the use of iodine therapy are applicable to ipodate.

Owing to the adrenergic component in thyrotoxicosis, various *adrenergic antagonists* have been employed in its management. Of these, propranolol is the agent of choice because of its relative freedom from side effects. In doses of 40 to 120 mg/d, propranolol alleviates such adrenergic manifestations as sweating, tremor, and tachycardia and may reduce to some extent the conversion of T_4 to T_3. However, propranolol should be used only as adjunctive therapy, since the underlying metabolic abnormalities are not affected. Moreover, although the diminution in heart rate and cardiac work may be beneficial, the blocking of adrenergic support of myocardial contractility requires caution in its use in the patient with coexisting heart failure, unless rate- or rhythm-related. As adjunctive therapy, propranolol is useful during the period when the response to conventional antithyroid agents or to radioiodine therapy is being awaited and in the management of thyrotoxic crisis. It has been employed as the sole agent in preparation for thyroidectomy, but its use in this setting is not recommended, since it does not render the patient euthyroid, with a likely greater risk of surgically induced crisis.

Radioactive iodine (^{131}I) affords a relatively simple, effective, and economical means of treating thyrotoxicosis. It can produce the ablative effects of surgery without the operative and postoperative complications. The principal disadvantage of ^{131}I therapy, in the dosage usually employed, is its tendency to produce hypothyroidism with a frequency that increases with time. As many as 40 to 70 percent of patients may develop this complication within 10 years after treatment. Although hypothyroidism is treatable, once diagnosed, the insidious onset may obscure the diagnosis until serious complications develop. Hence some recommend that all patients be treated with large doses of ^{131}I to ensure relief of thyrotoxicosis and then placed on permanent physiologic replacement doses of thyroid hormone.

There is no evidence of carcinogenic or leukemogenic effects of radioiodine when given to adults in the doses commonly used in treating hyperthyroidism. However, the susceptibility to carcinogenesis may be increased in the thyroids of children. Mutagenic effects have not been reported and would be difficult to document. For these reasons, many physicians prefer to reserve radioiodine therapy for patients over 30 years of age or those unlikely to have children subsequently. Moreover, the longer the life expectancy after ^{131}I therapy, the greater is the likelihood that hypothyroidism will develop. Among younger patients, therefore, only those with recurrent thyrotoxicosis following surgery, those who refuse surgery, and those with complicating illness that contraindicates surgery are candidates for radioiodine therapy. In elderly patients, treatment with large doses of radioiodine is the general method of choice so that the undesirable effects of incomplete treatment or recurrence can be avoided. In patients with significant ophthalmopathy, it may be prudent to administer glucocorticoids for approximately 2 weeks before and 6 weeks after the ^{131}I dose to reduce the likelihood of exacerbation of eye disease.

The usual therapeutic dose of ^{131}I [approximately 5.9 MBq (160 μCi) per gram of estimated gland weight] leads to a high frequency of hypothyroidism. As a result, some authorities continuing to use this dose regularly administer prophylactic replacement doses of thyroid hormone. Others have administered smaller doses [approximately 3.0 MBq/g (80 μCi/g)]. However, this does not diminish the frequency of late hypothyroidism but merely delays its onset. Moreover, the smaller dose is less likely to relieve thyrotoxicosis within a relatively short period. Antithyroid agents can be employed, however, to speed the attainment of a eumetabolic state, and propranolol can be given to relieve symptoms while the effect of the ^{131}I is taking hold. There is general agreement that patients with coexisting cardiac disease should receive ^{131}I in large doses in view of the hazard of recurrent thyrotoxicosis.

Radiation thyroiditis is an occasional immediate complication of ^{131}I therapy. It commonly appears within 7 to 10 days and is associated with accelerated release of hormone into the blood. Rarely, radiation thyroiditis may cause thyrotoxic crisis (see below), most commonly in the elderly thyrotoxic patient with other systemic illness. For these reasons, patients with severe hyperthyroidism or underlying heart disease should be rendered eumetabolic with antithyroid agents before ^{131}I is administered. Interruption of antithyroid therapy for 3 to 4 days before and after ^{131}I treatment suffices to permit adequate accumulation and retention of administered ^{131}I. Propranolol may be used as an adjunct both before and after ^{131}I administration but should not be relied on to provide adequate prophylaxis if given alone. The swelling that accompanies radiation thyroiditis may contraindicate the use of large doses of ^{131}I in patients with large retrosternal goiters.

Before radioactive iodine was introduced, *subtotal thyroidectomy* was the standard form of ablative therapy, and it is still employed in younger patients in whom antithyroid therapy is unsuccessful. Although precise preoperative programs differ, several general principles should be emphasized. Patients should first be rendered euthyroid by means of antithyroid agents. Only then should iodide (five drops of Lugol's solution a day for approximately 10 days) be administered concomitantly to effect an involutional response in the gland. Antithyroid drugs should not be discontinued merely because treatment with iodide is instituted. The response of the patient, and not the calendar, should dictate when surgery is performed.

Hazards of subtotal thyroidectomy include immediate complications, such as anesthetic accidents, hemorrhage sometimes leading to respiratory obstruction, and damage to the recurrent laryngeal nerve leading to vocal cord paralysis. Later complications include wound infection, hemorrhage, hypoparathyroidism, and hypothyroidism. Subtotal thyroidectomy should be performed by a surgeon experienced in this procedure; under this condition, surgery is effective and relatively safe. Postoperative recurrences are uncommon. However, carefully conducted follow-up studies reveal that hypothyroidism follows surgery more frequently than previously suspected, although not as commonly as with conventional doses of ^{131}I.

The *treatment of hyperthyroidism during pregnancy* is a subject of some disagreement. Most physicians believe that antithyroid therapy is preferable to surgery, which should not be performed in any event during the first and third trimesters. Antithyroid agents carry less risk to the patient and the pregnancy. Further, since they traverse the placental barrier, they have the theoretical advantage of preventing fetal and neonatal hyperthyroidism when maternal titers of TRAbs are high. As a clue to the risk of fetal hyperthyroidism, assays of such stimulators should be conducted in pregnant women with a history of Graves' disease, whether treated or not. On the other hand, the major disadvantage of antithyroid therapy is the possibility of inducing hypothyroidism in the fetus. T_4 and T_3 traverse the human placenta from mother to fetus only slowly, and simultaneous administration of thyroid hormone and antithyroid drugs to the mother will not protect the fetus from hypothyroidism. Hence the cardinal rule in using the antithyroid agents in pregnancy is that the dosage should be the smallest necessary to control hyperthyroidism in the mother. From the laboratory standpoint, the physician should aim to keep the serum TSH and the FT_4 concentration within the normal limits, remembering that pregnancy is normally associated with some elevation of the serum total T_4 owing to an increase in serum TBG concentration. Since pregnancy appears to attenuate the severity of hyperthyroidism, control can often be achieved with maintenance doses of 200 mg propylthiouracil daily or less. At this dose, fetal goiter or hypothyroidism has not been a problem. Patients who require doses of 300 mg/d or more during the first trimester should probably be treated by subtotal thyroidectomy during the middle trimester. The author believes that patients carried through pregnancy on antithyroid agents should not be given propranolol as adjunctive treatment, in view of reports that the agent may cause fetal growth retardation and neonatal respiratory depression. Propylthiouracil tends to be favored over methimazole, even though earlier reports of fetal anomalies with the latter agent have not been confirmed. Advantages of propylthiouracil include its effect on inhibiting conversion of T_4 to T_3 and its higher degree of protein binding, which retards its excretion into breast milk. Radioiodine should never be administered to a pregnant woman, and all women of childbearing age who are about to receive ^{131}I should have a pregnancy test performed first.

Ophthalmopathy, dermopathy When severe and progressive, ophthalmopathy is the most difficult component of Graves' disease to treat satisfactorily. Fortunately, in most patients the disorder runs a benign course that is largely independent of the hyperthyroidism. In most instances, the activity of even moderately severe disease declines and disappears with time, although some exophthalmos and ophthalmoplegia may persist. In mild disease, considerable benefit may be obtained from simple measures, such as elevating the head at night, administering diuretics to reduce edema, and providing tinted glasses for protection from sun, wind, and foreign bodies. A 1% solution of methylcellulose or plastic shields may prevent corneal drying in patients unable to oppose the lids during sleep. In more severe cases, as evidenced by progressive exophthalmos, chemosis, ophthalmoplegia, or loss of vision, large doses of prednisone (100 to 120 mg/d) should be administered, since this is usually effective in reducing the edematous and infiltrative components. With improve-

ment, the dosage is reduced to the lowest effective level to minimize the effects of glucocorticoid excess. Orbital radiation may be helpful in some patients with acute, severe infiltrative manifestations, particularly when administered concomitantly with glucocorticoids. In cases that progress despite these measures, orbital decompression, i.e., removal of part of the bony orbit, is required to relieve intraorbital pressure. The management must always be conducted in concert with an ophthalmologist.

In general, treatment of associated hyperthyroidism should be carried out as if ophthalmopathy were not present, since the mode of treatment of the hyperthyroidism does not influence the course of the ocular disease. Whether ^{131}I therapy may aggravate ophthalmopathy remains controversial. It is agreed, however, that hypothyroidism should be avoided.

Severe dermopathy can be alleviated by the topical application of glucocorticoids.

TOXIC MULTINODULAR GOITER

Toxic multinodular goiter is an occasional consequence of long-standing simple goiter, although the proportion of cases in which this complication arises is uncertain. In areas of nonendemicity, the cause of nontoxic multinodular goiter is usually indeterminate. Hence it is unclear whether a specific factor underlies those cases of nontoxic multinodular goiter that progress to thyrotoxic phase. Common to many nontoxic multinodular goiters, even in areas of iodine sufficiency, the iodine content of thyroglobulin is decreased, suggesting either a conditioned deficiency of iodine or an impairment of its normal incorporation into the protein. There is no pathologic feature to distinguish the nontoxic from the toxic multinodular goiter. However, the transition from nontoxic to toxic nodular goiter involves the development of functional autonomy, i.e., independence from TSH stimulation in one or more areas of the gland. Scattered foci of functional autonomy are demonstrable early in the disease process and increase in size and number as time passes so that approximately a fourth of seemingly euthyroid patients with nontoxic nodular goiter display, as evidence of functional autonomy, subnormal or absent responses to TRH administration. As judged from scintillation scanning, functional patterns may be of two types. In the more common, iodine accumulation occurs diffusely in patchy foci throughout the gland. The less common pattern is that of iodine accumulation in one or more discrete nodules within the gland, the remainder appearing to be essentially nonfunctional. Histologic and autoradiographic studies reveal marked heterogeneity of structure and function, the two being poorly correlated. In both endemic and sporadic nontoxic multinodular goiter, administration of iodides may lead to the development of thyrotoxicosis (jodbasedow), a complication consonant with the functional autonomy of this disorder.

Because it arises in long-standing simple goiter, toxic multinodular goiter is a disease of the aging or elderly. For this reason, and because of the nature of the underlying disease, the clinical presentation differs from that in Graves' disease. Ophthalmopathy is rare and would signal the emergence of Graves' disease superimposed on simple goiter. Some patients have typical thyrotoxicosis. Often, however, the degree of thyrotoxicosis is less severe than that in Graves' disease, although its physiologic impact on specific organ systems may be great. Notable among these is the cardiovascular system, in which arrhythmias or congestive failure may be precipitated or accentuated by thyrotoxicosis that may be manifested only by subtle findings in other areas (apathetic hyperthyroidism). Weakness and wasting may predominate, frequently with loss of appetite rather than hyperphagia, suggesting the presence of a carcinoma.

In some patients, a definitive diagnosis of toxic nodular goiter is difficult to establish. On the one hand, enlargement or nodularity of the gland may escape detection because the patient has a short neck or is kyphotic or because the thyroid is substernal. When this is the case, and when the clinical findings suggest thyrotoxicosis, RAIU and scintiscan are particularly helpful. On the other hand, even when a nodular goiter is palpable, the presence of mild but clinically significant thyrotoxicosis may be difficult to confirm, since values of the serum total T_4 and T_3, FT_4, and FT_4I are often only near or slightly above normal. For example, a value for the serum T_3 that would be normal for a young adult may represent an increase in the elderly patient, since serum T_3 usually declines with age. Despite their value in situations such as this, thyroid suppression tests should rarely be undertaken in the elderly patient because of the hazard of adverse cardiovascular responses. Unfortunately, although a normal response to TRH would exclude a diagnosis of thyrotoxicosis in a patient with a nodular goiter, subnormal responses do not establish the diagnosis. Responses to TRH decline in the elderly, especially in men, and seemingly euthyroid patients with nodular goiter may respond subnormally to TRH as a reflection of at least partial functional autonomy of the thyroid gland. An undetectable basal TSH and absent response to TRH by an ultrasensitive assay imply thyrotoxicosis (see Fig. 334-3). When laboratory findings do not permit a clear diagnosis of thyrotoxicosis but suggestive clinical findings are present, a therapeutic trial of antithyroid drugs may be indicated.

Radioactive iodine is the treatment of choice for toxic multinodular goiter. In contrast to Graves' disease, large doses [740 to 1110 MBq (20 to 30 mCi)] are usually required owing to the generally lower RAIU and to the variable degree of function throughout the gland. Moreover, the physiologic instability of the elderly patient makes definitive treatment urgent. For the same reason, it is usually wise to initiate therapy with antithyroid agents, withholding radioiodine until a euthyroid state is achieved, thereby forestalling an exacerbation of thyrotoxicosis should radiation thyroiditis occur. Unless contraindicated, propranolol is often useful in controlling manifestations of thyrotoxicosis both before and after radioiodine therapy, while its therapeutic effect is awaited. Hypothyroidism is an uncommon consequence of radioiodine treatment of toxic multinodular goiter owing to the variable activity of differing portions of the gland, which permits previously quiescent areas to function in place of those destroyed by ^{131}I.

UNUSUAL VARIETIES OF THYROTOXICOSIS

Thyrotoxicosis is also seen in other disorders, including follicular adenoma of the thyroid and various forms of thyroiditis, which are discussed in later sections. This section will consider still other unusual causes of thyrotoxicosis and unusual ways in which thyrotoxicosis may present.

UNUSUAL CAUSES OF THYROTOXICOSIS Rarely, hyperthyroidism and thyrotoxicosis are the result of sustained hypersecretion of TSH from either a *TSH-secreting pituitary adenoma* or a selective *resistance of the TSH-secretory mechanism* to feedback inhibition by thyroid hormones. The resistance syndromes in which both the pituitary and peripheral tissues are relatively resistant to thyroid hormones are discussed above. TSH-secreting pituitary adenomas can be distinguished, in many cases, by radiologic evidence of pituitary tumor, by the fact that the concentration of free α subunits of TSH in serum is elevated, and by the fact that the response of the serum TSH to TRH is negligible. In the variant caused by pituitary resistance, subunit concentrations are not grossly elevated, and the TSH response to TRH is usually normal.

Patients with *trophoblastic tumor*, either choriocarcinoma or hydatidiform mole, frequently display elevations, sometimes marked, of serum total and free T_4 and T_3 concentrations. In addition to signs of pregnancy, the usual manifestations of thyrotoxicosis may be present, but ophthalmopathy is absent. Thyroid hyperfunction is caused by a circulating thyroid stimulator of trophoblastic origin, which is human chorionic gonadotropin (hCG), and the diagnosis may be confirmed by the finding of extremely high blood or urine levels of βhCG. Abnormal thyroid function tests remit promptly after removal of the tumor.

Thyrotoxicosis factitia is a form of thyrotoxicosis without hyperthyroidism that results from purposeful or inadvertent ingestion of large amounts of thyroid hormone. The syndrome is usually a form of malingering and occurs most commonly in women with an underlying psychiatric disorder, usually paramedical personnel, or in patients who have taken thyroid hormones in the past or who have relatives who take thyroid hormones. In such patients, endogenous thyroid function is suppressed, as evidenced by subnormal values of the RAIU and serum thyroglobulin concentration. Serum TSH is suppressed, and both serum T_4 and T_3 concentrations are increased if the patient is taking a preparation that contains T_4, whereas the serum T_3 concentration is elevated and the serum T_4 depressed in patients taking T_3 alone. Factitious hyperthyroidism also has been described in people who ingest large quantities of ground meats contaminated with thyroid tissue.

Very rarely, thyrotoxicosis with a low RAIU is the result of excess hormone secretion by *ectopic thyroid tissue*, either widespread functioning metastases of thyroid carcinoma or struma ovarii.

The *jodbasedow phenomenon* refers to the induction of thyrotoxicosis in a previously euthyroid patient as a result of exposure to iodine. It typically occurs in areas of endemic iodine deficiency when measures to increase iodine intake or body iodine stores are implemented. The presumption is that the supplemental iodine permits functionally autonomous thyroid tissue to produce and secrete excessive hormone. A similar phenomenon can occur in patients with nontoxic multinodular goiter who receive large doses of iodide. Since such patients tend to be elderly with the danger of serious cardiovascular manifestations should thyrotoxicosis ensue, large doses of iodine should not be given to those with multinodular goiter. Similarly, in such patients, pharmaceuticals containing iodine, such as x-ray contrast media, should be used only when indicated and with consideration of the possible hazard of the jodbasedow phenomenon. When a contrast study is indicated under these conditions, it may be judicious to administer large doses of propylthiouracil (450 to 600 mg/d) prior to and for a week after the procedure. Some patients may develop hyperthyroidism following exposure to large quantities of iodine despite the fact that after iodine is withdrawn, they recover, thyroid function appears to be entirely normal, and evidence of functional autonomy is lacking.

UNUSUAL PRESENTATIONS OF THYROTOXICOSIS T_3 **toxicosis** Thyrotoxicosis in which serum T_4 is normal or low in the absence of a deficiency of TBG, while the serum T_3 is increased, is termed *T_3 toxicosis*. Although the production rate of T_3 is disproportionately increased relative to that of T_4 in hyperthyroidism, in some this discrepancy is exaggerated. This may occur in association with Graves' disease, multinodular goiter, or hyperfunctioning adenoma. The diagnosis should be suspected in a patient with clinical manifestations of thyrotoxicosis in whom the serum T_4 and FT_4 are normal or low and the RAIU is normal or increased. These features, together with the frequently palpable goiter, serve to differentiate this disorder from liothyronine-induced thyrotoxicosis factitia. In contrast to nonthyroidal disorders that mimic thyrotoxicosis, patients with this disorder demonstrate nonsuppressibility of thyroid function in response to exogenous T_3, undetectable serum TSH, and absent responses to TRH. In many patients, thyrotoxicosis with increased serum T_3 and normal serum T_4 precedes emergence of typical increases in both, either during an initial episode of hyperthyroidism or more commonly during recurrence after previous treatment. In some patients in whom symptoms of thyrotoxicosis fail to regress completely during antithyroid therapy despite return of the serum T_4 concentration to normal, the serum T_3 concentration is persistently elevated. Such patients are likely to experience a recurrence of thyrotoxicosis when antithyroid therapy is withdrawn.

T_4 toxicosis In most patients with hyperthyroidism, the serum T_3 is increased to a relatively greater extent than is the serum T_4. This reflects the fact that in hyperthyroidism, T_3 generated from T_4 peripherally is supplemented by release of substantial quantities of T_3 from the thyroid. However, thyrotoxicosis may sometimes be associated with a clear elevation of serum T_4 and a seemingly normal serum T_3 concentration. This syndrome of T_4 *toxicosis* occurs most commonly in the setting of prior excess iodine exposure in patients who are elderly, ill, or both and is, therefore, usually seen in a hospital setting. Increased iodine intake favors T_4 biosynthesis. In the absence of a history of excess iodine, the combination of high serum T_4 and normal serum T_3 concentration presumably reflects inhibition of peripheral T_3 generation from T_4, with persistence of T_3 secretion along with T_4 from the thyroid.

MAJOR COMPLICATIONS OF THYROTOXICOSIS

CARDIAC DISEASE Thyrotoxicosis causes increases in both systolic and diastolic cardiac function, probably secondary to effects on the expression of genes for the contractile protein, myosin. Untreated, the increased work eventually progresses to decompensation. As a consequence of this and peripheral effects of thyroid hormone, a variety of burdens are imposed on the heart. Hypermetabolism of the peripheral tissues increases both the metabolic and nonmetabolic (heat-loss) circulatory load, while direct effects of thyroid hormone on the myocardium cause rapid filling and increase the force, velocity, and rate of ventricular contraction. As a result, cardiac work and cardiac output are increased. Moreover, atrial irritability is enhanced, leading to arrhythmias, most importantly atrial fibrillation. In the patient with a normal heart, these burdens are usually tolerated. In the patient with underlying heart disease, however, cardiac insufficiency may be precipitated or aggravated. As would be expected, this complication is more common in the elderly patient and the patient with toxic multinodular goiter, sometimes as the most prominent manifestation of the thyrotoxic state. In patients with cardiac insufficiency, clues to the presence of thyrotoxicosis include atrial fibrillation, relatively rapid circulation time, increased cardiac output (high-output failure), and resistance to the usual therapeutic doses of digitalis.

Treatment is directed at rapid alleviation of thyrotoxicosis and restoration of cardiac compensation. The former objective is best met by treatment with large doses of an antithyroid agent, followed by iodine if the clinical situation is urgent. In less severe cases, radioiodine treatment is preceded by antithyroid drug treatment alone. The cardiac decompensation is managed in the usual manner, employing larger than usual doses of digitalis but with care to avoid digitalis intoxication as thyrotoxicosis is alleviated. Adrenergic antagonists should be used with caution in the presence of cardiac failure, unless failure is the consequence primarily of disturbance of cardiac rate or rhythm.

THYROTOXIC CRISIS Thyrotoxic crisis or storm causes a fulminating increase in the signs and symptoms of thyrotoxicosis. In the past, this disturbance usually occurred postoperatively in patients poorly prepared for surgery. However, with the preoperative use of antithyroid drugs and iodide and with appropriate therapy to control metabolic factors, weight, and nutritional status, postoperative thyrotoxic crisis should not occur. At present, so-called medical storm is more common and occurs in untreated or inadequately treated patients. It is precipitated by surgical emergency or complicating illness, usually sepsis. The syndrome is characterized by extreme irritability, delirium or coma, fever to 41°C or more, tachycardia, restlessness, hypotension, vomiting, and diarrhea. Rarely, the picture may be more subtle, with apathy, prostration, and coma, but with only slight elevation of temperature. Such postoperative complications as sepsis, septicemia, hemorrhage, and transfusion or drug reactions may mimic thyrotoxic crisis. The physiologic factor(s) that initiates thyrotoxic crisis is unknown. It does not appear to be an acute increase in the severity of thyroid hyperfunction. Rather, it may represent a shift from protein-bound to free hormone secondary to circulating inhibitors to binding in systemic illness.

Treatment consists of providing supportive therapy while undertaking measures to alleviate thyrotoxicosis as rapidly as possible.

Supportive therapy includes treatment of dehydration and the intravenous administration of glucose and saline, vitamin B complex, and glucocorticoids. The latter are indicated because of the increased glucocorticoid requirements in thyrotoxicosis and because adrenal reserve may be reduced. Patients should be placed in a cooled, humidified oxygen tent, and if hyperpyrexia is present, a cooling blanket should be used. Digitalization is required to control ventricular rate in those with atrial fibrillation. If shock exists, intravenous pressor agents should be employed. Therapy of the hyperthyroidism consists of blockade of hormone synthesis by the immediate and continued administration of large doses of an antithyroid agent (e.g., 100 mg propylthiouracil every 2 h). If the patient is unable to swallow the medication, the tablets should be triturated and given by nasogastric tube or per rectum, since parenteral preparations are unavailable. Following initiation of antithyroid therapy, hormone release is inhibited through the administration of large doses of iodine intravenously or by mouth. The iodinated x-ray contrast agent sodium ipodate can be administered instead of iodine and has the added action of inhibiting the peripheral conversion of T_4 to T_3. Doses of 1 g/d are effective. Adrenergic antagonists are an important, and perhaps critical, part of the therapeutic regimen in the absence of cardiac failure. Propranolol can be administered in doses of 40 to 80 mg every 6 h. If medications cannot be taken orally, 2 mg propranolol may be given intravenously, with careful electrocardiographic monitoring. Large doses of dexamethasone (e.g., 2 mg every 6 h) also should be administered, since they inhibit hormone release, impair the peripheral generation of T_3 from T_4, and provide adrenal support. Indeed, with the combined use of propylthiouracil, iodine, and dexamethasone, the serum T_3 concentration generally returns to normal within 24 to 48 h. Dexamethasone may be tapered thereafter, while antithyroid therapy and iodine must be continued until a normal metabolic state is approached, at which time iodine is progressively withdrawn and plans are made for definitive treatment.

NEOPLASMS

The prevalence of solitary nodules of the thyroid gland increases with age, averaging 6.4 percent of women and 1.5 percent of men. Many palpable thyroid nodules thought to be solitary are actually part of a multinodular thyroid gland. High-resolution ultrasound identifies nodules in a third of patients being evaluated for nonthyroid indications, and autopsy studies reveal thyroid nodules in as many as 50 percent of necropsies. In general, a nodule must reach a size of 1 cm in diameter to be detectable by palpation. In addition to thyroid neoplasms, the differential diagnosis of apparent thyroid nodules includes cysts, adenopathy, cystic hygroma, parathyroid tumors, and laryngocele. True intrathyroidal nodules usually represent colloid adenomas or simple follicular adenomas.

THYROID ADENOMAS True adenomas, as contrasted with localized adenomatous areas, are encapsulated and compress contiguous tissue. Adenomas vary in size and are classified into three histologic types: papillary, follicular, and Hürthle cell. The follicular adenomas can be subdivided according to the size of the follicles into colloid or macrofollicular, fetal or microfollicular, and embryonal varieties. There is variation in physiologic differentiation, as judged by the ability to concentrate radioiodine. The more highly differentiated adenomas (follicular) are the most common and are the most likely to mimic the function of normal thyroid tissue. Though the function may be responsive to TSH stimulation, it usually differs from that of normal thyroid tissue in being autonomous; i.e., the basal activity is independent of TSH stimulation. Adenomas of this type are usually unifocal, presenting as a single nodule. Often the patient reports that the nodule has grown slowly over many years. Initially, its function is insufficient to disturb hormonal equilibrium, though its capacity to accumulate radioiodine is evident in scintiscans as an area of increased density within the still-functioning extranodular tissue ("*warm*" *nodule*). At this stage, demonstration of the inherent autonomy requires scintiscanning while the patient is receiving suppressive doses of exogenous thyroid hormone (suppression scan). With time, the nodule grows larger, its function increasing until it is sufficient to suppress TSH secretion. Consequently, the remainder of the gland undergoes relative atrophy and loss of function, and the scintiscan reveals radioiodine accumulation only in the region of the nodule (''hot'' nodule). At this time, TSH is suppressed (''chemical'' thyrotoxicosis), but the patient may or may not be overtly thyrotoxic. Frank thyrotoxicosis usually supervenes eventually (toxic adenoma) and may be precipitated by iodine exposure such as from radiographic contrast dyes. Relative to its overall rate of occurrence, hyperfunctioning adenoma is a frequent cause of T_3 toxicosis. Hyperfunctioning adenomas are amenable to ablation by surgery or ^{131}I. Large doses of the latter are usually required to bring about prompt cure. Although it has been thought that radiation damage would be confined solely to the hyperfunctioning nodule being treated with ^{131}I, the remaining tissue being spared, this may not always be the case, since some patients with hyperfunctioning adenoma become euthyroid after treatment with ^{131}I only to become hypothyroid years later.

Hyperfunctioning nodules are rarely the seat of carcinoma. However, hyperfunctioning adenomas may undergo hemorrhagic necrosis. The resulting pain and nodularity may suggest subacute thyroiditis. Subsequently, there is loss of function and the appearance of a ''cold'' nodule on scintiscanning, since the remainder of the thyroid will have resumed function. When this happens, the nodule is likely to be mistaken for a carcinoma. Indeed, hypofunctioning, hemorrhagic adenomas and thyroid cysts account for the majority of cold nodules initially suspected of being carcinomas.

MALIGNANT TUMORS OF THE THYROID Due to its rich vascular supply, the thyroid is a common site of secondary or metastatic cancers from primary tumors elsewhere. Some common sources include malignant melanoma and carcinoma of the lung, breast, and esophagus. The thyroid also may be the site of lymphoproliferative disease, namely thyroid lymphoma, which constitutes about 5 percent of all thyroid malignancies. Of the latter, large cell histocytic (or immunoblastic) lymphoma is the most common and typically occurs in women between the ages of 55 and 75 who often have chronic lymphocytic thyroiditis with positive serum antithyroglobulin or anti-TPO antibodies. Indeed, the risk of this tumor is so much higher in elderly patients with Hashimoto's thyroiditis that an enlarging thyroid mass should be considered as thyroid lymphoma until an expedient evaluation rules out the diagnosis. Prognosis depends on cell type and the extent of disease beyond the neck. Variable success rates have followed therapy with combinations of surgery, radiation, and chemotherapy.

Primary thyroid carcinomas may be classified into two varieties depending on whether the lesion arises in thyroid follicular epithelium or from the parafollicular or C cells. The latter disorder, medullary thyroid carcinoma (MTC), may occur in four presentations: 80 percent are sporadic and 20 percent are familial, occurring as part of multiple endocrine neoplasia (MEN) types 2A or 2B or in a familial non-MEN setting. In familial forms, the diagnosis of early disease may be made in family members by screening measurements of serum calcitonin. The MEN syndromes are discussed separately below (see Chap. 343). The peak incidence of the sporadic form is in the sixth and seventh decades of life, and patients usually have cervical lymph node metastases at presentation. The tendency of the tumor and involved lymph nodes to calcify may be a clue to the diagnosis when calcification is noted on x-rays of the neck. Serum calcitonin serves as a tumor marker for residual disease after treatment, and the serum levels correlate with tumor burden. The mainstay of therapy is surgical excision; external radiation and chemotherapy have a palliative role for recurrent or residual disease.

Carcinomas of follicular epithelium Of the three general histologic types, papillary and follicular carcinomas tend to be slow growing and account for 70 and 15 percent, respectively, of all thyroid cancers, while anaplastic carcinoma is the least common, comprising approximately 5 percent of thyroid cancers. Anaplastic carcinoma usually occurs in the sixth to seventh decade of life. The tumor is histologically undifferentiated, largely composed of spindle and giant cells, rapidly growing, and highly malignant. Despite radical surgery, the prognosis is dismal, with survival in months rather than years but best in younger patients with early disease. The lesion is rapidly fatal owing to extensive local invasion which is refractory to external radiation and to radioiodine therapy because the tumor does not concentrate iodine. That many patients may have coexistent differentiated carcinoma suggests that anaplastic tumors arise from the former, and metastases of papillary or follicular carcinoma can undergo late malignant dedifferentiation. Anaplastic thyroid carcinoma may be confused with lymphoma and sarcoma, and positive immunocytochemical stains for keratin or the cytoskeletal protein vimentin help to confirm the diagnosis. While thyroglobulin staining may be positive due to entrapped follicular cells or colloid, measurements of serum thyroglobulin are of no diagnostic value as a tumor marker for this tumor in contrast to the situation in well-differentiated thyroid cancer. The lack of calcitonin immunoreactivity will differentiate anaplastic carcinoma from undifferentiated medullary thyroid carcinoma.

Follicular carcinoma tends to occur in older individuals, histologically resembles normal thyroid epithelium, is encapsulated, and differs from benign follicular adenoma only by the presence of capsular and/or vascular invasion. These tumors may be classified as minimally, moderately, or highly invasive, and prognosis varies accordingly. One subtype of follicular carcinoma, the Hürthle cell tumor, tends to be more invasive and have a less favorable clinical course. Follicular carcinoma undergoes early hematogenous spread, and the patient may present with a distant metastasis, usually in lung, bone, or the central nervous system. Lesions in bone are osteolytic. Like papillary carcinoma, large primary lesions are associated with worse prognosis, but even small lesions may metastasize widely. Rarely, the functioning mass of metastatic follicular carcinoma may be so great as to cause increased serum levels of thyroxine and/or triiodothyronine and clinical thyrotoxicosis. Follicular carcinoma or follicular elements in papillary carcinoma are responsible for those instances in which thyroid carcinoma, in situ or in metastases, accumulates significant quantities of ^{131}I. The third and most common type of tumor, papillary carcinoma, has a bimodal frequency, i.e., peaks occurring in the second or third decade and again in later life. This lesion is slowly growing, usually nonencapsulated, and typically may spread through the thyroid capsule to structures in the surrounding neck, especially the regional lymph nodes, where it may remain indolent for many years. Prognosis is a function of the size of the original lesion, with tumors of less than 2 cm having an excellent potential outcome. The presence of involved lymph nodes may be associated with greater risk for recurrence but not apparently with increased mortality. Acceleration of the disease may take place at any time. Follicular elements are usually present in both the primary lesion and its metastases. Papillary carcinoma is the most common thyroid malignancy after radiation exposure to the head and neck in childhood. Tumors in this setting are usually multicentric, thereby meriting more extensive thyroidectomy, but they are associated with a good prognosis.

DIAGNOSIS AND MANAGEMENT The diagnosis and management of thyroid carcinoma are interwoven with the management of the nodular goiter. In the past, this subject has evoked a wide disparity of views among authorities, stemming from seemingly contradictory data. On the one hand, surgically excised specimens of thyroid nodules, particularly solitary nodules, revealed a high frequency of carcinoma (as much as 20 percent in some series). On the other hand, despite the frequency of nodular goiter in the general population (approximately 4 percent), the frequency of thyroid carcinoma, either newly diagnosed or as a cause of death, is low. These respective data led either to vigorous or to conservative approaches to the management of nodular goiter. The discordance can be explained by the ability of the physician to select for surgery those patients who are at high risk of harboring thyroid carcinoma, with consequent weighting of statistics from surgical series. With the advent of fine-needle aspiration biopsy this capability has increased, bringing us closer to the as yet unrealized aim of operating only on those patients whose thyroids harbor carcinoma and avoiding surgery in patients whose thyroids do not.

Several features suggest the presence of carcinoma. Recent growth of a thyroid nodule or mass, especially if rapid and unaccompanied by tenderness and hoarseness, is a source of suspicion. Of particular importance is a history of x-ray to the head or neck or upper mediastinum in infancy or childhood, since this is associated with a high incidence of thyroid disease, including carcinoma, later in life. Nodular disease develops in approximately 20 percent of patients so exposed and may not be apparent until 30 years or more after the radiation exposure. Among patients in this group who have palpable nodules, approximately a third have thyroid carcinoma at surgery, often multicentric and sometimes metastatic. Risk for neoplasia correlates directly with younger age at exposure, female sex, and larger radiation dose. Patients who do not undergo surgery should be followed indefinitely and may be candidates for levothyroxine therapy.

Skillful palpation of the thyroid provides important information. A nodule in an otherwise normal gland (solitary nodule) creates more suspicion of thyroid tumor than does one nodule among many, since the latter is more likely to be part of a diffuse process, such as simple goiter. In addition, carcinomas are usually firm or hard in consistency and nontender. Fixation to surrounding structures and lymphadenopathy are late features, although patients may present with a midline mass above the thyroid isthmus (Delphian node) or lateral cervical adenopathy. Since purely cystic lesions, especially those which are less than a few centimeters in diameter, are less likely to reflect malignancy than solid lesions, transillumination is sometimes helpful, and ultrasonograms (see below) are particularly so. Age and sex of the patient also influence the clinical decision. Benign nodular lesions are more common in women than in men, malignant nodular lesions less so. Hence nodular lesions in men create more suspicion of carcinoma than in women.

Laboratory tests are of little assistance in differentiating between malignant and nonmalignant thyroid nodules. Overall thyroid function is usually normal. Except in patients with medullary thyroid carcinoma, in whom serum calcitonin concentrations may be elevated, tumor markers are of little value. Elevations of serum thyroglobulin are present in many patients with differentiated thyroid carcinoma but are not useful in the initial diagnosis, since they may be elevated in patients with benign adenoma, simple goiter, or Graves' disease. Soft-tissue x-rays of the neck may be of assistance, since finely stippled calcification within the thyroid suggests the presence of psammoma bodies within a papillary carcinoma and more dense calcifications may signify medullary carcinoma.

Fine-needle aspiration for cytology is the initial procedure of choice in the evaluation of most patients (Fig. 334-4). The technique is simple to learn, free of complications, and applicable to most nodules. Optimal application of that technique rests on obtaining a satisfactory specimen and the availability of experienced histopathologic interpretation of the specimen obtained. When such is available, aspiration biopsy provides a reliable means of differentiating between benign and malignant nodules in all except highly cellular lesions or follicular lesions, where evidence of vascular invasion may be required to differentiate benign from malignant forms. Needle aspirates of papillary carcinoma may reveal psammoma bodies, lymphocytes suggestive of Hashimoto's disease, and large pink follicular cells with large pale nuclei ("Orphan Annie cells") and numerous nucleoli. Despite the occasional occurrence of false-positive and -negative results, the procedure can reduce the number of operations performed for nodules that prove to be benign. Further, a diagnosis of carcinoma permits planning of the surgery to be undertaken preoperatively.

While fine-needle aspiration for cytology is the keystone in the approach to the management of the patient with nodular goiter, less specific measures such as ultrasonography or scintillation scanning also may be useful. Although only approximately 20 percent of nonfunctioning thyroid nodules prove to be malignant, demonstration that a nodule is "cold" on scintiscan adds substantial weight to the other factors suggesting carcinoma. Nodules that are hyperfunctioning are rarely malignant. Ultrasonograms of the thyroid have value in demonstrating whether nodules are cystic, solid, or a mixture of the two. Cystic nodules can be aspirated, a procedure that is often curative, and their contents should be subjected to cytopathologic examination. Solid or mixed lesions are consistent with tumor but may be either benign or malignant.

When the cytologic results are equivocal, the physician must decide whether to continue to observe the patient; to administer suppressive doses of thyroid hormone in the expectation that the suspect nodule will shrink or disappear—a hope that in the author's experience is usually unrealized; or to proceed to excisional biopsy and thyroidectomy. Patients in whom the author chooses the latter course include those with a history of radiation to the thyroid and one or more clearly palpable nodules, as well as young men and women with solitary cold nodules, particularly if hard, nontender, and changing rapidly in size. In the remainder, thyroid hormone

FIGURE 334-4 Diagnostic approach to the solitary nodule.

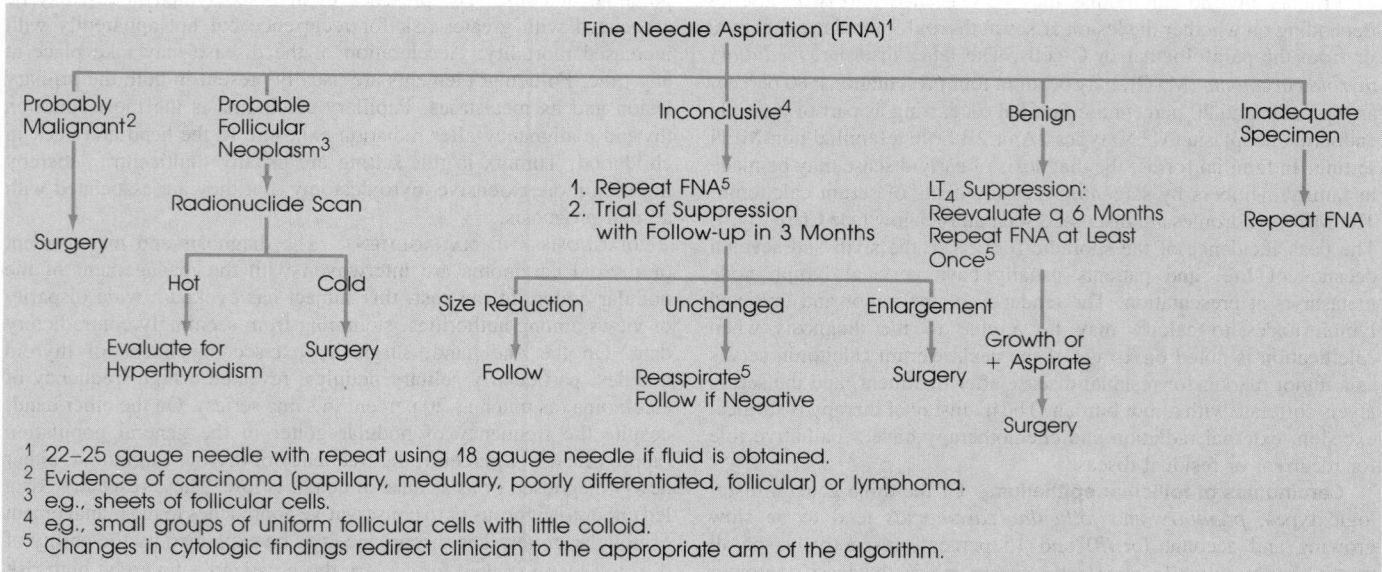

1 22–25 gauge needle with repeat using 18 gauge needle if fluid is obtained.
2 Evidence of carcinoma (papillary, medullary, poorly differentiated, follicular) or lymphoma.
3 e.g., sheets of follicular cells.
4 e.g., small groups of uniform follicular cells with little colloid.
5 Changes in cytologic findings redirect clinician to the appropriate arm of the algorithm.

therapy with repeat aspiration cytology in 3 to 6 months is recommended.

Regardless of the operative procedure planned, surgery for thyroid carcinoma should be performed by a surgeon experienced in the procedure. Should surgery be delayed, suppressive therapy with levothyroxine is often recommended preoperatively to facilitate the operative procedure and perhaps decrease the likelihood of tumor dissemination. In patients in whom a definitive preoperative diagnosis has not been made, the suspected lesion is removed en bloc with a wide margin of surrounding tissue and is examined by frozen section. Opinions vary as to the preferable procedure when carcinoma is found. For lesions of 2 cm or less that are not multicentric and that have not metastasized, some recommend ipsilateral lobectomy, isthmectomy, and possibly contralateral partial lobectomy. Despite its higher rate of morbidity, the author prefers a near-total thyroidectomy, especially for lesions >2 cm, in view of the frequency of seeding of tumor throughout the gland by transglandular lymphatic spread and of evidence that both recurrence rates and subsequent mortality are lower after the more extensive operation. Regional lymph nodes should be explored and removed if there is evidence of involvement, but radical neck dissection is not justified. If permanent sections reveal carcinoma when frozen sections had failed to do so and the initial procedure was limited, secondary surgery should be undertaken to remove residual thyroid tissue, preferably within a few days. A more complete thyroidectomy is warranted for follicular carcinoma in view of its tendency to metastasize to distant sites. This is so because the metastases do not concentrate adequate ^{131}I in the presence of residual normal thyroid tissue, which acts to both compete for the ^{131}I and restrain the increment in serum TSH required to stimulate uptake.

The postoperative necessity for thyroid remnant ablation with radioiodine and subsequent periodic radioisotopic scanning for residual or recurrent disease varies with the histologic type of cancer, size of lesion, presence of metastases, and other indications of invasiveness or aggressiveness. Radioiodine treatment of known residual disease is associated with clinical improvement and reduced recurrence rates, but it is not clear whether mortality rates are benefited by prophylactic postoperative ablation. Papillary cancers of <1.5 cm and unaccompanied by nodal metastases tend to have an excellent prognosis, and it is questionable whether ablation of residual normal thyroid bed and subsequent scanning are necessary. The author favors a more conservative approach in such cases, only administering levothyroxine suppression with periodic follow-up determinations of serum thyroglobulin levels.

Total-body scintiscanning with ^{131}I is the method employed to evaluate for residual normal or malignant thyroid tissue in the neck or distant metastases. Postoperatively, if replacement therapy is initiated with liothyronine (50 to 75 μ/d) rather than levothyroxine, a more rapid increase in TSH secretion is seen when the liothyronine is withdrawn some 3 weeks later. After an additional 2 or 3 weeks without any thyroid hormone replacement, when the serum TSH concentration has risen to the range of 50 mU/L, a large scanning dose of ^{131}I [185 to 370 MBq (5 to 10 mCi)] is administered and whole-body scans are obtained at 72 h. If residual thyroid tissue is found, as is usually the case, a thyroid ablating dose of 1850 MBq (50 mCi) of ^{131}I is administered, and if functioning metastases are present, the dose is doubled. Suppressive therapy with levothyroxine is reinstituted 24 to 48 h later. Approximately 1 week after administration of the second dose of ^{131}I, whole-body scans are repeated, since the larger dose of radioiodine may permit demonstration of functioning metastases not seen after the smaller initial dose. When this proves to be the case, some clinics withdraw suppressive therapy, administer an additional 3700 MBq (100 mCi) of ^{131}I, and then reinstitute suppressive therapy with levothyroxine. Future availability of recombinant human TSH for parenteral injection promises to obviate the discontinuation of thyroid hormone therapy for scanning. In some patients, only measurements of serum thyroglobulin before and after

TSH injection might be performed, with follow-up scanning solely in those in whom a significant rise in thyroglobulin is seen.

Patients are reexamined approximately 6 months after the initial operation and at least every 6 months for several years thereafter. At these examinations, the neck is palpated for evidence of recurrence of metastases, which often can be treated with selective surgical removal. Blood is drawn for a serum thyroglobulin measurement, since elevated values in patients receiving suppressive therapy signal the presence of metastatic disease. At the initial 6-month examination, patients in whom metastases had previously been found are prepared for a whole-body scan as described above. Those in whom no metastases had been demonstrated by earlier scans are not rescanned unless the serum thyroglobulin is elevated but are rescanned approximately 1 year after the initial surgery. Patients in whom whole-body scans are positive are reentered into the therapeutic algorithm, as described above. Those in whom scans are negative continue to be reexamined and have measurements of serum thyroglobulin concentrations at regular intervals. If both serum thyroglobulin concentrations and scans are unrevealing, patients are scanned for the last time after approximately 3 years, unless serum thyroglobulin concentrations rise. In some patients, serum thyroglobulin may be elevated despite the absence of demonstrable functioning metastases. Such patients obviously cannot be treated with ^{131}I but should be studied with x-rays and bone scans to ascertain the site of the thyroglobulin-secreting metastases and to determine whether they may be amenable to external radiation.

A program of this nature, involving near-total thyroidectomy, long-term suppressive therapy, and treatment of functioning metastases with radioiodine reduces the recurrence rate and prolongs survival in patients with papillary carcinoma of the thyroid. Follicular carcinoma should be treated with even greater vigor, since the results are generally less favorable. Because follicular carcinoma metastasizes to lung and bone, appropriate follow-up x-rays and measurements of serum thyroglobulin should be obtained. Mixed differentiated tumors with both follicular and papillary elements tend to behave biologically as papillary tumors and should be so managed. Radioiodine treatment of medullary thyroid carcinoma is usually not successful, those cases showing some reduction in serum calcitonin possibly representing a rare variant of mixed medullary and follicular cancer. Treatment of anaplastic carcinoma is largely palliative; most patients die within 6 months of diagnosis.

THYROIDITIS

Thyroiditis embraces disorders of differing etiology. *Pyogenic thyroiditis* and *chronic fibrosing (Riedel's) thyroiditis* are rare. Pyogenic thyroiditis is usually anteceded by a pyogenic infection elsewhere and is characterized by tenderness and swelling of the thyroid, redness and warmth of the overlying skin, and constitutional signs of infection. Treatment consists of antibiotic therapy and incisional drainage if a fluctuant area within the thyroid should occur. Patients with AIDS may present with thyroiditis due to unusual organisms such as *Pneumocystis carinii*. Riedel's thyroiditis is a disorder in which intense fibrosis of the thyroid and surrounding structures, leading to induration of the tissues of the neck, may be associated with mediastinal and retroperitoneal fibrosis. The principal importance of this disorder is that it requires differentiation from thyroid neoplasia. The other forms of thyroiditis, comprising subacute thyroiditis, chronic thyroiditis with transient thyrotoxicosis, and Hashimoto's thyroiditis, are more common. They are notable for their different clinical courses and for the fact that each can be associated, at one time or another, with a euthyroid, thyrotoxic, or hypothyroid state.

SUBACUTE THYROIDITIS This disorder, also termed *granulomatous, giant cell*, or *de Quervain's thyroiditis*, is viral in origin. Symptoms of thyroiditis usually follow those of an upper respiratory infection and include pronounced asthenia, malaise, and symptoms referable to stretching of the thyroid capsule, principally pain over the thyroid or pain referred to the lower jaw, ear, or occiput. Referred pain may predominate. These symptoms may smolder for weeks before the diagnosis is suspected. Less commonly, the onset is acute, with severe pain over the thyroid, fever, and occasionally symptoms of thyrotoxicosis. Physical findings include exquisite tenderness and nodularity of the thyroid, which may be unilateral but usually involves other areas of the gland. Although local or referred pain is usual, occasional patients have other features typical of the disease but no pain.

Two laboratory findings are characteristic: a high erythrocyte sedimentation rate (ESR) and a depressed RAIU. Values for the remaining tests depend on the stage of the disease in which they are obtained. Early, many patients are mildly thyrotoxic owing to leakage of hormone from the gland. The serum T_4 and T_3 are high, and TSH is undetectable. Later, as glandular hormone is depleted, the patient may pass through a hypothyroid phase, in which serum T_4 and T_3 are low and TSH is increased. Diagnosis of the thyrotoxic phase is especially troublesome in the painless variant because the patient may be thought to have Graves' disease or toxic nodular goiter and therapy inappropriate for subacute thyroiditis may be instituted. Demonstration of a low RAIU usually serves to differentiate subacute thyroiditis from these other causes of hyperthyroidism. Differentiation of painless subacute thyroiditis from chronic thyroiditis with transient thyrotoxicosis is discussed below.

The disorder may smolder for months but eventually subsides with a return of normal thyroid function. In mild cases, aspirin suffices to control the symptoms. In more severe cases, glucocorticoids (prednisone, 20 to 40 mg/d) are generally effective. Propranolol can be used to control associated thyrotoxicosis. When the RAIU and serum T_4 return to normal, therapy can be withdrawn without recurrence of symptoms.

CHRONIC THYROIDITIS WITH TRANSIENT THYROTOXICOSIS
This term denotes a disorder in which a self-limited episode of thyrotoxicosis is associated with a histologic picture of chronic lymphocytic thyroiditis that differs from that of Hashimoto's disease. This syndrome has been variously designated as painless thyroiditis, silent thyroiditis, hyperthyroiditis, chronic thyroiditis with spontaneously resolving hyperthyroidism, or, as the author prefers, chronic thyroiditis with transient thyrotoxicosis (CT/TT). Designations that imply the existence of hyperthyroidism are inappropriate, since ongoing production of thyroid hormone is negligible and the RAIU is decreased.

The syndrome occurs in patients of any age, although it occurs mainly in women. Manifestations of thyrotoxicosis are usually mild but may be severe. The thyroid is nontender, firm, symmetric, and enlarged slightly or moderately. Laboratory features include elevations of the serum T_4 and T_3 concentrations consonant with the thyrotoxicosis and a markedly depressed RAIU. The ESR is normal or slightly elevated, rarely exceeding 50 mm/h, and antithyroid antibodies, when present, are in low titer.

The etiology, pathogenesis, and pathophysiology of this disorder are unclear. Viral antibody titers show no characteristic patterns. It is presumed that thyrotoxicosis results from leakage of hormone from the gland, as in subacute thyroiditis. Low values for the RAIU, in turn, reflect hormonal suppression of TSH secretion and not increased plasma iodine, since urinary iodine excretion is not greatly elevated. Some degree of thyroid malfunction is indicated by failure of the RAIU to respond briskly to exogenous TSH stimulation.

Thyrotoxicosis in CT/TT usually abates within 2 to 5 months. Many patients have recurrent episodes of thyrotoxicosis of similar nature, sometimes following pregnancy (postpartum thyroiditis). The thyrotoxic phase may be followed in several months by a phase of self-limited hypothyroidism. The latter, particularly in the postpartum period, may be the only component of the disease that is diagnosed because the thyrotoxic phase may be very brief. While there appears to be wide geographic variation in incidence, on average, 4 to 8 percent of pregnant women may experience the syndrome post partum.

This disorder, in the thyrotoxic phase, can be differentiated from Graves' disease by demonstration of a depressed RAIU and absence of increased urinary iodine excretion. The latter serves also to exclude the jodbasedow syndrome. When these data are available, the disorder must be differentiated from other causes of thyrotoxicosis with a low RAIU, principally subacute thyroiditis. Lack of tenderness or nodularity of the thyroid and absence of marked elevation of the ESR tend to exclude the latter diagnosis. Patients with either functioning ectopic thyroid tissue or thyrotoxicosis factitia characteristically respond to exogenous TSH stimulation with a brisk increase in RAIU. Definitive diagnosis of CT/TT can be made by thyroid biopsy.

Since the thyroid is not hyperfunctioning in this disorder, measures used in the treatment of hyperthyroidism are useless. Propranolol and mild sedatives are administered until the thyrotoxicosis abates.

HASHIMOTO'S THYROIDITIS   This disorder, also termed *lymphadenoid goiter*, is a common chronic inflammatory disease of the thyroid in which autoimmune factors play a prominent role. It occurs most frequently in women of middle age and is the most common cause of sporadic goiter in children. Evidence of the participation of autoimmune factors includes the lymphocytic infiltration of the gland and the presence in the serum of increased concentrations of immunoglobulins and antibodies against several components of thyroid tissue. Of these, the most important from the clinical standpoint are the antithyroglobulin antibody detected by the tanned red cell agglutination and antithyroid peroxidase (anti-TPO or antimicrosomal) antibody detected by immunofluorescence, complement fixation, or the more sensitive immunosorbent (ELISA) technique. These autoantibodies probably reflect but do not cause the thyroid destruction noted in autoimmune thyroid disease. Hashimoto's thyroiditis also coexists with some frequency with other diseases of an autoimmune nature, including pernicious anemia, Sjögren's syndrome, chronic active hepatitis, systemic lupus erythematosus, rheumatoid arthritis, adrenal insufficiency, diabetes mellitus, and Graves' disease itself (see Chap. 343). These disorders, as well as Hashimoto's disease itself, also occur frequently in family members of patients with Hashimoto's disease. An association of HLA-DR3 and -DR5 with the atrophic and goitrous forms of Hashimoto's disease, respectively, has been noted.

Goiter is the outstanding feature. The enlargement involves the entire gland but not necessarily symmetrically. Typically, the consistency is rubbery, the margins are scalloped, and the general outline of the gland is preserved. The pyramidal lobe may be prominent. Early in the disease the patient is metabolically normal; however, even then decreased thyroid reserve is often manifest in an increase in serum TSH. The RAIU may be elevated early, reflecting the secretion of physiologically inactive iodoproteins, but the serum T_4 and T_3 are normal, and the patient is euthyroid. As the disease progresses, thyroid failure, at first subclinical, may supervene owing to progressive replacement of thyroid parenchyma by lymphocytes or fibrous tissue. The thyroid failure is evident first in a rise in serum TSH concentration. With time, the serum T_4 concentration declines, though the serum T_3 remains normal. Eventually, the serum T_3 concentration falls below normal, and frank hypothyroidism supervenes. Autoimmune thyroiditis including Hashimoto's disease may account for as many as 90 percent of cases of hypothyroidism. High titers of anti-TPO antibody are almost always present. High titers also may occur in other thyroid disorders, particularly primary thyroprivic hypothyroidism and Graves' disease, but with lesser frequency. Although the foregoing findings usually suffice to permit a diagnosis, histologic confirmation may be obtained by needle biopsy. In view of the frequency with which hypothyroidism is either present or eventually develops, treatment with replacement doses of levothyroxine is indicated. In some patients, such therapy is associated with regression of goiter. Pregnant women with high antibody titers may be at higher risk for miscarriage independent of the thyroid status.

Occasional patients present with hyperthyroidism in association with a thyroid gland that is unusually firm and with high titers of circulating antithyroid antibodies, a combination which suggests, probably correctly, the concurrence of Graves' disease and Hashimoto's thyroiditis (''Hashitoxicosis''). In others, hyperthyroidism may supervene in a patient known to have Hashimoto's thyroiditis, presumably due to the emergence of clones of lymphocytes that produce stimulatory anti-TSH receptor antibodies. Hyperthyroidism in association with Hashimoto's thyroiditis is treated in a conventional manner, but ablative therapy is less commonly employed, since the associated chronic thyroiditis tends to limit the duration of thyroid hyperfunction and also predisposes the patient to the development of hypothyroidism after surgical or radioiodine treatment.

REFERENCES

BLACK EG et al: Serial serum thyroglobulin measurements in the management of differentiated thyroid carcinoma. Clin Endocrinol 27:115, 1987

BURCH HB, WARTOFSKY L: Life-threatening thyrotoxicosis: Thyroid storm. Endocrinol Metab Clin North Am (in press)

————: Management of Graves' ophthalmopathy. Endocrinol Rev (in press)

CLARK OH, DUH Q-Y: Thyroid cancer. Med Clin North Am 75:211, 1991

DEGROOT LJ: Diagnostic approach and management of patients exposed to irradiation to the thyroid. J Clin Endocrinol Metab 69:925, 1989

FRADKIN JE, WOLFF J: Iodine-induced thyrotoxicosis. Medicine 62:1, 1983

HAMBURGER JI: The autonomously functioning thyroid nodule: Goetsch's disease. Endocrinol Rev 8:439, 1987

HASHIZUME K et al: Administration of thyroxine in treated Graves' disease: Effects on the level of antibodies to thyroid-stimulating hormone receptors and on the risk of recurrence of hyperthyroidism. N Engl J Med 324:947, 1991

HAY ID et al: American Thyroid Association assessment of current free thyroid hormone and thyrotropin measurements and guidelines for future clinical assays. Clin Chem 37:2002, 1991

HENNESSEY JV et al: L-Thyroxine dosage: A re-evaluation of therapy with contemporary preparations. Ann Intern Med 105:11, 1986

HEUFELDER AE, GORMAN CA: Radioiodine therapy in the treatment of differentiated thyroid cancer: Guidelines and considerations. Endocrinologist 1:273, 1991

MAHONEY KM, WARTOFSKY L: Significance of alterations in thyroid function tests in the critical care setting. J Intensive Care Med (in press)

MAXON HR, SMITH HS: Radioiodine-131 in the diagnosis and treatment of metastatic well differentiated thyroid cancer. Endocrinol Metab Clin North Am 19:685, 1990

MAZZAFERRI EL: Papillary thyroid carcinoma: Factors influencing prognosis and current therapy. Semin Oncol 14:315, 1987

MCDOUGAL IR: Graves' disease: Current concepts. Med Clin North Am 75:79, 1991

MOSEKILDE L et al: Effects of thyroid hormones on bone and mineral metabolism. Endocrinol Metab Clin North Am 19:35, 1990

NICOLOFF JT, SPENCER CA: The use and misuse of the sensitive thyrotropin assays. J Clin Endocrinol Metab 71:553, 1990

O'CONNOR G, DAVIES TF: Human autoimmune thyroid disease: A mechanistic update. Trends Endocrinol Metab 1:266, 1990

OPPENHEIMER JH et al: Advances in our understanding of thyroid hormone action at the cellular level. Endocrinol Rev 8:288, 1987

RIDGWAY EC: Clinician's evaluation of a solitary thyroid nodule. J Clin Endocrinol Metab 74:231, 1992

WARTOFSKY L: Use of sensitive TSH assay to determine thyroid hormone therapy and avoid osteoporosis. Annu Rev Med 42:341, 1991

335 DISEASES OF THE ADRENAL CORTEX

GORDON H. WILLIAMS / ROBERT G. DLUHY

BIOCHEMISTRY AND PHYSIOLOGY

STEROID NOMENCLATURE Steroids contain as their basic structure a cyclopentenoperhydrophenanthrane nucleus consisting of three 6-carbon hexane rings and a single 5-carbon pentane ring (Fig. 335-1). The carbon atoms are numbered in a sequence beginning with ring A. Adrenal steroids contain either 19 or 21 carbon atoms. The C_{19} steroids have methyl groups at C-18 and C-19. C_{19} steroids with a ketone group at C-17 are termed *17-ketosteroids*. The C_{19} steroids have predominant androgenic activity. The C_{21} steroids have a 2-carbon side chain (C-20 and C-21) attached at position 17 and methyl groups at C-18 and C-19. C_{21} steroids with a hydroxyl group at

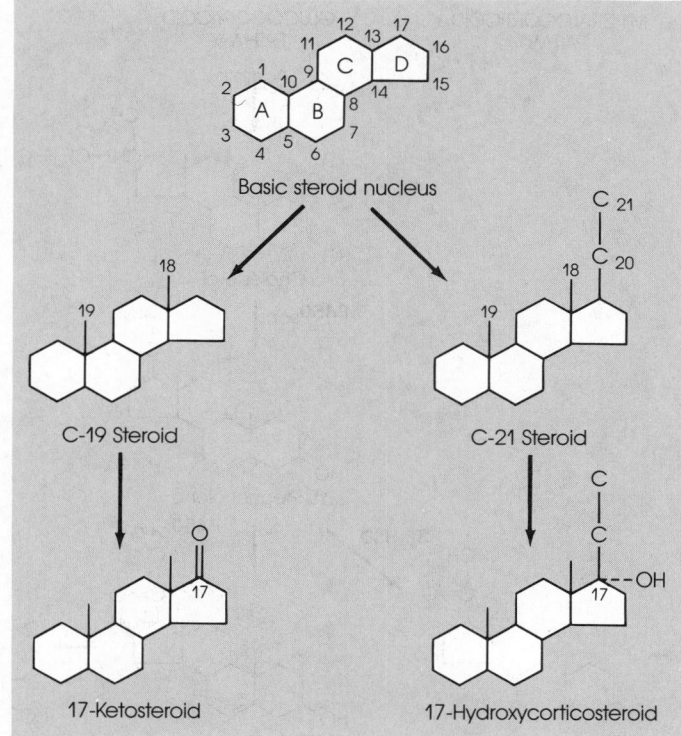

FIGURE 335-1 Basic steroid structure and nomenclature.

position 17 are termed *17-hydroxycorticosteroids*. The C_{21} steroids have either glucocorticoid or mineralocorticoid properties. *Glucocorticoid* signifies a C_{21} steroid with predominant action on intermediary metabolism; *mineralocorticoid* indicates a C_{21} steroid with predominant action on the metabolism of sodium and potassium.

BIOSYNTHESIS OF ADRENAL STEROIDS Cholesterol, derived from the diet and from endogenous synthesis, is the starting compound in steroidogenesis. Uptake of cholesterol by the adrenal cortex is mediated by the low-density lipoprotein (LDL) receptor. With long-term stimulation of the adrenal cortex by ACTH, the number of LDL receptors increases. The three major adrenal biosynthetic pathways lead to the production of glucocorticoids (cortisol), mineralocorticoids (aldosterone), and adrenal androgens (dehydroepiandrosterone). Separate zones of the adrenal cortex synthesize specific hormones; this reflects the enzymatic capacity of each zone to carry out certain transformations and hydroxylations (Fig. 335-2). The outer (glomerulosa) zone is mainly involved in aldosterone biosynthesis, and the inner (fasciculata-reticularis) zone is the site of cortisol and androgen biosynthesis.

STEROID TRANSPORT Some steroid hormones, e.g., testosterone and cortisol, circulate to a considerable extent bound to plasma proteins. Cortisol occurs in the plasma in three forms: free cortisol, protein-bound cortisol, and cortisol metabolites. *Free cortisol* refers to physiologically active hormone that is not protein-bound and, therefore, a form of cortisol acting directly on tissue sites. Normally, less than 5 percent of circulating cortisol is free. Only the unbound cortisol and its metabolites are filterable at the glomerulus. Increased quantities of free steroid are excreted in the urine in states characterized by hypersecretion of cortisol, as the unbound fraction of plasma cortisol rises. *Protein-bound cortisol* is reversibly bound to circulating plasma proteins. There are two cortisol-binding systems of plasma. One is a high-affinity, low-capacity alpha$_2$ globulin termed *transcortin* or *cortisol-binding globulin* (CBG), and the other is a low-affinity, high-capacity protein, *albumin*. The binding affinity of CBG for cortisol is reduced in areas of inflammation, thus increasing the local concentration of free cortisol. CBG in normal humans can bind approximately 700 nmol of cortisol per liter of plasma (25 μg/dL).

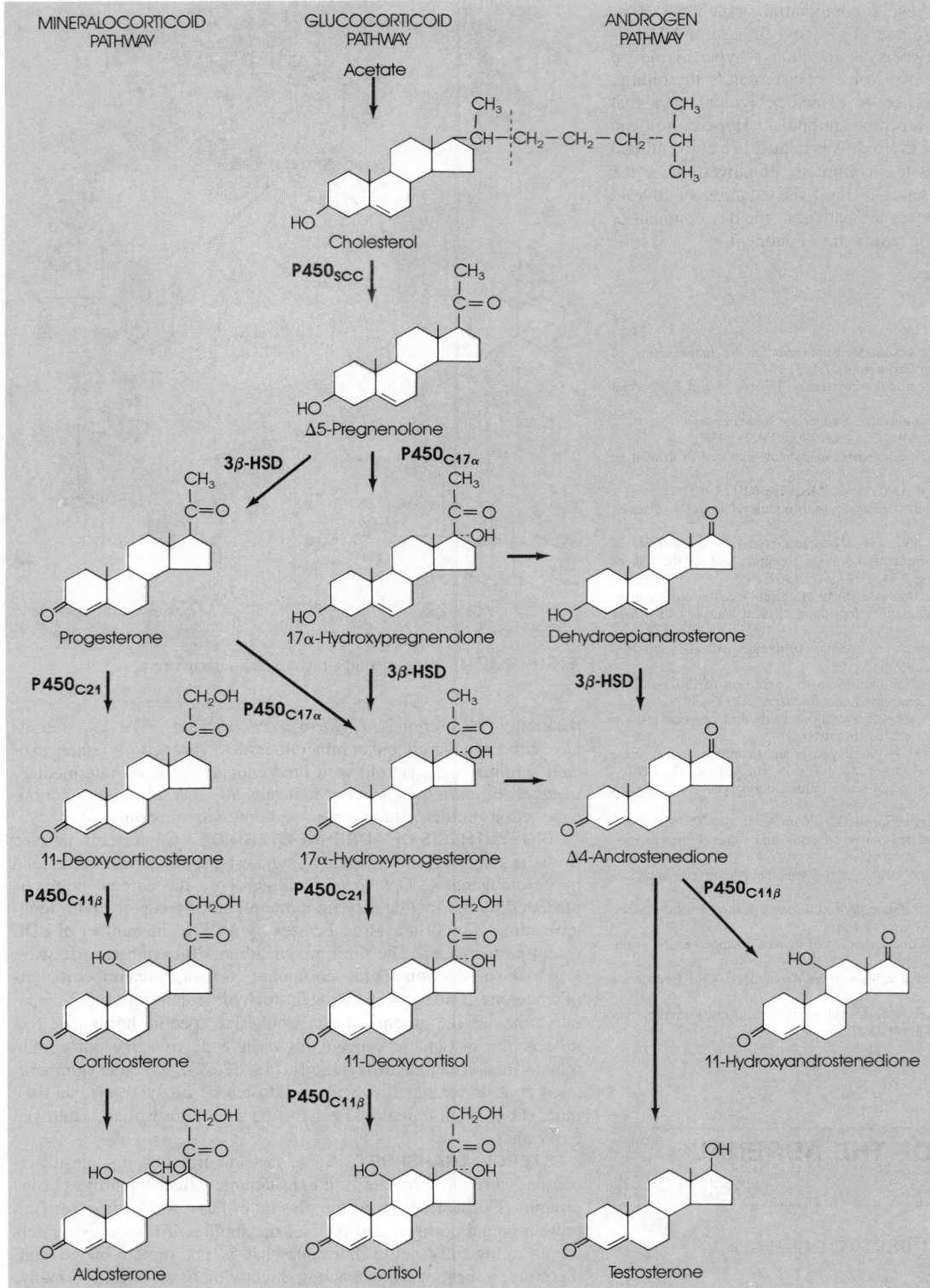

FIGURE 335-2 Biosynthetic pathways for adrenal steroid production; major pathways to mineralocorticoids, glucocorticoids, and androgens. Circled letters and numbers denote specific enzymes: $P450_{SCC}$ = cholesterol side chain cleavage enzyme; 3β-HSD = 3β-hydroxysteroid dehydrogenase; $P450_{C11β}$ = C-11 hydroxylase; $P450_{C17α}$ = C-17 hydroxylase; $P450_{C21}$ = C-21 hydroxylase.

When the concentration of cortisol exceeds this level, the excess becomes bound in part to albumin, and a greater proportion circulates unbound. For example, when the total cortisol level is 1400 nmol/L (50 μg/dL) 25 percent will be free. The CBG level is increased in high-estrogen states (e.g., pregnancy, oral contraceptive administration). The rise in CBG is accompanied by a parallel rise in protein-bound cortisol, with the result that the plasma cortisol concentration is elevated. However, the free cortisol levels probably remain normal, and manifestations of glucocorticoid excess are absent. Most synthetic glucocorticoid analogues bind less efficiently to CBG (approximately 70 percent binding). This may explain the propensity of some synthetic analogues to produce cushingoid effects at low dosage. *Cortisol metabolites* are biologically inactive and bind only weakly to circulating plasma proteins.

Aldosterone is bound to proteins to a smaller extent than either testosterone or cortisol, and an ultrafiltrate of plasma contains as much as 50 percent of the circulating aldosterone. The limited binding by plasma protein influences aldosterone metabolism.

STEROID METABOLISM AND EXCRETION Glucocorticoids

The daily secretion of cortisol ranges between 40 and 80 μmol (15 and 30 mg), with a pronounced diurnal cycle. Cortisol is distributed in a volume of body fluids approximating the total extracellular fluid space, with more than 90 percent in the protein-bound fraction. The plasma concentration of cortisol is determined by the rate of secretion, the rate of inactivation, and the rate of excretion of free cortisol. The liver is the major organ responsible for steroid inactivation. The major pathway is reduction of ring A and conjugation of the reduced products with glucuronic acid at position C-3 to form water-soluble compounds. The 11β-hydroxysteroid dehydrogenase converts cortisol to the inactive cortisone in the liver and kidney. The activity of this enzyme is influenced by the level of circulating thyroid hormone, the oxidative reaction being increased in hyperthyroidism.

Mineralocorticoids In normal subjects on a normal salt intake, the average daily secretion of aldosterone ranges between 0.1 and 0.7 μmol (50 and 250 μg). Since aldosterone is only weakly bound to proteins, its volume of distribution is larger than that of cortisol and approximates 35 L. During a single passage through the liver, more than 75 percent of circulating aldosterone is normally inactivated by ring A reduction and conjugation with glucuronic acid. However, under certain conditions, such as congestive failure, this inactivation is reduced.

From 7 to 15 percent of aldosterone is excreted in the urine as a glucuronide conjugate, from which free aldosterone is released on standing at pH 1. This *acid-labile conjugate* is formed in the liver and kidney. For average salt intake, the 24-h urine excretion of the acid-labile conjugate ranges from 15 to 50 nmol (5 to 19 μg), that of the reduced derivative from 70 to 100 nmol (25 to 35 μg), and that of the nonconjugated, nonreduced free aldosterone from 0.5 to 2 nmol (0.2 to 0.6 μg).

Adrenal androgens The major androgen secreted by the adrenal is dehydroepiandrosterone (DHEA) and its C-3 sulfuric acid ester. From 15 to 30 mg of these compounds is secreted daily. Smaller amounts of androstenedione, 11β-hydroxyandrostenedione, and testosterone are secreted. DHEA is the major precursor of the urinary 17-ketosteroids. Two-thirds of the urine 17-ketosteroids in the male are derived from adrenal metabolites, and the remaining one-third comes from testicular androgens. In the female, almost all urine 17-ketosteroids are derived from the adrenal.

Steroids passively diffuse through the cell membrane and bind to intracellular receptors (see Chap. 329). These receptors are part of a superfamily of transcription regulatory factors that include the thyroid hormone receptor. Glucocorticoid receptors are of two types: I and II. The type I receptor is the same as the mineralocorticoid receptor. Mineralocorticoids do not bind to the type II receptor, but most glucocorticoids bind to either receptor, although with different affinities. After the steroid binds to the receptor, the steroid-receptor complex is transported to the nucleus, where it binds to specific sites on steroid-regulated genes, modifying mRNA levels and then protein synthesis. Because cortisol binds to the mineralocorticoid (type I glucocorticoid) receptor with equal affinity to aldosterone, mineralocorticoid specificity is achieved by local metabolism of cortisol to the

inactive cortisone, which binds only minimally to the type I receptor. The glucocorticoid effects of other steroids, such as high-dose progesterone, correlate with their relative binding affinities for the type II glucocorticoid receptor. Inherited defects in the glucocorticoid receptor cause glucocorticoid resistance states. These individuals have high levels of cortisol but do not have manifestations of hypercortisolism.

ACTH PHYSIOLOGY ACTH (corticotropin) (see Chap. 331) is an unbranched polypeptide containing 39 amino acids. ACTH and a number of other peptides (lipotropins, endorphins, and melanocyte-stimulating hormones) are processed from a larger precursor molecule of 31,000 mol wt—pro-opiomelanocortin (POMC) (see Chap. 331 and Fig. 335-3). POMC is made in a variety of tissues, including brain, anterior and posterior pituitary, and lymphocytes. The actual peptide secreted varies depending on the tissue. In the anterior pituitary, ACTH is synthesized and stored in basophilic cells. The basophilic staining of the corticotrophs is the result of the glycosylation of ACTH and related peptides. Much of the potential for the corticotropic actions of ACTH is present in smaller polypeptide fragments; the N-terminal 18-amino-acid structure retains full biologic potency, and shorter N-terminal fragments exhibit partial biologic activity. Release of ACTH and related peptides from the anterior pituitary gland is governed by a "corticotropin-releasing center" in the median eminence of the hypothalamus, which upon stimulation releases a peptide with a chain of 41 amino acids (corticotropin-releasing hormone, CRH) that travels via the pituitary stalk portal bloodstream to the anterior pituitary, where it effects the release of ACTH (Fig. 335-4). Some related peptides such as β-lipotropin (β-LPH) are released in equimolar concentrations with ACTH, suggesting enzymatic cleavage from the parent POMC prior to or concomitant with the secretory process. However, β-endorphin levels may not correlate with circulating levels of ACTH depending on the nature of the stimulus. The functions and regulation of secretion of the related peptides derived from POMC are not understood.

The major factors controlling ACTH release include CRH, free cortisol concentration in plasma, stress, and the sleep-wake cycle (see Fig. 335-4). The plasma level of ACTH varies during the day as a result of its pulsatile secretion but roughly follows a diurnal pattern, with a peak just prior to waking and a nadir before retiring. After several days on a new sleep-wake cycle, the pattern is altered to conform to the new cycle. ACTH and cortisol levels also increase in response to eating. Stress (e.g., pyrogens, surgery, hypoglycemia, exercise, and severe emotional trauma) also can enhance ACTH release. Stress-related secretion of ACTH abolishes circadian periodicity but is, in turn, suppressed by prior high-dose glucocorticoid administration. The secretion of ACTH following stress and the normal pulsatile, diurnal ACTH release are regulated by CRH; this is the so-called open feedback loop. CRH secretion, in turn, is influenced by hypothalamic neurotransmitters. For example, serotoninergic and cholinergic systems stimulate the secretion of CRH and ACTH; there is contradictory evidence regarding the inhibitory effects of alpha-adrenergic agonists and gamma-aminobutyric acid (GABA) on CRH release. In addition, there may be direct pituitary effects

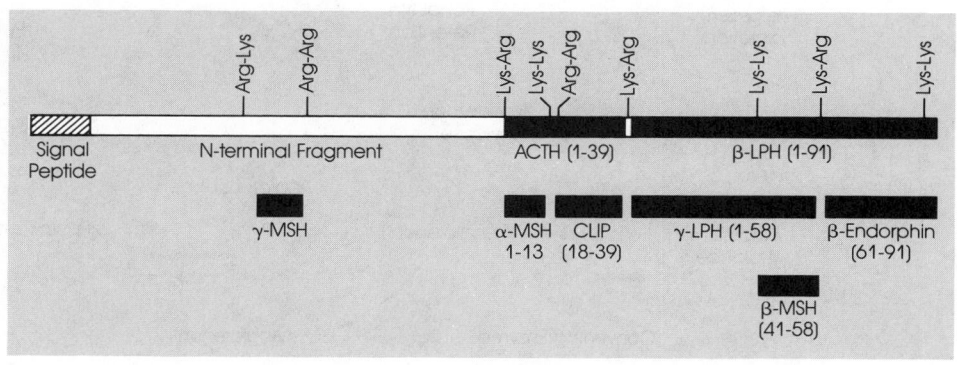

FIGURE 335-3 Schematic representation of the probable structure of the 31,000–mol wt pro-opiomelanocortin molecule. (*From DT Krieger, JB Martin, N Engl J Med 304:880, 1981. By permission of the New England Journal of Medicine.*)

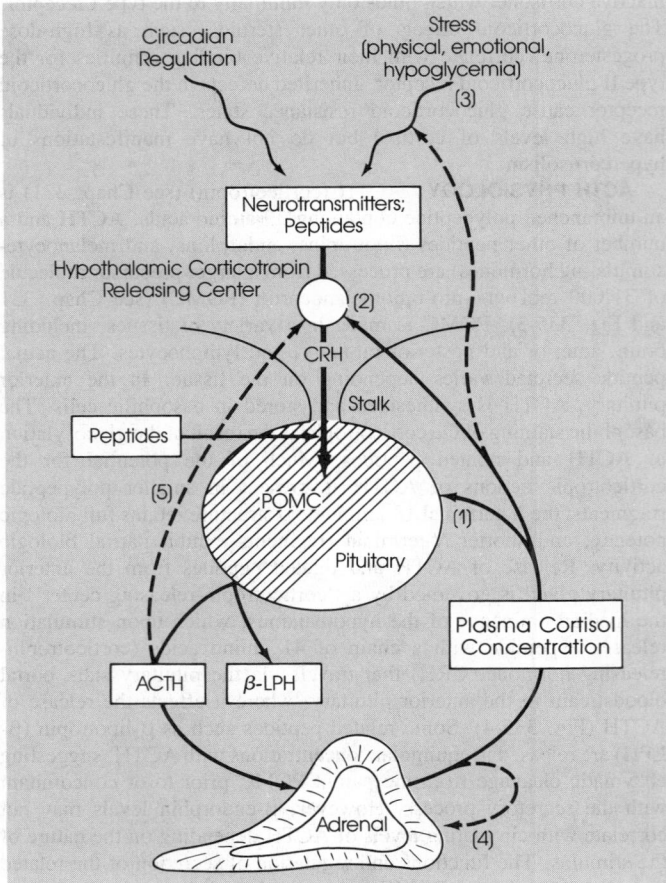

FIGURE 335-4 The hypothalamic-pituitary-adrenal axis. The dominant feedback control of plasma cortisol is on the pituitary gland (1) and on the hypothalamic corticotropin-releasing center (2). Feedback of plasma cortisol also may act on higher nerve centers (3) and/or on the adrenal gland itself (4). There also may be a short feedback inhibition of CRH by ACTH (5). Hypothalamic neurotransmitters influence CRH release; serotoninergic and cholinergic systems stimulate the secretion of CRH and ACTH; alpha-adrenergic agonists and gamma-aminobutyric acid (GABA) probably inhibit CRH release. The opioid peptides β-endorphin and enkephalin inhibit and vasopressin and angiotensin II augment the secretion of CRH and ACTH. CRH = corticotropin-releasing hormone; β-LPH = β-lipotropin; POMC = pro-opiomelanocortin.

of these neurotransmitters. There is also evidence for peptidergic regulation of ACTH release. For example, β-endorphin and enkephalin inhibit and vasopressin and angiotensin II augment the secretion of ACTH. The immune system also influences the hypothalamic-pituitary-adrenal axis. For example, the cytokine interleukin 1 (IL-1) stimulates CRH secretion. Finally, ACTH release is regulated by the free cortisol level in plasma. Cortisol decreases the responsiveness of adrenal corticotropic cells to CRH; i.e., in the presence of cortisol, more CRH is required to produce a given increment of ACTH. The response of the POMC mRNA to CRH is also inhibited by glucocorticoids. In addition, glucocorticoids inhibit CRH release. This servomechanism establishes the primacy of blood cortisol concentration in the control of ACTH secretion. The inhibition of ACTH occurs in two phases: (1) an early fast feedback, mediated via the type I glucocorticoid receptor, lasting less than 10 min and dependent on both the rate of increase of glucocorticoid levels and the specific glucocorticoid administered, and (2) a time-dependent delayed feedback, likely mediated by the type II glucocorticoid receptor, probably due to inhibition of synthesis of the precursor protein. The suppression of ACTH secretion that results in adrenal atrophy following *prolonged* glucocorticoid therapy may be primarily related to suppression of hypothalamic CRH release, since exogenous CRH administration in this circumstance produces a rise in plasma ACTH. Cortisol also exerts feedback on higher brain centers (hippocampus, reticular system, and septum) and perhaps on the adrenal cortex (see Fig. 335-4).

The biologic half-life of ACTH in the circulation is less than 10 min. The action of ACTH is also rapid; within minutes of its release, the concentration of steroids in the adrenal venous blood increases. ACTH stimulates steroidogenesis via activation of the membrane-bound adenyl cyclase. Adenosine-3′,5′-monophosphate (cyclic AMP), in turn, activates protein kinase enzymes, thereby resulting in the phosphorylation of proteins that activate steroid biosynthesis (see Chap. 69).

RENIN-ANGIOTENSIN PHYSIOLOGY (See also Chap. 209) Renin is a proteolytic enzyme that is produced and stored in the granules of the juxtaglomerular cells surrounding the afferent arterioles of glomeruli in the kidney. Renin exists both in active and inactive forms. Whether the inactive form is a precursor (''prorenin'') or is a product formed after release is uncertain. The juxtaglomerular apparatus consists of both the juxtaglomerular cells and the cells of the macula densa. Renin acts on the basic substrate angiotensinogen (a circulating alpha₂ globulin made in the liver) to form the decapeptide angiotensin I (Fig. 335-5). Angiotensin I is then enzymatically transformed by converting enzyme, present in many tissues, particularly in the pulmonary vascular endothelium, to the octapeptide

FIGURE 335-5 The interrelationship of the volume and potassium feedback loops on aldosterone secretion. Integration of signals from each loop determines the level of aldosterone secretion.

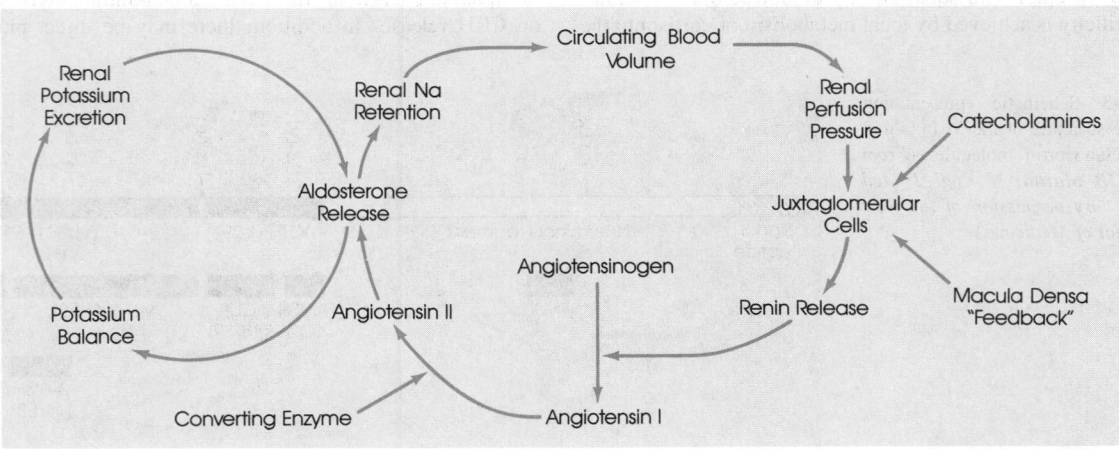

angiotensin II by splitting off the two *C*-terminal amino acids. Angiotensin II is a potent pressor agent and exerts its action by a direct effect on arteriolar smooth muscle. In addition, angiotensin II stimulates production of aldosterone by the zona glomerulosa of the adrenal cortex; the nonapeptide, angiotensin III, also may stimulate aldosterone production. Angiotensinases rapidly destroy angiotensin II (half-life approximately 1 min), while the half-life of renin is more prolonged (10 to 20 min). In addition to circulating renin-angiotensin, many tissues have a local renin-angiotensin system and the ability to produce angiotensin II. These include the uterus, placenta, vascular tissue, heart, brain, and particularly the adrenal cortex. While the role of locally generated angiotensin II is not established, it may be involved in growth and modulation of function of the adrenal cortex and vascular smooth muscle.

Renal renin release is controlled by four interdependent factors, and the amount of renin released is a composite of the effects of all four. The *juxtaglomerular cells*, which are specialized myoepithelial cells cuffing the afferent arterioles, act as miniature pressure transducers, sensing renal perfusion pressure and corresponding changes in afferent arteriolar perfusion pressures. For example, under conditions of a reduction in circulating blood volume, there is a corresponding reduction in renal perfusion pressure and, therefore, in afferent arteriolar pressure (see Fig. 335-5). This is perceived by the juxtaglomerular cells as a decreased stretch exerted on the afferent arteriolar walls. The juxtaglomerular cells then release increasing quantities of renin within the kidney circulation. This results in the formation of angiotensin I, which is converted in the kidney and peripherally to angiotensin II by converting enzyme. Angiotensin II influences sodium homeostasis via two major mechanisms: it changes renal blood flow so as to maintain a constant glomerular filtration rate, thereby changing the filtration fraction of sodium, and it stimulates the adrenal cortex to release aldosterone. Increasing plasma levels of aldosterone lead to increasing renal sodium retention and thus result in expansion of extracellular fluid volume, which, in turn, dampens the initiating signal for renin release. In this context, the renin-angiotensin-aldosterone system subserves volume control by appropriate modifications of renal hemodynamics and tubular sodium transport.

A second control mechanism for renin release centers in the *macula densa* cells, a group of distal convoluted tubular epithelial cells in direct apposition to the juxtaglomerular cells. They may function as chemoreceptors, monitoring the sodium (or chloride) load presented to the distal tubule, and such information may be conveyed to the juxtaglomerular cells, where appropriate modifications in renin release take place. Under conditions of increased delivery of filtered sodium to the macula densa, increasing release of renin is capable of decreasing glomerular filtration rate, thereby reducing the filtered load of sodium.

The *sympathetic nervous system* regulates release of renin in response to assuming the upright posture. The mechanism is either a direct effect on the juxtaglomerular cell to increase adenyl cyclase activity or an indirect effect on either the juxtaglomerular or the macula densa cells by way of a vasoconstrictive action on the afferent arteriole.

Finally, circulating factors influence renin release. Increasing dietary *potassium* directly decreases renin release; decreasing potassium intake increases renin release. The significance of this potassium effect is unclear. *Angiotensin II* itself can exert a negative feedback control on renin release independent of alterations in renal blood flow, pressure, or aldosterone secretion. *Atrial natriuretic peptides* also inhibit renin release. Thus the control of renin release is complex, consisting of both *intrarenal* (pressor receptor and macula densa) and *extrarenal* (sympathetic nervous system, potassium, angiotensin, etc.) mechanisms. A given level of renin secretion probably reflects all these factors, with the intrarenal mechanism predominating.

GLUCOCORTICOID PHYSIOLOGY The division of adrenal steroids into glucocorticoids and mineralocorticoids is arbitrary in that most glucocorticoids have some mineralocorticoid-like properties.

The descriptive term *glucocorticoid* is applied to those adrenal steroids with a predominant action on intermediary metabolism. The principal glucocorticoid is cortisol (hydrocortisone). This effect on intermediary metabolism is mediated by the type II glucocorticoid receptor. The physiologic actions of the glucocorticoids include the regulation of protein, carbohydrate, lipid, and nucleic acid metabolism. Glucocorticoids raise the blood glucose level by acting as an insulin antagonist and by suppressing the secretion of insulin, thereby inhibiting glucose uptake in peripheral tissues and promoting hepatic synthesis of glucose (gluconeogenesis). The actions on protein metabolism appear to be mainly catabolic in effect, with an increased protein breakdown and nitrogen excretion. Glucocorticoids increase hepatic glycogen content and promote hepatic gluconeogenesis. These actions are in large part explained by the mobilization of glycogenic amino acid precursors from peripheral supporting structures, such as bone, skin, muscle, and connective tissue, due to protein breakdown and inhibition of protein synthesis and amino acid uptake. Glucocorticoid-induced hyperaminoacidemia also facilitates gluconeogenesis by stimulating glucagon secretion. Glucocorticoids act directly on the liver to stimulate the synthesis of certain enzymes, such as tyrosine amino transferase and tryptophan pyrrolase. Glucocorticoids inhibit the synthesis of nucleic acids in most body tissues, but in the liver RNA synthesis is stimulated. Glucocorticoids regulate fatty acid mobilization by enhancing activation of cellular lipase by lipid-mobilizing hormones (e.g., catecholamines and pituitary peptides).

The actions of cortisol on structural protein and on adipose tissue vary in different parts of the body. For example, pharmacologic doses of cortisol can deplete the protein matrix of the vertebral column (trabecular bone), but long bones (primarily compact bone) are affected only minimally; peripheral adipose tissue mass decreases, whereas abdominal and interscapular fat may accumulate.

Glucocorticoids have anti-inflammatory properties, which are probably related to their actions on the microvasculature as well as to cellular effects. Cortisol maintains normal vascular responsiveness to circulating vasoconstrictor factors and opposes the increase in capillary permeability characteristic of acute inflammation. Glucocorticoids cause a polymorphonuclear leukocytosis; the circulating leukocyte mass is increased due to release from the bone marrow of mature cells as well as to inhibition of their egress through the capillary wall. Glucocorticoids produce a depletion of circulating eosinophils and of lymphoid tissue, specifically T cells (thymus-derived lymphocytes). The mechanism is by redistribution from the circulation into other compartments. Thus cortisol impairs cellular-mediated immunity. Glucocorticoids also inhibit the production or action of the local mediators of inflammation such as the lymphokines and prostaglandins. These actions occur via the type II glucocorticoid receptor, and the effects are blocked by inhibitors of RNA and protein synthesis. Glucocorticoids inhibit actions and production of immune interferon by T lymphocytes and the production of lymphocyte-activating factor (interleukin 1) by macrophages. The action of glucocorticoids in suppressing fever may be explained by the latter effect, since IL-1 appears to be identical to endogenous pyrogen, which can activate the hypothalamic fever center. Glucocorticoids also inhibit the production of T cell growth factor (IL-2) by T lymphocytes. Glucocorticoids reverse macrophage activation and antagonize the action of migration-inhibiting factor (MIF), leading to reduced adherence of macrophages to vascular endothelium. Glucocorticoids inhibit prostaglandin and leukotriene production by inhibiting the activity of phospholipase A_2, thus blocking release of arachidonic acid from phospholipids. Finally, glucocorticoids inhibit the inflammatory actions induced by bradykinin and serotonin, such as increased vascular permeability. It is probably only at pharmacologic dosages that antibody production is reduced and lysosomal membranes stabilized, thereby suppressing the release of proteolytic acid hydrolases stored in these cytoplasmic organelles.

Cortisol levels are responsive within minutes to a variety of physical (trauma, surgery, exercise) and psychological stresses (anxiety, depression). Hypoglycemia and fever are also potent stimuli of ACTH and cortisol secretion. The reasons why elevated glucocorticoid levels protect the organism under stress are not understood, but in the absence of glucocorticoids, such stresses may cause hypotension, shock, and death. For these reasons, glucocorticoid administration should always be increased in individuals with hypofunction of the pituitary-adrenal axis during stress.

Cortisol has a major action on the distribution and excretion of body water. It subserves the extracellular fluid volume by retarding the migration of water into cells. It promotes renal water excretion by suppressing the secretion of vasopressin, increasing the rate of glomerular filtration, and acting directly on the renal tubule, the consequence being to guard against water intoxication by increasing solute-free water clearance. Glucocorticoids also have weak mineralocorticoid-like properties, and increasing doses produce renal tubular sodium reabsorption and increased urine potassium excretion. Glucocorticoids also can influence behavior; emotional disorders may occur with either excesses or deficits of cortisol. Lastly, cortisol suppresses the secretion of pituitary POMC and peptides derived from this precursor molecule (ACTH, β-endorphin, and β-lipotropin) as well as the secretion of hypothalamic CRH and vasopressin.

MINERALOCORTICOID PHYSIOLOGY   The major mineralocorticoid, aldosterone, has two important activities: (1) It is a major regulator of extracellular fluid volume, and (2) it is a major determinant of potassium metabolism. These effects are mediated by binding of aldosterone to the type I glucocorticoid (mineralocorticoid) receptor in target tissues (see Chap. 329). Volume is regulated through a direct effect on the renal tubular transport of sodium. Aldosterone acts predominantly at the distal convoluted tubule, where it causes a decrease in the excretion of sodium and an increase in excretion of potassium. The reabsorption of sodium ions causes a fall in the transmembrane potential, thus enhancing the flow of positive ions out of the cell into the lumen. The major intracellular singly charged positive ion is potassium. Since its concentration in the cell is forty- to eightyfold greater than in the lumen, potassium passively follows this relative electric gradient to restore the normal positive charge to the lumen. The reabsorbed sodium ions are then transported out of the tubular epithelial cells into the interstitial fluid of the kidney and from there into the renal capillary circulation. Water passively follows the transported sodium.

Hydrogen ion is also abundant in the tubular epithelial cell. Since its concentration is greater in the lumen than in the cell, it is actively secreted, but the reduced intraluminal positivity allows more hydrogen to be secreted with the same amount of energy. Aldosterone and other mineralocorticoids also act on the epithelium of the salivary ducts, sweat glands, and gastrointestinal tract to cause reabsorption of sodium in "exchange" for potassium ions.

When normal individuals are given aldosterone (or deoxycorticosterone), an initial period of sodium retention is followed by a natriuresis, and sodium balance is reestablished after 3 to 5 days. As a result, edema does not develop. This phenomenon is referred to as the *escape phenomenon*, signifying an "escape" by the renal tubules from the sodium-retaining action of chronically administered aldosterone. While renal hemodynamic factors may play a role in the escape, the level of atrial natriuretic peptide also increases. Importantly, there is no evidence of escape from the potassium-losing effects of mineralocorticoids.

Three primary mechanisms control aldosterone release—the renin-angiotensin system, potassium, and ACTH (Table 335-1). The renin-angiotensin system is the major system for control of extracellular fluid volume, via regulation of aldosterone secretion (see Fig. 335-1). In effect, the renin-angiotensin system maintains the circulating blood volume constant by causing aldosterone-induced sodium retention during periods registered as volume deficiencies and by decreasing aldosterone-dependent sodium retention under conditions in which volume is registered as being ample.

Potassium ions directly regulate aldosterone secretion independently of circulating renin-angiotensin (see Fig. 335-5). However, potassium stimulates the adrenal production of angiotensin II, and

TABLE 335-1   Factors regulating aldosterone biosynthesis

Factors	Effects
Renin-angiotensin system	Stimulate
Sodium ion	Inhibit (?physiologic)
Potassium ion	Stimulate
Neurotransmitters	
Dopamine	Inhibit
Serotonin	Stimulate
Pituitary hormones	
ACTH	Stimulate
Non-ACTH pituitary hormones (e.g., growth hormone)	Permissive (for optimal response to sodium restriction)
Unidentified pituitary factors	Stimulate
β-Endorphin	Stimulate
γ-MSH	Permissive
Natriuretic factors	
Atrial peptide	Inhibit
Ouabain-like factors	Inhibit

administration of converting-enzyme inhibitors blocks the synthesis of locally generated angiotensin II and reduces the aldosterone response to potassium. In normal humans, oral potassium loading increases aldosterone secretion, excretion, and plasma levels. In addition, an increase in serum potassium of as little as 0.1 mmol/L increases plasma aldosterone levels under certain circumstances.

Physiologic amounts of ACTH stimulate aldosterone secretion acutely, but this action is not sustained if ACTH is infused for periods greater than 10 to 12 h. Most studies relegate ACTH to a minor role in the control of aldosterone. For example, subjects on long-term high-dose glucocorticoid therapy and with presumed complete suppression of ACTH have normal aldosterone secretory responses to sodium restriction. Therefore, chronic ACTH deficiency per se does not alter glomerulosa cell responsiveness.

The prior dietary intake of both potassium and sodium can alter the magnitude of the aldosterone response to acute stimulation. Increasing potassium intake or decreasing sodium intake sensitizes the response of the glomerulosa cells to acute stimulation by ACTH, angiotensin II, and/or potassium.

Neurotransmitters (dopamine and serotonin) and some peptides, such as atrial natriuretic peptide, γ-melanocyte-stimulating hormone (γ-MSH), β-endorphin, and an unidentified pituitary aldosterone-stimulating factor, also participate in the regulation of aldosterone secretion (see Table 335-1). Thus the control of aldosterone secretion involves both stimulatory and inhibitory factors.

ANDROGEN PHYSIOLOGY   Androgens regulate male secondary sexual characteristics and can cause virilizing symptoms in women. They produce these actions by binding to high-affinity cytoplasmic receptors.

Steroids with predominant androgenic activity have 19 carbon atoms (see Fig. 335-1). The principal adrenal androgens are dehydroepiandrosterone (DHEA), androstenedione, and 11-hydroxyandrostenedione. DHEA and androstenedione are weak androgens, and they exert their effects via conversion in extraglandular tissues to the potent androgen testosterone. The release of adrenal androgens is stimulated by ACTH, not by gonadotropins. With ACTH stimulation, 17-ketosteroids increase. It follows that adrenal androgens are suppressed by exogenous glucocorticoid administration.

LABORATORY EVALUATION OF ADRENOCORTICAL FUNCTION

The basic assumption in the measurement of plasma or urinary steroids is that they accurately reflect adrenal *secretory* rates of that steroid. A disadvantage of urine *excretion* values is that they may not truly reflect the secretion rate because of improper collection or altered metabolism. Measurement of the actual adrenal secretory rate of a given steroid would be preferable but is more difficult, involving

TABLE 335-2 Range of normal values for tests of adrenal function

Test	Normal value, range
Plasma cortisol, nmol/L (μg/dL):	
8 A.M.	140–690 (5–24)
4 P.M.	80–330 (3–12)
Cortisol secretory rate, nmol/d (mg/d)	14–69 (5–25)
Urinary free cortisol, nmol/d (μg/d)	55–275 (20–100)
17-Hydroxycorticosteroids, μmol/d (mg/d)	5.5–28 (2–10)
Plasma testosterone, nmol/L (ng/mL):	
Men	10–35 (3–10)
Women	<3.5 (<1)
Plasma dehydroepiandrosterone (DHEA), nmol/L (μg/L)	7–31 (2–9)
Plasma DHEA sulfate, μmol/L (μg/L)	1.3–6.7 (500–2500)
Plasma 11-deoxycortisol (S), nmol/L (μg/dL)	<30 (<1)
Plasma 17OH progesterone, nmol/L (μg/L):	
Women	
Follicular phase	0.6–3 (0.2–1)
Luteal phase	1.5–10.6 (0.5–3.5)
Men	0.2–9 (0.06–3)
Plasma aldosterone, pmol/L (ng/dL) (100 mmol Na, 60–100 mmol K, supine, 8 A.M.)	<240 (<8)
Aldosterone secretion, nmol/d (μg/d) (100 mmol Na, 600–100 mmol K)	140–690 (50–250)
Aldosterone excretion, nmol/d (μg/d) (100 mmol Na, 60–100 mmol K)	14–53 (5–19)
Plasma renin activity (μg/L)/h [(ng/mL)/h] (100 mmol Na, 60–100 mmol K, supine, 8 A.M.)	1–2.5 (1–2.5)
Plasma angiotensin II, ng/L (pg/mL) (100 mmol Na, 60–100 mmol K, supine, 8 A.M.)	10–30 (10–30)
Plasma ACTH, pmol/L (pg/mL) (8 A.M.)	<18 (<80)

isotope dilution techniques following administration of a radioactive steroid. Plasma levels reflect the level of secretion only at the time of measurement. The plasma level (PL) is dependent on two factors: the secretion rate (SR) of the hormone and the rate at which it is metabolized, i.e., its metabolic clearance rate (MCR). These three factors can be related mathematically as follows:

$$PL = \frac{SR}{MCR} \quad \text{or} \quad SR = MCR \times PL$$

BLOOD LEVELS (See Table 335-2) **Peptides** ACTH and angiotensin II can be measured by immunologic techniques. However, because of their low concentration and instability in plasma, special precautions are required when specimens are collected. In addition, ACTH levels fluctuate from moment to moment, and a circadian rhythm is superimposed on basal ACTH secretion, with lower levels in the early evening than in the morning. Angiotensin II levels also vary diurnally and are influenced by dietary sodium intake and posture. Both upright posture and sodium restriction elevate angiotensin II levels.

Most clinical determinations of the renin-angiotensin system, however, involve measurements of peripheral *plasma renin activity* (PRA) in which the renin activity is gauged by the generation of angiotensin I during a standardized incubation period. This method depends on the presence of sufficient angiotensinogen in plasma as substrate. The generated angiotensin I is then measured by radioimmunoassay. Plasma renin activity depends on dietary sodium intake and whether the patient is ambulatory. In normal humans, a diurnal rhythm for PRA is characterized by peak values in the morning with decreases in activity in the afternoon.

Steroids Cortisol and aldosterone are both secreted episodically, and levels generally vary during the day, with peak values in the morning and low levels in the evening. In addition, the plasma level of aldosterone, but not of cortisol, is increased by dietary potassium loading, sodium restriction, or assuming the upright posture. Measurement of the sulfate conjugate of DHEA is a useful index of adrenal androgen secretion, since little is formed in the gonads and the half-life is 7 to 9 h.

URINE LEVELS The urine *17-hydroxycorticosteroid* assay measures steroids with a "dihydroxyacetone" C-17 side chain, i.e., with

hydroxyl groups on C-17 and C-21 and a ketone group on C-20. Therefore, this determination includes cortisol, cortisone, tetrahydrocortisol, tetrahydrocortisone, and 11-deoxycortisol (see Fig. 335-2). Normally, daytime (7 A.M. to 7 P.M.) excretion exceeds night values (7 P.M. to 7 A.M.).

The urine *17-ketosteroids* contain a ketone group at C-17 (see Fig. 335-1). They originate either in the adrenal gland or the gonad. In normal women, 90 percent or more of total urinary 17-ketosteroids is derived from the adrenal gland, while in men only 60 to 70 percent is of adrenal origin. Urine 17-ketosteroid values are highest in young adults and decline with age.

The determination of urinary free cortisol is more useful than 17-hydroxysteroid measurements because elevated values correlate with states of hypercortisolism, reflecting changes in the unbound, physiologically active levels of circulating cortisol.

A carefully timed urine collection is a prerequisite for all excretory determinations. Urinary creatinine should be measured simultaneously to demonstrate the accuracy and adequacy of the collection procedure. Adjustments for body size can be made; e.g., normal subjects excrete 8 to 20 μmol (3 to 7 mg) of 17-hydroxycorticosteroids per gram of creatinine.

STIMULATION TESTS Stimulation tests are useful in documenting the existence of a hormonal deficiency state. A standardized and specific stimulus for the production and release of a given hormone is applied, and the quantity of the released hormone can then be measured.

Tests of glucocorticoid reserve Within minutes after initiation of an infusion of ACTH, cortisol levels increase in adrenal venous blood. This responsiveness of the adrenal gland to ACTH is utilized as an index of the "functional reserve" of the gland for production of cortisol. Under maximal ACTH stimulation, the cortisol secretion increases tenfold to 800 μmol/d (300 mg/d). Such maximal stimulation can be obtained only with prolonged ACTH infusions. For clinical purposes, the functional adrenal reserve for cortisol production is standardized with a 24-h ACTH infusion. Synthetic α^{1-24}-ACTH (cosyntropin) is usually given in 500 to 1000 mL normal saline at a rate of 2 units per hour for 24 h. Normal subjects increase 17-hydroxysteroid excretion rates to at least 70 μmol/d (25 mg/d), and plasma cortisol levels exceed 1100 nmol/L (40 μg/dL). In patients with secondary adrenal insufficiency, the maximal 17-hydroxysteroid excretion rate is 8 to 55 μmol/d (3 to 20 mg/d), and the plasma cortisol value at 24 h ranges between 280 and 1100 nmol/L (10 and 40 μg/dL). Patients with primary adrenal insufficiency have smaller responses.

A screening test (the so-called rapid ACTH stimulation test) involves the administration of 25 units (0.25 mg) of cosyntropin intravenously or intramuscularly and measurement of plasma cortisol levels before and 30 and 60 min later; the test can be performed at any time of the day. The most clear-cut criterion for a normal response is a stimulated cortisol level >500 nmol/L (18 μg/dL), and the minimal stimulated normal increment of cortisol is >200 nmol/L (7 mg/dL) above baseline. However, severely ill patients with elevated basal cortisol levels may show no further increases following acute ACTH administration.

Tests of mineralocorticoid reserve and stimulation of the renin-angiotensin system Stimulation tests utilize protocols of programmed volume depletion, such as sodium restriction, diuretic administration, or upright posture. A simple, potent test consists of severe sodium restriction and upright posture. After 3 to 5 days of a 10-mmol sodium intake, aldosterone secretion or excretion rates should increase two- to threefold over control. Supine morning plasma aldosterone levels usually increase three- to sixfold. In addition, plasma levels increase two- to fourfold in response to 2 to 3 h of upright posture.

Stimulation tests on normal dietary sodium intake may be carried out by the administration of a potent diuretic, such as 40 to 80 mg furosemide, followed by 2 to 3 h of upright posture. The normal response is a two- to fourfold rise in plasma aldosterone levels.

SUPPRESSION TESTS Suppression tests to document hypersecretion of adrenocortical hormones are based on the measurement of the target hormone response following standardized suppression of its tropic hormone.

Tests of pituitary-adrenal suppressibility The ACTH release mechanism is sensitive to the circulating blood level of glucocorticoids. When such blood levels are increased in the normal individual, less ACTH is released from the anterior pituitary and less steroid is produced by the adrenal gland. The integrity of this feedback mechanism can be tested clinically by giving a potent glucocorticoid and judging suppression of ACTH secretion by analysis of urine steroid excretory values and/or plasma cortisol and ACTH levels. A potent glucocorticoid such as dexamethasone is utilized so that the administered compound can be given in such small amounts that it does not contribute significantly to the steroids to be analyzed.

The best *screening* procedure is the overnight dexamethasone suppression test. This involves the measurement of plasma cortisol levels at 8 A.M. following the oral administration of 1 mg dexamethasone the previous midnight. The 8 A.M. value for plasma cortisol in normal subjects should be less than 140 nmol/L (5 μg/dL).

The definitive test of adrenal suppressibility is to administer 0.5 mg dexamethasone every 6 h for two successive days while collecting urine over a 24-h period for determination of creatinine, 17-hydroxysteroids, and/or free cortisol and/or measuring plasma cortisol levels. In a patient with a normal hypothalamic-pituitary ACTH release mechanism, a fall in the urine 17-hydroxycorticosteroids to less than 8 μmol/d (3 mg/d) on the second day of dexamethasone administration, urinary free cortisol to less than 80 nmol/d (30 μg/d), or plasma cortisol to less than 140 nmol/L (5 μg/dL) is seen.

Normal responses to either of the suppression tests implies that the ACTH control of the adrenal glands is physiologically normal. However, an isolated abnormal result, particularly when the overnight suppression test is being used, does not in itself imply pituitary and/or adrenal disease.

Tests of mineralocorticoid suppressibility Mineralocorticoid suppression procedures have been devised using saline infusions, oral salt loading, or deoxycorticosterone administration for expansion of the extracellular fluid volume. With expansion of extracellular fluid volume, there is a decrease in renal renin release, a decrease in circulating plasma renin activity, and a decrease in aldosterone secretion and/or excretion. Various tests differ in the rate at which extracellular fluid volume is expanded. One convenient suppression test is the intravenous infusion of 500 mL normal saline solution per hour for 4 h, which normally suppresses plasma aldosterone levels to <220 pmol/L (<8 ng/dL) on a sodium-restricted diet or to 140 pmol/L (<5 ng/dL) on a normal sodium intake. This test should not be performed in potassium-depleted subjects.

TESTS OF PITUITARY-ADRENAL RESPONSIVENESS Stimuli such as insulin hypoglycemia, arginine vasopressin, and pyrogen cause release of ACTH from the pituitary by an action on higher nerve centers, the hypothalamus, or the pituitary itself. By measuring plasma ACTH or plasma glucocorticoids, the status of pituitary ACTH can be evaluated. Insulin-induced hypoglycemia is particularly useful, since the release of growth hormone and ACTH is stimulated. In this test, 0.05 to 0.1 unit of regular insulin per kilogram of body weight is administered intravenously as a bolus to reduce fasting glucose levels at least 50 percent below basal. The normal cortisol response is a rise to more than 500 nmol/L (18 μg/dL).

One of the best ways to test the integrity of the pituitary-adrenal axis is the metyrapone test. Metyrapone is a drug that inhibits 11β-hydroxylase in the adrenal gland. As a result, the conversion of 11-deoxycortisol (compound S) to cortisol is interfered with, and increased amounts of 11-deoxycortisol accumulate while blood levels of cortisol decrease (see Fig. 335-2). The hypothalamic-pituitary axis responds to the declining cortisol blood levels by releasing more ACTH. The metabolites of 11-deoxycortisol are excreted in increasing amounts in the urine, where they are measured as 17-hydroxycorticosteroids. Alternatively, changes in plasma 11-deoxycortisol levels can

be measured. *Note that the adrenal glands must be capable of being stimulated by ACTH, since assessment of the response depends on both an intact hypothalamic-pituitary axis and adrenal steroid production.*

While modifications of the original metyrapone test have been described, we believe the best involves administering 750 mg of the drug by mouth every 4 h over a 24-h period and comparing the control and the postmetyrapone 17-hydroxysteroid excretion rates and/or plasma 11-deoxycortisol, cortisol, and ACTH levels. Normal individuals respond with at least a doubling of their basal 17-hydroxysteroid excretion; 11-deoxycortisol levels in the blood should exceed 290 nmol/L (10 μg/dL) following metyrapone administration. The metyrapone test does not accurately reflect ACTH reserve if subjects are ingesting exogenous glucocorticoids or drugs that accelerate the metabolism of metyrapone (e.g., phenytoin).

A direct and selective test of the pituitary corticotrophs can be achieved with the investigational agent corticotropin-releasing hormone (CRH). The bolus injection of 1 μg/kg of body weight of ovine CRH stimulates ACTH and β-lipotropin secretion in normal human subjects within 60 to 180 min. However, the magnitude of the ACTH response is less than that produced by the insulin tolerance test, which implies that additional factors (such as vasopressin) augment stress-induced increases in ACTH secretion.

Although the rapid ACTH stimulation test reliably diagnoses primary adrenal insufficiency, normal cortisol responsiveness may be seen in a subset of patients with secondary adrenocortical insufficiency in whom there is a partial ACTH deficit and absence of adrenal atrophy. These patients have inadequate pituitary ACTH reserve and fail to increase ACTH secretion in response to stress such as surgery or hypoglycemia. Since a bolus of exogenous ACTH does not invariably exclude a diagnosis of secondary adrenocortical insufficiency, direct tests of pituitary ACTH reserve (metyrapone, insulin tolerance testing) should be used in the appropriate clinical setting. On the other hand, the rapid ACTH test can distinguish between primary and secondary adrenal insufficiency, because aldosterone secretion is preserved in secondary adrenal failure by the renin-angiotensin system and potassium. Twenty-five units of cosyntropin is given intravenously or intramuscularly, and plasma cortisol and aldosterone levels are obtained before and 30 and 60 min later. Although the cortisol response is abnormal in both groups, patients with secondary insufficiency increase aldosterone levels above control by at least 140 pmol/L (5 ng/dL). No aldosterone response is seen in patients with primary adrenocortical insufficiency in whom the adrenal cortex is destroyed.

HYPERFUNCTION OF THE ADRENAL CORTEX

Distinct clinical syndromes are produced when excess adrenocortical hormones are secreted. Thus excess cortisol is associated with Cushing's syndrome, excess aldosterone causes aldosteronism, and excess adrenal androgens cause adrenal virilism. These syndromes do not always occur in the "pure" form but may have overlapping features.

CUSHING'S SYNDROME Etiology Cushing described a syndrome characterized by truncal obesity, hypertension, fatigability and weakness, amenorrhea, hirsutism, purplish abdominal striae, edema, glucosuria, osteoporosis, and a basophilic tumor of the pituitary. As awareness of this syndrome increased, the diagnosis of Cushing's syndrome has been broadened into the classification shown in Table 335-3. Regardless of etiology, all cases of endogenous Cushing's syndrome are due to increased production of cortisol by the adrenal gland. Most are due to *bilateral adrenal hyperplasia*; the cause may be adrenocortical stimulation due to hypersecretion of pituitary ACTH or production of ACTH by nonendocrine tumors. The incidence of pituitary-dependent adrenal hyperplasia in women is three times that in men, with the most frequent age of onset being the third or fourth decade. The cause of the hypersecretion of pituitary ACTH is still

TABLE 335-3 Causes of Cushing's syndrome

Adrenal hyperplasia
   A Secondary to pituitary ACTH overproduction
      1 Pituitary-hypothalamic dysfunction
      2 Pituitary ACTH-producing micro- or macroadenomas
   B Secondary to ACTH or CRH-producing nonendocrine tumors
      (bronchogenic carcinoma, carcinoid of the thymus, pancreatic
      carcinoma, bronchial adenoma)
Adrenal nodular hyperplasia
Adrenal neoplasia
   A Adenoma
   B Carcinoma
Exogenous, iatrogenic causes
   A Prolonged use of glucocorticoids
   B Prolonged use of ACTH

debated. Some speculate that the primary defect is the de novo development of a pituitary adenoma, since in some reports tumors are found in over 90 percent of patients with pituitary-dependent adrenal hyperplasia. Alternatively, the defect may reside in the hypothalamus or in higher nerve centers, leading to release of CRH inappropriate to the level of circulating cortisol. The consequence would be that a higher level of cortisol is required to reduce ACTH secretion to normal. This primary defect would lead to hyperstimulation of the pituitary, resulting in hyperplasia or tumor formation. As the pituitary tumor grows, it may become independent of the regulating influence of central nervous system factors and/or circulating cortisol levels. In surgical series, most individuals with hypersecretion of pituitary ACTH have a microadenoma (<10 mm; 50 percent are 5 mm or less in diameter), but a macroadenoma (>10 mm) of the pituitary or diffuse hyperplasia of the corticotropic cells (hypothalamic-pituitary dysfunction) also may be found. The common finding of a microadenoma in pituitary-dependent adrenal hyperplasia does not rule out dysregulation of hypothalamic CRH as the defect in Cushing's disease. Long-term follow-up to determine the rate of recurrence following successful surgical resection is necessary to answer this issue. In some studies, the recurrence rate is greater than 20 percent. Unfortunately, it may be difficult to distinguish between recurrence and inadequate primary therapy. Traditionally, only an individual who has an ACTH-producing pituitary tumor has been defined as having *Cushing's disease*. However, in many centers, anyone who has hypersecretion of pituitary ACTH regardless of whether a tumor is identified by radiographic procedures is classified as having Cushing's disease. In this chapter we will use the traditional definition, although these definitions may become less distinct as small tumors are more easily diagnosed by high-resolution scanning.

Nonendocrine tumors may secrete polypeptides that are biologically, chemically, and immunologically indistinguishable from either ACTH or CRH and that cause bilateral adrenal hyperplasia (see also Chap. 327). The ectopic production of CRH results in clinical, biochemical, and radiologic features indistinguishable from those caused by hypersecretion of pituitary ACTH. Often, but not invariably, the typical signs and symptoms of Cushing's syndrome are absent with ectopic ACTH production, and hypokalemic alkalosis and glucose intolerance are the prominent manifestations. The majority of these cases are associated with the primitive small cell (oat cell) type of bronchogenic carcinoma or with tumors of the thymus, pancreas, or ovary, medullary carcinoma of the thyroid, or bronchial adenomas. The onset of Cushing's syndrome may be sudden, particularly in patients with oat cell carcinoma of the lung, and this feature accounts in part for the failure of these patients to exhibit the classic physical findings. On the other hand, patients with carcinoid tumors or pheochromocytomas have longer clinical courses and usually exhibit the typical cushingoid features. The secretion of ACTH by nonendocrine tumors is also accompanied by the accumulation of ACTH fragments in plasma and by elevated plasma levels of ACTH precursor molecules. Since such tumors may produce large amounts of ACTH, baseline steroid values are usually markedly elevated, and

increased skin pigmentation may be present. Indeed, hyperpigmentation in patients with Cushing's syndrome almost always points to an extraadrenal tumor, either in an extracranial location or within the cranium.

Approximately 20 to 25 percent of patients with Cushing's syndrome have primary overproduction of cortisol and other adrenal steroids due to an adrenal neoplasm. These tumors are usually unilateral, and about half are malignant. Occasionally, patients have biochemical features both of hypersecretion of pituitary ACTH and of an adrenal adenoma. These individuals usually have micro- or macronodularity of both adrenal glands resulting in *nodular hyperplasia*. Two specific entities cause nodular hyperplasia: a familial autoimmune disorder in children or young adults (so-called pigmented multinodular cortical dysplasia) and hypersensitivity to gastric inhibitory polypeptide, probably secondary to enhanced expression of receptors for this peptide on the adrenal cortex.

The most common cause of Cushing's syndrome is *iatrogenic* administration of steroids for other reasons. While the clinical features bear some resemblance to those of individuals with an adrenal adenoma, these patients are usually readily distinguishable on the basis of history and initial laboratory studies.

Clinical signs, symptoms, and laboratory findings Many of the signs and symptoms of Cushing's syndrome logically follow from the known action of glucocorticoids (Table 335-4). As a result of mobilization of peripheral supportive tissue, muscle weakness and fatigability, osteoporosis, cutaneous striae, and easy bruisability result. The latter two signs are secondary to weakening and rupture of collagen fibers in the dermis. The osteoporosis may be so severe that collapse of vertebral bodies and pathologic fractures of other bones occur. Increased hepatic gluconeogenesis and insulin resistance can cause impaired glucose tolerance. Overt diabetes mellitus occurs in less than 20 percent of patients, probably in individuals with a familial predisposition to this disorder. Hypercortisolism promotes the deposition of adipose tissue in characteristic sites, notably in the upper part of the face, the typical "moon" facies; in the interscapular area, the "buffalo" hump; and in the mesenteric bed, where it produces the classic "truncal" obesity (Fig. 335-6). Rarely, there may be episternal fatty tumors and mediastinal widening secondary to fat accumulation. The reason for this peculiar distribution of adipose tissue is not known. The face appears plethoric, even in the absence of any increase in red blood cell concentration. Hypertension is common, and frequently there are profound emotional changes, ranging from irritability or emotional lability to severe depression, confusion, or even frank psychosis. In women, increased adrenal androgen secretion can cause acne, hirsutism, and oligomenorrhea or amenorrhea. The most common signs and symptoms in patients with hypercortisolism, i.e., obesity, hypertension, osteoporosis, and diabetes, are nonspecific and therefore less helpful in diagnosing this condition. On the other hand, easy bruising, typical striae, myopathy, and androgen effects (although less frequent) are, if present, more suggestive of Cushing's syndrome.

Except in iatrogenic Cushing's syndrome, plasma and urine cortisol and urinary 17-hydroxycorticosteroid levels are variably elevated. Occasionally, hypokalemia, hypochloremia, and metabolic alkalosis are present, particularly in individuals who have ectopic production of ACTH.

TABLE 335-4 Frequency of signs and symptoms in Cushing's syndrome, percent

Typical habitus	97	Amenorrhea	77
Increased body weight	94	Cutaneous striae	67
Fatigability and weakness	87	Personality changes	66
		Ecchymoses	65
Hypertension (>150/90)	82	Edema	62
		Polyuria, polydipsia	23
Hirsutism	80	Hypertrophy of clitoris	19

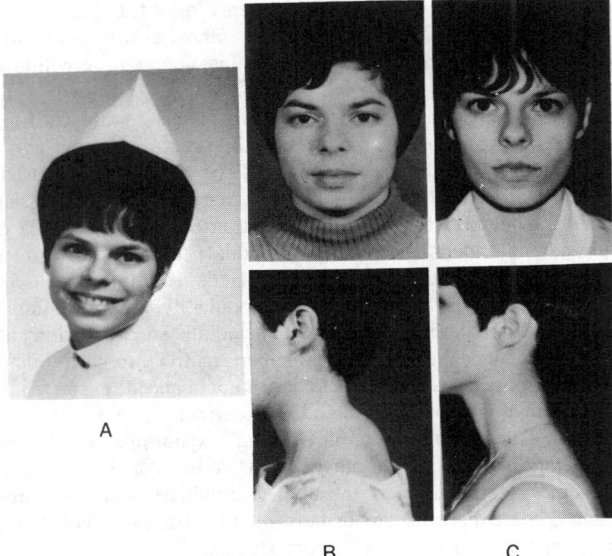

FIGURE 335-6 A 20-year-old woman with Cushing's syndrome due to a right adrenal cortical adenoma. *A*. Two years prior to surgery, age 18. *B*. One month prior to surgery, age 20. *C*. One year after surgery, age 21.

Diagnosis The diagnosis of Cushing's syndrome depends on the demonstration of increased cortisol production and the failure to suppress endogenous cortisol secretion normally when dexamethasone is administered. Once the diagnosis is established, further testing is designed to determine the etiology of the hypercortisolism (Fig. 335-7 and Table 335-5).

TABLE 335-5 Diagnostic tests to determine the type of Cushing's syndrome

Test	Pituitary macro-adenoma	Pituitary-hypothalamic dysfunction or micro-adenoma	Ectopic ACTH or CRH production	Adrenal tumor
Measurement of plasma ACTH	↑ to ↑↑	N to ↑	↑ to ↑↑↑	↓
Percent who respond to high-dose dexamethasone	<10	95	<10	<10
Percent who respond to CRH	>90	>90	<10	<10

NOTE: N, normal; ↑, elevated; ↓, decreased. See text for definition of a response.

For initial screening, the overnight dexamethasone suppression test is recommended (see above). In difficult cases (e.g., in obesity), measurement of a 24-h free cortisol excretion rate also can be used as a screening test. A level greater than 275 nmol/d (100 μg/d) is suggestive of Cushing's syndrome. The definitive diagnosis is then established by failure to suppress urinary cortisol to less than 80 nmol/d (30 μg/d), plasma cortisol to less than 140 nmol/L (5μg/dL), or 17-hydroxysteroid excretion to less than 8 μmol/d (3 mg/d) after a standard low-dose dexamethasone suppression test (0.5 mg every 6 h for 48 h). Owing to diurnal variability, plasma cortisol and, to a certain extent, ACTH determinations are not meaningful when performed in isolation, but demonstration that the normal fall in P.M. levels of plasma corticoid does not occur may be useful.

Determining the etiology of Cushing's syndrome is complicated by the lack of specificity of all tests available and the spontaneous,

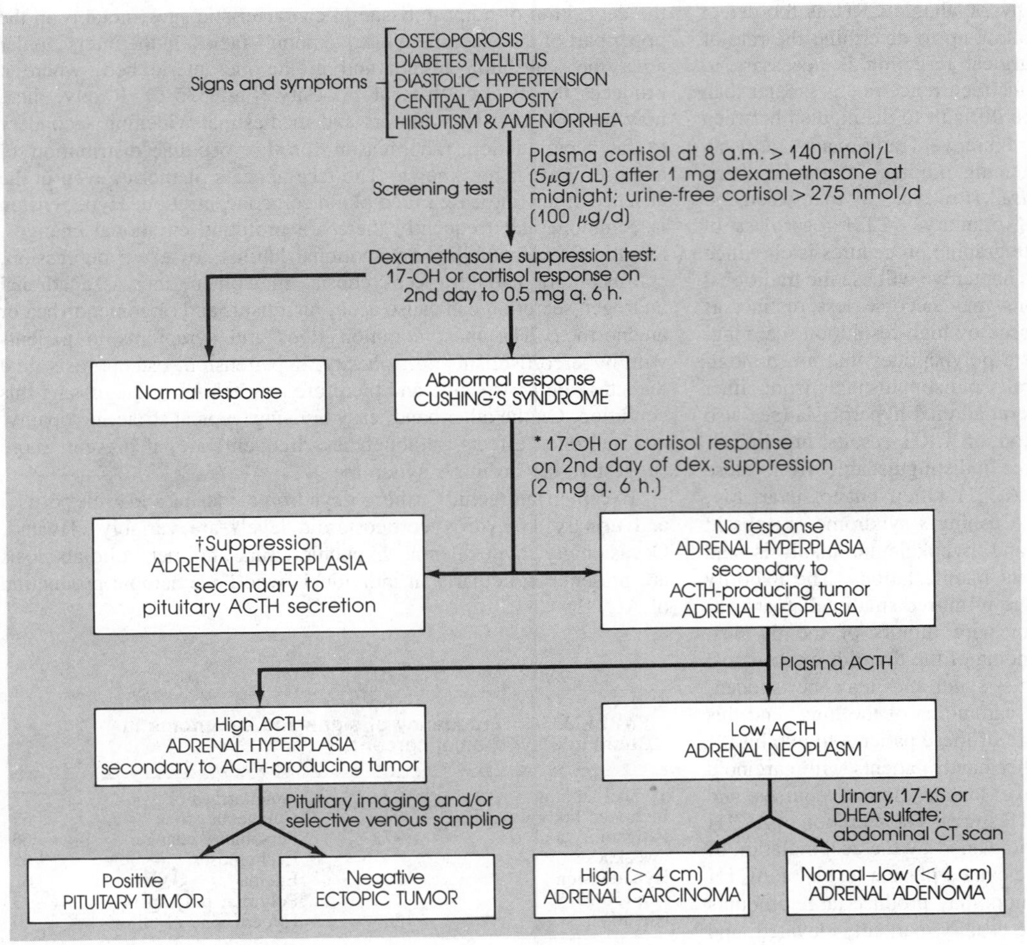

FIGURE 335-7 Diagnostic flowchart for evaluating patients suspected of having Cushing's syndrome.

*The 17-hydroxycorticosteroid response to metyrapone (750 mg given orally every 4 h for six doses) may be used as an alternative test to the high-dose dexamethasone test (2 mg given orally every 6 h). Increased urinary 17-hydroxycorticosteroid excretion following metyrapone occurs in the majority of patients with adrenal hyperplasia secondary to pituitary ACTH secretion; no response suggests an adrenal neoplasm or adrenal hyperplasia secondary to a nonendocrine ACTH-producing tumor.

†This group of patients probably contains subjects with both pituitary-hypothalamic dysfunction and pituitary microadenomas. In some instances, a pituitary microadenoma may be visualized by MRI scanning of the sella turcica.

Signs and symptoms — OSTEOPOROSIS / DIABETES MELLITUS / DIASTOLIC HYPERTENSION / CENTRAL ADIPOSITY / HIRSUTISM & AMENORRHEA

Screening test — Plasma cortisol at 8 a.m. > 140 nmol/L (5μg/dL) after 1 mg dexamethasone at midnight; urine-free cortisol > 275 nmol/d (100 μg/d)

Dexamethasone suppression test: 17-OH or cortisol response on 2nd day to 0.5 mg q. 6 h.

→ Normal response

→ Abnormal response CUSHING'S SYNDROME

*17-OH or cortisol response on 2nd day of dex. suppression (2 mg q. 6 h.)

†Suppression ADRENAL HYPERPLASIA secondary to pituitary ACTH secretion

No response ADRENAL HYPERPLASIA secondary to ACTH-producing tumor ADRENAL NEOPLASIA

Plasma ACTH

High ACTH ADRENAL HYPERPLASIA secondary to ACTH-producing tumor

Low ACTH ADRENAL NEOPLASM

Pituitary imaging and/or selective venous sampling

Urinary, 17-KS or DHEA sulfate; abdominal CT scan

Positive PITUITARY TUMOR

Negative ECTOPIC TUMOR

High (> 4 cm) ADRENAL CARCINOMA

Normal–low (< 4 cm) ADRENAL ADENOMA

sometimes clinical, changes in hormonal secretion, often dramatic, that may occur in the tumors producing this syndrome (periodic hormonogenesis). No test has a specificity greater than 95 percent, and it may be necessary to use a combination of tests to arrive at the correct diagnosis. A particularly useful step to distinguish patients with an ACTH-secreting pituitary microadenoma or hypothalamic-pituitary dysfunction from those with other forms of Cushing's syndrome is to determine the response of cortisol output to high-dose dexamethasone administration (2 mg every 6 h for 2 days). Indeed, when the diagnosis of Cushing's syndrome is clear-cut on the basis of baseline urinary and plasma assays, the high-dose dexamethasone suppression test may be utilized without performing the preliminary low-dose suppression test. The high-dose suppression test provides close to 100 percent specificity if the criteria are a suppression of urinary free cortisol by greater than 90 percent and/or 17-hydroxysteroid levels by greater than 65 percent. Occasionally, in individuals with bilateral nodular hyperplasia and/or ectopic CRH production, steroid output is also suppressed. Failure to suppress cortisol production after low- and high-dose dexamethasone administration (see Table 335-5) is usual in patients with adrenal hyperplasia secondary to an ACTH-secreting pituitary macroadenoma or ACTH-producing tumors of nonendocrine origin and in those with adrenal neoplasms.

Theoretically, plasma ACTH levels should be useful in distinguishing the various causes of Cushing's syndrome, particularly in separating the ACTH-dependent from the ACTH-independent causes. In general, this is true for the ACTH-independent etiologies of the syndrome, since most adrenal tumors have low or undetectable ACTH levels. Furthermore, ACTH-secreting pituitary macroadenomas and ACTH-producing nonendocrine tumors usually have elevated ACTH levels. In the ectopic ACTH syndrome, ACTH levels may be elevated above 110 pmol/L (500 pg/mL), with the majority above 40 pmol/L (200 pg/mL). In Cushing's syndrome, as the result of a microadenoma or pituitary-hypothalamic dysfunction, ACTH levels range from 10 to 30 pmol/L (50 to 150 pg/mL) [normal <18 pmol/L (<80 pg/mL)], with half of values within the normal range. However, two problems hinder the utilization of ACTH levels in the differential diagnosis of Cushing's syndrome. First, it is difficult to collect and measure ACTH levels, and second, ACTH levels may be similar in individuals with hypothalamic-pituitary dysfunction, pituitary microadenomas, ectopic CRH production, and ACTH production from some nonendocrine tumors (especially carcinoid tumors) (see Table 335-5).

Because of these difficulties, several additional tests have been advocated, e.g., the metyrapone and the CRH infusion tests. The rationales underlying these tests are similar: Steroid hypersecretion secondary to an adrenal tumor or the ectopic production of ACTH will suppress the hypothalamic-pituitary axis so that inhibition of pituitary ACTH release can be demonstrated by either test. Thus most patients with pituitary-hypothalamic dysfunction and/or a microadenoma have an increase in steroid or ACTH secretion in response to metyrapone and CRH administration, while most ectopic ACTH-producing tumors and adrenal tumors will not. Most pituitary macroadenomas also respond to CRH, while their response to metyrapone is variable. The utility of the CRH infusion test, however, is uncertain, since only a limited number of studies have been performed and since CRH is not clinically available for testing. In addition, false-positive and -negative CRH tests in patients with nonendocrine and pituitary tumors have been reported.

The major diagnostic dilemma in Cushing's syndrome is to distinguish between those individuals with microadenoma of the pituitary and/or pituitary-hypothalamic dysfunction from some paraendocrine tumors (e.g., carcinoids or pheochromocytoma) that ectopically produce CRH and/or ACTH. Clinical manifestations are similar unless the ectopic tumor produces other symptoms, such as diarrhea and flushing from a carcinoid tumor or episodic hypertension from a pheochromocytoma. Sometimes one can distinguish between ectopic and pituitary ACTH production by using metyrapone or CRH tests as noted above. In these situations, computed tomography (CT) scan of the pituitary gland is usually within normal limits. Magnetic

resonance imaging (MRI) with the enhancing agent gadolinium may be superior to CT scanning in demonstrating a pituitary microadenoma in some patients with Cushing's disease. However, finding a structural feature consistent with an adenoma does not prove that the lesion is secreting ACTH. In fact, as the resolution of scanners becomes greater, more variations of the normal pituitary anatomy will be imaged. For this reason, selective venous sampling for ACTH is employed in some centers. Demonstration of a gradient between ACTH level in the petrosal sinus and in peripheral blood localizes the source of ACTH overproduction to the pituitary gland but does not distinguish pituitary-dependent adrenal hyperplasia from pituitary hyperplasia secondary to a tumor producing CRH. CRH levels should be measured in the peripheral blood prior to petrosal sinus sampling. No reliable test is available to make this distinction if the ectopic tumor is not seen or if it produces no other hormones.

The diagnosis of *cortisol-producing adrenal adenoma* is suggested by disproportionate elevations in baseline urine 17-hydroxycorticosteroid or free-cortisol levels with only modest rises or suppression of urinary 17-ketosteroids or plasma DHEA sulfate. Adrenal androgen secretion is usually reduced in these patients owing to the cortisol-induced suppression of ACTH and subsequent involution of the androgen-producing zona reticularis.

The diagnosis of *adrenal carcinoma* is suggested by a palpable abdominal mass and by *markedly* elevated baseline values of *both* urine 17-hydroxysteroids and plasma DHEA sulfate. Plasma and urine cortisol levels are variably elevated. Adrenal carcinoma is usually resistant to both ACTH stimulation and dexamethasone suppression. Markedly elevated adrenal androgen secretion often leads to virilization in the female. Feminizing estrogen-producing adrenocortical carcinoma usually presents with gynecomastia in the male and dysfunctional uterine bleeding in the female. These adrenal tumors secrete increased amounts of androstenedione which is peripherally converted to the estrogens estrone and estradiol (see Chap. 341). Functioning adrenal carcinomas that produce Cushing's syndrome are most often associated with elevated values for the intermediates of steroid biosynthesis (especially 11-deoxycortisol), suggesting inefficient conversion of the intermediates to the final product. Approximately 20 percent of adrenal carcinomas are not associated with endocrine syndromes and are presumed to be nonfunctioning or to produce biologically inactive steroid precursors. In addition, the excessive production of gonadal steroids is not detectable in certain situations (e.g., androgens in adult men).

Differential diagnosis PSEUDOCUSHING'S SYNDROME A variety of groups may present problems in diagnosis; these are patients with obesity, chronic alcoholism, depression, and acute illness of any type. Extreme *obesity* is uncommon in Cushing's syndrome; furthermore, with exogenous obesity, the adiposity is generalized, not truncal. On adrenocortical testing, abnormalities in patients with exogenous obesity are usually modest. Basal urine steroid excretion levels in obese patients are either normal or slightly elevated, a finding similar to their cortisol secretory values. Some patients have elevated conversion of secreted cortisol into excreted metabolites. *Urinary* and *blood cortisol* levels are normal, and the diurnal pattern in blood and urine levels is normal. Patients with *chronic alcoholism* and *depression* share similar abnormalities in steroid output: modestly elevated urine cortisol and 17-hydroxysteroids, absent diurnal rhythm of cortisol levels, and resistance to suppression with dexamethasone (particularly overnight and low dose). In contrast to alcoholic subjects, depressed patients do not have clinical signs and symptoms of Cushing's syndrome. Following discontinuation of alcohol and/or improvement in the emotional status, steroid testing usually returns to normal. A normal cortisol response to insulin-induced hypoglycemia may distinguish these patients from subjects with Cushing's syndrome. *Acutely ill* subjects often have abnormal laboratory tests and fail to suppress with dexamethasone, since major stress (such as pain or fever) interrupts the normal regulation of ACTH secretion. A rare cause of hypercortisolism without cushingoid stigmata is *primary cortisol resistance*; the resistance is incomplete because patients do

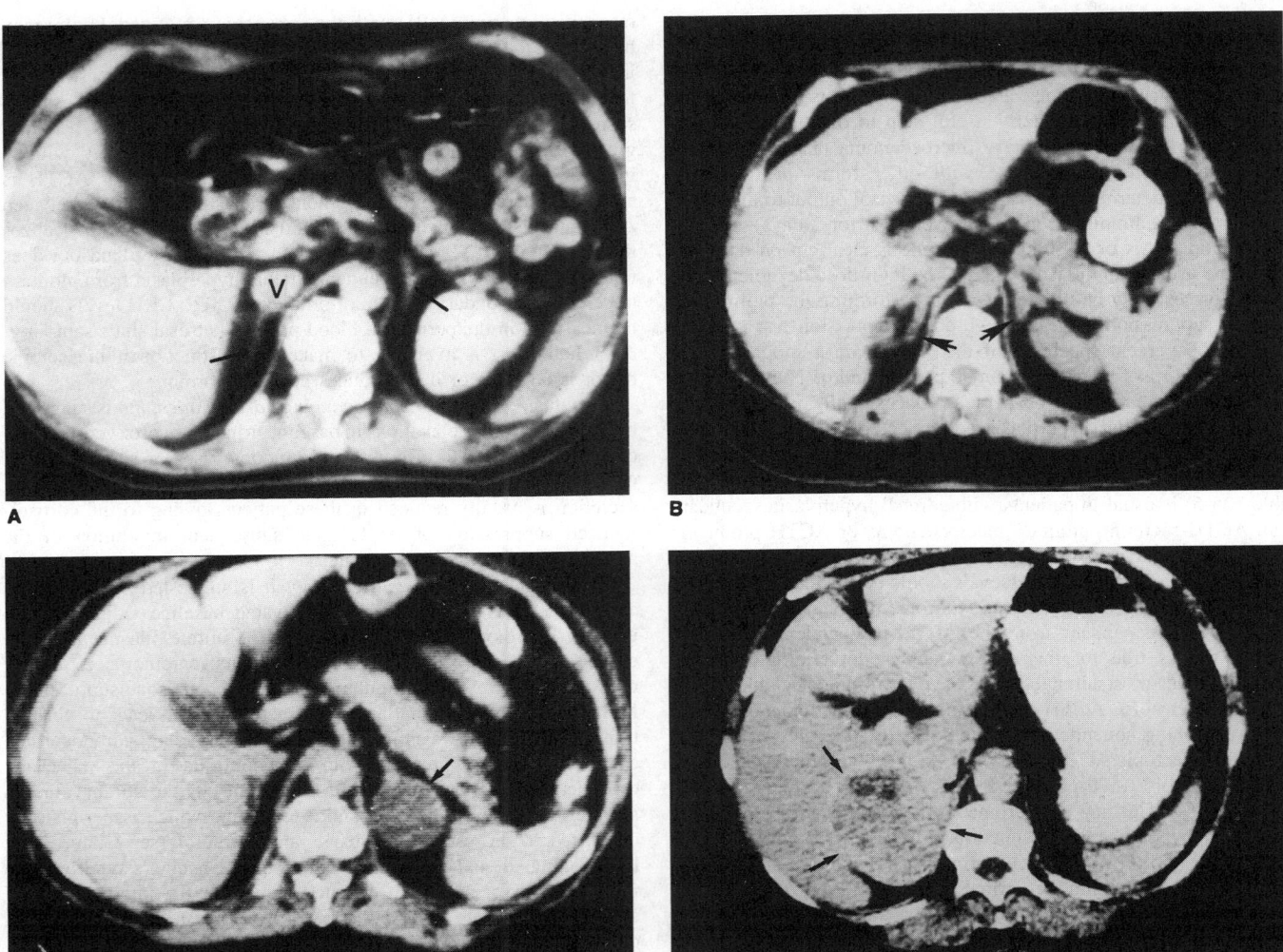

FIGURE 335-8 Computed tomography is the preferred method for visualizing the adrenal glands. The adrenal glands are indicated by arrows. *A*. The normal right adrenal gland is adjacent to the inferior vena cava (V) as it emerges from the liver. Approximately 90 percent of the right adrenal glands appear as linear structures extending posteriorly from the inferior vena cava into the space between the right lobe of the liver and the crus of the diaphragm. The normal left adrenal gland is lateral to the left crus of the diaphragm and below the stomach. The majority of left adrenal glands are shaped like an inverted V or Y. *B*. Adrenal CT scan of a patient with ectopic ACTH production. Both adrenal glands (*arrows*) are enlarged (compare with *A*). In contrast, only 50 percent of patients with bilateral adrenal hyperplasia secondary to pituitary ACTH hypersecretion show enlargement of the adrenals when imaged by CT scan. *C*. CT scan of a patient with Cushing's syndrome with biochemical evidence only of cortisol overproduction. The left adrenal has been replaced by a racquet-shaped 2-cm tumor (*arrow*). Attenuation of the tumor is low because of its high lipid content. *D*. CT scan in a patient with Cushing's syndrome and biochemical evidence of an adrenal carcinoma. In contrast to *C*, the right-sided mass has a heterogeneous appearance and is larger in size—usual characteristics of an adrenal carcinoma.

not exhibit signs of adrenal insufficiency. *Iatrogenic Cushing's syndrome*, induced by the administration of glucocorticoids, is indistinguishable by physical findings from endogenous adrenocortical hyperfunction. This situation can be distinguished by measuring blood or urine cortisol levels or urinary 17-hydroxysteroid excretion in a basal state where the levels are low secondary to suppression of the pituitary-adrenal axis. The severity of iatrogenic Cushing's syndrome is related to the total steroid dose, to the biologic half-life of the steroid preparation, and to the duration of therapy. Also, individuals on afternoon and evening doses of steroid develop Cushing's syndrome more readily and on smaller total daily steroid doses than do patients on a steroid program limited to morning doses only. The enzymatic disposition and binding of administered steroids also differ among patients.

Radiologic evaluation for Cushing's syndrome   The preferred radiologic study to visualize the adrenals is CT scan of the abdomen (Fig. 335-8). This procedure has largely replaced previous invasive procedures (such as selective adrenal arteriography and venography)

and 19-[¹³¹I]iodocholesterol scanning; the CT scan is of value both in localizing adrenal tumors and in differentiating them from bilateral hyperplasia. All patients believed to have hypersecretion of pituitary ACTH should have a pituitary MRI scan with the contrast agent gadolinium. Even with this technique small microadenomas may be undetectable; alternatively, false-positive masses due to nonsecretory variations of the normal pituitary anatomy may be imaged.

Evaluation of asymptomatic adrenal masses   With abdominal CT scanning, many incidental adrenal masses are discovered. This is not surprising, since 10 to 20 percent of subjects at autopsy have adrenocortical adenomas. The first step in evaluating such patients is to determine if the tumor is functioning by appropriate screening tests. However, in 90 percent of the cases, tumors detected incidentally at the time of abdominal CT scanning are nonfunctioning. Fortunately, they also are seldom malignant. Yet nonfunctioning tumors raise difficult therapeutic questions. Since 20 percent of adrenal carcinomas are nonfunctioning, one could argue that all such lesions should be removed. However, the frequency of adrenal carcinomas is low compared with the frequency of benign cortical adenomas (less than 1 percent), and surgery is not indicated in most cases. The size of the tumor sometimes is of value; adrenal carcinomas are rarely smaller than 3 cm in diameter, and adrenal adenomas are usually smaller than 6 cm (see Fig. 335-8). If surgery is not performed, a repeat CT scan in 3 to 6 months is usually required for followup.

Therapy ADRENAL NEOPLASMS When an adenoma or carcinoma is diagnosed, adrenal exploration is performed with excision of the tumor. Because of the possible atrophy of the contralateral adrenal, the patient is treated pre- and postoperatively as if for total adrenalectomy even when a unilateral lesion is suspected, the routine being similar to that for an Addisonian patient undergoing elective surgery (Table 335-11).

Despite operative intervention, most patients with adrenal carcinoma die within 3 years of diagnosis. Metastases occur most often to liver and lung. The principal antitumor drug used to treat metastatic adrenocortical carcinoma is mitotane (*o,p'*-DDD), an isomer of the insecticide DDT. This drug suppresses cortisol production and decreases plasma and urine steroid levels. Although its cytotoxic action is relatively selective for the glucocorticoid-secreting zone of the adrenal cortex, the zona glomerulosa also may be inhibited. Because mitotane also alters the extraadrenal metabolism of cortisol, plasma and urinary cortisol levels must be assessed to titrate the effect. The drug is usually given in divided doses three to four times a day, with the dose increased gradually to 8 to 10 g daily. At higher doses, almost all patients experience gastrointestinal side effects (anorexia, diarrhea, or vomiting) or neuromuscular side effects (lethargy, somnolence, or dizziness). All patients treated with mitotane should be placed on long-term maintenance glucocorticoid therapy, and in some, mineralocorticoid replacement is appropriate. In approximately one-third of patients, regression of both tumor and metastases occurs, but long-term survival is limited. In many patients, mitotane only inhibits steroidogenesis and does not cause regression of tumor metastases. Osseous metastases are usually refractory to the drug and should be treated with radiation therapy. Mitotane also can be given as adjunctive therapy after surgical resection of an adrenal carcinoma, although there is no evidence this improves survival.

BILATERAL HYPERPLASIA Patients with hyperplasia have a relative or absolute increase in ACTH levels. Since therapy would logically be directed at reducing ACTH levels, the ideal primary treatment for ACTH- or CRH-producing tumors, whether in the pituitary or ectopic, is surgical removal. Occasionally, this is not possible because the disease, particularly with ectopic ACTH production, is often far advanced. In this situation, "medical" or surgical adrenalectomy may be indicated to correct the hypercortisolism.

Controversy exists as to the proper treatment for bilateral adrenal hyperplasia when the source of the ACTH overproduction is not apparent. In some centers, these patients (especially patients with a positive high-dose dexamethasone suppression test) have surgical exploration of the pituitary via a transsphenoidal approach in anticipation of a microadenoma being found. These explorations prove fruitful in between 20 and 70 percent of the cases, depending on the skill of the surgeon and the ability of the radiologist to localize the microadenoma preoperatively. In equivocal circumstances, selective petrosal sinus venous sampling may be performed, or the patient may be referred to an appropriate center if the procedure is not locally available. In the event that a microadenoma is not found at the time of exploration, total hypophysectomy may be needed. Complications of transsphenoidal surgery include cerebrospinal fluid rhinorrhea, diabetes insipidus, panhypopituitarism, and optic or cranial nerve injuries. Furthermore, these pituitary neoplasms may recur if the primary abnormality actually resides in the hypothalamus.

In other centers, total adrenalectomy is the treatment of choice. Cure with this procedure is close to 100 percent. The adverse effects include the certain need for lifelong mineralocorticoid and glucocorticoid replacement therapy and a 10 to 20 percent probability of a pituitary tumor developing over the next 10 years, many requiring surgical therapy (Nelson's syndrome). It is uncertain whether in these

individuals (see Chap. 331) the tumor develops de novo or is present prior to bilateral adrenalectomy but is so small that it is not detected by routine procedures. Periodic radiologic evaluation of the pituitary gland by MRI and serial ACTH levels should be obtained in any individual who has undergone bilateral adrenalectomy for Cushing's syndrome. Often, such pituitary tumors become locally invasive and impinge on the optic chiasm or extend into the cavernous or sphenoid sinuses. Thus an aggressive surgical approach is often followed by postoperative irradiation.

In a few centers, pituitary radiation is the primary treatment for pituitary ACTH overproduction, with the use of either conventional external or alpha (proton-beam) radiation. The latter, while more effective, has a greater incidence of ocular motor palsy and hypopituitarism than does conventional radiation therapy. The long lag time between treatment and remission and the fact that the remission rate is less than 50 percent often contraindicate the use of external pituitary radiation in the presence of rapidly progressive or severe Cushing's syndrome.

Finally, in occasional patients in whom a surgical approach is not feasible, medical therapy directed at reducing hypothalamic CRH release either by administering the serotonin antagonist cyproheptadine or the inhibitor of GABA transaminase sodium valproate has been successful in reducing cortisol secretion. Bromocriptine, a dopaminergic agonist, also suppresses ACTH output in occasional patients.

If ACTH levels cannot be lowered successfully by any of the above treatment modalities, then "medical" or surgical adrenalectomy may be indicated (Table 335-6). Inhibition of steroidogenesis also may be indicated in severely cushingoid subjects prior to surgical intervention. Chemical adrenalectomy may be accomplished by the administration of the inhibitor of steroidogenesis, ketoconazole (600 to 1200 mg/d). In addition, mitotane (2 or 3 g/d) and/or the blockers of steroid synthesis aminoglutethimide (1 g/d) and metyrapone (2 or 3 g/d) have been effective either alone or in combination. Mitotane is slow in onset of action (over weeks). Hypoadrenalism is a risk with all these agents, and replacement steroids may be required.

ALDOSTERONISM Aldosteronism is a syndrome associated with hypersecretion of the major adrenal mineralocorticoid aldosterone. *Primary* aldosteronism signifies that the stimulus for the excessive aldosterone production resides within the adrenal gland; in *secondary* aldosteronism, the stimulus is extraadrenal.

Primary aldosteronism In the original case of excessive and inappropriate aldosterone production, the disease was the result of an *aldosterone-producing adrenal adenoma* (Conn's syndrome). The majority of cases involve a unilateral adenoma, usually small and occurring with equal frequency on either side. Rarely, primary aldosteronism occurs in association with adrenal carcinoma. It is twice as common in women as in men, occurs between the ages of 30 and 50, and is present in approximately 1 percent of unselected hypertensive patients. Many cases have clinical and biochemical features characteristic of primary aldosteronism, but a solitary adenoma is not found at surgery. Instead, these patients have *bilateral cortical nodular hyperplasia.* In the literature this disease has been alternatively termed "pseudo" primary aldosteronism, idiopathic hyperaldosteronism, or nodular hyperplasia. The cause is unknown.

TABLE 335-6 Treatment modalities for patients with adrenal hyperplasia secondary to pituitary ACTH hypersecretion

Reduce pituitary ACTH production
  A Transsphenoidal resection of microadenoma
  B Radiation
  C Treatment with hypothalamic serotonin antagonist (cyproheptadine) or GABA-transaminase inhibitor (sodium valproate)*
Reduce or eliminate adrenocortical cortisol secretion
  A Bilateral adrenalectomy
  B Medical adrenalectomy (metyrapone, mitotane, aminoglutethimide, ketoconazole)*

* Not curative but effective as long as chronically administered in selected patients.

SIGNS AND SYMPTOMS   The continual hypersecretion of aldosterone increases the renal distal tubular exchange of intratubular sodium for secreted potassium and hydrogen ions, with progressive depletion of body potassium and development of hypokalemia. Most patients have diastolic hypertension, usually not of marked severity, and complain of headaches. The hypertension is probably due to the increased sodium reabsorption and extracellular volume expansion. Potassium depletion is responsible for the muscle weakness and fatigue and is related to the effect of potassium depletion on muscle membrane. The polyuria results from impairment of concentrating ability and is often associated with polydipsia. Electrocardiographic and roentgenographic signs of left ventricular enlargement are secondary to the hypertension. Electrocardiographic signs of potassium depletion, such as prominent U waves, cardiac arrhythmias, and premature contractions, are common. In the absence of associated congestive heart failure, renal disease, or preexisting abnormalities (such as thrombophlebitis), edema is characteristically absent. In cases of long duration, nephropathy with azotemia may be associated with congestive heart failure and edema.

LABORATORY FINDINGS   Laboratory findings are dependent on both the duration and the severity of the potassium depletion. An overnight concentration test often reveals impaired ability to concentrate the urine, probably secondary to the hypokalemia. Urine pH is neutral to alkaline because of excessive secretion of ammonium and bicarbonate ions to compensate for a metabolic alkalosis. Tests of glucocorticoid and androgen secretion are within the normal range.

Hypokalemia may be severe (less than 3 mmol/L) and reflects significant body potassium depletion, usually in excess of 300 mmol. *Hypernatremia* is due to both sodium retention and a concomitant water loss from polyuria. Metabolic alkalosis and elevation of serum bicarbonate are a result of hydrogen ion loss into the urine and migration into potassium-depleted cells. The alkalosis is perpetuated by potassium deficiency, which increases the capacity of the proximal convoluted tubule to reabsorb filtered bicarbonate. If hypokalemia is severe, serum magnesium levels are also reduced. In the absence of azotemia, serum uric acid is normal.

Total-body sodium content and total exchangeable sodium usually are increased, while total exchangeable body potassium is reduced. The expanded extracellular fluid volume may be responsible for the reversed diurnal excretory pattern for salt and water, with predominant salt and water excretion occurring during the night.

DIAGNOSIS   The diagnosis is suggested by persistent hypokalemia in a nonedematous patient on a normal sodium intake who is not receiving potassium-wasting diuretics (furosemide, ethacrynic acid, thiazides). If hypokalemia occurs in a hypertensive patient on a potassium-wasting diuretic, the diuretic should be discontinued and the patient should be given potassium supplements. After 1 to 2 weeks, the potassium level should be remeasured, and if hypokalemia persists, the patient should be evaluated for a mineralocorticoid excess syndrome (Fig. 335-9).

The criteria for the diagnosis of primary aldosteronism are (1) diastolic hypertension without edema, (2) hyposecretion of renin (as judged by low plasma renin activity levels) that fails to increase appropriately during volume depletion (upright posture, sodium depletion), and (3) hypersecretion of aldosterone that fails to suppress appropriately during volume expansion (salt loading).

Patients with primary aldosteronism characteristically *do not have edema*, since they exhibit an "escape" phenomenon from the sodium-retaining aspects of mineralocorticoids. Rarely, pretibial edema may be present in patients with associated nephropathy and azotemia.

The estimation of plasma renin activity is of limited value in separating patients with primary aldosteronism from those with other causes of hypertension. While the failure of plasma renin activity to rise normally during volume-depletion maneuvers is a criterion for primary aldosteronism, suppressed renin activity also occurs in about 25 percent of patients with essential hypertension.

Since the determination of plasma renin responsiveness is not sufficient, the demonstration of lack of suppression of aldosterone

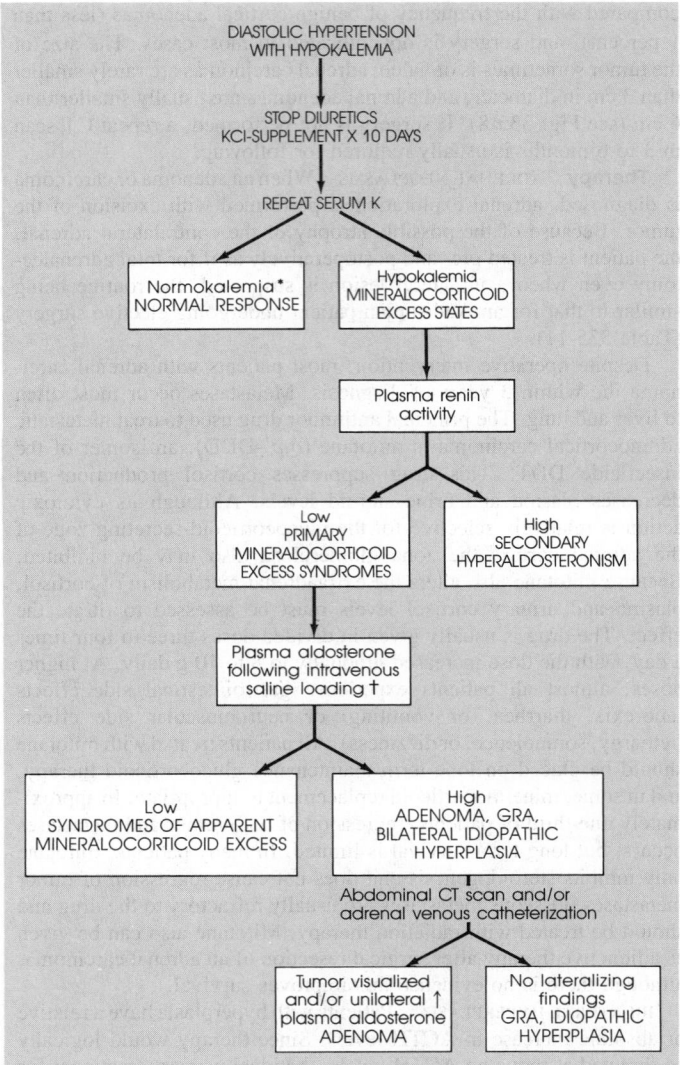

FIGURE 335-9 Diagnostic flowchart for evaluating patients with suspected primary aldosteronism.

*Serum K⁺ may be normal in some patients with hyperaldosteronism who are taking potassium-sparing diuretics (spironolactone, triamterene) or ingesting low sodium–high potassium intakes.

†This step should not be taken if hypertension is severe (diastolic pressure >115 mmHg) or if cardiac failure is present. Also, serum potassium levels should be corrected before the infusion of saline solution. Alternative methods producing comparable suppression of aldosterone secretion include oral sodium loading (200 mmol/d for 3 days) or 10 mg deoxycorticosterone acetate (DOCA) intramuscularly every 12 h for 3 days. (GRA = glucocorticoid-remediable aldosteronism.)

secretion is necessary to diagnose primary aldosteronism (see Fig. 335-9). The autonomy exhibited by aldosterone tumors in these patients refers only to the resistance to suppression of secretion during volume expansion; such tumors can and do respond in normal or above-normal fashion to the stimuli of potassium loading or ACTH infusion.

Once hyposecretion of renin and failure to suppress aldosterone secretion are demonstrated, localization of aldosterone-producing adenomas should be determined preoperatively by abdominal CT scan or by percutaneous transfemoral bilateral adrenal vein catheterization with simultaneous adrenal venography. The latter technique permits radiologic localization, and in addition, the adrenal vein sampling may demonstrate a two- to threefold increase in plasma aldosterone concentration on the involved side compared with the uninvolved side. In cases of hyperaldosteronism secondary to cortical nodular hyperplasia, no localization is found. It is important for samples to be obtained simultaneously if possible and for cortisol levels to be measured to ensure that false localization does not reflect an ACTH- or stress-induced rise in aldosterone levels.

DIFFERENTIAL DIAGNOSIS   Patients with hypertension and hypokalemia may have primary or secondary hyperaldosteronism (see Fig. 335-10). A useful maneuver to distinguish between them is the measurement of plasma renin activity. Secondary hyperaldosteronism in patients with accelerated hypertension is due to elevated plasma renin levels; in contrast, patients with primary aldosteronism have suppressed plasma renin levels.

Primary aldosteronism also must be distinguished from other *hypermineralocorticoid states*. The common problem is to distinguish between hyperaldosteronism due to an adenoma and that due to idiopathic bilateral nodular hyperplasia. This is of importance because hypertension associated with idiopathic hyperplasia is usually not benefited by bilateral adrenalectomy, whereas hypertension associated with aldosterone-producing tumors is usually improved or cured following removal of the adenoma. Although patients with idiopathic bilateral nodular hyperplasia tend to have less severe hypokalemia, lower aldosterone secretion, and higher plasma renin activity than do patients with primary aldosteronism, differentiation is impossible solely on clinical and/or biochemical grounds. An anomalous postural decrease in plasma aldosterone and elevated plasma 18-hydroxycorticosterone levels are present in most patients with a unilateral lesion. However, these tests are also of limited diagnostic value in the individual patient, since some adenoma patients have an increase in plasma aldosterone with upright posture. A definitive diagnosis is best made by radiographic studies, as noted above.

In a few instances, hypertensive patients with hypokalemic alkalosis have been found to have deoxycorticosterone (DOC)-secreting adenomas. Such patients have reduced plasma renin activity levels, but aldosterone measurements are either normal or reduced, suggesting the diagnosis of mineralocorticoid excess due to a hormone other than aldosterone. Rarely, hypermineralocorticoidism is due to a defect in cortisol biosynthesis, specifically 11- or 17-hydroxylation. ACTH levels are increased, with a resultant increase in the production of the mineralocorticoid 11-deoxycorticosterone. *Hypertension and hypokalemia can be corrected by glucocorticoid administration.* The definitive diagnosis is made by demonstrating an elevation of precursors of cortisol biosynthesis in the blood or urine. Occasionally, glucocorticoid administration produces normotension and normokalemia, although a hydroxylase deficiency cannot be identified (see Fig. 335-9). These patients have normal to slightly elevated aldosterone levels that do not fully suppress with saline but usually suppress after 2 weeks of dexamethasone (1 to 2 mg/d). The condition is inherited as an autosomal dominant trait and is termed *glucocorticoid-remediable aldosteronism* (GRA). This entity is secondary to a chimeric gene duplication whereby the 11β-hydroxylase promoter is fused to the aldosterone synthase coding sequence. Thus aldosterone synthase activity is expressed in the zona fasciculata and is regulated only by ACTH, similar to the regulation of cortisol secretion. Screening for this defect is best performed by assessing the presence or absence of the chimeric gene. Alternatively, the urinary 18-hydroxylated cortisol products can be measured. Since the abnormal gene may be present in the absence of hypokalemia, its frequency as a cause of hypertension is unknown. Individuals with juvenile-onset hypertension or a family history of early-onset hypertension and all patients with bilateral nodular hyperplasia should be screened for the disorder.

Another rare cause of hyperkalemia and hypertension is 11β-hydroxysteroid dehydrogenase deficiency in which cortisol cannot be converted to cortisone and hence binds to the glucocorticoid type I (mineralocorticoid) receptor and acts as a mineralocorticoid (see Chap. 329). This condition also has been termed *apparent mineralocorticoid excess syndrome*. The ingestion of candies or chewing tobacco containing certain forms of licorice produces a syndrome mimicking primary aldosteronism. The sodium-retaining principle in such agents is glycyrrhizinic acid, which inhibits the 11β-hydroxysteroid dehydrogenase and hence allows cortisol to act as a mineralocorticoid and causes sodium retention, expansion of the extracellular fluid volume, hypertension, depressed plasma renin levels, and suppressed aldosterone levels. The diagnosis is established or excluded by a careful history.

TREATMENT   Primary aldosteronism due to an adenoma is usually treated by surgical excision. However, dietary sodium restriction and the administration of an aldosterone antagonist, spironolactone, are effective in many cases. Hypertension and hypokalemia are usually controlled by doses of 25 to 100 mg spironolactone every 8 h. Some patients have been successfully managed medically for years, but chronic therapy in men is usually limited by the development of gynecomastia, decreased libido, and impotence.

When idiopathic bilateral hyperplasia is suspected, surgery is indicated only when significant, symptomatic hypokalemia cannot be controlled with medical therapy, e.g., by spironolactone, triamterene, or amiloride. Hypertension associated with idiopathic hyperplasia is usually not benefited by bilateral adrenalectomy.

Glucocorticoid-remediable hyperaldosteronism documented by genetic analysis may be treated with glucocorticoid administration or antimineralocorticoids, e.g., spironolactone, triamterene, or amiloride. Glucocorticoids should be used only in small doses to avoid inducing iatrogenic Cushing's syndrome. A combination approach is often necessary. Patients with 11β-hydroxysteroid dehydrogenase deficiency syndrome can be treated with small doses of dexamethasone. Although dexamethasone is a potent glucocorticoid that suppresses ACTH and endogenous cortisol production, it binds less well to the mineralocorticoid receptor than cortisol.

Secondary aldosteronism   *Secondary aldosteronism* refers to an appropriately increased production of aldosterone in response to activation of the renin-angiotensin system (see Fig. 335-10). The production rates of aldosterone are often higher in patients with secondary aldosteronism than in those with primary aldosteronism. Secondary aldosteronism usually occurs in association with the accelerated phase of hypertension or on the basis of an underlying edema disorder. Secondary aldosteronism in pregnancy is a normal physiologic response to estrogen-induced increases in circulating levels of renin substrate and plasma renin activity and to the antialdosterone actions of progestogens.

Secondary aldosteronism in hypertensive states either is secondary to a primary overproduction of renin (primary reninism) or is caused by an overproduction of renin which is secondary to a decrease in renal blood flow and/or perfusion pressure (see Fig. 335-10). Secondary hypersecretion of renin can be due to a narrowing of one or both of the major renal arteries either by an atherosclerotic plaque or by fibromuscular hyperplasia. Overproduction of renin from both kidneys also occurs in association with severe arteriolar nephrosclerosis (malignant hypertension) or secondary to profound renal vasoconstric-

FIGURE 335-10 Responses of the renin-aldosterone volume control loop in primary versus secondary aldosteronism.

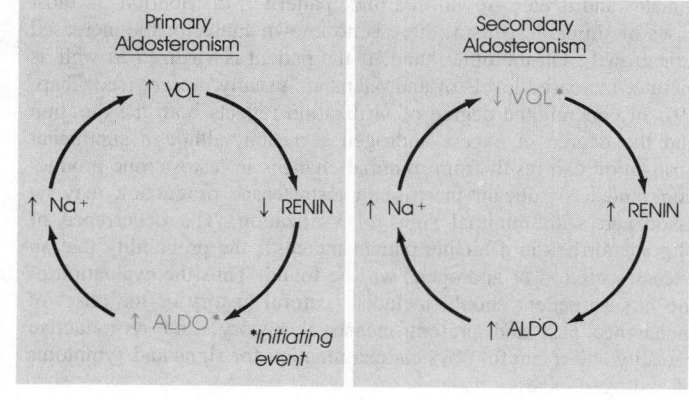

tion (accelerated phase of hypertensive disease). The secondary aldosteronism is characterized by hypokalemic alkalosis, moderate to severe increases in plasma renin activity, and moderate to marked increases in aldosterone levels (see Chap. 209).

Secondary aldosteronism with hypertension also can be caused by a rare renin-producing tumor in so-called primary reninism. These patients have the biochemical characteristics of renal vascular hypertension; however, the primary defect is renin secretion by a juxtaglomerular cell tumor. The diagnosis can be made by the absence of changes in renal vasculature and/or demonstration of a space-occupying lesion in the kidney by radiographic techniques and documentation of unilateral increases in renal vein renin activity. Rarely, these tumors arise in tissues such as the ovary.

Secondary aldosteronism is present in many forms of *edema*. Increased aldosterone secretion rates are usual in patients with edema as a result of either cirrhosis or the nephrotic syndrome. In congestive heart failure, elevated aldosterone secretion varies depending on the severity of cardiac decompensation. The stimulus for aldosterone release in these conditions appears to be *arterial hypovolemia* and/or hypotension. Diuretic therapy often exaggerates the secondary aldosteronism via volume depletion; when this happens, hypokalemia and, on occasion, alkalosis can become prominent features.

Secondary hyperaldosteronism rarely occurs without edema or hypertension (Bartter's syndrome). This syndrome is characterized by the signs of severe hyperaldosteronism (hypokalemic alkalosis) with moderate to marked increases in renin activity but normal blood pressure and absence of edema. Renal biopsy shows juxtaglomerular hyperplasia. The pathogenesis may be a defect in the renal conservation of sodium or chloride and/or an increased production of prostaglandins. The renal loss of sodium is thought to stimulate renin secretion and subsequent aldosterone production. Hyperaldosteronism produces potassium depletion, with the hypokalemia further elevating plasma renin activity. In some cases, the hypokalemia may be potentiated by a defect in renal conservation of potassium. Increased production of prostaglandins is present but is probably not a primary abnormality, since administration of inhibitors of prostaglandin synthesis only temporarily reverses the features of this syndrome (see Chap. 244).

SYNDROMES OF ADRENAL ANDROGEN EXCESS The syndromes of adrenal androgen excess result from excess production of dehydroepiandrosterone and androstenedione, which are converted to testosterone in extraglandular tissues; the elevated testosterone levels account for most of the androgenic effects. Adrenal androgen excess may be associated with the secretion of greater or smaller amounts of other adrenal hormones and may, therefore, present as "pure" syndromes of virilization or as "mixed" syndromes associated with excessive production of glucocorticoids and some characteristics of Cushing's syndrome.

Clinical signs and symptoms The signs and symptoms of androgen excess can be divided into four areas: hirsutism, oligomenorrhea, acne, and virilization. Clinically, it is important to distinguish between hypertrichosis, simple hirsutism, and hirsutism associated with virilization. Hypertrichosis is an increased hair growth in males or females anywhere on the body. In contrast, hirsutism is limited to females and is hair growth in a male pattern of distribution. In most cases of simple hirsutism, there is no known cause for the increased hair growth. On the other hand, if the patient is virilized as well as hirsute, increased levels of androgens are usually present (see Chap. 49). In general, the degree of virilization reflects both the duration and the degree of excess androgen secretion, although significant virilization can result from minimal changes in testosterone production, and a significant increase in testosterone production may be associated with minimal signs of virilization. The occurrence of oligomenorrhea in a hirsute patient increases the probability that an excess secretion of androgens will be found. Thus the evaluation of the hirsute patient should include a careful history of the onset of menarche, past and present menstrual history, and reproductive capacity and a careful physical examination for signs and symptoms of androgen excess.

Etiology As in other states of adrenocortical hyperfunction, the syndromes associated with androgen excess may result from hyperplasia, adenoma, or carcinoma (the latter two having been discussed above). Adrenal androgen overproduction also may arise from *congenital adrenal hyperplasia*, owing to enzymatic defects. In these patients, increased adrenal androgen production is associated either with excess or decreased secretion of mineralocorticoids or decreased production of glucocorticoids. Since, in humans, cortisol is the principal adrenal steroid regulating ACTH elaboration, and since the ACTH stimulates both cortisol and adrenal androgen production, an enzymatic interference with cortisol synthesis may result in the enhanced secretion of adrenal androgens. In severe congenital virilizing hyperplasia, the adrenal output of cortisol may be so compromised as to cause glucocorticoid deficiency despite anatomic adrenal hyperplasia.

Congenital adrenal hyperplasia is the most common adrenal disorder of infancy and childhood. These children usually have severe enzyme deficiencies (see Chap. 342). The deficiency of enzymes is the result of autosomal recessive mutations. Partial adrenal enzyme deficiencies can be expressed after adolescence, predominantly in women with hirsutism and oligomenorrhea but minimal virilization. Late-onset adrenal hyperplasia may account for 5 to 25 percent of women with hirsutism and oligomenorrhea, depending on the patient population.

Congenital adrenal hyperplasia is secondary to one of several defects in steroid synthesis. To date, defects have been described in the $P450_{C21}$, $P450_{C18}$, $P450_{C17\alpha}$, and $P450_{C11\beta}$ hydroxylases and in 3β-hydroxysteroid dehydrogenase (3β-HSD) (see Fig. 335-2). While the cDNAs for these enzymes have been cloned, the diagnosis of specific enzyme deficiencies with genetic techniques is not practical for routine use. These enzyme deficits usually occur singly. $P450_{C21}$ deficiency is closely linked to the histocompatibility leukocyte antigen (HLA-B) locus of chromosome 6 so that HLA typing and/or DNA polymorphism can be used to detect the heterozygous carriers and to diagnose affected individuals in some families (see Chap. 64). The clinical expression in the different disorders is variable, ranging from virilization of the female ($P450_{C21}$) to feminization of the male (3β-HSD). (See also Chap. 342.)

Adrenal virilization in the female at birth is associated with ambiguous external genitalia (*female pseudohermaphroditism*). The onset of virilization is most probably after the fifth month of embryonic development. At birth there may be enlarged genitalia in the male infant and enlargement of the clitoris, partial or complete fusion of the labia, and sometimes a urogenital sinus in the female. If the labial fusion is nearly complete, the female infant has external genitalia resembling a penis with hypospadias. In the *postnatal* period, congenital adrenal hyperplasia is associated with virilization in the female and isosexual precocity in the male. The excessive androgens result in accelerated growth, with bone age exceeding chronologic age. Since epiphyseal closure is hastened by excessive androgens, growth stops, but truncal development continues, giving the characteristic appearance of a child of short stature with a well-developed trunk.

The most common form of congenital adrenal hyperplasia (95 percent of cases) is a result of impairment of $P450_{C21}$. In addition to cortisol deficiency, there is an associated reduction in aldosterone secretion in approximately one-third of the patients. Thus, with $P450_{C21}$ deficiency, adrenal virilization occurs with or without an associated salt-losing tendency due to aldosterone deficiency (see Fig. 335-2).

$P450_{C11\beta}$ deficiency may cause a "hypertensive" variant of congenital adrenal hyperplasia. Hypertension and hypokalemia can occur because of the impaired conversion of 11-deoxycorticosterone to corticosterone, resulting in the accumulation of 11-deoxycorticosterone, a potent mineralocorticoid. The presence of hypertension is variable. Increased shunting again occurs into the androgen pathway.

$P450_{C17\alpha}$ deficiency is characterized by hypogonadism, hypokalemia, and hypertension. This rare disorder causes decreased production of cortisol and shunting of precursors into the mineralocorticoid pathway with hypokalemic alkalosis, hypertension, and suppressed plasma renin activity. Usually, 11-deoxycorticosterone production is elevated. Because $P450_{C17\alpha}$ hydroxylation is required for biosynthesis of adrenal androgens and for biosynthesis of gonadal testosterone and estrogen, this defect is associated with sexual immaturity, high urinary gonadotropin levels, and low urinary 17-ketosteroid excretion. Female patients have primary amenorrhea and lack of development of secondary sexual characteristics. Because of deficient androgen production, male patients either have ambiguous external genitalia or a female phenotype (male pseudohermaphroditism). Exogenous glucocorticoids can correct the hypertensive syndrome, and treatment with appropriate gonadal steroids results in sexual maturation.

With 3β-HSD deficiency, conversion of pregnenolone to progesterone is impaired, with the result that pathways to both cortisol and aldosterone are "blocked," with shunting then occurring into the adrenal androgen pathway via 17α-hydroxypregnenolone to dehydroepiandrosterone. Since dehydroepiandrosterone is a weak androgen, and because this enzyme deficiency is also present in the gonad, the genitalia of the male fetus may be incompletely virilized or feminized. Conversely, in the female, overproduction of dehydroepiandrosterone may produce partial virilization.

Diagnosis The diagnosis of *congenital adrenal hyperplasia* should be considered in all infants exhibiting "failure to thrive," particularly those having episodes of acute adrenal insufficiency or salt wasting or showing sustained hypertension. The diagnosis is further suggested by the finding of hypertrophy of the clitoris, fused labia, or urogenital sinus in the female and isosexual precocity in the male. In infants and children with a *$P450_{C21}$ block*, increased urine 17-ketosteroid excretion and increased plasma DHEA sulfate are typically associated with an increase in the blood levels of 17-hydroxyprogesterone and the excretion of its urinary metabolite pregnanetriol. Demonstration of elevated levels of 17-hydroxyprogesterone in amniotic fluid at 14 to 16 weeks of gestation allows prenatal detection of affected female infants.

The diagnosis of a *salt-losing form of congenital adrenal hyperplasia* due to defects in $P450_{C21}$ is suggested by episodes of acute adrenal insufficiency with hyponatremia, hyperkalemia, dehydration, and vomiting. These infants and children often crave salt and exhibit laboratory signs of concomitant deficits in both cortisol and aldosterone secretion.

With the *hypertensive form of congenital adrenal hyperplasia* due to $P450_{C11\beta}$ deficiency, 11-deoxycorticosterone and 11-deoxycortisol accumulate. Both urine 17-ketosteroid and 17-hydroxycorticosteroid excretion may be elevated, since 11-deoxycortisol is included in the analysis. The diagnosis is secured by demonstrating increased levels of 11-deoxycortisol in the blood or increased amounts of tetrahydro-11-deoxycortisol in the urine. Elevation of 17-hydroxyprogesterone levels does not imply a concomitant $P450_{C21}$ deficiency.

The finding of very high levels of urine dehydroepiandrosterone with low levels of pregnanetriol and of cortisol metabolites in urine is characteristic of children with 3β-HSD deficiency. Marked salt wasting may also occur.

Adults with *late-onset adrenal hyperplasia* (partial deficiency of $P450_{C21}$, $P450_{C11\beta}$, or 3β-HSD) are characterized by normal or moderately elevated urinary 17-ketosteroids and plasma DHEA sulfate. A high basal level of a precursor of cortisol biosynthesis (such as 17-hydroxyprogesterone, 17-hydroxypregnenolone, or 11-deoxycortisol) or elevation of the precursor after ACTH stimulation confirms the diagnosis of a partial deficiency. It is uncertain how long ACTH needs to be infused to unmask the enzyme deficiency, but measuring steroid precursors 60 min after the bolus administration of ACTH is usually sufficient. Adrenal androgen output is easily suppressed by the standard low-dose (2 mg) dexamethasone test.

Differential diagnosis The causes of hirsutism can be divided into four broad categories: familial, idiopathic, androgen excess, and drugs. In general, the first two conditions are not associated with other signs of androgen excess, i.e., oligomenorrhea, significant acne,

TABLE 335-7 Causes of hirsutism in women

Familial
Idiopathic
Ovarian
  A Polycystic ovaries; hilus cell hyperplasia
  B Tumor: arrhenoblastoma, hilus cell, adrenal rest
Adrenal
  A Congenital adrenal hyperplasia
  B Noncongenital adrenal hyperplasia (Cushing's)
  C Tumor: virilizing carcinoma or adenoma

or virilization. Likewise, drug-induced hirsutism is usually not associated with other signs and symptoms of androgen excess, unless the drug is an androgen. The drugs that produce an increase in body hair include phenothiazines, minoxidil, and phenytoin. Each of these drugs, particularly minoxidil, produces a generalized increase in hair growth, not just an increase in hair growth in androgen target areas. The mechanism may be related to the ability of these drugs to convert vellus into terminal hair follicles.

If drugs are excluded, the only known causes of hirsutism amenable to treatment are those secondary to excess production of androgens by either the adrenal or the ovary.

In the female, the differential diagnosis of hirsutism and virilization is between adrenal and ovarian etiologies (Table 335-7). *Sudden onset of progressive hirsutism and virilization* suggests an adrenal or ovarian neoplasm. *Adrenal adenomas and carcinomas* may cause a pure or mixed virilizing syndrome. Since adrenal androgens are weak compared with gonadal androgens, adrenal virilization is characterized by *large increments in urine 17-ketosteroid excretion*. Virilizing adrenal adenomas are rare. *Virilizing adrenal carcinomas*, the most common adrenal tumors causing virilization, are associated with high plasma DHEA sulfate levels and high urinary 17-ketosteroid excretion rates, and, as a rule, exceed 6 cm in size. Cortisol levels and 17-hydroxycorticosteroid excretion are normal or moderately elevated. Failure to reduce 17-ketosteroid levels and plasma DHEA sulfate levels to normal following dexamethasone suppression (0.5 mg given orally every 6 h for 2 days) further supports a diagnosis of virilizing adrenal tumor and excludes congenital adrenal hyperplasia. The most common virilizing *ovarian tumor* is the arrhenoblastoma, but other ovarian tumors, such as adrenal rest tumor, granulosa cell tumor, hilar cell tumor, and Brenner tumor, have been associated with virilization. Virilization due to ovarian tumors is usually characterized by normal levels of urinary 17-ketosteroids and DHEA sulfate, since the neoplasm usually secretes the potent androgen testosterone. Occasionally, increases in 17-ketosteroid excretion occur in some patients with ovarian neoplasms, but baseline 17-ketosteroid excretion in excess of 100 μmol/d (30 mg/d) is rare with the exception of adrenal rest tumors. Like adrenal neoplasms, ovarian tumors are not suppressed by dexamethasone. With the exception of adrenal rest tumors, these tumors are largely independent of ACTH stimulation. Elevations of plasma testosterone do not localize the neoplasm to the ovary, since testosterone can be elevated subsequent to peripheral conversion of adrenal precursors, such as DHEA (see Chap. 340).

The most common ovarian cause of excess androgen production is ovarian hyperthecosis or polycystic ovaries (see Chap. 340). As opposed to ovarian or adrenal tumors, virilization is less common with polycystic ovaries, whereas hirsutism is quite frequent. Many of these patients are obese and have hyperinsulinemia and glucose intolerance. Acanthosis nigricans may be present. Although the 17-ketosteroid excretion is partially reduced by dexamethasone, the residual level is often greater than in normal subjects. Plasma levels and production rates of androstenedione and, to a lesser extent, testosterone are usually increased. Follicle-stimulating hormone (FSH) levels tend to be lower than normal, and luteinizing hormone (LH) levels may be tonically elevated, leading to the characteristic increased LH/FSH ratio. The laboratory findings in patients with hirsutism-virilizing syndromes are summarized in Table 335-8.

TABLE 335-8   Laboratory evaluation of hirsutism-virilizing syndromes

	Ovarian		Adrenal			
	PCO	Ovarian tumor	CAH	Adrenal neoplasm	Cushing's syndrome	Idiopathic
Urinary 17-ketosteroids, plasma DHEA sulfate	N↑	N	N↑	↑↑↑	N↑	N
Plasma testosterone	N↑	↑↑	N↑	N↑	N↑	N
LH/FSH ratio	N↑	N	N	N	N	N
Precursors of cortisol biosynthesis:						
Basal	N	N	N↑	N↑	N	N
Following ACTH infusion	N	N	↑↑	N↑	N	N
Cortisol following overnight dexamethasone suppresion test	N	N	N	↑	↑	N

NOTE: CAH, congenital adrenal hyperplasia; PCO, polycystic ovary syndrome; N, normal; ↑, elevated.

Treatment   Treatment of adrenal virilism is dictated by the type of lesion. Patients with *congenital adrenal hyperplasia* have a fundamental defect of cortisol deficiency with resultant excessive ACTH secretion, producing hyperplasia of the adrenal glands and causing additional "shunting" into the adrenal androgen pathway. Therapy in these patients consists of daily administration of glucocorticoids to suppress pituitary ACTH secretion. Because of its cost and intermediate half-life, prednisone is the drug of choice except in infants, in whom hydrocortisone is usually used. In adults with late-onset adrenal hyperplasia, the smallest single bedtime dose of a long- or intermediate-acting glucocorticoid to suppress pituitary ACTH secretion should be administered. The amount of steroid required by children with congenital adrenal hyperplasia is approximately 1 to 1.5 times the normal cortisol production rate of 33 to 35 μmol (12 to 13 mg) cortisol per square meter of body surface area per day and is given in divided doses two or three times per day. The dosage schedule is governed by repetitive analysis of the urinary 17-ketosteroids, plasma DHEA sulfate, and/or precursors of cortisol biosynthesis. Skeletal growth and maturation also must be closely monitored, since overtreatment with glucocorticoid replacement therapy retards linear growth.

HYPOFUNCTION OF ADRENAL CORTEX

Adrenocortical hypofunction includes all conditions in which adrenal steroid hormone secretion falls below the requirements of the body. Adrenal insufficiency may be divided into two general categories: (1) those associated with primary inability of the adrenal to elaborate sufficient quantities of hormone and (2) those associated with a secondary failure due to a primary failure in the elaboration of ACTH (Table 335-9).

PRIMARY ADRENOCORTICAL DEFICIENCY (ADDISON'S DISEASE)   Addison's description of "general languor and debility, remarkable feebleness of the heart's action, irritability of the stomach, and a peculiar change of the color of the skin" summarizes the dominant clinical features. Advanced cases are usually easy to diagnose, but recognition of the disease in its early phases may present a real challenge.

Incidence   Primary adrenocortical insufficiency is relatively rare, may occur at any age, and affects both sexes equally. Because of increasing therapeutic use of steroids, secondary adrenal insufficiency is relatively common.

Etiology and pathogenesis   Addison's disease results from progressive adrenocortical destruction, which must involve more than 90 percent of the glands before signs of adrenal insufficiency appear. The adrenal is a frequent site for chronic granulomatous diseases, predominantly tuberculosis but also histoplasmosis, coccidioidomycosis, and cryptococcosis. In early series, tuberculosis was responsible for 70 to 90 percent of cases; however, the most frequent cause at present is *idiopathic* atrophy, and an autoimmune mechanism is probably responsible. Rarely, other lesions are encountered, such as bilateral hemorrhage, tumor metastases, amyloidosis, or sarcoidosis.

Half of patients have circulating adrenal antibodies. While some antibodies cause adrenal destruction, IgG antibodies can cause Addison's disease by blocking the binding of ACTH to its receptors. Some patients also have antibodies to thyroid, parathyroid, and/or gonadal tissue (see also Chap. 343). There is also an increased incidence of chronic lymphocytic thyroiditis and of premature ovarian failure, type I diabetes mellitus, and hyperthyroidism in patients with idiopathic adrenal insufficiency. The occurrence of two or more of these autoimmune endocrine disorders in the same individual defines the polyglandular autoimmune syndrome type II. Additional disorders include pernicious anemia, vitiligo, alopecia, nontropical sprue, and myasthenia gravis. Within families, multiple generations are affected by one or more of the above diseases. Type II polyglandular syndrome is the result of a mutant gene on chromosome 6 and is associated with the HLA alleles B8 and DR3.

The combination of parathyroid and adrenal insufficiency and chronic mucocutaneous moniliasis constitutes a distinct syndrome (type I polyglandular autoimmune syndrome). Other autoimmune diseases in these patients include pernicious anemia, chronic active hepatitis, alopecia, primary hypothyroidism, and premature gonadal failure. There is no HLA association; this syndrome is an autosomal recessive trait, often with multiple affected siblings. The type I syndrome usually presents during childhood, whereas the type II syndrome is usually expressed in adulthood. The mechanisms by which genetic predisposition and/or autoimmunity interact in the pathogenesis of these disorders are unknown.

Clinical suspicion of adrenal insufficiency should be high in patients with AIDS (see Chap. 279). Cytomegalovirus regularly involves the adrenal glands (so-called CMV necrotizing adrenalitis), and *Mycobacterium avium-intracellulare, Cryptococcus*, and Kaposi's sarcoma involvement of the adrenals also have been reported. Adrenal insufficiency in AIDS patients may not be manifest, but tests of adrenal reserve are frequently abnormal. When interpreting tests of

TABLE 335-9   Classification of adrenal insufficiency

Primary adrenal insufficiency
  A Anatomic destruction of gland (chronic and acute)
    1 "Idiopathic" atrophy (autoimmune)
    2 Surgical removal
    3 Infection (tuberculous, fungus, viral–especially in AIDS patients)
    4 Hemorrhage
    5 Invasion: metastatic
  B Metabolic failure in hormone production
    1 Congenital adrenal hyperplasia
    2 Enzyme inhibitors (metyrapone, ketoconazole, aminoglutethimide)
    3 Cytotoxic agents (mitotane)
  C ACTH-blocking antibodies
Secondary adrenal insufficiency
  A Hypopituitarism due to hypothalamic-pituitary disease
  B Suppression of hypothalamic-pituitary axis
    1 Exogenous steroid
    2 Endogenous steroid from tumor

TABLE 335-10 Frequency of symptoms and signs in Addison's disease, percent

Weakness	99	Pigmentation of mucous membranes	82
Pigmentation of skin	98		
Weight loss	97	Abdominal pain	34
Anorexia, nausea, and vomiting	90	Salt craving	22
		Diarrhea	20
Hypotension (<110/70)	87	Constipation	19
		Syncope	16
		Vitiligo	9

adrenocortical function, it is important to consider medications that might potentiate or cause adrenal failure (rifampin, phenytoin, ketoconazole, and opiates).

Clinical signs and symptoms Adrenocortical insufficiency caused by gradual adrenal destruction is characterized by an insidious onset of slowly progressive fatigability, weakness, anorexia, nausea and vomiting, weight loss, cutaneous and mucosal pigmentation, hypotension, and occasionally hypoglycemia (Table 335-10). However, the spectrum may vary, depending on the duration and degree of adrenal hypofunction, from a complaint of mild chronic fatigue to the fulminating shock associated with acute massive destruction of the glands described by Waterhouse and Friderichsen.

Asthenia is the cardinal symptom. Early it may be sporadic, usually most evident at times of stress; as adrenal function becomes more impaired, weakness progresses until the patient is continuously fatigued, necessitating bed rest.

Hyperpigmentation may be striking, but its absence does not exclude this diagnosis. It commonly appears as a diffuse brown, tan, or bronze darkening of both exposed and unexposed parts such as elbows or creases of the hand and of areas normally pigmented such as the areolas about the nipples. Bluish black patches may appear on the mucous membranes. Some patients develop dark freckles, and irregular areas of vitiligo may appear paradoxically. As an early sign, patients may notice persistent tanning following sun exposure.

Arterial hypotension with postural accentuation is frequent, and blood pressures may be in the range of 80/50 or less.

Abnormalities of gastrointestinal function often are the presenting complaint. Symptoms vary from mild anorexia with weight loss to fulminating nausea, vomiting, diarrhea, and ill-defined abdominal pain, which may be so severe as to be confused with an acute abdomen. In addition, patients frequently have personality changes, usually excessive irritability and restlessness. Enhancement of the sensory modalities of taste, olfaction, and hearing is reversible with therapy. Axillary and pubic hair may be decreased in women due to loss of adrenal androgen production.

Laboratory findings In the early phase of gradual adrenal destruction, there may be no demonstrable abnormalities in the routine laboratory parameters, but adrenal reserve is decreased, i.e., basal steroid output may be normal, but a subnormal increase occurs after stress. Adrenal stimulation with ACTH uncovers abnormalities in this stage of the disease with a subnormal response and/or failure of cortisol levels to rise over basal. In more advanced stages of adrenal destruction, serum sodium, chloride, and bicarbonate levels are reduced while the serum potassium level is elevated. The hyponatremia is due to both loss of sodium into the urine (due to aldosterone deficiency) and movement into the intracellular compartment. This extravascular sodium loss depletes extracellular fluid volume and accentuates hypotension. Elevated plasma vasopressin and angiotensin II levels may contribute to the hyponatremia through impairment of free water clearance. The hyperkalemia is due to a combination of aldosterone deficiency, impaired glomerular filtration, and acidosis. Basal levels of cortisol and aldosterone are subnormal and fail to increase following ACTH administration. Mild to moderate hypercalcemia occurs in 10 to 20 percent of patients for unclear reasons. The electrocardiogram may show nonspecific changes, and the electroencephalogram exhibits a generalized reduction and slowing. There may be a normocytic anemia, a relative lymphocytosis, and a moderate eosinophilia.

Diagnosis The diagnosis of adrenal insufficiency should be made only with ACTH stimulation testing to assess adrenal reserve capacity for steroid production (see above for ACTH test protocols). In *severe adrenal insufficiency*, the cortisol secretory rate is markedly decreased, and this may be ascertained indirectly by the finding of low to absent 24-h urine cortisol, 17-hydroxycorticosteroids, and 17-ketosteroids. With *mild adrenal insufficiency* (decreased adrenal reserve), urine and blood steroid values overlap the normal range; thus a diagnosis of adrenal insufficiency should never be excluded solely on the basis of normal basal urine steroid determinations. Plasma cortisol values vary from zero to the lower range of normal. Aldosterone secretion is usually low, resulting in salt wasting and rises in plasma renin levels. In primary adrenal insufficiency, plasma ACTH and associated peptides (β-lipotropin) are elevated because of loss of the usual cortisol-hypothalamic-pituitary feedback relationship, whereas in secondary adrenal insufficiency, plasma ACTH values are low or "inappropriately" normal (Fig. 335-11).

Differential diagnosis Since weakness and fatigue are common complaints, clinical diagnosis of early adrenocortical insufficiency is frequently difficult. However, mild gastrointestinal distress with weight loss, anorexia, and a suggestion of increased pigmentation make mandatory ACTH stimulation testing to rule out adrenal insufficiency, particularly before steroid treatment is begun. Weight loss is useful in evaluating the significance of weakness and malaise. Racial pigmentation may be a problem, but a *recent* and progressive *increase* is usually reported by the patient with gradual adrenal destruction. Hyperpigmentation is usually absent when adrenal destruction is rapid, as in bilateral adrenal hemorrhage. Hyperpigmenta-

FIGURE 335-11 Diagnostic flowchart for evaluating patients with suspected adrenal insufficiency. Plasma ACTH levels are low in secondary adrenal insufficiency. In adrenal insufficiency secondary to pituitary tumors or idiopathic panhypopituitarism, other pituitary hormone deficiencies are present. On the other hand, ACTH deficiency may be isolated, as seen following prolonged use of exogenous glucocorticoids.

Since the isolated blood levels obtained in these screening tests may not be definitive, the diagnosis should always be confirmed by a continuous 24-h ACTH infusion. Normal subjects and patients with secondary adrenal insufficiency may be distinguished by insulin tolerance or metyrapone testing.

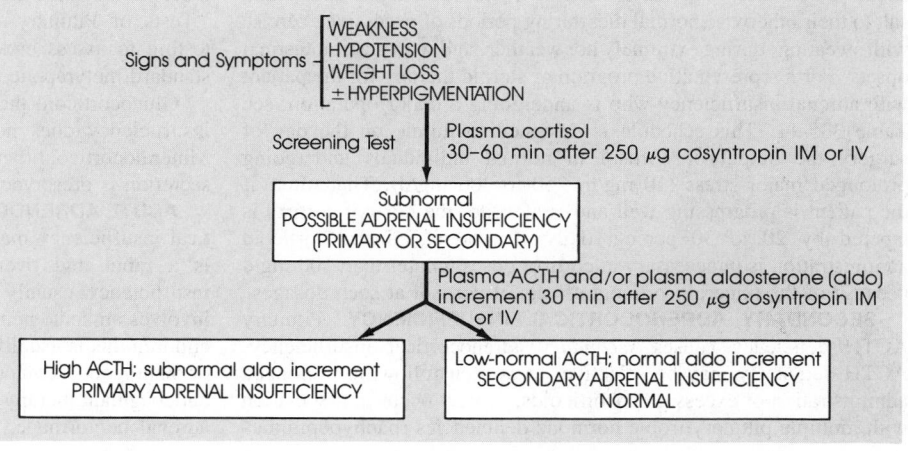

tion in other diseases also may present a problem, but the appearance and distribution of pigment in Addison's disease are usually characteristic. When doubt exists, measurement of ACTH levels and testing of adrenal reserve with the infusion of ACTH provide clear-cut differentiation.

Treatment   All patients with Addison's disease should receive specific hormone replacement. Like diabetics, these patients require careful education about their disease. Since the adrenal gland elaborates three general classes of hormones, of which two, glucocorticoids and mineralocorticoids, are of primary clinical importance, replacement therapy should correct both deficiencies. Cortisone (or cortisol) is the mainstay of treatment. Cortisone dosage varies from 12.5 to 50 mg/d, with the majority of patients taking 25 to 37.5 mg in divided doses. Cortisol (30 mg/d) or prednisone (7.5 mg/d) in divided doses also may be given for substitution therapy. Patients are advised to take their glucocorticoid replacement medication with meals or, if this is impractical, with milk or an antacid because the drugs may increase gastric acidity. This is particularly important because if the steroid is biologically active, e.g., cortisol, prednisolone, and dexamethasone, it may exert local effects on the gastric mucosa. In addition, the larger proportion of the dose (e.g., 25 mg cortisone) is taken in the morning, and the remainder (12.5 mg cortisone) is taken in the late afternoon to simulate the normal diurnal adrenal rhythm. Some patients exhibit insomnia, irritability, and mental excitement after initiation of therapy; in these, the dosage should be reduced. Other indications for smaller doses are hypertension, diabetes mellitus, or active tuberculosis.

Since this amount of cortisone or cortisol fails to replace the mineralocorticoid component of the adrenal gland, supplementary hormone is usually needed. This is accomplished by the daily oral administration of 0.05 to 0.1 mg fludrocortisone. Patients also should be instructed to ingest an ample intake of sodium (3 to 4 g/d). Adequacy of mineralocorticoid therapy can be assessed by measurement of blood pressure and serum electrolytes. Blood pressure should be normal and without postural change; serum sodium, potassium, creatinine, and urea nitrogen levels also should be normal.

Complications of glucocorticoid therapy, with the exception of gastritis, are *rare* in the dosage used in the treatment of Addison's disease. Complications of mineralocorticoid therapy occur more frequently and include hypokalemia, edema, hypertension, cardiac enlargement, or even congestive failure due to sodium retention. Periodic measurements of body weight, serum potassium level, and blood pressure are useful. All patients with adrenal insufficiency, including bilaterally adrenalectomized patients, should carry medical identification, should be instructed in the parenteral self-administration of steroids, and should be registered with a medical alerting system.

Special therapeutic problems   During periods of intercurrent illness, the dose of cortisone or cortisol should be increased to 75 to 150 mg/d. When oral administration is not possible, parenteral routes should be employed. Likewise, before surgery or dental extractions, supplemental glucocorticoids should be administered. Patients also should be advised to increase the dose of fludrocortisone and to add salt to their otherwise normal diet during periods of excessive exercise with sweating, during extremely hot weather, and with gastrointestinal upsets. For a representative program of steroid therapy for the patient with adrenal insufficiency who is undergoing a major operation, see Table 335-11. This schedule is designed to mimic on the day of surgery the output of cortisol in normal individuals undergoing prolonged major stress (10 mg/h, 250 to 300 mg/d). Thereafter, if the patient is progressing well and is afebrile, the dose of cortisol is tapered by 20 to 30 percent daily. Parenteral mineralocorticoid administration is unnecessary at cortisol doses greater than 100 mg/d because of the mineralocorticoid effects of cortisol at such dosages.

SECONDARY ADRENOCORTICAL INSUFFICIENCY   Pituitary ACTH deficiency causes *secondary* adrenocortical insufficiency. ACTH deficiency may be selective, as is seen following prolonged administration of excess glucocorticoids, or may occur in association with multiple pituitary tropic hormone deficiencies (panhypopituitar-

TABLE 335-11   Steroid therapy schedule for Addisonian patient undergoing a major operation*

	Cortisol infusion, continuous, mg/h		Cortisol (orally)		Fludro-cortisone (orally), 8 A.M.
			8 A.M.	4 P.M.	
Routine daily medication			20	10	0.1
Day before operation			20	10	0.1
Day of operation	10				
Postoperative:					
Day 1	5–7.5				
Day 2	2.5–5				
Day 3	2.5–5	or	40	20	0.1
Day 4	2.5–5	or	40	20	0.1
Day 5			40	20	0.1
Day 6			20	20	0.1
Day 7			20	10	0.1

* All steroid doses are given in milligrams. An alternative approach is to give cortisol as an IV bolus every 6 h on the day of operation (see text).

ism) (see Chap. 331). Patients with secondary adrenocortical hypofunction may have many symptoms and signs in common with Addisonian patients but are *characteristically not hyperpigmented*, since ACTH and related peptide levels are low. In fact, plasma ACTH levels distinguish between primary and secondary adrenal insufficiency, since they are elevated in the former and decreased to absent in the latter. Patients with total pituitary insufficiency also have manifestations of multiple hormone deficiencies. An additional feature distinguishing primary from secondary adrenocortical insufficiency is the *near-normal level of aldosterone secretion* seen in the presence of pituitary and/or isolated ACTH deficiencies (see Fig. 335-11). Patients with pituitary insufficiency may present with hyponatremia, which may be dilutional or secondary to subnormal increments in aldosterone secretion in response to severe sodium restriction. However, severe *dehydration, hyponatremia*, and *hyperkalemia* are characteristic of severe mineralocorticoid insufficiency and favor a diagnosis of primary adrenocortical insufficiency.

Patients receiving long-term steroid therapy, despite physical findings of Cushing's syndrome, develop adrenal insufficiency because of prolonged pituitary-hypothalamic suppression and adrenal atrophy secondary to the loss of endogenous ACTH. These patients have two deficits, a loss of adrenal responsiveness to ACTH and a failure of pituitary ACTH release. They are characterized by low blood cortisol and ACTH levels, low baseline steroid excretion, and abnormal ACTH and metyrapone responses. Most patients with steroid-induced adrenal insufficiency eventually recover normal hypothalamic-pituitary-adrenal responsiveness, but response time varies from days to months. The rapid ACTH test is a convenient assessment of recovery of hypothalamic-pituitary-adrenal function. Since the plasma cortisol concentrations after injection of cosyntropin and during insulin-induced hypoglycemia usually correlate closely, the rapid ACTH test assesses the integrated hypothalamic-pituitary-adrenal function (see "Tests of Pituitary-Adrenal Responsiveness," above). Additional testing to assess endogenous pituitary ACTH reserve includes the standard metyrapone and the insulin tolerance tests.

Glucocorticoid therapy in patients with secondary adrenocortical insufficiency does not differ from that for the primary disorder. Mineralocorticoid therapy is usually not necessary, since aldosterone secretion is preserved.

ACUTE ADRENOCORTICAL INSUFFICIENCY   Acute adrenocortical insufficiency may result from several processes. *Adrenal crisis* is a rapid and overwhelming intensification of chronic adrenal insufficiency, usually precipitated by sepsis or surgical stress. Another involves an acute hemorrhagic destruction of both adrenal glands. In children this is usually associated with septicemia with *Pseudomonas* or meningococcemia (Waterhouse-Friderichsen syndrome). In adults, anticoagulant therapy or a coagulation disorder may result in bilateral adrenal hemorrhage. Occasionally, bilateral adrenal hemorrhage in the newborn results from birth trauma. Hemorrhage has been observed during pregnancy, following idiopathic adrenal vein thrombosis, and as a complication of venography (e.g., infarction of an adenoma). A third, and probably the most frequent, cause of acute insufficiency results from the rapid withdrawal of steroids from patients with adrenal atrophy secondary to chronic steroid administration. Acute adrenocortical insufficiency also may occur in patients with congenital adrenal hyperplasia or those with decreased adrenocortical reserve when they are given drugs capable of inhibiting steroid synthesis (mitotane, ketoconazole) or increasing steroid metabolism (phenytoin, rifampin).

Adrenal crisis The long-term survival of patients with adrenocortical insufficiency largely depends on prevention and treatment of adrenal crisis. Consequently, the occurrence of infection, trauma (including surgery), gastrointestinal upsets, or other stress requires an immediate increase in hormone. In untreated patients, preexisting symptoms are intensified. Nausea, vomiting, and abdominal pain may become intractable. Fever may be severe or absent. Lethargy deepens into somnolence, and hypovolemic vascular collapse ensues. In contrast, patients previously maintained on chronic glucocorticoid therapy may not exhibit dehydration or hypotension until preterminally, since mineralocorticoid secretion is usually preserved. In all patients in crisis, a precipitating cause should be sought.

Treatment is primarily directed toward the repletion of circulating glucocorticoids and the replacement of the sodium and water deficits. Hence an intravenous infusion of 5% glucose in normal saline solution should be started with a bolus intravenous infusion of 100 mg cortisol followed by a continuous infusion of cortisol at a rate of 10 mg/h. An alternative approach is to administer a 100-mg bolus of cortisol intravenously every 6 h. However, only the continuous infusion maintains the plasma cortisol constantly at stress levels [>830 nmol/L (30 µg/dL)]. Effective treatment of hypotension consists of glucocorticoid replacement and aggressive repletion of sodium and water deficits. If the crisis was preceded by prolonged nausea, vomiting, and dehydration, several liters of saline solution may be required within the first few hours. Vasoconstrictive agents (such as dopamine) may be indicated in extreme conditions as adjuncts to volume replacement. With large doses of steroid, e.g., 100 to 200 mg cortisol, the patient receives a maximal mineralocorticoid effect, and supplementary mineralocorticoid is superfluous. Following improvement, the steroid dosage is tapered over the next few days to maintenance levels, and mineralocorticoid therapy is reinstituted if needed (see Table 335-11).

HYPOALDOSTERONISM

Isolated aldosterone deficiency accompanied by normal cortisol production occurs in association with hyporeninism, as an inherited biosynthetic defect, postoperatively following removal of aldosterone-secreting adenomas, during protracted heparin or heparinoid administration, in pretectal disease of the nervous system, and in severe postural hypotension.

The feature common to all patients with hypoaldosteronism is the inability to increase aldosterone secretion appropriately during salt restriction. Most patients have unexplained hyperkalemia often exacerbated by restriction of dietary sodium intake. In severe cases, urine sodium wastage occurs on a normal salt intake, whereas in milder forms, excessive losses of urine sodium occur only during salt restriction.

Most cases of isolated hypoaldosteronism occur in patients with a deficiency in renin production (so-called hyporeninemic hypoaldosteronism). This syndrome is seen most commonly in adults with mild renal failure and diabetes mellitus in association with hyperkalemia and metabolic acidosis out of proportion to the state of renal impairment. Plasma renin levels fail to rise normally following sodium restriction and postural changes. The pathogenesis is uncertain. Possibilities include renal disease (most likely), autonomic neuropathy, extracellular fluid volume expansion, and a defect in conversion of renin precursors to active renin. Aldosterone levels also fail to rise normally following salt restriction and volume contraction; this is probably related to the hyporeninism, since biosynthetic defects in aldosterone secretion cannot usually be demonstrated. In these patients, aldosterone secretion increases promptly following ACTH stimulation, but it is uncertain whether the magnitude of the response is normal. On the other hand, the level of aldosterone appears to be subnormal in relationship to the hyperkalemia.

Hypoaldosteronism also can be associated with high renin levels. In many of these subjects, there is an inability to transform the C-18 methyl group of corticosterone to the C-18 aldehyde of aldosterone probably due to a defect in corticosterone methyloxidase. These patients have low to absent aldosterone secretion, elevated plasma renin levels, and elevated values for the intermediates of aldosterone biosynthesis (corticosterone and 18-hydroxycorticosterone). Severely ill patients also may have hyperreninemic hypoaldosteronism. Patients with this syndrome have a high mortality rate (80 percent). Hyperkalemia is not part of this syndrome. Possible explanations for the hypoaldosteronism include adrenal necrosis (uncommon) or a shift in steroidogenesis from mineralocorticoids to glucocorticoids, possibly related to prolonged ACTH stimulation.

Before considering the diagnosis of isolated hypoaldosteronism in a patient with hyperkalemia, "pseudohyperkalemia" (e.g., hemolysis, thrombocytosis) should be excluded by measuring the plasma potassium level. The next step is to demonstrate a normal cortisol response to ACTH stimulation. Then stimulated (upright posture, sodium restriction) renin and aldosterone levels should be measured. Low renin–low aldosterone levels establish a diagnosis of hyporeninemic hypoaldosteronism. High renin–low aldosterone levels are consistent with an aldosterone biosynthetic defect or a selective unresponsiveness to angiotensin II. Finally, elevated renin and aldosterone levels suggest primary renal unresponsiveness to aldosterone, so-called pseudohypoaldosteronism.

The treatment of isolated hypoaldosteronism is to replace the mineralocorticoid deficiency. For practical purposes, the oral administration of 0.05 to 0.15 mg fludrocortisone daily should restore electrolyte balance if salt intake is adequate (e.g., 150 to 200 mmol/d). However, patients with hyporeninemic hypoaldosteronism usually require higher doses of mineralocorticoid to correct the hyperkalemia. This poses a risk in patients with hypertension and mild renal insufficiency and/or congestive heart failure. Therefore, an alternative approach is to administer furosemide, which can ameliorate acidosis and hyperkalemia, and reduce the salt intake. Occasionally, a combination of these two approaches is efficacious.

NONSPECIFIC CLINICAL USE OF ADRENAL STEROIDS

The widespread utilization of glucocorticoids emphasizes the need for a thorough understanding of the metabolic effects of these agents. Before instituting adrenal hormone therapy, the expected gains should be weighed against the undesirable actions.

HOW SERIOUS IS THE DISORDER? In a patient with unexplained shock or in whom other measures have failed, the physician need not hesitate to employ large-dosage steroid therapy. In contrast, one should exercise restraint in administering steroids to a patient with early rheumatoid arthritis who has not been tried on physiotherapy, analgesics, and general medical care.

HOW LONG WILL GLUCOCORTICOID THERAPY BE REQUIRED? The use of intravenous steroids for a period of 24 to 48 h for life-threatening situations such as status asthmaticus or pseudotumor cerebri has little or no contraindication, in contrast to the initiation of chronic steroid therapy for asthma, arthritis, or psoriasis. In the latter instances, the almost certain development of Cushing's syndrome of some degree must be weighed against the potential benefit. These side effects should be minimized by a careful choice of steroid preparations, alternate-day or interrupted therapy, and the judicious use of supplementary adjuvants.

WHICH PREPARATION IS PREFERABLE? Several considerations should be taken into account in deciding which steroid preparation to use:

1 The biologic half-life. The rationale behind every-other-day therapy is to decrease the metabolic effects of the steroids for a significant amount of time over the 2-day period and at the same time to produce pharmacologic effects of sufficient duration to induce remission. Too long a half-life would defeat the first purpose, and too short a half-life would defeat the second. In general, the more potent the steroid, the longer its biologic half-life.

2 The importance of the mineralocorticoid effects of the steroid. Most synthetic steroids have less mineralocorticoid effect than cortisol or cortisone (Table 335-12).

3 The biologically active form of the steroid. Cortisone and prednisone have to be converted to biologically active equivalents before anti-inflammatory effects can occur. Because of this, in a condition in which steroids are known to be effective and when an adequate dose has been given without response, one should consider substituting cortisol or prednisolone for cortisone or prednisone.

4 The cost of the medication. This is a serious consideration if chronic administration is to be undertaken. Prednisone is the least expensive of available steroid preparations.

5 The manner in which glucocorticoids are formulated. This factor may modify absorption. Thus it is advisable for a patient whose steroid dosage has been standardized to utilize the same preparation to avoid relapse or overdosage.

ACTH VERSUS STEROIDS In general, adrenal steroid therapy is effective by mouth and can be regulated more accurately than ACTH therapy. The amount of steroid produced in response to ACTH varies from day to day, depending on the rate and extent of absorption of ACTH and on the state of the adrenal cortex. ACTH therapy stimulates the secretion of adrenal androgens as well as of hydroxysteroids. Sodium retention with ACTH is often more marked than with cortisone or prednisone therapy.

While some studies imply that ACTH may be superior to oral steroid therapy in the treatment of certain disorders such as dermatomyositis and multiple sclerosis, it is generally believed that the two agents are equally effective (or ineffective). Both ACTH and steroid

therapy induce hypothalamopituitary suppression; however, in ACTH therapy adrenal gland size and activity are maintained, in contrast to the adrenal atrophy usually associated with steroid therapy.

EVALUATION OF PATIENT PRIOR TO INITIATING STEROID THERAPY (See Table 335-13) **Chronic infection** Three issues demand attention: (1) Any active infection, particularly tuberculosis, should be identified. If tuberculosis is present, steroid therapy should be employed, if indicated, in conjunction with antituberculous chemotherapy. (2) The chest film and tuberculin test provide baseline information for future comparison. Since high-dose steroids minimize the tuberculin reaction, serial chest roentgenograms may be necessary. (3) Infection due to "opportunistic" pathogens should be constantly considered in patients on steroid therapy, especially when combined with other immunosuppressive agents.

Diabetes mellitus Prolonged glucocorticoid therapy may unmask or aggravate diabetes mellitus. The presence of diabetes mellitus or the demonstration of impaired glucose tolerance may affect the decision to institute adrenal hormone therapy.

Osteoporosis All patients receiving long-continued steroid therapy are at risk for osteoporosis. Indeed, osteoporosis with vertebral fractures or compression is one of the dread complications of long-term steroid therapy for patients at high risk (postmenopausal women, elderly men, and patients with restricted physical activity). Alternate-day or interrupted steroid therapy minimizes this complication (Table 335-14), and adjunctive therapies may be effective in the therapy of steroid osteoporosis (see Chap. 362). Periodic assessment of spine density with CT or digital radiography should be done.

Peptic ulcer, gastric hypersecretion, or esophagitis In conventional doses (equivalent to 15 mg prednisone per day or less) glucocorticoids probably do not cause peptic ulceration; whether higher doses cause ulcer disease is not established and probably depends on duration and dose of treatment and predisposing factors such as hypoalbuminemia or cirrhosis. However, even in conventional doses patients with a history of ulcer may experience aggravation of symptoms while receiving glucocorticoids. Consequently, all individuals with a positive history or with known risk factors should be given a vigorous "ulcer combating" program (antacids, H-2

TABLE 335-13 A "checklist" for use prior to the administration of glucocorticoids in pharmacologic dosages

1 Presence of tuberculosis or other chronic infection (chest x-ray, tuberculin test)
2 Evidence of glucose intolerance or history of gestational diabetes mellitus
3 Evidence of preexisting osteoporosis (spine x-ray or bone density assessment, if available, in postmenopausal patients)
4 History of peptic ulcer, gastritis, or esophagitis (stool guaiac test)
5 Evidence of hypertension or cardiovascular disease
6 History of psychological disorders

TABLE 335-12 Glucocorticoid preparations

Commonly used name*	Estimated potency[†]	
	Glucocorticoid	Mineralocorticoid
SHORT-ACTING		
Cortisol	1	1
Cortisone	0.8	0.8
INTERMEDIATE-ACTING		
Prednisone	4	0.25
Prednisolone	4	0.25
Methylprednisolone	5	<0.01
Triamcinolone	5	<0.01
LONG-ACTING		
Paramethasone	10	<0.01
Betamethasone	25	<0.01
Dexamethasone	30–40	<0.01

* The steroids are divided into three groups according to the duration of biologic activity. Short-acting preparations have a biologic half-life of less than 12 h; long-acting, greater than 48 h; and intermediate, between 12 and 36 h. Triamcinolone has the longest half-life of the intermediate-acting preparations.

[†] Relative milligram comparisons with cortisol, setting the glucocorticoid and mineralocorticoid properties of cortisol as 1. Sodium retention is insignificant in usual doses employed of methylprednisolone, triamcinolone, paramethasone, betamethasone, and dexamethasone.

TABLE 335-14 Supplementary measures to minimize undesirable metabolic effects of glucocorticoids

1 Monitor caloric intake to prevent weight gain.
2 Restrict sodium intake to prevent edema and minimize hypertension and potassium loss.
3 Supplement potassium if necessary.
4 Give antacid therapy and/or H-2 receptor antagonist therapy.
5 Institute alternate-day steroid schedule if possible. Patients on steroid therapy over a prolonged period should be protected by an appropriate increase in hormone level during periods of acute stress. A rule of thumb is to *double* the maintenance dose.
6 Minimize osteopenia by (not proved effective):
   a Gonadal hormone replacement therapy: 0.625–1.25 mg conjugated estrogens given cyclically with progesterone, unless the uterus is absent; testosterone replacement for hypogonadal men
   b Calcium intake should be approximately 1200 mg/d
   c Consider supplemental vitamin D if blood levels of calciferol or 1,25(OH)$_2$ vitamin D are reduced
   d Consider calcitonin or diphosphonate therapy if fractures occur even with the above treatments

receptor antagonists) along with glucocorticoids. *The development of anemia in a patient receiving glucocorticoids should suggest gastrointestinal bleeding as a cause.*

Hypertension or cardiovascular disease In general, the sodium-retaining propensity of many adrenal steroid preparations requires that caution be used when they are given to patients with preexisting hypertension or cardiovascular or renal disease. Use of preparations in which sodium-retaining activity is minimal, restriction of dietary sodium intake, and the use of diuretic agents and supplementary potassium salts minimize the mineralocorticoid effects of steroid therapy. However, hypertension may be exacerbated by steroid-induced increases in renin substrate and consequently in angiotensin II levels and by reduction in vasodilator prostaglandin production. Steroids also accelerate atherogenesis by induction of hypertension, glucose intolerance, and unfavorable lipid profiles. Glucocorticoid-associated lipid abnormalities include hypertriglyceridemia, hypercholesterolemia, and increased LDL cholesterol levels.

Psychological difficulties Steroid therapy may cause psychological disturbances. In general, serious psychological disturbances are more closely related to the patient's personality than to the dose of hormone, although larger doses of hormone are associated with more frequent serious reactions. There is no reliable method of predicting beforehand a patient's psychological reaction to steroid therapy; moreover, previous tolerance of steroids does not necessarily ensure immunity to subsequent courses. Likewise, untoward psychological reactions on one occasion do not invariably mean that the patient will respond unfavorably to a second course of treatment. However, patients with depressive symptoms during a first course of steroids may benefit from prophylactic lithium prior to a second course.

Sleeplessness is common and can be minimized by using the shorter-acting steroids and by prescribing the total dose as a single early-morning medication.

ALTERNATE-DAY STEROID THERAPY The most effective measure to minimize the cushingoid effects of glucocorticoids is to administer the total 48-h dose as a *single* dose of *intermediate-acting steroid* in the morning, *every other day*. If symptoms of the underlying disorder can be controlled by this technique, the therapeutic program offers a distinct advantage. Three considerations deserve mention: (1) The alternate-day schedule may be approached through transition dose schedules that allow the patient to adjust to the ultimate program. (2) The physician should provide supplementary nonsteroid medications, if required, on the "off day" to minimize symptoms of the underlying disorder. (3) The physician and the patient should recognize that many symptoms during the off day (e.g., fatigue, joint pain, muscle stiffness or tenderness, and fever) are those of relative adrenal insufficiency rather than exacerbation of the underlying disease.

The alternate-day concept capitalizes on the fact that cortisol secretion and plasma levels normally are highest in the early morning and lowest in the evening. The normal pattern is mimicked by administering an intermediate-acting steroid in the morning (7 to 8 A.M.) (see Table 335-12).

Initially, the steroid program often requires daily or more frequent doses of steroid to accomplish the desired anti-inflammatory or immunity-suppressing action. *Only after this desired effect is achieved is an attempt made to switch to an alternate-day program.* A number of schedules may be employed for transferring from a daily to an alternate-day program. The key points to be considered are flexibility in arranging a program and the use of supportive measures on the off day. One may attempt a transition by a series of gradations rather than by an abrupt complete changeover. One approach is to keep the steroid dose constant on one day and gradually reduce the level on the alternate day. Alternatively, the steroid dose can be increased on one day and reduced on the alternate day. In any case, it is important to anticipate that some increase in pain or discomfort may occur in the 36 to 48 h following the last dose.

The general principles advocated in the long-term use of steroids and in implementing an alternate-day schedule are as follows:

1 Utilize intermediate-acting steroids such as prednisone or prednisolone.

2 Give the total daily steroid as a single morning dose.

3 Begin a transition program as soon as the manifestations of the diseases are under reasonable control.

4 If possible, eliminate steroid medication on the alternate day.

WITHDRAWAL OF GLUCOCORTICOIDS FOLLOWING LONG-TERM USE Complete withdrawal of steroids should be initiated by implementing an alternate-day schedule. Patients on an alternate-day program for a month or more experience less difficulty during a termination regimen. The dosage is gradually reduced and finally discontinued after a replacement dosage has been reached (e.g., 5 to 7.5 mg prednisone). Complications rarely ensue unless undue stress is experienced, and patients should understand that for 1 year or longer after withdrawal from long-term high-dosage steroid therapy, supplementary hormone should be given in the presence of serious infection, operation, or injury. A useful strategy in patients who have symptoms of adrenal insufficiency on every-other-day therapy is to measure plasma cortisol levels prior to the steroid dose. A level less than 140 nmol/L (5 μg/dL) indicates a continuing suppression of the pituitary-adrenal axis and that a more cautious tapering of steroids is indicated.

In patients on high-dose daily steroid therapy, it is advised to reduce dosage to approximately 20 mg prednisone daily as a single morning dose before beginning the transition to every-other-day therapy. If a patient cannot tolerate an alternate-day program, it is debatable whether complete discontinuance should be considered. Under these circumstances, a daily replacement dose should be continued, and at some future date another gradual transition to the alternate-day schedule should be attempted. These patients will not require mineralocorticoid therapy, since aldosterone secretion is usually adequate.

REFERENCES

ATKINSON AB: The treatment of Cushing's syndrome. Clin Endocrinol (oxf) 34:507, 1991

CUNEO RC et al: Chronic and acute volume expansion in normal man: Effect on atrial diameter and plasma atrial natriuretic peptide. Horm Metab Res 21:148, 1989

ELDAR-GEVA T et al: Secondary biosynthetic defects in women with late-onset congenital adrenal hyperplasia. N Engl J Med 323:855, 1990

FLACK MR et al: Urine-free cortisol in the high-dose dexamethasone suppression test for the differential diagnosis of Cushing's syndrome. Ann Intern Med 116:211, 1992

HOLLENBERG SM et al: Primary structure and expression of a functional human glucocorticoid receptor cDNA. Nature 318:635, 1985

IRONY I et al: Correctable subsets of primary aldosteronism: Primary adrenal hyperplasia and renin responsive adenoma. Am J Hypertens 3:576, 1990

KLIBANSKI A et al: Diagnosis and management of hormone-secreting pituitary adenomas. N Engl J Med 324:822, 1991

LACROIX A et al: Gastric inhibitory polypeptide-dependent cortisol hypersection: A new cause of Cushing's syndrome. N Engl J Med 327:974, 1992

LIFTON RP et al: A chimeric 11β-hydroxylase/aldosterone synthase gene causes glucocorticoid-remediable aldosteronism and human hypertension. Nature 355:262, 1992

LUTTON J-P et al: Clinical features of adrenocortical carcinoma, prognostic factors and the effect of mitotane therapy. N Engl J Med 322:1995, 1990

MAMPALAM TJ et al: Transsphenoidal microsurgery for Cushing disease: A report of 216 cases. Ann Intern Med 109:487, 1988

MELBY JC: Diagnosis of hyperaldosteronism. Endocrinol Metab Clin North Am 20:247, 1991

MUNCK et al: Physiological functions of glucocorticoids in stress and their relation to pharmacological actions. Endocr Rev 5:25, 1984

OLDFIELD EH et al: Petrosal sinus sampling with and without corticotropin-releasing hormone for the differential diagnosis of Cushing's syndrome. N Engl J Med 325:897, 1991

PEMBERTON PA et al: Hormone binding globulins undergo serpin conformational change in inflammation. Nature 336:257, 1988

QUINN SJ et al: Regulation of aldosterone secretion, in *The Adrenal Gland*, 2d ed, VHT James (ed). New York, Raven, 1992, p 152

RABINOWE SL et al: la-Positive T lymphocytes in recently diagnosed idiopathic Addison's disease. Am J Med 77:597, 1984

RAO RH et al: Bilateral massive adrenal hemorrhage: Early recognition and treatment. Ann Intern Med 110:227, 1989

SCHAMBELAN M et al: Prevalence, pathogenesis and functional significance of aldosterone deficiency in hyperkalemic patients with chronic renal insufficiency. Kidney Int 17:89, 1980

SCHLAGHECKE R et al: The effect of long-term glucocorticoid therapy on pituitary-adrenal responses to exogenous corticotropin-releasing hormone. N Engl J Med 326:226, 1992

SPEISER PW et al: Disease expression and molecular genotype in congenital adrenal hyperplasia due to 21-hydroxylase deficiency. J Clin Invest 90:584, 1992

STEWART PM et al: Mineralocorticoid activity of liquorice: 11-Beta-hydroxysteroid dehydrogenase deficiency comes of age. Lancet 2:821, 1987

―――― et al: Syndrome of apparent mineralocorticoid excess. A defect in the cortisol-cortisone shuttle. J Clin Invest 82:340, 1988

STRAUSS KW: Endocrine complications of the acquired immunodeficiency syndrome. Arch Intern Med 151:1441, 1991

SUDA T et al: Effects of corticotropin-releasing hormone and dexamethasone on proopiomelanocortin messenger RNA level in human corticotroph adenoma cells in vitro. J Clin Invest 82:110, 1988

ULICK S: Two uncommon causes of mineralocorticoid excess: Syndrome of apparent mineralocorticoid excess and glucocorticoid-remediable aldosteronism. Endocrinol Metab Clin North Am 20:269, 1991

―――― et al: Defective ring A reduction of cortisol as the major metabolic error in the syndrome of apparent mineralocorticoid excess. J Clin Endocrinol Metab 74:593, 1992

WILLIAMS GH, DLUHY RG: Diagnostic imaging of the adrenal gland, in *Endocrinology*, 2d ed, LG DeGroot et al (eds). Orlando, Grune & Stratton 1989, p 1633

WULFRATT NM et al: Immunoglobulins of patients with Cushing's syndrome due to pigmented adrenocortical micronodular dysplasia stimulate in vitro steroidogenesis. J Clin Endocrinol Metab 66:301, 1988

336   PHEOCHROMOCYTOMA

LEWIS LANDSBERG / JAMES B. YOUNG

Pheochromocytomas produce, store, and secrete catecholamines. They are usually derived from the adrenal medulla but may develop from chromaffin cells in or about sympathetic ganglia (extraadrenal pheochromocytomas or paragangliomas). Related tumors that secrete catecholamines and produce similar clinical syndromes include chemodectomas derived from the carotid body and ganglioneuromas derived from the postganglionic sympathetic neurons.

The clinical features and morbidity of these tumors are due predominantly to the release of catecholamines. Hypertension is the most common manifestation, and hypertensive paroxysms or crises, often spectacular and alarming, occur in over half the cases.

Pheochromocytoma occurs in approximately 0.1 percent of the hypertensive population but is, nevertheless, an important correctable cause of high blood pressure. Indeed, it is usually curable if properly diagnosed and treated but may be fatal if undiagnosed or mistreated. Postmortem series indicate that the majority of pheochromocytomas are unsuspected clinically even when the tumor is related to the fatal outcome.

PATHOLOGY   Location and morphology   In adults, approximately 80 percent are unilateral and solitary, 10 percent are bilateral, and 10 percent are extraadrenal. In children, a fourth of tumors are bilateral, and an additional fourth are extraadrenal. Solitary lesions inexplicably favor the right side. Although pheochromocytomas may grow to large size (over 3 kg), most weigh less than 100 g and are less than 10 cm in diameter. The tumors are highly vascular.

The tumors are made up of large, polyhedral, pleomorphic chromaffin cells. Less than 10 percent are malignant. As with other endocrine tumors, malignancy cannot be determined by the histologic appearance; local invasion of surrounding tissues or distant metastases indicate malignancy.

FAMILIAL PHEOCHROMOCYTOMA   In approximately 5 percent of cases, pheochromocytoma is inherited as an autosomal dominant trait either alone or in combination with other abnormalities such as multiple endocrine neoplasia (MEN) type 2a (Sipple's syndrome) or type 2b (mucosal neuroma syndrome) (see Chap. 343), von Recklinghausen's neurofibromatosis, or von Hippel–Lindau's retinal cerebellar hemangioblastomatosis. Bilateral adrenal pheochromocytomas are common in the familial syndromes; within MEN kindreds, over half of pheochromocytomas are bilateral. A familial syndrome should be suspected in any patient with bilateral pheochromocytomas.

EXTRAADRENAL PHEOCHROMOCYTOMAS   Extraadrenal pheochromocytomas usually weigh 20 to 40 g and are less than 5 cm in diameter. Most are located within the abdomen in association with the celiac, superior mesenteric, and inferior mesenteric ganglia. Approximately 1 percent are in the thorax, 1 percent are within the urinary bladder, and less than 1 percent are in the neck, usually in association with the sympathetic ganglia or the extracranial branches of the ninth or tenth cranial nerves.

Catecholamine synthesis, storage, and release   Pheochromocytomas synthesize and store catecholamines by processes resembling those of the normal adrenal medulla (Chap. 68). Little is known about the mechanisms of catecholamine release from pheochromocytomas, but changes in blood flow and necrosis within the tumor may be the cause in some instances. These tumors are not innervated, and catecholamine release does not result from neural stimulation. Pheochromocytomas also store and secrete a variety of peptides, including endogenous opioids, neuropeptide Y, and chromagranin A (see Chap. 68). These peptides may contribute to the clinical manifestations in selected cases, as noted below.

EPINEPHRINE, NOREPINEPHRINE, AND DOPAMINE   Most pheochromocytomas contain and secrete both norepinephrine and epinephrine, and the percentage of norepinephrine is usually greater than in the normal adrenal. Most extraadrenal pheochromocytomas secrete norepinephrine exclusively. Rarely, pheochromocytomas produce epinephrine alone, particularly in association with MEN. Although epinephrine-producing tumors may cause a preponderance of metabolic and beta-receptor effects, in general the major catecholamine secreted cannot be predicted from the clinical presentation. Increased production of dopamine and homovanillic acid (HVA) is uncommon with benign lesions but may occur with malignant pheochromocytoma.

CLINICAL FEATURES   Pheochromocytoma occurs at all ages but is most common in young to midadult life. Some series show a slight female preponderance. Most patients come to medical attention as a result of hypertensive crisis, paroxysmal symptoms suggestive of seizure disorder or anxiety attacks, or hypertension that responds poorly to conventional treatment. Less commonly, unexplained hypotension or shock in association with surgery or trauma will suggest the diagnosis. Most have hypertension in association with headaches, excessive sweating, and/or palpitations.

Hypertension   Hypertension is the most common manifestation. In approximately 60 percent of cases the hypertension is sustained, although significant blood pressure lability is usually present, and half of patients with sustained hypertension have distinct crises or paroxysms. The other 40 percent have blood pressure elevations only during an attack. The hypertension is often severe, occasionally malignant, and may be resistant to treatment with standard antihypertensive drugs.

Paroxysms or crises   The paroxysm or crisis occurs in over half of patients. In an individual patient the symptoms are often similar with each attack. The paroxysms may be frequent or sporadic, at intervals as long as weeks or months. With time, the paroxysms usually increase in frequency, duration, and severity.

The attack usually has a sudden onset. It may last from a few minutes to several hours or longer. Headache, profuse sweating, palpitations, and apprehension, often with a sense of impending doom, are common. Pain in the chest or abdomen may be associated with nausea and vomiting. Either pallor or flushing may occur during the attack. The blood pressure is elevated, often to alarming levels, and is usually accompanied by tachycardia.

The paroxysm may be precipitated by any activity that displaces the abdominal contents. In some cases a particular stimulus may induce an attack in a characteristic fashion, but in others no clearly defined precipitating event can be found. Although anxiety may accompany the attacks, mental or psychological stress does not usually provoke a crisis.

Other distinctive clinical features   Symptoms and signs of an increased metabolic rate, such as profuse sweating and mild to moderate weight loss, are common. Orthostatic hypotension is a consequence of diminished plasma volume and blunted sympathetic reflexes. Both these factors predispose the patient with unsuspected pheochromocytoma to hypotension or shock during surgery or trauma.

CARDIAC MANIFESTATIONS Sinus tachycardia, sinus bradycardia, supraventricular arrhythmias, and ventricular premature contractions all have been noted. Angina and acute myocardial infarction may occur even in the absence of coronary artery disease. Catecholamine-induced increase in myocardial oxygen consumption and, perhaps, coronary spasm may play a role in these ischemic events. Electrocardiographic changes, including nonspecific ST-T wave changes, prominent U waves, left ventricular strain patterns, and right and left bundle branch blocks may be present in the absence of demonstrable ischemia or infarction. Cardiomyopathy, either congestive with myocarditis and myocardial fibrosis or hypertrophic with concentric or asymmetric hypertrophy, may be associated with heart failure and cardiac arrhythmias. Noncardiogenic pulmonary edema may be due to either shifts in extracellular fluid, altered pulmonary capillary permeability, or increased pulmonary venous tone.

CARBOHYDRATE INTOLERANCE Over half of patients have impaired carbohydrate tolerance due to suppression of insulin and stimulation of hepatic glucose output. The impaired glucose tolerance rarely requires treatment with insulin and disappears after removal of the tumor.

HEMATOCRIT The elevated hematocrit is secondary to diminished plasma volume. Rarely, production of erythropoietin by the tumor may cause a true erythrocytosis.

OTHER MANIFESTATIONS Hypercalcemia has been attributed to the ectopic secretion of parathyroid hormone–related protein. Fever and an elevated sedimentation rate have been reported in association with the production of interleukin 6. Elevated temperature more commonly reflects catecholamine-mediated increases in metabolic rate and diminished heat dissipation secondary to vasoconstriction. Polyuria is an occasional finding, and rhabdomyolysis with myoglobinuric renal failure may result from extreme vasoconstriction with muscle ischemia.

PHEOCHROMOCYTOMA OF THE URINARY BLADDER Pheochromocytoma within the wall of the urinary bladder may result in typical paroxysms in relation to micturition. The location within the bladder wall is responsible for symptoms while the tumors are quite small, and consequently, catecholamine excretion may be normal or minimally elevated. Hematuria is present in over half, and the tumor can often be visualized at cystoscopy.

Adverse drug interactions Severe and occasionally fatal paroxysms have been induced by opiates, histamine, adrenocorticotropin, saralasin, and glucagon. These agents appear to release catecholamines directly from the tumor. Indirect-acting sympathomimetic amines, including methyldopa (when administered intravenously), may cause an increase in blood pressure by releasing catecholamines from the augmented stores within nerve endings. Drugs that block neuronal uptake of catecholamines, such as tricyclic antidepressants or guanethidine, may enhance the physiologic effects of circulating catecholamines. Indeed all medications should be carefully considered and cautiously administered in patients with known or suspected pheochromocytoma.

Associated diseases Pheochromocytoma is associated with medullary carcinoma of the thyroid in the MEN syndrome types 2a and 2b and with hyperparathyroidism in MEN 2a (see Chap. 343). Hypercalcemia, resolving after tumor resection, also has been described in the absence of parathyroid disease, as described above. Individuals at risk for MEN 2a and 2b should be screened periodically for pheochromocytoma by assay of a 24-h urine sample for catecholamines, including measurement of epinephrine. Pheochromocytoma should be excluded or removed before thyroid or parathyroid surgery.

The association of pheochromocytoma and neurofibromatosis is not common. Nevertheless, since incomplete forms of neurofibromatosis may be associated with pheochromocytoma, minor manifestations such as café au lait spots, vertebral abnormalities, or kyphoscoliosis should increase the suspicion of pheochromocytoma in a patient with hypertension. The incidence of pheochromocytoma in some

kindreds with von Hippel–Lindau disease may be as high as 10 to 25 percent. Many of these are unsuspected clinically and diagnosed postmortem.

The incidence of cholelithiasis is 15 to 20 percent. Cushing's syndrome is a rare association, usually a consequence of ectopic secretion of ACTH by the pheochromocytoma or, less commonly, by a coexistent medullary carcinoma of the thyroid.

DIAGNOSIS The diagnosis is established by the demonstration of increased excretion of catecholamines or catecholamine metabolites. The diagnosis can usually be made by the analysis of a single 24-h urine sample, provided the patient is hypertensive or symptomatic at the time of collection.

Biochemical tests The assays employed include vanillylmandelic acid (VMA), the metanephrines, and unconjugated or "free" catecholamines (Chap. 68). Although much has been written about the relative specificity and sensitivity of the different assays, they are probably equivalent provided they are properly performed. Accuracy of diagnosis is improved when two of the three determinations are employed, although this is not essential as a screening procedure. The following considerations apply to all the urinary tests: (1) Despite claims for the adequacy of determinations made on random urine samples, analysis of a full 24-h urine sample is preferable. Creatinine should be determined as well to assess the adequacy of collection. (2) Where possible, the collection should be made when the patient is at rest, on no medication, and without recent exposure to radiographic contrast media. Where it is not practical to discontinue all medications, drugs known specifically to interfere in the assays (as noted below) should be avoided. (3) The urine should be acidified and refrigerated during and after collection. (4) With high-quality assays, dietary restrictions are minimal and should be specified by the laboratory performing the analyses. (5) Although most patients with pheochromocytoma excrete increased catecholamines and catecholamine metabolites, the yield is increased in patients with paroxysmal hypertension if a 24-h urine collection is initiated during a crisis.

FREE CATECHOLAMINES The upper limit of normal for total catecholamines is between 590 and 885 nmol (100 and 150 μg) per 24 h. In most patients with pheochromocytoma, values in excess of 1480 nmol (250 μg) per day are obtained. Measurement of epinephrine is often of value, since increased epinephrine excretion [over 275 nmol (50 μg) per 24 h] is usually due to an adrenal lesion and may be the only abnormality in cases associated with MEN. False-positive increases in catecholamine excretion result from exogenous catecholamines and related drugs such as methyldopa, levodopa, labetalol, and sympathomimetic amines, which may elevate catecholamine excretion for up to 2 weeks. Endogenous catecholamines from stimulation of the sympathoadrenal system also may increase urinary catecholamine excretion. Relevant clinical situations include hypoglycemia, strenuous exertion, central nervous system disease with increased intracranial pressure, and clonidine withdrawal.

METANEPHRINES AND VMA In most laboratories, the upper limit of normal is 7 μmol (1.3 mg) of total metanephrine and 35 μmol (7.0 mg) of VMA excretion per 24 h. In most patients with pheochromocytoma, the increase in these urinary metabolites is considerable, often more than three times the normal range. Metanephrine excretion is increased by exogenous and endogenous catecholamines and by treatment with monoamine oxidase inhibitors; propranolol may cause a spurious increase in metanephrine excretion, since a propranolol metabolite interferes in the commonly utilized spectrophotometric assay. VMA is less affected by endogenous and exogenous catecholamines but is spuriously increased by a variety of drugs, including carbidopa. VMA excretion is decreased by monoamine oxidase inhibitors.

PLASMA CATECHOLAMINES Measurement of plasma catecholamines has a limited application. The care required in obtaining basal levels (Chap. 68); the lack of readily available, reliable plasma assays; and the satisfactory results with urinary determinations make measurement of plasma catecholamines unnecessary in most cases. Plasma catecholamine levels are affected by the same drugs and physiologic perturbations that increase urinary catecholamine excretion. In addition, alpha- and beta-adrenergic receptor blocking agents may elevate plasma catecholamines by impairing clearance.

When the clinical features suggest pheochromocytoma and the urinary assays are borderline, measurement of plasma catecholamines may be worthwhile. Markedly elevated basal levels of total catecholamines support the diagnosis, although approximately one-third of patients with pheochromocytoma have normal or slightly elevated basal values. The usefulness of plasma catecholamine determinations may be increased by agents that suppress sympathetic nervous system activity. Clonidine and ganglionic blocking agents (Chap. 68) reduce plasma catecholamine levels in normal subjects and in patients with essential hypertension. These drugs have little effect on catecholamine levels in patients with pheochromocytoma. In patients with elevated or borderline basal catecholamine values, failure to suppress plasma or urinary levels with clonidine supports the diagnosis of pheochromocytoma.

Pharmacologic tests   Reliable methods for the measurement of catecholamines and catecholamine metabolites in urine have rendered obsolete both the provocative and adrenolytic tests, which are nonspecific and entail considerable risk. A modified version of the adrenolytic test may be of some use, however, as a therapeutic trial in a patient in hypertensive crisis with features suggestive of pheochromocytoma. A positive response to phentolamine (5-mg bolus following a 0.5-mg test dose) is a reduction in blood pressure of at least 35/25 mmHg that becomes maximal after 2 min and persists for 10 to 15 min. The pharmacologic response is never diagnostic, and biochemical confirmation is essential. Provocative tests in normotensive patients are potentially dangerous and rarely indicated. However, a glucagon provocative test may be of use in patients with paroxysmal hypertension and nondiagnostic basal catecholamine levels. Glucagon has a negligible effect on blood pressure or plasma catecholamine levels in normal or hypertensive subjects. In patients with pheochromocytoma, on the other hand, glucagon may increase both blood pressure and circulating catecholamine levels. The elevation in plasma catecholamine concentration, moreover, may occur without a blood pressure response. It must be emphasized, however, that life-threatening pressor crises have occurred after administration of glucagon to patients with pheochromocytoma, so the test should never be performed casually. Careful continuous monitoring of the blood pressure is required, intravenous access must be adequate, and phentolamine must be at hand to terminate the test if a significant pressor reaction ensues.

Differential diagnosis   Since the manifestations may be protean, the diagnosis must be considered and excluded in many patients with suggestive clinical features. In patients with essential hypertension and "hyperadrenergic" features such as tachycardia, sweating, and increased cardiac output, and in patients with anxiety attacks associated with blood pressure elevations, analysis of a 24-h urine collection is usually decisive in excluding the diagnosis. Repeated determinations on urine collected during attacks may be necessary, however, before the diagnosis can be excluded with certainty. The clonidine suppression and glucagon stimulation tests may be helpful in excluding the diagnosis in difficult cases. Pressor crises associated with clonidine withdrawal or the use of monoamine oxidase inhibitors (Chap. 68) may mimic the paroxysms of pheochromocytoma. Factitious crises may be produced by self-administration of sympathomimetic amines in psychiatrically disturbed patients.

Intracranial lesions, particularly posterior fossa tumors or subarachnoid hemorrhage, may cause hypertension and increased excretion of catecholamines or catecholamine metabolites. While this is most common in patients with an obvious neurologic catastrophe, the possibility of subarachnoid or intracranial hemorrhage secondary to pheochromocytoma should be considered. Diencephalic or autonomic epilepsy may be associated with paroxysmal spells, hypertension, and increased plasma catecholamine levels. This rare entity may be difficult to distinguish from pheochromocytoma, but an aura, an abnormal electroencephalogram, and a beneficial response to anticonvulsant medications will often suggest the proper diagnosis.

MANAGEMENT   Preoperative management   The induction of stable alpha-adrenergic blockade is the basis of preoperative management and provides the foundation for successful surgical treatment. Once the diagnosis is established, the patient should be placed on phenoxybenzamine to induce a long-lived, noncompetitive alpha-receptor blockade. The usual initial dose is 10 mg every 12 h with increments of 10 to 20 mg added every few days until the blood pressure is controlled and the paroxysms disappear. Because of the long duration of action, the therapeutic effects are cumulative, and the optimal dose must be achieved gradually with careful monitoring of supine and upright blood pressures. Most patients require between 40 and 80 mg phenoxybenzamine per day, although 200 mg or more may be necessary. Phenoxybenzamine should be administered for at least 10 to 14 days prior to surgery. Over this time, the combination of alpha-receptor blockade and a liberal salt intake will restore the contracted plasma volume to normal. Before adequate alpha-adrenergic blockade with phenoxybenzamine is achieved, paroxysms may be treated with intravenous phentolamine. Prazosin, the selective alpha$_1$ antagonist, has been employed in the preoperative management of a small number of patients. Doses in the range of 1.5 to 2.5 mg every 6 h have effectively controlled blood pressure and paroxysms. The role of this and other longer-acting selective alpha$_1$ antagonists in the management of pheochromocytoma has not been established. They may be useful as antihypertensive agents in patients with suspected pheochromocytoma while workup is in progress, since they are usually better tolerated than phenoxybenzamine and will prevent serious pressor crises if pheochromocytoma is present. Nitroprusside, calcium channel blocking agents, and possibly angiotensin-converting enzyme inhibitors reduce blood pressure in patients with pheochromocytoma. Nitroprusside may be useful on occasion in the treatment of pressor crises.

Beta-adrenergic receptor blocking agents should be given only after alpha blockade has been induced, since administration of such agents by themselves may cause a paradoxic increase in blood pressure by antagonizing beta-mediated vasodilatation in skeletal muscle. Beta blockade is usually initiated when tachycardia develops during the induction of alpha-adrenergic blockade. Low doses often suffice, and a reasonable starting dose is 10 mg propranolol 3 to 4 times per day, increased as needed to control the pulse rate. Beta blockade is effective for catecholamine-induced arrhythmias, particularly those potentiated by anesthetic agents.

Preoperative localization of the tumor   Surgical removal of pheochromocytoma is facilitated if the location of the tumor or tumors can be established preoperatively. Once pheochromocytoma is diagnosed, localization should be undertaken while the patient is being prepared for surgery. Computed tomography (CT) or magnetic resonance imaging of the adrenals is usually successful in identifying intraadrenal lesions. Conventional roentgenograms and CT of the chest usually suffice to identify intrathoracic lesions. If these studies are negative, abdominal aortography (once alpha-adrenergic blockade is complete) may identify extraadrenal pheochromocytomas within the abdomen, since these lesions are often supplied by a large aberrant artery. If aortography and CT fail to localize the lesion, venous sampling at different levels of the inferior and superior vena cava may reveal catecholamine gradients in the region drained by the tumor; this area may then be restudied by selective angiography or scanning by CT. An additional localization technique involves a radionuclide scintiscan after administration of an investigational radiopharmaceutical [131I]metaiodobenzylguanidine (MIBG). This agent is concentrated by the amine uptake process and produces an external scintigraphic image at the site of the tumor. This type of scanning may be useful in characterizing lesions discovered by CT when biochemical confirmation is indeterminate, as well as in localizing extraadrenal pheochromocytomas. Percutaneous fine-needle aspiration of chromaffin tumors is contraindicated; indeed, pheochromocytoma should be considered before adrenal lesions are aspirated.

Surgery Surgery is best performed in centers with experience in the preoperative, anesthetic, and intraoperative management of pheochromocytoma. In experienced hands, surgical mortality is 2 or 3 percent.

Monitoring during the surgical procedure should include continuous recording of arterial pressure, central venous pressure, and electrocardiogram; in the presence of cardiac disease or if congestive failure has been present, pulmonary capillary wedge pressure should be monitored. Adequate fluid replacement is crucial. Intraoperative hypotension responds better to volume replacement than to vasoconstrictors. Hypertension and cardiac arrhythmias are most likely during induction of anesthesia, intubation, and manipulation of the tumor. Intravenous phentolamine is usually sufficient to control the blood pressure, but nitroprusside may be required. Propranolol may be given in the treatment of tachycardia or ventricular ectopy.

PHEOCHROMOCYTOMA IN PREGNANCY Spontaneous labor and vaginal delivery in unprepared patients are usually disastrous for mother and fetus. In early pregnancy, the patient should be prepared with phenoxybenzamine, and the tumor should be removed as soon as the diagnosis is confirmed. The pregnancy need not be terminated, but the operative procedure itself may result in spontaneous abortion. In the third trimester, treatment with adrenergic blocking agents should be undertaken; when the fetus is of sufficient size, cesarean section may be followed by extirpation of the tumor. Although the safety of adrenergic blocking drugs in pregnancy is not established, these agents have been administered in several cases without obvious adverse effect.

UNRESECTABLE AND MALIGNANT TUMORS In cases of metastatic or locally invasive tumor or in patients with intercurrent illness that precludes surgery, long-term medical management is required. When the manifestations cannot be adequately controlled by adrenergic blocking agents, the concomitant administration of metyrosine may be required. This agent inhibits tyrosine hydroxylase, diminishes catecholamine production by the tumor, and often simplifies chronic management. Malignant pheochromocytoma frequently recurs in the retroperitoneum and metastasizes most commonly to bone and lung. Although these are resistant to radiotherapy, combination chemotherapy has had limited success in malignant tumors. [131I]metaiodobenzylguanidine (MIBG) has had limited success in the treatment of malignant pheochromocytoma.

PROGNOSIS AND FOLLOW-UP The 5-year survival after surgery is usually over 95 percent, and the recurrence rate is less than 10 percent. After successful surgery, catecholamine excretion returns to normal in about 1 week and should be measured to ensure complete tumor removal. Catecholamine excretion should be assessed at the reappearance of suggestive symptoms or yearly for several years, if the patient remains asymptomatic. In malignant pheochromocytoma, the 5-year survival is less than 50 percent.

Complete removal cures the hypertension in approximately three-fourths. In the remainder, hypertension recurs but is usually well controlled by standard antihypertensive agents. In this group, either underlying essential hypertension or irreversible vascular damage induced by catecholamines may cause the persistence of the hypertension.

REFERENCES

AVERBUCH SD et al: Malignant pheochromocytoma: Effective treatment with a combination of cyclophosphamide, vincristine, and dacarbazine. Ann Intern Med 109:267, 1988

BRAVO EL, GIFFORD RW: Pheochromocytoma: Diagnosis, localization, and management. N Engl J Med 311:1298, 1984

BROWN MJ et al: Increased sensitivity and accuracy of phaeochromocytoma diagnosis achieved by use of plasma-adrenaline estimations and a pentolinium-suppression test. Lancet 1:174, 1981

DALY PA, LANDSBERG L: Phaeochromocytoma: Diagnosis and management. Baillieres Clin Endocrinol Metab 6:143, 1992

DUNCAN MW et al: Measurement of norepinephrine and 3,4-dihydroxyphenylglycol in urine and plasma for the diagnosis of pheochromocytoma. N Engl J Med 319:136, 1988

FUDGE TL et al: Current surgical management of pheochromocytoma during pregnancy. Arch Surg 115:1224, 1980

FUKUMOTO S et al: Pheochromocytoma with pyrexia and marked inflammatory signs: A paraneoplastic syndrome with possible relation to interleukin-6 production. J Clin Endocrinol Metab 73:877, 1991

GLUSHIEN AS et al: Pheochromocytoma: Its relationship to the neurocutaneous syndromes. Am J Med 14:318, 1953

HAMILTON BP et al: Measurement of urinary epinephrine in screening for pheochromocytoma in multiple endocrine neoplasia type II. Am J Med 65:1027, 1978

HORTON WA et al: Von Hippel–Lindau disease: Clinical and pathological manifestations in nine families with 50 affected members. Arch Intern Med 136:769, 1976

JONES DH et al: The biochemical diagnosis, localization and followup of phaeochromocytoma: The role of plasma and urinary catecholamine measurements. Q J Med 49:431, 1980

KHAIRI MRA et al: Mucosal neuroma, pheochromocytoma and medullary thyroid carcinoma: Multiple endocrine neoplasia type 3. Medicine 54:89, 1975

KREMPF M et al: Use of m-(131I) iodobenzylguanidine in the treatment of malignant pheochromocytoma. J Clin Endocrinol Metab 72:455, 1991

LAURSEN K, DAMGAARD-PEDERSON K: CT for pheochromocytoma diagnosis. AJR 134:277, 1980

MACDOUGALL IC et al: Overnight clonidine suppression test in the diagnosis and exclusion of pheochromocytoma. Am J Med 84:993, 1988

MANGER WM, GIFFORD RW JR: *Pheochromocytoma.* New York, Springer-Verlag, 1977

MCCORKELL SJ, NILES NL: Fine-needle aspiration of catecholamine-producing adrenal masses: A possibly fatal mistake. Am J Roentgenol 145:113, 1985

PALUBINSKAS AJ et al: Localization of functioning pheochromocytomas by venous sampling and radioenzymatic analysis. Radiology 136:495, 1980

REINIG JW, DOPPMAN JL: Magnetic resonance imaging of the adrenal. Radiologe 26:186, 1986

ROSS EJ et al: Preoperative and operative management of patients with pheochromocytoma. Br Med J 1:191, 1971

ST JOHN WM, GIFFORD RW JR: Prevalence of clinically unsuspected pheochromocytoma. Mayo Clin Proc 56:354, 1981

SHEMIN D et al: Pheochromocytoma presenting as rhabdomyolysis and acute mycoglobinuric renal failure. Arch Intern Med 150:2384, 1990

SISSON JC et al: Scintigraphic localization of pheochromocytoma. N Engl J Med 305:12, 1981

SJOERDSMA A et al: Pheochromocytoma: Current concepts of diagnosis and treatment. Ann Intern Med 65:1302, 1966

STEINER AL et al: Study of a kindred with pheochromocytoma, medullary thyroid carcinoma, hyperparathyroidism and Cushing's disease: Multiple endocrine neoplasia, type 2. Medicine 47:371, 1968

STEWART AF et al: Hypercalcemia in pheochromocytoma. Ann Intern Med 102:776, 1985

337 DIABETES MELLITUS

DANIEL W. FOSTER

Diabetes mellitus is the most common endocrine disease. The true frequency is difficult to ascertain because of differing standards of diagnosis but probably is between 1 and 2 percent if fasting hyperglycemia is the criterion for diagnosis. The disease is characterized by metabolic abnormalities and by long-term complications involving the eyes, kidneys, nerves, and blood vessels. The patient population is not homogeneous, and several distinct diabetic syndromes have been delineated.

DIAGNOSIS The diagnosis of symptomatic diabetes is not difficult. When a patient presents with signs and symptoms attributable to an osmotic diuresis and is found to have hyperglycemia, essentially all physicians agree that diabetes is present. There is likewise little disagreement about an asymptomatic patient with persistently elevated fasting plasma glucose concentrations. The problem arises with the asymptomatic patient who for one reason or another is considered to be a potential diabetic but has a normal fasting glucose concentration in plasma. Such patients are often given an oral glucose tolerance test, and if abnormal values are found, they are diagnosed as having impaired glucose tolerance or diabetes. There seems to be little question that normal glucose tolerance is strong evidence against the presence of diabetes; the predictive value of a positive test is less

TABLE 337-1   Classification of diabetes

Primary
1 Insulin-dependent diabetes mellitus (IDDM, type 1)
2 Non-insulin-dependent diabetes mellitus (NIDDM, type 2)
  a Nonobese NIDDM (type 1 IDDM in evolution?)
  b Obese NIDDM
  c Maturity-onset diabetes of the young (MODY)
Secondary
1 Pancreatic disease
2 Hormonal abnormalities
3 Drug or chemical induced
4 Insulin receptor abnormalities
5 Genetic syndromes
6 Other

certain. Much evidence suggests that the standard oral glucose tolerance test overdiagnoses diabetes to a remarkable degree, probably because a variety of stresses can produce an abnormal response. The operative mechanism is thought to be epinephrine discharge. Epinephrine blocks insulin secretion, stimulates glucagon release, activates glycogen breakdown, and impairs insulin action in target tissues such that hepatic glucose production is increased and the capacity to dispose of an exogenous glucose load is impaired. Even anxiety over venipunctures may generate sufficient epinephrine to produce an abnormal test. Concomitant illness, inadequate diet, and lack of physical exercise also contribute to false-positive examinations.

In an attempt to deal with these problems, the National Diabetes Data Group of the National Institutes of Health in 1979 provided revised criteria for the diagnosis of diabetes following a challenge with oral glucose:

1 *Fasting (overnight):* Venous plasma glucose concentration ≥ 7.8 mmol/L (140 mg/dL) on at least two separate occasions.[1]
2 *Following ingestion of 75 g of glucose:* Venous plasma glucose concentration ≥ 11.1 mmol/L (200 mg/dL) at 2 h and on at least one other occasion during the 2-h test; i.e., *two* values ≥ 11.1 mmol/L (≥200 mg/dL) must be obtained for diagnosis.

If the 2-h value is between 7.8 and 11.1 mmol/L (140 and 200 mg/dL) and one other value during the 2-h test period is equal to or greater than 11.1 mmol/L (200 mg/dL), a diagnosis of "impaired glucose tolerance" is suggested. The interpretation would be that persons in this category are at increased risk for the development of fasting hyperglycemia or symptomatic diabetes but that such progression is not predictable in an individual patient.

CLASSIFICATION A classification of diabetes is given in Table 337-1. The basic categories are those recommended by the National Diabetes Data Group except for division into primary and secondary types. *Primary* implies that no associated disease is present, while in the *secondary* category some other identifiable condition causes or allows a diabetic syndrome to develop. Insulin dependence in this classification is not equivalent to insulin therapy. Rather, the term means that the patient is at risk for ketoacidosis in the absence of insulin. Many patients classified as non-insulin-dependent require insulin for control of hyperglycemia, although they do not become ketoacidotic if insulin is withdrawn.

The term *type 1* is often used as a synonym for insulin-dependent diabetes (IDDM), and *type 2* diabetes has been considered equivalent to non-insulin-dependent disease (NIDDM). This probably is not ideal, since some patients with apparent non-insulin-dependent diabetes may in fact be destined to become fully insulin-dependent and prone to ketoacidosis. The subset of patients in this category are nonobese subjects who usually express HLA antigens associated with susceptibility to insulin-dependent diabetes and have evidence of an immune response to islet cell antigens (see "Pathogenesis," below). For this reason, it has been suggested that the classification shown in Table

337-1 be modified such that the terms *insulin-dependent* and *non-insulin-dependent* describe physiologic states (ketoacidosis-prone and ketoacidosis-resistant, respectively), while the terms *type 1* and *type 2* refer to pathogenetic mechanisms (immune-mediated and non-immune-mediated, respectively). Using such a classification, three major forms of primary diabetes would be recognized: (1) type 1 insulin-dependent diabetes, (2) type 1 non-insulin-dependent diabetes, and (3) type 2 non-insulin-dependent diabetes. Category 2 is an intermediate stage of autoimmune destruction in which sufficient insulin remains to prevent ketoacidosis but not to maintain normal blood glucose. The NIDDM stage of type 1 diabetes likely occurs when the autoimmune process begins at an older age and progresses at a slower rate. It is infrequently seen when IDDM appears in childhood or early adolescence.

Secondary forms of diabetes encompass a host of conditions. *Pancreatic disease*, particularly chronic pancreatitis in alcoholics, is a common cause. Destruction of the beta cell mass is the etiologic mechanism. *Hormonal causes* include pheochromocytoma, acromegaly, Cushing syndrome, and therapeutic administration of steroid hormones. "Stress hyperglycemia," associated with severe burns, acute myocardial infarctions, and other life-threatening illnesses, is due to endogenous release of glucagon and catecholamines. Mechanisms of hormonal hyperglycemia include varying combinations of impairment of insulin release and induction of insulin resistance. A large number of *drugs* can lead to hyperglycemia, but most simply produce impaired glucose tolerance. Hyperglycemia and even ketoacidosis may occur as a result of abnormalities at the level of the *insulin receptor*. The dysfunction may be due to quantitative or qualitative defects in the receptor itself or to antibodies directed against it. The mechanism is essentially pure insulin resistance. A number of *genetic syndromes* are associated with impaired glucose tolerance or hyperglycemia. The three most common are the lipodystrophies, myotonic dystrophy, and ataxia-telangiectasia. The final category, *other*, is poorly defined and is meant to include any condition which does not fit elsewhere in the etiologic scheme. The appearance of abnormal carbohydrate metabolism in association with any of the secondary causes does not necessarily indicate the presence of underlying diabetes, although in some cases a mild, asymptomatic primary diabetes may be made overt by the secondary illness.

PREVALENCE Prevalence of diabetes is difficult to determine because various standards, many no longer acceptable, have been used in diagnosis. The National Diabetes Data Group, utilizing the 75-g oral glucose tolerance test as the diagnostic criterion, has estimated the prevalence of diabetes at 6.6 percent, with 11.2 percent of the population having impaired glucose tolerance. These figures are almost certainly too high. Most subjects diagnosed with impaired glucose tolerance or diabetes by oral glucose tolerance testing, when followed longitudinally, never develop fasting hyperglycemia or symptomatic diabetes. For example, in a massive screening program (more than 300,000 subjects) in Cleveland, Ohio, only 31 percent of persons with 2-h glucose values of 10 mmol/L or higher in the glucose tolerance test progressed to overt diabetes after 5 years. Other studies confirm the propensity of oral glucose challenges to be imprecise in predicting or diagnosing diabetes—hence the estimates of 1 to 2 percent prevalence used here. Similar conclusions have been reached in Sweden, where a prevalence of 1.5 percent has been reported. Estimates for insulin-dependent diabetes are more reliable than for the non-insulin-dependent form because most patients are diagnosed after the abrupt appearance of symptoms. In England, prevalence of the type 1 illness has been estimated to be 0.22 percent by age 16, and a study in the United States suggested a prevalence of 0.26 percent by age 20. If the prevalence of diabetes is about 1 percent, it follows that about one-fourth of cases have insulin-dependent disease, while three-fourths are non-insulin-dependent. The relative frequency of insulin-dependent to non-insulin-dependent diabetes varies with age, being higher if a young population is studied and lower in the older age range. Frequently cited statements that the ratio of NIDDM to IDDM is 10 or more are based on inflated estimates

---

[1] Venous whole blood concentrations are 15 percent lower than plasma values. Capillary whole blood, utilized in patient self-monitoring, is equivalent to venous plasma.

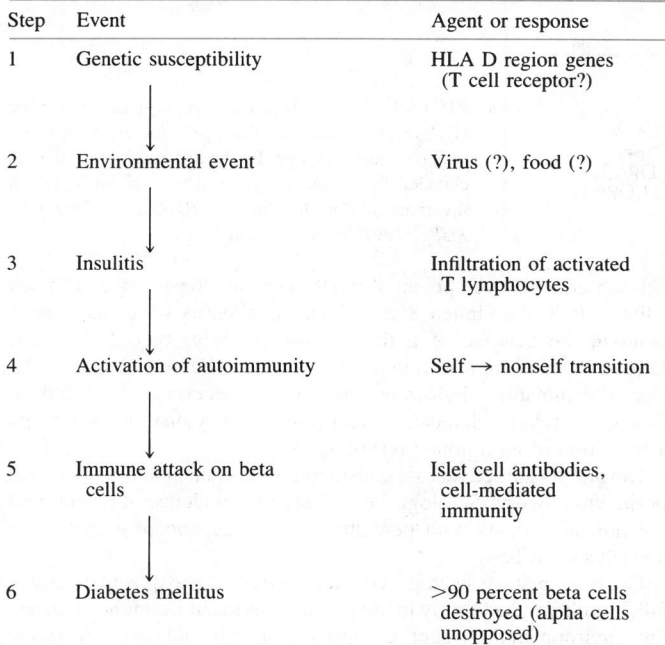

TABLE 337-2 The pathogenesis of type 1 diabetes mellitus

Step	Event	Agent or response
1	Genetic susceptibility	HLA D region genes (T cell receptor?)
2	Environmental event	Virus (?), food (?)
3	Insulitis	Infiltration of activated T lymphocytes
4	Activation of autoimmunity	Self → nonself transition
5	Immune attack on beta cells	Islet cell antibodies, cell-mediated immunity
6	Diabetes mellitus	>90 percent beta cells destroyed (alpha cells unopposed)

of NIDDM obtained with glucose tolerance testing. The cited prevalences are for populations as a whole. Certain subsets have different rates. For example, more than 40 percent of Pima Indians in the United States have type 2 NIDDM.

It has been argued that persons with asymptomatic, undiagnosed diabetes may develop complications despite the absence of fasting hyperglycemia. This has led to suggestions of large-scale screening with glucose tolerance tests. For the reasons given above, this seems unwise.

PATHOGENESIS OF INSULIN-DEPENDENT DIABETES MELLITUS By the time insulin-dependent diabetes mellitus appears, most of the beta cells in the pancreas have been destroyed. The destructive process is almost certainly autoimmune in nature, although details remain obscure. A tentative overview of the pathogenetic sequence is given in Table 337-2. *First,* genetic susceptibility to the disease must be present. *Second,* an environmental event ordinarily initiates the process in genetically susceptible individuals. Viral infection is believed to be one triggering mechanism, but noninfectious agents also could be involved. The best evidence that an environmental insult is required comes from studies in monozygotic twins, in whom the concordance rate for diabetes is less than 50 percent. If diabetes were a purely genetic illness, concordance rates would be approximately 100 percent. The *third* step in the sequence is an inflammatory response in the pancreas called *insulitis.* The cells that infiltrate the islets are monocyte/macrophages and activated T lymphocytes. The *fourth* step is an alteration or transformation of the beta cell such that it is no longer recognized as "self" but is seen by the immune system as a foreign cell or "nonself." The *fifth* step is the development of an immune response. Because the islets are now considered "nonself," cytotoxic antibodies develop and act in concert with cell-mediated immune mechanisms. The end result is the destruction of the beta cell and the appearance of diabetes. Rarely, type 1 diabetes may develop from an exclusive environmental insult. An example is the ingestion of Vacor, a rat poison. It is also possible that in some cases autoimmune diabetes develops in the absence of an environmental trigger; i.e., it is purely genetic. Usually, however, the pathogenetic sequence is genetic predisposition → environmental insult → insulitis → conversion of beta cell from "self" to "nonself" → activation of the immune system → destruction of the beta cell → diabetes mellitus.

Genetics Although insulin-dependent diabetes aggregates in families, the mechanism of inheritance is unclear in Mendelian terms. Transmission has been postulated to be autosomal dominant, recessive, and mixed, but none has been proven. The genetic predisposition is probably permissive and not causal.

Analysis of pedigrees shows a low prevalence of direct vertical transmission. In one series of 35 families in which there was a child with classic insulin-dependent diabetes, only four of the index cases had a parent with diabetes and two had a diabetic grandparent. Of the 99 siblings of these diabetic children, only 6 had overt disease. Overall, the chance of a child developing type 1 diabetes when another first-degree relative has the disease is only 5 to 10 percent. HLA identity of siblings (see below) increases the risk, while nonidentity decreases it. Haploidentity (sharing of one HLA genotype) is an intermediate risk. The presence of non-insulin-dependent disease in a parent increases the risk for insulin-dependent diabetes in the offspring. It is not known whether the intermixing of IDDM and NIDDM in the same family represents a single genetic trait (i.e., the apparent NIDDM is really type 1 NIDDM) or whether two common genetic predispositions coexist in the same family by chance, each perhaps influencing the expression of the other. Low rates of transmission of IDDM make it difficult to discern mechanisms of inheritance through study of families but are reassuring to diabetic parents who may wish to have children. Type 1 diabetes appears to be a disease in which *sexual imprinting* plays a role. The risk of diabetes is up to five times higher when the father has the disease than when the mother is diabetic.

One of the susceptibility genes in IDDM likely resides on the sixth chromosome in view of strong associations between diabetes and certain human leukocyte antigens encoded by the major histocompatibility region on this chromosome (see Chap. 64). Four loci designated by the letters A, B, C, and D are recognized with alleles at each site identified by numbers (e.g., DR3). A lowercase w indicates that identification is provisional (e.g., DQw8). Gene products of the A, B, and C regions are called *class I molecules*, while D-region products are called *class II molecules*. The D region (Fig. 337-1) is subdivided into DR, DP, and DQ and also contains several less well understood subregions. HLA gene products are located in the plasma membranes of cells and are best considered as recognition and/or programming signals for initiation and amplification of immune responses in the body. They are two-chain molecules, the light chain in class I HLA being beta₂ microglobulin, while in the D region the dimer is composed of α and β chains. Class I molecules are present on all nucleated cells and function primarily in defense against infections (especially viruses). They are also involved in immune surveillance against malignancy. Class II molecules are normally present on circulating and tissue macrophages, endothelial cells, B lymphocytes, and activated T lymphocytes. They function in the regulatory (helper-suppressor) T cell system. HLA genes are important in autoimmune diseases such as type 1 diabetes. Activation of the immune system is "MHC-restricted." This means that antigens are recognized only if they reach the cell surface in association with a "self" HLA allele which "fits" the receptor on the responding T cell. Thus activation of cytotoxic T lymphocytes to fight a viral infection requires that a viral antigen be presented by a class I molecule recognized by the responding cytotoxic T cell. Similar restriction applies to antigen presentation by macrophages to helper T cells.

While definite associations exist between class 1 alleles and type 1 diabetes (B8, B15), the D locus is considered of primary importance. Class 1 loci are involved through nonrandom associations with D (*linkage disequilibrium*). Because about 95 percent of white type 1 IDDM patients express either DR3 or DR4 or the heterozygous DR3/DR4 configuration, it was initially thought that a susceptibility gene might be located nearby. Focus has since shifted to the DQ locus. Originally, typing at D region sites was done by serologic methods but now can be carried out by analyzing DNA with allele-specific oligonucleotide probes. Certain class II alleles are associated with susceptibility to IDDM, while others are protective and still others

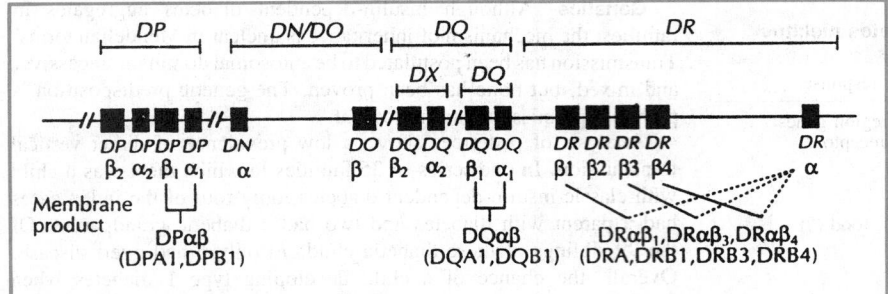

FIGURE 337-1 Schematic representation of the HLA D (class II) region. Gene products are determined by constituent α and β chains, each of which is encoded by a separate gene. The α chain at DR is invariant. *(From JM Baisch, JD Capra, Curr Biol 1:385, 1991, by permission.)*

are neutral. For example, HLA DQβ₁*0302 (which codes for one allele of the β chain of HLA DQ) is a susceptibility gene, while HLA DQβ₁*0301 is associated with a low risk for IDDM. HLA DQβ₁*0602 appears to be dominantly protective, overriding the high-risk DQβ₁*0302 gene when both are present. Terminology in the HLA field changes rapidly. DQβ₁*0301 was formerly known as DQw7 or DQw3.1, DQβ₁*0302 was previously known as DQw8 or DQw3.2, and DQβ₁*0602 was known as DQw1.2.

How might differing HLA alleles function in predisposition to or protection from IDDM? Probably by exhibiting varying affinity for diabetogenic peptides to be presented to the immune system. Thus HLA DQβ₁*0302 might bind a diabetogenic peptide with greater affinity for presentation on the cell surface than DQβ₁*0301. Conversely, a dominant protective allele (which presumably would not present antigen in such a way as to activate the immune system) might bind the diabetogenic peptide with such high affinity as to effectively "steal it" from a susceptibility gene even when both are present, thereby preventing the disease. Although the DQβ chain alleles appear to predict risk for diabetes most precisely, they may well be influenced by interaction with α chains. Thus T cell recognition of a DQβ₁*0302 is modified by the associated DQα allele. The situation is further complicated by the fact that α and β chains from different HLA molecules may interact to form new dimers, a process called *transcomplementation*. Some authors have found that susceptibility to autoimmune diabetes is linked to decreased expression of class I HLA molecules on splenocytes and lymphocytes in NOD mice (which get autoimmune diabetes) and in humans. The meaning of this finding and its reproducibility are not clear.

While emphasis has been placed on the HLA region as a site for regulatory genes and the development of type 1 diabetes, it is likely that one or more other genes are also involved. It also has been reported that HLA associations found in children may not operate when the disease begins in adults.

Environmental event   As noted earlier, the fact that a significant proportion of monozygotic twins remain discordant for diabetes (one twin with, the other without) has suggested that nongenetic factors are required for expression of diabetes in humans. Similar arguments derive from the fact that HLA identity or haploidentity does not ensure concordance.

The environmental factor in many cases is believed to be a virus capable of infecting the beta cell. A viral etiology was originally suggested by seasonal variations in the onset of the disease and what appeared to be more than a chance relationship between appearance of diabetes and preceding episodes of mumps, hepatitis, infectious mononucleosis, congenital rubella, and coxsackievirus infections. The viral hypothesis gained support from studies showing that certain strains of encephalomyocarditis virus cause diabetes in genetically susceptible mice. The isolation of a coxsackievirus B4 from the pancreas of a previously healthy boy who died following an episode of ketoacidosis and the induction of diabetes in experimental animals inoculated with the isolated virus also suggested that viruses can cause diabetes in humans. A rise in titer of neutralizing antibody to coxsackievirus over the weeks prior to death of the patient indicated that the virus was recently acquired. Further support for the viral theory comes from the observation that congenital rubella is associated

with subsequent development of IDDM in about 20 percent of affected individuals in the United States. Cytomegalovirus genes have been found in the genome of a fifth of patients with type 1 diabetes. Retroviral genes are also found consistently in the beta cells of NOD mice. Presumably viral infections of the pancreas could induce diabetes by two mechanisms: direct inflammatory disruption of islets or induction of an immune response.

Despite its attractiveness, considerable caution should be reserved for the viral theory. Serologic studies seeking evidence of recent viral infection in patients with new-onset insulin-dependent diabetes are inconclusive at best.

Great interest has been generated by reports that exposure to cow's milk or milk products early in life predisposes to autoimmune diabetes. The environmental trigger proposed is bovine albumin operating through the mechanism of molecular mimicry. In the initial study, diabetic subjects had antibodies to bovine albumin with a subset specific for a 17-amino acid epitope providing maximal association with the disease. The latter antibodies bind to a 69-kDa protein on the surface of the pancreatic beta cell. The idea would be that exposure to cow's milk induced an immune response to the 17-amino acid fragment in some infants. Cross-reactivity with the p69 antigen would destroy beta cells expressing this peptide. Not universally present on beta cells, p69 can be induced through the action of interferon-γ produced by intermittent viral infections. These results, while intriguing, have not been confirmed at the time of this writing.

Insulitis   In animals, macrophages and activated T lymphocytes infiltrate the pancreatic islets prior to or simultaneously with development of diabetes. Lymphocytes are also found in the islets of young persons dying from new-onset diabetes, and radioactively labeled lymphocytes localize in the pancreas in humans with IDDM. These findings are in accord with the observation that immune endocrinopathies in general are associated with lymphocytic infiltration of the affected tissue. It is not clear, however, that insulitis is primary to the destructive sequence in autoimmune diabetes. Some workers believe the cellular infiltration to be an epiphenomenon.

Conversion of the beta cell from "self" to "nonself" and activation of the immune system   There seems to be little doubt that the immune system mediates beta cell destruction in type 1 diabetes. The disease is frequently associated with other autoimmune endocrinopathies such as adrenal insufficiency and Hashimoto's thyroiditis; pancreas transplanted from a nondiabetic monozygotic twin into the diabetic twin is rapidly destroyed without evidence of rejection in the absence of immunosuppression, and temporary reversal of clinical symptoms occurs with early use of cyclosporine. Moreover, a majority of patients have antibodies directed against insulin and other beta cell antigens. Since the immune system normally does not attack "self" tissues, it is probably acceptable to define IDDM as an autoimmune disease.

The mechanism by which this occurs is not known. As noted earlier, an environmental trigger appears to be required (frequently, if not always). The putative environmental agent could be a virus, a toxin, or a food. The agent might act in one of several ways. Direct destruction of beta cells by a virus or toxin might expose cryptic antigens to the immune system, invoking an immune response. A relative deficiency of early complement components might impair clearing of islet cell viruses (analogous to persistent hepatitis B infection in some patients with chronic active hepatitis), thereby prolonging cryptic antigen stimulation of the immune system. Alternatively, the agent might form a neoantigen in association with normal membrane structures or newly expressed class II HLA molecules of the susceptibility type (see below). Another popular hypothesis is the aforementioned *molecular mimicry*, a term referring to chance homology between a foreign antigen and a short stretch of amino acids in normal tissue. The best-known example is acute rheumatic fever, where immune response to group A streptococci results in cross-reacting attack on the heart. Once cytotoxic T cells and plasma cells are activated against a particular antigenic epitope (armed), they seek and destroy any cell bearing the epitope. The bovine milk albumin hypothesis mentioned earlier invoked molecular mimicry. It is of interest that homology exists between a coxsackievirus protein and glutamic acid decarboxylase (GAD). Antibodies against GAD are common in subjects with type 1 diabetes.

A third possibility, currently less popular, is that viral infection, via cytokine release, induces HLA D-region molecules in the pancreas (where they are not normally present), converting one or more cell types into antigen-presenting cells.

It is possible that some patients may have a purely genetic form of the disease. In neonatal life, autoreactive T cells are normally destroyed in the thymus ("clonal deletion"). Any cells escaping the thymus are rendered anergic or suppressed in the periphery by regulatory T cells. Failure of either process could leave a repertoire of cells capable of responding to "self" antigens following cell injury. In support of the possibility that a contributing factor in autoimmune disease is suboptimal removal or regulation of autoreactive T cells, intrathymic injection of islets prevents diabetes in the BB rat, a species manifesting an autoimmune form of the disease. Presumably the presence of additional beta cell antigens in the thymus allows the removal of autoreactive lymphocytes capable of responding to islet tissue.

In summary, the precise mechanisms remain a mystery, but activated immune attack is believed to be the fundamental process causing IDDM.

Destruction of beta cells and development of IDDM Because persons developing insulin-dependent diabetes often have a rather abrupt onset of symptomatic hyperglycemia with polyuria and/or ketoacidosis, it was long assumed that beta cell damage occurred rapidly. It is now believed that in most cases there is a slow loss of insulin reserve over a few to many years. This insight came from studies of discordant monozygotic diabetic twins and triplets in whom one twin or triplet developed diabetes long after the index case. In the slow course the earliest sign of abnormality is the development of islet cell antibodies at a time when there is no elevation of the blood sugar and glucose tolerance is normal. Insulin responses to a glucose load are intact. A phase then ensues in which the only metabolic abnormality is decreased glucose tolerance. Fasting blood sugar remains normal. In the third stage fasting hyperglycemia develops, but ketosis does not occur even when the diabetes is poorly controlled. The clinical appearance is that of non-insulin-dependent diabetes mellitus. With time, however, insulin dependence and ketoacidosis may develop, especially with stress. Many nonobese patients with non-insulin-dependent diabetes mellitus may have a slow autoimmune form of the disease, as mentioned earlier.

The immune-directed destruction of beta cells probably involves both humoral and cell-mediated mechanisms, the latter being more important. Islet cell antibodies have different specificities. Originally, they were generically defined as cytoplasmic and surface (complement-fixing), but specific antigens have now been identified. These include insulin, proinsulin, two forms of glutamic acid decarboxylase (GAD 65 and GAD 67), carboxypeptidase H, two ganglioside antigens (GT3 and GM2-1), ICA 69 (an antibody reacting with the 69-kDa bovine albumin peptide), and antibodies directed against the glucose transporter of the beta cell (GLUT 2). The GAD 65 antibody is equivalent to the earlier described 64-kDa antibody. A subset of anti-GAD antibodies appears to react with human and rat but not mouse islets. These "restricted" islet cell antibodies appear to be linked to the protective HLA allele $DQ\beta_1*0602$ and thus may be a mark of resistance to development of diabetes rather than prediction that the disease will occur, as is usually the case.

A variety of cells appear to carry out the beta cell attack with natural killer cells, activated cytotoxic T lymphocytes (CD8), and macrophages each having a part. The final common pathway of cell destruction may be at least partially due to release of cytokines such as interleukin 1 (IL-1) and tumor necrosis factor alpha (TNFα) from activated macrophages. Experimentally, mixtures of cytokines (IL-1, TNFα, interferon-γ, and lymphotoxin) appear to act synergistically and are more potent than single agents. Purified beta cells are reported to be less sensitive to cytokine toxicity than beta cells in intact islets, suggesting that some effects may be indirect.

By the time overt diabetes appears, most insulin-producing cells have disappeared. In one study, pancreatic mass at autopsy averaged 40 g in type 1 diabetes versus 82 g in controls. Endocrine cell mass in subjects with IDDM decreased from 1395 to 413 mg, and beta cells, which averaged 850 mg in normal individuals, were unmeasurable. Since alpha cells remained essentially intact, the ratio of glucagon- to insulin-producing cells approached infinity.

PATHOGENESIS OF NON-INSULIN-DEPENDENT DIABETES
Little progress has been made in understanding the pathogenesis of non-insulin-dependent diabetes mellitus.

Genetics Although the disease runs in families, modes of inheritance are not known except for the variant known as *maturity-onset diabetes of the young* (MODY). MODY is usually manifested by mild hyperglycemia in young persons who are resistant to ketosis. Four lines of evidence suggest transmission as an autosomal dominant trait. First, three-generation direct transmission has been demonstrated in over 20 families. Second, a 1:1 ratio of diabetic to nondiabetic children is found when one parent has the disease. Third, about 90 percent of obligate carriers have diabetes. Fourth, direct male-to-male transmission excludes X-linked inheritance.

Genetic studies have shown a clear linkage between MODY and mutations in the glucokinase gene located on the short arm of chromosome 7. The abnormality is not found in ordinary NIDDM. A polymorphism in the glycogen synthase gene has been reported in some patients with typical NIDDM, but its significance is not known. Glycogen synthase is an attractive candidate because glycogen synthesis is impaired in NIDDM. However, the A_2 allele presumed to mark diabetes was present in only 30 percent of the study group of 107 patients (8 percent in controls). No HLA relationships have been identified, and autoimmune mechanisms are not thought to be operative. It is highly likely that more than one gene is involved in NIDDM, but a number of candidate molecules have proved unrewarding in the search for informative mutations. These include the glucose transporter molecules GLUT 2 and GLUT 4 (which transport glucose across the plasma membrane in pancreas/liver and muscle/fat, respectively), the insulin receptor, and the amyloidogenic peptide of islets called *amylin*. Whatever its nature, the genetic influence is powerful, since the concordance rate for diabetes in monozygotic twins with type 2 disease approaches 100 percent. Risk to offspring and siblings of patients with NIDDM is higher than in type 1 diabetes. Nearly four-tenths of siblings and one-third of offspring eventually develop abnormal glucose tolerance or frank diabetes.

Pathophysiology Patients with type 2 NIDDM have two physiologic defects: abnormal insulin secretion and resistance to insulin action in target tissues. Which of the abnormalities is primary is not known. Descriptively, three phases can be recognized in the usual clinical sequence. In the first, the plasma glucose remains normal despite demonstrable insulin resistance because insulin levels are elevated. In the second phase, insulin resistance tends to worsen so that despite elevated insulin concentrations, glucose intolerance becomes manifested by postprandial hyperglycemia. In the third phase, insulin resistance does not change, but insulin secretion declines, resulting in fasting hyperglycemia and overt diabetes.

Most authorities believe that insulin resistance is primary, with hyperinsulinemia being secondary; i.e., insulin secretion increases to compensate for the resistance state. However, it is possible that hypersecretion of insulin (and amylin?) causes insulin resistance; i.e., a primary islet cell defect causes insulin hypersecretion, and insulin hypersecretion, in turn, leads to insulin resistance. Explanatory hypotheses involve insulin-stimulated fat synthesis in the liver with fat transport (via very low density lipoproteins) leading to secondary fat storage in muscle. Increased fat oxidation would impair glucose uptake and glycogen synthesis. The late decline in insulin release could be due to toxic effects of glucose on the islets or result from an underlying genetic defect. Most patients with NIDDM are obese, and obesity per se causes insulin resistance. However, nonobese relatives of persons with NIDDM may have hyperinsulinemia and diminished insulin sensitivity, proving that obesity is not the sole cause of resistance. This is not to diminish the importance of excess fat, since a modest reduction in weight often results in major improvement in blood sugar control in obese subjects with NIDDM.

In summary, an insulin secretory defect and insulin resistance are characteristic of NIDDM. It is likely that both are required for diabetes to be expressed, since massively obese persons with marked insulin resistance may have normal glucose tolerance. Presumably, the beta cell lesion is not present in such persons. This might suggest that the primary defect resides in the insulin-producing cells. Beta cell mass is intact in type 2 NIDDM, in contrast to the situation with type 1 IDDM. The alpha cell population is increased, resulting in an elevated alpha to beta cell ratio. This accounts for the excess of glucagon relative to insulin that characterizes NIDDM and that is a feature of all hyperglycemic states.

Although insulin resistance in type 2 NIDDM is associated with decreased numbers of insulin receptors, the bulk of the resistance is postreceptor in type (see below). It has long been known that deposits of amyloid are found in the pancreas of patients with type 2 diabetes. This material is a 37-amino acid peptide termed *amylin*. Amylin is normally copackaged with insulin in secretory granules and is released simultaneously in response to insulin secretagogues. In animals, amylin has been reported to induce insulin resistance. Its deposition in the islets may be the consequence of overproduction secondary to the insulin resistance to which it contributes. Alternatively, accumulation of amylin in the islets might contribute to the late failure of insulin production with long-standing NIDDM. The safest conclusion is that a role for amylin is not established.

Regardless of the mechanism of insulin resistance, its physiologic consequences are clear. There is no major abnormality in either glucose uptake by the cell or its oxidative metabolism to CO_2, water, and lactate. Rather, the major metabolic block is in glycogen synthesis ("nonoxidative metabolism"). Impaired nonoxidative metabolism of glucose, like hyperinsulinemia and insulin resistance, may be seen in nonobese, normoglycemic relatives of subjects with NIDDM.

A rare form of type 2 NIDDM, clinically mild, is due to production of an abnormal insulin that does not bind well to insulin receptors. Such persons respond normally to exogenous insulin.

CLINICAL FEATURES   The manifestations of symptomatic diabetes mellitus vary from patient to patient. Most often medical help is sought because of symptoms related to hyperglycemia (polyuria, polydipsia, polyphagia), but the first event may be an acute metabolic decompensation resulting in diabetic coma. Occasionally, the initial expression is a degenerative complication such as neuropathy in the absence of symptomatic hyperglycemia. The metabolic derangements of diabetes are due to relative or absolute deficiency of insulin and relative or absolute excess of glucagon. Normally, it is a rise in the molar ratio of glucagon to insulin that leads to metabolic decompensation. Changes in this ratio can be caused by a fall in insulin or a rise in glucagon concentration, separately or together. Conceptually, alteration in biologic response to either hormone would have the same effect. Thus insulin resistance could cause metabolic effects expected of an elevated glucagon/insulin ratio even though the ratio assessed by immunoassay of the two hormones in plasma

TABLE 337-3   General characteristics of IDDM and NIDDM diabetes

	IDDM	NIDDM
Genetic locus	Chromosome 6	Unknown
Age of onset	<40	>40
Body habitus	Normal to wasted	Obese
Plasma insulin	Low to absent	Normal to high
Plasma glucagon	High, suppressible	High, resistant
Acute complication	Ketoacidosis	Hyperosmolar coma
Insulin therapy	Responsive	Responsive to resistant
Sulfonylurea therapy	Unresponsive	Responsive

was not markedly abnormal or even decreased (the glucagon being biologically active, the insulin relatively inactive). The relationship between metabolic abnormalities and degenerative complications will be discussed subsequently. Typically, the clinical features of IDDM and NIDDM are distinctive.

Insulin-dependent diabetes   Insulin-dependent diabetes usually begins before age 40; in the United States, peak incidence is around age 14. Some patients develop type 1 diabetes late in life, with a first episode of ketoacidosis occurring at age 50 or even later in rare instances. These patients, who on the basis of age should have type 2 NIDDM, are usually not obese. Onset of symptoms may be abrupt, with thirst, excessive urination, increased appetite, and weight loss developing over a several-day period. In some cases the disease is heralded by the appearance of ketoacidosis during an intercurrent illness or following surgery. As outlined in Table 337-3, type 1 patients vary from normal weight to wasted depending on the length of time between onset of symptoms and start of treatment. Characteristically, the plasma insulin level is low or immeasurable. Glucagon levels are elevated but suppressible with insulin. Once symptoms have developed, insulin therapy is required. Occasionally, an initial episode of ketoacidosis is followed by a symptom-free interval (the "honeymoon" period), during which no treatment is required. The likely explanation for this phenomenon is shown in Fig. 337-2.

FIGURE 337-2   Schematic representation of the "honeymoon" period. In this graph, insulin secretory capacity is shown gradually decreasing in a patient destined to develop diabetes. At approximately $13\frac{1}{2}$ years, insulin would become insufficient to maintain plasma glucose in the normal range. An initial episode of ketoacidosis, for example, in association with acute appendicitis, is shown occurring in the twelfth year. Presumably stress-induced epinephrine release blocks insulin secretion and causes the syndrome. In normal subjects, insulin reserve is such that hormone release is adequate, even in the face of stress. Following recovery from the stressful episode, insulin secretory capacity returns to the previous level and remains sufficient for an additional year, as indicated by the shaded area—the "honeymoon" period.

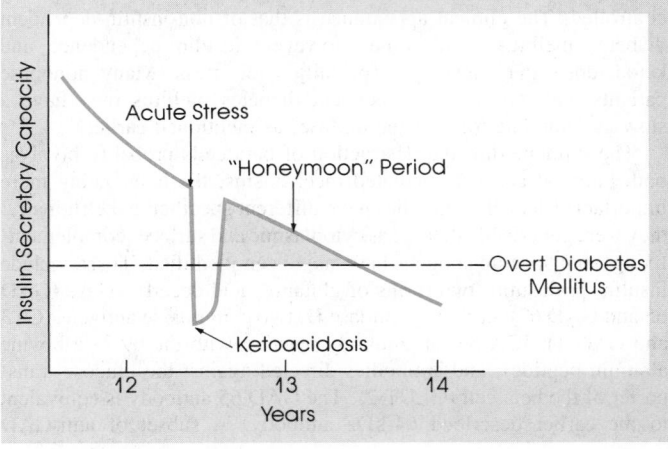

Non-insulin-dependent diabetes This disorder usually begins in middle life or beyond. The typical patient is overweight. Symptoms begin more gradually than in IDDM, and the diagnosis is frequently made when an asymptomatic person is found to have an elevated plasma glucose on routine laboratory examination. In contrast to insulin-dependent disease, plasma insulin levels are normal to high in absolute terms, although they are lower than predicted for the level of the plasma glucose; i.e., relative insulin deficiency is present. Stated in another way, if plasma glucose concentrations in nondiabetic subjects were raised to levels equivalent to those found in diabetic patients, insulin values would be higher in the normal group. This reflects the previously mentioned insulin secretory defect in NIDDM. Glucagon metabolism in non-insulin-dependent diabetes is complex. While the elevated fasting plasma concentrations can be lowered by large amounts of insulin, the exaggerated glucagon response to ingested nutrients cannot be suppressed; i.e., alpha cell function remains abnormal. For unknown reasons, patients with non-insulin-dependent diabetes do not develop ketoacidosis. In the decompensated state they are susceptible to the syndrome of hyperosmolar, nonketotic coma. One hypothesis to explain the absence of ketoacidosis during stress is that the liver is resistant to glucagon so that malonyl-CoA levels remain high, inhibiting the fatty acid oxidation–ketogenic pathway (see below). If weight loss can be induced, patients may be managed by diet alone. The majority of patients failing dietary therapy respond to sulfonylureas, but improvement of hyperglycemia in many is not sufficient for control of diabetes. For this reason, a high percentage of patients with NIDDM are treated with insulin.

TREATMENT   Diet An estimate is made of the total energy intake needed per day based on ideal body weight (determined from life insurance tables). A decision is then made regarding carbohydrate, fat, and protein content, and an appropriate diet is constructed from the exchange system provided by the American Diabetes Association. Caloric recommendations from the Food and Nutrition Board for adults carrying out "average" activity decrease with age and range from 175 kJ/kg of body weight (42 kcal/kg) in 18-year old men to 140 kJ/kg (33 kcal/kg) for 75-year-old women. Intakes slightly less than official recommendations are usually preferable; 150 kJ/kg (36 kcal/kg) for men and 140 kJ/kg (34 kcal/kg) for women are reasonable initial values in most patients, but upward or downward adjustments may be necessary to achieve desired weight.

The minimal protein requirement for good nutrition is about 0.9 g/kg of body weight per day. Recommended carbohydrate content is 40 to 60 percent of total energy intake, although fractional intakes as high as 85 percent have been prescribed. Protein and carbohydrate calories are supplemented with sufficient fat to bring energy intake to the desired level. Although sucrose is ordinarily not allowed in diabetic diets, a number of reports indicate that in moderation ordinary sugar does not exaggerate postprandial hyperglycemia. Currently, most diabetic diets emphasize polyunsaturated fats as an antiathero-genic measure. Alternatively, monounsaturated fats can be used and are thought preferable by some investigators. A 50 percent fat diet containing 33 percent monounsaturated fatty acids and 35 percent carbohydrate reportedly lowers glucose levels, insulin requirements, and very low density lipoprotein concentrations while raising plasma high-density lipoproteins. Fish oils containing omega 3 fatty acids also have been reported to be beneficial, but additional studies are required to draw firm conclusions. Increased amounts of fiber are often prescribed.

Once the desirable caloric intake and the fractional distribution between fat, protein, and carbohydrate are decided, a diet has traditionally been constructed using the exchange lists shown in Table 337-4.[2] For example, a 9200-kJ (2200-kcal) diet with 50 percent of the calories as carbohydrate and 1 to 1.5 g protein per kilogram of body weight can be met by providing 2 milk exchanges, 7 fruit exchanges, 12 bread exchanges, 8 meat exchanges, 4 fat exchanges,

[2] Copies of *Exchange Lists for Meal Planning* may be ordered from the American Diabetes Association, National Service Center, 1660 Duke Street, P.O. Box 25757, Alexandria, VA 22313, or from any local affiliate of the association.

TABLE 337-4   Composition of food exchanges*

Exchange	kJ (kcal)	Carbohydrate, g	Fat, g	Protein, g
Milk	711 (170)	12	10	8
Vegetable†	146 (35)	7	—	2
Fruit	167 (40)	10	—	—
Bread	293 (70)‡	15	—	2
Meat	314 (75)‡	—	5	7
Fat	188 (45)	—	5	—

* Composition listed for one exchange.
† Type A vegetables contain little carbohydrate, fat, or protein and can be eaten in any amount. Exchange values are for type B vegetables.
‡ Calculated value for bread exchange is 285 kJ (68 kcal) and for meat exchange is 306 kJ (73 kcal) using 17 kJ/g (4 kcal/g) for carbohydrate and protein and 38 kJ/g (9 kcal/g) for fat.

and unlimited type A vegetables (Table 337-5). In practice, precalculated diets of given caloric content prepared by the American Diabetes Association are usually used. Care must be taken to emphasize foods the patient likes and can obtain. As in any dietary regimen, it is important to emphasize that it is the long-term, overall dietary pattern that counts. Deviation for one or two meals does not matter much. Thus a teenage diabetic may be allowed to eat a dessert, ordinarily forbidden, as a special treat with the understanding that resumption of the diet will be necessary the next day. Even in adults the "treat" technique often ensures better dietary cooperation than more rigid demands. Ideally, patients should be trained by dieticians in a formal teaching program. Such classes are available in most large hospitals. If a patient is from a smaller community, it will probably be helpful to refer to a larger center for initial training.

In insulin-requiring patients, the distribution of calories is also important if hypoglycemia is to be avoided. A typical pattern might include 20 percent of the total for breakfast, 35 percent for lunch, 30 percent for dinner, and 15 percent as a late-evening feeding. Often, a midmorning and a midafternoon snack are necessary. Different distributions may be required for different life-styles; i.e., a person employed on a late-evening or night shift would not eat the major meal at noon. When regimes of meticulous control are attempted using multiple injections of insulin or insulin pumps, more frequent feedings are often prescribed. Thus one might recommend 20 percent of energy intake at both breakfast and lunch, 30 percent at dinner, and the remaining 30 percent as midmorning, midafternoon, and late-evening snacks depending on the pattern of plasma glucose level during the day.

The traditional approach to dietary therapy has come under question as a result of experiments designed to measure actual blood sugar responses to ingested foods. It is now clear that the exchanges are not necessarily equivalent; i.e., foods of the same weight and similar fat, carbohydrate, or protein content may result in different postprandial increases in the plasma glucose. The term *glycemic index* has been coined to express these differences. In calculating a glycemic index, the mean plasma glucose level is measured over a 2- to 3-h period after ingestion of a test food and compared with the response

TABLE 337-5   9400-kJ (2200-kcal) diabetic diet (50 percent carbohydrate)

Exchange	No.	kJ (kcal)	Carbohydrate, g	Fat, g	Protein, g
Milk	2	1420 (340)	24	20	16
Vegetable*					
Fruit	7	1170 (280)	70	—	—
Bread	12	3520 (840)	180	—	24
Meat	8	2510 (600)	—	40	56
Fat	4	750 (180)	—	20	—
Total		9370 (2240)	274 (50%)	80 (33%)	96 (17%)

* Type B vegetables include beets, carrots, onions, green peas, pumpkin, rutabagas, winter squash, and turnips. If these are desired, ½ to 1 cup can be substituted for one fruit exchange. All other common vegetables can be eaten as desired.

with a reference standard of defined composition such as bread. Although in principle the approach is attractive because it measures actual glycemic response to foods, its applicability to the general diabetic population is not established. One of the problems is that a glycemic index determined for a food ingested by itself may not apply in a normal mixed meal.

The importance of diet in the management of diabetes varies with type of disease. In insulin-dependent patients, particularly those on intensive insulin regimens, the composition of the diet is not of critical importance, since adjustment of insulin can cover wide variations in food ingestion. In non-insulin-dependent patients not treated with exogenous insulin, more rigorous adherence to a fixed diet is required, since endogenous insulin reserve is limited. Such patients cannot respond to increased demand produced by excess calories or increased intake of rapidly absorbed carbohydrate.

Insulin Insulin is required for treatment of all patients with IDDM and many patients with non-insulin-dependent disease. If the physician does not use oral agents (see below), all diet-unresponsive NIDDM subjects must be given the hormone. It is fairly easy to control the symptoms of diabetes with insulin, but it is difficult to maintain a normal blood sugar throughout 24 h even if one utilizes multiple injections of regular insulin or infusion pumps. In the Diabetes Control and Complications Trial (see below), where teams of health care workers attempted to return the blood glucose level to normal or near normal with much more frequent professional input than is usual in clinical situations, blood glucose levels and hemoglobin A_{1c} concentrations remained above normal in most subjects. It is even more difficult to maintain normal blood sugars utilizing traditional insulin therapy given as one or two injections a day. Nondiabetic subjects maintain the plasma glucose concentration within a narrow range at all times despite episodic food intake. When a meal is eaten, a prompt rise in insulin release occurs such that absorbed carbohydrate is rapidly transported into the liver and other tissues. Even after meals, therefore, the plasma glucose level in normal subjects does not rise into the hyperglycemic or glycosuric range. As the plasma glucose level falls under the influence of insulin, release of the hormone is damped, and counterregulatory hormones enter the circulation to prevent hypoglycemia, ensuring smooth control of plasma glucose throughout the absorptive process. The patient treated with insulin by injection cannot reproduce these physiologic responses. If enough insulin is given to keep the postprandial glucose normal, inevitably too much insulin will be present during the postabsorptive phase, and hypoglycemia will result.

No single standard exists for patterns of administration of insulin, and treatment plans vary from physician to physician and with a given physician in different patients. Three treatment regimes will be described: conventional, multiple subcutaneous injections (MSI), and continuous subcutaneous insulin infusion (CSII). MSI or CSII is required in intensive treatment schedules designed to protect against complications. *Conventional insulin therapy* involves the administration of one or two injections a day of intermediate-acting insulin such as zinc insulin (lente insulin) or isophane insulin (NPH insulin) with or without the addition of small amounts of regular insulin. If the newly diagnosed subject is not in acute distress, therapy can be started as an outpatient, provided instructions in diet, insulin use, and monitoring are adequate and the physician or nurse-clinician can be reached by telephone for consultation. Adults of normal weight may be started on 15 to 20 units a day (the estimated daily insulin production rate in nondiabetic subjects of normal size is about 25 units a day). Obese patients, because of insulin resistance, may be started on 25 to 30 units a day. It is preferable to use the same quantity of insulin for several days before changing, the one exception being the hypoglycemic patient, for whom the dose should be decreased immediately unless a nonrecurrent cause of hypoglycemia (such as excessive exercise) is present. Generally, changes should be no more than 5 or 10 units per step. It is probable that a single injection of insulin provides adequate control only in patients who have some residual capacity for insulin secretion. Poorly controlled

TABLE 337-6 Adjusting insulin dosage in conventional insulin therapy*

Blood glucose		Regular insulin, units	
mmol/L	mg/dL	Breakfast	Supper
		(to be mixed with intermediate dosage)	
2.8–5.5	51–100	8	4
5.6–8.3	101–150	10	5
8.4–11.1	151–200	12	6
11.2–13.9	201–250	14	7
14.0–16.6	251–300	16	8
>16.6	>300	20	10

* Once the patient has most blood sugars in the reasonable range, a prescription can be written for varying the regular insulin dosage as illustrated. The prescription in this case was for a patient in reasonable control on 25 units of NPH plus 10 units of regular before breakfast and 10 units of NPH plus 5 units of regular before supper. Change in metabolic status may require adjustments in both intermediate insulin and the sliding scale of regular insulin.

patients should be placed on split therapy, with about two-thirds of the total insulin given before breakfast and the remainder before supper. Two injections are almost always used when the total dose reaches 50 or 60 units a day but are helpful at smaller doses as well, since the peak action of intermediate insulins appears to be dose-related; i.e., a low dose may exhibit maximal activity earlier and disappear sooner than a large dose. Many physicians routinely add regular insulin to the intermediate dose even at initiation of therapy. Thus, in a single-dose schedule, one might begin with 20 units of intermediate and 5 units of regular insulin rather than 25 units of intermediate alone. This practice is based on the concept that the regular insulin lowers the plasma glucose level rapidly, after which the more slowly absorbed insulin maintains the lowered level. Most patients on twice-daily insulin injections are also treated with a mixture of intermediate and regular insulin; e.g., 25 units NPH plus 10 units of regular before breakfast and 10 units of NPH plus 5 units of regular before supper. Commercial premixed insulin (70/30 intermediate/regular) is acceptable and convenient for many patients. All patients should be taught to decrease insulin when significant extra activity or exercise is anticipated. The proper decrement must be determined by trial and error, although a reduction of 5 to 10 units is a reasonable first step. The blood glucose–lowering effect of exercise is due primarily to increased energy demands in previously noncontracting muscle. Extra regular insulin can be taken before a meal that contains extra calories or food ordinarily not allowed (e.g., when the diabetic must eat out at a banquet or the teenager goes out on a date). For patients willing to self-monitor plasma glucose level, an algorithm for adjusting insulin can be provided. A typical protocol is shown in Table 337-6. Patients with complicated control problems may require hospitalization, where frequent plasma glucose determinations can guide therapy.

The *multiple subcutaneous insulin injection technique* most commonly involves administration of intermediate- or long-acting insulin in the evening as a single dose together with regular insulin prior to each meal. Home glucose monitoring by the patient is necessary if the goal is the return of the plasma glucose level to normal. One approach to initiation of therapy involves administration of 25 percent of the previous daily insulin dose in the patient's conventional regimen at bedtime as intermediate insulin (NPH or lente insulin), with the other 75 percent given as regular insulin divided such that 40, 30, and 30 percent is given 30 min before breakfast, lunch, and supper, respectively. Alternatively, a three-injection schedule can be utilized by omitting the night intermediate insulin and giving a long-acting insulin, such as insulin zinc extended (ultralente insulin) or protamine zinc insulin (PZI insulin), before the evening meal. Adjustments of dosage depend on response of the plasma glucose. A number of different protocols have been utilized, all of which represent sliding scales of insulin based on the plasma glucose level. A typical schedule based on home monitoring of the plasma glucose level is shown in

TABLE 337-7 Adjusting insulin dosage in a multiple-injection schedule*

Initiation of therapy
1 0.6 to 0.7 units insulin per kilogram body weight
2 25% NPH at 9 P.M.; 75% regular in divided doses
   (40% before breakfast, 30% before lunch, 30% before supper)
3 Adjust NPH every 48 h based on fasting blood glucose
   <3.3 mmol/L (<60 mg/dL)   − 2 units
   >5.0 mmol/L (>90 mg/dL)   + 2 units
4 Adjust regular insulin every 48 h based on 1-h postprandial glucose
   <3.3 mmol/L (<60 mg/dL)   − 2 units
   >7.8 mmol/L (>140 mg/dL)   + 2 units

Daily therapy
   Preprandial glucose

mmol/L	mg/dL	Regular insulin, units
<3.3	<60	− 2
3.4–5.0	61–90	No change
5.1–6.7	91–120	+ 1
6.8–8.3	121–150	+ 2
8.4–11.0	151–200	+ 3
11.1–13.9	201–250	+ 4
>13.9	>250	+ 6

* With initiation of therapy insulin dosage is changed until target range is reached (see Table 337-8). After initial stabilization a variable insulin schedule is prescribed to maintain tight control. For example, if the patient after initiation is found to generally require 12 units of regular insulin before breakfast but has a prebreakfast blood sugar of 8.9 mmol/L (160 mg/dL), 15 units of regular insulin instead of the usual 12 would be taken.
SOURCE: Adapted from Schiffrin and Belmonte.

Table 337-7. Individual patients may require different dosages. For specific details, the reader should consult one of the published papers utilizing the technique (e.g., Schriffrin and Belmonte). MSI can be effective in controlling the plasma glucose level and in some studies appears to match goals achieved with CSII.

Continuous subcutaneous insulin infusion involves use of a small battery-driven pump that delivers insulin subcutaneously into the abdominal wall, usually through a 27-gauge butterfly needle. With CSII, insulin is delivered at a basal rate continuously throughout the day, with increased rates programmed prior to meals. Adjustments in dosage are made in response to measured capillary glucose values in a fashion similar to that used in MSI. Ordinarily, about 40 percent of the total daily dose is given at the basal rate, the remainder being administered as preprandial boluses. There is little question that CSII can improve diabetic control relative to conventional therapy. Most patients report positive feelings of well-being as control improves. The danger of hypoglycemia is real, especially during the night in patients who maintain the plasma glucose consistently below 5.5 mmol/L (100 mg/dL). A fall in plasma glucose of 2.7 mmol/L (50 mg/dL) may not be important if the starting value is 8.3 mmol/L (150 mg/dL) but may be fatal if it occurs against a steady-state level of 3.3 mmol/L (60 mg/dL). Several deaths from hypoglycemia have occurred in pump users. There is also an increased frequency of diabetic ketoacidosis in persons utilizing CSII. Pumps should be prescribed only in disciplined and motivated patients who are followed by physicians with extensive experience in their use.

In some centers, catheters for the insulin infusion pumps have been placed intravenously rather than subcutaneously. While few difficulties have been reported, this procedure appears unwise for routine use. Intraabdominal insulin pumps with reservoirs refillable from outside the body have been tried on experimental protocols. At present, no advantage is apparent except that a pump does not have to be worn externally. Administration of insulin by nasal insufflation, although attractive in principle, has not proved practical and is no longer under commercial development.

For surgical procedures in diabetic patients, intermediate insulin is omitted, and treatment is carried out with regular insulin alone. An effective method is to add 10 to 20 units of insulin to a liter of 5% glucose in water with infusion at a rate of 100 to 150 mL/h. Measurement of plasma glucose in capillary blood allows change of rate to avoid significant hypo- or hyperglycemia. It is also possible to administer 10 units of regular insulin subcutaneously and infuse 5% or 10% glucose at rates sufficient to avoid major changes in glucose concentration. Following surgery, a sliding scale can be constructed for use in postoperative management.

Types of Insulin A variety of insulins are available for use in the treatment of diabetes. Rapidly acting preparations are used in diabetic emergencies and in CSII and MSI programs. Intermediate-acting preparations are used in conventional and MSI regimens. Long-acting formulations are used almost exclusively in three-injection MSI schedules. Peak effects and duration vary from patient to patient and depend not only on route of administration but on dose. Insulin action in patients treated for long periods appears to be delayed, probably because of the presence of anti-insulin antibodies in plasma. In one study in diabetic subjects, regular insulin given subcutaneously had its onset of action at about 1 h, reached a peak at 6 h, and had measurable effects on average for 16 h, whereas in normal persons onset is within minutes, maximal action is around 2 h, and duration is only 6 to 8 h. With NPH insulin, diabetic patients exhibited an onset of action at 2.5 h, a peak at 11 h, and a total period of action of 25 h, more closely approximating values in normal subjects.

Commercial insulins are prepared in concentrations of 100 units per milliliter (U100), although higher concentrations can be obtained (e.g., U500). All animal insulins are purified such that proinsulin contamination is extremely low. Most patients are now treated with synthesized "human" insulin. The amino acid sequence is identical to that of the human hormone, and biologic activity appears to be equivalent. Complications of insulin therapy such as insulin allergy, fat atrophy, and fat hypertrophy are less common than with animal insulins but still occur.

Lente and NPH insulin are used in most conventional therapy and are roughly equivalent in biologic effects, although lente appears to be slightly more immunogenic and to mix less well with regular insulin than does NPH.

Self-monitoring of glucose For many years, effectiveness of treatment for diabetes was followed by reviewing symptoms (such as frequency of nocturia) and measurement of glucose in the urine by semiquantitative techniques. Since the renal threshold for glucose in normal persons is in the range of 10 to 11 mmol/L (180 to 200 mg/dL) plasma glucose and may increase with the appearance of renal disease, assessment of glycosuria is of little value. Most insulin-requiring patients now monitor control and alter therapy based on self-measurement of the capillary blood sugar. In addition to the fact that such measurements are necessary in all treatment schedules utilizing variable insulin dosage, the ability to assess the blood glucose as needed has other positive benefits. It bestows a sense of confidence and independence in the patient, has a reinforcing effect on therapeutic goals (e.g., the effect of dietary indiscretion can be immediately seen), serves to give early warning of incipient hypoglycemia, and allows documentation of hypoglycemia when suggestive symptoms are present.

Although the blood glucose level can be estimated visually utilizing reagent strips, it is generally preferable to use an instrument for readings. This is so because it is difficult for many patients to extrapolate accurately between the color changes and because subjective wishes may influence the extrapolation. It is harder to ignore a number appearing in a machine. A variety of glucose analyzers are available. Cost of equipment is reasonable, and many insurance carriers reimburse its purchase. The patient needs to have supervised training in the technique, and simultaneous checks of the blood sugar in a laboratory should be done periodically to test the accuracy of the self-analysis. Repeated studies show that patients can measure blood glucose accurately using these techniques.

Although urine testing for glucose is now rarely used to follow diabetes, the measurement of ketones in the urine remains important.

Goals of therapy Intensive insulin therapy designed to control the blood glucose level as near normal as possible has for many years been considered mandatory during pregnancy and after renal transplantation. Maintenance of a normal blood glucose level during pregnancy prevents fetal macrosomy, respiratory distress syndrome, and perinatal mortality. Prevention of congenital malformations probably requires that the blood glucose level be near normal at the time of conception, although one multicenter trial concluded that no relationship existed between control of diabetes and malformed fetuses. For maximal safety, however, intensive therapy should be started prior to conception, if at all possible.

The conclusion of the NIH-sponsored multicenter Diabetes Control and Complication Trial (DCCT) required broadening of the recommendation for intensive insulin therapy. This very large trial, involving more than 1400 patients with IDDM followed for 7 to 10 years, established that degenerative complications of diabetes are diminished by better control of the blood glucose level, although, as mentioned earlier, return of blood glucose level to normal was not achieved. Protection rates as high as 70 percent were seen in retinopathy. It follows that many more patients and their physicians will desire intensive insulin therapy than has been the case in the past. To do so will not necessarily be easy. It is clear from the DCCT that even with health care teams staffed with physicians, nutritionists, and experienced nurse-clinicians and with a dedicated group of participating volunteers, treatment goals were not met. There was a significant increase in frequency and severity of hypoglycemia, so therapy was not without risk. Patients with NIDDM were not studied. It thus remains to be seen whether the results of the DCCT can be applied widely under ordinary clinical circumstances.

My recommendations, which reflect the position of the American Diabetes Association, are as follows. If an experienced health care team familiar with both MSI and CSII is available, and if the patient is physically, emotionally, intellectually, and financially able to undergo the rigors of intensive therapy, it should be undertaken. Intensive therapy should not be offered under the age of 7 because of the danger of hypoglycemia to brain development. Older persons and those with comorbidity such as coronary artery disease or stroke should be excluded. Although subjects with NIDDM were not studied in the DCCT, there is no reason to believe that lowering the blood glucose level would not be beneficial in the prevention of complications, as is the case with IDDM. Insulin resistance may prove a problem in NIDDM, especially if hyperinsulinemia proves to be a risk factor for atherosclerosis and hypertension, as some investigators believe. The treatment group in DCCT also had significant weight gain, which likely will be a greater problem in NIDDM, since most patients are significantly overweight or obese. In short, persons with NIDDM should not be excluded, but considerable caution is required, especially in older persons with the disease.

Goals of therapy have not been defined. One set of standards for blood glucose is listed in Table 337-8. The "acceptable" category would apply in conventional therapy utilizing a two-dose schedule of intermediate and regular insulin. The upper limit of 11.1 mmol/L (200 mg/dL) postprandially is arbitrary but is based on the finding in the Pima Indian population that complications of diabetes are rare if the 2-h value in the oral glucose tolerance test is less than 11.1 mmol/L. The "ideal" column represents values targeted in meticulous control regimens. Although some authors are more stringent and prefer the 1-h postprandial value to be no more than 7.8 mmol/L (140 mg/dL),

the risk of hypoglycemia is greater under these circumstances. In general, avoidance of serious hypoglycemia is more important than avoidance of hyperglycemia, because the former has immediate consequences that may threaten the life of the patient or others (e.g., through an automobile accident), while the detrimental effects of hyperglycemia are long-term and less certain.

Hypoglycemia, the Somogyi effect, and the dawn phenomenon (See also Chap. 338)   The problem of hypoglycemia is common in insulin-dependent diabetics, particularly when aggressive efforts are made to keep both the fasting plasma glucose level and postprandial hyperglycemia within the normal range. Hypoglycemia may be caused by missing a meal or doing unexpected exercise but can occur in the absence of known precipitating events. Daytime episodes of hypoglycemia are usually recognized by autonomic symptoms, such as sweating, nervousness, tremor, and hunger. Hypoglycemia during sleep may produce no symptoms or cause night sweats, unpleasant dreams, and early-morning headache. In one study of insulin-dependent diabetic children monitored throughout 24 h, 18 percent had asymptomatic nocturnal hypoglycemia. If hypoglycemia is not aborted by counterregulatory hormone response or by ingestion of carbohydrate, central nervous system symptoms ensue: confusion, abnormal behavior, loss of consciousness, or convulsions.

Protection against hypoglycemia is normally provided by two mechanisms as blood glucose concentrations fall: cessation of insulin release and mobilization of counterregulatory hormones. The latter act to increase hepatic glucose production and decrease glucose utilization in nonhepatic tissues. Glucagon is the primary counterregulatory hormone, while epinephrine and norepinephrine released from the adrenal medulla and the sympathetic nervous system serve as the major backup. Catecholamines are not required for maintenance of the blood glucose level, provided glucagon is available, but they become critical in the absence of glucagon. Cortisol and growth hormone do not function acutely but come into play with prolonged fasting or sustained hypoglycemia. Diabetic patients are vulnerable to hypoglycemia because of both insulin excess and counterregulatory failure. Since insulin is given by injection or infusion, the capacity to decrease plasma concentrations of the hormone as glucose levels fall is not available. Very early on the diabetic subject with type 1 insulin-dependent disease loses the capacity to increase glucagon release in response to hypoglycemia. Protection is thus dependent on epinephrine. Unfortunately, many patients subsequently also lose the capacity to release epinephrine and norepinephrine in response to hypoglycemia. Since the initial signals of hypoglycemia are dependent on epinephrine (the other counterregulatory hormones are clinically silent), this results in the syndrome of *hypoglycemia unawareness*. This syndrome was originally thought due solely to autonomic neuropathy in patients with long-standing diabetes. It is now recognized that the syndrome may be *caused* by low blood glucose in the absence of neuropathy, with even a single episode of afternoon hypoglycemia having discernible effects the next day. Hypoglycemia does not prevent epinephrine release but lowers the level of glucose required to trigger response. The end result is that potentially dangerous hypoglycemia is unrecognized, and the defense against hypoglycemia is impaired.

Counterregulatory hormone failure is especially dangerous when intensive insulin therapy is prescribed. The incidence of hypoglycemia is inversely related to the mean level of blood glucose. There is no easy way to predict vulnerability. Experimentally, an insulin fusion test identifies persons at risk, but the procedure is too complicated for clinical practice. In this test, neuroglycopenic symptoms in the absence of autonomic signs or delay in return of the blood glucose level from nadir after infusion of a standard amount of insulin is used to identify defects in the response system. Perhaps the best clinical clue to counterregulatory failure is the presence of frequent hypoglycemia not explicable by change in diet or exercise.

An important question is whether hypoglycemic symptoms can occur in the absence of low plasma glucose levels. It has been believed traditionally that counterregulatory hormone release and autonomic

---

TABLE 337-8   Goals for blood glucose in the control of diabetes*

Goal	Acceptable		Ideal	
	mmol/L	mg/dL	mmol/L	mg/dL
Fasting	3.3–7.2	60–130	3.9–5.6	70–100
Preprandial	3.3–7.2	60–130	3.9–5.6	70–100
Postprandial (1 h)	<11.1	<200	<8.9	<160
3 A.M.	>3.6	>65	>3.6	>65

* Values for healthy patients below the age of 65. Goals may be shifted upward in older patients. *Acceptable* refers to goals for conventional therapy, while *ideal* indicates goals with intensive insulin therapy.

symptoms are not triggered until the plasma glucose level approaches 3 mmol/L (50 to 55 mg/dL). Careful studies in humans utilizing auditory or visual evoked potentials as a measure of cortical function in the brain have shown abnormalities at a glucose level of 4 mmol/L (70 to 72 mg/dL). A monitored drop in glucose level of only 0.5 mmol/L (10 mg/dL) resulted in delay of the evoked potential and, with time, release of counterregulatory hormones. These studies suggest that neuroglycopenic symptoms may occur in the presence of blood glucose levels not considered hypoglycemic.

From time to time, patients with diabetes report symptoms suggestive of catecholamine release in the presence of documented hyperglycemia. The cause of these episodes is unknown, but theories include simple anxiety, insulin-induced vascular permeability with hypotensive response, and sympathetic nervous system activation by insulin-enhanced carbohydrate utilization. Poorly controlled patients release counterregulatory hormones at higher concentrations of blood glucose than normal subjects or tightly controlled persons with diabetes. Thus insulin treatment affects counterregulatory response in two ways. With intensive therapy and tight control, especially with intermittent hypoglycemia, epinephrine release is impaired, and hypoglycemia unawareness may ensue. When control is less rigorous or poor, symptoms of hypoglycemia may occur in the absence of low blood glucose values because of a shift upward in the counterregulatory glucose threshold.

Hypoglycemia can occur in diabetic patients consequent to other mechanisms. Diabetic renal disease is not infrequently accompanied by diminished insulin requirements and may lead to frank hypoglycemia if adjustments in dosage are not made. The mechanism is not known. Although half-times for insulin in plasma are increased in diabetic nephropathy, other factors doubtless play a role. Uremia is known to impair gluconeogenesis, and this likely is important.

Hypoglycemia may be due to the development of autoimmune adrenal insufficiency as part of polyglandular autoimmune deficiency (see Chap. 343), which is more frequent in persons with diabetes than in the population as a whole. Some patients develop hypoglycemia in association with high levels of circulating insulin antibodies. The exact mechanism has not been established. Occasionally, an insulinoma may develop in a diabetic patient. Very rarely, permanent remission of apparently typical diabetes occurs. The reason is not known, but the initial sign may be frequent hypoglycemia in a previously well-controlled patient.

It must be emphasized that hypoglycemic attacks are dangerous and, if frequent, portend a serious or even fatal outcome. If the patient is conscious, sugar, candy, or a sugar-containing beverage can be given. If the patient is unarousable or unconscious, intravenous glucose is required. Patients should have a vial of glucagon available as well. If access to medical care is delayed, administration of 1 mg glucagon intramuscularly frequently aborts the attack.

The *Somogyi phenomenon* refers to rebound hyperglycemia following an episode of hypoglycemia due to counterregulatory hormone release. It should be suspected whenever wide swings in the plasma glucose occur over short time intervals even if symptoms are not reported. Such rapid changes contrast with the alterations seen following insulin withdrawal in previously well-controlled diabetic patients in whom hyperglycemia and ketosis develop gradually and smoothly over a 12- to 24-h period. Excessive hunger and weight gain occurring in the context of worsening hyperglycemia are clues that the insulin dosage may be too high, since poor control due to underinsulinization usually results in weight loss (because of osmotic diuresis and glucose wastage). If the Somogyi phenomenon is suspected, the insulin dose should be decreased as a trial, even when specific symptoms of overinsulinization are absent. The Somogyi phenomenon is probably rare in adults but may be more frequent in children.

The *dawn phenomenon* refers to an early morning rise in plasma glucose requiring increased amounts of insulin to maintain euglycemia. Although similar early morning hyperglycemia may result from hypoglycemia, as just described, the dawn phenomenon itself is thought to be independent of the Somogyi mechanism. The nocturnal surge of growth hormone release may be a factor. Increased clearance of insulin also occurs in the early morning hours, but the changes are probably not of major importance. Differentiation between the dawn phenomenon and posthypoglycemic hyperglycemia usually can be accomplished by measuring the blood glucose at 3 A.M. This is important, since the Somogyi phenomenon is avoided by decreasing insulin dosages for the critical time period, while the dawn phenomenon usually requires increased insulin to maintain glucose in the normal range.

Oral agents Non-insulin-dependent diabetes that cannot be controlled by dietary management often responds to sulfonylureas. The drugs are easy to use and appear to be safe. Fear that sulfonylureas might increase deaths from heart attacks, prompted by reports of the University Group Diabetes Program (UGDP), has largely dissipated because of questions about the design of that study and failure of other studies to confirm risks. On the other hand, use of the oral drugs has decreased concomitant with the emphasis on better control as a possible means of slowing the development of late complications. While some patients with relatively mild disease have return of plasma glucose to normal on oral drugs, those with significant hyperglycemia tend to improve but do not approach the normal range. Thus a high percentage of non-insulin-dependent diabetics are now treated with insulin.

Sulfonylureas act primarily by stimulating release of insulin from the beta cell. They have the capacity to increase the number of insulin receptors in target tissues and also enhance insulin-mediated glucose disposal independent of an increase in insulin binding, but these effects are physiologically unimportant. Mean levels of plasma insulin do not increase following treatment with sulfonylureas despite significantly improved mean plasma glucose concentrations. The paradox of improved glucose metabolism in the absence of higher steady state levels of insulin has been resolved by studies which show that elevation of plasma glucose to pretreatment values results in a rise of plasma insulin to levels higher than those seen pretreatment. Thus the initial action of the drugs is to increase insulin release with lowering of the blood glucose level. As glucose concentrations fall, insulin levels also decrease, since blood glucose is the major stimulus to insulin release, thereby masking the initial stimulation of insulin secretion. The insulinogenic effect can then be unmasked by raising the glucose to the previous elevated levels. The fact that sulfonylureas are ineffective in IDDM, where beta cell mass is diminished, supports the pancreatic effect as primary, although, as noted, extrapancreatic mechanisms may play a minor role.

The characteristics of the sulfonylureas are summarized in Table 337-9. The newer drugs such as glipizide and glyburide are effective in smaller doses but otherwise differ little from agents in long use such as chlorpropamide and tolbutamide. In patients who have significant renal disease, it is preferable to treat with tolbutamide or tolazamide, since these agents are exclusively metabolized and inactivated by the liver. Chlorpropamide has the capacity to sensitize the renal tubule to antidiuretic hormone. It thus is helpful in some patients with partial diabetes insipidus but may cause water retention in patients with diabetes mellitus. Hypoglycemia is less common with oral agents than with insulin, but when it occurs, it tends to be severe

TABLE 337-9 The sulfonylureas

Agent	Dose, mg/d	Doses per day	Duration of hyperglycemic action, h	Metabolism/ excretion
Acetohexamide	250–1500	1–2	12–18	Liver/kidney
Chlorpropamide	100–500	1	60	Kidney
Tolazamide	100–1000	1–2	12–14	Liver
Tolbutamide	500–3000	2–3	6–12	Liver
Glyburide	1.25–20	1–2	To 24	Liver/kidney
Glipizide	2.5–40	1–2	To 24	Liver/kidney
Glibornuride	12.5–100	1–2	To 24	Liver/kidney

and prolonged. Some patients have required massive glucose infusions for days following the last dose of sulfonylurea. For this reason, hospitalization is mandatory in patients with sulfonylurea-induced hypoglycemia.

The biguanides metformin and phenformin are oral agents used outside the United States. Phenformin was removed from the market by the Food and Drug Administration because of a possible association with lactic acidosis. Metformin has not been introduced in the United States. The drugs are thought to lower blood glucose by inhibiting hepatic gluconeogenesis, although they also may enhance insulin receptor number or activity. Biguanides should not be given to patients with renal disease and should be stopped if nausea, vomiting, diarrhea, or any intercurrent illness appears.

Another class of oral agents, thiazolidine derivatives, is currently under study for treatment of NIDDM. Pioglitazone, prototypical of the class, lowers blood glucose, free fatty acids, and triglycerides and appears to reduce insulin resistance, possibly by increasing insulin receptor kinase activity.

Two naturally occurring peptides are under investigation as adjuncts to treatment in NIDDM. Both insulin-like growth factor 1 (IGF-1, somatomedin C) and glucagon-like peptide 1 (GLP-1), a peptide derived from the proglucagon molecule, lower blood glucose level in normal subjects and in patients with diabetes. The GLP-1 (7-36) and (7-37) amides are the lead insulinotropins under development. Their ultimate usefulness is not established.

Monitoring control of diabetes   For those patients who measure blood glucose frequently for adjustment of insulin dosage, an estimate of mean ambient glucose concentrations is readily available. For other patients, and as a check on accuracy of the self measurements, most diabetologists measure hemoglobin A_{1c} to assess long-term control. Hemoglobin A_{1c}, a fast-moving minor hemoglobin component, is present in normal persons but increases in the presence of hyperglycemia. Its enhanced electrophoretic mobility is due to nonenzymatic glycation of the amino acids valine and lysine.

Glucose in the aldehyde (linear) configuration condenses with a free amino group to form a Schiff base (aldimine or pre-A_{1c}). The Schiff base undergoes a rearrangement to form hemoglobin A_{1c}, a ketoamine. Aldimine formation is reversible so that pre-A_{1c} is labile, while ketoamine formation is irreversible and thus stable. Pre-A_{1c} levels change rapidly with alterations in glucose concentrations and do not reflect long-term control, although they are measured in chromatographic methods for determining hemoglobin A_{1c}. Pre-A_{1c} must thus be removed to assess true Hb A_{1c} values accurately. Many laboratories employ high-performance liquid chromatography to make the measurement. A colorimetric method utilizing thiobarbituric acid also does not measure the labile pre-A_{1c} fraction. When properly assayed, the percent of glycated hemoglobin gives an estimate of diabetic control for the preceding 3-month period. Normal values must be obtained for each lab; on average, nondiabetic subjects have Hb A_{1c} values of less than 6 percent, while levels in poorly controlled patients may reach 10 to 12 percent. Measurement of glycated hemoglobin gives an objective assessment of metabolic control. Discrepancies between reported plasma glucose values and hemoglobin A_{1c} concentrations suggest either that measurement or reporting of the former is not accurate. Measurement of glycated albumin, because of its short half-life, can be used to monitor diabetic control over a 1- to 2-week period but clinically is rarely used.

ACUTE METABOLIC COMPLICATIONS   In addition to hypoglycemia, patients with diabetes are susceptible to two major acute metabolic complications: diabetic keotacidosis and hyperosmolar, nonketotic coma. The former is a complication of insulin-dependent diabetes, while the latter usually occurs in the setting of non-insulin-dependent disease. Ketoacidosis rarely, if ever, develops in true NIDDM.

Diabetic ketoacidosis   Diabetic ketoacidosis appears to require insulin deficiency coupled with a relative or absolute increase in glucagon concentration. It is often caused by cessation of insulin intake but may result from physical (e.g., infection, surgery) or emotional stress despite continued insulin therapy. In the former case, the concentration of glucagon rises secondary to insulin withdrawal, while in stress the operative stimulus for glucagon release is probably epinephrine. In addition to stimulating glucagon secretion, epinephrine presumably blocks release of the small amount of residual insulin found in some subjects with IDDM and inhibits insulin-induced glucose transport in peripheral tissues. These hormonal changes have multiple effects, but two are critical: (1) They induce maximal gluconeogenesis and impair peripheral utilization of glucose, causing severe hyperglycemia. Glucagon facilitates gluconeogenesis by inducing a fall in fructose-2,6-bisphosphate, an intermediate that stimulates glycolysis through activation of phosphofructokinase and blocks gluconeogenesis by inhibiting fructose bisphosphatase. When fructose-2,6-bisphosphate concentrations fall, glycolysis is inhibited, and gluconeogenesis is enhanced. The resultant hyperglycemia induces an osmotic diuresis that leads to the volume depletion and dehydration that characterize the ketoacidotic state. (2) They activate the ketogenic process and thus initiate development of metabolic acidosis. For ketosis to occur, changes must be produced in both adipose tissue and the liver. Free fatty acids from adipose stores represent the primary substrate for ketone body formation, and plasma levels of free fatty acids must rise if high rates of ketogenesis are to develop. However, fatty acids delivered to the liver are simply reesterified and stored as hepatic triglyceride or converted into very low density lipoproteins and transported back into the circulation unless the hepatic oxidative machinery for fatty acids is activated. While free fatty acid release is enhanced directly by insulin deficiency, accelerated fatty acid oxidation in the liver is primarily induced by glucagon, via action on the carnitine palmitoyltransferase system of enzymes responsible for the transport of fatty acids into the mitochondria. When long-chain fatty acids reach the liver, they are first esterified to coenzyme A (CoA). The fatty acyl CoA cannot traverse the mitochondrial membranes until it is transesterified with carnitine. As shown in Fig. 337-3, carnitine palmitoyltransferase I transesterifies fatty acyl-CoA to fatty acylcarnitine, which then traverses the inner mitochondrial membrane via translocase. Reversal of the reaction occurs internally under the influence of carnitine palmitoyltransferase II. In the fed state, carnitine palmitoyltransferase I is inactive, and as a consequence, long-chain fatty acids cannot reach the β-oxidative enzymes for ketone body production. During starvation or uncontrolled diabetes, the system is activated; under these circumstances, the rate of ketogenesis is a first-order function of the concentration of fatty acids reaching transferase I.

Glucagon (or a change in the glucagon/insulin ratio) activates the transport system in two ways. First, glucagon causes a rapid fall in hepatic malonyl-CoA content. It does so by interrupting the sequence glucose-6-phosphate $\rightarrow$ pyruvate $\rightarrow$ citrate $\rightarrow$ acetyl-CoA $\rightarrow$ malonyl-CoA via the previously mentioned decrease in fructose-2,6-bisphosphate. Glucagon also inhibits acetyl-CoA carboxylase, the enzyme that converts acetyl-CoA to malonyl-CoA. Malonyl-CoA, the first committed intermediate in the synthesis of fatty acids from glucose, is a competitive inhibitor of carnitine palmitoyltransferase I, and a fall in its concentration activates the enzyme. Second, glucagon causes a rise in hepatic carnitine concentration, which then drives the reaction toward fatty acylcarnitine formation by mass action. These events are summarized schematically in Fig. 337-4. At high plasma fatty acid concentrations, hepatic uptake of fatty acids is sufficient to saturate both oxidative and esterifying pathways, resulting in fatty liver, hypertriglyceridemia, and ketoacidosis. Overproduction of ketones by the liver is the primary event in ketotic states, but limitation of peripheral utilization also plays a role at high concentrations of acetoacetate and β-hydroxybutyrate.

Clinically, ketoacidosis begins with anorexia, nausea, and vomiting, coupled with an increased rate of urine formation. Abdominal pain may be present. If untreated, altered consciousness or frank coma may occur. Initial examination usually shows Kussmaul respiration, together with signs of volume depletion. Rarely, the latter is sufficient to cause vascular collapse and renal shutdown. Body temperature is

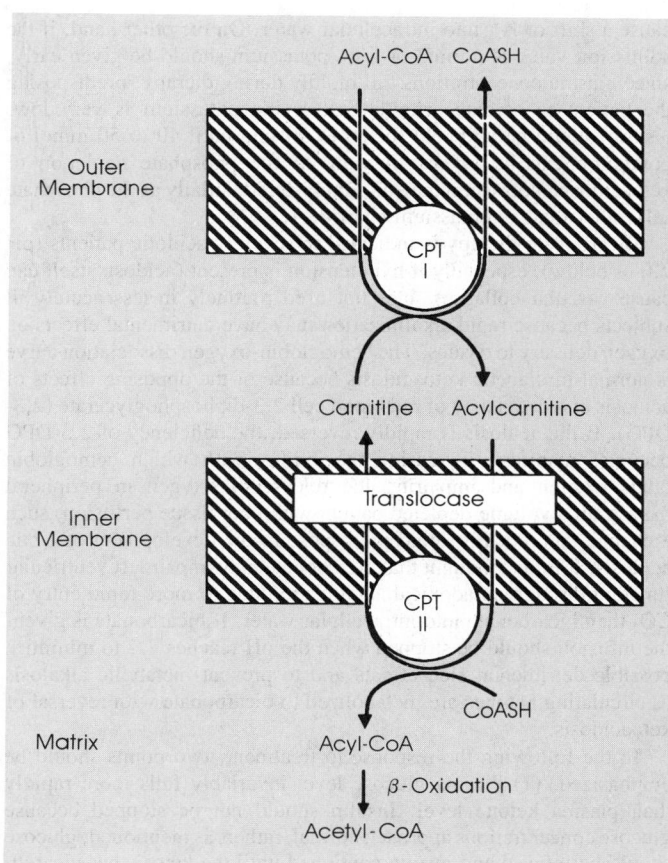

FIGURE 337-3 The carnitine palmitoyltransferase system. Long-chain fatty acyl-CoA molecules require transesterification to carnitine to traverse the inner mitochondrial membrane. Once across, the transesterification is reversed, and the fatty acyl-CoA is oxidized to either ketone bodies (liver) or CO_2 and water with the generation of ATP (nonhepatic tissues). CPT 1 is the rate-limiting step, controlled by malonyl-CoA levels in tissue. CPT 1, carnitine palmitoyltransferase 1; CPT II, carnitine palmitoyltransferase II.

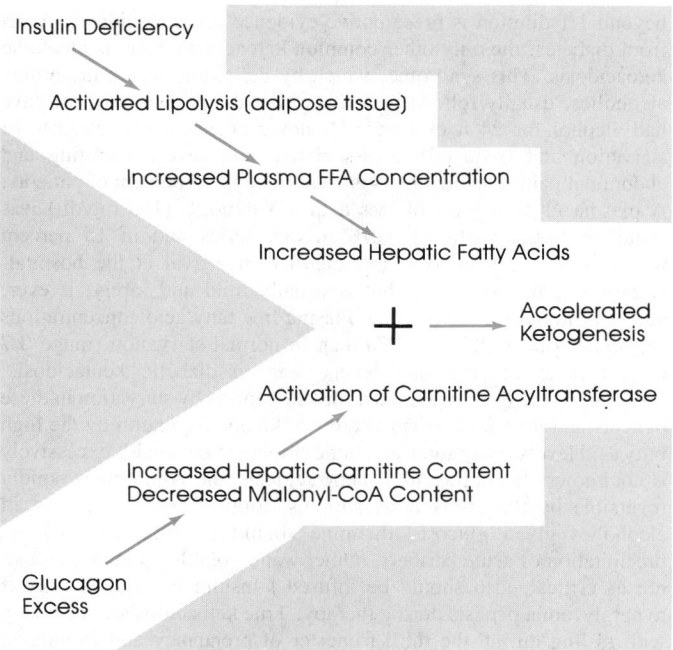

FIGURE 337-4 The regulation of ketogenesis. Significant production of acetoacetate and β-hydroxybutyrate by the liver requires provision of adequate free fatty acid substrate and activation of fatty acid oxidation. Lipolysis is primarily increased by insulin deficiency while the fatty acid oxidative sequence is activated primarily by glucagon. The immediate signal for oxidation is a fall in malonyl CoA content. *(After JD McGarry, DW Foster, Am J Med 61:9, 1976.)*

normal or below normal in uncomplicated keotacidosis: hence fever suggests the presence of infection. Leukocytosis, frequently very marked, is a feature of diabetic acidosis per se and may not indicate infection.

The characteristic metabolic abnormalities of diabetic coma are shown in Table 337-10. Several features deserve comment. The metabolic acidosis and anion gap are almost totally accounted for by the elevated plasma levels of acetoacetate and β-hydroxybutyrate, although other acids (e.g., lactate, free fatty acids, phosphates) contribute. Despite initial potassium concentrations that are normal to high, there is a total-body potassium deficit of several hundred millimoles. Similarly, initial serum phosphorus may be high despite depletion of body stores. Magnesium deficiency also may be present. The serum sodium concentration tends to be low in the face of modest osmolar concentration because of the hyperglycemia that draws intracellular water into the plasma space. A very low serum sodium level (e.g., 110 mmol/L) suggests an artifact due to severe hypertriglyceridemia. Newer autoanalyzers remove triglycerides before assay, eliminating this artifact. Hypertriglyceridemia is common in ketoacidosis and is the consequence of both impaired activity of lipoprotein lipase (a disposal defect) and the hepatic overproduction of very low density lipoproteins. If a fat meal has been ingested prior to the onset of keotacidosis, chylomicrons may make up a major portion of the circulating fat. Lipemia is usually visible if the triglyceride concentration is above 4.5 mmol/L (400 mg/dL). True hyponatremia may occur if the patient has vomited repeatedly and continued to drink water. Prerenal azotemia, reflecting volume depletion, is usually

modest in degree and reversible with treatment. The serum amylase level may be elevated, and frank pancreatitis can occur.

The diagnosis of ketoacidosis in a patient known to have insulin-dependent diabetes is not difficult. Its appearance in a patient not previously diagnosed requires differentiation from the other common causes of metabolic acidosis with an anion gap: lactic acidosis, uremia, alcoholic ketoacidosis, and certain poisonings. The first step is to test the urine for glucose and ketones. If urine ketones are negative, another cause for the acidosis is likely. If positive, plasma examination is required to be certain that something more than starvation ketosis is present. Since quantitative determinations of acetoacetate and β-hydroxybutyrate are not routinely available, semi-quantitative tests must be done using ketone reagent strips. Serial dilutions of plasma can be made and tested. A strong test may occur in undiluted plasma owing to starvation alone; a strong reaction

TABLE 337-10   Initial laboratory findings in diabetic ketoacidosis

Series:	Dallas*	Los Angeles†	Washington‡
Age, y	38	36	43
Glucose, mmol/L (mg/dL)	26(475)	37(675)	41(733)
Sodium, mmol/L	132	131	132
Potassium, mmol/L	4.8	5.3	6.0
Bicarbonate, mmol/L	<10	6	10
BUN, mmol/L (mg/dL)	9(25)	11(32)	15(42)
Acetoacetate, mmol/L	4.8	—	—
β-Hydroxybutyrate, mmol/L	13.7	—	—
Free fatty acids, mmol/L	2.1	—	2.3
Lactate, mmol/L	4.6	—	—
Osmolarity, mosmol/liter	310	323	331

* Eighty-eight consecutive episodes of ketoacidosis at Parkland Memorial Hospital (DW Foster, unpublished observations).
† Mean data from 308 episodes of nonfatal ketoacidosis (PM Beigelman, Diabetes 20:490, 1971).
‡ Mean data from 10 episodes of ketoacidosis (JE Gerich et al, Diabetes 20:228, 1971).

beyond 1:1 dilution is presumptive evidence for ketoacidosis. Apart from diabetes, the only other common ketoacidotic state is alcoholic ketoacidosis. This syndrome, which by definition occurs in chronic alcoholics, usually follows a debauch, but the patient may not have had alcohol for 24 h or longer. It never occurs in the absence of starvation and frequently is associated with severe vomiting and abdominal pain. Pancreatitis is present in up to 75 percent of patients. A plasma glucose level of less than 8.3 mmol/L (150 mg/dL) was found in three-fourths of cases in one series and in 15 percent was less than 2.8 mmol/L (50 mg/dL) on arrival at the hospital. Hyperglycemia may occur but is usually mild and rarely, if ever, above 17 mmol/L (300 mg/dL). Plasma free fatty acid concentrations are higher (mean 2.9 mmol/L) than in normal starvation (range 0.7 to 1.0 mmol/L), reaching levels seen in diabetic keotacidosis. Presumably the liver is activated for ketogenesis by starvation in these patients and driven to maximal rates of ketone formation by the high fatty acid levels. Why some alcoholics mobilize fatty acids excessively is not known. In contrast to diabetic acidosis, the syndrome is rapidly reversible by the intravenous administration of glucose. As in all alcoholics given glucose, thiamine should be supplied to avoid precipitation of acute beriberi. (Other water-soluble vitamins, though not as critical, also should be infused.) Insulin is required only if hyperglycemia persists during therapy. True ketoacidosis can develop with fasting during the third trimester of pregnancy and in nursing mothers who do not eat, but the complication is rare.

Diabetic ketoacidosis cannot be reversed without insulin. For decades, 50 or more units of insulin was given per hour until ketosis was reversed, but now most patients are treated by "low-dose" insulin schedules in which 8 to 10 units of insulin is infused intravenously each hour. Most diabetic acidosis can be reversed adequately with low-dose treatment, but some patients do not respond. Presumably the insulin resistance that is characteristic of diabetic ketoacidosis is more pronounced in these patients than in responsive subjects. The problem is that resistant subjects cannot be identified prospectively. For this reason, it is probably preferable to give 25 to 50 units of insulin as an initial intravenous bolus, followed by an infusion of 15 to 25 units an hour until ketoacidosis is reversed. There are no known toxic effects of larger insulin doses, since maximal physiologic response is obtained once insulin receptors are saturated regardless of how much insulin is given. The advantage of the higher dosage schedule is that it ensures saturation of the receptors in the face of competing antibodies or other resistance factors. High concentrations of insulin probably accelerate the reversal of ketoacidosis by acting via the IGF-1 receptor. Hormonal interaction with this receptor can lower the blood glucose level by a mechanism independent of the insulin receptor. Diabetic ketosis has been reversed by IGF-1 therapy in a patient with severe insulin resistance. If physicians choose to use the low-dose insulin schedule, they should be alert to the possibility of resistance. Should acidosis persist unabated after several hours of treatment, larger amounts of insulin are clearly indicated. Keotacidosis also can be treated adequately with intramuscular (but not subcutaneous) insulin.

Therapy of ketoacidosis also requires intravenous fluids. The usual fluid deficit is 3 to 5 L, and both salt solutions and free water are needed. Between 1 and 2 L of isotonic saline or Ringer's lactate should be given rapidly intravenously on arrival, with additional amounts determined by urine output and clinical assessment of the fluid state. When the plasma glucose level falls to about 17 mmol/L (300 mg/dL), 5% glucose solutions should be added, both as a source of free water and as a prophylactic measure to prevent the late cerebral edema syndrome. The latter is a rare complication of ketoacidosis occurring most often in children. It is suspected when the patient remains comatose or lapses into coma following reversal of acidosis.

Potassium replacement is always necessary, but the time of administration will vary. The initial potassium level is often high despite a total-body deficit because of the severe acidosis. In this case, the cation will ordinarily not be needed until 3 to 4 h after initiation of therapy when reversal of acidosis and the action of insulin

cause a shift of K^+ into intracellular water. On the other hand, if the admission value is normal or low, potassium should be given early, since plasma concentrations fall rapidly during therapy, predisposing the patient to cardiac arrhythmias. If the potassium is very low, insulin should be withheld for 60 to 90 min until 40 to 50 mmol of potassium can be given. In view of the phosphate depletion of ketoacidosis, potassium may be administered initially as the phosphate salt rather than as potassium chloride.

Bicarbonate therapy is indicated in severely acidotic patients (pH 7.0 or below), especially if hypotension is present (acidosis itself can cause vascular collapse). It is not used routinely in less acutely ill subjects because rapid alkalinization may have detrimental effects on oxygen delivery to tissues. The hemoglobin-oxygen dissociation curve is normal in diabetic ketoacidosis because of the opposing effects of acidosis and deficiency of red blood cell 2,3-diphosphoglycerate (2,3-DPG). If the acidosis is rapidly reversed, the deficiency of 2,3-DPG becomes manifest, increasing the avidity with which hemoglobin binds oxygen and impairing the release of oxygen in peripheral tissues. In a volume-depleted patient with poor tissue perfusion, such a change theoretically could predispose to the development of lactic acidosis. It is also thought that bicarbonate may impair left ventricular function through paradoxical acidification due to more rapid entry of CO_2 than bicarbonate into intracellular water. If bicarbonate is given, the infusion should be stopped when the pH reaches 7.2 to minimize possible detrimental side effects and to prevent metabolic alkalosis as circulating ketones are metabolized to bicarbonate with reversal of ketoacidosis.

In the following the response to treatment, two points should be emphasized. (1) Plasma glucose level invariably falls more rapidly than plasma ketone level. Insulin should not be stopped because glucose concentrations approach normal; rather, as mentioned, glucose should be infused and insulin continued until the ketosis has cleared. (2) Plasma ketone values are not very helpful. The testing materials measure acetoacetate and acetone but not β-hydroxybutyrate. Since β-hydroxybutyrate must be oxidized to acetoacetate prior to utilization, it is characteristic for the plasma ketones measured by reagent strip to remain stable or even rise early in therapy at a time when total ketone concentration (acetoacetate plus β-hydroxybutyrate) is falling. Because β-hydroxybutyrate and acetoacetate represent a redox couple in equilibrium with mitochondrial NADH/NAD concentrations, vascular collapse or severe hypoxia may mask the presence of ketoacidosis because acetoacetate is reduced to β-hydroxybutyrate. Under these circumstances, the β-hydroxybutyrate/acetoacetate ratio, normally about 3:1, may reach 7:1 or 8:1. Paradoxically, in such a situation ketosis may seem to worsen as the patient gets better because of conversion of β-hydroxybutyrate to acetoacetate when the circulation is reestablished and tissue oxygenation is restored. The key parameters to follow are the pH and the calculated anion gap, since these give a more accurate assessment of therapeutic progress. The usual picture is for the pH to rise and the anion gap to narrow even though the plasma bicarbonate level remains low. The persistently low bicarbonate is the consequence of hyperchloremia that develops because of rapid infusion of sodium chloride, the loss of potential bicarbonate from the body in urine as ketones, and exchanges with intracellular buffers. Some patients demonstrate a persistent anion gap despite clinical improvement and a rising pH. Presumably, the unmeasured anion derives from tissue buffers. If the anion gap remains elevated and pH is persistently low, this indicates insulin resistance and requires an aggressive increase in the amount of insulin administered. On the other hand, persistence of the anion gap does not indicate resistance when present in the face of clinical improvement, a rising pH, and clearing of urine ketones.

All patients should be followed with a flow sheet outlining amounts and timing of insulin and fluids together with a record of vital signs, urine volume, and blood chemistries. Without such a record, therapy tends to become chaotic.

Most patients with diabetic ketoacidosis recover when properly treated. While mortality in large series is reported to be around 10 percent, the majority of deaths result from late complications rather than from ketoacidosis itself. The major causes are myocardial infarction and infection, particularly pneumonia. Poor prognostic signs on admission include hypotension, azotemia, deep coma, and associated illness. In children, cerebral edema is a common cause of death (less frequent in adults). The cause of the brain swelling is not known. Theories include osmotic disequilibrium between brain and plasma as glucose is rapidly lowered, decreased plasma oncotic pressure due to infusion of large amounts of saline, and insulin-induced ion flux across the blood-brain barrier. Whatever the mechanism, mortality rates are high. Diagnosis is usually made by computed tomographic (CT) scan. Treatment involves the bolus infusion of 1 g mannitol per kilogram of body weight in the form of a 20% solution. Although of questionable benefit, dexamethasone is also usually given: 12 mg initially, then 4 mg every 6 h. If there is no response, hyperventilation to an arterial P_{CO_2} of about 28 mmHg should be carried out by an anesthesiologist or pulmonary specialist.

Other acute complications of ketoacidosis include vascular thrombosis and the adult respiratory distress syndrome. The former is induced by volume depletion, hyperosmolarity, increased viscosity of blood, and changes in clotting factors favoring thrombosis. The cause of the pulmonary lesion is not known; it is probably not related to the metabolic acidosis, since respiratory distress syndrome occurs in hyperosmolar coma as well. Acute gastric dilatation is another rare complication. An unusual infection associated with ketoacidosis is mucormycosis (see below). Table 337-11 summarizes the complications of diabetic ketoacidosis and its treatment.

Hyperosmolar coma Hyperosmolar, nonketotic diabetic coma is usually a complication of non-insulin-dependent diabetes. It is a syndrome of profound dehydration resulting from a sustained hyperglycemic diuresis under circumstances in which the patient is unable to drink sufficient water to keep up with urinary fluid losses. Commonly an elderly diabetic patient—often living alone or in a nursing home—develops a stroke or infection which worsens hyperglycemia and prevents adequate water intake. The full-blown syndrome probably does not occur until volume depletion has become severe enough to decrease urine output. Hyperosmolar coma also has been precipitated by therapeutic procedures such as peritoneal dialysis or hemodialysis, tube feeding of high-protein formulas, high-carbohydrate infusion loads, and the use of osmotic agents such as mannitol

and urea. Phenytoin, steroids, immunosuppressive agents, and diuretics also have been reported to initiate the disorder.

The absence of ketoacidosis is important in the pathophysiology. When ketoacidosis develops, nausea, vomiting, and air hunger bring the patient to the physician before extreme dehydration can occur. Such a protective mechanism is not operative in ketoacidosis-resistant, maturity-onset diabetes. Interestingly, hyperosmolar coma can occur in insulin-dependent diabetic patients given sufficient insulin to prevent ketosis but insufficient to control hyperglycemia. Although unusual, the same person may present on one occasion with ketoacidosis and on the next with hyperosmolar coma.

The reason for the absence of ketoacidosis in maturity-onset diabetes is not known. The hepatic ketogenic machinery is not impaired, since the patients frequently have ketone concentrations in the starvation range (2 to 4 mmol/L). Free fatty acid levels are lower in hyperosmolar coma than in ketoacidosis, and substrate deficiency may limit ketone formation. That this is the sole mechanism seems unlikely, since some patients with hyperosmolar coma have high levels of free fatty acids in plasma. A more likely explanation is that insulin concentrations in the portal vein of persons with NIDDM are higher than those of insulin-dependent subjects and prevent full activation of the hepatic carnitine palmitoyltransferase system. Other possibilities include glucagon resistance, previously mentioned, and maintenance of high malonyl-CoA levels via increased Cori cycle activity. The *Cori cycle* refers to conversion of circulating glucose to lactate in peripheral tissues with return of lactate to the liver for gluconeogenesis. Lactate is an excellent substrate for malonyl-CoA synthesis.

Clinically, patients present with extreme hyperglycemia, hyperosmolality, and volume depletion, coupled with central nervous system signs ranging from clouded sensorium to coma. Seizure activity—sometimes Jacksonian in type—is not unusual, and transient hemiplegia may be seen. Infections, particularly pneumonia and gram-negative sepsis, are common and indicate a grave prognosis. Pneumonia is often due to gram-negative organisms. A high index of suspicion for infection should be maintained, and routine culture of the blood and spinal fluid is indicated. Because of the extreme dehydration, plasma viscosity is high, and widespread in situ thrombosis has been found at post mortem. Bleeding, probably the consequence of disseminated intravascular coagulation, and acute pancreatitis may accompany the illness.

The laboratory findings in two large series are shown in Table 337-12. Plasma glucose is generally around 55 mmol/L (1000 mg/dL), about twice the value seen in ketoacidosis. The serum osmolality is extremely high, but because of the hyperglycemia, the absolute serum sodium concentration is often not elevated.[3] Prerenal azotemia with marked elevation of blood urea nitrogen (BUN) and creatinine is characteristic. A mild metabolic acidosis is present, plasma bicarbonate on average being about 20 mmol/L. The acidosis is due to a combination of starvation ketosis, retention of inorganic acids secondary to renal hypoperfusion, and a modest elevation of plasma lactate, the latter the consequence of volume depletion. If the bicarbonate is less than 10 mmol/L and plasma ketones are not elevated, it can be assumed that lactic acidosis is present.

The mortality rate in hyperosmolar coma is high (>50 percent). As a consequence, immediate treatment is urgent. The most important measure is rapid administration of large amounts of intravenous fluids to reestablish the circulation and urine flow. The average fluid deficit is 10 to 11 L. While free water will ultimately be needed, initial therapy should be with isotonic salt solutions, and 2 to 3 L should be given over the first 1 to 2 h. Subsequently, half-strength saline

---

TABLE 337-11 Clues to complications in diabetic ketoacidosis

Complication	Clues
Acute gastric dilatation or erosive gastritis	Vomiting of blood or coffee-ground material
Cerebral edema	Obtundation or coma with or without neurologic signs, especially if occurring after initial improvement
Hyperkalemia	Cardiac arrest
Hypoglycemia	Adrenergic or neurologic signs; rebound ketosis
Hypokalemia	Cardiac arrhythmias
Infection	Fever
Insulin resistance	Unremitting acidosis after 4–6 h of adequate therapy
Myocardial infarction	Chest pain, appearance of heart failure; appearance of hypotension despite adequate fluids
Mucormycosis	Facial pain, bloody nasal discharge, blackened nasal turbinates, blurred vision, proptosis
Respiratory distress syndrome	Hypoxemia in the absence of pneumonia, chronic pulmonary disease, or heart failure
Vascular thrombosis	Strokelike picture or signs of ischemia in nonnervous tissue

SOURCE: Adapted from DW Foster, in *Current Therapy in Endocrinology and Metabolism 1985–1986*, DT Krieger, CW Bardin (eds), Toronto/Philadelphia, Decker, 1985.

---

[3] Serum osmolality can be estimated from the formula Serum osmolality (mosmol/L) = $2 [Na^+ + K^+]$ + glucose (mmol/L) + BUN (mmol/L). Glucose and blood urea nitrogen (BUN) can be converted to milliosmoles per liter by dividing concentrations in milligrams per deciliter by 18 and 2.4, respectively. In practice, the contribution of the BUN is often ignored, since it contributes to total osmolality but does not reflect the free-water deficit. There are situations in which an increased osmolality is not equivalent to dehydration. Severe alcohol intoxication is one example, the ethanol itself providing the measured milliosmoles.

TABLE 337-12   Initial laboratory findings in hyperosmolar coma

Series:	Brooklyn*	Washington†
Age, y	60	57
Glucose, mmol/L (mg/dL)	65(1166)	54(976)
Sodium, mmol/L	144	142
Potassium, mmol/L	5	5
Chloride, mmol/L	99	98
Bicarbonate, mmol/L	17	22
BUN, mmol/L (mg/dL)	31(87)	23(65)
Creatinine, mmol/L (mg/dL)	490(5.5)	
Free fatty acids, mmol/L	0.73	0.96
Osmolarity, mosmol/L	384	374

* Mean data from 33 episodes of hyperosmolar coma (AA Arieff, HJ Carroll, *Medicine* 51:73, 1972).
† Mean data from 20 episodes of hyperosmolar coma (JE Gerich et al, *Diabetes* 20:228, 1971).

TABLE 337-13   Lesions of diabetic retinopathy

Background	Proliferative
Increased capillary permeability	New vessels
Capillary closure and dilatation	Scar (retinitis proliferans)
Microaneurysms	Vitreal hemorrhage
Arteriovenous shunts	Retinal detachment
Dilated veins	
Hemorrhages (dot and blot)	
Cotton-wool spots	
Hard exudates	

can be used. As the glucose level approaches normal, 5% dextrose can be given as a vehicle for free water. While hyperosmolar coma may be reversed by fluids alone, insulin should be given to control the hyperglycemia more rapidly. Many authors recommend small doses of insulin, but larger amounts may be necessary, particularly in the obese patient. Potassium salts are usually required earlier in the treatment of hyperosmolar coma than in ketoacidosis because the intracellular shift of plasma K^+ during therapy is accelerated in the absence of acidosis. If lactic acidosis is present, sodium bicarbonate should be given until tissue perfusion can be reestablished. Antibiotics are required if infection complicates the picture.

LATE COMPLICATIONS OF DIABETES The diabetic patient is susceptible to a series of complications that cause morbidity and premature mortality. While some patients may never develop these problems and others note their onset early, on average, symptoms develop 15 to 20 years following the appearance of overt hyperglycemia. A given patient may experience several complications simultaneously, or a single problem may dominate the picture.

Circulatory abnormalities Atherosclerosis occurs more extensively and earlier than in the general population. The cause for this accelerated atherosclerosis is not known, although, as discussed below, nonenzymatic glycation of lipoproteins may be important. The atherosclerotic lesion appears to be initiated by oxidized low-density lipoproteins (LDL) (not native LDL) in a complicated cascade that operates through the acetyl-LDL or scavenger receptor. Both high-density lipoproteins (HDL) and antioxidants have the capacity to impair LDL oxidation, thereby exerting an antiatherogenic action. In experimental animals, diabetes accelerates the oxidative process. Although lipoproteins are often in the normal range, HDL levels tend to be low, while LDL levels are high normal or high. A high LDL/HDL ratio favors atherogenesis, and with lower HDL levels reverse cholesterol transport (from established lesions) would be impaired. Lipoprotein (a) levels are elevated in IDDM but not NIDDM.

Other factors of potential importance are increased platelet adhesiveness, possibly due to enhanced thromboxane A_2 synthesis, and decreased prostacyclin synthesis. Hyperglycemia has been reported to increase secretion of endothelin-1 in vitro, and production of nitric oxide is diminished in aortas of diabetic rats and the coronary microvasculature of humans. These findings have not been confirmed in human diabetes. Endothelin is a powerful vasoconstrictor and is mitogenic for vascular smooth muscle, while nitric oxide is a vasodilator, is antimitogenic in vascular smooth muscle, and inhibits platelet aggregation. Advanced glycation end products may be important, as discussed below.

Atherosclerotic lesions produce symptoms in a variety of sites. Peripheral deposits may cause intermittent claudication, gangrene, and, in men, organic impotence on a vascular basis. Surgical repair of large-vessel lesions may be unsuccessful because of the simultaneous presence of widespread disease of the small vessels.

Coronary artery disease and stroke are common. Silent myocardial infarction is thought to occur with increased frequency in diabetes and should be suspected whenever symptoms of left ventricular failure appear suddenly. Diabetes also may be associated with the clinical picture of cardiomyopathy, in which heart failure occurs in the face of angiographically normal coronary arteries and the absence of other identifiable causes of heart disease. As in nondiabetic subjects, smoking is a major risk factor for both coronary and peripheral vascular disease and should be avoided. Hypertension is also a significant risk factor in many diabetic patients.

Retinopathy Diabetic retinopathy is a leading cause of blindness in the United States. On the other hand, most patients never become blind. Retinopathic lesions are divided into two large categories, *simple* (background) and *proliferative* (Table 337-13). The earliest sign of retinal change is an increased capillary permeability that is evidenced by leakage of dye into the vitreous humor after fluorescein injection. Occlusion of retinal capillaries follows, with subsequent formation of saccular and fusiform aneurysms. Arteriovenous shunts also occur. The vascular lesions are accompanied by proliferation of lining endothelial cells and a loss of the pericytes that surround and support the vessels. Hemorrhages into the inner retinal areas are dot-shaped, while bleeding into the more superficial nerve fiber layer causes flame-shaped, blot, or linear lesions. Preretinal hemorrhages characteristically have a boat-shaped appearance. Exudates are of two types. Cotton-wool spots can be shown by angiography to be microinfarcts—nonperfused areas surrounded by a ring of dilated capillaries. A sudden increase in the number of cotton-wool spots represents an ominous prognostic sign and may herald the appearance of rapidly advancing retinopathy. Hard exudates are more common than cotton-wool spots and probably represent leakage of protein and lipids from damaged capillaries. Retinal edema due to the previously mentioned increase in vascular permeability is most often seen in the posterior pole of the eye, often in association with hard exudates. If the edema is in the macular region, visual acuity may be seriously and permanently impaired. Macular edema should be suspected when loss of visual acuity is not corrected by glasses, especially if posterior pole exudates are seen. Edema is difficult to recognize without slit-lamp examination or stereoscopic fundal photographs. Consultation with a retinal surgeon should be sought early, since vision may be spared by laser therapy of the macular edema.

The fundamental characteristics of proliferative retinopathy are new vessel formation and scarring. The stimulus for neovascularization may be retinal hypoxia secondary to capillary or arteriolar occlusion. Two serious complications of proliferative retinopathy are vitreal hemorrhage and retinal detachment. Either may cause a sudden loss of vision in one eye.

The frequency of diabetic retinopathy appears to vary with the age of onset as well as the duration of the disease. Approximately 85 percent of patients eventually develop the complication, but some never develop lesions even after 30 years of disease. Retinopathy appears to develop earlier in older patients, but proliferative retinopathy is less common. Some 10 to 18 percent of patients with simple retinopathy progress to proliferative disease in a 10-year period. About half of patients with proliferative disease progress to blindness within 5 years. Proliferative retinopathy appears to be more common in insulin-treated patients than in those not treated with insulin.

Treatment for diabetic retinopathy is photocoagulation. Such treatment decreases the incidence of hemorrhage and scarring and is always indicated when new vessel formation occurs. Photocoagulation is also useful in treatment of microaneurysms, hemorrhages, and macular edema even if the proliferative stage has not begun. Panretinal photocoagulation is often used to diminish retinal demands for oxygen in the hope that the stimulus for neovascularization will be decreased. In this technique, several thousand lesions are produced over a 2-week period. Complications of photocoagulation are within the acceptable range. Some loss of peripheral vision is inevitable with extensive burns. Another surgical technique, pars plana vitrectomy, is utilized for treatment of nonresolving vitreal hemorrhage and retinal detachment. Postoperative complications are more frequent than with photocoagulation and include retinal tears, retinal detachment, cataracts, recurrent vitreal hemorrhage, glaucoma, infection, and loss of the eye. Hypophysectomy, once widely performed for diabetic retinopathy, is no longer recommended. There is hope that inhibition of angiogenesis by drugs such as the experimental heparin analogue beta-cyclodextrin tetradecasulfate may prevent proliferative retinopathy. All patients with diabetic retinopathy should be followed by retinal specialists.

Diabetic nephropathy Renal disease is a leading cause of death and disability in diabetes. About half of end-stage renal disease in the United States is now due to diabetic nephropathy. Approximately 35 percent of patients with insulin-dependent diabetes develop this complication. Prevalence in NIDDM varies from 15 to 60 percent depending on ethnic background. Pima Indians have the highest rates, while Europeans have the lowest. It is probable that nephropathy, like other complications, is influenced by the genetic background of the patient. Some families with multiple diabetic members rarely have renal disease, while in others more than 80 percent of persons at risk have nephropathy.

Diabetic nephropathy involves two distinct pathologic patterns that may or may not coexist: diffuse and nodular. The former, which is more common, consists of widening of the glomerular basement membrane together with generalized mesangial thickening. In the nodular form, large accumulations of PAS-positive material are deposited at the periphery of the glomerular tufts, the Kimmelstiel-Wilson lesion. In addition, there may be hyalinization of afferent and efferent arterioles, "drops" in Bowman's capsule, fibrin caps, and occlusion of glomeruli. Deposition of albumin and other proteins occurs in both glomeruli and tubules. The most specific lesions of diabetic glomerulosclerosis are hyalinization of afferent glomerular arterioles and the Kimmelstiel-Wilson nodules. Clinical renal dysfunction in diabetes does not correlate well with the histologic abnormalities.

Diabetic nephropathy may be functionally silent for long periods (10 to 15 years). At onset, the kidneys are usually enlarged with "superfunction" (i.e., glomerular filtration rates may be 40 percent above normal). The next stage is the appearance of *microproteinuria* (microalbuminuria), the excretion of albumin in the range of 30 to 300 mg/d. Normal persons excrete less than 30 mg/d. Microalbuminuria is not detected by reagent sticks for urinary protein, which generally become positive only when proteinuria is greater than 550 mg/d, a degree of leakage termed *macroproteinuria*. Microalbuminuria appears to be due primarily to decreased concentration of anionic heparan sulfate–proteoglycan in the glomerular basement membrane. Since microalbuminuria is initially transient and can be induced by mechanisms other than diabetes, diagnosis requires an excretion rate of albumin greater than 15 µg/h (30 mg/d) in two of three samples collected in a 6-month period. Persistent leakage of protein greater than 50 mg/d is predictive of subsequent macroproteinuria. Interestingly, microalbuminuria also appears to predict cardiovascular mortality in diabetes. Once the macroproteinuric phase begins, there is a steady decline in renal function, with glomerular filtration rate falling, on average, about 1 mL/min per month. A plot of the reciprocal of the serum creatinine against time usually results in a straight line and allows prediction of the rate of deterioration. Ordinarily, azotemia

begins about 12 years after diagnosis of diabetes. The nephrotic syndrome may occur prior to azotemia. Progression of renal disease is accelerated by hypertension.

There is no specific treatment for diabetic nephropathy. Meticulous control of diabetes can reverse microalbuminuria in some patients, and diabetic nephropathy may be slowed in its progression, as shown in the intensive treatment group of the DCCT. Hypertension must be treated aggressively whenever present. Angiotensin-converting enzyme inhibitors appear to be useful in slowing progression of diabetic nephropathy. They should be used in hypertensive patients with diabetes and may have a role in normotensive subjects with microalbuminuria. Low-protein diets may be useful, based on experimental studies in animals and humans. Once the azotemic phase is reached, treatment does not differ from that for other forms of renal failure. Chronic dialysis and renal transplantation are routine in patients with renal failure due to diabetes. Hyporeninemic hypoaldosteronism, which is associated with renal tubular acidosis, may require alkalinizing solutions (Shohl's solution) and avoidance of external potassium loads. Potassium tends to rise in parallel with hyperglycemia in the syndrome, since in the absence of aldosterone potassium loads must be disposed of intracellularly under the influence of insulin. Hyperglycemia, reflecting insulin deficiency, indicates impairment of the disposal pathway. Rarely, fludrocortisone may be required to control hyperkalemia.

Diabetic neuropathy Diabetic neuropathy may affect every part of the nervous system, with the possible exception of the brain. While it is rarely a direct cause of death, it is a major cause of morbidity. Distinct syndromes can be recognized, and several different types of neuropathy may be present in the same patient. The most common picture is that of *peripheral polyneuropathy*. Usually bilateral, the symptoms include numbness, paresthesias, severe hyperesthesias, and pain. The pain, which may be deep-seated and severe, is often worse at night. It is occasionally lancinating or lightning in type, resembling tabes dorsalis (pseudotabes). Fortunately, extreme pain syndromes are usually self-limited, lasting from a few months to a few years. Involvement of proprioceptive fibers leads to abnormalities of gait and development of typical Charcot joints, particularly in the feet. Loss of arch with multiple fractures of tarsal bones is a common finding by x-ray. On physical examination, absent stretch reflexes and loss of vibratory sense are early signs. Diabetic neuropathy also may cause delay in return of the ankle reflex identical to that seen in hypothyroidism. *Mononeuropathy*, though less common than polyneuropathy, also may occur. Characteristically, there is a sudden wrist drop, foot drop, or paralysis of the third, fourth, or sixth cranial nerves. Other single nerves, including the recurrent laryngeal, have been reported to be involved. Mononeuropathy is characterized by a high degree of spontaneous reversibility, usually over a several-week period. *Radiculopathy* is a sensory syndrome in which pain occurs over the distribution of one or more spinal nerves, usually in the chest wall or abdomen. The severe pain may mimic herpes zoster or an acute surgical abdomen. Like mononeuropathy, the lesion is usually self-limited. *Autonomic neuropathy* may present in a variety of ways. The gastrointestinal tract is a prime target, and there may be esophageal dysfunction with difficulty in swallowing, delayed gastric emptying, constipation, or diarrhea. The last is often nocturnal. Incompetence of the internal anal sphincter may mimic diabetic diarrhea. Orthostatic hypotension and frank syncope may occur. Cardiorespiratory arrest and sudden death, thought to be due solely to autonomic neuropathy, have been reported. Bladder dysfunction or paralysis is particularly distressing and often leads to the necessity of chronic catheter drainage. Impotence and retrograde ejaculation are additional manifestations in men. Erectile dysfunction is associated with a failure of nitric oxide generation in the penile vasculature. Deficiency of vasoactive intestinal polypeptide (VIP) may also be involved. Clues to autonomic neuropathy can be obtained by clinical tests such as measuring response of the heart rate to the Valsalva maneuver or standing. In both tests the subject has an electrocardiograph running for assessment of heart rate. In the former, the subject blows against an anaeroid or mercury manometer to 40 mmHg pressure for 15 s. The test is performed three times with a rest period of 1 min in between. Normally the heart rate speeds during Valsalva such that the ratio of the longest interval between beats after release to the shortest interval during the test is greater than 1.2. In autonomic neuropathy involving the parasympathetic system the ratio is less than 1.1. Similarly, the ratio at the thirtieth beat after standing relative to that at the fifteenth beat should be greater than 1.0. It is less than 1.0 in autonomic neuropathy. Diabetic *amyotrophy* is likely a form of neuropathy, although atrophy and weakness of the large muscles in the upper leg and pelvic girdle resemble primary muscle disease. Anorexia and depression may accompany amyotrophy. Because of the weight loss, such patients are often thought to have a paraneoplastic neuropathy.

Treatment of diabetic neuropathy is unsatisfactory in most respects. When pain is severe, it is easy for the patient to become habituated or addicted to narcotics or powerful nonnarcotic analgesics such as pentazocine. If the pain requires something stronger than aspirin, acetaminophen, or other nonsteroidal anti-inflammatory agents, codeine is the drug of choice. Phenytoin is used by some physicians, but others have not found it helpful. Combination therapy with amitriptyline and fluphenazine causes relief of pain in some patients and is worth trying. The recommended dosage is 75 mg amitriptyline at bedtime and 1 mg fluphenazine three times a day. Mononeuropathies and radiculopathies usually require no specific therapy because they are self-limited. Diabetic diarrhea often responds to treatment with diphenoxylate and atropine or loperamide. Orthostatic hypotension is best treated by having the patient sleep with the head of the bed elevated, avoidance of sudden assumption of the upright position, and the use of full-length elastic stockings. Occasionally, volume expansion with fludrocortisone is required, as in other forms of orthostatic hypotension.

Experimental therapy with aldose reductase inhibitors and myoinositol have failed to provide significant clinical benefit, although enhanced regeneration of nerves has been reported in humans treated with an aldose reductase antagonist. Topical application of capsaicin is occasionally helpful with burning pain syndromes and hyperesthesia.

Diabetic foot ulcers   A special problem in the diabetic patient is the development of ulcers of the feet and lower extremities. The ulcers appear to be due primarily to abnormal pressure distribution secondary to diabetic neuropathy. The problem is accentuated when there is bony distortion in the feet. Callus formation is usually the initial abnormality. Alternatively, the ulcer may be initiated by ill-fitting shoes which cause blister formation in patients whose sensory deficits preclude recognition of pain. Cuts and punctures from foreign bodies such as needles, tacks, and glass are common, and a foreign body of which the patient is unaware may be found in the soft tissue. For this reason, all patients with ulcers should have x-rays made of the feet. Vascular disease with diminished blood supply contributes to development of the lesion, and infection is common, often with multiple organisms. While no specific therapy is available for diabetic ulcers, supportive treatment often can lead to salvation of the leg without amputation. One approach is simply to put the patient to bed using hydrotherapy and debridement to remove nonviable tissue. Others recommend casting the leg with plaster to redistribute weight bearing and protect the lesion. Pending culture, initial antibiotic therapy for infected ulcers without systemic signs might be cefoxitin or ampicillin-sulbactam. If signs of sepsis are present, ampicillin-sulbactam plus gentamicin or aztreonam may be prescribed.

All patients should be instructed about proper foot care in an attempt to prevent ulcers. Feet should be kept clean and dry at all times. Patients with neuropathy should not be allowed to walk barefoot, even in the home. Properly fitted shoes are essential. This is a particular problem with women, since an adequate shoe is not often stylish. The feet should be carefully inspected daily for callus, infection, abrasions, or blisters and the physician consulted for any potentially troublesome lesion. Treatment with growth factors (e.g., fibroblast growth factor) may prove useful in the future.

What causes the complications of diabetes?   The cause of diabetic complications is not known and may be multifactorial. Major emphasis has been placed on the polyol pathway, wherein glucose is reduced to sorbitol by the enzyme aldol reductase. Sorbitol, which appears to function as a tissue toxin, has been implicated in the pathogenesis of retinopathy, neuropathy, cataracts, nephropathy, and aortic disease. The mechanism is perhaps best worked out in experimental diabetic neuropathy, where sorbitol accumulation is associated with a decrease in myoinositol content, abnormal phospho-inositide metabolism, and a decrease in Na^+, K^+-ATPase activity. In experimental models, primacy of the polyol pathway in initiating neuropathy was proven by showing that inhibition of aldol reductase prevented the fall in tissue myoinositol content and the decrease in ATPase activity. Myoinositol deficiency was not found in sural nerve biopsies from humans with diabetic neuropathy, in contrast to animals. Aldol reductase inhibition also has been shown to prevent experimental cataracts and retinopathy. It thus seems possible that neuropathy and retinopathy are primarily due to activation of the polyol pathway. It also may play a role in diabetic nephropathy.

A second mechanism of potential pathogenetic importance is glycation of proteins. (Current terminology uses *glycation* for nonenzymatic addition of hexoses to proteins and *glycosylation* for enzymatic addition.) The effect of such glycation on hemoglobin has been mentioned, but multiple proteins in the body are altered in the same way, often with disturbed function. Examples include plasma albumin, lens protein, fibrin, collagen, lipoproteins, and the glycoprotein recognition system of hepatic endothelial cells. Particularly intriguing is the effect of glycation on lipoproteins. Glycated LDL is not recognized by the normal LDL receptor, and its plasma half-life is increased. Conversely, glycated HDL turns over more rapidly than native HDL. It also has been reported that glycated collagen traps LDL at rates two to three times greater than normal collagen.

Glycated collagen is less soluble and more resistant to degradation by collagenase than native collagen. However, it is not clear that this is related either to the basement membrane thickening or to the tight, waxy skin syndrome with limited joint mobility (scleroderma-like) seen in some patients with insulin-dependent diabetes (see "Miscellaneous Abnormalities," below). Although it is attractive to presume that nonenzymatic glycation of protein plays a role in some degenerative complications, the evidence is less direct than with the polyol pathway. Linkage between the polyol pathway and the glycation sequence occurs as a result of the glycation of collagen and other proteins by fructose generated from sorbitol. The rate of glycation with fructose is seven or eight times faster than with glucose.

Glycated proteins also form *advanced glycation end products* (AGE) through a series of biochemical reactions that are poorly understood. Receptors for AGE are present on macrophages and endothelial cells. Binding of AGE to the receptors may induce the release of cytokines, endothelin-1, and tissue factor. The latter plays a preeminent role in the initiation of coagulation. Experimentally, AGE formation may be impaired or prevented by aminoguanidine, an agent currently in clinical trials in humans. In animals, it has a beneficial effect in prevention of retinopathy, nephropathy, and neuropathy (commonly called *microvascular complications*), but it is projected to have its major effect in atherosclerotic complications (commonly called *macrovascular complications*).

Increased blood flow has been postulated to play an initiating role in diabetic complications, possibly by increasing filtration of macromolecules that function as tissue toxins. There is supportive evidence for a role of hyperperfusion in diabetic nephropathy, but the hemodynamic hypothesis does not appear as attractive as the first two.

Can diabetic complications be prevented by meticulous control of diabetes?   As mentioned earlier, the strongest evidence that the answer is yes comes from the Diabetes Control and Complications Trial (DCCT). Additional clinical evidence supports the view that metabolic environment per se influences or causes complications independent of genetic factors. For example, kidneys from donors who have neither diabetes nor a family history of diabetes develop characteristic lesions of diabetic nephropathy within 3 to 5 years after transplantation into a diabetic recipient. Diabetic nephropathy did not develop when a kidney was transplanted into a diabetic subject whose disease had been reversed by pancreatic transplantation prior to renal transplantation. It also has been reported that kidneys manifesting diabetic nephropathy demonstrated reversal of the lesion when transplanted into normal recipients. All these findings suggest that hyperglycemia or some other aspect of the abnormal metabolism of diabetes causes or influences the development of complications. On the other hand, additional factors, probably genetic, must normally play a role. This follows from the fact that diabetic subjects with decades of poor control may escape the ravages of the late complications and from the fact that typical diabetic complications may be found in patients at the time of diagnosis of diabetes or even in the absence of hyperglycemia.

Meticulous control with insulin infusion pumps has been reported to decrease microalbuminuria, improve motor nerve conduction velocity, lower plasma lipoproteins, and decrease capillary leakage of fluorescein in the retina. Width of the capillary basement membrane in skeletal muscle also has been decreased. The changes are small in general, however, and of questionable biologic significance. Thus firm evidence does not exist to show that late complications can be *reversed* by long-term near-normalization of the plasma glucose level. Progression of retinopathy has been reported despite successful reversal of diabetes by pancreatic transplantation. The progression of diabetic complications after return of the plasma glucose level to normal or near normal has been termed *hyperglycemic memory*. Some investigators suggest that the mechanism is formation of advanced glycation end products during hyperglycemia which, being irreversible, continue their effects long term.

As discussed earlier, the question of intensive therapy for all patients with diabetes remains open at the time of this writing pending evidence that the results achieved in DCCT can be matched in the general population. Care of persons with diabetes is often delivered by nonspecialists who do not have available teams of support personnel, as was the case in the DCCT. There seems little question, however, that the thrust of treatment will be toward tighter control.

Miscellaneous abnormalities of diabetes Diabetes affects almost every system in the body. Space limitations preclude discussion of all associated features, but several deserve comment. *Infections* in persons with diabetes may not occur more frequently than in normal subjects, but they tend to be more severe. This may be due to impaired leukocyte function, a frequent accompaniment of poor control. In addition to common infections of the skin, urinary tract, lungs, and bloodstream, four unusual conditions appear to have specific relationship with diabetes. *Malignant external otitis*, usually due to *Pseudomonas aeruginosa*, tends to occur in older patients and is characterized by severe pain in the ear, drainage, fever, and leukocytosis. Soft tissues around the ear are swollen and tender. A mound of granulation tissue is characteristically present internally at the junction of the osseous and cartilaginous portions of the ear. The facial nerve becomes paralyzed in half the cases, and other cranial nerves also may be involved. Facial nerve paralysis is a poor prognostic sign, and mortality approximates 50 percent in this subset of patients. A 6-week course of ticarcillin or carbenicillin together with tobramycin is the treatment of choice. Ciprofloxacin, imipinem + cilastin, or third-generation parenteral antipseudomonal cephalosporin also may be used. Surgical debridement is often necessary. *Rhinocerebral mucormycosis* is a rare fungal infection which usually develops in patients during or following an episode of diabetic ketoacidosis. Organisms are from the genera *Mucor*, *Rhizopus*, and *Absidia*. Onset is sudden with periorbital and perinasal swelling, pain, bloody nasal discharge and increased lacrimation. The nasal mucosa and underlying tissues become black and necrotic. Cranial nerve palsies are not uncommon. There may be thrombosis of the internal jugular vein or

sinuses of the brain. Proptosis, chemosis, and retinal vein engorgement indicate cavernous sinus thrombosis. Untreated, death usually occurs in a week to 10 days. Amphotericin B and aggressive debridement are the indicated therapies. *Emphysematous cholecystitis* tends to affect diabetic men (in contrast to ordinary cholecystitis, a disease predominantly present in women). Gangrene of the gallbladder is 30 times more frequent than in the usual forms, accounting for high rates of perforation and a mortality rate 3 to 10 times higher than in ordinary cholecystitis. Diagnosis is made when gas is seen in the gallbladder wall on plain films of the abdomen. Clostridial species are frequently cultured from bile, but other organisms may be present. Treatment is cholecystectomy coupled with broad-spectrum antibiotics. Mezlocillin plus metronidazole is adequate initial coverage. *Emphysematous pyelonephritis* is signaled by the presence of gas in the kidney or perirenal space. Antibiotic therapy is usually ineffective, and nephrectomy may be required. Mortality rates of 80 percent have been reported.

Hypertriglyceridemia is common in diabetes and is usually due to insulin deficiency. Both overproduction of very low density lipoproteins in the liver and a disposal defect in the periphery appear to be operative. The latter is a consequence of lipoprotein lipase deficiency, an insulin-dependent enzyme. Some patients exhibit hyperlipemia even when diabetic control is adequate and likely have a primary familial hyperlipoproteinemia that is independent of diabetes. Patients who do not respond to dietary therapy should be treated for hypertriglyceridemia and hypercholesterolemia with drugs, as in nondiabetic subjects (see Chap. 344).

A variety of skin lesions occur in diabetes. *Necrobiosis lipoidica diabeticorum* is a plaquelike lesion with a central yellowish area surrounded by a brownish border. It is usually found over the anterior surfaces of the legs. Ulceration may occur. *Diabetic dermopathy* ("shin spots") is also usually located over the anterior tibial surface. The lesions are small rounded plaques with a raised border which may crust at the edges and ulcerate centrally. Several plaques may be arranged in linear fashion. Pigmentation is not prominent early, but as the lesion heals, a depressed scar occurs with diffuse brown discoloration. A rarer abnormality is *bullosis diabeticorum*. The bullae may be superficial with clear serum or may be mildly hemorrhagic. The cause is unknown. *Infestations of the skin* with *Candida* and dermatophytes are common, and bacterial infections of a variety of types occur. In women, *vaginal moniliasis* may be troublesome during hyperglycemic-glycosuric periods. While the symptoms respond to nystatin or gentian violet, recurrence is inevitable unless glycosuria is reversed. *Atrophy of adipose tissue* may occur at the site of insulin injections even with recombinant human insulin. *Hypertrophy* of fat also may occur, producing a lipoma-like lesion visible on physical examination.

Hyperviscosity occurs in diabetes, and *platelets aggregate abnormally*. The latter may be caused by increased thromboxane synthesis. *Wound healing* is impaired in experimental diabetes but probably is not a major factor clinically. An interesting accompaniment of insulin-dependent diabetes is the presence of *joint contractures* (Dupuytren's contracture) coupled with *tight, waxy skin* over the dorsum of the hands. The hands resemble those in patients with scleroderma. The cause of the tendon contractures is unknown, although alterations of cross-linking in collagen has been proposed. Patients with the joint contracture–waxy skin syndrome appear to have accelerated development of other diabetic complications. *Scleredema* is a common finding in diabetes. The lesion is a thickening of the skin over the shoulders and upper back that resembles scleroderma. The condition is benign.

Patients with diabetes may have additional illnesses. For example, there is a significant prevalence of eating disorders in young women with IDDM.

NONROUTINE THERAPY Transplantation with whole pancreas or segments has cured diabetes in a number of patients but is usually performed only when kidney transplantation is required. However, some isolated pancreas transplantations are done. There is no question that successful transplantation can normalize the blood glucose level. If the kidney is transplanted simultaneously, immunosuppression is required, and the pancreas is simply piggy-backed. The question is whether better control is worth the risk of immunosuppression when the pancreas alone is transplanted. This issue has not been addressed in clinical trials. Islet cell transplantation (as opposed to whole pancreas) also has been attempted, but results are poor. The possibility of utilizing nonpancreatic cells that have been genetically engineered to produce human insulin under glucose control is being studied.

Prevention of autoimmune diabetes by immunosuppressant agents is a desirable goal. Reversal of hyperglycemia without the need for insulin has been achieved in humans with new-onset diabetes using powerful drugs such as cyclosporine. The reversal is not permanent, however. Most physicians believe that prophylactic treatment with cyclosporine and similarly potent immunosuppressant agents such as FK506 is not warranted; i.e., the potential dangers are considered too great. Preventive trials are underway using insulin as prophylaxis in subjects predicted to develop diabetes in the near future based on the presence of islet cell antibodies and diminished insulin response to an intravenous glucose load. Scattered positive results have been reported. Other trials are testing the effect of nicotinamide as a possible protective and repair agent. Nicotinamide has been effective in some forms of experimental diabetes in animals.

INSULIN RESISTANCE Insulin resistance in diabetic subjects is arbitrarily defined as the requirement of 200 or more units of insulin per day to control hyperglycemia and prevent ketosis. Relative insulin resistance is present in essentially all persons with diabetes when carefully looked for using the glucose clamp technique. It is the consequence of near-complete insulin deficiency in IDDM, whereas in NIDDM the major problem is obesity.

Normal anabolic metabolism, mediated by insulin, requires the secretion of adequate amounts of normal hormone in response to meals. Insulin must then bind to a specific insulin receptor in target tissues (see Chap. 338). The insulin receptor is a tetrameric glycoprotein consisting of two α subunits and two β subunits linked by disulfide bonds. The β subunit is a tyrosine kinase that is activated when insulin binds to the α subunit. The tyrosine kinase autophosphorylates the insulin receptor and initiates subsequent intracellular phosphorylations that mediate the multiple actions of insulin. The only such action which is reasonably understood is glucose transport. Glucose enters the cell by facilitated diffusion utilizing "glucose transporter" molecules. While some of these are always present in the plasma membrane, insulin binding to the receptor initiates a rapid mobilization of intracellular stores of the transporter to the plasma membrane while simultaneously activating units already in place. In poorly controlled diabetes, the number of stored transporters appears to be deficient.

Insulin resistance is characterized as *prereceptor* (abnormal insulin or insulin antibodies), *receptor* (decreased receptor number or diminished binding of insulin), or *postreceptor* (abnormal signal transduction, especially failure to activate the receptor tyrosine kinase). Combinations may exist. The nature of the molecular defect is known in some syndromes of insulin resistance, but in many the defect has not been pinpointed.

In diabetic subjects with full-blown insulin resistance (>200 units of insulin per day), the problem is usually prereceptor resistance due to insulin antibodies. Insulin antibodies of IgG type are present in essentially all subjects within 60 days of the initiation of insulin therapy. The titer of these antibodies fluctuates for reasons that are not clear. Although the correlation between antibody titer and functional resistance is not close, insulin binding by high levels of antibody is presumed to be the primary mechanism in most cases. Probably less than 0.1 percent of insulin-treated patients ever have significant resistance. The problem may appear within a few weeks of the start of therapy or many years later. The onset may be abrupt, resulting in ketoacidosis, but usually is gradual, with uncontrollable hyperglycemia being the major problem. About 20 to 30 percent of

TABLE 337-14   Insulin-resistant states

Prereceptor resistance
A   Mutated insulins
B   Anti-insulin antibodies

Receptor and postreceptor resistance
A   Obesity
B   Type A syndrome (absent or dysfunctional receptor)
C   Type B syndrome (antibody to insulin receptor)
D   Lipodystrophic states (partial or generalized)
E   Leprechaunism
F   Ataxia-telangiectasia
G   Rabson-Mendenhall syndrome
H   Werner syndrome
I   Alström syndrome
J   Pineal hyperplasia syndrome

patients have concomitant insulin allergy. Therapy of the syndrome requires prednisone in large amounts—80 to 100 mg/d initially. Response often occurs in 48 to 72 h but may take longer. If no improvement has resulted after 3 to 4 weeks, it can be assumed that steroids will not be effective. Once insulin requirements begin to fall, prednisone dosage can be decreased rapidly by 10 to 20 mg every 3 to 7 days until a maintenance level of 5 to 10 mg/d is reached. These levels may be required for many months. Whether remission has occurred, allowing cessation of therapy, can only be determined by trial. Sulfated insulin may be of benefit. On rare occasions insulin resistance appears to be due to enhanced destruction of the hormone at the subcutaneous injection site. Such patients tend to respond normally to insulin given intravenously or intraperitoneally. In some patients, addition of a protease inhibitor (aprotinin) to the insulin mixture has been helpful. When resistance is extreme, U500 regular insulin should be used in order to control the volume of the injection.

Insulin resistance occurs in diseases other than diabetes. In such disorders, *acanthosis nigricans* is a physical sign of its presence. Acanthosis nigricans is a brown to black, velvety hyperpigmentation of the skin, most often present in the posterior and lateral folds of the neck. It is also found in the axilla, groin, umbilicus, and other areas. Acanthosis nigricans is common, occurring in 7 percent of 1412 children who made up the sixth and eighth grade populations of the public schools in one study. Higher prevalence was found in Hispanics and blacks than in whites. Although acanthosis nigricans may be a sign of occult malignancy, it is not associated with neoplasia in the insulin-resistance states. A list of the major syndromes of insulin resistance is given in Table 337-14.

Obesity is the most common cause of insulin resistance. It is associated with decreased receptor number, but the major problem is at the postreceptor level, where there is apparently a failure to activate the tyrosine kinase. *Werner's syndrome* is an autosomal recessive illness with a high incidence of hyperglycemia despite elevated concentrations of plasma insulin (see Chap. 343). There is little response to exogenous hormone. Other features include growth retardation, alopecia or premature graying of the hair, cataracts, hypogonadism, leg ulcers, atrophy of muscle, fat, and bone, soft tissue calcification, and a high frequency of sarcomas and meningiomas.

Of the rare conditions associated with acanthosis nigricans, women with *insulin receptor abnormalities* have attracted the greatest interest. Type A patients are tall young women with a tendency to hirsutism and abnormalities of the reproductive tract who most probably have polycystic ovaries. However, other causes of androgen excess are associated with the syndrome. Many mutations in the insulin receptor have been found in patients with the type A syndrome, most of which interfere with receptor activity by blocking or diminishing its tyrosine kinase activity. Type B subjects are older women with evidence of immunologic disease. The clinical picture includes arthralgias, alopecia, enlarged salivary glands, proteinuria, leukopenia, and antinuclear and anti-DNA antibodies. Insulin resistance in these patients is due to blocking antibodies to the insulin receptor (not to insulin itself). Interestingly, antireceptor antibodies also may cause hypoglycemia. The determinant of agonist (hypoglycemia) or antagonist (insulin resistance) activity presumably depends on the site of binding to the insulin receptor. Both A and B patients have high plasma insulin concentrations.

Generalized and *partial lipodystrophies* are fat depletion syndromes differing primarily in the extent of fat atrophy (see Chap. 355). In the generalized form, essentially all body fat is missing, while the more common partial type exhibits atrophy of fat in the face and trunk with normal or increased adiposity in the lower half of the body. The disease can be either congenital or acquired. Typically, the patients develop hyperglycemia at puberty, but ketoacidosis never occurs. Marked hypertriglyceridemia with eruptive xanthoma is a frequent finding. Characteristic features are hepatomegaly, splenomegaly, cardiomegaly, hirsutism, lymphadenopathy, hypertrophy of the external genitalia, varicose veins, and (in the congenital forms) muscle hypertrophy. Mental retardation is common, and renal disease may develop. The term *lipoatrophic diabetes* is synonymous with total lipodystrophy. All patients have elevated plasma insulin levels. Resistance may be due to decreased number of receptors, diminished affinity of the receptor for insulin, or a postreceptor defect.

The *pineal hypertrophy syndrome* is characterized by insulin resistance, early dentition with malformed teeth, dry skin, thick nails, hirsutism, and a peculiar sexual precocity with enlargement of the external genitalia. The latter may reach near adult size by age 3 or 4. The insulin resistance is severe, and ketoacidosis may occur despite high endogenous insulin levels. The *Alström syndrome* is a rare autosomal recessive disease characterized by childhood blindness due to retinal degeneration, nerve deafness, vasopressin-resistant diabetes insipidus, and, in males, hypogonadism with high plasma gonadotropin levels. The patients thus appear to have end organ resistance to multiple hormones. Other features include baldness, hyperuricemia, hypertriglyceridemia, and aminoaciduria. Superficially, the patients may resemble subjects with the Lawrence-Moon-Biedl syndrome but can be differentiated on initial examination by the absence of polydactyly and mental deficiency. Insulin resistance in the Alström syndrome is mild. *Ataxia-telangiectasia* is characterized by cerebellar ataxia, telangiectasia, and a variety of abnormalities in the immune system in addition to insulin resistance. The *Rabson-Mendenhall syndrome* consists of dental dysplasia, dystrophic nails, premature puberty, and acanthosis nigricans. The insulin resistance is probably due to an insulin receptor abnormality. *Leprechaunism* is characterized by an elfin appearance of the face, hirsutism, absence of subcutaneous fat, thickened skin, and insulin resistance. Defects are found in both α and β subunits of the insulin receptor so that expression in plasma membranes is markedly diminished. Not listed in Table 337-14 is insulin resistance due to hormone excess (acromegaly, Cushing syndrome), myotonic dystrophy, and thalassemia major. The insulin resistance in these conditions is usually not clinically significant.

INSULIN ALLERGY Insulin allergy is due to IgE antibodies to insulin. Manifestations include immediate reactions with local stinging or itching, delayed local reactions with brawny swelling lasting up to 30 h, and generalized urticaria or frank anaphylaxis. Systemic reactions are usually seen in patients who have stopped insulin therapy for one reason or another and have then resumed treatment. The allergic reaction may occur as early as the second injection on resumption of therapy. Mild reactions can be treated with antihistamines. If the problem is severe, desensitization procedures are required. A 1-day insulin desensitization procedure is shown in Table 337-15. Once the patient is desensitized, insulin therapy should not be interrupted.

THE EMOTIONAL RESPONSE TO DIABETES Acceptance of the fact that a person has a chronic disease that requires a change in lifestyle is always difficult. This is particularly true in the case of diabetes, since patients generally are aware that they are vulnerable to late complications and that life expectancy is shortened. It is not surprising that the emotional response to diabetes often hampers treatment. On the one hand, the primary reaction may be denial with an accompanying refusal to cooperate. At the other extreme is

TABLE 337-15 Insulin desensitization*

Time, h	Dose, U	Route	Time, h	Dose, U	Route
0	0.001	Intradermal	3.5	0.2	Subcut.
0.5	0.002	Intradermal	4	0.5	Subcut.
1	0.004	Subcut.	4.5	1	Subcut.
1.5	0.01	Subcut.	5	2	Subcut.
2	0.02	Subcut.	5.5	4	Subcut.
2.5	0.04	Subcut.	6	8	Subcut.
3	0.1	Subcut.			

* Following desensitization, use 2 to 10 units of regular insulin every 4 to 6 h for 24 to 36 h after the 6-h injection before switching to intermediate-acting insulin.
SOURCE: *Schedule of JA Galloway*. For detailed information see JA Galloway, R Bressler, Med Clin North Am 62:663, 1978.

excessive preoccupation with the illness. The physician should make every effort to define a middle ground wherein the patient acknowledges his or her disease and responds prudently without becoming obsessed. The goal is to live with diabetes not for it. Patients with diabetes are no different from other patients in that they may attempt to use their disease manipulatively with both family and physician. The problems are particularly acute with children and adolescents. While the psychiatric aspects of diabetes are not discussed here, most problems can be anticipated and handled if common sense is coupled with sympathy and firmness. It is also appropriate to offer cautious hope that the disease will be handled better in the future than is possible now.

REFERENCES

General review

UNGER RH, FOSTER DW: Diabetes mellitus, in *Williams' Textbook of Endocrinology*, 8th ed, JD Wilson, DW Foster (eds). Philadelphia, Saunders, 1992, pp 1255–1333

Genetics

BAISCH JM, CAPRA JD: Second class distinction. Curr Biol 1:385, 1991
BINGLY PJ et al: Can we really predict IDDM? Diabetes 42:213, 1993
DEFRONZO RA et al: Pathogenesis of NIDDM: A balanced overview. Diabetes Care 15:318, 1992
HARRISON LC et al: MHC molecules and β-cell destructive immune and nonimmune mechanisms. Diabetes 38:815, 1989
KARJALAINEN J et al: A bovine albumin peptide as a possible trigger of insulin-dependent diabetes mellitus. N Engl J Med 327:302, 1992
NEPOM GT: A unified hypothesis for the complex genetics of HLA associations with IDDM. Diabetes 39:1153, 1990
PALMER JP, McCULLOCH DK: Prediction and prevention of IDDM—1991. Diabetes 40:943, 1991
PERMUTT MA et al: Glucokinase and NIDDM: A candidate gene that paid off. Diabetes 41:1367, 1992
THAI AC, EISENBARTH GS: Natural history of IDDM. Diabetes Rev 1:1, 1993

Diabetic complications

BROWNLEE M: Glycation products and the pathogenesis of diabetic complications. Diabetes Care 15:1835 1992
CARROLL P, MATZ R: Uncontrolled diabetes mellitus in adults: Experience in treating diabetic ketoacidosis and hyperosmolar nonketotic coma with low-dose insulin and a uniform treatment regimen. Diabetes Care 6:579, 1983
DAGOGO-JACK SE et al: Hypoglycemia-associated autonomic failure in insulin-dependent diabetes mellitus: Recent antecedent hypoglycemia reduces autonomic responses to, symptoms of, and defense against subsequent hypoglycemia. J Clin Invest 91:819, 1993
FOSTER DW, McGARRY JD: The metabolic derangements and treatment of diabetic ketoacidosis. N Engl J Med 309:159, 1983
KITABCHI AE: Low-dose insulin therapy in diabetic ketoacidosis: Fact or fiction? Diabetes Metab Rev 5:337, 1989
ROSENSTOCK J, RASKIN P: Diabetes and its complications: Blood glucose control versus genetic susceptibility. Diabetes Metab Rev 4:417, 1988
SCHWARTZ CJ et al: Pathogenesis of the atherosclerotic lesion: Implications for diabetes mellitus. Diabetes Care 15:1156, 1992
SEQUIST ER et al: Familial clustering of diabetic renal disease: Evidence for genetic susceptibility and diabetic nephropathy. N Engl J Med 320:1161, 1989
SIPERSTEIN MD: Diabetic ketoacidosis and hyperosmolar coma. Endocrinol Metabol Clin North Am 21:915, 1992
VIBERTI J et al: Diabetic nephropathy: Future avenue. Diabetes Care 15:1216, 1992

Treatment

COUSTAN DR: Pregnancy in diabetic women. N Engl J Med 319:1663, 1988
GERICH JE: Oral hypoglycemic agents. N Engl J Med 321:1231, 1989

KOBAYASHI M et al: Pioglitazone increases insulin sensitivity by activating insulin receptor kinase. Diabetes 41:476, 1992

MARKS JB, SKYLER JS: Immunotherapy of type I diabetes mellitus. J Clin Endocrinol Metab 72:3, 1991

RAVID M et al: Long-term stabilizing effect of angiotensin-converting enzyme inhibition on plasma creatinine and on proteinuria in normotensive type II diabetic patients. Ann Intern Med 118:577, 1993

ROBERTSON RP: Pancreatic and islet transplantation for diabetes—Cures or curiosities? N Engl J Med 327:1861, 1992

SANTIAGO JV: Intensive management of insulin dependent diabetes: Risks, benefits, and unanswered questions. J Clin Endocrinol Metab 75:977, 1992

SCHIFFRIN A, BELMONTE MM: Comparison between subcutaneous insulin infusion and multiple injections of insulin: A one year prospective study. Diabetes 31:255, 1982.

SKYLER JS: Insulin pharmacology. Med Clin North Am 72:1337, 1988

Insulin resistance

FLIER JS: Syndromes of insulin resistance: From patient to gene and back again. Diabetes 41:1207, 1992

TAYLOR SI: Molecular mechanisms of insulin resistance: Lessons from patients with mutations in the insulin receptor gene. Diabetes 41:1473, 1992

338   HYPOGLYCEMIA

DANIEL W. FOSTER / ARTHUR H. RUBENSTEIN

Maintenance of the plasma glucose concentration within narrow bounds is essential for health. Hypoglycemia is dangerous (in the short run more serious than hyperglycemia) because glucose is the primary energy substrate of the brain. Its absence, like that of oxygen, produces deranged function, tissue damage, or even death if the deficit is prolonged. The vulnerability of the brain to hypoglycemia is due to the fact that it cannot utilize circulating free fatty acids as an energy source in contrast to other tissues of the body. Short-chain metabolites of the free fatty acids acetoacetic and β-hydroxybutyric acid (*ketone bodies, ketoacids*) are efficiently oxidized by the brain and can protect the central nervous system from damage by hypoglycemia when present at moderate concentrations in plasma. However, development of ketosis requires a number of hours. Ketogenesis is not, therefore, an effective protective mechanism against acute hypoglycemia. Preservation of central nervous system function in the early phases of fasting or during hypoglycemia thus requires a prompt increase in the production of glucose by the liver. At the same time, glucose utilization in other tissues is diminished by provision of free fatty acids as alternative substrate. These adaptive mechanisms are hormonally controlled and, under ordinary circumstances, are extremely effective. Occasionally, however, the system breaks down or is overwhelmed, resulting in the clinical syndrome of hypoglycemia.

DEFENSE AGAINST HYPOGLYCEMIA   The hypoglycemic states can best be understood as derangements of normal fuel metabolism. Under ordinary circumstances, energy needs are met by exogenous substrate derived from food. Oxidation of the constituent molecules of food to carbon dioxide and water is accompanied by the generation of adenosine triphosphate (ATP), the principal high-energy compound of the body. In one sense, life can be defined as the continued ability to generate ATP (and related high-energy nucleotides) for the preservation of cellular integrity in all its manifestations. When caloric intake is greater than immediate oxidative needs, as after the usual meal, excess substrate is stored as fat, structural protein, and glycogen. Substrate flux in this phase of metabolism, called *anabolic*, proceeds from intestine to liver to utilization and storage sites. Insulin is the primary hormone mediating the anabolic phase, and counterregulatory hormone levels are suppressed.

The *catabolic* phase of metabolism begins about 5 to 6 h after a meal. Normally, the only significant catabolic period is during the overnight fast, but under some circumstances, particularly serious illness, it may be prolonged. During fasting/catabolism, a series of metabolic adjustments maintains the plasma glucose in a safe range

for central nervous system metabolism and provides energy for other tissues in the body. First, the liver is activated for glucose production, and second, a lipid economy is established for most other tissues of the body. Initially, glucose from the liver is derived almost exclusively from hepatic glycogen. Because there are only about 70 g of glycogen stored in the human liver, glycogenolysis can only sustain the plasma glucose for a short time, ordinarily 8 to 10 h. Exercise may shorten the protective period, as may the stress of severe illness. To compensate for glycogen depletion, gluconeogenesis begins early, with flux of substrate from muscle and adipose tissue stores to liver and then to utilization sites.

The precursors for hepatic glucose synthesis are lactate/pyruvate and amino acids (primarily alanine) derived from muscle and glycerol released from adipose tissue by lipolysis. Amino acids constitute the primary substrate for gluconeogenesis. Most of the lactate is recycled from preformed glucose (*Cori cycle*), the only net contribution coming from the breakdown of muscle glycogen. Glycerol is initially a minor substrate but increases in importance with time. With prolonged fasting, the kidney also becomes a gluconeogenic organ and contributes to total glucose production. The primary renal substrate for gluconeogenesis is glutamine, not alanine. Proteolysis required to provide amino acids for gluconeogenesis accounts for the negative nitrogen balance of starvation. The same mechanism is operative in the stress of trauma, surgery, and severe infection. In quantitative terms, the liver produces about 11 μmol/kg per minute (2 mg/kg per minute) of glucose in the initial phases of fasting. Higher glucose turnover indicates increased utilization of glucose, an important consideration in the differential diagnosis of hypoglycemia.

The switch to fat metabolism is accomplished by activation of the hormone-sensitive lipase in adipose tissue, which hydrolyzes stored triglycerides to long-chain fatty acids and glycerol. The long-chain fatty acids have two fates. The bulk (normally about 120 g/d) is utilized directly, and the remainder (about 40 g/d) is oxidized in the liver to acetoacetic and β-hydroxybutyric acids. Ketoacids can be utilized efficiently as an energy source by most tissues (liver only minimally), but their primary importance is as backup substrate for the brain, as noted above. The shift of most tissues to lipid metabolism is important because the preferential oxidation of free fatty acids and ketones in place of glucose spares the latter for utilization by the central nervous system.

Catabolic metabolism is initiated by a fall in insulin concentration in plasma and secretion of the four counterregulatory hormones: glucagon, epinephrine, cortisol, and growth hormone. In addition, norepinephrine is released directly from sympathetic neurons. Glucagon is the primary hormone of glucose maintenance, and epinephrine plays a backup or secondary role. The latter is particularly important in the defense against hypoglycemia in diabetes mellitus, where the glucagon response is lost early (see Chap. 337). Cortisol and growth hormone function by antagonizing insulin action, and promoting mobilization of substrate and activation of gluconeogenesis.

The anabolic and catabolic phases of metabolism are summarized in Table 338-1. Breakdown in any of the adaptive mechanisms can lead to hypoglycemia.

SYMPTOMATOLOGY   Symptoms of hypoglycemia fall into two main categories: those induced by an *excessive secretion of epinephrine* and those due to *dysfunction of the central nervous system*. Rapid epinephrine release causes sweating, tremor, tachycardia, anxiety, and hunger. Central nervous system (CNS) symptoms include dizziness, headache, clouding of vision, blunted mental acuity, loss of fine motor skill, confusion, abnormal behavior, convulsions, and loss of consciousness. When the onset of hypoglycemia is gradual, CNS symptoms predominate, and the epinephrine phase may not be recognizable. With more rapid drops in plasma glucose (as in insulin reactions), adrenergic symptoms are prominent. In the diabetic subject, adrenergic symptoms may not be manifest if severe neuropathy is present.

The level of plasma glucose required to activate hormonal defenses and to produce symptoms varies. The literature is confusing because

TABLE 338-1   The feeding-fasting cycle

Phase	Primary hormone	Plasma substrates	Substrate flux	Active process

Anabolic*	Insulin	↑ Glucose
		↑ Triglycerides
		↑ Branched-chain amino
		   acids
		↓ Free fatty acids
		↓ Ketones
			Splanchnic bed → storage
			   and utilization sites
				Glycogen storage
				Protein synthesis
				Triglyceride formation

Catabolic†	Glucagon	↓ Glucose ↓ Triglycerides ↑ Alanine and glutamine‡ ↑ Free fatty acids ↑ Ketones	Storage sites → liver and utilization sites	Glycogenolysis Gluconeogenesis Proteolysis Lipolysis Ketogenesis

* Expected findings during the first several hours after ingestion of a mixed meal of fat, carbohydrate, and protein.
† The major catabolic phase occurs during the overnight fast, although partial catabolic cycles occur between meals.
‡ Arrows indicate plasma concentrations except for alanine and glutamine. While arterial concentrations of these amino acids are relatively constant, uptake by the liver and intestine
   is increased in the catabolic phase.

many experimental studies use "arterialized" venous blood samples (drawn from a hand vein in a heated box), while in clinical practice plain venous blood is ordinarily used. The latter may be as much as 1 mmol/L (18 mg/dL) lower than the arterialized sample. Clinically recognizable symptoms in persons without diabetes are regularly produced when venous plasma glucose concentrations fall below 2.5 m*M* (45 mg/dL) if the plasma glucose is lowered acutely, as by insulin injection. In the defense against acute hypoglycemia, progressive responses occur as the glucose levels fall. In one study in normal persons (arterialized venous samples), insulin secretion ceased at 4.6 mmol/L glucose (83 mg/dL), glucagon and epinephrine were released at 3.8 mmol/L (68 mg/dL), growth hormone at 3.7 mmol/L (67 mg/dL), and cortisol at 3.2 mmol/L (58 mg/dL). Thus protective mechanisms are activated before the symptomatic threshold is reached. Although overt symptoms are not present, evidence of CNS dysfunction may be demonstrable with minimal decrements of plasma glucose. In a study utilizing auditory evoked potentials as a sensitive indicator of CNS function, abnormalities were seen in normal persons with a drop in glucose in arterialized venous blood from 4.8 to 4.0 mmol/L (87 to 72 mg/dL). When blood glucose is sustained at 4.0 mmol/L (72 mg/dL), counterregulatory release eventually occurs (2 to 3 h) despite the fact that no symptoms are produced. Major symptoms of CNS dysfunction may not occur until plasma glucose concentrations approximate 1 mmol/L (20 mg/dL). This is so because normal persons have the capacity to increase cerebral blood flow sufficiently to deliver adequate glucose to the brain even with low concentrations. Cerebral atherosclerosis, with its nonelastic blood vessels, compromises this protective mechanism and allows symptomatic distress at higher glucose levels. Symptoms (adrenergic or CNS) due to hypoglycemia are unlikely with a plasma glucose above 2.8 mmol/L (50 mg/dL) in nondiabetic persons, recognizing that the physiologic sequence induced by hypoglycemia is subliminal CNS dysfunction, adrenergic symptoms, and then overt CNS dysfunction. Poorly controlled patients with diabetes mellitus appear to develop symptoms at higher glucose concentrations, and meticulously controlled diabetic patients have a lowering of the symptomatic threshold and may exhibit the syndrome of *hypoglycemia unawareness* (see Chap. 337). Some patients with insulinoma also have a lowering of the glucose threshold required to induce counterregulatory hormone release and epinephrine-induced symptoms.

A rare syndrome that mimics the CNS manifestations of hypoglycemia has been described in which blood glucose is normal but cerebrospinal fluid (CSF) glucose is low, presumably due to a defect in the glucose transporter molecule, GLUT 1. Seizures may result.

CLASSIFICATION   It is traditional to classify hypoglycemia as either *postprandial* (reactive) or *fasting*. Pathologically low plasma glucose concentrations occur in the former only in response to meals, while they occur in the latter only after fasting for a few to many hours. Patients with fasting hypoglycemia (particularly those with insulinomas) may exhibit a reactive component, but reactive patients

do not have symptoms when food is withdrawn. Fasting hypoglycemia usually means that a disease process is associated with the lowered plasma glucose, but symptoms suggestive of postprandial hypoglycemia are often found in the absence of recognizable disease.

CAUSES OF HYPOGLYCEMIA   Postprandial hypoglycemia The most common cause of postprandial hypoglycemia is alimentary hyperinsulinism (Table 338-2). Patients who have undergone gastrectomy, gastrojejunostomy, pyloroplasty, or vagotomy are subject to hypoglycemia following meals, presumably because of rapid gastric emptying with brisk absorption of glucose and excessive insulin release. Glucose concentrations fall more rapidly than insulin under these circumstances, and the resulting insulin-glucose imbalance leads to hypoglycemia. Ingestion of fructose or galactose induces hypoglycemia in children with fructose intolerance and galactosemia (see Chap. 354), respectively. Leucine intake rarely can cause the syndrome in susceptible infants. Diabetes mellitus in its early phase is usually listed as a cause of reactive hypoglycemia, but in our experience, symptomatic hypoglycemia as a premonitory symptom of diabetes is uncommon. Prediabetics, who by definition are normoglycemic, may have a late fall in plasma glucose after oral glucose tolerance testing, but this pattern is similar to that frequently present in asymptomatic, healthy individuals (see below).

Idiopathic alimentary hypoglycemia consists of two syndromes: *true hypoglycemia* and *pseudohypoglycemia*. In the former, adrenergic symptoms appear postprandially and are accompanied by a low plasma glucose at the time the symptoms appear spontaneously during everyday life. The symptoms are relieved by ingestion of carbohydrate, which raises the plasma glucose. Such patients are rare. The mechanism is unknown, although subtle dysfunction of the gastrointestinal tract might be operative. Some patients with true postprandial hypoglycemia turn out to have insulinomas (see below). *Pseudohypoglycemia* describes the condition of patients who reproducibly develop adrenergic symptoms suggestive of hypoglycemia 2 to 5 h after a meal but who do not have low plasma glucose concentrations when symptoms appear spontaneously in everyday life. The condition is often self-diagnosed, with "confirmation" coming from a 5-h glucose tolerance test that reveals a lower than "normal" plasma glucose between 2 and 5 h.

Two questions have to be asked about pseudohypoglycemia. First, what are the symptoms (which may be incapacitating) due to? Second,

TABLE 338-2   Causes of postprandial (reactive) hypoglycemia

A Alimentary hyperinsulinism
B Hereditary fructose intolerance
C Galactosemia
D Leucine sensitivity
E Idiopathic

can a valid diagnosis of hypoglycemia be made by a glucose tolerance test? The symptoms of nervousness, weakness, tremor, tachycardia, dizziness, and sweating reported by these patients are probably due to epinephrine release. Many otherwise normal persons experience similar symptoms at some time in their lives and may even have gained relief by eating. Patients with pseudohypoglycemia, on the other hand, develop the symptoms regularly and repetitively. In one study, 80 consecutive subjects with reproducible postprandial symptoms were studied by 5-h glucose tolerance testing. Hypoglycemia was considered to be present if (1) the plasma glucose fell below 3.3 mmol/L (60 mg/dL) during the test, (2) symptoms or signs compatible with hypoglycemia were present, and (3) at least a doubling of plasma cortisol occurred 39 to 90 min after the nadir of plasma glucose (suggesting hypoglycemia sufficient to activate the hypothalamic-pituitary-adrenal axis). Only 18 of the 80 (23 percent) who by history were candidates for postprandial hypoglycemia fulfilled these criteria. Twenty-five percent of asymptomatic matched normal controls also met all three criteria. When the patients and controls were tested after a mixed meal, no subject in either group had a plasma glucose below 3.3 mmol/L (60 mg/dL), yet 14 of the 18 patients (78 percent) had symptoms typical of those occurring after glucose tolerance testing. The absence of hypoglycemia after mixed meals despite the presence of typical symptoms has been observed in other studies. *Pseudohypoglycemia* appears to be an accurate descriptive term for the syndrome and is preferable to "idiopathic postprandial syndrome," which also has been used. Many such patients are thought to have stress or anxiety as a predisposing factor. Presumably they have enhanced catecholamine release following a meal, or they might be abnormally sensitive to normal postprandial norepinephrine/epinephrine release. Insulin can stimulate epinephrine release in humans if hypoglycemia is prevented. Whether enhanced insulin release plays a role in the pseudohypoglycemia syndrome is not known.

Fasting hypoglycemia The causes of fasting hypoglycemia are many, but in all there is an imbalance between the production of glucose by the liver and its utilization in peripheral tissues. In some, hypoglycemia is due primarily to a defect in glucose production, while in others, the problem is excess glucose utilization. Both defects may be present. For example, with insulin excess there is driven glucose utilization coupled with blunted hepatic glucose production. The latter is caused by insulin's capacity to block the glycogenolytic/gluconeogenic effects of the counterregulatory hormones. Dual defects are probably operative in disorders of fat oxidation and non-insulin-producing tumors as well.

Supply-side hypoglycemia (impaired production of glucose) characteristically requires much less glucose during therapy than does *demand-side hypoglycemia* (overutilization of glucose) (Table 338-3). As noted above, glucose production during a fast approximates 11 μmol/kg per minute (2 mg/kg per minute) in normal persons, but with insulin-induced hypoglycemia, glucose utilization increases to about 67 μmol/kg per minute (12 mg/kg per minute). Thus, if more than 56 mmol (10 g) of glucose per hour is required to prevent or reverse hypoglycemia, it can be assumed that overutilization is present.

UNDERPRODUCTION OF GLUCOSE As discussed earlier, the production of glucose by the liver initially involves the breakdown of stored glycogen and subsequently depends on gluconeogenesis, the synthesis of glucose from precursors delivered to the liver from peripheral tissues. The causes of inadequate production of glucose during fasting can be grouped into five categories: (1) hormone deficiencies, (2) defects in glycogenolytic or gluconeogenic enzymes, (3) inadequate substrate delivery, (4) liver disease, and (5) drugs. Hypopituitarism and adrenal insufficiency are the most common hormone deficiency states causing hypoglycemia. Defects in catecholamine or glucagon release are rare. Enzymic abnormalities causing hypoglycemia are generally seen in children and not adults. Glucose-6-phosphatase deficiency is the classic example of a defect in glycogen breakdown, but hypoglycemia may occur in young children with deficiencies of

TABLE 338-3 Major causes of fasting hypoglycemia

PRIMARILY DUE TO UNDERPRODUCTION OF GLUCOSE

A **Hormone deficiencies**
  1 Hypopituitarism
  2 Adrenal insufficiency
  3 Catecholamine deficiency
  4 Glucagon deficiency
B **Enzyme defects**
  1 Glucose-6-phosphatase
  2 Liver phosphorylase
  3 Pyruvate carboxylase
  4 Phosphoenolpyruvate carboxykinase
  5 Fructose-1,6-diphosphatase
  6 Glycogen synthetase
C **Substrate deficiency**
  1 Ketotic hypoglycemia of infancy
  2 Severe malnutrition, muscle wasting
  3 Late pregnancy
D **Acquired liver disease**
  1 Hepatic congestion
  2 Severe hepatitis
  3 Cirrhosis
  4 Uremia (probably multiple mechanisms)
  5 Hypothermia
E **Drugs**
  1 Alcohol
  2 Propranolol
  3 Salicylates

PRIMARILY DUE TO OVERUTILIZATION OF GLUCOSE

A **Hyperinsulinism**
  1 Insulinoma
  2 Exogenous insulin
  3 Sulfonylureas
  4 Immune disease with insulin or insulin receptor antibodies
  5 Drugs: quinine in falciparum malaria, disopyramide, pentamidine
  6 Endotoxic shock
B **Appropriate insulin levels**
  1 Extrapancreatic tumors
  2 Systemic carnitine deficiency
  3 Deficiency in enzymes of fat oxidation
  4 3-Hydroxy-3-methylglutaryl-CoA lyase deficiency
  5 Cachexia with fat depletion

hepatic glycogen phosphorylase and in other forms of glycogen storage disease (Chap. 350). The inability to make glycogen because of inadequate glycogen synthetase activity also renders the infant susceptible to fasting hypoglycemia. In addition to glucose-6-phosphatase, three other enzymes are necessary for gluconeogenesis: pyruvate carboxylase, phosphoenolpyruvate carboxykinase, and fructose-1,6-bisphosphatase (fructose-1,6-diphosphatase) (Fig. 338-1). Hypoglycemia can occur with decreased activities of any of these enzymes, often in association with lactic acidosis. The cause of lactic acidosis in these disorders is not known, although impaired hepatic lactate uptake due to the gluconeogenic defect probably plays a role. Substrate deficiency appears to be one of the mechanisms operative in ketotic hypoglycemia of infancy, since alanine turnover in such patients is low. Inadequate substrate supply also may contribute to hypoglycemia in malnutrition, muscle-wasting states, chronic renal failure, and late pregnancy. Acquired liver disease can cause serious hypoglycemia. Hepatic congestion due to right-sided heart failure is particularly troublesome, and severe viral hepatitis or cirrhosis also can cause hypoglycemia. Hypothermia, especially in association with alcohol, may cause very low levels of plasma glucose. Slowed enzymatic activity of the liver is the likely mechanism. The hypoglycemia of renal failure has multiple causes. In addition to impairing substrate delivery, uremic toxins may suppress hepatic gluconeogenesis, and decreased renal clearance of insulin and impairment of renal gluconeogenesis may contribute to the problem.

A number of drugs, in addition to insulin and sulfonylureas, cause hypoglycemia. Alcohol induces hypoglycemia only after a period of fasting sufficient to deplete liver glycogen stores. In this circumstance, hepatic glucose production is dependent on gluconeogenesis. The

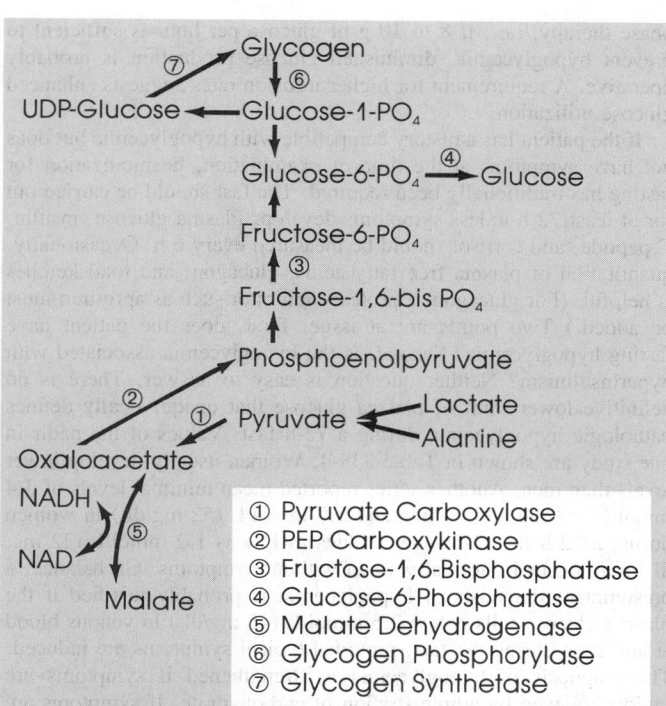

FIGURE 338-1 Scheme of hepatic carbohydrate metabolism. Only the sequences for gluconeogenesis, glycogen synthesis, and glycogenolysis are shown.

oxidation of ethanol in the liver generates high concentrations of NADH, the reduced form of nicotinamide adenine dinucleotide (NAD). The increased NADH/NAD ratio diverts oxaloacetate into malate formation, diminishing its availability to the gluconeogenic sequence via the action of phosphoenolpyruvate carboxykinase (see Fig. 338-1). The normal pathway of gluconeogenesis from pyruvate is thus blocked, leading to a drop in hepatic glucose output and hypoglycemia. Large amounts of ethanol are not required to produce this syndrome, and plasma alcohol concentrations may be as low as 5.4 mmol/L (25 mg/dL) at the time symptoms occur. Ethanol-induced hypoglycemia usually occurs in adults but can be seen in children who drink alcohol unknowingly. Salicylates (in children) and propranolol are the next most frequently involved drugs. Propranolol presumably causes difficulty in fasting patients or insulin-requiring diabetic subjects by impairing the glycogenolytic response. In diabetes the drug also may prevent recognition of impending hypoglycemia by blunting the symptomatic response to epinephrine release. Other drugs have been reported to cause hypoglycemia in isolated cases, but the relationship is often unproved. Some drugs enhance glucose utilization. Pentamidine and disopyramide cause hyperinsulinism, the former by beta cell cytolysis ("insulin leak") and the latter by an unknown mechanism, perhaps as a direct insulin secretagogue. Quinine given in falciparum malaria has been reported to cause hyperinsulinemic hypoglycemia, but the issue is clouded because hypoglycemia occurs in untreated malaria as well, possibly secondary to malnutrition, liver involvement, or cytokine release.

OVERUTILIZATION OF GLUCOSE Overutilization of glucose occurs in two settings: when hyperinsulinism is present and when plasma insulin concentrations are low. There are basically four causes of hyperinsulinemic hypoglycemia: insulinoma, exogenous insulin administration, sulfonylureas, and a peculiar form of insulin autoimmunity. *Insulinoma* is used generically here to include single solid tumors, microadenomatosis, and islet cell hyperplasia (nesidioblastosis), a rare syndrome in adults. Hypoglycemia in a diabetic taking prescribed insulin or oral agents is not a diagnostic problem. The difficulty comes when a nondiabetic subject induces hypoglycemia

deliberately and surreptitiously because of psychiatric disturbance, raising the possibility of an insulin-producing tumor. The differential diagnosis between insulinoma and factitious hypoglycemia is considered below. Rarely, hypoglycemia with hyperinsulinism occurs in autoimmune disease associated with antibodies to endogenous insulin. Mechanisms are not well understood, although dissociation of free insulin from hormone-antibody complexes at inappropriate times is probably most important. Idiotypic antibodies (antibodies against the anti-insulin antibodies) also might function as insulin agonists with the insulin receptor. By binding insulin, the antibodies also may induce excessive insulin release from the pancreas. Some patients have alternating insulin resistance/hyperglycemia and hypoglycemia. Insulin autoantibodies have been seen most frequently in subjects with hyperthyroidism treated with methimazole, but presumably they might arise in any autoimmune syndrome. Antibodies directed against the insulin receptor, usually a cause of insulin resistance, also may induce hypoglycemia with high plasma insulin levels. Under these circumstances, the configuration of the antibody is thought to allow it to activate the insulin receptor, simultaneously blocking access of native insulin and impairing its clearance.

Sepsis with endotoxinemia causes hyperglycemia followed by hypoglycemia in experiment animals. The excess insulin release is thought to be caused by sepsis-associated cytokine release, probably acting directly on the beta cell.

Hypoglycemia in the context of glucose overutilization and appropriately low plasma insulin concentrations occurs in two situations. The first is in association with solid extrapancreatic tumors, usually of large size. The most common are of mesothelial origin and include fibromas and sarcomas. The syndrome also can be seen with hepatomas, carcinomas of the gastrointestinal tract, renal cell carcinomas, and adrenal cancers. The mechanism of the hypoglycemia is not clear, although high levels of insulin-like growth factor (IGF-2) may play a role. The physiologic role of IGF-2 is not known, and it is not clear whether it produces hypoglycemia through its own receptor or by interacting with the insulin receptor. One patient with tumor-associated hypoglycemia was reported to have an increased number of insulin receptors in liver, muscle, and circulating mononuclear cells, but the significance of the finding is not clear.

Symptomatic hypoglycemia due to overutilization also may occur in situations where free fatty acids and ketones are not available for oxidation in muscle and other tissues. Patients with *systemic carnitine deficiency* can have severe hypoglycemia. In this condition, carnitine, which is necessary to transport fatty acids into mitochondria for oxidation, is low in plasma, muscle, liver, and other tissues. As a consequence, peripheral tissues cannot utilize fatty acids for energy production, and the liver cannot make ketone bodies as alternative substrate. The result is that all tissues become glucose-dependent, exceeding the capacity of the liver to meet the demand. Other features of systemic carnitine deficiency include nausea, vomiting, elevated blood ammonia levels, and hepatic encephalopathy. The illness thus constitutes one form of the Reye syndrome. (In *myopathic carnitine deficiency,* only muscle is involved, and a polymyositis-like syndrome without hypoglycemia is produced.) Nonketotic (or hypoketotic) hypoglycemia with secondary systemic carnitine deficiency and the Reye syndrome also may accompany *deficiencies of medium- and long-chain acyl-CoA dehydrogenases and 3-hydroxy-3-methylglutaryl-CoA lyase (HMG-CoA lyase).* The first two enzymes operate in the fatty acid oxidative sequence, while HMG-CoA lyase catalyzes the conversion HMG-CoA to acetoacetate and acetyl-CoA in the ketogenic cycle. Any time there is a block in fatty acid oxidation or ketone formation a secondary carnitine deficiency may develop. Accumulated acyl-CoA is transesterified to form acyl carnitine, which is then lost in the urine. Systemic carnitine deficiency in the absence of enzymic defect probably is due to a primary renal leak. It is not known whether the block in ketone production per se leads to hypoglycemia or whether secondary carnitine deficiency is required. If the former, ketones must become a primary (necessary) substrate during an extended fast. Hypoglycemia is less common with deficiency of *carnitine palmitoyltransferases*. Presumably, the defect is not complete in most patients, allowing some fatty acid oxidation to occur so that the tendency to hypoglycemia is minimized. The clinical picture is that of an exercise-induced myopathy with myoglobinuria. Hypoglycemia also occurs in patients with cachexia due to advanced cancer. At autopsy, no recognizable triglyceride stores are present in adipose tissue, suggesting free fatty acid deficiency as the primary mechanism.

Causes of hypoglycemia in hospitalized patients   Frequencies of diagnoses vary in different series. Drugs are the most common cause, the three most frequent being insulin, sulfonylureas, and alcohol. It has been estimated that 60 percent of the time one of these three agents is involved when hypoglycemia is diagnosed. Renal failure is responsible for about 15 percent of cases overall. Liver disease (about 15 percent), malnutrition (about 10 percent), and sepsis (about 5 percent) are also common causes. A high index of suspicion for insulinoma, solid tumors, enzymatic defects, or hormonal deficiencies should be engendered by the finding of hypoglycemia in nondiabetic persons without uremia, liver disease, cachexia, or history of alcohol intake.

DIAGNOSIS   Fasting hypoglycemia   If a person with diabetes mellitus presents with symptoms of hypoglycemia, it is usually safe to conclude that no special diagnostic tests are needed, since the hypoglycemia is almost always related to therapy. If a nondiabetic develops similar symptoms—particularly if confusion, loss of consciousness, or convulsions are present—it is critical to draw blood for assay before intravenous glucose is administered. *The best time to obtain diagnostic laboratory tests with spontaneous hypoglycemia is at presentation.* The goal is to assess plasma insulin level and counterregulatory hormone response while the plasma glucose is low. Assays should be carried out for glucose, insulin, insulin-connecting peptide (C peptide), cortisol, drugs, and toxins, especially sulfonylureas and alcohol. It is often wise to freeze a separate sample of plasma for subsequent tests (e.g., proinsulin, carnitine, insulin antibodies, lactate) should the diagnosis not be clear from initial evaluation. Demonstration that hypoglycemia is accompanied by inappropriate insulin levels sharply narrows the clinical possibilities. Routine laboratory examinations also may be helpful. For example, the absence of ketones or the presence of a metabolic acidosis may be clues to the primary problem.

Once the patient has become alert (assuming altered mental status is present on arrival), it is important to take a detailed history and carry out a physical examination. Special emphasis should be placed on food intake in the preceding 24 h and the possibility of drug ingestion. Signs of heart failure and hepatic congestion should be sought, and the presence and thickness of the adipose tissue mass should be noted. Pigmentation of the skin may suggest Addison's disease. Workup includes liver function studies and computed tomographic (CT) scanning or abdominal sonography (to look for solid tumors in the retroperitoneal space or abdominal cavity). Patients with enzyme defects and rare hormonal deficiencies (epinephrine, glucagon) usually require evaluation in referral centers, since definitive assays for these hormones and enzymes are not routinely available. For reasons cited above, it is important to quantitate the amount of glucose required to prevent recurrent hypoglycemia during acute phase therapy; i.e., if 8 to 10 g of glucose per hour is sufficient to prevent hypoglycemia, diminished glucose production is probably operative. A requirement for higher infusion rates suggests enhanced glucose utilization.

If the patient has a history compatible with hypoglycemia but does not have symptoms at the time of examination, hospitalization for fasting has traditionally been required. The fast should be carried out for at least 72 h unless symptoms develop. Plasma glucose, insulin, C peptide, and cortisol should be measured every 6 h. Occasionally, quantitation of plasma free fatty acids, glucagon, and total ketones is helpful. (For glucagon, a protease inhibitor such as aprotinin must be added.) Two points are at issue. First, does the patient have fasting hypoglycemia? Second, is the hypoglycemia associated with hyperinsulinism? Neither question is easy to answer. There is no definitive lower limit of plasma glucose that unequivocally defines pathologic hypoglycemia during a 72-h fast. Values of the nadir in one study are shown in Table 338-4. Women usually develop lower levels than men. Another series reported mean minimal levels of 3.4 mmol/L (62 mg/dL) in men and 2.9 mmol/L (52 mg/dL) in women during a 72-h fast. However, values as low as 1.2 mmol/L (22 mg/dL) may occur in normal women without symptoms. On balance, a presumptive diagnosis of hypoglycemia is probably justified if the plasma glucose falls below 2.5 mmol/L (45 mg/dL) in venous blood at any time during the fast, provided typical symptoms are induced. The diagnosis of hypoglycemia is strengthened if symptoms are rapidly relieved by administration of carbohydrate. If symptoms are not produced, the diagnosis of hypoglycemia should be made with caution.

Absolute insulin values are not always helpful in diagnosing hyperinsulinism. In normal subjects when glucose concentrations rise, insulin levels also increase, and when plasma glucose concentrations fall, insulin release is inhibited. This means that plasma insulin concentrations must be interpreted in the light of the simultaneously determined glucose value. Thus a "normal" absolute insulin level may be abnormal in the face of hypoglycemia, while high absolute levels may be appropriate if the glucose concentration is elevated.

Plasma insulin concentration generally reaches background levels for the assay when the plasma glucose falls below about 4.6 mmol/L (83 mg/dL), as noted earlier. While some studies have shown lower cutoff points, it is probable that any measurable insulin concentration should be considered suspicious if the venous plasma glucose is below 2.5 mmol/L (45 mg/dL). If hyperinsulinism is not demonstrated, one of the other causes of fasting hypoglycemia must be sought.

Some investigators screen for insulinoma utilizing outpatient tests. The C-peptide suppression test is based on the fact that suppression of the release of endogenous insulin and C peptide during insulin infusion is impaired in persons with insulinomas. The results are influenced by age and obesity. Less well standardized tests involve intravenous tolbutamide infusion and rigorous exercise in the fasted state. However, the 72-h fast remains the gold standard when the patient cannot be tested during a spontaneous hypoglycemic episode.

Should hypoglycemia not develop during fasting, insulinoma or other hypoglycemia-producing organic disease is unlikely, although insulinomas may rarely (~2 percent) exhibit no depression of the

---

TABLE 338-4   Mean plasma glucose and insulin during fasting

Assay	Subjects	Hours of fast				
		0*	24	36	48	72
Glucose mmol/L (mg/dL)	Men	4.7 (85)	4.6 (83)	4.3 (78)	4.3 (78)	3.9 (71)
	Women	4.6 (83)	3.5 (63)	2.8 (50)	2.6 (46)	2.7 (48)
Insulin pmol/L (μU/mL)	Men	100 (14)	64 (9)	57 (8)	57 (8)	43 (6)
	Women	86 (12)	43 (6)	29 (4)	21 (3)	29 (4)

* Zero values were obtained after overnight fast. Results are mean values for 20 normal men and 60 normal women.
SOURCE: TJ Merimee, JE Tyson, Diabetes 26:161, 1977.

plasma glucose even during a prolonged fast. Insulinomas rarely present solely as postprandial hypoglycemia. Diagnosis usually is suspected in such cases because inappropriate insulin levels are shown during the postmeal episodes.

Postprandial hypoglycemia   In patients presumed to have post-prandial hypoglycemia, the most widely used test has been a 5-h oral glucose tolerance examination. Since normal persons may have chemical hypoglycemia without symptoms in the glucose tolerance test while subjects with pseudohypoglycemia have symptoms in the absence of hypoglycemia following meal testing, the 5-h glucose tolerance test should be abandoned as a tool for diagnosis. The only unequivocal diagnostic test for true pseudohypoglycemia is the demonstration of a low plasma glucose concentration (less than 2.5 mmol/L, or 45 mg/dL) during spontaneously developed symptoms. Some physicians utilize a home glucose analyzer in diagnosis. If no hypoglycemia is demonstrated during one week of testing (on arising, 2 h after each meal, at bedtime, and during symptoms), the diagnosis of true postprandial hypoglycemia is rejected. Most authors consider home testing unreliable because of inaccuracies of measurements in the hypoglycemic range. Patients with pseudohypoglycemia usually have slightly elevated glucose concentrations during spontaneous attacks because of the hyperglycemic action of epinephrine, the stress hormone that induces the symptoms.

Insulinoma versus factitious hypoglycemia   The self-induction of hypoglycemia by the injection of insulin or the ingestion of sulfonylureas is so common as to equal or exceed the incidence of insulinoma. The demonstration of hyperinsulinism during hypoglycemia cannot, therefore, be taken as definitive evidence of the presence of an islet cell tumor. Factitious disease should always be suspected when hypoglycemic symptoms appear in medical personnel or families of diabetic patients. Several tests are helpful in distinguishing insulinoma from factitious hypoglycemia once hyperinsulinism has been established. Patients with insulinoma tend to have high concentrations of proinsulin in plasma (>20 percent of total insulin). Plasma proinsulin is not elevated by the administration of commercial insulin preparations or sulfonylureas. Measurement of the insulin connecting peptide (C peptide) will indicate whether the insulin circulating in plasma is of endogenous or exogenous origin. When insulin is cleaved from its precursor proinsulin molecule, C peptide is released into the portal vein in a 1:1 ratio with insulin. Thus, in patients with insulinoma, C-peptide concentrations should parallel the plasma insulin values. The characteristic pattern in factitious hypoglycemia due to insulin injection is a high circling level of insulin with relatively suppressed C-peptide values because exogenous insulin, which does not contain C-peptide, suppresses endogenous insulin release in normal persons, as described earlier. Antibodies to insulin are helpful if present because they usually indicate chronic insulin injection. Sulfonylureas elevate both the C-peptide and insulin concentrations in plasma. Therefore, factitious hypoglycemia due to oral agents can only be diagnosed by a high index of suspicion coupled with assay of the drug in plasma or urine. The differential characteristics of insulinoma and the two types of factitious hypoglycemia are shown in Table 338-5.

TREATMENT   The initial treatment of serious hypoglycemia (producing confusion or coma) is the intravenous administration of a bolus of 25 or 50 g glucose as a 50% solution followed by constant infusion of glucose until the patient is able to eat a meal. The importance of the meal is due to the fact that hepatic glycogen repletion is not effective with small quantities of intravenous glucose. Patients in the overutilization category may require large amounts of intravenous glucose to maintain consciousness. It is not enough to infuse 5% dextrose at a rate of 1 to 2 mL/min and assume the patient is protected (20% to 30% dextrose solutions may be required in some cases). Frequent measurement of capillary glucose concentrations should be carried out using glucose-sensitive reagent strips to assess effectiveness of glucose infusion rates. Intravenous glucose usually can be stopped once the patient has eaten, but this can only be determined by trial. Adrenergic reactions without central nervous

Test	Insulinoma	Exogenous insulin	Sulfonylurea
TABLE 338-5 Differential diagnosis of insulinoma and factitious hyperinsulinism			
Plasma insulin	High	Very high*	High
Insulin/glucose ratio	High	Very high	High
Proinsulin	Increased	Normal or low	Normal
C peptide	Increased	Normal or low[†]	Increased
Insulin antibodies	Absent	± Present[‡]	Absent
Plasma or urine sulfonylurea	Absent	Absent	Present

* Total plasma insulin in patients with insulinoma is rarely above 1435 pmol/L (200 μU/mL) in the basal state and often much lower. Values greater than 7175 pmol/L (1000 μU/mL) are highly suggestive of exogenous insulin injection.

[†] C peptide may be normal in absolute terms, but low in relation to the increased insulin value. See text for C peptide suppression test.

[‡] Insulin antibodies may not be present if only a few injections have been given, especially with purified insulin.

system abnormalities can be treated with oral carbohydrate and do not require parenteral therapy.

Hypoglycemia from sulfonylureas may last for prolonged periods (days) (Fig. 338-2). It is common for patients to lapse back into coma if glucose infusions are stopped too soon. The reason for the prolonged effect is not always clear, though drug interactions, hepatic disease, and renal failure may play a role in some cases.

Surgery is the treatment of choice for insulinoma. Localization of the tumor is best accomplished by ultrasound, and endoscopic ultrasound has the greatest sensitivity. Intraoperative ultrasound is also used if preoperative localization has not been possible. CT, magnetic resonance imaging, and arteriography are not as reliable. If the tumor cannot be found in the pancreas or located in an extrapancreatic site at the time of surgery, stepwise pancreatectomy (from tail to head) should be carried out with frozen sections made of sequential slices. Capillary glucose should be measured at each stage of the resection if the tumor is not obvious. A rise in plasma glucose may indicate removal of a small, nonpalpable lesion. In general, resection is stopped with an 85 percent pancreatectomy, even if the tumor is not found, to avoid malabsorptive complications. While a majority of patients are cured by surgery, as many as 15 percent have persistent hypoglycemia. Postoperative complications include acute pancreatitis, peritonitis, fistulas, pseudocyst formation, and chronic hyperglycemia (acquired diabetes).

Medical treatment is indicated in insulinoma only in preparation for surgery or after failure to find the tumor at operation. Two drugs are available, diazoxide and octreotide, a long-acting octapeptide analogue of somatostatin. Diazoxide can be given intravenously or orally in doses of 300 to 1200 mg/d. Because of its salt-retaining properties, it must be accompanied by a diuretic. Octreotide is given subcutaneously in divided doses of 100 to 600 μg/d. It may cause nausea and diarrhea and predispose to cholelithiasis. Treatment of metastatic insulin-producing carcinomas is unsatisfactory. It has been reported that streptozocin and doxorubicin are superior to streptozocin plus fluorouracil (median survival 2.2 and 1.4 years, respectively). Chlorozotocin, a nitrosourea-containing molecule similar to strepto-zocin, is currently under study. It appears to have fewer toxic side effects than streptozocin. Despite the generally poor prognosis, occasional patients with insulin-producing islet cell carcinomas survive for long periods.

Therapy of other forms of recurrent hypoglycemia, apart from hormone replacement in pituitary or adrenal insufficiency, is dietary. In most cases, avoidance of fasting is all that is required. This is critical in diseases of fat oxidation or ketone synthesis. If intercurrent illness prevents eating, hospitalization for intravenous glucose is absolutely required. A high-protein, low-carbohydrate diet often relieves symptoms in patients with pseudohypoglycemia. With true alimentary hypoglycemia, it is probably important to keep the size of the individual meals small. The practice of giving massive amounts

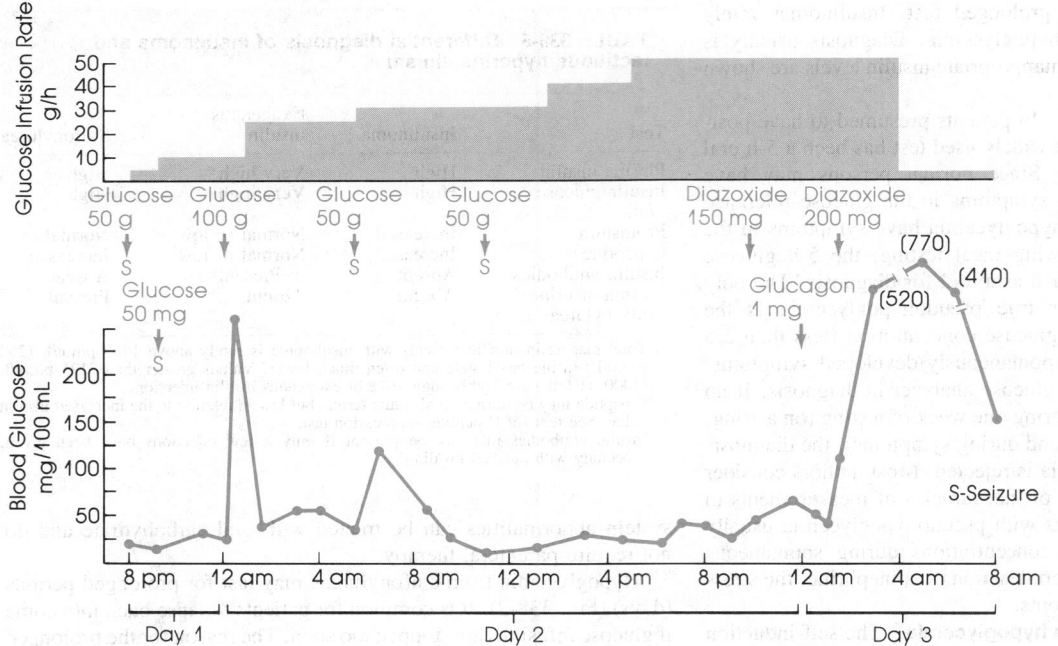

FIGURE 338-2 Prolonged and refractory hypoglycemia in factitious hypoglycemia due to chlorpropamide in an alcoholic. Note continued hypoglycemia despite the infusion of glucose at rates up to 50 g/h. (*From RM Jordan et al, Arch Intern Med 137:390, 1977. Copyright 1977, American Medical Association. Used by permission.*)

of vitamin E, crude adrenocortical extract, and trace metals to patients with pseudohypoglycemia is useless even if harmless (which has not been established).

REFERENCES

CHARLES MA et al: Comparison of oral glucose tolerance tests and mixed meals in patients with apparent idiopathic postabsorptive hypoglycemia: Absence of hypoglycemia after meals. Diabetes 30:465, 1981

CRYER PE: Glucose counterregulation: Prevention and correction of hypoglycemia in humans. Am J Physiol 264:E149, 1993

DAVIS SN, CHERRINGTON AD: The hormonal and metabolic responses to prolonged hypoglycemia. J Lab Clin Med 121:21, 1993

DE FEO P et al: Modest decrements in plasma glucose concentration cause early impairment in cognitive function and later activation of glucose counterregulation in the absence of hypoglycemic symptoms in normal man. J Clin Invest 82:436, 1988

FERNER RE, NEIL HAW: Sulphonylureas and hypoglycaemia. Br Med J 296:949, 1988

GRUNBERGER G et al: Factitious hypoglycemia due to surreptitious administration of insulin: Diagnosis, treatment, and long-term follow-up. Ann Intern Med 108:252, 1988

MARKS V: Recognition and differential diagnosis of spontaneous hypoglycemia. Clin Endocrinol 37:309, 1992

MERIMEE TJ: Insulin-like growth factors in patients with nonislet cell tumors and hypoglycemia. Metabolism 35:360, 1986

MOERTEL CG et al: Streptozocin-doxorubicin, streptozocin-fluorouracil, or chlorozotocin in the treatment of advanced islet-cell carcinoma. N Engl J Med 326:519, 1992

PANDIT MK et al: Drug-induced disorders of glucose tolerance. Ann Intern Med 118:529, 1993

SERVICE FJ: Hypoglycemias. J Clin Endocrinol Metab 76:269, 1993

——— et al: Insulinoma: Clinical and diagnostic features of 60 consecutive cases. Mayo Clin Proc 51:417, 1976

——— et al: C-peptide suppression test: Effects of gender, age, and body mass index; implications for the diagnosis of insulinoma. J Clin Endocrinol Metab 74:204, 1992

339 DISORDERS OF THE TESTES

JAMES E. GRIFFIN / JEAN D. WILSON

The testes produce sperm and the steroid hormones that regulate male sexual life. Both functions are under complex feedback control by the hypothalamic-pituitary system so that the testes have biosynthetic and regulatory features similar to those of the ovary and the adrenal. Testicular hormones are also responsible for the formation of the basic male phenotype during embryogenesis. The function of the embryonic testis and the disorders of sexual differentiation are described in Chap. 342.

PHYSIOLOGY AND REGULATION OF TESTICULAR FUNCTION

The testis consists of two components—clusters of interstitial or Leydig cells that produce androgenic steroids and a system of spermatogenic tubules for the production and transport of sperm.

THE LEYDIG CELL Testosterone synthesis The biochemical pathway by which the 27-carbon sterol cholesterol is converted to androgens and estrogens is depicted in Fig. 339-1. Cholesterol can either be synthesized de novo in the Leydig cell or derived from plasma lipoproteins. Five enzymatic transformations are required for the conversion of cholesterol to testosterone. In this process, the side chain of cholesterol is cleaved in two steps to reduce the size from 27 to 19 carbons, and the A ring of the steroid is converted to the Δ^4-3-keto configuration. The five enzyme reactions are cholesterol side chain cleavage ($P450_{SCC}$), 3β-hydroxysteroid dehydrogenase/isomerase (3β-HSD), 17α-hydroxylase ($P450_{17\alpha}$), 17,20-lyase ($P450_{17\alpha}$), and 17β-hydroxysteroid oxidoreductase (17β-HSOR). Both 17α-hydroxylase and 17,20-lyase activities are present in a single cytochrome $P450_{17\alpha}$. The first four reactions take place in the adrenal as well as the testis.

The rate-limiting process in testosterone synthesis is the conversion of cholesterol to pregnenolone by the $P450_{SCC}$; luteinizing hormone (LH) from the pituitary regulates the activity of this enzyme and of other enzymes in the pathway. Additional steroids including estradiol are synthesized in small amounts in the Leydig cell.

Testosterone secretion and transport Only about 70 nmol (20 μg) of testosterone is stored in the normal testes, so the total hormone content turns over about 200 times each day to provide the average of 17 to 20 μmol (5 to 6 mg) that is secreted into plasma in normal young men (Fig. 339-2). Testosterone is transported in plasma bound to protein, largely to albumin and to a specific transport protein, testosterone-binding globulin (TeBG, also called *sex hormone–binding globulin*, SHBG). The bound and unbound fractions in plasma are in dynamic equilibrium, only about 1 to 3 percent being unbound. The fraction of circulating testosterone available for entry into tissues approximates the sum of the free and albumin-bound fractions or about half the total plasma testosterone.

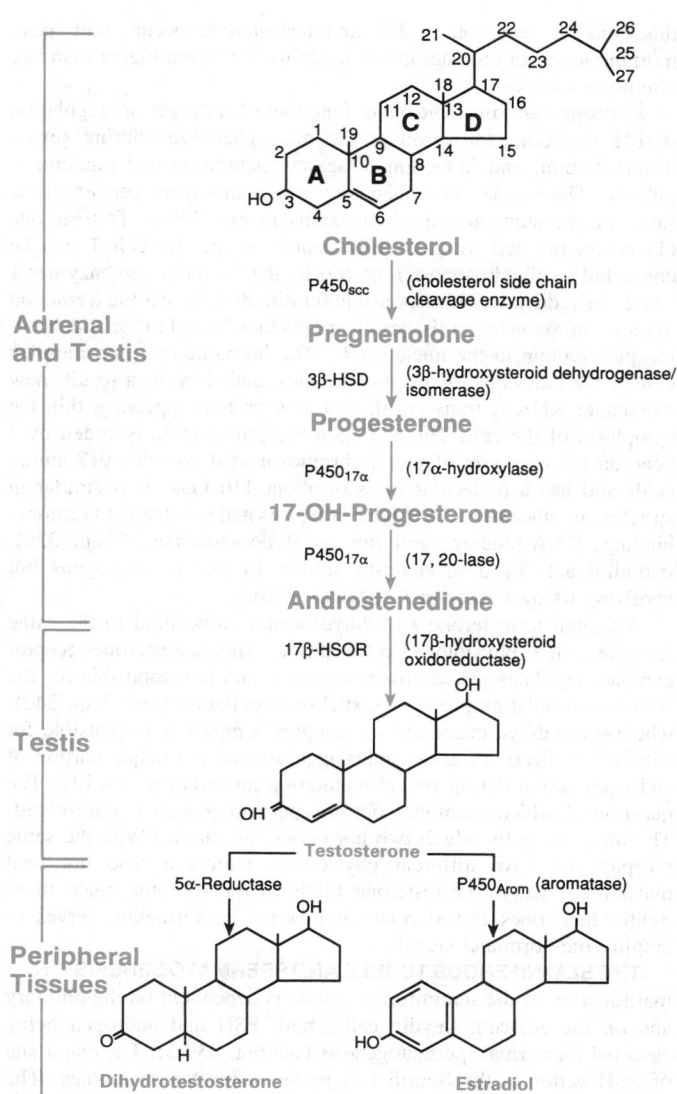

FIGURE 339-1 Pathways of androgen formation in the testis and the conversion of androgens to other active hormones in peripheral tissues.

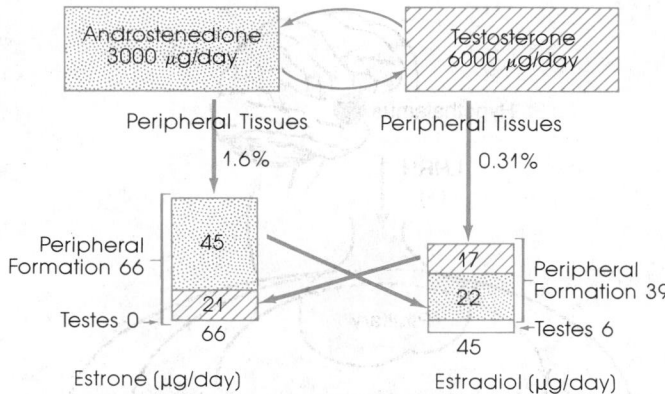

FIGURE 339-2 Androgen and estrogen production in normal young men. Average production of androstenedione and testosterone is shown in the top boxes, and mean daily production of estrone and estradiol is shown in the lower boxes. Estrogen is formed by extraglandular aromatization (*braces*) or by direct secretion from the testes. Vertical arrows indicate the rates of extraglandular aromatization of androgens, and the horizontal arrows indicate the interconversion of androgen and estrogens by 17β-hydroxysteroid dehydrogenase. Thus estradiol arises from plasma testosterone, from estrone, and from direct secretion by the testes. (*Adapted from PC MacDonald et al.*)

Peripheral metabolism of androgens Testosterone serves as a circulating precursor (or prohormone) for the formation of two other types of active metabolites that mediate many of the physiologic processes involved in androgen action (see Fig. 339-1). Testosterone can be 5α-reduced to dihydrotestosterone, which performs many of the differentiative, growth-promoting, and functional actions involved in male sexual differentiation and virilization. Circulating androgens in both sexes also can be converted to estrogens in extraglandular tissues. In men, estrogens act in some instances in concert with androgens but also can have effects independent of or opposite to those of androgens. Thus the physiologic effects of testosterone are the result of the combined effects of testosterone itself plus those of the active androgen and estrogen metabolites of the parent molecule. (In normal men, small amounts of estradiol and dihydrotestosterone are also derived by direct secretion from the testes and indirectly from the weak adrenal androgen androstenedione.)

The quantitative relation between circulating androgens and the formation of estrogen in normal young men is illustrated diagrammatically in Fig. 339-2. The production rates of testosterone and androstenedione average about 20 and 10 μmol (6 and 3 mg), respectively, per day. All estrone production [averaging about 240 nmol (66 μg) per day] can be accounted for by formation from circulating precursors. The mean estradiol production is approximately 170 nmol (45 μg)

per day; about 35 percent is derived from circulating testosterone, 50 percent is derived from the weak estrogen estrone, and 15 percent is secreted directly into the circulation by the testes. When gonadotropin levels are elevated, the amount of estradiol secretion by the testes is increased.

The 5α-reduced and estrogenic metabolites can exert local (paracrine) actions in the tissues in which they are formed or enter the circulation and act as hormones at other sites. Circulating dihydrotestosterone is formed principally in the androgen target tissues; estrogen formation takes place in many tissues, the most significant being adipose tissue. The overall rate of extraglandular estrogen formation increases with increasing amounts of adipose tissue and with age.

Plasma testosterone and its active metabolites are converted to inactive metabolites in the liver and excreted predominantly in the urine; approximately half the daily turnover is excreted in the form of urinary 17-ketosteroids (primarily androsterone and etiocholanolone), and the remainder is excreted as polar metabolites (diols, triols, and conjugates).

Gonadotropin regulation and testosterone secretion Testosterone secretion is regulated by pituitary LH (Fig. 339-3). (For the details of pituitary function, see Chap. 331.) Follicle-stimulating hormone (FSH) may augment testosterone secretion, possibly by inducing maturation of the Leydig cell. Testosterone also regulates the sensitivity of the pituitary to the hypothalamic-releasing factor luteinizing hormone–releasing hormone (LHRH, also called *gonadotropin-releasing hormone*, GnRH). Although the pituitary can convert testosterone to dihydrotestosterone and to estrogens, testosterone itself is the primary regulator of gonadotropin secretion. Testosterone also acts in the central nervous system to slow the rate of LHRH formation or secretion and consequently to decrease the frequency of pulsatile LH release. Under ordinary circumstances, LH secretion is exquisitely sensitive to the feedback effects of testosterone, with complete suppression following the administration of amounts of exogenous androgen that approximate the normal daily secretory rate of testosterone (about 20 μmol or 6 mg). However, prolonged elevation of plasma LH (as in testicular deficiency) renders the pituitary less sensitive to negative feedback control by exogenous androgen.

Neither the plasma concentration of testosterone nor that of LH is constant, each fluctuating in a pulsatile manner that reflects changes in secretory rates (Fig. 339-4). Major sleep-related surges in the pulsatile secretion of both LH and testosterone signal the initiation of male puberty. In young adults, diurnal variation in the magnitude of

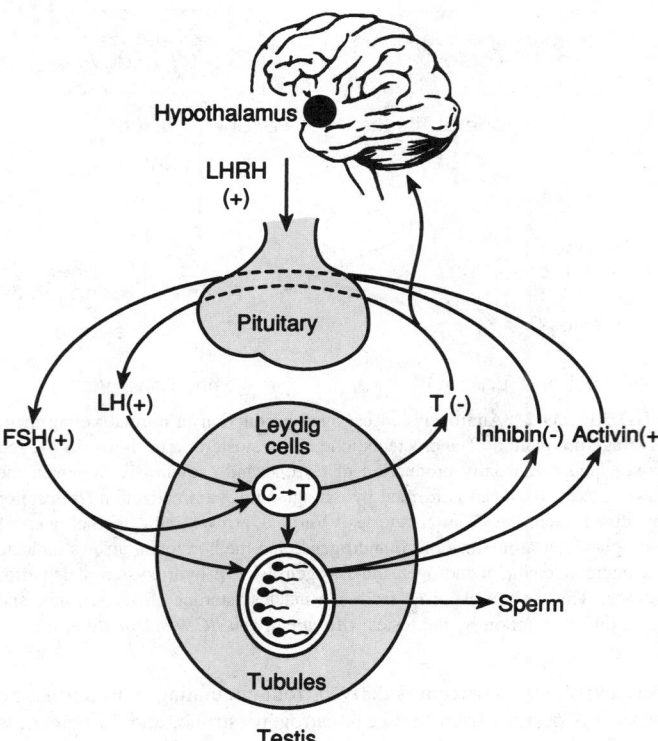

FIGURE 339-3 Regulation of testosterone and sperm production by LH and FSH. (C, cholesterol; T, testosterone.)

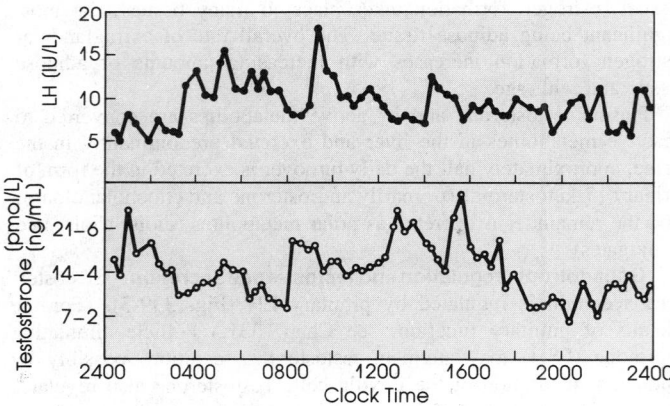

FIGURE 339-4 Twenty-four-hour pattern of plasma LH and testosterone in a normal man sampled every 20 min. *(Reprinted from Griffin and Wilson.)*

this episodic secretion of LH and testosterone occurs with peak morning levels of testosterone about 25 to 30 percent higher than late afternoon values.

Androgen action The major functions of androgen are regulation of LH secretion, formation of the male phenotype during sexual differentiation, and induction of sexual maturation and function at puberty. The cellular mechanisms by which androgens perform these functions are summarized schematically in Fig. 339-5. Testosterone (T) enters the cell by passive diffusion. Inside the cell T can be converted to dihydrotestosterone (D) by the 5α-reductase enzymes 1 and 2; 5α-reductase 2 is responsible for dihydrotestosterone formation in most androgen target tissues. T or D is then bound to the androgen-receptor protein in the nucleus (R). The hormone-receptor complex (TR or DR) attaches to specific chromosomal sites; as a result, new messenger RNA is transcribed, and new protein appears within the cytoplasm of the cell. The androgen receptor protein is coded by a gene on the long arm of the X chromosome; it contains 917 amino acids and has a molecular mass of about 110 kDa. It is similar in structure to other steroid hormone receptors and has distinct hormone-binding, DNA-binding, and functional domains (see Chap. 329). Estradiol acts by a mechanism similar to that of androgens but involving its own receptor (see Chap. 340).

Although testosterone and dihydrotestosterone bind to the same receptor, their physiologic roles differ. The testosterone-receptor complex regulates gonadotropin secretion and is responsible for the wolffian stimulation phase of sexual differentiation (see Chap. 342), whereas the dihydrotestosterone-receptor complex is responsible for external virilization during embryogenesis and the major portion of androgen action during sexual maturation and adult sexual life. The question of which hormone controls spermatogenesis is unresolved. The mechanism by which two hormones can interact with the same receptor but have different physiologic effects is also not well understood. Dihydrotestosterone binds to the receptor much more tightly than does testosterone, and hence its formation serves to amplify the hormonal signal.

THE SEMINIFEROUS TUBULE AND SPERMATOGENESIS Normal function of the seminiferous tubule is dependent on the pituitary and on the adjacent Leydig cells, both FSH and androgen being essential for normal spermatogenesis (see Fig. 339-3). The major site of FSH action is the Sertoli cell in the seminiferous tubules. The seminiferous tubule also contains androgen receptors. Androgen appears to be essential for spermatogenesis, whereas FSH is required for spermatid maturation. The normal adult testes produce more than 200 million sperm per day.

The Sertoli cell cannot synthesize steroid hormones de novo and is dependent on testosterone that diffuses in from adjacent Leydig cells. Sertoli cells can convert testosterone to estradiol and to dihydrotestosterone. The seminiferous tubules also produce the peptide hormones inhibin, which exerts a negative feedback control, and activin, which feeds back positively on FSH secretion by the pituitary (see Fig. 339-3). Testosterone and estradiol also can inhibit FSH secretion.

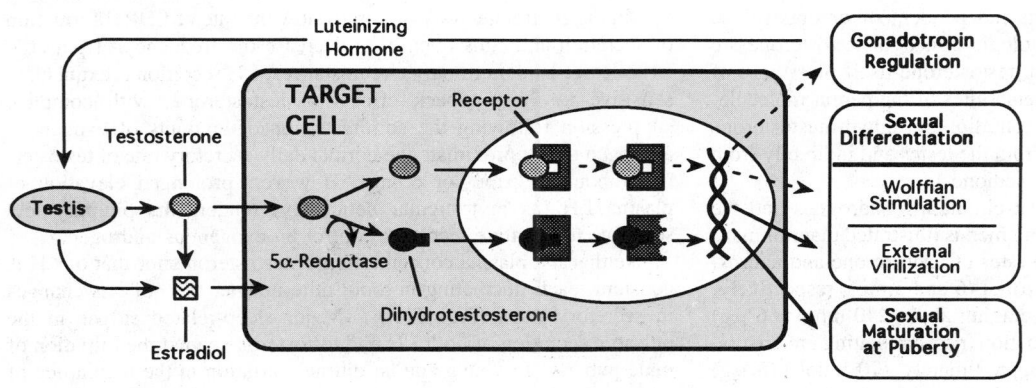

FIGURE 339-5 Current concepts of androgen action.

The interlocking system in which two pituitary hormones regulate testicular function provides a precise dual-control mechanism by hormonal signals from Leydig cells and the spermatogenic tubules that feed back on the hypothalamic-pituitary system to regulate their own function (see Fig. 339-3).

ASSESSMENT OF TESTICULAR FUNCTION

LEYDIG CELL FUNCTION   History and physical examination The assessment of Leydig cell function and androgen status should include inquiry about the presence at birth of developmental abnormalities of the urogenital tract, the timing and extent of sexual maturation at puberty, the rate of beard growth, and the current libido, sexual function, strength, and energy. Inadequate Leydig cell function or androgen action during embryogenesis may manifest by the presence of hypospadias, cryptorchidism, or microphallus. If Leydig cell failure occurs prior to puberty, sexual maturation will not occur, and the individual will develop the features termed *eunuchoidism*, including an infantile amount and distribution of body hair, poor development of skeletal muscles, and failure of closure of the epiphyses so that the arm span is more than 5 cm greater than the height and the lower body segment (heel to pubic) more than 5 cm longer than the upper body segment (pubic to crown). Detection of postpubertal Leydig cell failure requires a high index of suspicion and appropriate laboratory assessment. One reason is that decreased sexual function in adult men may be caused by nonendocrine as well as endocrine factors. The second is that certain functions that require androgens for initiation continue unabated when Leydig cell failure occurs, and functions that eventually regress may do so very slowly. For example, the frequency of shaving may not decrease for months or years because of slow decline in the rate of beard growth once established.

Plasma testosterone and dihydrotestosterone levels Plasma testosterone is measured by radioimmunoassay. Testosterone is secreted into plasma in a pulsatile fashion every 60 to 90 min (see Fig. 339-4); a single random sample provides a result within ±20 percent of the true mean value only two-thirds of the time, while three equally spaced samples 15 to 20 min apart provide a more accurate assessment. The samples do not need to be assayed separately, and aliquots of the three samples should be pooled for a single determination. The range of plasma testosterone in normal adult men is 10 to 35 nmol/L (3 to 10 ng/mL). In adult men, the plasma values vary somewhat throughout the day and at different times of the year, but these variations are not as great as those for plasma cortisol and are not significant in routine clinical assessment. Plasma levels of testosterone correlate in general with testosterone secretory rates as measured by isotope infusion. Estimation of TeBG concentration by radioimmunoassay is sometimes useful in the interpretation of total plasma testosterone levels. Bioavailable testosterone in plasma can be estimated by measuring the non-TeBG-bound fraction of testosterone.

The plasma testosterone value in prepubertal children is statistically higher in boys than in girls, the range in both being 0.2 to 0.7 nmol/L (0.05 to 0.2 ng/mL). The rise in plasma testosterone at the start of male puberty begins as a result of sleep-related nocturnal gonadotropin surges, so during the initial phases, plasma testosterone and LH are higher at night than during the day. Random daytime levels of plasma testosterone increase gradually as puberty progresses and reach adult levels at about age 17.

Dihydrotestosterone is also measured by radioimmunoassay. In young men, the plasma dihydrotestosterone level is about one-tenth the testosterone value and averages around 2 nmol/L (0.6 ng/mL). In older men with benign prostatic hyperplasia, plasma dihydrotestosterone levels average about 3 nmol/L (0.9 ng/mL).

Urinary 17-ketosteroids The measurement of urinary 17-ketosteroids is not a valid way to assess testicular function because testosterone contributes only about 40 percent of daily urinary 17-ketosteroids in men. The bulk of urinary 17-ketosteroids is derived from adrenal androgens.

Plasma LH Plasma LH is also measured by radioimmunoassay. LH is also secreted in a pulsatile fashion and fluctuates more widely than does plasma testosterone so that in adult men an isolated random plasma LH is likely to be within ±20 percent of true mean value only a third of the time. Again, assay of a pool of plasma composed of equal portions of three samples drawn 15 to 20 min apart as described above provides a value approaching the true mean. In early puberty, plasma LH secretion increases only during sleep, but the pulsatile secretion in the adult is of similar magnitude during sleep and waking periods. The normal plasma LH values should be established for a given laboratory. The usual normal range in adult men is 5 to 20 IU/L. Bioactive LH can be assessed in some laboratories by the rat interstitial cell assay and may be detectable at times when the immunoreactive LH is undetectable. A low plasma testosterone concentration can be interpreted correctly only if plasma LH is also measured simultaneously, and likewise, the "appropriateness" of a given plasma LH value must be interpreted in relation to the plasma testosterone value. For example, a low plasma testosterone coupled with a low LH implies hypothalamic or pituitary disease, whereas the finding of a low plasma testosterone and a high LH suggests primary testicular insufficiency (see Chap. 330).

Response to gonadotropin stimulation Leydig cell function is difficult to assess prior to puberty when both LH and testosterone levels are low, and it is common to measure response of plasma testosterone to gonadotropin stimulation as an index of Leydig cell capacity. Normal prepubertal boys respond to 3 to 5 days of injection of 1000 to 2000 IU human chorionic gonadotropin (hCG) with an increase in plasma testosterone to about 7 nmol/L (2 ng/mL); the magnitude of the response increases with the initiation of puberty and peaks in early puberty.

Response to luteinizing hormone–releasing hormone The responsiveness of the pituitary gland to luteinizing hormone–releasing hormone (LHRH) changes at the time of puberty. Prior to puberty, quantitative responses of LH and FSH are similar. With pubertal development, the LH response to acute administration of LHRH increases, while the FSH response remains the same. The amount of LH released following acute administration of LHRH probably reflects the amount of stored hormone in the pituitary. When 100 μg LHRH is given subcutaneously or intravenously to normal men, LH levels usually increase four- to fivefold, with the peak level at 30 min. However, the range of response is broad, some normal men having less than a doubling of LH levels. In general, the peak LH following a single LHRH injection correlates with the basal levels. In primary testicular failure, measurement of basal LH is usually sufficient, and measurement of LHRH response adds little to aid the diagnosis. Men with either pituitary disease or hypothalamic disease may have a normal or an abnormal LH response to acute administration of LHRH. Therefore, a normal response is of no diagnostic value either in determining the presence of disease or in distinguishing hypothalamic from pituitary disease. A subnormal response is of value in establishing that an abnormality exists, even though the site is not determined. The LHRH test is most useful in the evaluation of men with secondary hypogonadism and subnormal LH response to acute administration of LHRH. If daily infusions of LHRH for a week lead to the development of a normal acute LH response, a hypothalamic etiology is likely.

SEMINIFEROUS TUBULE FUNCTION   Examination of the testes Evaluation of the testes is an essential portion of the physical examination. The seminiferous tubules account for about 60 percent of testicular volume. The prepubertal testis measures about 2 cm in length and 2 mL in volume and grows during puberty to reach the adult proportions by age 16. When damage to the seminiferous tubules occurs prior to puberty, the testes are small and firm, whereas the testes are usually small and soft following postpubertal damage (the capsule, once enlarged, does not contract to its previous size). Testes in adults average 4.6 cm in length (range 3.5 to 5.5 cm), corresponding to a volume of 12 to 25 mL. Advanced age does not influence testicular size, so the significance of small testes is the same at all ages in the adult. Testis size varies among ethnic groups. Asian men have smaller testes than western Europeans, independent of differences in body size. Because of the possible causal role in infertility, the presence of varicocele should be sought by palpation with the patient standing.

Semen analysis Seminal fluid analysis is performed on samples obtained by masturbation into a glass container after 24 to 36 h abstinence. Analysis should be performed within an hour. The normal ejaculate volume is 2 to 6 mL. Immediately after ejaculation, the seminal fluid coagulates, followed within 15 to 30 min by liquefaction. Estimation of motility should be made on undiluted seminal fluid; more than 60 percent of the sperm should be motile and of normal morphology. The normal range for sperm density is generally considered to be greater than 20 million per milliliter, with a total count of more than 60 million per ejaculate, but the definition of a minimally adequate ejaculate is not clear. Some men with low sperm counts are nevertheless fertile. This uncertainty as to the lower level of sperm density, percent motility, and percent normal forms in fertile semen stems from two issues. First, many factors produce temporary aberrations in sperm count, and in men who present with semen of equivocal quality it is necessary to examine three or more ejaculates to determine whether abnormal findings are permanent or temporary. Second, the seminal fluid is routinely evaluated by tests that do not assess the functional capacity of sperm. Methods to measure sperm penetration of bovine cervical mucus and zona-free hamster ova are not sufficiently standardized to permit general use.

Plasma FSH Plasma FSH, as measured by specific radioimmunoassay, usually correlates inversely with spermatogenesis. In normal adult men, the range of plasma FSH is 5 to 20 IU/L. Men with intact hypothalamic-pituitary axes have elevations of FSH when damage to the germinal epithelium is severe.

Testicular biopsy Testicular biospy is useful in some patients with oligospermia and azoospermia both as an aid in diagnosis and as an indication of feasibility of treatment. For example, a normal testicular biopsy and a normal FSH in an azoospermic man suggest obstruction of the vas deferens, which may be surgically correctable.

ESTROGENIC FUNCTION **Examination of the breasts** Breast enlargement (gynecomastia) is the most consistent feature of feminizing states in men (see Chap. 341). Gynecomastia is due to the proliferation of both glandular and adipose tissue. The presence of gynecomastia should be sought by examining the sitting patient using the fingers to grasp glandular tissue. Palpation with the flat of the hand while the patient is supine may result in failure to detect early or minimal breast enlargement. In obese men it is important to try to define the edge of the rim of glandular tissue that separates it from adipose tissue of the chest wall.

Plasma estrogen As discussed above, most of the estradiol and all the estrone produced in normal men is formed by extraglandular aromatization of circulating androgens. Plasma estradiol is usually less than 180 pmol/L (50 pg/mL) in normal men; plasma estrone is somewhat higher but usually less than 300 pmol/L (80 pg/mL). Elevated estrogen production and elevated plasma levels can be due to elevations in plasma precursors (liver or adrenal disease), to increases in extraglandular aromatization (obesity), or to increased production by the testes (testicular tumors or androgen resistance).

PHASES OF NORMAL TESTICULAR FUNCTION

The phases of male sexual life can be defined in terms of the plasma testosterone value (Fig. 339-6). In the male embryo, the production of testosterone by the testes commences at about 7 weeks of gestation. Shortly thereafter plasma testosterone attains a high value that is maintained until it falls late in gestation so that at the time of birth plasma testosterone is only slightly higher in males than in females. Shortly after birth, plasma testosterone in the male infant again begins to rise and remains elevated for approximately 3 months, falling to low levels by age 6 months to 1 year. The concentration then remains

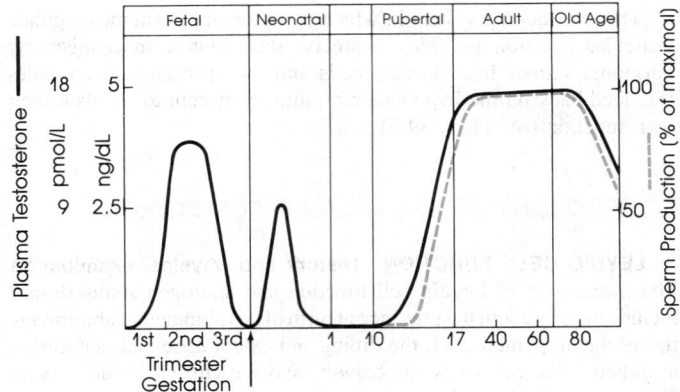

FIGURE 339-6 Phases of male sexual life. *(Reprinted from Griffin and Wilson.)*

low (but slightly higher in boys than in girls) until the onset of puberty, when it begins to rise in boys, reaching adult levels by about age 17. The mean plasma level remains more or less constant in the adult until late middle age and then declines slowly during the later decades of life. During the third, or adult, phase of male sexual life, sperm production becomes sufficient to allow reproduction to take place. The physiologic events that take place during these various phases differ, as do the pathologic consequences of derangements in testicular function at different stages of life. Male sexual differentiation during embryogenesis is considered in Chap. 342. The role of the surge of testosterone formation during the first year of life is not certain. However, in primates, neonatal activation of the hypothalamic-pituitary-testicular axis is important for subsequent normal pubertal development. The focus of this chapter is on testicular pathophysiology during puberty, adulthood, and old age.

ABNORMALITIES OF TESTICULAR FUNCTION

PUBERTY The factors that control the onset of puberty are poorly understood and may reside in the hypothalamic-pituitary system, the testes, or the adrenal. Prior to the onset of puberty, gonadotropin secretion by the pituitary is low but appears to be under regulatory control by the testes, since prepubertal castration results in a rise in plasma gonadotropin levels. This suggests that prior to puberty the negative feedback control of gonadotropin secretion is exquisitely sensitive to the small amount of circulating testosterone. The onset of puberty is heralded by sleep-associated surges in gonadotropin secretion. Later in puberty the rises in LH and FSH persist throughout the day. Thus, with maturation, the hypothalamic-pituitary system becomes less sensitive to negative feedback control, and the consequences are a higher mean plasma testosterone, maturation of the testes, and the onset of spermatogenesis. The rise in gonadotropin secretion is the consequence of both an increase in LHRH secretion and an increased sensitivity of the pituitary to LHRH. Plasma levels of bioactive LH increase even more than those of the immunoreactive hormone. The somatic changes at the time of puberty are secondary to the rise in plasma testosterone. Growth of the accessory organs of male reproduction (the penis, the prostate, the seminal vesicles, and the epididymides) accounts for about one-fourth of androgen-mediated nitrogen retention during puberty. Accelerated linear growth is accompanied by growth of muscle and connective tissue, accounting for the major portion of nitrogen retention at puberty. The principal androgen-sensitive muscles are those of the pectoral region and the shoulder. The characteristic hair growth of male puberty involves development of mustache and beard; regression of the scalp line; appearance of body, extremity, and perianal hair; and extension of the pubic hair upward into a diamond-shaped pattern. Growth of axillary and pubic hair is initiated under the control of adrenal androgens and is promoted by testicular androgens. The larynx enlarges, and the vocal cords become thickened, resulting in a lowering of the pitch of the voice. Hemoglobin levels increase about 10 g/L. These various androgen-mediated growth and maturation processes reach some limiting value so that once puberty is completed the administration of pharmacologic doses of androgen has no further effect. The entire process is heralded by testicular enlargement beginning at age 11 to 12 and is usually completed within 5 years, although some aspects of virilization, such as growth of the chest hair, may continue over a decade or more.

The events of normal male puberty are variable in onset, duration, and sequence. The central issue in dealing with disorders of puberty is separating instances of true absence or precocity from subjects at the extremes of normal variation. The use of staging criteria that correlate developmental and anatomic landmarks with chronologic age is useful in making this distinction. (See Marshall and Tanner.)

Sexual precocity Development of premature sexual characteristics appropriate for the phenotype, i.e., virilization in boys, is termed *isosexual precocity*. *Heterosexual precocity* refers to feminizing syndromes in boys.

ISOSEXUAL PRECOCITY Sexual development prior to age 9 in boys is generally considered abnormal. *True precocious puberty* or *complete isosexual precocity* occurs when both premature virilization and spermatogenesis take place, and *precocious pseudopuberty* or *incomplete isosexual precocity* refers to virilization unaccompanied by spermatogenesis, indicating that androgen formation is not the result of premature activation of the hypothalamic-pituitary system. This distinction is blurred in practice because pure virilizing syndromes may cause activation of gonadotropin secretion secondarily and thus be followed by development of spermatogenesis. Furthermore, local androgen production in the testis, as in Leydig cell tumors, can cause local areas of spermatogenesis around the tumor and limited sperm production. We therefore prefer a simple two-part classification: virilizing syndromes (in which hypothalamic-pituitary activity is appropriate for age) and premature activation of the hypothalamic-pituitary system.

Virilizing syndromes can result from Leydig cell tumors, human chorionic gonadotropin (hCG)–secreting tumors, adrenal tumors, congenital adrenal hyperplasia (most commonly 21-hydroxylase deficiency), androgen administration, or Leydig cell hyperplasia. In all these situations, plasma testosterone is inappropriately elevated for the age. Leydig cell tumors are rare in children but should be suspected when the testes are asymmetric in size (see Chap. 322). Virilizing adrenal tumors secrete large amounts of adrenal androgen (mainly androstenedione and dehydroepiandrosterone, some of which is converted to testosterone) and consequently cause elevated 17-ketosteroid secretion. Glucocorticoid administration does not suppress 17-ketosteroid excretion to normal in patients with testicular or adrenal tumors, in contrast to the prompt decrease that occurs following such treatment in congenital adrenal hyperplasia. Congenital adrenal hyperplasia leads to elevated 17-hydroxyprogesterone levels and as a consequence elevated androgen levels (see Chaps. 335 and 342). When this disorder is treated with glucocorticoids, true precocious puberty can then result if sufficient hypothalamic maturation has been produced by the increased androgen levels.

Gonadotropin-independent sexual precocity in boys may occur as a result of autonomous Leydig cell hyperplasia in the absence of Leydig cell tumor formation. The disorder is inherited as a male-limited autosomal disorder either from affected fathers to sons or from mothers who are unaffected carriers. Virilization begins usually by age 2. Testosterone levels are elevated, often to the adult male range; however, immunoreactive and bioactive LH levels and the LH response to LHRH are prepubertal. Many of these boys were mistakenly thought to have true precocious puberty in the past because of the presence of spermatogenesis.

Premature activation of the hypothalamic-pituitary system may be "idiopathic" or due to central nervous system (CNS) tumors, infections, or injuries. Such early hypothalamic-pituitary activation typically is associated with characteristics of normal puberty, i.e., sleep-related gonadotropin secretion, elevated plasma bioactive LH, and enhanced gonadotropin response to LHRH. Since the diagnosis of idiopathic true precocious puberty is one of exclusion, rare patients later prove to have been misclassified and to have an identifiable CNS abnormality. With improved means of diagnosis, such as computed tomographic scans and magnetic resonance imaging, delays in diagnosis will probably be less frequent.

Management of sexual precocity due to steroid- or gonadotropin-producing tumors, congenital adrenal hyperplasia, or CNS abnormality is directed toward the primary disease. In boys with Leydig cell hyperplasia, attempts have been made to lower plasma testosterone with medroxyprogesterone acetate or ketoconazole, but the long-term effectiveness of these agents is unknown. Idiopathic true precocious puberty and true precocious puberty due to inoperable CNS lesions are treated with LHRH analogue therapy, resulting in reversal of the pubertal maturation including decreased rate of skeletal development.

HETEROSEXUAL PRECOCITY Feminization in prepubertal boys can result from absolute or relative increases in estrogen due to a variety of causes (see Chap. 341).

Delayed or incomplete puberty The separation of failure of puberty from variants of normal is one of the most difficult problems in endocrinology. Some patients fail to show the normal spurt of growth and sexual development at the usual time but eventually commence puberty by age 16 or older. Adolescence may then either progress rapidly, or there may be a slow development and growth that continues until ages 20 to 22. Many men with delayed onset of puberty attain heights within the normal adult range. At times the history reveals that a parent or sibling has shown a similar pattern of development. The major problem is to separate this group of patients with delayed puberty from patients with organic disorders that impair puberty. Panhypopituitarism and hypothyroidism can cause pubertal failure in males (see Chaps. 331 and 334). Absent puberty also can result from primary disease of the testis, including defects in testicular development; this diagnosis is suspected on the basis of low plasma testosterone and elevated FSH and LH levels. Hereditary androgen resistance (in which plasma testosterone and LH levels are both high) usually results in hereditary male pseudohermaphroditism but in milder cases may be manifested by absent or incomplete puberty (see Chap. 342).

The most frequent finding in boys with absent puberty is both low plasma testosterone and low gonadotropin levels; in these patients it is necessary to distinguish boys with delayed puberty from those with isolated gonadotropin deficiency or idiopathic *hypogonadotropic hypogonadism* (*Kallman syndrome*). The manifestations of isolated gonadotropin deficiency vary from boys with eunuchoidal features and testes of prepubertal size to those with partial manifestations of LH and/or FSH deficiency and partial degrees of testicular enlargement and pubertal development. Anosmia or hyposmia and cryptorchidism are common. The disorder is inherited as an X-linked recessive trait or an autosomal dominant trait with variable expressivity. Serum FSH and LH levels are usually below the normal male range, and plasma testosterone levels are low for age. The secretion of other pituitary hormones is usually normal. The defect appears to be in the synthesis or release of LHRH with the resultant gonadotropin pattern ranging from absence of pulsatile LH secretion to defects in amplitude and frequency of LH secretion; the administration of synthetic LHRH for a sufficient period corrects the endocrine abnormalities and initiates spermatogenesis. If untreated, these patients usually remain in the prepubertal state indefinitely. A prepubertal manifestation is microphallus, in which the size of the penis is below the fifth percentile for the age. Indeed, a fourth or more of isolated prepubertal microphallus is due to hypogonadotropic hypogonadism. Distinction between this disorder and delayed puberty is particularly difficult in patients of early or midpubertal age; the presence of microphallus, anosmia, or a family history of hypogonadotropic hypogonadism may help to establish the diagnosis. In the absence of such evidence, differentiation of the two states may become clear only after several years of observation. In some cases the response of plasma LH to LHRH stimulation may be helpful in suggesting that puberty is imminent.

ADULT ABNORMALITIES OF TESTICULAR FUNCTION At the completion of puberty, plasma testosterone levels reach the adult level of 10 to 35 nmol/L (3 to 10 ng/mL) throughout the day, plasma gonadotropins are 5 to 20 IU/L each for LH and FSH, and sperm production is sufficient to allow reproduction. The adult set of the complex regulatory system (see Fig. 339-3) is sustained in the normal man for more than 40 years. However, the system is subject to a variety of influences, at the level of both the testes and the hypothalamic-pituitary system. Spermatogenesis is exquisitely sensitive to alterations in temperature, and brief increases either in systemic or local temperature (as in a hot bath) can be followed by temporary decreases in sperm production. The system is likewise subject to influence by diet, drugs, alcohol, environmental agents, and psychological stress, all of which may cause temporary decreases in sperm count.

Persistent abnormalities of testicular function in adults can be due to hypothalamic-pituitary disorders (see Chap. 331), testicular defects, or abnormalities of sperm transport. Certain of these conditions tend to affect Leydig cell function or spermatogenesis selectively, but most cause both underandrogenization and infertility (Table 339-1). The interlocking of defective Leydig cell function and infertility is a consequence of the dependence of spermatogenesis on androgen formation. Even partial decreases in testosterone production can cause infertility. Certain disorders (hyperprolactinemia, radiation, cyclophosphamide therapy, autoimmunity, paraplegia, androgen re-

sistance) can cause either isolated infertility or a combined defect in testicular function in different subjects.

Hypothalamic-pituitary disorders Disorders of the hypothalamus and pituitary can impair secretion of gonadotropins (and cause decreased androgen production and decreased spermatogenesis) either as a portion of generalized disease of the anterior pituitary (see Chap. 331) or as an isolated defect, usually hypogonadotropic hypogonadism, in which secretion of both LH and FSH are impaired; hypogonadotropic hypogonadism can be either congenital or, rarely, an acquired idiopathic defect. Alternatively, gonadotropin secretion can be altered by factors other than hypothalamic-pituitary pathology. For example, elevation of plasma cortisol in the *Cushing syndrome* can depress LH secretion independent of a space-occupying lesion of the pituitary. Some patients with *congenital adrenal hyperplasia* have suppressed gonadotropin secretion and consequent infertility. *Hyperprolactinemia* (as the consequence either of pituitary adenomas or of drugs such as phenothiazines) has been associated with combined Leydig cell and seminiferous tubule dysfunction, presumably the consequence of inhibition of LH and FSH secretion by prolactin. Occasionally, impaired fertility in hyperprolactinemia is associated with normal gonadotropin and androgen levels and is presumed to result from direct inhibition of spermatogenesis by prolactin. *Hemochromatosis* impairs testicular function most commonly as the result of effects on the pituitary; less often it affects the testis directly (see Chap. 345). The use of *androgens* for purposes other than replacement therapy is often associated with impaired sperm production (see below). In several other conditions, testosterone levels may be decreased in association with normal LH levels, and the mechanism is less clear. Men with massive obesity have decreased TeBG and decreased levels of total and bioavailable testosterone that return toward normal with weight loss. Obesity may be part of the mechanism for decreased testosterone levels in the subset of such men with Pickwickian syndrome (see Chap. 229). Some men with seizures of temporal lobe origin also have a hormonal pattern consistent with hypogonadotropic hypogonadism.

Testicular defects Abnormalities of testicular function in the adult can be grouped into several categories: developmental and structural defects of the testes, acquired testicular defects, and disorders secondary to systemic and/or neurologic disease.

DEVELOPMENTAL ABNORMALITIES The *Klinefelter syndrome* (both the classic and mosaic forms) and the *XX male syndrome* are usually not recognized until after the time of expected puberty (see Chap. 342). Some developmental defects cause infertility in the presence of normal androgen production. These include varicocele, germinal cell aplasia, and cryptorchidism. *Varicocele* may be of etiologic importance in as much as one-third of all male infertility. It is caused by retrograde flow of blood into the internal spermatic vein that eventuates in progressive, often palpable dilatation of the peritesticular pampiniform plexus of veins. Varicocele occurs in about 10 to 15 percent of men in the general population and in 20 to 40 percent of men with infertility and is thought to result from incompetence of the valve between the internal spermatic vein and the renal vein. It is more common on the left (85 percent). Unilateral varicocele increases the blood flow and the temperature of both testes as a result of the extensive anastomoses of the venous systems. The increased scrotal (and testicular) temperature is believed to be the cause of the poor-quality semen and infertility (the testes do not have the usual 2°C lower temperature than that of the abdominal cavity). The findings on semen analysis are usually nonspecific, with all parameters showing some abnormality. In some studies, surgical resection results in improved fertility, with the best results (70 percent pregnancy rate) obtained in men whose preoperative sperm counts are over 10 million per milliliter.

Some patients with *germinal cell aplasia* (the Sertoli cell–only syndrome) have a positive family history and may constitute a specific group in whom the germinal epithelium is missing with resulting azoospermia; plasma testosterone and LH values are normal, and plasma FSH levels are elevated. Other patients with identical histologic

---

TABLE 339-1 Abnormalities of adult testicular function	
Infertility with underandrogenization	Infertility with normal virilization
Hypothalamic-pituitary:	
Panhypopituitarism	
Isolated gonadotropin deficiency	Isolated FSH deficiency
Cushing's syndrome	Congenital adrenal hyperplasia
Hyperprolactinemia	Hyperprolactinemia
Hemochromatosis	Androgen use
Testicular:	
Developmental and structural defects	
Klinefelter's syndrome*	Germinal cell aplasia
XX male	Cryptorchidism
	Varicocele
	Immotile cilia syndrome
Acquired defects	
Viral orchitis*	*Mycoplasma* infection
Trauma	
Radiation	Radiation
Drugs	Drugs
(spironolactone, alcohol,	(cyclophosphamide)
ketoconazole,	
cyclophosphamide)	
Environmental toxins	Environmental toxins
Autoimmunity	Autoimmunity
Granulomatous disease	
Associated with systemic diseases	
Liver disease	Febrile illness
Renal failure	Celiac disease
Sickle cell disease	
Neurologic disease (myotonic	Neurologic disease (paraplegia)
dystrophy and paraplegia)	
Androgen resistance	Androgen resistance
Sperm Transport:	
	Obstruction of the epididymis or vas deferens (cystic fibrosis, diethylstilbesterol exposure, congenital absence)

* The common testicular causes of underandrogenization and infertility in adults—Klinefelter's syndrome and viral orchitis—are associated with small testes.

and clinical findings have androgen resistance or a history of viral orchitis or cryptorchidism. Consequently, a variety of conditions are commonly lumped under this term. The syndrome accounts for less than 10 percent of patients with azoospermia.

Unilateral *cryptorchidism*, even when corrected prior to puberty, is associated with abnormal semen in many individuals. This suggests that even in unilateral cryptorchidism the testicular abnormality is usually bilateral.

The *immotile cilia syndrome* is an autosomal recessive defect characterized by immotility or poor motility of the cilia of the airways and of the sperm. Kartagener's syndrome is a subgroup of the immotile cilia syndrome associated with situs inversus, chronic sinusitis, and bronchiectasis (see Chap. 221). The immotile sperm cannot fertilize. The structural abnormality leading to impaired motility of cilia can usually be defined by the electron-microscopic appearance. The specific defects that are known to cause the syndrome include defects in the dynein arms, spokes, or microtubule doublets. Cilia from epithelia and sperm tails from the same individual exhibit the same defects, but the pulmonary manifestations may be minor. *Other structural defects of sperm* that are less well understood can apparently lead to immotile sperm without involvement of cilia in the lung.

ACQUIRED TESTICULAR DEFECTS   The most common cause of acquired testicular failure in the adult is *viral orchitis*. The responsible viruses include mumps virus, echovirus, lymphocytic choriomeningitis virus, and group B arboviruses. The orchitis is due to actual infection of the tissue by virus rather than to indirect effects of the infection. Orchitis is the most common complication of mumps, occurring in as many as one-fourth of adult men with the disease. In about two-thirds the orchitis is unilateral, and in the remainder it is bilateral. Orchitis usually develops within a few days after the onset of parotitis but may precede it. The testis may return to normal size and function or undergo atrophy. Atrophy is believed to be due both to direct effects of the virus on the seminiferous tubules and to ischemia secondary to pressure and edema within the taut tunica albuginea. Semen analysis returns to normal in three-fourths of men with unilateral involvement and in only one-third of men with bilateral orchitis. Atrophy is usually perceptible within 1 to 6 months after the orchitis subsides, and the degree of atrophy is not necessarily proportional to the severity of the acute orchitis or the development of infertility. Unilateral atrophy occurs in approximately one-third of cases of mumps orchitis, and bilateral atrophy occurs in about one-tenth.

Trauma is the second most common cause of secondary atrophy of the testes. The exposed position of the testis in the scrotum renders it susceptible to both thermal and physical trauma—particularly in individuals with hazardous occupations.

The testes are sensitive to *radiation damage;* decreased secretion of testosterone appears to be a consequence of diminished testicular blood flow. Doses higher than 200 mGy (20 rad) cause increases in plasma FSH and LH levels and damage to the spermatogonia. After doses of about 800 mGy (80 rad), oligospermia or azoospermia develops. Higher doses may obliterate the germinal epithelium, except for occasional stem and Sertoli cells. Fractionated radiation may have a more profound effect than single-dose radiation. Recovery of sperm density occurs in a dose-related fashion, and complete recovery of sperm density to preradiation levels may require as long as 5 years. Permanent infertility can occur after radiation therapy of malignant lymphoma despite shielding of the testes. Permanent androgen deficiency in adult men is uncommon after doses of radiation in the therapeutic range; however, most boys receiving direct testicular radiation for acute lymphoblastic leukemia have permanently low plasma testosterone levels.

In general, *drugs* interfere with testicular function in one of four ways—inhibition of testosterone synthesis, blockade of the peripheral action of androgen, enhancement of estrogen levels, or direct inhibition of spermatogenesis. Certain drugs have multiple effects, and agents such as guanethidine that block the sympathetic nervous system can

impair sexual function in men whose pituitary-testicular axis is normal.

Spironolactone and ketoconazole block the synthesis of androgen by interfering with the late reactions in androgen biosynthesis. Spironolactone and cimetidine compete with androgen for the cytoplasmic receptor protein and thus interfere with androgen action in the target cell. Testosterone levels may be low and estradiol levels may be elevated in patients taking large amounts of marijuana, heroin, or methadone, although the exact reasons are unclear. Alcohol, when consumed in excess for prolonged periods, causes decreased plasma testosterone, independent of liver disease or malnutrition. Elevated plasma estradiol and decreased plasma testosterone levels have been reported in men taking digitalis.

Antineoplastic and chemotherapeutic agents commonly interfere with spermatogenesis. Cyclophosphamide causes azoospermia or extreme oligospermia within a few weeks after the initiation of therapy. Cessation of therapy is followed by a return of spermatogenesis within 3 years in about half of patients. Combination chemotherapy for acute leukemia, Hodgkin's disease, and other malignancies also may impair Leydig cell function. In pubertal boys this is manifested by decreased serum testosterone and elevated LH levels; in adult men testosterone levels do not decline, and the impaired Leydig cell function may only be detected as an enhanced LH response to LHRH. The alkylating agents in the chemotherapeutic regimens seem to be responsible for Leydig cell toxicity.

Because of the potentially toxic effects of many physical and chemical agents on spermatogenesis, the occupational and recreational history should be carefully evaluated in all men with infertility. Known environmental hazards include chemicals, such as the nematocide dibromochloropropane, cadmium, and lead, microwaves, and ultrasound.

Testicular failure also occurs as a part of a generalized disorder of *autoimmunity* in which multiple primary endocrine deficiencies coexist (Schmidt's syndrome) and in which circulating antibodies to the basement membrane of the testes are present (see Chap. 343). Sperm antibodies are also a cause of isolated male infertility. In some instances, such antibodies may be secondary phenomena resulting from duct obstruction or vasectomy. *Granulomatous diseases* also can destroy the testes, the most common such disorder being leprosy. Testicular atrophy occurs in 10 to 20 percent of men with lepromatous leprosy, the result of direct invasion of the tissue by the mycobacteria. The tubules are involved initially, followed by endarteritis and destruction of Leydig cells.

TESTICULAR ABNORMALITIES ASSOCIATED WITH SYSTEMIC DISEASE   The common systemic diseases that cause underandrogenization and infertility are liver disease and renal failure. In *cirrhosis of the liver*, a combined testicular and pituitary abnormality leads to decreased testosterone production independent of the direct toxic effects of ethanol. Although plasma LH is elevated, the level may be below the expected range given the degree of androgen deficiency. This is most likely the result of inhibition of LH secretion by estrogen in patients with chronic liver disease. Increased estrogen production results from impaired hepatic extraction of adrenal androstenedione and subsequent increased extraglandular conversion to estrone and estradiol. In effect, estrogen precursors are shunted to sites of extraglandular aromatization. Testicular atrophy and gynecomastia are present in about half of men with cirrhosis, and many such men are impotent.

In chronic *renal failure*, decreased androgen synthesis and diminution of sperm production develop in the setting of elevated plasma gonadotropins. The elevated LH is due to increased production as well as reduced clearance but is incapable of effecting normal testosterone production. In addition, about one-fourth of men with chronic renal failure have hyperprolactinemia. Low testosterone coupled with normal or increased plasma estrogen levels probably account for the presence of gynecomastia in about half of men on chronic hemodialysis. The role of the hyperprolactinemia in decreasing testosterone production is unclear. About half of men with renal failure on dialysis experience decreased libido and impotence. The etiology of the testicular abnormalities in renal failure is not well understood. Improvement in testosterone production with hemodialysis is incomplete, but successful transplantation may lead to return of testicular function to normal.

Men with *sickle cell anemia* usually have impaired secondary sexual development, and testicular atrophy is present in one-third. The defect may be either at the testicular or hypothalamic-pituitary level. Abnormalities in Leydig cell function, frequently accompanied by decreased sperm density, have been noted in a variety of chronic systemic diseases, including protein-energy *malnutrition*, advanced *Hodgkin's disease* and *cancer* prior to chemotherapy, and *amyloidosis*. Most of these disorders cause a lowered plasma testosterone level coupled with a normal to increased plasma LH level, suggesting combined hypothalamic-pituitary and testicular defects. The low plasma testosterone is not the result of inhibitors that interfere with the binding to TeBG and hence is not analogous to the sick euthyroid syndrome. Similar hormone changes occur following *surgery, myocardial infarction*, and severe *burns* and thus may be a nonspecific effect of illness.

The temporary decrease in sperm density after *acute febrile illness* usually occurs in the absence of any changes in testosterone production. Infertility in men with *celiac disease* is associated with a hormonal pattern typical of androgen resistance, namely elevated testosterone and LH levels. *Neurologic diseases* associated with altered testicular function include myotonic dystrophy and paraplegia. In myotonic dystrophy, small testes may be associated with abnormalities of both spermatogenesis and Leydig cell function. Spinal cord lesions resulting in paraplegia lead to a temporary decrease in testosterone levels and persistent defects in spermatogenesis; some patients retain the capacity to obtain erection and to ejaculate.

ANDROGEN RESISTANCE   Defects of the androgen receptor cause resistance to the action of androgen usually associated with defective male phenotypic development, infertility, and underandrogenization (see Chap. 342). A less severe form of androgen resistance, associated with infertility due to oligo- or azoospermia in otherwise phenotypically normal men, may cause a significant fraction of infertility previously classified as idiopathic azoospermia.

Impairment of sperm transport   Disorders of sperm transport may cause infertility in as many as 6 percent of infertile men with normal virilization. The obstruction may be unilateral or bilateral, congenital or acquired. In men with unilateral obstruction of sperm transport, the infertility may result from antisperm antibodies. Obstructive azoospermia at the level of the epididymis also occurs in association with chronic infections of the paranasal sinuses and lungs. Tuberculosis, leprosy, and gonorrhea are rare causes of acquired obstruction of ejaculatory structures. Congenital defects of the vas deferens can occur as an isolated abnormality associated with absence of the seminal vesicles (and consequently absence of fructose in the ejaculate), in patients with *cystic fibrosis* (on occasion the principal manifestation of the disease), or in men whose mothers received *diethylstilbestrol* during pregnancy.

At least 40 percent of infertile men have infertility of unknown etiology; none of the preceding conditions is found on careful search. The therapy in all forms of male infertility, except surgically correctable varicocele, vas deferens obstruction, or treatable endocrinopathy, is unsatisfactory. Empirical therapy with androgens or gonadotropins has no significant effect on fertility. Although the semen quality may improve with such treatment, the pregnancy rate is usually no greater than in infertile men given no therapy (25 percent fertility in patients followed for a year). This latter fact should be kept in mind, namely, that spontaneous resolution may occur in up to one-fourth of patients with idiopathic infertility followed with no treatment. Many forms of male infertility associated with some motile sperm in the semen can be treated by in vitro fertilization.

Fertility control in the male   A variety of approaches to fertility control in men have been tried, including use of the condom as a safe barrier method that also prevents sexually transmitted disease. Another widely used technique is ligation of the vas deferens, a procedure that has been successful in large numbers of men and can be performed on an outpatient basis. The time required for azoospermia to occur following the operation depends on the number of sperm in the terminal vas deferens and ejaculatory ducts at the time of surgery but is usually less than 40 days. Azoospermia should be documented in each case to prove effectiveness. No deleterious effects on either testosterone production or the hypothalamic-pituitary axis have been documented. Despite reports of immune-complex–associated accelerated atherosclerosis in vasectomized nonhuman primates, there does not appear to be any association between vasectomy and atherosclerosis in men. Vasectomy should only be recommended for men requesting permanent sterilization. Only about 30 to 40 percent of men subjected to vasovasostomy for reanastomosis of the vas subsequently achieve fertility.

OLD AGE   Beginning at about age 60, mean plasma total and bioavailable testosterone concentrations decline. Nevertheless, though statistically lower than levels in young men, the concentrations of testosterone in elderly men usually remain within the normal range. The cause of the decreased testosterone level is likely decreased Leydig cell numbers in the testes. There is also a decline in seminiferous tubule function and decreased sperm production in older men. Plasma LH and FSH levels are usually increased in elderly men, and an increase in the rate of conversion of androgen to estrogen in peripheral tissues results in a decrease in the effective ratio of androgen to estrogen. These latter endocrine changes may play a role in the development of prostatic hyperplasia and possibly in development of gynecomastia in aging men (see Chap. 341). Male sexual function gradually declines after early adulthood, but there is no convincing evidence that hormonal changes have any direct bearing on changes in sexual function with age.

Prostatic hyperplasia   See Chap. 323.

Cancer of the prostate   See Chap. 323.

DISORDERS OF ALL AGES   Testicular tumors (See Chap. 322) Chorionic gonadotropin is present in normal testes, and it is not surprising that plasma gonadotropins may be elevated in testicular tumors. Indeed, an elevated plasma level of the beta subunit of human chorionic gonadotropins (hCG-β) serves as a sensitive and specific marker of tumor activity in some men with germ cell tumors. Plasma levels of the beta subunit are elevated in all patients with choriocarcinoma, in one-third of embryonal carcinomas and teratocarcinomas, and rarely in seminomas. There is a good correlation between change in hCG-β levels and response to therapy.

Elevated estradiol and testosterone production in patients with testicular tumors can arise by at least two mechanisms. In trophoblastic tumors and in tumors of Leydig and Sertoli cells, production of both hormones occurs autonomously in the tumor tissue itself; in these instances, plasma gonadotropin levels and hormone production by the uninvolved portions of the testes are depressed, and azoospermia is common. However, when gonadotropins are secreted by the tumor, the gonadotropin acts to increase estradiol and testosterone production in the unaffected areas of the testes, and azoospermia is uncommon. When estrogens and androgens are formed (directly or indirectly) by the tumors, feminization, virilization, or no obvious change may result, depending on the pattern of hormones produced and the age of the patients. Other cellular markers of testicular tumor activity have been described in individual cases, including alpha fetoprotein.

Gynecomastia   See Chap. 341.

HORMONAL THERAPY

ANDROGENS   Pharmacologic preparations   Effective androgen therapy requires the use of chemically modified analogues of testosterone. When testosterone itself is administered by mouth, it is absorbed into the portal blood and degraded promptly by the liver so that insignificant amounts reach the systemic circulation; when injected parenterally, testosterone is rapidly absorbed from the injection vehicle and rapidly degraded. As a consequence, effective androgen therapy requires either the administration in a slowly absorbed form of testosterone (dermal patches or micronized oral preparation) or the administration of modified analogues. Such chemical modifications either retard the rate of absorption or catabolism, so as to sustain effective blood levels, or enhance the androgenic potency of each molecule, so that full androgenic effects can be achieved at a lower blood level of the drug. Three types of modification of the molecule have received widespread clinical application (Fig. 339-7), namely, esterification of the 17β-hydroxyl group, alkylation at the 17α position, and modification of the ring structure, particularly substitutions at the 2, 9, and 11 positions. Most agents actually contain combinations of ring structure alterations and either 17α-alkylation or esterification of the 17ß-hydroxyl. Esterification serves to decrease the polarity of the molecule. Consequently, the steroid is more soluble in the fat vehicles used for injection, and release of the steroid into the circulation is slowed. Most esters must be injected parenterally. The more carbon molecules in the acid esterified, the more prolonged is the action. Esters such as testosterone cypionate and testosterone enanthate can be injected every 1 to 3 weeks. Because the esters are hydrolyzed before the hormones act, the effectiveness of therapy can be monitored by assaying plasma testosterone level with time following administration.

The oral effectiveness of 17α-alkylated androgens (such as methyltestosterone and methandrostenolone) is due to slower hepatic catabolism than occurs with testosterone itself so that the alkylated derivatives escape degradation by the liver and reach the systemic circulation. For this reason, 17α-methyl or -ethyl substitution is a common feature of most orally active androgens. Unfortunately, all 17α-alkylated steroids may cause abnormalities of liver function, and for this reason they have a limited role in medicine.

Other alterations of the ring structure of the androgen molecule

FIGURE 339-7 Some of the androgen preparations available for pharmacologic use.

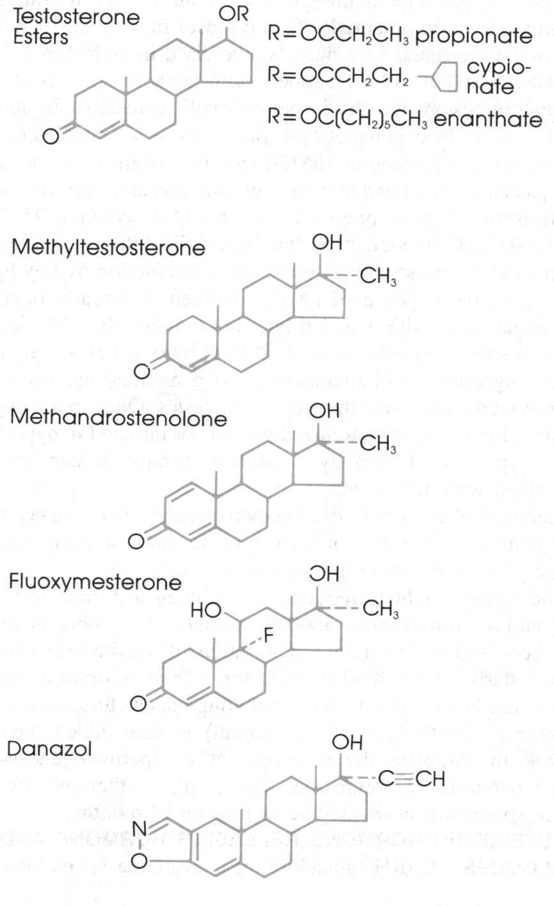

have been adopted empirically. In some instances the modification slows the rate of inactivation, in others it enhances the potency of a given molecule, and in still others it alters the conversion to other active metabolites. For example, the potency of fluoxymesterone may be due to the fact that, unlike most androgens, it is a poor precursor for conversion to estrogens in peripheral tissues. Transdermal preparations of testosterone in which a testosterone-loaded patch is applied each day are under evaluation. This therapy avoids the wide swings in serum testosterone values that occur between injections of testosterone esters.

Side effects of androgens All androgens carry the risk of inducing virilization in women. Early manifestations include acne, coarsening of the voice, hirsutism, and menstrual irregularities. If treatment is discontinued as soon as these effects develop, the manifestations may slowly subside. Long-term side effects such as male-pattern baldness, worsening of the hirsutism and voice changes, and hypertrophy of the clitoris are largely irreversible. There is considerable variation in the frequency and degree to which these signs develop in women, probably because of individual differences in susceptibility, in steady state blood levels of hormone, and in duration of therapy. In general, the younger the patient, the more striking are the virilizing signs; nevertheless, florid virilization also can occur in adult women. At physiologic replacement doses, testosterone esters have no known side effects in mature men. At supraphysiologic doses, however, gonadotropin secretion is inhibited, the testes decrease in volume, and the sperm count falls (indeed, low sperm counts may persist for as long as 9 months after cessation of androgen abuse). The so-called toxic side effects differ among the different agents and depending on the clinical setting in which they are used.

Retention of a limited amount of sodium is an inevitable consequence of androgen therapy, but in patients with underlying heart disease or renal failure or when androgens are administered in enormous amounts, the degree of sodium retention may lead to edema. Although androgens do not cause malignancy, they may promote growth of and intensify pain from carcinoma of the prostate and from breast carcinoma in men.

Feminizing side effects of androgen therapy in men are poorly understood. Testosterone itself can be converted (aromatized) in extraglandular tissues to estradiol. In contrast, 5α-reduction of the molecule precludes estrogen formation. The most common manifestation of feminization is the development of gynecomastia. Such breast enlargement is common in children given androgens and correlates with an increase in urinary estrogens, possibly because of a greater capacity to convert androgens to estrogens in childhood. The administration of testosterone esters to men results in an increase in plasma estrogen levels. In men with normal liver function, gynecomastia usually develops only after high doses of androgens.

All 17α-alkylated androgens can produce liver function abnormalities such as elevation of plasma alkaline phosphatase and conjugated bilirubin. The incidence of clinical liver disease probably depends on the previous integrity of the liver, but jaundice may occur in the absence of preexisting liver disease. 17α-Alkylated drugs also cause an increase in a variety of plasma proteins that are synthesized in the liver. The most serious complications of 17α-alkylated androgen therapy are the development of peliosis hepatis (blood-filled cysts in the liver) and hepatoma. These disorders were initially described in patients with aplastic anemia, many of whom had Fanconi anemia, itself a predisposing factor for the development of malignancy. However, both lesions also have been reported in patients who received substituted androgens for a variety of other causes, including use by athletes. There may be a similar increased incidence of hepatocellular neoplasms in women taking oral contraceptives. In some individuals these tumors regress and follow a benign course after discontinuation of the drugs; and in others the course is rapidly fatal.

One indication for the use of 17α-alkylated androgens is in hereditary angioedema; in this disorder the desired therapeutic benefit (increase in the level of the inhibitor of the first component of complement) may actually be a side effect of the 17-alkylated steroid rather than an effect of the parent androgen itself. As a consequence, weak androgens such as danazol are effective in this disorder (see Fig. 339-7). Danazol is also used in the management of endometriosis (see Chap. 48).

Replacement therapy   The aim of androgen therapy in hypogonadal men is to restore or bring to normal male secondary sexual characteristics (beard, body hair, external genitalia) and male sexual behavior and to mimic the hormonal effects on somatic development (hemoglobin, muscle mass, nitrogen balance, and epiphyseal closure). Since an assay for plasma testosterone is available for monitoring therapy, the treatment of androgen deficiency is almost universally successful. The parenteral administration of a long-acting testosterone ester such as 100 to 200 mg testosterone enanthate at 1- to 2-week intervals results in a sustained increase in plasma testosterone to the normal male range. Such esters act only through the release of testosterone itself into the circulation. If the hypogonadism is primary and of long duration (as in the Klinefelter syndrome), suppression of plasma LH to the normal range may not occur for many weeks, if at all. Considerable variability exists in the relation between plasma testosterone and male sexual behavior, but in postpubertal testicular failure (even of many years duration) resumption of normal sexual activity is usual following adequate replacement. Androgen does not restore spermatogenesis in hypogonadal states, but the volume of the ejaculate (derived largely from the prostate and seminal vesicles) and other male secondary sex characteristics return to normal. The effects of endogenous androgen on hemoglobin, nitrogen retention, and skeletal development are also reproduced.

In patients of all ages in whom hypogonadism developed prior to expected puberty (such as patients with hypogonadotropic hypogonadism), it is appropriate to bring plasma testosterone slowly into the adult range. When therapy is commenced at the time of expected puberty in such patients, the normal events of puberty proceed in the usual fashion. If therapy is delayed until after the time of usual puberty, the degree to which normal virilization will occur is variable, but many patients undergo a relatively complete anatomic and functional maturation. Intermittent low-dose androgen therapy is indicated in prepubertal hypogonadal boys with microphallus to bring the external genitalia into the normal range. If such patients are monitored closely and given androgens only for short periods, such therapy usually has no adverse effects on somatic growth.

In boys of pubertal age with either isolated hypogonadotropic hypogonadism or primary testicular deficiency, the usual practice is to institute androgen therapy between the ages of 12 and 14 years, depending on the subjective need for sexual development. The initial administration of small doses of testosterone esters followed by a gradual increase to 100 to 150 mg/m² of body surface area every 1 to 3 weeks should result in a normal pubertal growth spurt. The time from the start of treatment to the appearance of secondary sex characteristics is variable. Penile development, deepening of the voice, and other secondary sexual characteristics usually commence during the first year of treatment. In normal boys, puberty extends over several years, and treatment designed to replicate normal development does not shorten the process greatly.

Testosterone exerts its full action only in the presence of a balanced hormonal environment and, particularly, in the presence of adequate levels of growth hormone. Consequently, prepubertal boys with coexisting growth hormone and androgen deficiency exhibit a diminished response to androgens unless growth hormone is given simultaneously.

Pharmacologic uses   Androgens have been used for a variety of disorders unassociated with hypogonadism, in the hope that potential benefits from the nonvirilizing actions of the agents (such as increase in nitrogen retention and muscle mass, increased hemoglobin, etc.) would outweigh any deleterious actions of the drugs. The most common nonreplacement uses of androgen have been attempts to improve nitrogen balance in catabolic states, self-administration by

athletes in the belief that muscle mass and/or athletic performance will be improved, attempts to enhance erythropoiesis in refactory anemias including the anemia of renal failure, treatment of hereditary angioedema and endometriosis, and management of growth retardation of various etiologies. Most expectations of beneficial effects in these disorders have been illusory for two reasons. First, pharmacologic doses of androgens do little, if anything, in men beyond the normal testicular androgen, and in women the virilizing side effects of androgens are formidable. Second, no androgen has been devised that exhibits only the nonvirilizing effects of the hormone. This is not surprising in view of the fact that all actions of androgens are mediated by a single high-affinity receptor protein in the cytoplasm (see Fig. 339-5).

The most pervasive form of androgen abuse is by male athletes in the expectation that muscle development and athletic performance will be improved. In fact, however, in adequately controlled studies such therapy does not improve performance consistently. However, published trials of efficacy involve the administration of drugs at smaller doses than are usually taken by athletes; since the drugs at high dosage have multiple side effects, some of which preclude studies of efficacy in a double-blind fashion, it is not clear whether the question of efficacy can ever be resolved scientifically. Under no circumstances do putative benefits outweigh the risks associated with androgen abuse, a practice that cannot be condemned too harshly. The only established indications for androgen therapy outside of male hypogonadism are in selected patients with anemia due to bone marrow failure, hereditary angioedema, or endometriosis and as an adjunct to growth hormone therapy.

Parenteral administration of testosterone esters to normal men results in little effects of any kind, except for the suppression of gonadotropin secretion by the hypothalamic-pituitary system and a consequent decrease in the production of sperm. There is no established contraindication to their administration to men with those disorders (such as short stature) where their use has been advocated, but the efficacy is not yet established. However, in women, the virilizing side effects preclude androgen use in all except life-threatening situations. Even in potentially fatal diseases in women, such as bone marrow failure, great care must be exercised in androgen use.

GONADOTROPINS   Treatment with gonadotropins is utilized to establish or restore fertility in patients with gonadotropin deficiency of all causes. Two gonadotropin preparations are available: human menopausal gonadotropins (hMG) (purified from the urine of postmenopausal women) and human chorionic gonadotropin (hCG) (purified from the urine of pregnant women). hMG contains 75 IU FSH and 75 IU LH per vial. hCG has little FSH activity and resembles LH in its ability to stimulate testosterone production by Leydig cells. Because of the expense of hMG, treatment is usually begun with hCG alone, and hMG is added later to stimulate the FSH-dependent stages of spermatid development. A high ratio of LH to FSH activity and a long duration of treatment (3 to 6 months) are necessary to bring about maturation of the prepubertal testes. Once spermatogenesis is restored in hypophysectomized patients or initiated in hypogonadotropic hypogonadal men by combined therapy, it can usually be maintained with hCG alone.

Men with oligospermia of unknown etiology also have been treated with gonadotropins; the incidence of fertility in such patients is probably no greater than in untreated controls.

The dosage of hCG required to maintain a normal testosterone level varies from 1000 to 5000 IU weekly. A number of regimens have been utilized to induce maturation of spermatogenesis. Most involve starting with 2000 IU hCG three or more times a week until most of the clinical parameters, including plasma testosterone levels, are normal. hMG (usually one ampul) is then added three times a week to complete the development of spermatogenesis. After spermatogenesis has regressed, the length of therapy required to restore spermatogenesis may be as long as 12 months.

LUTEINIZING HORMONE–RELEASING HORMONE AND LHRH ANALOGUES   LHRH (gonadorelin) is available for endocrine testing. LHRH therapy is used by some physicians for chronic therapy of the infertility of hypogonadotropic hypogonadism. It is necessary to administer LHRH in frequent boluses (25 to 200 ng/kg of body weight every 2 h), requiring the use of portable infusion pumps or periodic nasal application. In general, LHRH does not appear to be more efficacious than gonadotropin in returning sperm counts to normal. LHRH analogues (leuprolide and nafarelin) are available for the suppression of gonadotropin secretion and induction of hypogonadism. In prostatic cancer, testicular androgen production can be blocked by monthly injection of 7.5 mg leuprolide in depot form.

REFERENCES

CARR BR, GRIFFIN JE: Fertility control and its complications, in *Williams' Textbook of Endocrinology*, 8th ed, JD Wilson, DW Foster (eds). Philadelphia, Saunders, 1992, pp 1007–1031

DAVIS JE: Male sterilization. Clin Obstet Gynaecol 6:97, 1979

DE KRETSER DM: The effects of systemic disease on the function of the testis. Clin Endocrinol Metabol 8:487, 1979

———, ROBERTSON DM: The isolation and physiology of inhibin and related proteins. Biol Reprod 40:33, 1989

GOLDZIEHER JW et al: Improving the diagnostic reliability of rapidly fluctuating plasma hormone levels by optimized multiple-sampling techniques. J Clin Endocrinol Metab 43:824, 1976

GRIFFIN JE, WILSON JD: Disorders of the testes and male reproductive tract, in *Williams' Textbook of Endocrinology*, 8th ed, JD Wilson, DW Foster (eds). Philadelphia, Saunders, 1992, pp 799–852

GRUMBACH MM, STYNE DM: Puberty: Ontogeny, neuroendocrinology, physiology, and disorders, in *Williams' Textbook of Endocrinology*, 8th ed, JD Wilson, DW Foster (eds). Philadelphia, Saunders, 1992, pp 1139–1221

LAUE L et al: Treatment of familial male precocious puberty with spironolactone and testolactone. N Engl J Med 320:496, 1989

MACDONALD PC et al: Origin of estrogen in normal men and in women with testicular feminization. J Clin Endocrinol Metab 49:905, 1979

MARSHALL WA, TANNER JM: Variation in the pattern of pubertal changes in boys. Arch Dis Child 45:13, 1970

MASSEY FJ et al: Vasectomy and health: Results from a large cohort study. JAMA 252:1023, 1984

NIESCHLAG E: Care for the infertile male. Clin Endocrinol (Oxf) 38:123, 1993

SANTORO N et al: Hypogonadotropic disorders in men and women: Diagnosis and therapy with pulsatile gonadotropin-releasing hormone. Endocr Rev 7:11, 1986

SIGMAN M, HOWARDS SS: Male infertility, in *Campbell's Urology*, 6th ed, PC Walsh et al (eds). Philadelphia, Saunders, 1992, pp 661–705

SNYDER PF, LAWRENCE DA: Treatment of male hypogonadism with testosterone enanthate. J Clin Endocrinol Metab 51:1335, 1980

WHITCOMB RN, CROWLEY WF: Hypogonadotropic hypogonadism: GnRH therapy, in *Current Therapy in Endocrinology and Metabolism*, 4th ed, CW Bardin (ed). Toronto, Decker, 1991, pp 273–275

WILSON JD: Androgen abuse by athletes. Endocr Rev 9:181, 1988

———, GRIFFIN JE: The use and misuse of androgens. Metabolism 29:1278, 1980

YING S-Y: Inhibins, activins, and follistatin: Gonadal proteins modulating the secretion of hormone. Endocr Rev 9:267, 1988

340 DISORDERS OF THE OVARY AND FEMALE REPRODUCTIVE TRACT

BRUCE R. CARR / JEAN D. WILSON

The ovary is the source of ova for reproduction and of the hormones that regulate female sexual life. The anatomic structure, response to hormonal stimuli, and secretory capacity of the ovary are different at different periods of life. This chapter will review normal ovarian physiology as a background for understanding abnormalities of the ovary and other tissues of the female reproductive tract.

DEVELOPMENT, STRUCTURE, AND FUNCTION OF THE OVARY

EMBRYOLOGY During the third week of gestation, the primordial germ cells arise from the endoderm lining the yolk sac at the caudal end of the embryo. The germ cells migrate to the genital ridge adjacent to the mesonephric kidney by the fifth week of gestation and undergo mitotic divisions. The gonads exist in an undifferentiated state until the seventh week of fetal life, at which time the primitive ovary can be differentiated from the testis (see Chap. 342). Estrogen formation in the ovary commences between weeks 8 and 10, and by 10 to 11 weeks of gestation, some oogonia in the developing ovarian cortex begin developing into primary oocytes. The ovary contains a finite number of germ cells, the maximal number of about 7 million oogonia being reached by the fifth to sixth month of gestation. Afterward, the germ cells decrease in number through a process of atresia such that only 1 million remain at birth, 400,000 are present at the time of menarche, and only a few remain at menopause. Two X chromosomes are required for normal development of the ovary; in individuals with a 45,X karyotype, ovarian development occurs, but the rate of atresia is accelerated so that only a fibrous streak remains at the time of birth (see Chap. 342).

After the oogonia cease to proliferate, meiosis commences, proceeds until the diplotene stage of the first meiotic division is completed, and remains stationary until the time of onset of ovulation at puberty. From the fifth month of fetal life, the primordial follicle consists of the primary oocyte arrested in meiosis, a single surrounding layer of granulosa cells, and a basement membrane that separates the primordial follicle from surrounding stromal (interstitial) tissues.

PUBERTAL MATURATION Final maturation of ovarian follicles commences during puberty. The two major hormones that regulate follicular development are the pituitary gonadotropins—follicle-stimulating hormone (FSH) and luteinizing hormone (LH) (Fig. 340-1). During the second trimester of fetal development, the plasma gonadotropins rise to levels equivalent to those at menopause. This peak in gonadotropin levels may be causally related to the simultaneous peak in replication of oocytes. The hypothalamic-pituitary axis (the so-called gonadostat) undergoes maturation and becomes sensitive after the second trimester to negative feedback by steroid hormones, particularly estrogen and progesterone produced in the placenta. The circulating gonadotropins decrease thereafter and are almost undetectable at the time of birth. In the neonate, concomitant with the decrease in estrogen and progesterone levels due to separation from the placenta at birth, there is a rebound increase in gonadotropin secretion that persists for the first few months of life. With continued maturation of the hypothalamic-pituitary system, the gonadostat becomes sensitive to negative feedback by the low levels of circulating steroid hormones, and plasma gonadotropins again decrease.

As the time of puberty nears, a decrease in the sensitivity of the gonadostat allows for increased secretion of FSH and LH, possibly secondary to increased episodic or pulsatile secretion of luteinizing hormone–releasing hormone (LHRH) by the hypothalamus (see Chap. 331). A sleep-induced, pulsatile pattern of LH secretion then ensues, the first step in the development of a cyclic pattern of gonadotropin secretion (see Fig. 340-1). The increase in estrogen secretion subsequently exerts a positive feedback which leads to an exaggeration of the pulsatile release of LH and eventually to ovulation and the menarche, after which mean plasma gonadotropin concentrations reach adult values in which day and night levels are similar. After the menopause, plasma gonadotropin levels rise, plateau 5 to 10 years later, and remain fairly constant until the eighth to ninth decade of life when the levels may fall. Although ovarian function is regulated primarily by LH and FSH, the ovary is a source of several peptide and protein hormones and growth factors that may play a role in ovarian function.

With the development at puberty of decreased sensitivity of the hypothalamic-pituitary centers to circulating steroid hormones, LHRH release by the hypothalamus increases, gonadotropin secretion by the pituitary is enhanced, ovarian estrogen secretion increases, and the anatomic changes of puberty ensue. At age 10 to 11, the first secondary sexual characteristics begin to appear in girls, namely, development of the breast buds (thelarche), followed by the development of pubic hair (pubarche), and later by the development of

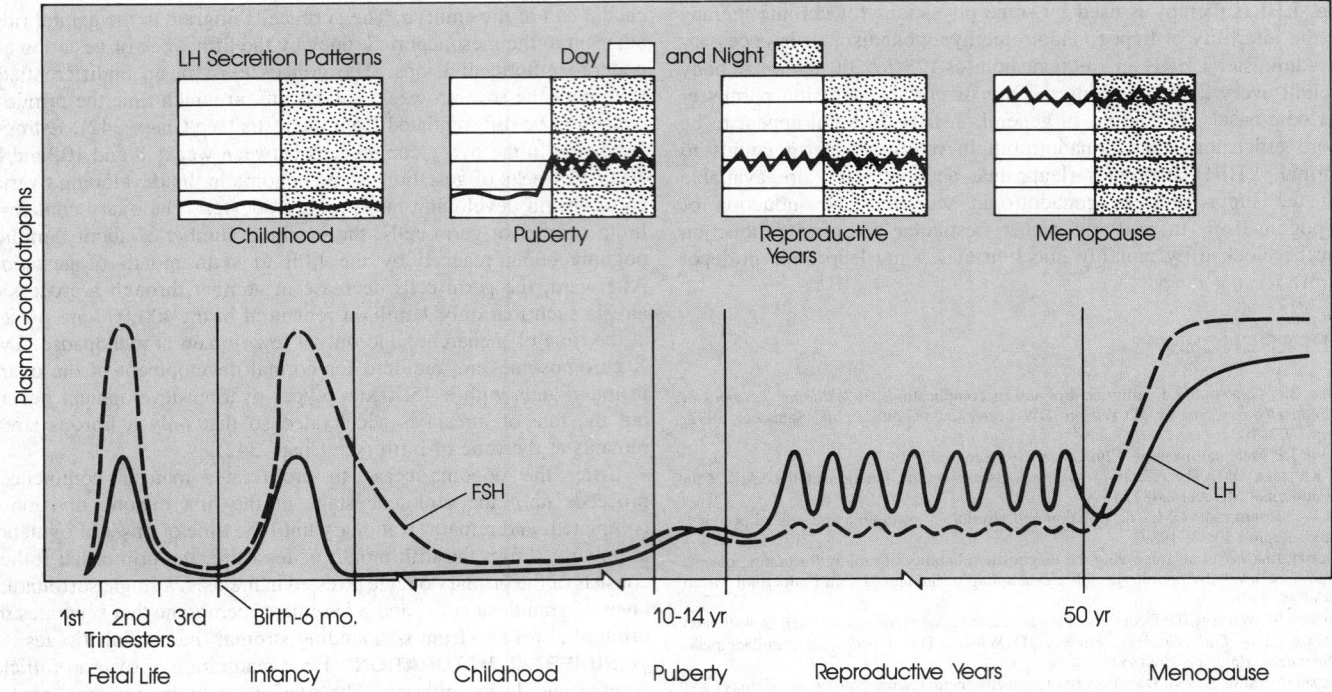

FIGURE 340-1 Pattern of gonadotropin secretion during different stages of life in women. FSH (follicle-stimulating hormone), LH (luteinizing hormone). The secretory patterns of LH during the waking hours (clear area) and night (stippled area) for each stage are indicated in the upper insets. (*After C Faiman et al.*)

axillary hair (adrenarche). The appearance of pubic and axillary hair is believed to be the result of an increase in adrenal androgens, commencing at approximately 6 to 8 years of age. A growth spurt ensues, and peak growth rate is attained at a mean age of 12 years.

The culmination of puberty is the onset of predictable, cyclic menses. The average time between the beginning of breast development and the onset of menses (menarche) is 2 years. During the first few years after menarche, menstrual cycles are often irregular and unpredictable due to anovulation. The age of menarche is variable and is determined in part by socioeconomic and genetic factors as well as general health. In the United States, the mean age of menarche is believed to have decreased at a rate of 3 to 4 months per decade over the last 100 years and is now around 13 years, a decrease believed to be due to an improvement in nutrition. A critical body weight of around 48 kg or a critical combination of weight, body water, and body fat is associated with development of hypothalamic insensitivity to circulating steroids that leads to increased secretion of gonadotropins and finally to menarche. Obese girls with a body weight 20 to 30 percent above ideal have earlier menarche than girls with normal weights. In contrast, participation in certain sports or ballet, malnutrition, and chronic debilitating disease can delay menarche.

MATURE OVARY Morphology The anatomic components and function of the adult ovary are illustrated schematically in Fig. 340-2. Under the influence of gonadotropins, a group of primary follicles is recruited, and by day 6 to 8 of the menstrual cycle, one follicle becomes mature or "dominant," a process characterized by accelerated growth of granulosa cells and enlargement of the fluid-filled antrum. The recruited follicles not destined to ovulate begin to undergo degeneration, similar to the atresia observed in other follicles during embryogenesis. Just prior to ovulation, meiosis resumes in the ova of the dominant follicle, and the first meiotic division is completed with formation of the first polar body. Rapid enlargement of the antrum (up to 10 to 25 mm in size) occurs with an associated increase in follicular fluid, followed by a thinning of the follicular surface and formation of a conical stigma. Ovulation from the dominant follicle occurs some 16 to 23 h after the LH peak or 24 to 38 h after the

onset of the LH surge as the result of rupture of the follicular wall at the area of the stigma, followed by expulsion of the ovum together with a mass of surrounding granulosa cells called *cumulus cells*. The rupture is believed to result from the action of hydrolyzing enzymes on the surface of the follicle, possibly under the control of prostaglandins. The second meiotic division begins after the egg is fertilized by a sperm, and the second polar body is then extruded. Following ovulation, the formation of the corpus luteum begins in the retained remnant of the ovulated follicle; the remaining granulosa and theca cells increase in size and accumulate lipids and a yellow pigment, lutein, to become "luteinized." The basement membrane that separated the granulosa cells from the stroma and blood vessels breaks, and capillaries, fibroblasts, and lymphatics from the theca invade the granulosa cells and reach the central cavity, thereby filling it with blood. After a period of 14 ± 2 days (the functional life of the corpus luteum), regression of vessels and atrophy of the corpus luteum commence and eventuate in replacement of the corpus luteum by a fibrous scar, the corpus albicans. The factors that limit the life span of the human corpus luteum are not known. However, if pregnancy occurs, the corpus luteum persists under the influence of placental or chorionic gonadotropins, and progesterone is produced by the corpus luteum for the support of early pregnancy.

Hormone formation STEROID HORMONES Like other steroid hormones, ovarian steroids are derived from cholesterol (Fig. 340-3). The ovary can synthesize cholesterol de novo from 2-carbon precursors and also can utilize cholesterol from circulating low-density lipoproteins (LDL) as substrate for steroid hormone formation (Fig. 340-4). Virtually all ovarian cells are believed to possess the complete enzymatic complement required for the conversion of cholesterol to estradiol (see Fig. 340-3); however, different cell types within the ovary contain different amounts of these enzymes so that the principal steroids produced differ in the various compartments. For example, the corpus luteum forms progesterone and 17-hydroxy-progesterone predominantly, whereas theca and stromal cells convert cholesterol to the androgens androstenedione and testosterone. Granulosa cells are particularly rich in the aromatase responsible for conversion of androgens to estrogen and utilize as substrates for this

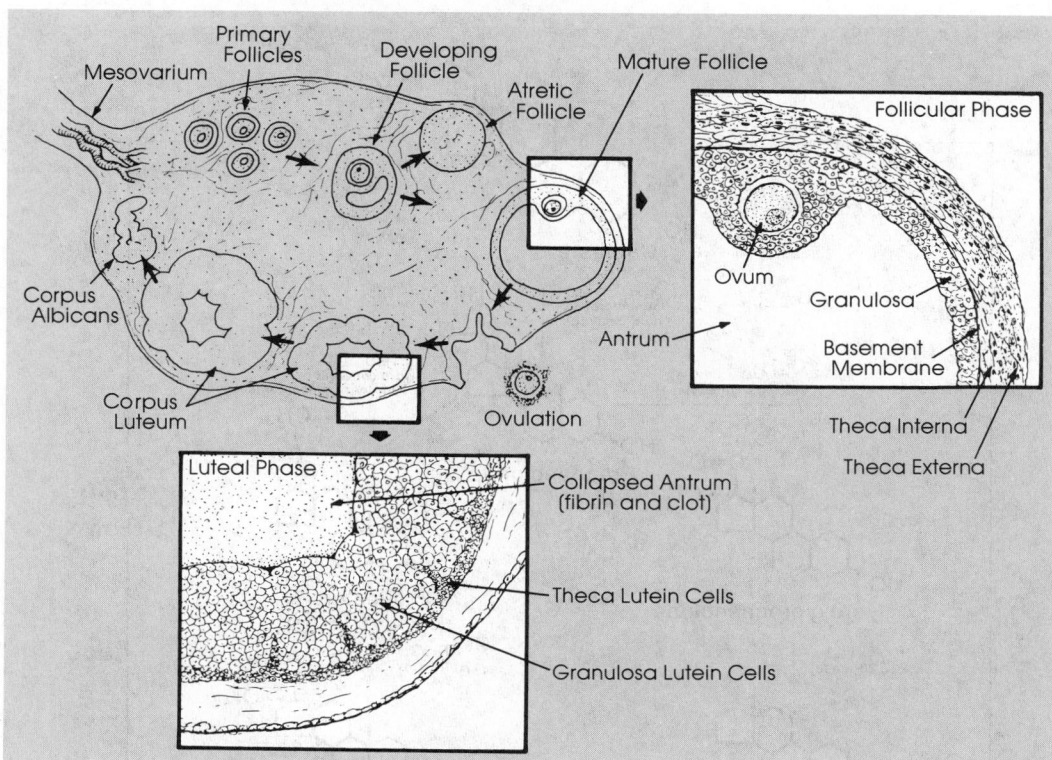

FIGURE 340-2 Developmental changes in the adult ovary during a complete 28-day cycle.

process androgens synthesized in the granulosa cells and the adjacent theca cells.

The principal sites of action of LH and FSH are also illustrated in Figs. 340-3 and 340-4. LH acts primarily to regulate the first step in steroid hormone biosynthesis, namely, the conversion of cholesterol to pregnenolone, and also induces subsequent enzymes in the pathway. FSH acts to regulate the final process by which androgens are aromatized to estrogens. As a consequence, in the absence of FSH, LH enhances substrate flow and the formation of androgens and/or progesterone, whereas FSH action is impeded in the absence of LH because of diminished substrate for aromatization.

Estrogens   Naturally occurring estrogens are 18-carbon steroids characterized by an aromatic A ring, a phenolic hydroxyl group at C-3, and either a hydroxyl group (estradiol) or a ketone (estrone) at C-17 (see Fig. 340-3). (For the numbering of the steroid ring, see Fig. 339-1.) The principal estrogen secreted by the ovary and the most potent naturally occurring estrogen is estradiol. Estrone is also secreted by the ovary, but the principal source of estrone is from extraglandular conversion of androstenedione in peripheral tissues. Estriol (16-hydroxyestradiol), the most abundant estrogen in urine, arises from the 16-hydroxylation of estrone and estradiol. Catechol estrogens are formed by hydroxylation of estrogens at the C-2 or C-4 position and may act as the intracellular mediators of some estrogen action. Estrogens promote development of the secondary sexual characteristics in women and cause uterine growth, thickening of the vaginal mucosa, thinning of the cervical mucus, and development of the ductular system of the breasts. The mechanism of estrogen action in target tissues is similar to that for other steroid hormones and involves the binding to a nuclear steroid receptor and enhancement of the transcription of messenger RNA, which in turn causes increased protein synthesis in the cell cytoplasm (see Chap. 329).

Progesterone   Progesterone, a 21-carbon steroid (see Fig. 340-3), is the principal hormone secreted by the corpus luteum and is responsible for progestational effects, namely, induction of secretory activity in the endometrium of the estrogen-primed uterus in preparation for implantation of the fertilized egg. Progesterone also induces a decidual reaction in endometrium. Other effects include inhibition of uterine contractions, increased viscosity of cervical mucus, glandular development of the breasts, and increase in basal body temperature (thermogenic effect).

Androgens   The ovary synthesizes a variety of 19-carbon steroids, including dehydroepiandrosterone, androstenedione, testosterone, and dihydrotestosterone, principally in stromal and thecal cells. The major ovarian 19-carbon steroid is androstenedione (see Fig. 340-3), part of which is secreted into plasma and the remainder of which is converted to estrogen in granulosa cells or to testosterone in the interstitium. In peripheral tissues, androstenedione also can be converted to testosterone and to estrogens. Only testosterone and dihydrotestosterone are true androgens that interact with the androgen receptor and induce virilizing signs in women (see Chaps. 49 and 339).

OTHER HORMONES   Other ovarian hormones play an uncertain role in human physiology. *Relaxin*, a polypeptide hormone produced by the human corpus luteum as well as by the decidua, causes softening of the cervix and loosening of the symphysis pubis in preparation for parturition in animals. *Oxytocin, vasopressin*, and other hypothalamic and pituitary hormones are also present in granulosa and/or luteal cells, but their function in these cells is unknown. *Follicular inhibin* or *folliculostatin* (the equivalent of testicular inhibin) is secreted by the follicle and is believed to inhibit the release of FSH by the hypothalamic-pituitary unit. *Activin* is also secreted by the follicle and may enhance FSH secretion. *Follicle regulatory protein* (FRP) of human follicular fluid inhibits granulosa secretion and growth. *Gonadocrinins*, peptides purified from rat follicular fluid, stimulate the release of both FSH and LH from the pituitary in vitro and in vivo. Granulosa cells secrete *oocyte maturation inhibitor* (OMI), a factor that prevents premature ovulation. In addition, in the gonads of both sexes a *meiosis-inducing substance* (MIS) triggers the onset of meiosis, an event that occurs earlier in ovarian than in testicular development. A variety of growth factors produced locally (including IGF1, IGF2, TGFα, and TGFβ) influence steroid secretion by the ovary.

The normal menstrual cycle   The menstrual cycle is usually divided into a follicular or proliferative phase and a luteal or secretory phase (Fig. 340-5). The secretion of FSH and LH is fundamentally under negative feedback control by ovarian steroids (particularly estradiol) and probably by inhibin, but the response of gonadotropins

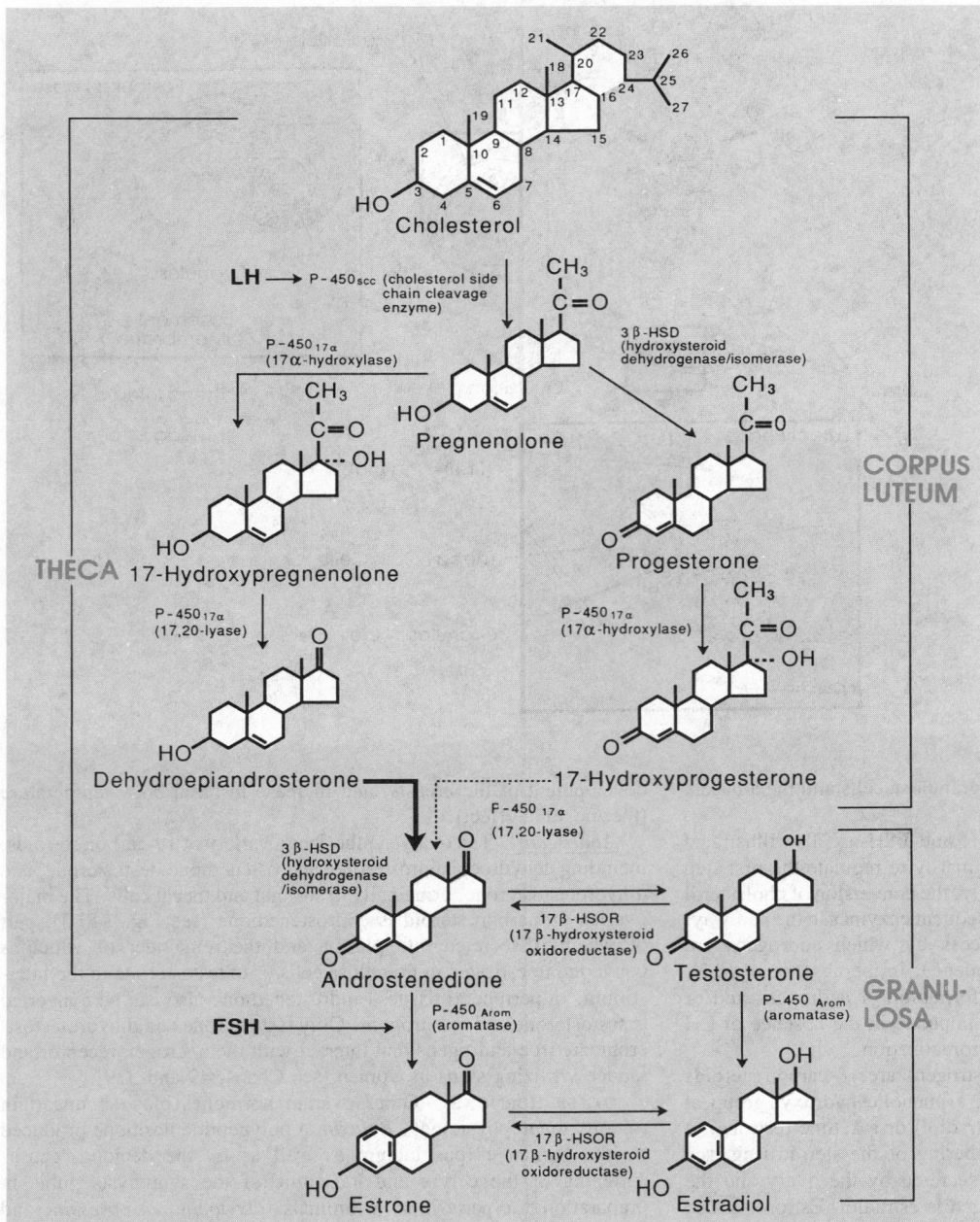

FIGURE 340-3 The principal pathway of steroid hormone biosynthesis in the ovary. Although every ovarian cell probably contains the complete enzyme complement required for the formation of estradiol from cholesterol, the amounts of the various enzymes and consequently the predominant hormones formed differ among the various cell types. The major enzyme complements for the corpus luteum, stroma, and granulosa cells are shown by the brackets; as a consequence these cells produce predominantly progesterone and 17-OH progesterone, androgen, and estrogen, respectively. The major sites of action of LH and FSH in mediating this pathway are shown in the horizontal arrows. The dotted line emphasizes that the metabolism of 17-hydroxyprogesterone is limited in the human ovary. (*From BR Carr, in JD Wilson and DW Foster, eds,* Williams' Textbook of Endocrinology, *8th ed, Philadelphia, Saunders, 1992.*)

to different levels of estradiol varies. FSH secretion is inhibited progressively as estrogen levels increase—typical negative feedback. In contrast, LH secretion is suppressed maximally by estrogen in low amounts and is enhanced in response to a rising and sustained elevation of estradiol—so-called positive feedback control. Negative feedback of estrogen involves both the hypothalamus and pituitary, whereas positive feedback operates primarily at the level of the pituitary.

The length of the normal menstrual cycle is defined as the time from the onset of one menstrual bleeding episode to onset of the next. In women of reproductive age, the menstrual cycle averages 28 ± 3 days, and the mean duration of flow is 4 ± 2 days. Longer menstrual cycles (usually characterized by anovulation) occur at menarche and prior to menopause. At the end of one menstrual cycle and in the face of a waning corpus luteum, plasma levels of estrogen and progesterone fall, and circulating levels of FSH increase concomitantly. Under the influence of increasing levels of FSH, follicular

recruitment is initiated to effect development of the follicle that will be dominant during the next cycle.

After the onset of menses, follicular development continues, but FSH levels decrease. Approximately 8 to 10 days prior to the midcycle LH surge, plasma estradiol levels begin to rise as the result of secretion of estradiol by the granulosa cells of the enlarging dominant follicle. During the second half of the follicular phase, LH levels also begin to rise (positive feedback). Just prior to ovulation, estradiol secretion reaches a peak and then falls. Immediately thereafter, a further rise in the plasma level of LH mediates the final maturation of the follicle, followed by follicular rupture and ovulation 16 to 23 h after the LH peak. Concomitant with the rise in LH is a smaller increase in the level of plasma FSH, the physiologic significance of which is unclear. Plasma progesterone also begins to rise just prior to midcycle and facilitates the positive feedback action of estradiol on LH secretion.

At the onset of the luteal phase, plasma gonadotropins decrease

Follicular Phase

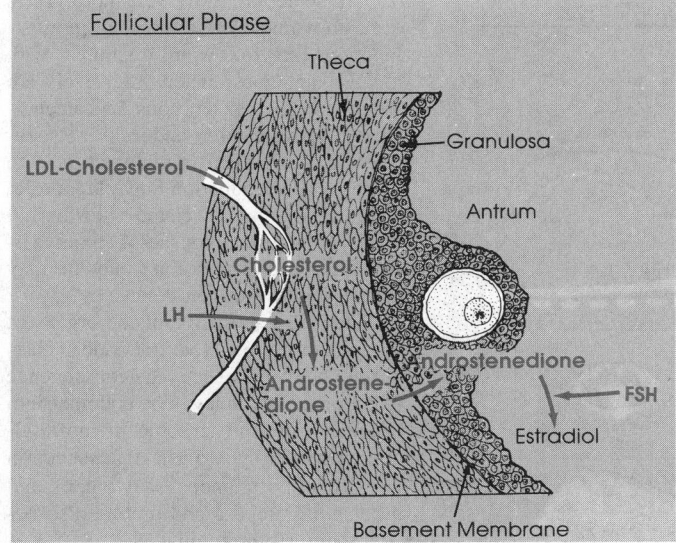

Luteal Phase

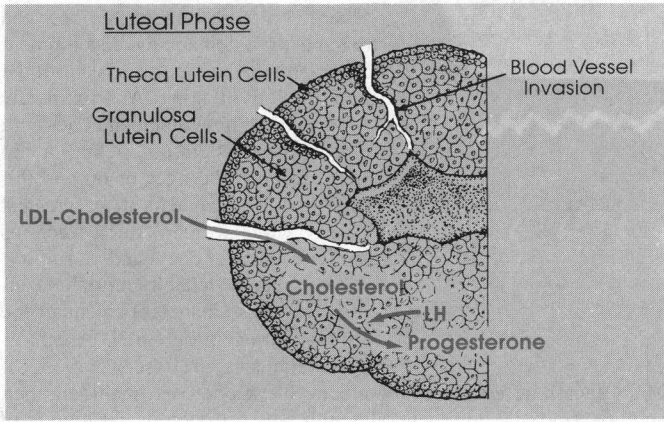

FIGURE 340-4 Cellular interactions in the ovary during the follicular phase (top) and luteal phase (bottom); LDL (low-density lipoprotein), FSH (follicle-stimulating hormone), and LH (luteinizing hormone). (*From BR Carr et al, 1982.*)

and plasma progesterone increases. A secondary rise in estrogens causes further gonadotropin suppression. Near the end of the luteal phase, progesterone and estrogen levels fall, and FSH levels begin to rise to initiate the development of the next follicle (usually in the contralateral ovary) and the next menstrual cycle.

The endometrium lining the uterine cavity undergoes marked alterations in response to the changing plasma levels of ovarian hormones (see Fig. 340-5). Concomitant with the decrease in plasma estrogen and progesterone and the decline of corpus luteum function in the late luteal phase, intense vasospasm occurs in the spiral arterioles supplying blood to the endometrium, followed by an ischemic necrosis, endometrial desquamation, and bleeding. This vasospasm is caused by locally synthesized prostaglandins. The onset of bleeding marks the first day of the menstrual cycle. By the fourth to fifth day of the cycle, the endometrium is thin. During the proliferative phase glandular growth of the endometrium is mediated by estrogen. After ovulation, increased progesterone leads to further thickening of the endometrium, but the rapid growth slows. The endometrium then enters the secretory phase characterized by tortuosity of the glands, curling of the spiral arterioles, and glandular secretion. As corpus luteum function begins to wane in the absence of conception, the sequence of events leading to menstruation is again set into action.

Biphasic changes in basal body temperature are characteristic of the ovulatory cycle and are mediated by alterations in progesterone

levels (see Fig. 340-5). An increase in basal body temperature of 0.3 to 0.5°C begins after ovulation, persists during the luteal phase, and returns to the normal baseline (36.2 to 36.4°C) after the onset of the subsequent menses (see Chap. 16).

Cellular interactions in the ovary during the normal cycle LH stimulates thecal cells surrounding the follicle to form androgens, and androstenedione diffuses across the basement membrane of the follicle into granulosa cells, where it is aromatized to estrogen (see Figs. 340-3 and 340-4).

The increase of FSH late in the preceding menstrual cycle stimulates growth and recruitment of the primary follicles by enhancing granulosa cell proliferation, resulting ultimately in the formation of the dominant follicle. In the granulosa cells, FSH also stimulates activity and the amount of aromatase that converts androstenedione to estrogen. Enhanced secretion of estradiol causes an increase in the number of estradiol receptors and further proliferation of granulosa cells. In the late follicular phase, FSH, in concert with estradiol, causes induction of LH receptors on the granulosa cells. LH acts via these receptors to increase progesterone secretion at midcycle. The amount of progesterone formed by the follicle is believed to be limited by the availability of LDL-cholesterol to serve as substrate for steroidogenesis and by the fact that most of the progesterone formed is converted to androstenedione by thecal cells. Prior to ovulation, the granulosa cells of the follicle are bathed in follicular fluid but have limited access to circulating blood and consequently to plasma LDL. As depicted in Fig. 340-4, the granulosa cells become vascularized after ovulation, and plasma LDL-cholesterol is made available to serve as the major substrate for progesterone synthesis by the corpus luteum. Thus increased progesterone synthesis by the corpus luteum is the consequence of increased substrate availability. The peak in progesterone secretion by the corpus luteum is attained 8 days after ovulation at the time of maximal vascularization of the granulosa cells.

MENOPAUSE The *menopause* is defined as the final episode of menstrual bleeding in women. However, the term is used commonly to refer to the period of the female climacteric that encompasses the transitional period between the reproductive years up to and beyond the last episode of menstrual bleeding. During this period, there is a gradual but progressive loss of ovarian function and a variety of endocrine, somatic, and psychological changes.

The median age of women at the time of cessation of menstrual bleeding is 50 to 51 years. Since the life expectancy in women is close to 80 years, approximately one-third of life occurs after cessation of reproductive function. Preceding the menopause, the pattern of menstrual cycles is variable, but the interval between menses usually becomes longer. In addition, there is an increase in the mean levels of plasma FSH and LH, despite the continuation of ovulatory cycles. Thus, the ovary appears to become less responsive to gonadotropins prior to the menopause.

The menopause is the consequence of the exhaustion of ovarian follicles. The decrease in the number of ova begins in intrauterine life; by the time of the menopause, few ova remain, and these appear to be nonfunctional. Only a small number of ova are lost as the result of ovulation during reproductive life, the majority of follicles and associated ova being lost by atresia. The cessation of follicular development results in a drop in the production of estradiol and other hormones, which, in turn, causes a loss of negative feedback on the hypothalamic-pituitary centers. In turn, the levels of plasma gonadotropins increase, with FSH levels rising earlier and to a greater extent than those of LH (Figs. 340-1 and 340-6). The higher concentration of FSH than LH in postmenopausal women may result from the decrease in inhibin secretion by the ovary, from the fact that FSH is cleared from plasma less rapidly than LH, and possibly from the loss of positive feedback on LH production by estradiol. Intravenous administration of LHRH to menopausal women results in a pronounced increase in the secretion of both FSH and LH, consistent with the enhanced hypothalamic-pituitary secretory activity in other forms of primary ovarian failure.

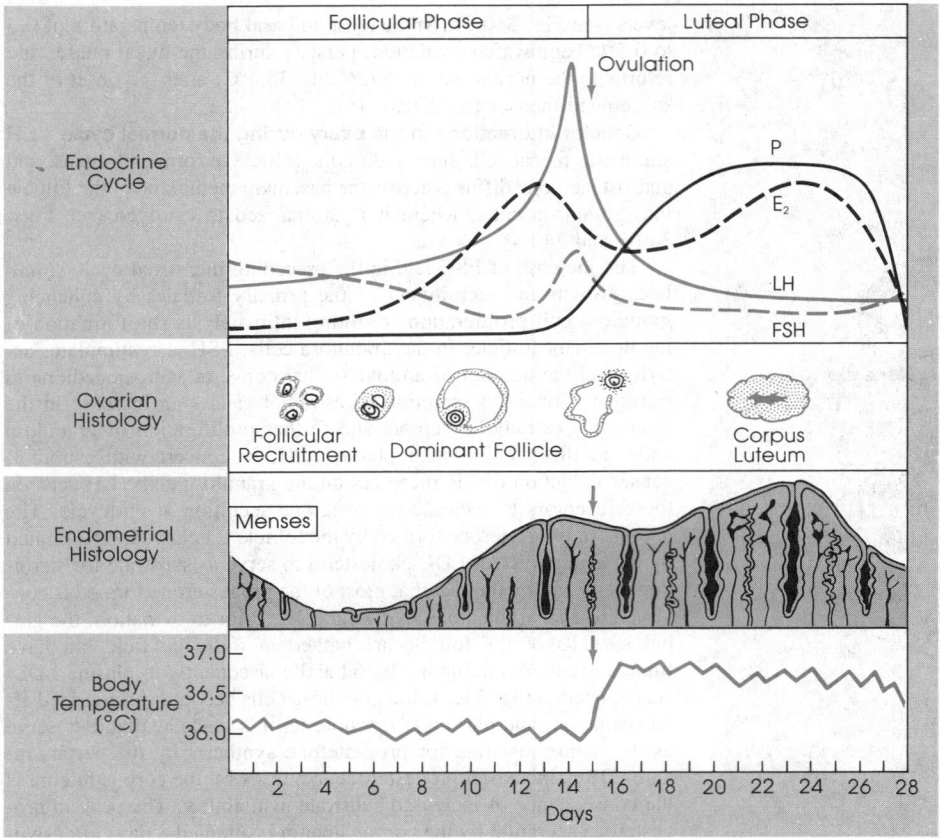

FIGURE 340-5   The hormonal, ovarian, endometrial, and basal body temperature changes and relationship throughout the normal menstrual cycle.

The ovaries of postmenopausal women are small, and the residual cells are predominantly stromal in type. Estrogen and androgen levels in plasma are reduced but not absent (see Fig. 340-6). Prior to the menopause, plasma androstenedione is derived almost equally from the adrenals and the ovaries; after menopause, the ovarian contribution ceases so that the plasma levels of androstenedione fall by 50 percent (see Fig. 340-6). However, the menopausal ovary continues to secrete testosterone, presumably formed in stromal cells.

Circulating estrogens in the ovulating woman are derived from two sources. Sixty percent of mean estrogen formation during the menstrual cycle is in the form of estradiol formed primarily by ovaries, and the remainder is estrone formed mainly in extraglandular tissues from androstenedione. After menopause, extraglandular estrogen formation is the major pathway for estrogen synthesis. Estrogen production by the menopausal ovary is minimal, and subsequent oophorectomy is not followed by any further decrease in estrogen levels. Plasma levels of estradiol, the principal estrogen secreted by the follicle, are lower in postmenopausal women than levels of estrone. The rate of peripheral formation of estrone increases somewhat in menopausal women so that estrone production is usually only slightly less than prior to the menopause despite the fall in plasma androstenedione. Because a major site of extraglandular estrogen production is adipose tissue, peripheral estrogen formation may actually be enhanced in obese postmenopausal women, so total estrogen production rates may be as great or greater than in premenopausal women. The predominant estrogen formed is estrone rather than estradiol.

The most common menopausal symptoms are those of vasomotor instability (hot flash), atrophy of the urogenital epithelium and skin, decreased size of the breasts, and osteoporosis. Approximately 40 percent of women in the postmenopausal period develop symptoms serious enough to seek medical assistance.

The pathogenesis of the hot flash is uncertain. There is a close temporal relationship between the onset of the hot flash and pulses of LH secretion; however, hot flashes occur in women with absence of pituitary function and following treatment with LHRH analogues, where LH levels are absent or low. Alterations in catecholamine, prostaglandin, endorphin, or neurotensin metabolism in conjunction with low estrogen production may play a role. Other symptoms associated with the hot flash, including nervousness, anxiety, irritability, and depression, may or may not be due to estrogen deficiency.

The decrease in size of the organs of the female reproductive tract and breasts during the menopause is the consequence of estrogen deficiency. The endometrium becomes thin and atrophic in most (although cystic hyperplasia may occur in one-fifth of postmenopausal women), and the vaginal mucosa and urethra also become thin and atrophic.

There is a close relationship between estrogen deprivation and the development of osteoporosis. Osteoporosis is one of the dread afflictions of aging. Approximately one-fourth of aging women and one-tenth of elderly men sustain a vertebral or hip fracture between the ages of 60 and 90, and the incidence appears to be greatest in elderly white women. Such fractures are a major cause of death and morbidity, and the fracture-related mortality increases from less than 10 percent in the 60- to 64-year age group to 30 percent or more in patients over 80 (see Chap. 358). Many factors affect the development of osteoporosis, including diet, activity, smoking, and general health, and estrogen deprivation is of particular importance in this regard. White postmenopausal women are more predisposed to osteoporosis and its consequences because bone density in such subjects is lower prior to menopause, so loss in bone density has more severe consequences in the group. Further evidence that osteoporosis is a disease of estrogen deprivation is suggested by early development of osteoporosis in women with premature menopause due either to natural causes or surgical castration.

FIGURE 340-6   Differences in hormone concentration in women during the reproductive years and in women during the menopause. FSH (follicle-stimulating hormone), LH (luteinizing hormone), E_2 (estradiol-17β), E_1 (estrone), Δ^4-A (androstenedione), T (testosterone). (*From SSC Yen and RB Jaffe, 1986, and from DR Mishell, Jr, and V Davajan.*)

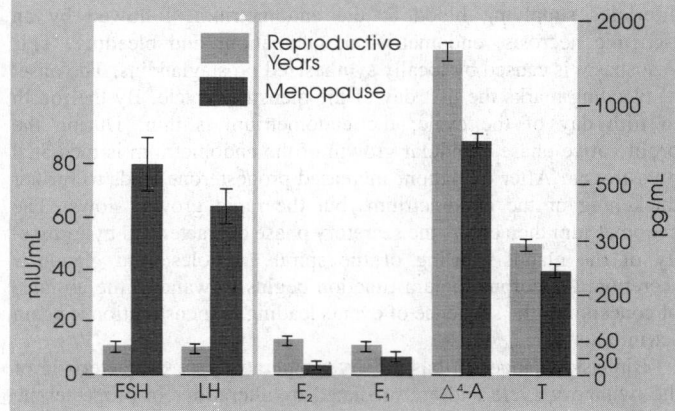

LABORATORY AND CLINICAL ASSESSMENT OF HORMONAL STATUS

The hormonal status of women can usually be assessed by obtaining a thorough history and physical examination. In general, the presence of secondary sexual characteristics such as normal female breast development indicates adequate estrogen secretion in the past, and the presence of regular, predictable, cyclic menses implies that ovulation and the production of gonadotropins, estrogen, progesterone, and androgens are adequate and that the outflow tract is intact. Such a history may be more valuable than laboratory tests in evaluating ovarian hormone status. However, laboratory tests provide valuable ancillary information in the workup of women with endocrine dysfunction or infertility.

PITUITARY GONADOTROPINS Plasma gonadotropins are assessed by radioimmunoassay (RIA), fluoroimmunoassay (FIA), or enzyme-linked immunosorbent assay (ELISA). Because both FSH and LH are secreted in pulsatile manner, the results obtained from a single serum sample may be difficult to interpret. Consequently, multiple samples at 20-min intervals for 2 h may be pooled to obtain a mean value. Serum gonadotropin measurements are of most use in evaluating women with suspected ovarian failure and in supporting the diagnosis of polycystic ovarian disease and hypogonadotropic hypogonadism. The normal ranges for serum LH and FSH in ovulating women are 5 to 25 and 5 to 30 IU/L, respectively. A persistent FSH above 40 IU/L is diagnostic of ovarian failure, and an LH value of less than 5 IU/L suggests hypogonadotropic hypogonadism. In practice, however, gonadotropin values may be equivocal and must be interpreted in light of the remainder of the findings.

OVARIAN HORMONES The mean plasma levels and production rates of the principal ovarian hormones are presented in Table 340-1. The production rate of a hormone is the sum of the amount of hormone produced by direct glandular secretion and by extraglandular conversion of prohormones.

Estrogen Normal secondary sexual characteristics imply that estrogen production was adequate in the past. The current estrogen status can be estimated by pelvic examination. The presence of a moist, rugated vagina with copious, clear, thin cervical mucus that can be stretched and that exhibits arborization or ferning when spread on a slide is strong evidence of adequate estrogen production. Cytologic demonstration of mature vaginal epithelial cells and abundant cornified squamous epithelial cells with pyknotic nuclei confirms the presence of adequate estrogen levels.

The progesterone-withdrawal test provides a functional assessment of estrogen status. If menses appear within a week to 10 days after the end of a trial of medroxyprogesterone acetate (10 mg by mouth once or twice a day for 5 days) or after a single intramuscular injection of progesterone (100 mg), then prior estrogen priming was adequate to allow withdrawal bleeding.

Due to its variable level in plasma during the normal cycle and the difficulty of estimating the day of the cycle in women with abnormal cycles, the determination of estrogen levels in plasma or urine by RIA, FIA, or ELISA is of little use in the routine assessment of estrogen status. Plasma estradiol is measured during attempts to induce ovulation with human menopausal gonadotropins to prevent the development of the ovarian hyperstimulation syndrome and is utilized along with ultrasound assessment to monitor follicular growth in women who are to undergo in vitro fertilization.

Progesterone Cyclic, predictable menses also imply that adequate progesterone is secreted during the luteal phase of the menstrual cycle. The indications for specific assay of progesterone are to document ovulation or evaluate the adequacy of the luteal phase in the evaluation of infertile women and to separate subjects with müllerian agenesis from those with the testicular feminization syndrome. Several functional assays of progesterone secretion can be utilized. The least expensive and most useful is the daily measurement of basal body temperature throughout a cycle. Due to the thermogenic properties of progesterone, documentation of the monthly biphasic curve with an elevated temperature for approximately 2 weeks after ovulation is a valid indication of progesterone secretion during the luteal phase (see Fig. 340-5). Presence of viscous cervical mucus that does not stretch or fern and of predominant intermediate cells on vaginal cytology or demonstration of a secretory epithelium in an endometrial biopsy during the luteal phase on days 20 to 22 of the cycle provides additional evidence of progesterone secretion. In addition, measurement of serum progesterone by RIA, FIA, or ELISA can be used to estimate progesterone secretion by the corpus luteum.

Androgen Under normal conditions, the ovary secretes androstenedione, testosterone, and dehydroepiandrosterone. In conditions of androgen excess, hirsutism and/or virilization are common. The evaluation of androgen excess is discussed in Chap. 49.

DIAGNOSIS OF PREGNANCY Pregnancy is usually suspected and diagnosed on the basis of the history and physical examination. That is, a woman with previous cyclic, predictable menses develops amenorrhea accompanied by breast tenderness, malaise, lassitude, and nausea, and on physical examination the uterus is soft and enlarged.

Laboratory assays of placental products excreted in urine facilitate the diagnosis of pregnancy. Human chorionic gonadotropin (hCG) is secreted by the trophoblastic cells of the placenta into the maternal plasma and excreted in the urine. Assays of urinary hCG make it feasible to detect the presence of functioning trophoblasts earlier than can be recognized by clinical assessments. Assays for measurement of hCG content of serum or urine utilize either antibody against hCG or receptor for hCG. With appropriate assays, it is possible to detect pregnancies 8 to 10 days after ovulation and before the first missed menstrual period. Assay of the β subunit of hCG in serum or urine makes it possible to differentiate between excess LH and hCG, an important distinction in evaluating women with trophoblastic disease such as hydatidiform mole or choriocarcinoma.

DISORDERS OF OVARIAN FUNCTION

PREPUBERTAL YEARS Puberty is said to be precocious if the onset of breast budding occurs before age 8 or if menarche commences before age 9. Those disorders in which the developing sexual characteristics are appropriate for the genetic and gonadal sex, i.e., feminization in girls or virilization in boys, are termed *isosexual precocity*, whereas *heterosexual precocity* occurs when sexual characteristics are not in accord with the genetic sex, namely, virilization in girls or feminization in boys. Pubertal disorders of boys are described in Chap. 339.

TABLE 340-1 Concentrations, metabolic clearance rates, and production rates of the major ovarian steroid hormones in blood of ovulatory women

Steroid	Binding	Phase of menstrual cycle	Plasma concentration nmol/L (ng/ml)	Production rate, μmol/d (mg/d)
Estradiol	TeBG and albumin	Follicular	0.07–2.6 (0.02–0.7)	0.3–3.6 (0.08–1.0)
		Luteal	0.7 (0.2)	0.9 (0.25)
Estrone	Albumin	Follicular	0.2–1.1 (0.05–0.3)	0.4–2.6 (0.1–0.7)
		Luteal	0.4 (0.1)	0.9 (0.24)
Progesterone	CBG and albumin	Follicular	3 (1)	6.4 (2)
		Luteal	16–80 (5–25)	80 (25)
Androstenedione	Albumin	—	5.6 (1.6)	10 (3)
Testosterone	TeBG and albumin	—	1.4 (0.4)	0.9 (0.25)

NOTE: TeBG, testosterone-binding globulin; CBG, cortisol-binding globulin; MCR, metabolic clearance rate.
SOURCE: Derived in part from MB Lipsett, in *Reproductive Endocrinology*, SSC Yen, RB Jaffe (eds). Philadelphia, Saunders, 1986.

TABLE 340-2 Differential diagnosis of sexual precocity

Isosexual precocity
  A True precocious puberty
    1 Constitutional
    2 Organic brain disease
    3 Congenital adrenal hyperplasia
  B Precocious pseudopuberty
    1 Ovarian tumors
    2 Adrenal tumors
    3 McCune-Albright syndrome
    4 Hypothyroidism
    5 Russell-Silver syndrome
    6 Estrogen-containing medications
  C Incomplete sexual precocity
    1 Premature thelarche
    2 Premature adrenarche
    3 Premature pubarche
Heterosexual precocity
  A Ovarian tumors
  B Adrenal tumors
  C Congenital adrenal hyperplasia

Isosexual precocious puberty   Isosexual precocious puberty in girls can be divided into three major categories (Table 340-2).

TRUE PRECOCIOUS PUBERTY   True precocious puberty is characterized by an early but otherwise normal sequence of pubertal development, including increased secretion of gonadotropins and ovulatory menstrual cycles. Constitutional or idiopathic precocious puberty comprises 90 percent of cases. In these individuals, no cause for the premature maturation of the central nervous system–hypothalamic-pituitary axis can be identified, and the diagnosis is one of exclusion. As many as half these individuals have abnormal electroencephalograms. Premature appearance of secondary sexual characteristics and of ovulatory cycles with the accompanying risk of fertility may result in significant emotional disturbances. Therefore, prompt initiation of therapy is imperative. LHRH analogues inhibit estrogen synthesis and thus inhibit precocious puberty, and they may prevent premature closure of the epiphyses and the resultant short stature.

About 10 percent of cases are due to organic brain diseases, including brain tumors (hypothalamic gliomas, astrocytomas, ependymomas, germinomas, and hamartomas), encephalitis, meningitis, hydrocephalus, head injury, tuberous sclerosis, and neurofibromatosis. It is essential to separate this group of patients from those with the idiopathic disorder, and patients designated as idiopathic occasionally prove to have such tumors. Fortunately, most patients with organic lesions serious enough to cause precocious puberty have obvious neurologic signs and symptoms. Evaluation of all patients with precocious puberty should include, at a minimum, skull films and computed tomographic (CT) scans or magnetic resonance imaging (MRI) of the brain. The success of treatment depends on the nature of the lesion, but surgical and radiation treatment of well-localized tumors is occasionally successful.

A rare cause of isosexual precocity is virilizing congenital adrenal hyperplasia due to 21-hydroxylase deficiency in girls in whom treatment is delayed until 4 to 8 years of age. After initiation of glucocorticoid replacement, such individuals may undergo true isosexual precocious puberty (see Chap. 335).

PRECOCIOUS PSEUDOPUBERTY   Precocious pseudopuberty occurs when girls feminize as a consequence of enhanced estrogen formation but do not ovulate or develop cyclic menses. Ovarian cysts or tumors that secrete estrogen (granulosa-theca cell tumors) are the most frequent cause of precocious pseudopuberty. Granulosa-theca cell tumors associated with intestinal polyps and pigmentation of the mucous membranes occur in the Peutz-Jeghers syndrome. Other ovarian tumors that secrete estrogens (or androgens that can be converted to estrogens at extraglandular sites) include dysgerminomas, teratomas, cystadenomas, and ovarian carcinomas (also see Chap. 321). Ovarian tumors usually can be detected by rectoabdominal examination, and sonography, CT scans, MRI, and/or laparoscopy also may be of help. Ovarian teratomas and choriocarcinomas and

other carcinomas that secrete hCG do not cause precocious puberty in girls unless there is concomitant secretion of estrogen by the tumor (hCG or LH in the absence of FSH does not induce ovarian estrogen production). Rarely, feminizing tumors of the adrenal cause isosexual precocious puberty, either by formation of estrogens directly or by secretion of weak androgens to serve as estrogenic precursors in extraglandular tissues.

Other causes of precocious pseudopuberty include the following: (1) The McCune-Albright syndrome (polyostotic fibrous dysplasia), characterized by café au lait spots, cystic fibrous dysplasia of bones, and sexual precocity. Some of these individuals have increased gonadotropin secretion, whereas others have functional ovarian cysts in the presence of low gonadotropins, which represents a form of gonadotropin-independent sexual precocity. Occasionally, this disorder leads to true precocious puberty (see Chap. 343). (2) Primary hypothyroidism in which secretion of thyrotropin-releasing hormone (TRH) as well as secretion of other hypothalamic hormones is enhanced, leading to increased FSH levels and ovarian estrogen secretion, frequently with galactorrhea. (3) The Russell-Silver syndrome, or congenital asymmetry associated with short stature and precocious feminization. (4) Estrogen-containing medications, including use of estrogen-containing creams for diaper rash or the ingestion of meat from estrogen-treated animals or poultry or any estrogen by mouth.

INCOMPLETE ISOSEXUAL PRECOCITY   This term is used to describe the premature development of a single pubertal event and encompasses several entities. The appearance of breast budding prior to the age of 8 (premature thelarche) without other evidence of estrogen secretion and without premature bone maturation is believed to be due to a transient increase in estrogen secretion or a temporary increase in sensitivity to the small amounts of circulating estrogens formed prior to puberty. Usually, the disorder is self-limited and resolves spontaneously. Occasionally, axillary hair and/or pubic hair (so-called *premature adrenarche* and *pubarche*) appear without any other secondary sexual development. The phenomenon is associated with adrenal androgen secretion in the range of normal puberty and can be distinguished from syndromes of virilization by the absence of clitoromegaly. It requires no treatment, and patients enter puberty at about the average time.

Heterosexual precocity   Virilization in a prepubertal female is usually due to congenital adrenal hyperplasia or to androgen secretion by an ovarian or adrenal tumor. The manifestations of virilization are described in Chap. 49. Virilization in girls with congenital adrenal hyperplasia usually takes place in a background of variable sexual ambiguity (see Chap. 342).

Evaluation of sexual precocity   The evaluation of sexual precocity involves a careful history and physical examination, including rectoabdominal examination, abdominal sonography, determination of bone age, and measurement of thyroid hormones, TSH, and gonadotropins (and androgen or estrogen levels when appropriate). Skull films and further diagnostic tests are indicated if a neurologic disorder is suspected and no evidence of ovarian or adrenal tumor is found.

REPRODUCTIVE YEARS Disorders of the menstrual cycle
ABNORMAL UTERINE BLEEDING   Between menarche and the menopause, almost every woman experiences one or more episodes of abnormal uterine bleeding, here defined as any bleeding pattern that differs in frequency, duration, or amount from the pattern observed during a normal menstrual cycle. A variety of descriptive terms (such as *menorrhagia*, *metrorrhagia*, and *menometrorrhagia*) have been used to characterize patterns of abnormal uterine bleeding. A more logical approach is to divide abnormal uterine bleeding into those patterns associated with ovulatory cycles and those associated with anovulatory cycles.

OVULATORY CYCLES   Normal menstrual bleeding with ovulatory cycles is spontaneous, regular, cyclic, and predictable and frequently associated with discomfort (dysmenorrhea). Deviations from this pattern associated with cycles that are still regular and predictable are most often due to organic disease of the outflow tract. For example, regular but prolonged and excessive bleeding episodes unassociated with bleeding dyscrasias (hypermenorrhea or menorrhagia) can result from abnormalities of the uterus such as submucous leiomyomas, adenomyosis, or endometrial polyps. Regular, cyclic, predictable menstruation characterized by spotting or light bleeding is termed *hypomenorrhea* and is due to obstruction of the outflow tract as from intrauterine synechiae or scarring of the cervix. Intermenstrual bleeding between episodes of regular, ovulatory menstruation is also often due to cervical or endometrial lesions. An exception to the association between organic disease of the uterus and abnormal uterine bleeding is the occurrence of episodes of regular bleeding more frequently than 21 days apart (polymenorrhea). These cycles may be a normal variant.

ANOVULATORY CYCLES Uterine bleeding that is unpredictable with respect to amount, onset, and duration and is usually painless is described as *dysfunctional uterine bleeding*. This disorder is not due to abnormalities of the uterus but rather to chronic anovulation and occurs when there is interruption of the normal progressive sequence of follicular and luteal phases under the influence of a dominant follicle and its resulting corpus luteum. As discussed above, normal uterine bleeding in ovulatory cycles is due to progesterone withdrawal and requires that the endometrium first be primed with estrogen (when castrates or postmenopausal women are given progesterone, withdrawal bleeding usually does not occur).

Dysfunctional uterine bleeding can occur in women who have a transient disruption of the synchronous hypothalamic-pituitary-ovarian patterns necessary for regular ovulatory cycles, most often at the extremes of the reproductive life, namely, in the early menarche and in the perimenopausal period, but also as the secondary consequence of temporary stresses or intercurrent illnesses.

On the other hand, primary *dysfunctional uterine bleeding* can result from at least three pathophysiologic mechanisms.

1 *Estrogen withdrawal bleeding* occurs when estrogen is given to a castrate or postmenopausal woman and then withdrawn. As in other types of dysfunctional uterine bleeding, this form of menstrual bleeding is usually painless.
2 *Estrogen breakthrough bleeding* occurs when there is prolonged continuous estrogen stimulation of the endometrium not interrupted by cyclic progesterone secretion and withdrawal. This is the most common type of dysfunctional uterine bleeding and is usually due to anovulation associated with chronic acyclic estrogen production as in women with polycystic ovarian disease. Such women may have histories of irregular, unpredictable menses, oligomenorrhea, or amenorrhea (see below). Alternatively, estrogen breakthrough bleeding can occur in hypogonadal women given estrogens chronically rather than intermittently or in women with estrogen-secreting tumors of the ovary. Estrogen breakthrough bleeding may be profuse and is unpredictable with respect to duration, amount of flow, and time of occurrence. The endometrium is typically thin because its repair between episodes of bleeding is incomplete.
3 *Progesterone breakthrough bleeding* occurs in the presence of abnormally high ratios of progesterone to estrogen, e.g., in women on continuous low-dose oral contraceptives.

The approach to a patient with dysfunctional uterine bleeding begins with a careful history of menstrual patterns and prior hormonal therapy. Since not all bleeding from the urogenital tract is from the uterus, rectal, bladder, and vaginal or cervical sources must be excluded by physical examination. If the bleeding is from the uterus, a pregnancy-related disorder such as abortion or ectopic pregnancy also must be excluded. Once the diagnosis of dysfunctional uterine bleeding is established, a rational approach to management is as follows: During a first episode of dysfunctional bleeding the patient can simply be observed, provided the bleeding is not copious and no evidence of bleeding dyscrasia is present. If bleeding is moderately severe, control can be achieved with relatively high dose estrogen oral contraceptives for 3 weeks. Alternatively, a regimen of three or

four low-dose oral contraceptive pills per day for 1 week followed by tapering to the usual dosage for up to 3 weeks is also effective. If uterine bleeding is more severe, hospitalization, bed rest, and intramuscular injections of estradiol valerate (10 mg) and hydroxyprogesterone caproate (500 mg) or intravenous or intramuscular conjugated estrogens (25 mg) usually control the bleeding. After initial treatment, iron replacement should be instituted, and recurrence can be prevented by cyclic oral contraceptives for 2 to 3 months (or more if pregnancy is not desired). Alternatively, menses should be induced every 2 to 3 months with medroxyprogesterone acetate, 10 mg by mouth once or twice a day for 10 days. If hormone therapy fails to control uterine bleeding, an endometrial biopsy, hysteroscopy, or dilatation and curettage may be required for diagnosis and therapy. Indeed, uterine sampling may be indicated prior to hormone therapy in women at risk for endometrial cancer (i.e., in women approaching the age of menopause or in the massively obese); endometrial cancer is rare in ovulatory women of reproductive age.

AMENORRHEA An acceptable definition of amenorrhea is failure of menarche by age 16, irrespective of the presence or absence of secondary sexual characteristics, or the absence of menstruation for 6 months in a woman with previous periodic menses. However, women who do not fulfill these criteria should be evaluated if (1) the subject and/or her family are greatly concerned, (2) no breast development has occurred by age 14, or (3) any sexual ambiguity or virilization is present (Chap. 342). Amenorrhea is usually categorized as either primary (in a woman who has never menstruated) or secondary (in a woman in whom menstruation is present for a variable time and then ceases); some disorders can cause either primary or secondary amenorrhea. For example, most women with gonadal dysgenesis have primary amenorrhea, but some have some follicles and ovulate for short periods so that pregnancies may rarely occur. Furthermore, patients with chronic anovulation (polycystic ovarian disease) most often have secondary amenorrhea but may present with primary amenorrhea. For these reasons, categorization of amenorrhea into primary and secondary types is less helpful in the differential diagnosis than a classification based on the major underlying physiologic derangements: (1) anatomic defects, (2) ovarian failure, and (3) chronic anovulation with or without estrogen present.

Anatomic defects A variety of anatomic or structural defects of the female genital tract can preclude menstrual bleeding. Starting from the caudal end of the female genital tract, labial agglutination or fusion is often associated with disorders of sexual development, particularly female pseudohermaphroditism (congenital adrenal hyperplasia or exposure to maternal androgens in utero) (see Chap. 342). Congenital defects of the vagina, imperforate hymen, and transverse vaginal septae also can cause amenorrhea. These women frequently have accumulation of menstrual blood behind the obstruction and may have cyclic, predictable episodes of abdominal pain.

More severe müllerian anomalies include müllerian agenesis (the Mayer-Rokitansky-Küster-Hauser syndrome; see Chap. 342), second in frequency only to gonadal dysgenesis as a cause of primary amenorrhea. Women with this syndrome have a 46,XX karyotype, female secondary sex characteristics, and normal ovarian function, including cyclic ovulation, but have absence or severe hypoplasia of the vagina. The uterus usually consists of only rudimentary bicornuate cords, but if the uterus contains endometrium, cyclic abdominal pain and accumulation of blood may occur as in other forms of outlet obstruction. One-third of patients have abnormalities of the urogenital tract, and one-tenth have skeletal anomalies, usually involving the spine. The major diagnostic problem is separating müllerian agenesis from complete testicular feminization, in which 46,XY genetic males with testes differentiate as phenotypic women with a blind vaginal pouch and an absent uterus. Women with testicular feminization have feminized breasts but a paucity of pubic and axillary hair. The disorder is due to a defect in the androgen-receptor protein that causes profound resistance to the action of testosterone (see Chap. 342). Testicular feminization can be diagnosed by demonstrating a male level of serum testosterone or a 46,XY karyotype, whereas demonstration of a 46,XX karyotype, biphasic basal body temperatures characteristic of ovulating women, and elevated levels of progesterone during the luteal phase establish the diagnosis of müllerian agenesis.

A rare cause of absence of the uterus in 46,XY phenotypic women who are sexually infantile is the so-called testicular regression syndrome or testicular agenesis (see Chap. 342).

Other abnormalities of the uterus that cause amenorrhea include obstruction due to scarring or stenosis of the cervix, often resulting from surgery, electrocautery, laser therapy, or cryosurgery. Destruction of the endometrium (Asherman's syndrome) may follow vigorous curettage, usually in association with postpartum hemorrhage or therapeutic abortion complicated by infection. This diagnosis is confirmed by hysterosalpingography or by direct vision of the endometrial scarring or synechiae using a hysteroscope.

Treatment of disorders of the outflow tract is surgical. Repair of vaginal agenesis results in normal menstruation and potential fertility only if an intact uterus is present.

Ovarian failure Primary ovarian failure is associated with elevated plasma gonadotropins and can result from several causes. The most frequent cause is *gonadal dysgenesis*, in which the germ cells are lacking and the ovary is replaced by a fibrous streak (also see Chaps. 62 and 342). Women with gonadal dysgenesis can be divided into two broad groups on the basis of chromosomal karyotype. The most common is due to deletion of genetic material in the X chromosomes and accounts for about two-thirds of gonadal dysgenesis. A 45,X karyotype is found in about half, and most have somatic defects, including short stature, webbed neck, shield chest, and cardiovascular defects, collectively termed the *Turner phenotype*. The remainder with identifiable abnormalities of the X chromosome have chromosomal mosaicism with or without associated structural abnormalities of the X chromosome. The most common form of mosaicism is 45,X/46,XX. Gonadal tumors are rare in 45,X patients, but gonadal malignancies may occur in women with chromosomal mosaicism involving the Y chromosome. Therefore, a chromosomal analysis should be obtained in all cases of amenorrhea associated with ovarian failure, and the streak gonad should be removed if a Y chromosome is present. Another means of identifying the presence of a Y chromosome is to amplify the sex-determining regions of the Y chromosome (SRY) by means of the polymerase chain reaction (see Chap. 342). Approximately 90 percent of individuals with gonadal dysgenesis associated with partial or complete deletion of the X chromosome never have menstrual bleeding, and the remaining 10 percent have sufficient follicles to experience menses and, rarely, fertility; the menstrual and reproductive lives of such individuals are invariably brief.

A tenth of subjects with bilateral streak gonads have a normal 46,XX or 46,XY karyotype and are said to have *pure gonadal dysgenesis*. These individuals have either normal or above-average stature due to failure of estrogen-mediated epiphyseal closure in the presence of a normal chromosomal constitution. Pure gonadal dysgenesis does not constitute a phenotypic or chromosomally homogeneous disorder (see Chap. 342). Approximately one-tenth of such individuals with a 46,XY karyotype develop signs of virilization, including clitoromegaly, and have an increased incidence of tumors in the gonadal streaks; as a consequence, gonadal streaks should be removed prophylactically as discussed above when a Y chromosome is present. Approximately two-thirds of women with 46,XX gonadal dysgenesis experience no menses, while the remainder have one or more menstrual episodes and are occasionally fertile.

Other causes of ovarian failure and amenorrhea include deficiency of the P450$_{17\alpha}$ enzyme that encodes 17α-hydroxylase and 17,20-lyase activities, premature ovarian failure, the resistant-ovary syndrome, and ovarian failure secondary to chemotherapy or radiation therapy for malignancy. *17α-Hydroxylase deficiency* is characterized by primary amenorrhea, sexual infantilism, and hypertension that is due to increased production of desoxycorticosterone (DOC), whereas women with *17,20-lyase deficiency* have primary amenorrhea and sexual infantilism with normal blood pressure (see Chaps. 335 and

342). The diagnosis of *premature ovarian failure* or *premature menopause* is applied to women who cease menstruating prior to age 40. The ovaries are similar to the ovaries of postmenopausal women, namely, paucity or absence of follicles as the result of accelerated follicular atresia. Premature ovarian failure due to ovarian antibodies may be one component of polyglandular failure together with adrenal insufficiency, hypothyroidism, and other autoimmune disorders (see Chap. 343). A rare form of ovarian failure is the *resistant-ovary syndrome*, in which the ovaries contain many follicles arrested in development prior to the antral stage, possibly because of resistance to the action of FSH in the ovary. To differentiate this disorder from the 46,XX variety of pure gonadal dysgenesis, both of which are associated with sexual immaturity, it is necessary to perform ovarian biopsy. However, such a distinction is not clinically useful, since the conventional treatment of infertility in both conditions is usually unsuccessful. Women with ovarian failure who desire pregnancy have been treated with hormone replacement and transfer of donor embryos to the uterine cavity or fallopian tubes.

CHRONIC ANOVULATION   At least 80 percent or more of gynecologic endocrine problems result from chronic anovulation. Women with chronic anovulation fail to ovulate spontaneously but may ovulate with appropriate therapy. The ovaries of such women do not secrete estrogen in a normal cyclic pattern; it is clinically useful to differentiate those women who produce sufficient estrogen to have withdrawal bleeding after progestogen therapy from those who fail to produce enough estrogen to have progesterone withdrawal bleeding and who often have hypothalamic-pituitary dysfunction.

Chronic anovulation with estrogen present   Women with chronic anovulation who experience withdrawal bleeding after progestogen administration are said to be in a state of "estrus" due to the acyclic production of estrogen, largely estrone, by extraglandular aromatization of circulating androstenedione. The most common term for this disorder is *polycystic ovarian disease* (PCOD), a syndrome characterized by infertility, hirsutism, obesity, and amenorrhea or oligomenorrhea. When spontaneous uterine bleeding occurs in subjects with PCOD, it is unpredictable with respect to time of onset, duration, and amount, and on occasion the bleeding can be severe. The dysfunctional uterine bleeding is usually due to estrogen breakthrough (see above).

The disorder, which may be transmitted as an autosomal dominant or X-linked trait, was originally described by Stein and Leventhal as characterized by enlarged, polycystic ovaries, but the syndrome and its accompanying endocrine abnormalities are now known to be associated with a variety of pathologic findings in the ovaries, only some of which result in enlargement of the ovaries and none of which are pathognomonic. The most common finding is a white, smooth, sclerotic ovary with a thickened capsule, multiple follicular cysts in various stages of atresia, a hyperplastic theca and stroma, and rare or absent corpora albicans. Other ovaries have hyperthecosis in which the ovarian stroma is hyperplastic and may contain lipid-laden luteal cells. Thus the diagnosis of PCOD is a clinical one, based on the coexistence of chronic anovulation and varying degrees of androgen excess.

In most women with PCOD, menarche occurs at the expected time, but uterine bleeding is unpredictable in onset, duration, and amount. Amenorrhea ensues after a variable time, although primary amenorrhea occurs in some women. Signs of androgen excess (hirsutism) usually become evident around the time of menarche. One formulation suggests that this disorder originates as an exaggerated adrenarche in obese girls (Fig. 340-7). The combination of elevated adrenal androgens and obesity would result in increased formation of extraglandular estrogen and lead to an acyclic positive feedback on LH secretion and negative feedback on FSH secretion so that the characteristic LH/FSH ratios in plasma would be greater than 2. The increased LH levels could then lead to hyperplasia of the ovarian stroma and theca cells and increased androgen production, which in turn would provide more substrate for peripheral aromatization and perpetuate the chronic anovulation. In the advanced state the ovary

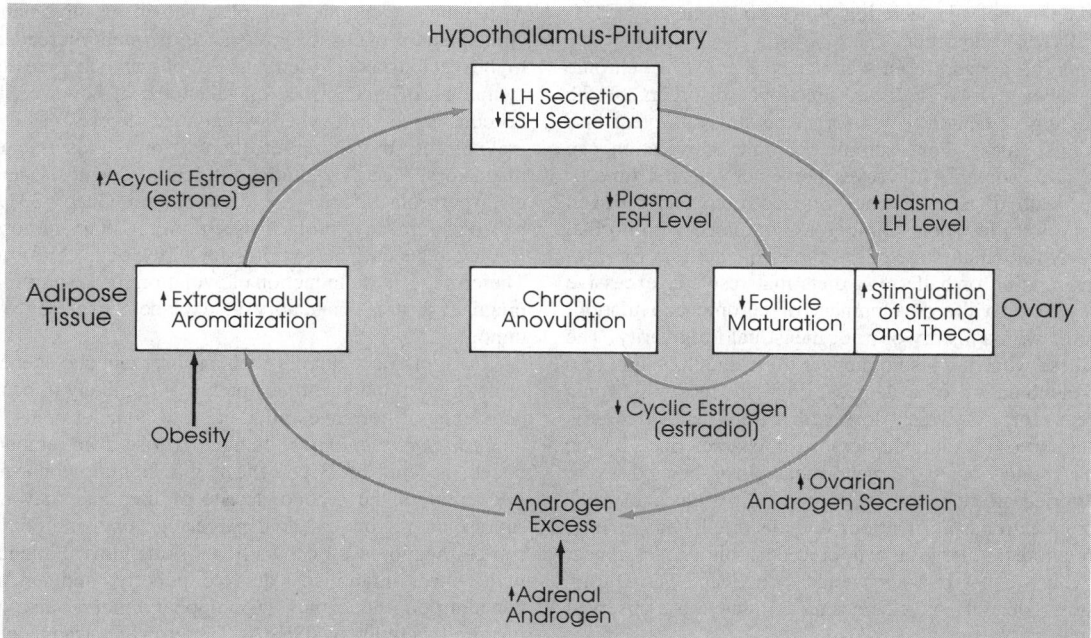

FIGURE 340-7   Proposed mechanism for the initiation and perpetuation of chronic anovulation in polycystic ovarian disease (PCOD). This cycle may be entered or initiated via adrenal androgen excess or obesity, both of which result in enhanced extraglandular formation of estrogens. The therapy of PCOD involves interruption of the cycle at various sites. (*From SSC Yen and RB Jaffe, 1986, and from U Goebelsmann in DR Mishell, Jr, and V Davajan.*)

is the major site of androgen production, but the adrenal may continue to secrete excess androgen as well. The greater the obesity, the more this sequence would be perpetuated because adipose tissue stromal cells aromatize androgens to estrogens, which in turn exaggerates inappropriate LH release by positive feedback.

Thus the fundamental defect in PCOD is viewed as one of inappropriate signals to the hypothalamus and pituitary. In fact, the hypothalamic-pituitary axis responds appropriately to high levels of estrogen, and ovulation can be induced with antiestrogens such as clomiphene citrate. Increased levels of plasma endorphins and inhibin may contribute to the perpetuation of the defect. The concept that the fundamental defect is one of inappropriate signals is supported by the findings in the ovary itself. Ovarian follicles from women with PCOD have low aromatase activity, but normal aromatase can be induced when the follicles are treated with FSH. In short, the anovulation is not due to an intrinsic abnormality in the ovary itself but rather the result of FSH deficiency and LH excess. An association exists between PCOD or hyperthecosis, virilization, acanthosis nigricans, and insulin resistance; in the ovary, insulin may interact via the insulin-like growth factor receptors to enhance androgen synthesis in insulin-resistant states.

Treatment of PCOD is directed toward interrupting this self-perpetuating cycle and can be accomplished in several ways, including decreasing ovarian androgen secretion (wedge resection or oral contraceptive agents), decreasing peripheral estrogen formation (weight reduction), and enhancing FSH secretion [administration of clomiphene, human menopausal gonadotropin (hMG), LHRH (gonadorelin) by portable infusion pump, or purified FSH (urofollitropin)]. The choice of therapy depends on the clinical findings and the needs of the patient. Attempt at weight reduction is appropriate in all who are obese. If the woman is not hirsute and does not desire pregnancy, periodic withdrawal menses can be induced with medroxyprogesterone acetate 10 days per month; such treatment prevents development of endometrial hyperplasia. If the woman is hirsute but does not desire pregnancy, the ovarian (and possibly the adrenal) component of androgen production can be suppressed with combined estrogen-progestogen oral contraceptive agents. Combined oral contraceptives are also indicated if prolonged or excessive menstrual bleeding is present. Once androgen excess is controlled,

treatment of previously existing hair growth by shaving, depilatories, or electrolysis may be indicated (see Chap. 49). If the woman wants to become pregnant, induction of ovulation is necessary. The drug of choice for this purpose is clomiphene, which promotes ovulation in three-fourths of cases, or treatment with hMG, urofollitropin, or gonadorelin. Pretreatment with LHRH analogues prior to hMG, urofollitropin, or gonadorelin has been utilized to improve ovulation and pregnancy rates. Wedge resection of the ovaries is rarely indicated today because of the development of adhesions but may be successful on occasion.

Chronic anovulation with estrogen present also may occur with tumors of the ovary. These include granulosa-theca cell tumors, Brenner tumors, cystic teratomas, mucous cystadenomas, and Krukenberg tumors (also see Chap. 321). These tumors can either secrete excess estrogen themselves or produce androgens that can then be aromatized in extraglandular sites. As a result, chronic anovulation and the clinical features of PCOD are produced. Occasionally, areas of the ovary not involved with tumors show the characteristic histologic changes of PCOD. Other causes of chronic anovulation with estrogen present include adrenal production of excess androgen (usually adult-onset adrenal hyperplasia due to partial $P450_{C21}$ deficiency) and various thyroid disorders.

Chronic anovulation with estrogen absent   Women with chronic anovulation who have low or absent estrogen production and do not experience withdrawal bleeding after progestogen treatment usually have hypogonadotropic hypogonadism due either to pituitary disease or to any of several organic or functional disorders of the central nervous system.

Isolated hypogonadotropic hypogonadism associated with defects of smell (olfactory bulb defects) is known as the *Kallman syndrome* (see Chaps. 331 and 339). Affected women are sexually infantile with a eunuchoid habitus and appear to have a defect in either the synthesis or release of LHRH. A variety of rare hypothalamic lesions also can impair LHRH production and cause hypogonadotropic hypogonadism; these include craniopharyngioma, germinoma (pinealoma), glioma, Hand-Schüller-Christian disease, teratomas, endodermal-sinus tumors, tuberculosis, sarcoidosis, and metastatic tumors that cause suppression or destruction of the hypothalamus. Central nervous system trauma and radiation also can cause hypothalamic amenorrhea and deficiencies in secretion of growth hormone, ACTH, vasopressin, and thyroid hormone.

More commonly, gonadotropin deficiency leading to chronic anovulation is believed to arise from functional disorders of the hypothalamus or higher centers. A history of a stressful event in a young woman is frequent. For example, chronic anovulation can begin suddenly in a woman who leaves home for the first time or experiences the death of a loved one. Gonadotropin and estrogen levels are in the low to low-normal range as compared with normal women in the early follicular phase of the cycle. In addition, rigorous exercise such as jogging or ballet and diets that result in excessive weight loss may lead to the development of chronic anovulation, particularly in girls with a history of prior menstrual irregularity. The amenorrhea in these women does not appear to be due to weight loss alone but to a combination of a decrease in body fat and chronic stress. An extreme form of weight loss with chronic anovulation is seen in anorexia nervosa. Anorexia nervosa is characterized by the development in a young woman of amenorrhea with associated severe weight loss, distorted attitudes toward eating and weight gain, self-induced vomiting, extreme emaciation, and distorted body image. Amenorrhea in anorexia nervosa can precede, follow, or appear coincidentally with the loss in body weight (see Chap. 74). During successful therapy, gonadotropin changes recapitulate those observed during normal puberty (see Fig. 340-1).

In addition, chronic debilitating diseases such as end-stage kidney disease, malignancy, or the malabsorption syndrome are believed to lead to development of hypogonadotropic hypogonadism via a hypothalamic mechanism.

Treatment of chronic anovulation due to hypothalamic disorders includes reversal of the stressful situation, reducing exercise, or correction of weight loss if appropriate. These women appear to be susceptible to the development of osteoporosis, and estrogen replacement therapy to induce and maintain normal secondary sexual characteristics and prevent bone loss is recommended in those who do not desire pregnancy, and gonadotropin or gonadorelin therapy is indicated when pregnancy is desired (see therapy section). When appropriate, therapy is directed at the primary disease of the hypothalamus.

Disorders of the pituitary can lead to the estrogen-deficient form of chronic anovulation by at least two mechanisms—direct interference with gonadotropin secretion by lesions that either obliterate or interfere with the gonadotropic cells (chromophobe adenomas, Sheehan's syndrome) or inhibition of gonadotropin secretion in association with excess prolactin (prolactinoma). *Pituitary tumors* make up approximately 10 percent of all intracranial tumors and may secrete no hormone, one hormone, or more than one hormone (see Chap. 331). In the past, most pituitary tumors were assumed to be nonfunctional chromophobe adenomas, but prolactin levels are elevated in 50 to 70 percent of cases, either because of prolactin secretion by the tumor (prolactinomas) or because of interference by tumor mass with the normal inhibitory influence of the hypothalamus on prolactin secretion.

Prolactinomas can be divided into microadenomas (less than 10 mm in diameter) and macroadenomas (greater than 10 mm). Prolactin excess associated with low levels of LH and FSH constitutes a specific subgroup of hypogonadotropic hypogonadism. One-tenth or more of amenorrheic women have increased levels of serum prolactin, and more than half of women with both galactorrhea and amenorrhea have elevated prolactin levels. The amenorrhea in this disorder is most often associated with decreased or absent estrogen production, but prolactin-secreting tumors may on occasion be associated with normal ovulatory menses or chronic anovulation with estrogen present. Most prolactin-secreting adenomas grow slowly, and some cease growth after attainment of a certain size. The increased frequency of diagnosis of prolactin-secreting adenomas is probably due to several factors, including increased awareness, improved radiographic detection methods, and availability of radioimmunoassays for prolactin. However, since in older autopsy series a 9 to 23 percent prevalence

of pituitary adenomas was observed in asymptomatic women, the clinical and prognostic significance of small microadenomas remains to be established. When tumors of any size are associated with symptoms of amenorrhea or galactorrhea, however, therapy should be considered, and when visual field defects or severe headaches are present, bromocriptine therapy or neurosurgical evaluation is mandatory. The evaluation, differential diagnosis, and management of hyperprolactinemia are described in Chap. 331. In the latter half of pregnancy, prolactin-secreting pituitary tumors may expand, leading to headaches, compression of the optic chiasm, and blindness. Therefore, prior to induction of ovulation for the purposes of achieving pregnancy, it is mandatory to exclude the presence of a pituitary tumor.

Large pituitary tumors such as chromophobe adenomas—whether or not hyperprolactinemia is present—are likely to be associated with deficiency of hormones in addition to gonadotropins (Chap. 331).

Craniopharyngiomas, thought to arise from remnants of Rathke's pouch, account for 3 percent of intracranial neoplasms, occur most frequently in the second decade of life, and may extend into the suprasellar region. A large percentage of these tumors calcify and can be diagnosed by conventional skull films. Patients often present with sexual infantilism, delayed puberty, and amenorrhea due to gonadotropin deficiency. Craniopharyngioma also may result in impaired secretion of TSH, ACTH, growth hormone, and vasopressin.

Panhypopituitarism may occur spontaneously, result from surgical or radiation treatment of pituitary adenomas, or develop after postpartum hemorrhage (Sheehan's syndrome). The latter patients exhibit characteristic clinical manifestations including failure to lactate or ovulate, loss of genital and axillary hair, hypothyroidism, and adrenal insufficiency (see Chap. 331).

Evaluation of amenorrhea   A general schema for the evaluation of women with amenorrhea is given in Fig. 340-8. In the initial physical examination, special attention should be given to three features: (1) degree of maturation of the breasts, the pubic and axillary hair, and the external genitalia, (2) the current estrogen status, and (3) the presence or absence of a uterus. All women with amenorrhea should be assumed to be pregnant until proven otherwise. Even when history and physical examination are not suggestive, it is prudent to exclude pregnancy by a suitable screening test. Once this is done, the cause of amenorrhea can frequently be diagnosed by history and physical examination. For example, Asherman's syndrome is suggested by a history of curettage in a woman who previously menstruated; in women with primary amenorrhea and sexual infantilism, the essential differential diagnosis is between gonadal dysgenesis and hypopituitarism, and the diagnosis of gonadal dysgenesis (Turner's syndrome) or of anatomic defects of the outflow tract (müllerian agenesis, testicular feminization, and cervical stenosis) is frequently suggested on the basis of physical findings. When a specific cause is suspected, it is appropriate to proceed directly to confirm the diagnosis (such as obtaining a chromosomal karyotype or measurement of plasma gonadotropins). It is also useful to measure serum prolactin level during the initial evaluation.

Estrogen status is evaluated by determining if the vaginal mucosa is moist and rugated and if the cervical mucus can be stretched and shown to fern upon drying. If these criteria are indeterminate, a progestational challenge is indicated, most often administration of 10 mg medroxyprogesterone acetate by mouth once or twice daily for 5 days or 100 mg progesterone in oil intramuscularly. (It should be emphasized that progestogen should never be administered until pregnancy is excluded.) If estrogen levels are adequate (and the outflow tract is intact), menstrual bleeding should occur within 1 week of ending the progestogen treatment. If withdrawal bleeding occurs, the diagnosis is chronic anovulation with estrogen present, usually polycystic ovarian disease.

If no withdrawal bleeding or only minimal vaginal spotting occurs, the nature of the subsequent workup is dependent on the results of the initial prolactin assay. If plasma prolactin is elevated, or if galactorrhea is present, radiography of the pituitary should be

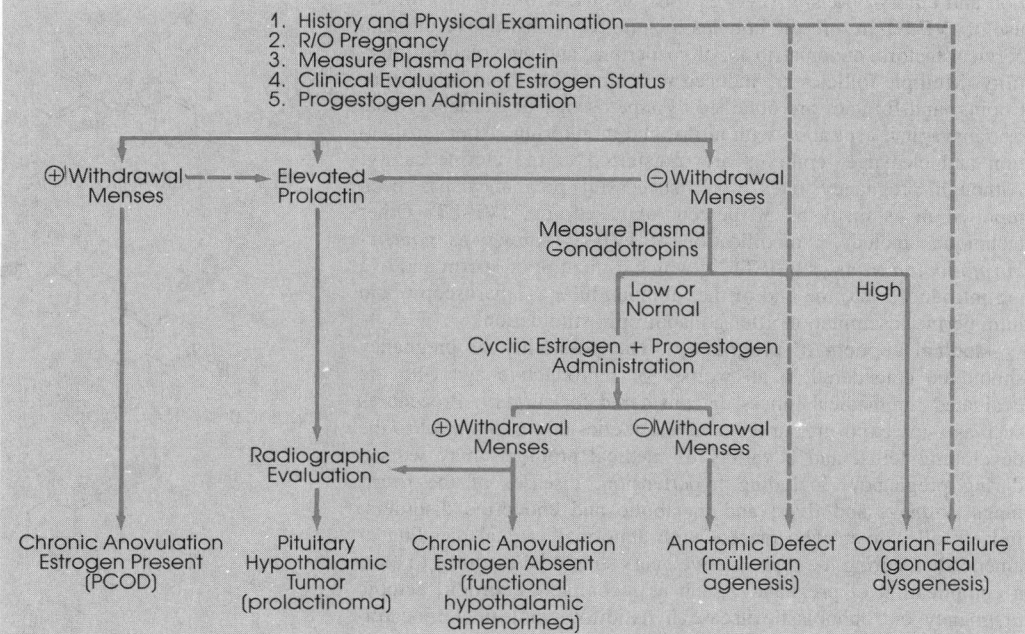

FIGURE 340-8 Flow diagram for the evaluation of women with amenorrhea. The most common diagnosis for each category is shown in parentheses. The dotted lines indicate that in some instances a correct diagnosis can be reached on the basis of history and physical exam alone.

undertaken. When the plasma prolactin level is normal in the anovulatory woman with estrogen absent, plasma gonadotropins should be measured. If the gonadotropin levels are elevated, the diagnosis is ovarian failure. If the gonadotropins are in the low or normal range, the diagnosis is either hypothalamic-pituitary disorder or anatomic defect of the outflow tract. As indicated previously, the diagnosis of outflow tract disorder is usually suspected or established on the basis of the history and physical findings. When the physical findings are not clear-cut, it is useful to administer cyclic estrogen plus progestogen (1.25 mg oral conjugated estrogens per day for 3 weeks with 10 mg medroxyprogesterone acetate added for the last 7 to 10 days of estrogen treatment), followed by 10 days of observation. If no bleeding occurs, the diagnosis of Asherman's syndrome or other anatomic defect of the outflow tract is confirmed by hysterosalpingography or hysteroscopy. If withdrawal bleeding occurs following the estrogen-progestogen combination, the diagnosis of chronic anovulation with estrogen absent (functional hypothalamic amenorrhea) is suggested. Radiologic evaluations of the pituitary-hypothalamic areas may be indicated in the latter cases—irrespective of the prolactin level—because of the danger of overlooking a pituitary-hypothalamic tumor and because the diagnosis of functional hypothalamic amenorrhea is one of exclusion (see Chap. 331).

Infertility Infertility, the failure to become pregnant after 1 year of unprotected intercourse, affects approximately 10 to 15 percent of couples and is one of the common complaints for which women seek gynecologic assistance. Male factors account for 40 percent of infertility problems (see Chaps. 47 and 339). In women, failure of ovulation accounts for 30 percent, pelvic factors such as tubal disease and endometriosis account for half, and a cervical factor is implicated in about one-tenth of infertility evaluations. In 10 to 20 percent of infertile women no etiology is found. An immunologic cause may explain a portion of infertility in these couples. Finally, infertility in women may be due to *luteal phase dysfunction* in which ovulation is assumed to occur but progesterone formation is insufficient to allow preparation of the endometrium for implantation; the disorder is believed to be due to inadequate FSH secretion or action and consequent inadequate estrogen formation by the dominant follicle during the follicular phase.

The first diagnostic step in evaluation of the infertile couple is to determine whether the man or woman is the infertile partner, ordinarily by first obtaining a semen analysis in the man (see Chap. 339) and

demonstration of presumed ovulation in the woman. Documentation of ovulatory cycles is obtained by daily measurement of basal body temperatures throughout the month. Occasionally, accurate basal body temperature records are not obtained, and demonstration of elevated serum progesterone levels during the luteal phase may be used as evidence of ovulation. Dating of endometrium by histologic examination of a biopsy sample is also useful for establishing ovulation or luteal phase dysfunction.

If the infertility is associated with amenorrhea, then the workup is that described in Fig. 340-8. If anovulation due to polycystic ovarian disease is the basis for infertility, ovulation can be induced utilizing clomiphene, gonadotropins, gonadorelin, or, on occasion, wedge resection of the ovaries. Bromocriptine is used to induce ovulation in cases of hyperprolactinemia. In the presence of prolactinomas, the appropriate therapy prior to induction of ovulation remains controversial. Recommended therapies in this situation include observation, reinstitution of bromocriptine therapy, radiation therapy, or surgical resection of the tumor (see Chap. 331).

Hysterosalpingograms may be obtained to evaluate the fallopian tubes and uterine cavity. Further evaluation of tubal and ovarian disease is obtained by diagnostic laparoscopy and the demonstration of dye spillage from the fimbria after transcervical injection of dye during laparoscopy. Microsurgical repair of damaged or previously ligated fallopian tubes has resulted in an apparent increase in pregnancy rates. Removal of peritubular and fimbrial adhesions utilizing laparoscopic surgery plus laser beam therapy is another treatment mode. Endometriosis can be diagnosed by laparoscopy, and treatment of endometriosis associated with infertility includes surgical resection of the endometrial implants or temporary gonadotropin suppression utilizing danazol (400 to 800 mg orally in divided doses for 4 to 6 months), LHRH analogues given by nasal spray or subcutaneous or depot injection, or continuous low-dose oral contraceptive agents to promote regression of the implants.

The cervical factor in infertility is evaluated by study of cervical mucus at an appropriate time after coitus, preferably just prior to ovulation (day 12 to 13) when cervical mucus is thin and stretches, and provides information as to the penetration and survival of the sperm in the female genital tract. Preferred treatment of infertility due to such abnormality is intrauterine insemination with washed sperm.

When other treatment modalities are unsuccessful, in vitro fertilization and embryo transfer (IVF-ET) may be tried. Indications for the use of IVF-ET in infertile couples include tubal obstructive disease, cervical factors, endometriosis, oligospermia, and unexplained infertility. Multiple follicles are induced with clomiphene and/or gonadotropins, and follicles are obtained by laparoscopy or transabdominal or transvaginal aspiration with ultrasound monitoring. After fertilization and cleavage, embryos are transferred to the uterine cavity. Although pregnancy rates vary, successful pregnancy has been reported in as many as 30 percent of cases after IVF-ET. Other techniques include a modification of IVF-ET known as *gamete-intrafallopian transfer* (GIFT), in which a mixture of sperm and ova are introduced into the end of the fallopian tube at laparoscopy, and intrauterine insemination after gonadotropin stimulation.

Medical aspects of pregnancy The possibility of pregnancy should be considered in all women of reproductive age who are evaluated for medical illness or considered for surgery. Procedures such as x-ray exposure, drugs, and anesthetics may be harmful to the developing fetus, and a variety of medical problems may worsen during pregnancy, including hypertension; diseases of the heart, lungs, kidney, and liver; and metabolic and endocrine disorders. Indeed, all women who present with abnormal vaginal bleeding or amenorrhea during the reproductive years should be assumed to have a complication of pregnancy, such as incomplete abortion, ectopic pregnancy, or trophoblastic disease (hydatidiform mole or choriocarcinoma). Women who present with these complications of pregnancy often have histories of abdominal pain and vaginal bleeding and may have evidence of intraabdominal hemorrhage.

Choriocarcinoma is a particular problem because of its protean manifestations. Half these malignancies follow pregnancies complicated by hydatidiform mole, and the remainder occur after spontaneous abortion, ectopic pregnancy, or normal deliveries. Patients may present with intraabdominal bleeding due to rupture of the uterus, liver, or ovary, with pulmonary manifestations (cough, hemoptysis, pleuritic pain, dyspnea, and respiratory failure) or gastrointestinal symptoms, usually chronic blood loss or melena. In addition, patients can present with cerebral metastases or renal involvement. The diagnosis can be established by demonstrating an elevated level of the β subunit of hCG in plasma. Treatment and cure are possible with chemotherapeutic agents (dactinomycin and/or methotrexate). (For manifestations of choriocarcinoma in men, see Chap. 322.)

Ovarian tumors See Chap. 321.

TREATMENT

PROGESTOGENS The major use of progestogen is in conjunction with estrogen to ensure the full maturation of the endometrium, both in combination birth control pills and in the therapy of hypogonadal states. In certain circumstances, however, progestogen therapy is appropriate by itself—to induce a progestational effect on the estrogen-primed endometrium (diagnostic tests for the evaluation of amenorrhea), to inhibit pituitary gonadotropins (the progestogen-only birth control pill or progestogen-containing implants) for contraception, for prophylaxis to prevent hyperplasia in PCOD, and for palliation in endometrial and breast carcinoma or treatment of endometriosis. Even when a direct progestational effect is desired, the available oral drugs substitute a synthetic derivative for the naturally occurring hormone. Oral progestogens include medroxyprogesterone acetate, megestrol acetate, norethindrone, norgestrel, and micronized progesterone. Parenteral agents include progesterone in oil, medroxyprogesterone acetate suspension, and 17-hydroxyprogesterone caproate. Vaginal progesterone suppositories are used for treatment of luteal phase defects, and progestogen implants are available for long-term contraception.

The most common undesirable side effect is breakthrough bleeding, which occurs when progestogens are used continuously. Other complications include nausea, vomiting, and hirsutism. Abnormal liver function is a side effect of those derivatives with alkyl substitution

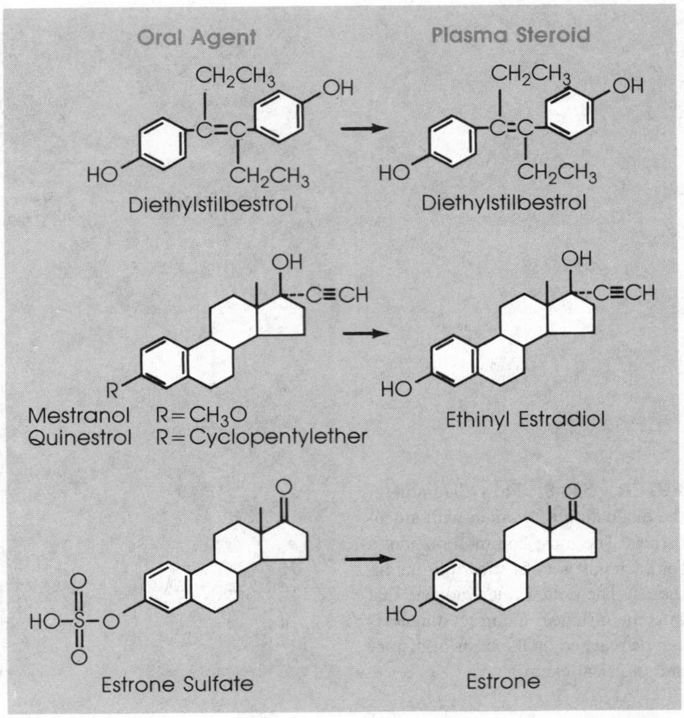

FIGURE 340-9 The circulating forms of administered estrogenic drugs.

in the 17α position. Progestogens are contraindicated if pregnancy is known or suspected because of the risk of birth defects.

ESTROGENS Estrogens are used for four purposes—the treatment of gonadal failure, control of fertility, management of dysfunctional uterine bleeding, and management of carcinoma of the breast. (The management of carcinoma of the breast is discussed in Chap. 319.) However, none of the presently available orally active or parenteral hormones replaces the pattern of concentration of estradiol characteristic of the normally cycling, premenopausal woman (see Fig. 340-5). Estrogens that can be given by mouth are either nonsteroidal agents (such as diethylstilbestrol) that mimic the action of estradiol, estrogen conjugates that must be hydrolyzed before they become active (estrogen sulfates, predominantly estrone sulfate from pregnant mare's urine), or estrogen analogues that cannot be metabolized to estradiol (mestranol, quinestrol) (Fig. 340-9). Even when micronized estradiol is given orally, it is rapidly converted in the body to estrone. Because oral therapy neither replaces nor mimics the daily secretory pattern of the lost hormone, such therapy must be viewed as a pharmacologic substitution rather than a physiologic replacement. Likewise, the use of parenteral estrogens rarely mimics the physiologic situation. Parenteral preparations of conjugated estrogens, like the oral derivatives, are poor precursors of estradiol, and estradiol esters (estradiol benzoate and valerate) rarely cause plasma estradiol levels that mimic the normal monthly secretory pattern of the hormone. Transdermal estrogen results in constant levels of blood estrogen and is effective in the treatment of menopausal symptoms. The side effects of estrogen substitution differ at various times of life.

Hypoestrogenism In women with decreased estrogen production, whether due to disease of the ovaries (gonadal dysgenesis) or to hypogonadotropic hypogonadism, treatment with cyclic estrogens should be instituted at the time of expected puberty for development and maintenance of female secondary sexual characteristics and prevention of osteoporosis. The most commonly used medications are conjugated estrogens (0.625 to 1.25 mg/d by mouth) or ethinyl estradiol or its precursors (0.02 to 0.05 mg/d by mouth). The addition of medroxyprogesterone acetate (5 to 10 mg/d) is recommended by most physicians during the last several days of monthly estrogen treatment to prevent development of endometrial hyperplasia during long-term estrogen treatment. Abnormal bleeding in women receiving estrogen replacement requires histologic evaluation of the endometrium. Such substitution therapy or the use of oral contraceptives (see below) also may be used for the purpose of suppressing pituitary gonadotropins, as in women with PCOD, in whom the major therapeutic aim is suppression of ovarian androgen production prior to the time when fertility is desired.

Temporary administration of estrogens in larger quantities (up to two times the usual adult maintenance dose) may be necessary to induce full development of secondary sexual characteristics in girls and for the control of menopausal symptoms. Even larger doses of parenteral estrogens (10 mg estradiol valerate or 25 mg conjugated estrogen) in conjunction with progestogen may be required in some instances of dysfunctional uterine bleeding. In addition to the potential long-term side effects of all estrogens (see below), high doses may cause specific problems, including nausea, vomiting, and edema.

Fertility control   Since the use of all contraceptive methods is associated with diverse side effects, an understanding of the use, methods of actions, and consequences of these agents is important to all physicians. Furthermore, since pregnancy may aggravate a variety of chronic illnesses, fertility control should be recommended in many patients.

To be effective, fertility control requires patient acceptance and compliance. The most widely utilized methods include (1) rhythm and withdrawal techniques, (2) barrier methods, including the condom, jellies, foam, suppositories, and diaphragms, (3) intrauterine devices (IUD), (4) hormonal contraceptives, (5) sterilization, and (6) abortion.

The rhythm and withdrawal technique and the barrier methods are effective if used correctly and consistently but in actual practice result in high failure rates because of imperfect compliance. Nevertheless, these methods carry the lowest incidence of side effects, and the side effects, when produced, are minor except for local allergic reactions. When the rhythm method is combined with self-evaluation of the preovulatory part of the menstrual cycle (i.e., evaluation of cervical mucus) plus home LH testing, it is an effective method of contraception. Use of these methods should be recommended when there is a relative or absolute contraindication to other therapy.

The most widely utilized nonsurgical methods of contraception, the IUD and birth control pills, are effective but may be associated with significant side effects.

IUD   The success rates of most IUDs are 95 to 98 percent. Only two devices are marketed in the United States. Both are T-shaped, cause minimal pain at insertion, and are associated with low expulsion rates. One of these IUDs contains copper, which enhances effectiveness, and is replaced at 8-year intervals. The other contains slow-release progesterone, which makes annual replacement necessary. The IUD is believed to prevent pregnancy by the induction of a chronic inflammatory reaction in the endometrium, resulting in an unfavorable environment for the implantation of the blastocyst, although some evidence suggests that IUDs prevent fertilization.

Once the IUD is inserted, it is necessary to check periodically to be certain that the device is in place. Both minor and serious side effects can occur. Intermenstrual spotting and increased bleeding and pain or cramps at the time of menses are frequent causes of discontinuation of the IUD. In addition, the device may be expelled spontaneously during a menstrual period without the subject being aware of its loss. The most serious side effect is pelvic infection, occasionally leading to the development of tuboovarian abscess and subsequent infertility. Pelvic infection is more frequent than in users of oral or barrier contraceptives but no more common than in women using no contraception. Women with multiple sex partners are at greatest risk for pelvic infection. For this reason, use in nulligravida women is not advocated by many gynecologists. In addition, pregnancy with an IUD in place is more likely to be ectopic because intrauterine but not extrauterine pregnancies are inhibited. Because of the increased incidence of spontaneous and septic abortions when IUDs are in place, the device should be removed if pregnancy is detected. Any user who develops persistent, severe bleeding, lower abdominal pain, fever, or discharge should have the IUD removed.

ORAL CONTRACEPTIVES   Oral contraceptive agents have been used by over 200 million women worldwide and by 1 of 4 women in the United States under age 45. These agents are popular because of ease of administration, low pregnancy rate (less than 1 percent), and a relatively low incidence of side effects.

The most widely utilized oral contraceptive pills are either combination tablets or triphasic formulations. A list of oral contraceptives marketed in the United States is given in Table 340-3. Combination oral contraceptive tablets contain one of two synthetic estrogens (mestranol or ethinyl estradiol) and one of five synthetic progestogens (norethindrone, norethindrone acetate, norethynodrel, norgestrel, ethynodiol diacetate desogestrel and norgestimate). The agents now available all contain no more than 50 μg ethinyl estradiol or its equivalent. The combination or triphasic tablets are taken for 21 consecutive days followed by 7 days' rest. Progestogen-only tablets are taken continuously on a daily basis. Presumably, the ideal contraceptive contains the lowest amount of steroid to minimize side effects but an amount that is at the same time sufficient to prevent pregnancy or breakthrough bleeding. The triphasic tablets, containing 35 μg or less of estrogen and less than 1 mg progestogen, come closest to this goal.

Oral contraceptives inhibit ovulation by suppressing FSH and LH secretion. As a consequence, the secretion of all ovarian steroids is also suppressed, including estrogen, progesterone, and androgen (Fig. 340-10). These agents also exert minor direct inhibitory effects on the reproductive tract, altering the cervical mucus and thereby decreasing sperm penetration and decreasing the motility and secretions of the fallopian tubes and uterus.

The death rates associated with oral contraceptives and other forms of birth control are summarized in Table 340-4. Up to age 40, the mortality rates in women using oral contraceptives and IUDs are lower than in women using no form of contraception (this difference results from the increased risk of death associated with pregnancy). The decrease in death rate below age 40 is even more striking in nonsmokers than in smokers using contraceptives. In fact, the death rates in nonsmoking women aged 15 to 24 who use oral agents are lower than those with other forms of fertility control. The increased death rates in women using rhythm or barrier techniques probably results from the higher failure rate and the consequent risk of pregnancy in such women. Oral contraceptive agents are not recommended for smoking women after age 35 and for women of all ages who are at increased risk for myocardial infarction.

Despite the overall safety of these agents, users are at risk for several serious side effects. In most retrospective and prospective studies, an increased incidence has been found for *deep vein thrombosis* and *pulmonary embolism*. The relative increased risk varies from two- to twelvefold and is greater for women taking tablets containing more than 50 μg estrogen. The use of oral contraceptives is also associated with an increased risk of thromboembolism after surgery, and for this reason, these agents should be discontinued at least 1 month prior to elective surgery. In retrospective studies there is a 3- to 9-times increased risk for *thromboembolic stroke* and a twofold greater risk for *hemorrhagic stroke* in users of oral contraceptives. However, three large prospective studies have demonstrated only a slight increase in hemorrhagic stroke in oral contraceptive users. Therefore, the drugs should be discontinued in women who experience visual complaints or severe headaches. Smoking and age increase the risk for stroke as well as the frequency of death from complications of deep venous thrombosis, pulmonary emboli, and myocardial infarction.

A small rise in blood pressure while taking oral contraceptives is common, and 5 percent of women develop significant *hypertension* (blood pressure greater than 140/90) after 5 years of continuous use. Estrogens induce the synthesis of a variety of proteins by the liver, including the renin substrate angiotensinogen. The resulting increased formation of angiotensin is believed to be involved in the development

TABLE 340-3 Composition of currently marketed oral contraceptives

Name	Estrogen	μg	Progestogen	mg
COMBINATION-TYPE				
Fixed type				
Estrogen content = 50 μg:				
Ortho-Novum 1/50	Mestranol	50	Norethindrone	1.0
Norinyl 1/50	Mestranol	50	Norethindrone	1.0
Ovcon 50	Ethinyl estradiol	50	Norethindrone	1.0
Ovral	Ethinyl estradiol	50	Norgestrel	0.5
Demulen	Ethinyl estradiol	50	Ethynodiol diacetate	1.0
Norlestrin 2.5/50	Ethinyl estradiol	50	Norethindrone acetate	2.5
Norlestrin 1/50	Ethinyl estradiol	50	Norethindrone acetate	1.0
Estrogen content <50 μg:				
Ortho-Novum 1/35	Ethinyl estradiol	35	Norethindrone	1.0
Norinyl 1 + 35	Ethinyl estradiol	35	Norethindrone	1.0
Modicon	Ethinyl estradiol	35	Norethindrone	0.5
Brevicon	Ethinyl estradiol	35	Norethindrone	0.5
Ovcon 35	Ethinyl estradiol	35	Norethindrone	0.4
Demulen 1/35	Ethinyl estradiol	35	Ethynodiol diacetate	1.0
Loestrin 1.5/30	Ethinyl estradiol	30	Norethindrone acetate	1.5
Loestrin 1/20	Ethinyl estradiol	20	Norethindrone acetate	1.0
Nordette	Ethinyl estradiol	30	Levonorgestrel	0.15
Lo-Ovral	Ethinyl estradiol	30	Norgestrel	0.3
Biphasic type				
Ortho-Novum 10/11				
First 10 days	Ethinyl estradiol	35	Norethindrone	0.5
Next 11 days	Ethinyl estradiol	35	Norethindrone	1.0
Triphasic type				
Ortho-Novum 7/7/7				
First 7 days	Ethinyl estradiol	35	Norethindrone	0.5
Second 7 days	Ethinyl estradiol	35	Norethindrone	0.75
Third 7 days	Ethinyl estradiol	35	Norethindrone	1.0
Tri-Norinyl				
First 7 days	Ethinyl estradiol	35	Norethindrone	0.5
Next 9 days	Ethinyl estradiol	35	Norethindrone	1.0
Next 5 days	Ethinyl estradiol	35	Norethindrone	0.5
Triphasil				
First 6 days	Ethinyl estradiol	30	Levonorgestrel	0.05
Second 5 days	Ethinyl estradiol	40	Levonorgestrel	0.075
Third 10 days	Ethinyl estradiol	30	Levonorgestrel	0.125
Tri-Levein				
First 6 days	Ethinyl estradiol	30	Levonorgestrel	0.05
Second 5 days	Ethinyl estradiol	40	Levonorgestrel	0.075
Third 10 days	Ethinyl estradiol	30	Levonorgestrel	0.125
PROGESTOGEN ONLY				
Micronor	None		Norethindrone	0.35
Nor Q.D.	None		Norethindrone	0.35
Ovrette	None		Norgestrel	0.075

of hypertension. Alternatively, the progestogen component of oral contraceptives may be associated with increased risk of hypertension. In most cases, blood pressure returns to normal when oral contraceptives are discontinued.

Serum lipids and lipoproteins are altered in women on oral contraceptives, the nature of the change depending on the specific components of the oral contraceptives. In general, estrogens increase serum high-density (HDL) and very low density lipoproteins (VLDL). Progestogens depress the concentration of HDL. However, with oral contraceptives containing less than 35 μg estrogen, lipoproteins change little if at all.

A few women taking oral contraceptives develop *impairment of glucose tolerance* as manifested by abnormal glucose levels and elevated plasma insulin after an oral glucose load, both of which usually return to normal after discontinuing the agents. Because juvenile-onset and adult-onset diabetes may be associated with increased incidence of cardiovascular disease, it is preferable to utilize other forms of contraception in these individuals.

Oral contraceptives should not be used by women with abnormal liver function tests or in women with acute or chronic liver disease. A rare complication linked to the long-term use of oral contraceptives is the development of peliosis hepatis, which can cause death due to sudden rupture and hemorrhage of the liver. Cholestatic jaundice may

occur in those women predisposed to the development of the syndrome of recurrent jaundice of pregnancy.

Oral contraceptives cause an increased concentration of cholesterol in the bile, which is probably the cause for the twofold increase in *cholelithiasis* and cholecystitis in women on oral contraceptives.

Estrogens induce elevation of a variety of proteins secreted by the liver, including cortisol-binding globulin (CBG), testosterone-binding globulin (TeBG), and thyroxine-binding globulin (TBG). Consequently, various laboratory tests of adrenal and thyroid function may be altered and must be interpreted with caution (see Chaps. 330 and 334). Oral contraceptives also slightly lower plasma ACTH levels, possibly due to an inhibitory effect on ACTH secretion or cortisol catabolism. Finally, serum prolactin levels are slightly elevated in women on oral contraceptives, but such treatment is not believed to play a role in the development of pituitary prolactinomas.

Other effects of oral contraceptive pills include minor dyspepsia, breast discomfort, weight gain, development of pigmentation of the face (chloasma), which is augmented by exposure to the sun, and a variety of psychological effects, such as depression and changes in libido. There is no convincing evidence that oral contraceptive use is associated with significant increase in the incidence of cancer of the uterus, cervix, or breast. In fact, oral contraceptives have many beneficial effects including control of dysmenorrhea and anovulatory

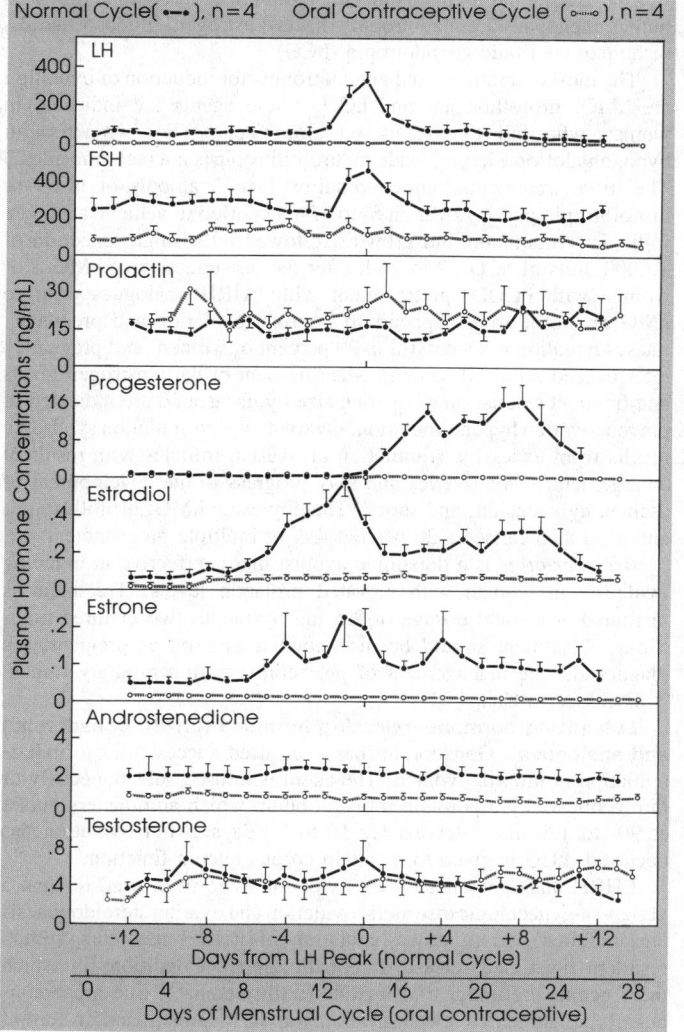

FIGURE 340-10 The mechanism of action of the birth control tablet. Mean daily plasma hormone concentrations during the ovarian cycle are shown for four ovulating women and four women treated with combination-type oral contraceptives. Data for the normal ovarian cycle are presented in relationship to the day of the LH peak; day 1 of the contraceptive cycle corresponds to the first day of uterine bleeding. The values are the mean ± SE obtained from four women. (*From BR Carr et al, 1979.*)

bleeding, prevention of sexually transmitted diseases, and decreased incidence of endometrial and ovarian cancer.

The absolute contraindications to the use of oral contraceptives include previous thromboembolic disorders, cerebral vascular or coronary artery disease, known or suspected carcinoma of the breast or estrogen-dependent neoplasia, undiagnosed abnormal genital bleeding, or known or suspected pregnancy. Relative contraindications must be weighed against the risk-versus-benefit ratio of the oral contraceptive pills and include hypertension, migraine headaches, diabetes mellitus, uterine leiomyomas, sickle cell anemia, hyperlipemia, and elective surgery.

OTHER STEROID CONTRACEPTIVES Types of steroid contraception other than the conventional oral contraceptives include (1) postcoital contraception and (2) injectable steroids, including progestogen-containing implants. Use of high-dose estrogen for 5 days during the fertile part of the cycle (the morning-after pill) is an effective method of contraception but is associated with significant side effects, particularly nausea. Administration of progestogens by injection or vaginal rings is used infrequently in the United States.

Estrogen treatment of the menopause The rationale for use of estrogens in postmenopausal women is based on the belief that such therapy may relieve many of the disorders of the menopause, including osteoporosis, and indeed of aging itself. In some parts of the United States, by the mid-1970s as many as half of women in the menopausal age group used one or more forms of estrogen replacement for a median period of 5 years, accounting for more than 30 million prescriptions per year.

The menopause is not associated with a simple state of estrogen deprivation, since some estrogens continue to be produced, but is instead a state of altered estrogen metabolism; the predominant estrogen becomes estrone formed by extraglandular conversion of prehormone rather than estradiol secretion by the ovary. As is true for all estrogen therapy, the estrogen treatment of the menopause is actually a pharmacologic substitution of one or another estrogen analogue for the physiologic estradiol rather than a physiologic replacement of the missing steroid. Estrogens available for replacement therapy include conjugated estrogens, estrogen substitutes (diethylstilbestrol), synthetic estrogen (ethinyl estradiol or derivatives), micronized estradiol, estrogen-containing vaginal creams, and estrogen-containing dermal patches. Regimens associated with low risk of complications include (1) cyclic estrogen therapy in the lowest effective dose for 25 days per month or continuous estrogens given each day of the month and (2) estrogens plus the addition of progestogen during the last 10 to 13 days of estrogen therapy, or low-dose continuous progestogen plus estrogen given daily.

The most clear-cut early benefit of estrogen therapy in the menopause is the relief of vasomotor instability (hot flashes) and of atrophy of the urogenital epithelium and skin. Estrogen therapy ameliorates these symptoms in the majority of cases. When estrogen therapy is designed to treat hot flashes alone, such therapy should be continued for only a few years, since hot flashes tend to diminish after 3 to 4 years in untreated women.

Several lines of evidence indicate that routine estrogen therapy is beneficial in preventing the complications of menopausal osteoporosis, especially in high-risk women (i.e., thin white women). First, in women undergoing premature menopause, the incidence and complication rates of osteoporosis are increased, and long-term estrogen replacement appears to be beneficial. Second, estrogen

TABLE 340-4 Annual death rates associated with fertility control per 100,000 women

Contraceptive techniques	Age group					
	15–19	20–24	25–29	30–34	35–39	40–44
None (birth-related)	7.0	7.4	9.1	14.8	25.7	28.2
Oral contraceptives						
Smokers	2.4	3.6	6.8	13.7	51.4	117.6
Nonsmokers	0.5	0.7	1.1	2.1	14.1	32.0
IUD	1.3	1.1	1.3	1.3	1.9	2.1
Abortion	0.5	1.1	1.3	1.9	1.8	1.1
Barrier methods (birth-related)	1.5	1.4	1.0	0.8	1.3	7.6

SOURCE: Adapted from Ory.

therapy has short-term positive effects on calcium balance and long-term beneficial effects on bone density. Third, in women given estrogen therapy, the incidence of fractures is decreased.

Of the potential side effects, the possibility of an increased risk of endometrial carcinoma is perhaps most worrisome. The relative risk of developing endometrial adenocarcinoma in estrogen users is between 6 and 8. The risk is increased with duration and dosage of estrogen but is less in women given combination estrogen-progestogen therapy.

Despite the large body of evidence linking endometrial carcinoma and estrogen use, two types of doubt have been raised about the clinical significance of the association. First, some epidemiologists have argued that the increased risk associated with estrogens has been exaggerated because of problems inherent in obtaining adequate controls in retrospective analyses. Second, despite an increased incidence of endometrial carcinoma in the United States, there was no concomitant increased mortality from this disease. Indeed, the increased incidence apparently involves low-grade malignancies which may be difficult to distinguish histologically from various forms of hyperplasia. These forms of malignancy have little effect on life expectancy.

Apprehension concerning worsening of hypertension and thromboembolic disease appears to be due to reports of the effects of estrogen-progestogen oral contraceptives during the reproductive years and not to estrogen use in menopausal women. There is no documented evidence that low-dose estrogen therapy in the menopause increases the incidence or the severity of thromboembolic disease, breast cancer, or hypertension. Low-dose estrogen treatment in the menopause does not appear to influence the development of atherosclerosis, myocardial infarction, or stroke. Strong evidence suggests that, in fact, estrogens may decrease the incidence of death from myocardial infarction. There is a slightly increased risk for the development of gallbladder disease with estrogen use in the menopause.

A reasonable approach to the use of estrogens in the menopause is as follows: (1) For long-term use, estrogens should be given in the minimal effective doses (0.625 mg conjugated estrogen orally or 0.01 to 0.02 mg ethinyl estradiol orally per day or transdermal estradiol 0.05 mg every 3 to 4 days). Except when hot flashes preclude intermittent use, the agents are often prescribed for 25 days each month followed by a rest period. (For women with an intact uterus, it is the practice in some clinics to give estrogens alone for 15 days, estrogen plus a daily progestogen for an additional 10 to 13 days, and nothing for a week. Other regimens include continuous estrogen treatment plus cyclic progestogens or low-dose continuous progestogens.) (2) Such replacement therapy is indicated routinely in women undergoing premature menopause (surgically induced or spontaneous) at least until the age of normal menopause. (3) Estrogen therapy is also indicated routinely in women of all ages who have severe hot flashes or symptomatic atrophy of the urogenital epithelium. Hot flashes rarely persist for longer than 4 years, so if given for this purpose, the duration of therapy can be limited. (4) In women who have had prior hysterectomy, potential benefits of treatment appear to outweigh the dangers. In women who do not have a uterus, cyclic or continuous estrogen without progestogen is recommended. Whether estrogens should be given routinely to all women with intact uteri is unsettled, but the authors prescribe it routinely in the absence of contraindications in hopes of ameliorating osteoporosis (in combination with calcium). (5) Each woman receiving estrogens must be monitored indefinitely at yearly intervals.

DRUGS TO INDUCE OVULATION   The most common treatment for ovulation induction in women with PCOD is *clomiphene*. This antiestrogen is believed to act as an antiestrogen in the hypothalamus and allow FSH to rise to stimulate follicular development and ultimately result in ovulation. Clomiphene therapy is usually begun in a dose of 50 mg by mouth daily for 5 days commencing on the fifth day of progestogen-induced uterine bleeding. If ovulation does not occur, the dose may be increased to 100 or 150 mg/d. Such treatment results in ovulatory cycles in 60 percent of women with PCOD. Additional regimens include clomiphene in combination with human menopausal gonadotropins (hMG), estrogen, glucocorticoids, or human chorionic gonadotropin (hCG).

The most commonly used gonadotropins for induction of ovulation are hMG, urofollitropin, and hCG. These agents are indicated in women who fail to ovulate on clomiphene. (For women with hypogonadotropic hypogonadism, urofollitropin is not recommended.) The usual treatment regimen requires 1 to 3 ampuls of hMG or urofollitropin per day over an 8- to 12-day period to achieve adequate follicular stimulation and growth, followed by a single injection of 10,000 units of hCG 12 to 24 h after the last injection of hMG. For women with PCOD, pretreatment with LHRH analogues prior to hMG or urofollitropin appears to improve ovulation and pregnancy rates. Ovulation is successful in 90 percent of women, and pregnancy rates exceed 50 to 60 percent. Measurement of daily estrogen levels and frequent evaluation of ovarian size by ultrasound are indicated to prevent ovarian hyperstimulation. Ovarian hyperstimulation syndrome results from excessive stimulation of ovarian follicles with resultant enlargement of the ovaries and may progress to the development of ascites, hypotension, and shock. Therapy using hMG, urofollitropin, and hCG also carries a 20 percent risk of multiple pregnancies.

Bromocriptine is a dopamine agonist that is effective in inducing ovulation in women with elevated prolactin levels. Treatment is instituted at a usual dosage of 2.5 mg by mouth two or three times a day. Treatment should be discontinued as soon as pregnancy is diagnosed. The management of prolactin-secreting pituitary tumors is discussed in Chap. 331.

Luteinizing hormone–releasing hormone (LHRH, gonadorelin) and analogues   Gonadorelin has been used successfully to induce ovulation in infertile women. The agent is infused subcutaneously or intravenously by a portable infusion pump which administers pulses at 90- to 120-min intervals for 10 to 20 days. After ovulation has occurred, hCG is given to maintain corpus luteum function.

LHRH analogues that block ovulation have been used to treat a variety of gynecologic disorders; ovulation and ovarian steroidogenesis are inhibited due to down-regulation of LHRH receptors with a resultant decreased release of gonadotropins. Conditions in which these agents are under trial include fertility control, true precocious puberty, endometriosis, uterine leiomyomas, hirsutism, and, in combination with gonadotropins, ovulation induction and in vitro fertilization.

OTHER DISORDERS OF THE FEMALE REPRODUCTIVE TRACT

VULVA   Most disorders of the vulva are due to venereal disease, most commonly syphilis (painless chancre), condylomata acuminata (venereal warts), and herpes vulvitis (painful ulcers) (see Chap. 88). All other lesions of the vulva, particularly in older women, must be biopsied. Early biopsy of cancer of the vulva is mandatory, because when it becomes symptomatic (pruritus and bleeding), it has often progressed to an advanced stage.

VAGINA   Infections of the vagina usually present as vaginal discharge and pruritus. The most frequent organisms are *Trichomonas*, *Candida albicans*, and *Gardnerella vaginalis* (also see Chap. 88). The diagnosis is made by microscopic examination of the discharge, and appropriate therapy can be instituted utilizing vaginal or oral antibiotics.

Abnormalities of the vagina and cervix in female offspring of women given diethylstilbestrol during pregnancy include adenosis of the vagina as well as structural abnormalities of the vagina, cervix, and uterus; the risk of developing a rare form of vaginal cancer (adenocarcinoma, clear cell type) is increased (2 per 10,000 exposed women). Periodic examination of women at risk should commence at ages 12 to 14, and reevaluation should be undertaken after any episode of abnormal bleeding.

CERVIX Preinvasive lesions of the cervix (also known as *cervical intraepithelial neoplasia*) as well as invasive carcinoma of the cervix can be detected reliably by obtaining a Papanicolaou smear (Pap smear). Current recommendations by the American Cancer Society are that a Pap smear be obtained every 3 years after 2 negative Pap smears were obtained at yearly intervals. However, many gynecologists recommend yearly Pap smears, especially in patients with more than one sexual partner.

UTERUS Only 40 percent of endometrial adenocarcinoma is detected by Pap smear. In women at high risk for endometrial carcinoma (obesity, history of chronic anovulatory cycles, diabetes, hypertension, estrogen treatment), yearly endometrial sampling should be performed. Low-dose oral estrogen therapy rarely causes breakthrough or withdrawal bleeding in menopausal women. Therefore, irrespective of whether the patient is on estrogen therapy, occurrence of postmenopausal bleeding makes it mandatory to obtain a tissue diagnosis to exclude endometrial cancer either by endometrial sampling or by curettage.

One of the most common disorders of the uterus and the most frequent tumor of women (1 of 4 women affected) is the uterine leiomyoma, or fibroid tumor. Three-fourths of women with leiomyoma are asymptomatic, and the diagnosis is made on routine pelvic examination. When associated with excessive menstrual blood loss, excessive size or rapid growth, or significant pelvic pain (see Chap. 48), the preferred treatment is surgical removal by hysterectomy if there is no desire for further childbearing. In young women, myomectomy may on occasion be indicated when infertility or repeated fetal wastage is a manifestation or where future childbearing is desired.

FALLOPIAN TUBES AND OVARIES Infectious pelvic inflammatory disease is a common disorder of the fallopian tubes and usually becomes symptomatic after a menstrual period; the symptoms include fever, chills, abdominal pain, and vaginal discharge, and pelvic tenderness on physical examination is common. The initiating organism most often is *Chlamydia trachomatis* or *Neisseria gonorrhoeae*, but tuboovarian abscess and sterility are probably caused by mixed aerobic and anaerobic superinfections and require wide-spectrum antibiotic treatment (see Chap. 89).

Endometriosis is a benign disorder characterized by the presence and proliferation of endometrial tissue (stroma and glands) outside the endometrial cavity. The clinical manifestations are variable. Endometriosis occurs most commonly between the ages of 30 and 40 and is found incidentally at the time of surgery in approximately one-fifth of all gynecologic operations. The fertility rate is significantly reduced in affected women. The disorder usually involves the posterior cul-de-sac or the ovaries and can give rise to ovarian enlargement (endometriomas), although it also may involve sites distant to the pelvis (lung, umbilicus). The most significant symptom is pelvic pain, characteristically dysmenorrhea (see Chap. 48). However, the frequency and degree of pelvic symptomatology correlate poorly with the extent of disease. Other symptoms include dyspareunia, pain with defecation, and infertility. The characteristic physical findings are multiple tender nodules palpable along the uterosacral ligament at the time of rectal-vaginal examination, a posteriorly fixed uterus, or enlarged cystic ovaries. The diagnosis can only be confirmed by direct visualization, usually at diagnostic laparoscopy. Treatment depends on the degree of involvement and the desires of the patient and includes observation for mild disease with no associated infertility or pain, hormonal suppressive therapy (see infertility), conservative surgery if fertility is desired, or removal of the uterus, tubes, and ovaries in severe disease. Endometriosis is rarely found after the menopause.

Any adnexal mass that persists for more than 6 weeks or is larger than 6 cm must be evaluated. Although ovarian cysts and neoplasms compose the largest group of pelvic adnexal masses (see above), tumors of the fallopian tubes, uterus, gastrointestinal tract, or urinary tract also should be considered. Sonography or radiographic evaluation is often helpful in identifying the nature of the adnexal mass prior to surgical exploration.

REFERENCES

ADASHI E: Putative intraovarian regulators. Semin Reprod Endocrinol 7:1, 1989

CARR BR: Disorders of the ovary and reproductive tract, in *Williams' Textbook of Endocrinology*, 8th ed, JD Wilson, DW Foster (eds). Philadelphia, Saunders, 1992, pp 733–798

——, BLACKWELL RE (eds): *Textbook of Reproductive Medicine*. Norwalk, Appleton & Lange, 1992

——, GRIFFIN JE: Fertility control and its complications, in *Williams' Textbook of Endocrinology*, 8th ed, JD Wilson, DW Foster (eds). Philadelphia, Saunders, 1992, pp 1007–1031

—— et al: Plasma levels of adrenocorticotropin and cortisol in women receiving oral contraceptive steroid treatment. J Clin Endocrinol Metab 49:346, 1979

—— et al: Plasma lipoprotein regulation or progesterone biosynthesis by human corpus luteum tissue in organ culture. J Clin Endocrinol Metab 52:875, 1981

—— et al: The role of lipoproteins in the regulation of progesterone secretion by human corpus luteum. Fertil Steril 38:303, 1982

CUNNINGHAM FG et al: *Williams' Obstetrics*, 18th ed. Norwalk, Appleton-Lange, 1989

D'ARMIENTO M et al: McCune-Albright syndrome: Evidence for autonomous multiendocrine hyperfunction. J Pediatr 102:584, 1983

DIZEREGA GS, HODGEN GD: Folliculogenesis in the primate ovarian cycle. Endocrinol Rev 2:27, 1981

DMOWSKI WP: Endocrine properties and clinical applications of danazol. Fertil Steril 31:237, 1979

ERICKSON GF et al: Functional studies of aromatase activity in human granulosa cells from normal and polycystic ovaries. J Clin Endocrinol Metab 49:514, 1979

—— et al: The ovarian androgen producing cells: A review of structure/function relationships. Endocr Rev 6:371, 1985

FAIMAN C et al: Patterns of gonadotropins and gonadal steroids throughout life. Clin Obstet Gynaecol 3:467, 1976

FILSHIE M, GUILLEBAND J (eds): *Contraception: Science and Practice*. London, Butterworths, 1989

FUTTERWEIT W: *Polycystic Ovarian Disease*. New York, Springer-Verlag, 1984

GEMZELL C, WANG CF: Outcome of pregnancy in women with pituitary adenoma. Fertil Steril 31:363, 1979

GLUCKMAN PD et al: The human fetal hypothalamus and pituitary gland, in *Maternal-Fetal Endocrinology*, D Tulchinksy, KJ Ryan (eds). Philadelphia, Saunders, 1980

GOLDZIEHER JW: Polycystic ovarian disease. Fertil Steril 35:371, 1981

GRUMBACH MM, CONTE FA: Disorders of sex differentiation, in *Williams' Textbook of Endocrinology*, 8th ed, JD Wilson, DW Foster (eds). Philadelphia, Saunders, 1992, pp 853–952

——, STYNE DM: Puberty: Ontogeny, neuroendocrinology, physiology and disorders, in *Williams' Textbook of Endocrinology*, 8th ed, JD Wilson, DW Foster (eds). Philadelphia, Saunders, 1992, pp 1139–1222

HATCHER RA et al: *Contraceptive Technology 1990–1992*. New York, Irvington, 1992

HERBST AL et al: *Comprehensive Gynecology*. 2d ed. St. Louis, Mosby, 1992

HSUEH AJW et al: Hormonal regulation of the differentiation of cultured ovarian granulosa cells. Endocr Rev 5:76, 1984

JONES HW JR et al (eds): *In Vitro Fertilization*. Baltimore, Williams & Wilkins, 1986

JUDD HL et al: Estrogen replacement therapy: Indications and complications. Ann Intern Med 98:195, 1983

KAPLAN SA (ed): *Clinical Pediatric Endocrinology*. Philadelphia, Saunders, 1990

KASE N, WEINGOLD A: *Principles and Practice of Clinical Gynecology*. New York, Wiley, 1983

KELCH RP: Management of precocious puberty. N Engl J Med 312:1057, 1985

KNOBIL E, NEILL JD (eds): *The Physiology of Reproduction*. New York, Raven, 1988

MISHELL DR JR, DAVAJAN V (eds): *Reproductive Endocrinology, Infertility, and Contraception*, 2d ed. Philadelphia, Davis, 1986

PIEPER DR et al: Ovarian gonadotropin-releasing hormone (GnRH) receptors: Characterization, distribution, and induction by GnRH. Endocrinology 108:1148, 1981

RIGGS BL et al: Effect of the fluoride/calcium regimen on vertebral fracture occurrence in postmenopausal osteoporosis. N Engl J Med 306:446, 1982

ROSS JL et al: A preliminary study of the effect of estrogen dose on growth in Turner's syndrome. N Engl J Med 309:1104, 1983

SCULLY RE: Ovarian tumors: A review. Am J Pathol 87:686, 1977

SEIBEL MM: A new era in reproductive technology. N Engl J Med 318:828, 1988

SHEARMAN RP (ed): *Clinical Reproductive Endocrinology*, Edinburgh, Churchill Livingston, 1985

SITTERI PK, MACDONALD PC: Role of extraglandular estrogen in human endocrinology, in *Handbook of Physiology*, sec 7, *Endocrinology*, SR Geiger et al (eds). Washington, American Physiological Society, 1973, p 615

SPEROFF L: Menopause. Semin Reprod Endocrinol 1:1, 1983

——: *Clinical Gynecologic Endocrinology and Infertility*, 4th ed. Baltimore, Williams & Wilkins, 1989

STEINGOLD KA et al: Treatment of hot flashes with transdermal estradiol administration. J Clin Endocrinol Metab 61:627, 1985

STUDD JWW, WHITEHEAD MI (eds): *The Menopause*. Oxford, Blackwell, 1988

STYNE DM, GRUMBACH MM: Disorders of puberty in the male and female, in *Reproductive Endocrinology*, SSC Yen, RB Jaffe (eds). Philadelphia, Saunders, 1991, pp 11–54

THOMPSON JD, ROCK JA: *Te Lindes Operative Gynecology*. Philadelphia, Lippincott, 1992

WALLACH EE, KEMPERS RD: *Modern Trends in Infertility and Contraception Control*, vol 3. Baltimore, Williams & Wilkins, 1985

WENTZ AC et al: *Gynecologic Endocrinology and Infertility*, Baltimore, Williams & Wilkins, 1988

YEN SSC: Neuroendocrine regulation of the menstrual cycle. Hosp Prac 14:84, 1979

————: Clinical application of gonadotropin-releasing hormone and gonadotropin-releasing hormone analogs. Fertil Steril 39:257, 1983

————, JAFFE RB (eds): *Reproductive Endocrinology*, 3d ed. Philadelphia, Saunders, 1991

YING SY et al: Gonadocrinins: Peptides in ovarian follicular fluid stimulating the secretion of pituitary gonadotropins. Endocrinology 108:1206, 1981

341 ENDOCRINE DISORDERS OF THE BREAST

JEAN D. WILSON

Examination of the breasts is an important part of the physical examination. The breasts are the site of fatal and preventable disease in women and provide clues to underlying systemic illness in both men and women. The internist frequently does not examine the male breast and is apt to refer the evaluation of the female breast to a gynecologist. It is the duty of every physician to distinguish the abnormal from the normal at the earliest possible stage and to call for assistance if there is any doubt. (For cancer of the breast see Chap. 319.)

ENDOCRINE CONTROL OF THE BREAST   There is no histologic or functional difference in the breasts of boys and girls prior to the onset of puberty, but a profound sexual dimorphism in breast development ensues at the time of puberty. The endocrine control of female breast development is illustrated in Fig. 341-1. The pubertal growth of the female breast is dependent primarily on the action of estradiol, which induces the growth, division, and elongation of the tubular duct system and maturation of the nipples. In men the administration of estrogen is equally effective in this regard. To produce true alveolar development at the ends of the ducts, however, the synergistic action of progesterone is required, a ratio of estrogen to progesterone of 1:20 to 1:100 being optimal. Once the anatomic development of the ducts and alveoli is complete, the continued action of estrogen and progesterone does not appear to be required for lactation itself.

The endocrine control of milk formation is complex, requiring, in addition to appropriate priming by estrogen and progesterone, specific lactogenic hormone and the permissive action of glucocorticoid, insulin, thyroxine, and, in some species, growth hormone. There are

FIGURE 341-1   Endocrine control of female breast development and function at various stages of life.

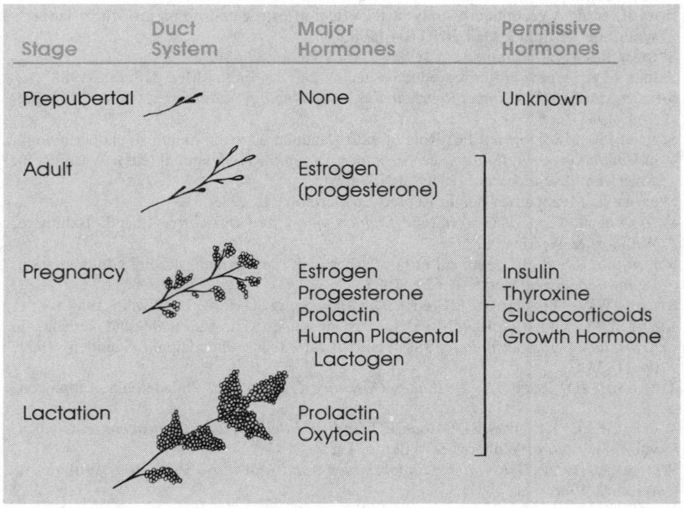

Stage	Duct System	Major Hormones	Permissive Hormones
Prepubertal		None	Unknown
Adult		Estrogen (progesterone)	
Pregnancy		Estrogen Progesterone Prolactin Human Placental Lactogen	Insulin Thyroxine Glucocorticoids Growth Hormone
Lactation		Prolactin Oxytocin	

two lactogenic hormones. Human placental lactogen (hPL or chorionic somatomammotropin) is secreted in large amounts by the placenta during the latter part of gestation and prepares the breast for milk production. hPL disappears from the fetal (and maternal) circulation shortly after termination of pregnancy. Pituitary prolactin (see Chap. 331) plays the critical role in the initiation and maintenance of lactation during the puerperium. The plasma level of prolactin rises during pregnancy; during late pregnancy and lactation, 60 to 80 percent of the anterior pituitary may consist of prolactin-secreting cells.

Unlike most pituitary hormones, the predominant regulation of prolactin secretion is negative, i.e., under ordinary basal conditions one or more inhibitory hypothalamic hormones, the most important being dopamine, is delivered to the pituitary via the hypothalamic portal system and inhibits the release of prolactin into the blood (see Chap. 331). Most factors that influence prolactin secretion do so by affecting the synthesis or release of the inhibiting factor(s). Basal prolactin levels fall following delivery, but prolactin secretion is enhanced by stimulation of the breasts, such as the act of nursing (the so-called sucking reflex), a phenomenon that is probably mediated by the reflex release of oxytocin. In the postgestational state, the normal woman is capable of forming about a liter of milk per day containing 38 g fat, 70 g lactose, and 12 g protein. Normal lactation can be suppressed by the administration of estrogens or diethylstilbestrol, which inhibit milk production by direct effects on the breast, or bromocriptine, which inhibits prolactin secretion by the pituitary. Alternatively, if a woman does not nurse or empty her breasts postpartum, lactation usually ceases of its own accord in 1 to 2 weeks.

GALACTORRHEA   Exactly what constitutes nonpuerperal or inappropriate lactation is not always clearly defined in the literature. According to the studies of Friedman and Goldfein, no breast secretion whatsoever can be demonstrated in normal, regularly menstruating nulligravid women, but breast secretions can be demonstrated in a fourth of normal women who have been pregnant in the past; thus breast secretions may be of no clinical significance in these instances. Spontaneous leakage of milk from the breasts is usually of more importance than milk that must be expressed. A second problem is related to the composition of the breast secretions. When the secretion is milky or white, it is safe to assume that it contains fat, casein, and lactose and is in fact milk; however, when the secretion is brown or greenish, it rarely contains normal milk constituents and consequently may not result from an underlying endocrinopathy. Milk also must be distinguished from blood or bloody discharges that may be due to neoplasms of the breast. It also should be kept in mind that the composition of milk constituents may increase upon repeated sampling from low, colostrum-like values to those typical of milk (see Chap. 319). With these problems in mind, galactorrhea can be defined as inappropriate production of milk that is persistent or worrisome to the patient, recognizing that in some instances no underlying pathology may be demonstrated.

Since the action of a lactogenic hormone is necessary for the initiation of milk production, it is logical to consider galactorrhea as a consequence of deranged prolactin physiology. However, as indicated above, a complex endocrinologic milieu is necessary for lactation, and in many instances in which prolactin is elevated, both in women who have not been appropriately primed and in men, no production of milk takes place. As a consequence, hyperprolactinemia is more common than galactorrhea. Furthermore, while enhanced prolactin secretion is necessary for the initiation of lactation, continued production can be maintained in the presence of minimally or intermittently elevated prolactin levels so that basal plasma prolactin levels are not always elevated in patients with galactorrhea. For example, repeated stimulation of the nipples of women who have previously been pregnant can cause galactorrhea with minimal elevations of basal prolactin (the wet nurse phenomenon). Perhaps the strongest evidence for a critical role for prolactin in galactorrhea is the fact that administration of bromocriptine, which suppresses plasma prolactin levels, causes a disappearance of galactorrhea even when the basal plasma prolactin levels are normal.

Differential diagnosis Galactorrhea is due either to a failure of the normal hypothalamic inhibition of prolactin release, to enhanced prolactin-releasing factor(s), or to autonomous prolactin secretion by tumors (Table 341-1). Pituitary stalk section results in a striking increase in prolactin secretion, as the result of the interruption of the delivery of prolactin inhibitory factors to the pituitary. Likewise, many drugs that influence the central nervous system (including virtually all psychotropic agents, methyldopa, reserpine, and antiemetics) cause enhanced prolactin release, presumably by inhibiting synthesis or release of dopamine or prolactin inhibitory factors such as dopamine. Estrogens enhance prolactin levels by an uncertain mechanism. Extrapituitary central nervous system diseases presumably cause galactorrhea by interfering with delivery of the inhibitory factors to the pituitary (central nervous system sarcoidosis, craniopharyngioma, pinealoma, encephalitis, meningitis, hydrocephalus, hypothalamic tumors).

In primary hypothyroidism, galactorrhea results from enhanced prolactin-releasing activity. Thyrotropin-releasing hormone (TRH) stimulates prolactin release, and thyroid hormone replacement cures the galactorrhea. A similar mechanism, as the result of enhanced secretion of oxytocin, may cause the galactorrhea of breast trauma.

Enhanced prolactin release also can occur from pituitary or nonpituitary tumors. Three types of pituitary tumors (see Chap. 331) may be associated with galactorrhea: pure prolactin-secreting tumors (micro- or macroadenomas), mixed tumors that secrete both growth hormone and prolactin and result in acromegaly with galactorrhea, and some null cell adenomas. The latter may interfere with the delivery of inhibitory factors to the pituitary. Prolactin also can be secreted by other malignancies such as bronchogenic carcinoma, and hydatidiform moles and choriocarcinomas may secrete placental lactogen.

In four published series totaling more than 500 carefully studied patients, a pituitary tumor was identified in about one-fourth of the patients, other known causes could be identified in another fourth or fifth, and the remaining half fall into the idiopathic category. Many patients prove ultimately to have prolactin-secreting pituitary tumors, some probably have subtle disorders of hypothalamic function, and in others a drug-related cause may have been missed, but the fact remains that no satisfactory diagnosis is reached in many patients. When normal menses and galactorrhea coexist, the likelihood of establishing a diagnosis is poor.

Galactorrhea is unusual in men, even in the presence of profound elevations of plasma prolactin; when it does occur, it is usually upon the background of a feminizing state (see below).

Diagnostic evaluation If hyperprolactinemia is present, the workup is fundamentally that of a pituitary tumor once drug causes and hypothyroidism are excluded (see Chap. 331). Even when a specific cause cannot be identified and the diagnosis of idiopathic galactorrhea is made by exclusion, it is necessary to remember that pituitary tumors may subsequently become manifest. The higher the prolactin values and the more persistent the galactorrhea, the greater is the likelihood of such a development.

Treatment Breast binders can be effective in patients with mild galactorrhea of unknown etiology, presumably by preventing stimulation of the nipple and the consequent perpetuation of lactation. The aim of treatment in other instances is to correct the elevated prolactin, and resection of pituitary tumor, cessation of causative drugs, or correction of hypothyroidism is often followed by the disappearance of galactorrhea. Bromocriptine, which suppresses plasma prolactin, has been used to treat idiopathic hyperprolactinemia, prolactin-secreting tumors of the pituitary (see Chap. 331), and even in women with normoprolactinemic galactorrhea. This drug not only suppresses lactation but also may cause resumption of menstrual cycles (and even fertility) in patients with amenorrhea and galactorrhea.

GYNECOMASTIA A central issue in the evaluation of breast tissue in adult men is the separation of the normal from the abnormal. The incidence of active gynecomastia in autopsy data is between 5 and 9 percent, but Nuttall and colleagues have reported that approximately 40 percent of normal men and up to 70 percent of hospitalized men have palpable breast tissue. The reason for this discrepancy is not clear. On the one hand, it may be difficult to distinguish true breast tissue from masses of adipose tissue without true breast enlargement (lipomastia); in such cases, true gynecomastia can be separated from lipomastia by mammography or by sonography. Alternatively, the incidence of gynecomastia may have increased, or the autopsy data may underestimate the frequency of palpable breast tissue. Regardless, we are left with major uncertainties; the finding of gynecomastia (distinct from lipomastia) could indicate underlying pathology or a normal variant. For the purposes of this discussion, we shall assume that any palpable breast tissue in men (except for the three so-called physiologic states) can be due to an underlying endocrinopathy and deserves a limited evaluation.

Early gynecomastia is characterized by proliferation of both the fibroblastic stroma and the duct system, which elongates, buds, and duplicates. As gynecomastia persists, progressive fibrosis and hyalinization are associated with regression of epithelial proliferation. Eventually, the number of ducts decreases. Resolution occurs by reduction in size and epithelial content with gradual disappearance of the ducts, leaving hyaline bands that eventually disappear.

Growth of the breast in men, as in women, is mediated by estrogen and results from disturbances of the normal ratio of active androgen to estrogen in plasma or within the breast itself. As described in Chap. 339 estradiol formation in the normal man occurs principally by the conversion of circulating androgens to estrogens in extraglandular tissues; the normal ratio of production of testosterone to estradiol in adult men is approximately 100:1 (6 mg versus 45 μg), and the normal ratio of the two hormones in plasma is about 300:1. Growth of the breast ensues in men when this effective ratio decreases significantly as the result of diminished testosterone production or action, enhanced estrogen formation, or both processes occurring simultaneously.

Enlargement of the male breast can be a normal physiologic phenomenon at certain stages of life or the result of several pathologic states (Table 341-2).

Physiologic gynecomastia In the *newborn*, transient enlargement of the breast is due to the action of maternal and/or placental estrogens. The enlargement usually disappears in a few weeks but may persist longer. *Adolescent* gynecomastia is common at some time during puberty. The median age of onset is 14; it is often asymmetric, occasionally unilateral for a portion of its course, and frequently tender, and it regresses so that by age 20 only a small number of men have palpable vestiges of gynecomastia in one or both breasts. Although the origin of the excess estrogen has not been identified, the onset of gynecomastia correlates with transient elevations of plasma estradiol prior to the completion of puberty so that the

---

TABLE 341-1   Classification of galactorrhea

Failure of normal hypothalamic inhibition of prolactin release
  A Pituitary stalk section
  B Drugs (phenothiazines, butyrophenones, methyldopa, tricyclic antide-
    pressants, opiates, reserpine, verapamil)
  C Central nervous system disease, including extrapituitary tumors and null
    cell adenomas of the pituitary
Enhanced prolactin-releasing factor
  Hypothyroidism
  Sucking reflex and breast trauma
Autonomous prolactin release
  A Pituitary tumors
    1 Prolactin-secreting tumors
    2 Mixed growth hormone and prolactin-secreting tumors
    3 Chromophobe adenomas
  B Ectopic production of human placental lactogen and/or prolactin
    1 Hydatidiform moles and choriocarcinomas
    2 Bronchogenic carcinoma and hypernephroma
Idiopathic

TABLE 341-2 Differential diagnosis of gynecomastia

PHYSIOLOGIC GYNECOMASTIA

Newborn
Adolescence
Aging

PATHOLOGIC GYNECOMASTIA

Deficient production or action of testosterone:
  Congenital defects:
    Congenital anorchia
    Klinefelter syndrome
    Androgen resistance (testicular feminization and Reifenstein syndrome)
    Defects of testosterone synthesis
  Secondary testicular failure:
    Viral orchitis
    Trauma
    Castration
    Neurologic and granulomatous diseases
    Renal failure
Increased estrogen production:
  Estrogen secretion:
    Testicular tumors
    True hermaphroditism
    Carcinoma of the lung and other tumors producing hCG
  Increased substrate for extraglandular aromatase:
    Adrenal disease
    Liver disease
    Malnutrition
    Hyperthyroidism
  Increase in extraglandular aromatase
Drugs:
  Estrogens (diethylstilbestrol, birth control pills, digitalis, estrogen-containing cosmetics, estrogen-contaminated foods, phytoestrogens)
  Drugs that enhance endogenous estrogen secretion (gonadotropins, clomiphene)
  Inhibitors of testosterone synthesis and/or action (ketoconazole, metronidazole, alkylating agents, cisplatin, spironolactone, cimetidine, flutamide, etomidate)
  Unknown mechanisms (busulfan, isoniazid, methyldopa, tricyclic antidepressants, penicillamine, diazepam, omeprazole, calcium-channel blockers, angiotensin-converting enzyme inhibitors, marijuana, heroin)
Idiopathic

---

androgen/estrogen ratio is low. *Gynecomastia of aging* also occurs in otherwise healthy men. Forty percent or more of aged men have gynecomastia. A likely explanation is the increase with age in the conversion of androgens to estrogens in extraglandular tissues. Abnormal liver function or drug therapy may be contributing causes in such men.

Pathologic gynecomastia Pathologic gynecomastia can result from one of three basic mechanisms: deficiency in testosterone production or action (with or without a secondary increase in estrogen production), increase in estrogen production, or drugs (Table 341-2). Most of the individual disorders that cause primary and secondary testicular failure have been discussed in Chap. 339. The fact that a deficiency in testosterone production by itself can cause gynecomastia is illustrated by the syndrome of congenital anorchia in which normal (or slightly low) estradiol production in the presence of profoundly decreased testosterone production results in florid gynecomastia. This mechanism is also responsible in some patients with Klinefelter syndrome and in men with testicular failure from other causes. In the inherited syndromes of androgen resistance, such as testicular feminization, deficient androgen action and increased testicular estrogen production are both present.

A primary increase in estrogen production can result from a variety of causes. Increased testicular estrogen secretion may result from elevations in plasma gonadotropins, for example, in cases of aberrant production of chorionic gonadotropin by testicular tumors or by bronchogenic carcinoma, from the ovarian elements in the gonads of men with true hermaphroditism, or as the result of direct secretion by testicular tumors (particularly Leydig cell and Sertoli cell tumors). Increased conversion of androgen to estrogens in extraglandular tissues can be due either to increased availability of substrate for

extraglandular estrogen formation or to increased amount of the enzymes of estrogen formation in peripheral tissues. Increased substrate availability for extraglandular conversion can result from increased production of androgens such as androstenedione (congenital adrenal hyperplasia, hyperthyroidism, and most feminizing adrenal tumors) or because of diminished catabolism of androstenedione by the usual pathways (liver disease). Increased amount of extraglandular aromatase can be caused by a rare hereditary abnormality or by tumors of the liver or adrenal gland.

Drugs can cause gynecomastia by several mechanisms. Many drugs either act directly as estrogens or cause an increase in plasma estrogen activity, for example, in men receiving diethylstilbestrol for prostatic carcinoma and in transsexuals in preparation for sex-change operations. Boys and young men are particularly sensitive to estrogen and can develop gynecomastia after the use of dermal ointments containing estrogen or after the ingestion of milk or meat from estrogen-treated animals. The gynecomastia of digitalis ingestion is usually attributed to an estrogen-like side effect of the drug, but in the experience of the author it usually occurs in men with abnormal liver function. A second mechanism of drug-induced gynecomastia is illustrated by gonadotropin, such as human chorionic gonadotropin, which causes enhanced testicular secretion of estrogen. Other drugs cause gynecomastia by interfering with testosterone synthesis (ketoconazole and alkylating agents) and/or testosterone action, for instance, by blocking the binding of androgen to its cytosol receptor protein in target tissues (spironolactone and cimetidine). Finally, drugs that cause gynecomastia by mechanisms which have not been defined include busulfan, ethionamide, isoniazid, methyldopa, tricyclic antidepressants, penicillamine, omeprazole, angiotensin-converting enzyme inhibitors, diazepam, marijuana, and heroin. In some instances, the feminization is due to effects of drugs on liver function.

Diagnostic evaluation The evaluation of patients with gynecomastia should include (1) a careful drug history, (2) measurement and examination of the testes (if both are small, a chromosomal karyotype should be obtained; if they are asymmetric, a workup for testicular tumor should be instituted), (3) evaluation of liver function, and (4) endocrine evaluation to include measurement of serum androstenedione or 24-h urinary 17-ketosteroids (usually elevated in feminizing adrenal states), measurement of plasma estradiol and hCG (helpful if elevated but usually normal), and measurement of plasma luteinizing hormone (LH) and testosterone. If LH is high and testosterone is low, the diagnosis is usually testicular failure; if LH and testosterone are both low, the diagnosis is most likely increased primary estrogen production (e.g., a Sertoli cell tumor of the testis); and if both LH and testosterone are elevated, the diagnosis is either an androgen-resistance state or a gonadotropin-secreting tumor.

A satisfactory diagnosis can be made in only half or less of patients referred for gynecomastia. This implies either that the diagnostic techniques are not sufficiently refined to recognize mild disturbances, that many causes of gynecomastia are as yet undefined, that the causes may be transient and difficult to diagnose, or, as suggested by Nuttall, that gynecomastia may in some instances be normal rather than due to a pathologic state. Because of the problem of separating the normal from the pathologic, gynecomastia should probably be routinely worked up only if the drug history is negative, if the breast is tender (indicating rapid growth), or if the breast mass is larger than 4 cm in diameter. In other instances, a decision to perform an endocrine evaluation depends on the clinical context. For example, gynecomastia associated with signs of underandrogenization should be evaluated.

Treatment When the primary cause can be identified and corrected, the breast enlargement usually subsides promptly and eventually disappears. For example, androgen replacement therapy may produce dramatic improvement in men with testicular insufficiency. However, if the gynecomastia is of long duration (and fibrosis has replaced the original ductal hyperplasia), correction of the primary defect may not be followed by resolution. In such instances and when the primary cause cannot be corrected, surgery is the only effective therapy. Indications for surgery include several psychologic and/or cosmetic problems, continued growth, or a suspected malignancy. Although the relative risk of carcinoma of the breast is increased in men with gynecomastia, it is rare nevertheless. Prophylactic radiation of the breasts prior to the institution of diethylstilbestrol therapy is effective in preventing gynecomastia and has a low complication rate in elderly men. In rare patients who have painful gynecomastia and who are not candidates for other therapy, treatment with antiestrogens such as tamoxifen may be indicated.

REFERENCES

Galactorrhea

CAVANAUGH J et al: Gynecomastia and cirrhosis of the liver. Arch Intern Med 150:563, 1990

CHOTINER HC et al: Lactose and casein content of nonpuerperal breast secretion. J Reprod Med 22:267, 1979

FRANTZ AG, WILSON JD: Endocrine disorders of the breast, in *Williams' Textbook of Endocrinology*, 8th ed, JD Wilson, DW Foster (eds). Philadelphia, Saunders, 1992, p 593

FRIEDMAN S, GOLDFEIN A: Breast secretions in normal women. Am J Obstet Gynecol 104:846, 1969

JOHNSON DG et al: Prolactin secretion and biological activity in females with galactorrhoea and normal circulating prolactin concentrations at rest. Clin Endocrinol 22:661, 1985

KLEINBERG DL et al: Galactorrhea: A study of 235 cases, including 48 with pituitary tumors. N Engl J Med 296:589, 1977

KOPPELMAN MCS et al: Hyperprolactinemia, amenorrhea, and galactorrhea. A retrospective assessment of twenty-five cases. Ann Intern Med 100:115, 1984

KULSKI JK et al: Changes in the milk composition of nonpuerperal women. Am J Obstet Gynecol 139:597, 1981

PADILLA SL et al: The efficacy of bromocriptine in patients with ovulatory dysfunction and normoprolactinemic galactorrhea. Fertil Steril 44:695, 1985

RUIZ-VELASCO V: Hyperprolactinemia and mammary prostheses. A report of eight cases. J Reprod Med 31:267, 1986

SAUER HJ: Physiology of lactation and factors affecting lactation. Obstet Gynecol Clin North Am 14:615, 1987

TURKSOY RN et al: Diagnostic and therapeutic modalities in women with galactorrhea. Obstet Gynecol 56:323, 1980

YAMAGUCHI M et al: Effects of nocturnal hyperprolactinemia on ovarian luteal function and galactorrhea. Eur J Obstet Gynecol 34:187, 1991

Gynecomastia

ANDERSON JA, GROOM JB: Male breast at autopsy. Acta Pathol Microbiol Immunol Scand 90:191, 1982

CIMORA GA et al: Percutaneous oestrogen-induced gynecomastia: A case report. Br J Plast Surg 35:209, 1982

DE GASPARO M et al: Antialdosterones: Incidence and prevention of sexual side effects. J Steroid Biochem 32:223, 1989

FASS D et al: Radiotherapeutic prophylaxis of estrogen-induced gynecomastia: A study of late sequela. Int J Radiation Oncology Bio Phys 12:407, 1986

FELDMAN D: Ketoconazole and other imidazole derivatives as inhibitors of steroidogenesis. Endocr Rev 7:409, 1986

FRANTZ AG, WILSON JD: Endocrine disorders of the breast, in *Williams' Textbook of Endocrinology*, 8th ed, JD Wilson, DW Foster (eds). Philadelphia, Saunders, 1992, p 953

KORENMAN SG: The endocrinology of the abnormal male breast. Ann NY Acad Sci 464:400, 1986

MABUCHI K et al: Risk factors for male breast cancer. J Natl Cancer Inst 74:371, 1985

MAHONEY CP: Adolescent gynecomastia: Differential diagnosis and management. Pediatr Clin North Am 37:1389, 1990

McDERMOTT MT et al: Tamoxifen therapy for painful idiopathic gynecomastia. South Med J 83:1283, 1990

NIEWOEHNER CV, NUTTALL FQ: Gynecomastia in a hospitalized male population. Am J Med 77:633, 1984

NUTTALL FQ: Gynecomastia as a physical finding in normal men. J Clin Endocrinol Metab 48:338, 1979

ROSE DP: Endocrine epidemiology of male breast cancer (review). Anticancer Res 8:845, 1988

342 DISORDERS OF SEXUAL DIFFERENTIATION

JEAN D. WILSON / JAMES E. GRIFFIN

Sexual differentiation is a sequential and ordered process. *Chromosomal sex,* established at the moment of fertilization, determines *gonadal sex,* and gonadal sex, in turn, causes the development of *phenotypic sex,* in which the male or female urogenital tract is formed (Table 342-1). A disturbance of any step in this process during embryogenesis may result in a disorder of sexual differentiation. Known causes of such disorders include environmental insults as in the ingestion of a virilizing drug during pregnancy, nonfamilial aberrations of the sex chromosomes as in 45,X gonadal dysgenesis, developmental birth defects of multifactorial etiology as in most cases of hypospadias, and hereditary disorders resulting from single gene mutations as in the testicular feminization syndrome.

Limitations of knowledge make it necessary to make empirical assignments as to the nature of the derangement in certain disorders. Nevertheless, a specific diagnosis usually can be made as the result of genetic, endocrine, phenotypic, and chromosomal assessment. As a consequence, appropriate gender assignment can be made, even in extreme instances of ambiguous genitalia, and tailoring of the phenotype can be undertaken when appropriate.

NORMAL SEXUAL DIFFERENTIATION

The first process in sexual differentiation is the establishment of chromosomal sex, the heterogametic sex (XY) being male and the homogametic sex (XX) female. The embryos of both sexes then develop in an identical fashion until approximately 40 days of gestation. The second phase of sexual differentiation is the conversion of the indifferent gonad into a testis or an ovary. The differentiation of the indifferent gonad into a testis is mediated by one or more sex-determining genes on the short arm of the Y chromosome (SRY); indeed, no matter how many X chromosomes are present (as in 47,XXY, 48,XXXY, etc.), a testis will develop as long as a Y chromosome is present. The final process, the translation of gonadal sex into phenotypic sex, is the consequence of the type of gonad formed and the endocrine secretions of the fetal gonads. The development of phenotypic sex results in the formation of the male and female urogenital tracts.

The internal urogenital tract is derived from the wolffian and müllerian ducts that exist side by side in early embryos of both sexes

---

TABLE 342-1 Classification of disorders of sexual development

Disorders of chromosomal sex
  Klinefelter syndrome
  XX male
  Gonadal dysgenesis
  Mixed gonadal dysgenesis
  True hermaphroditism
Disorders of gonadal sex
  Pure gonadal dysgenesis
  Absent testis syndrome
Disorders of phenotypic sex
  Female pseudohermaphroditism
    Congenital adrenal hyperplasia
    Nonadrenal female pseudohermaphroditism
    Developmental disorders of müllerian ducts
  Male pseudohermaphroditism
    Abnormalities in androgen synthesis
    Abnormalities in androgen action
    Persistent müllerian duct syndrome
    Development defects of male genitalia

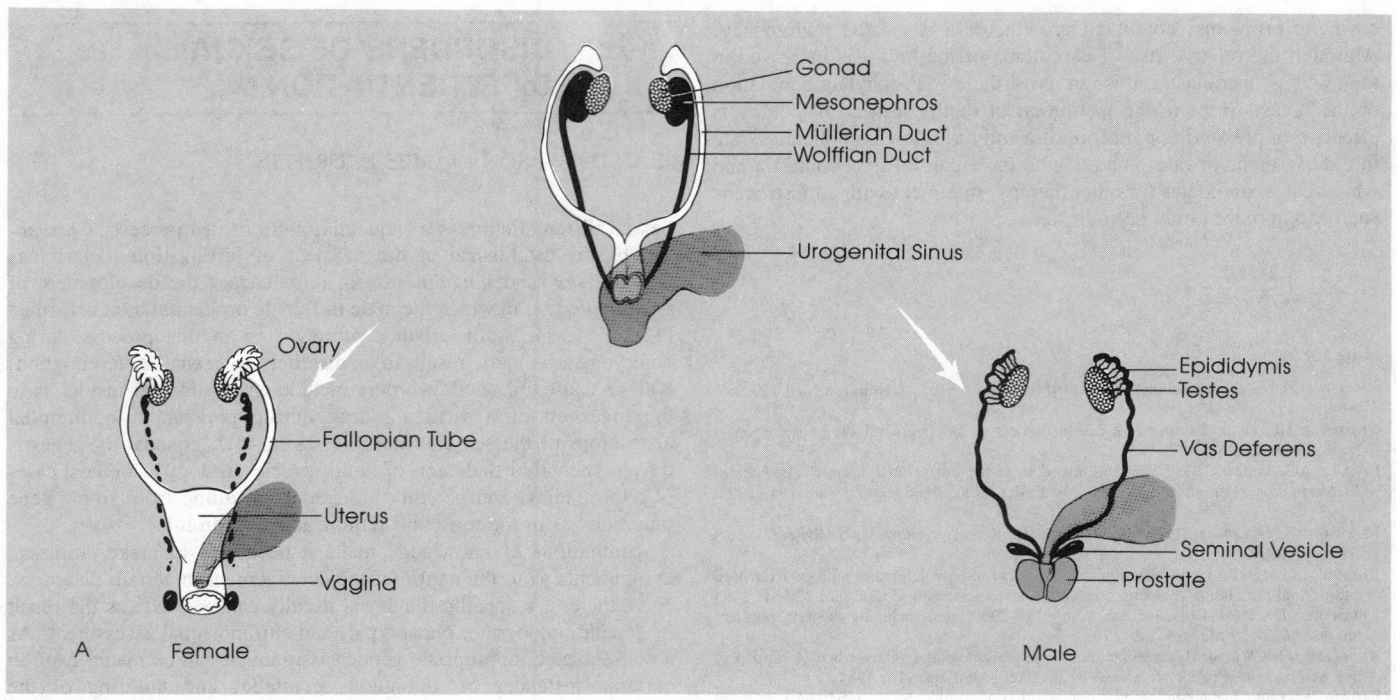

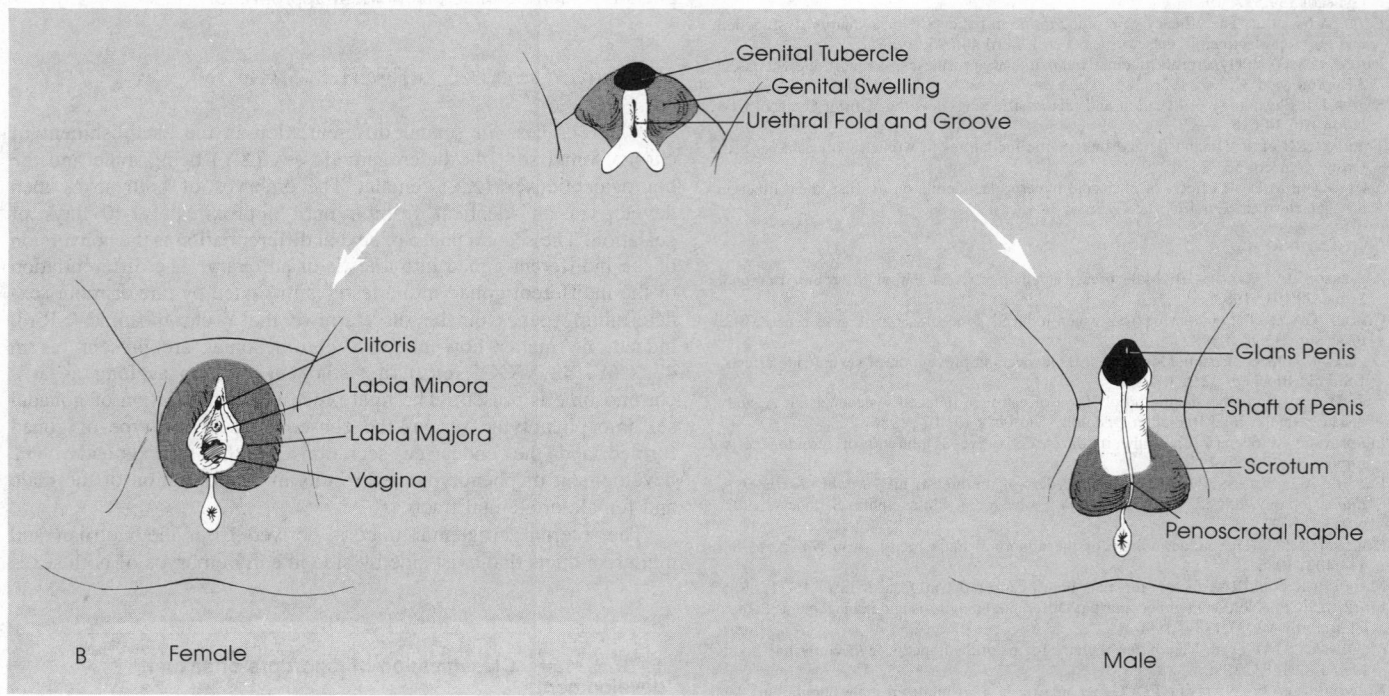

FIGURE 342-1   Normal sexual differentiation. *A*. Internal urogenital tract. *B*. External genitalia.

(Fig. 342-1*A*). In the male the wolffian ducts give rise to the epididymides, vasa deferentia, and seminal vesicles, and the müllerian ducts disappear. In the female the fallopian tubes, uterus, and upper vagina are derived from the müllerian ducts, and the wolffian ducts regress. The external genitalia and urethra in the two sexes develop from common anlage—the urogenital sinus and the genital tubercle, folds, and swellings (Fig. 342-1*B*). The urogenital sinus gives rise to the prostate and prostatic urethra in the male and to the urethra and lower portion of the vagina in the female. The genital tubercle is the origin of the glans penis in the male and the clitoris in the female. The urogenital swellings become the scrotum or the labia majora, and the urethral folds develop into the labia minora or fuse to form the shaft of the penis and the male urethra.

In the absence of the testis, as in the normal female or in the male embryo castrated prior to the onset of gonadal differentiation, phenotypic sex develops along female lines. Thus masculinization of the fetus is the positive result of action of hormones from the fetal testis, whereas female development does not require the presence of the ovary. Phenotypic sex normally conforms to chromosomal sex. That is, chromosomal sex determines gonadal sex, and gonadal sex, in turn, controls phenotypic sex.

The formation of the male phenotype is vested in the action of three hormones. Two—müllerian-inhibiting substance and testosterone—are secretory products of the fetal testis. Müllerian-inhibiting substance (MIS, also termed *antimüllerian hormone*, AMH) is a protein hormone that acts to suppress the müllerian ducts and prevent

TABLE 342-2 Clinical features of the disorders of chromosomal sex

Disorder	Common chromosomal complement	Gonadal development	External genitalia	Internal genitalia	Breast development	Comment
Klinefelter syndrome	47,XXY *or* 46,XY/47,XXY	Hyalinized testes	Normal male	Normal male	Gynecomastia	Most common disorder of sexual differentiation; tall stature.
XX male	46,XX	Hyalinized testes	Normal male	Normal male	Gynecomastia	Shorter than normal men; increased incidence of hypospadias. Similar to Klinefelter syndrome. May be familial.
Gonadal dysgenesis (Turner syndrome)	45,X *or* 46,XX/45,X	Streak gonads	Immature female	Hypoplastic female	Immature female	Short stature and multiple somatic abnormalities. May be 46,XX with structurally abnormal X chromosome.
Mixed gonadal dysgenesis	46,XY/45,X *or* 46,XY	Testis and streak gonad	Variable but almost always ambiguous; 60% reared as female	Uterus, vagina, and one fallopian tube	Usually male	Second most common cause of ambiguous genitalia in the newborn; tumors common.
True hermaphroditism	46,XX *or* 46,XY *or* mosaics	Testis and ovary or ovotestis	Variable but usually ambiguous; 60% reared as males	Usually a uterus and urogenital sinus; ducts correspond to gonad	Gynecomastia in 75%	May be familial.

development of the uterus and fallopian tubes in the male. Testosterone acts directly to stimulate virilization of the wolffian duct and is the precursor for the third embryonic male hormone, dihydrotestosterone (see Chap. 339). Dihydrotestosterone, which is formed from circulating testosterone, promotes development of the male urethra and prostate and formation of the penis and scrotum. Thus testosterone and dihydrotestosterone function during fetal life to induce formation of the male urogenital tract by the same intracellular machinery by which they act in postembryonic life (Chap. 339).

The secretion of testosterone by the fetal testis approaches a maximum by the eighth to tenth week of gestation, and formation of the sexual phenotypes is largely completed by the end of the first trimester. During the latter phases of gestation, the ovarian follicles develop and the vagina matures in the female and descent of the testes and growth of the external genitalia take place in the male.

DISORDERS OF CHROMOSOMAL SEX

Disorders of chromosomal sex (Table 342-2) occur when the number or structure of the X or Y chromosomes is abnormal (see Chap. 62).

KLINEFELTER SYNDROME Clinical features Klinefelter syndrome is characterized by small, firm testes, azoospermia, gynecomastia, and elevated levels of plasma gonadotropins in men with two or more X chromosomes. The common karyotype is either a 47,XXY chromosomal pattern (the classic form) or 46,XY/47,XXY mosaicism. The disorder is the most frequent major abnormality of sexual differentiation, the incidence being around 1 in 500 men.

Prepubertally, the testes are small but otherwise appear normal. After puberty, the disorder is manifest as infertility, gynecomastia, or occasionally underandrogenization (Table 342-3). Hyalinization of the seminiferous tubules and azoospermia are consistent features of the 47,XXY variety. The small, firm testes are characteristically less than 2 cm and always less than 3.5 cm in length (corresponding to 2- and 12-mL volume, respectively). The increased mean body height is the result of an increased lower body segment. Gynecomastia ordinarily develops during adolescence, is generally bilateral and painless, and may become disfiguring (see Chap. 341). Obesity and varicose veins occur in one-third to one-half, and mild mental deficiency, social maladjustment, abnormalities of thyroid function, diabetes mellitus, and pulmonary disease may be present. The risk of breast cancer is 20 times that of normal men (but only about a

fifth that in women). Most have a male psychosexual orientation and function sexually as normal men.

The mosaic variant comprises about 10 percent of the patients, as estimated by chromosomal karyotypes on peripheral blood leukocytes. The frequency of this variant may be underestimated, since chromosomal mosaicism may be present in the testes in subjects whose peripheral leukocyte karyotype is normal. The mosaic form is usually not as severe as the 47,XXY variety, and the testes may be normal in size (see Table 342-3). The endocrine abnormalities are less severe, and gynecomastia and azoospermia are less common. Indeed, occasional mosaic subjects may be fertile. In some the diagnosis may not even be suspected because of the minor manifestations.

Approximately 30 additional variants of Klinefelter syndrome have been described, including those with uniform cell lines (such as 48,XXYY, 48,XXXY, and 49,XXXXY) and a variety of mosaicisms of the X chromosome with or without associated structural abnormalities of the X. In general, the greater the degree of chromosomal abnormality (and in mosaic forms the more cell lines that are abnormal), the more severe are the manifestations.

Pathophysiology The classic form is due to meiotic nondisjunction of the chromosomes during gametogenesis (Fig. 342-2). About 40 percent of the responsible meiotic nondisjunctions occur during spermatogenesis, and 60 percent occur during oogenesis. Advanced maternal age is a predisposing factor. The mosaic form is thought to

TABLE 342-3 Characteristics of patients with classic versus mosaic Klinefelter syndrome*

	47,XXY, %	46,XY/47,XXY, %
Abnormal testicular histology	100	94[†]
Decreased length of testis	99	73[†]
Azoospermia	93	50[†]
Decreased testosterone	79	33
Decreased facial hair	77	64
Increased gonadotropins	75	33[†]
Decreased sexual function	68	56
Gynecomastia	55	33[†]
Decreased axillary hair	49	46
Decreased length of penis	41	21

* Table based on 519 XXY patients and 51 XY/XXY patients.
† Significantly different at $p < .05$ or better.
SOURCE: After Gordon et al.

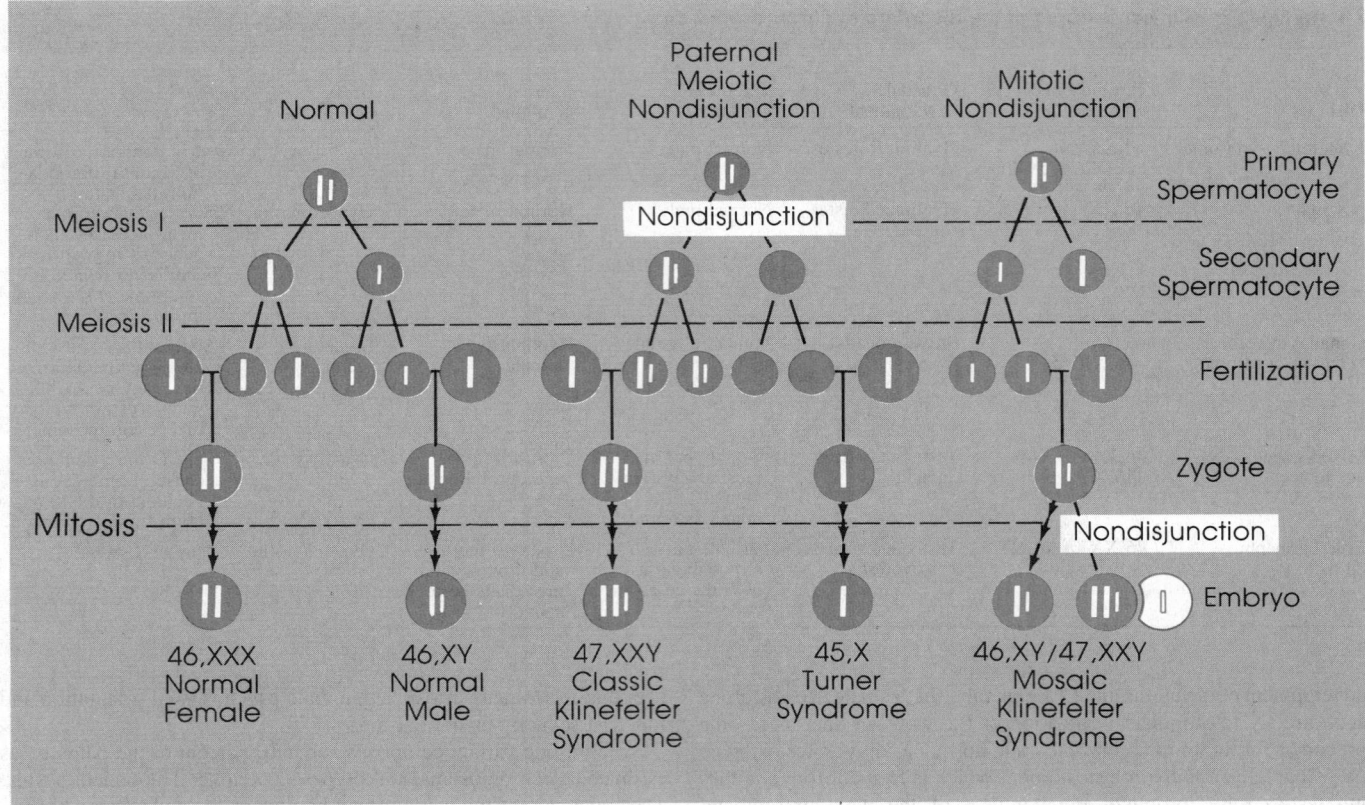

FIGURE 342-2   Schema for normal spermatogenesis and fertilization showing effects of meiotic and mitotic nondisjunction leading to classic Klinefelter syndrome, Turner syndrome, and mosaic Klinefelter. The schema would be similar if the abnormal events took place during oogenesis.

result from chromosomal mitotic nondisjunction after fertilization of the zygote and can take place either in a 46,XY zygote (see Fig. 342-2) or a 47,XXY zygote. The latter defect, or double nondisjunction (meiotic and mitotic), may be the usual cause and thus explain why the mosaic form is less frequent than the classic disorder.

Plasma follicle-stimulating hormone (FSH) and luteinizing hormone (LH) levels are usually high; FSH shows the best discrimination, and little overlap occurs with normal individuals, a consequence of the consistent damage to the seminiferous tubules. The plasma testosterone level averages half normal, but the range of values overlaps the normal range. Mean plasma estradiol levels are elevated, the cause of which is not entirely clear. Early, the testes may secrete increased amounts of estradiol in response to the elevated plasma LH level, but the testicular secretion of estradiol (and testosterone) eventually declines. Elevated plasma estradiol late in the course is probably due to a combination of a decreased metabolic clearance rate and an increased rate of conversion of testosterone to estradiol in extragonadal tissues. The net result both early and late is a variable degree of insufficient androgenization and enhanced feminization. The feminization, including gynecomastia, depends on the ratio of circulating estrogen to androgen (relative or absolute), and subjects with lower plasma testosterone and higher plasma estradiol levels are more likely to develop gynecomastia (see Chap. 341). The normal feedback inhibition of testosterone on pituitary LH secretion is diminished. Subjects with untreated Klinefelter syndrome may have enlarged or abnormal sella turcicas, presumably secondary to the persistent inadequate testosterone feedback and hyperplasia of the gonadotrophs. It is not known whether true adenoma formation occurs.

Management   No method is available for reversing the infertility, and surgical removal is the treatment for the gynecomastia. Some underandrogenized patients benefit from supplemental androgen, but such treatment may worsen the gynecomastia, presumably by providing increased androgen substrate for the conversion to estrogens in the peripheral tissues. Androgen should be administered in the form of testosterone cypionate or testosterone enanthate (see Chap. 339). Following the administration of testosterone, the plasma LH level returns to normal only after several months, if at all.

XX MALE SYNDROME   The incidence of a 46,XX karyotype in phenotypic males is approximately 1 in 20,000 to 24,000 male births. Affected individuals have absence of all female internal genitalia and male psychosexual identification. Indeed, the findings resemble those in Klinefelter syndrome: the testes are small and firm (generally less than 2 cm), gynecomastia is frequent, the penis is normal to small in size, azoospermia and hyalinization of the seminiferous tubules are usual, mean plasma testosterone level is low, plasma estradiol level is elevated, and plasma gonadotropin levels are high. Affected individuals differ from typical Klinefelter patients only in that average height is less than in normal men, the incidence of mental deficiency is not increased, and the incidence of hypospadias is increased.

The majority of XX males whose DNA is probed with Y-chromosome DNA fragments containing the SRY gene are positive for Y-related DNA; thus an X-Y interchange appears to be the common cause of the disorder. Other 46,XX males are negative for all Y-specific DNA, suggesting that these cases are the consequence of mutation in a downstream, autosomal or X-linked gene involved in development of the testes. The management is similar to that of Klinefelter syndrome.

GONADAL DYSGENESIS (TURNER SYNDROME)   Clinical features   Gonadal dysgenesis is characterized by primary amenorrhea, sexual infantilism, short stature, multiple congenital anomalies, and bilateral streak gonads in phenotypic women with any of several defects of the X chromosome. This condition should be distinguished from (1) mixed gonadal dysgenesis in which a unilateral testis and a contralateral streak gonad may be present, (2) pure gonadal dysgenesis in which bilateral streak gonads are associated with a normal 46,XX or 46,XY karyotype, normal stature, and primary amenorrhea, and (3) the Noonan syndrome, an autosomal dominant disorder of males and females characterized by webbed neck, short stature, congenital heart disease, cubitus valgus, and other congenital defects despite normal karyotypes and normal gonads.

The incidence is estimated at 1 in 2500 newborn females. The diagnosis is made either at birth because of the associated anomalies or more frequently at puberty when amenorrhea and failure of sexual development are noted in conjunction with the associated anomalies. Gonadal dysgenesis is the most common cause of primary amenorrhea, accounting for a third of such patients. The external genitalia are unambiguously female but remain immature, and there is no breast development unless the patient is treated with exogenous estrogen. The internal genitalia consist of infantile fallopian tubes and uterus and bilateral streak gonads located in the broad ligaments. Primordial germ cells are present transiently during embryogenesis but disappear as the result of an accelerated rate of atresia (see Chap. 340). After the age of expected puberty, these streaks lack identifiable follicles and ova but contain fibrous tissue that is indistinguishable from normal ovarian stroma.

The associated somatic anomalies primarily involve the skeleton and connective tissue. Lymphedema of the hands and feet, webbing of the neck, low hairline, redundant skin folds on the back of the neck, a shieldlike chest with widely spaced nipples, and a low birth weight are features that suggest the diagnosis in infancy. In addition, the facies may be characterized by micrognathia, epicanthal folds, prominent low-set or deformed ears, a fishlike mouth, and ptosis. Short fourth metacarpals are present in half, and 10 to 20 percent have coarctation of the aorta. In adults, the average height rarely exceeds 150 cm. Associated conditions include renal malformations, pigmented nevi, hypoplastic nails, tendency to keloid formation, perceptive hearing loss, unexplained hypertension, and autoimmune disorders. Hypothyroidism is present in 20 percent.

Pathophysiology About half have a 45,X karyotype, approximately one-fourth have mosaicism with no structural abnormality (46,XX/45,X), and the remainder have a structurally abnormal X chromosome with or without mosaicism (see Chap. 62). The 45,X variety may result from chromosome loss during gametogenesis in either parent or a mitotic error during one of the early cleavage divisions of the fertilized zygote (see Fig. 342-2). Short stature and other somatic features result from loss of genetic material on the short arm of the X chromosome. Streak gonads result when genetic material is missing from either the long or short arm of the X. In individuals with mosaicism or structural abnormalities of the X, phenotypes on average are intermediate in severity between that seen in the 45,X variety and the normal. In some patients with hypertrophy of the clitoris, there is an unidentified fragment of a chromosome present in addition to the X chromosome, assumed to be an abnormal Y; malignancy may develop in the streak gonads in this subset of patients. Rarely, familial transmission of gonadal dysgenesis can be the result of a balanced X-autosome translocation (see Chap. 62). Analysis of chromosomal karyotype is necessary to establish the diagnosis and to identify the fraction with Y chromosomal elements and a high chance of developing malignancy in the streak gonads.

Sparse pubic and axillary hair develop at the time of expected puberty, the breasts remain infantile, and no menses occur. Serum FSH is elevated in infancy, falls during midchildhood to the normal range, and increases to castrate levels at the age of 9 or 10. At this time, the serum LH level is also elevated, and plasma estradiol levels are low [<40 pmol/L (<10 pg/mL)]. Approximately 2 percent of 45,X subjects and 12 percent of mosaic subjects have sufficient residual follicles to allow some menstruation. Indeed, occasional pregnancy has been reported in minimally affected individuals; the reproductive life in such individuals is brief.

Management At the anticipated time of puberty, replacement therapy with estrogen should be instituted to induce maturation of the breasts, labia, vagina, uterus, and fallopian tubes (see Chap. 340). Linear growth and bone maturation rates are approximately doubled during the first year of treatment with estradiol, but the eventual height of patients rarely approaches the predicted height. Combination therapy with oxandrolone and/or growth hormone accelerates growth, but it is not established whether such therapy has an effect on final height (see Chap. 332).

Gonadal tumors are rare in 45,X patients but have occurred in several patients with mosaicism involving the Y chromosome; consequently, streak gonads should be removed in any patient with evidence of virilization or a Y-containing cell line.

MIXED GONADAL DYSGENESIS Clinical features Mixed gonadal dysgenesis is an entity in which phenotypic males or females usually have ambiguous genitalia and a testis on one side and a streak gonad on the other. Most have 45,X/46,XY mosaicism, but the clinical entity is not confined to that chromosomal pattern. The incidence is unknown, but in most hospitals the disorder is the second most common cause of ambiguous genitalia in the neonate after congenital adrenal hyperplasia.

About two-thirds of such children are reared as females. Many have ambiguous genitalia, including some degree of phallic enlargement, a urogenital sinus, and varying degrees of labioscrotal fusion. In most the testis is located intraabdominally; individuals with a testis in the inguinal or scrotal position are usually reared as males. A uterus, vagina, and at least one fallopian tube are almost invariably present.

The prepubertal testis appears relatively normal. The postpubertal testis contains abundant mature Leydig cells, but the seminiferous tubules lack germinal elements and contain only Sertoli cells. The streak gonad, a thin, pale, elongated structure located either in the broad ligament or along the pelvic wall, is composed of ovarian stroma. At puberty the testis secretes androgen, and virilization and phallic enlargement both occur. Feminization is rare; when it occurs, estrogen secretion from a gonadal tumor should be suspected.

Approximately a third of such patients exhibit the somatic features of 45,X gonadal dysgenesis, i.e., low posterior hairline, shield chest, multiple pigmented nevi, cubitus valgus, webbing of the neck, and short stature (height less than 150 cm).

Approximately two-thirds have the 45,X/46,XY karyotype, and the remainder have a 46,XY karyotype or a variant mosaicism. The 45,X/46,XY karyotype is not necessarily associated with abnormal sexual development, and it may be discovered incidentally in phenotypically normal men and women. In addition, females with bilateral streak gonads and males with bilateral dysgenetic testes may have this karyotype. The origin of 45,X/46,XY mosaicism is best explained by the loss of a Y chromosome during an early mitotic division of an XY zygote similar to the postulated loss of the X chromosome in the 46,XY/47,XXY mosaicism shown in Fig. 342-2.

Pathophysiology It has been assumed that the 46,XY cell line stimulates testicular differentiation, whereas the 45,X stem leads to the development of the contralateral streak gonad, but actual comparisons between karyotype and phenotypic expression have failed to substantiate such a relationship. Furthermore, there is no clear correlation between the percentage of cells cultured from blood or skin containing 45,X or 46,XY and the degree of gonadal development or of somatic anomalies.

Both masculinization and müllerian duct regression in utero are incomplete. Since Leydig cell function is normal at puberty, inadequate virilization in utero may be the result of delayed development of a testis that is ultimately capable of normal Leydig cell function. Alternatively, the fetal testis may simply be incapable of synthesizing adequate amounts of müllerian-inhibiting substance and androgen.

Management For the older child or adult in whom gender is fixed prior to diagnosis, the central issue in management is the possibility of tumor development in the gonads. The overall incidence of gonadal tumors is about 25 percent. Seminomas occur more frequently than gonadoblastomas, and the tumors may occur prior to puberty. The tumors occur most frequently in patients with a female phenotype who lack the somatic features typical of 45,X gonadal dysgenesis and are more common in intraabdominal testes than in the streak gonad. When the diagnosis is established in phenotypic females, early exploratory laparotomy and prophylactic gonadectomy should be undertaken both because gonadal tumors may occur in childhood and because the testis secretes androgen at puberty and thus causes virilization. Such subjects, like those with gonadal dysgenesis, are then given estrogen to induce and maintain feminization.

When the diagnosis is established in phenotypic males during late childhood or in adults, the management is more complicated. Phenotypic males with mixed gonadal dysgenesis are infertile (no germinal elements are present in the testes) and have a high risk of developing gonadal tumors. Which testes can be safely conserved? In general, the following observations apply: (1) tumors develop in scrotal streak gonads but not in scrotal testes, (2) tumors that develop in intraabdominal testes are always associated with ipsilateral müllerian duct structures, and (3) tumors in streak gonads are always associated with tumors in the contralateral abdominal testis. Based on these observations, it is recommended that (1) all streak gonads should be removed, (2) scrotal testes should be preserved, and (3) intraabdominal testes should be excised unless they can be relocated in the scrotum and are not associated with ipsilateral müllerian duct structures. Decisions as to reconstructive surgery of the phallus depend on the nature of the defect.

When the diagnosis is established in early infancy and the genitalia are ambiguous, gender assignment is usually female. Resection of the enlarged phallus and gonadectomy can then be accomplished in infancy, sometimes in one procedure. If the decision is for male gender assignment, the same criteria apply as to which testes should be removed in infants as in older males.

TRUE HERMAPHRODITISM   Clinical features   True hermaphroditism is a condition in which both an ovary and a testis or a gonad with histologic features of both (ovotestis) is present. To justify the diagnosis, there must be histologic documentation of both types of gonadal epithelium, the presence of ovarian stroma without oocytes not being sufficient. The incidence is unknown, but more than 400 cases have been reported. Three categories are recognized: (1) one-fifth are bilateral—testicular and ovarian tissue (ovotestes) on each side, (2) two-fifths are unilateral—an ovotestis on one side and an ovary or a testis on the other, and (3) the remainder are lateral—a testis on one side and an ovary on the other.

The external genitalia display all gradations of the male-to-female spectrum. Two-thirds are sufficiently masculinized to be reared as males. However, less than one-tenth have normal male external genitalia; most have hypospadias, and more than half have incomplete labioscrotal fusion. Two-thirds of phenotypic females have an enlarged clitoris, and most have a urogenital sinus. Differentiation of the internal ducts usually corresponds to the adjacent gonad. Although an epididymis usually develops adjacent to a testis, development of the vas deferens is complete in only one-third. Of the patients with an ovotestis, three-fourths have an epididymis, two-thirds have a fallopian tube, one-tenth have a vas deferens, and one-tenth have both a vas deferens and a fallopian tube. A uterus is usually present, although it may be hypoplastic or unicornuate. The ovary usually occupies the normal position, but the testis or ovotestis may be found at any level along the route of embryonic testicular descent, frequently associated with an inguinal hernia. Testicular tissue is present in the scrotum or the labioscrotal fold in one-third, in the inguinal canal in one-third, and in the abdominal area in one-third.

Variable feminization and virilization ensue at puberty, three-fourths develop gynecomastia, and about half menstruate. In phenotypic men, menstruation presents as cyclic hematuria. Ovulation occurs in approximately one-fourth and is more common than spermatogenesis. In men, ovulation may present as testicular pain. Fertility has been reported in women following removal of an ovotestis and in a man who fathered two children. Congenital malformations of other systems are rare.

Pathophysiology   About two-thirds of subjects have a 46,XX karyotype, a tenth have a 46,XY karyotype, and the remainder are chimeras or mosaics in which a Y cell line is present. The mechanism responsible for the gonadal development is unknown. Even though

not demonstrable with conventional karyotyping methods, it was assumed that sufficient genetic material from the Y chromosome was present (as the result of translocation, nondisjunction, or mutation) to induce the development of testicular tissue. Indeed, approximately a fourth of 46,XX true hermaphrodites have genetic sequences indicative of Y to X translocation. In rare instances, multiple sibs with a 46,XX karyotype are affected, possibly the result of an autosomal or X-linked mutation. The cause of the remaining instances of the 46,XX disorder is unknown.

Because corpora lutea are present in the ovaries of more than one-fourth of subjects, it can be deduced that a female neuroendocrine axis is present and functions normally in such individuals. Feminization (gynecomastia and menstruation) is the result of secretion of estradiol by the ovarian tissue present. In masculinized patients, secretion of androgen predominates over secretion of estrogen, and some produce sperm.

Management   When the diagnosis is made in a newborn or early infant, gender assignment depends on the anatomic features. In older children and adults, gonads and internal duct structures that are contradictory to the predominant phenotype (and the gender of rearing) should be removed, and when necessary, the external genitalia should be modified appropriately. Although gonadal tumors are rare in true hermaphroditism, a gonadoblastoma has been reported in an individual with an XY cell line. Consequently, the possibility of future tumor development must be taken into account when the decision regarding conservation of gonadal tissue is made.

DISORDERS OF GONADAL SEX

Disorders of gonadal sex result when chromosomal sex is normal, but for one of several reasons differentiation of the gonads is abnormal. Thus gonadal sex does not correspond to chromosomal sex.

PURE GONADAL DYSGENESIS   Clinical features   Pure gonadal dysgenesis is a disorder in which phenotypic females with gonads and genitalia characteristic of gonadal dysgenesis (bilateral streaks, infantile uterus and fallopian tubes, and sexual infantilism) have normal height, few if any somatic anomalies, and either a normal 46,XX or 46,XY karyotype. This disorder is only about one-tenth as common as gonadal dysgenesis. It is genetically distinct from gonadal dysgenesis, but it cannot be distinguished clinically from instances of gonadal dysgenesis associated with minimal somatic abnormalities. The height is normal or greater than normal, some subjects being over 170 cm. Estrogen levels vary from profound deficiency typical of 45,X gonadal dysgenesis to some breast development and appearance of menses that terminate in an early menopause. About 40 percent have some feminization. Axillary and pubic hair are scanty, and the internal genitalia consist of müllerian derivatives only.

Tumors may develop in the streak gonads, particularly dysgerminoma or gonadoblastoma in the 46,XY disorder. Such tumors may be heralded by the development of virilizing signs or a pelvic mass.

Pathophysiology   Although chromosomal mosaicisms have been described under this nosology, the designation here is restricted to subjects with uniform 46,XX or 46,XY karyotypes. (Those with mosaicism are variants of gonadal dysgenesis or mixed gonadal dysgenesis, as described above.) The rationale for this restricted definition is based on the fact that both the XX and XY varieties can result from single gene mutations that are presumed to involve gene(s) essential for gonadal development. Several sibships have been reported in which more than one individual is affected with the 46,XX type of the disorder, frequently the result of consanguineous matings, suggesting an autosomal recessive pattern of inheritance. Familial occurrence of the 46,XY variety also has been described; in some the mutation appears to be inherited in an X-linked recessive pattern, while in other families the occurrence is compatible with a male-limited autosomal recessive inheritance. In some sporadic patients with the 46,XY form of the disorder, the SRY region of the short arm of the Y chromosome is deleted, and in two 46,XY subjects, mutations in the SRY gene have been described. In both the 46,XX and the 46,XY forms the disorder prevents differentiation of ovary or testis, respectively; the development of the female phenotype is the consequence of the failure of gonadal development. As in all individuals with nonfunctional gonads, gonadotropin secretion is elevated and estrogen secretion is low.

Management The management of the estrogen deficiency is identical to that in gonadal dysgenesis; namely, appropriate estrogen replacement therapy is initiated at the time of expected puberty and maintained in adult life (see Chap. 340). Because of the high frequency of gonadal tumors in the 46,XY variety, the streak gonads should be removed once the diagnosis is made. The development of virilizing signs is indication for immediate surgery. The natural history of the gonadal tumors in this disorder is uncertain, but the prognosis after surgical removal is usually good.

THE ABSENT TESTES SYNDROME (ANORCHIA, TESTICULAR REGRESSION, GONADAL AGENESIS, AGONADISM) **Clinical features** A spectrum of phenotypes has been described in 46,XY males with absent or rudimentary testes but in whom unequivocal evidence exists that endocrine function of the testis (e.g., invariable müllerian duct regression and variable testosterone synthesis) was present at some time during embryonic life. This rare disorder can be distinguished from pure gonadal dysgenesis in which no evidence can be inferred for gonadal function during embryonic development. The disorder varies in its manifestations from complete failure of virilization through varying degrees of incomplete virilization of the external genitalia to otherwise normal males with bilateral anorchia.

The purest form is represented by 46,XY females with absent testes, sexual infantilism, and absence of both müllerian duct derivatives and accessory organs of male reproduction. Such individuals differ from 46,XY pure gonadal dysgenesis in that no gonadal remnant can be identified, including no streak gonad, and in the absence of müllerian derivatives. Testicular failure must have occurred between the onset of formation of müllerian-inhibiting substance and the secretion of testosterone, i.e., after development of the seminiferous tubules but before the onset of Leydig cell function.

In others, the testicular failure must have occurred later in gestation, and these individuals may constitute problems in gender assignment. In some, failure of müllerian regression is more pronounced than failure of testosterone secretion, but none exhibit normal müllerian development. In those with more extensive virilization, the external genitalia are phenotypically male, but rudimentary oviducts and vasa deferentia may coexist internally.

At the final extreme is the syndrome of bilateral anorchia in which phenotypic men have absence of müllerian structures and gonads but male development of the wolffian system and external genitalia. Microphallus implies that failure of androgen-mediated growth occurred late in embryogenesis after anatomic development of the male urethra was complete. Persistent gynecomastia may or may not develop.

Pathophysiology The pathogenesis is not understood. Sibships with multiple affected individuals have been described. The testicular regression could be the result of mutant genes, teratogen, or trauma. Multiple instances of agonadism in the same family have been reported, some of which are unilateral and others bilateral. Some subjects in whom no testes can be identified at laparotomy have blood testosterone values clearly above the castrate range, presumably derived from remnant testes.

Management The management of the two extremes is clear-cut. Sexually infantile, phenotypic females should be treated like gonadal dysgenesis; namely, they should be given adequate estrogen to ensure appropriate breast and female somatic development, and any coexisting vaginal agenesis should be treated by surgical or medical means. Likewise, phenotypic males with anorchia should be given androgen replacement to allow normal male secondary sexual development. The cases with incomplete virilization or ambiguous development of the external genitalia are more complex and require hormonal therapy at the time of expected puberty and individual assessment as to whether surgical therapy is appropriate.

DISORDERS OF PHENOTYPIC SEX

FEMALE PSEUDOHERMAPHRODITISM **Congenital adrenal hyperplasia** CLINICAL FEATURES The pathways by which glucocorticoids are synthesized in the adrenal gland and androgens are formed in the testis and adrenal are summarized in Fig. 342-3. Three

FIGURE 342-3 Pathways of glucocorticoid and androgen synthesis. Note abnormal conditions corresponding to impaired enzyme reactions.

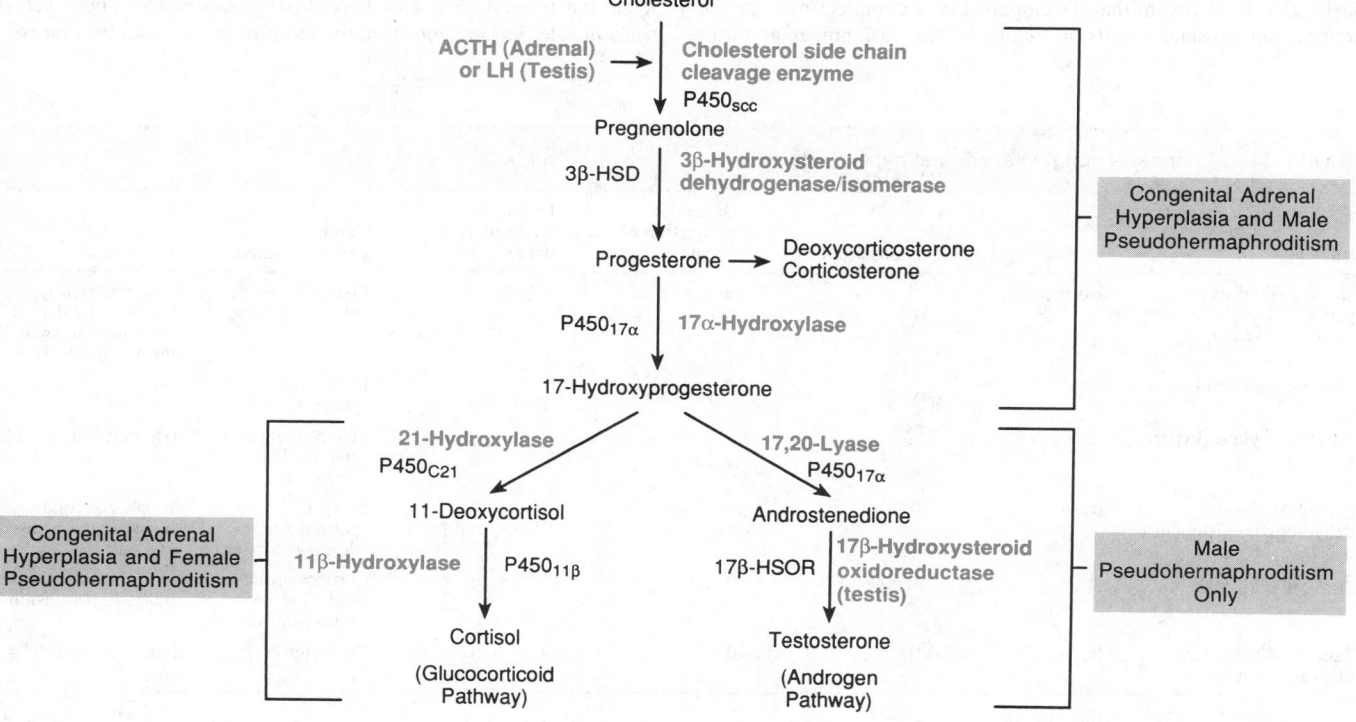

reactions are common to the formation of glucocorticoids and androgens (cholesterol side chain cleavage, 3β-hydroxysteroid dehydrogenase/isomerase, and 17α-hydroxylase); impairment of any of these reactions results in deficiency of glucocorticoid and androgen synthesis and consequently in both congenital adrenal hyperplasia (due to enhanced ACTH levels) and defective virilization of the male embryo (male pseudohermaphroditism). Two enzyme reactions are involved exclusively in androgen synthesis (17,20-lyase and 17β-hydroxysteroid oxidoreductase); deficiency in either results in pure male pseudohermaphroditism with normal glucocorticoid synthesis. Deficiency of either of the terminal two enzymes of glucocorticoid synthesis (21-hydroxylase and 11β-hydroxylase) results in defective formation of hydrocortisone; the compensatory increase in ACTH secretion causes adrenal hyperplasia and a secondary increase in androgen formation that results in virilization in the female or precocious masculinization in the male.

The *adrenal insufficiency* in these disorders may produce equally severe and life-threatening problems in both sexes and is described in detail in Chap. 335. The major features of congenital adrenal hyperplasia are listed in Table 342-4. From the standpoint of *abnormal sexual development,* some defects in steroidogenesis result in female pseudohermaphroditism, and some cause male pseudohermaphroditism. (3β-Hydroxysteroid dehydrogenase/isomerase deficiency can cause either male or female pseudohermaphroditism, but since incomplete virilization of the male is more common, it will be discussed as a form of male pseudohermaphroditism.)

Congenital adrenal hyperplasia due to classic 21-hydroxylase deficiency is the most common cause of ambiguous genitalia in the newborn, with an incidence of between 1 in 5000 and 1 in 15,000 lives births in Europe and the United States; it may or may not be associated with mineralocorticoid deficiency (salt loss) (see Table 342-4). Virilization is usually apparent at birth in the female and within the first 2 to 3 years of life in the male. Manifestations in females include hypertrophy of the clitoris with ventral binding (chordee), partial fusion of the labioscrotal folds, and variable virilization of the urethra. The internal female structures and ovaries remain unaltered, and the wolffian ducts regress normally, probably because adrenal function begins relatively late in embryogenesis. The external appearance of affected females is similar to that of a male with bilateral cryptorchidism and hypospadias. The labioscrotal folds are bulbous and rugated and resemble a scrotum. Rarely, the virilization is so severe that development of a complete male penile urethra and prostate results in errors in sex assignment at birth.

Radiography following the injection of radiopaque dye into the external genital orifice is helpful in demonstrating the presence of a vagina, uterus, and sometimes even fallopian tubes. In a few cases, virilization of the female is slight or absent at birth and becomes evident in later infancy, adolescence, or adulthood, presumably as the result of allelic variation of the mutant genes (the so-called nonclassic or late-onset form of the disorder). The untreated female with the classic disorder grows rapidly during the first year of life and has progressive virilization. At the time of expected puberty there is a failure of normal female sexual development and absence of menstruation. In both sexes, rapid somatic maturation results in premature epiphyseal closure and a short adult height.

Since male phenotypic differentiation is normal, the condition is usually not recognized in the male at birth in the absence of overt adrenal insufficiency. However, early growth and maturation of the external genitalia, appearance of secondary sex characteristics, coarsening of the voice, frequent erections, and excessive muscular development are noticeable in the first few years of life. Virilization in the male can follow either of two patterns. Excessive adrenal androgens can inhibit gonadotropin production so that the testes remain infantile in size despite the acceleration of masculinization. Such untreated adult men are capable of erection and ejaculation but have no spermatogenesis. Alternatively, adrenal androgen secretion can activate a premature maturation of the hypothalamic-pituitary axis and initiate a true precocious puberty including early maturation of spermatogenesis (see Chap. 339). The untreated male is also subject to the development of ACTH-dependent "tumors" of the testis composed of adrenal rest cells.

In classic 21-hydroxylase deficiency, which accounts for about 95 percent of congenital adrenal hyperplasia, decreased production of hydrocortisone leads to increased release of ACTH, enlargement of the adrenal glands, and partial or complete compensation of the defect in the secretion of hydrocortisone. In about half, the enzyme defect appears to be partial, and cortisol secretion is normal. This form is termed "simple virilizing." In the remainder, deficiency of the enzyme is more complete; the enlarged adrenal fails to produce adequate amounts of cortisol and aldosterone leading to severe salt wastage with anorexia, vomiting, volume depletion, and collapse within the first few weeks of life, the so-called salt-losing form of 21-hydroxylase deficiency. In all untreated patients, overproduction of the cortisol precursors prior to the 21-hydroxylase step occurs, leading to increase in plasma progesterone and 17-hydroxyprogesterone. These act as weak aldosterone antagonists at the receptor level and in the compen-

TABLE 342-4 Forms of congenital adrenal hyperplasia

Deficiency	Cortisol	Aldosterone	Degree of virilization of females	Failure of virilization in males	Dominant steroid secreted	Comment
Classic 21-hydroxylase, partial (simple virilizing or compensated)	Normal	↑	+ + + +	0	17-Hydroxyprogesterone	Most common type (¹95% of total); from one- to two-thirds salt losers
Severe (salt-losing)	↓	↓	+ + + +	0	17-Hydroxyprogesterone	
11β-Hydroxylase (hypertension)	↓	↓	+ + + +	0	11-Deoxycortisol and 11-deoxycorticosterone	Hypertension
3β-Hydroxysteroid dehydrogenase/isomerase	0	0	+	+ + + +	Δ⁵-3β-OH compounds (dehydroepiandrosterone)	Probably second most common, usually salt loss
17α-Hydroxylase	↓	↓	0	+ + + +	Corticosterone and 11-deoxycorticosterone	No feminization of female, hypertension
Cholesterol side chain cleavage enzyme	0	0	0	+ + + +	Cholesterol(?)	Rare, usually salt loss

sated form result in greater than normal aldosterone production to maintain normal sodium balance. Increased substrate availability is also responsible for the increase in androgen synthesis in the disorder.

Female pseudohermaphroditism also may occur in 11β-hydroxylase deficiency. In this disorder, a block in hydroxylation at the 11 carbon results in the accumulation of 11-deoxycortisol and deoxycorticosterone (DOC), a potent salt-retaining hormone that causes hypertension rather than salt loss. The clinical features that stem from glucocorticoid deficiency and androgen excess are similar to those in 21-hydroxylase deficiency.

PATHOPHYSIOLOGY Both disorders are due to autosomal recessive mutations. The carrier frequency for $P450_{C21}$ deficiency is about 1 in 50. Because the gene is located on the sixth chromosome close to the HLA-B locus, carriers of the disorder (as well as homozygotes) within a given family can be identified on the basis of the HLA haplotype. At the molecular level the mutations that give rise to 21-hydroxylase deficiency are even more polymorphic; indeed, deletions of portions of the gene (10 to 30 percent), conversion of the gene from a functional state to a form that is not transcribed normally (10 percent), and point mutations (60 to 75 percent) have been characterized in different families with the disorder. The classic disorder is due to mutations that severely reduce enzyme activity, and less severe mutations cause the nonclassic or late-onset variety. 11β-Hydroxylase activity is encoded by two genes on chromosome 8; the molecular biology of $P450_{11\beta}$ deficiency has not been characterized in extensive detail, but there are at least two variants, namely, the classic and late-onset types.

For discussion of the endocrine pathology see Chap. 335. In brief, urinary excretion of ketosteroids is elevated, as is the excretion of the major metabolites that accumulate proximal to the enzymatic blocks. Plasma ACTH is elevated. In $P450_{C21}$ deficiency, 17-hydroxyprogesterone accumulates in blood and is excreted predominantly as pregnanetriol. In $P450_{11\beta}$ deficiency, 11-deoxycortisol accumulates in blood and is excreted predominantly as tetrahydrocortexolone.

MANAGEMENT Gender assignment should correspond to the chromosomal and gonadal sex, and appropriate surgical correction of the external genitalia should be undertaken as early as possible. This is of importance because appropriately treated men and women are capable of fertility. However, if the correct diagnosis is made late (after 3 years of age), gender assignment should be changed only after careful consideration of the psychosexual background.

Treatment with appropriate glucocorticoids prevents the consequences of hydrocortisone deficiency, arrests the rapid virilization, and prevents premature somatic and epiphyseal maturation. The suppression of the abnormal steroid secretion results in cure of the hypertension in patients with 11β-hydroxylase deficiency and allows normal onset of menses and development of female secondary sex characteristics in both disorders. In males, glucocorticoid therapy suppresses adrenal androgens and results in normal gonadotropin secretion, testicular development, and spermatogenesis. Measurements of plasma 17-hydroxyprogesterone, androstenedione, ACTH, and renin levels have all been used to assess adequacy of replacement therapy. In severe 21-hydroxylase deficiency associated with salt loss or elevated plasma renin activity, treatment with mineralocorticoids is also indicated. In such patients, the monitoring of plasma renin is useful for determining the adequacy of mineralocorticoid replacement.

Other causes of female pseudohermaphroditism Female pseudohermaphroditism also may occur in babies born to mothers with virilizing tumors of the ovary (e.g., arrhenoblastomas or luteomas of pregnancy) and, rarely, to mothers with virilizing adrenal tumors. In the past, the administration to pregnant women of progestational agents with androgenic side effects (such as 17α-ethinyl-19-nortestosterone) to prevent abortion resulted in masculinization of female fetuses.

Developmental disorders of müllerian ducts (congenital absence of the vagina, müllerian agenesis) CLINICAL FEATURES Congenital hypoplasia or absence of the vagina in combination with abnormal or absent uterus (the Mayer-Rokitansky-Kuster-Hauser syndrome) is second to gonadal dysgenesis as a cause of primary amenorrhea. Most patients are ascertained after the time of expected puberty because of failure to menstruate. The height is normal, and the breasts, axillary and public hair, and habitus are feminine in character. The uterus can vary from almost normal, lacking only a conduit to the introitus, to the characteristic rudimentary bicornuate cords with or without a lumen. In some patients, cyclic abdominal pain indicates that sufficient functional endometrium is present to result in retrograde menstruation and/or hematometra.

About one-third have abnormal kidneys, most commonly agenesis, ectopy, fused kidneys of the horseshoe type, or solitary ectopic kidneys located in the pelvis. Skeletal abnormalities are present in one-tenth; two-thirds involve the spine, and limb and rib abnormalities account for the remainder. Specific bone abnormalities include wedge vertebrae, fused rudimentary or asymmetric vertebral bodies, and supernumerary vertebrae. The Klippel-Feil syndrome (congenital fusion of the cervical spine, short neck, low posterior hairline, and painless limitation of cervical movement) is a frequent association.

PATHOPHYSIOLOGY The karyotype is 46,XX. Familial occurrence has been described. The pattern of inheritance in most familial cases is consistent with a sex-limited autosomal dominant mutation. Sporadic cases may represent new mutations of the type responsible for the familial disorder or be multifactorial in etiology. In the familial cases, expressivity is variable; some affected family members have skeletal or renal abnormalities only, and some have other abnormalities of müllerian derivatives such as a double uterus. Bilateral renal aplasia in stillborn infants is commonly associated with absence of the uterus and vagina. Thus the family history should be probed for isolated skeletal and renal abnormalities and for stillbirths that might result from congenital absence of both kidneys. Ovarian function is normal, and successful pregnancies have occurred after corrective vaginal surgery in patients with normal uteri.

MANAGEMENT Vaginal agenesis can be treated by surgical or nonsurgical means. Surgical repair generally utilizes a split-thickness skin graft around a solid rubber mold for the creation of an artificial vagina. Medical treatment consists of the repeated application of pressure against the vaginal dimple with a simple dilator to cause development of adequate vaginal depth. In view of complication rates of 5 to 10 percent in surgical series, medical treatment should be tried in most, and surgery should be reserved for patients in whom a well-formed uterus is present and the possibility of fertility exists. Frequent coitus or instrumental dilatation is essential for maintaining the neovagina formed by either technique.

MALE PSEUDOHERMAPHRODITISM Defective virilization of the male embryo (male pseudohermaphroditism) can result from defects in androgen synthesis, defects in androgen action, defects in müllerian duct regression, and uncertain causes. Four-fifths of male pseudohermaphrodites have normal androgen synthesis.

Abnormalities in androgen synthesis CLINICAL FEATURES Enzymatic defects that result in defective testosterone synthesis (see Fig. 342-3) can cause incomplete virilization of the male embryo during embryogenesis (Tables 342-4 and 342-5). Each of the defects blocks a step in the conversion of cholesterol to testosterone. Three are common to the synthesis of other adrenal hormones as well: cholesterol side chain cleavage, 3β-hydroxysteroid dehydrogenase/isomerase, and 17α-hydroxylase or $P450_{17\alpha}$. Consequently, their deficiency results in congenital adrenal hyperplasia (see Table 342-4) as well as male pseudohermaphroditism. Two others (17,20-lyase and 17β-hydroxysteroid oxidoreductase) are unique to the pathway of androgen synthesis, and their deficiency results only in male pseudohermaphroditism. Since androgens are obligatory precursors of estrogens, synthesis of estrogen is also low in affected men and women in all but the terminal defect (17β-hydroxysteroid oxidoreductase deficiency).

The adrenal dysfunction is described in Chap. 335, and the present discussion concerns the abnormal sexual development. In 46,XY

TABLE 342-5 Anatomic, genetic, and endocrine profile of hereditary male pseudohermaphroditism

Disorder	Inheritance	Phenotype		Spermatogenesis	Urogenital sinus	External genitalia
		Müllerian ducts	Wolffian ducts			
DEFECTS IN TESTOSTERONE SYNTHESIS						
Five enzyme deficiencies	Autosomal or X-linked recessive	Absent	Variable development	Normal or decreased	Variable from male to female	Generally female
DEFECTS IN ANDROGEN ACTION						
Steroid 5α-reductase 2 deficiency	Autosomal recessive	Absent	Male	Normal or decreased	Female	Clitoromegaly
Receptor disorders:						
Complete testicular feminization	X-linked recessive	Absent	Absent	Absent	Female	Female
Incomplete testicular feminization	X-linked recessive	Absent	Male	Absent	Female	Clitoromegaly and posterior fusion
Reifenstein syndrome	X-linked recessive	Absent	Variable development	Absent	Variable from male to female	Incomplete male development
Infertile male syndrome	X-linked recessive	Absent	Male	Absent or decreased	Male	Male
Undervirilized fertile male	X-linked recessive	Absent	Male	Normal or decreased	Male	Male
DEFECTS IN MÜLLERIAN REGRESSION						
Persistent müllerian duct syndrome	Autosomal or X-linked recessive	Rudimentary uterus and fallopian tubes	Male	Normal	Male	Male

subjects there is usually no trace of uterus or fallopian tubes, indicating that the müllerian-inhibiting function of the testis during embryogenesis was normal. The masculinization of the urogenital tract and external genitalia and the degree of virilization at puberty vary from almost normal to absent, and therefore, the clinical picture spans the range from men with mild hypospadias to phenotypic women who prior to puberty resemble patients with complete testicular feminization. This variability is the consequence of varying severity of the enzymatic defects in different patients and of varying effects of the steroids that accumulate proximal to the metabolic blocks in the different disorders. In patients with partial defects and in whom the plasma testosterone level is normal, the diagnosis can only be made by measuring the steroids that accumulate proximal to the metabolic block.

Cholesterol side chain cleavage enzyme (P450$_{SCC}$) *deficiency (lipoid adrenal hyperplasia)* is an autosomal recessive disorder in which virtually no urinary steroids (either 17-ketosteroids or 17-hydroxycorticoids) can be detected. The defect is prior to the formation of pregnenolone and is assumed to involve the side-chain cleavage enzyme that is encoded on chromosome 15 and is responsible for the conversion of cholesterol to pregnenolone. The syndrome is associated with salt wasting and profound adrenal insufficiency, and most affected individuals die during infancy. At autopsy, the adrenals and testes are enlarged and infiltrated with lipid. Affected males are incompletely masculinized, whereas affected female infants have normal genital development. The gene for the human enzyme is located on chromosome 15.

3β-Hydroxysteroid dehydrogenase/isomerase deficiency is due to an autosomal recessive mutation of the 3β-HSD gene on chromosome 1 that causes varying failure of masculinization and development of a vagina in male infants. Female infants may be modestly virilized at birth due to the weak androgenic potency of dehydroepiandrosterone, the major steroid secreted. If the enzyme is absent in both the adrenal and testis, no urinary steroids contain a Δ^4-3-keto configura-

tion, whereas in patients in whom the defect is partial or affects only the testis, the urine may contain normal or elevated levels of Δ^4-3-ketosteroids. Most patients have marked salt wasting and profound adrenal insufficiency, and long-term survival in untreated cases occurs only in states of partial deficiency. Affected males may experience an otherwise normal male puberty except for profound gynecomastia. In these individuals, a low-normal blood testosterone level is accompanied by elevated Δ^5 precursors. The enzyme in different tissues must be under complex control, since deficiency of the enzyme in the testis may be less severe than in the adrenal and the enzyme activity in the liver appears to be encoded by a different gene.

17α-Hydroxylase-17,20-lyase (P450$_{17α}$) *deficiency* impairs the introduction of the 17-hydroxyl and the scission of the C-17,20 carbon bond that convert pregnenolone and progesterone to dehydroepiandrosterone and androstenedione, respectively. These reactions are mediated by a single cytochrome, P450$_{17α}$, encoded on chromosome 10, and it is unclear why both reactions occur in the ovary and testis, whereas in the adrenal 17-hydroxyprogesterone is largely converted to glucocorticoids and mineralocorticoids rather than the 19-carbon steroids. Likewise, it is unclear why some patients have selective impairment of either 17α-hydroxylase or 17,20-lyase activity; the distinction between these activities must be functional and may involve the relative concentration of steroid substrates and competing enzymes. Whatever the explanation, the clinical consequences of 17α-hydroxylase and 17,20-lyase deficiencies are different.

17α-Hydroxylase deficiency characteristically results in hypogonadism, absence of secondary sex characteristics, hypokalemic alkalosis, hypertension, and virtually undetectable hydrocortisone secretion in phenotypic women. The secretion of both corticosterone and desoxycorticosterone (DOC) by the adrenal is elevated, and urinary 17-ketosteroids are low. Aldosterone secretion is low due to high plasma DOC and depressed angiotensin levels and returns to normal after suppressive doses of hydrocortisone are administered. In 46,XX subjects, amenorrhea, absent sexual hair, and hypertension are

Breast	Endocrine profile relative to normal male		
	Testosterone production	Estrogen production	LH
Usually male	Normal to decreased	Variable	High
Male	Normal	Normal	Normal or increased
Female	High	High	High
Female	High	High	High
Female	High	High	High
Usually male	Normal or high	Normal or high	Normal or high
Usually male	Normal or high	Normal or high	Normal or high
Male	Normal	Normal	Normal

common, but since gonadal steroids are not required for female development during embryogenesis, the phenotype is that of a normal prepubertal woman. In males, the deficiency results in defective virilization that varies from complete male pseudohermaphroditism to ambiguous genitalia with perineoscrotal hypospadias and, in some, gynecomastia. Adrenal insufficiency does not develop, since the secretion of both corticosterone (a weak glucocorticoid) and DOC (a mineralocorticoid) is elevated. Hypertension and hypokalemia are prominent features of the disorder (even in the neonatal period) and remit after suppression of the DOC secretion by adequate glucocorticoid replacement.

17,20-lyase deficiency in males is associated with normal function of the adrenal cortex and a variable pattern of male pseudohermaphroditism. In the majority there is genital ambiguity at birth, with some virilization at the time of expected puberty. Rare 46,XY patients have had a female phenotype and no virilization at the time of expected puberty. The disorder has been recognized in one 46,XX woman with sexual infantilism. A number of mutations in the $P450_{17\alpha}$ gene on chromosome 10 have been described.

17β-Hydroxysteroid oxidoreductase (17β-HSOR) *deficiency* involves the final step in testosterone biosynthesis, reduction of the 17-keto group of androstenedione. This is the most common of the enzymatic defects in testosterone synthesis. Affected 46,XY males usually have a female phenotype with a blind-ending vagina and absence of müllerian derivatives, but inguinal or abdominal testes and virilized wolffian duct structures are present. At the time of expected puberty, both virilization (with phallic enlargement and development of facial and body hair) and a variable degree of female breast development take place. In some untreated patients, reversal of gender behavior from female to male occurs at puberty. Androgen and estrogen dynamics have not been elucidated in detail, but the 17-keto reduction of estrone to estradiol by the gonads is also low. 17β-Hydroxysteroid oxidoreductase is normally present in many tissues besides the gonads, and only the gonadal enzyme appears to be

defective in this disorder. Plasma testosterone level may be in the low-normal range, making it essential to document elevation in plasma androstenedione to make the diagnosis. It is not clear how many genes encode this activity.

PATHOPHYSIOLOGY These various disorders are inherited as autosomal recessive traits. The pattern of steroid secretion and excretion depends on the site of the various metabolic blocks (see Fig. 342-3). In general, gonadotropin secretion is high, and as a consequence, many individuals with incomplete defects are able to compensate so that the steady state levels of end products such as testosterone may be normal or almost normal.

In some cases of male pseudohermaphroditism, testosterone formation is deficient for reasons other than a single enzyme defect in androgen synthesis. These include disorders in which Leydig cell agenesis (possibly due to absence of the LH receptor) or the secretion of a biologically inactive LH molecule is thought to be the primary defect. In addition, as described above, in several disorders including familial 46,XY pure gonadal dysgenesis, sporadic dysgenetic testes, and the absent testis syndrome, deficient testosterone production is secondary to abnormal gonadal development.

MANAGEMENT Therapy with glucocorticoids and in some instances mineralocorticoids is indicated in those disorders causing adrenal hyperplasia. The decision as to the management of the genital abnormalities depends on the individual case. Fertility has not been reported, and its consideration does not enter into sex assignment. In genetic females there is no problem (except in diagnosis), in that affected individuals are raised appropriately as females and suitable estrogen replacement is administered at the time of expected puberty to promote development of normal secondary sex characteristics. The decision as to whether newborn males with ambiguous genitalia should be raised as males or females depends on the anatomic defect; in general, the more severely affected should be raised as females, and corrective surgery of the genitalia and removal of the testes should be undertaken as early as possible. In such subjects estrogen therapy is also indicated at the appropriate age to allow development of normal female secondary sex characteristics. In individuals raised as males, corrective surgery is indicated for any coexisting hypospadias, and monitoring of plasma androgens and estrogens should be undertaken at the time of expected puberty to determine whether supplemental testosterone therapy is appropriate.

Abnormalities in androgen action Several disorders of male phenotypic development result from abnormalities of androgen action. The spectrum of phenotypes is described in Tables 342-4 and 342-5. In these disorders, testosterone formation and müllerian regression are normal, but male development is impaired to a variable degree as a result of resistance to androgen action in the target cells.

STEROID 5α-REDUCTASE 2 DEFICIENCY This autosomal recessive disorder is characterized by (1) severe perineoscrotal hypospadias, (2) a blind vaginal pouch of variable size opening either into the urogenital sinus or into the urethra, (3) testes with normal epididymides, vasa deferentia, and seminal vesicles, and termination of the ejaculatory ducts into the blind-ending vagina, (4) a female habitus without female breast development but with normal axillary and pubic hair, (5) the absence of female internal genitalia, (6) normal male plasma testosterone, and (7) masculinization to a variable degree at the time of puberty.

The fact that virilization during embryogenesis is defective only in the urogenital sinus and the external genitalia provided insight into the fundamental abnormality. Testosterone, the androgen secreted by the fetal testis, is responsible for differentiation of the wolffian duct into the epididymis, vas deferens, and seminal vesicle, whereas dihydrotestosterone mediates virilization of the urogenital sinus and the external genitalia. Consequently, a failure of dihydrotestosterone formation in a male embryo would be expected to cause the phenotype observed in this disorder, normal male wolffian duct derivatives with defective masculinization of the external genitalia and urogenital sinus. Since testosterone itself regulates LH secretion (see Chap. 339), plasma LH level is normal or minimally elevated. As a result, testosterone and estrogen production rates are those of normal men, and gynecomastia does not develop.

The fact that 5α-reductase 2 enzyme is deficient in this disorder was established by assay of biopsied tissues and cultured fibroblasts from affected individuals. Deletions or point mutations in the gene encoding steroid 5α-reductase 2 have been identified in most families studied. Approximately 40 percent are compound heterozygotes.

RECEPTOR DISORDERS   The androgen receptor is a typical member of the steroid/thyroid family of receptors with steroid-binding, DNA-binding, and functional domains and is encoded by a gene on the long arm of the X chromosome. A variety of mutations of this gene impair receptor function and hence impair male phenotypic differentiation and/or virilization.

Clinical features   Complete testicular feminization is a common form of male pseudohermaphroditism; estimates of frequency vary from 1 in 20,000 to 1 in 64,000 male births. It is the third most common cause of primary amenorrhea in phenotypic women after gonadal dysgenesis and congenital absence of the vagina. The features are characteristic. Namely, a woman is ascertained either because of inguinal hernia (prepubertal) or primary amenorrhea (postpubertal). The development of the breasts after puberty, the general habitus, and the distribution of body fat are female in character so that most patients have a truly feminine appearance. Axillary and pubic hair is absent or scanty, but some vulval hair is usually present. Scalp hair is that of a normal woman, and facial hair is absent. The external genitalia are unambiguously female, and the clitoris is normal. The vagina is short and blind-ending and may be absent or rudimentary. All internal genitalia are absent except for testes that contain normal Leydig cells and seminiferous tubules without spermatogenesis. The testes may be located in the abdomen, along the course of the inguinal canal, or in the labia majora. Occasionally, remnants of müllerian or wolffian duct origin are present in the paratesticular fascia or in fibrous bands extending from the testis. Patients tend to be rather tall, and bone age is normal. Psychosexual development is unmistakably female with regard to behavior, outlook, and maternal instincts.

The major complication of undescended testes in this disorder, as in all forms of cryptorchidism, is the development of tumors (Chap. 322). Since affected individuals undergo a normal pubertal growth spurt and feminize successfully at the time of expected puberty, and since testicular tumors rarely develop until after puberty, it is usual to delay castration until after the time of expected puberty. Prepubertal castration is indicated if the testes are present in the inguinal region or the labia majora and result in discomfort or hernia formation. (If hernia repair is indicated prepubertally, most physicians prefer to remove the testes at the same time to limit the number of operative procedures.) If the testes are removed prepubertally, estrogen therapy is required at the appropriate age to ensure normal growth and breast development. When castration is performed postpubertally, menopausal symptoms and other evidence of estrogen withdrawal supervene, and suitable estrogen replacement is indicated (see Chap. 340).

Incomplete testicular feminization is about one-tenth as frequent as the complete form. In the incomplete disorder there is minor virilization of the external genitalia (partial fusion of the labioscrotal folds and/or some degree of clitoromegaly), normal pubic hair, and some virilization as well as feminization at the time of expected puberty. The vagina is short and blind-ending, but in contrast to the complete form, the wolffian duct derivatives are often partially developed. The management of patients with the complete and incomplete forms of testicular feminization differs. Since patients with the incomplete disorder virilize at the time of expected puberty, gonadectomy should be performed before the expected time of puberty in all prepubertal patients with clitoromegaly or posterior labial fusion.

Reifenstein syndrome is the term applied to forms of incomplete male pseudohermaphroditism initially described by a number of eponyms (Reifenstein syndrome, Gilbert-Dreyfus syndrome, Lubs syndrome). Each of these phenotypes was originally assumed to be a distinct entity, but these syndromes are now known to constitute

variable manifestations of mutations of the androgen receptor. The most common phenotype is a man with perineoscrotal hypospadias and gynecomastia, but the spectrum of defective virilization in affected families ranges from men with azoospermia to phenotypic women with pseudovaginas. Axillary and pubic hair is normal, but chest and facial hair is minimal. Cryptorchidism is common, the testes are small, and azoospermia is present. Some have defects in wolffian duct derivatives such as absence or hypoplasia of the vas deferens. Since the psychological development in most in unequivocally male, the hypospadias and cryptorchidism should be corrected surgically. The only successful form of treatment of the gynecomastia is surgical removal.

The *infertile male syndrome* may be the most common disorder of the androgen receptor and is not actually a form of male pseudohermaphroditism. Some such individuals are minimally affected subjects in families with Reifenstein syndrome with azoospermia as the only manifestation of the receptor abnormality. More commonly, subjects present with male infertility and have negative family histories; indeed, a disorder of the androgen receptor may be present in a fifth or more of men with idiopathic azoospermia. The *undervirilized fertile male* is another manifestation of an androgen receptor defect. In these families, affected men have gynecomastia and undervirilization, and some are fertile.

Pathophysiology   The karyotype is 46,XY, and the mutant gene is X-linked. The frequency of a positive family history varies from about two-thirds of patients with testicular feminization and Reifenstein syndrome to only occasional patients with the infertile male syndrome. The patients with a negative family history are believed to be the result of new mutations.

Hormone dynamics are similar in all disorders of the androgen receptor. Plasma testosterone levels and rates of testosterone production by the testes are normal or higher than normal. The elevated testosterone production is caused by the high mean plasma level of LH, which, in turn, is due to defective feedback regulation caused by resistance to the action of androgen at the hypothalamic-pituitary level. Elevated LH concentration is responsible also for the increased estrogen production by the testes (see Chap. 339). (In normal men, most estrogen is derived from peripheral formation from circulating androgens, but when the plasma LH level is elevated, the testes secrete increased amounts of estrogen into the circulation.) Thus resistance to the feedback regulation of LH secretion by circulating androgen results in elevated plasma LH levels, and this, in turn, results in the enhanced secretion of both testosterone and estradiol by the testes. Gonadotropin levels rise even higher (and menopausal symptoms may develop) when the testes are removed, indicating that gonadotropin secretion is under partial regulatory control. Presumably, in the steady state and in the absence of an androgen effect, estrogen alone regulates LH secretion, a control purchased at the expense of an elevated plasma estrogen concentration for a male. The hormonal changes in the infertile male syndrome are similar to those in the other receptor disorders but less marked. Some men with this syndrome do not have an elevation of plasma LH or plasma testosterone level.

Feminization in these disorders is the result of two interlocking phenomena. First, androgens and estrogens have antagonistic effects, and virilization occurs in normal men when the ratio of androgen to estrogen is 100:1 or greater; in the absence of androgen action, the cellular effect of estrogen is unopposed. Second, the testicular production of estradiol is greater than that of the normal male (although less than that of the normal female). Variable degrees of androgen resistance coupled with variably enhanced estradiol production result in different degrees of defective virilization and enhanced feminization in the four clinical syndromes.

Each of these syndromes is the result of an abnormality of the androgen receptor. In some families, the fundamental defect is due to the deletion of a portion of the gene; more commonly, the disorder is due to point mutations in the coding sequence leading to premature termination codons or amino acid substitutions in the hormone-binding domain. Some families with clinical syndromes typical of an androgen receptor disorder have normal androgen binding in fibroblasts. In many of these families, point mutations in the DNA-binding domain are responsible for the androgen resistance.

Persistent müllerian duct syndrome Men with this uncommon disorder have testes and normal phenotypic development and in addition have fallopian tubes, a uterus, an upper vagina, and variable development of the vas deferens. The disorder is heterogeneous. In one type, one or both testes are descended, and the uterus and ipsilateral fallopian tube are in the inguinal canal or scrotum; both testes and fallopian tubes may be present in the hernia sac or can be drawn into it. The other type is associated with high bilateral cryptorchidism and no hernias. In both types, the vasa deferentia are embedded in the wall of the uterus, a feature that complicates surgical procedures designed to preserve potential fertility. Most patients have uninformative family histories, but in some the condition is inherited as an autosomal recessive trait. Because the external genitalia are well developed and the patients masculinize normally at puberty, it is assumed that during the critical stage of embryonic differentiation the fetal testes produce a normal amount of androgen. However, müllerian regression does not occur. Utilizing immunoassays, subjects can be divided into two groups. In the MIS-positive group, levels of müllerian-inhibiting substance (MIS) in serum and testes are normal, and it is postulated that the MIS receptor is defective. In the MIS-negative group, serum MIS is absent or decreased, and one such patient has been shown to have single-nucleotide substitution that inserts a premature stop codon that results in a truncated hormone. To minimize the chance of tumor development and to maintain virilization, orchiopexy should be performed. Malignancy in the uterus or vagina has not been described, and because the vasa deferentia are closely associated with the broad ligaments, the uterus and vagina should be left in place to avoid disruption of the vasa deferentia during removal and consequently to preserve possible fertility.

Developmental defects of the male genitalia HYPOSPADIAS Hypospadias is a congenital anomaly in which the urethra terminates in an abnormal position along the midline of the ventral surface of the penis at some site between the normal urethral meatus and the perineum. This malformation is often associated with ventral contraction and bowing of the penis (chordee) and occurs in 0.5 to 0.8 percent of male births in the United States. It is common to categorize hypospadias as glandular (involving the glans penis), penile, or perineoscrotal. Since androgens control penile development, hypospadias is believed to result form some defect in androgen formation or androgen action during embryogenesis. Indeed, hypospadias occurs in most disorders of male sexual differentiation. A rare cause of hypospadias is maternal ingestion of progestational agents early in pregnancy. However, the known causes (single-gene defects, chromosomal abnormalities, and maternal drug ingestion) at best can account for only about one-fourth of cases, and the etiology of most remains unknown. The management is surgical.

CRYPTORCHIDISM The normal descent of the testis is perhaps the most poorly understood portion of male sexual differentiation, with regard both to the nature of the forces that result in the movement and to the hormonal factors that regulate the process. In anatomic terms, testicular descent can be divided into three phases: (1) transabdominal movement of the testis from its site of origin above the kidney to the inguinal ring, (2) formation of the opening in the inguinal canal (processus vaginalis) through which the testis exits the abdominal cavity, and (3) actual movement of the testis through the inguinal canal to its permanent site in the scrotum. This entire process occurs over a 6- to 7-month period during gestation, beginning at about the sixth week and not completed in some until after birth. Impairment of any of the above anatomic events can be responsible for the failure of descent of one or both testes. About 3 percent of full-term and 30 percent of premature male infants have at least one cryptorchid testis at birth, but completion of descent can occur within the first few weeks of life, so the incidence of failure of descent by

6 to 9 months of age is only 0.6 to 0.7 percent. It is this latter category of maldescent that requires intervention.

Permanent cryptorchidism can be classified as intraabdominal (10 percent), canalicular (in the inguinal canal) (20 percent), high scrotal (40 percent), or obstructed (30 percent), in which maldescent is due to a physical barrier between the inguinal pouch and the inlet of the scrotum. These disorders must be distinguished from the temporarily retracted normal testis.

The cryptorchid testis functions poorly after puberty, but the extent to which maldescent is the result of an abnormality of the testis or the cause of abnormal function is unknown. Two general theories have been advanced as to the etiology—inadequate intraabdominal pressure and deficient endocrine function of the testis either because of deficient testosterone synthesis or inadequate formation of müllerian-inhibiting substance. Indeed, defects that result in inadequate development of intraabdominal pressure of inadequate development of the testes can cause cryptorchidism. As is true for hypospadias, however, the known causes of cryptorchidism constitute only a small fraction of the cases, and the etiology in most remains to be identified. Two complications of cryptorchidism are important; spermatogenesis cannot occur at the temperature of the abdominal cavity, and it is therefore necessary to correct the process as early as possible to allow possible fertility. The fact that infertility is common in men who have been treated for unilateral as well as bilateral cryptorchidism suggests that maldescent is usually the consequence rather than the cause of the testicular malfunction. There is also a greater frequency of malignancy in undescended testes, and all should be surgically corrected for this reason (see Chap. 322).

REFERENCES

DE LA CHAPELLE A: The etiology of maleness in XX men. Hum Genet 58:105, 1981

DONAHOE PK et al: Mixed gonadal dysgenesis, pathogenesis and management. J Pediatr Surg 14:287, 1979

EDMAN CD et al: Embryonic testicular regression: A clinical spectrum of XY agonadal individuals. Obstet Gynecol 49:208, 1977

GEORGE FW, WILSON JD: Sex determination and differentiation, in *The Physiology of Reproduction*, E Knobil, JD Neill (eds). New York, Raven, 1988, vol 1, pp 3–26

GORDON DL et al: Pathologic testicular findings in Klinefelter's syndrome. 47,XXY vs 46,XY/47,XXY. Arch Intern Med 130:726, 1972

GRIFFIN JE: Androgen resistances: The clinical and molecular spectrum. N Engl J Med 336:611, 1992

———, WILSON JD: Disorder of sexual differentiation, in *Campbell's Textbook of Urology*, 6th ed, PC Walsh et al (eds). Philadelphia, Saunders, 1992, pp 1509–1542

——— et al: The androgen resistance syndromes: 5α-Reductase deficiency, and related disorders, in *The Molecular and Metabolic Basis of Inherited Disease*, 7th ed, CR Scriver et al (eds). New York, McGraw-Hill, in press

——— et al: Congenital absence of the vagina. The Mayer-Rokitansky-Kuster-Hauser syndrome. Ann Intern Med 85:224, 1976

GRUMBACH MM, CONTE FA: Disorders of sexual differentiation, in *Williams' Textbook of Endocrinology*, 8th ed, JD Wilson, DW Foster (eds). Philadelphia, Saunders, 1992, pp 853–951

GUERRIER D et al: The persistent müllerian duct syndrome: A molecular approach. J Clin Endocrinol Metab 68:46, 1989

JOSSO N et al: Anti-müllerian hormone and intersex states. Trends Endocrinol Metabol 2:227, 1991

LEONARD JM et al: The classification of Klinefelter's syndrome, in *Genetic Mechanism of Sexual Development*, HL Vallet, IH Porter (eds). New York, Academic, 1979

MCPHAUL MJ et al: The spectrum of mutations in the androgen receptor that causes androgen resistance. J Clin Endocrinol Metab 76:17, 1993

MILLER, WL: Molecular biology of steroid hormone synthesis. Endocrinol Rev 9:295, 1988

NEW M et al: Congenital adrenal hyperplasia and related conditions, in *The Metabolic Basis of Inherited Disease*, 6th ed, CR Scriver et al (eds). New York, McGraw-Hill, 1989, pp. 1881–1917

RAMSAY M et al: XX True hermaphroditism in Southern African blacks: An enigma of primary sexual differentiation. Am J Hum Genet Vol 43:4, 1988

SIMPSON JL: Gonadal dysgenesis and sex chromosome abnormalities: Phenotypic-karyotypic correlations, in *Genetic Mechanisms of Sexual Development*, HL Vallet, IH Porter (eds). New York, Academic, 1979

——— et al: XY gonadal dysgenesis: Genetic heterogeneity based upon clinical observations, H-Y antigen status and segregation analysis. Hum Genet 58:91, 1981

SINCLAIR AH et al: A gene from the human sex-determining region encodes a protein with homology to a conserved DNA-binding motif. Nature 364:240, 1990

WILSON JD et al: Steroid 5α-reductase 2 deficiency. Endocr Rev 14:577, 1993

YANASE T et al: 17α-Hydroxylase/17,20-lyase deficiency: From clinical investigation to molecular definition. Endocr Rev 12:91, 1991

ZAH W et al: Mixed gonadal dysgenesis. A case report and review of the world literature. Acta Endocrinol Suppl 197:3, 1975

343   DISORDERS AFFECTING MULTIPLE ENDOCRINE SYSTEMS

AUBREY E. BOYD / ROBERT F. GAGEL

NEOPLASTIC DISORDERS AFFECTING MULTIPLE ENDOCRINE ORGANS

In several familial disorders, neoplastic manifestations of multiple endocrine organs cause syndromes of hormone excess. Management of these disorders requires a broad understanding both of endocrine neoplasia and of the unique features associated with the manifestations of multiple hormone excess in a single patient. The genetic loci for the two major syndromes have been identified, and techniques for DNA-based genetic screening are now available.

MULTIPLE ENDOCRINE NEOPLASIA TYPE 1   Clinical manifestations   Multiple endocrine neoplasia type 1 (MEN 1), or Wermer's syndrome, is the association of neoplastic transformation of parathyroid, pituitary, and pancreatic islet cells (Table 343-1). The syndrome is inherited as an autosomal dominant trait; each child born to an affected parent has a 50 percent chance of inheriting the predisposing gene.

Several features of this syndrome have an impact on management. The first is the multicentric nature of the disease process within a single organ. Each tumor is derived from a single cell, and any endocrine cell within the affected organs may become transformed. Second, hyperplasia is the initiating lesion, followed later by adenomatous or carcinomatous changes. Third, a neoplastic process in one organ may affect the progression of a disease process in another organ. For example, hormone production by a pancreatic tumor may stimulate growth of a pituitary tumor. Fourth, this syndrome generally evolves over a 30- to 40-year period, and the manifestations will depend in large part on when the disorder is first identified.

Hyperparathyroidism is the most common manifestation. Hypercalcemia may be detected during the teenage years, and by age 40, most carriers of the gene are likely to be affected. Screening for hyperparathyroidism is enhanced by measurement of either an albumin-adjusted or ionized serum calcium. The diagnosis is established by the finding of elevated serum calcium and intact parathyroid hormone levels. Clinical features of hyperparathyroidism in MEN 1 do not differ substantially from those in sporadic hyperparathyroidism and may include calcium-containing kidney stones, bone abnormalities, and gastrointestinal and musculoskeletal complaints (see Chap. 356).

Other familial disorders associated with hypercalcemia include familial parathyroid hyperplasia, familial adenomatous hyperparathyroidism, and familial hypocalciuric hypercalcemia (FHH). Calcium excretion is usually elevated in the patient with MEN 1 or other forms of primary hyperparathyroidism and low in FHH. In addition, the serum calcium level is rarely elevated at birth in MEN 1 and frequently elevated at birth in FHH. Differentiation of hyperparathyroidism of MEN 1 from the other forms of familial primary hyperparathyroidism is usually based on family history, histologic analysis of parathyroid tissue, and, sometimes, long-term observation to determine whether other manifestations of MEN 1 develop.

Parathyroid hyperplasia is the most common cause of hyperparathyroidism in MEN 1, although single and multiple adenomas have been described. Hyperplasia of one or more parathyroid glands is common in younger patients; adenomas are generally found in older patients or those with long-standing disease.

Neoplasia of the pancreatic islets is the second most common manifestation of MEN 1, and these abnormalities tend to occur in parallel with parathyroid abnormalities. The syndromes of pancreatic islet cell hormone excess include pancreatic polypeptide (75 to 85 percent), gastrin (60 percent, Zollinger-Ellison syndrome), insulin (25 to 35 percent), vasoactive intestinal peptide (VIP) (3 to 5 percent, Verner-Morrison syndrome), glucagon (5 to 10 percent), and somatostatin (1 to 5 percent). The tumors may produce additional peptides, including adrenocorticotropin (ACTH) or corticotropin-releasing hormone (CRH), growth hormone–releasing hormone (GHRH), calcitonin gene products, neurotensin, gastric inhibitory peptide, and others. Many of the tumors produce more than one peptide.

The pancreatic neoplasms differ from the other components of MEN 1 in that approximately one-third of the tumors associated with MEN 1 display malignant features, including hepatic metastases. The differentiation of malignant from nonmalignant tumors is based either on histologic criteria or documentation of metastases.

Diagnosis of pancreatic islet cell tumors can be made by identification of a characteristic clinical syndrome, hormonal measurement with or without a provocative stimulus, or radiographic techniques. One approach utilizes annual screening studies of people at risk with measurement of basal hormone levels and a meal-stimulated measurement of pancreatic polypeptide to identify these tumors as early as possible. Implicit in this screening strategy is the concept that aggressive surgery to remove islet cell tumors at an early stage will be curative. Other groups recommend less aggressive screening to include measurement of a serum gastrin and pancreatic polypeptide level every 2 to 3 years with the understanding that pancreatic neoplasms will be detected at a later stage and managed medically, if appropriate, or by surgical removal. Magnetic resonance imaging (MRI) appears to be equivalent to other imaging techniques for identification of these tumors.

ZOLLINGER-ELLISON SYNDROME (ZES)   This syndrome, caused by excessive gastrin production, is found in over 50 percent of MEN 1 patients with pancreatic islet cell tumors (see Chap. 276). The clinical features include increased gastric acid production, recurrent multiple peptic ulcers, diarrhea, and esophagitis. The ulcer diathesis is frequently refractory to conservative therapy such as antacids. The

---

TABLE 343-1   Disease associations in the multiple endocrine neoplasia (MEN) syndromes

MEN 1	MEN 2	Mixed syndromes
Parathyroid hyperplasia or adenoma	**MEN 2A**	Familial pheochromocytoma and islet cell tumor
Pancreatic islet cell hyperplasia, adenoma, or carcinoma	Medullary thyroid carcinoma (MTC)	
Pituitary hyperplasia or adenoma	Pheochromocytoma	
Other less common manifestations: foregut carcinoid, pheochromocytoma, subcutaneous or visceral lipomas	Parathyroid hyperplasia or adenoma	
	MEN 2A with cutaneous lichen amyloidosis	von Hippel–Lindau syndrome, pheochromocytoma, and islet cell tumor
	Familial MTC	Neurofibromatosis with features of MEN 1 or 2
	MEN 2B	Myxomas, spotty pigmentation, and generalized endocrine overactivity in a single family
	MTC	
	Pheochromocytoma	
	Muscosal and gastrointestinal neuromas	
	Marfanoid features	

diagnosis is made by the finding of increased gastric acid secretion, an elevation of the basal gastrin concentration (generally greater than 115 pmol/L or 200 pg/mL), and an exaggerated stimulatory response to either secretin or calcium. Other causes of an elevated serum gastrin such as achlorhydria, treatment with H-2 receptor antagonists or omeprazole, retained gastric antrum, small-bowel resection, gastric outlet obstruction, or hypercalcemia should be excluded.

INSULINOMA Approximately one-third of MEN 1 patients with pancreatic islet cell tumors have insulin overproduction and hypoglycemia. The tumors may be benign or malignant (25 percent). Symptoms of nervousness, sweating, palpitations, excessive hunger or weight gain, seizures, and loss of consciousness in the fasting state should prompt an investigation for this disorder. On occasion, the diagnosis can be established by the documentation of hypoglycemia during a short fast with simultaneous inappropriate elevation of the serum insulin and C-peptide concentration. More commonly, it is necessary to subject the patient to a supervised 72-h fast to provoke hypoglycemia and measure glucose, insulin, and C-peptide levels at regular intervals during the fast. Insulin-secreting tumors may be localized by MRI or computed tomographic (CT) scanning, although small tumors may not be detected by radiographic techniques. Transhepatic venous catheterization with basal or calcium-stimulated sampling for insulin in the portal circulation may allow preoperative localization of the tumor. Intraoperative ultrasound also has been used to localize these tumors.

GLUCAGONOMA A small percentage of patients with pancreatic islet cell neoplasms have a syndrome consisting of hyperglycemia, a skin rash (necrolytic migratory erythema), anorexia, glossitis, anemia, depression, diarrhea, and venous thrombosis. In approximately half of these patients the plasma glucagon concentration is elevated, leading to its designation as the *glucagonoma syndrome*, although elevation of the plasma glucagon concentration is common in MEN 1 patients and not necessarily associated with this clinical syndrome. The glucagonoma syndrome may represent a complex interaction between glucagon overproduction and the nutritional status of the patient because the dermatologic manifestations sometimes respond to dietary manipulation.

THE VERNER-MORRISON OR WATERY DIARRHEA SYNDROME This syndrome consists of watery diarrhea, hypokalemia, hypochlorhydria, and systemic acidosis. The diarrhea can be voluminous and is almost always found in association with an islet cell tumor, prompting use of the term *pancreatic cholera*, although the syndrome is not restricted to pancreatic islet tumors and has been observed in association with carcinoid or other tumors. There is considerable evidence that this syndrome is caused by overproduction of VIP, although plasma concentrations of this peptide rarely may be normal. Hypercalcemia is common and is thought to be caused by VIP effects on bone.

PITUITARY TUMORS Over 50 percent of MEN 1 gene carriers develop pituitary tumors. These tumors are multicentric, making them difficult to treat by surgical methods (see Chap. 331). The most common manifestation is the galactorrhea-amenorrhea syndrome caused by a prolactinoma; diagnosis is established by the finding of a serum prolactin level greater than 200 µg/L with or without a pituitary mass detected by MRI. Values less than 200 µg/L may be due to a prolactin-secreting neoplasm or result from compression of the pituitary stalk. Acromegaly due to excessive growth hormone production is the second most common syndrome (see Chap. 331). Excessive production of GHRH by an islet cell tumor, although rare, should be considered in the differential diagnosis of acromegaly in MEN 1. Cushing's disease due to an ACTH-producing pituitary tumor also can occur. It is important to differentiate pituitary Cushing's disease from Cushing's disease due to ectopic production of ACTH or to ectopic production of CRH by other tumors in the MEN 1 syndrome. Diagnosis of pituitary Cushing's disease is generally best accomplished by a high-dose dexamethasone suppression test or by petrosal venous sinus sampling for ACTH after intravenous injection of CRH (see Chap. 335). Differentiation of a primary pituitary tumor from an ectopic CRH-producing tumor may be difficult because the

pituitary may be abnormal in both disorders; documentation of ectopic CRH production by a pancreatic islet or carcinoid tumor may be the only method of proving ectopic CRH production.

UNUSUAL MANIFESTATIONS OF MEN 1 Carcinoid tumors occur rarely in MEN 1. Most of the reported tumors are of the foregut type and are derived from thymus, lung, stomach, or duodenum; they may metastasize or be locally invasive. Most commonly, the tumors produce serotonin, calcitonin, or CRH; the classic carcinoid syndrome with flushing, diarrhea, and bronchospasm is rare (see Chap. 276). Subcutaneous or visceral lipomas and cutaneous leiomyomas also may be present. Malignant transformation of the latter tumors is rare.

Genetics and pathophysiology The gene responsible for MEN 1 is believed to belong to the category of oncogenes known as a *tumor suppressor gene*. Genes of this category play an important role in the regulation of cell growth. Each affected individual is believed to carry one mutated copy of the MEN 1 gene which is transmitted in an autosomal dominant manner (each child has a 50 percent chance of inheriting the gene). Tumor development begins when the normal copy, derived from the unaffected parent, is mutated as a result of errors in the replication of DNA. The MEN 1 locus has been mapped to a specific region on chromosome 11 (Fig. 343-1), but the gene itself has not been identified.

The "growth factor hypothesis" provides a second potential mechanism for development of MEN 1 tumors. There is evidence for production of a factor in MEN 1 patients that stimulates parathyroid gland growth. This factor is thought to be a member of the fibroblast growth factor family, although it has not been purified and the cell of origin is unknown.

Treatment Almost all individuals who inherit the mutant MEN 1 gene will develop abnormalities of at least one of the potentially affected organs. Most develop hyperparathyroidism, 80 percent develop pancreatic islet cell tumors, and more than half develop detectable pituitary tumors. In most cases, surgery is not curative. Indeed, most of these patients require surgery on two or more endocrine glands during a lifetime, and many require multiple surgical procedures. For this reason, it is important for the clinician to establish a clear set of goals with regard to management of these patients rather than casually recommending operation each time a tumor is discovered. In the following discussion, ranges for acceptable management will be discussed.

HYPERPARATHYROIDISM Most clinicians agree that individuals with a corrected serum calcium concentration greater than 3.0 mmol/L (12 mg/dL), evidence of calcium nephrolithiasis or renal dysfunction, neuropathic or muscular symptoms, or parathyroid hormone-induced bone abnormalities (including osteopenia) should

FIGURE 343-1 Schematic diagram of chromosomes 11 and 10 showing the MEN 1 and MEN 2 loci.

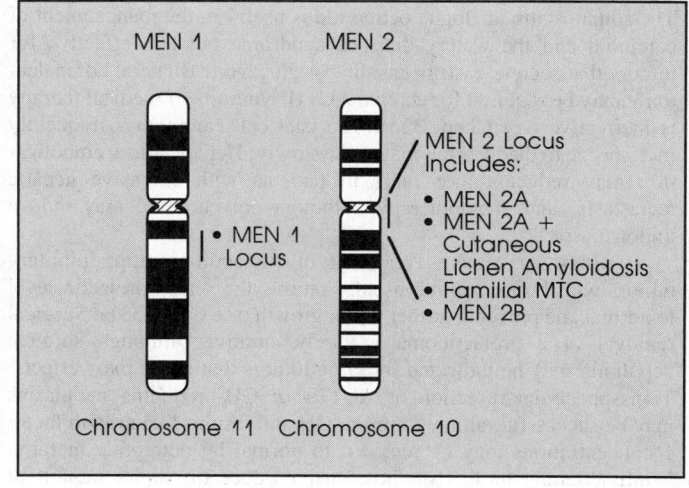

undergo parathyroid exploration. In MEN 1 there is, in addition, an additional criterion for operative intervention; hypercalcemia may stimulate gastrin overproduction and development of ZES in MEN 1, a feature that may be reversed by restoration of normocalcemia. There is less agreement regarding the necessity for parathyroid exploration in individuals who do not meet these criteria, and observation over a several-year period may be appropriate in a MEN 1 patient with asymptomatic hyperparathyroidism.

When surgery is indicated for hyperparathyroidism in MEN 1, the preferred procedure is to identify and remove all parathyroid tissue at the time of primary operation and to implant parathyroid tissue in multiple packets in the nondominant forearm. Consequently, if reoperation is necessary, surgical removal of single or multiple packets of tissue can be performed under local anesthesia with titration of tissue removal to return the serum calcium concentration to normal. A second approach is to remove $3\frac{1}{2}$ parathyroid glands from the neck, carefully marking the location of residual tissue so that the remaining tissue can be located easily during subsequent surgery.

PANCREATIC ISLET TUMORS   (See Chap. 276 for discussion of the treatment of pancreatic islet tumors not associated with MEN 1.) Two contradictory lines of thought exist as to the management of pancreatic islet cell tumors in MEN 1. First, the pancreatic islet cell tumors are multicentric, malignant about a third of the time, and result in the death of 10 to 20 percent of patients. Second, pancreatic islet tissue is required for insulin production and glucose homeostasis; removal of all pancreatic islets to prevent malignancy will result in diabetes mellitus, a disease with long-term complications equivalent to those of the potential malignancy. These contradictions make it difficult to formulate clear-cut guidelines, but several general concepts appear to be valid. First, surgical removal of islet cell tumors producing insulin, glucagon, VIP, GHRH, or CRH is appropriate, because medical therapy for these disorders is generally ineffective. Second, gastrin-producing islet cell tumors causing ZES can be managed by either surgical or medical approaches. The latter tumors are frequently multicentric, and the surgical cure rate is low. The availability of H-2 receptor antagonists (cimetidine or ranitidine) and an H^+,K^+-ATPase inhibitor (omeprazole) provides effective long-term alternatives to surgery for control of the ulcer diathesis, although high doses are required and the long-term safety of the drugs for this use has not been established. If a single tumor can be identified, a surgical approach seems reasonable in most cases. In patients with multicentric tumors or in those with hepatic metastasis, medical therapy is appropriate. Third, in families in which there is a high incidence of malignant islet cell tumors causing death, total pancreatectomy at an early age may be justified to prevent development of metastatic disease.

Long-term management of metastatic islet cell carcinoma is unsatisfactory. Hormonal abnormalities and their clinical sequelae can sometimes be controlled medically. For example, ZES can be effectively managed with H-2 receptor antagonists or omeprazole. The somatostatin analogue octreotide is useful in the management of carcinoid and the watery diarrhea syndrome but less effective for tumors that secrete gastrin, insulin, or glucagon. Bilateral adrenalectomy may be required for ectopic ACTH syndrome if medical therapy is ineffective (see Chap. 335). The islet cell carcinomas frequently metastasize to the liver but may grow slowly. Hepatic artery embolization may reduce tumor mass in patients with extensive hepatic metastasis, and chemotherapy, although not curative, may reduce tumor mass.

PITUITARY TUMORS   Treatment of prolactin-secreting pituitary tumors with bromocriptine usually returns the serum prolactin level to normal and prevents further tumor growth (see Chap. 331). Surgical removal of a prolactinoma is rarely curative, although surgical debulking may be indicated for large tumors that cause mass effects. Transsphenoidal resection of ACTH- or GH-producing neoplasms may be successful, although serum GH and insulin-like growth factor 1 concentrations may be returned to normal by octreotide therapy. Nonfunctioning tumors or those that produce the alpha subunit of the pituitary glycoprotein hormones are best managed surgically. Radiation therapy may be useful for large or recurrent tumors.

MULTIPLE ENDOCRINE NEOPLASIA TYPE 2   Clinical manifestations   The association of thyroid carcinoma and pheochromocytoma can be subcategorized into two major syndromes (see Table 343-1). Multiple endocrine neoplasia type 2A (MEN 2A) is the combination of medullary thyroid carcinoma, hyperparathyroidism, and pheochromocytoma. Two subvariants of MEN 2A are familial medullary thyroid carcinoma only (FMTC) and MEN 2A in association with cutaneous lichen amyloidosis. Multiple endocrine neoplasia type 2B is the combination of medullary thyroid carcinoma, pheochromocytoma, mucosal neuromas, intestinal ganglioneuromatosis, and marfanoid-like features.

MULTIPLE ENDOCRINE NEOPLASIA TYPE 2A   Medullary thyroid carcinoma is the most common manifestation. The fully developed neoplasm is located characteristically at the junction of the upper one-third and lower two-thirds of each lobe of the thyroid gland and appears grossly as chalky white to yellow lesions; tumors greater than 1 cm in size are frequently associated with local or distant metastasis. This tumor usually develops in childhood, beginning as hyperplasia of the C-cells, or calcitonin-producing cells, of the thyroid. Measurement of the serum calcitonin level after injection of a stimulator of release such as calcium or pentagastrin makes it possible to diagnose this disorder when the likelihood of metastasis is low.

Pheochromocytoma occurs in approximately 50 percent of MEN 2A patients and causes typical symptoms, including palpitations, nervousness, headaches, and sometimes sweating. About half the tumors are bilateral, and in the remainder, the contralateral adrenal normal. More than 50 percent of patients who have had unilateral adrenalectomy develop a pheochromocytoma in the contralateral gland over an 8- to 10-year period. A second characteristic of these pheochromocytomas is the disproportionate increase in epinephrine secretion relative to that of norepinephrine. Patients with minimal abnormalities of epinephrine secretion may be asymptomatic. Finally, capsular invasion is common in pheochromocytoma associated with MEN 2, but malignant behavior is rare.

Primary hyperparathyroidism occurs in 15 to 20 percent of MEN 2A gene carriers, with a peak incidence in the third or fourth decade. In a few families, hyperparathyroidism occurs early and may be significant. The clinical presentation of hyperparathyroidism does not differ from that in other forms of primary hyperparathyroidism (see Chap. 353), with renal nephrolithiasis being common. Diagnosis is established by the finding of hypercalcemia, hypophosphatemia, hypercalciuria, and an inappropriately high serum intact parathyroid hormone concentration. Multiglandular parathyroid hyperplasia is the most common histologic finding, although with long-standing disease adenomatous changes may be superimposed on hyperplasia.

MULTIPLE ENDOCRINE NEOPLASIA TYPE 2B   The association of medullary thyroid carcinoma, pheochromocytoma, mucosal neuromas, a marfanoid habitus, and the absence of hyperparathyroidism is designated MEN 2B. Medullary thyroid carcinoma in MEN 2B is similar to that in MEN 2A except that development of C-cell hyperplasia and microscopic carcinoma occurs early and metastatic disease may be present prior to 1 year of age. Indeed, medullary thyroid carcinoma with MEN 2B commonly causes death in the second or third decade of life. However, the prognosis is not invariably bad even in patients with metastatic disease; a number of multigenerational families with this disorder exist.

Pheochromocytoma occurs in more than half of MEN 2B patients and does not differ significantly from that in MEN 2A. Hypercalcemia is rare in MEN 2B, and most examples of hypercalcemia are thought to be caused by bone metastases.

The mucosal neuromas constitute the most distinctive feature. They are present on the tip of the tongue, under the eyelids, and throughout the gastrointestinal tract and are true neuromas and should be differentiated from the neurofibromas associated with neurofibromatosis. The presence of the neuromas and a marfanoid body habitus form a distinct clinical picture recognizable even in childhood. Children also may present with gastrointestinal symptoms, including increased gas, intermittent obstruction, and diarrhea caused by neuromas.

Genetics and pathophysiology The genetic locus for all four variants of the MEN 2 syndrome has been mapped to the pericentromeric region of chromosome 10, most likely on the proximal long arm (see Fig. 343-1). The nature of the genetic defect is unclear, but the mechanism of tumorigenesis differs from MEN 1 in that there is no evidence for involvement of a "tumor suppressor gene" in the pathogenesis. The hypothesis that best fits the experimental evidence is that a mutation in a single allele of the MEN 2 gene stimulates hyperplasia of the several cell types involved in this syndrome. Subsequent mutational events at other genetic loci on chromosome 1p, 22q, 3p, or 9 may be involved in the progression of the disease.

Treatment SCREENING FOR MULTIPLE ENDOCRINE NEOPLASIA TYPE 2 Death from medullary thyroid carcinoma can be prevented by early thyroidectomy. The currently accepted form of screening utilizes annual pentagastrin or combined pentagastrin-calcium stimulation of calcitonin release from the thyroidal C-cell to identify medullary thyroid carcinoma or its precursor lesion, C-cell hyperplasia, in children before development of metastatic disease. Screening of individuals at risk should begin in early childhood, preferably before age 5. The pentagastrin test involves measurement of serum calcitonin basally and 2, 5, 10, and 15 min after bolus injection of 5 μg pentagastrin per kilogram of body weight. Patients should be warned before injection of epigastric tightness, nausea, warmth, and tingling of extremities and reassured that the symptoms will last approximately 2 min. It is sometimes difficult to differentiate between a mildly abnormal test result in a normal child and the first evidence of abnormality in an affected child. This issue can be resolved either by repetitive pentagastrin testing or by genetic approaches to testing.

The identification of polymorphic DNA sequences closely linked to the MEN 2 locus has made it possible to identify gene carriers with 90 to 99 percent certainty. Genetic testing is not perfect because of the potential for recombination between the disease gene and closely linked polymorphic DNA sequences. For this reason, many investigators utilize both genetic and calcitonin testing to determine which children should undergo thyroidectomy.

Screening studies for pheochromocytoma in subjects at risk should be performed on a regular (usually annual) basis. The goal is to identify a pheochromocytoma before it causes significant symptoms or is likely to cause sudden death, an event most commonly associated with large tumors. The measurement of basal plasma or 12-h urine catecholamines can be performed easily in conjunction with pentagastrin testing. Radiographic studies, such as MRI or CT scans, are generally reserved for individuals with abnormal screening tests or with symptoms suggestive of pheochromocytoma (see Chap. 336).

Measurement of serum calcium and parathyroid hormone levels every 2 to 3 years provides an adequate screen for hyperparathyroidism, except in those families in which hyperparathyroidism is a prominent component, in whom measurements should be made annually.

TREATMENT OF MEDULLARY THYROID CARCINOMA Hereditary medullary thyroid carcinoma is a multicentric disorder. Total thyroidectomy with a central lymph node dissection should be performed in children with abnormal calcitonin responses. More than 90 percent of children in whom thyroidectomy was performed on the basis of calcitonin screening remain without evidence of disease more than 15 years after surgery, whereas 15 to 25 percent of patients in whom the diagnosis is made on the basis of clinical findings die from metastatic disease within 15 years.

In adults with medullary thyroid cancer greater than 1 cm in size, metastases to regional lymph nodes are common. Total thyroidectomy with central lymph node dissection and selective dissection of other regional chains provide the best chance for cure. In patients with significant local metastatic disease, external radiotherapy may prevent local recurrence or reduce tumor mass but does not alter the course. Chemotherapy is also not curative but may reduce tumor mass.

TREATMENT OF PHEOCHROMOCYTOMA The long-term goal for management of pheochromocytoma is to prevent death and cardiovascular complications. Pheochromocytomas detected by screening studies should be removed surgically through an anterior abdominal approach. The major question is whether to remove both adrenal glands at the time of primary surgery or to remove only the affected adrenal. Issues to be considered in making this decision include the possibility of malignancy (fewer than 10 reported cases), the likelihood of development of pheochromocytoma in the apparently unaffected gland (may occur over an 8- to 10-year period), and the risks of adrenal insufficiency caused by removal of both glands. Most but not all clinicians recommend removal only of the affected gland and leave the contralateral gland in place unless inspection during surgery reveals an abnormality. If both adrenals are removed, glucocorticoid and mineralocorticoid replacement is mandatory.

TREATMENT OF HYPERPARATHYROIDISM Hyperparathyroidism has been managed by one of two approaches. Removal of 3½ glands with maintenance of the remaining half gland in the neck is the usual procedure. In families in whom hyperparathyroidism is a prominent manifestation and recurrence is common, total parathyroidectomy with transplantation of parathyroid tissue into the nondominant forearm is the preferred approach. The advantage of the latter approach is the ease of subsequent removal of parathyroid tissue if hypercalcemia recurs.

OTHER GENETIC TUMOR SYNDROMES A number of mixed syndromes exist in which the neoplastic associations differ from those usually found in MEN 1 or 2 (see Table 343-1).

IMMUNOLOGIC SYNDROMES AFFECTING MULTIPLE ENDOCRINE ORGANS

The polyglandular autoimmune syndromes (PGA) are designated type I, type II, and type III (Table 343-2). The type I syndrome starts in childhood and is characterized by mucocutaneous candidiasis, hypoparathyroidism, and adrenal insufficiency. Hypoparathyroidism is unusual in the type II or III syndromes, which are seen in adults. All the syndromes may cause adrenal insufficiency.

POLYGLANDULAR AUTOIMMUNE SYNDROME TYPE I PGA type I usually is recognized in the first decade of life. Although the manifestations vary, ultimately, the triad of mucocutaneous candidiasis, hypoparathyroidism, and adrenal insufficiency is seen. This disorder is also called *autoimmune polyendocrinopathy-candidiasis-ectodermal dystrophy* (APECED). Other features include dystrophy of the dental enamel with hypoplasia of the teeth and nails, vitiligo and keratopathy, gonadal failure, and thyroid or gastric parietal cell dysfunction resulting in primary hypothyroidism or pernicious anemia. Destruction of the β cells of the pancreatic islets and development of insulin-dependent (type I) diabetes are less common than in the type II syndrome. Some patients develop autoimmune hepatitis or malabsorption. At the outset, only one organ

---

TABLE 343-2 Disease associations in polyglandular autoimmune syndromes (PGA)

PGA I	PGA II	PGA III
Mucocutaneous candidiasis	Adrenal insufficiency	Type I diabetes mellitus and autoimmune thyroid disease or adrenal insufficiency and autoimmune thyroid disease (Hashimoto's)
Hypoparathyroidism	Autoimmune thyroid disease	
Addison's	Type I diabetes mellitus	
Hypogonadism	Hypogonadism	
Alopecia	Myasthenia gravis	
Hypothyroidism	Vitiligo	
Malabsorption	Alopecia	
Chronic active hepatitis	Pernicious anemia	
Vitiligo	Celiac disease	
Pernicious anemia		

may be involved, but the number of systems involved increases with time so that patients eventually manifest two to five components of the syndrome.

In a Finnish series, 78 percent of patients had a nonendocrine presentation, with oral candidiasis the most common initial finding. Although candidiasis occurs in most patients, the symptoms are often mild and can easily be missed. Involvement of the parathyroid glands usually occurs before adrenal insufficiency develops. More than 60 percent of postpubertal women become hypogonadal, whereas only about 15 percent of men develop testicular failure. APECED is not a disease of childhood exclusively, since the endocrine components, including adrenal insufficiency or hypoparathyroidism, may not develop until the fourth decade. Thus patients and their families should be followed long term for early detection and treatment of new manifestations of this syndrome.

POLYGLANDULAR AUTOIMMUNE SYNDROME TYPE II Type I diabetes mellitus is the most common manifestation of PGA type II and occurs in approximately half of affected families. Mucocutaneous candidiasis does not occur. This disorder, which tends to develop later in life than PGA type I, was first described by Schmidt in patients who had lymphocytic infiltration of the adrenal and thyroid glands at autopsy and who had family members with type I diabetes and hypogonadism. The autoimmune thyroid disease causes either Hashimoto's thyroiditis or hyperthyroidism; however, many patients with antimicrosomal and antithyroglobulin antibodies never develop abnormalities of thyroid function. Thus these antibodies alone are poor predictors of future disease. Dermatologic manifestations, including vitiligo, alopecia totalis, and alopecia areata (alopecia occurring in scattered areas), are common. Antibodies against the melanocyte may explain the localized areas of depigmentation. A few patients develop transient hypoparathyroidism with hypocalcemia as the result of antibodies that block the action of parathyroid hormone. Up to 25 percent of patients with myasthenia gravis and an even higher percentage who have myasthenia and a thymoma have polyglandular autoimmune syndrome type II (see Chap. 386).

POLYGLANDULAR AUTOIMMUNE SYNDROME TYPE III In certain families, abnormalities of only two endocrine glands, either diabetes mellitus and autoimmune thyroid disease or adrenal insufficiency in association with Hashimoto's thyroiditis, occur in a heritable manner. In these families, the syndrome never extends to the full spectrum of organ involvement of the PGA type II syndrome.

GENETICS AND PATHOGENESIS Type I PGA syndrome shows no HLA associations and is inherited as an autosomal recessive trait. In contrast, the type II and III syndromes are usually associated with the DR3 or DR4 haplotypes, or both, and are inherited as autosomal dominant traits. Epidemiologic studies of twins with either type I diabetes mellitus or Graves' disease revealed that only about 50 percent of the noninvolved identical twins develop these diseases. Thus additional environmental factors must activate the immune disregulation, even in individuals who inherit the tendency to develop the disease. In type I diabetes mellitus and other autoimmune diseases, the concept of molecular mimicry has been advanced to explain how environmental factors may trigger the disease in a genetically susceptible individual. Certain foreign antigens such as rubella viral capsid proteins or cow's milk proteins may share an epitope with a common antigen expressed on the surface of the human β cell. Activation of the immune system by the foreign antigen would initiate an immune attack on both the antigens and result in destruction of the β cell. Anti-insulin and anti-islet cell antibodies have been used in research studies as markers to predict the later development of type I diabetes mellitus. Studies of monozygotic twins or relatives of patients with known type I diabetes have shown that the process of β cell failure may develop slowly, with up to 8 years from the time of antibody detection to the development of hyperglycemia. Patients with the PGA syndromes may have a variety of organ-specific autoantibodies directed against many different target antigens. Some of the antibodies are only markers of autoimmunity and recognize cytoplasmic components of various endocrine cells (antithyroglobulin and antimicrosomal antibodies). However, other antibodies may be disease-specific, like those that fix complement and destroy a particular target or those directed against the acetylcholine, TSH, or parathyroid hormone receptors that interfere with the function of the hormone and thus may cause the various disorders seen in these patients.

Diagnosis and treatment The clinical manifestations of adrenal insufficiency often develop slowly and may be difficult to detect. The disease can be fatal if not diagnosed and treated appropriately. Thus all patients and family members with the suspected PGA syndromes should be screened prospectively to diagnose and treat the various components of the syndrome in a timely manner. The most effective screening test for adrenal disease is a cosyntropin stimulation test (see Chap. 335). A fasting blood glucose level can be obtained to screen for hyperglycemia. Additional screening tests should include studies of thyroid function, including measurements of thyroid-stimulating hormone and serum thyroxine, measurements of luteinizing hormone (LH), follicle-stimulating hormone (FSH), and testosterone levels in men, and assessment of LH and FSH levels in women. In families with suspected type I PGA syndrome, calcium and phosphorus levels are also measured. These screening studies should be performed every 1 to 2 years up to about age 50 in families with PGA type II and III syndrome and until about age 40 in patients with type I syndrome.

With the exception of Graves' disease, the management of each of the endocrine components of the disease involves hormone replacement and is covered in detail in the chapters on adrenal, thyroid, gonadal, and parathyroid disease (Chaps. 334, 335, 339, 340, and 357). Because primary hypothyroidism can mask adrenal insufficiency by prolonging the half-life of cortisol, administration of thyroid hormone to a patient with unsuspected adrenal insufficiency can precipitate adrenal crisis. Thus one needs to screen for adrenal disease and, if present, to initiate treatment with glucocorticoids prior to or concurrently with the thyroid hormone replacement.

OTHER AUTOIMMUNE ENDOCRINE SYNDROMES Insulin receptor antibodies Insulin resistance, defined as a decrease in the biologic response to a given amount of insulin, occurs commonly in patients with obesity, severe infections, trauma, or surgery, as well as in individuals with acromegaly or Cushing's syndrome, in whom growth hormone or cortisol excess can antagonize the action of insulin. In contrast, rare insulin-resistance syndromes occur in patients who develop spontaneous antibodies directed against insulin receptor. These antibodies block the normal insulin signal transduction pathway. Conversely, other classes of anti-insulin receptor antibodies can activate the receptor and can cause hypoglycemia and must be considered in the differential diagnosis of fasting hypoglycemia (see Chap. 337).

Anti-insulin receptor antibodies with insulin resistance and acanthosis nigricans, type B insulin resistance These patients are typically middle-aged women who acquire insulin resistance in association with other autoimmune disorders such as systemic lupus erythematosus or Sjögren's syndrome. Vitiligo, alopecia, Raynaud's phenomenon, and arthritis also may be seen. Other autoimmune endocrine disorders, including hyper- or hypothyroidism and hypogonadism, occur rarely. A mossy, hyperpigmented, thickened skin lesion, typical of acanthosis nigricans, is prominent on the dorsum of the neck and other skin fold areas in the axillae or groin. However, acanthosis nigricans also may occur in patients with obesity or polycystic ovarian syndrome, also associated with insulin resistance, and thus is not diagnostic of this form of insulin resistance. This syndrome is called the *type B insulin resistance syndrome* and must be differentiated from type A insulin resistance syndromes, which are secondary to a variety of molecular defects in the insulin receptor gene that result in mutations which alter insulin receptor signaling.

The anti-insulin receptor antibodies block the interaction of the hormone with its receptor and impair its action to varying degrees. Activation of the receptor by the antibodies also may result in receptor down-regulation and impair insulin action. The degree of insulin resistance can be quite variable. Some patients with acanthosis nigricans show normal to mild glucose intolerance with a compensatory increase in insulin secretion that is only detected when insulin levels are measured. Others have severe diabetes mellitus requiring massive doses of insulin (several thousand units per day) to lower the blood glucose levels. The nature of the antibodies determines the manifestations. Although insulin resistance is more common, fasting hypoglycemia can be present from the first or develop during the course of the disease. The hypoglycemia results from interactions of insulinomimetic classes of antibodies with insulin receptor.

Anti-insulin antibodies and ataxia telangiectasia Ataxia telangiectasia is an autosomal recessive disorder with insulin-resistant diabetes mellitus, ataxia, telangiectasia, immune abnormalities, and an increased incidence of malignancies. This disorder is also associated with anti-insulin antibodies.

Autoimmune insulin syndrome with hypoglycemia Spontaneous polyclonal insulin-binding autoantibodies, typically found in patients with other autoimmune disorders, can bind the insulin released in response to meals and release it later to cause hypoglycemia, often several hours or more after a meal. Fasting hypoglycemia may be caused by release of insulin from these antibodies during a fast. Most cases of the syndrome have been described from Japan, and there may be a genetic component. The anti-insulin antibodies may interfere in the insulin assay and falsely elevate the insulin levels. A finding of normal C-peptide levels in this situation suggests a false-positive insulin measurement. In plasma cell dyscrasias such as multiple myeloma, the plasma cells may produce monoclonal antibodies against insulin and cause hypoglycemia by a similar mechanism.

Antithyroxine antibodies and hypothyroidism Circulating autoantibodies against thyroid hormones in patients with both immune thyroid disease and plasma cell dyscrasias such as Waldenström's macroglobulinemia can bind thyroid hormones, decrease their biologic activity, and result in primary hypothyroidism.

Plasma cell dyscrasia with polyneuropathy, organomegaly, endocrinopathy, M proteins, and skin changes (POEMS syndrome The features of this syndrome are highlighted by an acronyn that emphasizes its important features: *p*olyneuropathy, *o*rganomegaly, *e*ndocrinopathy, *M* proteins, and *s*kin changes (POEMS). The most important feature is a severe, progressive sensorimotor polyneuropathy associated with a plasma cell dyscrasia. Localized collections of plasma cells (plasmacytomas) can cause sclerotic bone lesions and produce monoclonal IgG or IgA proteins. Endocrine manifestations include amenorrhea in women and impotence and gynecomastia in men. Hyperprolactinemia, due to loss of normal inhibitory control of the lactotroph by the hypothalamus, may be associated with other central nervous system manifestations, including papilledema, and increased cerebrospinal fluid pressure and protein. Type II diabetes mellitus occurs commonly, whereas primary hypothyroidism and adrenal insufficiency are less frequent. Skin changes include hyperpigmentation, thickening of the dermis, hirsutism, and hyperhidrosis. Hepatomegaly and lymphadenopathy occur in about two-thirds of the cases, and splenomegaly is seen in about one-third. Other manifestations include peripheral edema, ascites, pleural effusions, and fever.

The systemic nature of the disorder may cause confusion with other connective tissue diseases. The endocrine manifestations suggest an autoimmune basis of the disorder, but circulating antibodies against endocrine cells have not been demonstrated. Thus the pathophysiologic basis for the POEMS syndrome is uncertain. Therapy directed against the plasma cell dyscrasia such as local radiation of bony lesions or chemotherapy may result in improvement.

TABLE 343-3 Other disorders with common polyglandular manifestations

Condition	Clinical features	Type of endocrine involvement						Inheritance/ molecular defect
		Hypothalamic-pituitary	Thyroid	Parathyroid	Pancreas	Adrenal	Gonads	
Ataxia-telangiectasia	Early ataxia Oculocutaneous telangiectasia Immunologic deficiency	Occasional diminished pituitary reserve			Diabetes mellitus	Cortical hypoplasia	Dysgenic gonads: gonadoblastomas in females	Autosomal recessive
Pseudo-hypoparathyroidism	Short stature Short metacarpals and metatarsals Round facies Ectopic calcification	Variable deficiency of all pituitary hormones including prolactin	Hypo- or hyper-thyroidism	Elevated parathyroid hormone levels with normo- or hypocalcemia	Diabetes mellitus		Ovarian failure	Mutation of the $GS_{s\alpha}$ subunit
Myotonic dystrophy	Muscular dystrophy Premature baldness Mental retardation	Gonadotropin and growth hormone abnormalities	Hypo-thyroidism		Diabetes mellitus		Primary gonadal failure	Insertion of unstable CTG repeat in myotonic dystrophy gene on chromosome 19
Noonan syndrome	Short stature Ptosis Webbed neck Pulmonary stenosis	Gonadotropin deficiency	Thyroiditis				Primary gonadal failure	Autosomal dominant
Fanconi syndrome	Short statuure Bone marrow hypoplasia Abnormal skin pigmentation Radial malformations	Panhypo-pituitarism			Diabetes mellitus	Adrenal atrophy	Gonadal atrophy	Autosomal recessive
Werner syndrome	Premature aging Atrophic skin Cataracts Early osteopenia		Papillary thyroid carcinoma		Diabetes mellitus		Gonadal atrophy	Autosomal recessive

Immune nodular adrenal hyperplasia   A rare form of Cushing's syndrome, nodular adrenal hyperplasia can occur due to several causes. Some patients have antibodies against the adrenal gland that stimulate adrenal cortical cell growth and result in hyperplasia and excess glucocorticoid production.

MISCELLANEOUS DISORDERS WITH ENDOCRINE MANIFESTATIONS

A variety of other clinical and genetic disorders are associated with multiple endocrine manifestations (Table 343-3).

REFERENCES

AHONEN P et al: Clinical variation of autoimmune polyendocrinopathy-candidiasis-ectodermal dystrophy (APECED) in a series of 68 patients. N Engl J Med 322:1829, 1990

BARDWICK PA et al: Plasma cell dyscrasia with polyneuropathy, organomegaly, endocrinopathy, M protein, and skin changes: The POEMS syndrome. Medicine 59:311, 1980

FRIEDMAN E et al: Clonality of parathyroid tumors in familial multiple endocrine neoplasia type 1. N Engl J Med 321:213, 1989

GAGEL RF: Multiple endocrine neoplasia, in *William's Textbook of Endocrinology*, 8th ed, JD Wilson, DW Foster (eds). Philadelphia, Saunders, 1992, pp 1537–1553

——— et al: The clinical outcome of prospective screening for multiple endocrine neoplasia type 2a: An 18-year experience. N Engl J Med 318:478, 1988

KAHN CR et al: The syndromes of insulin resistance and acanthosis nigricans: Insulin-receptor disorders in man. N Engl J Med 294:739, 1976

LARSSON C et al: Multiple endocrine neoplasia type 1 gene maps to chromosome 11 and is lost in insulinoma. Nature 322:85, 1988

NEUFELD M et al: Two types of autoimmune Addison's disease associated with different polyglandular autoimmune (PGA) syndromes. Medicine 60:355, 1981

RIZZOLI R et al: Primary hyperparathyroidism in familial multiple endocrine neoplasia type I: Long-term follow-up of serum calcium levels after parathyroidectomy. Am J Med 78:467, 1985

SIMPSON NE: The exploration of the locus or loci for the syndromes associated with medullary thyroid cancer (MTC) on chromosome 10, in *Hereditary Tumors*, ML Brandi, R White (eds). New York, Raven, 1991, pp 55–67

SKOGSEID B et al: Multiple endocrine neoplasia type 1: A 10-year prospective screening study in four kindreds. J Clin Endocrinol Metab 73:281, 1991

section 2   Disorders of intermediary metabolism

344   THE HYPERLIPOPROTEINEMIAS AND OTHER DISORDERS OF LIPID METABOLISM

MICHAEL S. BROWN / JOSEPH L. GOLDSTEIN

The *hyperlipoproteinemias* are disturbances of lipid transport that result from accelerated synthesis or retarded degradation of lipoproteins that transport cholesterol and triglycerides through plasma. Elevated plasma lipoprotein levels are important clinically because they can cause two life-threatening diseases: atherosclerosis and pancreatitis. A reduction in cholesterol-carrying lipoproteins, achieved by diet and drugs, reduces the risk of myocardial infarction in subjects with hyperlipoproteinemia. Some hyperlipoproteinemias are the direct result of *primary* defects in the synthesis or degradation of lipoprotein particles. Other hyperlipoproteinemias are *secondary;* that is, the elevated plasma lipoprotein level occurs as part of a constellation of abnormalities caused by an underlying disorder in a related metabolic system, such as thyroid hormone deficiency or insulin deficiency. The primary hyperlipoproteinemias can be divided into two broad categories: (1) *single-gene disorders* that are transmitted by simple dominant or recessive mechanisms and (2) *multifactorial disorders* with complex inheritance patterns in which multiple variant genes, each having a subtle effect, interact with environmental factors to produce varying degrees of hyperlipoproteinemia in members of a family.

ROLE OF LIPOPROTEINS IN LIPID TRANSPORT   The lipoproteins are globular particles of high molecular weight that transport nonpolar lipids (primarily *triglycerides* and *cholesteryl esters*) through the plasma. A general model for the structure of a lipoprotein particle is shown in Fig. 344-1. Each lipoprotein particle contains a nonpolar *core*, in which many molecules of hydrophobic lipid are packed to form an oil droplet. This hydrophobic core, which accounts for most

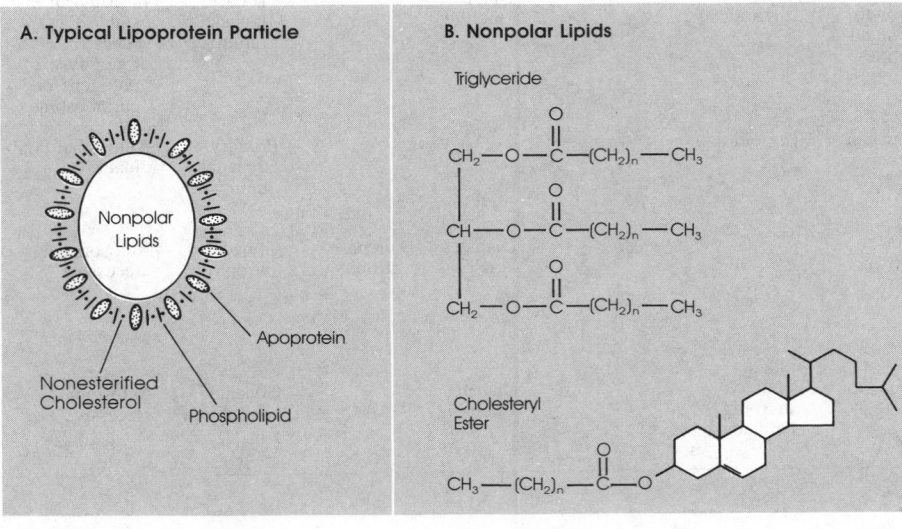

A. Typical Lipoprotein Particle

Nonpolar Lipids

Apoprotein

Nonesterified Cholesterol

Phospholipid

B. Nonpolar Lipids

Triglyceride

Cholesteryl Ester

FIGURE 344-1   *A.* Diagrammatic representation of the structure of a typical plasma lipoprotein particle. The *core* of the spherical lipoprotein particle is composed of two nonpolar lipids, triglyceride and cholesteryl ester, which are present in different lipoproteins in varying amounts. The nonpolar core is surrounded by a *surface coat* composed primarily of phospholipids. Apoproteins are exposed at the surface and extend into the core. Variable amounts of unesterified cholesterol are interdigitated with the phospholipids of the surface coat. The composition of the five major classes of lipoproteins in human plasma is summarized in Table 344-1. *B.* Two nonpolar lipids, triglyceride and cholesteryl ester. For them to be assimilated into tissues, the ester bonds between the fatty acids and either glycerol (triglycerides) or cholesterol (cholesteryl esters) must be broken by lipoprotein lipase and the lysosomal cholesterol esterase, respectively.

TABLE 344-1   Characteristics of the major classes of lipoproteins in human plasma

Lipoprotein class	Major lipids	Major apoproteins	Density, g/mL	Diameter, nm	Electrophoretic mobility
Chylomicrons and remnants	Dietary triglycerides	AI, AII, B48, CI, CII, CIII, E	<1.006	800–5000	Remains at origin
VLDL	Endogenous triglycerides	B48, CI, CII, CIII, E	<1.006	300–800	Pre-β
IDL	Cholesteryl esters, triglycerides	B100, CIII, E	<1.019	250–350	Slow pre-β
LDL	Cholesteryl esters	B100	1.019–1.063	180–280	β
HDL	Cholesteryl esters	AI, AII	1.063–1.210	50–120	α

of the mass of the particle, consists of triglycerides and cholesteryl esters in varying proportions. Surrounding the core is a polar *surface coat* of phospholipids that stabilize the lipoprotein particle so that it can remain in solution in the plasma. In addition to phospholipids, the polar coat contains small amounts of unesterified cholesterol. Each lipoprotein particle also contains specific proteins (termed *apoproteins*) that are exposed at the surface. The apoproteins bind to specific enzymes or transport proteins on cell membranes, thus directing the lipoprotein to its sites of metabolism.

Table 344-1 describes the characteristics of the five major classes of lipoproteins that normally circulate in human plasma. These lipoprotein classes differ in the composition of the nonpolar lipids in the core, in the composition of the apoproteins, and in density, size, and electrophoretic mobility.

Lipid transport: The exogenous pathway   Figure 344-2 shows the pathways by which lipoproteins transport lipids in plasma. The largest amounts of lipoproteins are involved in the transport of dietary fat, which amounts to more than 100 g triglyceride and about 1 g cholesterol per day. Within intestinal epithelial cells, dietary triglycerides and cholesterol are incorporated into large lipoprotein particles called *chylomicrons.* The chylomicrons are secreted into the intestinal lymph and pass into the general circulation for transport to the capillaries of adipose tissue and skeletal muscle, where they adhere to binding sites on the capillary walls. While bound to these endothelial surfaces, the chylomicrons are exposed to the enzyme *lipoprotein lipase.* The chylomicrons contain an apoprotein, apoprot-

FIGURE 344-2   Model for plasma triglyceride and cholesterol transport in humans. The details of this model are described in the text. VLDL, very low density lipoprotein; IDL, intermediate-density lipoprotein; LDL, low-density lipoprotein; HDL, high-density lipoprotein; LCAT, lecithin:cholesterol acyltransferase; LP lipase, lipoprotein lipase; FFA, free fatty acids. The major apoprotein for each class of lipoproteins is shown. Other apoproteins are also present, and these are listed in Table 344-1.

ein CII, that activates the lipase, liberating free fatty acids and monoglycerides (Fig. 344-3). The fatty acids pass through the endothelial cells and enter the underlying adipocytes or muscle cells, where they are either reesterified to triglycerides or oxidized.

After the core triglycerides have been removed, the remainder of the chylomicron dissociates from the capillary endothelium and reenters the circulation. It has now been transformed into a particle that is relatively poor in triglyceride and enriched in cholesteryl esters. It also has undergone an exchange of apoproteins with other plasma lipoproteins. The net result is the conversion of the chylomicron to a *chylomicron remnant particle,* enriched in cholesteryl esters and apoproteins B48 and E. This remnant travels to the liver, where it is taken up with great efficiency. This uptake is mediated by the binding of apoprotein E to specific receptors, called *chylomicron remnant receptors,* on the surface of the hepatocytes. The surface-bound remnants are taken into the cell and degraded within lysosomes by a process called receptor-mediated endocytosis (see Fig. 344-3). The overall result of the chylomicron transport process is to deliver dietary triglyceride to adipose tissue and cholesterol to the liver.

Some of the cholesterol that reaches the liver is converted to bile acids, which are excreted into the intestine to act as detergents and facilitate the absorption of dietary fat. In addition, some cholesterol is excreted into the bile without metabolism to bile acids. The liver also distributes cholesterol to other tissues by the endogenous pathway, which is discussed below.

Lipid transport: The endogenous pathway   Triglyceride synthesis in the liver is enhanced when the diet contains excess carbohydrates. The liver converts the carbohydrate to fatty acids, esterifies the fatty acids with glycerol to form triglycerides, and secretes the triglyceride into the bloodstream in the core of *very low density lipoprotein (VLDL).* The VLDL particles are relatively large, carry 5 to 10 times more triglycerides than cholesteryl esters, and contain a form of apoprotein B, designated B100, that differs from the apoprotein B48 of chylomicrons (see Table 344-1).

The VLDL particles are transported to tissue capillaries, where they interact with the same lipoprotein lipase enzyme that catabolizes chylomicrons. The core triglycerides of the VLDL particles are hydrolyzed, and the fatty acids are used for triglyceride synthesis within adipose tissue. The remnants generated from the action of lipoprotein-lipase on VLDLs are designated *intermediate-density lipoprotein (IDL).* A portion of the IDL particles is catabolized by the liver through binding to receptors called *low-density lipoprotein (LDL) receptors,* which are distinct from the chylomicron remnant receptors. The remaining IDLs remain in plasma, where they undergo a further transformation in which nearly all the residual triglycerides are removed. During this conversion, all the apoproteins are removed from the particle with the exception of apoprotein B100. The result is the transformation of the IDL particle into cholesterol-rich LDL. The core of LDL is composed almost entirely of cholesteryl esters, and the surface coat contains only one apoprotein, apoprotein B100. In humans, a relatively high fraction of IDL escapes hepatic uptake, and consequently, humans have relatively high circulating levels of LDL. Indeed, about three-fourths of the total cholesterol in normal human plasma is contained within LDL particles.

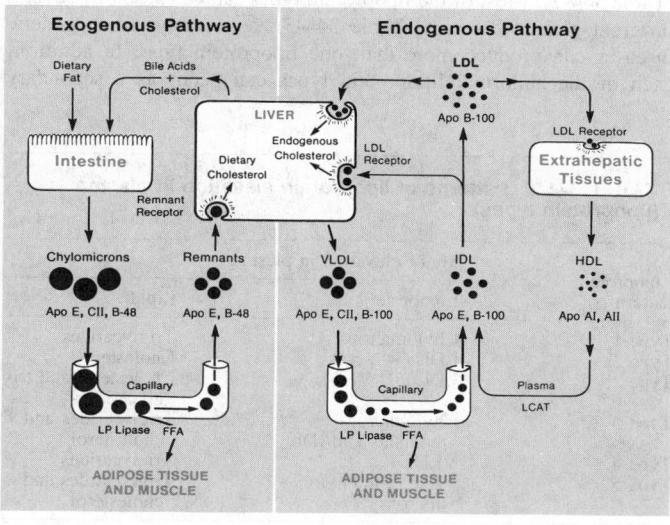

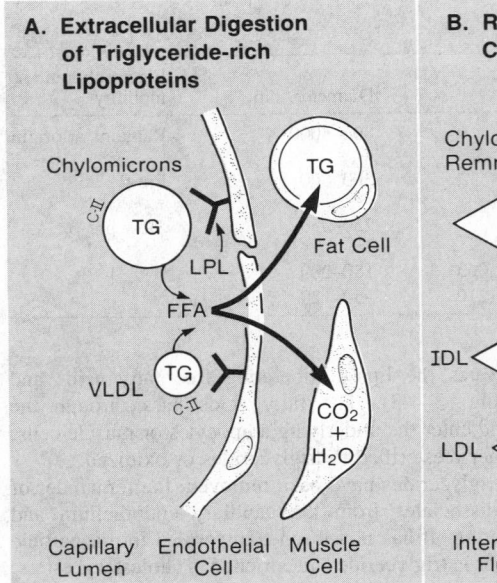

A. Extracellular Digestion of Triglyceride-rich Lipoproteins

B. Receptor-mediated Endocytosis of Cholesterol-rich Lipoproteins

FIGURE 344-3 Comparison of the mechanisms by which triglyceride-rich lipoproteins and cholesterol-rich lipoproteins deliver their core lipids to target tissues. Triglycerides are hydrolyzed by an extracellular enzyme (LPL) that is attached to endothelial cells and operates at the endothelial surface. Cholesteryl esters are hydrolyzed by an intracellular enzyme, acid lipase, that is located in lysosomes and cleaves the esters that enter cells via receptor-mediated endocytosis. TG, triglycerides; LPL, lipoprotein lipase; VLDL, very low density lipoproteins; CE, cholesteryl esters; IDL, intermediate-density lipoproteins; LDL, low-density lipoproteins; FFA, free fatty acid. The apoproteins responsible for the interactions (CII, B, and E) are indicated.

One function of LDL is to supply cholesterol to a variety of extrahepatic parenchymal cells, such as adrenal cortical cells, lymphocytes, and renal cells. These cells have *LDL receptors* localized on the cell surface. LDL that binds to this receptor is taken up by receptor-mediated endocytosis and digested by lysosomes within the cells (see Fig. 344-3). The cholesteryl esters of LDL are hydrolyzed by a lysosomal cholesteryl esterase (acid lipase), and the liberated cholesterol is used for membrane synthesis, as a precursor for steroid hormone synthesis, and as a regulatory molecule that suppresses the synthesis of new LDL receptors. Like extrahepatic tissues, the liver also has abundant LDL receptors; it uses the LDL-cholesterol for synthesis of bile acids and for generation of free cholesterol, which is secreted into the bile. In humans, 70 to 80 percent of LDL is removed from plasma by the LDL receptor pathway. Much of the remainder is degraded by a scavenger cell system in phagocytic cells in the reticuloendothelial system. In contrast to the receptor-mediated pathway for LDL degradation, the scavenger cell pathway is thought to function solely to degrade LDL when the lipoprotein reaches high concentrations in plasma rather than to supply cholesterol to cells.

As the membranes of parenchymal and scavenger cells undergo turnover and as cells die and are renewed, unesterified cholesterol is released into plasma, where it binds initially to *high-density lipoprotein (HDL)*. This unesterified cholesterol is then coupled to a fatty acid in an esterification reaction catalyzed by the plasma enzyme *lecithin:cholesterol acyltransferase (LCAT)*. The cholesteryl esters that are formed on the surface of HDL are transferred to VLDL and eventually appear in LDL. This establishes a cycle by which LDL delivers cholesterol to extrahepatic cells and by which cholesterol is returned to LDL from extrahepatic cells via HDL. Most of the cholesterol released from extrahepatic tissues is transported to the liver for excretion in the bile.

DIAGNOSIS OF HYPERLIPOPROTEINEMIA A number of diseases cause elevations in the concentrations of one or more lipoprotein classes in plasma. In general, these abnormalities are detected by the finding of an elevated concentration of triglycerides or cholesterol in fasting plasma, a condition called *hyperlipidemia*. The value for plasma cholesterol represents the total cholesterol, which includes both cholesteryl esters and unesterified cholesterol. The plasma cholesterol and triglyceride levels provide information regarding the nature of the lipoprotein particle that is increased. An isolated elevation in plasma triglycerides indicates that the concentrations of chylomicrons or VLDL are increased. On the other hand, an isolated elevation of plasma cholesterol nearly always indicates that the concentration of LDL is increased. Frequently, both triglycerides and

cholesterol are elevated. Such a combined abnormality may be produced by a marked elevation in chylomicrons or VLDL, in which case the ratio of triglyceride to cholesterol in plasma will be greater than 5:1. Alternatively, there may be an elevation of both VLDL and LDL, in which case the triglyceride/cholesterol ratio in plasma is usually less than 5:1.

The definition of hyperlipoproteinemia is arbitrary because plasma lipid and lipoprotein levels exhibit a bell-shaped distribution in the population, without clear separation between normal and abnormal values. Since lipoprotein concentrations are influenced by diet and other environmental factors, standards must be established for the population under consideration. Usually, arbitrary statistical limits of normal concentrations are selected, based on the examination of a large number of healthy-appearing subjects of different ages. The usual cut-off limit is the upper 5 to 10 percent of values (i.e., the 90th to 95th percentile values). However, analysis of blood lipid levels in individuals from industrialized and more agrarian cultures indicates that lipid and lipoprotein concentrations that are "normal" in a statistical sense are not necessarily healthy. As a working rule, hyperlipoproteinemia is considered to be present whenever the plasma cholesterol level exceeds 5.2 mmol/L (200 mg/dL) or the triglyceride level exceeds 2.2 mmol/L (200 mg/dL).

The various combinations of elevated lipoproteins that occur in disease states have been divided into six lipoprotein types or patterns (Table 344-2). Most of the lipoprotein types can be caused by several different genetic diseases (Table 344-3); conversely, some genetic diseases can produce more than one lipoprotein type. In addition, each of the abnormal lipoprotein types can occur as a secondary

TABLE 344-2 Patterns of lipoprotein elevation in plasma (lipoprotein types)

Lipoprotein pattern	Major elevation in plasma	
	Lipoprotein	Lipid
Type 1	Chylomicrons	Triglycerides
Type 2a	LDL	Cholesterol
Type 2b	LDL and VLDL	Cholesterol and triglycerides
Type 3	Chylomicron remnants and IDL	Triglycerides and cholesterol
Type 4	VLDL	Triglycerides
Type 5	VLDL and chylomicrons	Triglycerides and cholesterol

TABLE 344-3   Characteristics of the primary hyperlipoproteinemias resulting from single-gene mutations

Genetic disorder	Primary biochemical defect	Plasma lipoprotein elevation (pattern)	Typical clinical findings	Lipoprotein pattern in affected relatives	Drug therapy First choice	Other
Familial lipoprotein lipase deficiency	Deficiency of lipoprotein lipase	Chylomicrons (1)	Eruptive xanthomas, pancreatitis	1	None	None
Familial apoprotein CII deficiency	Deficiency of apoprotein CII	Chylomicrons and VLDL (1 or 5)	Pancreatitis	1 or 5	None	None
Familial type 3 hyperlipoproteinemia	Abnormal apoprotein E of VLDL	Chylomicron remnants and IDL (3)	Palmar and tuberous xanthomas; premature atherosclerosis	3, 2a, 2b, or 4	Gemfibrozil	Nicotinic acid; HMG CoA reductase inhibitor
Familial hypercholesterolemia	Deficiency of LDL receptor	LDL (2a, rarely 2b)	Tendon xanthomas; premature atherosclerosis	2a (rarely 2b)	Bile acid–binding resin plus HMG CoA reductase inhibitor	Nicotinic acid; probucol
Familial hypertriglyceridemia	Unknown	VLDL (rarely chylomicrons) (4, rarely 5)	Eruptive xanthomas; premature atherosclerosis	4 (rarely 5)	Gemfibrozil; nicotinic acid	
Multiple lipoprotein–type hyperlipidemia (familial combined hyperlipidemia)	Unknown	LDL and VLDL (2a, 2b, or 4, rarely 5)		2a, 2b, or 4 (rarely 5)	Gemfibrozil; nicotinic acid	HMG CoA reductase inhibitor

consequence of another metabolic disease (Table 344-4). Hence the lipoprotein type must be considered a shorthand notation to describe an abnormal lipoprotein pattern in plasma and not a designation of a specific disease.

Ordinarily, the simple measurement of plasma lipid levels, coupled with a clinical assessment, is sufficient to classify the type of lipoprotein abnormality present (see Table 344-2). Occasionally, electrophoresis of the plasma on agarose gels is useful either when an elevation in remnant particles is suspected (type 3 lipoprotein pattern giving a "broad beta" band on electrophoresis) or when chylomicronemia is a possibility (type 1 pattern). When the total cholesterol level exceeds 6.2 mmol/L (240 mg/dL), HDL levels should be measured, since low levels of this lipoprotein class are statistically associated with an increased risk of myocardial infarction (see Chap. 208). The level of HDL can be estimated in clinical laboratories using standardized lipoprotein separation techniques.

THERAPEUTIC APPROACHES   The first approach for treatment of all hyperlipoproteinemias is dietary. Individuals who are overweight should be placed on a weight-reducing regimen. Virtually all patients with hyperlipoproteinemia, either primary or secondary, can be treated with a single diet that is low in cholesterol and saturated animal fats and relatively (but not absolutely) high in polyunsaturated vegetable oils, which reduce concentrations of plasma LDL.

The second therapeutic aim is to eliminate aggravating factors, such as diabetes mellitus, alcoholism, or hypothyroidism. Patients with hyperlipoproteinemia also should be encouraged to reduce all other risk factors that predispose to atherosclerosis. These include cessation of smoking, treatment of hypertension, maintenance of a good exercise and physical fitness program, and control of blood glucose in subjects with diabetes mellitus (see Chap. 208).

The final aspect of therapy involves the use of drugs that lower plasma concentrations of lipoproteins, either by decreasing their production or by increasing their removal from plasma. The drugs available for this purpose are discussed below.

PRIMARY HYPERLIPOPROTEINEMIAS RESULTING FROM SINGLE-GENE MUTATIONS

FAMILIAL LIPOPROTEIN LIPASE DEFICIENCY   This rare autosomal recessive disorder is attributable to the absence or marked reduction in the activity of the enzyme lipoprotein lipase. This deficiency leads to a metabolic block in the metabolism of chylomi-

crons, causing these lipoproteins to accumulate to massive levels in plasma.

Clinical features   The disease usually presents in infancy or childhood with recurrent attacks of abdominal pain. The pain is caused by pancreatitis occurring as a consequence of the massive elevation of chylomicrons in plasma. Affected individuals intermittently develop eruptive xanthomas, small yellowish papules, frequently surrounded by an erythematous base, that appear predominantly on the buttocks and other pressure-sensitive surfaces. The xanthomas are caused by the deposition of large amounts of chylomicron triglycerides in cutaneous histiocytes. Triglycerides are also deposited in phagocytes of the reticuloendothelial system, producing hepatomegaly, splenomegaly, and foam cell infiltration of the bone marrow. When the level of chylomicrons in the blood is massively elevated [i.e., plasma triglyceride level greater than 22 mmol/L (2000 mg/dL)], the blood appears pale and creamy and is said to be *lipemic*. When viewed with the ophthalmoscope, the retina is pale, and the retinal vessels are white, producing the appearance of lipemia retinalis. Despite the massive elevation of plasma triglycerides, accelerated atherosclerosis does not occur.

Pathogenesis   Affected individuals have two copies of a mutant lipoprotein lipase gene. The activator of lipoprotein lipase, apoprotein CII, is present in normal amounts. The parents are obligate heterozygotes for the lipoprotein lipase defect, but they are usually normal clinically. As a result of the deficiency of lipoprotein lipase in homozygotes, chylomicrons cannot be metabolized normally, and the level of chylomicrons in the blood rises to high levels after a fat meal. In normal individuals, chylomicrons disappear from the blood after a 12-h fast. However, in affected patients, high levels of chylomicrons are found in the plasma even after several days of fasting or ingestion of a fat-free diet.

The circulating chylomicrons inflame the pancreas when they pass through its capillaries. Within the capillary lumen in the pancreas, chylomicrons are exposed to small amounts of pancreatic lipase that leaks from the tissue. Partial hydrolysis of the triglycerides and phospholipids of the chylomicron produces toxic products, including fatty acids and lysolecithin, that break down tissue membranes, produce further leakage of lipase from the pancreatic acinar cells, and eventually cause fulminant pancreatitis.

Diagnosis   The diagnosis of familial lipoprotein lipase deficiency is suggested by the finding of lipemic plasma in a young individual who has been fasting for at least 12 h. This lipemic plasma, when collected in the presence of EDTA, has a characteristic appearance

TABLE 344-4   Clinical disorders associated with secondary hyperlipoproteinemia

Underlying disorder	Plasma lipoprotein elevation				Lipoprotein type	Proposed mechanism for hyperlipoproteinemia	Associated abnormality of carbohydrate metabolism
	Chylomicrons	IDL	VLDL	LDL			
ENDOCRINE AND METABOLIC							
Diabetes mellitus	+		+ + +		4 (rarely 5)	Increased secretion of VLDL Decreased catabolism of VLDL and chylomicrons due to reduced lipoprotein lipase activity	Insulin deficiency or resistance
von Gierke's disease (glycogen storage disease, type I)	+		+ + +		4 (rarely 5)	Increased secretion of VLDL Decreased catabolism of VLDL and chylomicrons due to reduced lipoprotein lipase activity	Hypoglycemia with decreased insulin secretion
Lipodystrophies (congenital and acquired forms)			+ +		4	Increased secretion of VLDL	Insulin resistance
Cushing's syndrome			+	+ +	2a or 2b	Increased secretion of VLDL with conversion to LDL	Insulin resistance
Sexual ateliotic dwarfism (isolated growth hormone deficiency)			+ +	+ +	2b	Increased secretion of VLDL with conversion to LDL	Insulin deficiency or resistance
Acromegaly			+		4	Increased secretion of VLDL	Insulin resistance
Hypothyroidism		+		+ + +	2a (rarely 3)	Decreased catabolism of VLDL and IDL	
Anorexia nervosa			+ +		2a	Reduced biliary excretion of cholesterol and bile acids	
Werner's syndrome			+ +		2a	Unknown	Insulin resistance
Acute intermittent porphyria			+ +		2a	Unknown	
DRUG-INDUCED							
Alcohol	+		+ + +		4 (rarely 5)	Increased secretion of VLDL in individuals genetically predisposed to hypertriglyceridemia	
Oral contraceptives	+		+ + +		4 (rarely 5)	Increased secretion of VLDL in individuals genetically predisposed to hypertriglyceridemia	Insulin resistance
Glucocorticoids			+	+ +	2a or 2b	Increased secretion of VLDL with conversion to LDL	Insulin resistance
RENAL							
Uremia			+ + +		4	Decreased catabolism of VLDL due to reduced lipoprotein lipase activity	Insulin resistance
Nephrotic syndrome			+ +	+ + +	2a or 2b	Increased secretion of VLDL Direct secretion of LDL from liver Decreased catabolism of VLDL and LDL	
HEPATIC							
Primary biliary cirrhosis and extrahepatic biliary obstruction					↑ Cholesterol ↑ Phospholipids ↑ Lipoprotein X	Diversion of biliary cholesterol and phospholipids into bloodstream	
Acute hepatitis (nonfulminant)			+ + +		4	Decreased hepatic secretion of lecithin: cholesterol acyltransferase (LCAT)	

TABLE 344-4   Clinical disorders associated with secondary hyperlipoproteinemia (continued)

Underlying disorder	Plasma lipoprotein elevation				Lipoprotein type	Proposed mechanism for hyperlipoproteinemia	Associated abnormality of carbohydrate metabolism
	Chylomicrons	IDL	VLDL	LDL			
HEPATIC (continued)							
Hepatoma				+ +	2a	Lack of feedback inhibition of hepatic cholesterol synthesis by dietary cholesterol	
IMMUNOLOGIC							
Systemic lupus erythematosus	+ +				1	Presence of IgG or IgM that binds heparin, thereby decreasing activity of lipoprotein lipase	
Monoclonal gammopathies (myeloma, macroglobulinemia, lymphoma)	+ +	+ +	+ +		3 or 4	Presence of IgG or IgM that forms immune complex with chylomicron remnants and/or VLDL, thereby decreasing their catabolism	
STRESS-INDUCED							
Emotional stress, acute myocardial infarction, extensive burns, acute gram-negative sepsis			+ +		4	Increased secretion and decreased catabolism of VLDL	

after it has incubated overnight in a refrigerator at 4°C. A white layer of cream (which consists of chylomicrons) appears at the top of the tube. The layer beneath the cream is clear. The diagnosis of familial lipoprotein lipase deficiency is supported by the finding of a type 1 pattern on lipoprotein electrophoresis. It is confirmed by the demonstration that lipoprotein lipase levels in plasma fail to increase following the infusion of heparin. In normal individuals, intravenous heparin releases lipoprotein lipase from its binding sites within the capillary endothelium, and increased amounts of enzyme can then be assayed in the plasma. Gel electrophoresis of VLDL apoproteins in patients with lipoprotein lipase deficiency shows a normal amount of activator apoprotein CII, thus distinguishing these patients from those with the related disorder, familial apoprotein CII deficiency (see below).

Treatment   The symptoms and signs of the disease recede when the patient is placed on a fat-free diet. Every attempt should be made to maintain the fasting plasma triglyceride level below 11 mmol/L (1000 mg/dL) to prevent pancreatitis. It has been found empirically that the chronic fat intake in affected adults must be less than 20 g/d to prevent symptomatic hyperlipemia. Since medium-chain triglycerides are not incorporated into chylomicrons, they have been employed to help achieve normal caloric intake. The diet should be supplemented with fat-soluble vitamins.

FAMILIAL APOPROTEIN CII DEFICIENCY   This rare autosomal recessive disorder is due to the absence of apoprotein CII, an essential cofactor for lipoprotein lipase. Deficiency of this peptide creates a functional lipoprotein lipase deficiency, thus producing a syndrome that is similar but not identical to familial lipoprotein lipase deficiency (see above). Because of the apoprotein CII deficiency, lipoprotein lipase is not activated, and its two substrate lipoproteins, chylomicrons and VLDL, accumulate in the blood, thus causing hypertriglyceridemia (type 1 or type 5 lipoprotein pattern). The disorder is diagnosed in children or adults on the basis of recurrent attacks of pancreatitis or by milky plasma detected by chance. The diagnosis is made by showing an absence of apoprotein CII on gel electrophoresis of VLDL apoproteins. Transfusion of normal plasma (which contains abundant

apoprotein CII) into the patient is followed by a dramatic fall in plasma triglyceride levels. Heterozygotes, who have 50 percent reduction in apoprotein CII levels, may exhibit slightly elevated triglyceride concentrations but do not have pancreatitis. Treatment involves use of a fat-restricted diet throughout life. In case of severe pancreatitis, transfusion of 1 or 2 units of normal plasma is helpful. As compared with patients with familial lipoprotein lipase deficiency, subjects with homozygous apoprotein CII deficiency are generally detected at a later age, accumulate more VLDL in their plasma, and rarely show cutaneous eruptive xanthomas. The reason for these clinical differences is not known.

FAMILIAL TYPE 3 HYPERLIPOPROTEINEMIA   This is an inherited disorder in which the plasma concentrations of both cholesterol and triglycerides are elevated owing to the accumulation in plasma of remnant-like particles derived from the partial catabolism of VLDL. Also called *familial dysbetalipoproteinemia*, the disorder is transmitted by a single-gene mechanism, but its expression appears to require the presence of contributory environmental and/or genetic factors (discussed below).

Clinical features   Affected individuals characteristically do not manifest hyperlipidemia or any clinical feature of the disease until after age 20. A unique clinical feature is the occurrence of two types of cutaneous xanthomas: xanthoma striata palmaris, which appear as orange or yellow discolorations of the palmar and digital creases, and tuberous or tuberoeruptive xanthomas, which are bulbous cutaneous xanthomas that may vary from pea to lemon size. The tuberous xanthomas are characteristically located over the elbows and knees. Xanthelasmas of the eyelids also occur but are not unique to this disorder (see "Familial Hypercholesterolemia," below).

Severe and fulminant atherosclerosis involves the coronary arteries, the internal carotids, and the abdominal aorta and its branches. The sequelae include premature myocardial infarctions, strokes, intermittent claudication, and gangrene of the lower extremities. Patients who develop clinical manifestations of this disorder often have hypothyroidism, obesity, or diabetes mellitus as aggravating factors.

Pathogenesis   The hyperlipidemia is caused by the accumulation of large lipoprotein particles that contain both triglycerides and cholesteryl esters. These particles consist of chylomicron remnants produced from the catabolism of chylomicrons and IDL produced from the catabolism of VLDL through the action of lipoprotein lipase. In normal subjects, chylomicron remnant particles are rapidly taken up by the liver, and hence they are barely detectable in plasma. A portion of the IDL is also taken up by the liver, while the rest is converted to LDL. In patients with type 3 hyperlipoproteinemia, the uptake of IDL and chylomicron remnants by the liver is blocked, and these lipoproteins accumulate to high levels in plasma and tissues, producing xanthomas and atherosclerosis.

The mutation responsible for this disease involves the gene that encodes the structure of apoprotein E, a protein normally found in IDL and chylomicron remnants. This protein binds with very high affinity to both the chylomicron remnant receptor and the LDL receptor. Apoprotein E thus mediates the rapid uptake of chylomicron remnants and IDL by the liver. The gene for apoprotein E is polymorphic in the population. There are three common alleles, designated E^2, E^3, and E^4, with approximate frequencies of 0.12, 0.75, and 0.13 in the population. Each allele specifies a distinctive form of apoprotein E that differs from the others by a single amino acid substitution. This structural alteration allows each protein to be detected by isoelectric focusing. The three alleles create six genotypes: E^2/E^2, E^3/E^3, E^4/E^4, E^2/E^3, E^2/E^4, and E^3/E^4. Type 3 hyperlipoproteinemia occurs only in individuals who are homozygous for the E^2 allele (genotype E^2/E^2). The protein produced by the E^2 allele is defective in its ability to bind to the liver receptors that mediate uptake of chylomicron remnants and IDL, as a result of which these particles accumulate in plasma.

The frequency of the E^2/E^2 genotype in the population is about 1 in 100. Yet the frequency of type 3 hyperlipoproteinemia is only about 1 in 10,000. Thus only 1 percent of the individuals having genotype E^2/E^2 have symptomatic disease. Familial type 3 hyperlipoproteinemia occurs only in those individuals who are homozygous for the E^2 allele and who are also unable to compensate for the abnormal function of the E protein. The inability to compensate may be caused by the independent inheritance of another defect in lipoprotein metabolism, such as familial hypercholesterolemia or multiple lipoprotein–type hyperlipoproteinemia (see below). When an individual is a heterozygote for one of these dominant diseases and is also homozygous for the E^2 allele, he or she expresses the syndrome of type 3 hyperlipoproteinemia. The expression of hyperlipoproteinemia is also brought out when an individual of genotype E^2/E^2 develops hypothyroidism, diabetes mellitus, or obesity. It should be emphasized that heterozygotes for the E^2 allele never show the clinical syndrome of familial type 3 hyperlipoproteinemia.

In addition to the relatively common E^2 allele, rare mutant alleles also occur at the apo E locus. Some of these produce autosomal dominant as well as recessive forms of type 3 hyperlipoproteinemia.

Diagnosis   The diagnosis is suggested by the finding of palmar or tuberous xanthomas in a patient with elevated plasma levels of both cholesterol and triglyceride. Approximately 80 percent of symptomatic patients exhibit these xanthomas. The diagnosis is also suggested when a moderate elevation in the plasma concentration of both cholesterol and triglyceride occurs in such a way that the absolute concentrations of cholesterol and triglyceride are similar [e.g., the plasma cholesterol is about 7.8 mmol/L (300 mg/dL) and the triglyceride level is about 3.4 mmol/L (300 mg/dL)]. However, this finding does not always hold true and becomes especially unreliable when the disease is in severe exacerbation, in which case the plasma triglyceride level tends to rise higher than the cholesterol level.

The diagnosis is supported by the finding of a so-called broad beta band on lipoprotein electrophoresis (type 3 pattern). This appearance results from the presence of chylomicron remnants and IDL. The diagnosis can be established in specialized laboratories by two procedures. First, the plasma can be subjected to ultracentrifugation,

and the chemical composition of the VLDL fraction can be measured. In affected patients, the VLDL fraction contains IDL and chylomicron remnants that have a relatively high ratio of cholesterol to triglyceride. Second, the diagnosis can be confirmed by the finding of homozygosity for the E^2 allele on isoelectric focusing of the proteins extracted from the remnant particles.

Treatment   A vigorous search for occult hypothyroidism should be made, including measurement of plasma thyroid-stimulating hormone (TSH) levels. If hypothyroidism exists, levothyroxine should be instituted. Patients who have hypothyroidism show a dramatic lowering of lipid levels with treatment. In addition, attempts should be made to control obesity and diabetes mellitus through diet and insulin treatment. If these measures are not successful, patients with type 3 hyperlipoproteinemia should be treated with a fibric acid, such as gemfibrozil or clofibrate. Affected patients usually show a dramatic and sustained reduction in plasma lipid levels when treated with these drugs. Nicotinic acid may be effective in the severely hyperlipidemic patient who does not respond to gemfibrozil or clofibrate.

FAMILIAL HYPERCHOLESTEROLEMIA   This common autosomal dominant disorder affects approximately 1 in every 500 persons. It is caused by a mutation in the gene for the LDL receptor. Heterozygotes manifest a two- to threefold elevation in the concentration of total plasma cholesterol which is attributable to an elevation in the level of LDL. Patients with two mutant LDL receptor genes (called *familial hypercholesterolemia homozygotes*) have six- to eightfold elevations in plasma LDL-cholesterol levels.

Clinical features   Heterozygotes with familial hypercholesterolemia can be diagnosed at birth because their umbilical cord blood contains a two- to threefold increase in the concentration of LDL and hence a similar increase in total cholesterol. The elevated levels of plasma LDL persist throughout life, but symptoms typically do not develop until the third or fourth decade. The most important feature is the occurrence of premature and accelerated coronary atherosclerosis. Myocardial infarctions begin to occur in affected men in the third decade and peak in the fourth and fifth decades. By age 60, approximately 85 percent have experienced a myocardial infarction. In women, the incidence of myocardial infarction is also increased, but the mean age of onset is delayed 10 years as compared with men. Heterozygotes for this disorder constitute about 5 percent of all patients who have a myocardial infarction.

Xanthomas of the tendons constitute the second major clinical manifestation of the heterozygous state. These xanthomas are nodular swellings that typically involve the Achilles and other tendons about the knee, elbow, and dorsum of the hand. They are formed by the deposition of LDL-derived cholesteryl esters in tissue macrophages. The macrophages are swollen with lipid droplets and form foam cells. Cholesterol is also deposited in the soft tissue of the eyelid, producing xanthelasma, and within the cornea, producing arcus corneae. Whereas tendon xanthomas are essentially diagnostic of familial hypercholesterolemia, xanthelasma and arcus corneae also occur in many adults with normal plasma lipid levels. The incidence of tendon xanthomas in familial hypercholesterolemia increases with age, and up to 75 percent of heterozygotes display this sign. The absence of tendon xanthomas does not rule out familial hypercholesterolemia.

Approximately 1 in 1 million persons in the general population inherits two copies of the familial hypercholesterolemia gene and is a homozygote for the disorder. These individuals have marked elevations in the plasma level of LDL from birth. A unique type of planar cutaneous xanthoma is often present at birth and always develops within the first 6 years of life. These xanthomas are raised, yellow, plaquelike lesions at points of cutaneous trauma, such as the knees, elbows, and buttocks. Xanthomas are almost always present in the interdigital webs of the hands, particularly between the thumb and index finger. Tendon xanthomas, arcus corneae, and xanthelasma are also characteristic. Coronary artery atherosclerosis frequently has its clinical onset before age 10, and myocardial infarction has been reported as early as 18 months of age. In addition, cholesterol deposition in the aortic valve may produce symptomatic aortic stenosis. Homozygotes usually succumb to the complications of myocardial infarction before age 20.

Obesity and diabetes mellitus do not occur with increased frequency in familial hypercholesterolemia. A slender body habitus is the rule.

Pathogenesis The primary defect resides in the gene for the LDL receptor. Studies of DNA from affected individuals indicate that at least 150 mutant alleles occur at this locus. These mutant alleles can be grouped into three classes. The most common, designated *receptor-negative*, specifies a gene product that is nonfunctional. The second most frequent mutant, designated *receptor-defective*, produces a receptor that has 1 to 10 percent of normal LDL binding activity. The third type, designated *internalization-defective*, produces a receptor that binds LDL normally but is unable to transport the receptor-bound lipoprotein into the cell. This rare allele produces the so-called internalization defect.

Phenotypic homozygotes possess two mutant alleles at the LDL receptor locus, and hence their cells show a total or near-total inability to bind or take up LDL. Heterozygotes have one normal allele and one mutant allele at the LDL receptor locus, and hence their cells are able to bind and take up LDL at approximately half the normal rate.

Because of the reduction in LDL receptor activity, LDL catabolism is blocked, and the level of LDL in plasma rises in a manner that is inversely proportional to the reduction in LDL receptors. In addition to the impaired catabolism of LDL, LDL production is increased. Enhanced production of LDL has been attributed to the lack of an LDL receptor on liver cells. The liver fails to remove IDL from the plasma normally, with the result that an increased amount of IDL is converted to LDL. This overproduction of LDL, together with its inefficient catabolism, accounts for the high concentrations in affected patients. The elevated LDL levels causes an increase in the uptake of LDL by scavenger cells, which accumulate at various sites in the body, producing xanthomas.

The accelerated coronary atherosclerosis in familial hypercholesterolemia results from the high LDL levels, which lead to an enhanced infiltration of LDL into the artery wall following episodes of endothelial damage. The large amounts of LDL that penetrate the artery wall cannot be cleared from the interstitial space by the scavenger cells, and atherosclerosis ultimately results. Some of the lipids in LDL may undergo oxidation when the lipoprotein enters the artery wall, and the resultant products may be toxic to endothelial cells, thereby accelerating the damage. High LDL levels also may act to accelerate platelet aggregation at sites of endothelial injury, thereby enhancing the growth of the atherosclerotic plaque (see Chap. 208).

Diagnosis The diagnosis of heterozygous familial hypercholesterolemia is suggested by the finding of an isolated elevation of plasma cholesterol, with a normal concentration of plasma triglycerides. Such an isolated elevation in plasma cholesterol is usually due to an elevation in the plasma concentration of LDL alone (type 2a pattern). However, most individuals in the general population with type 2a hyperlipoproteinemia do not have familial hypercholesterolemia. Rather, they have a form of polygenic hypercholesterolemia that puts them on the upper end of the bell-shaped curve for the general population (see "Polygenic Hypercholesterolemia," below). Type 2a hyperlipoproteinemia is also caused by multiple lipoprotein–type hyperlipidemia and familial defective apo B100 (discussed below). In addition, a variety of metabolic disorders, including hypothyroidism and nephrotic syndrome, can cause type 2a hyperlipoproteinemia (see Table 344-4).

Among individuals who have a type 2a lipoprotein pattern, those with heterozygous familial hypercholesterolemia can be distinguished from those with polygenic hypercholesterolemia and multiple lipoprotein–type hyperlipidemia on several grounds. (1) In familial hypercholesterolemia the plasma cholesterol level tends to be higher. A plasma cholesterol level in the range of 9 to 10 mmol/L (350 to 400 mg/dL) is highly suggestive of heterozygous familial hypercholesterolemia.

However, many patients with heterozygous familial hypercholesterolemia have cholesterol levels of 7 to 9 mmol/L (285 to 350 mg/dL), a range in which the other disorders cannot be excluded. (2) The occurrence of tendon xanthomas virtually establishes the diagnosis of familial hypercholesterolemia, since such xanthomas usually do not occur in patients with other forms of hyperlipidemia. (3) In cases in which the diagnosis is in doubt, other family members should be surveyed. In familial hypercholesterolemia, half the first-degree relatives show an elevated plasma cholesterol level. Hypercholesterolemia in relatives is particularly informative when it occurs in children, since elevated levels of cholesterol in childhood are characteristic of familial hypercholesterolemia but not of the other disorders.

Approximately 10 percent of heterozygotes with familial hypercholesterolemia have a concomitant elevation in plasma triglyceride levels (type 2b pattern). In these cases, the disease is difficult to differentiate from multiple lipoprotein–type hyperlipidemia. The finding of a tendon xanthoma or a hypercholesterolemic child in the family establishes the diagnosis of familial hypercholesterolemia.

Differentiating heterozygous familial hypercholesterolemia from familial defective apo B100 is more difficult. The latter is caused by a missense mutation at amino acid 3500 in apo B100. This mutation interferes with the ability of apo B to bind to LDL receptors and thus results in hypercholesterolemia. Affected heterozygotes often have a positive family history of hypercholesterolemia, coronary atherosclerosis, and tendon xanthomas. The easiest way to distinguish this disorder from heterozygous familial hypercholesterolemia is by direct detection of the apo B100 mutation using polymerase chain reaction (PCR)–based molecular techniques (see Chap. 61).

The diagnosis of homozygous familial hypercholesterolemia ordinarily affords no problem, providing the physician is familiar with the clinical picture. Most patients are first seen by dermatologists in childhood because of the cutaneous xanthomas. Occasionally, the presentation is delayed until the onset of angina pectoris or until the child suffers a syncopal episode owing to the xanthomatous aortic stenosis. The finding of a cholesterol level greater than 16 mmol/L (600 mg/dL) with normal triglyceride values in a nonjaundiced child is highly suggestive of the diagnosis. Both parents should have elevated cholesterol levels and other features of heterozygous familial hypercholesterolemia.

In specialized laboratories, the diagnosis of both heterozygous and homozygous familial hypercholesterolemia can be made by direct measurement of the number of LDL receptors on cultured skin fibroblasts or freshly isolated blood lymphocytes. Homozygous familial hypercholesterolemia has been diagnosed in utero by the absence of LDL receptors on cultured amniotic fluid cells. The mutant genes for the LDL receptor also can be visualized directly in genomic DNA from affected individuals by using restriction enzyme digests, Southern blots, or the polymerase chain reaction (PCR) (see Chap. 61).

Treatment Inasmuch as the atherosclerosis in this disorder is a consequence of the long-standing elevation in plasma LDL levels, every effort should be made to lower the plasma LDL level into the normal range. Patients should be placed on a diet that is low in cholesterol, low in saturated fats, and high in polyunsaturated fats. This generally means the avoidance of milk, butter, cheese, chocolate, shellfish, and fatty meats and the addition of polyunsaturated cooking oils such as corn oil and safflower oil. With such a diet, heterozygotes usually show a 10 to 15 percent drop in plasma cholesterol level.

Bile acid–binding resins, such as cholestyramine, should be added to the regimen when dietary therapy fails to lower the cholesterol levels to the normal range. These resins trap the bile acids excreted by the liver into the intestine and prevent their reabsorption. The liver responds to bile acid depletion by converting additional cholesterol into bile acids. This leads to an enhanced production of LDL receptors by the liver, which, in turn, lowers the plasma level of LDL. Unfortunately, affected subjects also respond to bile acid depletion by enhancing cholesterol synthesis in the liver, and this compensatory response ultimately limits the long-term success of bile acid sequestrant therapy. With the combination of diet and bile acid–binding resins, the extent of reduction in plasma cholesterol level usually is in the range of 15 to 20 percent in heterozygotes. The addition of nicotinic acid may help to block the compensatory increase in hepatic cholesterol synthesis, thus allowing a further lowering of the cholesterol. Major side effects of bile acid–binding resins include gastrointestinal bloating, cramps, and constipation. The major side effect of nicotinic acid is hepatotoxicity; it also produces flushing and headaches in most patients. Probucol also has been used for the treatment of familial hypercholesterolemia. It is an antioxidant that retards the progression of atherosclerosis in animal models. Its effectiveness in humans is not established.

A new class of drugs shows great promise for treatment of hypercholesterolemia. These drugs inhibit 3-hydroxy-3-methylglutaryl coenzyme A (HMG CoA) reductase, an enzyme in the cholesterol biosynthetic pathway. This class includes lovastatin, pravastatin, and simvastatin. When cholesterol synthesis is inhibited, the production of LDL is diminished and the clearance of LDL by the liver is enhanced as a result of an increased production of LDL receptors. These two effects combine to lower plasma LDL levels by 30 to 50 percent. The HMG CoA reductase inhibitors are even more effective when given together with a bile acid–binding resin such as cholestyramine. The major side effects of this class of drugs are myopathy (0.5 percent) and asymptomatic but persistent increases in plasma transaminases (1.9 percent). A more severe myopathy with rhabdomyolysis is seen rarely in patients who are treated with reductase inhibitors plus immunosuppressive drugs, gemfibrozil, nicotinic acid, or erythromycin.

Heterozygotes often show a moderate to marked lowering of plasma cholesterol level in response to the creation of an intestinal anastomosis that bypasses the ileum. This operation has the same functional effect as bile acid–binding resins; i.e., it accelerates the loss of bile acids in the stool. In certain patients in whom drug therapy is not tolerated, the creation of an ileal bypass may be indicated.

Homozygotes tend to be more resistant to treatment, probably because they are unable to increase production of LDL receptors. In general, combination therapy consisting of diet, a bile acid–binding resin, nicotinic acid, and HMG CoA reductase inhibitors has little effect. Ileal bypass is uniformly ineffective. Several homozygous children have responded to surgical creation of a portacaval anastomosis. At least four homozygous children have been treated with liver transplantation, which provided LDL receptors and lowered LDL levels by 70 to 80 percent. The use of a continuous-flow blood cell centrifuge to perform plasma exchanges at monthly intervals lowers the cholesterol in all homozygotes. After each plasma exchange, the plasma cholesterol level drops to about 8 mmol/L (300 mg/dL) and then gradually rises over the ensuing 4 weeks to the pretreatment level. In one version of this procedure, plasma is exchanged with normal plasma or albumin. In another version, called LDL apheresis, plasma is passed extracorporeally over columns that remove apo B100–containing lipoproteins (VLDL, IDL, and LDL) but do not absorb HDL or other plasma proteins. The effluent is then returned to the patient. If facilities are available, plasma exchange is the treatment of choice for homozygotes.

Several studies have shown that cholesterol-lowering therapy retards the progression, and in some instances induces actual regression, of atherosclerotic plaques in the coronary arteries of patients with heterozygous familial hypercholesterolemia. The studies used serial coronary angiography to document these changes, which took place over periods of 2 to 3 years. Several different drug regimens and ileal bypass operations were employed to lower blood cholesterol, and the antiatherosclerotic effect seems to be independent of the regimen employed. These and other studies also documented a reduction in myocardial infarctions and other symptoms of coronary artery disease following such treatment. None of these studies has had sufficient statistical power to document a prolongation of life in treated patients.

FAMILIAL HYPERTRIGLYCERIDEMIA   This is a common autosomal dominant disorder in which the concentration of VLDL is elevated in the plasma, causing hypertriglyceridemia.

Clinical features   Affected individuals do not usually express hypertriglyceridemia until puberty or early adulthood. Thereafter, the fasting plasma triglyceride level tends to be moderately elevated in the range of 2 to 6 mmol/L (200 to 500 mg/dL) (type 4 lipoprotein pattern). The typical patient exhibits the clinical triad of obesity, hyperglycemia, and hyperinsulinemia. Hypertension and hyperuricemia are also frequent.

The incidence of atherosclerosis is increased. In one study, affected patients constituted 6 percent of all individuals with myocardial infarction. However, it has not been established that the hypertriglyceridemia per se causes the increased atherosclerosis. As discussed above, many patients with this disease have diabetes, obesity, and hypertension. Each of these disorders by itself may predispose to atherosclerosis. Hypertriglyceridemic subjects also tend to have reduced levels of HDL, which predisposes to atherosclerosis and which may account for the observed association of hypertriglyceridemia and myocardial infarction. Xanthomas are not a characteristic feature of familial hypertriglyceridemia.

Affected patients ordinarily have mild to moderate hypertriglyceridemia but may develop a severe exacerbation when exposed to a variety of precipitating factors. These include poorly controlled diabetes mellitus, excessive consumption of alcohol, ingestion of birth control pills containing estrogen, and the development of hypothyroidism. In response to any of these stimuli, the plasma triglyceride level can rise to more than 11 mmol/L (1000 mg/dL). During exacerbations, such patients develop *mixed hyperlipidemia;* that is, they show an elevation in the concentration of both VLDL and chylomicrons (type 5 lipoprotein pattern). Whenever the concentration of chylomicrons rises to high levels, patients are predisposed to the formation of eruptive xanthomas and the development of pancreatitis. With treatment of the exacerbating condition, the chylomicron-like particles disappear from plasma, and the concentration of triglycerides returns to the moderately elevated basal condition.

In certain families, some patients exhibit a severe mixed hyperlipidemia, even in the absence of known exacerbating factors. This is the so-called familial type 5 hyperlipidemia. Other individuals in the same family may have only the mild form of the disease with moderate hyperchylomicronemia and no hyperchylomicronemia (type 4 pattern).

Pathogenesis   Familial hypertriglyceridemia is transmitted as an autosomal dominant trait, implying a mutation in a single gene. However, the nature of the mutant gene and the mechanism by which it produces hypertriglyceridemia have not been identified. It is likely that the disorder is genetically heterogeneous; that is, the hypertriglyceridemia phenotype in different families may result from different mutations.

Some patients with familial hypertriglyceridemia seem to have an underlying defect in the ability to catabolize the triglycerides of VLDL. When VLDL production rates become elevated due to obesity or diabetes, they are unable to increase the catabolism of VLDL proportionately, and hypertriglyceridemia results. The reason for this defect in catabolism is not apparent. Lipoprotein lipase activity increases normally in plasma after the administration of heparin, and no abnormalities of lipoprotein structure have been identified.

The increased prevalence of diabetes mellitus and obesity in this syndrome is believed to be fortuitous, owing to the fact that both conditions tend to increase VLDL production and hence to exacerbate hypertriglyceridemia. In family studies, one can find relatives who have diabetes without hypertriglyceridemia and relatives who have hypertriglyceridemia without diabetes, indicating that the two are inherited by independent mechanisms. When an individual inherits the gene(s) for diabetes as well as the gene for hypertriglyceridemia, the hypertriglyceridemia is more severe, and such a person is more apt to come to medical attention. Similarly, an individual with familial hypertriglyceridemia who has a normal weight usually has mild hypertriglyceridemia and is less likely to come to medical attention. However, if obesity develops, the hypertriglyceridemia worsens, and a diagnosis is more likely to be made.

Diagnosis A moderate elevation in the plasma triglyceride level, together with a normal cholesterol level, raises the possibility of familial hypertriglyceridemia. In most patients, the plasma is clear to somewhat cloudy on inspection. Chylomicrons typically are not found at the top of the plasma after overnight refrigeration. Electrophoresis of the plasma reveals an increase in the pre-β fraction (type 4 lipoprotein pattern). As mentioned above, an occasional patient exhibits severe hypertriglyceridemia with an elevation in both chylomicrons and VLDL. In this case, a cream layer develops on top (chylomicrons) and a cloudy infranatant (VLDL) is present after overnight storage of plasma in the refrigerator (type 5 lipoprotein pattern).

Given an individual who has an elevation in VLDL levels with or without an elevation in chylomicrons, there is no simple test to determine whether this subject has familial hypertriglyceridemia or hypertriglyceridemia due to some other genetic or acquired cause, such as multiple lipoprotein–type hyperlipidemia or sporadic hypertriglyceridemia. In a typical case of familial hypertriglyceridemia, half the first-degree relatives have hypertriglyceridemia and no relatives have isolated hypercholesterolemia. Measurement of plasma lipid levels in children is not helpful inasmuch as the disease is typically not manifest until the time of puberty.

Treatment Attempts should be made to control all the exacerbating conditions. Caloric restriction is required in the obese subject. The dietary content of saturated fat also should be limited. Alcohol and oral contraceptives should be avoided. Diabetes mellitus, if present, should be treated vigorously. Thyroid function should be checked, and hypothyroidism should be treated if found. If the preceding measures fail, some patients respond to the administration of gemfibrozil or nicotinic acid. The mechanism of action of neither drug is well defined. Patients with severe hypertriglyceridemia frequently show a dramatic response to a fish oil diet. If a patient with hypertriglyceridemia has an especially low level of HDL-cholesterol, the prognosis for coronary artery disease is relatively poor, and therapeutic efforts must be especially vigorous.

MULTIPLE LIPOPROTEIN–TYPE HYPERLIPIDEMIA This common disorder, which is also called *familial combined hyperlipidemia*, is inherited as an autosomal dominant trait. Affected individuals in a single family characteristically show one of three different lipoprotein patterns: hypercholesterolemia (type 2a), hypertriglyceridemia (type 4), or both hypercholesterolemia and hypertriglyceridemia (type 2b). The level of HDL tends to be below normal

Clinical features Hyperlipidemia is not present in childhood. Elevations in the plasma cholesterol and/or triglyceride level appear at puberty and continue throughout life. The lipid elevations tend to be mild and vary from time to time so that affected individuals may have a mildly elevated cholesterol level at one examination and/or a mildly elevated triglyceride level at another time. Xanthomas are not a feature. However, premature atherosclerosis occurs, and the incidence of myocardial infarction in middle age is elevated in affected women as well as men.

Patients usually have a strong family history of premature coronary artery disease. This disorder is found in about 10 percent of all patients who have a myocardial infarction. The frequency of obesity, hyperuricemia, and glucose intolerance is increased in affected individuals, especially those with hypertriglyceridemia. However, this association is not as striking as in familial hypertriglyceridemia.

Pathogenesis The disease is transmitted within families as an autosomal dominant trait, implying a mutation in a single gene. Family studies show that about half the first-degree relatives of an affected individual have hyperlipidemia. However, blood lipid levels are variable among affected individuals in the same family as well as in the same individual at different times. About one-third of hyperlipidemic relatives have hypercholesterolemia (type 2a lipopro-

tein pattern), one-third hypertriglyceridemia (type 4), and one-third both hypercholesterolemia and hypertriglyceridemia (type 2b). In most affected relatives, the plasma lipid levels tend to be just above the 95th percentile for the population and to dip into the normal range intermittently.

While the extent (if any) of the genetic heterogeneity and the nature of the underlying biochemical mechanisms are not known, some affected individuals may have an elevated rate of secretion of VLDL by the liver. Others may be heterozygous for a mutation in the gene for lipoprotein lipase. Depending on the interplay of factors governing the efficiency of conversion of VLDL to LDL and the efficiency of catabolism of LDL, this overproduction of VLDL may manifest itself alternatively as an elevation in plasma VLDL levels (hypertriglyceridemia), an elevation in LDL levels (hypercholesterolemia), or both. The hyperlipidemia is worsened by diabetes, alcoholism, and hypothyroidism.

Diagnosis No clinical or laboratory methods exist by which to determine whether an individual with hyperlipidemia has the multiple lipoprotein–type disorder. The 2a, 2b, and 4 lipoprotein patterns can each occur in patients with several other diseases (see Tables 344-3 and 344-4). However, this disorder should be suspected in any individual whose hyperlipoproteinemia is mild and whose lipoprotein type changes with time. The diagnosis is supported by the finding of multiple abnormal lipoprotein types in relatives. The diagnosis can be ruled out by the finding of tendon xanthomas in the patient or the patient's relatives or by the finding of hypercholesterolemia in a relative under the age of 10 years.

Treatment Therapy should be directed at the predominant lipid elevated at the time of examination. General measures such as weight reduction, restriction of dietary saturated fat and cholesterol, and avoidance of alcohol and oral contraceptives are useful. Triglyceride elevations may respond to nicotinic acid or gemfibrozil. When only the cholesterol level is elevated, an HMG CoA reductase inhibitor should be given. Bile acid–binding resins should be avoided since lowering of cholesterol levels with such a drug is sometimes accompanied by an increase in triglyceride levels.

PRIMARY HYPERLIPOPROTEINEMIAS OF UNKNOWN ETIOLOGY

POLYGENIC HYPERCHOLESTEROLEMIA By definition, 5 percent of individuals in the general population have LDL-cholesterol levels that exceed the 95th percentile and therefore have hypercholesterolemia (type 2a or type 2b lipoprotein patterns). On average, among every 20 such hypercholesterolemic persons, 1 person has the heterozygous form of familial hypercholesterolemia, and 2 have multiple lipoprotein–type hyperlipidemia. The remaining 17 have a form of hypercholesterolemia, designated *polygenic hypercholesterolemia,* that owes its origin not to a single mutant gene but rather to a complex interaction of multiple genetic and environmental factors.

Most of the factors that place an individual in the upper part of the bell-shaped curve for cholesterol levels are not known. It is likely that subtle genetic differences exist among people with regard to many processes governing cholesterol metabolism. For example, among normal people there may be genetic polymorphisms in the proteins that govern the rates of intestinal cholesterol absorption, bile acid synthesis, cholesterol synthesis, and LDL synthesis or catabolism. Certain unfavorable combinations of these mildly altered proteins, coupled with an environmental challenge, such as a diet high in cholesterol or saturated fat, may raise the plasma cholesterol level.

Clinically, polygenic hypercholesterolemia can be distinguished from familial hypercholesterolemia and multiple lipoprotein–type hyperlipidemia in two ways: (1) family studies (hyperlipidemia is present in no more than 10 percent of first-degree relatives in polygenic hypercholesterolemia in contrast to 50 percent in the other two disorders) and (2) examination for tendon xanthomas (absent in both polygenic hypercholesterolemia and multiple lipoprotein–type hyperlipidemia but present in about 75 percent of adult heterozygotes with familial hypercholesterolemia).

Certain patients with polygenic hypercholesterolemia respond to dietary restriction of saturated fat and cholesterol. Other patients require drug therapy. An HMG CoA reductase inhibitor and a bile acid–binding resin with or without nicotinic acid also may be used.

FAMILIAL HYPERALPHALIPOPROTEINEMIA This entity is characterized by elevated plasma levels of HDL, also called *alpha lipoprotein*. The plasma levels of LDL, VLDL, and triglycerides are normal. The elevated HDL causes a slight elevation in the total plasma cholesterol level. Although a selective elevation in plasma HDL-cholesterol can be observed in individuals after exposure to chlorinated hydrocarbon pesticides, in alcoholism, and after administration of estrogen, most cases of hyperalphalipoproteinemia have a genetic basis. In some families, hyperalphalipoproteinemia is inherited as an autosomal dominant trait, while in others a multifactorial or polygenic basis is suspected. Individual subjects with familial hyperalphalipoproteinemia show no distinctive clinical features.

Hyperalphalipoproteinemia is associated with a slightly increased longevity and an apparent protection against myocardial infarction. The mechanism for the increase in plasma HDL levels in this disorder has not been determined.

SECONDARY HYPERLIPOPROTEINEMIAS

A number of clinical disorders produce secondary hyperlipoproteinemias. These are summarized in Table 344-4. The most frequently encountered forms of secondary hyperlipoproteinemia occur in association with diabetes mellitus, consumption of alcohol, and ingestion of oral contraceptives.

DIABETES MELLITUS Three distinct patterns of hypertriglyceridemia occur in patients with diabetes mellitus. Classic *diabetic hyperlipidemia* consists of a massive elevation in the plasma triglyceride level that occurs in patients who have suffered from insulin deficiency or insulin resistance for many weeks or months. Such insulin-deprived patients develop a progressive increase in concentration of plasma VLDL and eventually of chylomicrons as well. Triglyceride levels as high as 280 mmol/L (25,000 mg/dL) are seen. Eruptive xanthomas, lipemia retinalis, and hepatomegaly can occur. Ketosis is frequently present, but severe acidosis is not characteristic. This form of massive hyperlipoproteinemia is seen only in partial insulin deficiency. Patients with this form of diabetic hyperlipidemia usually respond to a fat-free diet and to the administration of insulin, although triglyceride levels may not return entirely to normal.

The second type of hypertriglyceridemia in diabetics is associated with acute ketoacidosis. Such patients usually exhibit a mild hyperlipidemia with elevations of VLDL but not chylomicrons. On occasion, however, marked elevations of triglyceride are seen with lipemia retinalis. In this case, both VLDL and chylomicrons are present.

The third type of hypertriglyceridemia is a mild to moderate elevation in plasma VLDL that persists even when patients appear to be adequately treated for their diabetes. This chronic triglyceride elevation generally occurs in patients who are obese. Inasmuch as most patients with well-controlled diabetes have normal plasma triglyceride levels, the occasional patient with persistent hypertriglyceridemia is likely to have an underlying familial hyperlipoproteinemic disorder. Indeed, family studies indicate that many of these patients have inherited the trait for familial hypertriglyceridemia in a pattern independent of the inheritance of diabetes mellitus.

The insulin deficiency or insulin resistance of diabetes produces a high VLDL level by two mechanisms. With acute insulin deprivation there is an increase in VLDL secretion from the liver as a secondary response to the increased mobilization of free fatty acids from adipose tissue. As the state of insulin deprivation becomes prolonged, the rate of removal of VLDL and chylomicrons from the circulation declines because lipoprotein lipase activity becomes diminished.

ALCOHOL CONSUMPTION In any individual, the daily consumption of large amounts of ethanol can produce a mild, asymptomatic elevation in the plasma triglyceride level due to an elevation of VLDL. However, in a subgroup ethanol ingestion regularly produces massive and clinically significant hyperlipidemia with elevations in both VLDL and chylomicrons (type 5 lipoprotein pattern). In most of this group, the VLDL level remains mildly elevated (type 4 lipoprotein pattern), even in the basal state after recovery from the severe alcoholic hyperlipidemia. This suggests that these individuals have a form of familial hypertriglyceridemia or multiple lipoprotein–type hyperlipidemia that is exacerbated and converted to a type 5 pattern by the ethanol ingestion.

Ethanol elevates the plasma triglyceride level primarily because it inhibits fatty acid oxidation and enhances fatty acid synthesis in the liver. The excess fatty acids are esterified to triglyceride. Some of this excess triglyceride accumulates in the liver, producing the characteristic enlarged fatty liver of alcoholics. The remainder of the newly formed triglyceride is secreted into plasma, resulting in an increased secretion of VLDL. In those who develop massive alcoholic hyperlipidemia, there appears to be a partial defect in the catabolism of these VLDL particles. As the concentration of VLDL increases, the lipoprotein begins to compete with chylomicrons for hydrolysis by lipoprotein lipase, and the plasma concentration of chylomicrons also rises.

In severe alcoholic hyperlipidemia, eruptive xanthomas and lipemia retinalis are frequent. The most serious complication, pancreatitis, may be difficult to diagnose, since elevated triglyceride levels can interfere with the estimation of serum amylase. There is no evidence to indicate that pancreatitis can cause hyperlipidemia; rather, the hyperlipidemia is the cause of the pancreatitis.

Plasma from patients with alcoholic hyperlipidemia is creamy in appearance. If a blood sample is drawn in calcium edetate and the plasma placed in the refrigerator at 4°C overnight, the chylomicrons float to the top, and the infranatant layer is turbid, owing to the combined elevation of VLDL and chylomicrons (type 5 pattern).

ORAL CONTRACEPTIVES The ingestion of estrogen-containing birth control pills causes an increase in the VLDL secretion rate from the liver. In most women the catabolism of VLDL also increases so that the overall increase in plasma triglyceride level is modest. However, in women who have an underlying genetic disorder (such as familial hypertriglyceridemia or multiple lipoprotein–type hyperlipidemia), the plasma VLDL-triglyceride level can increase markedly, and hyperchylomicronemia can develop when estrogen-containing medications are taken. These women generally have mild hypertriglyceridemia prior to the institution of oral contraceptive therapy, and they presumably are unable to increase VLDL catabolism in response to the stimulation of VLDL production. The elevated VLDL prevents the normal catabolism of chylomicrons by lipoprotein lipase, and secondary hyperchylomicronemia ensues. When the latter develops, severe pancreatitis can occur.

Ingestion of oral contraceptives may be a risk factor in promoting thromboembolic disease in young women, especially those with preexisting hypercholesterolemia. Thus it is important to measure the plasma cholesterol and triglyceride levels prior to the institution of birth control therapy. The finding of hyperlipidemia is a contraindication to the use of these drugs.

RARE DISORDERS OF LIPID METABOLISM

Table 344-5 summarizes the clinical and pathophysiologic features of five rare autosomal recessive disorders of lipid metabolism. In two—abetalipoproteinemia and Tangier disease—the major effect of the abnormality is to cause a decrease in lipid levels in plasma. In two—cerebrotendinous xanthomatosis and sitosterolemia—the major effect of the inborn error is to cause an accumulation of unusual sterols in tissues. In LCAT deficiency, the underlying mutation produces both an abnormal pattern of lipoproteins in plasma and an accumulation of unesterified cholesterol in tissues.

TABLE 344-5 Rare autosomal recessive disorders of lipid metabolism

Disorder	Typical age of onset	Plasma lipid abnormality	Major clinical manifestations	Pathogenesis	Treatment
Abetalipoproteinemia	Early childhood	Very low cholesterol and triglyceride levels	Malabsorption of fat, ataxia, neuropathy, retinitis pigmentosa, acanthocytosis	Defective synthesis of apoprotein B leads to absence of chylomicrons, VLDL, and LDL in plasma	Vitamin E
Tangier disease	Childhood	Low cholesterol; triglycerides, normal to slightly elevated	Large orange tonsils, corneal opacities, relapsing polyneuropathy. No premature atherosclerosis	Absence of HDL from plasma leads to generation of abnormal chylomicron remnants, which are taken up and stored as cholesteryl esters in phagocytic cells	None
Lecithin:cholesterol acyltransferase (LCAT) deficiency	Young adult	Total plasma cholesterol level variable with marked decrease in esterified cholesterol and increase in unesterified cholesterol; elevated VLDL level; structure of all lipoproteins is abnormal	Corneal opacities, hemolytic anemia, renal insufficiency, premature atherosclerosis	Decreased LCAT activity in plasma leads to accumulation of excess unesterified cholesterol in plasma and body tissues	Fat-restricted diet, kidney transplantation
Cerebrotendinous xanthomatosis	Young adult	None	Progressive cerebellar ataxia, dementia and spinal cord paresis, subnormal intelligence, tendon xanthomas, cataracts	Defective synthesis of primary bile acids in liver leads to increased hepatic synthesis of cholesterol and cholestanol, which accumulate in brain, tendons, and other tissues	None
Sitosterolemia	Childhood	Elevated levels of plant sterols in plasma, elevated or normal levels of cholesterol, normal triglyceride levels	Tendon xanthomas	Increased intestinal absorption of dietary cholesterol, sitosterol, and other plant sterols with accumulation in plasma and tendons	Diet low in plant sterols and cholesterol

REFERENCES

BROWN MS, GOLDSTEIN JL: A receptor-mediated pathway for cholesterol homeostasis. Science 232:34, 1986

——, ——: Drugs used in the treatment of hyperlipoproteinemias, in *Goodman and Gilman's The Pharmacological Basis of Therapeutics*, 8th ed, AG Gilman et al (eds). New York, Pergamon, 1990, chap 36

BRUNZELL JD: Familial lipoprotein lipase deficiency and other causes of the chylomicronemia syndrome, in *The Molecular and Metabolic Basis of Inherited Disease*, 7th ed, CR Scriver et al (eds). New York, McGraw-Hill, in press, chap 59

CONNOR WE et al: Reduction of plasma lipids, lipoproteins and apoproteins by dietary fish oils in patients with hypertriglyceridemia. N Engl J Med 312:1210, 1985

GOLDSTEIN JL et al: Familial hypercholesterolemia, in *The Molecular and Metabolic Basis of Inherited Disease*, 7th ed, CR Scriver et al (eds). New York, McGraw-Hill, in press, chap 62

HAVEL RJ: Lowering cholesterol, 1988: Rationale, mechanisms and means. J Clin Invest 81:1653, 1988

HOBBS HH et al: The LDL receptor locus and familial hypercholesterolemia: Mutational analysis of a membrane protein. Annu Rev Genet 24:133, 1990

KRAMSCH DM, BLANKENHORN DH: Regression of atherosclerosis: Which components regress and what influences their reversal? Wien Klin Wochenschr 104:2, 1992

MAHLEY RW, RALL SC: Type III hyperlipoproteinemia (dysbetalipoproteinemia): The role of apolipoprotein E in normal and abnormal lipoprotein metabolism, in *The Molecular and Metabolic Basis of Inherited Disease*, 7th ed, CR Scriver et al (eds). New York, McGraw-Hill, in press, chap 61

SCRIVER CR et al: *The Molecular and Metabolic Basis of Inherited Disease*, 7th ed. New York, McGraw-Hill, in press, chaps 56, 57, 63–65.

345 HEMOCHROMATOSIS

LAWRIE W. POWELL / KURT J. ISSELBACHER

DEFINITION Hemochromatosis is a disorder of iron storage in which an inappropriate increase in intestinal iron absorption results in deposition of excessive quantities of iron in parenchymal cells with eventual tissue damage and functional impairment of the organs involved, especially the liver, pancreas, heart, and pituitary. In 1889, von Recklinghausen named the disease *hemochromatosis* and the iron-storage pigment *hemosiderin* because he believed that the pigment was derived from the blood. The terms *hemosiderosis* and *siderosis* are often used to describe the presence of stainable iron in tissues, but quantitative measurement of tissue iron is necessary for accurate assessment of body iron status (see below and Chap. 303). *Hemochromatosis* implies present or potentially severe progressive iron overload leading to fibrosis and organ failure. Cirrhosis, diabetes mellitus, arthritis, cardiomyopathy, and hypogonadotrophic hypogonadism are the usual manifestations. Although there is debate about definitions, it seems logical to use the following terminology: (1) *genetic* or *hereditary hemochromatosis*—the disease now known to be due to the inheritance of a mutant gene that is tightly linked to the HLA-A6 locus on the short arm of chromosome 6, and (2) *acquired hemochromatosis*—iron overload and tissue injury secondary to other disease, usually an iron-loading anemia such as thalassemia or sideroblastic anemia, in which increased erythropoiesis is ineffective. In these acquired iron-loading disorders, massive iron deposits in parenchymal tissues can lead to the same clinical and pathologic features as in hereditary hemochromatosis.

The metabolic defect leading to increased iron absorption in hereditary hemochromatosis is unknown. The genetic disease can now be recognized during its early stages when the iron overload is of lesser degree and organ damage is minimal. At this stage the disease is best referred to as *early* or *precirrhotic hemochromatosis* (see Fig. 345-1).

PREVALENCE Hereditary hemochromatosis is one of the most common autosomal recessive disorders. In European populations, approximately 1 in 10 persons is a heterozygous carrier, and 0.3 percent of persons are homozygotes. However, expression of the disease is modified by several factors, especially blood loss associated with menstruation and pregnancies in women. The clinical expression of disease is 5 to 10 times more frequent in men than in women. Nearly 70 percent of patients develop the first symptoms between ages 40 and 60. The disease is rarely evident below age 20, although with family screening (see below) asymptomatic subjects with iron overload can be identified, including young menstruating women.

GENETICS AND MODE OF INHERITANCE The gene for hemochromatosis has not been identified. However, it is located in close proximity to the HLA-A locus on chromosome 6 (often but not always HLA-A3). This linkage has made possible the clarification of the mode of inheritance and prevalence. Thus siblings with overt hemochromatosis usually share the same HLA haplotypes and are homozygous for the autosomal recessive trait. Siblings who share only one haplotype with the proband are putative heterozygotes and unlikely to develop iron overload. The reason for the high prevalence of the mutant gene is unknown, but it may have conferred a selective advantage in protecting against iron deficiency.

FIGURE 345-1 Sequence of events in genetic hemochromatosis and their correlation with the serum ferritin concentration. Increased iron absorption is present throughout life. Overt, symptomatic disease usually develops between ages 40 and 60, but latent precirrhotic disease can be detected long before this.

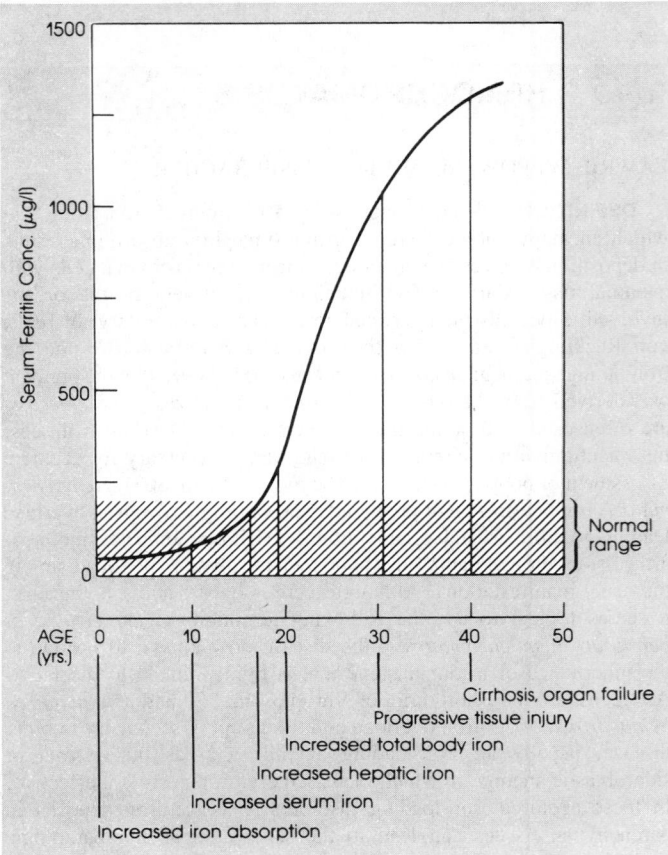

PATHOGENESIS Normally, the body iron content of 3 to 4 g is maintained such that intestinal mucosal absorption of iron is equal to loss. This amount is approximately 1 mg/d in men and 1.5 mg/d in menstruating women. In hemochromatosis, mucosal absorption is inappropriate to body needs, amounting to 4 mg/d or more. The resulting progressive accumulation of iron causes an early elevation in the plasma iron and an increased saturation of transferrin and progressive elevation of plasma ferritin level. The basic defect causing increased iron absorption is unknown. The genes for ferritin and transferrin receptor in the gut are coordinately regulated at the level of mRNA translation such that in iron overload, ferritin synthesis is increased and transferrin receptor synthesis is decreased. In iron deficiency, the reverse occurs. In hemochromatosis, this coordinate regulation is intact and responds normally to the usual influences, e.g., blood loss. An abnormally fast transport of iron out of the intestinal cell has been postulated. In advanced disease, the body may contain 20 g iron or more. This excess iron is deposited mainly in parenchymal cells of the liver, pancreas, and heart. Iron in the liver and pancreas may increase 50 to 100 times and in the heart, 5 to 25 times. Hypogonadotrophic hypogonadism occurs in both men and women due to iron deposition in the pituitary. Tissue injury may result from disruption of iron-laden lysosomes, from lipid peroxidation of subcellular organelles by excess iron, or from stimulation of collagen synthesis by the excess iron.

Parenchymal iron overload leading to *acquired* hemochromatosis occurs in association with chronic disorders of erythropoiesis, particularly in those with defects in hemoglobin synthesis or ineffective erythropoiesis such as sideroblastic anemia and thalassemia. In these disorders, the absorption of iron is increased, and such patients are also frequently treated with iron and blood transfusions. Porphyria cutanea tarda (PCT), a disorder characterized by a defect in porphyrin biosynthesis (Chap. 346), is also sometimes associated with excessive parenchymal iron deposits; however, the magnitude of the iron load is usually insufficient to produce tissue damage. The exact relationship between these two disorders is unclear, although iron may accentuate the inherited enzyme deficiency in PCT.

Alcoholic subjects with chronic liver disease and increased tissue iron stores can be divided into two groups. The first comprises patients with a mild to moderate increase in stainable hepatic iron but relatively normal body iron. These patients have alcoholic liver disease (usually cirrhosis) but not hemochromatosis. The increased iron may be due in part to cell necrosis and uptake of iron released from these cells. The second (less common) group of alcoholic subjects with increased hepatic iron have gross iron deposition and increased body iron stores and are usually found to have hereditary hemochromatosis with or without superimposed alcoholic liver disease. Hemochromatosis in a heavy drinker may be distinguished from alcoholic liver disease by two means: (1) measurement of hepatic iron concentration (see below and Table 345-1) and (2) studying relatives for evidence of the disease, including HLA typing.

Excessive iron ingestion over many years rarely, if ever, results in the clinical and pathologic features of hemochromatosis. The one important exception is South African blacks (Bantu), in whom the intake of excessive iron in an alcoholic beverage was due to the practice of brewing fermented beverages in vessels made of iron. In other populations, hemochromatosis has on occasion been described in apparently normal subjects who have taken medicinal iron over many years, but it is probable that such individuals have the genetic trait. Family studies may be helpful.

The common denominator in all patients with hemochromatosis is *excessive amounts of iron in parenchymal tissues*. Parenteral administration of iron in the form of blood transfusions or iron preparations results in predominantly *reticuloendothelial cell* iron overload. This appears to lead to less tissue damage than iron loading of parenchymal cells.

PATHOLOGY At autopsy, the enlarged, nodular liver and pancreas are rusty in color. Histologically, iron is increased in amount

TABLE 345-1 Representative iron values in normal subjects, patients with hemochromatosis, and patients with alcoholic liver disease

Determination	Normal	Symptomatic hemochromatosis	Homozygotes with early, asymptomatic hemochromatosis	Heterozygotes	Alcoholic liver disease
Plasma iron, µmol/L (µg/dL)	9–27 (50–150)	32–54 (180–300)	Usually elevated	Elevated or normal	Often elevated
Total iron-binding capacity, µmol/L (µg/dL)	45–66 (250–370)	36–54 (200–300)	36–54 (200–300)	Elevated or normal	45–66 (250–370)
Transferrin saturation, percent	22–46	50–100	50–100	Normal or elevated	27–60
Serum ferritin, µg/L	10–200	900–6000	200–500	Usually <500	10–500
Urinary iron,* mg/24 h	0–2	9–23	2.5	2–5	Usually <5
Liver iron, µg/gram dry wt	300–1400	6000–18,000	2000–4000	300–3000	300–2000
Hepatic iron index (µg/gram dry weight) / 56 × age	<1.0	>2	Usually >2	<2	<2

* After intramuscular administration of 0.5 g deferoxamine.

in many organs, particularly in the liver, heart, and pancreas and to a lesser extent in the endocrine glands. The epidermis of the skin is thin, and *melanin* is increased in the cells of the basal layer. Deposits of iron are present around the synovial lining cells of the joints, and calcium pyrophosphate crystals may be present within deposits of calcium in the synovial tissue.

Parenchymal iron in the liver of patients with hereditary hemochromatosis is in the form of ferritin and hemosiderin. In the early stages, these deposits are in the periportal parenchymal cells, especially within lysosomes in the pericanalicular cytoplasm of the hepatocytes. This stage progresses to perilobular fibrosis and eventually deposition of iron in bile duct epithelium, Kupffer cells, and fibrous septa. Inflammatory cells are few in contrast to prominent proliferation of bile ductules. Wedge biopsy specimens show a characteristic pattern of fibrosis with dense fibrous septa surrounding groups of lobules somewhat analogous to the pattern in chronic biliary disease. In the advanced stage, a macronodular or mixed macro- and micronodular cirrhosis develops.

CLINICAL MANIFESTATIONS The symptoms and signs include skin pigmentation, diabetes mellitus, liver and cardiac impairment, arthropathy, and hypogonadism. Initial symptoms include weakness, lassitude, weight loss, change in skin color, abdominal pain, loss of libido, and symptoms of diabetes mellitus. Hepatomegaly, pigmentation, spider angiomas, splenomegaly, arthropathy, ascites, cardiac arrhythmias, congestive heart failure, loss of body hair, testicular atrophy, and jaundice are prominent physical signs in advanced disease.

The *liver* is usually the first organ to be affected, and hepatomegaly is present in more than 95 percent of symptomatic patients. Hepatic enlargement may exist in the absence of symptoms or of abnormal liver function tests. Indeed, over half the patients with symptomatic hemochromatosis have little or no laboratory evidence of functional impairment of the liver, in spite of hepatomegaly and fibrosis. Loss of body hair, palmar erythema, testicular atrophy, and gynecomastia are common. Manifestations of portal hypertension and esophageal varices occur less commonly than in Laennec's cirrhosis. *Primary hepatocellular carcinoma* develops in about 30 percent of patients with cirrhosis. The incidence of this complication increases with age and is the most common cause of death in treated patients. However, it almost exclusively occurs in cirrhotic patients; hence the importance of early diagnosis and therapy. Splenomegaly is present in approximately half the symptomatic cases.

Excessive *skin pigmentation* is present in over 90 percent of symptomatic patients at the time of diagnosis. Melanin deposition in the skin usually gives rise to bronzing. The characteristic metallic or slate gray hue is believed to result from increased melanin or both melanin and iron in the dermis. Pigmentation usually is diffuse and generalized, but it may be more severe on the face, neck, extensor aspects of the lower forearms, dorsa of the hands, lower legs, genital regions, and in scars. In only 10 to 15 percent of cases is pigmentation demonstrable in the oral mucosa. Pigmentation of the hard palate and retina has been described.

Diabetes mellitus occurs in about 65 percent of patients and is more likely to develop in those with a family history of diabetes. The genetic predisposition and direct damage to the pancreas by iron deposition both contribute to the development of diabetes. The management of the diabetes is similar to that of other forms of diabetes except for a higher incidence of insulin resistance. Late degenerative sequelae are the same as in ordinary diabetes mellitus.

Arthropathy develops in 25 to 50 percent of patients. It usually occurs after the age of 50 but may occur at any time in the course, even as a first manifestation or long after therapy. The joints of the hands, especially the second and third metacarpophalangeal joints, are commonly the first joints involved. This manifestation helps to distinguish hemochromatotic chondrocalcinosis from the idiopathic form. A progressive polyarthritis involving wrists, hips, ankles, and knees also may ensue. Acute brief attacks of synovitis may be associated with deposition of calcium pyrophosphate (chondrocalcinosis or pseudogout), chiefly in the knees. Roentgenologic manifestations consist of cystic changes of sclerosis of the subchondral bones, loss of articular cartilage with narrowing of the joint space, diffuse demineralization, hypertrophic bone proliferation, and calcification of the synovium. The relation of these abnormalities to iron metabolism is not known. The arthropathy tends to progress despite removal of iron by phlebotomy. However, similar changes occur in other forms of iron overload, suggesting that iron plays some role.

Cardiac involvement is the presenting manifestation in about 15 percent of patients, the most common cardiac manifestation being congestive heart failure in about 10 percent of young adults with the disease. Symptoms of congestive failure may develop suddenly, with rapid progression to death if untreated. The heart is diffusely enlarged, and such cases may be misdiagnosed as idiopathic cardiomyopathy if other overt manifestations are absent. Cardiac arrhythmias include premature supraventricular beats, paroxysmal tachyarrhythmias, atrial flutter, atrial fibrillation, and varying degrees of atrioventricular block.

Hypogonadism is common in both sexes, and it may antedate other clinical manifestations. Manifestations include loss of libido, impotence, amenorrhea, testicular atrophy, and sparse body hair. Gynecomastia is less common than in other forms of cirrhosis. These changes are due to the decreased production of gonadotropins associated with impaired hypothalamic-pituitary function due to iron deposition. Symptoms may respond to therapy with gonadotrophins. Adrenal insufficiency, hypothyroidism, and hypoparathyroidism have been described.

DIAGNOSIS The association of (1) hepatomegaly, (2) skin pigmentation, (3) diabetes mellitus, (4) heart disease, (5) arthritis, and (6) evidence of hypogonadism should suggest the diagnosis. However, a parenchymal iron overload of comparatively short duration or modest degree may exist with none or only some of these manifestations [e.g., in young subjects (see Fig. 345-1)]. Therefore, a high index of suspicion is needed to make the diagnosis early, and hemochromatosis should be considered in any patient with unexplained hepatomegaly, cardiomyopathy, abnormal skin pigmentation, loss of libido, diabetes mellitus, or arthritis. This is particularly important because diagnosis and treatment before organ damage is irreversible can reverse the effects of iron toxicity and restore life expectancy to normal (see below).

The history should be particularly detailed in regard to disease in other family members, alcohol ingestion, iron intake, and ingestion of large doses of ascorbic acid, which promotes iron absorption. Appropriate tests should be performed to exclude iron loading secondary to hematologic disease. Confirmation of the presence of liver, pancreatic, cardiac, and joint disease should be obtained by physical examination, roentgenography, and standard function tests of these organs. It then remains to be demonstrated that there is an increase in total-body iron stores and, in particular, an increased parenchymal iron concentration with or without tissue damage.

The methods available for the demonstration of excessive parenchymal iron stores include (1) measurement of serum iron and determination of percent saturation of transferrin, (2) measurement of serum ferritin concentration, (3) liver biopsy (Table 345-1), (4) estimation of chelatable iron stores using the agent deferoxamine, and (5) computed tomography and/or magnetic resonance imaging of the liver. Each has its advantages and limitations. The serum iron level and percent saturation of transferrin are elevated early in the course of the disease, but their specificity is reduced by relatively high false-positive and false-negative rates. In particular, an increased serum iron concentration may be present in patients with alcoholic liver disease without iron overload; in this situation, however, the iron-binding capacity is usually not decreased as in hemochromatosis (Table 345-1). In otherwise healthy persons, a fasting serum transferrin saturation greater than 62 percent strongly suggests homozygosity for hemochromatosis.

The serum ferritin concentration is usually a good index of body iron stores, whether decreased or increased. In fact, each rise in serum ferritin level of 1 μg/L reflects an increase in body stores of some 65 mg. In most untreated patients with hemochromatosis, the serum ferritin level is greatly increased (Fig. 345-1 and Table 345-1).

These tests have therefore generally replaced the more cumbersome screening tests involving measurement of urinary iron excretion after the administration of an iron chelator such as deferoxamine. However, in patients with inflammation and hepatocellular necrosis, serum ferritin levels may be elevated out of proportion to body iron stores due to increased release from tissues. A repeat determination of serum ferritin should therefore be carried out when any concurrent acute hepatocellular damage has subsided, e.g., in alcoholic liver disease. In rare families, serum ferritin levels in symptomatic relatives are normal despite increased iron stores; the reason for this finding is unclear. In clinical practice, the *combined measurements* of the (1) percent transferrin saturation and (2) serum ferritin level provide the simplest and most reliable screening test for hemochromatosis, including the precirrhotic phase of the disease. If either of these tests is abnormal, liver biopsy should be performed, since it is the *definitive* test for the diagnosis of hemochromatosis. It permits histochemical estimation of tissue iron, measurement of hepatic iron concentration, and assessment of the extent of tissue damage. In addition, the calculation of the hepatic iron index (hepatic iron concentration ÷ age in years) is helpful in distinguishing early homozygous subjects

from heterozygotes (see Table 345-1). Computed tomography shows increased density of the liver due to iron deposition. However, dual-energy scanning and experienced personnel are required, and the lower limits for accurate detection of increased tissue iron are still unclear. Magnetic resonance imaging also may detect increased tissue iron, but the sensitivity requires further evaluation. A retrospective assessment of body iron storage is also provided by performing *weekly phlebotomy* and calculating the amount of iron removed before iron stores are exhausted (1 mL blood = 0.5 mg iron, approximately).

When the diagnosis of hemochromatosis is established, it is of importance to examine family members at risk. Asymptomatic as well as symptomatic family members with the disease usually have an increased saturation of transferrin and an increased serum ferritin concentration. These changes occur even before the iron stores are greatly increased (see Fig. 345-1). A liver biopsy should then be performed, since it is imperative to confirm the diagnosis and begin therapy before tissue damage occurs. As stated above, HLA typing is helpful in evaluating families with the disease. Affected siblings (homozygotes) usually have both HLA haplotypes identical with those of the proband, and where children of a proband are affected, a homozygote-heterozygote mating probably occurred. Siblings sharing only one HLA haplotype with a patient (heterozygotes) will probably not develop progressive iron overload. Thus HLA typing helps in predicting the probability of a sibling later developing the disease and therefore the desirable frequency of screening.

The distinction between hemochromatosis and alcoholic cirrhosis with increased tissue iron is usually not difficult if measurement is made of liver iron concentration and hepatic iron index (Table 345-1). Where biopsy is not possible, the deferoxamine excretion test can provide diagnostic information. It should be reemphasized that subjects with a history of excessive alcohol consumption and who have increased hepatic iron concentration are usually homozygotes for hereditary hemochromatosis.

TREATMENT The therapy of genetic hemochromatosis involves removal of the excess body iron and supportive treatment of damaged organs. Iron is best removed by weekly or twice weekly phlebotomy of 500 mL. Although there is an initial modest decline in the volume of packed red blood cells to about 35 mL/dL, the level stabilizes after several weeks. The plasma transferrin saturation remains increased until the available iron stores are depleted. In contrast, the plasma ferritin concentration falls progressively, reflecting the gradual decrease in body iron stores. Since one 500-mL unit of blood contains from 200 to 250 mg iron and about 25 g iron must be removed, weekly phlebotomy is usually required for 2 or 3 years. When the transferrin saturation and ferritin level become normal, phlebotomies are performed at such time intervals as required to maintain levels within the normal range. The measurements promptly become abnormal with iron reaccumulation. Usually one phlebotomy every 3 months will suffice.

Chelating agents such as deferoxamine, when given parenterally, remove 10 to 20 mg iron per day, less than half that mobilized by once weekly phlebotomy. Phlebotomy is also less expensive, more convenient, and safer for most patients. However, chelating agents are indicated when anemia or hypoproteinemia is severe enough to preclude phlebotomy. Subcutaneous infusion of deferoxamine using a portable pump is the most effective means of administration.

The management of the hepatic failure, cardiac failure, and diabetes mellitus differs little from conventional management of these conditions. Loss of libido and change in secondary sex characteristics are partially relieved by parenteral testosterone or gonadotropin therapy (see Chap. 339).

PROGNOSIS The principal causes of death in *untreated* patients are cardiac failure (30 percent), hepatocellular failure or portal hypertension (25 percent), and hepatocellular carcinoma (30 percent).

Life expectancy is improved by removal of the excessive stores of iron and maintenance of these stores at near-normal levels. The 5-year survival rate with therapy increases from 33 to 89 percent. With repeated phlebotomy, the liver and spleen decrease in size, liver function improves, pigmentation of skin decreases, and cardiac failure is reversed. Carbohydrate tolerance improves in about 40 percent. Removal of excess iron has little or no effect on hypogonadism or arthropathy. Hepatic fibrosis may decrease, but cirrhosis is irreversible. Hepatocellular carcinoma occurs as a late sequela in about one-third of patients who are cirrhotic at presentation despite adequate iron removal. The apparent increase in its incidence in treated patients is probably related in part to the increased life span. This complication does not appear to develop if the disease is treated in the precirrhotic stage, and the life expectancy of homozygotes diagnosed and treated before the development of cirrhosis is normal. Hence the importance of family screening and early therapy cannot be emphasized too strongly. Asymptomatic subjects who are detected by family studies should have phlebotomy therapy if iron stores are moderately to severely increased. Screening for increasing iron stores at appropriate intervals is also important. With this approach, most manifestations of the disease can be prevented.

REFERENCES

EDWARDS CQ et al: Prevalence of hemochromatosis among 11,065 presumably healthy blood donors. N Engl J Med 318:1355, 1988

GORDEUK V et al: Iron overload in Africa: Interaction between a gene and dietary iron content. N Engl J Med 326:95, 1992

KLAUSNER RD, HARFORD JB: Cis-trans models for post-transcriptional gene regulation. Science 246:870, 1989

LEGGETT BA et al: Factors affecting the concentration of serum ferritin in a healthy Australian population. Clin Chem 36:1350, 1990

NEIDERAU C ET AL: Survival and causes of death in cirrhotic and in noncirrhotic patients with primary hemochromatosis. N Engl J Med 313:1256, 1985

POWELL LW, KERR JFR: The pathology of liver in hemochromatosis, in *Pathobiology Annual*, H Joacim (ed). New York, Appleton-Century-Crofts, 1975

——— et al: Expression of hemochromatosis in homozygous subjects: Implications for early diagnosis and prevention. Gastroenterology 98:1625, 1990

SUMMERS KM et al: Identification of homozygous hemochromatosis subjects by measurement of hepatic iron index. Hepatology 12:20, 1990

---

346 THE PORPHYRIAS

ROBERT J. DESNICK

The porphyrias are inherited or acquired disorders of specific enzymes in the heme biosynthetic pathway (Fig. 346-1). These disorders are classified as either *hepatic* or *erythropoietic* depending on the primary site of overproduction and accumulation of the porphyrin precursor or porphyrin (Tables 346-1 and 346-2), but some have overlapping features. The major clinical manifestations of the hepatic porphyrias are neurologic symptoms, including abdominal pain, neuropathy, and mental disturbances, whereas patients with the erythropoietic porphyrias primarily have cutaneous photosensitivity. The reason for the neurologic involvement in the hepatic porphyrias is poorly understood. Cutaneous sensitivity to sunlight is due to the fact that excitation of excess porphyrins in the skin by long-wave ultraviolet light leads to cell damage, scarring, and deformation. Steroid hormones, drugs, and nutrition influence the production of porphyrin precursors and porphyrins, thereby precipitating or increasing the severity of some porphyrias. Thus these fall into the category of *ecogenic* disorders, in which environmental, physiologic, and genetic factors interact to cause disease manifestations.

Many symptoms of the porphyrias are nonspecific, and diagnosis is often delayed. Laboratory testing can confirm or exclude the diagnosis of a porphyria. Table 346-2 summarizes the major metabolites which accumulate in each porphyria. Urinary δ-aminolevulinic acid (ALA) and porphobilinogen (PBG) are easily quantitated by chemical methods, and the urinary porphyrin isomers can be separated

and quantitated by high-performance liquid chromatography. Fecal porphyrins can be extracted and analyzed semiquantitatively by thin-layer chromatography. Such studies, especially along with symptoms, make it possible to define the diagnostic profile of accumulated precursors and/or porphyrins in each disorder. However, a definite diagnosis requires demonstration of the specific enzyme deficiency. The isolation and characterization of the cDNAs encoding several of the heme biosynthetic enzymes have permitted the definition of the molecular lesions that cause specific porphyrias. Molecular analyses that take advantage of this information make it possible to provide prenatal diagnoses in families with known mutations.

HEME BIOSYNTHESIS   The first and last three enzymes in the heme biosynthetic pathway are in the mitochondrion, whereas the other four are in the cytosol (see Fig. 346-1). The first enzyme, δ-aminolevulinate synthase (ALA synthase), catalyzes the condensation of glycine, activated by pyridoxal phosphate and succinyl coenzyme A, to form ALA. In the liver, this rate-limiting enzyme for the pathway is inducible by a variety of drugs, steroids, and other chemicals. Distinct erythroid-specific and nonerythroid (i.e., housekeeping) forms of ALA synthase are encoded by separate genes. The occurrence of two ALA synthase genes provides the basis for the tissue-specific regulation of this pathway.

The second enzyme, δ-aminolevulinate dehydratase (ALA dehydratase), catalyzes the condensation of two molecules of ALA to form the pyrrole porphobilinogen (PBG). Four molecules of PBG condense to form the tetrapyrrole uroporphyrinogen III by a two-step process catalyzed by hydroxymethylbilane synthase (HMB synthase, also known as PBG deaminase or uroporphyrinogen I synthase) and uroporphyrinogen III synthase (URO synthase). HMB synthase catalyzes the head-to-tail condensation of four PBG molecules by a series of deaminations to form the linear tetrapyrrole hydroxymethylbilane (HMB). Uroporphyrinogen III synthase (URO synthase) catalyzes the rearrangement and rapid cyclization of HMB to form the asymmetric, physiologic, octacarboxylate porphyrinogen uroporphyrinogen III.

The fifth enzyme in the pathway, uroporphyrinogen decarboxylase (URO decarboxylase), catalyzes the sequential removal of the four carboxyl groups from the acetic acid side chains of uroporphyrinogen III to form coproporphyrinogen III, a tetracarboxylate porphyrinogen. This compound then enters the mitochondrion, where coproporphyrinogen oxidase (COPRO oxidase), the sixth enzyme, catalyzes the decarboxylation of two of the four propionic acid groups to form the two vinyl groups of protoporphyrinogen IX, a dicarboxylate porphyrinogen. Next, protoporphyrinogen oxidase (PROTO oxidase) oxidizes protoporphyrinogen IX to protoporphyrin IX by the removal of six hydrogen atoms. The product of the reaction is a porphyrin (oxidized form), in contrast to the preceding tetrapyrrole intermediates, which are porphyrinogens (reduced forms). The final step is the insertion of ferrous iron into protoporphyrin IX to form heme. This reaction is catalyzed by the eighth enzyme in the pathway, ferrochelatase (also known as heme synthetase or protoheme ferrolyase).

Each of the heme biosynthetic enzymes is encoded by a separate gene. Full-length human cDNAs for seven of the enzymes, including those for the erythroid and housekeeping forms of ALA synthase, have been isolated and sequenced, and the chromosomal locations of the genes have been identified (Table 346-3).

REGULATION OF HEME BIOSYNTHESIS   About 85 percent of heme is synthesized in erythroid cells to provide heme for hemoglobin, and most of the remaining heme is produced in the liver, where the heme biosynthetic pathway is under negative feedback control. "Free" heme in the liver regulates the synthesis and mitochondrial translocation of hepatic ALA synthase encoded by the housekeeping gene. Heme represses the synthesis of the ALA synthase mRNA and also interferes with the transport of the enzyme from the cysotol into mitochondria. ALA synthase is inducible by many of the same chemicals that induce the cytochrome P450 enzymes in the endoplasmic reticulum of the liver. Because most of the heme synthesized in

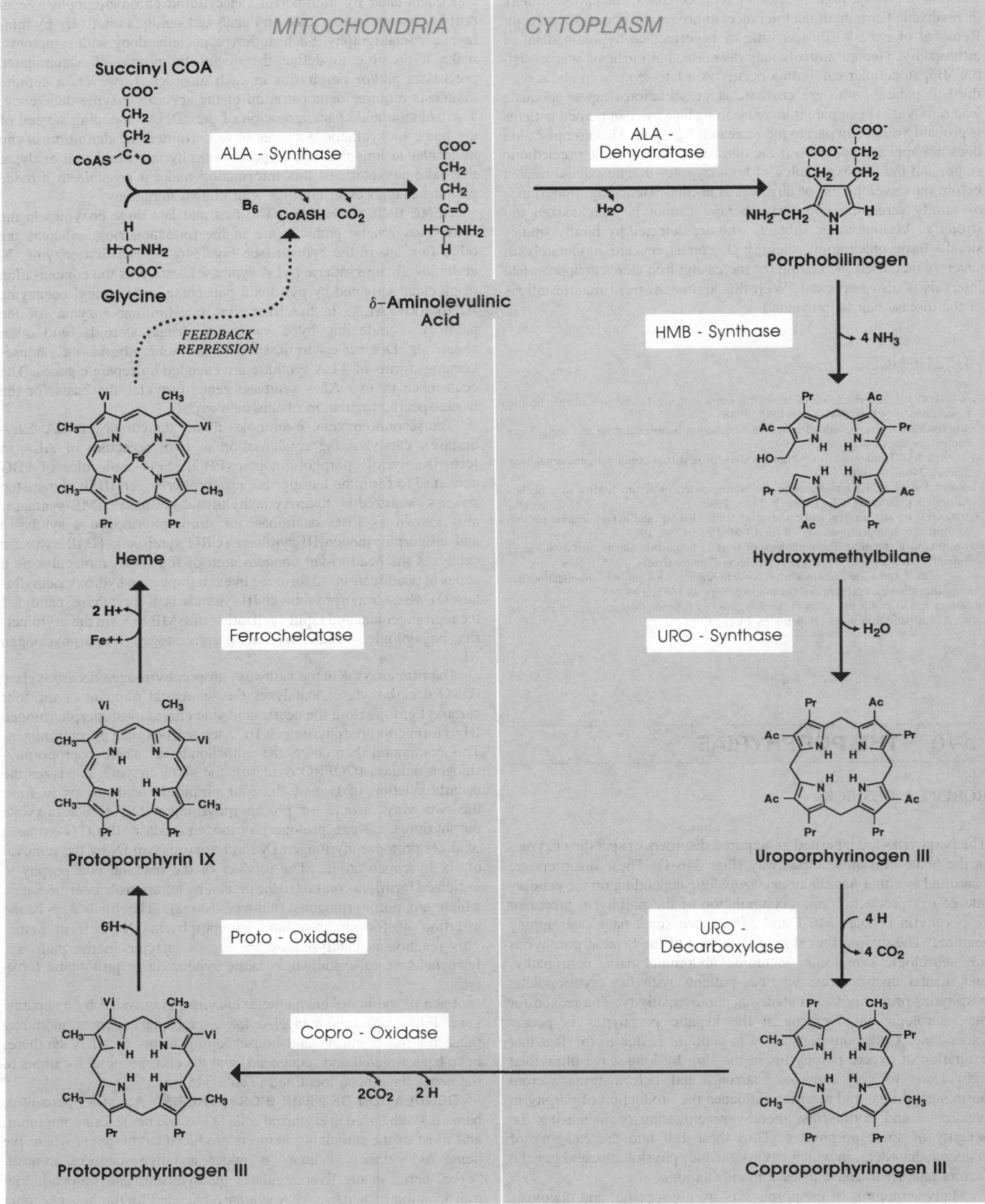

FIGURE 346-1   The human heme biosynthetic pathway.

TABLE 346-1 Classification of the human porphyrias

Type/porphyria	Deficient enzyme	Inheritance*	Photosensitivity	Neurovisceral symptoms
HEPATIC PORPHYRIAS				
ALA dehydratase deficiency	ALA dehydratase	AR	−	+
Acute intermittent porphyria (AIP)	HMB synthase	AD	−	+
Hereditary copro-porphyria (HCP)	COPRO oxidase	AD	+	+
Variegate porphyria (VP)	PROTO oxidase	AD	+	+
Porphyria cutanea tarda (PCT)	URO decarboxylase	AD	+	−
ERYTHROPOIETIC PORPHYRIAS				
X-linked sideroblastic anemia (XLSA)	ALA synthase	XLR	−	−
Congenital erythropoietic porphyria (CEP)	URO synthase	AR	+ + +	−
Erythropoietic protoporphyria (EPP)	Ferrochelatase	AD	+	−

* AR = autosomal recessive; AD = autosomal dominant; XLR = X-linked recessive.

the liver is used for the synthesis of the cytochrome P450 enzymes, hepatic ALA synthase and the cytochrome P450s are induced in a coordinated fashion.

In erythroid cells, different regulatory mechanisms control production of heme for hemoglobin. The erythroid-specific ALA synthase encoded on the X chromosome is expressed at higher levels than the hepatic gene encoded on chromosome 3. In addition, an erythroid-specific control mechanism regulates iron transport into erythroid

TABLE 346-2 The major metabolites accumulated in the human porphyrias

Type/porphyria	Increased erythrocyte porphyrins	Porphyrin excretion* Urine	Porphyrin excretion* Stool
HEPATIC PORPHYRIAS			
ALA dehydratase deficiency	—	ALA, COPRO III	—
Acute intermittent porphyria (AIP)	—	ALA, PBG	—
Hereditary copro-porphyria (HCP)	—	ALA, PBG, COPRO III	COPRO III
Variegate porphyria (VP)	—	ALA, PBG COPRO III	COPRO III, PROTO IX
Porphyria cutanea tarda (PCT)	—	URO I, 7-carboxylate, porphyrin	Isocopro
ERYTHROPOIETIC PORPHYRIAS			
X-linked sideroblastic anemia (XLSA)	—	—	—
Congenital erythropoietic porphyria (CEP)	URO I	URO I	COPRO I
Erythropoietic protoporphyria (EPP)	PROTO IX	—	PROTO IX

* ALA = δ-aminolevulinic acid; PBG = porphobilinogen; COPRO I = coproporphyrin I; COPRO III = coproporphyrin III; ISOCOPRO = isocoproporphyrin; URO I = uroporphyrin I; URO III = uroporphyrin III; PROTO = protoporphyrin IX

TABLE 346-3 The heme biosynthetic genes and their chromosomal locations

Structural gene	cDNA and genomic sequences characterized	Chromosomal assignment
ALA synthase		
Housekeeping	+	3p21
Erythroid	+	Xp11.21
ALA dehydratase	+	9q34
HMB synthase	+	11q23 → qter
URO synthase	+	10q25.3 → 26.3
URO decarboxylase	+	1p34
COPRO oxidase	−	9
PROTO oxidase	−	14q31 → q32
Ferrochelatase	+	18q21.3

cells. During erythroid differentiation, the activities of the heme biosynthetic enzymes increase in a coordinated fashion.

THE HEPATIC PORPHYRIAS

The rapid onset of neurologic symptoms is characteristic of the acute hepatic porphyrias. During an acute attack, individuals have markedly elevated plasma and urinary concentrations of the porphyrin precursors ALA and PBG, which originate from the liver.

ALA DEHYDRATASE–DEFICIENT PORPHYRIA This disease is a rare autosomal recessive trait that has been described in four unrelated males in Europe. Onset and severity of the disease are variable, presumably depending on the amount of residual ALA dehydratase activity. Treatment and prevention of the neurologic complications are the same as for other acute porphyrias (see below).

Clinical features The clinical presentation is variable. The first reported cases were two unrelated German men who had the onset during adolescence of abdominal pain and neuropathy, resembling acute intermittent porphyria (AIP; see below). The third patient, a Swedish infant, presented with failure to thrive and required transfusions and parenteral nutrition. Presumably, the earlier age of onset and more severe manifestations reflect a more complete enzyme deficiency. The fourth patient, a Belgian male, developed an acute motor polyneuropathy and polycythemia at age 63.

Diagnosis All four had increased urinary ALA and coproporphyrin levels. ALA dehydratase activity was reduced in erythrocytes (<5 percent of normal). It should be noted that both succinylacetone (which accumulates in hereditary tyrosinemia and is structurally similar to ALA) and lead inhibit ALA dehydratase and cause increased urinary excretion of ALA and manifestations that resemble those of the acute porphyrias. Therefore, lead intoxication and hereditary tyrosinemia (fumarylacetoacetase deficiency) should be considered in the differential diagnosis of the ALA dehydratase–deficient porphyria. Immunologic studies in the four reported cases demonstrated the presence of nonfunctional enzyme proteins that cross-reacted with anti-ALA dehydratase antibodies. DNA analysis revealed different missense mutations that resulted in the amino acid substitutions G133R and V275M in the infantile-onset case and R240W and A274T in one of the juvenile-onset cases.

Heterozygotes are clinically asymptomatic and do not excrete increased levels of ALA but can be detected by demonstration of intermediate levels of erythrocyte ALA dehydratase activity or by the presence of a specific mutation in the ALA dehydratase gene. The prenatal diagnosis of this disorder has not been made but should be possible by determination of the ALA dehydratase activity in cultured chorionic villi or amniocytes.

Treatment Treatment is similar to that in AIP (see below). The severely affected infant was supported by hyperalimentation and periodic blood transfusions. Continued failure to thrive led to a liver transplant, which did not improve the hematologic manifestations.

ACUTE INTERMITTENT PORPHYRIA This hepatic porphyria is an autosomal dominant condition resulting from the half-normal level of HMB synthase (formerly known as PBG deaminase) activity. The disease is widespread but more common in Scandinavia and perhaps Great Britain. The enzyme deficiency can be demonstrated in most heterozygous individuals, but clinical expression of this porphyria is highly variable. Activation of the disease is related to ecogenic factors, such as drugs, diet, and steroid hormones, which can precipitate the disease manifestations. Attacks can be prevented by avoiding known precipitating factors.

Clinical features Most heterozygotes remain clinically asymptomatic (latent) unless exposed to factors that increase the production of porphyrins. Endogenous and exogenous gonadal steroids, porphyrinogenic drugs, and a low caloric diet, usually instituted in an effort to lose weight, are the most common precipitating factors. The major drugs thought to be harmful in AIP [and in hereditary coproporphyria (HCP) and variegate porphyria (VP)] and drugs and anesthetic agents known to be safe are listed in Table 346-4. Although more extensive lists of drugs considered harmful or safe are available (see references), information is incomplete for many drugs. Attacks also can be provoked by infections and by surgery.

Because the neurovisceral symptoms rarely occur before puberty and are often nonspecific, a high index of suspicion is needed to suggest the proper diagnosis. The disease can be disabling but is rarely fatal. Abdominal pain, the most common symptom, is usually steady and poorly localized but may be cramping. Ileus, abdominal distention, and decreased bowel sounds are common. However, increased bowel sounds and diarrhea may occur. Abdominal tenderness, fever, and leukocytosis are usually absent or mild because the manifestations are neurologic rather than inflammatory. Nausea, vomiting, constipation, tachycardia, hypertension, mental symptoms, pain in the limbs, head, neck or chest, muscle weakness, sensory loss, dysuria, and urinary retention are characteristic. Tachycardia, hypertension, restlessness, tremors, and excess sweating are due to sympathetic overactivity.

The peripheral neuropathy is due to axonal degeneration (rather than demyelinization) and affects primarily motor neurons. Significant neuropathy does not occur with all acute attacks; abdominal symptoms are usually more prominent. Motor neuropathy affects the proximal muscles initially, more often in the shoulders and arms. The course and degree of involvement are variable. Deep tendon reflexes may be normal or hyperactive but are usually decreased or absent with advanced neuropathy. Motor weakness can be asymmetric and focal and can involve cranial nerves. Sensory changes such as paresthesias and loss of sensation are less prominent. Progressive muscle weakness leading to respiratory and bulbar paralysis and death may occur when diagnosis and treatment are delayed. Sudden death may result from sympathetic overactivity and cardiac arrhythmia.

Mental symptoms such as anxiety, insomnia, depression, disorientation, hallucinations, and paranoia can accompany acute attacks. Seizures can be due to direct neurologic effects or result from hyponatremia. Treatment of seizures is difficult because virtually all antiseizure drugs (except bromides) have at least some potential for exacerbating AIP (clonazepam may be less likely than phenytoin or barbiturates). Hyponatremia results from hypothalamic involvement and inappropriate vasopressin secretion or from electrolyte depletion due to vomiting, diarrhea, poor intake, or excess renal sodium loss. Persistent hypertension and impaired renal function may occur. When an attack resolves, abdominal pain may disappear within hours, and paresis begins to improve within days and may continue to improve over several years.

Diagnosis ALA and PBG are increased in plasma and urine during acute attacks. Urinary PBG excretion is usually 220 to 880 μmol/d (50 to 200 mg/d) [normal 0 to 18 μmol/d (0 to 4 mg/d)], and urinary ALA is 150 to 760 μmol/d (20 to 100 mg/d) [normal 8 to 53 μmol/d (1 to 7 mg/d)]. The excretion of these compounds generally decreases with clinical improvement, particularly after hematin infusions (see below). A normal urinary PBG level effectively excludes AIP as a cause for current symptoms. Fecal porphyrins are usually normal or minimally increased in AIP, in contrast to HCP and VP. Most asymptomatic ("latent") heterozygotes with HMB synthase deficiency have normal urinary excretion of ALA and PBG. Therefore, measurement of HMB synthase in erythrocytes is useful to confirm the diagnosis and to screen asymptomatic family members.

The enzyme deficiency is detectable in erythrocytes from most AIP heterozygotes (*classic AIP*). However, the activity is higher in young erythrocytes and may increase into the normal range in an AIP patient with increased erythropoiesis due to a concurrent condition. However, patients with the rare erythroid form of AIP (*erythroid AIP*) have normal erythrocyte enzyme activities and deficient activity in nonerythroid tissues (see below). The erythroid and housekeeping forms of HMB synthase are encoded by a single gene, which has two promoters. One encodes the messenger RNA for the housekeeping (i.e., ubiquitously expressed) form of the enzyme found in all tissues, and the other encodes the erythroid-specific transcript. Several deletions and over 20 different point mutations in the coding region of the gene have been found in unrelated AIP families (Fig. 346-2). These mutations alter the kinetic and/or stability properties of the mutant proteins or create premature termination codons. Mutations that cause erythroid AIP variants with half-normal enzyme in nonerythroid tissues but normal activity in erythrocytes include point mutations in the initiation methionine codon (that prevent translation) or in the 5' splice site of intron 1 (that cause abnormal splicing of the HMB synthase transcript).

Heterozygotes can be identified by RFLP studies in informative families using various polymorphic sites in the HMB synthase gene. Efforts are now underway to identify the specific mutations in the HMB synthase gene in all AIP families; this information will make possible the accurate identification of heterozygotes. Identified heterozygotes can be advised to avoid the factors known to cause acute attacks. The prenatal diagnosis of a fetus at risk can be made with cultured amniotic cells or chorionic villi.

Treatment During acute attacks, narcotic analgesics may be required for abdominal pain, and phenothiazines are useful for nausea, vomiting, anxiety, and restlessness. Chloral hydrate can be given safely for insomnia. Benzodiazepines in low doses are probably safe if a minor tranquilizer is required. Although intravenous glucose (at least 300 g/d) was recommended in the past for acute attacks of porphyria, a more complete parenteral nutritional regimen may be beneficial if oral feeding is not possible for a prolonged period. However, intravenous heme is more effective than glucose in reducing porphyrin precursor excretion and probably leads to more rapid recovery. The response to heme therapy is reduced if therapy is delayed. Therefore, 3 to 4 mg heme, in the form of hematin (Abbott Laboratories), heme albumin, or heme arginate (Leiras Oy, Turku, Finland), may be infused daily for 4 days beginning as soon as possible after onset of an attack. Heme arginate and heme albumin are chemically stable and less likely than hematin to produce phlebitis or an anticoagulant effect. The rate of recovery from an acute attack

TABLE 346-4 Categories of unsafe and safe drugs in AIP, HCP, and VP

Unsafe	Safe
Barbiturates	Narcotic analgesics
Sulfonamide antibiotics	Aspirin
Meprobamate	Acetaminophen
Glutethimide	Phenothiazines
Methyprylon	Penicillin and derivatives
Ethchlorvynol	Streptomycin
Mephenytoin	Glucocorticoids
Succinimides	Bromides
Carbamazepine	Insulin
Valproic acid	Atropine
Pyrazolones	
Griseofulvin	
Ergots	
Synthetic estrogens and progestogens	
Danazol	
Alcohol	

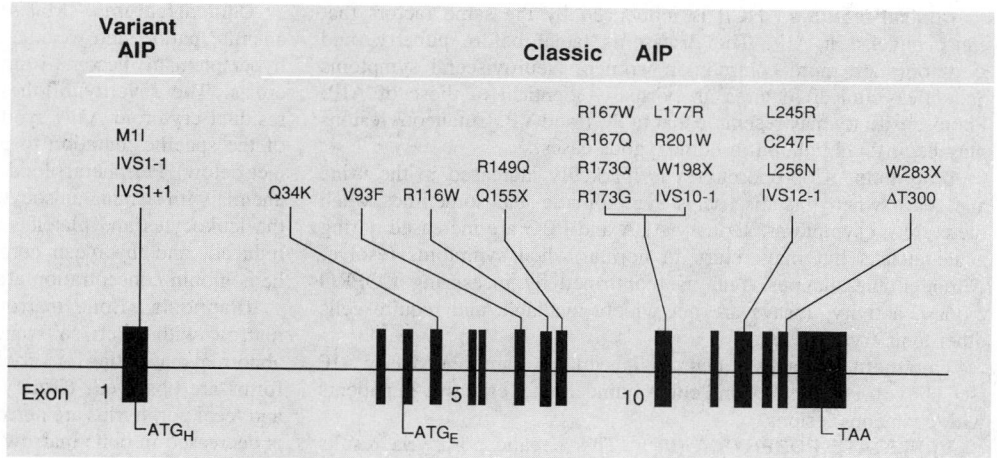

FIGURE 346-2 Mutations in the HMB synthase gene causing AIP. Mutation nomenclature: letters = one-letter code for amino acids; numbers = codon positions.

depends on the degree of neuronal damage and may be rapid (1 to 2 days) with prompt therapy. Recovery from severe motor neuropathy may continue for months or years. Identification of and avoidance of inciting factors can hasten recovery from an attack and prevent future attacks. Multiple inciting factors may contribute to a symptomatic episode. Frequent clear-cut cyclical attacks occur in some women and can be prevented with a luteinizing hormone–releasing hormone analogue (this indication is not approved by the U.S. Food and Drug Administration).

PORPHYRIA CUTANEA TARDA (PCT) The most common of the porphyrias can be sporadic (type I) or familial (types II and III) and also can develop after exposure to halogenated aromatic hydrocarbons. Hepatic URO decarboxylase is deficient in all types of PCT. In type I PCT, URO decarboxylase activity is normal in erythrocytes. In type II PCT, deficiency of the enzyme in erythrocytes and other tissues is inherited as an autosomal dominant trait. In type III PCT, inherited deficiency of the enzyme is limited to the liver. Deficient hepatic URO decarboxylase and a porphyrin pattern resembling PCT can be produced by exposure of normal individuals to a number of halogenated aromatic hydrocarbons. Hepatoerythropoietic porphyria (HEP) is an autosomal recessive form of porphyria that results from homozygous deficiency of URO decarboxylase.

Clinical features Cutaneous photosensitivity is the major clinical feature. Neurologic manifestations are not observed. Fluid-filled vesicles and bullae develop on sun-exposed areas such as the face, dorsa of the hands and feet, forearms, and legs. The skin in these areas is friable, and minor trauma may lead to the formation of bullae. Small white plaques, termed *milia*, may precede or follow vesicle formation. Bullae and denuded skin heal slowly and are subject to infection. Other features include hypertrichosis and hyperpigmentation, especially of the face, and thickening, scarring, and calcification resembling the cutaneous changes of systemic sclerosis.

A number of factors contribute to the development of hepatic URO decarboxylase deficiency, including excess alcohol, iron, and estrogens. PCT also can be induced by various chemicals. For example, an epidemic of PCT occurred in eastern Turkey in the 1950s as a result of consumption of wheat treated with the fungicide hexachlorobenzene. Hexachlorobenzene produces a disorder similar to PCT and induces hepatic URO decarboxylase deficiency in animals. A few cases of PCT in humans have occurred after exposure to other chemicals, including di- and trichlorophenols and 2,3,7,8-tetrachlorodibenzo-(ρ)-dioxin (TCDD, dioxin). Patients with PCT characteristically have mild to severe liver damage and are at risk for hepatocellular carcinoma. These carcinomas do not produce porphyrins.

Hepatoerythropoietic porphyria (HEP) resembles congenital erythropoietic porphyria (CEP) but also has erythropoietic features and usually presents with blistering skin lesions, hypertrichosis, scarring, and red urine in infancy or childhood.

Diagnosis Porphyrins are increased in the liver, plasma, urine, and stool. Urinary ALA may be slightly increased, but PBG is normal. Urinary porphyrins consist mostly of uroporphyrin and 7-carboxylate porphyrin with lesser amounts of coproporphyrin and 5- and 6-carboxylate porphyrins. Plasma porphyrins also are increased in a pattern that resembles that in urine. Isocoproporphyrins are increased in feces and sometimes also in plasma and urine. The finding of increased isocoproporphyrins is diagnostic for a deficiency of hepatic URO decarboxylase.

Type II PCT and HEP can be distinguished by finding low activity of URO decarboxylase in erythrocytes. URO decarboxylase activity in liver, erythrocytes, and cultured skin fibroblasts in type II PCT is approximately 50 percent of normal in clinically affected individuals and in family members with latent disease. In HEP, the URO decarboxylase activity is 3 to 28 percent of normal. Several point mutations have been identified in the coding region of the URO decarboxylase gene from unrelated type II PCT and HEP patients. Hepatic iron contributes to development of sporadic and familial forms of PCT. In the familial forms (types II and III), iron inhibits the residual normal enzyme so that enzymatic activity in liver is less than 50 percent of normal. In type I PCT the decreased hepatic URO decarboxylase activity is not accompanied by a decrease in the concentration of the enzyme protein, suggesting that the enzyme is present in an inactivated form and hepatic URO decarboxylase activity gradually increases after a remission is induced by phlebotomy.

Treatment If possible, alcohol, estrogens, iron supplements, and drugs that may contribute to exacerbation of the disease should be discontinued, but this does not always lead to improvement. A complete response can almost always be achieved by repeated phlebotomy to reduce hepatic iron. A unit (450 mL) of blood can be removed every 1 to 2 weeks. Because iron overload is not marked in most cases, a remission may occur after only five or six phlebotomies. Hemoglobin levels or hematocrits and serum ferritin should be followed closely to prevent development of iron deficiency and anemia. After remission, phlebotomies may not be needed even if ferritin levels return to normal. Relapses are successfully treated by additional phlebotomy.

PCT also can be treated with chloroquine or hydroxychloroquine, both of which complex with the excess porphyrins and promote their excretion. Small doses (e.g., 125 mg chloroquine phosphate twice weekly) should be given because standard doses can induce transient, sometimes marked increases in photosensitivity and hepatocellular damage. Hepatic imaging may be advisable to exclude complicating hepatocellular carcinoma. Treatment of PCT in patients with end-stage renal disease is facilitated by administration of erythropoietin.

HEREDITARY COPROPORPHYRIA (HCP) This hepatic porphyria results from deficiency of COPRO oxidase and is inherited as an autosomal dominant trait. Photosensitivity sometimes occurs. A few cases of homozygous HCP have been reported.

Clinical features   HCP is influenced by the same factors that cause attacks in AIP. The disease is latent before puberty, and symptoms are more common in women. Neurovisceral symptoms and other clinical features are virtually identical to those of AIP. Photosensitivity may resemble that in PCT and VP. Cutaneous lesions may begin in childhood in homozygous cases.

Diagnosis   Coproporphyrin is markedly increased in the urine and feces when this disease is symptomatic and sometimes when there are no symptoms. Urinary ALA and PBG are increased during acute attacks but may return to normal when symptoms resolve. Although the diagnosis can be confirmed by measuring COPRO oxidase activity, assays are not widely available and require cells other than erythrocytes.

Treatment   Attacks of neurologic symptoms are treated as in AIP (see above). Phlebotomy and chloroquine are not effective in patients with cutaneous lesions.

VARIEGATE PORPHYRIA (VP)   This hepatic porphyria results from the deficient activity of PROTO oxidase, is inherited as an autosomal dominant trait, and can present with neurologic symptoms, photosensitivity, or both.

Clinical features   Neurovisceral signs and symptoms develop after puberty and are indistinguishable from those of AIP or HCP (see above). Attacks are provoked by the same drugs, steroid hormones, and nutritional factors that are detrimental in AIP. Skin manifestations are more common than in HCP but usually occur apart from the neurovisceral symptoms. Since the skin lesions in VP, HCP, and PCT are not distinguishable by clinical examination or biopsy, these conditions must be diagnosed by measurements of porphyrins and porphyrin precursors in blood, urine, and feces.

VP is particularly common in South Africa, where 3 of every 1000 whites have the disorder. Most are descendants of a couple who emigrated from Holland to South Africa in 1688. Homozygous VP has been described; photosensitivity, neurologic symptoms, and developmental disturbances, including growth retardation, were noted in infancy or childhood. All cases had increased erythrocyte zinc protoporphyrin levels, a characteristic finding in all homozygous porphyrias so far described.

Dual porphyria, the simultaneous occurrence of VP and familial PCT, has been documented in several kindreds. *Chester porphyria* was described in a large family from Great Britain in which individuals had acute porphyric attacks and evidence of both PROTO oxidase and HMB synthase deficiencies. Photosensitivity was not observed. It is unclear whether Chester porphyria is a variant of VP or AIP.

Diagnosis   When VP is symptomatic, fecal protoporphyrin and coproporphyrin and urinary coproporphyrin are increased. Urinary ALA and PBG are increased during acute attacks. Plasma porphyrins are increased, particularly when there are cutaneous lesions. VP can be distinguished rapidly from all other porphyrias by examining the fluorescence emission spectrum of porphyrins in plasma at neutral pH. This is particularly useful for differentiating VP from PCT.

Assays of PROTO oxidase activity in cultured fibroblasts or lymphocytes are not widely available. Some latent cases of VP can be diagnosed by measurement of fecal porphyrins in relatives of VP patients.

Treatment   Acute attacks are treated with hematin as in AIP. Other than avoiding sun exposure, there are few effective measures for the skin lesions. β-Carotene, phlebotomy, and chloroquine are not helpful.

THE ERYTHROPOIETIC PORPHYRIAS

In the erythropoietic porphyrias, elevated bone marrow erythrocyte and plasma porphyrins become deposited in the skin and lead to cutaneous photosensitivity.

X-LINKED SIDEROBLASTIC ANEMIA (XLSA)   This anemia results from the deficient activity of the erythroid form of ALA synthase and is associated with ineffective erythropoiesis, weakness, and pallor.

Clinical features   Males with XLSA develop refractory hemolytic anemia, pallor, and weakness during infancy. They have secondary hypersplenism, become iron overloaded, and can develop hemosiderosis. The severity of these symptoms depends on the level of residual erythroid ALA synthase activity and on the responsiveness of the specific mutation to pyridoxal 5'-phosphate supplementation (see below). Peripheral blood smears reveal a hypochromic, microcytic anemia with striking anisocytosis, poikilocytosis, and polychromasia; the leukocytes and platelets appear normal. Hemoglobin content is reduced, and the mean corpuscular volume and mean corpuscular hemoglobin concentration are decreased.

Diagnosis   Bone marrow examination reveals a hypercellular marrow with a left shift and megaloblastic erythropoiesis with an abnormal maturation. A variety of Prussian blue–staining sideroblastic forms are observed. Urinary porphyrin precursors and both urinary and fecal porphyrins are normal. The level of erythroid ALA synthase is decreased in bone marrow, but this enzyme is difficult to measure in the presence of the normal housekeeping enzyme. Definitive diagnosis requires the demonstration of specific mutations in the erythroid ALA synthase gene.

Treatment   The severe anemia may respond to pyridoxine supplementation. This cofactor is essential for ALA synthase activity, and mutations in the pyridoxine binding site of the enzyme have been found in several responsive patients. Cofactor supplementation may obviate the need for periodic transfusions or reduce their frequency. Unresponsive patients may be transfusion-dependent and require chelation therapy.

CONGENITAL ERYTHROPOIETIC PORPHYRIA (CEP)   This autosomal recessive porphyria, also known as *Gunther's disease,* is due to deficiency of URO synthase and is associated with hemolytic anemia and cutaneous lesions. CEP is characterized by accumulation of the type I isomers of uroporphyrin and coproporphyrin.

Clinical features   Cutaneous photosensitivity is usually severe and begins in early infancy. The skin over sun-exposed areas is friable. Bullae and vesicles are prone to rupture and infection. Skin thickening, focal hypo- and hyperpigmentation, and hypertrichosis of the face and extremities are characteristic. Secondary infection can lead to disfiguring of the face and hands. Porphyrins are deposited in teeth and in bones. As a result, the teeth are reddish brown and fluoresce on exposure to long-wave ultraviolet light. Hemolysis is probably due to the marked increase in erythrocyte porphyrins and leads to splenomegaly. A milder form of the disease occurs with onset of symptoms in adulthood.

Diagnosis   Uroporphyrin and coproporphyrin (mostly isomer I) accumulate in the bone marrow, erythrocytes, plasma, urine, and feces. The diagnosis should be confirmed by demonstration of markedly deficient URO synthase activity. The disease can be detected in utero by measuring porphyrins in amniotic fluid and URO synthase activity in cultured amniotic cells or chorionic villi. Molecular analyses of the mutant alleles from over 20 unrelated patients have revealed the presence of gene rearrangements, an mRNA processing defect, and several point mutations that cause amino acid substitutions.

Treatment   Blood transfusions sufficient to suppress erythropoiesis appear to be the most effective form of treatment, but this strategy is complicated by iron overload. Splenectomy may reduce hemolysis and reduce transfusion requirements. Protection from sunlight and from minor skin trauma is important. β-Carotene may be of some value. Complicating bacterial infections should be treated promptly. Bone marrow transplantation has been reported in only one patient, who subsequently died from transplant complications.

ERYTHROPOIETIC PROTOPORPHYRIA (EPP)   This condition is due to the partial deficiency of ferrochelatase and is inherited as an autosomal dominant trait. Protoporphyrin accumulates in erythroid cells and plasma and is excreted in bile and feces. EPP is the most common erythropoietic porphyria and, after PCT, the second most common porphyria.

Clinical features   Skin photosensitivity usually begins in childhood. The skin manifestations of EPP differ from those of other porphyrias. Vesicular lesions are uncommon. Redness, swelling, burning, and itching can develop within minutes of sun exposure and resemble angioedema. Symptoms may seem out of proportion to visible skin lesions. Vesicles and bullae are absent or sparse and may occur in only 10 percent of cases. Chronic skin changes may include lichenification, leathery pseudovesicles, labial grooving, and nail changes. Severe scarring is rare, as are pigment changes, friability, and hirsutism.

The primary source of excess protoporphyrin is the bone marrow reticulocyte. Erythrocyte protoporphyrin is free (not complexed with zinc) and is mostly bound to hemoglobin. In plasma protoporphyrin is bound to albumin. Hemolysis and anemia are usually absent or very mild.

Liver function is usually normal. However, in some patients, accumulation of protoporphyrin causes chronic liver disease that can progress to liver failure and death. The hepatic complications are often preceded by increasing levels of erythrocyte and plasma protoporphyrin and probably result, in part, from protoporphyrin accumulation in the liver. Protoporphyrin is insoluble, forms crystalline structures in liver cells, and can decrease hepatic bile flow. Gallstones composed at least in part of protoporphyrin occur in some patients.

Some obligate heterozygotes are asymptomatic and have little or no increase in erythrocyte protoporphyrin. Thus there is phenotypic variation in this disease.

Diagnosis   Protoporphyrin concentrations are increased in bone marrow, circulating erythrocytes, plasma, bile, and feces. Urinary porphyrin and porphyrin precursors are normal. Decreased ferrochelatase activity can be demonstrated in cultured lymphocytes or fibroblasts.

Treatment   Oral β-carotene (Hoffman-LaRoche) (120 to 180 mg/d) improves tolerance to sunlight in many patients. Adjustment in dosage may be needed to maintain serum carotene levels in the recommended range of 10 to 15 μmol/L (600 to 800 μg/dL). Mild skin discoloration due to carotenemia is the only significant side effect. The beneficial effects of β-carotene may involve quenching of singlet oxygen or free radicals. Unfortunately, this drug appears less effective in other forms of porphyria associated with photosensitivity.

Treatment of hepatic complications is difficult. However, cholestyramine and other porphyrin absorbents such as activated charcoal may interrupt the enterohepatic circulation of protoporphyrin and promote its fecal excretion, leading to some improvement. Splenectomy may be helpful when the disease is accompanied by hemolysis and significant splenomegaly. Caloric restriction and drugs or hormone preparations that may induce the heme pathway in liver or impair hepatic excretory function should be avoided. Iron deficiency should be prevented or treated. Transfusions or intravenous heme therapy may suppress erythroid and hepatic protoporphyrin production and are sometimes clinically beneficial. Liver transplantation has been carried out in some patients with severe liver complications.

REFERENCES

ANDERSON KE et al: A GnRH analogue prevents cyclical attacks of porphyria. Arch Intern Med 150:1469, 1990

COTTER PD et al: Enzymatic defect in "X-linked" sideroblastic anemia: Molecular evidence for erythroid δ-aminolevulinate synthase deficiency. Proc Natl Acad Sci USA 89:4028, 1992

DESNICK RJ, ANDERSON KE: Disorders of heme biosynthesis: The porphyrias, in *Hematology: Basic Principles and Practices*, R Hoffman et al (eds). New York, Churchill Livingstone, 1991, pp 350–367

KAPPAS A et al: The porphyrias, in *The Metabolic Basis of Inherited Disease*, CR Scriver et al (eds). New York, McGraw-Hill, 1990, pp 1305–1366

MOORE MR et al: *Disorders of Porphyrin Metabolism*. New York, Plenum, 1987

MUSTAJOKI P, NORDMANN Y: Early administration of heme arginate for acute porphyric attacks. Ann Intern Med (in press)

PLEWINSKA M et al: δ-Aminolevulinate dehydratase deficient porphyria: Identification of the molecular lesions in a severely affected homozygote. Am J Hum Genet 49:167, 1991

WARNER CA et al: Congenital erythropoietic porphyria: Identification and expression of exonic mutations in the uroporphyrinogen III synthase gene. J Clin Invest 89:693, 1992

347   GOUT AND OTHER DISORDERS OF PURINE METABOLISM

ROBERT L. WORTMANN

Gout encompasses a heterogeneous group of disorders that occur alone or in combination and include (1) hyperuricemia, (2) attacks of acute, typically monarticular, inflammatory arthritis, (3) tophaceous deposition of urate crystals in and around joints, (4) interstitial deposition of urate crystals in renal parenchyma, and (5) urolithiasis. *Hyperuricemia,* the cardinal biochemical feature and prerequisite for gout, is defined as a plasma urate concentration greater than 420 μmol/L (7.0 mg/dL) and is an indication of increased total-body urate. Hyperuricemia can result from increased production of urate, decreased excretion of uric acid, or a combination of the two processes. When hyperuricemia exists, plasma and extracellular fluids are supersaturated with respect to urate and conditions exist that favor crystal formation and tissue deposition. These conditions may result in the clinical manifestations included in the term *gout.*

URIC ACID METABOLISM   Uric acid is the final breakdown product of purine degradation in humans. It is a weak acid with pK_a of 5.75 and 10.3. Urates, the ionized forms of uric acid, predominate in plasma, extracellular fluid, and synovial fluid, with approximately 98 percent existing as monosodium urate at pH 7.4. Monosodium urate is easily ultrafiltered and dialyzed from plasma. Binding of urate to plasma proteins has little physiologic significance.

Plasma is saturated with monosodium urate at a concentration of 415 μmol/L (6.8 mg/dL) at 37°C. At higher concentrations, plasma is therefore supersaturated with urate, and potential exists for urate crystal precipitation. However, precipitation does not occur even at plasma urate concentrations as high as 4800 μmol/L (80 mg/dL). Why urate forms stable supersaturated solutions in plasma is unclear but may relate to the presence of solubilizing substances.

Uric acid is more soluble in urine than in water, possibly because of the presence of urea, proteins, and mucopolysaccharides. The pH of urine greatly influences its solubility. At pH 5.0, urine is saturated with uric acid at concentrations ranging from 360 to 900 μmol/L (6 to 15 mg/dL). At pH 7.0, saturation is reached at concentrations between 9480 and 12,000 μmol/L (158 and 200 mg/dL). Ionized forms of uric acid in urine include mono- and disodium, potassium, ammonium, and calcium urates.

Although purine nucleotide synthesis and breakdown occur in all tissues, urate is produced only in tissues that contain xanthine oxidase, primarily liver and small intestine. The amount of urate in the body is the net result of the amount produced and the amount excreted (Fig. 347-1). Urate production varies with the purine content of the diet and the respective rates of purine biosynthesis, degradation, and salvage. Normally, two-thirds to three-fourths of urate produced is excreted by the kidneys, and most of the remainder is eliminated through the intestines. A three-component model that includes glomerular filtration and both tubular secretion and reabsorption is proposed for the renal handling of uric acid in humans (Fig. 347-2). Approximately 8 to 12 percent of urate filtered by the glomeruli is excreted in the urine as uric acid. After filtration, 98 to 100 percent of the urate is reabsorbed. Approximately half the reabsorbed urate is secreted back into the proximal tubule, and 40 to 44 percent of that is again reabsorbed.

Serum urate concentrations vary with age and sex. Most children have serum urate concentrations of 180 to 240 μmol/L (3.0 to 4.0 mg/dL). Levels begin to rise during puberty in males but remain low in females until menopause. Although the cause of this sex variation is not completely understood, it is in part due to higher functional excretion of urate in females and is attributable to hormonal influences. Mean serum urate values for adult men and premenopausal women are 415 and 360 μmol/L (6.8 and 6.0 mg/dL), respectively. After

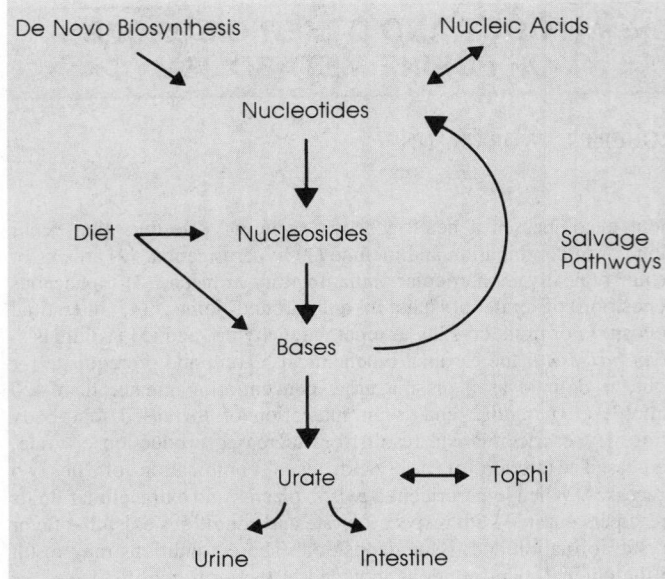

FIGURE 347-1 The total-body urate pool is the net result between urate production and excretion. Urate production is influenced by dietary intake of purines and the rates of de novo biosynthesis of purines from nonpurine precursors, nucleic acid turnover, and salvage by phosphoribosyltransferase activities. The formed urate is normally excreted by urinary and intestinal routes. Hyperuricemia can result from increased production, decreased excretion, or a combination of both mechanisms. When hyperuricemia exists, urate can precipitate and deposit in tissues as tophi.

menopause, values for women increase to approximate those of men. Adult concentrations rise steadily over time and vary with height, body weight, blood pressure, renal function, and alcohol intake.

HYPERURICEMIA

Hyperuricemia may be defined as a plasma (or serum) urate concentration greater than 420 μmol/L (7.0 mg/dL). This definition is based on physicochemical, epidemiologic, and disease-related criteria. Physicochemically, hyperuricemia is the concentration of urate in the blood that exceeds the solubility limits of monosodium urate in plasma, 415 μmol/L (6.8 mg/dL). In epidemiologic studies, hyperuricemia is defined by the mean plus 2 standard deviations of values determined from a randomly selected healthy population. In a major study, 95 percent of unselected individuals had serum urate concentrations below 420 μmol/L (7.0 mg/dL). Finally, hyperuricemia can be defined in relation to the risk of developing disease. The risk of developing gout or urolithiasis increases with urate concentrations greater than 420 μmol/L (7.0 mg/dL) and escalates in proportion to the degree of elevation. Hyperuricemia has a prevalence of between 2.0 and 13.2 percent in ambulatory adults and somewhat higher in hospitalized individuals.

CAUSES OF HYPERURICEMIA It is useful to classify hyperuricemia in relation to the underlying physiology, i.e., whether the hyperuricemia results from increased production, decreased excretion, or a combination of the two (Fig. 347-1, Table 347-1).

Increased urate production Diet provides an exogenous source of purines and, accordingly, contributes to the serum urate concentration in proportion to its purine content. Strict restriction of purine intake reduces the mean serum urate concentration by as little as 60 μmol/L (1.0 mg/dL) and urinary uric acid excretion by approximately 1.2 mmol/d (200 mg/d). Because about 50 percent of ingested RNA purine and 25 percent of ingested DNA purine appear in the urine as uric acid, foods high in nucleic acid content have a significant effect

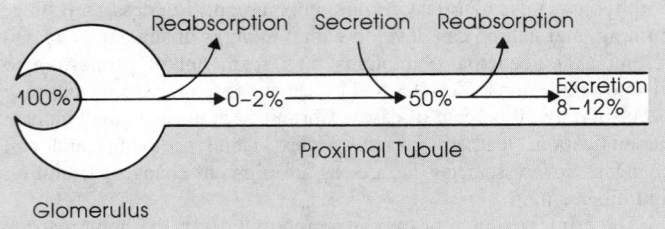

FIGURE 347-2 Schematic for handling of uric acid by the kidney. Components are illustrated with the percentage of filtered urate.

on the serum urate level. Such foods include liver, "sweetbreads" (i.e., thymus and pancreas), kidney, and anchovy.

Endogenous sources of purine production also influence the serum urate concentration (Fig. 347-3). De novo purine biosynthesis, the formation of a purine ring from nonring structures, is an 11-step process that results in formation of inosinate (IMP). The first step combines phosphoribosylpyrophosphate (PRPP) and glutamine and is catalyzed by amidophosphoribosyltransferase (amidoPRT) activity. The rate of purine biosynthesis and consequent urate production is determined, for the most part, by this enzyme. AmidoPRT is regulated by the substrate PRPP, which drives the reaction forward, and by the end products of biosynthesis (IMP and other ribonucleotides), which provide feedback inhibition. A second regulatory pathway is the salvage of purine bases by hypoxanthine phosphoribosyltransferase (HPRT). HPRT catalyzes the combination of the purine bases hypoxanthine and guanine with PRPP to form the respective ribonucleotides IMP and GMP. Increased salvage activity thus retards de novo synthesis by reducing PRPP levels and increasing concentrations of inhibitory ribonucleotides.

Serum urate concentrations are closely coupled to the rates of de novo purine biosynthesis. An X-linked disorder that causes an increase in activity of the enzyme PRPP synthetase causes increased PRPP production and accelerated de novo biosynthesis. PRPP is a substrate and allosteric activator of amidoPRT, the first enzyme in the de novo pathway. Individuals with this inborn error of metabolism have

TABLE 347-1 Classification of hyperuricemia

Urate overproduction	Decreased uric acid excretion	Combined mechanism
Primary idiopathic	Primary idiopathic	Glucose-6-phosphatase deficiency
HPRT deficiency	Renal insufficiency	Fructose-1-phosphate aldolase deficiency
PRPP synthetase overactivity	Polycystic kidney disease	Alcohol
Hemolytic processes	Diabetes insipidus	Shock
Lymphoproliferative diseases	Hypertension	
Myeloproliferative diseases	Acidosis	
Polycythemia vera	Lactic acidosis	
Psoriasis	Diabetic ketoacidosis	
Paget's disease	Starvation ketosis	
Glycogenosis III, V, and VII	Berylliosis	
Rhabdomyolysis	Sarcoidosis	
Exercise	Lead intoxication	
Alcohol	Hyperparathyroidism	
Obesity	Hypothyroidism	
Purine-rich diet	Toxemia of pregnancy	
	Bartter's syndrome	
	Down syndrome	
	Drug ingestion	
	Salicylates (>2 g/d)	
	Diuretics	
	Alcohol	
	Levodopa	
	Ethambutol	
	Pyrazinamide	
	Nicotinic acid	
	Cyclosporine	

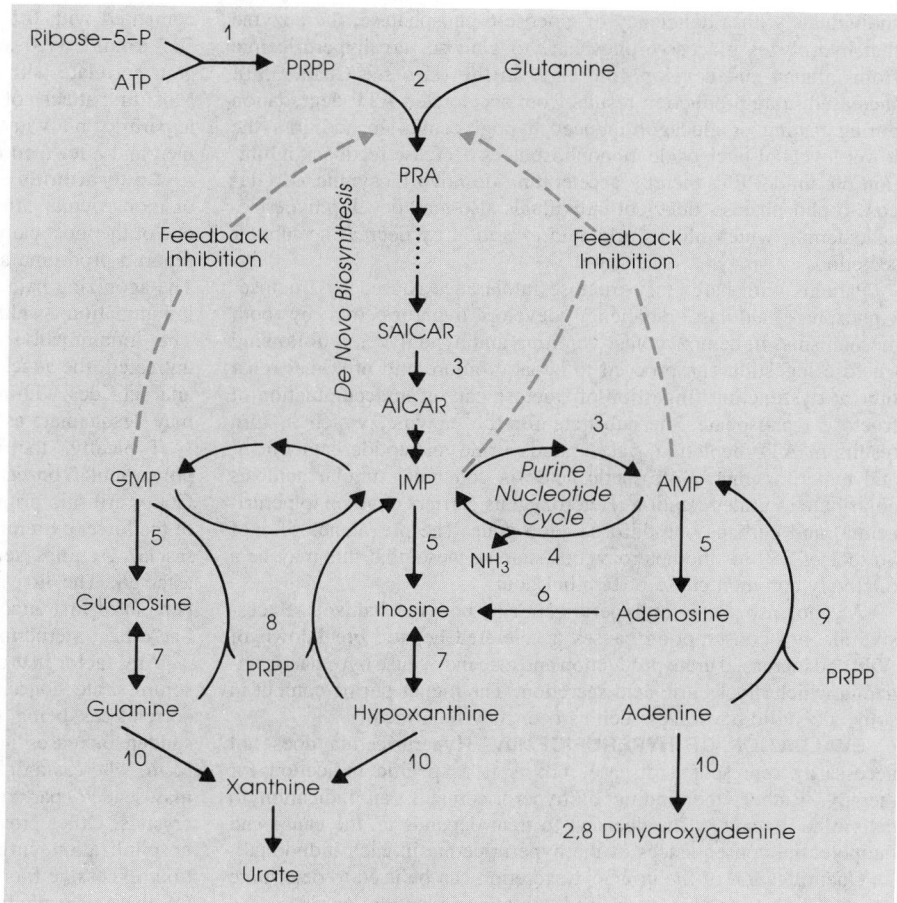

FIGURE 347-3 Abbreviated scheme of purine metabolism. (1) Phosphoribosylpyrophosphate (PRPP) synthetase, (2) amidophosphoribosyltransferase (amidoPRT), (3) adenylosuccinate lyase, (4) adenylate (AMP) deaminase, (5) 5'-nucleotidase, (6) adenosine deaminase, (7) purine nucleoside phosphorylase, (8) hypoxanthine phosphoribosyltransferase (HPRT), (9) adenine phosphoribosyltransferase (APRT), and (10) xanthine oxidase. PRPP, phosphoribosylpyrophosphate; PRA, phosphoribosylamine; SAICAR, succinylaminoimidazole carboxamide ribotide; AICAR, aminoimidazole carboxamide ribotide; GMP, guanylate; IMP, inosinate; AMP, adenylate.

overproduction of purines, hyperuricemia, and hyperuricaciduria and develop uric acid calculi and gout before age 20.

Similarly, individuals deficient in HPRT have hyperuricemia, hyperuricaciduria, uric acid calculi, and gout because of urate overproduction. HPRT deficiency is also X-linked. A complete deficiency of HPRT, the Lesch-Nyhan syndrome, is also associated with self-mutilation, choreoathetosis, and other neurologic problems. Individuals with partial HPRT deficiency, the Kelley-Seegmiller syndrome, only experience gout and renal calculi. HPRT deficiency enhances urate biosynthesis in two ways. PRPP is accumulated as a result of decreased utilization in the salvage pathway and, in turn, provides increased substrate for amidoPRT and de novo biosynthesis. In addition, decreased formation of the nucleoside monophosphates IMP and GMP via the salvage pathway decreases feedback inhibition on amidoPRT, further enhancing de novo biosynthesis.

Accelerated purine nucleotide degradation also can cause hyperuricemia, e.g., with conditions of rapid cell turnover, proliferation, or cell death, as in leukemic blast crises, cytotoxic therapy for malignancy, hemolysis, or rhabdomyolysis. Nucleic acids released from cells are hydrolyzed by the sequential activities of nucleases and phosphodiesterases, forming nucleoside monophosphates, and then are degraded to nucleosides, bases, and urate. Hyperuricemia can result from excessive degradation of skeletal muscle ATP after strenuous physical exercise or status epilepticus and in glycogen storage diseases types III, V, and VII. The hyperuricemia of myocardial infarction, smoke inhalation, and acute respiratory failure also may be related to accelerated breakdown of ATP.

Decreased uric acid excretion As many as 98 percent of individuals with primary hyperuricemia and gout have a defect in the renal handling of uric acid. This is evidenced as a lower than normal ratio of urate clearance to glomerular filtration rate (or urate to inulin clearance rate) over a wide range of filtered loads. As a result, gouty individuals excrete approximately 40 percent less uric acid than nongouty individuals for any given plasma urate concentration. Uric acid excretion increases in gouty and nongouty individuals when plasma urate levels are raised by purine ingestion or infusion, but in subjects with gout, plasma urate concentrations must be 60 to 120 μmol/L (1 to 2 mg/dL) higher than normal to achieve equivalent uric acid excretion rates.

Altered uric acid excretion could theoretically result from decreased glomerular filtration, decreased tubular secretion, or enhanced tubular reabsorption. Decreased urate filtration does not appear to cause primary hyperuricemia but does contribute to the hyperuricemia of renal insufficiency. Although hyperuricemia is invariable in chronic renal disease, the correlation between serum creatinine, urea nitrogen, and urate concentration is poor because although uric acid excretion per unit of glomerular filtration rate increases progressively with chronic renal insufficiency, tubular secretory capacity tends to be preserved, tubular reabsorptive capacity is reduced, and extrarenal clearance of uric acid increases as renal damage becomes more severe.

Decreased proximal tubular secretion of urate may cause the hyperuricemia in individuals with gout and no evidence of urate overproduction. Decreased tubular secretion of urate also causes the secondary hyperuricemia of acidosis. Diabetic ketoacidosis, starvation, ethanol intoxication, lactic acidosis, and salicylate intoxication are accompanied by accumulations of organic acids (β-hydroxybutyrate, acetoacetate, lactate, or salicylates) that compete with urate for tubular secretion. In some subjects with gout, hyperuricemia may be due to enhanced reabsorption of uric acid distal to the site of secretion, a mechanism known to be responsible for the hyperuricemia of extracellular volume depletion such as with diabetes insipidus or diuretic therapy.

Combined mechanisms Both increased urate production and decreased uric acid excretion may contribute to hyperuricemia.

Individuals with a deficiency of glucose-6-phosphatase, the enzyme that hydrolyzes glucose-6-phosphate to glucose, are hyperuricemic from infancy and develop gout early in life (also see Chap. 350). Increased urate production results from accelerated ATP degradation during fasting or glucagon-induced hypoglycemia. In addition, the lower levels of nucleoside monophosphates decrease feedback inhibition on amidoPRT, thereby accelerating de novo biosynthesis. Glucose-6-phosphatase–deficient individuals also may develop hyperlacticacidemia, which blocks uric acid excretion by decreasing tubular secretion.

Patients with hereditary fructose intolerance caused by fructose-1-phosphate aldolase deficiency develop hyperuricemia by both mechanisms. In hemozygotes, vomiting and hypoglycemia following fructose ingestion can proceed to hepatic failure and proximal renal tubular dysfunction. Ingestion of fructose causes an accumulation of fructose-1-phosphate, the substrate for the enzyme, which in turn results in ATP depletion, accelerated purine nucleotide catabolism, and hyperuricemia. Both lactic acidosis and renal tubular acidosis contribute to urate retention. Heterozygous carriers develop hyperuricemia, and perhaps one-third develop gout. The prevalence of 1 of 80 to 1 of 250 for the heterozygous state suggests that this may be a relatively common cause of familial gout.

Alcohol also promotes hyperuricemia by both mechanisms. Excessive alcohol consumption causes accelerated hepatic breakdown of ATP and increased urate production and also may cause hyperlacticacidemia which blocks uric acid secretion. The higher purine content in some alcoholic beverages such as beer may be a factor.

EVALUATION OF HYPERURICEMIA Hyperuricemia does not necessarily represent a disease, nor is it a specific indication for therapy. Rather, the finding of hyperuricemia is an indication to determine its cause. The decision to treat depends on the cause and the potential consequences of the hyperuricemia in each individual.

Quantification of the uric acid excretion can be used to determine whether hyperuricemia is caused by overproduction or decreased excretion. On a purine-free diet, men with normal renal function excrete less than 3.6 mmol/d (600 mg/d). Thus the hyperuricemia of individuals who excrete more uric acid per day while on a purine-free diet is due to purine overproduction, and that in those excreting less is due to decreased excretion. If the assessment is performed while the patient is on a regular diet, the level of 4.2 mmol/d (800 mg/d) can be used as the discriminating value. With renal insufficiency, less urate is filtered in the glomeruli and less uric acid appears in the urine. Consequently, in the presence of renal insufficiency, a lower 24-h urinary uric acid value does not necessarily rule out urate overproduction, but an elevated value provides strong evidence of urate overproduction. Spuriously high values can occur if the patient is taking a uricosuric agent at the time of urine collection. Glucocorticoids, ascorbic acid, salicylates in doses greater than 2 g/d, and other agents that promote urate excretion interfere with the interpretation of results.

Assessment of the ratio of uric acid to creatinine (or the ratio of uric acid clearance to creatinine clearance) in spot or random urine samples is not a reliable method to screen for urate overproduction. However, this is a useful tool for evaluating individuals with acute renal failure suspected of having acute uric acid nephropathy (see below).

COMPLICATIONS OF HYPERURICEMIA Although the manifestations of gout can occur in almost any combination, the typical sequence involves progression through asymptomatic hyperuricemia, acute gouty arthritis, interval or intercritical gout, and chronic or tophaceous gout. Nephrolithiasis can occur before or after the first attack of gouty arthritis.

The prevalence of hyperuricemia is estimated to range between 2.0 and 13.2 percent and the prevalence of gout varies between 1.3 and 3.7 percent in the general population. The higher the serum urate concentration, the more likely an individual is to develop gout. In one large study, the incidence of gout was 4.9 percent for individuals with serum urate concentrations of 540 μmol/L (9.0 mg/dL) or more

compared with 0.5 percent for those with values between 415 and 535 μmol/L (7.0 and 8.9 mg/dL). Similarly, the complications of gout correlate with the duration and severity of the hyperuricemia. Most first attacks of gouty arthritis follow 20 to 40 years of sustained hyperuricemia with a peak age of onset between 40 and 60 years for men and after menopause for women.

Gouty arthritis The benchmark feature of gout is the acute attack of monarticular arthritis. The first attack begins explosively and is one of the most painful events experienced. Occasionally, individuals report a prodrome or previous episodes of milder pain lasting hours. The agonizing pain of acute gout is accompanied by signs of intense inflammation: swelling, erythema, warmth, and exquisite tenderness. The inflammation may be accompanied by low-grade fever. If untreated, the attack usually peaks 24 to 48 h after the first symptoms and subsides within 7 to 10 days. The skin over the involved part may desquamate as the episode resolves.

Typically, the initial attack affects only one joint, although polyarticular onsets occur and may be more common in women. Gouty arthritis primarily affects peripheral joints, particularly those of the lower extremities. In addition, periarticular sites such as plantar fascia, Achilles tendon insertions, or other tenosynovia can be affected. The first metatarsophalangeal joint is involved in over 50 percent of first attacks and in 90 percent of individuals at some time. Sacroiliac, sternomanubrial, and spinal involvement occurs rarely.

Any factor that causes either an abrupt increase or decrease in the serum urate concentration may provoke an acute attack, the best correlations being with factors that cause a rapid fall. In theory, sudden increases in urate concentration may cause new crystals to form, whereas a drop in serum and extracellular urate concentrations may lead to partial dissolution and shedding of previously formed crystals. Other provocative factors include stress, trauma, infection, hospitalization, surgery, starvation, weight reduction, hyperalimentation, excessive food intake, alcohol, and medications (Table 347-2). Of these, hospitalization and medications are probably the most significant. Acute gouty attacks occur in 20 to 86 percent of individuals with a history of gout when they are hospitalized for medical or surgical reasons. The stress of a severe illness, changes in medication, shifts in fluid status or electrolytes, and general anesthesia probably contribute to the exacerbations. Attacks can follow the use of thiazide diuretics that cause hyperuricemia or after initiation of allopurinol or other therapies to lower serum urate.

Occasional attacks of acute gouty arthritis occur in the absence of hyperuricemia. Presumably most such attacks can be explained by factors that lower serum concentrations, temporarily altering the usual hyperuricemic state (and that perhaps triggered the attack). Occasionally, hyperuricemia cannot be documented despite repeated attempts. Gout could theoretically develop anytime synovial fluid is supersaturated with urate. Free water is cleared from the joint space more rapidly than urate, and if the amount of synovial fluid containing a normal concentration of urate increases because of trauma or edema, then the urate concentration within the joint would temporarily increase as the problem resolved and the water was more rapidly cleared. Supersaturated concentrations of urate could cause the formation of crystals and precipitate an attack.

TABLE 347-2 Medications with uricosuric activity

Acetohexamide	Glyceryl guaiacolate
ACTH	Glycopyrrolate
Ascorbic acid	Halofenate
Azauridine	Meclofenamate
Benzbromarone	Phenolsulfonphthalein
Calcitonin	Phenylbutazone
Chlorprothixene	Probenecid
Citrate	Radiographic contrast agents
Dicumarol	Salicylates (>2 g/2d)
Diflunisal	Sulfinpyrazone
Estrogens	Tetracycline that is outdated
Glucocorticoids	Zoxazolamine

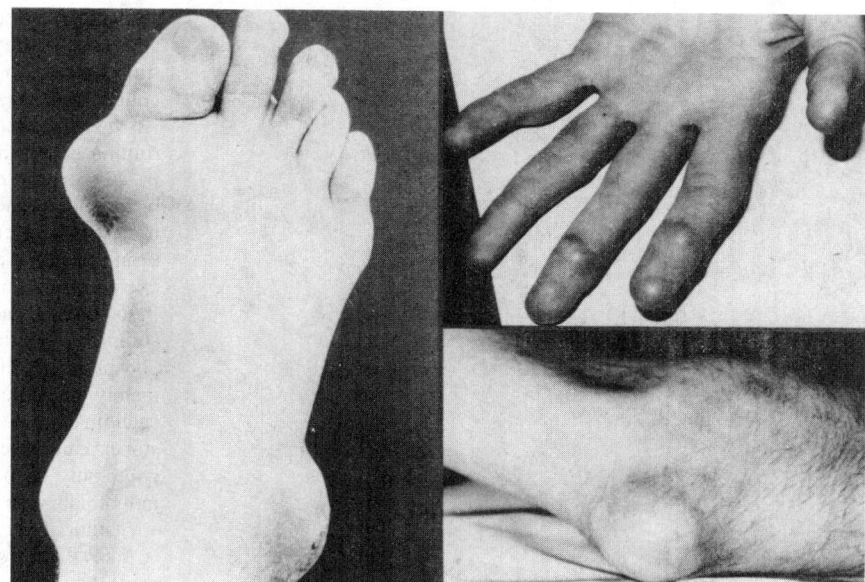

FIGURE 347-4 Chronic tophaceous gout. The left panel shows deformities of the foot in a 65-year-old man with a long history of gouty arthritis. On the right are tophi in an olecranon bursa and in the fingers of a 25-year-old man with Kelley-Seegmiller syndrome (partial HPRT deficiency).

Some individuals experience only a single gouty attack in their lifetime; others experience recurrence. Although the interval between first and second attacks may be over 40 years, three-fourths of individuals have a second attack within 2 years. The terms *interval gout* or *intercritical gout* describe the periods between attacks of acute arthritis when the individual has no joint complaints. In severe cases, unless therapeutic intervention occurs, chronic gouty arthritis develops with time. The pain-free intercritical periods shorten, and acute attacks occur with increased frequency, last longer, and involve more joints. The intensity of attacks may lessen somewhat, and involvement becomes polyarticular. Chronic gout is characterized by persistent polyarticular low-grade pain with superimposed acute or subacute inflammation. During this stage, tophi become apparent on physical examination (Fig. 347-4). Although there is individual variability, the rate of urate deposition in joint tissues and of articular destruction correlates with duration and severity of hyperuricemia. In general, approximately 10 years elapse between the first attack of the gouty arthritis and appearance of tophi. During the interim, however, destruction of cartilage and bone occurs, as evidenced by the radiographic changes (Fig. 347-5).

Pathogenesis   Acute gout results from the interaction between urate crystals and polymorphonuclear leukocytes (Fig. 347-6) and involves activation of humoral and cellular inflammatory mechanisms. Urate crystals activate complement through both the classic and alternate pathways. Hageman factor and the contact system of coagulation are also activated and result in generation of bradykinin, kallikrein, and plasmin. The interaction of urate crystals with neutrophils results in the release of lysosomal enzymes, oxygen-derived free radicals, leukotriene and prostaglandin metabolites, collagenase, and protease. Phagocytosis of crystals by neutrophils causes release of crystal-induced chemotactic factor (CCF). CCF, leukotriene B_4 (LTB_4), and the activated complement component C5a are all chemotactic and contribute to the marked polymorphonuclear leuko-cyte response in the initial phase of acute arthritis. With time, phagocytic mononuclear cells replace the polymorphonuclear cells. Urate crystals cause these cells to release prostaglandins (PGE_2), lysosomal enzymes, tumor necrosis factor alpha, and interleukins 1 and 6 (IL-1 and IL-6). Synovial lining cells also participate in the inflammatory response by releasing inflammatory mediators.

The inflammatory potential of urate crystals is greatly affected by the presence of absorbed proteins. Absorbed purified IgG causes enhanced crystal-induced platelet secretion, increased superoxide generation, and increased lysosomal enzyme release from polymor-phonuclear leukocytes. On the other hand, apoprotein B, a component

FIGURE 347-5 Radiographic changes in gout are the result of urate deposition. At first deposits are microscopic and are undetectable by x-ray. With persistent hyperuricemia, tophi enlarges to involve juxtaarticular bone and are apparent radiographically but not on physical examination. If unaltered by therapy, tophi continue to enlarge and become obvious in physical examination. The classic radiographic change of gout is a bony erosion. The location can be intraarticular, paraarticular, or at a distance from the joint. The erosions tend to be round and surrounded by a sclerotic border, giving a "punched out" appearance. There may be an "overhanging margin or lip." Nodular soft tissue prominence develops as the tophi enlarge. Joint spaces are typically preserved until late in the disease when secondary degenerative changes may occur. The left panel shows classic advanced changes of tophaceous gout including soft tissue distortion and erosion with sclerotic margins and overhanging edges. The right panel shows an erosive lesion in the interphalangeal joint in a patient with no tophi found on physical examination.

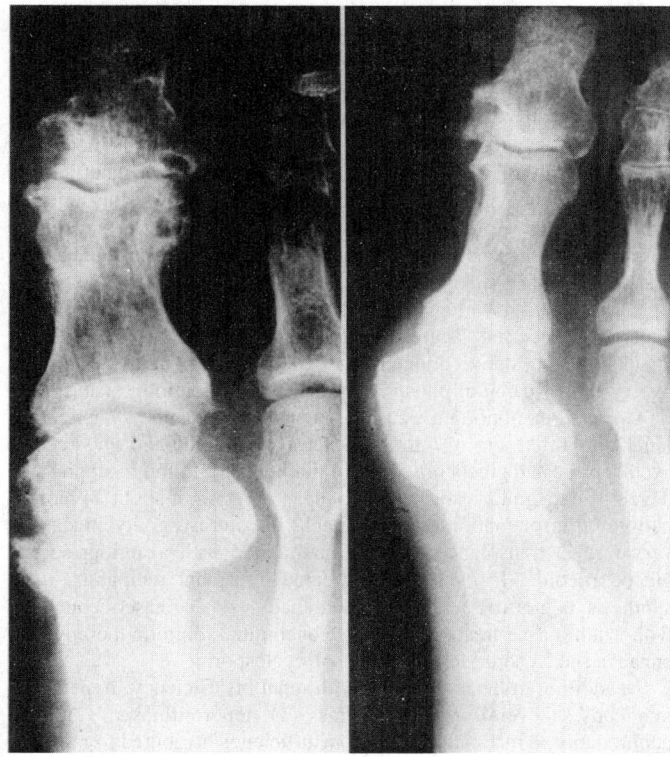

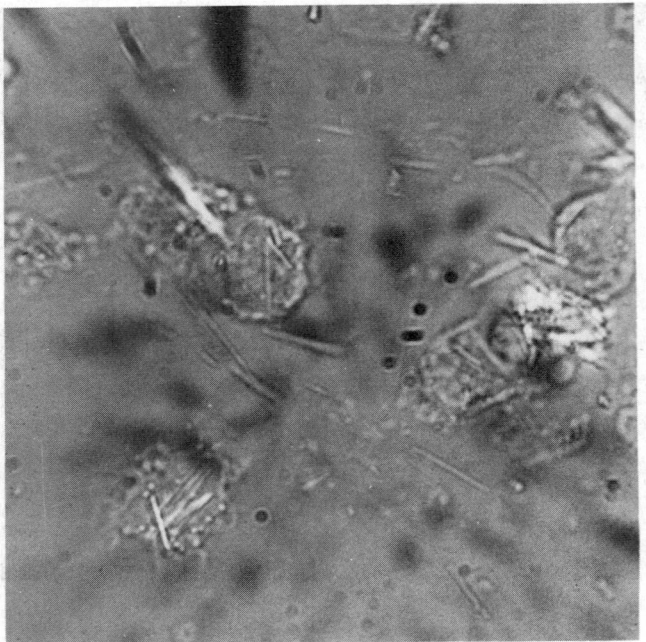

FIGURE 347-6 Crystals of monosodium urate in polymorphonuclear leukocytes and synovial fluid.

of very low density, low-density, and intermediate-density lipoproteins, inhibits urate crystal–induced stimulation of neutrophils. Apoprotein B is not normally present in synovial fluid and, because of its size, probably does not have access to that compartment under normal conditions. When synovitis develops, larger molecules, including lipoproteins, enter the joint space, bind to urate crystals, and, perhaps, play a role in terminating the attack.

Tophi are aggregates of monosodium urate monohydrate crystals that are generally surrounded by a giant cell, foreign body–type mononuclear cell inflammatory reaction. They can form in extraarticular and articular structures and cause deformity and destruction of hard and soft tissues. In joints, they lead to destruction of cartilage and bone, triggering secondary degeneration changes.

Renal disease Despite the invariable hyperuricemia in renal failure, gouty arthritis occurs in less than 1 percent of patients with chronic renal failure. Since most gouty arthritis follows 20 to 40 years of sustained hyperuricemia, most patients with renal failure are probably not hyperuricemic long enough to accumulate the necessary urate load. In addition, individuals with chronic renal insufficiency show diminished inflammatory responses to urate crystals injected subcutaneously. Polycystic disease of the kidneys is an exception, with a prevalence between 24 and 36 percent. The mechanism for this association is unknown.

Chronic renal failure patients on long-term hemodialysis can experience recurrent acute arthritis or periarthritis. Some of these attacks are gout due to urate crystal deposition, and others are caused by crystals of calcium phosphate (apatite) or calcium oxalate.

Gout is an important cause of morbidity in some recipients of renal allografts. From 7 to 12 percent of individuals who receive cyclosporine and glucocorticoids for maintenance immunosuppression develop acute gouty arthritis with a mean duration of about 24 months between transplantation and first attack. In contrast, gouty attacks are very rare in transplant recipients maintained with azathioprine and glucocorticoids. In cyclosporine-treated transplant recipients, urate synthesis is normal and urate clearances are decreased compared with azathioprine-treated controls. Concomitant diuretic therapy may enhance the hyperuricemic effects of cyclosporine.

In addition to the association with renal insufficiency, hyperuricemia causes several renal problems: (1) nephrolithiasis, (2) urate nephropathy, a rare cause of renal insufficiency attributed to monoso-dium urate crystal deposition in the renal interstitium, and (3) uric acid nephropathy, a reversible cause of acute renal failure resulting from deposition of large amounts of uric acid crystals in the renal collecting ducts, pelvis, and ureters.

NEPHROLITHIASIS Individuals with gout commonly develop nephrolithiasis. Nephrolithiasis may precede the onset of gouty arthritis in 40 percent of individuals with both conditions. In gout, the prevalence of nephrolithiasis correlates with the serum and urinary uric acid concentrations, reaching approximately 50 percent with serum urate levels of 770 μmol/L (13 mg/dL) or urinary uric acid excretion over 6.5 mmol/d (1100 mg/d).

Not all kidney stones that occur in individuals with gout are composed of uric acid. Stones composed of calcium oxalate, calcium phosphate, or those salts combined with uric acid occur in approximately 15 percent of cases. Uric acid may act as a nidus on which calcium oxalate can precipitate and grow. Furthermore, uric acid stones can develop in individuals with no other manifestations of gout, only 20 percent of whom are hyperuricemic. Some nongouty individuals with calcium oxalate stones have hyperuricemia or hyperuricaciduria.

URATE NEPHROPATHY Urate nephropathy, sometimes referred to as *urate nephrosis,* is a late manifestation of severe gout and is characterized histologically by deposits of monosodium urate crystals surrounded by a giant cell inflammatory reaction in the medullary interstitium and pyramids and can cause chronic renal insufficiency. The disorder is rare and cannot be diagnosed in the absence of gouty arthritis. Clinically, the lesions may be silent or associated with proteinuria, hypertension, and renal insufficiency.

Prior to the advent of antihyperuricemic agents and aggressive treatment for asymptomatic hypertension, renal failure was the cause of death in up to 25 percent of individuals with gout. Postmortem evaluations of kidneys from patients with gout frequently revealed urate crystals, pyelonephritis, and vascular changes. At present, aging or coexisting diseases that cause nephropathy, such as cardiovascular disease, hypertension, or independently occurring intrinsic renal disease, are usually responsible for the decreased renal function that may develop in gout.

URIC ACID NEPHROPATHY This reversible cause of acute renal failure is due to precipitation of uric acid in renal tubules and collecting ducts that causes obstruction to urine flow and is not a component of gout. Uric acid nephropathy develops following sudden urate overproduction and marked hyperuricaciduria. Factors that favor uric acid crystal formation include dehydration and acidosis. This form of acute renal failure occurs most often during an aggressive "blastic" phase of leukemia or lymphoma prior to or coincident with cytolytic therapy but also has been observed in individuals with other neoplasms, following epileptic seizures, and after vigorous exercise with heat stress. Autopsy studies have demonstrated intraluminal precipitates of uric acid, dilated proximal tubules, and normal glomeruli. Animal studies suggest that the initial pathogenic events include obstruction of collecting ducts with uric acid and obstruction of distal renal vasculature.

If recognized, uric acid nephropathy is potentially reversible. Appropriate therapy has reduced the mortality from 47 percent to practically nil. Serum levels cannot be relied on for diagnosis because this condition has developed in the presence of urate concentrations ranging from 720 to 4800 μmol/L (12 to 80 mg/dL). The distinctive clinical finding is the urinary uric acid concentration. In most forms of acute renal failure with decreased urine output, urinary uric acid content is either normal or reduced, and the ratio of uric acid to creatinine is less than 1. Because the decreased urine output in acute uric acid nephropathy is due to massive uricaciduria, the ratio of uric acid to creatinine in a random urine sample or 24-h specimen is greater than 1 and therefore is essentially diagnostic.

MANAGEMENT Asymptomatic hyperuricemia For many years, fear of adverse outcomes caused physicians to prescribe urate-lowering agents for asymptomatic hyperuricemia. Today, with perhaps one exception, no data indicate that treatment of asymptomatic hyperuricemia is cost-effective or beneficial. That exception is in individuals with neoplastic disease who are about to receive cytolytic therapy and are at risk for acute uric acid nephropathy.

Although hyperuricemic individuals are at risk for developing gouty arthritis, especially those with higher serum urate levels, treatment of asymptomatic hyperuricemia to prevent the first attack of gouty arthritis is not indicated because most people who are hyperuricemic never develop gout. Furthermore, organ damage does not appear to occur prior to a first gouty attack. Neither structural kidney damage nor tophi are identifiable before that event. Reduced renal function cannot be attributed to asymptomatic hyperuricemia, and treatment of asymptomatic hyperuricemia does not alter the progression of renal dysfunction in patients with renal disease. Although nephrolithiasis is common in gouty patients, and although a number of individuals with nephrolithiasis are hyperuricemic, the risk of stone formation in people with asymptomatic hyperuricemia is not established. Nor is hyperuricemia an independent risk factor for atherosclerotic cardiovascular disease.

Thus, other than for prevention of acute uric acid nephropathy, the routine treatment of asymptomatic hyperuricemia cannot be justified. In fact, routine screening for asymptomatic hyperuricemia is not recommended. If hyperuricemia is diagnosed, however, the cause should be determined. Causal factors should be corrected if the condition is secondary, and associated problems such as hypertension, hypercholesterolemia, diabetes mellitus, and obesity should be controlled. Treatment of asymptomatic hyperuricemia with antihyperuricemia agents entails inconvenience, cost, and potential toxicity and should not be prescribed.

Symptomatic hyperuricemia Initially, therapy should be directed toward relieving symptoms. Both gouty arthritis and nephrolithiasis are excruciatingly painful. Once the presenting symptoms are controlled, a decision must be made whether to initiate antihyperuricemic therapy.

Acute gouty arthritis As with any disease, appropriate and effective treatment requires accurate diagnosis. Few conditions can be diagnosed with more certainty or treated more successfully than gout. Thus a specific diagnosis provides insight into prognosis and treatment. A definitive diagnosis requires aspiration of the involved joint or tissue and demonstration of intracellular monosodium urate crystals in synovial fluid polymorphonuclear leukocytes or in tophaceous aggregates. Using polarized light microscopy with a first-order red compensator, the strong negative birefringence of the needle-shaped crystals can be appreciated easily. The triad of acute monarticular arthritis, hyperuricemia, and a dramatic response to colchicine provides presumptive evidence for gouty arthritis. These criteria, however, are a poor substitute for crystal identification, because some patients with gout are not hyperuricemic at the time of the attack. In addition, colchicine may be effective for other disorders, especially pseudogout (calcium pyrophosphate dehydrate crystal deposition disease) and calcific (basic calcium phosphate or apatite) tendinitis. These diseases that can mimic acute gout may occur in individuals who happen to be hyperuricemic. Finally, acute gouty arthritis can coexist with septic arthritis, psoriatic arthritis, systemic lupus erythematosus, rheumatoid arthritis, osteoarthritis, and pseudogout.

Once the diagnosis of gouty arthritis is secure, the choice of therapeutic agents includes colchicine, a nonsteroidal anti-inflammatory drug (NSAID), or intraarticular glucocorticoids. Regardless of the choice, the effectiveness of the agent is dependent on when it is used. Each will work if started early; none works quickly if initiated late in the course of the attack.

Colchicine, the traditional agent used, inhibits the release of leukocyte-derived crystal-induced chemotactic factor (CCF). Oral doses of 0.6 mg are given every hour until improvement is noted, gastrointestinal side effects develop, or 10 doses have been taken without relief (in which case the diagnosis may be questioned). Although highly effective, oral colchicine cannot be tolerated by up to 80 percent of people because of abdominal pain, diarrhea, and nausea. Colchicine also can be given intravenously, but administration by this route is potentially dangerous and should be used with extreme caution despite the fact that intravenous use can eliminate the gastrointestinal side effects (provided the drug is not also being taken orally). A single dose of 1 mg diluted in 20 mL normal saline is usually adequate. A second dose can be repeated 6 to 12 h later, but doses greater than 2 mg and repeated injections beyond 24 h are not recommended. Absolute contraindications for intravenous colchicine therapy include depressed bone marrow function, renal disease (creatinine clearance less than 10 mL/min, oliguria, or anuria), liver disease (liver function tests over twice the upper limit of normal), and sepsis.

Because of its relative specificity for acute gouty arthritis, oral colchicine is the agent of choice for the ambulatory patient in whom the diagnosis is not certain. If the diagnosis is certain, NSAID may be more appropriate because of better tolerance. Indomethacin is the usual agent, but ibuprofen, naproxen, tolmetin, sulindac, piroxicam, ketoprofen, and flurbiprofen have all been used effectively. The action of these agents is less specific for gout than that of colchicine, but they are effective, especially if used early in the attack. Treatment is begun with the highest approved dose of the selected agent and is continued until 3 to 4 days after all signs of inflammation have completely resolved. These agents are contraindicated in patients with active peptic ulcer disease; should be used in caution in patients with heart failure, other edematous states, or hypertension because of potential problems from sodium retention; and may precipitate hyperkalemia and renal insufficiency.

Intraarticular injection of glucocorticoids also may be used for acute gout. This is most useful when the patient cannot take oral medications, when colchicine and NSAIDs are contraindicated, or in refractory cases. ACTH injection and oral glucocorticoids have been employed for acute gouty arthritis but are not recommended for routine use.

Intercritical and chronic gout The term *intercritical* (or *interval*) *gout* applies to the period after the acute gouty attack has resolved and the patient is asymptomatic. It is at that time that the decision must be made whether to initiate antihyperuricemic therapy. All authors agree that hyperuricemia should be treated in patients with recurrent attacks, those with chronic gout or evidence of tophi, and individuals with gouty arthritis and nephrolithiasis. Some maintain that the first attack of acute gouty arthritis alone is sufficient indication. Others argue that first attacks are easily, inexpensively, and effectively treated and postpone urate-lowering therapy until one or more additional attacks occur.

Sustained hyperuricemia provides a definite risk to bone and cartilage for those with gouty arthritis. If hyperuricemia is not controlled, urate deposits enlarge and become radiographically evident before subcutaneous tophi develop. In a study of patients with intercritical gout, 42 percent had radiographic changes characteristic of bony tophi despite no evidence of tophi on physical examination (see Fig. 347-5). One cannot predict from the frequency of acute attacks, the history of therapy, or the serum urate levels at the time of evaluation which patients will show bony changes.

Before starting treatment with urate-lowering agents, the patient should be free of all signs of inflammation and have begun colchicine for prophylaxis. The sudden drop in serum urate with the initiation of allopurinol or uricosuric therapy may prolong or precipitate an acute attack. Colchicine, at a dose of 0.6 mg orally one to three times a day, is about 90 percent effective in preventing subsequent gout attacks. Rarely, a reversible colchicine-induced neuromuscular toxicity may be manifested by subacute myopathy and axonal neuropathy with elevated serum creatinine kinase levels. This toxicity is most common in individuals with renal insufficiency and is reversible when colchicine is discontinued.

Once antihyperuricemic therapy is initiated, the dosage used should maintain the serum urate at or below 300 μmol/L (5.0 mg/dL). Extracellular fluid is saturated with urate at a concentration of approximately 415 μmol/L (6.8 mg/dL). If the serum urate remains above this level, tissue deposition of urate crystals will continue. A reduction of the serum urate concentration from 600 to 480 μmol/L (10 to 8 mg/dL), for example, will not reduce the total-body urate pool but will only slow the rate at which the pool continues to increase. If, on the other hand, the urate concentration is reduced below 415 μmol/L (6.8 mg/dL), urate crystals can dissolve and the urate pool will decrease. Successful therapy will prevent future attacks of gout and also lead to resolution of tophi.

Treatment of hyperuricemia includes diet and specific urate-lowering agents. Diet plays a minor role in the treatment of hyperuricemia today because modern therapeutic agents are so effective. However, dietary counseling is important to the total management of the patient and should address obesity, hyperlipidemia, diabetes mellitus, hypertension, and the use of alcohol.

Allopurinol, a potent competitive inhibitor of xanthine oxidase, is the most widely used antihyperuricemic agent. It is also a substrate for the enzyme. Oxypurinol, the major metabolite of allopurinol, is also an effective inhibitor of xanthine oxidase. Allopurinol is efficiently absorbed from the gastrointestinal tract and has a half-life of 3 h. Oxypurinol excretion is enhanced by uricosuric agents and is reduced in renal insufficiency. Allopurinol is effective in the treatment of all types of hyperuricemia but is specifically indicated for the following: (1) Patients with gout and (a) evidence of urate overproduction [24-h urinary uric acid greater than 4.8 mmol (800 mg) with a general diet or greater than 3.6 mmol (600 mg) on a purine-restricted diet], (b) nephrolithiasis, (c) renal insufficiency (creatinine clearance less than 80 mL/min), (d) tophaceous deposits, (e) age over 60 years, or (f) inability to take uricosuric agents because of ineffectiveness or intolerance, (2) patients with nephrolithiasis of any type plus urinary uric acid excretion greater than 3.6 mmol/d (600 mg/d), (3) patients with renal calculi composed of 2,8-dihydroxyadenine, and (4) patients with, or at risk for, acute uric acid nephropathy.

Allopurinol administration decreases the serum urate concentration and the urinary excretion of uric acid in the first 24 h, with a maximum reduction occurring within 2 weeks. The average effective dose of allopurinol is 300 mg/d. However, the dosage required to control the serum urate concentration adequately depends on the severity of the tophaceous disease and on renal function. Failure of a 400-mg dose to produce an adequate antihyperuricemic effect is rare and suggests noncompliance. Allopurinol can be given once a day because of the long half-life of oxypurinol. The drug is effective in patients with renal insufficiency, but the dose should be reduced because of the prolonged half-life of oxypurinol.

Side effects, serious complications, and toxicity of allopurinol are unusual. The most frequent side effects are skin rash, gastrointestinal distress, diarrhea, and headache. The rash is usually maculopapular and erythematous, but exfoliative dermatitis and toxic epidermal necrolysis may occur. Desensitization with low doses of allopurinol may be useful in individuals with demonstrated hypersensitivity.

Serious adverse effects include alopecia, fever, lymphadenopathy, bone marrow suppression, hepatic toxicity, interstitial nephritis, renal failure, hypersensitivity vasculitis, and death. Such toxicity is fortunately rare but does occur in patients with renal insufficiency or in those taking thiazide diuretics.

Potential drug interactions must be considered when allopurinol is prescribed. Because 6-mercaptopurine and azathioprine are inactivated by xanthine oxidase, allopurinol prolongs the half-life of these agents and thus potentiates their therapeutic and toxic effects. Cyclophosphamide toxicity also may be enhanced by concomitant use. A threefold increase in ampicillin- and amoxicillin-related skin rashes has been reported in patients taking allopurinol.

Uricosuric agents also can effectively lower serum urate concentrations by the partial inhibition of proximal tubular reabsorption of filtered and secreted urate from the luminal side of the tubule at a site distal to the point of uric acid secretion.

Candidates for these agents are gouty patients who meet all the following criteria: (1) hyperuricemia attributable to decreased uric acid excretion [less than 4.8 mmol (800 mg) urinary uric acid per day while taking a regular diet or less than 3.6 mmol (600 mg) with a purine-restricted diet], (2) age under 60 years, (3) satisfactory renal function (a creatinine clearance greater than 80 mL/min), and (4) no history of nephrolithiasis.

Uricosuric agents are effective in 70 to 80 percent of patients. Failure to control the serum urate concentration may be attributed to drug intolerance, poor compliance, concomitant salicylate ingestion, or impaired renal function. Salicylates block the uricosuric effects of these agents, probably by inhibiting urate secretion. Uricosuric agents lose effectiveness as the creatinine clearance falls and are ineffective when glomerular filtration falls below 30 mL/min. The most commonly used uricosuric agents are probenecid and sulfinpyrazone. Probenecid therapy is begun at 250 mg twice a day and is increased as necessary up to 3.0 g/d. Because the half-life is 6 to 12 h, probenecid should be taken in two to three evenly spaced doses. Sulfinpyrazone therapy is initiated at a dose of 50 mg twice a day. The usual maintenance level is 300 to 400 mg/d in three or four divided doses.

By promoting uric acid excretion, uricosuric agents may precipitate nephrolithiasis. This rare complication can occur early in the course of treatment and may be prevented by initiating therapy at low doses, forcing hydration, and, possibly, alkalinizing the urine. Hypersensitivity, skin rash, and gastrointestinal complaints are the major side effects. Serious toxicity is rare, but hepatic necrosis and the nephrotic syndrome have been reported.

Nephrolithiasis Antihyperuricemic therapy is recommended for the individual who has both gouty arthritis and nephrolithiasis. Medical prophylaxis can be effective for hyperuricemic patients with either uric acid– or calcium-containing stones. Both types may occur in association with hyperuricaciduria. Regardless of the nature of the calculi, fluid ingestion should be sufficient to produce a daily urine volume greater than 2 L. Alkalinization of the urine with sodium bicarbonate or acetazolamide may be justified to increase the solubility of uric acid. Specific treatment of uric acid calculi requires reducing the urine uric acid concentration with allopurinol. Allopurinol is also useful in reducing the recurrence of calcium oxalate stones in gouty subjects and in nongouty individuals with hyperuricemia or hyperuricaciduria. Potassium citrate (30 to 80 mmol/d orally in divided doses) is an alternative to allopurinol therapy for patients with uric acid stones alone or mixed calcium/uric acid stones. Allopurinol is also indicated for the treatment of 2,8-dihydroxyadenine kidney stones.

Uric acid nephropathy Uric acid nephropathy is often preventable, and immediate, appropriate therapy has reduced the mortality rate to practically nil. Vigorous intravenous hydration and diuresis with furosemide dilute the uric acid in the tubules and promote urine flow to 100 mL/h or more. The administration of acetazolamide, 240 to 500 mg every 6 to 8 h, and sodium bicarbonate, 89 mmol/L, intravenously enhances urine alkalinity and thereby solubilizes more uric acid. It is important to ensure that the urine pH remains above 7.0 and to watch for signs of circulatory overload. In addition, antihyperuricemic therapy in the form of allopurinol in a single dose of 8 mg/kg is administered to reduce the amount of urate that reaches the kidney. If renal insufficiency persists, subsequent daily doses should be reduced to 100 to 200 mg because oxypurinol, the active metabolite of allopurinol, accumulates in renal failure. Despite these measures, hemodialysis may be required.

HYPOURICEMIA

Hypouricemia, defined as a serum urate concentration less than 120 μmol/L (2.0 mg/dL), may result from decreased production of urate, increased excretion of uric acid, or a combination of both mechanisms. This laboratory finding occurs in less than 0.2 percent of the general population and 0.8 percent of hospitalized individuals. Hypouricemia causes no recognized symptoms or pathology and therefore requires no therapy. It is, however, a sign of potential pathology, and its cause should be determined.

Most hypouricemia results from increased renal uric acid excretion. The finding of normal amounts of uric acid in a 24-h urine collection in an individual with hypouricemia is evidence for a renal cause. Medications with uricosuric properties (see Table 347-2) include aspirin (at doses over 2.0 g/d), x-ray contrast materials, and glyceryl-guaiacholate. Total parenteral nutrition by intravenous hyperalimentation also can cause hypouricemia, possibly a result of the high glycine content of the hyperalimentation infusions. Other causes of an increased urate clearance include neoplastic disease, hepatic cirrhosis, diabetes mellitus, inappropriate secretion of vasopressin, and defects in renal tubular transport such as primary Fanconi syndrome and Fanconi syndromes caused by Wilson's disease, cystinosis, multiple myeloma, heavy metal toxicity, and as isolated congenital defects in the bidirectional transport of uric acid.

Hypouricemia from decreased production of urate is accompanied by very low urinary uric acid levels. Accumulation of other purine nucleosides and bases may occur depending on the specific defect. Individuals treated with allopurinol and some subjects with neoplastic disease or severe hepatic dysfunction are hypouricemic and excrete increased quantities of hypoxanthine and xanthine in the urine. Xanthine oxidase deficiency can be inherited or acquired. Inherited forms include isolated xanthine oxidase deficiency and combined xanthine oxidase and sulfite oxidase deficiencies. Both cause hypouricemia and xanthinuria. Affected individuals excrete essentially no uric acid and may develop xanthine nephrolithiasis. Individuals with purine nucleoside phosphorylase deficiency, an inborn error of metabolism causing T cell–deficient immune dysfunction, are hypouricemic and excrete increased quantities of guanosine, deoxyguanosine, inosine, and deoxyinosine in the urine.

INBORN ERRORS OF PURINE METABOLISM
(See also Table 347-3, Fig. 347-3)

HPRT DEFICIENCY A complete deficiency of hypoxanthine phosphoribosyltransferase (HPRT), the Lesch-Nyhan syndrome, is characterized by hyperuricemia, self-mutilative behavior, choreoathetosis, spasticity, and mental retardation. A partial deficiency of HPRT, the Kelley-Seegmiller syndrome, is associated with hyperuricemia but no central nervous system manifestations. In each syndrome, the hyperuricemia results from urate overproduction and can cause uric acid crystalluria, nephrolithiasis, obstructive uropathy, and gouty arthritis. Early diagnosis and appropriate therapy with allopurinol can prevent or eliminate all the problems attributable to hyperuricemia but have no effect on the behavioral or neurologic activities.

HPRT catalyzes the condensation reaction which combines phosphoribosylpyrophosphate (PRPP) and the purine bases hypoxanthine and guanine to form the respective nucleoside monophosphate IMP or GMP and pyrophosphate. The functional enzyme is encoded by a single gene located on the X chromosome. Consequently, affected males are hemizygous for the trait and inherit the mutant allele from their asymptomatic mother, who is a carrier, or are the result of

spontaneous gene mutations. The deficiency state is generally the result of point mutations, deletions, insertions, or endoduplication of exons rather than major gene alterations.

INCREASED PRPP SYNTHETASE ACTIVITY Cells from individuals with increased PRPP synthetase activity contain elevated levels of PRPP. The high substrate content drives de novo purine synthesis causing overproduction of uric acid. Similar to the HRRT deficiency states, PRPP synthetase overactivity is X-linked and results in gouty arthritis and uric acid nephrolithiasis. Nerve deafness has been associated with PRPP synthetase overactivity in some families.

ADENINE PRT DEFICIENCY Individuals with a deficiency of adenine phosphoribosyltransferase (APRT) develop 2,8-dihydroxyadenine (DHA) kidney stones. APRT catalyzes the conversion of adenine to AMP. In the absence of APRT, adenine is converted by xanthine oxidase to 2,8-dihydroxyadenine, which is very insoluble in urine. Reports of 2,8-dihydroxyadenine stones are rare, most likely because of its chemical similarity to uric acid. Analysis by x-ray powder diffraction is necessary for correct identification. Because this technique is rarely employed, many 2,8-dihydroxyadenine stones are incorrectly called uric acid. The consequence of this misidentification is not too severe, because allopurinol therapy is the correct treatment for each type of stone.

APRT deficiency is inherited as an autosomal recessive trait. Caucasians with the deficiency have a complete deficiency (type I), whereas Japanese subjects have some measurable enzyme activity (type II). Expression of the defect is similar in the two populations, as is the frequency of the heterozygous state (0.4 to 1.1 per 100).

HEREDITARY XANTHINURIA A deficiency of xanthine oxidase causes all purine in the urine to occur in the form of hypoxanthine and xanthine. About two-thirds of deficient individuals are asymptomatic. The remainder develop kidney stones composed of xanthine. A very small number of symptomatic individuals also have experienced myopathy or recurrent polyarteritis. Xanthinuria appears to be inherited in an autosomal recessive pattern.

In a second form of inherited xanthinuria, the deficiency of xanthine oxidase is associated with a deficiency of sulfite oxidase. Neurologic symptoms attributable to the sulfite oxidase deficiency predominate over those of xanthinuria in individuals with the combined deficiency.

MYOADENYLATE DEAMINASE DEFICIENCY Adenylate (AMP) deaminase catalyzes the conversion of AMP to IMP with the release of ammonia and is an integral component of the purine nucleotide cycle. The purine nucleotide cycle plays an important role in skeletal muscle energy metabolism. A deficiency of myoadenylate deaminase, the isoform of AMP deaminase in skeletal muscle, is associated with myopathic syndromes.

Both primary (inherited) and secondary (acquired) forms of myoadenylate deaminase deficiency have been described. The primary form is inherited as an autosomal recessive trait. Clinically, this form tends to be a relatively benign disorder characterized by easy fatigability and postexercise cramps and myalgias. A number of individuals with this deficiency may be asymptomatic. Elevated serum

TABLE 347-3   Inborn errors of purine metabolism

Enzyme	Activity	Inheritance	Clinical features
Hypoxanthine phosphoribosyltransferase	Complete deficiency	X-linked	Self-mutilation, choreoathetosis, hyperuricemia, gout, and uric acid lithiasis
	Partial deficiency	X-linked	Hyperuricemia, gout, and uric acid lithiasis
Phosphoribosylpyrophosphate synthetase	Overactivity	X-linked	Hyperuricemia, gout, uric acid lithiasis, and deafness
Adenine phosphoribosyltransferase	Deficiency	Autosomal recessive	2,8-Dihydroxyadenine lithiasis
Xanthine oxidase	Deficiency	Autosomal recessive	Xanthinuria and xanthine lithiasis
Adenylosuccinate lyase	Deficiency	Autosomal recessive	Autism and psychomotor retardation
Myoadenylate deaminase	Deficiency	Autosomal recessive	Myopathy with exercise intolerance and myalgias
Adenosine deaminase	Deficiency	Autosomal recessive	Severe combined immunodeficiency disease and chrondro-osseous dysplasia
Purine nucleoside phosphorylase	Deficiency	Autosomal recessive	T cell–mediated immunodeficiency

creatine phosphokinase (CPK) levels are found in about half the individuals. In some cases, CPK values are normal at rest but become abnormal only after exercise. Electromyography and muscle histology are usually normal or show minor, nonspecific changes. The acquired deficiency occurs in association with a wide variety of neuromuscular diseases, including muscular dystrophies, neuropathies, inflammatory myopathies, and collagen vascular diseases. Measurement of plasma lactate and ammonia concentrations after forearm ischemic exercise can be used to screen for this disorder. Under these conditions, myoadenylate-deficient subjects can generate lactate but not ammonia. The diagnosis can be made only by documenting the absence of enzymic activity in a muscle biopsy specimen.

Myoadenylate deaminase is the only activity affected in the inherited form, whereas other muscle enzymes (creatine kinase and myokinase) are also decreased in the acquired deficiencies. Inherited deficiency is probably the result of point mutations, small deletions, or rearrangements. A single nonsense mutation has been identified in 11 unrelated families. In contrast, mRNA abundance is low in muscle from patients with acquired deficiencies, suggesting a different molecular basis for this form.

ADENYLOSUCCINATE LYASE DEFICIENCY   Adenylosuccinate lyase participates in the synthesis of purine nucleotides in two ways. It catalyzes the conversion of succinylaminoimidazole carboxamide ribotide (SAICAR) to aminoimidazole carboxamide ribotide (AICAR) in the de novo pathway and in the conversion of AMP succinate to AMP in the purine nucleotide cycle. A deficiency of this enzyme is transmitted by autosomal recessive inheritance and causes profound psychomotor retardation, seizures, and other movement disorders. All are mentally retarded and most are autistic.

ADENOSINE DEAMINASE DEFICIENCY AND PURINE NUCLEOSIDE PHOSPHORYLASE DEFICIENCY   See Chap. 278.

REFERENCES

Kelley WN, Wortmann RL: Hyperuricemia, in *Textbook of Rheumatology*, 4th ed, WN Kelley et al (eds). Philadelphia, Saunders, 1993

Levinson DJ, Becker MA: Clinical gout and the pathogenesis of hyperuricemia, in *Arthritis and Allied Conditions*, 12th ed, DJ McCarthy, WJ Koopman (eds). Philadelphia, Lea & Febiger, 1992, pp 1773–1806

McCarthy GM et al: Influence of antihyperuricemic therapy on the clinical and radiographic progression of gout. Arthritis Rheum 34:1489, 1991

Scriver CR et al: Purines and pyrimidines, in *The Molecular and Metabolic Basis of Inherited Disease*, 7th ed, CR Scriver et al (eds). New York, McGraw-Hill, in press

Wortmann RL: Management of hyperuricemia, in *Arthritis and Allied Conditions*, 12th ed, DJ McCarthy, WJ Koopman (eds). Philadelphia, Lea & Febiger, 1992, pp 1807–1818

Wyngaarden JB, Kelley WN: *Gout and Hyperuricemia*. New York, Grune & Stratton, 1976

348   WILSON'S DISEASE

I. HERBERT SCHEINBERG

Wilson's disease is an autosomal recessive abnormality in the hepatic excretion of copper that results in toxic accumulations of the metal in liver, brain, and other organs. The disease occurs in populations of every ethnic and geographic origin and has a worldwide prevalence of about 1 in 30,000. Deficiency of the plasma copper protein ceruloplasmin in a characteristic feature.

NATURAL HISTORY   Normal babies have low levels of plasma ceruloplasmin and high concentrations of hepatic copper. During the first year of life ceruloplasmin values rise, and hepatic copper concentrations fall to normal adult levels. In contrast, serum ceruloplasmin changes very little in subjects with Wilson's disease, and the concentration of hepatic copper remains elevated. However, clinical manifestations of copper excess are rare before age 6, and about half of untreated patients remain asymptomatic through adolescence.

Wilson's disease presents with hepatic involvement in about half of patients. Liver disease may be manifest in four ways: acute hepatitis, fulminant hepatitis, chronic active hepatitis, or cirrhosis. Acute hepatitis is often mistaken for viral hepatitis or infectious mononucleosis and is usually self-limited. Fulminant hepatitis, generally lethal, is characterized by progressive jaundice, malaise, ascites, hypoalbuminemia, and elevated plasma levels of liver enzymes. Sufficient copper may be released from necrosing hepatocytes to cause hemolytic anemia. Parenchymal liver disease may persist after acute hepatitis or develop insidiously without prior acute disease into a clinical and histologic picture indistinguishable from chronic active hepatitis and always accompanied by cirrhosis. Finally, decades may elapse with no sign or symptom of liver disease but with the insidious development of cirrhosis. A previous episode of hepatitis can be overlooked unless patients are questioned carefully.

In other patients the initial manifestations are extrahepatic. Neurologic or psychiatric disturbances are the first clinical signs in most of this group and are always accompanied by Kayser-Fleischer rings (Fig. A8-16). These golden deposits of copper in Descemet's membrane of the cornea do not interfere with vision but indicate that hepatic copper has been released and has probably caused brain damage. Rarely, Kayser-Fleischer rings may be accompanied by sunflower cataracts. If a patient with frank neurologic or psychiatric disease does not have Kayser-Fleischer rings when examined by a trained observer using a slit lamp, the diagnosis of Wilson's disease can be excluded.

The primary neurologic manifestations are those of a movement disorder. Resting and intention tremors, spasticity, rigidity, chorea, drooling, dysphagia, and dysarthria are common. Babinski responses may be present, and abdominal reflexes may be absent; sensory changes, save for headache, never occur. Psychiatric disturbances, primarily due to the toxic effects of copper on the brain, are present in most patients with symptomatic disease. Syndromes indistinguishable from schizophrenia, manic-depressive psychoses, and classic neuroses may occur, but some bizarre behaviors defy classification. Improvement in the psychiatric state can occur with pharmacologic reduction of the copper excess, but additional therapy may be required.

In occasional patients the clinical onset reflects neither a hepatic nor a central nervous system disturbance. For example, primary or secondary amenorrhea may be the first evidence in some young women; in others, repeated spontaneous abortions may be due to excess free copper in intrauterine secretions. Routine ophthalmologic examination in asymptomatic patients occasionally reveals Kayser-Fleischer rings, leading to the diagnosis.

PATHOGENESIS   The locus of Wilson's disease is on the long arm of chromosome 13 (within 13q14–q21), and the close linkage between this locus and other mapped markers on this chromosome makes it possible to identify carrier states and to make prenatal diagnosis in some families. The relation between the mutant gene and the metabolic defect has not been defined. The metabolic defect in Wilson's disease is an inability to maintain a near-zero balance of copper. Excess copper, small amounts of which are essential to life, accumulates possibly because hepatic lysosomes lack the normal mechanism to excrete into bile the copper that has been catabolically cleaved from the ceruloplasmin. This may cause deficiency of ceruloplasmin, since copper excess in vitro inhibits the formation of ceruloplasmin from apoceruloplasmin and copper. The capacity of hepatocytes to store copper is eventually exceeded, and release into blood and uptake in extrahepatic sites occurs (Table 348-1).

Under normal circumstances, essentially all tissue and plasma copper is present as the prosthetic element of copper proteins, including cytochrome oxidase, tyrosinase, superoxide dismutase, and ceruloplasmin. There is normally little or no free (non-protein-bound) copper. In Wilson's disease, more copper is present than can be bound by specific copper proteins; such copper is as toxic as non-protein-bound iron, zinc, mercury, or lead. Toxicity of these cations

TABLE 348-1 Summary of analytic data in patients with Wilson's disease, heterozygous carriers, and control subjects

Group	Serum ceruloplasmin		Hepatic copper concentration	
	No. of patients	Mean ± SD, mg/L	No. of patients	Mean ± SD, μg/g dry weight
Wilson's disease:				
Asymptomatic	31	36±53	36	983.5±368
Symptomatic	84	59±71	33	588.3±304
Heterozygous carriers	95*	284±85	14	117.0±51
Normal subjects	180	307±35	16	31.5±6.8

* 71 parents of patients with Wilson's disease and 24 children, each of whom had one parent with Wilson's disease.
SOURCE: Sternlieb and Scheinberg, 1968.

is probably effected by combinations with proteins that ordinarily do not contain metal.

The pathologic consequences of the accumulated copper occur first in the liver. Abnormal fat and glycogen deposits are the earliest findings by light microscopy (Fig. 348-1). With electron microscopy, mitochondrial abnormalities are observed early and appear to be specific for Wilson's disease (Fig. 348-2). Later, necrosis, inflammation, fibrosis, bile duct proliferation, and cirrhosis can be fatal. Abnormalities in liver chemistries, particularly aminotransferase elevations, may be seen in any of these stages.

Death can occur from central nervous system effects. In the brain, the excess copper is distributed ubiquitously. Necrosis of neurons with cavitation may be preceded by the appearance of Opalski and Alzheimer type II cells; however, neither is specific for Wilson's disease.

FIGURE 348-1 Fatty changes, glycogen deposits, and cellular infiltrates in a hematoxylin and eosin-stained section of liver from an asymptomatic boy with Wilson's disease.

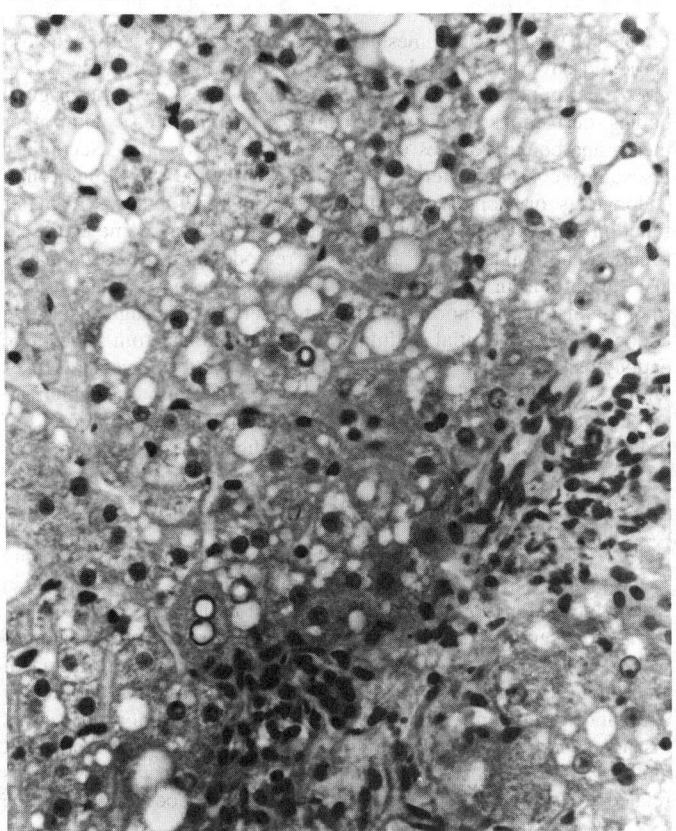

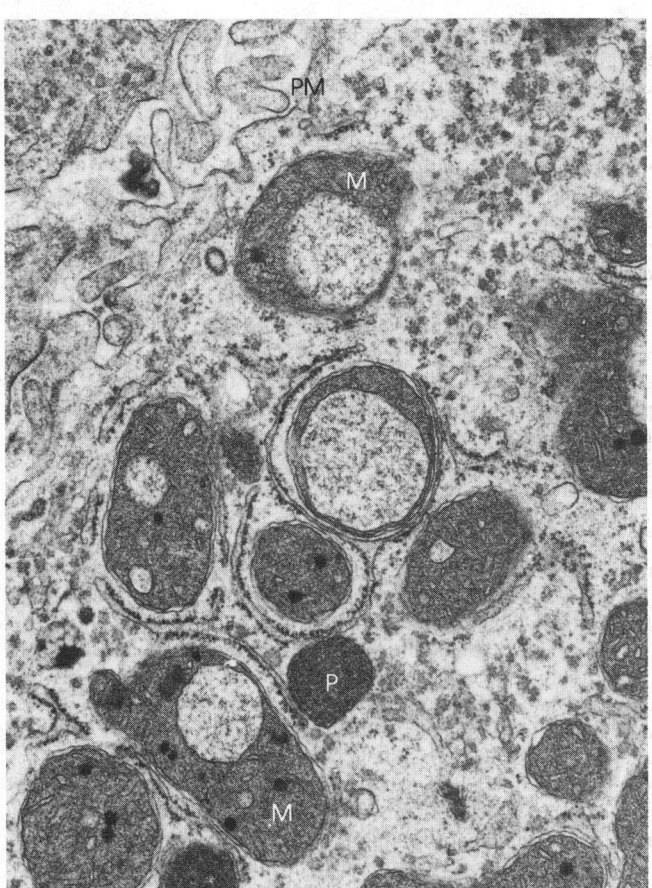

FIGURE 348-2 Electron micrograph of a liver biopsy sample from a 6-year-old asymptomatic boy. There are prominent vacuoles, containing granular material, in mitochondria (M). P, peroxisome; PM, plasma membrane.

Increased copper in the kidney produces little, if any, structural change and usually does not alter renal function. Hematuria, proteinuria, the Fanconi syndrome, and renal tubular acidosis, though commonly seen in untreated patients, almost never lead to clinical renal disease. Pathologic effects in other organs and tissues are minor.

DIAGNOSIS The diagnosis is easy—*provided it is suspected.* Wilson's disease should be considered in any patient under the age of 40 with an unexplained disorder of the central nervous system, signs or symptoms of hepatitis, chronic active hepatitis, unexplained persistent elevations of serum aminotransferase, hemolytic anemia in the presence of hepatitis, unexplained cirrhosis, or in any patient who has a near relative with Wilson's disease.

The diagnosis is confirmed in suspected cases by the demonstration of either (1) a serum concentration of ceruloplasmin less than 200 mg/L (20 mg/dL) and Kayser-Fleischer rings or (2) a serum ceruloplasmin less than 200 mg/L (20 mg/dL) and a concentration of copper in liver biopsy greater than 250 μg/g of dry weight. Most symptomatic patients also excrete more than 100 μg copper per day in urine and exhibit histologic abnormalities on liver biopsy.

About 5 percent of patients have a serum concentration of ceruloplasmin greater than 200 mg/L (20 mg/dL), and some patients with other hepatic disorders, chiefly primary biliary cirrhosis, have elevated hepatic copper levels and, rarely, Kayser-Fleischer rings. In either circumstance, measurement of the ability to incorporate radioactive copper into ceruloplasmin is useful as a discriminating test. Even in the presence of a normal concentration of ceruloplasmin, patients with Wilson's disease incorporate little or no isotope into the protein, while patients with other liver disorders and elevated hepatic copper incorporate the isotope normally.

TREATMENT Treatment consists of removing and detoxifying the deposits of copper as rapidly as possible and should be instituted once the diagnosis is secure whether the patient is ill or asymptomatic. Penicillamine is administered orally in an initial dose of 1 g daily, usually in divided doses 30 min before meals and at bedtime. Since penicillamine has an antipyridoxine effect in animals, 25 mg/d of vitamin B$_6$ is also given. Effectiveness of therapy should be assayed chemically and clinically. Initially, the 24-h urinary excretion of copper should increase fivefold or more over the pretreatment level, and 1 to 3 mg copper per day may be excreted during the first months of therapy.

White blood cell and platelet counts, urinalysis, and body temperature should be monitored several times weekly for the first month of therapy and at intervals thereafter. Sensitivity to penicillamine usually appears within the first 14 days of treatment and may cause rash, fever, leukopenia, thrombocytopenia, lymphadenopathy, or proteinuria. Discontinuation of treatment is required if sensitivity develops. Therapy can often be resumed if the drug is reinstituted in small and gradually increasing dosage, although reactions are less likely to recur if 20 mg prednisone is given daily for the first 2 weeks of reinstituted penicillamine treatment and subsequently gradually discontinued. Reactions requiring a desensitizing regimen may recur several times before penicillamine can be administered without a steroid.

Lifelong and continual treatment is required. Inadequate treatment or interruption of therapy causes relapse that may be irreversible. Thus, of 11 patients who voluntarily discontinued penicillamine after years of successful treatment, 8 died after an average survival of 2.6 years of noncompliance. When penicillamine is reinstituted after interruption of therapy sensitivity reactions may reappear. At any time—even after years of uneventful administration—granulocytopenia (or agranulocytosis), thrombocytopenia, the nephrotic syndrome, Goodpasture's syndrome, systemic lupus erythematosus, severe arthralgias, or myasthenia gravis may supervene. Toxicity is sometimes dose-related, and reduction of the dose to a level that is therapeutically effective but nontoxic may be possible. Continued low dosage of glucocorticoids may control penicillamine-associated lupus or arthralgias. After temporary interruption of the drug in patients with the nephrotic syndrome, it is sometimes possible to reinstitute therapy without recurrence of proteinuria. However, although irreversible intolerance to penicillamine is rare, the toxicity may be such that the drug must be withdrawn permanently and replaced by trientine.

After therapy with penicillamine has been successfully instituted, the patient should be seen indefinitely at 1- to 3-month intervals to detect drug toxicity and to manage the disease. Physical examination, including relevant neurologic assessment and inspection of the corneas with a slit lamp, and the patient's own evaluation provide the best indicators of the efficacy of treatment. Serial determinations of serum transaminase levels, albumin, and bilirubin are useful in following the course of liver function. Lack of clinical improvement or worsening of the disease may be due to irreversible damage present before therapy was begun, poor compliance, or inadequate dosage of penicillamine. Quantitative determinations of urinary copper excretion and of free copper in serum (total serum copper minus ceruloplasmin-bound copper) can help determine which is the case. After treatment for long periods, the level of urinary copper should be lower than at the onset of therapy and rarely exceeds 1.0 mg/d. Even more helpful, the concentration of free serum copper is generally less than 2 μmol/L (13 μg/dL) in the adequately treated patient. After a patient has remained asymptomatic with no laboratory evidence of liver dysfunction for a year and in patients with minimal residual disease that has not changed, the dose of penicillamine may be reduced to 0.75 g/d.

The simultaneous occurrence of fulminant hepatitis and Coombs-negative hemolytic anemia may be the initial clinical manifestation of Wilson's disease or may occur in a treated patient who has become noncompliant. The syndrome is almost always fatal unless the patient receives a liver transplant. Of 24 patients who received such transplants, 22 survived for more than a year.

Prophylactic treatment of more than 100 asymptomatic patients with a confirmed diagnosis has established that continued penicillamine therapy can prevent virtually every manifestation of this disease.

REFERENCES

Bowcock AM et al: Eight closely linked loci place the Wilson Disease locus within 13q14-q21. Am J Hum Genet 43:664, 1988

Cossu P et al: Prenatal diagnosis of Wilson's disease by analysis of DNA polymorphism. N Engl J Med 327:57, 1992

Figus A et al: Carrier detection and early diagnosis of Wilson's disease by restriction fragment length polymorphism analysis. J Med Genet 26:78, 1989

Scheinberg IH, Sternlieb I: Wilson's disease, in *Major Problems in Internal Medicine*. Philadelphia, Saunders, 1984

—— et al: The use of trientine in preventing the effects of interrupting penicillamine therapy in Wilson's disease. N Engl J Med 317:209, 1987

—— et al: Penicillamine may detoxify copper in Wilson's disease. Lancet 2:95, 1987

Sternlieb I: Evolution of the hepatic lesion in Wilson's disease (hepatolenticular degeneration), in *Progress in Liver Diseases*, H Popper et al (eds). New York, Grune & Stratton, 1972, vol IV, pp 511–526

——, Scheinberg JH: Prevention of Wilson's disease in asymptomatic patients. N Engl J Med 278:352, 1968

——, ——: Chronic hepatitis as a first manifestation of Wilson's disease. Ann Intern Med 76:59, 1972

Walshe JM: Wilson's disease (hepatolenticular degeneration), in *Handbook of Clinical Neurology*, PJ Vinken et al (eds). New York, American Elsevier, 1976, vol 27

349 LYSOSOMAL STORAGE DISEASES

ARTHUR L. BEAUDET

GENERAL FEATURES

DEFINITION Lysosomes are cytoplasmic organelles that enclose an acidic environment and contain enzymes capable of hydrolyzing most macromolecules (Fig. 349-1). Primary lysosomes, the original bodies derived from the Golgi apparatus, may fuse with other membrane-bound vesicles to form secondary lysosomes. Secondary lysosomes contain material derived from outside the cell through endocytosis or from within the cell through autophagy. A major function of the lysosome is degradation of used macromolecules as a part of normal turnover and tissue remodeling. The lysosome is also important in the uptake of molecules such as vitamin B$_{12}$, lipoproteins, peptide hormones, and growth factors through adsorptive endocytosis. The initial cellular vacuole resulting from adsorptive endocytosis is the receptosome or endosome, and this vacuole fuses with lysosomes. The lysosomal enzymes are glycoproteins which are synthesized within the endoplasmic reticulum. The initial products of protein synthesis undergo extensive modification, including proteolytic cleavage, addition of complex oligosaccharides, synthesis of recognition markers (mannose-6-phosphate in some instances), and compartmentalization into primary lysosomes. These processes occur in the endoplasmic reticulum, in the Golgi apparatus, and probably in the primary, if not secondary, lysosomes as well. (See Part 12 in Scriver et al. for more details of lysosomal biology.)

The concept of lysosomal storage diseases arose from the studies of type II (Pompe) glycogen storage disease. The demonstration of lysosomal accumulation of glycogen due to α-glucosidase deficiency and data from other disorders led Hers to define an inborn lysosomal disease as one in which (1) a single lysosomal enzyme is deficient and (2) abnormal deposits (of substrate) are present within vacuoles related to lysosomes. This definition has been modified to include

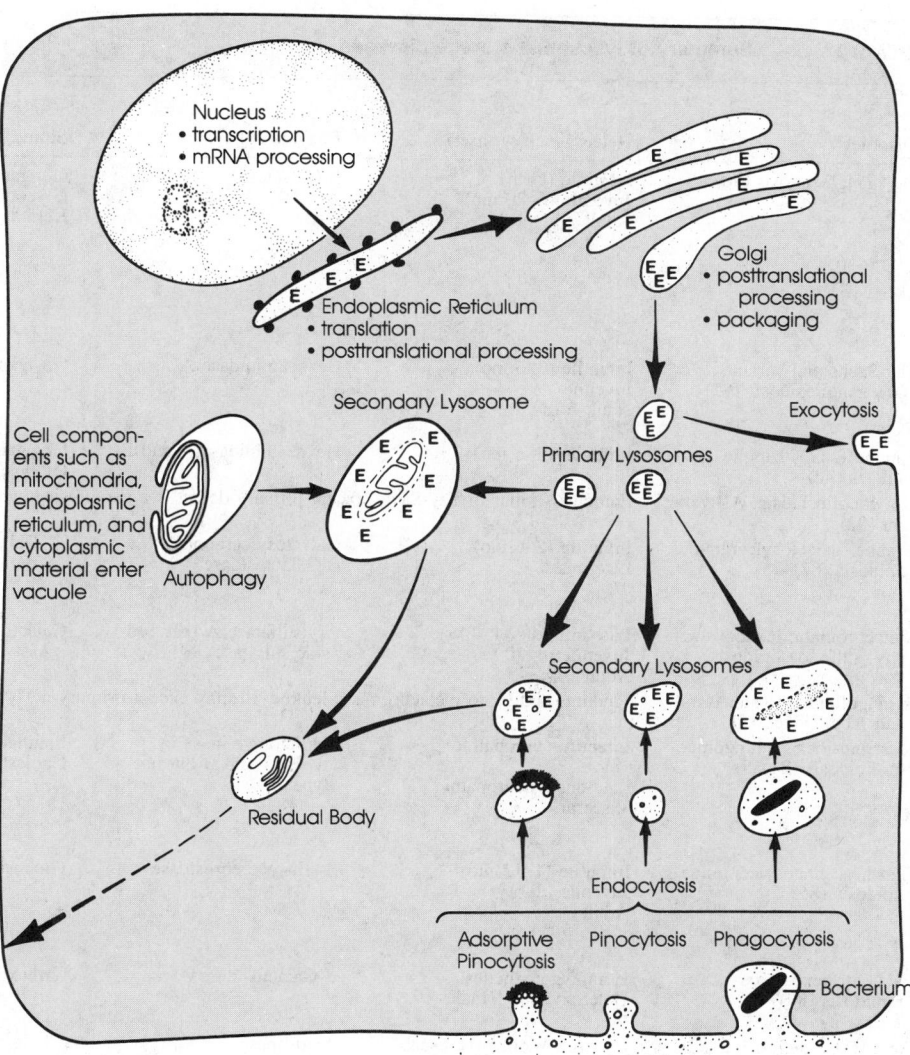

FIGURE 349-1 Biology of lysosomes. E represents lysosomal enzymes, including precursor forms. Lysosomal enzymes are synthesized in the endoplasmic reticulum and then undergo posttranslational processing that allows packaging into the primary lysosomes. The primary lysosomes can then undergo any of the several fates outlined.

single-gene defects affecting one or more lysosomal enzymes and thus encompasses disorders such as the mucolipidoses and multiple sulfatase deficiency. The concept also can be expanded to include the deficiency of other proteins necessary for lysosomal function, such as sphingolipid activator proteins. These activator proteins are essential for hydrolysis of some substrates. Disorders of lysosomal transport (e.g., transport of cysteine in cystinosis) do not conform as well to the conceptual framework for lysosomal enzyme deficiencies and are discussed elsewhere (see Chap. 352).

The lysosomal storage diseases include most of the lipid storage disorders, the mucopolysaccharidoses, the mucolipidoses, glycoprotein storage diseases, and others, as indicated in Table 349-1. The enzyme deficiencies have an autosomal recessive basis, with the exception of Hunter mucopolysaccharidosis II (MPS II), which is X-linked recessive, and Fabry disease, which is X-linked with frequent manifestations in females. The target organs are determined by the usual sites of degradation for a macromolecule. For example, cerebral white matter is affected with defects in degradation of myelin, hepatosplenomegaly develops with defects in degradation of glycolipids from red cell stroma, and generalized tissue involvement may occur with defects in the degradation of ubiquitous mucopolysaccharides. The accumulated material often causes visceromegaly or

macrocephaly, but secondary atrophy can occur, particularly in brain or muscle. In simple terms, the symptoms appear to be due to damage from stored material, but exactly how this causes cell death or dysfunction often is unclear. All the disorders are progressive, and many are fatal in childhood or adolescence. Definitive diagnosis is accomplished best by specific enzyme assays on serum, leukocytes, or cultured skin fibroblasts, selecting the appropriate tests on clinical grounds. There is extensive phenotypic variation within disorders with infantile, juvenile, and adult forms of many entities. In addition, varying combinations of visceral, skeletal, and neurologic involvement can occur with different mutations in a single gene.

DIAGNOSIS A lysosomal storage disease is usually suspected on the basis of progressive neurologic dysfunction, visceromegaly, skeletal dysostosis, or some more specific finding (Table 349-1). Progressive or degenerative disease is the hallmark of these disorders. The superimposition of degeneration on childhood development results in a slowing of progress prior to loss of previously acquired abilities. The history should focus on the course of childhood development, neurologic symptoms (including seizures and visual or auditory impairment), the course of physical growth, and specific findings such as coarsening facies, corneal clouding, exaggerated startle response, abdominal distention, joint pain, joint stiffness, hernias,

TABLE 349-1   Summary of lysosomal storage diseases

Disorder*	Heterogeneity (onset)	Enzyme deficiency	Stored material	Neurologic
G_{M1} gangliosidosis (90)	Infantile (birth) Juvenile (6–20 mo) Adult	β-Galactosidase	G_{M1} ganglioside Glycoproteins Keratan sulfate	Mental retardation, seizures, blindness; later in juvenile form, variable in adults
Tay-Sachs and variants, G_{M2} gangliosidosis (92)	Infantile (3–6 mo) Juvenile Adult forms	Hexosaminidase A	G_{M2} ganglioside	Mental retardation, seizures, blindness; later in juvenile form
Sandhoff, G_{M2} gangliosidosis (92)	Infantile (3–6 mo)	Hexosaminidase A and B	G_{M2} ganglioside Globoside	Mental retardation, seizures, blindness
G_{M2} gangliosidosis, AB variant (92)	Findings similar to Tay-Sachs except primary defect is a ganglioside activator protein.			
Krabbe, galactosylceramide lipidosis (87)	Infantile (2–6 mo) Late onset	Galactosylceramide β-Galactosidase	↑ Galactoscerebroside/sulfatide ratio	Mental retardation, leukodystrophy; variable in late onset
Metachromatic leukodystrophy, sulfatide lipidosis (88)	Late infantile (1–4 yr) Juvenile (4–20 yr) Adult	Arylsulfatase A (cerebroside sulfatase)	Galactosyl sulfatides	Mental retardation, leukodystrophy, psychosis and dementia in adults
Sphingolipid activator protein 1 deficiency (77)	Findings similar to metachromatic leukodystrophy except primary defect is activator protein.			
Niemann-Pick, sphingomyelin lipidosis (84,85)	Infantile neuropathic (1–4 mo) Late onset neuropathic Visceral	Sphingomyelinase in types A and B but not type C	Sphingomyelin Cholesterol	Mental retardation, ataxia, and seizures in neuropathic forms
Gaucher, glucosylceramide lipidosis (86)	Infantile (1–12 mo) Juvenile (2–6 yr) Adult	β-Glucocerebrosidase	Glucosylceramide	Mental retardation; spastic, later flaccid, ataxia in juvenile; no neurologic symptoms in adult form
Fabry, trihexosyl ceramidosis (89)	Hemizygous males Heterozygous females	α-Galactosidase A	Trihexosylceramide	Painful neuropathy
Acid lipase deficiency (82)	Infantile Wolman's disease (0–3 mo) Late onset cholesteryl ester storage disease (CESD)	Acid lipase	Cholesteryl ester Triglyceride	Mental retardation but mild related to growth failure in Wolman; none in CESD
Farber, ceramide deficiency (83)	Infantile (0–4 mo) Rare juvenile	Ceramidase	Ceramide	Occasional mental retardation, but may be secondary to somatic features
Pompe, glycogen storage type II (78)	Infantile (0–6 mo) Juvenile Adult	Acid maltase (α-1,4- and α-1,6-glucosidase)	Glycogen	Probably normal mentally
Fucosidosis (81)	Infantile (3–12 mo) Juvenile	α-Fucosidase	Glycopeptides Glycolipids Oligosaccharides	Mental retardation
Mannosidosis (81)	Infantile (6–18 mo) Milder form	α-Mannosidase	Oligosaccharides	Mental retardation
Aspartylglucosaminuria (81)	Young adult onset	Aspartylglucosamine amidase	Aspartylglucosamine Glycopeptides	Mental retardation
Mucopolysaccharidosis IH and IS (79)	Infantile Hurler (6–12 mo) Intermediate Adult Scheie	α-Iduronidase	Dermatan sulfate Heparan sulfate	Mental retardation, absent in Scheie
Hunter, mucopolysaccharidosis II (79)	Severe infantile (6–12 mo) Mild juvenile	Iduronosulfate sulfatase	Dermatan sulfate Heparan sulfate	Mental retardation, less in mild form

* Numbers in parentheses refer to the chapters in Scriver et al., 7th ed., in which the disorder is discussed in detail.

TABLE 349-1 Summary of lysosomal storage diseases (continued)

Liver and/or spleen enlargement	Skeletal dysplasia	Ophthalmic	Hematologic	Genetics	Unique manifestations
+ + + + Less in juvenile, variable in adult	+ + + + Variable in juvenile and adult forms	Cherry red spot in 50% of infantile; corneal clouding variable but more in adults	Foam cells Vacuolated lymphocytes	AR[†]	Coarse facies, edema, macroglossia, mucopolysacchariduria; early blindness in infantile, milder in juvenile; in adults often spondyloepiphyseal dysplasia ± mucopolysacchariduria
0	0	Cherry red spot in infantile form, rare in juvenile	0	AR	Macrocephaly, hyperacusis in infantile; increased in Ashkenazic Jews
0	0	Cherry-red spot	0	AR	Macrocephaly, hyperacusis, visceral histiocytosis
0	0	Optic atrophy	0	AR	Extreme irritability, ↑ CSF protein, fever, globoid cell neuropathology
0	0	Optic atrophy, less in juvenile and adult forms	0	AR	↑ CSF protein and early gait abnormalities in late infantile; peripheral neuropathy
+ + + + Less prominent in late onset forms	0	Macular degeneration and cherry red spot in neuronopathic forms	Distinctive foam cell Vacuolated lymphocytes	AR	Pulmonary infiltrates, brownish skin, infantile neuronopathic form increased in Ashkenazic Jews, sea-blue histiocytes
+ + + + Hypersplenism common	+ +	Usually normal	Distinctive foam cell	AR	Adult form includes ↑ acid phosphatase, pathologic fractures; Ashkenazic Jewish predilection
0	0	Corneal dystrophy, vascular lesions, cataracts	0	X-linked dominant	Cutaneous angiokeratoma, vascular thromboses, hypohidrosis
+ + +	0	0	Foam cells Vacuolated lymphocytes	AR	Adrenal calcification, anemia, vomiting and poor growth in Wolman; hepatic fibrosis and ↑ blood cholesterol in CESD
+/−	?	Mild macular degeneration	0	AR	Arthropathy—subcutaneous, periarticular and visceral nodules (lipogranulomatosis); ↑ CSF protein
Mild hepatomegaly	0	0	0	AR	Lethal skeletal and cardiac myopathy in infantile; primarily skeletal myopathy in adults
+ +	+ +	0	Vacuolated lymphocytes Foam cells	AR	Coarse facies, increased sweat electrolytes, angiokeratoma in juvenile
+ + +	+ +	Cataracts, corneal clouding	Vacuolated lymphocytes Granulated neutrophils	AR	Coarse facies, enlarged tongue
0	+ +	Lens opacities	Vacuolated lymphocytes	AR	Coarse facies, detectable by urine amino acid analysis
+ + +	+ + + +	Corneal clouding	Granulated lymphocytes	AR	Coarse facies, cardiovascular involvement, joint stiffness
+ + +	+ + + +	Retinal degeneration, no significant corneal clouding	Granulated lymphocytes	X-linked	Coarse facies, cardiovascular involvement, joint stiffness

[†] AR = autosomal recessive.

(Table continues next page)

TABLE 349-1 Summary of lysosomal storage diseases (continued)

Disorder*	Heterogeneity (onset)	Enzyme deficiency	Stored material	Neurologic
Sanfilippo A, muco-polysaccharidosis III A (79)		Heparan N-sulfatase (sulfamidase)		
Sanfilippo B, muco-polysaccharidosis III B (79)	Late infantile (1–4 yr)	N-Acetyl-α-glucosaminidase	Heparan sulfate	Severe mental retardation
Sanfilippo C, muco-polysaccharidosis III C (79)		Acetyl-CoA:α-glucosaminide N-acetyltransferase		
Sanfilippo D, mucopolysac-charidosis III D (79)		N-Acetylglucosamine-6-sulfate sulfatase		
Morquio, mucopolysacchar-idosis IV (79)	Some variation	N-Acetylgalactosamine-6-sulfate sulfatase	Keratan sulfate	0
Maroteaux-Lamy, muco-polysaccharidosis VI (79)	Variation in severity and cardiovascular involvement	N-Acetylhexosamine-4-sulfate sulfatase (arylsulfatase B)	Dermatan sulfate	0
β-Glucuronidase deficiency, mucopolysaccharidosis VII (79)	Few patients; infantile to adult forms	β-Glucuronidase	Dermatan sulfate ? Heparan sulfate	Mental retardation ? Absent in some adults
Multiple sulfatase deficiency (88)	Late infantile (1–4 yr)	Arylsulfatases A, B, and C Other sulfatases	Sulfatides Mucopolysaccharides	Mental retardation
Sialidosis (81)	Congenital, infantile, juvenile, cherry-red spot myoclonus	Glycoprotein neuraminidase (sialidase)	Sialyloligosaccharides	Mental retardation, myoclonus
Galactosialidosis (91)	Infantile Juvenile	Protective glycoprotein	Sialyloligosaccharides	Mental retardation
Mucolipidosis II, I cell disease (80)	Infantile (0–3 mo)	UDP-N-acetylglucosamine (GlcNAc):glycoprotein GlcNAc-1-phosphotransferase	Glycoproteins Glycolipids	Mental retardation
Mucolipidosis III, pseudo-Hurler polydystrophy (80)	Late infantile (>2 yr)		Glycoproteins Glycolipids	Mild mental retardation
Mucolipidosis IV	Infantile	? Ganglioside neuraminidase	? Multiple	Mental retardation
Neuronal ceroid lipofus-cinoses	Late infantile Juvenile Adult	Unknown	"Ceroid" "Lipofuscin"	Mental retardation, dementia variable in adults, seizures

* Numbers in parentheses refer to the chapters in Scriver et al., 7th ed., in which the disorder is discussed in detail.
† AR = autosomal recessive.

and recurrent infection. The family history may reveal similarly affected siblings or consanguinity in autosomal recessive disease or other affected male family members in X-linked disorders. Ethnic background may be helpful because several lipid storage diseases are more frequent in Ashkenazic Jews, and mannosidosis and aspartylglucosaminuria may occur with increased frequency in Scandinavian populations. The juvenile form of sialidosis is frequent in the Japanese.

On physical examination, the head circumference may be enlarged. Increased somatic growth may occur early in the course of some mucopolysaccharidoses and glycoprotein storage diseases, while short stature is a later finding in many disorders. Ophthalmologic examination should include slit-lamp and careful funduscopic examination. Enlargement of the tongue, coarsening of the facies, and hepatosplenomegaly may occur. Skeletal findings may include gibbus deformity, broadening of the long bones, and joint stiffness. Cutaneous findings are rare except in fucosidosis, sialidosis, Fabry disease, and Hunter disease. Careful neurologic examination should attempt to

distinguish the extent of involvement of gray matter, white matter, and peripheral nerves. Preliminary diagnostic studies should include examination of the peripheral blood smear for vacuolated or granulated leukocytes, urinary screening for mucopolysaccharide, and radiologic bone survey. The preferred method of diagnosis is to use the preceding information to select specific enzyme assays in serum, leukocytes, or cultured skin fibroblasts. If a mucopolysaccharide screening test is positive, or if clinical findings are suggestive, quantitative mucopolysaccharide analysis can be carried out. If a specific diagnosis is not readily established, biopsy of skin, bone marrow, rectal mucosa, liver, peripheral nerve, conjunctiva, or other tissue for light and electron microscopy can be helpful. Electron-microscopic findings can direct one toward or away from the general category of lysosomal storage diseases based on the presence or absence of engorged lysosomes. Again, enzyme assay is the proper method for diagnosis of the standard disorders. When significant evidence favors a lysosomal storage disease but no enzyme deficiency is demonstrable, chemical

TABLE 349-1 Summary of lysosomal storage diseases *(continued)*

Liver and/or spleen enlargement	Skeletal dysplasia	Ophthalmic	Hematologic	Genetics	Unique manifestations
+	+	0	Granulated lymphocytes	AR	Mild coarsening of facies
+	Severe, distinctive	Corneal clouding	Granulated neutrophils	AR	Severe deformity, odontoid hypoplasia, aortic regurgitation
+ +	+ + +	Corneal clouding	Granulated neutrophils and lymphocytes	AR	Mild coarsening of facies, joint stiffness, valvular heart disease
+ + +	+ + +	Corneal clouding	Granulated neutrophils	AR	Coarse facies, ↑ vascular involvement
+	MPS features	Retinal degeneration	Vacuolated and granulated cells	AR	Icthyosis, combined MPS and metachromatic leukodystrophy phenotype
+ + Less in late form	+ + Less or absent in late form	Cherry red spot	Vacuolated lymphocytes	AR	MPS phenotype in all but cherry red spot myoclonus
+ + Less in juvenile	+ +	Cherry red spot, corneal clouding	Vacuolated lymphocytes	AR	Angiokeratoma in juvenile; dysotosis multiplex
0/+	+ + +	Corneal clouding	Vacuolated and granulated neutrophils	AR	Coarse facies, inclusions in cultured fibroblasts, normal mucopolysacchariduria
0	+ + +	Corneal clouding	Vacuolated plasma cells	AR	Coarse facies, inclusions in cultured fibroblasts, joint contractures, valvular heart disease, normal mucopolysacchariduria
0	0	Corneal clouding, retinal degeneration	0	AR	Diagnosis based on electron microscopy; ? Ashkenazic Jewish predilection
0	0	Optic atrophy, macular degeneration, retinitis pigmentosa	Vacuolated lymphocytes Granulated neutrophils	AR	Electron microscopy helpful, degree of genetic heterogeneity unknown

analysis of biopsy tissue from liver or brain may be an appropriate research starting point.

The diagnosis of lysosomal storage diseases in adults is often difficult, although studies such as bone marrow aspiration in Gaucher disease and renal biopsy in Fabry disease may be pathognomonic. The diagnosis is difficult in the face of insidious, slowly progressive neurologic and psychiatric symptoms as described below for deficiencies of aryl sulfatase A, hexosaminidase A, or β-galactosidase. Erroneous diagnoses are common in these disorders, and a high index of suspicion is required. Lysosomal α-glucosidase deficiency mimics muscular dystrophy (see Chap. 385).

HETEROGENEITY There is extensive clinical, biochemical, and molecular heterogeneity within the lysosomal storage diseases. The biochemical genetic principles underlying this heterogeneity are reviewed in Chaps. 60 and 61. In general, structural genes for lysosomal enzymes produce propeptides that undergo posttranslational modification to become glycoproteins, often resulting in a series of

electrophoretic variants, or isozymes. These isozymes may hydrolyze one or a variety of substrates, and the substrate specificity of particular isozymes may vary. Differences in substrate specificity also arise from the occurrence of similar but genetically distinct enzymes, e.g., the β-galactosidases. Mutations within a gene may totally eliminate or reduce enzyme activity, alter posttranslational modification, or alter the activity of the enzyme for specific substrates.

In most instances, different mutations within the structural genes for lysosomal enzymes account for varying degrees of severity from individual to individual and for the diverse combinations of visceral, skeletal, neurologic, ocular, and other manifestations. The heterogeneity is increased further by the recessive nature of most of the conditions, and many affected individuals are compound heterozygotes. In this instance, either one or both genes may encode some form of residual enzyme activity for one or more substrates. Patients with intermediate clinical phenotypes for mucopolysaccharidosis type I (MPS I) are likely examples of compound heterozygotes. At a molecular level, the majority of lysosomal storage disease patients might prove to be compound heterozygotes. Although it is useful to characterize clinical phenotypes as infantile, juvenile, adult, neuropathic, or nonneuropathic, the existence of different mutant alleles and of compound heterozygotes provides an explanation for those occasional patients who appear aberrant or intermediate as compared with the usual phenotype. Another type of heterogeneity is illustrated by MPS III A, B, C, and D, which are very similar disorders caused by different gene defects. Thus biochemical heterogeneity can underlie apparent clinical homogeneity.

Further complexity results from the fact that certain enzyme activities are derived from complexes of nonidentical subunits. As a consequence, different mutations can cause deficiency of the same enzyme, e.g., hexosaminidase A deficiency in Tay-Sachs and Sandhoff diseases, and can explain multiple enzyme deficiencies due to a single-gene defect as in Sandhoff disease. Genetic disorders that affect the posttranslational modification of lysosomal enzymes and defects in the lysosome itself also may cause lysosomal storage diseases. The mucolipidoses II and III are situations in which a single-gene defect alters the ability of a number of lysosomal enzymes to enter the lysosome. Thus mutations outside the structural genes for the enzymes can account for further heterogeneity. Better understanding of the identity, subunit structure, posttranslational processing, and substrate specificities of lysosomal enzymes should provide further insight into phenotypic and genotypic heterogeneity.

Clinical diagnosis is facilitated but also somewhat complicated by the widespread use of synthetic substrates for measuring lysosomal enzyme activities. These substrates often measure a group of related activities attributable to different enzymes. Thus the activity of β-galactosidase using an artificial substrate may represent the sum of various β-galactosidases encoded by different structural genes and having different substrate specificities. Clinical reliability generally is achieved by manipulating in vitro conditions to reflect that enzyme activity whose deficiency is characteristic of a clinical disorder. Genetic heterogeneity has, however, resulted in individuals with a mutant enzyme that either hydrolyzes the natural substrate and not the artificial substrate or vice versa. This is exemplified by the normal individuals who have hexosaminidase A deficiency using artificial substrate and by patients with Tay-Sachs disease who have substantial levels of hexosaminidase A activity with artificial substrates. The presence or absence of disease correlates with ability to hydrolyze the natural G_{M2} ganglioside substrate. These phenomena have considerable significance for identification of affected patients, for heterozygote screening, and for prenatal diagnosis. They indicate the need to go beyond artificial substrate enzyme assays if normal results occur in the face of overwhelming clinical, electron-microscopic, or chemical evidence of a storage disease.

MANAGEMENT AND PREVENTION Specific therapy is rarely effective in lysosomal storage diseases at present (see ''Gaucher Disease,'' below, for some exceptions), and care is largely symptomatic. The relentless, progressive course in many instances represents a tragic burden. Splenectomy has been useful in type I Gaucher disease in the past, and transplantation is effective in reversing the renal failure in Fabry disease. Attempts at more specific therapy have focused on enzyme replacement, fibroblast transplantation, and bone marrow transplantation. The greatest success with enzyme replacement is in Gaucher disease, and the availability of recombinant enzymes offers somewhat more favorable prospects for additional enzyme replacement in the future. Bone marrow transplantation is primarily a research modality. Patients with life-threatening or severely disabling somatic manifestations who have an HLA-identical, unaffected sibling are the best candidates for bone marrow transplantation. The most distressing manifestations of the majority of lysosomal storage diseases involve the central nervous system and are less amenable to enzyme replacement or bone marrow transplantation.

Genetic counseling is important in the management of these disorders. All the lysosomal storage diseases in which the specific enzyme deficiency is known either have been or presumably could

be diagnosed in utero, since lysosomal enzyme activities are expressed in cultured amniotic fluid cells as well as in cultured skin fibroblasts. Prenatal diagnosis also can be made using chorionic villus biopsy, and the possibility of earlier diagnosis is attractive to families at high risk. Heterozygote detection in close relatives is sometimes possible, although it can be difficult to achieve adequate statistical confidence using biochemical methods. Molecular methods using mutation detection or linkage analysis are more reliable where applicable. Heterozygote detection is further complicated by random inactivation of X chromosomes in female carriers of X-linked diseases, and women at risk in such families should be counseled using molecular data where possible. More widespread approaches to prevention require identification of heterozygous couples prior to the birth of an affected offspring. The feasibility of this approach has been demonstrated by heterozygote testing programs for Tay-Sachs disease. Such programs could result in a decreased frequency of these disorders through extensive testing and appropriate reproductive decisions by the rare couples at risk for affected offspring; the high frequency of the heterozygous state in Ashkenazic Jews and reliable methods for carrier detection for Tay-Sachs disease have facilitated this program. Molecular analysis of mutations complements biochemical methods for Tay-Sachs testing and makes possible carrier detection for Gaucher disease in the Ashkenazic population. Efficient, accurate heterozygote detection methods would be needed to apply this approach to other diseases and to populations with lower heterozygote frequencies. Even under optimal conditions, genetic variants may cause false-positive or false-negative results in any screening process. Population-based carrier screening is not feasible for most lysosomal storage diseases.

MOLECULAR ANALYSIS Most of the genes encoding lysosomal enzymes have been cloned and sequenced. Many specific mutations are identified, and sometimes it is possible to correlate the genotype with the severity of the phenotype, as discussed for Tay-Sachs and Gaucher diseases below. There is extensive molecular heterogeneity, and many patients are compound heterozygotes. Molecular diagnosis generally can supplement but not replace enzymatic diagnosis. When a small number of mutations accounts for the majority of the defective gene copies, as in the case of Tay-Sachs and Gaucher diseases in the Ashkenazic population, mutation analysis is extremely valuable. Mutation detection and linkage analysis are also helpful in cases of prenatal diagnosis, where pseudodeficiency or biochemical difficulties can lead to diagnostic errors. The availability of the cloned cDNAs also improves the prospects for enzyme replacement using recombinant protein and for somatic gene therapy.

SPECIFIC DISORDERS

SPHINGOLIPIDOSES G_{M1} **gangliosidosis** G_{M1} gangliosidosis is due to deficiency of β-galactosidase. The features of the infantile form are summarized in Table 349-1. The juvenile form is characterized by a later onset, survival to the latter half of the first decade of life, neurologic impairment and seizures, and milder skeletal and ocular findings. In adults, one phenotype (sometimes called *Morquio B*) includes corneal clouding, normal intelligence, and spondyloepiphyseal dysplasia similar to that seen in MPS IV. Other adults have minimal bony abnormalities but exhibit spasticity, ataxia, or myoclonus. Patients with slowly progressive extrapyramidal signs with prominent dystonia, cerebral and caudate atrophy, and absence of visceral findings have been misdiagnosed as juvenile parkinsonism. A high index of suspicion is necessary to recognize the diverse phenotypes caused by β-galactosidase deficiency in juvenile and adult patients, since a wide range of skeletal, ocular, neurologic, and visceral findings can occur. Isozymes of β-galactosidase occur, but the diversity of phenotypes is believed to be due to different mutations in the same structural gene. All forms of G_{M1} gangliosidosis have an autosomal recessive inheritance. The frequency of the disease is low, with fewer than 50 patients reported for any given phenotype. Patients with isolated β-galactosidase deficiency must be distinguished from those with galactosialidosis, the combined deficiency of neuraminidase and β-galactosidase.

G_{M2} **gangliosidosis** Tay-Sachs disease is a relatively common inborn error of metabolism. Although it is clinically similar to Sandhoff disease, the two are genetically distinct, with deficiency of hexosaminidase A in the former and hexosaminidase A and B in the latter. An additional disorder, called the *AB variant* of G_{M2} gangliosidosis, is due to a deficiency of a protein factor (activator) necessary for activity of the enzyme against natural substrate. The presenting features are similar in all the infantile disorders and include a developmental delay beginning in the third to sixth month with subsequent, rapidly progressive neurologic deterioration. Macrocephaly, seizures, retinal cherry red spots, and an augmented startle response to sound suggest the diagnosis. The diagnosis is confirmed by enzyme assay. Most juvenile-onset patients with hexosaminidase deficiency present with dementia, seizures, and ocular findings, and some have an atypical spinocerebellar degeneration.

The neurologic manifestations of hexosaminidase A deficiency in adults are variable. Ataxia, dysarthria, lower motor neuron disease, pyramidal signs, and recurrent psychosis are common. Misdiagnoses have included Kugelberg-Welander spinal muscular atrophy, amyotropic lateral sclerosis, cerebellar or spinocerebellar ataxia, atypical Friedreich ataxia, muscular dystrophy, dementia, schizophrenia, and others. The manifestations are slowly progressive, and if considered, the diagnosis is easily established by serum enzyme assay.

Sandhoff disease is nonallelic with Tay-Sachs disease, whereas the juvenile forms of hexosaminidase deficiency are usually allelic with Tay-Sachs disease. Tay-Sachs disease is the most frequent form of hexosaminidase deficiency, the risk being about 100 times higher in Ashkenazic Jews than in other ethnic groups. All forms of G_{M2} gangliosidosis are autosomal recessive. Hexosaminidase B is composed of β subunits whose structural locus is on chromosome 5, while hexosaminidase A is composed of α and β subunits with the structural locus for the α subunit on chromosome 15. Thus there is a defect in the α subunit in Tay-Sachs disease and in the β subunit in Sandhoff disease.

Although no specific therapy is available, extensive programs for heterozygote detection have been carried out in which more than half a million people have been tested and hundreds of couples at risk have been identified. Almost 2000 prenatal diagnoses have been performed, and the frequency of affected births has been reduced by 80 to 90 percent in the Jewish population in the United States and Canada.

Molecular studies have identified four mutations that account for over 95 percent of the mutant genes in the Ashkenazic population; a large deletion mutation is common in the French Canadian population. Presently, mutational and enzyme analyses are both accurate for carrier detection in the Ashkenazic population, but the two together are slightly better than either alone; enzyme assays are preferable outside the Ashkenazic and French Canadian populations because of molecular heterogeneity. Most patients with adult G_{M2} gangliosidosis have the milder G269S mutation [substitution of glycine (G) for serine (S) at position 269] in a compound heterozygote state with a severe infantile allele.

LEUKODYSTROPHIES Krabbe galactosylceramide lipidosis or globoid cell leukodystrophy is an infantile disease due to deficiency of galactosylceramide β-galactosidase (see Table 349-1). Rapid neurologic deterioration and death occur within 1 to 2 years of onset. Premortem diagnosis is accomplished by enzyme assay. The presence of globoid cells in the brain is a characteristic postmortem finding. Galactosylceramide β-galactosidase is distinct from the β-galactosidase that is deficient in G_{M1} gangliosidosis. Krabbe disease is an autosomal recessive disorder, and diagnosis can be made prenatally. Juvenile or adult forms are rare.

Deficiency of arylsulfatase A (cerebroside sulfatase) is the basis of metachromatic leukodystrophy, a lipid storage disease with a frequency of 1 in 40,000. The age of onset is later than that in Tay-Sachs disease or Krabbe disease. Patients usually attain the ability to walk and frequently present with gait abnormalities in the second to fourth year of life. Initially the patients may be hypotonic with decreased deep tendon reflexes, the latter reflecting peripheral nerve involvement. The disease progresses over the first decade to include ataxia, increased muscle tone, decorticate or decerebrate posturing, and eventual loss of all contact with surroundings. Rare patients with a juvenile form of metachromatic leukodystrophy have the clinical onset between 4 and 20 years of age and progress more slowly.

The adult form deserves special mention as an example of the difficulties presented by subtle, slowly progressive forms of lysosomal storage disease. The onset is in the second to fifth decade with a slowly progressive dementia. Emotional difficulties, motor dysfunction, and indistinct speech are often present. Even though conduction velocity in peripheral nerves is usually diminished, the deep tendon reflexes are often increased. Typical misdiagnoses include organic dementia, multiple sclerosis, and schizophrenia; psychiatric hospitalization is common. Premortem diagnosis was rare in the past, but the presence of periventricular hypodensities of white matter on computed tomographic scan or abnormalities of periventricular white matter on magnetic resonance imaging of the brain may suggest the diagnosis, which should be confirmed by enzyme assay.

Although some diagnostic studies have been performed on urine, leukocytes or fibroblasts are preferable for diagnostic enzyme assay. Arylsulfatase A is measured using artificial substrate, but the assay is complicated by low levels of activity in normal individuals (psuedodeficiency) and moderate levels of residual activity in some patients. Analysis of mutations in the various forms of metachromatic leukodystrophy and delineation of a pseudodeficiency allele may be helpful in resolving diagnostic problems. A few patients with a phenotype similar to metachromatic leukodystrophy have deficiency of a sphingolipid activator protein. Arylsulfastase A deficiency also occurs in multiple sulfatase deficiency.

NIEMANN-PICK DISEASE Niemann-Pick disease is a sphingomyelin lipidosis. In disease types A and B, there is deficiency of sphingomyelinase, an enzyme that hydrolyzes sphingomyelin to yield ceramide and phosphorylcholine. The most common disorder, Niemann-Pick type A, begins shortly after birth with hepatosplenomegaly, failure to thrive, and neurologic impairment. Retinal cherry red spots occur, but seizures and hypersplenism are rare. The diagnosis is made by recognition of the distinctive Niemann-Pick cell in the bone marrow and is confirmed by enzyme assay. Niemann-Pick type B disease is a relatively benign disorder with hepatosplenomegaly, sphingomyelinase deficiency, and sometimes pulmonary infiltrates, but there is no neurologic involvement. Niemann-Pick type C disease is characterized by sphingomyelin lipidosis and progressive neurologic deterioration in childhood. Type C disease is not due to sphingomyelinase deficiency but is associated with a massive lysosomal accumulation of cholesterol due to an incompletely characterized defect in intracellular utilization of cholesterol.

GAUCHER DISEASE Gaucher disease is a glucosylceramide lipidosis caused by deficiency of β-glucocerebrosidase, commonly known as β-glucosidase. An infantile form is characterized by early onset, marked hepatosplenomegaly, and severe neurologic progression to early death. A juvenile form with milder neurologic involvement exists. The type 1, or nonneuronopathic, form (commonly called adult Gaucher) is the most common lysosomal storage disease. The diagnosis of Gaucher disease should be established by enzyme analysis, and mutational analysis also should be performed. All forms of Gaucher disease have an autosomal recessive genetic basis and are allelic disorders. Type 1 is about 30 times more frequent in Ashkenazic Jews, with an incidence in this group of at least 1 in 1000 births. Absence of neurologic involvement is the criterion for inclusion in the type 1 or adult category.

Clinical manifestations include incidental discovery of painless splenomegaly; thrombocytopenia, anemia, or leukopenia secondary to hypersplenism; and bone pain. The course is variable, ranging from confinement to a wheelchair early in life to asymptomatic diagnosis in the ninth decade. Most patients have a mild course with relatively normal life expectancy. Partial or total splenectomy may be required. Pneumococcal vaccine should be administered prior to splenectomy. Careful management of postsplenectomy infection risks is important, and prophylactic antibiotics are recommended. The extent of bone disease is variable and includes bone pain, pathologic fractures, vertebral collapse, and aseptic necrosis of the femoral head. Bone pain with fever is termed *psuedoosteomyelitis*. MRI is particularly effective in defining the bony abnormalities. Moderate hepatic dysfunction is common, and rarely, severe hepatic failure, portal hypertension, pulmonary infiltrates, and pulmonary hypertension may develop. Serum acid phosphatase is characteristically elevated. A distinctive storage cell is present in the bone marrow in all forms of Gaucher disease, but enzyme assay should be performed because the Gaucher cell also may be found in patients with granulocytic leukemia and myeloma.

Four mutations account for 96 percent of the mutations in the Ashkenazic population. These findings opened the way for genotype/phenotype correlations and carrier screening in that population. One mutation, designated N370S [substitution of serine (S) for asparagine (N) at position 370], is mild; a single copy of this mutation in a compound heterozygote does not cause neurologic involvement, and homozygosity for this mutation is associated with a particularly mild phenotype. In fact, homozygosity for the N370S phenotype was found in 2 of 453 "normal" Ashkenazic individuals.

A major change in the treatment for Gaucher disease is the availability of aglucerase for enzyme replacement therapy. Aglucerase is a modified form of β-glucosidase prepared from human placenta. Treatment improves anemia and thrombocytopenia, decreases organomegaly, and decreases bone pain. Although this treatment may reduce or eliminate the need for splenectomy, the cost is about $300,000 per year. Recombinant enzyme is undergoing clinical trials; however, cost is likely to remain a major obstacle, and the dosage and indications for treatment are subjects of current investigation.

FABRY DISEASE Fabry disease involves the accumulation of a trihexoside, galactosylgalactosylglucosylceramide, due to deficiency of α-galactosidase A. The disorder is X-linked. The most severe symptoms occur in hemizygous males, with an incidence of about 1 in 40,000; milder symptoms occur in heterozygous females. Painful neuropathy is the most prominent symptom in younger men. The pain may be constant or cause intermittent crises of burning pain particularly in the palms and soles. Painful crises may mimic appendicitis or renal colic, and associated low-grade fever may lead to misdiagnoses of inflammatory processes.

The diagnosis can be suggested by the astute dermatologist or ophthalmologist. Cutaneous manifestations include angiokeratoma and decreased sweating. The angiokeratoma occur as clusters of red angiectases in the superficial skin. They do not blanch with pressure and are located on the trunk, perineal area, penis, and scrotum. The anhidrosis or hypohidrosis can predispose to heat stroke with vigorous exercise, as in military training. A characteristic corneal opacity occurs in males and in most heterozygous females. Lenticular opacities and tortuosity of the conjunctival and retinal vessels also occur.

Cardiovascular manifestations include direct involvement of the myocardium with lipid deposition, arrhythmias, valvular dysfunction, and myocardial infarction. Cerebral vascular manifestations secondary to involvement of small vessels are not rare, and frank cerebral hemorrhage can occur. Deposition of lipid in the kidney results in progressive renal impairment with renal failure in middle age (see also Chap. 241). The mean age at death of males not treated for renal failure was 41 years in one study. The diagnosis is often recognized at renal biopsy on the basis of lipid vacuoles in glomerular and tubular epithelial cells.

Heterozygous females are affected more mildly, but corneal dystrophy and cutaneous manifestations may be present. Life expectancy is near normal in women, although the more serious complications occur rarely.

Therapeutic intervention of several types may be helpful. Counsel-

ing regarding the risks of hypohidrosis is important. Painful neuropathy frequently responds to administration of phenytoin. Renal failure can be treated by chronic dialysis, and the patients are acceptable candidates for transplantation because the donor kidney will not be impaired by the disease. Since the central nervous system is spared, the disease is a candidate for enzyme replacement therapy.

ACID LIPASE DEFICIENCY The infantile form of acid lipase deficiency, Wolman disease, is listed in Table 349-1. Cholesteryl ester storage disease in adulthood and adolescence is a rare disorder with mild phenotypic features by comparison. The usual features are hepatosplenomegaly, lipid deposition in the liver, and increased plasma cholesterol. Hepatic fibrosis, esophageal varices, and poor growth may occur.

GLYCOPROTEIN STORAGE DISORDERS Fucosidosis, mannosidosis, and aspartylglucosaminuria are rare, autosomal recessive disorders involving hydrolases that degrade polysaccharide linkages. Glycolipids as well as glycoproteins are accumulated in fucosidosis. All are characterized by neurologic impairment and varying somatic involvements (see Table 349-1). Fucosidosis and mannosidosis are most often lethal disorders in childhood, while aspartylglucosaminuria is a late-onset lysosomal storage disease with prominent mental retardation and a prolonged course. Abnormal sweat electrolytes and cutaneous angiokeratomas are distinctive in fucosidosis, and an unusual cartwheel-type cataract occurs in mannosidosis. Aspartylglucosaminuria is remarkable in that urinary amino acid analysis is diagnostic with an increase of aspartylglucosamine. The disorder is more frequent in the Finnish population. Sialidosis encompasses a group of phenotypes associated with glycoprotein neuraminidase (sialidase) deficiency. The phenotypes include an adult cherry red spot myoclonus syndrome, infantile and juvenile presentations with mucopolysaccharidosis-like phenotypes, and a congenital presentation with hydrops fetalis. Many patients previously classified as having mucolipidosis I have been proven to have mannosidosis or sialidosis. Some patients with sialidosis have β-galactosidase deficiency as well as neuraminidase deficiency. The combined β-galactosidase and neuraminidase deficiency is due to a defect in a "protective protein." Each of the glycoprotein storage diseases can be diagnosed by appropriate enzyme assay.

MUCOPOLYSACCHARIDOSIS (MPS) The mucopolysaccharidoses represent a broad spectrum of disorders due to deficiencies of one of a group of enzymes that degrade three classes of mucopolysaccharides: heparan sulfate, dermatan sulfate, and keratan sulfate. The MPS phenotype includes coarse facies, corneal clouding, hepatosplenomegaly, joint stiffness, hernias, dysostosis multiplex, mucopolysaccharide excretion in the urine, and metachromatic staining in peripheral luekocytes and bone marrow. Various components of the MPS phenotype are also found in the mucolipidoses, glycoprotein storage disorders, and other lysosomal storage diseases. Detailed clinical and radiologic evaluation and identification of the type of MPS excreted in the urine help to narrow the diagnostic possibilities. Diagnosis requires assay of specific enzymes in various tissues such as cultured skin fibroblasts.

Hurler or MPS IH disorder is the prototype MPS. Virtually all the components of the phenotype mentioned above are expressed in a severe degree. Nasal congestion and grossly visible corneal clouding are early features. Excessive growth during the first year of life is followed by poor growth late in the course. Radiologic features include enlargement of the sella turcica with a distinctive "shoe-shaped" fossa, broadening and shortening of the long bones, and hypoplasia and beaking of the vertebrae in the lumbar area. The vertebral beaking gives rise to an accentuated kyphosis or gibbus deformity. Death occurs within the first decade; postmortem findings include hydrocephalus and cardiovascular disease with occlusion of the coronary arteries. The biochemical defect is α-iduronidase deficiency with accumulation of heparan sulfate and dermatan sulfate.

MPS IS or Scheie syndrome, a clinically distinct disorder with childhood onset but adult survival, is characterized by joint stiffness, corneal clouding, aortic regurgitation, and usually normal intelligence.

Surprisingly, this much milder disorder is also the result of α-iduronidase deficiency; it is allelic with Hurler syndrome, as shown by lack of cross-correction of enzyme activity in cocultures of skin fibroblasts. Phenotypes occur that are clearly intermediate between Hurler and Scheie syndromes. It is believed that patients with an intermediate phenotype represent genetic compounds with one Hurler allele and one Scheie allele. Although genetic compounds must occur, in any one case their existence is difficult to distinguish from mutations of intermediate severity unless molecular analysis is performed.

Hunter or MPS II syndrome is distinguishable from the Hurler phenotype by the absence of gross corneal clouding and the X-linked recessive inheritance. The infantile form resembles the Hurler disease phenotype, and a milder form allows survival into adulthood. The severe and mild forms are allelic, and both are X-linked and share the same enzyme deficiency (iduronosulfate sulfatase).

Sanfilippo mucopolysaccharidoses (MPS III A, B, C, and D) are distinguished by the accumulation of heparan sulfate without dermatan or keratan sulfate and by the marked central nervous system involvement with milder somatic involvement. Sanfilippo mucopolysaccharidosis usually is diagnosed in the evaluation of mental retardation in childhood. Because the somatic features of this MPS are mild, the condition can be overlooked in the evaluation of an apparently isolated central nervous system problem. Death usually occurs during the second or third decade. The MPS III disorders are approximate genocopies. That is, four different enzyme deficiencies give rise to relatively indistinguishable clinical phenotypes with the same storage product. The four MPS III disorders can be diagnosed and distinguished by enzyme assay (see Table 349-1).

Morquio or MPS IV syndrome is distinguished by the absence of mental retardation and the presence of a distinctive bony dystrophy which can be classified as a spondyloepiphyseal dysplasia. Marked hypoplasia of the odontoid process can cause cervical dislocation and usually leads to some degree of spinal cord compression. Aortic regurgitation is frequent. The deficiency of N-acetylgalactosamine-6-sulfate sulfatase is the basis for this condition. Bone changes similar to those in Morquio syndrome also occur in one form of β-galactosidase deficiency. Maroteaux-Lamy or MPS VI disorder is characterized by prominent osseous involvement, corneal clouding, and normal intellect. Allelic forms with variable severity but the same deficiency of arylsulfatase B(N-acetylhexosamine-4-sulfate sulfatase) have been described. MPS VII, or β-glucuronidase deficiency, has been described in only a few patients with a rather complete MPS phenotype. Extreme variability from a lethal infantile form to a mild adult disease occurs.

MUCOLIPIDOSES *Mucolipidosis* is a general term for lysosomal storage diseases involving some combination of MPS, glycoprotein, oligosaccharide, and glycolipids. The category of mucolipidosis I probably can be abandoned, since most or all of these patients actually have a specific glycoprotein storage disease.

Mucolipidosis II, or I cell disease, is an early-onset disorder with mental retardation and an MPS phenotype. The distinctive features are striking inclusions in cultured skin fibroblasts and markedly elevated serum levels of lysosomal enzymes. The disorder has an autosomal recessive basis and is now known to represent a defect in the posttranslational processing of lysosomal enzymes. Mucolipidosis III, or pseudo-Hurler polydystrophy, is a milder disorder with many aspects of the MPS phenotype, particularly dysostosis multiplex. The disorder presents in the first decade with joint stiffness, the diagnosis of rheumatoid arthritis often being considered. The major handicaps are progressive physical disabilities, particularly claw hand deformity and hip dysplasia. Mild mental retardation is common. Aortic and/or mitral valvular disease is routinely present, although often not functionally significant. Survival into adult life with possible stabilization of the condition is characteristic, with greater disability in males than in females. Inclusions in cultured skin fibroblasts and elevation of serum lysosomal enzymes are essentially identical with the findings in mucolipidosis II, suggesting that these are allelic disorders. The primary defect in mucolipidosis II and III is deficiency of UDP-N-acetylglucosamine (GLcNAc):glycoprotein GLcNAc-1-phosphotransferase, an enzyme involved in posttranslational synthesis of the oligosaccharide portion of the lysosomal enzymes.

NEURONAL CEROID LIPOFUSCINOSES The neuronal ceroid lipofuscinosis disorders include a wide clinical spectrum with onset in childhood, juvenile, or adult periods. It is uncertain if these disorders are true lysosomal storage diseases, indeed whether single or multiple biochemical genetic disorders are present. The clinical features include central nervous system deterioration with cerebral atrophy, usually commensurate with the degree of impairment. Seizures, particularly myoclonic jerks, are prominent. Ocular involvement with optic atrophy, retinitis pigmentosa, and macular degeneration is present in the infantile and juvenile disorders but often absent in adult forms. Autosomal recessive inheritance is likely in most instances. The neuropathologic findings form the basis of the descriptive term for the disease. Electron microscopy demonstrates abnormal inclusions within lysosomes throughout a wide variety of tissues, despite the rather isolated clinical neurologic involvement. The presence of curvilinear bodies, electron-dense material, and fingerprint profiles on electron microscopy of white blood cells, liver biopsy, or muscle biopsy can be helpful diagnostically.

OTHER LYSOSOMAL STORAGE DISEASES Glycogen storage disease type II (Pompe disease) is the prototype lysosomal storage disease. The predominant clinical features of skeletal and cardiac myopathy are described in Chap. 350. Some rarer disorders are included in Table 349-1. Multiple sulfatase deficiency is an autosomal recessive disorder characterized by a deficiency of five or more cellular sulfatases: aryl sulfatase A, aryl sulfatase B, other mucopolysaccharide sulfatases, and a nonlysosomal steroid sulfatase. The clinical picture combines features of metachromatic leukodystrophy, an MPS phenotype, and ichthyosis. Other neurodegenerative diseases may eventually be classifiable as lysosomal storage diseases. Disorders such as juvenile dystonic lipidosis, neuroaxonal dystrophy, Hallervorden-Spatz disease, and other candidates exist. In addition, it is not unusual to identify patients with distinctive clinical features suggestive of lipidosis, mucolipidosis, or mucopolysaccharidosis, in which none of the present biochemically identifiable disorders can be identified. For these reasons, the number of distinct lysosomal storage diseases is likely to continue to increase.

REFERENCES

BEUTLER E: Gaucher's disease. N Engl J Med 325:1354, 1991

————: Gaucher disease: New molecular approaches to diagnosis and treatment. Science 256:794, 1992

DURAND P, O'BRIEN JS (eds): *Genetic Errors of Glycoprotein Metabolism.* Berlin, Springer-Verlag, 1982

NAVON R et al: Hexosaminidase A deficiency in adults. Am J Med Genet 24:179, 1986

NEUFELD EF: Lysosomal storage diseases. Annu Rev Biochem 60:257, 1991

SCRIVER CR et al (eds): *The Molecular and Metabolic Basis of Inherited Disease,* 7th ed. New York, McGraw-Hill, in press

WALTZ G et al: Adult metachromatic leukodystrophy. Arch Neurol 44:225, 1987

350 THE GLYCOGEN STORAGE DISEASES

ARTHUR L. BEAUDET

The glycogen storage diseases are a group of genetic disorders involving the pathways for storage of carbohydrate as glycogen and for its utilization to maintain blood sugar and to provide energy. Some forms are not associated with actual increases in glycogen content in tissues.

Glycogen is a highly branched polymer of glucose with the majority of residues in 1,4 linkage and with 7 to 10 percent of residues in 1,6 linkage. The treelike structure undergoes addition and removal of residues at its periphery. Glycogen synthesis begins by covalent attachment of glucose to a tyrosine residue on a protein, glycogenin. Through addition of glucose, individual particles can grow to include up to 60,000 glucose residues. Various forms of glycogen particles are distinguishable by electron microscopy. Liver generally contains less than 70 mg glycogen per gram of tissue, and muscle usually contains less than 15 mg/g, but these levels fluctuate as a consequence of feeding and hormonal stimuli. Abnormalities of glycogen structure can result either from decreased or increased branching.

The metabolic pathways involved in glycogen synthesis and breakdown are outlined in Fig. 350-1. These pathways differ among tissues; for example, certain reactions are active in liver but trivial or absent in muscle, and some enzyme functions are encoded by different genes in muscle and liver. Plasma glucose enters the cell and is phosphorylated by glucokinase or hexokinase. The former enzyme is found in liver where it accomplishes the majority of phosphorylation of glucose, while multiple hexokinases are distributed more widely in tissues. Glucose-6-phosphate (Glc-6-P) is converted to glucose-1-phosphate (Glc-1-P) in a reversible reaction catalyzed by phosphoglucomutase. Uridine diphosphate glucose (UDP-Glc) is synthesized from Glc-1-P and UTP by UDP-Glc pyrophosphorylase. Genetic deficiency has not been documented for any of these hepatic enzymes except that heterozygous glucokinase deficiency is a rare cause of type 2 diabetes mellitus (see Chap. 337). Glycogen is then elongated by the addition from UDP-Glc of individual glucose residues to an existing polymer. This reaction is catalyzed by glycogen synthase, which is encoded by separate genes in liver and muscle and is highly regulated, being stimulated by insulin and inhibited by epinephrine or glucagon. The regulation involves both phosphorylation of multiple sites to inhibit the enzyme and relief of the inhibition by the allosteric effect of Glc-6-P. Synthesis of a normally branched glycogen structure also requires the action of a branching enzyme (1,4-α-glucan:1,4-α-glucan-6-glucosyltransferase) which transfers a 1,4-linked oligosaccharide to a 1,6-linkage position.

Glucose is mobilized from glycogen by a complex group of enzyme reactions. Glycogen is acted on directly by the active form of phosphorylase, phosphorylase a, to remove individual glucose units and yield Glc-1-P. Phosphorylase is encoded by different gene products in muscle and liver. In both tissues, the enzyme can exist in an active phosphorylated form and in an inactive dephosphorylated form. Phosphorylase is a dimer of identical subunits, and both forms of the enzyme are subject to complex allosteric regulation. The inactive phosphorylase b is converted to the active form by phosphorylase b kinase. Phosphorylase b kinase also exists in an active phosphorylated form and in an inactive dephosphorylated form. Phosphorylase b kinase is a multimer of four nonidentical subunits ($\alpha,\beta,\gamma,\delta$)$_4$, and the δ chain is identical with the calcium-binding protein calmodulin. The rate of glucose mobilization by this system is regulated by a cascade of kinase reactions, including cyclic AMP-dependent protein kinase. Epinephrine and glucagon act to increase blood sugar via this cascade system by activation of phosphorylase and simultaneous inactivation of glycogen synthase. Glycogen also is acted on directly by a debranching enzyme which carries out the debranching process by first transferring an oligosaccharide from a branch point to leave a single 1,6-linked glucose residue and then hydrolyzing the 1,6 linkage. Thus the debrancher enzyme has both glucan transferase activity (oligo-1,4 $\rightarrow$ 1,4-transferase) and a glucosidase (amylo-1,6-glucosidase) activity and yields a single residue to glucose for each branch point removed. The Glc-1-P generated by phosphorylase, as mentioned above, must be further metabolized to Glc-6-P by phosphoglucomutase. In the liver, Glc-6-P is transported by a specific translocase to the inner surface of the endoplasmic reticulum for hydrolysis by Glc-6-P. The Glc-6-P system may require as many as six distinct proteins for proper function, including the catalytic protein, a Glc-6-P transport protein, and a phosphate transport protein. Free glucose derived from this system is able to exit the hepatic cell to maintain blood levels. Many genetic deficiencies occur in the enzymes required for the conversion of glycogen to free glucose in the liver, and these cause the hepatic-hypoglycemic forms of glycogen storage disease.

If glycogen is used as a direct energy source, as in muscle, Glc-6-P and Glc-1-P must enter the pathways for glycolysis. Again, numerous enzymes are required in muscle for proper breakdown of glycogen and entry into the glycolytic pathway and tricarboxylic acid cycle. The enzymatic steps associated with genetic deficiency states in muscle include muscle phosphorylase, debranching enzyme, muscle phosphofructokinase (PFK), and probably muscle phosphoglycerate mutase (PGAM) and lactate dehydrogenase (LDH) M subunit.

The lysosomal enzyme α-glucosidase, which is structurally and metabolically separate from the above-described pathways, is capable of degrading both 1,4 and 1,6 linkages in glycogen to give free glucose. This enzyme has widespread distribution in tissues, but its deficiency affects primarily skeletal and cardiac muscle.

CLASSIFICATION The clinical manifestations, diagnostic criteria, and therapy for glycogen storage diseases can be formulated in terms of the metabolic pathway outlined above (Table 350-1). According to this schema, two broad categories of disease can be delineated—those with a *hepatic-hypoglycemic* pathophysiology and those with a *muscle-energy* pathophysiology. Diseases with individualized pathophysiology also occur. It is suggested that disorders be designated by the specific protein deficiency, i.e., glucose-6-phosphatase deficiency. Although the roman numeral designations for types I through VII are in widespread use, numbering for higher types is confused and is to be avoided. Eponyms are of historical interest.

The hepatic-hypoglycemic disorders include glucose-6-phosphatase deficiency (type Ia), Glc-6-P microsomal translocase deficiency (type Ib), rarer type I subtypes, debrancher enzyme deficiency (type III), hepatic phosphorylase deficiency (type VI), and X-linked and autosomal forms of phosphorylase b kinase deficiency. Within this group, a distinction can be made between those disorders in which Glc-6-P and its metabolites are likely to be elevated (various forms of type I) and those disorders where Glc-6-P and related metabolites are likely to be decreased. This explains why increased glycolysis and lactic acidosis occur in type I disease but not in other forms of hepatic-hypoglycemic disease. Likewise, various forms of type I disease are distinct because gluconeogenesis, galactose, and fructose cannot contribute effectively to maintenance of blood sugar, in contrast to the other forms of hepatic-hypoglycemic disease. The glycemic response to epinephrine or glucagon tends to be blunted in the hepatic-hypoglycemic disorders. Dietary therapy with frequent feeding is a rational approach to the hepatic-hypoglycemic disorders and is tailored to reduce protein and to eliminate sources of galactose and fructose in type I disease.

The muscle-energy disorders include muscle phosphorylase deficiency (type V), phosphofructokinase deficiency (type VII), phosphoglycerate mutase deficiency, and LDH M-subunit deficiency. The clinical picture is one of muscle pain, myoglobinuria, and elevation of muscle enzymes in serum following vigorous exercise. The interruption of the pathway from glycogen to lactate with the accompanying failure to oxidize NADH is the unifying theme in these disorders. The failure of blood lactate to increase in response to exercise is a useful diagnostic test for the muscle-energy deficiency disorders. Debrancher enzyme deficiency constitutes an overlap syndrome; it presents primarily as a hepatic-hypoglycemic disorder in childhood, but serious muscle weakness occurs in some adults.

Two other disorders are best considered individually. Deficiency of lysosomal α-glucosidase is a lysosomal storage disease without major impact on either carbohydrate metabolism or maintenance of blood sugar (see Chap. 349). The major pathologic process in branching enzyme deficiency is a severe hepatic cirrhosis, possibly due to the harmful effects of the abnormal glycogen that accumulates. Glycogen content is generally normal, and the ability to maintain a normal blood sugar is not impaired.

HEPATIC-HYPOGLYCEMIC DISEASES Glucose-6-phosphatase deficiency, type Ia CLINICAL FEATURES Glucose-6-phosphatase deficiency, or von Gierke disease, is an autosomal recessive

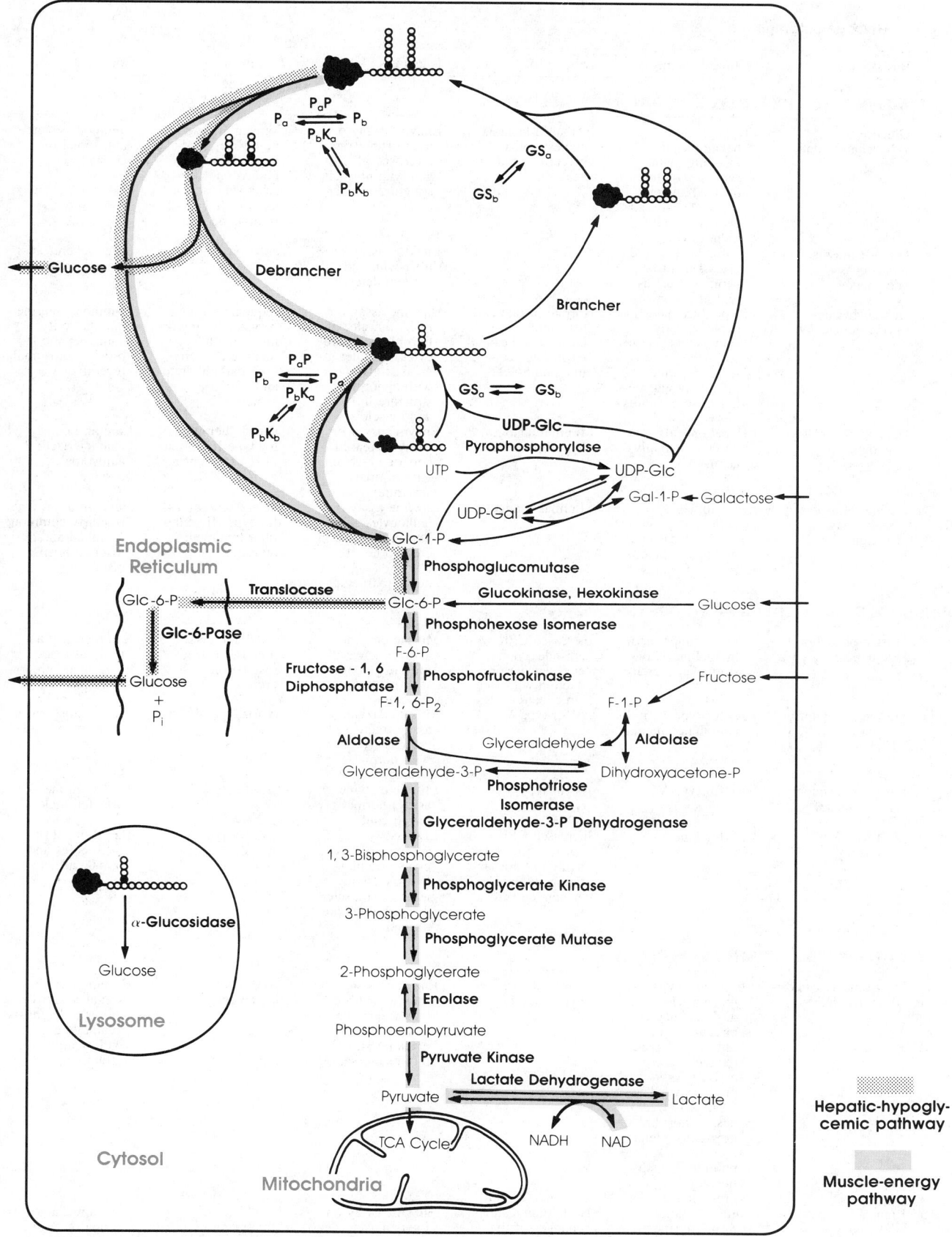

FIGURE 350-1 Metabolic pathways related to glycogen storage disease. A hypothetical composite cell is shown depicting both hepatic and muscle pathways. The shaded areas depict pathways that are blocked in the hepatic-hypoglycemic diseases or in the muscle-energy diseases. Nonstandard abbrevia-tions are as follows: GS_a, active glycogen synthase; GS_b, inactive glycogen synthase; P_a, active phosphorylase; P_b, inactive phosphorylase; P_aP, phosphorylase a phosphatase; P_bK_a, active phosphorylase b kinase; P_bK_b, inactive phosphorylase b kinase.

TABLE 350-1 Glycogen storage diseases

Type	Basic defect*	Clinical findings	Laboratory	Diagnosis	Treatment	Comments
DISORDERS WITH HEPATIC-HYPOGLYCEMIC PATHOPHYSIOLOGY						
Ia von Gierke	Glucose-6-phosphatase deficiency	Hypoglycemia, hepatomegaly, bleeding diathesis, short stature, delayed adolescence, hepatic adenomas, enlarged kidneys	Increased lactate, cholesterol, triglyceride, and uric acid	Enzyme assay on liver or intestine, increased glycogen with normal structure in liver	Cornstarch, and/or nighttime, feeding, 60–70% carbodhydrate, restrict sucrose and lactose, and allopurinol as needed	Common, severe, autosomal recessive
Ib	Glc-6-P microsomal translocase deficiency	As for Ia with addition of neutropenia and recurrent infection	As for Ia	Enzyme assay on liver with and without detergent	As for Ia	Rare, severe, autosomal recessive
III Cori	Debrancher enzyme deficiency	Hypoglycemia, hepatomegaly, some short stature and delayed adolescence, mild myopathy worsening in some adults	Normal lactate and uric acid; increased cholesterol, triglyceride, and SGOT	Enzyme assay on liver, muscle, or fibroblasts; leukocytes variable; increased glycogen with abnormal structure in liver and muscle	Frequent feeding, cornstarch, and/or nighttime tube feeding for some, 50% carbohydrate and 15–20% protein	Common, intermediate severity, some hepatic fibrosis, autosomal recessive
VI Hers	Hepatic phosphorylase deficiency	Hepatomegaly, variable hypoglycemia	Minimal changes, ? hyperlipidemia	Enzyme assay on liver, increased hepatic glycogen with normal structure	Dietary therapy as for type III, often little treatment required	Rare and poorly characterized; ? autosomal recessive
Formerly VIb, VIII, or IX	Hepatic phosphorylase b kinase deficiency	Hepatomegaly, variable hypoglycemia, occasional findings in heterozygous females	Minimal changes	Enzyme assay on leukocytes, fibroblasts, or liver; increased hepatic glycogen with normal structure	Dietary therapy as for type III, often little treatment required	Very mild but may be fairly common; X-linked and autosomal forms occur.
DISORDERS WITH MUSCLE-ENERGY PATHOPHYSIOLOGY						
V McArdle	Muscle phosphorylase deficiency	Pain, cramps, and mylgobinuria on strenuous exercise	Increased CPK with episodes, deficient lactate production with ischemic exercise test	Muscle enzyme assay, increased muscle glycogen with normal structure	Avoid exercise, glucose or fructose before exercise	Some clearly autosomal recessive, male preponderance
VII	Muscle phosphofructokinase deficiency	As for type V, mild hemolytic anemia	As for type V	Muscle enzyme assay, increased muscle glycogen with normal structure	As for type V	Rare, autosomal recessive
	Muscle phosphoglycerate mutase deficiency	As for type V	As for type V	Muscle enzyme assay, normal glycogen content	? As for type V	Based on one affected male
	LDH M-subunit deficiency	As for type V	Increased CPK with episodes; pyruvate but not lactate rises with ischemic exercise test	LDH isozymes on serum, erythrocytes or leukocytes; enzyme assay on muscle; ? glycogen content normal	? As for type V	Based on sibship of 3 males and 1 female affected
DISORDERS WITH INDIVIDUAL PATHOPHYSIOLOGY						
II Pompe	Lysosomal α-glucosidase deficiency	*Infantile:* hypotonia, muscle weakness, cardiac enlargement and failure, enlarged tongue, fatal early; *juvenile:* progressive skeletal muscle weakness; *adult:* progressive skeletal muscle weakness, pulmonary insufficiency presentation	Increased CPK, no hypoglycemia	Enzymes assay on muscle or fibroblasts, enzyme assay on leukocytes possible but pitfalls are serious	No effective treatment	Common, autosomal recessive, prenatal diagnosis available and widely utilized in infantile
VI Andersen	Brancher enzyme deficiency	Infantile failure to thrive, cirrhosis and liver failure, extreme hypotonia and weakness in some, fatal early	No hypoglycemia, changes of liver disease	Enzyme assay on liver, muscle, leukocytes or fibroblasts; glycogen content not remarkable but structure abnormal	No effective treatment	Very rare, autosomal recessive

* These defects provide the preferred nomenclature for the diseases.

genetic disorder with an incidence of 1 in 100,000 to 400,000. The disorder is usually manifested during the first 12 months of life by symptomatic hypoglycemia or by the recognition of hepatomegaly. Occasional patients experience hypoglycemia in the immediate neonatal period, and rare patients never have hypoglycemia. Characteristic findings include a full-cheeked, rounded facial appearance, a protuberant abdomen due to marked hepatomegaly, and thin extremities. Hyperlipidemia may cause eruptive xanthomas and lipemia retinalis. Splenomegaly is usually mild or absent, although massive enlargement of the left lobe of the liver may be mistaken for enlargement of the spleen. Growth is usually normal for the first few months of life; growth retardation then supervenes, and adolescence is delayed. Mental development is usually normal except for injury from hypoglycemia.

The characteristic profound symptomatic hypoglycemia may be associated with blood glucose levels below 0.8 mmol/L (15 mg/dL). Liver enzymes are mildly elevated if at all. The presence of lactic acidosis is helpful in diagnosing this disorder, although blood lactate may be normal in the fed state in young infants. However, these patients are relatively resistant to development of ketosis. Hyperlipidemia is frequent and involves elevation of both cholesterol and triglycerides. Hypertriglyceridemia can be extreme, with levels as high as 60 mmol/L (5000 mg/dL) or higher. Hyperuricemia due both to decreased renal excretion and increased production is frequent and often becomes more severe after adolescence. The rise in plasma glucose following administration of epinephrine or glucagon is impaired, as is the rise in blood glucose following administration of galactose by mouth. The pathogenesis of most of the metabolic abnormalities is not well understood; lactic acidosis may be due to increased glycolysis, and other abnormalities, including poor growth, may be the result of chronically altered levels of insulin and glucagon. Renal enlargement can be demonstrated by radiologic or sonographic techniques. Mild renal tubular dysfunction or the Fanconi syndrome may occur. Moderate anemia is usually due to recurrent nosebleeds and chronic acidosis but may become severe after prolonged acidosis. A bleeding diathesis is due to a platelet dysfunction.

Once type Ia disease is suspected clinically, the diagnosis is established by liver biopsy. Type Ia disease is suggested by lactic acidosis, an abnormal galactose tolerance test, or renal enlargement. Proper handling of biopsy material should be arranged to distinguish the various subtypes Ia, Ib, etc. Sufficient material for enzyme assay may be obtained by needle biopsy provided the bleeding time is normal, or alternatively, open liver biopsy provides more tissue for analysis. Microscopic examination of liver reveals increased glycogen in cytoplasm and nuclei; lipid vacuoles in hepatocytes are prominent, and fibrosis is usually absent.

The hypoglycemia and lactic acid acidosis may be life-threatening. Other troublesome features include short stature, delayed adolescence, and hyperuricemia. During adult years, uric acid nephropathy and glomerulosclerosis may lead to renal failure. Hepatic adenomata are common after adolescence. There is a significant risk of hepatic malignant degeneration, often during the third decade, and subjects who live long enough may be at increased risk for atherosclerosis.

TREATMENT The mainstay of management is frequent feeding. The most widely used approach in children has been the combination of frequent daytime feeding by mouth and continuous nighttime feeding by nasogastric tube (see Chap. 75). The regimen should include approximately 60 percent carbohydrate, and no significant portion of carbohydrate should come from sources containing galactose or fructose, which cannot be utilized effectively to maintain blood sugar. Uncooked cornstarch feeding provides a convenient, economical, and palatable source of slowly digested glucose polymer, and cornstarch therapy has become an important form of dietary treatment for this disease. The ability of a family to carry out such a program is a significant variable, but in some instances the metabolic abnormalities and the rate of growth have improved substantially. Optimal management requires a team attentive to the dietary and psychosocial needs of patient and family. Control of elevated plasma urate may require the addition of allopurinol. This regimen provides a reasonably optimistic short-term prognosis, and limited long-term follow-up data indicate that the risk of malignancy may be reduced. Portacaval anastomosis is no longer used in the management of glycogen storage disease. Prenatal diagnosis is not possible at present except by fetal liver biopsy.

Glc-6-P microsomal translocase deficiency, type Ib Glc-6-P microsomal translocase deficiency, historically referred to as *pseudo type I*, has an incidence of one-fifth to one-tenth that of type Ia. The term *microsomal translocase* describes the capacity to transport Glc-6-P into the endoplasmic reticulum. The clinical features are similar to those in type Ia, but unique features include neutropenia, impaired neutrophil migration, and recurrent pyogenic infections; in general, type Ib is more severe than Ia. Laboratory findings, responses to tolerance tests, and management are similar in the two disorders.

Type Ib disease was initially distinguished from type Ia by the presence of normal glucose-6-phosphatase activity on assay of biopsy tissue in the presence of detergent. However, glucose-6-phosphatase activity is low in type Ib disease when fresh tissue is homogenized and assayed in the absence of detergent. These results have been interpreted to imply a genetic deficiency of a microsomal Glc-6-P transport system as a primary defect in type Ib glycogen storage disease. The cause for the neutropenia and abnormal neutrophil migration is unknown, although the disease suggests a role for Glc-6-P transport in these cells.

Debrancher deficiency, type III CLINICAL FEATURES Debrancher enzyme deficiency, also known historically as *Cori disease*, is an autosomal recessive disorder and is one of the more frequent forms of glycogen storage diseases, occurring with a particularly high frequency in North African Jews. Symptomatic disease in the newborn period is unusual, and patients usually present with hypoglycemia or hepatomegaly during the first year of life. The physical findings are similar to those in type Ia, except that splenomegaly is more prominent, but the clinical course tends to be less severe. The skeletal or cardiac myopathy is usually mild or insignificant in childhood but may be disabling and progressive in adults. Some patients with myopathy are first diagnosed as adults because the features in childhood were mild and overlooked. Patients with enzyme deficiency in both liver and muscle are sometimes classified as type IIIa and those free of muscle involvement as type IIIb, but the molecular basis for the tissue specificity is unknown, since there is evidence for a single gene.

Fasting hypoglycemia occurs in about 80 percent of patients. The glucose response after glucagon or epinephrine is abnormal in the fasting state but may be normal shortly after eating because the terminal glucose residues in glycogen can be mobilized. The galactose tolerance test is usually normal. Ketosis is prominent, and blood lactate is normal. Serum transaminase is elevated, and further increases may occur with minor illnesses. Blood cholesterol and triglyceride are elevated in about two-thirds. Hyperuricemia is rare.

Two diagnostic modalities are used to establish the diagnosis—analysis of glycogen and measurement of debranching enzyme in tissue samples. The glycogen content of red blood cells and liver is increased in almost all, whereas glycogen content of muscle is increased only in some. Documentation of abnormal structure of glycogen with the use of spectrophotometric techniques is a more consistent finding than the increase in glycogen content. The establishment of the diagnosis by enzymatic assay is complicated by both methodologic problems and genetic heterogeneity. Both debrancher functions—the glucan transferase activity and glucosidase activity—are believed to reside in a single polypeptide, but various subtypes of the disease have been described. While the diagnosis can be made in some patients using red cells, leukocytes, or fibroblasts, it is generally preferable to document the abnormal glycogen structure and the enzyme deficiency directly in biopsy material from liver or muscle. The pathologic findings in liver are similar to those in type Ia except for less lipid deposition and more prominent fibrous septae.

With regard to growth retardation and abdominal protuberance, the course is one of progressive improvement following adolescence so that the adult appearance may be normal and hypoglycemia is less frequent. Liver tumors are not reported, and there is no information regarding the long-term risks of hyperlipidemia. The fraction of adult patients who develop a debilitating myopathy is probably low. Affected patients have had children.

TREATMENT   Frequent feeding is also the mainstay of therapy for type III in childhood. Gluconeogenesis is normal, and as described above, patients can ingest galactose, fructose, or protein to help maintain blood glucose. Thus dietary therapy can include a larger percentage of calories as protein, but carbohydrate intake should be 40 to 50 percent of the total. An evening feeding is often sufficient to avoid hypoglycemia, but nighttime nasogastric tube feeding or cornstarch therapy may be required in severely affected children. Attempts to lower blood lipids using dietary means are desirable. Prenatal diagnosis is possible.

Hepatic phosphorylase deficiency, type VI   The diagnosis of hepatic phosphorylase deficiency, or Hers disease, was previously applied to a diverse group of patients with reduced hepatic phosphorylase levels due to a variety of causes but is now limited to patients in whom deficiency of hepatic phosphorylase is the primary defect. This nosologic difficulty is a consequence of the fact that phosphorylase exists in both active and inactive forms, and many factors may inhibit activation of the enzyme secondarily. Consequently, diagnosis requires documentation that hepatic phosphorylase is deficient and that the phosphorylase *b* kinase responsible for its activation is normal. The disorder is probably due to an autosomal recessive mutation.

Most patients have features similar to those in type III but in a milder form. The diagnosis is suspected because of hepatomegaly or hypoglycemia, and patients generally respond to dietary management similar to that employed in type III disease.

Phosphorylase *b* kinase deficiency   Phosphorylase *b* kinase deficiency, now known to be a separate entity, was previously included in the type VI category. Various authors have designated this disorder as type VIa, type VIII, or type IX, but it is best termed *phosphorylase b kinase deficiency*. The best-characterized form of the disorder is the X-linked variety, but there is potential for genetic heterogeneity, since the enzyme is composed of four nonidentical subunits, and since autosomal recessive forms of the disorder have been described. This disorder is relatively benign and is manifested in affected males by hepatomegaly, occasional fasting hypoglycemia, and some growth retardation, all of which tend to resolve spontaneously at the time of adolescence. Mild hepatomegaly may occur in female heterozygotes. The diagnosis can be established by specific enzyme assay of leukocytes or liver. Muscle phosphorylase *b* kinase is believed to be normal in this condition. Dietary management similar to that employed in type III can be employed for hypoglycemia or growth retardation. It is possible that this condition is relatively common and passes undiagnosed. Healthy adults with a history of abdominal protuberance in childhood are often identified during family studies of patients with this condition.

MUSCLE-ENERGY DISEASES (See also Chap. 385)   In recognizing the various glycogen storage diseases that affect muscle, the *ischemic exercise test* is of particular use in the initial evaluation. A blood pressure cuff is inflated above arterial pressure, and the ischemic hand is exercised to maximum effort. The pressure cuff is released, and blood is drawn from the other arm at 2, 5, 10, 20, and 30 min for assay of lactate and pyruvate, muscle enzymes, and myoglobin.

Myophosphorylase deficiency, type V   Myophosphorylase deficiency, or McArdle disease, is uncommon. Symptoms of pain and cramps after exercise usually develop during the second or third decade. A history of myoglobinuria is present in most, and on occasion myoglobinuria can cause renal failure. Affected individuals are otherwise healthy, without evidence of hepatic, cardiac, or metabolic disturbance. Performance of an ischemic exercise test usually causes painful cramping, which is helpful diagnostically. In addition, blood lactate does not rise, whereas serum creatine

phosphokinase usually is elevated at rest but rises substantially after strenuous exercise.

The diagnosis is established by documentation of elevated glycogen content and reduced phosphorylase activity in biopsied muscle tissue. The glycogen is usually deposited in subsarcolemmal regions of the muscle. The gene for human myophosphorylase has been cloned and is located on chromosome 11, in keeping with the autosomal recessive nature of the disease. There is an excess of male patients, which may be due to better ascertainment in males, genetic heterogeneity, or other factors. A fatal infantile form of hypotonia in association with myophosphorylase deficiency also has been described.

Management of myophosphorylase deficiency requires the avoidance of strenuous exercise. Glucose or fructose ingestion prior to exercise can reduce symptoms.

Muscle phosphofructokinase deficiency, type VII   There are two genetically distinct forms of phosphofructokinase. Activity in muscle is due to a distinct muscle isoenzyme, whereas activity in red cells is due both to a red cell isoenzyme and to the muscle form of the enzyme. A small number of families have been identified with deficiency of the muscle isoenzyme. Symptoms similar to those in myophosphorylase deficiency were present with pain and cramps, myoglobinuria, and elevated muscle enzymes in serum after strenuous exercise. Lactate production was impaired, and a mild nonspherocytic hemolytic anemia was present. Other patients have the anemia but no muscle symptoms; the latter phenomenon might be due to a qualitatively abnormal, unstable enzyme that rapidly disappears from the anucleate red cell but is replaced effectively in muscle cells and consequently prevents muscle symptoms.

Other muscle-energy diseases   A group of even rarer familial metabolic disorders must be considered in the differential diagnosis of patients with myoglobinuria and elevated muscle enzymes in serum after exercise. These include phosphoglycerate mutase deficiency, LDH M-subunit deficiency, and carnitine palmityl transferase deficiency. (Older reports of phosphoglucomutase deficiency and phosphohexoseisomerase deficiency seem inconclusive by current standards.) When myophosphorylase, phosphofructokinase, or phosphoglycerate mutase are deficient, neither lactate nor pyruvate rises following exercise, whereas in deficiency of LDH M subunit there is a rise in pyruvate in the face of a failure of lactate production. Carnitine palmityl transferase deficiency is a disorder of lipid metabolism and is discussed in Chap. 338. Definitive diagnosis of these disorders must be established by enzyme assay of muscle tissue. Some patients with this clinical presentation have none of the above-mentioned enzyme deficiencies, and identification of other defects in muscle metabolism is likely in the future.

DISORDERS WITH INDIVIDUAL PATHOPHYSIOLOGY α-Glucosidase deficiency, type II   Alpha-glucosidase deficiency, or Pompe disease, is a lysosomal storage disease, and the pathophysiology is discussed in Chap. 349. The incidence is not known but may exceed 1 in 100,000. The disorder is not associated with hypoglycemia, ketosis, or other abnormalities of intermediary metabolism.

The infantile form presents within the first 6 months of life and may be manifested at birth. Clinical features include skeletal muscle hypotonia and weakness, massive cardiac enlargement, enlargement of the tongue, and varying degrees of hepatomegaly. Muscle enzymes such as creatine phosphokinase and aldolase are usually elevated, and the ECG may show large QRS complexes and a shortened PR interval. Motor weakness and developmental delay may be present. Death occurs in the first 2 to 3 years in most cases due to the cardiac involvement.

The juvenile form has features suggestive of a progressive form of muscular dystrophy. These patients have gait abnormalities but no cardiac symptoms. Plasma creatine phosphokinase and aldolase are elevated, and the length of survival is variable. An even milder adult form presents as skeletal muscle weakness in the third to the fifth decade. Again, cardiac symptoms are absent, and serum muscle enzymes are elevated. Some patients have respiratory failure due to involvement of the muscles of respiration and are often misdiagnosed as having some form of muscular dystrophy.

Vacuolization of muscle and increased glycogen content are demonstrable on muscle biopsy. Electron-microscopic studies demonstrate membrane-bound vacuoles containing glycogen, a finding strongly suggestive of the disorder. Excessive glycogen is also found in other tissues, including liver and central nervous system, particularly in the anterior horn cells of the spinal cord. Specific diagnosis is made by enzyme assay in biopsy material from muscle or liver or in cultured skin fibroblasts. In general, some residual enzyme activity is present in patients with the adult form of disease, but the exact level is not of prognostic significance. Prenatal diagnosis is reliable and has been used extensively for the infantile form. Various forms of enzyme infusion therapy have been tried but are ineffective.

Brancher deficiency, type IV   Brancher enzyme deficiency, or Andersen disease, is a rare, autosomal recessive disorder. Features in infants include hepatomegaly, failure to thrive, and hypotonia in the first few months of life with subsequent development of progressive cirrhosis. In other patients the predominant feature is cardiac involvement and/or extreme hypotonia similar to that observed in spinal muscular atrophy and anterior horn cell degeneration. Death usually occurs within the first 2 or 3 years, although a more benign course is possible.

The symptoms are thought to be related primarily to the abnormal glycogen structure that results from a generalized deficiency of brancher enzyme. The presence of long outer chains on the glycogen molecules has led to the designation of the disease as amylopectinosis. The laboratory findings are generally those associated with severe liver disease except that hypoglycemia usually does not occur. The absence of hypoglycemia and the presence of normal glycogen content in the liver make the diagnosis difficult to establish. The diagnosis is suggested by finding abnormally structured glycogen in biopsy material and is established by direct assay of the enzyme in liver, leukocytes, or cultured skin fibroblasts. No effective metabolic treatment is known, although liver transplantation has been performed. Prenatal diagnosis is possible using cultured amniotic cells.

Other possible disorders of glycogen metabolism   Deficiency of glycogen synthase has been reported in a small number of families. Affected patients usually have fasting hypoglycemia, seizures, and some degree of mental impairment. The presence of some hepatic glycogen, the increase in plasma glucose in response to glucagon or galactose, and the known lability of the activation system for glycogen synthase have all led to skepticism as to whether such a disorder actually exists. This syndrome may be confused with ketotic hypoglycemia of childhood (see Chap. 338).

There are also reports of more than one enzyme defect in the same patient and of different enzyme defects among siblings. Many of these reports may be related to difficulties inherent in measuring enzymes of glycogen metabolism in human pathologic tissue. At present no specific syndrome of multiple primary enzyme deficiency is documented.

REFERENCES

CHEN Y-T, BURCHELL A: Glycogen storage disease, in *The Molecular and Metabolic Basis of Inherited Disease*, 7th ed, CR Scriver et al (eds). New York, McGraw-Hill, in press

FERNANDES J et al: The glycogen storage diseases, in *Inborn Metabolic Diseases*, J. Fernandes et al (eds). Berlin, Springer-Verlag, 1990, p 69

SERVIDEI S, DiMAURO S: Disorders of glycogen metabolism of muscle. Neurol Clin 7:159, 1989

WOLFSDORF J et al: Glucose therapy for glycogenosis type 1 in infants: Comparison of intermittent uncooked cornstarch and continuous overnight glucose feedings. J Pediatr 117:384, 1990

351   HERITABLE DISORDERS OF CONNECTIVE TISSUE

DARWIN J. PROCKOP / HELENA KUIVANIEMI / GERARD TROMP

Heritable disorders that involve the major connective tissues of the body such as bone, skin, cartilage, blood vessels, and basement membranes are among the most common genetic diseases in human beings. Discoveries made over the last decade or so have expanded the number of such diseases so that they now include many clinical entities that were not previously recognized as either involving specific components of connective tissue or being genetically transmitted. Here we will focus primarily on the heritable disorders of connective tissue that can have severe manifestations, that are relatively common, and that are sufficiently understood at the molecular level to provide useful paradigms for a number of related diseases. Therefore, we will focus on osteogenesis imperfecta (OI), the Ehlers-Danlos syndrome (EDS), chondrodysplasias (CDs), the Marfan syndrome (MS), epidermolysis bullosa (EB), and the Alport syndrome (AS).

THE CHALLENGE OF CLASSIFYING THE DISEASES   The first comprehensive effort to classify diseases of connective tissue was made by McKusick in a series of reports and then in a monograph entitled *Heritable Disorders of Connective Tissue*, in which he drew attention to patients and families with connective tissue disorders in whom the changes appeared to be inherited as single-gene traits. He subsequently expanded the classification to include more than 12 major heritable diseases of connective tissue that were likely to be caused by single-gene defects on the basis of the pattern of inheritance, the cluster of signs and symptoms, the histologic changes in tissues, and limited information about the molecular defects in the tissues themselves. This classification was further developed and extended by a large number of investigators so that about a dozen types and subtypes were defined for OI, about the same number for the EDS, and over 150 for CDs.

For some of the original disease categories, most patients with the classical features of the disease have a mutation in a gene or genes coding for a single protein. For example, over 90 percent of patients with OI have a mutation in one of the two genes coding for type I procollagen. Similarly, most patients with MS have mutations in a gene for fibrillin. For other disease categories, the situation is more complex. In EDS, for example, most patients with the type IV variant have mutations in the gene for type III procollagen, most patients with the type VI variant have defects in the gene for the enzyme lysyl hydroxylase, and most patients with the type VII variant have defects that interfere with the processing of type I procollagen to type I collagen. Several limitations in the original classifications are now apparent.

One is that the same mutation in a gene does not always produce the same disease phenotype in terms of severity of the condition or its clinical course. Such phenotypic variation occurs in many genetic diseases, including the connective tissue disorders, in which some affected members of a family are severely affected, whereas others with the same gene mutation have a mild disorder.

Systems for classifying heritable disorders of connective tissue also probably overemphasize the etiologic differences between severe genetic diseases that are apparent in infants and the far more common diseases that appear much later in life. Single-gene defects may cause subsets of late-onset diseases such as osteoporosis, aneurysms, and osteoarthritis. For example, a small subset of patients with postmenopausal osteoporosis have mutations in the genes for procollagen I similar to the mutations in the same genes that produce lethal variants of OI. Also, a small subset of patients with familial aortic aneurysms have mutations in the gene for procollagen III similar to the mutations in the same gene that cause lethal variants of type IV

EDS, and a subset of patients with primary generalized osteoarthritis have mutations in the gene for procollagen II similar to the mutations in the same gene that cause lethal CDs. At the moment, there is still disagreement as to the best diagnosis for such patients in that some clinical investigators feel that after a mutation similar to those seen in the early-onset diseases is identified, the patients should be reclassified as having mild forms of OI, EDS, or CD even though they did not have definitive evidence of the early-onset diseases or seek medical attention until they were adults. The debate is fueled by the fact that many of the clinical classifications are based on variable clusters of signs and symptoms for which there are few objective criteria. However, some patients with late-onset diseases of connective tissue such as osteoporosis, osteoarthritis, and aneurysms inherit the disorders in a manner consistent with single-gene defects. Therefore, it may be necessary to expand greatly the category of diseases currently referred to as heritable disorders of connective tissues.

DEFINITION AND COMPOSITION OF CONNECTIVE TISSUES

The connective tissues are composed of distinctive macromolecules, many of which are also major constituents of the lung, the kidney, the walls of blood vessels, the vitreous gel of the eye, and the synovial fluid. Also, essentially all organs and tissues contain small amounts of the same macromolecules assembled into membranes and septa. Therefore, most of these structures are now regarded as connective tissues.

The distinguishing feature of connective tissues, however, is that they contain specific macromolecules that are assembled into an insoluble extracellular matrix (Table 351-1). The macromolecules include at least 18 different types of collagens, the related fiber-associated proteins known as *elastin* and *fibrillin*, a series of proteoglycans, and components whose structure and function have been only partially defined.

Differences in the connective tissues of bone, skin, and cartilage are in part explained by differences in their content of specific components (see Table 351-1). For example, tendons and ligaments consist primarily of type I collagen fibrils associated with small amounts of other components that probably help organize the type I collagen fibrils into larger fibers and fiber bundles. Cartilage consists primarily of fibrils of type II collagen in the form of arcade-like structures that are distended by the presence of highly charged proteoglycans. The extracellular matrix of large blood vessels such as the aorta contains collagens that provide tensile strength and elastin that provides elasticity. Differences among the connective tissues also depend on the three-dimensional organization of the molecular components. The type I collagen fibrils in tendon are packed into thick, parallel bundles of fibers. In skin, fibrils of the same type I collagen are randomly oriented in the plane of the skin. In cortical bone, type I collagen fibrils are deposited in intricate helical arrays around haversian canals.

BIOSYNTHESIS OF CONNECTIVE TISSUE

Assembly of the connective tissues is largely governed by the principle of self-assembly, whereby a molecular subunit of the correct size, shape, and surface properties binds to other molecules with the same structure, or with similar structures, in a spontaneous but ordered manner. The molecular mechanisms and driving forces are similar to those involved in the formation of large crystals from supersaturated solutions.

The principle of self-assembly in connective tissue is best illustrated by the assembly of collagen into fibrils. The molecule of a fibril-forming collagen is a long, thin rod consisting of three polypeptide α chains that are wrapped into a rigid, ropelike triple helix (Fig. 351-1). The molecule has a triple-helical conformation, because each of the three α chains has a simple, repetitive amino acid sequence of about 1000 amino acids in which glycine (Gly) appears as every third amino acid. Therefore, the sequence of each α chain can be designated as $(-Gly-X-Y-)_{333}$, where X and Y represent amino acids other than glycine. To fold into a triple helix, it is essential that every third amino acid in an α chain is glycine, the smallest amino acid, since this residue must fit in a sterically restricted space where the three chains of the triple helix come together. Many of the X- and Y-position amino acids are the ring amino acids proline and hydroxyproline that give rigidity to the triple-helical structure. The remaining X- and Y-position amino acids form clusters of hydrophobic and charged regions on the surface of the molecule that direct how one molecule

---

TABLE 351-1   Constituents of various connective tissues

Connective tissue	Known constituents	Approximate amounts (% dry wt)	Characteristics or functions
Skin, ligaments, tendons	Type I collagen	80	Bundles of fibrils
	Type III collagen	5–15	Thin fibrils
	Type IV collagen, laminin, nidogen	<5	In basal laminae under epithelium and in blood vessels
	Types V, VI, and VII collagens	<5	Functions unclear
	Elastin, fibrillin	<5	Provide elasticity
	Fibronectin	<5	Associated with collagen fibers and cell surfaces
	Proteoglycans* and hyaluronate	0.5	Provide resiliency
Bone (demineralized)	Type I collagen	90	Complex fibril network
	Type VI collagen	1–2	Function unclear
	Proteoglycans	1	Function unclear
	Osteonectin, osteocalcin, osteopontin, α2-glycoprotein, sialoproteins	1–5	Probably initial or regulate mineralization
Aorta	Type I collagen	20–40	Fibril network
	Type III collagen	20–40	Thin fibrils
	Elastin, fibrillin	20–40	Provide elasticity
	Type IV collagen, laminin, nidogen	<5	Form basal lamina
	Types V and VI collagens	<2	Functions unclear
	Proteoglycans	<3	Provide resiliency
Cartilage	Type II collagen	40–50	Arcades of thin fibrils
	Type IX collagen	5–10	Links type II fibrils
	Type X collagen	5–10	Surrounds hypertrophic cells
	Type XI collagen	<10	Function unclear
	Proteoglycans and hyaluronate	15–50	Provide resiliency

* As discussed in text, at least five proteoglycans have now been identified. They differ in the structures of their core proteins and their contents of mucopolysaccharide side chains of chondroitin-4-sulfate, chondroitin-6-sulfate, dermatan sulfate, and keratin sulfate. Basil lamina contain a proteoglycan with a side chain of heparan sulfate that resembles heparin.

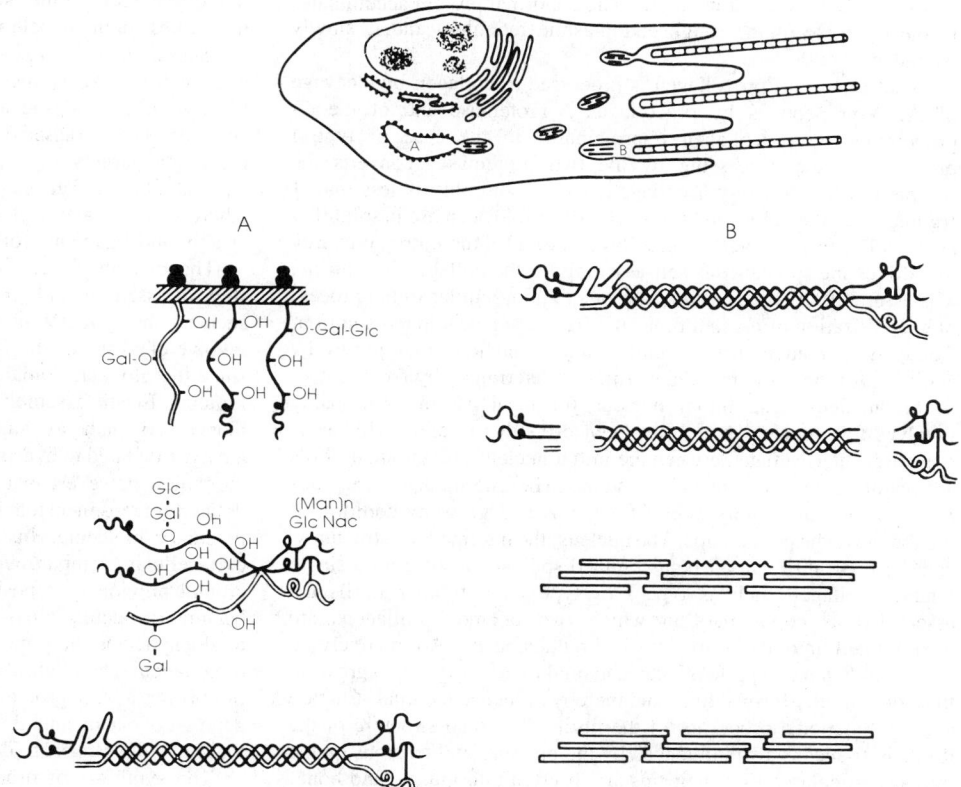

FIGURE 351-1 Schematic representation of synthesis of a type I collagen fibril by a fibroblast. *A*. Intracellular steps in the assembly of the procollagen molecule. Hydroxylations and glycosylations of the proα chains begin soon after the amino termini pass into the cisternae of the rough endoplasmic reticulum and continue after the three chains associate through their carboxy-terminal propeptides and become disulfide linked. *B*. Cleavage of procollagen to collagen, self-assembly of the collagen molecule into quarter-staggered fibrils, and cross-linking of the molecules in the fibrils. Cleavage of the propeptides may occur within crypts of the fibroblast, as shown here, or some distance from the cell. *(From DJ Prockop and KI Kivirikko. Used with permission.)*

spontaneously binds to other collagen molecules and thereby self-assembles into the large collagen fibrils found in tissues (see Fig. 351-1).

More than 18 different collagens have been identified. Most are minor constituents that probably have highly specialized functions. About one-third of fibrillar collagens are found in tissues as long, highly ordered fibrils with a characteristic banding pattern by electron microscopy. Type I collagen is the most abundant and is found as cross-striated fibrils in a large number of tissues (see Table 351-1). It is composed of two identical α chains called α1(I) and one α2(I) chain. Type II collagen, a similar fibrillar collagen in cartilage, is composed of three identical´ chains called α1(II). Type III collagen, the third most abundant fibrillar collagen, is found in smaller amounts in many tissues that contain type I collagen and in large amounts in large blood vessels and is composed of three identical chains called α1(III). The nonfibrillar collagens are similar to the fibrillar collagens in that they contain -Gly-X-Y- sequences of amino acids that form triple-helical domains, but they also contain large globular domains. Self-assembly of most of the nonfibrillar collagens usually involves binding together of the globular domains to form network-like structures. For example, the type IV collagen in basement membranes self-assembles into a complex three-dimensional network that provides a diffusion barrier in the renal glomerulus and pulmonary alveolus and provides support for epithelial and endothelial cells in these tissues and in skin, the gastrointestinal tract, and blood vessels.

Because fibrillar collagens spontaneously self-assemble into fibrils, they are first synthesized as larger and more soluble precursors called *procollagens*. The procollagen forms of type I, II, and III collagens are 1.5 times the mass of the corresponding collagens due to the presence of amino acid sequences that are called *propeptides* and are located at both the *N* terminus and the *C* terminus of the proα chains of the procollagens.

The biosynthesis of procollagens involves a large number of intracellular processing steps (see Fig. 351-1) and an unusual self-assembly whereby the three chains fold into a triple-helical conforma-

tion. As the proα chains of procollagen are translated from mRNAs on ribosomes, they pass into the cisternae of the rough endoplasmic reticulum. Hydrophobic signal peptides at the *N* terminus are cleaved, and a series of additional posttranslational reactions begin. Proline residues in the Y position of the repeating -Gly-X-Y- sequences are converted to hydroxyproline by prolyl hydroxylase, requiring oxygen, iron, and ascorbic acid. Lysine residues in the Y position are similarly hydroxylated to hydroxylysine by a specific lysyl hydroxylase. Many of the hydroxylysine residues are further modified by glycosylation with galactose or with galactose and glucose. A large mannose-rich oligosaccharide is assembled on the *C*-terminal propeptide of each chain. As the last amino acids are incorporated into the proα chains, they are released into the cisternae of the rough endoplasmic reticulum. At this stage two proα1(I) and one proα2(I) chains associated through their *C*-propeptides. The association of the proα chains is directed by the structure and the surface properties of the globular *C*-propeptides. After the *C*-propeptides assemble correctly, the structure is locked in place by the formation of interchain disulfide bonds. Posttranslational modifications of the proα chains continue until each chain acquires a critical level of about 100 hydroxyproline residues. Then a few of the -Gly-X-Y- sequences at the *C* terminus of the protein that are very rich in hydroxyproline fold into a triple-helical conformation. The short region of triple helix becomes a nucleus for self-assembly of the triple helix of the whole protein, much like a nucleus for crystallization, in that the triple-helical conformation in one -Gly-X-Y- sequence induces the next -Gly-X-Y- sequence to fold into the same conformation. As a result, the conformation is propagated in a zipper-like fashion from the *C* terminus to the *N* terminus of the molecule and the entire α-chain domain becomes a continuous triple helix. Once the protein is folded, it passes from the rough endoplasmic reticulum to other membranous compartments and is secreted. The requirement for ascorbic acid in the hydroxylation of prolyl residues by prolyl hydroxylase explains why wounds fail to heal in scurvy (see Chap. 72). If a sufficient number of proline residues are not converted to hydroxyproline, the protein cannot fold into a triple helix that is stable at body temperature. The abnormal protein accumulates in the cisternae of the rough endoplasmic reticulum and is slowly degraded.

After secretion, procollagen is processed to collagen by cleavage of the N-propeptides by procollagen N-proteinase and of the C-propeptides by procollagen C-proteinase. In the case of type I procollagen, the processing by the two proteinases converts the soluble precursor to type I collagen, whose solubility is less than 1 μg/mL under the same conditions. The 1000-fold decrease in solubility as procollagen is converted to collagen provides the entropic energy that drives the spontaneous self-assembly of the collagen into fibrils. The assembly of collagen into fibrils is, again, similar to the process of crystallization of a small molecule from a supersaturated solution. Collagen monomers first assemble into a nucleus that grows by addition of monomers in a manner that is determined by the structure of the nucleus. The initial nucleus for fibril assembly probably involves few molecules and has been difficult to define. However, structures intermediate between the initial nucleus and the final fibrils are readily detected in in vitro systems. The intermediate structures have pointed and highly symmetrical tips and grow by addition of monomers to the pointed tips. The nucleus, the intermediate structures, and the final fibril can all be assembled spontaneously from a single kind of collagen such as type I or type II, but other fibrils are assembled as copolymers in which two or more collagens are incorporated into the same fibril simultaneously. Alternatively, a second collagen or a proteoglycan can bind to the surface of a growing fibril or to a fully formed fibril and thereby influence the final structure and the functional properties of the fibrils. The final structure of the fibrils in tissues is also influenced by the pressure and tensions on the fibrils, particularly after their tips are inserted into muscle and bone. The tension on tendons, for example, probably makes the thin fibrils that are initially assembled to coalesce into large fiber bundles. The initial self-assembly of collagen into fibrils, however, involves a large number of specific interactions along the surface of each rodlike molecule and therefore can only be altered by molecules that bind either to the surface of the large, rodlike monomer or to the surfaces of the growing fibrils. For this reason, assembly of collagen fibrils is less subject to influence of other components than the crystallization of small molecules.

Self-assembled collagen fibers have considerable tensile strength, and the strength is increased by cross-linking reactions that form covalent bonds between α chains in one molecule and α chains in adjacent molecules. The first step in cross-linking is oxidation by lysyl oxidase of amino groups on a few lysine or hydroxylysine residues to form aldehydes. The aldehydes then interact to form a complex series of stable covalent bonds that may or may not involve enzymic reactions.

Collagen fibers in most tissues of normal adults undergo very little metabolic turnover. One exception to this is the collagen fibrils that undergo repeated degradation and synthesis as part of the continual remodeling of bone. During growth and development, however, the collagen fibrils in all tissues undergo repeated synthesis, degradation, and resynthesis. The degradation of collagen fibers in tissues is initiated by collagenase in leukocytes, fibroblasts, synovial cells, or related cell types. The collagenases cleave the collagen molecule at a point about three-quarters of the distance from its N terminus. The cleavage apparently triggers unfolding of the molecules on the surface of a fibril and further degradation by other proteinases.

Although the collagen in many adult tissues is metabolically stable, the turnover changes under some circumstances. In starvation, a large fraction of the collagen in skin and other connective tissues is degraded, thus providing amino acids for gluconeogenesis. Large losses of collagen also occur in most connective tissues during immobilization or prolonged periods of low-gravitational stress. In rheumatoid arthritis, pannus invasion of articular cartilage causes a rapid degradation of the collagen in the tissue, and prolonged or excessive treatment with glucocorticoids decreases the collagen content of most connective tissues, including bone, by decreasing the

rate of collagen synthesis. The decreases in collagen content weaken the tissues. In many pathologic states, however, collagen is deposited in excess. With injury to any tissue, the inflammatory response is usually followed by increased deposition of collagen fibrils in the form of fibrotic tissue and scars that primarily consist of type I collagen. The increased deposition of collagen fibrils during the repair process is largely irreversible and therefore is a major feature of the pathologic changes in hepatic cirrhosis, pulmonary fibrosis, atherosclerosis, and nephrosclerosis and in the scarring in tissues such as skin and ligaments following surgery or trauma.

The biosynthesis of all collagens involves essentially the same steps of assembly and processing. Assembly of nonfibrillar collagens such as the type IV of basement membranes does not, however, involve cleavage of the globular domains at the ends of the protein, since the globular domains are required for the self-assembly of the proteins. Elastin assembly appears to be closely related to the collagen biosynthetic pathway, since a few of the prolyl residues in the protein are hydroxylated to hydroxyproline by prolyl hydroxylase. The elastin monomer, however, is a single polypeptide that does not fold into a defined three-dimensional structure and is not synthesized as a larger precursor molecule. Instead, it is slowly secreted from cells into extracellular compartments, where it forms amorphous deposits around previously deposited microfibrils. The elastin deposits then become covalently cross-linked through oxidation of lysine residues to aldehydes by the same lysyl oxidase that initiates the cross-linking of collagen. The microfibrils in elastin deposits are largely composed of fibrillin, a large protein that forms beadlike strands. The amorphous deposits of elastin and fibrillin also may contain additional components that have not yet been identified.

The synthesis of proteoglycans begins with assembly of a core protein in the cisternae of the rough endoplasmic reticulum. The core protein then undergoes modifications by a series of sugar and sulfate transferases that generate large side chains of glycosaminoglycans. At least five proteoglycans have been identified by differences in the structures of their core proteins. The major proteoglycan of cartilage, called *aggrecan*, has a core protein of about 2000 amino acids to which are bound multiple side chains of chondroitin sulfate and keratin sulfate, distinctive mucopolysaccharides consisting of highly charged and repetitive disaccharide sequences. After secretion from cells, the aggrecan monomer binds to a smaller protein called a *link protein*. The complex of core protein and link protein then spontaneously binds to a long chain of hyaluronic acid to form a huge copolymer called a *proteoglycan aggregate*. The large and highly charged proteoglycan aggregate binds water and small ions and thereby provides a large swelling pressure and resiliency to cartilage. Smaller proteoglycans such as decorin, biglycan, and fibromodulin have smaller core proteins with somewhat different mucopolysaccharide side chains. They do not form large aggregates with hyaluronate but bind to fibrils of collagens or fibronectin and may thereby help regulate the assembly of fibrils or their spatial orientation. One group of small proteoglycans known as *syndecans* are bound to the plasma membranes of cells and may have a role in migration of cells along fibrils or in signal transduction.

The assembly of bone follows much the same principles as the assembly of other connective tissues (see also Chap. 356). The first step is deposition of osteoid tissue that consists largely of type I collagen fibrils (see Fig. 351-1). Mineralization of osteoid occurs by steps that are still incompletely defined; proteins such as osteopontin and osteocalcin probably bind to the collagen fibrils and chelate calcium to initiate mineralization. Small proteoglycans such as decorin or fibromodulin also may have a role in mineralization.

MUTATIONS THAT PRODUCE DISEASES OF CONNECTIVE TISSUES   Because of the large number of tissue-specific macromolecules present in connective tissues, a large number of gene-protein systems are candidates for mutations that might cause pathologic changes in the tissues. However, the situation appears to be simpler than originally assumed in that most forms of the diseases are caused by mutations in the genes for the structural proteins of connective tissues, and many are in the genes for collagens. Because most of the diseases involve defects in structural proteins, most are inherited as autosomal dominant traits. Also, many involve synthesis of structurally abnormal proteins instead of simply a decrease in the amount of the protein synthesized. The deleterious effects of the structurally abnormal proteins are largely explained by the consequences they have for the assembly of macromolecules into the insoluble extracellular matrix.

The most complete data on mutations causing heritable disorders of connective tissue are available on OI. Over 90 percent of patients with OI have mutations in either the gene for the proα1(I) chain or the gene for the proα2(I) chain of type I procollagen (the COL1A1 and COL1A2 genes). In patients with mild disease, some of the mutations decrease expression of protein from one allele of the genes. Most of the mutations in patients with severe OI cause synthesis of a structurally abnormal but partially functional proα chain (Figs. 351-2 and 351-3). The mutations that cause synthesis of structurally abnormal proα chains include partial gene deletions, partial gene duplications, and RNA splicing mutations. The most common mutations, however, are single-base mutations that substitute amino acids with bulkier side chains for the obligate glycine residues that appear as every third amino acid in the triple-helical domain of a proα chain (Fig. 351-4). The structurally abnormal proα chains exert their effects primarily through one of three molecular mechanisms (see Fig. 351-2). First, the presence of an abnormal proα chain in a procollagen molecule containing two normal proα chains can prevent folding of the protein into a triple-helical conformation and lead to degradation of the whole molecule in a process called *procollagen suicide*. Similar dominant negative mutations are seen with other multisubunit proteins. The net result of procollagen suicide is a marked reduction in the amount of collagen available for fibril assembly. Second, the presence of one abnormal proα chain in a procollagen molecule can interfere with cleavage of the *N*-propeptide from the protein by procollagen *N*-proteinase. The persistence of the *N*-propeptide on a fraction of the molecules produced by fibroblasts interferes with the self-assembly of normal collagen synthesized by the same cell so that thin and irregular collagen fibrils are formed. Third, the substitution of a bulkier amino acid for glycine can produce a change in the conformation of the molecule. Because the abnormal collagen can copolymerize with normal collagen, a small amount of collagen with an abnormal conformation can cause assembly of collagen fibrils that are abnormally branched (see Fig. 351-3) or abnormally thick and short. Also, copolymerization of the mutated collagen with normal collagen can

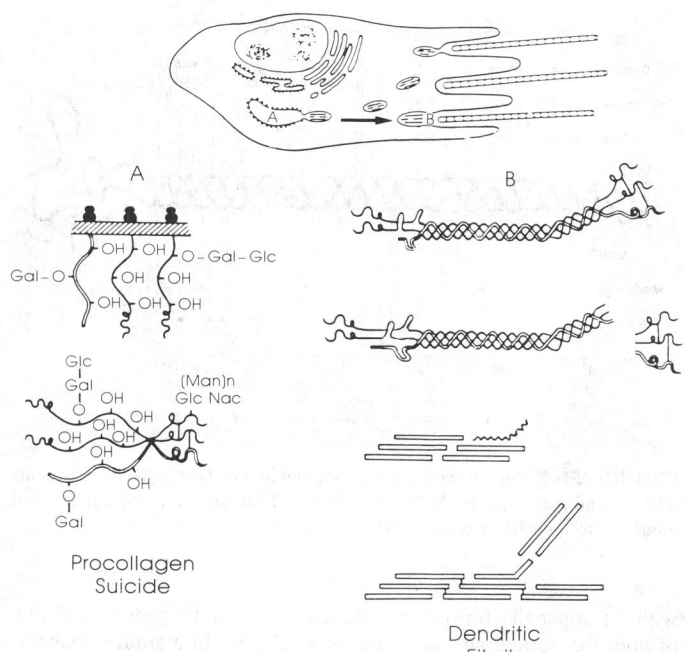

FIGURE 351-2 Schematic summary of three mechanisms (see text) whereby mutations that cause biosynthesis of structurally abnormal proα1(I) or proα2(I) chains of type I procollagen interfere with either the assembly of the protein (*A*) or its processing to normal collagen fibrils (*B*). (*From DJ Prockop et al, Am J Med Genet 34:60, 1989. Used with permission.*)

slow fibril assembly and decrease the total amount of collagen incorporated into fibrils.

There are several reasons why the type I procollagen genes harbor most of the mutations that cause OI. One, because collagen fibrils are a principal source of the strength of bone, the structure is weakened by any mutation that reduces the amount or distorts the normal geometry of collagen. The self-assembly of collagen fibrils is easily disrupted by a defective subunit that can participate in the assembly process but has the wrong structure. For example, the substitution of a bulky amino acid for a single glycine in one proα chain can interfere

FIGURE 351-3 Space-filling model showing a cysteine substitution of glycine α1-748 of type I procollagen (*on the left*) and dark-field light micrographs (*on the right*) of fibrils formed from control type I collagen at 32°C (*A*) and from the mixture of normal and mutated type I collagen containing the same cysteine substitution (*B*). (*From A Vogel et al, J Biol Chem 263:19249, 1988; and KE Kadler et al, Biochemistry 30:5081, 1991. Used with permission.*)

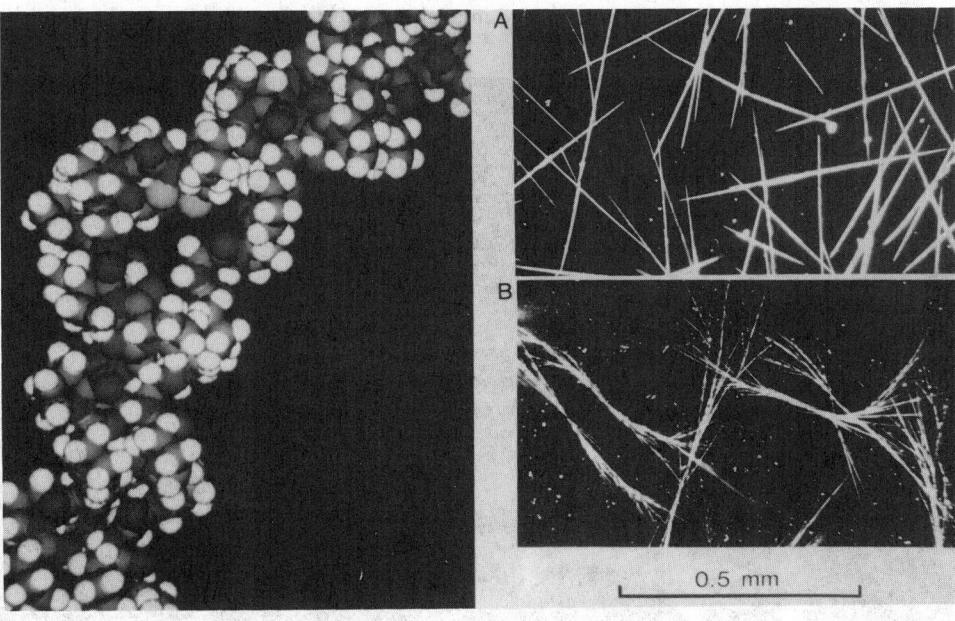

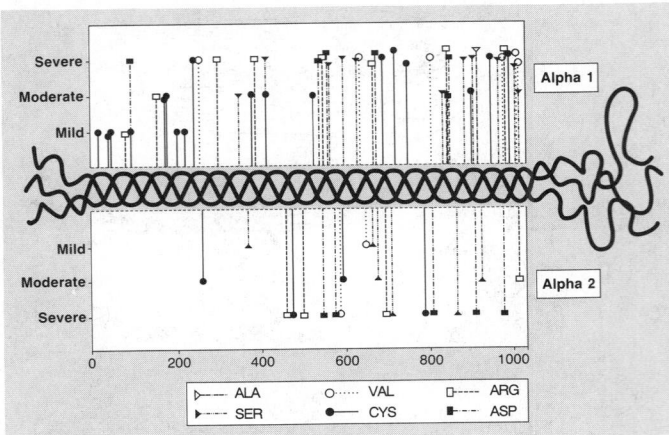

FIGURE 351-4   Single-base mutations found in type I procollagen in patients with OI and osteoporosis. Mild refers to type I OI, severe to type II OI, and moderate to type III or type IV OI.

with the zipper-like formation of the triple helix and trigger degradation of both the normal and abnormal proα chains. In a similar manner, the presence of a few incompletely processed or flawed collagen monomers can interfere with the self-assembly of normal collagen into fibrils. Hence a mutation at any one of a large number of different sites can either decrease the amount of collagen available for fibril assembly or interfere with the process of fibril assembly so as to markedly decrease the strength of bone and other connective tissues.

Over 100 mutations in the two genes for type I procollagen have been found in patients with OI (see Fig. 351-4). Initially, there was concern that many of the mutations might be neutral variations in the structure of the genes and not the cause of the disease phenotypes. However, the causal relationship between most of the mutations and the disease has now been demonstrated by several kinds of evidence: (1) DNA linkage studies in families with mild variants of OI demonstrated that specific mutated alleles coinherited with the disease phenotypes. (2) Probands with lethal variants of OI were shown to have new or sporadic mutations not found in their normal parents or in only a few cells from a mosaic parent (see below). (3) Studies with cultured skin fibroblasts from a series of patients demonstrated that the mutations produced either specific disruptions in the biosynthesis of type I procollagen or caused synthesis of a type I procollagen that generated abnormal collagen fibrils (see Fig. 351-2). (4) The mutations in probands with OI were not found in a large number of

normal alleles for the genes. (5) Expression of several of the mutated genes for type I procollagen in transgenic mice generated disease phenotypes essentially the same as the phenotypes seen in patients who inherited the mutated genes (Fig. 351-5).

The data on mutations in type I procollagen that cause OI have been used as a paradigm for defining mutations in other procollagen and collagen genes that cause other heritable disorders of connective tissue. For example, similar mutations in the gene for type III procollagen occur in patients with the type IV variant of EDS, which causes early death because of rupture of the aorta or other hollow organs (Fig. 351-6). Also, similar mutations in the gene for type II procollagen (COL2A1) are found in about half of patients with a series of CDs (Fig. 351-7). In addition, transgenic mice expressing mutated genes for type II procollagen develop phenotypes resembling several CDs. Although the data are not as extensive, it appears that similar mutations in the gene for type VII collagen (COL7A1) are found in patients with the dystrophic form of EB and that similar mutations in one of the five genes for type IV collagen (COL4A5) are found in many patients with AS. As discussed below, the paradigm developed for defining the consequences of mutations in procollagen genes helps explain findings on mutations in a fibrillin gene that cause the MS and mutations in keratin genes that cause the simplex variant of EB.

Several general trends are apparent. One is that unrelated patients rarely have the same mutation in the same gene. Mutations that produce the most severe disease are largely sporadic mutations in one allele that occur either during the generation of the germline of one of the parents or during meiosis in the fertilized egg. Most of the milder variants are caused by mutations that are specific or "private" to a given family. There are, in effect, no common mutations responsible for the disorders in unrelated patients and no "hot spots" that contain most of the mutations.

Another general trend is that similar mutations in the same gene can produce different disease syndromes in terms of both severity and the major tissues involved. One reason for heterogeneity in pathologic manifestations is that different regions of a large molecule may be more important for its function in some connective tissues than in others. For example, some regions of the type I collagen molecule may be essential for the binding of mineralizing proteins in bone so that mutations in these regions cause fragile bones but do not impair function in skin and other nonmineralizing tissues. It is more difficult, however, to explain how the same mutation can produce a severe phenotype in some members of a family and a mild phenotype in other members of the same family. Such phenotypic variation appears to be particularly dramatic in OI, where some subjects are short and have multiple fractures from minor trauma,

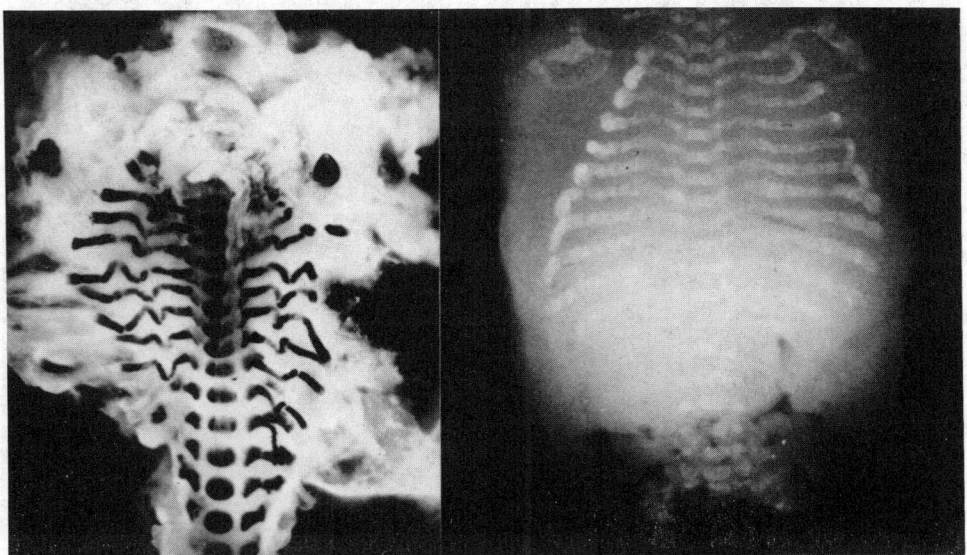

FIGURE 351-5   Similarities of the phenotypes in transgenic mice with mutated type I procollagen and in an OI child. Note in both pictures the waviness of the ribs due to fractures in utero.

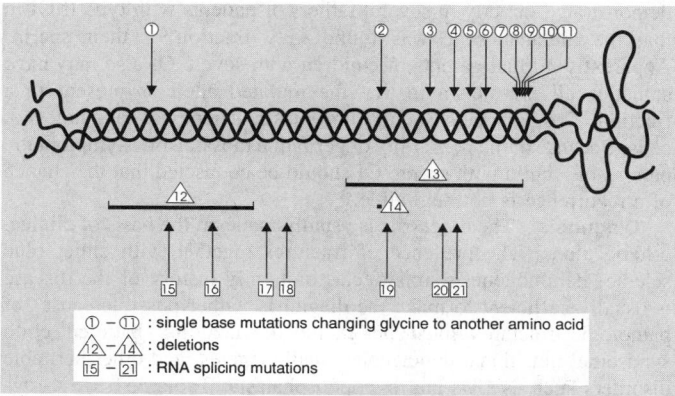

FIGURE 351-6 Mutations in the gene for the proα1(III) chain of type III procollagen that cause EDS IV and familial aneurysms.

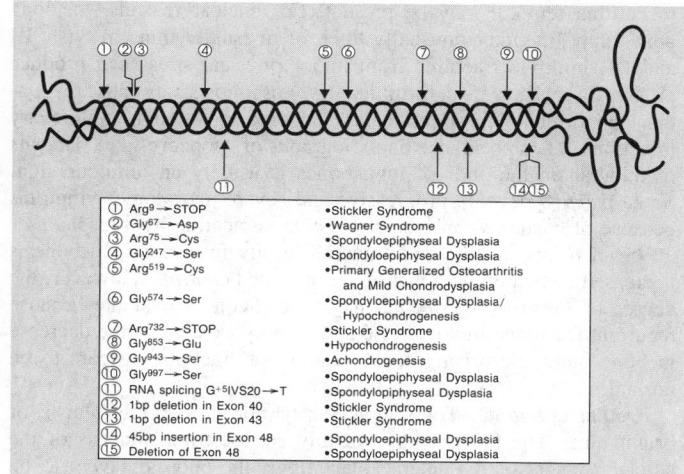

FIGURE 351-7 Mutations in the gene for the proα1(II) chain of type II procollagen that cause CD and related disorders.

whereas others in the same family are of normal stature and free of fractures. In the past, such phenotypic variation was explained by undefined variations in the genetic background of different family members. Studies in transgenic mice, however, demonstrated similar phenotypic variation with expression of a mutated collagen gene in an inbred strain of mice in whom the genetic background is uniform. Therefore, the phenotypic variation is probably caused by undefined stochastic or chance events during embryonic and fetal development. Fortunately, dramatic phenotypic variation is relatively rare in OI and related disorders, but it is important to consider in counseling families about the consequences of inherited mutations.

Still another feature is that these diseases are rarely due to mutations in genes for nonstructural proteins. An exception to this conclusion is that two forms of EDS are caused by mutations in the genes for two of the procollagen processing enzymes (see below). Such enzyme deficiencies appear to be relatively rare causes of connective tissue diseases because, as with most enzyme deficiencies, a homozygous state in which the patient inherited two defective alleles of a gene is necessary to reduce enzyme activity sufficiently to cause symptoms. Unless heterozygous carriers of mutated alleles are common in a population, homozygotes are rare. In addition, complete deficiency of critical enzymes such as prolyl hydroxylase may be lethal.

OSTEOGENESIS IMPERFECTA Osteogenesis imperfecta (OI) is a heritable defect that makes bones brittle because of a generalized decrease in bone mass (osteopenia). The disorder is frequently associated with blue sclerae, dental abnormalities (dentinogenesis imperfecta), progressive hearing loss, and a positive family history. The most severe forms of OI produce death in utero, at birth, or shortly thereafter. The clinical course of mild and moderate forms is more variable. Some patients appear normal at birth and then become progressively worse. Some patients have multiple fractures in infancy and childhood, improve after puberty, and fracture more frequently later in life. Women are particularly prone to fracture during pregnancy and after menopause. A few women from families with mild variants of OI do not develop fractures until after menopause, and their disease may be difficult to distinguish from postmenopausal osteoporosis.

Classification into types The most commonly used classification scheme for OI is the one developed by Sillence (Table 351-2). Type

I is the mildest form of the disease and is inherited as an autosomal dominant trait. Most patients have distinctly blue sclerae. Type I OI is subdivided into types IA and IB depending on whether or not dentinogenesis imperfecta is also present. Type II is lethal in utero or shortly after birth. Radiographic criteria can be used to subdivide type II OI into five groups, with subgroup 1 showing the most severe changes and subgroup 5 the least. Types III and IV OI are intermediate in severity between types I and II. They differ from type I because of greater severity and because the sclerae are only slightly bluish in infancy and white in adulthood. Type III is distinguished from type IV in that it tends to become progressively severe with age. Also, type III OI is inherited either as an autosomal recessive or autosomal dominant trait, whereas type IV is always dominant. The clinical courses are variable, and the mode of inheritance in types III and IV OI is frequently difficult to establish because many patients have sporadic mutations and because many couples with one severely affected OI child elect not to have additional children. For these and related reasons, some think that the distinction between type IV OI and more severe variants of type I OI is not helpful. Therefore, it may be sufficient to classify patients simply as mild with blue sclerae (type I), lethal (type II), and moderately severe (type III).

Incidence Type I OI has a population frequency of about 1 in 30,000. Type II OI has a birth incidence of about 1 in 60,000. Types III and IV are less common, but the incidence of the three severe forms clearly recognizable at birth (types II, III, and IV) may be as high as 1 in 20,000. Therefore, the overall incidence of the disease may be as high as 5 in 60,000 or about 1 in 12,000.

Skeletal changes In type I OI, the fragility of bones may be severe enough to limit many physical activity or so mild that individuals are largely unaware of any disability. Radiographs of the skull of some patients with mild disease show a mottled or wormian appearance, apparently because of small islands of irregular ossification. In type II OI, bones and other connective tissues are fragile so that massive injuries can occur in utero or during delivery (see Fig. 351-5). Ossification of many bones is frequently incomplete. Continuously beaded or broken ribs and crumpled long bones

TABLE 351-2 Classification of osteogenesis imperfecta (OI)

Type	Bone fragility	Blue sclerae	Abnormal dentition	Hearing loss	Inheritance*
I	Mild	Present	Absent in IA, present in IB	Present in most	AD
II	Extreme	Present	Present in some	Unknown	AR or S
III	Severe	Bluish at birth	Present in some	High incidence	AR or AD
IV	Variable	Absent	Absent in IVA, present in IVB	High incidence	AD

* AD, autosomal dominant; AR, autosomal recessive; S, sporadic.

(accordina femora) may be present. For unclear reasons, the long bones may be either unusually thick or unusually thin. In types III and IV, multiple fractures from minor physical stress can produce progressive and severe deformities. Kyphoscoliosis may cause respiratory impairment, cor pulmonale, and predisposition to pulmonary infections. The appearance on radiographs of "popcorn-like" deposits of mineral on the ends of long bones is usually an ominous sign. Some patients develop progressive and severe neurologic symptoms because of basilar compression and communicating hydrocephalus.

In all forms of OI, bone mineral density in unfractured bone is decreased compared with that of age-matched controls. However, the degree of intrinsic osteopenia may be difficult to evaluate because recurrent fractures limit exercise and thereby exacerbate the decrease in bone mass. Surprisingly, the healing of fractures appears to be normal.

Ocular changes   The sclerae can be normal, slightly bluish, or bright blue. The blueness is probably caused by a thinness of the collagen layers of the sclerae that allows the choroid layers to be seen. Blue sclerae, however, are an inherited trait in some families without evidence of increased bone fragility.

Dentinogenesis imperfecta   The teeth may be normal, moderately discolored, or grossly abnormal. The enamel generally appears normal, but the teeth may have a characteristic amber, yellowish brown, or translucent bluish gray color because of improper deposition or deficiency of dentin. The deciduous teeth are usually smaller than normal, whereas permanent teeth are frequently bell-shaped and restricted at the base. In some patients, the teeth readily fracture and need to be extracted. The defect in dentin is directly attributable to the fact that normal dentin is rich in type I collagen. Similar tooth defects, however, occur in some families without any evidence of OI.

Hearing loss   Hearing loss is common. It usually begins during the second decade of life and can be detected in 90 percent of subjects over age 30. The loss can be conductive, sensorineural, or mixed and ranges widely in severity. The middle ear usually exhibits maldevelopment, deficient ossification, persistence of cartilage in areas that are normally ossified, and abnormal calcium deposits.

Associated features   Many patients and families show involvement of other connective tissues. Some have thin skin that scars extensively. Others have extreme joint laxity with permanent dislocations indistinguishable from those of EDS. A few have cardiovascular manifestations such as aortic regurgitation, floppy mitral valves, mitral incompetence, and fragility of large blood vessels. For unknown reasons, some patients develop a hypermetabolic state with elevated serum thyroxine levels, hyperthermia, and excessive sweating.

Molecular defects   Most patients with OI have mutations in one of the two genes for type I procollagen. A third or more of the patients with type I OI have as yet undefined mutations in the proα1(I) gene that decrease the steady state levels of the mRNA for proα1(I) chains and decrease the rates of synthesis of proα1(I) chains relative to those for proα2(I) chains. In more severe forms (types II, III, and IV), most of the mutations cause synthesis of structurally abnormal proα chains whose effects are amplified by the three molecular mechanisms discussed above (see Fig. 351-2). The mutations that change the structure of the protein near the N-proteinase cleavage site cause accumulation of a partially processed procollagen and produce lax joints more characteristic of type VII EDS rather than OI. Mutations that change the structure in the middle or near the C terminus tend to produce severe or lethal variants of OI. It is difficult, however, to deduce a more precise correlation between the site or nature of the mutation and the clinical phenotype (see Fig. 351-4). Rare patients are homozygous with two mutated alleles for proα1(I) or proα2(I) chains.

Mosaicism in germ line cells and in somatic cells   Most of the lethal variants of OI are the result of new autosomal dominant mutations. The frequency of a second child with lethal OI in the same family, however, is about 7 percent because of germ line mosaicism in one of the parents. The presence of germ line mosaicism was demonstrated directly in several fathers of patients with type II OI in that the mutated gene was found in a fraction of their sperm. Apparently normal parents of children with severe OI also may have somatic cell mosaicism in that the mutated allele is present in a fraction of somatic cells such as fibroblasts, leukocytes, and hair root cells. Because of the possibility of germ line mosaicism, asymptomatic parents of a child with severe OI should be counseled that the chance of a recurrence is not negligible.

Diagnosis   The diagnosis is usually made on the basis of clinical criteria alone. The presence of fractures together with either blue sclerae, dentinogenesis imperfecta, or family history of the disease is usually sufficient to make the diagnosis. Other possible causes of pathologic fractures must be excluded, including battered child syndrome, nutritional deficiencies, malignancies, and other heritable disorders such as CDs and hypophosphatasia (Table 351-3). X-rays usually reveal a decrease in bone density that can be verified by photon or x-ray absorptiometry. There is no consensus, however, as to whether the diagnosis can be made by microscopy of bone specimens. With research procedures, a molecular defect in type I procollagen can be demonstrated in half or more of patients by incubating skin fibroblasts with radioactive amino acids and then analyzing the proα chains by polyacrylamide gel electrophoresis. The analysis detects decreases in the rate of synthesis of proα1(I) chains relative to proα2(I) chains, abnormally long pro-α chains, abnormally short proα chains, and proα chains that are posttranslationally overmodified because of an amino acid substitution that delays folding of the triple helix. The mutations themselves can be defined in most patients by DNA sequencing of mRNA-derived cDNAs or sequencing of genomic DNAs. Because each proband and family usually has a "private" mutation, extensive analysis of 5000 or more bases in each of the two genes is required to identify the exact mutation. After a mutation in a type I procollagen gene is identified, a test based on the polymerase chain reaction can be used to screen family members at risk and for prenatal diagnosis.

Treatment   Treatment is ineffective. Many patients have successful careers despite severe deformities. Patients with mild disorder may need little treatment when fractures decrease after puberty, but women require special attention during pregnancy and after menopause, when fractures again increase. More severely affected children require a comprehensive program of physical therapy, surgical management of fractures and skeletal deformities, and vocational education.

Many of the fractures are only slightly displaced and have little soft tissue swelling. Therefore, they can be treated with minimal support or traction for a week or two followed by a light cast. If fractures are relatively painless, physical therapy can be initiated early. A judicious amount of exercise is obviously important to

TABLE 351-3 Differential diagnosis of OI

Age	Diagnosis	Distinguishing features
At birth	Hypophosphatasia	Unmineralized skull
	Achondrogenesis	Unmineralized vertebrae
	Thanatophoric dwarfism	H-shaped vertebrae
	Asphyxiating thoracic dystrophy	Cylindrical thorax
	Achondroplasia	Large head, short, tubular bones
Infancy	Battered child syndrome	Skull and rib fractures more common
	Immobilization osteogenesis	
	Scurvy	
	Congenital syphilis	
Childhood	Homocystinuria	Marfanoid appearance and mental deficiency
	Celiac disease	Steatorrhea, anemia
	Adrenal cortical tumor	
	Glucocorticoid therapy	

SOURCE: After R Smith et al, *The Brittle Bone Syndrome: Osteogenesis Imperfecta*, London, Butterworths, 1983, p 128.

prevent loss of bone mass secondary to physical inactivity. Some physicians advocate insertion of steel rods into long bones to correct limb deformities; the risk/benefits and cost/benefits of such procedures are difficult to evaluate. Aggressive conventional intervention is usually warranted for pneumonia and cor pulmonale. For severe hearing loss, excellent results have been reported with stapedectomy or replacement of the stapes with a prosthesis. Moderately to severely affected patients probably should be evaluated periodically to anticipate possible neurologic problems. About half of patients have a substantial increase in growth if treated during childhood with growth hormone. Treatment with bisphosphorates and related agents to decrease bone loss has been discussed, but no controlled studies have been reported.

A program for careful orthotic management developed by Bleck and a program for compressive management developed by Marini are useful guides. Counseling and emotional support for patients and parents is important, and lay organizations to provide help in these areas have now been formed in most countries. Prenatal ultrasonography will detect severely affected fetuses at about 16 weeks of pregnancy. Diagnosis by analysis for synthesis of abnormally migrating proα chains or by DNA sequencing can be carried out in chorionic villa biopsies at 8 to 12 weeks of pregnancy.

EHLERS-DANLOS SYNDROME The Ehlers-Danlos syndrome (EDS) is a group of heritable disorders characterized by hyperelasticity of the skin and hypermobile joints (Fig. 351-8).

Classification into types Beighton initially identified five types of EDS based primarily on the extent to which the skin, joints, and other tissues are involved (Table 351-4). Type I is the classical, severe form of the disease, with both severe joint hypermobility and skin changes that make it velvety in texture, hyperextensible, and easily scarred. Type II is similar to type I but milder. In type III, joint hypermobility is more prominent than the skin changes, and in type IV, the skin changes are far more prominent than the joint changes. A striking feature of type IV, however, is that the patients have a strong predisposition to sudden death from rupture of large blood vessels or the large bowel. Type V is similar to type II but characterized by X-linked inheritance. Type VI usually can be distinguished by the presence of scoliosis, ocular fragility, and a cone-shaped deformity of the cornea (keratoconus). Type VII is characterized by marked joint hypermobility that is difficult to distinguish from type III except by the specific molecular defects in the processing of type I procollagen to collagen. Type VIII is distinguished by periodontal changes. The remaining types IX, X, and XI were defined on the basis of preliminary biochemical and clinical data, but these classifications have not proven useful. Because of overlapping signs and symptoms, many patients and families cannot be assigned to any of the nine defined types of EDS.

Incidence Figures on the incidence of EDS have been difficult to develop, largely because patients with mild skin or joint symptoms rarely seek medical attention. Also, it is difficult to define the normal range of variation for features such as joint mobility or skin elasticity. An incidence of about 1 in 5000 births is gaining acceptance, although a higher value has been reported for a predominantly black population. Types I, II, and III account for most of the diagnosed patients.

Skin The changes vary from unusually thin and velvety skin to skin that is either dramatically hyperextensible ("rubber man" syndrome) or easily torn or scarred. Patients with type I develop characteristic "cigarette-paper" scars. In type IV, extensive scars and hyperpigmentation develop over bony prominences, and the skin may be so thin that subcutaneous blood vessels become visible. In type VIII, the skin is more fragile than hyperextensible, and it heals with atrophic, pigmented scars. Easy bruisability is a feature of several types of EDS.

Ligament and joint changes Laxity and hypermobility of joints vary from mild to unreducible dislocations of hips and other large joints. In milder forms, patients learn to reduce dislocations themselves and to avoid them by limiting physical activity. In more severe forms, surgical repair is required. Some patients have progressive difficulty

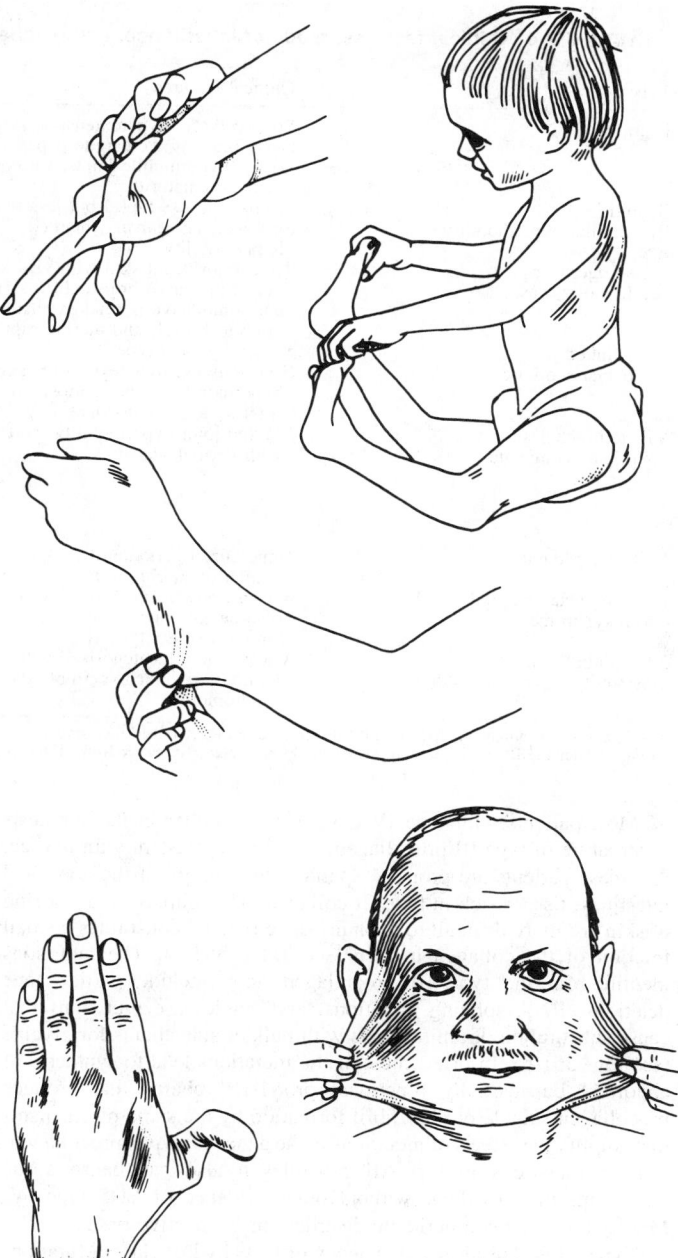

FIGURE 351-8 Schematic representation of the skin and joint changes in EDS. Girl in upper right has type VII EDS with dislocations of both hips that were not correctable by surgery. *(From DJ Prockop and NA Guzman, Hosp Pract 12(12):61, 1977. Used with permission.)*

with age, but severe joint laxity is compatible with a normal life span.

Associated changes Mitral valve prolapse occurs, particularly in type I. Pes planus and mild to moderate scoliosis are common. Extreme joint laxity and repeated dislocations may lead to degenerative arthritis. Hernias are frequent in patients with type I. In type VI, the eye may rupture with minimal trauma, and kyphoscoliosis can produce respiratory impairment. Sclerae are frequently blue in type VI.

Molecular defects The molecular defects in the type I, type II, and type III variants of EDS are unknown. Electron microscopy of the skin from some patients has shown an unusual morphology of collagen fibers, but similar features are seen occasionally in normal skin.

TABLE 351-4   Clinical features, mode of inheritance, and biochemical defects in EDS

Type	Clinical features	Inheritance*	Biochemical defect
I, gravis	Soft, velvety, hyperextensible skin; easy bruising; "cigarette paper" scars; hypermobile joints; varicose veins; prematurity	AD	Not known
II, mitis	Similar to EDS type I but less severe	AD	Not known
III, familial hypermobility	Soft skin, no scarring, marked hypermobility	AD	Not known
IV, acrogeric, ecchymotic, vascular	Thin, translucent skin with visible veins; increased bruisability, skin and joints have normal extensibility; arterial, bowel, and uterine rupture	AD	Mutations in type III procollagen (see Fig. 351-6)
V, X-linked	Similar to EDS type II	XLR	Not known
VI, ocular-scoliotic	Soft, velvety, hyperextensible skin; hypermobile joints; scoliosis; ocular fragility and keratoconus	AR	Lysyl hydroxylase deficiency
VII, arthrochalasis multiplex congenita	Marked joint hypermobility, soft skin with normal scarring	AD	A. Structural defect in the proα1(I) chain
		AD	B. Structural defect in the proα2(I) chain
		AR	C. Procollagen N-proteinase deficiency
VIII, periodontal	Generalized periodontitis, skin similar to EDS type II	AD	Not known
IX, cutis laxa occipital horn syndrome	Vacant, now recategorized as a disorder of copper transport		
X	Similar to EDS type II	AR	Possible defect in fibronectin
XI, familial joint instability	Vacant, now recategorized with familial articular hypermobility syndromes		

* AD, autosomal dominant; AR, autosomal recessive; XLR, X-linked recessive.
SOURCE: After PH Byers, in *Clinical Medicine*, Philadelphia, Harper & Row, 1983, p. 1; and P Beighton et al, Am J Med Genet 29:581, 1988.

Most patients with type IV have a defect either in the synthesis or structure of type III procollagen, a finding consistent with the fact that these patients are prone to spontaneous rupture of the aorta and intestines, tissues rich in type III collagen. The thinness and scarring of skin are more difficult to explain, since type III constitutes a small fraction of the collagen in skin (see Table 351-1). The mutations identified in the type III procollagen gene include partial gene deletions, RNA splicing mutations, and single-base mutations that cause substitution of amino acids with bulkier side chains for glycine (see Fig. 351-6). In brief, most of the mutations lead to synthesis of abnormal but partially functional proα1(III) chains that produce procollagen suicide or alter fibril formation by the same mechanisms that amplify the effects of mutations in the genes for type I procollagen. Similar mutations in type III procollagen also can cause aortic aneurysms in individuals without other evidence of EDS type IV, MS, or other defined heritable disorders of connective tissue.

Type VI is caused by a deficiency of lysyl hydroxylase. Mutations in the gene for this enzyme have been defined in two families. In one family, the mutation produced a premature stop codon, and in the other the mutation produced a large duplication of the gene. Deficiency of lysyl hydroxylase causes synthesis of a collagen that is deficient in its content of hydroxylysine and as a result does not form stable cross-links.

Type VII is a defect in the conversion of procollagen to collagen in patients with marked joint hypermobility. The defect can be caused either by mutations that make type I procollagen resistant to cleavage by procollagen N-proteinase or by mutations that decrease the activity of the enzyme. In type VIIA, the mutations alter the cleavage site in the proα1(I) chain. In type VIIB, the mutations alter the cleavage site in the proα2(I) chain. Both types are dominantly inherited. Type VIIC is caused by mutations that decrease the activity of procollagen N-proteinase. It is inherited as an autosomal recessive trait. In all three forms of type VII EDS, the persistence of the N-propeptide on the molecule causes the formation of fibrils that are thin and irregular in cross section. Since most patients do not have clinical osteopenia, the thin and irregular fibrils apparently suffice for the mineralization of bone but do not provide the necessary tensile strength for ligaments and joint capsules.

The cause of type VIII is unknown. Type IX is a disorder of copper transport. The syndrome, also referred to as *Menkes' syndrome*, is due to an X-linked defect and is associated with cutis laxa, hypopigmentation, unusual hair ("kinky"), vascular aneurysms, neurologic degeneration, and mental retardation. Mutations in a gene coding for a copper-transporting ATPase cause the disease. Type X EDS may be caused by defects in fibronectin, but no specific mutations have been defined. (See also Chaps. 78 and 353.)

Diagnosis   The diagnosis of EDS is based primarily on clinical criteria. Biochemical assays and gene analyses for known molecular defects in EDS are difficult and time-consuming, but specific diagnostic tests should be available in the future for families in which the mutations have been defined.

Treatment   There is no specific therapy. Surgical repair and tightening of joint ligaments require careful evaluation of individual patients, since the ligaments frequently will not hold sutures. Patients with easy bruisability should be evaluated for other bleeding disorders. Patients with type IV EDS and members of their families probably should be evaluated at regular intervals by sonography and related techniques for early detection of aneurysms. Surgical repair of aneurysms may be difficult because of increased friability of tissues, and there is limited experience with elective surgery in such patients. Also, women with type IV EDS should be counseled about the increased risk of uterine rupture, bleeding, and other complications of pregnancy.

CHONDRODYSPLASIAS   The chondrodysplasias (CDs) are heritable disorders of skeletal growth that produce dwarfism with abnormal body proportions. The category also includes some individuals with normal stature and body proportions who have features such as characteristic ocular changes or cleft palate that are common in more severe CDs. Also, many patients with CD develop degenerative joint changes that are difficult to distinguish from osteoarthritis. Therefore, mild CDs in adults may be difficult to differentiate from primary generalized osteoarthritis. Some authors refer to the disorders as "skeletal dysplasias," but CD is a more widely used term because most of the diseases produce changes in cartilage and because the effects on the bony skeleton appear to be secondary to effects on cartilage.

Classifications of the diseases Over 150 distinct types of CDs with 8 major subtypes have been defined in the literature (Table 351-5). The classifications have been based on a variety of criteria such as "bringing death" (thanatophoric), causing "twisted" bones (diastrophic), primarily affecting metaphyses (metaphyseal), primarily affecting epiphyses (epiphyseal), and producing characteristic histologic changes such as an apparent increase in the fibrous material seen in the epiphyses (fibrochondrogenesis). Also, a number of eponyms have been introduced based on the first or most comprehensive case reports. Severe forms of the diseases produce gross distortions of most cartilaginous structures and of the eye (see Table 351-1). Mild forms are more difficult to classify. Among the features are cataracts, degeneration of the vitreous and retinal detachment, high forehead, hypoplastic facies, cleft palate, short and thin extremities, and gross distortions of the epiphyses, metaphyses, and joint surfaces.

Incidence Data on the frequency of most CDs are not available, but the incidence of the Stickler syndrome has been estimated as high as 1 in 10,000. Therefore, the diseases are probably among the more common heritable disorders of connective tissue.

Molecular defects Because most CDs produce dramatic changes in the appearance of cartilage, most are probably caused by a mutation in a gene for one of the structural proteins in the matrix of cartilage (see Table 351-1). To date, however, the only gene explored extensively for such mutations is the gene for type II procollagen (COL2A1) (see Fig. 351-7).

DNA linkage studies with the COL2A1 gene demonstrated that specific alleles of the gene were frequently coinherited with the Stickler syndrome and with arthroophthalmopathy, a condition characterized by myopia and lattice degeneration of the vitreous and frequently associated with cleft palate, hypoplastic facies, variable skeletal changes, and early-onset degenerative arthritis. In one series,

---

TABLE 351-5 Classifications of chondrodysplasias

Achondrodysplasia family
  Achondroplasia
  Hypochondroplasia
  Thanatophoric dysplasia
Spondyloepiphyseal dysplasia (SED) family
  Achondrogenesis type IA
  Achonodrogenesis type IB
  Achondrogenesis type II
  Hypochondrogenesis
  SED congenita
  Strudwick syndrome
  Stickler syndrome
  Kniest dysplasia
Chondrodysplasia punctata family
  Rhizomelic chondrodysplasia punctata
  Conradi-Hünermann disease
  X-linked dominant chondrodysplasia punctata
  Chondrodysplasia punctata associated with Xp
Short rib (-polydactyly) family
  Ellis-van Creveld syndrome
  Asphyxiating thoracic dysplasia
  Short rib–polydactyly syndrome type I
  Short rib–polydactyly syndrome type II
Metatropic dysplasia family
  Metatropic dysplasia
  Metatropic-like dysplasia
Metaphyseal chondrodysplasia family
  Metaphyseal chondrodysplasia, Jansen type
  Metaphyseal chondrodysplasia, Schmid type
  Metaphyseal chondrodysplasia, McKusick type
Brachyolmia family
  Brachyolmia, Hobaek type
  Brachyolmia, Maroteaux type
  Brachyolmia, autosomal dominant type
Acromelic dysplasia family
  Peripheral dysostosis
  Achodysplasia
  Trichorhinophalangeal syndrome type I
  Trichorhinophalangeal syndrome type II

SOURCE: After Spranger J. Eur J Pediatr 151:407, 1992; WA Horton and JT Hecht.

---

half of families demonstrated linkage to the COL2A1 gene. Subsequently, direct analysis of the COL2A1 gene demonstrated that four unrelated families had different mutations that produced premature termination codons for translation of the mRNA. The consequences of premature termination codons were not explicitly defined, but they probably caused synthesis of shortened proα1(II) chains that lack *C*-terminal propeptides and therefore are not incorporated into type II procollagen and do not contribute to the assembly of type II collagen fibrils. A decrease in the amount of type II collagen in the eye is consistent with the lattice degeneration of the vitreous and retinal detachment. A decrease in type II collagen fibers also explains the cleft palate, the skeletal changes, and the degenerative arthritis of joints. As with OI, however, it is less clear why other mutations in the same COL2A1 gene cause other phenotypes (see Fig. 351-7). For example, a mutation that substituted an aspartate for a glycine codon was seen in a family defined as having the Wagner syndrome because they had the ocular changes characteristic of the Stickler syndrome but no evidence of extraocular tissue involvement.

Defects of the COL2A1 gene in more severe CDs include one exon deletion, one partial gene duplication, one RNA splicing mutation, and five glycine substitutions (see Fig. 351-7). The clinical phenotypes range from lethal at birth (hypochondrogenesis and achondrogenesis II/hypochondrogenesis) to severe spondyloepiphyseal dysplasia. Again, there is no apparent relationship between the site or nature of the mutation and the phenotype. Although the data are incomplete, about half of patients with severe CDs have mutations in the gene for type II procollagen, and the remainder are likely to have mutations in genes for other molecules.

Of special interest, two different mutations in the COL2A1 gene replace arginine codons in the triple-helical domain with codons for cysteine. Cysteine is not found in the triple-helical domain of type II collagen from any species, and the presence of cysteine in the type II collagen introduces an abnormal disulfide cross-link in collagen. One of the cysteine-for-arginine substitutions was found in affected members of a large family with primary generalized osteoarthritis and minimal evidence of a CD. The other was found in a family with a mild spondyloepiphyseal dysplasia. In brief, mutations in the COL2A1 gene, like mutations in the genes for type I and type III procollagen, can cause a spectrum of diseases from lethal conditions to common disorders such as osteoarthritis.

Diagnosis The diagnosis of severe forms of CD is made on the basis of analysis of the physical appearance, x-ray findings, histologic changes, and clinical course (Table 351-5).

Treatment No definitive therapy is available. Symptomatic treatment is directed toward secondary features such as degenerative arthritis. Many patients require joint replacement surgery and corrective surgery for cleft palates. Ocular changes should be monitored carefully for the development of cataracts and for the need for laser therapy to prevent retinal detachment. Patients probably should be advised to avoid obesity and contact sports. Counseling for the serious psychological problems of short stature is critical, and support groups have formed in many countries. Ultrasonography is sometimes successful for prenatal diagnosis but less frequently than with OI. Specific tests should be available in the future for the CDs caused by mutations in the COL2A1 gene.

MARFAN SYNDROME Severe Marfan syndrome (MS) is characterized by a triad of features: (1) long, thin extremities frequently associated with other skeletal changes, (2) reduced vision as the result of dislocations of the lenses (ectopia lentis), and (3) aortic aneurysms that typically begin at the base of the aorta. Milder forms of the disorder, particularly those with only the skeletal changes, are difficult to classify.

Classification The severe form is usually due to a mutation in a single allele of the fibrillin gene (FBN1). At the same time, MS must be distinguished from related syndromes: (1) homocystinuria that frequently causes ectopia lentis and some of the same skeletal changes as the MS, (2) congenital contractural arachnodactyly that causes similar skeletal changes but none of the other features of MS,

(3) familial ectopia lentis not associated with other features of MS, and (4) familial aortic aneurysms that result from a more common autosomal dominant disorder not associated with other features of MS, type IV EDS, or other known disorders of connective tissue.

Incidence and inheritance   MS has an incidence of about 1 in 10,000 in most racial and ethnic groups. The disorder is inherited as an autosomal dominant trait, but at least one-quarter of patients do not have an affected parent and therefore their disorders probably are due to new mutations.

Skeletal changes   Patients are usually tall compared with other members of the same family and have long limbs. The ratio of the upper segment (top of the head to top of the pubic ramus) to the lower segment (top of the pubic ramus to the floor) is usually 2 standard deviations below mean for age, race, and sex. The fingers and hands are long and slender and have a spider-like appearance (arachnodactyly). Many patients have severe chest deformities, including depression (pectus excavatum), protrusion (pectus carinatum), or asymmetry. Scoliosis is usually accompanied by kyphosis. High-arched palate and high pedal arches or pes planus are common. A few patients have joint hypermobility similar to that in mild EDS, but joint mobility is usually normal.

Cardiovascular changes   Cardiovascular abnormalities are the major source of morbidity and mortality. Mitral valve prolapse develops early in life and in about one-quarter progresses to mitral valve regurgitation of increasing severity because of redundancy of the leaflets, stretching of the chordae tendinae, and dilatation of the valvulae annulus. Dilatation of the root of the aorta and the sinuses of Valsalva may be detected by echocardiography in utero. The rate of dilatation is unpredictable, but the dilatation can cause aortic regurgitation, dissection of the aorta, and rupture. Dilatation is probably accelerated by physical and emotional stress, as well as by pregnancy.

Ocular changes   The dislocation of the lens may be readily apparent, but diagnosis usually requires pupillary dilatation and slit-lamp examination. The displacement is usually not progressive but may contribute to the formation of cataracts. The ocular globe is frequently elongated, most patients are myopic, and some develop retinal detachment. A few patients have lattice degeneration and retinal tears; most have adequate vision.

Associated changes   Striae may occur over the shoulders and buttocks. Otherwise the skin is normal. A number of patients develop spontaneous pneumothorax. Inguinal and incisional hernias are common. Marked dilatation of the dural sac is seen frequently in CT scans, but the condition is usually asymptomatic. Characteristically, patients are thin with little subcutaneous fat, but adults may develop centripetal fat accumulation.

Molecular defects   Most patients with the classical features of MS have mutations in a gene for fibrillin, a glycoprotein of 350 kDa that is a major component of elastin-associated microfibrils. These microfibrils are abundant in large blood vessels and the suspensory ligaments of the lens. Patients are heterozygous for the mutations, and many of the mutations appear to change amino acid codons at various sites along the protein. The function of fibrillin has not been defined, but the data suggest that fibrillin self-assembles into a fibrillar structure and that the conformation and surface properties of the entire molecule are critical for normal assembly. Therefore, the functional consequences of mutations that change the amino acid sequence of fibrillin may be similar to the effects of mutations that change the conformation of a fibrillar collagen (see Figs. 351-2, 351-4, 351-6, and 351-7). Although only a few mutations have been specifically identified, most patients with the classical syndrome are thought to have mutations in the same gene located on the long arm of chromosome 15 (FBN1), since extensive studies demonstrated linkage of the mutated genes to the same site. In addition, DNA linkage studies indicate that the gene causing familial ectopia lentis without any other signs of MS is also located on chromosome 15, but it is unclear whether the gene is identical with FBN1. Two families with a Marfan-related syndrome characterized by congenital contractural

arachnodactyly demonstrate linkage to a second fibrillin gene located on chromosome 5 (FBN2). A third fibrillin gene (FBN3) is presented on chromosome 17, but no defect has yet been linked to the gene. Also, two patients with atypical forms of the syndrome apparently have defects in the proα2(I) chain of type I procollagen. Therefore, patents with classical MS have mutations in genes other than the FBN gene on chromosome 15.

Diagnosis   The diagnosis is easily established if the patient and other members of the family have dislocated lenses, aortic dilatation, and long and thin extremities together with kyphoscoliosis or other chest deformities. The diagnosis is frequently made if ectopia lentis and an aneurysm of the ascending aorta occur in the absence of a Marfan habitus or a positive family history. All patients in whom the diagnosis is suspected should have a slit-lamp examination and an echocardiogram. Also, homocystinuria (see Table 351-3) should be ruled out by a negative cyanide-nitroprusside test for disulfides in the urine. A few patients with types I, II, and III EDS have ectopia lentis but lack the Marfan habitus and instead have characteristic skin changes not present in MS. Patients with familial aortic aneurysms tend to develop aneurysms at the base of the abdominal aorta. The location of the aneurysms, however is, variable, and the high incidence of aortic aneurysms (1 in 100) makes the differential diagnosis difficult unless other features of MS are clearly present. A few families with familial aortic aneurysms have mutations in the gene for type III procollagen (see Fig. 351-6).

Treatment   There is no established treatment, but several investigators have recommended use of propranolol or other beta-adrenergic blocking agents to delay or prevent aortic dilatation. Surgical replacement of the aorta, aortic valve, and mitral valve has been successful in some patients, and all patients should be followed carefully with echocardiography and other techniques for evaluation of cardiovascular changes. Patients probably should be advised of the risks of severe physical and emotional stress and of pregnancy.

The scoliosis tends to be progressive and should be treated by mechanical bracing and physical therapy if greater than 20 degrees or by surgery if it progresses to greater than 45 degrees. Estrogen has been tried in girls with scoliosis, but the results are inconclusive. Dislocated lenses rarely require surgical removal, but patients should be followed closely for retinal detachment. Pyeritz has summarized current protocols for the management of patients.

Diagnostic tests based on detection of fibrillin defects in cultured skin fibroblasts or DNA analysis of the gene may be available in the near future.

EPIDERMOLYSIS BULLOSA   Epidermolysis bullosa (EB) is a group of disorders in which the skin and related epithelial tissues break and blister as the result of minor trauma. As with most heritable disorders of connective tissues, the clinical manifestations range from lethal to mild disorders.

Classifications   Three major categories are defined on the basis of the level at which blistering occurs: EB simplex for blistering in the epidermis, EB junctional for blistering in the dermal-epidermal junction, and EB dystrophica for blistering in the dermis. More than 20 subtypes have been separated on the basis of the clinical findings together with ultrastructural and immunohistologic changes in skin.

Incidence   The incidence of EB in the United States is estimated to be 1 in 50,000.

Molecular defects   The molecular basis of several specific variants of EB has been defined. Some of the first information came from experiments with transgenic mice in which mice expressing a gene for a truncated keratin (keratin 14) developed intraepidermal blistering similar to that seen in patients with EB simplex. Subsequently, point mutations in the same gene were found in two patients with the herpetiformis variant of EB simplex. In addition, point mutations in another keratin gene (keratin 5) were identified in several other patients with EB simplex. The structure-function relationships of the multiple keratins found in the epithelium have not been defined. The findings in transgenic mice and in patients suggest that the proteins are similar to collagens in that a large part of the conformation and surface properties of the monomers must be preserved for normal function.

In EB dystrophica, DNA linkage studies established that both dominantly and recessively inherited forms of the disease are coinherited with specific alleles of the genes for type VII collagen (COL7A1). Type VII collagen is seen in electron micrographs of skin as strandlike fibrils that anchor the basal lamina to the collagen fibrils of the dermis. Anchoring fibrils are decreased in number or absent in skin from patients with EB dystrophica. Therefore, mutations in the gene for type VII collagen can account for the clinical syndrome.

The gene or genes at fault in EB junctional are still unknown.

Diagnosis The diagnosis is based on skin that readily breaks and forms blisters. EB simplex, which affects only the epidermis, is generally milder than either EB junctional or EB dystrophica. EB dystrophica variants are generally associated with large and prominent scars. Classification within specific subtypes usually requires ultrastructural microscopy.

Treatment The treatment is symptomatic. Bruckner-Tuderman has reviewed the diagnostic criteria and management.

ALPORT SYNDROME (See also Chaps. 234 and 241) The Alport syndrome (AS) is a heritable disorder characterized by hematuria. Two forms of the disease are now recognized: (1) classic AS, which is inherited as an X-linked disorder with hematuria, sensorineural deafness, and conical deformation of the anterior surface of the lens (lenticonus), and (2) nonclassical AS, which is inherited as an autosomal trait that causes hematuria but not deafness or lenticonus.

Incidence The incidence of AS is about 1 in 10,000 in the general population and as high as 1 in 5000 in some ethnic groups.

Molecular defects Electron microscopy of kidneys from patients with classic AS demonstrated that the glomerular basement membrane was up to five times thicker than normal and that the lamina densa was distorted and split. DNA linkage studies demonstrated that the gene at fault is located on the long arm of the X chromosome (Xq22). The subsequent discovery that the $\alpha5(IV)$ chain of type IV collagen is also encoded on the long arm of the X chromosome spurred extensive analysis of the gene in the disease, and several mutations were identified. Most of the mutations are large deletions or gene rearrangements that probably cause decreased synthesis of $\alpha5(IV)$ chains. In the hemizygous male who inherits only the mutated gene, therefore, none of these chains is likely to be synthesized. The absence of the $\alpha5(IV)$ chains probably explains the manifestations. The most abundant type IV collagen in most basement membranes consists of two $\alpha1(IV)$ chains and one $\alpha2(IV)$ chain in the form of a large, rodlike molecule with globular ends and a long triple-helical domain that is interrupted by short sequences that do not form triple helices. The molecules self-assemble through both the globular ends and the triple-helical domains to form a complex, three-dimensional network. Since $\alpha5(IV)$ chains are similar in structure to $\alpha1(IV)$ or $\alpha2(IV)$ chains, they probably are assembled into monomers of a similar type IV collagen, either as homotrimers of $\alpha5(IV)$ chains or together with the $\alpha3(IV)$ and $\alpha4(IV)$ chains found in some basement membranes. No disease-causing mutations in the genes for $\alpha1(IV)$, $\alpha2(IV)$, $\alpha3(IV)$, or $\alpha4(IV)$ chains have been identified.

The cause of nonclassic AS with hematuria but without deafness is unknown.

Diagnosis The diagnosis of classic AS is based on X-linked inheritance of hematuria, sensorineural deafness, and lenticonus. Because of the X-linked transmission, women are usually less severely affected than men and are generally underdiagnosed. The hematuria progresses to nephritis and may cause renal failure in late adolescence in affected males and at older ages in some women. The sensorineural deafness is primarily in the high-tone range. It frequently can be detected only by an audiogram and usually is not progressive. The lenticonus rarely occurs without nephritis and is considered to be pathognomonic of classic AS.

Treatment There is no known treatment. DNA tests should soon be available for prenatal diagnosis.

REFERENCES

BARKER DF et al: Identification of mutations in the COL4A5 collagen gene in the Alport syndrome. Science 248:1224, 1990

BLECK EE: Non-operative treatment of osteogenesis imperfecta: Orthotic and mobility management. Clin Orthop 159:115, 1981

BOYE E et al: Major rearrangements in the α5(IV) collagen gene in three patients with Alport syndrome. Genomics 11:1125, 1991

BRUCKNER-TUDERMAN L: Epidermolysis bullosa, in *Connective Tissue and Its Heritable Disorders*, PM Royce, B Steinmann (eds). New York, Wiley-Liss, 1993, p. 507

BYERS PH: Osteogenesis imperfecta, in *Connective Tissue and Its Heritable Disorders*, PM Royce, B Steinmann (eds). New York, Wiley-Liss, 1993, p 317

FLINTER FA et al: Genetics of classic Alport's syndrome. Lancet 2:1005, 1988

HORTON WA, HECHT JT: The chondrodysplasias, in *Connective Tissue and Its Heritable Disorders*, PM Royce, B Steinmann (eds). New York, Wiley-Liss, 1993 p 641

KUIVANIEMI H et al: Mutations in collagen genes: Causes of rare and some common diseases in humans. FASEB J 5:2052, 1991

MARINI JC: Osteogenesis imperfecta: Comprehensive management. Adv Pediatr 35:391, 1988

——— et al: Evaluation of growth hormone axis and responsiveness to growth stimulation of short children with osteogenesis imperfecta. Am J Med Genet 45:21, 1993

McKUSICK VA: *Heritable Disorders of Connective Tissue*, 4th ed. St Louis, Mosby, 1972

PROCKOP DJ: Mutations in collagen genes as a cause of connective-tissue diseases. N Engl J Med 326:540, 1992

———, KIVIRIKKO KI: Heritable diseases of collagen. N Engl J Med 311:376, 1984

PYERITZ RE: The Marfan syndrome, in *Connective Tissue and Its Heritable Disorders*, PM Royce, B Steinmann (eds). New York, Wiley-Liss, 1993, p 437

SILLENCE DO: Osteogenesis imperfecta: An expanding panorama of variance. Clin Orthop 191:11, 1981

STEINMANN B et al: The Ehlers-Danlos syndrome, in *Connective Tissue and Its Heritable Disorders*, PM Royce, B Steinmann (eds). New York, Wiley-Liss, 1993, p 351

UITTO J, CHRISTIANO AM: Molecular genetics of the cutaneous basement membrane zone: Perspectives on epidermolysis bullosa and other blistering skin disorders. J Clin Invest 90:687, 1992

352 INHERITED DISORDERS OF AMINO ACID METABOLISM AND STORAGE

LEON E. ROSENBERG

All polypeptides and proteins are polymers of 20 different amino acids. Eight of these, referred to as *essential*, cannot be synthesized by humans and must be obtained from dietary sources. The others are formed endogenously. Although most of the body's amino acids are "tied up" in proteins, small intracellular pools of *free* amino acids are in equilibrium with extracellular reservoirs in plasma, cerebrospinal fluid, and the lumina of the gut and kidney. Physiologically, amino acids are more than mere "building blocks." Some (glycine, glutamate, γ-aminobutyric acid) are neurotransmitters. Others (phenylalanine, tyrosine, tryptophan, glycine) are precursors of hormones, coenzymes, pigments, purines, or pyrimidines. Each has a unique degradative pathway by which its nitrogen and carbon components are used for the synthesis of other amino acids, carbohydrates, and lipids.

Current concepts of inherited metabolic diseases are based to a considerable degree on investigations of amino acid disorders. More than 70 such disorders are now known, the catabolic defects (approximately 60) discussed in this chapter far outnumbering the transport abnormalities (approximately 10) considered in Chap. 353. Each of these disorders is rare—the incidences range from 1 in 10,000 for cystinuria or phenylketonuria to 1 in 200,000 for homocystinuria or alkaptonuria. Collectively, however, they occur in perhaps 1 in 500 to 1 in 1000 live births.

The salient features of inherited disorders of amino acid catabolism are summarized in Table 352-1. In general, these disorders are named for the compound that accumulates to highest concentration in blood (*-emias*) or urine (*-urias*). For many conditions (often called *aminoacidopathies*), the parent amino acid is found in excess; for

TABLE 352-1   Inherited disorders of amino acid catabolism

Amino acid(s) affected	Disorder or condition	Enzyme defect	Clinical manifestations*			
			Mental retardation	Neuropsychiatric dysfunction	Protein intolerance	Metabolic ketoacidosis
AROMATIC—HETEROCYCLIC						
Phenylalanine	Classic phenylketonuria	Phenylalanine hydroxylase	+	+	−	−
	Benign hyperphenylalaninemia	Phenylalanine hydroxylase	−	−	−	−
	Transient hyperphenylalaninemia	Phenylalanine hydroxylase	−	−	−	−
	Malignant hyperphenylalaninemia	Dihydropteridine reductase	+	+	−	−
	Malignant hyperphenylalaninemia	GTP cyclohydrolase	+	+	−	−
	Malignant hyperphenylalaninemia	6-Pyruvoyltetrahydrobiopterin synthase	+	+	−	−
Tyrosine	Hypertyrosinemia	Tyrosine aminotransferase (cytosol)	+	−	−	−
	Tyrosinosis	Tyrosine aminotransferase (?)	−	−	−	−
	Hereditary tyrosinemia	Fumarylacetoacetate hydrolase	−	−	−	−
	Alkaptonuria	Homogentisic acid oxidase	−	−	−	−
	Albinism (oculocutaneous)	Tyrosinase	−	−	−	−
	Albinism (ocular)	Unknown	−	−	−	−
Tryptophan	Tryptophanuria	Unknown	+	+	−	−
	Xanthurenic aciduria	Kynureninase	?	−	−	−
Histidine	Histidinemia	Histidine-ammonia lyase	±	±	−	−
	Urocanic aciduria	Urocanase	+	+	−	−
	Formiminoglutamic aciduria	Formiminotransferase	?	+	−	−
GLYCINE-IMINO ACIDS						
Glycine	Hyperglycinemia	Glycine cleavage	+	+	−	−
	Sarcosinemia	Sarcosine dehydrogenase	−	−	−	−
	Hyperoxaluria (type I)	Alanine: glyoxylate aminotransferase	−	−	−	−
	Hyperoxaluria (type II)	D-Glyceric acid dehydrogenase	−	−	−	−
Imino acids	Hyperprolinemia (type I)	Proline oxidase	−	−	−	−
	Hyperprolinemia (type II)	Δ′-Pyrroline dehydrogenase	−	−	−	−
	Hyperhydroxyprolinemia	Hydroxyproline reductase	−	−	−	−
	Iminopeptiduria	Prolidase	+	−	−	−
SULFUR-CONTAINING						
Methionine	Hypermethioninemia	Methionine adenosyltransferase	−	−	−	−
Homocystine	Homocystinuria	Cystathionine β-synthase	±	±	−	−
	Homocystinuria	5,10-Methylenetetrahydrofolate reductase	+	+	−	−
	Homocystinuria and methylmalonic acidemia (cblC, D)‡	Cobalamin (vitamin B_{12}) reductase (cytosol)	+	+	−	−
	Homocystinuria and methylmalonic acidemia (cblF)	Lysosomal efflux	+	+	−	−
	Homocystinuria (cblE, G)	Methyltransferase-associated cobalamin reductase (?)	+	+	−	−
Cystathionine	Cystathioninuria	Cystathionase	−	−	−	−
Cystine	Cystinosis	Lysosomal efflux	−	−	−	−
S-Sulfo-L-cysteine	*S*-Sulfo-L-cysteine, sulfite, and thiosulfaturia	Sulfite oxidase	+	+	−	−
CATIONIC						
Lysine	Hyperlysinemia	α-Aminoadipic semialdehyde synthase			−	
	Saccharopinuria	δ-Aminoadipic semialdehyde synthase	−	−	−	
	α-Ketoadipic aciduria	α-Ketoadipic acid dehydrogenase			−	−
	Glutaric aciduria (type I)	Glutaryl CoA dehydrogenase	−	+	−	−
	Glutaric aciduria (type II)	Electron transfer flavoprotein; or ETF-ubiquinone oxidoreductase	−	+	−	+

* +, Regularly present; ±, sometimes present; −, absent; ?, uncertain; all designations refer to manifestations in untreated disorder.
† AR, autosomal recessive; XL, X-linked; (AR), probably autosomal recessive.
‡ Designations in parentheses refer to complementation groups assigned by genetic analysis with cultured cells.

Ammonia intoxication	Other	Inheritance pattern[†]
−	Hypopigmented skin and hair, eczema	AR
−		AR
−		AR
−		AR
−		AR
−		AR
−	Palmar keratosis, corneal dystrophy	AR
−	Myasthenia gravis	?
−	Cirrhosis, hepatic failure, renal tubular dysfunction	AR
−	Ochronosis, arthritis	AR
−	Hypopigmentation of hair, skin, and optic fundus	AR
−	Hypopigmentation of optic fundus	XL, AR
−	Photosensitive skin rash	AR
−		?
−	Hearing and speech deficit	AR
−		?
−		(AR)
−		AR
−		AR
−	Calcium oxalate nephrolithiasis, renal failure	AR
−	Calcium oxalate nephrolithiasis, renal failure	AR
−		AR
−		AR
−		AR
−	Crusting erythematous, ecchymotic dermatitis, recurrent infections	AR
−		?
−	Dislocated lenses, osteoporosis, thrombotic vascular disease	AR
−		AR
−	Megaloblastic anemia	AR
−		(?)
−	Megaloblastic anemia	AR
−		AR
−	Fanconi syndrome, renal failure, photophobia	AR
−	Dislocated lenses	AR
−		AR
−		?
−		?
−		AR
−	Hypoglycemia, fatty degeneration of liver, kidney, heart	

(Table continues next page)

others, generally referred to as *organic acidemias*, products in the catabolic pathway accumulate. Which compound(s) accumulates depends, of course, on the site of the enzymatic block, the reversibility of the reactions proximal to the lesion, and the availability of alternative pathways of metabolic "runoff." For some amino acids, such as the sulfur-containing or branched-chain molecules, defects have been described at nearly each step in the catabolic pathway. For others, only small numbers of defective reactions have been described. Biochemical and genetic heterogeneity is common among the aminoacidopathies and organic acidemias. Five distinct forms of hyperphenylalaninemia, seven forms of homocystinuria, and seven types of methylmalonic acidemia are recognized. Such heterogeneity reflects the presence of an even larger array of molecular defects and is of clinical importance as well as scientific interest.

The manifestations of these conditions differ widely (see Table 352-1). Some, such as sarcosinemia or hyperprolinemia, produce no clinical consequences. At the other extreme, complete deficiency of ornithine transcarbamylase or of branched-chain keto acid dehydrogenase is lethal in the untreated neonate. Central nervous system dysfunction, in the form of developmental retardation, seizures, alterations in sensorium, or behavioral disturbances, occurs in more than half the disorders. Protein-induced vomiting, neurologic dysfunction, and hyperammonemia occur in many disorders of urea cycle intermediates. Metabolic ketoacidosis, often accompanied by hyperammonemia, is a frequent presenting finding in the disorders of branched-chain amino acid metabolism. Occasional disorders produce focal tissue or organ involvement such as liver disease, renal failure, cutaneous abnormalities, or ocular lesions.

The clinical manifestations in many of these conditions can be prevented or mitigated if diagnosis is achieved early and appropriate treatment (i.e., dietary protein or amino acid restriction or vitamin supplementation) is instituted promptly. For this reason, several aminoacidopathies and organic acidemias are screened for in mass newborn surveys that analyze blood or urine with an array of chemical and microbiologic techniques. Once a presumptive diagnosis is made, confirmation can be provided by direct enzyme assay on extracts of leukocytes, erythrocytes, or cultured fibroblasts. DNA-based diagnostic capability is possible for several disorders. For example, substitutions, deletions, and insertions can be identified to diagnose and characterize phenylketonuria, ornithine transcarbamylase deficiency, citrullinemia, gyrate atrophy of the retina, propionic acidemia, and methylmalonic acidemia (see also Chap. 61). As additional genes are cloned, DNA-based analysis will become more common.

Several of these disorders (including branched-chain ketoaciduria, isovaleric acidemia, propionic acidemia, methylmalonic acidemia, homocystinuria, cystinosis, phenylketonuria, ornithine transcarbamylase deficiency, citrullinemia, argininosuccinic aciduria) can be diagnosed prenatally by chemical analysis of amniotic fluid or by chemical, enzymatic, or DNA-based studies of fresh or cultured amniotic fluid cells. In addition to permitting selective termination of at-risk pregnancies, such diagnosis has led to improved postnatal treatment.

The remainder of this chapter focuses on selected disorders that illustrate the principles, properties, and problems presented by the disorders of amino acid metabolism.

THE HYPERPHENYLALANINEMIAS

DEFINITION The hyperphenylalaninemias (see Table 352-1) result from impaired conversion of phenylalanine to tyrosine. The most common and clinically important is phenylketonuria, which is characterized by an increased concentration of phenylalanine in blood, increased concentrations of phenylalanine and its by-products (notably phenylpyruvate, phenylacetate, phenyllactate, and phenylacetylglutamine) in urine, and severe mental retardation.

ETIOLOGY AND PATHOGENESIS Each of the hyperphenylalaninemias results from reduced activity of *phenylalanine hydroxylase*. In humans, this complete enzyme system is expressed only in liver. Phenylalanine and molecular oxygen are substrates, and a reduced

TABLE 352-1   Inherited disorders of amino acid catabolism (continued)

Amino acid(s) affected	Disorder or condition	Enzyme defect	Clinical manifestations*			
			Mental retardation	Neuropsychiatric dysfunction	Protein intolerance	Metabolic ketoacidosis
CATIONIC (continued)						
Ornithine	Hyperornithinemia-hyperammonemia-homocitrullinuria	Mitochondrial ornithine translocator (?)	+	+	+	−
	Hyperornithinemia	Ornithine-D-aminotransferase	−	−	−	−
UREA CYCLE						
Carbamylphosphate	Hyperammonemia (type I)	Carbamylphosphate synthetase I	+	+	+	−
N-acetylglutamate	Hyperammonemia (type IA)	N-acetylglutamate synthetase	?	+	+	−
Ornithine	Hyperammonemia (type II)	Ornithine transcarbamylase	±	+	+	−
Citrulline	Citrullinemia	Argininosuccinate synthetase	+	+	+	−
Argininosuccinic acid	Argininosuccinic aciduria	Argininosuccinase	+	+	+	−
Arginine	Argininemia	Arginase	+	+	+	−
BRANCHED-CHAIN						
Valine	Hypervalinemia	Valine aminotransferase	+	+	+	−
Leucine, isoleucine	Hyperleucine-isoleucinemia	Leucine-isoleucine aminotransferase	+	+	+	−
Valine, leucine, isoleucine	Classic branched-chain ketoaciduria	Branched-chain ketoacid dehydrogenase	+	+	+	
	Intermittent branched-chain ketoaciduria	Branched-chain ketoacid dehydrogenase	±	−	+	+
Leucine	Isovaleric acidemia	Isovaleryl CoA dehydrogenase	±	±	+	+
	β-Methylcrotonyl glycinuria	β-Methylcrotonyl CoA carboxylase	+	+	−	+
	β-Hydroxy-β-methylglutaric aciduria	β-Hydroxy-β-methylglutaryl CoA lyase	−	+	+	+
Isoleucine, valine	α-Methylacetoacetic aciduria	β-Ketothiolase	±	±	+	+
	Propionic acidemia (pcc A, B, C)‡	Propionyl CoA carboxylase	±	±	+	+
	Propionic acidemia (bio)‡	Holocarboxylase synthetase; biotinidase	+	±	+	+
	Methylmalonic acidemia (mut)‡	Methylmalonyl CoA mutase	±	±	+	+
	Methylmalonic acidemia (cbl A)‡	Cobalamin (vitamin B_{12}) reductase (mitochondrial) (?)	±	±	+	+
	Methylmalonic acidemia (cbl B)‡	Cobalamin (vitamin B_{12}): ATP adenosyltransferase	±	±	+	+

* +, Regularly present; ±, sometimes present; −, absent; ?, uncertain; all designations refer to manifestations in untreated disorder.
† AR, autosomal recessive; XL, X-linked; (AR), probably autosomal recessive.
‡ Designations in parentheses refer to complementation groups.

pteridine, tetrahydrobiopterin, is cofactor (Fig. 352-1). Tyrosine and dihydrobiopterin are the products of this catalytic system, the latter being reconverted to tetrahydrobiopterin by a second enzyme, dihydropteridine reductase. In classic phenylketonuria, activity of the hydroxylase apoenzyme, encoded by a gene in the q22–q24.1 region of chromosome 12, is almost totally deficient. Six different mutations leading to such complete deficiency are recognized. These include missense changes, splicing defects, and partial deletions. Benign hyperphenylalaninemia results from a less complete deficiency, and transient hyperphenylalaninemia (sometimes called *transient phenylketonuria*) is caused by a delayed maturation of the hydroxylase apoenzyme. In "malignant" hyperphenylalaninemia, however, persistent impairment of hydroxylating activity results not from abnormality in the apohydroxylase but from tetrahydrobiopterin deficiency due to blocks in the pathway by which tetrahydrobiopterin is synthesized from GTP or deficiency of dihydropteridine reductase, the enzyme that regenerates tetrahydrobiopterin from dihydrobiopterin (see Fig. 352-1). This reductase system is also utilized by tyrosine hydroxylase and tryptophan hydroxylase.

The hyperphenylalaninemias are autosomal recessive traits that occur in about 1 in 10,000 births. Classic phenylketonuria, which accounts for nearly two-thirds of these, is widely distributed among whites and Orientals. It is rare in blacks. Phenylalanine hydroxylase activity in obligate heterozygotes is low but higher than in affected homozygotes. Heterozygous carriers are clinically well but may have slightly increased phenylalanine concentrations in plasma.

Phenylalanine accumulation in blood and urine and reduced tyrosine formation are direct consequences of the impaired hydroxylation. In untreated phenylketonuria and in its tetrahydrobiopterin-deficient variants, plasma concentrations of phenylalanine become sufficiently high [greater than 1200 μmol/L (20 mg/dL)] to activate alternative pathways of metabolism and lead to formation of phenylpyruvate, phenylacetate, phenyllactate, and other derivatives that are rapidly cleared by the kidney and excreted in urine. Plasma concentrations of several other amino acids are moderately reduced, probably secondary to inhibition of gastrointestinal absorption or impairment of renal tubular reabsorption by excess phenylalanine. The severe brain damage is due to several consequences of phenylalanine

Ammonia intoxication	Other	Inheritance pattern[†]
+		AR
−	Gyrate atrophy of choroid and retina	AR
+		AR
+		?
+		XL
+		AR
+		AR
+		AR
−		?
−		?
−	"Maple syrup" odor	AR
−		AR
±	"Sweaty feet" odor	AR
−	"Cat's urine" odor	AR
−		?
+		AR
+		AR
−		AR
+		AR
+		AR
+		AR

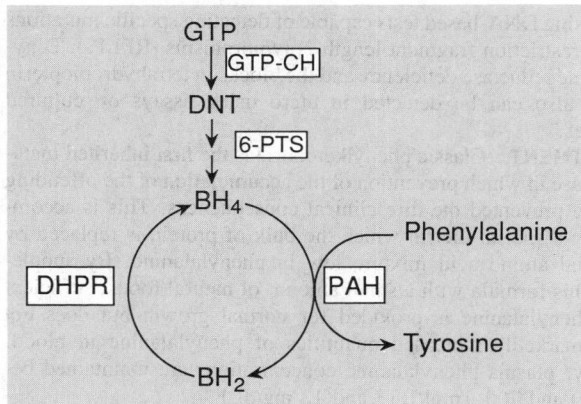

FIGURE 352-1 Pathways, enzymes, and coenzymes involved in the hyperphenylalaninemias. Blocked-in symbols highlight points of etiologic or therapeutic significance to the various genetic defects underlying these disorders. Abbreviations: GTP, guanosine triphosphate; GTP-CH, guanosine triphosphate cyclohydrolase; DNT, dihydroneopterin triphosphate; 6-PTS, 6-pyruvoyltetrahydropterin synthase; BH_4, tetrahydrobiopterin; BH_2, dihydrobiopterin; DHPR, dihydropteridine reductase; PAH, phenylalanine hydroxylase.

accumulation: competitive inhibition of transport of other amino acids required for protein synthesis, impaired polyribosome formation or stabilization, reduced myelin synthesis, and inadequate formation of norepinephrine and serotonin. Phenylalanine is a competitive inhibitor of tyrosinase, a key enzyme in the pathway of melanin synthesis. This block, plus reduced availability of the melanin precursor tyrosine, accounts for the hypopigmentation of hair and skin.

CLINICAL MANIFESTATIONS   No abnormalities are apparent at birth, but untreated children with classic phenylketonuria fail to attain early developmental milestones and demonstrate progressive impairment of cerebral function. Most require chronic institutionalization within a few years of birth because of the hyperactivity, seizures, and severe mental retardation. Electroencephalographic abnormalities, "mousy" odor of skin, hair, and urine (due to phenylacetate accumulation), and a tendency to hypopigmentation and eczema complete the devastating clinical picture. In contrast, affected children who are detected at birth and treated promptly show none of these abnormalities. Children with transient hyperphenylalaninemia or with the benign variant are not at risk for the clinical consequences of untreated

classic phenylketonuria. Children with tetrahydrobiopterin deficiency, however, are the most unfortunate. Seizures appear early, followed by progressive cerebral and basal ganglia dysfunction (rigidity, chorea, spasms, hypotonia). Most succumb to secondary infection within a few years despite early diagnosis and vigorous treatment.

A number of women with phenylketonuria who have been treated since infancy have reached adulthood and become pregnant. More than 90 percent of their offspring are markedly retarded, and many have additional congenital anomalies such as microcephaly, growth retardation, and congenital heart defects. Since these children are heterozygous, not homozygous for a phenylketonuria mutation, the clinical manifestations must be attributed to damage produced by the elevated maternal concentrations of phenylalanine to which they have been exposed in utero. This alarming syndrome is called *maternal phenylketonuria*.

DIAGNOSIS   Plasma phenylalanine concentrations are usually normal at birth in the hyperphenylalaninemias but rise rapidly after institution of protein feedings and are usually abnormal by day 4. Since diagnosis and initiation of dietary treatment of classic phenylketonuria must occur before the child is 30 days of age if developmental retardation is to be prevented, most newborns in North America and Europe are screened by determinations of blood phenylalanine concentration using the Guthrie bacterial inhibition assay. Infants with abnormal values are followed up with more quantitative fluorometric or chromatographic assays. In classic phenylketonuria and in tetrahydrobiopterin deficiency, values greater than 1200 μmol/L (20 mg/dL) are regularly observed. In transient or benign hyperphenylalaninemia, concentrations are usually lower but above control values of less than 60 μmol/L (1 mg/dL). Separation of classic phenylketonuria from its benign variants depends on following serial plasma phenylalanine concentrations as a function of age and dietary restriction. In transient hyperphenylalaninemia, plasma values return to normal within 3 to 4 months. In benign hyperphenylalaninemia, dietary restriction produces a more profound fall in plasma phenylalanine than in classic phenylketonuria. Deficiency of tetrahydrobiopterin must be considered in any child with hyperphenylalaninemia who develops progressive neurologic impairment despite prompt diagnosis and dietary treatment. These variants, which account for 1 to 5 percent of phenylketonuric children, can be diagnosed by enzyme assay on cultured fibroblasts. Administration of oral tetrahydrobiopterin loads also can distinguish children with classic phenylketonuria (who show no chemical response) from those with tetrahydrobiopterin deficiency (who exhibit a sharp fall in plasma phenylalanine). Prenatal diagnosis of classic phenylketonuria is now feasible using DNA-based tests capable of detecting specific mutations or linked restriction fragment length polymorphisms (RFLPs). Dihydropteridine reductase deficiency and the blocks in tetrahydrobiopterin synthesis also can be detected in utero using assays on cultured amniocytes.

TREATMENT   Classic phenylketonuria is the first inherited metabolic disease in which prevention of the accumulation of the offending metabolite prevented the dire clinical consequences. This is accomplished by a special diet in which the bulk of protein is replaced by an artificial amino acid mixture low in phenylalanine. By supplementing this formula with a small amount of natural foods, sufficient dietary phenylalanine is provided for normal growth but does not produce markedly increased quantities of phenylalanine in blood. Ordinarily, plasma phenylalanine concentrations are maintained between 180 and 700 μmol/L (3 and 12 mg/dL).

Such diet therapy must be instituted during the first month of life. Even then, modest nervous system dysfunction is often seen. Because uncontrolled hyperphenylalaninemia results in brain damage throughout childhood (and perhaps in adults), dietary restriction should be continued indefinitely in classic phenylketonuria. The transient and benign forms of hyperphenylalaninemia do not require long-term dietary restriction. As mentioned earlier, children with tetrahydrobiopterin deficiency deteriorate despite dietary phenylalanine restriction; efficacy of pteridine cofactor replacement is under study. Such patients may be helped, however, by a regimen in which dietary phenylalanine restriction is combined with supplements of levodopa and 5-hydroxytryptophan. Finally, the deleterious consequences of maternal phenylketonuria can be minimized by instituting dietary phenylalanine restriction prior to conception and continuing such treatment throughout gestation. This means that women with phenylketonuria should stay on a phenylalanine-restricted diet from birth through the childbearing years.

THE HOMOCYSTINURIAS

The homocystinurias are seven biochemically and clinically distinct disorders (see Table 352-1), each characterized by increased concentration of the sulfur-containing amino acid homocystine in blood and urine. The most common form results from reduced activity of cystathionine β-synthase, an enzyme in the transsulfuration pathway by which methionine is converted to cysteine. The other forms are the result of impaired conversion of homocysteine to methionine, a reaction catalyzed by homocysteine:methyltetrahydrofolate methyltransferase and two essential cofactors, methyltetrahydrofolate and methylcobalamin (methyl–vitamin B_{12}). Depending on the underlying disorder, some patients show chemical and, in some instances, clinical improvement following administration of specific vitamin supplements (pyridoxine, folate, or cobalamin).

CYSTATHIONINE β-SYNTHASE DEFICIENCY   Definition   Deficiency of this enzyme leads to increased concentrations of methionine and homocystine in body fluids and to decreased concentrations of cysteine and cystine. The clinical hallmark is dislocated optic lenses. Mental retardation, osteoporosis, and thrombotic vascular disease are frequent.

Etiology and pathogenesis   The sulfur atom of the essential amino acid methionine is transferred ultimately to cysteine by the transsulfuration pathway (Fig. 352-2). In one of these steps, homocysteine condenses with serine to form cystathionine. This reaction is catalyzed by the pyridoxal phosphate–dependent enzyme cystathionine β-synthase. The gene for this homodimeric enzyme has been mapped to the q21 region of chromosome 21. The condition is common in Ireland (1 in 40,000 births) but rare elsewhere (less than 1 in 200,000 births).

Homocysteine and methionine accumulate in cells and body fluids; cysteine synthesis is impaired, resulting in reduced concentrations of this amino acid and its disulfide form cystine. In approximately half of patients, synthase activity in liver, brain, leukocytes, and cultured fibroblasts is undetectable. In the remaining patients, tissues retain 1 to 5 percent of normal activity, and this residual activity often can be stimulated by pyridoxine supplementation. Heterozygous carriers of this autosomal recessive trait show no reproducible chemical abnormalities in body fluids but have reduced tissue synthase activity.

Homocysteine interferes with the normal cross-linking of collagen, an effect that likely plays an important role in the ocular, skeletal, and vascular complications. Altered collagen in the suspensory ligament of the optic lens and in bone matrix may account for the dislocated lenses and osteoporosis. Similarly, interference with normal ground substance metabolism in vascular walls may predispose to the arterial and venous thrombotic diathesis. Increased platelet adhesiveness may result from homocysteine accumulation, thereby contributing to the thrombotic occlusive disease so often observed. Recurrent cerebrovascular accidents secondary to thrombotic disease may account for the mental retardation, but direct chemical effects on cerebral cell metabolism have not been excluded.

Clinical manifestations   More than 80 percent of homozygotes for complete synthase deficiency have dislocated optic lenses. This abnormality usually appears by 3 to 4 years of age and often results in glaucoma and impaired visual acuity. Mental retardation occurs in about half of such patients, often accompanied by ill-defined behavioral disturbances. Osteoporosis is a common radiologic finding (seen in two-thirds of patients by age 15) but rarely causes clinical disease. Life-threatening vascular complications, probably initiated by damage to vascular endothelium, are the major cause of morbidity and mortality. Occlusion of coronary, renal, and cerebral arteries with attendant tissue infarction can occur during the first decade of life. Nearly one-quarter of patients die of vascular disease before age 30. These vascular complications seem to be exacerbated by angiographic procedures. Importantly, pyridoxine-responsive patients have milder clinical manifestations in all regards. Heterozygous carriers for synthase deficiency (about 1 in 70 in the population) and others with high concentrations of plasma homocysteine may be at increased risk for premature coronary, peripheral, and cerebral occlusive vascular disease.

Diagnosis   The cyanide-nitroprusside test is a simple way of demonstrating increased excretion of sulfhydryl-containing compounds in urine. Since cystine and S-sulfocysteine also give a positive test, other disorders of sulfur metabolism must be excluded, but this is usually possible on clinical grounds. Distinction of cystathionine β-synthase deficiency from other causes of homocystinuria usually can be accomplished by measurements of plasma methionine, which tend to be increased in synthase-deficient patients and normal or low in those with impaired methionine formation (see below). Diagnostic confirmation depends on measurements of synthase activity in tissue extracts. Heterozygotes can be identified by measurement of peak serum homocystine after an oral methionine load and by measurement of tissue synthase activity.

Treatment   As with classic phenylketonuria, effective treatment depends on early diagnosis. A number of infants diagnosed in the newborn period have been treated successfully with methionine-restricted, cystine-supplemented diets. Their clinical course is benign compared with that of untreated affected siblings. In approximately half of patients, oral pyridoxine (25 to 500 mg/d) produces a fall in plasma and urinary methionine and homocystine and an increase in cystine concentration in body fluids. This effect probably reflects a modest increase in synthase activity in cells of patients in whom the defect is characterized either by reduced affinity for cofactor or by accelerated degradation of mutant enzyme. Since such vitamin supplementation is apparently harmless, it should be tried in all patients. There are no reports of the effect of the initiation of pyridoxine supplementation soon after birth. Similarly, there are no data regarding pyridoxine supplements in heterozygous carriers.

5,10-METHYLENETETRAHYDROFOLATE REDUCTASE DEFICIENCY   Definition   In this form of homocystinuria, methionine concentrations in body fluids are normal or decreased because deficiency of 5,10-methylenetetrahydrofolate reductase leads to im-

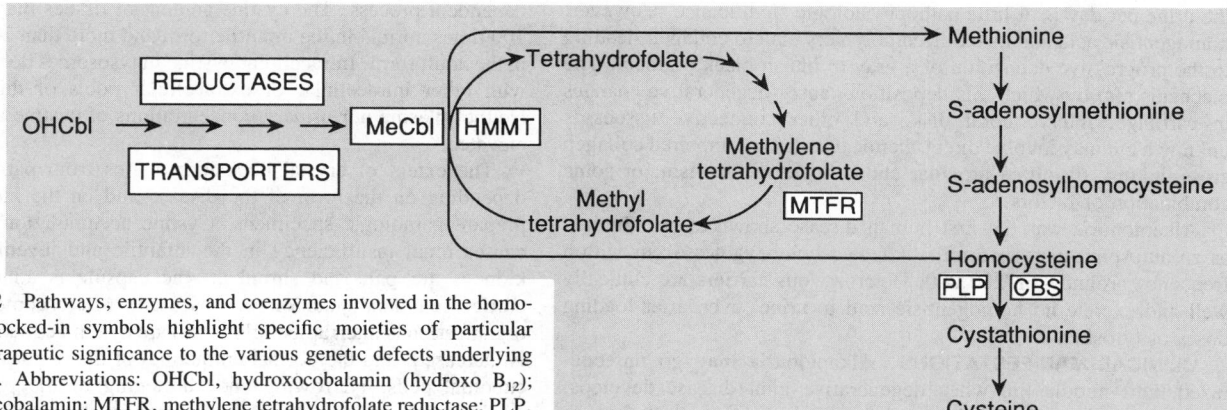

FIGURE 352-2 Pathways, enzymes, and coenzymes involved in the homocystinurias. Blocked-in symbols highlight specific moieties of particular etiologic or therapeutic significance to the various genetic defects underlying these disorders. Abbreviations: OHCbl, hydroxocobalamin (hydroxo B_{12}); MeCbl, methylcobalamin; MTFR, methylene tetrahydrofolate reductase; PLP, pyridoxal phosphate; CBS, cystathionine β-synthase.

paired synthesis of 5-methyltetrahydrofolate, a cofactor in the enzymatic formation of methionine from homocysteine (see Fig. 352-2). Central nervous system dysfunction occurs in most patients.

Etiology and pathogenesis 5-Methyltetrahydrofolate:homocysteine methyltransferase catalyzes the conversion of homocysteine to methionine. The methyl group transferred in this reaction comes from 5-methyltetrahydrofolate, which is converted to tetrahydrofolate in the process. 5-Methyltetrahydrofolate, in turn, is synthesized enzymatically from 5,10-methylenetetrahydrofolate by 5,10-methylenetetrahydrofolate reductase. Thus reductase activity controls both methionine synthesis and tetrahydrofolate generation. This series of reactions is critical to normal DNA and RNA synthesis. A primary defect in the reductase activity results, secondarily, in deficient methyltransferase activity and impaired conversion of homocysteine to methionine. Methionine deficiency and impaired nucleic acid synthesis may contribute to the central nervous system dysfunction. The disorder appears to be inherited as an autosomal recessive trait.

Clinical manifestations More than 25 children with homocystinuria due to reductase deficiency have been reported. The most severely affected have developmental retardation and cerebral atrophy early in life. Others have behavioral disturbances (catatonia) during the second decade or mild retardation. Presumably the severity of the clinical manifestations reflects the severity of the reductase deficiency.

Diagnosis and treatment The combination of increased concentrations of homocystine in body fluids with normal or decreased concentrations of methionine should suggest this entity. Serum folate concentrations are low in some patients. Confirmation requires direct reductase assays in tissue extracts (brain, liver, cultured fibroblasts). Although therapeutic experience is limited, one teenage girl with a catatonic psychosis responded dramatically, both chemically and clinically, to folate supplements (5 to 10 mg/d). When the folate was withdrawn, behavior worsened. This observation suggests that early diagnosis followed by folate supplementation may forestall neurologic or psychiatric disturbances.

DEFICIENCY OF COBALAMIN (VITAMIN B_{12}) COENZYME SYNTHESIS Definition Five other forms of homocystinuria also reflect impaired conversion of homocysteine to methionine. The primary defects in these entities, however, are in the synthesis of methylcobalamin, a cobalamin (vitamin B_{12}) coenzyme required by methyltetrahydrofolate:homocysteine methyltransferase (see Fig. 352-2). In some, methylmalonic acid accumulates in body fluids because of impaired synthesis of a second coenzyme, adenosylcobalamin, required for isomerization of methylmalonyl coenzyme A (CoA) to succinyl CoA. These disorders are designated cblC, D, E, F, and G.

Etiology and pathogenesis As with 5,10-methylenetetrahydrofolate reductase deficiency, each disorder impairs remethylation of homocysteine. Since methylcobalamin is required for methyl-group transfer from methyltetrahydrofolate to homocysteine, impaired cobalamin metabolism leads to deficient methyltransferase activity. The

defects responsible for impaired synthesis of methylcobalamin involve one of several steps in lysosomal or cytosolic activation of the vitamin precursor (see Fig. 352-2). In the cblF disorder, the transport of cobalamins out of lysosomes is impaired. In cblC and D, a reductase needed for formation of both methylcobalamin and adenosylcobalamin is deficient. In cblE and G, some component required to maintain a reduced form of cobalamin on the methyltransferase apoenzyme is impaired. Somatic cell genetic studies indicate that each of these abnormalities is distinct and imply that all are inherited as autosomal recessive traits.

Clinical manifestations More than 25 patients—mostly children—with these defects in cobalamin metabolism have been described. Although clinical manifestations vary, abnormalities include developmental delay, dementia, spasticity, megaloblastic anemia, and pancytopenia. It is not possible to define a specific clinical syndrome for each of the defects in cobalamin metabolism.

Diagnosis and treatment Homocystinuria, homocystinemia, and hypomethioninemia are the chemical hallmarks. Methylmalonic acidemia, too, has been noted in those defects resulting from defective synthesis of both cobalamin coenzymes. These findings also may be present in juvenile- or adult-onset pernicious anemia in which intestinal cobalamin absorption is impaired. Measurement of serum cobalamin concentrations, low in pernicious anemia and normal in patients with defective conversion of cobalamin vitamin to coenzymes, helps in the differential diagnosis. Definitive diagnosis depends on demonstrating impaired coenzyme synthesis in cultured cells. Treatment of affected children with cobalamin supplements (1 to 2 mg/d) causes homocystine and methylmalonate excretion to fall to near normal values; the hematologic and neurologic deficits also have lessened to a variable degree in several patients. Intervention early in life seems to offer the best long-term prognosis.

ALKAPTONURIA

DEFINITION Alkaptonuria is a rare disorder of tyrosine catabolism in which deficiency of homogentisic acid oxidase leads to excretion of large amounts of homogentisic acid in urine and accumulation of oxidized homogentisic acid pigment in connective tissues (ochronosis). After many years, ochronosis produces a distinctive form of degenerative arthritis.

ETIOLOGY AND PATHOGENESIS Homogentisic acid is an intermediate in the catabolism of tyrosine. Activity of homogentisic acid oxidase, the enzyme that catalyzes the opening of the phenolic ring yielding maleylacetoacetic acid, is deficient in liver and kidney of patients with alkaptonuria, and homogentisic acid accumulates in cells and body fluids. Patients have minimally increased concentrations of homogentisic acid in blood because it is rapidly cleared by the kidney. The excretion of as much as 3 to 7 g homogentisic acid in the urine per day is of little pathophysiologic significance. However, homogentisic acid and its oxidized polymers bind to collagen, leading to the progressive deposition of a gray to bluish black pigment. The mechanism(s) by which this deposition causes degenerative changes in cartilage, intervertebral disk, and other connective tissues is unknown but may involve direct chemical irritation, impaired collagen cross-linking, disturbed articular chondrocyte metabolism, or some combination of factors.

Alkaptonuria was the first human disease shown to be inherited as an autosomal recessive trait. Affected homozygotes occur with a frequency around 1 in 200,000. Heterozygous carriers are clinically well and excrete no homogentisic acid in urine, even after loading doses of tyrosine.

CLINICAL MANIFESTATIONS Alkaptonuria may go unrecognized until middle life when degenerative joint disease develops. Prior to this time, the tendency of the patient's urine to darken on standing may go unnoticed, as may slight discoloration of the sclerae and ears. The latter manifestations are generally the earliest external evidence of the disorder and develop after age 20 to 30. Foci of gray-brown scleral pigment and generalized darkening of the concha, anthelix, and finally, helix of the ear are typical. Ear cartilages may be irregular and thickened. *Ochronotic arthritis* is heralded by pain, stiffness, and some limitation of motion of the hips, knees, and shoulders. Acute arthritis may resemble rheumatoid arthritis, but small joints are usually spared. Limitation of motion and ankylosis of the lumbosacral spine are common late manifestations. Pigmentation of heart valves, larynx, tympanic membranes, and skin occurs, and occasional patients develop pigmented renal or prostatic calculi. Degenerative cardiovascular disease may be increased in older patients.

DIAGNOSIS A patient whose urine darkens to blackness on standing must be suspected of having alkaptonuria but, because of modern plumbing conditions, is not often observed. The diagnosis is usually made from the triad of degenerative arthritis, ochronotic pigmentation, and urine that turns black upon alkalinization. Homogentisic acid in urine may be identified presumptively by other tests: upon addition of ferric chloride, a purple-black color is observed; treatment with Benedict's reagent yields a brown color; addition of a saturated silver nitrate solution produces an immediate black color. These screening tests can be confirmed by chromatographic, enzymatic, or spectrophotometric determinations of homogentisic acid. X-rays of the lumbar spine are virtually pathognomonic. They show degeneration and dense calcification of the intervertebral disks and narrowing of the intervertebral spaces.

TREATMENT There is no specific treatment for ochronotic arthritis. Joint manifestations might be mitigated if homogentisic acid accumulation and deposition could be curbed by dietary restriction of phenylalanine and tyrosine, but the long course of the disease has discouraged such therapeutic attempts. Ascorbic acid impedes oxidation and polymerization of homogentisic acid in vitro, but the efficacy of this form of treatment has not been established. Symptomatic treatment is similar to that for osteoarthritis (Chap. 296).

CYSTINOSIS

DEFINITION Cystinosis is a rare disorder characterized by the intralysosomal accumulation of free cystine in body tissues. This results in the appearance of cystine crystals in the cornea, conjunctiva, bone marrow, lymph nodes, leukocytes, and internal organs. Three variants have been identified: an infantile (nephropathic) form leading to the Fanconi syndrome and renal insufficiency in the first decade, a juvenile (intermediate) form in which renal disease is manifest during the second decade, and an adult (benign) form characterized by deposition of cystine in the cornea but not in the kidney.

ETIOLOGY AND PATHOGENESIS The basic defect involves impaired efflux of cystine from lysosomes rather than an abnormality in cystine catabolism. Lysosomal cystine efflux is an active, ATP-

dependent process. The cystine content of tissues may be more than 100 times normal in the infantile form and more than 30 times normal in the adult form. Intracellular cystine in lysosomes does not exchange with other intracellular or extracellular pools of this amino acid. Neither plasma nor urinary concentrations of cystine are particularly elevated.

The extent of crystal deposition varies from patient to patient, depending on the form of the disease and on the methods used to prepare pathologic specimens. Cystine accumulation in the kidney causes renal insufficiency in the infantile and juvenile forms. The kidneys are pale and shrunken, the capsule is adherent, and the corticomedullary junction is obscured. Microscopically, nephron organization is interrupted, glomeruli are hyalinized, connective tissue is increased, and the normal epithelium of the tubules is replaced by cuboidal cells. Narrowing and shortening of the proximal tubule produce the swan neck deformity that is characteristic of but not specific for cystinosis. Patchy depigmentation and degeneration of the peripheral retina occurs in the infantile and juvenile forms. Cystine crystals also may be deposited in the cornea, ocular conjunctiva, or uvea.

Each form appears to be inherited as an autosomal recessive trait. Obligate heterozygotes have intracellular cystine concentrations intermediate between those of normal persons and affected patients but are free of clinical abnormalities.

CLINICAL MANIFESTATIONS In the infantile form, abnormalities are usually apparent by 4 to 6 months of age. Growth retardation, vomiting, fever, vitamin D–resistant rickets, polyuria, dehydration, and metabolic acidosis are prominent. Generalized proximal tubular dysfunction (the Fanconi syndrome) leads to hyperphosphaturia and hypophosphatemia, renal glycosuria, generalized aminoaciduria, hypouricemia, and often hypokalemia. Pyelonephritis may contribute, along with interstitial fibrosis, to progressive glomerular insufficiency. Death due to uremia or intercurrent infection usually occurs before age 10. Ocular manifestations are prominent. Photophobia is usually demonstrable within the first few years of life due to cystine deposits in the cornea, and retinal degeneration may appear even earlier.

In contrast, patients with the adult form have only ocular abnormalities. Photophobia, headache, and burning or itching of the eyes are major complaints. Glomerular and tubular function and the integrity of the retina are preserved. The findings in the juvenile variant fall between these extremes. Ocular and renal manifestations do not become significant until the second decade. The renal lesion, albeit milder than that in the infantile form, eventually leads to renal insufficiency.

DIAGNOSIS Cystinosis must be considered in any child with vitamin D–resistant rickets, the Fanconi syndrome, or glomerular insufficiency. Hexagonal or rectangular cystine crystals can be detected in the cornea (by slit-lamp examination), in leukocytes from peripheral blood or bone marrow, or in biopsies of rectal mucosa. Diagnosis can be confirmed by quantification of cystine in peripheral blood leukocytes or cultured fibroblasts. The infantile form has been diagnosed prenatally by the demonstration of increased cystine content in cultured amniotic fluid cells.

TREATMENT The adult form is benign and requires no treatment. Symptomatic treatment of renal disease in the infantile or juvenile form does not differ from that of other forms of chronic renal insufficiency: maintenance of adequate fluid intake to prevent dehydration; correction of the metabolic acidosis; and ingestion of supplementary calcium, phosphate, and vitamin D to heal the rickets. Such measures are effective in maintaining growth, development, and well-being in affected children for a time. Two specific therapies have been attempted. Cystine-restricted diets do not prevent progression of renal disease. This is not surprising given the nature of the primary defect and the large amount of cystine produced endogenously by cellular protein turnover. Whereas the early use of thiol reagents such as penicillamine and dimercaprol yielded no long-term benefits, administration of the free thiol cysteamine slows the progression of renal dysfunction, improves growth, and dissolves corneal cystine crystals. This compound acts in lysosomes by forming a mixed disulfide with cysteine that can be transported out of the organelle by a different transporter from that deficient in the disease.

The most successful form of therapy for nephropathic cystinosis is renal transplantation. Hundreds of affected children with end-stage renal disease have been so treated. Those patients who tolerated the procedure and did not develop immunologic problems have had return of kidney function toward normal. The transplanted kidneys have not developed the functional abnormalities typical of cystinosis (i.e., the Fanconi syndrome or glomerular insufficiency). Patients may, however, continue to accumulate cystine in the cornea and other ocular tissues. Because the usual life span of a transplanted kidney is generally 15 to 20 years, some patients with the infantile form of cystinosis have received two or more transplanted kidneys.

PRIMARY HYPEROXALURIA

DEFINITION Primary hyperoxaluria is the designation for two rare disorders characterized by chronic excessive urinary excretion of oxalic acid and by calcium oxalate nephrolithiasis and nephrocalcinosis. Typically, patients with both forms develop renal insufficiency early in life and die of uremia. At postmortem examination, calcium oxalate deposits are widespread in renal and extrarenal tissues, a condition referred to as *oxalosis*.

ETIOLOGY AND PATHOGENESIS The metabolic basis for the primary hyperoxalurias involves pathways of glyoxylate metabolism. In type I hyperoxaluria, urinary excretion of oxalate and of the oxidized and reduced forms of glyoxylate is increased. The excessive synthesis of these substances results from a block in glyoxylate metabolism. The primary defect in most patients is deficiency of the hepatic peroxisomal enzyme alanine:glyoxylate amino transferase. In the remainder the transferase is misdirected to mitochondria and is, thereby, nonfunctional. The resulting expansion of the glyoxylate pool leads to enhanced oxidation of glyoxylate to oxalate and to enhanced reduction of glyoxylate to glycolate. Each of these 2-carbon acids is then excreted in excess in the urine. In type II hyperoxaluria, L-glyceric acid is excreted in excess along with oxalate. In this condition, activity of D-glyceric acid dehydrogenase, which catalyzes the reduction of hydroxypyruvate to D-glyceric acid in the catabolic pathway of serine metabolism, is absent in leukocytes (and presumably other tissues). The accumulated hydroxypyruvate is instead reduced by lactic dehydrogenase to the L-isomer of glycerate, which is excreted in the urine. The reduction of hydroxypyruvate is coupled in some way to the oxidation of glyoxylate to oxalate, thus causing the formation of increased oxalate. Both disorders appear to be inherited as autosomal recessive traits. Heterozygotes are asymptomatic.

Stone formation, nephrocalcinosis, and oxalosis are due to insolubility of calcium oxalate. Extrarenal deposits of oxalate are prominent in the heart, walls of arteries and veins, male urogenital tract, and bone.

CLINICAL MANIFESTATIONS Nephrolithiasis and oxalosis may be manifest during the first year of life. Most patients experience renal colic or hematuria between ages 2 and 10 and succumb to uremia before age 20. With the onset of uremia, patients may develop severe peripheral arterial spasm and necrosis with resulting vascular insufficiency. Oxalate excretion falls as renal failure worsens. In patients with delayed onset of symptoms, survival to age 50 or 60 has been reported, despite recurrent nephrolithiasis.

DIAGNOSIS Oxalate excretion in normal children or adults is less than 0.5 mmol (60 mg) per 1.73 m² surface area per day. Patients with type I or type II hyperoxaluria generally excrete two to four times this amount. Distinction between the two types depends on measurements of the other organic acids that identify them: glycolic acid in type I and L-glyceric acid in type II. Since patients with pyridoxine deficiency or chronic ileal disease may excrete excessive amounts of oxalate, these conditions must be excluded.

TREATMENT There is no satisfactory treatment. Urinary oxalate concentration can be transiently reduced by increasing the urinary flow rate. Large doses of pyridoxine (100 mg/d) may reduce urinary oxalate, but long-term effects are not dramatic. A diet high in phosphate content seems to reduce the frequency of attacks of renal colic, but oxalate excretion is unaffected. Finally, after renal transplantation renal function is lost because of calcium oxalate deposition in the transplanted kidney. The beneficial effects of combined liver-kidney transplantation observed in a single patient warrant additional study.

REFERENCES

BOERS GHJ et al: Heterozygosity for homocystinuria in premature peripheral and cerebral occlusive arterial disease. N Engl J Med 313:709, 1985

EISENSMITH RC, WOO SLC: Molecular basis of phenylketonuria and related hyperphenylalaninemias: Mutations and polymorphisms in the human phenylalanine hydroxylase gene. Hum Mutat 1:13, 1992

FENTON WA, ROSENBERG LE: Inherited disorders of cobalamin transport and metabolism, in *The Molecular and Metabolic Basis of Inherited Disease*, 7th ed, CR Scriver et al (eds). New York, McGraw-Hill, in press

GAHL WA et al: Lysosomal transport disorders, in *The Molecular and Metabolic Basis of Inherited Disease*, 7th ed, CR Scriver et al (eds). New York, McGraw-Hill, in press

HILLMAN RE: Primary hyperoxalurias, in *The Molecular and Metabolic Basis of Inherited Disease*, 7th ed, CR Scriver et al (eds). New York, McGraw-Hill, in press

LADU BN: Alcaptonuria, in *The Molecular and Metabolic Basis of Inherited Disease*, 7th ed, CR Scriver et al (eds). New York, McGraw-Hill, in press

MUDD SH et al: Natural history of homocystinuria due to cystathionine β-synthase deficiency. Am J Hum Genet 37:709, 1985

—— et al: Disorders of transsulfuration, in *The Molecular and Metabolic Basis of Inherited Disease*, 7th ed, CR Scriver et al (eds). New York, McGraw-Hill, in press

PLATT LE et al: Maternal phenylketonuria collaborative study, obstetric aspects and outcome: The first 6 years. Am J Obstet Gynecol 166:1150, 1992

PURDUE PE et al: Mistargeting of peroxisomal L-alanine:glyoxylate aminotransferase to mitochondria in primary hyperoxaluria patients depends upon activation of a cryptic mitochondrial targeting sequence by a point mutation. Proc Natl Acad Sci USA 88:10900, 1991

ROSENBERG LE, SCRIVER CR: Disorders of amino acid metabolism, in *Metabolic Control and Disease*, 8th ed, PK Bondy, LE Rosenberg (eds). Philadelphia, Saunders, 1980, pp 583–776

SCRIVER CR et al: The hyperphenylalaninemias, in *The Molecular and Metabolic Basis of Inherited Disease*, 7th ed, CR Scriver et al (eds). New York, McGraw-Hill, in press

353 INHERITED DEFECTS OF MEMBRANE TRANSPORT

LEON E. ROSENBERG / ELIZABETH M. SHORT

The passage of many molecules across plasma cell membranes depends on transport systems that owe their specificity to membrane receptor and "carrier" proteins. These membrane constituents recognize individual molecules or structurally related substances and catalyze their transmembrane movement by mechanisms poorly understood. The disorders considered in this chapter have three features in common: each is characterized by a specific defect in the transport of one or more compounds; each is inherited as a dominant or recessive trait, implying that a single genetic locus is involved; and each is presumed to reflect a primary alteration in a specific membrane protein. Many of these defects have been well characterized physiologically. The mutation in one of these disorders has been identified, namely, the intestinal glucose transporter gene in a family with glucose-galactose malabsorption syndrome.

More than 20 inherited disorders of membrane transport have been described (Table 353-1). Most affect the gut and/or kidney only. Classes of substrates represented include amino acids, sugars, cations, anions, vitamins, and water. Some are discussed elsewhere in this text. Those impairing the transport of amino acids, hexoses, urate, and chloride are discussed here as examples of the abnormalities encountered.

TABLE 353-1   Genetic disorders of membrane transport

Class of substance and disorder	Individual substrates	Tissues manifesting transport defect	Proposed molecular basis of defect	Major clinical manifestations	Mode of inheritance	Location of discussion
AMINO ACIDS						
Classic cystinuria	Cystine, lysine, arginine, ornithine	Proximal renal tubule, jejunal mucosa	Mutation of shared dibasic-cystine transport protein	Cystine nephrolithiasis	Autosomal recessive	Chap. 353
Dibasicamino-aciduria	Lysine, arginine, ornithine	Proximal renal tubule, jejunal mucosa	Mutation of dibasic transport protein	Type I: Benign Type II: Protein intolerance, hyperammonemia, retardation	Autosomal recessive	Chap. 353
Hypercystinuria	Cystine	Proximal renal tubule	Mutation of cystine transport protein	Some risk of cystine nephrolithiasis	Autosomal recessive	Chap. 353
Lysinuria	Lysine	Proximal renal tubule, jejunal mucosa	Mutation of lysine transport protein	Seizures, physical and mental retardation	Possible autosomal recessive	Chap. 353
Hartnup disease	Neutral amino acids	Proximal renal tubule, jejunal mucosa	Mutation of shared neutral amino acid transport protein	Constant neutral aminoaciduria, intermittent symptoms of pellagra	Autosomal recessive	Chap. 353
Tryptophan malabsorption	Tryptophan	Jejunal mucosa	Mutation of tryptophan transport protein	Indoluria, ?hypercalcemia, ?nephrocalcinosis	Probable autosomal recessive	Chap. 353
Methionine malabsorption	Methionine	Jejunal mucosa	Mutation of methionine transport protein	α-Hydroxy-butyricaciduria, white hair, mental retardation, convulsions, hyperpneic attacks, edema	Probable autosomal recessive	Chap. 353
Histidinuria	Histidine	Proximal renal tubule, jejunal mucosa	Mutation of histidine transport protein	Mental retardation	Autosomal recessive	Chap. 353
Iminoglycinuria	Glycine, proline, hydroxyproline	Proximal renal tubule, jejunal mucosa	Mutation of shared glycine–imino acid transport protein	None	Autosomal recessive	Chap. 353
Dicarboxylic-aminoaciduria	Glutamic acid, aspartic acid	Proximal renal tubule, jejunal mucosa	Mutation of shared dicarboxylic amino acid transport protein	None	Probable autosomal recessive	Chap. 353
Cystinosis	Cystine	Lysosomal membranes	Mutation of cystine transport protein	Renal failure, hypothyroidism, blindness	Autosomal recessive	Chap. 352
HEXOSES						
Renal glycosuria	D-Glucose	Proximal renal tubule	Mutation of D-glucose transport protein	Glycosuria with normal blood glucose	Autosomal recessive	Chap. 353
Glucose-galactose malabsorption	D-Glucose D-Galactose	Jejunal mucosa, proximal renal tubule	Mutation of shared Na$^+$-dependent glucose-galactose transport protein	Watery diarrhea on feeding glucose, lactose, sucrose, or galactose	Autosomal recessive	Chaps. 254, 353
LIPIDS						
Familial hypercholesterolemia	Cholesterol	Fibroblasts, lymphoid lines, leukocytes	Mutation of membrane LDL–cholesterol receptor protein	Hypercholesterolemia, tendon xanthomas, arcus corneae, coronary artery atherosclerosis	Autosomal dominant	Chap. 344
URATE						
Hypouricemia	Uric acid	Proximal renal tubule	Mutation of urate transport protein	Hypouricemia, hyperuricosuria, ?hypercalcinuria	Autosomal recessive	Chap. 353
ANIONS						
Familial hypophosphatemic rickets	Inorganic phosphate	Proximal renal tubule, jejunal mucosa	Mutation of inorganic phosphate transport protein	Hypophosphatemia, phosphaturia, phosphatopenic rickets/osteomalacia	X-linked dominant	Chap. 358

TABLE 353-1 Genetic disorders of membrane transport *(continued)*

Class of substance and disorder	Individual substrates	Tissues manifesting transport defect	Proposed molecular basis of defect	Major clinical manifestations	Mode of inheritance	Location of discussion
ANIONS *(continued)*						
Congenital chloridorrhea	Chloride	Ileal and colonic mucosa	Mutation of Cl^-/H^+ uptake pump of Cl^-/HCO_3 exchange pump carrier protein	Hydramnios, watery diarrhea, elevated fecal chloride, achloriduria, metabolic alkalosis with volume depletion, hyperaldosteronism	Autosomal recessive	Chaps. 254, 353
Cystic fibrosis	Chloride	Lung, pancreas, sweat gland	Mutation of ion channel protein	Pulmonary, pancreatic destruction	Autosomal recessive	Chap. 222
Familial goiter	Inorganic iodide	Thyroid gland, salivary gland, gastric mucosa	Mutation of iodide transport protein	Congenital hypothyroidism (cretinism), goiter	Probable autosomal recessive	Chap. 334
CATIONS						
Distal renal tubular acidosis (type I—gradient)	Hydrogen ion	Distal renal tubule	Mutation of distal tubule H^+ pump carrier protein	Hyperchloremic acidosis, hypokalemia, acquired nephrocalcinosis, and hypercalcinuria	Autosomal dominant	Chap. 244
Proximal renal tubular acidosis (type II—HCO_3^- wasting)	Hydrogen ion	Proximal renal tubule	Mutation of proximal tubule H^+ pump carrier protein	Hyperchloremic acidosis, bicarbonate wasting	Probable autosomal recessive	Chap. 244
Menkes' disease	Copper	Duodenal and jejunal intestinal cells	Possible serosal transport protein or intracellular transport defect	Severe mental retardation, pili torti (kinky hair), typical facies, arterial tortuosity, excess Wormian bones, thermal instability	X-linked recessive	Chaps. 78
Lethal diarrhea	Sodium ion	Jejunal intestinal cells	Mutation of Na^+/H^+ proton exchange pump	Watery diarrhea, severe sodium depletion, and acidosis	Recessive?	Chap. 254
WATER						
Nephrogenic diabetes insipidus (AVP-resistant)	Water	Distal renal tubule	Lack of activation of AVP-responsive luminal membrane adenylate cyclase, possible defect in receptor or enzyme protein	Polyuria, polydipsia, hyposthenuria	X-linked recessive	Chap. 244
VITAMINS						
Juvenile pernicious anemia	Cobalamin (vitamin B_{12})	Ileal mucosa	Mutation of receptor for intrinsic factor–cobalamin complex	Megaloblastic anemia	Autosomal recessive	Chap. 304
Folate malabsorption	Folic acid	Small bowel	Mutation of folate transport protein	Megaloblastic anemia	Autosomal recessive	Chap. 304
OTHER						
Sialic acid storage	Sialic acid (monosaccharide)	Lysosomes	Mutation of sialic acid transport protein	Retardation	Autosomal recessive	Chap. 349

DISORDERS OF AMINO ACID TRANSPORT

As noted in Table 353-1, 10 disorders of amino acid transport have been described. Five (cystinuria, dibasicaminoaciduria, Hartnup disease, iminoglycinuria, and dicarboxylicaminoaciduria) show transport abnormalities for structurally related amino acids, thereby implying the existence of group-specific membrane receptors or carriers. With the exception of iminoglycinuria and dicarboxylicaminoaciduria, the defects have important clinical consequences. The remaining five disorders affect the transport of only one amino acid, implying the existence of substrate-specific transport systems. Each of these conditions affects transport in the kidney, gut, or both; none has been shown to alter transport in other tissues.

CYSTINURIA Definition Cystinuria, the most common inborn error of amino acid transport, is characterized by impaired tubular reabsorption and excessive urinary excretion of the dibasic amino acids lysine, arginine, ornithine, and cystine. A similar transport defect exists in the intestinal mucosa. Because cystine is the least soluble of the naturally occurring amino acids, its overexcretion predisposes to the formation of renal, ureteral, and bladder stones. Such stones are responsible for the signs and symptoms of the disorder.

Etiology and pathogenesis Massive excretion of cystine and the other dibasic amino acids occurs only in classic cystinuria. The disorder, inherited as an autosomal recessive trait, is believed to result from alterations in a membrane carrier protein essential for transport of this group of amino acids in the apical brush border of proximal renal tubule and small intestinal cells. The protein has a greater affinity for ornithine and arginine than for lysine and cystine. Although the renal clearance of all four amino acids is increased in homozygotes, the presence of some residual transport capacity for these compounds plus the existence of three other disorders marked by selective excretion of members of this group (dibasicaminoaciduria, hypercystinuria, lysinuria) argues for the existence of at least three discrete renal transport systems for these amino acids: one for each amino acid alone; one shared by lysine, arginine, and ornithine; and one for all four amino acids.

Whereas urinary excretion patterns and renal clearance abnormalities in all homozygotes are similar, evidence for three variants has come from studies of intestinal transport in homozygotes and of urinary excretion in heterozygotes. Type I homozygotes lack intestinal transport of cystine, lysine, arginine, and ornithine; heterozygotes have normal urinary amino acid excretion patterns. Type II homozygotes lack mediated lysine transport in the gut but retain some capacity for cystine transport; heterozygotes have moderately increased urinary excretion of each of the four amino acids. Type III homozygotes retain some capacity for mediated intestinal transport of the four involved substrates; heterozygotes have modestly increased urinary lysine and cystine.

Clinical manifestations Cystinuria is among the most common inborn errors, with a frequency of 1 in 10,000 to 1 in 15,000 in many ethnic groups. Two-thirds of adults with cystinuria are type I homozygotes. Cystine stones account for 1 to 2 percent of all urinary tract calculi. The maximum solubility of cystine in the physiologic urinary pH range of 4.5 to 7.0 is about 1200 μmol/L (300 mg/L). Since affected homozygotes regularly excrete 2400 to 7200 μmol (600 to 1800 mg) daily, crystalluria and stone formation are a constant threat. Stone formation usually becomes manifest in the second or third decade but may occur in the first year of life. Symptoms and signs are those typical of urolithiasis: hematuria, flank pain, renal colic, obstructive uropathy, and infection (see Chap. 245). Recurrent urolithiasis may lead to progressive renal insufficiency.

Diagnosis The presence of cystine in a urinary tract stone is pathognomonic of cystinuria. However, since half the stones in cystinuric subjects are of mixed composition, and since as many as 10 percent may contain *no* detectable cystine, a urinary nitroprusside test should be done on all patients with urolithiasis to exclude this diagnosis. The nitroprusside test is also positive (appearance of a cherry red color) in some heterozygotes for cystinuria; in patients with hypercystinuria, homocystinuria, and cysteine β-mercaptolactate disulfiduria; and in the presence of acetone in the urine. When cystine content exceeds 1000 μmol/L (250 mg/L), cystine crystals may be seen in the sediment of acidified, concentrated, chilled urine. These hexagonal crystals are pathognomonic of cystine overexcretion in patients not taking sulfonamides.

Diagnostic confirmation of cystinuria depends on demonstration of the characteristic amino acid excretion pattern in the urine. Selective excretion of cystine, lysine, arginine, and ornithine can be demonstrated by paper chromatography or electrophoresis, and quantitative determinations can be made by column chromatography. Quantitation is important for differentiating some heterozygotes from homozygotes and for documenting the reduction of free cystine excretion during therapy.

Treatment Management is aimed at reducing the concentration of cystine in urine. The most important treatment is maintenance of a large urine volume. Fluid ingestion in excess of 4 L/d is essential, and 5 to 7 L/d is optimal. Urinary cystine excretion should measure less than 1000 to 1200 μmol/L (250 to 300 mg/L). The daily fluid ingestion necessary to maintain this dilution of excreted cystine should be spaced over the waking hours, with one-quarter to one-third of the total volume ingested at bedtime. Stones can be prevented and even dissolved by such hydration. It must be made clear to the cystinuric subject that water is a drug. Solubility of cystine rises sharply in urine above pH 7.5, and urinary alkalinization can be therapeutic in some situations. Vigorous administration of sodium bicarbonate, acetazolamide, and polycitrates is required to maintain a persistently alkaline pH, but this measure introduces the danger of inducing formation of calcium oxalate, calcium phosphate, and magnesium ammonium phosphate stones and of producing nephrocalcinosis.

Another treatment involves administration of penicillamine, which undergoes sulfhydryl-disulfide exchange with cystine to form the mixed disulfide of penicillamine and cysteine. Since this disulfide is more than 50 times as soluble as cystine, penicillamine (in doses of 1 to 3 g/d) reduces free cystine excretion markedly, thereby preventing new stone formation and promoting dissolution of existing calculi. Unfortunately, side effects include acute serum sickness, agranulocytosis, pancytopenia, immune glomerulitis, and the Goodpasture syndrome. Thus its use should be reserved for patients who fail to respond to hydration alone or who are in a high-risk category (one remaining kidney, renal insufficiency). Those patients unable to tolerate penicillamine may benefit from α-mercaptopropionylglycine, an experimental drug whose mechanism of action is similar to that of penicillamine but whose structure, and hence toxicity, is different. As many as two-thirds of patients unable to tolerate penicillamine may take α-mercaptopropionylglycine without ill effects. Captopril, a sulfhydryl-containing antihypertensive agent, is ineffective in reducing cystine excretion. When medical management fails, urologic surgery is required. An occasional patient may require renal transplantation because of renal failure.

DIBASICAMINOACIDURIA This disorder is characterized by a defect in renal tubular reabsorption of lysine, arginine, and ornithine but *not* of cysteine. The disorder almost surely reflects mutations in the gene(s) coding for a widely distributed transport protein used solely by the three dibasic amino acids. Two variants are each apparently inherited as an autosomal recessive trait. Manifestations are related to the losses of ornithine, arginine, and perhaps lysine.

In the common form of dibasicaminoaciduria (type II), also known as *lysinuric protein intolerance* and more common in Finland (1 in 60,000) than elsewhere, homozygotes show defective intestinal transport of dibasic amino acids as well as exaggerated renal losses. The transport defect affects basolateral rather than luminal membrane transport. Uptake of these substances is also defective in cultured fibroblasts and hepatocytes. Affected patients present in childhood with hepatosplenomegaly, protein intolerance, and episodic ammonia intoxication. Plasma concentrations of lysine, arginine, and ornithine are reduced. The clinical findings have been attributed to hyperammonemia resulting from insufficient amounts of arginine and ornithine to maintain proper function of the urea cycle. Treatment includes dietary protein restriction and supplementation with citrulline, a neutral amino acid whose intestinal and hepatic transport are unimpaired, and which, when metabolized to arginine and ornithine, fuels the urea cycle. With 2.0 to 8.0 g of oral citrulline daily, dietary protein intake can be increased and growth improved in children. Obligate heterozygotes are healthy and show no excess urinary loss of dibasic amino acids.

Type I dibasicaminoaciduria has been described in a large French-Canadian kindred. The proband was moderately mentally retarded. Her urinary losses of dibasic amino acids were not as great as those seen in type II homozygotes. The condition differed from type II by the presence of modest excesses of dibasic amino acids in urine of both asymptomatic parents. Several chemically affected members of the family also were symptom-free. Other families containing asymptomatic heterozygotes have been identified by urinary screening programs. Type I disease may involve the same transport system as that impaired in the more common type II disorder.

HARTNUP DISEASE Pellagra-like skin lesions, variable neurologic manifestations, and aminoaciduria for the monoaminomonocarboxylic amino acids with neutral or aromatic side chains characterize this disease. Alanine, serine, threonine, valine, leucine, isoleucine, phenylalanine, tyrosine, tryptophan, glutamine, asparagine, and histidine are excreted in urine in quantities 5 to 10 times normal, and intestinal transport for these same amino acids is defective. The clinical manifestations result from nutritional deficiency of the essential amino acid tryptophan, caused by the combination of intestinal malabsorption and renal loss. Manifestations are episodic, related, at least in part, to metabolic demands for tryptophan. Only a small fraction of patients with the chemical findings of this disorder develop a pellagra-like syndrome, implying that manifestations depend on factors over and above the transport defect.

The major pathway of tryptophan metabolism leads to the synthesis of niacin and nicotinamide-adenine dinucleotide (NAD). This pathway supplies about half the daily niacin needs. In patients with Hartnup disease, the renal and intestinal transport defect for tryptophan leads to niacin deficiency. The transport defect likely reflects abnormalities of a group-specific system for neutral amino acids. Some residual reabsorptive capacity persists for each involved amino acid. This suggests that they are transported by other carrier systems as well, a conclusion supported by the identification of patients with substrate-specific transport errors for tryptophan, methionine, and histidine.

Hartnup disease is inherited as an autosomal recessive trait. Homozygotes occur with a frequency of about 1 in 24,000 births. Heterozygotes exhibit no clinical or chemical abnormalities.

Pellagra is the clinical syndrome produced by dietary niacin deficiency, and its features are those of Hartnup disease (see Chap. 77). The diagnosis of Hartnup disease should be suspected in any patient with pellagra without a history of dietary niacin deficiency. The neurologic and psychiatric manifestations range from attacks of cerebellar ataxia to mild emotional lability to frank delirium and usually accompany exacerbations of the erythematous, eczematoid skin rash. Fever, sunlight, stress, and sulfonamide therapy provoke clinical relapses. Diagnosis is made by detection of the neutral aminoaciduria that does not occur in dietary niacin deficiency. Treatment is directed at niacin repletion and includes a high-protein diet and daily nicotinamide supplementation (50 to 250 mg). Tryptophan ethyl esters also can bypass the absorption defect.

IMINOGLYCINURIA This benign autosomal recessive trait is characterized by excessive urinary excretion of glycine and the imino acids proline and hydroxyproline. Homozygotes occur with a frequency of about 1 in 16,000. The enhanced excretion of glycine, proline, and hydroxyproline reflects a defect in the tubular transport system shared by these three compounds. An intestinal transport defect also may be present. This suggests that more than one mutation may lead to iminoglycinuria, a thesis corroborated by the demonstration that obligate heterozygotes from some but not all families have glycinuria. No consistent clinical abnormalities have been reported in homozygotes, who are usually detected by urinary amino acid screening programs. Individuals with iminoglycinuria should be reassured as to the benign nature of the disturbance.

DICARBOXYLICAMINOACIDURIA Selective urinary loss and exaggerated endogenous renal clearance of glutamic and aspartic acids have been described in two unrelated children. Intestinal absorption of these dicarboxylic amino acids was impaired in one. This patient suffered from recurrent hypoglycemia; the other was asymptomatic.

SUBSTRATE-SPECIFIC DEFECTS IN AMINO ACID TRANSPORT Rare pedigrees exist in which individuals have defective renal tubular reabsorption and/or impaired intestinal absorption of a single free amino acid. These disorders, each apparently inherited as an autosomal recessive trait, suggest that transport of amino acids is catalyzed by substrate-specific as well as group-specific transport mechanisms.

Hypercystinuria Two siblings exhibited modest cystinuria without excessive urinary excretion of lysine, arginine, or ornithine. Fractional tubular reabsorption of cystine was reduced to about 80 percent of the filtered load, and up to 250 mg/d was excreted in the urine. Intestinal absorption of cystine was normal. Both were clinically well, although the cystine excretion places them at risk for cystine urolithiasis. Cystine excretion by the parents was normal.

Lysinuria A child with selective impairment of renal tubular reabsorption of lysine has been described. Endogenous lysine clearance was increased; intestinal transport was impaired; plasma lysine was reduced. Mental and growth retardation and seizures were present. A lysine-supplemented diet stimulated growth. Urinary lysine excretion was normal in the parents.

Histidinuria Two siblings, each with mental retardation, exhibited a selective renal transport defect for histidine. Urinary loss of histidine approached 40 to 50 percent of the filtered load, and intestinal transport of histidine also was defective. The clinically normal parents had normal urinary excretion but a modest defect in intestinal absorption of histidine. In two additional cases of isolated histidinuria myoclonic seizures occurred.

Methionine malabsorption Children from two pedigrees have shown an intestinal transport defect for methionine. One may have had a renal transport defect as well. This disorder was detected because of urinary excretion of α-hydroxybutyric acid, a by-product of the intestinal bacterial breakdown of the unabsorbed methionine. This compound, which gives an odor resembling malt or dried celery to the urine, appears to be responsible for the white hair, attacks of hyperpnea, convulsions, edema, and mental retardation. Treatment of one of these children with a methionine-restricted diet caused improvement in all clinical manifestations.

Tryptophan malabsorption An isolated defect in intestinal absorption of tryptophan has been described in two siblings. The renal tubular reabsorption of tryptophan was normal. A number of indoles were excreted in stool and urine. These compounds result from chemical degradation of unabsorbed tryptophan by intestinal bacteria and may be present in patients with Hartnup disease as well. Because of concomitant renal disease, hydrolytic enzymes were released into the urine, acted on the indoles found there, and led to the formation of a blue pigment, indigotin. This sequence of events earned this condition the sobriquet "blue-diaper syndrome." No pellagra-like symptoms were described. The mother also excreted indole compounds, suggesting that she is a carrier of this trait.

DISORDERS OF HEXOSE TRANSPORT

Nondiabetic melituria occurs in a number of conditions. Pentoses, hexoses, heptoses, and disaccharides have been identified in the urine; all except sucrose yield a positive test for reducing substances. Some meliturias result from diffuse renal injury, others from ingestion of nonmetabolizable sugars. In still others the sugars accumulate in blood owing to deficient activity of catabolizing enzyme systems and "spill" into the urine. Only among the hexoses have specific inherited disorders of sugar transport been identified. The existence of renal glycosuria and intestinal glucose-galactose malabsorption as heritable, autosomal recessive disorders points to the existence of at least two specific carrier proteins for hexoses in human jejunal and renal brush border membranes: one for glucose and one shared by glucose and galactose.

RENAL GLYCOSURIA To avoid confusion with diabetes mellitus, Marble's criteria for the diagnosis of renal glycosuria should be followed: (1) glycosuria in the absence of hyperglycemia, (2) constant glycosuria with little fluctuation related to diet, (3) normal (or slightly flat) oral glucose tolerance test, (4) identification of urinary reducing substance as glucose, and (5) normal storage and utilization of carbohydrates. The Fanconi syndrome, in which renal glycosuria occurs as part of generalized proximal tubular dysfunction, also should be excluded. The condition is benign, but occasionally glycosuria may be great enough to cause polyuria and polydipsia. Even more rarely, dehydration or ketosis may develop under conditions of stress such as pregnancy or starvation.

In normal persons, glucose is present in the glomerular filtrate at a concentration equal to that in plasma water and is reabsorbed throughout the proximal renal tubule by a sodium-dependent, phlorizin-inhibitable transport process. Reabsorptive capacity exceeds normal plasma glucose concentration. Thus glucose does not appear in the urine until the threshold for reabsorption is reached. The plasma concentration at which filtered glucose begins to escape proximal tubular reabsorption is usually around 10 mmol/L (200 mg/dL). Maximal renal reabsorptive capacity is exceeded at a filtered load of around 2 mmol (325 mg)/min per 1.73 m² body surface area, and this value is defined as the tubular maximum for glucose (TmG).

Two patterns of glycosuria are recognized: type A, characterized by a reduced tubular maximum reabsorptive capacity, and type B, showing a reduced threshold for glycosuria, an increased "splay" in the titration curve, and a normal TmG. Renal glycosuria occurs in homozygotes for either of these recessively inherited mutations and in compound heterozygotes for these presumably allelic mutations. Modest reduction in renal threshold or TmG is present in heterozygotes in some families; modest glycosuria occurs in such family members when plasma glucose is elevated. The gene responsible for renal glycosuria segregates with the HLA haplotype, suggesting that it is located on chromosome 6. No linkage disequilibrium was observed, and no specific HLA antigens have been associated with renal glycosuria.

GLUCOSE-GALACTOSE MALABSORPTION In this condition, infants develop a profuse, watery diarrhea when fed milk or foods containing lactose, sucrose, glucose, or galactose. Fructose or carbohydrate-free formulas are well tolerated. A specific defect in intestinal absorption of glucose and galactose can be demonstrated by oral tolerance tests that produce little or no increase in plasma glucose or galactose. The primary defect involves the sodium/hexose cotransporter in the intestinal and renal brush border. Active D-glucose and D-galactose transport is absent in affected children, and intermediate transport capacity is present in their parents. These findings confirm the specificity and the autosomal recessive inheritance of the disorder. Treatment with a glucose- and galactose-free diet leads to resolution of symptoms in childhood. Although the basic transport defect is present throughout life, most patients show an improved tolerance for glucose and galactose with age.

A number of these patients have renal glycosuria at normal plasma glucose concentrations. Renal titration studies generally demonstrate a reduced threshold for glucose reabsorption (type B renal glycosuria) and a normal TmG. Urinary glucose loss is not as severe as in isolated renal glycosuria. This finding suggests the presence of multiple glucose transport proteins in the kidney. One, responsible for the bulk of glucose reabsorption and specific for glucose only, is affected in renal glycosuria; another, shared by glucose and galactose and responsible for transporting less of the filtered load of glucose, is affected in glucose-galactose malabsorption. Either the former is not present in intestinal mucosa, or the shared system is more important in that tissue. In both disorders, transport of sugars in all other tissues is normal, reflecting the multiplicity and tissue specificity of membrane transport proteins.

DEFECTIVE URATE TRANSPORT: HYPOURICEMIA

Individuals with a selective defect in renal tubular reabsorption of sodium urate have marked hypouricemia. Since little serum urate is bound to plasma proteins, failure to reabsorb filtered urate results in a serum urate ranging from 12 to 110 μmol/L (0.2 to 1.8 mg/dL). Moderate uricosuria is present, and 25 percent of patients have renal calculi.

Renal urate clearance normally averages 15 percent of glomerular filtration rate, and the excreted urate is composed both of filtered urate that has escaped reabsorption and of secreted urate. Subjects with isolated hypouricemia have urate clearances averaging from 33 to 85 percent of the filtration rate; in some, urate clearance exceeds the glomerular filtration rate. Studies with probenecid, which blocks tubular reabsorption of urate, and pyrazinamide, which blocks tubular secretion, reveal that 11 of the 16 families described have a presecretory urate reabsorptive defect, and 5 have defective transport affecting the entire tubule. In 4 families hypercalciuria due to enhanced intestinal calcium absorption is also present, but in others only uricosuria has been demonstrated. The defect is inherited as an autosomal recessive trait. Urate transport appears to be normal in nonrenal tissue. Obligate heterozygotes have moderately increased urate clearance. The defect is presumed to reflect mutation of one or both of the proximal renal tubular membrane proteins that transport sodium urate. The findings in these families support the hypothesis that renal urate reabsorption is controlled by more than one transport protein.

DEFECTIVE ANION TRANSPORT: CHLORIDORRHEA

This rare, autosomal recessive disease results from impairment of active transport of chloride in the ileum and colon. Absence of chloride-bicarbonate ion exchange causes profound symptoms even before birth (polyhydramnios and absence of meconium). Massive watery diarrhea is apparent from the first days of life. This fluid loss, with its attendant impairment of electrolyte homeostasis, is life-threatening. A hypokalemic, hypochloremic, hyponatremic metabolic alkalosis develops with dehydration and secondary hyperaldosteronism. Fecal fluid contains an excess of chloride ion over the sum of the accompanying cations sodium and potassium. Fecal chloride concentration always exceeds 90 mmol/L when volume and serum electrolyte disturbances are corrected, and this chloridorrhea is diagnostic. Renal chloride transport is normal. Decreased urine chloride results from the kidney's attempts to conserve salt and water.

Treatment requires adequate, lifelong repletion of electrolyte and fluid losses. Exact replacement of water, sodium chloride, and potassium chloride can prevent the growth and psychomotor retardation and the development of progressive renal damage. The renal lesion, with hyalinized glomeruli, juxtaglomerular hyperplasia, calcifications, and arteriolar changes, is probably a result of chronic volume depletion. Treatment of hyperreninemia and hypokalemia with prostaglandin inhibitors may reduce renal damage but does not alter intestinal symptoms or the need for chronic sodium chloride repletion.

REFERENCES

DESJEUX JF: Congenital selective Na⁺ D-glucose cotransport defects leading to renal glycosuria and congenital selective intestinal malabsorption of glucose and galactose, in *The Molecular and Metabolic Basis of Inherited Disease*, 7th ed, CR Scriver et al (eds). New York, McGraw-Hill, in press

ELSAS LJ, ROSENBERG LE: Renal glycosuria, in *Strauss and Welt's Diseases of the Kidney*, 3d ed, LE Earley, CW Gottschalk (eds). Boston, Little, Brown, 1979, pp 1021–1028

HOLMBERG C, PERHEENTUPA J: Congenital chloride diarrhoea (CCD), in *Population Structure and Genetic Disorders*, AW Erikson et al (eds). New York, Academic, 1980, pp 596–599

KAMOUN PP et al: Renal histidinuria. J Inherited Metab Dis 4:217, 1981

LEVY HL: Hartnup disorder, in *The Molecular and Metabolic Basis of Inherited Disease*, 7th ed, CR Scriver et al (eds). New York, McGraw-Hill, in press

MILLINER DS: Cystinuria. Endocrinol Metab Clin North Am 19:889, 1990

ROSENBERG LE: Intestinal hexose transport in familial glucose-galactose malabsorption, in *Membranes and Disease*, L Bolis et al (eds). New York, Raven, 1976, pp 253–262

———, SCRIVER CR: Disorders of amino acid metabolism, in *Metabolic Control and Disease*, 8th ed, PK Bondy, LE Rosenberg (eds). Philadelphia, Saunders, 1980, pp 616–645

SEGAL S, THIER SO: Cystinurias, in *The Molecular and Metabolic Basis of Inherited Disease*, 7th ed, CR Scriver et al (eds). New York, McGraw-Hill, in press

SHORT EM, ROSENBERG LE: Renal aminoaciduria, in *Strauss and Welt's Diseases of the Kidney*, 3d ed, LE Earley, CW Gottschalk (eds). Boston, Little, Brown, 1979, pp 975–1020

SIMELL O: Lysinuric protein intolerance and other cationic aminoacidurias, in *The Molecular and Metabolic Basis of Inherited Disease*, 7th ed, CR Scriver et al (eds). New York, McGraw-Hill, in press

SPERLING O: Hereditary renal hypouricemia, in *The Molecular and Metabolic Basis of Inherited Disease*, 7th ed, CR Scriver et al (eds). New York, McGraw-Hill, in press

WEITZ R, SPERLING O: Hereditary renal hypouricemia: Isolated tubular defect of urate reabsorption. J Pediatr 96:850, 1980

354 GALACTOSEMIA, GALACTOKINASE DEFICIENCY, AND OTHER RARE DISORDERS OF CARBOHYDRATE METABOLISM

KURT J. ISSELBACHER

DEFINITION *Galactosemia* refers to any of three inborn errors of galactose metabolism. *Classic galactosemia* is due to the deficiency of galactose-1-phosphate uridyl transferase (GALT) and is typically associated with cataract formation, mental retardation, and cirrhosis. The second disorder, *galactokinase deficiency*, leads primarily to cataract formation. The third, *UDP-galactose-4-epimerase deficiency*, is the rarest of the group; few cases have been described, and the eventual outcome is uncertain.

PATHOGENESIS Lactose, the main carbohydrate in milk, is a disaccharide containing galactose and glucose; when ingested, it is hydrolyzed by intestinal lactase. Normally, the absorbed galactose is converted to glucose in the liver. The first reaction in this pathway is the phosphorylation of galactose to galactose-1-phosphate by galactokinase (specified by a gene on chromosome 17):

$$\text{Galactose} + \text{ATP} \xrightarrow{\text{galactokinase}} \text{galactose-1-phosphate}$$

The next step involves the conversion of galactose-1-phosphate to glucose-1-phosphate by GALT (the gene for which is on chromosome 9):

$$\text{Galactose-1-phosphate} + \text{UDP-glucose} \xrightarrow{\text{GALT}}$$
$$\text{UDP-galactose} + \text{glucose-1-phosphate}$$

The uridine diphosphate (UDP) sugars can be reversibly interconverted by an epimerase reaction (UDP-galactose-4-epimerase):

$$\text{UDP-galactose} \rightleftharpoons \text{UDP-glucose}$$

Galactose also can be metabolized by alternative pathways. It can be converted (reduced) in the presence of NADPH (or NADH) to galactitol (dulcitol) by aldose reductase. It also can be oxidized to a limited extent by galactose dehydrogenase, leading to the formation of galactonic acid, xyulose, and CO_2. These pathways account for limited galactose metabolism in patients with galactosemia.

In galactokinase deficiency, galactose accumulates in the blood and tissues. In the lens, galactose is converted by aldose reductase to galactitol, a sugar to which the lens is impermeable. As a consequence, excessive hydration occurs which, together with a decrease in glutathione in the lens, leads to cataract formation.

In classic galactosemia, GALT deficiency results in tissue accumulation of galactose-1-phosphate and galactose. As in galactokinase deficiency, cataracts develop secondary to galactitol accumulation in the lens. It is assumed that the cirrhosis and mental retardation of classic galactosemia are related to increased amounts of galactose-1-phosphate in these tissues. Elevated blood galactose levels may lead to a decreased hepatic output of glucose and hence to hypoglycemia. In the kidney and intestine, accumulation of galactose and galactose-1-phosphate appears to lead to an inhibition of amino acid transport. In female homozygotes there is an increased incidence of hypergonadotrophic hypogonadism in which ovarian failure develops at an early age, and this complication may persist despite dietary therapy.

Both galactokinase and GALT deficiencies are transmitted as autosomal recessive traits. Heterozygotes for these disorders have half-normal enzyme levels but are asymptomatic. Maternal deficiency of galactokinase, together with lactose intake during pregnancy, may contribute to cataract formation during fetal development. However, not all persons with decreased GALT enzyme activity in their cells are carriers of classic galactosemia. Some individuals homozygous for another gene, called the *Duarte variant*, normally have half-normal GALT levels and are asymptomatic. This group can be differentiated from classic galactosemia heterozygotes on the basis of the electrophoretic properties of the mutant enzyme. In both galactokinase deficiency and classic galactosemia there is a functional deficiency or absence of the involved enzyme. Classic galactosemia is due to a variety of mutations in regions of the gene that are highly conserved throughout evolution. This molecular heterogeneity may help to explain diverse clinical outcomes in patients. Mutations in the variable (less conserved) regions of the gene contribute to polymorphisms accounting for normal function of GALT but with altered electrophoretic mobility.

The incidence of classic galactosemia is about 1 per 50,000 births in the white population. Approximately 0.8 to 1.3 percent of the population are heterozygotes for the GALT gene, and about 10 percent carry the Duarte variant. During screening of newborns for galactosemia, the most frequent cause of an abnormal result is compound heterozygosity for the Duarte variant and for classic galactosemia in which GALT levels are about 17 percent of normal. Such individuals are clinically asymptomatic.

CLINICAL FEATURES Symptoms of classic galactosemia usually begin within days to weeks after birth. The infant usually is reluctant to ingest breast milk or milk formulas, develops vomiting, shows poor nutrition, and fails to thrive. Jaundice, hepatomegaly, and evidence of liver disease may develop. Cataracts are usually not present at birth but develop gradually over weeks to months. Mental retardation becomes evident after 6 to 12 months and is usually not reversible. Infants with classic galactosemia are subject to bacterial sepsis (especially with *Escherichia coli*), and this may be the leading cause of death in the neonatal period. The only consistent feature of galactokinase deficiency is cataract formation.

DIAGNOSIS Galactokinase deficiency should be suspected in infants or children with cataract formation who have non-glucose-reducing substances in the urine. The diagnosis is made by demonstrating the deficiency of galactokinase in red blood cells.

Classic galactosemia must be considered when one or more of the clinical features described above are found. If the patient is ingesting milk, reducing sugar is present in the urine but gives a negative glucose oxidase reaction (i.e., is not glucose) and is identified as galactose by other techniques, such as chromatography. If the child is vomiting, has a poor food intake, or is on intravenous glucose feedings, galactose may not be present in the urine. The definitive diagnosis is made by demonstrating a lack or deficiency of red cell GALT by one of several techniques. The disease also can be diagnosed prenatally by enzyme studies on culture amniocentesis cells or by demonstrating increased galactitol in amniotic fluid. A nonenzymatic glycosylation of hemoglobin, analogous to that in diabetes mellitus, can be detected in patients with galactosemia as manifested by increased concentrations in the blood of Hb A_{lab} rather than Hb A_{lc}.

In the neonatal period galactosemia needs to be differentiated from primary liver disease. With liver damage, galactose removal from the blood is impaired, and elevated blood galactose levels and galactosuria

TABLE 354-1   Some other disorders of carbohydrate metabolism

Metabolic defect	Manifestations
HEREDITARY FRUCTOSE INTOLERANCE	
Deficiency of fructose-1-phosphate aldolase leads to accumulation of fructose-1-PO$_4$ in tissues.	Liver disease, renal tubular damage, and hypoglycemia.
FRUCTOSE-1,6-DIPHOSPHATASE DEFICIENCY	
Deficiency of the enzyme prevents gluconeogenesis from its normal precursors, lactate, glycerol, and alanine. Thus maintenance of blood sugar is dependent on exogenous glucose.	Lactic acidosis leads to hyperventilation, somnolence, and coma, usually with hypoglycemia and ketosis.

may be present. However, GALT levels are normal in patients with liver damage.

TREATMENT   The treatment of galactosemia consists of the removal of galactose-containing foods from the diet, especially milk. Milk substitutes such as Nutramigen are often used. Although soybean preparations contain polysaccharide-bound galactose, they appear to be well tolerated because the bound galactose is not readily liberated. In general, the red cell levels of galactose-1-phosphate are not increased in affected infants fed soybean formulas.

The institution of a galactose-free diet usually leads to a dramatic improvement in all clinical features except for mental retardation. Patients should be kept on galactose-free diets indefinitely or at least until they have attained adequate physical and neurologic development.

OTHER DISORDERS OF CARBOHYDRATE METABOLISM   Features of hereditary fructose intolerance and fructose-1,6-diphosphatase deficiency, two autosomal recessive disorders of fructose metabolism that lead to hypoglycemia, are summarized in Table 354-1 (also see Chaps. 338 and 350).

REFERENCES

ALLEN TJ et al: Evidence of galactosemia in utero. Lancet 1:603, 1980

BEUTLER E: Galactosemia: Screening and diagnosis. Clin Biochem 24:293, 1991

GITZELMANN R et al: Disorders of fructose metabolism, in *The Molecular and Metabolic Basis of Inherited Disease*, 7th ed, CR Scriver et al (eds). New York, McGraw-Hill, in press, Chap 23

KAUFMAN FR et al: Correlation of ovarian function with galactose-1-phosphate uridyl transferase levels in galactosemia. J Pediatr 112:754, 1988

NG WG et al: Transferase-deficiency galactosemia and the Duarte variant. JAMA 257:187, 1987

REICHARDT JKV, WOO SLC: Molecular basis of galactosemia: Mutations and polymorphisms in the gene encoding human galactose-1-phosphate uridyltransferase. Proc Natl Acad Sci USA 88:2633, 1991

SEGAL S: Disorders of galactose metabolism, in *The Metabolic Basis of Inherited Disease*, 6th ed, CR Scriver et al (eds). New York, McGraw-Hill, 1989, p 453

WAGGONER D et al: Long-term prognosis in galactosemia: Results of a survey of 350 cases. J Inherited Metab Dis 13:802, 1990

355   THE LIPODYSTROPHIES AND OTHER RARE DISORDERS OF ADIPOSE TISSUE

DANIEL W. FOSTER

This chapter is concerned with abnormalities in adipose tissue. The disorders are rare, and the pathophysiology is frequently not clear.

THE LIPODYSTROPHIES

The lipodystrophies are characterized by generalized or partial loss of body fat and metabolic abnormalities, including insulin resistance, hyperglycemia, and hypertriglyceridemia. A classification is shown in Table 355-1. In *generalized lipodystrophy* essentially all body fat is lost, while in *partial lipodystrophy* fat atrophy is limited. The common acquired form of partial lipodystrophy ordinarily involves half the body, usually the upper segment. Dominantly transmitted partial lipodystrophy tends to spare the face. One variant is associated with eye and tooth malformations, the Rieger anomaly. *Localized lipodystrophy* may be either inflammatory or noninflammatory. The best-studied syndrome is *centrifugal lipodystrophy*, in which fat atrophy begins in the groins or axillae of children under the age of 3 and spreads centrally to involve the entire abdomen. The edge of the lesion is red and scaly, with an inflammatory infiltrate demonstrable on histologic examination. Fat atrophy usually disappears spontaneously when the patient is around 13 years of age.

GENERALIZED LIPODYSTROPHY   Generalized lipodystrophy (also called *lipoatrophic diabetes*) may be either congenital or acquired. The congenital form is transmitted as an autosomal recessive trait. Males and females are equally affected. Rates of parental consanguinity are high. Loss of fat is usually obvious at birth, but the rest of the clinical picture may not appear until later (up to 30 years). The acquired disease often develops after some other illness. Measles, chicken pox, whooping cough, and infectious mononucleosis are common precipitating events, but hypothyroidism, hyperthyroidism, and pregnancy have been implicated. Some cases begin with the appearance of painful nodular swellings of adipose tissue resembling acute panniculitis (see below). The congenital and acquired forms are similar in clinical manifestations (Table 355-2).

Fat atrophy   Loss of body fat is the central feature. In congenital cases the skin of the face is tightly drawn over the bony structures, and the entire body appears to be devoid of adipose tissue on physical examination. However, whole-body magnetic resonance imaging (MRI) has shown preservation of some fat in the orbits, palms, soles, and juxtaarticular and epidural regions where support and cushioning functions of adipose tissue are primary. In the acquired form the face may be spared. In atrophic areas adipose tissue cells can be identified microscopically, but they contain no triglyceride stores. Paradoxically, the liver is engorged with fat, and the reticuloendothelial system contains lipid-laden macrophages (foam cells). The cause of the fat

TABLE 355-1   The lipodystrophies

Generalized lipodystrophy
   Congenital (familial or sporadic)
   Acquired (sporadic)
Partial lipodystrophy
   Common (sporadic)
   Dominant (familial)
      Limb and trunk
      With Rieger anomaly
Localized lipodystrophy
   Inflammatory
   Noninflammatory

TABLE 355-2   Characteristics of the lipodystrophies

Finding	Congenital general	Acquired general	Acquired partial	Dominant partial
Inheritance	Autosomal recessive	Sporadic	Usually sporadic	Autosomal dominant
Age of onset	Infancy	Childhood to adult	Childhood to adult	Puberty
Sex incidence	Males and females equal	Female preponderance	Female preponderance	Female preponderance
Lipoatrophy	Face, trunk, limbs	Face, trunk, limbs	Face, upper trunk, upper limbs	Trunk and limbs
Liver involvement	+	+ +	Rare	0
Renal disease	+	+	+ +	0
Insulin resistance	+	+	+	+
Hyperglycemia	+	+	+	+
Hypertriglyceridemia	+	+	+	+
Acanthosis nigricans	+	+	Rare	+
Genital hypertrophy	+	+	Rare	+
Bone age	Accelerated	Normal to accelerated	Normal	Normal

atrophy is not known. Fat-mobilizing polypeptides have been described in the urine of patients with generalized lipodystrophy, but their role in the disease is uncertain.

A candidate molecule for the induction of lipodystrophy would be a compound similar to tumor necrosis factor alpha (TNF-α), a potent inhibitor of lipoprotein lipase that causes fat depletion and hypertriglyceridemia when injected into animals. Lipoprotein lipase activity is low in generalized lipodystrophy, as would be predicted if TNF-α or a similar cytokine were the cause. However, plasma levels of TNF were normal in two of the author's patients. Hepatic lipase is not impaired. Since triglyceride content of the adipocyte is the result of a balance between fat synthesis and fat breakdown, an alternative mechanism might involve activation of the hormone-sensitive lipase that catalyzes hydrolysis of triglycerides in the fat cell. For example, a defect in a natural inhibitor of the lipase, such as adenosine, could result in enhanced response to physiologic (nonelevated) concentrations of lipolytic hormones. Enhanced lipolysis also could be due to sympathetic nervous system activity. Release of free fatty acids into plasma following norepinephrine infusion is impaired, but this may simply reflect the depleted triglyceride stores.

Although an inducing molecule could act as a circulating hormone in generalized lipodystrophy, such a cause is unlikely in partial lipodystrophy, where autotransplantation of adipocytes from an affected area to a nonaffected site resulted in reaccumulation of fat and reverse transplantation from normal to affected site resulted in fat atrophy. An autocrine or paracrine function may be involved. In the former a cellular product would act on the cell of origin, while in the latter a cellular product would act on adjacent cells, but in neither case would the putative inducer of lipodystrophy enter the circulation to act as a typical hormone.

Growth and maturation   Linear growth is accelerated in the first few years of life in the congenital disorder and in acquired disease that begins early in childhood. Epiphyses close early, however, so that the final height is usually normal. True muscular hypertrophy is present, and patients may have an acromegalic appearance with coarse facial features and large hands and feet. The ears tend to be prominent in the congenital form. Many viscera are enlarged, and generalized lymphadenopathy may be present. The cause of the growth disorder is not known. Levels of growth hormone (GH) and insulin-like growth factor I (IGF-I, somatomedin C) are normal or low. Insulin-like growth factor II has not been systematically assessed. It is likely that abnormal growth and pseudoacromegaly are due to high concentrations of insulin in plasma secondary to insulin resistance (see below). Insulin binds to the IGF-I receptor and at high concentrations could mimic the acromegalic sequence (GH → IGF-I → growth) by activating the IGF-I receptor.

Liver   Enlargement of the liver causes protuberance of the abdomen. Fatty liver may progress to cirrhosis, especially in the acquired disorder. Several patients have died from bleeding esophageal varices. Splenomegaly does not occur in the absence of portal hypertension.

Kidneys   The kidneys are usually enlarged. Subjects with the acquired disorder may have proteinuria and the nephrotic syndrome, although not as frequently as in partial lipodystrophy. Moderate hypertension is common.

Genitalia   The external genitalia (penis and testes in males, clitoris and labia majora in females) are usually hypertrophied in children with the congenital disease. In women, polycystic ovaries are common, resulting in the clinical picture of Stein-Leventhal syndrome. The cause of the genital abnormalities is not known. Systematic investigation of gonadotropin, estrogen, and androgen metabolism has not been carried out.

Skin   Acanthosis nigricans is present in most. Hypertrichosis of face, neck, trunk, and limbs is frequent. Scalp hair is usually thick and curly, particularly early in life.

Central nervous system   Mental retardation is present in about half the congenital cases. It appears to be less common in the acquired form. Pneumoencephalography suggested that structural abnormalities in the third ventricle and basal cisternae were present in several patients studied a number of decades ago, but only a few patients have had computed tomographic (CT) or MRI scans. Three patients at the author's institution have had normal brain MRI scans.

Other abnormalities   Osteolytic lesions resulting in bone cysts may be present, and occasionally, the skeleton appears sclerotic. Cystic bone lesions are also seen in membranous lipodystrophy (Nasu disease), which is associated with presenile dementia. Despite its name, membranous lipodystrophy appears to be associated with fat necrosis and is more properly classified as a panniculitis (see below). Cardiomegaly is common, but heart failure appears to be rare. Goiter is frequent. The associated abnormalities in generalized lipodystrophy are summarized in Table 355-3.

Metabolic and endocrine abnormalities   Three major metabolic disturbances are characteristic.

1 *Insulin resistance.* Insulin resistance may be mild or severe. When severe, the hyperglycemia may be difficult to control. Insulin and C-peptide concentrations are relatively or absolutely elevated, and response to exogenous insulin is impaired. Resistance is due to several causes, and affected siblings may exhibit different mechanisms. Increased insulin clearance, decreased numbers of

TABLE 355-3   Accompanying abnormalities of lipodystrophy

Bone	Sclerosis, cystic angiomatosis
Brain	Mental retardation, third ventricle dilatation
Genitalia	Clitoromegaly, polycystic ovaries, penile hypertrophy
Heart	Cardiomegaly
Kidneys	Hypertrophy without renal failure
Liver	Hepatomegaly, fatty liver, cirrhosis, hepatic failure
Lymph nodes	Generalized lymphadenopathy
Skin	Acanthosis nigricans, hypertrichosis
Thyroid	Goiter, euthyroid state

insulin receptors, diminished affinity of the receptor for insulin, and postreceptor defects have all been reported. Mutations in the insulin receptor have been identified in some patients. Insulin in the plasma of affected subjects is biologically active. Although glucagon levels are high (indicating insulin resistance in the alpha cell of the islets of Langerhans) and free fatty acid concentrations are elevated, ketoacidosis is unusual. One patient had recurrent episodes of metabolic acidosis considered to be ketoacidosis, but concentrations of acetoacetate and β-hydroxybutyrate were characteristic of fasting ketosis, not diabetic ketoacidosis; presumably lactate or other organic acids were involved.

True ketoacidosis may be infrequent because insulin resistance is less severe in liver and skeletal muscle than in adipose tissue. Glycogen levels in the liver are high (insulin stimulates glycogen synthesis), and branched-chain amino acids fall normally or near normally in response to injected insulin. Elevated insulin levels in portal vein plasma would counteract the actions of glucagon in the insulin-responsive hepatocyte (see Chap. 338). This would prevent activation of ketone body synthesis in liver and ensure utilization of incoming fatty acids for triglyceride/VLDL synthesis. The elevated long-chain fatty acids in the plasma are of dietary origin and fall toward normal with restriction of dietary fat. Diabetes mellitus accompanying lipodystrophy appears to be typical apart from insulin resistance, including the propensity to develop late degenerative complications. High levels of insulin in plasma and resistance to ketoacidosis distinguish this condition from type I (autoimmune) insulin-dependent diabetes mellitus, although both conditions begin in childhood or early adult life.

2 *Hypertriglyceridemia with accumulation of both chylomicrons and very low density lipoproteins in the blood.* Eruptive xanthomas, lipemia retinalis, and recurrent pancreatitis may be seen. Although lipoprotein lipase is low, as noted, and there is a defect in disposal of triglycerides in the atrophied fat tissue, the major cause for the hypertriglyceridemia is overproduction of VLDL in the liver. This overproduction is probably driven by the elevated free fatty acids in blood, since dietary fat restriction results in a fall of VLDL production rates toward normal. Hyperinsulinemia may contribute by enhancing hepatic fat synthesis.

3 *A hypermetabolic state with normal thyroid function.* Basal metabolic rates are usually elevated, although thyroid hormone values (thyroxine, triiodothyronine, reverse triiodothyronine) are normal. Patients do not gain weight with excessive caloric intake, indicating a facile capacity to waste calories as heat. Food intakes as high as 21,000 kJ (5000 kcal)/d are not unusual. One 16-month-old child ate 10,000 kJ (2400 kcal) daily. Following thyroidectomy in one patient, the basal metabolic rate decreased but did not return to normal; symptoms and signs of hypothyroidism supervened, requiring treatment with thyroid hormone despite continued high metabolic rates. It thus seems clear that hypermetabolism is not due to hyperthyroidism. There is also no evidence of mitochondrial disease. The most likely explanation for the increased metabolic rate is enhanced "futile" cycles with wastage of ATP. Increased sympathetic nervous system activity may play a role. There is no evidence for adrenal medullary dysfunction.

Course and treatment   Patients with generalized lipodystrophy may die at an early age. Hepatic failure, hemorrhage from esophageal varices, and renal failure are common causes of death. Despite the almost constant hypertriglyceridemia, symptomatic coronary artery disease is rare. Recurrent pancreatitis may be life-threatening. There is no specific treatment for lipodystrophy, although dietary fat restriction is generally recommended. Medium-chain triglyceride supplementation has been reported to be of benefit. Because of insulin resistance, large amounts of insulin are often required to control the plasma glucose. Gemfibrozil is usually prescribed to lower triglycerides but is often ineffective. In patients with recurrent pancreatitis, nicotinic acid may be prescribed to lower triglycerides.

ACQUIRED PARTIAL LIPODYSTROPHY   This is the most common of the lipodystrophies and usually affects women. Fat atrophy occurs in the upper half of the body, including the face, but spares the lower extremities. Rarely, the lower half of the body is affected, leaving the upper torso intact. Occasionally, the lesion affects only one side. The other anatomic features of generalized lipodystrophy are usually absent, and liver disease is unusual. Proteinuria, with or without the nephrotic syndrome, occurs more frequently than in other forms. The complement system is abnormal, and C3 levels tend to be low. C3 nephritic factor, a polyclonal IgG immunoglobulin that interacts with alternative pathway convertase (C3b Bb) to augment C3 activation, is present in serum. C3 levels may be low in unaffected first-degree relatives, but C3 nephritic factor is absent. Complement abnormalities disappeared after renal transplantation in one subject. Dermatomyositis and Sjögren's syndrome may occur. Rarely, partial lipodystrophy progresses to the generalized form of the disease.

An unusual form of partial lipodystrophy is mandibuloacral dysplasia, a syndrome with typical features of lipodystrophy, including insulin resistance, hypermetabolism, and increased glucose production. Other features include hypoplasia of the mandibles and clavicles with lytic bone lesions, wrinkled skin, and joint contractures. Some patients have hypogonadism, short stature, and alopecia.

LIPODYSTROPHY WITH DOMINANT TRANSMISSION   This variant is characterized by fat atrophy of the limbs and trunk with sparing of the face, which may actually be rounded. The neck also may be exempt. The disease usually begins at puberty but may not appear until middle age. Males are rarely affected. In families with the Rieger anomaly, onset tends to be in infancy. Insulin resistance and hyperglycemia are usual, and severe hypertriglyceridemia with eruptive xanthomas may occur. The labia majora are hypertrophied, and polycystic ovaries may be seen. Acanthosis nigricans is usually present. Liver and renal disease do not occur.

LOCALIZED LIPODYSTROPHY   Localized lipodystrophy takes several patterns. Centrifugal lipodystrophy (*lipodystrophia centrifugalis abdominalis infantilis*) has been mentioned already. Annular lipoatrophy is a bandlike ring of fat atrophy encircling a limb or the ankles. Occasionally, only half the limb is involved, in which case the term often used is *lipoatrophia semicircularis*. On biopsy, inflammatory infiltrates are usually present in the areas of fat atrophy. Localized lipodystrophy also may occur secondary to injection of insulin, iron dextrans, triamcinolone, and diphtheria/pertussis/tetanus vaccine.

MULTIPLE SYMMETRIC LIPOMATOSIS

Multiple symmetric lipomatosis, a disease found predominantly in men, is characterized by formation of nonencapsulated lipomas in various areas. Two patterns of distribution are noted. In the *type I* variant, lipomas are primarily in the nape of the neck and in the supraclavicular and deltoid regions, resulting in an extraordinary bull-necked appearance (*Madelung collar*). Extension into the mediastinum may produce obstruction of the trachea or vena cava. Fat over the remainder of the body appears normal. In the *type II* pattern, lipomas are not localized to the neck but extend down over the body, giving the appearance of simple obesity. Correct diagnosis requires recognition that the fat masses are symmetric and that the distal arms and legs are spared. Deep lipomatosis is absent in type II disease, and vena caval and tracheal compression do not occur.

Multiple symmetric lipomatosis may occur sporadically or in families. Autosomal dominant transmission has been postulated in the latter. Alcoholism is common. Coexisting folate deficiency, macrocytic anemia, and abnormal liver function may be due to alcohol and not lipomatosis. Neuropathy, which may be sensory, motor, or autonomic, is prominent, and neuropathic foot ulcers may be present. Histologic evidence from sural nerve biopsies suggests that the neuropathy is integral to the disease and not due to alcohol. The lesion is a chronic distal atrophy without the axonal degeneration and demyelination characteristic of alcohol injury.

Metabolic abnormalities include hyperuricemia, hypertriglyceridemia (VLDL, chylomicrons), and paradoxically, an elevation of high-density lipoproteins (HDL) as well. Diabetes mellitus has not been reported, although hyperinsulinism may be present. A few patients have had renal tubular acidosis.

The cause of multiple symmetric lipomatosis is not known. The fat cells are slightly smaller than normal, suggesting hyperplasia. Isolated adipocytes appear to have a marked increase in lipoprotein lipase activity and a defect in adrenergic lipolysis. Lipolytic response to cyclic AMP is intact, suggesting an abnormality at the hormone receptor/adenylate cyclase unit. The biochemical abnormalities are not present in all cases.

There is no treatment except for surgical removal of lipomas that cause compression. They also may be removed for cosmetic reasons.

OTHER LIPOMATOSES

MEDIASTINOABDOMINAL This lipomatosis may be a variant of multiple symmetric lipomatosis. The syndrome comprises (1) exertional dyspnea due to compression of airways by lipomas of the mediastinum, (2) massive enlargement of the abdomen (pseudoascites) due to intraperitoneal and retroperitoneal fat, and (3) abnormal glucose tolerance or diabetes mellitus. The metabolic abnormalities and enzymatic changes in adipocytes are identical with those in multiple symmetric lipomatosis except that HDL levels are not elevated.

PELVIC Pelvic lipomatosis is characterized by nonmalignant overgrowth of dense, unencapsulated fat in pelvic spaces enveloping the pelvic viscera. The disease is almost always present in men, the male-to-female ratio being 18:1. Symptoms are of bladder dysfunction (frequency, dysuria, hematuria), constipation, and vague abdominal pain. The constricting pelvic fat may cause bilateral ureteral obstruction with hydronephrosis and renal failure. Hypertension is common. Radiographic studies show a deformed bladder, deviation of the ureters, displacement of rectosigmoid junction, and hydronephrosis in advanced cases. MRI examination or CT scan reveals the compressing fat. The cause is not known. There is no treatment except surgery to remove the fat and relieve upper urinary tract obstruction.

EPIDURAL Epidural lipomatosis is a syndrome of spinal cord compression due to adipose tissue. It causes back pain, radicular pain, or compression of the cord. The syndrome is most often seen with chronic glucocorticoid therapy and may occur in Cushing's syndrome. Cord compression requires laminectomy, but otherwise a trial of decreased steroid dosage should be undertaken.

ACUTE PANNICULITIS (NODULAR FAT NECROSIS)

The appearance of single or multiple crops of tender nodules in subcutaneous fat with a histologic picture of fat cell necrosis, infiltration of inflammatory cells, and development of fat-filled macrophages (foam cells) is the hallmark of acute panniculitis. The nodules range in size from 0.5 to 10 cm and may be firm or fluctuant. They are usually, but not always, tender. On occasion they drain an oily solution, and suppuration may occur. Individual lesions last from 1 to 8 weeks before disappearing, and a pigmented depressed area may be left at the involved site. While some patients have only nodular panniculitis, which may or may not be relapsing, others develop fever, abnormal liver function, involvement of the bone marrow with leukemoid response, bleeding tendencies, nodular pulmonary lesions, and evidence of pancreatic disease with elevated plasma amylase and lipase levels. In the past this constellation of findings was called *Weber-Christian disease*. However, since painful or nonpainful panniculitis may result from a variety of conditions,

Weber-Christian disease is not a specific entity, and the term should probably be abandoned.

It is not possible to develop a firm classification of acute panniculitis since the lesions may appear in sporadic fashion with many conditions. One classification system is given in Table 355-4.

Panniculitis without systemic disease is usually due to trauma (sometimes factitiously induced) or cold. For example, in equestrian cold panniculitis the lesions appear in the outer thighs of persons riding horseback for several hours in icy weather. One variant, subcutaneous fat necrosis of the newborn, may be due to a combination of obstetric trauma and hypothermia.

Panniculitis with systemic disease can be divided into several large categories. Collagen vascular disease is a frequent cause, although few patients with connective tissue disorders develop this complication. Lupus is probably most common, and scleroderma is second. Nodular fat necrosis occurs in about 2 to 3 percent of patients with lupus and is more common in discoid than in systemic lupus. Lymphomas and histiocytosis represent a second category. Histiocytic cytophagic panniculitis (HCP) is characterized by fever, serositis (pleural effusions), hepatosplenomegaly, panniculitis, anemia, leukopenia, thrombocytopenia, and coagulation defects. The characteristic lesion is the "beanbag" histiocyte containing ingested lymphocytes, red cells, and platelets. While some patients have a benign course, the majority have a fatal outcome due to hemorrhagic complications. Malignant T cell lymphoma occasionally involves subcutaneous tissue directly and may mimic HCP. Infiltrating T lymphocytes in HCP are of clonal origin, suggesting that subcutaneous T cell lymphomas are a malignant counterpart or late transformation phase of HCP. Deficiencies of α_1-antitrypsin have been found in a number of patients with acute panniculitis. It is postulated that the α_1-antitrypsin deficiency predisposes to panniculitis secondary to trauma and induces a hyperactive immune response. Panniculitis with systemic symptoms, including fever and hepatitis, also has been seen with light chain paraproteinemia and acquired deficiency of C_1 inhibitor in the classic complement-generating sequence. Severe pancreatic disease also may cause acute panniculitis. One distinct syndrome has been called *disseminated fat necrosis* and is described below. Panniculitis rarely may be associated with generalized lipodystrophy, especially the acquired type. Rare causes of panniculitis include gout, familial Mediterranean fever, Nasu disease (see above), drugs (glucocorticoids, aspartame), renal failure, atheromatous emboli, and infection. Eosinophilic panniculitis may be seen with vasculitis, parasitic infestation, lymphomas, and atopic dermatitis.

Acute panniculitis can only be diagnosed histologically. Once the lesion is identified, a search for the cause must be made. If systemic symptoms are present and the course is rapidly downhill, the primary differential diagnosis is between collagen vascular disease, lymphoproliferative disorder, and pancreatitis or pancreatic cancer. Milder cases raise the possibility of α_1-antitrypsin deficiency.

Treatment is often unsatisfactory. Some patients with histiocytic cytophagic panniculitis respond to combined chemotherapy with cyclophosphamide, bleomycin, and prednisone. Patients with α_1-antitrypsin deficiency may respond to dapsone but should be given

---

TABLE 355-4 Causes of panniculitis

Panniculitis without systemic disease
  Trauma
  Cold
  Subcutaneous fat necrosis of the newborn
Panniculitis with systemic disease
  Connective tissue disorders (lupus erythematosus, scleroderma)
  Lymphoproliferative disease (lymphoma, histiocytosis)
  α_1-Antitrypsin deficiency
  Pancreatic disease (cancer, pancreatitis)
  Generalized lipodystrophy
  Paraproteinemia with C1 inhibitor deficiency
  Miscellaneous (see text)

α_1-antiprotease concentrate (60 mg/kg body weight weekly) if this fails.

DISSEMINATED FAT NECROSIS

Disseminated fat necrosis (also called *metastatic fat necrosis*) is a syndrome in which patients with pancreatitis (two-thirds) or carcinoma of the pancreas (one-third) develop lesions that appear to be similar to or identical with nodular panniculitis. The fat necrosis has a predilection for periarticular sites. Fever is almost invariably present. Arthritis occurs in about 60 percent of cases and may be severe, resulting in destruction of the joint. Often there are sinus tracts running from the site of subcutaneous fat necrosis into the joint space, leading to deposition of necrotic material. Lytic bone lesions may underlie the site of fat necrosis. Polyserositis and vasculitis may be present. Since complement levels are low and immunofluorescent staining shows deposition of complement and IgG, the syndrome resembles, in some respects, lupus-associated panniculitis. Serologic studies for lupus have not been systematically carried out. However, antinuclear antibody (ANA) and rheumatoid factor are undetectable in some patients.

Disseminated fat necrosis may be due to release of pancreatic enzymes into blood or lymph, and these enzymes may initiate fat necrosis at distal sites. Presumably, free fatty acids released by pancreatic lipase and phospholipase A_2, both of which may be elevated in serum, induce tissue necrosis, with trypsin playing an ancillary role. Experimentally, necrosis can be induced in pericardial, subpleural, and subcutaneous fat by ligation of pancreatic ducts. Amylase and lipase levels may be elevated in pleural, pericardial, and ascitic fluid. These enzymes also have been found in fluid aspirated from subcutaneous nodules. The possibility that release of aberrant pancreatic enzyme into the blood is the cause is supported by the occurrence of disseminated fat necrosis in patients with pancreatic–portal vein fistulas. On the other hand, an immune mechanism cannot be ruled out, given that polyserositis is common and that low complement levels and vasculitis may be present. The meaning of the eosinophilia that frequently accompanies disseminated fat necrosis is not known.

Mortality rates are high (even in the absence of pancreatic carcinoma), and death may occur in weeks to months. No treatment is known. Infusion of the protease inhibitor aprotinin appeared to have beneficial effects in one patient.

ADIPOSIS DOLOROSA

Adiposis dolorosa (Dercum's disease) is characterized by painful circumscribed adipose tissue deposits in subcutaneous tissues of the extremities and of other parts of the body. Juxtaarticular areas, particularly the knees, are the most common sites. Lesions vary from 0.5 to 5.0 cm. Pain and paresthesias may occur spontaneously or result from pressure. Affected subjects are frequently women (30:1). They are usually obese. The syndrome is associated with weakness, fatigue, emotional instability, and occasional dementia. The condition rarely begins until after menopause. Most cases are sporadic, but familial occurrence has been noted with a presumed dominant inheritance. Multiple associations have been reported, but they are probably chance phenomena. Autopsy reports from early in the century suggested abnormalities of the pituitary and other endocrine glands, but modern endocrinologic evaluations have not been undertaken.

Biopsy of affected sites may show no abnormalities, but granulomas with giant cell formations are usually seen. Fat necrosis is rare, thus separating the condition from acute panniculitis.

Treatment is unsatisfactory, although intravenous lidocaine has apparently provided relief in two cases.

REFERENCES

Lipodystrophy

BILLINGS JK et al: Lipoatrophic panniculitis: A possible autoimmune inflammatory disease of fat. Report of three cases. Arch Dermatol 123:1662, 1987

CHUN SI et al: Membranous lipodystrophy: Primary idiopathic type. J Am Acad Dermatol 24:844, 1991

CUTLER DL et al: Insulin-resistant diabetes mellitus and hypermetabolism in mandibulo-acral dysplasia: A newly recognized form of partial lipodystrophy. J Clin Endocrinol Metab 73:1056, 1991

DUNNIGAN MG et al: Familial lipoatrophic diabetes with dominant transmission: A new syndrome. Q J Med 43:33, 1974

FRANKLIN B et al: Very low-density lipoprotein metabolism in an unusual case of lipoatrophic diabetes. Metabolism 33:814, 1984

GARG A et al: Peculiar distribution of adipose tissue in patients with congenital generalized lipodystrophy. J Clin Endocrinol Metab 75:358, 1991

KLEIN S et al: Generalized lipodystrophy: In vivo evidence for hypermetabolism and insulin-resistant lipid, glucose, and amino acid kinetics. Metabolism 41:893, 1992

LILLYSTONE D, WEST RJ: Lipodystrophy of limbs associated with insulin resistance Arch Dis Child 50:737, 1975

SEIP M: Generalized lipodystrophy, in *Ergebnisse der Inneren Medizin und Kinderheilkunde*, P Frick et al (eds). Berlin, Springer-Verlag, 1971, pp 59–95

WACHSLICHT-RODBARD H et al: Heterogeneity of the insulin-receptor interaction in lipoatrophic diabetes. J Clin Endocrinol Metab 52:416, 1981

WILSON DE et al: Eucaloric substitution of medium chain triglycerides for dietary long chain fatty acids in acquired total lipodystrophy: Effects on hyperlipoproteinemia and endogenous insulin resistance. J Clin Endocrinol Metab 57:517, 1983

Multiple symmetric lipomatosis

ENZI G: Multiple symmetric lipomatosis: An updated clinical report. Medicine 63:56, 1984

LEUNG NWY et al: Multiple symmetric lipomatosis (Launois-Bensaude syndrome): Effect of oral salbutamol. Clin Endocrinol 7:601, 1987

POLLOCK M et al: Neuropathy in multiple symmetric lipomatosis. Madelung's disease. Brain 111:1157, 1988

RUZICKA T et al: Benign symmetric lipomatosis Launois-Bensaude. Report of ten cases and review of the literature. J Am Acad Dermatol 17:663, 1987

Mediastinoabdominal lipomatosis, pelvic lipomatosis, and epidural lipomatosis

ENZI G et al: Mediastino-abdominal lipomatosis: Deep accumulation of fat mimicking a respiratory disease and ascites. Clinical aspects and metabolic studies *in vitro*. Q J Med 53:453, 1984

FESSLER RG et al: Epidural lipomatosis in steroid-treated patients. Spine 17:183, 1992

HEYNS CF: Pelvic lipomatosis: A review of its diagnosis and management. J Urol 146:267, 1991

Acute panniculitis

ALEGRE VA, WINKELMANN RK: Histiocytic cytophagic panniculitis. J Am Acad Dematol 20:177, 1989

ARONSON IK et al: Panniculitis associated with cutaneous T-cell lymphoma and cytophagocytic histiocytosis. Br J Dermatol 112:87, 1985

HYTIROGLOU P et al: Histiocytic cytophagic panniculitis: Molecular evidence for a clonal T-cell disorder. J Am Acad Dermatol 27:333, 1992

PASCUAL M et al: Recurrent febrile panniculitis and hepatitis in two patients with acquired complement deficiency and paraproteinemia. Am J Med 83:959, 1987

PATTERSON JW: Differential diagnosis of panniculitis, in *Advances in Dermatology*, 6th ed, JP Callen et al (eds). St Louis, Mosby–Year Book, 1991, pp 309–330

PETERS MS, SU WPD: Panniculitis. Dermatol Clin 10:37, 1992

SMITH KC et al: Panniculitis associated with severe α_1-antitrypsin deficiency: Treatment and review of the literature. Arch Dermatol 123:1655, 1987

WINKELMANN RK: Panniculitis in connective tissue disease. Arch Dermatol 119:336, 1983

Disseminated fat necrosis

PHILLIPS MR JR et al: Inflammatory arthritis and subcutaneous fat necrosis associated with acute and chronic pancreatitis. Arthritis Rheum 23:355, 1980

POTTS JR: Pancreatic–portal vein fistula with disseminated fat necrosis treated by pancreaticoduodenectomy. South Med J 84:632, 1991

WILSON HA et al: Pancreatitis with arthropathy and subcutaneous fat necrosis. Evidence for the pathogenicity of lipolytic enzymes. Arthritis Rheum 26:121, 1983

Adiposis dolorosa

ATKINSON RL: Intravenous lidocaine for the treatment of intractable pain of adiposis dolorosa. Int J Obes 6:351, 1982

section 3   Disorders of bone and mineral metabolism

356   CALCIUM, PHOSPHORUS, AND BONE METABOLISM: CALCIUM-REGULATING HORMONES

MICHAEL F. HOLICK / STEPHEN M. KRANE / JOHN T. POTTS, JR.

BONE STRUCTURE AND METABOLISM (See also Chap. 358) Bone is a dynamic tissue that is constantly remodeled throughout life. The arrangement of compact and cancellous bone provides a combination of strength and density suitable for mobility. In addition, bone provides a reservoir for calcium, magnesium, phosphorus, sodium, and other ions necessary for the support of homeostatic functions. The skeleton is highly vascular and receives about 10 percent of the cardiac output.

The properties of bone are a function of its extracellular components. The structure consists of a solid mineral phase in close association with an organic matrix, of which 90 to 95 percent is type I collagen (see Chap. 351). The noncollagenous portion of the organic matrix contains proteins derived from serum (albumin and α_2-HS glycoproteins), α-carboxyglutamic acid (GLA)-containing proteins (*bone GLA protein*, or *BGP*, or *osteocalcin* and a matrix GLA protein), the glycoprotein *osteonectin*, the phosphoprotein *osteopontin*, sialoproteins, *thrombospondin*, and other less well characterized proteins. Some of these proteins may function in initiating mineralization and in binding of the mineral phase to the matrix. The mineral phase is made up of calcium and phosphate, best characterized as a poorly crystalline hydroxyapatite, although the calcium/phosphate molar ratio is less than the 1.67 molar ratio of hydroxyapatite [empirical formula $Ca_{10}(PO_4)_6(OH)_2$]. In addition, other ions are present, predominantly in the surface layers. The mineral phase of bone is deposited initially in intimate relation to the collagen fibrils and is found in specific locations within the "holes" between the collagen fibrils. This architectural arrangement of mineral and matrix results in a two-phase material uniquely suited to withstand mechanical stresses. The formation and the localization of the inorganic phase are determined in part by the organic matrix.

Cells of mesenchymal origin, *osteoblasts,* synthesize and secrete the organic matrix. Mineralization of the matrix, largely in *osteons* (haversian systems), begins soon after the matrix is secreted (primary mineralization) but is not completed until after several weeks (secondary mineralization). Osteoblasts are characterized by their location and morphology, the presence of a specific skeletal form of alkaline phosphatase, the presence of receptors for parathyroid hormone (PTH) and 1,25-dihydroxyvitamin D [$1,25(OH)_2D$], and the ability to synthesize specific matrix proteins such as type I collagen, osteocalcin, and osteopontin. As an osteoblast secretes matrix, which is then mineralized, the cell becomes surrounded by matrix and becomes an *osteocyte,* still connected with its blood supply through a series of canaliculi. Resorption of bone is carried out mainly by *osteoclasts.* Osteoclasts are multinucleated cells formed by fusion of precursor hematopoietic stem cells related to the mononuclear phagocyte series. Resorption of bone takes place in scalloped spaces (Howship's lacunae) where the osteoclasts are attached through a specific $\alpha v\beta 3$ integrin to components of the bone matrix such as osteopontin. This

zone (clear zone) contains contractile proteins. The resorbing end of the cell forms a specialized ruffled border. Mineral and matrix are removed in this space where the ruffled border is folded and is in contact with the bone. Proteins, including a specialized proton pump ATPase, are found in the ruffled border membrane, which contributes to the production of a unique acid environment in the enclosed extracellular compartment and results in solubilization of the mineral phase. This area is also rich in protein encoded by the oncogene c-*src* and in the src phosphorylation substrate p80/85. In addition to the proton pump, carbonic anhydrase (type II isoenzyme) is required to maintain the acid pH. Other features of osteoclasts include the presence of tartrate-resistant acid phosphatase, cell surface receptors for calcitonin, sodium pumps of the kidney type, bicarbonate/chloride exchanger of the band 3 family, and an ability to resorb mineralized bone. The bone matrix is resorbed in the acid environment adjacent to the ruffled border by acid hydrolyases following solubilization of the mineral phase. Several soluble ligands modulate the differentiation of osteoblasts or osteoclasts from precursor cells and modulate the function of the differentiated cells, particularly the colony stimulating factors and interleukins 6 and 11 (IL-6 and IL-11). Bone is a storehouse for growth regulatory factors. Some that affect osteoblast function include transforming growth factors (TGFβ I and II), acidic and basic fibroblast growth factors (FGF), platelet-derived growth factors (PDGF), and insulin-like growth factors (IGF-1 and -2). In addition, several proteins have the capacity to induce ectopic bone formation and may have a role in bone remodeling, e.g., osteoinductive factor, osteogenin, and bone morphogenic proteins. Other cytokines modulate resorption through effects on osteoclasts, e.g., interleukin 1 (IL-1), tumor necrosis factor (TNF), interferon-γ, and colony stimulating factors (CSFs). Some of these effects on osteoclasts are mediated by osteoblasts and adjacent stromal fibroblasts in the marrow. For example, PTH receptors are not found on mature osteoclasts, and PTH increases osteoclastic bone resorption by first acting on osteoblasts or stromal fibroblasts. $1,25(OH)_2D$ receptors are found in precursor cells, which can differentiate into monocytes or osteoclasts, and $1,25(OH)_2D$ promotes differentiation along the osteoclast pathway. Some cytokines such as IL-1 and TGFα may induce local production of prostaglandins and other cytokines such as IL-6 and CSFs. What had initially been termed *osteoclast-activating factor* is currently thought to reflect the presence of cytokines such as IL-1, TNFα, TNFβ (lymphotoxin), and probably others as well.

In the embryo and in the growing child, bone develops by remodeling and replacing previously calcified cartilage (endochondral bone formation), or it is formed without a cartilage matrix (intramembranous bone formation). New bone, whether in infants or in adults during repair, has a relatively high ratio of cells to matrix and is characterized by coarse fiber bundles of collagen that are interlaced and randomly dispersed (woven bone). In adults, the more mature bone is organized with fiber bundles regularly arranged in parallel or concentric sheets (lamellar bone). In long bones, deposition of lamellar bone in a concentric arrangement around blood vessels forms the haversian systems. Growth in length of bones is dependent on proliferation of cartilage cells and on the endochondral sequence at the growth plate. Growth in width and thickness is accomplished by formation of bone at the periosteal surface and by resorption at the endosteal surface with the rate of formation exceeding that of resorption. In adults, after the epiphyses close, growth in length and endochondral bone formation cease, except for some activity in the cartilage cells beneath the articular surface. Even in adults, however, remodeling of bone (remodeling of haversian systems as well as trabecular bone) continues through life. Newly forming surfaces are characterized by smooth character, by uptake of tetracycline, and by relatively low mineral density and are covered by active osteoblasts. The osteoid seam that results from the lag in mineralization of the newly formed organic matrix is about 12 μm in width. An index of the rate of bone formation can be obtained by examination of undemineralized sections of bone biopsies from individuals who have received tetracycline for two periods separated by a drug-free interval. The distance between the fluorescent bands on the sections reflects the new bone formed. Resorption areas are characterized by irregular configurations and the presence of osteoclasts (Fig. 356-1). Resorption precedes formation and is more intense, but it does not persist as long as formation. In adults, approximately 4 percent of the surface of trabecular bone (such as iliac crest) is involved in active resorption, whereas 10 to 15 percent of trabecular surfaces is covered with osteoid. Radioisotope studies indicate that as much as 18 percent of the total skeletal calcium is deposited and removed each year. Thus bone is an active metabolizing tissue that requires an intact blood supply. The remodeling of bone is somehow related to the mechanical stresses to which it is subjected. Bone also serves as an important reservoir of mineral ions such as calcium, which are critical for a variety of processes.

The response of bone to fractures, infection, and interruption of blood supply and to expanding lesions is relatively limited. Dead bone must be resorbed, and new bone must be formed, a process carried out in association with growth of new blood vessels into the involved area. In injuries that disrupt the organization of the tissue, such as a fracture in which apposition of fragments is poor and motion exists at the fracture site, the progenitor stromal cells differentiate into cells with functional capacities different from those of osteoblasts, and varying amounts of fibrous tissue and cartilage are formed. When

there is good apposition with fixation and little motion at the fracture site, repair occurs predominantly by formation of new bone without other scar tissue. Remodeling of this bone occurs along lines of force determined by mechanical stresses that are somehow translated into biologic response.

Expanding lesions in bone, such as tumors, induce resorption at the surface in contact with the tumor. A bowing deformity causes increased new bone formation at the concave surface and resorption at the convex surface, all seemingly designed to produce the strongest mechanical structure. Even in a disorder as architecturally disruptive as Paget's disease, remodeling is dictated by mechanical forces. Thus the plasticity of bone is due to cells interacting with each other and with the environment.

Mechanisms of bone formation and resorption Bone formation is an orderly process in which inorganic mineral is deposited in relation to an organic matrix. The mineral phase is composed of calcium and phosphorus, and the concentration of these ions in the plasma and extracellular fluid (ECF) influences the rate at which mineral is formed. In vitro, mineralization can proceed, and crystals of hydroxyapatite can grow at concentrations of calcium and phosphorus similar to those in an ultrafiltrate of plasma. However, the concentration of these ions at the sites of mineralization is unknown, and the cells involved (osteoblasts, osteocytes) may determine the local concentration of calcium, phosphorus, and other ions. Collagens from a variety of sources can catalyze the nucleation of a mineral phase of calcium and phosphorus from solutions of these ions, and the initial mineral phase is deposited in specific locations in the holes produced by the particular packing arrangement of the collagen molecules. The organization of collagen probably influences the amount and type of mineral phase formed in bone. The primary structures of type I collagen in skin and bone tissues are similar. There are differences, however, in posttranslational modifications of type I collagen such as hydroxylation, glycosylation, and the type, number, and distribution of intermolecular cross-links. In addition, the "holes" in the packing structure of the collagen are larger in mineralized collagen of bone and dentin than in unmineralized collagens such as tendon. The fact that single amino acid substitutions in the helical portion of either the α1 or α2 chains of type I collagen due to mutations in the COL1A1 or COL1A2 genes in osteogenesis imperfecta disrupt the organization of bone indicates the importance of the fibrillar matrix in the structure of bone (see also Chap. 351). The noncollagenous organic components such as osteocalcin, osteonectin, or osteopontin also may play a role in the formation of the mineral phase of bone. Alkaline phosphatase is a marker for osteoblasts, and cellular levels of this enzyme correlate with mineralization potential of osteoblasts. Although mineralization defects occur in individuals with mutations in the alkaline phosphate gene that cause decreased alkaline phosphatase activity (hypophosphatasia), the function of alkaline phosphatase in mineralization is not completely understood. Inorganic pyrophosphate is a potent inhibitor of mineralization at concentrations below those necessary to bind calcium ions. Since alkaline phosphatase in osteoblasts and other cells can catalyze the hydrolysis of inorganic pyrophosphate a neutral pH, this enzyme could regulate mineralization by controlling the concentrations of pyrophosphate. In addition, macromolecular inhibitors such as proteoglycan aggregates also may influence mineralization. In cartilage undergoing calcification, mineralization may be initiated in membrane-bound vesicles outside the cells.

In bone, the calcium phosphate solid phase at the inception of mineralization is brushite ($CaHPO_4 \cdot 2H_2O$). As mineralization progresses, the solid phase is a poorly crystalline hydroxyapatite with a relatively low (~1.2) calcium/phosphate molar ratio. With age and maturation, the perfection of the crystal and the calcium/phosphate ratio increase. Fluoride ions, when incorporated into the mineral phase, decrease the proportion of amorphous calcium phosphate and enhance the crystal structure.

There is a limit for the concentration of calcium and phosphorus ions in the ECF below which mineralization will not occur. A "solubility product" for bone mineral is difficult to calculate because

FIGURE 356-1 Schematic representation of bone remodeling surfaces in trabecular bone. Most bone surfaces in adults are involved in neither formation nor resorption. Such surfaces are usually smooth, have no osteoid seam, and are covered either by no visible cells or by flattened cells. Active formation surfaces are smooth and covered by osteoblasts which have an osteoid seam (*clear*), normally no thicker than 12 μm. The calcification front is located at the junction of the osteoid seam and mineralized bone (*stippled*). Inactive formation surfaces are not covered by osteoblasts but by only a few flattened cells. Active resorption surfaces are irregular or scalloped and contain multinucleated osteoclasts. The latter are not seen on inactive resorption surfaces.

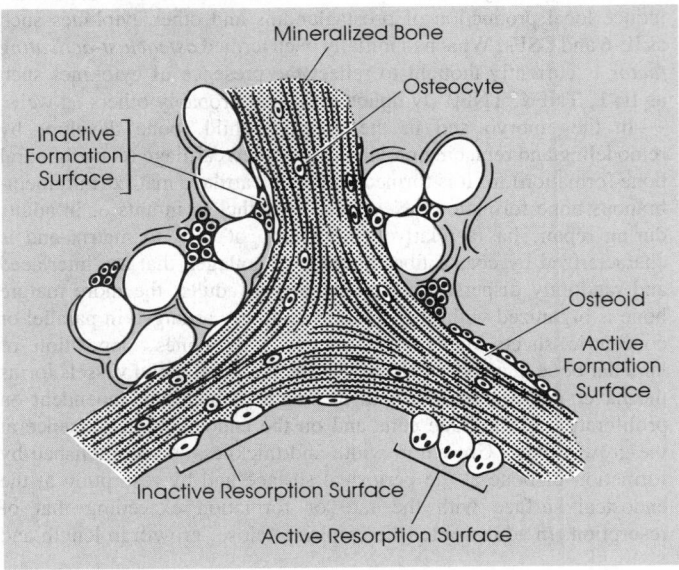

the mineral phase itself is of variable composition and the various components in ECF that regulate this solubility product are not known. Nevertheless, when the concentrations of calcium and phosphorus in ECF are excessive, a mineral phase may form in areas that are not normally mineralized.

When bone is resorbed, calcium and phosphorus ions are released into the ECF, and the organic matrix is then resorbed. The fact that bone resorption takes place in the region of the osteoclast adjacent to the bone surface, where the extracellular pH is low, suggests that an acid environment is required for solubilization of bone mineral. The alkaline phosphatase of bone cells is an ectoenzyme that is released into the ECF. Increased circulating levels of the bone-derived enzyme are correlated with rates of bone formation. Other circulating markers of bone formation include osteocalcin and type I procollagen carboxy-terminal peptides. Urinary markers for bone resorption are hydroxyproline, hydroxylysine and its glycosides, and the bone-specific hydroxypyridinium collagen cross-links.

CALCIUM METABOLISM There are about 1 to 2 kg calcium in the average adult body, over 98 percent of which is in the skeleton. The calcium of the mineral phase at the surface of the crystals is in equilibrium with the ECF, but only a minor proportion of the total calcium (about 0.5 percent) is exchangeable. The calcium in ECF is critical for a variety of functions, and it is remarkably constant. In normal adults, the range of plasma concentration is 2.2 to 2.6 mmol/L (8.8 to 10.4 mg/dL). The calcium in plasma is in three forms: as free ions, bound to plasma proteins, and, to a small extent, as diffusible complexes. The concentration of free calcium ions, mean 1.2 mmol/L (4.8 mg/dL), influences many cellular functions and is subjected to tight hormonal control, especially through parathyroid hormone (PTH), as described below. The concentration of serum proteins is an important determinant of calcium ion concentration; most is bound to albumin. Ionized calcium can be measured directly with the use of calcium-specific electrodes. If ionized calcium cannot be measured, certain approximations can be utilized to distinguish the protein bound from the ionized fraction. One formula that approximates the amount of calcium bound to protein is

$$\% \text{ protein-bound Ca} = 0.8 \times \text{albumin (g/L)}$$
$$+ 0.2 \times \text{globulin (g/L)} + 3$$

A simplified correction is sometimes used to indicate whether a stated total serum calcium concentration is abnormal when serum proteins are low. The correction is to add 1 mg/dL to serum calcium for every g/dL that serum albumin is below 4.0 g/dL. If the serum calcium, for example, is 7.8 mg/dL (a subnormal value) and the serum albumin is only 3.0 mg/dL, then the stated serum calcium is corrected by adding 1 mg/dL; the corrected value of 8.8 mg/dL is within the normal range. These rough approximations generally agree with measurements of ionized calcium in patients with subnormal serum proteins.

Calcium ions inside the cell mediate a variety of cellular functions (see also Chap. 69). Most of the cellular calcium is in the form of insoluble complexes. The concentration of free calcium within the cell, which is critical for functional regulation, is low, approximately 0.1 μmol/L; thus the gradient between plasma and intracellular free calcium is about 10,000 to 1. This gradient is tightly regulated. The concentration of calcium ions in the ECF is kept constant by processes that constantly feed calcium into and withdraw calcium from the extracellular fluid. Calcium enters the plasma via absorption from the intestinal tract and by resorption of ions from the bone mineral. Calcium leaves the ECF via secretion into the gastrointestinal tract (~100 to 200 mg/d), urinary excretion (~50 to 300 mg/d), deposition in bone mineral, and losses in sweat (up to 100 mg/d). Bone resorption and formation are tightly coupled, approximately 12 mmol (500 mg) calcium entering and leaving the skeleton daily (Fig. 356-2).

The average dietary calcium intake for most adults in the United States is approximately 15 to 20 mmol/d (0.6 to 0.8 g/d). However, with the heightened awareness of the role of adequate calcium intake for the prevention of osteoporosis, many adults on supplements have

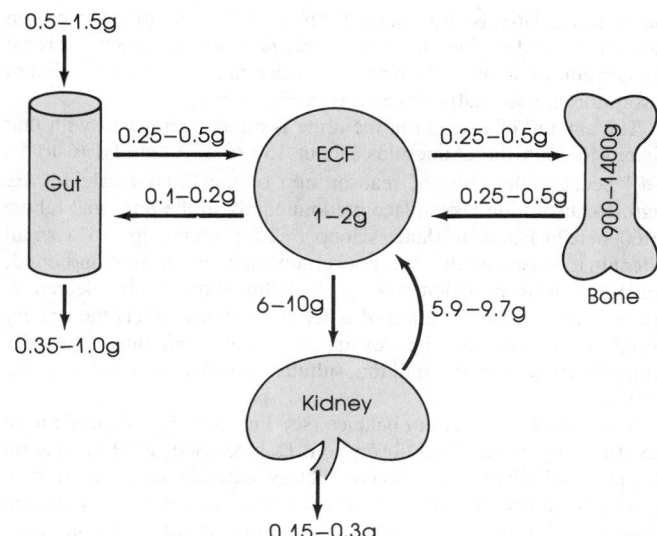

FIGURE 356-2 Calcium homeostasis. Schematic illustration of calcium content of extracellular fluid (ECF) and bone as well as of diet and feces; magnitude of calcium flux per day as calculated by various methods is shown at sites of transport in intestine, kidney, and bone. Ranges of values shown are approximate and chosen to illustrate certain points discussed in text. In intestine, absorption efficiency varies inversely with dietary calcium (chronic adaptation). This is reflected in typical quantities absorbed and excreted in feces; with 0.5-g intake, 50 percent absorption is depicted to occur (0.25 g), but at 1.5 g only 30 percent (0.5 g). Endogenous fecal calcium, the 0.1 to 0.2 g secreted into the intestinal lumen daily, is constant and does not vary with calcium intake or absorption. Quantities of calcium depicted as filtered, reabsorbed, and excreted at the kidney are chosen arbitrarily to indicate that at lower rates of filtration of calcium (expected at lower glomerular filtration rates), most is reabsorbed (e.g., 5.85 of 6 g), leading to urinary excretion of 150 mg; at higher rates of filtration (at high dietary calcium intake), slightly less is reabsorbed (e.g., 9.7 of 10 g), leading to a higher urinary excretion, 300 mg. In all situations, renal calcium reabsorption exceeds 95 percent of filtered load. Urinary calcium excretion is seen, therefore, to increase by only 150 mg despite a 1-g increase in dietary intake. In conditions of calcium balance, rates of calcium release from and uptake into bone are equal.

an intake of 20 to 37 mmol/d (0.8 to 1.5 g/d). In adults, less than half of dietary calcium is absorbed. Calcium absorption increases during periods of rapid growth in children, in pregnancy, and in lactation and decreases with advancing age. Most of the calcium is absorbed in the proximal small intestine, and the efficiency of absorption decreases in the more distal intestinal segments. Both active transport and diffusion-limited absorption are involved; the former is more important in the upper and the latter is more important in the lower intestine. Both processes are influenced by vitamin D through the action of its metabolites. All forms of calcium in the diet may not be equally absorbed; calcium as the chloride is probably absorbed more efficiently than that in other preparations.

Calcium is also secreted into the lumen of the gastrointestinal tract. When radioactive calcium is administered intravenously, it appears in the feces, making possible calculations of *endogenous fecal calcium* (see Fig. 356-2). Higher estimates of calcium losses in intestinal juices have been made by other techniques. Secretion of calcium into the intestinal lumen is constant and independent of absorption. If calcium availability in the diet is low [<12 mmol/d (500 mg/d)], positive calcium balance requires an efficiency of absorption greater than 30 to 40 percent.

The urinary calcium excretion of normal adults on average calcium intakes ranges between 2.5 and 10 mmol/d (100 and 400 mg/d). When the dietary calcium is below 5 mmol/d (200 mg/d), urinary calcium excretion is usually less than 5 mmol/d (200 mg/d). However, in most normal individuals, the level of dietary intake over a wide range has relatively little effect on urinary calcium. Hence, in individuals on diets low in calcium, this relative inefficiency of renal calcium conservation leads to negative calcium balance unless calcium absorption is maximally efficient (see Fig. 356-2).

The amount of calcium in the urine is minute compared with that filtered through the glomerulus [about 150 to 250 mmol/d (6 to 10 g/d)] because the rates of reabsorption of the filtered calcium are high. Reabsorption takes place predominantly in the proximal tubule (~60 percent) and in Henle's loop (~25 percent) and to a small extent in the distal tubule. It is not certain whether non-protein-bound, nonionic forms of calcium (e.g., calcium citrate) are cleared at different rates. The excretion of other electrolytes affects the urinary excretion of calcium. For example, urinary calcium is usually proportional to urinary sodium; sulfate also increases calcium excretion.

Maintenance of calcium balance (see Fig. 356-2) is dependent on the efficiency of intestinal absorption. Deficiency of PTH or vitamin D, intestinal disease, or severe dietary calcium deprivation may provide challenges to calcium homeostasis that cannot be compensated adequately by renal calcium conservation, resulting in negative calcium balance. Increased bone resorption may protect against ECF calcium depletion even in states of chronic negative calcium balance but only at the expense of progressive bone loss.

Pathophysiology Decrease in the concentration of free calcium ions in plasma results in increased neuromuscular irritability and tetany. This syndrome is characterized by peripheral and perioral paresthesias, carpal spasm, pedal spasm, anxiety, seizures, bronchospasm, laryngospasm, Chvostek's, Trousseau's, and Erb's signs, and lengthening of the QT interval of the electrocardiogram. In infants, tetany may be manifested only by irritability and lethargy. The level of calcium ions that determines which features of tetany will be manifested varies among individuals. Tetany is also influenced by the concentration of other components of the ECF. For example, hypomagnesemia and alkalosis lower whereas hypokalemia and acidosis raise the threshold for tetany.

Increases in total serum calcium are usually accompanied by increases in calcium ions and may be associated with anorexia, nausea, vomiting, constipation, hypotonia, depression, and occasionally lethargy and coma. Persistent hypercalcemia, especially when accompanied by normal or elevated levels of serum phosphate, may cause ectopic deposition of a solid phase of calcium and phosphate in walls of blood vessels, connective tissue about the joints, gastric mucosa, cornea, and renal parenchyma. Hypercalcemia per se alters renal function in addition to the pathologic effects of calcium phosphate deposition.

PHOSPHORUS METABOLISM Phosphorus is a major component of bone and of all other tissues and in some form is involved in almost all metabolic processes. The total amount of phosphorus in the normal adult is about 32 mol (1 kg), of which about 85 percent is in the skeleton.

In fasting plasma, most of the phosphorus is present as inorganic orthophosphate in concentrations of approximately 0.9 to 1.3 mmol/L (2.8 to 4 mg/dL). In contrast to calcium, where about 50 percent is bound, only about 12 percent of the phosphorus in plasma is bound to proteins. Free HPO_4^{2-} and $NaHPO_4^-$ normally are about 75 percent of the total phosphorus, and free $H_2PO_4^-$ is 10 percent. Since so many species are present, depending on pH and other factors, it is the convention to express concentrations in terms of mass of elemental phosphorus, i.e., millimoles per liter or milligrams per deciliter. Total phosphorus levels are higher in children and in women after the menopause. There is a circadian variation in phosphorus concentration even during a 24-h fast, mediated in part by the adrenal cortex. The nadir occurs between 9 A.M. and 12 noon, followed by an increase to a plateau in the afternoon and another small peak after midnight. The magnitudes of the peaks and troughs vary with phosphorus intake but occur regardless of whether the intake is high or low. Dietary restriction of phosphorus that only modestly decreases the morning fasting levels may abolish the afternoon rise. Despite changes in

serum phosphorus levels of nearly twofold, serum ionized calcium levels do not change significantly.

During phosphate depletion, phosphaturia decreases before serum phosphorus declines. This adaptive response of increasing tubular transport when luminal concentrations are decreasing is an intrinsic property of these cells. There is also heterogeneity of phosphorus transport among different segments of proximal renal tubules. Tubular fluxes of phosphorus rather than hypophosphatemia per se may be critical in modulating effects of hypophosphatemia such as the stimulation of 25(OH)D-1α-hydroxylase. Conversely, increased phosphorus loads and increased renal tubular phosphorus fluxes result in decreased renal tubular reabsorption and increased clearance of phosphorus and suppress the activity of 25(OH)D-1α-hydroxylase (see below). Ingestion of carbohydrate depresses serum phosphorus acutely by 0.3 to 0.5 mmol/L (1 to 1.5 mg/dL), presumably as the result of cellular uptake and formation of phosphate esters. Ingestion of phosphorus per se increases serum levels. Therefore, for the interpretation of serum levels and urinary clearances, samples should be obtained in the fasting state. Decreases in plasma phosphorus also occur during induction of alkalosis.

Whereas dietary calcium is inefficiently absorbed from the intestine, phosphorus absorption is remarkably efficient. At low levels of intake (less than 2 mg/kg of body weight per day), 80 to 90 percent of ingested phosphorus is absorbed. Even with levels of intake greater than 10 mg/kg of body weight per day in the form of dairy products, cereals, eggs, and meat, absorption is about 70 percent. Hypophosphatemia due to deficient intestinal absorption is unusual except when nonabsorbable antacids are consumed; the antacids bind phosphorus and prevent absorption from the intestinal lumen.

The major control of phosphorus economy is exerted at the level of the kidney. Phosphorus filtered through the glomerulus is largely reabsorbed in the proximal tubule (there is homeostatically important distal reabsorption as well) so that only about 10 to 15 percent of the filtered load is normally excreted. When filtered loads of phosphorus decrease, proximal tubular reabsorption increases. Conversely, when phosphorus loads are increased, tubular reabsorption decreases and clearance rises. Thus the urinary excretion of phosphorus normally reflects dietary intake, and conservation or elimination of excessive amounts depends on adequate renal handling (Fig. 356-3). There is no good evidence for renal tubular phosphate secretion. Proximal reabsorption of phosphorus is dependent on parallel sodium reabsorption, but whereas the sodium rejected by the proximal tubule may be reabsorbed distally, the rejected phosphorus is not. Therefore, volume expansion and decreased sodium reabsorption increase phosphorus clearance; similarly, diuretics that act proximally, such as acetazolamide, are phosphaturic parallel to the degree to which they are natriuretic.

Pathophysiology No direct symptoms result from hyperphosphatemia. When high levels are maintained for long periods, however, the driving force for mineralization is increased, and calcium phosphate may be deposited in abnormal sites. Ectopic calcification of this type is encountered in untreated chronic renal failure, with severe hypercalcemia, and in vitamin D intoxication. *Tumoral calcinosis* is a rare heritable disorder in which ectopic calcification is associated with hyperphosphatemia and normal glomerular filtration rates (GFR). The disorder is characterized by high ratio of phosphorus tubule maximum (TmP) to GFR and increased serum levels of 1,25(OH)$_2$D. The latter is a paradoxical finding and presumably is related to the abnormal renal tubular phosphate fluxes. In contrast, severe acute hypophosphatemia may cause anorexia, dizziness, bone pain, proximal muscular weakness, and waddling gait. Significant hypophosphatemia is encountered in severe alcoholics and may be aggravated after repletion of nutrients, in the course of therapy of diabetic ketoacidosis, and for various reasons in severely ill, hospitalized elderly patients (see also Chap. 359). Myopathy in severe hypophosphatemia may be accompanied by elevations in serum creatinine kinase levels and by rhabdomyolysis. Severe congestive cardiomyopathy may occur with chronic hypophosphatemia, and restoration of phosphorus

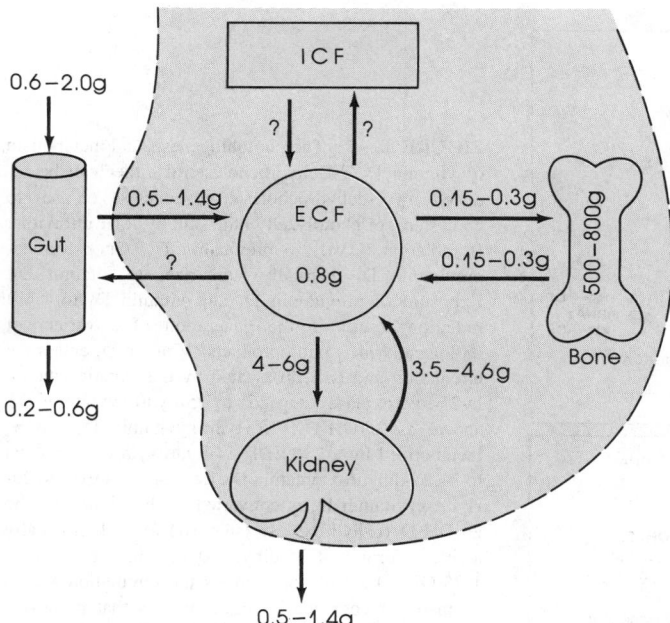

FIGURE 356-3 Phosphate homeostasis. Schematic illustration of inorganic phosphorus content (termed here *phosphate*) in extracellular fluid (ECF) and bone as well as diet and feces; magnitude of phosphorus flux per day as estimated by various methods is shown at transport sites in intestine, kidney, and bone. Range of values shown illustrates special features of phosphorus metabolism discussed in text. Intestinal phosphorus absorption is highly efficient, 85 percent at a lower intake (0.5 g of a 0.6-g intake) and 70 percent at a higher intake (1.4 g of a 2.0-g intake). Estimates of magnitude of endogenous fecal phosphate are less well established than for calcium. Contribution of at least 0.15 g is estimated to be added to the nonabsorbed phosphorus to provide a total of 0.2 g fecal phosphorus at the low intake level. At high phosphorus dietary intakes, no correction for endogenous fecal phosphate is calculated. Higher quantities of phosphorus are excreted in urine at all levels of dietary intake than for corresponding intakes of calcium; quantities excreted match closely the quantities absorbed, thereby maintaining phosphorus balance (no correction in this illustration is made for endogenous fecal phosphorus). Note that renal phosphorus reabsorption, in contrast to high and relatively invariant renal calcium reabsorption, varies from a low of 75 percent of filtered load to greater than 85 percent. The compartment labeled ICF refers to intracellular phosphorus, both organic and inorganic; rapid shifts of phosphorus into cells (and corresponding, possibly slower, efflux of phosphorus from cells) contribute to changes in ECF phosphorus. These shifts between ECF and ICF and phosphorus release from and uptake by bone are equal in conditions of phosphorus balance.

deficits leads to prompt reversal. Respiratory muscle weakness in severe hypophosphatemia also may improve with phosphate repletion. The bone pain and waddling gait are attributed to the osteomalacia that develops as a result of phosphate depletion. The muscular weakness may be due either to direct effects of hypophosphatemia on nerves and muscle or, in some instances, to the effects of hyperparathyroidism (either primary or secondary) which may have a role in the etiology of the hypophosphatemia. Phosphorus depletion in children may cause defective growth. Hypophosphatemia results in decreased levels of 2,3-diphosphoglyceric acid and adenosine triphosphate (ATP) in erythrocytes, which in turn alter the dissociation of oxyhemoglobin so that less oxygen is delivered to tissues. Hemolytic anemia may result from impairment of the ability of erythrocytes to deform in small vessels.

VITAMIN D

Vitamin D is a hormone, not a vitamin. With adequate exposure to sunlight, no dietary supplements are needed. The active principle of vitamin D is synthesized under metabolic control via successive hydroxylations in the liver and kidney and is transported through the blood to its target tissues (the small intestine and bone), where it regulates calcium homeostasis. Calcium and phosphate ions, parathyroid hormone, and possibly other peptide and steroid hormones regulate the renal metabolism of vitamin D. Analysis of hereditary and acquired defects in these processes has provided new insights into the pathophysiology of several disorders involving calcium, phosphorus, and bone metabolism. These discoveries culminated in the chemical synthesis of active vitamin D metabolites and analogues, the clinical use of $1\alpha,25$-dihydroxyvitamin D_3 [$1,25(OH)_2D_3$] (calcitriol) in many vitamin D–resistant disorders, and the development of assays for measuring vitamin D metabolites in blood to define suspected abnormalities in vitamin D metabolism.

PHOTOBIOGENESIS OF VITAMIN D Vitamin D_3 is a derivative of 7-dehydrocholesterol (provitamin D_3), the immediate precursor of cholesterol. When skin is exposed to sunlight or certain artificial light sources, the ultraviolet radiation enters the epidermis and causes transformation of 7-dehydrocholesterol to vitamin D_3. Wavelengths between 290 and 315 nm are absorbed by the conjugated double bonds at C_5 and C_7 of 7-dehydrocholesterol and fragment the B ring between C_9 and C_{10} to yield a 9,10-secosterol (*seco* means "split"), previtamin D_3 (Fig. 356-4). Previtamin D_3 is biologically inert but spontaneously undergoes a temperature-dependent molecular rearrangement of its conjugated triene system (three double bonds) to form the thermally stable 9,10-secosterol, vitamin D_3 (see Fig. 356-4). At body temperature it takes approximately 24 h for previtamin D_3 to convert completely into vitamin D_3. Wide changes in skin surface do not affect the rate of this conversion because the process occurs in the actively growing layers of the epidermis, where the temperature is relatively constant; changes in the core body temperature also have little effect on this reaction. Once vitamin D_3 is synthesized, it is translocated from the epidermis to the circulation by the vitamin D–binding protein. Thus vitamin D_3 is made in the skin from previtamin for many hours after a single sun exposure (see Fig. 356-4). Although melanin in the skin competes with 7-dehydrocholesterol for ultraviolet photons and thus can limit the synthesis of previtamin D_3, the photochemical isomerization of previtamin D_3 and vitamin D_3 to biologically inert products appears to be more important in preventing excessive production of previtamin D_3 and vitamin D_3 during prolonged exposure to the sun.

Aging decreases the capacity of the skin to produce vitamin D_3; greater than fourfold reduction occurs after the age of 70 years. Topical sunscreens can reduce or prevent the cutaneous vitamin D_3 production by absorbing the solar radiation responsible for previtamin D_3 synthesis in the skin. Other factors that affect the cutaneous synthesis of vitamin D_3 include altitude, geographic location, time of day, and area of exposure. Latitude has profound effects on the cutaneous synthesis of vitamin D_3. As the zenith angle of the sun increases with approaching winter, more of the high-energy ultraviolet photons responsible for previtamin D_3 synthesis are absorbed by the ozone layer. In Boston (42°N) and in Edmonton (52°N), the absorption of these photons is so complete that essentially no vitamin D_3 is made in the skin between the months of November through February and October through March, respectively. When the entire body is exposed to sufficient sunlight to cause mild erythema, the increase in the blood vitamin D is about equivalent to consuming an oral dose of 10,000 to 25,000 international units (1 IU = 0.025 µg) of vitamin D. Only when skin irradiation is insufficient to produce the required quantities of vitamin D_3 is dietary supplementation needed to prevent skeletal mineralization defects. Fish liver oils, a natural source of vitamin D, were used widely for the treatment of rickets early in this century. The fortification of milk and some cereals with either crystalline vitamin D_2 (see Fig. 356-4) or vitamin D_3 prevents rickets and osteomalacia. However, a survey of the vitamin D content in milk from five Eastern states revealed that 71 percent did not contain 80 to 120 percent of the amount of vitamin D on the label and 20 percent of samples of skim milk did not contain detectable vitamin D. Although

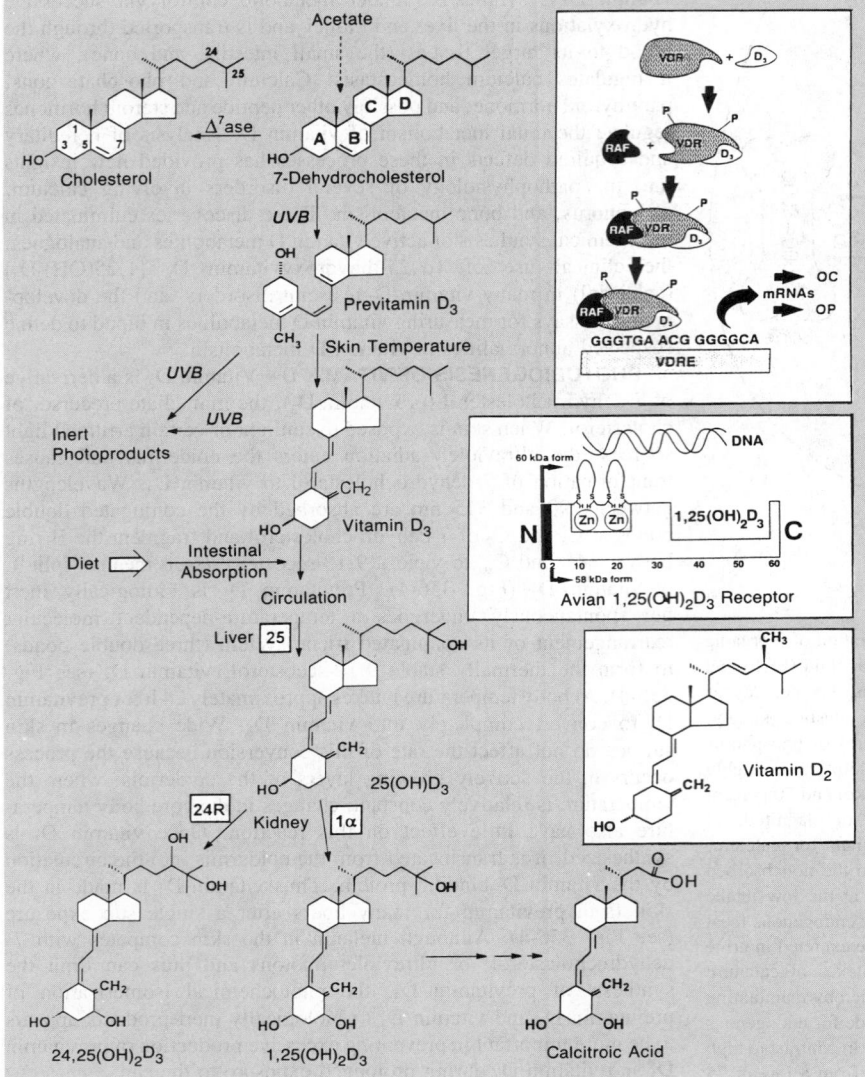

FIGURE 356-4 The photobiogenesis and metabolism of vitamin D. 7-Dehydrocholesterol either can be reduced by 7-dehydrocholesterol reductase (Δ^7ase) to cholesterol or photolyzed in the skin by solar ultraviolet B radiation (UVB) to previtamin D_3. Once formed, previtamin D_3 thermally isomerizes to vitamin D_3. Exposure of previtamin D_3 and vitamin D_3 to UVB radiation results in the generation of a variety of biologically inert photoproducts. Vitamin D_3 enters the circulation and is hydroxylated by the hepatic vitamin D-25-hydroxylase (step 25) to 25-hydroxyvitamin D_3, shown as $25(OH)D_3$. 25-Hydroxyvitamin D_3 can be metabolized by a $25(OH)D$-24-hydroxylase (step 24R) to 24,25-dihydroxyvitamin D_3, i.e., $24,25-(OH)_2D_3$. 25-Hydroxyvitamin D_3 is converted in the kidney by the 25-OH-D-1α-hydroxylase (step 1α) to its biologically active form, 1,25-dihydroxyvitamin D_3, i.e., $1,25(OH)_2D_3$. This form enters the circulation and is ultimately recognized by target tissues that possess a specific nuclear receptor (VDR) for it.

As shown in the top two inserts, the VDR, a member of the steroid superfamily of receptors, interacts with $1,25(OH)_2D_3$ (identified as D_3), resulting in the phosphorylation of the $1,25(OH)_2D_3$-VDR complex. This complex interacts with a receptor accessory factor (RAF) to form a heterodimer which, in turn, interacts with the vitamin D-responsive element (VDRE) in the targeted nuclei. In the bone, this interaction increases the expression of mRNAs for osteocalcin (OC) and osteopontin (OP).

1,25-Dihydroxyvitamin D_3 can undergo multiple hydroxylations in its side chain that may ultimately result in the formation of the water-soluble biologically inactive calcitroic acid.

The lower insert is the structure for vitamin D_2. It is structurally different from vitamin D_3 in having a double bond between C_{22} and C_{23} and a methyl group on C_{24}.

the National Research Council of the United States recommends an intake of 200 IU/d for adults, this amount may be inadequate if there is little cutaneous production of vitamin D_3. In the absence of sunlight, between 400 and 600 IU of vitamin D is required to satisfy the daily requirement.

METABOLISM OF VITAMIN D Once vitamin D enters the circulation, either by its absorption from the diet or through the skin, it is transported to the liver bound to a specific alpha$_1$ globulin (vitamin D-binding protein). In the liver, vitamin D is metabolized to 25-hydroxyvitamin D [25(OH)D] by hepatic mitochondrial and/or microsomal enzyme(s) (see Fig. 356-4). 25(OH)D is one of the major circulating metabolites, and its half-life is estimated to be about 21 days. The concentrations of 25(OH)D and some of its metabolites in the serum are measured using competitive binding assays. The normal serum 25(OH)D varies among different laboratories from 20 to 200 nmol/L (8 to 80 ng/mL). Individuals exposed to excessive sunlight may have concentrations of 25(OH)D up to 250 nmol/L (100 ng/mL) without adverse effects on calcium metabolism. Assays that employ chromatographic separation prior to binding analysis often have a lower normal range, possibly because other vitamin D metabolites simulate 25(OH)D in this assay. The normal range, apparently independent of method, is lower in Great Britain, where additions of vitamin D to foods are not routine and where exposure to sunlight is less than in most regions of the United States. The serum 25(OH)D levels usually reflect both 25-hydroxyvitamin D_2 [25(OH)D$_2$] and 25-hydroxyvitamin D_3 [25(OH)D$_3$]. The ratio of these two 25-hydroxylated derivatives depends on the relative amounts of vitamins D_2 or D_3 present in the diet and the amount of previtamin D_3 produced by exposure to sunlight.

The hepatic 25-hydroxylation of vitamin D is regulated by a product feedback mechanism. This regulation, however, is not tight; an increase in dietary intake or endogenous production of vitamin D_3 causes increases in 25(OH)D levels in the serum. The levels can rise to greater than 1200 nmol/L (500 ng/mL) when the intake of vitamin D is increased. Serum 25(OH)D levels are reduced in severe chronic liver disease (Table 356-1).

25(OH)D is not biologically active at physiologic levels in vivo but is active in vitro at high concentrations. Normally, after formation in the liver, 25(OH)D is bound by the vitamin D-binding protein and transported to the kidney for an additional stereospecific hydroxylation on either C_1 or C_{24} (see Fig. 356-4). The kidney plays a pivotal role in the metabolism of 25(OH)D to the biologically active metabolite. The renal mitochondrial 25(OH)D-1α-hydroxylase activity is enhanced by hypocalcemia so that the rate of conversion of 25(OH)D to $1,25(OH)_2D$ increases. Hypocalcemia may not control this hydroxylation directly, however. Any decrease in the serum concentration of calcium below normal is a stimulus for increased secretion of PTH. PTH acts physiologically to increase the synthesis of $1,25(OH)_2D$ in the renal proximal convoluted tubule. The mechanism by which PTH exerts its influence on the renal metabolism of 25(OH)D is not

TABLE 356-1 Serum concentrations of 25(OH)D in disorders of calcium, phosphorus, and bone metabolism

Disease states	Serum 25(OH)D
Vitamin D deficiency	↓
Intestinal malabsorption syndromes	↓
Liver disorders (chronic and severe)	↓
Nephrotic syndrome	↓
Osteopenia in the aged	N or ↓
Vitamin D intoxication	↑

NOTE: ↓ = decreased; N = normal; ↑ = increased.

established; however, the renal production of 1,25(OH)₂D enhances the effects of PTH in lowering circulating concentrations (and presumably renal intracellular concentrations) of phosphate (Fig. 356-5). 1,25(OH)₂D also influences the renal metabolism of 25(OH)D by diminishing 25(OH)D-1α-hydroxylase activity and enhancing the metabolism of 24R,25-dihydroxyvitamin D [24,25(OH)₂D].

24,25(OH)₂D is a circulating metabolite of 25(OH)D normally present in serum at a concentration of 1 to 10 nmol/L (0.5 to 5.0 ng/mL). 24,25(OH)₂D is also a substrate for renal 25(OH)D-1α-hydroxylase and is converted to 1α,24R,25-trihydroxyvitamin D [1,24,25(OH)₃D], which, in turn, is metabolized to the biologically inactive calcitroic acid (see Fig. 339-4). Cultured cells that possess nuclear receptors for 1,25(OH)₂D, such as chondrocytes, skin keratinocytes and fibroblasts, and intestinal and melanoma cells, also metabolize 25(OH)D to 24,25(OH)₂D. Although 24,25(OH)₂D may play a role in the expression of vitamin D action, it is more likely, that the C₂₄ hydroxylation is the first step in the degradation of both 25(OH)D and 1,25(OH)₂D to water-soluble inactive metabolites including calcitroic acid (see Fig. 339-4). More than 35 metabolites originate from 25(OH)D or 1,25(OH)₂D. Most of the metabolites appear to be degradation products.

PHYSIOLOGY OF VITAMIN D 1,25(OH)₂D, produced by the kidney and the placenta, is the only known important metabolite of vitamin D; the potential roles of other metabolites have not been clarified. 1,25(OH)₂D bound to a vitamin D–binding protein is delivered to the intestine, where the free form is taken up by the cells and transported to a specific nuclear receptor protein. The 1,25(OH)₂D receptor belongs to the superfamily of steroid receptors that are related to the oncogene v-erbA (see Chap. 329). The vitamin-receptor complex interacts with a nuclear accessory factor and becomes phosphorylated to enhance the transcription of genes; in the intestine calcium-binding protein is synthesized, and in bone osteocalcin, osteopontin, and alkaline phosphatase are produced. 1,25(OH)₂D also may have nonnuclear effects on its target tissues; 1,25(OH)₂D increases the transport of calcium from the extracellular to intracellular space, and it can mobilize calcium from intracellular calcium pools and enhance phosphotidylinositol metabolism. In the intestine, the net effect of 1,25(OH)₂D is to stimulate calcium and phosphate transport from the lumen of the small intestine into the circulation (see Fig. 356-5). The effect of 1,25(OH)₂D on the enhancement of bone resorption is believed to be synergistic with PTH. Mature osteoclasts do not possess receptors either for PTH or 1,25(OH)₂D, and the two hormones may increase bone resorption activity by stimulating immature osteoclastic precursors that possess receptors for both to become mature osteoclasts and/or by interacting with osteoblasts and bone marrow stromal cells to produce cytokines that enhance the activity of mature osteoclasts. The role of 1,25(OH)₂D in the renal handling of calcium and phosphorus remains uncertain.

Receptors for 1,25(OH)₂D are present in intestine, bone, and kidney and in tissues and cells that have not classically been recognized as target organs for this hormone, including skin, breast, pituitary, parathyroids, beta cells of the pancreatic islets, gonads, brain, skeletal muscle, circulating monocytes, and activated B and T lymphocytes. Although its physiologic role in these cells remains to be determined,

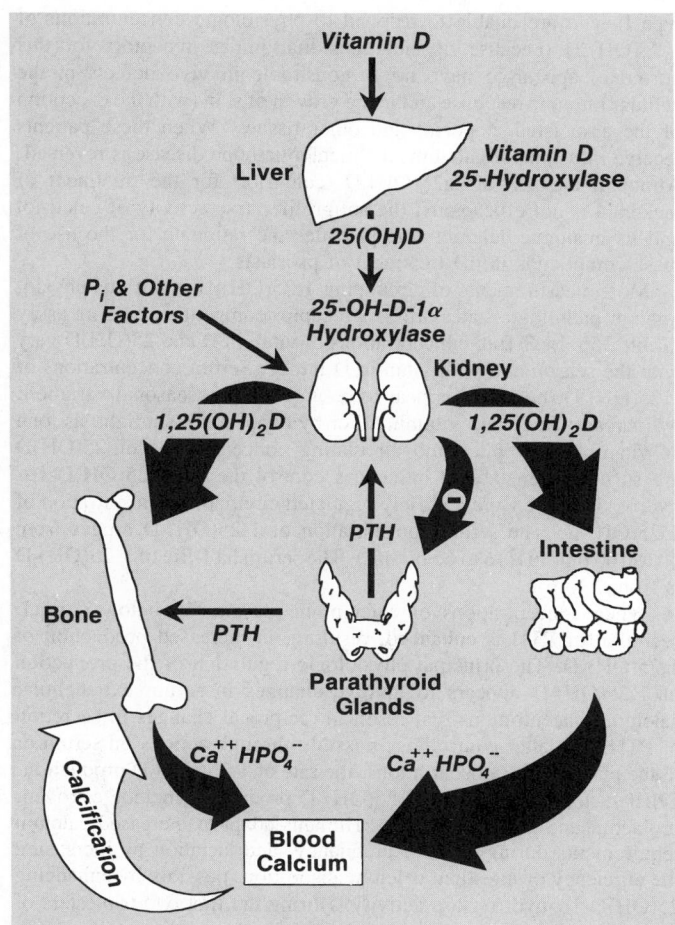

FIGURE 356-5 Schematic representation of the hormonal control loop for vitamin D metabolism and function. A reduction in the serum calcium below approximately 2.2 mmol/L (8.8 mg/dL) prompts a proportional increase in the secretion of PTH and so mobilizes additional calcium from the bone. PTH promotes the synthesis of 1,25(OH)₂D in the kidney, which, in turn, stimulates the mobilization of calcium from bone and intestine and regulates the synthesis of PTH by negative feedback.

in vitro 1,25(OH)₂D inhibits proliferation of keratinocytes and fibroblasts, stimulates terminal differentiation of keratinocytes, induces monocytes to produce IL-1 and to mature into macrophages and osteoclast-like cells, inhibits the production of PTH, and inhibits IL-2 and immunoglobulin production by activated T and B lymphocytes, respectively.

In addition, a variety of tumor cell lines, including breast carcinomas, melanomas, and promyeloblasts, possess receptors for 1,25(OH)₂D. Tumor cell lines that have receptors for 1,25(OH)₂D respond to the hormone by decreasing the rate of proliferation and by enhancing differentiation. For example, when malignant receptor-positive human promyelocytic cells (HL-60) are exposed to 1,25(OH)₂D, the cells mature into functioning macrophages within 1 week. Although the mechanism of induction of maturation is unknown, 1,25(OH)₂D decreases the expression of c-*myc* oncogene coincident with decreasing replication. This effect, however, is not a lasting one; when the metabolite is removed from maturing HL-60 promyelocytes, the cells revert to their original malignant state, and expression of c-*myc* oncogene is no longer suppressed.

The role of 1,25(OH)₂D in the regulation of differentiation and immunoregulation is unknown. However, it may regulate PTH synthesis by negative feedback (see Fig. 356-5). This is the rationale for giving 1,25(OH)₂D₃ intravenously to suppress PTH in patients with chronic renal failure. Patients with vitamin D–dependent rickets type II who are unable to respond to physiologic concentrations of $1,25(OH)_2D$ (because of mutations that impair receptors for this hormone) appear to have no demonstrable in vivo defects in the cellular immune response and in the growth of skin (with the exception of the associated alopecia) and other tissues. When these patients receive infusions of calcium, the metabolic bone disease is reversed. Although the use of $1,25(OH)_2D$ (calcitriol) for the treatment of leukemia is not efficacious, the antiproliferative activity of calcitriol and its analogue calcipotriene provides the rationale for the use of these compounds in the treatment of psoriasis.

Most measurements of circulating $1,25(OH)_2D$ in various physiologic or pathologic states utilize a receptor/competitive binding assay (Table 356-2). Serum concentrations of vitamin D and $25(OH)D$ vary with the season and with vitamin D intake. Serum concentrations of $1,25(OH)_2D$, however, appear to be unaltered by seasonal variation, by increases in dietary vitamin D, or by exposure to sunlight; as long as vitamin D supplies and circulating concentrations of $25(OH)D$ are sufficient, metabolic influences control the renal $25(OH)D$-1α-hydroxylase to ensure a closely regulated circulating concentration of $1,25(OH)_2D$. The serum concentration of $1,25(OH)_2D$ ranges from 40 to 160 pmol/L (16 to 65 pg/mL). The serum half-life of $1,25(OH)_2D$ is from 3 to 6 h.

When concentrations of calcium in plasma fall below normal, secretion of PTH is enhanced, resulting in increased production of $1,25(OH)_2D$. The principal physiologic regulation of the production of $1,25(OH)_2D$ appears to involve changes in serum extracellular calcium concentrations that result in reciprocal changes in secretion of PTH, the latter controlling, possibly through actions on serum or tissue phosphorus concentrations, the rate of $1,25(OH)_2D$ production. Other factors that enhance $1,25(OH)_2D$ production include estrogen, prolactin, and growth hormone. Humans adapt to increased calcium requirements during growth, pregnancy, and lactation by increasing the efficiency of intestinal calcium absorption, possibly by enhancing $25(OH)D$-1α-hydroxylase activity. During the first two trimesters of pregnancy, the concentrations of $1,25(OH)_2D$ increase in proportion to the concentrations of the vitamin D–binding protein; concentrations of free $1,25(OH)_2D$ do not change. During the last trimester, the need for calcium for mineralization of the fetal skeleton is met by an increase in the free concentrations of $1,25(OH)_2D$, which in turn enhance maternal intestinal calcium absorption.

PATHOPHYSIOLOGY OF DISORDERS OF VITAMIN D NUTRITION AND METABOLISM *Hypovitaminosis D* results from inadequate endogenous production of vitamin D_3 in the skin, insufficient dietary supplementation, and/or the inability of the small intestine to absorb adequate amounts of vitamin D from the diet. Resistance to the effects of vitamin D can result from (1) use of drugs that antagonize vitamin D action, (2) alterations in the metabolism of vitamin D, or (3) deficient or defective receptors for $1,25(OH)_2D$. The consequences of hypovitaminosis D include (1) disturbances of mineral ion metabolism and secretion of PTH and (2) mineralization defects in the skeleton (e.g., rickets in children, osteomalacia in adults). The changes in the skeleton are described in Chap. 358. With regard to calcium metabolism, lack of vitamin D action leads to insufficient intestinal calcium absorption and hypocalcemia. The latter stimulates the secretion of PTH (secondary hyperparathyroidism), which enhances calcium release from bone and decreases calcium clearance by the kidney and tends to blunt the hypocalcemia. (Late in the course of untreated hypovitaminosis D, severe hypocalcemia develops.) Hypophosphatemia is more marked than hypocalcemia, especially in early stages of vitamin D deficiency. The efficiency of intestinal phosphate absorption is also decreased. The increased secretin of PTH, although partially effective in minimizing hypocalcemia, leads to urinary phosphate wasting through decreases in renal tubular reabsorption. This latter effect is the most significant factor in causing hypophosphatemia. With an adequate GFR, the predominant changes are hypophosphatemia, moderate or slight hypocalcemia, increased levels of PTH, and low levels of $25(OH)D$ (see Table 356-1). As discussed in Chap. 358 defects in skeletal mineralization may accompany these disturbances in mineral ion metabolism.

Although the conversion of vitamin D to $25(OH)D$ is impaired in severe chronic liver disease, there is no strong correlation between low serum $25(OH)D$ levels and osteopenia. Patients with nephrotic syndrome with more than 4 g/d of proteinuria may have low $25(OH)D$ levels due to the loss in the urine of the vitamin D-binding protein with its associated tightly bound $25(OH)D$. Circulating levels of $25(OH)D$ also may be decreased when the catabolism of $25(OH)D$ is increased, as in sarcoidosis and hyperparathyroidism. Chronic anticonvulsant therapy also can cause the development of osteomalacia or rickets; mineralization defects are worse in patients on multiple drug therapy and when vitamin D intake or exposure to sunlight is inadequate. Anticonvulsant drugs have multiple effects on calcium metabolism. Phenobarbital induces hepatic microsomal enzymes, alters the kinetics of the vitamin D-25-hydroxylase, and stimulates bile secretion, which result in decreased serum concentrations of vitamin D and $25(OH)D$. Phenytoin and phenobarbital inhibit intestinal calcium transport and bone mineral mobilization, independent of effects of vitamin D metabolism.

Glucocorticoids in high doses cause disturbances in calcium metabolism and osteoporosis but do not induce osteomalacia and rickets. Glucocorticoids directly inhibit vitamin D–mediated intestinal calcium absorption and bone mineral mobilization and enhance the sensitivity of bone cells to $1,25(OH)_2D$ by stabilizing the $1,25(OH)_2D$ receptor or by increasing the affinity or number of receptors. Patients receiving glucocorticoids chronically may have depressed circulating levels of $1,25(OH)_2D$; the mechanism(s) is unknown.

A genetic defect in the hepatic 25-hydroxylation of vitamin D has not been described, but in one inherited disorder of calcium and bone metabolism renal production of $1,25(OH)_2D$ is defective. In the syndrome of pseudovitamin D–deficient rickets (also known as vitamin D–dependent rickets type I; see Chap. 358), circulating levels of $1,25(OH)_2D$ are low, but the therapeutic response to physiologic doses of calcitriol (0.25 to 1.0 µg/d) is normal. These findings are accounted for by a deficiency in renal $25(OH)D$-1α-hydroxylase activity. In patients with a similar phenotype, pseudovitamin D–resistant rickets (vitamin D–dependent rickets type II), mutations that impair the $1,25(OH)_2D$ receptors alter hormone binding or DNA

TABLE 356-2 Serum concentrations of $1,25(OH)_2D$ in disorders of calcium, phosphorus, and bone metabolism

Disease states	Serum $1,25(OH)_2D$
Vitamin D deficiency	↓ *
Renal failure:	
GFR > (30 mL/min)/1.7 m²	↓ or N
GFR < (30 mL/min)/1.7 m²	↓
Hypoparathyroidism	↓ or N
Pseudohypoparathyroidism	↓ or N
Vitamin D–dependent rickets:	
Type I	↓
Type II	↑
X-linked vitamin D–resistant rickets	↓ or N
Tumor-induced osteomalacia	↓
Oncogenic hypercalcemia	↓
Some lymphomas	↑
Hyperparathyroidism	↑
Sarcoidosis, tuberculosis, silicosis	↑
Idiopathic hypercalciuria	N or ↑
Williams' syndrome	↑
Vitamin D intoxication	N or ↑

* Serum $1,25(OH)_2D$ concentrations are normal or elevated in occasional patients with biopsy-proven osteomalacia and undetectable or low circulating concentrations of $25(OH)D$. These patients also have secondary hyperparathyroidism, and they may represent a partially treated state; if a small amount of vitamin D is obtained from the diet or generated in the skin in these patients, the vitamin is efficiently converted to $1,25(OH)_2D$. The net effect is low or undetectable circulating concentrations of $25(OH)D$ along with normal or elevated concentrations of $1,25(OH)_2D$. However, in extreme vitamin D deficiency, circulating concentrations of $1,25(OH)_2D$ are low or undetectable.

NOTE: ↓ = decreased; N = normal; ↑ = increased; GFR = glomerular filtration rate.

binding of the receptor-hormone complex. Individuals with this disorder have high circulating levels of $1,25(OH)_2D$; administration of high doses of vitamin D produce further increases in the levels of $1,25(OH)_2D$.

In patients with X-linked hypophosphatemic rickets, serum concentrations of $1,25(OH)_2D$ are normal or low. Since hypophosphatemia is a potent stimulator of the renal $25(OH)D$-1α-hydroxylase, levels of $1,25(OH)_2D$ should be high. In this syndrome there is a functional defect in the $25(OH)D$-1α-hydrolase even in the presence of normal circulating levels of $1,25(OH)_2D$. Therefore, the combination of calcitriol and phosphate supplements is superior to therapy with phosphate supplements alone (Chap. 358). In patients with mild to moderate chronic renal failure [GFR > 0.5 mL/s (> 30 mL/min)] and decreased phosphate clearance, hyperphosphatemia and acidosis play important roles in suppressing the renal production of $1,25(OH)_2D$ despite high circulating concentrations of PTH. With progressive destruction of the renal cortex, the reserves of the $25(OH)D$-1α-hydroxylase are depleted to a point at which the kidney is unable to produce sufficient $1,25(OH)_2D$ to maintain calcium homeostasis, even when serum phosphorus concentrations are normal. Under these circumstances, replacement therapy with calcitriol is most beneficial (Chap. 358). Aging decreases the responsiveness of the renal $25(OH)D$-1α-hydroxylase to PTH, results in small decreases in circulating levels of $1,25(OH)_2D$, and may contribute to decreased calcium absorption in the elderly.

Patients with hypocalcemia due to hypoparathyroidism or pseudohypoparathyroidism have lower than normal mean serum concentrations of $1,25(OH)_2D$, although individual values may be in the normal range. In these patients, small replacement doses of calcitriol (0.25 to 1.0 μg/d; see Chap. 357) are effective even when the serum $25(OH)D$ concentrations are elevated. These observations suggest that absent or ineffective action of PTH decreases the activity of renal $25(OH)D$-1α-hydroxylase. It is not known to what extent serum $1,25(OH)_2D$ concentrations would be restored if the hyperphosphatemia were adequately controlled.

Patients with tumor-induced (oncogenic) osteomalacia have low levels of serum phosphorus and $1,25(OH)_2D$. These tumors presumably secrete a substance(s) that causes renal phosphorus wasting and inhibits the synthesis of $1,25(OH)_2D$; after removal of the tumor, the serum phosphorus and $1,25(OH)_2D$ levels return to normal.

In disorders such as sarcoidosis (and other chronic granulomatous disorders), lymphomas, idiopathic hypercalciuria, and Williams' syndrome there is enhanced synthesis of $1,25(OH)_2D$ from $25(OH)D$ (see Table 356-2). Hypercalcemia and hypercalciuria in sarcoidosis are associated with elevated circulating concentrations of $1,25(OH)_2D$; granulomas and pulmonary alveolar macrophages from patients with sarcoidosis synthesize $1,25(OH)_2D$. Normal pulmonary macrophages also can be induced to metabolize $25(OH)D$ to $1,25(OH)_2D$ in vitro when exposed to lipopolysaccharides from the cell wall of gram-negative bacteria or to interferon-γ. Most patients with tumor-induced hypercalcemia have low circulating concentrations of $1,25(OH)_2D$ (see Table 356-2). The exceptions are patients with several types of lymphoma (including T cell, mixed histiocytic-lymphocytic, and B cell immunoblastic lymphomas) where hypercalcemia is associated with elevated concentrations of $1,25(OH)_2D$. In one report, surgical excision of a solitary splenic lymphoma resulted in rapid return of elevated serum $1,25(OH)_2D$ and calcium levels to normal, suggesting that the lymphoma metabolized $25(OH)D$ to $1,25(OH)_2D$ in an unregulated manner. Patients with hypercalcemia and elevated blood levels of $1,25(OH)_2$ due to unregulated extrarenal production of the hormone respond to glucocorticoids with a decrease in the circulating concentrations of $1,25(OH)_2D$ and calcium. Patients with primary hyperparathyrodisim, hypercalciuria, and renal stones, on average, have elevated circulating levels of $1,25(OH)_2D$. Similarly, in some instances of idiopathic hypercalciuria, intestinal calcium absorption is inappropriately increased. Approximately one-third of these patients have elevated circulating $1,25(OH)_2D$. These findings are consistent with the hypothesis that excessive $1,25(OH)_2D$ production is responsible for the hyperabsorption of calcium by the small intestine. Infants with hypercalcemia associated with supravalvular aortic stenosis, mental retardation, and elfin facies (*Williams' syndrome*) also have elevated serum concentrations of $1,25(OH)_2D$. It is not clear whether the increased levels result from abnormal synthesis or degradation of $1,25(OH)_2D$.

PHARMACOLOGY AND SOURCES OF VITAMIN D AND ITS METABOLITES Casual exposure to sunlight provides most humans with their vitamin D requirement. For the elderly who wish to take advantage of this natural source of vitamin D, exposure of hands, face, and arms to a suberythemal dose of sunlight two to three times a week is usually adequate. If the patient plans to remain outdoors in sunlight after the initial exposure, a sunscreen with a protection factor of at least 15 (SPF-15) should be applied to help prevent the damaging effects caused by excessive chronic overexposure to sunlight. A variety of over-the-counter vitamin preparations contain 400 IU of either vitamin D_2 or vitamin D_3. More potent preparations of vitamin D (calciferol) are available in capsule and tablet form (50,000 IU), as oil (500,000 IU/mL), and in oral solution (8000 IU/mL). A single oral dose of 50,000 IU of vitamin D_2 increases the circulating concentrations of vitamin D from less than 25 nmol/L (10 ng/mL) to 130 to 260 nmol/L (50 to 100 ng/mL) within 12 to 24 h; the plasma half-life is about 2 days. Serum concentrations of $25(OH)D$ and $1,25(OH)_2D$ are not changed by these doses of vitamin D. For treatment of vitamin D deficiency, 50,000 IU of vitamin D twice a week for several weeks raises the circulating concentration of $25(OH)D$ into the normal range; in the presence of secondary hyperparathyroidism, the circulating concentrations of $1,25(OH)_2D$ can increase to supranormal levels [up to 600 pmol/L (250 pg/mL)]. $25(OH)D_3$ (calcifediol) is available in capsules containing either 20 or 50 μg. This drug may be useful in treating vitamin D deficiency [low $25(OH)D$ concentrations] in patients with severe liver dysfunction. Pharmacologic doses are used to treat disorders of $25(OH)D$ metabolism; in pharmacologic doses, $25(OH)D_3$ is believed to act via interaction with the receptor for $1,25(OH)_2D$. $1,25(OH)_2D$ (calcitriol) is available in capsules containing 0.25 or 0.5 μg and as a solution for intravenous use (1.0 and 2.0 μg/mL). Calcitriol is efficacious in a variety of disorders (see Chap. 357). 1α-Hydroxyvitamin D_3 [$1(OH)D_3$] is a potent $1,25(OH)_2D_3$ agonist that is used in Europe and Japan. The structure of this analogue is identical to that of the natural renal hormone with the exception that it lacks a C_{25} OH (Fig. 356-6). In humans, this analogue is rapidly metabolized by the liver to $1,25(OH)_2D_3$. Topical preparations of calcitriol (3 μg/g) and calcipotriene (50 μg/g) are available in Europe for the treatment of psoriasis. When used over a large surface area, both can cause hypercalcemia.

When vitamin D is chemically manipulated to rotate the A ring through 180 degrees, the C_3 β-OH assumes a geometric position that mimics the C_1 α-OH (see Fig. 356-6). These compounds, called *pseudo-1α-hydroxyvitamin D analogues,* include the clinically useful dihydrotachysterol (DHT). This analogue is less effective in stimulating intestinal calcium transport on a weight basis than either vitamin D or $1,25(OH)_2D$, but because it does not require 1α-hydroxylation to be active on intestinal calcium transport, it is 3 to 10 times more potent than vitamin D in disease states that impair renal $25(OH)D$-1α-hydroxylase, such as hypoparathyroidism and chronic renal failure. Dihydrotachysterol is efficiently metabolized in the liver to 25-hydroxy-DHT, which is the biologically active form.

PARATHYROID HORMONE Physiology The function of PTH is to maintain ECF calcium concentration. The hormone acts directly on bone and kidney and indirectly on intestine through its effects on synthesis of $1,25(OH)_2D$ to increase serum calcium concentrations; in turn, PTH production is closely regulated by the concentration of serum ionized calcium. This feedback system is the critical homeostatic mechanism for maintenance of ECF calcium. Any tendency toward hypocalcemia, as might be induced by calcium-deficient diets, is counteracted by an increased secretion of PTH. This in turn (1) acts to increase the rate of dissolution of bone mineral, thereby

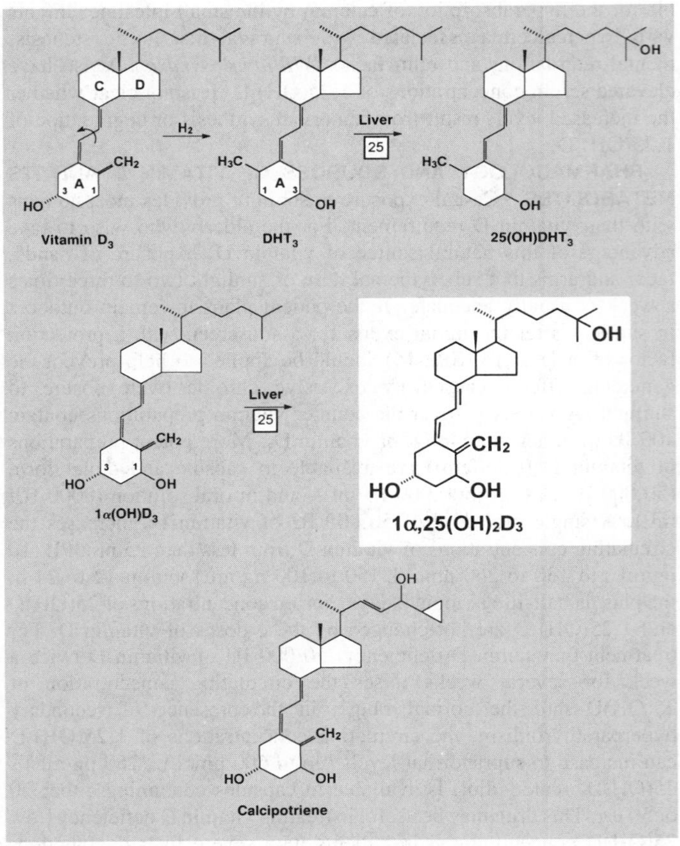

FIGURE 356-6   Structure of 1,25-dihydroxyvitamin D$_3$, i.e. 1α,25(OH)$_2$D$_3$, and some of its clinically important analogues. When vitamin D$_3$, is hydrogenated, its A ring is rotated 180°, placing the 3β-OH in a pseudo 1α spatial orientation. This analogue, dihydrotachysterol (DHT$_3$) is metabolized by a liver 25-hydroxylase (step 25) to 25-hydroxydihydrotachysterol, i.e., 25(OH)DHT$_3$. It is believed that 25(OH)DHT$_3$ is the biologically active form that mimics 1,25(OH)$_2$D$_3$ in its activity. Two clinically important analogues of 1α,25(OH)$_2$D$_3$ include its 25-deoxy derivative 1α-hydroxyvitamin D$_3$, i.e., 1α(OH)D$_3$, and calcipotriene. 1α(OH)D$_3$ is metabolized in the liver by 25-hydroxylase to 1α,25(OH)D$_3$. Calcipotriene is an analogue that is currently being used in Europe for the topical treatment of psoriasis.

increasing the flow of calcium from bone into blood, (2) reduces the renal clearance of calcium, returning more of the calcium filtered at the glomerulus into ECF, and (3) increases the efficiency of calcium absorption in the intestine. The relative physiologic importance in minute-to-minute calcium homeostasis of stimulation of calcium transport in bone, kidney, and intestine is not established, but immediate control of blood calcium is probably due to effects of the hormone on bone and, to a lesser extent, on renal calcium clearance. Maintenance of steady state calcium balance, on the other hand, probably results from the effects of the hormone on 1,25(OH)$_2$D levels and hence on the efficiency of intestinal calcium absorption. As much as 12 mmol (500 mg) calcium is transferred between ECF and bone each day (a large amount in relation to the total ECF calcium pool), and PTH has a major effect on this transfer. The homeostatic role of the hormone serves to preserve calcium concentration in blood acutely at the cost of bone destruction. The action of PTH on kidney to increase the reabsorption of filtered calcium also may contribute to rapid regulation of blood calcium concentration.

PTH has a dual action on bone, the *calcium replacement* and the *bone remodeling* effects. There is an increased rate of release of calcium from bone into blood after administration of PTH, the time needed to observe the change varying with the dose of hormone and the overall metabolic status (influenced by age, diet, etc.). Usually

30 min to 1 h is required to detect a significant increase in blood calcium, but with the use of radioisotopes, changes in bone calcium release can be seen within minutes. When studied carefully in animals, a rapid efflux of calcium out of blood into bone, presumably into bone cells, precedes the release of calcium from bone. On the other hand, the chronic effects of PTH, mainly an increase in the number of osteoclasts and a general increase in the remodeling of bone, are apparent only hours after the hormone is given. These latter actions, which involve increased protein synthesis, persist for hours after PTH has been given. The administration of PTH intermittently over days in animals leads to a net stimulation of bone formation rather than bone breakdown. Human studies in vitro and in vivo confirm that chronic intermittent hormone administration can lead to anabolic actions in skeleton rather than merely increased turnover. This skeletal anabolic action of PTH is being studied in clinical trials, but the extent and mechanism of the effect are still poorly understood. Osteoblasts mediate principally the bone-forming response of PTH and indirectly stimulate osteoclasts. Osteoclasts are the principal bone-resorbing cells.

Osteoblastic cells but not osteoclasts have receptors for PTH. The action of PTH on osteoclasts is indirect, through cytokines released from osteoblasts to activate osteoclasts; e.g., osteoblasts must be present along with osteoclasts for PTH to activate osteoclasts to resorb bone. The nature of the cytokines that stimulate osteoclasts is a subject of major interest. IGF-1, interleukin-6, GM-CSF, and possibly other agents are candidates, but the definitive messenger(s) has not been determined.

Chemistry   The complete amino acid sequences of PTH from cow, pig, rat, and human have been defined. The peptides consist of a single-chain structure composed of 84 amino acids. The molecules lack cysteine or cystine; the sequences of the four forms of the hormone are similar. The sequence of chicken PTH has been deduced from the nucleotide sequence of the cloned cDNA. This molecule differs from the mammalian hormones. One large sequence deletion in the middle of the molecule, and a larger addition near the carboxyl terminus result in a molecule of 88 rather than 84 amino acids. There is, however, marked conservation in the amino-terminal portion needed for biologic actions of the molecule.

Some structural requirements for the binding of the hormone to receptors and hence for its biologic activity have been defined. Synthetic fragments containing the amino-terminal sequence residues 1–34 (or even shorter sequences, 2–26 being minimally active) exert the known biologic actions of the hormone on mineral ion transport in kidney and bone and, by stimulating the renal 25-hydroxyvitamin D-1α-hydroxylase, stimulate intestinal calcium absorption.

Fragments shortened at the amino terminus lose binding affinity more slowly than capacity to stimulate biologic response. The peptide composed of sequences 7–34 is a competitive inhibitor of the binding of active hormone to receptors in vitro but is a weak inhibitor in vivo.

Biosynthesis, secretion, and metabolism and mode of action   Several larger molecular forms have been identified in the biosynthetic sequence leading from gene transcription and translation to final packaging of the 84-amino acid peptide in secretory granules prior to secretion. The earliest detected precursor, *preproparathyroid hormone,* consists of 115 amino acids; this molecular form is converted to an intermediate form of 90 amino acids termed *proparathyroid hormone,* and then to the secreted product of 84 amino acids, PTH. PTH shares with other polypeptides and proteins destined for secretion from cells this complex pattern of initial synthesis as a larger molecule which is then reduced in size by several cleavages prior to secretion. The regulation of these sequential steps in PTH biosynthesis is poorly understood except by analogy with regulatory steps in biosynthesis, transport, and packaging of other proteins destined for secretion. The hydrophobic regions of the preproparathyroid hormone are similar to preprotein-specific regions of other cell-secreted proteins and serve a role in guiding transport of the polypeptide from sites of synthesis on polyribosomes through the endoplasmic reticulum to secretory granules. In one kindred with hypoparathyroidism, a mutation disrupts the critical hydrophobic sequence and interferes with hormone secretion.

The genes for bovine, rat, and human PTH have been cloned, and the gene structures from these three species are highly homologous. Studies with cloned and expressed PTH genes in vitro have demonstrated regions for control of gene expression at the transcriptional level, including sites for interaction and regulation by $1,25(OH)_2D$ and its receptor and "upstream" silencer elements as well as sites in which ambient calcium concentration regulates transcription. These in vitro observations are not well understood in terms of physiologic regulation of PTH biosynthesis and secretion; the rate of processing of hormone precursors and the proteolytic destruction and turnover of the hormone itself (posttranslational regulation of hormone production) may be more central to hormone availability than changes in rates of transcription. It does not appear that changes in transcriptional activity of the PTH gene in the normal physiologic range of levels of blood calcium and $1,25(OH)_2D$ nor in short-term environmental stresses (e.g., fasting for 24 h) are important in control of blood levels of the hormone. Control is exerted by precise and rapid variation of rates of processing of preformed hormone under the control of ECF calcium.

Blood calcium concentration over wide ranges controls the secretion of PTH; the ionized fraction of blood calcium is the important determinant of hormone secretion. Hormone secretion increases steeply to a maximum value of fivefold above basal rates of secretion as calcium concentration falls from normal to the range of 1.9 to 2.0 mmol/L (7.5 to 8.0 mg/dL) (measured as total calcium). Beta-adrenergic agonists such as epinephrine and H-2 agonists also may increase hormone secretion, but the physiologic significance of these secretagogues is not established. Furthermore, drugs such as propranolol or cimetidine do not reproducibly decrease circulating PTH levels.

Magnesium may influence hormone secretion in the same direction as calcium but is a less potent secretagogue. It is unlikely that physiologic variations in magnesium concentration affect PTH secretion, but severe intracellular magnesium deficiency impairs PTH secretion.

The hormone secreted in vivo by normal bovine and human parathyroid glands and from parathyroid adenomas is indistinguishable by immunologic criteria and by molecular size from the 84-amino acid peptide (molecular weight 9500) extracted from glands. However, much of the immunoreactive material found in the circulation of humans and animals (cow, dog) is smaller than the extracted or secreted hormone. The principal circulating fragments of immunoreactive hormone (approximate molecular weight 7000) lack a portion of the critical amino-terminal sequence required for biologic activity and, hence, are biologically inactive fragments (so-called middle- and carboxyl-terminal fragments). Study of these fragments suggests that an endopeptidase cleaves the molecule into at least two types of pieces. Much of the proteolysis of hormone occurs in the liver and kidney.

The proteolytic process should result in formation of a second fragment (molecular weight 2000 to 3000) representing the amino-terminal, biologically active portion of the hormone. Hormone fragments as well as intact hormone are also released from the gland. However, fragments corresponding only to the middle- and carboxyl-terminal portions have been detected so far in effluent blood. If biologically active fragments do actually survive hormone proteolysis within the gland or in peripheral sites, such amino-terminal fragments could be alternative active hormonal species. After much study, certain conclusions can be drawn. There is no convincing evidence for circulating amino-terminal fragments. Circulating biologically active fragments are also not detected after analysis of products produced by peripheral metabolism. Peripheral metabolism of PTH does not appear to be regulated by physiologic states (high versus low calcium, etc.); hence peripheral metabolism of hormone, although responsible for rapid clearance of secreted hormone, appears to be a high-capacity, metabolically invariant catabolic process.

The rate of clearance of the secreted 84-amino acid peptide from blood is more rapid than the rate of clearance of the biologically inactive fragment(s) corresponding to the middle- and carboxyl-terminal regions of the molecules that result from peripheral metabolism or glandular secretion. Hence measurements of PTH in blood by most earlier immunoassays provided only an overall index of parathyroid gland activity rather than a direct measure of biologically active hormone. Changes in the rate of production or clearance of fragments can change the concentration of immunoreactive hormone without influencing the rate of hormone secretion. Such discordance between concentrations of immunoreactive hormone and biologically active peptide occurs, for example, in renal failure, since the kidney seems to be the principal route of excretion of inactive hormone fragments. The problems inherent in accurate measurements of PTH in blood due to the heterogeneity of circulating forms of the molecule are now circumvented by use of double-antibody assays that detect only the intact molecule (as discussed in Chap. 357).

Parathyroid hormone–related protein The application of the techniques of molecular biology together with careful physiologic and clinical studies led to the cloning and subsequent physiologic evaluation of the parathyroid hormone–related protein (PTHrP) responsible for hypercalcemia in cancer patients, a syndrome that resembles hyperparathyroidism. This protein, now appreciated to be a paracrine or autocrine factor, plays a role both in fetal development and in adult physiology. Many different cell types produce PTHrP, including brain, pancreas, heart, lung, mammary tissue, placenta, endothelial cells, and smooth muscle.

PTH and PTHrP, although distinctive proteins and products of different genes, share considerable functional and structural homology (Fig. 356-7) and may have evolved from an ancestral gene. The

FIGURE 356-7 Schematic diagram to illustrate similarities and differences in structure of human PTH and human PTHrP. Close structural (and functional) homology exists between the first 30 amino acids of hPTH and hPTHrP. The PTHrP sequence may be 144 amino acid residues in length or longer. PTH is only 84 residues long; after residue 30, there is little structural homology between the two. Dashed lines in the PTHrP sequence indicate homology; underlined residues, although different from those of PTH, still represent conservative changes (charge or polarity preserved). Eleven amino acids are identical, and a total of 21 of 30 are homologues.

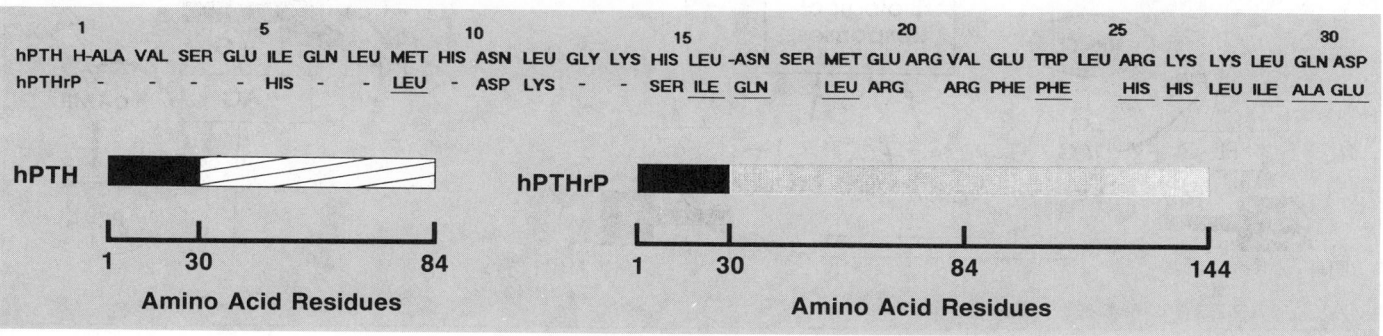

structure of the gene for human PTHrP, however, is more complex than that of PTH, containing multiple exons and multiple sites for alternate splicing patterns during formation of the messenger RNA. Protein products of 141, 139, and 173 amino acids are produced. The varying molecular forms have multiple potential internal cleavage sites, and the biologic roles of these various molecular species and the nature of the circulating forms of PTHrP are unclear. The assays currently available are based on a variety of immunologic methods. Furthermore, multiple PTHrP products are synthesized, and other molecular forms may result from tissue-specific degradation at accessible internal cleavage sites. In fact, it is uncertain whether PTHrP circulates at all in normal human adults; as a paracrine factor, PTHrP may be produced, act within, and be destroyed locally within tissues.

PTHrP may have little to do with calcium homeostasis, except in disease states (Chap. 357), when large tumors, especially of the squamous cell type, lead to massive overproduction of PTHrP, which then circulates. PTHrP (see Fig. 356-7) shares a significant homology with PTH in the critical amino terminus that allows it to bind to the PTH receptor; synthetic molecules corresponding to the first 34 amino acids of PTHrP bind to and activate the PTH receptor indistinguishably from effects seen with PTH. This finding explains much of the confusion in earlier clinical studies of the humoral hypercalcemia of malignancy (Chap. 357).

PTHrP exerts important developmental influences in calcium and bone biology. Gene knockout studies in mice reveal a lethal deformity in the fetuses made homozygous for deletion of the PTHrP gene in which animals are born with a severe skeletal deformity of the chondrodysplastic type. In fetal animals, PTHrP directs transplacental calcium transfer, and high concentrations of PTHrP are produced in mammary tissue and secreted into milk. Human and bovine milk, for example, contains very high concentrations of the hormone. The

biologic significance of the latter is unknown. PTHrP also may play a role in uterine contraction.

HORMONE ACTION   The action of PTH at the biochemical level involves receptor-mediated effects on second messengers in target cells (see also Chap. 69). Stimulation of enzyme activity (adenyl cyclase, phospholipase C) during hormone–target cell membrane interaction leads to an increase in second messengers, including intracellular cAMP, products of polyphosphoinositol metabolism, and transmembrane and intracellular fluxes of calcium. PTH interacts with a specific receptor/adenylate cyclase complex on plasma membranes of target cells consisting of hormone receptor, enzyme catalytic unit (adenylate cyclase), and a guanyl nucleotide (GTP or GDP)–binding regulatory protein (G protein). The latter protein consists of α subunits that bind GTP and dissociate from the remainder of the G protein complex. The α subunit with bound GTP complexes with adenylate cyclase, thereby activating the enzyme to increase the rate of cAMP production from ATP. Hydrolysis of the GTP to GDP on the α subunit leads to reassociation of the G units and reduction in adenylate cyclase activity. The receptor, when activated by hormone binding, drives the G protein cycle by binding the α subunit portion and catalyzing the GDP/GTP exchange. Other G proteins link hormone action to phospholipase C; rapid changes in intracellular calcium concentrations within cells may be independent of phospholipase C stimulation.

The multiplicity of PTH actions on target cells in kidney and bone and the variety of second messengers—cAMP, IP$_3$, DAG, and Ca^{2+}—raise obvious questions as to the mechanism whereby specific responses are mediated. With many other hormonal systems, several different, although related, receptor subtypes direct hormone responses to individual second-messenger pathways by favoring coupling to one versus another G protein species; the concept is illustrated for PTH in Fig. 356-8A.

FIGURE 356-8   Schematic models of possible mechanisms of PTH action. Depicted in *A* is the hormone response systems seen with numerous hormones and predicted for PTH before cloning of the receptor; namely, several distinctive but closely related receptor types each mediate PTH–binding effects on distal cellular biological responses by coupling preferentially to different G proteins—G$_s$, G$_q$, etc.—which, in turn, activate a particular cellular second messenger such as cyclic AMP (cAMP), diacylglycerol (DAG), inositol triphosphate (IP$_3$), calcium Ca^{++}), or other specific receptor pathways indicated by ? Certain cells preferentially express one receptor type and, hence, one biological response is predominant.

Depicted in *B* is the actual result found so far with the cloning of the PTH receptor from several species. Only one receptor is present, which couples to multiple G proteins and effector pathways; in this model, cellular specificity or other factors (hormone levels, receptor expression levels) determine which pathway is activated predominantly in one cell type versus another. Although one form of receptor so far has been identified with PTH and PTHrP, multiple receptors of the type shown in *A* may yet be identified, and both mechanisms of control of PTH action may be used in vivo, varying from one target organ or cell to another.

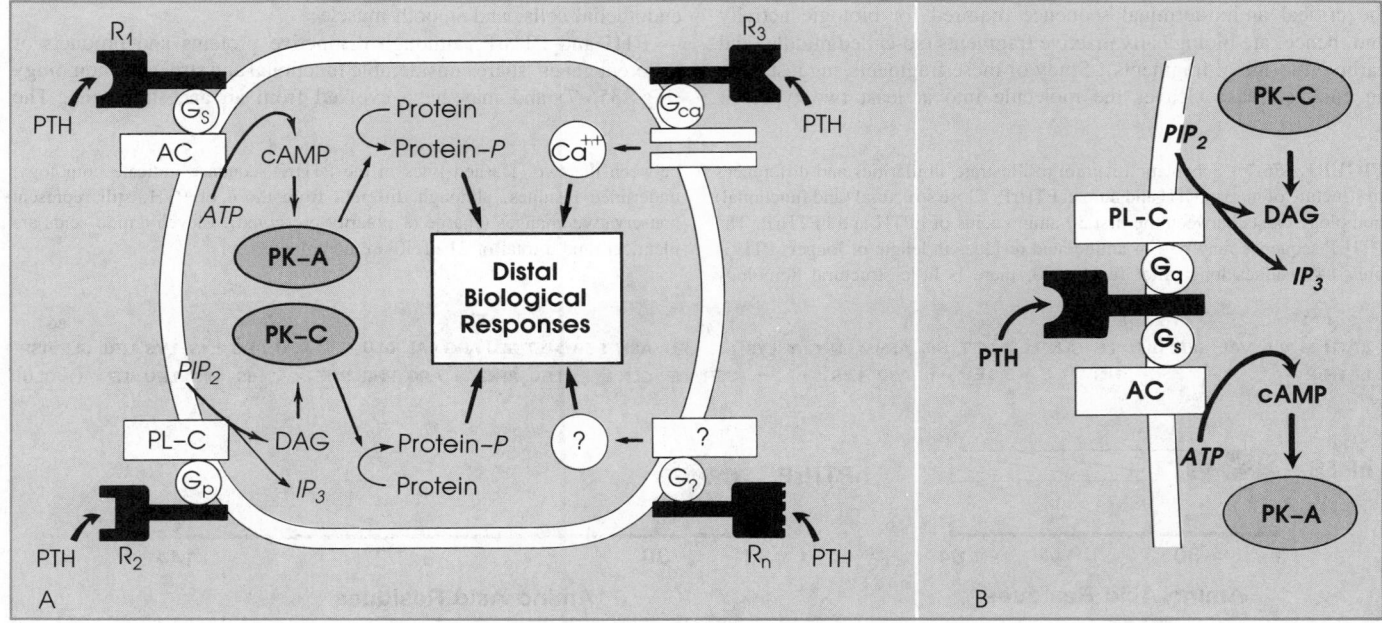

However, only one molecular species has been detected in kidney and bone in human, rat, and other animal species, suggesting that a single PTH receptor (Fig. 356-8B) can be coupled to more than one G protein second-messenger kinase pathway. The receptors for PTH and calcitonin (the two receptors share close homology) are polypeptides of 500 to 600 amino acids. The primary amino acid sequence predicts the structures illustrated in Fig. 356-9: an extracellular domain, seven hydrophobic membrane-spanning domains connected by three extracellular and three intracellular loops, and a carboxyl-terminal intracellular domain. The extracellular regions are involved in hormone binding, and the intracellular domains, after hormone activation, bind G protein subunits to transduce hormone signaling into cellular responses through stimulation of second messengers by activated G protein subunits.

The details of the biochemical steps by which an increased intracellular concentration of cAMP, IP_3, or DAG lead to changes in calcium and phosphate ion translocation are unknown. Stimulation of protein kinases (protein kinase A, cAMP; protein kinase C, DAG) and calcium transport channels is associated with a variety of hormone-specific tissue responses, some of which are cAMP-dependent and others cAMP-independent. These responses include inhibition of phosphate and bicarbonate transport and stimulation of calcium transport and renal 1α-hydroxylase in the kidney. The responses in bone include effects on collagen synthesis; alkaline phosphatase activity; ornithine decarboxylase, citrate decarboxylase, and glucose-6-phosphate dehydrogenase activity; DNA, protein, and phospholipid synthesis; and calcium and phosphate transport. Ultimately, these cellular biochemical events lead to an integrated hormonal response in bone turnover and calcium homeostasis.

Pathophysiology In hyperparathyroidism, PTH is overproduced by tumors of the parathyroid or hyperplasia involving all glands. The excess hormone results in hypercalcemia secondary to increased intestinal calcium absorption [increased synthesis of 1,25(OH)$_2$D], reduced renal calcium clearance, and increased bone calcium release. Bone turnover increases in all patients, and resorption exceeds formation in many. Individual patients respond to the excess hormone variably at intestinal, renal, and bone target sites; the factors influencing the response from patient to patient are not known.

Hypophosphatemia results from the actions of the excessive PTH on renal tubular phosphate reabsorption. Hypophosphatemia in turn aggravates the hypercalcemia by increasing the synthesis of 1,25(OH)$_2$D and by increasing the sensitivity of the bone to PTH. Hypophosphatemia also may interfere with the normal mineralization

of bone, leading to a mixed picture of increased resorption and deficient mineralization in adjacent skeletal sites.

Hypoparathyroidism causes hypocalcemia and hyperphosphatemia, a reversal of the response seen with hormone excess. See Chap. 357 for details of the clinical syndromes.

CALCITONIN (See also Chap. 343) Calcitonin is a hypocalcemic peptide hormone that, in many ways, acts as the physiologic antagonist to parathyroid hormone. The hypocalcemic activity of calcitonin is accounted for primarily by inhibition of osteoclast-mediated bone resorption and secondarily by stimulation of renal calcium clearance. These effects are mediated by receptors on osteoclasts and renal tubular cells. Calcitonin exerts additional effects presumably through binding to receptors present in brain, gastrointestinal tract, and the immune system (Fig. 356-9). The hormone, for example, has analgesic effects exerted directly on cells in the hypothalamus and related structures, possibly by interacting with receptors for related peptide hormones, such as calcitonin gene–related peptide (CGRP) or amylin. The latter ligands have specific high-affinity receptors and also can bind to and trigger calcitonin receptors. The calcitonin receptors as deduced from the nucleotide sequences of the cDNA, contain seven transmembrane α-helical domains similar to the G protein–coupled receptors. The calcitonin, PTH, and PTHrP receptors are sufficiently different from other G protein–coupled receptors as to constitute a distinct subfamily. Other members of this subfamily include receptors for secretin, vasoactive intestinal peptide, growth hormone–releasing hormone, and gastric inhibitory peptide. Interaction of calcitonin with its receptors activates signal transduction pathways that, like those for PTH, involve distinct G proteins. Thus calcitonin can stimulate adenylyl cyclase and protein kinase A as well as protein kinase C and induce calcium transients as well. These specific G protein interactions probably involve distinct amino acid sequences in a single receptor protein.

The thyroid is the major source of the hormone, and the cells involved in calcitonin synthesis arise from neural crest tissue. During embryogenesis, these cells migrate into the ultimobranchial body, derived from the last branchial pouch. In submammalian vertebrates, the ultimobranchial body constitutes a discrete organ, anatomically separate from the thyroid gland, but in mammals, the ultimobranchial gland fuses with and is incorporated into the thyroid gland.

The naturally occurring calcitonins consist of a peptide chain of 32 amino acids. There is a considerable variability in sequence among species. The entire chain of 32 amino acids appears to be required for biologic activity in the intact animal, although fragments function

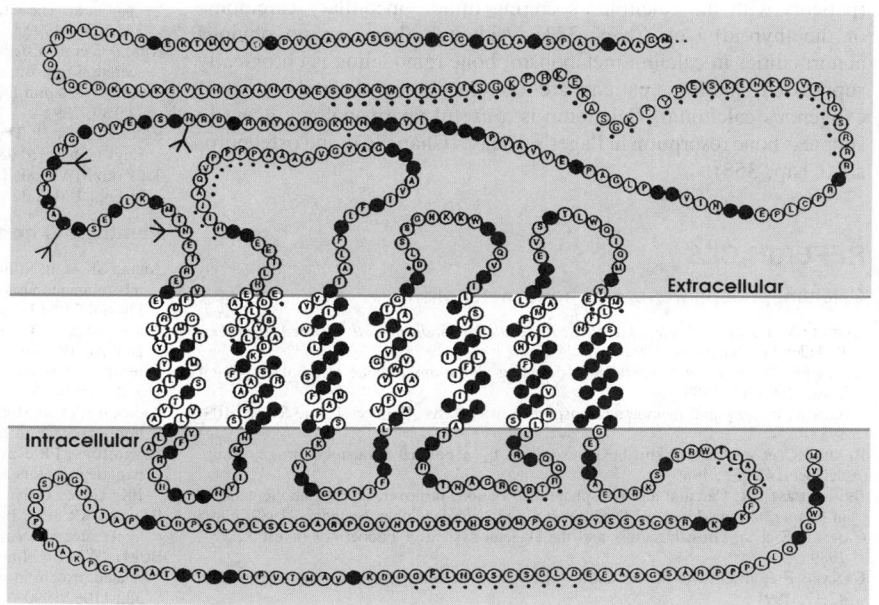

FIGURE 356-9 Schematic illustration of predicted structure of PTH and calcitonin receptors contains one large extracellular domain, seven membrane-spanning domains, three extracellular loops connecting the membrane-spanning domains on the cell surface, one large intracellular domain, and three intracellular loops. Backbone structure is of the PTH receptor; shaded residues are common between PTH and the CT receptor.

in in vitro systems. Calcitonin from salmon is 10 to 100 times more potent than mammalian forms in lowering serum calcium in animals; eel calcitonin is also potent. Slow turnover may in part explain the greater potency of salmon calcitonin, but the hormone binds more tightly to receptor sites as well. Calcitonin is synthesized as a precursor molecule that is four times larger than calcitonin itself. Analysis of the sequence of the coding portions of the gene for rat calcitonin indicates that at least two peptides flank calcitonin, from which they are separated by basic residues. It is likely (in analogy with the common precursor for ACTH and endorphin) that these peptides are released along with calcitonin. There is no known biologic function for these noncalcitonin peptides.

There are two calcitonin genes, α and β, located on chromosome 11 in the general region of the beta globulin and parathyroid hormone genes. The two genes are sometimes called calcitonin/CGRP-1 and / CGRP-2. The transcription of these genes is complex. Two different messenger RNA molecules are transcribed from the α gene; one is translated into the precursor for calcitonin, and the other message is transcribed into an alternate product, calcitonin gene–related peptide (CGRP). CGRP is synthesized wherever the calcitonin message is expressed, e.g., in medullary carcinoma of the thyroid. The β, or CGRP-2, gene is transcribed into the messenger RNA for CGRP in the central nervous system (CNS) in animals; this gene is silent for calcitonin production. CGRP has cardiovascular actions and may serve a neurotransmitter or developmental role in CNS.

The secretin of calcitonin is under the direct control of blood calcium: An increase in calcium causes an increase and a decrease in calcium causes a decrease in calcitonin levels. Once secreted, calcitonin disappears from the circulation with a half-life of 2 to 15 min.

The concentration of calcitonin in the peripheral blood of normal humans is lower than that in many other species. Basal and stimulated immunoreactive calcitonin levels are lower in women than in men and tend to decrease with age to a greater extent in women.

In animals, calcitonin acts to lower both blood calcium and blood phosphate by inhibiting bone resorption and by increasing urinary calcium and phosphate clearance. The actions of calcitonin on kidney and bone are in turn modulated by the regulation of calcitonin production by serum calcium. The view that calcitonin serves to protect against hypercalcemia is thus explained by the hypocalcemic effects of calcitonin triggered in response to hypercalcemia.

In humans, changes in calcium and phosphate metabolism are not seen despite extreme variations in hormone production; no definite effects are attributable to calcitonin deficiency (totally thyroidectomized patients receiving only replacement thyroxine) or excess (patients with the calcitonin-secreting tumor, medullary carcinoma of the thyroid) (see Chap. 343). Although there are no obvious abnormalities in calcium metabolism, bone remodeling is chronically suppressed, and these patients are refractory to the skeletal actions of exogenous calcitonin. Calcitonin is a useful pharmacologic agent to suppress bone resorption in Paget's disease (Chap. 361) and osteoporosis (Chap. 358).

REFERENCES

Calcium, phosphorous, and bone metabolism

AVIOLI LV, KRANE SM (eds): *Metabolic Bone Disease and Clinically Related Disorders.* Philadelphia, Saunders, 1990

AZRIA M: The value of biomarkers in detecting alterations in bone metabolism. Calcif Tissue Int 45:7, 1989

BARON R: Polarity and membrane transport in osteoclasts. Connect Tissue Res 20:109, 1988

BLAIR HC et al: Osteoclastic bone resorption by a polarized vacuolar proton pump. Science 245:855, 1989

BRINGHURST FR: Calcium and phosphate distribution, turnover, and metabolic actions, in *Endocrinology,* 2d ed, LJ DeGroot et al (eds). Philadelphia, Saunders, 1989, p 805

CANALIS E et al: Growth factors and the skeletal system. J Endocrinol Invest 12:577, 1989

CANALIS E et al: Growth factors and cytokines in bone cell metabolism. Annu Rev Med 42:17, 1991

COHN DV et al (eds): *Calcium Regulating Hormones and Bone Metabolism: Bone and Clinical Aspects.* Amsterdam, Excerpta Medica, 1992

DELMAS PD: Clinical use of biochemical markers of bone remodeling in osteoporosis. Bone 13:S17, 1992

EPSTEIN S: Serum and urinary markers of bone remodeling: Assessment of bone turnover. Endocrine Rev 9:437,1988

ERICKSEN EF: Normal and pathological remodeling of human trabecular bone: Three dimensional reconstruction of the remodeling sequence in normals and in metabolic bone disease. Endocrine Rev 7:379, 1986

EVERED D, HARNETT S (eds): *Cell and Molecular Biology of Vertebrate Hard Tissues.* Chichester, Wiley, 1988

HOROWITZ MC: Cytokines and estrogen in bone: Anti-osteoporotic effects. Science 260:626, 1993

KANDERS B et al: Interaction of calcium nutrition and physical activity on bone mass in young women. J Bone Min Res 3:145, 1988

KATZ EP et al: The structure of mineralized collagen fibrils. Connect Tissue Res 21:149, 1989

KLEEREKOPER M, KRANE SM (eds): *Clinical Disorders of Bone and Mineral Metabolism.* New York, Mary Ann Liebert, 1989

MARCUS R: Biochemical markers of bone remodeling, in *Clinical Disorders of Bone and Mineral Metabolism,* M Kleerekopper, SM Krane (eds). New York, Mary Ann Liebert, 1989, p 49

MUNDY GR: Identifying mechanisms for increasing bone mass. J Natl Inst Health Res 1:65, 1989

PARFITT AM: The coupling of bone formation: A critical analysis of the concept and of its relevance to the pathogenesis of osteoporosis. Metab Bone Dis Relat Res 4:1, 1982

———: The cellular basis of bone remodeling: The quantum concept reexamined in light of recent advances in the cell biology of bone. Calcif Tissue Int 36:S37, 1984

PORTALE AA et al: Physiologic regulation of the serum concentration of 1,25-dihydroxyvitamin D by phosphorus in normal men. J Clin Invest 83:1494, 1989

POUILLES JM et al: Sensitivity of dual-photon absorptiometry in spinal osteoporosis. Calcif Tissue Int 43:329, 1988

RAISZ LG, KREAM BE: Regulation of bone formation. N Engl J Med 309:29, 1983

ROBEY PG: The biochemistry of bone. Endocrinol Metab Clin North Am 18:859, 1989

ROODMAN GD: Interleukin-6: An osteotropic factor? J Bone Miner Res 7:474, 1992

SAGE EH, BORNSTEIN P: Extracellular proteins that modulate cell-matrix interactions. SPARC, tenascin, and thrombospondin. J Biol Chem 266:14831, 1991

SLAVKIN H, PRICE P (eds): *Chemistry and Biology of Mineralized Tissues.* Amsterdam, Excerpta Medica, 1992

SORIANO P et al: Targeted disruption of the c-*src* proto-oncogene leads to osteopetrosis in mice. Cell 64:693, 1991

SUDA T et al: Modulation of osteoclast differentiation. Endocr Rev 13:66, 1992

UEBELHART D et al: Urinary excretion of pyridinium crosslinks: A new marker of bone resorption in metabolic bone disease. Bone Miner 8:87, 1990

——— et al: Effect of menopause and hormone replacement therapy on the urinary excretion of pyridinium cross-links. J Clin Endocrinol Metab 7:367, 1991

URIST MR et al: Bone cell differentiation and growth factors. Science 220:680, 1983

WOZNEY JM et al: Novel regulators of bone formation: molecular clones and activities. Science 242:1528, 1988

Vitamin D

ADAMS JS et al: A role for endogenous arachidonate metabolites in the regulated expression of the 25-hydroxyvitamin D 1-hydroxylation reaction in cultured alveolar macrophages from patients with sarcoidosis. J Clin Endocrinol Metab 70:595, 1990

BARAN D et al: 1α,25-Dihydroxyvitamin D₃–induced increments in hepatocyte cytosolic calcium and lysophosphatidylinositol: Inhibition by pertussis toxin and 1β,25-dihydroxyvitamin D₃. J Bone Miner Res 5:517, 1990

HOLICK MF: Vitamin D: biosynthesis, metabolism, and mode of action, in *Endocrinology,* LJ DeGroot et al (eds). New York, Grune & Stratton, 1989, vol 2, pp 902–926

——— et al: The vitamin D content of fortified milk and infant formula. N Engl J Med 326:1178, 1992

KRALL E et al: Effect of vitamin D intake on seasonal variation in parathyroid hormone secretion in postmenopausal women. N Engl J Med 321:1777, 1989

PIKE JW: Vitamin D₃ receptors: Structure and function in transcription. Annu Rev Nutr 11:189, 1991

REICHEL H et al: The role of the vitamin D endocrine system in health and disease. N Engl J Med 320:981, 1989

TILYARD MW et al: Treatment of postmenopausal osteoporosis with calcitriol or calcium. N Engl J Med 326:356, 1992

Parathyroid hormone and calcitonin

ABBAS SK et al: Stimulation of ovine placental calcium transport by purified natural and recombinant parathyroid hormone–related protein (PTHrP) preparations. Q J Exp Physiol 74:549, 1989

ABOU-SAMRA AB et al: Expression cloning of a common receptor for parathyroid hormone and parathyroid hormone–related peptide from rat osteoblast-like cells: A single receptor stimulates intracellular accumulation of both cAMP and inositol triphosphates and increases intracellular free calcium. Proc Natl Acad Sci USA 89:2732, 1992

ARNOLD A et al: Mutation of the signal peptide-encoding region of the preproparathyroid hormone gene in familial isolated hypoparathyroidism. J Clin Invest 86:1094, 1990

BRINGHURST FR et al: Cloned, stably expressed parathyroid hormone (PTH)/PTH–related peptide receptors activate multiple messenger signals and biological responses in LLC-PK₁ kidney cells. Endocrinology 132:2090, 1993

BUDAYR AR et al: Increased serum levels of PTH-like protein in malignancy-associated hypercalcemia. Ann Intern Med 111:807, 1989

BURTIS WJ et al: Immunochemical characterization of circulating parathyroid hormone–related protein in patients with humoral hypercalcemia of malignancy. N Engl J Med 322:1106, 1990

DEMAY MB et al: Sequences in the human parathyroid hormone gene that bind the 1,25-dihydroxyvitamin D_2 receptor and mediate transcriptional repression in response to 1,25-dihydroxyvitamin D_3. Proc Natl Acad Sci USA 89:8097, 1992

FORCE T et al: A cloned porcine renal calcitonin receptor couples to adenyl cyclase and phospholipase C. Am J Physiol 262:F1110, 1992

GARDELLA TJ et al: Mutational analysis of the receptor activating region of human parathyroid hormone. J Biol Chem 266:13141, 1991

GORN AH et al: The cloning characterization and expression of a human calcitonin receptor from an ovarian carcinoma cell line. J Clin Invest 90:1726, 1992

GRILL V et al: PTH-related protein: Elevated levels in both humoral hypercalcemia of malignancy and hypercalcemia complicating breast cancer. J Clin Endocrinol 73:1309, 1991

HAYMAN JA et al: Expression of parathyroid hormone–related protein in normal skin and in tumors of skin and skin appendages. J Pathol 158:293, 1989

HENDERSON JR et al: Circulating concentrations of PTH-like peptide in malignancy and in hyperparathyroidism. J Bone Miner Res 5:105, 1990

JUPPNER H et al: A G-protein–linked receptor for parathyroid hormone and parathyroid hormone–related protein. Science 254:1024, 1991

KAO PC et al: PTH-related peptide in plasma of patients with hypercalcemia and malignancy lesions. Mayo Clin Proc 65:1399, 1990

KARAPLIS AC et al: Gene-encoding parathyroid hormone–like peptide: Nucleotide sequence of the rat gene and comparison with the human homolog. Mol Endocrinol 4:441, 1990

———— et al: Disruption of parathyroid hormone–related peptide gene leads to a multitude of skeletal abnormalities and preinatal mortality. J Bone Miner Res 7(suppl 1):abst 1, 1992

LIM SK et al: Full-length chicken parathyroid hormone: Biosynthesis in *Escherichia coli* and analysis of biological activity. J Biol Chem 266:3709, 1991

LIN HY et al: Expression cloning of an adenylate cyclase–coupled calcitonin receptor. Science 254:1022, 1991

MARTIN TJ et al: Parathyroid hormone–related protein: Biochemistry and molecular biology. CRC Crit Rev Biochem Mol Biol 26:377, 1991

NIKOLS GA et al: Hypotension and cardiac stimulation due to the parathyroid hormone–related protein, humoral hypercalcemia of malignancy factor. Endocrinology 125:834, 1989

———— et al: Hypercalcemia and ectopic secretion of PTH by an ovarian carcinoma with rearrangement of the gene for PTH. N Engl J Med 323:1324, 1990

NUSSBAUM SR, POTTS JT JR: Immunoassays for parathyroid hormone 1–84 in the diagnosis of hyperparathyroidism. J Bone Miner Res 6:543, 1991

POTTS JT JR: Chemistry of the calcitonins. Bone Miner 16:169, 1992

RATCLIFFE WA et al: Immunoreactivity of plasma parathyrin-related peptide. Clin Chem 37:1781, 1991

SCHIPANI E et al: Identical complementary deoxyribonucleic acids encode a human renal and bone parathyroid hormone (PTH)/PTH–related peptide receptor. Endocrinology 132:2157, 1993

SUVA LJ et al: A parathyroid hormone–related protein implicated in malignant hypercalcemia: Cloning and expression. Science 237:893, 1987

THIEDE M et al: Human renal carcinoma expresses two messages encoding a parathyroid hormone–like peptide: Evidence for the alternative splicing of a single copy gene. Proc Natl Acad Sci USA 85:4605, 1988

WIMALAWANSA SJ: Calcitonin: Molecular biology, physiology, pathophysiology and its therapeutic uses, in *Advances in Bone Regulatory Factors: Morphology, Biochemistry, Physiology and Pharmacology*, AB Pecile (ed). London, Plenum Press, 1990, p 121

YAMAMOTO M et al: Suckling-mediated increases in urinary phosphate and $3',5'$-cyclic adenosine monophosphate excretion in lactating rats: Possible systemic effects of parathyroid hormone–related protein. Endocrinology 129:2614, 1991

ZAIDI M et al: Evidence that the action of calcitonin on rat osteoclasts is mediated by two G proteins acting via separate post-receptor pathways. J Endocrinol 126:473, 1990

ZAJAC JD et al: Regulation of gene transcription and proliferation by parathyroid hormone is blocked in mutant osteoblastic cells resistant to cyclic AMP. Mol Cell Endocrinol 87:69, 1992

evaluation? What are the most probable causes of hypercalcemia, and how can they be diagnosed?

Whenever hypercalcemia is confirmed, a definitive diagnosis must be established. Although hyperparathyroidism, a frequent cause of asymptomatic hypercalcemia, is a chronic disorder in which manifestations, if any, may be expressed only over months or years, hypercalcemia also can be the earliest clue to the presence of malignancy, the second most common cause of hypercalcemia in the adult. The causes of hypercalcemia are numerous (Table 357-1), but hyperparathyroidism and cancer account for 90 percent of cases. Diagnosis can usually be established. However, the optimal management of asymptomatic hyperparathyroidism is still unsettled, and treatment of the hypercalcemia of cancer is difficult.

Before undertaking an evaluation of hypercalcemia, it is essential to be sure that true hypercalcemia, not a false-positive laboratory test, is present. Hypercalcemia is a chronic problem, and it is cost-effective to obtain several serum calcium measurements; these tests need not be in the fasting state. False-positive calcium tests are usually the result of inadvertent hemoconcentration during blood collection or elevation in serum proteins, particularly albumin. Measurement of ionized calcium is technically feasible, but there is no advantage, except in research applications, to measurement of ionized rather than total calcium.

Clinical features alone are helpful in differential diagnosis. Hypercalcemia in an adult who is asymptomatic is usually due to primary hyperparathyroidism. In most cases of malignancy-associated hypercalcemia the disease is not occult; rather, symptoms of the underlying malignancy bring the patient to the physician, and hypercalcemia is discovered during the workup. In patients with malignancy, the interval between detection of hypercalcemia and death is often less than 6 months. Accordingly, if an asymptomatic individual has had hypercalcemia or some manifestation of hypercalcemia, such as kidney stones, for more than 1 or 2 years, it is unlikely that malignancy is the cause. As discussed below, however, differentiating primary hyperparathyroidism from *occult* malignancy can occasionally be a problem, and careful evaluation of patients is required, particularly when the duration of the hypercalcemia is unknown.

Hypercalcemia not due to hyperparathyroidism or malignancy can result from excessive vitamin D action, high bone turnover from any of several causes, or from renal failure (Table 357-1). The sensitivity and specificity of various diagnostic tests for the differential diagnosis were previously not optimal, but newer parathyroid hormone (PTH) immunoassays based on double-antibody methods are reliable. Dietary history and a history of ingestion of vitamins and drugs are often helpful in recognizing some of the less frequent causes. Except in malignancy-associated hypercalcemia, acute management of the hypercalcemia is usually successful prior to the institution of definitive

357 DISEASES OF THE PARATHYROID GLAND AND OTHER HYPER- AND HYPOCALCEMIC DISORDERS

JOHN T. POTTS, JR.

HYPERCALCEMIA

Hypercalcemia can be a manifestation of a serious illness such as malignancy or can be detected coincidentally by laboratory testing in a patient with no obvious illness. Management is a particular problem when the patient is asymptomatic. The number of patients recognized with asymptomatic hypercalcemia has increased severalfold in the last two decades. Does the hypercalcemia always require further

TABLE 357-1 Classification of causes of hypercalcemia

Parathyroid-related:
1. Primary hyperparathyroidism
   a. Solitary adenomas
   b. Multiple endocrine neoplasia
2. Lithium therapy
3. Familial hypocalciuric hypercalcemia

Malignancy-related:
1. Solid tumor with metastases (breast)
2. Solid tumor with humoral mediation of hypercalcemia (lung, kidney)
3. Hematologic malignancies (multiple myeloma, lymphoma, leukemia)

Vitamin D–related:
1. Vitamin D intoxication
2. ↑ $1,25(OH)_2D$; sarcoidosis and other granulomatous diseases
3. Idiopathic hypercalcemia of infancy

Associated with high bone turnover:
1. Hyperthyroidism
2. Immobilization
3. Thiazides
4. Vitamin A intoxication

Associated with renal failure:
1. Severe secondary hyperparathyroidism
2. Aluminum intoxication
3. Milk-alkali syndrome

therapy. The type of treatment is based on the severity of the hypercalcemia and the nature of associated symptoms.

Hypercalcemia from any cause can result in fatigue, depression, mental confusion, anorexia, nausea, vomiting, constipation, reversible renal tubular defects, increased urination, alteration in the electrocardiogram (a short QT interval), and, in some patients, cardiac arrhythmias. There is a variable relation between the severity of hypercalcemia and the presence or absence of symptoms from one patient to the next. Generally, symptoms are more common at calcium levels above 2.9 to 3 mmol/L (11.5 to 12.0 mg/dL), but some patients, even at this level, are asymptomatic. When calcium exceeds 3.2 mmol/L (13 mg/dL), renal insufficiency and calcification in kidneys, skin, vessels, lungs, heart, and stomach may occur, particularly if blood phosphate levels are normal or elevated due to impaired renal function. Severe hypercalcemia, usually defined as 3.7 mmol/L (15 mg/dL) or above, is a medical emergency. When serum calcium is 3.7 to 4.5 mmol/L (15 to 18 mg/dL) or higher, coma and cardiac arrest can occur.

PARATHYROID-RELATED HYPERCALCEMIA   Primary hyperparathyroidism

NATURAL HISTORY AND INCIDENCE   Primary hyperparathyroidism is a generalized disorder of calcium, phosphate, and bone metabolism that results from an increased secretion of parathyroid hormone. The excessive concentration of circulating hormone usually leads to hypercalcemia and hypophosphatemia. There is great variation in the clinical presentation. Patients may present with multiple signs and symptoms, including recurrent nephrolithiasis, peptic ulcers, mental changes, and, less frequently, extensive bone resorption. However, with greater awareness of the disease and wider use of multiphasic screening tests, including blood calcium determinations, the diagnosis is frequently made in patients who have no symptoms and minimal, if any, signs of the disease other than hypercalcemia and elevated levels of parathyroid hormone. The annual incidence of the disease is estimated to be as high as 0.2 percent in patients over age 60, with an estimated prevalence due to undiscovered asymptomatic patients of 1 percent or higher. The clinical manifestations may be subtle, and the disease may have a benign course for many years or a full lifetime. Rarely, the disease seems to appear abruptly, and patients may exhibit severe complications, such as marked dehydration and coma, so-called hypercalcemic parathyroid crisis. The disease is most common in adults, with peak incidence between the third and fifth decades, but it occurs in young children and in the elderly.

ETIOLOGY AND PATHOLOGY *Solitary adenomas*   The cause of hyperparathyroidism is one or more hyperfunctioning glands. The traditional view has been that a single abnormal gland is the cause in approximately 80 percent of patients; the abnormal gland is usually a benign neoplasm or adenoma and rarely a malignant tumor or parathyroid carcinoma. In a second group, approximately 15 percent, all glands are hyperfunctioning; this is termed *chief cell parathyroid hyperplasia*. Most, but not all, of the second group are hereditary and associated with other endocrine abnormalities. The remaining few percent seem to have more than one but not necessarily all glands involved, as in hyperplasia; this disorder is labeled *double or multiple adenoma*. There is considerable disagreement about this etiologic classification, particularly about the frequency of disorders involving single, several, and all glands. This uncertainty has led to an associated disagreement about surgical management, in particular about how much tissue to remove to cure the disease and restore the euparathyroid state (discussed below).

Benign neoplasms were thought to be monoclonal, and direct genetic evidence for monoclonality has been obtained for parathyroid adenoma. Monoclonality implies one originally abnormal cell, losing growth control but still functioning, even if abnormally; an abnormal gland mass or adenoma results. Chief cell hyperplasia was thought to be polyclonal, with all parathyroid cells becoming abnormal in response to an extrinsic stimulus. The gene locus on chromosome 11 that is responsible for the familial syndrome of parathyroid hyperplasia and associated pancreatic and pituitary tumors, the multiple endocrine

neoplasia syndrome type 1 (MEN 1), appears to function normally as an antioncogene (Figure 351-1; see also Chap. 343). Such genes, identified in retinoblastoma and other hereditary cancer syndromes, appear normally to control cell growth; loss of both alleles leads to abnormal growth. In these syndromes, one gene is usually defective in the germ line; a second mutation or loss of the portion of the chromosome that carries the normal allele in a single cell then leads to a monoclonal expansion. In women, studies using X chromosome markers that undergo random inactivation permit direct tests of monoclonality versus polyclonality of excised parathyroid tumors and indicate that many adenomas are monoclonal. In other patients, the evidence is insufficient to allow deductions as to clonality. Other lines of evidence have shed new light on possible mechanisms of abnormal cellular growth. The synthesis of parathyroid hormone (PTH) is under the control of a promoter that has evolved to drive high rates of hormone gene transcription in the parathyroid cell. In a reciprocal translocation involving chromosome 11, the PTH promotor drives overexpression of a gene product termed PRAD-1. The gene product is D-cyclin, a protein that plays a critical role in regulation of normal cell division and that, if overexpressed (or mutated), contributes to abnormal rates of cellular replication, characteristic of the neoplastic phenotype.

Parathyroid enlargement in the syndrome of chief cell hyperplasia and MEN 1 is probably due to a monoclonal expansion and thus is similar to that in adenomas. Loss of both copies of a functional MEN 1 gene can be deduced by tumor analyses and genetic screening in families with informative restriction fragment length polymorphisms.

FIGURE 357-1   Schematic diagram indicating concept of autosomal recessive rather than autosomal dominant inheritance of tumor susceptibility. In somatic cells, generally represented by circulating lymphocytes (*L*), the patient with the hereditary abnormality (multiple endocrine neoplasia, or MEN) is envisioned as having one defective gene (*X*) inherited from the affected parent, the father (♂), but one copy of the normal gene is present from the mother (♀). In the monoclonal tumor [an enlarged parathyroid gland (*T*)], a somatic event, here partial chromosomal deletion, removes the normal gene from a cell. The cell, deprived of growth-regulating influence from this gene, has unregulated growth and becomes a tumor. The numbers adjacent to the chromosome (*1, 2, 1*) refer to restriction fragment length polymorphisms which allow the identification of which chromosome/gene came from which parent. The fact that the normal gene copy is invariably lost in the tumor leads to the deduction that the MEN 1 gene is an antioncogene; the inheritance pattern resembles the 50 percent incidence expected of an autosomal dominant pattern.

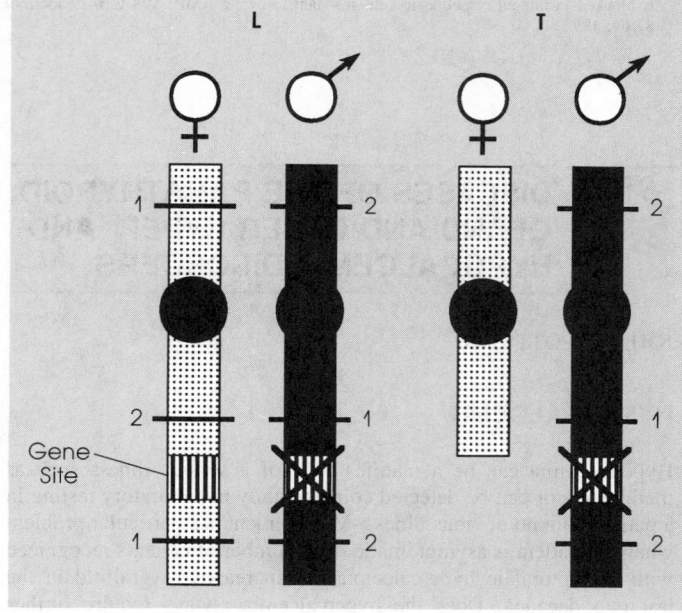

Only the abnormal allele is preserved in the tumor; the presumably normal allele from the unaffected parent is deleted in the tumor but not in normal cells. The tumor then has no functioning copy of the MEN 1 gene, the presumed growth-controlling gene. Interestingly, loss of at least one copy of the MEN 1 gene can be detected by chromosomal analyses in some sporadic adenomas; whether both copies are defective (as by a mutation in the second allele) is not known. It also remains unsettled whether hereditary chief cell hyperplasia characterstically begins as polyclonal expansions. Detailed analyses of the status of the chromosome region around the MEN 1 gene locus in all glands in sufficient numbers of patients will be required to determine if all or only the larger glands are monoclonal.

Thus the genetic and somatic basis of cellular defects in hyperparathyroidism is understood in some detail, but it is not yet feasible to use the data to determine how to treat patients with the disorder. Many of the management issues depend on clinical judgment and clinicopathologic correlations.

Adenomas are most often located in the inferior parathyroid gland, but in 6 to 10 percent of patients, parathyroid adenomas may be located in the thymus, the thyroid, the pericardium, or behind the esophagus. Adenomas are usually 0.5 to 5 g in size but may be as large as 10 to 20 g (normal glands weigh 25 mg on average). Chief cells are predominant in both hyperplasia and adenoma. The adenoma is sometimes encapsulated by a rim of normal tissue. Chief cell hyperplasia is especially common in familial cases of hyperparathyroidism and those that are part of the multiple endocrine neoplasia (MEN) syndromes (see Chap. 343). With hyperplasia, the enlargement may be so asymmetric that some involved glands appear grossly normal. If hyperplasia is present, histologic examination reveals a uniform pattern of chief cells and disappearance of fat even in the absence of an increase in gland weight. Thus microscopic examination of biopsy specimens of several glands is essential to interpret findings at surgery. When an adenoma is present, the other glands are usually normal and contain a normal distribution of all cell types (rather than only chief cells) and normal amounts of fat.

Parathyroid carcinoma is usually not aggressive in character. Long-term survival without recurrence is common if at initial operation the entire gland is removed without rupture of the capsule. Even recurrent parathyroid carcinoma is usually slow-growing with local spread in the neck, and surgical correction of recurrent disease may be feasible. Occasionally, however, parathyroid carcinoma is more aggressive in character, with distant metastases (lung, liver, and bone) found at the time of initial operation. It may be difficult to appreciate initially that a primary tumor is carcinoma; increased numbers of mitotic figures and increased fibrosis of the gland stroma may precede invasive features. The diagnosis of carcinoma is often made in retrospect. Hyperparathyroidism from a parathyroid carcinoma may be clinically indistinguishable from other forms of primary hyperparathyroidism; a potential clue to the diagnosis, however, is provided by the degree of calcium elevation. Calcium values of 3.5 to 3.7 mmol/L (14 to 15 mg/dL) are frequent with carcinoma; this finding may alert the surgeon to remove the abnormal gland with care to avoid capsular rupture. A genetic defect may be a central factor in the disregulated cellular growth in parathyroid carcinoma. Defects in function of the retinoblastoma gene have been identified in a number of patients with parathyroid carcinoma, suggesting that a different type of antioncogene than that suspected in parathyroid adenomas is lost.

Multiple endocrine neoplasia Hyperparathyroidism may occur in a familial pattern without other endocrinologic abnormality. More often, however, hereditary hyperparathyroidism is part of a multiglandular endocrinopathy (see Chap. 343). There are several distinct MEN syndromes. The type 1 disorder (MEN 1, Wermer's syndrome) consists of hyperparathyroidism and tumors of the pituitary and pancreatic islet cells, often associated with peptic ulcer and gastric hypersecretion (the Zollinger-Ellison syndrome). A mitogenic factor for parathyroid tissue is present in the sera of patients with MEN 1. Another distinct constellation of endocrinologic abnormalities consists of hyperparathyroidism associated with pheochromocytoma and medullary carcinoma of the thyroid (MEN 2a). The pattern of inheritance is autosomal dominant. Tumors of the thyroid and adrenal medulla are not found in patients with MEN 1, and pancreatic and pituitary tumors do not occur in patients with MEN 2a. Since the different endocrine tumors can develop at widely separated intervals, hyperparathyroidism and the related endocrine disorders should be carefully and repeatedly searched for in kindreds afflicted with the MEN syndromes.

SIGNS AND SYMPTOMS   Half or more of patients with hyperparathyroidism are asymptomatic. In series in which patients are followed without operation, as many as 80 percent can be classified as without symptoms; the number may be smaller if mild manifestations, such as silent bone deterioration or reduced renal function, are considered. Manifestations of hyperparathyroidism involve primarily the kidneys and the skeletal system. Kidney involvement, due either to deposition of calcium in the renal parenchyma or to recurrent nephrolithiasis, was present in 60 to 70 percent of patients prior to 1970. With the earlier detection of asymptomatic persons, renal complications are much less common.

Renal stones are usually composed of either calcium oxalate or calcium phosphate. Repeated episodes of nephrolithiasis or the formation of large calculi may lead to urinary tract obstruction and infection and loss of renal function. Nephrocalcinosis also may cause decreased renal function and phosphate retention.

The unique bone involvement in hyperparathyroidism is osteitis fibrosa cystica. In the past, osteitis fibrosa cystica occurred in 10 to 25 percent of patients with hyperparathyroidism. Histologically, the pathognomonic features are a reduction in the number of trabeculae, an increase in the giant multinucleated osteoclasts in scalloped areas on the surface of the bone (Howship's lacunae), and a replacement of the normal cellular and marrow elements by fibrous tissues. Other bone changes include resorption of the phalangeal tufts and a replacement of the usually sharp cortical outline of the bone in the digits by an irregular outline (subperiosteal resorption). Loss of the lamina dura of the teeth is less specific. Tiny "punched-out" lesions may cause the so-called salt-and-pepper appearance in the skull.

Osteitis fibrosa cystica is now uncommon, even though the disease may be of long standing. The reduced frequency has not been explained. Other manifestations of bone disease, however, are frequent. Histomorphometric analyses of biopsied bone reveal an abnormality in bone turnover in most patients, even in those who do not have progressive loss of net bone mass; in such patients, rates of bone formation and bone restoration must be increased but balanced. In some patients, however, who do not have symptomatic bone disease or osteitis fibrosa cystica, rates of formation and resorption are not balanced so that a progressive loss of bone mineral mass causes osteopenia. There are no pathognomonic criteria to separate unequivocally parathyroid-dependent osteopenia from "high-turnover" osteoporosis, as occurs in patients who are not hyperparathyroid.

Improved techniques are not available for monitoring bone mineral density. Computed tomography and quantitative digital radiography (DEXA) of the spine provide reproducible quantitative estimates (within a few percent) of spinal bone density. Similar, highly reproducible quantitation is also possible by single-photon densitometry for measurement of cortical bone density in the extremities. Serial measurements with these techniques can provide early evidence of whether or not osteopenia is progressive. Considerable attention has been addressed to the problem of asymptomatic hyperparathyroidism. In the absence of evidence of organ deterioration (bone, kidney), many patients are followed without surgery (see below). Bone disease with primary hyperparathyroidism can be quite variable. In general, cortical bone mass is lost selectively in hyperparathyroidism.

In symptomatic patients, dysfunctions of the central nervous system, peripheral nerve and muscle, the gastrointestinal tract, and the joints also occur. An awareness of the signs and symptoms that may be seen in hyperparathyroidism may give the initial clue in the diagnosis. In some instances, severe neuropsychiatric manifestations are reversed by parathyroidectomy; in these patients there appears to be a cause-and-effect relationship. Generally, however, the fact that hyperparathyroidism is common in elderly patients, in whom there are often other problems, suggests the possibility that such problems as hypertension, renal deterioration, and depression may not be parathyroid-related and suggests caution in recommending surgery as a cure for these conditions in hyperparathyroid patients. It is not apparent why some patients with hyperparathyroidism have no symptoms, while others with similar biochemical abnormalities develop symptomatic disease.

Neuromuscular manifestations include proximal muscle weakness, easy fatigability, and atrophy of muscles. The clinical signs in these patients may be so striking as to suggest a primary neuromuscular disorder. The distinguishing feature is the complete regression of neuromuscular disease after surgical correction of the hyperparathyroidism.

Gastrointestinal manifestations of hyperparathyroidism are sometimes subtle and include vague abdominal complaints and disorders of the stomach and pancreas. Again, cause and effect are unclear, except in certain situations, such as the multiple endocrine syndromes. In MEN 1 patients with hyperparathyroidism, duodenal ulcer is a result of the associated pancreatic tumors that secrete excessive quantities of gastrin (the Zollinger-Ellison syndrome). Pancreatitis has been reported in association with hyperparathyroidism, but the incidence and the mechanism are not established.

Chondrocalcinosis and pseudogout are said to be sufficiently frequent in hyperparathyroidism that screening of such patients is warranted. Occasionally, pseudogout is the initial manifestation.

DIAGNOSIS   The diagnosis is made primarily on clinical grounds. The newer immunoassays for PTH are reliable and cost-effective. Since hypercalcemia can be the presenting evidence for malignancy or other serious disease, a thorough evaluation of possible etiologies, including hyperparathyroidism, is indicated even in asymptomatic subjects. If the diagnosis of hyperparathyroidism is suspected after such an evaluation, a decision may be made to follow the patient rather than to recommend surgery.

Hypercalcemia is the most common manifestation—either sustained or intermittent hypercalcemia. Careful consideration must be given to the justification for surgical exploration in the absence of hypercalcemia. So-called normocalcemic hyperparathyroidism, i.e., surgically proven hyperparathyroidism accompanied by a normal calcium level but elevated values of immunoreactive PTH (iPTH), is rare in the absence of renal failure or gastrointestinal disease. If such patients have coexisting conditions that interfere with the calcium-elevating actions of PTH, such as chronic renal failure, severe malabsorption, or vitamin D deficiency, then the lack of calcium elevation need not argue against the presence of true hyperparathyroidism. Confusing situations can arise, however, in patients with recurrent kidney stones who are suspected of having hyperparathyroidism because of elevated iPTH levels but who have normal serum calcium. These patients may have true normocalcemic hyperparathyroidism. In situations in which the symptoms call for an early definitive diagnosis, it may be useful to search for postabsorptive hypercalcemia (detectable in certain patients when fasting hypercalcemia is absent) or to use a provocative test with benzothiadiazides (see below).

Hypercalciuria is common in hyperparathyroidism. However, PTH actually reduces calcium clearance, and the daily excretion of calcium in urine is lower than in patients with equivalent degrees of hypercalcemia from nonparathyroid causes.

Serum phosphate is usually low but may be normal, especially if renal failure has developed. Hypophosphatemia is a less useful diagnostic finding than hypercalcemia for two reasons. First, phosphate levels are influenced by dietary intake, diurnal variations, and other factors; to be useful, samples must be obtained in the morning under fasting conditions. Second, patients with severe hypercalcemia of all causes may have a low serum phosphate.

Many tests based on renal responses to excess parathyroid hormone (renal calcium and phosphate clearance; blood phosphate, chloride, magnesium; urinary or nephrogenous cyclic AMP) have been proposed and used in the past. These tests have low specificity for hyperparathyroidism, are not cost-effective, and have been replaced by the improved PTH immunoassays.

TREATMENT   *Medical treatment*   Medical treatment involves two separate issues. If hypercalcemia is severe and symptomatic, then the calcium must be lowered (the measures are described below). Hypercalcemia is not symptomatic in most patients with hyperparathyroidism, and it is usually not difficult to control the hypercalcemia. Simple hydration will often suffice to lower the calcium concentration to values below 2.9 mmol/L (11.5 mg/dL). There have been discussions in the past about whether chronic management of the hypercalcemia of hyperparathyroidism should be undertaken with oral phosphate therapy. Lowering the calcium concentration by phosphate is accompanied by an increase in iPTH levels in blood; it is unclear whether the increased PTH levels would cause more or less organ deterioration. There have been no systemic trials to evaluate the effects of medical therapy for hypercalcemia.

Rather, the usual issue is to decide whether surgical intervention is required. If not, medical management consists of following the patient without specific therapy but monitoring bone and renal function periodically to ensure that silent osseous and renal deterioration does not occur. In postmenopausal women with hyperparathyroidism who are either unwilling or unable to undergo parathyroid surgery, estrogen therapy may retard demineralization of the skeleton and reduce blood and urinary calcium levels.

The natural history of the disease has been studied in several centers. Several hundred patients have been followed in attempts to afford a rational explanation for the benefits of surgery versus the risks of medical observation. Large-scale randomized, prospective clinical trials have not been undertaken, however. Rather, the long-term effects of hyperparathyroidism have been assessed in patients who do not have kidney stones, osteitis fibrosa cystica, or other clear-cut symptoms. Of principal concern is the possibility of progressive loss of bone density, a worrying problem in women who face the problem of age-dependent and estrogen-deficient bone loss in the absence of hyperparathyroidism. The concern is that such patients, even though asymptomatic, will suffer a degree of bone loss due to PTH excess that will leave them more vulnerable later in life to developing symptomatic osteoporosis.

The importance of the topic of asymptomatic hyperparathyroidism led the National Institutes of Health to hold a Consensus Conference on Management of Asymptomatic Hyperparathyroidism in 1991. *Asymptomatic hyperparathyroidism* was defined as the clinical profile of patients with documented (presumptive) hyperparathyroidism without signs or symptoms attributable to the disease. It was emphasized that surgery to correct the hyperparathyroidism is always an acceptable approach, if feasible medically, but surveillance may be justified in patients over the age of 50 with minimal calcium elevation when renal function and bone mass are close to normal and remain so during careful monitoring.

Three of the important questions addressed were: (1) *What is the most accurate, cost-effective method of diagnosing hyperparathyroidism?* (2) *Are there patients with asymptomatic hyperparathyroidism who can safely be followed, and should they be?* (3) *If not operated on, how should asymptomatic patients be monitored and managed?*

The recommendation was that the diagnosis of primary hyperparathyroidism can best be established by demonstrating persistent hypercalcemia (artifactual elevation in serum calcium concentration should be eliminated) and an elevated serum PTH concentration. The panel agreed that the improved PTH assay is sensitive, specific, and reliable and that other tests are usually unnecessary.

As to which asymptomatic patients should be followed medically, the consensus was that a subgroup of patients over age 50 is appropriate for medical monitoring if certain criteria are met and the patients wish to avoid surgery.

Patients under age 50 should be routinely operated on, given the long surveillance that would be required. Other guidelines for recommending surgery in patients with asymptomatic hyperparathyroidism include the following:

1 Elevation of serum calcium, more than 0.25 to 0.40 mmol/L (1 to 1.6 mg/dL) above the upper limit of normal for the laboratory.

2 History of an episode of life-threatening hypercalcemia, such as an episode induced by dehydration and recurring illness.

3 Reduction of creatinine clearance by greater than 30 percent compared with age-matched controls (the author finds it difficult to use this criterion as an absolute, given the multiplicity of factors that affect creatinine clearance with age).

4 Presence of kidney stones detected by abdominal radiograph.

5 Elevation of 24-h urinary calcium excretion above 400 mg.

6 Reduction of bone mass more than 2 standard deviations below normal by one of several noninvasive methods of measuring bone mass.

Practical considerations that favor surgery include concern that consistent follow-up would be unlikely or that coexistent illness would complicate management. Asymptomatic patients should be monitored regularly. Surgical correction of hyperparathyroidism can always be undertaken when indicated, since the success rate is high (greater than 90 percent), mortality is low, morbidity is minimal, and cure is common. The goals of monitoring are early detection of worsening hypercalcemia, deteriorating bone or renal status, or other complications of hyperparathyroidism. Cortical bone mass is principally at risk in untreated primary hyperparathyroidism. Some data indicate that there is also an increased risk of vertebral bone fracture in patients with untreated hyperparathyroidism, suggesting that cancellous bone is also at risk. Cancellous bone loss may be a particular problem when vitamin D and calcium intakes are low.

Although patients have reduced bone mass at the time of initial detection, there may be little further loss over years of subsequent follow-up. It is not clear which technique of bone mass monitoring should be used routinely and how much reduction from normal or change should be considered an indication for surgery. The use of single-photon absorptiometry to follow cortical bone is relatively easy and inexpensive; in the United States at least, increased loss of cancellous bone and increased risk of vertebral fractures are unusual. Consequently, the monitoring of spinal bone mass by dual-energy x-ray absorptiometry need not be undertaken. The consensus panel did not make a recommendation as to estrogen use in patients for whom surgery was not elected because there was too little cumulative experience with such therapy.

Surgical treatment Parathyroid exploration is best undertaken by an experienced surgeon with the help of an experienced pathologist. Certain features help in predicting the pathology; for example, in familial cases multiple abnormal glands are likely. However, some critical decisions regarding management can be made only during the operation. The examination by frozen section of tissue removed at surgery helps direct the subsequent course of the operation.

As discussed under etiology, there are many unresolved issues to consider in surgery for hyperparathyroidism. At the extreme of conservatism, the surgical approach is based on the view that typically only one gland (the adenoma) is abnormal. If an enlarged gland is found, a normal gland should be sought. If a biopsy of a normal-sized second gland confirms its histologic and therefore presumed functional normality, no further exploration, biopsy, or excision is needed. At the other extreme is the minority viewpoint that not only should all four glands be sought but also most of the total parathyroid tissue mass should be removed.

The concern with the former approach is that the rate of recurrence of hyperparathyroidism may be high because a second abnormal gland will sometimes be missed; the latter approach could involve unnecessary surgery and an unacceptable rate of hypoparathyroidism.

The majority viewpoint, judged by surgical reviews, is in favor of conservative surgery, i.e., removal of what is usually only one enlarged gland but only after four-gland exploration to eliminate the possibility that more than one gland is abnormal. When normal glands are found in association with one enlarged gland, excision of the single adenoma leads to cure or symptom-free disease in most such patients.

Known hyperplasia, as predicted in familial cases, poses more difficult questions of surgical management. Once a diagnosis of hyperplasia is established, it is necessary to identify all the glands. Two different schemes for surgical management have been proposed. One is that three glands be totally removed and the fourth gland be partially excised; care is taken to leave a good blood supply for the remaining gland. Other surgeons advocate total parathyroidectomy with immediate transplantation of a portion of a removed, minced parathyroid gland into the muscles of the forearm with the view that even if recurrence of residual gland enlargement and hyperfunction is seen, surgical excision is easier from the ectopic site in the arm. Cryopreservation is also being explored, but functional survival of the glands is unclear. When parathyroid carcinoma is encountered, the tissue should be widely excised; care must be taken to avoid rupture of the capsule to prevent local seeding of the tumor.

If no glandular abnormalities are found in the neck, the issue of further exploration must be decided. There are documented cases of five or six parathyroid glands and, therefore, of unusual locations for adenomas. A variety of techniques have been developed to aid in the preoperative localization of the abnormal parathyroid tissue; usually these techniques are used only in patients with unsuccessful neck explorations before further surgery is undertaken. The early techniques featured either selective intraarterial angiography or selective venous catheterization of the thyroid venous plexus and adjacent areas coupled with radioimmunoassay for PTH. The techniques were often successful but not better than the rate of success of an experienced parathyroid surgeon in finding the abnormal tissue at the first operation, so such procedures are not warranted. Less invasive techniques also have been utilized for preoperative localization, including ultrasound, computed tomography of the neck and mediastinum, differential scanning after simultaneous radiothallium and technetium administration, and intraarterial digital angiography; the yield for these procedures in preoperative localization is also insufficiently high to warrant their use except when the initial surgery is unsuccessful.

Ultrasound is reported to detect abnormal parathyroid tissue in 60 to 70 percent of cases and has been advocated for lesions in the vicinity of the thyroid; it is less successful for lesions in the anterior mediastinum. The technique may assist the surgeon even in the initial operation by directing the surgery to the side of the neck where the abnormal gland is located. Computed tomography has a similar success rate and is more helpful with mediastinal glands, although false-positive results are noted. The subtraction of the technetium image, which targets the thyroid, from the radiothallium image, which targets both thyroid and parathyroid, has led to successful preoperative localization in approximately half of patients undergoing a second exploration.

Several generalizations seem warranted. Localization and removal of a single abnormal parathyroid gland at the first operation are usually successful depending on the experience of the surgeon (greater than 90 percent success for experienced surgeons). Preoperative localization techniques, therefore, which are less than 90 percent successful, should be reserved for patients in whom initial exploration is unsuccessful. When a second parathyroid exploration is indicated, ultrasound, computed tomography, and thallium-technetium scanning should probably be combined with selective digital arteriography in one of the centers specializing in these techniques. At one center, long-term cures have been achieved with selective embolization or injection of large amounts of contrast material into the end-arterial circulation feeding the parathyroid tumor.

A decline in serum calcium occurs within 24 h after successful surgery; usually blood calcium falls to low-normal values for 3 to 5 days until the remaining parathyroid tissue resumes hormone secretion. Intraoperative monitoring of PTH levels by rapid PTH immunoassays may be useful in guiding the surgery, especially in patients who are reexplored after an initial unsuccessful operation. Severe postoperative hypocalcemia is likely only if osteitis cystica is present or if injury to all the normal parathyroid glands has occurred during surgery.

In general, patients with good renal and gastrointestinal function, who do not have symptomatic bone disease and a large deficit in bone mineral, have few problems with postoperative hypocalcemia. The extent of postoperative hypocalcemia varies with the surgical approach. If all glands are biopsied, hypocalcemia may be more prolonged and may be transiently symptomatic. Symptomatic hypocalcemia is more likely to occur after second parathyroid explorations, when normal parathyroid tissue may have been removed at the unsuccessful initial operation and when the manipulation and/or biopsy of the remaining normal gland has been more extensive in the search for the missing adenoma. Patients with hyperparathyroidism have efficient intestinal calcium absorption due to the increased levels of $1,25(OH)_2D$ stimulated by parathyroid excess. Once hypocalcemia signifies successful surgery, patients can be put on a high calcium intake or be given oral calcium supplements. Despite manifestations of mild hypocalcemia, most patients do not require parenteral therapy and do not experience severe symptoms. If the serum calcium falls below 2 mmol/L (8 mg/dL), *in particular if the phosphate level simultaneously rises*, the possibility of hypoparathyroidism must be considered. Coexistent hypomagnesemia should be checked for, since it interferes with PTH secretion and causes a relative hypoparathyroidism. Parenteral calcium replacement at a low level should be instituted if symptomatic hypocalcemia supervenes. Such symptoms include a general sense of anxiety and positive Chvostek and Trousseau signs coupled with serum calcium consistently below 2 mmol/L (8 mg/dL). For parenteral therapy, calcium (gluconate or chloride) solutions are prepared at a concentration of 1 mg/mL in 5% dextrose in water. The rate and duration of intravenous therapy are determined by the severity of the symptoms and the response of the serum calcium. A rate of infusion of 0.5 to 2 (mg/kg)/h or 30 to 100 mL/h of a 1 mg/mL solution usually suffices to relieve symptoms. Generally, parenteral therapy is required for only a few days. If symptoms become severe or if the need for parenteral calcium continues for more than 2 to 3 days, replacement therapy with a vitamin D analogue and/or oral calcium (2 to 4 g/d) should be started (see below). It is cost-effective to use calcitriol (doses of 0.5 to 1.0 μg/d) because of the rapidity of onset and rapidity of cessation of action, in contrast to vitamin D per se (see below). A sudden rise in blood calcium after several months of vitamin D replacement may indicate restoration of parathyroid function to normal. It is also appropriate to monitor serum PTH serially to estimate gland function in such patients.

Magnesium deficiency also may complicate the postoperative course. Magnesium deficiency impairs the secretion of PTH, and therefore, hypomagnesemia should be corrected whenever detected. Magnesium chloride is effective by mouth, but this compound is not widely available. Accordingly, repletion is usually parenteral. Since the depressant effect of magnesium on central and peripheral nerve functions does not occur below 2 mmol/L (normal range 0.8 to 1.2 mmol/L), parenteral replacement can be given rapidly. A cumulative dose as great as 0.5 to 1 mmol/kg of body weight can be administered if severe hypomagnesemia is present; often, however, total doses of 12 to 12 mmol are sufficient. The magnesium is given either as an intravenous infusion over 8 to 12 h or in divided doses intramuscularly (magnesium sulfate, USP).

LITHIUM THERAPY Lithium, used in the management of bipolar depression and other psychiatric disorders, causes hypercalcemia in approximately 10 percent of patients. The parathyroids are involved in mediation of the hypercalcemia, and PTH levels may be elevated. The hypercalcemia is dependent on continued lithium treatment, remitting and recurring when lithium is stopped and restarted. In a few patients, parathyroid adenomas were present. Histologic findings in the remaining parathyroid glands in these patients have not been described, but the implication is that there is a single abnormal gland.

The presence of hypercalcemia does not correlate with plasma lithium level, but the frequency with which hypercalcemia occurs is sufficiently high to support a causal relationship between lithium and the hypercalcemia, particularly the dependence of the hypercalcemia on the continuation of the lithium. It is presumed that in most cases an adenoma is not present, merely hyperfunctioning glands. Lithium, at the levels achieved in blood in treated patients, can be shown in vitro to shift the curve describing PTH secretion as a function of calcium level to the right; i.e., higher calcium levels are required to lower PTH secretion. It is logical to assume that this effect can cause elevated PTH and consequent hypercalcemia in otherwise normal individuals. If careful studies were done, elevated PTH levels might be found in more patients treated with lithium than the 10 percent in whom frank hypercalcemia is detected. The adenomas reported in some hypercalcemic patients with lithium therapy may reflect the presence of an independently occurring parathyroid tumor; a permanent effect of lithium on parathyroid gland growth need not be implicated, since the majority of patients have complete reversal of hypercalcemia when lithium is stopped. On the other hand, evidence suggesting monoclonality in large parathyroid glands in some patients with renal failure and secondary hyperparathyroidism implies that long-standing stimulation of parathyroid cell replication may predispose to development of adenomas such as those seen in primary hyperparathyroidism; hence chronic lithium stimulation of the parathyroids may be risk factor for adenoma formation. Long-term follow-ups have not been reported; many patients are continued on lithium to treat psychiatric problems. These patients are presumably best managed according to the principles used in asymptomatic hypercalcemia independent of lithium administration. If troubling symptoms or signs, such as rising blood calcium levels, progressive bone demineralization, or kidney stones, develop, it may be necessary to try alternate psychotropic medication. It does not seem wise to recommend parathyroid surgery unless hypercalcemia and elevated PTH persist after lithium is discontinued.

Familial hypocalciuric hypercalcemia Familial hypocalciuric hypercalcemia (familial benign hypercalcemia; FHH) is inherited as an autosomal dominant trait. Affected individuals are frequently discovered because of asymptomatic hypercalcemia; surgical exploration of the parathyroids is not indicated because parathyroidectomy does not cure the disorder. It is therefore important to separate such patients from those with primary hyperparathyroidism.

The pathophysiology is not understood, and there is no single biochemical marker to distinguish these patients from patients with primary hyperparathyroidism. The genetic defect maps to a locus on chromosome 3. A defect in a calcium channel or a calcium signaling mechanism is suspected. The aggregate evidence serves to separate FHH clinically from primary hyperparathyroidism. The majority of patients with primary hyperparathyroidism have less than 99 percent renal calcium reabsorption, and most patients with FHH exceed 99 percent reabsorption. The hypercalcemia may be detectable in affected members of the kindreds in the first decade of life, whereas hypercalcemia rarely occurs in primary hyperparathyroidism and the MEN syndromes under the age of 10 years. The iPTH values may be elevated in FHH, but the values are usually normal or lower for the same degree of calcium elevation than in patients with primary hyperparathyroidism. Recurrent surgery in a few patients led to permanent hypoparathyroidism, but hypocalciuria persisted nevertheless; the hypocalciuria, therefore, is not PTH-dependent. Serum magnesium levels are, on average, higher in FHH than in primary hyperparathyroidism.

Few clinical signs or symptoms are present in patients with FHH. Unlike the MEN syndromes, other endocrine abnormalities are not present. Most patients are detected as a result of family screening after the diagnosis has been made in one member of the kindred. All too commonly, the initial patient is operated on without reversal of the hypercalcemia. At operation, the glands appear normal, or a moderate degree of hyperplasia of all parathyroid glands is seen. No patient has had reversal of hypercalcemia by surgery unless all the parathyroid tissue has been inadvertantly removed, rendering the patient hypoparathyroid, a most undesirable result. The high renal calcium reabsorption (parathyroid independent) and the prompt recurrence of hypercalcemia as long as any parathyroid tissue remains establish that there is some abnormality in the regulation of the ratio of extracellular to intracellular calcium concentration or some abnormal mechanisms of calcium sensing in cell membranes in the kidney and parathyroid gland. The exact nature of this disorder and its natural history are not clear yet, but since the parathyroid glands are permissive rather than responsible for the syndrome, parathyroid surgery is not appropriate, nor, in view of the lack of symptoms, is medical treatment needed to lower the calcium.

MALIGNANCY-RELATED HYPERCALCEMIA Clinical syndromes and mechanisms of hypercalcemia Hypercalcemia due to malignancy is common (occurring with 10 to 15 percent of certain types of tumor, such as lung carcinoma), often severe and difficult to manage, confusing as to etiology, and sometimes difficult to distinguish from primary hyperparathyroidism. Traditionally, hypercalcemia in malignancy was thought to be due to a local invasion and destruction of bone by tumor cells; many cases are now known to result from the elaboration by the malignant cells of humoral mediators of hypercalcemia.

Although the presence of malignancy is often clinically obvious, hypercalcemia can occasionally be due to an occult tumor. With occult malignancy, diagnosis and definitive treatment must be accomplished quickly if the patient is to be protected from the complications of the underlying malignancy.

Humoral hypercalcemia of malignancy occurs in patients with cancers of the lung and kidney in which bone metastases are absent, minimal, or not detectable clinically. The clinical picture resembles primary hyperparathyroidism (hypophosphatemia accompanies hypercalcemia), and elimination or regression of the primary tumor leads to disappearance of the hypercalcemia. Ectopic production of PTH by the tumor was initially felt to be responsible, but the disorder is in fact due to humoral mechanisms unrelated to ectopic PTH production.

Many patients with the humoral hypercalcemia of malignancy have elevated urinary nephrogenous cyclic AMP excretion, hypophosphatemia, and increased urinary phosphate clearance, findings compatible with the actions of a humoral agent that emulates PTH action. On the other hand, these patients generally have lower iPTH levels than patients with hyperparathyroidism. Using double-antibody assays of greater specificity, in fact, patients with the hypercalcemia of malignancy have either undetectable or suppressed immunoreactive PTH levels, consistent with non-PTH mechanisms. Other features of the syndrome differ from true hyperparathyroidism. Patients may have high, rather than low, renal calcium clearance (relative to serum calcium when compared to true hyperparathyroidism) and low to normal levels of 1,25-dihydroxyvitamin D [1,25(OH)$_2$D], all consistent with mediation by humoral factors distinct from PTH.

The histologic character of the tumor is more important than the extent of skeletal metastases in predicting hypercalcemia. Small cell carcinoma (oat cell) and adenocarcinoma of lung, although the most common lung tumors associated with skeletal metastases, rarely cause hypercalcemia. By contrast, as many as 10 percent of patients with squamous cell carcinoma of the lung develop hypercalcemia. Histologic studies of bone in patients with squamous cell or epidermoid carcinoma of the lung, in sites invaded by tumor as well as areas remote from tumor invasion, reveal bone remodeling, including osteoclastic and osteoblastic activity. In contrast, minimal evidence of skeletal metabolic activation is seen despite extensive skeletal metastases of small cell (oat cell) carcinoma.

Agents other than PTH are responsible for hypercalcemia, and only certain tumor types produce these factors. At least two general mechanisms of hypercalcemia are suspected. Most solid tumors associated with hypercalcemia, particularly squamous cell and renal tumors, produce and secrete cellular factors that are believed to cause increased bone resorption and to mediate the hypercalcemia through systemic actions on the skeleton as a whole by stimulation of bone resorption. On the other hand, direct bone marrow invasion occurs with other tumors, both hematologic malignancies such as leukemia, lymphoma, and multiple myeloma and solid tumors such as breast carcinoma. Substances produced by cells involved in the marrow response to the tumors promote resorption of bone through local destruction and may be identical or analogous to some of the known lymphokines and cytokines.

A classification of the hypercalcemia of malignancy is given in Table 357-2. Multiple myeloma and other hematologic malignancies involving the bone marrow have been typically considered as one group; bone destruction and hypercalcemia are believed to be caused through local mechanisms of malignant cells spread widely throughout the marrow spaces. Breast carcinoma is typical of solid tumors that cause hypercalcemia through *localized osteolytic destruction*, probably mediated by locally secreted tumor products that may differ from those involved in multiple myeloma or lymphoma. Finally, solid tumors not involving bone may cause hypercalcemia by secretion of a humoral mediator. In other instances, etiologic mechanisms may overlap.

In addition to the bone-resorbing factors elaborated by malignant cells in patients with hypercalcemia of malignancy, there may be variable synergism and antagonism between various bone-active agents secreted by the tumors. In some patients with the humoral hypercalcemia of malignancy, osteoclastic resorption may be generalized, and there is an absence of an osteoblastic or bone-forming response to the surge of bone resorption, implying some inhibition of the normal coupling of formation and resorption. Cooperativity and antagonism in the skeletal actions of locally released cytokines may include blockade of cytokine-induced bone resorption by interferon or related cytokines, both the bone-resorbing and bone-resorbing-blocking cytokines being secreted in response to interactions among tumor cells and host inflammatory cells. Thus the interaction of more than one substance may determine whether hypercalcemia develops in a particular patient.

Several hormones, hormone analogues, cytokines, and growth factors have been implicated as the result of clinical assays, in vitro tests, or chemical isolation. In some lymphomas, typically B cell lymphomas, there is an increased blood level of 1,25(OH)$_2$D. It is not clear whether the increased 1,25(OH)$_2$D is produced by stimulation of the renal 1α-hydroxylase or by lymphocytes; the latter seems likely, based on studies with the malignant cells. The search for etiologic mechanisms in hematologic malignancies has focused on the production of distinctive bone-resorbing factors by activated normal lymphocytes and by myeloma and lymphoma cells. This factor(s), termed *osteoclast activation factor* (OAF), now appears to represent the biologic action of several different cytokines, probably interleukin 1 and lymphotoxin or tumor necrosis factor, two closely related cytokines.

More than one factor may be responsible for humorally mediated hypercalcemia in patients with solid tumors, but as discussed in the

---

TABLE 357-2 Classification of tumor hypercalcemia

HEMATOLOGIC MALIGNANCIES

A Local bone destruction (OAF, interleukin 1, tumor necrosis factor, lymphotoxin)
  Multiple myeloma
  Lymphomas
B Humoral mediation [1,25(OH)$_2$D, PTH-rP]
  Lymphomas

SOLID TUMORS

A Local bone destruction (prostaglandin, E series)
  Some breast cancers
B Humoral mediation (PTH-rP, ?other agents)
  Lung (squamous cell)
  Kidney
  Urogenital tract
  Other breast cancers

preceding chapter, a specific factor termed *parathyroid hormone–related protein* (PTH-rP) that resembles but is distinct from PTH fulfills criteria of a humoral agent for the hypercalcemia syndrome. This factor binds equivalently to the PTH receptor and activates the receptor in a manner indistinguishable from PTH itself. As discussed in Chap. 356, immunoassays for PTH-rP are complicated by the heterogeneity of the circulating forms of the peptide. Nonetheless, elevated levels of PTH-rP are present in patients with the typical syndrome of humoral hypercalcemia of malignancy. The complexity of the etiologic mechanisms, however, are illustrated by several findings. For example, some breast carcinoma cells produce high levels of PTH-rP, and a distinctive type of T cell lymphoma/leukemia syndrome due to HTLV-I infection is also associated with severe hypercalcemia and high levels of circulating PTH-rP. In most instances, in contrast, breast carcinoma is believed to cause hypercalcemia by local stimulation of osteoclasts directly by products secreted by the metastatic breast carcinoma cells and associated inflammatory cells. Breast carcinoma cells produce and secrete prostaglandins of the E series, which are potent local stimulators of bone-resorbing cells.

Several aspects of the hypercalcemia of malignancy remain unclear. Levels of urinary cyclic AMP rise in test animals treated with synthetic PTH-rP, but $1,25(OH)_2D$ levels also rise, which is at variance with the fact that many patients with the humoral hypercalcemic syndrome have normal or depressed levels of $1,25(OH)_2D$. Tumor-derived growth factors, believed to act as autocrine regulators to maintain the transformation and growth of tumor cells, and cellular growth factors produced by nonmalignant cells are also potent bone-resorbing agents in vitro. Still other factors potentially involved in tumor hypercalcemia are known only by their bone-resorbing properties and lack of stimulation of renal or bone cell cyclic AMP production. Several of these factors stimulate production of prostaglandins of the E_2 type.

Assays to detect PTH-rP using different approaches (single-antibody, double-antibody, different epitopes) give similar results, but there are discrepancies perhaps relating to the methodologic difficulties listed above. Most data indicate undetectable (or low) levels in normal subjects, elevated levels in many cancer patients with the humoral syndrome, and high levels in human milk. Thus, although identification of PTH-rP represents a singular advance, it is not established to what extent the substance constitutes the sole pathophysiologic mechanism in the humoral hypercalcemia of malignancy.

Diagnostic issues and treatment   Ordinarily, the diagnosis of hypercalcemia secondary to tumor is not difficult to make because the tumor symptoms are prominent at the time the hypercalcemia is detected. Indeed, the hypercalcemia may be noted incidentally during the workup of a patient with known or suspected malignancy. Patients with malignancy and hypercalcemia may have a coexistent parathyroid adenoma, some reports suggesting an incidence as high as 10 percent.

Laboratory testing becomes critical when occult carcinoma is a possibility. Levels of iPTH by the newer double-antibody technique are undetectable or extremely low in tumor hypercalcemia, as would be expected with the mediation of the hypercalcemia by a nonparathyroid agent (the hypercalcemia suppressing the normal parathyroid glands). This improvement in the usefulness of the PTH assay is a significant advance in laboratory diagnosis. (Earlier assays gave equivocal results.) Assays for PTH-rP should be helpful; low or undetectable PTH and elevated PTH-rP would focus attention on the presence of an occult malignancy.

Clinical suspicion that malignancy is the cause of the hypercalcemia is heightened when symptoms associated with the paraneoplastic syndromes, such as weight loss, fatigue, muscle weakness, and unexplained skin rash, or symptoms specific for a particular tumor are present. Squamous cell tumors are most frequently associated with hypercalcemia, and the tumors most frequently arise in the lung, kidney, and urogenital tract. X-ray examinations can focus on these areas when clinical evidence is unclear. Bone scans with technetium-labeled diphosphonate are useful for detection of osteolytic metastases; the sensitivity is high, but specificity is low; results must be confirmed by conventional x-rays to be certain that areas of increased uptake are due to osteolytic metastases per se. Bone marrow biopsies are helpful in patients with anemia or abnormal peripheral blood smears.

Treatment of the hypercalcemia of malignancy must be considered in the perspective of the individual patient. Control of the tumor is the principal objective, and reduction of tumor mass is usually also the key to satisfactory control of hypercalcemia. If a patient has severe hypercalcemia yet has an excellent chance for effective tumor therapy, treatment of the hypercalcemia should be vigorous. If hypercalcemia, on the other hand, is an accompaniment of the late stages of a tumor that is resistant to therapy, the treatment of the hypercalcemia should not be vigorous, since hypercalcemia can have a mild sedating effect. Standard therapies for hypercalcemia (discussed below) are applicable to patients with malignancy.

VITAMIN D–RELATED HYPERCALCEMIA   Hypercalcemia related to abnormal vitamin D action can be due to *excessive ingestion* of vitamin D or *abnormal metabolism* of the vitamin. Abnormal metabolism of the vitamin is usually acquired in association with some widespread granulomatous disorder, but one rare hereditary form of vitamin D sensitivity in infants is associated with other developmental anomalies. As discussed in Chap. 356, vitamin D metabolism is carefully regulated, particularly the activity of the renal 1α-hydroxylase responsible for the production of $1,25(OH)_2D$. Many details of the regulation of 1α-hydroxylase remain unclarified, but the normal feedback suppression by $1,25(OH)_2D$ on the enzyme seems to work less well in infants than in adults and operates poorly, if at all, in ectopic sites, as distinct from the renal tubule; these facts explain the occurrence of hypercalcemia secondary to excessive $1,25(OH)_2D_3$ production in certain infants (Williams' syndrome) and in adults with granulomatous disease (sarcoidosis) or certain lymphomas.

Vitamin D Intoxication   The chronic ingestion of large doses of vitamin D, usually at least 50 to 100 times the normal physiologic requirement (doses in excess of 50,000 to 100,000 units per day), is required to produce hypercalcemia in normal individuals. In animals, vitamin D intoxication causes increased bone resorption as well as increased intestinal calcium absorption. In humans, excessive vitamin D action leads to an increase in intestinal calcium absorption, but it is not known whether increased bone resorption contributes to the hypercalcemia.

The immediate mechanism for the hypercalcemia is presumed to be an excessive production of $1,25(OH)_2D$ as a consequence of an increase in the substrate for the renal 1α-hydroxylase; namely, $25(OH)D$ production is less tightly regulated than is the production of $1,25(OH)_2D$. Hence concentrations of $25(OH)D$ average 5 to 10 times above normal in patients on high-dose vitamin D, whether therapeutically, as in hypoparathyroidism, or accidentally, as in vitamin D intoxication. $25(OH)D$ has a definite, if low, biologic activity in intestine and bone. Hence part of vitamin D intoxication may be attributable to the high levels of $25(OH)D$ itself, as well as supernormal levels of $1,25(OH)_2D$.

The diagnosis is substantiated by documenting elevated levels of $25(OH)D$. Hypercalcemia is usually controlled by restriction of dietary calcium intake and appropriate attention to hydration. These measures, plus discontinuation of vitamin D, usually lead to satisfactory management, but vitamin D stores in fat may be substantial, and vitamin D intoxication may persist for weeks after vitamin D ingestion is terminated. Such patients are responsive to glucocorticoids, which in doses of 100 mg of hydrocortisone per day, or its equivalent, usually return calcium levels to normal over several days; severe intoxication may require intensive therapy.

Sarcoidosis and other granulomatous diseases   Normal relations between $25(OH)D$ and the product, the active metabolite $1,25(OH)_2D$, are not maintained in patients with sarcoidosis and other granulomatous diseases. There is a positive correlation between $25(OH)D$ levels (reflecting vitamin D intake) and the circulating concentrations of $1,25(OH)_2D$; normally there is no increase in $1,25(OH)_2D$ with increasing $25(OH)D$ levels due to multiple feedback controls on the activity of the renal 1α-hydroxylase (see Chap. 356). In patients with sarcoidosis, the site of synthesis of $1,25(OH)_2D$ is believed to be in macrophages or other cells associated with granulomatous deposits. Hypercalcemia has been reported in an anephric sarcoidosis patient in association with increased $1,25(OH)_2D$ levels. Macrophages obtained from granulomatous tissue form $1,25(OH)_2D$ at an increased rate when $25(OH)D$ is provided as substrate. The usual regulation of active metabolite production by calcium or PTH does not operate in these patients; hypercalcemia does not lead to a reduction in the blood levels of $1,25(OH)_2D$ in patients with sarcoidosis. PTH-independent production of $1,25(OH)_2D$ is indicated by reports of normal $1,25(OH)_2D$ production in a patient with sarcoidosis and hypoparathyroidism. Clearance of $1,25(OH)_2D$ from blood may be decreased in sarcoidosis as well.

Even normocalcemic patients with sarcoidosis have unregulated production of $1,25(OH)_2D$ in response to vitamin D loading. Exposure to sunlight or administration of as little as 9000 units of vitamin D daily is followed by increased levels of the active metabolite. Treatment with moderate doses of glucocorticoids leads to a reversal of the hypercalcemia, as in other cases of excessive vitamin D action such as vitamin D intoxication, and reversal of the abnormal responsiveness of $1,25(OH)_2D$ levels to vitamin D challenge. Presumably, glucocorticoid administration causes multiple effects in the disease, and both excessive production of the metabolite and the responsiveness to it in target organs are blocked.

Variation in reported frequency of hypercalcemia in sarcoidosis (10 percent or less in recent reports, 60 percent or more in older reports) is probably explained in part by the common use of glucocorticoids to control pulmonary complications and other manifestations of the granulomatous disease. Lytic lesions also occur in bone so that increased bone resorption could play a role in some cases. In most, however, hypercalcemia is directly related to an increased intestinal calcium absorption. Clinically, hypercalcemia is usually a manifestation of disseminated disease. Hence pulmonary involvement is usual; chest x-ray may reveal a diffuse fibronodular infiltrate and/or prominent hilar adenopathy. Levels of angiotensin converting enzyme are elevated; blood gamma globulin also may be elevated. The most useful diagnostic procedure is demonstration of noncaseating granulomas in liver or lymph node biopsy. Hypercalcemia due to sarcoidosis can be elusive when many of the typical features of the disease are lacking (see section on differential diagnosis).

Management of the hypercalcemia in these patients can be accomplished by avoiding excessive sunlight exposure and by limiting vitamin D and calcium intake; glucocorticoids in the equivalent of 100 mg hydrocortisone per day or less usually are sufficient to control hypercalcemia when it occurs. Presumably, however, the abnormal sensitivity to vitamin D and abnormal regulation of $1,25(OH)_2D$ synthesis will persist as long as the disease is active. PTH levels are usually suppressed and $1,25(OH)_2D$ levels are elevated, but primary hyperparathyroidism and sarcoidosis may occur in some patients.

Idiopathic hypercalcemia of infancy This unusual disorder, sometimes referred to as *Williams' syndrome*, consists of multiple congenital development defects, including supravalvular aortic stenosis, mental retardation, and an elfin facies, in association with hypercalcemia due to abnormal sensitivity to vitamin D. The syndrome was first recognized in England after the commencement of fortification of milk with vitamin D. Hypercalcemia develops with vitamin D intakes as small as 2000 to 4000 units per day. Levels of $1,25(OH)_2D$ are elevated, ranging from 46 to 120 nmol/L (150 to 500 pg/mL). The mechanism of the abnormal sensitivity to vitamin D and of the increased circulating levels of $1,25(OH)_2D$ is unclear. The children become hypercalcemic because of excessive intestinal calcium absorption. The abnormality in vitamin D metabolism and the increased sensitivity to vitamin D intake do not occur after the first year of life. Treatment is restriction of calcium intake. Occasionally, the hypercalcemia can be severe, and calcium values

above 4 mmol/L (16 mg/dL) are recorded. Treatment with glucocorticoids in the doses used for vitamin D intoxication or sarcoidosis, adjusted for body weight, rapidly reverses the hypercalcemia.

HYPERCALCEMIA ASSOCIATED WITH HIGH BONE TURNOVER

Hyperthyroidism As many as 20 percent of hyperthyroid patients have high-normal or mildly elevated serum calcium concentrations; hypercalciuria is even more common. The hypercalcemia seems due to increased bone turnover, with bone resorption exceeding bone formation. Severe calcium elevations are not typical, however, and the presence of such suggests a concomitant disease such as hyperparathyroidism. Indeed, patients with thyrotoxicosis are more sensitive to the hypercalcemic effects of PTH. Usually, the diagnosis is obvious, but signs of hyperthyroidism may occasionally be occult, particularly in the elderly. Hypercalcemia is managed by specific therapy of the hyperthyroidism.

Immobilization Immobilization in adults is rarely associated with hypercalcemia in the absence of an associated disease but may cause hypercalcemia in children and adolescents, particularly after spinal cord injury and paraplegia or quadriplegia. With resumption of some ambulation, the hypercalcemia in children usually returns to normal spontaneously.

The mechanism appears to involve a disproportion between rates of bone formation and bone resorption. Hypercalciuria and increased mobilization of skeletal calcium can be seen in normal volunteers subjected to extensive bed rest, although hypercalcemia does not usually occur. Immobilization in an adult with an underlying disease associated with high bone turnover, such as Paget's disease, may cause hypercalcemia.

Thiazides Administration of benzothiadiazines (thiazides) can cause hypercalcemia in patients with high rates of bone turnover, such as patients with hypoparathyroidism treated with high doses of vitamin D. Traditionally, thiazides are associated with aggravation of hypercalcemia in primary hyperparathyroidism but this effect can be seen in other high-bone-turnover states as well. The mechanism of action of the drugs is complex, but the overall result seems to be to impose a challenge to calcium homeostasis by actions on renal calcium excretion, on bone-calcium turnover, and on parathyroid action. Thiazide administration in normal individuals causes a transient increase in blood calcium (but usually within the high normal range) which reverts to preexisting levels after a week or more of continued administration. If hormonal function and calcium and bone metabolism are normal, homeostatic controls are reset to counteract the calcium-elevating effect of the thiazides. In the presence of hyperparathyroidism or increased bone turnover from another cause, homeostatic mechanisms are ineffective. The abnormal effects of the thiazide on calcium metabolism disappear within days of cessation of the drug.

Many aspects of the action of the thiazides on calcium metabolism remain unclear. The drug clearly augments PTH responsiveness of target cells of bone and renal tubule. Chronic thiazide administration leads to reduction in urinary calcium excretion; the hypocalciuric effect of the drug appears to reflect the enhancement of proximal tubular resorption of sodium and calcium in response to sodium depletion. Some of this renal action reflects augmentation of PTH actions and is more pronounced in subjects with intact parathyroid secretion. However, a substantial hypocalciuric effect can be achieved in hypoparathyroid patients on high-dose vitamin D and oral calcium replacement if sodium intake is restricted. This finding is the rational for the use of thiazides as an adjunct to therapy in hypoparathyroid patients as discussed below.

Vitamin A intoxication Vitamin A intoxication is a rare cause of hypercalcemia. Most vitamin A intoxication is a side effect of excessive intake of the vitamin. Calcium levels can be elevated into the 3 to 3.5 mmol/L (12 to 14 mg/dL) range after the ingestion of 50,000 to 100,000 units of vitamin A daily (10 to 20 times the minimum daily requirement). The patients have typical features of severe hypercalcemia, which include fatigue and anorexia. They may have severe muscle and bone pain. The excess vitamin A intake is presumed to increase bone resorption.

Diagnosis can be established by history and by measurements of vitamin A levels in serum, which may be increased severalfold above normal. Occasionally, skeletal x-rays reveal periosteal calcifications, particularly in the hands. Withdrawal of the vitamin is usually associated with the prompt disappearance of the hypercalcemia and reversal of the skeletal changes. As in vitamin D intoxication, administration of 100 mg/d hydrocortisone or its equivalent leads to a rapid return of the serum calcium to normal.

HYPERCALCEMIA ASSOCIATED WITH RENAL FAILURE Severe secondary hyperparathyroidism Secondary hyperparathyroidism occurs when partial resistance to the metabolic actions of the hormone leads to excessive PTH production. Parathyroid gland hyperplasia occurs because resistance to the normal level of the hormone leads to hypocalcemia, which, in turn, is a stimulus to enlargement of the parathyroid glands with resultant increased secretion of PTH. This concept is based on studies in experimental animals with renal failure and phosphate retention and studies of the treatment of patients with diphosphonates that block skeletal resorptive response. In Fig. 357-2 is illustrated the pathophysiology of hormone production in secondary hyperparathyroidism. When the parathyroid secretory reserve is tested by deliberately lowering blood calcium, the extent of rise in PTH for each decrement of plasma calcium is greater with parathyroid hyperplasia than with normal glands. There is, therefore,

FIGURE 357-2 The relation between blood calcium and iPTH in normal subjects and subjects with secondary (2°) hyperparathyroidism. This model of secondary hyperparathyroidism assumes that there is an increased mass of parathyroid tissue. The lower line represents normal secretory patterns, and the upper line describes the exaggerated secretion (steeper slope) typical of secondary hyperparathyroidism. When calcium level in blood is raised by calcium infusion and multiple measurements of PTH and calcium are made, some portion of hormone secretion in normals is constant despite high calcium levels in blood (nonsuppressible secretion), and this secretion is higher in hyperparathyroidism. An elevation of blood calcium from low normal levels [(2 mmol/L (8 mg/dL)] to high normal levels [(2.2 mmol/L (9 mg/dL)] results in a reduction in PTH in both normal and hyperparathyroid individuals, but true involution of secondary hyperparathyroidism with treatment can be confirmed only by showing a return of the exaggerated response curve to normal.

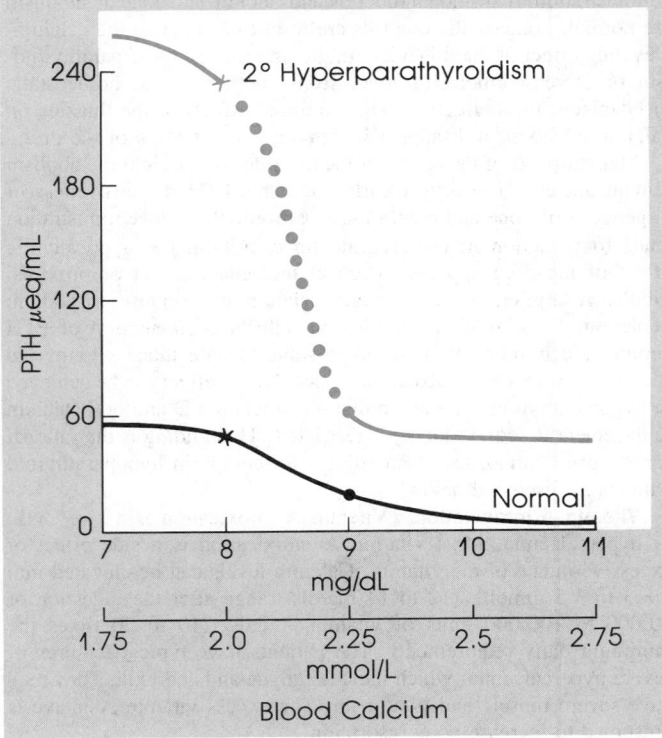

a higher concentration of hormone at any given level of calcium concentration. Since a portion of PTH secretion by each individual parathyroid cell is not suppressible by any degree of elevation of blood calcium concentration, larger glands (more cells) have a higher hormone output at the hypercalcemic end of the dose-response curve.

Secondary hyperparathyroidism occurs in patients with renal failure, osteomalacia (vitamin D deficiency), and pseudohypoparathyroidism (deficient response to PTH at the level of the receptor). The clinical manifestations of secondary hyperparathyroidism vary in these states. Hypocalcemia seems to be the common denominator in secondary hyperparathyroidism. Primary and secondary hyperparathyroidism can be distinguished conceptually by the autonomous nature of the growth of the parathyroid glands in primary hyperparathyroidism (presumably irreversible) and the adaptive increase in parathyroid gland size in secondary hyperparathyroidism (presumably reversible). In fact, reversal over weeks from an abnormal pattern of secretion, presumably accompanied by an involution of parathyroid gland mass to a normal pattern of function, can be monitored in patients treated with bisphosphonate after the drug is withdrawn (see Fig. 357-2). In some patients with secondary hyperparathyroidism, enlarged glands are monoclonal in origin. This phenomenon must mark conversion of the parathyroid glands from a state of reversible hyperplasia (polyclonal) to an irreversible growth defect (monoclonal); presumably, a more serious state of glandular hyperfunction occurs after the monoclonal transformation. Clinically, this concept has been referred to as *tertiary hyperparathyroidism.*

In progressive kidney disease, the initial tendency to hypocalcemia seems attributable to two causes: phosphate retention that develops because of the reduced excretion of phosphate and reduced concentrations of 1,25(OH)$_2$D associated with progressive renal damage. The two disturbances reduce skeletal responsiveness to PTH. The deficiency of 1,25(OH)$_2$D also interferes with the absorption of calcium from the intestine, already impaired in uremia. The ultimate pathophysiologic consequences in any given patients with chronic renal failure represent the outcome of competing physiologic adaptations, stimuli that cause parathyroid gland hyperplasia (tendency toward hypercalcemia and excessive bone resorption) versus those which modify the hormonal responsiveness of the end organs—bone, gut, and residual renal tubules (tendency toward hypocalcemia, hyperphosphatemia, and reduced bone resorption). Typically patients with renal failure exhibit hyperphosphatemia (renal retention and increased bone breakdown) and a low normal or moderately low blood calcium (calcium-lowering action of the phosphate level and reduced availability of calcium from bone and gut). In patients with severe secondary hyperparathyroidism, hypercalcemia and hyperphosphatemia both develop due to an increase in bone resorption; parathyroid hypersecretion "overshoots" the degree of resistance to hormone action; the monoclonal expansion of parathyroid gland mass may play a role in the "overshoot" and hypercalcemia.

In addition to hypercalcemia and hyperphosphatemia, patients with secondary hyperparathyroidism may develop bone pain, ectopic calcification, and pruritus. The bone disease in patients with secondary hyperparathyroidism and renal failure is usually termed *renal osteodystrophy*. Concomitant osteomalacia (vitamin D and calcium deficiency) and osteitis fibrosa cystica (excessive PTH action on bone) may occur. In fact, osteitis fibrosa cystica is now more common in untreated renal failure than in primary hyperparathyroidism.

Judicious medical therapy, which includes reduction of excessive blood phosphate by dietary phosphate restriction plus the use of nonabsorbable antacids (or, to avoid excess aluminum ingestion, calcium-containing antacids, either of which tie up phosphate in the gut) and careful, selective addition of calcitriol (0.25 to 2.0 µg/d), may reverse severe secondary hyperparathyroidism. Intravenous administration of calcitriol has been reported to cause long-term involution of secondary hyperparathyroidism (this experimental approach is designed, in part, to suppress PTH synthesis). As illustrated in Fig. 357-2, involution of the parathyroids then occurs; reduction of increased cellular mass causes the exaggerated secretory response to return to normal. The level of PTH at any given level of blood calcium is now more appropriate, and excessive parathyroid action is reversed. Somewhat paradoxically, during successful medical reversal of secondary hyperparathyroidism, elevated serum calcium (and phosphate) levels return to normal despite the administration of increased amounts of calcium and vitamin D metabolites that might have been expected to aggravate the hypercalcemia.

Aluminum intoxication Aluminum intoxication occurs in patients on chronic dialysis; manifestations include acute dementia and unresponsive and severe osteomalacia. Bone pain, multiple nonhealing fractures, particularly of the ribs and pelvis, and a proximal myopathy may occur. Hypercalcemia develops when attempts are made to treat these patients as one treats those with severe secondary hyperparathyroidism and renal osteodystrophy due to renal failure, as discussed above, namely, by administration of vitamin D or calcitriol. Acute hypercalcemia occurs after administration of vitamin D because of impaired skeletal responsiveness. Aluminum is present at the site of osteoid mineralization, and osteoblastic activity is minimal. Presumably, these patients are unable to incorporate the increased blood calcium into the skeleton. Prevention is accomplished by avoidance of aluminum excess in the dialysis regimen; treatment involves mobilizing aluminum through the use of the chelating agent deferoxamine. Aluminum is mobilized from bone and, being tightly bound to the chelating agent, can be removed via dialysis. After aluminum toxicity is reversed, patients may show typical features of renal osteodystrophy and secondary hyperparathyroidism. They can then be managed like other patients with secondary hyperparathyroidism with renal disease. A failure to recognize the syndrome is associated with persistence of the disabling bone disease and a fatal course due to progressive features or to hypercalcemia inadvertently induced by treatment with vitamin D.

Milk-alkali syndrome The milk-alkali syndrome can cause several clinical presentations—acute, subacute, and chronic—all of which feature hypercalcemia, alkalosis, and renal failure. The disorder is due to an excessive ingestion of calcium and absorbable antacids such as milk or calcium carbonate and is less frequent since nonabsorbable antacids and H-2 receptor antagonists such as cimetidine and ranitidine became available for the treatment of peptic ulcer disease.

Individual susceptibility must be important in pathogenesis, since many patients are treated with calcium carbonate without developing the syndrome. One variable is the fractional calcium absorption as a function of calcium intake. Some individuals absorb a high fraction of calcium, even with intakes as high as 2 g and more of elemental calcium per day, instead of reducing calcium absorption with high intake, as occurs in most normal subjects. Resultant mild hypercalcemia after meals in such patients is postulated to be the critical factor in the generation of alkalosis. With the development of hypercalcemia, increased sodium excretion and some depletion of total-body water occur. These phenomena and perhaps, additionally, some suppression of endogenous PTH secretion due to mild hypercalcemia would lead to increased bicarbonate resorption. This bicarbonate retention then would lead to alkalosis in the face of continued calcium carbonate ingestion. Alkalosis per se causes selective enhancement of calcium resorption in the distal nephron, thus aggravating the hypercalcemia. The cycle of mild hypercalcemia → bicarbonate retention → alkalosis → renal calcium retention → severe hypercalcemia perpetuates and aggravates hypercalcemia and alkalosis as long as calcium and absorbable alkali are ingested.

Acute hypercalcemia and alkalosis occurring within days of beginning calcium and alkali ingestion, *acute milk-alkali syndrome*, is manifested by weakness, myalgia, irritability, and apathy. The impairment of renal function, including reduced renal concentrating ability and tubular dysfunction as well as hypercalcemia and alkalosis, reverses rapidly upon stopping the intake of calcium and alkali.

The far-advanced milk-alkali syndrome, sometimes referred to as *Burnett's syndrome*, is due to long-standing calcium and alkali ingestion. Severe hypercalcemia, irreversible renal failure, and phos-

phate retention may be accompanied by ectopic calcification. Some improvement may result when the ingestion of calcium and alkali is reduced, but prior to the availability of renal dialysis, renal failure led to death. There is an intermediate or subacute form in which the renal failure is reversible over a period of weeks after withdrawal of excessive calcium and alkali intake.

DIFFERENTIAL DIAGNOSIS: SPECIAL TESTS Differential diagnosis of hypercalcemia is best achieved by using clinical criteria, but the radioimmunoassay for PTH, as now modified, is useful in distinguishing among major causes. The clinical features that deserve major emphasis are the presence or absence of symptoms or signs of disease and evidence of chronicity. If one discounts fatigue or depression, patients with *asymptomatic hypercalcemia* have primary hyperparathyroidism in well over 90 percent of instances; symptoms of malignancy are usually present when hypercalcemia is due to cancer. Disorders other than hyperparathyroidism and malignancy cause no more than 10 percent of cases of hypercalcemia, and some of the nonparathyroid causes are associated with clear-cut manifestations such as renal failure.

Chronicity is the second most important clinical criterion. If hypercalcemia has been manifest for more than 1 year, malignancy can usually be excluded as the cause of hypercalcemia. A striking feature of malignancy-associated hypercalcemia is the rapidity of the course, whereby signs and symptoms of the underlying malignancy are evident within months of the detection of hypercalcemia. Hyperparathyroidism is the likely diagnosis in patients with *chronic hypercalcemia*. Diseases such as sarcoidosis are rare causes of chronic hypercalcemia. A careful *history* of dietary supplements and drug use will often readily reveal intoxication with vitamins D or A or the use of thiazides.

Although clinical considerations are helpful in arriving at the correct diagnosis of the cause of hypercalcemia, appropriate laboratory testing is essential for definitive diagnosis (Table 357-3). Theoretically, the radioimmunoassay for PTH should separate hyperparathyroidism from all other causes of hypercalcemia, those with hyperparathyroidism having elevated levels of iPTH despite hypercalcemia and patients with malignancy and the other causes of hypercalcemia (except for other disorders mediated by PTH such as lithium-induced hypercalcemia) having levels of hormone below normal or undetectable. Early assays sometimes gave equivocal results, but assays based on the double-antibody method separate from those with primary hyperparathyroidism hypercalcemic patients with malignancy (Fig. 357-3), thus establishing the method as possessing the relevant specificity and sensitivity to serve the central test in the differential diagnosis (see Table 357-3). $1,25(OH)_2D$ levels are elevated in many (but not all) patients with primary hyperparathyroidism and are also increased in states of vitamin D intoxication, particularly sarcoidosis. In other disorders associated with hypercalcemia, concentrations of $1,25(OH)_2D$ are low or, at the most, normal. Since not all patients with hyperparathyroidism, however, have elevated $1,25(OH)_2D$ levels, and since not all nonparathyroid hypercalcemic patients have suppressed $1,25(OH)_2D$, the test is of low specificity and not cost-effective in

---

TABLE 357-3 Differential diagnosis of hypercalcemia

Clinical issues alone

>90% due to hyperparathyroidism or cancer

If asymptomatic or chronic	Hyperparathyroidism most likely

Use of PTH assay

If PTH level increased (or rarely normal)	Hyperparathyroidism confirmed
If PTH level decreased (or undetectable)	*Acute presentation*—with or without symptoms—screen carefully for malignancy *Chronic*—malignancy unlikely, sarcoidosis or other rarer cause

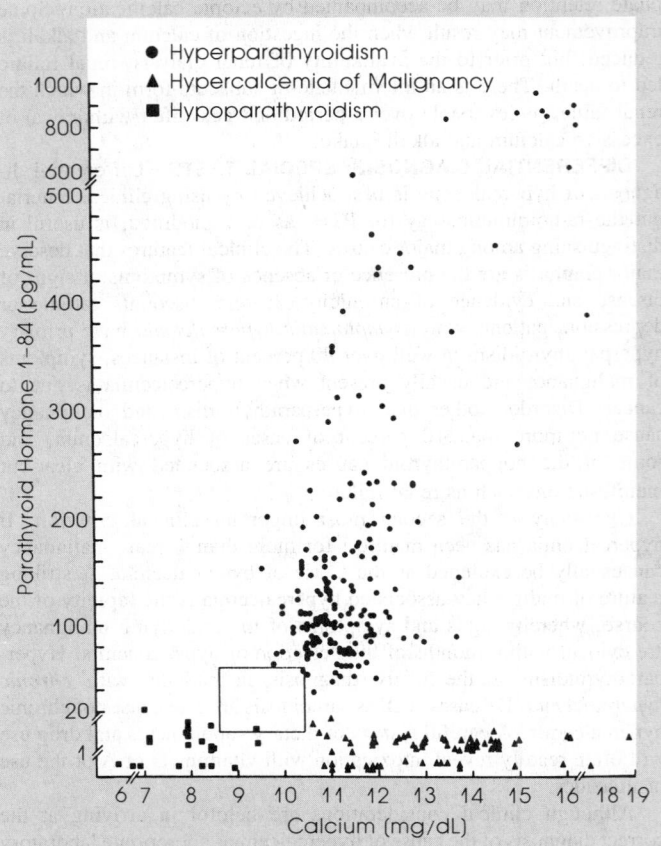

FIGURE 357-3 Levels of iPTH detected in patients with primary hyperparathyroidism, hypercalcemia of malignancy, and hypoparathyroidism. *(From Nussbaum and Potts.)*

differential diagnosis per se; measurement of 1,25(OH)₂D is of critical value in establishing the cause of hypercalcemia in sarcoidosis and certain B cell lymphomas.

PTH levels are elevated in chronic renal failure; the elevation seen in early assays reflects, in part, accumulation of fragments secondary to renal failure rather than true parathyroid oversecretion. Results with the double-antibody assay correlate well with independent evidence for parathyroid gland overactivity. Patients with sarcoidosis have low or undetectable levels of iPTH. No systematic surveys have been reported of the results of double-antibody PTH radioimmunoassays in many of the other non-parathyroid-related causes of hypercalcemia shown in Table 357-1 largely because of the infrequency with which the disorders are encountered, but it is predicted that they will be low or undetectable.

In summary, iPTH values are elevated in greater than 90 percent of parathyroid-related causes of hypercalcemia, undetectable or low in malignancy-related hypercalcemia, and undetectable or normal in vitamin D-related and high-bone-turnover–related causes of hypercalcemia (although there is a paucity of data for these latter categories).

Measurements of nephrogenous cyclic AMP are of limited value in distinguishing primary hyperparathyroidism and malignancy. Elevation of nephrogenous cyclic AMP occurs in some patients with malignancy and in essentially all patients with primary hyperparathyroidism. Specific laboratory tests are of utility in diagnosing particular disorders (such as thyrotoxicosis), and the newer immunoassays for PTH-rP are helpful in diagnosing certain types of malignancy-associated hypercalcemia.

Some general recommendations can be made as to the differential diagnosis of hypercalcemia. Two independent causes of hypercalcemia in the same person, although reported, are rare. If a specific disease traditionally associated with hypercalcemia (see Table 357-1) is

clinically evident, it is reasonable to assume that the disease is responsible for the hypercalcemia. It is cost-effective, in view of the specificity and speed of the PTH radioimmunoassay and the high frequency of hyperparathyroidism in hypercalcemic patients, to measure the iPTH level in all hypercalcemic patients unless malignancy is clinically evident or a specific diagnosis of a nonparathyroid disease is obvious. If hypercalcemia disappears in response to control of hyperthyroidism or after reduction of excessive intake of fat-soluble vitamins or alkali and calcium, in the cases of vitamin D intoxication and milk-alkali syndrome, respectively, there is no need to search for a second cause of hypercalcemia. If specific treatment does not lead to a reversal of the hypercalcemia, a search for an additional cause, by detailed laboratory testing, must be undertaken. It also follows that the management of the patient with the hypercalcemia of malignancy focuses on management of the malignancy.

When the diagnosis is unclear, either because the patient is asymptomatic or because chronic illness obscures manifestations that might indicate the presence of malignancy, the following general approach can be used: If the patient is *asymptomatic* and there is evidence by history of *chronicity* to the hypercalcemia, hyperparathyroidism is almost certainly the cause. If iPTH levels (usually measured at least twice) are elevated, little additional evaluation is necessary. Hyperparathyroidism is never confirmed until abnormal parathyroid tissue is removed surgically and hypercalcemia is corrected, but patients with asymptomatic hypercalcemia can be presumed to have the diagnosis on the basis of elevated concentration of iPTH. If there is a family history suggestive of other endocrine abnormalities, screening for multiple endocrine neoplasia should be undertaken in the patient and family.

If the patient does not have clear-cut symptoms and there is only a short history or no clue as to the duration of the hypercalcemia, *occult malignancy* must be considered. If the iPTH levels with the double-antibody technique are increased, the diagnosis of asymptomatic hyperparathyroidism is established.

If patients with recent-onset hypercalcemia have clear-cut systemic symptoms and/or the iPTH levels are not elevated, then a thorough workup must be undertaken for malignancy, including chest x-ray, computed tomography of chest and abdomen, and bone scan. Attention also should be paid to clues for underlying hematologic disorders such as anemia, increased plasma globulin, and abnormal serum immunoelectrophoresis; bone scans can be negative in patients with multiple myeloma.

Finally, if a patient with *chronic hypercalcemia* is *asymptomatic* but iPTH values are not elevated, and if malignancy seems unlikely on clinical grounds (*chronicity*), it is useful to search for other chronic causes of hypercalcemia, such as occult sarcoidosis. Table 357-3 summarizes the approach.

MEDICAL TREATMENT OF HYPERCALCEMIA   The acute treatment of hypercalcemia is usually successful. The serum calcium concentration can be decreased by 0.7 to 2.2 mmol/L (3 to 9 mg/dL) within 24 to 48 h in most patients, enough to relieve acute symptoms, prevent death from hypercalcemic crisis, and permit diagnostic evaluation. However, the chronic medical management of hypercalcemia is less satisfactory unless the underlying cause can be corrected because available therapies are inconvenient and may be toxic.

Hypercalcemia develops because of excessive skeletal calcium release, increased intestinal calcium absorption, or inadequate renal calcium excretion. Understanding the particular pathogenesis helps guide therapy. For example, hypercalcemia in patients with osteolytic metastases or acute immobilization is primarily due to excessive skeletal calcium release and is, therefore, minimally improved by restriction of dietary calcium. On the other hand, patients with vitamin D hypersensitivity or vitamin D intoxication have excessive intestinal calcium absorption, and restriction of dietary calcium is beneficial. Decreased renal function or extracellular fluid depletion decreases urinary calcium excretion. If additional abnormalities, such as increased bone breakdown, are present, hypercalcemia will develop. This may happen, for example, when patients with resorptive bone disease become dehydrated. In such situations, rehydration may rapidly reduce or reverse the hypercalcemia, even though bone resorption and urinary calcium excretion are increased.

Hydration, increased salt intake, mild and forced diuresis The first principle of treatment is to restore *normal hydration*. Many hypercalcemic patients are dehydrated because of vomiting, inanition, and/or hypercalcemia-induced defects in urinary concentrating ability. The resultant drop in glomerular filtration rate is accompanied by an additional decrease in renal tubular sodium and calcium clearance. Restoring a normal extracellular fluid volume corrects these abnormalities and increases urine calcium excretion by 2.5 to 7.5 mmol/d (100 to 300 mg/d). Increased urinary sodium excretion to 400 to 500 mmol/d increases urinary calcium excretion even further than simple rehydration. After rehydration has been achieved, saline can be administered or furosemide or ethacrynic acid can be given twice daily to depress the tubular reabsorptive mechanism for calcium (care must be taken to prevent dehydration). The combined use of these therapies can increase urinary calcium excretion to 12.5 mmol/d (500 mg/d) or higher in most hypercalcemic patients. Since this is a substantial percentage of the exchangeable calcium pool, the serum calcium concentration usually falls 0.25 to 0.75 mmol/L (1 to 3 mg/dL) within 24 h. Precautions should be taken to prevent potassium and magnesium depletion; calcium-containing renal calculi are a potential complication.

Under life-threatening circumstances, the preceding approach can be pursued more aggressively, giving as much as 6 L isotonic saline (900 mmol sodium) daily plus furosemide or equivalent in doses up to 100 mg every 1 to 2 h or ethacrynic acid in doses to 40 mg every 1 to 2 h. Urinary calcium excretion may exceed 25 mmol/d (1000 mg/d), and the serum calcium may decrease by 1 mmol/L (4 mg/dL) or more within 24 h. Depletion of potassium and magnesium is inevitable unless replacements are given; pulmonary edema can be precipitated. The potential complications can be reduced by careful monitoring of central venous pressure and plasma or urine electrolytes; a bladder catheter may be necessary. This treatment approach should be immediately supplemented with agents to block bone resorption

that become effective within a few days, since forced diuresis is difficult to sustain even in patients with good cardiopulmonary and renal function.

Bisphosphonates The bisphosphonates are analogues of pryophosphate, with high affinity for bone, especially in areas of increased bone turnover. These bone-seeking compounds are stable in vivo because phosphatase enzymes cannot hydrolyze the central carbon-phosphorus-carbon bond. The bisphosphonates are concentrated in areas of high bone turnover and are taken up by and inhibit osteoclast action; the detailed mechanism of action is not well understood. Bisphosphonates may alter proton pump function or impair the release of acid hydrolases into the excellular lysosomes contiguous with mineralized bone. They also may inhibit the differentiation of monocyte-macrophage precursors into osteoclasts.

Etidronate, a first-generation bisphosphonate, is poorly absorbed and, like most bisphosphonates, generally must be given intravenously to be effective. At times, the continuation of oral etidronate after intravenous therapy may be useful to control hypercalcemia.

A newer class of bisphosphonates has more favorable efficacy and longer duration of action (Table 357-4). Pamidronate is a potent inhibitor of osteoclast-mediated skeletal resorption yet does not cause mineralization defects as ordinary doses. (Pamidronate is approved by the FDA for intravenous use for hypercalcemia of malignancy.) Several additional bisphosphonates (alendronate, toludronate, and risidronate) that are highly potent and have a favorable ratio of blocking resorption over inhibiting bone formation are undergoing clinical trials in the United States. Between 60 and 90 mg pamidronate, given as a single intravenous dose, returns serum calcium to normal in 80 to 100 percent of patients for weeks or months.

While the bisphosphonates have similar structures, efficacy, toxicity, and side effects vary. Etidronate therapy results in hyperphosphatemia, through a direct renal mechanism, whereas hypophosphatemia is seen following therapy with other bisphosphonates. Toxicities of the aminobisphosphonates include low-grade fever in as many as 20 percent of patients, likely related to release of cytokines from osteoclasts, monocytes, and macrophages, and possibility,

TABLE 357-4 Therapies for severe hypercalcemia

Treatment	Onset of action	Duration of action	Advantages	Disadvantages
MOST USEFUL THERAPIES				
Hydration with saline	Hours	During infusion	Rehydration invariably needed	
Forced diuresis; saline + loop diuretic	Hours	During treatment	Rapid action	Cardiac decompensation, intensive monitoring electrolyte disturbance hypokalemia, hypomagnesemia
Bisphosphonates				
1st generation: etidronate	1–2 days	5–7 days in doses used	First available bisphosphonate; intermediate onset of action	Hyperphosphatemia; 3-day infusion
2d generation: pamidronate	1–2 days	10–14 days after high dose	High potency; intermediate onset; prolonged duration of action	Fever in 20%; hypophosphatemia hypocalcemia, hypomagnesemia
Calcitonin	Hours	2–3 days	Rapid onset of action; useful as adjunct in severe hypercalcemia	Often limited calcium lowering, rapid tachyphylaxis
OTHER THERAPIES				
Gallium nitrate	Day after 5-day administration	7–10 days	High potency	Length of IV administration; cannot be used with renal failure
Plicamycin	3–4 days	Days	Potent antiresorptive	Liver, kidney, and marrow toxicity; bleeding
Phosphate				
Oral	24 h	During use	Low toxicity if P < 4 mg/dL	Limited use except as adjuvant or chronic therapy
Intravenous	Hours	During use and 24–48 h afterward	Rapid action, highly potent	Ectopic calcification; severe hypocalcemia
Glucocorticoids	Days	Days, weeks	Oral therapy, antitumor agent	Active only in certain malignancies; glucocorticoid side effects
Dialysis	Hours	During use and 24–48 h afterward	Useful in renal failure; onset of effect in hours; can immediately reverse life-threatening hypercalcemia	Complex procedure, reserved for extreme or special circumstances

reversible hepatocellular injury (Table 357-4). Overall, second-generation bisphosphonates are now the agents of choice in several hypercalcemia, particularly that associated with malignancy.

Calcitonin Calcitonin acts within minutes of its administration, through receptors on osteoclasts, to decrease the release of skeletal calcium, phosphorus, and hydroxyproline. In addition, inhibition of renal tubular calcium reabsorption may, in part, contribute to its rapid onset of action. In various reports, however, the administration of 2 to 8 U/kg of body weight intravenously, subcutaneously, or intramuscularly every 6 to 12 h caused variable and minimal lowering of calcium in some patients. Tachyphylaxis, a well-known phenomenon with this drug, may explain the variable results. This escape from the hypocalcemic effects of calcitonin is seen in vitro, where it can be prevented by glucocorticoids. In vivo in humans, administration of glucocorticoids in combination with calcitonin may augment or prolong the action of calcitonin; in some patients, particularly those with lymphoproliferative malignancies, continued lowering of calcium may last for as long as 10 days. In other studies, however, the prevention of tachyphylaxis by glucocorticoids was not impressive. Calcitonin therapy with the salmon, porcine, and human sequences, as currently used, rarely returns serum calcium to normal and can best be viewed as a nontoxic therapy with a very rapid onset of action and definite, although limited, efficacy. However, in life-threatening hypercalcemia, calcitonin can be used while waiting for a more sustained effects from plicamycin, gallium, or bisphosphonate. Calcitonin therapy may be associated with transient nausea, cramping, abdominal pain, and flushing.

Plicamycin For the acute management of hypercalcemia, plicamycin (mithramycin), which inhibits bone resorption, has been a useful therapeutic agent. Plicamycin must be given intravenously, either as a bolus injection or by slow infusion. The usual dose is 25 μg/kg of body weight. In some patients, 10 μg/kg of body weight can be given twice a week for chronic therapy. Treatment should not be repeated until hypercalcemia recurs, because the toxicity of the drug is dependent on the frequency of treatment and the total dosage. Careful monitoring is needed if repeated doses are used. The major side effects are thrombocytopenia, hepatocellular necrosis with increased lactic acid dehydrogenase (LDH) and aspartate aminotransferase (AST) levels, and decreased levels of clotting factors with resultant epistaxis, bruising, hemorrhage, and bleeding gums. Azotemia, proteinuria, and hypocalcemia may occur. Hypophosphatemia, hypokalemia, nausea, vomiting, stomatitis, and facial swelling may occur. Toxicity is rare when only one or two doses are used and can be minimized by repeating single doses only when hypercalcemia recurs. Toxic effects other than hemorrhage can usually be reversed by stopping the drug. Use of plicamycin has been largely replaced by the less toxic second-generation bisphosphonates.

Gallium nitrate Gallium nitrate exerts a hypocalcemic action by inhibiting bone resorption and altering the structure of bone crystals. The major disadvantages appear to be the 5-day duration of infusion and the potential for nephrotoxicity. Alternative, shorter-dosage regimens have not been reported. (Gallium nitrate is approved by the FDA for the treatment of hypercalcemia; further clinical experience should help define its ultimate role.)

Other therapies Glucocorticoids increase urinary calcium excretion and decrease intestinal calcium absorption when given in pharmacologic doses (e.g., 40 to 200 mg prednisone daily in divided doses), but they also cause negative skeletal calcium balance. In normal subjects and in patients with primary hyperparathyroidism, glucocorticoids neither increase nor decrease the serum calcium concentration. In patients with hypercalcemia due to certain osteolytic malignancies, however, glucocorticoids may be effective as a result of antitumor effects. The malignancies in which hypercalcemia responds to glucocorticoids include hematologic malignancies such as multiple myeloma, leukemia, Hodgkin's disease, other lymphomas, and carcinoma of the breast, at least early in the course. Glucocorticoids are also effective in treating hypercalcemia due to vitamin D intoxication and sarcoidosis. In all the preceding situations, the hypocalcemic effect develops over several days, and the usual glucocorticoid dosage is 40 to 100 mg prednisone (or its equivalent) daily in four divided doses. The side effects of chronic glucocorticoid therapy may be acceptable in some circumstances.

Hypercalcemia complicated by renal failure is difficult to manage; dialysis is often the treatment of choice. Peritoneal dialysis with calcium-free dialysis fluid can remove 5 to 12.5 mmol (200 to 500 mg) of calcium in 24 to 48 h and lower the serum calcium concentration by 0.7 to 3 mmol/L (3 to 12 mg/dL). Large quantities of phosphate are lost during dialysis, and serum inorganic phosphate concentrations usually fall, thus aggravating hypercalcemia. Therefore, the serum inorganic phosphate concentration should be measured after dialysis, and phosphate supplements should be added to the diet or to dialysis fluids if necessary.

Phosphate therapy, oral or intravenous, has a role in certain circumstances. Patients with primary hyperparathyroidism are frequently hypophosphatemic, and hypercalcemia of other causes also may be complicated by hypophosphatemia. Hypophosphatemia decreases the rate of calcium uptake into bone, increases intestinal calcium absorption, and directly and indirectly stimulates bone breakdown. These effects aggravate hypercalcemia, and correcting hypophosphatemia lowers the serum calcium concentration. The usual treatment is 1 to 1.5 g phosphorus per day for several days, given in four divided doses to minimize the chances of developing hyperphosphatemia. Such therapy has been administered for prolonged periods in selected patients. It is generally believed but not established that toxicity will not occur if the phosphate therapy is limited to restoring serum inorganic phosphate concentrations to normal rather than making them supranormal.

Raising the serum inorganic phosphate concentration above normal does decrease serum calcium levels, sometimes strikingly. Intravenous phosphate is one of the most dramatically effective treatments available for severe hypercalcemia but is toxic and even dangerous so that it is used rarely and *only* in severely hypercalcemic patients with cardiac or renal failure. A dose of 1500 mg phosphate phosphorus or more intravenously over 6 to 8 h leads to a prompt decrease in serum calcium of as much as 1.2 to 2.5 mmol/L (5 to 10 mg/dL) in patients with initially normal serum inorganic phosphate concentrations. This therapy should be employed only in extreme emergencies for two reasons. First, fatal hypocalcemia can be produced by excessive dosage; serum calcium should be measured frequently if intravenous phosphate is administered. Second, unlike sodium chloride, sodium phosphate does not remove calcium from the body. In fact, urine calcium generally declines, and fecal calcium declines or remains the same. The decline in serum calcium reflects a redistribution of calcium within the body. There is a rapid efflux of calcium with no change in calcium influx to the circulation, findings indicative of precipitation of calcium phosphate salt. The calcium precipitates in bone, and metastatic calcification also may occur in patients receiving oral or intravenous phosphate therapy for hypercalcemia. Indeed, hyperphosphatemia can cause metastatic calcification in normocalcemic animals. Thus administration of intravenous phosphate in patients with compromised renal function who cannot have diuretic therapy is justifiable only as an emergency treatment.

Inorganic phosphate is commercially available for oral use in liquid, powder, and capsule form and as a liquid for intravenous use. It is important to calculate doses in terms of phosphate phosphorus (see Table 357-5).

Summary The various therapies for hypercalcemia are listed in Table 357-4. The choice depends on the underlying disease, the severity of the hypercalcemia, the serum inorganic phosphate level, and the renal, hepatic, and bone marrow function. Mild hypercalcemia [3 mmol/L (12 mg/dL) or less] can usually be managed by the sequence of hydration followed by intravenous sodium chloride and, if needed, small doses of furosemide or ethacrynic acid. Severe hypercalcemia [3.7 mmol/L (15 mg/dL)] requires rapid correction. Calcitonin should be given for its rapid, albeit short-lived, blockade of bone resorption, and intravenous pamidronate should be administered,

TABLE 357-5 Commercially available phosphate preparations

	1000 mg P	mmol Na	mmol K
ORAL PREPARATIONS			
Neutraphos (1250-mg capsule)	4 caps	28.5	28.5
Neutraphos-K (1450-mg capsule)	4 caps	—	57
Phos-Tabs (860-mg tablet)	6 tabs	—	51
Fleets Phospho-Soda (liquid)	6.7 mL	40	—
INTRAVENOUS PREPARATIONS			
In-Phos	40 mL	65	8
Hyper-Phos-K	15 mL	—	50

SOURCE: After RM Neer and JT Potts Jr, in *Endocrinology*, LJ DeGroot et al (eds), 2d ed, Philadelphia, Saunders, 1989, with permission.

although its onset of action is delayed for 1 to 2 days. Hence aggressive sodium-calcium diuresis with intravenous saline and large doses of furosemide and ethacrynic acid works but should be initiated only if appropriate monitoring is available and cardiac function is adequate.

There is a role for oral phosphate therapy in chronic management of hypercalcemia, but its utility may be superseded by the bisphosphonates. Phosphate supplements should only be administered if hyperphosphatemia is not present.

Severe dietary calcium restriction should be employed and glucocorticoids should be administered judiciously if intestinal absorption is enhanced (in sarcoidosis, vitamin D intoxication). Dialysis is appropriate for hypercalcemia complicating acute or chronic renal failure.

Chronic therapy of hypercalcemia poses greater problems of toxicity. One satisfactory regimen for chronic use is a combination of dietary calcium restriction, administration of sodium chloride with or without furosemide or ethacrynic acid to maintain high urinary calcium, and moderate-dose oral phosphate (the patient is kept normophosphatemic). Some of the effective remedies (plicamycin, glucocorticoids, high-dose oral phosphate) may have significant toxicity when used chronically. Oral bisphosphonates, if proven nontoxic, may become the chronic treatment of choice in cases of hypercalcemia where increased bone resorption is responsible for the disturbance in calcium metabolism.

HYPOCALCEMIA

PATHOPHYSIOLOGY OF HYPOCALCEMIA: CLASSIFICATION BASED ON MECHANISM *Chronic hypocalcemia* is less common than hypercalcemia; causes include chronic renal failure, hereditary and acquired hypoparathyroidism, vitamin D deficiency, pseudohypoparathyroidism, and hypomagnesemia.

Critically ill patients may have *transient hypocalcemia* in association with severe sepsis, burns, acute renal failure, and extensive transfusions with citrated blood. Acute hypocalcemia in association with certain medications is also usually transient and may have no symptoms. Although as many as half of patients in intensive care setting are reported to have calcium concentrations below 2.1 mmol/L (8.5 mg/dL), less than 10 percent have a reduction in ionized calcium. Patients with severe sepsis may have a decrease in ionized calcium (true hypocalcemia), but in other severely ill subjects, hypoalbuminemia is the cause of the reduced total calcium concentration. Alkalosis, however, increases calcium binding to proteins, and in this setting, direct measurements of ionized calcium should be made.

Medications such as protamine, heparin, and glucagon may cause transient hypocalcemia. These forms of hypocalcemia, apparent or real, are usually not associated with tetany and resolve with improvement in the overall medical condition. The hypocalcemia after repeated transfusions of citrated blood also usually resolves quickly.

Patients with acute *pancreatitis* have hypocalcemia that persists during the acute inflammation and varies in degree with the severity of the pancreatitis. The cause of hypocalcemia in pancreatitis remains unclear. PTH values are variously reported to be low, normal, or elevated, and both resistance to PTH and impaired PTH secretion have been postulated. Occasionally, a chronic low total-blood calcium and low ionized calcium concentration are detected in an elderly patient without obvious cause and with a paucity of symptoms of hypocalcemia; the pathogenesis is unclear.

Chronic hypocalcemia, however, is usually symptomatic and requires treatment. Neuromuscular and neurologic manifestations of chronic hypocalcemia include muscle spasms, carpopedal spasm, facial grimacing, and in extreme cases, laryngeal spasm and convulsions. Respiratory arrest may occur. Increased intracranial pressure occurs in some patients with long-standing hypocalcemia, often in association with papilledema. Mental changes include irritability, depression, and psychosis. The QT interval on the electrocardiogram is prolonged, in contrast to its shortening with hypercalcemia. Arrhythmias occur, and digitalis effectiveness may be reduced. Intestinal cramps and chronic malabsorption may occur. Chvostek's or Trousseau's sign can be used to confirm latent tetany.

The classification of hypocalcemia shown in Table 357-6 is based on the premise that PTH is responsible for minute-to-minute regulation of plasma calcium concentration within narrow limits and, therefore, that the occurrence of hypocalcemia must mean a failure of the homeostatic action of PTH. Failure of the PTH response can occur if PTH is absent due to hereditary or acquired gland failure, if the hormone is ineffective at target organs, or if the action of the hormone is overwhelmed by the loss of calcium from the extracellular fluid at a rate faster than it can be replaced.

PTH ABSENT Hypoparathyroidism, whether hereditary or acquired, has a number of common components. Acute and chronic symptoms of untreated hypocalcemia are shared by both types of hypoparathyroidism, although typically the onset of hereditary hypoparathyroidism is more gradual and hereditary hypoparathyroidism is associated with developmental defects. In earlier decades, acquired hypoparathyroidism secondary to surgery in the neck was

TABLE 357-6 Functional classification of hypocalcemia (excluding neonatal conditions)

PTH ABSENT

A Hereditary hypoparathyroidism
B Acquired hypoparathyroidism
C Hypomagnesemia

PTH INEFFECTIVE

A Chronic renal failure
B Active vitamin D lacking
   1 ↓ dietary intake or sunlight
   2 Defective metabolism:
     Anticonvulsant therapy
     Vitamin D–dependent rickets type I
C Active vitamin D ineffective
   1 Intestinal malabsorption
   2 Vitamin D–dependent rickets type II
D Pseudohypoparathyroidism

PTH OVERWHELMED

A Severe, acute hyperphosphatemia
   1 Tumor lysis
   2 Acute renal failure
   3 Rhabdomyolysis
B Osteitis fibrosa after parathyroidectomy

more common than hereditary hypoparathyroidism, but the frequency of surgically induced parathyroid failure has diminished as a result of parathyroid gland preservation and the use of nonsurgical treatment of hyperthyroidism. Basal ganglia calcification and extrapyramidal syndromes are more common and earlier in onset in hereditary hypoparathyroidism. Pseudohypoparathyroidism, an example of ineffective PTH action rather than a failure of parathyroid gland production, shares several features with hypoparathyroidism, including extraosseous calcification and extrapyramidal manifestations such as choreoathetotic movements and dystonia. Papilledema and raised intracranial pressure occur in both states, as do chronic changes in fingernails and hair and lenticular cataracts, the latter usually reversible with treatment of hypocalcemia. Certain skin manifestations, including alopecia and candidiasis, occur exclusively in hereditary hypoparathyroidism.

Hypocalcemia associated with hypomagnesemia is associated with both deficient PTH release and impaired responsiveness to the hormone (see also Chap. 360). Patients with hypocalcemia secondary to hypomagnesemia have absent or low levels of circulating PTH, indicative of diminished hormone release despite maximum physiologic stimulus by hypocalcemia. Plasma PTH levels return to normal with correction of the hypomagnesemia. Thus hypoparathyroidism associated with low levels of PTH in blood can be due to hereditary gland failure, acquired gland failure, or acute but reversible gland dysfunction (hypomagnesemia). Patients with acquired or hereditary hypoparathyroidism also have hyperphosphatemia and absent or low levels of $1,25(OH)_2D$.

Hereditary hypoparathyroidism Hypoparathyroidism can occur as an isolated entity without other endocrine or dermatologic manifestations (idiopathic hypoparathyroidism) or, more typically, in association with other abnormalities such as defective development of the thymus or failure of function of other endocrine organs such as the adrenal thyroid or ovary (see also Chap. 343). Idiopathic and hereditary hypoparathyroidisms are often manifest within the first decade but may appear later.

One rare form of hypoparathyroidism due to congenital aplasia of the parathyroid glands is manifested shortly after birth; there is a linkage between defective development of the thymus and the parathyroid glands. The disorder is termed the *DiGeorge syndrome*, or the *third and fourth branchial pouch syndrome*, is associated with congenital cardiovascular and other developmental defects. Most patients die in early childhood with severe infections, hypocalcemia and seizures, or cardiovascular complications. Some patients survive into adulthood. Milder, incomplete forms are recognized. Most cases are sporadic. Cytogenetic abnormalities involving chromosome 22 are reported.

Hypoparathyroidism can occur in association with other diverse developmental defects or as part of a complex hereditary autoimmune syndrome involving failure of the adrenals, the ovaries, and the parathyroids in association with recurrent mucocutaneous candidiasis, alopecia, vitiligo, and pernicious anemia (see Chap. 343). In many cases, antibodies to endocrine organs are present; there is, in addition, a failure of cell-mediated immunity. The inheritance of the autoimmune syndrome appears to be autosomal recessive, and some unaffected family members show antibodies to endocrine tissue without evidence of endocrine failure. The disorder is usually referred to as autoimmune polyglandular deficiency.

Hereditary hypoparathyroidism occurs also as an isolated entity without any other defects. The mechanism of inheritance varies from one kindred to another. Autosomal dominant, autosomal recessive, and X-linked inheritance patterns have all been identified. In one family in which the disorder was transmitted as an autosomal dominant trait, a structural abnormality in the PTH gene has been identified. The defect in the signal sequence needed for processing of the hormone before secretion rather than in the structural portion interferes with PTH secretion. In one kindred with autosomal recessive inheritance, the homozygous mutant allele has a mutation in the first gene intron which causes a splicing defect in mRNA production. Most

kindreds, however, have no clue as to the genetic origin of the hypoparathyroidism.

Treatment of hypoparathyroidism is similar to that for acquired hypoparathyroidism and pseudohypoparathyroidism, although specific features of each disease require additional treatments. Replacement therapy with vitamin D or calcitriol combined with a high oral calcium intake usually suffices to regulate blood calcium and phosphate levels satisfactorily. Oral calcium and vitamin D restore the overall calcium-phosphate balance but do not reverse the lowered urinary calcium reabsorption typical of hypoparathyroidism. Therefore, care must be taken to avoid excessive urinary calcium excretion after vitamin D and calcium replacement therapy; otherwise, kidney stones can develop. Thiazide diuretics lower urine calcium by as much as 100 mg/d in hypoparathyroid patients on vitamin D, provided patients are maintained on a low-sodium diet. Use of thiazides seems to be of benefit in mitigating hypercalciuria.

Acquired hypoparathyroidism *Acquired chronic hypoparathyroidism* is usually the result of inadvertent surgical removal of all the parathyroid glands; in some instances, not all the tissue is removed, but the remainder undergoes compromise of vascular supply secondary to fibrotic changes in the neck after surgery. In the past, the most frequent cause of acquired hypoparathyroidism was surgery for hyperthyroidism. Hypoparathyroidism now usually occurs after surgery for hyperparathyroidism when the surgeon, facing the dilemma of removing too little tissue and thus not curing the hyperparathyroidism, removes too much.

Parathyroid function is not totally absent in all patients with postoperative hypoparathyroidism, but suitable therapy varies greatly from patient to patient irrespective of the type of hypoparathyroidism or the question of residual parathyroid activity.

Even rarer causes of acquired chronic hypoparathyroidism include radiation-induced damage subsequent to radioiodine therapy of hyperthyroidism or glandular damage in patients with hemochromatosis or hemosiderosis after repeated blood transfusions. Chronic infections may involve one or more of the parathyroids but usually do not cause permanent hypoparathyroidism because all four glands are not usually involved.

Transient hypoparathyroidism is frequent following surgical exploration for hyperparathyroidism. Often, after a variable period of hypoparathyroidism, normal parathyroid function returns due to hyperplasia or recovery of remaining tissue. Occasionally, recovery occurs months after surgery. The management of transient postoperative hypoparathyroidism is discussed under the surgical treatment of hyperparathyroidism. The treatment of chronic acquired hypoparathyroidism is similar to that used with idiopathic hypoparathyroidism: replacement with calcitriol and oral calcium.

Hypomagnesemia Hypomagnesemia of a severe degree is associated with severe hypocalcemia (see also Chap. 360). Restoration of the total-body magnesium deficits leads to rapid reversal of hypocalcemia. There are least two causes of the hypocalcemia—impaired secretion and reduced responsiveness to PTH.

Hypomagnesemia is generally classified as primary or secondary; primary hypomagnesemia is due to hereditary defects in intestinal absorption or renal reabsorption of magnesium. Secondary hypomagnesemia, a more common condition, occurs on a nutritional basis or as a result of acquired intestinal or renal disorders. The most common causes of the secondary disorder are chronic alcoholism with poor nutritional intake, intestinal malabsorption syndromes, and parenteral nutrition in which magnesium replacement is omitted.

Magnesium in extracellular fluid has effects similar to those of calcium on secretion of PTH; hypermagnesemia suppresses and hypomagnesemia stimulates PTH secretion. Effects of magnesium on hormone secretion are normally of little physiologic significance, however, because the effects of calcium dominate. Greater change in magnesium than in calcium is needed to influence hormone secretion. Nonetheless, hypomagnesemia, if it influences hormone secretion at all, might be expected to increase hormone secretion. It is therefore surprising to find that severe hypomagnesemia is associated with blunted secretion of PTH. The explanation for the paradox is that severe, chronic hypomagnesemia reflects intracellular magnesium deficiency; severe intracellular magnesium deficiency interferes with secretion and peripheral responses to PTH. The mechanism of the cellular defects due to hypomagnesemia is unknown, although a defective adenylate cyclase response (for which magnesium may serve as a cofactor) has been proposed.

Severe hypocalcemia is often seen when serum magnesium is substantially below the normal range of 0.8 to 1.2 mmol/L (2 to 3 mg/dL). In most cases in which hypomagnesemia is associated with hypocalcemia, serum magnesium is below 0.4 mmol/L (1.0 mg/dL).

PTH levels are usually undetectable or inappropriately low despite the extreme stimulus of severe hypocalcemia, and acute repletion of magnesium leads to a rapid increase in PTH concentration. The overall data indicate that PTH secretion is blunted in virtually all patients with severe hypomagnesemia; thus absolute or relative hypoparathyroidism seems to be the rule in patients with hypocalcemia secondary to hypomagnesemia.

In addition, diminished peripheral responsiveness to administered PTH occurs in some patients, as manifested by subnormal response in urinary phosphorus and urinary cyclic AMP excretion after administration of exogenous PTH to hypomagnesemic patients who are hypocalcemic. Both blunted PTH secretion and lack of renal response to administered PTH can occur in the same patient. When acute magnesium repletion is undertaken, the restoration of PTH concentrations to normal or supranormal levels may precede by several days the restoration of normal serum calcium.

Overall, blunted PTH secretory response in hypomagnesemia seems the real cause of hypocalcemia. The fact that impaired peripheral responsiveness, particularly renal response, is more variable from patient to patient suggests that an even greater degree of magnesium deficiency is required to induce end-organ resistance than to impair hormone secretion.

Several other features have been noted. The brisk response in hormone secretion following magnesium repletion, sometimes demonstrable within minutes of giving a large parenteral dose of magnesium, indicates that hormone biosynthesis is not impaired, only secretion. Serum phosphate levels are often not elevated, as they usually are in patients with acquired or idiopathic hypoparathyroidism, probably because phosphate deficiency is a frequent accompaniment of hypomagnesemia. Magnesium wasting may occur in chronic renal disease; magnesium is usually elevated in acute renal failure but is usually normal in chronic renal failure.

Repletion of magnesium is the cure of the condition, and attention must be given to restoring the intracellular deficiency, which may be considerable. After intravenous magnesium administration, serum magnesium may return transiently to the normal range, but unless replacement therapy is adequate, serum magnesium will rapidly fall to subnormal levels again. If renal function is normal, a useful indicator of restoration of magnesium deficiency is the urinary magnesium excretion; magnesium is retained by the kidney until magnesium deficiencies are repleted. Intracellular deficits can be as great as 50 mmol or more. Parenteral administration of 10 to 14 mmol magnesium usually reverses the signs of magnesium deficiency. If the cause of the hypomagnesemia is renal magnesium wasting, treatment may have to be administered chronically to prevent recurrence.

PTH INEFFECTIVE PTH can be considered ineffective when the hormone receptor–guanyl nucleotide-biding protein complex is defective or when PTH action to promote calcium absorption from the diet is interfered with because of a primary deficiency of vitamin D or because of conditions in which vitamin D is ineffective (receptor or synthesis defects) or in chronic renal failure in which the calcium-elevating action of PTH is opposed by several different processes associated with uremia.

Despite diverse pathophysiologic mechanisms, these latter conditions involving ineffectiveness of PTH (excluding the rare condition of defective PTH-receptor response) often involve, but are not limited to, the unavailability of vitamin D as a cofactor for PTH. Hypocalcemia is usually mild and is accompanied by hypophosphatemia. Typically, hypophosphatemia is more severe than hypocalcemia due to the increased secretion of PTH. Increased PTH is only partly effective in elevating blood calcium, but its ability to promote renal phosphate excretion is only slightly impaired in vitamin D deficiency. Varying degrees of bone disease with impaired mineralization and/or frank osteomalacia are the more frequent and harmful consequences of chronic renal failure or inadequate or ineffective vitamin D action due to the hypophosphatemia.

Pseudohypoparathyroidism, on the other hand, has a distinct pathophysiology from the other disorders of ineffective PTH action. Pseudohypoparathyroidism most closely resembles conditions in which there is an absence of PTH synthesis and secretion and is manifested, in the untreated state, by hypocalcemia and hyperphosphatemia. The cause of the disease, however, is defective hormone binding to the receptor or deficient activation of guanyl nucleotide-binding proteins, resulting in failure to increase intracellular cyclic AMP (see below).

Chronic renal failure Severe abnormalities in mineral and bone metabolism occur in chronic renal failure, and improved medical management of chronic renal failure and/or a more indolent course of the renal disease allow many patients to survive long enough for renal osteodystrophy, the mixed bone disease associated with renal failure, to became an important feature. The roles of phosphate retention and impaired production of 1,25(OH)$_2$D are recognized as the principal factors responsible for inducing calcium deficiency, secondary hyperparathyroidism, and frequently a picture of severe bone disease. The uremic state appears to be associated also with impairment of intestinal absorption by factors other than defects in vitamin D metabolism. Nonetheless, treatment with supraphysiologic amounts of vitamin D or calcitriol leads to satisfactory calcium absorption.

Hyperphosphatemia per se in renal failure tends to lower blood calcium concentration by several actions; these include extraosseous deposition of calcium and phosphate, impaired sensitivity of the skeleton to the bone-resorbing action of PTH, reduced 1,25(OH)$_2$D production by surviving renal tissue, and reduction in calcium absorption due to trapping of calcium in insoluble form as calcium phosphate complexes. In animals, prevention of hyperphosphatemia by dietary means can block the development of secondary hyperparathyroidism, emphasizing the importance of phosphate retention in the pathogenesis of secondary hyperparathyroidism and the associated disorders of mineral and bone metabolism in renal failure. Low levels of 1,25(OH)$_2$D are due to hyperphosphatemia and to destruction of renal tissue and are critical in the hypocalcemia.

Therapy of chronic renal failure (see Chaps. 237 and 238) involves careful management of patients prior to dialysis as well as adjustment of dialysis regimens once this becomes necessary. Attention should be paid to restriction of phosphate in the diet, use of phosphate-binding antacids such as those based on aluminum hydroxide or calcium-containing salts which serve as phosphate binders and as a source of needed calcium supplementation and which avoid the problem of aluminum intoxication, provision of an adequate calcium intake by mouth, usually 1 to 2 g/d, and supplementation with 0.25 to 1.0 μg/d calcitriol. Each patient must be monitored closely. The aims of therapy are to restore normal calcium balance to prevent osteomalacia and secondary hyperparathyroidism. Renal osteodystrophy, as discussed earlier, is the principal disabling feature of chronic renal failure related to calcium metabolism. Reduction of hyperphosphatemia and restoration of normal intestinal calcium absorption by calcitriol can improve blood calcium concentration and reduce the manifestations of secondary hyperparathyroidism.

Vitamin D deficiency due to inadequate diet and/or sunlight Vitamin D deficiency is more common in the United States than previously recognized. Biopsies of bone in elderly patients with hip fracture (documenting osteomalacia) and abnormal concentrations of vitamin D metabolites, PTH, calcium, and phosphate have established that vitamin D deficiency may occur in as many as 25 percent of elderly patients, particularly in areas where there is little ambient sunlight. Concentrations of 25(OH)D are at the lower limits of normal or below normal in these patients. Quantitative histomorphometry of bone biopsy specimens reveals widened osteoid seams consistent with osteomalacia. PTH hypersecretion compensates for a tendency of the blood calcium level to fall, but with the consequence of inducing renal phosphate wasting and a combined mineral ion abnormality that results in osteomalacia.

The genesis of vitamin D deficiency is impaired intake of dairy products that are enriched with vitamin D, lack of vitamin supplementation, and reduced sunlight exposure in the elderly, particularly in winter in northern latitudes.

Treatment involves the administration of vitamin D and provision of 1 to 1.5 g calcium in the diet. Vitamin D supplementation should aim to provide several times the recommended daily requirement in younger people, which is probably a safe recommendation; a dosage of 1000 to 2000 units of vitamin D per day is satisfactory. Vitamin D is usually not available in small-dose forms. Hence the administration of a capsule containing 50,000 units of vitamin D once monthly is safe in elderly patients who have osteomalacia. The increased awareness of the importance of calcium supplementation, particularly in women, even without supplementation of vitamin D, may lessen the frequency of this problem. Severe hypocalcemia is rarely seen in the moderately severe vitamin D deficiency of the elderly, but vitamin D deficiency needs to be considered in the differential diagnosis of mild hypocalcemia.

Defective vitamin D metabolism ANTICONVULSANT THERAPY Anticonvulsant therapy with any of several agents induces a state of acquired vitamin D deficiency by increasing the conversion of vitamin D into inactive compounds. The more marginal the degree of vitamin D intake in the diet, the more likely that anticonvulsant therapy will lead to abnormalities in mineral and bone metabolism. The syndrome at its extreme involves severe rickets with bone fractures, hypocalcemia, hypophosphatemia, and on occasion severe proximal myopathy. More often, frank hypocalcemia is not detected, and mild osteomalacia is the only clinical symptom. In other patients on long-term anticonvulsant therapy, no symptoms or signs are present, but bone density is lower than normal and responds favorably to vitamin D supplementation.

Anticonvulsants stimulate the hepatic microsomal mixed-oxidase enzymes and hence increase the rate of clearance of vitamin D and its metabolites. Phenytoin also impairs intestinal calcium absorption independent of effects on vitamin D; the drug also has deleterious effects on bone cell function in vitro, including inhibition of collagen synthesis. All manifestations of the syndrome can nevertheless be reversed with adequate vitamin D supplementation.

Although 1,25(OH)$_2$D levels are lower for the degree of vitamin D intake in patients treated with chronic anticonvulsants than in the normal population, there is a great deal of variation. The greater prevalence of the disorder in some European populations and in children in homes for the mentally retarded probably reflects the lower vitamin D intake of those groups. Restoration of bone mineral mass and reversal of hypocalcemia, when seen, can be accomplished with vitamin D replacement plus added oral calcium. Adjustments in dose are indicated depending on the age and body size of the patient, but approximately 50,000 units of vitamin D weekly plus 1 g elemental calcium per day for several months is usually sufficient. Alternatively, administration of one 50,000-unit capsule of vitamin D monthly may be preventive if anticonvulsant therapy must be given chronically.

VITAMIN D–DEPENDENT RICKETS TYPE I Rickets can be due to *resistance* to the *action* of vitamin D as well as to vitamin D deficiency. Vitamin D–dependent rickets type I, previously termed *pseudo-vitamin D–dependent rickets*, differs from vitamin D–resistant rickets in that it is less severe and the biochemical and radiographic abnormalities can be reversed with large doses of the vitamin.

Clinical features include hypocalcemia, often with tetany or convulsions, hypophosphatemia, secondary hyperparathyroidism, and osteomalacia, often associated with skeletal deformities and increased alkaline phosphatase. Doses of vitamin D or calcifediol, 100 to 1000 times above the usual amounts, are required to heal the bone disease, whereas physiologic amounts of calcitriol cure the disease. This finding fits with the pathophysiology. The disorder, an autosomal recessive trait, is due to a defect in conversion of 25(OH)D to 1,25(OH)$_2$D. Plasma levels of 1,25(OH)$_2$D are low or undetectable even after administration of large doses of vitamin D or calcifediol. Response to high doses of vitamin D or calcifediol is probably due to direct actions of high levels of 25(OH)D. Treatment requires careful adjustment of calcitriol dose, particularly during growth periods.

Active vitamin D ineffective INTESTINAL MALABSORPTION Mild hypocalcemia, secondary hyperparathyroidism, severe hypophosphatemia, and a variety of nutritional deficiencies occur with gastrointestinal diseases. Hepatocellular dysfunction can lead to reduction in 25(OH)D levels, as in portal or biliary cirrhosis of the liver. Malabsorption of vitamin D and its metabolites, including 1,25(OH)$_2$D, may occur in a variety of intestinal diseases, hereditary or acquired. Hypocalcemia itself can lead to steatorrhea, due to deficient production of pancreatic enzymes and bile salts. Depending on the disorder, vitamin D or its metabolites can be administered parenterally, thereby guaranteeing adequate blood levels of active metabolites.

VITAMIN D–DEPENDENT RICKETS TYPE II Pseudo-vitamin D–dependent rickets can be due to defective response as well as to defective production of 1,25(OH)$_2$D. This disorder, vitamin D–dependent rickets type II, results from any of several types of end-organ resistance to the active metabolite, including absence or qualitative defects of the intracellular receptor protein for the hormone and postreceptor blocks in hormone action (see Chap. 329). The clinical features are similar to those with the type I disorder and include hypocalcemia, hypophosphatemia, secondary hyperparathyroidism, and rickets. Plasma levels of 1,25(OH)$_2$D are elevated at least three times above normal, in keeping with the refractoriness of the end organs. Severe alopecia totalis may commence early in life. Patients with this disorder usually require much higher doses of vitamin D or vitamin D metabolites than with the type I disorder.

Pseudohypoparathyroidism Pseudohypoparathyroidism (PHP) is a hereditary disorder characterized by symptoms and signs of hypoparathyroidism, typically in association with distinctive skeletal and developmental defects. The hypoparathyroidism is due to a deficient end-organ response to PTH. Excessive secretion of PTH is the consequence of hyperplasia of the parathyroids, a response to the resistance to hormone action. The entity is actually a syndrome in which various individuals and kindreds exhibit different aberrancies in hormone receptor complex response. Studies, both clinical and basic, have clarified some aspects of this still confusing syndrome, including the variable spectrum of the clinical features, the pathophysiology, the genetic defects, and the hereditary patterns.

Most patients show a characteristic phenotype usually referred to as *Albright's hereditary osteodystrophy* (AHO). Short stature, round face, skeletal anomalies (brachydactyly), and heterotopic calcification constitute the AHO phenotype. The patients have low calcium and high phosphate, as do patients with true hypoparathyroidism. PTH levels, however, are elevated, and resistance to hormone action can be demonstrated as, for example, by defective urinary cyclic AMP response to PTH administration. The cases are commonly familial; not all kindreds show the AHO phenotype but only the abnormal mineral metabolism. A few patients are resistant to PTH but exhibit normal urinary cyclic AMP response (responses in calcium and phosphate seemingly blocked after the adenyl cyclase step).

At least part of the defect is attributable in the majority of patients (those with the AHO phenotype) to inheritance of one defective allele that must encode the α subunit of the guanyl nucleotide–binding protein (G$_{s\alpha}$). This defect seems to account for a diminished response to PTH (approximately 50 percent of normal, consistent with one defective allele). However, in some kindreds there are individuals with a distinctive AHO phenotype who, while unaffected with symptoms or signs of defective mineral metabolism, still have a demonstrable 50 percent reduction in assays of $G_{s\alpha}$ subunits (so-called pseudopseudohypoparathyroidism). Hence the defective guanyl nucleotide subunit concentration is not itself sufficient to explain the pathophysiology. Perhaps another independently inherited allelic defect so far undetected is needed to provide full expression of the disordered mineral metabolism.

Since the defective $G_{s\alpha}$ subunit function was recognized, attention has focused on the molecular mechanism of the defective guanyl nucleotide–binding protein function. The gene encoding this subunit has been cloned (chromosome 20); multiple defects have now been identified, including abnormalities in splice junctions associated with deficient mRNA production and point mutations that would result in a protein unit with defective function. The commonly held view that the disease is an X-linked disorder has given way, with a combination of careful family and molecular genetic studies, to the view that the subset with hereditary osteodystrophy is due to an autosomal dominant mode of inheritance (chromosome 20). The inheritance of the variant disorder in which individuals have no abnormalities in mineral metabolism despite an abnormal gene for $G_{s\alpha}$ is not understood.

A working classification of the various forms of pseudohypoparathyroidism is given in Table 357-7. The classification scheme is based on the signs of ineffective parathyroid hormone action (low calcium and high phosphate), urinary cyclic AMP response to exogenous PTH, the presence or absence of Albright's hereditary osteodystrophy (AHO), and assays of the concentration of the $G_{s\alpha}$ subunit of the adenylate cyclase enzyme (see Chap. 69). Using these criteria, there are four types: pseudohypoparathyroidism (PHP) type I, subdivided into a and b categories; PHP-II; and pseudopseudohypoparathyroidism (PPHP). Individuals with PHP-I, the most common of the disorders, show a deficient response in urinary cyclic AMP following administration of exogenous parathyroid hormone. Pseudohypoparathyroidism type II refers to patients with hypocalcemia and hyperphosphatemia who have a normal urinary cyclic AMP response to PTH. These patients are assumed to have a defect in the response to PTH at a locus beyond that of cyclic AMP production, although at least some patients reported to have PHP-II may instead have occult vitamin D deficiency. It is disputed whether PHP-II is a discrete phenotypic and genotypic entity because vitamin D deficiency and an associated hypocalcemia can result in a clinical picture of enhanced cyclic AMP response to administered PTH yet a blunted phosphatemic response (the hallmark of the PHP-II syndrome). Patients with the PHP-I syndrome are divided into type a, with reduced activity of the stimulatory G-protein subunit ($G_{s\alpha}$) in in vitro assays, and type b, with normal amounts of $G_{s\alpha}$ in erythrocytes. Subjects with PHP-Ia have shortened metacarpals and metatarsals and the other features of Albright's hereditary osteodystrophy syndrome and commonly show resistance to hormones in addition to PTH. Patients with PHP-Ib have a normal phenotype without the AHO syndrome. Fibroblasts cultured from the skin of some patients with PHP-Ib show a much reduced response of cyclic AMP accumulation to PTH, consistent with the presence of a defective receptor. A subset of these patients, however, have a normal response to cyclic AMP production in fibroblasts in vitro.

Patients with PPHP have typical features of the hereditary osteodystrophy syndrome despite normal serum calciums and normal response of urinary cyclic AMP to exogenous PTH. These individuals are usually first-degree relatives of patients with PHP-Ia, and patients initially classified as having PPHP have subsequently developed mild hypocalcemia. Patients with PPHP on average have levels of $G_{s\alpha}$ subunits that are half normal. These various features suggest that PPHP is a mild variant of PHP-Ia and illustrate the heterogeneity of the defect in PTH responsiveness. Further studies will be necessary to clarify the pathogenesis of these disorders.

The mineral deposits in ectopic sites may include true bone, whereas bone formation in ectopic sites never occurs in idiopathic hypoparathyroidism. Amorphous deposits of calcium and phosphate are found in the basal ganglia in about half of patients. The defects in metacarpal and metatarsal bones are sometimes accompanied by abnormal phalanges as well, possibly reflecting premature closing of the epiphyses. The typical findings are abnormally short fourth and fifth metacarpals and metatarsals. The defects are usually bilateral. Exostoses and radius curvus are frequent. Impairments in olfaction and taste and unusual dermatoglyphic abnormalities have been reported. There is little improvement in mental status even after adequate therapy with calcium and vitamin D.

The diagnosis can usually be made without difficulty. Positive family history for developmental defects and/or the presence of developmental defects characteristic of PHP-Ia, including brachydactyly, in association with the signs of hypoparathyroidism, low calcium, and high phosphate, make the diagnosis likely on clinical grounds. On the other hand, patients with PHP-Ib or PHP-II do not have phenotypic abnormalities. Here the clue is hypocalcemia with high PTH levels. In PHP-Ib, administration of exogenous parathyroid hormone can lead to detection of the blunted cyclic AMP response; such tests are usually used to confirm the diagnosis even in PHP-Ia. Low levels of $G_{s\alpha}$ subunits in erythrocyte membranes can also distinguish patients with PHP-Ia from those with PHP-Ib. Patients in both categories have elevated serum PTH, particularly if they are hypocalcemic. The diagnosis of PHP-II is more complex, in that cyclic AMP responses in urine are, by definition, normal. Since vitamin D deficiency itself can result in dissociation between phosphaturic and urinary cyclic AMP responses to exogenous PTH, vitamin D deficiency must be excluded before diagnosis of PHP-II can be made.

Treatment of PHP is similar to that of hypoparathyroidism, except that the dose of vitamin D and calcium is usually lower than that required in true hypoparathyroidism, presumably because the defect in PHP is only partial (a 50 percent reduction in $G_{s\alpha}$). Variations in individual responses make it necessary to establish the optimal therapeutic program for each patient, based on maintaining the appropriate blood calcium concentration and urinary calcium excretion.

PTH overwhelmed Occasionally, loss of calcium from the extracellular fluid is so severe that PTH cannot compensate. Such situations include severe, acute hyperphosphatemia, often in association with renal failure, or acute pancreatitis, conditions in which there is rapid efflux of calcium from extracellular fluid. Severe hypocalcemia can occur quickly; PTH rises in response to hypocalcemia but does not

---

TABLE 357-7 Classification of pseudohypoparathyroidism (PHP) and pseudopseudohypoparathyroidism (PPHP)

Type	Hypocalcemia, hyperphosphatemia	Response of Urinary cAMP to PTH	Serum PTH	G_s subunit deficiency	AHO	Resistance to hormones in addition to PTH
PHP-Ia	Yes	↓	↑	Yes	Yes	Yes
PHP-Ib	Yes	↓	↑	No	No	No
PHP-II	Yes	Normal	↑	No	No	No
PPHP	No	Normal	Normal	Yes	Yes	±

NOTE: ↓ = decreased; ↑ = increased; AHO = Albright's hereditary osteodystrophy.

return blood calcium to normal. The chance of hypocalcemia is enhanced when renal failure is present.

Severe, acute hyperphosphatemia   Severe hyperphosphatemia occurs in situations associated with extensive tissue damage or cell destruction (see also Chap. 359). The combination of an increased release of phosphate from muscle and an impaired ability to excrete phosphorus secondary to the renal failure causes moderate to severe hyperphosphatemia, the latter causing calcium loss from the blood and hypocalcemia of mild to moderate severity. Hypocalcemia is usually reversed with tissue repair and restoration of renal function as phosphorus and creatinine values return to normal. There may even be a mild hypercalcemic period in the oliguric phase of recovery of renal function. This sequence, severe hypocalcemia followed by mild hypercalcemia, reflects widespread deposition of calcium in muscle with subsequent redistribution of some of the calcium to the extracellular fluid after restoration of phosphate levels to normal.

Other causes of hyperphosphatemia that lead to hypocalcemia include hypothermia, massive hepatic failure, and hematologic malignancies, either because of high cell turnover as part of the malignancy or because of cell destruction when chemotherapy is instituted.

Treatment is directed toward lowering of blood phosphate by the administration of phosphate-binding antacids or dialysis, often needed for the management of renal failure. Although calcium replacement may be necessary if hypocalcemia is severe and symptomatic, calcium administration during the hyperphosphatemic period may increase extraosseous cellular calcium deposition, thereby aggravating ultimate tissue damage. Although the levels of $1,25(OH)_2D$ may be low during the hyperphosphatemic phase and may return to normal during the oliguric phase of recovery, mineral ion imbalance per se seems to be the principal pathophysiologic mechanism.

Osteitis fibrosis after parathyroidectomy   Severe hypocalcemia after parathyroid surgery is less common now that osteitis fibrosa cystica is an infrequent manifestation of hyperparathyroidism. When osteitis fibrosa cystica is severe, however, bone mineral deficits can be large, and after parathyroidectomy, blood calcium levels can fall to the hypocalcemic range and remain depressed for days if calcium replacement is inadequate. The mechanism of the hypocalcemia is complex. Increased cellularity of bone in severe osteitis fibrosa cystica involves both osteoblastic and osteoclastic cells. High levels of PTH enhance bone-blood exchange, with resorption favored over formation; an abrupt decrease in PTH levels with surgery leaves bone formation favored over resorption. Calcium loss from blood is increased, and temporary hyporesponsiveness of bone to the bone-resorbing actions of PTH (lowered hormone levels after parathyroid surgery in the presence of receptor down-regulation) may add to the imbalance between bone resorption and bone formation. Treatment may require parenteral administration of calcium; addition of calcitriol and oral calcium supplementation may hasten the ability to withdraw parenteral calcium supplementation and/or reduce the amount needed.

DIFFERENTIAL DIAGNOSIS   Care must be taken to ensure that true hypocalcemia is present; in addition, acute transient hypocalcemia can be a manifestation of a variety of severe, acute illnesses, as discussed above. *Chronic hypocalcemia*, however, can usually be ascribed to a few disorders associated with an absence of PTH or its ineffectiveness. Important clinical criteria include the duration of the illness, signs or symptoms of associated disorders, and the detection of features that suggest a hereditary abnormality in calcium and bone metabolism. A nutritional history can be helpful in detecting a low intake of vitamin D and calcium in the elderly, and a history of excessive alcohol intake can be the clue to magnesium deficiency.

Hypoparathyroidism and pseudohypoparathyroidism are typically lifelong illnesses; hence a recent onset of hypocalcemia in an adult is usually due to nutritional deficiencies, renal failure, or intestinal disorders that result in vitamin D deficiency or ineffective vitamin D action. A history of seizure disorder raises the issue of anticonvulsive medication. Neck surgery, even long past, can be associated with a delayed onset of postoperative hypoparathyroidism. Developmental defects, particularly in childhood and adolescence, may point to the diagnosis of pseudohypoparathyroidism. Rickets and a variety of neuromuscular syndromes and deformities may indicate ineffective vitamin D action, either due to hereditary defects in vitamin D metabolism or, rarely, to vitamin D deficiency.

A pattern of *low calcium* with *high phosphorus* in the absence of renal failure or massive tissue destruction almost invariably means hypoparathyroidism or pseudohypoparathyroidism. A *low calcium* and a *low phosphorus* points to absent or ineffective vitamin D, thereby rendering the action of PTH on calcium metabolism ineffective. The relative ineffectiveness of PTH in vitamin D deficiency, anticonvulsant therapy, gastrointestinal disorders, and hereditary defects in vitamin D metabolism leads to secondary hyperparathyroidism as a compensation. The relatively unopposed action of the excess PTH on renal tubule phosphate transport, less dependent on vitamin D sufficiency than calcium transport, accounts for renal phosphate wasting and hypophosphatemia.

Exceptions to these patterns may occur. Most forms of hypomagnesemia are due to long-standing nutritional deficiency, and despite the fact that the hypocalcemia is due principally to an acute absence of PTH, phosphate levels are usually low rather than elevated as in hypoparathyroidism. Chronic renal failure is often associated with hypocalcemia and hyperphosphatemia, despite secondary hyperparathyroidism.

Diagnosis is usually established by application of the PTH radioimmunoassay, tests for vitamin D metabolites, and measurements of the urinary cyclic AMP response to exogenous PTH. In hereditary and acquired hypoparathyroidism and severe hypomagnesemia, PTH is either undetectable or in the normal range, especially with double-antibody assays; this result in a hypocalcemic patient is supportive of hypoparathyroidism, as distinct from ineffective PTH action, in which even mild hypocalcemia is associated with elevated PTH levels. Hence a failure to detect elevated PTH levels establishes the diagnosis of hypoparathyroidism; elevated levels suggest the presence of secondary hyperparathyroidism, as found in many of the situations in which the hormone is ineffective due to associated abnormalities in vitamin D action. Assays for $25(OH)D$ and $1,25(OH)_2D$ can be quite helpful. Low or low normal $25(OH)D$ indicates vitamin D deficiency due to lack of sunlight, inadequate vitamin D intake, or intestinal malabsorption. A low level of $1,25(OH)_2D$ in the presence of elevated concentrations of PTH suggests ineffective PTH action, including chronic renal failure, severe vitamin D deficiency, vitamin D–dependent rickets type I, and pseudohypoparathyroidism. Recognition that mild hypocalcemia, rickets, and hypophosphatemia are due to chronic anticonvulsant therapy is made by history.

TREATMENT OF HYPOCALCEMIA   The chronic management of hypoparathyroidism or pseudohypoparathyroidism, chronic renal failure, and hereditary defects in vitamin D metabolism features the use of vitamin D or vitamin D metabolites and calcium supplementation. Vitamin D itself is the least expensive form of vitamin D replacement and is frequently used in the management of uncomplicated hypoparathyroidism and disorders associated with ineffective vitamin D action. When vitamin D is used prophylactically, as in the elderly or in those with chronic anticonvulsant therapy, there is a wider margin of safety than with the more potent metabolites. On the other hand, most of the conditions in which vitamin D is administered for chronic management of hypocalcemia require the use of 50 to 100 times the daily replacement doses because the formation of $1,25(OH)_2D$ is deficient. In such situations, vitamin D is no safer than the active metabolite because intoxication does occur with high-dose vitamin D therapy. Calcitriol is more rapid in onset of action and also has a short biologic half-life; in high doses, vitamin D is stored in body tissues and is cleared slowly.

One to five micrograms per day of vitamin D or calcifediol and slightly lower doses of calcitriol (0.25 to 1.0 µg/d) are required to prevent rickets in normal subjects. In contrast, 500 to 3000 µg of vitamin D_2 or D_3 is typically required in hypoparathyroidism; doses of calcifediol are also high (several hundred micrograms per day) compared with doses required in euparathyroid individuals. The dose of calcitriol is unchanged in hypoparathyroidism, since the defect is in hydroxylation by the 1α-hydroxylase.

The slightly greater therapeutic efficacy of calcifediol than vitamin D_3 when the metabolism of the vitamin is impaired may be due to superior metabolic availability for the renal 1α-hydroxylase or to direct action directly by 25(OH)D at receptors in target tissues. Vitamin D is metabolized to a variety of compounds other than the principal product, 25(OH)D. Calcifediol bypasses these alternate pathways and is directly available for metabolism to 1,25(OH)$_2$D. In hypoparathyroidism and in hereditary defects in renal 1α-hydroxylase, the efficiency of formation of 1,25(OH)$_2$D from 25(OH)D is low, but some formation does occur with high substrate levels. Calcifediol has about 1 percent of the potency of calcitriol in vivo and in vitro tests of vitamin D responsiveness.

Unless a loading dose is given, 2 to 4 weeks or even longer are required to achieve the maximum calcium replacement action of vitamin D or calcifediol; again, the onset of action of calcifediol is slightly more rapid. Calcitriol can be given for hypoparathyroidism at the same dose required for the prevention of rickets in euparathyroid individuals, 0.2 to 1.0 μg/d. Its onset of action is days rather than weeks. When vitamin D or calcifediol is withdrawn, weeks are required for the disappearance of the biologic effects, compared with a few days for calcitriol.

Patients with hypoparathyroidism should be given 2 to 3 g elemental calcium by mouth each day. The two agents, vitamin D (or vitamin D metabolites) and oral calcium, can be varied independently. Higher doses of vitamin D or its metabolites increase the efficiency of intestinal calcium absorption; higher intakes of oral calcium permit adequate calcium assimilation despite a lower efficiency of intestinal calcium absorption. When hypercalcemia occurs during the treatment of chronic hypocalcemia, the withdrawal of the supplemental oral calcium is effective in lowering calcium within 24 h, even more rapidly than withdrawal of calcitriol. Most patients with hypoparathyroidism can be managed with high-dose vitamin D therapy combined with 2 to 3 g oral calcium per day. If hypocalcemia alternates with episodes of hypercalcemia, then administration of calcitriol will often make management easier.

The administration of thiazide diuretics in the usual antihypertensive doses and sodium restriction in patients with hypoparathyroidism lowers urinary calcium excretion. This hypocalciuric effect allows the calcium and vitamin D supplementation to be reduced. Patients will have a lower urinary calcium excretion at any given level of blood calcium on thiazides. The treatment also may protect against the development of kidney stones, a potential complication of the long-term management of hypoparathyroidism. If on dialysis, patients with chronic renal failure and hypocalcemia can have adjustments in dialysate calcium concentrations as an alternative to vitamin D and calcium supplementation. The doses of vitamin D and calcium required for the management of pseudohypoparathyroidism are usually lower than those required for hypoparathyroidism, reflecting incomplete resistance to the action of PTH in pseudohypoparathyroidism. The acute treatment of hypomagnesemia is discussed above.

REFERENCES

AHN TG et al: Familial isolated hypoparathyroidism: A molecular genetic analysis of 8 families with 23 affected persons. Medicine 65:73, 1986

ARNOLD A et al: Mutation of the signal peptide-encoding region of the preproparathyroid hormone gene in familial isolated hypoparathyroidism. J Clin Invest 86:1084, 1990

BENSON L et al: Hyperparathyroidism presenting as the first lesion in multiple endocrine neoplasia type 1. Am J Med 82:731, 1987

BILEZIKIAN JP: Etiologies and therapy of hypercalcemia. Endocrinol Metab Clin North Am 18:389, 1989

BUDAYR AR et al: Increased serum levels of PTH-like protein in malignancy-associated hypercalcemia. Ann Intern Med 111:807, 1989

BURTIS WJ et al: Immunochemical characterization of circulating parathyroid hormone–related protein in patients with humoral hypercalcemia of malignancy. N Engl J Med 322:1106, 1990

CHOU YH et al: The gene responsible for familial hypocalciuric hypercalcemia maps to chromosome 3 in four unrelated families. Nature Genet 1:295, 1992

FIBISON WJ et al: Molecular studies of DiGeorge syndrome. Am J Hum Genet 46:888, 1990

FITCH N: The identification and inheritance of Albright's hereditary osteodystrophy. Am J Med Genet 11:11, 1982

FLEISCH H: Bisphosphonates: Pharmacology and use in the treatment of tumor-induced hypercalcemia and metastatic bone disease. Drugs 42:919, 1991

FRIEDMAN E et al: Clonality of parathyroid tumors in familial multiple endocrine neoplasia type 1. N Engl J Med 321:213, 1989

FUKAGAWA M et: Suppression of parathyroid gland hyperplasia by 1,25(OH)$_2$D$_3$ pulse therapy. N Engl J Med 315:421, 1990

GEJMAN PV et al: Genetic mapping of the Gs-alpha subunit gene (GNAS1) to the distal long arm of chromosome 20 using a polymorphism detected by denaturing gradient gel electrophoresis. Genomics 9:782, 1991

GIDDING SS et al: Unmasking of hypoparathyroidism in familial partial DiGeorge syndrome by challenge with disodium edentate. N Engl J Med 319:1589, 1988

GRILL V et al: PTH-related protein: Elevated levels in both humoral hypercalcemia of malignancy and hypercalcemia complicating metastatic breast cancer. J Clin Endocrinol 73:1309, 1991

HENDERSON JR et al: Circulating concentrations of PTH-like peptide in malignancy and in hyperparathyroidism. J Bone Miner Res 5:105–112, 1990

JAMESON JL, ARNOLD A: Recombinant DNA strategies for determining the molecular basis of endocrine disorders. J Endocrinol Metab 70:301, 1990

KAO PC et al: PTH-related peptide in plasma of patients with hypercalcemia and malignancy lesions. Mayo Clin Proc 65:1399, 1990

LEVINE MA, DEILY JR: Identification of multiple mutations in the gene encoding the alpha subunit of Gs in patients with pseudohypoparathyroidism Ia. Abstracts of the Annual Meeting of the American Society for Bone and Mineral Research, Atlanta, GA, 1990

MALLETTE LE, EICHORN E: Effects of lithium carbonate on human calcium metabolism. Arch Intern Med 146:770, 1986

MARX SJ: Familial hypocalciuric hypercalcemia, in Primer on the Metabolic Bone Diseases and Disorders of Mineral Metabolism, MJ Favus (ed). Richmond, VA, William Byrd Press, 1990, p 113

MAYNARD FM: Immobilization hypercalcemia following spinal cord injury. Arch Phys Med Rehabil 67:41, 1986

MOTOKURA T et al: Cloning and characterization of human cyclin D3, a cDNA closely related in sequence to the PRAD1/cyclin D1 proto-oncogene. J Biol Chem 267:20412, 1992

MUDDE AH et al: Ectopic product of 1,25-dihydroxyvitamin D by B-cell lymphoma as a cause of hypercalcemia. Cancer 59:1543, 1987

NEUFELD M et al: Autoimmune polyglandular syndromes. Pediatr Ann 9:43, 1980

NUSSBAUM SR, POTTS JT Jr: Immunoassays for parathyroid hormone 1-84 in the diagnosis of hyperparathyroidism. J Bone Miner Res 6(suppl 2):S43, 1991

ORWOLL ES: The milk-alkali syndrome: Current concepts. Ann Intern Med 97:242, 1982

PARFITT AM et al: Asymptomatic primary hyperparathyroidism discovered by multichannel biochemical screening: Clinical course and considerations bearing on the need for surgical intervention. J Bone Miner Res 6(suppl 2):S97, 1991

PARKINSON DB, THAKKER RV: A donor splice site mutation in the parathyroid hormone gene is associated with autosomal recessive hypoparathyroidism. Nature Genet 1:149, 1992

PATTEN JL et al: Mutation in the gene encoding the stimulatory G protein of adenylyl cyclase in Albright's hereditary osteodystrophy. N Engl J Med 322:1412, 1990

POTTS JT Jr et al (eds): Proceedings of the NIH Consensus Development Conference on Diagnosis and Management of Asymptomatic Primary Hyperparathyroidism. J Bone Miner Res 6(suppl 2):S1–S166, 1991

RALSTON SH et al: Comparison of aminohydroxypropylidene diphosphonate, mithramycin and corticosteroids/calcitonin in treatment of cancer-associated hypercalcemia. Lancet 2:907, 1985

——— et al: Cancer-associated hypercalcemia: Morbidity and mortality. Ann Intern Med 12:499, 1990

RATCLIFFE WA et al: Immunoreactivity of plasma parathyrin-related peptide. Clin Chem 37:1781, 1991

ROSENBERG CL et al: Coding sequence of the overexpressed transcript of the putative oncogene PRAD1/cyclin D1 in two primary human tumors. Oncogene 8:519, 1993

SCHWINDINGER WF et al: Identification of a novel missense mutation in the gene encoding the alpha subunit of the stimulatory G protein of adenylyl cyclase in a subject with Albright hereditary osteodystrophy. Abstracts of the 74th Annual Meeting of the Endocrine Society, San Antonio, TX, 1992

STUCKEY BGA et al: Fasting calcium excretion and parathyroid hormone together distinguish familial hypocalciuric hypercalcaemia from primary hyperparathyroidism. Clin Endocrinol 27:525, 1987

THAKKER RV et al: Association of parathyroid tumors in multiple endocrine neoplasia type 1 with loss of alleles on chromosome 11. N Engl J Med 321:218, 1989

——— et al: Mapping the gene causing X-linked recessive idiopathic hypoparathyroidism to Xq26–Xq27 by linkage studies. J Clin Invest 86:40, 1990

WARRELL RP et al: A randomized double-blind study of gallium nitrate compared with etidronate for acute control of cancer related hypercalcemia. J Clin Oncol 9:1467, 1991

WEINSTEIN LS et al: Mutations of the Gs alpha-subunit gene in Albright hereditary osteodystrophy detected by denaturing gradient gel electrophoresis. Proc Natl Acad Sci USA 87:8287, 1990

WILSON DI et al: A prospective cytogenetic study of 36 cases of DiGeorge syndrome. Am J Hum Genet 51:957, 1992

WINTER WE et al: Autosomal dominant hypoparathyroidism with variable, age-dependent severity. J Pediatr 103:387, 1983

358   METABOLIC BONE DISEASE

STEPHEN M. KRANE / MICHAEL F. HOLICK

OSTEOPOROSIS

GENERAL CONSIDERATIONS   *Osteoporosis* is the term used for diseases of diverse etiology that cause a reduction in the mass of bone per unit volume. The reduction in mass is not accompanied by a significant decrease in the ratio of the mineral to the organic phase, nor by any known abnormality in bone mineral or organic matrix. Histologically, the disorder is characterized by a decrease in cortical thickness and in the number and size of the trabeculae of cancellous bone. Individual trabecular plates are abnormally perforated and may be fractured, and trabecular connectivity is reduced. The osteoid seams, however, are of normal width. Osteoporosis is the most common of the metabolic bone diseases (disorders in which all the skeleton is involved) and is an important cause of morbidity in the elderly.

The remodeling of bone (its formation and resorption) is a continuous process. In osteoporosis, the bone mass *is* decreased, indicating that the rate of bone resorption must exceed that of bone formation. Bone formation is higher in cortical than in cancellous bone. This difference is exaggerated by the normal menopause and exaggerated further in patients with osteoporosis because rates of formation of cancellous bone tend to be lower in patients with osteoporosis, particularly in women after the menopause. The fact that about a third of postmenopausal women have high skeletal turnover, assessed by whole-body retention of ^{99m}Tc-methylene diphosphonate and by other biochemical markers, could reflect the greater relative contribution of cortical remodeling in this group. After closure of epiphyses and cessation of longitudinal growth, there is a period of consolidation with a decrease in cortical porosity. When peak adult bone mass is reached at about age 30 to 35 for cortical bone and probably earlier for trabecular bone, rates of bone formation and resorption are relatively low (compared with the period of growth spurt) and approximately equal. The normal balance between bone formation and resorption results in maintenance of skeletal mass. The rates of remodeling differ, however, not only in cortical compared with trabecular bone but also in individual bones or portions of bones. Most of the bone surfaces are "inactive" and not involved at any given time either in formation or resorption. Active surfaces may be distributed randomly, but formation and resorption are locally coupled as units. Resorption areas are covered by osteoclasts if active; bone formation surfaces are characterized by the presence of osteoid seams and are covered by active osteoblasts. Resorption precedes formation and is probably more intense, but it does not last as long as formation. As a consequence, there are normally more sites of active formation than of resorption. Bone turnover is high when there are many units active and low when there are few. Unless formation compensates for resorption, bone mass decreases. In both sexes after age 40 to 50 there is a slow rate of loss of cortical bone of about 0.3 to 0.5 percent per year. In women around the menopause, an accelerated loss of cortical bone is superimposed on the age-related loss. Loss of trabecular bone begins at an earlier age in both sexes but is probably greater in degree in women. The rate of bone loss in women also may be accelerated around the time of menopause. The cumulative losses of bone mass range from 20 to 30 percent in men and 40 to 50 percent for some women. In general, the bone loss involves predominantly trabecular bone in the spine and distal radius in women and the spine and hip in both women and men. The fact that loss is not uniform has been documented with techniques such as single- and dual-photon absorptiometry, quantitative computed tomography, x-ray–based dual-energy densitometry, and neutron activation analysis of total-body calcium. For example, the rate of loss is greater in the metacarpals, the femoral neck, and the vertebral bodies than in the midshaft of the femur, the tibia, and the skull.

Although, as noted, skeletal turnover may be increased, turnover is usually normal or low. Bone formation is low in the majority, but the degree of reduction varies with the different bone surfaces. The major remodeling abnormalities in patients with vertebral crush fractures are a reduced frequency of activation of remodeling units and a decrease in the function of osteoblasts. Even in those individuals with increased bone resorption, however, bone formation does not compensate. At some critical point if the difference between rates of formation and resorption is maintained, loss of bone substance may become so marked that the bone can no longer resist the normal mechanical forces to which it is subjected, and fracture results. This problem is most evident following perforation of bony trabecular plates. The template for formation of new bone is lost, and loss of bone is rapid as bone resorption continues and is even more uncoupled from resorption. Osteoporosis usually becomes a clinical problem following fracture. Although the level of reduction in bone mass sufficient to result in fractures after minimal trauma is variable, the bone mineral density as measured by x-ray–based dual-energy absorptiometry (DEXA) is an excellent predictor of fracture risk. The strength of bones such as vertebrae depends on "quality" (e.g., trabecular connectivity and arrangement) as well as mineral density. For example, horizontal trabeculae of the cancellous bone of vertebrae are preferentially lost in osteoporosis. Additional factors such as the adequacy of ligamentous support and the age-related changes in the intervertebral disks influence the susceptibility to fracture. Microfractures are frequent. In elderly individuals with osteoporosis, age- or drug-related impairments of vision, hearing, and other neurologic and intellectual functions are additional contributions to the occurrence of fractures.

In the process of remodeling lamellar bone in adults, most of the net resorption occurs at the corticoendosteal surface. The abnormal remodeling in osteoporosis follows the same pattern; the bone loss includes cancellous bone, cortical bone at the endosteal surface, and intracortical bone, resulting in enlargement of the medullary cavity and thinning of the cortex. Since bone formation at the periosteum continues at a slow rate, the diameter of the bone does not decrease, and the periosteal surface retains its smooth configuration. In addition, the cancellous bone also undergoes progressive resorption, with some trabeculae being resorbed at rates faster than others, particularly those vertebral trabeculae with horizontal orientation.

The age-related loss of bone begins earlier and proceeds more rapidly in women, and there is a trend toward acceleration of bone loss before the menopause. All the reasons for this age-associated bone loss are not known, although several risk factors have been identified. In general, white women have a greater risk than black women, and white men have a greater risk than black men. One explanation for these population differences is that the bone mass at skeletal maturity is one determinant of the bone mass at subsequent ages. The lower incidence of osteoporosis and hip fracture in black men and women has been attributed to a higher bone mineral content in blacks than in whites despite the fact that bone formation is lower in blacks. Since formation and resorption are usually coupled, and since bone mass is increased, bone resorption (and turnover) also must be reduced. Osteoporotic subjects are frequently less muscular and have lower average body weight. Patients who are kept at complete bed rest and astronauts in microgravity can lose approximately 1 percent of their bone mass each month. Exercise may have a beneficial effect in maintaining bone mass. The facts that accelerated bone loss accompanies the menopause in some women and that premature osteoporosis occurs after premature surgical menopause suggest that estrogens play a major role in preventing bone loss. Furthermore, osteoporotic women as a group may have an earlier menopause than age-matched nonosteoporotic women. Osteoporotic women also have a higher incidence of smoking; cigarette smoking might directly affect bone remodeling or have secondary effects on ovarian function. Excessive alcohol consumption, which can result in decreased bone formation, also is a risk factor for osteoporosis. Dietary calcium intake during the first three decades of life influences the ultimate peak bone mass. Calcium intake during adult life also has a small effect on bone mass and risk of fracture. Inability to synthesize adequate amounts of $1\alpha,25$-dihydroxyvitamin D [$1,25(OH)_2D$] may play a role in the decreased calcium absorption, possibly because of decreased sensitivity of the $25(OH)D$-1α-hydroxylase to parathyroid hormone or impaired activity of the renal $25(OH)D$-1α-hydroxylase.

Local production of selected cytokines appears to mediate the effects of estrogen deficiency in enhancing osteoclast-mediated bone resorption. Peripheral blood monocytes from patients with osteoporosis secrete more interleukin 1 (IL-1), and in women with postmenopausal osteoporosis the increased production of IL-1 is suppressed by estrogen treatment. IL-1 and other cytokines such as tumor necrosis factor α (TNF-α) stimulate production of IL-6 by osteoblasts and other mesenchymal cells. IL-6 is probably the most important cytokine in the excessive recruitment of osteoclasts that is a common feature of the abnormal bone remodeling in postmenopausal osteoporosis. Although osteoporosis occurs with Cushing's syndrome, there is no established role for adrenal steroids in the osteoporosis associated with the menopause or advancing age.

Excessive acid intake, particularly in the form of high-protein diets, may contribute to "dissolution" of bone in an attempt to buffer the extra acid. Acidosis also may increase osteoclast function directly. Prolonged use of heparin as an anticoagulant is also associated with osteoporosis, and heparin potentiates bone resorption in vitro. Subjects with osteoporosis have increased numbers of mast cells, presumably capable of producing heparin and other substances that modulate bone cell function, in the bone marrow. Circumscribed and diffuse areas of osteoporosis occur in patients with systemic mastocytosis.

As mentioned earlier, the remodeling of bone is responsive to mechanical forces. The early response to immobilization in the normal skeleton is an increase in bone resorption while bone formation remains normal or is decreased; later there is a compensatory increase in bone formation. In osteoporosis, immobilization tends to aggravate the defect by increasing the gap between formation and resorption. A sedentary life may reduce mechanical forces exerted on the skeleton and increase the tendency to bone loss.

CLASSIFICATION (See Table 358-1)   In some instances, osteoporosis is a feature of another disease such as Cushing's syndrome. Osteoporosis is also characteristic of certain heritable diseases of connective tissue such as osteogenesis imperfecta (see Chap. 351). In most cases of osteoporosis, however, no other disease is apparent. One form occurs in children or young adults of both sexes and with normal gonadal function and is frequently termed *idiopathic osteoporosis*, although most of the other forms are also of unknown pathogenesis. So-called *type I osteoporosis* occurs in a subset of postmenopausal women who are between 51 and 75 years of age and is characterized by an accelerated and disproportionate loss of trabecular bone. Fractures of vertebral bodies and the distal forearm are common complications. Decreased parathyroid gland function may be compensatory to increased bone resorption. So-called *type II osteoporosis* is found in a large proportion of women and men over the age of 70 and is associated with fractures of the femoral neck, proximal humerus, proximal tibia, and pelvis. These skeletal sites contain both cortical and trabecular bone. Circulating levels of parathyroid hormone (PTH) tend to be high. Both groups have decreased mean circulating levels of $1,25(OH)_2D$.

GENERAL CLINICAL FEATURES   Although osteoporosis is a generalized disorder of the skeleton, its major clinical sequelae result from fractures of the vertebrae, wrist, hip, humerus, and tibia. The most frequent symptoms from vertebral body fractures are pain in the back and deformity of the spine. Pain usually results from collapse of the vertebrae especially in the dorsal and lumbar regions, is typically acute in onset, and often radiates around the flank into the abdomen. Such episodes may occur after sudden bending, lifting, or jumping movements that may seem to have been trivial; on some occasions they cannot be related to trauma. The pain may be increased

---

TABLE 358-1   Classification of osteoporosis

Common forms, unassociated with other disease
  A Idiopathic osteoporosis (juvenile and adult)
  B Type I osteoporosis
  C Type II osteoporosis
Osteoporosis as a common feature
  A Hypogonadism
  B Hyperadrenocorticism
  C Chronic glucocorticoid administration
  D Hyperparathyroidism
  E Thyrotoxicosis
  F Malabsorption
  G Scurvy
  H Calcium deficiency
  I Immobilization
  J Chronic heparin administration
  K Systemic mastocytosis
  L Adult hypophosphatasia
  M Associated with other metabolic bone diseases
Osteoporosis as a feature of heritable disorders of connective tissue
  A Osteogenesis imperfecta
  B Homocystinuria due to cystathionine synthase deficiency
  C Ehlers-Danlos syndrome
  D Marfan's syndrome
Osteoporosis is associated but pathogenesis is not understood
  A Rheumatoid arthritis
  B Malnutrition
  C Alcoholism
  D Epilepsy
  E Primary biliary cirrhosis
  F Diabetes mellitus
  G Chronic obstructive pulmonary disease
  H Menkes' syndrome

---

even with slight movements such as turning in bed or the Valsalva maneuver. Bed rest may relieve the pain temporarily, only for it to recur in spasms of variable duration. Radiation of pain down one leg is uncommon, and symptoms or signs of spinal cord compression are rare. The acute episodes of pain also may be accompanied by abdominal distention and ileus, thought to be due to retroperitoneal hemorrhage, but the use of narcotics also contributes to the ileus. Loss of appetite and muscular weakness also may be present. Episodes of pain usually subside after several days to a week, and by 4 to 6 weeks patients may be fully ambulatory and able to resume normal activities. Although acute pain may be minimal, nagging, deep, dull, uncomfortable sensations may be localized to the area of fracture and brought about by straining or sudden changes in position. Patients may be unable to sit up in bed and have to arise by rolling over on the side and then propping themselves up. Most patients have disappearance or diminution of pain between episodes of vertebral body collapse. Others do not have acute episodes but complain of backache made worse by standing or sudden movement. Tenderness is common over involved areas of the spinous processes or rib cage. Some patients have an associated disease such as osteoarthritis of facet joints to account for chronic back pain. When collapse fractures of vertebral bodies do occur, they are usually anterior, producing a wedge-shaped deformity and contributing to loss in height. This is particularly common in the middorsal region, where collapse may be unassociated with pain but may result in a dorsal kyphosis and exaggerated cervical lordosis described as a "dowager's" or "widow's" hump. Postural slumping with increase in existing curves also contributes to the loss of height. Scoliosis is also common. Generalized skeletal pain is uncommon, and between fractures most patients are free of pain. Although recurrent episodes of vertebral collapse, increasing spine deformity, and loss of height are common, the course in any one subject is not predictable, and there may be intervals of several years between fractures.

RADIOLOGIC FEATURES   Prior to fracture and collapse, the osteoporotic vertebral body shows a decrease in mineral density, increase in prominence of vertical striations due to a relatively greater loss of the horizontally oriented trabeculae, and prominence of the end plates. The bodies may become increasingly biconcave because of weakening of the subchondral plates, microfractures, and expansion of the intervertebral disks, resulting in the so-called codfish vertebrae. When collapse occurs, it usually produces a decrease in the anterior height of the vertebral body and irregularity in the anterior cortex (Fig. 358-1). Older compression fractures may show reactive changes and osteophytes about the anterior margins. Most osteoporotic fractures occur in the middle and lower thoracic and upper lumbar vertebral bodies. Fractures of isolated vertebral bodies of T4 or higher should suggest malignancy. Although the cortices of long bones may be thin because of excessive endosteal resorption, the outer margins are sharp in contrast to the typical effects of the subperiosteal resorption of hyperparathyroidism. Pseudofractures or Looser's zones do not occur in the absence of osteomalacia, but it may be impossible to distinguish osteoporosis from osteomalacia on radiologic grounds alone. In the absence of fractures, standard roentgenograms are insensitive indicators of bone loss, since as much as 30 percent decrease in bone mass may not be appreciated. Other procedures are required to establish whether a given individual has a sufficient decrease in bone mass to be at risk for fracture. Dual-energy x-ray absorptiometry is an excellent technique because of its sensitivity, ability to scan the entire skeleton, low radiation exposure, and short scanning time. Single- and dual-photon absorptiometry and quantitative computed tomography (CT) also can detect small (1 to 2 percent) changes in the bone mineral density of the hip and lumbar spine.

LABORATORY FINDINGS The concentrations of calcium and inorganic phosphorus in the blood are usually normal. Slight hyperphosphatemia occurs in women who are past the menopause. The alkaline phosphatase in uncomplicated instances is normal but may increase after fractures. About 20 percent of postmenopausal women with osteoporosis have hypercalciuria. Urinary excretion of peptides containing hydroxyproline, an index of bone resorption, is usually normal or slightly increased in those with high-turnover osteoporosis. Serum levels of osteocalcin (bone GLA protein), urinary excretion of hydroxypyridinium cross-link compounds, and uptake of ^{99m}Tc-methylene diphosphonate also correlate with the rate of bone turnover.

DIFFERENTIAL DIAGNOSIS Since decrease in skeletal mass is a universal feature of aging, it is difficult to evaluate asymptomatic decreased bone density, determined radiographically, in older women, especially when unaccompanied by marked increase in biconcavity of vertebral bodies or fractures. Quantitative measurement of bone mass is, however, a predictor of future fractures. In the presence of bone pain with or without fracture or deformity, it is important to establish the presence or absence of known causes of osteoporosis as listed in Table 358-1 and to be certain that osteoporosis is the correct diagnosis. Malignancies of various types, particularly *multiple myeloma, lymphoma, leukemia,* and *metastatic carcinoma,* may result in diffuse loss of bone, especially the trabecular bone of the vertebral column, even in the absence of hypercalcemia. The absence of anemia, elevated erythrocyte sedimentation rate, abnormal electrophoretic patterns of serum proteins, and Bence Jones proteinuria is helpful in eliminating the possibility of multiple myeloma. However, needle bone biopsy or marrow aspiration may be appropriate in instances of severe osteoporosis with fractures. Quantitative histomorphometry on standard biopsy samples from the iliac crest is a research tool but is available in some referral laboratories. Bone biopsy samples must be properly fixed, not demineralized, and embedded in plastic to rule out osteomalacia, however.

Radiologic evidence of osteoporosis is common in patients with primary *hyperparathyroidism,* who may not have osteitis fibrosa (discrete lytic lesions of varying size and subperiosteal resorption) or elevation of serum alkaline phosphatase. Although mild asymptomatic primary hyperparathyroidism is not a major risk factor in osteoporosis, it does contribute to accelerated bone loss. An element of secondary hyperparathyroidism may be present in some elderly patients with type II osteoporosis and in others with impairment of renal function, inadequate oral calcium intake, or decrease of intestinal calcium absorption. Increased numbers of osteoclasts may be present in bone biopsy specimens from such patients.

Osteomalacia may mimic osteoporosis or coexist with it, yet specific radiologic signs of osteomalacia may not always be present. Although the presence of abnormalities such as low or undetectable circulating levels of 25-hydroxyvitamin D [25(OH)D] and/or hypophosphatemia suggests the possibility of osteomalacia, bone biopsy may be essential for diagnosis, as discussed below. Since osteomalacia is more responsive to therapy (e.g., vitamin D in hypovitaminosis D or phosphate supplements in phosphate depletion) than the usual case of osteoporosis, such diagnostic procedures are often warranted. Subclinical vitamin D deficiency with associated secondary hyperparathyroidism may be more common in elderly women than previously recognized, and treatment of postmenopausal women with small doses of vitamin D_3 (20 µg or 800 IU daily) may reduce the risk of hip fractures and other nonvertebral fractures.

In an occasional patient with *Paget's disease,* the radiologic features may be almost purely lytic and be confused with osteoporosis. However, high alkaline phosphatase levels and moderately or markedly increased urinary excretion of hydroxyproline-containing peptides are clues to the presence of Paget's disease. Scanning procedures with bone-seeking isotopes are not helpful in differential diagnosis if fractures are present because fractures cause preferential uptake of isotope. However, in the absence of fractures, "hot spots" suggest tumor or early Paget's disease, particularly if present in the appendicular skeleton.

IDIOPATHIC OSTEOPOROSIS *Idiopathic osteoporosis* occurs in younger men and in premenopausal women in whom no other etiologic factor is detected. These patients probably have a number of different disorders with superficial resemblances. In some women, the onset of the disease appears to be related to pregnancy and may represent a transient failure in homeostatic mechanisms, such as failure to increase circulating levels of $1,25(OH)_2D$ and hence to protect the

FIGURE 358-1 Lateral views of the lumbar spine of a 54-year-old man with idiopathic osteoporosis. A typical anterior compression fracture is indicated by the arrow.

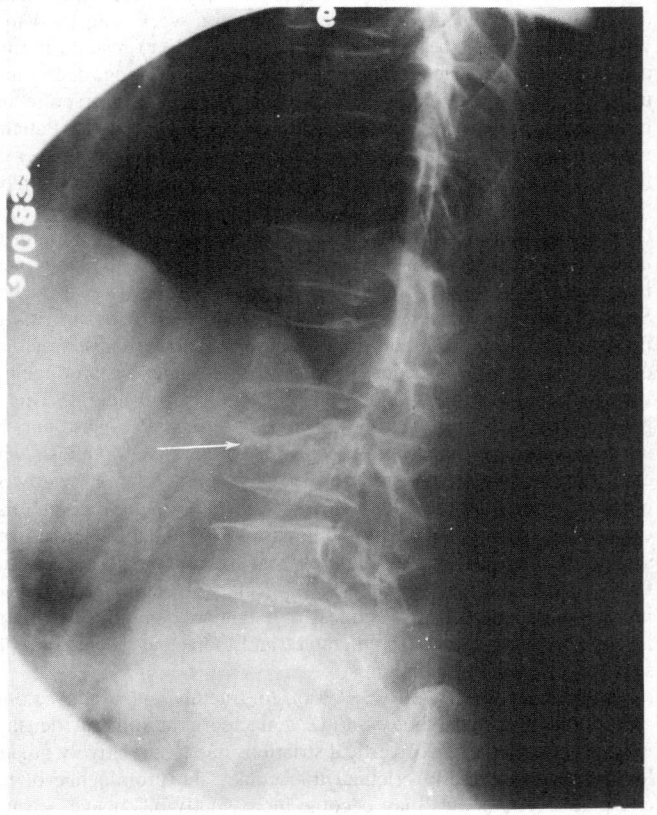

maternal skeleton from the stresses of childbirth (see Chap. 356). Some patients have low levels of serum alkaline phosphatase, though not low enough to fulfill diagnostic criteria for *hypophosphatasia*. Estrogens are ineffective in therapy. Losses of calcium and phosphorus are probably excessive, and it is unwise to permit women with osteoporosis to breast-feed because calcium losses via lactation are appreciable. Some patients have a disorder similar to mild forms of osteogenesis imperfecta and may thus have defects in type I collagen genes, although such features as family history, blue sclerae, and deafness are lacking. The course is variable; although recurrent episodes of fractures are characteristic, progressive deterioration does not occur in all patients, and in some the clinical problem is benign. Juvenile osteoporosis is a rare disorder with onset usually between the ages of 8 and 14 years and is characterized by the abrupt appearance of bone pain and fractures after minimal trauma. In many cases the disorder is self-limited, and recovery takes place spontaneously within 4 or 5 years.

GLUCOCORTICOID EXCESS Glucocorticoid excess does not appear to be involved in osteoporosis of the idiopathic variety or in the type I or II disorder. Osteoporosis, however, commonly accompanies Cushing's syndrome, both endogenous and exogenous, and in some instances is rapidly progressive, especially in children and in women over age 50. Bone loss of glucocorticoid excess is accounted for by a combination of low rates of bone formation (depressed osteoblastic oppositional rate) and high rates of bone resorption reflected in the hypercalciuria that accompanies increased activation frequency of bone remodeling units. A part of the latter may be the result of glucocorticoid-induced secondary hyperparathyroidism, although increases in circulating PTH are not found consistently. Glucocorticoids, however, potentiate the effects of PTH and $1,25(OH)_2D$ on bone cells in vitro. Glucocorticoids depress collagen synthesis in many tissues, as evidenced by delayed wound healing, thinning of the dermis, striae, and tendency to blue sclerae. In some disorders in which glucocorticoids are administered in pharmacologic doses, such as rheumatoid arthritis, a tendency to thin skin and osteoporosis is initially present, and the skeletal effects of the glucocorticoids may become particularly apparent. Even low dosages of glucocorticoids may accelerate bone loss in postmenopausal women and men with rheumatoid arthritis. Blood levels of $25(OH)D$ are normal or slightly decreased, and blood levels of $1,25(OH_2)D$ are usually normal. Glucocorticoids inhibit intestinal calcium absorption by a direct, vitamin D-independent action on the intestine. Osteomalacia is not observed histologically. Once osteoporosis develops in adults with Cushing's syndrome, the abnormality may persist indefinitely following alleviation of the glucocorticoid excess. In children, however, cure of the Cushing's syndrome may result in striking improvement in the appearance of the spine due to new endochondral bone formation around the less dense, older osteoporotic bone. Likewise, increase in bone mass, increase in serum osteocalcin levels (indicative of increased osteoblastic function), and decrease in urinary hydroxyproline excretion may occur in young adults following therapy of Cushing's syndrome. Withdrawal of glucocorticoids or decrease of the dose by alternate-day schedule is important to halt progression of the osteoporosis. Anabolic steroids are not effective in this regard. The defect in intestinal calcium absorption may be overcome by administering calcitriol $[1,25(OH)_2D_3]$ in oral doses of 0.5 to 1.0 µg/d plus 1 g supplemental oral calcium daily. Such regimens with or without calcitonin (e.g., 400 IU/d intranasally) are effective in preventing glucocorticoid-induced bone loss. Vitamin D metabolites such as calcifediol $[25(OH)D]$ also may be effective. It is important to monitor serum and urinary calcium levels at intervals of 2 to 4 months. In Cushing's syndrome, spontaneous, symptomless fractures may occur in ribs and pubic and ischial rami even in the absence of marked osteoporosis of the spine. These fractures often heal partially with an exuberant calcified callus surrounding a radiolucent zone of nonunion, superficially resembling the pseudofractures of osteomalacia. If they appear in the thorax superimposed on the lungs, they may be confused with nodules suggesting primary or metastatic tumor.

GONADAL DEFICIENCY Receptors for estrogens are in osteoblasts, and estrogens may function in these cells by stimulating production of substances that are anabolic for bone such as somatomedin C (insulin-like growth factor 1) or by reducing the production of catabolic cytokines by osteoblasts and mononuclear phagocytes. Estrogen is deficient in the postmenopausal woman, and the administration of estrogen to such an individual reduces the negative calcium balance and decreases urinary hydroxyproline excretion. Estrogens are particularly useful in retarding the bone loss in women who have oophorectomy at an early age and in preventing the development of osteoporosis following the menopause. Bone mass is also decreased in women athletes who are amenorrheic, such as marathon runners. Such women are particularly prone to tibial stress fractures. In patients of either sex castrated at an early age, the adult skeleton is smaller to begin with, and therefore, age-related losses are more significant. Bone density is also decreased in women with hyperprolactinemia and in men with hypogonadism of all types.

THYROTOXICOSIS In many patients with hyperthyroidism, excessive bone resorption, occasionally marked in degree and far exceeding that in the usual patient with osteoporosis, can be associated with increased excretion of calcium and phosphorus in urine and feces. The excessive bone resorption is usually accompanied by a compensatory increase in bone formation. PTH secretion is decreased, and levels of $1,25(OH)_2D$ are normal or low. If the hyperthyroidism is of short duration, skeletal losses are inconsequential. In patients with chronic hyperthyroidism, however, especially in women after the menopause, this accelerated bone loss becomes significant, and it is important to eliminate hyperthyroidism as a contributing cause of osteoporosis. Hypothyroid patients treated with excessive doses of levothyroxine also may have accelerated loss of bone mass. Although typical osteitis fibrosa (resorption lacunae containing osteoclasts and a fibrous stroma) may be seen on biopsy, the skeletal lesions have the radiologic appearance of osteoporosis.

ACROMEGALY Hypercalciuria and overall net negative calcium balance occur in acromegaly, and occasionally, osteoporosis is an associated finding. The secondary panhypopituitarism and the associated gonadal insufficiency may be factors in production of the osteoporosis. In adult animals, growth hormone decreases endosteal resorption and stimulates bone formation, and it is therefore unlikely that excessive secretion of growth hormone in itself produces osteoporosis.

DIABETES MELLITUS Individuals with juvenile or adult-onset diabetes mellitus have a decreased bone mass. In some series, the incidence of hip fractures is increased, but studies of large groups of diabetic subjects have not revealed abnormal calcium metabolism or significant bone disease specifically attributable to the diabetes.

CALCIUM DEFICIENCY AND MALABSORPTION Although calcium deficiency may be a factor, it cannot be the sole or major cause in idiopathic, senile, or postmenopausal osteoporosis. Osteoporosis is an associated finding in a significant number of cases of steatorrhea, prolonged obstructive jaundice, and lactose intolerance and in patients following gastrectomy. Other patients may have a specific defect in calcium absorption or a failure to adapt adequately to a low-calcium diet either by increasing the percentage of dietary calcium absorbed or by decreasing urinary calcium excretion. Presumably, vitamin D is adequate in these instances to prevent osteomalacia.

HERITABLE DISORDERS OF CONNECTIVE TISSUE In the strict sense, the bone disease of osteogenesis imperfecta is osteoporosis (see Chap. 351). *Osteogenesis imperfecta* is clinically, genetically, and biochemically heterogeneous. Type I osteogenesis imperfecta is the autosomal dominant form, characterized by mild to moderate bone fragility, blue sclerae, and premature deafness. The frequency of fractures tends to decrease around puberty, and another period of increased incidence occurs in women after the menopause. Type II is the lethal perinatal disorder. Type III is characterized by severe bone fragility, progressive bone deformity, and white sclerae. In type IV, sclerae are white, but other features are similar to those of type I disease. Many instances of osteogenesis imperfecta of all types have been linked to mutations in the *COL1A1* and *COL1A2* genes that encode type I collagen. In other individuals, defects in these genes may predispose to what is now diagnosed as idiopathic or postmenopausal osteoporosis, in the absence of other features of osteogenesis imperfecta. Osteoporosis also occurs in patients with *homocystinuria* due to cystathionine synthase deficiency, an autosomal recessive trait associated with ectopia lentis, various deformities of the extremities, mental retardation, decreased pigmentation of hair and skin, and thromboembolism. The diagnosis is established by the finding of homocystine in urine. The osteoporosis may be due to the effect of homocysteine or other metabolites in interfering with the cross-linking of collagen.

THERAPY In considering treatment, it should be emphasized that one is dealing with a group of disorders rather than a single entity. Even in patients within the same category, e.g., those with idiopathic osteoporosis, the etiologies may be different. It is also difficult to predict the course, especially in patients seen because of pain and collapse-fracture. Many patients in the idiopathic, postmenopausal (type I), and senile (type II) groups have a few episodes of vertebral body collapse but then go for many years without symptoms or further loss in height. Furthermore, the acute pain associated with vertebral body fracture tends to subside in weeks, and *any* treatment administered at that time might be considered efficacious. Although accurate estimation of bone mass can help determine efficacy of therapy, clinical benefit (diminution of bone pain, decrease in incidence of fractures) is more difficult to assess in view of variability in disease progression. It is generally agreed, however, that estrogen replacement in women is effective in preventing bone loss after oophorectomy or early in the menopause.

General measures Patients with acute pain secondary to fracture of vertebral bodies frequently require rest in bed in a position of maximum comfort, local heat, adequate analgesics, and avoidance of constipation. Use of traction or plaster jacket splints is not indicated. As soon as pain permits, the patient should attempt to move out of bed, slowly at first, perhaps with support of a walker or crutches. Braces are commonly employed, but their efficacy in preventing progression of spinal deformity is not established. A well-made corset may provide support and comfort. Exercises to correct postural deformity and increase muscle tone are useful. Patients should be taught to avoid sudden painful movements such as jumping and how to lift and carry objects with minimal back strain. After the fractures have healed, a supervised exercise program that includes daily walking may be helpful in preventing further skeletal losses.

Estrogens and androgens The administration of estrogens to postmenopausal women causes a decrease in urinary calcium and hydroxyproline excretion, especially during the first few months of treatment (see Chap. 340). Estrogens may have direct effects on osteoblasts and mononuclear phagocytes and decrease the rate of bone resorption, but bone formation usually does not increase and eventually decreases. Nevertheless, estrogens produce significant calcium retention, decrease the different between bone formation and resorption, and retard bone loss. Although any restoration of skeletal mass is minimal, the use of estrogens effectively prevents bone loss following castration and in the menopause and decreases the incidence of osteoporotic fracture in postmenopausal women. The major role of estrogens is in preventing osteoporosis in menopausal women rather than treating clinical disease already developed, although they also may be effective in mild or moderate disease during the first 10 years following cessation of ovarian function. The common dosage is 0.625 mg/d as conjugated estrogens, usually in a cyclic fashion, for the first 25 days of each month. (Lower doses are usually ineffective.) Estradiol also can be administered in a percutaneous patch or gel for transdermal absorption (see Chap. 340). In women after hysterectomy, progestogens are not necessary, but in women with a uterus, a progestogen (e.g, medroxyprogesterone 5 mg/d) may be added for the last 12 days of estrogen administration (see Chap. 340). Estrogen (e.g., conjugated estrogens 0.625 mg/d) and a progestogen (e.g., medroxyprogesterone 2.5 mg/d) also may be administered continu-

ously and will prevent the menstrual cycle. Testosterone preparations are useful in treatment of osteoporotic men with gonadal deficiency, but there is no evidence of efficacy in men with normal gonadal function. There is also no proven advantage to combinations of estrogens and androgens.

Calcium supplements, vitamin D metabolites, and thiazide diuretics Women who are estrogen-deprived require an average oral intake of 1500 mg/d of elemental calcium to remain in calcium equilibrium. The recommendation of the National Institutes of Health of 1000 mg elemental calcium per day for women on estrogen replacement and for men is reasonable. In postmenopausal women unable to take estrogens, the use of 1500 mg/d of oral calcium may have minor benefit in preserving cortical bone but has no effects on trabecular bone mass. Adequate calcium intake before age 30 to 35 may enhance peak bone mass, however. The content of elemental calcium of available preparations varies depending on the accompanying anion and the composition (Table 358-2). Vitamin D preparations have been used in osteoporosis because calcium absorption is impaired and levels of the active metabolite, $1,25(OH)_2D$, are marginally low in serum.

Subclinical vitamin D deficiency and associated secondary hyperparathyroidism are common in elderly women, particularly those confined to nursing homes. In these women, low doses of vitamin D (20 μg or 800 IU daily) combined with calcium supplements (1 to 1.5 g elemental calcium daily) are effective in maintaining bone mass and decreasing incidence of hip fractures. Oral administration of calcitriol [$1,25(OH)_2D$] also may improve intestinal calcium absorption, suppress bone resorption, and prevent bone loss in postmenopausal osteoporosis. Bone formation is not increased, however, and the dose used in one study (mean, 0.8 μg/d) caused hypercalcemia and hypercalciuria. Thiazide diuretics are useful in patients with high-turnover osteoporosis associated with hypercalciuria and secondary hyperparathyroidism. In the absence of secondary hyperparathyroidism, the thiazide diuretics lower urinary calcium excretion, suppress parathyroid gland function, inhibit synthesis of $1,25(OH)_2D$, and reduce intestinal calcium absorption.

Calcitonin Calcitonin decreases bone resorption, and the use of salmon calcitonin in established osteoporosis has been recommended in doses of 50 units subcutaneously every other day. Patients with high-turnover osteoporosis (elevated levels of serum osteocalcin, increased urinary hydroxyproline excretion, and increased total-body retention of ^{99m}Tc-methylene diphosphonate) appear to respond best with improvement in bone mass. Another approach involves the use of salmon calcitonin administered by nasal spray (200 units per day) to avoid injections.

Bisphosphonates The bisphosphonate etidronate has been used cyclically, alternating with calcium and vitamin D, to inhibit bone resorption without producing osteomalacia. In the studies reported, the effects of etidronate on bone mass were similar to those of estrogen and calcitonin. It is not yet certain, however, whether therapy with etidronate prevents fractures. Bisphosphonates that do not inhibit mineralization of bone may prove to be more useful antiresorptive agents.

Fluoride Fluoride ions are deposited in the skeleton, where they become incorporated into the crystal lattice of hydroxyapatite,

TABLE 358-2 Elemental calcium content of various oral calcium preparations

Calcium preparation	Elemental calcium content
Calcium citrate	40 mg/300 mg
Calcium carbonate	400 mg/g
Calcium lactate	80 mg/600 mg
Calcium gluconate	40 mg/500 mg
Calcium carbonate + 5 μg vitamin D_2 (Os-Cal 250)	250 mg/tablet

substituting for hydroxyl ions. This process results in a mineral phase of greater crystallinity. Sodium fluoride or intermittent low doses of PTH (currently in therapeutic trials) are the only agents that can stimulate osteoblastic proliferation and function and increase bone formation. Indeed, chronic ingestion of high amounts of fluoride, usually in endemic areas where fluoride content of drinking water is high, produces a form of hyperostosis, with dense bones, exostoses, neurologic complications due to bony overgrowth, and ligament ossification. Increased amount of bone with excessive osteoid is evidence of stimulation of bone formation. When sodium fluoride is used to treat osteoporosis, there is a continuous increase in bone mass of the spine. In some series this increase in bone mass is accompanied by decreased incidence of spinal fractures, but the therapy may result in an increased risk of fractures of the hip as well as other nonvertebral fractures. Even in series in which a satisfactory effect of sodium fluoride is observed, some patients do not respond at all. Some patients do develop side effects, including knee, foot, and ankle pain attributed to microfractures; other patients cannot tolerate the drug because of nausea. An oral slow-release form is better tolerated with fewer gastrointestinal and rheumatologic complications. In any case, calcium supplements with or without vitamin D are necessary to prevent bone mineralization defects that accompany the use of sodium fluoride alone. Lower doses of sodium fluoride may be effective in lowering fracture risk in subjects with osteoporosis without loss of bone quality.

RICKETS AND OSTEOMALACIA

Rickets and *osteomalacia* are disorders in which mineralization of the organic matrix of the skeleton is defective (Table 358-3). In *rickets*, the growing skeleton is involved; defective mineralization occurs both in bone and in the cartilaginous matrix of the growth plate. The term *osteomalacia* is usually reserved for the disorder in the adult, in whom the epiphyseal growth plates are closed. A number of conditions result in rickets and/or osteomalacia, such as inadequate dietary intake of vitamin D, inadequate exposure to solar ultraviolet radiation to form endogenous vitamin D, intestinal malabsorption of vitamin D, acquired and inherited disorders of vitamin D metabolism, inherited defects in the receptor for 1,25(OH)$_2$D in target tissues, chronic acidosis, renal tubular defects which produce hypophosphatemia or acidosis, aluminum intoxication, and chronic administration of anticonvulsants. In the renal tubular disorders, rickets and osteomalacia develop in the presence of normal intestinal function and are not cured by treatment with doses of vitamin D adequate to cure deficiency rickets. Thus the term *vitamin D-resistant* (or *refractory*) *rickets* has been applied in these instances. Renal insufficiency, especially in children, and chronic hemodialysis per se are also associated with rickets or osteomalacia.

PATHOGENESIS AND HISTOPATHOLOGY For skeletal mineralization, sufficient calcium and phosphate must be present at the mineralization sites. Other conditions required for normal mineralization include intact metabolic and transport functions of osteoblasts and chondrocytes, adequate collagen matrix, possibly phosphorylation or other modifications of matrix components, and low concentrations of inhibitory substances such as proteoglycan aggregates or inorganic pyrophosphate. A specific function in the mineralization process for the noncollagenous matrix proteins (e.g., osteocalcin, osteonectin, and phospho-sialoproteins) synthesized by bone cells has not been demonstrated, although they bind calcium ions. In cartilage, the initial mineral phase is in membrane-bound extracellular vesicles. If the osteoblast continues to produce matrix components that cannot be mineralized adequately, rickets and osteomalacia result. If calcification continues to be inadequate, the production of organic matrix (osteoid) also gradually decreases. In bone, there will be an increase in the fraction of the forming surface covered by incompletely mineralized osteoid, an increase in osteoid volume and thickness (the latter normally less than 12 to 14 μm), and a decrease in the calcification

TABLE 358-3 Classification of rickets and osteomalacia

Vitamin D deficiency
 A Dietary deficiency
 B Deficient endogenous synthesis
Gastrointestinal
 A Small-intestinal diseases with malabsorption
 B Partial or total gastrectomy
 C Hepatobiliary disease
 D Chronic pancreatic insufficiency
Disorders of vitamin D metabolism
 A Hereditary: pseudovitamin D deficiency or vitamin D dependency, types I and II
 B Acquired
  1 Anticonvulsants
  2 Chronic renal failure
Acidosis
 A Distal renal tubular acidosis (classic or type I)
 B Secondary forms of renal acidosis
 C Ureterosigmoidostomy
 D Drug-induced disease
  1 Chronic acetazolamide ingestion
  2 Chronic ammonium chloride ingestion
Chronic renal failure
Phosphate depletion
 A Dietary: low phosphate intake plus ingestion of nonabsorbable antacids
 B Impaired renal tubular phosphate reabsorption
  1 Hereditary
   a X-linked hypophosphatemic rickets (vitamin D–resistant rickets)
   b Adult-onset vitamin D–resistant hypophosphatemic osteomalacia
  2 Acquired
   a Sporadic hypophosphatemic osteomalacia (phosphate diabetes)
   b Tumor-associated (oncogenous) rickets and osteomalacia
   c Neurofibromatosis
   d Fibrous dysplasia
Generalized renal tubular disorders (Fanconi's syndrome)
 A Primary renal
 B Associated with systemic metabolic abnormality
  1 Cystinosis
  2 Glycogenosis
  3 Lowe's syndrome
 C Systemic disorder with associated renal disease
  1 Hereditary
   a Inborn errors
    (1) Wilson's disease
    (2) Tyrosinemia
   b Neurofibromatosis
  2 Acquired
   a Multiple myeloma
   b Nephrotic syndrome
   c Transplanted kidney
  3 Intoxications
   a Cadmium
   b Lead
   c Outdated tetracycline
Primary mineralization defects
 A Hereditary: hypophosphatasia
 B Acquired
  1 Diphosphonate (disodium etidronate) treatment
  2 Fluoride treatment
States of rapid bone formation with or without a relative defect in bone resorption
 A Postoperative hyperparathyroidism with osteitis fibrosa cystica
 B Osteopetrosis
Defective matrix synthesis: fibrogenesis imperfecta ossium
Miscellaneous
 A Magnesium-dependent conditions
 B Axial osteomalacia
 C Parenteral alimentation
 D Aluminum intoxication

or mineralization front. The latter is detected in undemineralized sections by the fluorescence of previously ingested tetracycline or by special stains. There is a marked decrease in the rate of apposition of mineralized bone. A number of methods are available to measure the thickness of the osteoid seams and the calcification front. In histologic sections stained with hematoxylin and eosin, the more heavily mineralized areas tend to appear violet or blue, whereas the osteoid seams appear pink. Subtle degrees of osteomalacia may not be appreciated with routine preparations, and undecalcified, thin sections (3 to 5 μm) stained, for example, with Goldner's trichrome method are necessary to establish its presence (Fig. 358-2). Rickets

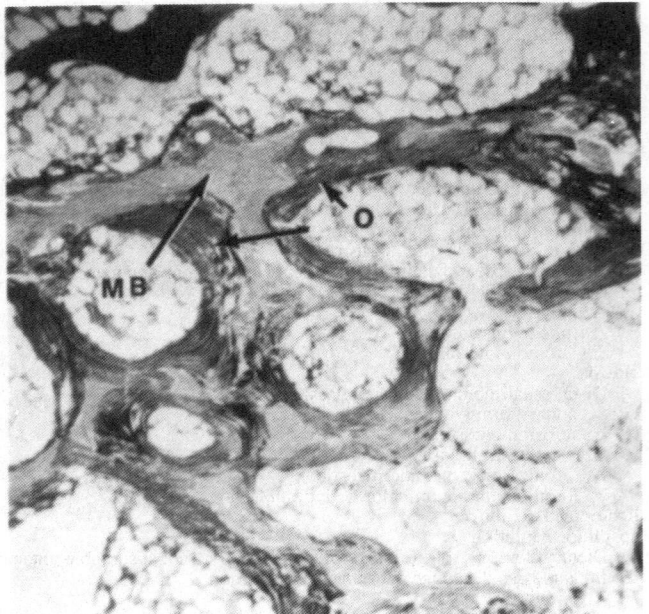

FIGURE 358-2 Photomicrograph of an undemineralized section stained with Goldner method of an iliac crest bone biopsy from a 45-year-old man with chronic renal failure maintained on hemodialysis. Almost the entire surface is covered by osteoid (O) readily distinguished from mineralized bone (MB). The thickness of the osteoid seams exceeds 100 μm in several areas.

is also characterized by inadequate mineralization of the matrix of cartilage in the growing epiphyseal plate. Calcification in the interstitial regions of the hypertrophic zone is defective, the growth plate increases in thickness, the columns of cartilage cells (usually highly ordered) are disorganized, and there is a variable cupping of the epiphyses. The rachitic bones are often incapable of withstanding usual mechanical stresses and tend to undergo bowing deformities. If rickets is untreated, growth at the epiphyseal plates is slowed, and the eventual length of the long bones is diminished.

It has not been established whether vitamin D, through one of its metabolites, has a major direct effect on mineralization as long as the supply of mineral ions is adequate. Its primary roles after metabolic conversion to 25(OH)D and 1,25(OH)₂D are to regulate and enhance absorption of calcium ions from the intestinal lumen and, possibly, to enhance differentiation of stem cells to form osteoclasts. Insufficiency of the active metabolites of vitamin D leads to decreased intestinal absorption of calcium and decreased mobilization of calcium from bone, resulting in hypocalcemia. This stimulates increased synthesis and secretion of PTH and hyperplasia of the parathyroid glands. The increased circulating concentration of PTH tends to increase plasma calcium and enhances renal phosphate clearance, which, in turn, produces hypophosphatemia. When the concentration of phosphorus in the extracellular fluid falls below a critical level, mineralization cannot proceed normally. In severe vitamin D deficiency, normal levels of serum calcium cannot be maintained, and the driving force for mineralization is further decreased. The absence of some critical metabolite of vitamin D that acts directly on the skeleton also may play a role in the defective mineralization of rickets and osteomalacia.

Phosphate depletion alone can produce osteomalacia, as in patients consuming large amounts of nonabsorbable antacids and in persons with excessive renal loss of phosphate due to decreased tubular reabsorption. Secondary hyperparathyroidism is usually not present in these patients. Hypophosphatemia per se produces mineralization defects despite its effect on increasing the activity of the renal 25(OH)D-1α-hydroxylase, but it cannot account for the osteomalacia in all the disorders listed in Table 358-3. In chronic renal failure, for example, plasma phosphate levels are not decreased and usually are increased. Similarly, plasma phosphorus levels are not depressed in infants and children with osteomalacia secondary to hypophosphatasia, a hereditary deficiency in alkaline phosphatase. Osteomalacia in some patients with chronic renal failure is associated with accumulation of aluminum in bone, and the aluminum probably plays a role in production of the mineralization defect.

CLINICAL FINDINGS The clinical manifestations of rickets are the result of skeletal deformities, susceptibility to fractures, weakness and hypotonia, and disturbances in growth. In extreme instances of vitamin D-deficiency rickets, hypocalcemia may cause tetany which, when severe, may be accompanied by laryngeal spasm and seizures. In infants and young children, features include listlessness, irritability, and often profound hypotonia and muscular weakness. As the disorder progresses, children become unable to walk without support. Abnormal parietal flattening and frontal bossing develop in the skull. The calvaria are softened (craniotabes), and sutures may be widened. Prominence of the costochondral junctions is called the "rachitic rosary," and the indentation of the lower ribs at the site of attachment of the diaphragm is known as *Harrison's groove*. If untreated, deformities of the pelvis and extremities progress, with bowing particularly common in the tibia, femur, radius, and ulna. Fractures are frequent, dental eruption is often delayed, and enamel defects are common.

The presentation of osteomalacia in adults is usually more insidious. The skeletal deformities may be overlooked, and the features of the underlying disorder may dominate, as, for example, in the vitamin D deficiency of adult celiac disease. Symptoms, when they occur, include diffuse skeletal pain and bony tenderness. Pain about the hips may result in an antalgic gait. Muscular weakness may be difficult to distinguish from hesitancy to move because of skeletal pain. Proximal weakness may mimic that of primary muscle disorders and contribute to the waddling gait. Pain and weakness may cause patients to be confined to bed and chair. Many factors, including secondary hyperparathyroidism, contribute to the myopathy. Clinical improvement in the myopathy usually results from specific therapy such as vitamin D repletion in nutritional osteomalacia, phosphate replacement in renal hypophosphatemia, or correction of acidosis. Fractures of the involved bones may occur with minimal trauma. When the ribs are involved, severe deformities may develop in the thoracic cage, and the collapse of vertebral bodies may produce loss of height.

RADIOLOGIC FEATURES In rickets, radiologic alterations are most evident at the epiphyseal growth plate, which is increased in thickness, cupped, and hazy at the metaphyseal border due to decreased calcification of the hypertrophic zone and inadequate mineralization of the primary spongiosa. The trabecular pattern of the metaphyses is abnormal, the cortices of the diaphyses may be thinned, and the shafts may be bowed.

In osteomalacia, decrease in bone density is usually associated with loss of trabeculae and thinning of the cortices. The radiologic changes may be indistinguishable from those in osteoporosis. Trabecular patterns may be blurred, producing a homogeneous ground glass appearance. The specific finding that suggests osteomalacia is the presence of radiolucent bands ranging from a few millimeters to several centimeters in length, usually perpendicular to the surface of the bones. They are particularly common at the inner aspects of the femur, especially near the femoral neck, in the pelvis, in the outer edge of the scapula, in the upper fibula, and in the metatarsals (Figs. 358-3 and 358-4). These radiolucent bands, called *pseudofractures* or *Looser's zones*, occur most often at sites where major arteries cross the bones and are thought to be due to the mechanical stress of the pulsation of these vessels. On radionuclide bone scans the pseudofractures appear as hot spots. Subperiosteal erosions along the diaphyseal cortices are sometimes seen in secondary hyperparathyroidism.

Increased rather than decreased density of bones may be observed in patients with renal tubular disorders rather than with vitamin D deficiency and may produce a striking thickening of the cortices and trabeculae of spongy bone. Despite the increase in mass of bone per

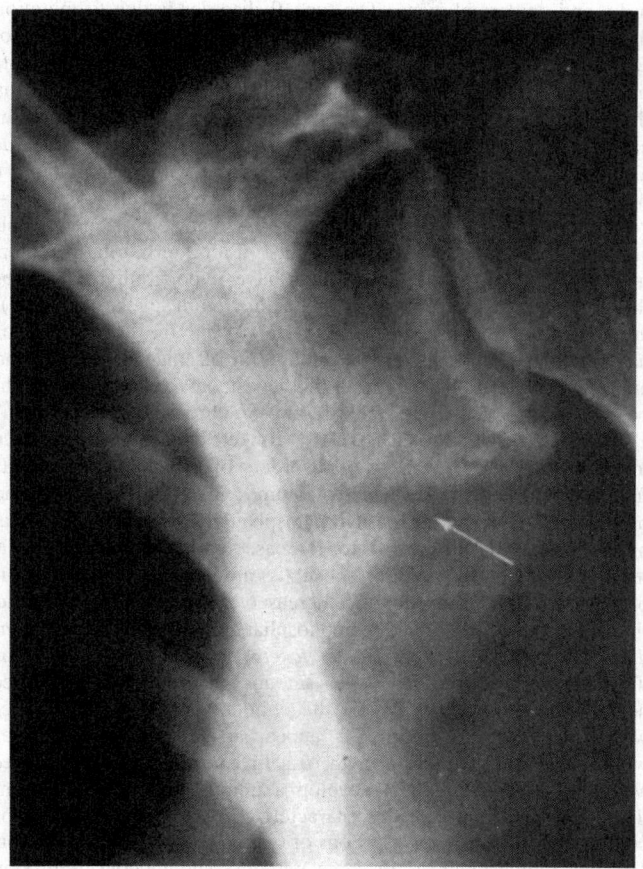

FIGURE 358-3 Radiographs of the scapula of a 58-year-old woman with phosphate diabetes. The presence of a pseudofracture or Looser's zone is indicated by the arrow.

unit volume, the trabeculae are covered with thickened osteoid seams typical of osteomalacia. Similar findings may occur in patients with chronic renal failure. The reason for the hyperostosis is unknown; the bone is architecturally abnormal and subject to fracture with minimal trauma.

LABORATORY FINDINGS Changes in serum concentrations of calcium, inorganic phosphorus, 25(OH)D, and 1,25(OH)$_2$D vary with the different disorders (see Chap. 356). In vitamin D deficiency, whether due to dietary lack, inadequate sunlight exposure, or intestinal malabsorption, serum calcium levels are normal or low, whereas phosphorus and 25(OH)D levels are consistently low, the latter usually <20 nmol/L (<8 ng/mL) depending on the assay. In contrast, levels of 1,25(OH)$_2$D may be normal or elevated due to secondary hyperparathyroidism. Eventually, when levels of 25(OH)D become so low that there is inadequate substrate for the renal 25(OH)D-1α-hydroxylase, then the serum level of 1,25(OH)$_2$D also declines. In adults, the lower limit of serum phosphorus concentration is around 0.9 mmol/L (2.8 mg/dL); in children, the lower limit of normal is closer to 1.3 to 1.5 mmol/L (4.0 to 4.5 mg/dL). In *severe* vitamin D depletion, hypocalcemia may be sufficient to produce tetany. Mild acidosis and generalized aminoaciduria result from secondary hyperparathyroidism. As a rule, patients with renal tubular disorders have normal serum calcium levels and hypophosphatemia. Other laboratory findings, such as glucosuria, aminoaciduria, acidosis, and hypouricemia, reflect variable degrees of disturbance of proximal tubular function or features of the underlying disease (e.g., low plasma ceruloplasmin in Wilson's disease or abnormalities of immunoglobulins in multiple myeloma). In chronic renal failure, hyperphosphatemia and hypocalcemia are usually accompanied by normal 25 (OH)D and low 1,25(OH)$_2$D levels. In nephrotic syndrome, serum 25(OH)D levels can be low due primarily to urinary losses of protein-bound 25(OH)D. Serum phosphorus levels are also normal or elevated in hypophosphatasia. Increased excretion of hydroxyproline-containing peptides occurs when secondary hyperparathyroidism and excessive bone resorption are associated with the defect in mineralization. Alkaline phosphatase levels in plasma are usually elevated in rickets or osteomalacia, but typical and even severe osteomalacia, especially that due to renal tubular disorders, may be accompanied by normal levels or borderline elevations. Levels may increase during the early phases of therapy.

DIETARY VITAMIN D DEFICIENCY AND INADEQUATE ENDOGENOUS SYNTHESIS Most foods unfortified with vitamin D contain insufficient amounts of the vitamin to prevent rickets in growing children or osteomalacia in adults living in temperate-zone cities. As discussed in Chap. 356, in the absence of supplements, vitamin D must be formed endogenously through the ultraviolet irradiation of precursor 7-dehydrocholesterol in the skin. Many factors decrease the formation of vitamin D$_3$ from its precursor: increased melanin pigmentation, hyperkeratosis, sunscreens, limited exposure of the body, short days of sunlight, oblique angle of ultraviolet irradiation, and factors in the atmosphere, such as smog, which prevent adequate penetration of solar ultraviolet radiation. Since fortification of milk and routine use of vitamin D supplements for infants have been in

FIGURE 358-4 Radiograph of the femurs of a 47-year-old woman with Fanconi's syndrome of adult onset. The presence of multiple pseudofractures is indicated by the arrows.

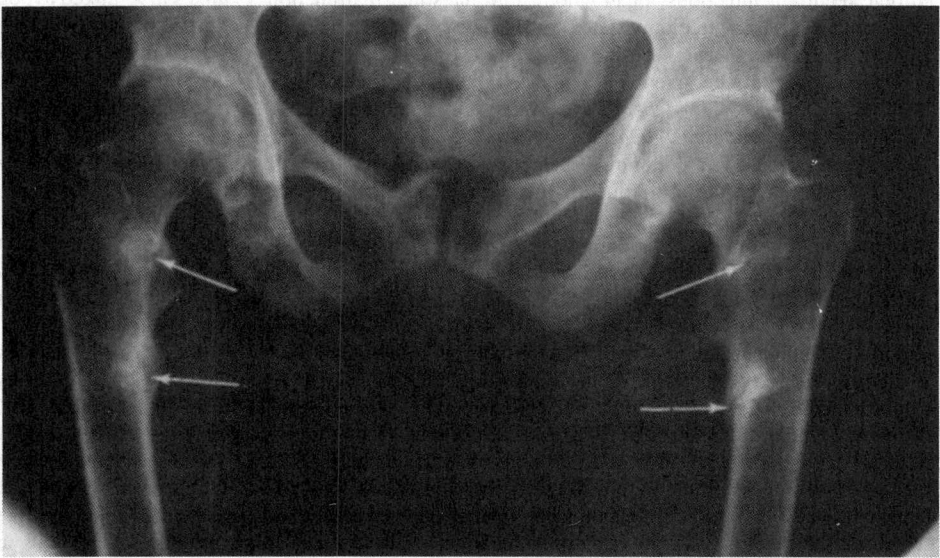

effect, deficiency is unusual in the United States. Poor, dark-skinned infants living in crowded northern cities are most susceptible. Furthermore, elderly individuals with insufficient sun exposure, particularly those who are housebound or in nursing homes, drink no milk, and receive no vitamin D supplements, may have low serum levels of 25(OH)D, secondary hyperparathyroidism, and increased frequency of hip fractures. Intestinal absorption of vitamin D is normal in the elderly.

VITAMIN D LOSS AND INTESTINAL MALABSORPTION Osteomalacia may occur with intestinal malabsorption such as in adult celiac disease and regional enteritis. Prior to the discovery of gluten sensitivity in some of these cases, celiac disease was among the more common disorders underlying osteomalacia. Vitamin D absorption, which normally occurs via chylomicrons, is impaired in diseases causing steatorrhea, such as chronic biliary obstruction. Patients with cholestatic liver disease or extrahepatic biliary obstruction may have low serum levels of 25(OH)D and osteomalacia due not only to poor vitamin D absorption but also to decreased hepatic production of 25(OH)D. Osteomalacia is less frequent in chronic pancreatic insufficiency. Patients who have had gastric surgery for peptic ulcer disease or gastric bypass for obesity also may develop osteomalacia, possibly due to malfunction of the proximal small bowel. Additional factors may contribute to the osteomalacia in patients with small-bowel disease, such as inadequate absorbing surface and failure of intestinal cells to respond to the active metabolites of vitamin D. Secondary hyperparathyroidism is usually present in intestinal malabsorption, as in dietary lack of vitamin D, and may be particularly severe in patients who develop osteomalacia following intestinal bypass surgery. Some patients who lack vitamin D, usually associated with intestinal malabsorption, have normal circulating levels of 1,25(OH)$_2$D despite low or undetectable levels of 25(OH)D. In these individuals, the normal levels of 1,25(OH)$_2$D may be accounted for by ingestion of sufficient vitamin D in hospital diets to produce substrate 25(OH)D for 1α-hydroxylation by the renal enzyme that is increased in activity due to secondary hyperparathyroidism. In other patients, circulating 1,25(OH)$_2$D levels may not reflect levels at critical target cells.

ABNORMAL METABOLISM OF VITAMIN D Serum 25(OH)D levels are reduced in some instances of parenchymal and obstructive liver disease, but these findings have not been correlated with quantitative histologic studies of bone. Patients consuming anticonvulsant drugs such as phenobarbital, phenytoin, or carbamazepine may develop rickets or osteomalacia. For a given intake of vitamin D, patients on chronic anticonvulsant therapy have lower serum levels of calcium and 25(OH)D. Consumption of anticonvulsants may be especially important in individuals whose intake of vitamin D is marginal, who are nonambulatory and confined indoors, who have chronic recurrent infections, or in whom mild intestinal malfunction exists as in the postgastrectomy state. As discussed in Chap. 356, the anticonvulsant drugs have multiple actions on calcium homeostasis.

Two autosomal recessive syndromes associated with rickets have been termed *vitamin D–dependent rickets* (also see Chap. 329). Features of *type I vitamin D–dependent rickets* include hypocalcemia, hypophosphatemia, short stature, skeletal deformities of rickets, dental enamel hypoplasia, frequently marked elevations of serum alkaline phosphatase activity, generalized aminoaciduria, and secondary hyperparathyroidism. Circulating levels of 1,25(OH)$_2$D are low or undetectable. Treatment with massive doses of vitamin D or small doses of calcitriol reverses the abnormal biochemical findings, induces healing of the rickets, and restores the rate of skeletal growth. The abnormalities are due to mutations that impair the renal 25(OH)D-1α-hydroxylase. By linkage analysis, the disorder has been mapped to chromosome 12q14. Lifelong replacement therapy with calcitriol is required. *Type II vitamin D–dependent rickets*, also termed *hereditary resistance to 1,25(OH)$_2$D*, has many clinical features of the type I syndrome. Rickets is usually of early onset but varies in severity in different kindreds. Distinguishing features include alopecia, which may develop during the first few months of age, and multiple

milia and epidermal cysts. The type II disorder is due to mutations that impair structure and function of the 1,25(OH)$_2$D receptor. Different molecular abnormalities in different kindreds include mutations that impair binding of the receptor to DNA, mutations that cause the formation of incomplete receptor molecules, and mutations that cause single amino acid substitutions in the protein. This disorder also maps by linkage analysis to chromosome 12 in a locus close to but distinct from that for type I vitamin D–dependent rickets.

Abnormalities in vitamin D metabolism, not on a genetic basis, and osteomalacia may occur in patients on long-term total parenteral nutrition. Some of these individuals have hypoparathyroidism, but this cannot account for the osteomalacia. Serum levels of 25(OH)D are normal, although levels of 1,25(OH)$_2$D may be low. Aluminum has been detected in increased amounts in plasma, urine, and bone and may play a role in genesis of the osteomalacia similar to that postulated in patients with renal failure on chronic hemodialysis.

RENAL TUBULAR DISORDERS Rickets and osteomalacia occur in association with a variety of disorders of proximal renal tubular function. These disorders have in common increased renal clearance of inorganic phosphorus and hypophosphatemia with normal or near-normal glomerular filtration rate. Increased phosphate clearance with resultant hypophosphatemia is usually an isolated defect with no other abnormalities except for increased urinary glycine excretion (hyperglycinuria). X-linked hypophosphatemia (also called *phosphate diabetes* or *vitamin D–resistant rickets*) is an X-linked dominant disorder characterized by rickets in an otherwise well-nourished, healthy-appearing child. When the child begins to walk and bear weight, lower limb deformities appear and become progressively worse. The rate of linear growth is at first normal and then slowed. Many of these individuals develop a unique disorder of tendons, ligaments, and joint capsules characterized by calcification or, more probably, ossification of insertions of tendons and ligaments and joint capsules (enthesopathy). In some patients, spontaneous remissions may be followed by recurrences in adult life, e.g., with pregnancy and lactation. Hypophosphatemia is due to defective renal conservation of phosphate, which in turn is due to defective phosphate transport across the luminal membrane of proximal renal tubular cells. [A model of the human disease occurs in a strain of hypophosphatemic (Hyp) mice.] On the basis of analysis of restriction fragment polymorphism studies in several kindreds of X-linked hypophosphatemia, the gene has been mapped to the short arm of the X chromosome (Xp22.31-p21.3). The responsible gene has not been identified. In affected individuals, the serum levels of 25(OH)D are normal, and the levels of 1,25(OH)$_2$D are in the low-normal range. Whereas the induction of hypophosphatemia in normal individuals results in stimulation of 25(OH)D-1α-hydroxylase and an increase in the levels of 1,25(OH)$_2$D, altered renal tubular cellular phosphate fluxes in X-linked hypophosphatemia fail to stimulate the hydroxylase. Thus levels of 1,25(OH)$_2$D, although in the normal range, are inappropriately low relative to the phosphate depletion. The skeletal mineralization defect is due both to the low ambient phosphate levels and to an intrinsic defect in osteoblast function possibly related to that in the renal tubular cells. Effective therapy therefore requires both phosphate repletion with large amounts of oral phosphate and treatment with calcitriol (see below). Such combined therapy reverses the osteomalacia of trabecular bone surfaces, corrects the microscopic periosteocytic mineralization defects, and results in improvement in longitudinal growth. After the rickets is healed, however, defects in phosphate clearance and hypophosphatemia persist, and medical therapy is still required. The effects of excessive calcitriol administration, such as nephrocalcinosis and nephrolithiasis, must be avoided. Adults with X-linked hypophosphatemia frequently have pseudofractures; osteoarthritis in the sacroiliac joints, wrists, knees, hips, and feet; and marked enthesopathy. Another variant of hereditary rickets has been termed *hereditary hypophosphatemic rickets with hypercalciuria*. Muscular weakness, not a feature of X-linked hypophosphatemia, may be present. These individuals, whose disorder is probably inherited as an autosomal recessive trait, have normocalcemia, hypophosphatemia, and striking absorptive hypercalciuria; the latter disappears after fasting and returns after oral calcium loading. Levels of 1,25(OH)$_2$D in serum are elevated, in contrast to low-normal levels in X-linked hypophosphatemia. These elevations of serum 1,25(OH)$_2$D are an appropriate response of the 25(OH)D-1α-hydroxylase to phosphate depletion. Phosphate replacement induces healing of the rachitic lesions.

Sporadic cases of hypophosphatemia also have been described in adults in whom family histories are negative and proximal muscle weakness is a prominent feature (see also Chap. 359). These patients also are best treated with a combination of calcitriol and inorganic phosphorus. As mentioned above, secondary hyperparathyroidism is not present in most untreated patients with renal tubular disorders associated with rickets and osteomalacia.

In other patients, the disorder in tubular function may be more widespread, involving (besides phosphorus) glucose, potassium, amino acids, and uric acid; the various combinations are termed the *de Toni-Debré-Fanconi syndrome*. The more complete renal tubular defects may occur sporadically or in families. In some instances, the lesion is part of a more widespread disorder, as in Wilson's disease and cystinosis. Fanconi syndrome also may be a feature of plasma cell myeloma, where it is attributed to toxic effects of deposited Bence Jones protein. Similarly, osteomalacia and renal tubular acidosis have been observed in Sjögren syndrome with increased urinary excretion of beta$_2$ microglobulin and retinol-binding protein. The acidosis of proximal tubular defects also plays a role in development of osteomalacia, possibly by altering metabolism of vitamin D or the renal handling of calcium and phosphorus. In this regard, osteomalacia has accompanied the hyperchloremic acidosis or ureterocolic anastomosis.

TUMOR-ASSOCIATED (ONCOGENOUS) OSTEOMALACIA Osteomalacia and hypophosphatemia with high renal phosphate clearance occur with a variety of mesenchymal tumors, including giant cell tumors (benign or malignant), reparative granulomas, hemangiomas, fibromas, and other mesenchymal neoplasms. A similar syndrome occurs in patients with prostatic carcinoma. In some instances, removal of the tumor resulted in return of renal phosphorus clearance to normal, rise in serum phosphorus levels, and healing of the osteomalacia (or rickets in children). Serum 1,25(OH)$_2$D levels are low or undetectable, although chronic administration of sufficient calcitriol to raise circulating levels of this metabolite to normal does not alter renal phosphorus clearance or serum phosphorus concentrations. Humoral factors released by these tumors may impair proximal tubular functions such as 1α-hydroxylation of 25(OH)D *and* phosphate transport.

CHRONIC RENAL FAILURE Osteomalacia is common in patients with chronic renal failure; it tends to be the predominant type of renal osteodystrophy in younger patients and is more frequent in those with the lower plasma levels of calcium and phosphorus. A component of secondary hyperparathyroidism and osteitis fibrosa is almost always present. The defect itself probably involves a decreased conversion of 25(OH)D to 1,25,(OH)$_2$D either because of insufficient viable renal cortical tissue or the inhibitory effect of hyperphosphatemia on renal 25(OH)D-1α-hydroxylase activity. In addition, there may be a primary defect in intestinal calcium absorption. Part of the secondary hyperparathyroidism also may be due to decreased phosphate clearance and subsequent hyperphosphatemia. Under circumstances of hyperphosphatemia and near-normal plasma concentration of calcium, the presence of inhibitors probably causes the defective mineralization. In some patients, the osteomalacia responds to large doses of vitamin D or dihydrotachysterol or to small doses of calcitriol or calcifediol. However, some patients with renal osteodystrophy do not respond to pharmacologic doses of vitamin D or to calcitriol. In some, accumulation of aluminum in the bone accounts for the vitamin D–refractory osteomalacia. Aluminum deposits can be identified at the mineralization fronts, and bone apposition rates are low. These individuals have high levels of aluminum and uncoupling of matrix deposition and mineralization. Individuals with lower amounts of aluminum develop

a form of "aplastic" bone disease where matrix deposition and mineralization are more closely coupled. Deferoxamine can mobilize aluminum from bone and other tissues and is effective therapy. In some patients with renal osteodystrophy, the total bone mass may be increased (osteosclerosis), resulting in increased density of bone. This is particularly evident in the spine, where a characteristic appearance is that of dense bone at the superior and inferior margins of the vertebral bodies with more radiolucent central portions ("rugger jersey sign"). Histologically, although there is more bone per unit area, each trabecula is covered by a wide osteoid seam.

HYPOPHOSPHATASIA Rickets is a feature of a deficiency of alkaline phosphatase in infants and children termed *hypophosphatasia*. There are four forms of hypophosphatasia, i.e., lethal perinatal, infantile, childhood, and adult. Rickets occurs in the infantile and childhood forms. In adults, the disorder may not be recognized until middle age, but there is frequently a history of early loss of deciduous or permanent teeth. Osteomalacia and calcium pyrophosphate deposition disease occur in the adult form. The severe perinatal and infantile forms are inherited as autosomal recessive traits; the pattern of inheritance in the other forms is uncertain. The low levels of circulating alkaline phosphatase activity are explained by a deficiency of the tissue-nonspecific enzyme (bone-liver-kidney). Missense mutations have been demonstrated in the alkaline phosphatase gene.

Although alkaline phosphatase is abundant in osteoclasts, its function in mineralization is not established. In hypophosphatasia, there is increased urinary excretion of phosphoethanolamine and increased circulating levels of pyridoxal-5'-phosphate. The metabolic origin of the phosphoethanolamine is not established. Concentrations of pyridoxal-5'-phosphate are not elevated intracellularly, and the extracellular increases are consistent with the function of alkaline phosphatase as an ectoenzyme; whether alterations of pyridoxal-5'-phosphate metabolism contribute to the clinical abnormalities is not known. Inorganic pyrophosphate (PPi) is a substrate for alkaline phosphatase, which accounts for increased levels of PPi in urine and plasma and for the increased incidence of calcium pyrophosphate deposition disease in hypophosphatasia. Since PPi also can function to inhibit growth of the calcium-phosphate mineral phase, excessive concentrations of PPi may cause the rickets and osteomalacia. There is no effective therapy.

OTHER DISORDERS ASSOCIATED WITH DEFECTIVE MINERALIZATION Disturbances in mineralization may be seen in patients consuming high doses of fluoride ion and in patients with Paget's disease treated with diphosphonates such as etidronate. Some decrease in mineralization of newly forming matrix, increase in surface covered by osteoid, and increase in the width of the osteoid seams may occur in conditions that are not usually considered as osteomalacia except by these criteria. Examples include patients with the osteitis fibrosa of hyperparathyroidism following surgical cure. In these circumstances, there is a temporary imbalance between the rate at which mineral is supplied to bone and the rate at which bone matrix is formed. Biopsies in some of these conditions show a normal calcification front. Wide osteoid seams and hypophosphatemia are also seen in children with osteopetrosis, in whom there is inadequate resorption of bone and calcified cartilage but active bone formation.

A condition that resembles osteomalacia and is associated with a coarsened, mottled bony trabecular pattern, pseudofractures, and bone pain but normal plasma levels of calcium and phosphorus is *fibrogenesis imperfecta ossium*. The bone has a distinctive histologic appearance, with wide osteoid seams, distortion of the birefringent pattern of normal bone, and abnormal collagen fibers by electron microscopy. The nature of the abnormality is not known.

TREATMENT OF RICKETS AND OSTEOMALACIA In rickets and osteomalacia due to dietary absence of vitamin D or inadequate exposure to sunlight, vitamin D$_2$ (ergocalciferol) or vitamin D$_3$ (cholecalciferol) is given orally in doses of 800 to 4000 IU (0.02 to 0.1 mg) daily for 6 to 12 weeks, followed by daily supplements of 200 to 400 IU, which are adequate to prevent the development of the disorder in otherwise normal subjects. In infants and children, such treatment causes improvement in muscle tone and strength, increase in serum calcium and phosphorus levels, and decrease in alkaline phosphatase levels after several weeks. Radiologic evidence of healing is evident within weeks and may be complete by a few months. Calcium supplements and larger initial doses of vitamin D may be necessary in infants and children with tetany. In adults with nutritional osteomalacia, healing of pseudofractures may be evident within 3 to 4 weeks after therapy with as little as 2000 IU (0.5 mg) vitamin D daily. Healing is complete usually by 6 months.

Patients with osteomalacia due to intestinal malabsorption do not respond to small doses of vitamin D. In the presence of active steatorrhea, daily oral doses of vitamin D of 50,000 to 100,000 IU (1.25 to 2.5 mg) and large doses of calcium (e.g., 15 g calcium lactate or 4 g calcium carbonate orally per day) may be required. In some instances, oral vitamin D is ineffective, and the parenteral route is required (e.g., 10,000 IU/d intramuscularly). Another approach is the use of artificial ultraviolet B radiation or exposure to sunlight in addition to supplemental calcium. Small doses of calcitriol (0.5 to 1.0 μg daily) are usually effective in this form of osteomalacia. Inorganic phosphate therapy is not indicated either in deficiency or in intestinal malabsorption of the vitamin, since hypocalcemia will develop and intestinal calcium absorption will remain inadequate. In all patients in whom large doses of vitamin D are used, serum calcium and 25(OH)D levels should be monitored periodically. Semiquantitative urinary calcium measurements are inadequate.

In patients on anticonvulsants, it is usually necessary to continue the drugs while adding 4000 to 40,000 IU/d of vitamin D and to monitor levels of serum calcium and serum 25(OH)D until a therapeutic response (evidence of radiologic healing, improvement in symptoms) is obtained.

Treatment of rickets and osteomalacia in the presence of renal tubular disorders is more difficult. In the past, the X-linked form of hypophosphatemic osteomalacia was treated with large doses of vitamin D (from 50,000 to several hundred thousand IU/d), but skeletal responses were rarely complete. The use of dihydrotachysterol, a pseudo-1α(OH)D analogue, 0.2 to 0.6 mg orally per day, in place of vitamin D had the advantage of shorter onset and duration of action and more consistent skeletal healing. With such therapy, radiologic evidence of healing in many patients is incomplete; some hypophosphatemia persists, linear skeletal growth remains abnormally slow, and bony deformities continue to develop. In addition, hypercalcemia and its consequences are potential hazards. Currently, oral supplements of inorganic phosphate in divided doses of phosphorus, 1.0 to 3.6 g/d, and calcitriol, 0.5 to 2.0 μg/d, constitute the best regimen to restore skeletal growth and heal the bone disease. In some adults therapy with inorganic phosphate alone abolishes muscle weakness and bone pain and produces radiologic and histologic healing. The addition of calcitriol improves calcium balance and helps decrease secondary hyperparathyroidism and maintain a sufficient level of serum phosphorus to permit complete healing. In some patients there may be temporary increase in bone pain and rise in serum alkaline phosphatase during the early phases of treatment. In the osteomalacia associated with the chronic acidosis of renal tubular disorders, the use of alkali may be of value in supplementing therapy with phosphate and calcitriol. In patients with ureterosigmoidostomy, oral sodium bicarbonate can reverse acidosis, improve serum phosphate level, and heal the bone disease; with maintenance doses of alkali, recurrence of symptoms can be prevented.

Patients with nephrotic syndrome and low serum 25(OH)D levels benefit from modest vitamin D supplementation. In chronic renal failure, high doses of vitamin D, similar to those needed to treat osteomalacia of renal tubular disorders, are used. Dihydrotachysterol at doses of 0.2 to 1.0 mg daily and small doses of calcitriol are equally effective in treating hypocalcemia and osteodystrophy resulting from chronic renal failure. The recommended initial dose of calcitriol is 0.25 μg/d. If after 2 to 4 weeks on this dose the biochemical parameters are unaltered, the dose is increased by 0.25 μg/d every 2 to 4 weeks until a satisfactory clinical biochemical response (including elevation of serum calcium levels and decrease in PTH levels) is obtained. The usual dose is 0.5 to 1.0 μg/d. Calcitriol also may be administered intravenously (1.0 to 2.5 μg three times weekly) in patients on dialysis, particularly to treat refractory osteitis fibrosa. Because there are no regulatory mechanisms to control the biological responses to calcitriol, there is a high incidence of transient hypercalciuria and hypercalcemia, especially initially. Thus serum calcium should be monitored frequently during the first 1 to 2 months of therapy and less frequently once a stable dose has been established. Since calcitriol has a short duration of action and is not stored in fat depots, hypercalcemia usually resolves in 2 to 7 days after the dose is discontinued or decreased. Phosphate supplements are, of course, contraindicated in the usual patient with chronic renal failure. Occasionally, however, hypophosphatemia may result from the excessive use of nonabsorbable antacids or from excessive removal of phosphate through hemodialysis.

In patients who have had rickets in childhood, the abnormal mechanical stress of severe deformities may contribute to the development of degenerative joint disease, particularly in hips and knees. Osteotomies at the proper time after healing may prevent this complication and the requirement for more extensive arthroplasties later in life.

REFERENCES

Osteoporosis

AVIOLI LV, KRANE SM (eds): *Metabolic Bone Disease and Clinically Related Disorders*. Philadelphia, Saunders, 1990

BERGKVIST L et al: The risk of breast cancer after estrogen and estrogen-progestin replacement. N Engl J Med 321:293, 1989

BILLER BMK et al: Mechanisms of osteoporosis in adult and adolescent women with anorexia nervosa. J Clin Endocrinol Metab 68:548, 1989

BOIVIN G et al: Fluoride content in human iliac bone: Results in controls, patients with fluorosis, and osteoporotic patients treated with fluoride. J Bone Miner Res 3:497, 1988

BUCHANAN JR et al: Effect of excess endogenous androgens on bone density in young women. J Clin Endocrinol Metab 67:937, 1988

CHEEMA C et al: Effects of estrogen on circulating "free" and total 1,25-dihydroxyvitamin D and on the parathyroid–vitamin D axis in postmenopausal women. J Clin Invest 83:537, 1989

CIVITELLI R et al: Bone turnover in postmenopausal osteoporosis: Effect on calcitonin treatment. J Clin Invest 82: 1268, 1988

COLE WG et al: New insights into the molecular pathology of osteogenesis imperfecta. Q J Med 70, 1, 1989

DEMPSTER DW: Bone histomorphology in glucocorticoid-induced osteoporosis. J Bone Miner Res 4:137, 1989

——, LINDSAY R: Pathogenesis of osteoporosis. Lancet 341:797, 1993

DIAMOND T et al: Ethanol reduces bone formation and may cause osteoporosis. Am J Med 86:282, 1989

DRINKWATER BL et al: Bone mineral content of amenorrheic and eumenorrheic athletes. N Engl J Med 311:277, 1984

EASTELL R et al: Colles' fracture and bone density of the ultradistal radius. J Bone Miner Res 4:607, 1989

ETTINGER B et al: Postmenopausal bone loss is prevented by treatment with low-dosage estrogen with calcium. Ann Intern Med 106:40, 1987

FINKELSTEIN JS et al: Osteoporosis in men with idiopathic hypogonadotropic hyogonadism. Ann Intern Med 106:354, 1987

GALLAGHER JC et al: Epidemiology of fractures of the proximal femur in Rochester, Minnesota. Clin Orthop 150:163, 1980

HEANEY RP et al: Thinking straight about calcium. N Engl J Med 328:503, 1993

HEDLUND LR, GALLAGHER JC: Increased incidence of hip fracture in osteoporotic women treated with sodium fluoride. J Bone Miner Res 4:223, 1989

HODSMAN AB, DROST DJ: The response of vertebral bone mineral density during the treatment of osteoporosis with sodium fluoride. J Clin Endocrinol Metab 69:932, 1989

HOLBROOK TL et al: Dietary calcium and risk of hip fracture: 14-year prospective population study. Lancet 2:1046, 1988

HOROWITZ MC: Cytokines and estrogen in bone: Anti-osteoporotic effects. Science 260:626, 1993

HUPPERT LC: Hormonal replacement therapy: Benefits, risks, doses. Med Clin North Am 71:23, 1987

JENSEN J et al: Cigarette smoking, serum estrogens, and bone loss during hormone-replacement therapy early after menopause. N Engl J Med 313:973, 1985

KRANE SM, SCHILLER AL: Metabolic disease, in *Endocrinology*, 2d ed, LJ DeGroot et al (eds). Philadelphia, Saunders, 1989, vol 2, p 1151

LINDSAY R: Prevention and treatment of osteoporosis. Lancet 341:801, 1993

—— et al: Prevention of spinal osteoporosis in oophorectomised women. Lancet 2:1151, 1980

MAMELLE N et al: Risk-benefit ratio of sodium fluoride treatment in primary vertebral osteoporosis. Lancet 2:361, 1988

MARIE PJ et al: Osteocalcin and deoxyribonucleic acid synthesis in vitro and histomorphometric indices of bone formation in postmenopausal osteoporosis. J Clin Endocrinol Metab 69:272, 1989

NABULSI AA et al: Association of hormone-replacement therapy with various cardiovascular risk factors in postmenopausal women. N Engl J Med 328:1069, 1993

NAGANT DE DEUXCHAISNES C: Therapy for skeletal disorders. Curr Opin Rheumatol 1:98, 1989

PAK CYC et al: Safe and effective treatment of osteoporosis with intermittent slow release sodium fluoride: Augmentation of vertebral bone mass and inhibition of fractures. J Clin Endocrinol Metab 68:150, 1989

PARFITT AM: Dietary risk factors for age-related bone loss and fractures. Lancet 2:1181, 1983

——— et al: Relationship between surface, volume, and thickness of iliac trabecular bone in aging and in osteoporosis: Implications for the microanatomic and cellular mechanisms of bone loss. J Clin Invest 72:783, 1985

POCOCK NA et al: Recovery from steroid-induced osteoporosis. Ann Intern Med 107:319, 1987

PRIOR JC et al: Spinal bone loss and ovulatory disturbances. N Engl J Med 323:1221, 1990

PROCKOP DJ: Mutations that alter the primary structure of type I collagen. J Biol Chem 265:15349, 1990

REGINSTER JY et al: Relationship between whole plasma calcitonin levels, calcitonin secretory capacity, and plasma levels of estrone in healthy women and postmenopausal osteoporotics. J Clin Invest 83:1073, 1989

REID IR et al: Effect of calcium supplementation of bone loss in postmenopausal women. N Engl J Med 328:460, 1993

RIGGS BL, MELTON LJ III: Evidence for two distinct syndromes of involutional osteoporosis. Am J Med 75:899, 1983

———, ——— Involutional osteoporosis. N Engl J Med 314:1676, 1986

——— et al: Incidence of hip fractures in osteoporotic women treated with sodium fluoride. J Bone Miner Res 2:123, 1987

——— et al: Effect of fluoride treatment on the fracture rate in postmenopausal women with osteoporosis. N Engl J Med 322:802, 1990

———, ——— The prevention and treatment of osteoporosis. N Engl J Med 327:620, 1992

RIIS B et al: Does calcium supplementation prevent postmenopausal bone loss? N Engl J Med 316:173, 1987

RYAN PJ et al: Osteoporosis and chronic back pain: A study with single-photon emission computed tomography bone scintigraphy. J Bone Miner Res 7:1455, 1992

SAMBROOK P et al: Prevention of corticosteroid osteoporosis: A comparison of calcium, calcitriol, and calcitonin. N Engl J Med 328:1747, 1993

SEEMAN E et al: Risk factors for spinal osteoporosis in men. Am J Med 75:977, 1983

——— et al: Effect of early menopause on bone mass in normal women and patients with osteoporosis. Am J Med 85:213, 1988

SILVERBERG SJ et al: Abnormalities in parathyroid hormone secretion and 1,25-dihydroxyvitamin D_3 formation in women with osteoporosis. N Engl J Med 320:277, 1989

SMITH R et al: Osteoporosis of pregnancy. Lancet 1:1178, 1985

SPENCER H et al: Chronic alcoholism: Frequently overlooked cause of osteoporosis in men. Am J Med 80:393, 1986

STEINBERG KK et al: Sex steroids and bone density in premenopausal and perimenopausal women. J Clin Endocrinol Metab 69:533, 1989

STEPAN JJ et al: Castrated men exhibit bone loss: Effect of calcitonin treatment on biochemical indices of bone remodeling. J Clin Endocrinol Metab 69:523, 1989

STEWART AF et al: Calcium homeostasis in immobilization: An example of resorptive hypercalciuria. N Engl J Med 306:1136, 1982

STORM T et al: Effect of intermittent cyclical etidronate therapy on bone mass and fracture rate in women with postmenopausal osteoporosis. N Engl J Med 322:1265, 1990

TILYARD MW et al: Treatment of postmenopausal osteoporosis with calcitriol or calcium. N Engl J Med 326:357, 1992

WATTS et al: Intermittent cyclical etidronate treatment of postmenopausal osteoporosis. N Engl J Med 323:73, 1990

WEINSTEIN RS, BELL NH: Diminished rates of bone formation in normal black adults. N Engl J Med 319:1698, 1988

WHITEHEAD MI, FRASER D: Controversies concerning the safety of estrogen replacement therapy. Am J Obstet Gynecol 156:1313, 1987

WILSON RJ et al: Mild asymptomatic primary hyperparathyroidism is not a risk factor for vertebral fractures. Ann Intern Med 109:959, 1988

Osteomalacia

ANDRESS DL et al: Osteomalacia and aplastic bone disease in aluminum-related osteodystrophy. J Clin Endocrinol Metab 65:11, 1987

ANDRESS DL et al: Intravenous calcitriol in the treatment of refractory osteitis fibrosa of chronic renal failure. N Engl J Med 321:274, 1989

BONKOVSKY HL et al: Prevalence and prediction of osteopenia in chronic liver disease. Hepatology 12:273, 1990

BURNSTEIN MI et al: The enthesopathic changes of hypophosphatemic osteomalacia in adults: Radiologic findings. AJR 153:785, 1989

CHARHON SA et al: Effects of parathyroidectomy on bone formation and mineralization in hemodialyzed patients. Kidney Int 27:426, 1984

CHINES A, PACIFICI R: Antacid and sucralfate-induced hypophosphatemic osteomalacia: A case report and review of the literature. Calcif Tissue Int 47:291, 1990

COLLINS N et al: A prospective study to evaluate the dose of vitamin D required to correct low 25-hydroxyvitamin D levels, calcium, and alkaline phosphatase in patients at risk of developing antiepileptic drug-induced osteomalacia. Q J Med 78:113, 1991

DAWSON-HUGHES B et al: Effect of vitamin D supplementation on wintertime and overall bone loss in healthy postmenopausal women. Ann Intern Med 115:505, 1991

DELVIN EE et al: Vitamin D nutritional status and related biochemical indices in an autonomous elderly population. Am J Clin Nutr 48:373, 1988

DIAMOND TH: Metabolic bone disease in primary biliary cirrhosis. J Gastroenterol Hepatol 5:66, 1990

FRASER D, SCRIVER CR: Hereditary rickets and osteomalacia associated with abnormalities in vitamin D metabolism (calcipenic rickets) or phosphate homeostasis (phosphopenic rickets), in *Endocrinology*, 2d ed, LJ DeGroot et al (eds). Philadelphia, Saunders, 1989, vol 2, p 1080

GALLAGHER JC: Vitamin D metabolism and therapy in elderly subjects. South Med J 85:2S43, 1992

GLORIEUX FH: Disturbances of phosphate metabolism—Effects on bone, in *Metabolic Bone Disease: Cellular and Tissue Mechanism*, CS Tam et al (eds). Boca Raton, Fla, CRC Press, 1988, p 215

———: Rickets, the continuing challenge. N Engl J Med 325:1875, 1991

GODSALL JW et al: Vitamin D metabolism and bone histomorphometry in patients with antacid-induced osteomalacia. Am J Med 77:747, 1984

HARDY DC et al: X-linked hypophosphatemia in adults: Prevalence of skeletal radiographic and scintigraphic features. Radiology 171:403, 1989

HARRELL RM et al: Healing of bone disease in X-linked hypophosphatemic rickets/osteomalacia: Induction and maintenance with phosphorus and calcitriol. J Clin Invest 75:1858, 1985

HARVEY JA et al: Lack of effect of 24,25-dihydroxyvitamin D_3 administration on parameters of calcium metabolism. J Clin Endocrinol Metab 69:467, 1989

HENDERSON JB et al: Blunted seasonal variation in serum 25-hydroxy vitamin D and increased risk of osteomalacia in vegetarian London Asians. Eur J Clin Nutr 46:509, 1992

HENTHORN PS et al: Different missense mutations at the tissue-nonspecific alkaline phosphatase gene locus in autosomal recessively inherited forms of mild and severe hypophosphatasia. Proc Natl Acad Sci USA 89:9924, 1992

HOCKBERG Z et al: 1,25-dihydroxyvitamin D resistance, rickets, and alopecia. Am J Med 77:805, 1984

HODSMAN AB et al: Vitamin D-resistant osteomalacia in hemodialysis patients lacking secondary hyperparathyroidism. Ann Intern Med 94:629, 1981

——— et al: Bone aluminum and histomorphometric features of renal osteodystrophy. J Clin Endocrinol Metab 54:439, 1982

HUTCHISON FN, BELL NH: Osteomalacia and rickets. Semin Nephrol 12:127, 1992

KLEEREKOPER M, KRANE SM (eds): *Clinical Disorders of Bone and Mineral Metabolism*. New York, Mary Ann Liebert, 1989

KLEIN GL, COLVURN JW: Metabolic bone disease associated with total parenteral nutrition. Adv Nutr Res 6:67, 1984

——— et al: Bone disease in burn patients. J Bone Miner Res 8:337, 1993

KONISHI K et al: Hypophosphatemic osteomalacia in von Recklinghausen neurofibromatosis. Am J Med Sci 301:322, 1991

KUMAR R: Hepatic and intestinal osteodystrophy and the hepatobiliary metabolism of vitamin D. Ann Intern Med 98:662, 1983

LABUDA M et al: Two hereditary defects related to vitamin D metabolism map to the same region of human chromosome 12q13–14. J Bone Miner Res 7:1447, 1992

LEICHT E et al: Tumor-induced osteomalacia: Pre- and postoperative biochemical findings. Horm Metab Res 22:640, 1990

LIPS P et al: The effect of vitamin D supplementation on vitamin status and parathyroid function in elderly subjects. J Clin Endocrinol Metab 67:644, 1988

MALLOY PJ et al: Abnormal binding of vitamin D receptors of deoxyribonucleic acids in a kindred with vitamin D–dependent rickets, type II. J Clin Endocrinol Metab 68:263, 1989

MCELDUFF A, POSEN S: Parathyroid hormone sensitivity in familial X-linked hypophosphatemic rickets. J Clin Endocrinol Metab 69:386, 1989

MIYAUCHI A et al: Hemangiopericytoma-induced osteomalacia: Tumor transplantation in nude mice causes hypophosphatemia and tumor extracts inhibit renal 25-hydroxyvitamin-1-hydroxylase activity. J Clin Endocrinol Metab 67:46, 1988

MONTE NESTO JT et al: Osteomalacia secondary to renal tubular acidosis in a patient with primary Sjögren's syndrome. Clin Exp Rheumatol 9:625, 1991

NORDAL KP, DAHL E: Low dose calcitriol versus placebo in patients with predialysis chronic renal failure. J Clin Endocrinol Metab 67:929, 1988

PARFITT AM et al: Metabolic bone disease with and without osteomalacia after intestinal bypass surgery: A bone histomorphometric study. Bone 6:211, 1985

PETERSON DJ et al: X-linked hypophosphatemic rickets: A study (with literature review) of linear growth response to calcitrol and phosphate therapy. J Bone Miner Res 7:583, 1992

POLISSON RP et al: Calcification of entheses associated with X-linked hypophosphatemic osteomalacia. N Engl J Med 313:1, 1985

PORTALE AA et al: Physiologic regulation of the serum concentration of 1,25-dihydroxyvitamin D by phosphorus in normal men. J Clin Invest 83:1494, 1989

RALPHS JR et al: Ultrastructural features of the osteoid of patients with fibrogenesis imperfecta ossium. Bone 10:243, 1989

SCRIVER CR et al: X-linked hypophosphatemia: An appreciation of a classic paper and a survey of progress since 1958. Medicine 70:218, 1991

STONE MD et al: A neuroendocrine cause of oncogenic osteomalacia. J Pathol 167:181, 1992

SULLIVAN W et al: A prospective trial of phosphate and 1,25-dihydroxyvitamin D_3 therapy in symptomatic adults with x-linked hypophosphatemic rickets. J Clin Endocrin Metab 75:879, 1992

VILLAREAL DT et al: Subclinical vitamin D deficiency in postmenopausal women with low vertebral bone mass. J Clin Endocrinol Metab 72:6281, 1991

WEBB AR et al: An evaluation of the relative contributions of exposure of sunlight and of diet on the circulating concentrations of 25-hydroxyvitamin D in an elderly nursing home population in Boston. Am J Clin Nutr 51:1075, 1990

WEIDNER N: Review and update: oncogenic osteomalacia-rickets. Ultrastruct Pathol 15:317, 1991

WHYTE MP: Hypophosphatasia, in *The Molecular and Metabolic Basis of Inherited Disease*, 7th ed, CR Scriver et al (eds). New York, McGraw-Hill, in press, chap 136

359 DISORDERS OF PHOSPHORUS METABOLISM

JAMES P. KNOCHEL

Phosphorus is the most abundant intracellular anion and is critical for membrane structure, transport, and energy storage. The role of phosphate ions in tissues explains the systemic nature of cellular injury consequent to phosphorus deficiency.

At a plasma pH of 7.4, inorganic phosphate in plasma is a 4:1 mixture of HPO_4^{2-} and $H_2PO_4^{2-}$. The sum of the products of the valences of these ions $(4 \times 2^- + 1 \times 1^-)$ divided by the sum of the ions $(4 + 1)$ is equal to 9/5 or an average valence of 1.8. Of the average 700 g of phosphorus in the body, 85 percent is in the skeleton, about 15 percent is in soft tissues, and 0.1 percent is in extracellular fluid. The phosphorus in extracellular fluid is in a freely diffusible form that (1) permits excretion of hydrogen ions as phosphate buffer into the urine and (2) is in diffusion equilibrium with cytosolic inorganic phosphate in cells.

A normal adult consumes approximately 1 g phosphorus each day. Soluble phosphates in dairy products and meat are almost completely absorbed, predominantly in the midjejunum. Insoluble phosphates, in vegetables and seeds, are absorbable provided the phosphate can be digested from its ligand. For example, phosphorus in corn and oats is partly in the form of phytic acid; these foods contain little phytase, which splits phytic acid (inositol hexaphosphate) into phosphate and inositol, and hence phosphorus from this source may be poorly absorbed. Thus corn and oats may be rachitogenic in man if they are the major components of the diet. Addition of rye bran to the diet, which contains phytase, increases the bioavailability of phosphorus from these sources.

Phosphorus absorption is under the influence of vitamin D, and phosphorus excretion is under the control of parathyroid hormone. Parathyroid hormone decreases tubular phosphate reabsorption and increases excretion into the urine. The effect of vitamin D on phosphate reabsorption by the kidney is relatively minor. The quantity of soluble phosphorus available for absorption from the diet varies, and excretion of phosphorus in the urine on a given day depends directly on absorption. Accordingly, the range for phosphorus excretion in health is very broad.

HYPOPHOSPHATEMIA

CAUSES   Hypophosphatemia has many causes (Table 359-1). The finding of hypophosphatemia is not always a reliable indicator of deficiency, since a total-body deficit of phosphorus may exist in the face of hyperphosphatemia, such as, for example, in diabetic ketoacidosis.

Hypophosphatemia can be moderate or severe. Decreased dietary intake is an unusual cause of hypophosphatemia because of the ubiquitous and abundant distribution of the mineral in foods. Decreased absorption of phosphorus from the small intestine occurs in a variety of malabsorptive states, but simple diarrhea is usually not a cause. One of the most common causes of hypophosphatemia is respiratory alkalosis. Indeed, discovery of hypophosphatemia should lead to a search for potentially serious causes of hyperventilation such as sepsis or otherwise unsuspected alcohol withdrawal. Reduction of intracellular P_{CO_2} and elevation of pH increase the activity of phosphofructokinase, the rate-limiting enzyme of glycolysis. Phosphorylation of glucose intermediates causes cellular uptake of phosphorus and hypophosphatemia. Administration of insulin and consumption of nutrients that stimulate insulin release are also common causes of hypophosphatemia. Insulin stimulates phosphorus uptake by cells. Cellular phosphorus uptake also occurs in patients recovering from hypothermia as a result of reactivation of metabolism. Certain rapidly

TABLE 359-1   Causes of hypophosphatemia

Decreased dietary intake
Decreased intestinal absorption
  A Vitamin D deficiency
  B Malabsorption
  C Steatorrhea
  D Secretory diarrhea
  E Vomiting
  F PO_4-binding antacids
Shifts from serum into cells
  A Respiratory alkalosis
    1 Sepsis
    2 Alcohol withdrawal
    3 Heat stroke
    4 Neuroleptic malignant syndrome
    5 Hepatic coma
    6 Salicylate poisoning
    7 Gout
    8 Panic attacks
    9 Psychiatric depression
  B Hormonal effects
    1 Insulin
    2 Glucagon
    3 Epinephrine
    4 Androgens
    5 Glucocorticoids
    6 Anovulatory hormones
  C Nutrient effects
    1 Glucose
    2 Fructose
    3 Glycerol
    4 Lactate
    5 Amino acids
    6 Xylitol
  D Cellular uptake syndromes
    1 Recovery from hypothermia
    2 Burkitt's lymphoma
    3 Histiocytic lymphoma
    4 Acute myelomonocytic leukemia
    5 Acute myelogenous leukemia
    6 Treatment of pernicious anemia
    7 Hungry bone syndrome
      a Following parathyroidectomy
      b Acute leukemia
Increased excretion into the urine
  A Hyperparathyroidism
  B Renal tubular defects
    1 Renal rickets
    2 Polyostotic fibrous dysplasia
    3 Postrenal transplantation
    4 Oncogenic osteomalacia
  C Aldosteronism
  D Licorice ingestion
  E Volume expansion
  F Inappropriate secretion of vasopressin
  G Mineralocorticoid administration
  H Glucocorticoid therapy
  I Diuretics

growing malignancies may take up enough phosphate to cause hypophosphatemia. Deposition of bone mineral following parathyroidectomy also may be a cause. Hypocalcemia consequent to saline infusion causes release of parathyroid hormone. Thus volume expansion and parathyroid hormone both reduce tubular reabsorption of phosphorus. A number of other conditions associated with chronic volume expansion may cause hypophosphatemia.

Severe hypophosphatemia is defined as phosphorus levels in serum below 0.3 mmol/L (1.0 mg/dL). Many of the conditions that result in such low levels are associated with prolonged hyperventilation with respiratory alkalosis or reflect rapid cellular uptake (Table 359-2). Respiratory alkalosis does not cause phosphorus deficiency but may reduce serum phosphorus values to 0.1 mmol/L (0.3 mg/dL) and urinary phosphorus excretion to virtually undetectable levels. Severe hypophosphatemia and severe total-body deficiency of phosphorus occur in patients with poor dietary intake who consume phosphate-binding antacids. Similarly, treatment of diabetic ketoacidosis results in hypophosphatemia. Reduction of serum phosphorus below 0.3 mmol/L (1.0 mg/dL) suggests, but does not prove, the existence of

TABLE 359-2 Causes of severe hypophosphatemia

Chronic alcoholism and alcohol withdrawal
Dietary deficiency and phosphate-binding antacids
Severe thermal burns
Recovery from diabetic ketoacidosis
Hyperalimentation
Nutritional recovery syndrome
Respiratory alkalosis
Therapeutic hyperthermia
Neuroleptic malignant syndrome
Recovery from exhaustive exercise
Renal transplantation
Acute renal failure

serious phosphorus depletion. In chronic alcoholics, reduction of phosphorus content of skeletal muscle may occur because of a renal phosphate leak. The resulting phosphorus deficiency may cause a reduction of muscle magnesium and potassium and accumulations of calcium, sodium, chloride, and water. These findings are not necessarily associated with elevations of creatine phosphokinase activity that would reflect acute muscle damage. However, during withdrawal from alcohol, phosphorus is often taken up rapidly into skeletal muscle or liver, resulting in severe hypophosphatemia, and in this instance hypophosphatemia may precipitate acute rhabdomyolysis.

Most patients with diabetic ketoacidosis are not severely depleted of phosphorus. Although, on the one hand, metabolic acidosis and insulin deficiency mobilize intracellular phosphate stores and lead to their excretion into the urine, most patients have not been sick long enough for severe phosphorus deficiency to occur. On the other hand, patients with hypophosphatemia and hypokalemia, in the presence of severe diabetic ketoacidosis, are likely severely depleted of phosphorus and potassium and require treatment. The history usually shows that this type of patient with diabetic ketoacidosis has been sick for many days, has not had significant vomiting, has maintained a good intake of fluids, and has excreted phosphorus briskly for a period of many days, thus establishing severe deficiency. Such patients probably represent no more than 5 percent of cases of diabetic ketoacidosis.

MANIFESTATIONS The manifestations of phosphorus deficiency are listed in Table 359-3; many of these can occur simultaneously.

Phosphate trapping is an acute disorder resulting from reduction of intracellular inorganic phosphate concentration. The most common cause is administration of intravenous fructose. Fructose is metabolized by only three tissues in the body—the liver, the small bowel epithelium, and the proximal tubule of the kidney. When glucose is taken up into liver cells and phosphorylated by hexokinase, the resulting glucose-6-phosphate inhibits hexokinase, producing a smoothly regulated uptake of glucose that does not deplete or trap stores of inorganic phosphate. When fructose is administered intravenously, it is taken up into liver cells, where it is converted to fructose-1-phosphate by the enzyme fructokinase. Fructose-1-phosphate does not inhibit fructokinase, thus permitting rapid uptake of fructose into liver cells and consumption or trapping of available stores of inorganic phosphate. Reduced intracellular phosphate concentration activates AMP deaminase and nucleotidase. The consequent reduction of adenylate compounds is reflected by increased uric acid production and hyperuricemia. Acute reduction of ATP, which is bound to magnesium, is heralded by a modest rise of magnesium in serum. Acute liver cell damage may occur. Disturbances of renal function also may occur after intravenous fructose. Hepatic and renal metabolic disturbances that follow fructose administration are preventable by infusing inorganic phosphate. Whether oral fructose affects intestinal epithelium in a similar manner is not known.

Rhabdomyolysis predictably occurs in chronic alcoholics who become acutely hypophosphatemic during the course of alcohol withdrawal. Hypophosphatemic rhabdomyolysis also occurs rarely during treatment for diabetic ketoacidosis, during the course of hyperalimentation, or while refeeding patients with malnutrition. In alcoholics, evidence of muscle cell injury precedes the occurrence of

hypophosphatemia. Presumably, severe hypophosphatemia triggers induction of acute rhabdomyolysis. This syndrome can be reproduced experimentally. It does not occur if hypophosphatemia is prevented during hyperalimentation.

Cardiomyopathy occurs in severe phosphorus depletion. The manifestations include reduction in cardiac output, hypotension, impaired pressor responsiveness to cathecholamines, and a reduced threshold to ventricular arrhythmias.

Respiratory insufficiency occurs in malnourished patients receiving intravenous nutrients with inadequate phosphorus who become progressively hypophosphatemic over 8 or 10 days. Profound weakness causes failure of diaphragm function, hypoxia, and respiratory acidosis. Despite severe hypophosphatemia, these patients rarely develop rhabdomyolysis, presumably because they had no preexistent muscle damage. The initial clue may be an inability to extubate a patient from a ventilator at the anticipated time. This syndrome is seldom seen in chronic alcoholics because rhabdomyolysis in such patients may correct hypophosphatemia spontaneously. Rapid correction of chronic respiratory acidosis also may cause hypophosphatemia and diaphragm weakness. In these patients, administration of phosphorus rapidly corrects muscle weakness and respiratory insufficiency.

Erythrocyte dysfunction is due to a decrease in 2,3-diphosphoglycerate (2,3-DPG) content. The red cell is the only tissue in the body that produces this substance. Both 2,3-DPG and ATP facilitate dissociation of oxyhemoglobin and promote oxygen delivery to tissue. Reduced 2,3-DPG and ATP both enhance affinity of oxygen for hemoglobin and reduce tissue oxygenation. This mechanism may explain central nervous system dysfunction in hypophosphatemia. Hemolysis due to phosphorus deficiency probably does not occur.

Leukocyte dysfunction due to phosphorus deficiency results in impaired phagocytosis and opsonization. As a result, chronic hypophosphatemia increases susceptibility to bacterial and fungal infections.

Skeletal demineralization is an important effect of phosphorus deficiency, especially in patients with a poor dietary intake who simultaneously ingest phosphate-binding antacids. Under conditions of increased bone turnover, in normal children or in adults with Paget's disease, hyperparathyroidism, or bony metastases, demineralization may occur at such a rate as to cause hypercalcemia. Osteopenia, bone pain, and a syndrome resembling osteomalacia occur in chronic phosphorus deficiency.

Metabolic acidosis may occur in children or adults with phosphorus deficiency due to vitamin D deficiency. Reduced phosphorus intake results in mobilization of hydroxyapatite from bone that serves to maintain normal levels of serum phosphorus. Hypercalciuria occurs normally as a result of phosphorus deprivation. Severe hypophosphatemia has two important metabolic effects on the kidney. First, inorganic phosphate excretion into the urine falls so that hydrogen excretion as NaH_2PO_4 into the urine is eliminated. Second, phosphorus deficiency also elevates renal intracellular pH, which results in a profound decrease in ammonia production. The reduction in ammonia production eliminates hydrogen excretion as ammonium ions (NH^{4+}). Since excretion of hydrogen as phosphate buffer or ammonium accounts for nearly all the kidney's capacity to secrete acid, it is surprising that phosphorus deficiency is only rarely associated with metabolic acidosis. The explanation lies in the fact that mobilization

TABLE 359-3 Hypophosphatemic syndromes

Phosphate trapping
Rhabdomyolysis
Cardiomyopathy
Respiratory insufficiency
Erythrocyte dysfunction
Leukocyte dysfunction
Skeletal demineralization
Metabolic acidosis
Nervous system dysfunction

of hydroxyapatite from bone provides carbonate ions, which, in turn, buffer the retained hydrogen ions that otherwise would be excreted in the urine. Under conditions in which hydroxyapatite cannot be mobilized during phosphorus deprivation (e.g., vitamin D deficiency, severe magnesium deficiency, and perhaps aluminum poisoning), buffer cannot be mobilized adequately, and metabolic acidosis ensues.

Nervous system dysfunction is a distinctive and predictable feature of severe hypophosphatemia and phosphorus deficiency. This syndrome usually occurs in the setting of refeeding or hyperalimentation-induced hypophosphatemia that develops over the course of 8 to 10 days. Such patients become irritable and apprehensive and hyperventilate sufficiently to cause paresthesias and numbness. Profound muscular weakness is followed by dysarthria, confusion, obtundation, convulsive seizures, coma, and death. Alternatively, ascending motor paralysis with or without sensory disturbances may resemble the Guillain-Barré syndrome. In such cases, the cerebrospinal fluid is normal. Ophthalmoplegia, diplopia, and dysphagia suggest botulism, and poorly defined defects in color perception (metachromatopsia) suggests cerebral cortical dysfunction. In these patients, as in those with respiratory failure, spontaneous rhabdomyolysis does not occur despite severe hypophosphatemia.

TREATMENT   Before initiating treatment for hypophosphatemia, the cause should be ascertained. Measurement of arterial pH and blood gases and of phosphorus concentration in the urine is helpful.

Milk is an excellent source of phosphorus, containing 33 mmol/L (100 mg/dL). Phosphate salts are also available for oral use. They are less likely to cause diarrhea in phosphorus-deficient patient than in a normal person. Phosphorus salts cannot be given by intramuscular or subcutaneous injection, but sodium phosphate and potassium phosphate are available for intravenous use. The potassium salt should be given when hypokalemia and hypophosphatemia coexist. A safe dosage regimen for treatment of alcoholics who are hypophosphatemic, hypokalemic, and hypomagnesemic is the infusion each 8 to 12 h of 1 L of 0.5 normal NaCl in 5% glucose containing 9 mmol of potassium phosphate and 4.2 mmol $MgSO_4$ (2.0 mL of 50% $MgSO_4$ solution). Serum concentrations of potassium, magnesium, and phosphate should be monitored closely. Such infusions should be stopped when oral intake becomes possible.

Hyperphosphatemia should be avoided because it can cause severe hypocalcemia and crystal deposition in important structures, including blood vessels, the eye, lung, heart, and kidney. Fatal alveolar diffusion block has occurred, especially if the patient is alkalotic.

HYPERPHOSPHATEMIA

Defined in adults as an elevation of serum phosphorus above 1.67 mmol/L (5 mg/dL), hyperphosphatemia is a common finding with many causes (Table 359-4). Abnormal positively charged serum proteins, as in plasma cell dyscrasias, may cause marked elevations of phosphorus. In one instance, the serum concentration was 4.5 mmol/L (13.5 mg/dL), and each millimole of myeloma protein bound 15 molecules of phosphate.

Decreased renal excretion of phosphorus is the most common cause of hyperphosphatemia. Since parathyroid hormone (PTH) is phosphaturic, hyperphosphatemia is a cardinal feature of hypoparathyroidism, either as a primary disorder or in patients whose renal cAMP response to PTH is abnormal (pseudohypoparathyroidism type I) or those whose phosphaturic response to PTH is suppressed (pseudohypoparathyroidism type II).

Of interest, severe hypomagnesemia causes marked suppression of PTH in plasma despite hypocalcemia but does not cause hyperphosphatemia. Hyperphosphatemia occurs in tumoral calcinosis, pseudoxanthoma elasticum, infantile hypophosphatasia, and hyperostosis because of decreased renal excretion. Untreated severe hyperthyroidism apparently increases cellular catabolism sufficiently to elevate serum phosphorus despite increased phosphorus loss in the urine. Acromegaly or administration of growth hormone causes modest hyperphosphatemia. Presumably, the higher phosphorus levels in

TABLE 359-4   Causes of hyperphosphatemia

BINDING TO SERUM PROTEINS

Plasma cell dyscrasias

DECREASED RENAL EXCRETION

Renal insufficiency
Hypoparathyroidism
Pseudohypoparathyroidism, types I and II
Tumoral calcinosis
Pseudoxanthoma elasticum
Infantile hypophosphatasia
Hyperostosis
Hyperthyroidism
Growth hormone activity
Adrenal insufficiency
Bisphosphonate therapy

INCREASED INTESTINAL ABSORPTION

Phosphorus-containing cathartics
Medication with vitamin D compounds
Granulomatous diseases producing vitamin D
   Sarcoidosis
   Tuberculosis

INTERNAL REDISTRIBUTION

Acute metabolic acidosis
Acute respiratory acidosis
Reduced insulin level
Clonidine administration

CELLULAR RELEASE

Rhabdomyolysis
Organ infarction
Tumor lysis
   Burkitt's lymphoma
   Lymphoblastic lymphoma
   Metastatic small cell carcinoma
Thyrotoxicosis
Acute hemolysis

PARENTERAL ADMINISTRATION

Intravenous phosphate salts
Lipid (phospholipid) infusion

children partly reflect growth hormone activity. Hyperphosphatemia occurs in untreated adrenal insufficiency because of volume contraction, metabolic acidosis, and possibly reduced glomerular permeability. Mild hyperphosphatemia may occur with biphosphonate therapy because of increased tubular reabsorption of phosphorus.

Hyperphosphatemia secondary to increased absorption from the gut occurs during administration of excess phosphate salts by mouth or from the colon as a result of enemas that contain phosphorus. Overmedication with vitamin D and production of vitamin D by granulomatous tissue such as sarcoidosis and tuberculosis can cause hyperphosphatemia. Both acute metabolic and acute respiratory acidosis may decompose cellular organic phosphates, reduce phosphorylation, and result in diffusion of phosphorus from the cell and hyperphosphatemia. Reduced insulin levels or clonidine administration also can cause hyperphosphatemia. Cellular release of phosphorus may cause hyperphosphatemia, particularly in rhabdomyolysis, infarction of other tissues, tumor lysis, or hemolysis. Severe hyperphosphatemia after intravenous infusion of phosphate salts is a particular danger in patients who are acidotic or oliguric. Finally, infusion of compounds containing phospholipids for parenteral nutrition has caused hyperphosphatemia.

REFERENCES

ANGELI P et al: Hypophosphatemia and renal tubular dysfunction in alcoholics. Gastroenterology 100:502, 1991

Blachley J et al: Fluid and electrolyte disorders associated with alcoholism and liver disease, in *Fluid and Electrolytes*, JP Kokko, RL Tannen (eds). Philadelphia, Saunders, 1990, chap 11, pp 649–688

Davis SV et al: Reversible depression of myocardial performance in hypophosphatemia. Am J Med Sci 295:183, 1988

Fuller TJ et al: Reversible depression in myocardial performance in dogs with experimental phosphorus deficiency. J Clin Invest 62:1194, 1978

Johnson MA et al: Adenosine triphosphate turnover in humans. J Clin Invest 84:990, 1989

Knochel JP: Hypophosphatemia and phosphorus deficiency, in *The Kidney*, 4th ed, B Brenner, F Rector (eds). Philadelphia, Saunders, 1991

————: Central nervous system manifestations of hypophosphatemia and phosphorus depletion, in *Metabolic Brain Dysfunction in Systemic Disorders*, AC Arief, RC Griggs (eds). Boston, Little, Brown, 1992, chap 10, pp 183–204

————: Hypophosphatemia and rhabdomyolysis. Am J Med 92:455, 1992

Kotanko P: Hyperphosphatemia in multiple myeloma. N Engl J Med 326:1781, 1992

Levi M et al: Disorders of phosphate and magnesium metabolism, in *Disorders of Bone and Mineral Metabolism*, FC Coe, MJ Favus (eds). New York, Raven, 1992, chap 28, pp 587–610

Veech RL et al: Cytosolic phosphorylation potential. J Biol Chem 254:6538, 1979

360   DISORDERS OF MAGNESIUM METABOLISM

JAMES P. KNOCHEL

Magnesium is the most abundant intracellular divalent cation. The total magnesium content of a normal man is 12.4 mmol (0.3 g) per kilogram of body weight. Of this, 1 percent is extracellular, 31 percent is in cells, and 67 percent is in bone. Serum magnesium ranges between 0.8 and 1.2 mmol/L (2 and 3 mg/dL). Of this, the unbound diffusible concentration is about 0.6 mmol/L (1.4 mg/dL). It exists in two forms in cells, one in solution which is in equilibrium with the diffusible form in plasma and a larger quantity bound to organic components. Since most magnesium inside cells is bound to ATP, in accordance with the principle of mass action, MgATP is in equilibrium with free magnesium ions. Thus shifts in free magnesium concentration may help regulate stores of ATP. From the opposite viewpoint, if ATP is acutely reduced, e.g., by infusion of fructose intravenously, freed magnesium ions diffuse from the cell, and serum magnesium rises. Since ATP is critical to nearly all metabolic transformations, a normal concentration of serum magnesium is essential to maintain adequate stores of this important nucleotide.

The ideal intake of magnesium for an adult is 15 to 20 mmol/d (36 to 48 mg/d). Foods rich in magnesium include seed grains, nuts, peas, and beans. Fresh meat, fish, and most fresh fruits contain relatively small amounts of magnesium. Magnesium is absorbed primarily in the jejunum and ileum, and healthy persons absorb about 30 to 40 percent of ingested magnesium. This may increase to 70 percent when intake is low or magnesium deficiency exists. Vitamin D deficiency reduces magnesium absorption. When magnesium intake is restricted, fecal excretion becomes negligible, and urinary excretion decreases to 0.5 to 1 mmol/d (12 to 24 mg/d). Thus magnesium retention by the kidney is very efficient. Magnesium excretion depends on glomerular filtration of the unbound fraction, of which 25 percent is reabsorbed in the proximal tubule and 50 to 60 percent is reabsorbed in the loop of Henle. Loop diuretics, such as ethacrynic acid, bumetanide, or furosemide, cause greater excretion of magnesium than do diuretics such as thiazides that act on the distal tubule. Magnesium excretion is increased by expanding extracellular fluid volume by ingestion of water and salt, and aldosterone decreases reabsorption of magnesium by the renal tubule. Magnesium excretion increases sharply when the concentration in serum exceeds 0.8 mmol/L (2 mg/dL).

Slight hypomagnesemia occurs in athletically trained individuals, hypermetabolic states such as pregnancy and cold acclimatization, or after experimental administration of thyroid hormone.

MAGNESIUM DEFICIENCY

When any of the three major intracellular elements is deprived or lost, whether magnesium, potassium, or phosphorus, losses of the others usually follow. For this reason, deficiency of a single intracellular component almost never occurs. A diet devoid of magnesium causes depletion of phosphorus and potassium in skeletal muscle. Selective potassium deficiency may cause reductions in magnesium and phosphorus. Phosphorus deficiency may cause reductions in potassium and magnesium contents of tissue. The usual somatic responses to selective deprivation of one major intracellular element are anorexia, cellular atrophy, a negative nitrogen balance, and net loss of the other two major intracellular elements. Shrinkage of the cell and expulsion of the elements not deprived help to maintain a normal intracellular composition.

During hyperalimentation, a different situation prevails. Provision of a diet that is otherwise replete but deficient in one major intracellular element promotes an anabolic state, and the protoplasm that is synthesized has a major deficit of the ion being deprived. In these situations, serious derangements of cellular composition include accumulations of sodium, chloride, calcium, and water, suggesting a major interference with cellular ion transport. Indeed, elevation of cellular calcium, by activating proteases and phospholipases, may be an important cause of cellular injury under these conditions.

As in deficiencies of other major intracellular elements, deficiency of body magnesium can exist even when serum values are normal. In addition, certain tissues become deficient before others. The definition of a true deficit of an intracellular element is reduction of its ratio to nitrogen in tissue. In muscle, this ratio is about 0.3 mmol (7 mg) magnesium per gram of nitrogen. Red cell magnesium content decreases in all species during magnesium deficiency, whereas muscle magnesium content remains normal in some species. Because of the inconsistency of tissue levels, and because measurement of tissue magnesium is difficult, the clinician must rely on serum magnesium levels to detect magnesium deficiency or excess.

THE CLINICAL PHYSIOLOGY OF MAGNESIUM DEFICIENCY

Volunteers fed a diet deficient in magnesium eventually develop characteristic symptoms and findings. Within 3 to 7 days after reducing dietary magnesium intake to less than 0.5 mmol (12 mg) per day, renal excretion of magnesium declines to below 0.5 mmol (12 mg) per day. Anorexia, nausea, vomiting, lethargy, and weakness develop within weeks. Characteristic symptoms of magnesium deficiency consist of paresthesias, muscular cramps, irritability, decreased attention span, and mental confusion. These complaints may require months to appear.

The physical findings are manifestations of the associated hypocalcemia. These are positive Trousseau and Chvostek signs, peculiar movements of the fingers best described as athetoid tetany, and, on occasion, convulsions. Muscle fasciculations may be precipitated by a blow with a neurologic hammer to muscle. About half of patients with selective magnesium depletion become hypokalemic. In animals, rhabdomyolysis may occur. Cardiac arrhythmias, disturbances of conduction, and even ventricular fibrillation and cardiac arrest can occur in patients with coexisting hypokalemia and hypomagnesemia. In such instances, hypokalemia may be the cause of the associated ECG abnormalities. Digitalis potentiates the severity and potential danger of arrhythmias. In the presence of QT prolongation, polymorphic ventricular tachycardia (torsades des pointes) may occur that responds to magnesium salts. The causes of magnesium deficiency are shown in Table 360-1.

Hypocalcemia usually does not develop until serum magnesium falls below 0.5 mmol/L (1.2 mg/dL). Although mild magnesium deficiency may increase release of parathyroid hormone, severe hypomagnesemia [levels below 0.4 mmol/L (1 mg/dL)] blocks release of parathyroid hormone. The resulting hypocalcemia may be severe. In addition, magnesium deficiency impairs the normal calcemic response to parathyroid hormone at the level of the skeleton. Hypocalcemia can become sufficiently severe to cause tetany. Al-

TABLE 360-1 Causes of hypomagnesemia

Primary nutritional disturbances
  A Inadequate intake
  B Total parenteral nutrition
  C Refeeding syndrome
Gastrointestinal disorders
  A Specific absorptive defects
  B Malabsorption syndromes
    1 Enteric fistulas
    2 Nontropical sprue
    3 Whipple's disease
    4 Intestinal lymphoma
    5 Chronic pancreatic insufficiency
    6 Biliary diversion
    7 Giardiasis
    8 Short bowel syndrome
  C Prolonged diarrhea
  D Prolonged nasogastric suction
  E Pancreatitis
Endocrine disorders
  A Hyperparathyroidism
  B Hypoparathyroidism
  C Hyperthyroidism
  D Primary hyperaldosteronism
  E Bartter's syndrome
  F Diabetic ketoacidosis
  G Alcoholic ketoacidosis
  H Administration of epinephrine
  I Syndrome of inappropriate secretion of antidiuretic hormone
  J "Hungry bone" syndrome after parathyroidectomy
Chronic alcoholism, alcoholic withdrawal
Increased renal excretion
  A Ethanol ingestion
  B Idiopathic
  C Following renal transplantation
  D Cisplatin therapy
  E Aminoglycoside therapy
  F Amphotericin B therapy
  G Capreomycin therapy
  H Viomycin therapy
  I Diuretic administration
    1 Furosemide
    2 Ethacrynic acid
    3 Acetazolamide
    4 Thiazides
    5 Chlorthalidone
    6 Osmotic agents
  J Recovery phase of acute tubular necrosis
  K Pentamidine therapy
  L Theophylline toxicity
  M Colony stimulating factor therapy

though tetany has been reported in patients with hypomagnesemia independently of hypocalcemia, both conditions usually exist in patients with this finding. In most cases the tetany with hypomagnesemia does not respond to infusions of calcium and requires correction of magnesium levels. The hypocalcemia also responds only to magnesium replacement therapy, usually requiring 2 to 7 days for correction. In patients whose hypomagnesemia is caused by steatorrhea, administration of magnesium salts intravenously can cause prompt and sometimes explosive release of parathyroid hormone. In rare instances, acute hypercalcemia can occur.

Hypokalemia in patients with magnesium deficiency is less well understood. Aldosterone production may be enhanced, thus permitting loss of potassium into the urine. It is difficult to correct the potassium deficiency with supplemental potassium salts. However, administration of magnesium salts sufficient to correct the hypomagnesemia promptly reduces potassium excretion and corrects the hypokalemia. For this reason, it should be kept in mind that hypokalemia refractory to potassium supplements may be due to magnesium deficiency.

GASTROINTESTINAL CAUSES OF MAGNESIUM DEFICIENCY
Familial hypomagnesemia is manifested during childhood and is caused by reduced absorption of dietary magnesium. The most common cause of magnesium deficiency in adults is intestinal malabsorption and steatorrhea, as in nontropical sprue, the short

bowel syndrome, chronic pancreatic insufficiency, or biliary diversion. Because of unabsorbed fat, complexes of nonabsorbable magnesium–fatty acid soaps form in the intestinal lumen. When long-standing, hypomagnesemia in such cases is often associated with hypocalcemia, hypokalemia, and hypophosphatemia. Because of steatorrhea, disorders related to malabsorption of fat-soluble vitamins, especially vitamins K, A, and D, may coexist. It is important to recognize that vitamin D deficiency associated with hypomagnesemia can cause weakness due to proximal myopathy in association with pain in the lower back and hips resulting from osteomalacia.

Magnesium deficiency also occurs after prolonged nasogastric suction in patients who have not received adequate magnesium salts. Acute hypomagnesemia, along with acute hypocalcemia, can occur in acute hemorrhagic pancreatitis when magnesium– and calcium–fatty acid soaps form in situ as a result of tissue necrosis.

ENDOCRINE CAUSES OF HYPOMAGNESEMIA   Mild hypomagnesemia occurs in poorly controlled diabetes mellitus. Moderate hypomagnesemia may occur in hyperparathyroidism, hypoparathyroidism, hyperthyroidism, and primary hyperaldosteronism, as well as during recovery from diabetic ketoacidosis. In primary hyperaldosteronism, aldosterone enhances magnesium excretion directly and acts via volume expansion to cause net losses of magnesium. These effects can be reversed by spironolactone. Hypomagnesemia may occur in hypokalemic and hyponatremic patients with the syndrome of inappropriate secretion of vasopressin (antidiuretic hormone). Presumably, this is the result of increased aldosterone production and overexpansion of extracellular volume. Epinephrine and other potent beta agonists may cause transient hypomagnesemia, presumably because of uptake of magnesium ions into adipose tissue as fatty acids are released. Furthermore, as catecholamines cause release of fatty acids into the blood, insoluble fatty acid–magnesium and fatty acid–calcium complexes form in serum. If serum is centrifuged, the precipitates settle to the bottom of the tube, and spurious hypomagnesemia and hypocalcemia can be diagnosed.

HYPOMAGNESEMIA ASSOCIATED WITH ALCOHOLISM   Ethanol causes a transient loss of magnesium into the urine. Alcoholics with a reasonably normal nutrient intake and normal intestinal function usually have normal or only slightly depressed magnesium levels in blood. The total-body deficit of magnesium in chronic alcoholics is modest, amounting to 100 to 150 mmol (2.4 to 3.6 g). However, during alcoholic withdrawal, hypomagnesemia may occur in association with acute hypophosphatemia and acute hypokalemia. Simultaneously, urinary excretion of magnesium, PO_4, and potassium falls. Thus hypomagnesemia occurs both because of net deficit and because of a shift into cells during withdrawal. In animals, sustained ethanol administration in intoxicating doses causes severe depletion of phosphorus, moderate depletion of magnesium and potassium, and increases in intracellular sodium, chloride, water, and calcium. Selective depletion of phosphorus also causes magnesium wasting and muscle magnesium deficiency. The same findings occur in muscle of severely alcoholic patients. In acute alcohol withdrawal, respiratory alkalosis and insulin release stimulated by administration of nutrients act in concert to incorporate phosphate into cells. Increased ATP synthesis as a result of phosphate movement into cells may cause increased magnesium binding and worsen hypomagnesemia.

In alcoholics with intestinal malabsorption and steatorrhea, hypomagnesemia can be severe in association with hypocalcemia, hypophosphatemia, and hypokalemia. Although a relationship between hypomagnesemia and alcoholic withdrawal seizures has been suggested, alcoholics in a withdrawal state display prominent respiratory alkalosis, which lowers the threshold for seizure activity. Thus the relationship of hypomagnesemia to seizures in this setting is not clear. Furthermore, correction of hypomagnesemia in a withdrawing alcoholic appears to have no favorable effect on the withdrawal syndrome.

Magnesium deficiency may play a role in the temporary hypertension that occurs during alcohol withdrawal. Independently of alcohol, magnesium deficiency causes accumulation of calcium in smooth muscle and increases vascular tone. Magnesium salts reduce arteriolar tone by reducing cytosolic calcium. Accumulation of calcium potentiates the pressor response to circulating catecholamines. Withdrawing alcoholics nearly always have elevations of circulating catecholamines. Thus the combined effects of magnesium depletion, calcium accumulation in cells, and elevated levels of catecholamines may explain the occurrence of hypertension and the favorable effect of calcium channel blocking drugs under such circumstances.

MAGNESIUM DEFICIENCY DUE TO INCREASED RENAL EXCRETION Hypomagnesemia also can result from impaired renal tubular reabsorption. Most of these states are associated with renal potassium wasting and hypokalemia, and some patients are hypercalciuric. Transient hypomagnesemia due to reduced renal tubular reabsorption may follow renal transplantation.

Aminoglycosides, cisplatin, diuretics, and cyclosporine can cause magnesium wasting in the urine. Aminoglycosides cause hypomagnesemia and hypokalemia as a result of impaired tubular reabsorption. Hypomagnesemia develops after prolonged treatment and usually in patients who have received more than 8.0 g of aminoglycosides. Total recovery is the rule after the drug is stopped. Most patients treated with cisplatin develop hypomagnesemia that can be severe; hypokalemia is less common. Renal tubular mitochondrial injury may be responsible for these events. Even after cisplatin is withdrawn, the nephron defect may persist for months, years, or for life. Of interest, calcitriol may enhance magnesium wasting in patients with cisplatin nephrotoxicity who are also hypomagnesemic and hypocalcemic. About a fourth of patients treated with cyclosporine and prednisone after renal transplantation develop serum magnesium levels below 0.5 mmol/L (1.2 mg/dL). Loop diuretics are potent magnesuric agents, but hypomagnesemia is frequent in patients medicated with diuretics. Patients who receive large doses of diuretics or who receive two or more diuretics that act at different sites in the nephron are more likely to develop hypomagnesemia. Treatment with pentamidine, theophylline, and granulocyte-macrophage colony stimulating factor has each caused hypermagnesuria and hypomagnesemia.

TREATMENT OF HYPOMAGNESEMIA AND MAGNESIUM DEFICIENCY Treatment of hypomagnesemia and its associated disorders should be aimed at correcting the cause. Patients with inadequate dietary intake or with disorders that reduce intestinal absorption or cause excessive losses into the urine can often be corrected by oral administration of magnesium salts. Patients with potentially serious cardiac arrhythmias or with nausea and vomiting should be given intravenous magnesium sulfate. Magnesium sulfate heptahydrate ($MgSO_4 \cdot 7H_2O$) has a molecular weight of 234; thus 1 mL of a 50% solution contains 2.1 mmol (50 mg) of magnesium. The usual adult dose of 50% magnesium sulfate is 2 mL every 6 h on the first day and half this quantity on each of the following 3 to 4 days. Magnesium sulfate may be given intramuscularly, but this is painful and may cause elevation of creatine phosphokinase levels, reflecting muscle damage and thus blunting the value of measurements of the enzyme to detect rhabdomyolysis. It is preferable to infuse magnesium in a dose of 4.1 mmol (1 g) magnesium sulfate every 6 h. Patients who require intravenous magnesium sulfate are often hypokalemic and hypophosphatemic. Potassium phosphate and potassium chloride may be included with magnesium sulfate in 0.5% saline containing 5% glucose. The total potassium content in each infusion bottle should represent one-fourth the amount determined to be necessary each day. In patients with adequate urine flow, such solutions can be given in a quantity of 750 mL every 6 h until nausea and vomiting disappear and oral intake becomes possible. In patients with tetany due to magnesium deficiency, although hypocalcemia coexists, calcium is generally ineffective, and infusions of magnesium salts usually require 2 h or more to relieve the tetany. Up to a full day may be required for all signs of latent tetany, such as the Chvostek and Trousseau signs, to disappear completely. Several oral preparations of magnesium salts are available. Thus 5 mL of magnesium hydroxide–containing antacids (Maalox, Gelusil, Mylanta) each contains 14 mmol (340 mg) of magnesium. However, there are two theoretical objections to the use of these preparations: they contain aluminum salts that may be hazardous if renal impairment is present, and they bind phosphate in the gut, which by itself promotes loss of magnesium. Other preparations include magnesium chloride tablets, magnesium gluconate tablets, and commercially available magnesium oxide powder. Since both spironolactone and triamterene cause retention of magnesium and potassium, these drugs may be useful adjuncts to maintain normal serum magnesium balance in patients taking diuretics.

Considerable attention has been focused on the role of hypomagnesemia or magnesium deficiency in cardiac arrhythmias under a variety of circumstances, including alcoholic withdrawal, open-heart surgery, coronary angioplasty, myocardial infarction, congestive heart failure, and the multiple organ failure syndrome. In some of these situations, there appears to be an inverse relationship between serum magnesium levels and potentially dangerous ventricular arrhythmias. Although therapeutic and prophylactic treatment with $MgSO_4$ appears to be efficacious, it is controversial whether these patients are actually magnesium deficient. The favorable effect of magnesium under these conditions is probably the result of nonspecific antiarrhythmic properties and electrical stabilization of membranes.

HYPERMAGNESEMIA

Patients with end-stage renal disease frequently have modest hypermagnesemia that can be aggravated by ingesting magnesium-containing compounds such as antacids or cathartics. Surreptitious ingestion of magnesium salts as a cathartic may be identified by demonstration of hypermagnesemia in serum and fecal magnesium concentration above 25 mmol/L (60 mg/dL). Rhabdomyolysis causes hypermagnesemia because of release from injured muscle. Adrenal insufficiency also may cause modest hypermagnesemia. Half of patients with familial benign hypocalciuric hypercalcemia have modest hypermagnesemia. Pronounced hypermagnesemia (6.5 mmol/L) has been described in patients with near-drowning in the Dead Sea in Jordan or Basque Lake in British Columbia. Magnesium concentrations in water from these sources average 164 and 174 mmol/L, respectively. In the Dead Sea, survivals in near-drowning cases have been attributed to pronounced hypercalcemia because of the extreme calcium levels in this water.

Symptomatic hypermagnesemia is uncommon and is usually precipitated by inadvertent overdosage with magnesium salts or is deliberately induced to treat patients with eclampsia. Infants born of eclamptic mothers treated with magnesium may be hypermagnesemic. Magnesium can reduce neuromuscular transmission and act as a central nervous system depressant. Symptoms of hypermagnesemia usually correspond to serum levels. Nausea usually appears at between 2 and 4 mmol/L (5 and 10 mg/dL). Sedation, hypoventilation with respiratory acidosis, decreased deep tendon reflexes, and muscle weakness appear at levels between 8 and 14 mmol/L (20 and 34 mg/dL). Hypotension, bradycardia, and diffuse vasodilatation appear at 10 to 20 mmol/L (24 to 48 mg/dL). Areflexia, coma, and respiratory paralysis occur at 20 to 30 mmol/L (48 to 72 mg/dL). Patients treated for eclampsia must be observed very carefully for signs of magnesium intoxication. If this occurs, symptoms and findings can generally be reversed promptly by infusion of calcium salts, since these ions electrically oppose one another at their sites of action. Administration of saline and furosemide may help promote excretion of magnesium. Hemodialysis is also effective.

REFERENCES

ALFREY AC et al: Evaluation of body magnesium stores. J Lab Clin Med 84:153, 1974

ANDERSON R et al: Skeletal muscle phosphorus and magnesium deficiency in alcoholic myopathy. Miner Electrolyte Metab 4:106, 1980

BRADY HR et al: Mitochondrial injury: An early event in cisplatin toxicity to renal proximal tubules. Am J Physiol 258:F1181, 1990

CRONIN RE et al: Skeletal muscle injury after magnesium depletion in the dog. Am J Physiol 243:F113, 1982

———, et al: Magnesium deficiency, in *Advances in Internal Medicine*, GH Stollerman (ed). Chicago, Year Book Medical Publishers, 1983, chap 28, pp 509–533

D'ANGELO EKG et al: Magnesium relaxes arterial smooth muscle by decreasing intracellular Ca^{2+} without changing intracellular Mg^{2+}. J Clin Invest 89:1988, 1992

FINE KD et al: Diagnosis of magnesium-induced diarrhea. N Engl J Med 324:1012, 1991

KNOCHEL JP: Hypophosphatemia in the alcoholic. Arch Intern Med 140:613, 1980

KROENKE K et al: The value of serum magnesium determination in hypertensive patients receiving diuretics. Arch Intern Med 147:1553, 1987

MOSSERI M et al: Electrocardiographic manifestations of combined hypercalcemia and hypermagnesemia. J Electrocardiol 23:235, 1990

PORATH A et al: Dead Sea water poisoning. Ann Emerg Med 18:121, 1989

RALSTON MA et al: Serum and tissue magnesium concentrations in patients with heart failure and serious ventricular arrhythmias. Ann Intern Med 113:841, 1990

SHILES ME: Magnesium in health and disease. Annu Rev Nutr 8:429, 1988

TZIVONI D et al: Treatment of torsade de pointes with magnesium sulfate. Circulation 77:392, 1988

VELOSO D et al: The concentrations of free and bound magnesium in rat tissues. J Biol Chem 248:4811, 1973

VICTOR M: The role of hypomagnesemia and respiratory alkalosis in the genesis of alcohol withdrawal symptoms. Ann NY Acad Sci 215:235, 1973

WHANG R et al: Frequency of hypomagnesemia in hospitalized patients receiving digitalis. Arch Intern Med 145:655, 1985

361 PAGET'S DISEASE OF BONE

STEPHEN M. KRANE

Paget's disease of bone (osteitis deformans) is usually focal but may be widespread. The initial event is excessive resorption of bone by cells such as osteoclasts, followed by the replacement of normal marrow by vascular, fibrous connective tissue. At some stage and to a variable degree, the resorbed bone is replaced by coarse-fibered, dense trabecular bone organized in haphazard fashion. The irregular and often rapid deposition of this new bone, to a great extent still lamellar, causes an increase in the number of prominent, irregular cement lines that give the bone its characteristic "mosaic" pattern. Most lesions show both excessive resorption and chaotic new bone formation.

INCIDENCE The prevalence is difficult to determine because the disease is often asymptomatic and is frequently detected when roentgenograms are obtained for other reasons or because of a high level of alkaline phosphatase on routine blood screening. On the basis of autopsy examination, the incidence is estimated to be about 3 percent in individuals over age 40; there is increased likelihood of occurrence with increasing age. The incidence varies in different parts of the world. Figures based on radiologic surveys indicate less than a 1 percent frequency in the adult populations in the United States, Great Britain, and Australia. In India, Japan, the Middle East, and Scandinavia, the disease is rare.

ETIOLOGY The cause is unknown. No convincing evidence of endocrine abnormality has been produced. Likewise, although pagetic bone can be exceedingly vascular, it has not been established that the vascular abnormality is primary. Some of the manifestations can be suppressed with glucocorticoids, salicylates, and cytotoxic drugs, but there is no convincing evidence that the fundamental lesion is inflammatory. Intranuclear inclusions have been found by electron microscopy in osteoclasts in pagetic bone but not in osteoclasts or other bone cells in normal persons or patients with other bone diseases with the exception of pyknodysostosis. Some of the inclusions resemble nucleocapsids of viruses belonging to the measles group. Indirect immunofluorescence and immunoperoxidase studies using antibodies to measles virus support the suggestion that the inclusions are indeed measles virus nucleocapsids. Measles virus nucleocapsid mRNA also has been detected by in situ hybridization in bone cells from patients with Paget's disease. Other evidence suggests that the inclusions are due to respiratory syncytial virus. In one area of England, ownership of dogs is more common in pagetic subjects than in controls, suggesting that a canine virus (e.g., canine distemper) might be the infective agent. Thus different viral agents might be responsible for Paget's disease in different patients.

PATHOPHYSIOLOGY The characteristic feature is increased resorption of bone accompanied by an increase in bone formation, which is usually adequate to compensate. In the early phase bone resorption predominates (e.g., in the variant *osteoporosis circumscripta*), and the bones are exceedingly vascular. This has been termed the *osteoporotic, osteolytic,* or *destructive phase* of disease in which the external calcium balance may be negative. Commonly, the excessive resorption is followed closely by formation of new pagetic bone. In this so-called mixed phase of the disease, the rate of bone formation is so geared to that of bone resorption that the magnitude of the increase in bone turnover is not reflected in the overall calcium balance.

As the activity decreases, a progressive decrease in resorptive rate relative to formation rate may occur, eventually leading to the occurrence of hard, dense, less vascular bone (the so-called *osteoplastic* or *sclerotic phase*) and a positive external calcium balance. The rates of bone turnover may be increased enormously in patients with active Paget's disease, occasionally more than 20 times normal. Quantitative histomorphometry of bone biopsies confirms the extent of remodeling with marked increase in resorption surfaces and deep scalloped lacunae containing osteoclasts and increased numbers of osteoblasts lining the edges. Increased generation and overactivity of osteoclasts are considered the major abnormality. The osteoclasts are larger than normal and contain multiple pleomorphic nuclei and nuclear and cytoplasmic inclusions that resemble viral nucleocapsids. Increased numbers of osteoclast-like multinucleated cells are generated from hematopoietic precursors in long-term marrow cultures from individuals with Paget's disease compared with normal individuals. Production of the cytokine interleukin 6 (IL-6) by the pagetic marrow cells is increased. Thus IL-6 could act as a local factor that contributes to the increased osteoclast formation and activity in this disease. The calcification rate is also increased. The normal hematopoietic marrow is replaced by a loose stroma which may be highly vascular. The magnitude of the increase in turnover varies with the extent as well as the activity of the disease. The increase correlates with the increased plasma levels of bone alkaline phosphatase, which are higher in Paget's disease than in any other condition with the exception of hereditary hyperphosphatasia. Although increased bone resorption enhances release of calcium and phosphate ions from bone, utilization of these ions for new bone formation and, presumably, feedback control of parathyroid hormone secretion usually maintain the concentration of calcium ions in the plasma at normal levels. The concentration of phosphate in the plasma is normal or slightly elevated. When marked imbalance between bone formation and resorption occurs in favor of resorption, as after prolonged immobilization or fractures, urinary calcium excretion may be increased, and rarely, hypercalcemia may occur. If, on the other hand, bone formation exceeds resorption (relatively uncommon), circulating levels of parathyroid hormone may be increased. Significant increases in trabecular bone resorption and osteoid surfaces in normal bone from patients with Paget's disease may be due to compensatory, secondary hyperparathyroidism. Resorption involves the organic phase of bone as well as the mineral phase. While the inorganic ions of the mineral phase are reutilized for bone formation, amino acids such as hydroxyproline and hydroxylysine and the hydroxypyridinium cross-link compounds are released during resorption of the collagen matrix of bone and are not reutilized for collagen biosynthesis. The urinary excretion of small peptides containing hydroxyproline is increased, reflecting the increased bone resorption. Peptides of about 1500 to 5000 mol wt containing hydroxyproline and other amino acids in proportions characteristic of collagen are also excreted in increased amounts in the urine and are correlated with increased bone formation. Other markers for increased matrix synthesis include elevated levels of osteocalcin (bone-GLA protein) (see Chap. 356) and procollagen extension fragments in plasma.

RADIOLOGIC CHANGES The radiologic findings reflect the underlying pathology and the phase of the disease that predominates at the time of the examination. The pelvic bones are most commonly involved, followed by the femur, skull, tibia, lumbrosacral spine, dorsal spine, clavicles, and ribs; small bones are not as frequently diseased. The lytic phase of the disease may be overlooked except when it occurs in the skull as *osteoporosis circumscripta,* with areas of sharply demarcated radiolucency in the frontal, parietal, and occipital bones. In the long bones, the lytic areas are usually first seen at one end, from which they progress toward the other end with a V-shaped advancing edge. The lesion may produce expansion of the cortex and exhibit features suggesting malignancy. Usually the lytic area is followed by a zone of increased density, representing the new bone formation of the mixed phase of the disease. In general, the bone shows enlargement with irregularly widened cortex in a coarse, striated pattern and increased density, occasionally focal in distribution. Perpendicular lines of radiolucency (cortical infractions) are frequent and occur on the convex side of bowed long bones, particularly the femur and tibia. Transverse fractures also may occur, some initiated at the sites of these cortical infractions. The remodeling of the pagetic bone usually follows the lines of stress produced by muscle pull or gravity, accounting for the characteristic lateral bowing of the femur or anterior bowing of the tibia and the tendency for most of the dense bone to be deposited on the concave side of the bowed bone. In the skull, in the mixed stage, there is enlargement and thickening, especially of the outer table, with irregular areas of increased density, often spotty (Fig. 361-1). Basilar invagination is common with involvement of the base of the skull. The changes in the pelvis also consist of bone resorption and new bone formation and are frequently accompanied by a characteristic thickening of the pelvic brim. In the sclerotic phase of the disease, the bone may show uniform increase in density, often in the absence of striations. This is common in the facial bones but is occasionally seen as well in the vertebrae, where a homogeneous, dense pattern gives an "ivory" appearance similar to that typical of Hodgkin's disease, although the involved vertebrae are not enlarged in Hodgkin's disease. Computed tomography is useful in defining atypical lesions, particularly where neoplastic involvement is suspected. Technetium 99m diphosphonate bone scans are indicated to document the extent of disease when therapy is contemplated or to confirm the diagnosis when radiologic findings are inconclusive. Gallium 67 scans also have been used to define the extent of bone involvement.

FIGURE 361-1 Lateral roentgenogram of the skull from a 58-year-old woman with Paget's disease of bone.

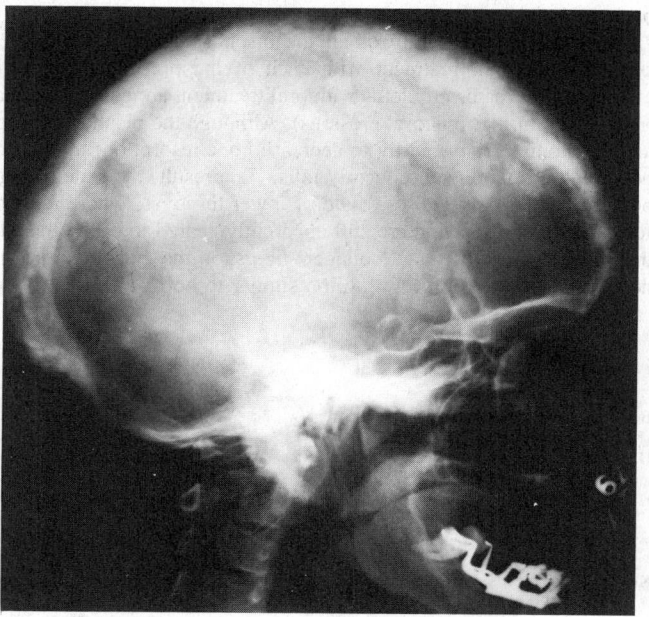

CLINICAL PICTURE The clinical presentation is a function of the extent of the disease, the particular bones involved, and the presence of complications. Many patients are asymptomatic. In these individuals, the disorder is discovered during radiologic examination of the pelvis or spine for an unrelated disease or complaint or because of the finding of an elevated level of plasma alkaline phosphatase. Other individuals may gradually become aware of a swelling or deformity of a long bone or develop a disturbance in gait due to unequal length of and change in the distribution of mechanical forces in the lower extremities. Enlargement of the skull is often not noticed by the patients, or they may be aware of increasing hat size. Pain in the face and headache are initial complaints in some; backache and pain in the lower extremities are common. The pain is usually dull but may be shooting or knifelike. Back pain is most common in the lumbar region and may radiate into the buttocks or lower extremities. This pain is probably due to the pagetic process itself, to distortion of articular facets, and to secondary osteoarthritis. Pain in the lower extremities may be associated with the transverse cortical infractions along the convex lateral surface of the femur or the anterior surface of the tibia. Often the new lytic lesions detected on bone scan are the most painful. Pain also may be due to involvement of the hip joint resembling degenerative joint disease and characterized by narrowing of the joint space, bony lipping at the margin of the acetabulum, and deepening of the acetabulum. Angioid streaks may be present in the retina. Hearing loss is due to direct involvement of the ossicles of the inner ear or of bone in the region of the cochlea or to impingement by bone on the eighth cranial nerve in the auditory foramen. More serious neurologic complications can result from overgrowth of bone at the base of the skull (platybasia) and compression of the brainstem. Compression of the spinal cord with paraplegia has been observed, particularly with involvement of the middorsal spine. Pathologic fractures of vertebrae also may produce spinal cord lesions.

COMPLICATIONS Blood flow may be markedly increased in extremities involved with Paget's disease. There is proliferation of blood vessels in pagetic bone, but anatomic and functional studies have not confirmed the presence of arteriovenous fistulas. Although blood flow is increased in bone, cutaneous vasodilatation in the pagetic extremities accounts for the increased warmth noted clinically. When the disease is widespread, involving one-third or more of the skeleton, the increased blood flow may be associated with *high cardiac output* and rarely with so-called high-output heart failure. However, heart disease in individuals with Paget's disease is usually due to the same conditions that occur in other patients of similar age. *Pathologic fracture* may occur in the destructive phase of the disease. In the weight-bearing bones fractures are often incomplete, multiple, and on the convex side of the bone. They may occur spontaneously or follow slight trauma; the lesions are painful but heal spontaneously with no major disability. More serious fractures also may occur. Complete fractures are often transverse as if the bone were snapped like a piece of chalk. Under these circumstances the fracture may upset the delicate balance between bone formation and resorption in favor of resorption. At this stage the imbalance may be reflected by increased urinary calcium excretion, and in rare instances the serum calcium level may rise to dangerous levels.

There is no characteristic level of urinary calcium excretion, although calcium excretion tends to be higher when the resorptive phase predominates. This may be a factor which accounts for the somewhat higher incidence of *urinary stone* in these patients. Secondary changes in the cartilage of the hip joints and knees may result in articular symptoms. Hyperuricemia and gout commonly occur in men with Paget's disease, and calcific periarthritis may occur.

Sarcoma is the dread complication. The incidence is probably no greater than 1 percent, although higher incidence has been noted in some series that include many patients with polyostotic involvement. The sarcomas most frequently arise in the femur, humerus, skull, facial bones, and pelvis and rarely in the vertebrae. In about 20 percent the tumors are multicentric. Histologically, they are usually osteosarcomas, although fibrosarcomas and chondrosarcomas also have been found. Increase in pain and swelling are the common complaints that lead to recognition of the sarcomas. The extent and character of the neoplastic involvement are established by computed tomography and/or magnetic resonance imaging. The level of alkaline phosphatase in the serum of patients with sarcomas usually reflects the activity and extent of the Paget's disease. In occasional patients, an "explosive rise" of the phosphatase level may accompany the growth of the sarcoma, whereas in patients with limited Paget's disease, phosphatase levels may be only slightly elevated and give no clue to the development of the malignant lesion. The prognosis is poor following the development of sarcomas, and ablative surgery is rarely successful. Although chemotherapy is successful for treatment of some osteosarcomas in children, such regimens have little effect on survival of patients in whom osteosarcomas develop on the background of Paget's disease. Reparative granulomas resembling giant cell tumors may be locally destructive, but they do not metastasize.

THERAPY Most patients require no treatment, since the disease is localized and does not cause symptoms. Indications for therapy include persistent pain in involved bones, neural compression, rapidly progressive deformity resulting in disabling disturbance of posture and/or gait, high-output congestive heart failure, hypercalcemia, severe hypercalciuria with or without formation of renal stones, repeated fractures or nonunion, and preparation for major orthopedic surgery. Nonsteroidal anti-inflammatory drugs such as *indomethacin*, 25 mg three or four times daily, may relieve pain, especially in the presence of hip involvement. *Glucocorticoids* suppress the disease but only in large doses (greater than 60 mg prednisone per day), which are usually not tolerated and, therefore, are not recommended. It is of interest that the high cardiac output of some patients may be reduced significantly after only a few days of glucocorticoid treatment. Orthopedic procedures also have a role in the management of selected cases. Total hip replacement may be indicated, and osteotomy may correct marked bowing deformities, particularly of the tibia. In patients with fractures or orthopedic procedures or in patients immobilized for any reason, urinary and serum calcium levels should be measured at intervals to anticipate the development of hypercalciuria and hypercalcemia. Early ambulation and adequate fluid intake are essential. If hypercalcemia does occur under these circumstances, intravenous infusion of the bisphosphonate pamidronate disodium (see below) is recommended in dosage of 20 mg over 2 to 6 h repeated each day for 3 to 4 days.

Several agents reduce the excessive bone resorption of Paget's disease and are of possible therapeutic value. The administration of porcine, salmon, and human *calcitonins* for prolonged periods to pagetic patients causes a decrease in plasma alkaline phosphatase and in urinary hydroxyproline excretion. Treatment with calcitonin causes variable decrease in bone pain due to suppression of the pagetic lesion and an independent, centrally mediated analgesic effect. Calcitonin also induces improvement in neurologic symptoms and decrease in elevated cardiac output. Some patients have not continued to respond to porcine and salmon calcitonins, possibly because of the development of neutralizing antibodies. These individuals usually continue to exhibit a satisfactory response to human calcitonin. In others, the development of secondary hyperparathyroidism has been postulated as the cause for a diminished response, although this cannot account for resistance in all cases. The calcitonins are probably most useful in patients with pain in areas of pagetic involvement not due to associated joint disease. The dose of salmon calcitonin (the form available in the United States) is 50 to 100 MRC units daily given subcutaneously. In most cases, it is possible to reduce the dose to three times weekly. In severe cases, alkaline phosphatase levels decrease, but not to the normal range. The disorder relapses after weeks or months when the calcitonin is discontinued. Some patients develop a sensation of warmth and/or nausea 30 min to several hours after injection. This may occur after initiating treatment or after months or years of therapy. The etiology is unknown, but the symptoms may be severe enough to discontinue the medication. The use of nasal spray formulations of calcitonin is under investigation.

Although cytotoxic drugs such as plicamycin and dactinomycin have been used in the past to treat Paget's disease, they no longer have a place in therapy, since other agents are safer and more effective. *Etidronate*, a bisphosphonate compound, given orally in doses up to 20 mg/kg body weight per day, is effective in reducing bone resorption in almost all affected individuals and in producing clinical improvement in some. Biochemical indices may be brought to normal, but in most the responses are incomplete. Serum alkaline phosphatase and urinary hydroxyproline excretion remain decreased for several months after withdrawal of the drug and only gradually return to pretreatment levels. In doses of 20 mg/kg of body weight per day for periods of 6 months or longer and even with lower doses, mineralization of new bone may be inhibited (osteomalacia), predisposing to fracture. Some patients develop disabling pain over pagetic lesions within weeks or months of starting treatment that may be severe enough to warrant discontinuing the drug. Radiographs in some instances show an increase in bone lysis that heals when the drug is stopped. It is therefore recommended that doses of 5 mg or occasionally 10 mg/kg of body weight per day be used for 6-month periods. Treatment should be reinstituted within 3 to 12 months if biochemical relapse occurs.

Newer bisphosphonates that result from substitutions at R_1 and R_2 of the

$$\begin{array}{c} R_1 \\ | \\ -P-C-P- \\ | \\ R_2 \end{array}$$

bond are now used in therapy in Europe, and several should soon be available in the United States. These compounds (alendronate, clodronate, pamidronate, risendronate, and tiludronate) are more potent than etidronate and in doses that are effective in completely suppressing the pagetic lesions do not inhibit mineralization. Pamidronate, as already discussed, is approved for treatment of hypercalcemia. These drugs should replace etidronate in the therapy of Paget's disease. Several dosage schedules have been used, such as 15 to 20 mg pamidronate intravenously over 2 to 6 h daily or several times per week for 4 to 10 treatments. Higher intravenous doses may produce fever and flulike symptoms. With such a program, urinary hydroxyproline excretion returns to normal within weeks, and serum alkaline phosphatase becomes normal within months. Remission usually lasts for more than 12 months and for up to 5 years in some patients.

The oral bioavailability of all the bisphosphonates is poor (~ 1 percent), but oral treatment with each of the preceding agents is effective. The major problems with oral treatment are gastrointestinal (nausea, vomiting, mucosal erosions). Although the bisphosphonates and calcitonins act primarily to decrease bone resorption, the rate of new bone formation subsequently falls. As a result, the state of high bone turnover is shifted to a state of lower turnover, where rates of formation and resorption are still apparently geared to each other. In this lower turnover state, collagen fibers of the bone matrix are deposited in a more orderly fashion similar to normal bone.

REFERENCES

BONE HG, KLEEREKOPER M: Clinical review 39: Paget's disease of bone. J Clin Endocrinol Metab 75:1179, 1992

HARINCK HIJ et al: Relation between signs and symptoms in Paget's disease of bone. Q J Med 226:133, 1986

HUVOS AG: Osteogenic sarcoma of bones and soft tissues in older persons. Cancer 57:1442, 1986

——— et al: Osteogenic sarcoma associated with Paget's disease of bone: A clinicopathologic study of 65 patients. Cancer 52:1489, 1983

KRANE SM: Paget's disease of bone, in *Current Therapy of Endocrinology and Metabolism*, CW Bardin (ed). Philadelphia, BC Decker, 1991, pp 456–460

McDonald DJ, Sim FH: Total hip arthroplasty in Paget's disease. J Bone Joint Surg 69A:766, 1987

Nagant de Deuxchaisnes C, Krane SM: Paget's disease of bone: Clinical and metabolic observations. Medicine 43:233, 1964

Rebel A (ed): Symposium on Paget's disease. Clin Orthop 217:1, 1987

Roodman GR et al: Interleukin 6: A potential autocrine/paracrine factor in Paget's disease of bone. J Clin Invest 89:46, 1992

Seret P et al: Sarcomatous degeneration of Paget's bone disease. J Cancer Res Clin Oncol 113:392, 1987

Singer FR, Krane SM: Paget's disease of bone, in *Metabolic Bone Disease*, LV Avioli, SM Krane (eds). Philadelphia, Saunders, 1990, pp 546–615

———, Wallach S (eds): *Paget's Disease of Bone*. New York, Elsevier 1991, pp 1–313

Strickberger SA et al: Association of Paget's disease of bone with calcific aortic valve disease. Am J Med 82:953, 1987

362 HYPEROSTOSIS, NEOPLASMS, AND OTHER DISORDERS OF BONE AND CARTILAGE

STEPHEN M. KRANE / ALAN L. SCHILLER

HYPEROSTOSIS

A number of disease states have in common an increase in the mass of bone per unit volume (hyperostosis) (Table 362-1). Such increase in bone mass is detected radiologically as increased density of the bone, often associated with a variable disturbance in the architecture of the tissue. In the basence of quantitative histomorphometric data, it is usually not possible to distinguish between an increase in bone mass due to excessive formation of new bone or to decreased resorption of bone already formed. When bone deposition is rapid, the new bone may be of the woven type, but if the process is more chronic, true lamellar bone is formed. The additional bone may be located at the periosteum, within the compact bone of the cortex, or in the trabeculae of the cancellous regions. In the medullary area, the new bone is deposited on and between the trabeculae and encroaches on the medullary spaces. Typical examples of such responses are seen in areas adjacent to tumors or in association with infection. In some diseases, the increase in bone mass may be spotty, as in osteopoikilosis, whereas in others, most of the skeleton may be involved, as in the malignant form of osteopetrosis in children. The increase in mass is usually not due to an excessive amount of mineral relative to matrix, except in disorders such as osteopetrosis, where islands of calcified cartilage may persist. (The mineral density of calcified cartilage is greater than that of bone.) In some diseases, such as the osteosclerosis of renal insufficiency, the bone mass and radiodensity may be increased, even though the new bone formed is poorly mineralized and contains widened osteoid seams. Hyperostosis could be due to dysfunction of osteoblasts or osteoclasts. It is of interest, therefore, that infection of newborn mice produces an osteopetrosis-like phenotype in which osteoblast progenitors appear to induce increased bone formation. In human osteopetrosis of the relatively benign and sporadic type, however, viral nucleocapsid particles have been found in osteoclasts, and it is possible that viral infection causes disordered function in these cells to account for the excessive bone mass.

Several of these conditions are discussed in more detail in other chapters, although some generalizations are pertinent. Bone that is denser than normal may be seen occasionally in the osteitis fibrosa associated with hyperparathyroidism. When the hyperparathyroidism is successfully treated, the rate of bone resorption decreases abruptly out of proportion to the rate of bone formation; this imbalance may

TABLE 362-1 Causes of hyperostosis

1 Endocrine disorders
  a Primary hyperparathyroidism
  b Hypothyroidism
  c Acromegaly
2 Radiation osteitis
3 Chemical poisoning
  a Fluoride
  b Elemental phosphorus
  c Beryllium
  d Arsenic
  e Vitamin A intoxication
  f Lead
  g Bismuth
4 Osteomalacic disorders
  a Renal tubular osteomalacia (vitamin D resistance or phosphate diabetes)
  b Chronic renal glomerular failure
5 Osteosclerosis (localized) associated with chronic infection
6 Osteosclerotic phase of Paget's disease
7 Osteoscleorsis associated with carcinomatous metastases, malignant lymphoma, and hematologic disorders (myeloproliferative disorders, sickle cell disease, leukemia, multiple myeloma, systemic mastocytosis)
8 Osteosclerosis of erythroblastosis fetalis
9 Osteopetrosis
  a Infantile (malignant, autosomal recessive form)
  b Adult (benign, dominant form)
  c Intermediate form with carbonic anhydrase II deficiency and renal tubular acidosis
10 Unclassified diseases
  a Pyknodysostosis
  b Osteomyelosclerosis
  c Hyperostosis corticalis generalisata
  d Hyperostosis generalisata with pachydermia
  e Hereditary hyperphosphatasia
  f Progressive diaphyseal dysplasia (osteopathia hyperostotica multiplex infantilis; Camurati-Engelmann disease)
  g Melorheostosis
  h Osteopoikilosis
  i Hyperostosis frontalis interna

lead to the production of areas of bone density greater than in the surrounding skeleton, especially in the healing of brown tumors. In addition, intermittent low levels of parathyroid hormone act directly on osteoblasts, to increase bone formation. In hypothyroidism, the rates of both bone formation and resorption may be decreased, but when the balance is in favor of formation, bones are of increased density but normal architecture. Increased bone density also occurs in some instances of osteomalacia associated with disturbances in renal tubular function. The increased mass of bone occurs together with widened osteoid seams, as in chronic renal glomerular insufficiency. In the vertebral bodies, the bone appears denser in transverse bands at the upper and lower margins, with a relatively radiolucent center. This "sandwich" appearance is similar to that seen in some patients with osteopetrosis and has been termed by the British the *rugger jersey sign*. Skeletal hyperostosis, including cortical hyperostoses, periostitis, and tendon and ligament ossification, is also a complication of long-term therapy with synthetic retinoids such as isotretinoin.

OSTEOPETROSIS Osteopetrosis (Albers-Schönberg or marble bone disease) is clinically, biochemically, and genetically heterogeneous. Although osteopetrosis has multiple causes, a defect in bone resorption is always the underlying mechanism. Several genetically determined forms of osteopetrosis in rodents may serve as models for the human diseases. Some can be cured by bone marrow transplantation from a normal littermate and probably represent stem cell defects. Two other forms of osteopetrosis, in *op/op* mice and *tl/tl* toothless rats, are not cured by bone marrow transplantation, however. These animals have few osteoclasts, and those which are present express osteoclast enzymes weakly. The *op/op* mice have a defect in the coding region of the gene for colony stimulating factor 1 (CSF-1, also known as M-CSF, the M standing for macrophage), and the skeletal defects in these animals and in *tl/tl* rats can be reversed by treatment with CSF-1. Another form of osteopetrosis has been produced in transgenic mice by "knockout" of the c-src gene by homologous recombination; c-src and its phosphorylation substrate, P80/85 are expressed at high levels in osteoclasts. Human homologues of these rodent diseases have not yet been demonstrated. The most severe form in human infants is also due to defects in differentiation and/or function of osteoclasts. Infantile osteopetrosis is manifested in utero and progresses after birth with anemia, hepatosplenomegaly, hydrocephalus, cranial nerve involvement, and death, often due to infections. The disorder is usually inherited as an autosomal recessive trait. Several attempts to transplant bone marrow from normal donors to provide normal osteoclast precursor cells have been successful, and osteopetrotic bone has been repopulated with functioning osteoclasts of donor origin that produce radiologic and/or bone biopsy evidence of bone resorption. One infant received a bone marrow transplant from a brother with successful response lasting more than 4 years, although vision was not restored. In other individuals with osteopetrosis, peripheral blood monocyte function is defective. In still other cases of osteopetrosis, clinical improvement has been obtained using high doses of calcitriol.

Less fulminant forms of osteopetrosis occur in older children and adults. In some of the latter, the disorder appears to be sporadic. In others, the osteopetrosis is inherited as an autosomal dominant trait and is progressive with increasing age; anemia is not as severe, neurologic abnormalities are not as frequent, and recurrent pathologic fractures are the main feature. Although most cases are in infants and children, many are discovered first in adult life when roentgenograms are obtained because of fractures or unrelated diseases. There is no predilection for either sex. Even the inherited adult disorder is heterogeneous. Type I is characterized by increased thickness of the cranial vault, whereas rugger jersey sign and "endo bones" in the pelvis are features of type II. A defect in modeling of endosteal bone is present in both types, and there is an additional defect in the remodeling of trabecular bone in type II osteopetrosis.

An "intermediate" form of osteopetrosis has been described in several kindreds in which the skeletal abnormality is associated with renal tubular acidosis and cerebral calcification. This form, which is inherited as an autosomal recessive defect, is compatible with long survival and is associated with a virtual absence of one of the isoenzymes of carbonic anhydrase (carbonic anhydrase II). Carbonic anhydrase II is a major component of the enzyme system required for generation of the unique acid environment adjacent to the ruffled border of the osteoclast, and deficiency of carbonic anhydrase results in disordered bone resorption. Bone resorption is depressed. In some instances, islands of unresorbed calcified cartilage are encased in bone. The defect in remodeling results in disorganization of bone structure with thickened cortices and lack of funnelization of metaphyses. Despite increased density, the bone is abnormal mechanically and fractures readily. Osteomalacia or rickets is sometimes a component of the osteopetrosis in children (Fig. 362-1).

The histologic changes are reflected in the roentgenograms (Fig. 362-2), which reveal uniformly dense, sclerotic bone often without distinction between the cortical and cancellous regions. In the severe infantile form, there is persistence of the primary spongiosa with central calcified cartilage cores surrounded by woven bone. Osteoclasts are often increased in number but apparently do not function properly. Osteoclasts may be morphologically normal or have loss of the ruffled borders, suggesting that a spectrum of changes may occur. The variability may reflect heterogeneity in this syndrome, as in the osteopetrosis in rodents. The long bones are usually involved, with increased density along the entire shaft. Foci of increased density may be seen in the epiphyses corresponding to regions of unresorbed calcified cartilage. The metaphyses have a characteristic clubbed or splayed appearance. Horizontal bandings of increased density alternating with zones of decreased density in the long bones and vertebrae suggest that the defect is intermittent during periods of growth. The skull, pelvis, ribs, and other bones may be involved. The phalanges and the distal humerus may appear normal.

Encroachment of bone on the marrow cavity, particularly in the malignant infantile disorder, is associated with anemia of the myelophthisic type with foci of extramedullary hematopoiesis in liver, spleen, and lymph nodes and enlargement of these organs. Neurologic abnormalities are associated with encroachment on cranial nerves and include optic atrophy, nystagmus, papilledema, exophthalmos, and impairment of extraocular motility. Facial paralysis and deafness are frequent; trigeminal lesions and anosmia are less common. In infants, macrocephaly, hydrocephalus, and convulsions may occur, and

FIGURE 362-2   Roentgenogram of the spine and pelvis of a 55-year-old man with the more benign, dominant form of osteopetrosis.

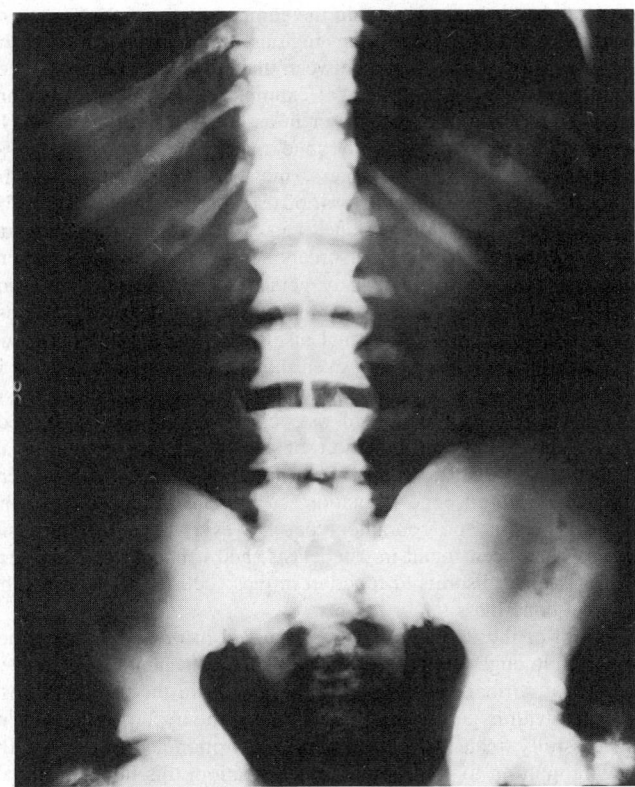

FIGURE 362-1   Lateral roentgenogram of the thorax of a 9-month-old boy with the "malignant" form of osteopetrosis. Note the uniform increase in mineral density of the vertebral bodies and the marked flaring of the ends of the ribs (arrows), indicative of rickets.

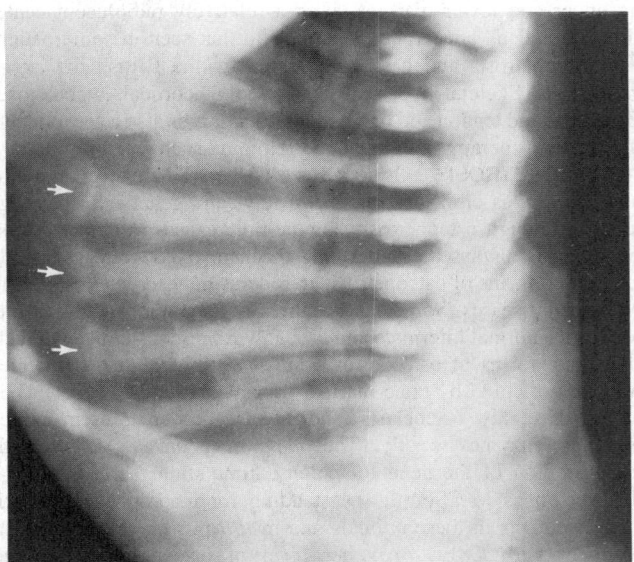

infections such as osteomyelitis are frequent. Renal tubular acidosis is a feature of the osteopetrosis associated with a deficiency in carbonic anhydrase II.

In the milder dominant osteopetrosis, about half the patients have no symptoms, and the disorder is discovered incidentally on roentgenograms. Other patients present because of fractures, bone pain, osteomyelitis, and cranial nerve palsies.

Fractures are a complication even with trivial trauma. Healing of such fractures is usually satisfactory, although delayed union may occur. When the disease is manifested first in adult life, fractures may be the only clinical problem. Levels of calcium and alkaline phosphatase in the plasma are usually normal in adults, although in children hypophosphatemia and moderate hypocalcemia have been noted. Serum acid phosphatase levels are usually increased.

The skeletal defect is not the same in all forms of osteopetrosis, and within a clinical subtype, genetic and biochemical heterogeneity is common. As mentioned, in several children with severe osteopetrosis, bone marrow transplants from HLA-identical siblings have resulted in histologic and radiologic increases in bone resorption and variable improvement in anemia, vision, hearing, and growth and development.

Unfortunately, it is not always possible to find appropriate donors, or patients may not be good candidates for bone marrow transplantation. In patients with the lethal forms, calcitriol therapy is associated with the appearance of osteoclasts with normal ruffled borders and other evidence for increased bone resorption.

PYKNODYSOSTOSIS *Pyknodysostosis* is a form of osteosclerosis that superficially resembles osteopetrosis. It is one of the types of short-limbed dwarfism associated with bone fragility and a tendency to fracture with minimal trauma. Nevertheless, life span is usually normal. In addition to a generalized increase in bone density, features include short stature, separated cranial sutures, hypoplasia of the mandible, kyphoscoliosis and deformities of the trunk, persistence of deciduous teeth, progressive acroosteolysis of the terminal phalanges, high, arched palate, proptosis, blue sclerae, and a pointed, beaked nose. Life span is usually unaffected, and the patient usually presents because of frequent fractures. Pyknodysostosis is inherited as an autosomal recessive trait. In one case, levels of plasma calcitonin were intermittently elevated, and the response of the plasma calcitonin to infusions of calcium and glucagon was exaggerated. The gene that causes this disorder may be located on the short arm of a small acrocentric chromosome.

OSTEOMYELOSCLEROSIS *Osteomyelosclerosis* is a disorder in which the marrow cells are replaced by diffuse fibroplasia, occasionally accompanied by osseous metaplasia. When the latter is prominent, increased skeletal density is seen on roentgenograms. In early stages woven bone may be found in intratrabecular locations, whereas in more advanced stages woven bone is observed in the medulla. The disorder is probably a phase in the course of the myeloproliferative disorders and is characteristically accompanied by extramedullary hematopoiesis.

Hyperostosis corticalis generalisata (van Buchem's disease) is characterized by osteosclerosis of the skull (base and calvaria), lower jaw, clavicles, and ribs and thickening of the diaphyseal cortices of the long and short bones. Alkaline phosphatase levels in the serum are elevated, and the disorder may be due to increased formation of bone of normal structure. The major manifestations are due to neural compression and consist of optic atrophy, facial paralysis, and perception deafness. In *hyperostosis generalisata with pachydermia* (Uehlinger), the sclerosis is due to increased formation of subperiosteal spongy bone and involves the epiphyses, metaphyses, and diaphyses. Pain, swelling of joints, and thickening of the skin of the lower arms are common.

HEREDITARY HYPERPHOSPHATASIA This disorder is characterized by severe structural deformities of the skeleton with increase in thickness of the calvaria, large homogeneous areas of increased density at the base of the skull, and widening and loss of normal architecture of the shafts and the epiphyses of the long and short bones. There is a failure to deposit normal bone, with haphazard

orientation of lamellae suggesting active remodeling that resembles Paget's disease of bone. Osteoclasts with multiple nuclei characteristic of Paget's disease and the typical "mosaic" pattern of faceted units of lamellar bone are not found, however. Levels of plasma alkaline phosphatase and urinary excretion of hydroxyproline peptides and other collagen degradation products are markedly increased. The disorder is apparently inherited as an autosomal recessive trait. Calcitonin therapy may be of value in some of these patients.

PROGRESSIVE DIAPHYSEAL DYSPLASIA A disorder in which a symmetric thickening and increased diameter of the diaphyses of long bones occurs, particularly in femurs, tibias, fibulas, radii, and ulnas, has been termed *progressive diaphyseal dysplasia* (Camurati-Engelmann disease). Pain over affected areas, fatigue, abnormal gait, and muscle wasting are the major manifestations. Serum alkaline phosphatase levels may be elevated, and on occasion, hypocalcemia and hyperphosphatemia may be found. Other abnormalities include anemia, leukopenia, and elevated erythrocyte sedimentation rate. Clinical and biochemical improvement may result from the use of glucocorticoids.

MELORHEOSTOSIS This rare condition usually begins in childhood and is characterized by a slowly progressive linear hyperostosis in one or more bones of one limb, usually in a lower extremity. All segments of the bone may be involved, with sclerotic areas that have a "flowing" distribution. The involved limb is often extremely painful. Soft tissue masses, not connected to bone, are often mineralized and are composed of osseous or cartilaginous tissue. Other types of soft tissue masses are associated with joint contractures or consist of fibrofatty, lymphatic, or vascular tissue.

OSTEOPOIKILOSIS This benign autosomal dominant trait is usually discovered by chance. It is characterized by dense spots of trabecular bone less than a centimeter in diameter, usually of uniform density, that are located in the epiphyses and adjacent parts of the metaphyses. All bones may be involved except the skull, ribs, and vertebrae.

HYPEROSTOSIS FRONTALIS INTERNA *Hyperostosis frontalis interna* is an abnormality of the inner table of the frontal bones of the skull consisting of smooth, rounded enostoses covered by dura and projecting into the cranial cavity. These enostoses are usually less than 1 cm at their greatest diameter and usually do not extend posteriorly beyond the coronal suture. The abnormality is found almost exclusively in women, who are frequently obese, hirsute, and have a variety of neuropsychiatric complaints (Morgagni-Stewart-Morel syndrome). However, hyperostosis frontalis interna also occurs in women with no obvious illness or particular associated disease. The finding in the skull may be a manifestation of a generalized metabolic disorder.

NEOPLASMS OF BONE

Primary neoplasms of the skeletal system reflect in their histology the cellular and extracellular components of the skeleton. However, it is not always possible to prove that a tumor arises from the same type of tissue that it produces. The precursor cells of bone tissue are derived from distinct cell lines in which the osteoclasts arise from hematopoietic stem cells and the osteoblasts arise from stromal stem cells. The primitive stromal stem cells can differentiate into chondroblasts and fibroblasts as well as osteoblasts. Neoplasms can arise from all these cell types. Each of these cells can produce its characteristic extracellular matrix, and neoplasms arising from them may thus be recognized. Primary neoplasms of bone can arise also from other hematopoietic, vascular, and neural elements.

PATHOPHYSIOLOGY Neoplasms in bone induce resorption of skeletal tissue. This bone resorption results from production by the tumor cells of factors that stimulate osteoclast function and/or recruitment and differentiation of the osteoclast hematopoietic precursor cells. One of the factors produced by the tumor cells is the parathyroid hormone-related protein (PTHrP) that interacts with the

PTH receptor (see also Chap. 357). Other factors that induce bone resorption by modulating recruitment, differentiation, and/or activation of osteoclasts include cytokines such as transforming growth factor alpha; interleukins 1, 6, and 11; tumor necrosis factor alpha; lymphotoxin; and tumor necrosis factor beta derived from the tumor, resident bone cells, or infiltrating mononuclear inflammatory cells. What was initially termed "osteoclast activating factor" is now known to include cytokines such as interleukin 1 and lymphotoxin produced by monocytes and lymphocytes. Prostaglandin or other eicosanoid production by some tumors also may mediate bone resorption. T lymphocytes infected with some viruses can metabolize circulating 25(OH)D to 1,25(OH)$_2$D, which also may stimulate bone resorption. Tumors also may alter blood supply to bone by obstructing vessels or inducing angiogenesis. Tumors also may produce reaction in surrounding bone and alter the normal contour. The epiphyseal plate, articular cartilage, cortex, and periosteum of bone often offer a barrier to the spread of neoplastic tissue. Alteration of the contour of the cortex is not due to "expansion" but to remodeling of the bone in the area and formation of new bone with the new contour. Some tumors induce primarily an osteoblastic or sclerotic reaction in surrounding bone, which results in increased radiodensity. Primary neoplasms may be less radiopaque than surrounding bone or more radiopaque depending on the degree of calcification or ossification of the matrix and the density of the tissue. Bone tumors may be recognized because of (1) the presence of a mass in the soft tissues, (2) deformity of a bone, (3) pain and tenderness, or (4) pathologic fractures. Tumors of bone also may be detected incidentally on roentgenograms obtained for other reasons. Although it is usually possible to classify bone tumors as benign or malignant, prediction of the clinical outcome on histologic and radiologic criteria is not always possible.

The extent of the lesions should be defined by standard and computed tomographic techniques and magnetic resonance imaging, if available. Lesions also can be assessed by bone scans utilizing ^{99m}Tc polyphosphonate. There are numerous pitfalls in the clinical diagnosis and interpretation of histologic features of tumors of bone. However, proper evaluation and selection of therapy require evaluation of both radiographic and histologic features. Management, therefore, requires cooperation of the orthopedist, oncologist, radiologist, radiotherapist, and pathologist.

BENIGN TUMORS   The most common benign tumors are *osteochondromas* (exostoses) and *endochondromas* (which may be multiple in Ollier's disease), *giant cell tumors, unicameral bone cysts, osteoid osteomas, and nonossifying fibromas* (fibrous cortical defects). As a rule, benign tumors are not painful except for osteoid osteomas, chondroblastomas, and chondromyxoidfibroma. The usual clinical problem is that of slowly progressing mass, pathologic fracture, or deformity. Treatment is usually accomplished by resection or curettage and bone grafting. When wide resection of tissue is necessary, insertion of metal and plastic prostheses or allograft transplantation may preserve limb function.

MALIGNANT TUMORS   The most common malignant tumor of bone is multiple myeloma (see Chap. 280). Primary lymphoma also may arise locally in bone. Malignant tumors of nonhematopoietic origin include osteosarcomas, chondrosarcomas, fibrosarcomas, and Ewing's tumor. Giant cell tumors may be included here because they may metastasize, especially after incomplete curettage, and are locally destructive. *Osteogenic sarcomas* are presumed to arise from osteoprogenitor cells and have a wide variation in histopathology, with at least 12 histologic types. These tumors always contain woven bone, at least in small foci, and may contain in addition cartilaginous and fibrous elements. They are most common in the second and third decades and are less common under age 10 and over age 40. Genetic factors are important in the genesis of osteosarcomas particularly in children. Between 30 and 40 percent of patients with retinoblastoma have a hereditary predisposition to the tumor as well as to other cancers, particularly osteosarcomas. This predisposition has been mapped to chromosome 13q14, the locus of the retinoblastoma (*Rb*)

gene. The *Rb* gene, which functions normally as a tumor suppressor by forming complexes with several viral-encoded oncoproteins, is inactivated on one allele in these patients as well as in others with sporadic neoplasms, where the gene inactivation is derived from somatic events. Thus homozygosity for the mutant *Rb* allele in the osteoblast precursor could lead to osteosarcoma in the same way that homozygosity at the same allele in a retinoblast could lead to retinoblastoma. Other tumor suppressor genes also may predispose to osteosarcoma. For example, in patients with the multifocal osteosarcoma subtype, mutations have been identified in a highly conserved region of the p53 gene. When osteosarcomas occur in older individuals, e.g., in those with Paget's disease of bone or prior exposure to ionizing radiation, it is probable that mutations in the *Rb*, p53, or other genes are responsible for the abnormal growth and other features of the malignant osteoblasts. In primary osteogenic sarcomas, the lesions usually arise in the metaphyseal region of long bones, especially in the distal femur, proximal tibia, and proximal humerus. The most common symptoms are pain and swelling which may be present for weeks or months. The roentgenographic features of osteosarcomas depend on the degree of bone destruction, the extent to which mineralized bone is formed by and within the tumor, and the type of reaction in the surrounding bone. Thus the lesions may vary from purely lytic lesions to dense areas containing radiopaque lumps, clouds, or spicules of tumor bone in varying patterns of organization. Discontinuities may occur in the cortex surrounding the lesion. In other cases, hyperostotic periosteal reactions may involve grossly layered bone. If the tumor grows rapidly, it may destroy the cortex and penetrate the soft tissue surrounding the bone; it leaves only a cuff of periosteal new bone at the peripheral margin of the tumor, just at the point of penetration (Codman's triangle). High plasma alkaline phosphatase levels in those sarcomas which are predominantly osteogenic parallel the course of the tumor. In general, high levels of serum alkaline phosphatase activity correlate with a poor prognosis. When lesions are adequately treated by amputation or wide resection, chemotherapy, or radiation, the level of alkaline phosphatase falls, and when metastases appear, the level rises again, often reaching values higher than those present initially. When values are initially high, the course is often rapidly fatal. Metastases occur primarily by the hematogenous route, especially to the lung.

The prognosis of osteosarcoma was very poor prior to development of effective chemotherapy, with radiologic evidence of pulmonary metastases usually occurring within a year following surgical excision that was potentially curative. The course varies with the type of tumor; for example, a high-grade histologic variant has a very poor prognosis unless treated with aggressive chemotherapy, whereas the less common low-grade intramedullary type has a better prognosis. In the typical intramedullary type of osteosarcoma, death occurs within 6 months from the onset of detectable pulmonary metastases, suggesting that the lesions in the lungs were present at the time of surgery or that cells were shed from the tumor during the operation.

The management of bone tumors in general has been improved by the introduction of a reliable staging system. The staging is based on the histologic grade of the lesion, flow cytometric analysis of tumor DNA content, and assessment as to whether the lesion is confined to a skeletal compartment or has metastasized. Several chemotherapeutic programs are efficacious. The disease-free and overall survival rates after 4 to 5 years in patients with no demonstrable metastases have increased from about 20 percent with ablative surgery alone to 80 percent or higher with current treatment programs. Since microscopic metastatic foci must be present when the bone tumors are first recognized, aggressive adjuvant chemotherapy is now routine. Chemotherapeutic programs include high-dose methotrexate with leucovorin rescue and various combinations of doxorubicin, cisplatin, bleomycin, cyclophosphamide, and dactinomycin. Amputation or surgical resection of the sarcoma leaving a wide margin of normal tissue is generally carried out. More frequently, a limb-sparing procedure is attempted, particularly in distal femoral osteosarcomas, with allograft bone and cartilage transplants and/or prosthetic devices used to preserve the joint. Resection of isolated pulmonary metastases combined with chemotherapy also may improve survival in younger individuals with primary osteosarcomas. The prognosis of osteosarcoma occurring on the background of Paget's disease in adults is still poor despite chemotherapy.

Chondrosarcomas are distinguishable from osteogenic sarcomas. In contrast to the latter, chondrosarcomas usually arise in adulthood and old age, with the peak incidence in the fourth, fifth, and sixth decades. Most are located in the pelvic girdle, ribs, and diaphyseal portions of the femur and humerus; distal portions of the extremities are involved rarely. Chondrosarcomas probably arise by malignant transformation in enchondromas and more rarely in the cartilaginous cap of osteochondromas. As a rule, chondrosarcomas are slow growing and slow to recur. Radiographically, the lesions appear destructive, with mottled increases in radiodensity which reflect the variable degree of calcification of cartilaginous matrix and ossification. Radical excision is the treatment of choice. Histologic grading of the tumor can be valuable for predicting prognosis and determining appropriate surgical therapy.

Ewing's tumor   This is a malignant sarcoma composed of small, round cells that occurs most frequently in the first three decades of life. Most are located in the long bones, although any bone may be involved. No specific tumor marker is available for Ewing's sarcoma, and light and electron microscopy are most useful tools in diagnosis. A characteristic cytogenetic feature in Ewing's sarcoma is a reciprocal translocation of the long arms of chromosomes 11 and 22. Although Ewing's sarcoma is highly malignant, it responds to chemotherapy and radiation with overall survival rates approaching 60 to 70 percent. Limb-sparing surgery with resection of the involved bone is coupled with chemotherapy, and radiation is used for metastatic disease or if the surgical margins contain tumor cells. Chemotherapy with doxorubicin, cyclophosphamide, vincristine, and dactinomycin improves survival of patients with Ewing's sarcoma, including some with metastatic disease.

TUMORS METASTATIC TO BONE   The skeleton is a common site for metastases from carcinomas and occasionally even from sarcomas. Skeletal metastases may be silent or produce symptoms by the same mechanisms as primary tumors, i.e., pain, swelling, deformity, encroachment on hematopoietic tissue in the marrow, compression of spinal cord or nerve roots, and pathologic fractures. In addition, rapidly lytic skeletal metastases can result in hypercalcemia. The bones involved most commonly are the vertebrae, proximal femur, pelvis, ribs, sternum, and proximal humerus, in that order of frequency. The carcinomas that most frequently metastasize to bone arise in prostate, breast, lung, thyroid, kidney, and bladder. Malignant cells reach the skeleton via the bloodstream. Those which survive may proliferate and distort the normal architecture, probably by production of substances that cause dissolution of both mineral phase and organic matrix.

Osteolysis most often results from modulation of osteoprogenitor cells to osteoclasts in the surrounding bone. Some mediators involved in induction of osteoclasts were described earlier in this section. Some carcinoma cells also may act directly to resorb bone. Carcinomatous metastases (which are usually predominantly osteolytic) arise from thyroid, kidney, and lower bowel. Other tumors induce an *osteoblastic* response in which the new bone does not arise from the tumor itself but is induced from normal skeletal cells by some product(s) of the tumor cells. The resulting lesion may be more dense than the surrounding tissue. Occasionally, the increase in radiodensity is uniform, simulating osteosclerosis. Carcinoma of the prostate characteristically produces osteoblastic metastases. Carcinoma of the breast can cause both osteolytic and osteoblastic metastases. Malignant carcinoid tumors arising from the embryonic foregut and hindgut metastasize to bone with high frequency, producing an osteoblastic reaction. Hodgkin's disease in bone also produces an osteoblastic response both focal and diffuse. More malignant lymphomas in bone produce predominantly destructive lesions. As a rule, osteolytic metastases are the ones associated with hypercalcemia, hypercalciuria,

and increased excretion of hydroxyproline-containing peptides (reflecting matrix destruction); they are usually associated with normal or only slightly increased levels of serum alkaline phosphatase. Osteoblastic metastases, on the other hand, may cause more marked elevations of serum alkaline phosphatase and may be associated with hypocalcemia. With some metastases (as in carcinoma of the breast), there may be phases in which osteolysis predominates (with hypercalciuria, hypercalcemia, and normal alkaline phosphatase levels) alternating with phases in which alkaline phosphatase levels rise and the skeletal lesions become more sclerotic.

Treatment of skeletal metastases is usually palliative. In slowly growing localized lesions (as in some instances of carcinoma of the thyroid or occasionally in carcinoma of the kidney), local radiation is useful to relieve pain or reduce compression of surrounding structures. Many patients with carcinomas of breast or prostate survive for years even after extensive skeletal metastases are recognized. Castration and estrogen therapy or receptor antagonists may slow the progress of the lesions in patients with metastatic prostatic carcinoma (see Chap. 323). When patients with mammary cancer are treated with estrogens or androgens, the character of the reaction to the metastases may temporarily shift from a predominantly osteoblastic to a lytic phase with resultant hypercalcemia (see Chap. 319).

Intravenous administration of bisphosphonates such as pamidronate diminishes bone pain and reduces the incidence of fracture and indices of excessive bone resorption in patients with osteolytic metastases, e.g., from breast cancer. Pamidronate also alleviates bone pain in patients with metastatic prostate carcinoma. The bone pain in patients with metastatic carcinoma also may be relieved by the use of levodopa. Hypercalcemia in patients with malignant tumors is not due solely to skeletal metastases, although this is the most common cause. Production of circulating stimulators of osteoclast differentiation, such as PTHrP, is another cause of the humoral hypercalcemia of malignancy. Hypercalcemia per se, whether spontaneous or induced by therapy, may produce anorexia, polyuria, polydipsia, depression, and eventually coma. In addition, nephrocalcinosis can result from hypercalcemia, and death may result from renal insufficiency. Intravenous pamidronate is effective in treatment of the hypercalcemia of malignancy due either to humoral factors such as PTHrP or to local factors produced by metastases in bone.

OTHER DISORDERS OF BONE AND CARTILAGE

FIBROUS DYSPLASIA (McCUNE-ALBRIGHT SYNDROME)   This syndrome is characterized by osteitis fibrosa disseminata, areas of pigmentation, and endocrine dysfunction, with precocious puberty in females. The bony lesions, called *fibrous dysplasia*, may occur in the absence of the other features. The fundamental nature of the disorder is unknown; the disease does not appear to be heritable, although it has been reported to affect monozygotic twins. The disease occurs with equal frequency in both sexes.

Incidence   The disease may be divided into three main categories: (1) monostotic, (2) polyostotic, and (3) McCune-Albright syndrome and its variants. The monostotic form is the most common. The lesions can be asymptomatic, associated with local pain, or predispose to pathologic fracture. The majority of the lesions are in the ribs or in the craniofacial bones, especially the maxillas. Many other bones may be affected, however, such as metaphyseal or diaphyseal portions of the proximal femurs or tibias. Monostotic fibrous dysplasia is most often diagnosed between 20 and 30 years of age. There are usually no associated skin lesions. Approximately a quarter of the individuals with the polyostotic form have more than half the skeleton involved by disease. One side of the body may be affected, and the lesions may be distributed segmentally in a limb, particularly in the lower extremities. Craniofacial lesions are present in approximately half of patients with the polyostotic form. Whereas the monostotic form is usually detected in young adults, fractures and skeletal deformities occur in childhood in the polyostotic form; the disease is generally more severe and deforming with early clinical onset. Lesions, especially monostotic lesions, may become quiescent around the time of puberty and may worsen during pregnancy. McCune-Albright syndrome (polyostotic fibrous dysplasia, multiple café au lait spots, and sexual precosity) is more common (10:1) in females. Short stature is ascribed to premature closure of the epiphyses. The most frequent extraskeletal manifestations are the skin lesions.

Pathology All forms of fibrous dysplasia have a similar histologic appearance, although cartilage is more commonly involved in the polyostotic form. The marrow cavity is filled by gritty, gray-pink, rubbery tissue that replaces the normal cancellous bone. Often, the endosteal cortical surface is scalloped. Histologically, the lesions contain benign-appearing fibroblastic tissue arranged in a loose whorled pattern (Fig. 362-3). The grittiness is due to irregularly arranged woven bone spicules, most of which lack osteoblastic palisading or rimming, which are embedded in the fibrous tissue. These bone spicules also may have prominent cement lines. In approximately 10 percent of cases, islands of hyaline cartilage are present, and more rarely, myxoid tissue may predominate in young patients. Examination by polarized light and with the use of special stains indicates a contiguity of collagen fibers of the osseous and marrow tissue. In the polyostotic form, cystic degeneration may be characterized by the presence of hemorrhage with hemosiderin-containing macrophages and osteoclast-type giant cells in the periphery of the cyst. Malignant transformation of either monostotic or polyostotic fibrous dysplasia occurs but with a frequency of less than 1 percent. The malignant change is usually detected in the third or fourth decades in individuals who have had lesions first identified in childhood. In about a third of the cases the neoplasms arise in previously radiated lesions. Ossifying fibroma of long bones is a peculiar fibroosseous cortical lesion which may be a variant of fibrous dysplasia. It is most common in the tibial shaft of teenagers. Although benign, the lesion has a tendency to recur if not adequately excised.

Radiologic changes The roentgenographic appearance of the lesions is that of a radiolucent area with a well-delineated, smooth or scalloped border, typically associated with focal thinning of the cortex of the bone (Fig. 362-4). Fibrous dysplasia and Paget's disease of bone are two disorders that can cause a bone to become larger than normal. The lesions of fibrous dysplasia are not usually cysts in the strict sense, since they are not fluid-filled cavities. They occasionally appear multiloculate. The so-called ground glass appearance reflects the content of the thin spicules of calcified, woven bone. Frequently, deformities are present such as coxa vara, shepherd's-crook deformity of the femur, bowing of the tibia, Harrison's grooves, and protrusio acetabuli. Involvement of facial bones, usually with lesions of increased radiodensity, may create a leonine appearance (leontiasis ossea). Fibrous dysplasia of the temporal bones can cause progressive

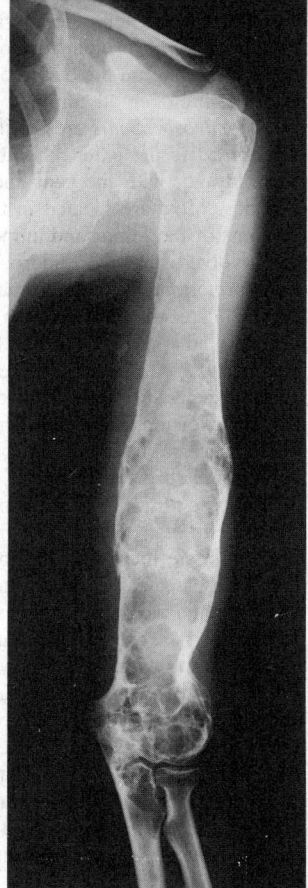

FIGURE 362-4 Roentgenogram of the upper extremity from a 33-year-old woman with fibrous dysplasia of bone. Typical lesions involve the entire humerus as well as the scapula and proximal ulna.

loss of hearing and obliteration of the external ear canal. Advanced skeletal age in females is correlated with sexual precocity but also may be seen in males without sexual precocity. The lesions tend to spare the epiphyseal regions before puberty, but in older individuals fibrous dysplasia may develop in the epiphyses. Occasionally, a focus of fibrous dysplasia may undergo cystic degeneration with an enormous distortion of the shape of the bone and mimic the so-called aneurysmal bone cyst.

Clinical picture The clinical course is variable. Skeletal lesions are usually detected because of localized pain, deformities, or fractures. Other symptoms ascribable to bone involvement are headache, seizures, cranial nerve abnormalities, hearing loss, narrowing of the external ear canal, or even spontaneous scalp hemorrhages if there is craniofacial bone disease. In some females and even less commonly in males, sexual precocity is the presenting complaint, occasionally before the appearance of skeletal symptoms. Serum calcium and phosphorus values are usually normal. In approximately one-third of patients, levels of serum alkaline phosphatase may be elevated to high values, and urinary hydroxyproline excretion is often increased. In some subjects, high cardiac output similar to that in extensive Paget's disease may be found. In general, patients with extensive involvement have widespread disease when symptoms first appear, whereas when disease is mild at the onset, extensive disease does not usually develop.

The cutaneous pigmentation in most patients with McCune-Albright syndrome consists of isolated dark-brown to light-brown macules which tend to remain on one side of the midline (Fig. 362-5). The border is usually, although not always, irregular or jagged ("coast of Maine") in contrast to the smooth borders of the pigmented macules of neurofibromatosis ("coast of California"). As a rule, there are fewer than six of the lesions, which range in size from 1 cm to those covering very large areas, particularly the back, buttocks, or

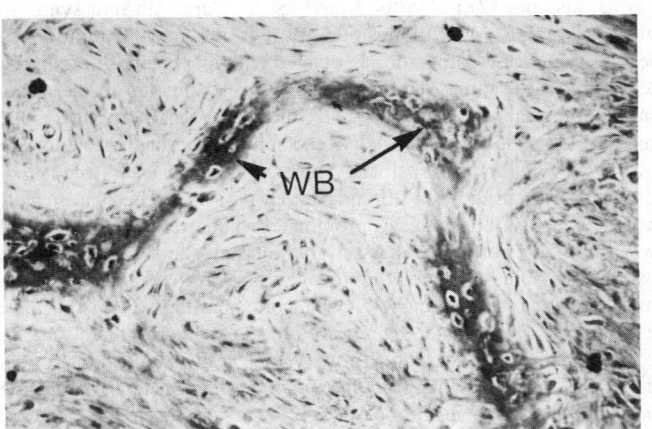

FIGURE 362-3 Photomicrograph of the lesion of fibrous dysplasia. Note spicules of dark-staining woven bone (WB) surrounded by loose fibroblastic tissue.

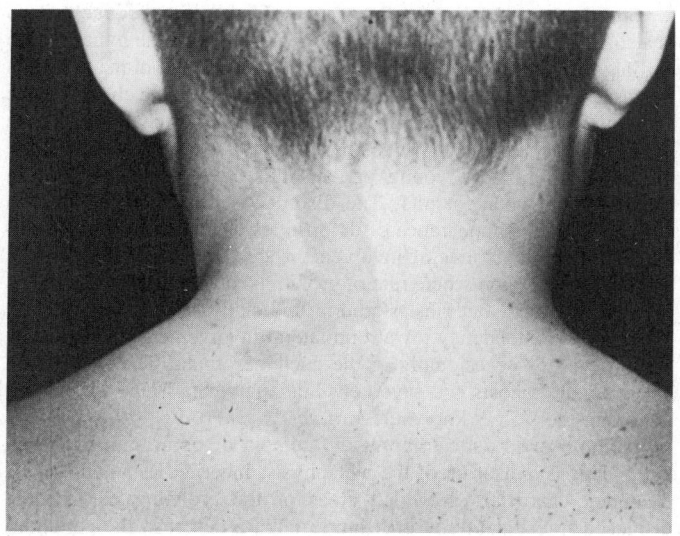

FIGURE 362-5 Typical pigmented café au lait lesion of the skin in an 11-year-old boy with polyostotic fibrous dysplasia. The border has the jagged "coast of Maine" appearance that is characteristic of McCune-Albright's syndrome. Note that the lesion is limited to one side (left) of the body.

sacral regions. When the lesions are present in the scalp, the overlying hair may be more deeply pigmented than that over the remainder of the scalp. Localized alopecia is associated with osteomas of the skin, and such lesions tend to have concordance with the skeletal lesions. The pigmentation tends to be on the same side as the skeletal lesions and actually overlie them. Occasionally, neurofibromatosis and fibrous dysplasia coexist.

The sexual precocity occurs more commonly in females than in males (see also Chaps. 339 and 340). Premature vaginal bleeding and development of axillary and pubic hair and of breasts are the main features. In the few ovaries that have been examined, no corpora lutea have been seen. In the few cases where measurements have been reported, the girls have high estrogen levels and low or undetectable gonadotropins. Estrogen receptors have been measured in the bone lesions. It is therefore not surprising that precocious sexuality is not limited to patients with cranial involvement. The characteristic pigmented macules are usual but not invariable. Another endocrine abnormality that occurs with increased frequency is hyperthyroidism. Rarer associations include Cushing's syndrome, acromegaly, possibly hypogonadotropic hypogonadism, and soft tissue myxomas. Hypophosphatemic osteomalacia also may accompany fibrous dysplasia and resembles the disorder associated with other skeletal and nonskeletal tumors. Sexual precocity and adrenal and thyroid hyperfunction in association with fibrous dysplasia are due to autonomous end-organ activity, not to pituitary or hypothalamic dysfunction. Thus luteinizing hormone (LH) or follicle-stimulating hormone (FSH) levels are low and do not show the expected early pubertal nocturnal rise and are not responsive to luteinizing hormone–releasing hormone (LHRH). Furthermore, treatment with LHRH analogues does not suppress gonadal steroid secretion or reverse sexual precocity. The multiple endocrine hyperfunction and possibly the fibrous dysplasia lesions in the disorder may be due to defects in the G protein–cyclic AMP–protein kinase A–dependent pathway. Activating mutations have been identified in the G protein that stimulates adenylyl cyclase ($G_{s\alpha}$) by nucleotide sequence analysis of $G_{s\alpha}$ cDNA in tissues from affected patients. The mutations presumably result in constitutive activation of signal transduction pathways and induce end-organ hyperfunction. Since germ line mutations might be lethal, somatic mutations may occur early in embryogenesis in patients with McCune-Albright syndrome so that affected individuals are mosaics. It is of interest that the error in Albright's hereditary osteodystrophy (pseudohypoparathyroidism) is the converse of that found in the McCune-Albright syndrome (fibrous dysplasia). In the former, mutations in $G_{s\alpha}$ proteins result in *deficient* activity and decreased responsiveness to hormones that function through cAMP-mediated signal transduction pathways.

Although the lytic lesions of fibrous dysplasia resemble the brown tumors of hyperparathyroidism, the age of the patient, normal calcium levels, increased density of bone in the skull, and areas of cutaneous pigmentation identify the former condition. Fibrous dysplasia and hyperparathyroidism may coexist, however. Neurofibromas may involve bone and produce cutaneous pigmentation as well as nodules in the skin. The pigmented macules of neurofibromatosis are more numerous and more widely distributed than in fibrous dysplasia, usually have smooth borders, and tend to involve areas such as the axillary folds. Other lesions that have roentgenographic features similar to those of isolated fibrous dysplasia are unicameral bone cysts, aneurysmal bone cysts, and nonossifying fibromas. Leontiasis ossea is most often due to fibrous dysplasia, although other disorders also may produce this appearance, such as craniometaphyseal dysplasia, hyperphosphatasia, and, in adults, Paget's disease.

Treatment Fibrous dysplasia is not curable. The symptoms, however, can be managed using a variety of orthopedic procedures such as casting, osteotomy with internal fixation, curettage, and bone grafting depending on the lesion and the age of the patient. Indications for such procedures include progressive deformity, nonunion of fractures, and pain unresponsive to conservative treatment. Calcitonin may be effective in treatment of widespread disease associated with bone pain and high serum alkaline phosphatase levels (see Chap. 361).

DYSPLASIAS AND CHONDRODYSTROPHIES A variety of diseases of bone and cartilage have been called *dystrophies* or *dysplasias*. The *osteochondrodysplasias* are heritable disorders of connective tissue that are characterized by primary abnormalities of cartilage that lead to disturbances in cartilage and bone growth and development. They comprise more than 100 distinct entities, which can be distinguished based on clinical, genetic, and radiologic features. The biochemical (and genetic) defects have been identified in few of these conditions. Genetic errors have been demonstrated at various steps in the metabolism of glycosaminoglycans (mucopolysaccharides) to account for the abnormal phenotypes in the Hunter and Hurler syndromes (also see Chap. 349), and mutations in collagen genes have been identified in several forms of the skeletal dysplasias. For example, mutations in the type II collagen gene have been found in Stricker syndrome, Kniest dysplasia, other chondrodysplasias associated with osteoarthritis, and in a related syndrome, spondyloepiphyseal dysplasia, and deletion in one type X collagen allele has been found in a form of metaphyseal chondrodysplasia. Mutations in several genes, e.g., types II, IX, and X collagen genes, in transgenic mice result in phenotypes that resemble several of the human disorders (also see Chap. 351). Eventually, it should be possible to classify many of these disorders based on the genetic and biochemical defects. At present, however, a useful scheme is that proposed by Rubin based on the consideration of errors in modeling of bone and cartilage (Table 362-2). Other clinical and genetic features form the basis of a classification by Rimoin. Pathologic processes in the skeletal dysplasias may be expressed as a deficiency (hypoplasia) or excess (hyperplasia) in relation to normal development.

Spondyloepiphyseal dysplasia The *spondyloepiphyseal dysplasias* are disorders in which abnormalities of growth occur in various bones, including the vertebrae, pelvis, carpal and tarsal bones, and the epiphyses of tabular bones. On the basis of roentgenographic findings, this group can be divided into (1) those with generalized platyspondyly, (2) those with multiple epiphyseal dysplasias, and (3) those with epiphysometaphyseal dysplasias. *Morquio's syndrome*, in which there is a defect in degradation of glycosaminoglycans (therefore a "mucopolysaccharidosis"), is inherited as an autosomal recessive trait and is associated with corneal opacities, dental defects, variable disturbances in intellect, and increased urinary excretion of keratosulfate, and it belongs to the first group. Other forms of spondyloepiphy-

TABLE 362-2 Working classification of bone dysplasias

Epiphyseal dysplasias
  A Epiphyseal hypoplasias
     1 Failure of articular cartilage: spondyloepiphyseal dysplasia, congenita and tarda
     2 Failure of ossification of center: multiple epiphyseal dysplasia, congenita and tarda
  B Epiphyseal hyperplasia
     1 Excess of articular cartilage: dysplasia epiphysialis hemimelica
Physeal (growth plate) dysplasias
  A Cartilage hypoplasias
     1 Failure of proliferating cartilage: achondroplasia, congenita and tarda
     2 Failure of hypertrophic cartilage: metaphyseal dysostosis, congenita and tarda
  B Cartilage hyperplasias
     1 Excess of proliferating cartilage: hyperchondroplasia
     2 Excess of hypertrophic cartilage: enchondromatosis
Metaphyseal dysplasias
  A Metaphyseal hypoplasias
     1 Failure to form primary spongiosa: hypophosphatasia, congenita and tarda
     2 Failure to absorb primary spongiosa: osteopetrosis, congenita and tarda
     3 Failure to absorb secondary spongiosa: craniometaphyseal dysplasia, congenita and tarda
  B Metaphyseal hyperplasia
     1 Excessive spongiosa: familial exostosis
Diaphyseal dysplasias
  A Diaphyseal hypoplasias
     1 Failure of periosteal bone formation: osteogenesis imperfecta, congenita and tarda
     2 Failure of endosteal bone formation: idiopathic osteoporosis
  B Diaphyseal hyperplasias
     1 Excessive periosteal bone formation: Engelmann's disease
     2 Excessive periosteal bone formation: hyperphosphatasia

seal dysplasia, some of which are accounted for by defects in type II collagen, may not be recognized until late in childhood or young adult life. Flat vertebral bodies are associated with other abnormalities in shape and alignment. The disordered development of the capital femoral epiphyses leads to irregularities in shape and flattening of the femoral heads and early onset of osteoarthritis of the hips.

Achondroplasia *Achondroplasia* is a physeal dysplasia in which dwarfism results from decrease in the proliferation of cartilage in the growth plate. This disorder is among the more common types of dwarfism and is inherited as an autosomal dominant trait. Histologic sections through the growth plate show a thin zone of cartilage cells with absence or abbreviation of the normal columnar arrangement and zone of provisional calcification, although endochondral ossification may not be completely disorganized. Formation of the primary spongiosa is reduced, since there is often a transverse bar of bone sealing off the plate from further endochondral ossification. Formation and maturation of the secondary ossification centers and articular cartilage are not disturbed, however. Appositional growth at the metaphysis continues, with resulting flare in this region of the bone; intramembranous bone formation at the periosteum is normal. The abnormal proliferation at the growth plate, leaving other areas relatively unaffected in the tubular bones, causes production of short bones that are proportionately thick. The length of the spine is almost always normal. The appearance of short limbs with a normal trunk is characteristically accompanied by a large head, saddlenose, and an exaggerated lumbar lordosis. The disease is usually recognized at birth. Those who survive the period of infancy usually have normal mental and sexual development, and life span may be normal. Spinal deformity nevertheless may lead to a cord compression and nerve root encroachment, especially in those with kyphoscoliosis. Homozygous achondroplasia is a more serious disorder and a cause of neonatal death. In view of the observations in spondyloepiphyseal dysplasia, several of the achondroplasias also may eventually be explained on the basis of defects in genes encoding extracellular matrix components of cartilage such as proteoglycan core protein, types II, IX, or X collagens, or link protein.

Enchondromatosis (dyschondroplasia, Ollier's disease) This is also a disorder affecting the growth plate in which the hypertrophic cartilage is not resorbed and ossified in a normal fashion. It results in masses of cartilage with disorderly arrangement of the chondrocytes showing variable proliferative and hypertrophic changes. These masses are located in the metaphyses in close association with the growth plate in very young patients but often are diaphyseal in teenagers and young adults. The disorder is usually recognized in childhood by the appearance of deformities or retardation in growth. The most common sites of involvement are the ends of long bones, usually in the region where rate of growth is most marked. The pelvis is often involved, but ribs, sternum, and skull are seldom affected. There is also a tendency toward unilateral involvement. Chondrosarcoma develops occasionally in the enchondromata. The association of enchondromatosis and cavernous hemangiomata in the soft tissues including the skin is known as *Maffucci's syndrome*.

Multiple exostoses (diaphyseal aclasis or osteochondromatosis) This is a disorder of the metaphysis, inherited as an autosomal dominant character, in which areas of the growth plate become displaced, presumably by growing through a defect in the perichondrium or so-called ring of Ranvier. The spongiosa forms within the mass as vessels invade the cartilage. Therefore, the diagnostic radiographic finding is the direct continuity of the mass to the marrow cavity of the parent bone with absence of underlying cortex. Usually the growth of these exostoses ceases when growth of the adjacent plate ceases. The lesions may be solitary or multiple and are usually located in the metaphyseal areas of long bones with the apex of the exostosis directed toward the diaphysis. Often the lesions produce no symptoms, but occasionally, interference with the function of a joint or tendon or compression of nerves may result. Dwarfism may occur. The metacarpals may be shortened, resembling those seen in Albright's hereditary osteodystrophy. Multiple exostoses are sometimes seen in patients with pseudohypoparathyroidism.

An exostosis may suddenly begin to enlarge long after growth should have ceased, and rarely, chondrosarcomas may develop from the cartilage cap of an exostosis. Although pregnancy may stimulate growth of an exostosis that clinically may mimic malignancy, the lesion merely undergoes exuberant endochondral ossification and cartilage hyperplasia without malignant changes.

RELAPSING POLYCHONDRITIS See Chap. 299.

TIETZE'S SYNDROME (COSTOCHONDRAL SYNDROME) See Chap. 299.

REFERENCES

Hyperostosis

BENLI IT et al: Epidemiological, clinical and radiological aspects of osteopoikilosis. J Bone Joint Surg 74B:504, 1992

BOLLERSLEY J et al: Structural and histomorphometric studies of iliac crest trabecular and cortical bone in autosomal dominant osteopetrosis: A study of two radiological types. Bone 10:19, 1989

BOSTMAN OM et al: Osteosarcoma arising in a melorheostoric femur. J Bone Joint Surg 69A:1232, 1987

BYERS PH et al: Research perspectives in heritable disorders of connective tissue. Matrix 12:333, 1992

CAUDLE RJ et al: Melorheostosis of the hand: A case report with long-term follow-up. J Bone Joint Surg 69A:1229, 1987

CHAN Y-L et al: Dialysis osteodystrophy: A study involving 94 patients. Medicine 64:296, 1985

COCCIA PF et al: Successful bone-marrow transplantation for infantile malignant osteopetrosis. N Engl J Med 302:701, 1980

——— et al: Cells that resorb bone. N Engl J Med 310:456, 1984

COINDRE JM et al: Histomorphometric analysis of sclerotic bone from idiopathic myeloid metaplasia (nine cases). J Pathol 144:163, 1984

CRISP AJ, BRENTON DP: Engelmann's disease of bone - a systemic disorder? Ann Rheum Dis 41:183,1982

DiGIOVANNA JJ et al: Extraspinal tendon and ligament calcification associated with long-term therapy with etretinate. N Engl J Med 315:1177, 1986

EDELSON JG et al: Pycnodysostosis: Orthopedic aspects with a description of 14 new cases. Clin Orthop 280:263, 1992

EINHORN TA et al: Hyperphosphatasemia in an adult: Clinical, roentgenographic, and histomorphometric findings and comparison to classical Paget's disease. Clin Orthop 204:253, 1986

GEBHARDT MC, MANKIN HJ: The diagnosis and management of bone tumors, in *Metabolic Bone Disease*, LV Avioli, SM Krane (eds). Philadelphia, Saunders, 1990, pp 753–792

GENANT HK et al: Osteosclerosis in primary hyperparathyroidism. Am J Med 59:104, 1975

GOLDMAN AB et al: Case report 778. Skeletal Radiol 22:206, 1993

IAVARONE A et al: Germ-line and somatic p53 gene mutations in multifocal osteogenic sarcoma. Proc Natl Acad Sci USA 89:4207, 1992

JACCOBSON HG: Dense bone—too much bone: Radiological considerations and differential diagnosis, part II. Skeletal Radiol 13:97, 1985

JOHNSON CC et al: Osteopetrosis: A clinical, genetic, metabolic and morphologic study of the dominantly inherited benign form. Medicine 47:149, 1968

KAPLAN FS et al: Successful treatment of infantile malignant osteopetrosis by bone-marrow transplantation. J Bone Joint Surg 70A:617, 1988

KEY L et al: Treatment of congenital osteopetrosis with high-dose calcitriol. N Engl J Med 310:409, 1984

KRAEMER KH et al: Prevention of skin cancer in xeroderma pigmentosum with the use of oral isotretinoin. N Eng J Med 318:1633, 1988

KUIVANIEMI H et al: Mutations in collagen genes; causes of rare and some common diseases in humans. FASEB J 5:2052, 1991

MARKS SC et al: Administration of colony stimulating factor-1 corrects some macrophage, dental, and skeletal defects in an osteopetrotic mutation (toothless, *tl*) in the rat. Bone 13:89, 1992

MAJZOUB JA, SCULLY RE: A six-year-old boy with multiple bone lesions, repeated fractures, and sexual precocity. N Engl J Med 328:496, 1993

SCHOTLAND HM et al: Neurofibromatosis 1 and osseous fibrous dysplasia in a family. Am J Med Gen 43:815, 1992

SHAPIRO F et al: Variable osteoclast appearance in human infantile osteopetrosis. Calcif Tissue Int 43:67, 1988

SHELDON J et al: Englemann's disease (progressive diaphyseal dysplasia): A review and presentation of two cases with abnormal phosphate retention. Metab Bone Dis Rel Res 2:307, 1981

SINGER FR: Osteopetrosis. Semin Nephrol 12:191, 1992

SLAVKIN H, PRICE P (eds): Chemistry and Biology of Mineralized Tissues. Amsterdam, Excerpta Medica, 1992, pp 1–550

SLY WS et al: Carbonic anhydrase II deficiency in 12 families with the autosomal recessive syndrome of osteopetrosis with renal tubular acidosis and cerebral calcification. N Engl J Med 313:139, 1985

THOMPSON RC JR et al: Hereditary hyperphosphatasia. Am J Med 47:209, 1969

TRICHE T, CAVAZZANA A: Round cell tumors of bone, in *Bone Tumors*, KK Unni (ed). New York, Churchhill Livingstone, 1988, pp 199–223

ULLRICH SJ et al: the p53 tumor suppressor protein, a modulator of cell proliferation. J Biol Chem 267:15259, 1992

VAN BUCHEM FSP et al: Hyperostosis corticalis generalisata. Am J Med 33:387, 1962

WEINBERG RA: Tumor suppressor genes. Science 254:1138, 1991

WEINSTEIN LS et al: Activating mutations of the stimulatory G protein in the McCune-Albright syndrome. N Engl J Med 325:1688, 1991

WHYTE MP, MURPHY WA: Osteopetrosis and other sclerosing bone disorders, in *Metabolic Bone Disease*, LV Avioli, SM Krane (eds). Philadelphia, Saunders, 1990, pp 616–658

WULFSBERG EA et al: Chondrodysplasia punctata: A boy with X-linked recessive chondrodysplasia punctata due to an inherited X-Y translocation with a current classification of these disorders. Am J Med Genet 43:823, 1992

Neoplasms of bone

BACCI G et al: Therapy for primary non-Hodgkin's lymphoma of bone and comparison of results with Ewing's sarcoma: Ten years' experience at the Istituto Ortopedico Rizzoli. Cancer 57:1468, 1986

——— et al: Neoadjuvant chemotherapy for osteosarcoma of the extremity. Clin Orthop 224:268, 1987

ETTINGER LJ et al: Adjuvant adriamycin and cisplatin in newly diagnosed, nonmetastatic osteosarcoma of the extremity. J Clin Oncol 4:353, 1986

GEBHARDT MC, MANKIN HJ: The diagnosis and management of bone tumors, in *Metabolic Bone Disease*, LV Avioli, SM Krane (eds). Philadelphia, W.B. Saunders Co., pp 753–792, 1990

GOORIN AM et al: Osteosarcoma: Fifteen years later. N Engl J Med 313:165, 1985

HAN M-T et al: Aggressive thoractomy for pulmonary metastatic osteogenic sarcoma in children and young adolescents. J Pediatr Surg 16:928, 1981

HAYES FA et al: Metastatic Ewing's sarcoma: Remission induction and survival. J Clin Oncol 5:1199, 1987

VAN HOLTEN-VERZANTVOORT AT et al: Reduced morbidity from skeletal metastases in breast cancer patients during long-term bisphosphonate (APD) treatment. Lancet 2:983, 1987

HUVOS AG: Osteogenic sarcoma of bones and soft tissues in older persons. A clinicopathologic analysis of 117 patients older than 60 years. Cancer 57:1442, 1986

——— et al: Osteogenic sarcoma associated with Paget's disease of bone. A clinicopathologic study of 65 patients. Cancer 52:1489, 1983

IAVARONE A et al: Germ-line and somatic p53 gene mutations in multifocal osteogenic sarcoma. Proc Natl Acad Sci USA 89:4207, 1992

KLEEREKOPER M, KRANE SM (EDS): *Clinical Disorders of Bone and Mineral Metabolism*. New York, Mary Ann Liebert, pp 1--649, 1989

MANKIN HJ et al: The use of frozen cadaveric allografts in the management of patients with bone tumors of the extremities. Orthop Clin North Am 18:275, 1987

MISER JS et al: Preliminary results of treatment of Ewing's sarcoma of bone in children and young adults: Six months of intensive combined modality therapy without maintenance. J Clin Oncol 6:484, 1988

SCHILLER AL: Diagnosis of borderline cartilage lesions of bone. Semin Diag Pathol 2:42, 1985

SIMON MA, NACHMAN J: The clinical utility of preoperative therapy for sarcomas. J Bone Joint Surg 68A:1458, 1986

——— et al: Limb-salvage treatment versus amputation for osteosarcoma of the distal end of the femur. J Bone Joint Surg 68A:1331, 1986

SUIT HD et al: Treatment of the patient with stage M_o soft tissue sarcoma. J Clin Oncol 6:854, 1988

SUTOW WW et al: Survival after metastasis in osteosarcoma. Natl Cancer Inst Monogr 56:227, 1981

UNNI KK et al: Conditions that stimulate primary neoplasms of bone. Pathol Ann 15(Part 1):91, 1986

WINKLER K et al: Neoadjuvant chemotherapy of osteosarcoma: Results of a randomized cooperative trial (COSS-82) with salvage chemotherapy based on histological tumor response. J Clin Oncol 6:329, 1988

YUNIS EJ, BARNES L: The histologic diversity of osteosarcoma. Pathol Ann 21(Part 1):121, 1986

Other disorders of bone and cartilage

AKESON WH et al: *Symposium on Heritable Disorders of Connective Tissue*. St. Louis, Mosby, 1982

ALBRIGHT FA et al: Syndrome characterized by osteitis fibrosa disseminata, areas of pigmentation and endocrine dysfunction, with precocious puberty in females. Report of five cases. N Engl J Med 216:727, 1937

BENEDICT PH et al: Melanotic macules in Albright's syndrome and in neurofibromatosis. JAMA 205:618, 1968

GRABIAS SL, CAMPBELL CJ: Fibrous dysplasia. Orthop Clin North Am 8:771, 1977

HARRIS RI: Polyostotic fibrous dysplasia with acromegaly. Am J Med 78:539, 1985

HARRIS WH et al: The natural history of fibrous dysplasia: An orthopaedic, pathological and roentgenographic study. J Bone Joint Surg (BR) 44A:207, 1962

KAPLAN FS et al: Estrogen receptors in bone in a patient with polyostotic fibrous dysplasia (McCune-Albright syndrome). N Engl J Med 319:421, 1988

LEE B et al: Identification of the molecular defect in a family with spondyloepiphyseal dysplasia. Science 244:978, 1989

NAGER GT et al: Fibrous dysplasia: A review of the disease and its manifestations in the temporal bone. Ann Otol Rhinol Laryngol 91(suppl 92):1, 1982

PALOTIE A et al: Predisposition to familial osteoarthrosis linked to type II collagen gene. Lancet 1:924, 1989

RIMOIN DL: The chondrodystrophies. Adv Hum Genet 5:1, 1975

RUBIN P: Dynamic Classification of Bone Dysplasias. Chicago, Year Book, 1964

SAMBROOK PN et al: Synovial complications of spondylepiphyseal dysplasia of late onset. Arthritis Rheum 31:282, 1988

SILLENCE DO et al: Neonatal dwarfism. Pediatr Clin North Am 25:431, 1978

STEPHENSON RB et al: Fibrous dysplasia. An analysis of options for treatment. J Bone Joint Surg 69A:409, 1987

TRICHE T, CAVAZZANA A: Round cell tumors of bone, in *Bone Tumors*, KK Unni (ed). New York, Churchhill Livingstone, 1988, pp 199–223

WEINBERG RA: Tumor suppressor genes. Science 254:1138, 1991

YABUL SM et al: Malignant transformation of fibrous dysplasia. A case report and review of the literature. Clin Orthop 281, 1988

363 APPROACH TO THE PATIENT WITH NEUROLOGIC DISEASE

JOSEPH B. MARTIN*

Symptoms and signs of disordered nervous system function are among the most frequent in clinical medicine. Because neurologic disorders may affect cognitive function with disturbances in language, perception, and memory, as well as produce specific symptoms referable to subcortical structures, spinal cord, peripheral nerve, or muscle, the symptoms and signs presented to the physician are numerous and diverse. A careful assessment of the character and pattern of the symptoms, their temporal profile, and associated complaints, together with a focused neurologic examination, permit a conclusion to be reached among various alternatives.

These considerations are made more complicated by the difficulties that often arise in distinguishing so-called neurologic from psychiatric diseases. In general, the neurologist has defined disease of the nervous system as any condition that produces a visible anatomic or definable biochemical lesion. However, it is now recognized that many primary neurologic disorders, some of which present with severe clinical manifestations, fail to show any demonstrable neuropathologic or neurochemical abnormality, even when scrutinized by the most modern techniques of neurobiology. Torsion dystonia, tardive dyskinesia, and Gilles de la Tourette's syndrome, for example, are considered to be neurologic disorders, some with a clear-cut genetic basis, yet no defined structural abnormality has been reported. The possibility that such disorders are caused by abnormalities of neurotransmitter release or of receptor function is currently viewed as likely because they occur after drug treatment or show partial response to various neuropharmacologic agents. In other disorders traditionally treated by the psychiatrist, in particular the major psychoses of schizophrenia and of manic-depressive disease, accumulated evidence based on genetic analysis, responses to neuroactive agents, and documented neuroendocrine-biochemical abnormalities suggest that these, too, are primary disorders of nervous system function (see Chap. 389). This conclusion is supported further by observations that similar psychotic symptoms can be observed in patients with readily identifiable lesions of the nervous system (chronic complex partial seizures, brain tumor) or after the administration of certain drugs, such as lysergic acid or amphetamines.

Despite the importance of these areas of overlap between neurology and psychiatry, most neurologic conditions for which a patient seeks general medical care are due to readily demonstrated disease processes. It is the task of the clinician to develop a neurologic method of analysis that will result in accurate diagnosis of the site of the disorder and of its likely cause. Only then can effective approaches to management and treatment be developed.

In this and the subsequent sections, neurology and psychiatry are considered separately because many of the approaches to diagnosis and treatment remain distinct even today. In the chapters that follow, neurologic disorders and diseases are described as they present to the

neurologist or general internist. Currently accepted explanations in terms of anatomy, physiology, pharmacology, and chemistry are offered. The section on psychiatric disorders is found in Chap. 389. Dependency syndromes are described in Chaps. 390 to 393.

THE NEUROLOGIC METHOD OF CLINICAL EVALUATION The strategy used in evaluating a patient with neurologic illness is to begin with the question, What portion of the neural axis is likely to be involved in causing the neurologic symptoms? The first clues to defining the anatomic area of involvement appear in the history, and the examination is then directed to confirm or rule out these impressions and to clarify uncertainties suggested by the history. A more detailed examination of a particular region of the central nervous system (CNS) or peripheral nervous system is often indicated. For example, optokinetic nystagmus may be an important part of the examination in a patient with a left hemiparesis and dressing apraxia but irrelevant to the examination of a patient complaining of burning feet. In a patient who presents with a history of ascending paresthesia and weakness, the examination should be *directed* toward deciding, among other things, if the location of the lesion is the spinal cord or peripheral nerves. Notations regarding muscle stamina or endurance might be crucial to the examination of a patient with myasthenia gravis, as opposed to the usual tests of peak muscle power. What one does in the neurologic examination depends on what the questions are; the questions are formulated by a properly taken history.

Deciding "where the lesion is" accomplishes the task of delimiting the number of possible etiologies to a manageable, finite size. In addition, this strategy safeguards against making really tragic errors. Symptoms of recurrent vertigo, diplopia, and nystagmus should not trigger "multiple sclerosis" as an answer (etiology) but "brainstem" or "pons" (location); then a diagnosis of brainstem arteriovenous malformation will not be missed because it is not considered. Similarly, the combination of optic neuritis and spastic ataxic paraparesis should not suggest only multiple sclerosis; CNS syphilis and vitamin B_{12} deficiency (both treatable) also can cause these findings. When the question, "Where is the lesion?" is answered, then the question, "What is the lesion?" can be addressed.

The neurologic history A bewildering array of clinical abnormalities requires documentation and interpretation during the neurologic evaluation of a patient. The analysis becomes difficult because similar symptoms and signs may present in a patient with any of several disorders. A number of general principles relevant to obtaining a complete neurologic history are important for the physician, whether a generalist or a specialist. Careful attention to the description of the symptoms as experienced by the patient and substantiated by family members or friends permits, in many instances, an accurate localization and determination of the probable cause of the complaints even before an examination of the patient has been undertaken. Two principles should be followed. First, each complaint ought to be pursued as far as possible in an effort to delineate (before the examination) where the lesion might be or, more important, *to formulate a set of questions to be answered by the examination.* A patient complains of weakness of the right upper limb. What are the associated features? Is this weakness for brushing the hair or opening a twist-top can? Second, in neurology—where many of the diseases are due to *anatomically restricted* lesions—*negative* associations may be crucial. A patient with a right hemiparesis without a language

* The author acknowledges the prior contributions of Raymond D. Adams to this chapter.

deficit likely has a different lesion (and likely etiology) than a patient with a right hemiparesis and aphasia. Additional important factors that aid in defining the nature of the neurologic disorder include:

1 *Temporal course of the illness.* It is particularly important to ascertain the precise rate of appearance and progression of the symptoms experienced by the patient. A paroxysmal onset of a neurologic complaint, occurring within seconds or minutes, usually indicates a cerebrovascular lesion or a seizure. Attention to the temporal march of symptoms may help define a focal seizure, a transient cerebral ischemic attack (TIA), or the onset of a migraine. For example, the onset of sensory symptoms located in one extremity that spread over a few seconds to adjacent portions of that extremity and then to the other limb or to the face suggests a seizure. A more gradual onset involving less discrete regions of the extremities points to the possibility of a TIA. A similar but slower progression of sensory change occurring in a young person together with other symptoms of headache, nausea, or visual disturbance suggests migraine. In general, the march of a migraine is slower than that of seizure, and a TIA tends to be more generalized in location on the side of the body or extremities. The presence of positive sensory symptoms or motor movements suggests a seizure; in contrast, transient loss of a function (negative symptom) suggests a TIA. A stuttering onset where symptoms appear, stabilize, regress, and then progress over hours or days also suggests the presence of impending vascular ischemia. In some cases, a demyelinating process may produce new symptoms over the course of a few hours. Progressing symptoms associated with the systemic manifestation of fever, stiff neck, and altered level of consciousness or awareness suggest the possibility of an infectious process. The course of the illness over years in terms of remissions and exacerbations offers additional clues to the nature of the process. Recurrent neurologic symptoms involving any level of the neuraxis with partial or complete recovery suggest the possibility of multiple sclerosis. Slowly progressive disorders without remissions tend to be characteristic of a neurodegenerative disorder.

2 *Subjective descriptions of the complaint.* Patient vocabularies are often limited, and symptoms are interpreted within the experience of the patient. Descriptions are highly introspective and subject to the patient's degree of intelligence and general familiarity with medical terminology. The same words often mean very different things to individual patients. For example, "dizziness" may be a description applied by the patient to impending syncope, to a sense of giddiness, or to true vertigo. "Numbness" may mean a complete loss of feeling, a positive sensation of tingling, or paralysis. "Blurring of vision" may be used to describe unilateral visual loss, as in amaurosis fugax, or diplopia. It is important to determine the level of understanding that the patient exhibits with respect to the complaint in order to assess accurately the precise significance of the symptom.

3 *Corroboration of the history by other close associates.* It is often useful to obtain additional information from family, friends, or observers to corroborate or expand the patient's description. Memory loss, personality change, drug abuse, excess alcohol intake, and other factors may severely impair the ability of patients to describe accurately their subjective experiences or prevent them from being completely open and forthright about the factors that have contributed to the illness. Complaints of loss of consciousness that may be due to syncope or seizures necessitate seeking details from patients and family to ascertain the exact circumstances. Major manifestations of depression and anxiety may mask or color the presentation given by the patient. Failure to note these underlying factors that interfere with the patient's performance may result in the incorrect interpretation that the complaints are actually due to structural disease of the brain.

4 *Family history.* Many neurologic disorders, particularly those presenting in childhood or early adulthood, are familial or inherited conditions. It is important to ascertain the familial frequency of occurrence of systemic diseases such as hypertension, heart disease, or stroke, which may affect the nervous system. It is essential to inquire about the possibility of consanguinity of the parents or of the existence of similar symptoms in other members of the family. These may provide clues to a propensity toward a hereditary neurologic condition. It is critical to distinguish between a *negative* family history and an *incomplete* family history. It is insufficient to simply ask, Is there any similar illness in any member of your family? A negative response to such an inquiry may mean that there is, in fact, no such illness in the patient's family, but it also may mean that the patient is unfamiliar with relatives or their medical histories. It is wise to elicit specific positive or negative data about relatives as follows: Are your parents living? If so, are they well? If not, what illness did they have, and how did they die? It should always be remembered that maternity is a fact, but paternity is only an assumption.

It is also important to elicit family history data regarding all illnesses rather than just neurologic and psychiatric disorders. Many familial neurologic illnesses are associated with signs and symptoms in other systems (e.g., the phakomatoses, hepatocerebral disorders, neuroophthalmic syndromes, etc.).

5 *Medical illnesses.* Many neurologic illnesses occur in the context of systemic disorders. A history of allergy and asthma may suggest the onset of polyarteritis, with mononeuritis multiplex. Previous or current medical illnesses such as diabetes mellitus, hypertension, and abnormalities of blood lipids may be relevant to evolving symptoms that affect the nervous system. Similarly, the presence of systemic diseases that have an increased association with peripheral neuropathy should be explored. Most patients with coma in a hospital setting can be shown to have a metabolic, toxic, or infectious process.

6 *The patient's perception of the disease.* It is frequently helpful to ask patients what they perceive to be wrong. Patients who complain of failing memory are often concerned that they have early symptoms of Alzheimer's disease. Patients with headaches may fear that a tumor or an impending stroke is a possibility. Patients with sensory symptoms frequently are concerned about the possibility of multiple sclerosis. The patient may seek medical attention because a relative or friend has been diagnosed with a serious neurologic illness.

7 *Drug use and abuse and toxin exposure.* It is essential to inquire about the history of drug use, both prescribed and illicit. Complaints of yellow vision may occur with digitalis administration. Excessive vitamin administration may lead to peripheral neuropathy, as has been demonstrated in the case of pyridoxine. Aminoglycoside antibiotics may exacerbate symptoms of weakness in patients with disorders of neuromuscular transmission, such as myasthenia gravis. Dizziness may be secondary to ototoxicity caused by the aminoglycosides. In eliciting a history of drug use it is often necessary to be quite specific and to use lay terminology. Most patients are, for example, unaware that over-the-counter sleeping pills, cold preparations, and diet pills are actually drugs. Alcohol, the most prevalent neurotoxin, is often not recognized as such by patients. History of environmental or industrial exposure to neurotoxins may provide the essential clue; consultation with the patient's family or employer may be required.

8 *History of malignancy.* Patients with prior malignancy can present with unexpected and unusual neurologic complications. Malignant tumors may present with nervous system metastases or occasionally with a paraneoplastic syndrome. In a patient with history of malignancy, it is important to ask whether chemotherapy or radiotherapy was given.

9 *Formulating an impression of the patient.* Use the opportunity while taking the history to form an impression of the patient. Is there evidence of anxiety, depression, hypochondriasis? Are there any clues to defects of language, memory, inappropriate behavior, or secondary gain? The neurologic assessment begins as soon as the patient walks into the room and the first introduction is made.

The neurologic examination After obtaining a complete medical and neurologic history, the physician should have reliable clues to the portions of the nervous system to be examined. By the elicitation of specific signs it is then determined whether the nervous system is affected and, if so, to what degree and which part. The anatomic localization of the lesion assumes special significance in neurology, since certain diseases are known to affect certain regions of the nervous system and not to involve others. Recognition of a constellation of symptoms and signs (a syndrome) points to the possible existence of certain diseases and to the exclusion of others.

A systematic neurologic examination should encompass a survey of all functions from the cerebrum to peripheral nerve and muscle, i.e., from the mental status examination to the simplest reflexes. Such a detailed examination requires the performance of a series of physical tests aimed at eliciting the functional capacities of each part of the nervous system. The examiner must acquire skills that come only from the repeated use of the same techniques and instruments on a large number of normal and abnormal individuals. Errors and serious omissions are avoided if the examination procedure is orderly and systemic, beginning with mental (cerebral) functions and continuing with cranial nerves, then with motor, reflex, and sensory functions of the arms, trunk, and legs, and finishing with an analysis of posture and gait.

The mental status is already appreciated while the history is being taken. But rather profound disorders of recent memory or of spatial organization may be missed unless specifically tested for. Faults of memory, incoherence of thought, dominating ideas, peculiarities of mood and outlook, aphasic errors, problems of articulation, and loss of insight and judgment should be sought. If abnormalities are noted, a more formal analysis of these functions is undertaken along the lines suggested in Chaps. 25, 27, and 28. The function of each cranial nerve is then examined in order, beginning with olfaction (see Chaps. 18, 19, 20, and 380). Examination of the motor system should include estimates of power of each of the major muscle groups, evidence of atrophy or fasciculation, and assessment of the tone of the musculature during passive manipulations, looking for signs of spasticity, rigidity, or hypotonia (as outlined in Chaps. 21 and 382). Speed and coordination of the limbs are assessed. Next, prevailing postures and the stance and gait are evaluated (Chap. 22). The tendon reflexes are examined for evidence of increased or decreased (or absent) response or of asymmetry between right and left sides or between arms and legs. The superficial cutaneous reflexes, abdominal and plantar, are then evaluated. Touch, pain, vibration, and joint-position sense are tested as the final part of the examination (see Chap. 24).

This detailed neurologic examination is undertaken only if there are symptoms of disturbed nervous system functioning. If none are present, it suffices to do an abbreviated examination which includes evaluation only of pupils, ocular movements, optic fundi, facial movements, speech, strength of arm and leg muscles, tendon and plantar reflexes, pain and vibratory sensation in hands and feet, and gait. All this can be completed in 3 to 5 min. The findings, even in the short examination, should be recorded in the patient's record for future reference.

Two additional points about the examination are worth noting. First, in recording observations, it is important for the physician to describe what is found rather than to apply a poorly defined medical term (i.e., ''patient groans to sternal rub'' rather than ''obtunded''). Second, if the patient's complaint is brought out by some activity, reproduce the activity in the office. If the complaint is of dizziness when raising the right arm and turning the head to the left, have the patient do it. If pain occurs after walking two blocks, have the patient demonstrate it, and repeat the examination.

Experience teaches that the neurologic examination may be normal even in patients with a serious neurologic disease, such as one which causes seizures or syncope. Or the patient may arrive in a coma with no available history, and the examination proceeds along the lines described in Chap. 26. An inadequate history may to some extent be replaced by a succession of examinations from which the course of the illness may be plotted.

The formulation of the problem and establishment of an etiologic diagnosis The clinical data obtained from the history and the examination are assembled into one of the known syndromes and are interpreted and translated in terms of neuroanatomy and neurophysiology. From the syndrome the physician should be able to determine the anatomic localization(s) that best explains the clinical findings. The anatomic localization, mode of onset and course of illness, other medical data, and laboratory findings are then integrated. Finally, the etiologic diagnosis is reached, and therapy appropriate for the disorder is proposed.

Laboratory tests The proper selection of tests is important to arrive at an anatomic, but more particularly an etiologic, diagnosis. The laboratory assessment of a patient with positive neurologic findings may include (1) serum electrolytes, complete blood count, and renal, liver, and endocrine studies, (2) cerebrospinal fluid (CSF) examination, (3) imaging studies of the CNS (see Chap. 365), or (4) electrophysiologic studies (see Chap. 366).

Lumbar puncture Lumbar puncture should be considered (1) to measure CSF pressure and to obtain a sample for cellular, chemical, and bacteriologic examination, (2) to administer spinal anesthetics, antibiotics, or antineoplastic agents, and (3) to inject contrast substances for myelography or a radioactive substance [e.g., indium or radioactive iodinated serum albumin (RISA)] for the study of CSF dynamics and to aid in the diagnosis of hydrocephalus or CSF leak.

Lumbar puncture carries a risk if the CSF pressure is high (evidenced by headache and papilledema), for it increases the possibility of fatal cerebellar or tentorial herniation. In patients in whom this possibility exists, it is wise first to obtain a CT or MRI scan to exclude a mass lesion before proceeding to a lumbar puncture. However, if it seems important in a given case of suspected increased intracranial pressure to have the information yielded by CSF examination, the lumbar puncture may be performed with a fine-bore (22- or 24-gauge needle). If the pressure is over 400 mmHg, one should obtain the necessary sample of fluid, remove the needle, and then, according to the suspected clinical disease and the patient's condition, administer mannitol in a dose of 0.75 to 1.0 mg/kg. Unless contraindicated, dexamethasone should be started in a dose of 4 to 6 mg every 6 h in cases of tumor, cerebral trauma, hemorrhage, and certain types of encephalitis (acute hemorrhagic leukoencephalitis, herpes simplex encephalitis).

Cisternal puncture and lateral cervical puncture (C1–C2) are safe procedures in the hands of the expert but should not be performed by those without experience. Cisternal puncture is sometimes necessary in instances of spinal block to perform myelography above a lesion.

Lumbar puncture should always be done under sterile conditions. If local anesthetic is injected into and beneath the skin, the procedure should be painless. Failure to enter the lumbar subarachnoid space after two or three trials can usually be corrected by doing the puncture with patients in the sitting position and then assisting them to lie on their side for pressure measurements and fluid removal. The ''dry tap'' is more often due to an improperly placed needle than to a pathologic obliteration of subarachnoid space by a compressive lesion of the spinal cord or by chronic adhesive arachnoiditis. A bloody tap due to penetration of a meningeal vessel may result in confusion of the diagnosis if it is wrongly interpreted as indicating hemorrhage into the subarachnoid space. Lumbar puncture should be undertaken with particular care in patients with thrombocytopenia or disorders of blood coagulation because serious hemorrhage into the extradural or intradural space may occur.

CSF should be studied for (1) pressure and ''dynamics,'' (2) color, including centrifugation, if blood is present, to examine the supernatant for xanthochromia, (3) number and type of cells and presence of microorganisms, (4) protein, sugar, and other chemical measurements, (5) exfoliative cytology using Millipore filters, (6) VDRL determination and appropriate serologic precipitation reactions (including cryptococcal antigen in patients with immunologic suppression, e.g., AIDS), (7) protein immunoelectrophoresis for determination of gamma globulin levels and other special biochemical tests (for NH_3, pH, CO_2, enzymes, etc.), and (8) bacteriologic cultures and virus isolation. Normal values of CSF constituents are shown in the Appendix.

The principal complication of lumbar puncture is a headache caused by a drop in CSF pressure. Such headaches are worsened by an upright posture and usually disappear in a few hours. Severe cases may require nonsteroidal anti-inflammatory drugs or epidural injection of an autologous "blood patch."

REFERENCES

ADAMS RD, VICTOR M: *Principles of Neurology*, 5th ed. New York, McGraw-Hill, 1993
DEJONG RN: *The Neurologic Examination.* New York, Harper & Row, 1979
FISHMAN RA: *Cerebrospinal Fluid in Diseases of the Nervous System*, 2d ed. Philadelphia, Saunders, 1992
SWANSON PD: *Symptoms and Signs in Neurology.* Philadelphia, Lippincott, 1984

section 1   The central nervous system

364 IMPACT OF NEUROBIOLOGY AND MOLECULAR GENETICS ON NEUROLOGY

JOSEPH B. MARTIN

Advances in molecular genetics, neurobiology, and brain imaging are having a major impact on neurology and psychiatry. These advances are changing our understanding of how the brain is constructed and of the way it functions. They are also expanding the repertoire of experimental approaches, some of which may be successful in solving clinical problems and offering new therapeutic approaches. Molecular genetic discoveries have made possible a more rational taxonomy for many of the inherited diseases that affect the central and peripheral nervous systems, enable new approaches for understanding the molecular basis of development (and degeneration) of the nervous system, and permit presymptomatic or prenatal diagnosis.

The advances have occurred on several fronts, which are now beginning to coalesce. The identification of genes responsible for several of the inherited neurologic diseases has provided insight into their pathogenesis (Table 364-1). Research in molecular structure has disclosed several proteins that subserve receptor and membrane channel functions. Elucidation of the genes that encode for neurotransmitters and their receptors has led to new understanding of neurotransmitter signal transduction and of intercellular and intracellular communication. These discoveries have major implications for drug development by permitting identification of more selective receptor agonists and antagonists. There is also new insight into the mechanisms of cellular injury and neuronal death. The ability to analyze neuronal structure and function extends also to the intact brain. Positron emission tomography (PET), magnetoencephalography, and in vivo magnetic resonance spectroscopy now provide powerful techniques for analysis of the functional organization of the brain (see also Chap. 365).

MOLECULAR GENETICS Applications of molecular biology have already had a major effect on the clinical neurosciences. In the case of inherited neurologic diseases, the use of DNA probes that demonstrate restriction fragment length polymorphisms (RFLPs), combined with linkage analysis in affected pedigrees, have made possible the chromosomal localization of the mutant gene in Huntington's disease (see Chap. 370), familial Alzheimer's disease (see Chap. 370), neurofibromatosis types I and II (see Chap. 370), Friedreich's ataxia (see Chap. 370), spinal muscular atrophy, torsion dystonia, Wilson's disease, and several types of familial CNS tumors including retinoblastoma and von Hippel-Lindau disease (see Table 364-1). The use of linkage analysis with chromosome-specific RFLPs is the first step toward localization and eventual characterization of the abnormal

gene product, a process referred to as *reverse genetics*, i.e., analysis of gene structure to study the abnormal cellular protein, an approach more correctly referred to as *positional cloning*.

In several conditions this approach has already affected clinical practice. In Duchenne's dystrophy, and Becker's X-linked disorders, the muscle abnormality results from failure to encode for a membrane-attached protein, *dystrophin*, which is absent from skeletal muscle in virtually all patients with the Duchenne variant of the disorder (see Chap. 385). In Becker's dystrophy dystrophin is present but is abnormal in amount or in size. Dystrophin is also present in smooth muscle, cardiac muscle, and brain. Its presence in the brain presumably accounts in some way yet to be defined for the frequent occurrence of mental retardation in individuals with Duchenne's dystrophy. The discovery of dystrophin demonstrates elegantly the power of molecular genetics. Decades of effort attempting to define the protein abnormality in Duchenne's dystrophy had been unsuccessful. The quantities of dystrophin present in muscle are so minute that it could not have been characterized by current biochemical approaches.

In retinoblastoma, identification of the protein encoded by the normal allele of the gene (a growth suppressor gene) that is absent from the tumor has provided insight into cellular growth. It is postulated that an inherited mutation affects one allele of the normal gene. If this is followed by a "second hit" mutation that eliminates the function of the second allele in one of the cells in the developing retina, the cell growth suppressor cannot be synthesized. The consequence is the abnormal division of cells in the retina and tumor formation (see also Chap. 63). Another tumor associated with hereditary retinoblastoma is osteosarcoma. A similar mechanism for tumor formation may be involved in Wilms' tumor (on chromosome 11) and in the von Hippel-Lindau syndrome, which leads to hemangioblastoma, pheochromocytoma, and renal cell carcinoma (see Table 364-1).

The application of DNA diagnostics has provided new approaches to presymptomatic and prenatal diagnosis of Huntington's disease, Duchenne's dystrophy, retinoblastoma, and von Hippel-Lindau disease (Table 364-1).

CHARACTERIZATION OF NEW NEUROTRANSMITTER CANDIDATES More than 60 neurotransmitter candidates have been identified in the brain based upon localization within synaptic vesicles, release with depolarization, and interactions with postsynaptic receptors. The functions of these agents, many of which are small-molecular-weight peptides (neuropeptides), remain obscure in many cases. But some are known to modulate functions such as pain transmission (opioid peptides), satiety (cholecystokinin), and thirst (angiotensin).

The discovery of these molecules has made possible new approaches to defining neuronal populations in the human brain by immunohistochemical staining, autoradiography, and in situ messenger RNA hybridization. This information has made it possible to delineate the subclasses of cells affected in neurodegenerative diseases, such as Alzheimer's, Parkinson's, and Huntington's disease. Realiza-

TABLE 364-1 Molecular genetics of neurologic disorders

Chromosome location	Disorder	Principal clinical findings/phenotype	Mode of inheritance	Genotype/gene product	Genetic testing?	Ref. (or Chap.)
1p36.2-p36.1	Neuroblastoma	Related to tumor location and metastases, opsoclonus, myoclonus.	Usually sporadic.	Tumors commonly show hemizygous (one copy) of regions of chromosome 1p. Genomic amplification of N-*myc* occurs.	Tumor analysis for hemizygous state possible.	369
1q21.2-q23	Charcot-Marie-Tooth peripheral neuropathy, Type IB	Onset 2d-3d decade. Distal weakness in legs, less affected in arms. Decreased reflexes, minimal sensory changes. Demyelinating disorder with hypertrophic neuropathy.	AD	Unknown.	Not available.	383
1q21	Gaucher's disease	Infantile, juvenile, and adult forms. Mental retardation, spasticity or ataxia.	AR	Mutations in gene encoding ß-glucocerebrosidase.	Available.	349
2p24	Hypobetalipoproteinemia	Fat malabsorption, neuropathy, sensory loss, ataxia, retinitis pigmentosa, acanthocytosis.	AR	Defect in apolipoprotein B-100. Genetic basis unknown.	Not available.	383
2q33-qter	Cerebrotendinous xanthomatosis	Progressive cerebellar ataxia, dementia, weakness, mental retardation, tendon xanthomas.	AR	Defective synthesis in bile acids in liver.	Not available.	344
2q35	Waardenburg's syndrome, type I	Deafness, white forelock, abnormal pigmentation due to developmental defect caused by defective neural crest migration.	AD	Mutant gene is a member of the paired box-containing (PAX-3) gene family; DNA binding proteins.	Possible in selected families.	54, Tassabehji et al (1992)
3p25	von Hippel-Lindau disease	Retinal vascular malformations, hemangioblastomas, renal cell carcinoma.	AR	Tumor suppressor gene identified.	Possible in selected families.	378, Latif et al
3p14.2	G$_{M1}$-gangliosidosis	Mental retardation, seizures, blindness.	AR	Mutations in gene for ß-galactosidase.	Widely available.	349
3q	Retinitis pigmentosa 1	Night blindness, peripheral field loss, blindness, abnormal EEG.	AD	Mutations in gene that encodes rhodopsin.	Possible in families with identified mutations.	19
4p16.3	Huntington's disease	Chorea, dementia.	AD	CAG triplet repeats 5' end of gene that encodes a novel protein huntingtin.	Yes.	370, MacDonald et al (1993)
4p16.1	Wolf-Hirschhorn syndrome	Mental retardation, peculiar facies.	Sporadic	Deletion 4p16.	No.	
4q35	Facioscapulohumeral muscular dystrophy	Typical weakness atrophy. Face and shoulder muscles.	AD	Unknown.	Possible by linkage testing in large families.	385
5q12.2-q13.3	Spinal muscular atrophy (SMA) type 1,2,3	Weakness, muscle atrophy, diminished or absent reflexes.	AR	Unknown.	Linkage testing possible.	372
5q1.13	G$_{M2}$-gangliosidosis (Sandhoff disease)	Mental retardation, seizures, blindness.	AR	Mutations in A-B hexosaminidase.	Widely applied.	349
6p21.3	Epilepsy, juvenile myoclonic	Tonic-clonic seizures, myoclonus, onset 8–20 years, EEG abnormal.	AD	Unknown.	Linkage testing possible in some pedigrees.	367
6p24-23	Spinocerebellar ataxia 1 (SCA1)	Ataxia, progressive dementia, spasticity.	AD	Expansion of CAG repeats in gene.	Possible.	372/381
6p21.1-cen	Retinitis pigmentosa, peripherin-related	Night blindness, peripheral visual loss leading to blindness.	AD	Mutations in RDS/peripherin gene, a rod photoreceptor membrane protein.	Possible in families with identified mutations.	Kajiwara et al (1993)
7q35	Myotonia congenita (Thomsen disease)	Myotonia, symptoms variable in severity	AD	Mutation in muscle chloride channel gene.	Possible.	385
9p.13	Galactosemia	Cataracts, mental retardation, cirrhosis.	AR	Deficiency of galactose-1-phosphate uridyl transferase.	Prenatal diagnosis by measuring enzyme.	354
9q12-13	Friedreich's ataxia	Onset in puberty; ataxia; dysarthria; absent DTRs; decreased vibration, joint position sense; 1/50,000 incidence.	AR	Unknown.	97% reliable.	370
9q31-33	Familial dysautonomia Riley-Day syndrome	Sensory and autonomic dysfunction, occurs in Ashkenazi-Jewish population.	AR	Unknown.	Possible.	163

(continued)

TABLE 364-1   Molecular genetics of neurologic disorders (continued)

Chromosome location	Disorder	Principal clinical findings/Phenotype	Mode of inheritance	Genotype/gene product	Genetic testing?	Ref. (or Chap.)
9q34	Tuberous sclerosis 1	1/10,000 births, mental retardation, seizures, adenoma sebaceum.	AD	Unknown.	Not reliable.	378
9q34	Torsion dystonia	Dystonia, torticollis, occurs in both Ashkenazi-Jewish and non-Jewish pedigrees.	AD	Unknown.	97% reliable.	370
11q22.3-q23.1	Ataxia telangiectasia	Cerebellar degeneration, oculocutaneous telangiectasia, immunodeficiency, endocrinopathy.	AR	Unknown.	Not available.	278
11q24.1-q24.2	Acute intermittent porphyria	Confusion, coma, peripheral neuropathy with proximal weakness.	AD	Defect in porphobilinogen deaminase. Gene defect not defined.	Not available.	346
12q23-24.1	Spinocerebellar ataxia 2 (SCA2)	Ataxia, clinically indistinguishable from SCA1.	AD	Unknown.	Possible by linkage.	372
13q14.1-q14.2	Retinoblastoma	40% hereditary, 60% nonhereditary, multiple tumors in inherited form.	AR	*Rb* gene mutations or deletions cause disease. Rb protein is 105-kDa tumor suppressor.	Detection of carriers and presymptomatic diagnosis.	19, 60
13q14-q21	Wilson's disease	Kayser-Fleischer ring in cornea, movement disorder, progressive neurologic deficit if untreated.	AR	Unknown.	Not available.	348
14q21-q31	Krabbe's disease	Mental retardation, leukodystrophy.	AR	Enzyme defect, galactosylceramide, ß-galactoside.	Possible.	349
14q24.3	Alzheimer's disease, early onset	Dementia, memory loss, typical AD.	AD	Unknown.	Not available.	370
15q11	Prader-Willi/Angelman syndrome	Prader-Willi: hypotonia, hypogonadism, hyperphagia, hypopigmentation. Angelman: movement disorder, ataxia, reverse mental retardation.	Sporadic	Deletion mutation defect due to unequal expression of maternal or paternal alleles. Prader-Willi due to active paternal allele, Angelman to active maternal allele.	Cytogenetics in individual patients.	Wagstaff et al
15q23-q24	Tay-Sachs disease, G_{M2}-gangliosidosis	Mental retardation, delayed development, seizures, blindness.	AR	Mutations in hexosaminidase A.	Widely available.	349
16p12.1	Batten disease—Juvenile neuronal lipofuscinosis	Dementia, paralysis, white matter disease.	AD	Unknown.	Possible.	Mitchison et al
16p3	Tuberous sclerosis 2	Hamartomas, epilepsy, mental retardation.	AD	Unknown.	Not available.	378
17p13.3	Miller-Dieker lissencephaly syndrome	Microcephaly, micrognathia, epilepsy, pathology shows smooth brain (agyria) due to failure of cortical neuronal migration.	AD	17p13 deletion, gene of homologue of ß-transducin.	Cytogenetics possible.	Reiner et al
17p11.2	Charcot-Marie-Tooth Type 1A	Motor and sensory neuropathy, distal muscle atrophy, areflexia, pes cavus, decreased nerve conduction velocities.	AD	Mutation or duplication in peripheral myelin protein gene, PMP-22.	Possible in families with demonstrated mutations.	383, Pentao et al (1992)
17q11.2	Von Recklinghausen neurofibromatosis, NF1	Multiple neurofibromas, 1/3500 individuals, café au lait spots, malignant gliomas, Lisch nodules.	AD	Encodes neurofibromin, a member of the GTPase activating protein (GAP) family.	Possible in families with demonstrated mutations.	378
17q23.1-q25.3	Hyperkalemic periodic paralysis	Myotonia, periodic areflexic paralysis.	AD	Point mutation sodium channel.	Possible.	387
18q11.2-q12.1	Familial amyloid neuropathy due to mutations in transthyretin	Sensorimotor cardiac neuropathy.	AD	Over 40 different point mutations in gene for transthyretin.	Yes.	383
18q22.1	Tourette's syndrome	Familial, but not all cases linked to this chromosomal site.	AD?	Unknown.	No.	370
19q13.3	Myotonic dystrophy	Multisystem disorder, cataracts, myotonia, weakness, frontal baldness, mental retardation.	AD, anticipation	CTG repeats 3' end of myotonin protein kinase.	Yes.	385
19q13.1	Malignant hyperthermia	Sensitivity to volatile anesthetics, muscle contraction.	AD	Mutation in ryanodine receptor.	Yes.	398

(continued)

TABLE 364-1   Molecular genetics of neurologic disorders (*continued*)

Chromosome location	Disorder	Principal clinical findings/Phenotype	Mode of inheritance	Genotype/gene product	Genetic testing?	Ref. (or Chap.)
19q12-q13.2	Central core disease of muscle	Hypotonia, weakness.	AD	Mutation in ryanodine receptor.	Yes.	385
19q13.2	Alzheimer's disease, late-onset	Memory loss, dementia.	AD	Apolipoprotein E4 association.	Not available.	370
20pter-p12	Gerstmann-Straussler disease	Spongioform encephalopathy with dementia, myoclonus.	AD	Prion protein mutation.	Yes.	375
20pter-p12	Familial Creutzfeldt-Jakob disease	Spongioform encephalopathy with dementia, myoclonus.	AD	Prion protein mutation.	Yes.	375
20q	Benign neonatal familial epilepsy	Onset early in life, remits by 1 year, small percentage have mental retardation.	AD	Unknown.	Not available.	367
21q21.3-q22.05	Familial Alzheimer's disease with amyloid precursor protein mutation	Rare cause of early onset Alzheimer's disease.	AD	Mutation in amyloid precursor protein.	Possible.	370
21q22.1-q22.2	Familial amyotrophic lateral sclerosis	Weakness, muscle atrophy, spasticity, increased DTRs. About 5% of cases are familial.	AD	Point mutations in Cu, Zn-superoxide dismutase (SOD1). In 40 percent of families.	Possible.	370, Rosen et al (1993)
21q21.3-q22.05	Familial cerebral amyloid angiopathy (Dutch type)	Cerebral hemorrhage.	AD	Point mutation in amyloid precursor protein (APP).	Possible.	370
21q22.3	Epilepsy, progressive myoclonic	Rare, dementia and other neurologic findings.	AD (probably)	Unknown.	Not available.	367
22q1.11	Neurofibromatosis type II (NFII)	Acoustic neuromas, bilateral.	AD	Deletions in the gene that encodes for merlin, a 587 amino acid cytoskeletal protein.	Yes.	378, Trofatter et al (1993)
22q11.21-q13.1	Acoustic neuroma, meningioma	Acoustic neuromas, bilateral. Meningiomas.	AD	Deletions in merlin gene.	Yes.	369
22q13-13qter	Metachromatic leukodystrophy	Mental retardation, leukodystrophy, dementia.	AR	Several mutations in gene encoding for arylsulfatase A have been identified.	Enzyme measurement available, DNA diagnosis possible.	383
Xp22.3	Kallmann syndrome	Anosmia with hypogonadism (GnRH deficiency), syndrome due to failure of neuronal migration.	X-LR	Mutations in gene (*KALIG-1*) which encodes protein with homology to neural cell adhesion (N-CAM) molecules.	Possible.	339/340
Xp21.2	Duchenne's muscular dystrophy and Becker's muscular dystrophy	Onset of muscular weakness in early life, progressive. Becker's is more benign.	X-LR	Mutations in the dystrophin-encoding gene.	Widely available.	385, Ahn and Kunhal (1993)
Xp11.4	Norrie disease	Failure of normal brain development.	X-LR	Gene encodes small protein with homology to glycosylated mucins.	Possible.	Meindl et al
Xq12-q13	Menkes disease	Progressive neurologic deterioration, kinky or steely hair, pallor, death in childhood.	X-LR	Mutations in a gene (*MCI*) that encodes a protein that regulates cation transport (probably including copper).	Possible.	Vulpe et al (1993)
Xq21.3-q22	Spinal muscular atrophy; Kennedy disease	Muscular weakness.	X-LR	Trinucleotide repeats in androgen receptor gene.	Possible.	372
Xq22	Pelizaeus-Merzbacher disease	Progressive neurologic deterioration.	X-LR	One-quarter of patients have mutation in proteolipid protein gene.	Not available.	Strautnieks et al
Xq22	Fabry disease	Painful neuropathy.	X-LR	Enzyme defect in α-galactosidase A	Possible.	241/349
Xq13	Charcot-Marie-Tooth, X-linked-1 dominant	Neuropathy, with weakness and sensory loss.	X-LR	Unknown.	Not available.	383
Xq21.2	Choroideremia	Retinitis pigmentosa, visual loss due to degeneration of pigment epithelium and choroid.	X-LR	Gene isolated encodes geranylgeranyl transferase that prenylates several proteins.	Possible.	Cremers et al
Xq21-q22	Spastic paraplegia, X-linked	Midlife onset, spasticity, weakness, urinary frequency.	X-LR	Unknown.	Not available.	370
Xq26-q27.2	Lesch-Nyhan syndrome	Mental retardation.	X-LR	HPRT deficiency.	90% have point mutation in exon 9 of HPRT gene.	347

(*continued*)

TABLE 364-1   **Molecular genetics of neurologic disorders** (*continued*)

Chromosome location	Disorder	Principal clinical findings/Phenotype	Mode of inheritance	Genotype/gene product	Genetic testing?	Ref. (or Chap.)
Xq27.3	Fragile-X syndrome	Decreased head size, prominent forehead, large ears, macro-orchidism, mental retardation.	X-LR	Gene characterized by trinucleotide 5′ repeats of CGG. Gene identified as *FMR*-1.	Yes.	62 and 378
Xq28	Adrenoleukodystrophy	Mild neuropathy, spastic paraparesis, baldness, hypogonadism, hypoadrenalism.	X-LR	Gene characterized.	Possible.	377
Xq28	Emery-Dreifuss muscular dystrophy	Onset before age 10, benign course characterized by slowly progressive proximal weakness, cardiac arrhythmias may occur.	X-LR	Unknown.	Not available.	385

Abbreviations: AD, autosomal dominant; AR, autosomal recessive; X-LR, X-linked recessive; HPRT, hypoxanthine-guanine phosphoribosyltransferase.
SOURCE: Martin JB, Ann Neurol, vol. 34, 1993.

tion that dopamine cells are affected in Parkinson's disease led to therapy with levodopa. In Huntington's disease, it has been possible to define the subsets of neurons affected by the degenerative process in the striatum and to show selective sparing of other cell types (see Chap. 370). Although this has not led yet to specific theories about the mechanisms of cell death, it has resulted in speculations about potentially beneficial therapeutic strategies.

Many of these newly discovered neuropeptides appear to share nerve terminals and often even secretory vesicles with conventional neurotransmitters. It appears likely that neuropeptides exert profound modulatory effects on the actions of the primary neurotransmitter. In other cases the peptide may influence neuronal plasticity, growth, or differentiation. A most surprising discovery was the recognition that nitric oxide (NO), synthesized in neurons by the enzyme nitric oxide synthase, acts after cellular release to exert a variety of effects on neural tissues. First recognized as an endothelial cell–derived muscle cell relaxant (nitrates dilate blood vessels, as in the treatment for angina), NO can be both beneficial and toxic to brain cells. Subclasses of neurons contain NO synthase, as for example do NADPH diaphorase-positive neurons of the striatum, and NO release in normal quantities can activate other neurons. Excessive release can prove toxic. Other gases, such as carbon monoxide, may also serve modulatory roles in nervous tissue.

BIOCHEMICAL CLASSIFICATION OF RECEPTOR SUBTYPES Some of the most important insights from neurobiology have resulted from the cloning of the genes of several neurotransmitter and hormone receptors that are critical to brain function. Based on pharmacologic analysis alone it was difficult to account for the diverse effects mediated by molecules of low molecular weight. For example, pharmacologic analysis of acetylcholine disclosed muscarinic and nicotinic effects. With the biochemical elucidation of acetylcholine receptor subtypes and by means of molecular cloning techniques and molecular probes, it is now established that multiple forms of muscarinic (M1, M2, M3, M4, and M5) and nicotinic (N1 and N2) receptors exist in the brain and that their distribution varies from region to region. Thus, differences in receptor subtypes expressed in different regions of the brain can account for the complex multiple effects of the medications acting on cholinergic receptors. The molecular specificities of the various receptor subtypes provide sensitive systems with which to search for selective agonists and antagonists. For example, M1 agonists may facilitate memory. Regional differences in the distribution of the subtypes of the nicotinic cholinergic receptor in the central nervous system make it possible to explore the neurologic basis of nicotine addiction.

Identification of the subclasses of the alpha- and beta-adrenergic, serotoninergic, gamma-aminobutyric acid (GABA), and glutamatergic receptors makes it possible to correlate structure and function and to

provide a rational basis for molecular classification of drug actions. In the case of the GABA receptor, structural features that account for the interaction of barbiturates and benzodiazepines can now be recognized.

Subclasses of glutamate receptors mediate excitatory amino acid neurotransmitter effects. Glutamate, one of the most abundant of all neurotransmitters in the brain, functions to promote rapid neurotransmitter depolarization by opening membrane channels that permit diffusion of sodium and potassium ions. These rapid effects are mediated by two receptor subtypes, identified by ligand binding with kainate and AMPA. The identification of an additional subtype of glutamate receptor which binds *N*-methyl-D-aspartate (the *NMDA receptor*) made possible identification of additional glutamate functions. The NMDA receptor appears to mediate other functions that heretofore were classed in the category of plasticity, a process considered important, for example, in memory and learning. The NMDA subtype of glutamate receptor is linked to a voltage-sensitive channel that responds to repetitive activation by the opening of an ion channel. The actions of calcium permit transduction of electrical events into molecular changes that can alter neuronal function permanently, i.e., change cellular function to subserve a memory or learning response.

Based on definitive experimental results, it is now clear that activation of the NMDA receptor can also have deleterious effects on the cell, whereby calcium entry induces *neurotoxicity* that, if sufficiently severe, can lead to neuronal cell death. This mechanism may explain some of the extensive neuronal cell damage that occurs in ischemia, hypoxia, epilepsy, and, perhaps, neurodegenerative diseases (see Choi).

These findings have resulted in great interest in the development of new drugs that might selectively block the NMDA receptor, thereby minimizing the effects of ischemia or hypoxia that occur in stroke or after cardiorespiratory arrest. The profound potential of this work is illustrated by the demonstration that NMDA receptor blockade induced even several hours after the neuronal insult may be ''neuroprotective.''

Cloning of cellular membrane channels (sodium, potassium, calcium) also has had a profound effect on defining mechanisms of neuronal excitability. It is anticipated that these findings will lead to the discovery of more effective drugs for epilepsy, neuroprotection, and migraine.

BRAIN IMAGING The development of computed tomography and proton imaging by magnetic resonance has revolutionized our ability to define lesions in the brain and spinal cord (see Chap. 365). Other techniques have been developed to make it possible to study brain function as well as structure by the application of positron emission tomography (PET), single photon emission computed tomography (SPECT), magnetoencephalography, and nuclear magnetic resonance spectroscopy (NMRS).

PET scanning involves the use of positron-emitting radionuclides with short half-lives in which particle disintegration is captured in a three-dimensional array by multiple sensors positioned about the head. With the use of radioisotopes for carbon (^{13}C), oxygen (^{15}O), and fluorine (^{18}F), it is possible to measure cerebral blood flow, cerebral oxygen metabolism, and cerebral glucose uptake (with ^{18}F-labeled deoxyglucose). The last technique employs the principles developed by Sokoloff and colleagues, who first used the technique of labeled deoxyglucose combined with tissue section autoradiography. PET scanning also can define regional changes in cerebral function associated with stroke, Alzheimer's disease, Huntington's disease, and schizophrenia, and it identifies foci of hyperactivity associated with epilepsy.

Perhaps the most creative use of PET techniques has been analysis of cognitive function. Two theories of language had emerged from studies in neurology and linguistics. The first proposed that language function occurs serially, i.e., an object is first seen in the occipital lobes, its name is recalled by the temporal lobes, and the information is then sent to the frontal lobes, which direct formation of speech. PET studies have now confirmed the second of these hypotheses, which suggested from linguistic analysis that language occurs in a parallel array. Posner and colleagues, using subtraction techniques to isolate activity associated with a particular language task, have shown clearly that brain processing occurs simultaneously in several of the regions underlying a set of neurologic functions. These kinds of analyses now permit regionalized functional study of the brain in a manner not hitherto expected by the physical limits set by three-dimensional imaging using positron emitters. Regional studies of this kind have also shown that brain blood flow changes that occur in panic disorder and anticipatory anxiety correlate with anatomic loci in the temporal lobes.

There have also been important advances in the use of radioligands for neurotransmitter receptors. The imaging of dopamine and of dopamine receptors in the basal ganglia has been achieved in both normals and in patients with Parkinson's disease and with 1-methyl-4-phenyl-1,2,3,6-tetrahydropyridine (MPTP) poisoning. In the latter case deficits in basal ganglion function in asymptomatic subjects exposed to MPTP raise the possibility of identifying subclinical deficits and of following subjects over time to determine eventual outcome and prognosis. MRI techniques can also be applied to functional studies in the brain. Blood flow changes, measured in real time, have been detected by MRI in the visual cortex in subjects exposed to visual stimulation. Mapping of the brain by MRI, PET, and magnetoencephalography is now being actively pursued in many laboratories.

SPECT imaging has been made possible by refinements in detection systems for single photon emitters. The resolution of SPECT does not yet reach the capacity of PET, but the longer half-lives of the isotopes and the simplicity of the detection systems make it less expensive and potentially more widely available. Its potential includes measurement of radioligand binding to receptors and determination of cerebral blood flow. Thus far, studies with SPECT have delineated regional changes in brain metabolism and blood flow in the neurodegenerative diseases.

NMR spectroscopy offers an opportunity to assess brain function at the subcellular molecular level. The technique uses natural emissions from atomic nuclei activated by magnetic fields to measure endogenous molecules. Potential nuclei include ^{31}P, ^{13}C, ^{23}Na, ^{7}Li, in addition to ^{1}H. The promise of analysis of ^{31}P is the closest to realization. It is possible to quantitate several phosphate-containing compounds (phosphocreatine, ATP, ADP, and inorganic phosphorus). The combination of spectral analysis with topical NMR permits localization within superficial regions of the brain. It can be anticipated that further refinements of this technique will make possible measurement of brain metabolism with spatial resolution that may exceed that of PET.

REFERENCES

AHN AH, KUNKEL LM: The structural and functional diversity of dystrophin. Nature Genet 3:283, 1993

BLUMENFELD A et al: Localization of the gene for familial dysautonomia on chromosome 9 and definition of DNA markers for genetic diagnosis. Nature Genet 4:160, 1993

BREAKEFIELD XO, CAMBI F: Molecular genetic insights into neurologic diseases, in *Annual Review of Neuroscience*, vol 10, WM Cowan et al (eds). Palo Alto, Annual Reviews, 1987, pp 535–594

BROWN GG et al: In vivo ^{13}P NMR profiles of Alzheimer's disease and multiple subcortical infarct dementia. Neurology 39:1423, 1989

BUCKLEY NJ et al: Antagonist binding properties of five cloned muscarinic receptors expressed in CHO-K1 cells. Molec Pharmacol 35(4):469, 1989

CHOI D: Glutamate neurotoxicity and diseases of the nervous system. Neuron 1:623, 1989

COOPER JR et al: *The Biochemical Basis of Neuropharmacology*. New York, Oxford University Press, 1986

CREMERS FPM et al: An autosomal homologue of the choroideremia gene colocalizes with the Usher syndrome type II locus on the distal part of chromosome 1q. Hum Mol Gen 1:71, 1992

GUSELLA JF et al: DNA markers for nervous system diseases. Science 225:1320, 1984

KAJIWARA K et al: A null mutation in the human peripherin RDS gene in a family with autosomal dominant retinitis punctata albescens. Nature Genet 3:208, 1993

KATIF F et al: Identification of the von Hippel-Lindau disease tumor suppressor gene. Science 260:1317, 1993

KAUPPINEN RA et al: Applications of magnetic resonance spectroscopy and diffusion-weighted imaging to the study of brain biochemistry and pathology. Trends Neurosci 16:88, 1993

MacDONALD M et al: A novel gene containing a trinucleotide repeat that is expanded and unstable on Huntington's disease chromosomes. Cell 72:971, 1993

MARTIN JB: Molecular genetics: Applications to the clinical neurosciences. Science 238:765, 1987

————: Molecular genetic studies in the neuropsychiatric disorders. Trends Neurosci 12:130, 1989

MARTIN JB: Molecular genetics in neurology. Ann Neurol vol. 34, 1993

MEINDL A et al: Norrie disease is caused by mutations in an extracellular protein resembling C-terminal globular domain of mucins. Nature Genet 2:139, 1992

MEISSEN GJ et al: Predictive testing for Huntington's disease with use of a linked DNA marker. N Engl J Med 318:535, 1988

MITCHISON HM et al: Fine genetic mapping of the Batten disease locus (CLN3) by haplotype analysis and demonstration of allelic association with chromosome 16p microsatellite loci. Genomics 16:455, 1993

PENTAO L et al: Charcot-Marie-Tooth type-1A duplication appears to arise from recombination at repeat sequences flanking the 1.5 Mb monomer unit. Nature Genet 2:292, 1992

PETTEGREW JW et al: ^{31}P nuclear magnetic resonance studies of phosphoglyceride metabolism in developing and degenerating brain: Preliminary observations. J Neuropathol Exp Neurol 46:419, 1987

POSNER EM et al: Localization of cognitive operations in the human brain. Science 240:1627, 1988

REINER O et al: Isolation of a Miller-Dieker lissencephaly gene containing G-protein β-subunit-like repeats. Nature 364:717, 1993

ROSEN DR et al: Mutations in Cu/Zn superoxide dismutase gene are associated with familial amyotrophic lateral sclerosis. Nature 362:59, 1993

REIMAN EM et al: Neuroanatomical correlates of anticipatory anxiety. Science 243:1071, 1989

ROWE CC et al: Localization of epileptic foci with postictal single photon emission computed tomography. Ann Neurol 26:660, 1989

SHULMAN RG et al: Nuclear magnetic resonance imaging and spectroscopy of human brain function. Proc Natl Acad Sci USA 90:3127, 1993

SNYDER SH: Drug and neurotransmitter receptors: New perspectives with clinical relevance. JAMA 261:3126, 1989

————, BREDT DS: Biological roles of nitric oxide. Sci Amer May 1992:68

STRAUTNIEKS S et al: Pelizaeus-Merzbacher disease: Detection of mutations Thr 181-Pro and Leu 223-Pro in the proteolipid protein gene, and prenatal diagnosis. Am J Hum Genet 51:871, 1992

TASSABEHJI M et al: Waardenburg's syndrome patients have mutations in the human homologue of the Pax-3 paired box gene. Nature 355:635, 1992

TROFATTER JA et al: A novel Moesin-like, Ezrin-like, Radixin-like gene is a candidate for the neurofibromatosis-2 tumor suppressor. Cell 72:791, 1993

VULPE C et al: Isolation of a candidate gene for Menkes disease and evidence that it encodes a copper-transporting ATPase. Nature Genet 3:273, 1993

WAGSTAFF J et al: Maternal but not paternal transmission of 15q11-13-linked nondeletion syndrome leads to phenotypic expression. Nature Genet 1:291, 1992

365   IMAGING OF THE NERVOUS SYSTEM

KENNETH R. DAVIS / JOSEPH B. MARTIN

Advances in imaging have revolutionized the ability to visualize brain and spinal cord lesions that cause neurologic dysfunction. These developments have followed the application to clinical problems of computed tomography (CT) in the 1970s, magnetic resonance imaging (MRI) in the 1980s, and positron emission tomography (PET) and single-photon emission computed tomography (SPECT) in the past decade. Magnetic resonance spectroscopy (MRS), as well as MR perfusion and diffusion studies, have promise for the study of function in the central nervous system (CNS) like that currently possible with PET and SPECT.

COMPUTED TOMOGRAPHY   CT scanning provides a sensitive and reproducible method for evaluating suspected lesions in the CNS. It has been replaced by MRI as the procedure of choice for imaging of the brain and spinal cord, although it remains more widely available than MRI. Its principal utility is when rapid information about the state of the CNS is desired, and it is particularly important for decisions related to emergent surgical versus medical management of patients with the sudden onset of a neurologic deficit. Such conditions include acute head or spinal trauma, stroke where a differentiation between hemorrhage and infarction is important, and other circumstances where a decision as to immediate operative intervention is important. CT continues to have an advantage over MRI in emergency settings in patients with acute neurologic deterioration. It has high specificity, particularly for the demonstration of acute hemorrhage, where its imaging capacity exceeds that of MRI.

CT is also widely used for the evaluation of lesions that involve bone, such as metastatic disease at the base of the skull. However, the radionuclide bone scan provides a more sensitive generalized evaluation for bone metastases than CT or MRI. Calcification within lesions of the brain is demonstrated best by CT rather than MRI. CT is also the better imaging method for fractures of the face, temporal bone, and base of the skull. It is also an important imaging technique for evaluating fractures of the spine, although soft tissue encroachment upon the spinal cord is better visualized by MRI.

MAGNETIC RESONANCE IMAGING   MRI is useful in the following circumstances:

1 Screening for metastatic disease. With the administration of intravenous MRI contrast material containing gadolinium, metastatic tumors can be visualized within the brain parenchyma, as well as primary tumors that cause a breakdown of the blood-brain barrier (Fig. 365-1). Imaging with gadolinium-DTPA is more sensitive for these conditions than noncontrast MR or CT with contrast. It is also preferred for visualization of pituitary tumors, acoustic neurinomas (Fig. 365-2), and other posterior fossa tumors, where CT artifacts from dental fillings on coronal scans of the sellar region and from nearby bony structures in the posterior fossa may prevent clear delineation of the lesion.

2 Imaging of demyelinating diseases such as multiple sclerosis (MS) and other white matter disorders of the brain and spinal cord (Fig. 365-3). It is possible to visualize small (2 to 5 mm) white matter lesions and to watch their progress over time. Contrast enhancement may make it possible to determine the acute perivascular involvement of new active lesions in MS. It is also the method of choice for evaluation of the leukodystrophies and for other white matter diseases such as senescent white matter ischemia (leukoariosis or Binswanger's disease) (see Chap. 368).

3 Screening for the presence of arteriovenous malformation (AVM) and aneurysms, particularly when family members at risk require evaluation (Fig. 365-4). MRI is followed by angiography if more detailed visualization is necessary in preparation for surgical intervention, or if the findings are equivocal. Development of MRI methods for evaluation of blood flow (MR angiography) promises to improve the ability to delineate blood flow and vascular lesions, including encroachment upon the lumen by atheromatous plaques in the carotid and vertebral basilar systems (Fig. 365-5).

4 Evaluation of congenital and developmental abnormalities of the CNS. These include the Chiari malformation, porencephalic cysts, mesial temporal sclerosis (as a cause of epilepsy), as well as a variety of inherited abnormalities affecting the CNS (e.g., tuberous sclerosis).

5 Detection of posterior fossa vascular lesions. Small lacunes can be visualized within the brainstem that are not visible on CT scan (see Chap. 368). It is also the procedure of choice for the demonstration of small hemorrhages more than several days old in the posterior

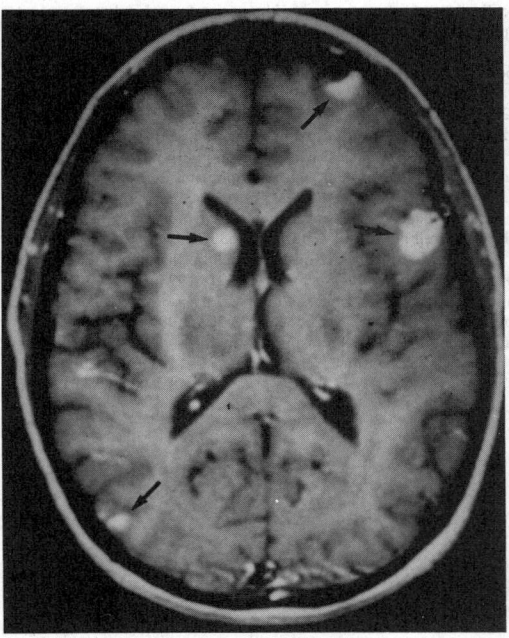
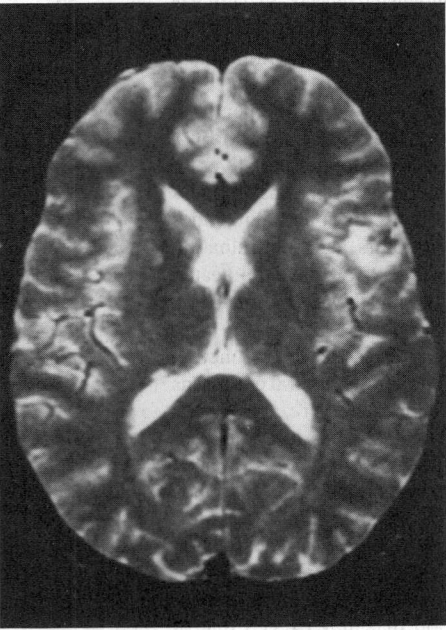

FIGURE 365-1 Cerebral metastases. Magnetic resonance scan of the brain showing many more obvious enhancing lung metastases on the T1-weighted image (*arrows*) with intravenous contrast material (*A*) than on the T2-weighted image prior to contrast injection (*B*).

A   B

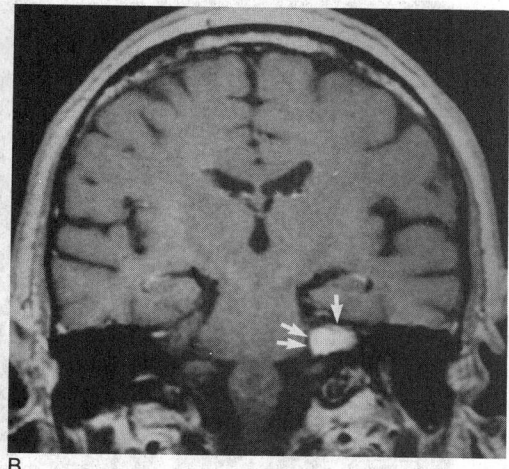

FIGURE 365-2 Acoustic neurinoma. MRI with intravenous contrast material clearly depicts the intracanalicular (*arrow*) and cerebellopontine angle cistern (*double arrows*) components of an acoustic neurinoma on axial (*A*) and coronal (*B*) views. (*Courtesy of R.G. Gonzalez, M.D.*)

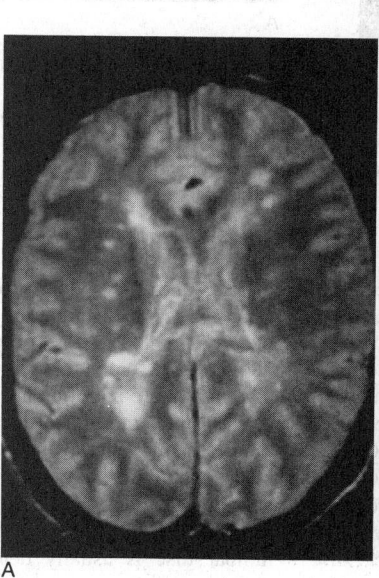

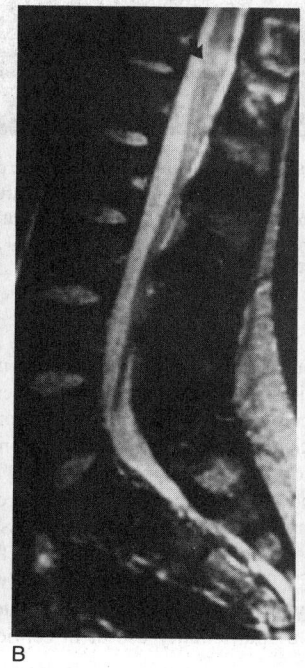

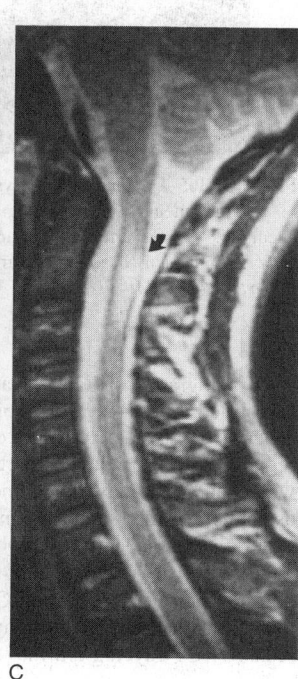

FIGURE 365-3 Multiple sclerosis. *A.* Proton-density MRI reveals multiple periventricular hyperintense multiple sclerosis plaques. T2-weighted MRI of the spine shows a hyperintense plaque within the conus medullaris (*B*) and the upper cervical cord (*C*), respectively (*arrows*), in different patients. (*Courtesy of S. Sweriduk, M.D.*)

fossa. MR angiography is capable of visualizing basilar and vertebral artery flow (Fig. 365-5).

6 Lesions intrinsic to the spinal cord. Particularly advantageous is the ability to examine the entire spinal cord and canal, a technique that has led to improved management, particularly of thoracic disc syndromes. Myelopathy should be evaluated first with an MRI to differentiate intramedullary from extramedullary lesions. Metastatic disease affecting the spinal cord from an epidural location is easily visualized by MRI. It is also the best method for the demonstration of intrinsic spinal cord lesions including tumors (Fig. 365-6), syringomyelia, and areas of demyelination (Fig. 365-3). Use of intravenous contrast material may provide increased sensitivity or improved characterization of a lesion (Fig. 365-7). As compared to the myelogram, MRI allows visualization within and around the entire cord. The postmyelography CT scan is limited in the full evaluation of the spine because a large number of slices, and hence excessive time, are required. MRI is the choice for acute spinal cord syndromes caused by extramedullary lesions, including epidural abscess and metastases. Leptomeningeal metastases are also best evaluated by gadolinium-enhanced MR scans. Osteomyelitis of the spine and secondary abscess are readily visualized by MRI (Fig. 365-8).

7 Although MRI is useful in the evaluation of all vertebral disc and

spondylosis problems, it is particularly valuable for patients who have had previous back surgery. Following the administration of intravenous contrast material, it is possible to visualize extradural granulation tissue and to determine whether fibrosis (scarring) or recurrent disc protrusion is contributing to root symptoms. Fibrous granulation tissue usually shows early enhancement following intravenous contrast material, whereas a disc fragment may show delayed slight enhancement 15 to 20 min after injection.

8 Developmental lesions of the spinal cord such as syringomyelia, tethered cord, lipomas, and cavernous hemangiomas. MRI can demonstrate vascular lesions that subsequently may require angiography for definition, but may also demonstrate small intramedullary lesions that are not visible on the angiogram.

However, the problems of taking care of patients in the MRI scanner, particularly those who are unconscious on life-support systems, who have gunshot wounds, or who are in MRI-incompatible tongs or halos for spinal traction or immobilization, limit the use of MRI. In these circumstances, it may be necessary to obtain a myelogram performed with a water-soluble, nonionic contrast material that permits a subsequent CT-myelogram.

MYELOGRAPHY If the MRI is insufficient to account for the clinical presentation, it may be necessary to perform a myelogram or

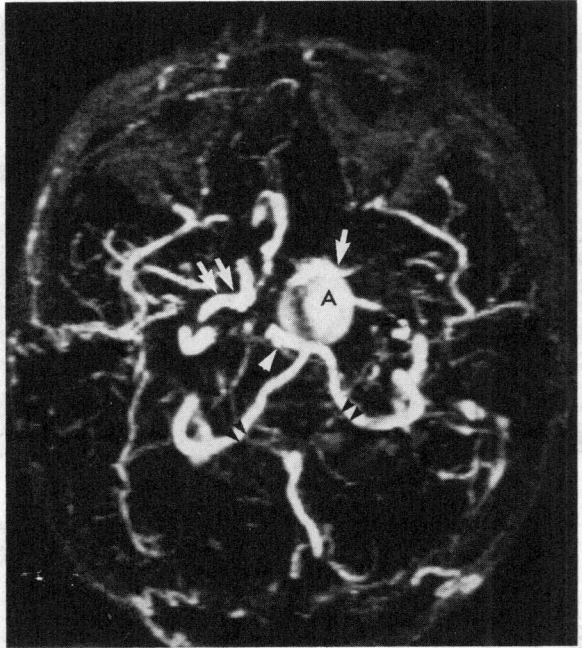

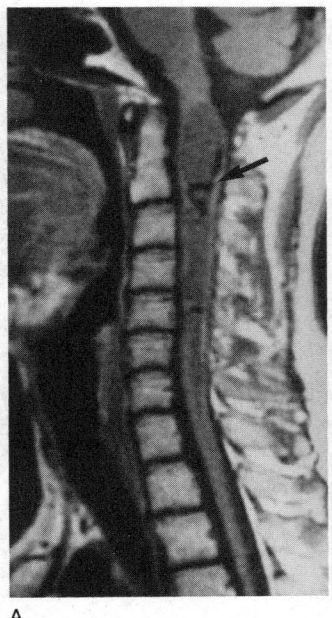
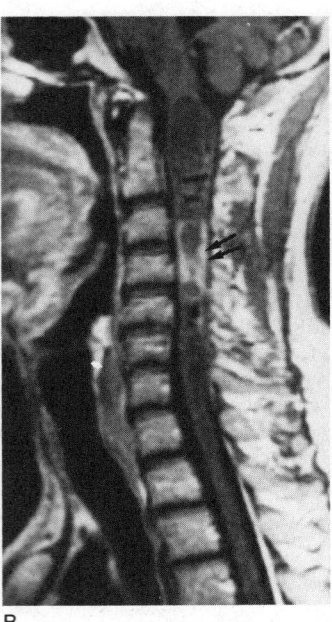

A   B

FIGURE 365-4 Cerebral aneurysm. MR angiography indicates the presence of a large aneurysm originating from the left internal carotid artery. A, aneurysm. Single arrow: left carotid artery. Double arrows: right carotid artery. Angle arrowhead: basilar artery. Double arrowheads: vertebral arteries. (*Courtesy of D. Mikulis, M.D.*)

FIGURE 365-6 Ependymoma. *A.* T1-weighted sagittal MRI of the cervical spine made without intravenous contrast shows expansion of the cervical cord by an ependymoma (*arrow*) with mixed hypointense signal intensities. *B.* Following intravenous injection of gadolinium-DTPA contrast, the T1 image shows enhancement of a portion of the tumor (*double arrows*) that would be most likely to yield a positive biopsy.

CT-myelogram in which a water-soluble, nonionic contrast material is instilled into the subarachnoid space. Films are usually taken at the time of contrast injection and followed by a CT scan of the appropriate regions. The procedure is particularly useful in cervical spondylosis where an MRI may not demonstrate detail of a herniated disc or osteophyte. The safety of new nonionic, water-soluble contrast materials has made myelography a more feasible procedure associated with less risk. Iophendylate myelography, no longer performed, did not permit subsequent CT evaluation. Furthermore, residual iophendylate after myelography produced artifacts on subsequent MR scans. A CT-myelogram may be particularly useful in cervical disc

disease and spondylosis to demonstrate narrowing of the neural foramen and to differentiate an osteophyte (hard disc) from soft disc material, if this is not optimally visualized on MRI. For tumors of the vertebral foramen, such as neurofibromas, a myelogram and CT-myelogram are not often necessary, given the availability of MRI and use of intravenous contrast material (see Fig. 365-7). Seeding of tumors along roots in the cauda equina is often visualized on MRI, but such tumors may be too small to be identified or not enhance with intravenous contrast material. In this circumstance, a myelogram followed by a CT-myelogram may be the best choice. Herniated lumbar disc is usually detected by MRI (Fig. 365-9), but some physicians still prefer to have the anatomic details confirmed by CT and myelography prior to surgery. If the MRI is normal or equivocal, a myelogram or CT-myelogram may demonstrate enlarged veins in cases of suspected spinal AVM prior to deciding on spinal angiography. MRI may detect flow voids of the AVM and an abnormal signal within the cord. Where AVM is suspected a CT-myelogram followed by a spinal angiogram is the next step after an unremarkable MRI. Finally, a CT-myelogram may be the examination of choice in spinal cord injury where ferromagnetic metal stabilization has been used and MRI-incompatible life-support systems are required. In these circumstances, it is difficult to perform an adequate MRI.

INTERVENTIONAL RADIOLOGY It is now possible to navigate into small vessels using maneuverable microcatheters and to visualize the vasculature and tip of the microcatheter by high-resolution digital fluoroscopic equipment with real-time roadmapping capabilities. The decrease in the time required for microcatheter entry and visualization of target vessels results in faster studies at lower risk. The studies are usually performed by transfemoral retrograde catheterization using specialized coaxial microcatheters that can enter small vessels in the distribution of the anterior, middle, and posterior cerebral, vertebral, basilar, external carotid, or spinal circulations. This technique, along with availability of polymerizing glues such as *n*-butyl-cyanoacrylate, microcoils, and various particulate agents, such as polyvinyl alcohol (PVA) and gelfoam, makes endovascular embolization treatment of AVMs possible. Treatment is usually partial, to facilitate surgical

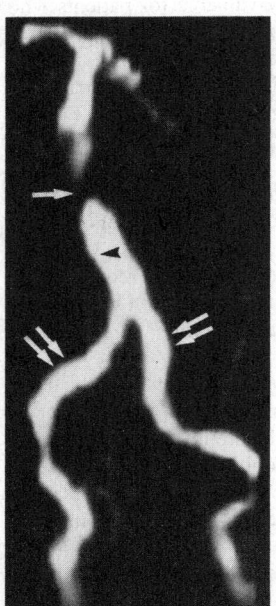

FIGURE 365-5 Basilar artery stenosis. MR angiogram of the vertebral basilar circulation showing stenosis of the midbasilar artery (*arrow*) with turbulent flow artifact above the stenosis. Double arrows: vertebral arteries. Arrowhead: normal lower basilar artery. (*Courtesy of Gilbert Vezina, M.D.*)

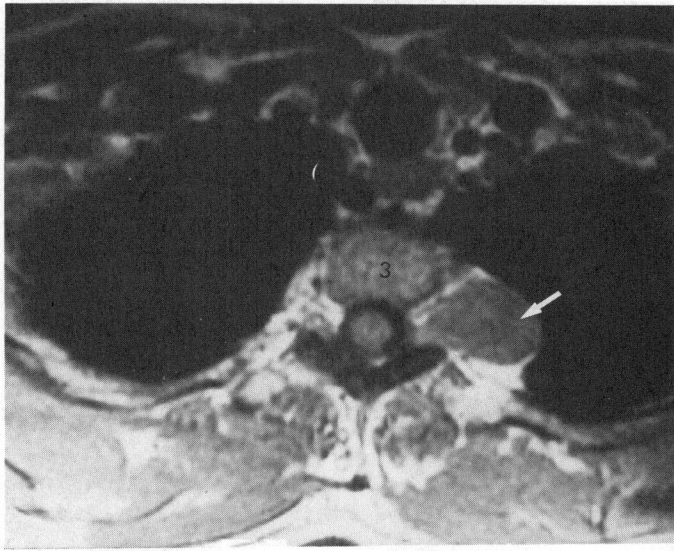

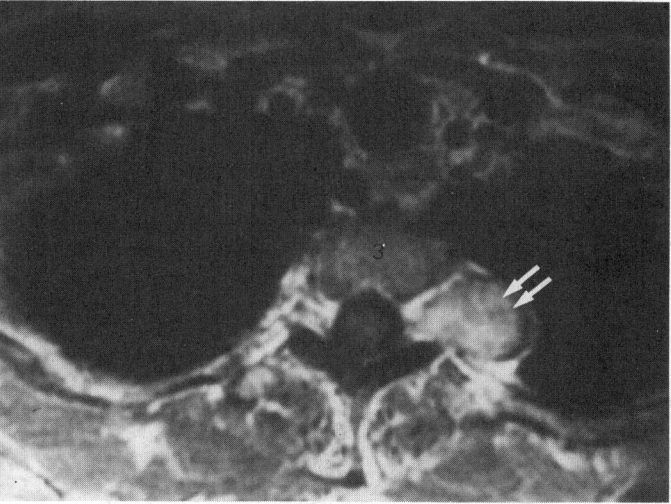

FIGURE 365-7 Neurofibroma. T1-weighted axial MRI of the spine through the D2-3 neural foramen reveals a hypointense foraminal and extraforaminal neurofibroma (*arrow*) extending into the left paraspinal region (*A*) that enhances (*double arrows*) with intravenous contrast (*B*).

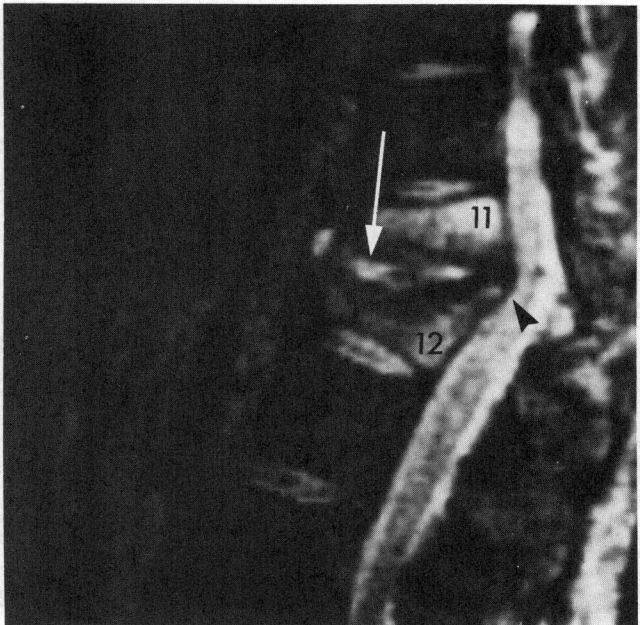

FIGURE 365-8 Osteomyelitis of the spine. T2-weighted sagittal MRI indicates hyperintense signal of the remaining D11-12 disc space (*arrow*) between the collapsed, slightly hyperintense surrounding vertebral bodies. These findings are caused by disc space infection and surrounding osteomyelitis. Posterior extension of the epidural mass represents epidural granulation tissue and abscess (*arrowhead*).

resection, but occasionally is primary and definitive. The development of detachable balloons that are attached to microcatheters has made possible the endovascular treatment of fistulas, such as carotid-cavernous or vertebral-venous fistulas. Detachable balloons and platinum coils, such as the thermoelectric detachable type, can be used to occlude intracranial and cavernous aneurysms or the parent feeding vessel. Temporary inflation of nondetachable balloons is used to predict deficiencies of neurologic function that may follow permanent surgical or balloon occlusion of vessels. Selective microcatheterization of a vessel supplying an AVM followed by injection of amobarbital also can be used to test for adverse neurologic effect prior to embolization. Nondetachable balloons may be used to dilate and treat certain cases of vasospasm secondary to subarachnoid hemorrhage from an aneurysm. Finally, preoperative embolization is often used to reduce vascularity in tumors such as meningiomas, glomus jugulare, and angiofibromas prior to surgical removal.

POSITRON EMISSION TOMOGRAPHY PET is based upon three-dimensional reconstruction of brain sections using positron-emitting radionuclides. By utilization of a number of individual radionuclides and radiolabeled moieties, it provides an opportunity to measure quantitatively: regional cerebral blood flow, blood volume, oxygen metabolism, glucose transport and metabolism, and neurotransmitter metabolism; and it permits neurotransmitter receptor localization. PET can provide spatial resolution approaching 3 to 5 mm definition in sequential slices.

Cerebrovascular disease In acute ischemic injury to the brain, PET studies demonstrate functional alterations in blood flow and oxygen metabolism when the CT scan may be normal; however, the difficulty in obtaining emergency PET studies limits its usefulness in this setting. MRI scans do show acute changes in stroke more readily than CT and are now widely used. In the assessment of long-term neurologic dysfunction after a stroke, PET scanning with deoxyglucose may show focal abnormalities that extend well beyond the lesions seen on CT or MRI. Analysis in such circumstances may provide insight into neural connections important for cognition.

Epilepsy The PET application most useful in epilepsy is assessment of glucose metabolism by measurement of brain uptake and phosphorylation of [18F]fluorodeoxyglucose (FDG). The methods are based on those developed by Sokoloff and colleagues for 2-deoxyglucose autoradiography in tissue sections. The PET scan summates approximately 40 min of local cerebral glucose metabolism and allows assessment of regional variations. PET studies have been most useful in patients with focal seizures. About 70 percent of patients with partial (focal) seizures that are refractory to medical treatment show zones of decreased glucose metabolism in the interictal state. The site of hypometabolism correlates with the epileptic focus in many patients. The same region often shows enhanced glucose metabolism if it is measured during a seizure discharge. In patients with temporal lobe seizures, it is common to find hypometabolism in one lobe.

The application of FDG-PET to evaluation of epilepsy patients undergoing consideration for surgical treatment is useful for confirming the unilaterality of sites producing electrical discharges and, in some cases, rendering intracerebral recordings unnecessary (Fig. 365-10).

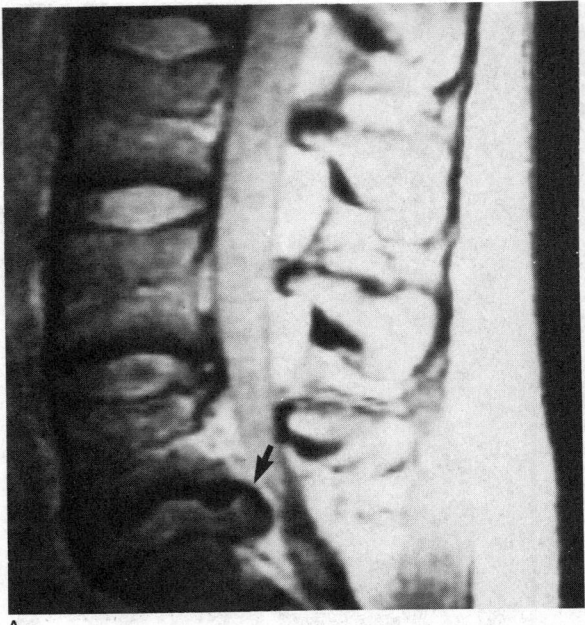

A   B

FIGURE 365-9 Herniated and extruded disc at L5-S1. *A*. The sagittal proton density MRI shows the abnormal hypointense disc (*arrow*) producing a large extradural defect. *B*. Using a 110-degree flip angle, the axial multiplanar gradient echo image shows the disc lateralized to the left (*double arrows*) compressing the S1 root sleeve and thecal sac as well as extruding caudally into the lateral recess of S1.

Neurodegenerative diseases Parkinson's nigrostriatal disease, caused by degeneration of the dopaminergic nigrostriatal pathway, can be demonstrated by [¹⁸F]6-fluoro-L-dopa (¹⁸F-FD) and PET. Decreased accumulation of ¹⁸F-FD occurs in the striatum in Parkinson's disease and during normal aging. 6-Fluoro-L-dopa is decarboxylated to 6-fluoro-L-dopamine by the enzyme aromatic L-amino acid decarboxylase, and the product then enters nerve terminals. PET allows visualization of the entrapped labeled dopamine. Decreased

FIGURE 365-10 Preoperative CT, MRI, and FDG-PET images of a patient with infantile spasms (epilepsy). Right side of the brain is to the viewer's left. CT and MRI failed to show abnormalities. Interictal PET studies revealed right occipitotemporal hypometabolism, matching the surface EEG localization of interictal discharges. (*Used with permission of Harry Chugani and Annals of Neurology.*)

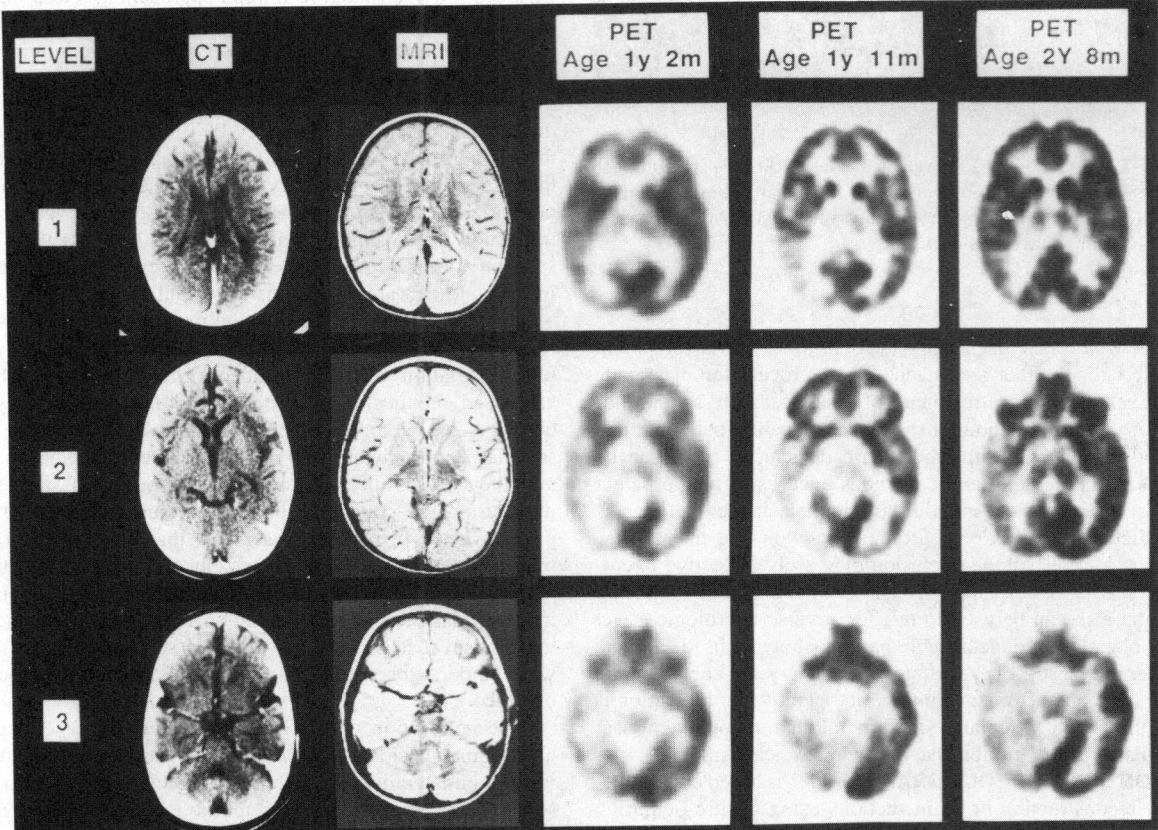

dopamine levels have been demonstrated in patients with Parkinson's disease induced by 1-methyl-4-phenyl-1,2,3,6-tetrahydropyridine and in asymptomatic drug addicts exposed to the drug, who presumably have subclinical degeneration of the nigrostriatal pathway.

Abnormalities also can be detected by FDG-PET in the basal ganglia in Huntington's disease (decreased metabolism) and in the brainstem and cerebellum in degenerative diseases such as olivopontocerebellar degeneration and Friedreich's ataxia (decreased metabolism). Decreased oxygen extraction and metabolism in the cerebral cortex may be demonstrated in Alzheimer's disease and in schizophrenia. Abnormalities in dopamine receptors have also been documented in schizophrenia. PET studies are also valuable in neuropsychological studies.

Although PET is at present primarily a research tool, its increasing availability in medical centers for cardiac imaging (see Chap. 191) makes likely more widespread application to other neurologic and psychiatric disease.

SINGLE-PHOTON EMISSION COMPUTED TOMOGRAPHY

SPECT depends on gamma-emitting radionuclides attached to molecules that can readily cross the blood-brain barrier. SPECT allows for concurrent blood flow determination and visualization of neurotransmitter receptors. For example, $[^{123}I]$isopropyl amphetamine (IMP) and $[^{99}Tc]$m-d, 1-hexamethyl-propylene-amine-oxime–labeled iodoamphetamine have been used to demonstrate abnormalities in epilepsy, Alzheimer's disease, and Parkinson's disease. However, present SPECT technology is relatively nonquantitative and insensitive in demonstrating changes, and its spatial resolution is considerably less than that of PET. On the other hand, SPECT is less expensive and more widely available. It is now widely acknowledged as a potentially important diagnostic tool for differentiation of dementia caused by Alzheimer's disease from that caused by vascular disease (multi-infarct dementia) (see Chap. 25).

MAGNETIC RESONANCE SPECTROSCOPY MRS offers the potential of assessing brain function at metabolic and molecular levels. MRS uses naturally occurring nonradioactive measurements of ^{31}P, ^{13}C, ^{23}Na, ^{7}Li, and ^{1}H. The ^{31}P MR spectrum can detect tissue concentrations of the phosphomonoesters phosphocholine and inorganic orthophosphate, the phosphodiesters glycerol-3-phospho-ethanolamine and glycerol-3-phosphocholine, the triphosphate ATP, and other phosphorus-containing molecules including phosphocreatinine. The ^{31}P MR spectrum gives quantitative analysis of these compounds in vivo with the potential of three-dimensional resolution within the brain. ^{1}H spectroscopy offers the ability to measure lactate concentrations and neuronal markers such as *N*-acetyl aspartate. At present, much of the work in this area is experimental.

MAGNETIC SOURCE IMAGING Magnetic source imaging (MSI) is based on electromagnetic field shifts created by brain electrical activity. MSI provides a new, still largely experimental method to map activity in the brain.

REFERENCES

ATLAS SW (ed): *Magnetic Resonance Imaging of the Brain and Spine*. New York, Raven, 1991

CHUGANI HT et al: Infantile spasms: I. PET identifies focal cortical dysgenesis in cryptogenic cases for surgical treatment. Ann Neurol 27:406, 1990

DUARA R et al: Positron emission tomography in Alzheimer's disease. Neurology 36:879, 1986

EDELMAN R, HESSELINK, J (eds): *Clinical Magnetic Resonance Imaging*. Philadelphia, Saunders, 1990

———, WARACH S: Magnetic resonance imaging. N Engl J Med 328:708, 1993

FELIX R et al: Brain tumors: MR imaging with gadolinium-DTPA. Radiology 156:681, 1985

JOHNSON KA et al: Single photon emission computed tomography in Alzheimer's disease: Abnormal iofetamine I 123 uptake reflects dementia severity. Arch Neurol 45:392, 1988

JUNCK L et al: PET imaging of human gliomas with ligands for the peripheral benzodiazepine binding site. Ann Neurol 26:752, 1989

LATCHAW RE (ed): *MR and CT Imaging of the Head, Neck and Spine*. 2d ed. Chicago, Mosby Year Book, 1991

LEE SH et al (eds): *Cranial MRI and CT*, 3d ed. New York, McGraw-Hill, 1992

McCARTHY G et al: Echo-planar magnetic resonance imaging studies of frontal cortex activation during word generation in humans. Proc Natl Acad Sci USA 90:4952, 1993

McGEER PL et al: Positron emission tomography in patients with clinically diagnosed Alzheimer's disease. Can Med Assoc J 134:597, 1986

MODIC MT et al (eds): *Magnetic Resonance Imaging of the Spine*. Chicago, Year Book, 1989

PETTEGREW JW et al: ^{31}P nuclear magnetic resonance study of the brain in Alzheimer's disease. J Neuropath Exp Neurol 47:235, 1988

PHELPS ME, MAZZIOTTA JC: Positron emission tomography: Human brain function and biochemistry. Science 228:799, 1985

PRICHARD JW, BRASS LM: New anatomical and functional imaging methods. Ann Neurol 32:395, 1992

QUAST MJ et al: The evolution of acute stroke recorded by multimodal magnetic resonance imaging. Magn Reson Imaging 11:465, 1993

ROSS JS et al: Magnetic resonance angiography of the extracranial carotid arteries and intracranial vessels: A review. Neurology 39:1369, 1989

SMITH ME et al: Clinical worsening in multiple sclerosis is associated with increased frequency and area of gadopentetate dimeglumine enhancing magnetic resonance imaging lesions. Ann Neurol 33:480, 1993

WILLIAMS AL, HAUGHTON VM (eds): *Cranial Computed Tomography. A Comprehensive Text*. St. Louis, Mosby, 1985

WONG DF et al: Positron emission tomography reveals elevated D_2 dopamine receptors in drug-naive schizophrenics. Science 234:1558, 1986

ZAWADZKI MB, NORMAN D: *Magnetic Resonance Imaging of the Central Nervous System*. New York, Raven, 1987

---

366 ELECTROPHYSIOLOGIC STUDIES OF THE CENTRAL AND PERIPHERAL NERVOUS SYSTEMS

MICHAEL J. AMINOFF

ELECTROENCEPHALOGRAPHY

The electrical activity of the brain (the electroencephalogram or EEG) is easily recorded from electrodes placed on the scalp. The potential difference between pairs of electrodes on the scalp (bipolar derivation) or between individual scalp electrodes and a relatively inactive common reference point (referential derivation) is amplified and displayed on paper or the screen of an oscilloscope. The findings depend on the patient's age and level of arousal. The rhythmic activity normally recorded represents the postsynaptic potentials of vertically oriented pyramidal cells of the cerebral cortex, and is characterized by its frequency. In normal awake adults lying quietly with the eyes closed, an 8–13 Hz alpha rhythm is seen posteriorly in the EEG, intermixed with a variable amount of generalized faster (beta) activity, and it is attenuated when the eyes are opened (Fig. 366-1). During drowsiness, the alpha rhythm is also attenuated; with light sleep, slower activity in the theta (4–7 Hz) and delta (<4 Hz) ranges becomes more conspicuous.

The EEG is best recorded from several different electrode arrangements (montages) in turn, and activating procedures are generally undertaken in an attempt to provoke abnormalities. Such procedures commonly include hyperventilation (for 3 or 4 min), photic stimulation, sleep, and the deprivation of sleep on the night prior to the recording.

Electroencephalography is relatively inexpensive and may aid clinical management in several different contexts.

THE EEG AND EPILEPSY The EEG is most useful in evaluating patients with suspected epilepsy. The presence of *electrographic seizure activity*, i.e., of abnormal, repetitive, rhythmic activity having an abrupt onset and termination, clearly establishes the diagnosis. The absence of such electrocerebral accompaniment does not exclude a seizure disorder, however, because there may be no change in the scalp-recorded EEG during simple or complex partial seizures. It is often not possible to obtain an EEG during clinical events that may represent seizures, especially when such events occur unpredictably or infrequently. The development of portable equipment to record the EEG continuously on cassettes for 24 h or longer in ambulatory patients

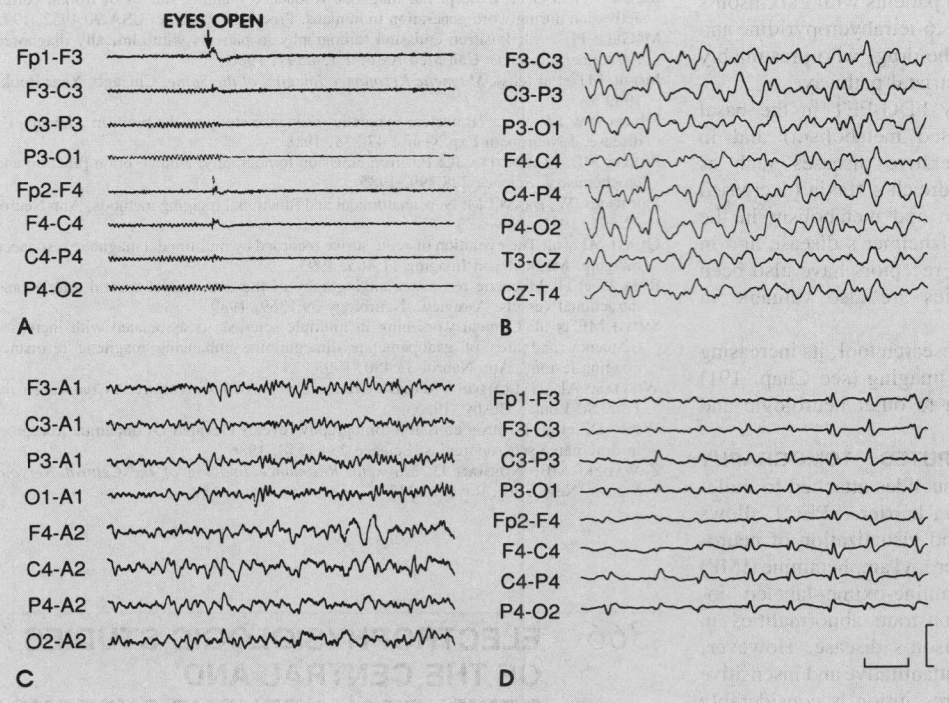

FIGURE 366-1 *A*. Normal EEG showing a posteriorly situated 9-Hz alpha rhythm that attenuates with eye opening. *B*. Abnormal EEG showing irregular diffuse slow activity in an obtunded patient with encephalitis. *C*. Irregular slow activity in the right central region, on a diffusely slowed background, in a patient with a right parietal glioma. *D*. Periodic complexes occurring once every second in a patient with Creutzfeldt-Jakob disease. Horizontal calibration: 1 s; vertical calibration: 200 μV in A, 300 μV in other panels. (*From Aminoff, 1992.*) In this and the following figure, electrode placements are indicated at the left of each panel and accord with the international 10:20 system. A, earlobe; C, central; F, frontal; Fp, frontal polar; P, parietal; T, temporal; O, occipital. Right-sided placements are indicated by even numbers, left-sided placements by odd numbers, and midline placements by Z.

has made it easier to capture the electrocerebral accompaniments of such clinical episodes, and monitoring by this means is sometimes helpful in confirming that seizures are occurring, characterizing the nature of clinically equivocal episodes, and determining the frequency of epileptic events.

The EEG findings may also be helpful in the interictal period by showing certain abnormalities that are strongly supportive of a diagnosis of epilepsy. Such *epileptiform activity* consists of bursts of abnormal discharges containing spikes or sharp waves. The presence of epileptiform activity is not specific for epilepsy, but it has a much greater prevalence in epileptics than normal subjects. When epileptiform activity is found in the EEG of a patient with episodic behavioral disturbances that clinically might be epileptic in nature, the likelihood that epilepsy is the correct diagnosis is markedly increased.

The EEG findings also have been used in classifying seizure disorders and selecting appropriate anticonvulsant medication for individual patients (Fig. 366-2). The episodic generalized spike-wave activity that occurs both during and between seizures in patients with typical absences (petit mal epilepsy) contrasts with the normal findings, focal interictal epileptiform discharges, or ictal patterns found in patients with complex partial seizures. These latter seizures may have no correlates in the scalp-recorded EEG or may be associated with abnormal rhythmic activity of variable frequency, a localized or generalized distribution, and a stereotyped pattern that varies with the patient. Focal or lateralized epileptogenic lesions are important to recognize, especially if surgical treatment is contemplated. Intensive long-term monitoring of clinical behavior and the EEG is required for operative candidates, however, and this generally also involves recording from intracranially placed electrodes (which may be subdural, extradural, or intracerebral in location).

The findings in the routine scalp-recorded EEG may indicate the prognosis of seizure disorders: in general, a normal EEG implies a better prognosis than otherwise, whereas an abnormal background or profuse epileptiform activity suggests a poor outlook. The EEG findings are not helpful in determining which patients with head injuries, stroke, or brain tumors will go on to develop seizures, because in such circumstances epileptiform activity is commonly encountered regardless of whether seizures occur. The EEG findings

are sometimes used to determine whether anticonvulsant medication can be discontinued in epileptic patients who have been seizure-free for several years, but the findings provide only a general guide to prognosis: further seizures may occur after withdrawal of anticonvulsant medication despite a normal EEG or, conversely, may not occur despite a continuing EEG abnormality. The decision to discontinue anticonvulsant medication is made on clinical grounds, and the EEG does not have a useful role in this context except for providing guidance when there is clinical ambiguity or the patient requires reassurance about a particular course of action.

The EEG has no role in the management of tonic-clonic status epilepticus except when there is clinical uncertainty whether seizures are continuing in a comatose patient. In patients treated by pentobarbital-induced coma for refractory status epilepticus, the EEG findings are useful in indicating the level of anesthesia and whether seizures are occurring. During status epilepticus, the EEG shows repeated electrographic seizures or continuous spike-wave discharges. In nonconvulsive status epilepticus, a disorder which may not be recognized unless an EEG is performed, the EEG may also show continuous spike-wave activity ("spike-wave stupor") or, less commonly, repetitive electrographic seizures (complex partial status epilepticus).

THE EEG AND COMA The EEG tends to become slower as consciousness is depressed, regardless of the underlying cause (Fig. 366-1). Other findings may also be present and may suggest diagnostic possibilities, as when electrographic seizures are found or there is a focal abnormality indicating a structural lesion. The response of the EEG to external stimulation is helpful prognostically because electrocerebral responsiveness implies a lighter level of coma than a nonreactive EEG. Serial records provide a better guide to prognosis than a single record and supplement the clinical examination in following the course of events. As the depth of coma increases, the EEG becomes nonreactive and may show a burst-suppression pattern, with bursts of mixed-frequency activity separated by intervals of relative cerebral inactivity. In other instances there is a reduction in amplitude of the EEG until eventually electrocerebral activity cannot be detected. Such electrocerebral silence does not necessarily reflect irreversible brain damage, because it may occur in hypothermic patients or with drug overdose. The prognosis of electrocerebral

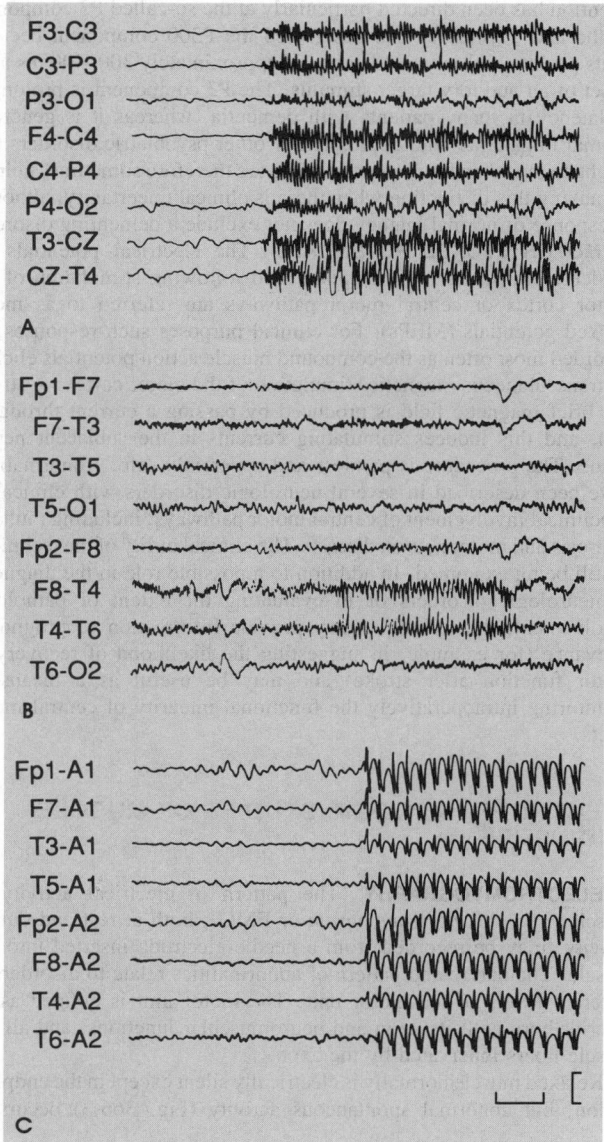

FIGURE 366-2 Electrographic seizures. *A.* Onset of a tonic seizure showing generalized repetitive sharp activity with synchronous onset over both hemispheres. *B.* Burst of repetitive spikes occurring with sudden onset in the right temporal region during a clinical spell characterized by transient impairment of external awareness. *C.* Generalized 3-Hz spike-wave activity occurring synchronously over both hemispheres during an absence (petit mal) attack. Horizontal calibration: 1 s; vertical calibration: 400 μV in A, 200 μV in B, and 750 μV in C. (*From Aminoff, 1992.*)

silence, when recorded using an adequate technique, depends upon the clinical context in which it is found. In patients with severe cerebral anoxia, for example, electrocerebral silence in a technically satisfactory record implies that useful cognitive recovery will not occur.

The EEG is usually normal in patients with locked-in syndrome and helps in distinguishing this disorder from the comatose state with which it is sometimes confused clinically.

THE EEG IN OTHER NEUROLOGIC DISORDERS In the developed countries, CT scanning and MRI have taken the place of EEG as a noninvasive means of screening for focal structural abnormalities of the brain, such as tumors, infarcts, or hematomas (Fig. 366-1). Nonetheless, the EEG is still used for this purpose in many parts of the world, although infratentorial or slowly expanding lesions may fail to cause any abnormalities. Focal slow-wave disturbances,

a localized loss of electrocerebral activity, or more generalized electrocerebral disturbances are common findings, but provide no reliable indication about the nature of the underlying pathology.

The EEG is also helpful for diagnostic purposes when it reveals the characteristic but nonspecific abnormalities found in certain neurologic disorders. The presence of complexes occurring with a regular repetition rate (so-called periodic complexes) in dementing disorders, for example, supports a diagnosis of Creutzfeldt-Jakob disease (Fig. 366-1) or subacute sclerosing panencephalitis, depending upon the appearance and frequency of the complexes and the clinical context. Focal or lateralized periodic slow-wave complexes, sometimes with a sharpened outline, in patients with an acute encephalopathy suggest a diagnosis of herpes simplex encephalitis, and periodic lateralized epileptiform discharges are commonly found with acute hemispheric pathology such as a hematoma, abscess, or rapidly expanding tumor.

The EEG generally slows in metabolic encephalopathies, and triphasic waves may be present. The findings do not permit differentiation of the underlying metabolic disturbance but help to exclude other encephalopathic processes by indicating the diffuse extent of cerebral dysfunction.

The EEG findings in dementia are nonspecific and usually do not distinguish between the different causes of cognitive decline except in rare instances when Creutzfeldt-Jakob disease or subacute sclerosing panencephalitis is responsible. The EEG may be normal or diffusely slowed, and the EEG findings alone cannot indicate whether a patient is demented or distinguish between dementia and pseudodementia.

EVOKED POTENTIALS

SENSORY EVOKED POTENTIALS The noninvasive recording of spinal or cerebral potentials elicited by stimulation of specific afferent pathways is an important means of monitoring the functional integrity of these pathways, but does not indicate the pathologic basis of lesions involving them. Such evoked potentials (EPs) are so small compared to the background EEG activity that the responses to a number of stimuli have to be recorded and averaged with a computer in order to permit their recognition and definition. The background EEG activity, which has no fixed temporal relationship to the stimulus, is averaged out by this procedure.

Visual evoked potentials (VEPs) are elicited by monocular stimulation with a reversing checkerboard pattern, and are recorded from the occipital region in the midline and on either side of the scalp. The component of major clinical importance is the so-called P100 response, a positive peak having a latency of approximately 100 ms. Its presence, latency, and symmetry over the two sides of the scalp are noted. Amplitude may also be measured, but changes in size are much less helpful for the recognition of pathology. VEPs are most useful in detecting dysfunction of the visual pathways anterior to the optic chiasm. In patients with acute severe optic neuritis the P100 is frequently lost or grossly attenuated; as clinical recovery occurs and visual acuity improves, the P100 is restored but with an increased latency that generally remains abnormally prolonged indefinitely. The VEP findings are therefore helpful in indicating previous or subclinical optic neuritis. They may also be abnormal with ocular abnormalities and with other causes of optic nerve disease, such as ischemia or compression by a tumor. Normal VEPs may be elicited by flash stimuli in patients with cortical blindness.

Brainstem auditory evoked potentials (BAEPs) are elicited by monaural stimulation with repetitive clicks, and are recorded between the vertex of the scalp and the mastoid process or ear-lobe. A series of potentials, designated by roman numerals, occur in the first 10 ms after the stimulus, and represent in part the sequential activation of different structures in the pathway between the auditory nerve (wave I) and the inferior colliculus (wave V) in the midbrain. The presence, latency, and interpeak latency of the first five positive potentials recorded at the vertex are evaluated. The findings are helpful in screening for acoustic neuromas, detecting brainstem pathology, and evaluating comatose patients. The BAEPs are normal in coma due to metabolic/toxic disorders or bihemispheric disease, but abnormal in the presence of brainstem pathology.

Somatosensory evoked potentials (SEPs) are recorded over the scalp and spine in response to electrical stimulation of a peripheral (mixed or cutaneous) nerve. The configuration, polarity, and latency of the responses depend on the nerve that is stimulated and on the recording arrangements. SEPs are used to evaluate proximal (otherwise inaccessible) portions of the peripheral nervous system and the integrity of the central somatosensory pathways.

Clinical utility of sensory evoked potentials   EP studies may detect and localize lesions in afferent pathways in the CNS. They have been used particularly to investigate patients with suspected multiple sclerosis, the diagnosis of which requires the recognition of lesions involving several different regions of the central white matter. In patients with clinical evidence of only one lesion, the electrophysiologic recognition of abnormalities in other sites helps to suggest or support the diagnosis, but does not establish it unequivocally. In patients with suspected multiple sclerosis (or other neurologic disorders) who have vague, ill-defined complaints, the organic basis of symptoms may be supported by the presence of EP abnormalities in the appropriate afferent pathway. MRI is also helpful in detecting lesions in patients with possible multiple sclerosis, but electrophysiologic studies are cheaper and monitor the functional rather than anatomic status of the afferent pathways under study. Moreover, the electrophysiologic studies occasionally reveal abnormalities missed by MRI or vice versa. The two techniques therefore complement each other. Normal electrophysiologic (or imaging) findings do not exclude multiple sclerosis when this is a clinical possibility. In established multiple sclerosis, the use of EP studies to follow the disorder or its response to treatment is of uncertain value and unjustified at the present time.

EP abnormalities occur in disorders other than multiple sclerosis that involve the afferent pathways under test. Even multimodality EP abnormalities are not specific for MS; they may occur in AIDS, Lyme disease, systemic lupus erythematosus, neurosyphilis, spinocerebellar degenerations, familial spastic paraplegia, and deficiency of vitamin E or B_{12}. The diagnostic utility of the electrophysiologic findings therefore depends upon the circumstances in which they are found. Abnormalities may aid in the localization of lesions to broad areas of the CNS, but attempts at precise localization on electrophysiologic grounds are misleading because the generators of many components of the EP are unknown.

The EP findings are sometimes of prognostic relevance. Bilateral loss of those SEP components that are generated in the cerebral cortex implies that cognition may not be regained in posttraumatic or postanoxic coma, and EP studies may also be useful in evaluating patients with suspected brain death. In patients with spinal cord injuries, SEPs have been used to indicate the completeness of the lesion—the presence or early return of a cortically generated response to stimulation of a nerve below the injured segment of the cord indicates an incomplete lesion and thus a better prognosis for functional recovery than otherwise. Intraoperative monitoring of function in neural structures placed at risk by the surgical procedure may permit the early recognition of dysfunction, but whether this enables any permanent deficit to be averted or minimized by alteration of the responsible operative manipulation has not been established.

Visual and auditory acuity have been determined by ophthalmologists and audiologists using EP techniques in patients whose age or mental state precludes their cooperation for behavioral testing.

COGNITIVE EVOKED POTENTIALS   Certain EP components depend upon the mental attention of the subject and the setting in which the stimulus occurs, rather than simply on the physical characteristics of the stimulus. Such "event-related" or "endogenous" potentials (ERPs) are related in some manner to the cognitive aspects of distinguishing an infrequently occurring target stimulus from other stimuli occurring more frequently. For clinical purposes,

attention has been directed particularly at the so-called P3 component of the ERP, which is also designated the P300 component because of its positive polarity and latency of approximately 300–400 ms after onset of an auditory target stimulus. The P3 component is prolonged in latency in many patients with dementia, whereas it is generally normal in patients with depression or other psychiatric disorders that might be mistaken for dementia. ERPs are therefore sometimes helpful in making this distinction when there is clinical uncertainty, although a response of normal latency does not exclude a dementing disorder.

MOTOR EVOKED POTENTIALS   The electrical potentials recorded from muscle or the spinal cord following stimulation of the motor cortex or central motor pathways are referred to as motor evoked potentials (MEPs). For clinical purposes such responses are recorded most often as the compound muscle action potentials elicited by transcutaneous magnetic stimulation of the motor cortex. A strong but brief magnetic field is produced by passing a current through a coil, and this induces stimulating currents in the subjacent neural tissue. The procedure is painless and apparently safe. Abnormalities have been described in several neurologic disorders with clinical or subclinical involvement of central motor pathways, including multiple sclerosis and motor neuron disease. The clinical utility of the technique is still being examined. In addition to a possible role in the diagnosis of neurologic disorders or in evaluating the extent of pathologic involvement, the technique may provide information of prognostic relevance (for example, in suggesting the likelihood of recovery of motor function after stroke) and may be useful as a means of monitoring intraoperatively the functional integrity of central motor tracts.

ELECTROPHYSIOLOGIC STUDIES OF MUSCLE AND NERVE

ELECTROMYOGRAPHY   The pattern of electrical activity in muscle (i.e., the *electromyogram* or EMG), both at rest and during activity, may be recorded from a needle electrode inserted into the muscle. The nature and pattern of abnormalities relate to disorders at different levels of the motor unit. The motor unit is defined as an anterior horn cell, its axon and neuromuscular junctions, and all the muscle fibers innervated by the axon.

Relaxed muscle normally is electrically silent except in the endplate region, but abnormal spontaneous activity (Fig. 366-3) occurs in

FIGURE 366-3   Activity recorded during EMG. *A*. Spontaneous fibrillation potentials and positive sharp waves. *B*. Complex repetitive discharges recorded in partially denervated muscle at rest. *C*. Normal triphasic motor unit action potential. *D*. Small, short-duration, polyphasic motor unit action potential such as is commonly encountered in myopathic disorders. *E*. Long-duration polyphasic motor unit action potential such as may be seen in neuropathic disorders.

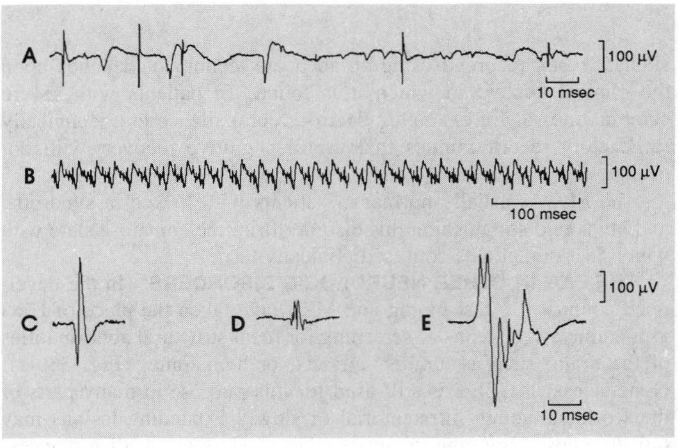

various neuromuscular disorders. Fibrillation potentials and positive sharp waves (which reflect muscle fiber irritability) and complex repetitive discharges are most often—but not always—found in denervated muscle and may also occur after muscle injury and in certain myopathic disorders, especially inflammatory disorders such as polymyositis. Fasciculation potentials (which reflect the spontaneous activity of individual motor units) are characteristic of neuropathic disorders, especially those with degeneration of anterior horn cells (such as amyotrophic lateral sclerosis). Myotonic discharges—high-frequency discharges of potentials derived from single muscle fibers that wax and wane in amplitude and frequency—are the signature of myotonic disorders such as myotonic dystrophy or myotonia congenita, but occur occasionally in polymyositis or other, rarer, disorders.

Slight voluntary contraction of a muscle leads to activation of a small number of motor units. The potentials generated by any muscle fibers of these units that are within the pick-up range of the needle electrode will be recorded (Fig. 366-3). The parameters of normal motor unit action potentials depend on the muscle under study and age of the patient, but their duration is normally between 5 and 15 ms, amplitude is between 200 µV and 2 mV, and most are bi- or triphasic; the number of units activated depends on the degree of voluntary activity. The incidence of small, short-duration, polyphasic motor unit action potentials (i.e., having more than four phases) is usually increased in myopathic muscle, and an excessive number of units is activated for a specified degree of voluntary activity. By contrast the loss of motor units that occurs in neuropathic disorders leads to a reduction in number of units activated during a maximal contraction and an increase in their firing rate; the configuration and dimensions of the potentials may also be abnormal depending on the duration of the neuropathic process and on whether reinnervation has occurred.

Electromyography (EMG) enables disorders of the motor units to be detected and characterized as either neurogenic or myopathic. In neurogenic disorders, the pattern of affected muscles may localize the lesion to the anterior horn cells or to a specific site as the axons traverse a nerve root, limb plexus, and peripheral nerve to their terminal arborizations. The findings do not enable a specific etiologic diagnosis to be made, however, except in conjunction with the clinical findings and results of other laboratory studies.

The findings may provide a guide to the severity of an acute disorder of a peripheral or cranial nerve (by indicating whether denervation has occurred and the completeness of the lesion), and whether the pathologic process is active or progressive in chronic or degenerative disorders such as amyotrophic lateral sclerosis. Such information is important for prognostic purposes.

Various quantitative EMG approaches have been developed. The most common is to determine the mean duration and amplitude of 20 motor unit action potentials using a standardized technique. The technique of macro-EMG provides information about the number and size of muscle fibers in a larger volume of the motor unit territory, and has also been used to estimate the number of motor units in a muscle. Scanning EMG is a computer-based technique that has been used to study the topography of motor unit action potentials and, in particular, the spatial and temporal distribution of activity in individual units. Both of these latter approaches are of limited interest except to specialists and merit no further discussion. The technique of single-fiber EMG is of immediate clinical relevance, however, and is discussed separately below.

NERVE CONDUCTION STUDIES Recording of the electrical response of a muscle to stimulation of its motor nerve at two or more points along its course (Fig. 366-4) permits conduction velocity to be determined in the fastest-conducting motor fibers between the points of stimulation. Similarly, sensory nerve conduction studies are performed by determining the conduction velocity and amplitude of action potentials in sensory fibers when these fibers are stimulated at one point and the responses are recorded at another point along the course of the nerve. In adults, conduction velocity in the arms is

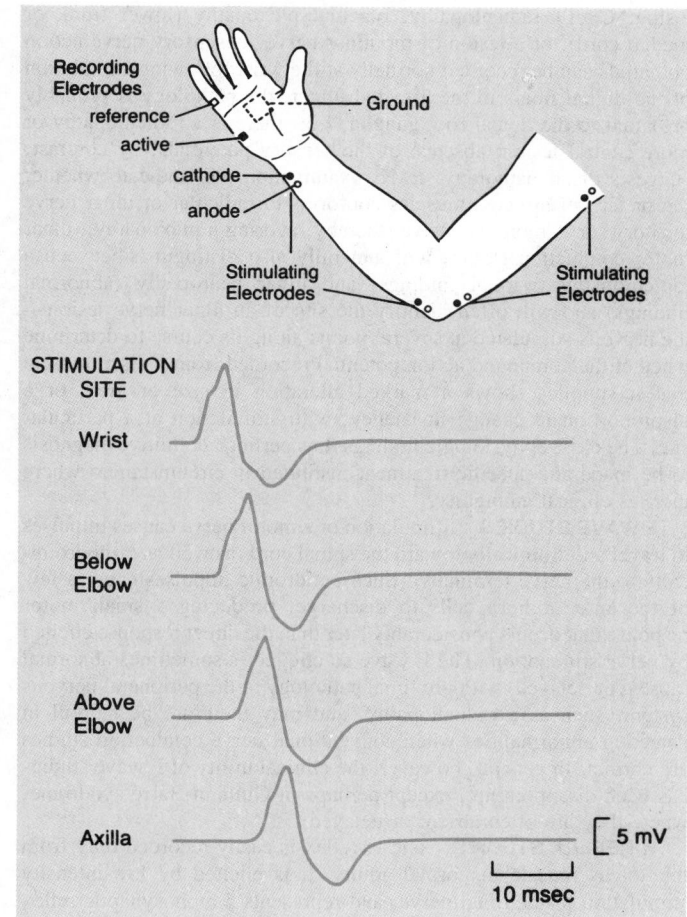

FIGURE 366-4 Arrangement for motor conduction studies of the ulnar nerve. Responses are recorded with a surface electrode from the abductor digiti minimi muscle to supramaximal stimulation of the nerve at different sites, and are shown in the lower panel. (*From Aminoff, 1987.*)

normally between 50 and 70 m/s, and in the legs is between 40 and 60 m/s.

Nerve conduction studies complement the EMG examination, enabling the presence and extent of peripheral nerve pathology to be determined. They are particularly helpful in determining whether sensory symptoms are arising from pathology proximal or distal to the dorsal root ganglia (in the former instance, peripheral sensory conduction studies will be normal) and whether neuromuscular dysfunction relates to peripheral nerve disease. In patients with a mononeuropathy, they are invaluable as a means of localizing a focal lesion, determining the extent and severity of the underlying pathology, providing a guide to prognosis, and detecting subclinical involvement of other peripheral nerves. They enable a polyneuropathy to be distinguished from a mononeuropathy multiplex when this is not possible clinically, an important distinction because of the etiological implications. Nerve conduction studies provide a means of following the progression and therapeutic response of peripheral nerve disorders, and may suggest the underlying pathologic basis in individual cases. Conduction velocity is often markedly slowed and conduction block may occur in the acquired demyelinating neuropathies, whereas conduction velocity is normal or slowed only mildly, sensory nerve action potentials are small or absent, and there is EMG evidence of denervation in axonal neuropathies.

The utility and complementary role of EMG and nerve conduction studies are best illustrated by reference to a common clinical problem. Numbness and paresthesias of the little finger and associated wasting of the intrinsic muscles of the hand may result from a spinal cord lesion, C8/T1 radiculopathy, brachial plexopathy (lower trunk or medial cord), or a lesion of the ulnar nerve. If sensory nerve action potentials can be recorded normally at the wrist following stimulation of the digital fibers in the affected finger, the pathology is probably proximal to the dorsal root ganglia, i.e., there is a radiculopathy or more central lesion; absence of the sensory potentials, by contrast, suggests distal pathology. EMG examination will indicate whether the pattern of affected muscles conforms to radicular or ulnar nerve territory, or is more extensive (thereby favoring a plexopathy); ulnar motor conduction studies will generally also distinguish between a radiculopathy (normal findings) and ulnar neuropathy (abnormal findings) and will often identify the site of an ulnar nerve lesion— the nerve is stimulated at several points along its course to determine whether the compound action potential recorded from a distal muscle that it supplies shows a marked alteration in size or area, or a disproportionate change in latency, with stimulation at a particular site. The electrophysiologic findings thus permit a definitive diagnosis to be made and specific treatment instituted in circumstances where there is clinical ambiguity.

F WAVE STUDIES   Stimulation of a motor nerve causes impulses to travel antidromically toward the spinal cord (as well as orthodromically to the nerve terminals). Such antidromic impulses cause a few of the anterior horn cells to discharge, producing a small motor response that occurs considerably later than the direct response elicited by nerve stimulation. The F wave so elicited is sometimes abnormal (absent or delayed) with proximal pathology of the peripheral nervous system, such as a radiculopathy, and may therefore be helpful in detecting abnormalities when conventional nerve conduction studies are normal. In general, however, the clinical utility of F wave studies has been disappointing, except perhaps in Guillain-Barré syndrome, where they are often absent or delayed.

H REFLEX STUDIES   The H reflex is easily recorded only from the soleus muscle in normal adults. It is elicited by low-intensity stimulation of the tibial nerve, and represents a monosynaptic reflex in which spindle (Ia) afferent fibers constitute the afferent arc and alpha motor axons the efferent pathway. The H reflexes are often absent bilaterally in elderly patients or with polyneuropathies, and may be lost unilaterally in S1 radiculopathies.

MUSCLE RESPONSE TO REPETITIVE NERVE STIMULATION   The size of the electrical response of a muscle to supramaximal electrical stimulation of its motor nerve relates to the number of muscle fibers that are activated. Neuromuscular transmission can be tested by several different protocols, but the most helpful is to record with surface electrodes the electrical response of a muscle to supramaximal stimulation of its motor nerve by repetitive (2 to 3 Hz) shocks delivered before and at selected intervals after a maximal voluntary contraction.

There is normally little or no change in size of the compound muscle action potential following repetitive stimulation of a motor nerve at 2 to 3 Hz with stimuli delivered at intervals after voluntary contraction of the muscle for about 20 to 30 s, even though preceding activity in the junctional region influences the release of acetylcholine and thus the size of the endplate potentials elicited by a test stimulus. This is because more acetylcholine is normally released than is required to bring the motor endplate potentials to the threshold for generating muscle fiber action potentials. In disorders of neuromuscular transmission this safety factor is reduced. Thus, in myasthenia gravis repetitive stimulation, particularly at a rate of between 2 and 5 Hz, may lead to a depression of neuromuscular transmission, with a decrement in size of the response recorded from affected muscles. Similarly, immediately after a period of maximal voluntary activity, single or repetitive stimuli of the motor nerve may elicit larger muscle responses than before, indicating that more muscle fibers are responding. This postactivation facilitation of neuromuscular transmission is followed by a longer-lasting period of depression, maximal between 2 and 4 min after the conditioning period and lasting for as long as 10 min or so, during which responses are reduced in size.

Decrementing responses to repetitive stimulation at 2 to 5 Hz are common in myasthenia gravis but may also occur in the congenital myasthenic syndromes. In Lambert-Eaton myasthenic syndrome, in which there is defective release of acetylcholine at the neuromuscular junction, the compound muscle action potential elicited by a single stimulus is generally very small. With repetitive stimulation at rates of up to 10 Hz, the first few responses may decline in size, but subsequent responses increase. If faster rates of stimulation are used (20 to 50 Hz), the increment may be dramatic so that the amplitude of compound muscle action potentials eventually reaches a size that is several times larger than the initial response. In patients with botulism, the response to repetitive stimulation is similar to that in Lambert-Eaton syndrome, although the findings are somewhat more variable and not all muscles are affected.

SINGLE-FIBER ELECTROMYOGRAPHY   The technique of single-fiber EMG is particularly helpful in detecting disorders of neuromuscular transmission. A special needle electrode is placed within a muscle and positioned to record action potentials from two muscle fibers belonging to the same motor unit. The time interval between the two potentials will vary in consecutive discharges, and this is called the *neuromuscular jitter*. The jitter can be quantified as the mean difference between consecutive interpotential intervals, and is normally between 10 and 50 µs. This value is increased when neuromuscular transmission is disturbed for any reason, and in some instances impulses in individual muscle fibers may fail to occur because of impulse blocking at the neuromuscular junction. Single-fiber EMG is more sensitive than repetitive nerve stimulation or determination of acetylcholine receptor antibody levels in diagnosing myasthenia gravis.

Single-fiber EMG can also be used to determine mean fiber density of motor units (i.e., mean number of muscle fibers per motor unit within the recording area) and to estimate the number of motor units in a muscle, but this is of less immediate clinical relevance.

BLINK REFLEXES   Electrical or mechanical stimulation of the supraorbital nerve on one side leads to two separate reflex responses of the orbicularis oculi—an ipsilateral R1 response having a latency of approximately 10 ms and a bilateral R2 response with a latency in the order of 30 ms. The trigeminal and facial nerves constitute the afferent and efferent arcs of the reflex, respectively. Abnormalities of either nerve or intrinsic lesions of the medulla or pons may lead to uni- or bilateral loss of the response, and the findings may therefore be helpful in identifying or localizing such pathology.

TESTS OF AUTONOMIC FUNCTION

Noninvasive tests of autonomic function are becoming increasingly important for the recognition of small-fiber peripheral neuropathies and in defining central dysautonomias, such as the Shy-Drager syndrome. Invasive tests, such as microneurography, provide information of considerable academic importance, but because of their specialized nature and limited clinical utility they are not discussed further.

Tests of *heart-rate responses* to various maneuvers are easy to perform, safe, reproducible, and provide clinically relevant information. One such test is to record the heart-rate response to deep breathing for 1 min at a rate of approximately six breaths per minute. In normal persons a tachycardia occurs during inspiration and a bradycardia during expiration. The difference in heart rate between inspiration and expiration is age-dependent, but is usually more than about 15 beats per minute. Heart-rate variation of less than 10 is clearly abnormal, and suggests vagal dysfunction. The Valsalva ratio, which depends on both vagal and sympathetic function, is also a sensitive indicator of autonomic dysfunction. It is determined from the maximum heart rate generated during a forced expiratory maneuver and the slowest heart rate following the maneuver. It is conveniently recorded with an electrocardiograph—the longest interbeat interval after the maneuver is divided by the shortest interbeat interval during it. Another approach is to record the heart-rate changes that occur with change from a supine to erect posture; the heart rate increases in the first 15 s or so and then slows. The ratio of the heart rates or the R-R intervals at the 30th and 15th beats after standing, which is age-dependent, has therefore been used as an index of vagal function.

Sudomotor function has been evaluated in various ways. Perhaps the easiest is the thermoregulatory sweat test, in which the patient's body temperature is increased by 1°C by radiant heat from a heat cradle, and the presence and distribution of sweat is noted by a change in color of an indicator powder placed on the skin. This provides information about the integrity of pre- and postganglionic sympathetic fibers, and the distribution of abnormalities may suggest the underlying pathology. Because it is so time consuming, however, alternative approaches have been favored. One simple approach is to measure the skin potential in response to electrical stimulation. This depends upon activation of sweat glands, but is of limited utility because only an absent response, and not the latency or size of the response, indicates an abnormality. The test is therefore nonquantitative, and the response habituates rapidly, further complicating interpretation. The quantitative sudomotor axon reflex test (QSART) is more complicated, but is sensitive, specific, and reproducible. The function of postganglionic sudomotor fibers is evaluated in selected sites in the limbs by accurate determination of sweat output in response to iontophoresed acetylcholine.

Adrenergic function can be tested most easily by recording the blood pressure with the patient supine and then tilted into a 60° head-up position. Other approaches include recording the rise in systolic and diastolic blood pressure, and in heart rate, to sustained hand grip. Sympathetic efferent activity can also be evaluated qualitatively by determining whether peripheral blood flow is reduced, or arterial blood pressure is increased, by emotional stress (such as from a sudden loud noise or attempted mental arithmetic despite being distracted).

REFERENCES

AMINOFF MJ: *Electromyography in Clinical Practice: Electrodiagnostic Aspects of Neuromuscular Disease*, 2d ed. New York, Churchill Livingstone, 1987

AMINOFF MJ (ed): *Electrodiagnosis in Clinical Neurology*, 3d ed. New York, Churchill Livingstone, 1992

DALY DD, PEDLEY TA (eds): *Current Practice of Clinical Electroencephalography*, 2d ed. New York, Raven Press, 1990

EBERSOLE JS (ed): *Ambulatory EEG Monitoring*. New York, Raven Press, 1988

KIMURA J: *Electrodiagnosis in Diseases of Nerve and Muscle*, 2d ed. Philadelphia, Davis, 1989

NIEDERMEYER E, LOPES DA SILVA F (eds): *Electroencephalography*, 3d ed. Baltimore, Urban & Schwarzenberg, 1993

367 THE EPILEPSIES AND CONVULSIVE DISORDERS

MARC A. DICHTER

The *epilepsies* are a group of disorders characterized by chronic, recurrent, paroxysmal changes in neurologic function caused by abnormalities in the electrical activity of the brain. They are estimated to affect between 0.5 and 2 percent of the population and can occur at any age. Each episode of neurologic dysfunction is called a *seizure*. Seizures may be *convulsive* when they are accompanied by motor mainfestations or may be manifest by other changes in neurologic function (i.e., sensory, cognitive, emotional events). Epilepsy can be acquired as a result of neurologic injury or a structural brain lesion and also can occur as a part of many systemic medical diseases.

Epilepsy also occurs in an *idiopathic* form in an individual with neither a history of neurologic insult nor other apparent neurologic dysfunction and may have a genetic cause. Isolated, nonrecurrent seizures may occur in otherwise healthy individuals for a variety of reasons, and under these circumstances, the individual is *not* said to have epilepsy.

CLASSIFICATION OF SEIZURES AND EPILEPSY SYNDROMES

The neurologic manifestations of epileptic seizures are varied, ranging from a brief lapse of attention to a prolonged loss of consciousness with abnormal motor activity. The proper classification of the kinds of seizures which an individual is experiencing is important for an appropriate diagnostic workup, prognostic evaluation, and selection of therapy. The classification of epileptic seizures provided in this chapter is based on the International League Against Epilepsy (ILAE) classification of epileptic seizures. It emphasizes the clinical seizure type and ictal (seizure-associated) and interictal (between-seizure) electroencephalographic pattern (Table 367-1), whereas etiology, anatomic substrate, and pathways of spread are not major considerations. The older terminology of grand mal, petit mal, and psychomotor or temporal lobe epilepsy has been integrated into the current scheme. In addition to identifying the seizure types which an individual is experiencing, it is also useful to categorize the clinical context within which the seizures occur. Epilepsy syndromes which take into account the age of the patient, types of seizures, presence of underlying neurologic lesion, etc. help define groups of patients with relatively predictable prognoses and for whom specific therapies are indicated. A detailed description of these syndromes is beyond the scope of this chapter. However, Table 367-2 summarizes the ILAE classification of the epilepsies and epilepsy syndromes.

The major underlying premise of the seizure classification is that some seizures (partial or focal seizures) start in one area of brain (cortex) and either remain localized or secondarily generalize (i.e., spread throughout the brain), whereas other seizures appear to be generalized from their earliest manifestation.

PARTIAL OR FOCAL SEIZURES Partial or focal seizures begin with the activation of neurons in one area of cortex. The specific clinical symptoms depend on the area of cortex involved and imply

---

TABLE 367-1 Classification of epileptic seizures

PARTIAL OR FOCAL SEIZURES

Simple partial seizures (with motor, sensory, autonomic, or psychic signs)
Complex partial seizures (psychomotor or temporal lobe seizures)
Secondary generalized partial seizures

PRIMARY GENERALIZED SEIZURES

Tonic-clonic (grand mal)
Tonic
Absence (petit mal)
Atypical absence
Myoclonic
Atonic
Infantile spasms

STATUS EPILEPTICUS

Tonic-clonic status
Absence status
Epilepsia partialis continua

RECURRENCE PATTERNS

Sporadic
Cyclic
Reflex (photomyoclonic, somatosensory, musicogenic, reading epilepsy)

TABLE 367-2 Classification of epilepsies and epileptic syndromes

LOCALIZATION-RELATED (FOCAL, LOCAL, PARTIAL) EPILEPSIES AND SYNDROMES

Idiopathic, with age-related onset
  Benign childhood epilepsy with centrotemporal spike
  Childhood epilepsy with occipital paroxysms
Symptomatic—syndromes of great individual variability based on anatomic
  localization, clinical features, seizure types, and etiologic factors (if
  known)

GENERALIZED EPILEPSIES AND SYNDROMES

Idiopathic, with age-related onset
  Benign neonatal familial convulsions
  Benign neonatal convulsions
  Benign myoclonic epilepsy in infancy
  Childhood absence epilepsy (pyknolepsy)
  Juvenile absence epilepsy
  Juvenile myoclonic epilepsy (impulsive petit mal)
  Epilepsy with grand mal seizures (GTCS) on awakening
Idiopathic and/or symptomatic
  West syndrome (infantile spasms)
  Lennox-Gastaut syndrome
  Epilepsy with myoclonic-astatic seizures
  Epilepsy with myoclonic absences
Symptomatic
  Nonspecific etiology—early myoclonic encephalopathy
  Specific syndromes—epileptic seizures may complicate many diseases

EPILEPSIES AND SYNDROMES UNDETERMINED AS TO WHETHER THEY ARE FOCAL OR GENERALIZED

With both generalized and focal seizures
  Neonatal seizures
  Severe myoclonic epilepsy in infancy
  Epilepsy with continuous spikes during slow wave sleep
  Acquired epileptic aphasia (Landau-Kleffner syndrome)
Without unequivocal generalized or focal features

SPECIAL SYNDROMES

Situation-related seizures
  Febrile convulsions
  Seizures related to other identifiable situations such as stress, hormonal
    changes, drugs, alcohol, or sleep deprivation
Isolation, apparently unprovoked epileptic events
Epilepsies characterized by specific modes of seizure precipitation
Chronic progressive epilepsia partialis continua of childhood

---

dysfunction in a limited area of the cortex. The seizures may be due to birth injury, postnatal trauma, tumor, abscess, infarction, vascular malformation, or some other structural abnormality. The abnormal area of cortex underlying the seizure activity can be identified by the specific neurologic phenomena observed during the focal seizure. Partial seizures are classified as *simple* if there is no alteration of consciousness or awareness of the environment and *complex* if there is such a change.

Simple partial seizures Simple partial seizures can occur with motor, sensory, autonomic, or psychic symptoms. A simple partial seizure with motor signs consists of recurrent contractions of the muscles of one part of the body (finger, hand, arm, face, etc.) without loss of consciousness. Each muscular contraction is caused by the discharge of neurons in the corresponding area of the contralateral motor cortex.

The initial symptoms of a partial seizure (*ictus*) may remain confined to one area or may spread from the affected area to involve contiguous ipsilateral body parts (i.e., right thumb to right hand to right arm to right side of the face). This "Jacksonian march," first described by Hughlings Jackson, is caused by a demonstrable progression of epileptiform discharges in the contralateral motor cortex and may occur over seconds or minutes. The electroencephalographic manifestations of this form of seizure are often very striking and consist of regularly occurring spike discharges in the appropriate area

of motor cortex. Between seizures (*interictal period*) this region may give rise to irregular spike discharges in the EEG.

Simple partial seizures may have other behavioral manifestations if the seizure discharges occur in other cortical regions. Thus sensory symptoms (i.e., paresthesias, vertiginous feelings, simple auditory or visual hallucinations) occur with epileptiform discharges in the contralateral sensory cortex, and autonomic and psychic symptoms [i.e., the sensation of having experienced something before (déjà vu), unwarranted sense of fear or anger, illusions, and even complex hallucinations] occur with discharges in temporal and frontal lobes.

Complex partial seizures (temporal lobe or psychomotor seizures) Complex partial seizures are episodic changes in behavior in which an individual loses conscious contact with the environment. The onset of these seizures may consist of any of a variety of auras: an unusual smell (as of burning rubber), a feeling that the current experience has happened before (déjà vu), a sudden intense emotional feeling, a sensory illusion such as that of objects growing smaller (micropsia) or larger (macropsia), or a specific formed sensory hallucination. Patients may come to recognize these as heralding their seizures, or the memory of the aura may be lost in the postictal amnesia that often occurs if the seizure becomes generalized. During complex partial seizures, there may be a cessation of activity with some minor motor activity, such as lip smacking, swallowing, walking aimlessly, or picking at one's clothes (automatisms). Complex partial seizures also may be accompanied by the unconscious performance of highly skilled activities such as driving a car or playing complicated musical pieces. When the seizure ends, the individual is amnesic for events which took place during the seizure and may take minutes or hours to recover full consciousness.

Patients with complex partial seizures have EEGs which exhibit unilateral or bilateral spikes, sharp waves, or slow wave discharges over temporal or frontotemporal regions both interictally and during seizures. Most of these seizures originate from epileptiform activity in the temporal lobes—especially the hippocampus or amygdala—or other parts of the limbic system, but others have been shown to originate from mesial parasagittal or orbital frontal regions. Epilepsy manifest by these kinds of seizures is also referred to as *temporal lobe epilepsy* and *psychomotor epilepsy* in older classification schemes.

Although often showing spike discharges or focal slowing during complex partial seizures, exceptionally, the surface EEG may be normal. Sphenoidal electrodes may record the abnormal discharges, but in some cases only depth electrodes in the hippocampus or amygdala or other limbic structures will show seizure discharges. The occasional discrepancy between surface and depth electrophysiologic events is a particularly difficult problem when trying to use the surface EEG to determine the nature of an abnormal behavior in an individual suspected of having complex partial seizures (see "Differential Diagnosis of Seizures," below).

Secondary generalization of partial seizures Simple or complex partial seizures can progress to generalized seizures with loss of consciousness and often with convulsive motor activity. This may occur immediately or after many seconds or a minute or two. In addition, many patients with focal seizures have generalized seizures without an obvious initial focal component which are difficult to distinguish from primary generalized seizures. The presence of an aura or the observation of any focal feature (twitching of one extremity, aphasia, tonic eye deviation) at the onset of the generalized seizure or the presence of a postictal focal neurologic deficit (Todd's paralysis) is an important clue to a focal origin to the seizure.

PRIMARY GENERALIZED SEIZURES **Tonic-clonic (grand mal)** One of the most common kinds of epileptic paroxysms is the generalized tonic-clonic seizure. Some of these appear to be primary generalized seizures, and others are the result of secondary generalization from partial seizures. In either case, the seizures follow a common pattern. The primary generalized seizures usually start without warning, although some individuals sense a vague, nonspecific sense of the impending event. The onset is heralded by a sudden loss of consciousness, a *tonic* contraction of the muscles, a loss of postural control, and a cry produced by a forced expiration caused by contraction of the respiratory muscles. The individual falls to the floor in an opisthotonic posture, often sustaining injury, and remains rigid for many seconds. There may be cyanosis as respiration is inhibited. Soon a series of rhythmic contractions of all four limbs occurs. This *clonic* phase can last for a variable period of time and ends when the muscles relax. The individual may remain unconscious for a period of minutes or longer. There is usually a gradual return to consciousness and a period of disorientation during recovery. The patient may even be combative if restrained. During the seizure, urinary or fecal incontinence and tongue biting may occur. Postictally, there is amnesia for the seizure and sometimes a retrograde amnesia as well. Headache and drowsiness are common sequelae, and the individual may not return to baseline functioning for days.

The EEG in patients with tonic-clonic seizures shows low-voltage fast (10 Hz or more) activity during the tonic phase, which converts gradually to slower, larger sharp waves throughout both hemispheres. During the clonic phase, there are bursts of sharp waves associated with the rhythmic muscular contractions and slow waves coincident with the pauses. Often the excessive muscular activity of the seizure causes artifacts which interfere with ictal EEG recordings. Interictally, the EEG is often abnormal, with polyspike (or spike) and wave or occasionally sharp and slow wave discharges; interictal EEGs also may be normal.

Tonic seizures Tonic seizures are a less common form of primary generalized seizure which consist of the sudden occurrence of a rigid posturing of the limbs or torso, often with deviation of the head and eyes toward one side. They are not followed by a clonic phase and are often of shorter duration than tonic-clonic seizures.

Absence seizures (petit mal) Pure absence seizures consist of the sudden cessation of ongoing conscious activity without convulsive muscular activity or loss of postural control. Such seizures may be so brief as to be inapparent. Usually they last for seconds and occasionally as long as several minutes. The brief lapses of consciousness or awareness may be accompanied by minor motor manifestations such as eyelid fluttering, small chewing movements of the mouth, or mild shaking of the hands. During longer absences, automatisms may occur which may be difficult to distinguish from complex partial seizures. At the end of the absence seizure, the patient regains awareness of the environment very quickly, and there is usually no period of postictal confusion.

Absence seizures almost always begin in young children (6 to 14 years of age), although occasionally they appear for the first time in older adults. These brief seizures may occur hundreds or more times per day and go on for weeks or months before it is recognized that the child is having seizures. Absence seizures may first be recognized when the child begins having learning difficulties in school.

The EEG is pathognomonic in this form of seizure disorder. Brief 3-Hz spike and wave discharges, which appear synchronously throughout all the leads, occur interictally but become clinically significant as absence seizures when they last more then several seconds. Interictal EEG background activity is otherwise normal. Often the EEG demonstrates that the child is having more seizures than was thought from clinical observation alone.

Absence seizures usually occur in otherwise neurologically normal children. These seizures are usually sensitive to antiepileptic drugs (see below). Children with this condition often do quite well once it is treated. Approximately one-third outgrow the seizure disorder, one-third continue to have only absence seizures, and one-third have concomitant generalized tonic-clonic seizures.

Absence seizures can be differentiated from absence-like attacks which occasionally occur in complex partial seizures by the lack of aura, immediate recovery from the absence, and typical 3-Hz spike and wave EEG pattern.

Atypical absence Atypical absence seizures are similar to absence seizures but coexist with other forms of generalized seizures, such as tonic seizures, myoclonic seizures or atonic seizures (see below). The EEG is more heterogeneous, containing spike and wave discharges at 2 or 4 Hz during the absence attacks and poorly developed background with spike or polyspike activity during interictal periods.

Atypical absence seizures commonly occur in children with some other form of underlying neurologic dysfunction and tend to be resistant to medication. In the most severe form of this disorder, the Lennox-Gastaut syndrome, children have several kinds of generalized seizures and often have intellectual impairment.

Myoclonic seizures Myoclonic seizures are sudden, brief, single or repetitive muscle contractions involving one body part or the entire body. In the latter case, the seizure is accompanied by a violent fall, without a loss of consciousness. Myoclonic seizures often coexist with other seizure types but may occur alone. The EEG shows polyspike and wave discharges or sharp and slow waves, both ictally and interictally. Although often idiopathic, myoclonic seizures occur as a major neurologic symptom in a variety of medical conditions, including uremia, hepatic failure, Creutzfeldt-Jakob disease, subacute leukoencephalopathies, and a hereditary degenerative condition, Lafora body disease.

Juvenile myoclonic epilepsy (of Janz) (JME) has been identified as a distinct syndrome which begins in adolescence and which has a genetic component. Its specific mode of inheritance has not been absolutely delineated (autosomal dominant or recessive), but the gene for JME has been possibly localized to the short arm of chromosome 6. JME ofens begins with postawakening myoclonic seizures, and later in its course, these may be followed by generalized tonic-clonic seizures.

Atonic seizures Atonic seizures are brief losses of consciousness and postural tone not associated with tonic muscular contractions. The individual may simply drop to the floor without apparent cause. Atonic seizures usually occur in children and are often accompanied by other forms of seizures. The EEG contains polyspikes and slow waves. The "drop attacks" of atonic seizures need to be distinguished from cataplexy seen in narcolepsy (where the patient remains conscious), transient brainstem ischemia, or sudden rises in intracranial pressure.

Infantile spasms or hypsarrhythmia These primary generalized seizures occur in infants between birth and approximately 12 months of age and consist of several types of brief synchronous contractions of the neck, torso, and both arms (usually in flexion). Infantile spasms often occur in children with underlying neurologic diseases, such as anoxic encephalopathy or tuberous sclerosis, but can occur rarely in an otherwise apparently normal infant. The prognosis for children with this form of seizure disorder is grave, and approximately 90 percent develop mental retardation in addition to their seizures. The EEG is characterized by a very disorganized background, random high-voltage slow waves, spikes, and burst suppression (hypsarrhythmia). The spasms and hypsarrhythmia tend to disappear over the first 3 to 5 years of life only to be replaced by other forms of generalized seizures. Infantile spasms sometimes respond to treatment with ACTH or valproic acid.

STATUS EPILEPTICUS Prolonged or repetitive seizures without a period of recovery between attacks can occur with all forms of seizures and is defined as *status epilepticus*. When tonic-clonic seizures are involved, this state can be life-threatening (see "Treatment of Seizures"). Absence status, on the other hand, may proceed for some time before it is recognized because the patient does not lose consciousness or have convulsive movements. Status epilepticus of partial seizures is called *epilepsia partialis continua* and may occur with partial motor, sensory, or visceral seizures. Complex partial seizures also may present as status epilepticus.

RECURRENCE PATTERNS All classes of recurrent seizures can occur sporadically or randomly, with no apparent triggering event, or can occur cyclically, i.e., in concert with the sleep-waking cycle or the menstrual cycle (catamenial epilepsy). Epileptic seizures also can occur as evoked reactions to a specific stimulus (reflex epilepsy), although this is relatively infrequent. Examples are seizures triggered by photic stimulation (photomyoclonic or photoconvulsive epilepsy), specific musical compositions (musicogenic epilepsy), tactile stimulation (somatosensory-induced epilepsy), or reading (reading or language epilepsy). The latter usually consists of brief myoclonic jerks of the jaw, cheek, and tongue which occur during silent or oral reading and may progress to generalized tonic-clonic seizures.

PATHOPHYSIOLOGY OF EPILEPSY

Epileptic seizures can be induced in any normal human (or vertebrate) brain with a variety of different electrical or chemical stimuli. The ease and rapidity with which these seizures can occur and the stereotyped nature of the seizures produced suggest that the normal brain, particularly the cerebral cortex, contains within its fine anatomic and physiologic structure a mechanism which is inherently unstable and which can be influenced in many different ways to produce a seizure. Thus many different kinds of metabolic abnormalities and anatomic lesions of brain can produce seizures, and conversely, there is no pathognomonic lesion of the epileptic brain.

The hallmark of the altered physiologic state of epilepsy is a rhythmic and repetitive hypersynchronous discharge of many neurons in a localized area of the brain. A reflection of this hypersynchronous discharge can be observed in the EEG. The EEG records the integrated electrical activity generated by synaptic potentials in neurons in the superficial layers of a localized area of cortex. Normally, the EEG records unsynchronized activity during periods when the mind is actively working or mildly synchronized activity when the mind is in a restful state (i.e., alpha waves during relaxation with closed eyes) or during various stages of sleep. In the epileptic focus, neurons in a small area of the cortex are activated for a brief period (50 to 100 ms) in an unusually synchronized manner and are then inhibited. This produces a larger, sharper waveform in the EEG—the spike discharge—followed by a slow wave. If the synchronous neuronal discharge occurs repetitively over several seconds, a focal seizure follows; if it spreads through the brain and lasts for many seconds or minutes, a complex partial or generalized seizure (the ictus) will occur, and the EEG can have a variety or appearances depending on which areas of brain are involved and how the primary discharging areas project to the superficial cortex. During the seizure, the EEG may display low-voltage fast activity or high-voltage spikes or spike and wave discharges throughout both hemispheres.

During the interictal spike discharge, the neurons in the epileptic focus undergo a large membrane depolarization (the depolarizing shift, or DS) accompanied by action potential generation. After the DS, the neurons hyperpolarize and stop firing for several seconds. In areas around the discharging focus, the neurons are inhibited throughout the spike discharge. Thus it appears as if the epileptic discharge is limited to a localized area of cortex by a ring of inhibition around the focus and slightly delayed inhibition within the focus. When the epileptic focus undergoes a transition from the isolated discharges to a seizure, the post-DS inhibition disappears and is replaced by a depolarizing potential. Neurons in contiguous areas and in synaptically connected distant areas are then recruited into the seizure and become activated. Local cortical circuits, long association pathways (including callosal), and subcortical pathways are all utilized for the spread of the discharges. Thus a focal seizure can spread locally or generalize throughout the brain. Widely ramifying thalamocortical pathways are likely to be responsible for the rapid generalization of some forms of focal epilepsy and primary generalized epilepsy as well.

A number of metabolic events occur within the brain during the epileptic discharges which may contribute to the development of the focus, to the transition to seizures, or to postictal dysfunction. During the discharges, extracellular potassium concentration increases and extracellular calcium concentration decreases. Both these changes have profound effects on neuronal excitability and neurotransmitter release and on neuronal metabolism. Neurotransmitters and neuropeptides are also released in unusually large amounts during seizure discharges. Some of these substances can have prolonged actions on

central neurons and may be responsible for prolonged postictal phenomena such as Todd's paralysis. In addition to the ionic effects, seizures produce increases in cerebral blood flow to the primary involved areas, increases in glucose utilization, and alterations in oxidative metabolism and local pH. It is possible that these events are not just consequences of the seizures but actually contribute to the development of the seizure activity and that manipulation of such factors could become an effective means for controlling seizures.

There are many mechanisms by which seizures can develop in either normal or pathologic brains. Three common mechanisms include (1) diminution of inhibitory mechanisms [especially synaptic inhibition due to gamma-aminobutyric acid (GABA)], (2) enhancement of excitatory synaptic mechanisms [especially those mediated by the N-methyl-D-aspartate (NMDA) component of glutamate responses], and (3) enhancement of endogenous neuronal burst firing (usually by enhancing voltage-dependent calcium currents). Different forms of human epilepsy may be caused by any one or combination of these mechanisms. For example, in some forms of chronic focal epilepsy, inhibitory interneurons appear to be preferentially lost or inhibitory efficacy is reduced; in other models, and possibly in cases of human hippocampal sclerosis, aberrant recurrent excitatory connections may form among surviving neurons; under other circumstances, neurons may develop enhanced burst firing either because of injury or secondary to genetic factors. In primary generalized absence epilepsy, thalamic neurons with large, low-threshold, transient, voltage-dependent calcium currents may be responsible for generating the diffusely synchronous cortical spike and wave activity.

Currently available antiepileptic drugs appear to operate on several of these mechanisms. Phenytoin, carbamazepine, barbiturates, and valproic acid all appear able to block voltage-dependent sodium channels in a use- and/or voltage-dependent manner such that individual action potentials are relatively unaffected but high-frequency repetitive firing is reduced. The barbiturates and benzodiazepines can enhance GABA-mediated inhibition. Ethosuximide appears to block a low-threshold, transient calcium current in neurons. At present, no drugs are available for clinical use which specifically block excitatory synaptic systems, but much effort is being expended in this direction.

There are a number of animal models in which epilepsy is caused by genetic factors. The best characterized of these is a group of mice in which single-gene mutations cause either absence or tonic-clonic seizures. It is clear from studies of these mice that alterations in a single gene can cause an entire epilepsy syndrome, including multiple seizure types, that different genotypes can produce very similar epilepsy phenotypes, and that interactions between genes can produce intermediate phenotypes. In no case, however, is the genetic basis of the epileptic activity yet understood. Given how many ways seizures can be induced in normal animals, it is likely that a great variety of genetic lesions will produce epilepsy as part of their phenotypic expressions. At the level of human epilepsy, several genetic syndromes have been localized to specific chromosomes (JME possibly to chromosome 6, benign familial neonatal convulsions to chromosome 20, myoclonic epilepsy of the Unverricht-Lundborg type to chromosome 21), and one complex syndrome (myoclonic epilepsy with ragged red fibers) has been localized to a single mutation in mitochondrial DNA.

Electrical stimulation is another mechanism by which seizures can easily be produced in a normal brain. At certain current strengths and stimulus frequencies, seizure discharges are produced and become self-sustaining beyond the original stimulus. Generalized tonic seizures result. At lower stimulus parameters, only brief afterdischarges may occur. However, if afterdischarge-eliciting stimuli are repeated at regular intervals (which may even be as infrequent as one stimulation per day), the afterdischarge duration and spread throughout the brain will increase until generalized seizures occur to the same stimulus which was originally subthreshold. Eventually, spontaneous seizures may occur without any further electrical stimulation. This phenomenon has been called *kindling*. Its relationship to the development of epilepsy, after either an early lesion or trauma, or to the issue of whether the occurrence of seizures themselves tends to foster the continued development of a seizure focus in man has not been resolved.

THE CAUSES OF EPILEPSY

The likely cause of a given seizure depends on the age of the patient and the type of seizure (Table 367-3). In young infants, anoxia or ischemia before or during birth; intracranial birth injury; metabolic disturbances such as hypoglycemia, hypocalcemia, and hypomagnesemia; congenital malformations of the brain; and infections are the most common causes of seizures. In the young child, trauma and infections are common causes of epilepsy, although idiopathic seizures (possibly caused by genetic factors) account for the majority of patients.

Genetic factors can influence the development of epilepsy and also have been shown to affect EEG patterns in general. Patients with primary generalized seizures, especially absence and myoclonic seizures, have a higher familial incidence of epilepsy than is found in the normal population, and relatives of such patients have higher incidences of dysrhythmic EEGs, even when they do not have seizures. The mode of inheritance of epilepsy susceptibility appears complicated for many syndromes and probably represents multiple genes with variable penetrance.

Young children also frequently (approximately 2 to 5 percent of the population) develop seizures with febrile illnesses. These febrile convulsions are short, generalized tonic-clonic convulsions which occur during the early phases of a febrile illness in children between the ages of 3 months and 5 years. Febrile seizures must be distinguished from seizures which are triggered by central nervous system infections which coincidentally produce fever (meningitis or encephalitis). There is minimal likelihood that the child will develop epilepsy or any neurologic impairment from the febrile convulsion if the seizure lasts less than 5 min, is generalized rather than focal, and is not associated with any interictal EEG abnormalities or abnormalities on neurologic examination. There may be a family history of this kind of febrile seizure. Febrile seizures of this kind are probably best treated with quick and relatively vigorous attempts to keep children from developing excessive fevers during various childhood illnesses but without specific antiepileptic medication. Some pediatricians prefer to maintain children susceptible to febrile convulsions on phenobarbital

TABLE 367-3 The causes of seizures

Infant (0–2)	Perinatal hypoxia and ischemia
	Intracranial birth injury
	Acute infection
	Metabolic disturbances (hypoglycemia, hypocalcemia, hypomagnesemia, pyridoxine deficiency)
	Congenital malformation
	Genetic disorders
Child (2–12)	Idiopathic
	Acute infection
	Trauma
	Febrile convulsion
Adolescent (12–18)	Idiopathic
	Trauma
	Drug, alcohol withdrawal
	Arteriovenous malformations
Young adult (18–35)	Trauma
	Alcoholism
	Brain tumor
Older adult (>35)	Brain tumor
	Cerebrovascular disease
	Metabolic disorders (uremia, hepatic failure, electrolyte abnormality, hypoglycemia)
	Alcoholism

medication; others advocate administration of benzodiazepines at the first sign of illness. On the other hand, if the febrile convulsion is prolonged or focal or is associated with an abnormal EEG, or if the child has a neurologic abnormality, there is a significant risk of subsequent epilepsy. These children should be treated with chronic antiepileptic therapy.

In adolescents and young adults, head trauma is a major cause of focal epilepsy. Epilepsy can be caused by any kind of serious head injury, with the likelihood of developing recurrent seizures being proportional to the extent of the damage. Injuries which either cause dural penetration or produce posttraumatic amnesia of more than 24 h duration may result in a 40 to 50 percent incidence of later epilepsy, while the incidence with closed head injuries with cerebral contusion varies from 5 to 25 percent. Brief concussions or nonpenetrating head injuries without loss of consciousness are not usually epileptogenic. Seizures which occur immediately or within the first 24 h of injury are not associated with a poor prognosis, whereas seizures occurring after the first day and within the first 2 weeks indicate a high likelihood of posttraumatic epilepsy. Most recurring seizures develop by 2 years after the injury. Approximately 50 percent of patients with posttraumatic seizures spontaneously recover, 25 percent have medically controllable seizures, and 25 percent have seizures that are much more intractable to antiepileptic medication. The effectiveness of prophylactic anticonvulsant medication after head trauma still requires adequate documentation.

In the adolescent or young adult age group, generalized tonic-clonic seizures tend to be idiopathic or are associated with drug abuse (especially cocaine) or alcohol use or withdrawal. Arteriovenous malformations may present as focal seizures in this age group. Between the ages of 30 and 50 years, brain tumors become more common causes of seizures and may be present in 30 percent of patients with new focal seizures. In general, the incidence of seizures is higher with slowly growing brain tumors involving the cerebrum, such as meningiomas or low-grade gliomas, than with the more malignant types. However, seizures can occur in individuals with any kind of central nervous system mass lesion.

Above age 50, cerebrovascular disease is the most common cause of focal or generalized seizures. Seizures can occur acutely in patients with an embolus, hemorrhage, or, more rarely, a thrombosis but more often as a late sequel to these lesions. Seizures also can result from "silent" cerebral infarctions in patients with no known cerebrovascular disease. Brain tumors, either primary or metastatic, also present with seizures in the older age group.

At any age, a variety of medical diseases can produce metabolic disturbances which may present as seizures. Uremia, hepatic failure, hypo- or hypercalcemia, hypo- or hyperglycemia, and hypo- or hypernatremia may be associated with myoclonic seizures or generalized tonic-clonic seizures.

EVALUATION OF THE PATIENT WITH A SEIZURE

Individuals with seizures present to physicians either in an emergency room setting during the acute attack or in an office setting days after the epileptic event. In the former case, the seizure may be the presenting symptom of serious central nervous system disorder which requires immediate diagnosis and therapy. In the latter case, the seizure may be a symptom of a more chronic neurologic dysfunction, and a different approach is warranted.

Initial emergency evaluation is directed toward ensuring adequate ventilation and perfusion and stopping the seizure (see "Treatment"). Once the patient is medically stable, the investigation is directed at determining the cause of the seizure. Often a careful history (either from the patient, if recovered, or from a friend or relative), a physical examination, and a few blood studies can provide the diagnosis.

A history indicating a focal component to the seizure [e.g., an aura, a focal motor or sensory symptom at onset, a postictal focal deficit (Todd's paralysis)] indicates a high likelihood of an underlying structural/pathologic etiology of the seizure and directs the evaluation accordingly. A recent febrile illness accompanied by headaches, change in mental status, or confusion suggests an acute central nervous system infection (either meningitis or encephalitis) and indicates the need for urgent examination of the cerebrospinal fluid. In this context, a complex partial seizure may be the presenting symptom of herpes simplex encephalitis. A history of headache and/or change in mental functioning preceding the seizure, coupled with signs of either increased intracranial pressure or a focal neurologic deficit, suggests an underlying mass lesion (tumor, abscess, arteriovenous malformation) or a chronic subdural hematoma. A magnetic resonance imaging (MRI) or computed tomographic (CT) scan (both without and with contrast) should be performed for a more definitive diagnosis.

The general physical examination may provide important etiologic information. Gum hyperplasia is usually the result of chronic phenytoin therapy. Exacerbation of a chronic seizure disorder due to intercurrent infection, alcohol, or cessation of therapy is a common cause of patients presenting to an emergency room. Skin examination may reveal the port wine facial stain of Sturge-Weber disease (with accompanying cerebral calcifications) or the stigmata of tuberous sclerosis (adenoma sebaceum and shagreen patches) or neurofibromatosis (subcutaneous nodules, café au lait spots). Body or limb asymmetries may indicate hypotrophic somatic development contralateral to a congenital or infantile cerebral lesion.

The history or physical examination also may reveal evidence of chronic alcoholism. Heavy alcohol users commonly have seizures for any of several reasons—old cerebral contusion (secondary to trauma), chronic subdural hematoma, metabolic derangements of undernutrition and liver disease, central nervous system infection, or alcohol withdrawal ("rum fits"). Seizures occurring during alcohol use or withdrawal, in the absence of other causes, are usually brief, generalized tonic-clonic seizures which occur singly or in a flurry of two or three. Once the flurry is over, chronic antiepileptic treatment is unnecessary, since they are usually self-limiting. Seizures in alcoholics which occur at other times should be treated, but this group of patients presents a particular challenge because of lack of compliance and metabolic problems which complicate drug therapy.

Routine blood studies will indicate if the seizure was caused by hypoglycemia, hypo- or hypernatremia, or hypo- or hypercalcemia. These biochemical abnormalities should be corrected and the cause determined. In addition, other less common causes of seizures can be sought with appropriate tests: thyrotoxicosis, acute intermittent porphyria, and lead or arsenic intoxication.

In the older patient, a seizure may indicate an acute cerebrovascular accident or may be a delayed effect of an old cerebral infarct (even a silent one). The manner in which further evaluation proceeds is dictated by the patient's age, cardiovascular status, and accompanying symptoms.

Generalized tonic-clonic seizures can occur in neurologically normal individuals after moderate sleep deprivation. Such seizures can be seen in individuals working double shifts, in college students around examination time, and in soldiers returning from short leaves of absence. Similarly, brief myoclonic jerks or a generalized tonic-clonic seizure can occur after a vasovagal syncopal episode. In these situations, if all investigations are normal, such individuals do not require further treatment.

If the patient's history, physical examination, and blood chemistries are all normal after a seizure, it is likely that the seizure was "idiopathic" and was not caused by a serious underlying CNS lesion. However, tumors or other mass lesions may be entirely asymptomatic, and every older child and adult with an unexplained seizure should have an EEG and an MRI or CT scan (both without and with contrast) and should be reevaluated at regular intervals (3 to 6 months).

The EEG is important in relation to the differential diagnosis of the seizure, the determination of the cause of the seizure, and the proper classification of the seizure. When the diagnosis of a seizure is in doubt, such as, for example, when trying to distinguish seizures from syncope, the presence of a paroxysmal EEG abnormality supports the diagnosis of epilepsy. For this purpose, special activation procedures (sleep recording, photic stimulation, or hyperventilation), special EEG leads (sphenoidal, nasopharyngeal, nasoethmoidal) for recording from deep structures, or prolonged monitoring, even on an ambulatory basis, can be employed. The EEG also can reveal focal abnormalities (spikes, sharp waves, or focal slow waves) which would indicate the possibility of a focal neurologic lesion even if the seizure symptomatology appeared generalized from the outset.

The EEG is also used to help classify seizures. It can distinguish focal seizures with secondary generalization from primary generalized seizures and is especially useful in the differential diagnosis of brief lapses of consciousness. Absence seizures are always accompanied by bilateral spike and wave discharges, whereas complex partial seizures are accompanied by either focal paroxysmal spikes or slow waves or by a normal surface EEG. In cases of absence seizures, the EEG may reveal that the patient is having many more small seizures than was clinically apparent and may help in monitoring antiepileptic drug therapy.

Lumbar puncture is performed in those situations where acute or chronic CNS infections or subarachnoid hemorrhage is suspected. MRI and CT scans provide definitive information about anatomic lesions. MRI is capable of demonstrating hippocampal sclerosis and/or atrophy in a subset of patients with complex partial seizures. Positron emission tomography (see Chap. 365) can identify seizure foci, but the technique remains primarily experimental. Similarly, magnetoencephalography is undergoing experimental assessment for its efficacy to localize seizure discharges.

DIFFERENTIAL DIAGNOSIS OF SEIZURES

SYNCOPE VERSUS SEIZURE   Sudden loss of consciousness, usually without convulsive movements, presents a common diagnostic problem in both children and adults (see Chap. 17). Faints are often preceded by a feeling of light-headedness, of the room spinning, of a flush and are often, but not always, precipitated by an environmental stimulus such as prolonged standing in a hot, crowded area, the sight of blood, a fright, etc. In older people, pure syncope is most often secondary to cardiovascular problems, such as Stokes-Adams attacks, tachyarrhythmias, or orthostatic hypotension, and these may occur with or without a warning. A clear focal onset of the event (i.e., abnormal smell, head turning, staring, etc.) favors seizure as the cause. In addition, convulsive muscular contractions, tongue biting, or incontinence commonly accompany seizures but are much less common with fainting spells. Occasionally, vasovagal or other types of fainting episodes can be accompanied by either clonic movements or brief generalized tonic-clonic seizures. If the original loss of consciousness can be ascribed to a clear nonepileptic cause (e.g., the patient was having blood drawn or a dental procedure at the time), it is not necessary to regard the episode as a manifestation of epilepsy, and antiepileptic drug therapy is not indicated.

When the origin of a syncopal episode is in doubt, the patient should undergo a complete cardiovascular evaluation, an EEG with sleep recording, and, if available, prolonged ambulatory EEG monitoring. If the EEG shows paroxysmal activity (which is often brought out by drowsiness and sleep onset) and the patient has no signs of cardiac arrhythmia with electrocardiographic monitoring or of valvular disease on echocardiogram, it is likely that the syncopal episode represented a seizure, and the patient should be evaluated and treated accordingly.

TRANSIENT ISCHEMIC ATTACKS AND MIGRAINE   Transient ischemic attacks (TIAs) and migraine episodes can present as a transient alteration in neurologic function (usually without loss of consciousness) which may be confused diagnostically with focal seizures. Neurologic dysfunction due to ischemia (TIA or migraine) is often a negative symptom (i.e., loss of feeling, numbness, visual field deficit, paralysis), whereas deficits due to focal seizure activity are often positive (twitching, paresthesias, visual distortion, or hallucination), although this distinction is not absolute. Brief stereotyped episodes which conform to dysfunction in a single vascular territory in an individual with either known vascular disease, heart disease, or risk factors for vascular disease (diabetes, hypertension) are more likely TIAs. However, since cerebral infarcts are a common cause of subsequent seizures in older patients, a paroxysmal EEG focus should be sought.

Classic migraine headaches with a visual aura, unilateral headache, and gastrointestinal upset are usually easy to distinguish from seizures. However, some migraine patients have only "migraine equivalents" such as a hemiparesis, numbness, or aphasia and may not have subsequent headache. These episodes, especially when they occur in older individuals, are hard to distinguish from TIAs but also may represent focal seizures. The presence of loss of consciousness after some forms of vertebrobasilar migraine and the common occurrence of headaches after seizures make this differential diagnosis more difficult. The slower development of neurologic dysfunction in migraine (often occurring over minutes) is the most helpful point. Nevertheless, occasionally such patients need to be investigated for all three problems with an MRI or CT scan, carotid studies, and specialized EEG procedures before a diagnosis can be made. In some cases, a therapeutic trial with antiepileptic drugs (which, interestingly, can prevent migraines as well as seizures in some patients) will be necessary for the final diagnosis.

PSEUDOSEIZURES AND "HYSTERICAL" SEIZURES Some patients with complex partial seizures may have bizarre behavioral manifestations of their seizures. These may consist of abrupt changes in personality, feelings of impending doom or of undirected fear, abnormal bodily sensations, episodic forgetfulness, or brief repetitive motor activities such as picking at one's clothes or stamping a foot. Some of these patients also have personality disorders, and a significant proportion have had psychiatric treatment. It is common, especially if these patients do not have tonic-clonic seizures or loss of consciousness and when these patients appear emotionally disturbed, for these episodes of complex partial seizures to be called *pseudoseizures, psychopathic fugues,* or *"hysterical" seizures.* This incorrect diagnosis is often reinforced by a "normal" EEG interictally or even during one of these episodes. It must be emphasized that seizures (as well as interictal discharges) can arise from foci deep in temporal lobe structures with *no* surface EEG manifestations. This has been demonstrated repeatedly with depth electrode recordings. Moreover, deep temporal seizures can be manifest only by the kinds of phenomena described above and may be free of the usual seizure phenomena of motor convulsions and loss of consciousness.

In a small number of cases, individuals present with seizure-like events which upon investigation turn out to be pseudoseizures or, rarely, frank malingering. Often these individuals have had true seizures in the past or are acquainted with an individual with epilepsy. Such pseudoseizures can be quite difficult to distinguish from true seizures. They are characterized by nonphysiologic events such as a progression of twitching from one hand to the other without spread to subjacent ipsilateral face or leg areas, twitching of all four extremities without loss of consciousness (or with surreptitious loss of consciousness), or careful attention to avoiding injury by moving away from a wall or bed edge while having motor convulsions. In addition, pseudoseizures, especially in adolescent girls, may have frankly sexual overtones, with pelvic thrusting or genital manipulation. While many forms of complex partial seizures can occur with normal surface EEGs, generalized tonic-clonic seizures always produce abnormal EEGs both during and after the seizure. In addition, most generalized tonic-clonic seizures and many complex partial seizures of moderate duration are accompanied by rises in serum prolactin (during a 30-min postictal period), whereas pseudoseizures are not. Although not an absolute distinguishing point, such measurements, especially if positive, can be very helpful in characterizing the origin of a given "spell." After careful observation, especially with video-EEG monitoring, and after establishing a relationship with the patient,

pseudoseizures can sometimes be elicited by suggestion. Frequently, when patients are appropriately confronted with this diagnosis, they respond well, and the pseudoseizures are eliminated or greatly reduced in frequency.

TREATMENT OF SEIZURES

Treatment of the patient with a seizure disorder is directed at eliminating the cause of the seizures, suppressing the expression of the seizures, and dealing with the psychosocial consequences which may occur as a result of the neurologic dysfunction underlying the seizure disorder or from the presence of a chronic disability.

If the seizure disorder is a result of a metabolic disturbance, such as hypoglycemia or hypocalcemia, restoration of normal metabolic function is usually accompanied by cessation of the seizures. If the seizures are caused by a structural brain lesion, such as a brain tumor, arteriovenous malformation, or cerebral cyst, removal of the offending lesion may eliminate the seizures. However, long-standing lesions, even nonprogressive ones, can result in gliosis and chronic denervation. These changes may lead to chronic epileptic foci which will not be eliminated by the subsequent removal of the original lesion. In such cases, surgical extirpation of the epileptic brain regions may be necessary for control of the epilepsy (see "Neurosurgical Approaches to Epilepsy," below).

There is complex interrelationship between the limbic system and neuroendocrine function which may have significant implications for patients with epilepsy. Normal hormonal fluctuations may influence the frequency of seizures. Some women have a marked change in the pattern of their seizures during particular parts of the menstrual cycle (catamenial epilepsy), while others may have changes in seizure frequency in response to oral contraceptives or pregnancy. In general, estrogens tend to exacerbate seizures, while progesterones tend to be more protective.

In addition, epilepsy can cause changes in neuroendocrine function. Some patients with epilepsy, especially those with complex partial seizures, also may have an associated reproductive endocrine dysfunction. Disorders in sexual interest, especially hyposexuality, are frequently observed. In addition, women may have polycystic ovary disease, and men may have disturbances in potency. Interestingly, some patients with these endocrine disorders have not had clinical seizures but have significantly abnormal EEGs (often with temporal discharges). Whether the epilepsy causes the endocrine and/or behavioral dysfunction or whether the two conditions are separate manifestations of a common underlying neuropathologic process is not known. However, endocrine manipulation can sometimes be useful in controlling some forms of seizures, and antiepileptic medication may be a useful adjunct for treating some forms of endocrine dysfunction.

PHARMACOLOGIC CONTROL OF EPILEPSY The fundamental modality for the treatment of epilepsy is pharmacologic therapy. The goal is to protect the patient from having seizures without interfering with normal cognitive function (or, in the child, with development of normal intellectual function) and without producing harmful systemic side effects. If possible, the individual should be treated with the lowest possible dose of a single antiepileptic medication. Precise knowledge of the kind of seizure the patient is having, the spectrum of action of the available antiepileptic medications, and a few basic pharmacokinetic principles can result in the complete control of seizures in approximately 60 percent of patients with epilepsy. Many patients appear to be resistant to medications or develop unnecessary side effects because the medications chosen are not appropriate for the kind(s) of seizure or are not administered in the optimal doses.

The availability of serum levels of antiepileptic drugs makes it possible to optimize dosage regimens for individual patients and to monitor drug compliance. Thus patients can be placed on a medication, and after a suitable equilibration period (usually several weeks, but at least five "half-lives"), the amount of medication in the serum can be determined and compared with standard "therapeutic ranges" established for each drug. Utilizing blood levels to adjust doses can compensate for individual patient variability in absorption or metabolism of drugs.

Many antiepileptic drugs are bound by serum proteins, and it is the unbound, or "free," drug which is in equilibrium with extracellular spaces within the brain; this level correlates best with seizure control. However, "total" drug is measured in the serum by conventional

TABLE 367-4 Commonly used antiepileptic drugs

Generic name	Trade name	Principal uses	Dosage	Half-life	Therapeutic range	% Protein bound	Toxic effects Neurologic	Toxic effects Systemic	Drug interactions
Phenytoin (PTN) (diphenyl-hydantoin)	Dilantin	Tonic-clonic (grand mal) Partial	300–400 mg/d (3–5 mg/kg, adult) (4–7 mg/kg, child)	24 h (with wide variation)	10–20 μg/mL	90	Ataxia Incoordination Confusion Cerebellar Skin rash	Gum hyperplasia Lymphadenopathy Hirsutism Osteomalacia	Level increased by INH, dicoumarol, sulfonamides Level decreased by CBZ, phenobarbital Altered folate metabolism Folate interferes with effects
Carbamazepine CBZ	Tegretol	Tonic-clonic Partial	600–1200 mg/d (20–30 mg/kg, child)	13–17 h	4–12 μg/mL	80	Ataxia Dizziness Diplopia Vertigo	Bone marrow suppression Gastrointestinal irritation Hepatotoxicity	Level decreased by phenobarbital, PTN Level increased by erythromycin
Phenobarbital	Luminol	Tonic-clonic Partial	60–120 mg/d (1–5 mg/kg, adult) (3–6 mg/kg, child)	90 h (shorter in children)	10–50 μg/mL	40–60	Sedation Ataxia Confusion Dizziness Decreased libido Depression	Skin rash	Level increased by VPA, PTN Enhances metabolism of other drugs via liver enzyme induction
Primidone	Mysoline	Tonic-clonic Partial	750–1000 mg/d (10–25 mg/kg)	Primidone, 8 h PEMA, 24–48 h Phenobarbital, 90 h	Primidone, 2–10 μg/mL Phenobarbital, 10–50 μg/mL	Small for primidone or PEMA	Same as phenobarbital		
Sodium valproate (valproic acid, VPA)	Depakene Depakote	Absence Atypical absence Myoclonic Tonic-clonic (Partial)	750–1250 mg/d (30–60 mg/kg)	15 h	50–100 μg/mL	80–94	Ataxia Sedation Tremor	Hepatotoxicity Bone marrow suppression Gastrointestinal irritation Weight gain Transient alopecia Hyperammonemia	May precipitate absence status if given with clonazepam Increases free PTN Decreases phenobarbital Increases active CBZ metabolites
Felbamate	Felbatol	Partial Second. generalized Lennox-Gastaut synd.	3600 mg/d	20–23 h	Unknown	25%	Insomnia Headache Dizziness	Gastrointestinal irritation, nausea Anorexia	Increase PTN level Increase VPA level Dec. CBZ level but inc. CBZ epoxide PTN, CBZ dec. Fel.
Ethosuximide	Zarontin	Absence (petit mal)	750–1250 mg/d (20–40 mg/kg)	60 h, adult 30 h, child	40–100 μg/mL	Small	Ataxia Lethargy	Gastrointestinal irritation Skin rash Bone marrow suppression	
Methsuximide	Celontin	Absence (complex partial)	600–1200 mg/d	38–50 h	10–30 μg/mL (N-desmethyl methsuximide)	Small	Ataxia Lethargy	Same as ethosuximide	Increases PTN level Increases phenobarbital from primidone
Clonazepam	Clonopin	Absence Atypical absence Myoclonic	1–12 mg/d (0.1–0.2 mg/kg)	24–48 h	5–70 ng/mL	50	Ataxia Sedation Lethargy	Anorexia	May precipitate absence status if given with VPA
Trimethadione	Tridione	Absence Atypical absence (use only with intractable seizures)	900–2100 mg/d (20–60 mg/kg)	6–13 days (for dimetha-dione)	700 μg/mL (for dimetha-dione)	Small	Sedation Blurred vision	Skin rash Bone marrow suppression Nephrosis Hepatitis	
Lamotrigine	Lamictal	Partial	300–500 mg/d (depends on concomitant AEDs)	25 h 13 h (with PTN, CBZ, PHB, PRIM) 60–70 h (with VPA)	Unknown	55%	Headache Dizziness Ataxia Diplopia	Skin rash Nausea	PTN, CBZ, Barbiturates shorten half life VPA prolongs half life Decrease VPA level
Gabapentin	Neurontin	Partial	900–1200 mg/d (up to 2400 mg/d if necessary and tolerated)	5–7 h	Unknown	None	Dizziness Somnolence Ataxia	Gastrointestinal irritation	None

assays. Under most circumstances, this is adequate for determining if the antiepileptic drug is in the therapeutic range. Occasionally, serum antiepileptic drug levels will be high, yet the patient continues to have seizures without any "physiologic" side effects of the drug. In these cases, it is possible that serum protein binding is higher than expected and that the patient is "undermedicated" in relation to the "free" drug available. Increase in dose may produce control without any untoward side effects (despite a blood level above "therapeutic range"). Similarly, individuals with impaired liver or renal function may have low serum proteins or circulating "toxins" which reduce drug binding. In these cases, toxicity may appear at unusually low serum levels because of a relatively higher "free" level of drug.

Intensive long-term EEG and video monitoring has demonstrated that careful characterization of seizures and selection of antiepileptic drugs can significantly increase seizure control in many patients whose seizures had previously been considered intractable to conventional antiepileptic drugs. In fact, often these patients can have one or more of their multiple drugs removed while still achieving better control.

INDICATIONS FOR USE OF SPECIFIC DRUGS Generalized tonic-clonic seizures (grand mal) There are four medications which are of proven value in this very common form of seizure—phenytoin (or diphenylhydantoin), carbamazepine, phenobarbital (and other long-acting barbiturates), and valproic acid (Table 367-4). Most patients will be controlled by adequate doses of any one of these, although individual patients may respond better to one or another. The choice among them often relates to minimizing undesirable side effects.

Phenytoin often can produce effective control with no sedation and very little, if any, intellectual impairment. However, phenytoin produces gum hyperplasia in some individuals, coarsening of facial features, and mild hirsutism, all of which can lead to long-term changes in appearance, which is especially unpleasant for young women. Phenytoin may produce lymphadenopathy and, in very high doses, may be toxic to the cerebellum.

Carbamazepine is equally effective and does not have many of the side effects seen with phenytoin. Cognitive function is well preserved. However, carbamazepine may exacerbate generalized spike-wave discharges in the EEG and absence seizures, even in patients who had only previously experienced generalized tonic-clonic seizures. Carbamazepine can cause gastrointestinal upset and may cause bone marrow suppression with mild to moderate falls in peripheral white count (3.5 to 4 × 10³ per microliter) which can occasionally become severe and which must be watched carefully. In addition, carbamazepine can produce hepatotoxicity. For these reasons, a complete blood count and liver function tests should be performed before starting carbamazepine and at 2-week intervals for a period after initiating therapy.

Phenobarbital is also effective against tonic-clonic seizures and has none of the systemic side effects mentioned above. It commonly causes sedation and a dulling of intellect, however, especially early in its use, and this may lead to poor compliance. The sedation is dose-dependent and may limit the amount of drug which can be given to achieve complete control. However, if control can be achieved with nonsedative doses of phenobarbital, it can be a safe regimen. Primidone is a barbiturate which is metabolized to phenobarbital and phenylethylmalonamide (PEMA). In children, the barbiturates can produce a state of hyperactivity and hyperirritability which will limit their usefulness. Barbiturates also may exacerbate depression.

Valproic acid (sodium valproate) is also effective for tonic-clonic seizures and does not produce sedation or interfere with cognitive function. It can cause gastrointestinal irritation, patchy hair loss, excessive weight gain, bone marrow suppression (especially thrombocytopenia), hyperammonemia, and hepatic dysfunction (including rare instances of fatal progressive hepatic failure which appear to be idiosyncratic rather than dose-related and more common in children under 2 years of age). A complete blood count with platelet count and liver function tests should be performed before beginning therapy and at biweekly intervals after initiating therapy for a suitable

period until the safety of the drug is established in the individual patient.

In addition to their systemic side effects, all four of these drugs have neurologic toxicities at higher doses. Nystagmus is common at therapeutic blood levels, but ataxia, dizziness, tremor, intellectual dulling, forgetfulness, confusion, and even stupor may occur with increasing blood concentrations. These are reversible when blood levels fall back to therapeutic levels.

Partial seizures, including complex partial seizures (temporal lobe epilepsy) Three of the four groups of drugs which are useful for tonic-clonic seizures are also effective for partial seizures. Carbamazepine and phenytoin are the drugs of choice, while the barbiturates also may be effective. Valproic acid has more variable effects. Felbamate is a new drug recently approved by the FDA for use in partial seizures with or without secondary generalization and in children with multiple seizure types associated with the Lennox Gastaut syndrome. Its side effects include gastrointestinal upset, anorexia, and insomnia, but in general it is well tolerated. Felbamate has important interactions with some other antiepileptic drugs (see Table 367-4). At present, two other anti-epileptic drugs (lamotrigine and gabapentin) have also been approved by the FDA Advisory Panel for use in partial seizures. The relevant pharmacologic data for both are included in Table 367-4.

In general, complex partial seizures are difficult to control, and such patients may require more than one medication (i.e., carbamazepine and phenobarbital, or phenytoin and phenobarbital, or any one of the primary drugs and high doses of methsuximide) and may become candidates for neurosurgical intervention. These are the kinds of seizures for which many epilepsy centers are conducting trials of new antiepileptic drugs.

Other primary generalized seizures [absence (petit mal), atypical absence, myoclonic] These seizures respond to different classes of medications than either tonic-clonic or focal seizures. For simple absence, ethosuximide and valproic acid are the drugs of choice. Side effects of ethosuximide include gastrointestinal upset, behavior changes, dizziness, and lethargy, but these are not often troublesome. For more difficult to control atypical absence seizures and for myoclonic seizures, valproic acid is the drug of choice. Clonazepam (a benzodiazepine) also can be used for atypical absence and myoclonic seizures, but its effectiveness is often limited by the development of tolerance. It can cause drowsiness and irritability but usually does not cause other systemic side effects. Trimethadione was one of the first antiabsence drugs, but it is now rarely used because of its potential toxicity.

Approximately one-third of children who present with "pure" absence seizures also have tonic-clonic seizures at some later time. The question of whether these children should be treated prophylactically with an anti–tonic-clonic seizure medication has not been resolved. Since valproic acid is effective against both classes of seizures, its use has been increasing in children with absence. The concurrent use of phenobarbital with antiabsence drugs for this purpose should be avoided because it may interfere with therapy for the absence. Clinical trials are underway with several new antiepileptic drugs, including lamotrigine, felbamate, and vigabatrin. None is approved for clinical use in the United States.

Status epilepticus Generalized tonic-clonic status epilepticus is a life-threatening medical emergency, but overzealous and incautious treatment can produce more harm than good. Patients are in danger from hyperpyrexia and acidosis (from prolonged muscle activity) and, less commonly, hypoxia or compromise of respiratory function. Immediate treatment for status is protection of the airway, protection of the tongue (with a soft object, large enough not to be swallowed, between the clenched teeth), protection of the head, and then establishment of a secure parenteral (IV) access. A bolus of 50% glucose in water (after blood is drawn for analysis), even if hypoglycemia is not expected, may stop the seizures. All further intravenous medication should be given after respiratory and circulatory support are available.

Phenytoin, 1000 to 1500 mg (18 to 20 mg/kg) in a slow IV "push" (not in 5% dextrose in water—phenytoin precipitates in this low-pH solution), no faster than 50 mg/min, is one of the drugs of choice. It does not depress respiration but may produce mild atrioventricular block and, if given too rapidly, can cause a serious fall in blood pressure. Blood pressure and ECG should be monitored.

The benzodiazepines, diazepam (10 mg) or lorazepam (4 mg, followed by another 4 mg if necessary), are also effective in stopping status epilepticus when administered intravenously. These drugs may depress respiratory function (or even cause respiratory arrest), and measures for respiratory support should be available before they are administered. The use of a benzodiazepine after phenobarbital administration carries a particular risk. The benzodiazepines are short-acting drugs in these circumstances, and after they are administered, a second, longer-acting antiepileptic such as phenytoin is usually required to prevent recurrence of seizures.

Phenobarbital, in a dose of 10 to 20 mg/kg (up to 1 g), divided into two to four doses at 30- to 60-min intervals, also can be administered for status epilepticus. Phenobarbital causes respiratory depression and should not be used immediately after treatment with IV diazepam.

If tonic-clonic seizures cannot be controlled within 30 to 60 min with the above sequence, the likelihood of serious neurologic sequelae or death becomes very high. These patients often have a serious underlying cause for the status epilepticus, such as cerebral hypoxia, sepsis, or some metabolic derangement. Serious consideration needs to be given to anesthetizing the patient with barbiturates or inhalation anesthetics, with EEG monitoring, to ensure that cessation of electrical seizure activity accompanies cessation of motor convulsions.

After stopping the seizures, it is imperative to determine the cause of the status epilepticus in order to prevent its recurrence. In most adults, the cause can be determined and is usually tumor, vascular disease, infection, cerebral damage, or precipitous withdrawal from alcohol or antiepileptic medication. In children, the incidence of idiopathic status is higher (approximately 50 percent), and the remaining cases are divided between acute brain illnesses such as purulent meningitis, encephalitis, and dehydration with electrolyte disturbances and chronic encephalopathies. Tonic-clonic status epilepticus is a dangerous condition; the mortality may be over 10 percent, with another 10 to 30 percent of patients being left with permanent neurologic sequelae.

NEUROSURGICAL TREATMENT OF EPILEPSY   If a structural lesion (i.e., tumor, cyst, abscess, etc.) is causing recurrent seizures, the removal of that lesion and nearby diseased brain will often eliminate the seizures or make them easier to control. Some patients, however, have uncontrollable seizures without a demonstrable structural lesion. These are often complex partial seizures with ictal and interictal EEG abnormalities emanating from one or both temporal lobes. Some patients have demonstrable lesions in the hippocampus (sclerosis or atrophy) visible by high-resolution MRI. Many surgical series have shown that if the epileptogenic lesion can be clearly localized to the depths of one temporal lobe, neurosurgical removal of that temporal lobe can result in complete elimination of the seizures or significant improvement in 60 to 95 percent of the patients. Individuals with epileptic foci in temporal neocortex or other neocortical areas often have a somewhat lower chance of such success but may still be helped significantly. Localization often depends on intensive EEG monitoring and may require intracranial recordings from the temporal or frontal lobes. In a high percentage of cases, the removed temporal lobe can be shown to have microscopic pathology, such as hippocampal (or "Ammon's horn") sclerosis (loss of pyramidal cells in the hippocampus), a hamartoma, or cortical ectopia.

Some individuals with complex partial seizures also develop a psychiatric illness characterized most often as a borderline personality disorder with certain specific behavioral manifestations, including hypergraphia, hyperreligiosity, lack of sense of humor, and disordered sexuality. The psychiatric aspects of this illness may result from the epilepsy or may be produced independently by the same underlying brain lesion which produces the epilepsy. The personality disorder may not significantly change after epilepsy surgery, even if the seizures are controlled.

TREATMENT OF A SINGLE SEIZURE   Some individuals present with a single, brief, generalized tonic-clonic seizure and, after complete evaluation, are found to have a normal EEG and no underlying cause for the seizure. Some of these individuals (between 40 and 70 percent, depending on the series) go on to have recurrent seizures. The decision to treat such a patient with several years (at least) of antiepileptic medication must be made on an individual basis, considering the patient's life style, risks from a sudden loss of consciousness, and feelings about medications.

CESSATION OF ANTIEPILEPTIC DRUG THERAPY   Many patients with epilepsy require antiepileptic drug therapy for life. However, a large proportion of epileptic patients become seizure-free on appropriate medication, and approximately half of such patients can eventually stop their medications and remain seizure-free. Individuals with the best chance of remaining seizure-free after medication discontinuation meet the following criteria: no seizures for 2 to 4 years, relatively few seizures before control was attained, only required a single medication for control, normal neurologic examination, no structural lesion causing the seizures, normal EEG at the end of the therapeutic period. (An abnormal EEG is not, however, a contraindication to discontinuing medication.) When considering the discontinuance of antiepileptic therapy, the consequences of the recurrence of seizures must be considered carefully. One inopportune seizure in a previously well-controlled patient who is not used to taking precautions may be a life-threatening event or lead to loss of a driver's license or loss of employment. Nevertheless, since all medications carry some risk of toxicity, and since medication compliance in a healthy individual is often variable, it is worth a careful trial of medication tapering in individuals who meet the above criteria and are willing to accept the risk.

EPILEPSY AND PREGNANCY   Most women with epilepsy can undergo uneventful pregnancies and deliver healthy babies—even those taking antiepileptic medications. During the pregnant state, however, body metabolism changes, and close attention must be given to antiepileptic drug levels. Sometimes relatively high doses have to be given to ensure therapeutic levels. Most women who are well controlled before pregnancy will remain so during pregnancy and delivery. Women whose seizures are not under good control before becoming pregnant are at higher risk for having increased difficulties during the pregnancy.

One of the most serious complications of pregnancy, toxemia, often presents as a generalized tonic-clonic convulsion in the third trimester. This seizure is a symptom of a severe neurologic disturbance and is not a manifestation of epilepsy, nor is it more common in epileptic women. The toxemic state must be treated in order to control the seizures.

There is a two- to fivefold higher incidence of significant fetal malformations in offspring of epileptic women, and this is likely due to a combination of a genetic predisposition in this population as well as a low, but real, incidence of medication-induced malformations. Among those malformations which do occur, a syndrome consisting of cleft lip and palate, heart defects, digital hypoplasia, and nail dysplasia has been identified which was initially ascribed to phenytoin ("fetal-hydantoin syndrome") but also has been associated with other antiepileptic drugs.

Although it would be ideal for women contemplating pregnancy to have their antiepileptic drugs discontinued, it is likely that for a large number of women this would result in recurrence of seizures, which would, in the long run, be more harmful for both mother and baby. If patients meet the criteria for discontinuance of medication, this should be done with a suitable interval before pregnancy is to occur. Other patients should be tapered to a minimal effective dosage and, if possible, be maintained on only one medication. There are no clear data indicating differences in safety for phenobarbital, phenytoin, or carbamazepine when used alone. Less experience is available for valproate. Phenobarbital, primidone, and phenytoin can cause transient and reversible deficiency in vitamin K–dependent clotting factors in the neonate, and this should be treated promptly. Babies exposed to chronic barbiturates in utero are often transiently sluggish, hypotonic, jittery, and may show signs of barbiturate withdrawal. These babies should be considered at risk for neonatal problems and should be withdrawn slowly from barbiturates and closely observed in the nursery during the neonatal period.

DRIVING AND EPILEPSY Each state has its own regulations for determining when an individual with epilepsy can obtain a driver's license, and several states have laws about the physician's obligations in either reporting epileptic patients to the registry or informing the patients of their responsibilities to do so. In general, patients can drive after a seizure-free interval (on or off medications) which ranges from 6 months to 2 years. In some states there is no fixed interval, but the individual is required to have a physician's letter attesting to seizure control. It is the physician's responsibility to warn the patient with epilepsy of the risks of driving when seizures are not under control.

SOCIAL AND EDUCATIONAL REHABILITATION Many people with epilepsy attain adequate control of their seizures and are able to attend school, obtain employment, become involved in relationships, and live relatively normal lives. Some individuals are more disabled by the fact that they have epilepsy than by the seizures themselves and unduly restrict their activities or withdraw from social interactions. These individuals need to have their psychosocial concerns professionally treated. Children with epilepsy tend to have more problems in school than their peers, but every effort should be made to keep these children integrated into the mainstream of the educational process while supplying additional help in the form of academic tutoring or psychological counseling.

REFERENCES

BERKOVIC SF et al: Hippocampal sclerosis in temporal lobe epilepsy demonstrated by magnetic resonance imaging. Ann Neurol 29:175, 1991

CALLAGHAN N et al: Withdrawal of anticonvulsant drugs in patients free of seizures for two years. N Engl J Med 318:942, 1988

CENDES F et al: MRI volumetric measurement of amygdala and hippocampus in temporal lobe epilepsy. Neurology 43:719, 1993

COMMISSION ON CLASSIFICATION AND TERMINOLOGY OF THE ILAE: Proposal for revised clinical classification of epileptic seizures. Epilepsia 22:489, 1981

————: Proposal for revised clinical classification of epilepsies and epileptic syndromes. Epilepsia 30:3898, 1989

DELGADO-ESCUETA A, JANZ D: Consensus guidelines: Preconception counseling, management, and care of the pregnant woman with epilepsy. Neurology 42(suppl 5):149, 1992

DICHTER M, AYALA GF: Cellular mechanisms of epilepsy: A status report. Science 237:157, 1987

————, BUCHHALTER J: The genetic epilepsies, in The Molecular and Genetic Basis of Neurological Diseases, R Rosenberg et al (eds). Boston, Butterworth, 1993, pp 925–950

EMERSON R et al: Stopping medication in children with epilepsy. N Engl J Med 304:1125, 1981

ENGEL J: Clinical neurophysiology, neuroimaging, and the surgical treatment of epilepsy. Curr Opin Neurol Neurosurg 6:240, 1993

ENGEL J JR: Seizures and Epilepsy. Philadelphia, Davis, 1989

———— (ed): Surgical Treatment of the Epilepsies. New York, Raven, 1987

HAJEK M et al: Mesiobasal versus lateral temporal lobe epilepsy—Metabolic differences in the temporal lobe shown by interictal F-18-FDG positron emission tomography. Neurology 43:79, 1993

LAIDLAW J, RICHENS A (eds): A Textbook of Epilepsy, 3d ed. London, Churchill Livingstone, 1988

LEHESJOKI AE et al: Localization of a gene for progressive myoclonus epilepsy to chromosome 21q22. Proc Natl Acad Sci (USA) 88:3696, 1991

LEPPERT M et al: Benign familial neonatal convulsions linked to genetic markers on chromosome 20. Nature 337:647, 1989

LEPPIK IF et al: Felbamate for partial seizures: Results of a controlled clinical trial. Neurology 41:1785, 1991

LEVY R et al (eds): Antiepileptic Drugs, 3d ed. New York, Raven, 1989

MATTSON R, CRAMER J: Epilepsy, sex hormones and antiepileptic drugs. Epilepsia 26(S):S40, 1985

———— et al: Comparison of carbamazepine, phenobarbital, phenytoin, and primidone in partial and secondarily generalized tonic-clonic seizures. N Engl J Med 313:145, 1985

NOBELS JL: Molecular genetics and epilepsy, in Recent Advances in Epilepsy, T Pedley, B Meldrum (eds). Edinburgh, Churchill Livingstone, 1992, pp 1–13

SO EL: Update on epilepsy. Med Clin North Am 77:203, 1993

TEMKIN N et al: A randomized, double-blind study of phenytoin for the prevention of post-traumatic seizures. N Engl J Med 323:497, 1990

368 CEREBROVASCULAR DISEASES

J. PHILIP KISTLER / ALLAN H. ROPPER / JOSEPH B. MARTIN

Cerebrovascular disease, the third leading cause of death after heart disease and cancer in developed countries, has an overall prevalence of 794 per 100,000. In the United States, it is estimated that more than 400,000 patients are discharged each year from hospitals after a stroke. The loss of these patients from the work force and the extended hospitalization they require during recovery make the economic impact of the disease one of the most devastating in medicine.

PATHOGENESIS AND PATHOLOGY OF STROKE Cerebrovascular disease is caused by one of several pathologic processes involving the blood vessels of the brain. The process may (1) be intrinsic to the vessel, as in atherosclerosis, lipohyalinosis, inflammation, amyloid deposition, arterial dissection, developmental malformation, aneurysmal dilation, or venous thrombosis; (2) originate remotely, as occurs when an embolus from the heart or extracranial circulation lodges in an intracranial vessel; (3) result from decreased perfusion pressure or increased blood viscosity with inadequate cerebral blood flow; or (4) result from rupture of a vessel in the subarachnoid space or intracerebral tissue.

A *stroke* is the acute neurologic injury occurring as a result of one of these pathologic processes and is manifested either as brain infarction or hemorrhage. Approximately 80 percent of strokes are due to ischemic cerebral infarction and 20 percent to brain hemorrhage. An infarcted brain is pale initially. Within hours to days, the gray matter becomes congested with engorged, dilated blood vessels and minute petechial hemorrhages. When an embolus blocking a major vessel migrates, lyses, or disperses within hours, recirculation into the ischemic area causes hemorrhagic infarction that may aggravate edema formation from blood-brain barrier disruption. A primary intracerebral hemorrhage damages the brain directly at the site of the hemorrhage by compressing the surrounding tissue.

The brain is unable to repair itself and only forms fibrogliotic scar tissue at the site of infarction or hemorrhage; therefore, the most effective therapy for stroke is prevention. After a stroke, therapy is directed toward minimizing subsequent worsening of the infarction or hemorrhage, preventing a second stroke, or decreasing edema. Therapy in ischemic stroke is aided by a precise diagnosis that determines the primary vascular pathology, the extent and location of the stroke, and the collateral circulation. The clinical presentation and temporal profile of a stroke often suggests the cause. Diagnosis includes imaging studies (CT and MRI) and noninvasive laboratory tests (carotid and transcranial Doppler ultrasonography and magnetic resonance angiography).

Primary risk factors for stroke include hypertension, hypercholesterolemia, and smoking as the most important for arteriosclerotic cerebrovascular disease, atrial fibrillation or recent myocardial infarction for cardiogenic embolism, and hypertension for primary intracerebral hemorrhage. Hypertension also causes lipohyalinosis, the primary pathologic lesion of lacunar stroke. Virtually every type of cardiac disease is associated with increased risk for stroke.

ISCHEMIC CEREBROVASCULAR DISEASE: GENERAL REMARKS

Ischemic cerebrovascular disease is divided into two broad categories, thrombotic and embolic (Table 368-1). Cerebral embolic strokes usually occur abruptly but may present with stuttering, fluctuating symptoms. Thrombotic strokes are heralded in 50 to 75 percent of patients by transient symptoms, transient ischemic attacks (TIAs), or a minor stroke leading to a more devastating event.

TABLE 368-1 Causes of ischemic stroke

THROMBOSIS

A Atherosclerosis
B* Arteritis: Temporal arteritis, granulomatous arteritis, polyarteritis,
    Wegener's granulomatosis, granulomatous arteritis of the great vessels
    (Takayasu's arteritis, syphilis)
C* Dissections: Carotid, vertebral, or intracranial arteries at the base of the
    brain (spontaneous or traumatic)
D* Hematologic disorders: Polycythemia first-degree or second-degree,
    sickle cell disease, thrombotic thrombocytopenic purpura, etc.
E* Cerebral mass effect compressing intracranial arteries: Tentorial
    herniation—post-cerebral artery; giant aneurysm—middle cerebral
    artery compression
F* Miscellaneous: Moyamoya disease, fibromuscular dysplasia,
    Binswanger's disease

VASOCONSTRICTION

A* Cerebral vasospasm following subarachnoid hemorrhage
B* Reversible cerebral vasoconstriction: Etiology unknown, following
    migraine, trauma, eclampsia of pregnancy

EMBOLISM

A Atherothrombotic arterial source: Bifurcation common carotid artery,
    carotid siphon, distal vertebral artery, aortic arch
B* Cardiac source
    1 Structural heart disease
        a Congenital: mitral valve prolapse, patent foramen ovale, etc.
        b Acquired: following myocardial infarction, marantic vegetation,
            etc.
    2 Dysrhythmia, atrial fibrillation, sick sinus syndrome, etc.
    3 Infection: acute bacterial endocarditis
C* Unknown source
    1 Healthy child or adult
    2 Associations: hypercoagulable state secondary to systemic disease,
        carcinoma (especially pancreatic), eclampsia of pregnancy, oral
        contraceptives, lupus, anticoagulants, factor C deficiency, factor S
        deficiency, etc.

* May occur in patients under 30.

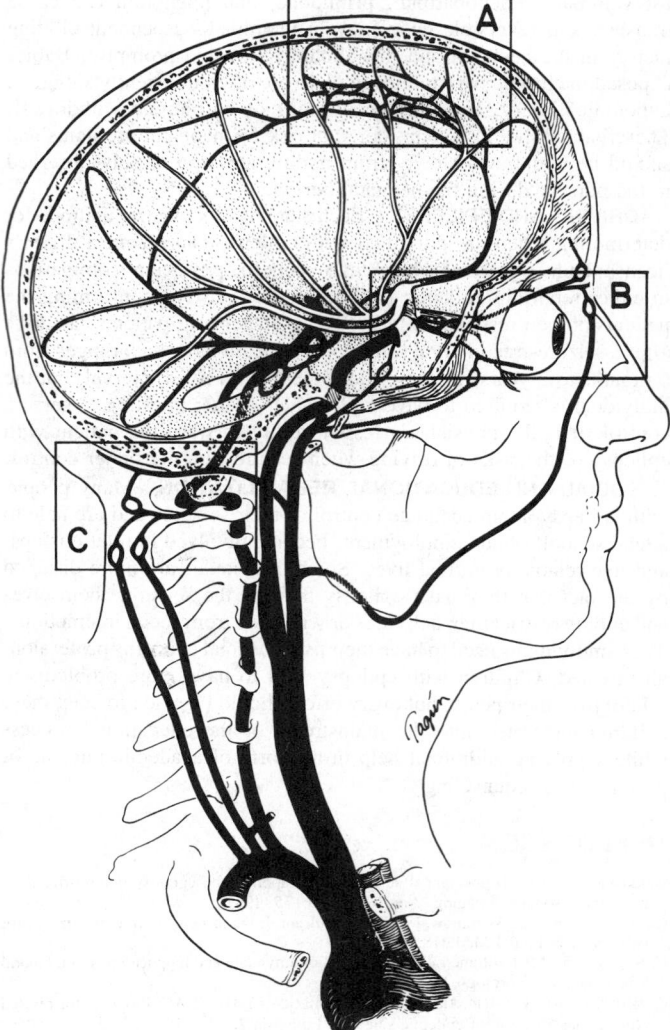

TIA SYNDROME TIAs can be conveniently divided into three types: (1) large vessel low-flow TIA, (2) embolic TIA, and (3) lacunar or small penetrating vessel TIA. *Low-flow TIAs* are brief (usually minutes to a few hours), recurrent, and stereotyped. They are often associated with a tightly stenotic atherosclerotic lesion at the internal carotid artery origin or in the intracranial portion of the internal carotid artery (siphon) when collateral flow from the circle of Willis to the ipsilateral middle or anterior cerebral artery is impaired (Figs. 368-1 and 368-2). Other important causes include atherosclerotic stenotic lesions in the middle cerebral artery stem or at the junction of the vertebral and basilar artery (see Fig. 368-2). Any obstructive vascular process listed in Table 368-1 in the extra- or intracranial arteries can cause a low-flow TIA syndrome if collateral flow to the potentially ischemic brain is also impaired (see Figs. 368-1*A–C* and 368-2).

Embolic TIAs are characterized by discrete, usually single, more prolonged (hours) episodes of focal neurologic symptoms. The embolus may arise from a pathologic process in an artery, usually extracranial, or from the heart. If symptoms or signs persist beyond 24 h, an ischemic stroke with infarction has occurred. However, symptoms that last less than 24 h also may be associated with ischemic infarction. If the primary pathologic process is thought to be embolic, a diligent search for its source is necessary before therapy to prevent future stroke is initiated. *Lacunar or penetrating vessel TIAs* occasionally occur due to transient cerebral ischemia from stenosis of one of the intracerebral penetrating vessels arising from the middle cerebral artery stem, the basilar or vertebral artery, or the circle of Willis (see Fig. 368-2). Occlusion of these small intracerebral penetrating vessels is usually due to lipohyalinosis from hypertension but also may arise from atheromatous disease at their origin. Occasionally, recurrent stereotyped TIAs occur. In this case, the term *lacunar* or *small-vessel TIAs* seems appropriate.

FIGURE 368-1 Arrangement of the major arteries of the right side carrying blood from the heart to the brain. Also shown are vessels of collateral circulation that may modify the effects of cerebral ischemia (*A,B,C*). Not shown is the circle of Willis, which also provides a source for collateral circulation. *A.* The anastomotic channels between the distal branches of the anterior and middle cerebral artery, termed borderzone or watershed anastomotic channels. Note that they also occur between the posterior and middle cerebral arteries and the anterior and posterior cerebral arteries. *B.* Anastomotic channels occurring through the orbit between branches of the external carotid artery and ophthalmic branch of the internal carotid artery. *C.* Wholly extracranial anastomotic channels between the muscular branches of the ascending cervical arteries and muscular branches of the occipital artery that anastomose with the distal vertebral artery. Note that the occipital artery arises from the external carotid artery, thereby allowing reconstitution of flow in the vertebral from the carotid circulation. (*Courtesy of C.M. Fisher, M.D.*)

STROKE SYNDROME The clinical characteristics and temporal course of ischemic stroke are produced by the same pathophysiologic mechanism responsible for TIAs: (1) large vessel thrombosis with low flow, (2) artery-to-artery, cardiogenic, or unknown-source embolism, or (3) small intracerebral penetrating vessel occlusion producing a lacuna. Of the many causes of primary thrombotic and embolic stroke listed in Table 368-1, thrombosis complicating atherosclerosis accounts for most cases of thrombotic stroke, and embolus of an unknown or cardiac source accounts for most cases of embolic stroke. The symptoms and signs resulting from an ischemic stroke differ depending on the precise location of the occlusion and the extent of the spared collateral flow. The following descriptions apply to

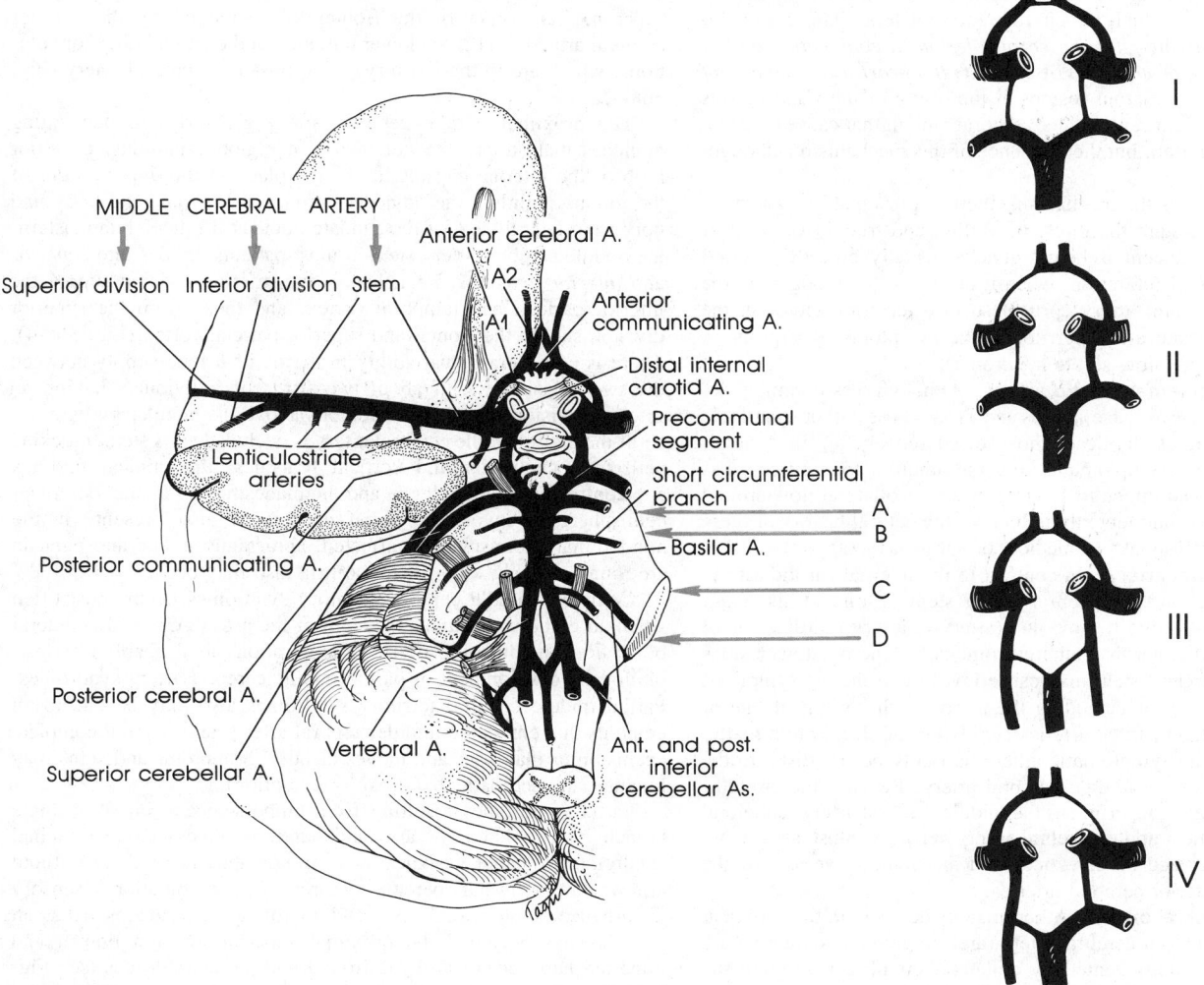

FIGURE 368-2 Diagram of the brainstem, cerebellum, inferior right frontal lobe, and temporal lobe transected. Principal branches of the vertebral basilar arterial system are pictured. Small branches of the vertebral and basilar artery that penetrate the medulla and pons are not pictured. The stem of the middle cerebral artery with its small, deep penetrating lenticulostriate arteries and the circle of Willis with its small, deep penetrating branches are shown. Roman numerals I, II, III, and IV represent some of the possible variations of the circle of Willis due to atresia of one or more of its arterial components. *A, B, C,* and *D* arrows point to the four cross sections of the brainstem diagrammed below (*D* = Fig. 368-7, *A* = Fig. 368-8, *B* = Fig. 368-9, *C* = Fig. 368-10). Although typical vascular syndromes of the pons and medulla have been designated by the shaded areas in Figs. 368-7 to 368-10, the shading is arbitrary. Great variability in infarct size and location occurs when the basilar or vertebral arteries or one of their penetrating branches becomes occluded. This variability is because of variation in arterial anatomic location and available collateral circulation. Thus the stroke syndromes produced are often atypical, incomplete, or merge with one another. (*Courtesy of C.M. Fisher, M.D.*)

infarction and ischemia in specific arteries due to atherothrombosis, although similar syndromes may occur with other types of arterial pathology, after primary embolic stroke, and occasionally after primary intracerebral hemorrhage.

ATHEROTHROMBOTIC DISEASE OF THE INTERNAL CAROTID ARTERY AND ITS BRANCHES

PATHOPHYSIOLOGY The origin of the internal carotid artery is the most common site of atherosclerosis and superimposed atherothrombosis that leads to TIA or stroke. Less often, disease at the siphon (S-shaped portion of the internal carotid artery in the cavernous sinus) or in the proximal segment (stem) of the middle or anterior cerebral arteries may be responsible. Rarely, the origin of the common carotid artery may be the site.

Internal carotid artery Atherosclerosis in the proximal internal carotid artery is usually most severe in the first 2 cm and arises from the posterior wall, often extending downward into the common carotid artery. Atherosclerosis at this site is often heralded by a minor stoke or TIA caused by embolism or, less frequently, low flow.

Emboli arising from a stenotic or ulcerated atherosclerotic lesion at the origin of the internal carotid artery may cause occlusion of the ophthalmic artery, the middle cerebral artery stem or one of its branches, or, less often, the anterior cerebral artery. Small platelet emboli that occlude the ophthalmic artery branches cause transient monocular blindness (*amaurosis fugax*). Larger emboli composed of platelet-fibrin clot may occlude the primary and secondary branches of the middle cerebral artery leading to discrete and easily recognizable neurologic syndromes. Large emboli may occlude the proximal "stem" of the middle cerebral artery, leading to devastating ischemia of the entire middle cerebral territory (deep white matter, lenticular nuclei, and cortical surface). In some instances, only deep infarction occurs because collateral flow through the cortical surface is sufficient (see Fig. 368-1*A*). Large emboli may partially occlude a major vessel or may migrate or lyse and disperse, causing a neurologic deficit that fluctuates (stroke in evolution) or resolves.

In some patients, an ulcerated plaque may be the only lesion in the carotid bifurcation, but more often there is an accompanying stenosis with a residual lumen diameter of less than 2 mm. *A nonstenotic or slightly stenotic carotid lesion in conjunction with a stroke or a single prolonged TIA suggests the heart as the source of the embolus.* Atheromatous lesions at the origin of the great vessels in the aortic arch also can produce cerebral emboli that cause transient ischemia or infarction, but the incidence of this mechanism is thought to be low.

When *low flow* is the mechanism, there is presumably inadequate collateral flow through the circle of Willis, and true TIAs, with or without retinal transient ischemic attacks, usually precede cerebral infarction. Cerebral infarction, when it occurs, usually begins in the distal middle cerebral artery cortical surface territory and/or in the distal lenticulostriate artery territory. The symptoms may progress slowly or fluctuate (slow stroke syndrome).

Intracranial internal carotid artery   Although less common, lesions in the siphon can cause strokes and TIAs whose pathophysiologic and clinical features duplicate those discussed above. In general, siphon stenosis is asymptomatic until the atheromatous process has reduced the residual lumen to 1.5 mm or less. Collateral flow around the circle of Willis undoubtedly influences the natural history of these lesions and their response to medical or surgical therapy.

Middle cerebral artery   In contrast to the internal carotid artery, occlusion of the middle cerebral artery stem or one of its major branches is usually due to embolus (artery-to-artery, cardiac, or of unknown source) rather than atherothrombosis. Atheromatous lesions in the middle cerebral stem may cause low-flow ischemic symptoms either by narrowing or occluding the artery or the origin of one or more of the lenticulostriate arteries supplying the deep white matter and basal ganglia. Symptomatic atheroma rarely occurs distal to the first bifurcation of the middle cerebral artery. Because the circle of Willis is proximal to the origin of the middle cerebral artery, collateral blood flow to the middle cerebral artery territory must arise from small cortical surface border zones and anastomotic vessels of the anterior and posterior cerebral arteries.

Anterior cerebral artery   Atheromatous deposits in the proximal segment of the anterior cerebral artery rarely cause symptoms because the occlusion is circumvented by collateral circulation through the anterior communicating artery. However, if the anterior communicating artery is congenitally atretic or if the atheromatous lesion occurs distal in the anterior cerebral artery, TIAs and stroke may occur.

CLINICAL SYNDROMES   Middle cerebral artery   The cortical branches of the middle cerebral artery supply the lateral surface of the hemisphere except for (1) the frontal pole and a strip along the superomedial border of the frontal lobe supplied by the anterior cerebral artery and (2) the lower temporal and occipital pole convolutions, which are in the territory of the posterior cerebral artery (Fig. 368-3).

The proximal middle cerebral artery gives rise to penetrating branches that supply the putamen, outer globus pallidus, posterior limb of the internal capsule above the plane of the upper border of the globus pallidus, the adjacent corona radiata, and the body and upper and lateral head of the caudate nucleus. In the sylvian cistern, the middle cerebral artery stem in most patients divides into *superior* and *inferior divisions.* Branches of the inferior division supply the inferior parietal and temporal cortex, and those from the superior division supply the frontal and superior parietal cortex (Fig. 368-4). There is considerable variability in the parietal lobe supply between the two divisions, with about two-thirds of individuals having an inferior division that supplies regions above the angular gyrus.

If the entire middle cerebral artery is occluded at its stem, blocking both the penetrating and cortical branches, the clinical findings are contralateral hemiplegia and hemianesthesia. If the dominant hemisphere is involved, global aphasia is also present. If the nondominant hemisphere is affected, apractagnosia and anosognosia are found (see Fig. 368-4). Dysarthria also may occur.

Complete middle cerebral territory syndromes occur most often when an embolus occludes the stem of the artery. Cortical collateral blood flow and differing arterial configurations are probably responsible for the development of partial middle cerebral artery syndromes. Partial middle cerebral territory syndromes also may be due to an embolus that enters the middle cerebral artery stem without complete occlusion or that lyses and moves distally. Symptoms and signs may fluctuate in such patients (stroke in evolution).

Partial syndromes resulting from embolic occlusion of a single branch include hand, or arm and hand, weakness alone (brachial syndrome) or facial weakness with motor aphasia, with or without arm weakness (frontal opercular syndrome). A combination of sensory disturbance, motor weakness, and motor aphasia suggests that an embolus has occluded the proximal superior division branch and infarcted large portions of the frontal and parietal cortices (see Fig. 368-4). If Wernicke's aphasia occurs without weakness, the inferior division of the middle cerebral artery supplying the posterior part (temporal cortex) of the dominant hemisphere is probably involved (see Fig. 368-4). Jargon speech and an inability to comprehend written and oral language are prominent features, often accompanied by a

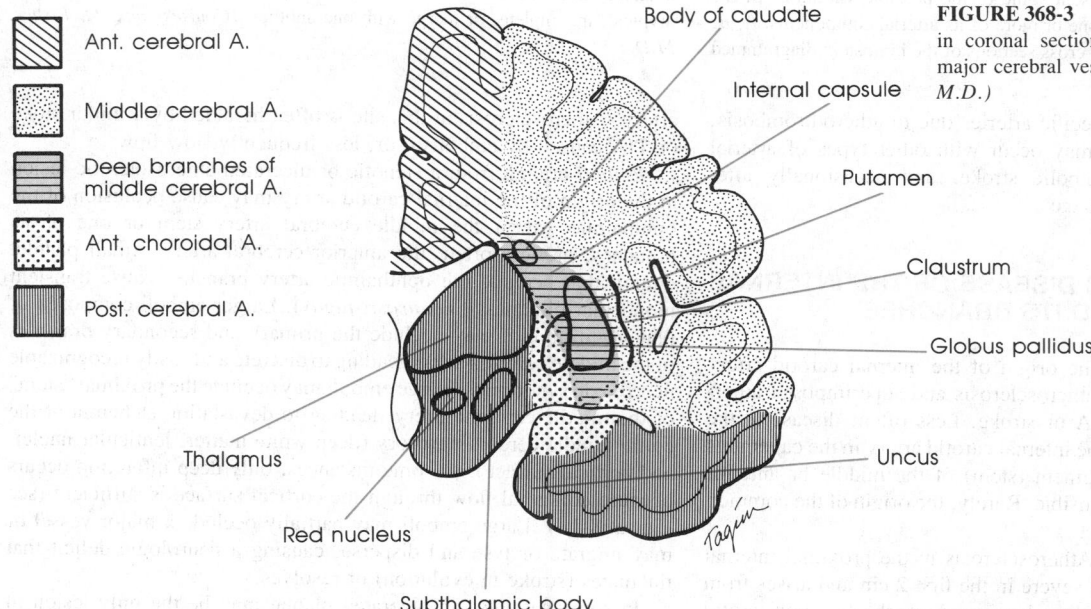

Ant. cerebral A.

Middle cerebral A.

Deep branches of middle cerebral A.

Ant. choroidal A.

Post. cerebral A.

Body of caudate

Internal capsule

Putamen

Claustrum

Globus pallidus

Uncus

Thalamus

Red nucleus

Subthalamic body

FIGURE 368-3   Diagram of a cerebral hemisphere in coronal section showing the territories of the major cerebral vessels. *(Courtesy of C. M. Fisher, M.D.)*

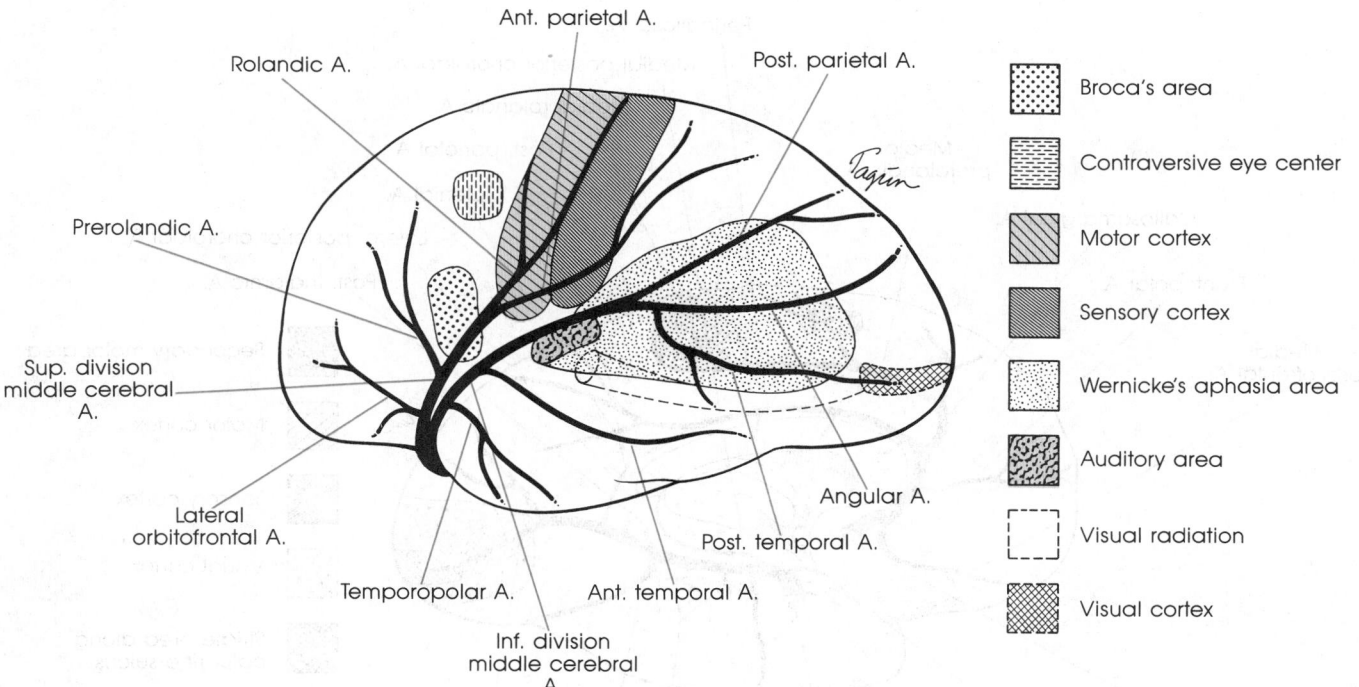

FIGURE 368-4 Diagram of a cerebral hemisphere, lateral aspect, showing the branches and distribution of the middle cerebral artery and the principal regions of cerebral localization. Note the bifurcation of the middle cerebral artery into a superior and inferior division (*Courtesy of C. M. Fisher, M.D.*)

Signs and symptoms	Structures involved
Paralysis of the contralateral face, arm, and leg; sensory impairment over the same area (pinprick, cotton touch, vibration, position, two-point discrimination, stereognosis, tactile localization, barognosis, cutaneographia)	Somatic motor area for face and arm and the fibers descending from the leg area to enter the corona radiata and corresponding somatic sensory system
Motor aphasia	Motor speech area of the dominant hemisphere
Central aphasia, word deafness, anomia, jargon speech, sensory agraphia, acalculia, alexia, finger agnosia, right-left confusion (the last four comprise the Gerstmann syndrome)	Central, suprasylvian speech area and parietooccipital cortex of the dominant hemisphere
Conduction aphasia	Central speech area (parietal operculum)
Apractognosia of the minor hemisphere (amorphosynthesis), anosognosia, hemiasomatognosia, unilateral neglect, agnosia for the left half of external space, dressing "apraxia," constructional "apraxia," distortion of visual coordinates, inaccurate localization in the half field, impaired ability to judge distance, upside-down reading, visual illusions (e.g., it may appear that another person walks through a table)	Nondominant parietal lobe (area corresponding to speech area in dominant hemisphere); loss of topographic memory is usually due to a nondominant lesion, occasionally to a dominant one
Homonymous hemianopsia (often homonymous inferior quadrantonopsia)	Optic radiation deep to second temporal convolution
Paralysis of conjugate gaze to the opposite side	Frontal contraversive field or fibers projecting therefrom

contralateral superior quadrantanopsia. Hemineglect or spatial agnosia without weakness indicates that the inferior division of the middle cerebral artery in the nondominant hemisphere is involved.

Anterior cerebral artery The anterior cerebral artery is divided into two segments: the precommunal (A1) circle of Willis, or stem, which connects the internal carotid artery to the anterior communicating artery, and the postcommunal (A2) segment distal to the anterior communicating artery (see Fig. 368-2). The A1 segment of the anterior cerebral artery gives rise to several deep penetrating branches that supply the anterior limb of the internal capsule, the anterior perforate substance, amygdala, anterior hypothalamus, and the inferior part of the head of the caudate nucleus (see Fig. 368-3).

Infarction in the territory of the anterior cerebral artery is uncommon and most often due to embolism rather than atherothrombosis. Occlusion of the A1 segment of the anterior cerebral artery is usually well tolerated because of collateral flow. If both A2 segments arise from a single anterior cerebral stem (contralateral A1 segment atresia), then the occlusion affects both hemispheres. Profound abulia (a delay in verbal and motor response) and bilateral pyramidal signs with paraplegia result. Occlusion of a single A2 segment of the anterior

cerebral artery results in the contralateral symptoms noted in the legend of Fig. 368-5.

Anterior choroidal artery This artery arises from the internal carotid artery and supplies the posterior limb of the internal capsule and the white matter posterolateral to it, through which pass some of the geniculocalcarine fibers (Figs. 368-3 and 368-6). The complete clinical syndrome of anterior choroidal artery occlusion consists of contralateral hemiplegia, hemianesthesia (hypesthesia), and homonymous hemianopsia. However, because this territory is also supplied by penetrating vessels of the middle cerebral stem and the posterior communicating and posterior choroidal arteries, syndromes with minimal deficits may occur, and patients frequently recover partially or completely.

Internal carotid artery The clinical picture of internal carotid occlusion varies depending on whether the cause of ischemia is propagated thrombus, embolism, or low flow. The cortex supplied by the middle cerebral territory is most often affected. With a competent circle of Willis, however, occlusion can be entirely asymptomatic. Less often, there is massive infarction of the deep white matter and cortical surface from propagation of a thrombus up

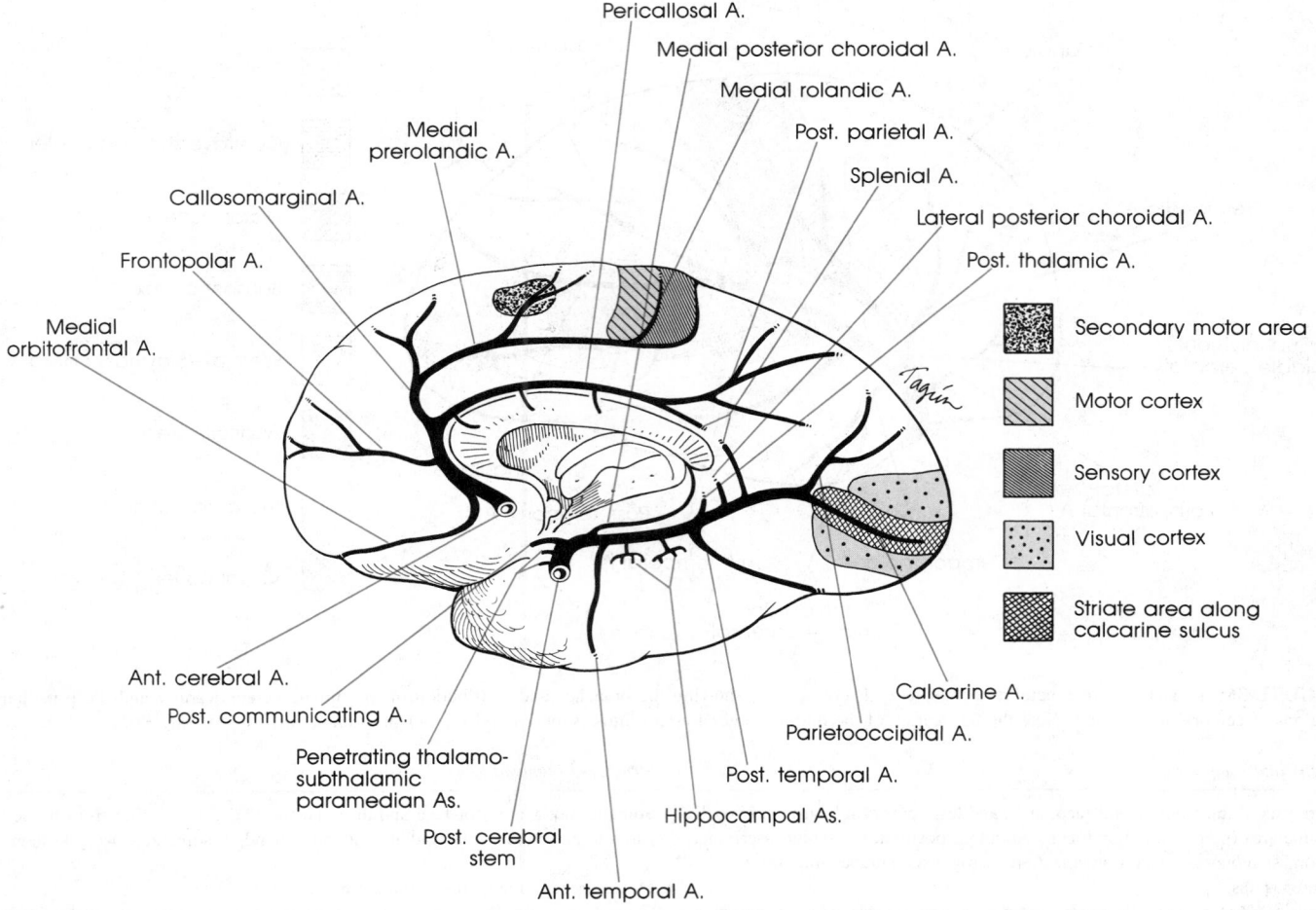

FIGURE 368-5   Diagram of a cerebral hemisphere, medial aspect, showing the branches and distribution of the anterior cerebral artery and the principal regions of cerebral localization. (*Courtesy of C. M. Fisher, M.D.*)

Signs and symptoms	Structures involved
Paralysis of opposite foot and leg	Motor leg area
A lesser degree of paresis of opposite arm	Involvement of arm area of cortex or fibers descending to corona radiata therefrom
Cortical sensory loss over toes, foot, and leg	Sensory area for foot and leg
Urinary incontinence	Sensorimotor area in paracentral lobule
Contralateral grasp reflex, sucking reflex, gegenhalten (paratonic rigidity)	Medial surface of the posterior frontal lobe (?) supplemental motor area
Abulia (akinetic mutism), slowness, delay, intermittent interruption, lack of spontaneity, whispering, reflex distraction to sights and sounds	Uncertain localization—probably cingulate gyrus and medial inferior portion of frontal, parietal, and temporal lobes
Impairment of gait and stance (gait apraxia)	Frontal cortex near leg motor area
Dyspraxia of left limbs, tactile aphasia in left limbs	Corpus callosum

the internal carotid artery, into the middle cerebral stem, or from embolization to the stem of the middle cerebral artery. Symptoms are identical to middle cerebral stem occlusion (see above). When the origins of both the anterior and middle cerebral arteries are occluded by embolus to the top of the carotid artery, abulia and/or stupor occurs with hemiplegia, hemianesthesia, and aphasia or anosognosia. When the posterior cerebral artery arises from the internal carotid artery (an unusual configuration called a *fetal posterior cerebral artery*), it also may become occluded and give rise to symptoms referable to its peripheral territory (see Figs. 368-5 and 368-6).

Carotid occlusion may cause low-flow infarction if the circle of Willis is incomplete. The territory of the distal cortical branches of the middle cerebral artery tends to be involved, giving rise to transient or stepwise, progressive hip, shoulder, or arm weakness. Other TIAs suggestive of carotid insufficiency include recurrent unilateral tongue, lip, cheek, or hand numbness, with or without motor weakness.

In addition to supplying the ipsilateral brain, the internal carotid artery perfuses the optic nerve and retina via the ophthalmic artery (see Fig. 368-1). In about 25 percent of symptomatic internal carotid disease, transient recurrent monocular blindness (TMB or amaurosis fugax) warns of the lesion. Patients may describe a shade that seems to sweep up, down, or across the field of vision or may say that the periphery of vision fades away. They also may complain that their vision was blurred in that eye or that the upper or lower half of vision disappeared. In most cases, these symptoms last only a few minutes. Rarely, ophthalmic or central retinal artery occlusion develops at the time of stroke.

Common carotid artery   All the neurologic symptoms and signs of internal carotid occlusion also may be present with occlusion of the common carotid artery. Bilateral common carotid arterial occlusion at their origin may occur in "pulseless disease," or the aortic arch syndrome (see Chap. 210). Clues to this condition are absence of

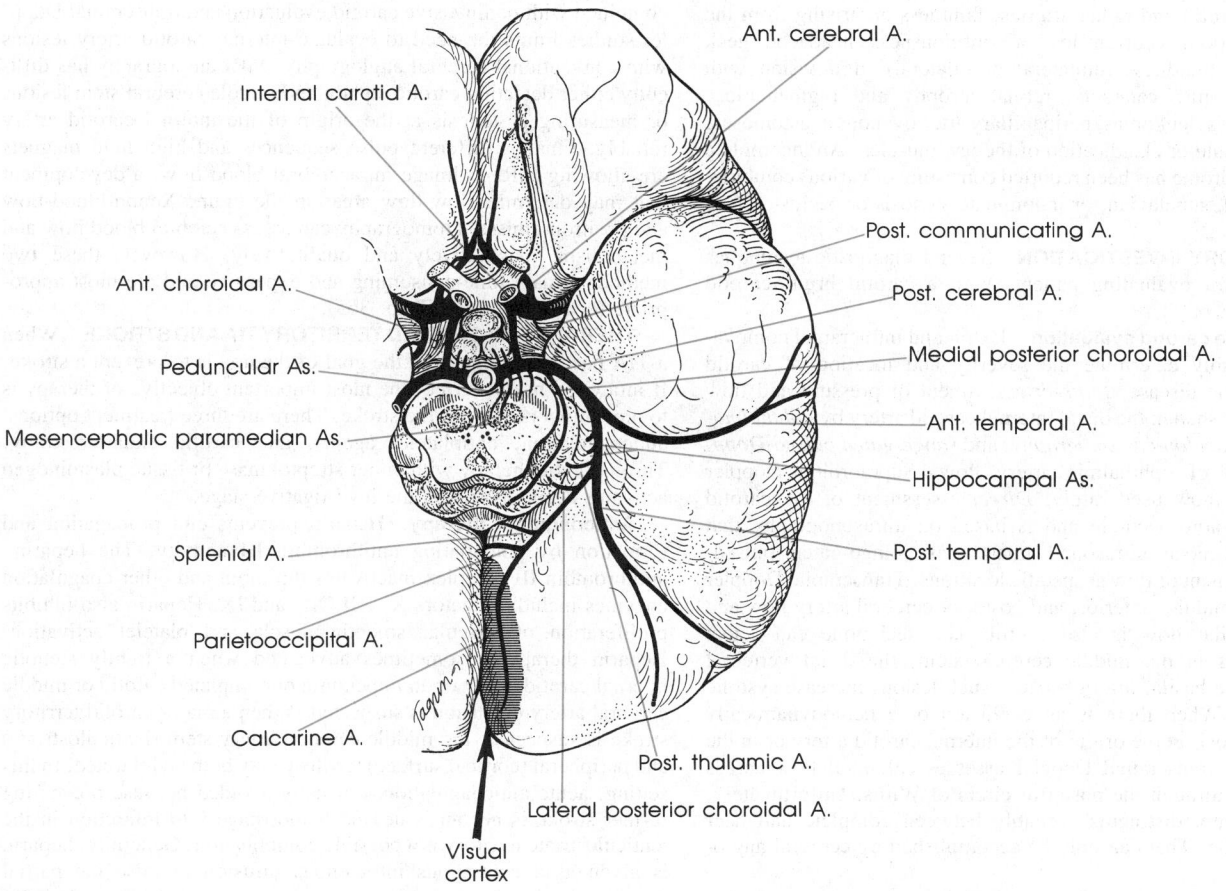

FIGURE 368-6 Inferior aspect of the brain with the branches and distribution of the posterior cerebral artery and the principal anatomic structures shown. (*Courtesy of C. M. Fisher, M.D.*)

Signs and symptoms	Structures involved
Peripheral territory (see also Fig. 368-5)	
Homonymous hemianopsia (often upper quadrantic)	Calcarine cortex or optic radiation nearby
Bilateral homonymous hemianopsia, cortical blindness, awareness or denial of blindness; tactile naming, achromatopsia (color blindness), failure to see to-and-fro movements, inability to perceive objects not centrally located, apraxia of ocular movements, inability to count or enumerate objects, tendency to run into things which the patient sees and tries to avoid	Bilateral occipital lobe with possibly the parietal lobe involved.
Verbal dyslexia without agraphia, color anomia	Dominant calcarine lesion and posterior part of corpus callosum
Memory defect	Hippocampal lesion bilaterally or on the dominant side only
Topographic disorientation and prosopagnosia	Usually with lesions of nondominant, calcarine, and lingual gyrus
Simultagnosia, hemivisual neglect	Dominant visual cortex, contralateral hemisphere
Unformed visual hallucinations, peduncular hallucinosis, metamorphopsia, teleopsia, illusory visual spread, irreminiscence, paliopsia, distortion of outlines, central photophobia	Calcarine cortex
Complex hallucinations	Usually nondominant hemisphere
Central territory	
Thalamic syndrome: sensory loss (all modalities), spontaneous pain and dysesthesias, choreoathetosis, intention tremor, spasms of hand, mild hemiparesis	Posteroventral nucleus of thalamus; involvement of the adjacent subthalamus body or its afferent tracts
Thalamoperforate syndrome: crossed cerebellar ataxia with ipsilateral third nerve palsy (Claude's syndrome)	Dentatothalamic tract and issuing third nerve
Weber's syndrome: third nerve palsy and contralateral hemiplegia	Third nerve and cerebral peduncle
Contralateral hemiplegia	Cerebral peduncle
Paralysis or paresis of vertical eye movement, skew deviation, sluggish pupillary responses to light, slight miosis and ptosis (retraction nystagmus and "tucking" of the eyelids may be associated)	Supranuclear fibers to third nerve, interstitial nucleus of Cajal, nucleus of Darkschewitsch, and posterior commissure
Contralateral rhythmic, ataxic action tremor; rhythmic postural or "holding" tremor (rubral tremor)	Dentatothalamic tract (?)

pulsation in carotid and radial arteries, faintness on arising from the horizontal position, recurrent loss of consciousness, headache, neck pain, transient blindness (unilateral or bilateral), dim vision with exercise, premature cataracts, retinal atrophy and pigmentation, atrophy of the iris, leukomas, peripapillary arteriovenous anastomoses, optic atrophy, and/or claudication of the jaw muscles. An incomplete aortic arch syndrome has been reported consisting of various combinations of carotid, subclavian, or innominate stenosis or occlusion (see below).

LABORATORY INVESTIGATION   Several diagnostic techniques are available for evaluating patients with a carotid bruit, carotid territory stroke, or TIA.

Noninvasive carotid evaluation   Extra- and intracranial noninvasive tests reliably determine the severity and location of carotid atherothrombotic disease. *Indirect* assessment of pressure and flow can be accomplished in the distal internal carotid artery by *ophthalmodynamometry, oculoplethysmography*, and *range-gated pulsed-Doppler assessment* of ophthalmic artery flow. Supraorbital Doppler examination is now used rarely. *Direct* assessment of the carotid bifurcation is more accurate and is based on ultrasonography that combines a B-mode ultrasound image with range-gated pulsed-Doppler assessment of flow at specific locations. Transcranial Doppler assessment of middle, anterior, and posterior cerebral artery flow and of vertebrobasilar flow is also useful. This technique can detect stenotic lesions in the middle cerebral stem, the distal vertebral arteries, and the basilar artery because such lesions increase systolic flow velocity. When there is an occlusion or a hemodynamically significant stenosis at the origin of the internal carotid artery or in the carotid siphon, transcranial Doppler assesses collateral flow across the anterior or through the posterior circle of Willis. Unfortunately, these tests cannot distinguish reliably between complete and near carotid occlusion. That can only be accomplished by cerebral angiography.

Cerebral angiography   Cerebral angiography performed by selective extracranial dye injection after transfemoral catheterization remains the most reliable method of assessing the cerebrovascular system. It can (1) detect ulcerative lesions, severe stenosis, and formation of mural thrombus at the bifurcation of the common carotid artery, (2) visualize atherothrombotic disease or dissection in the carotid siphon or intracranial vessels, (3) demonstrate collateral circulation around the circle of Willis and on the cortical surface, and (4) show embolic occlusion of cerebral branch vessels. Although angiography cannot measure blood flow directly, the timing of dye arrival reflects relative pressures in major vessels and may demonstrate compromised flow in the internal carotid artery system.

The advantages of selective cerebral angiography must be balanced in each patient against complications that occur in 2 to 12 percent. The principal risks are aortic or carotid artery dissection and embolic stroke. Cholesterol emboli from aortic arch atheroma rarely can cause watershed cerebral infarction and renal failure. A skilled angiographer and careful attention to hydration reduce these risks. Because of the risks, attention is now being directed to the development of magnetic resonance angiographic imaging (see Chap. 365).

Brain imaging   Brain imaging remains the most important acute test once a stroke has occurred. *Computed tomographic* (CT) *scans* immediately exclude hemorrhage as the cause of stroke, but they may fail to show small ischemic strokes in the posterior fossa or be imprecise because of bone artifact. CT scans also may miss infarction on the cortical surface. Furthermore, they cannot detect cerebral infarction reliably for the first 24 to 48 h (see Chap. 365).

Magnetic resonance imaging (MRI) reliably documents the extent and location of infarction not only in the cortical surface, but also in the deep white matter and in the posterior fossa within 1 h of its onset. It also documents primary intracranial hemorrhage. The higher the field strength, the more reliable and precise the image will be. Using high field strengths (1.5 Tesla) and different pulse sequencing, blood flow may be imaged in the extracranial arteries and in the large intracranial extracerebral vessels. In many cases, *MRI angiography*

combined with noninvasive carotid evaluation and transcranial Doppler studies limits the need to evaluate internal carotid artery lesions with conventional cerebral angiography. MRI angiography has difficulty either detecting carotid siphon and middle cerebral stem lesions or measuring a stenosis at the origin of the internal carotid artery reliably. Finally, different pulse sequences and high field magnets are allowing MRI to image intracerebral blood flow, a development that may determine low-flow areas in the brain. Xenon-blood-flow and positron-emission tomography can assess cerebral blood flow and metabolism quantitatively and qualitatively. However, these two methods remain time-consuming and expensive and are most appropriate for research (see Chap. 365).

THERAPY FOR CAROTID TERRITORY TIA AND STROKE   When a TIA has been diagnosed, the goal of therapy is to prevent a stroke. If infarction has occurred, the most important objective of therapy is to prevent worsening of the stroke. There are three treatment options: anticoagulation, antiplatelet agents, and carotid endarterectomy. Thrombolytic therapy with either streptokinase or tissue plasminogen activator agents is still in the investigative stage.

Anticoagulant therapy   Heparin prevents clot propagation and formation by potentiating antithrombin III activity. The heparin–antithrombin III complex inactivates thrombin and other coagulation enzymes including factors X, XII, XI, and IX. Heparin also inhibits proliferation of vascular smooth muscle and platelet activation. Heparin therapy is sometimes advocated when a tightly stenotic internal carotid artery or an impending or completed carotid or middle cerebral artery occlusion is suspected. When a major carotid territory stroke is suspected, the middle cerebral artery stem (lenticulostriate) and peripheral (cortical surface) territory may both be infarcted. In this setting, acute anticoagulation is usually avoided because preventing further stroke is not an issue and hemorrhage into infarction in the lenticulostriate territory is a possible complication. Generally, heparin is given as a continuous intravenous infusion to raise the partial thromboplastin time to 1.5 to 2.5 times control. A 1000- to 10,000-unit bolus may be given prior to initiating the continuous infusion.

Sodium warfarin (Coumadin) inhibits the activation of vitamin K, the essential cofactor in the activation of the vitamin K–dependent coagulation proteins. Chronic oral anticoagulation with sodium warfarin is considered in patients when an embolic or low-flow TIA or stroke is related to carotid siphon or middle cerebral stem stenosis. It is also considered for 6-month trial to prevent subsequent embolism when the internal carotid artery is known to have been occluded recently. Although several studies have suggested that sodium warfarin is effective in these clinical settings, a randomized study is required to document conclusively the effectiveness of either oral anticoagulation or antiplatelet agents. It is well established that the risk of hemorrhage is directly related to the intensity of anticoagulation. Therefore, low-intensity warfarin anticoagulation (prothrombin time ratio 1.2 to 1.5 times control or international normalized ratio 1.5 to 2.7 or 2 to 3) is usually used (see "Embolism," below). When the standard medical contraindications are present, antiplatelet therapy becomes the only option.

Antiplatelet therapy   Studies of the effect of antiplatelet agents on the natural history of TIAs and minor stroke all suffer from a lack of precise understanding of the pathophysiologic condition underlying the ischemic event. Aspirin has been the most widely studied antiplatelet agent. Paradoxically, aspirin has dual effects: It inhibits platelet formation of thromboxane A_2, a platelet-aggregating, vasoconstricting prostaglandin, but it also inhibits the formation of prostacyclin, an antiaggregating, vasodilating prostaglandin derived from endothelial cells. Aspirin in low doses predominantly inhibits the production of thromboxane A_2; therefore, many physicians recommend aspirin in doses of 300 mg or less per day.

Dipyridamole acts by inhibiting platelet phosphodiesterase, which is responsible for the breakdown of cyclic adenosine monophosphate (AMP). The resulting elevation in cyclic AMP inhibits the aggregation of platelets. There is no reliable evidence to suggest that dipyridamole alone prevents ischemic stroke. In one study in patients with prosthetic valves, there was a nonstatistically significant suggestion that warfarin in combination with dipyridamole helped prevent embolism. Ticlopidine is thought to inhibit platelet binding to fibrinogen, and recent studies have shown it to be comparable to aspirin in preventing stroke in patients with TIAs or stroke. Unfortunately, these studies also suffer from failure to define precisely the pathophysiologic cause of the cerebral symptoms. Ticlopidine has the disadvantage of incurring a small risk of leukopenia, diarrhea, and rash. It is recommended for use as an antiplatelet agent only if aspirin is contraindicated or fails.

Carotid endarterectomy Carotid endarterectomy is the treatment of choice for patients who have had a low-flow or embolic TIA or minor stroke resulting from a tightly stenotic (>70 percent stenosis) arteriosclerotic lesion at the origin of the internal carotid artery. Its efficacy has been documented by three randomized trials. However, none of them found a statistically significant improvement in subsequent ipsilateral stroke when endarterectomy is performed on lesions that are not tightly stenotic. One of the trials is continuing to randomize patients with a 30 to 70 percent stenotic internal carotid artery origin lesion and ipsilateral carotid territory symptoms. Each trial has had a combined surgery and angiography complication rate of less than 4 percent. It is clear that the morbidity is lowest when patients are properly selected from a cardiac/medical risk point of view and an experienced team of surgeons, physicians, and nurses manages the patients. Reliable guidelines have now been developed to exclude patients with an unacceptable cardiac risk. Unless the combined anesthesia and surgical morbidity and mortality are less than 5 percent, medical therapy is probably the best choice. Because in one study endarterectomy carried a 26 percent benefit for stroke reduction compared with aspirin, the latter might not be the best medical therapy. Low-intensity warfarin anticoagulation may be better. It is often considered in patients with symptomatic tightly stenotic carotid stenosis who carry too high a risk for surgery.

Antiedema and general medical therapy Cerebral edema occurs in most ischemic infarctions but is rarely a problem unless large middle cerebral stem territory infarction occurs. When edema with mass effect is evident on CT or MRI and the patient becomes drowsy, it is best to keep the patient slightly dehydrated with a normal or elevated serum sodium level. If symptoms worsen, therapy with mannitol to keep the serum osmolarity above 300 mosmol/L is helpful. Serious cerebral edema usually begins 48 to 72 h after the stroke and begins to resolve by the second week. In all patients with acute carotid territory ischemic stroke and hypertension, it is best not to lower the blood pressure rapidly. The expanded use of anticoagulant therapy to prevent subsequent stroke has the added advantage of helping to prevent phlebitis in patients with a hemiparesis.

Experimental therapies Therapies designed to protect the brain under conditions of extreme ischemia are being actively studied. Therapies designed to reduce blood viscosity have been effective in the laboratory setting but have not been clearly effective in the clinical setting of prolonged ischemia. Nonetheless, they carry little risk and may be of benefit. It is probably best to keep the hematocrit slightly low, at 35 percent, if there is prolonged cerebral ischemia in the stroke process. Calcium channel antagonists have not convincingly limited infarct size. Experimental studies with glutamate receptor antagonists (specifically the NMDA subtype; see Chap. 364), show promise of reducing stroke size.

ASYMPTOMATIC CAROTID BIFURCATION STENOSIS WITH A BRUIT The natural history of asymptomatic atherosclerotic lesions of the carotid bifurcation that produce a bruit is uncertain. There is evidence that the tighter the stenotic lesion, the more likely symptoms are to occur over time. Patients with tightly stenotic lesions that are hemodynamically significant (residual lumen diameter 1.5 mm or less, 75 percent stenosis) may be at higher risk of embolic stroke. Although such patients have reduced flow in the distal internal carotid artery, they remain asymptomatic because of adequate collateral flow in circle of Willis. Clot may form in the low-flow carotid and may be associated with artery-to-artery embolism.

A high-pitched prolonged carotid bruit fading into diastole is often associated with such tightly stenotic lesions. As the stenosis grows tighter and flow distal to the stenosis becomes reduced, the bruit becomes fainter and finally disappears when occlusion is imminent. Noninvasive carotid testing combined with transcranial Doppler assessment of collateral flow across the anterior circle of Willis helps identify such lesions and document progression.

Medical therapy (aspirin 325 mg/d) generally has been recommended for patients with asymptomatic carotid stenosis. However, patients with hemodynamically significant lesions, particularly if they have progression in severity, may benefit from low-morbidity carotid endarterectomy. However, surgery should be considered only in the absence of significant cardiac disease and when the physiologic age of the patient will allow the benefits of endarterectomy over time. Randomized trials comparing medical and surgical therapy may reliably identify patients with tightly stenotic hemodynamically significant lesions and establish criteria for choosing one treatment over the other.

ATHEROTHROMBOTIC DISEASE OF THE VERTEBROBASILAR–POSTERIOR CEREBRAL ARTERY SYSTEM

The two vertebral arteries join to form the basilar artery at the pontomedullary junction. The basilar artery divides into two posterior cerebral arteries in the interpeduncular fossa (see Fig. 368-2). Each of these major arteries gives rise to long and short circumferential branches and to smaller deep penetrating branches that supply the cerebellum, medulla, pons, midbrain, subthalamus, thalamus, hippocampus, and medial temporal and occipital lobes. Atherosclerosis has a predilection for the origin and the distal segments of the vertebral arteries, the proximal basilar artery, and the origin of the major and minor branches of the vertebral, basilar, and posterior cerebral arteries. Predictably, atheromatous disease at each site carries its own unique natural history, produces its own clinical syndromes, and has its own specific therapeutic implications.

POSTERIOR CEREBRAL ARTERY **Pathophysiology** In 70 percent of cases, both posterior cerebral arteries arise from the bifurcation of the basilar artery; in 22 percent, one or the other comes from the ipsilateral internal carotid artery; in 8 percent, both come from the ipsilateral internal carotid artery (see Fig. 368-2) via the posterior communicating arteries. The precommunal segment (mesencephalic portion) of the true posterior cerebral artery is atretic in such cases (see Fig. 368-2).

Atheroma formation at the top of the basilar artery or along the precommunal segment of the posterior cerebral artery may cause symptoms by narrowing one or more of the small brainstem-penetrating branches (see Figs. 368-2 and 368-6) that supply the middle cerebral peduncles, the substantia nigra, red nucleus, oculomotor nuclei, midbrain reticular formation, subthalamic nucleus of Luys, decussation of superior cerebellar peduncles, the medial longitudinal fasciculus, and the medial lemniscus. The artery of Percheron (the posterior thalamosubthalamoparamedian artery) is a single artery that arises from either the right or the left precommunal segment of the posterior cerebral artery. It divides in the subthalamus to supply the inferomedial and anterior portions of the thalamus and subthalamus bilaterally. The thalamogeniculate branches, which also originate from the precommunal portion of the posterior cerebral artery, supply the dorsal, dorsomedial, anterior, and inferior thalamus and the medial geniculate body. The medial posterior choroidal artery supplies the superior dorsomedial and dorsoanterior thalamus and the medial geniculate body in addition to the tela choroidea of the third ventricle. The lateral posterior choroidal artery supplies the choroid plexus of the lateral ventricle.

Atheroma in the posterior cerebral artery distal to the junction with the posterior communicating artery (see Fig. 368-6) may occlude small circumferential branches that course around the midbrain to supply the lateral part of the cerebral peduncles, medial lemniscus, tegmentum of the midbrain, superior colliculi, lateral geniculate body, and posterolateral nucleus of the thalamus, choroid plexus, and hippocampus. On the rare occasions when atheroma occur more distally in the posterior cerebral artery (see Fig. 368-6), occlusion may produce ischemia and infarction in the inferomedial temporal lobe, parahippocampal and hippocampal gyri, and occipital lobe—including the calcarine cortex and the visual association areas 18 and 19.

Clinical manifestations The site of atheromas and the degree of narrowing determine the clinical syndrome. Although factors of collateral circulation or serum viscosity may play a role in some cases, embolic occlusion is the usual cause of stroke in this vascular territory. Two syndromes are commonly observed: (1) midbrain, subthalamic, and thalamic signs, which are due to disease of the precommunal segment of the posterior cerebral artery or of its penetrating branches and (2) cortical temporal and occipital lobe syndromes, due to occlusion of the postcommunal segment.

PROXIMAL PRECOMMUNAL SYNDROMES (CENTRAL TERRITORY) If the proximal posterior cerebral artery is occluded, infarction usually occurs in the ipsilateral or bilateral subthalamus and medial thalamus and in the ipsilateral cerebral peduncle and midbrain, producing concomitant signs (see Fig. 368-6). If the posterior communicating artery is atretic, the peripheral territory supplied by posterior cerebral artery is also affected (see Fig. 368-6). If the posterior cerebral artery is completely occluded at its origin, hemiplegia secondary to infarction of the cerebral peduncle occurs. Involvement of the red nucleus and/or dentatorubrothalamic tract can produce contralateral ataxia. A third nerve palsy with contralateral ataxia (Claude's syndrome) or with contralateral hemiplegia (Weber's syndrome) may result. If the subthalamic nucleus of Luys is involved, contralateral hemiballismus may occur. Occlusion of the artery of Percheron produces paresis of upward gaze and drowsiness and is often associated with abulia. Extensive infarction in the midbrain of the subthalamus occurring with bilateral posterior cerebral stem occlusion is usually secondary to embolism. Coma, bilateral pyramidal signs, and "decerebrate rigidity" occur in this setting.

Atheromatous occlusion of the penetrating branches of the thalamic and thalamogeniculate arteries produces less extensive thalamic and thalamocapsular lacunar syndromes. The *thalamic syndrome of Déjerine and Roussy* is the best known. Its main feature is contralateral hemisensory loss of both superficial sensation (pain and temperature) and deep sensation (touch and proprioception). Occasionally, it may affect only pain and temperature or vibration and joint position sense. After a few weeks or months, an agonizing, searing pain may develop in the affected areas. Patients describe the pain as tight, drawing, icy, and knifelike. It is devastatingly persistent and responds poorly to analgesics. Occasionally, anticonvulsants are beneficial. If the posterior limb of the internal capsule is involved, hemiparesis or hemiplegia may accompany the hemisensory syndrome. Other associated motor signs include hemiballismus, choreoathetosis, intention tremor, incoordination, and posturing of the hand and arm, particularly while walking.

POSTCOMMUNAL SYNDROMES (PERIPHERAL OR CORTICAL TERRITORY) (See also Fig. 368-6) Occlusion of the posterior cerebral artery causes infarction of the cortical surface of the medial temporal and occipital lobes. Contralateral homonymous hemianopsia is the usual manifestation. Occasionally, only the upper quadrant of the visual field is involved. If the visual association areas are spared and only the calcarine cortex is involved, the patient is aware of visual defects. Central vision may be spared if middle cerebral artery branches supply the macular region of the occipital pole. Medial temporal lobe and hippocampal involvement may cause an acute disturbance in memory, particularly if it occurs in the dominant hemisphere, but the defect usually clears because memory has bilateral representation. If the dominant hemisphere is affected and the infarct extends to involve the splenium of the corpus callosum, the patient may demonstrate alexia without agraphia. Visual agnosia for faces, objects, mathematical symbols, and colors and anomia with paraphasic

errors (amnestic aphasia) also may occur in this setting even without callosal involvement. Occlusion of the posterior cerebral artery can produce peduncular hallucinosis (visual hallucinations of brightly colored scenes and objects).

Bilateral infarction in the distal posterior cerebral arteries produces cortical blindness. The patient is often unaware of the blindness. The clinical clue to the site is a finding of normal pupillary reaction to light. Tiny islands of vision may persist, and the patient then reports that vision fluctuates as images are captured in the preserved portions. Rarely, only peripheral vision is lost and central vision is spared, resulting in "gun-barrel" vision. A constellation of symptoms termed *Balint's syndrome* can occur with unilateral or bilateral visual association area lesions. It includes optic ataxia (inability to visually guide limb movements), ocular ataxia (inability to direct eyes to a precise point in the visual field), inability to enumerate objects in a picture or extract meaning from a picture, and inability to avoid objects seen in one's path. Balint's syndrome is seen most often with bilateral infarctions, secondary to low flow in the distal posterior and/or middle cerebral "watershed" territories as occurs after arrest. Embolic occlusion of the top of the basilar artery can produce a clinical picture that includes any or all of the central or peripheral territory symptoms. Its hallmark is suddenness of onset and bilaterality of symptoms, including ptosis and somnolence (see above in the discussion of the artery of Percheron).

Laboratory evaluation Infarction in the peripheral territory of the posterior cerebral artery can be documented easily by CT or MRI. Infarction in the central territory of the posterior cerebral artery, particularly in territories supplied by the penetrating branches of the posterior cerebral artery, is not reliably detected by CT scanning. MRI can detect infarctions greater than 0.5 cm in this area. MRI angiography and intracranial Doppler may identify atherosclerotic stenotic lesions in the proximal posterior cerebral artery.

Therapy Because infarction in the territory of the posterior cerebral artery is usually secondary to embolism from the vertebrobasilar system or from the heart, treatment with anticoagulants to prevent further embolic events is appropriate. Transient ischemic symptoms in the territory of the posterior cerebral artery may result from atherothrombotic stenosis of its proximal portion or one of its penetrating branches (lacunar TIA). The natural history of such atheromatous disease is unknown. Thus the efficacy of anticoagulants versus antiplatelet therapy is still uncertain.

VERTEBRAL AND POSTERIOR INFERIOR CEREBELLAR ARTERIES The *vertebral artery*, which arises from the innominate artery on the right and the subclavian artery on the left, divides into four anatomic segments. The first segment extends from its origin to its entrance into the sixth or fifth transverse vertebral foramen. The second segment traverses the vertebral foramina from C6 to C2. The third segment passes through the transverse foramen and circles around the arch of the atlas to pierce the dura at the foramen magnum. The fourth segment courses upward to join the other vertebral artery to form the basilar artery; only the fourth segment gives rise to branches that supply the brainstem and cerebellum. The *posterior inferior cerebellar artery* in its proximal segments supplies the lateral medulla and, in its distal branches, the inferior surface of the cerebellum. Anastomotic channels exist among the ascending cervical arteries, the thyrocervical arteries, the occipital artery (branch of the external carotid artery), and the second segment of the vertebral artery (see Fig. 368-1). In 10 percent of patients, one vertebral artery is too small to contribute significant blood to the brainstem.

Atherothrombotic lesions have a predilection for the first and fourth segments of the vertebral artery. Although the atheromatous narrowing in the first segment (the origin) may be significant, it seldom produces brainstem ischemic strokes. Collateral flow from the contralateral vertebral artery or the ascending cervical and ascending thyrocervical or occipital arteries is usually sufficient to prevent ischemia (see Fig. 368-1D). When one vertebral artery is atretic and an atherothrombotic lesion threatens the origin of the other, the only avenues for collateral circulation are through the ascending cervical artery, the thyrocervical artery, and the occipital artery or by retrograde flow down the basilar artery via the posterior communicating artery (see Fig. 368-2 and 368-6). In this setting, low flow in the vertebrobasilar system exists and TIAs may occur. In addition, incipient thrombosis in the proximal basilar or distal vertebral system may occur. If the subclavian is blocked proximal to the origin of the vertebral artery, exercise of the left arm may draw blood from the vertebrobasilar insufficiency (*subclavian steal*). It rarely leads to significant vertebrobasilar ischemia.

Atheroma in the fourth segment of the vertebral artery can occur proximal to or distal to the origin of the posterior inferior cerebellar artery, as well as at the junction with the other vertebral artery to form the basilar artery. When it is proximal to the origin of the posterior inferior cerebellar artery, a critical narrowing can threaten the lateral medulla and posteroinferior surface of the cerebellum.

Although atheromatous disease rarely narrows the second and third segments of the vertebral artery, this region is subject to dissection, fibromuscular dysplasia, and, rarely, encroachment by osteophytic spurs within the vertebral foramina.

Clinical manifestations *True transient cerebral ischemic attacks* resulting from vertebral artery insufficiency cause dizziness or vertigo, numbness of the ipsilateral face and contralateral limbs, diplopia, hoarseness, dysarthria, and dysphagia. Hemiparesis is rare. Such TIAs are usually short (up to 10 to 15 min) and repetitive.

When *infarction* ensues, it most often affects the lateral medulla with or without the posteroinferior cerebellum (Wallenberg's syndrome). Its features are listed in Fig. 368-7. In 70 to 80 percent of the cases, the syndrome occurs after ipsilateral vertebral artery occlusion; in the remainder, it results from posterior inferior cerebellar artery occlusion. Atherothrombotic occlusion of the medullary penetrating branches of the vertebral or posterior inferior cerebellar artery results in partial syndromes of the ipsilateral, lateral, or medial medulla.

Rarely, a medial medullary syndrome occurs in which the pyramid becomes infarcted, causing a contralateral hemiparesis of the arm and leg, sparing the face. If the medial lemniscus and emerging hypoglossal nerve fibers are involved, contralateral loss of joint position sense and ipsilateral tongue weakness occur.

Cerebellar infarction with edema formation can lead to *sudden respiratory arrest* due to raised intracranial pressure in the posterior fossa. Drowsiness, Babinski signs, dysarthria, and bifacial weakness may be absent or present only briefly before respiratory arrest ensues. Gait unsteadiness, dizziness, nausea, and vomiting may be the only early symptoms and signs and should arouse suspicion of this impending complication.

Laboratory evaluation When true TIAs occur in the territory of the lateral medulla, it becomes important to determine the adequacy of blood flow in the distal vertebral artery and the posterior inferior cerebellar artery. CT scanning may detect a large cerebellar infarction in the territory of the posterior inferior cerebellar artery. MRI can detect cerebellar infarction earlier and, with high-resolution scanning, can detect lateral medullary infarction. MRI angiography can determine the patency of the vertebral artery and occasionally the posterior inferior cerebellar artery. Cerebral angiography is rarely necessary if MRI angiography is available in evaluating stroke in this territory. Transcranial Doppler analysis of flow in the vertebral artery determines its patency, but its sensitivity in detecting distal vertebral artery stenotic lesions is limited.

Therapy Four important therapeutic issues arise in managing patients with ischemia or infarction in the territory of the vertebral or posterior inferior cerebellar artery. First, the ensuing edema may be life-threatening. It should be treated with osmotic agents (mannitol); surgical decompression may be necessary. Second, thrombosis of the fourth segment of the vertebral artery may send clots into the basilar artery or emboli into the basilar or posterior cerebral arteries. Symptoms or signs of basilar insufficiency may ensue. Acute anticoagulation with heparin is advocated in such cases in an effort to prevent

clot propagation. Third, some physicians argue for the prophylactic use of heparin in acute vertebral artery occlusion whether or not basilar artery symptoms have occurred. Chronic anticoagulation has not been recommended after the acute phase of the stroke has passed. Fourth, when one vertebral artery is symptomatic with atheromatous disease and the contralateral vertebral is congenitally atretic or already occluded, basilar ischemia may ensue and proximal basilar thrombosis may develop. Despite its potential hazards, acute anticoagulation with heparin, followed by chronic warfarin anticoagulation, is recommended in such patients. When the same circumstance occurs but the symptomatic vertebral atherothrombotic lesion lies immediately proximal to the posterior inferior cerebellar artery, occipital to posterior inferior bypass grafting has been recommended. The efficacy of this surgery is unproven, and it should be considered only after anticoagulation therapy has failed.

BASILAR ARTERY Pathophysiology Branches of the basilar artery supply the base of the pontis and superior cerebellum and fall into three groups: (1) paramedian, 7 to 10 in number, which supply a wedge of pons on either side of the midline, (2) short circumferential branches, 5 to 7 in number, which supply the lateral two-thirds of the pons and middle and superior cerebellar peduncles, and (3) 2 bilateral long circumferential arteries (superior cerebellar and anterior inferior cerebellar arteries) which course around the pons to supply the cerebellar hemispheres.

Atheromatous lesions can occur anywhere along the basilar trunk but are most often in the proximal basilar and distal vertebral segments. Typically, lesions occlude either the proximal basilar and one or both vertebral arteries. The clinical picture varies depending on the availability of retrograde collateral flow from the posterior communicating arteries.

Although atherothrombosis occasionally occludes the top of the basilar artery, emboli from the heart or proximal vertebral or basilar segments are more common.

Clinical manifestations Because the brainstem contains many structures in close approximation, a diversity of clinical syndromes may emerge with ischemia. Involvement of the corticospinal tracts, corticobulbar tracts, medial and superior cerebellar peduncles, spinothalamic tracts, and cranial nerve nuclei causes the common symptoms and signs (Figs. 368-8 to 368-10).

Unfortunately, the symptoms of transient ischemia or infarction in the territory of the basilar artery often do not indicate whether the basilar artery itself or one of its branches is diseased, yet the distinction has important implications for therapy. The picture of complete basilar insufficiency, however, is easy to recognize. A combination of bilateral long tract signs (sensory and motor) with signs of cranial nerve and cerebellar dysfunction suggests this diagnosis. A "locked-in" state of quadriplegia occurs with bilateral basis pontis infarction. Coma due to dysfunction of the reticular activating system and quadriplegia with cranial nerve signs suggest complete and devastating pontine and upper midbrain infarction. The therapeutic goal, however, is to recognize impending basilar occlusion before such a devastating infarction occurs. A series of TIAs and a slowly progressive, fluctuating stroke become extremely significant when they herald an atherothrombotic occlusion of the distal vertebral or proximal basilar artery.

TRANSIENT ISCHEMIC ATTACKS Transient ischemic attacks in the proximal basilar distribution may produce dizziness (often described by patients as "swimming," "swaying," "moving," "unsteadiness," or "light-headedness"). Patients may complain that the room is upside down or that the floor seems to move toward them. Other symptoms that warn of basilar thrombosis include diplopia, dysarthria, facial or circumoral numbness, and hemisensory symptoms. In general, symptoms of basilar branch TIAs affect one side of the brainstem, whereas symptoms of basilar artery TIAs usually affect both sides, though a "herald" hemiparesis has been emphasized as an initial symptom of basilar occlusion. Most often TIAs, whether due to impending occlusion of the basilar artery or of a basilar branch, are short-lived (5 to 30 min) and repetitive, occurring several times a

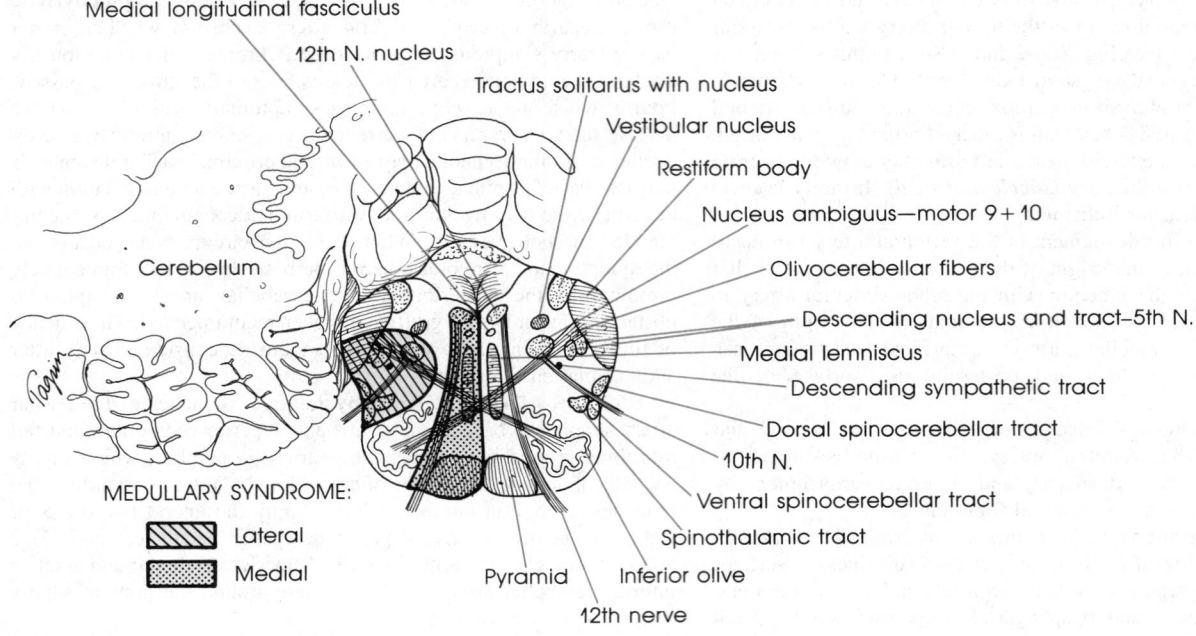

Medial longitudinal fasciculus
12th N. nucleus
Tractus solitarius with nucleus
Vestibular nucleus
Restiform body
Nucleus ambiguus—motor 9 + 10
Cerebellum
Olivocerebellar fibers
Descending nucleus and tract–5th N.
Medial lemniscus
Descending sympathetic tract
Dorsal spinocerebellar tract
10th N.
Ventral spinocerebellar tract
MEDULLARY SYNDROME:
Spinothalamic tract
Lateral
Medial
Pyramid   Inferior olive
12th nerve

FIGURE 368-7   *(Courtesy of C. M. Fisher, M.D.)*

Signs and symptoms	Structures involved
1 Medial medullary syndrome (occlusion of vertebral artery or of branch of vertebral or lower basilar artery)	
On side of lesion:	
Paralysis with atrophy of half the tongue	Ipsilateral twelfth nerve
On side opposite lesion:	
Paralysis of arm and leg sparing face; impaired tactile and proprioceptive sense over half the body	Contralateral pyramidal tract and medial lemniscus
2 Lateral medullary syndrome (occlusion of any of five vessels may be responsible—vertebral, posterior inferior cerebellar, superior, middle, or inferior lateral medullary arteries)	
On side of lesion:	
Pain, numbness, impaired sensation over half the face	Descending tract and nucleus fifth nerve
Ataxia of limbs, falling to side of lesion	Uncertain—restiform body, cerebellar hemisphere, cerebellar fibers, spinocerebellar tract (?)
Nystagmus, diplopia, oscillopsia, vertigo, nausea, vomiting	Vestibular nucleus
Horner's syndrome (miosis, ptosis, decreased sweating)	Descending sympathetic tract
Dysphagia, hoarseness, paralysis of palate, paralysis of vocal cord, diminished gag reflex	Issuing fibers ninth and tenth nerves
Loss of taste	Nucleus and tractus solitarius
Numbness of ipsilateral arm, trunk, or leg	Cuneate and gracile nuclei
On side opposite lesion:	
Impaired pain and thermal sense over half the body, sometimes face	Spinothalamic tract
3 Total unilateral medullary syndrome (occlusion of vertebral artery): Combination of medial and lateral syndromes	
4 Lateral pontomedullary syndrome (occlusion of vertebral artery): Combination of lateral medullary and lateral inferior pontine syndromes	
5 Basilar artery syndrome (the syndrome of the lone vertebral artery is equivalent): A combination of the various brainstem syndromes plus those arising in the posterior cerebral artery distribution	
Bilateral long tract signs (sensory and motor; cerebellar and peripheral cranial nerve abnormalities)	Bilateral long tract; cerebellar and peripheral cranial nerves
Paralysis or weakness of all extremities, plus all bulbar musculature	Corticobulbar and corticospinal tracts bilaterally

day. The pattern suggests intermittent reduction of flow rather than recurrent embolism.

INFARCTION   Atherothrombotic occlusion of the basilar artery with brainstem infarction usually causes *bilateral* brainstem signs. Sometimes only gaze paresis or internuclear ophthalmoplegia associated with ipsilateral hemiparesis, i.e., a particular combination of cranial nerve and long tract (sensory and/or motor) deficits, signifies

bilateral brainstem ischemia. More often, bilateral basis pontis signs coexist with unilateral or bilateral pontine tegmental signs.

Symptomatic atherothrombotic occlusion of a branch of the basilar artery usually causes *unilateral* symptoms and signs involving motor, sensory, and cranial nerves. Occlusion of the long circumferential branches of the basilar artery produces specific clinical syndromes depending on the artery involved.

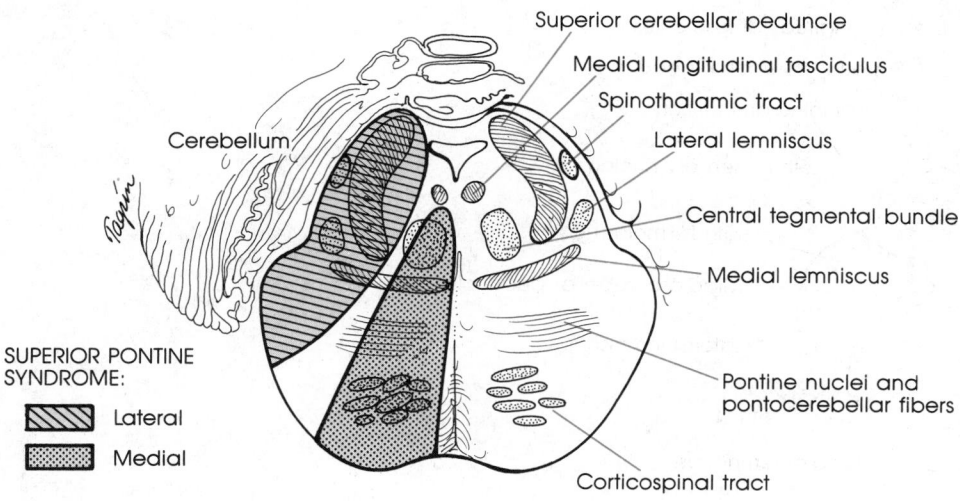

Superior cerebellar peduncle
Medial longitudinal fasciculus
Spinothalamic tract
Lateral lemniscus
Central tegmental bundle
Medial lemniscus
Pontine nuclei and pontocerebellar fibers
Corticospinal tract
Cerebellum

SUPERIOR PONTINE SYNDROME:

▨ Lateral

▦ Medial

FIGURE 368-8 (*Courtesy of C. M. Fisher, M.D.*)

Signs and symptoms	Structures involved
1 Medial superior pontine syndrome (paramedian branches of upper basilar artery)	
On side of lesion:	
Cerebellar ataxia (probably)	Superior and/or middle cerebellar peduncle
Internuclear ophthalmoplegia	Medial longitudinal fasciculus
Myoclonic syndrome, palate, pharynx, vocal cords, respiratory apparatus, face, oculomotor apparatus, etc.	Localization uncertain—central tegmental bundle (?), dentate projection (?), inferior olivary nucleus (?)
On side opposite lesion:	
Paralysis of face, arm, and leg	Corticobulbar and corticospinal tract
Rarely touch, vibration, and position are affected	Medial lemniscus
2 Lateral superior pontine syndrome (syndrome of superior cerebellar artery)	
On side of lesion:	
Ataxia of limbs and gait, falling to side of lesion	Middle and superior cerebellar peduncles, superior surface of cerebellum, dentate nucleus
Dizziness, nausea, vomiting; horizontal nystagmus	Vestibular nucleus
Paresis of conjugate gaze (ipsilateral)	Pontine contralateral gaze
Skew deviation	Uncertain
Miosis, ptosis, decreased sweating over face (Horner's syndrome)	Descending sympathetic fibers
Static tremor reported in one case	Dentate nucleus (?), superior cerebellar peduncle (?)
On side opposite lesion:	
Impaired pain and thermal sense on face, limbs, and trunk	Spinothalamic tract
Impaired touch, vibration, and position sense, more in leg than arm (there is a tendency to incongruity of pain and touch deficits)	Medial lemniscus (lateral portion)

SUPERIOR CEREBELLAR ARTERY Occlusion of the superior cerebellar artery results in severe ipsilateral cerebellar ataxia (middle and/or superior cerebellar peduncles), nausea and vomiting, dysarthria, and contralateral loss of pain and temperature sensation over the extremities, body, and face (spino- and trigeminothalamic tract). Partial deafness, ataxic tremor of the ipsilateral upper extremity, Horner's syndrome, and palatal myoclonus may occur rarely. Partial syndromes occur frequently (see Fig. 368-8).

ANTERIOR INFERIOR CEREBELLAR ARTERY Occlusion of the anterior inferior cerebellar artery produces variable degrees of infarction because the size of this artery and the territory it supplies vary inversely with those of the posterior inferior cerebellar artery. The principal symptoms include ipsilateral deafness, facial weakness, true vertigo (whirling dizziness), nausea and vomiting, nystagmus, tinnitus and cerebellar ataxia, Horner's syndrome, and paresis of conjugate lateral gaze. The opposite side of the body loses pain and temperature sensation. An occlusion close to the origin of the artery may cause corticospinal tract signs (see Fig. 368-10).

Occlusion of one of the five to seven short circumferential branches of the basilar artery affects the lateral two-thirds of the pons and/or middle or superior cerebellar peduncle, whereas occlusion of one of the 7 to 10 paramedian branches of the basilar artery affects a wedge-shaped area on either side of the medial pons (see Figs. 368-8 to 368-10). Many brainstem syndromes with cranial nerve abnormalities and crossed hemiplegia have been given eponyms, e.g., Weber, Claude, Benedict, Foville, Raymond-Cestan, Millard-Gubler.

Laboratory evaluation MRI scanning can detect brainstem infarction due to either basilar artery or basilar branch occlusion. MRI angiography combined with transcranial Doppler analysis may eventually replace conventional angiography in documenting basilar artery potency. CT scanning is not reliable in detecting brainstem infarcts but can show hemorrhages and assess mass effect after large cerebellar infarctions.

Selective cerebral arteriography remains the best method to define atherothrombotic disease of the basilar artery. Arteriography entails potential morbidity and may precipitate the very stroke one is seeking

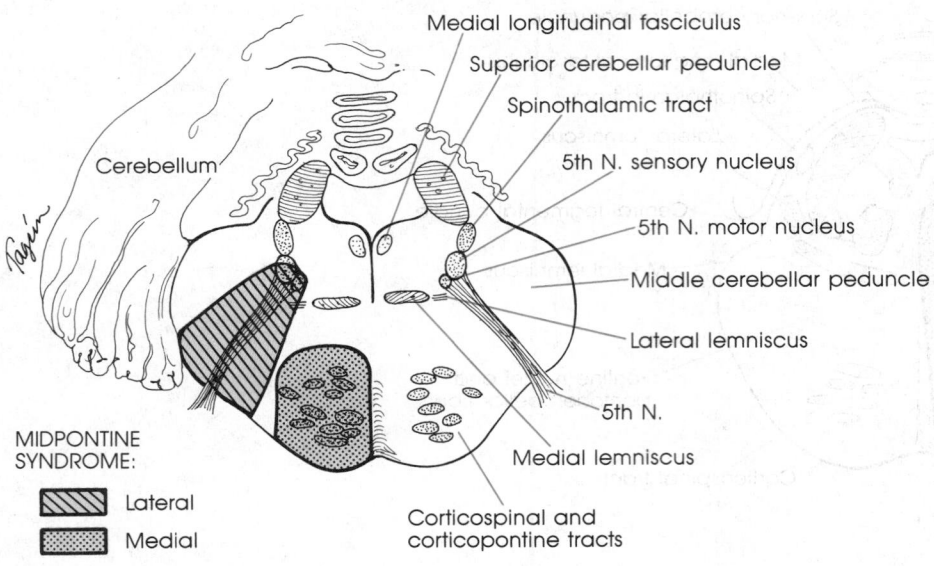

Medial longitudinal fasciculus
Superior cerebellar peduncle
Spinothalamic tract
5th N. sensory nucleus
5th N. motor nucleus
Middle cerebellar peduncle
Lateral lemniscus
5th N.
Medial lemniscus

Cerebellum

MIDPONTINE SYNDROME:

Lateral

Medial

Corticospinal and
corticopontine tracts

FIGURE 368-9 *(Courtesy of C. M. Fisher, M.D.)*

Signs and symptoms	*Structures involved*
1 Medial midpontine syndrome (paramedian branch of midbasilar artery)	
On side of lesion:	
Ataxia of limbs and gait (more prominent in bilateral involvement)	Pontine nuclei
On side opposite lesion:	
Paralysis of face, arm, and leg	Corticobulbar and corticospinal tract
Variable impaired touch and proprioception when lesion extends posteriorly	Medial lemniscus
2 Lateral midpontine syndrome (short circumferential artery)	
On side of lesion:	
Ataxia of limbs	Middle cerebellar peduncle
Paralysis of muscles of mastication	Motor fibers or nucleus of fifth nerve
Impaired sensation over side of face	Sensory fibers or nucleus of fifth nerve
On side opposite lesion:	
Impaired pain and thermal sense on limbs and trunk	Spinothalamic tract

to prevent. It is recommended only when MRI angiography fails to detect the clinically suspected basilar arterial lesion that, if known, would influence patient management. Occasionally, injection of angiographic dye in the posterior circulation precipitates a delirious state sometimes associated with cortical blindness. This reversible state can last for 24 to 38 h or, rarely, several days.

Therapy Impending basilar occlusion causing transient or fluctuating symptoms should be treated with short-term anticoagulation with intravenous heparin, after MRI or CT scanning has excluded hemorrhage. When basilar artery stenosis or occlusion is associated with minor or improving stroke, long-term anticoagulation with warfarin is recommended. If, on the other hand, basilar branch disease is the cause, then the rationale for using warfarin is uncertain. While embolism from the heart or from atheroma in the distal vertebral system may occlude a penetrating basilar branch, this is unlikely. Therefore, long-term control of blood pressure and antiplatelet therapy are recommended as preventive measures in the management of small-vessel basilar branch disease. Because of the long-term accumulative risk of anticoagulation therapy, it is generally reserved for symptomatic large-vessel atherothrombotic disease.

LACUNAR DISEASE

The term *lacunar infarction* refers to infarction following atherothrombotic or lipohyalinotic occlusion of *one* of the penetrating branches

of the circle of Willis, middle cerebral artery stem, or vertebral and basilar arteries.

PATHOPHYSIOLOGY The middle cerebral artery stem, the arteries comprising the circle of Willis (A1 segment of the anterior cerebral artery, anterior and posterior communicating arteries, and precommunal segment of the posterior cerebral arteries), and the basilar and vertebral arteries all give rise to 100- to 300-μm-diameter branches that penetrate the deep gray and white matter of the cerebrum or brainstem (see Fig. 368-2). Each of these small branches can be thrombosed either by atherothrombotic disease at its origin or by the development of lipohyalinotic thickening. Thrombosis of these vessels causes small infarcts that are referred to as *lacunes*. They range in size from as small as 3 to 4 mm to 1 to 2 cm. Hypertension is the principal risk factor for such small-vessel disease. Lacunar infarcts represent approximately 20 percent of all strokes.

CLINICAL MANIFESTATIONS Lacunar infarcts cause recognizable stroke syndromes that usually evolve over hours or longer. Transient symptoms (lacunar TIAs) may herald a lacunar infarct; they may occur several times a day and last only a few minutes. When infarction occurs, it usually causes a sudden deficit, but it may evolve in a progressive fashion over a few days. Recovery often begins within hours or days after the infarct and over weeks or months may be complete or result in minimal residual deficit. In some cases, significant disability persists.

The most common lacunar syndromes are the following:

1 Pure motor hemiparesis from an infarct in the posterior limb of

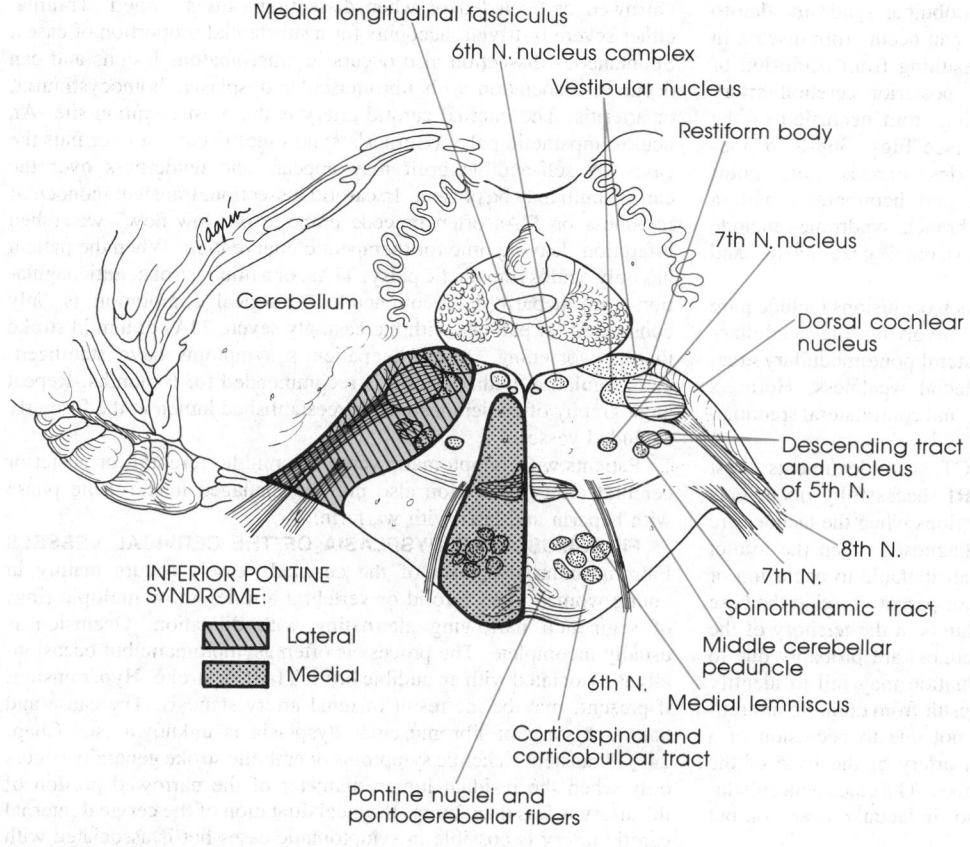

Medial longitudinal fasciculus
6th N. nucleus complex
Vestibular nucleus
Restiform body
7th N. nucleus
Dorsal cochlear nucleus
Cerebellum
Descending tract and nucleus of 5th N.
8th N.
7th N.
Spinothalamic tract
Middle cerebellar peduncle
Medial lemniscus
6th N.
Corticospinal and corticobulbar tract
Pontine nuclei and pontocerebellar fibers

INFERIOR PONTINE SYNDROME:
Lateral
Medial

FIGURE 368-10 *(Courtesy of C. M. Fisher, M.D.)*

Signs and symptoms	Structures involved
1 Medial inferior pontine syndrome (occlusion of paramedian branch of basilar artery)	
On side of lesion:	
Paralysis of conjugate gaze to side of lesion (preservation of convergence)	"Center" for conjugate lateral gaze
Nystagmus	Vestibular nucleus
Ataxia of limbs and gait	Middle cerebellar peduncle (?)
Diplopia on lateral gaze	Abducens nerve
On side opposite lesion:	
Paralysis of face, arm, and leg	Corticobulbar and corticospinal tract in lower pons
Impaired tactile and proprioceptive sense over half of the body	Medial lemniscus
2 Lateral inferior pontine syndrome (occlusion of anterior inferior cerebellar artery)	
On side of lesion:	
Horizontal and vertical nystagmus, vertigo, nausea, vomiting, oscillopsia	Vestibular nerve on nucleus
Facial paralysis	Seventh nerve
Paralysis of conjugate gaze to side of lesion	"Center" for conjugate lateral gaze
Deafness, tinnitus	Auditory nerve or cochlear nucleus
Ataxia	Middle cerebellar peduncle and cerebellar hemisphere
Impaired sensation over face	Descending tract and nucleus fifth nerve
On side opposite lesion:	
Impaired pain and thermal sense over half the body (may include face)	Spinothalamic tract

the internal capsule or basis pontis. Here, the face, arm, leg, foot, and toes are almost always involved. The weakness may be intermittent (TIA), progress in a stepwise manner, or appear abruptly and may progress to complete paralysis, but improvement occurs in many cases.

2 Pure sensory stroke from an infarct in the ventrolateral thalamus.

3 Ataxic hemiparesis from an infarct in the base of the pons or *dysarthria and a clumsy hand or arm* due to infarction in the base of the pons or in the genu of the internal capsule.

4 Pure motor hemiparesis with "motor aphasia" due to thrombotic occlusion of a lenticulostriate branch supplying the genu and anterior limb of the internal capsule and adjacent white matter of the corona radiata.

Before the advent of hypertensive therapy, multiple lacunes often caused *pseudobulbar palsy* with emotional instability, a slowed abulic state, and bilateral pyramidal signs. This syndrome is now uncommon. Other lacunar syndromes have been described, some not correlated with arterial occlusion. An anarthric pseudobulbar syndrome due to bilateral infarctions in the internal capsule can occur from disease in the lenticulostriate arteries. Syndromes resulting from occlusion of the penetrating arteries of the proximal posterior cerebral artery were discussed above. Syndromes resulting from occlusion of the penetrating arteries of the basilar artery (see Figs. 368-8 to 368-10) include ipsilateral ataxia and crural (leg) paresis, pure motor hemiparesis with horizontal gaze palsy, and hemiparesis with a crossed sixth nerve palsy. Lower basilar branch syndromes include sudden internuclear ophthalmoplegia, horizontal gaze palsy, and appendicular cerebellar ataxia.

Syndromes resulting from vertebral branch occlusions include pure motor hemiparesis sparing the face by involving the medullary pyramid and syndromes that involve the lateral pontomedullary area, which may include vertigo, vomiting, facial weakness, Horner's syndrome, ipsilateral trigeminal numbness, and contralateral spinothalamic sensory loss.

LABORATORY EVALUATION The CT scan documents most supratentorial lacunar infarctions, and MRI successfully documents both supratentorial and infratentorial infarctions when the lacunes are 5 mm or greater. Lacunar infarction is diagnosed when the infarct size is less than 2 cm, and its location is attributable to occlusion of a small penetrating arterial branch of a major parent vessel at the base of the brain. Larger deep white matter infarcts in the territory of the middle cerebral artery (so-called giant lacunes) are probably due to embolism. The CT scan and clinical evaluation may fail to identify cortical surface infarction. *Giant lacunes* result from embolic infarctions in a large-vessel territory. They are not due to occlusion of a single penetrating vessel arising from an artery at the base of the brain. Hence they should not be called lacunes. The electroencephalogram (EEG) is usually normal, or nearly so, in lacunar infarction but abnormal in cortical surface infarction.

THERAPY Lacunar strokes may present with a fluctuating progressive course, and acute reduction in blood pressure may worsen symptoms. Antihypertensive therapy is begun after the patient's symptoms become stable. Whether anticoagulant or antiplatelet agents benefit patients with lacunar TIAs and fluctuating stroke is unknown. Some studies suggest that thalamic lacunes may be associated with minor hemorrhage, since hemosiderin-laden macrophages are sometimes seen at autopsy. This circumstance increases the risk of using heparin. On the other hand, some patients with fluctuating hemiparesis from atherothrombotic disease of a basilar branch or of the middle cerebral stem lenticulostriate arteries may improve coincident with heparin administration. Most physicians, however, do not use anticoagulation in patients with typical lacunar strokes. Long-term therapy after lacunar stroke requires careful control of hypertension to prevent progression of vascular disease.

OTHER CAUSES OF CEREBRAL INFARCTION

VENOUS THROMBOSIS (See also Table 368-1) Lateral or sagittal sinus thrombosis or thrombosis of small cortical veins occurs as a complication of sepsis, intracranial infections (meningitis), conditions associated with hypercoagulable states such as polycythemia and sickle cell anemia, or during pregnancy or administration of oral contraceptives. Venous thromboses may cause an increase in intracranial pressure, headaches, focal seizures, and focal neurologic signs affecting the legs more than the arms. Massive venous infarction with secondary edema may be fatal. The CT scan shows hemorrhagic infarction underlying the occluded veins and may show clot in the posterior sagittal sinus, but the definitive diagnosis is made with angiography.

DISSECTION OF THE CERVICOCEREBRAL ARTERIES Dissection of the large extracranial arteries may cause cerebral infarction and is a frequent cause of stroke in children and young adults. The dissection divides the media of the vessel or separates the intima from the media. TIAs and infarction occur when the vessel is critically

narrowed or occluded or when dissection causes emboli. Trauma, either severe or trivial, accounts for a substantial proportion of cases. Spontaneous dissection also occurs in atheromatous lesions and can occur in association with fibromuscular dysplasia, homocystinuria, or arteritis. The internal carotid artery is the most common site. An oculosympathetic palsy (Horner's syndrome) occurs in over half the cases. A self-audible bruit may appear, and tenderness over the carotid bulb may be present. In carotid dissection, transient monocular blindness or TIAs often precede embolic or "low-flow" watershed infarction, leaving time for therapeutic intervention. When the patient has only oculosympathetic palsy, TIAs, or a minor stroke, anticoagulation with heparin is recommended. Surgical exploration is only considered for patients with increasingly severe TIAs or a mild stroke that is worsening. After the patient's symptoms have stabilized, anticoagulation with warfarin is recommended for 6 months. Repeat angiography often demonstrates a reestablished lumen in the formerly occluded vessel.

Patients with symptomatic vertebral, middle cerebral, or posterior cerebral artery dissection also may be managed in the acute phase with heparin and later with warfarin.

FIBROMUSCULAR DYSPLASIA OF THE CERVICAL VESSELS Fibromuscular dysplasia of the cervical vessels occurs mainly in young women. The carotid or vertebral arteries show multiple rings of segmental narrowing alternating with dilatation. Occlusion is usually incomplete. The process is often asymptomatic but occasionally is associated with an audible bruit, TIAs, or stroke. Hypertension, if present, may be the result of renal artery stenosis. The cause and natural history of fibromuscular dysplasia is unknown (see Chap. 243). Transient ischemic symptoms or embolic stroke generally occurs only when the residual lumen diameter of the narrowed portion of the artery is less than 2 mm. Surgical dilatation of the cervical internal carotid artery is possible in symptomatic cases but is associated with considerable morbidity. Anticoagulation may be more successful than surgery in patients with TIAs of increasing severity.

ARTERITIS Arteritis due to bacterial or syphilitic infection is no longer a common cause of cerebral thrombosis. Other arteritides are rare but can cause cerebral thrombosis (see below and Chaps. 284 and 291). Necrotizing or granulomatous arteritis, occurring alone or in association with generalized polyarteritis nodosa or Wegener's granulomatosis, involves the distal small branches (<2 mm diameter) of the main intracranial arteries and produces small ischemic infarcts in the brain, optic nerve, or spinal cord. The disease, although rare, is relentlessly progressive. The cerebrospinal fluid often has cells. In some cases, glucocorticoid therapy (prednisone, 40 to 60 mg/d) has been helpful, and recently, immunosuppressive drugs have been used with some success (see Chap. 291). Idiopathic giant cell arteritis involving the great vessels arising from the aortic arch (Takayasu's syndrome) may, on rare occasions, cause carotid or vertebral thrombosis. It is an infrequent cause of the aortic arch syndrome in the western hemisphere (see Chap. 210).

TEMPORAL ARTERITIS (CRANIAL ARTERITIS) (See also Chap. 291) This is a relatively common affliction of elderly persons in which the external carotid system, particularly the temporal arteries, is the site of a subacute granulomatous inflammation with an exudate of lymphocytes, monocytes, neutrophilic leukocytes, and giant cells. Usually the most severely affected parts of the artery become thrombosed. Headache or head pain is the chief complaint. Systemic manifestations include anorexia, loss of weight, malaise, and polymyalgia rheumatica. The inflammatory nature of the illness is indicated by one of the following: fever, slight leukocytosis, increased erythrocyte sedimentation rate, and anemia. Occlusion of branches of the ophthalmic artery results in blindness in one or both eyes in over 25 percent of patients. Occasionally, an ophthalmoplegia due to involvement of ocular nerves occurs. An arteritis of the aorta and its major branches, including the carotid, subclavian, coronary, and femoral arteries, has been found at postmortem examination in some cases. Significant inflammatory involvement of intracranial arteries is rare, but strokes occur occasionally on the basis of occlusion of the internal carotid, middle cerebral, or vertebral arteries. The diagnosis depends on the finding of a tender thrombosed or thickened cranial artery and demonstration of the lesion in a biopsy specimen. Glucocorticoids bring striking subjective relief and often prevent blindness. Prednisone is most often used, beginning with large daily doses of 80 to 120 mg and then tapering after 2 to 4 weeks using the erythrocyte sedimentation rate as a guide.

MOYAMOYA DISEASE Moyamoya disease is a poorly understood occlusive disease involving large intracranial arteries, especially the internal carotid artery and the stem of the middle and anterior cerebral arteries. The lenticulostriate arteries develop a rich collateral flow circulation around the middle cerebral occlusive lesion that on cerebral angiography gives the impression of a puff of smoke (*moyamoya*). Other collaterals include transdural anastomoses between the cortical surface branches of the middle cerebral artery and the scalp arteries. The disease mainly occurs in the oriental population but should be suspected when TIAs or stroke occur in children or young adults. Its etiology is unknown. Few pathologic studies have been made; they suggest that hyalinotic fibrous-type material is associated with the arterial narrowing. Because of the occurrence of subarachnoid hemorrhage from rupture of the transdural anastomotic channels, anticoagulation is not recommended in all symptomatic cases. Extracranial-intracranial (EC/IC) bypass grafting has been recommended in some cases, but its efficacy is not established.

ISCHEMIC DISEASES ASSOCIATED WITH HYPERCOAGULATION STATE Certain diseases have been associated with ischemic infarction in special clinical circumstances through a mechanism of a hypercoagulable state (see Chaps. 314 and 315). They include polycythemia vera, thrombotic thrombocytopenic purpura, idiopathic thrombocytosis, hyperproteinemia, sickle cell anemia, and familial clotting abnormalities, e.g., protein C deficiency. Furthermore, circulation of anticardiolipin antibodies ("lupus anticoagulant") has been associated with stroke in young adults, although its relative frequency is controversial. Some cases may be due to cerebral embolism (see below), but others seem to be caused by local arterial thrombosis.

REVERSIBLE CEREBRAL SEGMENTAL VASOCONSTRICTION Reversible, widespread cerebral segmental vasoconstriction has been noted in patients with severe headache and fluctuating neurologic symptoms and signs. Sometimes cerebral infarction has ensued. The cause is unknown. Eclampsia, the postpartum period, head injury, migraine, and sympathomimetic intoxication have all been associated with this entity. Angiography is the only means of establishing the diagnosis. The cerebrospinal fluid is normal in most cases, but an elevated protein and slight lymphocytic pleocytosis has been found in some cases. No effective therapy is known. Maintenance of normal systemic arterial pressure or even increasing it modestly with adequate hydration seems important on empirical grounds. Glucocorticoids and vasodilators such as calcium channel blocking agents or intravenous nitroglycerin may be considered.

BINSWANGER'S DISEASE Binswanger's disease (chronic progressive subcortical encephalopathy) is a rare condition in which the subcortical white matter becomes subacutely infarcted. The CT or MRI scan detects periventricular areas of white matter disruption and gliosis. There is lipohyalinosis in the small arteries of the deep white matter, as in hypertension. There are usually associated lacunar or embolic strokes. Binswanger's disease may represent a type of border zone ischemic infarction in the deep white matter between the penetrating arteries of the circle of Willis and of the cortex. Unfortunately, the pathophysiologic basis of the disease remains unknown, and the underlying microvascular pathology may be different in younger patients without hypertension and typical cases in older patients with severe long-standing hypertension. Binswanger's disease is one of the causes of gait disability and abulia in the elderly.

ORAL CONTRACEPTIVE AGENTS Oral contraceptive agents have been associated with an increased incidence of stroke in young women (13.2:100,000 among women who take oral contraceptives compared with 2.8:100,000 among those who do not). In most cases,

there is no vascular occlusion on angiography, or if there is occlusion, it is found to have opened later, suggesting embolism as the cause of the stroke. The source of the embolus, however, is uncertain. Pathologic examination has shown that the affected arteries and the heart are normal. Migraine and cigarette smoking have been associated with increased frequency of strokes in young women on oral contraceptives and suggest that hypercoagulability may predispose to thrombosis formation and/or embolization.

CEREBRAL EMBOLISM

PATHOPHYSIOLOGY Cerebral embolism is the most common cause of ischemic stroke. The heart is the most common source of embolic material, with artery-to-artery embolism, usually arising from an atherothrombotic lesion in the carotid or vertebrobasilar system or ascending aorta, a somewhat less frequent source (see above). Other causes, such as thrombus in the pulmonary vein, fat emboli, tumor emboli, marantic endocarditis, air emboli, paradoxical emboli, and complications of neck or thoracic surgery (see Table 368-1), may occasionally be responsible. Frequently, however, embolic cerebral infarction occurs without an obvious source.

The term *cerebral embolism of unknown source* is used when a sudden stroke occurs and cardiac monitoring, echocardiography, and carotid, vertebral, and transcranial Doppler studies fail to disclose an obvious source. About 40 percent of ischemic strokes fall into this category. The etiology of these presumed emboli poses one of the most perplexing problems in cerebrovascular disease. Sophisticated analyses of activity of the hemostatic system, blood coagulation factors, and autoantibodies show that patients with hypercoagulable states are prone to cerebral embolism. Hypercoagulability may be induced by anticardiolipid antibodies, protein C deficiency, protein S deficiency, antithrombin III deficiency, metastatic tumor, and even surgery. The association of cerebral embolism with these pathophysiologic conditions is suspected, but its incidence is uncertain. Transesophageal echocardiography has identified atheromatous plaques in the ascending aorta as a possible source of central embolism. The incidence and natural history of this lesion are uncertain.

Cardiogenic cerebral embolism is presumed to have occurred when cardiac arrhythmias or structural abnormalities are found or known to be present. Of the cardiac arrhythmias, atrial fibrillation is commonly associated with cerebral embolism. Prospective evidence suggests that independent of other cardiac disease, including mitral stenosis, persistent or paroxysmal atrial fibrillation is the most important cause of cerebral embolism from the heart. The presumed mechanism is thrombus formation in the fibrillating atrial appendage with subsequent embolization. Recent therapeutic trials and natural history studies suggest that age over 60 years is an important risk factor for such embolization. Mitral annulus calcification, left ventricular aneurysm, and left atrial size also may be risk factors.

The most common cause of cerebral embolism from structural heart disease occurs with atherothrombotic cardiovascular disease. *Left ventricular myocardial infarction*, either subendocardial or transmural, represents an important risk for embolus, especially in the first few weeks when mural thrombus formation and maturation usually occur in younger patients (see Chaps. 202 and 203). *Congenital septal defects* have long been associated with cerebral embolism. The deep peripheral venous system is usually the source of *paradoxical emboli*. Transesophageal and bubble echocardiographic techniques can demonstrate a patent foramen ovale as a conduit for cerebral embolism. Mitral valve prolapse is considered a potential source of emboli, but the incidence and natural history require further assessment. Mitral annulus calcification independent of atrial fibrillation has been shown to be a risk factor for ischemic stroke. Cardiogenic embolization during or following coronary artery surgery or intracardiac surgery is a well-recognized complication.

Vegetations of acute and subacute bacterial endocarditis give rise to septic emboli (see Chaps. 200 and 201) that cause large areas of infarction. Small septic infarcts of microscopic size may appear in the brain. Large brain abscesses, however, are not commonly associated with embolism from subacute bacterial endocarditis. Large septic emboli pose a greater risk of hemorrhage into the infarction than nonseptic embolism. Mycotic aneurysms caused by septic emboli may give rise to subarachnoid or intracerebral hemorrhage. Therefore, endocarditis should always be considered when cerebral embolism is suspected. Vegetations on the aortic and mitral valves from rheumatic or marantic endocarditis are also associated with systemic or cerebral emboli. Typically, flat vegetations under the mitral and, to a lesser extent, aortic valve leaflets have been noted in patients with systemic lupus erythematosus (Libman-Sacks vegetations). These may give rise to cerebral embolism and may be a nidus for bacterial endocarditis.

Atrial myxoma may give rise to tumor emboli from the endocardial surface. Signs of pulmonary hypertension or a high erythrocyte sedimentation rate, together with signs of systemic illness (fever, malaise), may help in the differential diagnosis. Thoracic surgery (pulmonary vein embolism) and head and neck surgery (aortic or carotid artery-to-artery emboli) have an uncommon, but definite, association with cerebral embolism.

Embolic infarction depends on the size of the embolic fragment and where it lodges, resulting from the size, location, and clinical findings. Emboli from the heart lodge in the middle cerebral artery or one of its branches 80 percent of the time, in the posterior cerebral artery or its branches 10 percent of the time, and in the vertebral artery or its branches in the remainder. Cardiac emboli rarely reach the anterior cerebral artery. Emboli large enough to occlude the stem of the middle cerebral artery (3 to 4 mm) lead to a large stroke, one that involves both deep gray and white matter and some portion of the cortical surface and its underlying white matter. A smaller embolus may occlude a small cortical or penetrating arterial branch. Characteristically, embolic platelet fibrin clot has a tendency to migrate, lyse, and disperse, accounting for fluctuation in symptoms and, in some cases, complete recovery of the ischemic deficit. The location and size of an infarct also depend on the extent of the spared collateral circulation.

Because emboli migrate and lyse, recirculation into the infarcted brain may cause petechial hemorrhages (*hemorrhagic infarction*). On rare occasions, petechial hemorrhages coalesce to form a significant hemorrhage mass (*hemorrhage into infarction*). This is more likely to occur when the stem of the middle cerebral artery is occluded and large areas of infarction develop in the territory of the lenticulostriate arteries before recirculation occurs.

CLINICAL MANIFESTATIONS   The onset of the neurologic deficit from embolism is sudden and usually maximal. This temporal profile with a neurologic syndrome corresponding to the distribution of a major branch vessel points to cerebral embolism. Sometimes, however, the neurologic deficit may not be complete and, after its sudden onset, may fluctuate. The neurologic signs may wax and wane, lasting only a few minutes or hours, and then partially or completely disappear, suggesting an embolic TIA, or a mild deficit may progress to complete major infarction over hours. The neurologic deficit corresponds to the cerebral cortex supplied by the affected artery. The resulting deficits resemble those caused by occlusive atheromatous lesions (see sections on atherothrombosis and lacunar stroke). Certain neurologic syndromes strongly suggest embolism as their cause. In the middle cerebral artery territory these include (1) the frontal opercular syndrome, in which there is facial weakness and severe aphasia or dysarthria, (2) the brachial or hand plegia syndrome, in which the arm and hand or the hand is paralyzed with or without cortical sensory abnormalities, (3) the syndromes of Broca's or Wernicke's aphasia alone, when the dominant hemisphere is involved, or (4) the syndrome of left visual neglect, when the nondominant parietal lobe is involved. Sudden hemianopic field defect suggests a posterior cerebral artery embolus; sudden foot incoordination or weakness suggests an anterior cerebral territory embolus. Sudden gait unsteadiness may suggest a cerebellar embolus. Sudden sleepiness

and an inability to look up associated with bilateral ptosis suggest an embolus to the top of the basilar artery, specifically to the artery of Percheron (the small vessel supplying both sides of the medial subthalamus and thalamus arising from the top of the basilar artery).

Seizures following cerebral infarction occur most often after embolic infarction and are not associated with deep white matter lacunar infarction. They are associated with supratentorial cortical surface infarction but are infrequent at the onset and are more often the result of gliotic scar that matures months or more after stroke. Seizures after infarction are rare before 6 months and peak in incidence at 12 to 18 months. Many cases of idiopathic epilepsy in the elderly are probably the result of silent cortical infarction.

LABORATORY EVALUATION   Although early CT scanning is usually negative in embolic stroke, it serves to exclude hemorrhage. MRI scanning is better to document the extent and location of the embolic infarction, both supratentorially and infratentorially. Although endocarditis is rarely the cause of cerebral embolism, laboratory evaluation should include a sedimentation rate and blood cultures. Noninvasive carotid studies combined with transcranial Doppler analysis can exclude hemodynamically significant carotid stenosis as the source of emboli if there is any clinical reason to consider this source. Cerebral angiography is considered only when endarterectomy is considered and/or noninvasive tests for significant carotid stenosis have produced equivocal results. An ECG may show an arrhythmia or myocardial infarction that may have been the source of embolism. Echocardiography (conventional or transesophageal) is used to determine whether a cardiac thrombus or ascending aorta lesion was the source of embolism. These techniques are generally insensitive to small clots and are positive in less than 20 percent of patients who have had cerebral emboli.

THERAPY   Therapy of patients with embolic cerebral infarction consists of managing the stroke itself, in both the acute and chronic phases, and of preventing further embolic strokes. When cerebral embolism is suspected, the immediate goal is to keep cerebral perfusion in the ischemic area as adequate as possible. The blood pressure should not be lowered even if hypertension is found unless it is malignant hypertension (see Chap. 209). If the blood pressure is low, raising it is probably advisable in the hours after stroke. An excessive rise above normal may, however, aggravate edema formation. Approximately 5 percent or less of patients with embolic strokes have enough *secondary cerebral edema* to cause clinical problems. Edema seldom becomes problematic until the second or third day but can then cause mass effect for up to 10 days. Two observations governing the severity of the edema associated with cerebral embolism seem to apply. First, in instances of supratentorial embolic infarction, the larger the area of infarct, the more likely it is that edema formation will become a problem. Emboli that lodge in the middle cerebral artery stem are much more likely to cause symptomatic edema formation that leads, in a few patients, to coma and death than are emboli in a distal branch of the middle cerebral artery. Second, small amounts of edema formation in the cerebellum following embolic infarction, usually in the territory of the posterior inferior cerebellar artery (inferior cerebellum), can lead to an acute increase in intracranial pressure in the posterior fossa. The resulting compression of the brainstem may result in sudden coma and respiratory arrest requiring emergency surgical decompression. Water restriction and agents that raise the serum osmolality should be considered early in both instances. Intravenous mannitol is most frequently used to raise the serum osmolarity to approximately 300 mosmol/L; it is given as often as every 2 to 4 h. The acute management of artery-to-artery embolus, in either the carotid or vertebral territory, is discussed above (see "Ischemic Cerebrovascular Disease").

When the deficit is large enough to suggest that the embolus has lodged in the middle cerebral artery stem with corresponding infarction of the basal ganglion, deep white matter, and cortical surface, acute anticoagulation with heparin is generally avoided. On rare occasions, symptomatic basal ganglion hemorrhage into infarcted tissue occurs. But when the stroke is smaller and involves the cortical surface, or when the deficit fluctuates, suggesting partial arterial occlusion, then acute anticoagulation should be considered. For future stroke prevention, chronic anticoagulation with warfarin is general recommended beginning 2 to 5 days after the stroke. A second embolism is rare in the first 3 days. Anticoagulation is usually continued for 6 months. Chronic ventricular failure or a ventricular aneurysm, if present, may indicate a need for longer treatment. Antiplatelet as opposed to anticoagulation therapy has not been assessed adequately in this setting. Lifelong anticoagulation with warfarin may be legitimately considered in patients who have evidence of recurrent embolism or embolism associated with chronic intermittent or sustained atrial fibrillation. Low-intensity anticoagulation (PT 1.2 to 1.5 times control or international normalized ratio, INR, 1.5 to 2.7 or 2 to 3) for patients with chronic, intermittent, or sustained atrial fibrillation has been proven conclusively to be safe and to prevent cerebral embolism. The rate of significant hemorrhage under careful anticoagulation control is the same for warfarin-treated and untreated groups. Aspirin, by contrast, did not demonstrate consistent efficacy for preventing cerebral embolism in this setting. Thus low-intensity warfarin anticoagulation is generally recommended for patients with atrial fibrillation who are over age 60. Higher intensities of anticoagulation (INR > 3) have been used for prosthetic heart valve patients, but they are associated with higher incidence of hemorrhagic complications. It is possible, though as yet unproven, that in nonvalvular atrial fibrillation patients, a lower intensity of anticoagulation (INR 1.4 to 1.9), may be as effective and require less monitoring.

INTRACRANIAL HEMORRHAGE: GENERAL REMARKS

Of the many causes of nontraumatic intracranial hemorrhage, four are particularly common: deep hypertensive and spontaneous lobar intracerebral hemorrhages, ruptured saccular aneurysm, and bleeding from an arteriovenous malformation. Hemorrhage associated with a bleeding disorder and rupture of a mycotic aneurysm are less common. Rare causes include idiopathic brain purpura, brainstem (Duret) hemorrhages associated with brainstem compression during herniation, and small multifocal hemorrhages associated with hypertensive encephalopathy.

HYPERTENSIVE INTRACEREBRAL HEMORRHAGE

PATHOPHYSIOLOGY Hypertensive hemorrhages typically occur in one of four sites: (1) the putamen and adjacent internal capsule, (2) the thalamus, (3) the pons, and (4) the cerebellum. They rarely originate in the central white matter of the hemispheres. A penetrating artery arising from the middle cerebral artery stem, basilar artery, or circle of Willis is generally the source of hemorrhage, the same vessels that are known to be damaged by hypertension.

The hemorrhage begins as a small oval mass and then spreads by dissection, growing in volume and displacing and compressing adjacent brain tissue. Rupture or seepage into the ventricular system may occur. Primary intraventricular hemorrhage is rare.

Most hypertensive intracerebral hemorrhages develop over a few minutes, but some evolve over 30 to 60 min, and others, particularly those associated with anticoagulant therapy, may evolve for as long as 24 to 38 h. Once bleeding stops, it has generally been thought not to start again. Edema in the compressed tissue around the hemorrhage often leads to increasing mass effect and, in some cases, worsening of the clinical state. Within 48 h, macrophages begin to phagocytize the hemorrhage at its outer surface. After 1 to 6 months, the hemorrhage mass is generally resolved to a slitlike orange cavity lined with glial scar tissue and hemosiderin-laden macrophages.

CLINICAL MANIFESTATIONS Hypertensive intracerebral hemorrhages are most common in patients with prolonged, sustained hypertension. Although not particularly associated with exertion, intracerebral hemorrhages almost always occur while the patient is awake and sometimes when under stress. Unlike the sudden onset of embolism, these strokes usually evolve over a few minutes, with the neurologic signs and symptoms dependent on the site and size of the extravasation. Vomiting and headache are hallmarks of acute hemorrhages that distinguish them from other strokes. Seizures are uncommon but occur in a few instances.

Putamenal hemorrhage, the most common hypertensive hemorrhage, invariably disrupts the internal capsule adjacent to the basal ganglia. Contralateral hemiplegia is therefore the sentinel sign, but when these hemorrhages are large, the patient may become comatose within a few minutes. In milder cases, over 5 to 30 min, the face sags on one side, speech becomes slurred, the arm and leg gradually weaken, and *the eyes deviate away from the side of the hemiparesis*. The paralysis may worsen until the affected limbs become flaccid or extend rigidly with a Babinski sign on the same side. In the worst case, drowsiness gives way to stupor as signs of upper brainstem compression appear. Coma ensues, accompanied by deep, irregular, or intermittent respiration, a dilated and fixed ipsilateral pupil, bilateral Babinski signs, and decerebrate rigidity. Edema formation in the adjacent brain may cause progressive deterioration over 12 to 72 h.

Thalamic hemorrhages also produce a hemiplegia or hemiparesis from pressure on or dissection through the internal capsule adjacent to the thalamus. A prominent sensory deficit involving all modalities is usually present. Aphasia, often with preserved verbal repetition, may occur after hemorrhage into the dominant (left) thalamus, and apractagnosia or mutism occurs in some cases of nondominant hemorrhage. There also may be a transient homonymous visual field defect. Thalamic hemorrhages cause several typical ocular disturbances by virtue of extension medially into the upper midbrain. These include, most characteristically, deviation of the eyes downward and inward so that they appear to be looking at the patient's nose, unequal pupils with absence of light reaction, skew deviation with the eye opposite the hemorrhage displaced downward and medially, ipsilateral ptosis and miosis (Horner's syndrome), absence of convergence, paralysis of vertical gaze, an assortment of lateral gaze abnormalities (paresis or pseudoparesis of the sixth nerve), and retraction nystagmus.

In *pontine hemorrhages*, deep coma with quadriplegia usually occurs over a few minutes. There is often prominent decerebrate rigidity and small (1-mm) pupils that react to light. There is impairment of reflex horizontal eye movements evoked by head turning (doll's-head or oculocephalic maneuver) or by irrigation of the ears with cold water (see Chap. 26). Hyperpnea, severe acute hypertension, and hyperhidrosis are common. Death usually occurs within a few hours, but there are exceptions where consciousness is retained because the hemorrhage is limited to the tegmentum.

Cerebellar hemorrhages usually develop over several hours with repeated vomiting and inability to walk or stand. In mild cases there may be no other neurologic signs; therefore, it is imperative to test gait. Occipital headache and dizziness or vertigo may be prominent symptoms. There is often paresis of conjugate lateral gaze toward the side of the hemorrhage, forced deviation of the eyes to the opposite side, or an ipsilateral sixth nerve palsy. Other less frequent ocular signs include blepharospasm, involuntary closure of one eye, ocular bobbing, and skew deviation. There may be little or no evidence of the usual signs of cerebellar disease, and only a minority of cases show nystagmus or ataxia of the limbs. A mild ipsilateral facial weakness and a diminished corneal reflex are common. Dysarthria and dysphagia may occur. There are no Babinski signs until late in the evolution of the hemorrhage as it expands to the brainstem. As the hours pass, and occasionally with unanticipated suddenness, the patient becomes stuporous, then comatose as a result of brainstem compression, at which point reversal of the syndrome by surgical removal of the clot is seldom successful.

In summary, ocular signs have been highlighted as a method of rapidly localizing hemorrhages. In putamenal hemorrhage, the eyes are deviated to the side opposite the paralysis; in thalamic hemorrhage, the eyes are deviated downward and the pupils may be 3 to 4 mm and unreactive; in pontine hemorrhage, the reflex lateral eye movements are impaired and the pupils are less than 1 mm yet reactive; and in cerebellar hemorrhage, the eyes may be deviated laterally (to the side opposite the lesion) in the absence of paralysis.

LABORATORY EVALUATION   The CT scan reliably detects all acute hemorrhages of 1 cm or more in diameter in the cerebral or cerebellar hemispheres. After the first 2 weeks, x-ray attenuation values of clotted blood diminish until they become isodense with surrounding brain. Mass effect and edema may remain. In some cases, a surrounding rim of contrast enhancement appears after 2 to 4 weeks and may persist for months. Small pontine hemorrhages may not be identified because of motion and bone artifact that obscure structures in the posterior fossa. MRI, though more sensitive for delineating posterior fossa lesions, is not necessary in most instances. Images of flowing blood on MRI scan may identify arteriovenous malformations as the cause of the hemorrhage. Angiography is used when the cause of intracranial hemorrhage is uncertain, particularly if the hematoma is not in one of the four usual sites for hypertensive hemorrhage. For example, hemorrhage into the temporal lobe suggests rupture of a middle cerebral artery berry aneurysm. Lumbar puncture carries considerable risk after intracerebral hemorrhage and should generally be avoided unless CT scanning is not available.

THERAPY   The size and location of the hematoma determine the treatment and prognosis. Supratentorial hematomas greater than 5 cm in largest diameter generally have a poor prognosis, and infratentorial pontine hematomas greater than 3 cm in size are usually fatal. The occurrence of edema in the week after the intracerebral hemorrhage often worsens the prognosis. The tissue surrounding the hematoma is displaced and compressed but not necessarily infarcted. Hence, in survivors, improvement can result as the hematoma is reabsorbed and the tissue regains its function. Careful management of the patient during the critical acute phase of the cerebral hematoma can lead to considerable recovery.

Surgical removal of an acute supratentorial clot is controversial, but most surgeons have found it necessary on rare occasions. In stuporous patients who still have reflex eye movements and some pupillary reaction, surgery may prevent temporal lobe herniation and irreversible brainstem compression. One important randomized trial has shown a benefit of surgery, though marginal, only in patients in this state. Lifesaving surgery may nonetheless leave major neurologic residua. In contrast, surgical treatment of acute cerebellar hemorrhage is nearly always recommended because it prevents secondary brainstem compression that is the mechanism of death and it offers an excellent prognosis for recovery. If patients are alert without focal brainstem signs and if the cerebellar hematoma is small, acute surgical removal may not be necessary.

Mannitol and other osmotic agents reduce intracranial pressure that has been raised by the volume of the hematoma and edema (see Chap. 376). Glucocorticoids are of uncertain value in curtailing edema from intracerebral hematoma. Monitoring of the intracranial pressure may help to assess medical therapy. Both excessive hypo- and hypertension should be avoided. Toxemia of pregnancy and malignant hypertension associated with acute hemorrhage should be treated cautiously to avoid excessive or precipitous lowering of the blood pressure.

LOBAR INTRACEREBRAL HEMORRHAGE

As control of hypertension in the general population has improved, the relative proportion of hemorrhages outside the basal ganglia and thalamus has increased. These "lobar hemorrhages" appear on CT scan as oval or circular clots in the subcortical white matter. The role of chronic hypertension in their genesis is controversial, but many occur without a history of increased blood pressure. A number of other underlying conditions are found in almost half the cases, the most common being arteriovenous malformation. Others are due to bleeding diathesis, often associated with warfarin administration; hemorrhages into tumor, usually a melanoma or glioma; and aneurysms of the circle of Willis that bleed into brain substance; and there are a large number whose causes remain undetermined even after extensive study including arteriography. Many of these are presumed to be from arteriovenous malformations or venous angiomas that have become obliterated or are angiographically occult.

Amyloid angiopathy, a cause of both single and recurrent lobar hemorrhages in the elderly, can only be diagnosed by postmortem demonstration that cerebral vessels stain strongly with Congo red. Amyloid is deposited in the walls of the cerebral arteries but not elsewhere in the body. Patients may have multiple hemorrhages, with months between occurrences.

CLINICAL MANIFESTATIONS   The neurologic symptoms and signs of lobar hemorrhage appear suddenly, over one to several minutes. Most lobar hemorrhages are small enough to cause a restricted clinical syndrome that simulates an embolus to a vessel supplying one lobe. For example, the major neurologic deficit of occipital hemorrhage is hemianopsia; of left temporal hemorrhage, aphasia and delirium; of parietal hemorrhage, thalamic-like hemisensory loss; and of frontal hemorrhage, arm weakness. Large hemorrhages may be associated with stupor or coma if they secondarily compress the lower thalamus and midbrain, but the greater distance of lobar clots from these vital structures makes coma result less frequently than from putamenal or thalamic hemorrhages.

Most patients with lobar hemorrhages have focal headaches that are attributable to the innervation of adjacent dural vessels; occipital hemorrhage causes pain over the ipsilateral eye; temporal hemorrhage, over the area around or anterior to the ipsilateral ear; frontal hemorrhage, over the forehead or diffusely in the frontal quadrant; and parietal hemorrhage, over the temple region. Stiff neck or seizures are uncommon, but more than half the patients vomit or are initially drowsy.

TREATMENT   In awake or drowsy patients, surgical evacuation offers little benefit over medical management with fluid restriction and osmotic agents. Stuporous or comatose patients who do not respond rapidly to medical therapy for raised intracranial pressure should generally have the clot evacuated.

SUBARACHNOID HEMORRHAGE—SACCULAR ANEURYSM

Rupture of an intracranial saccular aneurysm is the most common cause of subarachnoid hemorrhage, followed by arteriovenous malformation. Although autopsy studies have estimated that 5 percent of the population harbor aneurysms, the incidence of bleeding is about 4:100,000 per year. This devastating disease causes a greater than 10 percent mortality during the first day, and another 25 percent succumb in the first 3 months. Of those who survive, more than half are left with major neurologic deficits as a result of the initial hemorrhage or of a delayed complication, such as rehemorrhage, infarction from cerebral vasospasm, or hydrocephalus. Given these alarming figures, the major therapeutic emphasis should be on preventing the initial rupture and, if rupture occurs, preventing the predictable early complications.

PATHOPHYSIOLOGY   Saccular aneurysms occur at the bifurcations of the large arteries at the base of the brain and rupture into the subarachnoid space of the basal cisterns. The common sites of saccular aneurysms include the junction of the anterior communicating artery with the anterior cerebral artery, the junction of the posterior communicating artery and the internal carotid artery, the bifurcation of the middle cerebral artery, the top of the basilar artery, the junction of the basilar artery and the superior cerebellar artery or the anterior inferior cerebellar artery, or the junction of the vertebral artery and the posterior inferior cerebellar artery. Approximately 85 percent of cases occur in the anterior circle of Willis; 10 to 30 percent of patients have multiple aneurysms; 10 to 20 percent occur in bilateral identical locations.

As an aneurysm develops, it often forms a neck with a dome. The length of the neck and the size of the dome, factors that are important in planning microsurgical obliteration, vary greatly. The arterial internal elastic lamina disappears at the base of the neck. The media thins, and connective tissue replaces smooth-muscle cells. At the site of rupture (most often the dome), the wall thins to less than 0.3 mm, and the tear that allows bleeding is often no more than 0.5 mm long.

It is not possible to determine which aneurysms are likely to rupture, but limited data suggest that those larger than 7 mm may warrant prophylactic surgical obliteration.

CLINICAL SYMPTOMS, EVOLUTION, AND MANAGEMENT   Prodromal symptoms   Prodromal symptoms may suggest the location of an unruptured aneurysm and suggest that it is progressively enlarging. A third nerve palsy, particularly when associated with pupillary dilatation, loss of light reflex, and focal pain above and behind the eye, indicates an expanding aneurysm at the junction of the posterior communicating artery and the internal carotid artery. Prompt surgery is indicated. A sixth nerve palsy may indicate an aneurysm in the cavernous sinus, and visual field defects can occur with an expanding supraclinoid carotid aneurysm. Occipital and posterior cervical pain may signal a posterior inferior cerebellar artery (PICA) or anterior inferior cerebellar artery (AICA) aneurysm. Pain in or behind the eye and in the low temple can occur with an expanding middle cerebral aneurysm.

It is not known for certain if an aneurysm can cause small intermittent bleeding into the subarachnoid space—so-called warning leaks. However, the importance of recognizing the smallest aneurysmal rupture or leak is undeniable. Sudden unexplained headache at any location should raise suspicion of subarachnoid hemorrhage and be investigated by a CT scan to look for blood in the basal cisterns. Often a small subarachnoid hemorrhage will not be seen by CT scan, necessitating a lumbar puncture to detect subarachnoid blood.

Initial clinical presentation: Acute major subarachnoid hemorrhage   At the moment of aneurysmal rupture with major subarachnoid hemorrhage, the intracranial pressure approaches the mean arterial pressure, and cerebral perfusion pressure falls. This may account for the sudden transient loss of consciousness that occurs in up to 45 percent of cases. Sudden loss of consciousness may be preceded by a brief moment of excruciating headache, but most patients first complain of headache upon regaining consciousness. In 10 percent of cases, aneurysmal bleeding may be severe enough to cause loss of consciousness for several days. In about 45 percent of cases, severe headache, usually associated with exertion, is the presenting complaint. The headache is often called by the patient "the worst headache of my life." Words like *explode* and *burst* may be used. It may be "all over" or "in the back of the head and neck." Vomiting is a prominent symptom and when coupled with sudden headache should always raise the question of acute subarachnoid hemorrhage.

Although sudden headache in the absence of focal neurologic symptoms is the hallmark of aneurysmal rupture, focal neurologic deficits may occur (in addition to direct cranial nerve compression by the enlarging aneurysm as noted above). Anterior communicating artery aneurysms or middle cerebral bifurcation aneurysms may rupture into the subdural space, into the basal cisterns of the subarachnoid space, or directly into the underlying brain and form a clot large enough to produce a localized mass effect. The common deficits that result include hemiparesis, aphasia, anosognosia (hemineglect), memory loss, and abulia. An unusual acute unilateral hemispheric swelling with associated focal neurologic signs and stupor occurs rarely, immediately following aneurysmal rupture. Transient interruption of the cerebral circulation, possibly from acute vascular spasm, may underlie this complication.

Initial evaluation   Over 75 percent of cases have evidence of a subarachnoid clot on a noncontrast CT scan obtained within 72 h of aneurysmal rupture. The extent and location of subarachnoid blood may help locate the underlying aneurysm and identify the cause of the initial neurologic deficit. The clot in the subarachnoid space also may help predict the delayed neurologic deficits due to cerebral vasospasm. *A noncontrast CT scan should be done first because arterial enhancement in the basal cisterns may be mistaken for clotted blood.* If the CT scan neither establishes the diagnosis of subarachnoid hemorrhage nor demonstrates a mass lesion or obstructive hydrocephalus, a lumbar puncture should be performed to establish the presence of subarachnoid blood. Lumbar puncture prior to scanning is indicated only if the CT scan is not available at the time of the suspected subarachnoid hemorrhage. Once the diagnosis of subarachnoid hemorrhage from ruptured saccular aneurysm has been established, four-vessel angiography is generally performed to localize and define the anatomic details of the aneurysm and to determine if other unruptured aneurysms exist.

The ECG frequently shows ST-segment and T-wave changes similar to those associated with ischemic coronary heart disease. Prolonged QRS complex, increased QT interval, and prominent "peaked" or deeply inverted symmetric T waves, although suggesting primary cardiac disease, are usually secondary to the intracranial hemorrhage. The cause of these changes is debated, but there is evidence that structural myocardial lesions may occur after acute hemorrhage.

Serum electrolytes are obtained because hyponatremia may develop from urinary sodium loss, possibly due to natriuretic peptides released by the brain or heart.

Initial management   Following subarachnoid hemorrhage, a stuporous or comatose patient may have increased intracranial pressure. Care is required to maintain adequate cerebral perfusion pressure while avoiding excessive elevation of mean arterial pressure. Frequent arterial blood gas determinations are helpful to assess alveolar ventilation. If hypercapnia exists, mechanically assisted ventilation is necessary. If a subdural or intracerebral hematoma mass is causing neurologic deterioration, its surgical removal and, if feasible, obliteration of the aneurysm are undertaken.

Because rebleeding is possible, all patients are put on bed rest in a quiet, preferably darkened room and are given adequate stool softeners to prevent constipation. If headache or neck pain is severe, mild sedation and analgesics are prescribed. Aspirin, an antiplatelet agent, is inappropriate, but acetaminophen, meperidine, and phenobarbitol or other sedatives may be used. Extreme sedation is generally avoided because it can obscure the assessment of initial or delayed neurologic deficits.

Seizures are uncommon at the onset of aneurysmal rupture. The quivering, jerking, and extensor posturing that usually accompany loss of consciousness are probably related to the sharp rise in intracranial pressure. However, phenytoin or phenobarbitol is sometimes given as prophylactic therapy, since a seizure may cause rebleeding.

Glucocorticoids may help reduce the head-and-neck ache caused by the irritative effect of blood in the subarachnoid space, but there is no evidence to suggest they help in treatment of the cerebral edema that is sometimes seen in patients immediately after a subarachnoid hemorrhage, and they are generally omitted.

DELAYED NEUROLOGIC DEFICITS   There are three major causes of delayed neurologic deficits: *rerupture, hydrocephalus,* and *cerebral vasospasm.* Recognizing each of these depends on knowing precisely the cause and character of the initial neurologic findings.

Rerupture   The incidence of rerupture in the first 3 weeks following subarachnoid hemorrhage is 10 to 30 percent. Because rerupture is associated with a 60 percent mortality and poor outcome, early surgery is now generally recommended for stable patients. In the event surgery cannot be accomplished, antifibrinolytic agents may be considered. They have been associated with a reduced incidence of aneurysmal rerupture but are also associated with an increased incidence of secondary cerebral infarction, presumably due to vasospasm. Hence antifibrinolytic agents are an option only when the early CT scan suggests that cerebral vasospasm is not likely to follow (see below).

Hydrocephalus   Acute hydrocephalus can cause stupor and coma and requires emergency ventricular drainage. More often, subacute hydrocephalus over a few days or a few weeks causes progressive drowsiness or abulia with incontinence. Differentiating hydrocephalus from symptomatic cerebral vasospasm in the anterior communicating arteries is often difficult. It may clear spontaneously or require temporary ventricular drainage. Permanent ventricular drainage, if necessary, is usually done at the time of aneurysmal surgery. Chronic hydrocephalus similar to normal-pressure hydrocephalus may appear a few weeks to months after subarachnoid hemorrhage. It may present with gait difficulty, incontinence, or slowed mentation (abulia). The clue to the diagnosis may be a lack of initiative in conversation or a failure to recover independence after the aneurysm has been surgically clipped. Ventricular shunting is the treatment of choice.

Cerebral vasospasm   Narrowing of the arteries at the base of the brain following subarachnoid hemorrhage from ruptured saccular aneurysm (*cerebral vasospasm*) can lead to delayed cerebral ischemia and infarction. This *symptomatic cerebral vasospasm* after subarachnoid hemorrhage occurs in approximately 30 percent of patients and is the major cause of delayed morbidity or death. Signs of ischemia usually appear 4 to 14 days after the initial subarachnoid hemorrhage, most frequently at about 7 days. The new deficits may fluctuate and correspond to ischemia in specific arterial territories. The severity and distribution of vasospasm determine whether cerebral infarction will develop. Although the precise mechanism of cerebral vasospasm is uncertain, it seems related to the presence of clotted blood surrounding an artery. Because there are no vasa vasorum around the arteries at the base of the brain, clotted blood prevents cerebrospinal fluid from nourishing the vessels. The current hypothesis suggests that spasmogenic hemoglobin breakdown products from the clot induce vasospasm in the underlying vessel, and reduction in local ATP may then prevent the artery from relaxing.

Clinical evidence suggests that the extent and location of clotted blood on CT scans can be used to predict the incidence, location, and severity of cerebral vasospasm in patients after subarachnoid hemorrhage. A high incidence of symptomatic cerebral vasospasm in the middle and anterior cerebral artery territories has been found in patients with early CT scans showing globular subarachnoid clots larger than 5×3 mm in the basal cisterns or layers of blood 1 mm thick or greater in the cerebral fissures. CT scans less reliably predict vasospasm in the vertebral, basilar, or posterior cerebral arteries. For this purpose, the CT scan should be obtained between 24 and 96 h following subarachnoid hemorrhage, since blood present initially can disappear or "wash out" on a scan obtained after 24 h. With the further passage of time, x-ray attenuation values of clotted blood diminish so that its full extent and location may not be reliably detected after 96 h.

CLINICAL SYNDROMES   Symptomatic severe cerebral vasospasm presents with symptoms referable to the specific arterial territories involved. For example, spasm of the middle cerebral stem or its main branches causes contralateral hemiparesis, dysphasia (dominant hemisphere), anosognosia, or apractagnosia (nondominant hemisphere). Even severe vasospasm may not produce ischemic symptoms if sufficient collateral blood flow develops through border zone anastomotic channels (see Fig. 368-1A). Proximal anterior cerebral artery vasospasm is associated with abulia and incontinence, while severe vasospasm of the posterior cerebral artery is associated with hemianopic visual field defects. Severe spasm of the basilar or vertebral arteries occasionally produces focal brainstem ischemia. All these focal neurologic symptoms may develop over a few days, fluctuate, or present abruptly. Transcranial Doppler assessment of proximal middle, anterior, and posterior cerebral and basilar artery flow can now reliably detect the onset of vasospasm prior to symptoms and follow its course and response to therapy.

TREATMENT   Therapeutic efforts to prevent or treat symptomatic cerebral vasospasm have been universally disappointing. The failure to find a satisfactory therapy for cerebral vasospasm has prompted a search for prophylactic measures to prevent or minimize its occurrence.

Treatment with the calcium channel blocking agent nimodipine has been reported in several studies to have beneficial effects, but patients in both the treated and untreated groups developed symptomatic vasospasm.

The most commonly accepted form of therapy for symptomatic cerebral vasospasm is to increase the cerebral perfusion pressure by raising mean arterial pressure through plasma volume expansion and the judicious use of pressor agents, ordinarily phenylephrine or dopamine. Raised perfusion pressure has been associated with symptomatic improvement in some patients, but high arterial pressure may risk rebleeding. The therapies generally require monitoring the central venous pressure, arterial pressure, and, in severe cases, the intracranial and pulmonary artery wedge pressure. If symptomatic vasospasm persists despite optimal medical therapy, then percutaneous intraarterial angioplasty, if available, is considered. It can effectively relieve focal severe symptomatic vasospasm in the arteries at the base of the brain, but it carries the risk of precipitating further ischemic stroke or arterial rupture and requires a highly skilled, experienced team.

Severe cerebral edema in patients with infarction from vasospasm may increase the intracranial pressure enough to reduce cerebral perfusion pressure. Treatment, as outlined in Chap. 376, is with mannitol and hyperventilation. Plasma osmolality is usually raised to approximately 300 mosmol/L. As a last resort, barbiturate-induced coma has been used to reduce intracranial pressure in some patients; it has not been proven to improve outcome.

Surgical interventional neuroradiologic treatment of saccular aneurysm   The advent of the operating microscope has made surgical obliteration of a ruptured saccular aneurysm the safest and most effective means of preventing disastrous rerupture. Recently, acute (day 1 to day 3) surgical management has been advocated, eliminating the problem of rerupture and allowing more aggressive medical treatment of symptomatic cerebral vasospasm. Interventional neuroradiologic techniques, including balloon occlusion of the aneurysm or of the internal carotid artery in a patient with inoperable aneurysm and angioplasty for cerebral vasospasm, are now possible. These new therapeutic strategies hold promise for improving management of patients with subarachnoid hemorrhage.

Giant aneurysms   Giant aneurysms larger than 2 cm in diameter occur at the same sites as small aneurysms. The three most common locations are the intracranial internal carotid, middle cerebral bifurcation, and top of the basilar arteries. Although they can bleed, they usually cause symptoms by compressing the adjacent brain or cranial nerves. Edema formation in the compressed brain can be relentless, compounding the mass effect. It is resistant to treatment and may be fatal. This progression is particularly likely if a giant aneurysm occurs at the bifurcation of the middle cerebral artery. Surgical decompression, until recently, was the only adequate therapy. It is extremely difficult technically and carries a high morbidity in the presence of edema. Newer interventional neuroradiologic procedures may prove helpful (see Chap. 365).

Mycotic aneurysms   Mycotic aneurysms are located distal to the first bifurcation of major arteries of the circle of Willis. Emboli from bacterial endocarditis should be suspected and appropriate blood cultures taken. Because of their distal location in the arterial tree, they rarely leave significant amounts of clotted blood in the basal cisterns, and severe cerebral vasospasm is infrequent. Mycotic aneurysms, however, are subject to rerupture. Although antibiotic therapy may reduce this risk, surgical obliteration may be required.

OTHER CAUSES OF INTRACRANIAL HEMORRHAGE

ARTERIOVENOUS MALFORMATION   An angioma, or hemangioma, consists of a tangle of abnormal vessels forming an abnormal communication between the arterial and venous systems. Most are developmental arteriovenous fistulas in which the constituent vessels enlarge and grow with the passage of time. Angiomas vary in size from a small blemish a few millimeters in diameter to a huge mass of tortuous channels composing an arteriovenous shunt of sufficient magnitude to raise the cardiac output. Hypertrophic dilated arterial "feeders" approach the main lesion, disappear below the cortex, and break up into a network of thin-walled blood vessels which connect directly with draining veins. These often form huge, dilated, pulsating channels carrying away arterial blood. The blood vessels forming the tangle interposed between arteries and veins are usually abnormally thin and do not have a normal structure. Angiomas occur in all parts of the brain, brainstem, and spinal cord, but the larger ones are most frequently in the posterior half of the hemispheres, commonly forming a wedge-shaped lesion extending from the cortex to the ventricular lining.

Angiomas are more frequent in men and may occur in more than one member of a family in the same or successive generations. Although the lesion is present from birth, bleeding or other complaints are most common between the ages of 10 and 30, occasionally as late as the fifties.

The chief clinical symptoms and signs are headache, seizures, and those associated with rupture. When headache occurs (without bleeding), it may be hemicranial and throbbing, like migraine, or diffuse. There may be hemiplegia with headache, resembling hemiplegic migraines. Focal seizures that become generalized occur in about 30 percent of cases and are usually well managed with anticonvulsants. In half of cases, arteriovenous malformations become evident as intracerebral hemorrhages. In most of these cases, the hemorrhage is mainly intraparenchymal with a small amount of spillage into the subarachnoid space. Blood is usually not deposited in the basal cistern, and symptomatic cerebral vasospasm is therefore rare. The threat of rerupture in the first 3 weeks is low, so there is no need to consider the use of antifibrinolytic agents. The hemorrhage may be massive, leading to death acutely, or may be as small as 1 cm in diameter, leading to minor focal symptoms or no deficit. In either case, the hemorrhagic mass may compress the arteriovenous malformation so completely that angiography cannot detect the malformation. Hence, when arteriovenous malformation (AVM) is suspected, angiography is best postponed until the hematoma has completely resolved, i.e., after 6 to 8 weeks. Rarely the angioma is large enough to steal blood away from adjacent normal brain tissue, rendering the surrounding brain ischemic. This deprivation is most often seen when large AVMs in the middle cerebral–posterior cerebral system or middle cerebral–anterior cerebral system extend from the cortical surface to the ventricular system. Hydrocephalus may result when the vein of Galen enlarges as a channel for drainage from the AVM.

Large AVMs of the carotid–middle cerebral system may be associated with a systolic and diastolic bruit (sometimes self-audible) over the eye, forehead, or neck where a bounding, forceful carotid pulse may be perceived. Headache at the onset of AVM rupture is not as prominent or as common as it is with a ruptured saccular aneurysm. Contrast CT scan can often detect the channels of an AVM prior to rupture; newer MRI techniques may prove more sensitive.

Small AVMs, 0.5 cm or less, are usually low-pressure venous angiomas that can bleed slowly. If they have bled, surgical obliteration or resection should be considered.

The management of patients with arterial AVMs is best accomplished by a team approach. Many cases are first assessed and may be treated by interventional neuroradiology. Each case requires a unique approach that takes into account the extent and location of the lesion, the feasibility and safety of the various therapeutic options, and the assumption of a risk of 3 percent per year rate of hemorrhage.

TRAUMA Head injury can result in intracerebral (especially temporal lobe and inferior frontal) hematoma and infratentorial hematomas, subarachnoid bleeding, acute and chronic subdural hematoma formation, and acute epidural hematoma formation. Trauma must be considered in any patient with an unexplained acute neurologic deficit (hemiparesis, stupor, or confusion), particularly if the deficit occurred in the context of a fall. These entities and their

distinction from spontaneous hemorrhage are discussed more fully in Chap. 376.

HEMATOLOGIC DISORDERS Intracerebral hemorrhage associated with hematologic disorders (leukemia, aplastic anemia, thrombocytopenic purpura) can occur at any intracranial site and may present as multiple intracerebral hemorrhages. Skin and mucous membrane bleeding is usually evident and offers a diagnostic clue. Intracerebral hemorrhage associated with anticoagulant therapy can occur at any location, often lobar, and may evolve slowly over 24 to 48 h. Fresh frozen plasma and vitamin K are usually given immediately. When intracerebral hemorrhage is associated with aspirin, fresh platelet transfusions may be required.

BRAIN TUMORS Hemorrhage into a brain tumor may be the first manifestation of neoplasm. Choriocarcinoma, malignant melanoma, renal cell carcinoma, and bronchogenic carcinoma are among the most common metastatic tumors associated with intracerebral hemorrhage. Glioblastoma multiforme in adults and medulloblastoma in children also may have areas of intracerebral hemorrhage.

OTHER CAUSES Primary intraventricular hemorrhage is rare. It usually begins intraparenchymally and dissects into the ventricular system without leaving signs of intraparenchymal hemorrhage. Sepsis can cause small petechial hemorrhages through the cerebral white matter. There is no blood in the spinal fluid, and this condition should not be confused with a stroke. Inflammatory disease of the arteries and veins, especially polyarteritis nodosa and lupus erythematosus, can produce hemorrhage into the central nervous system. Most of the time it is associated with hypertension. An intensely inflammatory and hemorrhagic white matter process termed *Hurst's hemorrhagic leukoencephalitis* is probably a type of hyperacute multiple sclerosis. Moyamoya, mainly an obliterative disease that causes ischemic symptoms, also may have multiple small aneurysms that rupture in a small percentage of patients. Hemorrhages into the spinal cord are usually the result of an AVM or metastatic tumor. Epidural spinal hemorrhage usually compresses the cord rapidly and produces a transverse myelopathy (see Chap. 381).

HYPERTENSIVE ENCEPHALOPATHY (See Chap. 209)

In this acute syndrome, severe hypertension is associated with headache, nausea, vomiting, convulsions, confusion, stupor, and coma. Focal or lateralizing neurologic signs, either transitory or lasting, may occur but are infrequent and always suggest some other form of vascular disease (hemorrhage, embolism, or atherosclerotic thrombosis). By the time neurologic manifestations appear, the hypertension has usually reached the malignant state, with retinal hemorrhages, exudates, papilledema (hypertensive retinopathy grade IV), and evidence of renal and cardiac disease. In many, but not all, cases the cerebrospinal fluid pressure and the protein values are both elevated. The hypertension may be essential or due to chronic renal disease, acute glomerulonephritis, acute toxemia of pregnancy, pheochromocytoma, Cushing's syndrome, or ACTH toxicity. Lowering of the blood pressure with hypotensive drugs may reverse the process in several days if permanent damage is not severe. Neuropathologic examination may reveal a cerebral swelling or hemorrhages of various sizes from massive to petechial. A cerebellar pressure cone reflects increased pressure in the posterior fossa, and in some instances lumbar puncture has been fatal. Microscopically, there are small hemorrhages, clusters of microglial cells, minute cerebral infarcts, and necrosis of arterioles.

The term *hypertensive encephalopathy* should be reserved for this syndrome and not for chronic recurrent headaches, dizziness, epileptic seizures, recurrent TIAs, or small strokes which often occur in association with high blood pressure.

REFERENCES

AMARENCO P et al: The prevalence of ulcerated plaques in the aortic arch in patients with stroke. N Engl J Med 326:221, 1992

BAUER KA, ROSENBERG RD: The pathophysiology of the prethrombotic state in humans: Insights gained from studies using markers of hemostatic system activation. Blood 70:343, 1987

BOSTON AREA ANTICOAGULATION TRIAL FOR ATRIAL FIBRILLATION INVESTIGATORS: The effect of low-dose warfarin on the risk of stroke in patients with nonrheumatic atrial fibrillation. N Engl J Med 323:1505, 1990

BOUSSER MG et al: "AICLA" controlled trial of aspirin and dipyridamole in the secondary prevention of athero-thrombotic cerebral ischemia. Stroke 14:5, 1983

CALL GK et al: Reversible cerebral segmental vasoconstriction. Stroke 19:1159, 1988

CANADIAN COOPERATIVE STUDY GROUP: A randomized trial of aspirin and sulfinpyrazone in threatened stroke. N Engl J Med 299:53, 1978

CEREBRAL EMBOLISM STUDY GROUP: Immediate anticoagulation of embolic stroke: Brain hemorrhage and management complications. Stroke 15:779, 1984

CHAMBERS BR et al: Outcome in patients with asymptomatic neck bruits. N Engl J Med 315:860, 1986

EAGLE KA, BOUCHER CA: Cardiac risk of noncardiac surgery. N Engl J Med 321:1330, 1989

EC/IC BYPASS STUDY GROUP: Failure of extracranial-intracranial arterial bypass to reduce the risk of ischemic stroke: Results of an international randomized trial. N Engl J Med 313:1191, 1985

EUROPEAN CAROTID SURGERY TRIALISTS' COLLABORATIVE GROUP: MRC European Carotid Surgery Trial: Interim results for symptomatic patients with severe (70–99%) or with mild (0–29%) carotid stenosis. Lancet 337:1235, 1991

EZEKOWITZ MD et al: Warfarin in the prevention of stroke associated with nonrheumatic atrial fibrillation. N Engl J Med 327:1406, 1992

FALKEBORN M et al: Hormone replacement therapy and the risk of stroke—follow-up of a population-based cohort in Sweden. Arch Intern Med 153:1201, 1993

FISHER CM: Clinical syndromes in cerebral thrombosis, hypertensive hemorrhage, and ruptured saccular aneurysm. Clin Neurosurg 22:117, 1975

————: Concerning transient ischemic attacks. Cleve Clin J Med 54:3, 1987

————: Lacunar strokes and infarcts: A review. Neurology 32:871, 1982

————: Late-life migraine accompaniments as a cause of unexplained transient ischemic attacks. Can J Neurol Sci 7:9, 1980

————: Occlusion of the internal carotid artery. Arch Neurol Psychiatry 65:346, 1951

———— et al: The arterial lesions underlying lacunes. Acta Neuropathol (Berl) 12:1, 1969

———— et al: Atherosclerosis of the carotid and vertebral arteries: Extracranial and intracranial. J Neuropathol Exp Neurol 24:455, 1965

———— et al: Cerebral vasospasm with ruptured saccular aneurysm: The clinical manifestations. Neurosurgery 1:245, 1977

———— et al: Lateral medullary infarction: The pattern of vascular occlusion. J Neuropathol Exp Neurol 20:323, 1961

———— et al: Spontaneous dissection of cervico-cerebral arteries. Can J Neurol Sci 5:9, 1978

HINTON RC et al: Symptomatic middle artery stenosis. Ann Neurol 5:152, 1979

HIRSH J et al: Optimal therapeutic range for oral anticoagulants. Chest (Suppl) 95:5S, 1989

KISTLER JP et al: Carotid endarterectomy: Specific therapy based on pathophysiology. N Engl J Med 325:505, 1991

———— et al: The relation of cerebral vasospasm to the extent and location of subarachnoid blood visualized by CT scan: A prospective study. Neurology 33:424, 1983

———— et al: Therapy of ischemic cerebral vascular disease due to atherothrombosis. N Engl J Med 311:27, 100, 1984

KOUDSTAAL PJ et al: Predictors of major vascular events in patients with a transient ischemic attack or nondisabling stroke. Stroke 24:527, 1993

MAYBERG MR et al: For the Veterans Affairs Cooperative Studies Program 309 Trialist Group: Carotid endarterectomy and prevention of cerebral ischemia in symptomatic carotid stenosis. JAMA 266:3289, 1991

NORTH AMERICAN SYMPTOMATIC CAROTID ENDARTERECTOMY TRIAL COLLABORATORS: Beneficial effect of carotid endarterectomy in symptomatic patients with high-grade carotid stenosis. N Engl J Med 325:445, 1991

PETERSEN P et al: Placebo-controlled, randomized trial of warfarin and aspirin for prevention of thromboembolic complications in chronic atrial fibrillation: The Copenhagen AFASAK study. Lancet 1:175, 1989

ROPPER AH, DAVIS KR: Lobar cerebral hemorrhages: Acute clinical syndromes in 26 patients. Ann Neurol 8:141, 1980

WELIN L et al: Analysis of risk factors for stroke in a cohort of men born in 1913. N Engl J Med 317:521, 1987

WOLF PA et al: Atrial fibrillation as an independent risk factor for stroke: The Framingham study. Stroke 22:983, 1991

369　NEOPLASTIC DISEASES OF THE CENTRAL NERVOUS SYSTEM

FRED HOCHBERG / AMY PRUITT

Tumors of the brain, of its meningeal coverings, and of the spinal cord are estimated to cause 90,000 deaths in the United States each year. *Primary* tumors arising within the meninges or the parenchyma of the brain or spinal cord are common at all ages of life. Yet, more than three-quarters of central nervous system (CNS) tumors are *secondary* metastases arising in patients undergoing treatment for systemic cancer. CNS neoplasms claim a disproportionate share of hospital beds, diagnostic tests, and other medical resources. One-fourth of the annual $4 billion cost for the care of cancer patients in the United States is allocated to patients with neoplasms of the CNS.

Although the specialized care of such patients is usually delegated to the neurosurgeon, radiotherapist, or neurooncologist, with the advent of new imaging techniques, the internist is increasingly involved in the initial diagnosis. Late in the course of the disease, such patients again may come under the care of a general physician. The proper care of patients with primary or metastatic tumors of the CNS requires a systematic approach that enables the physician to (1) distinguish tumor from other causes of neurologic dysfunction such as infection, immunosuppression, metabolic derangement, pseudotumor cerebri, or subdural hematoma; (2) make proper use of sophisticated diagnostic techniques, such as magnetic resonance imaging (MRI) and computed tomography (CT), and of more invasive tests, such as spinal fluid evaluation and arteriography; (3) provide early therapy to control cerebral edema and avoid seizure activity; (4) exclude systemic malignancy prior to referring the patient for a brain biopsy; and (5) recognize the medical complications of the tumor and of its therapy.

APPROACH TO THE PATIENT WITH CNS TUMORS

CLASSIFICATION OF TUMORS Both benign and malignant primary CNS tumors are capable of producing neurologic impairment. Primary tumors arise from glial cells (astrocytoma, oligodendroglioma, glioblastoma), ependymal cells (ependymoma), or supporting tissue (meningioma, schwannoma, papilloma of the choroid plexus). In childhood, tumors arise from more primitive cells (medulloblastoma, neuroblastoma, chordoma). Malignant astrocytoma or glioblastoma is the most common type of primary tumor in adults over age 20. A classification of intracranial tumors is given in Table 369-1.

CLINICAL MANIFESTATIONS OF INTRACRANIAL TUMOR Intracranial tumors may be located within the brain substance (intraaxial) or in close proximity to the brain (extraaxial). The latter produce symptoms by compression of the brain. Many of the symptoms caused by intracranial masses reflect tumor expansion within a fixed bony vault into space normally occupied by brain, blood, and cerebrospinal fluid (CSF). The nature and severity of these symptoms depend on the location of the tumor and the rate of its growth. Although brain tissue can accommodate the presence of slowly growing tumors, masses larger than 3 cm in diameter compress the brain, its blood supply, and CSF pathways. This compression is increased by peritumoral edema (vasogenic cerebral edema). Neurologic deterioration occurs as the tumor infiltrates or displaces normal brain structures; as the tumor develops areas of hemorrhage, necrosis, or cyst formation; or as the tumor obstructs the normal flow of CSF, producing hydrocephalus.

TABLE 369-1　Classification of intracranial tumors

Type of tumor	Percent of total
Glioma:	40
Glioblastoma	20
Astrocytoma grades I and II	10
Ependymoma	6
Medulloblastoma	2
Oligodendroglioma	1
Papilloma of choroid plexus	1
Metastases	23
Meningioma	17
Pituitary adenoma	5
Schwannoma	5
Lymphoma	3
Miscellaneous (congenital tumors, PNETs*)	7

*Primitive neuroectodermal tumors.

Symptoms of intracranial tumor may develop in patients with previously diagnosed systemic cancer or in those not known to harbor a malignancy. Patients with intracranial tumor usually present with one or more of the following groups of symptoms: (1) headache with or without evidence of increased intracranial pressure, (2) progressive generalized decline in cognitive abilities or impairment of specific neurologic functions affecting speech and language, gait, or memory, (3) adult-onset seizures or increased frequency or severity of previously documented seizure activity, or (4) focal neurologic symptoms reflecting the particular anatomic site of the tumor, such as those caused by acoustic schwannoma (neuroma) in the cerebellopontine angle, by meningioma of the olfactory groove, sella, or parasellar areas, or by pineal area masses which abut the diencephalon.

Headache is the initial symptom in half of patients with brain tumors. Traction on the dura, blood vessels, or cranial nerves results from local compression, elevation of intracranial pressure, edema, or hydrocephalus. In most patients with supratentorial tumor, pain radiates to the side of the tumor mass, whereas patients with posterior fossa masses describe retroorbital, retroauricular, or occipital pain. Emesis and hiccups, often without nausea, signal development of increased intracranial pressure and are especially common in patients with masses located beneath the tentorium.

Tumors of the frontal lobes may attain considerable size before symptoms develop, and then symptoms often are nonspecific. Subtle, progressive disturbances of mentation, slowness of comprehension, loss of acuity in business affairs, memory disorders, or apathy, lethargy, and drowsiness may be reported. Spontaneity of thought and activity is lost. Incontinence of urine and disordered gait may be seen by family members. The development of a true dysphasia and/or motor weakness signal progression of the tumor or its associated edema into motor cortex and speech areas of the frontoparietal region. Papilledema, choking of the optic nerve head, or loss of retinal venous pulsations follows.

Masses in the temporal lobes are associated with personality changes that may resemble affective or psychotic thought disorders. Various combinations of auditory hallucinations, abrupt shifts in mood, and altered sleep, appetite, and sexual functions are soon interspersed with complex partial seizures, possibly accompanied by visual field defects in the superior quadrants contralateral to the tumor. Temporal tumors force the medial temporal lobe (uncus) through the tentorial notch (uncal herniation). The third cranial nerve is compressed against the diencephalon. The pupil dilates, followed shortly by hemiparesis on the opposite side.

Disorders of communication and vision characterize parietooccipital masses. Receptive aphasia with contralateral hemianopsia characterizes left parietal tumors, while a combination of spatial disorientation, constructional apraxia, and left homonymous hemianopsia bespeaks right parietal tumors.

Seizures occur as the initial symptom in 20 percent of patients with brain tumors. Patients with new onset of epilepsy after the age of 35 must be evaluated for brain tumor. Similar high-risk groups of new seizure patients include those with previously diagnosed systemic cancer, longstanding neurologic diseases (including such neuroectodermal disorders as von Recklinghausen's disease and tuberous sclerosis), or acute or atypical psychiatric disorders. A carefully obtained history may uncover disordered time perceptions (déjà vu or déjà jamais), paroxysms of fear, and clinging "viscous" personality changes in addition to obvious features such as "complex partial" (temporal lobe) seizures or personality changes that antedate the diagnosis by years. Occasionally, the first symptom simulates a transient ischemic attack with no residual deficit or discernible seizure, but more commonly the pattern of clinical seizures provides localizing information. Thus, the "Jacksonian march" of tonic-clonic seizure points to frontal tumors and a sensory march characterizes tumors of the sensory parietal cortex. Metastatic tumors, occupying the junction of gray and white matter, are more likely than are primary tumors to produce acute symptoms evolving in days to weeks. Even more rapid onset of symptoms reflects hemorrhage in tumors of lung, melanoma,

renal cell, choriocarcinoma, or thyroid origins. In contrast, with the exception of oligodendroglioma and malignant astrocytoma, primary brain tumors are unlikely to hemorrhage.

PHYSICAL EXAMINATION OF THE PATIENT WITH SUSPECTED CNS TUMORS When the physician examines a brain tumor suspect who is not previously known to have a systemic cancer, the general examination should include (1) survey of the skin for stigmata of neurocutaneous syndromes or melanoma, (2) a search for enlarged lymph nodes, (3) an examination of the abdomen for hepatic or splenic enlargement, (4) a rectal examination with stool guaiac test, (5) a breast and pelvic examination in female patients, and (6) a cardiopulmonary examination.

The neurologic examination of the patient with suspected brain tumor should focus first on an evaluation of the mental status. The examiner should look for evidence of specific localizing cognitive deficits, such as dysphasia, dyspraxia, or memory loss, in addition to gleaning a sense of any personality change which has occurred. The patient is examined for increased intracranial pressure (papilledema or sixth cranial nerve paresis) and for other cranial nerve abnormalities. Asymmetries of strength, sensation, visual fields, and reflex activity should be sought. Combinations of cranial nerve abnormalities and corticospinal or lumbosacral radicular signs raise suspicion of leptomeningeal metastases (see below).

INVESTIGATION OF THE PATIENT WITH INTRACRANIAL TUMOR Advances in neuroradiology have contributed greatly to the diagnosis and management of patients with suspected neoplastic disease of the CNS. A plan for appropriate diagnostic studies based on the initial MRI or CT scan results is outlined in Table 369-2. The language of neurooncology differs from that of medical oncology, familiar terms such as "benign," "malignant," and "metastasizing" taking on different connotations when the tumor involves the CNS. Benign and malignant tumors are not differentiated in the scheme of Table 369-2 because the initial clinical approach is identical. Although many primary CNS tumors exhibit microscopic characteristics classifiable as "benign" because they are well-differentiated histologically and grow slowly, they are, nevertheless, often incurable. Tumors of identical histology may have very different prognoses, depending on their location and amenability to resection and on the patient's age. Secondary CNS tumors are malignant in the conventional sense, since they represent metastases and invade normal tissue. Both benign and malignant tumors may produce profound, irreversible neurologic impairment. Primary brain tumors, with rare exceptions, do not metastasize outside the CNS; however, virtually all primary brain tumors are capable of diffuse seeding to the leptomeninges. Thus, the approach to *all* intracranial tumors, summarized in Table 369-2, relies on the clinical history and physical examination and on information provided by MRI and CT.

The laboratory evaluation of intracranial tumors Contrast-enhanced and unenhanced MRI and CT have now largely replaced the combination of skull x-ray, electroencephalogram, radionuclide brain scan, and arteriography as the principal tests for the evaluation of patients with suspected brain tumor.

MAGNETIC RESONANCE IMAGING (MRI) MRI is the procedure of choice for the evaluation of neurologic dysfunction in a patient suspected of having cancer. MRI delineates most metastatic and primary tumors of the nervous system (see also Chap. 365). Lesions of the skull base and those in the brainstem, cerebellum, and spinal cord are visualized with greater detail with MRI than with CT, myelographic, or radionuclide images (Fig. 369-1). In addition to great sensitivity and delineation of anatomic detail, MRI offers the advantages of requiring no radiation exposure. The "flow-void" characteristic of MRI images provides a measure of tumor vascularity and may be reconstructed to create an MRI angiogram that may obviate preoperative arteriography (Fig. 369-2). Hemorrhage, seen in metastatic melanoma and glioblastoma, is easily identified as hemoglobin products or as ferritin. Tumors which contain fat (epidermoid, lipoma, craniopharyngioma) are recognized by their "bright" T2 signals as are those growths with cysts containing high concentra-

TABLE 369-2   Evaluation following MRI or CT scan of the patient with suspected neoplastic disease of the brain and spinal cord

CT/MRI result	Possible diagnosis	Pretreatment evaluation	Primary treatment	Secondary treatment
KNOWN SYSTEMIC CANCER: BRAIN				
Normal				
No focal deficits on examination	Infection, metabolic abnormality	Lumbar puncture, exclude infection	See text	——
Focal deficits on examination	Vascular disease, carcinomatous meningitis, seizure, paraneoplastic syndrome, complications of therapy	Lumbar puncture, follow-up MRI 4–6 weeks, gadolinium MRI	See text	Glucocorticoids as needed
Solitary mass	Radioresistant or radiosensitive tumor, unrelated tumor	MRI (Gd-DTPA), metastatic evaluation, surgical opinion	Glucocorticoids, radiation if radiosensitive tumor or active systemic disease found	Glucocorticoids as needed
Multiple masses	Metastases	None	Glucocorticoids, radiation	Glucocorticoids as needed, radiation, chemotherapy as indicated
NO KNOWN SYSTEMIC CANCER: BRAIN				
Normal	No disease	Repeat MRI (Gd-DTPA) in 8–12 weeks if symptoms persist	——	——
Solitary mass	Neoplastic disease, primary or secondary tumor, benign or malignant tumor	Metastatic evaluation, surgical opinion, MRI (Gd-DTPA)	Glucocorticoids, biopsy, radiation	Glucocorticoids as needed
Multiple masses	Neoplastic disease, primary or secondary tumor	Metastatic evaluation	Glucocorticoids and radiation if systemic tumor identified. Glucocorticoids, biopsy, and radiation if no systemic tumor is found	See text
KNOWN SYSTEMIC CANCER: SPINAL CORD				
Normal	Nonneoplastic disease Carcinomatous meningitis Paraneoplastic	CSF analysis CSF cytology CT/myelogram	See text	See text
Abnormal	Metastases vs. tumor vs. nonneoplastic	CSF cytology, CT/myelogram, metastatic evaluation, surgical opinion	Glucocorticoids, chemotherapy (meningeal disease), Radiation	See text
NO KNOWN SYSTEMIC CANCER: SPINAL CORD				
Normal	No disease	Further evaluation in 8–12 weeks if symptoms persist (EMG)	See text	——
Abnormal	Metastases vs. primary tumor vs. nonneoplastic	Metastatic evaluation, CSF analysis and cytology, angiography, CT/myelogram, MRI (Gd-DTPA)	See text	——

tions of protein. The interpretation of MRI abnormalities can be very vexing, however. Many patients harbor unexplained white matter abnormalities ("unidentified bright objects," of UBOs) in close proximity to the ventricular system. Extensive areas of T2 signal abnormality on MRI are not clearly correlated with the extent of tumor on CT nor with the histologic tumor margin. These areas reflect cerebral edema, infarction, tumor necrosis, and the effects of prior irradiation and surgery.

Paramagnetic contrast with intravenous gadolinium diethylenetri-amine pentaacetic acid (gadolinium DTPA) produces contrast changes in MRI similar to those observed following the use of organic iodides in CT. The combination of paramagnetic agents and higher energy MRI units provides better separation of tumor from nontumor tissue and better resolution of the spinal cord, nerve roots, and brachial plexus. Contrast MRI provides definition of an altered blood-brain barrier. It is useful for targeting stereotactic surgical procedures, delineating the extent of the tumor mass, and measuring tumor volume for longitudinal assessment of the response to therapy. Reconstruction in the coronal and sagittal planes allows detection of masses larger than 5 mm. Contrast-enhanced tumor margins are defined to within 1 cm of the tumor's histologic border. Echoplanar MRI (fast MRI) provides assessment of blood volume within tumors (see Chap. 365). Gadolinium DTPA administration occasionally produces hypotension and nausea or emesis. The agent is cleared through the kidneys and must be used with caution in hepatic failure because of altered iron metabolism. Because red cell morphology may be altered, gadolinium DTPA should be used with caution in hemolytic anemia.

CT SCAN   The virtues of CT remain those of speed, cost, and the delineation of bony density. Contrast-enhanced CT imaging delineates intracranial masses as small as 0.5 cm in diameter. Certain tumors whose density exceeds that of normal brain parenchyma, including meningioma, melanoma, and primary lymphoma, and tumors with spontaneous hemorrhage can be visualized without contrast enhancement. CT scanning may be better than MRI for definition of calcium-containing meningiomas, oligodendrogliomas and pineal region tumors. Tumors commonly appear as homogeneous or ring-enhancing masses surrounded by variable amounts of edema.

Initial unenhanced CT or MRI studies may show no abnormality

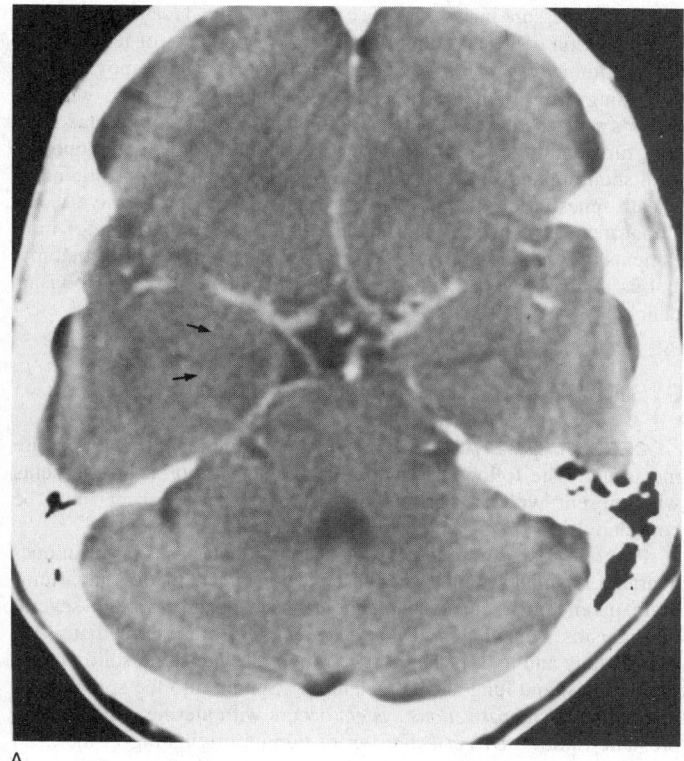

A

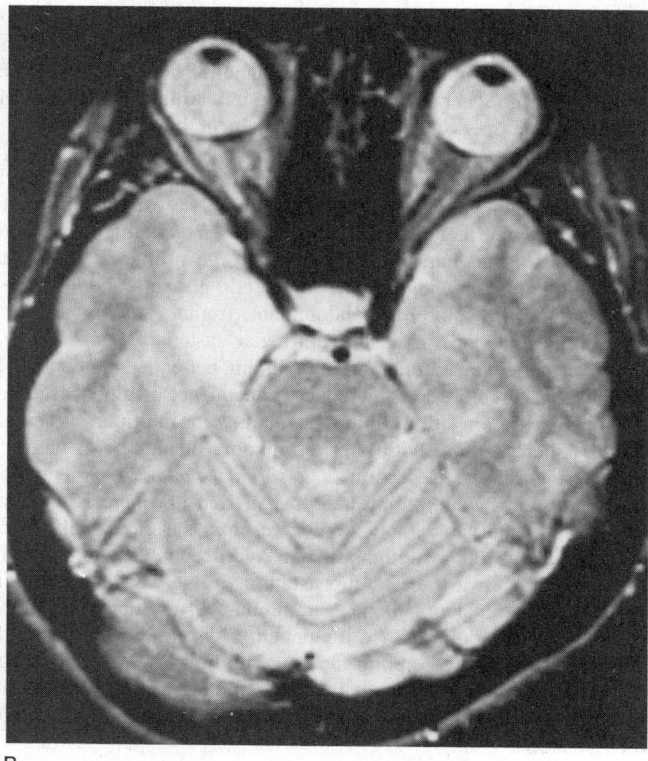

B

FIGURE 369-1   CT and MRI scans in a 57-year-old woman with a long history of temporal lobe epilepsy. *A*. Contrast-enhanced CT scan showed decreased absorption in the medial left temporal lobe (arrows) with no sign of contrast enhancement. Lesion was present on a CT scan taken 5 years earlier. *B*. Recent T2-weighted image shows a hyperintense circumscribed mass in the same lobe. Biopsy revealed a low-grade astrocytoma.

in meningeal carcinomatosis, small metastases, primary brain lymphoma, or some glial tumors that emerge in the setting of chronic seizure activity. Repeat CT scanning, using single or double doses of contrast, or enhanced MRI, 4 to 5 weeks later, usually provides tumor detection. Enhanced MRI should be performed if the initial CT scan is negative or uncertain and a CNS cancer is suspected. The clinician should be wary of attributing all CT or MRI scan masses to tumor, as ringlike abnormalities may occur in abscesses, in recent cerebral infarction, in the plaques of multiple sclerosis, as a consequence of encephalitis, and in certain vascular malformations with or without hemorrhage. Asymptomatic meningioma and aneurysm are sometimes detected incidentally during evaluation for brain tumors.

Before MRI, brainstem, cerebellar, and spinal cord masses could be further defined by a combination of CT and subarachnoid administration of water-soluble contrast agents. MRI has largely supplanted this procedure except for the preoperative delineation of intradural lesions of the spinal cord.

ANGIOGRAPHY   Transfemoral arteriography provides selective visualization of internal carotid and vertebral arteries and their branches. Vessels of malignant tumors are characterized by an angiographic "blush" with enlarged early draining veins, features not seen in association with an intracerebral hemorrhage, infarction, or abscess. The identification on MRI of "flow-voids" has diminished the requirement for arteriograms. Preoperative neurosurgical planning is often aided by knowledge of the vascular anatomy or by embolization of excessively vascularized tumors such as meningioma (see Chap. 365).

MANAGEMENT OF INTRACRANIAL TUMORS   Surgery: biopsy and resection   Surgical exploration allows tumor identification in patients with either solitary or multiple intracranial masses. Surgical exploration may be necessary to obtain a diagnosis in patients with

FIGURE 369-2   Meningioma. Gadolinium-enhanced T1 magnetic resonance scan reveals a homogeneous mass attached to the midline falx and superior sagittal sinus. A magnetic resonance angiogram (not shown) revealed patency of the sinus circulation.

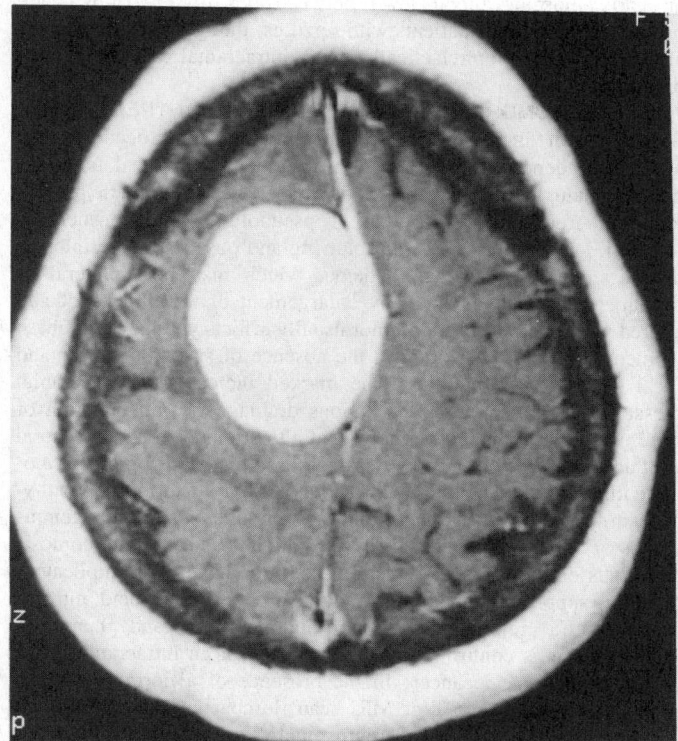

multiple CT masses in whom a thorough systemic evaluation, including hemogram, liver function studies, carcinoembryonic antigen, chest x-ray, sputum cytology, radionuclide bone and liver scans, and perhaps intravenous pyelography is unrewarding. Of patients with multiple CNS metastatic lesions, 20 percent have no evidence of systemic cancer.

Tumor biopsy is performed through an open craniotomy or with MRI or CT-guided stereotaxic techniques. The establishment of a diagnosis is important to determine prognosis and treatment. *Resection* is undertaken and may be curative for some primary tumors such as meningioma, ependymoma, oligodendroglioma, and low-grade astrocytoma (see below) in nondominant, frontal, anterior temporal, or occipital locations or in the ventricular system. *Partial resection* improves patient symptoms, often including better seizure control; by diminishing cerebral edema, it reduces dependence on glucocorticoids. Although resection offers little to patients with multiple intracranial lesions, such as those with brain lymphoma, it may be of value for solitary metastases. Resection of a *solitary tumor* in patients with known systemic cancer may be considered if (1) there is a greater than 2-year interval without known residual systemic malignancy, (2) relief of specific symptoms such as hydrocephalus is required, (3) the tumor is known to be radioresistant as in the case of melanoma, sarcoma, and renal or colonic carcinomas, (4) symptomatic tumor recurs after radiation, and (5) the patient's systemic disease is under good control and the cerebral tumor is the limiting factor in quality of survival. For selected patients, this approach offers survival free of neurologic disease of more than 1 year and is superior to radiation therapy alone.

Acute treatment of intracranial tumors Clinical evidence of acute or subacute deterioration, such as stupor, focal neurologic signs, or evidence of transtentorial herniation, requires aggressive management. Treatment is directed to reducing cerebral edema, lowering intracranial pressure, and reducing the risk of seizures. Treatment with daily doses of dexamethasone 30 to 60 mg or methylprednisolone 120 to 200 mg in four to six divided doses reduces cerebral edema and associated surgical morbidity. Glucocorticoids may not control symptoms caused by obstruction of the ventricular system, and emergency ventricular drainage may be required. Anticonvulsant medications, such as phenytoin (to achieve an early morning blood level between 15 to 20 μg/dL) or carbamazepine (to achieve an early morning blood level between 9.5 to 11 μg/dL), are usually prescribed for patients with seizures, though many physicians administer them prophylactically when intracranial tumor has been diagnosed.

PSEUDOTUMOR—BENIGN INTRACRANIAL HYPERTENSION
Symptoms of increased intracranial pressure may occur in the absence of demonstrable parenchymal or leptomeningeal tumor or hydrocephalus. However, little distinguishes the symptomatic presentation of true tumor from that of pseudotumor, which includes headache, neck stiffness, visual blurring and obscurations, diplopia, nausea, and vomiting. Papilledema, which may be unilateral or asymmetric, is accompanied by enlargement of the blind spot and altered visual acuity. Pseudotumor usually afflicts young, often obese women; it occurs most often in the absence of systemic cancer and focal neurologic difficulties. The marked increases in intracranial pressure may reflect impaired venous drainage within the brain or skull or may accompany the hormonal alterations of pregnancy, oral contraceptive use, or obesity. Less-common predisposing endocrinologic illnesses include both hypo- and hyperthyroidism, hypoparathyroidism, adrenal insufficiency, and both endogenous and exogenous excess of adrenocorticoids. Rare associations occur with sarcoidosis and lupus erythematosus. A variety of drugs have been implicated, including supplemental vitamin A, tetracycline, nalidixic acid, nitrofurantoin, sulfa preparations, lithium, indomethacin, and phenytoin. The diagnosis is confirmed by the exclusion of an intracranial mass lesion or meningeal cancer. In the presence of a normal or small ventricular system on CT or MRI scan, lumbar puncture carries no risk for brain herniation. Cerebrospinal fluid is invariably under

increased pressure but is otherwise unremarkable. Treatment is aimed at prevention of visual deficits and lasting symptoms of reducing the CSF volume by repetitive lumbar punctures. The removal of an offending drug or metabolic cause will reverse symptoms within 1 week's time. Patients refractory to this may benefit from acetazolamide, furosemide, or short-term glucocorticoid therapy. Lumboperitoneal shunting and surgical subtemporal decompression or optic nerve sheath fenestration are reserved for patients with progressive visual impairment who have failed medical therapy. The outlook for most patients is excellent—fully 80 percent respond to conservative therapy, but as many as 10 percent experience permanent or recurrent visual deficits.

SYSTEMIC CANCER AND THE CNS

CEREBRAL METASTASES The most common CNS tumors are metastatic. The following section discusses the approach to patients who present with a CNS tumor where systemic cancer must be considered.

Pathogenesis and pathology Cerebral metastases occur in one-quarter of patients with systemic cancer. Spread to the calvarium, brain parenchyma, and subarachnoid space occurs through several mechanisms. *Hematogenous tumor embolism* from intermediate sites such as lung and liver is the most common mechanism in solid tumors of the breast and lung and in melanoma. Spread into the spinal canal via the *perivertebral venous system* occurs with uterine, colonic, and prostatic tumors. *Direct extension* of tumors originating in the head and neck may occur through the base of the skull. *Paraspinal direct* infiltration may occur with lymphoma and with prostate and breast carcinomas. *Tumor passage from the eye* or through the choroid plexus to the brain and subarachnoid space occurs in lymphoma and leukemia.

Clinical manifestations Sixty percent of cerebral metastases occur in the setting of diagnosed systemic cancer. Cancers of lung in men and of breast in women account for the largest percentage, although melanoma is the tumor with highest likelihood of spread to the CNS. Of patients with a cerebral metastasis (most often arising in the lung) 20 percent develop neurologic symptoms before discovery of the primary malignancy. At some point after diagnosis of systemic cancer, 25 percent of patients with lung carcinoma, 6 to 20 percent of patients with breast carcinoma, and about 50 percent of those with melanoma (when this last tumor has already metastasized to a site outside the CNS) develop tumors in brain or spinal cord. Patients with recurrent sarcoma or ovarian or colorectal cancer who survive beyond 3 years after the original diagnosis face a heightened risk of neurologic involvement. These tumors rarely accounted for cerebral metastases in the past. In the majority of patients, cerebral metastases occur with systemic relapse (Table 369-3). An exception occurs in patients with lung cancer, where the CNS is frequently either the initial site of presentation or of first demonstrated recurrence in otherwise apparently well-controlled disease. As systemic treatment continues to improve survival, the incidence of CNS involvement can be expected to rise for virtually all tumors.

Diagnosis of cerebral metastases More often than is the case with primary brain tumors, those of metastatic origin occur in a setting of seizure activity, increasingly severe head pain, and motor weakness. These difficulties often evolve in days to weeks. MRI or contrast-enhanced CT scan is the procedure of choice for evaluating patients with known systemic cancer and new neurologic symptoms (Table 369-2). Tumors appear with equal frequency as multiple ring-shaped lesions or solitary masses. Three categories of patients without neurologic symptoms or signs are initially evaluated by MRI or CT. First, patients with lung carcinoma for whom attempted cure with pulmonary lobectomy is planned should have a scan preoperatively, since 5 percent of such patients will have clinically unsuspected cerebral metastases. Second, prophylactic brain radiation for small cell carcinoma of the lung should be preceded by a scan. Third,

TABLE 369-3 Interval between diagnosis of cancer and occurrence of brain metastases

| Tumor | Patients with brain metastases, percent | | | Interval from diagnosis of primary tumor to diagnosis of brain metastasis, percent |
	At diagnosis of primary	Sometime during course of tumor growth	At autopsy	
Lung tumor	10–15	20–30	15–30	90 after 3 months
Breast tumor	1	6–20	15–30	90 after 1 year
Melanoma	6	50	40–80	80 after 1 year
Renal tumor	4	11–13	8–20	90 after 1 year
Colorectal tumor	1	—	1	75 after 2 years
Sarcoma	1	36	—	90 after 1 year

SOURCE: L Weiss et al, *Brain Metastases*, Boston, Hall, 1980; M Deutsch et al, Cancer 34:1607, 1974.

patients with widely disseminated cancer due to breast or testicular tumors, sarcoma, or melanoma who are about to receive systemic chemotherapy often with bone marrow transplantation or as part of experimental treatment should have a scan to stage the disease.

Ten percent of patients with cancer develop neurologic difficulties in the absence of an intracranial mass on CT scan. Most of these will be found to have an abnormality on MRI scan. Focal motor or cranial nerve symptoms, headache, or impaired intellectual performance may reflect cerebrovascular lesions known to be associated with systemic cancer, unwitnessed seizures, meningeal carcinomatosis, paraneoplastic syndromes, or complications of tumor therapy.

Patients with systemic neoplasms can develop several types of cerebrovascular disease. Multiple cerebral infarctions are the most frequent in patients with solid tumors. Patients with lymphoma or leukemia may develop diffuse encephalopathic difficulties from infarcts due to disseminated intravascular coagulation; or may develop focal findings from emboli of nonbacterial thrombotic endocarditis, hemorrhage in the setting of clotting abnormalities, or thrombocytopenia. If the cause is unknown, laboratory studies should be done to exclude a circulating anticoagulant.

Focal deficits in patients with negative MRI or CT scans may result from seizures due to undetectable metastatic disease or may be manifestations of meningeal carcinomatosis or paraneoplastic syndromes (see Chap. 328). Gadolinium-enhanced MRI or repeat CT scan in 4 to 6 weeks often discloses the tumor if present. A lumbar puncture with cytologic examination is mandatory in such patients both to exclude infection and to search for leptomeningeal tumor (see below). CSF pleocytosis with mild elevation of protein may be found with paraneoplastic disorders.

Treatment The common assumption that brain metastases represent a uniform disease has proven invalid. Therapeutic decisions must be based on the type, extent, and radiosensitivity of the primary tumor, the morbidity produced, and the number and location of metastases.

Patients with solitary lesions and little or no active systemic disease should be considered for surgical resection or stereotactic radiosurgical therapy, whereas for those with advanced, widespread systemic cancer, comfort is the prime consideration. Glucocorticoids may be used in such patients to maximize neurologic function and to reduce headache (see "Acute Treatment of Intracranial Tumors").

RADIATION THERAPY After acute symptoms are treated, most patients with multiple cerebral metastases or unresectable solitary lesions receive radiation therapy. Patients with small (<3 cm) metastases are increasingly provided focused *stereotactic radiosurgery* using linear accelerators, "gamma knife," or cyclotron sources. Eighty percent of lesions so treated are rendered necrotic but still appear as enhanced abnormalities on contrast scans. For multiple or larger metastases a common approach is palliative whole-brain radiation totaling about 30 Gy (3000 rad) given in 10 to 15 equal fractions. Three-quarters of patients improve clinically and by CT; over one-half are able to discontinue their glucocorticoid medication for a time. However, only 30 percent of patients who complete radiation therapy survive 6 months and fewer than 20 percent are alive at 1 year. Two-thirds of the latter patients die from recurrent

systemic tumor and not from cerebral disease. Treatment is less effective in the elderly, in those with advanced systemic cancer, and in patients with radiation-resistant tumors such as melanoma and gastrointestinal and lung tumors. Reinstitution of glucocorticoids may be useful when progressive neurologic deterioration recurs.

CHEMOTHERAPY Systemic (intravenous or intraarterial) chemotherapy has been used with some success to treat cerebral metastases of lung (small cell), breast, and testicular origin. Anecdotal reports of brain metastases of breast origin responding to tamoxifen or other systemic chemotherapy have appeared.

LEPTOMENINGEAL METASTASES Pathogenesis and pathology Eight percent of patients with cancer develop diffuse infiltration of the meninges. The cranial and spinal nerve roots are usually affected. Tumors that commonly invade the meninges include non-Hodgkin's lymphoma, leukemia, melanoma, and adenocarcinoma of breast, lung, or gastrointestinal origin.

Clinical manifestations The common symptoms are headache, alteration in mentation, cranial nerve abnormalities, and lumbosacral radiculopathies. Patients may also present with seizures. The MRI or CT scan usually is normal, but may reveal enlarged ventricles. With contrast injections, scans may reveal diffuse enhancement of the meninges over the cerebral hemispheres and at the base of the brain.

A lumbar puncture is required for diagnosis. Three-quarters of patients show a modest CSF mononuclear pleocytosis of 5 to 100 cells. Elevation of protein and lowered glucose content may occur, but demonstration of malignant cells is required to confirm the diagnosis. Repeat lumbar or cervical subarachnoid punctures may be necessary to obtain positive cytology. In the past, myelography was often done in such patients because of back pain and radicular symptoms; it often disclosed multiple small nodules on the nerve roots. MRI studies using surface coils provide equal sensitivity providing that arachnoiditis is not present. Larger lesions can be detected and treated with radiation.

Treatment Treatment of meningeal carcinomatosis usually requires a combination of cranial radiation and intrathecal administration of chemotherapeutic agents. Chemotherapy is given either into the lumbar subarachnoid space or (more effectively) into a reservoir connected to the lateral ventricle. Agents commonly used include methotrexate, triethylenethiophosphoramide (thio-TEPA), cytosine arabinoside, and methylprednisolone either alone or in combination.

About one-half of patients with breast carcinoma respond initially to these treatments, but the median survival is only 7 months. The prognosis is particularly grave for meningeal carcinomatosis of melanoma or lung tumor origin; few responses are seen. A much better prognosis is expected in patients with lymphoma or leukemia with control for 2 or more years being common. Treatment failures reflect tumor drug resistance, poor circulation of drug within the subarachnoid space, and complications arising from chemotherapy and radiation.

TOXIC EFFECTS OF CANCER TREATMENT Chemotherapy Chronic glucocorticoid therapy may induce insulin-dependent diabetes mellitus, myopathy, and aseptic necrosis of the hip and may predispose to thrombophlebitis. In the early stages, the muscle changes reverse with steroid taper and intensive physical therapy. Administration of anticonvulsants is associated with cutaneous allergies. Anticonvulsant doses may need to be adjusted in patients receiving glucocorticoids. Allergy to an anticonvulsant may be masked while the patient receives glucocorticoids and revealed later when the steroid medication is tapered. Confusion and altered mentation may accompany glucocorticoid, L-asparaginase, nitrosourea, and methotrexate treatment. Ataxic syndromes may follow the use of 5-fluorouracil and cytosine arabinoside. Neuropathies of the cranial nerves may occur after nitrosourea and cisplatin administration. Vinca alkaloids may produce cranial and peripheral neuropathies.

Radiation therapy Radiation therapy may cause toxic effects on the CNS. Acute changes include lethargy, loss of appetite, alterations in mental status, or exacerbation of previous symptoms and signs. These develop within 1 to 2 weeks of its initiation. These effects are usually attributable to worsening cerebral edema and are best treated with increased doses of glucocorticoids. Subacute changes that develop between 3 and 18 months after treatment are ascribed to radiation-induced demyelination and are unresponsive to glucocorticoids. Reappearance of previous neurologic impairment and the appearance of a mass which is indistinguishable from recurrent tumor on MRI or CT scan may occur. These areas of radiation necrosis may be visualized by hypometabolism following the injection of positron-emitting ^{18}F-deoxyglucose (PET scan). Patients who have received spinal radiation may develop Lhermitte's phenomenon with tingling in the back and legs following flexion of the neck.

Between 18 and 60 months after radiation, still other less reversible changes occur. These include retarded growth rate and impaired intellectual development in children who have received more than 30 Gy (3000 rad) of whole-brain radiation. At doses above 50 Gy (5000 rad), adults may exhibit cortical atrophy, communicating hydrocephalus, and hypothalamic dysfunction with elevated prolactin levels and amenorrhea or impotence. Dementia resulting from these changes is irreversible and in the case of hydrocephalus is usually unimproved by ventricular shunting.

The peripheral nervous system also can be affected by radiation therapy. Localized dysfunction of the brachial or lumbosacral plexus may follow radiation in excess of 40 Gy (4000 rad), usually appearing more than 1 year after treatment (see Chap. 383). Unlike peripheral nerve problems due to tumor invasion, radiation plexopathy is commonly painless. Additional tests, including CT scan, may be necessary to distinguish tumor invasion from radiation toxicity. Glucocorticoids may afford some benefit.

PRIMARY BRAIN TUMORS

In the following section, the most common primary brain tumors in adults are discussed by histologic type. Other tumors which occur in characteristic locations and whose presenting symptoms therefore reflect site rather than specific histology are then discussed by location. These include tumors located in the diencephalon-third ventricle, the posterior fossa, and the skull base.

MALIGNANT ASTROCYTOMA (GLIOBLASTOMA) Definition Malignant astrocytoma or glioblastoma (also known as malignant glioma or grade 3 or 4 astrocytoma) and the less malignant anaplastic astrocytoma account for about one-quarter of the 5000 intracranial gliomas diagnosed yearly in the United States; 75 percent of gliomas in adults are of this category. Because of its profound and uniform morbidity, it contributes more to the cost of cancer on a per capita basis than does any other tumor. The patient, commonly stricken in the fifth decade of life, enters a cycle of repetitive hospitalizations and operations while experiencing the progressive complications associated with relatively ineffective treatments of radiation and chemotherapy.

Pathogenesis and pathology Epidemiology studies offer few clues to the etiology of malignant astrocytoma. Some tumors arise in patients with long-standing seizure disorders or personality disorders resulting from temporal lobe dysfunction and in scars incurred from head trauma, suggesting that in certain instances the malignant cells emerge from a more benign glial proliferation. There are rare instances of malignant tumors occurring in families, suggesting a genetic propensity. At least four human oncogenes (*sis*, *myc*, *src*, n-*myc*) have been identified in cell lines derived from primary brain tumors, and there is overexpression for the receptors of both platelet-derived (PDGF) and epidermal (EGF) growth factors. Small clusters of tumors have appeared in certain occupational settings, notably in the petroleum processing industry. The tumor has an appearance similar to that produced by a variety of viral agents inoculated into animals. On gross examination, the surrounding normal brain is distorted and infiltrated by yellow tumor tissue containing areas of necrosis, cysts, and hemorrhage. Microscopic examination reveals a highly cellular composite of heterogeneous glial cells with elongated or rounded astrocytes whose processes stain for glial fibrillary acidic protein. Giant cells may be seen along with mitotic figures and the proliferation of small capillaries.

Clinical manifestations Patients commonly present with a subacute progresssive neurologic deficit exhibiting either focal signs or personality changes. Prior mental changes or seizures may antedate tumor diagnosis by months to years. Clinical symptoms may occur abruptly with seizures or with sudden deficits secondary to tumor hemorrhage. CT or MRI reveals a heterogeneous pattern of tumor enhancement interspersed with hypodense foci presumably corresponding to tumor necrosis and edema. Multiple tumors can occur but are uncommon. MRI scans often define more extensive tumor involvement than is indicated on the CT scan.

Malignant astrocytoma can arise in the brainstem, cerebellum, or spinal cord in addition to the more common locations within the white matter of the cerebral hemispheres. The prognosis for any site, unfortunately, has not changed greatly in the last 20 years. Following treatment, less than 6 months of useful function can be expected for most patients before progression of symptoms signals recurrent tumor. Death results in 80 percent of patients from tumor recurrence within 6 to 12 months. Progressive neurologic deterioration is followed by stupor and coma. In patients who survive over 1 year, often young adults, CNS dissemination can occur to the meninges or the ventricular ependyma. Metastasis outside the CNS is extremely rare.

Treatment Confirmation of histology by biopsy should be performed in most patients; debulking of tumor is recommended if the tumor is located in an area that permits an extensive operation. Large tumor resections are more likely than biopsies to disclose small glioblastoma tumor foci within anaplastic astrocytoma.

Therapeutic modalities are not highly effective. The average life expectancy of 17 weeks for untreated patients is improved by postoperative external beam radiation alone to 47 weeks and by radiation combined with chemotherapy to 62 weeks. A subgroup of young patients under age 50 obtains significant improvement in quality and duration of life. Such patients have a 20 percent 2-year survival after cranial radiation of 55 to 60 Gy (5500 to 6000 rad) combined with adjunctive chemotherapy with the nitrosoureas carmustine (BCNU) or lomustine (CCNU).

Efforts to improve prognosis for this malignancy include trials of implanted radiation sources of isotopic iodine (^{125}I brachytherapy) and twice daily (hyperfraction) radiation. Current chemotherapeutic trials are often based on the localized nature of the tumor and of its recurrence. No superiority over intravenous BCNU has been seen as a result of experimental approaches including the modification of the blood-brain barrier, the administration of oxygen carriers, or the local or arterial instillation of chemotherapeutic agents.

ASTROCYTOMA Definition Low-grade astrocytomas occur throughout the brain and spinal cord. The subcortical white matter is the most common site in adults. In children and young adults astrocytomas arise in the optic nerves, cerebellum (cystic, juvenile, pilocytic astrocytoma), and brainstem (pontine glioma). These tumors are also associated with neurofibromatosis (type II) and tuberous sclerosis and are found in 20 percent of patients undergoing temporal lobectomy for control of chronic seizure disorders.

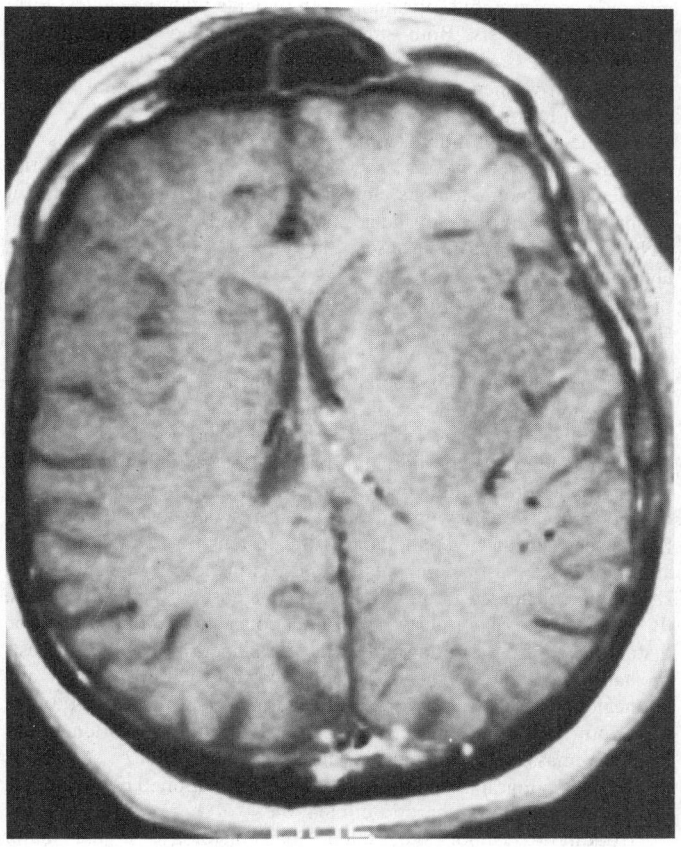

A

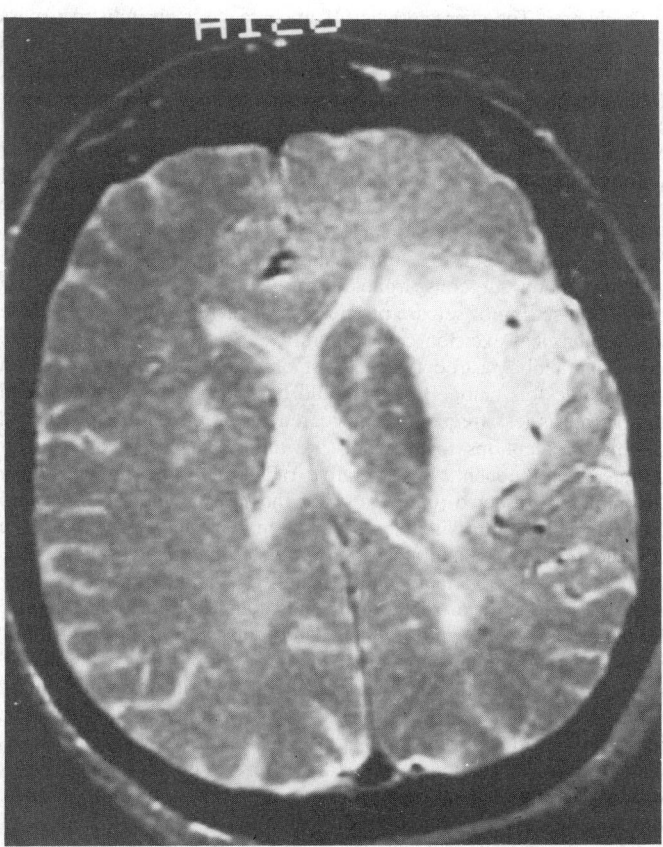

B

FIGURE 369-3   *A*. Gadolinium-DTPA-enhanced T1-weighted axial image demonstrating a decreased signal in the right temporoparietal region with no evidence of contrast enhancement. Mild effacement of the body of the left lateral ventricle without midline shift is present. Biopsy showed low-grade glioma. *B*. T2-weighted axial MRI of same tumor showed area of hyperintense signal corresponding to low signal area seen on T1 study.

Pathogenesis and pathology   The tumors are avascular without necrosis and contain homogeneous populations of well-differentiated astrocytes. Progress to malignancy is associated with the appearance of mitotic figures and necrotic zones. The astrocytomas are divided into those with good prognosis (80 percent survivorship at 5 years) (cystic cerebellar, "juvenile" pilocytic, giant cell subependymoma) and those with likely recurrence after surgery (infiltrating, gemisto-cytic, and anaplastic).

Clinical manifestations   The tumors evolve slowly over several years, producing symptoms by displacement of normal brain or by invasion of white matter tracts. Optic nerve gliomas cause progressive, monocular or bitemporal visual field defects leading eventually to blindness and sometimes proptosis. Hypothalamic compression may cause endocrine dysfunction. Hydrocephalus is rare. In the brainstem, such tumors typically involve several cranial nerves (often the abducens, facial, and trigeminal) and later impinge on corticospinal fibers and medial lemniscal and spinothalamic tracts. These symptoms must be distinguished from those caused by multiple sclerosis, arteriovenous malformations, cysts of cysticercosis and echinococcal origin, and extramedullary tumors such as schwannomas or meningiomas. Cerebellar astrocytomas cause progressive incoordination and gait ataxia combined with abnormalities of eye movements. In supratentorial locations, these tumors may produce seizures before any focal abnormality appears on clinical examination. In *gliomatosis cerebri*, slow infiltration of white matter occurs with atypical individual astrocytes without evidence of localized tumor.

Early use of MRI may allow for earlier diagnosis and intervention (see Figs. 369-1, 369-3, 369-4). MRI often demonstrates white matter abnormalities in patients with normal CT scans and is the preferred procedure for early diagnosis and follow-up. A stable clinical course is common with astrocytoma and repeat radiologic studies may show

FIGURE 369-4   Brainstem glioma in a 9-year-old boy. The medulla and cervical spinal cord are twice as wide as normal. Focal areas of cystic degeneration are seen as hypodense T1 signals. Biopsy revealed an astrocytoma.

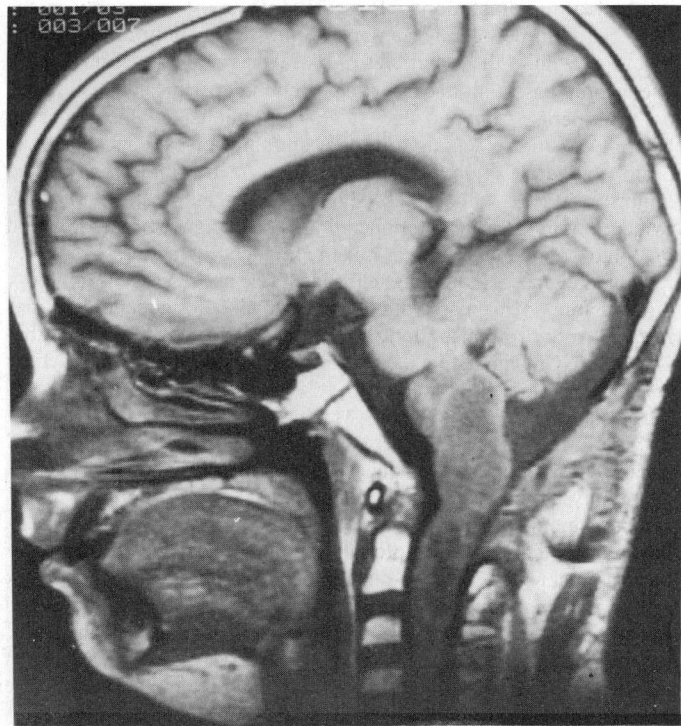

little change. The characteristic CT appearance is an indistinct mass that is hypodense with respect to surrounding brain and exhibits little or no contrast enhancement, calcification, or evidence of edema. Malignant degeneration of astrocytomas is heralded by rapid progression of symptoms and signs, evidence of expanded size or altered MRI T2 or CT signal, or the presence of new enhancement on MRI with gadolinium DTPA or CT with iodine contrast. Echoplanar MRI reveals areas of increased "blood flow" in malignant zones while PET studies identify foci of increased glucose uptake.

Treatment As astrocytomas may contain areas of aggressive gliomas, many surgeons argue for early biopsy. This is especially true in the setting of seizure progression or increase in the size of the lesion. Surgical excision can be curative for some cerebellar, optic nerve, and lobar astrocytomas. Cyst drainage and partial resection are feasible for many. Biopsy should be obtained for supratentorial tumors but is less frequently considered for brainstem or spinal cord gliomas. Exceptions to the latter are tumors that have a cystic or extraaxial component. Postoperative radiation is recommended for incompletely resected tumors and for those involving the brainstem (for which multiple daily doses are often provided). Its role in the treatment of excised supratentorial tumors is less clear. The possible benefits of radiation therapy are weighed against the known long natural course of the astrocytoma and the complications of irradiation. Radiation is recommended when symptoms and signs progress or areas of enhancement or enlargement on CT or MRI are observed. Radiation may be safely delayed for several years in apparently totally resected tumors because of the accuracy of MRI and CT scans. The judicious use of glucocorticoids during radiation or when symptoms recur improves function. The median life expectancy is 67 months for supratentorial tumors and 89 months for cerebellar tumors. Average survivals of 15 months after radiation are reported for patients with brainstem tumors. However, the 5-year survival is only 30 percent. Chemotherapy, currently under investigation for brainstem tumors, may offer some improvement in survival.

OLIGODENDROGLIOMA   Definition This tumor may develop in isolation or may be mixed with other glial cells. An uncommon tumor, it represents less then 10 percent of all gliomas.

Pathology Microscopic examination discloses rounded cells containing darkly staining nuclei with poorly staining cytoplasm, the "fried egg" appearance. The tumor is prone to spontaneous hemorrhage. Both "benign" and "malignant" forms are seen.

Clinical manifestations Presentation is most commonly in the third or fourth decade and tumors are most frequently in the frontal lobes or within the ventricles. CT reveals a well-defined, low-attenuation mass with fine speckled calcium deposits and small cysts.

Treatment Although the oligodendroglioma is histologically benign, resection is curative in only one-third of patients. Formerly postoperative radiation was recommended for incompletely resected tumors or those with mixed glial or malignant features or with evidence of progression after operation. The malignant transformation of "pure" oligodendroglial or mixed oligodendroglial tumors is more readily diagnosed if contrast-enhanced CT or MRI is used. Fully three-quarters of patients with "pure" or mixed oligodendrogliomas respond to the administration of chemotherapy with PCV (procarbazine, CCNU, vincristine) prior to irradiation. This approach is currently the subject of study.

MENINGIOMA   Definition Meningiomas account for 20 percent of brain tumors. They can arise in either the cranium or the spinal canal. They occur more frequently at all sites in women. They are commonly found as asymptomatic tumors at postmortem. When symptomatic they usually present in the fifth or sixth decades.

Pathogenesis and pathology Meningiomas arise from cells of the pia-arachnoid. Common sites include the midline along the falx cerebri and the lateral cerebral convexity, the olfactory groove and along the sphenoid ridge, the tuberculum sellae, foramen magnum, and tentorium of the cerebellum. They also arise on occasion within the ventricles, where on radiographic examination they are indistinguishable from a papilloma of the choroid plexus. Meningio-

mas may coexist with schwannomas in patients with the central form of neurofibromatosis. Both tumor types are related to the loss of a "tumor suppressor" gene on chromosome 22. They occur more frequently in women with breast cancer; some meningiomas contain estrogen and progesterone receptors.

On the basis of microscopic characteristics, meningiomas are divided into seven categories: syncytial, transitional, fibroblastic, microcystic, psammomatous, angioblastic, and malignant. Malignant tumors display mitoses, invade normal brain, and occasionally develop CNS and extraneural metastases. Angioblastic and malignant forms are prone to recur.

Clinical manifestations The clinical presentation reflects the slow expansion of tumor within the skull and spine, with neurologic deficits evolving over many years. Tumors of the parasellar region produce a combination of second, third, fourth, fifth, and sixth cranial nerve deficits. Cerebellopontine tumors may produce a syndrome similar to that of acoustic schwannomas (see "Tumors of the Posterior Fossa," below). Early hearing loss is not a typical finding in meningioma. Parasagittal and frontal tumors may produce seizures or may be entirely asymptomatic, often growing to enormous size before they are discovered. Parasagittal lesions that attain sufficient size may cause spastic paraparesis and incontinence. Falx meningioma should be considered in the differential diagnosis of gait disorders in the middle-aged and elderly. In all locations, meningiomas must be distinguished from similar-appearing dural metastases from breast, prostate, and lung. CT often discloses calcium within a tumor and delineates the close relation between the mass and the dura, falx, or tentorium, as well as the altered bony calvarium. MRI often shows isodense masses that enhance with gadolinium-DTPA. Magnetic resonance angiography identifies tumor vessels supplied by meningeal vessels of the external carotid circulation.

Treatment Tumor site, rather than histology, is the major determinant of outcome. Intraventricular or parasagittal tumors are usually resectable and recurrence is rare. Those in the olfactory groove, sphenoid ridge, and parasellar locations are more difficult to resect completely and are prone to recur. Tumors of the foramen magnum may be totally removed with microneurosurgical techniques (see "Spinal Tumors," below). Radiation, often using beams of small focus, is advocated for malignant meningiomas and for incompletely excised symptomatic tumors of other histologic subtypes. Chemotherapy is without apparent efficacy; but antiprogestational agents are under evaluation.

PAPILLOMA OF THE CHOROID PLEXUS   Definition Neoplasms derived from choroid plexus epithelium are rare, representing only 0.5 percent of all intracranial tumors.

Pathogenesis and pathology In children most such tumors occur as aggressive tumors in the lateral ventricles, whereas in adults the fourth ventricle is the most common site. The histologic structure resembles normal choroid plexus, with a connective tissue core covered by a single layer of cuboidal epithelium.

Clinical manifestations Very rare examples of malignant transformation have been described. Metastases to the leptomeninges may occur. The tumor may secrete excessive CSF leading to communicating hydrocephalus.

Treatment Surgery is the treatment of choice and is usually highly successful.

LIPOMA Lipoma can develop anywhere within the brain or spinal cord, though the corpus callosum is the most common location. The association of lipomas with partial or complete agenesis of this structure and with other dysplastic or hamartomatous anomalies such as ectopias, colloid cysts, and epidermoids supports the theory that they are the result of disorders of development. Intraspinal lipomas are most common in the thoracic region and are associated with spina bifida in one-third of cases. All lipomas can be easily demonstrated by MRI. The treatment of symptomatic cranial and spinal lipomas is excision.

DERMOID AND EPIDERMOID TUMOR   Definition The distinction between dermoid tumors and epidermoids (true cholesteatomas) is often difficult. Both result from inclusion of ectodermal tissue at the time of closure of the neural groove and soon thereafter.

Pathology and pathogenesis Cholesteatomas are slowly growing tumors that most often afflict young adults, occurring commonly in lateral or midline locations within the skull, i.e., the cerebellopontine angle, the suprasellar region, the fourth ventricle, the pineal region, and over the hemispheres. No clear relationship has been established between cholesteatoma of the cerebellopontine angle and middle ear infection. Dermoid tumors, which are frequently cystic, occur largely in the posterior fossa or in the lumbosacral region. Rarely they are found in suprasellar or pineal regions.

Clinical manifestations Symptoms vary according to the location of these tumors, the general pattern being slow evolution of defects attributable to the specific area with seizures interspersed when the tumor occupies cortical regions. MRI provides excellent delineation.

Treatment Treatment of the cholesteatoma is total surgical removal of the tumor together with its capsule. Dermoid tumors similarly are curable if total surgical excision is possible.

PRIMARY LYMPHOMA OF THE CNS **Definition** Primary lymphomas are now recognized to be relatively common in the CNS. Before 1972, fewer than 25 cases had been identified at the Massachusetts General Hospital over a 50-year period. Since 1980 the tumor has tripled in frequency. Primary lymphoma is distinguished from the more frequent secondary involvement of the meninges that occurs in patients with poorly differentiated non-Hodgkin's lymphomas.

Pathogenesis and pathology The tumor is uncommon in patients without immunologic compromise. It is usually seen in patients with mixed humoral and cellular immune deficits. Three such disorders are recognized: inherited disorders of immunity such as combined immunodeficiency disease, selective IgM deficiency, or selective IgA abnormalities seen with combined immunodeficiency and Wiskott-Aldrich syndrome; AIDS; and therapeutic immunosuppression following organ transplantation or treatment of autoimmune disorders. Epstein-Barr virus (EBV) DNA has been demonstrated within primary lymphoma in 80 percent of immunosuppressed patients, raising the possibility that this agent may play a role in the pathogenesis of this disease.

The tumor may be focal or multicentric in the subcortical white matter, the walls of the ventricles, or the subarachnoid space. Tumor cells are always found in a perivascular distribution. At biopsy, tumor cells are often indistinguishable from normal lymphocytes, leading to an erroneous early diagnosis of "encephalitis" or "nonspecific perivascular inflammation." The B cell populations may be characterized as malignant by the immunohistochemical demonstration of monoclonal immunoglobulin surface proteins. The tumors contain cells defined histologically as immunoblastic or large cell (see Chap. 311). Burkitt-type lymphomas are rarely reported.

Clinical manifestations A history of personality change, focal deficits, or seizures evolving over several weeks in an immunosuppressed patient should raise the suspicion of cerebral lymphoma. Obviously, in these circumstances infection must be excluded. Patients with HIV infection are often treated presumptively for toxoplasmosis and brain lymphoma. In immunosuppressed and nonsuppressed populations, MRI and CT typically reveal multiple periventricular masses which enhance with contrast. T2-weighted MRI abnormalities have disappeared. A characteristic feature, rarely observed with other types of intracranial tumor, is the marked reduction or disappearance of lesions after a few weeks of high-dose glucocorticoid therapy (dexamethasone 5 to 10 mg four times daily). When both symptoms and CT abnormalities resolve after glucocorticoid therapy, remissions lasting several months are common, and steroids can be tapered. Spontaneous remissions without glucocorticoid therapy have been described. The usual clinical course is recurrence after 4 to 6 months, with resistance to steroid administration. Staging of patients should include HIV serologic testing, enhanced MRI or CT, slit lamp eye examination, and immunohistologic examination of CSF cell populations. The tumor may seed the meninges in one-quarter of patients. Systemic lymphoma is found in less than 10 percent of

patients and occurs late in the course of the disease. However, uveitis or vitreitis may occur at the time of presentation or early in the evolution of the disease; when present, it is helpful in the initial diagnosis.

Treatment After biopsy or diagnosis by CSF cytology, the recommended treatment is chemotherapy consisting of high-dose methotrexate and glucocorticoids, alone or in combination with cyclophosphamide, doxorubicin, and vincristine, followed by radiation. Chemotherapy provides therapeutic drug levels in brain parenchyma and most importantly, in the CSF. Partial or complete remission occurs in over three-quarters of patients. When methotrexate is administered prior to radiation, there is a reduced risk of radiation or drug-induced white matter damage. The median survival following chemotherapy and irradiation is in excess of 2 years. Radiation treatment is recommended for immunosuppressed patients with brain lymphoma.

TUMORS OF THE THIRD VENTRICLE AND PINEAL REGION Tumors of the diencephalon often present with a combination of failure of pupillary constriction to light, failure of upward gaze, and neuroendocrine abnormalities. Hydrocephalus due to obstruction to CSF flow at the level of the third ventricle leads to headache. Masses which push down on the diencephalon create the picture of *central herniation:* altered consciousness, Cheyne-Stokes respiration with reserved pupillary reaction. Masses below the diencephalon affect eye movement and pupillary responses. Several categories of tumors occur in close proximity to the diencephalon, hypothalamus, and third ventricle; these are pituitary adenoma, craniopharyngioma, germ-cell neoplasms, pineal tumors, and glial, meningeal, or metastatic tumors.

Uncommon tumors of the pineal region include astrocytomas, glioblastomas, meningiomas, and metastases. Nonneoplastic masses occurring in this region include colloid cysts of the third ventricle (see "Colloid Cysts," below) and parasitic cysts (cysticercosis).

Pituitary adenomas These tumors are described in Chap. 331.

Craniopharyngiomas These tumors arise from remnants of Rathke's pouch, derived from the primitive stomatodeum. They are usually suprasellar in location and cause symptoms by compressing hypothalamus or the optic chiasm (see also Chap. 331). They are easily identified by a "bright" T2 signal on MRI (Fig. 369-5).

Germ-cell tumors DEFINITION Germ-cell tumors, which account for half of all pineal region neoplasms, arise primarily during childhood or early adolescence and include germinoma, teratoma, embryonal carcinoma, endodermal sinus tumor, and choriocarcinoma.

CLINICAL MANIFESTATIONS The most common of these germ-cell tumors is the germinoma. It may occur in the pineal region or at the base of the hypothalamus. It occurs more frequently in males, who present with findings of diabetes insipidus and other neuroendocrine deficiencies, bitemporal visual field defects, paralysis of upward gaze (see Chap. 19), and sometimes hydrocephalus. The typical features of pineal masses occur more commonly with nongerminomatous germ cell tumors. Findings include Parinaud's syndrome—a failure of upward gaze and pupillary dilatation with deficiencies in response to light. Rarely, other signs such as nystagmus retractorius or brainstem signs due to compression may occur. Diagnosis may be assisted by the finding of elevated serum and CSF levels of alpha-fetoprotein (AFP) and of human chorionic gonadotropin (hCG) in germinomas. MRI and CT scans identify tumors of the pineal region *but offer no histologic differentiation.*

TREATMENT Following CT stereotactic biopsy by transcallosal or suboccipital route, radiation is given. Germinomas are radiosensitive; up to 80 percent are cured by doses of cranial radiation sufficient to produce disappearance of the MRI mass while avoiding damage to surrounding hypothalamic tissue. Craniospinal irradiation is provided when the tumor invades the ventricles or subarachnoid space, or is found outside the pineal region. Other histologic subtypes have poorer prognoses and recurrence is common, often with seeding of the cranial nerves and meninges. Recurrences sometimes respond to drug treatment with bleomycin, cisplatin, and vinblastine, which are beneficial in testicular tumors of similar histology.

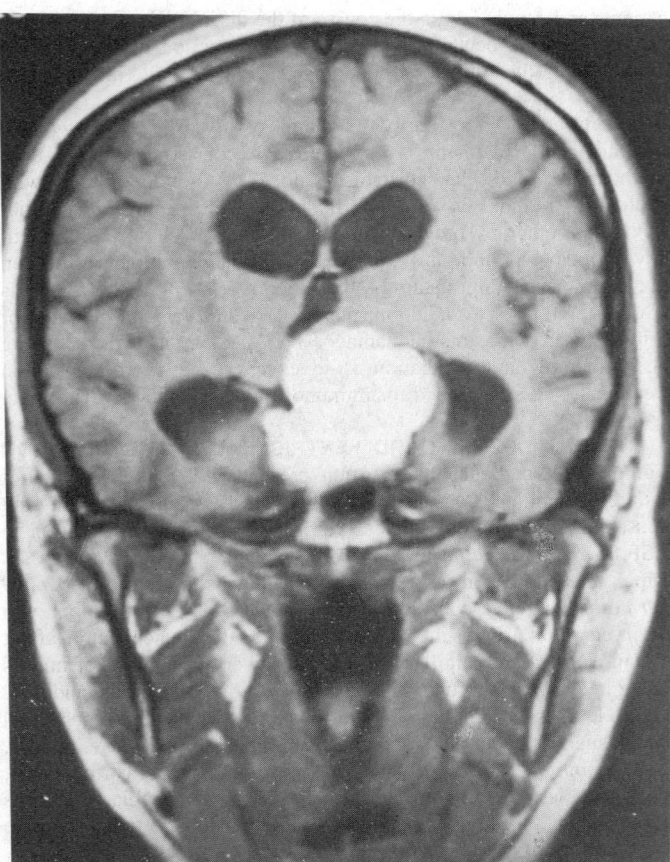

FIGURE 369-5 This 39-year-old woman presented with headaches and gait disturbance (caused by a craniopharyngioma). On a T1-weighted coronal MRI, a large, lobulated hyperdense mass is visualized in the suprasellar cistern compressing the inferior third ventricle. There is enlargement of the frontal and temporal ventricles.

Pineoblastoma and pineocytoma These tumors account for 20 percent of growths in the pineal region.

PATHOGENESIS AND PATHOLOGY Pineoblastoma and pineocytoma arise from pineal organ cells. The pineoblastoma is a primitive malignant tumor of childhood and early adult life and is indistinguishable both in appearance and natural history from primitive neuroectodermal tumors that arise elsewhere in the CNS. The tumor may contain astrocytic or neuronal elements. Recurrence is invariable and dissemination through the ventricular system and subarachnoid space is frequent.

TREATMENT Brain and neuraxis radiation are recommended, and chemotherapy as outlined above for germ cell tumors has been successful in producing remissions in a few patients. Chemotherapy prior to irradiation is reserved for pineoblastoma. The pineocytoma is a more slowly growing tumor which is often well-demarcated and resembles the normal structure of the pineal. Although histologically benign, it tends to recur, probably because of incomplete removal. It is resistant to radiation.

Colloid cysts PATHOGENESIS AND PATHOLOGY Colloid cysts arise within the anterior third ventricle and are considered to develop from the anlage of the paraphysis, a component of the third ventricle, or possibly from the ependyma itself. The cysts are well-encapsulated and consist of a layer of connective tissue covered with columnar ciliated cells. The cyst is filled with glycoproteinaceous material which stains with periodic acid Schiff (PAS).

CLINICAL MANIFESTATIONS Symptoms occur usually in adults and may be dramatic, with episodes of headache, weakness of the limbs, and loss of consciousness. These symptoms are attributed to intermittent acute hydrocephalus due to blockage of the foramen of

Monro by the mobile cyst. Diagnosis follows MRI identification of the cyst and the visualization of either intact or obstructed CSF flow. Treatment is removal of the cyst.

TUMORS OF THE POSTERIOR FOSSA Tumors of the posterior fossa pose special problems in diagnosis and treatment. Rapidly growing tumors hindering CSF flow in the fourth ventricle or aqueduct of Sylvius may cause obstructive hydrocephalus, and even small mass lesions in the posterior fossa may result in vomiting, lethargy, headache, and papilledema. Slowly growing tumors give rise to progressive signs which are recognized by rather specific syndromes. These include progressive unilateral hearing loss, facial weakness, pain or numbness, and a unilateral sixth nerve deficit occurring with tumors in the cerebellopontine angle. (See Chap. 380 for discussion of cranial nerve symptoms and signs.) Gait ataxia and unilateral cerebellar signs occur with hemangioblastoma, medulloblastoma, or cystic astrocytoma of the cerebellum. Progressive diplopia, cranial nerve abnormalities, and crossed corticospinal tract and reflex abnormalities occur in brainstem glioma. Nuchal and occipital pain are common with all tumors of the posterior fossa. Corticospinal signs develop with further tumor enlargement and encroachment on the brainstem. Cerebellar tumors force the cerebellar tonsils into the foramen magnum. This *tonsil herniation* is accompanied by bradycardia, hypertension and respiratory irregularities when medullary compression occurs.

Acoustic schwannoma DEFINITION The acoustic schwannoma (synonymous with acoustic neuroma) is composed of myelin-forming Schwann cells that cover the acoustic nerve fibers. Schwann cells normally replace oligodendroglia as the nerve leaves the brainstem to enter the internal auditory meatus.

PATHOGENESIS AND PATHOLOGY Schwannomas are slow-growing masses that compress rather than invade normal tissue. When bilateral, they represent an inherited form of schwannoma which is diagnostic of "central" neurofibromatosis (NFII). Other CNS tumors associated with neurofibromatosis or von Recklinghausen's disease are schwannomas of spinal and other cranial nerves, intracranial and spinal meningiomas, gliomas, and ependymomas (see Chap. 378).

CLINICAL MANIFESTATIONS AND TREATMENT Early detection of acoustic schwannomas at a time of minimal hearing deficit and minimal facial motor difficulty is essential, as hearing may be spared by microneurosurgical intervention while the tumor is still restricted to the canal. Brainstem auditory evoked responses, CT and MRI studies, especially with contrast injection, have replaced metrizamide cisternography by enhancing the physician's ability to detect these tumors in their early stages. Recurrent masses are increasingly treated with small field radiation approaches (radiosurgery or gamma knife).

Hemangioblastoma DEFINITION The cerebellar hemangioblastoma is an uncommon tumor that may be solitary but is frequently multiple. When the tumors are multiple, they are considered part of von Hippel-Lindau disease. This autosomal dominant disorder, linked to chromosome 3, typically consists of retinal, cerebellar, and spinal hemangioblastomas and visceral lesions, usually renal and/or pancreatic tumors or cysts. Polycythemia may be present.

PATHOGENESIS AND PATHOLOGY Hemangioblastomas are well-circumscribed and often cystic. The tumor may consist solely of a small nodule attached to the wall of a large cyst. The lesion is usually highly vascular and may be mistaken for an arteriovenous malformation. The microscopic appearance is one of numerous capillary vessels separated by sheets of clear cells with an abundance of intracytoplasmic vacuoles. The tumors are probably derived from capillary endothelial cells.

CLINICAL MANIFESTATIONS Dizziness, ataxia of gait or of the limbs, and symptoms of raised intracranial pressure are characteristic features of the cerebellar hemangioblastoma. The tumors may bleed spontaneously, resulting in a paroxysmal onset of headache and neurologic deficit. The MRI may show vascular "flow voids" or ferritin suggesting old hemorrhage in the wall of a cyst.

TREATMENT Craniotomy with opening of the cerebellar cyst and excision of the mural tumor may be curative. Though the tumor is histologically benign, postoperative recurrences and the appearance of less operable spinal lesions worsen the prognosis. Patients with the von Hippel-Lindau syndrome should have periodic ophthalmologic evaluation for the appearance of retinal angiomas and general medical follow-up for early detection of renal tumors.

Ependymoma PATHOGENESIS AND PATHOLOGY These are glial tumors that occur chiefly in childhood and young adulthood, with a typical cranial location in the fourth ventricle. The tumor is composed of uniform ependymal cells surrounding a central lumen. Spinal ependymomas, which are more common, arise within the dura of the lumbar spine and represent more than half of spinal intramedullary gliomas. In this location, the prognosis is excellent. Supratentorial tumors are often more aggressive in rate of growth.

TREATMENT Resection and radiation to the tumor site results in 5-year survival in excess of 80 percent for spinal cord lesions and between 30 and 50 percent for posterior fossa tumors. The role of chemotherapy in the treatment of local recurrences and of seeding within the subarachnoid space is not established.

PRIMITIVE NEUROECTODERMAL TUMORS (PNET) Several histologic varieties of tumor arise from primitive neuroectodermal tumors (PNET) which contain dense aggregates of small cells with a capacity to differentiate into medulloblasts, astrocytes, oligodendrocytes, ependyma, ganglion cells, or skeletal muscle. Some tumors have several cell types, but all PNETs of the posterior fossa share a propensity for local invasion, subarachnoid dissemination, and extraneural metastases. The initial evaluation should include enhanced MRI scan of the brain and lumbosacral nerve roots as well as cytologic evaluation of CSF.

Medulloblastoma DEFINITION The *medulloblastoma* is the most common variety of PNET. It accounts for 25 percent of childhood brain tumors. However, one-fourth of medulloblastomas occur in patients over age 20.

PATHOGENESIS AND PATHOLOGY In children the tumor is usually located in the midline, in the inferior portion of the vermis of the cerebellum. In adults the cerebellar hemisphere is most often the site of occurrence. It is composed of small, densely staining cells which elicit a brisk glial response. Invasion of the meninges, ventricles, and subarachnoid space is common.

CLINICAL MANIFESTATIONS The common presentation is occipital headache, vomiting and truncal ataxia. Hydrocephalus is frequent. With enlargement of the tumor other signs of brainstem compression emerge. As spinal axis dissemination occurs in one-third of patients, initial evaluation should include CSF cytologic examination and either MRI of the cauda equina or myelography.

TREATMENT Resection of the tumor is usually attempted, followed by radiation in doses of 45 to 50 Gy (4500 to 5000 rad) to the posterior fossa, together with 40 Gy (4000 rad) to the whole brain and 35 to 40 Gy (3500 to 4000 rad) to the spinal cord. Chemotherapy prior to irradiation is under investigation for children and those whose tumors invade the ventricle or have disseminated. Drugs have been used with some success in recurrent tumors. Nitrosourea, procarbazine, and vincristine combined with prednisone and intrathecal methotrexate are advocated. Five-year survival is nearly 75 percent. The posterior fossa remains the major site for recurrence. A pessimistic outlook exists for children under 3 years, those with large tumors, and those with subarachnoid spread. Metastases to lung, liver, vertebrae, and pelvis are reported. Some medulloblastomas may take on features reminiscent of neuroblastoma.

Neuroblastoma DEFINITION The neuroblastoma, a relatively common adrenal tumor, can rarely occur as a primary CNS tumor. Eighty percent of cases present during the first decade of life.

CLINICAL MANIFESTATIONS The most important clue to the presence of neuroblastoma is opsoclonus (see Chap. 328), the presence of which confers a better prognosis.

PATHOGENESIS AND PATHOLOGY Microscopically, neuroblastoma resembles medulloblastoma because of its small dense cells. Variations in pathology occur. Some tumors show differentiation to ganglion cells but do not have a better prognosis. These tumors appear to form a spectrum of tumors of embryonal origin, ranging from the aggressive, poorly differentiated PNETs to the very well differentiated and quite slow growing neurocytomas. The intraparenchymal tumors found in children resemble in clinical behavior the PNETs, with neuraxis spread and occasional extraneural metastases. CT reveals a hypodense mass with dense uniform enhancement after contrast administration as well as variable hemorrhage and calcification. These tumors may present as slowly growing intraventricular masses in adults and may grow to large size before discovery.

TREATMENT The rarity of these tumors has prevented any randomized therapeutic trials. Optimal treatment may consist of radical excision with postoperative radiation, though definitive evidence that radiation increases survival is lacking. Because of the frequency of local recurrence and CSF metastases, prophylactic spinal irradiation may be justified. A trial of chemotherapy, either pre- or postirradiation may be worthwhile, especially in younger patients with more aggressive-appearing tumors. Long-term follow-up is complete but appears to have a greater than 30 percent 5-year survival. The survival of adults with intraventricular tumors may be better than that of other primitive CNS tumors.

TUMORS OF THE SKULL BASE Tumors in this region produce characteristic clinical presentations that pose unique diagnostic difficulties even with advanced neuroradiologic procedures. Meningiomas, tumors of bone (including epidermoid and dermoid tumors and osteomas), chordomas, schwannomas (neurofibromas) of the cranial nerves, nasopharyngeal carcinoma, and metastases may all present with pain localized to the lower face, ear, or occiput and with involvement of one or more cranial nerves making exit from the skull. Metastases arise commonly from the lung, breast, nasopharynx, testicle, and prostate. Multiple myeloma and occasionally lymphoma may appear at this site. The mass may be palpable or may be visualized on enhanced CT scan, or MRI. These studies usually differentiate successfully other erosive processes of the skull base, including fibrous dysplasia, Paget's disease, xanthomatosis, and osteitis fibrosa cystica. Enlargement of specific cranial nerve foramens may be the first evidence of schwannomas or of *glomus* tumors of the chromaffin cells in the jugular bulb. These last tumors invade temporal and occipital bone and produce hearing abnormalities and lower cranial nerve deficits.

Chordomas arise from remnants of the notochord. Of these, 60 percent are localized in the clivus, 30 percent in the sacral region, and the remaining 10 percent along the extent of the spine and skull base. The chordoma is not easily distinguished in appearance from radiation-sensitive chondrosarcomas and chondroid chordoma. They are highly invasive, expanding along the skull base and causing serial cranial nerve compression, sometimes with invasion of the nasopharynx. Up to one-third may metastasize via the subarachnoid space. A cauda equina syndrome (see ''Spinal Tumors'') results from sacral tumors. Clivus tumors may be difficult to visualize adequately on CT scan but are clearly delineated by MRI. Complete removal is rarely feasible and postoperative radiation therapy is recommended. Radiation with cyclotron-derived protons is followed by 80 percent survival at 5 years and 63 percent at 10 years with minimal complications.

Metastases to the skull base are treated with radiation therapy. In the presence of characteristic patterns of pain and cranial nerve deficit, radiation may be considered to treat presumptive metastases in patients with known systemic malignancy even when radiographic examinations are inconclusive.

SPINAL TUMORS Pathogenesis and pathology Tumors of the spinal canal and of the cord are only one-quarter as common as are intracranial tumors. Spinal neoplasms arise from the same types of cells as their counterparts in the cerebrum. They are classified according to location as intramedullary (within the substance of the spinal cord), extramedullary (or intradural), and extradural. Some tumors, such as schwannomas, may be both extradural and intradural. The most frequent location for all types of spinal neoplasms is in the thoracic cord, presumably reflecting its greater total length. These tumors arise from cells of the spinal cord, nerve roots, meninges, vascular structures, or the vertebral column. Tumors of the spinal cord parenchyma are relatively infrequent compared to lesions arising outside the substance of the cord. In one large series, nerve sheath tumors (schwannomas) accounted for 29 percent of all spinal tumors, meningiomas for 25.5 percent, gliomas for 22 percent, and sarcomas for 12 percent. Metastatic lesions represent about 13 percent of all spinal tumors, but as with intracranial tumors, these figures reflect neurosurgical service statistics and metastases are likely to be underrepresented.

Clinical manifestations   Any lesion that narrows the spinal canal sufficiently to encroach on neural structures can give rise to neurologic symptoms. Dysfunction may arise from direct compression of the spinal cord and its nerve roots or from interference with blood supply. The rapid growth of metastatic lesions leads to motor and sensory symptoms over a period of days to weeks, whereas slowly growing astrocytomas and ependymomas produce symptoms over a period of months to years.

Extramedullary tumors (both intradural and epidural) cause symptoms by compressing the spinal cord or nerve roots. The initial symptoms are usually focal back pain and paresthesias followed by sensory loss below the level of the pain, weakness, and bladder and bowel dysfunction. Intramedullary lesions usually extend over several spinal cord segments, and their symptoms and signs are more varied than those of extramedullary tumors. A common pattern is dissociated sensory loss, with pain and temperature sensation impairment in the segments of tumor origin and with sparing of posterior column sensory function. Later, as the tumor grows peripherally, spinothalamic tracts may be involved. Since, in the thoracic and cervical regions, the sacral pain and temperature fibers lie superficial to those fibers representing more rostral regions, the sacral segments may be spared. Atrophy in the appropriate segments due to anterior horn cell involvement may combine with corticospinal tract signs.

These clinical presentations are not diagnostic of spinal cord neoplasm. Transverse myelitis from multiple sclerosis or other causes can lead to rapid onset of spinal cord dysfunction associated with pain, paresthesias, and weakness (see Chap. 381). A similar syndrome can occur as a paraneoplastic process, resulting from a necrotic myelopathy (see Chap. 328). Syringomyelia can produce a chronic syndrome indistinguishable from that produced by intramedullary neoplasms. Other diseases that can lead to a progressive spinal cord syndrome include combined system degeneration due to vitamin B_{12} deficiency, amyotrophic lateral sclerosis, cervical spondylosis, arachnoiditis, vascular anomalies, meningeal carcinomatosis, and spinal stenosis due to a combination of degenerative disk disease and hypertrophy of the ligamentum flavum (see Chap. 381).

Additional specific clinical syndromes occur in two other locations within the spinal canal. *Foramen magnum tumors* may extend into the cervical region or rostrally into the posterior fossa. A combination of signs and symptoms referrable to lower cranial nerves, sensory loss in the distribution of the second cervical segment, posterior headache, and asymmetric sensory and motor involvement of the limbs leads to the suspicion of such a tumor, most commonly a meningioma. *Tumors of the conus medullaris or cauda equina* produce pain in the back, rectum, and/or both legs and may mimic lumbosacral disk disease. With tumor growth, muscle atrophy in the legs associated with sphincter dysfunction and reflex changes usually point to the correct site of involvement.

Diagnosis of spinal cord tumors   MRI has replaced all other modalities in the evaluation of patients suspected to have cancer outside or within the dura of the spinal canal (Fig. 369-6 and 369-7) In most centers MRI can be performed as an emergency procedure. With or without gadolinium, these studies delineate the site, number, and extent of *extradural* deposits, while providing definitive information concerning the enlargement of neural foramens (which occurs with schwannomas), distortion of paraspinal tissues with masses that have grown into the spinal canal from extraneural sites (as with lymphomatous spread), and the intricate anatomy of the cervicomedul-

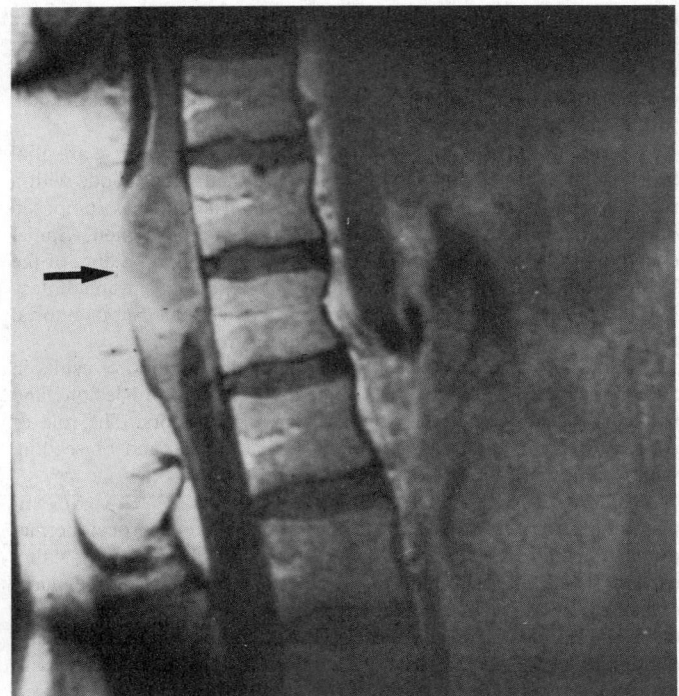

FIGURE 369-6   Sagittal T1-weighted MRI image of the conus medullaris (arrow) in a 26-year-old male with malignant primitive neuroectodermal tumor.

lary junction (as with meningioma or skull-base chordoma or nasopharyngeal metastases). MRI pictures have supplanted confusing arguments regarding "complete" or "incomplete" myelographic block. By identifying multiple extradural lesions needless surgery can be avoided and irradiation fields appropriately applied. Intradural, leptomeningeal metastases or tumors within the spinal cord or its roots are equally amenable to MRI visualization, especially when used following injection of gadolinium.

Myelography following the subarachnoid injection of nonionic contrast materials is often used to complement MRI studies or when MRI is unavailable. A small amount of contrast injected prior to CT

FIGURE 369-7   Sagittal MRI of the thoracic spinal cord in a patient with metastatic breast cancer reveals destruction of a vertebral body with epidural tumor mass compressing the spinal cord.

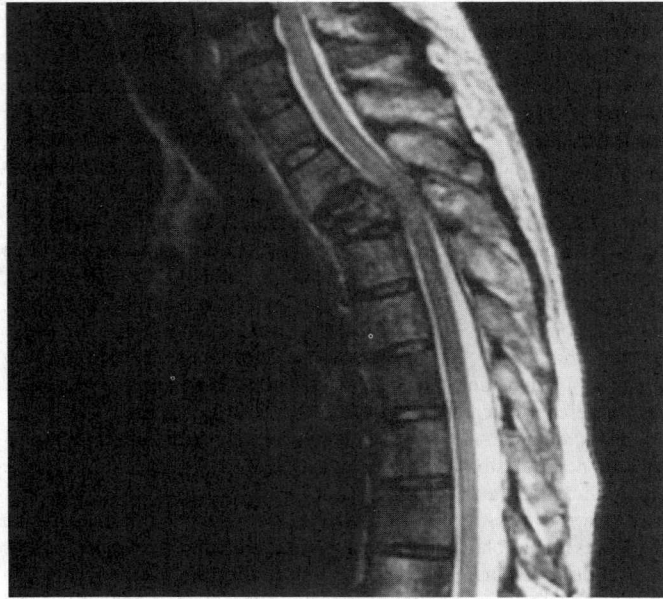

evaluation of the spine is used to elucidate the coexistence of extradural tumor *and* calcified disk fragment, compression fracture of the bony vertebrae, osteomyelitis, or defects from prior surgery or irradiation. Similarly these CT studies identify intradural processes including arachnoiditis, lipomatous masses, and syrinx for which MRI experience remains scanty.

Cerebrospinal fluid removed at the time of myelography should be analyzed for cell count, protein content, and cytology. A specimen stained with Wright's stain should be analyzed and cells examined further after cytocentrifugation. The cell count is usually normal in spinal tumors unless there is meningeal tumor, but protein content is increased in virtually all cases of high-grade spinal cord block. The CSF glucose is usually normal unless there is meningeal tumor invasion.

Treatment   Once the diagnosis of spinal cord tumor is established, rapid treatment is mandatory to maximize neurologic recovery. Extramedullary primary neoplasms are treated with microneurosurgery, and complete resection is usually possible. The most common intramedullary tumors, ependymomas and astrocytomas, usually can only be partially resected and are likely to recur. The role of radiation therapy for slowly growing tumors of this class is not well established; for high-grade astrocytomas a course of postoperative radiation is recommended. Glucocorticoids may improve function temporarily. There is no established role for chemotherapy of spinal neoplasms.

EPIDURAL CANCER: THE PATIENT WITH CANCER AND BACK PAIN   Spinal epidural cancer should be suspected in patients with back pain and known systemic malignancy even in the absence of neurologic signs. Progressive paraparesis with bladder dysfunction and development of a sensory deficit may be avoided by timely MRI imaging of the spine followed by surgical or radiation therapy. The MRI identification of tumor anterior to the spinal cord may pave the way for surgical anterior decompression (Fig. 369-7). High doses of glucocorticoids (up to 100 mg dexamethasone per day) are administered immediately and radiation therapy is usually recommended. The results of treatment in the large series of patients with epidural cancer reported by Gilbert has led to the conclusion that radiation therapy is as effective as surgery in the relief of symptoms. The clinical condition of the patient at the time of diagnosis is the most important factor in prognosis; only 3 percent of patients paraplegic at the time of treatment, regardless of type of therapy, regain ambulation. Reconsideration is being given to surgical decompression as a primary mode of treatment in patients with radioresistant malignancies such as melanoma and lung, prostatic, and colonic cancers and in the setting of paraparesis of recent onset.

REFERENCES

BLACK P McL: Brain tumors. N Engl J Med 324:1471, 1555, 1991

BULLARD DE et al: Oligodendroglioma. An analysis of the value of radiation therapy. Cancer 60:2179, 1987

BYRNE TN, WAXSMAN SG: *Spinal Cord Compression; Diagnosis and Principles of Management.* Philadelphia, FA Davis, 1990

CONSTINE LS et al: Hypothalamic pituitary dysfunction after radiation for brain tumors. N Engl J Med 328:87, 1993

CORBETT JJ et al: Visual loss in pseudotumor cerebri. Arch Neurol 39:461, 1982

GLANTZ MJ et al: Influence of the type of surgery on the histologic diagnosis in patients with anaplastic gliomas. Neurology 41:1741, 1991

GOWLAND P et al: Dynamic studies of gadolinium uptake in brain tumors using inversion-recovery echo-planar imaging. Magn Reson Med 26:241, 1992

GUTIN PH: Recurrent malignant gliomas: Survival following interstitial brachytherapy with high activity iodine 125 sources. J Neurosurg 67:864, 1987

HELWEG-LARSEN S: Recovery of gait following radiation therapy in paralyzed patients with metastatic epidural spinal cord compression. Neurology 40:1234, 1990

HOCHBERG FH et al: The therapy of primary brain lymphoma. J Neuro-Oncol 10:191, 1991

HOCHBERG FJ, MILLER DC: Primary central nervous system lymphoma. J Neurosurg 68:835, 1988

HUGHES EN et al: Medulloblastoma at the Joint Center for Radiation Therapy between 1968 and 1984. The influence of radiation dose on the patterns of failure and survival. Cancer 61:1992, 1988

JANUS TJ et al: Use of [F-18] fluorodeoxyglucose positron emission tomography in patients with primary malignant brain tumors. Ann Neurol 33:540, 1993

JENNINGS MT et al: Intracranial germ cell tumors: Natural history and pathogenesis. J Neurosurg 63:155, 1985

KORNBLITH PL, WALKER M: Chemotherapy for malignant gliomas. J Neurosurg 68:1, 1988

LEVINE AJ, SCHMIDEK HH (eds): *Molecular Genetics of Nervous System Tumors.* New York, Wiley-Liss, 1993

MAHALEY MS: Neuro-oncology index and review—adult primary brain tumors. J Neuro-Oncol 11:85, 1991

PATCHELL R: A randomized trial of surgery in the treatment of single metastases to the brain. N Engl J Med 322:494, 1990

SIDRANSKY D et al: Clonal expansion of P53 mutant cells associated with brain tumor progression. Nature 355:846, 1992

SMOKER WR et al: The role of MR imaging in evaluating metastatic spinal disease. Am J Radiol 149:1241, 1987

WASSERSTROM WR: Diagnosis and treatment of leptomeningeal metastases from solid tumors. Cancer 49:759, 1982

YOUNG DP: Neurology complications of chemotherapy, in *Neurological Complications of Therapy,* A Silverstein (ed). Mount Kisco, NY, Futura Publishing, 1982, p 57

370   ALZHEIMER'S DISEASE AND OTHER DEMENTIAS

M. FLINT BEAL / EDWARD P. RICHARDSON, JR. / JOSEPH B. MARTIN

In classifying diseases of the nervous system, it is customary to designate a group of them as *degenerative*, indicating that they are characterized by gradually evolving, relentlessly progressive neuronal death occurring for reasons that are still largely unknown. The identification of these diseases depends on exclusion of such possible causative factors as infections, metabolic derangements, and intoxications. A considerable proportion of the disorders classed as degenerative are genetic, with either dominant or recessive inheritance. Others, however, occur only sporadically—as isolated instances in a given family.

Classification of the degenerative diseases cannot be based on any exact knowledge of cause or pathogenesis; their subdivision into individual syndromes rests on descriptive criteria based largely on neuropathologic and clinical aspects. This group of diseases presents as several distinct clinical syndromes, the recognition of which can assist the clinician in arriving at a diagnosis.

GENERAL CONSIDERATIONS   The degenerative disorders usually begin insidiously and run a gradually progressive course over many years. Their course is generally more protracted than that of the hereditary metabolic diseases of the nervous system (see Chap. 377). The earliest changes may be so subtle that it often is impossible to assign any precise time of onset. At times the history suggests an abrupt onset of disability—particularly when an injury or some other event in the patient's life has occurred to which illness might conceivably be related. By careful questioning, it is frequently evident that the patient or family has suddenly become aware of a condition that had, in fact, already been present but had passed unnoticed.

The family history is of great importance, and denial of familial occurrence cannot always be taken at face value. Some patients or their relatives are hesitant to disclose that a neurologic disease afflicts the family. In other cases, the extent of the disease affecting other family members may be so slight as to go unnoticed by the family—as may occur, for instance, in the group of the hereditary ataxias. Moreover, small sibships in a family may prevent well-established hereditary diseases from being recognized. Familial occurrence, of course, does not always mean that a disease is hereditary; it may indicate instead that there has been a common exposure to an infective or toxic agent.

Many of the degenerative nervous system diseases progress uninfluenced by therapeutic measures. Caring for such patients is often an anguishing experience for all concerned. In others, such as persons with Parkinson's disease, symptoms can often be alleviated by wise and skillful management. The physician's caring attention may be of great help even when curative measures cannot be offered.

The symptoms and signs of this group of diseases tend to have a bilaterally symmetric distribution. This aspect alone may help to distinguish the disorder from other varieties of neurologic disease. In some patients, in the early stages, one side of the body or one limb may become involved in the presence of normal findings elsewhere. Eventually, despite the asymmetric beginning, the inherently bilateral nature of the process generally asserts itself.

A striking characteristic of the degenerative disorders is that particular anatomic or physiologic systems of neurons may be selectively affected, leaving others entirely intact. This is exemplified in amyotrophic lateral sclerosis, in which the disease process is limited to cerebral and spinal motor neurons, and in some forms of progressive ataxia, in which only the Purkinje cells of the cerebellum are affected. In Friedreich's ataxia and some other syndromes, the disease process affects multiple neuronal systems.

In this respect, certain degenerative neuronal diseases resemble others of known cause, particularly intoxications, where similarly circumscribed effects occur. Diphtheria toxin, for example, produces selective breakdown of peripheral nerve myelin, triorthocresyl phosphate affects the corticospinal tracts in the spinal cord together with the peripheral nerves, and the neurotoxin 1-methyl-4-phenyl-1,2,3,6-tetrahydropyridine (MPTP) brings about death of dopamine-containing neurons in the substantia nigra. Selective involvement of particular neuronal systems is not, however, characteristic of all the degenerative diseases; some are characterized by pathologic changes that are diffuse and unselective.

Typically, the pathologic process in the nervous system is one of slow involution of nerve cell bodies or their axonal extensions, unaccompanied by any intense tissue reaction or cellular response, although the loss of neurons and fibers is often accompanied by hyperplasia of fibrillary astrocytes (gliosis). The cerebrospinal fluid (CSF) shows little, if any, change—at most a slight elevation of protein, without abnormalities in specific proteins, cell count, or other constituents. Moreover, since these diseases invariably result in tissue loss, rather than in new tissue formation, radiologic visualization of the brain, the ventricular system, or subarachnoid space shows either no change or an enlargement of the CSF compartments. These negative laboratory findings thus help to distinguish the degenerative disorders from the other large classes of progressive diseases of the nervous system—tumors and infections.

CLASSIFICATION Since etiologic classification is impossible, subdivision of the degenerative diseases into individual syndromes rests on descriptive criteria based largely on their clinical aspects and pathologic anatomy. Many of these syndromes are named after distinguished neurologists and neuropathologists. A useful classification is outlined in Table 370-1.

SYNDROMES IN WHICH PROGRESSIVE DEMENTIA PREDOMINATES

In the disease entities that follow, the clinical picture is dominated by gradual loss of intellectual capacities, i.e., by dementia. Other neurologic abnormalities, except in the terminal stages, are absent or relatively insignificant. (For further discussion of dementia, including its clinical evaluation, Chaps. 25 and 27 should be consulted.)

ALZHEIMER'S DISEASE Alzheimer's disease is perhaps the most important of all the degenerative diseases because of its frequent occurrence and devastating nature. It is the most common cause of dementia in the elderly, with all that this implies in the way of distress for patients and families and economic loss in the form of the costs entailed in the long-term care of patients totally disabled by the disease. Historically, the term *Alzheimer's disease* was applied to progressive dementia coming on in late middle life but preceding the senile period, following the original description by Alois Alzheimer in 1907, in which the illness of a woman dying at the age of 55 was depicted clinically and pathologically. It became usual to classify cases of this kind under the heading of *presenile dementia*. Meanwhile, it became increasingly apparent that very old people dying with progressive mental deterioration, generally referred to as *senile dementia*, showed cerebral lesions that were identical to those found in cases of presenile dementia. Such cases are now designated as *senile dementia of the Alzheimer type*. Current evidence indicates that the disease process is the same, regardless of the age of onset. At the same time, Alzheimer's disease is clearly age-related. It is extremely uncommon in young people and rare in middle age; as age advances, however, it is increasingly frequent, such that its prevalence in persons over 85 years old is estimated to be as high as 47 percent. Advancing age is unmistakably a predisposing factor, but it is incorrect to consider Alzheimer's disease as the inevitable accompaniment of aging. Many elderly people remain mentally unimpaired into the ninth and tenth decades. Genetic predisposition to Alzheimer's disease emerges as a clear-cut pattern in some families; however, these cases comprise less than 20 percent of all cases. There are well-documented familial cases, some following an autosomal dominant pattern of inheritance with linkage to either chromosome 21 or 19. An exception to the statement that Alzheimer's disease is rare in young people occurs in the instance of Down's syndrome (trisomy 21), which leads to the development of the characteristic lesions of Alzheimer's disease in the majority of the patients after 40 years of age.

Pathology The outstanding pathologic feature is death and disappearance of nerve cells in the cerebral cortex. This leads

---

TABLE 370-1   Clinical classification of the degenerative diseases of the nervous system

Progressive dementia in the absence of other prominent neurologic signs
- A   Alzheimer's disease
- B   Senile dementia of the Alzheimer type
- C   Pick's disease (lobar atrophy)

Syndromes combining progressive dementia with other prominent neurologic abnormalities
- A   Mainly in adults
  - 1   Huntington's disease
  - 2   Multiple system atrophy combining dementia with ataxia and/or manifestations of Parkinson's disease
  - 3   Progressive supranuclear palsy (Steele-Richardson-Olszewski)
  - 4   Diffuse Lewy body disease
  - 5   Corticodentatonigral degeneration
- B   Mainly in children or young adults
  - 1   Hallervorden-Spatz disease
  - 2   Progressive familial myoclonic epilepsy

Syndromes of gradually developing abnormalities of posture and movement (see Chap. 371)
- A   Paralysis agitans (Parkinson's disease)
- B   Striatonigral degeneration
- C   Progressive supranuclear palsy (see II, A, 3 above)
- D   Torsion dystonia (torsion spasm; dystonia musculorum deformans)
- E   Spasmodic torticollis and other restricted dyskinesias
- F   Familial tremor
- G   Gilles de la Tourette syndrome

Syndromes of progressive ataxia (see Chap. 372)
- A   Cerebellar degenerations
  - 1   Cerebellar cortical degeneration
  - 2   Olivopontocerebellar atrophy (OPCA)
- B   Spinocerebellar degenerations (Friedreich's ataxia and related disorders)

Central autonomic nervous system failure (Shy-Drager syndrome) (see Chap. 379)

Syndromes of muscular weakness and wasting without sensory changes (motor neuron disease) (see Chap. 372)
- A   Amyotrophic lateral sclerosis
- B   Spinal muscular atrophy
  - 1   Infantile spinal muscular atrophy (Werdnig-Hoffmann)
  - 2   Juvenile spinal muscular atrophy (Wohlfart-Kugelberg-Welander)
  - 3   Other forms of familial spinal muscular atrophy
- C   Primary lateral sclerosis
- D   Hereditary spastic paraplegia

Syndromes combining muscular weakness and wasting with sensory changes (progressive neural muscular atrophy; chronic familial polyneuropathies) (see Chap. 383)
- A   Peroneal muscular atrophy (Charcot-Marie-Tooth)
- B   Hypertrophic interstitial polyneuropathy (Dejerine-Sottas)
- C   Miscellaneous forms of chronic progressive neuropathy

Syndromes of progressive visual loss
- A   Pigmentary degeneration of the retina (retinitis pigmentosa)
- B   Hereditary optic atrophy (Leber's disease)

ultimately to extensive convolutional atrophy, especially in the frontal, parietal, and medial temporal regions. There is a corresponding enlargement of the ventricular system, but this is usually not extreme.

Two kinds of microscopic lesions are distinctive for the disease. The first, originally described by Alzheimer, consists of intraneuronal accumulations of filamentous material in the form of loops, coils, or tangled masses—referred to as *Alzheimer neurofibrillary tangles*. The neuropathologic evidence strongly suggests that these fibrillar masses are of major importance in bringing about the death of neurons. Neurofibrillary tangles and loss of synapses are the neuropathologic features most closely linked to dementia. Electron microscopy reveals accumulations of paired helical filaments that differ from normal neurofilaments and microtubules. Recent studies have shown that a major component is an abnormally phosphorylated form of the microtubule protein tau. Alzheimer neurofibrillary tangles also contain ubiquitin, a protein that marks cells for proteolysis.

Neurofibrillary tangles tend to be most abundant, together with the most extreme degrees of neuronal loss, in the hippocampus and adjacent parts of the temporal lobe—structures that have been found to be of greatest importance in memory function.

The other histopathologic change that characterizes Alzheimer's disease is the presence of intracortical clusters of thickened neuronal processes, both axons and dendrites (collectively referred to as *neurites*), generally in the form of an irregular ring surrounding a spherical deposit of amyloid fibrils. These lesions, which had been recognized before Alzheimer's description of the neurofibrillary change, were termed *senile plaques*. Recent elucidation of their structure has led to their current designation as *neuritic plaques*. They have been shown to contain paired helical filaments identical to those found in the perinuclear cytoplasm of the diseased neurons. One form of plaque, the *diffuse plaque*, consists of amorphous amyloid without neurites.

In many, but not all, cases, identical amyloid deposits may be found in the walls of small meningeal and intracortical arteries, and the question has arisen as to whether this cerebrovascular amyloidosis (often called *cerebral amyloid angiopathy* or *congophilic angiopathy* because of the characteristic staining of amyloid with the dye Congo red) has a close relationship, perhaps even causative, to plaque amyloidosis. Antibodies against the cerebrovascular amyloid cross-react with the amyloid in neuritic plaques. It is as yet unclear where the amyloid in plaques originates—whether from neurons or blood vessels; most investigators favor the former. The amyloid in the blood vessels in Alzheimer's disease, as well as that in the core of neuritic plaques, has been isolated and sequenced. It consists of a 42 to 43 amino acid peptide. Some recent evidence suggests that it may exert neurotoxic effects. The amyloid peptide (β- or A$_4$-peptide) gene is on chromosome 21, on which the familial Alzheimer's disease gene also has been localized in some families. A recent advance has been the finding that in a handful of families with familial Alzheimer's disease there are point mutations in the amyloid precursor protein. This observation suggests that Alzheimer's disease can be linked to a primary defect in amyloid production or processing, but most cases of familial and sporadic Alzheimer's disease do not have a clear cause (see Chap. 364).

Biochemical studies show that choline acetyltransferase, the key enzyme required for the synthesis of acetylcholine, is decreased in the cerebral cortex in Alzheimer's disease. The major source of neocortical cholinergic innervation is a group of neurons situated in the basal part of the forebrain just beneath the corpus striatum—the nucleus basalis of Meynert. Careful neuropathologic investigations have shown that in Alzheimer's disease this nucleus is a site of major neuronal loss and of frequent Alzheimer neurofibrillary tangles. These studies suggest that impairment of cholinergic transmission may play a part in the clinical expression of the disease. However, attempted therapy with cholinomimetic agents has been largely unsuccessful. Less consistent reductions in cortical norepinephrine and serotonin appear to be caused by neuronal loss in the locus coeruleus and raphé nucleus, respectively. Loss of peptidergic neurons in the cerebral cortex is associated with reduced cortical concentrations of somato-statin and corticotropin releasing factor.

It is anticipated that investigations of the biochemistry of the cerebral lesions in Alzheimer's disease will lead ultimately to an understanding of their pathogenesis. The remarkable discovery that one form of progressive dementia, Creutzfeldt-Jakob disease, is the result of infection with a transmissible virus-like agent has led to the question as to whether Alzheimer's disease and other neuronal degenerations might be due to a similar form of infectious agent (see Chap. 375). All attempts to transmit Alzheimer's disease have failed, however, so that currently an infective basis is thought unlikely.

Clinical manifestations The onset is insidious and subtle, with changes most noticeable first in memory for recent happenings and in other aspects of mental activity. Psychiatric disturbances such as depression, anxiety, or odd, unpredictable quirks of behavior, delusions, and hallucinations may be salient features in the early stages. Progression is usually slow and gradual, and unless other medical conditions supervene, it may smolder on for 10 or more years.

In the milder cases, including those of the senile period, the noteworthy features are those of simple dementia, as described in Chap. 25. More unusual disorders of thought and intellect, including aphasia, apraxic disturbances, and abnormalities of space perception, may be seen, especially in the presenile group. Exceptionally, and only in the advanced stages of the disease, extrapyramidal signs appear; the patient walks in a shuffling manner with short steps, and there is a generalized stiffness of the musculature with slowness and awkwardness of all movements. In some patients, sudden jerklike contractions of various muscles (myoclonus) may occur in the presence of otherwise typical Alzheimer's disease, but this is unusual and should immediately raise the suspicion of Creutzfeldt-Jakob disease (Chap. 375). Terminally, the patient may become nearly decorticate, losing all ability to perceive, think, speak, or move.

Laboratory investigations, including blood and CSF determinations, do not yield any conclusive or pertinent data. There is a diffuse slowing in the electroencephalogram in the more advanced stages of the disease. Enlargement of the ventricular system and subarachnoid space resulting from brain atrophy can be demonstrated by computed tomography (CT) and by magnetic resonance imaging (MRI). These imaging procedures, however, are not decisive for making the diagnosis, especially in the earlier stages, because the degree of cerebral atrophy demonstrated may be no more than that seen in patients of a similar age group who are functioning normally. Recent studies with positron-emission tomography have shown decreased glucose metabolism in the temporal and parietal lobes. During the course of the illness, occasional convulsive seizures may occur, but they are relatively rare and should raise suspicion of other diseases. Terminally, the patient dies from intercurrent disease, in a state of total helplessness. Institutional care is usually necessary long before the end.

Differential diagnosis The physician should recognize that treatable conditions may at first appear to be dementia of the Alzheimer type. Space-occupying lesions, such as chronic subdural hematoma or slowly growing frontal neoplasms (meningioma or glioma), should be excluded. CT and MRI usually demonstrate mass lesions of these kinds, as well as an unsuspected hydrocephalus, which, when treated by a shunt procedure for ventricular decompression, may lead to dramatic improvement in the patient's state. Other treatable conditions producing a dementia-like state include metabolic derangements (liver disease), vitamin B$_{12}$ deficiency, and hypothyroidism. Elderly people may be unusually susceptible to the sedative effects of medications, so chronic drug intoxication may need to be considered. Cerebrovascular disease is not ordinarily a cause of uncomplicated dementia, but finding multiple small infarcts by CT or MRI raises the possibility of multi-infarct dementia. Depression can mimic dementia, particularly in the elderly, in whom it may be all too easy to attribute deficits in thinking, motivation, and memory to cerebral disease (see Chap. 25). Depression may show a most gratifying response to appropriate treatment (see Chap. 389).

The evidence that cholinergic innervation may be impaired in Alzheimer's disease has led to attempts to correct the deficiency pharmacologically. The most recent of these is the acetylcholinesterase inhibitor tetrahydroaminoacridine, which produces limited improvement in some mental status tests but which is compromised by liver toxicity.

Practical measures that may help in the management of cases of Alzheimer's disease are suggested in Chap. 25.

PICK'S DISEASE (LOBAR ATROPHY)   This remarkable form of cerebral disease, characterized by circumscribed cerebal atrophy (lobar sclerosis), enters in the differential diagnosis of dementia in the presenile period. It is, however, an extremely rare condition as compared with diffuse cerebral atrophy of the Alzheimer type. Hereditary transmission (as a dominant trait) is frequent in Pick's disease, and women are more frequently affected than men. The age distribution is similar in both these varieties of progressive dementia.

Pathology   So striking are the gross pathologic changes in the brain that in typical cases the diagnosis can be made at a glance. Severe atrophy of the anterior portions of the frontal and temporal lobes occurs, and there is a curiously sharp line of demarcation between the atrophied portions and the remainder of the brain, which appears normal or nearly so. In some cases, the frontal atrophy is more prominent; in others, the temporal lobes are more severely involved; in general, both regions are affected. Rarely, the disorder has a predominantly unilateral localization—as in cases described originally by Pick. Atrophic changes also occur in subcortical structures, i.e., the caudate nucleus, putamen, thalamus, and substantia nigra, and in the descending frontopontine fiber system. There are striking changes in nerve cells in the affected regions in most cases. These consist of fibrillary deposits within the cytoplasm—masses of straight fibrils, differing from the paired helical filaments of Alzheimer's disease. In some neurons, densely packed spherical aggregates (Pick bodies) can be seen with silver-impregnation methods. In other affected neurons, the fibrils are more widely dispersed, and the neuronal cytoplasm takes on a rounded, distended appearance, forming "ballooned" cells. Recent evidence suggests that despite the morphologic differences, these neuronal changes are biochemically related to those in Alzheimer's disease, as indicated by common antigenic properties. In rare instances of Alzheimer's disease, disproportionate atrophy of the frontal and temporal lobes may suggest Pick's disease, but in such cases the distinguishing feature is the presence of the characteristic plaques and neurofibrillary tangles, which are not found in Pick's disease.

Clinical manifestations   If Pick's disease has any distinctive clinical features, they consist of unusually severe signs of frontal lobe or temporal lobe dysfunction (see Chap. 27). Typical early manifestations are a general impoverishment of mental function, changes in behavior patterns, and a striking lack of insight. Some patients have an early impairment of language with difficulty naming objects or people. The later phases of the disease are characterized by loss of retentive memory (with temporal lobe involvement), loss of all language functions, and, when the frontal lobes are mainly affected, prominent grasp and sucking reflexes. In CT and MRI scans the shrinkage of the cortex and the low density of the white matter in the affected lobes may be diagnostic. Progression, as in Alzheimer's disease, is slow and relentless, the average duration being about 7 years. In the late stages, rigidity, dystonic postures, and perhaps tremor may be prominent features; these can be ascribed to extension of the disease process into the basal ganglia.

Differential diagnosis   The considerations already noted with regard to Alzheimer's disease apply to Pick's disease as well.

SYNDROMES COMBINING DEMENTIA WITH OTHER NEUROLOGIC SIGNS

HUNTINGTON'S DISEASE   This disorder, characterized by a combination of choreoathetotic movements and progressive dementia usually beginning in midadult life, is transmitted as an autosomal dominant disease. The determining gene is located on the terminal segment of the short arm of chromosome 4. The classic description is that of George Huntington, who, together with his father and grandfather, all physicians, made clinical observations on familial cases living near their home on Long Island, New York. Huntington, writing in 1872, entitled his paper "On Chorea"; subsequently, the disorder described by him came to be known as *Huntington's chorea*. The more general term used in this chapter—Huntington's disease—is preferable, since the disease state comprises more than abnormal movements, and the motor abnormalities often are more complex than would be implied by the unqualified term *chorea*.

Because of its distressing and incapacitating nature and its implications for members of any family in which it appears (50 percent risk in each child of an affected parent), the disease has attracted attention in recent years and has been found to be considerably more frequent and widely distributed than once was thought. It is estimated that there are approximately 25,000 cases in the United States alone. In virtually all cases that come to the notice of a physician, there is a family history of the disease, although occasionally patients present with typical symptoms and no documentable family history; no proven case of a new mutation has occurred. Some of these cases are classified as senile chorea, where family members have died of other causes before the disease became manifest. Genetic testing of at-risk patients with a known family history is now available in many clinical settings.

Pathology   Distinctive for Huntington's disease is atrophy of the caudate nucleus and, to a lesser extent, other structures of the basal ganglia (putamen and globus pallidus), out of proportion to any other changes in the brain. The degree of atrophy is directly related to the severity and duration of the disease. In the late stages, the caudate nucleus, which normally forms a convexly rounded eminence in the lateral wall of the lateral ventricle, takes on instead a flattened or concave appearance. As the result of the tissue loss, the ventricular system becomes correspondingly widened, especially the frontal horns. Along with these changes in the basal ganglia, there characteristically is diffuse gyral atrophy, most severe over the convex aspect of the brain.

The atrophy of the caudate nucleus and putamen is seen microscopically to be due to extensive loss of neurons, which stands out in contrast to the intactness of adjacent structures such as the nucleus accumbens septi, the nucleus basalis of Meynert (so strikingly involved in Alzheimer's disease), and the thalamus. Recent studies also show loss of neurons in the cerebral cortex.

There are no morphologically distinctive or characteristic cytopathologic alterations in the neurons in Huntington's disease such as occur in Alzheimer's and some other diseases. Neurochemical studies have shown a striking decrease of γ-aminobutyric acid (GABA) and of its synthesizing enzyme, glutamic acid decarboxylase, in the caudate nucleus, putamen, globus pallidus, and pars reticulata of the substantia nigra, as well as some decrease in choline acetyltransferase in the caudate nucleus. The loss of GABA can be attributed to depletion of the abundant medium-sized *spiny* neurons within the striatum. Spiny neurons are characterized in Golgi studies by a large number of dendritic spines and have been shown to constitute the projection neurons of the striatum. They provide efferents to both the globus pallidus and substantia nigra. In contrast, *aspiny* neurons, with few dendritic spines, are striatal interneurons with locally arborizing axons. In addition to GABA, other neurotransmitters contained within striatal spiny neurons, including substance P, enkephalins, and dynorphin, are similarly depleted in the striatum and its sites of projection.

Recent observations indicate that the peptide neurotransmitters somatostatin and neuropeptide y are relatively increased in the caudate nucleus and putamen in Huntington's disease, and cells identifiable as somatostatin–neuropeptide y neurons (*aspiny* neurons) are selectively preserved—in striking contrast to the loss of other neurons in the same regions. The large aspiny neurons containing acetylcholine are also preserved. The pathophysiologic meaning of this sparing is not clear as yet; its occurrence emphasizes the fact that in Huntington's disease, as in other neuronal system degenerations, selective vulnerability of neurons occurs in a particular region with preservation of others. The pattern of resistance of certain neuronal groups has provided clues to a possible underlying pathogenesis of the disease. The susceptible spiny neurons have dense glutamate inputs from the cerebral cortex. The pattern of cell death can be reproduced experimentally by glutamate receptor agonists that act on the *N*-methyl-D-aspartate subclass of glutamate receptors (see Chap. 364). Recent work shows that the spared aspiny neurons produce nitric oxide, a new neurotransmitter candidate (see Chap. 364). These observations have led to the hypothesis that striatal neurons die as a result of glutamate-induced neurotoxicity.

Clinical aspects   The disorder has a prevalence in Europe and North America of 7 to 10 per 100,000 population. The movement disorder generally makes its appearance in early to middle adult years (average age of onset about 35 to 40 years). It is characteristic of the disease that younger patients, with onset of symptoms in the age group of 15 to 40 years, suffer a more severe form of the disorder than older patients, with onset in the 50s and 60s, and the neuropathologic changes in the brain are correspondingly more extensive and severe in the younger as compared with the older patients. Huntington's disease is occasionally manifest in childhood (even before the age of 4); in such cases, transmission usually occurs through the father. Such cases are rare and tend to be characterized more by rigidity than by chorea and by other atypical features such as convulsive seizures and cerebellar ataxia (Westphal variant).

The involuntary movements (bizarre grimacing, respiratory irregularity, faulty articulation of speech, and irregular, arrhythmic, unpatterned movements of the limbs, imparting to the gait a peculiar dancing quality) tend to be less quick and more athetoid than in Sydenham's chorea (see Chap. 21). Some reported cases that on genealogic and pathologic grounds must be classified with Huntington's chorea have shown progressive rigidity rather than choreiform movements, even in the adult. As a general rule, dementia runs parallel with the motor disorder. Occasionally it may appear before or after chorea; very rarely it may be slight or lacking altogether. Neuropsychiatric manifestations of depression, erratic behavior, and emotional outbursts often seriously handicap the patient before dementia or the movement disorder is severe. The advance of the disease is slow, with death occurring, on average, 15 to 20 years after onset of symptoms. Increasing disability from involuntary movements and mental changes result in death from intercurrent infection or, not rarely, suicide.

Differential diagnosis   There is no difficulty in the recognition of typical cases. Midlife onset of chorea in a patient with a positive family history together with the slowly progressive course and prominent dementia make the diagnosis straightforward. In patients with a negative family history, the diagnosis is more difficult. Genetic testing is of no benefit in isolated cases because it remains dependent on linkage analysis in affected families. Lack of association with rheumatic fever helps to exclude Sydenham's chorea. Patients with Parkinson's disease, when overdosed with levodopa, may develop a widespread chorea or choreoathetosis, and this, combined with the early dementia that occurs in some patients, can reproduce the picture of Huntington's disease. Phenothiazine drugs may induce generalized chorea, unassociated with dementia, and the movement disorder may persist for months or years after the medication is discontinued (tardive dyskinesia). Typically, tardive dyskinesia spares the forehead and does not impair gait, in contrast to the findings in Huntington's disease. Finally, there is a form of self-limited chorea, which, like other localized dyskinesias, may appear in older persons without identifiable cause. Hepatolenticular degeneration (Wilson's disease) and nonfamilial forms of hepatocerebral degeneration may display clinical abnormalities resembling those of Huntington's disease, but the specific changes characteristic of these disorders, including liver disease, corneal Kayser-Fleischer rings (in Wilson's disease), and the

typical biochemical abnormalities, are absent in Huntington's disease (see Chap. 348). Choreoathetosis appearing during the second postnatal year and lasting throughout life is due to hypoxic birth injury or kernicterus. Sporadic cases of choreiform movements beginning in middle or late life may present a difficult problem in exact diagnosis. The occasional cases of violent choreiform movements produced by vascular lesions, classically in the subthalamic region, are characterized by sudden onset, unilateral distribution (hemiballismus), and a tendency to improve after a period of initial severity. A few cases of acute choreoathetosis have accompanied hyperthyroidism. Virus encephalitis may occasionally be associated with choreiform movements; acute development, fever, and pleocytosis in the CSF help in recognition of such cases. Hereditary acanthocytosis is a rare condition which can mimic Huntington's disease.

Treatment   No form of treatment has as yet been devised that halts the relentless progression of this disease, and therapeutic attempts to alleviate the abnormal movements have generally been unsatisfactory. Dopamine receptor antagonists (butyrophenones or phenothiazines) may partially ameliorate the chorea, but the side effects characteristic of this class of drugs limit their use. The depression, which is so common in many patients, usually responds to tricyclic antidepressants. The application of molecular genetic probes for presymptomatic and prenatal testing is available in several centers. However, until the gene itself is discovered, testing can only be performed in families by linkage analysis (see Chaps. 61 and 364).

MULTIPLE-SYSTEM ATROPHY   General experience has indicated that cases of multiple affection of neuronal systems may occur in which progressive dementia is combined with varying degrees of ataxia, dysarthria, parkinsonian dyskinesia, and autonomic dysfunction depending on the pattern of anatomic distribution of the pathologic changes (see Chap. 379). For cases of this kind, the general term *multiple-system atrophy* or *degeneration* has been applied. In some, loss of neurons in the cerebellar cortex and in the pontine nuclei and inferior olivary nuclei results in the predominating picture of *olivopontocerebellar degeneration*, to be discussed as one of the syndromes of progressive ataxia. These changes may be combined with similar neuronal loss in the substantia nigra (and in the striatum in striatonigral degeneration), resulting in parkinsonian features (discussed under ''Parkinson's Disease''). Cases with loss of neurons in the intermediolateral columns are termed *Shy-Drager syndrome* (see Chap. 379). Pathologically, the disease process is characterized by death and disappearance of the affected cells and an accompanying reactive gliosis, without intracellular inclusions or other distinctive features. The cerebral cortex generally shows little discernible change, so it may be difficult to ascribe a definite pathoanatomic basis for the dementia, which, for this reason, is sometimes designated as *subcortical*. Typically, multiple-system atrophy is a disorder of late adult life, occurring sporadically in some instances and genetically transmitted in others. Further details of individual syndromes are given in later sections.

PROGRESSIVE SUPRANUCLEAR PALSY (STEELE-RICHARDSON-OLSZEWSKI SYNDROME)   This disorder is discussed in Chap. 371 among the syndromes characterized by gradually developing abnormalities of posture and movement. It is mentioned here because progressive dementia may accompany the other neurologic abnormalities, although it appears late in the course and generally is not severe.

DIFFUSE LEWY BODY DISEASE   Diffuse lewy body disease is a rare illness that presents with progressive dementia or psychosis. Confusional episodes with pronounced impairment of attention occur early. Agitation, hallucinations, and delusions may be prominent features. Parkinsonian signs, which may be absent or mild at the onset, eventually become common, and rigidity is usually severe. Tremor is often absent. Other features include involuntary movements, myoclonus, quadriparesis in flexion, orthostatic hypotension, and dysphagia in some cases. Lewy bodies are found profusely in the brainstem, basal forebrain, hypothalamic nuclei, and neocortex. The course of the illness is relentlessly progressive over several years.

CORTICODENTATONIGRAL DEGENERATION   Corticodentato-nigral degeneration with neuronal achromasia is a rare illness which also has been termed *cortical-basal ganglionic degeneration*. Watts and colleagues have studied seven cases. The illness begins between the ages of 55 and 75, and the initial symptoms are loss of dexterity in one limb (usually an arm) combined with rigidity and often a tremor in the limb. The illness then progresses steadily over several months to involve the other limbs, with rigidity, postural imbalance, and masked facies. Dyspraxia is a prominent clinical feature, but dementia is usually mild or absent until late in the clinical course. The findings at autopsy are severe neuronal loss and gliosis in the cerebral cortex, which is greatest in the perirolandic regions, and mild neuronal loss and gliosis in the substantia nigra. In cortical areas, many of the pyramidal neurons are swollen with indistinct nuclei and poorly stained pale cytoplasm ("achromasia").

HALLERVORDEN-SPATZ DISEASE   This unusual disorder, often affecting several siblings in a family in a manner suggesting an autosomal recessive trait, is associated with a rather variable clinical picture in which abnormalities of posture and muscle tone, involuntary movements, and progressive dementia predominate. Pathologically, there are characteristic abnormalities in the basal ganglia, suggesting a localized disorder of metabolism. The features of the condition were classically described in an affected family by Hallervorden and Spatz (1922).

Pathology   Distinctive for this condition is the accumulation of large amounts of pigmented material in the globus pallidus and pars reticulata of the substantia nigra, resulting in grossly visible brownish discoloration of these regions. Microscopically, there are irregular pigmented, ferruginous concretions and granules of varying brownish or greenish hues depending on the stains used. Although much of this pigment contains iron, serum iron and ferritin are normal, and there is no systemic disorder of iron metabolism. There also is loss of nerve cells. Another feature of the disease is the presence of focal swelling of axons, most probably in their terminal portions; this is especially pronounced in the regions affected by the pigmentary disorder but typically can be found at all levels of the central nervous system, including the cerebral cortex. This neuroaxonal change may link the disease with childhood neuroaxonal dystrophy.

Clinical aspects   The disorder typically makes its appearance in childhood or adolescence, with abnormalities in muscle tone and movements, such as rigidity and choreoathetosis. Abnormal postures of the trunk characteristic of torsion spasm (dystonia) may be seen, or the clinical picture may be reminiscent of parkinsonism. Cerebellar ataxia is also present in some instances. Speech becomes indistinct, and there is progressive intellectual impairment. Eventually, the involuntary movements give way to increasing generalized rigidity, and death comes as a rule about 10 years after onset. A few cases of late onset have shown a parkinsonian syndrome.

Differential diagnosis   No feature of the clinical picture serves to distinguish this particular disorder from other conditions showing dementia with extrapyramidal motor abnormalities. Wilson's disease must be excluded by appropriate laboratory tests. The clearly progressive course sets this condition apart from clinically similar abnormalities resulting from accidents or illnesses at birth or in the neonatal period. It has lately been demonstrated that following intravenous injection of labeled ferrous citrate, there is a selective uptake of radioactive iron in the region of the basal ganglia; possibly a study of this kind would be helpful in diagnosis. In an advanced case, CT scanning may show extreme atrophy of the brain, especially including the structures of the basal ganglia, but the pigmented deposits do not show any increased radiographic density. In some cases there is lucency in the putamen and globus pallidus. MRI scans show a characteristic pattern of increased density in the globus pallidus surrounded by low density on T2-weighted images. This sign has been termed "eye of the tiger." At present, no effective treatment is known. Treatment with a chelating agent, deferoxamine mesylate, has not shown definite benefit, and levodopa and other antiparkinsonian

medications, tryptophan, and megavitamin therapy have been of only temporary and questionable help.

PROGRESSIVE FAMILIAL MYOCLONIC EPILEPSY   There are several neurologic disorders that can result in a syndrome of convulsive seizures, myoclonic jerklike contractions of the musculature, and progressive dementia. Those most frequently encountered in practice are subacute sclerosing panencephalitis in children, adolescents, and young adults (Chap. 375) and subacute spongiform encephalopathy (Creutzfeldt-Jakob disease) in older adults (Chap. 375). The syndrome also can occur in some of the rare forms of metabolic familial disorders: neuraminidase deficiency associated with macular cherry red spots (Chap. 349) and ceroid-lipofuscinosis (Chap. 355). When these and other disorders of known cause can be excluded from consideration, there remain some clinicopathologic entities which can appropriately be considered under the heading of the hereditary degenerative diseases. Several families presenting this syndrome have been carefully studied in northern Europe (Sweden and Finland), but there is no specific geographic distribution.

Lafora's disease   This variety of recessively inherited progressive myoclonic epilepsy is characterized by distinctive intracytoplasmic inclusions in cerebral neurons, called *Lafora bodies* following their original description by Gonzalo Lafora (1911). These have been found to be composed of polymers of glucose (polyglucosans) and thus indicate a disorder of carbohydrate metabolism, but the biochemical defect that leads to their accumulation is unknown. The Lafora bodies are widely distributed, but they are most numerous in the thalamus, substantia nigra, and dentate nucleus of the cerebellum. Subsequent to Lafora's reports, similar polysaccharide deposits have been found in myocardial and skeletal muscle fibers, skin, and the liver, and it is now possible to establish the diagnosis in the presymptomatic phase by skin or liver biopsy.

The disorder characteristically makes its appearance during childhood or adolescence in the form of recurrent seizures (generalized or restricted), uncontrollable myoclonic jerks, or combinations of the two. With the passage of time, the myoclonic phenomena become increasingly severe, and there is deterioration of all intellectual functions. Death from intercurrent infection generally occurs before age 25. Anticonvulsive treatment may help in controlling the seizures, but there currently is no effective treatment for the underlying disease.

Unverricht-Lundborg disease   This is a rare autosomal recessive illness with onset in adolescence of myoclonic and tonic-clonic seizures. Dementia is mild or absent at the outset, but eventually there is a gradual intellectual decline as well as dysarthria, ataxia, and intention tremor. Survival into adulthood is usual. Pathologic studies show widespread degenerative changes without evidence of storage material.

Other varieties of myoclonic epilepsy   When Lafora's disease and the metabolic and infective disorders mentioned above have been excluded, there remains a rather heterogeneous group of progressive neurologic illnesses having in common autosomal recessive inheritance, myoclonic phenomena, convulsive seizures, and mild dementia. Ataxia of stance, gait, and limb movements is a prominent feature in most cases—so much so that the term introduced by Ramsay Hunt, *dyssynergia cerebellaris myoclonica*, is often applied. In a few cases, including some of those originally described by Hunt, there is an overlap with Friedreich's ataxia, or with chronic sensorimotor neuropathies (see Chaps. 381 and 383). The neuropathologic changes in the few cases that have come to postmortem examination have varied from case to case. In some, atrophy of the dentate nucleus and its fiber projections has been prominent; in others, there has been loss of neurons, especially Purkinje cells, in the cerebellar cortex; in still others, changes have been confined to long-tract degeneration (posterior columns and spinocerebellar tracts) in the spinal cord; a few patients have had cortical, basal-ganglionic, or retinal lesions. Variations also occur in the age of onset and the rate of progression. Until more is known about the biochemistry and genetics of this group of disorders, no satisfactory classification is possible. For further details of these syndromes, general reference works on neurology, such as that of Adams and Victor, should be consulted.

Treatment with appropriate anticonvulsant medications has been helpful in some mild cases, but phenytoin is contraindicated. l-Tryptophan and carbidopa or valproic acid have ameliorated myoclonus in a few cases.

NORMAL-PRESSURE HYDROCEPHALUS Normal-pressure hydrocephalus (NPH) is a syndrome of communicating hydrocephalus in which intracranial hypertension is either absent or not recognized.

Pathology and pathophysiology Although it is recognized that delayed hydrocephalus can occur after meningitis, head injury, or subarachnoid hemorrhage, the majority of patients presenting with NPH give no history of such an illness. Studies of isotope cisternography indicate that NPH is a communicating hydrocephalus presumed to be due to partial obliteration of the subarachnoid space with defective CSF reabsorption through the arachnoid villi. Whether episodes of increased intracranial pressure occur during the course of the illness is debated. Some patients monitored continuously show fluctuations in CSF pressure including so-called plateau waves.

Clinical manifestations Typically, the patient or family describes a subacute onset, over weeks, months, or sometimes years, of progressive intellectual deterioration accompanied by slowness and restriction of movements, particularly of gait. No single diagnostic gait disorder occurs (see description, Chap. 22). A broad-based stance with hesitant initiation of walking is common. In some patients, ataxic features are present. Hyperreflexia in the legs and extensor plantar responses may be found. Urinary incontinence is noted in less than one-half of patients.

Differential diagnosis Parkinson's disease can be differentiated by its clinical features and the response to carbidopa-levodopa (Sinemet). Bifrontal disease due to tumor (butterfly glioma), metastases, or cerebral infarction can be identifed by CT or MRI. Multi-infarct dementia with gait disorder can be recognized by focal, often asymmetric, neurologic signs and by CT changes. Aqueductal stenosis may present occasionally in late adulthood with hydrocephalus, headaches, dementia, and incontinence. The CT or MRI usually will demonstrate an enlarged third ventricle with normal fourth ventricle.

Treatment The diagnosis can be difficult because of the common association of ventricular enlargement in patients with degenerative brain conditions, particularly Alzheimer's disease. The characteristic gait disorder is the most reliable clinical feature of NPH. CSF pressure in NPH is usually in the normal range of 80 to 150 mmH$_2$O. Isotope cisternography demonstrating reflux into the ventricular system has not proved to determine reliably which patients are likely to improve following a surgical shunt. Temporary benefit in the gait disorder after removal of 25 to 30 mL of CSF has been noted in some patients. When the history of dementia and gait disorder is subacute in onset and accompanied by considerable ventricular dilatation, surgical shunting is warranted. Ventricular-peritoneal shunting is the procedure most commonly performed. Between 40 and 70 percent of patients show benefit after surgery. The gait disorder tends to show a better response to shunting than the dementia (see Black et al. for review).

REFERENCES

General

ADAMS JH et al (eds): *Greenfield's Neuropathology*, 5th ed. New York, Wiley, 1992
ADAMS RD, VICTOR M: *Principles of Neurology*, 5th ed. New York, McGraw-Hill, 1993
ASBURY AK et al: *Diseases of the Nervous System*, vols I and II, 2d ed. Philadelphia, Ardmore Medical Books, Saunders, 1992

Alzheimer's disease

ARRIAGADA PV et al: Neurofibrillary tangles but not senile plaques parallel duration and severity of Alzheimer's disease. Neurology 42:631, 1992
BRAAK H, BRAAK E: Neuropathological staging of Alzheimer-related changes. Acta Neuropathol 82:239, 1991
EVANS DA et al: Prevalence of Alzheimer's disease in a community population of older persons: Higher than previously reported. JAMA 262:2551, 1989

FARRER LA et al: Segregation analysis reveals evidence of a major gene for Alzheimer disease. Am J Hum Genet 48:1026, 1991
GOATE A et al: Segregation of a missense mutation in the amyloid precursor protein with familial Alzheimer's disease. Nature 349:704, 1991
HANSEN L et al: The Lewy body variant of Alzheimer's disease: A clinical and pathologic entity. Neurology 40:1, 1990
KATZMAN R, SAITOH T: Advances in Alzheimer's disease. FASEB J 5:278, 1991
KOSIK KS: Alzheimer's disease: A cell biological perspective. Science 256:780, 1992
MCKEE AC et al: Neuritic pathology and dementia in Alzheimer's disease. Ann Neurol 30:156, 1991
PERICAK-VANCE MA et al: Linkage studies in familial Alzheimer disease: Evidence for chromosome 19 linkage. Am J Hum Genet 48:1034, 1991
SELKOE DJ: Amyloid protein and Alzheimer's disease. Sci Am 265:68, 1991
SKOOG I et al: A population-based study of dementia in 85-year-olds. N Engl J Med 328:153, 1993
ST. GEORGE-HYSLOP PH et al: Genetic linkage studies suggest that Alzheimer's disease is not a single homogeneous disorder. Nature 347:194, 1990
YANKNER BA, MESULAM M-M: β-Amyloid and the pathogenesis of Alzheimer's disease. N Engl J Med 325:1849, 1991.

Huntington's disease

BEAL MF: Does impairment of energy metabolism result in excitotoxic neuronal death in neurodegenerative illness? Ann Neurol 31:119, 1992
CHAPMAN MA: Canadian experience with predictive testing for Huntington disease: Lessons for genetic testing centers and policy makers. Am J Med Genet 42:491, 1992
DAWSON T et al: A novel neuronal messenger molecule in brain: The free radical, nitric oxide. Ann Neurol 32:297, 1992
HARPER P (ed): *Huntington's disease*. Philadelphia, Saunders, 1992
HUGGINS M et al: Ethical and legal dilemmas arising during predictive testing for adult-onset disease: The experience of Huntington's disease. Am J Hum Genet 47:4, 1990
KOROSHETZ W ET AL: The neurology of Huntington's disease, in *Movement Disorders in Neurology and Neuropsychiatry*, AB Joseph and RR Young (eds). Cambridge, 1992. pp 167–177
MARTIN JB, GUSELLA JF: Huntington's disease: Pathogenesis and management. N Engl J Med 315:1267, 1986
MEISSEN GJ et al: Predictive testing for Huntington's disease with use of a linked DNA marker. N Engl J Med 318:535, 1988
VONSATTEL JP et al: Neuropathological classification of Huntington's disease. J Neuropathol Exp Neurol 44:559, 1985

Miscellaneous

BLACK PM et al: CSF shunts for dementia, incontinence and gait disturbance. Clin Neurosurg 32:632, 1985
BRION S et al: Maladie de pick point de vue anatomo-clinique. Rev Neurol 147:693, 1991
BRYNE EJ et al: Diffuse Lewy disease: Clinical features in 15 cases. J Neurol Neurosurg Psychiatry 52:709, 1989
CRYSTAL HA et al: Antemortem diagnosis of diffuse Lewy body disease. Neurology 40:1523, 1990
GIBB WRG: Cortical Lewy body dementia. Behav Neurol 3:189, 1990
SNOWDEN JS et al: Progressive language disorder due to lobar atrophy. Ann Neurol 31:174, 1992
TISSOT R et al: *La Maladie de Pick*. Paris, Masson, 1975
VANNESTE J et al: Shunting normal-pressure hydrocephalus: Do the benefits outweigh the risks? A multicenter study and literature review. Neurology 42:54, 1992

---

371 PARKINSON'S DISEASE AND OTHER EXTRAPYRAMIDAL DISORDERS

M. FLINT BEAL / J. STEPHEN FINK / JOSEPH B. MARTIN*

PARKINSON'S DISEASE This is a common condition first named and described by James Parkinson in 1817. His remarkably complete account gives this definition:

Involuntary tremulous motion, with lessened muscular power, in parts not in action and even when supported; with a propensity to bend the trunk forward, and to pass from a walking to a running pace, the senses and intellects being uninjured.

Typically, Parkinson's disease is a disorder of middle or late life, with very gradual progression and a prolonged course. Although it

* The authors acknowledge the contribution of E.P. Richardson and R.D. Adams in previous editions.

has been seen to occur in families (the estimated familial incidence is 1 to 2 percent), it usually is sporadic. It is well recognized, however, that the epidemic encephalitis of von Economo, which occurred in a worldwide distribution in the years following World War I, was followed by a syndrome clinically almost indistinguishable from paralysis agitans. It is usual in such instances to speak of postencephalitic parkinsonism, whereas the term *Parkinson's disease* should be reserved for true paralysis agitans of unknown cause. Parkinson's disease bears no consistent relation to any known disease process such as arteriosclerosis, trauma, or intoxication (except for MPTP, see below), although such conditions have often been invoked as etiologically significant and may at times produce somewhat similar clinical manifestations.

Pathology   The most regularly observed changes have been in the aggregates of melanin-containing nerve cells in the brainstem (substantia nigra, locus coeruleus), where there are varying degrees of nerve cell loss with reactive gliosis (most pronounced in the substantia nigra) along with distinctive eosinophilic intracytoplasmic inclusions (Lewy bodies). Similar changes are seen in the nucleus basalis of Meynert. Lesions in pigmented nuclei, but without Lewy bodies, characterize the pathologic findings in postencephalitic parkinsonism, in striatonigral degeneration, and in the Shy-Drager syndrome (discussed below).

Biochemical studies show a decrease of dopamine in the caudate nucleus and putamen, emphasizing the point that Parkinson's disease can be considered an example of neuronal system disease, involving mainly the nigrostriatal dopaminergic system. Confirmation of the importance of the nigrostriatal dopaminergic system arose from observations of the effects of accidental intoxication of drug users by self-injection with 1-methyl-4-phenyl-1,2,3,6-tetrahydropyridine (MPTP), which selectively destroys dopaminergic neurons of the substantia nigra. The typical clinical manifestations of this disease resemble closely those of Parkinson's disease. The pathologic features of MPTP-induced Parkinson's disease, however, differ from those of idiopathic cases in the absence of Lewy bodies and the lack of neuronal loss in the locus coeruleus. The mechanism by which the drug kills substantia nigra neurons may provide new insights about the pathogenesis of the idiopathic illness. Recent studies show that a metabolite of MPTP blocks mitochondrial function. The possibilities of either mitochondrial impairment or excess free-radical formation are leading theories of causation in Parkinson's disease.

Clinical aspects   In its fully developed form, Parkinson's disease is easily recognized. The stooped posture, the stiffness and slowness of movement, the fixity of facial expression, and the rhythmic tremor of the limbs, which subsides on active willed movement or complete relaxation, are familiar to every clinician. Although symmetric in the later stages, the disorder typically begins asymmetrically, e.g., as a slight tremor of the fingers of one hand or in one leg. Also typical are more or less general hypokinesia and stiffness of the musculature so that even where tremor is inapparent, the disease may betray itself by a somewhat staring and immobile facial expression, a monotonous voice, a general slowness and diminution of all motor activity, and a curious lack of the little spontaneous movements of postural adjustment that are so characteristic of the normal individual. When tremor is minimal, patients often are able to alleviate it by relaxation or by movement or to hide it by keeping their hands in their pockets. The tremor is generally most pronounced in the hands but may involve the legs (and thus secondarily the trunk), lips, tongue, and neck muscles and is easily seen in the eyelids when they are lightly closed. Its frequency is 4 to 5 per second, but another faster (action) tremor (7 to 8 per second) predominates in some patients (see Chap. 21). There is never total paralysis, although this is implied by the name of the disease; nevertheless, general enfeeblement of voluntary movement is characteristic of the fully developed disorder. Generally accompanying the stopped attitude is the typical festinating gait, whereby the patient, prevented by the abnormality of postural tone from making the appropriate reflex adjustments required for effective walking, progresses with quick shuffling steps at an accelerating pace

as if to catch up with the body's center of gravity. Clinical examination of the tendon and plantar reflexes discloses no abnormalities. There are no sensory changes, although deep aching in joints and muscles may occur. Eventually, even with maximal drug therapy, patients may become so incapacitated by rigidity and tremor as to be helpless in caring for themselves. It has often been observed, however, that even severely disabled patients may, when excited or under great emotional stress, perform complex motor acts quickly and efficiently. Although the temporary alleviation under extreme provocation can never be long maintained, it is nevertheless true that the severity of the symptoms is considerably influenced by emotional factors. Despite the inherently progressive nature of the condition, much can be achieved with good medical management, and patients may continue for years to live effective, happy lives.

Although intellectual deterioration is not a consistent feature of early Parkinson's disease, dementia has been increasingly recognized to be a feature of advanced Parkinson's disease. It eventually afflicts up to one-quarter of all cases.

Differential diagnosis   In typical cases, this is not difficult. The extrapyramidal syndromes associated with most diseases of known cause or established nature, such as cerebrovascular disease, cerebral hypoxia (including carbon monoxide asphyxia), or metallic poisoning, differ from Parkinson's disease in a number of respects, such as atypical behavior or tremor, presence of signs of corticospinal tract deficit, or early onset of dementia. These clinical conditions which resemble idiopathic Parkinson's disease are collectively termed *Parkinson syndromes* or *parkinsonism*. The differentiation from postencephalitic parkinsonism may be difficult; a clear history of an attack of epidemic encephalitis (prolonged somnolence, disturbance of consciousness, diplopia) and relatively early age of onset of the disorder, little or no progression of symptoms, relative sensitivity to levodopa, and oculogyric crises may be the only clues to this diagnosis. A neurologic disorder similar to some degree to Parkinson's disease occurs with the prolonged administration of large amounts of reserpine and neuroleptic drugs as the result of their blocking action on dopaminergic transmission. This drug-induced syndrome usually subsides on discontinuation or decrease in the dosage of the drug. MPTP-induced parkinsonism persists because of the destructive effects of the drug on the nigral dopaminergic neurons. Chronic manganese poisoning and other toxins (carbon monoxide, cyanide) also may produce parkinsonism. Parkinsonism very rarely is produced by cerebral neoplasms or other focal lesions, but then only when the nigrostriatal system has been largely destroyed, with relative sparing of the corticospinal projections.

Some Parkinson-like postural and motor abnormalities may be seen following the repeated blows to the head sustained by boxers—in the "punch drunk" syndrome, in which lesions of the substantia nigra are one of the neuropathologic components. In this condition, dementia, ataxia, dysarthria, and inappropriate behavior are prominent, and neuronal cell loss with neurofibrillary tangles is evident in the cerebral cortex.

Multiple bilateral infarcts in the corticospinal pathways and central structures of the brain may produce parkinsonism (so-called arteriosclerotic parkinsonism), but careful clinical assessment of the history and findings, particularly the deep tendon reflexes, serves to distinguish this disorder from true Parkinson's disease. In their fully developed form and with adequate history, other akinetic-rigid syndromes are usually differentiated from idiopathic Parkinson's disease (see below). However, in early stages, idiopathic Parkinson's disease may be indistinguishable from other Parkinson syndromes in up to one-quarter of cases.

Treatment   An important part of any therapeutic program is the maintenance of optimal general health and neuromuscular efficiency by planned programs of exercise, activity, and rest; expert physical therapy may be of great help in achieving these ends. In addition, the patient often needs much emotional support in meeting the stress of the illness, in comprehending its nature, and in carrying on courageously in spite of it. Along with these general supportive measures, which are applicable to many chronic illnesses, patients generally require a carefully thought-out program of treatment specifically aimed at counteracting the pathophysiologic disorder that produces their disabilities.

Drug therapy should be adapted to the patient's needs, which vary with the stage of the disease and the predominant manifestation(s). Usually, anticholinergic drugs are most effective in suppressing tremor at rest, and propranolol or primidone is best for action tremor. Levodopa improves akinesia and postural imbalance; anticholinergic drugs have little effect on these two abnormalities.

The decision about whether to treat with a drug and the choice of drug(s) are influenced by the stage of the disease. The scale of Hoehn and Yahr is recommended:

Stage I: Unilateral involvement.
Stage II: Bilateral involvement but no postural abnormalities.
Stage III: Bilateral involvement with mild postural imbalance; the patient leads an independent life.
Stage IV: Bilateral involvement with postural instability; the patient requires substantial help.
Stage V: Severe, fully developed disease; the patient is restricted to bed and chair.

A recent advance in the therapy of Parkinson's disease has been the observation that treatment with deprenyl, a monoamine oxidase B inhibitor, may slow the progression of the illness. Because the drug has some symptomatic benefits, it is not possible to unequivocally conclude that it exerts a neuroprotective effect. Most clinicians now treat patients with mild disease (stages I and II) with deprenyl at a dose of 5 mg bid. The mechanism by which deprenyl is effective is uncertain; a leading theory is that it reduces free-radical formation generated from the oxidation of catecholamines.

Once a patient develops significant disability (stages III, IV, and V), the initiation of therapy with levodopa is required. Levodopa is the most effective drug available for treatment of Parkinson's disease and remains the mainstay of treatment. Levodopa is the precursor of dopamine. Treatment increases dopamine levels in the striatum and restores neurotransmitter balance between dopamine and acetylcholine. It is particularly effective in improving akinesia and rigidity; often, concurrent administration of anticholinergic medications is required to optimally control rest tremor. Postural instability frequently does not respond to levodopa. The initiation of levodopa is predictably accompanied by a rapid and dramatic reduction of symptoms and signs. A lack of response to levodopa (at doses greater than 1,000 mg/d) suggests a clinical condition other than Parkinson's disease. Levodopa is given in combination with a dopa-carboxylase inhibitor (carbidopa) which prevents destruction of levodopa in the bloodstream and peripheral tissues but does not pass the blood-brain barrier. This combination therefore makes it possible to achieve optimal effects with a smaller dosage of levodopa than would otherwise need to be used. In this way, some of the side effects of levodopa, particularly nausea and vomiting, can be greatly reduced. The combination (Sinemet) is available in ratios of 1:4 carbidopa to levodopa (25 mg/100 mg) or 1:10 (10 mg/100 mg, 25 mg/250 mg). At all stages of disability it is desirable to use the lowest dose of levodopa that gives satisfactory benefit; this decreases the chances of unwanted side effects such as dyskinesias and hallucinations. A controlled-release formulation (Sinemet CR) is now available consisting of 50 mg carbidopa and 200 mg levodopa. This formulation has a slower onset of effect but lasts for 4 to 6 h, resulting in more sustained clinical benefit. Initial therapy is started with one-half tablet bid (at least 6 h apart) and titrated upward as needed. Some patients are dissatisfied with the delayed onset of response, particularly in the morning. In this instance, the addition of a small amount of standard Sinemet, such as half a 25 mg/100 mg tablet, may be useful. A total daily dosage of levodopa from 200 to 2000 mg can be used. Although levodopa is the cornerstone of therapy, it can be combined with dopamine receptor agonists or anticholinergic drugs.

Direct-acting dopamine receptor agonists are the next most effica-cious agents. Bromocriptine and pergolide are available in the United States, while lisuride is available in some other countries. When used alone in patients with mild disease, a dose of bromocriptine of 15 to 30 mg daily is often effective. Pergolide mesylate was found to be efficacious at a mean dose of 2.6 mg daily as sole therapy. Uncontrolled trials of dopamine agonists indicate that the use of low doses of these agents in the early phase of symptomatic therapy, in combination with lower doses of levodopa, results in fewer clinical fluctuations, particularly end-of-dose loss of efficacy, and dyskinesias than with levodopa alone. The major disadvantage of the early use of agonists is the high cost of dopamine receptor agonists. The side effects of dopamine agonists are much the same as those with levodopa.

Anticholinergics and amantadine are weaker antiparkinsonian agents, but they are useful in the early stages of the illness or as adjuvant drugs later in the disease. Anticholinergics appear to be particularly useful in patients whose tremor is not completely relieved by levodopa and the dopaminergic agonists. Anticholinergic drugs reduce cholinergic transmission by blocking muscarinic receptors. Amantadine releases dopamine from presynaptic terminals and may prove useful in enhancing the effects of levodopa in patients with mild symptoms. The usual dosage is 100 mg bid; larger doses may produce side effects such as skin changes (livedo reticularis), ankle edema, and mental confusion.

Currently available anticholinergic drugs are trihexyphenidyl, benztropine, biperiden, and procyclidine. The usual dose of trihexy-phenidyl is 1 to 2 mg qid. Benztropine has both anticholinergic and antihistaminic properties; the usual dose is 0.5 to 1.0 mg tid. The optimal dose of all these medications varies for each patient and often needs to be adjusted. Low doses of these drugs cause dry mouth but few, if any, other side effects. Larger doses should be given with caution, for in the elderly they may cause confusion, visual and tactile hallucinations, narrow-angle glaucoma, and urinary retention. Anticholinergic drugs may exacerbate dementia and should be withdrawn when dementia becomes clinically evident.

It must be said that although the modern treatment of Parkinson's disease is more successful than any that was available before the introduction of levodopa, including stereotactic surgery, there are still many problems. Underlying much of the difficulty undoubtedly is the fact that none of these therapeutic measures has an effect on the underlying disease process, which consists of neuronal degeneration. Ultimately, a point seems to be reached where pharmacotherapy can no longer compensate for the loss of basal ganglia dopamine. The major difficulties consist of fluctuations or sudden variations in the response to the drugs used (the on-off response), the development of weakness or immobility (akinesia), and dyskinesias. Hallucinations, particularly in the elderly, become more frequent in some patients with moderate to advanced disease. Initial treatment is dosage reduction; however, if this is unsuccessful, the atypical neuroleptic clozapine has been used successfully. Clozapine has little or no extrapyramidal effects, but neutropenia can occur. As time passes, the therapeutic window between an effective dose of levodopa and a dose producing dyskinesias lessens. The dyskinesias consist of choreiform or choreoathetotic movements, which in the advanced stages of the disease alternate with paralyzing akinesia depending on a very narrow dosage variation (50 to 100 mg) of levodopa. Interference with absorption of levodopa may be partially responsible, since continuous intravenous infusions of levodopa result in a stable clinical state. Loss of therapeutic efficacy also occurs: a single dose which at one time was effective for 5 to 6 h may last only an hour or so. Giving smaller amounts of medication more frequently is sometimes efficacious or using a sustained-release preparation of levodopa (Sinemet CR). In addition, agents acting directly on the postsynaptic receptor, such as bromocriptine or pergolide, are sometimes more effective. It has been shown recently that temporary levodopa withdrawal, advocated as a method of dealing with the long-term complications of Parkinson's disease, carries some risk and does not result in sustained improvement in efficacy of levodopa.

As many as one-half of patients with Parkinson's disease have depressive symptoms. They should be treated along the lines suggested in Chap. 389.

The introduction of stereotactic surgery, with the placement of precisely localized focal lesions in central structures in the brain—mainly the ventrolateral thalamus or globus pallidus contralateral to the side of the major symptoms—was an important advance in the attempt to relieve the symptoms of Parkinson's disease. The success that has been achieved with levodopa has largely supplanted these procedures, which, although very beneficial in well-chosen cases, were not without risk and at times were followed by severe disability. Neurosurgical treatment of this kind can still be recommended for patients who are relatively young and who have a severe unilateral disabling or disfiguring tremor unresponsive to medication. Recent interest has focused on adrenal medullary transplants to the striatum. Although initial reports indicated favorable responses, subsequent experience in many centers has failed to confirm the earlier report. Fetal tissue transplants containing substantia nigra neurons may be more effective, but remain experimental.

OTHER AKINETIC-RIGID SYNDROMES   In addition to parkinsonism resulting from encephalitis, drugs or toxins, head trauma, or structural causes, akinetic-rigid syndromes may occur in other uncommon degenerative diseases. Often, these akinetic-rigid syndromes are accompanied by other extrapyramidal signs such as chorea, dystonia, ballism, dyskinesias, or myoclonus. The most common of these akinetic-rigid syndromes are *progressive supranuclear palsy (PSP)* and a group of disorders collectively referred to as *multiple-system degenerations*. The latter group of disorders includes the clinically heterogeneous *olivopontocerebellar atrophy (OPCA), striatonigral degeneration*, and the *Shy-Drager syndrome*; the exact clinical designation depends on the predominant clinical features. The multiple-system degenerations have in common lesions within the cerebellum, inferior olives, basal ganglia, pigmented nuclei, pontine nuclei, and spinal cord. In patients with these akinetic-rigid syndromes there is little or no clinical improvement with levodopa. Parkinsonism accompanied by ataxia, corticobulbar signs, and corticospinal deficits would be considered a type of OPCA (see Chap. 372). Signs of autonomic failure (such as orthostatic hypotension, urinary incontinence, and sexual dysfunction) are prominent in the Shy-Drager syndrome (see Chap. 379). In patients in whom parkinsonism progresses more rapidly than idiopathic Parkinson's disease, akinesia/rigidity and postural disturbances but not tremor are prominent, and in those in whom there is little or no clinical improvement with levodopa, the diagnosis of striatonigral degeneration should be considered. Usually it is not possible to clinically distinguish with certainty striatonigral degeneration from idiopathic Parkinson's disease or other akinetic-rigid syndromes. Confirmation of clinical diagnosis of striatonigral degeneration can only be made by postmortem examination of brain. Progressive supranuclear palsy is considered in more detail below. The Shy-Drager syndrome is considered in more detail in Chapter 379.

Parkinsonism may be present in other less common degenerative diseases. Hepatolenticular degeneration (Wilson's disease, Chap. 348) and acquired hepatocerebral degeneration (Chap. 377) are often accompanied by rigidity and bradykinesia. Parkinsonism accompanied by prominent apraxia, asymmetric severe rigidity, action tremor, and preserved intellect suggests the diagnosis of corticobasal ganglionic degeneration (Chap. 370). Parkinsonism also may be present in other degenerative diseases in which dementia is a prominent feature. These disorders include Alzheimer's disease, Pick's disease, Parkinson-dementia-amyotrophic lateral sclerosis (ALS) complex of Guam, Creutzfeldt-Jakob disease, normal-pressure hydrocephalus, a rigid form of Huntington's disease, progressive supranuclear palsy, Hallervorden-Spatz disease, Wilson's disease, and some metabolic diseases (Lafora body disease, ceroid lipofuscinosis) (see Chaps. 370 and 372).

PROGRESSIVE SUPRANUCLEAR PALSY (STEELE-RICHARDSON-OLSZEWSKI SYNDROME)   This disorder, first clearly described in 1963 by Richardson, Steele, and Olszewski, occurs in elderly individuals in approximately the same age period as Parkinson's disease. Moreover, it is among the group of parkinsonian patients that most of the examples of this disease are to be found.

Pathology   A loss of neurons and gliosis are found on postmortem examination in the tectum and tegmentum of the midbrain, the subthalamic nuclei of Luys, the vestibular nuclei, and to some extent the ocular nuclei. A characteristic finding is the presence of neurofibrillary tangles similar to those of Alzheimer's disease on light-microscopic examination but differing from them on electron microscopy in that they are composed of straight rather than paired helical filaments. The cause of the disease is unknown. A slow virus has been suspected, but attempts to transfer it to monkeys by the intracerebral inoculation of brain tissue have failed.

Clinical manifestations   The clinical features are quite distinctive: disturbances of balance and gait with unexpected falls; rigidity of the neck and other trunk muscles, resembling Parkinson's disease; "masking" of the face; reduction in the volume of the voice; extreme flexion or extension dystonia of the neck; and difficulty in looking down—all these are early symptoms, and any one of them may first bring the patient to a physician. In contrast to idiopathic Parkinson's disease, rest tremor is usually absent in progressive supranuclear palsy. Ophthalmoplegia has been regarded as the cardinal clinical sign of the disease. Typically there is initial impairment of vertical saccadic movements and a loss of the fast component of optokinetic nystagmus usually affecting downward more than upward gaze. With progression of the disease, horizontal eye movements are affected, with oculovestibular reflexes preserved. Symptoms progress over months and years, until the patient becomes virtually anarthric with total loss of voluntary control of eye movements and severe cervical and truncal rigidity. Dementia is usually mild, with forgetfulness, slowing of thought processes, apathy, and impaired ability to manipulate acquired knowledge. There are no impairments of vision, hearing, somatic sensation, or voluntary power, and signs of corticospinal involvement are minimal or absent. The diagnosis should be considered whenever an elderly patient begins to fall repeatedly and inexplicably and has extrapyramidal symptoms with a rigid neck and paralysis of conjugate or vertical gaze.

Treatment   Treatment has been largely unsuccessful. Relatively little benefit comes from the administration of the antiparkinsonian group of drugs, although they should be tried. Occasionally, levodopa, or a combination of levodopa with an anticholinergic drug, has helped to diminish some of the symptoms. Idazoxan, which increases norepinephrine neurotransmission, improves motor function in some patients, but it is not available for clinical usage.

TORSION DYSTONIA (TORSION SPASM; DYSTONIA MUSCULORUM DEFORMANS)   This is a syndrome of sustained muscular contraction frequently causing twisting and repetitive movements that result in abnormal, at times bizarre, postures of the limbs and trunk. Eventually these postures become more or less fixed. Recent studies using segregation analysis have shown that in Jewish and non-Jewish families, idiopathic early-onset generalized dystonia is transmitted as an autosomal dominant disorder with variable penetrance. Genetic studies have shown linkage to a region on chromosome 9. It is to these cases, both hereditary and sporadic, that the term *torsion dystonia* (torsion spasm, dystonia musculorum deformans) is correctly applied. When this disorder occurs in late-adult life, it tends to be focal in onset. In cases of early onset, dystonia tends to generalize. The cause and pathogenesis remain unknown.

Dystonias in which the etiology is known are called *secondary dystonias*. Underlying the secondary dystonias may be any of several pathologic conditions, including lesions of neonatal hypoxia, strokes, Wilson's disease, the pigmented lesions of Hallevorden-Spatz, GM_1 gangliosidosis, ataxia-telangiectasia, or kernicterus.

Pathology   Few cases of torsion dystonia not due to one of the definable disease processes indicated above have been adequately studied neuropathologically. Reported results from these cases have led to uncertainty as to what the pathologic-anatomic basis of the clinical state might be, although it was generally assumed that the basal ganglia were diseased. A careful study by Zeman and Dyken, which included comparison of the findings in patients with the disease with control material, failed to demonstrate any neuropathologic abnormality to which the clinical changes could reasonably be attributed. These negative findings, which are perhaps surprising, must not be interpreted as indicating that there is "no disease" in the brain, but rather that the pathologic state is not one that can be disclosed by the usual histopathologic techniques. It may well be that more careful quantitative assessments of certain populations of neurons and studies of the pathophysiology of neurotransmitters will result in further elucidation of this disease.

Clinical manifestations   A descriptive classification of the motor abnormalities of dystonia is given in Chap. 21. In the early stages, the involuntary muscular contractions are intermittent and variable in location and severity, but they typically interfere with motor performance by superimposing an unwanted posture on parts in use. One leg may briefly be pulled into a flexed or extended position or one shoulder elevated. Later the lingual, pharyngeal, neck, and thoracic muscles participate, and grimacing may occur. These latter also may be the first and only signs of disease for several years. Progression may be relatively rapid in cases with onset during early childhood but is slow in those beginning in late childhood or adult life. The end result is extreme disability, with grossly distorted postures of the trunk and contractures of the limbs. Affection of face and tongue muscles results in faulty articulation of speech, which eventually becomes incomprehensible. The tendon and plantar reflexes are normal.

Early-onset dystonia characteristically makes its appearance in childhood after a preceding period of normalcy. Typically it becomes evident first in the lower limbs and then evolves, sometimes relatively rapidly, into the generalized state of severe incapacity described above. When onset is in adulthood, it tends to appear first in the upper limbs and to remain more restricted in its extent than the early-onset variety, and progression is less relentless. The late-life sporadic cases are generally similar in character.

A rare form is *dopa-responsive dystonia*. This syndrome appears to be inherited in an autosomal dominant manner with reduced penetrance. Onset is in childhood, with dystonia usually affecting gait. There is diurnal fluctuation with worsening as the day progresses. Most individuals later develop parkinsonism. There is a dramatic response to levodopa therapy.

FOCAL DYSTONIAS   In addition to the generalized dystonias noted above, there is a group of focal or segmental dystonias which appear sporadically in adult life. Their clearly involuntary nature and lack of susceptibility to willed control by the patient distinguish them from common tics, habit spasms, and mannerisms. They have often been erroneously interpreted as manifestations of hysteria. If the muscle contraction is frequent and prolonged, aching pain accompanies it—for which the spasm may mistakenly be blamed.

The most frequent and familiar type of focal dystonia is *spasmodic torticollis*. This is a disorder of adults that afflicts women somewhat more frequently than men. It consists of an involuntary turning of the head to one side—intermittent at first, then gradually worsening to the point of being more or less continuous. In some cases, torticollis is the first manifestation of a generalized dystonia, but more usually it remains focal and segmental.

Another frequent focal dystonia of adults is exemplified by *writer's cramp*, in which the dystonic postures and movements occur only during the performance of specific acts, to the extent that carrying out the act in the usual way, such as writing with a pen or pencil, becomes impossible, while other motor activities using the same musculature are unimpaired. An analogous disorder sometimes afflicts musicians.

The combination of blepharospasm and oromandibular dystonia—*cranial dystonia*—is sometimes referred to as Meige's syndrome. When the throat and respiratory muscles are involved, this interferes with speech production, resulting in spasmodic dysphonia. The

muscles of the neck are variably affected. It should be recalled that similar dystonic states (facial-cervical and more extreme dyskinesias) can result from the use of phenothiazine and similar drugs. This sometimes persists after discontinuation of the medication as *tardive dystonia*—a troublesome condition that may resist all forms of treatment.

Differential diagnosis   The treatable condition of hepatolenticular degeneration (Wilson's disease) should be seriously considered in any case presenting these motor symptoms, and appropriate measures should be undertaken for its investigation (see Chap. 348). The progressive course and possibly, the family history differentiate the degenerative group of dystonias from the "secondary" dystonias resulting from infections or metabolic disorders occurring at birth or later and structural lesions of the brain such as occur following trauma, strokes, or neoplasms. Hallervorden-Spatz disease, however, cannot be distinguished on clinical grounds alone (see Chap. 370). Rare instances of GM_1 gangliosidosis or other lipid storage diseases may begin in adult life with a dystonic syndrome, and drug-induced (tardive) dystonia must be considered in all cases of focal or generalized dystonia in adults, especially if they have or have had a psychiatric illness.

Treatment   This is extremely difficult and often unsatisfactory. In the generalized dystonias, pharmacotherapy should certainly be attempted and, in most patients, needs to be individualized. Marsden and Fahn, whose experience with this disorder is extensive, suggest beginning with an anticholinergic agent such as trihexyphenidyl or ethopropazine and very gradually increasing the dosage until either benefit ensues or intolerable side effects appear. They found that the response in children (who may be able to take as much as 80 mg/d of trihexyphenidyl) was better than in adults, who tolerated the high doses less well, generally because of mental disturbances. In their experience, the next best group of drugs for ameliorating dystonic spasms are the benzodiazepines (such as diazepam or clonazepam), which likewise are used in high dosage after a very gradual introduction and increase (up to 80 mg diazepam daily). Again, children are more tolerant of the side effects (mainly drowsiness). A combination of anticholinergics and benzodiazepines may work out best. Other drugs—both dopaminergic agonists and antagonists, as well as carbamazepine—have been used, occasionally with success. Neuroleptics (dopaminergic antagonists) such as haloperidol, perhaps together with dopamine-depleting drugs (reserpine, tetrabenazine) and anticholinergics, may be useful in the treatment of some refractory dystonias. Dopa-responsive dystonia shows a dramatic response to levodopa, which may warrant a therapeutic trial if this diagnosis is suspected.

The symptoms of the focal dystonias, if not severe, may be more acceptable to the patient than prolonged trials with various drugs or surgical intervention. The most promising therapy for focal dystonia has been injections of botulinum toxin, which blocks acetylcholine release at the neuromuscular junction. Beneficial effects last on average 2 to 6 months. The most responsive of the focal dystonias to botulinum toxin treatments is blepharospasm. Denervative surgical procedures may in some cases be beneficial if only a restricted group of muscles is involved (as in torticollis). Medical management must be adapted to the individual patient's needs. The medications used for the treatment of generalized dystonias also may be useful for some focal dystonias; however, some focal dystonias (e.g., writer's cramp) are uniformly unresponsive to medications.

FAMILIAL TREMOR   One of the most common hereditary disorders of the human nervous system is that which gives rise to a fast-frequency (6 to 8 per second) action tremor. This may appear at any age but more often during adolescence and adult years; once started, it lasts throughout life. The heredity is dominant. Probably all cases are not the same, for some patients have tremors of slower frequency, looking more like those of Parkinson's disease, but lacking the slowness of movement, rigidity, and flexed postures of that disorder. In patients of advanced age it is called *senile tremor*. Consumption of alcohol suppresses the fast-frequency forms, as does a beta-adrenergic blocking agent (propranolol) in doses of 20 to 40 mg three times daily. The slightly slower rhythmic action tremors with frequencies of approximately 6 per second do not consistently respond to propranolol or alcohol. Primidone 50 mg at bedtime has recently been found to be effective and has been advocated for use as initial therapy. If there is no response after 1 week, the dose should be increased gradually up to 250 mg at bedtime.

GILLES DE LA TOURETTE SYNDROME This condition, of unknown cause and uncertain pathology, presents with multiple tics, associated with snorting, sniffing, and involuntary vocalizations. It begins in childhood, usually as isolated tics, which are at first difficult to distinguish from habit spasms. Progression occurs over years, and other behavioral findings appear; compulsive touching of others, repeating of words or phrases, and explosive utterance of obscenities (coprolalia). Careful attention to other members of the family has given evidence that the disease is hereditary, with an autosomal dominant pattern of transmission. Obsessive compulsive disorder appears to be an alternate phenotypic expression of the gene in these families.

The course of the illness is unpredictable. In some cases associated mild neurologic abnormalities are found with hyperactivity, disorders of attention, and abnormal psychologic tests. Dementia does not occur. In some patients the condition abates, in others it progresses, leading to serious disability. Treatment is only partially satisfactory. Haloperidol has received the most clinical attention, but side effects are often unacceptable and it should be used only in severe cases and in the smallest effective dosage: 0.25 to 0.5 mg daily. Pimozide has recently been approved for treatment of Gilles de la Tourette. It causes fewer side effects than haloperidol but can cause widening of the QT interval and sudden death at high doses. Therefore, the electrocardiogram should be followed and the dose limited to 0.3 mg/kg per day. Clonidine has proved effective in some cases.

REFERENCES

General

ADAMS JH et al (eds): *Greenfield's Neuropathology*, 5th ed. New York, Wiley, 1992
ADAMS RD, VICTOR M: *Principles of Neurology*, 5th ed. New York, McGraw-Hill, 1993
ASBURY AK et al: *Diseases of the Nervous System*, vols 1 and 2, 2d ed. Philadelphia, Ardmore Medical Books, Saunders, 1992
MARSDEN CD, FAHN S (eds): *Movement Disorders*. London, Butterworth, 1987
WEINER WJ, LANG AE: *Movement Disorders: A Comprehensive Survey*. Mt. Kisco, N.Y., Futura, 1988

Parkinson's disease

BEAL MF: Does impairment of energy metabolism result in excitotoxic neuronal death in neurodegenerative illnesses? Ann Neurol 31:119, 1992
BLOEM BR et al: The MPTP model: Versatile contributions to the treatment of idiopathic Parkinson's disease. J Neurol Sci 97:273, 1990
FAHN S et al (eds): *Recent Advances in Parkinson's Disease*. New York, Raven Press, 1986
FRIEDMAN JH, LANNON MC: Clozapine in the treatment of psychosis in Parkinson's disease. Neurology 39:1219, 1989
HOEHN MN, YAHR MD: Parkinsonism: Onset, progression and mortality. Neurology 17:427, 1967
HUGHES AJ et al: Accuracy of clinical diagnosis of idiopathic Parkinson's disease: A clinico-pathological study of 100 cases. J Neurol Neurosurg Psychiatry 55:181, 1992
LINDVALL O et al: Transplantation of fetal dopamine neurons in Parkinson's disease: One-year clinical and neurophysiological observations in two patients with putaminal implants. Ann Neurol 31:155, 1992
MARSDEN CD: Parkinson's disease. Lancet 1:948, 1990
MOURADIAN MM et al: Modification of central dopaminergic mechanisms by continuous levodopa therapy for advanced Parkinson's disease. Ann Neurol 27:18, 1990
PARKINSON STUDY GROUP: Effect of deprenyl on the progression of disability in early Parkinson's disease. N Engl J Med 321:1364, 1989
RIEDERER P et al: Recent advances in pharmacological therapy of Parkinson's disease. Adv Neurol 60:626, 1993
STANDAERT DG, STERN MB: Update on the management of Parkinson's disease. Med Clin North Am 77:169, 1993

Miscellaneous

ADAMS RD et al: Striatonigral degeneration. J Neuropathol Exp Neurol 23:584, 1964
BERKOVIC SF et al: Progressive myoclonic epilepsies: Specific causes and diagnosis. N Engl J Med 315:296, 1986
CHAN J et al: Idiopathic cervical dystonia: Clinical characteristics. Movement Dis 6:119, 1991

GHIKA J et al: Idazoxan treatment in progressive supranuclear palsy. Neurology 41:986, 1991
GILMAN S: Medical progress: Advances in neurology. N Engl J Med 326:1608, 1992
GOETZ CG et al: Adult tics in Gilles de la Tourette's syndrome: Description and risk factors. Neurology 42:784, 1992
GREENE P et al: Double-blind, placebo-controlled trial of botulinum toxin injections for the treatment of spasmodic torticollis. Neurology 40:1213, 1990
IIVANAINEN M, HIMBERG J-J: Valproate and clonazepam in the treatment of severe progressive myoclonus epilepsy. Arch Neurol 39:236, 1982
JANKOVIC J et al: Cervical dystonia: Clinical findings and associated movement disorders. Neurology 41:1088, 1991
————, SCHWARTZ K: Botulinum toxin injections for cervical dystonia. Neurology 40:277, 1990
KRAMER PL et al: Dystonia gene in Ashkenazi Jewish population is located on chromosome 9q32-34. Ann Neurol 27:114, 1990
LOGIGIAN EL et al: Myoclonus epilepsy in two brothers: Clinical features and neuropathology of a unique syndrome. Brain 190:411, 1986
MCGEER PL, MCGEER PL: The dystonias. Can J Neurol Sci 15:447, 1988
MESULAM MM, PETERSEN RC: Treatment of Gilles de la Tourette syndrome: Eight-year, practice-based experience in predominantly adult population. Neurology 37:1828, 1987
NYGAARD TG et al: Dopa-responsive dystonia: Long-term treatment response and prognosis. Neurology 41:174, 1991
SETHI KD et al: Hallervorden-Spatz syndrome: Clinical and magnetic resonance imaging correlations. Ann Neurol 24:692, 1988
SINGER HS, WALKUP JT: Tourette syndrome and other tic disorders: Diagnosis, pathophysiology, and treatment. Medicine 70:15, 1991
STEELE JC: Progressive supranuclear palsy. Brain 95:693, 1972
WATTS RL et al: Corticobasal ganglionic degeneration. Neurology 35:178, 1985
ZEMAN W, DYKEN P: Dystonia musculorum deformans: Clinical, genetic and pathoanatomical studies. Psychiatr Neurol Neurochir 70:77, 1967

372   MOTOR NEURON DISEASE AND THE PROGRESSIVE ATAXIAS

ROBERT H. BROWN, JR.

MOTOR NEURON DISEASE (MUSCULAR WEAKNESS AND WASTING WITHOUT SENSORY CHANGES)

AMYOTROPHIC LATERAL SCLEROSIS Amyotrophic lateral sclerosis (ALS) is the most common form of progressive motor neuron disease (Table 372-1). It is a prototypic example of a neuronal system disease and is arguably the most devastating of the neurodegenerative disorders.

Pathology The pathology of the motor neuron degenerative disorders affects two classes of neurons: lower motor neurons (consisting of anterior horn cells in the spinal cord and their brainstem homologues innervating bulbar muscles) and upper motor neurons (emanating from layer five of the motor cortex to descend via the corticospinal and corticobulbar tracts to synapse directly with lower motor neurons or indirectly via interneurons) (see Chap. 21). Typical ALS is characterized by progressive loss of both categories of motor neurons, although variants may involve specific subsets of motor neurons, particularly early in the course of the illness. Thus, in *bulbar palsy* and *spinal muscular atrophy* (or progressive muscular atrophy), the lower motor neurons of brainstem and spinal cord, respectively, are most severely involved, whereas *pseudobulbar palsy* and *primary lateral sclerosis* affect predominantly upper motor neurons innervating the brainstem and spinal cord. The loss of motor neurons is not accompanied by any distinctive or unique cytopathologic features. The affected cells undergo shrinkage, often with some excessive accumulation of the pigmented lipid (lipofuscin) that normally develops in these cells with advancing age, and they eventually disappear. Focal enlargement of proximal motor axons is frequently seen; ultrastructurally, these "spheroids" are composed of accumulations of neurofilaments. Beyond some astroglial proliferation, which is the inevitable accompaniment of all degenerative processes in the central nervous system (CNS), the interstitial and supportive tissues and the macrophage system remain inactive, and there is no inflammation.

TABLE 372-1   Classification of motor neuron disorders

SPORADIC

Upper and lower motor neurons
   Amyotrophic lateral sclerosis
Predominantly upper motor neurons
   Primary lateral sclerosis
Predominantly lower motor neurons
   Multifocal motor neuropathy with conduction block
   Motor neuropathy with paraproteinemia
   Motor-predominant peripheral neuropathies
Other
   Associated with other degenerative disorders
      Olivopontocerebellar atrophy
      Azorean (Machado-Joseph) disease
   Secondary motor neuron disorders (see Table 372-2)

FAMILIAL

Familial amyotrophic lateral sclerosis
   Autosomal dominant
   Autosomal recessive (juvenile)
Spinal muscular atrophies
   SMA I: Infantile: Werdnig-Hoffman disease
   SMA II: Childhood onset
   SMA III: Adolescent onset: Wohlfart-Kugelberg-Welander disease
Familial spastic paraparesis (FSP)
   Familial HTLV-I myelopathy
   Isolated FSP
   Complicated FSP
Hereditary biochemical disorders
   Superoxide dismutase deficiency
   Hexosaminidase A and B deficiency
   Androgen receptor mutation (Kennedy's syndrome)
Miscellaneous
   Arthrogryposis multiplex congenita
   Progressive juvenile bulbar palsy (Fazio-Londe)

The death of the peripheral motor neurons in the brainstem and spinal cord leads to denervation and consequent atrophy of the corresponding muscle fibers. Histochemical and electrophysiologic evidence indicates that in the early phases of the illness denervated muscle may be reinnervated by sprouting of preserved nearby distal motor axon terminals, although reinnervation in this disease is less extensive than in other disorders affecting motor neurons (e.g., poliomyelitis, peripheral neuropathy). As denervation progresses, there is shrinkage of the musculature and muscle fiber atrophy. This muscular atrophy is designated *amyotrophy* in the name for the disease. The loss of upper motor neurons in the cortex results in disappearance of their long axons and myelin sheaths in the corticospinal and corticobulbar tracts (see Chap. 21). The loss of fibers in the corticospinal tracts of the spinal cord, together with the accompanying astrogliosis, imparts a firmness (sclerosis) to the spinal cord (lateral sclerosis). Nerve fiber loss is more extensive in the distal parts of the affected tracts in the lower spinal cord than in the more proximal parts, such as the internal capsule, suggesting that affected neurons undergo a process of ''dying back.'' The disease clearly affects both large pyramidal neurons (Betz cells) of the motor cortex in the precentral gyrus and other long projection neurons involved in voluntary movement and located in the cerebral cortex and selected subcortical nuclei.

The remarkable selectivity of neuronal cell death entirely spares the sensory systems, the neural systems that control coordination of movement, and the components of the brain that are needed for cognition. However, immunostaining indicates that neurons bearing ubiquitin, a marker for degeneration, are also detected in nonmotor systems. Selectivity within the motor system is also seen; motor neurons required for ocular motility (oculomotor, trochlear, and abducens) remain unaffected, as do the parasympathetic neurons in the sacral spinal cord (the nucleus of Onufrowicz or Onuf) which innervate the sphincters of the bowel and bladder.

Clinical manifestations   The manifestations of motor neuron disease are variable depending on whether upper or lower motor neurons are more prominently involved. With lower motor neuron cell death and early denervation, the first evidence of the disease typically is insidiously developing asymmetric weakness, usually first evident distally in one of the limbs. A careful history will often disclose the recent development of cramping with volitional movements, typically in the early hours of the morning (e.g., while stretching in bed). Weakness caused by denervation is associated with progressive wasting and atrophy of muscles and, particularly early in the illness, spontaneous twitching of motor units, or *fasciculations*. In the hands, a preponderance of extensor over flexor weakness is very common. When the initial denervation involves bulbar rather than limb muscles, the first symptoms are difficulty with chewing, swallowing, and movements of the face and tongue. Early involvement of the muscles of respiration may lead to respiratory compromise before the disease is far advanced elsewhere.

With prominent corticospinal involvement, there is hyperactivity of the muscle stretch reflexes (tendon jerks) and, often, spastic resistance to passive movements of the affected limbs. The patient complains of muscle stiffness. Involvement of corticobulbar projections innervating the brainstem results in dysarthria and exaggeration of the motor expressions of emotion leading to involuntary weeping or laughing (*pseudobulbar affect*).

Virtually any muscle group may be the first to show signs of the disease, but as time passes, more and more muscles become involved, until ultimately the disorder takes on a symmetric distribution in all regions. It is characteristic of ALS that, regardless of whether the initial disease involves upper or lower motor neurons, both categories are eventually implicated. Indeed, in the absence of clear involvement of both types of motor neurons, the diagnosis of ALS is questionable. Even in the late stages of the illness, sensory, bowel and bladder, and cognitive functions are preserved. Dementia is not usually a component of ALS, although it may occur in a small subset of patients. Similarly, even when there is severe brainstem disease, ocular motility is spared until the very late stages of the illness.

The illness is relentlessly progressive, leading ultimately to death (usually from respiratory paralysis). In most large series, median survival is from 3 to 5 years. There are rare reports of stabilization or even regression of ALS.

Epidemiology   There are approximately 1 to 3 per 100,000 new cases and about 3 to 5 per 100,000 total cases per year in populations worldwide. Several endemic foci of higher prevalence are described in the western Pacific (e.g., in specific regions of Guam and Papua New Guinea). In the United States and Europe, it is agreed that males are somewhat more frequently affected than females. Although ALS is overwhelmingly a sporadic disorder, approximately 5 to 10 percent of cases are inherited as an autosomal dominant trait.

Differential diagnosis   Because ALS is currently untreatable, it is imperative that potentially remediable causes of motor neuron dysfunction be excluded (Table 372-2). Atypical features that should alert the physician include (1) restriction of disease to either upper or lower motor neurons, (2) involvement of neurons other than motor neurons, and (3) evidence of motor neuronal conduction block on electrophysiologic testing (see Chap. 366). *Compression of the cervical spinal cord* or *cervicomedullary junction* from tumors in the cervical spinal canal or at the foramen magnum or from cervical spondylosis with osteophytes can give rise to weakness, wasting, and fasciculations in the upper limbs and spasticity in the legs, thus closely resembling ALS. The absence of cranial nerve involvement may be helpful in differentiation, although some compressive lesions in the foramen magnum may implicate the twelfth cranial (hypoglossal) nerve as well, with weakness and atrophy of the tongue. Absence of pain or of sensory changes, normal function of bowel and bladder, normal imaging studies of the spine, and absence of changes in cerebrospinal fluid (CSF) all favor ALS rather than spinal cord compression. If doubt exists, magnetic resonance imaging (MRI) and contrast myelography should be performed to visualize the cervical spinal cord and the cervicomedullary junction.

Another entity in the differential diagnosis of ALS is multifocal *motor neuropathy with conduction block* (MMCB). In this disorder, lower motor neuron function is regionally and chronically disrupted

TABLE 372-2   Etiology and investigation of secondary motor neuron disorders

Diagnostic categories	Investigations
Structural lesions	MRI scan head (including
Parasagittal or foramen magnum tumors	foramen magnum), cervical spine
Cervical spondylosis	
Chiari malformation or syrinx	
Spinal cord arteriovenous malformation	
Infections	CSF examination, culture
Bacterial–tetanus, Lyme	Serum Lyme titers
Viral–poliomyelitis, herpes zoster	Antiviral antibody titers
Retroviral myelopathy	HTLV-I
Intoxications, physical agents	24-h urine for heavy metals;
Toxins–lead, aluminum, other metals	serum, urine for lead or aluminum
Drugs–strychnine, phenytoin	
Electric shock	
X-irradiation	
Immunologic mechanisms	Complete blood count,
Plasma cell dyscrasias	sedimentation rate,
Autoimmune polyradiculoneuropathy	immunoprotein electrophoresis, anti-G_{M1} antibodies
Paraneoplastic	Anti-Hu antibody, bone marrow
Paracarcinomatous	biopsy
Paralymphomatous	
Metabolic	Fasting blood sugar (FBS),
Hypoglycemia	routine chemistries, including
Hyperparathyroidism	calcium
Hyperthyroidism	Thyroid functions
Deficiency of folate, vitamins B_{12}, E	Vitamin B_{12}, folate levels
Malabsorption	24-h stool fat, carotene, prothrombin time
Hereditary biochemical disorders	
Superoxide dismutase	Red cell SOD1 deficiency
Androgen receptor defect (Kennedy's disease)	Abnormal –CAG– repeat insert
Hexosaminidase deficiency	Lysosomal enzyme screen
Infantile α-glucosidase deficiency (Pompe's disease)	
Hyperlipidemia	Lipid electrophoresis
Hyperglycinuria	Urine and serum amino acids

by remarkably focal blocks in nerve conduction. Many cases have associated elevations in serum titers of mono- and polyclonal antibodies to ganglioside G_{M1}; it is hypothesized that the antibodies may selectively produce focal, paranodal demyelination of motor neurons. MMCB is not typically associated with corticospinal signs. In contrast to ALS, MMCB may respond dramatically to intravenous gamma globulin or chemotherapy; it is thus imperative that MMCB be excluded when considering the diagnosis of ALS.

A diffuse *lower motor axonal neuropathy* mimicking ALS sometimes evolves as a component of hematopoietic disorders such as lymphoma. The underlying marrow pathology is often signaled by the presence of an M-component in serum, which, in this clinical setting, should prompt consideration of a bone marrow biopsy. Lyme disease also may cause an axonal lower motor neuropathy.

Other treatable disorders that occasionally can mimic ALS are *chronic lead poisoning* and *thyrotoxicosis*. These disorders may be suggested by the patient's social or occupational history or by unusual clinical features. When the family history is positive, *inherited enzyme disorders* such as hexosaminidase A or α-glucosidase deficiency must be excluded (see Chap. 349). These are readily identified by appropriate laboratory tests. *Benign fasciculations* are commonly a source of concern to the patient. On inspection, they may resemble the fascicular twitchings that accompany motor neuron degeneration. Absence of weakness, atrophy, or denervation on clinical and electrophysiologic examination excludes ALS or other serious neurologic disease. *Poliomyelitis* may lead to a delayed, progressive deterioration of motor neurons which presents clinically with progressive weakness, atrophy, and fasciculations. Its cause is unknown but is thought to reflect sublethal prior injury to motor neurons by poliovirus (see Chap. 375).

Rarely, ALS develops concurrently with features indicative of more widespread neurodegeneration. Thus otherwise typical ALS patients may present with a parkinsonian movement disorder or dementia. It remains unclear whether this reflects the unlikely simultaneous occurrence of two disorders or a primary defect triggering two forms of neurodegeneration. The latter is suggested by the observation that multisystem neurodegenerative diseases may be inherited; rare families are reported with ALS and parkinsonism or ALS and dementia with features of Pick's disease (see Chap. 371).

Familial ALS   Several forms of motor neuron disease are inherited (see Table 372-1). Two disorders selectively involve corticospinal and lower motor neurons. The most common is familial ALS. Inherited as an autosomal dominant trait, it is clinically indistinguishable from sporadic ALS. Family linkage studies with DNA probes suggest that there is more than one gene for autosomal dominant ALS; one gene, superoxide dismutase, is on chromosome 21 (see also Chap. 364). There is also a recessive form of hereditary ALS. Unlike sporadic ALS, this begins in childhood and entails very prolonged survival; a locus for this disease has been genetically mapped to the long arm of chromosome 2. *Kennedy's syndrome* is another familial, adult-onset disorder that may mimic ALS (see below).

Treatment   There is no treatment for ALS. However, several of the disorders listed in Table 372-2 which resemble ALS are treatable; for this reason, a careful search for such forms of secondary motor neuron disease is warranted. Recently, several motor neuron trophic factors have been cloned and biologically characterized; at least two, ciliary neurotrophic factor (CNTF) and insulin-like growth factor 1 (IGF-1), are in clinical trials in ALS. A variety of rehabilitative aids may substantially assist ALS patients. Foot-drop splints facilitate ambulation by avoiding tripping and by obviating excessive hip flexion. Finger-extension splints can potentiate grip. Respiratory support may be life-sustaining. For patients electing against long-term ventilation by tracheostomy, positive-pressure ventilation by mouth or nose may provide transient (several weeks) relief from hypercarbia and hypoxia.

OTHER LOWER MOTOR NEURON DISORDERS   In the varieties of motor neuron disease grouped under this heading, the peripheral motor neurons are affected without evidence of involvement of the corticospinal motor system (Table 372-1).

X-linked spinobulbar muscular atrophy (Kennedy's disease) Kennedy's disease is an X-linked lower motor neuron disorder in which progressive weakness and wasting of limb and bulbar muscles begins in midadult life and is conjoined with androgen insensitivity manifested by gynecomastia and reduced fertility (see Chap. 339). A critical finding distinguishing this disorder from ALS is the absence of signs of hyperreflexia and spasticity. The molecular defect is an expanded trinucleotide repeat (–CAG–) in the first exon of the androgen receptor gene on the X chromosome; this abnormality is readily demonstrated on a small sample of DNA obtained from peripheral blood leukocytes. An inverse correlation appears to exist between the number of –CAG– repeats and the age of onset of the disease.

Adult Tay Sach's disease   Hexosaminidase enzyme mutations may cause adult-onset, predominantly lower motor neuronopathies that closely mimic ALS. The condition is slowly progressive. Dysarthria and cerebellar atrophy may occur. The latter may be accompanied by signs of cerebellar incoordination. Rarely, spasticity also may be present (Chap. 349).

Spinal muscular atrophy   The spinal muscular atrophies (SMA) are a group of familial disorders all associated with selective lower motor neuron diseases with early age of onset. Despite some phenotypic variability (largely in age of onset), the defect in the majority of families with SMA is genetically linked to a locus on the proximal long arm of chromosome 5 (see also Chap. 364). Each disorder is transmitted as an autosomal recessive trait. Neuropathologically, SMA is characterized by extensive loss of large motor neurons; biopsied muscle reveals evidence of denervation atrophy. *Infantile SMA (SMA I, Werdnig-Hoffmann disease)* has an early onset and is rapidly fatal. In some instances it is apparent even before birth, as indicated by decreased fetal movements late in the third trimester. Although alert, afflicted infants are weak and floppy (hypotonic) and lack muscle stretch reflexes. Death generally ensues within the first year of life. When the family history is unclear, it is difficult in the early weeks and months to distinguish SMA I from benign congenital hypotonia. An electromyogram is helpful by showing denervation, which does not occur in the congenital hypotonias. *Chronic childhood SMA (SMA II)* begins in childhood and progresses slowly. *Juvenile SMA (SMA III, Wohlfart-Kugelberg-Welander disease)* manifests during late childhood or early adolescence and runs a slow, indolent course. Unlike most denervating diseases, in this chronic disorder weakness is greatest in the proximal muscles; indeed, the pattern of weakness may suggest a primary myopathy such as limb girdle dystrophy (see Chap. 385). Electrophysiologic and muscle biopsy evidence of denervation distinguish SMA III from the myopathies.

Miscellaneous forms of lower motor neuron disease In individual families, other syndromes characterized by selective lower motor neuron dysfunction in an SMA-like pattern have been described. There are rare X-linked and autosomal dominant forms of SMA. There is also an ALS variant of juvenile onset, the Fazio-Londe syndrome, which involves mainly the musculature innervated by the brainstem. A component of lower motor neuron dysfunction is also found in some patients with multisystem degenerative disorders such as Machado-Joseph's disease and the related olivopontocerebellar degenerations (see below).

UPPER MOTOR NEURON DISORDERS   Primary lateral sclerosis (PLS) This exceedingly rare disorder arises sporadically in adults in middle to late life. It is characterized by progressive spastic weakness of the limbs, preceded or followed by spastic dysarthria and dysphagia, indicating combined involvement of the corticospinal and corticobulbar tracts. Fasciculations, amyotrophy, and sensory changes are absent; neither electromyography nor muscle biopsy show denervation. On neuropathologic examination there is selective loss of the large pyramidal cells in the precentral gyrus and degeneration of the corticospinal and corticobulbar projections. The lower motor neurons and other neuronal systems are spared. The course of PLS is variable; while long-term survival is documented, the course may be as aggressive as in ALS with approximately 3-year survival from onset to death. Early in its course, PLS raises the question of a diagnosis of multiple sclerosis or other demyelinating diseases such as adrenoleukodystrophy. A myelopathy suggestive of PLS occurs rarely with CNS infection with the retrovirus HTLV-I (see Chap. 375). The clinical course and laboratory testing will distinguish these possibilities. The myelopathy associated with HIV infection occasionally may cause spasticity without sensory changes.

Familial spastic paraplegia (FSP) This disorder is transmitted in most families as an autosomal dominant trait. It is characterized by progressive spastic weakness beginning in the distal lower extremities. It first causes symptoms in the third or fourth decades and typically has long survival with slow progression and with minimal involvement of the arms or of the respiratory musculature. Late in the illness there is commonly urinary urgency and incontinence, sometimes as well as fecal incontinence, but with preservation in males of sexual function. In pure forms of autosomal dominant FSP, ataxia, posterior column sensory loss, and amyotrophy are absent or minimal; however, in some patients, minor sensory changes (impaired vibration and position sense) may be observed in late stages. Mild involvement in some family members may be manifest only as spasticity without noticeable symptoms. Neuropathologically, FSP is associated with degeneration of the corticospinal tracts, which appear nearly normal in the brainstem but show increasing atrophy at more caudal levels in the spinal cord.

Rarely, patients with FSP have involvement of other regions of the nervous system, including lower motor neuron involvement (amyotrophy), mental retardation or mental retardation with skin thickening, optic atrophy, and sensory neuropathy (see review by Harding). In some cases, there is loss of fibers in the ascending posterior columns and the spinocerebellar tracts, features reminiscent of Friedreich's ataxia. These complicated forms of FSP emphasize the challenge inherent in classifying the neurodegenerative disorders until the precise genetic abnormalities are identified; there may be considerable overlap of the clinical phenotypes in diseases otherwise classified as distinct.

MUSCULAR WEAKNESS AND WASTING ASSOCIATED WITH SENSORY CHANGES

PROGRESSIVE NEURAL MUSCULAR ATROPHY Degenerative disorders characterized by progressive weakness and wasting of skeletal muscles combined with sensory changes are usually due to chronic diseases of peripheral nerves; many are hereditary. The most frequent form of hereditary peripheral neuropathy is Charcot-Marie-Tooth (CMT) disease. In its usual form, it occurs as a dominantly inherited demyelinating neuropathy with striking motor and sensory findings on physical examination and slowing of conduction on electrophysiologic studies (see Chap. 383). Many families with dominant CMT show linkage to a duplicated locus on chromosome 17p11.2 containing a gene for a peripheral myelin protein. Some variants of CMT are recessively inherited and predominantly axonal with corresponding motor neuron manifestations. Such cases can be impossible to distinguish from true lower motor neuronopathies on clinical grounds; genetic studies linking affected individuals to known SMA (chromosome 5q) or CMT (e.g., chromosome 17p, chromosome 1, or X) loci may distinguish these entities. Similarly, some forms of Friedreich's ataxia and adrenomyeloneuropathy may have prominent lower motor neuron signs; usually either genetic, radiographic, or biochemical studies will distinguish these from isolated lower motor neuropathy syndromes.

SYNDROMES OF PROGRESSIVE VISUAL LOSS Some neurodegenerative disorders are accompanied by concomitant impairment of the visual system. Thus, in Friedreich's ataxia, there may be slowing of conduction in the optic nerves. Two broad categories of visual pathology have been described: selective degeneration of retinal ganglion cells with secondary optic atrophy and a more diffuse degeneration involving all retinal components. The latter entails subsequent migration of melanin-containing cells of the pigment epithelium into the superficial retinal layers, resulting in pigmentary degeneration of the retina. Historically, this has been described as "retinitis pigmentosa," a misnomer because there is no inflammation within the retina. Some disorders causing retinitis pigmentosa are now documented to arise from genetic defects in mitochondrial DNA or in autosomal genes encoding mitochondrial proteins (see Chap. 385). An important implication of these findings, as yet not firmly established, is that mitochondrial lesions may be implicated in the associated neurodegenerative sensory and motor syndromes. Other inherited forms of retinitis pigmentosa are due to mutations in the photoreceptor rhodopsin (see Chaps. 19 and 364).

THE HEREDITARY ATAXIAS

These conditions present with progressive unsteadiness in standing and walking, along with impaired coordination of the limbs. In the pediatric age group, such conditions are often associated with metabolic disturbances that may give rise to either remitting or chronic progressive imbalance. A detailed review of these metabolic disorders is beyond the scope of this chapter, but an outline of the major entities is included in Table 372-3. In adults, the major diseases of progressive unsteadiness are characterized pathologically by degeneration of the cerebellum and/or its related fiber systems and thus constitute classic examples of the system degenerations. Although sporadic instances occur, hereditary transmission is the outstanding feature in most cases. Accordingly, this group of disorders is often referred to as the *hereditary ataxias*. As with other neurodegenerative disorders, it has

TABLE 372-3   Selected major syndromes of progressive ataxia in adults

INHERITED DEGENERATIVE DISORDERS

Disease	Chromosome
Friedreich's ataxia	9q13-21
Spinocerebellar atrophy 1	6p22-23
Spinocerebellar atrophy 2	12q23-24
Spinocerebellar atrophy 3	Unknown
Machado-Joseph disease	14q24.3-31
Ataxia with vitamin E deficiency	8q

SYSTEMIC DISORDERS

Metabolic disorders
  Mitochondrial disorders
  Abnormal amino and organic acid metabolism
  Urea cycle defects
  Vitamin and cofactor deficiencies
  Enzyme defects
    Hexosaminidase deficiency
    Gamma-glutamyl cysteine synthetase deficiency
    Glutamate dehydrogenase deficiency
  Lipid metabolism disorders
    A- and hypobetalipoproteinemia
    Refsum's disease
    Cerebrotendinous xanthomatosis
DNA repair defects
  Ataxia telangiectasia
  Xeroderma pigmentosum
Inflammatory autoimmune disorders
  Paraneoplastic cerebellar degeneration
  Multiple sclerosis and related disorders
Infections
  Prion or "slow-viral" infection
  Postinfectious cerebellar inflammation

OTHER

Post-hyperthermia
Post-anoxia
Drug-induced disorders
  Phenytoin
  Chronic ethanol abuse
Structural lesions
  Posterior fossa tumors
  Hydrocephalus

proved difficult to devise an absolute classification scheme for these diseases based either on their clinical presentation or on neuropathologic findings. Nonetheless, the following clinicopathologic subdivision of the adult ataxic diseases is useful: (1) cerebellar cortical degeneration, (2) olivopontocerebellar atrophy, and (3) spinocerebellar degenerations, including Friedreich's ataxia.

CEREBELLAR CORTICAL DEGENERATION The principal neuropathologic finding in this disorder is loss of neurons (mainly Purkinje cells) in the cerebellar cortex. The onset of symptoms usually occurs in late adult life. In the majority of patients it is inherited as an autosomal dominant trait, although apparently sporadic cases have been described.

Pathology The loss of Purkinje cells is usually most severe in the superior vermis and adjacent parts of the cerebellar cortex but can be more widely distributed. The granule layer neurons are less affected. In long-standing cases, there is an associated atrophy of neurons in the olivary nuclei of the medulla, apparently representing a transsynaptic retrograde degeneration resulting from the loss of Purkinje cells, to which the olivocerebellar fibers project. In advanced cases, atrophy of the cerebellar cortex can be readily demonstrated by computed tomographic (CT) or MRI scanning. In the purest forms of this disorder, as exemplified by the cases of late onset, slow progression, and dominant inheritance, other neuronal systems remain relatively intact.

Clinical manifestations Incoordination first appears in the legs, resulting in abnormal stance and an unsteady, wavering, lurching gait typical of cerebellar ataxia (see Chap. 22). This gait disturbance is a consequence of degenerative changes in the superior vermis of the cerebellum and adjacent parts of the cerebellar cortex. With more extensive cerebellar involvement, a disturbance in articulation and rhythm of speech occurs, and the arms also become ataxic. There may be nystagmus. The illness progresses gradually, often extending over two or three decades, without appreciably curtailing the life span. Dementia may occur, but it tends to be mild or is a late feature. Cerebellar cortical degeneration with similar features may occur as a component of other ataxic disorders.

In addition to this slowly evolving cerebellar cortical degeneration, there is a subacute diffuse cerebellar cortical degeneration that affects all parts of the cerebellar cortex indiscriminately, often in association with inflammatory changes. This disorder occurs in the presence of malignant neoplastic diseases of various kinds and is referred to as *subacute cortical cerebellar degeneration* (see Chap. 328). This is one of several paraneoplastic neurologic degenerative syndromes that result from an indirect effect of the neoplasm on the CNS.

OLIVOPONTOCEREBELLAR ATROPHY (OPCA) Grouped under this category are a number of similar disorders characterized by a combination of cerebellar cortical degeneration, atrophy of the inferior olivary nuclei secondary to this, and degeneration and disappearance of neurons of the pontine nuclei and their fiber projections in the basis pontis and middle cerebellar peduncles. Five subtypes have been described on the basis of differences in hereditary transmission and in the extent of other abnormalities both within and outside the nervous system. Most instances of OPCA can now be considered to represent a form of multiple system degeneration in which admixtures of parkinsonism, dementia, spasticity, choreoathetosis, retinal degeneration, myelopathy, and peripheral neuropathy may be encountered, these associated findings sometimes obscuring the ataxic component.

Pathology The variants of OPCA provide yet another example of selective premature neuronal death, affecting vulnerable neuronal systems while sparing others. It is not certain what pathologic change results in the dementia that so often accompanies them. It has been generally assumed that abnormalities occur in the cerebral cortex, but examination in typical cases fails to disclose sufficient abnormalities to account for the cognitive and behavioral alterations. The lesions in the basal ganglia and substantia nigra (equivalent to striatonigral degeneration) underlie the features of parkinsonism and of other postural movement disorders that are so frequently seen as manifestations of OPCA. Involvement of the peripheral motor neurons, similar to that encountered in motor neuron diseases, produces the muscular weakness and atrophy that may be encountered. The site of degeneration that leads to the disturbances of ocular motility that typify some cases has not been elucidated.

Clinical manifestations There is considerable variation in the clinical findings of OPCA. Some patients present with a picture of a relatively pure cerebellar ataxia indistinguishable from that seen in patients with atrophy of the cerebellar cortex. Others are characterized by parkinsonian features. Superimposed is an evolving dementia. Accounts of the varied forms of clinical expression can be found in the monographs by Duvoisin and Plaitakis and by Harding.

Genetics and pathogenesis Autosomal dominant inheritance is characteristic in many families. Genetic linkage analysis has localized the mutant gene to the short arm of chromosome 6 in several large families [spinocerebellar atrophy type 1 (SCA1)]. In a large Cuban family, the disease was linked to chromosome 12q23-24 (SCA2). The defect in SCA1 is an expanded -CAG- repeat in a gene expressed in muscle, brain, and other tissues. The function of the protein encoded by this gene has not been fully defined. Data indicate that in some forms of OPCA there may be a reduction in levels of glutamic acid dehydrogenase (GDH) as assayed in fibroblasts and leukocytes. This occurs either as a sporadic disorder or on a familial basis with either dominant or recessive inheritance. The dominant GDH deficiency cases are often of childhood onset with clinical features resembling other types of OPCA. Peripheral neuropathy and slowed saccadic eye movements may be prominent. The observation of GDH deficiency in OPCA has led to the hypothesis that the loss of Purkinje cells and other neurons may be a consequence of elevated levels of glutamate. The possibility that mitochondrial function is deranged in OPCA is supported by reports of individuals with mitochondrial complex I deficiency or myoclonic epilepsy with ragged red fibers (MERRF) who develop degeneration of selected populations of olivary, pontine, dentate, and other neurons with associated long tract (spinocerebellar, posterior column, corticospinal) degeneration. While these features are reminiscent of pathologic findings in OPCA (see below), a specific biochemical defect has yet to be delineated for any form of OPCA or indeed any of the progressive ataxias.

SPINOCEREBELLAR DEGENERATION (FRIEDREICH'S ATAXIA)

This group of ataxic disorders is characterized by degeneration of long ascending and descending fiber systems in the spinal cord, including the spinocerebellar tracts, and concomitant degeneration of peripheral axons and myelin sheaths in the form of chronic peripheral neuronopathy. There is considerable overlap in the clinical and neuropathologic findings of the spinocerebellar and OPCA disorders. The principal clinical feature justifying separation of these groups is the relative sparing of brainstem function in the spinocerebellar disorders. The classic form of hereditary spinocerebellar ataxia is Friedreich's disease, usually inherited as an autosomal recessive trait. First depicted by Nikolaus Friedreich in 1863, it constitutes a relatively distinct symptom complex that generally is inherited in a phenotypically recognized form. In some families, the disorder occurs with dominant inheritance. Recent studies have linked the recessive form of the disease to the long arm of chromosome 9; a specific gene has not been identified (see Chap. 364).

Pathology The principal changes are cell loss in the dorsal root ganglia and secondary degeneration in the posterior columns and spinocerebellar tracts of the cord and in peripheral nerves. Degeneration is also evident in the corticospinal tracts in most cases. The cerebellum is variably affected. In addition to these neuropathologic changes, there occurs in some cases a peculiar form of cardiomyopathy resulting in muscle fiber loss and fibrosis. There are no other associated visceral lesions.

Clinical manifestations As with other progressive ataxias, the disorder first appears in the legs, affecting the individual during late childhood. The patient begins to stagger and lurch in walking and is unsteady on standing. Clumsiness and cerebellar tremor of the hands and arms appear later along with dysarthria and an abnormal rhythm (scanning) of speech. These symptoms result from changes in the dorsal root ganglia, the spinocerebellar tracts, and the cerebellum. The limbs, in addition to being ataxic, generally show considerable weakness. Examination usually discloses nystagmus and skeletal deformities such as kyphoscoliosis, the basis of which is not certain, and a peculiar foreshortening of the feet (pes cavus) with cocking of the toes, best ascribed to atrophy and contractures of the musculature of the feet at a time when the bones of the feet are malleable. Typically, there is an unusual combination of total absence of tendon reflexes with extensor plantar reflexes (Babinski sign). This results from the degeneration of the corticospinal tracts together with the involvement of peripheral sensory neurons that relay afferent signals from muscle spindles. Impairment of position and vibration sense in the extremities is prominent, and in some patients, sensation of pain, temperature, and light touch is diminished in a distal and roughly symmetric distribution consistent with an axonal neuropathy affecting small nerve fibers. Mentation is usually preserved, though a few patients have been of low intelligence or have become demented late in the course of the disease. Survival beyond early adult life is rare, with death frequently the result of associated cardiomyopathy. Survival is somewhat better in families with the dominantly inherited forms of the illness.

Occasionally, mild or fragmentary forms of the disorder (such as pes cavus and absent or hyperactive tendon reflexes) may be encountered with little, if any, disability or progression. Such abnormalities are most likely to be seen in other members of the family of a patient afflicted with the fully developed form of the disease. A related syndrome, the Roussy-Levy syndrome, shows similarities to Friedreich's ataxia and to peroneal muscular atrophy. Mild ataxia, pes cavus, absent ankle and knee tendon jerks, and atrophy of lower leg muscles occur. In some well-documented cases, the peripheral nerves show hypertrophy due to proliferation of Schwann cells (see Chap. 383). Chronic familial polyneuropathies are particularly difficult to distinguish because they also give rise to sensory ataxia (see Chap. 383). Hereditary forms of ataxia with corticospinal signs (hyperactive tendon reflexes) and sensory disturbances are also known to occur in the adolescent or adult. Familial spastic paraplegia with or without optic atrophy (Behr's syndrome) is another closely related disease. In the absence of a family history and with atypical clinical findings, further diagnostic studies are necessary to exclude congenital malformation, spinal cord compression, foramen magnum tumor, and multiple sclerosis.

Treatment No treatment is of proven value. Because the myocardium may be involved, regular evaluation of cardiac function is prudent.

DIFFERENTIAL DIAGNOSIS OF THE ATAXIAS The slow but relentless progression in the absence of abnormalities in other parts of the nervous system and in the CSF distinguishes the hereditary group from other diseases and other forms of cerebellar ataxia such as may occur with hereditary metabolic diseases, with neoplastic, infectious, or demyelinative disease, or with drug intoxication (e.g., phenytoin) or hyperpyrexia. The degenerative disorders under discussion tend to develop slowly over many years in a setting of otherwise good general health and in the absence of other neurologic symptoms and signs; this, together with the other clinical differences, distinguishes them from such hereditary metabolic diseases as juvenile Gaucher's disease, juvenile Niemann-Pick disease, juvenile hexosaminidase deficiency, and alcoholic cerebellar ataxia or nutritional deficiency disease with or without Wernicke-Korsakoff syndrome. Alcoholic cerebellar degeneration usually develops over a few days to weeks and then may remain more or less unchanged (see Chap. 377). A prolonged deficiency of vitamin E, sometimes arising as an inherited defect, can result in progressive ataxia, incoordination of the limbs, areflexia, and distal loss of proprioception and vibratory sense, mimicking the spinocerebellar degeneration of Friedreich's ataxia (see Chap. 377). Most cases are associated with fat malabsorption.

In the cases associated with carcinoma, the tempo of evolution of the process is relatively rapid, with severe disability coming on within a period of months. Vertigo, diplopia, and nausea may be prominent. In an occasional patient, the neurologic symptoms appear before any evidence of carcinoma. Opsoclonus (rapid side-to-side jerking of the eyes) and oscillopsia (rhythmic movement back and forth of perceived objects) may be conjoined (see Chap. 328). In contrast to the consistently normal CSF findings in the forms of cerebellar degeneration noted above, the CSF in paraneoplastic degeneration may show increased lymphocytes and elevated protein. Finally, the serum and CSF in patients with paracarcinomatous cerebellar degeneration may have high titers of antibodies seen specifically in the paraneoplastic syndromes (e.g., anti-Hu and anti-Yo) (see Chap. 328).

A dominantly inherited, progressive ataxia termed *Machado-Joseph* or *Azorean disease* occurs in Portuguese families of Azorean descent and is linked to a marker on chromosome 14q. This adult-onset disorder shows considerable clinical variability. Its central characteristic is progressive ataxia with eye movement weakness, nystagmus, and eyelid retraction resulting in a prominent stare. Additionally, early-onset patients have a more rapid course with superimposed pyramidal (spasticity) and extrapyramidal (dystonia and rigidity) manifestations. Late-onset patients may show distal amyotrophy and neuropathic sensory loss in addition to the ataxia and eye movement abnormalities. In all ages, memory and cognition are usually spared. Pathologic studies document that this is a multisystem degenerative disorder with features overlapping both the olivopontocerebellar and the spinocerebellar degenerations. There is degeneration of the spinocerebellar tracts and Clarke's columns and loss of brainstem (vestibular nuclei, pontine, dentate nucleus) and spinal motor neurons. Cerebellar Purkinje neurons are spared. The genetic basis for Machado-Joseph disease remains unclear; it is linked to chromosome 14q24 and thus is distinct from SCA1, ataxia with vitamin E deficiency, Friedreich's ataxia, and SCA2, respectively, at loci on chromosomes 6, 8, 9, and 12. It also has been established that Machado-Joseph disease is not an allelic form of Huntington's disease.

NEURODEGENERATIVE DISORDERS ASSOCIATED WITH AUTONOMIC FAILURE (SHY-DRAGER SYNDROME)

Abnormalities of central autonomic nervous system functions, manifest principally by failure to maintain blood pressure and by urinary incontinence, are now recognized to be caused in some cases by a progressive degenerative disorder of the CNS that affects several systems (see Chap. 379). In some patients, the peripheral nervous system is also involved (postganglionic sympathetic neurons). Bradbury and Eggleston in 1925 called attention to the combination of postural hypotension, incontinence, impotence, and abnormality of sweating (anhidrosis). Symptoms of central neurologic origin develop later in many of these patients, consisting predominantly of extrapyramidal or cerebellar dysfunction.

Pathogenesis and pathology   The cause of the disorder is unknown. In 1960, Shy and Drager described neuropathologic changes in the brainstem and basal ganglia, and subsequently, others showed a prominent loss of neurons in central regions of the autonomic nervous system, affecting in particular the cells of the intermediolateral column of the thoracic spinal cord. Abnormalities also have been found in peripheral autonomic ganglia (cell loss). In the brainstem and basal ganglia there is widespread symmetric neuronal degeneration affecting the caudate nucleus, substantia nigra, locus coeruleus, olivary nuclei, dorsal vagal nuclei, and, in some cases, the cerebellum. Cell loss is accompanied by gliosis; Lewy bodies typical of Parkinson's disease are present in some cases. For these reasons, many neurologists consider the Shy-Drager syndrome to be a unique form of multisystem degeneration resembling but distinct from either Parkinson's disease or OPCA.

Clinical manifestations   The onset is insidious, usually in the sixth or seventh decade. Men are more frequently affected than women. Disturbances of urinary bladder function, including hesitancy and incontinence, postural dizziness and syncope, impotence, and decreased sweating are the presenting manifestations. Symptoms of extrapyramidal dysfunction resembling parkinsonian or cerebellar findings may emerge. The condition becomes severely disabling over the course of 5 to 7 years in most patients. The hallmark of the condition is postural hypotension, defined as a fall in blood pressure greater than 30/20 mmHg on standing upright from a supine position (see Chap. 379). Despite this fall in blood pressure, there is usually a total failure of compensatory tachycardia; the pulse rate fails to change. Autonomic signs of pupillary asymmetry, partial Horner's syndrome, or partial parasympathetic denervation occur in some patients. Anhidrosis is common and can be demonstrated by placing the individual in a warm room after application of a starch-iodine mixture to the skin. The parkinsonian manifestations may be identical to those of idiopathic parkinsonism, although in many patients rigidity and bradykinesia are more prominent than tremor. Cerebellar gait ataxia may be evident. Other findings include laryngeal paralysis and sleep apnea, which may herald the onset of the disease. MRI may demonstrate T2-weighted signal hypointensity in the putamen, globus pallidum, and substantia nigra. Positron emission tomography shows decreased uptake of dopamine derivatives in the putamen and caudate, probably reflecting a loss of nigrostriatal dopaminergic neurons.

Treatment   The treatment is symptomatic. The postural hypotension is usually the most disabling initial symptom. Antigravity stockings to minimize pooling of venous blood in the legs are recommended. A leotard that covers the lower abdomen may provide additional benefit. Pharmacologic agents are given to expand blood volume and enhance vascular responsivity. Increased NaCl intake combined with fludrohydrocortisone, 0.05 to 0.2 mg twice daily, is usually beneficial (see Chap 379). In severe cases, adrenergic drugs such as ephedrine, levodopa, or amphetamine may improve the disability. The parkinsonian symptoms often respond initially to Sinemet or bromocriptine, but later in the course most patients become refractory to these agents. Centrally acting alpha agonists (e.g., yohimbine or clonidine or the investigational drug xamoterol) also may be beneficial.

REFERENCES

Motor neuron diseases

BRZUSTOWICZ LM et al: Genetic mapping of chronic childhood-onset spinal muscular atrophy to chromosome 5q11.2–13.3. Nature 344:540, 1990

DALAKAS M, ILLA I: Post-polio syndrome: Concepts in clinical diagnosis, pathogenesis, and etiology. Adv Neurol 56:495, 1991

LA SPADA AR et al: Androgen receptor gene mutations in X-linked spinal muscular atrophy. Nature 352:77, 1991

MUNSAT TL: Poliomyelitis—New problems with an old disease. N Engl J Med 324:1206, 1991

PRADAS J et al: The natural history of amyotrophic lateral sclerosis and the use of natural history controls in therapeutic trials. Neurology 43:751, 1993

ROSEN DR et al: Association of mutations in Cu/Zn cytosolic superoxide dismutase with familial amyotrophic lateral sclerosis. Nature 362:59, 1993

ROWLAND LP (ed): *Advances in Neurology,* vol. 56: *Amyotrophic Lateral Sclerosis and Other Motor Neuron Diseases.* New York, Raven, 1991

SIDDIQUE TS et al: Linkage of a gene causing familial amyotrophic lateral sclerosis to chromosome 21 and evidence of genetic locus heterogeneity. N Engl J Med 324:1381, 1991

SMITH RA (ed): *Handbook of Amyotrophic Lateral Sclerosis.* New York, Marcel Dekker, 1992

Progressive ataxias

CARSON WJ et al: The Machado-Joseph disease locus is different from the spinocerebellar ataxia locus (SCA1). Genomics 13:852, 1992

DUVOISIN RC, PLAITAKIS A (eds): *Advances in Neurology,* vol. 41: *The Olivopontocerebellar Atrophies.* New York, Raven Press, 1984

GILMAN S et al: *Disorders of the Cerebellum.* Philadelphia, Davis, 1981

GISPERT S et al: Chromosomal assignment of the second locus for autosomal dominant cerebellar ataxia (SCA2) to human chromosome 12q23-24.1. Nature Genet 4:295, 1993

HARDING AE: *The Hereditary Ataxias and Related Diseases.* London, Churchill Livingstone, 1984

KAGEYAMA Y et al: An autopsy case of mitochondrial encephalomyopathy with prominent degeneration in olivo-ponto-cerebellar system. Acta Neuropathol 83:99, 1991

KEATS BJ et al: ''Acadian'' and ''classical'' forms of Friedreich ataxia are most probably caused by mutations at the same locus. Am J Med Genet 33:266, 1989

KONIGSMARK BW, WEINER LP: The olivopontocerebellar atrophies: A review. Medicine 49:227, 1970

PLAITAKIS A: Olivopontocerebellar atrophy with glutamate dehydrogenase deficiency, in *Handbook of Clinical Neurology,* vol 16: *Hereditary Neuropathies and Spinal Ataxias,* JMBV de Jong (ed). New York, Elsevier Science Publishers, 1991, p 551

RANUM LP et al: Autosomal dominant spinocerebellar ataxia: Locus heterogeneity in a Nebraska kindred. Neurology 42:344, 1992

SUDARSKY L et al: Machado-Joseph disease in New England: Clinical description and distinction from the olivopontocerebellar atrophies. Mov Disord 7:204, 1992.

TAKIYAMA Y et al: The gene for Machado-Joseph disease maps to human chromosome 14q. Nature Genet 4:300, 1993

Miscellaneous

BROOKS DJ et al: The relationship between locomotor disability, autonomic dysfunction, and the integrity of the striatal dopaminergic system in patients with multiple system atrophy, pure autonomic failure, and Parkinson's disease, studied with PET. Brain 113:1539, 1990

LUPSKI JR et al: DNA duplication associated with Charcot-Marie-Tooth disease type IA. Cell 66:219, 1991

MCLEOD JG, TUCK RR: Disorders of the autonomic nervous system: 2. Investigation and treatment. Ann Neurol 21:519, 1987

OBARA A et al: Effect of xamoterol on Shy-Drager syndrome. Circulation 85:606, 1992

SANDRONI P et al: Autonomic involvement in extrapyramidal and cerebellar disorders. Clin Auton Res 1:147, 1991

STEPHEN L. HAUSER

The demyelinating diseases occupy a unique place in neurology, arising from their frequency and tendency to strike young adults, the diversity of manifestations that challenge the most skilled clinician, and the range of fundamental questions in neurobiology, immunology, virology, and genetics that arise regarding their pathogenesis. These disorders share the common feature of inflammation and selective destruction of central nervous system (CNS) myelin. Their course may be chronic (multiple sclerosis) or acute (acute disseminated encephalomyelitis and acute hemorrhagic leukoencephalitis). The peripheral nervous system (PNS) is generally spared. No specific tests for the demyelinating diseases exist, and diagnosis is based on recognition of the distinctive clinical patterns of CNS injury they produce.

MULTIPLE SCLEROSIS

Multiple sclerosis (MS) is characterized by chronic inflammation, demyelination, and gliosis (scarring). Lesions of MS are classically said to be disseminated in time and space. MS affects 350,000 Americans and is, with the exception of trauma, the most frequent cause of neurologic disability in early to middle adulthood. Indirect evidence supports an autoimmune etiology for MS, perhaps triggered by a viral infection in a genetically susceptible host. As in other chronic inflammatory disorders, the manifestations of MS are variable and range from a benign illness to a rapidly evolving and incapacitating disease. Complications from MS may affect multiple body systems and may require profound adjustments in life-style and goals for patients and their families; hence a multidisciplinary approach is necessary to optimize clinical care.

PATHOLOGIC FEATURES MS derives its name from the multiple scarred areas visible on macroscopic examination of the brain. These lesions, termed *plaques*, are well-demarcated gray or pink areas easily distinguished from surrounding white matter. Occasionally, plaques are also present in gray matter. Plaques vary in size from 1 or 2 mm to several centimeters. The acute MS lesion, rarely found at autopsy, is characterized by perivenular cuffing and tissue infiltration by mononuclear cells, predominantly T lymphocytes and macrophages, and by demyelination. B cells and plasma cells are rarely found. The inflammatory infiltrates appear to mediate the loss of myelin sheaths that surround axis cylinders. As the lesion progresses, large numbers of macrophages and microglial cells (specialized CNS phagocytes of bone marrow origin) scavenge the myelin debris, and proliferation of astrocytes (gliosis) occurs. Proliferation of oligodendrocytes, the myelin-producing cells, is also present initially, but these cells appear to be destroyed as the infiltration and gliosis progress. Gliosis is more severe in MS lesions than in most other neuropathologic conditions. In chronic MS lesions, complete or nearly complete demyelination, dense gliosis, and loss of oligodendroglia are present. In some plaques (chronic active lesions), gradations in histologic findings from the center to the lesion edge suggest that lesions expand by concentric outward growth.

Lesions of MS are typically more numerous than anticipated on the basis of clinical criteria. Selective demyelination with sparing of axon cylinders is the hallmark of the disease, yet partial or total axonal destruction, and in extreme cases cavitation, may occur. Although partial remyelination (shadow plaques) is occasionally present, in most lesions significant remyelination does not occur. The correlation of plaque number and size with clinical symptoms is poor.

Hence an extensive plaque burden may be associated with only mild symptoms, or conversely, minor pathologic findings may be present in some individuals severely disabled during life. Approximately 35 percent of cases are clinically silent with evidence of MS only at autopsy.

PATHOPHYSIOLOGY AND PATHOGENESIS **Pathophysiology** Experimental studies indicate that demyelination may result in either negative or positive effects on axonal conduction. *Negative conduction abnormalities* consist of slowed axonal conduction, variable conduction block that occurs in the presence of high- but not low-frequency trains of impulses, or complete conduction block. Conduction block in demyelinated fibers also may occur in response to raised temperature or with metabolic changes in the extracellular milieu of axons. *Positive conduction abnormalities* include ectopic impulse generation, spontaneously or following mechanical stress, and abnormal "cross-talk" between demyelinated axons. While the degree to which these negative and positive changes occur in MS is unknown, their presence may explain several characteristics of the disease. For example, conduction block may account for the fluctuations in function that vary from hour to hour and from day to day in MS and for the worsening that follows elevation in core body temperature. Ectopic impulse generation or "crosstalk" might give rise to Lhermitte's symptom, paroxysmal symptoms, or parasthesias (see below). Experimental therapies based on postulated conduction abnormalities in MS have included the use of calcium blockers to reduce the threshold for impulse generation and pharmacologic blockage of voltage-dependent potassium channels (4-aminopyridine) that are exposed in the internodal axon membrane following myelin loss.

Epidemiology MS is approximately twofold more common in females than in males. MS is unusual before adolescence, then rises steadily in incidence from the teens to age 35, and declines gradually thereafter. There is a slightly later age of onset in men than in women. MS beginning as early as age 2 or as late as age 74 is rare but well documented.

Marked differences in the prevalence of MS exist between different populations and ethnic groups. The highest known prevalence (250 per 100,000) occurs in the Orkney islands, located north of the mainland of Scotland, and MS is also common in Scandinavia and throughout northern Europe. In the United States, the prevalence of MS is higher in Caucasians than in other racial groups, consistent with observations in other parts of the world. MS is extremely rare in Japan (2 per 100,000) and is essentially unknown in black Africa, yet Japanese-Americans and black Americans are at significant risk for MS, with respective prevalence rates estimated at one-quarter and one-third that of Caucasian Americans.

MS is in general a disease of temperate climates. In both hemispheres, its prevalence decreases with decreasing latitude. Comparison of North American and European populations indicates that similar prevalence rates and north-south gradients are observed. Migration data in well-defined ethnic populations also support an effect of environment on risk. Children born to parents who have migrated from a high-risk to a low-risk area for MS have a lower lifetime risk than their parents. Conversely, migration from a low-risk to a high-risk area confers an increased risk for MS in the children. Some migration studies, notably those from South Africa and Israel, suggest that a critical environmental exposure in MS occurs prior to the age of 15 years, but these data are based on small numbers of individuals who have migrated at different ages. Other evidence for an environmental effect on MS is derived from apparent point epidemics that have occurred, e.g., the cluster of MS that appeared in the Faroe Islands off the coast of Denmark following the British occupation during World War II.

Genetics Compelling data indicate that susceptibility to MS is inherited. Familial aggregation is known to occur, and first-, second-, and third-degree relatives of patients are at increased risk for the disease. Siblings of MS patients have a 2 to 5 percent lifetime risk for MS, whereas the risk to parents or children of patients is somewhat lower. Concordance of MS is also increased in monozygotic compared with dizygotic twins. The risk of MS to a monozygotic twin of an MS patient is approximately 30 percent, whereas the risk to a dizygotic twin approximates the risk to a nontwin sibling.

Pedigree study of multiple-affected-member families is consistent with the hypothesis that multiple unlinked genes confer susceptibility. Genetic heterogeneity, i.e., independent major genes, also may be present in MS. The major histocompatibility complex (MHC) on chromosome 6 has been identified as one genetic determinant for MS. This complex encodes genes for the histocompatibility antigens (the HLA system) that serve in the context of antigen presentation to T cells. Linkage disequilibrium studies suggest that MS susceptibility is linked to the class II (DR, DQ, and DP) region of the MHC. The DR2(15) DQw1 haplotype is common in Caucasian populations at risk for MS, and some family studies support a genetic effect of the DR2-bearing haplotype on susceptibility. Other HLA haplotypes may be associated with MS in other ethnic populations, but family studies supporting their role have been negative or are lacking. The MHC locus contributes only a small fraction to the genetic effect on MS. Other studies have implicated a role for other genes in MS, including T cell receptor, immunoglobulin heavy chain, and MBP genes.

Immunology Attention has focused on the role of thymus-derived or T lymphocytes in the pathogenesis of MS. T cells reactive against myelin proteins, either myelin basic protein (MBP) or myelin proteolipid protein (PLP), mediate CNS inflammation in experimental allergic encephalomyelitis (EAE), a laboratory model for demyelinating diseases. This has been proven by adoptive transfer experiments in which sensitized T cells from an animal with EAE can transfer disease to a healthy syngeneic recipient. EAE is induced in genetically susceptible animals by immunization with CNS tissue homogenized in an adjuvent. Chronic relapsing/remitting forms of EAE have been described that pathologically resemble human MS. Occasional laboratory accidents have resulted in human inoculation with an EAE homogenate that was followed by development of an acute EAE-like illness, indicating that humans are also susceptible.

Evidence that myelin-reactive T cells play a role in MS is only indirect. The frequency of MBP-reactive T cells appears to be increased in peripheral blood of patients, and such cells carry a high frequency of mutations, indicating that they may have undergone chronic stimulation in vivo. Perhaps more significant, T cells reactive against MBP and PLP are concentrated in CSF in MS compared with their frequency in peripheral blood.

One remarkable feature of the T cell response to MBP in EAE concerns the repertoire of antigen receptor molecules that are present on disease-inducing (encephalitogenic) cells. In rodents, a restricted number of different families of T cell receptor (TCR) genes are expressed by encephalitogenic T cells, and if these cells are removed or rendered inactive, the animal is protected from EAE. This has been accomplished both by passive and active immunization against these families of TCR genes. The majority of T cells do not express TCR genes that are targeted by therapy; hence cellular immunity is preserved and selective immunotherapy achieved. In MS patients, analysis of the T cell response to MBP has revealed that similar restrictions of the T cell repertoire occur in some individuals, although the identity of the TCR genes appears to differ between different patients. Thus specific therapy against MBP-reactive T cells may require that it be tailored to the individual immune response that is present.

Elevated levels of CNS immunoglobulin (Ig) are also characteristic of MS. Some of this antibody can be shown to be oligoclonal, indicating that it is comprised of a small number of different molecules. Oligoclonal Ig is also detected in other chronic inflammatory responses, including infections, and thus is not specific to MS. It is synthesized locally by plasma cells that are present within the CNS. The specific pattern or fingerprint is unique to each patient. Numerous attempts to identify an antigen against which the majority of oligoclonal Ig is directed have been unsuccessful. The appearance of oligoclonal Ig may thus represent a secondary event resulting from chronic inflammation or tissue injury.

It is possible that tissue damage in MS is mediated by cytokine products of activated T cells, macrophages, or astrocytes. For example, the cytokine tumor necrosis factor (TNF) has been found to be selectively toxic to myelin and to oligodendrocytes in vitro. TNF is present in lesions of MS, CSF levels are reported to parallel MS disease activity, and antibodies to TNF have been found to block acute EAE.

Virology Epidemiologic evidence supports the role of an environmental exposure in MS. MS risk also correlates with high socioeconomic status, which may reflect improved sanitation and delayed initial exposures to infectious agents. Some viruses, e.g., poliomyelitis and measles, produce neurologic sequelae that are more common when the age of initial infection is delayed. Despite many claims, no specific virus has been identified in MS. Reports of infection with a human retrovirus related to HTLV-I have not been confirmed. Elevated antibody titers to measles virus are found in different populations of MS patients, but proof of persistent infection has not followed, and MS may occur in individuals with no evidence of prior measles exposure. In animals, the most widely studied model of virus-induced demyelinating disease has been Theiler virus, a murine coronavirus similar to measles and canine distemper virus. Infection with some Theiler strains results in a chronic infection of oligodendrocytes with multifocal perivascular lymphocytic infiltration and demyelination. As is the case for EAE, genetic factors—both MHC-linked and other loci—influence susceptibility to demyelinating disease due to Theiler virus, in part by determining the magnitude of the immune response against viral determinants that occurs.

CLINICAL MANIFESTATIONS (See also Table 373-1) The onset of MS may be dramatic or so mild as to not cause a patient to seek medical attention. In most published series, the most common initial symptoms include weakness in one or more limbs, visual blurring due to optic neuritis, sensory disturbances, diplopia, and ataxia.

Weakness of the limbs may present insidiously as fatigue with exertion, difficulty in climbing stairs, or loss of dexterity associated with increased muscle tone. Patients may report injury and stubbing of the great toe due to a subtle foot drop. At an early stage of the disease, weakness may not be detectable on testing. Increased motor tone (spasticity), hyperreflexia, an extensor plantar response, Hoffmann reflex, and absent superficial abdominal reflex, all indicative of pyramidal tract disease, may be present. Occasionally, a tendon reflex, e.g., a triceps jerk, may be lost due to a focal lesion in the dorsal root entry zone through which the afferent fibers of the motor reflex arc traverse, simulating a peripheral nerve lesion.

Sensory symptoms include paresthesia (tingling, "pins and needles," or, less commonly, pain) or hypesthesia (numbness or a "dead" feeling). The sensory attack may begin in one foot, typically in a great toe, and ascend over hours or several days; at a variable time into the attack, ascending numbness in the other leg appears, and involvement of the perineum and lower trunk may be noted. Involvement of the trunk with a "cord level" is diagnostically helpful because it distinguishes the sensory attack from peripheral neuropathies due to Guillain-Barré syndrome, mononeuropathy multiplex, or toxins. In patients with established sensory deficits, unpleasant

TABLE 373-1 Initial symptoms of MS

Symptom	Percent cases	Symptom	Percent Cases
Weakness	35	Lhermitte	3
Sensory loss	37	Pain	3
Paresthesias	24	Dementia	2
Optic neuritis	36	Visual loss	2
Diplopia	15	Facial palsy	1
Ataxia	11	Impotence	1
Vertigo	6	Myokymia	1
Paroxysmal	4	Epilepsy	1
Bladder	4	Falling	1

SOURCE: After Matthews et al.

complaints of "swollen," "wet," or "tightly wrapped" body parts are common.

Cerebellar involvement results in ataxia of gait and limbs. In advanced MS, dysarthria of cerebellar origin (scanning speech) is common. In individual patients, the contribution of cerebellar involvement to specific symptoms may be difficult to define when motor and sensory deficits are also present.

Optic neuritis, a core symptom of demyelinating disease, produces variable visual loss. It usually begins as visual blurring that may remain mild or progress to severe visual loss, or, rarely, to complete loss of light perception. Symptoms are generally monocular, but attacks may be bilateral. Pain, localized to the orbit or supraorbital area, is typically present and may precede visual symptoms. The pain may worsen with eye movement. Examination may reveal an enlarged pupil, diminished visual acuity, and a paracentral blind spot (scotoma). The optic disc may be visually swollen (papillitis), and a Gunn phenomenon—pupillodilatation on exposure to direct light following constriction by indirect light—may be detected by a swinging flashlight test (see Chap. 19). Funduscopic examination also may detect venous sheathing of retinal vessels. Residual pallor of the optic disc (optic atrophy) commonly follows bouts of optic neuritis. Rarely, uveitis also has been present in patients with otherwise typical MS.

Visual blurring in MS may result from optic neuritis or diplopia. These two causes are distinguished by asking the patient to sequentially cover each eye and observing whether the visual difficulty clears. Diplopia in MS is often due to the development of an internuclear ophthalmoplegia (INO) or to a sixth nerve palsy; ocular muscle palsies due to involvement of the third or fourth cranial nerves are rare. An INO consists of a delay or complete loss of adduction on attempted horizontal gaze to one side accompanied by nystagmus in the abducting eye. Convergence is preserved, distinguishing INO from medial rectus palsy. An INO results from involvement of the crossed medial longitudinal fasciculus that connects contralateral third and sixth cranial nerve nuclei; involvement is usually on the side of the adducting eye. The presence of bilateral INO in an awake patient is virtually diagnostic of MS. Other gaze deficits include horizontal gaze palsy due to ipsilateral lesions of the lateral pontine tegmentum and the "one and a half" syndrome, consisting of a horizontal gaze palsy to one direction and an INO to the other (see Chap. 19).

Trigeminal neuralgia, a lancinating shocklike facial pain, may occur. Typically, trigeminal neuralgia occurs in patients over 50 years of age and is only rarely due to MS (see Chap. 380). Clinical features that raise a question of underlying MS include onset at a young age; bilaterality, if present; objective signs of sensory loss on the affected side; and prolonged pain lasting minutes or hours.

Interruption of motor innervation to the face may result in several clinical syndromes. Facial palsy due to MS may be difficult to distinguish from idiopathic Bell's palsy. In MS, facial palsy is usually not associated with ipsilateral loss of taste sensation or retroaural pain, two characteristics of Bell's palsy. Chronic flickering contractions of the facial musculature, termed *facial myokymia,* are thought to arise from involvement of corticobulbar tracts and, if chronic, are characteristic of MS. Facial hemispasm, while less common than other motor syndromes, also may occur.

Vertigo may appear suddenly and in dramatic fashion with gait unsteadiness and vomiting, and an incorrect diagnosis of labyrinthitis may be made. A brainstem rather than end-organ origin of vertigo may result in associated "neighborhood" signs, including ipsilateral trigeminal or facial nerve involvement, vertical nystagmus, or the presence of type 3 nystagmus on Barany testing (i.e., no latency, no direction reversal, and no fatigue) (see Chap. 18). Hearing loss also may occur in MS but is unusual.

Urinary bladder, and less frequently bowel, urgency or incontinence occurs in most MS patients at some time and may be present at disease onset.

Cognitive dysfunction is common in advanced MS but also may occur in early or mild disease. Rarely, cognitive symptoms are the initial manifestation of the disease. Memory loss is the most common cognitive change in MS, and impaired judgment or inappropriate jocularity may be noted. Uncontrollable episodes of laughter or crying, occurring either spontaneously or triggered by emotional stimuli (pseudobulbar palsy), may occur. Depression is also common and is generally secondary to the clinical devastation of MS.

Ancillary symptoms   Other clinical accompaniments, when present, support consideration of MS in a patient with neurologic complaints of uncertain cause. *Lhermitte's symptom* is a momentary electric-like sensation evoked by neck flexion, other neck movement, or cough. The symptom typically is experienced as a shooting phenomenon that travels down the spine and into the legs. Variants of Lhermitte's symptom include other tingling or painful sensations induced by neck movements, spread to the arms, or induction by movements of the lumbar spine.

Heat sensitivity, i.e., the appearance or worsening of symptoms upon exposure to heat (typically a hot shower), occurs in most patients with MS. One characteristic form of heat sensitivity is Uhthoff's symptom, in which transient visual blurring, generally monocular, occurs with exercise or upon exposure to heat.

Fatigue is present in the majority (up to 88 percent) of MS patients. Fatigue is typically present in midafternoon and may take the form of increased motor weakness with effort, mental fatigue, or lassitude and sleepiness.

Paroxysmal attacks consist of brief, stereotyped, recurrent phenomena. These underrecognized symptoms frequently occur at the onset of MS or early in its course. Typical are "tonic seizures," in which an unpleasant tingling or other sensory sensation is associated with tonic contraction of a limb, face, or trunk. Others consist of paroxysmal dysarthria and ataxia, diplopia, or transient unilateral paralysis, paresthesias, or pain. Attacks may be momentary or persist for 30 s or longer. They generally begin in clusters, occurring many times daily, and the patient may identify precipitating factors, such as particular movements, that trigger attacks.

DISEASE COURSE   McAlpine's illustration of the clinical course characteristics of MS are shown in Fig. 373-1. The course may be stratified into three general categories. The first, *relapsing MS,* is characterized by recurrent attacks of neurologic dysfunction. MS attacks generally evolve over days to weeks and may be followed by complete, partial, or no recovery. Recovery from attacks generally occurs within weeks to several months from the peak of symptoms, although rarely some recovery may continue for 2 or more years. The second form of the disease, *chronic progressive MS,* results in gradually progressive worsening without periods of stabilization or remission. This form develops most often in individuals with a prior history of relapsing MS, although in 20 percent of patients no relapses can be recalled. Acute relapses also may occur during the progressive course. A third form, *inactive MS,* is characterized by fixed neurologic deficits of variable magnitude. Most patients with inactive MS have an earlier history of relapsing MS.

While the clinical course of MS is highly variable, some general prognostic indicators can be defined. In one study that assessed function 25 years after the initial diagnosis of MS, 25 percent of patients remained capable of work, and 50 percent were still ambulatory. Other studies have reported a less favorable long-term prognosis, and in general, the longer that a population is followed, the smaller is the proportion of patients with mild disease. Despite these discouraging data, MS may be present for many decades and produce little or no disability in 5 to 10 percent of patients. Favorable prognostic factors include early onset (excluding childhood), a relapsing course, and little residual disability 5 years after onset. By contrast, poor prognosis is associated with a late age of onset (age 40 or older) and a progressive course; these variables are interdependent, since chronic progressive MS tends to begin at a later age than relapsing MS. Disability from chronic progressive MS is usually due to progressive paraplegia or quadriplegia, and in individual patients, the tempo of worsening, once established, tends to persist throughout the disease course. In relapsing MS, disability results from poor or incomplete recovery from attacks in approximately half

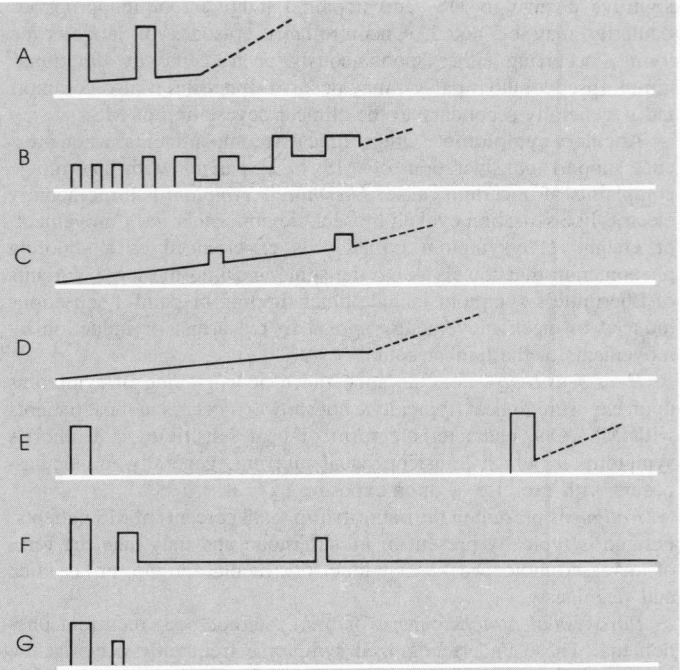

FIGURE 373-1 The clinical course of MS. *A.* Severe relapses, increasing disability and early death. *B.* Many short attacks, tending to increase in duration and severity. *C.* Slow progress from onset, superimposed relapses, and increasing disability. *D.* Slow progression from onset without relapses. *E.* Abrupt onset with good remission followed by long latent phase. *F.* Relapses of diminishing frequency and severity; slight residual disability only. *G.* Abrupt onset; few if any relapses after first year; no residual disability. *(From McAlpine, with permission.)*

of patients and from an evolution to chronic progressive MS in the other half.

DIAGNOSIS   The diagnosis of MS is usually easily made in young adults with relapsing and remitting symptoms referable to different areas of CNS white matter. Diagnosis is more difficult in a patient with recent onset of neurologic complaints or in a patient with a primary progressive course. In such situations, the patient should be questioned carefully for history of prior attacks that may not be recalled initially. Other presentations that may cause diagnostic uncertainty include symptoms with a rapid or even explosive onset, suggesting a cerebrovascular accident; progressive brainstem syndromes, raising a question of brainstem glioma; cervical myelopathy in the setting of degenerative disk disease; or mild symptoms unaccompanied by objective signs on examination. Rarely, a mass lesion resulting from intense inflammation and swelling may occur in MS and falsely suggest a primary or metastatic tumor.

Examination reveals objective evidence of neurologic disease in the great majority of patients. Abnormal signs on examination are often more widespread than expected from the interview. For example, the MS patient may present with symptoms in one leg and signs in both. This is helpful when it permits exclusion of a single focal lesion as the source of a symptom complex. Other MS patients may experience symptoms unaccompanied by objective neurologic findings on examination. They are frequently misdiagnosed as suffering from a conversion reaction, a label that should be avoided unless rigid diagnostic criteria for that condition are met.

The differential diagnosis of MS will vary depending on the specific clinical situation. Numerous diagnostic formulas have been proposed (see Table 373-2) that, while useful, should not be used in place of sound clinical judgment. No clinical sign or diagnostic test is unique to MS. The appearance of symptoms that are uncommon or rare in MS should call the diagnosis into question; these include

TABLE 373-2   Diagnostic criteria for MS

1 Examination must reveal *objective* abnormalities of the CNS.
2 Involvement must reflect predominantly disease of white matter long tracts, usually including (a) pyramidal pathways, (b) cerebellar pathways, (c) medial longitudinal fasciculus, (d) optic nerve, and (e) posterior columns.
3 Examination or history must implicate involvement of two or more areas of the CNS.
   a MRI may be used in patients below the age of 40 to document a *second* lesion when only one site of abnormality has been demonstrable on examination. A confirmatory MRI must have either four lesions involving the white matter or three lesions if one is periventricular in location. Acceptable lesions must be greater than 3 mm in diameter.
   b Evoked response testing may be used to document a *second* lesion.
4 The clinical pattern must consist of (a) two or more separate *episodes* of worsening involving different sites of the CNS, each lasting at least 24 h and occurring at least 1 month apart or (b) gradual or step-wise *progression* over at least 6 months if accompanied by increased CSF IgG synthesis or two or more oligoclonal bands.
5 Age of onset between 15 and 60 years of age.
6 The patient's neurologic condition could not be better attributed to another disease. Laboratory testing that may be advisable in specific cases includes (a) CSF analysis, (b) MRI of the head or spine, (c) serum B_{12} level, (d) human T cell lymphotropic virus type I (HTLV-I) titer, (e) sedimentation rate, (f) rheumatoid factor, antinuclear, anti-DNA antibodies (SLE), (g) serum VDRL, (h) angiotensin-converting enzyme (sarcoidosis), (i) *Borrelia* serology (Lyme disease), (j) very long chain fatty acids (adrenoleukodystrophy), and (k) serum or CSF lactate, muscle biopsy, or mitochondrial DNA analysis (mitochondrial disorders).

DIAGNOSTIC CATEGORIES

1 Definite MS: All six criteria fulfilled.
2 Probable MS: All six criteria fulfilled except (a) only one objective abnormality despite two symptomatic episodes or (b) one symptomatic episode and unrelated signs detected on examination.
3 At risk for MS: All six criteria fulfilled except one symptomatic episode and corresponding signs detected on examination.

aphasia, extrapyramidal syndromes suggesting Parkinson's disease, chorea, isolated dementia, amyotrophy with fasciculations, peripheral neuropathy, seizures, or coma. In patients with mild symptoms, there is often little to be gained by making a diagnosis of "definite MS," and a wise course of action may be to exclude other, potentially treatable causes of the presenting symptoms.

Systemic lupus erythematosus (SLE) may on rare occasions result in a relapsing or progressive CNS disorder that mimics MS. Other signs of SLE are usually present, including an elevated erythrocyte sedimentation rate (ESR), autoantibodies, and evidence of systemic disease. Neurologic involvement in SLE may simulate optic neuritis or transverse myelitis; the two may occur in succession (neuromyelitis optica; see below). Myelopathy in SLE may be acute or progressive and is due to vasculitis or infarction rather than to primary demyelination. Behçet's disease (see Chap. 290) also may result in a chronic CNS illness with optic neuropathy and myelopathy but more often resembles acute disseminated encephalomyelitis (see below) in its presentation; the characteristic oral and genital lesions, associated uveitis, and predilection for men are distinguishing features. Relapsing/remitting CNS disease also has been described in Sjögren's syndrome (see Chap. 288). Sarcoidosis may produce relapsing/remitting cranial nerve palsies (particularly of the seventh nerve), progressive optic atrophy, or myelopathy that raises a question of MS; associated lymphadenopathy, pulmonary or hepatic involvement, an elevated angiotensin-converting enzyme, and hypercalcemia may be present. Lyme disease (see Chap. 137) may involve the optic nerve, brainstem, or spinal cord in the absence of characteristic rash, fever, or meningoradiculitis. Other chronic infections, notably meningovascular syphilis, may need to be considered. CSF examination may aid in distinguishing these disorders from MS when marked lymphocytosis, polymorphonuclear leukocytes, or a raised protein level is present. MS is a common disorder, and in individual patients it may be difficult to exclude the coexistence of two different diseases.

The acute onset of a focal CNS disturbance in a previously healthy individual may suggest a vascular etiology, either cerebrovascular disease or migraine. Progressive focal deficits should always prompt consideration of a compressive lesion. Primary CNS lymphoma may produce solitary or multiple lesions that enhance by MRI and may resemble acute lesions of MS. The development of a progressive or relapsing brainstem disturbance may be due to a vascular malformation in the posterior fossa. Pontine glioma is distinguished from MS by its tendency to produce progressive deficits that involve contiguous structures. Arnold-Chiari malformation presenting in adulthood may cause cerebellar ataxia, nystagmus, and spastic weakness of the limbs. Headache, a short neck, lower cranial nerve palsies, and a syringomyelic syndrome are useful distinguishing features.

Patients who present with primary progressive myelopathies unaccompanied by relapses may present a diagnostic uncertainty. Focal lesions of the spinal cord may result from cervical spondylosis, extradural tumor, or arteriovenous malformation. Subacute necrotic myelopathy (Foix-Alajouanine) is a rare disorder that presents as a spinal cord syndrome that progresses over weeks to months, may appear to ascend, and generally results in complete loss of function below the level of the lesion; pathology reveals necrosis, venous thrombosis, and in some cases vascular malformation within the substance of the cord.

HTLV-I–associated myelopathy (HAM; tropical spastic paraparesis) is a chronic illness that evolves over years and is characterized by back pain, progressive spasticity affecting predominantly the lower limbs, and bladder symptoms (see Chap. 279). It is caused by a human retrovirus that is endemic to certain parts of the world, including southern Japan and the Caribbean, but cases also have been identified from nonendemic regions, including the United States. Clinical examination invariably confirms evidence of pyramidal tract disease, and signs of posterior column, cerebellar, or cranial nerve involvement also may be present. Peripheral neuropathy, when present, is a useful distinguishing feature. CSF pleocytosis is present in up to 20 percent of cases. Diagnosis is based on identification of specific antibody to HTLV-I in serum and CSF and by direct virus isolation.

Inherited and other degenerative disorders also may be questioned, particularly where familial occurrence or a progressive course is present. Asymmetric clinical signs, a sharply demarcated spinal cord level, an intact peripheral nervous system, and CSF inflammatory changes may point to a correct diagnosis of MS. Subacute combined degeneration may on occasion develop in the absence of characteristic megaloblastic anemia and can be excluded by a normal serum B_{12} level and a Schilling test. Two related inherited defects, cobalamin G mutation and plasma R binder deficiency, are reported to result in MS-like syndromes (see Chap. 77). Mitochondrial disorders, including subacute necrotic encephalopathy (Leigh's disease), mitochondrial encephalopathy with acidosis and stroke (MELAS), and Leber's hereditary optic neuropathy, may be excluded by blood and CSF lactate levels, by muscle biopsy, and by biochemical or DNA identification of the specific deficit (see Chap. 385). Heredity ataxias produce symmetric involvement of posterior columns and corticospinal and spinocerebellar tracts, with or without involvement of the peripheral nervous system. Other single-gene disorders that may present in adulthood and resemble MS include the autosomal recessive disorders metachromatic leukodystrophy and Krabbe disease and the X-linked disorders Fabry disease and adrenoleukodystrophy (ALD). ALD is of particular interest because it is associated with an intense CSF inflammatory response.

Neuromyelitis optica (Devic's syndrome) is an unusual condition characterized by the development of acute bilateral optic neuritis, followed within days to weeks by transverse myelitis, in a previously healthy individual. On occasion, optic neuritis may be unilateral or occur after an initial bout of myelitis. CNS lesions may be necrotizing and severe. CSF findings are variable but in some cases consist of polymorphonuclear pleocytosis and an increase in the protein content. Neuromyelitis optica may present as an initial manifestation of MS but also may occur in ADEM, SLE, or Behçet's disease.

LABORATORY DIAGNOSIS Laboratory support for MS may be derived from CSF analysis, evoked response testing, and neuroimaging. CSF abnormalities consist of mononuclear cell pleocytosis, an elevation in the level of total Ig, and the presence of oligoclonal Ig. In one large series, CSF pleocytosis (>5 cells per microliter) was present in 25 percent of MS patients. CSF cell counts are generally less than 20 cells per microliter in MS, and counts above 50 cells per microliter are unusual but may occur at the onset of disease. Pleocytosis of >75 cells per microliter or a finding of polymorphonuclear leukocytes in CSF makes the diagnosis of MS unlikely. Pleocytosis is present more commonly in young patients with relapsing MS than in older patients with chronic progressive MS or inactive MS. In relapsing MS, CSF cell counts correlate poorly with clinical disease activity, indicating that an inflammatory response may be ongoing even at times of clinical remission.

In approximately 80 percent of patients, the CSF content of IgG is increased in the presence of a normal concentration of total protein. This results from the selective production of IgG within the CNS. Occasional MS patients exhibit mild elevations in the total CSF protein content. Various formulas are employed in different laboratories to quantitate the selective increase of IgG that is present and to distinguish local synthesized IgG from serum IgG that may have passively entered the CNS across an abnormal blood-brain barrier. This is important because, under normal conditions, the proportion of total protein that is IgG is lower in CSF than in serum. One useful formula expresses CSF IgG as a ratio to that of CSF albumin.

Oligoclonal banding of CSF IgG is detected by agarose gel electrophoresis techniques (Fig. 373-2A). Two or more oligoclonal bands are found in 75 to 90 percent of MS patients. The presence of oligoclonal banding correlates with an elevated total IgG level in MS. Oligoclonal banding may be absent at the onset of MS, and in individual patients the number of bands present may increase with time. Other Ig abnormalities in MS CSF include free kappa or lambda light chains and elevated levels of other Ig isotypes including IgA. It is important that paired serum samples be studied in order to exclude a systemic origin to the abnormal CSF protein that is detected.

Metabolites derived from myelin breakdown also may be detected in CSF. Elevated levels of MBP or its fragments may be detected by radioimmunoassay both in MS and in some patients with other neurologic diseases. The sensitivity of different assays employed to detect CSF MBP varies.

Evoked response testing may detect slowed or abnormal conduction in visual, auditory, somatosensory, or motor pathways. These tests employ computer averaging techniques to record the electrical response evoked in the nervous system following repetitive sensory or motor stimuli (see Fig. 373-2B). One or several evoked responses are abnormal in 80 to 90 percent of patients with MS. Testing is of greatest value when it provides evidence of a second lesion in a patient with a single clinically apparent lesion or when it demonstrates an objective abnormality in a patient with subjective complaints and a normal examination. Slowing of evoked response latencies in MS is thought to result from loss of saltatory conduction along the course of demyelinated axons. Nonetheless, these changes, when present, are etiologically nonspecific and are also present in other conditions, including vascular disease, in which selective demyelination does not occur.

Neuroimaging has assumed an important role in the diagnosis and longitudinal assessment of MS and has modified basic concepts of the disease. Computed tomographic (CT) scanning is abnormal in a proportion of patients and may reveal ventricular enlargement, low-density periventricular abnormalities, or focal regions of enhancement following injection of a contrast agent. Magnetic resonance imaging (MRI) is the most useful imaging method available, and abnormal scans are present in greater than 90 percent of patients with definite MS. On inversion-recovery (T1-weighted) imaging, the CNS may appear normal or show darkened punctate foci corresponding to white matter structures. Characteristic changes of MS are best appreciated

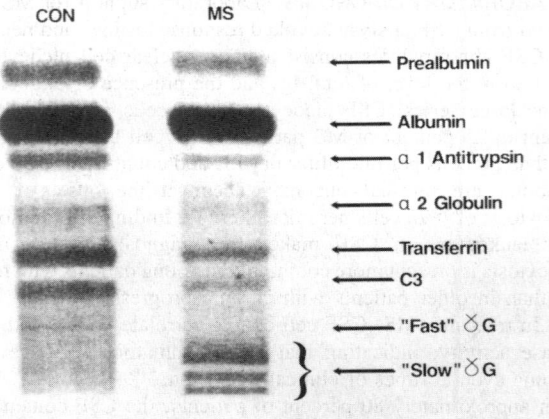

A

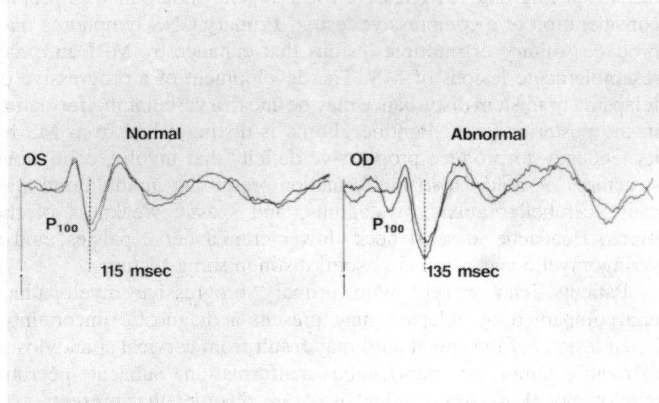

B

FIGURE 373-2 *A*. Agarose gel electrophoresis of CSF in MS reveals multiple bands in the "slow" IgG region. No banding is present in control (CON) CSF. *B*. Pattern stimulation visual evoked responses recorded from an

MS patient reveals a mononuclear latency abnormality. Left eye (OS) response was normal at 115 ms; right eye (OD) response was abnormal with P100 peak delayed in latency at 135 ms. *(Courtesy of Keith Chiappa, MD.)*

with spin-echo (T2-weighted) MRI sequences, in which abnormal areas stand out brightly from the surrounding brain substance (Fig. 373-3*A*). Some T2-weighted bright foci may appear to arise from the ventricular surface and extend in a linear fashion corresponding to a pattern of perivenous demyelination that is observed pathologically (Dawson's fingers). Abnormal foci also may be detected in the spinal cord (Fig. 373-3*B*). Following administration of the contrast agent gadolinium DPTA, enhancement of "active" lesions may be visualized as a result of extravasation of the injected substance across a disrupted blood-brain barrier; these are best appreciated on T1-weighted sequences. Serial MRI studies in relapsing MS indicate that new T2-weighted bright foci appear and may disappear far more frequently than anticipated on the basis of clinical criteria alone. More surprising, similar changes are also present in chronic progressive MS, although abnormal foci in these patients tend to be more confluent than in relapsing MS. These data indicate that in both forms of MS frequent flares of disease activity may be ongoing in the absence of clinical symptoms or signs.

MANAGEMENT   Management may be divided into two categories consisting of (1) treatment designed to arrest the disease process and (2) symptomatic management. The importance of longitudinal staging of the status of MS cannot be overemphasized as an aid to decisions

FIGURE 373-3 *A*. Spin-echo MRI sequence in MS demonstrates extensive bright signal abnormalities in periventricular and other white matter areas. *B*. In a different patient, two discrete abnormal areas are present in the cervical cord.

A

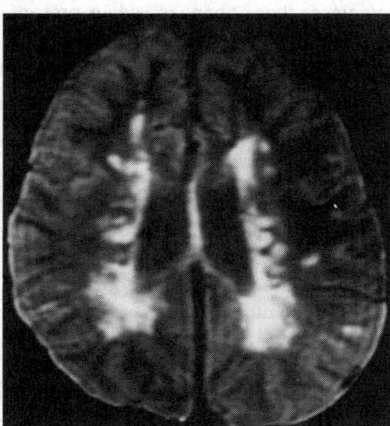

B

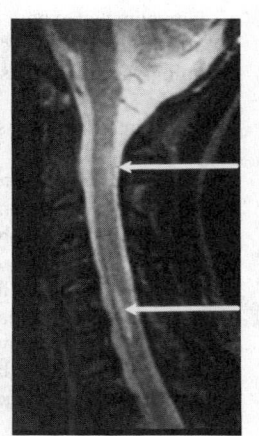

regarding therapy. Many disease scoring systems have been proposed. For gait assessment, one simple and reliable measure is the ambulation index (Table 373-3), which can be rapidly performed in an office or bedside setting.

Treatment designed to arrest the disease process   Immunosuppressive drugs remain the cornerstone of therapy, although their efficacy is limited and their chronic use entails considerable risk. It is thus not surprising that differences in opinion exist as to their specific indications. One practical approach to therapy is summarized in Fig. 373-4.

Long the mainstay of MS therapy, ACTH and glucocorticoids are used for their anti-edema and anti-inflammatory effects. Pulse therapy with these agents speeds the tempo of recovery from acute attacks and may modestly improve the degree of recovery that occurs. They are useful as short-term therapy for relapsing MS. There is no evidence that their use alters the long-term course of the disease.

When neurologic symptoms arise in relapsing MS, it is useful to consider whether they result from new inflammatory lesions in the CNS or whether old MS symptoms have reappeared as a nonspecific consequence of infection or other intercurrent illness. The decision whether or not to treat acute attacks with new neurologic symptoms depends on their severity. Mild deficits, which do not impede functioning, can go untreated, while moderate attacks may benefit from a course of intravenous methylprednisolone followed by oral prednisone. In the past, moderate attacks were most frequently treated with oral prednisone alone on an outpatient basis, but a recent trial of acute optic neuritis indicated that the relapse rate was increased

TABLE 373-3   Ambulation index

0   Asymptomatic; fully active
1   Walks normally but reports fatigue that interferes with athletic or other demanding activities
2   Abnormal gait or episodic imbalance; gait disorder is noticed by family and friends; able to walk 25 ft (8 m) in 10 s or less
3   Walks independently; able to walk 25 ft in 20 s or less
4   Requires unilateral support (cane or single crutch) to walk; walks 25 ft in 20 s or less
5   Requires bilateral support (canes, crutches, or walker) and walks 25 ft in 20 s or less, or requires unilateral support but needs more than 20 s to walk 25 ft
6   Requires bilateral support and more than 20 s to walk 25 ft; may use wheelchair on occasion
7   Walking limited to several steps with bilateral support; unable to walk 25 ft; may use wheelchair for most activities
8   Restricted to wheelchair; able to transfer self independently
9   Restricted to wheelchair; unable to transfer self independently

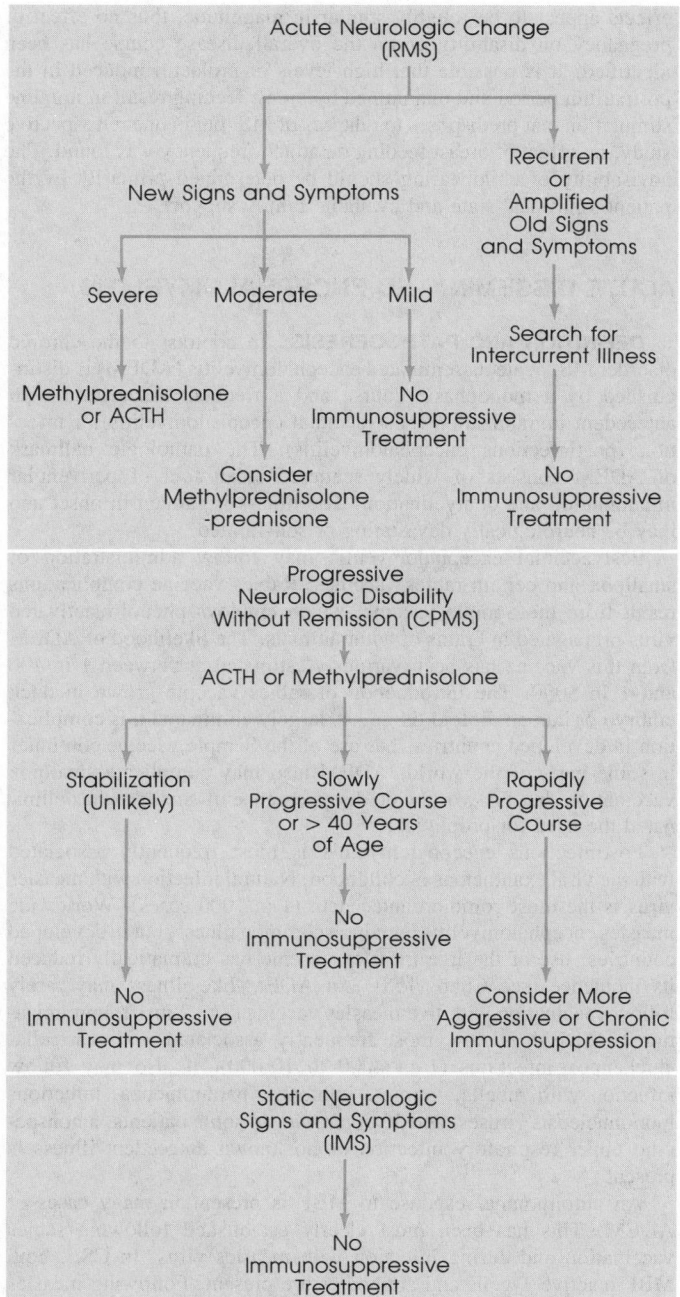

FIGURE 373-4 Therapeutic strategies for MS.

TABLE 373-4 Therapeutic regimens for MS

ACTH

1 Aqueous ACTH (20 U/mL), 80 U is given IV in 500 mL of 5% dextrose and water over 6–8 h for 3 days
2 ACTH gel (40 U/mL) is then given IM in a dose of 40 U every 12 h for 7 days. The dose is then reduced every 3 days as follows:
    35 U bid for 3 days
    30 U bid for 3 days
    50 U qd for 3 days
    40 U pd for 3 days
    30 U qd for 3 days
    20 U qd for 3 days
    20 U every other day for 3 doses

METHYLPREDNISOLONE

Methylprednisolone is mixed in 500 mL D₅W and administered slowly, over 4 to 6 h, preferably in the morning:
    1000 mg daily for 3 days
    500 mg daily for 3 days
    250 mg daily for 3 days

METHYLPREDNISOLONE-PREDNISONE

Methylprednisolone, 1000 mg IV daily for 3 days, followed by oral prednisone (1 mg/kg per day) for 14 days

progressive MS in patients with rapid neurologic deterioration. The chronic use of glucocorticoids has not proved useful in the treatment of MS, although clinical trials have employed only low dosages. The antimetabolite azathioprine given orally on an outpatient basis is a relatively safe and well-tolerated form of chronic immunosuppression. Its beneficial effect is modest in controlled trials and must be weighed against potential risks that include hepatitis, susceptibility to infection, and a possible increased cancer risk. Pulse therapy with the alkylating agent cyclophosphamide is of benefit to young (<40 years) ambulatory patients with rapidly progressive MS. The side effects associated with treatment are considerable and include nausea, hair loss, a risk of hemorrhagic cystitis, and temporary profound immunosuppression. A modest effect of cyclosporine on the course of chronic progressive MS is also present, but side effects, notably hypertension and reversible renal dysfunction, have limited its widespread use.

More than 100 other therapies have been proposed for treatment of MS. Most represent variants of nonspecific immunosuppression strategies. Conversely, others have attempted to stimulate immunity on the assumption that MS may be caused by a chronic viral infection. One such trial employed interferon-γ (immune), which appeared to trigger attacks of MS in a chronic progressive MS population. One effect of interferon-γ is to increase expression of MHC molecules on the surface of antigen-presenting cells, thus facilitating antigen presentation to T cells. This might have resulted in amplification of an autoimmune response in MS. MHC expression induced by interferon-γ can be abrogated by interferon-β. A recently completed 3-year trial of interferon-β therapy in relapsing-remitting MS indicated that this treatment lessened the frequency of MS attacks by one-third, and reduced by 80 percent disease activity as assessed by MRI. Patients enrolled in this trial were ambulatory without support and had experienced at least two MS attacks in the previous 2 years. This subgroup of MS patients should thus be considered as candidates for chronic treatment with subcutaneously administered interferon-β, which was approved for use in 1993. Whether the beneficial effect of interferon-β on MS is due to its antiviral or immunosuppressive properties is not known.

Patients should be discouraged from seeking out costly studies or potentially hazardous therapies carried out by well-meaning but naive practitioners. The National Multiple Sclerosis Society remains the best source for information on therapeutic options for MS.

Symptomatic therapy Spasticity with stiffness, flexor spasms, and clonus can be functionally disabling and painful. Acute worsening of spasticity may occur with underlying infection (frequently of the urinary tract), obstipation, bedsores, other painful lesions, or injuries.

by prednisone but not by methylprednisolone-prednisone therapy. Whether these data are generally applicable to the relapsing MS population is unknown, but caution in the use of oral prednisone alone is warranted. Severe MS attacks, which are functionally disabling, may require hospitalization for intravenous treatment with methylprednisolone or ACTH. The effect of ACTH on MS is likely due to stimulation of endogenous cortisol production rather than to direct effects of ACTH itself. One clinical trial found a similar response to intravenous methylprednisolone or ACTH in acute MS attacks. Specific treatment regimens are outlined in Table 373-4, but varied recommendations with respect to dosage and duration of treatment have been proposed. Because of the high incidence of hypomanic reactions to corticosteroids or ACTH in MS, coadministration of lithium carbonate (300 mg two or three times daily) is routinely employed in all the above regimens.

More aggressive therapies have been employed in attempts to limit the number or severity of relapses in relapsing MS or halt chronic

These precipitants should be sought out and treated specifically. All medications for spasticity have limited efficacy and may produce symptomatic worsening in patients who require stiffness in order to ambulate. Baclofen (15 to 80 mg/d in divided dosages) is the most useful drug available. In refractory cases, oral baclofen in higher dosages (up to 240 mg/d) or intrathecal administration via an indwelling catheter may be effective. Diazepam (2 mg bid or tid) is useful in patients who tolerate its sedative effect, and a single bedtime dose may be especially effective for nocturnal spasms. Dantrolene may produce unacceptable weakness, and its use is reserved for nonambulatory patients. A course of glucocorticoids may be given in exceptional cases where other agents have failed; a beneficial effect may last for several months.

Pain, including trigeminal neuralgia and painful dysesthesias, may respond to carbamazepine (100 to 1200 mg/d in divided, escalating dosages), phenytoin (300 mg/d), or amitriptyline (50 to 200 mg/d). The distinction between dysesthesias due to MS and radiculopathy due to lumbar disk disease may be difficult in patients with unilateral leg pain. Conservative (e.g., *nonsurgical*) therapy is often justified in the absence of convincing signs of nerve root compression.

Paroxysmal symptoms respond to acetazolamide (125 to 250 mg tid) or carbamazepine (up to 1200 mg in divided doses). No treatment for tremor is satisfactory. Isoniazid (up to 1200 mg in divided doses) is reported to benefit postural tremor but is of little practical value for most patients; pyridoxine should be administered concomitantly to prevent peripheral neuropathy. Stereotaxic thalamotomy may be considered in rare cases of disabling tremor in which a unilateral reduction in symptoms is required.

Because specific symptoms of bladder dysfuntion correlate poorly with physiologic findings, urodynamic evaluation is often required. The pathophysiology of abnormal micturition also may change over time in MS. Bladder hyperreflexia is treated with anticholinergics (oxybutynin, 5 mg bid or tid, or propantheline, 7.5 to 15 mg qid). Urinary retention due to bladder hyporeflexia may respond to the cholinergic drug bethanecol (10-50 mg tid or qid). Dyssynergia between detrusor and external sphincter muscles is common in MS, is difficult to treat, and may require a combination of anticholinergic medication to decrease bladder contractions, as well as intermittent catheterization. Supravesical urinary diversion or a chronic indwelling catheter may be required in cases of severe bladder disturbance. Ascorbic acid may reduce the risk of urinary tract infections.

Bowel dysfunction, including constipation and urge incontinence, can be ameliorated by regimentation of bowel function with laxatives and enemas. A low-fiber diet to decrease bulk may be advised for incontinence. Sexual dysfunction may be treated in males by penile implantation, or erections may be achieved pharmacologically using papaverine and phentolamine injections in the corpora cavernosa. Women may experience vaginismus, which may respond to antispasticity medications, or decreased vaginal lubrication leading to dyspareunia, which may be simply treated with lubricants.

Afternoon fatigue may benefit from a shift to an early work schedule or by a regular afternoon nap. Amantadine (100 mg bid) may transiently benefit a small proportion of patients. Emotional lability responds to amitriptyline (25 to 75 mg/d) or to other tricyclic antidepressant medications. It is essential that signs of reactive depression be sought out and specifically treated. Suicide is an important cause of death in MS. Occupational counseling and other support services may assist patients and their families in coping with the effects of the disease. Health maintenance should be emphasized, including stress reduction, a balanced diet, avoidance of rapid weight loss, and adequate rest. There is little evidence linking vaccination with relapses of MS, yet it would be prudent to avoid unnecessary immunizations. Swimming is an ideal form of exercise for many patients because of the buoyant support and hypothermia that is achieved.

Pregnancy may affect the course of MS. Compared with nonpregnant MS patients, pregnant patients experience fewer attacks during gestation but more attacks in the first 3 months postpartum. Both effects appear to be roughly similar in magnitude; thus no effect of pregnancy on disability or on the overall disease course has been identified. It is possible that high levels of prolactin induced in the postpartum period and maintained by breast feeding result in immune stimulation that predisposes to relapses of MS, but in one retrospective study, no effect of breast feeding on attack frequency was found. The advisability of childbearing should be determined primarily by the patient's physical state and available family support.

ACUTE DISSEMINATED ENCEPHALOMYELITIS

DEFINITION AND PATHOGENESIS   In contrast to the chronic disorder MS, acute disseminated encephalomyelitis (ADEM) is distinguished by a monophasic course and a frequent association with antecedent immunization (postvaccinial encephalomyelitis) or infection (postinfectious encephalomyelitis). The pathologic hallmark of ADEM consists of widely scattered small foci of perivenular inflammation and demyelination. The illness is sudden in onset and may be neurologically devastating or self-limited.

Postvaccinial encephalomyelitis may follow administration of smallpox and certain rabies vaccines. Rabies vaccine complications result from the Semple vaccine, which employs phenol-inactivated virus propagated in brains of adult animals. The likelihood of ADEM from this vaccine has been variously estimated at between 1 in 400 and 1 in 5000. The introduction of rabies vaccine grown in duck embryo or human diploid tissue has largely eliminated this complication in developed countries, but use of the Semple vaccine continues in some parts of the world. ADEM also may complicate smallpox vaccination, but the worldwide disappearance of smallpox has eliminated the need for prophylaxis.

Postinfectious encephalomyelitis is most frequently associated with the viral exanthemas of childhood. Natural infection with measles virus is the most common antecedent (1 in 1000 cases). Worldwide measles encephalomyelitis remains a common illness, but in developed countries, use of the live measles vaccine has dramatically reduced its incidence (see Chap. 155). An ADEM-like illness may rarely follow vaccination with live measles vaccine (1 to 2 in 10^6 immunizations). ADEM is now most frequently associated with varicella-chickenpox infections (1 in 4000 to 10,000). It also may follow infection with rubella, mumps, influenza, parainfluenza, infectious mononucleosis viruses, and *Mycoplasma*. In some patients, a nonspecific upper respiratory infection or no known antecedent illness is present.

An autoimmune response to MBP is present in many cases of ADEM. This has been most clearly established following rabies vaccination and during infection with measles virus. In CSF, both MBP-reactive T cells and antibodies are present. Following measles infection, induction of immune responses to a variety of CNS constituents may occur, but only the response to MBP correlates with development of ADEM. As noted earlier, many cases of postvaccinial encephalomyelitis almost certainly result from sensitization with brain material that contaminates the viral vaccines. Postinfectious ADEM generally begins late in the course of the viral illness as the exanthem is fading. Many attempts to demonstrate direct viral invasion of the CNS have been unsuccessful. The molecular mechanism responsible for virus-induced triggering of an autoimmune response to MBP is not known but may include molecular mimicry due to common antigens shared between the virus and host protein, CNS injury with secondary sensitization to MBP, or nonspecific effects of virus infection on immune regulation.

CLINICAL MANIFESTATIONS   The severity of ADEM is variable. In severe cases, the onset is abrupt, and progression is rapid, over the course of hours to days. In postinfectious ADEM, fever that may have faded reappears, and headache, meningismus, and lethargy progressing to coma may develop. Seizures are common. Signs of disseminated neurologic disease are consistently present. Motor findings may include hemiparesis or quadriparesis and extensor plantar responses. Tendon reflexes may be lost initially, later to become hyperactive. Variable degrees of sensory loss and of brainstem involvement may occur. In ADEM due to complications from chickenpox, cerebellar involvement is often prominent and may dominate the clinical picture. CSF protein is modestly elevated (50 to 150 mg/dL). Lymphocytic pleocytosis, generally 200 cells per microliter or less, occurs in 80 percent of cases. Occasional patients may have higher counts or a mixed polymorphonuclear-lymphocytic pattern during the initial days of the illness. Transient CSF oligoclonal banding has been reported in some patients. MRI scanning may reveal extensive gadolinium enhancement of white matter in brain and spinal cord. Electrophysiologic studies indicate involvement of the peripheral nervous system in a proportion of patients.

Prognosis reflects the severity of the underlying acute illness. Measles encephalomyelitis is associated with an estimated mortality of 5 to 20 percent, and permanent neurologic residua occur in the majority of survivors. Children with encephalopathy may have persistent seizures and behavioral and learning disorders. On rare occasions, recovery from apparent ADEM has been followed by development of a chronic or relapsing/remitting CNS disorder.

DIAGNOSIS Correct diagnosis is easily established in settings of recent vaccination or exanthemous illness. In severe cases with predominantly cerebral involvement, acute encephalitis due to infection with herpes simplex or other viruses may be difficult to exclude. In the absence of a specific viral prodrome or immunization, it may not be possible to distinguish ADEM from acute MS. The simultaneous onset of disseminated symptoms and signs indicating optic nerve, brain, and spinal cord involvement is common in ADEM and rare in MS. Similarly, meningismus, drowsiness or coma, or seizures suggest ADEM. Optic nerve involvement is generally bilateral in ADEM and unilateral in MS, and transverse myelopathy is usually complete in the former and partial in the latter. CSF protein is normal in the great majority of MS patients, lymphocyte counts are rarely above 50 cells per microliter, and polymorphonuclear leukocytes are not present. MRI findings that may support a diagnosis of ADEM include extensive and relatively symmetric white matter abnormalities that also involve the posterior fossa and diffuse gadolinium enhancement of all abnormal areas, indicating active disease and a monophasic course. It is worth emphasizing that MS may on occasion present in an explosive fashion, particularly in children. The clinician is often best advised to classify such cases as "acute demyelinating disease," reflecting this uncertainty.

TREATMENT Treatment consists of intravenous methylprednisolone or methylprednisolone-prednisone in an analogous fashion as employed for MS (see Table 373-4). ACTH also has been reported in uncontrolled studies to be of benefit. Occasional patients may show evidence of relapse shortly following termination of therapy, and in such cases, reinstitution of therapy may be useful.

ACUTE HEMORRHAGIC LEUKOENCEPHALITIS

Acute hemorrhagic leukoencephalitis (AHL) of Weston Hurst is a rare, devastating, and hyperacute demyelinating disorder of unknown etiology. CNS lesions of AHL are characterized by perivenous demyelination and intense infiltration by mononuclear and especially polymorphonuclear inflammatory cells. Vasculitis results in necrosis of the walls of venules, fibrin deposition, and innumerable small hemorrhages scattered throughout the white matter of the hemisphere, brainstem, and spinal cord. Large necrotic foci may form by coalescence of smaller lesions.

The clinical course resembles that of severe forms of ADEM but may be even more explosive in onset and progression. The CSF profile consists of marked pleocytosis (up to 3000 cells per microliter), variable numbers of red blood cells, and elevated protein content. Peripheral blood may show an elevated ESR and leukocytosis. Occasional cases may display mixed features of both ADEM and AHL or evolve from one form to the other during the course of the

acute illness. As in ADEM, immune sensitization to MBP also has been described in AHL. Thus AHL may represent a form of ADEM in which a hyperacute inflammatory response is superimposed on lymphocyte-mediated perivenular demyelination. In animal models of EAE, demyelinating lesions also may be either lymphocytic or polymorphonuclear/hemorrhagic depending on the genetic background of the animal, the immunization regimen, and the adjuvent employed.

The differential diagnosis of AHL includes viral encephalitis, acute bacterial cerebritis, venous thrombosis, or multiple embolic infarctions. Prognosis is generally poor. Death may occur within 2 to 4 days of onset. In some patients, complete neurologic recovery has been observed, and as for ADEM, occasional reports describe the subsequent development of a chronic disease similar to MS. These observations further highlight the diagnostic uncertainties and possible overlap between the clinically defined demyelinating diseases. Therapy for AHL consists of methylprednisolone or methylprednisolone-prednisone regimens (see Table 373-4).

REFERENCES

ADAMS CWM et al: Pathology, histochemistry and immunocytochemistry of lesions in acute multiple sclerosis. J Neurol Sci 92:291, 1989

BECK RW et al: A randomized, controlled trial of corticosteroids in the treatment of acute optic neuritis. N Engl J Med 326:581, 1992

GOODKIN DE et al: Diagnostic criteria for multiple sclerosis research involving multiply affected families. Arch Neurol 48:805, 1991

HARDING AE et al: Occurrence of a multiple sclerosis-like illness in women who have a Leber's hereditary optic neuropathy mitochondrial DNA mutation. Brain 115:979, 1992

HARTUNG HP: Immune-mediated demyelination. Ann Neurol 33:563, 1993

HEMACHUDHA T et al: Myelin basic protein as an encephalitogen in encephalomyelitis and polyneuritis following rabies vaccination. N Engl J Med 316:369, 1987

IFNB MULTIPLE SCLEROSIS STUDY GROUP: Interferon beta-1b is effective in relapsing-remitting multiple sclerosis. I. Clinical results of a multicenter, randomized, double-blind, placebo-controlled trial. Neurology 43:655, 1993

JOHNSON RT et al: Measles encephalomyelitis: Clinical and immunologic studies. N Engl J Med 310:137, 1984

KESSELRING J et al: Acute disseminated encephalomyelitis: MRI findings and the distinction from multiple sclerosis. Brain 113:291, 1990

KURTZKE JF, HYLLESTED K: Multiple sclerosis in the Faroe Islands: II. Clinical update, transmission, and the nature of MS. Neurology 36:307, 1986

MATTHEWS WB et al: McAlpine's Multiple Sclerosis. New York, Churchill Livingstone, 1991

McALPINE D et al: Multiple Sclerosis: A Reappraisal. Edinburgh, Livingstone, 1965

MYRIANTHOPOULOS NC: Genetic aspects of multiple sclerosis, in Handbook of Clinical Neurology, vol. 3: Demyelinating Diseases, JC Koetsier (ed). New York, Elsevier Science Publishers, 1985

PATY DW et al: Interferon beta-1b is effective in relapsing-remitting multiple sclerosis. II. MRI analysis results of a multicenter, randomized, double-blind, placebo-controlled trial. Neurology 43:662, 1993

——— et al: MRI in the diagnosis of MS: A prospective study with comparison of clinical evaluation, evoked potentials, oligoclonal banding, and CT. Neurology 38:180, 1988

SADOVNICK AD et al: Parent-child concordance in multiple sclerosis. Ann Neurol 29:252, 1991

WAKSMAN SG: Clinical course and electrophysiology of multiple sclerosis, in Advances in Neurology, vol 47: Functional Recovery in Neurological Disease, SG Waksman (ed). New York, Raven, 1988.

WEINER HL et al: Intermittent cyclophosphamide pulse therapy in progressive multiple sclerosis: Final report of the Northeast Cooperative Multiple Sclerosis Treatment Group. Neurology 43:910, 1993

YUDKIN PL et al: Overview of azathioprine treatment in multiple sclerosis. Lancet 338:1051, 1991

ZAMVIL SS and STEINMAN L: The T lymphocyte in experimental allergic encephalomyelitis. Annu Rev Immunol 8:579, 1990

374 BACTERIAL MENINGITIS AND BRAIN ABSCESS

W. MICHAEL SCHELD

ACUTE BACTERIAL MENINGITIS

DEFINITION Bacterial meningitis may be defined as an inflammatory response to bacterial infection of the pia-arachnoid and the cerebrospinal fluid (CSF) of the subarachnoid space. Since the subarachnoid space is continuous through the brain, spinal cord, and optic nerves, infection in this space extends throughout the cerebrospinal axis unless there is obstruction of the subarachnoid space. Ventriculitis is nearly uniformly present in patients with bacterial meningitis.

EPIDEMIOLOGY Bacterial meningitis remains a common disease worldwide. Although precise figures are unavailable, the incidence of bacterial meningitis is between 4.6 and 10 per 100,000 people per year in the United States. More than 2000 deaths due to bacterial meningitis are reported annually in the United States. Approximately 25,000 cases of bacterial meningitis occur annually, of which about 70 percent occur in children under 5 years of age. The disease is even more common in developing countries. The relative frequency of isolation of various bacterial species as a cause of meningitis is age related (Table 374-1). Gram-negative bacilli (principally *Escherichia coli,* of the K1 capsular type), other enteric bacilli, *Pseudomonas* sp., *Listeria monocytogenes,* and group B streptococci are the major causative agents during the neonatal period. *Haemophilus influenzae* and *Neisseria meningitidis* are the major causes in children beyond 1 month of age. Meningitis in adults is due primarily to meningococci and pneumococci, although disease due to aerobic gram-negative bacilli is observed with increasing frequency, especially in the elderly. *N. meningitidis* is the only major cause of epidemics of bacterial meningitis. Recent trends indicate an increase in the proportion of cases due to gram-negative bacilli and *L. monocytogenes.*

In 1981, it was estimated that *H. influenzae* meningitis developed in approximately 1 in every 500 children during the first 4 years of life. The Centers for Disease Control and Prevention estimate that 29,000 cases due to *H. influenzae,* 4800 cases of pneumococcal meningitis, and 4600 cases of meningococcal disease occurred in the United States during 1973. Similar figures for the 1978–1981 period were reported recently, and the incidence may be increasing, particularly in adults. The overall incidence per 10^5 population per year in the United States during 1986 was 2.9, 1.35, and 1.0 for meningitis due to *H. influenzae* (with significant variability by geographic region), *N. meningitidis,* and *Streptococcus pneumoniae,* respectively (Table 374-2). These most recent figures are derived from a prospective laboratory-based surveillance project in an area with a population of 34 million, 14 percent of the U.S. population. A similar overall incidence for neonatal meningitis of 2.8 cases per 100,000 population

per year was observed in western Sweden during a comparative time period. It is hoped that widespread usage of *H. influenzae* polysaccharide-conjugate vaccines will lead to a marked decline in the incidence of invasive disease due to this pathogen, as observed in the greater Helsinki area since extensive trials with conjunctive vaccines began in 1986.

Meningitis is a major international health problem, as is evident by the recent experience in Africa and South America; explosive and highly fatal outbreaks may occur. At least 30 countries worldwide, including the United States, have reported serious outbreaks of meningococcal meningitis in recent years. During one decade (1973–1982), 4100 cases of meningitis were admitted to a single hospital in Salvador, Brazil, and this disease accounted for 27 percent of all admissions in this interval. The differences in etiology among various studies performed on four different continents are shown in Table 374-3. Worldwide, the three major meningeal pathogens (*H. influenzae, N. meningitidis,* and *S. pneumoniae*) account for approximately 75 to 80 percent of cases, but the proportion due to each organism is somewhat variable by geographic region.

ETIOLOGY At the present time, *H. influenzae* is the most common isolate from cases of bacterial meningitis in the United States. Nearly all cases occur in children under 6 years of age, and more than 90 percent are due to capsular type b strains (see Chap. 112). Meningitis usually follows nasopharyngeal acquisition of a virulent organism with subsequent systemic invasion. *H. influenzae* accounts for only about 0.5 percent of total CSF isolates after 6 years of age, and isolation of this organism from older age groups should suggest the presence of certain predisposing factors, including sinusitis, epiglottitis, pneumonia, otitis media, head trauma with a CSF leak, diabetes mellitus, alcoholism, splenectomy or other asplenic states, and immune deficiency (including hypogammaglobulinemia and AIDS).

Meningitis due to *N. meningitidis* is most often encountered in children and young adults and may occur in epidemics (Chap. 109). Epidemic meningococcal meningitis is usually due to serogroups A or C, although the potential for epidemic spread of any serogroup exists. Type B strains are isolated most frequently in sporadic cases, accounting for approximately 50 percent of all isolates in the United States. Type Y strains are associated with pneumonia. The meningococcus is isolated from approximately 20 percent of all cases of bacterial meningitis in the United States. Nasopharyngeal carriage of virulent organisms also accounts for the initiation of infection. Infection is more likely in patients who have deficiencies in the terminal complement components (C5 to C8, and perhaps C9), the so-called membrane attack complex. Persons with these deficiencies have an 8000-fold increased risk of *Neisseria* infections, although the mortality rates appear to be lower than in patients with an intact complement system. Meningococcal meningitis also may occur in properdin-deficient individuals.

Pneumococcal meningitis is the most frequently observed agent in adults over the age of 30 years and accounts for approximately 15 percent of the total cases of meningitis in the United States (see Chap. 101). Mortality rates remain high, in the 19 to 30 percent range.

TABLE 374-1 Bacterial etiology of meningitis, by age

Organism	Neonates (≤1 month), %	Children (1 month to 15 years), %	Adults (>15 years), %
H. influenzae	0–3	40–60	1–3
S. pneumoniae	0–5	10–20	30–50
N. meningitidis	0–1	25–40	10–35
Gram-negative bacilli	50–60	1–2	1–10
Streptococci	20–40*	2–4	5
Staphylococci	5	1–2	5–15
Listeria species	2–10	1–2	5

* Nearly all isolates are group B streptococci.
SOURCE: After Roos et al.

TABLE 374-2 Bacterial meningitis in five states and Los Angeles County, 1986

Organism	Percent of total cases	Case fatality rate (%)
H. influenzae	45	3
S. pneumoniae	18	19
N. meningitidis	14	13
Group B streptococci	5.7	12
L. monocytogenes	3.2	22
Others	15	18

SOURCE: After Wenger et al.

TABLE 374-3 Etiology of bacterial meningitis in four geographic areas (% of total cases)

Organism	United States, 1978–1981	United Kingdom, 1980–1984	Dakar, Senegal, 1970–1979	Salvador, Brazil, 1973–1982
H. influenzae	48	29	20	23
S. pneumoniae	13	20	29	17
N. meningitidis	20	25	11	32
Group B streptococcus	3	7	4	2
L. monocytogenes	2	2	<0.5	—
Other	8	16	9	8
Unknown	6	—	26	19

SOURCE: After Roos et al.

Pneumococcal infection of the meninges is often associated with distant foci such as pneumonia, otitis media, mastoiditis, sinusitis, or endocarditis. Serious pneumococcal infections may be observed in patients with predisposing conditions, including splenectomy or asplenic states, multiple myeloma, hypogammaglobulinemia, alcoholism, cirrhosis, and the Wiskott-Aldrich syndrome. *S. pneumoniae* is the most common meningeal isolate in head trauma patients who have suffered a basilar skull fracture with subsequent CSF leak.

Although *L. monocytogenes* represents only a small minority of cases of bacterial meningitis in the United States, mortality remains high (see Table 374-2). *Listeria* infection is more likely in neonates, the elderly, alcoholics, cancer patients, and immunosuppressed adults (e.g., renal transplant patients). The incidence of *Listeria* meningoencephalitis may be declining in renal transplant populations due to the frequent use of trimethoprim-sulfamethoxazole prophylaxis. However, up to 30 percent of adults and 50 percent of children with listeriosis have no apparent underlying condition. Serious *Listeria* infections have been associated with several foodborne outbreaks involving contaminated cole slaw, milk, and cheese.

Meningitis due to aerobic gram-negative bacilli is unusual except at the extremes of life. *E. coli* is isolated from 30 to 50 percent of neonates with bacterial meningitis. *Klebsiella* sp., *E. coli,* and *Pseudomonas aeruginosa* also may be isolated following head trauma, neurosurgical procedures, in the elderly, in immunosuppressed patients, and in patients with gram-negative bacteremia. Despite the relative low frequency of meningitis due to this group of microorganisms, the mortality rates remain high. Many of these infections are nosocomial in origin, although community-acquired gram-negative bacillary meningitis appears to be increasing in frequency, particularly among the elderly and in debilitated, alcoholic, or diabetic adults. Staphylococcal meningitis is rare except in patients with indwelling CSF shunts, in whom *Staphylococcus epidermidis* is the most common organism. Meningitis due to *S. aureus* is unusual and accounts for about 1 to 8 percent of cases in various surveys. *S. aureus* is the second most common cause of CSF shunt infections and is also a nosocomial pathogen. Although secondary meningitis in the setting of infective endocarditis is relatively uncommon, most of these infections are due to *S. aureus*. Other important associated conditions include head trauma, abscesses in other organs, neurosurgical procedures, sinusitis, osteomyelitis, pneumonia, cellulitis, decubitus ulcers, and infected intravascular grafts or shunts. Many patients have concomitant conditions, including diabetes mellitus, malignancy, renal failure, and immunosuppression. The mortality of staphylococcal meningitis remains high (about 50 percent in adults), although the prognosis for CSF shunt infections is more favorable.

Group B streptococci are an important cause of neonatal meningitis. These infections may occur as early-onset septicemia associated with premature rupture of the membranes and low-birth-weight or late-onset meningitis more than 7 days after birth. The early-onset form is acquired from the maternal genital tract, whereas the source of the group B streptococci in late-onset disease is more controversial; at least 40 percent of infected infants are born to culture-negative mothers. Rare cases of group B streptococcal meningitis have been reported in adults, including postpartum females following vaginal delivery. Bacteremic infections, usually in older adults, unrelated to

pregnancy occur in the setting of underlying risk factors in the following approximate order of decreasing frequency: diabetes mellitus, malignancy, liver failure or history of alcoholism, neurologic impairment, renal failure, congestive heart failure, use of intravenous catheters, glucocorticoid administration, asplenia, and AIDS. Nevertheless, this is a rare disease in the adult.

Meningitis due to anaerobic bacteria is rare, accounting for less than 1 percent of pyogenic cases. Recovery of anaerobic bacteria from CSF should suggest intraventricular rupture of a brain abscess. Most other cases arise from spread of infection secondary to a contiguous focus of disease and are seen in patients predisposed to focal suppurative intracranial processes.

A plethora of microorganisms have been documented as the cause of meningitis in isolated case reports or in small numbers of patients. Meningitis due to *Flavobacterium meningosepticum* may be a problem in certain neonatal intensive care units, and nosocomial meningitis due to other gram-negative bacilli or *Acinetobacter* sp. appears to be increasing in frequency. Polymicrobial bacterial meningitis with simultaneous recovery of two or more bacterial species from CSF is unusual and accounts for less than 1 percent of cases. The majority of cases occur in adults with a wide spectrum of etiologic agents. Many patients have had tumors in close proximity to the neuraxis, rectal carcinoma, or a fistulous communication with the CNS. Simultaneous isolation of viruses and bacteria from the CSF is rare; only seven well-documented cases have been reported since 1988. Nevertheless, CSF samples are infrequently cultured for both groups of microorganisms, and this occurrence may be a gross underestimate of the actual problem.

PATHOGENESIS AND PATHOPHYSIOLOGY Since most cases of bacterial meningitis are hematogenous in origin, pathogenesis involves sequential steps related to the expression of several different bacterial virulence factors that overcome host defense mechanisms and allow the pathogen to reach, invade, and replicate in the CSF. These pathogenic steps include the following: (1) nasopharyngeal colonization, (2) nasopharyngeal epithelial cell invasion, (3) bloodstream invasion, (4) bacteremia with intravascular survival, (5) traversal across the blood-brain barrier and entry into CSF, and (6) survival and replication within the subarachnoid space.

Nasopharyngeal mucosal colonization and invasion by meningeal pathogens require evasion of secretory IgA, avoidance of ciliary clearance mechanisms, adhesion to the apical epithelial cell membrane, and passage to the basolateral side of the cell. Virtually all clinical isolates of the three major meningeal pathogens secrete IgA proteases that cleave the hinge region of IgA and render it nonfunctional, thereby facilitating bacterial adhesion to the epithelium. Studies using a human nasopharyngeal organ culture model have elucidated the distinct mechanisms of adhesion and invasion by the human pathogens *H. influenzae* and *N. meningitidis*. Infection of human nasopharyngeal organ cultures with either organism results in injury to ciliated epithelial cells with ciliostasis and selective adherence to nonciliated epithelial cells. Meningococcal binding is dependent on expression of cell surface pili, and the organism interacts with epithelial cell microvilli. Meningococci enter nonciliated epithelial cells by an endocytotic process and proceed to the abluminal side by a transcellular route within membrane-bound vacuoles. *H. influenzae,* in contrast, creates separations between apical tight junctions of columnar epithelial cells and invades primarily via an intercellular route. After adhesion to and invasion of the nasopharyngeal epithelium, pathogenic bacteria must enter and survive within the intravascular space prior to penetration of the CNS. Evasion of the host's alternative complement pathway is an important strategy of meningeal pathogens to sustain intravascular survival; this virulence property is largely dependent on expression of capsular polysaccharide. The actual molecular basis for this complement evasion strategy differs among the major meningeal pathogens and has been attributed to meningococcal capsular sialic acid and the *H. influenzae* type b polysaccharide capsule (polyribosoyl-ribose-phosphate). *H. influenzae* is capable of replication within the intravascular space.

Once bacteremia occurs, the bacterial pathogens must invade the CNS. The site and mechanism of meningeal invasion by bacteria, however, are poorly understood. Early studies in an experimental infant rat model of *H. influenzae* meningitis suggested that the dural venous sinuses were the major route of CNS invasion. More recent studies, however, suggest that a nonspecific sterile focal inflammation above the cribriform plate facilitates CNS invasion at this site. Experimental studies also have demonstrated that bacteria may enter the CSF via the choroid plexus related to its exceptional high rate of blood flow and fenestrated capillaries. Three hypotheses are proposed to account for the observed neurotropism of meningeal pathogens and for their entry into the CNS: (1) meningitis is secondary to a sustained bacteremia that must be of sufficient duration and magnitude, (2) adhesion to critical blood-brain barrier components may mediate CNS invasion, supported by the potential role of adhesion of *E. coli* strains to the luminal surface of microvascular cerebral endothelium and the epithelial lining of the choroid plexus and ventricles, and (3) microorganisms are transferred within macrophages or other phagocytic cells entering the CNS by normal cellular trafficking pathways.

Once bacteria cross the blood-brain barrier and enter the CNS, host humoral defense mechanisms, particularly dependent on immunoglobulin and complement activity, are virtually absent, resulting in a significant advantage for the pathogen. Since opsonic activity is often undetectable even in infected CSF, phagocytosis of the encapsulated bacterial pathogens in the fluid medium of the CSF is inefficient. Thus bacterial meningitis represents an infection in an area of impaired host resistance commonly leading to very large bacterial densities in the CSF and mandating the use of bactericidal agents for optimal response to therapy.

Once bacteria enter and replicate within the CSF, subarachnoid space inflammation ensues. This inflammation is largely responsible for the pathophysiologic consequences that contribute to the clinical syndrome of bacterial meningitis, including the following: increased permeability of the blood-brain barrier, cerebral edema (vasogenic, interstitial, and cytotoxic in origin), increased outflow resistance to CSF, cerebral vasculitis, increased intracranial pressure, decreased cerebral blood flow and/or loss of autoregulation of cerebral blood flow, cortical hypoxia, and CSF acidosis.

CSF neutrophilic pleocytosis is a hallmark of subarachnoid space inflammation. Nevertheless, the pathway of neutrophil traversal into the CSF is largely unknown. Adhesion of neutrophils to vascular endothelial cells is a necessary prerequisite for this traversal; pretreatment of endothelial cells in tissue culture with various inflammatory cytokines induces formation of specific adhesion molecules [e.g., endothelial leukocyte adhesion molecule 1 (ELAM-1)], although some of these adhesion molecules have yet to be demonstrated in cerebral endothelium. Leukocyte endothelial cell adhesion is mediated by specific transmembrane glycoproteins expressed on the endothelial cells that interact with specific counterparts on neutrophils. Three families of adhesion molecules may mediate these important interactions, including the immunoglobulin superfamily (e.g., ICAM-1 and ICAM-2), the integrin family (e.g., the CD11/CD18 subfamily), and the selectin family (ELAM-1). The complex interrelationships among these three families, including the inducibility of neutrophil adhesion, and the participation of multiple glycoproteins in diapedesis and the

induction of inflammation are considered in greater detail in Chap. 79. Important for consideration is evidence that blockage of neutrophil adhesion to endothelium by the systemic administration of a monoclonal antibody (IB4) against the CD11/CD18 family of receptors leads to absence of CSF pleocytosis in experimental animal models of meningitis. The CSF pleocytosis following challenge with live microorganisms and cell wall components is prevented. Combination treatment with dexamethasone and monoclonal antibody IB4 is more effective than either agent alone in the prevention of CSF pleocytosis.

Subarachnoid space inflammation is induced by constituents of bacteria. Capsular polysaccharides are remarkably noninflammatory, although bacterial capsule is crucial for intravascular and subarachnoid space survival of meningeal pathogens. Experimental animal studies have documented that the cell wall of gram-positive microorganisms and the endotoxin (lipopolysaccharide, or LPS, or lipooligosaccharide) of gram-negative organisms induce subarachnoid space inflammation. In the case of pneumococcus, intracisternal injection of the major components of the cell wall, teichoic acid and peptidoglycan, induces inflammation. In gram-negative meningitis, the lipid A region of LPS is responsible for the induction of inflammation. CSF inflammatory changes are also invoked following the intracisternal inoculation of *H. influenzae* type b outer membrane vesicles, which may serve as a relevant nonreplicating vehicle for the delivery of the toxic moieties of LPS to host cells in vivo. Pneumococcal cell wall and *H. influenzae* type b LPS elicit subarachnoid space inflammation through the release of various inflammatory mediators within the CNS. Both interleukin 1 (IL-1) and tumor necrosis factor (TNF) appear within CSF rapidly following the intracisternal inoculation of pneumococcal cell wall or LPS from gram-negative bacteria. These proinflammatory cytokines induce subarachnoid space inflammation independently and appear to act synergistically in this effect. In addition, increased CSF concentrations of TNF may be specific for bacterial meningitis, since elevated levels are found in bacterial but not viral meningitis in both experimental animals and humans. The role of other inflammatory cytokines in the induction of subarachnoid space inflammation is less clear. Although interleukin 6 (IL-6) and platelet-activating factor (PAF) are present at increased concentrations in the CSF during the disease, the precise contribution of these inflammatory cytokines within the CNS is unknown. Nevertheless, higher CSF concentrations of TNF and PAF are associated with increased severity of the disease in children.

One of the major pathophysiologic consequences of bacterial meningitis is increased permeability of the blood-brain barrier, which leads to vasogenic cerebral edema. After the intracisternal inoculation of bacterial pathogens in experimental animals, a uniform host response to experimental meningitis at the level of the cerebral capillary endothelium is observed, characterized morphologically by an early and sustained increase in pinocytotic vesicle formation and a progressive increase in separation of intercellular tight junctions. These morphologic alterations correlate with a functional penetration of a marker protein (albumin) across the blood-brain barrier. CSF leukocytes augment changes in permeability late in the disease course. Intracisternal inoculations of pneumococcal cell walls, *H. influenzae* type b LPS, outer membrane vesicles prepared from *H. influenzae*, and various proinflammatory cytokines all induce increased blood-brain permeability in vivo. Encapsulation of *H. influenzae* is not essential for blood-brain barrier injury but facilitates its progression by allowing the organism to escape host clearance mechanisms within the CSF in vivo. Studies that utilize an in situ perfusion protocol of albumin–colloidal gold as tracer as well as complementary immunogold detection of perfused monomeric albumin have localized the site of albumin traversal to the postcapillary venule in the subarachnoid space during bacterial meningitis. Albumin traversal occurs primarily via a paracellular pathway through open intercellular junctions in venular segments, since transcytosis to the abluminal side of the endothelium is minimal. Although gram-negative cell wall components in addition to LPS (e.g., peptidoglycan) may induce subarachnoid space inflammation, the effect is minimal when compared with

LPS alone. The precise primary and secondary messengers governing alterations in blood-brain barrier permeability and the paracellular leak of albumin remain unknown, but ongoing development of in vitro systems of isolated cerebral microvascular endothelial cells may assist in delineating this event at the cellular level. Furthermore, the recent demonstration of elevated concentrations of excitatory amino acids within CSF suggests a role for these substances in the altered blood brain-barrier permeability as well as altered CNS homeostasis.

Another important pathophysiologic consequence of subarachnoid space inflammation is the development of increased intracranial pressure (ICP) caused primarily (but not exclusively) by the development of cerebral edema that may be vasogenic, cytotoxic, and/or interstitial in origin. Vasogenic cerebral edema is primarily a result of increased blood-brain barrier permeability. Cytotoxic cerebral edema results from swelling of the cellular elements of the brain, most likely due to the release of toxic factors from neutrophils and/or bacteria. Interstitial cerebral edema occurring during meningitis is largely due to obstruction of normal CSF pathways with resultant increased CSF outflow resistance. Cerebral edema is always found in experimental animal models of meningitis, as measured by increased brain water content. The attenuation of the observed cerebral edema, raised ICP, and increased CSF outflow resistance with glucocorticoid administration in experimental animal models of meningitis led directly to a reexamination of the potential adjunctive roles for these agents in the treatment of this disease (see below). Cerebral blood flow alterations also have been documented in animal models and in patients with bacterial meningitis. In an infant rhesus monkey model of *H. influenzae* meningitis, certain areas of the cortex (postcentral, temporal, and occipital) were hypoperfused relative to the hypothalamus and midbrain, while the brainstem was hyperperfused, suggesting cerebral cortical hypoperfusion with resultant relative cerebral anoxia as an early physiologic change during *H. influenzae* meningitis. Loss of cerebral autoregulation has been documented in an experimental rabbit model of pneumococcal meningitis. It has been suggested that even minor fluctuations of mean arterial blood pressure may have adverse consequences for patients with meningitis, since autoregulation may be lost, resulting in an increased risk of brain injury from either transient hypotension or hypertension. The blood flow alterations may lead to regional hypoxia, increased brain lactate concentrations secondary to utilization of glucose by anaerobic pathways, and CSF acidosis, which may be a precursor to encephalopathy. It is possible that generation of reactive oxygen intermediates in the microvasculature potentiates these changes in regional cerebral blood flow. Infusion of superoxide dismutase modifies the early alterations in cerebral blood flow in experimental models of pneumococcal meningitis.

PATHOLOGY The pathologic hallmark of bacterial meningitis is a subarachnoid space exudate. On gross examination, the exudate has a typical grayish yellow or yellowish green appearance. It is most abundant in the cisterns at the base of the brain and over the convexities of the cerebral hemispheres in the rolandic and sylvian fissures. Purulent exudate accumulates in the basal cisterns and also, in the absence of obstruction, extends along the spinal cord and nerve sheaths and into the ventricular system. Microscopic examination of the subarachnoid exudate in the early stages demonstrates large numbers of neutrophils and bacteria. Within 2 to 3 days of infection, evidence of inflammation in the wall of the small and medium-sized subarachnoid blood vessels appears. Subintimal arterial infiltration by lymphocytes and neutrophils is relatively unique to infection of the meninges. The meningeal veins become distended and develop mural infection, which may be complicated by focal necrosis of the vessel wall, mural thrombus formation in the lumen, or involvement of the dural sinuses. Hemorrhagic cortical infarction may be the result of cortical venous and dural sinus thrombosis. By the end of the first week of meningeal inflammation, a change in the cellular composition of the subarachnoid exudate occurs. Neutrophils begin to degenerate and are removed by macrophages, derived from meningeal histiocytes. The nuclei of affected neurons and glia cells become shrunken,

pyknotic, and darkly staining. Further infiltration of subependymal tissues and perivascular spaces by neutrophils and lymphocytes occurs. Blockage of normal CSF pathways, particularly in the fourth ventricle through the midline foramen of Magendie and the lateral foramina of Luschka may result in noncommunicating or obstructive hydrocephalus. Interference of CSF absorption via the arachnoid villi may result from accumulation of the fibrinopurulent exudate. Diffuse cerebral edema and/or increased intracranial pressure may lead to life-threatening herniation. Cranial and spinal nerve deficits, focal neurologic deficits, seizure disorders, encephalopathy, and subdural effusions are all recognized complications of meningitis.

CLINICAL MANIFESTATIONS The classic clinical presentation of adults with bacterial meningitis includes headache, fever, and meningismus, often with signs of cerebral dysfunction; these are found in more than 85 percent of patients. Nausea, vomiting, rigors, profuse sweats, weakness, myalgias, and photophobia are also common. The meningismus may be subtle or marked, accompanied by Kernig's and/or Brudzinski's signs. These signs are elicited in only about 50 percent of adults with bacterial meningitis, and their absence does not rule out this possibility. Cerebral dysfunction is manifested primarily by confusion, delirium, or a declining level of consciousness ranging from lethargy to coma. Cranial nerve palsies, especially involving cranial nerves IV, VI, and VII, are found in 10 to 20 percent of cases, occasionally in concert with focal neurologic deficits such as visual field defects, dysphasia, and hemiparesis in a small minority of patients. Seizures occur in about 40 percent of cases. The presence of bilateral sixth nerve palsies, manifested as weakness of the lateral rectus muscles, suggests raised ICP. Papilledema is rare (<1 percent of patients) and should suggest an alternative diagnosis, such as an intracranial mass lesion. Later in the disease course patients may develop signs of increased ICP, including coma, hypertension, bradycardia, and third nerve palsy; these findings are ominous prognostic signs. Focal neurologic deficits, seizure activity, and encephalopathy may arise from cortical and/or subcortical ischemia and/or infarction, raised ICP, or the development of a subdural effusion.

Certain symptoms and/or signs may suggest a specific etiologic diagnosis in patients with meningitis. Meningococcemia with or without meningitis presents with a prominent rash, principally of the extremities, in about 50 percent of patients. Early in the disease process, the rash is often erythematous and macular but typically evolves quickly into a petechial phase with further coalescence into a purpuric form with gun metal gray necrosis in the center of the purpuric regions. This rash often matures rapidly, sometimes with the appearance of new petechial lesions during the performance of the physical examination. A similar rash also may be seen in other forms of meningitis (e.g., due to echovirus type 9, *S. aureus, Acinetobacter* sp., and, rarely, *S. pneumoniae* or *H. influenzae*), Rocky Mountain spotted fever or other rickettsioses, *S. aureus* endocarditis, rapidly overwhelming sepsis due to encapsulated bacteria in splenectomized patients, or noninfectious disorders such as vasculitis or thrombotic thrombocytopenic purpura. An additional suppurative focus of infection, typically otitis media, sinusitis, or pneumonia, may be seen in approximately 30 percent of patients with pneumococcal or *H. influenzae* meningitis. Patients with meningitis following a CSF leak may demonstrate rhinorrhea or otorrhea due to a persistent defect.

Conversely, certain subgroups of patients may not manifest many of the classic signs and/or symptoms of bacterial meningitis. Meningismus and/or fever are commonly absent in neonates, and the only clinical clues may be listlessness, high-pitched crying, refusal to feed, irritability, or other nonspecific manifestations. Elderly patients often present insidiously with lethargy or obtundation and with variable signs of meningeal inflammation and no fever. In this subgroup of patients, an altered mental status should not be ascribed to other causes until bacterial meningitis has been excluded by CSF examination. Many of the signs of bacterial meningitis, including alteration in consciousness, are present in patients following neurosurgery and/or head trauma. The diagnosis of meningitis is difficult in this situation, and the physician should have a low threshold for CSF examination if any clinical deterioration occurs.

DIAGNOSIS The diagnosis of bacterial meningitis rests on examination of the CSF, usually following lumbar puncture. When papilledema and/or focal neurologic findings suggestive of an intracranial mass lesion are present, lumbar puncture should be deferred until a computed tomographic (CT) scan or magnetic resonance imaging (MRI) study is performed. Nevertheless, if meningitis remains an important consideration, empirical antimicrobial therapy should be started during the performance of the neuroimaging study. Although CSF cultures may be rendered sterile, the CSF profile will still be suggestive of bacterial meningitis despite empirical antimicrobial therapy during the performance of the procedure.

The typical CSF findings in acute bacterial meningitis consist of an elevated opening pressure, neutrophilic pleocytosis, elevated protein concentration, and hypoglycorrhachia. The opening pressure is elevated in virtually all cases. Values exceeding 600 mL of water suggest cerebral edema, communicating hydrocephalus, or the presence of intracranial suppurative foci. The gross appearance of the fluid may be cloudy or turbid if the white cell count is elevated. Occasionally, the fluid may appear turbid due to the presence of microorganisms in the absence of significant CSF pleocytosis; this is an ominous prognostic sign. Traumatic lumbar puncture may produce a bloody CSF initially but should clear as flow continues. Xanthochromia may occur during meningitis but should suggest the possibility of subarachnoid hemorrhage and in patients with heart valve disease raises the possibility of ruptured mycotic aneurysm. The CSF leukocyte concentration is usually elevated in untreated bacterial meningitis, ranging from 10 to $> 1000 \times 10^3$ per liter with a neutrophilic predominance. Approximately 10 percent of patients present initially with a predominance of lymphocytes in CSF. A very low CSF white cell concentration in bacterial meningitis often has been associated with poor prognosis. Therefore, Gram's stain and culture should be performed on all CSF specimens even in the absence of a CSF pleocytosis. The CSF protein concentration is elevated in virtually all cases of bacterial meningitis, sometimes to an extreme degree when spinal block is present, presumably due to disruption of the blood-brain barrier and/or generation of protein from leukocytes or microorganisms in the subarachnoid space. The CSF glucose concentration is less than 40 mg/dL (<2.2 mmol/L) in approximately 60 percent of patients with bacterial meningitis, and the CSF to serum glucose ratio is less than 0.31 in about 70 percent of patients. The CSF glucose concentration must be compared with simultaneous serum glucose concentration for proper evaluation. A recent analysis found that a CSF glucose level less than 34 mg/dL (1.9 mmol/L), a CSF/blood glucose ratio of less than 0.23, a CSF protein level of greater than 2.2 g/L (220 mg/dL), and more than 2000×10^6 CSF leukocytes per liter or more than 1180×10^6 CSF neutrophils per liter were individual predictors of bacterial as opposed to viral meningitis with 99 percent certainty or better.

CSF examination by Gram's stain should always be performed and permits a rapid and accurate identification of the etiologic agent in approximately 60 to 90 percent of cases of bacterial meningitis (overall sensitivity is approximately 75 percent). The probability of organism detection correlates with bacterial concentrations in CSF. False-positive findings may occur as a result of contamination of collection tubes or the staining reagents. Negative CSF Gram's stains are usually related to prior antimicrobial therapy and low CSF concentrations of microorganisms. The CSF culture is positive in approximately 70 to 85 percent of patients with bacterial meningitis. The probability of identifying an organism may decrease in patients who have received prior antimicrobial therapy. Blood cultures also should be obtained because they are positive in a variable proportion of patients with bacterial meningitis depending on the pathogen.

Many other rapid diagnostic tests have been developed to aid in the diagnosis of bacterial meningitis when the Gram's stain is negative. Countercurrent immunoelectrophoresis (CIE) may be helpful in the detection of specific microbial antigens in CSF with a sensitivity of approximately 62 to 95 percent with high specificity. Nevertheless, newer techniques employing staphylococcal coagglutination or latex agglutination are more rapid and sensitive than CIE (ability to detect bacterial antigen concentrations of approximately 1 ng/mL of CSF). It must be emphasized that a negative test does not rule out infection due to a particular meningeal pathogen. The limulus lysate test is highly sensitive in the detection of LPS within CSF, although it does not distinguish between gram-negative organisms that may be present and the results often do not alter decisions on therapeutic regimen.

Neuroimaging techniques such as CT and MRI have little role in the diagnosis of acute bacterial meningitis but may detect complications and/or a parameningeal source of infection. CT or MRI may be useful in patients with prolonged fever several days after initiation of antimicrobial therapy, with prolonged obtundation or coma in the presence of new or recurrent seizure activity, with signs of increased ICP, or with focal neurologic deficits. MRI is more sensitive than CT for the evaluation of subdural effusions, cortical infarction, and cerebritis but is more difficult to obtain in a critically ill patient. The vast majority of patients with suspected or proven bacterial meningitis do not require a neuroimaging study.

Most patients with suspected bacterial meningitis deserve initial evaluation in an intensive care setting. Multiple complications may ensue, including shock, disseminated intravascular coagulation, the syndrome of inappropriate secretion of vasopressin (antidiuretic hormone), and others. In addition to frequent monitoring, blood cultures and tests for coagulation factors and electrolytes, including renal function, are essential. A chest x-ray may reveal a coexistent pneumonia. Stains of petechiae or purpuric lesions may reveal intracellular cocci in approximately 70 percent of meningococcemia cases. In the presence of frank arthritis, arthrocentesis with culture and stains may yield the etiologic agent.

DIFFERENTIAL DIAGNOSIS Multiple infectious and noninfectious processes may be responsible for an acute meningitis syndrome and can be confused with acute bacterial meningitis, including parameningeal foci of infection (e.g., brain abscess, subdural empyema, and epidural abscess; see below), viral meningitis or encephalitis, CSF syphilis, the neurologic manifestations of Lyme disease, tuberculous meningitis, fungal meningitis, bacterial endocarditis, rickettsial infections such as Rocky Mountain spotted fever, CNS neoplasms, cerebral vasculitis, granulomatous angiitis, sarcoidosis, cyst-related meningitis, subarachnoid hemorrhage, neuroleptic malignant syndrome, chemical meningitis due to drugs, radiocontrast agents, or anesthetics, and various poorly understood chronic or recurrent meningeal syndromes.

TREATMENT **Antimicrobial therapy** The initial procedure in a patient with suspected bacterial meningitis is performance of a lumbar puncture to obtain CSF for analysis. Patients should receive emergent empirical antimicrobial therapy based on age and underlying disease status if no etiologic agent is identified by Gram's stain or rapid diagnostic tests and the diagnosis of bacterial meningitis is likely. In those few patients who present with focal signs on neurologic examination, a CT scan should be obtained prior to a lumbar puncture. However, if meningitis is a strong possibility, empirical antimicrobial therapy should be instituted immediately. The empirical regimens for presumed bacterial meningitis are based primarily on the age of the host and the likely infecting pathogens. For neonates under 1 month of age, the most likely pathogens are *E. coli*, *S. agalactiae*, and *L. monocytogenes*. Empirical therapy commonly consists of ampicillin plus a third-generation cephalosporin, usually cefotaxime due to the concerns of albumin binding by ceftriaxone and bilirubin metabolism in this age group. An alternative treatment regimen is ampicillin plus an aminoglycoside. In older infants (ages 4 to 12 weeks), infections with either *H. influenzae* or *S. pneumoniae* join the typical neonatal pathogens, and the regimen of choice is ampicillin plus a third-generation cephalosporin. From ages 3 months to 6 years, *H. influenzae* is by far the most common etiologic agent, and empirical therapy with a third-generation cephalosporin may be used. Some authorities still recommend ampicillin plus chloramphenicol or chloramphenicol alone in this age group, but cefuroxime should be avoided. In younger adults, most cases of meningitis are due to *N. meningitidis* or *S. pneumoniae,* and penicillin G or ampicillin are often used. Because of the prevalence of gram-negative aerobic bacilli in older adults (over 50 years of age) and the possibility of *L. monocytogenes* infection, the empirical regimen should consist of ampicillin in combination with a third-generation cephalosporin. In postneurosurgical patients or in those with CSF shunts or foreign bodies in place, the likely infecting organisms include staphylococci, diphtheroids, or gram-negative bacilli, including *P. aeruginosa.* Empirical antimicrobial therapy in these situations should consist of vancomycin plus ceftazidime until culture results are available.

Once the infecting microorganism has been isolated in culture (or identified by other means), antimicrobial therapy can be modified for optimal treatment based on susceptibility results. For bacterial meningitis due to *S. pneumoniae* or *N. meningitidis,* penicillin G or ampicillin remain the drugs of choice, but recent developments may modify these recommendations. "Relatively" penicillin-resistant pneumococci have increased in frequency in recent years. Thus susceptibility testing of pneumococcal isolates from sterile body fluids is mandatory. For relatively resistant strains, a third-generation cephalosporin should be used, and for meningitis due to "highly" penicillin-resistant pneumococci (MIC $\geqslant$ 2 µg/mL), vancomycin is commonly recommended, although failures may occur. Meningococcal strains that are relatively resistant to penicillin also have been reported from several areas, particularly Spain. Although most patients harboring these strains have recovered with standard penicillin therapy, a third-generation cephalosporin may be indicated for empirical treatment for adults with meningitis where these strains are prevalent. Approximately 33 percent of *H. influenzae* isolates in the United States produce β-lactamase and are resistant to ampicillin. Fortunately, chloramphenicol resistance is rare in the United States, but it may be found in more than 50 percent of CSF isolates in some countries. Recently, the American Academy of Pediatrics has endorsed the use of the third-generation cephalosporins as empirical therapy in children with bacterial meningitis. Ceftriaxone is clearly superior to cefuroxime in this age group. The third-generation cephalosporins have revolutionized the treatment of gram-negative enteric bacillary meningitis. Cure rates of 78 to 94 percent have been obtained with these agents, and one, ceftazidime, may be used in monotherapy or as part of combination regimens for the care of patients with *Pseudomonas* meningitis. Intrathecal or intraventricular aminoglycoside therapy should be considered for patients with gram-negative aerobic bacillary meningitis if there is no response to systemic therapy alone. The quinolone agents (e.g., ciprofloxacin, pefloxacin, and ofloxacin) have been used in some patients with gram-negative meningitis but should only be considered for adult patients with meningitis due to multi-drug-resistant gram-negative bacilli or in patients failing conventional therapy. The third-generation cephalosporins are, however, inactive against *L. monocytogenes;* therefore, ampicillin is often added empirically for treatment of this organism. In documented *Listeria* meningitis, consideration should be given to a combination of an aminoglycoside and ampicillin to achieve synergy in vivo. In the penicillin-allergic patient, systemic trimethoprim-sulfamethazole, which is bactericidal against *Listeria* in vitro, can be used. Patients with *S. aureus* meningitis should be treated with nafcillin, oxacillin, or vancomycin. Since *S. epidermidis* is the most likely isolate in patients with CSF shunt infection, vancomycin is the drug of choice; rifampin may be added if the patient fails to improve. Shunt removal is often required to optimize therapy.

The duration of therapy for bacterial meningitis is based largely on tradition in the absence of rigorous scientific data. In general, the following treatment durations are recommended: *N. meningitidis:* 7 days; *H. influenzae:* 7 to 10 days; *S. pneumoniae:* 10 to 14 days; and gram-negative aerobic bacilli: 3 weeks. Therapy should be individualized and based on the clinical response; some patients may require longer courses of treatment.

Adjunctive therapy Despite the availability of bactericidal antimicrobial therapy, the morbidity and mortality from bacterial meningitis remain at unacceptably high levels. Recent studies have focused on the pathogenesis and pathophysiology of bacterial meningitis, since the introduction of newer antimicrobial agents may not improve this situation. However, rapidly bactericidal therapy, the desired result of the initiation of antimicrobial agents, may result in accentuated release of proinflammatory bacterial cell wall components into the CSF. Initiation of treatment with bacteriolytic agents in experimental meningitis results in an increase in CSF leukocyte concentration. Antibiotic therapy also results in higher concentrations of free LPS in the CSF of children with *H. influenzae* meningitis during the first day of treatment. Hence anti-inflammatory agents, particularly glucocorticoids or nonsteroidal anti-inflammatory agents, have been shown to decrease the inflammatory response in the subarachnoid space in experimental models of infection (as assessed by CSF pleocytosis) with resultant improvement in many of the pathophysiologic consequences, including blood-brain barrier permeability, cerebral edema, and ICP. Based on these studies and the known effects of glucocorticoids on cytokine generation, these agents have been reevaluated in patients with bacterial meningitis. Several prospective, double-blind, randomized clinical trials have now evaluated dexamethasone as an adjunctive therapy for children with meningitis. Although mortality was not affected, CSF inflammatory indices normalized faster, fever disappeared more rapidly, and the incidence of moderate to severe bilateral sensorineural hearing loss and/or overall neurologic sequelae was reduced. Dexamethasone also reduced mortality in adults and children with pneumococcal meningitis treated in one Egyptian trial. Although concerns have been raised about the routine use of dexamethasone in all patients with bacterial meningitis and virtually no information exists in neonates or older adults, this adjunctive therapy is potentially beneficial in children, particularly those with proven or suspected *H. influenzae* disease. Close monitoring of the hematocrit and stool guaiac for blood loss is essential during therapy. The mechanism of the beneficial effect of dexamethasone is incompletely defined, but CSF concentrations of IL-1β fall more rapidly in children receiving dexamethasone when compared with a placebo control. If dexamethasone is used, it should be administered shortly before or simultaneously with the first dose of antimicrobial agents to maximally attenuate the CSF inflammatory response. The recommended dose of dexamethasone is 0.15 mg/kg per dose, administered four times daily (total of 0.6 mg/kg per day) for 4 days. Studies on the potential role of adjunctive dexamethasone in neonates and adults are in progress.

Other adjunctive therapies may be useful in critically ill patients with bacterial meningitis. Patients with signs of increased ICP may benefit from the insertion of an intracranial pressure monitoring device and vigorous treatment of raised ICP. Elevation of the head of the bed to 30°, hyperventilation to a Pa_{CO_2} of 27 to 30 mmHg, hyperosmolar agents such as mannitol, intravenous lidocaine to reduce transient increases in ICP during endotracheal suctioning, and glucocorticoids may be tried alone or in combination (see Chap. 376). Seizures should be treated promptly to avoid status epilepticus with appropriate agents such as lorazepam or diazepam and/or phenytoin. Occasionally, barbiturates are necessary for control of seizure activity. Another important adjunctive therapy in children with bacterial meningitis is fluid restriction to combat excess secretion of antidiuretic hormone if the patient is not hypotensive. Treatment of shock and/or disseminated intravascular coagulation may be necessary (see Chap. 83). Plasma exchange or plasmapheresis has proven lifesaving in some patients with fulminant meningococcemia, but this treatment modality must be considered experimental at the present time.

PROGNOSIS The overall case fatality rates of the major meningeal pathogens in cases of meningitis encountered in the United States in 1986 are shown in Table 374-2. The mortality rate for *H. influenzae* meningitis is less than 5 percent but may exceed 20 to 25 percent in some developing countries. Meningococcemia without meningitis is associated with a worse prognosis than meningitis alone due to this organism. Pneumococcal meningitis, among the three major pathogens, is associated with the highest mortality rate. Gram-negative aerobic bacillary meningitis is often refractory to therapy, and relapses may occur. In addition, permanent neurologic sequelae are encountered in approximately one-third to one-half of survivors of bacterial meningitis. The major sequelae include hearing loss or language delay, mental retardation, cerebral palsy, seizures, and behavioral problems. Prospective studies have documented persistent sensorineural hearing loss in approximately 10 percent of survivors of bacterial meningitis (approximately 31 percent following pneumococcal meningitis), a finding with critical implications for growth and educational development. Despite an apparent recent decline in the incidence of severe neurologic sequelae among children surviving bacterial meningitis, as measured by learning patterns upon school entry, the public health problems as a result of this disease are significant worldwide.

BRAIN ABSCESS

DEFINITION   Brain abscess is a focal suppurative process within the brain parenchyma of diverse pathogenesis and etiology.

EPIDEMIOLOGY   The incidence of brain abscess has remained relatively stable in the antibiotic era; nevertheless, it is generally regarded as a rare disease, with large autopsy series reporting an occurrence rate of 0.18 to 1.3 percent. It has been estimated that brain abscess accounts for approximately 1 out of every 10,000 general hospital admissions, and about 4 to 10 cases are seen yearly on active neurosurgical services in hospitals of developed countries. Although some series have noted a slightly increased incidence in recent years, this may represent a bias derived through more sensitive diagnostic techniques. In addition, brain abscess remains a significant problem in the developing world, particularly in children in lower socioeconomic regions. Focal suppurative processes of the brain have emerged as an important type of intracranial infection in patients with AIDS. For example, estimates of the prevalence of toxoplasma encephalitis alone have ranged from 2.6 to 30.8 percent in patients with AIDS.

In most series, the male/female ratio has been approximately 2:1, with the median age at presentation of 30 to 40 years. Approximately 25 percent of brain abscesses occur in children less than 15 years of age. Brain abscess in a child less than 2 years of age is distinctly unusual and suggests an associated gram-negative bacillary (especially *Citrobacter diversus*) meningitis. In some series, brain abscess secondary to otitis media displays a bipolar age distribution, with peaks in the pediatric age group and after age 40. In contrast, brain abscess secondary to paranasal sinusitis occurs more commonly between 10 and 30 years of age.

ETIOLOGY   In the preantibiotic era, the most common etiologic agents isolated from brain abscesses were *S. aureus*, streptococci, and coliform bacteria, although no growth was recorded in up to 50 percent of patients. With proper attention to anaerobic culture techniques, the role of anaerobic bacteria in brain abscess has become apparent, and sterile abscesses are less frequently encountered. Microbial isolates from brain abscesses are dependent to a significant degree on the immune status of the host. The etiology of focal CNS infections in patients with AIDS is addressed in Chaps. 279 and 375.

Currently, pyogenic brain abscesses are often (30 to 60 percent) mixed infections. In a summary of 12 separate series of patients with brain abscess, excluding AIDS patients, 61 percent of the isolates were aerobic bacteria, while 32 percent were anaerobic bacteria. Aerobic or microaerophilic streptococci accounted for about one-half of the aerobic isolates and have been noted to be present in approximately 70 percent of all brain abscess patients. The most frequently isolated streptococci include organisms belonging to the *S. milleri* group (*S. anginosus*, *S. constellatus*, *S. intermedius*, etc.). *S. aureus* is isolated from about 15 percent of patients with brain abscess, especially following head trauma or neurosurgery. Aerobic

gram-negative bacilli (e.g., *Proteus* sp., *E. coli*, *Klebsiella* sp., *Enterobacter* sp., and *P. aeruginosa*) have been observed with increased frequency in recent studies, often in mixed culture, and are isolated from 16 to 30 percent of patients. Anaerobes most recently encountered include *Bacteroides* sp. (including *B. fragilis*), *Fusobacterium* sp., anaerobic streptococci, and *Clostridium* sp. Anaerobic bacteria are particularly prevalent pathogens in the setting of underlying chronic otitis or pulmonary disease.

The location of a given brain abscess and its underlying predisposing cause often suggest the most likely etiologic agent(s). Frontal lobe abscesses resulting from a preexisting sinusitis often yield an organism of the *S. milleri* group in pure culture. Furthermore, brain abscess in association with chronic sinusitis is often a mixed infection with an aerobic/anaerobic ratio of approximately 1 to 1.5 in most series. Posttraumatic or postoperative brain abscesses are usually caused by staphylococci. Temporal lobe abscesses are often a complication of otitis media and almost always yield multiple agents upon culture, including streptococci, *Bacteroides* sp., and gram-negative aerobic bacilli. Approximately 33 percent of chronically infected ears yields anaerobes on culture. In contrast to the role of *S. pneumoniae*, *H. influenzae*, and *M. catarrhalis* in acute otitis media, other streptococci, gram-negative aerobes including *P. aeruginosa*, anaerobic cocci, and *Bacteroides* sp. are the most common isolates from chronic otitis media and its intracranial complications. Pneumococci, meningococci, and *H. influenzae* very rarely cause brain abscess, even in association with a purulent meningitis.

In addition, the microbiology of a brain abscess is fundamentally influenced by the immune status of the host. Immunocompromised patients may develop brain abscess due to fungi, and *Toxoplasma gondii* is a major cause of focal CNS lesions in patients with AIDS. Brain abscess in neutropenic patients is usually due to aerobic gram-negative bacteria, *Candida* sp., *Aspergillus* sp., or zygomycosis. Conversely, focal brain abscess in patients with abnormal cell-mediated immunity is commonly due to *T. gondii*, *Nocardia asteroides*, *L. monocytogenes*, *Mycobacterium* sp., or *Cryptococcus neoformans*. *Pseudallescheria boydii* abscess may follow a near-drowning episode. Multiple other fungi, protozoa, and helminths may cause brain abscess.

PATHOGENESIS AND PATHOPHYSIOLOGY   Brain abscesses occur most commonly in association with three distinct clinical settings: (1) a contiguous focus of infection, particularly otitis, sinusitis, or dental infection, (2) hematogenous spread from a distant focus of infection, especially chronic pyogenic lung disease, and (3) following cranial trauma or surgery. The predisposing factor remains undefined in approximately 15 to 20 percent of cases.

A review of multiple series encompassing more than 3500 cases of brain abscess in the past half century reveals that about 45 percent of cases were associated with a contiguous focus of infection (predominantly otitis or sinusitis). Recent data suggest that otogenic brain abscesses are decreasing in frequency, perhaps related to the availability and common use of antimicrobial agents for upper respiratory tract infections. Frequent but inadequate courses of antimicrobial agents for ear or sinus infections have, however, altered the natural history of brain abscess, resulting in puzzling or more subtle clinical presentations. Otogenic brain abscesses are most commonly located in the temporal lobe or cerebellum; conversely 85 to 95 percent of cerebellar abscesses are associated with ear or mastoid infections. Sinusitis as a cause of brain abscess also appears to be decreasing in overall incidence. Rhinogenic abscesses are rare in children and in adults over the age of 60 years. Most brain abscesses in the setting of sinusitis are localized in the frontal lobe. Sphenoid sinusitis is notable for both the frequency and severity of its potential intracranial complications. The diagnosis of this form of sinusitis is often difficult and may lead to therapeutic delay. Cocaine inhalation is an additional risk factor for sphenoid sinusitis and subsequent brain abscess development. Dental infections, often overlooked as a cause of brain abscess, have been implicated in about 10 percent of patients with brain abscess. Periapical abscesses surrounding the teeth are often detected in patients with "cryptogenic brain abscess." Brain abscesses rarely complicate the course of bacterial meningitis in adolescents or adults. Nevertheless, the presence of a brain abscess should be strongly considered in neonates with gram-negative meningitis, particularly due to *Citrobacter* or *Proteus* sp.

Brain abscess is a rare complication of neurosurgical procedures or cranial trauma. CNS infections occur in only 0.6 to 1.7 percent of clean neurosurgical procedures, and brain abscess accounts for only 10 percent of these infections. Brain abscess may, however, complicate penetrating cranial injuries, with an increased risk noted in the setting of gunshot wound complications. Retained bone fragments have been consistently noted as an important risk factor.

Hematogenous brain abscess arising from distant foci of infections account for about 25 percent of cases. These lesions are associated most commonly with pulmonary infections and share the following characteristics: (1) location in the distribution of the middle cerebral artery, (2) initial location at the gray matter–white matter junction, (3) poor encapsulation, and (4) higher mortality. Hematogenous brain abscesses are most likely to present as multiple lesions. Multiple brain abscesses was reported in only 1 to 15 percent in older series; however, with the advent of CT scanning, multiple lesions are now detected in 10 to 50 percent of patients. Important preceding processes have included chronic lung infections (lung abscess, bronchiectasis, and empyema), osteomyelitis, cholecystitis, intraabdominal infection, and/or pelvic sources. Brain abscess has been observed following endoscopic sclerosis of esophageal varices or dilatation of esophageal strictures. Although a transient bacteremia may follow these procedures and is instrumental in the development of a brain abscess, macroscopic CNS lesions are rare complications of bacterial endocarditis. *S. aureus* is the most common cause of endocarditis complicated by intracranial involvement. Hereditary hemorrhagic telangiectasia is an important risk factor for brain abscess, especially in affected patients with clubbing, cyanosis, and/or polycythemia. This condition (Osler-Rendu-Weber syndrome) may be underrecognized in patients with brain abscess. Cyanotic heart disease is recognized in 3 to 14 percent of brain abscess cases and may be the most common underlying process found within brain abscess in children. Tetralogy of Fallot is the most commonly cited anomaly; however, brain abscess may complicate patent foramen ovale, ventricular septal defect, and transposition of the great vessels. The presence of a right-to-left shunt appears to be critical for the development of brain abscess in these patients.

Brain abscess development in any of the above-described clinical settings appears to require a compromised area of brain as the final common pathway. Experimental data suggest that brain is remarkably resistant to infection. Brain abscess development from an area of contiguous infection usually follows two major mechanisms: (1) direct extension through areas of associated osteitis or osteomyelitis and (2) retrograde thrombophlebitic spread via diploic or emissary veins into the intracranial compartment. The polycythemia and systemic hypoxia observed in cyanotic congenital heart disease and hereditary hemorrhagic telangiectasia increase blood viscosity, which may, in concert with a reduction in brain capillary blood flow, result in microinfarction or reduced tissue oxygenation in brain as a nidus for ensuing infection.

PATHOLOGY A solitary brain abscess involves the following brain regions in approximate decreasing order of frequency: frontal ≥ frontoparietal > parietal > cerebellar > occipital. This distribution reflects the associated, often contiguous foci of infection. Brainstem, intrasellar, basal ganglia, and thalamic abscesses are rare.

The pathologic evolution of brain abscess has been documented most convincingly in experimental models of infection and appears to involve four histopathologic stages. Importantly, the histopathologic features may correlate with specific findings on CT, which has direct implications for subsequent therapy. The four stages include (1) early cerebritis (days 1 to 3 following intracerebral inoculation of animals), characterized by a perivascular inflammatory response surrounding a developing necrotic center, with profound edema, (2) late cerebritis, with maximal extent of the well-formed necrotic center and the appearance of fibroblasts and neovascularity in the periphery of the necrotic zone, (3) early capsule formation (days 10 to 13 following intracerebral inoculation of experimental animals), characterized by a well-developed layer of fibroblasts with persistent cerebritis and neovascularity, and (4) late capsule formation, with thickening of the capsule and an abundance of reactive collagen. It should be noted, however, that these stages are somewhat stereotyped, are best described for abscess following infection with alpha-hemolytic streptococci, and may not reflect the sequence in abscesses caused by other microorganisms. Nevertheless, encapsulation is frequently more complete on the cortical side of the abscess when compared with the ventricular side and is often less extensive in abscesses resulting from hematogenous spread than in those arising from a contiguous focus of infection. These observations may explain the propensity for abscesses to rupture medially into the ventricular system rather than into the subarachnoid space. Brain abscess formation is a continuum from cerebritis to a well-encapsulated necrotic focus. Maturity of the lesion(s) is dependent on multiple factors, including local oxygen concentration, the offending microorganism, and the host immune response.

CLINICAL MANIFESTATIONS (See also Table 374-4) The clinical course of a patient with a brain abscess may range from indolent to fulminant; however, the duration of symptoms is 2 weeks or less in about 75 percent of patients. In most cases, the prominent clinical manifestations of brain abscess reflect the expanding intracerebral mass rather than systemic signs of infection. Furthermore, the clinical manifestations are often nonspecific and depend on several variables (e.g., the virulence of the infecting organisms, the patient's immune status, and the location of the abscess or abscesses). Only a minority of patients display the classic triad of fever, headache, and focal neurologic deficits. Headache is most consistently observed (70 percent of patients), but fever is documented in only one-half of patients. Focal neurologic deficits are encountered in about half the cases, and the specific features are dependent on the number and location of the brain abscesses. Focal deficits may include hemiplegia, hemianopsia, cranial nerve abnormalities, and others depending on location. Cerebellar abscess often results in nystagmus, ataxia, vomiting, and dysmetria, whereas frontal lobe abscess is often dominated by headache, drowsiness, inattention, and a generalized deterioration in mental function. Hemiparesis with unilateral motor signs and/or a speech disorder are frequent findings. Seizures are observed in 25 to 45 percent of patients and, when present, are usually generalized. The presence of nausea and vomiting correlates to some degree with the ICP. A change in mental status (lethargy to coma) occurs in most patients, but frank coma on presentation is now infrequently noted and may reflect the availability of improved diagnostic modalities such as CT. Papilledema is observed with varying frequency, does not correlate with the size of the abscess, but appears to be associated closely with the presence of headache and vomiting. Nuchal rigidity (about 25 percent of patients) is observed more commonly with a shorter duration of illness and may lead to confusion with bacterial meningitis. Intrasellar abscess often simulates a pituitary tumor, presenting with headache, visual field defects, and endocrine disturbances.

TABLE 374-4 Clinical manifestations of brain abscess

Symptom/sign	Percent
Headache	70
Triad of fever, headache, focal deficit	<50
Fever	40–50
Focal neurologic deficit	~50
Seizures	25–40
Nausea/vomiting	22–50
Nuchal rigidity	~25
Papilledema	~25

NOTE: Other symptoms/signs are dependent on location.
SOURCE: After Wispelwey et al, 1991.

Since the clinical presentation may be nonspecific and fever is often absent, brain abscess may be confused with several other processes, and the following should be considered in the differential diagnosis: pyogenic meningitis, subdural empyema, epidural abscess, encephalitis, mycotic aneurysm, complicated migraine headache, intracerebral or subarachnoid hemorrhage, cerebral infarction, cerebral venous sinus thrombosis, and primary or metastatic malignancies of the CNS.

DIAGNOSIS Routine studies of the blood and urine are rarely helpful in the diagnosis of a brain abscess. A moderate peripheral blood leukocytosis may be present, but 40 percent of patients display a completely normal peripheral leukocyte count. The erythrocyte sedimentation rate is often elevated but may be normal in the setting of cyanotic congenital heart disease. Serum C-reactive protein concentrations have been used to differentiate brain abscess from intracranial neoplasms but are inadequate for this purpose. Blood cultures are only occasionally ($\leq$10 percent) positive in patients with a brain abscess.

Although the CSF is often abnormal in patients with brain abscess, the findings are nonspecific, and lumbar puncture is usually contraindicated in a patient with a suspected parenchymal abscess. The diagnostic yield is poor, and the risk of subsequent herniation after the procedure has been reported to be as high as 20 percent. The poor diagnostic yield and significant morbidity of lumbar puncture in the presence of a brain abscess necessitate that this procedure be delayed in patients with a febrile CNS disorder with focal neurologic signs. However, if pyogenic meningitis is also a strong consideration in the individual patient, blood cultures should be obtained and appropriate antimicrobial agents started parenterally before obtaining a neuroradiologic study. Although abnormalities may be noted, skull roentgenograms, electroencephalograms, arteriography, ventriculography, and/or technetium 99m brain scans are rarely necessary in the evaluation of a patient with a suspected brain abscess. Radionuclide brain scans are, however, useful in facilities lacking CT scan or MRI technology.

The introduction of CT and MRI has revolutionized the diagnostic and therapeutic approach to brain abscess. CT is superior to other, older radiologic techniques in the evaluation of paranasal sinuses, mastoids, and the middle ear and should be obtained, along with a chest roentgenogram, in all patients with suspected brain abscess. CT is sensitive (over 95 percent) in the detection of a brain abscess but can give additional crucial information such as the extent of the surrounding edema, the presence of hydrocephalus and/or a midline shift, and the precise localization of the lesion. The typical CT appearance of a brain abscess is a hypodense lesion surrounded by a uniformly enhancing ring upon contrast administration. A variable hypodense area of edema extends beyond the ring. Unfortunately, this CT appearance is not specific for a brain abscess, and other processes, including neoplasm, granuloma, cerebral infarction, or resolving hematoma, may give a similar finding on CT. Furthermore, glucocorticoid use may alter the typical appearance on CT; only about 40 to 60 percent of brain abscesses in patients on glucocorticoid therapy reveal ring enhancement on CT scan. Indium 111–labeled leukocyte scintigraphy may prove complementary to CT in the diagnosis of abscesses in the CNS. However, necrotic tumors may be confused with brain abscess by this methodology, and the concomitant use of glucocorticoids also may produce a false-negative scan.

The data regarding the utility of MRI in the diagnosis and evaluation of a patient with a brain abscess continue to accumulate. MRI permits multiplanar imaging, accentuates the contrast between gray and white matter, and affords a variety of imaging techniques to elucidate pathologic changes. In addition, bony artifact, which may hinder CT interpretation, is not a problem with MRI techniques. MRI appears to be more sensitive than CT in the cerebritis phase of brain abscess development, as well as in the detection of associated cerebral edema. Therefore, MRI may detect early satellite lesions not demonstrated by CT and is often more useful for demonstration of

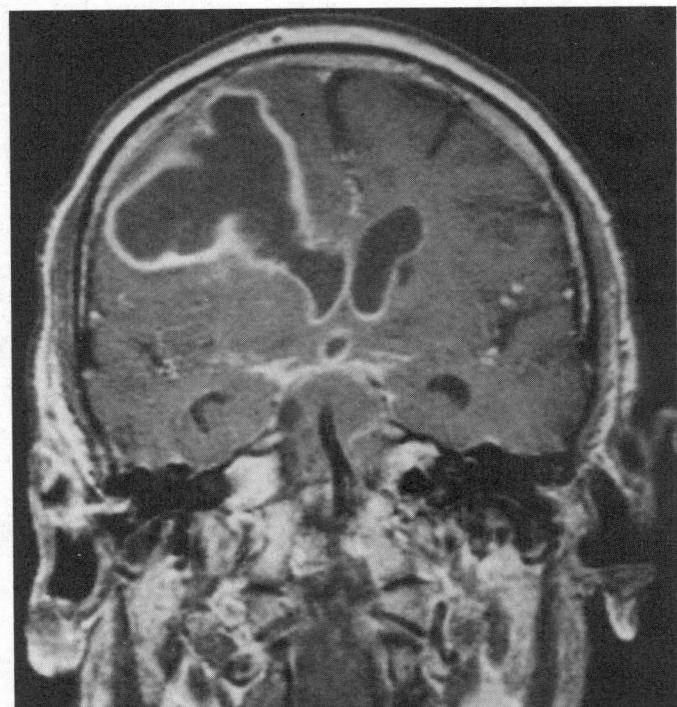

FIGURE 374-1   MRI of brain abscess. Coronal T_1-weighted spin-echo image following gadolinium-DTPA enhancement demonstrating large necrotic right frontal lobe mass with intense peripheral enhancement and surrounding edema. Multiple complications are also evident: ependymal enhancement in lateral and third ventricles and enhancement of subarachnoid space reflecting ventricular rupture, ventriculitis, and meningitis, and mass effect with midline shift. Aspiration revealed pus and *S. milleri* in pure culture.

extraparenchymal extension of an abscess (i.e., ventricular rupture) than CT (Fig. 374-1). The lack of ionizing radiation, greater tissue characterization, lack of bone artifact, increased sensitivity in follow-up evaluations, and less toxic contrast agents make MRI the procedure of choice in the evaluation of a patient with suspected brain abscess.

THERAPY The optimal management of most patients with a bacterial brain abscess requires both administration of antimicrobial agents and surgical intervention. CT scanning or MRI should be performed without delay in the patient with neurologic complaints and a predisposing condition suggesting brain abscess, as described above. Results in animal models and humans suggest that focal bacterial infections of the brain parenchyma may be "staged" by a sequential CT scan. Cerebritis is characterized by an area of low density surrounded by ring enhancement (often thick and diffuse) that does not decay on delayed contrast scans obtained 1 h later. In contrast, an encapsulated abscess is characterized by a faint ring on the unenhanced scan and ring enhancement that decays in the delayed CT scan. These parameters may prove useful in planning a combined medical-surgical approach. Since 1971, it has been recognized that early antimicrobial therapy alone, in the absence of surgical intervention, could cure cerebritis without the later development of encapsulated abscess. Subsequent cases claiming "cure" of an encapsulated abscess share many of the following features: (1) the initial diagnosis and resolution of brain abscess(es) were documented by sequential CT scans, usually without aspiration or histopathology; (2) prolonged courses (e.g., $\geq$8 weeks) of high-dose antibiotic therapy were administered, and (3) evidence of encapsulation often was lacking. Based on experimental animal models of brain abscess and the well-defined CT appearance of the cerebritis stage, medical "cures" of established brain abscess may represent successful resolution of bacterial cerebritis. In general, close cooperation between medical and surgical disciplines is essential for the optimal management of a given patient with suspected brain abscess.

The antimicrobial regimens recommended for the empirical (and specific) therapy of a brain abscess reflect considerations of the microbiology as well as evidence from both animal and human studies evaluating the penetration of a given antimicrobial agent into brain parenchyma and/or brain abscess pus. Unfortunately, no prospective, randomized clinical trials exist to guide the clinician in the choice of an optimal antimicrobial regimen. If CT scanning suggests cerebritis and the patient is neurologically stable, antibiotics can be started and the patient observed. Since the early 1960s, a combination of penicillin G (20 to 24 million units per day IV) plus chloramphenicol (1.0 to 1.5 g IV every 6 h) has been advocated in adults. Penicillin remains a mainstay of therapy because of (1) excellent activity against streptococci, including the *S. milleri* group, complicating contiguous foci of infection, and pyogenic lung disease, (2) activity against most anaerobes encountered in brain abscess patients, (3) favorable results obtained in experimental animal models of brain abscess, and (4) a marked reduction in brain abscess mortality observed after the introduction of penicillin in the 1940s. Chloramphenicol often has been administered concurrently with penicillin in the past because of its high lipid solubility, resulting in brain tissue concentrations often exceeding those present in plasma, and good activity against anaerobic bacteria, including *B. fragilis*. The use of metronidazole for the therapy of brain abscess has increased greatly in recent years and has generally supplanted chloramphenicol because (1) metronidazole is bactericidal against *B. fragilis*, whereas chloramphenicol may be bacteriostatic, (2) metronidazole attains reproducibly excellent concentrations in brain abscess pus, (3) entry of metronidazole into brain abscess pus is not affected by concomitant steroid treatment in contrast to several other antibiotics, (4) chloramphenicol may be degraded by deacylation in pus, as shown in experimental intraabdominal abscess, and (5) metronidazole may have had a salutary affect on mortality, as suggested by several recent retrospective studies. Metronidazole, when substituted for chloramphenicol, may lead to more rapid healing and a lower mortality rate; however, these two agents have never been compared in a prospective, randomized clinical trial. Nevertheless, an antianaerobic agent such as metronidazole is indicated for the treatment of brain abscess complicating otitis media, mastoiditis, or pyogenic lung abscess because anaerobes are often present. Metronidazole should never be used alone to treat a patient with suspected brain abscess. Antianaerobic therapy may not be necessary in addition to penicillin for patients with frontal or ethmoidal sinusitis and brain abscess because *B. fragilis* is an uncommon isolate; however, empirical therapy with at least two agents is mandatory prior to culture confirmation. When staphylococci are proven or suspected, as in posttraumatic or postneurosurgical brain abscess, nafcillin or oxacillin (1.5 to 2 g IV every 4 h) is indicated. Vancomycin may be substituted if either the patient is allergic to penicillin or a methicillin-resistant strain is isolated. The frequent isolation of aerobic gram-negative bacilli in brain abscesses of otitic origin prompts many to add a third-generation cephalosporin or trimethoprim-sulfamethoxazole to the antimicrobial regimen pending culture results. Since *P. aeruginosa* is encountered in this setting of chronic middle ear infection, ceftazidime is a logical empirical choice. Recent data suggest that cefotaxime may be adequate for the majority of streptococcal isolates as well, thereby replacing penicillin as the standard regimen (i.e., cefotaxime plus metronidazole as empirical therapy). Installation of antibiotics into the abscess cavity during aspiration, although frequently employed, has never been studied systematically and has no proven additional benefit.

The relative role of aspiration alone or total excision of a brain abscess in the individual patient remains problematic. Given the current availability of stereotactic CT-guided aspiration and its attendant low morbidity while obtaining an accurate microbiologic and pathologic diagnosis, operative therapy should remain the definitive approach for most patients with brain abscess. If the CT scan or MRI suggests the presence of cerebritis and the patient is neurologically stable, antibiotic therapy as previously outlined should be initiated and the patient observed. If the patient remains stable and the abscess is accessible, CT-guided aspiration is then desirable to facilitate a specific pathologic and microbiologic diagnosis. Although this delay may render subsequent cultures negative, aspiration during the cerebritis stage may be associated with an unacceptable risk of hemorrhage, especially in children. If the lesion appears encapsulated by CT scan criteria, antibiotic therapy should be started and aspiration for diagnosis and drainage performed immediately. Subsequent management will depend on both clinical and radiologic assessments. Multiple aspirations may be required to drain the abscess successfully, and this is a potential disadvantage relative to total excision. Neurologic deterioration or failure of the lesion to resolve on follow-up imaging studies is an indication for further surgery, often excision if feasible. The duration of antimicrobial therapy is empirical and also may relate to the initial surgical procedure. Lesions treated by total excision may require a shorter duration of antimicrobial therapy than those treated with aspiration only. In general, most authorities recommend that patients be treated with at least 4 to 6 weeks of parenteral therapy. Metronidazole may be an exception to this rule because of the high oral bioavailability facilitating oral regimens. Prolonged therapy with oral regimens, if a suitable agent(s) is available against the isolated pathogen(s), is often continued for 2 to 6 months following parenteral therapy but is of no proven benefit when compared with shorter treatment regimens. A cured brain abscess may continue to exhibit contrast enhancement on CT scans for 4 to 10 weeks to up to 6 to 9 months after completion of successful therapy. The management of a focal CNS process in an HIV-infected patient requires a different approach and is discussed in Chap. 375. Empirical therapy for toxoplasmosis is often started if the CT appearance is characteristic in a seropositive patient. Brain biopsy for diagnosis may be considered in patients with a negative toxoplasmosis serology, atypical findings on the CT, or evidence of a disseminated process due to another pathogen.

Adjunctive glucocorticoids are often employed during management of patients with brain abscess, but their role remains controversial. Glucocorticoids may reduce antibiotic entry into the CNS, decrease collagen formation and glial response, and therefore lessen the degree of encapsulation of the brain abscess, or they may alter the CT scan appearance of ring enhancement as inflammation subsides, which may obscure information from sequential CT studies from the assessment of cure. Experimental animal models do not suggest that glucocorticoids alter mortality. Glucocorticoids should be employed in patients with proven or suspected raised ICP. In this circumstance, ICP monitoring may be advisable, and elevation may be controlled with steroids, hyperventilation, mannitol, or a combination of these methods. Anticonvulsants are frequently administered empirically to patients with suspected brain abscess.

PROGNOSIS The mortality rate of brain abscess was about 40 to 60 percent in the preantibiotic era and has remained high until relatively recently. The major reduction of the mortality rate (to about 10 percent) coincides with the advent of CT. The incidence of neurologic sequelae, however, ranges between 30 and 55 percent, and late seizures have been documented in as many as 90 percent of survivors. The relative contributions of medical and surgical approaches to the individual patients continue to be refined. Earlier diagnosis through improved technology and an aggressive medical-surgical approach remain essential for the successful management of this unforgiving CNS infection.

SUBDURAL EMPYEMA

DEFINITION Subdural empyema is a collection of pus in the space between the dura mater and the arachnoid membrane. Subdural empyema accounts for about 20 percent of all localized intracranial infections. Prior to the advent of antimicrobial therapy, the disease was almost always fatal, but with current methods of diagnosis and treatment, mortality rates range from 10 to 30 percent.

EPIDEMIOLOGY Although precise incidence figures are unavailable, subdural empyemas are most often a complication of otorhinologic infection. Males predominate by a ratio of approximately 3:1, and about 70 percent of patients are in the second or third decade of life.

ETIOLOGY In the majority of cases, a single microorganism is responsible for subdural empyema, but many cultures obtained at surgery are sterile because patients are often receiving antimicrobial therapy. In addition, the precise role of anaerobic bacteria in this infection has not been studied carefully because anaerobic techniques are often inadequate or not performed at surgery. Nevertheless, the major pathogens include aerobic and anaerobic streptococci (about 50 percent), staphylococci (about 16 percent), aerobic gram-negative bacilli (3 to 8 percent), and other anaerobic bacteria (about 5 percent). As with brain abscess, the causative organism is somewhat predictable based on the anatomic focus of contiguous infection. Otorhinogenic subdural empyemas are usually caused by streptococci (including members of the *S. milleri* group), whereas staphylococci and anaerobes are unusual. Infections arising from head trauma, surgery, or indwelling foreign devices commonly involve staphylococci and/or aerobic gram-negative bacilli. Subdural empyema rarely complicates meningitis but cases due to *S. pneumoniae* or *H. influenzae* have been described. Rare etiologic agents including *Salmonella* sp., *Campylobacter fetus*, *N. meningitidis*, *Pasterella* sp., and *Actinomyces* sp.

PATHOGENESIS AND PATHOPHYSIOLOGY The subdural space, normally a potential space rather than an actual space, is divided anatomically into several large compartments by the foramen magnum, tentorium cerebelli, base of the brain, and falx cerebri. Since these spaces are confined anatomically, a developing empyema can quickly evolve into a fatal expanding mass lesion. The pathogenesis usually involves spread of infection to the subdural space via valveless emissary veins in association with thrombophlebitis or by extension of an osteomyelitis of the skull with accompanying epidural abscess. Paranasal sinusitis overwhelmingly predominates as the major precipitating factor in patients with subdural empyema. The frontal sinuses are almost always involved, often with other sinuses as well. The frontal and sphenoid sinuses are intimately associated with the dura mater and are often separated by only a thin bony layer. Only about 10 percent of subdural empyemas are found infratentorially. The lesion may communicate with the contralateral side via the inferior free margin of the falx cerebri. The mastoid or middle ear is the source of subdural empyema in 10 to 20 percent of patients, especially in geographic areas (e.g., Sri Lanka) where delay in therapy of otitis media may be complicated by this event. Otitis or mastoiditis may extend directly into the subdural space via erosion of the tegmen tympani or bone adjacent to the dura mater and air cells or may spread indirectly by way of a progressive thrombophlebitis of the perforating veins. Otitis-induced subdural empyema is localized initially on or around the tentorium. Bacterial meningitis in adults is a very unusual cause of subdural empyema. Nevertheless, this lesion complicates about 2 percent of bacterial meningitis cases in infants and may follow an initially sterile subdural effusion. Other predisposing conditions include cranial trauma, neurosurgical procedures, or infection of a preexisting subdural hematoma. Subdural empyema is metastatic in origin in a small minority of cases (about 5 percent), principally from chronic infection in the chest. Once infection develops in the subdural space, spread along the falx and over the convexities may occur. Septic thrombophlebitis of the cortical veins may evolve and lead to hemorrhage, cerebral infarction, brain edema, and fatal transtentorial herniation.

CLINICAL MANIFESTATIONS Subdural empyema may present as a rapidly progressive life-threatening condition. The symptoms and signs relate to the presence of increased ICP, meningeal irritation, or focal cortical inflammation. In addition, the majority of patients (60 to 90 percent) have evidence of their antecedent infection (e.g., sinusitis or otitis). In general, patients often have a nonspecific illness for days to weeks prior to an acutely ill presentation. The most common symptoms and signs include headache, fever, stiff neck, and focal neurologic deficits. Headache, initially localized to the infected sinus or ear, is a prominent complaint and can become generalized

as the infection progresses. Vomiting is common as ICP rises. Early during the course, about one-half of patients have altered mental status, which can progress to obtundation and/or coma in the absence of treatment. Fever above 39°C is present in most cases. Focal neurologic findings appear after 24 to 48 h of illness and progress rapidly to involvement of the entire cerebral hemisphere. Hemiparesis or hemiplegia are the most common focal findings; although ocular palsy is common, dysphasia, homonymous hemianopsia, cerebellar signs, dilated pupils, and other focal presentations also have been observed. Seizures, either focal or generalized, are found in more than 50 percent of cases. Meningeal irritation (particularly meningismus) is found in 70 to 80 percent of patients, although Kernig's and/or Babinski's signs are less frequently noted. In the absence of treatment, neurologic deterioration occurs rapidly with signs of increased ICP and cerebral herniation. Papilledema develops in less than 50 percent of patients. This fulminant picture may not be seen in several clinical settings, including patients with subdural empyema following cranial surgery and/or trauma, where the presentation may be subacute and subtle, in patients receiving prior antimicrobial therapy, after infection of a subdural hematoma, and/or following a metastatic infection to the subdural space from a chronic focus elsewhere. The clinical manifestations of subdural empyema in infants are similar to those found in adults, except that a bulging anterior fontanelle is a common finding.

DIAGNOSIS As with brain abscess, routine studies of blood, urine, and CSF are of limited value in the evaluation of patients with suspected subdural empyema. Most patients have a peripheral blood leukocytosis, and plain films of the skull may be useful in the demonstration of sinusitis or mastoiditis. Since a high clinical suspicion and rapid diagnosis of this condition are critical for a successful outcome, subdural empyema should be suspected in any patient with a CNS syndrome with fever and focal neurologic findings. Lumbar puncture is contraindicated in this setting because of the risk of cerebral herniation. When performed, CSF findings are nonspecific and include an elevated opening pressure, a moderate neutrophilic pleocytosis, and an increased protein concentration. Unless the course is complicated by coexistent bacterial meningitis, CSF Gram's stain and cultures are negative. Cerebral arteriography was the diagnostic procedure of choice prior to the development of CT scans.

At the present time, CT scan with contrast enhancement and MRI are the diagnostic procedures of choice in patients with suspected subdural empyema. The typical CT appearance is of a crescentic or elliptically shaped area of hypodensity below the cranial vault or adjacent to the falx cerebri. Loculations may be seen, and associated mass effect with displacement of midline structures is common. After the administration of contrast material, a fine intense line of enhancement is seen between the subdural collection and the cerebral cortex. However, false-negative CT scans have been reported; MRI provides greater clarity for morphologic detail and may detect empyema not seen clearly on CT. MRI is of particular value in identifying subdural empyema located at the base of the brain, along the falx cerebri, or in the posterior fossa. On the basis of signal intensity, extraaxial empyemas can be differentiated from sterile effusions and/or chronic hematomas. Both CT and MRI can be useful for the demonstration of sinusitis and otitis, although CT is superior to MRI in bone imaging and should be used in cases of penetrating injury or when osteomyelitis is a consideration. Cerebral arteriography should be employed on an emergent basis when MRI is unavailable and subdural empyema is strongly suspected despite a normal CT scan. Arteriography may establish the presence of a subdural avascular mass and detect spread of the lesion to the contralateral or parafalcine subdural space. As stated above, subdural empyema shows a striking sex and age predilection and should be strongly considered in young males in the second and third decades with appropriate clinical findings.

TREATMENT Subdural empyema is a surgical emergency. While awaiting operative intervention, antibiotics should be chosen based on the suspected source of infection, the known organisms associated with that focus of infection, and the host immune status. A combined medical-surgical approach is optimal for the management of these patients. As with brain abscess, no controlled clinical trials have evaluated different antimicrobial regimens for the treatment of subdural empyema. Empirical therapy often includes penicillin G and/or chloramphenicol in the doses as for brain abscess described above. If staphylococci are suspected, a β-lactamase–stable penicillin (e.g., nafcillin, 1.5 g IV every 4 h) should be used, with vancomycin (about 1 g IV every 12 h in adults) reserved for patients allergic to penicillin or when methicillin resistant *S. aureus* (MRSA) are suspected Metronidazole is often substituted for chloramphenicol at a loading dosage of 15 mg/kg, followed by 7.5 mg/kg IV every 6 h. Many authorities add a third-generation cephalosporin (often cefotaxime or ceftriaxone) in combination until culture results are available. Ceftazidime is useful in patients in whom *P. aeruginosa* is a consideration (after neurosurgery or trauma, etc.). The duration of therapy is empirical; however, parenteral antibiotics should be continued for 3 to 4 weeks after drainage, depending on the patient's clinical response. Longer periods of intravenous therapy and/or continuation as an oral regimen may be required if an associated osteomyelitis is present.

Although case reports have suggested that subdural empyema may respond to antimicrobial agents alone, the optimal approach requires surgical drainage. The comparative efficacy of multiple burr holes versus an open craniotomy has not been subjected to rigorous clinical trial. All cases should involve close cooperation with a neurosurgical service. Previous studies documenting a lower mortality rate in patients undergoing craniotomy may merely reflect a larger percentage of gravely ill patients treated with burr hole drainage alone because of the greater surgical risk associated with an open craniotomy. Unfortunately, burr holes may be inadequate due to the thickened pus during the course of the infection. Craniotomy is often essential for posterior fossa subdural empyemas and is also needed in the 10 to 20 percent of patients who are initially treated with trephination. When craniotomy is performed, wide exposure should be afforded to allow adequate exploration of all areas where subdural pus is suspected. Although antibiotic irrigation at the time of surgery has become common, there are no data on the potential benefits of this practice. Drains or catheters are often left in the subdural space after the initial drainage, but this practice may increase the risk of nosocomial superinfection. Finally, surgical correction of the antecedent otorhinologic infection also may be necessary on an emergent basis. Adjunctive measures to control raised ICP are also essential. Preoperative use of mannitol, dexamethasone, and/or hyperventilation may be effective in controlling ICP. Glucocorticoids should, however, be tapered rapidly after surgical therapy because of the risk of secondary infection. Anticonvulsants are indicated in patients with seizures.

PROGNOSIS The overall mortality of subdural empyema averages 15 to 25 percent, with severe neurologic sequelae (chiefly disabling hemiparesis or aphasia) found in 5 to 25 percent of survivors. Seizures are documented on follow-up in 8 to 46 percent of patients.

SPINAL SUBDURAL EMPYEMA This rare condition, with approximately 20 to 30 cases reported in the literature, is far less common than spinal epidural abscess. The signs and symptoms include fever, back pain, and subsequent manifestations of spinal cord compression, but tenderness to palpation or percussion along the spine is often absent, in contrast to spinal epidural abscess. Most cases occur following hematogenous dissemination from a distant site of infection, and *S. aureus* is the most common etiologic agent. The presentation may resemble transverse myelitis. MRI is the diagnostic procedure of choice for the detection of suspected spinal subdural empyema, since the extent of the lesion is defined more favorably by MRI when compared with CT. Metrizimide spinal CT is also useful in the diagnosis of this condition. Myelography should be performed when MRI and CT are not available. Myelography may not detect the entire length of the empyema if complete blocks are present within

the spinal canal at multiple levels. Treatment should consist of empirical antibiotics initially directed at *S. aureus*, streptococci, and gram-negative enteric bacilli in association with prompt laminectomy for drainage of the empyema. The antimicrobial regimen is commonly administered for 2 to 4 weeks following surgical drainage.

EPIDURAL ABSCESS

SPINAL EPIDURAL ABSCESS This type of abscess possesses unique clinical features and constitutes an important neurologic and neurosurgical emergency. It is discussed in Chap. 381.

INTRACRANIAL EPIDURAL ABSCESS An *epidural abscess* is defined as a suppurative infection in the epidural space. This space is located between the dura mater and the overlying bone. Cranial epidural abscess often crosses the cranial dura along the emissary veins, so subdural empyema is also often present. Therefore, the etiology, pathogenesis, and bacteriology of intracranial abscess are usually similar to those described for subdural empyema, with an initial focus on infection in the paranasal sinuses, middle ear, or mastoids. The overall incidence of cranial epidural abscess is unknown. In general, it is the third most common localized intracranial infection following brain abscess and subdural empyema in frequency. Only about 10 percent of all epidural abscesses arise in the intracranial epidural space. Unlike the striking sex and age distribution of subdural empyema, intracranial abscesses are rare in young children and have been reported over a wide age range. Above the foramen magnum, the epidural space represents only a potential space, since the dura is essentially adherent to the inner lining of the skull. Infections of the intracranial epidural space result primarily from an extension of a contiguous focus of infection, including sinusitis, mastoiditis, scalp or orbital cellulitis, and rhinocerebral mucormycosis, or as a result of an intracranial defect caused by a skull fracture, neurosurgical procedure, or as a complication of fetal monitoring. In general, epidural abscess is a slowly growing mass, which accounts for its insidious clinical presentation. Intracranial abscesses rarely dissect beyond the base of the skull. Similar to subdural empyema, the organisms responsible for intracranial epidural abscesses are dependent on the underlying mechanism. Aerobic and microaerophilic streptococci predominant in infections of the paranasal sinuses, whereas *S. aureus* or *S. epidermidis* and aerobic gram-negative bacilli are associated with cranial trauma. Many other organisms have been isolated from localized intracranial abscesses, including *Salmonella* sp., *Eikenella corrodens, Aspergillus* sp. and the agents of mucormycosis. The onset of symptoms is often insidious and may be overshadowed by the primary focus of infection (e.g., sinusitis or otitis). Headache is a usual complaint, but the patient may otherwise be asymptomatic unless the clinical course is complicated by the development of subdural empyema or involvement of deeper intracranial structures because the epidural abscess usually enlarges slowly and does not produce sudden major neurologic deficits unless complicated by deep extension. However, focal neurologic signs and/or focal generalized seizures may develop ultimately. Without treatment, papilledema or other signs of increased ICP develop as the abscess enlarges. An epidural abscess localized near the petrous bone may present as Gradenigo's syndrome, characterized by involvement of cranial nerves V and VI with unilateral facial pain and weakness of the lateral rectus muscle. If cranial osteomyelitis is present, edema and cellulitis of the face and/or scalp may be present. Attention may be focused on the primary process, such as sinusitis, cellulitis, or skull fracture, allowing a developing intracranial abscess to remain undetected. Thus the striking manifestations of the complications, including an alteration in mental status and a declining level of consciousness (including coma and/or meningismus), may be the first indication of an intracranial process. As with patients with suspected subdural empyema, CT scanning and MRI are the diagnostic procedures of choice for the detection of intracranial epidural abscess. Both studies usually demonstrate a superficial circumscribed area of diminished density, often with contrast enhancement. This rim enhancement is usually thicker and more irregular with an epidural abscess than with subdural empyema. Subgaleal or subperiosteal abscesses, calvarial osteomyelitis, and frontal sinusitis are often associated with intracranial abscesses. MRI offers several advantages over CT scanning in the evaluation of patients with suspected intracranial epidural abscess. Small collections are often identified more accurately with MRI, and streak artifacts from bone are absent. In addition, MRI readily differentiates postoperative and posttraumatic abscesses from sterile effusions and/or chronic extraaxial hematomas with far greater accuracy than CT scanning.

As is the case with other focal suppurative infections of the CNS, a combined medical-surgical therapeutic approach is optimal for management of intracranial epidural abscess. In adults, where 60 to 90 percent of intracranial abscesses are a direct result of extension from paranasal sinusitis or mastoiditis, empirical antimicrobial therapy should be directed against aerobic streptococci, staphylococci, and anaerobic bacteria and commonly involves a combination of agents. When cranial defects are suspected or proven, an antistaphylococcal agent such as a penicillinase-resistant penicillin or vancomycin should be added in the dosages discussed above. All intracranial epidural collections should be drained surgically. Furthermore, appropriate stains and cultures should be obtained at the time of surgery, including investigation for acid-fast bacteria and/or fungi if clinically warranted. The actual procedure employed, e.g., burr holes versus craniotomy or craniectomy, depends on the extent of the lesion and involvement of overlying bone. Dural grafting may be necessary if the dura has been breached by infection, and communications between sinus cavities and the epidural space may require surgical closure later. Perhaps due to its insidious clinical presentation, improved diagnostic accuracy of the CT scan and MRI, and the availability of potent antimicrobial agents, the morbidity and mortality of intracranial epidural abscess are low.

SUPPURATIVE INTRACRANIAL THROMBOPHLEBITIS

EPIDEMIOLOGY AND ETIOLOGY Suppurative intracranial thrombophlebitis is defined by the simultaneous presence of venous thrombosis and suppuration in the intracranial compartment. The process may begin within veins and/or venous sinuses following infection of the paranasal sinuses, middle ear, mastoid, facial skin, or oropharynx and may involve additional vessels by propagation of clot or discontinuous spread. Septic intracranial thrombophlebitis also may complicate the presence of epidural abscess, subdural empyema, or bacterial meningitis. Occasionally, but rarely, metastatic spread of infection from a distant site may lead directly to suppurative intracranial thrombophlebitis. Conditions that increase blood viscosity or coagulability, including dehydration, pregnancy, oral contraceptive use, sickle cell disease, polycythemia, malignancy, or trauma, all increase the likelihood of intracranial thrombosis and suppurative complications. Intracranial venous sinus thrombosis depends, to a large extent, on the close proximity of the dural venous sinuses to other structures involved by antecedent conditions. The usual predisposing conditions for the development of cavernous sinus thrombosis are paranasal sinusitis (especially frontal, ethmoidal, or sphenoidal) or infections of the face or mouth. The most common bacterial pathogens depend on the initial source of infection as follows: (1) staphylococci, aerobic and/or microaerophilic streptococci, gram-negative bacilli, and/or anaerobes with sinusitis, and (2) *S. aureus* secondary to facial infections. Otitis media or mastoiditis may be complicated by the development of lateral sinus thrombosis and/or infection of the superior and inferior petrosal sinuses. Infections of the face, scalp, subdural space, epidural space, or meningitis are associated with suppurative thrombophlebitis of the superior sagittal sinus. Again, the most likely infecting microorganisms depend on the associated primary condition. *S. aureus* is the most important

associated pathogen in patients with cavernous sinus thrombosis and is isolated in more than two-thirds of cases. This predominance reflects the importance of this organism in the associated infections of the face and scalp and in acute sphenoid sinusitis. Less common isolates in patients with cavernous sinus thrombosis include streptococci, pneumococci, gram-negative bacilli, and *Bacteroides* sp.

CLINICAL MANIFESTATIONS Not unexpectedly, the clinical presentation of suppurative cortical thrombophlebitis depends on the location of involvement. In addition, if the cortical venous system is involved, the appearance of neurologic deficits is dependent on the adequacy of collateral venous drainage. Patients with inadequate collateral flow present with impairment of consciousness, focal or generalized seizures (often alternating in character), symptoms of increased ICP, and various focal neurologic findings (e.g., hemiparesis). Aphasia is common when the dominant cerebral hemisphere is involved. The most common complaints in patients with cavernous sinus thrombosis include periorbital swelling (73 percent) and headache (52 percent). Headache is more common when the antecedent condition is sinusitis rather than a facial cellulitis. Other prominent symptoms include diplopia, tearing, photophobia, drowsiness, and ptosis. Fever is present in over 90 percent of patients with cavernous sinus thrombosis. Upon examination, proptosis, chemosis, periorbital edema, and weakness of the extraocular muscles due to involvement of the cranial nerves III, IV, or VI are common. Since the abducens nerve is the only cranial nerve traversing the inferior portion of the cavernous sinus, a lateral gaze palsy may be an early neurologic finding. Papilledema or venous engorgement and a change in mental status are observed in approximately 65 and 55 percent of patients, respectively. Meningitis, often confusing the diagnostic issues, is present in about 40 percent of cases, usually secondary to retrograde spread of thrombophlebitis. About 25 percent of patients also have dilated or sluggishly reactive pupils, decreased visual acuity (frequently progressing to blindness), and dysfunction of cranial nerve V. With spread of the infection to the opposite cavernous sinus, these findings may be duplicated in the opposite eye. In addition, septic cavernous sinus thrombosis may present in two ways. In the acute presentation, the onset between the primary infection (usually a facial cellulitis) and cavernous sinus thrombosis is less than 1 week. The patient appears seriously ill, with a rapid development of symptoms and signs described above and progression to bilateral eye signs. In contrast, some patients present with a more indolent form of cavernous sinus thrombosis, usually secondary to dental infections, otitis media, or paranasal sinusitis. The orbital manifestations are less impressive, and involvement of the contralateral eye is a late and inconsistent finding. Headache is the most prominent finding (> 80 percent) in patients with septic lateral sinus thrombosis, but earache, vomiting, nausea, and vertigo are often present, since otitis media is a common predisposing condition. Fever and abnormal ear findings are observed in the majority of patients (about 80 and 98 percent, respectively); facial pain, altered facial sensation, papilledema, mild nuchal rigidity, and/or a sixth nerve palsy also may be present. Thrombosis of the superior sagittal sinus produces an abnormal mental status progressing to coma, motor deficits, nuchal rigidity, and papilledema. Seizures occur in more than 50 percent of patients. The onset may be subacute, particularly in patients with sinusitis. Involvement of the inferior petrosal sinus may produce ipsilateral facial pain and lateral rectus muscle weakness (Gradenigo's syndrome).

DIAGNOSIS MRI is the diagnostic procedure of choice for the evaluation of patients with suspected suppurative intracranial thrombophlebitis. MRI is far superior to CT in differentiating thrombosis from normal flowing blood. MRI also can reveal the evolution and resolution of the entire venoocclusive process. CT scanning, with and without intravenous contrast enhancement, also permits diagnosis of venous sinus thrombosis, but it is considerably less sensitive and reliable than MRI. The CT appearance usually reveals unilateral or bilateral multiple irregular filling defects in the enhancement of the cavernous sinus with or without orbital inflammatory change. Both MRI and CT can reliably evaluate the paranasal sinuses and provide information concerning subdural and epidural infection, cerebral infarction, cerebritis, hemorrhage, and/or cerebral edema. In the unusual case in which MRI and CT are negative but suspicion of thrombophlebitis is high, carotid arteriography with venous phase studies should be performed. Arteriography reveals narrowing of the intracavernous segment of the carotid sinus in cavernous sinus thrombosis. Orbital venography also may be useful and is the most definitive method of demonstrating cavernous sinus thrombosis. As with other focal suppurative intracranial processes, the lumbar puncture usually demonstrates a mild pleocytosis and an elevated protein concentration. In septic thrombosis of the superior sagittal sinus, however, the CSF finding may be consistent with a frank meningitis, and the causative organism is often isolated on CSF culture. Blood cultures may be positive, especially in patients with a rapidly progressing course. Chest radiographs may reveal evidence of septic pulmonary emboli following propagation of thrombus into the inferior petrosal sinus and the jugular vein.

TREATMENT Analogous to subdural empyema and epidural abscess, empirical therapy should be directed toward gram-positive organisms, including staphylococci, aerobic gram-negative bacilli, and anaerobes. In cavernous sinus thrombosis, a potent antistaphylococcal agent should always be included in the antimicrobial regimen. Nafcillin should be used, with vancomycin reserved for the penicillin-allergic patient and when methicillin-resistant organisms are suspected or proven. Combination regimens including nafcillin or vancomycin plus metronidazole plus a third-generation cephalosporin are often used. Surgical intervention may be required for optimal therapy. Surgical drainage of infected sinuses is necessary when antimicrobial therapy alone is ineffective. Operative intervention for patients with cavernous sinus thrombosis is often employed, especially in the setting of sphenoid sinusitis. Internal jugular vein ligation and thrombectomy have been utilized in patients with lateral sinus vein thrombosis, but the efficacy of these procedures is poorly defined. Surgical therapy also may be necessary for other contiguous foci of infection, e.g., dental abscess. Anticoagulation is controversial. Although anticoagulation may prevent the spread of the thrombus, the benefit is most apparent when initiated early during the course. However, the hazards of intracranial hemorrhage, including bleeding from sites of cortical venous infarction, must be recognized. In the absence of definitive data and specific contraindications, anticoagulation is most likely to be useful early in the course of cavernous sinus thrombosis. Anticoagulation is not recommended for septic lateral sinus thrombophlebitis because the cortical veins overlying the infected mastoid may become occluded, resulting in small venous hemorrhagic infarcts and leading to the consequences of intracerebral hemorrhage.

REFERENCES

CAMPBELL S: Amebic brain abscess and meningoencephalitis. Semin Neurol 13:153, 1993

DiNUBILE MJ et al: Septic cortical thrombophlebitis. J Infect Dis 161:1216, 1990

FEIGIN RD et al: Diagnosis and management of meningitis. Pediatr Infect Dis J 11:785, 1992

HELFGOTT DC et al: Subdural empyema, in *Infections of the Central Nervous System*, WM Scheld et al (eds). New York, Raven, 1991, pp 487–498

KILPI T et al: Severity of childhood bacterial meningitis and duration of illness before diagnosis. Lancet 2:406, 1991

KUMAR P, VERMA IC: Antibiotic therapy for bacterial meningitis in children in developing countries. Bull World Health Organ 71:183, 1993

LEBELL MH et al: Dexamethasone therapy for bacterial meningitis: Results of two double-blind, placebo-controlled trials. N Engl J Med 319:964, 1988

ODIO CM et al: The beneficial effects of early dexamethasone administration in infants and children with bacterial meningitis. N Engl J Med 324:1525, 1991

PELTOLA H et al: Rapid disappearance of *Haemophilus influenzae* type b meningitis after routine childhood immunization with conjugate vaccines. Lancet 340:592, 1992

PFISTER HW et al: Spectrum of complications during bacterial meningitis in adults—Results of a prospective clinical study. Arch Neurol 50:575, 1993

PINNER RW et al: Meningococcal disease in the United States—1986. J Infect Dis 164:368, 1991

POMEROY LS et al: Seizures and other neurologic sequelae of bacterial meningitis in children. N Engl J Med 323:1651, 1990

QUAGLIARELLO V, SCHELD WM: Bacterial meningitis: Pathogenesis, pathophysiology, and progress. N Engl J Med 327:864, 1992

ROOS KL et al: Acute bacterial meningitis in children and adults, in *Infections of the Central Nervous System*, WM Scheld et al (eds). New York, Raven, 1991, pp 335–409

SAEZ-LLORENS X et al: Molecular pathophysiology of bacterial meningitis: Current concepts and therapeutic implications. J Pediatr 116:671, 1990

SCHELD WM: Recent advances in the pathophysiology and management of bacterial meningitis. J Infect Dis (in press)

SEYDOUX CH, FRANCIOLI P: Bacterial brain abscesses: Factors influencing mortality and sequelae. Clin Infect Dis 15:394, 1992

SOUTHWICK FS et al: Septic thrombosis of the dural venous sinuses. Medicine 65:82, 1985

SPANOS A et al: Differential diagnosis of acute meningitis. JAMA 262:2700, 1989

STEPHENS DS, FARLEY MM: Pathogenetic events during infection of the human nasal pharynx with *Neisseria meningitidis* and *Haemophilus influenzae*. Rev Infect Dis 13:22, 1991

TUNKEL AR et al: Bacterial meningitis: Recent advances in pathophysiology and treatment. Ann Intern Med 112:610, 1990

TUNKEL AR, SCHELD WM: Pathogenesis and pathophysiology of bacterial meningitis. Ann Rev Med 44:103, 1993

TUREEN JH et al: Effect of hydration status on cerebral blood flow and cerebrospinal fluid lactate acidosis in rabbits with experimental meningitis. J Clin Invest 89:947, 1992

TYLER K, MARTIN JB: *Infectious Diseases of the Central Nevous System*. Philadelphia, FA Davis, 1993

WENGER JD et al: Bacterial meningitis in the United States, 1986: Report of a multistate surveillance study. J Infect Dis 162:1316, 1990

WISPELWEY B, SCHELD WM: Brain abscess, in *Principles and Practices of Infectious Diseases*, 4th ed. GL Mandell et al (eds). New York: Churchill Livingstone, in press

——— et al: Brain abscess, in *Infections of the Central Nervous System*, WM Scheld et al (eds). New York, Raven, 1991, pp 457–486

ZIMMERMAN RD, WEINGARTEN K: Evaluation of intracranial inflammatory disease by CT and MRI, in *Clinical Neuroimaging*, WH Theodore (ed). New York, Liss, 1988, pp 75–100

375   VIRAL AND PRION DISEASES OF THE NERVOUS SYSTEM

KENNETH L. TYLER

Hundreds of viruses have been reported to produce acute infection and injury to the central or peripheral nervous systems. Many aspects of the clinical characteristics of these diseases are determined by whether the infection is limited primarily to the meninges (*meningitis*) or extends to involve the parenchyma of the brain (*encephalitis*) and/or spinal cord (*myelitis*). Although there are a number of similarities in the basic epidemiology and diagnostic approaches to these disorders, they are discussed separately. Viruses also can produce chronic or persistent infections of the central nervous system (CNS). These disorders are sufficiently different from acute viral infections and from each other as to merit separate consideration. Special emphasis is given to HIV infection of the nervous system, both because of its obvious epidemiologic importance and because of its capacity to produce myriad neurologic syndromes as it attacks virtually every part of the nervous system. An additional group of neurologic disorders, commonly discussed in the context of viral infections, shares the characteristics of being transmissible neurodegenerative diseases (TNDs), although the brunt of recent evidence indicates that they are caused by a novel class of agents, commonly referred to as *prions* ("proteinaceous infectious particles").

ACUTE VIRAL INFECTIONS

VIRAL MENINGITIS   Clinical picture The syndrome of viral meningitis consists of fever, headache, and signs of meningeal irritation coupled with an inflammatory cerebrospinal fluid (CSF) profile typically consisting of a lymphocytic pleocytosis, a slightly elevated protein level, and a normal glucose level. Fever may be accompanied by malaise, myalgia, anorexia, nausea and vomiting, abdominal pain, or diarrhea. It is not uncommon to see a mild degree

TABLE 375-1 Viruses causing aseptic meningitis*

Common	Less common	Rare
Enteroviruses	HSV-1	Adenoviruses
Arboviruses	LCMV	CMV
HIV	Mumps	EBV
HSV-2		Influenza A, B; measles; parainfluenza; rubella; VZV

* CMV = cytomegalovirus; EBV = Epstein-Barr virus; HIV = human immunodeficiency virus; HSV = herpes simplex virus; LCMV = lymphocytic choriomeningitis virus; VZV = varicella-zoster virus.

of lethargy or drowsiness. The presence of more profound alterations in consciousness such as stupor, coma, or marked confusion should prompt consideration of alternative diagnoses. Similarly, the presence of seizures, cranial nerve palsies, or other focal neurologic signs or symptoms suggests parenchymal involvement and is not typical of uncomplicated viral meningitis. The headache associated with viral meningitis is typically frontal or retro-orbital in location and often associated with photophobia and pain on moving the eyes. Nuchal rigidity is present in the majority of cases but may be mild in nature and present only in the terminal portion of neck anteflexion. Evidence of severe meningeal irritation, such as Kernig's and Brudzinski's signs, are generally absent.

Etiology Comprehensive attempts to identify the etiology of individual cases of viral meningitis are rarely made in general practice. In large series, using routine serologic and culture techniques, a specific viral cause can be found in 30 to 70 percent of cases (Table 375-1).

Epidemiology It is impossible to determine the exact incidence of viral meningitis in the United States, since the majority of cases go unreported to public health authorities. There is a striking increase in cases during the summer months, reflecting the seasonal predominance of enterovirus and arbovirus infections, with a peak monthly incidence of about 1 reported case per 100,000 population. The striking seasonal predilections of some of the viruses causing meningitis can provide a valuable clue to diagnosis (Table 375-2), although it is important to recognize that seasonal distributions are relative rather than absolute indicators of frequency.

Laboratory diagnosis CSF EXAMINATION The most important laboratory test in the diagnosis of meningitis is examination of the CSF. The typical profile in cases of viral meningitis is a lymphocytic pleocytosis, slightly elevated protein level, and normal glucose level. Organisms *cannot* be seen on Gram's or acid-fast stained smears or india ink wet mounts of CSF. Polymorphonuclear neutrophils (PMNs) may predominate in the first 48 h of illness, especially in some enteroviral infections, and may last longer when infection is due to echovirus 9 or Eastern equine virus (EEV). Patients with suspected viral meningitis and a PMN pleocytosis should have a follow-up CSF examination after 8 to 12 h to look for the presence of a shift toward mononuclear cells. The presence of a PMN pleocytosis always should prompt consideration of bacterial meningitis or parameningeal infections. The total CSF cell count per microliter in viral meningitis rarely exceeds 1000. The CSF glucose level is typically normal in viral infections, although it may be decreased in cases due to mumps (10 to 30 percent), lymphocytic choriomeningitis virus (LCMV) and, less frequently, echovirus and other enteroviruses, herpes simplex

virus type 2 (HSV-2), or varicella-zoster virus (VZV). As a general rule, a lymphocytic pleocytosis with a low glucose level ($\leq$25 mg/dL) should suggest the presence of fungal, listerial, or tuberculous meningitis or of noninfectious disorders (e.g., sarcoid, neoplastic meningitis).

A number of tests measuring levels of various CSF proteins, enzymes, and mediators, including C-reactive protein, lactic acid, lactate dehydrogenase, neopterin, interleukin 1β (IL-1β), IL-6, soluble IL-2 receptor, beta$_2$ microglobulin, and tumor necrosis factor (TNF), have been proposed as potential discriminators between viral and bacterial meningitis or as markers of specific types of viral infection (e.g., human immunodeficiency virus, HIV), but most appear to lack sufficient sensitivity and specificity to be truly useful. It has been suggested recently that the presence of detectable TNF-α in the CSF is indicative of bacterial infection and is not found in cases of viral meningitis, although this observation requires further confirmation. Patients with HIV CNS infection often have elevated CSF levels of p24 antigen, and this may be useful in diagnosis.

CSF CULTURE The overall results of CSF culture for the diagnosis of viral infection are disappointing (Table 375-3), presumably reflecting the generally low concentration of infectious virus present and the need to customize isolation procedures for individual viruses. For viral isolation, 2 mL of CSF should be obtained and brought promptly to the microbiology laboratory, where it should be refrigerated and processed as speedily as possible. As a general rule, CSF specimens for viral isolation should never be stored in a freezer (-20°C), since viruses are often unstable at this temperature, and most modern freezers have "frostfree" warmup cycles that are detrimental to viral stability. Storage for more than 24 h is probably best done in a -70°C freezer.

OTHER SOURCES FOR VIRAL ISOLATION It is important to remember that viruses also may be isolated from sites and body fluids other than CSF. Enteroviruses and adenoviruses may be found in feces; arboviruses, some enteroviruses, and LCMV, in blood; mumps and cytomegalovirus (CMV), in urine; and enteroviruses, mumps, and adenoviruses, in throat washings. During enteroviral infections, viral shedding in stool may persist for several weeks. The presence of enterovirus in stool is not diagnostic and may result from residual shedding from a previous enteroviral infection and also can occur in some asymptomatic individuals during enteroviral epidemics.

NUCLEIC ACID AMPLIFICATION Amplification of viral-specific DNA or RNA from CSF using polymerase chain reaction (PCR) amplification or related techniques appears to have great promise as a diagnostic tool. HSV-1 DNA has been amplified from the CSF of patients with herpes simplex encephalitis and recurrent (Mollaret) meningitis even when standard culture techniques have been negative. Successful genomic amplification and detection of picornaviruses (coxsackie, polio) in the CSF of patients with meningitis also have been reported. These techniques will undoubtedly become more widely available in the future.

SEROLOGIC STUDIES In most cases, definitive diagnosis of viral infection depends on documentation of seroconversion between acute phase and convalescent sera (typically obtained after 2 to 4 weeks). Antiviral antibodies also may be measured in CSF (see below). The timing of the antibody response often means that the utility of serologic data is primarily in retrospective establishment of a specific diagnosis, and their value in initial diagnosis and management is limited. Most viral infections of the CNS are associated with

TABLE 375-2 Seasonal prevalence of viruses commonly causing meningitis

Summer–early fall	Fall and winter	Winter and spring	Nonseasonal
Arboviruses Enteroviruses	LCMV	Mumps	HIV HSV

NOTE: Abbreviations as in Table 375-1.

TABLE 375-3 Possibility of culturing specific viruses from CSF

Excellent	Fair	Poor or none
Coxsackie, echo, LCMV, mumps	HIV, adeno, arboviruses (most), HSV-2, VZV, rabies	Polio, HSV-1, EBV, CMV

NOTE: Abbreviations as in Table 375-1.

intrathecal synthesis of antiviral antibody. This results in an elevation in the CSF/serum antibody ratio. Similar elevations also may occur as a result of breakdown in the blood-brain barrier (BBB), but this is typically associated with elevation in the CSF/serum albumin ratio. Obtaining paired CSF and sera for serologic testing may provide additional evidence that an antibody response is the result of CNS infection. The sensitivity of CSF/serum antibody ratio studies may be enhanced by correcting for breakdown of the BBB using the CSF/serum albumin ratio or using CSF/serum antibody ratios of other viruses as controls. Although use of CSF/serum antibody ratio determinations may enhance the sensitivity of diagnosis, the technique still suffers from the delay between onset of infection and appearance of the host's antibody response.

Agarose electrophoresis or isoelectric focusing of CSF gamma globulins may reveal the presence of oligoclonal bands. These have been found in association with a number of viral infections, including HIV, HTLV-I, mumps, subacute sclerosing panencephalitis (SSPE), and progressive rubella panencephalitis. The associated antibodies are often directed against viral proteins. The finding of oligoclonal bands may be of some diagnostic utility, since they are not seen with arbovirus, enterovirus, or HSV infections. It is important to recognize that oligoclonal bands are commonly encountered in certain noninfectious neurologic diseases (e.g., multiple sclerosis) and may be found in nonviral infections (e.g., syphilis, Lyme borreliosis).

OTHER LABORATORY STUDIES All patients with suspected viral meningitis should have a complete blood count and differential, platelet count, hematocrit, erythrocyte sedimentation rate (ESR), electrolytes, glucose, liver function tests, BUN, creatinine, creatine kinase, aldolase, amylase, and lipase. Abnormalities in specific tests may provide a clue suggesting particular etiologic diagnoses. Magnetic resonance imaging (MRI), computed tomography (CT), electroencephalography (EEG), evoked response studies, electromyography (EMG), and nerve conduction studies are not necessary in the majority of cases and should not be ordered routinely. Their use is best tailored to individual circumstances when atypical presentations or unusual features of particular cases present diagnostic problems.

Differential diagnosis Perhaps the most important issue in the differential diagnosis is the exclusion of nonviral causes that can mimic viral encephalitis. The major categories of disease that should always be specifically considered and excluded are (1) parameningeal infections or partially treated bacterial meningitis, (2) nonviral infectious meningitides where cultures may be negative (e.g., fungal, tuberculous, or syphilitic disease), (3) neoplastic meningitis, and (4) meningitis secondary to noninfectious inflammatory diseases such as sarcoid, Behçet disease, and the uveomeningitic syndromes. Although the diagnosis of a specific viral etiology in a particular case of viral meningitis can rarely be made on clinical grounds alone, proper attention to epidemiologic, clinical, and laboratory features may substantially narrow the diagnostic possibilities. Statistically, *enteroviruses* (see Chap. 154) are the most common cause of viral meningitis (>80 percent of cases with etiology identified) and should be considered the leading candidates when a typical case occurs in the summer months, especially in a child (<15 years of age) (Table 375-4). However, despite their summer prevalence, it is important to recognize that sporadic cases of enteroviral CNS infection are seen year-round. The physical examination should include a careful search for exanthemata, hand-foot-mouth disease, herpangina, pleurodynia, myopericarditis, and hemorrhagic conjunctivitis, which may be stigmata of enterovirus infections.

Mumps (see Chap. 157) should be considered when meningitis occurs in the late winter or early spring, especially in males (male/female ratio 3:1). With the widespread use of the live attenuated mumps vaccine in the United States, the incidence of mumps meningitis has fallen dramatically. Rare cases of mumps vaccine–associated meningitis have been reported, but they are not usually seen after vaccination with the Jeryl-Lynn strain of virus used in the United States. The presence of orchitis, oophoritis, parotitis, or pancreatitis or elevations in serum lipase and amylase are suggestive

TABLE 375-4 Enteroviruses causing aseptic meningitis

	Polio	Coxsackie	Echo	Entero
Common		A7,9 B2–5	4,6,9,11,16 30	
Less common	1–3	A1–6,8,10, 11,14,16– 18,22,24 B1,6	1–3,5,7,8 12–15,17–23 25,27,28,30 31,33	70,71

but can be found with other viruses. Mumps infection confers lifelong immunity, so a previous history of documented infection excludes this diagnosis. The presence of hypoglycorrhachia (10 to 30 percent) may be an additional diagnostic clue, once other causes have been excluded (see above).

Development of meningitis in the late fall or winter associated with a history of exposure to house mice (*Mus musculus*), pet or laboratory rodents (e.g., hamsters), or their excreta should suggest the possibility of *LCMV infection* (see Chap. 160). Some patients have an associated rash, pulmonary infiltrates, alopecia, parotitis, orchitis, or myopericarditis. Laboratory clues to the diagnosis may include the presence of leukopenia, thrombocytopenia, abnormal liver function tests, or pulmonary infiltrates. Some cases present with a marked CSF pleocytosis (>1000 cells per microliter) and hypoglycorrhachia (<30 percent).

HSV-2 (see Chap. 143) *meningitis* should be suspected in any patient with concomitant primary genital infection, but it also occurs less commonly with recurrent (secondary) episodes of genital disease. Both *HSV-1* and *HSV-2* should be considered in patients with recurrent episodes of aseptic meningitis (Mollaret meningitis), although special techniques, such as PCR amplification of viral genomic material from the CSF, may be required to establish the diagnosis in these cases. *Epstein-Barr virus (EBV) infections* also may produce aseptic meningitis, with or without accompanying evidence of the infectious mononucleosis syndrome. The diagnosis may be suggested by the presence of atypical lymphocytes in the CSF or an atypical lymphocytosis in peripheral blood. *VZV meningitis* should be suspected in the presence of concurrent chickenpox or shingles. Some patients develop a distinctive syndrome of acute cerebellar ataxia. This typically occurs in children and presents with the abrupt onset of limb and truncal ataxia. A similar syndrome occurs less commonly in association with EBV and enteroviral infection.

Arbovirus infections typically occur in the summer months, have clear geographic localization, and occur in epidemics, all factors reflecting the ecology of their transmission through infected insect vectors (see Fig. 375-1 and Table 375-6; see also Chap. 159). Arboviral meningitis should be considered when clusters of meningitis cases occur in a restricted geographic region during the summer or early fall. A history of tick exposure or travel or residence in the appropriate geographic area should suggest the possibility of Colorado tick fever virus (CTFV) or Powassan virus infection, although nonviral diseases producing meningitis (e.g., Lyme disease) or headache with meningismus (e.g., Rocky mountain spotted fever) also may present this way.

HIV infection is discussed more fully below and in Chap. 279. HIV meningitis should be suspected in any patient with known or identified risk factors for HIV infection. Aseptic meningitis appears to be a common manifestation of primary exposure to HIV and may be associated with HIV seroconversion (see Chap. 279). In some patients, seroconversion may be delayed for several months, and in seronegative patients, serology should be repeated after 3- and 6-month intervals. Cranial nerve palsies are more common in HIV meningitis than in other viral infections, most commonly involving cranial nerves V, VII, or VIII.

Treatment In the usual case of viral meningitis, treatment is symptomatic, and hospitalization is not required. Exceptions to this rule include patients with deficient humoral immunity, neonates with

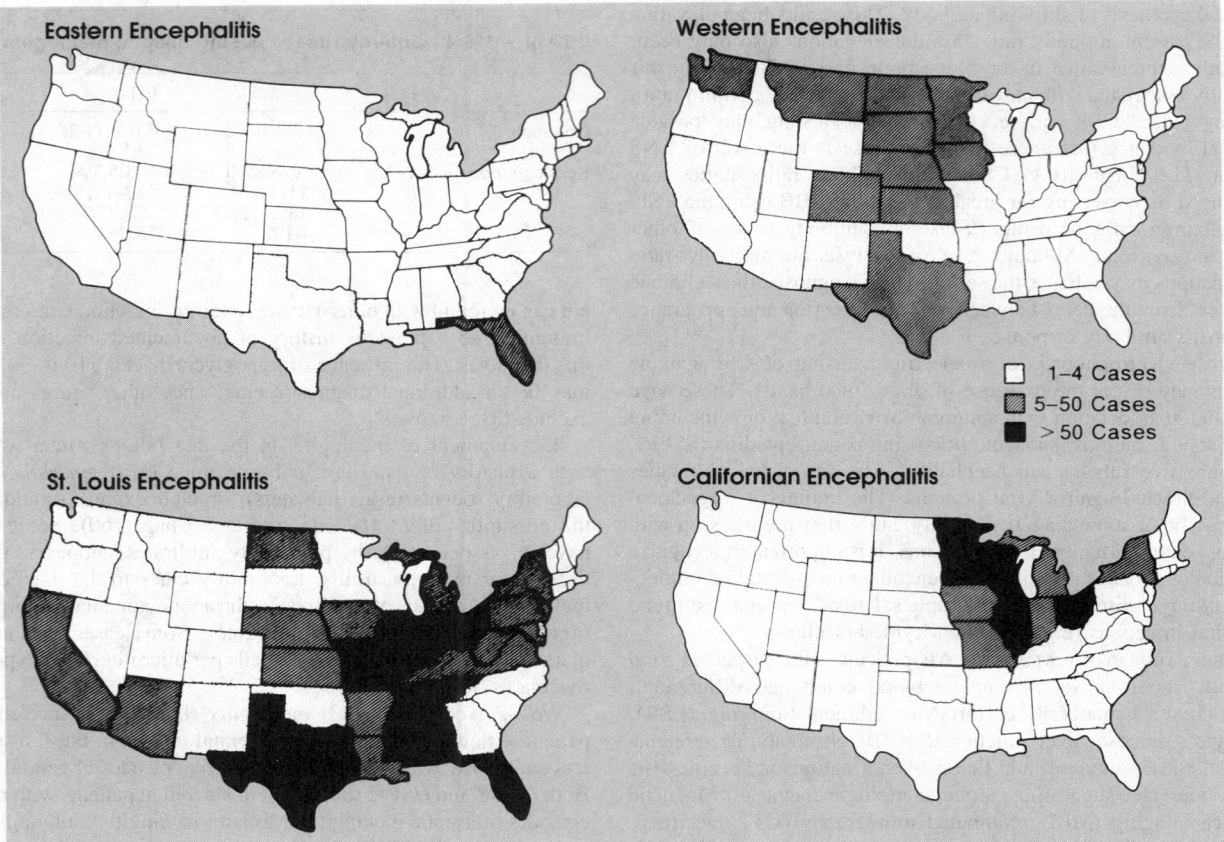

FIGURE 375-1 Geographic distributions of the most commonly encountered arbovirus encephalitides in the United States. (*From RT Johnson, with permission.*)

overwhelming infection, and patients in whom the clinical or CSF profile suggests the possibility of bacterial or other nonviral causes of infection. Patients with suspected bacterial meningitis should receive appropriate empirical therapy pending culture results (see Chap. 374). Patients with deficient humoral immunity may benefit from a trial of intravenous gamma globulin. Oral or intravenous acyclovir may be beneficial to patients with meningitis caused by HSV-1 or HSV-2 and, although rarely indicated, would theoretically be of value in cases of severe EBV or VZV infection. Zidovudine (AZT) or didanosine (formerly dideoxyinosine; ddI) presumably would be of value in the treatment of HIV meningitis, although no clinical trials have been performed. Patients usually prefer to rest undisturbed in a quiet, darkened room. Analgesics can be used to relieve headache, which is often reduced by the initial diagnostic lumbar puncture. Antipyretics may help to reduce fever, which rarely exceeds 40°C. Hyponatremia may develop as a result of the syndrome of inappropriate vasopressin secretion (SIADH), so fluid and electrolyte status should be monitored. Repeat lumbar puncture is only indicated in patients whose fever and symptoms fail to be resolving after a few days or if there is doubt about the initial diagnosis. Vaccination is an effective method of preventing the subsequent development of meningitis and other neurologic complications associated with poliovirus, mumps, and measles infection.

Prognosis In adults, the prognosis for full recovery from viral meningitis is excellent. Rare patients continue to complain of persisting headache, mild mental impairment, incoordination, or generalized asthenia for weeks to months. The outcome in infants and neonates (<1 year of age) is less certain. Intellectual impairment, learning disabilities, hearing loss, and other lasting neurologic sequelae have been reported in some but not all studies; however, their frequency is uncertain.

VIRAL ENCEPHALITIS Definition In distinction to meningitis, where the brunt of the infectious process and associated inflammatory response is limited to the meninges, in encephalitis there is, in addition, involvement of the brain parenchyma.

Clinical picture In addition to the acute febrile illness with evidence of meningeal involvement characteristic of meningitis, the patient with encephalitis commonly has an altered level of consciousness, an abnormal mental state, and evidence of either focal or diffuse neurologic signs and symptoms. All degrees of altered consciousness may occur, ranging from mild lethargy to deep coma. A patient with encephalitis is not mentally alert and is frequently confused, delirious, and disoriented. Mental aberrations may include hallucinations, agitation, personality change, behavioral disorders, and at times, a frankly psychotic state. Focal or generalized seizures occur in more than 50 percent of patients with severe encephalitis. Virtually every possible type of focal neurologic disturbance has been reported in viral encephalitis, the signs and symptoms reflecting the sites of infection and inflammation. The most commonly encountered focal findings are aphasia, ataxia, hemiparesis (with hyperactive tendon reflexes and extensor plantar responses), involuntary movements (e.g., myoclonic jerks), and cranial nerve deficits (e.g., ocular palsies, facial weakness). Involvement of the hypothalamic-pituitary axis may result in temperature dysregulation, diabetes insipidus, or the development of SIADH. Despite the clear neuropathologic evidence that viruses differ in the regions of the CNS they injure, it is often impossible to reliably distinguish on clinical grounds alone one type of viral encephalitis (e.g., that caused by HSV) from others (see "Differential Diagnosis").

Etiology The number of viruses reported to cause encephalitis is legion. In the United States, there are approximately 20,000 reported cases per year. The same organisms responsible for aseptic meningitis are also responsible for encephalitis, although their relative frequencies differ (Table 375-5).

Laboratory diagnosis CSF EXAMINATION CSF examination should be performed in all patients with suspected viral encephalitis unless contraindicated by the presence of severely increased intracranial pressure (ICP). The characteristic CSF profile is indistinguishable from that of viral meningitis and consists of a lymphocytic pleocytosis, a mildly elevated protein level, and a normal glucose level. A CSF pleocytosis (>5 cells per microliter) occurs in more than 95 percent of patients with documented viral encephalitis, and its absence should prompt a careful search for other causes of an encephalopathy. In rare cases, a pleocytosis may be absent on the initial lumbar puncture, but present subsequently. Patients who are severely immunocompromised by radiation, chemotherapy, or certain lymphoreticular malignancies may fail to mount a CSF inflammatory response. The cell count exceeds 500 cells per microliter in only about 10 percent of patients. Infections with certain arboviruses (Eastern equine encephalitis or California encephalitis), mumps, and LCMV occasionally may result in more than 1000 cells per microliter, but this degree of pleocytosis should suggest the possibility of nonviral infections or other inflammatory processes. Atypical lymphocytes in the CSF may be seen in EBV infection and less commonly with other viruses, including CMV and HSV. The presence of substantial numbers of PMNs after the first 48 h should prompt consideration of bacterial infection, leptospirosis, amebic infection, and noninfectious processes such as acute hemorrhagic leukoencephalitis; however, large numbers of PMNs in the CSF are occasionally present with Eastern encephalitis, echovirus 9, and other enteroviral infections. About 20 percent of patients with encephalitis will have a significant (>500 cells per microliter) number of red blood cells in the CSF in a nontraumatic tap. The pathologic correlate of this may be the presence of a hemorrhagic encephalitis of the type seen with HSV, Colorado tick fever virus (CTFV), and occasionally California encephalitis virus (CEV). A decreased CSF glucose level is distinctly unusual in viral encephalitis and should suggest the possibility of fungal, tuberculous, parasitic, leptospiral, syphilitic, sarcoid, or neoplastic meningitis. Rare patients with mumps, LCMV, or late in the stage of HSV encephalitis may have hypoglycorrhachia.

CSF CULTURE   Attempts to culture viruses from the CSF in cases of encephalitis are often disappointing (see Table 375-3). In particular, it should be noted that cultures are invariably negative in cases of HSV-1 encephalitis.

NUCLEIC ACID AMPLIFICATION   Early reports indicated that this may be an extremely promising approach to the diagnosis of certain types of viral encephalitis. Most studies have focused on PCR amplification of HSV DNA from the CSF of patients with suspected HSV encephalitis, although successful amplification of enteroviral RNA also has been reported (see "Viral Meningitis").

SEROLOGIC STUDIES AND ANTIGEN DETECTION   The basic approach to the serodiagnosis of viral encephalitis is identical to that discussed earlier for viral meningitis. In the case of HSV encephalitis, attention has focused on the detection of HSV antibodies in the CSF. In one large series, antibodies to HSV-1 glycoprotein B were found in 97 percent of biopsy-proven cases of HSV encephalitis. The specificity was 100 percent if the assay was corrected for leakage across the blood-brain barrier using adenovirus antibodies as a marker. In another study, virus glycoprotein antigens (gB, gC, gD, and gE) were found in the CSF of 92 percent of patients with biopsy-proven cases of HSV encephalitis and had a specificity of 82 percent. Unfortunately, the best results with these types of assays occur after the first week of illness. This limits their utility to retrospective diagnostic confirmation rather than acute diagnosis.

CT, MRI, EEG   Patients with suspected encephalitis almost invariably undergo structural imaging studies and often EEG. The utility of these tests is to identify or help exclude alternative diagnoses and to help establish the existence of a focal, as opposed to a diffuse, encephalitic process. The presence of focal findings should always raise the possibility of HSV encephalitis. These are (1) periodic focal spikes on a background of slow or low-amplitude ("flattened") activity with a temporal predominance of EEG, (2) temporoparietal areas of low absorption, mass effect, and contrast enhancement on CT, or (3) areas of increased signal intensity in the frontotemporal,

TABLE 375-5   Viruses causing encephalitis

Common	Less common	Rare
Arboviruses, enteroviruses, HSV-1, mumps	CMV, EBV, HIV, measles, VZV	Adenoviruses, CTFV, influenza A, LCMV, parainfluenza, rabies, rubella

NOTE: Abbreviations as in Table 375-1. Also CTFV = Colorado tick fever virus

cingulate, or insular regions of the brain on T_2-weighted spin-echo MRI images.

BRAIN BIOPSY   The isolation of HSV from brain tissue obtained at biopsy has been considered the gold standard for the diagnosis of HSV encephalitis and has been employed in the major trials of HSV encephalitis therapy conducted by the National Institutes of Allergy and Infectious Diseases Collaborative Antiviral Study Group (NIAID-CASG). Biopsy tissue is cultured for virus and examined histopathologically and ultrastructurally. Biopsy is typically carried out under general anesthesia through a craniectomy. Tissue should be taken from a site that appears to be significantly involved based on clinical and laboratory criteria. The most common practice is to obtain tissue (1 cm³) from the anterior portion of the inferior temporal gyrus through a subtemporal craniectomy. The sensitivity of brain biopsy exceeds 95 percent, and its specificity is probably greater than 99 percent. Although brain biopsy is not an innocuous procedure, the mortality rate is low (<0.2 percent). Potential morbidity, in addition to that related to general anesthesia, includes local bleeding and edema, the development of a seizure focus, and wound dehiscence or infection. From a practical viewpoint, the incidence of serious morbidity appears to be between 0.5 and 2 percent.

Although brain biopsy was widely employed when vidarabine was the primary therapeutic agent for the treatment of HSV encephalitis, its use has declined substantially with the recognition that empirical acyclovir treatment is safe and associated with minimal complications (see below). The decision about whether to biopsy patients suspected of HSV encephalitis prior to instituting therapy with acyclovir remains controversial. Advocates of the biopsy approach stress the fact that biopsy can lead to identification of potentially treatable non-HSV-related diseases, although the frequency with which this occurs remains controversial. One recent decision-analysis model based on data from the NIAID-CASG trials suggested that as many as 40 percent of biopsy-negative patients may have alternative non-HSV diseases identifiable by brain biopsy, of which 40 percent represent treatable illnesses. These estimates appear excessively high and are not consistent with more recent data or the personal experiences of many neurologists. These data were compiled prior to the widespread use of MRI. It is difficult to believe that these numbers, which included diseases such as tumors, subdural hematomas, adrenoleukodystrophy, subdural empyema, and brain abscess, would be nearly as high if all patients had MRI and CT scans with new-generation scanners. As a general principle, the higher the likelihood that a patient has HSV encephalitis, the easier it is to justify empirical acyclovir therapy without biopsy. Conversely, the lower the probability of HSV encephalitis, the greater is the potential rationale for biopsy. The work of the NIAID-CASG clearly indicates that the capacity of physicians to distinguish between HSV and non-HSV encephalitis on the basis of clinical criteria alone is little better than chance. Among the laboratory tests widely employed to help this differentiation are imaging studies (MRI, CT, brain scan) and EEG. The presence of focally abnormal imaging studies in a patient over age 30 with a CSF lymphocytic pleocytosis (>5 cells per microliter) would seem sufficient to justify empirical therapy. Conversely, a young patient with no evidence of focal process on CT or MRI and a nonfocal EEG may be a candidate for biopsy, because of the diminished prior probability of having HSV encephalitis and the possibility that biopsy may lead to a treatable diagnosis.

Differential diagnosis The initial step in diagnosis is to exclude nonviral causes of the encephalitis syndrome. These can include both infections and noninfectious diseases. Although the list of possibilities is extensive, insight into some of the most common illnesses masquerading as viral encephalitis comes from a list of alternative diagnoses made in patients referred for entry into the NIAID-CASG trials as cases of suspected HSV encephalitis. Among the nonviral diagnoses that mimicked HSV encephalitis were vascular diseases; abscess and empyema; fungal, parasitic, rickettsial, and tuberculous infections; tumors; Reye's syndrome; toxic encephalopathy; subdural hematoma; and systemic lupus erythematosus. Of the nonviral infections, particular attention should be paid to *Listeria, Mycoplasma, Cryptococcus,* and *Mucor* infections, as well as toxoplasmosis and tuberculosis.

Once nonviral causes of encephalitis have been excluded, the major diagnostic impetus is to distinguish HSV from other causes of encephalitis. This distinction is particularly important because in virtually every other instance the therapy is supportive, whereas specific and effective antiviral therapy is available for HSV, and its efficacy is enhanced when therapy is instituted early in the course of infection. HSV encephalitis should be considered when clinical features suggesting involvement of the inferomedial frontotemporal regions of the brain, including prominent olfactory or gustatory hallucinations, anosmia, unusual or bizarre behavior or personality alterations, or memory disturbance, are present. Unfortunately, the results from the NIAID-CASG studies suggest that clinical criteria alone are not reliable in differentiating HSV and non-HSV encephalitis.

Epidemiologic factors may provide important clues that help to limit or focus the diagnostic possibilities. Particular attention should be paid to the season of the year (see Table 375-2), the age of the patient (Table 375-6), the geographic location and travel history (see Fig. 375-1 and Table 375-6), and possible exposure to animal bites, rodents, ticks. *Morbidity and Mortality Weekly Reports* provides regular information about the prevalence of particular viruses causing encephalitis by season and region of the country. State public health authorities provide another valuable resource concerning isolation of particular agents in individual regions.

Treatment Specific antiviral therapy should be initiated when appropriate (see below). Vital functions, including respiration and blood pressure, should be monitored continuously and supported as required. In the initial stages of encephalitis, many patients will require ICU care. Basic management and supportive therapy should include careful monitoring of ICP, fluid restriction and avoidance of hypotonic intravenous solutions, and suppression of fever. Seizures should be treated with standard anticonvulsant regimens, and prophylactic therapy is probably indicated in view of the high frequency of seizures in severe cases of encephalitis (>50 percent). Like all seriously ill, immobilized patients with altered consciousness, encephalitis patients are at risk for aspiration pneumonia, stasis ulcers and decubiti, contractures, deep venous thrombosis and its complications, and infections of indwelling lines and catheters.

Acyclovir (ACV) is of benefit in the treatment of HSV encephalitis and is also useful in selected cases of severe encephalitis due to infection with EBV or VZV. These viruses encode an enzyme, deoxypyrimidine (thymidine) kinase, that phosphorylates ACV to produce ACV-5'-monophosphate (AMP). Host cell enzymes then phosphorylate AMP to form a triphosphate derivative. It is the triphosphate that acts as an antiviral agent by inhibiting viral DNA polymerase and by causing premature termination of nascent viral DNA chains. The specificity of action of ACV depends on the fact that uninfected cells do not phosphorylate significant amounts of ACV to AMP. A second level of specificity is provided by the fact that the ACV triphosphate is a more potent inhibitor of viral DNA polymerase than of the analogous host cell enzymes.

Patients should receive a dose of 10 mg/kg of acyclovir IV every 8 h for a 10-day course. The drug should be diluted to a concentration not exceeding 7 mg/mL. (A 70-kg person would receive a dose of 700 mg, which would be diluted in a volume ≥100 mL.) Each dose should be infused slowly over 60 min rather than by rapid or bolus infusion to minimize the risk of renal dysfunction. Care should be taken to avoid extravasation or intramuscular or subcutaneous administration. The alkaline pH of ACV can cause local inflammation and phlebitis (9 percent). Dose adjustment is required in patients with impaired renal glomerular filtration. CSF penetration is excellent, with average drug levels approximately 50 percent of serum levels. Complications of therapy include elevations in BUN and creatinine levels (5 percent), thrombocytopenia (6 percent), gastrointestinal toxicity (nausea, vomiting, diarrhea) (7 percent), and neurotoxicity, (lethargy or obtundation, disorientation, confusion, agitation, hallucinations, tremors, seizures) (1 percent). ACV resistance may be mediated by changes in either the viral deoxypyrimidine kinase or DNA polymerase. To date, ACV-resistant isolates have not been a significant clinical problem in immunocompetent individuals. However, there has been an increasing number of reports of clinically virulent ACV-resistant HSV isolates from immunocompromised individuals, including those with AIDS.

Sequelae There is considerable variation in the incidence and severity of sequelae in patients surviving viral encephalitis. In the case of Eastern equine encephalitis virus infection, nearly 80 percent of survivors have severe neurologic sequelae. At the other extreme are infections due to EBV, California encephalitis virus, and Venezuelan equine encephalitis virus, where sequelae are extremely rare. Detailed information about sequelae in patients with HSV encephalitis treated with ACV are available from the NIAID-CASG trials. Twenty-six of 32 ACV-treated patients survived (81 percent). Of the 26 survivors, 12 (46 percent) had no or only minor sequelae, 3 (12 percent) were moderately impaired (gainfully employed but not functioning at their previous level), and 11 (42 percent) were severely impaired (requiring continuous supportive care). The incidence and severity of sequelae were directly related to the age of the patient and the level of consciousness at the time of initiation of therapy. Patients with severe neurologic impairment (Glasgow coma score ≤ 6) at initiation of therapy either died or survived with severe sequelae. Young (≤30 years old) patients with good neurologic function at initiation of therapy did substantially better (100 percent survival, 62 percent

TABLE 375-6 Features of selected arbovirus encephalitides

	Virus*				
	WEE	EEE	VEE	SLE	CE
Region	West, midwest	Atlantic and Gulf	South	All	East, and North Central
Age	Infants, adults > 50	Children	Adults	Adults > 50	Children
Deaths	5–15 percent	50–75 percent	1 percent	2–20 percent	<1 percent
Sequelae	Low–moderate	80 percent	Rare	20 percent	Rare
Vector	Mosquito	Mosquito	Mosquito	Mosquito	Mosquito
Animal host	Birds	Birds	Horses, small mammals	Birds	Rodents

* CE = California encephalitis virus; EEE = Eastern equine encephalitis virus; SLE = St. Louis encephalitis virus; VEE = Venezuelan equine encephalitis virus; WEE = Western equine encephalitis virus.
SOURCE: After Whitley, 1990 with permission.

normal or mild sequelae) compared with their older (≥30 years) counterparts (64 percent survival, 57 percent normal or mild sequelae).

MYELITIS AND RADICULITIS

The prototypical viral myelitis is the syndrome of acute anterior poliomyelitis caused by polioviruses and rarely by other enteroviruses and possibly EBV and mumps virus. A distinctive syndrome is produced by enterovirus 70. Patients develop acute hemorrhagic conjunctivitis, followed days to weeks later by a poliomyelitis-like syndrome (see below). Some cases of rabies present with an acute ascending paralysis with areflexia which can resemble poliomyelitis or the Guillain-Barré syndrome. Paralytic polio is a rarity in the United States (<20 cases per year), although it remains a major problem in some other regions of the world. Most cases of paralytic polio in the United States occur as a result of the exceedingly rare reversion of vaccine strains to virulence. The cases are divided among those recently vaccinated and unvaccinated nonimmune adults exposed to recently vaccinated children. Occasional outbreaks have occurred in nonimmunized populations such as the Amish in Pennsylvania. Illness typically begins with prodromal symptoms, including fever, headache, myalgia, pharyngitis, nausea and vomiting, and meningeal signs. These are associated with the typical CSF profile of aseptic meningitis. In some patients these symptoms are followed by the development of muscle weakness. The incidence, severity, and pattern of weakness are age-dependent, with more severe disease being seen with increasing age. Young children often develop weakness of one leg, older children weaknesss of both legs, and adults asymmetric quadriparesis often with associated urinary retention. Weakness is associated with fasciculations, loss of deep and superficial reflexes, and the development of atrophy. Involvement of the brainstem (bulbar polio) can result in dysphagia, dysarthria, respiratory impairment, and vasomotor disturbances. Although some patients complain of paresthesias, objective sensory loss is not present.

Viruses also may affect both the anterior and posterior portions of the spinal cord over a considerable longitudinal extent, producing the syndrome of "transverse" myelitis. The clinical syndrome is one of acutely developed muscle weakness, which may be of the flaccid hyporeflexic type initially but usually develops into spastic paralysis with hyperreflexia and extensor plantar responses. Sensory loss is almost invariably present and typically involves both pain-temperature and position-vibration, producing a sensory level. Urinary symptoms (retention, overflow incontinence, or in milder cases, hesitancy or decreased voiding sensation) and constipation or even fecal incontinence are present in virtually all patients. Although this syndrome can be caused by a variety of viruses, most cases are due to HSV-2, CMV, VZV, or EBV. Pathologic evidence of myelitis is commonly encountered in severe cases of St. Louis, Eastern, and Western encephalitis. A milder form of the syndrome may be encountered in patients with episodes of herpes genitalia. Especially during the primary outbreak, patients may develop an aseptic meningitis syndrome associated with urinary retention or other symptoms; dysesthesia, paresthesias, or neuralgia in the legs, buttocks, or genital area; and weakness in one or both legs. A chronic viral myelitis is associated with infection by HIV (vacuolar myelopathy) and by HTLV-I (tropical spastic paraparesis, or TSP, and HTLV-I–associated myelopathy, or HAM) (see Chaps. 151 and 279).

HERPES ZOSTER A distinctive clinical syndrome consisting of paresthesias or dysesthesias in a dermatomal distribution followed by a localized cutaneous eruption ("shingles," "zoster") is commonly associated with VZV infection and rarely may be produced by HSV. Zoster occurs in patients previously infected with chickenpox (varicella). During the initial varicella infection, virus in the skin travels up the sensory nerves to become latent in the sensory ganglia. The mechanisms that account for maintenance of latency and subsequent reactivation remain unknown. Reactivation results in active viral replication in sensory ganglia followed by spread of virus

through nerves to the skin, where a dermatomal vesicular eruption occurs. The incidence of zoster increases with age and is higher in patients with compromised cellular immunity. The typical history is one of several days of itching, tingling, burning, or pain in a dermatomal distribution that is followed after several days by a vesicular eruption consisting of clear vesicles on an erythematous base. The vesicles become cloudy, dry, and crust over after 1 to 2 weeks. The lesions are most commonly found in the thoracic dermatomes, with T5–T10 accounting for approximately two-thirds of cases. Most patients will have hypalgesia and hypesthesia in the affected dermatome. About 5 percent of patients develop motor weakness and atrophy (zoster paresis) in the associated myotome. Forty-five percent of patients over age 50 who develop shingles will experience pain persisting for more than 6 weeks after disappearance of the rash, i.e., *postherpetic neuralgia* (PHN). PHN is almost never seen in children who develop zoster and is rare (6 percent) in adults younger than 50. PHN may benefit from topical therapy with capsaicin ointment, as well as systemic therapy with amitriptyline and carbamazepine. Characteristic syndromes result from zoster eruptions involving the trigeminal and geniculate distribution. In 10 to 15 percent of cases, reactivation of virus in the trigeminal ganglia results in rash in the distribution of the ophthalmic division of the trigeminal nerve (ophthalmic zoster). Vesicular eruption may be conjoined with conjunctivitis, keratitis, ocular muscle palsies, ptosis, and mydriasis. Rare cases are followed by the development of cerebral angiitis involving the ipsilateral carotid and/or middle cerebral arteries. Vascular compromise may lead to hemiplegia, aphasia, or other focal deficits contralateral to the side of the facial eruption. Reactivation of virus in the geniculate ganglion is reported to produce the Ramsay Hunt syndrome, consisting of facial palsy often associated with loss of taste in the anterior tongue, tinnitus, hearing loss, and vertigo. Zoster eruptions are found in the external auditory meatus.

HIV AND OTHER VIRAL NEUROPATHIES Isolated virus-induced peripheral or cranial neuropathies or plexopathies are unusual, with the exception of those associated with HIV infection (see below). CMV has been reported to produce both peripheral neuropathy and brachial plexus neuropathy. A similar syndrome may be seen with EBV. The incidence of CMV neuropathy is clearly increased in patients with AIDS. In some cases there has been evidence for direct viral infection, whereas in others the mechanism appears to be one of virus-induced segmental demyelination. CMV, HSV, EBV, VZV, mumps, and hepatitis B virus (HBV) also have been associated with Guillain-Barré syndrome. An almost identical syndrome can be seen in association with HIV infection, although these patients typically have a CSF pleocytosis rather than the classic albuminocytologic dissociation (elevated protein, no or few cells). Isolated cranial nerve palsies, especially of the facial (VII) nerve (Bell's palsy), have been attributed to VZV (Ramsay Hunt syndrome), HIV, EBV, enteroviruses, mumps, and HSV, although in many cases the etiologic relationship appears rather tenuous. Mumps, measles, and VZV may produce unilateral or bilateral nerve deafness. Seroepidemiologic studies also suggest a possible role for parainfluenza, adenoviruses, and HSV in acute hearing loss.

CHRONIC AND PERSISTENT VIRAL CNS DISEASE

GENERAL CONSIDERATIONS From a practical point of view, chronic and persistent CNS viral diseases can be divided into those caused by conventional viruses and those caused by unconventional agents such as prions (Table 375-7).

HIV A complete discussion of the virologic aspects of HIV infection, of specific complications of HIV infection such as associated opportunistic infections, and of HIV therapy can be found in Chap. 279. We will focus here on the consequences of direct HIV infection on the central and peripheral nervous system.

Neurologic manifestations of HIV infection differ at different stages of illness (Fig. 375-2). Primary HIV infection can be associated

TABLE 375-7   Chronic and persistent CNS diseases caused by viruses and prions

Disease	Agent	Disease	Agent
Progressive multifocal leukoencephalopathy	JC virus	Creutzfeldt-Jakob	Prion
Subacute sclerosing panencephalitis	Measles virus	Gerstmann-Straussler-Scheinker	Prion
Progressive rubella panencephalitis	Rubella virus	Kuru	Prion
Tropical spastic paraparesis	HTLV-I	Fatal familial insomnia	Prion
AIDS	HIV	Alper's	Prion?

with aseptic meningitis and more rarely with an acute encephalopathy. No clinical features clearly differentiate HIV aseptic meningitis from other viral meningitides, although the diagnosis should be strongly considered in patients with known risk factors for HIV infection. The syndrome is characterized by fever, headache, meningeal signs, and in some patients cranial nerve palsies (V, VII, VIII). The CSF shows a mononuclear pleocytosis, elevated protein level, and normal glucose level. HIV can be isolated from CSF, and p24 core protein may be present, which establishes the diagnosis. More commonly, the diagnosis is established by documenting HIV antibody seroconversion and intrathecal HIV antibody synthesis. In suspected cases, follow-up HIV serology should be obtained at 1, 2, and 3 months because seroconversion may be delayed.

Persisting CSF pleocytosis also has been found in otherwise asymptomatic HIV-seropositive individuals. Seropositive individuals also may develop Guillain-Barré syndrome (GBS), chronic inflammatory demyelinating polyneuropathy (CIDP), or myopathy. HIV-associated GBS appears clinically indistinguishable from the syndrome that occurs in non-HIV-infected individuals. Patients present with acute onset of progressive extremity weakness, which may progress to respiratory failure. Bifacial weakness is common. Sensory symptoms may occur, but sensory signs are far less conspicuous than motor findings. All patients are areflexic or severely hyporeflexic. Findings in CIDP are similar but generally progress chronically rather than acutely and are not typically as severe. A diagnostic clue to HIV-associated GBS or CIDP may be the presence of a CSF

FIGURE 375-2 The relative frequency and timing of major neurologic complications of direct HIV infection. Diseases that affect the CNS are shaded with diagonal lines; those which affect the peripheral nervous system are cross-hatched. The height of the boxes is a relative indicator of the frequency of each type of disease. (*From RT Johnson et al, FASEB J 2:2970, 1988, with permission.*)

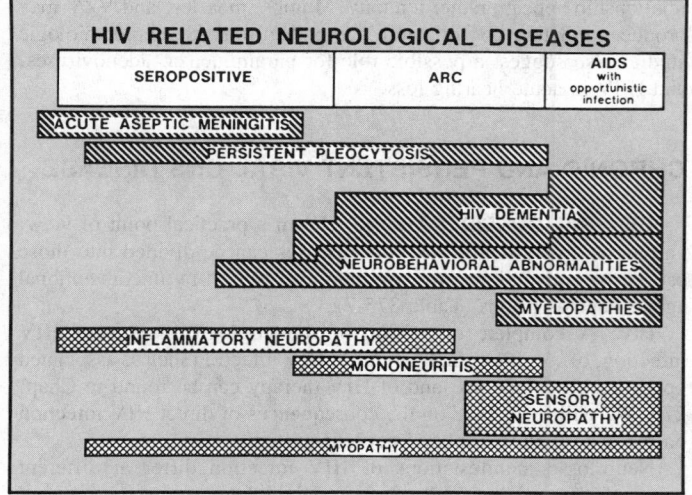

pleocytosis in place of the typical albuminocytologic dissociation (no or few cells, elevated protein) seen in non-HIV cases. Electrophysiologic studies are consistent with demyelination (slowed conduction velocities, prolonged or absent F responses and distal motor latencies, etc.). Extensive controlled trials of therapy in HIV-associated GBS and CIDP are not available. Plasmapheresis is the standard therapy for non-HIV-associated CIDP and GBS. Recent studies suggest that intravenous high-dose immunoglobulin may also be effective and associated with few side effects, although some patients relapse following treatment. Both these treatments should be considered in HIV-positive individuals.

Progression of HIV infection from the asymptomatic state to more clinically advanced disease is associated with an increased incidence of neuropsychological abnormalities, including the development of HIV encephalopathy and dementia, also referred to as *AIDS-dementia complex*. Common early symptoms of cognitive impairment include difficulty concentrating, memory loss, slowness of thought, apathy, depression, social withdrawal, and personality changes. In distinction to "cortical" dementias such as Alzheimer disease, aphasia, apraxia, and agnosia are uncommon, leading some investigators to classify HIV encephalopathy as a "subcortical dementia." At least 50 percent of patients will have associated signs or symptoms of motor dysfunction, including leg weakness, balance difficulty, ataxia, tremor, or pyramidal tract signs (hyperreflexia, extensor plantars). The illness progresses slowly over months, although mean survival time from the onset of severe dementia rarely exceeds 6 months. Laboratory studies are helpful in excluding or diminishing the possibility of other treatable processes. Twenty percent of patients will have CSF lymphocytic pleocytosis (<50 cells per microliter), and 60 percent will have an elevated protein level. Hypoglycorrhachia is rare. CSF beta$_2$ microglobulin concentrations appear to correlate with the severity of HIV encephalopathy and may serve as a useful marker of disease progression or response to antiviral therapy. CT and MRI typically show evidence of diffuse cerebral atrophy with widened sulci and ex vacuo ventricular enlargement. T2-weighted MRI spin-echo images show either patchy or diffuse white matter lesions. EEG findings are nonspecific, although some degree of generalized slowing is almost invariably present.

The neuropathologic hallmarks of AIDS encephalopathy are the presence of multinucleated giant cells (MGC) seen throughout the cortex and white matter, microglial nodules, white matter pallor, and reactive gliosis. The MGCs have been shown to contain HIV particles by electron microscopy and copious amounts of viral antigen and genome by immunocytochemistry and in situ hybridization. They appear to arise by syncytial fusion of infected monocyte-macrophage-microglial cells. These cells contain the bulk of HIV antigen and genome found in brain material. Endothelial cells and oligodendroglia may be found to contain HIV antigen or genome; neurons are rarely, if ever, positive. Neuronal dysfunction is not the result of productive infection with subsequent cell destruction. The mechanism by which HIV infection indirectly produces neuronal injury has not yet been established. Neurons may be injured as a result of cytokines, excitatory neurotoxins, or other soluble factors released by infected immune cells, macrophages, or glia. Alternatively, binding of gp120 or other viral proteins to neurons may result in alterations in ion channel conductance (e.g., Ca^{2+}) or neurotransmitter levels leading to cell injury (see also Chap. 279).

No definitive therapy is available. Both AZT and didanosine have been reported to lead to improvement in some patients, although didanosine's limited CSF penetration may limit its usefulness.

Symptomatic HIV-infected patients also may develop CIDP or mononeuropathy multiplex (MM). MM typically presents with asymmetric multifocal peripheral and/or cranial nerve lesions. These may appear acutely as isolated regions of sensory loss or weakness in a peripheral nerve distribution. The pathogenesis appears to be ischemic injury to nerves resulting from arteritis of the vasa nervorum. In distinction to CIDP, the electrophysiologic studies suggest an axonal rather than a demyelinating lesion.

A distal symmetric painful sensory neuropathy is the most common form of neuropathy encountered in patients with clinically advanced AIDS and is present in at least one-third of patients. Most patients complain of painful distal paresthesias in the feet ("burning feet"), which are often induced in causalgia-like fashion by pressure or contact. Walking may be difficult or impossible, and even minimal contact with blankets or sheets can produce severe discomfort. Findings on examination include a stocking-type sensory loss to pin, temperature, and touch and loss of ankle reflexes. The knee jerks are usually intact. Motor changes (weakness, atrophy) are mild compared with the prominence of sensory signs and symptoms and are usually limited to weakness of the intrinsic foot muscles. Trophic changes, including atrophy of the skin, loss of hair, nail abnormalities, edema, and vasomotor disturbances, may be found. Patients with advanced HIV infection also may develop an autonomic neuropathy characterized by diarrhea, postural hypotension, and cardiac arrhythmias.

Electrophysiologic studies are indicative of a distal sensorimotor axonopathy, which is consistent with findings on nerve biopsy. Conduction velocities and distal latencies are normal, but compound muscle action potentials in the legs and the sural sensory action potential are diminished in amplitude. HIV has been isolated from nerve biopsy specimens, although the source of virus (Schwann cells, axons, inflammatory cells) has not been established definitively. A similar neuropathy has been associated with CMV infection, and CMV antigen and genome can be detected in some biopsy specimens by immunocytochemistry, in situ hybridization, or PCR. The relative importance of HIV and CMV infection in the production of this syndrome remains to be established. Patients receiving either didanosine or dideoxycytidine also may develop neuropathic symptoms, and this should be considered in the differential diagnosis. No adequate therapy exists. Patients with evidence to suggest CMV infection should be treated with ganciclovir. Analgesics, tricyclic antidepressants, anticonvulsants (including phenytoin and carbamazepine), and topical capsaicin ointment may be useful in the control of pain. Mineralocorticoids such as fludrocortisone may help control postural hypotension in patients with autonomic neuropathy.

A chronic progressive myelopathy affecting the posterior and lateral columns of the spinal cord may be seen in 10 to 25 percent of AIDS patients. Patients develop a spastic ataxic paraparesis with diminished position and vibratory sense and urinary incontinence. Tibial somatosensory evoked responses are abnormal in virtually all patients. The clinical features resemble those seen in subacute combined degeneration secondary to vitamin B_{12} deficiency and those of nitrous oxide–induced myelopathy. Most patients (>90 percent) have associated HIV encephalopathy or dementia. Pathologic changes consist of vacuolar degeneration of the white matter of the lateral and posterior columns, typically maximal in the thoracic cord. The vacuolar areas result from severe edema within the myelin sheaths of nerve fibers and contain axonal spheroids and lipid-laden macrophages. HIV has been isolated from the spinal cord of affected individuals, and HIV genome has been found by in situ hybridization, although the role of direct viral infection versus indirect mechanism(s) of injury has not been established. No definitive therapy is available, and treatment with either AZT or didanosine is generally of little benefit.

In addition to vacuolar myelopathy, a variety of other myelopathic syndromes may occur in HIV-infected individuals. Ganglionitis of the lumbar and sacral dorsal root ganglia can result in secondary degeneration of the fasciculus gracilis within the posterior column of the spinal cord. The resulting clinical syndrome includes paresthesias and sensory loss (vibration, position sense) in the legs. Transverse myelitis also may result from infection with HSV, CMV, or both viruses simultaneously. Concurrent HIV and HTLV-I infection can occur, with the latter producing a spastic myelopathy (see next section).

Patients at any stage of HIV infection may develop myopathy. This is typically characterized by slowly progressive polymyositis-like proximal muscle weakness, myalgia, elevated muscle enzymes

(creatine kinase, aldolase, lactate dehydrogenase, SGOT), and a myopathic pattern (brief low-amplitude motor unit potentials) on EMG testing. Muscle biopsy may show inflammation and/or myofiber degeneration and necrosis. Some patients have additional histologic changes, including nemaline rod and cytoplasmic bodies, mitochondrial abnormalities, and ragged red fibers. The pathogenesis of the syndrome has not been established. Direct HIV infection of muscle has not been detected, although HIV-infected monocytes, macrophages, and multinucleated giant cells may surround muscle fibers.

HIV-associated myopathy should be distinguished from myopathy as a complication of AZT therapy. Most patients with AZT myopathy have been on therapy for 6 months or more and often have higher enzyme levels and more pain than non-AZT cases. Biopsy may help with the differential diagnosis, since AZT-related cases show more muscle fiber necrosis and less inflammation than patients with HIV myopathy. Discontinuation of AZT results in resolution of symptoms. Concurrent glucocorticoid therapy may allow continuation of AZT treatment.

TROPICAL SPASTIC PARAPARESIS (TSP), HTLV-I–ASSOCIATED MYELOPATHY (HAM) TSP and HAM are characterized by the development of slowly progressive spastic paraparesis, often associated with a neurogenic bladder (see Chap. 151). Symptoms of these diseases typically appear during the third or fourth decades, and women are affected far more frequently than men. The majority of reported cases have been from Japan (HAM), the Caribbean basin, parts of South America (Panama, Colombia, Peru, Brazil), the Seychelles Islands, and western Africa. Isolated cases have occurred in the southeastern United States and in many other locations. Neurologic examination shows a spastic paraparesis or paraplegia with hyperactive tendon reflexes, clonus, and extensor plantar responses. Although some patients have paresthesias, dyesthesias, or pain in the legs, sensory findings are usually mild (e.g., mild diminution in vibratory sense), and a true sensory level is only rarely found. Additional findings are seen in 5 to 20 percent of cases and can include brisk reflexes in the upper extremities, frontal release responses, cranial nerve abnormalities (optic neuropathy, deafness, nystagmus, diplopia, facial paresis), and cerebellar signs (tremor, dysmetria).

Tropical spastic myelopathies are multifactorial in nature and may be caused by a wide variety of toxic and nutritional factors. Several epidemiologic studies have unequivocally shown that infection with HTLV-I is the cause of an important subset of this disorder. Infection appears to be acquired through blood transfusion, sexual contact, intravenous drug use, and vertical transmission from mother to fetus. HTLV-I–associated cases are characterized by the presence of serum and CSF anti-HTLV-I antibodies. The CSF/serum antibody ratio is elevated, indicative of intrathecal antibody synthesis. HTLV-I–specific CSF oligoclonal bands are often present. Between 25 and 60 percent of patients will have a mild lymphocytic pleocytosis (<50 cells per microliter), and a higher percentage will have a mild elevation in protein. HTLV-I genome can be found in CSF and peripheral blood lymphocytes using Southern blot hybridization or PCR amplification. Virus also can be isolated from CSF and blood of affected individuals.

A number of abnormalities may be found on laboratory tests, although specific diagnosis requires viral isolation or positive serology. MRI of the spinal cord may show evidence of demyelination, and similar findings are occasionally found in the periventricular white matter in the cerebrum. Somatosensory evoked response studies may show evidence of posterior column dysfunction, even when clinical findings are mild or absent. Some patients have evidence of a demyelinating peripheral neuropathy with slowed conduction velocities, increased distal latencies, and slow or absent F waves. Pathologic examination of the spinal cord typically shows symmetrical degeneration of the lateral columns encompassing the corticospinal tracts. Degenerative changes also may involve the posterior columns and spinocerebellar and spinothalamic tracts. There is an associated inflammatory infiltrate in the spinal leptomeninges, cord parenchyma, and surrounding vessels. Myelin destruction may at times resemble the vacuolar myelopathy seen in association with AIDS.

The pathogenesis of the spinal cord disease has not been completely established. Both direct viral injury and immune-mediated processes may play a role in the spinal cord pathology. Recent evidence suggests that HTLV-I–specific cytotoxic T lymphocytes (CTLs) may be important in the production of immune-mediated spinal cord injury.

Definitive therapy is not currently available. Many patients benefit from oral prednisolone or equivalent glucocorticoid therapy. AZT would be expected to be beneficial in limiting viral replication and associated direct cell injury.

PROGRESSIVE MULTIFOCAL LEUKOENCEPHALOPATHY (PML)   As the name implies, PML is a progressive disorder characterized pathologically by multifocal areas of demyelination varying greatly in size and scattered throughout the CNS. In addition to demyelination, there are characteristic cytologic alterations in both astrocytes and oligodendrocytes. Astrocytes are tremendously enlarged and contain hyperchromatic, deformed and bizarre nuclei, and frequent mitotic figures. Oligodendrocytes have enlarged, densely staining nuclei that contain viral inclusions formed by crystalline arrays of JC virus (JCV) particles. Patients often present with visual deficits (45 percent), typically a homonymous hemianopia, and mental impairment (38 percent) (dementia, confusion, personality change). Motor weakness may not be present early but eventually occurs in 75 percent of cases.

CT and MRI remain the most valuable diagnostic studies in suggesting the diagnosis of PML. CT shows hypodense nonenhancing white matter lesions without associated edema or mass effect. Lesions are typically located periventricularly, in the centrum semiovale, in the parietal-occipital region, and in the cerebellum. MRI is more sensitive than CT and reveals hyperintense signal in the white matter on T2-weighted spin-echo images. EEG almost always shows focal or diffuse slowing, and abnormalities may occasionally precede those seen by CT. The CSF is typically normal, although mild elevation in protein and/or IgG may be found. Pleocytosis occurs in less than 25 percent of cases, is predominantly mononuclear, and rarely exceeds 25 cells per microliter. The presence of oligoclonal bands, a substantial pleocytosis, or PMNs or red cells in the CSF should suggest such possibilities as acute multiple sclerosis, acute hemorrhagic leukoencephalitis, HIV-associated leukoencephalomyelopathy, multifocal VZV leukoencephalitis, or postinfectious or vaccinal immune-mediated encephalomyelitis.

Almost all patients (>95 percent) have an underlying immunosuppressive disorder. Prior to the HIV epidemic, common associated diseases included lymphoproliferative disorders, immune deficiency states, myeloproliferative disease, and chronic infectious or granulomatous diseases. Since 1984, the importance of these associated disorders has been dwarfed by that of AIDS. According to some recent estimates, more than 60 percent of currently diagnosed PML cases occur in patients with AIDS. Conversely, it has been estimated that nearly 1 percent of AIDS patients will develop PML. Early indications suggest that the basic clinicopathologic features of AIDS-associated PML do not differ significantly from those of non-AIDS-associated PML. Some patients with AIDS-associated PML have shown significant spontaneous improvement in the absence of therapy. Unfortunately, this appears to be the exception rather than the rule, and most cases pursue the same relentless downhill course to a fatal termination that characterizes almost all reported cases of non-AIDS-associated PML.

Definitive diagnosis depends on identification of the characteristic neuropathologic abnormalities at biopsy or necropsy. The presence of JCV antigen and genomic DNA can be confirmed by immunocytochemistry, in situ hybridization, and PCR amplification on brain tissue. However, detection of JCV antigen or genomic material is not diagnostic of PML unless accompanied by characteristic pathologic changes, since both antigen and genomic material can be found in the brains of normal patients. Between 80 and 90 percent of the population is seropositive for JCV by middle adult life. Virus may remain latent in brain or other tissues and become reactivated during immunosuppression. PML also may result from primary exposure to JCV in an immunocompromised host, since 10 to 20 percent of individuals are seronegative at the time of disease diagnosis. JCV DNA has been amplified from the CSF of patients using PCR, but initial results suggest that this test is relatively insensitive as a diagnostic tool.

SUBACUTE SCLEROSING PANENCEPHALITIS (SSPE)   This is a rare disease, with less than 10 cases per year reported in the United States. The incidence has declined substantially since the introduction of a measles vaccine. Most patients give a history of primary measles infection at an early age (≤2 years), which is followed after a latent interval of 6 to 8 years by the development of a progressive neurologic disorder. Eighty-five percent of cases are between 5 and 15 years of age at diagnosis. Initial manifestations include poor school performance and mood and personality changes. As the disease develops, these nonspecific symptoms give way to progressive intellectual deterioration, focal and/or generalized seizures, myoclonus, ataxia, and visual disturbances. In the late stage of the illness, patients are unresponsive, quadriparetic, and spastic, with hyperactive tendon reflexes and extensor plantar responses. The EEG shows a characteristic periodic pattern with bursts every 3 to 8 s of high-voltage sharp slow waves, followed by periods of attenuated (''flat'') background. The CSF pattern may be diagnostic. The fluid is acellular with a normal or mildly elevated protein level and a markedly elevated gamma globulin level (>20 percent of total CSF protein). CSF antimeasles antibody levels are invariably elevated, and oligoclonal antimeasles antibodies are often present. CT and MRI show evidence of multifocal white matter lesions, cortical atrophy, and ex vacuo ventricular enlargement. Measles virus can be cultivated from brain tissue using special cocultivation techniques. Viral antigen can be identified immunocytochemically, and viral genome can be detected by in situ hybridization or PCR amplification. No definitive therapy is currently available. Treatment with Inosiplex (isoprinosine) (100 mg/kg per day) remains controversial but has been reported to prolong survival and produce clinical improvement in some patients.

The pathogenesis of SSPE remains unclear. Almost all patients with SSPE fail to make an antibody response to the measles virus M (matrix) protein despite an adequate antibody response to other viral proteins. The failure to make antibody apparently results from a lack of viable M protein in infected cells. The M protein is essential for complete virion assembly and release of virus by budding from infected cells. Electron microscopy of virus-infected cells from SSPE patients reveals nucleocapsids but no complete or budding viral particles. Genomic sequencing suggests that viral isolates from SSPE patients contain the gene encoding the M protein. Absence of M protein could theoretically result from transcriptional or translational errors or the production of an unstable protein, although none of these abnormalities has been documented consistently in SSPE. It has been hypothesized that lack of M protein results in intracellular accumulation of incomplete measles virions in brain cells. The host immune response is unable to clear the intracellular infection, and the persisting accumulation leads to neuronal dysfunction.

PROGRESSIVE RUBELLA PANENCEPHALITIS   This is an extremely rare disorder that predominantly affects children with congenital rubella syndrome, although isolated cases have been reported following childhood rubella. All the approximately 20 cases reported to date have been in male children. After a latent period of 8 to 19 years, patients develop progressive neurologic deterioration. The initial manifestations are similar to those seen in SSPE and include decline in school performance, behavioral alterations, and seizures. These are followed by severe progressive dementia, prominent ataxia, pyramidal signs (spasticity, hyperreflexia, extensor plantar responses), and visual deterioration. Myoclonus may be present but is less prominent than in SSPE, whereas cerebellar signs are a great deal more prominent. In the terminal stages of the illness, patients are globally demented, mute, and quadriparetic, often with associated ophthalmoplegia. CSF shows a mild lymphocytic pleocytosis (<40 cells per microliter), slightly elevated protein level (<150 mg/dL), markedly increased gamma globulin level (35 to 50 percent of total protein), and oligoclonal bands. The oligoclonal antibodies are specific for rubella virus antigens. The CSF/serum antirubella antibody ratio is markedly elevated, indicating high levels of intrathecal antirubella antibody synthesis. CT scans show ex vacuo ventricular enlargement with associated cortical atrophy. There may be hypodensity in the white matter, especially in the centrum semiovale. Cerebellar atrophy and associated fourth ventricle enlargement may be especially prominent. The EEG is nondiagnostic but is almost invariably abnormal with diffuse slowing. A few patients have a burst-suppression pattern similar to that encountered in SSPE. Biopsy or autopsy material shows perivascular lymphocytic and plasma cell cuffing in the white matter, leukomalacia of the centrum semiovale, and the atrophic and ex vacuo ventricular changes described above. Virus particles are not seen by electron microscopy, although rubella virus has been isolated from explant and cocultivation cultures of brain biopsy material in one reported case. The pathogenesis of the disease remains unclear. No therapy is currently available. Isoprinosine and amantadine are of no benefit. Universal prevention of both congenital and childhood rubella through the use of the available live attenuated rubella vaccine would be expected to eliminate the disease.

PRION DISEASES

Although traditionally included in discussions of viral diseases of the CNS, a substantial and rapidly accumulating body of research suggests that the transmissible neurodegenerative diseases (TNDs), e.g., kuru, Creutzfeldt-Jakob disease, Gerstmann-Straussler-Scheinker (GSS) syndrome, are not viral diseases at all. The leading hypothesis for the etiology of these diseases suggests that they are caused by a proteinaceous infectious particle (*prion*) devoid of nucleic acid that is encoded by a single-copy host gene (designated *PRNP*) present on the short arm of chromosome 20. The function of the normal cellular isoform of the PRNP gene (*PrP^c*) is unknown, although both membrane-associated and secreted forms exist. Neurons contain high concentrations of PrP^c, which is developmentally regulated. Substantial amino acid homology exists between PrP^c and a chicken protein (*ARIA*) produced by motor neurons that induces acetylcholine receptor activity.

A modified form, *PrP^Sc*, which is resistant to proteolytic digestion and spontaneously aggregates to produce rodlike or fibrillary particles (scrapie-associated fibrils, prion rods) can be isolated from the brains of animals and humans with TNDs. The exact mechanism by which the normal cellular protein (PrP^c) is modified to its pathologic isoform (PrP^Sc), the method by which PrP^Sc replicates itself, and the way PrP^Sc accumulation leads to neuronal degeneration remain unknown.

Epidemiologic and clinical studies indicate that human TNDs can be sporadic (Creutzfeldt-Jakob disease), infectious (kuru, rare cases of Creutzfeldt-Jakob), or genetic (GSS syndrome, familial Creutzfeldt-Jakob disease) in origin. The basic clinical features of each of these diseases are discussed below.

KURU This disease was previously endemic among members of the Fore linguistic tribal group of the Eastern Highlands area of Papua New Guinea. At its peak, the disease affected close to 1 percent of the population, although currently less than 10 cases per year are reported. The cardinal features of the illness were severe cerebellar ataxia with associated involuntary movements, including choreoathetosis, myoclonus, and tremor. These were associated with the subsequent development of mental impairment and frontal release signs. Brain material from affected individuals transmits the disease to primates. No new cases of the disease have been reported among individuals born since the cessation of ritual cannibalism in the affected areas. It has been suggested that ingestion of infected brain material during these rituals was responsible for disease transmission.

CREUTZFELDT-JAKOB DISEASE Most cases are sporadic in nature, although 5 to 15 percent are familial with an autosomal dominant pattern of inheritance. Regions of high incidence and prevalence are scattered throughout the world, most prominently in parts of Libya and North Africa and in Slovakia. Creutzfeldt-Jakob disease is not contagious, but person-to-person spread of the disease has occurred following transplantation of corneas or dural grafts obtained from infected individuals. Isolated cases also have been attributed to improperly decontaminated neurosurgical instruments and stereotactic intracerebral depth electrodes. Approximately 25 cases have been reported in patients with panhypopituitarism who received supplemental cadaveric human growth hormone therapy and in patients who received cadaveric human gonadotropins for treatment of infertility.

Creutzfeldt-Jakob disease typically presents as a rapidly progressive dementia with prominent associated myoclonus. Clinical manifestations are protean and often include combinations of severe and progressive dementia, pyramidal and extrapyramidal motor disturbances, and signs and symptoms of cerebellar dysfunction. Clinical and pathologic subtypes with predominant involvement of specific regions of the brain have been described (e.g., occipital, thalamic, and cerebellar types). Early signs of mental impairment may be manifested as slowness in thinking, difficulty concentrating, impaired judgment, and memory loss. Mood changes and emotional lability may be combined with visual or other types of hallucinations. About a third of patients present initially with prominent cerebellar or visual disturbances, which may initially overshadow the mental impairment. Myoclonus occurs in more than 90 percent of patients and may be provoked or aggravated by startle. Additional motor signs and symptoms can include tremor, clumsiness, and choreoathetosis. As the disease progresses, about two-thirds of patients will develop a parkinsonian extrapyramidal syndrome with hypokinesia and rigidity. Hyperreflexia, spasticity, and extensor plantar responses occur in about half of patients. The clinical presentation of Creutzfeldt-Jakob disease associated with use of cadaveric human pituitary hormone therapy may differ from that of classic Creutzfeldt-Jakob disease. Patients are typically younger and often present with a kuru-like illness in which cerebellar features may be more prominent initially than dementia.

Laboratory tests are helpful in excluding other causes of rapidly progressing dementia. The CSF is typically unremarkable, although the protein level may be mildly elevated. A pleocytosis is unusual and should prompt a thorough search for other processes. It has been suggested recently that two-dimensional isoelectric focusing of CSF proteins may show abnormal protein species, two of which (proteins designated 130 and 131) may be typical of Creutzfeldt-Jakob disease. This test has recently become commercially available; however, additional studies of sensitivity and specificity will be required to establish its diagnostic utility. CT and MRI may show evidence of generalized cortical atrophy, but more typically the degree of clinical dementia appears disproportionate to the amount of tissue loss seen on CT and MRI. In some patients, sequential studies performed at biweekly or monthly intervals may show rapidly progressive loss of brain tissue and ex vacuo ventricular enlargement. The EEG may be quite useful in suggesting the diagnosis. The typical pattern of periodic sharp wave complexes consists of a generalized slow background interrupted by bilaterally synchronous sharp wave complexes occurring at intervals of 0.5 to 2.5 s and lasting for 200 to 600 ms. The classic EEG pattern is found in 75 to 95 percent of cases, although it may not be present very early or in the terminal stages of the disease. Sequential EEG studies may be useful if the initial recording fails to reveal the typical pattern.

The gold standard for diagnosis remains the histologic study of brain material obtained at biopsy or necropsy and the subsequent demonstration of transmissibility to susceptible rodents. The pathologic hallmarks of Creutzfeldt-Jakob disease are spongiform changes (small round vacuoles) within the neuropil, neuronal loss, hypertrophy and proliferation of glial cells, and absence of significant inflammation or white matter involvement. Pathologic changes are maximal in the cortex but are often prominent in the basal ganglia, cerebellum, and thalamus. The brainstem and spinal cord are usually spared. Recent studies suggest that the demonstration of prion proteins in immunoblots of brain material is a sensitive and apparently specific marker for the presence of Creutzfeldt-Jakob disease or related TNDs. The finding of prion rods or scrapie-associated fibrils which may be seen in electron micrographs of prepared brain material also appears to be pathognomonic for TNDs.

Creutzfeldt-Jakob disease is invariably fatal, and no specific therapy is available. A number of drugs, including amantadine, have been reported to slow disease progression in isolated anecdotal case reports; however, the results have not been consistently reproducible.

Recent molecular genetic studies have established an unequivocal linkage between mutations in the PRNP gene and familial cases of Creutzfeldt-Jakob disease. Several mutations have been described, which may correlate with variations in the clinical phenotype of the disease in individual familial clusters. Among the commonly reported mutations are a Lys for Glu substitution in codon 200 and an Asn for Asp substitution in codon 178. Inserts in the PRNP gene also occur in several families with Creutzfeldt-Jakob disease. No consistent PRNP gene mutation has been identified in cases of sporadic Creutzfeldt-Jakob disease. Some recent reports suggest that homozygosity at a polymorphic amino acid residue at codon 129 of the PRNP gene occurs with greater than expected frequency in cases of sporadic and iatrogenic Creutzfeldt-Jakob disease and kuru, although this requires further confirmation.

GERSTMANN-STRAUSSLER-SCHEINKER SYNDROME   This is a rare hereditary spinocerebellar degeneration. Patients develop signs and symptoms of progressive cerebellar dysfunction in midlife, evidenced by unsteadiness, clumsiness, incoordination, and progressive gait difficulty. As the illness progresses, the cerebellar findings become increasingly severe and include ataxia, dysarthria, and nystagmus. Some patients have additional findings, which can include parkinsonian, pyramidal and extrapyramidal findings, deafness, blindness, and gaze palsies. In distinction to their prominence in Creutzfeldt-Jakob disease, dementia and myoclonus are either absent or minor features and are overshadowed by the cerebellar dysfunction.

Molecular genetic studies of GSS syndrome families have consistently demonstrated mutations in the PRNP gene. The most common abnormality is a Leu for Pro substitution at codon 102. Additional mutations have included a Val for Ala substitution at codon 117, as well as a point mutation in codon 198. Although the clinical material is limited because of the rarity of the disease, it appears that ataxia is the dominant feature of the disease in families with the codon 102 mutation, whereas ataxia plus dementia is seen in those with the codons 117 and 198 mutations.

PUTATIVE TNDs   Fatal familial insomnia (FFI) is a rapidly progressive autosomal dominant disease of middle or later life characterized by intractable insomnia, sympathetic hyperactivity and other autonomic and endocrine disturbances, dysarthria, and motor system abnormalities, including myoclonus, tremor, ataxia, hyperreflexia, and spasticity. Dementia is not prominent, although mild memory and attention deficits are common. Patients often experience complex hallucinations with the characteristics of "enacted dreams." A variety of endocrine abnormalities also may occur, including loss of the normal circadian fluctuations in melatonin, prolactin, and growth hormone secretion, decreased ACTH secretion, and elevated cortisol secretion. Pathologic changes include atrophy and gliosis of specific thalamic nuclei, cerebellar cortex, and inferior olives. One patient has been described who had spongiform changes in the involved areas and periodic sharp wave complexes on EEG, but this appears exceptional rather than typical. Sequencing of the PRNP gene from patients in two families with FFI has shown an Asn for Asp mutation in codon 178, similar to that reported in some cases of familial Creutzfeldt-Jakob disease. Brain material from patients in these two families was found to contain the protease-resistant PrP^{Sc} isoform. There have been no reports to date of successful transmission of the disease from brain material of infected cases.

There is one reported case of transmission of a scrapie-like disease to rodents using brain material from a 2½-year-old child diagnosed as having Alper's disease (progressive infantile poliodystrophy). This has not been confirmed, and no molecular genetic studies on the PRNP gene have been reported from patients with Alper's disease.

REFERENCES

BALE JF: Viral encephalitis. Med Clin North Am 77:25, 1993

BERGER JR et al: Progressive multifocal leukoencephalopathy associated with human immunodeficiency virus infection. Ann Intern Med 107:78, 1987

BOOSS J, ESIRI MM: *Viral Encephalitis*. Oxford, Blackwell Scientific, 1986

BUCHER B et al: Tropical neuromyelopathies and retroviruses: A review. Rev Infect Dis 12:890, 1990

CONNOLLY KJ, HAMMER SM: The acute aseptic meningitis syndrome. Infect Dis Clin North Am 4:599, 1990

GABUZDA DH, HIRSCH MS: Neurologic manifestations of infection with the human immunodeficiency virus. Ann Intern Med 107:383, 1987

GILLESPIE SM et al: Progressive multifocal leukoencephalopathy in persons infected with human immunodeficiency virus, San Francisco 1981–1989. Ann Neurol 30:597, 1991

JEFFERY DR et al: Transverse myelitis—Retrospective analysis of 33 cases, with differentiation of cases associated with multiple sclerosis and parainfectious events. Arch Neurol 50:532, 1993

JOHNSON RT: *Viral Infections of the Nervous System*. New York, Raven, 1982

MANETTO V et al: Fatal familial insomnia: Clinical and pathologic study of five new cases. Neurology 42:312, 1992

MCARTHUR JC: Neurological manifestations of AIDS. Medicine 66:407, 1987

MCKENDALL RR (ed): *Viral Disease, (Handbook of Clinical Neurology)*, vol 56/12. Amsterdam, Elsevier, 1989

MEDORI R et al: Fatal familial insomnia, a prion disease with a mutation at codon 178 of the prion protein gene. N Engl J Med 326:444, 1992

PRUSINER SB: Molecular biology of prion diseases. Science 252:1515, 1991

————: Molecular biology and genetics of neurodegenerative diseases caused by prions. Adv Virus Res 41:241, 1992

ROOS KL (ed): Central nervous system infections. Semin Neurol 12:155, 1992

ROSENBLUM ML et al (eds): *AIDS and the Nervous System*. New York, Raven, 1988

SCHELD WM et al: *Infections of the Central Nervous System*. New York, Raven, 1991

TSAI TF: Arboviral infections in the United States. Infect Dis Clin North Am 5:73, 1991

TYLER KL: Diagnosis and management of acute viral encephalitis. Semin Neurol 4:480, 1984

————, Martin JB: *Infectious Diseases of the Central Nervous System*. Philadelphia, F.A. Davis, 1993

VINKEN PJ et al (eds): *Infections of the Nervous System (Handbook of Clinical Neurology)* vol 34. Amsterdam, North-Holland, 1978

WHITEMAN MLH et al: Progressive multifocal leukoencephalopathy in 47 HIV-seropositive patients—Neuroimaging with clinical and pathologic correlation. Radiology 187:233, 1993

WHITLEY RJ: Viral encephalitis. N Engl J Med 323:242, 1990

———— et al: Vidarabine versus acyclovir therapy in herpes simplex encephalitis. N Engl J Med 314:144, 1986

WOOD M, ANDERSON M: *Neurological Infections (Major Problems in Neurology)*, vol 16. Philadelphia, Saunders, 1988

376   TRAUMA OF THE HEAD AND SPINE

ALLAN H. ROPPER

Head injuries are frequent in industrialized countries, affecting many patients in the prime of life. To appreciate the medical and social magnitude of this problem, it needs only to be recognized that almost 10 million Americans have head injuries yearly, about 20 percent serious enough to cause brain damage. Among men under 35 years old, accidents, usually motor vehicle collisions, are the chief cause of death, and over 70 percent of these involve head injury. Minor head injuries are so common that almost all physicians encounter patients requiring immediate care or suffering from various sequelae. Traumatic spinal cord injuries often occur in conjunction with head injury. The two are best considered together in the context of trauma to the nervous system.

Declining mortality from head and spinal cord injuries can be attributed mainly to public health measures, such as use of seat belts and motorcycle helmets, and the development of ambulance systems with trained personnel. A systematic approach to the evaluation of patients with head and spine trauma, beginning at the scene of the accident, has improved outcome. Understanding the pathologic lesions produced by trauma, essential for diagnosis and management, has been revolutionized by the wide availability of computed tomography (CT) scanning.

TYPES OF HEAD INJURIES

SKULL FRACTURES A blow to the skull causes fractures if the elastic tolerance of the bone is exceeded. Significant intracranial lesions accompany two-thirds of skull fractures, and the presence of a skull fracture increases manyfold the chances of an underlying subdural or epidural hematoma. Consequently, fractures assume importance primarily as markers of the site and severity of injury. They also cause cranial nerve injuries and produce entry pathways to the cerebrospinal fluid (CSF) for bacteria (meningitis) and air (pneumocephalus) or for leakage of CSF. Fractures are classified as linear, basilar, compound, or depressed; linear fractures account for 80 percent of all skull fractures and are most often associated with subdural or epidural hematomas. Linear fractures usually extend from the point of impact toward the base of the skull.

Basilar skull fractures are often extensions of adjacent fractures over the convexity of the skull but may occur independently due to stresses on the floor of the middle cranial fossa or occiput. They are usually located parallel to the petrous bone or along the sphenoid bone toward the sella turcica and ethmoidal groove. Most are uncomplicated, but they may cause CSF leak, pneumocephalus, or cavernous-carotid fistula. Fractures of the basal skull bones are often accompanied by signs of hemotympanum (blood behind the tympanic membrane), delayed ecchymosis over the mastoid process (Battle's sign), or periorbital ecchymosis ("racoon sign"). Because routine x-ray examination can fail to disclose basilar fractures, they should be suspected in the presence of these clinical signs. Cerebrospinal fluid also may leak through the cribriform plate or the adjacent sinus and present as a watery discharge from the nose (CSF rhinorrhea). Persistence of rhinorrhea or recurrent meningitis is an indication for a surgical repair of torn dura underlying the fracture. The site of the leak is often difficult to determine, but useful diagnostic tests include metrizamide instillation into the CSF with subsequent CT scans and radionuclide or fluorescein injection into the CSF followed by assessment of uptake by absorptive nasal pledgets. The site of intermittent leaks is rarely delineated; most resolve spontaneously. Sellar fractures also can be radiologically occult, although they are sometimes associated with serious neuroendocrine dysfunction. Occasionally, fractures of the dorsum sella cause sixth or seventh nerve palsies or optic nerve damage. An air-fluid level in the sphenoid sinus suggests a fracture of the sellar floor.

About 20 percent of petrous bone fractures, usually along the long axis of the bone, are associated with facial palsy. Disruption of ear ossicles and CSF otorrhea are other complications. Transverse petrous fractures are less common, almost always damaging the cochlea or labyrinths and often the facial nerve. External bleeding from the ear can result from petrous bone fractures, although local laceration of the external canal from abrasions is more common. Frontal bone fractures are often depressed, involving the frontal and paranasal sinuses and the orbits; anosmia frequently follows if the olfactory filaments in the cribriform plate are disrupted.

Depressed skull fractures are often compound but are commonly neurologically asymptomatic because the impact energy is dissipated in breaking the bone; however, some cause brain contusions and focal signs from the underlying cortical area. Surgical repair and bone elevation with exploration of the dura are required in most cases. Delayed or incomplete debridement of the wound leads to a high incidence of infection. If the skin is lacerated over a skull fracture and the underlying meninges are torn, or if the fracture passes through the posterior wall of a nasal sinus, bacteria or air may enter the cranial cavity resulting in meningitis, abscess formation, or pneumocephalus.

CRANIAL NERVE INJURIES Cranial nerves liable to injury with basilar skull fractures are the olfactory, optic, oculomotor, trochlear, first and second branches of the trigeminal, facial, and auditory. Anosmia and an apparent loss of taste (actually a loss of perception of aromatic flavors, with elementary tastes retained) occurs in approximately 10 percent of serious head injuries, particularly with falls on the back of the head. This results from displacement of the brain and shearing of the olfactory nerve filaments. Recovery usually occurs with residual hyposmia, but if bilateral anosmia persists for several months, the prognosis is poor. Fractures of the sphenoid bone may bruise or transect the optic nerve, resulting in unilateral partial or complete blindness and an unreactive pupil, usually equal in size to the other side, with a preserved consensual light response. Partial optic nerve injuries from closed trauma result in blurring of vision, central or paracentral scotomas, or sector defects. Direct orbital injury may cause short-lived blurred vision for close objects because of reversible iridoplegia. Oculomotor nerve injury causes the globe to turn outward with loss of adduction and vertical movement and a fixed dilated pupil; vision is preserved. Diplopia only on looking down, which suggests trochlear nerve damage from fracture of the lesser sphenoid wing, occurs as an isolated problem from minor injury and may be delayed in appearance for several days. Patients report correction of the diplopia by tilting the head away from the affected eye. Direct facial nerve injury by a basal fracture is present immediately in 3 percent of severe injuries or also may be delayed 5 to 7 days. Petrous fractures, particularly the less common transverse type, are liable to produce this injury. Delayed facial palsy has a good prognosis; its mechanism is not known. Injury to the eighth cranial nerve with fractures of the petrous bone causes loss of hearing, vertigo, and nystagmus immediately after injury; the nystagmus is frequently positional. Deafness due to nerve injury must be distinguished from rupture of the eardrum, blood in the middle ear, or disruption of the ossicles from fracture through the middle ear. A high-tone hearing loss occurs with direct cochlear concussion.

CONCUSSION Concussion refers to an immediate but transient loss of consciousness often described as dazed or "star struck" and associated with a short period of amnesia. It typically occurs after blunt impact or deceleration of the frontal or occipital areas that creates sudden movement of the brain within the skull. In severe cases, a brief convulsion or autonomic symptoms and signs such as facial pallor, bradycardia, faintness with mild hypotension, or sluggish pupillary reaction may occur, but most patients are neurologically normal. Higher primates are particularly susceptible to concussion; in contrast, billy goats, rams, and woodpeckers can tolerate impact velocity and deceleration a hundred times greater than that experienced by humans. The mechanism of loss of consciousness in concussion is believed to be transient electrophysiologic dysfunction of the reticular activating system in the upper midbrain caused by rotation of the cerebral hemispheres on the relatively fixed brainstem. The mechanism of the associated amnesia is not known. Gross and light microscopic changes in the brain are usually absent after concussion, but biochemical and ultrastructural changes such as mitochondrial ATP depletion and local disruption of the blood-brain barrier suggest that complex abnormalities occur. The CT and magnetic resonance (MRI) scans are usually normal, and there are usually no red blood cells in the CSF, as occurs with more severe injuries. Approximately 3 percent of patients who have had concussions will have an intracranial hemorrhage (subdural, epidural, or parenchymal), but the presence of a skull fracture increases the risk.

Amnesia after concussion typically follows a few moments of unresponsiveness after impact. Rarely there is no loss of consciousness. The memory loss spans the time of, and moments before, mild impact injuries but may encompass previous weeks (rarely months) in more severe trauma. Any anterograde amnesia is usually brief and disappears rapidly in alert patients. The extent of retrograde amnesia has been suggested as a rough measure of the severity of injury.

Improvement usually occurs in an orderly progression from most distant to recent memories, with islands of amnesia occasionally remaining in severe cases. Hysterical posttraumatic amnesia is not uncommon and should be suspected when abnormalities of behavior occur, such as a tendency to recount events that cannot be recalled on later testing, bizarre affect, forgetting one's own name, or exaggerated anterograde deficit in comparison with the degree of injury.

A single uncomplicated head injury has not been shown to produce permanent neurobehavioral changes in most patients who are free of preexisting psychiatric problems and substance abuse. In some patients, however, there has been increasing attention to minor problems in memory and concentration that may have an anatomic correlate in small shearing or other microscopic lesions (see below).

CONTUSION, BRAIN HEMORRHAGES, AND SHEARING LESIONS Hemispheral lesions Contusions on the surface of the brain and deeper hemorrhages result from mechanical forces that move the hemispheres relative to the skull. Deceleration of the brain against the inner skull causes contusions, either under a point of impact (coup lesion) or in the antipolar area (contrecoup lesion). Trauma sufficient to cause prolonged unconsciousness usually produces contusions varying from small superficial cortical petechiae to hemorrhagic and necrotic destruction of large portions of a hemisphere. Because the motion of the hemispheres brings them into contact with the prominences of the sphenoid and other frontal basal bones, blunt impact, as from an automobile dashboard, typically causes contusions on the orbital surfaces of the frontal lobes and the anterior and basal portions of the temporal lobes. The anterior corpus callosum also may be bruised from striking the falx. With lateral forces, as from the doorframe of a car, contusions occur on the convexity of the hemispheres.

Contusions are visible on CT scan, appearing early as inhomogeneous hyperlucencies from scattered cortical and subcortical blood with mass effect that distorts the lateral ventricles. After several hours, the surrounding edematous tissue appears as a ring of lower density. Confluent, roughly spherical contusions can be distinguished from cerebral hemorrhages because contusions extend to the cortical surface. After a week, some contusions have a surrounding ringlike contrast-enhancing density that may be mistaken for tumor or abscess. Glial and macrophage reactions begin within 2 days, years later resulting in scarred hemosiderin-stained depressions on the surface (*plaques jaune*) that are one source of posttraumatic epilepsy. Large single hemorrhages after minor trauma may occur in patients with a bleeding diathesis or in the elderly, sometimes related to cerebrovascular amyloidosis.

The clinical signs produced by contusions vary with their location and size; most often a hemiparesis or gaze preference is seen, similar to a middle cerebral artery stroke. Bilateral large contusions produce coma with extensor posturing; when contusions are limited to the frontal lobes, an abulic-taciturn state or inappropriate jocularity and indifference occur. Contusions of the temporal lobes cause an aggressive combative syndrome, described below. With large contusions, the secondary effect of progressive edema is the most threatening aspect of the injury. Coma and signs of secondary brainstem compression (pupillary enlargement) then dominate. Seizures soon after trauma are rare with contusions, as indeed they are for several weeks after most acute head injuries.

Deep hemorrhages in the central white matter may result from confluent contusions in the depths of a sulcus. However, ganglionic, diencephalic, and other deep hematomas due to torsion or shearing forces in the brain infrequently occur independently of surface damage. The areas around these hematomas can become edematous, resulting in enlargement of the affected region and progressively raised intracranial pressure.

Another type of white matter, or ''shearing,'' lesion consists of widespread acute disruption of axons at the time of impact. The affected areas of white matter are replaced with glial proliferation over a period of several months. There are characteristically small areas of tissue disruption in the corpus callosum and dorsolateral pons. Widespread axonal shearing lesions in the deep white matter of both hemispheres may explain persistent coma or vegetative state, but small hemorrhages in the midbrain and low diencephalon are as often the cause. Only severe shearing lesions are visualized by CT scanning, as small hemorrhages of the corpus callosum and centrum semiovale; MRI is able to show them throughout the white matter.

On occasion, head trauma causes diffuse brain swelling within a few hours after injury, although CT scanning fails to reveal focal lesions or hemorrhage, particularly in children. The swelling creates a mass effect with disastrous consequences. This problem is probably due to microvascular disruption and greatly increased cerebral blood flow.

Deep cerebral hemorrhages may be delayed several days after severe injury. Sudden neurologic deterioration, often in already comatose patients, or a sustained and unexplained rise in intracranial pressure should therefore prompt a CT scan.

Brainstem hemorrhages A syndrome with coma, midposition or larger pupils unreactive to light, and impaired or absent oculocephalic reflex eye movements results from small linear or oval-shaped hemorrhages in the high midbrain, visible on CT scan, although often delayed in appearance. Although extensor posturing occurs with stimulation, the limbs are otherwise flaccid. This clinical syndrome should be suspected even in the initial absence of a hemorrhage on CT scan. These acute midbrain hemorrhages may be the result of primary injury from rotational forces in the upper midbrain. They also occur from secondary compression of the brainstem by supratentorial hematomas and lateral tissue shifts or pressure from the adjacent temporal lobes. MRI shows many other small brainstem and hemispheric white matter lesions that are related to mechanical disruption of tissue, similar to shearing. In pathologic material from severe, acutely fatal injuries, small linear and oval hemorrhages are found in the low thalamic and subthalamic regions and throughout the midline of the brainstem (*Duret hemorrhages*).

Residual symptoms and signs of primary or secondary brainstem hemorrhages or ischemic lesions include tremor, pupillary enlargement, eye movement abnormalities, or the ''locked-in'' syndrome (see Chap. 26). Midbrain or diencephalic hemorrhages are the only well-defined direct traumatic brainstem lesions responsible for coma. Most other lesions causing coma and subsequent persistent vegetative state that are unexplained by CT scan are probably due to diffuse axonal shearing injuries in the cerebral hemispheres or severe anoxia-ischemia at the time of trauma.

SUBDURAL AND EPIDURAL HEMATOMAS In severe head injury, hemorrhages beneath the dura (subdural) or between the dura and skull (epidural) may be combined with contusions and other injuries, making it difficult to determine their relative contribution to the clinical state. However, subdural and epidural hematomas often occur as the primary lesion, each with a characteristic clinical and radiologic appearance. Because the mass effect of the hemorrhage and rise in intracranial pressure may be life-threatening, it is important to make an immediate diagnosis by CT scan and carry out surgical evacuation.

Acute subdural hematoma Acute subdural hematomas become symptomatic within minutes to hours after injury. Up to one-third of patients have a lucid interval before coma supervenes, but the majority are drowsy or comatose from the moment of injury. Arousable patients complain of unilateral headache and frequently have a slightly enlarged pupil on that side. Stupor or coma and unilateral pupillary enlargement are the major signs in larger hematomas. Pupillary dilation is usually ipsilateral, but 5 to 10 percent are contralateral to the hematoma. Lateralizing signs such as a hemiparesis are helpful but may be ipsilateral to the clot. The CT scan shows the clot, allowing early evacuation. The degree of midline shift is often disproportionately greater than the size of the clot in one CT scan axial section, but in general, rules relating shift to the level of consciousness, outlined in Chap. 26, remain useful. MRI may fail to demonstrate an acute clot. In an acutely deteriorating patient with diminished alertness and pupillary enlargement, burr holes or an emergency craniotomy are appropriate at times without prior radiographic confirmation of subdural hematoma. A subacute syndrome with drowsiness, headache, confusion, or mild hemiparesis occurring days to 2 weeks after injury is seen in alcoholics and in the elderly.

Direct trauma or surface contusions are not required for acute subdural hemorrhage; acceleration forces alone, as from whiplash, are adequate, especially in the elderly. Most subdural hematomas are small crescentic collections over the hemispheral convexity, adjacent to variable degrees of surface hemorrhagic contusions. Larger clots are thought to be primarily venous in origin, although additional arterial bleeding sites are often found, and some, when explored surgically, appear to be exclusively arterial. Most are located over the frontotemporal region, less often in the inferior middle fossa or over the occipital poles. Less common instances of interhemispheric, posterior fossa, or bilateral convexity clots are difficult to diagnose clinically, although drowsiness and the signs expected for each region can be detected. Small subdural hematomas may be asymptomatic and usually do not require therapy.

Acute epidural hematoma Epidural hematomas evolve more rapidly than subdural hematomas and therefore can be more treacherous. They occur in 1 to 3 percent of all head injuries, in up to 10 percent of severe cases, and are less often associated with underlying cortical damage than subdural hematomas. The majority of patients are unconscious when first seen. A "lucid interval" of several minutes to hours before coma supervenes is said to be most characteristic of epidural hemorrhage, although it is not common and by no means the only cause of this temporal profile.

The location of an epidural hematoma overlying the lateral temporal convexity is explained by its origin from torn dural vessels, most commonly the middle meningeal artery. The majority of patients have fractures of the squamous portion of the temporal bone, through the path of the torn vessel. Frontal, inferior temporal, or occipitoparietal epidural hematomas are less frequent, occurring when fractures disrupt branches of the middle meningeal artery. Dural laceration over the sagittal or lateral sinuses and rupture of small diploic veins are rarer causes. Epidural hematomas strip the tightly attached dura from the inner table of the skull, producing a characteristic lenticular-shaped clot on CT scan. They may be relatively less frequent in the elderly because of the tighter attachment of dura to skull that occurs with aging. Posterior fossa epidural hematomas are rare and difficult to detect clinically (most result from surgery such as resection of an acoustic neuroma).

Chronic subdural hematoma In chronic subdural hematoma, a preceding traumatic cause is less often clear; 20 to 30 percent of patients fail to give a history of injury, particularly elderly patients or those with a bleeding diathesis. The causative injury may be trivial (striking the head against the branch of a tree, a sudden stop in a car with lurching forward, or minor head contact during a fall or faint) and is often forgotten because it was remote in time. A period of weeks, or even months, follows when headaches (common but not invariable), slowed thinking, confusion, changes in personality, seizures, and/or a mild hemiparesis emerges. Fluctuation in the severity of the headache is typical, often with positional changes. Many chronic subdural hematomas are bilateral and give particularly misleading clinical syndromes. The initial clinical impression is often a stroke, brain tumor, drug intoxication, or a depressive, senile, or other type of dementia, the latter because drowsiness, inattentiveness, or incoherence of thought is more prominent than focal signs such as hemiparesis. Hemianesthesia or hemianopia is seldom observed, probably because the anatomic structures subserving these functions are deep and not easily compressed. The diagnosis should be considered in dementias of rapid onset, particularly if headache is present. The condition does not usually progress unless acute bleeding is superimposed on the chronic hematoma, making the patient comatose with fluctuations of alertness and pupillary dilation. Occasionally patients present with "spells" of hemiparesis or aphasia typically lasting more than 10 min and indistinguishable from transient ischemic attacks. Patients with undetected small bilateral subdural hematomas seem to tolerate surgery, anesthesia, and nervous system depressive drugs poorly, often remaining drowsy or confused for long periods postoperatively.

Skull x-rays are usually normal except for a shift of a calcified pineal body to one side or an occasional unexpected fracture. The CT scan without contrast infusion typically shows a low-density mass over the convexity of the hemisphere, but between 2 to 6 weeks after the initial bleeding may show only a shift of the midline structures and compression of the lateral ventricles because the clot is isodense to adjacent brain. Bilateral chronic hematomas are often missed because of the absence of lateral tissue shifts. A "hypernormal" CT scan with full cortical sulci and small ventricles in an older patient should suggest the diagnosis of bilateral isodense hematomas. Contrast infusion demonstrates a chronic fibrous capsule surrounding the clot. MRI is reliable in identifying a subacute clot. Lumbar puncture is not recommended for diagnosis because of risk of worsening tissue shifts but, if performed, shows xanthochromia and a variable number of red blood cells. Chronic subdural hematomas can gradually expand and then behave clinically like a tumor. Treatment with glucocorticoids alone is sufficient in some cases, but surgical evacuation is most often successful. Fibrous membranes (pseudomembranes) that grow from the dura and encapsulate the region require surgical resection to prevent recurrent fluid accumulation. Small hematomas are largely resorbed, and only the organizing membranes remain, becoming calcified after many years.

PENETRATING INJURIES, COMPRESSIONS, AND LACERATIONS Tangential scalp wounds from bullets can produce neurologic signs or delayed seizures due to small hemorrhages or contusions, even in the absence of missile penetration. Bullets entering the brain cause considerable damage because of tremendous kinetic energy. A cylindrical area of necrosis surrounds the bullet track. Injuries differ with varying projectiles; soft civilian bullets typically shatter on impact and leave a track of metallic fragments with moderate parenchymal damage. Military bullets, because of high velocity and energy, disrupt tissue at great distances from the track and produce massive brain destruction.

Penetrating bullet injuries cause a rapid increase in intracranial pressure for several minutes followed by a drop depending on the volume of secondary hemorrhage and the degree of developing edema. Infection is a risk mainly from shell fragments, shrapnel, grenades, and mines, because such small projectiles carry surface bacteria and dirt into the brain. Most neurosurgeons administer systemic antibiotics prophylactically and perform local debridement in all types of penetrating injuries. Traumatic aneurysms can form as a result of disruption of vessel walls from the shock wave of the projectile; facial-orbital entrance wounds have the highest incidence. The aneurysms have an unpredictable course, but most that rupture do so in the first month. The prognosis for survival after missile injuries is good if consciousness is preserved and poor if coma is present from the outset.

Other intracranial foreign bodies from knives, picks, studguns, or high-speed tool bits may be missed unless skull x-rays are taken after minor penetrating injuries. Surgical removal, debridement, and extensive exploration for hemorrhage and necrotic tissue are required.

TRAUMATIC VASCULAR OCCLUSION AND DISSECTION Minor, sometimes unnoticed, neck trauma can produce dissection (stripping of the intima or the media) of the internal carotid or vertebral arteries. Chiropractic neck manipulation accounts for some cases. Severe blunt trauma to the neck can initiate a dissection several centimeters above the origins of the internal carotid or vertebral arteries. In awake patients there is usually local neck pain over the internal carotid artery, a Horner's syndrome, and headache over the ipsilateral anterior cranium. Some patients with carotid dissection subsequently have large middle cerebral artery strokes with hemiplegia. In drowsy or comatose patients, evidence of dissection or subsequent stroke is difficult to discern but is suggested by unexplained hemiplegia, unilateral miosis, or appearance of cerebral infarction on

CT scan. Angiography demonstrates either the typical "string sign" characterized by an elongated, narrowed lumen extending over 5 to 10 cm or complete occlusion of the carotid artery beginning several centimeters distal to the bifurcation. On rare occasions, basilar skull fractures cause carotid dissection beginning at the point of entry of the artery into the skull. Traumatic "false" aneurysms of the cervical carotid artery result from deep penetrating, and occasionally from nonpenetrating, blunt trauma of the neck. A pulsatile mass and bruit over the artery establish the diagnosis. Traumatic vertebral artery dissection can produce vertigo, vomiting, suboccipital or supraorbital headache, and other signs of lateral medullary ischemia. These symptoms are frequently attributed to vestibular concussion. In comatose patients, the only indication of vertebral artery occlusion may be inferior cerebellar infarction on CT scan.

Preexisting saccular aneurysms may rupture after basilar skull fractures, and this diagnosis should be considered if subarachnoid hemorrhage is profuse and inadequately explained by accompanying subdural blood on CT scan. Vasospasm from traumatic subarachnoid blood may be involved in the development of infarction after head injury.

Cavernous sinus arteriovenous fistulas are serious complications in patients surviving severe head injury. They are first evident as a self-audible bruit (many are also audible to the examiner), proptosis, conjunctival injection, or visual impairment. Angiography shows early filling of the cavernous sinus and its draining tributaries. The fistula generally enlarges, causing increasingly severe local changes around the eye and orbit and decreased chances of visual recovery. About 10 percent, mostly small fistulas, resolve spontaneously. Many surgical approaches have been tried, including ligation of the carotid artery, direct obliteration of the fistula or cavernous sinus, and angiographic-guided balloon embolization. A detachable balloon technique has proved successful in many cases (see Chap. 365).

INTRACRANIAL PRESSURE AND CEREBRAL BLOOD FLOW

Intracranial pressure (ICP) regulation and its relationship to cerebral blood flow (CBF), which is applicable to many pathologic processes including cerebral hemorrhage, encephalitis, and brain edema after stroke, is best understood in the context of head trauma. The components of the intracranial compartment are brain, CSF, and blood. Because the skull limits total intracranial content, the volume of these compartments is compromised by expanding lesions within the cranial cavity. The brain is virtually incompressible; therefore, CSF and blood serve as the main buffers of increasing intracranial volume. The relationship between increments in intracranial volume and the associated rises in ICP, termed *compliance*, approximates an exponential function. ICP is normally between 2 and 12 mmHg. Raised ICP in the range 15 to 40 mmHg, while not harmful by itself, can rapidly result in secondary damage, either by precipitously decreasing cerebral perfusion when ICP approaches blood pressure in the cranium or by associated shifts of brain tissue that damage the upper brainstem. The global damage from increased ICP is therefore ischemic in nature and related to the difference between ICP and blood pressure in the major cerebral arteries. When this pressure difference, termed *cerebral perfusion pressure* or *CPP*, is below 40 to 60 mmHg, raised ICP becomes detrimental to nerve cells; therapy is therefore directed toward maintaining perfusion above this range. The rationale for keeping CPP even higher (i.e., bringing ICP below 15 to 20 mmHg) is to afford a margin of safety should transient increases in ICP occur. Physiologic changes or medications that increase blood pressure do not necessarily improve CPP because increased vascular pressures can exacerbate brain edema in damaged areas, resulting in further increases in ICP that ultimately lower perfusion.

The most important secondary nervous system complication of head injury is raised intracranial pressure arising from the added volume of contusions, hematomas, and the progressive edema surrounding them. A close relationship exists between clinical outcome and ICP in patients with closed head injury. At least 50 percent of patients who die as a result of head injury do so because of uncontrolled rises in ICP, and outcome is inversely related to the level of ICP after acute injury. Aggressive treatment of raised ICP in modern intensive care units is believed to improve survival after severe head injury. The role of direct monitoring of ICP to guide therapy is more controversial.

Resting ICP, CPP, and compliance are spontaneously interrupted by rises in ICP termed *plateau waves* that may be precipitated by iatrogenic maneuvers such as suctioning, physical therapy, excess fluid administration, or pain. Plateau waves are due to a loss of cerebrovascular tone with a resultant increase in cerebral blood volume. Some apparently spontaneous plateau waves are due to mild, often unnoticed hypotension that causes cerebrovascular dilation. Such plateau waves (lasting 1 to 10 min and ranging from 25 to 60 mmHg) are most pronounced in patients with diminished intracranial compliance. They are best appreciated with continuous trend recordings of ICP. Signs of apparent transtentorial herniation such as pupillary enlargement may occur after plateau waves (they more often do not), and occasionally, brain death ensues.

There is little consensus about the importance of alterations in cerebral blood flow caused by head injury. For several minutes to an hour after acute head injury, cerebral blood flow may increase in some patients, although metabolic demands and oxygen consumption are diminished. Autoregulation, the ability of the cerebral vasculature to keep blood flow constant in response to decreased or increased perfusion pressure, is also impaired in damaged regions. Vascular factors have been found to account for approximately two-thirds of the rise in ICP after severe head injury. The blood-brain barrier also becomes more permeable after head injury in badly damaged regions, making edema formation more likely.

There is a complex relationship between raised ICP and clinical signs such as coma and pupillary enlargement that accompany supratentorial masses. ICP represents the accommodation of intracranial contents to additional mass; clinical signs are a parallel barometer of tissue shifts, particularly affecting structures around the tentorial opening. Raised ICP per se does not cause signs until it reaches levels that preclude cerebral perfusion; it then causes global ischemia in a fashion similar to acute hypotension. Coma and other secondary signs resulting from tissue shifts in the region of the tentorial opening are described in Chap. 26. Horizontal midline shift at the level of the pineal body is closely related to the level of consciousness with acute unilateral mass lesions.

Other secondary phenomena after severe head injury cause brain damage and alter outcome. Hypoxia or coagulopathy, for example, are common from a number of causes and, when severe, are associated with a poorer outcome.

CLINICAL SYNDROMES AND TREATMENT OF HEAD INJURY

MINOR INJURY A fully alert and attentive patient presenting after head injury with one or more symptoms of headache, faintness, nausea, a single episode of emesis, difficulty with concentration, or slight blurring of vision has a good prognosis with little risk of subsequent deterioration. Such patients have sustained a concussion or have been dazed and have a brief amnestic epoch surrounding the moment of impact. Occasionally, vasovagal syncope occurs several minutes to an hour after the injury and causes concern. Constant generalized or frontal headache is common in the days following trauma; it is often throbbing or hemicranial in nature, like migraine. The majority of patients with a minor syndrome do not have a skull fracture on skull x-ray or hemorrhage on CT scan. The decision to obtain these tests depends largely on the availability of CT or MRI scanning and clinical signs suggesting that the impact was severe (e.g., prolonged concussion, periorbital or mastoid hematoma, repeated vomiting, etc). Children and young adults are particularly prone to drowsiness, vomiting, and irritability, sometimes delayed for several hours after apparently minor injuries. After a period of observation for several hours, arrangements may be made for the patient to be accompanied home to be observed by family or friends.

Persistent severe headache and repeated vomiting in the context of normal alertness and no focal neurologic signs are usually benign, but CT or MRI scanning and/or skull x-rays should be obtained. Skull fractures increase the likelihood of a subdural or epidural hematoma. Skull x-ray is an acceptable screening method in areas without access to CT scanning. Patients with these exaggerated signs, even if they follow minor injury, deserve observation in the hospital for 24 h. Clinical judgment, the presence of associated noncranial injuries, the availability of others at home, and the examiner's certainty of a normal neurologic examination should guide the need for further surveillance.

INJURY OF INTERMEDIATE SEVERITY Patients who are not comatose but who have persistent confusion, behavioral changes, less than normal alertness, extreme dizziness, or focal neurologic signs such as hemiparesis should be admitted to the hospital and have a CT scan. The clinical syndromes most common in this group, in addition to postconcussive headache and dizziness, unsteadiness, photophobia, and vomiting of minor injury, include (1) delirium with a disinclination to be examined or moved, expletive speech, and resistance if disturbed, often associated with anterior temporal lobe contusions; (2) a quiet, disinterested, slowed mental state (abulia) with dull facial appearance and slight irascibility if bothered, the patient lying quietly with eyes closed when undisturbed, seen with inferior and frontopolar frontal contusions; (3) severe memory loss with poor retrograde and anterograde performance, headache, and photophobia, with medial temporal lobe contusions or diffuse injury; (4) a focal deficit such as aphasia or mild hemiparesis (hemianopsia is rare as an isolated posttraumatic finding), suggesting subdural hematoma or convexity contusion, or rarely, carotid artery dissection and stroke; (5) global confusion with inattention, poor performance on simple mental tasks, fluctuating or slightly erroneous orientation, associated with several types of injuries including the first two described above as well as medial frontal contusions and interhemispheric subdural hematoma; (6) repetitive vomiting, nystagmus, drowsiness, and unsteadiness, usually from a labyrinthine concussion, but occasionally due to a posterior fossa subdural hematoma or vertebral artery dissection; (7) drowsiness alone or with muteness, often unassociated with significant CT scan abnormalities; and (8) diabetes insipidus with or without a frontal-temporal lobe syndrome, from damage to the median eminence or pituitary stalk and adjacent medial cortex.

The syndromes of intermediate severity are usually preceded by brief loss of consciousness, and many are associated with skull fractures. A CT scan is required to exclude surgically remediable subdural or epidural hematomas and to define areas of contusion that later enlarge with edema or coalesce to form intraparenchymal hemorrhages. Paroxysmal or rhythmic EEG abnormalities, in contrast to acute convulsions, are common over the region of a large contusion. Many intermediate injuries are complicated by drug or alcohol intoxication, making toxic screening important.

Close clinical observation in a well-staffed setting is advisable in order to detect increasing drowsiness and change in respiratory pattern or pupillary enlargement and to ensure fluid restriction. Fully awake or slightly drowsy patients with small subdural hematomas may be treated with glucocorticoids and fluid restriction; larger clots, especially with fluctuating or worsening alertness, require surgery. Follow-up CT scanning is advisable. Epidural hematomas causing compression of adjacent brain should be evacuated in patients who have a reasonable chance of recovery from other injuries. Free water intake should be limited, allowing serum osmolarity to rise spontaneously toward 290 mosmol/L. Fever must be treated assiduously with antipyretics or a cooling blanket, and its source must be identified

(usually aspiration). So-called central fever is rare. The routine, acute administration of phenytoin is controversial. About half of neurosurgeons advocate its use, particularly in children and young adults, in the belief that it may reduce the incidence of posttraumatic epilepsy, but the best randomized trial has shown no benefit beyond the first week of drug administration. Glucocorticoids may be useful if there is a contusion, hemorrhage, or edema on the CT scan; otherwise, they complicate management and should be omitted. The possibility of associated cervical spine injuries should be considered in all patients with syndromes of intermediate severity. The neck should be immobilized, and adequate x-rays of the spine should be obtained.

The majority of patients with intermediate injury improve over 1 to 6 weeks. During the first week, alertness, irascibility, memory, and mental performance fluctuate. Behavioral changes such as agitation are most evident at night and sometimes seem to be worsened by large doses of glucocorticoids or CNS-depressant drugs. Haloperidol is useful when used sparingly. Subtle abnormalities of intellectual function, particularly attention, spontaneity, and memory, tend to return toward normal later, and sometimes do so abruptly. Persistent intellectual difficulties are discussed below.

SEVERE HEAD INJURY AND COMA Patients who are stuporous or comatose from the outset require immediate neurologic attention and, often, resuscitation. There is often pupillary enlargement or asymmetry. Persistent unresponsiveness is a grave sign. After the patient is intubated and the blood pressure is stabilized, attention is given to life-threatening noncranial injuries, followed by a survey neurologic examination. The possibility of cervical injuries should not be overlooked, and the cervical spine must be immobilized during the initial assessment. The depth of coma and the size of the pupils are most important. Extensor limb posturing and bilateral Babinski signs, combined with apparently purposeful movements, are common. Asymmetry in limb posture, limb movement, or gaze preference suggests a subdural or epidural hematoma or a large contusion.

As soon as vital functions permit and cervical spine x-rays and a CT scan have been obtained, the patient should be taken to a critical care unit. The finding of an epidural or subdural hematoma or large intracerebral hemorrhage is usually an indication for surgery and intracranial decompression. In one large series, the time between injury and evacuation of acute subdural hematomas was the major determinant of outcome. If such lesions are not present and the patient is still comatose and critically ill, attention is directed toward treating raised ICP. Patients with abnormal CT scans showing contusions, hemorrhages, or tissue shifts are the best candidates for ICP monitoring. The lumbar CSF pressure does not accurately reflect the intracranial pressure and lumbar puncture may increase the risk of brain herniation; therefore, the practice in most head injury treatment centers is to use one of several devices inserted intracranially to measure ICP. The pressure can be monitored continuously, disturbances in compliance and falling CPP can be identified, and appearance of plateau waves can be noted.

The treatment of raised ICP is best guided by direct measurement but may proceed on a presumptive basis using clinical status and CT scan as guides. All potentially exacerbating factors must be eliminated. Hypoxia, hyperthermia, hypercarbia, awkward head positions, and high mean airway pressures from mechanical ventilation all increase cerebral blood volume and ICP. Many, but not all, patients will have lower ICPs when the head and trunk are elevated. If raising the patient's head lowers blood pressure, then cerebral perfusion pressure may be optimal in the supine position. Active management of raised ICP includes induced hypocarbia to an initial level of 28 to 33 mmHg P_{CO_2} and hyperosmolar dehydration with 20% mannitol (0.25 to 1 g/ kg every 3 to 6 h), preferably using directly measured ICP as a guide. Otherwise, a serum osmolality of 305 to 315 mosmol/L is desirable, as is ventricular or subarachnoid fluid drainage when possible.

Persistently raised ICP after inception of this conservative therapy generally indicates a poor outcome, but the addition of high-dose barbiturates may further lower ICP. In many instances, barbiturates cause a parallel reduction in ICP and blood pressure without resulting in net improvement in cerebral perfusion. The beneficial effects of barbiturates, aside from their sedative and anticonvulsant activities, are not established, and they can cause disastrous hypotension, so their routine use in severe head injury is not recommended. Further details of treatment of raised ICP are given in Chap. 26. Systolic blood pressure should be maintained above 100 mmHg by vasopressor agents, if necessary, but when pressors are required to support barbiturate use, there is usually little improvement in CPP. Mean blood pressure levels above 110 to 120 mmHg may exaggerate brain edema and are associated with plateau waves; hypertension may be treated with diuretics and beta-adrenergic blocking agents, angiotensin-converting enzyme inhibitors, or intermittent doses of barbiturates. A number of other antihypertensive drugs, including some calcium-channel blockers, are relatively contraindicated because they may raise ICP. Fluid and electrolytes must be administered cautiously, and free water administration should be limited. Administration of phenytoin to prevent seizures is recommended by many neurosurgeons. Antacids by nasogastric tube or directly acting drugs should be administered to keep gastric pH above 3.5 and prevent gastrointestinal bleeding. The use of large doses of glucocorticoids in severe head injury does not improve outcome. Several recent studies suggest that early nutritional support results in earlier neurologic recovery from head injury. If the patient remains comatose, it is worthwhile to repeat the CT scan to exclude a delayed surface or intracerebral hemorrhage. Intensive care salvages some critically ill head-injured patients by concentrating efforts on simple treatments that avoid medical complications, particularly pneumonia and sepsis and preventable increases in ICP. Whether more assiduous control of ICP and CPP will produce better results remains to be proved.

ASSOCIATED DERANGEMENTS OCCURRING WITH SEVERE HEAD TRAUMA   Injuries outside the cranium should be searched for at the outset, because they are likely to be forgotten if not initially noted. In particular, associated spinal, long bone, and abdominal injuries may cause delayed difficulties in management. However, secondary medical complications dominate the intermediate-term intensive care of head trauma patients.

Fluids and electrolytes   Over half of patients who persist in coma for 24 h after head injury develop abnormalities of electrolytes or fluid balance. Frequently these are a consequence of therapy, but the metabolic responses to head trauma are similar to those produced by trauma elsewhere and are important in planning treatment. Daily input-output records and body weights, when possible, are useful. Water restriction and osmotic agents render most patients hyperosmolar and hypovolemic, requiring monitoring of serum osmolality and sodium concentrations. Diabetes insipidus should be suspected if urine output increases and urine specific gravity is low. Replacement of water losses suffices for mild cases, but vasopressin may be required in persistent cases. Serum osmolality above approximately 325 mosmol/L should be avoided because of the associated decrease in cardiac output.

Aldosterone and antidiuretic hormone (vasopressin, AVP) secretion in response to stress favor sodium and free water retention, respectively. The latter usually predominates, leading to mild hypervolemic hyponatremia in untreated patients, but is obscured by concomitant administration of osmotic agents. Severe hyponatremia results from excessive AVP secretion, which may occur with raised ICP, basilar skull fractures, and after prolonged mechanical ventilation. Potassium is lost in head injury because of trauma-induced aldosterone hypersecretion, therapeutic osmotic diuresis, and glucocorticoids. Because potassium is predominantly an intracellular ion, hypokalemia is frequently manifested as a hypochloremic alkalosis with normal or minimally depressed serum potassium and requires adequate replacement therapy with KCl.

Respiratory complications   Some patients with head injuries have hypoxia acutely after injury without obvious pulmonary infiltrates. Aspiration pneumonia presents a great risk; acid burn injury from aspirated gastric contents, infection, and atelectasis may combine to produce the adult respiratory distress syndrome (ARDS) and severe arteriovenous shunting. Some evidence suggests that agents that coat the gastric lining without reducing pH, such as sucralfate, are associated with less aspiration pneumonia than are conventional prophylactic agents for gastric bleeding. ARDS also can occur due to disseminated intravascular coagulopathy, fat embolism, or, rarely, "neurogenic" pulmonary edema. Treatment is similar to other cases of ARDS with positive end-expiratory pressure (PEEP) to allow lowered inspired oxygen concentrations and to prevent further atelectasis. The effect of PEEP on ICP is complex, but PEEP should not be withheld if necessary for oxygenation.

Atelectasis is common in all poorly responsive patients and is treated with chest physical therapy and adequate ventilator tidal volumes. Pulmonary embolism is also a major threat to bedridden patients, and intermittent pneumatic calf compression or modest doses of subcutaneous heparin may be useful prophylaxis. The latter has not predisposed to intracerebral or gastrointestinal bleeding. Early recognition of deep leg vein thrombosis and aggressive treatment by occlusion of the inferior vena cava may prevent later emboli.

Gastrointestinal hemorrhage   The majority of patients with severe head injuries develop gastric erosions, but only a few have clinically significant hemorrhages. Gastrointestinal bleeding usually occurs in the first days to 1 week. Unlike most patients in shock or with stress ulceration, head-trauma patients often have elevated gastric acidity. The synergistic effect of glucocorticoids in causing upper tract hemorrhage has been questioned, but the incidence of viscus perforation, particularly of the cecum, is elevated. Prophylactic treatment with gastric coating agents, as discussed above, with H-2 blockers or with frequent antacid administration to keep gastric pH high, probably reduces gastric hemorrhage in other stress states and is commonly used in head trauma.

Fat embolism   Patients with severe long bone injuries are subject to widespread cerebral fat embolism. This complication is seen less often than previously, perhaps due to better fluid replacement. In the typical case, head injury is a minor part of the overall trauma; in a few, severe cranial injury masks the syndrome. Several days after the bone fractures, restlessness, delirium, or drowsiness progressing to coma in severe cases, seizures, generalized brain edema, and/or hypoxia develops. About half the patients have retinal and conjunctival punctate hemorrhages or visible fat in retinal vessels. A petechial rash, prominent in the anterior axillary folds and supraclavicular fossae, diffuse interstitial infiltrates on the chest x-ray, fat in the urine, and/or renal failure occurs in some patients. Severe reduction in arterial oxygen content is common from widespread lung injury (ARDS). Cerebral fat embolism causes cerebral purpura, mainly in the white matter, due to capillary occlusion by fat globules. There is evidence that cases recognized and treated early have a better prognosis. Massive doses of glucocorticoids, reduction of ICP, and administration of positive-pressure ventilation with high end-expiratory pressures have been claimed to be useful. Heparin or intravenous alcohol are no longer recommended.

Cardiovascular changes   Acute head trauma may cause transient apnea and cardiac arrest. In the absence of overwhelming brain damage, recovery from the arrest is the rule. Subsequently, a sympathoadrenal discharge or raised ICP may cause systemic hypertension, either with the classically associated bradycardia (Cushing response) or, almost as frequently, with tachycardia. Cardiac arrhythmias are common, most notably sinus bradycardia, supraventricular tachycardias, nodal rhythm, and heart block. T-wave inversion and alterations in the ST segment may simulate subendocardial ischemia.

Neurogenic pulmonary edema is a form of ARDS in which the alveoli fill with fluid as they would in congestive heart failure but left ventricular end-diastolic pressure (measured by pulmonary capillary wedge pressure) is normal. A pulmonary vascular leak may be produced when a sudden shift of intravascular volume occurs from the systemic to pulmonary circulation, as occurs transiently with suddenly raised ICP, or there may be a direct neurogenic influence of hypothalamic function on the pulmonary microvasculature. Once

TABLE 376-1 Glasgow Coma Scale for head injury	
Eye opening (E):	
Spontaneous	4
To loud voice	3
To pain	2
Nil	1
Best motor response (M):	
Obeys	6
Localizes	5
Withdraws (flexion)	4
Abnormal flexion posturing	3
Extension posturing	2
Nil	1
Verbal response (V):	
Oriented	5
Confused, disoriented	4
Inappropriate words	3
Incomprehensible sounds	2
Nil	1

NOTE: Coma score = E + M + V. Patients scoring 3 or 4 have an 85 percent chance of dying or remaining vegetative, while scores above 11 indicate 5 to 10 percent likelihood of death or vegetative state and 85 percent chance of moderate disability or good recovery. Intermediate scores correlate with proportional chances of patients recovering.

the pulmonary vasculature has been damaged, an alveolar capillary leak may continue despite return of pulmonary vascular pressure to normal. The result is pulmonary edema with normal central venous and wedge pressures after the initial injury.

Hematologic complications   A large number of patients demonstrate a mild coagulopathy, and 5 to 10 percent have various degrees of disseminated intravascular coagulation, a harbinger of poor outcome. A correlation may exist between the severity of injury and the level of increased fibrin degradation products in blood. One cause of the coagulopathy is thought to be the release of highly thromboplastic material into the systemic circulation from the damaged brain.

PROGNOSIS   Extensive work by Jennet's group in Glasgow and from the Traumatic Coma Data Bank has provided data on the outcome in severe head injury (Table 376-1). Verbal output, eye opening, and the best motor response are important predictors of ultimate outcome. Eighty-five percent of patients with aggregate Glasgow Coma Scale scores of 3 or 4 die 24 h after injury. Yet a number of patients with a poor initial prognosis, including absent pupillary light responses, survive, suggesting that aggressive management is justified in virtually all patients. Patients below approximately 20 years of age, particularly children, may make remarkable recoveries after grave early neurologic signs. In one large study of severe head injury, 55 percent of children had a good outcome at 1 year, compared with 21 percent of adults. Increased intracranial pressure, older age, and signs of cisternal compression and midline shift on CT scan all have poor prognostic significance.

Evoked potentials also have prognostic value in head injury, and their accuracy probably exceeds clinical observations. Somatosensory evoked potentials are the most useful, with bilaterally absent cortical potentials (with more caudal potentials present) being predictive of death or a vegetative state in 85 to 95 percent of patients. Prediction of a good functional outcome in the presence of normal or mildly abnormal tests is less certain.

NEUROPSYCHOLOGICAL OUTCOME AFTER HEAD INJURY

Traumatic damage and cognitive sequelae of head injury both occur in a continuum, but most patients recover to normal after mild injury. There is probably a high rate of temporary inattention and memory and other subtle deficits after all but the mildest injuries. Attention has recently been directed toward a structural basis for the fatigue, dizziness, headache, and difficulty in concentration after mild injury,

termed the *postconcussion syndrome*. Based on experimental models, some investigators believe that subtle axonal shearing lesions or biochemical alterations account for these symptoms despite normal brain imaging, evoked potentials, and EEG. In moderate and severe trauma, neuropsychological changes are found routinely; however, formal testing often shows deficits that are not important in daily functioning. This is partly due to the type of testing and the nature of the control groups. Test scores tend to improve rapidly during the first 6 months after injury, then more slowly for years.

SPINAL CORD TRAUMA

Approximately 10,000 patients a year in the United States, mostly young and otherwise healthy, become paraplegic or quadriplegic because of spinal cord injuries. There are an estimated 200,000 quadriplegics in the country. The majority of cord injuries in civilian life result from damage to the surrounding vertebral column from fracture, dislocation, or both. Vertical compression with flexion is the main mechanism of injury in the thoracic cord, and hyperextension or flexion is the main cause of injury in the cervical cord. Preexisting spondylosis, a congenitally narrowed spinal canal, hypertrophied ligamentum flavum (see Chap. 381), and instability of the apophyseal joints of adjacent vertebrae from diseases such as rheumatoid arthritis predispose to severe spinal cord damage after minor degrees of injury.

PATHOPHYSIOLOGY AND PATHOLOGY OF CORD INJURY   Much damage to the spinal cord is due to secondary phenomena in the minutes and hours following injury. Even when a complete transverse myelopathy is evident immediately after impact, some secondary changes are avoidable, and the resultant damage may be reversible. The immediate injury causes pericapillary hemorrhages that coalesce and enlarge, particularly in the gray matter. Infarction of gray matter and early white matter edema are evident within 4 h of experimental blunt injury. Eight hours after injury there is global infarction at the injured level, and only at this point does necrosis of white matter and paralysis below the level of the lesion become irreversible. The necrosis and central hemorrhages enlarge to occupy one or two levels above and below the point of primary impact. Gliosis in these regions results in necrotic areas over several months and may cavitate causing a progressive syringomyelic syndrome.

The early phases of injury are associated with reduced regional blood flow from direct capillary damage and a more prolonged secondary ischemia. A number of interventions, including opiate antagonists, thyrotropin-releasing hormone, local cord cooling, dextran infusion, adrenergic blockade, and hyperbaric oxygen, have been of uncertain clinical usefulness. A large randomized trial has shown the benefit of high doses of methylprednisolone administered within 8 h of injury. This effect may result from inhibition of lipid peroxidation rather than a direct anti-inflammatory action. The critical factor for recoverable function is the time from injury to institution of any therapy. Complete axonal disruption from the immediate trauma or secondary phenomena precludes recovery.

TYPES OF SPINAL CORD INJURY AND THEIR MANAGEMENT   Any patient with severe head injury potentially has an associated instability of the spinal column. The care of such patients begins at the scene of the accident. The neck should be immobilized to prevent cord damage, and care should be taken during transport and during the physical and radiologic examinations to avoid neck extension or rotation and to prevent torsion-rotation of the thoracic spine. Blood pressure, respiratory status, and systemic injuries are attended to rapidly. Most patients can be intubated, if necessary, by blind nasotracheal technique without neck extension. High thoracic or cervical cord trauma regularly cause mild hypotension and bradycardia because of functional sympathectomy that responds to infusion of crystalloid or colloid (often corroborated by bilateral ptosis and miosis—Horner's syndrome).

The neurologic examination in the awake patient focuses on neck or back pain, diminished limb power, a sensory level on the trunk, and deep tendon reflexes, usually absent below the level of an acute cord injury. Injuries above C5 cause quadriplegia and respiratory failure. At C5 and C6 the biceps are also weak, and at C4 and C5 the deltoid and supra- and infraspinatus are weak. C7 injuries cause weakness of the triceps, wrist extensors, and forearm pronators. Injuries at T1 and below cause paraplegia; the precise level can be determined from the level of sensory loss. Compression in the low thoracic and lumbar region causes a conus medullaris or cauda equina syndrome (see Chap. 381). Cauda equina injuries are usually incomplete, involving peripheral nerves rather than spinal cord, and therefore are surgically remediable for longer periods after injury than spinal cord compression. In a comatose patient, absent reflexes, especially with small pupils or paradoxical breathing, signify a high cervical cord injury.

The next priority is to exclude a surgically remediable and potentially reversible cord compression due to dislocation of a vertebral body. Many traumatic myelopathies have no clearly associated fracture or dislocation. If x-rays suggest any aberration in the position of vertebrae, then reduction should be undertaken quickly. The role of myelography is controversial, but many neurosurgeons instill a few drops of water-soluble contrast media into the spinal subarachnoid space to demonstrate a block to the flow of CSF by CT scan or conventional myelography. Examination by MRI, when available, can be more useful. Decompression within 2 h of severe injury may lead to some recovery of cord function. With incomplete myelopathies, especially if the limbs are becoming progressively weaker, early decompression is strongly recommended, even many hours after injury. Surgical approaches to decompressing the spinal column depend on the specific nature of the injury. In complete transverse myelopathies beyond 6 to 12 h in duration, decompressive laminectomies are usually unsuccessful in restoring function.

The concerns with spinal column fractures, with or without myelopathy, are threefold: (1) detection of vertebral dislocations causing cord compression, (2) instability caused by fractures that will lead to misalignment and cord compression in the future, and (3) the proper treatment of fractures through the pedicles, facets, or vertebral bodies. Some fractures heal with immobilizaton and time, usually 2 to 3 months; others require surgical fusion to ensure stability.

Atlantoaxial dislocations can cause immediate death from respiratory failure, an event that may occur with no neurologic signs. Rheumatoid arthritis predisposes to this injury. Atlantooccipital dislocations occur predominantly in children and are almost always fatal. "Jefferson's fractures" are burst fractures of the ring of the atlas resulting from a force descending on the vertex of the skull as in diving accidents; they are usually asymptomatic. "Hangman's fractures" are produced by hyperextension and longitudinal distraction of the upper cervical spine, as occurs with penal hanging or striking the chin on a steering wheel in head-on collisions. These are usually fractures through the pedicles of C2 with subluxation anteriorly of C2 on C3. Traction reduction and immobilization allow proper healing.

Hyperflexion dislocation of the cervical vertebrae commonly causes traumatic quadriplegia. Occasionally, a markedly displaced injury is unassociated with neurologic dysfunction, presenting only with neck pain. In most cases, however, minor subluxation is associated with a severe neurologic deficit. Ligamentous disruption presumably allows compression of the cord at the moment of impact, but the vertebral bodies return closer to their original stations afterward. Therefore, any degree of subluxation must be treated as potentially unstable.

Compression fractures of the cervical spine can cause neurologic damage if a bone fragment is driven backward (burst fracture) into the spinal cord. "Teardrop fractures" with crushing of a vertebral body, leaving a fragment of bone anteriorly, are usually associated with ligamentous disruption and spinal instability. Single compression fractures of the thoracic spine are usually stable because the thoracic cage provides support, but they may be associated with anterior cord

compression and require decompression and stabilization with the insertion of metal rods.

Mild hyperextension injuries may cause only disruption of supporting ligamentous structures and be well tolerated. More severe injuries cause vertebral displacement and cord compression. The "central cord syndrome" is produced by brief compression of the cervical cord and disruption of the central gray matter, usually occurring in patients with an already narrow spinal canal, either congenitally or from cervical spondylosis. There is weakness of the arms, often with pinprick loss over the arms and shoulders, and relative sparing of leg power and sensation on the trunk and legs. Abnormality of bladder function is variable. The prognosis for recovery is good.

Thoracolumbar fractures are produced by impact in the high or midback, usually while the patient is bent over. Impingement on the spinal canal results in a complex combination of cauda equina and conus medullaris dysfunction. Pure lumbar fractures produce cauda equina compression. Myelography, MRI, or CT scan allows precise localization, and surgical decompression is usually recommended, even with complete deficits, because the potential for recovery of peripheral nerves is great.

The subsequent care of patients with spinal cord injury is best undertaken in specialized centers. General principles of medical and urologic management are discussed in Chap. 381.

REFERENCES

ADAMS JH et al: Diffuse brain damage of the immediate impact type. Brain 100:489, 1977

BAKAY L, GLASSAUER FE: *Head Injury*. Boston, Little, Brown, 1980

DACEY RG et al: Neurosurgical complications after apparently minor head injury. J Neurosurg 65:203, 1986

EISENBERG HM et al: Report of the Traumatic Coma Data Bank. J Neurosurg 75 (suppl) S1, 1991

GOLDSTEIN M: Traumatic brain injury: A silent epidemic. Ann Neurol 27:327, 1990

LANGFITT TW, GENARELLI TA: Can the outcome from head injury be improved? J Neurosurg 56:19, 1982

LEVIN HS et al: Neurobehavioral outcome following minor head injury: A three center study. J Neurosurg 66:234, 1987

REINUS WR et al: Practical selection criteria for noncontrast cranial computed tomography in patients with head trauma. Ann Emerg Med 22:1148, 1993

ROPPER AH et al (eds): *Neurological and Neurosurgical Intensive Care*, 2d ed. Baltimore, Aspen, 1988

RUFF RM et al: Predictors of outcome following severe head trauma: Follow-up data from the Traumatic Coma Data Bank. Brain Inj 7:101, 1993

STEIN SC et al: Delayed and progressive brain injury in closed-head trauma: Radiological demonstration. Neurosurgery 32:25, 1993

377 NUTRITIONAL AND METABOLIC DISEASES OF THE NERVOUS SYSTEM

MAURICE VICTOR / JOSEPH B. MARTIN

Included under this title are a large and diverse number of disorders of the nervous system. They fall readily into two groups—acquired and inherited. Here the emphasis will be on the *acquired* diseases, since they are essentially disorders of adult life and a major concern to both internists and neurologists. The *inherited* metabolic and nutritional diseases, on the other hand, are predominantly disorders of infancy and childhood and are more appropriately considered in a textbook of pediatrics (see also Chaps. 349 to 352). However, a small number of the inherited diseases permit survival to adolescence or early adult life or may even have their onset during these periods. These latter instances, which need to be differentiated from certain degenerative and acquired metabolic diseases, will be discussed briefly in this chapter and in others, to which the reader will be referred.

DISEASES DUE TO NUTRITIONAL DEFICIENCY

The general aspects of deficiency disease have been presented in Chap. 77, which should be reviewed as an introduction to the deficiency diseases of the nervous system. The term *deficiency*, used here in its strictest sense, designates those diseases or syndromes resulting from the *lack of an essential nutrient in the diet or from a conditioning factor that increases the need for that nutrient*. This category comprises the following neurologic diseases:

1 Wernicke's disease and Korsakoff's psychosis
2 "Alcoholic" cerebellar degeneration
3 Nutritional polyneuropathy
4 Pellagra
5 Deficiency amblyopia (nutritional optic neuropathy)
6 The syndrome of amblyopia, painful neuropathy, and orogenital dermatitis (Strachan's syndrome)
7 Subacute combined degeneration of the spinal cord (vitamin B_{12} deficiency)
8 Folic acid deficiency
9 Vitamin E deficiency

A number of general principles are applicable to all the above diseases. Of the known vitamin deficiencies, the B deficiencies (rarely, vitamin E deficiency) are most important in neurologic disease. Thiamine chloride, nicotinic acid, pyridoxine, pantothenic acid, and possibly folic acid and riboflavin each plays a role in carbohydrate metabolism, upon which the CNS depends for its principal source of energy. These vitamins function as coenzymes in the Krebs tricarboxylic acid cycle; in addition, thiamine is involved in the hexosemonophosphate shunt. Vitamin B_{12} is required for the conversion of methylmalonyl to succinyl coenzyme A and for the conversion of homocysteine to methionine.

Except for subacute combined degeneration of the spinal cord secondary to vitamin B_{12} deficiency and the ocular signs of Wernicke's disease resulting from thiamine deficiency, it is rarely possible to relate the deficiency diseases in humans to the lack of one particular vitamin. For example, polyneuropathy may result from any one of several vitamin deficiencies [thiamine chloride (vitamin B_1), pyridoxine (vitamin B_6), pantothenic acid, and probably B_{12}]. Pellagra, beriberi, and Strachan's syndrome are probably related to a deficiency of several vitamins. It is noteworthy that chronic pyridoxine (vitamin B_6) intoxication also causes a sensory polyneuropathy similar to that caused by its deficiency.

In the western world, deficiency diseases of the nervous system occur most often in the alcoholic population of large urban centers. Alcohol acts mainly by displacing food in the diet, but it also increases the demand for B vitamins, which are necessary to metabolize the carbohydrate furnished by alcohol itself, and it may impair the gastrointestinal absorption of vitamins. Dietary faddism, impaired absorption of dietary nutrients (as occurs in sprue or after gastric plication for the treatment of obesity or resection of the stomach and small bowel), and the use of certain drugs (e.g., isoniazid and hydralazine, which interfere with the enzymatic function of pyridoxine) account for a small number of cases of deficiency disease.

Each of the deficiency diseases may occur in pure form and will be so described. More often they occur in various combinations. Stated in another way, deficiency diseases usually involve both the central and peripheral nervous systems, an attribute that they share with few other categories of disease. Also, the examination of patients with deficiency disease frequently discloses nonneurologic signs of malnutrition such as general wasting, lesions of the skin and mucous membranes, and circulatory abnormalities.

WERNICKE'S DISEASE OR ENCEPHALOPATHY Wernicke originally described an illness of acute onset characterized by mental disturbance, paralysis of eye movements, and ataxia of gait. Swelling of the optic discs and retinal hemorrhages also were present, and there was a progressive depression of the state of consciousness, leading to death, so that a fatal outcome was at one time considered a universal feature of this disease. Wernicke observed focal vascular lesions in the gray matter around the third and fourth ventricles and aqueduct of Sylvius; he regarded them as inflammatory in nature and named the disease *acute superior hemorrhagic polioencephalitis*. Since Wernicke's time, views regarding this disease have undergone considerable modification.

Symptoms and signs   The most readily recognized abnormalities are the ocular motor signs, and it is difficult to make the clinical diagnosis without them. The usual abnormality is a weakness or paralysis of abduction (abducens palsy) which is invariably bilateral (though rarely symmetric) and accompanied by horizontal diplopia, strabismus, and nystagmus. Three types of nystagmus may occur, horizontal or vertical gaze–evoked nystagmus being the most frequent. A horizontal gaze–evoked nystagmus limited to the abducting eye is characteristic of internuclear ophthalmoplegia. Rarely, one sees an upbeat or downbeat nystagmus in the primary position, accompanied by oscillopsia. Each of these abnormalities may be present alone, but far more often a constellation of signs of disordered motility is present, including supranuclear paralysis of gaze. Horizontal gaze palsy is more frequent than vertical gaze palsy. Rarely an isolated paralysis of downgaze or an isolated paralysis of convergence or divergence occurs. In advanced disease there may be complete loss of ocular movement, and the pupils, which ordinarily are spared, may become miotic and nonreacting. Ptosis is rare. The parenteral administration of thiamine in the early stages results in dramatic improvement of ocular motility although horizontal nystagmus may persist indefinitely.

The *ataxia* affects stance and gait predominantly and may be so severe that the patient cannot stand or walk without support. With specific treatment the disorder of equilibrium improves, and the patient is left with a wide-based, uncertain gait. The mildest degree of ataxia is brought out only by heel-to-toe walking. In contrast to the gross disorder of locomotion, an intention (cerebellar) tremor of the limbs is relatively infrequent. The latter abnormality, when present, affects the legs more than the arms. Scanning speech is present only in isolated cases.

A derangement of mental function is found in about 90 percent of patients and takes one of several forms: (1) The most common is a *global confusional-apathetic state*, characterized by profound listlessness, inattentiveness, indifference to the surroundings, and disorientation. Unconsciousness or deep stupor as the initial abnormality is distinctly rare, but drowsiness is common. Spontaneous speech is minimal. Many questions directed to the patient go unanswered, or the patient may fall asleep while being questioned, a state from which he or she can be readily roused, however. Whatever questions the patient answers betray disorientation in time and place, misidentification of those nearby and an inability to grasp the meaning of the illness or immediate situation. Many of the patient's remarks are irrational and show no consistency from one moment to another. Under these circumstances, a more extensive evaluation of intellectual function is seldom possible. (2) Some patients show a disproportionate disorder of retentive memory, i.e., the Korsakoff amnesic state (see Chap. 25 and further on in this chapter). (3) A relatively small number of patients (less than 20 percent in our series) show the symptoms of alcohol withdrawal, either delirium tremens or a variant thereof.

The symptoms of Wernicke's disease may appear simultaneously and rather acutely, but more often ophthalmoplegia and/or ataxia precede the mental signs by days or weeks.

Wernicke's disease is usually associated with other manifestations of nutritional disease, both neurologic and nonneurologic. In more than 80 percent of patients, a *polyneuropathy* of varying degrees of severity is evident. Rarely, *amblyopia* or *spinal spastic ataxia* may be present. Many patients in the chronic stage demonstrate impaired olfactory discrimination, a defect that is most likely related to the diencephalic lesions (see below). Hypothermia may complicate acute Wernicke's disease.

Full-blown beriberi heart disease occurs only rarely in patients with Wernicke's disease, although indications of *disordered cardiovascular function* such as tachycardia, exertional dyspnea, postural hypotension, and minor electrocardiographic abnormalities are common. Occasionally, the patient dies suddenly, the mode of death suggesting "cardiovascular collapse." Wernicke's disease is characterized by a state of high cardiac output, which is out of proportion to the oxygen consumption. This is probably due to peripheral vasodilatation, which, in turn, may be related to thiamine deficiency. Postural hypotension and syncope are related to impaired function of the automatic nervous system, more specifically to a defect in sympathetic regulation.

Ancillary findings Vestibular function, as measured by the response to standard caloric testing, is always impaired bilaterally and more or less symmetrically in the acute stages of Wernicke's disease (*vestibular paresis*). The cerebrospinal fluid (CSF) is normal or shows only a modest elevation of protein content; protein values above 1.0 g/L (100 mg/dL) or a pleocytosis should always suggest the presence of a complicating illness. In untreated cases of Wernicke's disease, there is invariably an elevation of the *blood pyruvate* and a marked reduction in the *blood transketolase* (a thiamine-dependent enzyme of the hexose monophosphate shunt). Diffuse slowing of the EEG, mild to moderate in degree, occurs in about one-half of patients. On the other hand, total cerebral blood flow and cerebral oxygen and glucose consumption may be greatly reduced in the acute stages and persist for several weeks after the institution of treatment.

Course of the illness Death occurs in 15 to 20 percent of hospitalized patients and is usually due to hepatic failure or to a complicating infection (pneumonia, pulmonary tuberculosis, and septicemia being the most common).

Patients who recover do so in a characteristic manner. Ocular palsies may *begin to improve* within hours after the administration of thiamine and practically always within several days. Failure to respond in this manner raises doubts about the diagnosis of Wernicke's disease. Sixth nerve palsies, ptosis, and vertical gaze palsies recover completely, within a week or two in most cases, but vertical gaze–evoked nystagmus may persist for months. Horizontal gaze palsies recover completely as a rule, but a fine horizontal gaze–evoked nystagmus often remains as a permanent sequela of the disease.

Ataxia improves somewhat more slowly than the ocular motor abnormalities. Approximately half the patients recover incompletely and are left with a slow, shuffling, wide-based gait and an inability to walk tandem. The residual gait disturbance and horizontal nystagmus provide a means of identifying obscure and chronic cases of dementia as alcoholic-nutritional in origin. Vestibular function, as measured by caloric testing, improves at about the same rate as the ataxia of stance and gait, i.e., over a period of weeks or months, and recovery is usually but not always complete.

The symptoms of apathy, drowsiness, and confusion recede gradually, and as they do, the *defect in retentive memory and learning* stands out more clearly (*Korsakoff's psychosis*; see Chap. 25). It needs to be emphasized that Wernicke's disease and Korsakoff's psychosis are not separate diseases, but that the changing ocular and ataxic signs and the transformation of the global confusion state into an amnesic syndrome are successive stages in the recovery of a single disease process. Stated in another way, Korsakoff's psychosis is the psychic component of Wernicke's disease. Hence the symptom complex should be called *Wernicke's disease* when the amnesic state is not evident and the *Wernicke-Korsakoff syndrome* when both the ocular-ataxic and amnesic symptoms are present.

The outcome of the Korsakoff amnesic state varies. Complete or almost complete recovery occurs in less than 20 percent of patients. In the remainder, recovery is slow and incomplete. Depending on the severity of the residual symptoms, the patient may or may not be able to lead a supervised existence out of a hospital. The residual mental state is characterized by large gaps in memory, usually without

confabulation, and an inability of the patient to sort out events in their proper temporal sequence. This late stage of the disease, when the ocular and ataxic signs have receded or are not recognized, is often loosely referred to as "alcoholic deteriorated state" or "alcoholic dementia."

Pathologic findings In patients who die in the acute stages of Wernicke-Korsakoff disease there are symmetrically placed lesions in the paraventricular regions of the thalamus and hypothalamus, the mammillary bodies, periaqueductal region of the midbrain, floor of the fourth ventricle, and anterosuperior folia of the cerebellum, particularly of the vermis. Lesions are invariably found in the mammillary bodies and less consistently in the other areas. Microscopically, the principal change consists of varying degrees of necrosis of parenchymal structures. Many nerve cells and fibers are destroyed; others remain intact and are seen against a background of reactive glial elements, both astrocytes and microgliocytes. The blood vessels are prominent, owing to adventitial and endothelial proliferation. Hemorrhagic lesions are present in a small proportion of cases and are usually of recent origin. The oculomotor and vestibular nuclei are regularly involved, but to a lesser degree.

Clinical-pathologic correlations The ocular motor signs are attributable to lesions in the brainstem affecting the abducens nuclei and eye movement centers in the pons and rostral midbrain (see Chap. 19). The lesions of the vestibular nuclei are probably responsible for the loss of caloric responses and the gross abnormality of equilibrium that characterize the initial stage of the disease. The lack of significant destruction of nerve cells in these lesions accounts for the rapid improvement in oculomotor and vestibular function.

The persistent ataxia of stance and gait is related to the loss of neurons in the superior vermis of the cerebellum; extension of the lesion into the anterior parts of the anterior lobes accounts for the ataxia of individual movements of the legs. These cerebellar lesions are indistinguishable from those of so-called *alcoholic cerebellar degeneration* (see below).

The amnesic defect is related to lesions in the diencephalon, more specifically to those in the medial dorsal nuclei of the thalami. Lesions in the mammillary bodies are probably not critical in respect to memory function since they are found in patients with Wernicke's disease who had shown no disorder of memory during life.

Etiology and pathogenesis The specific factor responsible for most, if not all, of the symptoms of the Wernicke-Korsakoff syndrome is a deficiency of thiamine. The marked sensitivity of the ocular abnormalities to the administration of thiamine accounts for their rapid abatement after the ingestion of a meal or two. The quality of prompt reversibility indicates that the ocular signs are due to a biochemical abnormality and not to irreversible structural changes. On the other hand, the slow and incomplete recovery of the memory defect suggests that this symptom is due to irreversible structural changes, presumably in the medial dorsal nuclei.

The mechanism whereby thiamine deficiency causes brain lesions is not fully understood. Thiamine is a cofactor for several enzymes, including transketolase, pyruvate dehydrogenase, and α-ketoglutarate dehydrogenase. Thiamine deficiency produces a diffuse decrease in cerebral glucose utilization, and lesions in thiamine-deficient experimental animals are diminished by antagonists that block N-methyl-D-aspartate–preferring glutamic acid receptors. This latter finding suggests that the neurotoxicity of thiamine deficiency may be mediated by excitotoxicity evoked by glutamic acid release (see also Chaps. 364 and 370).

The selective vulnerability of certain periventricular regions to a deficiency of thiamine also remains to be explained. McEntee and Mair have pointed out that the lesions lie in the monoamine-containing pathways and have presented evidence that 3-methoxy-4-hydroxyphenylglycol (MHPG), the primary brain metabolite of norepinephrine, is decreased in the CSF of alcoholic patients with Korsakoff's psychosis; moreover, the administration of clonidine, an alpha$_2$-adrenergic agonist, seemed to improve the memory disorder in these patients. These authors have theorized that damage to the ascending norepinephrine-containing neurons in the brainstem and diencephalon is the basis for the amnesia.

The topography of the lesions caused by thiamine deficiency has been studied in rhesus monkeys. Witt and Goldman-Rakic found that the severity and number of brain nuclei affected are related to the duration and number of bouts of thiamine deficiency.

Treatment of the Wernicke-Korsakoff syndrome Wernicke's disease represents a medical emergency, and its recognition demands the immediate administration of thiamine. A delay of a few hours may be crucial in determining whether the patient with ocular and ataxic signs will be prevented from developing an amnesic state and whether the patient with early Korsakoff changes will be restored to a state of mental competency. Although 2 to 3 mg of thiamine may modify the ocular signs, much larger doses are needed to replenish the thiamine stores—50 mg intravenously and 50 mg intramuscularly, the latter dose being repeated each day until the patient resumes a normal diet. The other B vitamins may be given by mouth in the dosages outlined in Chap. 77. If the patient cannot or will not eat, parenteral feeding and administration of B vitamins become necessary.

A particular danger attends the treatment of the severely depleted alcoholic patient with intravenous glucose solutions. Such infusions may exhaust the patient's reserve of B vitamins and either precipitate Wernicke's disease in a previously unaffected patient or cause a rapid worsening of an early form of the disease. For this reason, B vitamins must be administered to all alcoholic patients requiring parenteral glucose. The cardiovascular status of each patient should be monitored carefully. Since these patients are confused and forgetful, they must be supervised continually.

A special problem arises when the patient recovers from the acute phase of the illness and the amnesic psychosis becomes prominent. The disposition of the patient to family, nursing home, or mental institution should be made on the basis of the severity of the mental illness as well as the capacity of the family unit and social circumstances.

NUTRITIONAL POLYNEUROPATHY (See also Chaps. 77 and 383) In the United States, nutritional polyneuropathy is usually a disease of alcoholics. As mentioned above, it is present in most patients with the Wernicke-Korsakoff syndrome, but it often occurs as the sole manifestation of deficiency disease. The peripheral neuropathy of alcoholics ("alcoholic polyneuropathy") does not differ in any fundamental way from neuropathic beriberi. The clinical features of nutritional polyneuropathy and its identity with beriberi are discussed in Chaps. 77 and 383. A deficiency of thiamine chloride, pyridoxine, pantothenic acid, vitamin B_{12}, and perhaps folic acid has been demonstrated in individual cases to cause nutritional polyneuropathy. In the alcoholic patient it is usually not possible to incriminate a particular vitamin.

"ALCOHOLIC" CEREBELLAR DEGENERATION This is the term applied to a common, stereotyped, nonfamilial form of cerebellar ataxia that occurs on a background of prolonged ingestion of alcohol. Usually the symptoms evolve in subacute fashion, i.e., over several weeks or months, sometimes more rapidly. In some patients the symptoms are present in mild but stable form and worsen after an attack of pneumonia or delirium tremens.

The signs are those of cerebellar dysfunction, affecting stance and gait predominantly. The legs are involved more severely than the arms, and nystagmus and speech disturbances occur infrequently. Once established, the signs change very little, although some improvement of gait may follow the cessation of drinking, due probably to improvement in general nutrition and recovery from an associated polyneuropathy.

The pathologic changes consist of degeneration of varying severity of all the neurocellular elements of the cerebellar cortex, particularly of the Purkinje cells, with a striking topographic restriction to the anterior and superior aspects of the vermis and adjacent parts of the anterior lobes of the cerebellum. The disorder of stance and gait is related to the lesion in the vermis, and the ataxia of the limbs to the involvement of the anterior lobes. A similar clinical-pathologic

syndrome is observed occasionally in nutritionally depleted nonalcoholic patients.

CNS disorders in alcoholics not associated with vitamin deficiency Alcoholics are vulnerable to a number of CNS disorders that are attributable neither to nutritional deficiency nor to trauma. There appears to be an increased incidence of hypertension in alcoholics and probably of strokes, both ischemic infarction and spontaneous subarachnoid hemorrhage. Alcoholics as a group also show dilatation of the lateral ventricles and widening of sulci on CT scans or MRI. The nature of these changes is obscure. They do not correlate with mental abnormality, nor do they represent cerebral atrophy insofar as partial and sometimes complete reversal occur with sustained abstinence. Some believe that alcohol can cause intellectual deterioration separate from effects due to nutritional deficiency, but an entity of "alcoholic dementia" has never been established on the basis of clinical and neuropathologic studies. A syndrome of progressive myelopathy occurring in alcoholics also has been described. Such patients are said to show no evidence of nutritional deficiency (B_{12} or folic acid) or of liver disease. The nature of the spinal cord disease is unknown, and a causal relationship to the toxic effects of alcohol remains to be established.

PELLAGRA This disease is described in Chap. 77. Neurologic manifestations are quite diverse. Pellagra is essentially an encephalopathy, although involvement of the spinal cord and peripheral nerves may occur. The early mental symptoms—insomnia, fatigue, anxiety, nervousness, irritability, and depression—may be mistaken for a psychiatric disorder. However, as the disease advances, slowing and inefficiency of mental processes and impairment of memory become apparent. Pellagra may not only cause psychiatric manifestations but occasionally also may result from them because certain mental illnesses, including alcoholism, cause anorexia and dietary deficiency.

The spinal cord involvement in pellagra has not been clearly delineated, perhaps because the mental state of the patients has precluded accurate testing. In general, there is both posterior and lateral column involvement, predominantly the former. Neuropathic signs are difficult to distinguish from other types of nutritional polyneuropathy. Other manifestations such as tremor, extrapyramidal rigidity, suck and grasp reflexes, and coma (referred to in the past as "nicotinic acid–deficiency encephalopathy") have been included in the pellagra syndrome on uncertain grounds, as have various disorders of the special senses.

A *spastic spinal syndrome*, apart from the other symptoms and signs of pellagra, may be a rare manifestation of nutritional deficiency. The chief signs are spastic weakness of the legs with absent abdominal and increased tendon reflexes, clonus, and extensor plantar responses. These signs are usually accompanied by other manifestations of nutritional deficiency, such as Wernicke's disease, amblyopia, and peripheral neuropathy.

Pathologic features The distinctive neuropathologic changes in pellagra are most readily discerned in the large Betz cells of the motor cortex, although the same changes are seen to a lesser extent in the smaller pyramidal cells of the cerebral cortex and cells of the basal ganglia, cranial motor and dentate nuclei, and anterior horns of the spinal cord. The affected cells appear swollen and rounded with eccentric nuclei and loss of Nissl staining. This *central neuritis of pellagra*, as it is called, probably represents a primary affection of the motor cell and not a reaction to interruption of the corticospinal tracts. The spinal cord lesions take the form of a symmetric degeneration of the dorsal columns, especially the fasciculus gracilis, and to a lesser extent of the corticospinal tracts. The posterior column degeneration is probably secondary to degeneration of specific dorsal root ganglion cells.

DEFICIENCY AMBLYOPIA (NUTRITIONAL OPTIC NEUROPATHY, "TOBACCO-ALCOHOL AMBLYOPIA") These terms refer to a characteristic form of visual impairment that complicates nutritional deficiency. The lesion responsible for the visual loss lies in the optic nerve, more or less confined to the zone of the papillomacular bundle; the cornea and other parts of the refractive mechanism are uninvolved.

The main symptoms are dimness or blurring of vision for near and distant objects and impairment of color vision, which worsens progressively and insidiously for several days or weeks. In addition to a reduction in visual acuity, examination discloses the presence of bilateral and roughly symmetric central or centrocecal scotomas, which are larger for colored than for white test objects. Pallor of the temporal portion of the optic disc is observed in some cases. Untreated, this condition progresses to irreversible optic atrophy.

Deficiency amblyopia was common among prisoners of war in the Far East. Although this form of amblyopia had previously been described in association with beriberi (due to thiamine deficiency) and pellagra (due to niacin deficiency), the peak incidence among prisoners coincided with neither of these syndromes but with the syndrome of orogenital dermatitis and ''burning feet'' (Strachan's syndrome, see below).

In the United States, most, if not all, of the cases of retrobulbar neuropathy attributed to the toxic effects of alcohol or tobacco—so-called tobacco-alcohol amblyopia—are of nutritional origin. Optic neuropathy may occur as the only manifestation of vitamin deficiency, but often it is combined with other evidence of nutritional deficiency, such as peripheral neuropathy and the Wernicke-Korsakoff syndrome.

Although the nutritional origin of this type of amblyopia has been established, a specific vitamin deficiency can rarely be identified. Observations in both humans and experimental animals indicate that a deficiency of thiamine (vitamin B_1), vitamin B_{12}, or perhaps riboflavin may cause lesions in the optic nerves. The notion that cyanide or other substances in tobacco smoke have a toxic effect on the optic nerves is not supported by experimental data.

Treatment consists of the administration of a balanced diet, supplemented with B vitamins, and the interdiction of alcohol where this is the cause of nutritional deficiency.

SYNDROME OF AMBLYOPIA, PAINFUL NEUROPATHY, AND OROGENITAL DERMATITIS (STRACHAN'S SYNDROME) This is a neurologic syndrome that is probably nutritional in origin but which does not fit readily within the boundaries of beriberi or pellagra. Strachan attributed the disorder to malaria. Originally known as ''Jamaican neuritis,'' the syndrome occurs among the undernourished populations of many tropical countries. Large numbers of patients with this syndrome also were observed in the besieged population of Madrid during the Spanish Civil War and among prisoners of war during World War II in the Middle and Far East. In the United States, this syndrome is observed occasionally in alcoholic patients.

Strachan's syndrome is essentially a disorder of the peripheral and optic nerves. The peripheral nerve disorder results in sensory symptoms and signs (painful paresthesias of the feet, loss of superficial and deep sensation, and ataxia); foot drop and muscle weakness occur rarely. Failing vision, which may go on to complete blindness and pallor of the optic discs, may also occur. Deafness and vertigo are rare; in these respects the syndrome differs from beriberi. Along with the neurologic signs there may be an *orogenital syndrome* consisting of stomatoglossitis, corneal degeneration, and genital dermatitis.

The few pathologic studies of this syndrome show damage to the papillomacular bundle in the optic nerve, and a loss of myelinated fibers in the posterior columns (fasciculus gracilis) of the spinal cord, the latter indicating degeneration of the central processes of the large bipolar sensory neurons of the lumbosacral spinal ganglia. Degeneration of the peripheral processes of small sensory neurons probably accounts for the loss of pain and temperature sensation.

SUBACUTE COMBINED DEGENERATION (SCD) OF THE SPINAL CORD (See also Chap. 77) This term designates the spinal cord disease that is due to vitamin B_{12} deficiency. The white matter of the brain, optic nerves, and peripheral nerves also may be affected but far less often than the spinal cord. The neurologic and hematologic manifestations (pernicious anemia) of vitamin B_{12} deficiency are distinctive insofar as they are caused not by a lack of this vitamin in the food but by an inability to transfer minute amounts of this nutrient across the intestinal mucosa. Such a nutritional disorder is referred to as a *conditioned deficiency*, since it depends on the lack of an intrinsic factor in the gastric secretions (see Chap. 304). Rarely, neurologic symptoms due to vitamin B_{12} deficiency occur in patients with disease of the distal small intestine (Crohn's disease, lymphoma) or after surgical resection.

Clinical manifestations Neurologic symptoms are present in the majority of patients with vitamin B_{12} deficiency. The patient first notices general weakness and paresthesias, consisting of tingling, ''pins-and-needles'' feelings, or other vaguely described sensations in the distal parts of the limbs; either the lower or the upper extremities may be involved first. The paresthesias tend to be persistent, to progress steadily, and to be the source of much distress. As the illness progresses, the gait becomes unsteady, and movements of the limbs, especially the legs, become stiff and awkward.

Early in the course of the illness, when only paresthesias are present, there may be no objective signs. Later, the neurologic examination discloses a disorder of the posterior and lateral columns of the spinal cord, predominantly the former. Loss of vibration sense, the most consistent sign, is more pronounced in the legs than in the arms, and frequently it extends over the trunk. Position sense is involved to a somewhat lesser extent. The motor defects are usually limited to the legs and include weakness, spasticity, changes in the tendon reflexes, clonus, and extensor plantar responses. At first the patellar and Achilles reflexes may be diminished, increased, or absent. With treatment, the reflexes may return to normal or become hyperactive. The gait at first is predominantly ataxic, later ataxic and spastic. If the disease remains untreated, an ataxic paraplegia with variable degrees of spasticity and contracture develops.

A loss of superficial sensation below a segmental level on the trunk, implicating the spinothalamic tracts, occurs rarely, but such a finding should always suggest the possibility of some other disease of the spinal cord. More often the sensory defect takes the form of a blunting of tactile, painful, and thermal sensation over the distal segments of the lower limbs, implicating the peripheral nerves, but such findings are uncommon.

The nervous system involvement in vitamin B_{12} deficiency is characteristically, though not perfectly, symmetric. A definite asymmetry of motor or sensory findings, maintained over a period of weeks or months, should always cast doubt on the diagnosis.

Mental signs are frequent, ranging from irritability, apathy, somnolence, suspiciousness, and emotional instability to a marked confusional or depressive psychosis, or even to intellectual deterioration. Optic neuropathy with impaired acuity and cecocentral scotomas has been reported with all forms of vitamin B_{12} deficiency; variable improvement in acuity occurs once systemic vitamin B_{12} is administered. Dementia and amblyopia are relatively uncommon manifestations of vitamin B_{12} deficiency, but each may occasionally be the initial manifestation of the disease.

Pathology and pathogenesis The pathologic process takes the form of a diffuse, though uneven, degeneration of the white matter of the spinal cord and sometimes of the brain. At first there is swelling of myelin sheaths, characterized by separation of the myelin lamellae and formation of intramyelinic vacuoles. This is followed by a coalescence of small foci of tissue destruction into larger ones, giving the tissue a vacuolated appearance. The myelin sheaths and the axis cylinders are both affected, the former perhaps earlier and to a greater extent than the latter. Astrocytic gliosis is minimal in the early lesions, but in the more chronic ones gliosis is pronounced. The changes begin in the posterior columns of the lower cervical and upper thoracic cord and spread from this region up and down the cord, as well as forward into the lateral columns. The lesions are not limited to specific systems of fibers within the posterior and lateral funiculi but are scattered irregularly through the white matter. The changes in the optic nerves are similar to those in other types of nutritional neuropathy, i.e., a bilateral degeneration of myelinated fibers in the territory of the papillomacular bundles.

The *pathogenesis* of the nervous system lesions in vitamin B_{12} deficiency is not fully known. Impairment of DNA synthesis probably accounts for the hematologic abnormalities and the production of megaloblasts; however, since neurons do not divide, this mechanism cannot be invoked to explain the central nervous system changes. One of the better-understood functions of vitamin B_{12} is its role as a coenzyme in the methylmalonyl CoA mutase reaction. Impairment of this metabolic step may lead to the production of abnormal fatty acids, which are important building blocks of cell membranes and of myelin. However, Carmel and his colleagues have described a hereditary form of cobalamin deficiency, in which methylmalonyl CoA mutase activity was normal despite the presence of typical neurologic abnormalities. These authors attributed the neurologic abnormalities to an impairment of methionine synthase activity. These and other hypotheses have been reviewed by Beck.

Diagnosis and treatment The chief obstacle to early diagnosis is the lack of parallelism between the hematologic and neurologic signs. This is particularly true of patients who have received folic acid, which serves to maintain a hematologic remission for an indefinite period while the neurologic signs worsen, often to an irreversible stage. Under these circumstances the most reliable diagnostic procedures are the measurement of the serum B_{12} concentration and the two-stage Schilling test (see Chap. 304). In rare instances, even these tests may be inconclusive, in which case the finding of high serum concentrations of cobalamin metabolites—methylmalonic acid and homocysteine—may be diagnostically useful.

The treatment of the neurologic manifestations of vitamin B_{12} deficiency differs in no way from the treatment of the hematologic ones. Patients whose vitamin B_{12} stores have been depleted require large doses of cobalamin—1000 μg intramuscularly each day during hospitalization, then weekly for a month, and then monthly for the remainder of the patient's life.

The most important factor influencing the *response to treatment* is the duration of the neurologic symptoms. Recovery may be complete if therapy is instituted within a few weeks of their onset. For this reason, SCD and the other neurologic complications of vitamin B_{12} deficiency represent medical emergencies. If symptoms have been present for longer than a month or two, only partial recovery can be expected, and in long-standing cases the best that can be expected is the arrest of progression of the disease.

FOLIC ACID DEFICIENCY Despite the frequent occurrence of folic acid deficiency, its role in the pathogenesis of nervous system disease has not been established beyond doubt. The polyneuropathies that occasionally complicate sprue and other malabsorption syndromes and the chronic administration of phenytoin have been attributed, on uncertain grounds, to folate deficiency. With respect to folate deficiency and spinal cord disease, the data are equally limited. Cases have been described in which the neurologic signs of subacute combined degeneration were attributed to folic acid deficiency (see Pincus). In these cases there was no evidence of vitamin B_{12} deficiency, but there was a resolution of both the hematologic and neurologic abnormalities after the institution of folate therapy.

VITAMIN E DEFICIENCY A rare neurologic disorder of childhood, consisting essentially of a spinocerebellar degeneration in association with a polyneuropathy and pigmentary retinopathy, has been related to vitamin E deficiency developing after prolonged intestinal malabsorption (Satya-Murti et al.; Sokol et al.). The same mechanism has been proposed to explain the neurologic disorders that sometimes complicate abetalipoproteinemia, fibrocystic disease, and extensive intestinal resections (Harding et al.). Vitamin E deficiency also occurs in young children with chronic cholestatic hepatobiliary disease. Ataxia, loss of tendon reflexes, ophthalmoparesis, proximal muscle weakness with elevated serum creatine phosphokinase, and decreased sensation are the usual manifestations. These symptoms are referable to parts of the nervous system and musculature known to be involved in animals deprived of vitamin E—degeneration of Clarke's columns, spinocerebellar tracts, posterior columns, nuclei of Goll and Burdach, and sensory roots (Nelson et al.). In affected children, neurologic function improves after the long-term correction of vitamin E deficiency.

NEUROLOGIC SYNDROMES CAUSED BY HYPERVITAMINOSIS

Acute toxicity with vitamin A causes symptoms of headache, dizziness, irritability, and drowsiness. Chronic hypervitaminosis A can give rise to chronic increased intracranial pressure or pseudotumor cerebri (see Chap. 77).

The ingestion of pyridoxine in excessive amounts (2 g or more daily) can cause a sensory neuropathy characterized clinically by progressive ataxia, impairment of position and vibration sense, and loss of deep tendon reflexes. Motor function is preserved. The syndrome is reversible with discontinuation of pyridoxine.

ACQUIRED (SECONDARY) METABOLIC DISEASES OF THE NERVOUS SYSTEM

In this important category of neurologic disease, disturbance of cerebral function is due to disease in some other organ system—heart (and circulation), lungs (and respiration), kidneys, liver, endocrine glands, and possibly pancreas. Each of these diseases affects the nervous system in somewhat different ways.

ANOXIC-ISCHEMIC ENCEPHALOPATHY This common and often disastrous condition is caused by a lack of oxygen to the brain, resulting from hypotension or respiratory failure. Sometimes both are responsible, and one cannot say which predominates—hence the ambiguous reference, in clinical records, to "cardiorespiratory failure." The conditions that most often lead to anoxic-ischemic encephalopathy are (1) myocardial infarction; (2) cardiac arrest; (3) hemorrhage, with shock and circulatory collapse; in these situations vascular supply to the brain is compromised before respiration; (4) shock; (5) suffocation (from drowning, strangulation, aspiration of vomitus or blood, compression of the trachea by hemorrhage or a surgical pack, or a foreign body in the trachea); (6) diseases that paralyze the muscles of respiration or compromise the CNS respiratory drive (trauma, vascular disease of the brain, epilepsy), causing respiratory failure followed by cardiac failure; and (7) carbon monoxide (CO) poisoning. In circumstances (4) through (7) respiration fails first and then cardiovascular functions. Hypoxia alone may induce different clinicopathologic consequences than a combination of hypoxia and hypoperfusion (ischemia).

Clinical manifestations Mild degrees of hypoxia cause inattentiveness, impaired judgment, and motor incoordination but have no lasting effects. With severe hypoxia or anoxia, as occurs with cardiac arrest, consciousness is lost within seconds, but recovery will be complete if breathing, oxygenation of blood, and cardiac action are restored within 3 to 5 min. If anoxia persists beyond this time, there is serious and permanent injury to the brain, particularly to those parts in which the efficiency of circulation is marginal (globus pallidus, cerebellum, hippocampus, and the "borderzone regions" of the parietooccipital lobes). Clinically, it is difficult to judge the precise degree of hypoxia-ischemia, since slight heart action or an imperceptible blood pressure may serve to maintain the circulation to some extent. Hence some individuals have made an excellent recovery after cerebral anoxia that allegedly lasted 8 to 10 min or longer. *An important clinical rule is that degrees of hypoxia that at no time abolish consciousness rarely if ever cause permanent damage to the nervous system.* P_{O_2} as low as 2.7 kPa (20 mmHg) is well tolerated if it develops gradually and blood pressure is normal. Also, subjects who demonstrate intact brainstem function (as indicated by normal ciliospinal, oculovestibular, and pupillary light responses and intact doll's-head eye movements) usually have a better outlook for recovery of consciousness and perhaps all their faculties. Conversely, absence of these reflexes and the presence of pupils that are persistently fixed to light indicate a grave prognosis.

Extreme or sustained global ischemia causes brain death (see Chap. 26). Immediately after resuscitation from cardiorespiratory arrest, the physical findings may suggest brain death (dilated, unresponsive pupils, absent brainstem reflexes and respiration, and isoelectric EEG), yet full recovery may occur. However, persistence of the unresponsive state for more than an hour or two invariably carries a poor prognosis. The diagnosis of brain death must be made with caution because anesthesia, drug intoxication, and hypothermia also may cause deep coma, absent brainstem reflexes, and an isoelectric EEG but permit recovery. The problem of brain death is being constantly brought to public attention because of ethical and moral issues that surround the question of discontinuing supportive medical therapy.

Issues of management are most difficult in the patient who has suffered severe anoxic encephalopathy, but one that falls short of causing "brain death." Often breathing and heart action have stabilized by the time the patient is seen by a physician. Neurologic evaluation shows the patient to be profoundly comatose, with eyes slightly divergent and motionless but with reactive pupils, flaccid or intensely rigid limbs, and diminished tendon reflexes. Within a few minutes after cardiac action and breathing have been restored, generalized convulsions and isolated or grouped twitches of muscles (myoclonus) may supervene. Decerebrate or decorticate postures may be present or can be brought out by pinching the limbs, and bilateral Babinski signs can be evoked. Death may occur in the first 24 to 48 h, in a setting of rising temperature, deepening coma, and circulatory collapse. Or, with somewhat lesser degrees of injury, in which the cerebral and cerebellar cortices are partly or completely destroyed but brainstem-spinal structures remain intact, the individual may survive in a state referred to as "irreversible coma" or "persistent vegetative state" (see Chap. 26). The latter patients remain mute, unresponsive, and unaware of their environment for weeks, months, or even years. Criteria that accurately predict the outcome of anoxic encephalopathy early in the comatose period have been developed (see Chap. 26). If intoxication can be excluded, the presence of fixed dilated pupils and paralysis of eye movement for 24 to 48 h, along with marked slowing of the EEG, usually signifies irreversible cerebral damage. Deep coma of this type, lasting more than a few days, is rarely attended by full recovery.

Patients with lesser degrees of injury improve after a period of coma. Consciousness is regained, and then varying degrees of confusion, visual agnosia, extrapyramidal rigidity, or movement disorder (action or intention myoclonus, choreoathetosis, cerebellar ataxia) become manifest. Some of these patients pass quickly through this posthypoxic phase and proceed to make full recovery; others are left with permanent neurologic sequelae. The *posthypoxic syndromes* observed most frequently are (1) *persistent coma or stupor*, and, with lesser degrees of cerebral injury, (2) *dementia*, with or without extrapyramidal signs, (3) *visual agnosia*, (4) *parkinsonism*, (5) *choreoathetosis*, (6) *cerebellar ataxia*, (7) *intention or action myoclonus*, and (8) the *Korsakoff amnesic state*. *Seizures* may continue to be a problem but are uncommon.

A relatively uncommon and unexplained phenomenon is *delayed postanoxic encephalopathy*. Initial improvement, which appears to be complete, is followed after a variable period of time (several days to a week or longer) by a relapse, characterized by apathy, confusion, irritability, and occasionally agitation or mania. A few patients have recovered from this second episode, but in most the neurologic syndrome is a progressive one, with shuffling gait, diffuse rigidity and spasticity, coma, and death after 1 to 2 weeks. Postmortem examination of these patients has shown the major abnormality to be widespread cerebral demyelination. Even more rare is a syndrome in which a period of hypoxia is followed by a slow, deteriorating state, affecting basal ganglia more than cerebral cortex and white matter and progressing for weeks to months until the patient is mute, rigid, and helpless.

The essential *mechanism* in hypoxic encephalopathy is a neuronal lack of oxygen and an arrest of all aerobic metabolic processes necessary to sustain the Krebs tricarboxylic cycle and the electron transport system. Lactic acid accumulates in the tissues. The pathophysiology of delayed progression is not understood. Recent experimental observations suggest that excitatory neurotransmitters, and particularly glutamate, released from hypoxic-ischemic brain tissue

are instrumental in the rapid destruction of neurons (see Choi and Rothman). The restoration of oxygen to the ischemic brain, e.g., following cardiac arrest, may result in reperfusion injury probably related to the effects of oxygen-derived free radicals upon membrane phospholipids.

Diagnosis The diagnosis depends on the history of a hypoxic-ischemic event and evidence of (1) reduced oxygenation of arterial blood [P_{O_2} < 5.3 kPa (40 mmHg)], (2) CO intoxication (indicated by its spectroscopic band or cherry red color of the skin for a few minutes to hours after the episode), (3) blood pressures below 9.3 kPa (70 mmHg) systolic, or (4) cardiac arrest. The typical clinical sequence of events after a possible hypoxic-ischemic episode has terminated as outlined above, confirm the diagnosis. Renal damage (anuria) and myocardial infarction also may have occurred and provide corroborative evidence of the hypoxic-ischemic event.

Treatment The treatment of anoxic encephalopathy is directed mainly at the prevention of a critical degree of hypoxic injury. After a clear airway is secured, artificial respiration, external thoracic cardiac massage, the use of a cardiac defibrillator or pacemaker, and open chest surgery all have their place, and every second counts in their prompt utilization. Once cardiac and pulmonary function are restored, there is no evidence that any pharmacologic measure enhances recovery. Barbiturates, glucocorticoids, dimethyl sulfoxide, and benzodiazepines have been given without clear proof of benefit. A small proportion of patients develop diffuse brain swelling after cardiac arrest; this condition is more common in children. This is evidenced by compression of the lateral ventricles and cisterns on CT scan or by very high lumbar CSF pressure. Seizures should be controlled by anticonvulsants. Posthypoxic myoclonus may respond to oral administration of clonazepam 1.5 to 10 mg/d. Other details of treatment are considered in Chap. 26.

HYPERCAPNIC ENCEPHALOPATHY Chronic emphysema and fibrosing lung disease and, in rare instances, an inadequacy of central respiratory drive lead to chronic respiratory acidosis, with an elevation of P_{CO_2} and a reduction in arterial P_{O_2}. Secondary polycythemia and cor pulmonale are common sequelae of these pulmonary diseases.

Clinical manifestations The clinical syndrome consequent on hypercapnia (and hypoxia) consists of generalized or bilateral frontal or occipital headache, often intense and persistent for hours; papilledema; mental dullness, drowsiness, confusion, stupor, and coma; a fast-frequency action tremor and coarse twitching of all the muscles, which are in a state of sustained contraction; and an inability to maintain a fixed posture or interruption of a voluntary movement because of brief lapses of sustained muscle contraction (asterixis). Intermittent drowsiness, indifference and inattention to the environment, reduction of psychomotor activity, imperception of the sequence of events, and forgetfulness constitute the more subtle manifestations of this syndrome.

In fully developed cases, the CSF is under increased pressure, P_{CO_2} may exceed 10 kPa (75 mmHg), and oxygen saturation of the arterial blood ranges from 85 to 40 percent. The EEG reveals slow activity in the delta and theta range, sometimes bilaterally synchronous. The cerebral disorder is said to be due to CO_2 narcosis, but the biochemical mechanism is not known. The danger of administering morphine or sedatives, which blunt the respiratory drive (already depressed by the CO_2 retention), or inhaled O_2, which removes the sole stimulus (low P_{O_2}) to the respiratory center, is now widely recognized.

Treatment Forced ventilation with an intermittent positive-pressure respirator, treatment of heart failure with digitalis and diuretics, venesection to reduce the viscosity of the blood, and antibiotics to combat pulmonary infection are the most effective therapeutic measures. If stupor or coma persists, the arterial O_2 level should be rechecked; it may be critically reduced, and it needs to be raised by controlled O_2 administration to a point [6.7 to 7.3 kPa (50 to 55 mmHg)] where consciousness is improved but the stimulus to respiratory drive is not removed. Also, the pH of the CSF may be very low, in the range of 7.15 to 7.25. In CO_2 narcosis, correction of the acidosis of blood is easier than that of CSF, which tends to lag. The management of respiratory failure is discussed in detail in Chap. 223.

Differential diagnosis   Unlike pure hypoxic encephalopathy, hypercapnia rarely causes prolonged coma and is not a cause of irreversible brain damage. Papilledema and asterixis are important diagnostic features. (Asterixis is also characteristic of liver failure and uremia, and occasionally it is observed in other metabolic disorders.) The syndrome of hypercapnia is apt to be mistaken for brain tumor, a confusional psychosis of nondescript type, or a chronic extrapyramidal syndrome causing myoclonus or chorea.

HYPOGLYCEMIC ENCEPHALOPATHY (See also Chaps. 337 and 338)   This condition is an important cause of episodic confusion, convulsions, coma, and sometimes of hemiparesis and other focal neurologic signs. The essential biochemical abnormality is a critical lowering of the blood glucose concentration to usually less than 1.4 mmol/L (25 mg/dL) (lower in infants), which, if it lasts for many minutes, leads to exhaustion of the cerebral glucose reserve. As cerebral oxidation proceeds without exogenous glucose, the lipid and protein components of neurons are metabolized, and irreversible damage occurs. The severely hypoglycemic patient becomes deeply comatose before permanent damage occurs; consequently, prompt treatment is important.

Etiology   The most common causes of hypoglycemic encephalopathy are (1) accidental or deliberate overdose of insulin or an oral antidiabetic agent, (2) insulin-secreting islet cell tumor or retroperitoneal sarcoma, (3) rare cases of protracted ethanol intoxication, (4) acute, nonicteric hepatic encephalopathy of childhood (Reye's syndrome), and (5) an idiopathic syndrome occurring in the neonatal period. Hypoglycemic encephalopathy was a frequent complication of "insulin shock" therapy of schizophrenia, a form of treatment fortunately no longer used.

Clinical manifestations   As the concentration of blood glucose decreases to about 1.7 mmol/L (30 mg/dL), the initial symptoms (reflecting norepinephrine release) appear—nervousness, hunger, flushed facies, headache, palpitation, anxiety, sweating, and trembling—and these gradually or rapidly give way to signs of cerebral glucopenia, i.e., confusion, drowsiness, focal neurologic signs, and occasionally excitement or overactivity. In the next stage, forced sucking, grasping, motor restlessness, muscular spasms, and finally decerebrate rigidity occur, in that sequence; myoclonic twitching and convulsions frequently develop in this stage. Blood levels of approximately 0.6 mmol/L (10 mg/dL) are associated with deep coma, dilatation of the pupils, pallor, shallow respirations, bradycardia, and hypotonicity of limb musculature—the so-called medullary phase of hypoglycemia. If glucose is administered before the medullary phase is reached, the patient is restored to normal within a few minutes, retracing the aforementioned steps in reverse order. Once the medullary phase appears, and particularly if it persists for a time before the hypoglycemia is corrected, neurologic recovery is delayed for a period of days or weeks and may be incomplete.

A huge dose of insulin that produces severe hypoglycemia, even of relatively brief duration (30 to 60 min), is more dangerous than a series of less severe hypoglycemic episodes from smaller doses of insulin, presumably because the counterregulation mechanisms are likely to be less effective in the former situation. Massive amounts of glucose may have to be infused in order to maintain plasma glucose levels in the normal range (see Chap. 338).

Pathology   The major *neuropathologic effect* is on the cerebral cortex; nerve cells degenerate and are replaced by microgliocytes and astrocytes. The distribution of lesions is similar though not identical to that in hypoxic encephalopathy (the cerebellar cortex is relatively spared in hypoglycemic encephalopathy). The neurologic sequelae of the two disorders are also much alike.

Episodes of chronic hypoglycemia may give rise to two other syndromes, both relatively uncommon. One, termed *subacute hypoglycemia*, is characterized by drowsiness and lethargy, diminution in psychomotor activity, deterioration of social behavior, and confusion.

Oral or intravenous glucose immediately alleviates the symptoms. In the other, *more chronic syndrome*, there is gradual deterioration of intellectual function, raising the question of a presenile dementia, and in some reported instances there have been tremor, chorea, rigidity, cerebellar ataxia, and rarely signs of lower motor neuron involvement ("hypoglycemic amyotrophy"). These subacute and chronic forms of hypoglycemia have been observed with islet cell hyperplasia or tumor, as well as with carcinoma of the stomach, fibrous mesothelioma, carcinoma of the cecum, and hepatoma.

Differential diagnosis   The major clinical differences between hypoglycemia and hypoxia reflect the clinical setting and mode of evolution of the neurologic disorder. With hypoglycemia, the disturbance of cerebral function evolves more slowly than with hypoxia, over a period of 30 to 60 min rather than in a few seconds or minutes. The recovery phase and sequelae of the two conditions are much the same. *Recurrent hypoglycemia*, as occurs with an islet cell tumor, may masquerade for some time as an episodic confusional psychosis or seizure disorder, and diagnosis awaits a period of demonstrably low blood glucose or hyperinsulinism (see Chap. 338).

Correction of the hypoglycemia at the earliest moment is the obvious therapy. It is not known whether hypothermia or other measures will increase the safety period of hypoglycemia or alter the outcome.

HYPERGLYCEMIC COMA   Two coma-producing hyperglycemic syndromes occur, mainly in the diabetic: (1) hyperglycemia with ketoacidosis and (2) hyperosmolar nonketotic hyperglycemia. These are described in Chap. 337.

HEPATIC ENCEPHALOPATHY   Chronic hepatic insufficiency with portacaval shunting of blood is often punctuated by episodes of stupor, coma, and other neurologic symptoms, a state referred to as *hepatic coma* or *portal-systemic encephalopathy*. Also, hereditary hyperammonemic syndromes of infancy may lead to episodic coma with or without seizures. A special type of nonicteric hepatic encephalopathy (Reye's syndrome) occurs in children, presenting as acute brain swelling, in conjunction with rapid enlargement of the liver, fine droplets of fat in hepatocytes, high serum aspartate aminotransferase (AST, SGOT) and other liver enzymes, and very high levels of serum ammonia (see Chap. 270).

Clinical features   The central feature of hepatic encephalopathy in the adult is a derangement of consciousness, presenting first as mental confusion with increased or decreased psychomotor activity, followed by progressive drowsiness, stupor, and coma. Severe brain edema, which can be visualized by MRI, occurs commonly. The confusional state before coma intervenes is frequently combined with characteristic lapses of sustained muscle contraction (asterixis). The EEG becomes abnormal during the earliest stages of the confusional state. Paroxysms of bilaterally synchronous delta waves, characteristically triphasic and prominent in the frontal regions, are at first interspersed with alpha activity and later, as the coma deepens, displace all normal activity. A variable, fluctuating rigidity of the trunk and limbs, grimacing, suck and grasp reflexes, exaggeration or asymmetry of tendon reflexes, Babinski signs, and focal or generalized seizures round out the clinical picture. An elevated CSF glutamine level is found in most patients with severe hepatic encephalopathy, reflecting its synthesis by astrocytes in response to elevated plasma ammonia levels.

The syndrome usually evolves subacutely, over a period of days to weeks, and often terminates fatally. At times it does not advance beyond the stage of drowsiness and confusion with asterixis and EEG changes. This relatively mild form needs to be differentiated from other forms of acute confusional psychosis and delirium. If the metabolic disorder persists for months and years, a mild dementia and a persistent disorder of posture and movement may gradually appear (grimacing, tremor, dysarthria, ataxia of gait, choreoathetosis), and the condition must then be distinguished from other dementing and extrapyramidal syndromes (see later). Hepatic coma is rapidly reversed following successful hepatic transplantation.

Pathology and pathogenesis The striking *neuropathologic finding* in patients who die in a state of hepatic coma is a diffuse increase in the number and size of the protoplasmic astrocytes (Alzheimer type II astrocytes) in the deep layers of the cerebral cortex and in the lenticular nuclei, with little or no alteration in the nerve cells or other parenchymal elements. Brain edema is seen as well, often sufficient to cause cerebellar herniation.

The *pathogenesis* of hepatic encephalopathy is not fully understood. The most plausible theory relates it to an abnormality of nitrogen metabolism, wherein ammonia and/or other amines, which are formed in the bowel by the action of urease-containing organisms on dietary protein and are carried in the portal circulation to the liver, fail to be converted into urea, either because of hepatocellular disease or portal-systemic shunting of blood, or both. As a result, these substances reach the systemic circulation, where they interfere with cerebral metabolism in some obscure way. Other theories of causation have been discussed in Chap. 268 and have been reviewed in detail by Zieve, by Cooper and Plum, and by Butterworth and his colleagues.

Treatment Despite an incomplete understanding of the genesis of hepatic coma, the most effective means of treating this disorder consists of restriction of dietary protein, mechanical cleansing of the colon, oral administration of antibiotics that suppress or eliminate urease-producing organisms in the bowel, and the use of lactulose, an inert sugar that acidifies the colonic contents. Liver transplantation has proved highly efficacious in some patients. Additional methods of treatment, the practicality of which remain to be established, are discussed in Chap. 268.

In *acute fulminant hepatitis*, delirious, confusional, and comatose states also occur, but their mechanisms are not understood. Blood ammonia levels are usually elevated but of unclear significance because of other associated metabolic abnormalities.

CHRONIC HEPATIC ENCEPHALOPATHY (ACQUIRED HEPATO-CEREBRAL DEGENERATION) Clinical manifestations Patients who survive one or more episodes of hepatic coma are occasionally left with residual neurologic abnormalities, such as tremor of the head or arms, asterixis, grimacing, choreatic twitching of the limbs, dysarthria, ataxia of gait, or impairment of intellectual function, and these symptoms may worsen with repeated attacks of stupor and coma. In other patients with hepatic failure, these neurologic abnormalities become manifest in the absence of discrete episodes of hepatic coma. In either event, patients thus afflicted deteriorate neurologically over a period of months or years. As the condition evolves, a characteristic dysarthria, mild ataxia, wide-based, unsteady gait, and choreoathetosis, mainly of the face, neck, and shoulders, are joined in a common chronic syndrome. Mental function is slowly altered—a simple dementia evolves, with indifference to the illness. A coarse rhythmic tremor of the arms, appearing with certain sustained postures, mild corticospinal tract signs, and diffuse EEG abnormalities complete the clinical picture. Other less frequent signs are muscular rigidity, grasp reflexes, tremor in repose, nystagmus, asterixis, and action or intention myoclonus. Many of the neurologic abnormalities that occur as part of acute or subacute hepatic encephalopathy also may be observed in patients with chronic hepatocerebral degeneration, the only difference being that the abnormalities are transient in the former and irreversible in the latter.

The chronic cerebral symptoms, like the transient ones, may occur with all varieties of chronic liver disease. Portacaval or intrahepatic shunts are always present; jaundice, ascites, and esophageal varices are manifest in most of the cases.

Pathology Chronic hepatocerebral degeneration, like acute and subacute hepatic encephalopathy, is characterized by a widespread hyperplasia of protoplasmic astrocytes in the deep layers of the cerebral and cerebellar cortices as well as in the thalamic and lenticular nuclei and many other nuclear structures of the brainstem. In addition, in the chronic disease, medullated fibers and nerve cells are destroyed in the affected areas, and polymicrocavitation is prominent at the corticomedullary junction, in the striatum (particularly in the superior pole of the putamen), and in the cerebellar white matter. Protoplasmic

astrocytic nuclei contain periodic acid Schiff (PAS)–positive glycogen granules. Nerve cells may appear swollen and chromatolyzed, accounting for the so-called Opalski cells. The similarity of these lesions to those observed in the familial form of hepatocerebral disease (Wilson's disease) suggests a common hepatogenesis.

UREMIC ENCEPHALOPATHY Episodic confusion and stupor and other neurologic symptoms may accompany any form of severe renal disease. In addition, a number of neurologic syndromes complicate chronic hemodialysis and kidney transplantation. Chronic polyneuropathy, the most common neurologic complication of renal failure, is discussed in Chap. 383.

Acute uremic encephalopathy The initial cerebral symptoms attributable to uremia consist of apathy, fatigue, inattentiveness, and irritability; later, confusion, disturbances of sensory perception, hallucinations, and stupor supervene. The later symptoms are practically always associated with twitching of the muscles, myoclonic jerks, and asterixis, and the patient may convulse.

Uremic encephalopathy, if associated with irreversible and progressive renal disease, can only be managed with dialysis or renal transplantation (see Chap. 238). Convulsive seizures, which occur in about one-third of cases, often preterminally, respond to relatively low plasma concentrations of phenytoin and phenobarbital.

The brains of patients with uremic encephalopathy and the twitch-convulsive syndrome show hyperplasia of protoplasmic astrocytes in some cases but never to the degree observed in hepatic encephalopathy. Cerebral edema is notably absent. Restoration of renal function corrects the neurologic syndrome, attesting to a biochemical rather than a structural abnormality. Whether this is caused by the retention of organic acids, elevation of phosphate in the CSF, or the action of other toxins has never been settled.

"Disequilibrium syndrome" and dialysis encephalopathy These terms refer to syndromes that commonly complicate hemodialysis or peritoneal dialysis. These treatments induce an acute intracellular shift of water. Intracellular osmolality becomes transiently greater than that of the serum. This gradient induces a syndrome akin to water intoxication. The *disequilibrium syndrome* is characterized by headaches, nausea, muscular cramps, nervous irritability, agitation, drowsiness, convulsions, and intracranial hypertension. The headache develops in approximately 70 percent of patients, while the other symptoms are observed in 5 to 10 percent, usually in those undergoing rapid dialysis or in the early stages of a dialysis program. The symptoms tend to occur in the third or fourth hour of dialysis and last for several hours. Sometimes the symptoms appear 8 to 48 h after completing dialysis (see Chap. 238).

Dialysis encephalopathy or *dialysis dementia* is a now uncommon complication of chronic hemodialysis. It begins with stuttering and dysarthria, coupled with a predominantly motor aphasia, to which are added facial and generalized myoclonus, focal and generalized seizures, personality changes and psychotic episodes, intellectual decline, progressive aphasic disorder, and EEG abnormalities. The last consist of bisynchronous, predominantly frontal or multifocal bursts of slow wave discharges, associated with spikes and sharp waves. The CSF is usually normal. At first these symptoms are intermittent, occurring during or immediately after dialysis and lasting for only a few hours, but gradually they become more persistent and eventually permanent. Once established, the syndrome is usually steadily progressive over a 1- to 15-month period (average survival of 6 months in 42 cases analyzed by Lederman and Henry). A few patients have a waxing and waning course and survive for several years. In some patients the myoclonus and seizures subside for several months under the influence of clonazepam or diazepam.

The neuropathologic changes are subtle and consist of a mild microcavitation of the upper layers of the cerebral cortex. Although the changes are diffuse, some neuropathologic studies indicate that the left (dominant) hemisphere is affected more than the right, and the left frontotemporal operculum more than other parts of the cortex (Winkelman). These findings may explain the striking disturbance of speech and language. Alfrey and his associates found that the cerebral gray matter of patients who died with dialysis encephalopathy contained a much greater amount of aluminum than analogous tissue from dialysis patients without encephalopathy. The aluminum was derived from both the dialysate and orally administered aluminum gels. The concept that dialysis encephalopathy represented a form of aluminum intoxication was supported by the observations that (1) the frequency of dialysis dementia was related to the concentrations of aluminum in the dialysate and (2) deionization of the water used in the dialysate prevented the occurrence of new cases. The possibility that other trace elements contribute to the syndrome has not been excluded.

Kidney transplantation is associated with an increased risk of developing primary cerebral lymphoma, Wernicke's encephalopathy (if not given thiamine), and central pontine myelinolysis. Systemic fungal infections are common at autopsy in patients who have had renal transplants and long periods of immunosuppressive treatment, and in some of these patients there is involvement of the CNS. *Cryptococcus, Aspergillus, Candida, Nocardia*, and *Histoplasma* are the usual organisms. Other CNS infections that complicate transplantation are toxoplasmosis and cytomegalic inclusion disease.

ENCEPHALOPATHIES DUE TO ELECTROLYTE AND ENDO-CRINE DISTURBANCES Only brief reference to these important groups of metabolic encephalopathies can be made here. Detailed accounts are found in the cross-referenced chapters.

Metabolic acidosis (arterial pH <7.30, P_{CO_2} <35 mmHg, HCO_3^- <10 mmol/L) due to diabetes mellitus, renal failure, lactic acidosis, or poisoning with an acid substance produces a syndrome characterized by drowsiness, stupor, and coma with dry skin and Kussmaul breathing, described in Chap. 46. Extreme degrees of *hyperosmolality* of the blood may develop in the course of diabetes mellitus [blood glucose > 22 mmol/L (>400 mg/dL)] and in extreme hypernatremia, resulting in either case in tremulousness, seizures, and coma. The patient may present with focal motor seizures (epilepsia partialis continua). In some instances the movement disorder resembles chorea or the myoclonic twitching of uremia. *Hypokalemia* is characterized by extreme muscular weakness (see Chap. 387) without any abnormality in cerebral function.

Hyponatremia, usually with water intoxication, is another cause of episodic coma, especially in infants. Among the many causes, the syndrome of inappropriate secretion of antidiuretic hormone (SIADH) is of special importance, since it commonly complicates neurologic diseases of many types—head trauma, bacterial meningitis and encephalitis, cerebral infarction and subarachnoid hemorrhage, neoplasm, and sometimes Guillain-Barré disease (see Chap. 333). The diagnosis of SIADH should be suspected in any critically ill neurologic or neurosurgical patient who excretes urine that is hypertonic relative to the plasma. As the hyponatremia develops, there is a decrease in alertness, which progresses through stages of confusion to coma, often with convulsive seizures. Lack of recognition of this state may allow the serum Na^+ to fall to dangerously low levels, 100 mmol/L or lower. Treatment is described in Chap. 333. Replacement with intravenous NaCl in severe cases must be done cautiously because vigorous and rapid correction of severe hyponatremia has been incriminated in the pathogenesis of central pontine myelinolysis (CPM) and related brainstem, cerebellar, and cerebral lesions. Firm therapeutic guidelines for the restoration of severe hyponatremia have yet to be established, but the most careful studies to date indicate that the serum sodium should be raised by no more than 12 mmol/L in the first 24 h and by no more than 20 mmol/L in the first 48 h (Laureno and Karp).

In children more than adults, cholera being an exception, extremely *severe diarrhea* may be attended by an encephalopathy. Irritability, weakness, headache, seizures, stupor, and coma may develop over a period of 2 to 3 days. Presumably this is a metabolic encephalopathy due to loss of fluids and electrolytes and can be corrected by their replacement. This metabolic disturbance carries a grave prognosis unless promptly relieved.

In the *endocrine encephalopathies* the clinical phenomena are even more abstruse. Confusional states may be combined with agitation, hallucinations, delusions, anxiety, and depression. And the duration of the illness may be measured in weeks and months rather than days. Derangement of higher cerebral function may follow the *administration of ACTH or glucocorticoids*, and the same symptoms have been reported in *Cushing's disease* (see Chap. 335). The neurologic manifestations of *thyrotoxicosis* are particularly elusive. Allusions to thyrotoxic psychosis are widely recorded in the medical literature; mental confusion, seizures, manic or depressive attacks, delusions, and chorea occur in various combinations with muscular weakness and atrophy, periodic paralysis, and myasthenia (see Chap. 334). Treatment of the hyperthyroidism gradually restores the patient to a normal mental state. *Myxedematous patients* may show slow mentation and depression, and in a small proportion there is a major change in cerebral function, taking the form of inattentiveness, apathy, and drowsiness or extreme somnolence. These symptoms can usually be reversed within weeks to months by thyroid medication. The association of myxedema and cerebellar ataxia is well documented, but the neuropathologic basis of this disorder remains unclear. In *hyperparathyroidism*, when the serum calcium levels reach 3.7 mmol/L (15 mg/dL) or higher, the patient sinks into a quiet state of inattentiveness, lethargy, and confusion. Stupor, coma, and death may be caused by extreme degrees of *hypercalcemia* such as occur occasionally in cases of hypervitaminosis D and metastatic tumors of the bones. Chronic *hypoparathyroidism*, either idiopathic or following thyroid or parathyroid resection, may rarely give rise to intracranial calcifications and an extrapyramidal motor syndrome. *Adrenal insufficiency* may be attended by episodic confusion, stupor, or coma, without special identifying features (see Chap. 335).

The term *pancreatic encephalopathy* describes a syndrome of agitation and confusion, sometimes with hallucinations and clouding of consciousness, dysarthria, and changing rigidity of the limbs, in association with acute pancreatic disease. The status of this entity is uncertain, and a uniform neuropathologic change has not been discerned. We agree with Pallis and Lewis, who suggest that before such a diagnosis can be entertained in a patient with acute pancreatitis, one needs to exclude delirium tremens, the cerebral effects of shock, renal or hepatic failure, hypoglycemia, diabetic acidosis, hyperosmolality, hypokalemia, hypo- or hypercalcemia, any one of which may complicate the underlying disease(s).

Lactic acidosis may be the cause of an encephalopathy in patients who undergo jejunoileostomy for treatment of morbid obesity. Such patients report episodes of confusion, ataxia, and slurred speech. D-Lactate, an isomer not normally found in the blood and a product of intestinal bacteria, is present in the serum, urine, and stool of these patients. D-Lactate causes encephalopathy by interfering with pyruvate metabolism. Diagnosis is dependent on recognition of metabolic acidosis associated with hyperchloremia and measurement of elevated D-lactate (see Dahlquist; Cross). A more common cause of encephalopathy in patients with jejunoileal shunting is hepatic failure (see Chap. 73).

HEREDITARY METABOLIC DISEASES OF LATE ONSET

Inherited metabolic disorders affecting amino acid metabolism (Chap. 352), lysosomal enzyme functions (Chap. 349), and cerebral lipids (Chap. 349) are generally rare and usually become manifest during infancy or childhood. In this chapter are described a small number of hereditary metabolic disorders that may have their onset in late adolescence and adulthood and may present diagnostic problems because of the similarity of clinical presentation to other more common acquired and degenerative diseases of the nervous system. Noteworthy attributes of these diseases are their chronicity and progressive nature.

METACHROMATIC LEUKODYSTROPHY (See Chap. 349) Probably the most common member of this category is *adult metachromatic leukodystrophy (MLD)*. While the majority of cases appear in early childhood, approximately 25 percent manifest their first symptoms after age 21. Men outnumber women 2:1. The mode of inheritance is autosomal recessive in almost all instances. The onset is insidious, and the course is protracted, over 20 or more years.

Mental symptoms tend to dominate the clinical picture. Failing scholastic performance, forgetfulness, and irrationality occur early in the illness but may be obscured by peculiarities of personality, such as suspiciousness, delusional thinking, and bizarre actions. These latter qualities may raise the question of schizophrenia or immature (''borderline'') personality development. Sooner or later a mild cerebellar ataxia presenting as awkwardness and falling, mild pyramidal signs, masked facies, and bizarre postures stamp the illness as neurologic. Eventually, mental processes deteriorate to the point where the patient is helpless, demented, mute, incontinent, and bedfast.

Specific diagnostic tests include (1) the demonstration of a diminished arylsulfatase A activity in white blood cells, serum, and urine, (2) increased excretion of sulfatides in the urine, (3) slowed conduction velocity in nerves, and (4) deposits of metachromatic material in nerve biopsies. No treatment is available.

ADRENOLEUKODYSTROPHY   In this X-linked metabolic disorder, either adrenal insufficiency or cerebral symptoms may be the initial manifestation. The cerebral lesions may present as a homonymous hemianopia, cortical blindness, hemiparesis, aphasia, or dementia. The signs are usually asymmetric at first and progress intermittently. Relatively pure polyneuropathic and myelopathic forms also have been described. The diagnosis is usually made by finding a low blood cortisol level in a male with cerebrospinal demyelinating disease, although a purely spinal type, taking the form of a progressive spastic paraparesis, has been described in the heterozygote (female carrier). Increased urinary concentration of C22–C26 fatty acids is diagnostic. Glucocorticoid replacement therapy helps the symptoms of adrenal insufficiency but has no effect on the neurologic disorders. The latter progress intermittently over a few years, and the outcome is usually fatal.

ADULT LIPID STORAGE DISEASES G_{M2} *gangliosidosis* (hexosaminidase A deficiency) has been observed in young adults. Many are from non-Jewish families, and males and females in the same generation are equally affected. Generalized seizures may mark the beginning of a cerebral disorder that later is evidenced by alterations of behavior and intellectual decline. A progressive ataxia and mild signs of corticospinal disease, the combination of which interferes with independent locomotion, clarifies the diagnosis. The fundi and visual function are normal in most cases, but typical cherry red macular spots are seen occasionally. The liver and spleen are normal or slightly enlarged. The CSF protein is normal. CT scans of the brain reveal a modest ventricular enlargement. A slowly developing dementia, cerebellar ataxia, polymyoclonus, and failing vision may characterize the clinical picture in some cases. In yet others, the presenting syndrome has consisted of prominent motor neuron involvement accompanied by muscle cramps, suggesting a diagnosis of spinal muscular atrophy or amyotrophic lateral sclerosis (see Chap. 372). G_{M2} ganglioside is increased in tissue obtained by cerebral biopsy. Membranous cytoplasmic bodies are visualized by electron microscopy of rectal, appendicular, and cortical neurons. *Gaucher's* and *Niemann-Pick* diseases are yet other storage diseases that may present in adult life (see Chap. 349).

Ceroid lipofuscinosis   The Kufs type of *ceroid lipofuscinosis* is a lipid storage disease that only becomes evident in adolescence or early adult life. Usually the disease begins with mental deterioration, followed by seizures, ataxia, increasing rigidity, athetotic posturing, and corticospinal signs. Skin and conjunctival biopsies, examined by electron microscopy, show lipofuscin storage material in fibroblasts and endothelial cells.

SUBACUTE   NECROTIZING   ENCEPHALOMYELOPATHY (LEIGH'S DISEASE)   This disease, now classified as a disorder of mitochondrial metabolism, sometimes begins in adolescence and takes the form of a progressive polymyoclonus with seizures and cerebellar ataxia and relatively mild impairment of intellectual function.

SUMMARY   These rare forms of hereditary metabolic disease should be considered whenever an adolescent or young adult becomes demented, shows a psychiatric syndrome with decline in cognitive functions, or has seizures (especially with polymyoclonus), failing vision, and cerebellar ataxia in combination with corticospinal signs or a progressive polyneuropathy.

REFERENCES

ADAMS RD, VICTOR M: *Principles of Neurology*, 5th ed. New York, McGraw-Hill, 1993, chaps 38 and 39

ALFREY AC et al: The dialysis encephalopathy syndrome: Possible aluminum intoxication. N Engl J Med 294:184, 1976

ALLEN RH et al: Diagnosis of cobalamin deficiencies: I. Usefulness of serum methylmalonic acid and total homocysteine concentrations. Am J Hematol 34:90, 1990

BECK WS: Neuropsychiatric consequences of cobalamin deficiency. Adv Intern Med 36:33, 1991

BUTTERWORTH RF: Pathophysiology of cerebellar dysfunction in the Wernicke-Korsakoff syndrome. Can J Neurol Sci 20(Supplement 3):123, 1993

——— et al: Ammonia: Key factor in the pathogenesis of hepatic encephalopathy. Neurochem Pathol 6:1, 1987

CARMEL R: Subtle and atypical cobalamin deficiency states. Am J Hematol 34:108, 1990

——— et al: Hereditary defect of cobalamin metabolism (*cblG* mutation) presenting as a neurologic disorder in adulthood. N Engl J Med 318:1738, 1988

CHOI DW, ROTHMAN SM: The role of glutamate neurotoxicity in hypoxic-ischemic neuronal death. Annu Rev Neurosci 13:171, 1990

COOPER AJL, PLUM F: Biochemistry and physiology of brain ammonia. Physiol Rev 67:440, 1987

FLEMING JL et al: Whipple's disease: Clinical, biochemical, and histopathologic features and assessment of treatment in 29 patients. Mayo Clin Proc 63:539, 1988

FRANCIS GS et al: Metachromatic leukodystrophy: Multiple nonfunctional and pseudodeficiency alleles in a pedigree: Problems with diagnosis and counseling. Ann Neurol 34:212, 1993

HARDING AE et al: Spinocerebellar degeneration associated with a selective defect of vitamin E absorption. N Engl J Med 313:32, 1985

HORNBEIN TF et al: The cost to the central nervous system of climbing to extremely high altitude. N Engl J Med 321:1714, 1989

KERTESZ A et al: The structural determinants of recovery in Wernicke's aphasia. Brain Lang 44:153, 1993

KOLODNY EH, BOUSTANY RM: Storage diseases of the reticuloendothelial system, in Nathan D, Oski F (eds): *Hematology of Infancy and Childhood*, 3d ed. Philadelphia, Saunders, 1986

LAURENO R: Central pontine myelinolysis following rapid correction of hyponatremia. Ann Neurol 13:232, 1983

———, KARP BI: Pontine and extrapontine myelinolysis following rapid correction of hyponatremia. Lancet 1:1439, 1988

LEDERMAN RS, HENRY CE: Progressive dialysis encephalopathy. Ann Neurol 4:199, 1978

LINDENBAUM J et al: Neuropsychiatric disorders caused by cobalamin deficiency in the absence of anemia or macrocytosis. N Engl J Med 318:1720, 1988

MULLEN KD: Benzodiazepine compounds and hepatic encephalopathy. N Engl J Med 325:509, 1991

NELSON JS et al: Progressive neuropathologic lesions in vitamin E–deficient rhesus monkeys. J Neuropathol Exp Neurol 40:166, 1981

NORENBERG MD: The role of astrocytes in hepatic encephalopathy. Neurochem Pathol 6:13, 1987

PALLIS CA, LEWIS PD: *The Neurology of Gastrointestinal Disease*. Philadelphia, Saunders, 1974

PINCUS JH: Folic acid deficiency: A cause of subacute combined system degeneration, in Botez MI, Reynolds EH (eds): *Folic Acid in Neurology, Psychiatry, and Internal Medicine*. New York, Raven Press, 1979, pp 427–433

PLUM F, POSNER JB: *Diagnosis of Stupor and Coma*, 3d ed. Philadelphia, Davis, 1980

RAO RVL et al: Glutamatergic synaptic dysfunction in hyperammonemic syndromes. Metab Brain Dis 7:1, 1992

RASKIN NH, FISHMAN RA: Neurologic disorders in renal failure. N Engl J Med 294:143, 1976

RIZZO JF, LESSELL S: Tobacco amblyopia. Am J Ophthalmol 116:84, 1993

SATYA-MURTI S et al: The spectrum of neurologic disorders from vitamin E deficiency. Neurology 36:917, 1986

SCHAUMBURG HH et al: Sensory neuropathy from pyridoxine abuse: A new megavitamin syndrome. N Engl J Med 309:445, 1983

SERDARU M et al: The clinical spectrum of alcoholic pellagra encephalopathy. Brain 111:829, 1988

SOKOL RJ et al: Vitamin E deficiency neuropathy in children with fat malabsorption: Studies in cystic fibrosis and chronic cholestasis. Ann NY Acad Sci 570:156, 1989

VICTOR M: Polyneuropathy due to nutritional deficiency and alcoholism, in Dyck PJ et al (eds): *Peripheral Neuropathy*, 2d ed. Philadelphia, Saunders, 1984, pp 1899–1940

———, ROTHSTEIN J: Neurologic manifestations of hepatic and gastrointestinal diseases, in Asbury AK et al (eds): *Diseases of the Nervous System*, 2d ed. Philadelphia, Saunders, 1992, pp 1442–1455

——— et al: The acquired (nonwilsonian) type of chronic hepatocerebral degeneration. Medicine 44:345, 1965

———— et al: *The Wernicke-Korsakoff Syndrome and Related Disorders Due to Alcoholism and Malnutrition.* Philadelphia, Davis, 1989

WILKINSON DS, PROCKOP LD: Hypoglycemia: Effects on the nervous system, in Vinken PJ, Bruyn BW (eds): *Handbook of Clinical Neurology,* vol 27. Amsterdam, North-Holland, 1976, pp 53–78

WINKELMAN MD, RICANATI ES: Dialysis encephalopathy: Neuropathologic aspects. Hum Pathol 17:823, 1986

WITT ED, GOLDMAN-RAKIC PS: Intermittent thiamine deficiency in the rhesus monkey: I. Progression of neurological signs and neuroanatomical lesions. Ann Neurol 13:376, 1983

ZIEVE L: Pathogenesis of hepatic encephalopathy. Metab Brain Dis 2:147, 1987

378 NEUROCUTANEOUS SYNDROMES AND OTHER DEVELOPMENTAL DISORDERS OF THE CENTRAL NERVOUS SYSTEM

VERNE S. CAVINESS, JR.*

Developmental disorders that involve the nervous system and are encountered in adult life are the emphasis of this chapter. The discussion is arranged according to broad phenotypic groupings, namely *neurocutaneous* syndromes in which abnormalities of the nervous system are associated with abnormalities of osseous structures and the skin, *developmental* disorders principally affecting the nervous system, and *neuroskeletal* disorders.

NEUROCUTANEOUS SYNDROMES

A large number of neurocutaneous disorders (also known as *phakomatoses*, from phakos, "lentil," "mole," or "freckle") are expressed in a patchy fashion in affected tissues. The most commonly encountered of these, reviewed below, are transmitted by autosomal dominant inheritance. In each of these disorders the severity of expression is highly variable. Where mild, the disorder will be overlooked; telltale features must be sought diligently among family members of affected patients. The chromosomal linkage group has been (provisionally) identified for four of these dominantly transmitted forms (Table 378-1).

NEUROFIBROMATOSIS (VON RECKLINGHAUSEN'S DISEASE) The dominating feature of this disorder is the neurofibroma, a tumor that arises from the Schwann cells and fibroblasts of the neurilemmal sheath of the peripheral nerve. Two nonallelic heritable forms are now recognized. *Neurofibromatosis type 1* (NF1), carried on chromosome 17, is the classic autosomal dominant neurocutaneous disorder in which tumors involving the sheaths or peripheral nerves are associated with characteristic cream-brown cutaneous lesions (café au lait spots). The neurofibromas themselves are only occasionally symptomatic, as when they result in entrapment of a nerve root at intervertebral foramina or in the unusual instances when they are sarcomatous. The disorder may be associated with other tumors of the central nervous system (CNS) including optic glioma, glioblastoma, and meningioma and rarely with pheochromocytoma (see also Chap. 336). Other associated aberrations include hamartomas of the iris (Lisch nodules), freckling concentrated around the nipples and in the axillae, macrocephaly unassociated with hydrocephalus, stenosis of the aqueduct of Sylvius, leading to obstructive hydrocephalus, and mild degrees of mental retardation, which has been ascribed to dysplasia of the cerebral cortex.

The structure of the NF1 gene is now known. The deduced structure of the encoded protein, *neurofibromin*, suggests that it

* This chapter is in part a revision of one for the 11th edition by G.R. DeLong and R.D. Adams.

TABLE 378-1 Chromosomal locations of dominant mutant genes in the phakomatoses*

Disorder	Chromosome	Phenotypic signature	Mental retardation	Tumors
NF1	17	Café au lait spots, neurofibromas	Occasionally	Multiple types: CNS, PNS, viscera
NF2	22	Bilateral acoustic neuromas	No	Acoustic neuromas; other CNS
TS	9, 16	White spots, adenoma sebacea	Frequent	CNS: tubers, gliomas; viscera
VH-L	3	Cerebral hemangioblastomas, retinal angiomas	No	Angiomas of viscera; renal cell carcinomas

* NF1 and NF2 are neurofibromatosis types 1 and 2; TS, tuberosclerosis; VH-L, von Hippel-Lindau. See also Chap. 364.

should have GTPase activating properties. Neurofibromin under normal circumstances appears to have tumor suppressor properties which are impaired or lost with mutation. The tumor suppressor function is currently thought to be exercised through modulation of the state of phosphorylation of *ras*, a proto-oncogene involved in regulation of cell division and differentiation.

Neurofibromatosis type 2, carried on chromosome 22, is also an autosomal dominant disorder in which neurofibromas involve the acoustic nerves exclusively and usually bilaterally. The acoustic neurinomas may produce deafness and other symptoms and signs of a cerebellopontine angle lesion. They may also be associated with meningiomas and astrocytomas.

TUBEROUS SCLEROSIS (BOURNEVILLE'S DISEASE) In this condition, cutaneous lesions of multiple types are associated with malformation and tumors of the CNS. Mental deficiency, though not invariable, may be profound and associated with a remarkably intractable seizure disorder. The earliest lesions to emerge are leaf-shaped hypopigmented spots ("white spots") scattered over the trunk and limbs. These are seen most clearly under ultraviolet light (Wood's lamp). The adenoma sebaceum, a hallmark of the disorder, is an angiofibroma, distributed in a butterfly pattern over the cheeks, chin, and forehead. The individual adenomas vary in size from 0.1 to 1.0 cm and are elevated and pinkish or pinkish yellow in color. The skin over the lumbosacral region of the back may be marked by a rough thickening which is yellowish in color like sharkskin or pigskin (shagreen patch). The cutaneous lesions may provide the earliest clue to the causation of mental retardation or infantile epilepsy. Rhabdomyoma of the heart and tumorous malformations (angioleiomyomas) of the kidney, liver, adrenal glands, and pancreas are also characteristic of this disorder. The cardiac rhabdomyoma may be imaged by ultrasound in utero. The disorder is inherited as an autosomal dominant trait: linkage studies with RFLPs in some pedigrees have located the mutant gene to chromosome 9 but in other pedigrees to chromosome 16.

In the brain multiple nodular tumors, composed of abnormal neurons and glial cells, often lie in the plane of the cerebral cortex itself. These can be diagnosed accurately in T2 weighted magnetic resonance scans. If calcified, they may also be visualized by CT scans or skull x-rays. Calcified nodules occur in brain subependymal regions adjacent to the ventricles. If large, they may obstruct the foramen of Monro, causing a unilateral or bilateral hydrocephalus. Masses of subependymal glial tissue forming nodules are likened to "candle gutterings" on the walls of the ventricles. The electroencephalogram is usually abnormal but without specific pattern. The only treatment is symptomatic. When severe epilepsy and mental retardation are present, prognosis for life beyond the third decade is poor. Death is usually due to seizures, associated tumors, or intercurrent diseases.

CEREBELLORETINAL HEMANGIOBLASTOMATOSIS (VON HIPPEL-LINDAU SYNDROME)   This syndrome of retinal and cerebellar hemangioblastoma is inherited as an autosomal dominant disorder (encoded on chromosome 3). (See Table 378-1) The retinal lesions are capillary angiomas, usually multiple, causing progressive loss of vision. The cerebellar hemangioblastomas, which may occur multiply, are slowly growing cystic tumors. These may also occur in the medulla or in the spinal cord where they may be associated with a syrinx. Enlargement of cerebellar tumor may lead to obstructive hydrocephalus with headache, papilledema, and cerebellar ataxia. Only rarely do tumors become symptomatic before adolescence but the diagnosis must be considered in all adults with a cerebellar tumor. Tumors of the CNS are a part of a constellation including angiomas and cysts of the liver, pancreas, and kidneys, and tumors of the epididymis and kidney. The latter may be lethal. Pheochromocytomas may occur in this as in other of the phakomatoses (see Chap. 336). An association with renal cell carcinoma led to localization of the mutant gene on chromosome 3. The mutant gene has recently been identified (see Chap. 364). Polycythemia, presumably the consequence of ectopic production of erythropoietin by the hemangioblastoma, may disappear after excision of the tumor.

ENCEPHALOTRIGEMINAL SYNDROME (STURGE-WEBER DISEASE)   Capillary or cavernous hemangiomas, within but not always limited to the cutaneous distribution of the trigeminal nerve, occur along with a predominantly venous hemangioma that can spread through subjacent leptomeninges. The adjacent cerebral cortex is progressively destroyed, perhaps as a consequence of interruption of local blood flow. The first neurologic symptom is usually a focal seizure on the side opposite the skin lesion. Sensorimotor paralysis or permanent visual field defect, the most common sequelae, may be either of sudden or insidious onset with progression. In time calcium is deposited within the area of involved cortex and may be visualized as a characteristic "railroad track" in conventional x-ray or CT scans. If the skin lesion is within the area of supply of the ophthalmic division of the trigeminal nerve, the occipital lobes are more commonly involved. A facial nevus is more often associated with involvement of the parietal and frontal lobes. The intracranial and cutaneous lesions may also occur separately. The disease is usually sporadic; a familial occurrence consistent with autosomal dominant inheritance is exceptional. Deeply situated arteriovenous malformations rarely coexist. Blindness in the eye on the side of the nevus is nearly always due to glaucoma. Most patients with this malformation survive for many years, often with mental defects and hemiparesis. Intractable seizures and cognitive functions may in some instances be substantially improved by resection of large blocks of involved cerebrum.

Hemangioma of the trunk or upper or lower extremity may be associated with a spinal cord vascular malformation (Klippel-Trenaunay syndrome) and with hypertrophy of the involved extremity. The cord lesion may cause infarction in nervous tissue, producing a spinal sensorimotor paralysis. Surgical exploration and decompression are seldom beneficial.

DEVELOPMENTAL DISORDERS OF THE CNS

Developmental disorders expressed largely or even exclusively as disturbance of neurologic functions afflict a substantial portion of the population. Certain of these, particularly when neurologic disability is severe, are complicated secondarily by restricted general somatic growth, articulatory contractures, and general medical disorders resulting from limited mobility and poor personal care. The discussion will be focussed upon developmental disorders expressed predominantly as malfunction of the forebrain, in particular, of the cerebral hemispheres. Three general syndromes are emphasized: mental retardation where the disability is predominantly in the domains of cognition, language, and memory; autism where socialization is prominently defective; and "cerebral palsy" where disability largely relates to motor function.

MENTAL RETARDATION   Mental retardation specifies an IQ less than 70 resulting from pathophysiologic processes affecting the cerebrum during the developmental period. If IQ is normal, the diagnosis is not applied to more restricted learning disabilities including dyslexia, incompetence with mathematics, and a variety of developmental language disorders. Mental retardation, even if the predominant disability, is conjoined with a complex of other disabilities which include disordered motor function, abnormalities of special senses, such as hearing and sight, and a variety of medical problems.

Etiology and pathogenesis   The specific cause of abnormal cerebral development cannot be defined for as many as half of all mentally retarded persons. For many, the disorder is familial and may be due either to single-gene defects or polygenic inheritance. Among the remaining half in whom the cause can be identified, the recognized causes include the 21 trisomy and fragile X syndromes and intrauterine exposure to alcohol (see Chap. 62). Collectively these few disorders are responsible for a third of mental retardation in this country. Prevalence for each approximates 1:1000 live births. Other identifiable causes include encephaloclastic processes, such as infection, hypoxia/ischemia, trauma, and hydrocephalus, occurring either before or after birth. Intrauterine exposures to infectious and pharmacologic teratogenic agents are also common, e.g., herpes simplex and human immunodeficiency virus (HIV), other viral and protozoal infectious agents, or cocaine and other "recreational" drugs. Malnutrition, hypothyroidism, and other metabolic disorders also may cause mental retardation during intrauterine and postnatal life. Among the general medical conditions is a substantial list of heritable disorders of metabolism. The list is long and includes enzymopathies relating to amino acid, carbohydrate, organic acid, and lipid processing such as phenylketonuria (see Chap. 349), galactosemia (see Chap. 354), propionic aciduria, and disorders of lysosomal enzyme function such as neuronal ceroid lipofuscinosis, the gangliosidoses, and the mucopolysaccharidoses (see also Chaps. 349 and 351).

Many chromosomal and single-gene disorders of metabolism may be diagnosed prenatally. Where diagnosis is made postnatally, it may be critical to do so expeditiously in the case of treatable CNS infections and correctable or manageable metabolic disorders, i.e., cretinism or phenylketonuria. During the first 2 years of life diagnosis and intervention are also critical for malnutrition, a state usually coupled to other socioeconomic deprivations. These deprivations may result in retarded brain growth and mental development that persist into adult life. If, however, such children are "rescued" by refeeding and placement in a stimulating and supportive environment, the effects of early malnutrition are largely reversible, and normal mental development can result.

Clinical manifestations   The defining characteristic of this domain of cerebral disturbance, subnormal IQ, is an inexact but a meaningful predictor of behavioral capabilities. Severely retarded children, those with IQs of less than 20, are virtually unable to look after themselves. Often they never sit up, walk, or stand. Language is rudimentary; at most a few words are understood and uttered. They exhibit only primitive emotional reactions and sphincteric control may never be achieved. Motor mannerisms such as rhythmic rocking, rolling, head banging, and bouncing movements are typical and often are accompanied by bleating sounds and squeals. Music may encourage rhythmic movements. Their physical appearance may be unremarkable. However, if the insult to the brain occurs in utero or early in postnatal life, a variety of physical deformities, particularly microcephaly and variable degrees of joint contracture, are common in this group.

If the mental defect is less pronounced (IQ of 20 to 50), and if specific motor defects do not coexist, then sitting, walking, and speech are acquired, often after a delay. The existence of a cerebral defect may be noted for the first time when the child fails to speak normally during the second and third year of life and seems not to be able to learn the usual household tasks and play activities as well as other children. However, delay in speech development by itself is not a mark of mental retardation, for some children who are intelligent and show remarkable talent in communicating by gesture are slow in talking. Also the deaf child may be singled out by indifference to noise and reduced vocalization but otherwise normal development. Toilet training also may be difficult to accomplish in the retarded child, but again it may be delayed in an otherwise normal child.

The least severely retarded of these individuals (IQ of 50 to 70) grows and develops in many ways not different from the normal child during the early years of life. Their abilities and adaptations merge imperceptibly with those of the general population. Often there is neither somatic nor other specific neurologic abnormality. That the child is handicapped may not be evident until it is apparent that scholastic pursuits are relatively unsuccessful. There may be manifest inability to learn, with poor school progress, and the child with an IQ of 60 to 70 is generally unable to pass the sixth grade. Vocational training is of more value than other types of education. The mildly retarded child may be able to acquire useful occupational skills and to work under careful supervision.

Whereas IQ is a useful index of competence, the clinical and behavioral characteristics of individuals with retarded development cannot be adequately described by this single attribute. In particular, the social competence, which may vary in ways that are not predicted by IQ, may largely determine the life expectations of retarded children. This aspect of behavior should be an organizing theme for education and training. Some mentally retarded persons are pleasant and amiable and achieve a satisfactory social adjustment. At the opposite extreme is the poorly understood syndrome of autism, associated with varying degrees of retardation, in which the child or older person fails to manifest any kind of interpersonal, social contact (see "Autism," below). Many retarded individuals are dull, apathetic, and underactive. Others display an incessant hyperactivity, characterized by a very short attention span, a restless inquisitive searching of the environment, and low frustration tolerance; they may be destructive or recklessly fearless and may seem strangely impervious to injury. As with the mentally normal but hyperactive, inattentive child, improvement in these children can often be achieved by using stimulants and desipramine.

Three specific disorders associated with mental retardation deserve separate description.

Fetal alcohol syndrome The *fetal alcohol* syndrome may be the most prevalent cause of defective cerebral development in industrialized nations. Its estimated frequency in the United States, 1:700 live births, is probably less than the actual occurrence and is even greater than the occurrences of trisomy 21 (Down's syndrome) and the fragile X syndrome. The fully developed disorder includes marked growth retardation, microcephaly, and cardiac valvular lesions. Characteristic facial features include hypotelorism, small palpebral fissures, small nasal bridge, and reduction of the vermilion border of the upper lip. Mental retardation may be profound. However, the less severely affected may have IQs in the normal range but be significantly disabled by attention deficit disorder with hyperactivity and learning disabilities. The severity of the disorder is related to alcohol dose, and the threshold for clinical expression appears to lie in mother's ingestion of 30 to 60 mL of absolute alcohol equivalent per day. Additional risk factors including exposure to multiple drugs or venereally transmitted infectious agents may interact with alcohol abuse. The potential risk to successive offspring is obvious.

Fragile X syndrome The *fragile X chromosome anomaly* is a phenotype that combines dysmorphic somatic characteristics with mental retardation. Cytogenetic analysis shows constriction of the terminal segment of the long arm of the affected X chromosome, and the fragile link is subject to breakage. Expression of the anomaly in standard tissue culture conditions is enhanced by folate deficiency and other modifications. The characteristic phenotype, which generally becomes evident only after puberty, is expressed in approximately 80 percent of males and in 35 percent of females carrying a single affected X chromosome. The mother of an affected male is always a carrier; paradoxically, within a lineage carrying the genetic disorder, there is increasing risk of expression with successive generations.

Stigmata include macro-orchidism in males, possibly large ovaries in females, prognathism, and large everted ears. The skull is narrow and elongate. Mental retardation is usually mild to moderate and associated with dysphonic, sometimes echolalic speech. The association of the fragile X chromosome anomaly and autism in males (see below) has been estimated to be as high as 10 to 15 percent. The fragile X phenotype reflects disruption in the function of the FMR-I gene which is located at the fragile site; the gene becomes disabled through a succession of modifications, rather than just a single modification. These include both the methylation and acquisition of multiple repetitions of a CpG sequence located approximately 150 base pairs 5′ to the gene. Susceptibility to this sequence of modifications is acquired during meiosis as a germline "premutation." The repetitions accumulate in successive generations, a phenomenon which explains the increasing expression through successive generations within a lineage. Approximately 60 to 79 repeats correspond to the threshold for clinical expression; 100 percent expression is associated with 90 to 200 repeats. A therapeutic response to treatment with folate has not been substantiated.

Down's syndrome (See Chap. 62) *Down's syndrome* accounts for about 1 percent of all retardation. Trisomy of chromosome 21 or translocation of parts of this chromosome is responsible for the disorder. Older mothers are more apt to have babies with Down's syndrome than are young mothers. The mean age of the mother is 37.

The degree of mental retardation in Down's syndrome varies from mild to severe and is associated with a characteristic facial appearance and small stature. Many stigmata can be recognized in the neonatal period. The head tends to be small and round, with sloping forehead. The ears are set low and are oval, with small lobules. The eyes slant slightly upward and outward owing to the presence of a medial epicanthal fold, which partly covers the angle of the palpebral fissure. The bridge of the nose is poorly developed. The mouth tends to hang open, and the tongue is usually enlarged, heavily fissured, and protruding. Gray-white specks of depigmentation are seen in the iris (Brushfield's spots). The little fingers are often short and curved inward (clinodactyly), owing to a hypoplastic middle phalanx. The hands are broad with a single transverse palmar crease. Lenticular opacities and congenital heart lesions (septal defects) are found in some cases. At birth these children are of average size, but at later periods of life they are characteristically small. The brain is of reduced weight with a relatively simple convolutional pattern. Of the patients who survive to puberty, many live to middle adult life and may develop a premature Alzheimer's type cerebral degeneration (onset in the majority by the age of 40) (see Chap. 370).

CRETINISM (See also Chap. 334) Cretinism and childhood hypothyroidism occur endemically in parts of the world where there is iodine deficiency and in infants everywhere with congenital disorders of thyroid function. The frequency is greater than that of phenylketonuria. For iodine deficiency to produce cretinism the mother must be lacking in iodine during the pregnancy, especially in the first trimester. Diagnosis rests with the clinical picture, for in the iodine-deficient state routine measures of thyroid function may be normal. Jaundice, umbilical hernia, noisy respirations, hypotonia, depression of reflexes, and lethargy are present at birth. Coarse facial features, large tongue, and constipation become manifest later. Among those with endemic cretinism, the neurologic abnormality consists of mental deficiency, deaf-mutism (or lesser degrees of hearing loss), and a combination of flexed posture with spasticity and rigidity of proximal limb musculature. These deficits persist throughout adult life.

AUTISM Autism is a mysterious and provocative condition. Long considered primarily psychiatric or a childhood form of schizophrenia, it is now generally thought to represent an organic defect in brain development characterized by failure to develop communicative language or other form of social communication. The incidence is at least 2 to 5 per 10,000 births; the disorder is approximately 1.5 times as prevalent in males as in females. The essence of the cognitive disorder has been formulated as a defect in "the theory of mind," that is, an impairment in the ability to appreciate what is going on in the minds of other people. In normal children this ability is well developed by age 4. Some autistic persons often show motor and other skills far beyond that expected of a mentally retarded person. Often they are obsessively preoccupied with inanimate objects, such as lights, running water, or spinning objects. Most children with autism prove later to be retarded, and the ultimate level of disability depends largely on the IQ. Some gradually acquire language and may then exhibit certain exceptional talents, such as in mathematics (idiot savant). Up to 30 percent of autistic children eventually manifest temporal lobe epilepsy. Upon reaching adult life they retain all the above characteristics. Not more than 1 in 20 improves significantly. Anecdotal pathologic reports draw attention to structural abnormalities of the limbic part of the forebrain. A blighting of the neocerebellar vermis, although visualized in the sagittal plane by MRI in a limited series of autistic subjects, is now recognized from more extensive study not to be characteristic of the disorder. The cause of autism is unknown and is likely to be multiple. There is no specific therapy.

ABNORMALITIES OF MOTOR FUNCTION (CEREBRAL PALSY)

Cerebral palsy carries the connotation of a developmental disorder of motor function that is present from infancy or early childhood and that is due to a nonprogressive cerebral disorder. The more commonly encountered conditions are spastic diplegia (affecting the legs), hemiplegia (affecting the arm and leg on the same side), and heterogeneous extrapyramidal syndromes. Cerebral infarction resulting from hypoxia and/or ischemia is one determinant of these disorders. For most the abnormal state has its origins before birth in events that go unrecognized. The insult may occur perinatally as a result of obstetrical mishap in 20 percent or less of cases. For some few an encephaloclastic event occurs in early childhood.

Spastic diplegia resulting from a prenatal or perinatal insult to the brain may not attract attention until several weeks or months after birth. There may be a delay in all normal developmental sequences, especially those that depend on the motor system. Once walking is attempted, usually much later than in the normal child, the characteristic stance and gait become manifest. The legs are advanced stiffly in short steps, each describing part of the arc of a circle: adduction is often so strong as to lead to actual crossing (scissors gait), with lower legs slightly splayed out and the feet flexed and turned in, the heels not touching the ground. Crural paraparesis is the rule, though in general associated with at least a mild affection of the arms as well. In the adolescent and adult, the legs tend to be short and small, but the muscles are not markedly atrophic, as in infantile muscular atrophy and dystrophy. Less commonly there may also be pseudobulbar dysarthria and athetosis.

Hemiplegia is a not uncommon condition of infancy and childhood, and a difference in function of the right and left extremities may be noticed soon after birth or during the first 6 to 12 months of life. The parents may be the first to notice that movements of prehension and exploration are carried out with only one arm. The affection of the leg is usually recognized later, i.e., during the first attempt to stand and walk. Mental defect is even less common than with cerebral diplegia and less common than in bilateral hemiplegia. Convulsions occur in 35 to 50 percent of children with congenital hemiplegia and may persist throughout life. If the hemiplegia is acquired during childhood, seizures often accompany the onset. They may be generalized but are frequently unilateral and limited to the hemiplegic side. Often, after a series of seizures, the affected side will be weak for several hours or longer (Todd's paralysis).

In *double hemiplegia*, a less frequent condition, the bilateral weakness of face, arms, and legs arises at any age under conditions of more severe acquired cerebral disease. The arms are severely affected, in contrast to their minimal involvement in cerebral diplegia. A quadriplegic state may occur without bulbar involvement. The condition is relatively rare and may result from a bilateral cerebral lesion or a high cervical cord lesion. Although this may occasionally result from cysts, tumors, and other malformations, it is usually produced in the infant by fracture-dislocation of the cervical spine, induced during a difficult breech delivery. Similarly, in paraplegia, with weakness or paralysis limited to the legs, the lesion may be either a cerebral form of diplegia or a spinal one. Sphincteric disturbances and a loss of sensation below a certain level on the trunk favor a spinal localization.

The spastic and rigid cerebral diplegias discussed above shade almost imperceptibly into the congenital extrapyramidal syndromes. Many such patients are found in every cerebral palsy clinic and ultimately reach adult medical clinics. Pyramidal tract signs may be absent. The nonprogressive extrapyramidal cases considered here are generally attributable to severe perinatal hypoxia; others represent separate diseases such as erythroblastosis fetalis with kernicterus. These are to be distinguished from the progressive acquired or hereditary postnatal syndromes such as familial athetosis, dystonia musclorum deformans, and cerebellar ataxia.

Congenital choreoathetosis (double athetosis) is probably the most frequent representative of this group. Like the spastic states, it may be recognized only after several months or a year have elapsed. Syndromes may be mixed, however. All combinations of chorea, athetosis, ballismus, myoclonus, and dystonia may be found in a single case, or one or another type of movement disorder may predominate. However, in all instances there is, in addition, a primary defect in voluntary movement. Choreoathetosis varies in severity. In some the disorder is so mild that the abnormal movements are misinterpreted as restlessness or "the fidgets"; in others, every voluntary act is marred by intense involuntary movements, leaving the patient nearly helpless. The severely handicapped patients, even with the help of rehabilitation clinics and corrective orthopedic operations, rarely achieve a degree of motor control that permits them to lead an independent life, and they need supportive treatment and help as adults. In selected patients dorsal rhizotomy may diminish spasticity without augmenting the motor disability and, thus, facilitates a rehabilitative program. Intelligence may be preserved.

Kernicterus was a more common cause of abnormal cerebral development prior to the contemporary practice of restraining early postnatal serum bilirubin concentrations to levels below 250 μmol/L (15 mg/dL). The majority of infants with this disorder die within the first week or two of life, and those who survive are often mentally retarded, deaf, and totally unable to sit, stand, or walk. However, exceptional patients, obviously less damaged, are mentally normal or at most only slightly backward. Either athetosis or ataxia may be present. A few have rigid limbs and a picture not too different from that of cerebral spastic diplegia with involuntary movements. Kernicterus should always be suspected if an extrapyramidal syndrome is accompanied by bilateral deafness and palsy of upward gaze.

NEUROSKELETAL DISORDERS

The skull and vertebral column normally enlarge coordinately with growth of the central nervous system. Abnormalities in the size of the skull can occur secondary to underlying abnormalities of brain development. Abnormalities resulting primarily from derangements of osseous development may lead to aberrations in skull shape and to entrapment of the enclosed nervous system, as in the Chiari and related malformations. Abnormalities of nervous and skeletal systems are characteristically associated with disorders of body configuration and size and with the viscera. The majority of disorders with the neuroskeletal spectrum appear to arise as a consequence of pathologic processes set in motion from the earliest phases of organ formation and CNS development. These pathologic processes, though not well understood, are recognized to have both genetic and nongenetic causes. Among those which have their origins in gene mutation are those which appear to be segmental or multisegmental in their developmental affects; mutation or overexpression of homeotic genes in experimental animals provides models for certain of these complex and mysterious disorders.

SECONDARY MACROCRANIA AND MICROCRANIA Alterations in the circumference of the head greater than (macrocrania) or less than (microcrania) the 98th percentile are considered abnormal. Macrocrania may result from potentially correctable hydrocephalus and is associated with headache, mental dullness, depression, visual blurring, difficulty walking and urinary incontinence. Limited ability to elevate the eyes, ataxia of gait, hyperreflexia in the legs, and Babinski responses are common signs.

Developmental causes of *noncommunicating hydrocephalus* include aqueductal stenosis, the Dandy-Walker malformation in which the CSF escape from the 4th ventricle is obstructed, and the Chiari malformations (see below). Neoplasms or cysts, particularly when located within the ventricular system or impinging upon structures of the posterior fossa, must be excluded. *Communicating hydrocephalus* may develop after recovery from disorders that cause scarring of the leptomeninges, such as intraventricular hemorrhage in the perinatal period, especially in premature infants, and meningitis. Localized head enlargement, associated with mental slowing and contralateral long tract signs, may complicate porencephalic cerebral defects resulting from a focal cerebral injury in the perinatal period of early childhood.

Macrocrania may also be the result of an abnormally large brain (macrocephaly). Benign, or asymptomatic, macrocephaly may be familial. Macrocephaly associated with a characteristic triangular face, moderate impairment of cognitive functions and macrosomia constitute the syndrome of cerebral gigantism (Soto), which in some families appears to be transmitted by autosomal dominant inheritance. Symmetric or asymmetric macrocephaly, seizures, and cognitive impairment may occur with neurofibromatosis. Macrocephaly can also occur in certain lysosomal storage disorders that affect the brain, but such individuals rarely reach adulthood.

Microcrania is most commonly secondary to microcephaly. Typically this is a consequence of lack of brain growth and may result from virtually any heritable or acquired disorder that affects the developing brain. *Microcephaly vera* is a rare but distinctive disorder transmitted by autosomal recessive inheritance and associated mental retardation and brain weight less than 500 g. The face and facial features are distinctively prominent in relation to the small cranium.

PRIMARY DISORDER OF SKELETAL DEVELOPMENT The Chiari malformations are among the most prevalent and complex neuroskeletal malformations. The characteristic feature is entrapment and compression of the rhombencephalon within an underdeveloped posterior cranial fossa (see Marin-Padilla). In the severest forms, typically apparent at birth, the cerebellar vermis, medulla, and 4th ventricle are herniated or extruded into the upper cervical canal (Chiari Type II) or protrude exteriorly as an occipital encephalocele at the base of the skull (Chiari type III). Hydrocephalus and hydromyelia may be associated with meningomyelocele arising from the lumbosacral spinal cord. Milder degrees of herniation of the posteroinferior region of the cerebellum ("tonsils") into the cervical canal with little or no downward displacement of the 4th ventricle (Chiari Type I) or milder degrees of the Chiari II deformity may become symptomatic only in adolescence or adult life. Symptoms typical of adult expression of the Chiari malformation include pain that is localized to the cranial-cervical junction, which is aggravated by head movement or Valsalva maneuver. There may be unsteadiness of gait, dysarthria and dysphagia, corresponding to compromise of cerebellar related connections and lower cranial nerve paresis. Downbeat nystagmus is characteristic.

Syringomyelia or *syringobulbia* occur in association with the Chiari malformations. Syringomyelia, a disorder of the cervical region of the spinal cord, can be viewed as a progressive destructive expansion of a central cavitation of the spinal cord. A variable number of segments of the upper cervical and thoracic cord, or of the medulla and pons in the case of syringobulbia, may be involved. Typically, the commissure and the posterior horns of the central gray and the axonal fascicles of the posterior and lateral columns of the cord are damaged. The neurologic manifestations include impairment of pain and temperature perception in a cape-like distribution and impairment of perception of vibration and joint displacement and spasticity in the lower extremities. To the extent that anterior horn cells are destroyed at cervical segmental levels, muscle atrophy and weakness appear in the upper extremities (see Chap. 381). Extension of the cystic cavity upward into the brainstem can cause facial pain, nystagmus, and lower cranial nerve deficits.

Other disorders of the axial skeleton and the lower spinal cord and cauda equina are also characteristically associated with the Chiari malformation but may occur independently. The osseous anomalies include aberrations of the primary pattern of formation (absence or fusion) or the size of vertebrae, hemivertebra, or fusion of vertebra and scapula (Sprengel deformity). The Klippel-Feil deformity is a complex of osseous and visceral anomalies that include low hair line, platybasia, fusion of cervical vertebra with short neck, and deafness. These malformations may entrap and damage the brain and spinal cord. The disorders of the lower vertebral region may become symptomatic with rapid growth in adolescence or in adult life. Diastematomyelia, the protrusion of a bony spur into the vertebral canal, is of particular importance in adults because it represents a treatable form of deficit. Intermittent, generally progressive disturbances of somatic and visceral motor function, typically associated with pain, may be subtle clues to the diagnosis.

A cauda equina syndrome, that is, impairment of both somatic and visceral sensory and motor functions referable to the lower lumbar and sacral roots, may result from lipomas or dermoid cysts within the lower vertebral canal. A dimple or tuft of hair near the midline in the lumbar region or within the gluteal crease may suggest the persistence of a sinus tract or a deeper lying anomaly affecting vertebral canal and spinal roots. Tethering of the cord to the lower end of the vertebral canal by fibrous bands may result in traction that becomes symptomatic with growth in adolescence. Stenosis of the lumbar vertebral elements may be associated with claudication, that is, symptoms of a cauda equina syndrome that develop with walking.

Computed tomography and magnetic resonance imaging, particularly when utilized in conjunction with myelography for syrinx and other spinal disorders, are sensitive and efficient diagnostic procedures. Images obtained in the midsagittal plane are particularly appropriate for diagnosis of the Chiari malformation and syrinx and for abnormalities of the lumbosacral region. In principle, treatment is surgical. Decompression is appropriate for entrapment and compression, shunting is required for hydrocephalic (or syringomyelic) states. Mass lesions and bony spurs are excised.

SYNOSTOSES AND CRANIOFACIAL DEFORMITIES Cranial synostosis and some other craniofacial anomalies affect principally the rostral region and the vault of the skull. Premature closure of the sagittal suture results in an elongate (scaphocephalic) skull, and premature closure of the coronal sutures causes a broad and foreshortened (brachycephalic) skull. If all major sutures close prematurely, a tower (turricephalic) skull manifests itself by shallow orbits with bulging eyes. Other combinations may affect one or more sutures. Synostosis, particularly when generalized, may result in cerebral compression and hydrocephalus. Less extensive disorders are cosmetically disfiguring. Early surgical correction of the disorders is appropriate.

REFERENCES

ADAMS RD: Neurocutaneous disease, in *Dermatology in General Medicine*, 3d ed, TB Fitzpatrick et al (eds). New York, McGraw-Hill, 1986

————, LYON G: *Neurology of Hereditary Metabolic Diseases of Children*. New York, McGraw-Hill, 1982

BALLING R et al: Undulated, a mutation affecting the development of the mouse. Cell 55:531, 1988

BENSON PF, FENSOM AH: *Genetic Biochemical Disorders*. New York, Oxford Medical Publications, 1986

BERG BO: Current concepts of neurocutaneous disorders. Brain Dev 13:9, 1991

CASKEY CT et al: Triplet repeat mutations in human disease. Science 256:784, 1992

CHASNOFF IJ et al: Cocaine use in pregnancy. N Engl J Med 313:666, 1985

COPP AJ et al: The embryonic development of mammalian neural tube defects. Prog Neurobiol 35:363, 1990

DENCKLA MB, JAMES LS (eds). *An Update on Autism: A Developmental Disorder*. Pediatrics, vol 87, 1991

FRITH U et al: The cognitive basis of a biological disorder: Autism. Trends Neurosci 14:433, 1991

GOMEZ MR: Phenotypes of the tuberous sclerosis complex with revision of diagnostic criteria, in *Tuberous Sclerosis and Allied Disorders*, WG Johnson, MR Gomez (eds). Ann NY Acad Sci, Vol 615, 1991

HARRIS RM et al: Physical mapping within the tuberous sclerosis linkage group in region 9q32-q34. Genomics 15:265, 1993

HUGHES I, NEWTON R: Genetic aspects of cerebral palsy. Dev Med Child Neurol 34:80, 1992

LATIF F et al: Identification of the von Hippel-Lindau disease tumor suppressor gene. Science 260:1317, 1993

LUFKIN T et al: Disruption of the Hox-1.6 homeobox gene results in defects in a region corresponding to its rostral domain of expression. Cell 66:1105, 1991

MARIN-PADILLA M: Clinical and experimental rachischisis, in *Handbook of Clinical Neurology*, PJ Vinken, GW Bruyn (eds). Amsterdam, North Holland Publishing, 1978, pp 159–191

MARTUZA RL, ELDRIDGE R: Neurofibromatosis 2 (bilateral acoustic neurofibromatosis). N Engl J Med 318:684, 1988

ROWLAND LP et al (eds). *Molecular Genetics in Diseases of Brain, Nerve, and Muscles*. New York, Oxford University Press, 1989

SMITH DW: *Recognizable Patterns of Human Malformation*, 3d ed. Philadelphia, Saunders, 1982

SWAIMAN KF: *Pediatric Neurology: Principles and Practice*. St. Louis, Mosby, 1989

VISKOCHIL D et al: The neurofibromatosis type-1 gene. Annu Rev Neurosci 16:183, 1993

VOLPE JJ: *Neurology of the Newborn*. Philadelphia, Saunders, 1987

WALLACE MR, COLLINS FS: Molecular genetics of von Recklinghausen neurofibromatosis, in *Advances in Human Genetics* vol. 20, J Harris, K Hirschhorn (eds). New York, Plenum, 1991, pp 267–307

379   DISORDERS OF THE AUTONOMIC NERVOUS SYSTEM

RONALD J. POLINSKY / JOSEPH B. MARTIN

The regulation of homeostatic functions throughout the body is accomplished by the autonomic nervous system (ANS). An extensive peripheral innervation network combined with central vigilance provides rapid adjustments in vital physiologic mechanisms that are critical to survival. The importance of this regulation is emphasized by the extent and severity of disability resulting from compromised ANS function. The functional anatomy and relevant pharmacology of the sympathetic and parasympathetic components of the ANS are discussed in Chap. 68. This chapter describes the clinical manifestations, diagnosis, and treatment of ANS disorders. Hypothalamic disorders that cause disturbances in homeostasis are discussed in Chaps. 16 and 331.

CLINICAL MANIFESTATIONS   **Classification**   Disorders of the ANS may result from central or peripheral causes; they may be generalized, segmental, or focal. In many instances, the clinical signs and symptoms are due to interruption of reflex control of autonomic responses. For example, a lesion of the medulla oblongata in the brainstem may paralyze blood pressure responses to postural changes (orthostatic hypotension). Lesions of afferent connections (as in tabes dorsalis or diabetes mellitus) or of the efferent portion of the reflex arc (spinal cord disease, postganglionic autonomic insufficiency) may produce similar effects. Segmental disorders or focal deficits occur in spinal cord disease, in reflex sympathetic dystrophy (causalgia), and in Horner's syndrome (Table 379–1). Diagnosis of the site of reflex interruption is dependent on associated clinical findings, autonomic nervous system tests, and neural imaging.

Another approach to the classification of ANS disorders is based on the presence (or absence) of central nervous system (CNS) signs. The primary value of this approach is that pathophysiology and prognosis differ between these two groups. Subdivision of the two groups is based on special characteristics, e.g., the presence of a positive family history, pathologic characteristics, and the association with sensory/motor neuropathy. Unfortunately, some syndromes do

TABLE 379-1   Classification of ANS Disorders

GENERALIZED ANS DISORDERS

A   **With CNS signs**
1. Multiple system atrophy (Chap. 372)
2. Shy-Drager syndrome (Chap. 372)
3. Olivopontocerebellar degeneration (Chap. 372)
4. Striatonigral degeneration (Chap. 371)
5. Parkinson's disease (Chap. 337)
6. Huntington's disease (Chap. 370)
7. Hypothalamic disorders (Chap. 331)

B   **Without CNS signs**
1. Pure autonomic failure (Bradbury and Eggleston)
2. Guillain-Barré syndrome (occasionally accompanied by CNS signs) (Chap. 383)
3. Chronic idiopathic anhidrosis
4. Postural orthostatic tachycardia syndrome (POTS)
5. Raynaud's syndrome (Chap. 211)
6. Familial dysautonomia—Riley-Day syndrome

SEGMENTAL ANS DISORDERS

A   **Afferent loop disorders**
1. Tabes dorsalis (Chap. 381)
2. Diabetes mellitus (Chap. 337)
3. Spinal cord and root disorders (Chap. 381)
4. Guillain-Barré syndrome (Chap. 383)

B   **Efferent loop disorders**
1. Diabetes mellitus (Chap. 337)
2. Peripheral neuropathy (Chap. 383) (amyloidosis, porphyria, alcoholism)
3. Lambert-Eaton syndrome (Chap. 386)

FOCAL ANS DISORDERS

A   **Reflex sympathetic dystrophy (Chap. 299)**
1. Shoulder-hand syndrome
2. Causalgia

B   **Horner's syndrome (Chap. 19)**

C   **Reinnervation anomalies**
1. "Crocodile" tears (Chap. 380)

not fit easily into any classification scheme. Included in this category are chronic idiopathic anhidrosis, postural orthostatic tachycardia syndrome, and reflex sympathetic dystrophy of which little is known about their causes, pathology, or treatment (see Table 379–1).

Symptoms of autonomic dysfunction   The clinical manifestations of autonomic lesions depend on a number of factors including the organ involved and its normal balance of sympathetic-parasympathetic innervation, the nature of the underlying illness, and the severity and stage of progression (see Table 379–2). However, some generalizations can be made about evolution of autonomic symptoms. *Impotence* often heralds autonomic failure in men and may precede the appearance of other symptoms by more than a decade, making its relevance apparent only in retrospect (see Chap. 47). A decrease in the frequency of spontaneous erections may occur months before loss of nocturnal penile tumescence and development of total impotence. *Bladder dysfunction* also appears early in men and women, particularly in those with CNS involvement. As with other autonomic symptoms, there can be overactivity or loss of function; however, neurogenic bladder with frequency and incontinence is more common than retention. *Gastrointestinal dysfunction* is typically manifested as severe constipation, although diarrhea can occur in some disorders such as diabetes mellitus. Impairment of glandular secretory function may cause difficulty with food intake (decreased salivation) and eye irritation (decreased lacrimation). Occasionally, temperature elevation and vasodilation can result from *anhidrosis* since sweating is an important form of heat dissipation (see Chap. 16).

Orthostatic hypotension is the most disabling feature of autonomic dysfunction. Generally accepted criteria for diagnosis are a postural decrease of 20 mmHg in systolic or 10 mmHg in diastolic blood pressure sustained for at least 3 minutes in the standing position to differentiate autonomic failure from sluggish baroreflex responses that are common in the elderly. Postural hypotension can cause a variety of symptoms including headache, neck/shoulder pain, dimming or

TABLE 379-2 Major clinical manifestations in some generalized autonomic failure syndromes

Disorder	Postural hypotension	Genitourinary dysfunction	Gastrointestinal involvement	Sweating deficit	Other manifestations
Aging	+ +	+	+	+/−	Postprandial hypotension
Alcoholism	+	+			Tachycardia
Amyloidosis	+ + +	+	+ +	+ +	Dissociated sensory loss
Diabetes mellitus	+ + +	+ +	+ + + +	+	Distal neuropathy
Familial dysautonomia	+ +	+	+ + +	+	Abdominal crises, fevers, ↓ sensitivity to pain
Holmes-Adie syndrome	+ +		+ +	+	Tonic pupils, areflexia, supine hypertension
Multiple system atrophy	+ + + +	+ + +	+ + +	+ + +	Parkinsonian and/or cerebellar dysfunction
Parkinson's disease	+ +	+	+ +	+/−	Sweating may be increased
Progressive supranuclear palsy	+	+ +	+ + +	+	Rigidity, gaze palsies
Pure autonomic failure	+ + + +	+	+ + +	+ + +	

Abbreviations: ± = Inconsistent or minimal; + = mild; + + = moderate; + + + = severe; + + + + = disabling lack of adrenergic output. Also, insulin can cause profound hypotensive effects.

loss of vision, and weakness. Syncope results when the drop in systemic pressure impairs cerebral perfusion (see Chap. 17). Other manifestations of impaired cardiovascular control from baroreflex dysfunction include supine hypertension, fixed heart rate, and postprandial hypotension.

Autonomic testing The organizational and functional characteristics of the ANS can be assessed by physiologic and pharmacologic tests. Physiologic methods offer the advantage of ease but are useful primarily for demonstrating the presence of an autonomic lesion, whereas pharmacologic tests can elucidate pathophysiologic abnormalities and guide the development of rational therapy.

VALSALVA RESPONSE Investigation of blood pressure (BP) control is particularly valuable in eliciting evidence of ANS disorders. The Valsalva response assesses the afferent limb, central integrity, and efferent limb of the baroreceptor reflex. An abnormal Valsalva response indicates a lesion in the pathways responsible for BP control, and analysis of the type of abnormal response can help define the site of the defect. With the use of continuous noninvasive BP recordings using plethysmographic techniques, the integrity of the efferent limb of the baroreflex arc can be evaluated by measuring the BP response to immersion of the hand in ice water (cold pressor test). This test may be invalid if spinothalamic function (pain and temperature) is abnormal. *The presence of an afferent or central lesion can be inferred when a normal cold pressor efferent response is evoked in the presence of an abnormal Valsalva response.* Central vasomotor function can be assessed by examining the BP response to hyperventilation. Sinus arrhythmia and the heart rate response to deep breathing provide physiologic indices of parasympathetic function. These are assessed by measuring the changes in RR interval on the electrocardiogram during phases of respiration.

QUANTITATIVE SUDOMOTOR AXON REFLEX TEST (QSART) Sweating is induced by release of acetylcholine (ACh) from sympathetic postganglionic fibers. The *sudomotor axon reflex* can be activated by a constant current generator, and ACh-induced sweat release can be quantified (see Low). A reduced or absent response indicates a lesion of the postganglionic sudomotor axon. Abnormalities may be identifiable in patients with autonomic dysfunction (diabetes mellitus, amyloidosis) before clinical symptoms emerge.

ORTHOSTATIC BLOOD PRESSURE RECORDINGS Beat-to-beat BP measurements determined in supine, 80° tilt, and tilt-back are useful to quantitate orthostatic failure in BP control. It is important to allow a 20-min period of supine rest before assessing changes in BP during tilting.

PHARMACOLOGIC TESTS Pharmacologic assessments are based on responses to the administration of selectively active drugs. Neurochemical investigations typically provide the rationale for selecting various drugs as probes. For example, low plasma norepinephrine (NE) levels reflect postganglionic involvement in peripheral autonomic disorders. Further definition of specific abnormalities in noradrenergic neuronal function can be achieved by using drugs with

pressor activity. Tyramine, an indirect sympathomimetic, increases blood pressure if neuronal NE stores are adequate and the uptake mechanisms are intact. Up-regulation of postsynaptic noradrenergic receptors, a manifestation of denervating lesions, can be demonstrated by measuring the BP response to NE. Supersensitivity is reflected by a leftward shift of the dose-response curve in contrast to the increased slope that results from decentralization. The chronotropic response to BP elevation using a pure alpha-adrenergic agonist (e.g., phenylephrine) serves as an index of afferent baroreflex function. Measurement of BP and heart rate responses to isoproterenol provide measures of beta$_2$- and beta$_1$-adrenergic cardiovascular functions, respectively.

SPECIFIC SYNDROMES OF ANS DYSFUNCTION Two neurodegenerative disorders (pure autonomic failure and multiple system atrophy) have been intensively studied in an effort to clarify the distinction between central and peripheral ANS lesions (see Table 379–1).

Pure autonomic failure This syndrome of isolated, generalized autonomic dysfunction was described by Bradbury and Eggleston in 1925. The etiology is unknown. It occurs in the absence of peripheral neuropathy and is not inherited. The disorder generally begins in the middle decades with insidious onset and affects women more than men. The symptoms, particularly postural hypotension, can be disabling, but the disease does not appear to shorten the life-span. Although the pathologic changes have not been characterized in detail, the clinical and neuropharmacologic characteristics are consistent with primary involvement of postganglionic sympathetic neurons. Low plasma NE, reduced NE response to tyramine, decreased neuronal uptake of NE, and noradrenergic supersensitivity reflect peripheral sympathetic noradrenergic dysfunction.

Multiple system atrophy The clinicopathologic and neurochemical features of multiple system atrophy differ from those in pure autonomic failure. *The term refers to several overlapping clinical disorders including striatonigral degeneration and olivopontocerebellar atrophy* (see Chap. 372). *Shy-Drager syndrome* is a well-characterized form of multiple system atrophy that is accompanied by autonomic failure. Most patients present with autonomic dysfunction, and somatic neurologic manifestations usually develop within 5 years. Patients with the striatonigral variant exhibit a form of parkinsonism in which bradykinesia and rigidity are more prominent than tremor. Patients with either a pure cerebellar syndrome or striatonigral degeneration may also develop pyramidal tract involvement. Some patients, particularly those with Shy-Drager syndrome, have features of both subtypes (see Chap. 372).

These disorders progress relentlessly to death 7 to 10 years after onset. Normal or elevated plasma NE, defective baroreflex modulation of BP, and low CSF monoamine metabolite levels (MHPG, 5HIAA) are consistent with CNS involvement in this syndrome. From a neuropathologic standpoint, these disorders are classified as primary neuronal degenerations with loss of neurons and gliosis in many

CNS regions including the brainstem, cerebellum, striatum, and intermediolateral zone of the spinal cord.

Pure autonomic failure and multiple system atrophy are relatively uncommon. ANS disorders occurring in Parkinson's disease, Huntington's disease, and progressive supranuclear palsy are more common (see Chap. 371).

Peripheral nerve disorders Peripheral neuropathies are the most common cause of chronic autonomic insufficiency (see Chap. 383). Neuropathies that affect small myelinated and unmyelinated fibers of the sympathetic and parasympathetic nerves occur in diabetes mellitus, amyloidosis, chronic alcoholism, porphyria, and Guillain-Barré syndrome.

DIABETES MELLITUS Autonomic involvement in diabetes may begin at any stage in the disease and often presents with altered vagal function (see Chap. 337). Loss of myelinated fibers in the splanchnic innervation, carotid sinus, and vagus nerves characterize the disorder. Widespread enteric neuropathy can cause profound disturbances in gut motility, achlorhydria, and rectal incontinence and may result in failure of the typical signs of hypoglycemia to appear when sympathetic efferents to the adrenal gland are impaired. Insulin excess may also cause profound hypotension in patients with abnormal blood pressure regulation. Autonomic dysfunction may lengthen the QT interval and enhance the risk of sudden death. The cause of the neuropathy in diabetes is unknown. Hyperglycemia appears to be one risk factor for autonomic involvement. Biochemical and pharmacologic studies in diabetic neuropathy reveal low plasma NE, decreased responses to tyramine and edrophonium, and enhanced pressor responsivity to phenylephrine.

AMYLOID POLYNEUROPATHY Autonomic neuropathy occurs in both sporadic and familial forms of amyloidosis (see Chap. 383). Although patients usually present with a painful neuropathy accompanied by a dissociated sensory loss, autonomic insufficiency can precede the development of the sensorimotor neuropathy. Cardiac and renal impairment are the usual causes of death. Postmortem studies reveal amyloid deposition in many organs including two sites that contribute to autonomic failure: intraneural blood vessels and neurons in autonomic ganglia.

ALCOHOLIC NEUROPATHY Abnormal parasympathetic vagal and efferent sympathetic function occur in chronic alcoholics, and pathologic changes can be demonstrated in the vagus nerves, sympathetic fibers, and ganglia. Impotence is a major problem, but concurrent abnormalities in gonadal hormones may obscure the parasympathetic contribution to this symptom. Autonomic failure generally appears after the onset of peripheral neuropathy, although orthostatic hypotension may be prominent in Wernicke's encephalopathy. Alcoholics with liver disease are more likely to develop autonomic neuropathy. Autonomic involvement may contribute to the high mortality rates in alcoholism.

PORPHYRIA Although each of the porphyrias can cause autonomic dysfunction, the condition is most extensively documented in the acute intermittent type (see Chap. 346). Prominent symptoms include abdominal pain, nausea, vomiting, tachycardia, sweating abnormalities, urinary retention, and hypertension. Abnormal autonomic function can occur both during acute attacks and during remissions. Elevated catecholamine levels during acute attacks correlate with the degree of tachycardia and hypertension. Interestingly, several heme precursors inhibit NE uptake in platelets from patients with acute porphyria.

GUILLAIN-BARRÉ SYNDROME Blood pressure fluctuations and arrhythmias can be severe in acute demyelinating polyradiculoneuropathy. Abnormal sweating, sphincter disturbance, and pupillary dysfunction also occur. Fortunately, autonomic dysfunction is minimal in most patients and is rare in the chronic form of the disorder. Pathologic changes have been described in the vagus and glossopharyngeal nerves, the sympathetic chain, and the white rami communicans.

Segmental involvement of the ANS REFLEX SYMPATHETIC DYSTROPHY Reflex sympathetic dystrophy, also referred to as the *shoulder-hand syndrome* or *causalgia*, is characterized by pain, loss of function, and localized autonomic impairment. Myocardial infarction, limb paralysis, and shoulder trauma can be precipitating events. The pain has a neuropathic character, and the autonomic dysfunction causes localized sweating and changes in blood flow. Abnormal hair and nail growth may accompany edema or atrophy of the skin. Although the pathophysiology is not completely understood, the changes in blood flow and sweating appear to result from localized noradrenergic and cholinergic supersensitivity. An analogous defect, perhaps involving endogenous opioids, could underlie the pain. Treatment of reflex sympathetic dystrophy is a difficult therapeutic challenge (see Chap. 11).

SPINAL CORD LESIONS Spinal cord transection may be attended by autonomic hyperreflexia. The increased autonomic discharge can be elicited by bladder pressure or by other stimuli. This phenomenon affects 85 percent of patients with a spinal cord lesion above the C6 level. Sudden, dramatic increases in blood pressure can lead to intracranial hemorrhage and death.

MULTIPLE SCLEROSIS A variety of abnormalities in autonomic function occur in multiple sclerosis. Abnormal sweating occurs in approximately 40 percent of cases. Impairment of cardiovascular control is less common and usually minor. There does not appear to be any relationship between the severity of the disease and degree of autonomic involvement. However, the sympathetic nervous system can modulate immune mechanisms that could contribute to disease progression.

Inherited disorders Riley-Day syndrome (familial dysautonomia) is an autosomal recessive disorder occurring in Ashkenazic Jews which is associated with decreased tearing, reduced sensitivity to pain, and absent fungiform papillae on the tongue. Episodic abdominal crises and fever are common. Increased sensitivity to intraocular methacholine and absent axon flare response to intradermal histamine injection are useful diagnostic markers. Normal resting plasma NE levels that do not increase upon standing are consistent with an afferent lesion. The mechanism of the increased urinary excretion of homovanillic acid is unclear (see Chap. 364).

A syndrome of dopamine-β-hydroxylase deficiency has been described in siblings and may be hereditary. This rare syndrome is an important model for the development of rational pharmacotherapy. Patients with this condition have a variety of sympathetic failure. Plasma levels of NE and epinephrine are virtually absent while dopamine levels are extremely high. Administration of an unnatural NE precursor, L-dihydroxyphenylserine (L-DOPS), increases plasma NE and greatly improves the symptoms. This compound bypasses the enzymatic block in NE synthesis resulting from the deficiency of dopamine-β-hydroxylase.

Miscellaneous Other conditions associated with autonomic failure include autoimmune disease, infections, toxins, malignancy, and aging. Disorders of the hypothalamus can affect autonomic function and produce, in addition to the symptoms already discussed, abnormalities in temperature control, satiety, sexual function, and circadian rhythms (see Chap. 331).

TREATMENT In most conditions, management of autonomic failure is limited to alleviating the disability caused by the symptoms. If possible, the primary disorder, e.g., diabetes mellitus, should be treated, but this will not generally improve autonomic function. Orthostatic hypotension is the main focus of treatment because it can drastically impair function. Other aspects of autonomic failure may also affect blood pressure control. For example, severe constipation leads to excessive straining that can precipitously lower blood pressure.

Orthostatic hypotension only requires treatment if it causes symptoms. Supine hypertension presents a therapeutic dilemma in some patients. In the early stages patients can maintain normal function by using good judgment and a few precautions. For example, small meals are better tolerated because they mitigate the shunting of blood towards the splanchnic circulation during digestion. Alcohol intake and excessive environmental temperatures should be avoided because vasodilation can precipitously lower blood pressure in patients with deficient baroreflex activity. Drugs that affect blood pressure should be used with caution; many nonprescription medicines contain sympathomimetic agents.

Salt intake should be increased to the maximum tolerated. Sleeping in a reverse Trendelenburg position (head-up tilt) reduces nocturnal diuresis in these patients and helps to minimize supine hypertension. Compressive garments are of questionable value but may be tried; they present a number of practical problems, particularly for individuals with neurogenic bladder and/or neurologic impairment.

Eventually, most patients require drug therapy for management of hypotension. Fludrocortisone, which enhances renal sodium conservation, is the initial drug of choice; potassium supplements are necessary with chronic administration. Inhibitors of prostaglandin synthesis (e.g., ibuprofen) have potent pressor effects in patients with autonomic dysfunction. Other pharmacologic agents have been used with variable success to elevate blood pressure. These include beta-blockers (propranolol, pindolol, xamoterol), sympathomimetics (ephedrine, midodrine), dopamine antagonists (metoclopramide), and venoconstrictors (dihydroergotamine). Other approaches include the vasopressin analogue desmopressin and the somatostatin analogue octreotide. Desmopressin minimizes fluid loss which may play an important role in exacerbating the hypotension in patients with autonomic failure. Octreotide inhibits release of gut peptides, some of which have profound vasodilator and hypotensive effects. Since these substances are typically released after a meal, octreotide is most effective in alleviating postprandial hypotension.

Many patients with ANS failure exhibit exaggerated sensitivity to various drugs. Compounds with hypotensive actions should generally be avoided. Hence, anticholinergic agents are a better initial choice than dopaminergic compounds for parkinsonism. Anesthetic management poses unique problems since these patients have atypical physiologic and pharmacologic responses, abnormal fluid balance, and adrenal medullary insufficiency. More important than the choice of anesthetic is awareness by the physician of the implications autonomic failure may have for peri- and postoperative monitoring and management.

REFERENCES

ARNOLD JMO et al: Increased venous alpha-adrenoceptor responsiveness in patients with reflex sympathetic dystrophy. Ann Intern Med 118:619, 1993

BANNISTER R (ed): *Autonomic Failure*, 3d ed. London, Oxford University Press, 1992

———, OPPENHEIMER DR: Degenerative diseases of the nervous system associated with autonomic failure. Brain 95:457, 1972

BRADBURY S, EGGLESTON C: Postural hypotension: A report of three cases. Am Heart J 1:73, 1925

DAGOGOJACK SE et al: Hypoglycemia-associated autonomic failure in insulin-dependent diabetes-mellitus—Recent antecedent hypoglycemia reduces autonomic responses to, symptoms of, and defense against subsequent hypoglycemia. J Clin Invest 91:819, 1993

HIRAYAMA M et al: Postprandial hypotension—Hemodynamic differences between multiple system atrophy and peripheral autonomic neuropathy. J Auton Nerv Syst 43:1, 1993

JOHNSON RG: Autonomic involvement in systemic diseases. Curr Opinion Neurol Neurosurg 5:468, 1992

LOW PA, PFEIFER MA: Standardization of autonomic function, in PA Low (ed): *Clinical Autonomic Disorders: Evaluation and Management*. Boston, Little Brown, 1992

MAN IN'T VELD AJ et al: Congenital dopamine-β-hydroxylase deficiency: A novel orthostatic syndrome. Lancet 1:183, 1987

MCLEOD JG: Autonomic dysfunction in peripheral nerve disease. Muscle Nerve 15:3, 1992

———, TUCK RR: Disorders of the autonomic nervous system. Ann Neurol 21:419(1), 519(2), 1987

POLINSKY RJ: Clinical autonomic neuropharmacology. Neurol Clin 8:77, 1990

———: Autonomic dysfunction in neurological illness, in *Textbook of Clinical Neuropharmacology*, HL Klawans et al (eds). New York, Raven Press, 1992, pp 537–557

Proceedings of a consensus development conference on standardized measures in diabetic neuropathy: Autonomic nervous system testing. Neurology 42:1823, 1992

ROBERTSON D et al: Isolated failure of autonomic noradrenergic neurotransmission. Evidence for impaired β-hydroxylation of dopamine. N Engl J Med 314:1494, 1986

SHY GM, DRAGER GA: A neurologic syndrome associated with orthostatic hypotension. Arch Neurol 2:511, 1960

380 DISORDERS OF THE CRANIAL NERVES

MAURICE VICTOR / JOSEPH B. MARTIN

The cranial nerves are susceptible to disorders that rarely affect the spinal peripheral nerves and, for this reason, deserve to be considered separately. This chapter describes the principal syndromes of disordered cranial nerve function and the diseases that cause them. Disorders of taste and smell, vision and ocular movement, and vertigo and deafness are discussed in Chaps. 18 to 20.

OLFACTORY NERVE (See Chap. 20)

OPTIC NERVE

TRANSIENT MONOCULAR BLINDNESS (AMAUROSIS FUGAX) (See also Chap. 368) **Definition** These terms are used interchangeably to designate an attack of transient painless loss of vision in one eye. Frequently it is recurrent.

Clinical manifestations Amaurosis fugax is a common clinical symptom indicative of transient retinal ischemia, usually associated with ipsilateral internal carotid artery stenosis or embolism of the retinal arteries. In some cases the basis for the symptom cannot be discerned.

Typically, the episode of blindness evolves swiftly, in a matter of 10 to 15 s, and is described as a shade that falls smoothly and painlessly over the field of vision until the eye is completely blind. Or a similar obliteration of the visual field may occur from below. The blindness lasts for a few seconds or minutes, sometimes longer, then clears slowly and uniformly, the patient's vision returning in the reverse direction from that in which it was lost. Sometimes there is only a generalized dimness of vision, rather than a complete loss, or only a segment of the visual field may be involved. Many patients who experience amaurosis fugax on the basis of carotid stenosis also have transient attacks of contralateral hemiparesis, but it is uncommon for the two types of attack to occur simultaneously.

Diagnosis The transient visual loss that accompanies classic migraine is of a different type. Often it begins with unformed flashes of light (photopsia) or dazzling zigzag lines (fortification spectra or teichopsia) which move across the visual field for several minutes, leaving scotomatous or hemianopic defects. The patient with migraine may complain of blindness in one eye, but examination usually shows the visual loss to be bilateral and homonymous, i.e., to occupy corresponding halves of both visual fields. The latter abnormality points to an origin in the visual cortex of one occipital lobe. In so-called basilar migraine, in which the neurologic symptoms are referable to the territory of the basilar artery, the transient visual disturbances may occupy the whole of both visual fields.

Investigation and treatment Amaurosis fugax is most commonly a manifestation of ipsilateral internal carotid artery disease. Carotid bruits should be sought, and noninvasive tests for carotid blood flow and lumen diameter should be carried out in every case. The decision of when to proceed to angiography is discussed in Chap. 368. Definitive treatment is dependent on the results of these investigations. In the absence of carotid disease, possible sources of emboli (cardiac or aortic) should be sought. Amaurosis fugax may sometimes herald occlusion of the central retinal artery or anterior ischemic optic neuropathy due to giant cell arteritis or to nonarteritic (atherosclerotic) disease. The sedimentation rate is usually elevated in giant cell arteritis (Chap. 291).

RETROBULBAR OPTIC NEUROPATHY OR NEURITIS Definition This syndrome is characterized by the rapid development (hours or days) of impaired vision in one or both eyes. In the latter case the eyes may be affected either simultaneously or sequentially. The visual loss in such cases is usually the result of acute demyelinative disease of optic nerves, although several other causes of unilateral or bilateral optic nerve disease need also to be considered (see below).

Clinical manifestations   The most frequent setting is one in which a child, adolescent, or young adult notes a rapid diminution of vision in one eye (as though a veil or haze covered every object seen). Within a few days the condition may progress to severe loss of vision, but complete blindness is rare. The optic disc and retina may appear normal, but in some patients the disc is hyperemic and elevated with blurring of the disc margins (papillitis). Peripapillary hemorrhages are seen infrequently, and the veins are not engorged. *Papillitis* is distinguished from *papilledema* due to increased intracranial pressure by the acute and often marked reduction of visual acuity that accompanies the former. Also, in retrobulbar neuropathy, movement of the eye or pressure on the globe is often painful. After a few days or weeks the other eye may become similarly involved, with loss, typically, of central vision but with some preservation of peripheral vision. The pupillary light reflex is impaired. With complete or nearly complete interruption of one optic nerve, the pupil fails to react to direct light stimulation but does constrict when light is shone in the healthy eye (consensual reflex). With lesser degrees of optic nerve damage, there may be a failure to sustain pupillary constriction in response to a steady light stimulus (''pupillary escape'' or Gunn pupil sign) (see Chap. 19, Fig. 19-3).

In a high percentage of patients, no cause can be found, and after a few days or weeks there is spontaneous recovery of vision. Sometimes a small central scotoma persists. The optic disc later becomes slightly pale due to demyelination, most prominent in the temporal region. The CSF may be normal or may contain from 10 to 20 lymphocytes, and the protein content, particularly the gamma globulin portion, may be increased. Oligoclonal bands are found in some patients.

More than half of such patients will develop the symptoms and signs of multiple sclerosis within 10 to 15 years, and an even higher percentage will do so if the patients are observed for longer periods (see Chap. 373). The prognosis for children with retrobulbar neuropathy is considerably better than that for adults. Multiple sclerosis is the most common cause of a *unilateral retrobulbar neuritis*. Bilateral optic neuritis may occur in association with or slightly in advance of an attack of transverse myelitis, a combination referred to as neuromyelitis optica or Devic disease (Chap. 373).

Diagnosis   Other causes of unilateral optic neuropathy include postinfectious or disseminated encephalomyelitis, posterior uveitis, and, much more commonly (particularly in persons > 50 years of age), vascular lesions of the optic nerve. *Anterior ischemic optic neuropathy (AION)* is a condition caused by interruption of blood supply to the optic nerve secondary to atherosclerotic or inflammatory disease of the ophthalmic artery or its posterior ciliary branches (see Chap. 19). It presents clinically as acute, painless, visual loss in one eye, often accompanied by an altitudinal visual field defect. In severe cases, visual loss is complete and permanent. The fundus shows a markedly swollen optic disc surrounded by splinter-shaped peripapillary hemorrhages. Investigations are directed toward excluding temporal arteritis (see Chap. 291). Rarely, microemboli can cause occlusion of the posterior ciliary arteries and AION, following open heart or coronary artery bypass surgery, for example.

Central retinal artery occlusion (CRAO) also presents with sudden blindness. In this entity the optic disc initially appears normal. The retina is infarcted and appears pale with accentuation of the macular cherry red spot. In all cases of unilateral involvement of the optic nerve, tumor (glioma, von Recklinghausen neurofibromatosis, meningioma) needs to be ruled out.

Treatment   Acute optic neuropathy due to demyelinative disease usually resolves without specific treatment. Severe visual loss is commonly treated with intravenous methylprednisolone or ACTH as outlined in the section on multiple sclerosis (see Chap. 373), but it should not be treated with oral prednisone alone (see Lessell).

Treatment may hasten recovery from an individual attack but does not prevent further attacks or modify their severity.

TOXIC-NUTRITIONAL OPTIC NEUROPATHY   Simultaneous impairment of vision in the two eyes, with central or centrocecal scotomas, occurring over a period of days or weeks, is usually due to a toxic or nutritional disorder rather than to a demyelinative process (see Chap. 377). Impairment of vision due to *methyl alcohol intoxication* is abrupt in onset and is characterized by large symmetric central scotomas, as well as by symptoms of systemic disease and acidosis (see Chap. 395). The lesion is in the retinal ganglion cells and their axons, which constitute the optic nerve. The most important therapeutic measure is the immediate intravenous administration of sodium bicarbonate. Hemodialysis is a useful adjunct because of the slow rate of oxidation of methyl alcohol. Other drugs with proven but less devastating toxic effects on the optic nerve include chloramphenicol, ethambutol, isoniazid, streptomycin, sulfonamides, digitalis, ergot, disulfiram, and heavy metals (see also Chap. 19).

Degenerative diseases may affect the retina or the optic nerves, taking the form of optic atrophy. There are several types of hereditary optic atrophy, a common one being the Leber type, which has been shown to be due to a point mutation in mitochondrial DNA and is therefore maternally inherited (see Chap. 385). An autosomal dominant form of congenital or early infantile optic atrophy and optic atrophy with diabetes mellitus and deafness are equally common. Senile macular degeneration and various forms of retinitis pigmentosa are important causes of visual loss (see Chap. 19).

BITEMPORAL HEMIANOPIA   This type of visual disorder is usually related to suprasellar extension of a pituitary adenoma (often with an enlarged sella), but it also may be due to a craniopharyngioma, saccular aneurysm of the circle of Willis, meningioma of the tuberculum sellae (normal sella or thickened tuberculum by radiography), and rarely sarcoidosis, metastatic carcinoma, and Hand-Schüller-Christian disease (see Chap. 331). The lesion involves the decussating nasal fibers from each retina.

OCULOMOTOR, TROCHLEAR, AND ABDUCENS NERVES (See Chap. 19)

TRIGEMINAL NERVE

The trigeminal nerve supplies sensation to the skin of the face and anterior half of the head. Its motor part innervates the masseter and pterygoid masticatory muscles.

PAROXYSMAL FACIAL PAIN (TRIGEMINAL NEURALGIA, TIC DOULOUREUX)   Definition   The most striking disorder of trigeminal nerve function is tic douloureux, a condition characterized by excruciating paroxysms of pain in the lips, gums, cheek, or chin and, very rarely, in the distribution of the ophthalmic division of the fifth nerve. The disorder occurs almost exclusively in middle-aged and elderly persons. The pain seldom lasts more than a few seconds or a minute or two but may be so intense that the patient winces, hence the term *tic*. The paroxysms recur frequently, both day and night, for several weeks at a time. Another characteristic feature is the initiation of pain by stimuli applied to certain areas on the face, lips, or tongue (''trigger zones'') or by movement of these parts. Sensory loss cannot be demonstrated. In studying the relations between stimuli applied to a trigger zone and the paroxysm of pain, it is found that the adequate stimulus for precipitating an attack is a tactile one and possibly tickle, rather than a noxious or thermal stimulus. Usually a spatial and temporal summation of impulses is necessary to trigger an attack, which is followed by a refractory period of up to 2 or 3 min.

The *diagnosis* of this disorder rests on these strict clinical criteria, and the condition must be distinguished from other forms of facial and cephalic neuralgia and pain arising from diseases of the jaw, teeth, or sinuses (see Chap. 14). Tic douloureux is usually without assignable cause; occasionally, when it appears in younger adults, it may be due to a demyelinative plaque at the root entry zone of the fifth nerve. Very rarely it may occur with herpes zoster or a tumor. To a degree that remains uncertain, pain of tic douloureux may be caused by a redundant or tortuous blood vessel in the posterior fossa, causing an irritative lesion of the nerve or its root. Usually, however, lesions such as aneurysms, neurofibromas, or meningiomas affecting the nerve produce a loss of sensation (trigeminal neuropathy, see below).

Treatment The initial treatment of tic douloureux is pharmacologic. Carbamazepine is the drug of choice and is effective initially in 75 percent of patients. Carbamazepine should be started gradually, 100 mg with food, as a single dose, and increased to 200 mg qid. Doses greater than 1200 mg daily provide no additional benefit. Unfortunately, not all patients can tolerate the drug in the doses required to alleviate pain, in which case phenytoin, 300 to 400 mg daily, can be substituted.

If drug treatment fails, surgical therapy should be offered. The most widely applied procedure is percutaneous retrogasserian rhizotomy accomplished by radiofrequency lesions. Injection of glycerol in Meckel's cave is a method preferred by some surgeons. Relief is obtained by either of these procedures in more than 95 percent of patients. The pain recurs in 7 to 31 percent of patients. Complications and morbidity are infrequent in experienced hands. These procedures result in partial numbness of the face and carry a risk of corneal denervation with secondary keratitis when used for rare instances of first-division trigeminal neuralgia.

A third treatment, microvascular decompression, requires a suboccipital craniectomy, a major procedure requiring several days of hospitalization. It has an 80 percent efficacy rate, but the pain may recur, and in a small number of cases, there may be damage to the eighth or seventh nerve. A rare but most troublesome complication of all surgical treatments is the development of anesthesia dolorosa or denervation hypersensitivity. This condition responds poorly to treatment. Tricyclic antidepressants or phenothiazines are usually given with only partial success in alleviating the discomfort.

TRIGEMINAL NEUROPATHY A variety of diseases may affect the trigeminal nerve in addition to those mentioned above. Most present with sensory loss on the face or with weakness of the jaw muscles. Deviation of the jaw on opening indicates weakness of the pterygoids of the side to which the jaw deviates. Tumors of the middle cranial fossa (meningiomas), of the trigeminal nerve (schwannomas), or of the base of the skull (metastatic) may cause a combination of motor and sensory signs. Lesions in the cavernous sinus can affect the first and second divisions of the trigeminal nerve, and lesions of the superior orbital fissure can affect the first (ophthalmic) division. The accompanying corneal anesthesia increases the risk of ulceration (neurokeratitis).

Anesthesia and analgesia of the face have been reported after treatment with stilbamidine (formerly used in the treatment of kala azar and multiple myeloma). Pain and itching may occur during recovery. Rarely, an idiopathic form of trigeminal neuropathy is observed. It is characterized by feelings of numbness and paresthesias, sometimes bilaterally, with loss of sensation in the territory of the trigeminal nerve but without weakness of the jaw. Recovery is the rule, but the symptoms may be troublesome for many months, or even years. Leprosy may involve the trigeminal nerves.

Tonic spasm of the masticatory muscles, known as *trismus*, is symptomatic of tetanus (see Chap. 106). It also may occur as an idiosyncratic reaction in patients treated with phenothiazine drugs; lesser degrees may be associated with disease of the pharynx, temporomandibular joint, teeth, and gums.

FACIAL NERVE

FACIAL PALSY AND FACIAL SPASM The seventh cranial nerve supplies all the muscles concerned with facial expression. The sensory component is small (the nervus intermedius of Wrisberg); it conveys taste sensation from the anterior two-thirds of the tongue and probably cutaneous impulses from the anterior wall of the external auditory canal. The motor nucleus of the seventh nerve lies anterior and lateral to the abducens nucleus. After leaving the pons, the seventh nerve enters the internal auditory meatus with the acoustic nerve. The nerve continues its course in its own bony channel, the facial canal, and exits from the skull via the stylomastoid foramen. It then passes through the parotid gland and subdivides to supply the facial muscles.

A complete interruption of the facial nerve at the stylomastoid foramen paralyzes all muscles of facial expression. The corner of the mouth droops, the creases and skin folds are effaced, the forehead is unfurrowed, and the eyelids will not close. Upon attempted closure of the lids, the eye on the paralyzed side is seen to roll upward (Bell's phenomenon). The lower lid sags also, and the punctum falls away from the conjunctiva, permitting tears to spill over the cheek. Food collects between the teeth and lips, and saliva may dribble from the corner of the mouth. The patient complains of a heaviness or numbness in the face, but sensory loss is rarely demonstrable and taste is intact.

If the lesion is in the middle ear portion, taste is lost over the anterior two-thirds of the tongue on the same side. If the nerve to the stapedius is interrupted, there is hyperacusis (painful sensitivity to loud sounds). Lesions in the internal auditory meatus also may affect the adjacent auditory and vestibular nerves, causing deafness, tinnitus, or dizziness. Intrapontine lesions that paralyze the face usually affect the abducens nucleus as well, and often the corticospinal and sensory tracts.

If the peripheral facial paralysis has existed for some time and recovery of motor function has begun but is incomplete, a kind of contracture (actually a continuous diffuse contraction) of facial muscles may appear. The palpebral fissure becomes narrowed, and the nasolabial fold deepens. With the passage of time, the face and even the tip of the nose become pulled to the unaffected side. Attempts to move one group of facial muscles may result in contraction of all of them (associated movements, or *synkinesis*). Facial spasms may develop and persist indefinitely, being initiated by every facial movement (*hemifacial spasm*). This condition may represent a transient or permanent sequela to a Bell's palsy but also may be due to an irritative lesion of the facial nerve (e.g., an acoustic neuroma, an aberrant artery that compresses the nerve and is relieved by surgery, or a basilar artery aneurysm). However, in the most common form of hemifacial spasm, the cause and pathology are unknown. Anomalous regeneration of the seventh nerve fibers may result in other troublesome phenomena. If fibers originally connected with the orbicularis oculi come to innervate the orbicularis oris, closure of the lids may cause a retraction of the mouth, or if fibers originally connected with muscles of the face later innervate the lacrimal gland, anomalous tearing (crocodile tears) may occur with any activity of the facial muscles, such as eating. Yet another unusual facial synkinesia is one in which jaw opening causes a closure of the eyelids on the side of the facial palsy (jaw-winking).

BELL'S PALSY **Definition** The most common form of facial paralysis is idiopathic, i.e., *Bell's palsy*. The incidence rate of this disorder is about 23 per 100,000 annually, or about 1 in 60 or 70 persons in a lifetime. The pathogenesis of the paralysis is unknown. The few autopsied cases of this disease have shown only nondescript changes in the facial nerve and not inflammatory changes, as is commonly presumed.

Clinical manifestations The onset of Bell's palsy is fairly abrupt, maximal weakness being attained by 48 h as a general rule. Pain behind the ear may precede the paralysis for a day or two. Taste sensation may be lost unilaterally, and hyperacusis may be present. In some cases there is mild CSF lymphocytosis. Fully 80 percent of patients recover within a few weeks or months. Electromyography may be of value in distinguishing a temporary conduction defect from a pathologic interruption in the continuity of nerve fibers. Evidence of denervation after 10 days indicates that there has been axonal degeneration and that there will be a long delay (3 months, as a rule) before regeneration occurs and that it may be incomplete. The presence of incomplete paralysis in the first week is the most favorable prognostic sign.

Treatment   Protection of the eye during sleep, massage of the weakened muscles, and a splint to prevent drooping of the lower part of the face are the measures generally employed in the management of such cases. A course of prednisone beginning with 60 to 80 mg daily during the first 5 days and then tapered over the next 5 days may be beneficial. Unroofing of the nerve in the facial canal has been practiced, but there is no evidence that this measure is helpful, and it may be harmful.

Differential diagnosis   There are many other causes of facial palsy. Tumors that invade the temporal bone (carotid body, cholesteatoma, dermoid) may produce a facial palsy, but the onset is insidious and the course progressive. The *Ramsay Hunt syndrome*, presumably due to herpes zoster of the geniculate ganglion, consists of a severe facial palsy associated with a vesicular eruption in the pharynx, external auditory canal, and other parts of the cranial integument; often the eighth cranial nerve is affected as well. *Acoustic neuromas* frequently involve the facial nerve by local compression (see Chap. 369). Infarcts and tumors are the common pontine lesions that interrupt the facial nerve fibers. Bilateral facial paralysis (facial diplegia) occurs in acute inflammatory polyradiculoneuritis (*Guillain-Barré syndrome*) and in a variety of sarcoidosis known as *uveoparotid fever* (*Heerfordt syndrome*). The *Melkersson-Rosenthal syndrome* consists of a rarely encountered triad of recurrent facial paralysis, recurrent—and eventually permanent—facial (particularly labial) edema, and less constantly, plication of the tongue; many causes of this rare syndrome have been suggested, but none has been established. Leprosy frequently involves the facial nerve.

A puzzling disorder is the *facial hemiatrophy of Romberg*. It occurs mainly in females and is characterized by a disappearance of fat in the dermal and subcutaneous tissues on one side of the face. It usually begins in adolescence or early adult years and is slowly progressive. In its advanced form, the affected side of the face is gaunt, and the skin is thin, wrinkled, and rather brown. The facial hair may turn white and fall out, and the sebaceous glands become atrophic. The muscles and bones are not involved as a rule. Sometimes the atrophy becomes bilateral. The condition is a form of lipodystrophy, and the localization within a dermatome suggests a disorder of some neural trophic factor of unknown nature. There is no treatment other than transplantation of skin and subcutaneous fat by a plastic surgeon.

Facial myokymia refers to a fine rippling activity of the facial muscles; it may be caused by a plaque of multiple sclerosis. *Blepharospasm* is an involuntary recurrent spasm of both eyelids that occurs in elderly persons as an isolated phenomenon or with varying degrees of spasm of other facial muscles (see Chap. 21). Relaxant and sedative drugs are of little help, although in many patients this disorder subsides spontaneously. Severe persistent cases of blepharospasm or hemifacial spasm are now successfully treated by local injection of botulinus toxin into the orbicularis oculi; the spasms are relieved for 3 to 4 months, and the injections can be repeated without morbidity.

All these forms of nuclear or peripheral facial palsy must be distinguished from the supranuclear type. In the latter, the frontalis and orbicularis oculi muscles are involved less than those of the lower part of the face, since the upper facial muscles are innervated by corticobulbar pathways from both motor cortices, whereas the lower facial muscles are innervated only by the opposite hemisphere. In supranuclear lesions there may be a dissociation of emotional and voluntary facial movements, and often some degree of paralysis of the arm and leg or an aphasia (in dominant hemisphere lesions) is conjoined.

VESTIBULAR NERVE

The eighth cranial nerve has two components, vestibular and auditory. Symptoms and signs of involvement of the vestibular portion are discussed in Chap. 18 and in this section. The auditory nerve and its disorders are discussed in Chap. 20.

MÉNIÈRE'S SYNDROME   Definition and clinical manifestations   Ménière's disease, or Ménière's syndrome, is the name applied to recurrent vertigo associated with tinnitus and progressive deafness. Tinnitus and/or deafness may be absent during the initial attack(s) of vertigo, but they invariably appear as the disease progresses and are increased in severity during an acute attack. With milder forms of the syndrome the patient may complain more of head discomfort, slight instability, and difficulty in concentration than of vertigo and may be considered to be anxious or depressed. Provided that deafness is not complete, the recruitment phenomenon can be demonstrated (see Chap. 20).

Ménière's disease has its onset most frequently in the fifth decade of life, although younger adults and the elderly are not spared. The pathologic changes are said to consist of a dilatation of the endolymphatic system which leads to a degeneration of the delicate vestibular and cochlear hair cells. The relation of these pathologic changes to the paroxysmal disorder of labyrinthine function is unknown.

Treatment   During an acute attack, rest in bed is the most effective treatment, since the patient can usually find a position in which vertigo is minimal. Dimenhydrinate, cyclizine, or meclizine in doses of 25 to 50 mg tid is useful in treating more protracted attacks. A low-salt diet is still used in treatment, but its value is difficult to judge. Mild sedative drugs may help the anxious patient between attacks. Usually the deafness is unilateral and progressive, and when it is complete, the vertiginous attacks cease. However, the course is variable, and if the attacks persist in a severe manner, permanent relief can be obtained by surgical destruction of the labyrinth or section of the vestibular portion of the eighth nerve intracranially.

BENIGN POSITIONAL VERTIGO   Another disorder of labyrinthine function is characterized by the occurrence of paroxysmal vertigo and nystagmus with the assumption of certain critical positions of the head. This is the positional vertigo of Bárány, of the so-called benign paroxysmal type (see Chap. 18). In refractory cases, in which attacks continue, vestibular exercises may be beneficial.

DIFFERENTIAL DIAGNOSIS OF VERTIGO   There are many other causes of acute vertigo, such as purulent labyrinthitis complicating meningitis, serous labyrinthitis due to infection of the middle ear, "toxic labyrinthitis" due to drug intoxication (e.g., with alcohol, quinine, streptomycin, gentamicin, and other antibiotics), motion sickness, trauma, and hemorrhage into the internal ear. In these instances, the attacks of vertigo tend to last longer than in the recurrent form, but in other respects the symptoms are similar. Aminoglycoside antibiotics may damage the fine hair cells of the vestibular end organs and cause a permanent disorder of equilibrium (as well as hearing), especially in older patients (see also Chap. 18).

There has been described a dramatic clinical syndrome, characterized by the abrupt onset of severe vertigo, nausea, and vomiting without tinnitus or hearing loss. The vertigo persists for several days or weeks, and labyrinthine function is permanently ablated on one side. Occlusion of the labyrinthine division of the internal auditory artery would logically explain this syndrome, but pathologic or angiographic confirmation of this hypothesis has so far not been obtained.

Vertigo of vestibular nerve origin may occur with diseases that involve the nerve in the petrous bone or the cerebellopontine angle. Except that it is less severe and is less frequently paroxysmal, it has many of the characteristics of labyrinthine vertigo. The adjacent auditory division of the eighth cranial nerve also may be affected, which explains the frequent association of vertigo with tinnitus and deafness. The function of the eighth cranial nerve may be disturbed by tumors of the lateral recess (especially acoustic neuroma), less frequently by meningeal inflammation in this region and, rarely, by an abnormal vessel that compresses the nerve.

Vestibular neuronitis and *benign recurrent vertigo* are the names applied to a clinical syndrome that occurs mainly in middle-aged and young adults (sometimes in children) and is characterized by the abrupt onset of vertigo, nausea, and vomiting without impairment of hearing. The attacks are brief and leave the patient for some days with a mild positional vertigo. They may occur only once or recur in varying degrees of severity. The cause is unknown. The medical treatment is the same as for Ménière's disease.

A particular variety of paroxysmal vertigo affects children. The attacks occur in a setting of good health and are of sudden onset and brief duration. Pallor, sweating, and immobility are prominent manifestations, and occasionally vomiting and nystagmus occur. No relation to posture or movement of the head has been observed. The attacks are recurrent but tend to cease spontaneously after a period of several months or years. The outstanding abnormality is demonstrated by caloric testing, which shows impairment or loss of vestibular function, bilateral or unilateral, frequently persisting after the attacks have ceased; cochlear function is unimpaired, however. The pathologic basis of this disorder has not been determined.

GLOSSOPHARYNGEAL NERVE

GLOSSOPHARYNGEAL NEURALGIA This form of neuralgia resembles trigeminal neuralgia in many respects but is much less common. The pain is intense and paroxysmal; it originates in the throat, approximately in the tonsillar fossa. In some cases the pain is localized in the ear or may radiate from the throat to the ear because of implication of the tympanic branch of the glossopharyngeal nerve. Spasms of pain may be initiated by swallowing. There is no demonstrable sensory or motor deficit. Cardiac symptoms—bradycardia, hypotension, and fainting—have been reported. A trial of

carbamazepine or phenytoin is the recommended therapy, but if this is unsuccessful, division of the glossopharyngeal nerve near the medulla is the definitive treatment. Percutaneous rhizotomy of glossopharyngeal and vagal fibers in the jugular foramen alleviates pain in some patients.

Very rarely, herpes zoster may involve the glossopharyngeal nerve. Glossopharyngeal neuropathy in conjunction with vagus and accessory nerve palsies may occur with a tumor or aneurysm in the posterior fossa or in the jugular foramen. Hoarseness due to vocal cord paralysis, some difficulty in swallowing, deviation of the soft palate to the intact side, anesthesia of the posterior wall of the pharynx, and weakness of the upper part of the trapezius and sternocleidomastoid muscles make up the syndrome (see Table 380-1, jugular foramen syndrome).

VAGUS NERVE

DYSPHAGIA AND DYSPHONIA Complete interruption of the intracranial portion of one vagus nerve results in a characteristic paralysis. The soft palate droops ipsilaterally and does not rise in phonation. There is loss of the gag reflex on the affected side, as well as the "curtain movement" of the lateral wall of the pharynx, whereby the faucial pillars move medially as the palate rises in saying "ah." The voice is hoarse, slightly nasal, and the vocal cord lies immobile in the cadaveric position, i.e., midway between abduction and adduction. There also may be a loss of sensibility at the external auditory meatus and back of the pinna. Usually no change in visceral function can be demonstrated.

Complete interruption of both vagi is said to be incompatible with life, and this is probably true if the nuclei are involved in the medulla by poliomyelitis or some other disease. However, in the cervical region, both vagi have been blocked with procaine (Novocain), for the treatment of intractable asthma, without mishap. The pharyngeal branches of both vagi may be affected in diphtheria; the voice has a nasal quality, and regurgitation of liquids through the nose occurs during the act of swallowing.

The vagus nerve may be implicated at the meningeal level by neoplastic and infectious processes and within the medulla by tumors, vascular lesions (e.g., the lateral medullary syndrome of Wallenberg), and by motor neuron disease. This nerve may be involved by the inflammatory lesion of herpes zoster. Polymyositis and dermatomyositis, which cause hoarseness and dysphagia by direct involvement of laryngeal and pharyngeal muscles, may be confused with diseases of the vagus nerves. Also, dysphagia is a symptom in some patients with myotonic dystrophy (see Chap. 37 for discussion of nonneurologic forms of dysphagia).

The recurrent laryngeal nerves, especially the left, are most often damaged as a result of intrathoracic disease. Aneurysm of the aortic arch, an enlarged left atrium, and tumors of the mediastinum and bronchi are much more frequent causes of an isolated vocal cord palsy than are intracranial disorders.

When confronted with a case of laryngeal palsy, the physician must attempt to determine the site of the lesion. If it is intramedullary, there are usually other signs, such as ipsilateral cerebellar dysfunction, loss of pain and temperature sensation over the ipsilateral face and contralateral arm and leg, and an ipsilateral Horner syndrome. If the lesion is extramedullary, the glossopharyngeal and spinal accessory nerves are frequently involved (see jugular foramen syndrome, Table 380-1). If it is extracranial in the posterior laterocondylar or retroparotid space, there may be a combination of ninth, tenth, eleventh, and twelfth cranial nerve palsies and a Horner syndrome. Combinations of these lower cranial nerve palsies have a variety of eponymic designations, listed in Table 380-1. If there is no sensory loss over the palate and pharynx and no palatal weakness or dysphagia, the lesion is below the origin of the pharyngeal branches, which leave the vagus nerve high in the cervical region; the usual site of disease is then the mediastinum.

TABLE 380-1 Cranial nerve syndromes

Site	Cranial nerves involved	Eponymic syndrome	Usual cause
Sphenoid fissure (superior orbital)	III, IV, first division V, VI	Foix	Invasive tumors of sphenoid bone; aneurysms
Lateral wall of cavernous sinus	III, IV, first division V, VI, often with proptosis	Foix Tolosa-Hunt	Aneurysms or thrombosis of cavernous sinus; invasive tumors from sinuses and sella turcica; benign granuloma responsive to steroids
Retrosphenoid space	II, III, IV, V, VI	Jacod	Large tumors of middle cranial fossa
Apex of petrous bone	V, VI	Gradenigo	Petrositis; tumors of petrous bone
Internal auditory meatus	VII, VIII		Tumors of petrous bone (dermoids, etc.); infectious processes; acoustic neuroma
Pontocerebellar angle	V, VII, VIII, and sometimes IX		Acoustic neuroma; meningioma
Jugular foramen	IX, X, XI	Vernet	Tumors and aneurysms
Posterior laterocondylar space	IX, X, XI, XII	Collet-Sicard	Tumors of parotid gland, carotid body, and metastatic tumor
Posterior retroparotid space	IX, X, XI, XII and Horner syndrome	Villaret Mackenzie Tapia	Tumors of parotid gland, carotid body, lymph nodes; metastatic tumor; tuberculous adenitis

ACCESSORY NERVE

Isolated involvement of the accessory, or eleventh cranial, nerve can occur anywhere along its route, resulting in partial or complete paralysis of the sternocleidomastoid and trapezius muscles. More commonly, involvement occurs in combination with deficits of the ninth and tenth cranial nerves in the jugular foramen or after exit from the skull (see Table 380-1). An idiopathic form of accessory neuropathy, akin to Bell's palsy, has been described, and it may be recurrent in some cases. Most but not all patients recover.

HYPOGLOSSAL NERVE

The twelfth cranial nerve supplies the ipsilateral muscles of the tongue. The nucleus of the nerve or its fibers of exit may be involved by intramedullary lesions such as tumor, poliomyelitis, or most often motor neuron disease. Lesions of the basal meninges and the occipital bones (platybasia, invagination of occipital condyles, Paget's disease) may compress the nerve in its extramedullary course or in the hypoglossal canal. Isolated lesions of unknown cause can occur. Atrophy and fasciculation of the tongue develop weeks to months after interruption of the nerve.

MULTIPLE CRANIAL NERVE PALSIES

Several cranial nerves may be affected by the same disease process. In this situation, the main clinical problem is to determine whether the lesion lies within the brainstem or outside it. Lesions that lie on the surface of the brainstem are characterized by involvement of adjacent cranial nerves (often occurring in succession) and late and rather slight involvement of the long sensory and motor pathways and segmental structures lying within the brainstem. The opposite is true of intramedullary, intrapontine, and intramesencephalic lesions. The extramedullary lesion is more likely to cause bone erosion or enlargement of the foramens of exit of cranial nerves. The intramedullary lesion involving cranial nerves often produces a crossed sensory or motor paralysis (cranial nerve signs on one side of the body and tract signs on the opposite side).

Involvement of multiple cranial nerves outside the brainstem is frequently the result of trauma (sudden onset), localized infections such as herpes zoster (acute onset), granulomatous disease such as Wegener's granulomatosis (subacute onset), Behçet's disease, or tumors and enlarging saccular aneurysms (chronic development). Of the tumors, neurofibromas, meningiomas, chordomas, cholesteatomas, carcinomas, and sarcomas have all been observed to implicate a succession of lower cranial nerves. Owing to their anatomic relationships, the multiple cranial nerve palsies form a number of distinctive syndromes, listed in Table 380-1. Sarcoidosis has been found to be the cause of some cases of multiple cranial neuropathy, and chronic glandular tuberculosis (scrofula) the cause of a few others. Malignant granuloma of the nasopharynx also may affect multiple cranial nerves, as do nasopharyngeal tumors, platybasia, basilar invagination of the skull, and the Chiari malformation that becomes evident in adult life. A purely motor disorder without atrophy always raises the question of myasthenia gravis (see Chap. 386). Guillain-Barré syndrome commonly affects the facial nerves bilaterally (facial diplegia). In the Fisher variant of the Guillain-Barré syndrome, oculomotor paresis occurs with ataxia and areflexia in the limbs. Wernicke encephalopathy can cause a severe ophthalmoplegia combined with other brainstem signs (see Chap. 377).

An idiopathic form of multiple cranial nerve involvement on one or both sides of the face is occasionally seen. The disease may recur over a period of years with variable degrees of recovery between attacks. The clinical features overlap those of the Tolosa-Hunt orbitocavernous sinus syndrome (Juncos and Beal).

REFERENCES

ADAMS RD, VICTOR M: *Principles of Neurology*, 5th ed. New York, McGraw-Hill, 1993, chap 47

BRODAL A: The cranial nerves, in *Neurological Anatomy in Relation to Clinical Medicine*, 3d ed. New York, Oxford, 1980, chap 7, pp 448–577

BROWNSTONE PK et al: Bilateral superior laryngeal neuralgia. Arch Neurol 37:525, 1980

CHALK C, ISAACS H: Recurrent spontaneous accessory neuropathy. J Neurol Neurosurg Psychiatry 53:621, 1990

DEVINSKY O, FELDMANN E: *Examination of the Cranial and Peripheral Nerves*. New York, Churchill Livingstone, 1988

DURELLI L et al: The Melkersson-Rosenthal syndrome: A case with increased CNS IgG synthesis. Ann Neurol 18:623, 1985

EISEN A, BERTRAND G: Isolated accessory nerve palsy of spontaneous origin: A clinical and electromyographic study. Arch Neurol 27:496, 1972

GROVES J: Bell's (idiopathic) facial palsy, in *Scientific Foundations of Otolaryngology*, R Hinchcliffe, D Harrison (eds). London, Heinemann, 1976, pp 446–459

HAUSER WA et al: Incidence and prognosis of Bell's palsy in the population of Rochester, Minnesota. Mayo Clin Proc 46:258, 1971

JANKOVIC J, BRIN MF: Therapeutic uses of botulinum toxin. N Engl J Med 324:1186, 1991

JANNETTA PJ: Posterior fossa neurovascular compression syndrome other than neuralgias, in *Neurosurgery*, Wilkins RH, Rengachary SS (eds). New York, McGraw-Hill, 1985, pp 1901–1906

JUNCOS JL, BEAL MF: Idiopathic cranial polyneuropathy. Brain 110:197, 1987

KARNES WE: Diseases of the seventh cranial nerve, in *Peripheral Neuropathy*, 3d ed, PJ Dyck et al (eds). Philadelphia, Saunders, 1993, chap 43, pp 818–836

LECKY BRF et al: Trigeminal sensory neuropathy. Brain 110:1463, 1987

LESSELL S: Corticosteroid treatment of acute optic neuritis. N Engl J Med 326:634, 1992

MAYO CLINIC AND MAYO FOUNDATION: *Clinical Examinations in Neurology*, 6th ed., St. Louis, Mosby Yearbook, 1991

SAWLE GV et al: The natural history of non-arteritic anterior ischemic optic neuropathy. J Neurol Neurosurg Psychiatry 53:830, 1990

SELBY G: Diseases of the fifth cranial nerve, in *Peripheral Neuropathy*, 3d ed, PJ Dyck et al (eds). Philadelphia, Saunders, 1993, chap 42, pp 801–817

SWEET WH: The treatment of trigeminal neuralgia (tic douloureux). N Engl J Med 315:174, 1986

———: Percutaneous methods for the treatment of trigeminal neuralgia and other faciocephalic pain; comparison with microvascular decompression. Semin Neurol 8:272, 1988

381   DISEASES OF THE SPINAL CORD

ALLAN H. ROPPER / JOSEPH B. MARTIN

Diseases of the spinal cord are frequently devastating, causing permanent and severe neurologic disability. Small lesions can produce quadriplegia, paraplegia, and sensory deficits far beyond the damage they would inflict elsewhere in the nervous system because the spinal cord contains, in a small cross-sectional area, almost the entire motor output and sensory input systems. Many spinal diseases are reversible, particularly extrinsic cord compression, making acute spinal cord lesions among the most critical of neurologic emergencies.

The stereotypic organization of the spinal cord, innervating the limbs and trunk segmentally through 31 pairs of spinal nerves, makes anatomic diagnosis relatively straightforward. A sensory level, paraplegia, or other typical syndromes usually permit recognition of a spinal cord process. Full assessment of cord disease requires a careful examination supplemented by laboratory tests, including magnetic resonance imaging (MRI), computed tomographic (CT) scanning, myelography, analysis of cerebrospinal fluid (CSF), electromyography, and somatosensory evoked responses. Most deficiencies in evaluating patients with signs of spinal cord disease result from cursory physical examination or inadequate x-rays. Computed tomography and MRI have replaced conventional myelography because of their ease of performance and better resolution; MRI gives particularly valuable information about intrinsic cord structure.

SPINAL COLUMN AND SPINAL CORD ANATOMY RELEVANT TO CLINICAL SIGNS   The spinal cord is organized in a uniform somatotopic fashion throughout its length, giving rise to easily identifiable syndromes (see Chaps. 11, 21, and 24). The longitudinal location of lesions is established by the uppermost level of sensory and motor dysfunction. However, the relationship between the vertebral bodies of the spinal column (or their surface markers, the vertebral spines) and the cord segments that underlie them complicates the anatomic interpretation of signs of spinal cord diseases. The level of a spinal cord syndrome is described according to the cord segment affected rather than by the surrounding vertebrae. During embryologic development, growth of the cord lags behind that of the spinal column so that the cord ends behind the first lumbar vertebral body and the lower nerves must take an increasingly downward course to exit in the appropriate vertebral foramen. The upper cervical cord segments lie behind the same numbered vertebral body, whereas the lower cervical segments are located one above each corresponding vertebral body, the upper thoracic cord two segments higher, and the lower thoracic cord, three segments higher. The lumbar and sacral cord segments, which form the conus medullaris, are located behind the ninth thoracic to first lumbar vertebrae. The cervical roots (except C8) exit from neural foramina above their respective vertebral bodies, while thoracic and lumbar roots exit below each body.

CLINICAL SYNDROMES OF SPINAL CORD DISEASE The principal clinical signs of spinal cord damage are a "sensory level," i.e., loss of sensation below a circumferential horizontal line on the trunk, and weakness in the extremities innervated by the descending corticospinal fibers. Sensory symptoms, particularly paresthesias, may begin in the feet (or in one foot) and ascend, giving the impression early on of a polyneuropathy before a fixed sensory level is apparent. Lesions that disrupt descending corticospinal and bulbospinal tracts at a single cord level cause paraplegia or quadriplegia, with increased muscle tone, enhanced deep tendon reflexes, and Babinski signs. A careful examination often also elicits segmental signs that are approximate indicators of the location of a transverse lesion, such as a band of altered sensation at the upper extent of the sensory level (hyperalgesia or hyperpathia), and isolated flaccidity, atrophy, or a single diminished deep tendon reflex. The sensory level to pinprick and temperature sensation is generally one or two segments below the level of an asymmetric lesion but is at the level of the lesion when bilateral. This is a result of the course of sensory fibers that synapse in the dorsal horn and then ascend and cross to the opposite spinothalamic tract. Midline back pain is also an accurate localizing sign, particularly in the thoracic region, where aching interscapular pain may be the first sign of cord compression. Radicular pain marks the primary site of a more laterally placed spinal lesion. Pain from lower cord (conus medullaris) lesions is often referred to the low back.

Early in the course of a severe and acute transverse lesion there may be flaccidity of the limbs rather than spasticity, due to so-called spinal shock. This state may last for several days, rarely for weeks, and may be mistaken for extensive segmental damage or a polyneuropathy, but the reflexes later become increased. Brief clonic or myoclonic limb movements often precede paralysis in acute transverse lesions, particularly those due to infarction. Autonomic dysfunction, mainly urinary retention, is another prominent sign in transverse spinal lesions and should call attention to cord disease.

Much is made of the clinical distinction between intramedullary (within the cord) and extramedullary compressive lesions, but most rules are approximations that do not distinguish one from the other dependably. Features that favor extramedullary lesions include radicular pain, a Brown-Séquard hemicord syndrome (see below), asymmetric lower motor neuron signs in one or two segments, early corticospinal signs, marked sacral sensory loss, and early, prominent CSF abnormalities. On the other hand, poorly localized burning pain, dissociated loss of pain sensation with sparing of joint position sensation, sparing of sensation in the perineal and sacral areas, late corticospinal signs, and normal or minimally altered CSF generally favor an intramedullary lesion. *Sacral sparing* refers to the preservation of pinprick and temperature sensation in the sacral dermatomes, usually S3 to S5, with more rostral areas affected up to the sensory

level. This is usually a dependable sign of intrinsic cord disease damaging the innermost fibers of the spinothalamic tracts while sparing those placed more laterally which subserve sacral sensation.

The *Brown-Séquard syndrome* is an eponym given to an idealized hemicord syndrome consisting of ipsilateral mono- or hemiplegia and loss of joint position and vibration sense, with contralateral loss of pain and temperature (spinothalamic) sensation. The segmental level for pain and temperature loss is sometimes one or two levels below the anatomic lesion. Segmental signs, such as radicular pain, muscle atrophy, or decreased tendon reflexes when they occur, are unilateral.

Lesions limited to or primarily within the central portion of the cord preferentially damage gray matter neurons and segmental tracts crossing at that level. Traumatic contusion, developmental syringomyelia, tumors, and vascular lesions in the territory of the anterior spinal artery are the most common lesions localized to the central cord. Inflammatory diseases occur in this distribution less frequently. In the cervical cord, the central cord syndrome gives arm weakness out of proportion to leg weakness and a "dissociated" sensory loss signifying analgesia (loss of pin sensation) in a cape distribution over the shoulders, lower neck, and upper trunk without anesthesia (loss of touch sensation) or pallanesthesia (loss of vibration sense).

Lesions located in the region of the first lumbar vertebral body or below compress the spinal nerves of the cauda equina and cause a flaccid, areflexic, asymmetric paraparesis usually accompanied by bladder and bowel dysfunction. A sensory level is found in a saddle distribution up to L1, corresponding to the roots carried in the cauda equina. The Achilles and patellar reflexes are diminished or absent. Pain is common and projected to the perineum or thighs. With conus medullaris lesions, pain is less prominent than in cauda equina lesions, and bladder and prominent bowel symptoms occur earlier. Compressive lesions may involve both the cauda equina and conus medullaris, causing a combined syndrome of lower motor neuron signs and hyperflexia or a Babinski sign.

The classic syndrome of the foramen magnum is weakness of the shoulder and arm followed by weakness of the ipsilateral leg, then contralateral leg, and finally, contralateral arm. Masses in this region sometimes produce suboccipital pain spreading to the neck and shoulders. A Horner's syndrome is another clue to a high cervical cord lesion; it does not occur with lesions below T2.

A few nontraumatic diseases are capable of producing sudden "strokelike" myelopathy without preceding symptoms. They include epidural hemorrhage, hematomyelia, cord infarction, nucleus pulposus embolism, and compression by spinal subluxation.

SPINAL CORD COMPRESSION Tumors of the cord Tumors in the spinal canal may be primary or metastatic and are classified as extradural ("epidural") or intradural, and the latter as intra- or extramedullary (inside or outside the cord) (see Chap. 369). The majority of neoplastic lesions are epidural, arising from metastases to the adjacent spinal column. Neoplasms originating in the prostate, breast, and lung, and lymphoma and plasma cell dyscrasias are particularly common, although virtually every malignant tumor has been reported to cause metastatic epidural cord compression. The initial symptom in epidural compression is usually local back pain, often worse in the recumbent position and causing the patient to awaken at night. Radiating radicular pain exacerbated by coughing, sneezing, or straining may accompany the back pain. Pain and local tenderness may precede other symptoms by many weeks. Neurologic signs commonly evolve over several days to a few weeks. The cord syndrome begins with progressive weakness, eventually acquiring all the hallmarks of a transverse myelopathy with paraparesis and a sensory level. A plain radiograph may show lytic or blastic changes or a compression fracture at the level appropriate to the cord syndrome; radionuclide bone scans are frequently positive. CT scan, myelography, and particularly MRI provide the optimal way of demonstrating cord compression. A horizontally widened and flattened cord from extrinsic compression is seen at the margins of the subarachnoid block, and the adjacent vertebral body is usually abnormal (Fig. 381-1).

In the past, emergency laminectomies were considered necessary to treat epidural cord compression by tumor, but treatment with high-dose glucocorticoids and rapid, fractionated radiation therapy has been as successful. Outcome is most closely related to the tumor type and its radiosensitivity. Paraparesis frequently improves within 48 h of the administration of glucocorticoids. Some incomplete or early transverse cord syndromes may still be better treated surgically, but each case must be analyzed individually, taking into account the radiosensitivity of the tumor, distribution of other metastases, and the patient's general medical condition. Whichever therapy is chosen, it is wise to proceed quickly and use glucocorticoids as soon as the diagnosis of cord compression is suspected.

Intradural, extramedullary tumors are a less frequent cause of spinal cord compression and evolve more slowly than extradural lesions. Meningiomas and neurofibromas are the most common causes. Symptoms usually begin with radicular sensory changes and an asymmetric spinal cord syndrome. Radiologic studies show dislocation of the cord to one side and an outline of the tumor within the subarachnoid space. Primary intramedullary tumors of the spinal cord are discussed in Chap. 369.

Compressive myelopathies of all types initially cause moderate elevation of CSF protein concentration, but with complete block of the subarachnoid space, CSF protein concentration rises to the 1 to 10 g/L (100 to 1000 mg/dL) range due to impaired CSF circulation from the caudal sac to the intracranial subarachnoid space. There are usually few or no cells, cytology for malignant cells is usually negative, and CSF glucose concentration remains normal unless there is accompanying widespread carcinomatous meningitis (see Chap. 369).

Epidural abscess   This is a treacherous lesion, often misdiagnosed at first (see Chap. 374). The predisposing clinical settings are

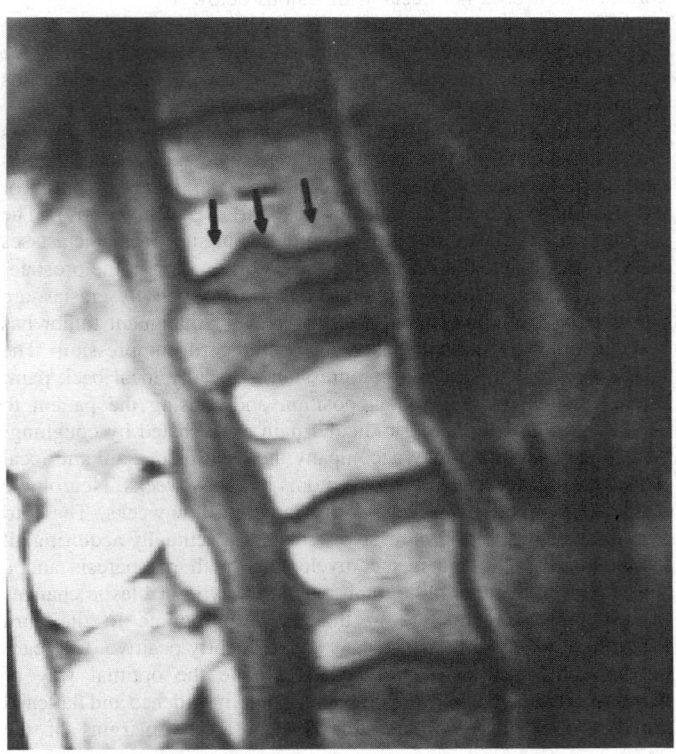

FIGURE 381-1   Sagittal section MRI showing compression deformity of the T12 vertebral body from metastatic adenocarcinoma (*below arrows*) and compression and displacement of the spinal cord. (*Courtesy of Greg Shoukimas, M.D., Department of Radiology, Massachusetts General Hospital.*)

furunculosis of the back or scalp, bacteremia, or minor back injury. The condition can occur as a complication of local operation or very rarely after lumbar puncture. Spinal osteomyelitis acts as the nidus for the formation of an abscess that subsequently enlarges to compress the cord. The osteomyelitis is usually small and may not be evident on plain radiographs. For several days to 2 weeks there may be only unexplained fever and mild spinal ache with local tenderness; later, radicular pain occurs. As the abscess expands, it rapidly causes cord compression with a transverse syndrome. The proper treatment is rapid decompression by laminectomy and drainage, followed by appropriate antibiotics determined from culture of the purulent material. Incomplete drainage is not uncommon, resulting in a chronic granulomatous and fibrous reaction that may be sterilized with antibiotics but continues to act as a compressing mass. Tuberculous pyogenic abscess formation is still a common cause of epidural abscess in developing countries.

Epidural hemorrhage and hematomyelia   Hemorrhage into the spinal cord (hematomyelia) or epidural space produces an acute transverse myelopathy evolving over minutes or hours, accompanied by severe pain. Although these hemorrhages may originate from an arteriovenous malformation, hemorrhage into a tumor, or from anticoagulation with warfarin or another coagulopathy, they are commonly spontaneous. Epidural hematoma may occur in the setting of minor trauma or lumbar puncture. Back and radicular pain precedes weakness by several minutes to hours. Patients may appear to be exaggerating their difficulties if back pain is severe but there are minimal or no neurologic signs. Lumbar epidural hematoma results in loss of both knee and ankle reflexes, whereas retroperitoneal hematomas usually cause only absence of the knee reflexes. A myelogram or MRI defines the mass; CT scan is sometimes normal because the clot cannot be distinguished from adjacent bone. Subdural and subarachnoid clots occur spontaneously or under circumstances similar to those causing epidural hemorrhages. The CSF with epidural hemorrhage is usually clear or contains a few red blood cells; in subarachnoid or subdural hemorrhage the CSF is grossly bloody at first and later becomes discolored to a deep yellow-brown characteristic of blood pigments present in the CSF. There may be, in addition, a pleocytosis and lowered CSF glucose, giving the impression of bacterial meningitis.

Acute disk protrusion   Lumbar disk herniation, a common disorder, is discussed in Chap. 15. Thoracic or cervical disk protrusion is less often a cause of spinal cord compression, usually occurring after direct trauma to the spinal column. Degeneration of cervical disk spaces with adjacent osteoarthritic hypertrophy causes a subacute spondylytic compressive myelopathy in the cervical and, less often, the thoracic region (discussed below). Embolism from nucleus pulposus material causing acute spinal cord infarction is also described below.

Other unusual compressive lesions   Patients with iatrogenic or primary Cushing's syndrome have a tendency to form foci of epidural fat tissue that rarely can reach a size sufficient to compress the thoracic cord. Extramedullary hematopoiesis also has caused cord compression in hematologic diseases. Eroding aortic aneurysms, echinococcal or other parasitic cysts, gummas, lymphomatoid-granulomatosis, mucopolysaccharidoses, and other rare lesions also can compress the cord.

Arthritic diseases of the spine occur in two clinical forms: a lumbar or cauda equina compression from *ankylosing spondylitis* or cervical cord compression from destruction of the cervical apophyseal or atlantoaxial joints in *rheumatoid arthritis*. Spinal complications arising as one component of severe generalized joint disease in rheumatoid arthritis are often overlooked. Forward subluxation of cervical vertebral bodies or of the atlas on the axis can cause a devastating, even fatal, acute cord compression after minor trauma such as whiplash, or it may present as a chronic compressive myelopathy similar to cervical spondylosis. Separation of the odontoid process from the axis may narrow the upper spinal canal compressing the cervicomedullary junction, particularly during flexion movements.

NONCOMPRESSIVE NEOPLASTIC MYELOPATHIES   Intramedullary metastasis, paracarcinomatous myelopathy, and radiation myelopathy   In the context of known cancer, most myelopathies are compressive. However, when radiologic studies fail to show compression, there is often difficulty distinguishing between several less common entities: intramedullary metastasis, paraneoplastic myelopathy, and radiation myelopathy. In a patient with metastatic cancer and a noncompressive myelopathy, intramedullary metastasis is the most likely diagnosis (see Chap. 328). Back pain is the most common initial symptom, although it is not invariable, followed by progressive spastic paraparesis and, less often, paresthesias. Dissociated sensory loss or sacral sparing, which is characteristic of intrinsic compression, is uncommon, and asymmetric paraparesis with incomplete sensory loss is typical. Myelography, CT scan, or MRI may show a swollen cord without extrinsic compression; in almost half of patients CT or myelography are normal; MRI is more successful in outlining a metastatic mass or primary intramedullary tumor (Fig. 381-2). Intramedullary metastases usually arise from bronchogenic carcinoma and less often from breast cancer and other solid tumors. Metastatic melanoma, an uncommon cause of extrinsic cord compression, more often presents as an intramedullary mass. The pathology of the metastasis is usually a single eccentrically placed nodule that presumably arises from hematogenous dissemination. Radiation therapy may be helpful in appropriate circumstances.

Carcinomatous meningitis, a common form of CNS invasion in malignancy, does not cause a myelopathy unless there is extensive subpial infiltration from adjacent roots causing nodules with secondary compression or infiltration of the cord. An incomplete, painless cauda equina syndrome can result from carcinomatous root infiltration (see Chap. 369). Headache is common, and repeated CSF examinations eventually reveal malignant cells, an elevated protein, and, in some cases, reduced CSF glucose concentration.

A progressive necrotic myelopathy associated with a paucity of inflammation can occur as a remote effect of cancer, usually with solid tumors (paraneoplastic myelopathy). The radiologic studies and CSF are normal, or there may be slightly elevated protein. A subacute progressive spastic paraparesis evolves over days or weeks, usually asymmetrically, with distal paresthesias ascending to establish a sensory level, and late bladder dysfunction. Several adjacent segments of cord are involved (see Chap. 328).

Radiation may produce a delayed subacute progressive myelopathy due to microvascular hyalinization and vascular occlusion (see Chap. 369). It frequently presents a differential diagnostic problem when the cord lies within radiation portals used to treat other structures such as the mediastinal lymph nodes. Differentiation from paraneoplastic myelopathy or intramedullary metastasis is difficult except by circumstantial history of prior radiation.

INFLAMMATORY MYELOPATHIES   Acute myelitis, transverse myelitis, and necrotic myelopathy   These related diseases are characterized by intrinsic inflammation of the cord and a clinical syndrome evolving over several days to 2 or 3 weeks. There may be a virtually complete spinal syndrome (transverse myelitis) or incomplete variants such as a posterior column myelopathy with ascending paresthesias and a sensory level for vibration; ascending, predominantly spinothalamic findings; or a Brown-Séquard syndrome with leg paresis and contralateral spinothalamic-type sensory changes. Many cases follow a viral illness. The most common presenting findings in transverse myelitis are back pain, progressive paraparesis, and asymmetric ascending paresthesias in the legs, later affecting the hands if the disease progresses, creating confusion with Guillain-Barré syndrome. Radiologic studies are necessary to exclude a compressive lesion. The CSF contains 5 to 50 lymphocytes per microliter in most patients, and rarely, polymorphonuclear cells predominate. The inflammatory process is most common in the middle and low thoracic regions, but any level of the cord may be affected. A chronic progressive cervical myelitis has been described, predominantly in older women, and is believed to be a form of multiple sclerosis (see Chap. 373).

In some cases necrosis is profound and may progress intermittently for several months to involve contiguous portions of the cord, reducing much of it to a thin gliotic ribbon. The term *progressive necrotic myelopathy* has been given to this condition. Severe cases of necrotic myelopathy progress to involve virtually the entire cord (necrotic panmyelopathy). When a transverse necrotic lesion occurs before or shortly after optic neuritis, it has been termed *Devic's disease* or *neuromyelitis optica*. All these processes appear to be variants of multiple sclerosis. It is not clear what proportion of patients will ultimately be found to have multiple sclerosis after a single episode of acute transverse myelitis. Estimates have been 15 to 80 percent, a range similar to multiple sclerosis after optic neuritis. The postinfectious demyelinating disorders are usually monophasic and only rarely recur, although fluctuation of symptoms related to a single level of the cord is common (see Chap. 375). Systemic lupus erythematosus and other autoimmune disorders also have been associated with myelitis.

Infectious myelopathy   Several neurotropic viruses can cause myelitis. In the past, the most common form was poliomyelitis. Herpes zoster, preceded by radicular symptoms and rash, is presently the most common cause of viral myelitis. The pathologic process is not restricted to the gray matter and causes a transverse myelopathy. Lymphocytes are always found in the CSF.

The human retroviruses HTLV-I and HIV may be associated with myelopathies (see Chaps. 151 and 375). HTLV-I causes a chronic progressive, noninflammatory cord syndrome with symmetric spastic paraparesis and mild sensory and bladder disturbances. The disease is endemic in several areas, including areas of the Caribbean, South America, and southern Japan. It was identified as *tropical spastic paraparesis* before the virus was known. A myelopathy with vacuolar pathologic changes occurs with HIV infections. There is generally no clear sensory level in the retroviral myelopathies. An inflammatory cauda equina neuritis caused by cytomegalovirus is described in AIDS patients.

Intramedullary cord abscesses caused by bacteria or mycobacteria

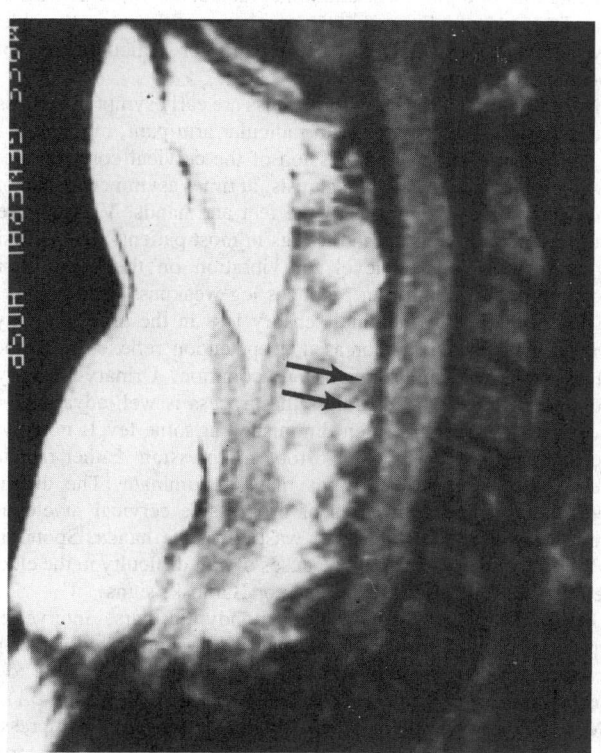

FIGURE 381-2   Sagittal MRI showing intrinsic fusiform enlargement of the cervical spinal cord from an intramedullary tumor. The tumor displays a low-density signal (*arrows*). *(Courtesy of Greg Shoukimas, M.D., Department of Radiology, Massachusetts General Hospital.)*

may occur after systemic infections. Chronic meningitic lesions due to syphilis may produce a secondary subpial myelitis and radiculitis that evolve slowly (see below). An intense granulomatous, necrotic, and inflammatory myelitis is peculiar to infestation by *Schistosoma mansoni*, caused by a local response to tissue-digesting enzymes produced by ova from the parasite. Toxoplasmosis also may rarely cause a focal myelopathy.

Toxic myelopathy   A toxic noninflammatory myelopathy, sometimes with optic atrophy, has been reported mainly in Japan and has been linked to ingestion of iodochlorhydroxyquinoline. Most patients have recovered, but many have persistent paresthesias.

Arachnoiditis   This is a nonspecific term referring to inflammation, scarring, and fibrous thickening of the arachnoid membrane that is capable of compressing nerve roots or, rarely, the spinal cord. It is usually a postoperative complication or results from instillation of radiographic dye, antibiotics, or noxious chemicals into the subarachnoid space. The CSF contains cells and an elevated protein concentration soon after the inciting event, but the inflammation then subsides. Bilateral asymmetric radicular limb pain is the most prominent feature, with additional signs of root compression, such as reflex loss. There may be slight fever in acute cases. Back pain and radicular symptoms are attributed to lumbar arachnoiditis more often than justified. Congenital meningeal cul-de-sacs or arachnoid cysts along nerve roots may produce severe radicular pain in midadulthood when the cysts enlarge and distort or exert traction on spinal nerve roots or ganglia. An unexplained delayed paraplegia has been reported after the use of chymopapain for the treatment of disk herniation.

SPINAL CORD INFARCTION   Because the anterior or posterior spinal arteries are not usually involved by atherosclerosis, and only occasionally are affected by angiitis or emboli, most infarctions of the spinal cord are due to distant vascular occlusions or severe hypotension. Aortic thrombosis or dissection causes cord infarction by interrupting the entire radicular and direct arterial supply to the anterior and posterior spinal arteries. The infarction typically occurs in a vascular watershed region of the thoracic cord between the large tributary to the spinal cord arising from the lower aorta, the artery of Adamkiewicz, and the anterior spinal artery arising from the vertebral arteries. The anterior spinal artery syndrome usually appears abruptly, like a stroke, or emerges postoperatively if the proximal aorta has been clamped. In some cases, however, symptoms progress over 24 to 72 h, making diagnosis difficult. Spinal infarction has been reported rarely with systemic arteritis, immune reactions of serum sickness, and after intravascular contrast injection, in the latter heralded by severe back pain at the time of injection.

Cord infarction caused by microscopic fragments of herniated nucleus pulposus may occur after minor trauma, frequently during athletic activities. There is sharp local pain followed by a rapid paraplegia and a transverse cord syndrome evolving over several minutes to an hour. Pulposus tissue is found in small intramedullary vessels and often within the marrow of the adjacent vertebral body. The route from the disk space to marrow and thence to the cord is uncertain. This entity should be suspected in young adults with catastrophic transverse cord syndromes after back injury or exercise.

VASCULAR MALFORMATION OF THE SPINAL CORD   Arteriovenous malformations (AVM) of the spinal cord are rare but may simulate multiple sclerosis, transverse myelitis, spinal cord stroke, or neoplastic compression. They are difficult lesions to detect because of their great clinical variability. AVMs are most often found in the low thoracic or lumbar cord in middle-aged men. The majority begin with an incomplete progressive cord syndrome that may advance subacutely or episodically, like multiple sclerosis, producing bilateral corticospinal, spinothalamic, and posterior column symptoms and signs in any combination. About a third of patients have an abrupt syndrome with a single acute transverse myelopathy from bleeding, which simulates acute myelitis; others present with several acute exacerbations. About half have back or radicular pain, a few have a claudication syndrome similar to lumbar canal stenosis, and rare

patients describe an acute onset with severe, localized back pain. Fluctuation of pain or neurologic signs with exercise, posture, or menses is helpful in suspecting the diagnosis. Bruits over the lesion are rare but should be sought at rest and after exercise. Most patients have mild elevation of CSF protein and a few show CSF pleocytosis. Myelography, CT, or MRI shows a lesion in 75 to 90 percent of cases. The anatomic details of most AVMs can be demonstrated with selective spinal angiography, and simultaneous interventional neuroradiologic embolization has been a major advance in the treatment of the disorder.

The myelopathy caused by AVMs appears to be a noninflammatory gliotic and sometimes necrotic process consistent with ischemia. A special type of dorsal AVM with a prominent progressive intramedullary syndrome (Foix-Alajouanine disease) has been reported with an adjacent necrotic myelopathy. The abnormal vessels have a characteristic thickened, hyalinized wall. Since any necrotic process within the cord may give rise to neovascularization and thick-walled vessels, the pathologic interpretation of this vascular malformation remains controversial. Arteriovenous fistulas outside the spinal cord, including in visceral organs such as the kidney, have been associated with a vascular myelopathy due to large draining veins that traverse the spinal canal.

CHRONIC MYELOPATHIES   Spondylosis   This is a general term for several related degenerative changes of the spine giving rise to compression of the cervical cord and adjacent roots. Cervical spondylosis is primarily a disease of older patients, affecting men more often than women, and consisting of a combination of (1) narrowing of intervertebral disk spaces with nucleus pulposus herniation or annulus bulging, (2) osteophytic spur formation on the dorsal (posterior) aspect of the vertebral bodies, (3) partial subluxation of vertebrae, and (4) hypertrophy of the dorsal spinal ligament and dorsolateral facet articulations (see Chap. 15). The bony changes are reactive in nature, but there is no true arthritis. The most important feature causing spinal cord symptoms and signs is usually a "spondylitic bar" formed by osteophytes arising from the dorsal surfaces of adjacent vertebral bodies resulting in a horizontal compression of the ventral cord (Fig. 381-3A and B). The sagittal diameter of the spinal canal may be narrowed further during neck extension. Extension of the bar laterally and articulatory hypertrophic changes that encroach on the neural foramina cause additional radicular symptoms. Although the radiographic findings of spondylosis are common in the elderly, only a few patients develop myelopathy or radiculopathy, often dependent on a congenitally narrow canal.

Neck and shoulder pain with stiffness are early symptoms; pressure on nerve roots is associated with radicular arm pain, most often in a C5 or C6 distribution. Compression of the cervical cord produces a slowly progressive spastic paraparesis, at times asymmetric, and often accompanied by paresthesias in the feet and hands. Vibratory sense is substantially diminished in the legs in most patients, and occasionally there is a sensory level for vibration on the upper thorax. Coughing or straining often produces leg weakness or radiating arm or shoulder pain. Dermatomal sensory loss in the arms, atrophy of intrinsic hand muscles, increased deep tendon reflexes in the legs, and asymmetric Babinski signs are common. Urinary urgency or incontinence do not occur unless the process is well-advanced. The reflexes in the arms are often diminished at some level, notably the biceps, corresponding to C5–C6 root compression. Either radicular, myelopathic, or combined signs may predominate. The diagnosis should be considered in cases of progressive cervical myelopathy, paresthesias of feet or hands, or wasting of the hands. Spondylosis is also one of the most common causes of gait difficulty in the elderly, often causing increased leg reflexes or Babinski signs.

Plain radiographs demonstrate spondylitic bars, intervertebral narrowing and subluxations, reversal of the normal cervical spine curvature, and reduction of the sagittal diameter of the canal to less than 11 mm, or to 7 mm with neck extension (see Fig. 381-3A). CT or MRI are the preferred methods of demonstrating cord compression. The CSF is usually normal or shows a slightly elevated protein

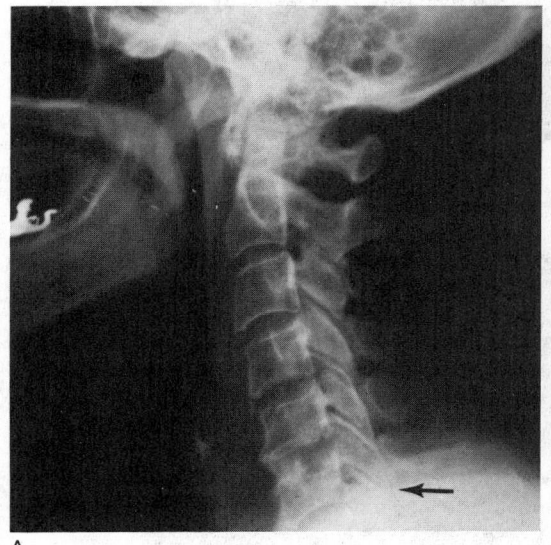
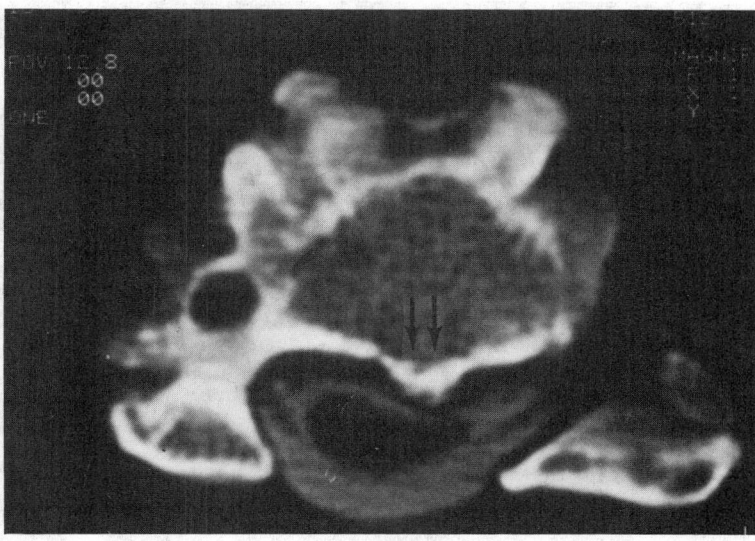

A   B

FIGURE 381-3 *A.* Lateral x-ray of the cervical spine showing spondylitic "bar" formation from the junction of adjacent osteophytes at C6–C7 (*arrow*). *B.* Horizontal CT section at C6 from patient shown in *A* after instillation of water-soluble dye into the subarachnoid space. A spur of the bony osteophyte compresses and distorts the spinal cord (*arrows*).

concentration. Electromyography also may be useful in demonstrating radicular compression.

Cervical spondylosis is both an under- and overdiagnosed disease. Many patients with intrinsic cord processes, particularly amyotrophic lateral sclerosis, multiple sclerosis, and subacute combined degeneration, have had cervical laminectomies in the belief that spondylosis was responsible. There may be temporary improvement, suggesting that there was an element of spondylitic compression, but the underlying intrinsic myelopathy soon progresses. A mild progressive gait disorder with sensory symptoms in the feet and hands caused by cervical spondylosis also may be incorrectly attributed to peripheral neuropathy.

Rest and cervical immobilization with a soft collar are helpful in minor cases, traction may be helpful in others, but an operation is advisable if there are advanced symptoms of gait difficulty, severe hand weakness, or bladder difficulty.

Lumbar stenosis (also discussed in Chap. 15) is an intermittent and chronic compression of the cauda equina usually based on congenital narrowing of the lumbar spinal canal, which is further compromised by disk protrusion or spondylitic changes. Exercise brings about an aching pain in the buttocks, thighs, and calves, frequently sciatic in distribution, ceasing with rest and thereby simulating vascular-induced claudication. During the peak of pain, deep tendon reflexes and sensation may be reduced as compared with the resting state; peripheral vascular studies are normal. Lumbar stenosis and cervical spondylosis commonly occur together, the former probably explaining occasional lower extremity fasciculations in cervical spondylosis.

Degenerative and inherited myelopathies The prototype of the inherited disorders causing spinal cord syndromes is Friedreich's ataxia, a progressive, recessively inherited leg and truncal ataxia of late childhood onset. Intention tremor, clumsiness of the arms, and, later, dysarthria occur. Kyphoscoliosis and pes cavus are common. Areflexia, Babinski signs, and severely impaired vibratory and joint position sense loss are found on examination. Fragmentary or milder forms of the illness occur and overlap with other syndromes, including spastic paraparesis (Strümpell-Lorrain), cerebellar cortical degeneration with ataxia, and olivopontocerebellar atrophy (see also Chap. 372).

Amyotrophic lateral sclerosis (motor neuron disease) must be considered in patients with symmetric spastic paraparesis without sensory findings. It causes a pure motor syndrome with combined corticospinal, corticobulbar, and anterior horn cell involvement. Clinical or electromyographic evidence of widespread muscle fasciculations and denervation, in contrast to the limited segmental denervation of spondylosis, confirms the diagnosis (see Chaps. 372 and 382).

Subacute combined degeneration due to vitamin B₁₂ deficiency This treatable myelopathy causes a progressive spastic and ataxic paraparesis and neuropathy, usually with prominent distal paresthesias of the feet and hands. It should be considered in cases simulating cervical spondylosis, late-onset degenerative myelopathies, and symmetric late-onset spinal multiple sclerosis. The disease also can involve the peripheral and optic nerves and the brain. The diagnosis is confirmed by low B_{12} serum concentration and a positive Schilling test. This entity and related nutritional degenerations are discussed in Chap. 377. Whether folate or vitamin E deficiencies can produce a similar syndrome is controversial.

Syringomyelia *Syringomyelia* is a progressive myelopathy characterized pathologically by cavitation of the central spinal cord. It is often idiopathic or developmental (see Chap. 378) but may result from trauma, primary intramedullary tumors, extrinsic compression with central cord necrosis, arachnoiditis, hematomyelia, or necrotic myelitis. The developmental type usually begins in the midcervical cord and extends upward to the medulla or downward as low as the lumbar cord. It commonly takes an eccentric position, often causing unilateral long tract signs or reflex asymmetries. Many cases occur in association with craniovertebral abnormalities, most commonly the Arnold-Chiari malformation, but also including myelomeningocele, basilar skull impression (platybasia), atresia of the foramen of Magendie, or Dandy-Walker cysts (see Chap. 378).

The cardinal signs of syringomyelia correspond to a central high cervical cord syndrome and depend on the extent of the syrinx and associated abnormalities such as the Arnold-Chiari malformation. The classic presentation is (1) sensory loss, usually of a dissociated type (loss of pain and temperature and preservation of touch and vibration senses), which is "suspended" over the nape of the neck, shoulders, and upper arms (cape distribution), and eventually extends to the hands, (2) wasting of muscles in the lower neck, shoulders, arms, and hands, with asymmetric or absent reflexes, and (3) high thoracic kyphoscoliosis. The majority begin asymmetrically with unilateral sensory loss. A number of patients develop loss of pin sensation on the face from damage to the descending tract of the trigeminal nerve in the upper cervical cord. Cough-induced headache and neck pain are common with associated Arnold-Chiari malformations.

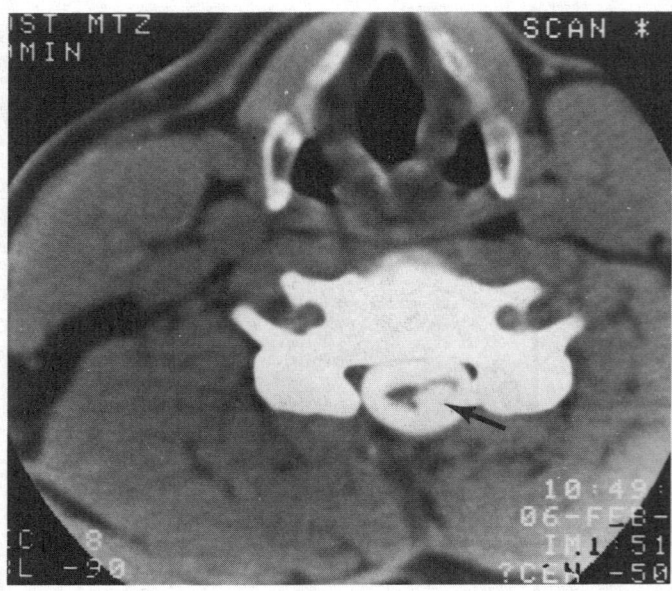

A

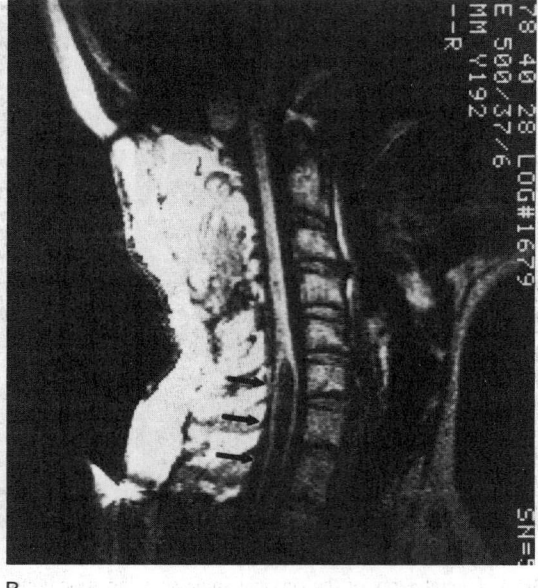

B

FIGURE 381-4 *A.* Horizontal CT section 1 h after subarachnoid instillation of water-soluble contrast medium showing the cervical spinal cord surrounded by contrast and dye in a large intramedullary syrinx cavity (*arrow*). *B.* Sagittal MRI of same patient as in *A* showing the syrinx cavity and enlargement of the spinal cord (*arrows*). *(Courtesy of Greg Shoukimas, M.D., Department of Radiology, Massachusetts General Hospital.)*

Symptoms in idiopathic cases begin in adolescence or early adulthood, progress irregularly, and frequently arrest for several years. A few patients escape major disability, but over half become wheelchair-bound. Analgesia leads to injuries, burns, and trophic ulcers in the fingertips. Charcot joints in the shoulders, elbows, or knees are common in advanced cases. Prominent lower extremity weakness or hyperreflexia suggests an associated abnormality at the craniovertebral junction. Syringobulbia results from extension of the cavity into the medulla, or rarely the pons, usually occupying the lateral medullary tegmentum. Palatal and vocal cord paralysis, dysarthria, nystagmus, episodic dizziness, tongue weakness, and Horner's syndrome may occur.

The diagnosis can be made dependably from the clinical features, confirmed by finding an enlarged cervical cord on delayed CT images several hours after subarachnoid instillation of metrizamide or another water-soluble contrast material (Fig. 381-4*A*), but syrinx cavities are shown to greatest advantage by MRI (Fig. 381-4*B*). The cervicomedullary junction should be examined for associated developmental abnormalities. Therapy is directed at decompressing the cavity to prevent progression of damage and decompressing the spinal canal if the cord is distended. Laminectomies and suboccipital decompression are sometimes recommended when an Arnold-Chiari malformation accompanies an enlarged cervical cord.

Tabes dorsalis   *Tabes* and *meningovascular syphilis* of the spinal cord are presently rare but at one time had to be considered in the differential diagnosis of most spinal cord syndromes. The most common symptoms of tabes are characteristic fleeting and repetitive, lancinating pains occurring mostly in the legs, less commonly in the back, thorax, abdomen, arms, and face. Severe gait and leg ataxia due to loss of position sense occurs in half of patients. Paresthesias, bladder disturbances, and acute abdominal pain with vomiting (visceral crisis) occur in 15 to 30 percent. The cardinal signs of tabes are loss of reflexes in the legs, impaired position and vibratory sense, Romberg's sign, and bilateral Argyll Robertson pupils, which fail to constrict to light but react with accommodation.

Traumatic spinal cord lesions are discussed in Chap. 376.

GENERAL CARE OF THE PATIENT WITH ACUTE PARAPLEGIA OR QUADRIPLEGIA   Protection from secondary damage to the urinary tract is a high priority in the acute stages of paraplegia. The bladder is areflexic, retains urine, and the patient is unaware of bladder distention, making damage to the detrusor muscle from overdistention possible. Urologic rehabilitation requires bladder drainage and avoidance of urinary infection. This is best accomplished by intermittent catheterization by trained personnel. Continuous closed system urinary drainage, which is associated with a higher infection rate than intermittent catheterization, and suprapubic drainage are less desirable alternatives. Patients with acute lesions, especially those causing spinal shock, frequently need special cardiovascular care because of paroxysmal hypertension or hypotension. Ileus and gastric stress ulcers are other potential acute medical problems in patients with complete transverse cord lesions. Cimetidine, ranitidine, or sucralfate may be useful in these circumstances. Pulmonary embolism due to immobilization is a grave early risk occurring in up to one-third of patients after acute cord trauma. Subcutaneous heparin may reduce the risk of early embolic complications. Rarely, spinal injury patients have become hypercalcemic from immobilization.

High cervical cord lesions cause varying degrees of mechanical respiratory failure requiring artificial ventilation. In cases of incomplete respiratory failure with forced vital capacities of 10 to 20 mL/kg, chest physical therapy is useful, and a negative-pressure cuirass may be used to alleviate atelectasis, particularly if the major lesion is below C4. With severe respiratory failure, tracheal intubation (performed over an endoscope if the spine is unstable), followed by tracheostomy, provides tracheal access for ventilation and suctioning. Phrenic nerve pacing may be useful in some patients with lesions at C5 or above.

As clinical signs stabilize, attention should be directed to the psychological state of the patient and the development of a rehabilitation plan framed by realistic expectations. An aggressive program is often remarkably successful with younger and middle-aged patients, allowing return to home and a productive lifestyle.

Chronic nursing care problems can be handled by patients with varying degrees of assistance. The major issues are related to immobilization: skin breakdown over pressure points, urinary sepsis, autonomic instability, and the potential for pulmonary embolism. Early care includes frequent repositioning, application of skin emollients, and soft bed coverings. Specialized beds turn the patient or distribute body weight evenly rather than predominantly on bony prominences. If the sacral cord segments are undamaged, then a large degree of automatic voiding can be entrained. Patients initially void reflexly between catheterizations and later learn to induce voiding with various maneuvers. If residual urinary volumes lead to infection, surgical procedures or an indwelling catheter may be necessary. Bowel regimens and disimpaction are necessary in most patients to ensure at least biweekly evacuation and avoid colonic distention or obstruction.

Severe hypertension and bradycardia occur in response to noxious superficial stimuli, bladder or bowel distention, or surgery, particularly in patients with cervical and high thoracic cord lesions. Flushing and diaphoresis above the level of the lesion may accompany the hypertension. The mechanism of this dysautonomia is not well understood. A potent antihypertensive agent may be necessary, particularly during surgery, but beta-blocking drugs should probably be avoided. Some patients become severely bradycardic with tracheal suctioning; this can be prevented with small doses of atropine.

Detailed aspects of the physical therapy, rehabilitation, and orthotics related to severe spinal cord diseases may be found in specialized texts.

REFERENCES

AMINOFF MJ, LOGUE V: Clinical features of spinal vascular malformations. Brain 97:197, 1974

BAKER AS et al: Spinal epidural abcess. N Engl J Med 293:463, 1975

BERNS DH et al: Magnetic resonance imaging of the spine. Clin Orthop 244:78, 1989

BYRNE TN, WAXMAN SG: Spinal cord compression. Contemporary Neurology Series, vol 33. Philadelphia, Davis, 1990

CHOUCAIR AK: Myelopathies in cancer patients: Incidence, presentation, diagnosis and management, part 1. Oncology 5:71, 1991

GILBERT RW et al: Epidural cord compression from metastatic tumor: Diagnosis and treatment. Ann Neurol 3:40, 1978

GREENBERG HS et al: Epidural spinal cord compression from metastatic tumor: Results with a new treatment protocol. Ann Neurol 8:361, 1980

HACKING HG et al: Factors related to the outcome of inpatient rehabilitation in patients with neoplastic epidural spinal cord compression. Paraplegia 31:367, 1993

JACOBSON S et al: Isolation of HTLV-II from a patient with chronic, progressive neurological disease clinically indistinguishable from HTLV-I-associated myelopathy/tropical spastic paraparesis. Ann Neurol 33:392, 1993

JEFFERY DR et al: Transverse myelitis. Retrospective analysis of 33 cases, with differentiation of cases associated with multiple sclerosis and parainfectious events. Arch Neurol 50:532, 1993

JOHNSON RT, MCARTHUR JC: Myelopathies and retroviral infections. Ann Neurol 21:113, 1987

LOGUE V, EDWARDS MR: Syringomyelia and its surgical treatment. J Neurol Neurosurg Psychiatr 44:273, 1981

MCILROY WJ, RICHARDSON JC: Syringomyelia: A clinical review of 75 cases. J Can Med Assoc 93:731, 1965

ROPPER AH, POSKANZER DC: Prognosis of acute and subacute transverse myelopathy based on early signs and symptoms. Ann Neurol 4:51, 1978

SNOW RB, WEINER H: Cervical laminectomy and foraminotomy as surgical treatment of cervical spondylosis: A follow-up study with analysis of failures. J Spinal Disord 6:245, 1993

UMBACH I, HEILPORN A: Review article: Post-spinal cord injury syringomyelia. Paraplegia 29:219, 1991

section 2

Disorders of nerve and muscle

382 APPROACH TO THE PATIENT WITH NEUROMUSCULAR DISEASE

ROBERT C. GRIGGS / WALTER G. BRADLEY*

The neuromuscular diseases are disorders of the *motor unit* and of the sensory and autonomic peripheral nerves. Each motor unit consists of (1) the *motor neuron cell body*, located in either the spinal cord anterior horn (for muscles innervated by the spinal cord) or a cranial nerve nucleus (for ocular, facial, bulbar musculature), (2) the *axon* of the motor neuron in the peripheral (or cranial) nerve, (3) the *neuromuscular junction*, and, (4) the *muscle fibers* innervated by the motor neuron. The sensory peripheral nerves comprise (1) the *sensory neuron* cell body in the posterior root ganglion, (2) the *central axon* passing to the spinal cord in the posterior root, (3) the *distal axon* in the peripheral nerve, and (4) the *sensory nerve terminal* in skin, muscle, joint capsule, etc. The autonomic nerves are divided into *sympathetic* and *parasympathetic* fiber systems. The sympathetic preganglionic fibers arise from cell bodies in the intermediolateral column of the spinal cord and enter the sympathetic ganglia, where postganglionic fibers arise to innervate blood vessels or viscera. The parasympathetic preganglionic neurons lie in the brainstem and sacral spinal cord, and axons terminate in the viscera, special sensory organs, or skin, which contain the postganglionic neurons and their nerve terminals. Neuromuscular diseases are classified into four groups depending on which portion of the motor unit is involved (see Table 382-1).

The major symptoms of diseases of the motor unit are muscle weakness, wasting, fatigue, cramps, pain, or stiffness. Symptoms of peripheral nerve disease include, in addition, decreased sensation (hypesthesia or hypalgesia), abnormal sensations (paresthesias), or painful sensations (dysesthesias) (see Chap. 24). Symptoms of autonomic nervous system disease include postural dizziness; abnormal cardiac, visceral, and ocular function; and changes in sweating (see also Chap. 379). The symptoms of neuromuscular disease, particularly those of weakness or sensory disturbance, do not necessarily distinguish disorders of the peripheral nervous system from those of the central nervous system. Most neuromuscular diseases are relatively symmetric in contrast to the asymmetry of many central nervous system diseases.

CLINICAL ASSESSMENT

History and physical examination will lead to a diagnosis in a majority of patients with neuromuscular disease. Failure to arrive at a diagnostic impression before routine and sophisticated laboratory studies often leads to diagnostic inaccuracy and confusion. Few of the biochemical, histologic, and electrodiagnostic studies used to evaluate patients with neuromuscular disease are pathognomonic, since nerve and muscle can respond to disease processes in only a limited number of ways.

CLINICAL HISTORY **Weakness and fatigue** (See Chap. 21) The patient with weakness, particularly when of gradual onset, may not recognize it, emphasizing the useful axiom that "signs of muscle weakness precede symptoms of weakness." Words such as "numbness," "deadness," "tiredness," or "fatigue" may be used by a patient with weakness who is unfamiliar with what is taking place. On the other hand, some complaints of "weakness" result from systemic rather than neuromuscular disease. In such patients,

---

* The authors acknowledge the contributions of Robert Young and Bhagwan Shahani to this chapter in previous editions.

TABLE 382-1 Classification of neuromuscular disease	
Site of involvement	Typical example
Anterior horn cell	
Without upper motor neuron involvement	Spinal muscular atrophy
With upper motor neuron involvement	Amyotrophic lateral sclerosis
Peripheral nerve	
Unifocal	Carpal tunnel syndrome
Multifocal	Mononeuritis multiplex (e.g., polyarteritis nodosa)
Diffuse	Diabetic neuropathy
Neuromuscular junction	Myasthenia gravis
Muscle	Duchenne's muscular dystrophy

strength is often normal or only mildly reduced, since the complaint is usually loss of stamina and endurance. The patient with fatigue should be asked to distinguish between true weakness and the less specific symptoms of lassitude and asthenia. If the patient is unable to perform a normal activity, true weakness is suggested. Objective evidence of weakness is established if symptoms exceed the bounds of normal variation (e.g., double vision, drooping eyelids, difficulty in swallowing, aspiration of food or liquids into the airway) as opposed to the more subjective complaints of inability to lift, carry, or push an object.

The time-course and severity of weakness must be quantitated by questions concerning alterations in functional abilities: for the legs, difficulty in rising from a chair or commode, rising from a squatting position, or climbing up and down stairs and a history of frequent tripping, stumbling, or falling; for the trunk, difficulty in sitting up from supine in bed; or for the arms, difficulty in washing the hair, opening jars, fastening buttons, or raising objects onto a shelf.

Abnormalities of sensation (See Chaps. 24 and 383) Sensory symptoms suggest peripheral nerve disease, although, as with weakness, sensory abnormalities can occur with disease at any level of the nervous system. The characteristics and localization of sensory symptoms in the various peripheral nerve syndromes and diseases are discussed in Chap. 24. In contradistinction to weakness, it is axiomatic that "sensory symptoms precede objective sensory signs."

Muscle pain (See Chap. 23) Muscle aches and pains may suggest inflammatory or metabolic muscle disease but are far more common in bone, joint, and nerve disease. Persistent muscle pain in a patient with normal strength usually results from a cause other than myopathy. Intermittent muscle pain, however, particularly when precipitated by exercise, should raise a consideration of a substrate utilization defect such as a glycogen or lipid storage myopathy. It is important to determine if other factors, such as fasting, precipitate pain and then to inquire about associated findings such as dark urine which may be indicative of myoglobinuria.

Autonomic dysfunction The most common complaint is "dizziness" or "blackouts," which prove to be precipitated by the patient standing up from sitting or lying (see Chap. 17). Loss of potency in the male is frequent in autonomic neuropathies. Explosive diarrhea or cyclical diarrhea-constipation are sometimes present, as is partial urinary retention.

PHYSICAL EXAMINATION Strength testing Reliable testing of strength requires that the examiner have an adequate frame of reference for normal strength and that the patient be motivated and able to cooperate with testing. As with history taking, it is helpful to quantitate the ability to perform tasks required in daily living. The legs are particularly easy to test by observing walking on heels and toes; rising from a chair, noting whether there is a need to use the arms; rising from a squat; and stepping up onto a chair. It is also important to examine the legs for a *knee-extension lag*, the inability to fully extend the leg against gravity. The number of degrees of extension lag can be measured with a goniometer. Patients with even a minor extension lag almost invariably report frequent tripping and falling. The converse is also true: Patients with muscle weakness

who report frequent falls usually have quadriceps muscle weakness producing a knee-extension lag. Trunk and neck muscles can be tested by having the patient sit up from supine; extending the head over the edge of an examining table is a sensitive method of detecting neck weakness. The arms are not as easily evaluated with function testing: inspection of shoulders for scapular winging as the arms are elevated and watching the patient lift the arms above the head test shoulder girdle function. Hand strength can be judged by determining the degree of difficulty in extracting two fingers from the grip of the patient and by noting the ability of the patient to blanch the knuckles when making a tight fist. When the lesion affects a specific region, e.g., the brachial plexus or the ulnar nerve, it is essential to test each individual muscle of the arm or hand.

Formal muscle testing, assigning a numerical grade to muscle strength, is usually based on the MRC (Medical Research Council of Great Britain) 0 to 5 scale:

5—normal
4—able to oppose gravity plus resistance
3—able to move fully against gravity but not resistance
2—able to move with gravity eliminated
1—trace movement
0—no movement

An important assessment is whether a muscle is indeed *weaker than one would expect*, after making allowances for age, male-female differences, inactivity, or generalized illness. If one has a limited time for the testing of muscle strength, the assessment of function is likely to be of more value than formal muscle testing.

Muscle bulk Muscle atrophy and hypertrophy are often difficult to recognize because of wide variation among normal individuals. The problem is accentuated in young children and in obese patients because of overlying adipose tissue. Atrophy is easier to appreciate when asymmetric. Muscle enlargement or hypertrophy is a normal accompaniment of physical activity. It is occasionally a sign of disease in patients with long-standing spasticity or myotonic disorders. So-called pseudohypertrophy, in which the muscles become enlarged by replacement with connective tissue and fat, may be prominent in certain of the muscular dystrophies but is also seen with spinal muscular atrophy and other denervating conditions. Actual hypertrophy of muscle fibers also may be present in these patients. Muscle enlargement also may be caused by infiltration with substances such as amyloid or by parasitic infestation (e.g., cysticercosis).

Focal muscle swelling may be due to inflammatory infiltrates, calcium deposits, localized myositis, sarcoidosis, ectopic calcification, neoplasms, or tendon rupture. Preservation of some parts of a muscle, while other parts atrophy, may occur in spinal muscular atrophy and some forms of muscular dystrophy, giving an appearance of a focal swelling during muscle contraction ("belly hypertrophy"). Single or multiple muscle masses in a patient without weakness may indicate a neoplastic process.

Pathologic fatigue Patients with disorders of neuromuscular transmission such as myasthenia gravis usually can be shown to fatigue on examination. Sustained upward gaze produces gradual ptosis of the eyelids (curtain sign); eye movements become disconjugate on sustained horizontal gaze; the voice may become hoarse, slurred, or nasal with prolonged speech; or a smile may rapidly become a sneer when the patient cannot maintain facial muscle activity. Inability to sustain limb activity is less easily quantitated, since patients who are weak from any cause may have decreased endurance.

Sensory testing Patients with peripheral neuropathy usually have sensory loss. The distribution of sensory disturbance and the modalities affected are often of diagnostic importance (see Chaps. 24 and 383).

Autonomic testing A fall of systolic blood pressure of more than 20 mmHg from lying to standing indicates impaired autonomic control of peripheral blood vessels. A greater fall often occurs with exercise in the erect position. The pulse rate does not increase

TABLE 382-2   Presenting clinical features of the neuromuscular diseases

	Anterior horn cell	Peripheral nerve	Neuromuscular junction	Muscle
Distribution of weakness	Asymmetric limb or bulbar	Symmetric distal	Extraocular, bulbar, proximal limb	Symmetric limb (bulbar in some)
Atrophy	Marked and early	Moderate	None	Slight early; marked later
Sensory involvement	None	Paresthesias, hypesthesia	None	None
Characteristic features	Fasciculations, cramps	Combined sensory and motor abnormality	Diurnal fluctuation	
Reflexes	Variable (depending on degree of upper motor neuronal involvement)	Decreased out of proportion to weakness	Normal	Decreased in proportion to weakness

normally in response to this hypotension if there is an autonomic neuropathy. Similarly, there is no slowing of the heart rate following a sustained Valsalva maneuver (see Chap. 379).

Other findings Myotonia, fasciculations, myokymia, and other spontaneous activity (Chap. 23) should be sought. Certain disorders such as myotonic dystrophy and facioscapulohumeral dystrophy have distinctive and virtually pathognomonic facial features. Less diagnostic but significant facial weakness is found in other myopathies and in myasthenia gravis. Contractures, particularly of the Achilles tendons, limitation of hip joint movement, and scoliosis may indicate that weakness is of long duration.

DIFFERENTIAL DIAGNOSIS Weaknesses produced by diseases of the motor unit are distinguishable from each other by their distribution, by the time-course of the illness, and by accompanying clinical findings such as muscle bulk and tone, reflexes, and sensory findings. The portion of the motor unit involved by a disease process is usually evident from clinical findings (Table 382-2). Motor neuron diseases (Chap. 372) are suggested in the patient whose weakness is accompanied by prominent atrophy, fasciculations, and lack of sensory involvement. The reflexes may be disproportionately depressed if anterior horn cell disease alone is present or pathologically increased if there is coexistent upper motor neuron disease, such as amyotrophic lateral sclerosis. Peripheral neuropathy (Chap. 383) is suggested by the presence of distal weakness associated with sensory involvement. In general, patients with peripheral neuropathy have depressed reflexes; preservation of reflexes in the presence of significant weakness suggests a cause other than neuropathy. Neuromuscular junction disorders (Chap. 386) are suggested if ocular and bulbar weakness is prominent, particularly if there is *diurnal variation*, with the patient becoming weaker as the day progresses. Pathologic fatigue usually can be demonstrated. Reflexes are preserved in most neuromuscular junction disorders, particularly myasthenia gravis.

Myopathy versus other neuromuscular disease Clinical features which suggest myopathy in contrast to other motor unit diseases include a proximal distribution of weakness, relative preservation or increase of muscle bulk, and the preservation of reflexes. Table 382-3 presents a classification of primary muscle diseases. Many patients with muscle symptoms, however, do not have a primary myopathy, and clinical evaluation discloses disease in another portion of the motor unit or in another system (see Chap. 21). For example, a patient with a denervation produced by nerve root damage from a lumbar disk protrusion may have muscle cramps, pain, and weakness in muscles innervated by those nerve roots. Furthermore, fatigue, weakness, and pain are common accompaniments of derangements of cardiac, hematologic, gastrointestinal, pulmonary, renal, or hepatic function. Despite complaints of weakness and fatigue and the finding of atrophy, it is relatively infrequent for patients with pulmonary or cardiac disease to be mistaken for those with primary muscle disease.

Proximal weakness is so characteristic of myopathies that, by a somewhat circular argument, proximal weakness is usually attributed to "myopathy." In fact, neuropathies such as acute or chronic inflammatory polyneuropathy, the neuromuscular junction disorders, and many anterior horn cell diseases have predominantly proximal weakness. Proximal weakness, occurring in disorders such as hyperthyroidism and hyperparathyroidism and as a result of glucocorticoid administration, is often termed "myopathic," despite the fact that the underlying pathophysiology of the muscle disorders in these conditions has not been defined.

Acute generalized weakness Weakness developing over the course of less than an hour is usually caused by a metabolic or toxic disorder affecting either the neuromuscular junction or muscle. A sudden alteration in circulating levels of potassium, calcium, sodium, magnesium, or phosphate may result in partial or complete paralysis of muscle. Acute failure of neuromuscular junction transmission may occur with botulism and other toxins, hypermagnesemia, aminoglycoside antibiotics, and other medications. Weakness developing over the course of 24 h may occur in electrolyte, metabolic, and toxic disorders; in periodic paralysis (Chap. 387); and in acute inflammatory myopathies, particularly those related to viral and parasitic infection (Chap. 384) and certain acute polyneuropathies (Chap. 383). Occasionally, patients with more chronic disorders first realize that they are weak when the insidious progression of their weakness produces an abrupt change in function.

Subacute weakness Weakness developing over days is more common in peripheral nerve or neuromuscular junction diseases than in muscle or anterior horn cell disease. Acute inflammatory polyneuropathy (Guillain-Barré syndrome) and porphyric, diphtheritic, and toxic neuropathies are of subacute onset. Myasthenia gravis and other neuromuscular junction diseases also must be considered in the differential diagnosis. Subacute weakness can occur in severe polymyositis and dermatomyositis (see Chap. 384). Weakness from endocrine disorders and certain muscle toxins (see Table 382-3) also

TABLE 382-3   Classification of primary muscle diseases

Hereditary
- A Muscular dystrophy (Chap. 385): Duchenne's, myotonic, facioscapulohumeral, limb-girdle, oculopharyngeal, scapuloperoneal, congenital, distal, and ocular
- B Congenital myopathies (Chap. 385): Central core, nemaline, centronuclear, fiber-type disproportion
- C Metabolic myopathies (Chap. 385):
  - 1 Glycogen: Deficiencies of phosphorylase, phosphofructokinase, phosphoglyceromutase, acid maltase, others
  - 2 Lipid: Defective synthesis or transport of carnitine; deficiency of carnitine palmitoyl transferase
  - 3 Purine nucleotide cycle: Deficiency of myoadenylate deaminase
- D Myotonia (Chap. 385 and 387): Congenita, paramyotonia
- E Periodic paralysis (Chap. 23 and 387): Hypokalemic, hyperkalemic, normokalemic

Inflammatory (Chap. 384)
- A Collagen disease: Systemic lupus erythematosus, rheumatoid arthritis, scleroderma, mixed-connective tissue
- B Sarcoidosis, carcinoid
- C Infections: Numerous, especially viral (influenza B), protozoal (toxoplasmosis), parasitic (trichinosis)
- D Idiopathic: Polymyositis, dermatomyositis, inclusion body myositis

Endocrine and metabolic (Chap. 385)
- A Electrolyte abnormalities: Calcium, phosphate, magnesium, sodium, potassium
- B Endocrine: Hypo- and hyperfunction of thyroid, adrenal, parathyroid, pituitary

Toxic (Chap. 385): Alcohol, opiates, pentazocine, clofibrate, others

Tumors and masses: Primary and metastatic neoplasms, infection, sarcoidosis, myositis ossificans, calcinosis, muscle rupture and hemorrhage may develop subacutely (Chap. 385). Of the anterior horn cell disorders, only infections with poliomyelitis and other viruses commonly evolve subacutely. Amyotrophic lateral sclerosis occasionally pursues a subacute, severe course.

Slowly progressive weakness *Slowly progressive proximal weakness* evolving over weeks to months may be caused by polymyositis or dermatomyositis or an unsuspected endocrinopathy. When the course has extended for a year or more, however, one of the muscular dystrophies, spinal muscular atrophy, or a neuromuscular junction defect such as myasthenia gravis may be present. Neuropathies are seldom proximal, the major exceptions being acute and chronic inflammatory polyneuropathy, porphyric neuropathy, and diabetic proximal mononeuropathy. *Slowly progressive distal weakness* is more characteristic of peripheral nerve or anterior horn cell disorders than of disorders of muscle or the neuromuscular junction. The only commonly encountered distal myopathy is myotonic dystrophy. Less common disorders such as distal muscular dystrophy, nemaline and centronuclear myopathies, and a variant of polymyositis known as *inclusion body myositis* may present with distal weakness. Prominent distal lower limb weakness is also present in the facioscapulohumeral and scapuloperoneal muscular dystrophies, but proximal involvement is invariably also present in such patients. *Slowly progressive bulbar weakness* is more typical of anterior horn cell or neuromuscular junction disorders than of myopathies. Bulbar weakness (difficulty in speaking, coughing, and swallowing) occurs commonly in motor neuron disease (especially amyotrophic lateral sclerosis) and neuromuscular junction disorders. It is also seen in oculopharyngeal dystrophy, myotonic dystrophy, and polymyositis or dermatomyositis. *Ocular muscle weakness and ptosis* do not occur in motor neuron disease and are uncommon in peripheral neuropathy. Ophthalmoparesis is typical of myasthenia gravis and may occur in myotonic and oculopharyngeal dystrophies. Weakness limited to or predominantly ocular in location (*progressive external ophthalmoplegia*) occurs in disorders such as the Kearns-Sayre syndrome (Chap. 385).

LABORATORY ASSESSMENT

Patients with significantly impaired strength and sensation merit thorough diagnostic study. The sequence of investigations should be based on the test's diagnostic specificity and sensitivity, level of patient discomfort, and cost. Hematologic, renal, and hepatic function and serum electrolytes should be evaluated. In many instances, thyroid, adrenal, and other endocrine studies may be indicated. Other useful diagnostic tests are the serum creatine kinase (CK) level, nerve conduction studies, electromyography, and in many instances muscle biopsy. Nerve biopsy is a more specialized technique with a relatively small number of specific indications (see Chap. 383). Repetitive stimulation of nerve with recording from muscle should be obtained when a neuromuscular junction defect is suspected. Since many diagnostic tests are uncomfortable and expensive, it is important to consider what information is being sought in requesting each test. Confounding features in the investigations also must be understood. For instance, muscle necrosis and inflammation and an elevated serum CK level may occur after minor muscle trauma such as is caused by electromyography and intramuscular injection. Electromyography and muscle biopsy obtained from a muscle affected by past nerve root disease (e.g., from a herniated disk) may show neuropathic abnormalities unrelated to a new disease process. A patient complaining of weakness and fatigue who is found on examination to have no weakness should be examined during exercise. Some of these patients have a metabolic myopathy. Others may have a neuromuscular junction, central nervous system, or psychological problem requiring appropriate investigations.

BIOCHEMICAL EVALUATION OF NEUROMUSCULAR DISEASE Certain enzymes, especially CK, occur in high concentrations in the sarcoplasm of muscle and may leak into blood to serve as an indicator of muscle damage. The serum CK, lactic dehydrogenase (LDH), aspartate aminotransferase (AST, SGOT), and alanine aminotransferase (ALT, SGPT) levels may be elevated in patients with active muscle destruction. Since several of these enzymes are used for screening for abnormalities of organs other than muscle, it is not uncommon for a patient with muscle disease to be first identified by an unexpected elevation in one of these enzymes. The clue to the muscle origin of the increased enzyme levels is that the degree of abnormality decreases in the order CK > LDH > SGOT > SGPT. The serum CK level is the most sensitive test and may be very high (raised more than tenfold) in diseases with muscle fiber necrosis, such as the muscular dystrophies, polymyositis, and rhabdomyolysis. It is frequently slightly elevated in spinal muscular atrophy, amyotrophic lateral sclerosis, and other motor neuron disorders and is usually normal in peripheral neuropathies and neuromuscular junction disorders. Strenuous exercise in normal individuals can elevate the level of serum CK for 6 h or more. Three isoenzymes of CK occur: MM, MB, and BB. MM predominates in skeletal muscle, MB occurs mainly in cardiac muscle, and BB is mainly in brain. Elevations of CK-MB levels are used to indicate the presence of myocardial damage. CK elevation caused by acute muscle injury is usually due to the MM isoenzyme. However, in many patients with long-standing necrotizing muscular diseases and in athletes, the proportion of MB in skeletal muscle rises, and in consequence, the proportion of CK-MB in blood is elevated.

MUSCLE COMPOSITION AND MASS Computed tomography and magnetic resonance imaging can differentiate between muscle fibers, fat, and connective tissue and may show distinctive differences between muscular dystrophy and the other forms of muscle disease. The high cost and the nonspecificity of the findings limit the role of these techniques. Estimations of total muscle mass are of some importance in metabolic studies. A simple decline in muscle mass without weakness is indicative of a process other than a neuromuscular disease, e.g., aging, neoplasm, impaired nutrition, renal or hepatic disease. The 24-h urinary creatinine excretion is the most widely available technique used to estimate muscle mass; it is decreased in patients with wasting from any cause.

METABOLIC, ENDOCRINE, AND OTHER STUDIES Hypo- and hyperkalemia, hypernatremia, hypo- and hypercalcemia, hypophosphatemia, and hypermagnesemia can all cause severe, usually acute, weakness. Serum potassium levels are labile and subject to rapid shifts induced by acidosis or alkalosis. The intracellular concentration of potassium is high, so hemolysis during blood collection may spuriously elevate the potassium level. The extensive muscle damage in rhabdomyolysis may produce a true hyperkalemia. Such elevations in serum potassium level are generally not greater than 0.1 mmol/L, however, unless the serum is stained with hemoglobin, as occurs with hemolysis, or the urine is stained with myoglobin, as occurs with rhabdomyolysis.

Chronic endocrine disorders, either hypo- or hyperfunction of thyroid, adrenal, or parathyroid glands, may cause weakness in the absence of other clinical evidence of endocrinopathy. Rheumatoid arthritis, systemic lupus erythematosus, scleroderma, and the polymyalgia rheumatica syndrome may be complicated by muscle weakness. Tests for these diseases are usually indicated in the evaluation of unexplained muscle pain and weakness. The weakness in most of these disorders is related to disuse atrophy and joint pain; muscle inflammation and evidence of muscle destruction are uncommon. Disorders of muscle mitochondrial function may cause a high plasma lactate level. Other laboratory investigations that may be indicated in patients with peripheral neuropathy include tests for diabetes mellitus; levels of serum vitamin B_{12}, folate, and lipids; serum protein electrophoresis; urinary and serum immunoelectrophoresis; lipoprotein electrophoresis; and urinary porphyrins and heavy metal levels. Diagnostic enzyme determinations are available in white blood cells in certain neuromuscular disorders, such as aryl sulfatase and acid maltase deficiencies.

MYOGLOBINURIA Acute muscle destruction, *rhabdomyolysis* associated with myoglobinuria, occurs with acute toxic, metabolic, inflammatory, infectious, and traumatic muscle damage (see Chap. 384). The molecular weight of myoglobin is lower than that of hemoglobin, so the urine rather than the serum changes color in extensive rhabdomyolysis. Myoglobinuria causes a positive urine test for blood in the absence of urinary erythrocytes. Confirmatory testing for myoglobin uses a specific immunoassay.

EXERCISE TESTING (See Chap. 385) Patients with substrate utilization defects characteristically have decreased exercise tolerance and muscle pain and weakness during or following exercise. Most defects in the enzymatic pathways of glycolysis result in the failure of muscle to generate adenosine triphosphate (ATP) from glycogen and a diminished or absent production of lactic acid. Patients with these disorders can be evaluated with forearm exercise determining the level of venous lactic acid. Patients with disturbance of fatty acid metabolism (such as carnitine palmitoyl transferase deficiency, in which long-chain fatty acids cannot be transferred into mitochondria for beta oxidation) generate lactic acid normally. Patients with myoadenylate deaminase deficiency generate lactate in normal or increased amounts but fail to produce ammonia in the exercise test (Chap. 385). Measurement of specific muscle enzymes can define the cause of the disorder.

ELECTROPHYSIOLOGIC STUDIES OF NEUROMUSCULAR DISEASE

NORMAL MOTOR UNIT PHYSIOLOGY The motor unit is the final common pathway for motor activity of the nervous system, and muscle is the final effector of the motor unit. All movement, posture, and reflex activity results from integrated discharge of large numbers of motor units by spinal and supraspinal mechanisms. The strength of a muscle contraction depends on the number of motor units recruited, the frequency of motor unit discharge, the speed of contraction of muscle fibers in the motor unit, and the nature of the motor unit (whether fatigue-resistant or fatigue-prone). The number of motor units varies greatly among muscles, ranging from as few as 10 in the extraocular muscles, to approximately 100 in the intrinsic muscles of the hands, to several thousand in leg muscles such as the gastrocnemius. The number of muscle fibers per muscle varies up to a thousandfold, from 1000 in extraocular muscles to over 1 million in large leg muscles. The muscle fibers of the motor unit are dispersed randomly within an area of muscle, and fibers innervated by the same anterior horn cell are generally not contiguous. An understanding of the organization of motor units and their patterns of firing is important in the interpretation of clinical and laboratory findings in normal and diseased muscle.

The physiologic characterization of the muscle fibers relates importantly to the exercise capacity of muscle. Motor units that consist of type 1 slow-twitch muscle fibers are designed for continuous and prolonged activity, since their energy supply is derived from the oxidative metabolism of mitochondria. These motor units are smaller and are activated (*recruited*) by low-intensity efforts. High-intensity effort or rapid muscle contraction, such as lifting of a heavy weight or sprinting, recruits larger motor units that consist of rapid-twitch type 2 muscle fibers, which derive their energy supply from anaerobic glycolysis.

As muscles relax, the cessation of firing of individual motor units occurs in a groupwise fashion so that a patient exerting an inadequate effort owing to functional weakness (e.g., malingering), lack of motivation, or pain will frequently have a ratchet-like or "give-way" quality on muscle testing. This may permit the distinction between true and feigned weakness.

ELECTROMYOGRAPHY The normal electromyogram The measurement of electrical activity arising from muscle fibers is usually performed by inserting a needle electrode percutaneously into a muscle. The electrical activity from this electrode is then displayed on a cathode-ray oscilloscope and can be made audible through a loudspeaker. Such studies provide only an average picture of the local

electrical activity of muscle, and normal electrical activity in one area does not exclude the possibility of pathologic phenomena close by.

In a single muscle fiber, as the action potential travels from the neuromuscular junction toward the ends of the muscle fiber, current flows outward through the normally polarized region of the muscle membrane (*sarcolemma*) toward the depolarized zone (zone A, Fig. 382-1). The recording electrode initially becomes slightly positive relative to the reference electrode (wave A). When the depolarized region moves under the recording electrode (zone B), a negative deflection (wave B) occurs. As the active region moves away from the electrode (zone C), the membrane under the electrode become repolarized (wave C). The net result is a triphasic action potential (see Fig. 382-1). The motor unit comprises many such fibers, and hence firing of many fibers of the motor unit produces a more complex waveform (*the motor unit action potential*) resulting from summation of individual single-fiber action potentials. Normal muscle is electrically silent when at rest, once *insertional activity*, produced by the trauma of placing the needle, has died down. When a muscle is voluntarily contracted, motor unit action potentials appear. With increasing strength of contraction, the number and size of the motor unit action potentials increase, until with full contraction individual motor unit potentials can no longer be distinguished, and a *complete recruitment (interference) pattern* is produced.

The abnormal electromyogram SPONTANEOUS ACTIVITY DURING COMPLETE RELAXATION Persistent insertional activity occurs in myotonic disorders, in polymyositis, and in denervated muscles. Spontaneous activity of a single muscle fiber is called *fibrillation*, and of part of or an entire motor unit, *fasciculation*. Triphasic fibrillation potentials and biphasic positive sharp waves can be seen 7 to 25 days after denervation of muscle fibers (depending on the distance of denervated muscle fibers from the site of the nerve lesion) and may persist for several years unless reinnervation occurs. Fibrillation appears with destruction of the motor neuron or its axon and in muscle diseases where a portion of a muscle fiber is separated from its innervated portions by segmental necrosis.

FIGURE 382-1 The single muscle fiber action potential. The shaded area represents the zone of the action potential at each of three positions, A, B, and C, as it sweeps along the muscle fiber from left to right. When the action potential reaches zone A, wave A is seen in the cathode-ray oscilloscope (*CRO*), reflecting the positive potential difference between the active (*vertical arrow*) and the reference (*Ref.*) electrodes. When the action potential reaches zone B, wave B occurs, and when it reaches zone C, wave C is recorded at the active electrode.

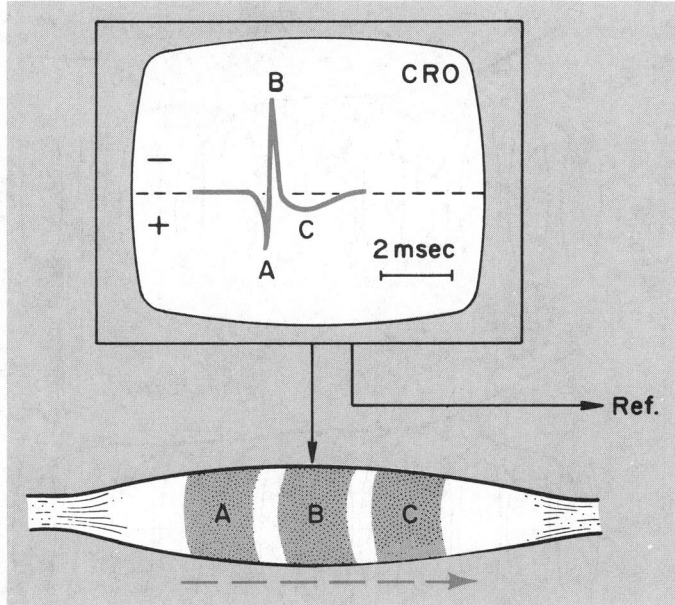

Fasciculations are seen with slowly progressive disease of the anterior horn cells such as amyotrophic lateral sclerosis and progressive spinal muscular atrophy, with compressive nerve root lesions, and in some motor neuropathies. In the syndrome of *benign fasciculations*, the same motor unit tends to fire at a regular rate that is usually faster than that of fasciculations indicative of disease.

In *myotonia*, the sarcolemma is irritable, and repeated muscle depolarization and contraction occur despite voluntary relaxation (see Chap. 385). Such patterns occur in myotonia congenita, myotonic dystrophy, and the periodic paralyses. On electromyography (EMG), myotonia causes high-frequency repetitive discharges that wax and wane in amplitude and frequency, producing a "dive bomber" or "motorcycle" sound on the loudspeaker. *Bizarre, repetitive high-frequency discharges* without waxing and waning are seen in many disorders affecting the motor neurons or muscle. *Coupling of action potentials* into doublets, triplets, or higher multiples of single units occurs in tetany, hemifacial spasm, and myokymia and indicates

FIGURE 382-2 Motor unit potentials. The shaded muscle fibers are functional members of one motor unit; the axon, which enters from the upper left, branches terminally to innervate the appropriate muscle fibers. The motor unit action potential produced by each motor unit is seen in the upper right; its duration is measured between the two small vertical lines. The normal-appearing but unshaded fibers belong to other motor units. *A.* The normal situation, with five muscle fibers in the active unit. *B.* In this myopathic unit, only two fibers remain active; the other three (shrunken and unshaded) have been destroyed by a muscle disease. *C.* Four fibers which belonged to other motor units and had been denervated have now been reinnervated by terminal axon sprouting from the healthy motor unit. Both the motor unit and its action potential are now larger than normal. Note that only under these abnormal circumstances do fibers in the same unit lie next to one another.

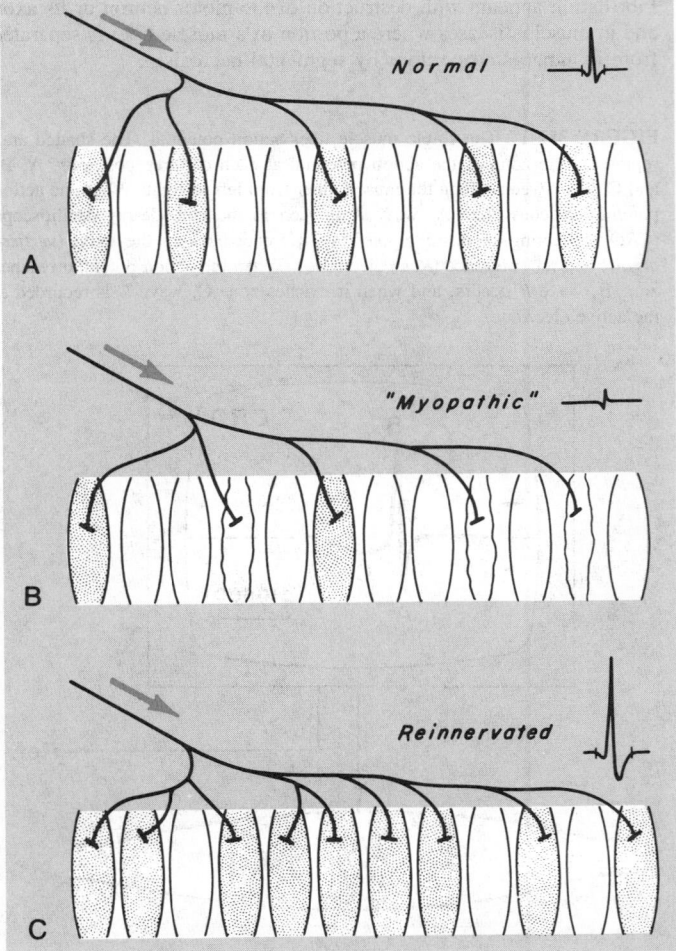

instability in repolarization of the nerve fiber. Electrical silence characterizes *contracture*, as in McArdle's disease and malignant hyperthermia.

ABNORMALITIES IN MOTOR UNIT POTENTIALS Early in the course of denervation, the remaining motor units are normal, but with the development of reinnervation, the remaining motor units increase in amplitude and become longer in duration and polyphasic (see Fig. 382-2). Conversely, in diseases such as polymyositis, the muscular dystrophies, and other myopathies that destroy scattered fibers within a motor unit (Fig. 382-2), the motor unit action potentials are of lower amplitude and shorter duration and are polyphasic.

In diseases of the central or peripheral nervous system, a *reduced recruitment (interference) pattern* results from maximum voluntary effort because fewer motor units are activated. Conversely, in patients with primary muscle disease, submaximal voluntary effort produces a *full recruitment pattern* despite marked weakness. Because fewer muscle fibers are active, however, the amplitude of the pattern is reduced from normal.

A number of advanced electromyographic techniques, such as single-fiber EMG and macro EMG (see Chap. 366), have been developed to investigate the stability of neuromuscular junction and motor unit reinnervation; their description is beyond the scope of this presentation.

Nerve conduction studies Stimulation of the larger peripheral motor and sensory nerves permits the recording of their action potentials and provides objective quantitative data of *latency* and *conduction velocity*. The technique is performed by stimulating the nerve with surface electrodes placed over the nerve. The resulting *compound action potential* is recorded by electrodes placed over the nerve proximally in the case of large sensory nerve fibers or over the muscle distally in the case of motor nerve fibers in a mixed motor sensory nerve (see Fig. 382-3). The normal maximum motor and sensory nerve conduction velocities vary from 40 to 80 m/s in different peripheral nerves. Values are approximately half in newborn infants and reach the adult range by 3 to 4 years of age. Normal values have been defined for *distal* or *peripheral latencies* that represent conduction time from the most distal stimulating electrodes, measured in milliseconds from the stimulus artifact to the onset of the response. It is important that the limb be kept warm during nerve conduction studies because subnormal temperatures cause slower conduction velocity. The *compound muscle action potential* obtained by stimulating a mixed motor nerve is of relatively high amplitude (5 to 10 mV) because of the amplification produced by the large number of muscle fibers in each motor unit. Sensory nerve action potentials, lacking this amplification, are of low amplitude (10 to 50 μV) and hence are more difficult to record. In abnormal nerves, sensory nerve action potentials may be small or absent, and sensory conduction measurements may be impossible to record. In contrast, reliable measurement of motor conduction velocities are usually possible even though only a few functional motor nerve fibers remain intact.

Maximum nerve conduction velocity measurements reflect the status of the best surviving of the largest myelinated nerve fibers and may be normal despite extensive loss of nerve fibers. Hence nerve conduction velocity is normal or only slightly below normal in many neuropathies, although the amplitude of the evoked action potential is often reduced. In diseases of peripheral nerves causing severe segmental demyelination, such as chronic inflammatory polyneuropathy, diphtheria, metachromatic leukodystrophy, and the hereditary demyelinating hypertrophic neuropathies, the maximum nerve conduction velocities may be reduced to below half normal. Focal compressions of nerve, as in entrapment syndromes, produce localized slowing of conduction because of demyelination and narrowing of axons at the site of compression. The conduction of proximal segments of the nerves and nerve roots can be studied by F waves and H reflexes (see Chap. 366), or by stimulation of nerve roots by a needle electrode or magnetic stimulator.

Repetitive stimulation tests In myasthenia gravis, a disorder of the neuromuscular junction, the size of the initial compound muscle

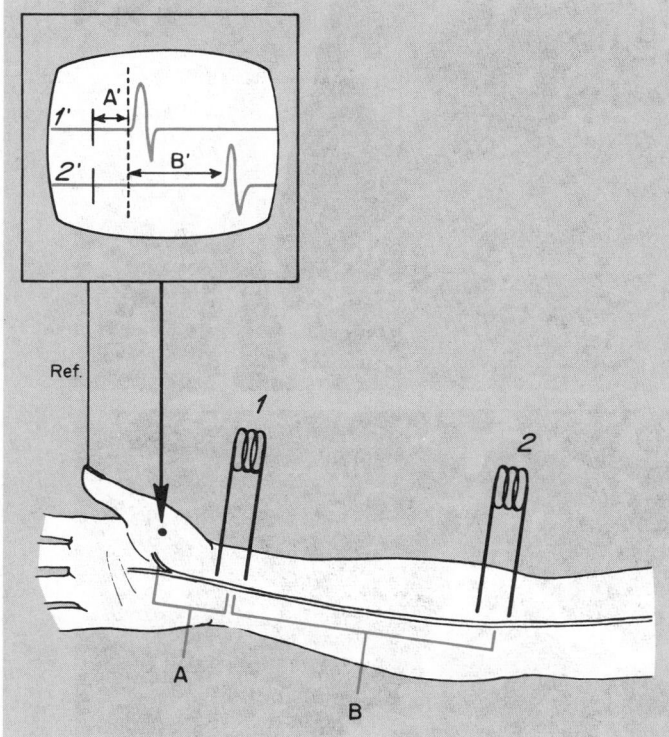

FIGURE 382-3 Measurement of nerve conduction velocity. The median nerve is stimulated through the skin at the wrist (1) or in the antecubital fossa (2), and the resultant compound muscle action potential is recorded as the potential difference between a surface electrode over the thenar eminence (*vertical arrow*) and a reference electrode (*Ref.*) more distally. Sweep 1′ on the cathode-ray oscilloscope (*CRO*) depicts the stimulus artifact (moment of stimulation at 1) followed by the muscle potential. The distal latency is the time A′ on the CRO sweep (3.0 ms, for example) which corresponds to conduction over distance A in the hand. The same is true for sweep 2′ where stimulation is at point 2, and the time from artifact to response is A′ + B′. The maximal motor conduction velocity from points 2 to 1 is obtained by dividing distance B by time B′.

action potential produced by a supramaximal electrical stimulus to the nerve may be normal. However, after a few stimuli at rates of 2 to 3 Hz, the amplitude of compound muscle action potential declines. It then increases again after the fourth or fifth stimulus. This pattern of decrement followed by increment is characteristic of myasthenia gravis. This defect resembles the partial blockade produced by curare and reflects a postjunctional disorder of synaptic function. The defect is reversed by administration of anticholinesterase medications such as intravenous edrophonium hydrochloride (5 to 10 mg). A progressive decline in the compound muscle action potential with repetitive stimulation also may occur in poliomyelitis, amyotrophic lateral sclerosis, myotonia, and other diseases of the motor unit. Usually, the typical pattern of decrement-increment seen in myasthenia gravis is not present in other disorders.

In the Lambert-Eaton (myasthenic) syndrome, repetitive stimulation causes a facilitation of transmission. Rapid stimulation of nerve (20 to 30 Hz) results in a progressive increase in the amplitude of the muscle action potential, which is small at the first stimulus, to a nearly normal amplitude. This facilitation response is not affected by anticholinesterase drugs.

HISTOPATHOLOGY OF MUSCLE AND NERVE

MUSCLE BIOPSY Biopsy is useful in (1) distinguishing between neurogenic and myopathic processes, (2) recognizing specific disorders of muscle such as muscular dystrophy or the congenital myopa-

thies, (3) identifying specific metabolic defects of muscle by histochemical or biochemical techniques, and (4) diagnosing diseases of connective tissue and blood vessels, such as polyarteritis nodosa, and infections such as trichinosis.

Muscle biopsy is performed under local anesthesia. In children and in adults with diffuse conditions, an adequate specimen often can be obtained by needle biopsy. Open biopsy may be necessary to obtain sufficient tissue to diagnose focal, patchy processes such as myositis or vasculitis. In all instances, the muscle chosen for sampling must be appropriate for the condition suspected, and the specimen must be handled by a laboratory skilled in the evaluation of muscle biopsies. Muscles to be biopsied should generally be only slightly weak. If the biopsy is taken from a muscle that has recently been traumatized by an EMG needle or that has been affected by a preexisting disease (e.g., coincidental nerve root compression), misleading information will be obtained.

Muscle fibers are subdivided into two types which have different staining characteristics with the myosin ATPase reaction at pH 9.4. Type 1 fibers (fatigue-resistant and rich in oxidative enzymes) stain lightly with this reaction, and type 2 fibers (fast-contracting, fatigue-prone, and rich in glycolytic enzymes) stain darkly. Normal muscle has a random distribution of fibers of the two histochemical types.

Denervation, reinnervation A denervated muscle fiber undergoes atrophy, and in the initial stages myofibrils are lost to a greater degree than is sarcoplasm containing the mitochondria, so the muscle fibers appear "super dark" with stains for oxidative enzymes (Fig. 382-4). Such denervated fibers are squeezed by adjacent innervated fibers and therefore become angulated and atrophic. In the initial stages of denervation, because of motor unit overlap, denervated atrophic fibers are distributed randomly throughout the muscle. Remaining motor axons sprout to reinnervate such fibers, eventually producing fiber type grouping. With subsequent death of such enlarged motor units, grouped fiber atrophy occurs. The typical appearance of a denervated and reinnervated muscle is shown in Fig. 382-4B and C. The fiber diameter distribution in chronically denervated and reinnervated muscle is bimodal, with the atrophic denervated fibers making up one population and the normal-sized (or hypertrophied) innervated fibers making up the other population.

Muscle fiber necrosis and regeneration Damage of the sarcolemma of the muscle fiber allows entry of calcium at high extracellular concentration into the low-calcium environment of the sarcoplasm. Calcium entry activates a neutral protease, initiating proteolysis. Calcium also poisons mitochondrial function and can cause cell death. Invading macrophages phagocytize the muscle fibers. Satellite cells, which provide the basis for regeneration of muscle fibers, are spared in most of the processes that damage muscle. They proliferate and fuse to produce multinuclear myotubes leading to regeneration of the muscle fiber. Characteristically, regenerating fibers are small, are basophilic owing to an increased concentration of RNA, and have large vesicular internalized nuclei. The distribution of muscle fiber diameters in a typical chronic myopathy is broad and unimodal, very different from the bimodal diameter distribution of denervated and reinnervated muscle.

Muscle fiber necrosis and regeneration are common in trauma, Duchenne's muscular dystrophy, polymyositis, and dermatomyositis. Eventually, if the necrosis is sufficiently chronic, regeneration may fail, causing progressive loss of muscle fibers and replacement with fat and fibrous tissue. A chronic myopathy, Duchenne's muscular dystrophy, is illustrated in Fig. 382-5. Differences in the extent and tempo of these processes allow histologic distinction among the muscular dystrophies, inflammatory myopathies, and acute rhabdomyolysis.

Structural changes in muscle fibers Degeneration of muscle fibers without frank necrosis produces structural alteration of individual muscle fibers; disorganization of myofibrils and sarcoplasm produces target fibers (Fig. 382-4C), ringbinden (appearance of a portion of the myofibrils wrapped circumferentially around the remaining longitudinal myofibrils), central cores, cytoid bodies, and

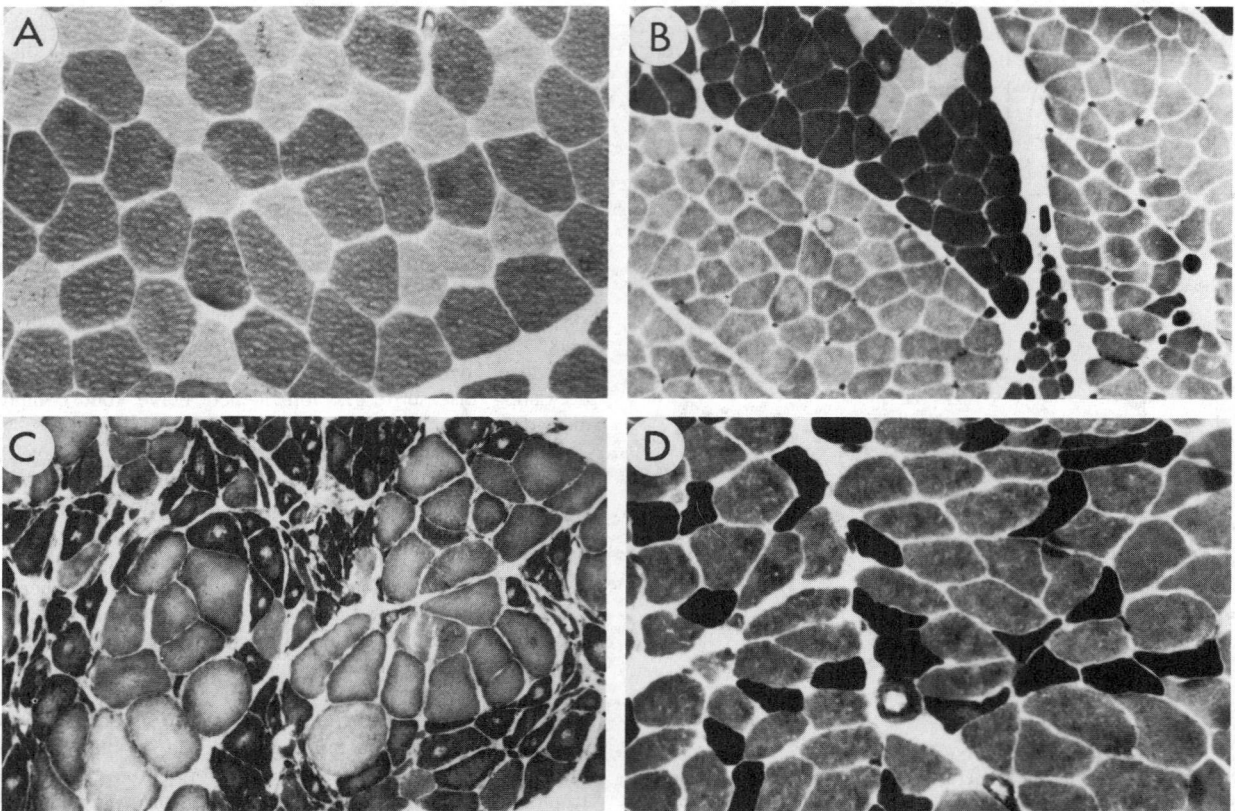

FIGURE 382-4 *A*. Normal skeletal muscle biopsy stained for myosin ATPase, pH 9.4. Type 1 fibers are light and type 2 dark. *B*. Chronic denervation-reinnervation showing fiber type grouping. Myosin ATPase, pH 9.4. *C*. Chronic denervation-reinnervation in amyotrophic lateral sclerosis, preparation stained for mitochondrial enzyme, NADH-TR. There are groups of reinnervated type 2 fibers (*light*), and of denervated angulated atrophic fibers, many of them ''superdark'' and showing target-fiber changes. *D*. Type 2 fiber atrophy. Myosin ATPase, pH 9.4.

nemaline bodies. In one congenital myopathy, the fibers resemble myotubes (centronuclear myopathy). In others, abnormal mitochondria suggest an abnormality of mitochondrial biochemistry, while the presence of vacuoles suggests a disturbance of glycogen or lipid metabolism. Rimmed vacuoles (accumulations of degenerating phospholipid material between myofibrils) occur particularly in oculopharyngeal muscular dystrophy and inclusion-body myositis.

Inflammatory changes   Perivascular and interstitial inflammatory cell infiltration with lymphocytes and macrophages is characteristic of polymyositis and dermatomyositis. Necrosis and regeneration of muscle fibers are also present. In some instances, atrophy of the fibers located on the periphery of muscle fasciculi (*perifascicular atrophy*) is prominent and can be an indicator of inflammatory myopathy, even

though a focus of inflammation is not present in the muscle taken at biopsy. Muscle biopsy may show vasculitis in patients with collagen diseases or granulomas in patients with sarcoidosis.

Changes specific to fiber type   Pathologic changes may be restricted to one fiber type in the muscle. The most common such condition is type 2 fiber atrophy (Fig. 382-4*D*), which occurs in a wide range of disorders that limit activity such as disuse, muscle pain, joint pain, and upper motor neuronal dysfunction. Atrophy of type 1 fibers is less frequent and occurs in myotonic dystrophy, rheumatoid arthritis, and some congenital myopathies.

NERVE BIOPSY   Nerve biopsy is more difficult and more traumatic than muscle biopsy and is useful in only a limited number of specific circumstances (see Chap. 383). The sural nerve in the leg or

FIGURE 382-5 *A*. Normal muscle (hematoxylin-eosin). *B*. Duchenne's muscular dystrophy, showing hyalin fibers, fiber degeneration, loss of fibers and fibrosis (hematoxylin-eosin).

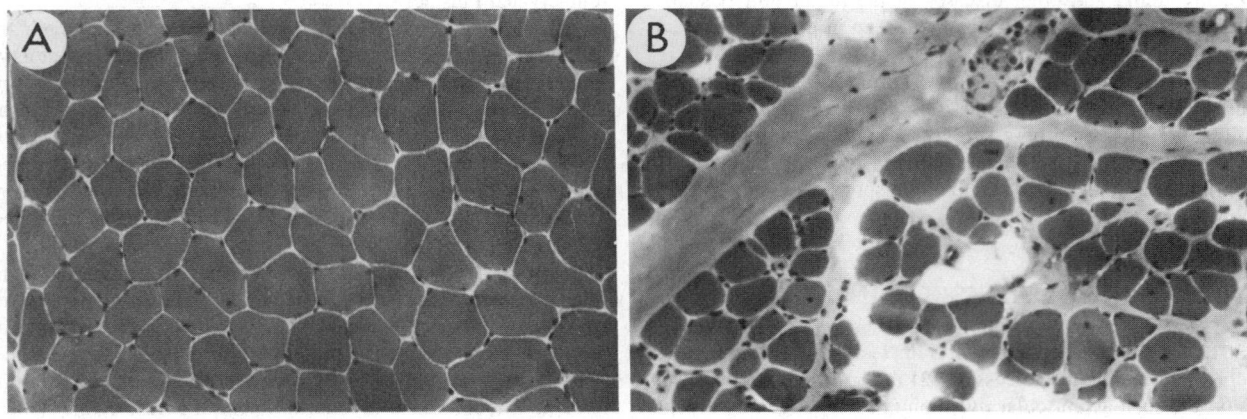

the superficial radial nerve at the wrist are the usual biopsy sites. Both are sensory nerves and may show no changes in pure motor neuropathies. The biopsy procedure is performed under local anesthesia, and specimens are obtained for light and electron microscopy and for teasing of individual nerve fibers. Nerve biopsy aids in (1) distinguishing between segmental demyelination and axonal degeneration, (2) identifying inflammatory neuropathies, and (3) establishing specific diagnoses such as amyloidosis, sarcoidosis, leprosy, vasculitis, and several metabolic neuropathies. Full evaluation of the nerve biopsy requires the facilities of a laboratory with special interest and experience in peripheral nerve pathology. Light microscopic examination of biopsied nerves is of limited value, showing only gross changes such as vasculitis, inflammation, infiltration by granuloma or amyloid, loss of axons, and axonal degeneration. More information is obtained by electron microscopy and studies of single teased nerve fibers. Some diseases affect specific nerve fiber types. For instance, large myelinated fibers are affected in Friedreich's ataxia and unmyelinated fibers in familial amyloidosis. Quantitative morphometry (measurement of the number of nerve fibers and the distribution of their diameters) can therefore be of additional help. Two basic pathologic processes may be seen in nerve biopsies.

Segmental demyelination Diseases may attack either myelin or the Schwann cell, causing the myelin sheath to undergo degeneration but leaving the axon essentially unchanged. Healing of this segmental demyelination proceeds through a phase of abnormally thin myelin sheaths, which may eventually return to normal thickness. However, even after apparent recovery of segmental demyelination, single teased nerve fiber studies demonstrate short and variable lengths of the internodes (distance between the nodes of Ranvier). If this process is progressive, *onion-bulb formation* occurs, with thinly remyelinated fibers lying at the center of concentric lamellae of redundant Schwann cell cytoplasm.

Axonal degeneration Death of the nerve cell body or section of the axon at any level will lead to degeneration of the distal parts of the axon with secondary degeneration of the myelin sheath. If the nerve cell body remains intact proximally, there is attempted axonal regeneration with sprouting. Such nerve sprouts (*clusters*) are characteristic of degenerating and regenerating axonal neuropathy.

Pathologic changes in neuropathies Axonal degeneration is most common in toxic, inherited, traumatic, and ischemic diseases. Segmental demyelination may occur in the inherited and autoimmune inflammatory disorders; in the latter condition, inflammatory cell infiltration may be seen. A mixed picture of axonal degeneration and segmental demyelination, together with a vasculopathy, is characteristic of diabetes mellitus. Some specific pathologic changes may indicate the probable etiology of a neuropathy. The deposition of IgM on the myelin-associated glycoprotein of the myelin sheaths in IgM gammopathies can be detected by immunofluorescence techniques. The deposition leads to an increase in myelin periodicity. Amyloid fibrils are present in amyloid neuropathy. Specific inclusions may be seen in the Schwann cells in metachromatic leukodystrophy and adrenomyeloleukodystrophy.

GENERAL THERAPEUTIC CONSIDERATIONS

Cardiac Most disorders of skeletal muscle also involve cardiac muscle. Symptomatic cardiac dysfunction is relatively uncommon, however, perhaps because the limited exercise capacity of the patient with weakness decreases demands on cardiac performance. Relatively specific electrocardiographic abnormalities occur in Duchenne's dystrophy and infantile acid maltase deficiency. Cardiac conduction disorders including complete heart block occur in patients with myotonic dystrophy. An electrocardiogram should be obtained in all patients with neuromuscular disease, particularly in patients with myopathies.

Respiratory Diminished pulmonary function in patients with acute or chronic neuromuscular disease may progress to ventilatory failure. The earliest manifestation of respiratory muscle weakness is a decrease in maximum expiratory and inspiratory pressures. Diaphragmatic weakness in particular may be substantial in patients with neuromuscular disease and should be evaluated by examining pulmonary function while the patient is both supine and sitting. Diaphragmatic weakness causes a decrease in pulmonary function when measured in the supine compared with the erect position. Paradoxical abdominal movements may be evident. Patients with chronic respiratory failure may be maintained with home respiratory support. The possible occurrence of cor pulmonale from insidious respiratory failure should be considered in any patient with neuromuscular disease who develops ankle edema or other signs of heart failure.

Physical therapy Physical therapy is of greatest value in patients with muscle weakness when joint contractures are developing and when enforced immobility, such as an injury, results in decreased activity. Exercises may increase strength in muscles weakened by disease just as in normal persons, but there is little evidence that exercise improves functional abilities. However, therapeutic standing in patients with marginal leg and trunk function has considerable psychological benefit and may help to preserve bone mineralization and cardiovascular reflexes.

Dietary modification Dietary restriction is often necessary in patients with muscle weakness, since caloric expenditure is decreased because of immobility and loss of muscle mass. Development of obesity further compromises already reduced mobility, worsens pulmonary function, and may depress ventilatory drive. Unless there is specific evidence for malabsorption of vitamin B_{12} or vitamin E, neither these nor any other vitamin has a specific role in the treatment of neuromuscular disease. Certain vitamins are hazardous in excessive dosages, including vitamins B_6, A, and D (see Chaps. 77 and 357).

Bracing In patients with distal leg weakness, particularly of foot dorsiflexion, ankle-foot orthoses can restore gait to nearly normal. With more proximal weakness, however, leg braces diminish mobility and are of value only in enabling patients who are unable to walk to perform therapeutic standing. In most adults, even this use of braces is impractical because such standing in braces usually requires assistance.

Scoliosis Spinal deformity complicates many neuromuscular diseases, particularly those which occur before puberty. Duchenne's dystrophy, spinal muscular atrophy, and congenital myopathies are particularly liable to this complication. Once full long-bone growth has been achieved, many of these patients should have surgical correction of the scoliosis. Severely impaired pulmonary function is a contraindication to such therapy; therefore, patients with progressive scoliosis need careful sequential follow-up to determine the appropriate timing for surgery.

GENETIC EVALUATION AND COUNSELING (See also Chap. 385) Management of the patient with hereditary muscle disease should include careful family pedigree analysis and genetic counseling. The family history may initially be negative in many patients with autosomal dominant diseases such as Charcot-Marie-Tooth disease, myotonic dystrophy, and facioscapulohumeral dystrophy because of the variable expressivity of the disorders. The availability of chromosomal markers for linkage analysis and of specific tests for gene abnormalities has made carrier detection, antenatal diagnosis, and early diagnosis of disease feasible in most hereditary neuromuscular diseases (e.g., in Duchenne's and myotonic dystrophy). The availability of therapy for disorders such as periodic paralysis, myotonia, and certain metabolic myopathies and of preventive measures in disorders such as malignant hyperthermia provides a strong impetus for early diagnosis. History alone is often inadequate for family evaluation. Physical examination or inspection of photographs of family members will often identify mildly afflicted individuals, providing clues to the characteristic facial or other features of the disorder. Molecular biologic techniques now permit specific diagnosis of certain neuromuscular diseases by identification of an abnormal or missing gene product. Thus the protein dystrophin is lacking in muscle of patients with Duchenne's dystrophy (see Chap. 385), and the sodium channel is abnormal in hyperkalemic periodic paralysis (see Chap. 387).

REFERENCES

BROOKE MH: *A Clinician's View of Neuromuscular Disease*, 2d ed. Baltimore, Williams and Wilkins, 1986

CARPENTER S, KARPATI G: *Pathology of Skeletal Muscle*. New York, Churchill Livingstone, 1984

DYCK PJ et al (eds): *Peripheral Neuropathy*, 3d ed. Philadelphia, Saunders, 1993

ENGEL AG, FRANZINI-ARMSTRONG C (eds): *Myology*, 2d ed. New York, McGraw-Hill, 1994

KIMURA J: *Electrodiagnosis in Diseases of Nerve and Muscle*, 2d ed. Philadelphia, Davis, 1989

OH SJ: *Electromyography; Neuromuscular Transmission Studies*. Baltimore, Williams and Wilkins, 1988

383   DISEASES OF THE PERIPHERAL NERVOUS SYSTEM

ARTHUR K. ASBURY

The basic processes affecting nerve and muscle and the approach to diseases of nerve and muscle are set forth in Chap. 382. The first purpose here is to build upon that base by providing an overview of the wide array of peripheral neuropathies that afflict humans. Peripheral neuropathy is a general term indicating disorder of peripheral nerve of any cause; the manifestations may be so bewildering and complex that it is difficult for the physician to know where to begin and how to proceed. Therefore the second purpose here is to develop a logical approach and assessment scheme (summarized in Fig. 383-1) which

will guide the examiner to correct diagnoses and management decisions.

GENERAL DESCRIPTION OF NEUROPATHIC SYNDROMES

The prototypical picture of polyneuropathy occurs with acquired toxic or metabolic neuropathic states. From a symptom standpoint, the first noticeable features tend to be sensory and consist of tingling, prickling, burning, or bandlike dysesthesias in the balls of the feet or tips of the toes, or in a general distribution over the soles. Symmetry of symptoms and findings in a distal graded fashion is the rule, but occasionally dysesthesias appear in one foot a brief time before the other or may be more pronounced in one foot. Some care and judgment is needed to avoid confusion with mononeuropathy multiplex. If the polyneuropathy remains mild, no objective motor or sensory signs may be detectable.

With progression, pansensory loss is usually found over both feet, ankle jerks are lost, and weakness of dorsiflexion of the toes, best demonstrated in the great toe, may be present. In some instances, the process begins with weakness in the feet, usually dorsiflexion of the toes and feet without subjective sensory symptoms. As worsening occurs, sensory loss moves centripetally in a graded "stocking" fashion, and the patient may complain that the feet have a numb or "wooden" feeling or may say "I feel as though I'm walking on stumps." Patients experience difficulty walking on their heels during examination and their feet may slap while walking. Later, the knee jerk reflex disappears and foot drop becomes more apparent. By the time sensory disturbance has reached the upper shin, dysesthesias are usually noticed in the tips of the fingers. The degree of spontaneous pain varies, but is often considerable. Light stimuli to hypesthetic areas, once perceived, may be experienced as extremely uncomfortable (hyperpathia). Unsteadiness of gait may be out of proportion to muscle weakness because of proprioceptive loss.

FIGURE 383-1   Flowchart approach to the evaluation of peripheral neuropathies. (*After Asbury, 1983.*)

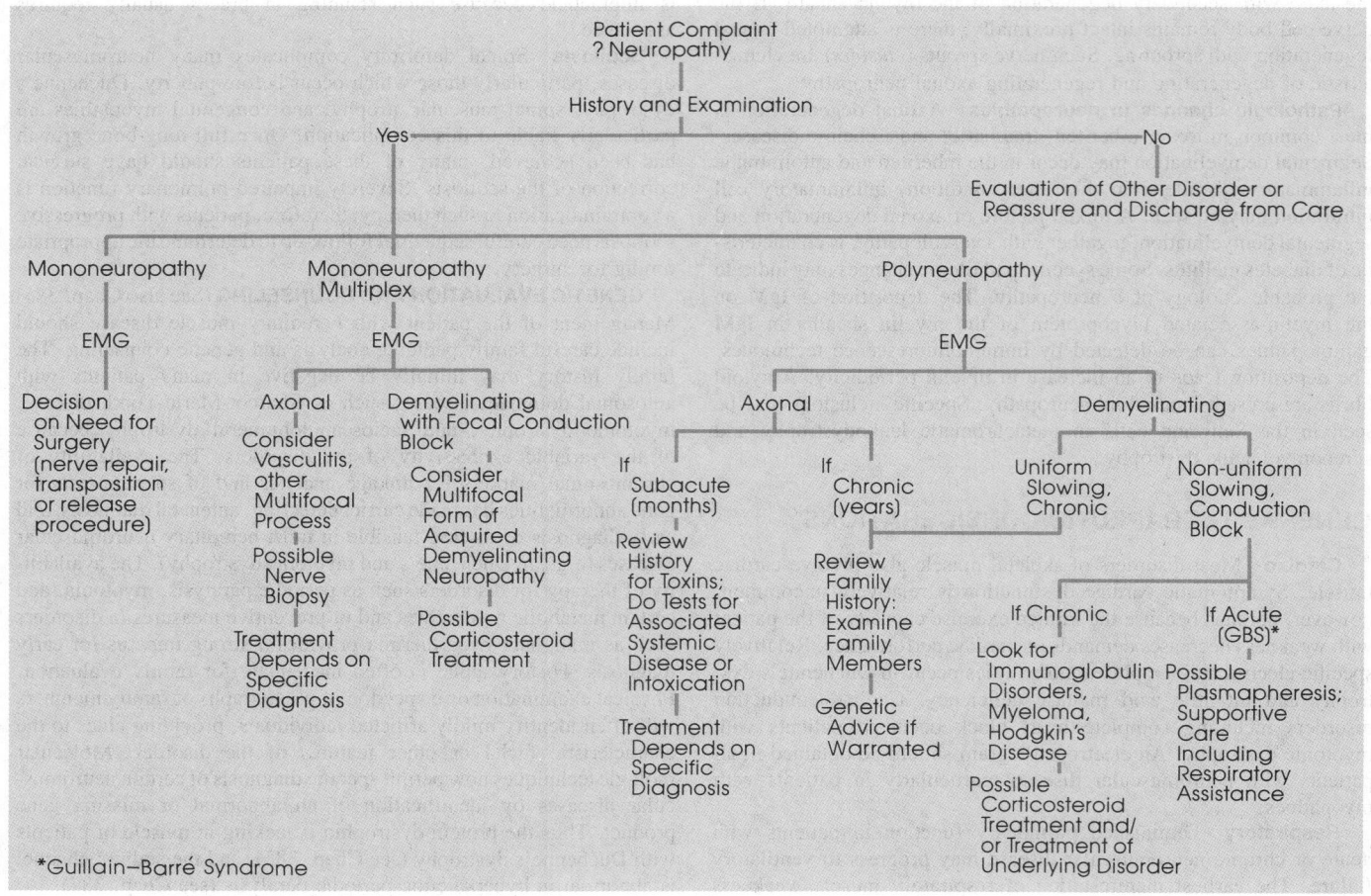

*Guillain–Barré Syndrome

Worsening proceeds in a centripetal, symmetrically graded manner with muscle atrophy, pansensory loss, and areflexia and with motor weakness that is usually greater in the extensor muscles than in corresponding flexor groups. When the sensory disturbance reaches mid thigh, generally a tent-shaped area of hypesthesia on the lower abdomen may be demonstrated. This will grow broader, and the apex will extend rostrally toward the sternum as the neuropathy worsens. By this time, patients generally cannot stand or walk or hold objects in their hands.

In the most extreme cases, ventilatory capacity may be impaired along with sphincteric function. Hypesthesia at the crown of the scalp may be present and spread radially into both the trigeminal and C2 distribution. Considering the entire sequence, nerve fibers are affected according to length of axon without regard to root or nerve trunk distribution—hence, the aptness of the term ''stocking-glove'' to describe the pattern of sensory deficit. In general, the motor deficit is also graded, distal, and symmetric.

Variations on the general sequence outlined above are manifold and explain the diversity of clinical syndromes encountered. Variations include the rate of evolution; fluctuations in the course; the eventual degree of severity; the presence or absence of positive motor and sensory symptoms; the symmetry of features and their distribution in terms of proximal versus distal, arms versus legs, and motor versus sensory; the relative proportion of dysfunction attributable to large fiber deficit and to small fiber deficit; and the determination, mainly by electrodiagnostic examination, of axonal versus demyelinating processes.

ASSESSMENT AND DIAGNOSIS OF NEUROPATHY **Taking the first step** Clues to the diagnosis of specific peripheral neuropathies often lie in unnoted or readily forgotten events occurring weeks or months prior to the onset of symptoms. Inquiry should be made about recent viral illnesses; other systemic symptoms; institution of new medications; potentially toxic exposures to solvents, pesticides, or heavy metals; the occurrence of similar symptoms in family members or coworkers; habits concerning alcohol; and the presence of known preexisting medical disorders. It is also useful to ask patients if they would otherwise feel well if free of their neuropathic symptoms, to obtain an idea of the presence or absence of an underlying systemic illness.

It is important to learn how symptoms first appeared. Even with distal polyneuropathies, symptoms may appear in the sole of one foot a few days or a week before the other, but usually the patient will describe a distal graded disturbance that moves evenly and symmetrically in centripetal fashion. Tingling dysesthesias will appear in the fingertips only when similar symptoms have reached the level of the knees. It is important to determine whether symptoms first appeared in the distribution of individual digital nerves involving only one-half of a digit at a time and then gradually spread to become coalescent. This pattern of onset raises strong suspicions of a multifocal process (mononeuropathy multiplex) such as might be encountered with a systemic vasculitis or cryoglobulinemia.

The evolution of neuropathy ranges from rapid worsening over a few days to an indolent process extending many years. Polyneuropathies with a slowly progressive course lasting more than 5 years are most likely to be genetically determined, particularly if the major manifestations are distal atrophy and weakness with few or no positive sensory symptoms. Exceptions are diabetic polyneuropathy and paraproteinemic neuropathies in which the progression may be insidious over 5 to 10 years. Axonal degenerations of toxic or metabolic origin tend to evolve over several weeks to a year or more, and the rate of progression of demyelinating neuropathies is highly variable, ranging from a few days in Guillain-Barré syndrome to many years in others.

Major fluctuations in the course of neuropathy raise two possibilities: (1) relapsing forms of neuropathy; or (2) repeated toxic exposures. A slow fluctuation in symptoms taking place over weeks or months (reflecting changes in the activity of neuropathy) should not be confused with day-to-day variation or diurnal undulation of symptoms.

The latter are common to all neuropathic disorders. An example is carpal tunnel syndrome in which dysesthesias may be prominent at night but absent during the day.

In polyneuropathies, the findings are symmetric on both sides of the body. If only one foot slaps when the patient walks, the process is not symmetric and the possibility of a multifocal process is raised. In addition, in acquired symmetric polyneuropathies, the muscles of extension and abduction tend to be weakened to a greater extent than the muscles of flexion and adduction. Hence, weakness in lower legs often affects the peronei and anterior tibial muscles, with attendant foot drop and weakness of eversion, more than the gastrocnemius group or foot inverters. In most polyneuropathies the legs are more severely affected than the arms and the distal muscles more than the proximal ones. There are exceptions to this rule, as in lead neuropathy, in which manifestation of bilateral wrist drop may predominate, and occasionally in porphyric neuropathy, in which arms may be more affected than legs and proximal muscles more than distal.

Palpation of the nerve trunk to detect enlargement is a frequently forgotten part of the neurologic examination. In mononeuropathies, the entire course of the nerve trunk in question should be explored manually for focal thickening; the presence of neurofibroma, point tenderness, or Tinel's phenomenon (generation of a tingling sensation in the sensory territory of the nerve by tapping along the course of the nerve trunk); and elicitation of pain by putting the nerve trunk on stretch. In leprous neuritis, fusiform thickening of nerve trunks is frequent, and beading of nerve trunks may be encountered in amyloid polyneuropathy. In genetically determined hypertrophic neuropathies uniform thickening of all nerve trunks may occur, often to the caliber of a clothesline or larger.

Most neuropathies involve nerve fibers of all sizes, but on occasion selective damage may be restricted either to large or to small fibers. In a polyneuropathy affecting mainly small fibers, diminished pinprick and temperature sensation, often with burning painful dysesthesias, may predominate along with autonomic dysfunction but with relative sparing of motor power, balance, and tendon jerks. Selected cases of amyloid and distal diabetic polyneuropathies fall into this category. In contrast, large-fiber polyneuropathy is characterized by areflexia, imbalance, relatively minor cutaneous sensory deficit, and variable but often severe motor dysfunction.

In addition to a history and a physical examination, other measures need to be undertaken routinely in the evaluation of a patient with neuropathy. Electrodiagnostic examination is a key procedure in all patients. For patients with polyneuropathy or mononeuropathy multiplex, standard tests should include a complete blood count and erythrocyte sedimentation rate, urinalysis, chest x-ray, postprandial blood glucose, and serum protein electrophoresis. Further tests should be dictated by the formulation arrived at via the combined history and physical and electrodiagnostic examination (see Fig. 383-1).

Taking the next step The next step is electrodiagnostic examination. It is not generally possible to make the distinction between axonal versus demyelinating disorders on clinical examination alone; here electrodiagnostic analysis is particularly useful. Electrodiagnostic features of demyelination are slowing of nerve conduction velocity (NCV), dispersion of evoked compound action potentials (CAPs), conduction block (major decrease in amplitude of muscle CAP upon proximal stimulation of its nerve as compared to distal stimulation), and marked prolongation of distal latencies. In contrast, axonal neuropathies are characterized by a reduction in amplitude of evoked CAPs with relative preservation of NCV. The distinction between a primarily demyelinating neuropathy from one that is primarily axonal is crucial because of the differing approaches to diagnosis and management.

If in a particular instance of progressive polyneuropathy of subacute or chronic evolution the electrodiagnostic findings are those of an axonopathy, a long list of metabolic states and exogenous toxins comes into consideration (see Tables 383-1 and 383-2). If the course is protracted over several years, it raises the likelihood of the neuronal (axonal) form of peroneal muscular atrophy (HMSN-II); family

TABLE 383-1   Polyneuropathy associated with systemic diseases

Systemic disease/Occurrence	Axonal*			Demyelinating*			Sensory vs. motor†	Autonomic*	Comment
	Acute	Subacute	Chronic	Acute	Subacute	Chronic			
Diabetes mellitus/Common	−	±	+	−	±	+	S, SM, rarely M	± to +	See Table 383-4
Uremia/Sometimes	±	+	+	−	−	−	SM	±	Controllable with proper dialysis; curable with successful renal transplant
Porphyria (3 types)/Rare	+	±	−	−	−	−	M or SM	± to +	May be proximal > distal and may have atypical proximal sensory deficits
Hypoglycemia/Rare	±	+	±	−	−	−	M	−	Usually with insulinoma; arms often > legs
Vitamin deficiency, exclude B$_{12}$/Sometimes	−	+	+	−	−	−	SM	±	Involves thiamine, pyridoxine, folate, pantothenic acid; probably others
Vitamin B$_{12}$ deficiency/Sometimes	−	±	+	−	−	−	S	−	Neuropathy overshadowed by myelopathy
Critical illness (sepsis)/Common	−	+	±	−	−	−	M > S	−	Severely ill, sepsis patients, often on ventilator
Chronic liver disease/Sometimes	−	−	−	−	−	+	S or SM	−	Usually mild or subclinical
Primary biliary cirrhosis/Rare	−	±	+	−	−	−	S	−	Intraneural xanthomas
Primary systemic amyloidosis/Rare	−	±	+	−	−	−	SM	+	Also in amyloidosis with myeloma or macroglobulinemia
Hypothyroidism/Rare	−	−	−	−	±	+	S	−	May respond to thyroid replacement
Chronic obstructive lung disease/Rare	−	±	+	−	−	−	S or SM	−	Severe pulmonary insufficiency
Acromegaly/Rare	−	−	+	−	−	−	S	−	Carpal tunnel syndrome also frequent
Malabsorption (sprue, celiac disease)/Sometimes	−	±	+	−	−	−	S or SM	±	Basis for neuropathy unclear; deficiency?
Carcinoma (sensory)/Rare	−	+	+	−	−	−	Pure S	−	Due to gangliitic neuronopathy; mostly small cell lung or breast carcinoma; paraneoplastic
Carcinoma (sensorimotor)/Sometimes	−	+	±	−	−	−	SM	±	Sensorimotor axonal neuropathy; mostly with lung carcinoma
Carcinoma (late)/Common	−	+	+	−	−	−	S > M	±	Mild, probably related to weight loss and wasting
Carcinoma (demyelinating)/Sometimes	−	−	−	+	+	±	SM	−	Acute or relapsing demyelinating neuropathy
HIV infection/Sometimes	−	±	+	−	−	−	S ≫ M	−	Late stages of AIDS; other neuropathies occur; see text
Lyme disease/Sometimes	−	±	+	−	−	−	S > M	−	Variable picture; see text
Lymphoma including Hodgkin's/Sometimes	−	+	+	+	+	±	See above	±	Same as with carcinomatous types
Polycythemia vera/Rare	−	±	+	−	−	−	S	−	Also many CNS manifestations; often shooting pains in limbs
Multiple myeloma lytic type/Sometimes	−	±	+	−	−	−	S, M, or SM	±	Symptomatic neuropathy uncommon, subclinical neuropathy frequent
Multiple myeloma‡: osteosclerotic or solitary plasmacytoma/Sometimes	−	−	±	−	±	+	SM	−	May show severe slowing of nerve conduction velocity
Benign monoclonal gammopathy:									
IgA	−	±	+	−	−	−	SM	−	IgM$_\kappa$ (or occasionally IgM$_\lambda$) may bind to myelin-associated glycoprotein or glycolipids
IgG	−	±	+	−	−	−	SM	−	
IgM /Sometimes	−	−	−	−	±	+	SM or S	−	
Cryoglobulinemia/Rare	−	±	+	−	−	−	SM	−	May be mononeuropathy multiplex in presentation

*± = sometimes; + = usual.
†S = sensory; M = motor; SM = sensorimotor.
‡Some cases associated with POEMS syndrome (see text).

members must be examined and additional attention given to the family history. Alternatively, if the electrodiagnostic findings indicate primary demyelination of nerve, the approach is entirely different. The possibilities then include acquired demyelinating neuropathy, thought to be immunologically mediated, and genetically determined neuropathies, some of which are marked by uniform and drastic slowing of nerve conduction velocities.

The flowchart in Fig. 383-1 summarizes the clinical and electrodiagnostic approach to evaluation and management of a neuropathic disorder. Using this scheme, the clinician determines for each patient the tempo, distribution, severity, and functional impairment, and other features previously discussed, making a clinical judgment as to whether the problem represents a mononeuropathy, a mononeuropathy multiplex, or a polyneuropathy. Often this distinction is obvious.

TABLE 383-2 Polyneuropathy associated with drugs or environmental toxins

	Axonal*			Demyelinating*			Sensory vs. motor†	Autonomic*	CNS*	Comment
	Acute	Subacute	Chronic	Acute	Subacute	Chronic				
DRUGS										
Amiodarone (anti-arrhythmic)	−	−	+	−	−	+	SM	−	−	Dose-dependent neuropathy, reversible by decreasing dose
Aurothioglucose (antirheumatic)	±	±	−	+	+	−	SM	−	−	Idiosyncratic reaction, ? immune-mediated
cis-Platinum (antineoplastic)	−	+	+	−	−	−	S	−	−	Severe sensory neuropathy, also ototoxicity; dose-related
Dapsone (dermatologic including leprosy)	−	±	+	−	−	−	M	−	−	Dose-related pure motor neuropathy
Disulfiram (antialcohol)	±	+	+	−	−	−	SM	−	±	Usually occurs after months of treatment
Hydralazine (antihypertensive)	−	±	+	−	−	−	S > M	−	−	A pyridoxine antagonist
Isoniazid	−	±	+	−	−	−	SM	±	−	A pyridoxine antagonist; neurotoxic in slow acetylators
Metronidazole (antiprotozoal)	−	−	±	−	−	−	S or SM	−	+	Dose-related central-peripheral distal axonopathy
Misonidazole (radiosensitizer)	−	±	+	−	−	−	S or SM	−	+	Neurotoxicity is the limiting factor
Nitrofurantoin (urinary antiseptic)	−	±	+	−	−	−	SM	−	−	Generally total dose-related; renal failure enhances toxicity
Nucleoside neuropathies (ddC, ddI, d4T) (antiretrovirus)	±	+	+	−	−	−	S >> M	−	?	Dose-related; painful
Phenytoin (anticonvulsant)	−	−	+	−	−	−	S > M	−	−	After 20-30 years of phenytoin use
Pyridoxine (vitamin)	−	±	+	−	−	−	S	−	−	Occurs with large intake: >500 mg/d
Vincristine (antineoplastic)	−	+	+	−	−	−	S > M	−	−	Sensory symptoms common, hands > feet; motor signs ominous; should stop treatment
TOXINS										
Acrylamide (flocculant; grouting agent)	−	±	+	−	−	−	S > M	±	+	Large-fiber neuropathy; sensory ataxia
Arsenic (herbicide; insecticide)	±	+	+	−	−	−	SM	±	±	Skin changes, Mees' lines in nails; painful; systemic effects
Diphtheria	−	−	−	+	+	−	SM	−	−	Clinically very rare; can be confused with GBS
γ-Diketone hexacarbons (solvents)	−	±	+	−	−	+	SM	±	+	Neurofilamentous swelling of axons; these solvents now in restricted use
Inorganic lead	−	−	+	−	−	−	M > S or M	−	±	Selective motor neuropathy with prominent wrist drop
Organophosphates	−	±	+	−	−	−	SM	−	+	Brain and spinal cord also affected, the latter irreversibly
Thallium (rat poison)	−	+	+	−	−	−	SM	−	+	Also alopecia, Mees' lines in nails; painful

* ± = sometimes, + = usual.
† S = sensory; M = motor; SM = sensorimotor.
The following drugs and environmental toxins are also neurotoxic, mainly to the peripheral nervous system.

Drugs	Environmental toxins
Amitriptyline, chloramphenicol, colchicine, ethambutol, glutethimide, nitrous oxide, perhexiline maleate, sodium cyanate, suramin, thalidomide, L-tryptophan, vinarabine	Allyl chloride, buckthorn berry, carbon disulfide, dimethylaminoproprionitrile, (DMAPN), ethylene oxide, methyl bromide, polychlorinated biphenyls, styrene, trichlorethylene, vacor

With the sum of clinical and electrodiagnostic information in hand, the differential diagnostic possibilities and management options will have been narrowed to only a few. The remainder of this chapter deals with the details of this formulation.

Electrodiagnosis As seen in Fig. 383-1, electrodiagnosis is a key part of the evaluation of any neuropathy. See Chap. 382 for details of technique and interpretation. For example, electrodiagnosis helps one to be certain about the presence or absence of a sensory involvement when this is not clear by clinical examination alone. It provides information about the distribution of subclinical findings, thus sharpening the diagnostic focus. The general questions that may be posed by the clinician to the electrodiagnostician include

1 The distinction between disorders primary to nerve or to muscle (neuropathy versus myopathy).

2 The distinction between root or plexus involvement and more distal nerve trunk involvement.

3 The distinction between generalized polyneuropathic processes and widespread multifocal nerve trunk affection.

4 The distinction between upper and lower motor neuron weakness.

5 The distinction, in a given generalized polyneuropathic process, between primary demyelinating neuropathy and axonal degeneration.

6 The assessment, in both primary axonal and demyelinating neuropathies, of many factors bearing on the nature, activity, and likely prognosis of the neuropathy.

7 The assessment, in mononeuropathies, of the site of the lesion and its major effect on nerve fibers, especially the distinction between demyelinating conduction block and wallerian degeneration.

8 The characterization of disorders of the neuromuscular junction.

9 The identification, often in muscle of normal bulk and strength, of important features such as chronic partial denervation, fasciculations, and myotonia.

10 The analysis of cramp, and its distinction from physiologic contracture.

Nerve biopsy The sural nerve at the ankle is the preferred site for cutaneous nerve biopsy. There are few indications to employ this invasive technique. The main one is in asymmetric and multifocal neuropathic disorders producing a clinical picture of mononeuropathy multiplex, the basis of which is still unclear after other laboratory investigations are complete. Diagnostic considerations include vasculitis, amyloidosis, leprosy, and occasionally sarcoidosis. Nerve biopsy is also helpful when one or more cutaneous nerves are palpably enlarged. Another clinical application is in establishing the diagnosis in some genetically determined childhood disorders such as metachromatic leukodystrophy, Krabbe's disease, giant axonal neuropathy, and infantile neuroaxonal dystrophy. In all of these recessively inherited diseases, both the central nervous system (CNS) and the peripheral nervous system (PNS) are affected.

There is a tendency to carry out sural nerve biopsy in distal symmetric polyneuropathies of subacute or chronic evolution. This practice is discouraged because it is a low-yield measure. Nerve biopsy in this situation is only useful as part of an approved research protocol when the biopsy will provide crucial information not otherwise obtainable.

POLYNEUROPATHY Although this term connotes a widespread symmetric process, usually distal and graded, polyneuropathies present a high degree of diversity because of the extreme variability of tempo, severity, mix of sensory and motor features, and presence or absence of positive symptoms. The patient with a fulminant, severely dysesthetic sensory neuropathy and alopecia who is in the early phases of thallium intoxication bears little similarity to the patient with a 40-year history of insidiously progressive clumsiness of gait whose findings are foot drop, lower leg atrophy, pes cavus, and minimal asymptomatic distal sensory deficit (i.e., peroneal muscular atrophy, either type I or II; see Table 383-3). These two patients fall near opposite ends of the spectrum of polyneuropathy.

The classification of peripheral neuropathies has become increasingly complex as the capacity to discriminate new subgroups and identify new associations with toxins and systemic disorders improves. Further, our grasp of the pathophysiologic basis for the clinical phenomena observed in neuropathy has increased rapidly (see Chap. 382). But these advances are primarily descriptive; little or no progress has been made in understanding the fundamental pathogenic events in nervous tissue that eventuate in any one of the polyneuropathies.

The important features of each major grouping of polyneuropathies are summarized below and key aspects of specific polyneuropathies may be found in Tables 383-1 to 383-5.

Acute axonal polyneuropathy In this setting the term acute means evolution over days, making these neuropathies relatively uncommon. Included are porphyric neuropathy and massive intoxications, often suicidal or homicidal in intent. For example, an individual receiving a large dose of arsenic (e.g., 100 mg of arsenous oxide) will become violently ill in a few hours with vomiting, diarrhea, and circulatory collapse. In 1 to 3 days serious renal and liver failure will ensue, and between 14 and 21 days painful polyneuropathy will appear, often as the systemic disorder abates. Progression occurs for 2 or 3 weeks, but following a plateau, recovery requires months.

Subacute axonal polyneuropathy Subacute, meaning to evolve in weeks, characterizes many instances of toxic and metabolic polyneuropathy, but perhaps even more of these are chronic in evolution (months to years). Scanning the appropriate columns in Tables 383-1 and 383-2 provides many possibilities. Management in almost all instances involves removing from contact the offending agent or treating the associated systemic order.

Chronic axonal polyneuropathy This category includes many more types of polyneuropathy, in part because the term chronic subsumes neuropathies that have progressed over a period as short as 6 months to as long as 60 years. As a rough approximation, slow worsening for more than 5 years, absence of positive symptoms, mainly motor deficit, and absence of systemic disorder all favor a genetically determined neuropathy. Although these are mostly autosomal dominant in inheritance pattern, recessively inherited and X-linked varieties also occur, including a form phenotypically resembling dominantly inherited peroneal muscular atrophy (HMSN-II) and also adrenomyeloneuropathy (Table 383-3). To complete the picture, an array of rare autosomal recessive neuropathies occur in childhood (Table 383-3).

Acute demyelinating polyneuropathy For all practical purposes, this category is synonymous with Guillain-Barré syndrome (GBS). This acute, frequently severe and fulminant polyneuropathy occurs at a rate of one case per million population per month, or approximately 3500 cases per year in the United States and Canada. Incidence patterns are similar worldwide. In over two-thirds, an infection, usually viral, either clinically overt or evidenced by serum titer rise, precedes the onset of neuropathy by 1 to 3 weeks. Herpes infections [cytomegalovirus, Epstein-Barr virus (EBV)] account for a large proportion of virus-triggered cases. Some cases appear to be triggered by *Campylobacter jejuni* gastroenteritis. A small proportion, less than 5 percent, occur within 1 to 4 weeks of a surgical procedure. GBS occurs on a background of lymphoma, including Hodgkin's disease, and in lupus erythematosus more frequently than can be attributed to chance alone. Although the weight of evidence suggests that GBS is immune-mediated, the immunopathogenesis remains obscure. In 1976 to 1977, a flurry of some 500 cases followed in the wake of the national swine flu vaccination program in the United States. This exceeded by severalfold the baseline incidence expected in this period in those vaccinated. The epidemiologic features of this outbreak resembled a point-source epidemic with an "incubation" period of 1 to 6 weeks. The reason why swine flu vaccine appears to have triggered GBS in 1976 to 1977 has never been discovered. In subsequent annual flu vaccine programs in the United States, no excess cases of GBS have been identified.

The clinical features of GBS typically include areflexic motor paralysis with mild sensory disturbance coupled with an acellular rise of total protein in the cerebrospinal fluid by the end of the first week of symptoms. Most patients with GBS require hospitalization, and about 30 percent will need ventilatory assistance at some point during the illness. The prognosis is good; approximately 85 percent of patients will make a complete or nearly complete recovery. The mortality rate is 3 to 4 percent. Management is generally supportive care, but plasmapheresis also has a role. Large, multicenter, controlled trials in North America and Europe have demonstrated a beneficial effect of plasmapheresis, if initiated in the first 2 weeks of illness. Intravenous administration of high-dose immunoglobulin (2 g/kg body weight given over 5 days) is probably as effective as plasmapheresis. In contrast, glucocorticoid treatment has not been shown to be effective.

TABLE 383-3 Genetically determined neuropathies

Genetic disorder	Inheritance pattern	Age of onset	Basic process	Other features*	Other systems involved	Metabolic defect	Comment
Peroneal muscular atrophy (HMSN-I)[†]	Dominant; large duplication on chr. 17 in most families	Decades 2–3	Demyelinating	Hypertropic change with onion bulbs; marked ↓ NCV	Rare; bony defects	Defective myelin protein?	Pes cavus, motor deficit predominates
Peroneal muscular atrophy (HMSN-II)[†]	Dominant	Decades 3–5	Axonal	Marked ↓ NAP; NCV sl. decreased	–	Unknown	Same as HSMN-I
Hereditary amyloid neuropathies	Dominant	Decades 3–6	Axonal	Small fiber involvement; endoneurial amyloid deposition	Some families—cornea; kidneys	Point mutations in transthyretin (prealbumin) in most families	Dysautonomia often prominent. Genetic defect on chromosome 18.
Hereditary sensory neuropathy (HSN-I)	Dominant	Decades 1–3	Neuronopathic	DRG neurons selectively involved	Sensorineural deafness, some families	Unknown	Frequent distal mutilation—hands and feet
Porphyric neuropathy	Dominant	Adult life	Axonal	Neuropathy part of attacks; may be recurrent	Widespread cellular abnormality	Enzyme defects in porphyrin pathway	Acute intermittent porphyria, variegate porphyria, and erythropoietic porphyria
Hereditary liability to pressure palsy	Dominant	Decades 2–3	? Demyelinating	Tomaculous changes in myelin	–	Unknown	Mostly ulnar, peroneal, and brachial plexus
Fabry's disease	X-linked	Young males	Neuronopathic	Sensory neuronopathy, small DRG neurons	Kidney, skin, lung	Accumulation of ceramidetrihexoside	Neuropathy painful; often die of renal failure
Peroneal muscular atrophy	X-linked	Infancy to 2d decade	Axonal or demyelinating	Heterozygote females may have symptoms	–	Unknown	Localizes to long arm of X chromosome
Adrenomyeloneuropathy	X-linked	Young males	? Axonal	Mild neuropathy, spastic paraparesis, baldness, hypogonadism	Adrenal cortex, cerebral white matter, spinal cord	Accumulation of very long chain fatty acids	Phenotypic variant of adrenoleukodystrophy: dietary therapy possible
Hereditary sensory neuropathy (HSN-II)	Recessive	Decades 1–3	Neuronopathic	DRG neurons selectively involved	–	Unknown	May be less severe than HSN-I
Déjerine-Sottas neuropathy (HMSN-III)	Recessive	1st decade	Demyelinating	Hypertrophic change with onion bulb formation	May be mentally retarded	Unknown	Marked nerve trunk enlargement
Refsum's disease	Recessive	1st or 2d decade	Demyelinating	Hypertropic change with onion bulb formation	Retinitis pigmentosa, ichthyosis, sensorineural deafness	Defect in α-oxidation of β-methylated fatty acids	Low phytanate diet, plasmapheresis therapy
Ataxia-telangiectasia	Recessive	Decade 1 or 2	Axonal	Neuropathy moderate	Cell nuclear aneuploidy, skin and scleral telangiectasia, cerebellar atrophy, immunopathy	Basic defect unknown	High incidence of early neoplasia
Abetalipoproteinemia	Recessive	Decade 1 or 2	Neuronopathic	Large DRG neurons	Retinitis pigmentosa, acanthocytosis of red blood cells	Absence of all lipoprotein-containing apo B	Proprioceptive disturbance marked, minimal small fiber deficit
Giant axonal neuropathy	Recessive	1st decade	Axonal	Massive segmented accumulation of neurofilaments in axons	Slowly progressive encephalopathy with Rosenthal fibers	Generalized disorder of 10-nm filaments	Intermediate filament masses in other cell types
Metachromatic leukodystrophy	Recessive	1st decade	Demyelinating	Schwannopathy with cerebroside accumulation	Cerebral white matter disease predominates	Defect of arylsulfatase A	Infantile, juvenile, and adult onset forms
Globoid cell leukodystrophy	Recessive	1st decade	Demyelinating	Schwannopathy with galactocerebroside accumulation	Cerebral white matter disease predominates	Defect of β-galactosidase	Characteristic clefts in Schwann cell cytoplasm
Friedreich's ataxia	Recessive linked to chr. 9	1st decade	Axonal	Spinocerebellar and corticospinal tracts involved; also 1° sensory neuron	Cardiomyopathy; usual cause of death	Controversial	Ataxia is both sensory and cerebellar

* chr. = chromosome; DRG = dorsal root ganglia; NAP = nerve action potential; NCV = nerve conduction velocity; sl = slightly; HMSN = hereditary motor-sensory neuropathy; HSN = hereditary sensory neuropathy.
[†] Both forms are also collectively referred to as Charcot-Marie-Tooth neuropathy.

Other acute demyelinating polyneuropathies are rare and include buckthorn berry intoxication and diphtheritic polyneuritis (see Table 383-2).

Subacute demyelinating polyneuropathy Neuropathies in this category are heterogeneous in origin, although all are acquired. Most common is a relapsing and remitting neuropathy which has many clinical features in common with GBS, but differs from GBS in tempo, course, and absence of discernible triggering events (see "Acquired Demyelinating Neuropathies," below). Previously mentioned toxins (buckthorn berry, diphtheria toxin, aurothioglucose) may also induce a picture of widespread subacute demyelination of peripheral nerves (see Table 383-2).

TABLE 383-4   Classification of diabetic neuropathies

Symmetric
 1 Distal, primarily sensory polyneuropathy
   a Mainly large fibers affected
   b Mixed*
   c Mainly small fibers affected*
 2 Autonomic neuropathy
 3 Chronically evolving proximal motor neuropathy*†
Asymmetric
 1 Acute or subacute proximal motor neuropathy*†
 2 Cranial mononeuropathy†
 3 Truncal neuropathy*†
 4 Entrapment neuropathy in the limbs

---

*Often painful.
†Recovery, partial or complete, is likely.

Chronic demyelinating polyneuropathy   Although more common than the subacute neuropathies, chronic polyneuropathy with demyelinating features encompasses a wide diversity of disorders, including hereditary neuropathies, inflammatory neuropathies, and other acquired neuropathies associated with diabetes mellitus, dysproteinemias, other metabolic states, and some chronic intoxications. To complicate matters, many of these disorders present an electrodiagnostic picture of mixed axonal-demyelinative findings. Frequently it is difficult to determine which process, axonal degeneration or demyelination, is the primary event. Aspects of many of these neuropathies are included in Table 383-1 to 383-5 and in the sections below.

SPECIAL CATEGORIES OF NEUROPATHY   Hereditary neuropathies   The major characteristics of this highly variegated group of disorders are summarized in Table 383-3. With the exception of the porphyric neuropathies, the onset of neuropathic dysfunction is insidious and progression is indolent over years or decades. Most of these diseases are quite rare with the striking exception of the dominantly inherited peroneal muscular atrophies (HMSN-I and HMSN-II; see Table 383-3). In peroneal muscular atrophy, phenotypic expression is often variable, so that affected family members of a propositus may have no symptoms and minimal neurologic findings but (in HMSN-I) may still show severe reduction of nerve conduction velocity.

Acquired demyelinating neuropathies   These fall into two major groups, the acute form called Guillain-Barré syndrome and more chronic forms, usually referred to as chronic inflammatory demyelinat-

ing polyradiculoneuropathy (CIDP). The entire group of acquired demyelinating neuropathies constitutes a significant proportion of all cases of polyneuropathy and shares a distinctive clinical, electrophysiologic, and pathologic pattern. The diagnosis rests upon recognition of the clinical pattern and of other features, including elevated cerebrospinal fluid protein level, electrophysiologic changes (marked slowing of conduction velocities, delayed late responses, prolonged distal latencies, dispersion of evoked responses, and evidence of conduction block), and pathologic changes of low-grade inflammation, endoneurial edema, and demyelination-remyelination of peripheral nerves. The course of GBS is acute and monophasic, whereas the more chronic forms pursue either a slowly progressive or a relapsing course. Cases with an intermediate course occur frequently enough to blur the diagnostic delimitation of GBS from the more chronic type of acquired demyelinating neuropathy (CIDP).

Pathogenically, this group of neuropathies is generally agreed to be immune-mediated, but the specific antigens involved and the crucial events of the immune response and why it is activated are uncertain. Also unknown is whether GBS and CIDP share a common immunopathogenesis.

Management of CIDP involves a judicious mix of glucocorticoid therapy; plasmapheresis; immunosuppressants such as azathioprine, cyclophosphamide or cyclosporine; and high-dose intravenous immunoglobulin. These powerful agents are used only if the disorder is severe enough to threaten walking.

Diabetic neuropathies   Classifications of the neuropathies of diabetes mellitus are found in Table 383-4. Although this provides a satisfactory frame of reference, the limitations inherent in classifying diabetic neuropathies should be understood. The most serious limitation is that most patients will not fit neatly into any single category, but rather will have overlapping clinical features of several. For instance, many diabetics with distal, primarily sensory polyneuropathy also can be shown to have autonomic dysfunction, usually in the form of vasomotor disturbance in the limbs and abnormalities of sweating. Similarly, patients who develop a proximal motor syndrome may have dysautonomic features (including sexual impotence in males) and some degree of distal sensory polyneuropathy. To compound matters, such patients appear at risk to develop a cranial mononeuropathy.

Classifying the diabetic neuropathies tells us nothing of the pathogenesis of the neuropathic lesion. Rather, attempts at classification represent an educated guess at identifying the apparent anatomic sites of disorder and the critical clinical features. Pain is a frequent

---

TABLE 383-5   Sensory neuropathies

Cause or association	Course	Fiber size affected		Neuronopathy	Comment
		Small	Large		
TOXINS/DRUGS					
cis-Platinum (antineoplastic)	Sub/Chr	+	+ +	+	Dose-related
Pyridoxine (megadose)	Sub/Chr	+	+ +	+/−	Dose-related
Taxol (antineoplastic)	Acu/Sub	+ +	+	−	NGF may be protective
SYSTEMIC DISEASES					
Paraneoplastic	Sub	+	+ +	+ +	Most SCLC and breast
Sjögren syndrome	Sub/Chr	+/−	+	+ +	Variable presentation
Dysproteinemia (mainly IgMk)	Chr	+	+ +	−	Demyelinating; may bind to MAG
IDIOPATHIC					
Sporadic	Acu	+/−	+ +	+ +	Poor recovery
Sporadic	Chr	+/−	+ +	?	Sensory ataxia
HEREDITARY					
Many varieties (see Table 383-3)	Chr	Variable		Some	Progressive

Abbreviations: + + = most; + = some; ± = occasionally; Acu = acute; Sub = subacute; Chr = chronic; NGF = nerve growth factor; MAG = myelin-associated glycoprotein; SCLC = small cell lung carcinoma.

feature of diabetic neuropathies (see Table 383-4) but is variable in incidence and degree and is subjective in nature. The term diabetic amyotrophy should be avoided because of its ambiguity.

Diabetic neuropathies tend to occur in the setting of long-standing hyperglycemia (decades) whether insulin-dependent or not. By far the most common neuropathies related to diabetes mellitus are the diffuse sensory and autonomic types (categories 1 and 2 under "Symmetric" in Table 383-4). Sensory and autonomic polyneuropathy, chronic and indolent in evolution, may first be noticed in the third or fourth decade in patients with juvenile-onset diabetes but tends to occur after age 50 in patients with adult-onset diabetes. Focal and multifocal types of neuropathy are less common but quite dramatic (categories 1, 2, and 3 under "Asymmetric" in Table 383-4). They rarely occur before the age of 45 and are usually subacute or acute in onset. Cranial mononeuropathies refer to isolated sixth or third nerve palsies. The latter spares the pupil in three-fourths of cases, and some local pain or headache occurs in one-half. Truncal, or thoracoabdominal, neuropathy is painful, involves one or more intercostal or lumbar nerves unilaterally, and frequently coexists with the asymmetric proximal motor neuropathy. Femoral and obturator nerve–innervated muscles (quadriceps femoris, iliopsoas, adductor magnus) and loss of knee jerk on that side are the most evident features of asymmetric proximal motor neuropathy. Sensory deficit is minor, but pain in the hip and anterior thigh may predominate. Common to all of these multifocal and focal neuropathies is the strong likelihood of subsidence of pain within weeks to a year and partial or complete recovery of function. The same is true of symmetric proximal motor neuropathy (category 3 under "Symmetric" in Table 383-4).

Focal and multifocal diabetic neuropathies are considered to be ischemic in origin, and the basis for symmetric polyneuropathies, thought by some to involve abnormality of nerve metabolism, includes the possibility of ischemia.

Management of diabetic neuropathies is directed toward optimal control of hyperglycemia and symptomatic pain suppression. The role of aldose reductase inhibitors in preventing or reversing diabetic complications, including neuropathy, remains unclear. Entrapment neuropathies are frequently amenable to surgical decompression procedures.

Neuropathies with dysproteinemia An association between polyneuropathy and both multiple myeloma and macroglobulinemia has been recognized for many years. With commonly encountered multiple myeloma (MM) having either lytic or diffuse osteoporotic bone lesions, clinically overt polyneuropathy is relatively infrequent, occurring in approximately 5 percent of patients. These neuropathies are sensorimotor, may be severe, and generally do not reverse with successful suppression of the myeloma. In most cases, electrodiagnostic and pathologic features are consistent with a process of axonal degeneration.

In contrast, myeloma with osteosclerotic features, although representing only 3 percent of all myelomas, is associated with polyneuropathy in almost one-half of cases. These neuropathies, which may also occur with solitary plasmacytoma, seem to be different from those linked to MM in that they (1) often respond to radiation or removal of the primary lesion, (2) are more frequently demyelinating in character, (3) are associated with different monoclonal proteins and light chains (almost all lambda as opposed to mostly kappa in MM), and (4) frequently occur in association with other systemic findings. These include skin thickening, hyperpigmentation, hypertrichosis, organomegaly, endocrinopathy, anasarca, papilledema, and clubbing of fingers (POEMS syndrome: *p*olyneuropathy, *o*rganomegaly, *e*ndocrinopathy, *m* protein, and *s*kin changes). A great deal of attention has been paid to this curious syndrome in Japan, where it is more prevalent, but the underlying mechanism remains unknown, other than abnormality of lambda light chains.

Benign monoclonal gammopathy with an IgM serum spike, and usually with kappa light chains, is described in association with demyelinating polyneuropathy that often follows a protracted course

and indolent progression. In about one-quarter of cases, the monoclonal serum protein binds to normal human peripheral myelin, specifically to myelin-associated glycoprotein. Immunocytochemical studies show binding of IgM to nerve obtained at biopsy or autopsy of these patients, but in a pattern different from that seen following incubation of sections of nerve with the IgM serum. Incubated nerves show uniform staining of the entire expanse of compact myelin sheath, but in vivo deposited IgM can be demonstrated to localize more selectively, probably at sites of myelin splitting, the latter a phenomenon characteristic of most dysglobulinemic neuropathies. Whether the IgM bound to nerve in vivo plays a role in damaging nerve is unresolved.

Neuropathies with HIV infection Neuropathies are common in HIV infection, but different types of neuropathy are seen according to the stage of the disease. GBS or CIDP are the neuropathies likely to occur following conversion to seropositivity and during the asymptomatic phase of HIV infection. Treatment is the same as for HIV-negative patients. In later, symptomatic stages, subacute to chronic mononeuritis multiplex, axonal in nature, can occur. In some cases, vasculitis of the vasa nervorum has been demonstrated.

The most common neuropathy is a distal symmetrical mainly sensory polyneuropathy that evolves slowly in the late symptomatic stages of HIV infection, and frequently coexists with symptomatic encephalopathy and myelopathy (see Table 383-1 and Chap. 279). Improvement of this polyneuropathy with zidovudine treatment has been claimed. Also in the late stages, a severe, destructive subacute polyradiculopathy involving the cauda equina may be seen; it is caused by an opportunistic infection of roots with cytomegalovirus. Ganciclovir, started early, can arrest the disorder.

Neuropathies with Lyme disease In the aftermath of primary infection by the tick-borne spirochete *Borrelia burgdorferi*, a focal or multifocal radiculoneuropathy may occur weeks, months, or even years later. Although usually sensory and either dysesthetic or painful, the distribution is variable, affecting cranial nerves and spinal roots or nerves in a patchy asymmetrical fashion. Neuropathy is often chronic and persistent; CSF pleocytosis is the rule. In many, improvement occurs spontaneously, but the course is shortened by treatment with antibiotics, usually intravenous ceftriaxone (see Chap. 137).

Autonomic neuropathy The autonomic nervous system regulates the visceral organs and vegetative functions. Many pharmacologic agents modify specific autonomic functions, but autonomic neuropathy (dysautonomia) with structural changes in pre- and postganglionic neurons can also occur. Usually autonomic neuropathy is a manifestation of a more generalized polyneuropathy also affecting somatic peripheral nervous function, as in diabetic neuropathy, GBS, and alcoholic polyneuropathy, but occasionally syndromes of pure pandysautonomia are encountered. Symptoms of dysautonomia are mainly negative (i.e., loss of function) and include postural hypotension with faintness or syncope, anhidrosis, hypothermia, bladder atony, obstipation, dry mouth and dry eyes from failure of salivary and lacrimal glands to secrete, blurring of vision from lack of pupillary and ciliary regulation, and sexual impotence in males. Positive phenomena (hyperfunction) may also occur and include episodic hypertension, diarrhea, hyperhidrosis, and either tachycardia or bradycardia.

Pure motor neuropathy Disorder affecting any level of the motor unit—anterior horn cell (can be called *motor neuronopathy*), motor axon, or neuromuscular junction—can result in a purely lower motor syndrome without sensory disturbance. Distinguishing anterior horn cell disorders from motor axonopathies may be difficult clinically because they share manifestations (weakness, muscle denervation atrophy, hypo- or areflexia, fasciculations). Electrodiagnostic examination may also fail to localize the primary site of the lesion (neuropathic versus neuronopathic) unless the lesion is demyelinative in nature, in which case it is by definition neuropathic.

Examples of motor neuronopathies include the lower motor form of amyotrophic lateral sclerosis, poliomyelitis, hereditary spinal muscular atrophies, and adult variant of hexosaminidase A deficiency. Motor neuropathies may be seen with lead or dapsone intoxication, occasionally with porphyria, and also with multifocal motor neuropathy. The latter is a chronic asymmetrical disorder of midlife that may be associated with high titers of antiganglioside antibodies (particularly anti-G_{M_1}), persistent conduction block electrodiagnostically, or both. Neuromuscular junction disorders (e.g., Lambert-Eaton myasthenic syndrome, tick bite paralysis, other toxic neuromuscular blockade) can be recognized and localized electrodiagnostically. Some motor-sensory polyneuropathies have predominant motor symptoms and signs, such as hereditary motor-sensory neuropathies, GBS, and CIDP, but the subclinical sensory component is readily demonstrated electrodiagnostically or by quantitative sensory testing.

Pure sensory neuropathy   Clinical presentations involving primary sensation only (see Chap. 24) are not uncommon. Manifestations may: (1) be pansensory; (2) reflect mainly large afferent fiber involvement with deficits of vibratory and proprioceptive sense, areflexia, and sensory ataxia with or without tingling dysesthesias; or (3) reflect mainly small afferent fiber involvement with numbness and cutaneous hypesthesia to pin-prick and temperature stimuli, often with painful burning dysesthesias. The pattern of distribution, although variable, is often distal and symmetrical, particularly for large-fiber neuropathies.

The most severe and widespread of these pure sensory syndromes exhibit poor or no recovery, suggesting irreversible lesions of nerve cell bodies or dorsal root and trigeminal ganglion cells. These are frequently referred to as *sensory neuronopathies*. With sensory neurotoxins, moderate doses lead to potentially reversible neuropathy, but high doses appear to cause neuronopathy (see Table 383-5).

Plexopathy   This term refers to disorders of either the brachial or lumbosacral plexus. Lesions of the brachial plexus are characterized by motor and sensory signs different from those expected either in mononeuropathies of the upper limb or in polyneuropathies. The usual causes are direct trauma to the plexus, idiopathic brachial neuritis (also called neuralgic amyotrophy), cervical rib or band, infiltration by malignant tumor, or prior radiation therapy. When the upper parts of the brachial plexus, arising from cervical roots 5 through 7, are affected, weakness and atrophy of shoulder girdle and upper arm muscles occur. Injuries to the lower brachial plexus, arising from the eighth cervical and first thoracic roots, produce distal arm weakness, atrophy, and focal sensory deficit in the forearm and hand. In general, idiopathic brachial neuritis, radiation damage greater than 60 Gy (6000 rad), and particular types of trauma (arm jerked downward) result in damage to the upper portions of the brachial plexus. In contrast, infiltration by malignant tumor, cervical rib or band, and certain other types of trauma (arm jerked upward) cause damage to the lower brachial plexus. Lumbosacral plexopathies are less common; they may be due to idiopathic lumbosacral plexitis, retroperitoneal hemorrhage, malignant tumor infiltration, or occur in association with long-standing diabetes mellitus.

Miscellaneous causes of neuropathy   Ischemia of nerve severe enough to produce clinical symptoms has as its basis the widespread compromise of blood flow in the vasa nervorum. Typically, this is the result of small-vessel disease involving the vasa nervorum directly, as occurs with vasculitis, rather than large-vessel disease, such as atherosclerosis. Clinically, widespread disease of the vasa nervorum produces mononeuropathy multiplex, which electrodiagnostically has the features of a patchy axonal process.

Cold exerts deleterious effects on peripheral nerve directly without an intermediate step of ischemia being necessary. Cold injury to nerve occurs after prolonged exposure, usually of a limb, to moderately low temperatures, as with immersion of the feet in seawater; actual freezing of tissue is not required. Axonal degeneration of myelinated fibers is the pathologic expression of cold injury. Frequently limbs affected by cold injury to nerve show sensory deficit and dysesthesias, cutaneous vasomotor instability, pain, and marked sensitivity to minimal cold exposure, which persist for many years. The pathophysiology of these phenomena is uncertain.

TROPHIC CHANGES IN SEVERE NEUROPATHY   The array of observable changes in completely denervated muscle, bone, and skin, including hair and nails, is well known, if incompletely understood. It is unclear what portion of the changes is due purely to denervation versus that caused by disuse, immobility, lack of weight bearing, and particularly recurrent, unnoticed, painless trauma. Considerable evidence favors the view that ulceration of skin, poor healing, tissue resorption, neurogenic arthropathy, and mutilation are the result of repeated heedless injury to insensitive parts. This sequence of events is avoidable with proper attention to and care of the insensitive parts by both patient and physician.

RECOVERY FROM NEUROPATHY   In contrast to axons in the CNS, peripheral nerve fibers have an excellent capability to regenerate under proper circumstances. The process of regeneration following axonal degeneration may take from 2 months to more than a year, depending on the severity of the neuropathy and the length of regeneration required. Whether regeneration takes place depends upon the subsidence of the initial basis for neuropathy. This could be removal from contact with a neurotoxic substance or correction of an abnormal metabolic state. A deficit secondary to demyelination may recover rapidly since intact axons may remyelinate in just a few weeks. For example, a patient with GBS, in whom demyelination but no secondary axonal degeneration has occurred, may recover to normal strength from bedfastness and paralysis of arms and legs in as little as 3 to 4 weeks.

MONONEUROPATHY MULTIPLEX (MULTIFOCAL NEUROPATHY)   This term means simultaneous or sequential involvement of individual noncontiguous nerve trunks, either partially or completely, evolving over days to years. Since the disease process underlying mononeuropathy multiplex involves peripheral nerves in a multifocal and random fashion, there is a tendency, as worsening occurs, for the neurologic deficit to become less patchy and multifocal and more confluent and symmetric. Some patients present initially with a distal symmetric neuropathy. Attention to the pattern of early symptoms is therefore important in making the judgment that a particular neuropathy is indeed a mononeuropathy multiplex.

Once that issue is settled, the next question is whether the process is primarily axonal or demyelinating. Almost one-third of all adults with the clinical syndrome of mononeuropathy multiplex have a clear-cut picture of a demyelinating disorder usually with multiple foci of persistent conduction block by electrodiagnostic examination. More intensive study of this subgroup suggests that the multifocal demyelinating neuropathy represents part of the spectrum of chronic acquired demyelinating neuropathy, that is, CIDP. Management of this multifocal subgroup is the same as for CIDP. (See ''Acquired Demyelinating Neuropathies,'' above.)

The remaining two-thirds of patients with mononeuropathy multiplex have a picture by electrodiagnostic examination of axonal involvement that is heterogeneously distributed. Although ischemia would be suspected as the basis of neuropathy in these patients, only about one-half can be shown to have a process, usually vasculitis, affecting the vasa nervorum. Management of those with proven vasculitis of vasa nervorum is the same as treatment for systemic vasculitis (see Chap. 291). The others remain undiagnosed even on follow-up, and the basis for their mononeuropathy multiplex is uncertain. Management in this group is conservative and many patients will stabilize or recover, at least partially.

In individuals in whom vasculitic change in vasa nervorum can be demonstrated, any one of a large number of underlying disorders may be responsible. The primary vasculitides of the polyarteritis nodosa group constitute the most frequent basis, followed closely by the vasculitis syndrome occurring in the course of other connective tissue disorders. In descending order of frequency, the latter are rheumatoid arthritis, systemic lupus erythematosus, and mixed connective tissue disease. Other rarer causes of mononeuropathy multiplex due to nerve ischemia from occlusion of vasa nervorum include mixed cryoglobulinemia, Sjögren's syndrome, Wegener's granulomatosis, progressive systemic sclerosis, Churg-Strauss allergic granulomatosis, and hypersensitivity angiitides. Management of the neuropathy in each instance is predicated upon the appropriate treatment of the responsible disease.

Mononeuropathy multiplex syndrome may also be seen as a manifestation of leprosy, sarcoidosis, certain types of amyloidosis, hypereosinophilia syndrome, cryoglobulinemia, and multifocal types of diabetic neuropathy.

MONONEUROPATHY Mononeuropathy means focal involvement of a single nerve trunk and therefore implies a local causation. Direct trauma, compression, and entrapment are the usual causes. Ulnar neuropathies, due to lesions either at the ulnar groove or in the cubital tunnel, and median neuropathy due to compression in the carpal tunnel constitute the great majority of mononeuropathies encountered in clinical practice. These are described below, and other common mononeuropathies are listed in Table 383-6.

In the absence of a history of trauma to the nerve trunk, factors favoring conservative management include sudden onset, no motor deficit, few or no sensory findings even though pain and sensory symptoms might be present, and no evidence of axonal degeneration by electrodiagnostic criteria. Factors favoring surgical intervention include chronicity and worsening neurologic deficit on examination, particularly if motor, and electrodiagnostic evidence that the lesion has produced a degree of wallerian degeneration.

Ulnar nerve   Complete ulnar paralysis results in a characteristic claw-hand deformity owing to wasting and weakness of many of the small hand muscles and hyperextension of the fingers at the metacarpophalangeal joints and flexion at the interphalangeal joints. The flexion deformity is most pronounced in the fourth and fifth fingers. Sensory loss occurs over the fifth finger, the ulnar aspect of the fourth finger, and the ulnar border of the palm. The superficial

TABLE 383-6   Some common mononeuropathies

Nerve	Origin (spinal segments)	Muscles innervated	Usual site of lesion	Clinical features	Comments
UPPER EXTREMITY					
Suprascapular	C5, C6	Supraspinatus Infraspinatus	Suprascapular notch of scapula	Weakness of lateral rotation of the humerus	No sensory deficit
Long thoracic	C5–C7	Serratus anterior	Variable	Winging of scapula	No sensory deficit
Axillary	C5, C6	Deltoid, teres minor	Near shoulder joint	Weakness of shoulder abduction; atrophy of shoulder	Sensory deficit similar to C5 dorsal root lesion (see Figs. 24-2 and 24-3)
Radial	C5–T1	Triceps, brachioradialis, wrist, finger, and thumb extensors	Spiral groove of humerus	Wrist drop most obvious, also finger and thumb extensors paralyzed	Saturday night palsy (acute compression) is frequent cause
Posterior interosseous branch	C7, C8	Finger and thumb extensors	Edge of supinator muscle below elbow	Finger drop; wrist relatively spared	No sensory deficit
Ulnar	C8, T1	Ulnar flexor of the wrist, long flexors of 4th and 5th digits, and most intrinsic hand muscles	Ulnar groove at the elbow	Weakness of finger adduction and abduction and thumb adduction (see text); interosseous atrophy, claw-hand	May be acute or insidious; sensory symptoms/signs are distinctive (Figs. 24-2 and 24-3); see also text
			Cubital tunnel	Same as above	Often pain over medial proximal forearm (cubital tunnel)
			Medial base of palm	Intrinsic hand muscles only, interosseous atrophy	No sensory deficit
Median	C6–T1	Abductor pollicis brevis; more proximal muscles include forearm pronator, long finger and thumb flexors	Carpal tunnel	Characteristic sensory symptoms and deficit and inability to make a circle with thumb and index finger	Sensory deficit as per Figs. 24-2 and 24-3 (see text); known as carpal tunnel syndrome
Anterior interosseous branch	C7–T1	Long flexors of thumb and index and middle fingers	Anterior interosseus branch below the elbow	Weakness of pinch; pain in volar forearm	No sensory deficit
LOWER EXTREMITY					
Femoral	L2–L4	Iliopsoas (hip flexor) and quadriceps femoris (knee extensor)	Proximal to inguinal ligament	Knee buckling; absent knee jerk; weak anterior thigh muscles with atrophy	Association with diabetes mellitus; sensory disturbance as per Fig. 24-2
Lateral femoral cutaneous branch	L2, L3	None	Inguinal ligament	Dysesthetic hyperpathia of lateral thigh	Known as meralgia paresthetica
Obturator	L3, L4	Thigh adductors	Intrapelvic or at pubis	Weakness of hip adduction	Sensory deficit on medial thigh
Sciatic	L4–S3	Hamstring muscles, hip abductor and all muscles below the knee	Near sciatic notch	Severe lower leg and hamstring weakness; flail foot; severe disability	Uncommon except from war wounds
Posterior tibial	L5–S2	Calf muscles (proximally), toe flexors and other intrinsic foot muscles	Tarsal tunnel, near medial malleolus	Pain and numbness of sole, weak toe flexors	Known as tarsal tunnel syndrome
Peroneal	L4–S1	Dorsiflexors of toes and foot, evertors of foot	At neck of fibula	Foot drop and weakness of foot eversion	Sensory deficit is similar in distribution to L5, S1 sensory roots

location of the nerve at the elbow makes it a common site of pressure palsy. The ulnar nerve may also become entrapped just distal to the elbow in the cubital tunnel formed by the aponeurotic arch linking the two heads of the flexor carpi ulnaris. Also, prolonged pressure on the base of the palm, as occurs with use of hand tools or bicycle riding, may result in damage to the deep palmar branch of the ulnar nerve, causing weakness of the small hand muscles but no sensory loss.

Median nerve The median nerve in the carpal tunnel lies in close quarters with nine tendons. Entrapment of the nerve at the wrist (carpal tunnel syndrome) may be secondary to excessive use of the wrist, tenosynovitis with arthritis, or local infiltration, for example, by a thickening of connective tissue as in acromegaly or by deposit of amyloid or by one of the mucopolysaccharidoses. Other systemic diseases associated with an increased incidence of carpal tunnel syndrome are hypothyroidism, rheumatoid arthritis, and diabetes mellitus, but underlying diseases account for only a small fraction of all cases. The main symptoms of carpal tunnel syndrome are nocturnal paresthesias of thumb, index, and middle fingers. With worsening, numbness demonstrable by pin examination occurs in that distribution, and eventually weakness and atrophy of the abductor pollicis brevis (thenar eminence) becomes evident. Treatment of carpal tunnel syndrome is surgical section of the carpal ligament to relieve entrapment. Incomplete lesions of the median nerve between the axilla and wrist may result in causalgia (a particularly severe type of burning pain; see Chap. 11).

OTHER FOCAL NEUROPATHIES Peripheral nerve tumors These are mostly benign and can arise on any nerve trunk or twig. Although peripheral nerve tumors occur anywhere in the body including the spinal roots and cauda equina, many are subcutaneous in location and present as a soft swelling, sometimes with a purplish discoloration of the skin. Two major categories of peripheral nerve tumors are recognized: neurilemmoma (schwannoma) and neurofibroma. Neurilemmomas are usually solitary and grow within the nerve sheath, rendering the tumor relatively easy to dissect free. In contrast, neurofibromas tend to be multiple, grow within the endoneurial substance, rendering them difficult to dissect, may undergo malignant changes, and are the hallmark of von Recklinghausen's neurofibromatosis (NF1). This disease is characterized by an autosomal dominant inheritance pattern, any number of neurofibromas from one to thousands, five or more café au lait–pigmented skin lesions greater than 1.5 cm (80 percent of patients), axillary freckles (93 percent of patients), an increased incidence of seizure disorder and mental retardation and an exceptionally high rate of spontaneous mutation (see Chap. 378). The gene for NF1 is on chromosome 17, and its protein product, neurofibromin, is a large, widely expressed protein that appears to regulate the proto-oncogene *ras*.

Herpes zoster This is a sensory neuritis due to varicella-zoster infection and is characterized by acute inflammation of one or more dorsal root ganglia. Lancinating pain and hyperalgesia over the skin surface supplied by affected roots occur for 3 to 4 days, followed by the appearance of herpetic eruption in the same segment characterized by painful raised blisters on reddened bases. If the inflammatory process spreads to involve adjacent motor roots of anterior horns of the cord, segmental motor weakness and wasting appear. Paralysis of the oculomotor nerves may occur in conjunction with ophthalmic division involvement of the trigeminal ganglion (ophthalmoplegic zoster). Facial paralysis may occur with involvement of the geniculate ganglion and herpetic eruption on the ipsilateral tympanic membrane or external ear canal (Ramsay Hunt syndrome).

In less than 5 percent, neuropathic pain persists in the dermatomal distribution of the affected ganglia. The pain, known as *postherpetic neuralgia,* is intense, burning, hyperpathic, unrelenting, and often dominates the lives of those affected. Advancing age is a risk factor for this outcome. In some patients blunting of the pain to tolerable levels is achieved by use of carbamazepine or a tricyclic antidepressant such as desipramine (see also Chap. 11).

Leprous neuritis This is a major worldwide cause of neuropathy. *Mycobacterium leprae* organisms readily invade Schwann cells in cutaneous nerve twigs, particularly those associated with unmyelinated nerve fibers. Two major forms of leprous neuritis are recognized, tuberculoid and lepromatous, which actually represent the far ends of a spectrum of disease, the middle of which is called dimorphous leprosy (patchy and multifocal involvement of skin and nerve). Treatment depends upon where in the spectrum a given case is classified (see Chap. 131). Tuberculoid (high-resistance) leprosy is restricted to a single patch of hypesthetic or anesthetic skin in any location. The skin patch is frequently thickened, reddened, or hypopigmented. If a superficially placed nerve trunk, typically a cutaneous nerve, courses just beneath the area of affected skin, it may be engulfed in the inflammatory reaction, resulting in an associated mononeuropathy. Such a nerve may be palpably enlarged and beaded. Lepromatous (low-resistance) leprosy is marked by immunologic tolerance and widespread skin thickening, cutaneous anesthesia, and anhidrosis, sparing only the warmest parts of the body, notably the axilla, groin, and beneath the scalp hair. Motor signs (focal weakness and atrophy) result from damage to mixed nerves lying close to the skin, particularly the median, ulnar, peroneal, and facial nerves.

Bell's palsy This seventh nerve palsy is due to inflammation of the facial nerve in the facial canal, the basis for which remains obscure. Edema may play a part leading to compression of nerve fibers, with resulting acute unilateral paralysis of facial muscles (see Chap. 380).

Sarcoidosis This may involve single or multiple peripheral nerves, producing asymmetric mononeuritis or polyneuritis. Unilateral or bilateral facial paralysis is described in association with parotitis and uveitis (Heerfordt's syndrome).

Polyneuritis cranialis This is a relapsing and remitting mononeuropathy multiplex restricted to cranial nerves. It is usually associated with indolent tuberculous cervical adenitis (scrofula) or sarcoidosis. Treatment of the underlying condition will halt the cranial nerve palsies.

Acknowledgment

By arrangement with the publishers, portions of this section also appear in substantially the same form in Asbury AK: Diseases of peripheral nerve, in *Diseases of the Nervous System,* 2d ed, AK Asbury, GM McKhann, WI McDonald (eds). Philadelphia, Saunders, 1992.

REFERENCES

ASBURY AK: New aspects of disease of the peripheral nervous system, in *Harrison's Textbook of Internal Medicine, Update IV.* McGraw-Hill, New York, 1983, pp 211–229

———, GILLIATT RW: *Peripheral Nerve Disorders: A Practical Approach.* London, Butterworth, 1984

BAROHN RJ et al: Peripheral nervous system involvement in a large cohort of human immunodeficiency virus infected individuals. Arch Neurol 50:167, 1993

CHANCE PF et al: DNA deletion associated with hereditary neuropathy with liability to pressure palsies. Cell 72:143, 1993

DAWSON DM et al: *Entrapment Neuropathies,* 2d ed. Boston, Little, Brown, 1991

DYCK PJ et al (eds): *Peripheral Neuropathy,* 3d ed. Philadelphia, Saunders, 1992

HELLER S, WARD JD: Neurologic consequences of hypoglycemia and pathogenic mechanisms involved in diabetic neuropathy. Curr Opin Neurol Neurosurg 6:423, 1993

———: *Diabetic Neuropathy.* Philadelphia, Saunders, 1987

LAYZER RB: *Neuromuscular Manifestations of Systemic Disease,* vol 25: *Contemporary Neurology Series.* Philadelphia, Davis, 1984

RAIVICH G, KREUTZBERG GW: Nerve growth factor and regeneration of peripheral nervous system. Clin Neurol Neurosurg 95:S84, 1993

ROPPER AH et al: *Guillain Barré Syndrome.* Philadelphia, FA Davis, 1991

STEWART JD: *Focal Peripheral Neuropathies.* New York, Elsevier, 1987

SUTER U et al: Progress in the molecular understanding of hereditary peripheral neuropathies reveals new insights into the biology of the peripheral nervous system. Trends Neurosci 16:50, 1993

384 DERMATOMYOSITIS AND POLYMYOSITIS

RUP TANDAN / WALTER G. BRADLEY

Dermatomyositis and polymyositis are conditions of presumed autoimmune etiology in which the skeletal muscle is damaged by a nonsuppurative inflammatory process dominated by lymphocytic infiltration. The term *polymyositis* is applied when the condition spares the skin and the term *dermatomyositis* when polymyositis is associated with a characteristic skin rash. One-third of cases are associated with various connective tissue disorders, such as rheumatoid arthritis, lupus erythematosus, mixed connective tissue disorder, and progressive systemic sclerosis, and one-tenth with a malignancy.

ETIOLOGY The precise cause of these diseases is unknown, but interplay between host genetic factors, viral infection of muscle, and autoimmune mechanisms is probably contributory. Familial occurrence of these diseases, and the increased frequency of HLA-DR3 and -DRw52 antigens in patients, suggest an underlying genetic and immunologic predisposition. Experimental viral myositis can be induced in animals by coxsackie virus. A mild inflammatory myopathy can occur with influenza and coxsackie viruses in humans. However, the several electron-microscopic observations of virus-like particles in muscle fibers in dermatomyositis or polymyositis have not been confirmed by virus isolation or demonstration of rising viral antibody titers, and the disease has not been passed into animals by injection of extracts of skeletal muscles. Nevertheless, the presence of serum antibodies to several cytoplasmic ribonucleoproteins involved in translation (especially histidyl tRNA synthetase or Jo-1 and signal recognition particle, SRP) may result from an immune response to an altered virus that serves as an immunogen in polymyositis. These antibodies probably represent a cross-reactive phenomenon.

A lymphocyte-mediated disease resembling polymyositis has been reported in laboratory animals injected with muscle antigens together with Freund's adjuvant (experimental allergic myositis). Recent immunohistochemical and muscle co-culture studies indicate that muscle fiber necrosis in polymyositis and inclusion body myositis probably derive from activation of T cells of the cytotoxic-suppressor types, accompanied by T helper-inducer cells and macrophages present in the inflammatory infiltrates. In dermatomyositis, deposition of immunoglobulins and the C_{5b-9} complement membrane attack complex (MAC) has been demonstrated on intramuscular blood vessels even in unaffected or minimally involved regions of muscle, suggesting that humorally mediated blood vessel damage initiates the angiopathy that precedes muscle destruction. The final pathway for muscle fiber damage in dermatomyositis may be T helper cell-dependent stimulation of B cells, with resultant antibody-mediated cytotoxicity.

CLASSIFICATION The classification of the dermatomyositis-polymyositis group that is most widely used and which was proposed before the recent advances in the understanding of the immunology of these diseases, is given in Table 384-1. This classification is based partly on known differences in etiology and has a number of drawbacks, as noted below. Other uncommon associations of polymyositis are sarcoidosis, giant cell myositis with thymoma, and myositis

TABLE 384-1 Classification of polymyositis-dermatomyositis

Group I:	Primary idiopathic polymyositis
Group II:	Primary idiopathic dermatomyositis
Group III:	Dermatomyositis (or polymyositis) associated with neoplasia
Group IV:	Childhood dermatomyositis (or polymyositis) associated with vasculitis
Group V:	Polymyositis (or dermatomyositis) with associated collagen vascular disease

SOURCE: Classification suggested by Bohan et al.

in systemic infections due to viruses, toxoplasma, or parasites. A focal infective myositis due to streptococcal or staphylococcal infection is mostly seen in the tropics. Focal nodular myositis is a variant of polymyositis where focal areas of myositis cause hot, often painful, multifocal muscle masses. Inclusion body myositis is an inflammatory myopathy with characteristic clinical and pathologic features (see below).

INCIDENCE Current estimates that the annual incidence of the inflammatory myopathies is about five per million of the population are probably too low; we estimate that the incidence may be as high as two to three per hundred thousand population.

CLINICAL MANIFESTATIONS Group 1: Primary idiopathic polymyositis This group comprises about one-third of all cases of inflammatory myopathy. It is usually insidiously progressive over weeks, months, or even years. Rarely the disease is acute, producing severe muscle weakness in a matter of days or even rhabdomyolysis. The disease may develop at any age and in either sex. Females outnumber males 2:1.

The patients first become aware of weakness of the proximal limb muscles, especially the hips and thighs, and find difficulty in arising from the squatting or kneeling position and in climbing or descending stairs. When shoulder girdle muscles are involved, placing an object on a high shelf or combing the hair becomes difficult. Occasionally the disease is more restricted, affecting only the neck, the shoulder, or the quadriceps muscles. Pain of an aching type in the buttocks, thighs, and calves is experienced in about 10 percent of the cases, and tenderness on palpation in another 20 percent. Early symptoms of dysphagia and weakness of flexor muscles of the neck in a patient with a chronic myopathy suggest the diagnosis of polymyositis.

When the patient is first seen, there may be weakness of the muscles of the trunk, the pectoral and pelvic girdles, the upper arms and thighs, the anterior neck, more so than the posterior, and the pharynx. Ocular muscles are almost never affected except in a rare association with myasthenia gravis. The distal muscles are spared in about 75 percent of cases. Muscle atrophy, contractures, and diminished tendon reflexes are rare in early myositis and never as pronounced as in muscular dystrophies and denervating conditions. When the reflexes are disproportionately reduced, carcinoma with polymyositis and polyneuropathy or the Lambert-Eaton syndrome should be considered. Occasionally, the reflexes may be paradoxically brisk in dermatomyositis-polymyositis, perhaps due to irritation of muscle spindle receptors by the inflammation.

At presentation about 25 percent of patients have dysphagia, about 5 percent have significant respiratory impairment, and 5 percent are unable to walk. Dysphagia is due to involvement of striated muscles of the pharynx and upper esophagus. At some time in the course of the disease cardiac abnormalities are observed in about 30 percent of cases; these include ECG changes, arrhythmias, and heart failure secondary to myocarditis. About half of the fatal cases have pathologic evidence of cardiac disease with necrosis of myocardial fibers, usually with only modest inflammatory reaction. The frequency of myocardial infarction may be increased in those treated for long periods with glucocorticoids. In a few cases there is dyspnea due to lymphocytic pneumonitis, obliterating bronchiolitis, pulmonary edema, or pulmonary fibrosis. Arthralgia, Raynaud's phenomenon, and rarely, low-grade fever may also be present.

Group II: Primary idiopathic dermatomyositis This group comprises just over one-third of all cases of myositis. The skin changes may precede or follow the muscle syndrome and include a localized or diffuse erythema, maculopapular eruption, scaling eczematoid dermatitis, or, rarely, an exfoliative dermatitis. The classic lilac-colored (heliotrope) rash is on the eyelids, bridge of the nose, cheeks (butterfly distribution), forehead, chest, elbows, knees and knuckles, and around the nail beds. Itching may be troublesome in some cases. The skin lesions may be subtle and easily overlooked. Periorbital edema is frequent, particularly in acute cases. The skin lesions may occasionally ulcerate. Subcutaneous calcification may occur, especially in children.

The typical rash and myositis allow a diagnosis of dermatomyositis, and such cases may be placed in this category (group II, Table 384-1) if idiopathic and into groups III, IV, and V if there are other features, namely malignancy, vasculitis in children, and an established collagen vascular disease. There should be concern about an underlying malignancy in patients with dermatomyositis over the age of 60.

Group III: Polymyositis or dermatomyositis with neoplasia This syndrome, which comprises about 8 percent of all cases of myositis, is categorized separately, although muscle and skin changes are indistinguishable from those in the other groups. Malignancy, however, is uncommon in myositis seen in children and in association with a connective tissue disorder. The malignancy may antedate or postdate the onset of the myositis by up to 2 years. The incidence of this paraneoplastic syndrome is higher in patients with dermatomyositis over the age of 60; therefore, in such patients a thorough history and clinical examination (including breast and rectal) must be supplemented by hemogram, biochemical profile, serum protein electrophoresis and immunofixation, screening for carcino-embryonic antigen, urine analysis for blood and cytology, stool samples for occult blood, chest x-ray, sputum for cytology, and bone scan seeking clues for an underlying malignancy. This relatively inexpensive search often uncovers most malignancies; undirected radiologic screening procedures are costly and unhelpful in improving the yield. The most common malignancies are lung, ovary, breast, gastrointestinal tract, and myeloproliferative disorders. The myositis is a paraneoplastic syndrome, the cause of which may lie in an altered immune status or an occult viral infection of the muscle.

Group IV: Childhood polymyositis and dermatomyositis associated with vasculitis This group comprises about 8 to 20 percent of all cases of myositis in various series. Inflammatory myopathy in childhood is frequently associated with skin involvement and clinical or pathologic evidence of vasculitis in skin, muscles, gastrointestinal tract, and other organs. Degeneration and loss of capillaries in a perifascicular distribution occur in the skeletal muscles; often necrotizing lesions of the skin, and ischemic infarction of kidneys, gastrointestinal tract, and rarely brain may be seen. Consequently, some authors have reported mortality rates of up to one-third in childhood dermatomyositis, though most have found that the prognosis is better than in adult dermatomyositis-polymyositis. One limitation of the classification of Bohan et al. is that it is not clear whether or not all cases of childhood myositis should be included in group IV. Subcutaneous calcification is frequently present in childhood dermatomyositis.

Group V: Polymyositis or dermatomyositis with an associated connective tissue disorder This "overlap group" of myositis comprises about one-fifth of all cases that occur in association with several connective tissue diseases. Progressive systemic sclerosis, rheumatoid arthritis, mixed connective tissue disease (the rheumatologic overlap disorder), and lupus erythematosus are the most common associated conditions; polyarteritis nodosa and rheumatic fever are more rarely associated. Criteria for placement in the "overlap group" combine the demonstration of the appropriate clinical and laboratory abnormalities required for the diagnosis of the connective tissue disorder together with clinical and laboratory evidence of myositis. The diagnosis of myositis is often difficult in patients with a connective tissue disorder producing arthritis, since this may often produce muscle weakness with type II fiber atrophy. Moreover, perivascular inflammatory foci are common in muscle in connective tissue disorders. Demonstration of increased serum creatine kinase (CK), electromyography (EMG), and muscle biopsy are often required to make this diagnosis. Though patients in this overlap group usually respond to glucocorticoid therapy, the prognosis for recovery of function is poorer than in pure dermatomyositis-polymyositis. Dysphagia in group V patients with progressive systemic sclerosis is often due to involvement of the smooth muscle of the distal third of the esophagus.

Other disorders associated with myositis SARCOIDOSIS AND POLYMYOSITIS The skeletal muscle contains noncaseating granulomas with Langhans-type multinuclear giant cells in at least one-quarter of patients with sarcoidosis. Symptomatic polymyositis is, however, uncommon. Regenerating multinuclear myoblasts resemble Langhans' giant cells, which has led to misdiagnosis in many of the cases reported in the literature to have "sarcoid myositis." Giant cell or granulomatous polymyositis and myocarditis, sometimes associated with myasthenia gravis, have been recorded in patients with thymomas.

FOCAL NODULAR MYOSITIS A syndrome of acutely developing and painful focal inflammatory nodules, sometimes occurring sequentially in different muscles, has been termed *focal nodular myositis*. The pathologic appearance and response to therapy are similar to those in generalized polymyositis. The differential diagnosis includes, when single, a muscle tumor (sarcoma or rhabdomyosarcoma) or proliferative fasciitis and myositis and, when multiple, muscle infarcts such as can occur in polyarteritis nodosa.

INFECTIOUS POLYMYOSITIS Rare cases of polymyositis have clear-cut evidence of being due to known pathogens such as toxoplasma (Chap. 177), viruses (Chap. 154), and spirochetes (Lyme disease). Antibody screening will suggest the diagnosis in such cases. Trichinosis may be confused with idiopathic polymyositis, particularly if the history of raw pork ingestion is not obtained. The symptoms of trichinosis are variable and depend upon the parasitic load. Low-grade fever, muscle pain of variable degree, conjunctival and periorbital edema, and fatigue are frequent. Weakness is generally mild. Heavy infestation is often associated with central nervous system symptoms of delirium, coma, or focal neurologic deficit. The frequent myocardial involvement is manifested by tachycardia and ECG changes. The diagnosis is made by the history of ingestion of undercooked pork, marked eosinophilia, sensitivity to intradermal *Trichina* antigen, and the appearance of serum antibodies to *Trichina* during the course of the disease. Occasionally the diagnosis is not recognized until a muscle is biopsied. Pyomyositis, a suppurative inflammation of muscle due to staphylococci or streptococci, is mainly seen in the tropics but has recently been reported in patients with AIDS. The presentation is that of a diffuse abscess of the muscle.

MYOPATHY IN HIV INFECTION Polymyositis occurs in AIDS, which is caused by infection with the human immunodeficiency virus (HIV) (see Chap. 279). It may be the presenting manifestation of the disorder or, rarely, be due to therapy with zidovudine (AZT). Profound weight loss greater than 10 percent of baseline body weight with associated chronic diarrhea or weakness characterizes the HIV wasting syndrome; a myopathy, among other causes, may underlie this entity. Raised serum CK, EMG evidence of myopathy, and muscle fiber necrosis with or without inflammatory infiltrates occur in AIDS myopathy. HIV-antigens are detectable in macrophages in muscle inflammatory infiltrates but are absent in muscle fibers. The inflammatory myopathy associated with early HIV infection usually responds to glucocorticoids. Polymyositis also occurs in patients displaying the spectrum of diseases associated with human T lymphotropic virus type I (HTLV-I) infection, especially in the Caribbean islands and Japan.

AZT myopathy is dose related and usually improves upon discontinuation of the drug or after reduction of the dose. Structural and functional mitochondrial abnormalities are usually associated with AZT myopathy.

INCLUSION BODY MYOSITIS The clinical features of this typically sporadic, but rarely familial disorder, are similar to those of chronic idiopathic polymyositis, except that onset is at an older age, focal and distal muscle involvement are more frequent, and disease duration is longer. Muscle biopsy shows interstitial and occasional perivascular inflammatory infiltrates, necrosis, and regeneration of muscle fibers, but in addition there are "rimmed vacuoles" in the fibers that stain positively with Congo-red, like amyloid. Electron microscopy reveals paramyxovirus-like 15- to 18-nm filaments in the nuclei and sarcoplasm that show immunoreactivity to ubiquitin and β-amyloid protein. The nature of the inflammatory infiltrate and the mechanism of muscle fiber damage are similar to that in polymyositis. Recent immunocytochemical and in-situ hybridization studies suggest that a previously reported etiologic link with the mumps virus seems unlikely. This disorder usually responds poorly to glucocorticoids and immunosuppressive therapy, and the prognosis is for a chronically progressive disorder with loss of ambulation about 5 to 10 years after presentation.

Eosinophilic myositis This rare disease probably represents one manifestation of the spectrum of hypereosinophilic syndrome. There are a number of subtypes. Subacute onset of muscle pain and proximal weakness, elevated serum CK, myopathic features on electromyogram, and histologic appearances of a myositis with an eosinophilic inflammatory infiltrate are characteristic. Some patients may respond to glucocorticoids, methotrexate, or leukapheresis.

EOSINOPHILIA-MYALGIA SYNDROME A syndrome that is more common in women has recently been associated with ingestion of the essential amino acid L-tryptophan. Fever, rash, arthralgia, cough, dyspnea, and edema are commonly accompanied by eosinophilia (more than 1000 cells per microliter), peripheral neuropathy and myositis with endomysial, perimysial, and fascial infiltration of lymphocytes and eosinophils. A di-L-tryptophan aminal of acetaldehyde, a contaminating by-product of the manufacture of some batches of L-tryptophan, has been incriminated. Cell-mediated immunologic muscle damage produced by cytotoxic T cells alone or with accompanying macrophages has been reported.

EOSINOPHILIC FASCIITIS This disorder is characterized by painful swelling and thickening of the skin in the extremities, limitation of movement due to contractures, and mild muscle weakness. Raised sedimentation rate, peripheral eosinophilia, hypergammaglobulinemia, and mildly elevated CK are seen. The EMG may show myopathic features. Histologically there is marked thickening and infiltration of the deep fascia with mononuclear cells and eosinophils, some involvement of the epimysium and perimysium, and varying but not striking degeneration of muscle. Most patients respond to treatment with glucocorticoids.

RELAPSING EOSINOPHILIC PERIMYOSITIS In this disease there are recurrent painful and tender areas in the neck or lower extremities, but without muscle weakness. Raised sedimentation rate and peripheral eosinophilia are frequent, serum CK is sometimes raised, and pathologically there is eosinophilic infiltration of the perimysium. Response to glucocorticoids is usually good.

LABORATORY FINDINGS In all forms of polymyositis there may be elevated serum levels of the enzymes present in skeletal muscle, such as CK, aldolase, serum glutamic oxaloacetic transaminase (SGOT), lactic acid dehydrogenase (LDH), and serum glutamic pyruvate transaminase (SGPT). The degree of rise decreases from the first to the last in this series of enzymes, and the pattern is the reverse of that seen in liver disease. The erythrocyte sedimentation rate is elevated in about two-thirds of cases. Tests for circulating rheumatoid factor are positive in less than one-half and antinuclear antibodies in about three-quarters of the cases. Several autoantibodies seem to be associated with clinically distinct groups of patients. Anti-Jo-1 antibodies are more common in polymyositis, especially in patients with interstitial lung disease, and anti-nRNP antibodies are often associated with polymyositis seen in lupus erythematosus. Other antibodies seen in patients with dermatomyositis and polymyositis in association with connective tissue diseases include anti-Scl-70 (progressive systemic sclerosis), anti-Sm (lupus erythematosus), anti-Ro and anti-La (Sjögren's syndrome and lupus erythematosus), and anti-ENA (mixed connective tissue disease). Myoglobin can be found in the urine when muscle destruction is acute and extensive; rarely, acute polymyositis causes the full syndrome of rhabdomyolysis and myoglobinuria. Most other hematologic indexes are normal. In about 40 percent of cases the electromyogram reveals a markedly increased insertional activity (muscle irritability), together with the typical myopathic triad of motor unit action potentials which are of low amplitude, are polyphasic, and have an abnormally early recruitment. In a further 40 percent of the patients only myopathic changes are present. The ECG is abnormal in about 5 to 10 percent of the cases at presentation. Since the pathologic process in myositis is patchy,

greater diagnostic yield is obtained by taking the biopsy from two clinically affected muscles and by skip serial sectioning of all specimens. Magnetic resonance imaging may serve to identify sites of muscle involvement. Muscles recently used for EMG or intramuscular injection must be avoided as these procedures can produce inflammatory changes and muscle fiber damage, leading to false-positive results. In about two-thirds of cases, the biopsies will demonstrate the typical pathologic changes of myositis, but despite following the above recommendations, about 10 percent of cases have normal muscle biopsy.

Skeletal muscle pathology The principal changes in muscle consist of infiltrates of inflammatory cells (lymphocytes, macrophages, plasma cells, and rare eosinophils and neutrophils) and destruction of muscle fibers with a phagocytic reaction. Perivascular (usually perivenular) inflammatory cell infiltration is the hallmark of polymyositis. Interstitial inflammatory cell infiltration is also a prominent feature of the disease, but lesser degrees of it may be seen in other conditions as a secondary reaction (e.g., in facioscapulohumeral and Becker's muscular dystrophy). Evidence of muscle fiber degeneration and regeneration is almost invariably present. Many of the residual muscle fibers are small, with increased numbers of sarcolemmal nuclei. Either the degeneration of muscle fibers or the infiltration of inflammatory cells may predominate in any given biopsy specimen. Blood vessel changes and perifascicular atrophy are prominent in childhood dermatomyositis, but less so in adult dermatomyositis and polymyositis. Capillary loss due to endothelial cell necrosis occurs particularly in the periphery of fascicles and may explain the perifascicular atrophy. Other features include reduplication of capillary basement membrane and the presence of tubular inclusions within endothelial cells. Type II muscle fiber atrophy and muscle infarcts also may be found. Vasculitis is also seen in polymyositis or dermatomyositis associated with connective tissue disorders.

DIAGNOSIS Patients with dermatomyositis showing the characteristic skin rash, muscle weakness, and evidence of muscle damage by EMG and elevation of serum CK may not require a muscle biopsy to confirm the diagnosis. In the case of idiopathic polymyositis, however, a firm diagnosis must be based on the presence of a typical clinical picture, a typical EMG, elevation of serum CK, and a diagnostic muscle biopsy. All four criteria are required to be certain of the diagnosis, since inflammatory changes may occasionally occur in other myopathies (e.g., facioscapulohumeral muscular dystrophy) and in other connective tissue disorders without clear muscle weakness. However, in less than one-third of cases of polymyositis are *all* these criteria satisfied. It may be particularly difficult to obtain a diagnostic muscle biopsy because of the patchy nature of the disease. Thus, a therapeutic trial of glucocorticoids should be given when full investigation of a patient with significant disability leaves a diagnosis of "possible polymyositis," usually because of a nondiagnostic muscle biopsy.

DIFFERENTIAL DIAGNOSIS The clinical picture of skin rash and proximal or diffuse muscle weakness has few causes other than dermatomyositis. However, proximal muscle weakness without skin involvement can be due to many conditions other than polymyositis and necessitates detailed investigation to establish the correct diagnosis.

Subacute or chronic progressive muscle weakness This may be due to denervating conditions such as the spinal muscular atrophies or amyotrophic lateral sclerosis. Upper motor neuron signs in the latter in addition to the muscle weakness aid in the diagnosis. The muscular dystrophies, such as those of Duchenne and Becker and the limb-girdle and facioscapulohumeral types, may appear similar to polymyositis (Chap. 385). However, the muscular dystrophies usually develop more slowly, rarely present after the age of 30, usually involve the pharyngeal and posterior neck muscles only in their later course, and have a pattern of muscle involvement which is selective, involving some muscles, such as the biceps and brachioradialis, early in the course of the disease, and sparing others, such as the deltoid. Nevertheless, in rare patients it may be difficult, even with a muscle biopsy, to distinguish chronic polymyositis from a rapidly advancing muscular dystrophy. This is particularly true of facioscapulohumeral muscular dystrophy, where interstitial inflammatory cell infiltration is commonly found early in the disease. Such doubtful cases should always be given an adequate trial of glucocorticoid therapy. Dystrophia myotonica produces a characteristic facies with ptosis, facial myopathy, temporalis muscle wasting, and grip myotonia (Chap. 385). Some of the metabolic myopathies, including glycogen storage disease due to myophosphorylase deficiency and the lipid storage diseases due to carnitine and carnitine palmityltransferase deficiency, produce exertional cramps, rhabdomyolysis, and muscle weakness; diagnosis rests upon biochemical studies of the muscle biopsy (Chap. 385). Glycogen storage disease due to acid maltase deficiency also requires muscle biopsy for diagnosis. The endocrine myopathies such as those due to hypercorticosteroidism, hyper- and hypothyroidism, and hyper- and hypoparathyroidism require the appropriate laboratory investigations for diagnosis. Muscle wasting in patients with an underlying neoplasm may be true polymyositis, but it can be due to a protein-wasting state (cachexia), a paraneoplastic neuropathy, or type II fiber atrophy.

Muscle weakness with marked exercise-induced fatigue Fatigue without much muscle wasting may be due to the neuromuscular junction disorders, myasthenia gravis, or the Lambert-Eaton syndrome. Repetitive nerve stimulation studies aid in the diagnosis of these conditions (Chap. 386).

Acute muscle weakness This may be caused by an acute neuropathy such as that due to the Guillain-Barré syndrome or a neurotoxin. When combined with painful muscle cramps, rhabdomyolysis, and myoglobinuria, it may be due to known metabolic disorders including some of the glycogen storage diseases such as myophosphorylase deficiency (McArdle's disease), carnitine palmityltransferase deficiency, and myoadenylate deaminase deficiency. Acute viral infections may cause a similar syndrome. Chronic alcoholics may develop a painful myopathy with myoglobinuria after a bout of heavy drinking or may present with a painless acute hypokalemic myopathy which is completely reversible, or may show an asymptomatic elevation of serum CK and myoglobin. Acute muscle weakness with myoglobinuria may occur in prolonged severe hypokalemia due to potassium loss, or with hypophosphatemia and hypomagnesemia, often seen in chronic alcoholics and in patients on nasogastric suction receiving parenteral hyperalimentation. An acute necrotizing myopathy with myoglobinuria can rarely accompany hypernatremia and hyponatremia.

Drug-induced myopathies Rhabdomyolysis and myoglobinuria have been associated with intake of amphotericin B, ϵ-aminocaproic acid, fenfluramine, heroin, and phencyclidine. A predominantly hypokalemic myopathy may result from prolonged use of diuretics, carbenoxolone, and azathioprine. Penicillamine has been reported to produce a myositis. The use of clofibrate, cimetidine, chloroquine, colchicine, carbimazole, cyclosporine, emetine, lovastatin, phenytoin, and, recently, AZT has been associated with a myopathy. Toxic myopathies usually have a different pathology from polymyositis and require a careful drug history for diagnosis. In other cases investigation reveals no etiology, and these may be due to a true acute autoimmune polymyositis or to an as yet undiscovered metabolic defect.

Pain on movement and muscle tenderness Patients with muscle pain and little or no weakness may be thought to be neurotic or hysterical. A number of conditions including *polymyalgia rheumatica* (Chap. 291) and arthritic disorders of adjacent joints enter into the differential diagnosis of polymyositis. The muscle biopsy either is normal or discloses type II fiber atrophy, but in polymyalgia rheumatica the temporal artery biopsy may show giant cell arteritis (Chap. 291). *Fibrositis* and *fibromyalgia* are syndromes which frequently enter into the differential diagnosis of polymyositis. Patients complain of focal or diffuse muscle tenderness, aching, and weakness, which is sometimes poorly separated from joint pain. In other patients there may be minor signs of a collagen vascular disorder, such as an increased erythrocyte sedimentation rate, antinuclear antibody (ANA),

or rheumatoid factor, and occasionally there is slight elevation of the serum CK. The muscle biopsy occasionally shows a few interstitial inflammatory cells. Where there is a focal "trigger point," biopsy may show inflammatory infiltration of the connective tissue. Rarely does this syndrome develop into frank polymyositis, and the prognosis is therefore more benign than that of polymyositis (see below). Many such patients show some response to nonsteroidal anti-inflammatory agents, though most continue to have indolent complaints.

TREATMENT Glucocorticoids in high dosage are the accepted treatment for severe dermatomyositis-polymyositis, though there is no controlled trial to prove their effectiveness. The best results are obtained from the use of prednisone, starting at a dose of 1 to 2 mg/kg body weight per day (60 to 100 mg/d for adults). Improvement may begin within 1 to 4 weeks, though in some patients treatment may need to be continued for 3 months before improvement occurs. When there is significant improvement in the weakness, the daily dose may be reduced by 5 mg every 4 weeks. Repeated manual muscle testing and serum CK determinations should be performed to ensure that the myositis does not relapse. At about 40 mg/d, the schedule is changed gradually to 80 mg every other day in order to reduce the incidence of glucocorticoid side effects. There is some evidence that the use of alternate-day glucocorticoids from the outset may be effective, particularly in patients with milder disease. Children and patients with acute to subacute dermatomyositis-polymyositis tend to improve more rapidly than those with chronic polymyositis. If the dose is reduced too rapidly, or to too low a level, relapse will occur, necessitating return to high dosage. Prednisone therapy may have to be continued for several years, but an attempt should be made every year to withdraw the therapy from patients who are clinically stable in order to determine if the disease is still active.

Cytotoxic drugs should be tried when the disease is severe, when the response to glucocorticoids is inadequate after 1 to 3 months, or when relapses are frequent. Azathioprine (2.5 to 3.5 mg/kg body weight per day in divided doses) is the most commonly used cytotoxic drug in this disease, and in combination with glucocorticoids in preliminary studies has shown a better response than glucocorticoids alone. Cyclophosphamide, methotrexate, and cyclosporine also have been used with benefit in uncontrolled reports. The aim of cytotoxic therapy with azathioprine or cyclophosphamide (usual dose about 2 mg/kg body weight per day) is to lower the total lymphocyte count to about 750 per microliter, while maintaining the hemoglobin level above 12 g/dL, the total white cell count above 3000 per microliter, and the platelet count about 125,000 per microliter. Weekly blood counts are required to monitor the cytotoxic drug therapy. Methotrexate is effective at doses that do not produce lymphopenia (usual dose about 0.5 mg/kg body weight per week, attained by slowly increasing to that dose). The combined use of prednisone and a cytotoxic drug usually allows a lower dose of prednisone to be used. In preliminary studies total-body irradiation has been successfully used in some patients with disease refractory to glucocorticoids and immunosuppressants, but long-term follow-up and controlled studies are lacking for this potentially dangerous therapy. A recent controlled trial of plasma exchange and leukapheresis in a small number of patients with dermatomyositis-polymyositis resistant to glucocorticoids showed no benefit over sham pheresis. High-dose intravenous immunoglobulin therapy has produced improvement in patients otherwise refractory to glucocorticoids, immunosuppressive drugs, and plasma exchange, but controlled trials need to be undertaken. Bed rest has been recommended in the acute phase of the disease but is harmful in the long term. Physiotherapy and rehabilitative devices are important in the long-term treatment of patients with dermatomyositis-polymyositis.

Elderly patients, particularly those with dermatomyositis, should be followed closely for the possibility of malignant disease, and any new symptoms or signs must be appropriately investigated by a directed approach. If a malignant lesion is found, it should be treated, since the muscle weakness may disappear if the neoplasm is eradicated. However, a response to glucocorticoids can usually be obtained even in patients with dermatomyositis-polymyositis associated with a malignancy.

The serum CK activity is useful for following patients during reduction of immunosuppressive therapy, since a rise in level generally indicates an incipient clinical relapse. However, it cannot be used to indicate initial response in patients being treated with prednisone for dermatomyositis-polymyositis, since this drug lowers the serum CK activity in a way which is not fully understood, but which is not related to the suppression of muscle inflammation.

Side effects of high-dose daily glucocorticoid therapy (see Chap. 335) are relatively common in patients treated for polymyositis, and these may limit therapy. However, these can be minimized by appropriate use of alternate-day therapy. When patients who have been stable on a static dose of prednisone develop increasing muscle weakness, this may be due to either a relapse of the myositis or to glucocorticoid myopathy. An EMG, serum CK measurement, and, rarely, muscle biopsy may help in differentiating these two conditions if the changes of myositis are present. However, often the only way to separate them is to reduce the dose of prednisone slowly; if glucocorticoid myopathy is the cause of the weakness, it will improve as the dose is reduced; if a relapse of the myositis is responsible, the weakness will increase with reduction in the dose.

Side effects of cytotoxic drugs include marrow suppression, alopecia, gastrointestinal tract disorders, damage to the testes and ovaries (including potential genetic damage), disorders of chronic immunosuppression, and potential for malignancy.

PROGNOSIS The overall mortality rate of individuals with dermatomyositis-polymyositis is about four times that of the general population; death is due usually to pulmonary, renal, and cardiac complications. Females, blacks, and those severely affected at presentation or treated after long delays have a worse prognosis. Unfavorable outcome is also seen in patients with significant dysphagia, associated cancer or connective tissue diseases, and serum antibodies to Jo-1 and SRP. Evidence from several series suggests that patients seen at tertiary referral centers may have less favorable outcome when compared with patients seen at smaller community hospitals, probably because they represent a population with more severe disease which shows poorer response to therapy. Nevertheless, the 5-year survival rate is about 75 percent overall, and is better than this in children. The majority of patients improve with therapy. Many patients make a full functional recovery, though some weakness of the shoulders and hips, usually not disabling, remains at the conclusion of treatment. Relapse may occur at any time. Glucocorticoids should not be discontinued too soon, for the relapse which may follow is often more difficult to treat than the original presentation. About one-half of the patients with this disease recover and can discontinue therapy within 5 years after the onset of the symptoms; about 20 percent still have active disease requiring continued therapy. The remaining 30 percent have inactive disease but residual muscle weakness.

REFERENCES

BANKER BQ, ENGEL AG: The polymyositis and dermatomyositis syndromes, in *Myology,* 2d ed, AG Engel, Franzini-Armstrong C (eds). New York, McGraw-Hill, 1994

BOHAN A et al: A computer-assisted analysis of 153 patients with polymyositis and dermatomyositis. Medicine 56:255, 1977

BRADLEY WG, TANDAN R: Inflammatory diseases of muscle, in *Textbook of Rheumatology,* 3d ed, WN Kelly et al (eds). Philadelphia, Saunders, 1988, chap 72

CACCAMO DV et al: Fulminant rhabdomyolysis in a patient with dermatomyositis. Neurology 43:844, 1993

CARPENTER S, KARPATI G: *Pathology of Skeletal Muscle.* New York, Churchill Livingstone, 1984, pp 515–592

DALAKAS MC: Polymyositis, dermatomyositis and inclusion-body myositis. N Engl J Med 325:1487, 1991

DEVERE R, BRADLEY WG: Polymyositis: Its presentation, mortality, and morbidity. Brain 98:637, 1975

EMSLIE-SMITH AM, ENGEL AG: Microvascular changes in early and advanced dermatomyositis: A quantitative study. Ann Neurol 27:343, 1990

LEONMONZON M et al: Search for HIV proviral DNA and amplified sequences in the muscle biopsies of patients with HIV polymyositis. Muscle Nerve 16:408, 1993

MARTIN RW et al: The clinical spectrum of the eosinophilia-myalgia syndrome associated with L-tryptophan ingestion. Ann Intern Med 113:124, 1990

MILLER FW: Myositis-specific autoantibodies: Touchstones for understanding the inflammatory myopathies. JAMA 270:1846, 1993

SIGURGEIRSSON B et al: Risk of cancer in patients with dermatomyositis or polymyositis: A population-based study. N Engl J Med 326:363, 1992

385 INHERITED, METABOLIC, ENDOCRINE, AND TOXIC MYOPATHIES

JERRY R. MENDELL / ROBERT C. GRIGGS

The muscle disorders discussed in this chapter include diseases that cause acute, subacute, or chronic muscle weakness. Some also cause pain in addition to or instead of weakness. The differential diagnosis of neuromuscular disease is discussed in Chap. 382. Dermatomyositis and polymyositis are discussed in Chap. 384 and periodic paralysis in Chap. 387.

HEREDITARY MYOPATHIES

Muscular dystrophy refers to a group of hereditary progressive diseases. Each type of muscular dystrophy has unique phenotypic and genetic features (Table 385-1).

DUCHENNE MUSCULAR DYSTROPHY This X-linked recessive disorder, sometimes also called *pseudohypertrophic muscular dystrophy,* occurs with an incidence of about 30 per 100,000 live born males. The disease bears the name of the French neurologist Duchenne because he established criteria for diagnosis and accurately described muscle biopsies.

Clinical features Duchenne dystrophy is present at birth, but the disorder usually becomes apparent between ages 3 and 5. The boys fall frequently and have difficulty keeping up with their friends when playing. Running, jumping, and hopping are invariably abnormal. By age 5, muscle weakness is obvious by muscle testing. On getting up from the floor, the patient uses his hands to climb up himself (Gowers' maneuver). In younger children, the calf muscles may feel firm and rubbery and are usually enlarged from true muscle hypertrophy; later calf enlargement is appropriately called *pseudohypertrophy* since muscle is replaced by fat and connective tissue. Contractures of the heel cords and iliotibial bands become apparent by age 6, when toe walking is associated with a lordotic posture. Loss of muscle strength is progressive, with predilection for proximal limb muscles and the neck flexors; leg involvement is more severe than arm involvement. Between ages 8 and 10 walking may require the use of braces; joint contractures and limitations of hip flexion, knee, elbow, and wrist extension are made worse by prolonged sitting. By age 12, most patients are confined to a wheelchair. Contractures become fixed and a progressive scoliosis often develops which may be associated with considerable discomfort. The chest deformity associated with scoliosis impairs the pulmonary function already diminished by muscle weakness. By age 16 to 18, patients are predisposed to serious, sometimes fatal pulmonary infections. Other causes of death include aspiration of food and acute gastric dilatation.

A cardiac cause of death is uncommon despite the existence of a cardiomyopathy in almost all patients. Congestive heart failure seldom occurs except with severe stress such as pneumonia. Cardiac arrhythmias are rare. The typical ECG shows an increase net RS in lead V_1; deep narrow Q waves in the precordial leads; and RSR' or polyphyasic R waves in V_1. Intellectual impairment in Duchenne dystrophy is common; the average intelligent quotient (IQ) is approximately one standard deviation below the mean. Impairment of

TABLE 385-1   Progressive muscular dystrophies

Type	Genetics	Clinical features	Other organ system involvement
Duchenne	X-linked recessive mutation of dystrophin gene	Onset before age 5 Progressive weakness of girdle muscles Inability to walk after age 12 Kyphoscoliosis Respiratory failure in second to third decade	Cardiomyopathy Mental impairment
Becker	X-linked recessive mutation of dystrophin gene	Onset in early to late childhood Slowly progressive weakness of girdle muscles Ability to walk after age 15 Respiratory failure after fourth decade	Cardiomyopathy
Myotonic	Autosomal dominant Expansion of unstable region of DNA at chromosome 19q13.3	Onset any decade Slowly progressive weakness of eyelids, face, neck, distal limb muscles Myotonia	Cardiac conduction defects Mental impairment Cataracts Frontal baldness Gonadal atrophy
Facioscapulohumeral	Autosomal dominant Frequent mutations at chromosome 4q35	Onset before age 20 Slowly progressive face, shoulder girdle, foot dorsiflexion weakness	Hypertension Deafness
Limb-girdle (may include several disorders)	Autosomal recessive or autosomal dominant	Onset in early childhood to adulthood. Slowly progressive weakness of shoulder and hip girdle muscles	Cardiomyopathy
Oculopharyngeal	Autosomal dominant (French-Canadian or Hispanic background)	Onset fifth to sixth decade Slowly progressive weakness of extraocular, eyelid, face, and pharyngeal muscles Cricopharyngeal achalasia	
Congenital (includes several disorders including Fukuyama and cerebro-ocular-dysplasia types)	Autosomal recessive	Onset at birth Hypotonia, contractures, and delayed milestones Early respiratory failure in some, static course in others	Cerebral Eye

intellectual function appears to be nonprogressive and affects verbal ability more than performance. IQs of Duchenne patients are lower than children with comparably disabling and chronic disorders, indicating mental subnormality in Duchenne dystrophy is not solely the reflection of physical limitations. The basis for intellectual impairment in Duchenne dystrophy has not been established.

Laboratory investigation   Serum CK levels are invariably elevated between 20 and 100 times normal. The levels are abnormal at birth but decline late in the disease because of inactivity and loss of muscle mass.

Electromyography (EMG) demonstrates features typical of myopathy. The muscle biopsy shows muscle fibers of varying size as well as small groups of necrotic and regenerating fibers. Connective tissue and fat replace lost muscle fibers. A definitive diagnosis of Duchenne dystrophy can be established on the basis of dystrophin deficiency in biopsied muscle tissue or mutation analysis on peripheral blood leukocytes as discussed below.

Genetics   Duchenne dystrophy, inherited as an X-linked recessive trait, is caused by a mutation of the gene responsible for producing dystrophin. The latter is a 427 kDa protein localized to the inner surface of the sarcolemma of the muscle fiber. The dystrophin gene, an estimated 2000 kb in size, is one of the largest identified human genes. It is localized to the short arm of the X chromosome at the Xp21 site. At the present time, mutations of the gene can be identified (in approximately two-thirds of Duchenne patients) using a battery of cDNA probes. Deletions are not uniformly distributed over the gene, but rather occur with a higher frequency near the middle of the gene. Deletion size does not correlate with severity of disease. Gene duplication represents another type of mutation, although less common, leading to Duchenne dystrophy. Identification of a specific mutation provides for an unequivocal diagnosis and makes possible accurate testing of potential carriers and for use of amniotic fluid cells or chorionic villi in prenatal diagnosis. In families without deletions or duplications, linkage analysis using probes recognizing restriction fragment length polymorphisms is also available.

Dystrophin determination of muscle tissue represents an accurate method of diagnosis of Duchenne dystrophy. The amount and alteration in the size of dystrophin can be determined by western blot analysis of muscle biopsy specimens. In addition, immunocytochemical staining of muscle, using antibodies raised against dystrophin, can be used to demonstrate absence or deficiency of dystrophin localizing to the sarcolemmal membrane. Carriers of the disease may demonstrate a mosaic pattern, but dystrophin analysis of muscle biopsies for carrier detection is not reliable.

Treatment   Prednisone in a dose of 0.75 mg/kg per day has been shown to significantly alter the progression of Duchenne dystrophy for up to 3 years. Despite these favorable results, there are patients who clearly cannot tolerate glucocorticoid therapy. The weight gain represents a significant deterrent for some boys. Treatment must be tailored to the individual.

BECKER MUSCULAR DYSTROPHY   This less severe form of X-linked recessive muscular dystrophy was described by Becker and Keiner in 1955. It is often called the benign form of pseudohypertrophic muscular dystrophy. Until recently it was not known whether Duchenne and Becker muscular dystrophies represented genetically distinct disorders. Molecular genetic studies now indicate that Duchenne and Becker dystrophies result from allelic defects of the same gene. Becker muscular dystrophy is approximately 10 times less frequent than Duchenne, with an incidence of about 3 per 100,000.

Clinical features   The pattern of muscle wasting in Becker muscular dystrophy closely resembles that seen in Duchenne. Proximal muscles, especially of the lower extremities, are prominently involved. As the disease progresses, weakness becomes more generalized. Significant facial muscle weakness is not a feature. Hypertrophy of muscles, particularly the calves, is an early and prominent finding.

The majority of Becker patients first experience difficulties between ages 5 and 15 years, although an onset in the third or fourth decade or even later can occur. By definition, Becker patients ambulate beyond age 15, allowing for a clinical distinction between Becker and Duchenne dystrophy. Becker dystrophy patients have a reduced life expectancy, but the majority survive into the fourth or fifth decade.

Mental retardation may be seen in Becker dystrophy, but not as frequently as in Duchenne. Cardiac involvement occurs in Becker dystrophy and may result in heart failure.

Laboratory features   The serum CK, EMG, and muscle biopsy features closely resemble Duchenne dystrophy. The diagnosis of Becker muscular dystrophy requires western blot analysis of muscle biopsy samples demonstrating dystrophin of reduced amount or abnormal size. In addition, in Becker dystrophy mutation analysis of DNA from peripheral blood leukocytes recognizes deletions and duplications of the dystrophin gene in approximately the same number (65 percent) as seen in Duchenne. In both Becker and Duchenne, the size of the DNA deletion does not predict clinical severity; however, in about 95 percent of Becker dystrophy patients DNA deletions do not alter the translational reading frame of messenger RNA. This "in-frame" mutation allows for production of some dystrophin, and accounts for the presence of altered rather than absent dystrophin on western blot analysis.

Phenotypic variations on dystrophin deficiency   The preceding discussion implies a clear delineation between typical Duchenne and Becker patients, but in actuality there is a spectrum of muscle weakness ranging from very severe to very mild. A well-recognized subgroup of patients have clinical characteristics intermediate between Duchenne and Becker dystrophy patients. On western blot studies of muscle biopsy, intermediate phenotypic patients show dystrophin of reduced amounts or abnormal size similar to Becker dystrophy.

Treatment   The use of prednisone has not been adequately studied in Becker dystrophy and other mild dystrophin-deficiency disorders.

MYOTONIC DYSTROPHY   This condition was originally described by Steinert in 1909 and represents the most common adult muscular dystrophy. This disorder has an incidence of 13.5 per 100,000 live births and involves an equal proportion of males and females.

Clinical features   The clinical expression of myotonic dystrophy varies widely and affects many systems other than muscle. Myotonic dystrophy patients have a typical "hatchet-faced" appearance due to temporalis, masseter, and facial muscle atrophy and weakness. Men have frontal baldness and women often have a balding hair pattern. Neck muscles, including the flexors and sternocleidomastoids, become involved early as do distal limb muscles. Weakness of wrist extensors, finger extensors, and intrinsic hand muscles impairs function. Ankle dorsiflexor weakness may cause footdrop. Proximal muscles remain stronger throughout the course, although preferential atrophy and weakness of quadriceps muscles occurs in many patients. Palatal, pharyngeal, and tongue involvement produces a dysarthric speech, nasal voice, and swallowing problems. Some patients have diaphragm and intercostal muscle weakness, resulting in respiratory insufficiency.

Myotonia, which usually appears by age 5, is demonstrable by percussion of thenar eminence, tongue, and wrist extensor muscles. Myotonia causes a slow relaxation of hand grip following a forced voluntary closure. Advanced muscle wasting makes myotonia more difficult to detect.

Congenital myotonic dystrophy is a more severe form of the disease occurring in approximately 25 percent of infants of affected mothers. It is characterized by severe facial and bulbar weakness and neonatal respiratory insufficiency. Most patients will recover from respiratory distress. Congenital myotonic dystrophy patients usually have impaired intelligence.

Cardiac disturbances occur in the majority of patients with myotonic dystrophy. Electrocardiographic abnormalities are common, including first degree heart block or more extensive conduction system involvement. Complete heart block and sudden death can occur. Congestive heart failure occurs infrequently, but may result from cor pulmonale secondary to respiratory failure. Mitral valve prolapse also occurs commonly in myotonic dystrophy patients.

Other features associated with myotonic dystrophy include intellectual impairment, hypersomnia, posterior subcapsular cataracts, gonadal atrophy, insulin resistance and decreased esophageal and colonic motility.

Laboratory features   The diagnosis of myotonic dystrophy can usually be made on clinical grounds alone and seldom requires laboratory studies. Serum CK levels may be normal or mildly elevated. EMG evidence of myotonia will be found readily in most cases by EMG. Muscle biopsy shows muscle atrophy, selectively involving type 1 fibers in 50 percent of cases. Typically, increased numbers of central nuclei can be seen. Necrosis of muscle fibers and increased connective tissue, common in other muscular dystrophies, do not usually occur in myotonic dystrophy.

Genetics   Myotonic dystrophy is an autosomal dominant disorder. Evidence indicates that new mutations do not contribute to the pool of affected individuals. The disorder is transmitted by a mutant gene on the long arm of chromosome 19. Studies now indicate that, at 19q13.3, patients with myotonic dystrophy demonstrate an unstable region of DNA characterized by an increased number of trinucleotide CTG repeats. An increase in the severity of the disease phenotype in successive generations (genetic anticipation) is accompanied by an increase in the number of trinucleotide repeats. A similar type of mutation has been identified in fragile X syndrome (see Chap. 378). The unstable triplet repeat in myotonic dystrophy can be used for prenatal diagnosis. The greater severity of disease in the affected infants of mothers with myotonic dystrophy remains unexplained.

The protein encoded by the myotonic dystrophy gene has an amino acid composition homologous to a protein kinase (referred to as myotonin-protein kinase).

Treatment   Myotonia in other forms of myotonic disorders such as myotonia congenita responds well to treatment. Myotonia in myotonic dystrophy, however, rarely warrants treatment. Phenytoin represents the preferred agent for the occasional patient who requires an antimyotonia drug; other agents, particularly quinine and procainamide may worsen cardiac conduction. Cardiac pacemaker insertion should be considered for patients with unexplained syncope or advanced conduction system abnormalities with evidence of second degree heart block or trifascicular conduction disturbances with marked prolongation of the PR interval.

Molded ankle-foot orthoses, for controlling footdrop and stabilizing the ankle, will help prevent patients with distal lower extremity weakness from falling.

FACIOSCAPULOHUMERAL MUSCULAR DYSTROPHY   This form of muscular dystrophy, also called *Landouzy-Dejerine dystrophy*, has an incidence of approximately 1 in 20,000.

Clinical features   The condition typically has an onset in childhood and young adult years. In most cases, facial weakness represents the initial manifestation, appearing as an inability to smile, whistle, or fully close the eyes. Weakness of the shoulder girdles, rather than facial muscles, usually brings the patient to medical attention. Loss of scapular stabilizer muscles makes arm elevation difficult. Scapular winging becomes apparent with attempts at abduction and forward movement of the arms. Biceps and triceps muscles may be severely affected with relative sparing of the deltoid muscles. Weakness of wrist extension invariably exceeds that of wrist flexion and weakness of the anterior compartment muscles of the legs may lead to footdrop.

In the majority of patients, the weakness remains restricted to facial, upper extremity, and distal lower extremity muscles. In 20 percent of cases, weakness progresses to involve the pelvic girdle muscles and severe functional impairment and possible wheelchair confinement result.

Characteristically, patients with facioscapulohumeral dystrophy do not have involvement of other organ systems, although labile hypertension is common and there is an increased incidence of nerve deafness.

Laboratory features   Serum CK may be normal or mildly elevated. EMG usually indicates a myopathic pattern. The muscle biopsy shows nonspecific features of a myopathy. A prominent inflammatory infiltrate, which is often multifocal in distribution, is present in some biopsies. The cause or significance of this finding is unknown.

Genetics   An autosomal dominant inheritance pattern with almost complete penetrance has been established, but requires examination of each family member for confirmation since approximately 30 percent of those affected will be unaware of involvement. The gene for facioscapulohumeral dystrophy is on the distal long arm of chromosome 4. A genetic probe localized to the site of the gene has been found so that carrier detection and prenatal diagnosis are possible. Studies with this probe indicate that most sporadic cases represent new mutations.

Treatment No specific treatment is available; ankle-foot orthoses are helpful for those with footdrop. Scapular stabilization procedures improve scapular winging, but may not improve function.

LIMB-GIRDLE DYSTROPHY This term which encompasses more than one disorder, is used to describe muscle weakness occurring in both males and females with onset ranging from late in the first decade to the fourth decade. Both autosomal recessive and autosomal dominant inheritance are found, and variable rates of progression occur. From a practical viewpoint, limb-girdle dystrophy groups together patients who defy classification into one of the better defined groups.

Clinical features In limb-girdle dystrophy, the initial symptoms of weakness of the proximal leg muscles usually begin in the second or third decade. Upper limb involvement with scapular winging appears later. The onset may be delayed until the third or fourth decade. Respiratory insufficiency from diaphragm weakness may occur. Distribution of weakness and rate of progression varies from family to family.

In some patients, cardiac involvement results in congestive heart failure or arrhythmias; occasional patients may present with a cardiomyopathy. Intellectual function remains normal.

Laboratory features Elevated serum CK, a myopathic EMG, and muscle biopsy features indicative of myopathy represent the characteristic changes in limb-girdle dystrophy. Careful attention to exclude phenotypically similar disorders such as spinal muscular atrophy and metabolic and inflammatory myopathies is required. The availability of western blot analysis for dystrophin allows for definite distinction of limb-girdle dystrophy from Becker muscular dystrophy.

Genetics Autosomal recessive or autosomal dominant inheritance may occur, depending on individual families. One variety of autosomal dominant limb-girdle dystrophy has been linked to chromosome 5. In another, inherited as a childhood autosomal recessive condition, a deficiency has been identified in one of the dystrophin-associated glycoproteins, which are a large complex of sarcolemmal glycoproteins linking dystrophin to the extracellular matrix.

Treatment No specific treatment can be offered.

OCULOPHARYNGEAL DYSTROPHY The term *progressive external ophthalmoplegia* (PEO) describes disorders characterized by slowly progressive ptosis and limitation of eye movements with sparing of pupillary reactions for light and accommodation. Patients usually do not complain of diplopia, in contrast to conditions with a more acute onset of ocular muscle weakness (e.g., myasthenia gravis). Oculopharyngeal muscular dystrophy represents one of the distinct disorders presenting with PEO. Two other disorders, centronuclear myopathy and mitochondrial myopathies with PEO, are discussed below.

Clinical features Oculopharyngeal muscular dystrophy usually presents with ptosis and/or dysphagia in the fourth to sixth decade. The swallowing problem may become debilitating and result in pooling of secretions and repeated episodes of aspiration. Mild neck and extremity weakness also occur.

Laboratory features The serum CK may be 2 to 3 times normal. A myopathic EMG is typical. On biopsy muscle fibers contain vacuoles, which by electron microscopy are shown to contain membranous whorls, accumulation of glycogen, and other nonspecific debris related to lysosomes. A distinct feature of oculopharyngeal dystrophy is the presence of tubular filaments, 8.5 nm in diameter, within muscle nuclei.

Genetics Oculopharyngeal dystrophy has an autosomal dominant inheritance pattern with complete penetrance. French-Canadians repre-

sent a commonly affected ethnic group. The disorder also occurs with increased frequency in Spanish-American families of the southwest United States. A large Jewish kindred of eastern European background has been reported.

Treatment Dysphagia can cause inanition and makes oculopharyngeal muscular dystrophy a potentially life-threatening disease. Cricopharyngeal myotomy may improve swallowing, although it does not prevent aspiration. Eyelid crutches can improve vision in patients in whom ptosis obstructs vision; candidates for ptosis surgery must be carefully selected; those with severe facial weakness are not suitable.

CONGENITAL MUSCULAR DYSTROPHY This rare disorder includes one or more genetic diseases; clinically, cases can be divided into a group having associated central nervous system involvement and one with only skeletal muscle disease.

Clinical features One form of congenital muscular dystrophy presents at birth or in the first few months of life with hypotonia, proximal limb weakness, and joint contractures at the elbows, hips, knees, and ankles. Contractures present at birth are referred to as *arthrogryposis*. Weakness of facial muscles may occur, but other cranial nerve musculature is spared. Severity varies greatly, but about half of the affected never achieve the ability to stand independently. Death may ensue because of respiratory insufficiency early in life. Some patients learn to walk, although difficulty in motor activities (e.g., running) persist.

In other forms of congenital muscular dystrophy patients have CNS involvement. A well-defined type is *Fukuyama congenital muscular dystrophy* associated with generalized tonic-clonic seizures and developmental delay in both verbal and mental spheres. Microcephaly and enlarged ventricles occur. A third variant, *cerebro-ocular-dysplasia muscular dystrophy*, has corneal abnormalities, cataracts, retinal dysplasia, and hypoplasia of the optic nerve. Hypomyelination of the cerebral white matter may be seen in patients with congenital muscular dystrophies.

Laboratory features Serum CK elevations range from normal to 20 times normal. The EMG shows a myopathic pattern and muscle biopsy features are nonspecific but demonstrate dystrophic features. Dystrophin analysis must be done on all cases of congenital muscular dystrophy to permit distinction from early-onset Duchenne muscular dystrophy.

Genetics Sporadic occurrences account for most of the cases of congenital muscular dystrophy without CNS involvement. Autosomal recessive inheritance has been established as the major mode of transmission for Fukuyama congenital muscular dystrophy and cerebro-ocular-dysplasia muscular dystrophy. In the Fukuyama-type, there is abnormal expression of dystrophin-associated proteins.

Treatment Supportive care and especially stretching to improve joint range of motion is important for congenital muscular dystrophies. Infants and very young children require special wheelchair modifications and adaptive seating to maximize functional capabilities.

DISTAL MYOPATHIES Patients with predominantly distal weakness and histologic evidence favoring muscular dystrophy are difficult to classify. Four of these disorders fulfill the definition of "muscular dystrophy" because of their hereditary nature and progressive course, although in the literature they are referred to as distal myopathies.

These distal myopathies can be separated into two late adult-onset types and two early adult-onset types.

The most familiar late-onset form was described by Welander. This disorder is seen predominantly in Scandinavian families. It is inherited as an autosomal dominant condition with onset in the fifth decade. Weakness begins in the hands with distal leg muscle involvement occurring later in the course. The lower extremity involvement begins in muscles of the distal anterior compartment (anterior tibial and peroneal muscle groups). The serum CK is either normal or mildly increased in this condition. Muscle biopsy changes are myopathic with some muscle fibers showing vacuoles.

Another late adult-onset form of distal myopathy is also inherited as an autosomal dominant trait but occurs in non-Scandinavian patients. Weakness begins in the anterior compartment of the distal lower extremities. Serum CK is normal or mildly elevated. Muscle biopsies from these patients reveal a myopathy with many fibers showing vacuoles.

Both of the early adult-onset distal myopathies have autosomal recessive inheritance. In one type, the weakness begins in the anterior compartment of the distal lower extremities, although in some cases it may begin in the hands. The serum CK is moderately elevated (less than 10 times normal) and muscle biopsies reveal a myopathy with many fibers showing vacuoles. The other form of early adult-onset distal myopathy is distinguished by weakness beginning in the posterior compartment, i.e., the gastrocnemius muscle. Serum CK is markedly elevated in this latter form (greater than 10 times normal) and biopsy shows a myopathy without vacuolated fibers. This condition with predilection for gastrocnemius weakness has been referred to as *Miyoshi myopathy*.

CONGENITAL MYOPATHIES

These rare disorders are distinguished from muscular dystrophies by the presence of specific histochemical and structural abnormalities in muscle. The description was originally introduced to distinguish nonprogressive muscle disease present at birth from muscular dystrophy which is progressive. Congenital myopathies can be severe and even fatal. Three major types are described: *central core disease, nemaline (rod) myopathy,* and *centronuclear (myotubular) myopathy.* Other rare types such as multicore disease, fingerprint body myopathy, and sarcotubular myopathy are not discussed here (see Banker).

CENTRAL CORE DISEASE   Clinical features Patients with central core disease may have decreased fetal movements and breech presentation. Skeletal abnormalities include congenital hip dislocation, scoliosis, and pes cavus; clubbed feet also occur. Hypotonia and delayed motor milestones, particularly walking, occur. Later in childhood, patients develop problems with stair climbing, running, and getting up from the floor. On examination there is mild facial and neck flexor weakness as well as weakness of the proximal extremity muscles, particularly in the legs. Most cases are nonprogressive but exceptions are well documented.

Laboratory features Serum CK is usually normal. Needle EMG demonstrates a myopathic pattern. The muscle biopsy is diagnostic, showing fibers with single or multiple central or eccentric discrete zones (cores) devoid of oxidative enzymes, and diminished PAS staining.

Genetics Autosomal dominant inheritance is characteristic; sporadic cases also occur. The gene for central core disease has been localized to the long arm of chromosome 19.

Treatment Patients with central core disease usually do not require specific treatment; however, recognition of the disease is important since there is a well-established predisposition for malignant hyperthermia during general anesthesia.

NEMALINE MYOPATHY The term *nemaline* refers to the distinctive presence of rods or coils of thread-like structures (*nema* = thread in Greek) in muscle fibers.

Clinical features Severe neonatal hypotonia with early respiratory distress may occur. A delay in motor milestones is common. The physical appearance may be striking because of the long, narrow facies or head, high arched palate, and open-mouthed appearance due to a prognathous jaw. Other skeletal abnormalities include pectus excavatum, kyphoscoliosis, pes cavus, and clubbed foot deformities. Facial and generalized muscle weakness commonly occur. The course is variable; some exhibit a static or nonprogressive course while others progress to wheelchair confinement. The disease may be fatal in infancy or childhood.

Myocardial involvement represents an unusual manifestation of nemaline myopathy which has been associated with an adult-onset form of the disease.

Laboratory features Serum CK is usually normal or slightly elevated. The EMG in weak muscles demonstrates a myopathic pattern with occasional fibrillation potentials. The muscle biopsy is diagnostic, demonstrating clusters of small rods or nemaline bodies. Rods occur preferentially, but not exclusively, in type 1 muscle fibers and the biopsies often show type 1 muscle fiber predominance. Rods originate from the Z disk material of the muscle fiber.

Genetics Evidence favors autosomal dominant inheritance with incomplete penetrance; sporadic cases also occur.

Treatment No specific treatment exists for this condition; some patients require bracing or surgery for the scoliosis as well as ankle-foot orthoses for distal lower extremity weakness.

CENTRONUCLEAR MYOPATHY   Clinical features Three distinct variants of the disease occur. *A neonatal form of centronuclear myopathy* presents with severe hypotonia and weakness at birth. Respiratory assistance may be required and swallowing difficulties may necessitate a feeding tube. This form of the disease carries a poor prognosis, often with a fatal outcome. The *late infantile–early childhood form of centronuclear myopathy* presents without difficulty at birth, but delayed motor milestones, especially walking, occur. Later, difficulty with running and stair climbing become apparent. Ptosis and varying degrees of ophthalmoplegia represent important distinguishing features of this congenital myopathy. A marfanoid appearance, slender body habitus, long narrow face, and high arched palate are typical. Scoliosis and clubbed feet may be present. The condition may be static or progress to weakness, requiring a wheelchair. A third rare variant, the *late childhood–adult type of centronuclear myopathy* has an onset in the second or third decade. Patients have full extraocular muscle movements and rarely exhibit ptosis. Patients have mild, nonprogressive limb weakness and no associated skeletal abnormalities.

Laboratory features Normal or slightly elevated CK levels occur in each of the forms of centronuclear myopathy. EMG studies are distinctive, showing positive sharp waves and fibrillation potentials, complex and repetitive discharges and myotonic discharges. Muscle biopsy in longitudinal section demonstrates rows of central nuclei, often surrounded by a halo. In transverse sections, central nuclei are found in 25 to 80 percent of muscle fibers.

Genetics Indisputable evidence for X-linked recessive inheritance exists in the neonatal form of centronuclear myopathy. The gene for the X-linked form has been localized to Xq28 allowing for identification of carriers. In the late infantile–early childhood disorder evidence favors autosomal recessive inheritance, and the late childhood–adult form of centronuclear myopathy has an autosomal dominant inheritance pattern.

Treatment Patients with a neonatal form of centronuclear myopathy require careful management for respiratory support and gastric feeding. For patients with the late infantile–early childhood disorder, ambulatory aids and orthotic devices and less often wheelchairs may be necessary. Occasional patients benefit from scoliosis surgery.

DISORDERS OF MUSCLE ENERGY METABOLISM

Skeletal muscle utilizes two principal sources of energy—fatty acids and glucose. Abnormalities in either glucose or lipid utilization can be associated with distinct clinical presentations. The clinical presentation can range from an acute painful syndrome with rhabdomyolysis and myoglobinuria to a chronic progressive muscle weakness simulating muscular dystrophy.

GLYCOGEN STORAGE AND GLYCOLYTIC DEFECTS There are four major disorders of glycogen metabolism (types II, III, IV, and V) and four disorders of glycolysis (types VII, IX, X, and XI) associated with significant skeletal muscle manifestations (see Chap. 350).

ACID MALTASE DEFICIENCY (TYPE II GLYCOGENOSIS) Acid maltase is an acid hydrolase lysosomal enzyme, with α-1,4- and α-1,6- glucosidase activity that breaks down glycogen to glucose.

Clinical features   Three clinical forms of acid maltase deficiency can be distinguished. *Infantile acid maltase deficiency* is the most common, with onset of symptoms in 3 months of life. Infants develop severe muscle weakness, cardiomegaly, hepatomegaly, and respiratory insufficiency. Glycogen accumulation in motor neurons of the spinal cord and brainstem contributes to muscle weakness. Death usually occurs by 1 year of age. In *childhood acid maltase deficiency* the picture resembles muscular dystrophy. Delayed motor milestones result from proximal limb muscle weakness and involvement of respiratory muscles. The heart may be involved, but the liver and brain are unaffected. The *adult form of acid maltase deficiency* begins in the third or fourth decade. Respiratory failure and diaphragmatic weakness are often initial manifestations heralding progressive proximal muscle weakness. The heart and liver are not involved.

Laboratory findings   Serum CK is usually elevated (2 to 10 times normal). EMG examination demonstrates a myopathic pattern, but other features are especially distinctive including: myotonic discharges; trains of fibrillation and positive waves; and complex repetitive discharges. At times, these special EMG discharges are very prominent in the lumbosacral paraspinal muscles. The muscle biopsy shows vacuoles containing glycogen and the lysosomal enzyme acid phosphatase. By electron microscopy, membrane-bound and free tissue glycogen are found. Definitive diagnosis is established by enzyme determination in muscle.

Genetics   The three forms of acid maltase deficiency are all transmitted as an autosomal recessive trait. The gene, localized to the long arm of chromosome 17, has been isolated and sequenced making possible prenatal diagnosis for acid maltase deficiency.

Treatment   No adequate method of replacing enzyme has been established, nor is dietary treatment of proven efficacy.

DEBRANCHER ENZYME (TYPE III GLYCOGENOSIS)   The complete degradation of glycogen via the phosphorylytic pathway requires debranching enzyme. Absence of this enzyme results in a lesser proportion of muscle glycogen availability.

Clinical features   The most common presentation of debrancher enzyme deficiency is the appearance of hepatomegaly, growth retardation, and hypoglycemia. Muscle involvement is often inconspicuous, although hypotonia and delayed motor milestones may be present. These findings usually diminish or disappear after puberty and a slowly progressive form of muscle weakness can develop in adult life. Rarely, myoglobinuria may be seen.

Laboratory features   Serum CK is elevated. Forearm exercise test shows no rise in venous lactate. The muscle biopsy demonstrates subsarcolemmal and intermyofibrillar accumulation of glycogen. The definitive diagnosis is established by enzyme analysis of muscle (or liver).

Genetics   Debrancher enzyme deficiency is inherited as an autosomal recessive trait.

Treatment   No specific form of treatment for debrancher enzyme deficiency has been identified. Avoidance of hypoglycemia during episodes of intercurrent infection is necessary. Occasional patients require treatment for congestive heart failure.

BRANCHING ENZYME DEFICIENCY (TYPE IV GLYCOGENOSIS)   This is a rare and fatal glycogen storage disease.

Clinical features   This disorder is characterized by failure to thrive and hepatomegaly. Hypotonia and muscle wasting may be present, but the skeletal muscle manifestations are relatively minor compared to liver failure.

Laboratory features   Diagnosis is usually established by demonstrating branching enzyme deficiency in skin fibroblasts or peripheral blood leukocytes.

Genetics   The disorder is inherited as an autosomal recessive trait.

Treatment   One patient has been successfully treated by liver transplantation.

MUSCLE PHOSPHORYLASE DEFICIENCY (TYPE V GLYCOGENOSIS)   The clinical description of myophosphorylase deficiency, in 1951 by McArdle, led to later identification of enzyme defect.

Clinical features   Exercise intolerance is the dominant feature of the disorder. Symptoms usually occur first in adolescence with muscle pain and fatigue following intense exercise such as running or lifting heavy objects. Many patients report a "second-wind phenomenon" if they rest briefly or reduce intensity during the exercise, allowing them to continue activities for a longer period of time. Overexertion may lead to rhabdomyolysis and myoglobinuria, and renal failure can result. Variance of the classic presentation occurs, with some patients reporting only fatigability, others, having progressive weakness, and rare patients presenting with severe weakness and respiratory failure in infancy.

In the usual patients with McArdle's disease, examination between attacks is normal. Other organs are not affected.

Laboratory findings   Serum CK levels fluctuate widely and may be elevated even during symptom-free periods. The forearm exercise test shows no rise in lactic acid; such testing is an important part of the evaluation of patients with myoglobinuria. The EMG is often normal except when taken after an episode of rhabdomyolysis, when muscle irritability (fibrillation potentials and positive waves) may be present. Muscle biopsy often shows subsarcolemmal blebs, containing glycogen, and absence of histochemical myophosphorylase staining; findings should be confirmed biochemically.

Genetics   Myophosphorylase deficiency is usually inherited as an autosomal recessive trait with an unexplained predilection for men. The gene for muscle phosphorylase has been localized to the long arm of chromosome 11.

Treatment   Patients can remain moderately active once they establish their limitations. Dietary supplementation with either glucose or fructose has not alleviated symptoms.

PHOSPHORYLASE b KINASE DEFICIENCY   Muscle phosphorylase exists in two forms: phosphorylase a, the active enzyme initiating glycogen breakdown; and the inactive form, phosphorylase b. Phosphorylase b kinase converts inactive to active phosphorylase. Phosphorylase b kinase deficiency is a rare disorder with heterogeneous presentations. Children have weakness and liver enlargement and adults may have exercise intolerance and myoglobinuria. The inheritance pattern of muscle phosphorylase b kinase deficiency has not been established.

PHOSPHOFRUCTOKINASE DEFICIENCY (TYPE VII GLYCOGENOSIS)   This condition is less common than McArdle's disease but has similar manifestations.

Clinical features   Myalgias and fatigue occur following exercise and represent the predominant clinical manifestations. Unlike McArdle's disease, patients with phosphofructokinase (PFK) deficiency may worsen with carbohydrate ingestion. Patients present with rhabdomyolysis and myoglobinuria. Permanent limb weakness is less common than in McArdle's disease. Because of erythrocyte deficiency of PFK, a mild hemolytic anemia often occurs and may be useful in diagnosis.

Laboratory findings   Elevated serum CK is often found. Reticulocytosis is a common feature, as is slight anemia and elevated bilirubin. The muscle biopsy shows subsarcolemmal blebs containing glycogen. A histochemical stain for phosphofructokinase can demonstrate the deficiency, but the definitive diagnosis requires biochemical analysis of muscle.

Genetics   PFK deficiency is transmitted as an autosomal recessive trait. The disorder has an unusually strong male predominance and has an over representation in Ashkenazic Jews.

Treatment   The anemia of PFK deficiency usually requires no treatment. Dietary manipulation does not alter muscle symptoms.

PHOSPHOGLYCERATE KINASE DEFICIENCY (TYPE IV GLYCOGENOSIS)   **Clinical features**   The clinical features of phosphoglycerate kinase (PGK) deficiency usually manifest as a nonspherocytic hemolytic anemia. Central nervous system dysfunction with mental retardation and seizures has been described. A rare variant of

PGK deficiency can also present with exercise intolerance and myoglobinuria.

Laboratory features   Serum CK levels can be elevated. The forearm exercise test shows reduced levels of venous lactate compared to controls. The muscle biopsy shows a mild increase in glycogen. Muscle biochemistry confirms the diagnosis.

Genetics   PGK deficiency is transmitted as an X-linked recessive trait. The gene is located on the short arm of the X chromosome.

Treatment   No specific treatment is available. In patients with hemolytic anemia, splenectomy may be beneficial.

PHOSPHOGLYCERATE MUTASE DEFICIENCY (TYPE X GLYCOGENOSIS)   Clinical features   In this rare disorder, patients present with myalgia, muscle cramping, and myoglobinuria following intense exercise. No other organ system involvement occurs.

Laboratory findings   Serum CK levels are elevated and the forearm exercise test reveals a reduced rise in venous lactate.

Genetics   The inheritance pattern is probably autosomal recessive, although no multigeneration families or sibs have yet been described.

Treatment   No specific treatment is available.

LACTIC DEHYDROGENASE DEFICIENCY (GLYCOGENOSIS TYPE XI)   Lactic dehydrogenase (LDH) is a tetrameric enzyme composed of two subunits, M and H. M-subunit isoenzymes predominate in skeletal muscle, while H-subunit–containing isoenzymes are the main components of LDH in heart.

Clinical features   Patients with LDH-M deficiency have exercise intolerance, muscle pain, and myoglobinuria in the teenage years. No other organ system is involved.

Laboratory findings   Serum CK is expectedly high during myoglobinuria, but there is a failure of serum LDH to rise. This corresponds to the defect of LDH-M. Forearm exercise test produces a minimal rise of lactic acid, but serum pyruvate rises substantially, pointing to the defect involved in conversion of pyruvate to lactate. The diagnosis can be confirmed by the biochemical analysis of muscle tissue showing markedly decreased LDH-M subunit. The M subunit can also be shown to be decreased in erythrocytes and leukocytes, although these other tissues are composed of combinations of the two subunits, M and H of LDH.

Genetics   The disease appears to be inherited as an autosomal recessive trait. The M subunit of LDH is localized to chromosome 11. A deficiency of the H subunit of LDH, the cardiac isoform, has been described but is not associated with skeletal muscle symptoms.

Treatment   Currently no treatment is available for this disorder.

DISORDERS OF LIPID METABOLISM

Lipid is an important muscle energy source during rest and prolonged, submaximal exercise. Fatty acids are derived from circulating very low density lipoprotein (VLDL) in the blood or from triglycerides stored in muscle fibers. Oxidation of fatty acids occurs in the mitochondria. In order to enter the mitochondria, fatty acids must first be converted to an "active fatty acid," acyl-CoA. The fatty acid acyl-CoA must be linked with carnitine by the enzyme carnitine palmityoltransferase 1 (CPT 1) for transport into the mitochondria. CPT 1 is present on the inner side of the outer mitochondrial membrane. Carnitine is removed by CPT 2, an enzyme attached to the inside of the inner mitochondrial membrane, allowing transport of acyl-CoA into the mitochondrial matrix for β-oxidation.

CARNITINE DEFICIENCY   Deficiency of this important substrate results in a myopathic and systemic disorder.

Myopathic carnitine deficiency is associated with generalized muscle weakness, usually beginning in childhood. The clinical features overlap with muscular dystrophy and polymyositis. Patients develop progressive, painless proximal weakness. A severe cardiomyopathy may be present. Serum CK levels may be mildly to markedly (greater than 10 times) elevated. The muscle biopsy shows striking lipid accumulation. Serum carnitine is normal. The cause for decreased muscle carnitine is not understood. Most cases are sporadic, but the inheritance pattern is thought to be autosomal recessive. Some patients respond to oral carnitine supplement; this should be tried in all cases. Other patients have responded to prednisone, riboflavin, or propranolol. A diet substituting medium-chain for long-chain triglycerides has been helpful in some cases.

Systemic carnitine deficiency usually presents in infancy and early childhood and is characterized by progressive weakness and episodes of hepatic encephalopathy with nausea, vomiting, confusion, coma, and early death. Carnitine levels are reduced in muscle, liver, kidney, and heart, but the low serum carnitine levels are especially useful in distinguishing this condition from the myopathic form. No single cause has been identified to explain the low serum carnitine levels. Decreased hepatic synthesis explains some cases, while increased urinary excretion is seen in others. Serum CK levels may be slightly elevated. The muscle biopsy may show lipid storage. In some cases, the liver, heart, and kidney will show increased lipid. Treatment with oral carnitine supplements or glucocorticoid has helped some, but not all, patients.

Secondary carnitine deficiency accompanies a variety of disorders in which carnitine deficiency is accounted for by decreased synthesis (cirrhosis), insufficient intake (parenteral nutrition), and excessive loss (renal dialysis, Fanconi's syndrome, or organic acidemia). Carnitine deficiency may also be seen in the muscular dystrophies, thought to be a nonspecific result of loss of muscle tissue. Carnitine treatment has not been shown to clearly benefit patients with these secondary syndromes.

CARNITINE PALMITYOLTRANSFERASE DEFICIENCY (CPT)   This disorder is the most common recognizable cause of recurrent myoglobinuria, more common than the glycolytic defects.

Clinical features   This disorder usually has its onset in teenage years or in the early twenties. Muscle pain and myoglobinuria occur after prolonged exercise. Fasting predisposes to the development of symptoms. In contrast to defects in glycolysis where muscle cramps follow short intense bursts of exercise, the muscle pain in CPT deficiency does not occur until the limits of utilization have been exceeded and muscle breakdown has already begun. Episodes of rhabdomyolysis may produce severe weakness. In contrast to carnitine deficiency, strength is normal between attacks.

Laboratory findings   Serum CK and EMG are both usually normal between episodes. Normal rise of venous lactate during forearm exercise distinguishes this condition from glycolytic defects, especially phosphorylase deficiency. The muscle biopsy does not show lipid accumulation and is usually normal between attacks. The diagnosis requires direct measurement of muscle CPT.

Genetics   CPT deficiency is most commonly a sporadic condition of men although the disorder is thought to be transmitted as an autosomal recessive trait.

Treatment   It has been suggested that frequent meals and a low-fat, high-carbohydrate diet can prolong exercise tolerance. Others suggest substituting medium-chain triglycerides in the diet. Neither approach has proven benefits.

MYOADENYLATE DEAMINASE DEFICIENCY   The muscle enzyme myoadenylate deaminase converts 5′ adenosine monophosphate (5′AMP) to inosine monophosphate (IMP) with liberation of ammonia. Myoadenylate deaminase may play a role in regulating adenosine triphophosphate (ATP) levels in muscle. In 1978, a group of patients with myalgias and exercise intolerance were found to be deficient in myoadenylate deaminase. The deficiency, however, has been found to occur as an incidental finding in as many as 1 percent of muscle biopsies detected by histochemical staining of muscle tissue. Muscle ammonia production is decreased following forearm exercise in patients deficient in myoadenylate deaminase.

Most subjects with myoadenylate deaminase deficiency have no symptoms. In patients with myalgia and fatigue associated with myoadenylate deaminase deficiency, the cause-and-effect relationship between muscle symptoms and enzyme deficiency remains unclear. There have been numerous questions raised about the clinical effects of myoadenylate deaminase deficiency and specifically the relationship to exertional myalgia and fatigability. No consistent agreement exists. There have been a few patients described with myoglobinuria and a report of two brothers with exercise-exacerbated myalgia and myoglobinuria. At present, it can only be concluded that the full clinical significance of myoadenylate deaminase deficiency has not been established.

MITOCHONDRIAL MYOPATHIES

The mitochondrial myopathies represent a heterogeneous group of diseases recognized by abnormal muscle fibers, called *ragged red fibers,* which have accumulations of abnormal mitochondria. The name "ragged red fiber" is derived from characteristics observed in modified trichrome staining of fresh frozen muscle in which mitochondria accumulations appear red. By electron microscopy, the mitochondria in ragged red fibers are enlarged, often bizarre-shaped, and have distorted cristae and crystalline inclusions.

Mitochondria play a key role in energy production. Oxidation of the major food stuffs derived from carbohydrate, fat, and protein leads to the generation of reducing equivalents (2H). The latter are transported through the respiratory chain in the process known as oxidative phosphorylation, responsible for the generation of ATP. The respiratory chain is composed of four multienzyme complexes: complex I (NADH, coenzyme Q oxidoreductase); complex II (succinate, coenzyme Q oxidoreductase); complex III (coenzyme Q, cytochrome c oxidoreductase); and complex IV (cytochrome c oxidase). In addition, there are two low molecular weight redox carriers, coenzyme Q and cytochrome c. The energy generated by the oxidation-reduction reactions of the respiratory chain is stored in an electrochemical gradient coupled to ATP synthesis from ADP by the enzyme ATP synthetase or complex V.

A novel feature of mitochondria is their genetic composition. Each mitochondrion possesses DNA genomes that are distinct from nuclear DNA. Mitochondrial DNA (mtDNA) consists of a double-stranded, circular DNA molecule composed of 16,569 base pairs. mtDNA codes for 22 transfer RNAs, 2 ribosomal RNAs, and 13 polypeptides of the respiratory chain enzymes. Complex I, made up of 25 polypeptides, has 7 encoded by mtDNA; complex III has 1 of 11 encoded from mtDNA; complex IV includes 13 polypeptides, 3 derived from mtDNA; 2 of the 12 polypeptides of complex V arise from mtDNA. Only polypeptides of complex II have no mtDNA contribution.

The genetics of mitochondrial diseases differ from those of chromosomal disorders. The DNA of mitochondria is directly inherited from the cytoplasm of germline cells, mainly the oocyte. The sperm contributes very little of its mitochondria to the offspring at the time of fertilization. Thus, mitochondrial genes are derived almost exclusively from the mother, accounting for maternal inheritance of mitochondrial disorders.

PROGRESSIVE EXTERNAL OPHTHALMOPLEGIA (PEO) SYNDROMES AND RAGGED RED FIBERS   Most patients with fixed, nonfluctuating, insidiously progressive ptosis and ophthalmoplegia have a mitochondrial myopathy.

Kearns-Sayre syndrome   This disorder has its onset before age 20, and importantly, has no family history. The characteristic findings are a triad of clinical features: PEO, pigmentary degeneration of the retina, and heart block. The Kearns-Sayre syndrome may also include other features: ataxia, hearing loss, dementia, short stature, delayed secondary sexual characteristics, hypoparathyroidism, hypothyroidism, and peripheral neuropathy.

The diagnosis is established by muscle biopsy which demonstrates ragged red fibers. In addition, the mtDNA extracted from the muscle may demonstrate two populations (heteroplasmy): one demonstrates variable size mtDNA deletions and the other is normal in size.

The size of the mtDNA deletions do not correlate with clinical manifestations.

Kearns-Sayre syndrome represents a sporadic, noninherited disease. Mutations leading to an affected individual are thought to take place in the fertilized ovum.

Familial PEO syndrome   The clinical features of this disorder, in contrast to the Kearns-Sayre syndrome, are restricted to muscle without other organ system involvement. Varying degrees of PEO and proximal limb weakness occur. Rarely, the weakness may advance to wheelchair confinement. Mutations of mtDNA responsible for this condition have not as yet been identified.

A rare form of familial PEO has been found to be inherited as an autosomal dominant trait. The patients have ragged red fibers on muscle biopsy and multiple mtDNA deletions. The mutation accounting for the autosomal dominant inheritance occurs in a *nuclear* gene that encodes a protein involved in the control of mtDNA replication. A failure or disruption of binding of this nuclear-encoded protein during mtDNA replication results in multiple deletions.

MYOCLONIC EPILEPSY AND RAGGED RED FIBERS   This disorder, called the *MERRF syndrome,* consists of mitochondrial myopathy, myoclonus, generalized seizures, intellectual deterioration, ataxia, and hearing loss. PEO does not occur in MERRF. As with other mitochondrial disorders, individuals display varying manifestations of the disease. MERRF syndrome is maternally inherited. In most patients, a defect in mtDNA has been identified as a point mutation in the transfer RNA gene for lysine (tRNA^{lys}) of mtDNA. This abnormality can be detected in mtDNA isolated from peripheral blood leukocytes or skeletal muscle and is useful for clinical diagnosis and genetic counseling.

MITOCHONDRIAL MYOPATHY, ENCEPHALOPATHY, LACTIC ACIDOSIS, AND STROKE-LIKE EPISODES   This disorder is usually referred to by the acronym MELAS. It is a multisystem mitochondrial encephalomyopathy that begins in childhood after normal birth and early development. Patients have stunted growth and recurrent stroke-like episodes manifesting as hemiparesis, hemianopsia, or cortical blindness. Episodic vomiting may occur and some patients have hearing loss. Focal or generalized seizures and myoclonic epilepsy may be present. Full expression of the disease leads to dementia, a bedridden state, and death often before age 20. MELAS may be maternally inherited, but sporadic cases are more common. No large pedigrees have been reported. In most patients, a point mutation of the transfer RNA gene for leucine (tRNA^{leu}) of mtDNA has been identified. Mutation analysis provides a specific diagnostic test that can be performed on peripheral blood leukocytes or skeletal muscle.

SUCCINIC DEHYDROGENASE (COMPLEX II) DEFICIENCY   This disorder presents in childhood with exercise intolerance. Physical exertion, even of a modest degree, causes exhaustion associated with shortness of breath and palpitations. If physical activity persists, rhabdomyolysis may occur with painful, stiff and swollen muscles associated with myoglobinuria. Physical examination is usually normal, although some patients may have enlarged calf muscles. Exercise-induced dyspnea and tachycardia can be demonstrated by having patients climb a flight of stairs. The diagnosis is established by muscle biopsy which shows ragged red fibers and deficiency of succinic dehydrogenase in muscle fibers. Biochemical analysis of muscle reveals markedly impaired succinate oxidation.

Complex II of the respiratory chain is encoded for entirely by nuclear DNA. The disease is inherited as an autosomal recessive trait.

CYTOCHROME C OXIDASE (COMPLEX IV DEFICIENCY)   There are three established clinical syndromes of cytochrome c oxidase (COX) deficiency: two infantile myopathies and a disorder predominantly affecting the brain (subacute necrotizing encephalopathy, also referred to as Leigh disease). A fatal form of COX deficiency inherited as an autosomal recessive trait presents clinically as a myopathy in the neonatal period with respiratory failure. No CNS involvement is seen. These patients have a renal tubular defect leading to aminoaciduria (DeToni-Fanconi-Debré syndrome). Muscle biopsy demonstrates

COX deficiency by histochemistry and biochemistry. Antibodies to the subunits of COX show a selective loss of subunit 7a,b of COX representing a defect in a nuclear-encoded polypeptide of the respiratory chain.

A benign form of infantile myopathy due to COX deficiency is initially indistinguishable from the fatal form of COX deficiency. Patients with the benign form have no renal tubular defect. Spontaneous recovery often occurs during the first year of life, and the child is normal by age 2 to 3.

The muscle biopsy changes during the neonatal period resemble those of fatal COX deficiency. Immune staining, however, demonstrates that in addition to the absence of nuclear-encoded subunit 7a,b of COX, there is a loss of subunit 2 of mtDNA. Immune staining of these subunits returns to normal as the clinical condition improves. Recognition of this distinction on immune staining between the fatal and benign forms of COX deficiency is of great importance in diagnosis.

Leigh disease This disease, also known as *subacute necrotizing encephalomyelopathy,* has more than one cause. At least one form, however, is caused by COX deficiency. A typical presentation occurs in the neonatal period with hypotonia and recurrent vomiting. Later visual and hearing loss occurs and seizures develop. In some cases, the onset of Leigh disease may be delayed until walking begins. In these patients, ataxia and loss of intellectual development accompanies muscle weakness. Patients with Leigh disease have elevated lactate and pyruvate levels in cerebrospinal fluid and blood. COX deficiency can be recognized on muscle biopsy. In addition, immune staining demonstrates that all subunits of COX, both mitochondrial- and nuclear-encoded polypeptides are absent.

Most cases of Leigh disease are sporadic, but the disorder also occurs in siblings suggesting autosomal recessive inheritance.

ENDOCRINE AND METABOLIC MYOPATHIES

Many endocrine disorders cause weakness. Muscle fatigue is more common than true weakness. The cause of weakness in these disorders is not well defined. It is not even clear that weakness results from disease of muscle as opposed to another part of the motor unit since the serum CK level is often normal (except for hypothyroidism), and the muscle histology is characterized by atrophy rather than destruction of muscle fibers. Nearly all endocrine myopathies respond to treatment.

THYROID DISORDERS (See Chap. 334) Abnormalities of thyroid function can cause a wide array of muscle disorders. These conditions relate to the important role of thyroid hormones in the metabolism of carbohydrates and lipids as well as in accelerating protein synthesis and enzyme production. Thyroid hormones also stimulate calorigenesis in muscle, increase muscle demand for vitamins, and enhance muscle sensitivity to circulating catacholamines.

Hypothyroidism Hypothyroid patients have frequent muscle complaints, but definite muscle weakness occurs in only about one-third of patients. Weakness when present, is predominantly proximal. Muscle cramps, pain, and stiffness occur commonly. The so-called myotonoid features characterized by slow muscle contraction and relaxation occur in 25 percent of patients and are often accompanied by myoedema (local contraction produced by tapping or pinching the muscle). The relaxation phase of muscle stretch reflexes is characteristically prolonged. The serum CK levels are often elevated (up to 10 times normal) even with minimal clinical evidence of muscle disease.

In both children and adults, a distinct syndrome has been described. Severe hypothyroid children, especially boys, may have the Debré-Kocher-Sémélaigne syndrome, characterized by weakness, slowness of movement, and striking muscle hypertrophy, causing an "infant Hercules appearance." In adult hypothyroidism, Hoffman's syndrome results in prominent muscle enlargement and weakness with muscle stiffness. The cause of muscle enlargement in these two syndromes

has not been determined. The muscle biopsy shows only muscle atrophy.

Hyperthyroidism Thyrotoxic patients commonly have muscle weakness on clinical examination, but rarely complain of the deficit. Proximal weakness and atrophy with preserved and often brisk muscle stretch reflexes characterize thyrotoxic myopathy. Prominent shoulder-girdle atrophy associated with scapular winging can occur. Bulbar, respiratory and even esophageal muscles may occasionally be affected, causing dysphagia, dysphonia, and aspiration. When bulbar involvement occurs, it is usually accompanied by chronic proximal limb weakness, but may occasionally present in the absence of generalized thyrotoxic myopathy. Other neuromuscular disorders occur in association with hyperthyroidism and include periodic paralysis (see Chap. 387), myasthenia gravis, and a progressive ocular myopathy associated with proptosis (Graves' ophthalmopathy). Serum CK levels are low in thyrotoxic myopathy. The muscle histology usually shows only atrophy of muscle fibers.

PARATHYROID DISORDERS (See Chap. 357) **Hyperparathyroidism** Muscle weakness is an integral part of primary and secondary hyperparathyroidism. Proximal muscle weakness, muscle wasting, and brisk muscle stretch reflexes are the main features of this endocrinopathy. Serum CK levels are usually normal or slightly elevated. Serum calcium and phosphorus levels show no correlation with the clinical neuromuscular manifestations. Muscle biopsies show only varying degrees of atrophy without muscle fiber degeneration.

Hypoparathyroidism An overt myopathy due to hypocalcemia is rarely seen. Neuromuscular symptoms are usually related to localized or generalized tetany. Serum CK levels may be increased secondary to muscle damage following tetany. Hyporeflexia or areflexia is usually present and contrasts with hyperreflexia seen in hyperparathyroidism.

ADRENAL DISORDERS (See Chap. 335) Conditions associated with glucocorticoid excess cause a myopathy and, in fact, steroid myopathy is the most commonly diagnosed endocrine muscle disease. Steroid excess, either endogenous or exogenous, produces varying degrees of proximal limb weakness. Muscle wasting may be striking. A cushingoid appearance invariably precedes or accompanies clinical signs of myopathy. Serum CK level is normal in steroid myopathy. The muscle biopsy shows atrophy predominantly affecting type 2 fibers. Muscle fiber degeneration is usually not seen.

Adrenal insufficiency commonly causes muscle fatigue. Objective weakness occurs less commonly and is typically only mild. Patients with myopathy and adrenal insufficiency usually have hypo- or hyperkalemia. In some cases this may result from adrenal gland destruction, affecting both glucocorticoid and mineralocorticoid production.

In primary hyperaldosteronism or Conn's syndrome, neuromuscular complications are due to potassium depletion. The clinical picture is one of persistent muscle weakness. Long-standing hyperaldosteronism may lead to proximal limb weakness and wasting. Serum CK may be elevated and a muscle biopsy may demonstrate degenerating fibers, some with vacuoles. These changes relate to hypokalemia and are not a direct effect of aldosterone on skeletal muscle.

PITUITARY DISORDERS (See Chap. 331) Muscle weakness and acromegaly develop insidiously and represent a relatively late manifestation of endocrinopathy. Patients usually show mild proximal weakness without muscle atrophy. Muscles often appear enlarged, but have decreased forced generation. The duration of acromegaly, rather than the serum growth hormone levels, correlates with the degree of myopathy.

DIABETES MELLITUS (See Chap. 337) Neuromuscular complications of diabetes mellitus are most often related to neuropathy with cranial and peripheral nerve palsies or distal sensorimotor polyneuropathy. "Diabetic amyotrophy" is sometimes thought to be a primary muscle complication, but there is overwhelming evidence that this is a type of neuropathy affecting the proximal major nerve trunks and lumbosacral plexus. More appropriate terms for this disorder include diabetic proximal neuropathy, lumbosacral plexopathy, or the eponymic designation Bruns-Garland syndrome.

The most notable myopathy of diabetes mellitus is ischemic infarction of thigh muscles. This condition occurs in poorly controlled diabetics and presents with acute onset of pain, tenderness, and edema of one thigh with a palpable mass. Muscles most often affected include the vastus lateralis, thigh adductors, and biceps femoris. Computed tomography or magnetic resonance imaging can demonstrate focal abnormalities in the affected muscle. Imaging of the muscle may avoid muscle biopsy.

VITAMIN DEFICIENCY   Vitamin D offers the best evidence that a myopathy occurs as an integral part of vitamin deficiency. Vitamin D deficiency (see Chaps. 77 and 356) from either decreased intake or decrease absorption, as well as impaired vitamin D metabolism as it occurs in renal disease, may lead to chronic muscle weakness. Pain reflects the underlying bone disease (osteomalacia).

It has not been established that deficiency of other vitamins causes a myopathy.

MYOPATHIES OF SYSTEMIC ILLNESS   Systemic illnesses such as chronic respiratory, cardiac, or hepatic failure are frequently associated with severe muscle wasting and complaints of weakness. Strength testing often demonstrates mild weakness in such patients. Lack of endurance is a more significant problem.

Myopathy may be a manifestation of chronic renal failure, separate and distinct from the better known uremic polyneuropathy. Abnormalities of calcium and phosphorus homeostasis and bone metabolism in chronic renal failure result from a reduction in 1,25-dihydroxyvitamin D leading to decreased intestinal absorption of calcium. Hypocalcemia, further accentuated by hyperphosphatemia due to decreased renal phosphate clearance, leads to secondary hyperparathyroidism. Renal osteodystrophy results from the compensatory hyperparathyroidism leading to osteomalacia from reduced calcium availability, and to osteitis fibrosa from the parathyroid hormone excess. The clinical picture of the myopathy of chronic renal failure is identical to that of primary hyperparathyroidism and osteomalacia. There is proximal limb weakness with bone pain.

Gangrenous calcification represents a separate, rare, and sometimes fatal complication of chronic renal failure. In this condition widespread arterial calcification occurs and results in ischemia. Extensive skin necrosis may occur along with painful myopathy and even myoglobinuria.

The term *carcinomatous myopathy* has been used to explain the frequent occurrence of muscle atrophy in patients with malignancy. In the usual patient with cancer, weakness is mild. In patients with severe weakness, other disorders should be considered and include: inflammatory myopathies, hormone-producing tumors resulting in hypercalcemia, ectopic ACTH production, or Eaton-Lambert syndrome. The last is caused by a defect in release of acetylcholine from the neuromuscular junction and is not a myopathy (see Chaps. 328 and 386).

TOXIC MYOPATHIES

The classification of toxic myopathies is shown in Table 385-2. Drugs and chemicals may produce focal or generalized damage of skeletal muscle.

The most common cause of focal damage is the injection of narcotic analgesics. Three agents in particular, pentazocine, meperidine, and heroin, may cause a severe fibrotic reaction in muscle. Common injection sites include deltoid, triceps, gluteus maximus, and quadriceps muscles. The muscles become indurated and may have local abscess formation. Cutaneous ulcerations and depressions may occur. Severe joint contractures may develop.

Other drugs may induce generalized muscle weakness, particularly affecting the proximal muscles. In most cases the exact mechanism of drug toxicity is poorly understood. D-Penicillamine induces a condition simulating the clinical and pathologic picture of polymyo-

---

TABLE 385-2   Toxic myopathies

Focal myopathies: Pentazocine, meperidine, heroin
Generalized myopathies
  A Inflammatory: cimetidine, D-penicillamine, procainamide
  B Muscle weakness and myalgias: zidovudine, chloroquine, clofibrate, colchicine, glucocorticoids, emetine, ε-aminocaproic acid, labetalol, perhexilene, propranolol, vincristine, niacin, cyclosporine
  C Rhabomyolysis and myoglobinuria: alcohol, heroin, amphetamine, clofibrate, lovastatin, gemfibrozil, ε-aminocaproic acid, phencyclidine, barbiturates, cocaine
  D Malignant hyperthermia: halothane, ethylene, diethyl ether, methoxylflurane, ethyl chloride, trichloroethylene, gallamine, succinylcholine, lidocaine, mepivacaine

---

sitis. A similar condition has been reported with cimetidine. Procainamide may cause myositis as part of a systemic lupus-like reaction.

Zidovudine, used in the treatment of AIDS, produces proximal weakness and pain. On muscle biopsy, zidovudine demonstrates a distinctive pathologic alteration of skeletal muscle resembling ragged red fibers. In some patients, reintroduction of zidovudine in lower doses may be tolerated.

Chloroquine administration may cause a vacuolar myopathy.

The cholesterol-lowering agents including clofibrate, lovastatin, gemfibrozil, and niacin have all been implicated as causes of myopathy. Lovastatin alone or in combination with gemfibrozil has caused rhabdomyolysis and myoglobinuria. Emetine hydrochloride (used for treatment of amebiasis) ε-aminocaproic acid (an antifibrinolytic agent), and perhexilene (used for angina pectoris) have all been observed to cause muscle weakness and muscle fiber necrosis following several weeks of therapy.

Drug-induced myopathy accompanied by proximal weakness occurs with glucocorticoid therapy. Those fluorinated in the 9α-position, such as triamcinolone, dexamethasone, and betamethasone, are most likely to cause weakness, but chronic administration of all glucocorticoids including prednisone causes weakness. Divided-dose as opposed to single-morning-dose therapy produces more severe weakness. A single-dose, alternate-day regimen is still less toxic. The clinical diagnosis of steroid-induced muscle weakness can be difficult if medication is being used to treat an underlying inflammatory myopathy. The presence of a normal serum CK level, minimal or no changes of myopathy on EMG, and type 2 muscle fiber atrophy on biopsy are helpful in suggesting steroid-induced weakness.

Alcohol causes acute muscle weakness with rhabdomyolysis and myoglobinuria by several different mechanisms including prolonged obtundation, seizures, hypokalemia, and hypophosphatemia. Chronic myopathy causing slowly progressive weakness is controversial. Alcoholics are often weak, but the clinical picture usually results from neuropathy, poor nutrition, and other processes.

A very serious drug-induced condition, *malignant hyperthermia* (Chap. 398), occurs in susceptible individuals following exposure to certain general anesthetic and depolarizing muscle relaxants (Table 385-2). The local anesthetic, amides including lidocaine, and mepivacaine have been implicated as precipitating agents.

REFERENCES

BANKER BQ: The congenital myopathies, in *Myology* AG Engel, BQ Banker (eds). New York, McGraw-Hill, 1986, vol. 2

BAROHN RJ et al: Autosomal recessive distal dystrophy. Neurology 41:1365, 1991

BROOKE MH: *A Clinician's View of Neuromuscular Disease*, 2d ed. Baltimore, Williams & Wilkins, 1985

CARROLL JE: Myopathies caused by disorders of lipid metabolism. Neurol Clinics, 6:563, 1988

DALAKAS MC et al: Mitochondrial myopathy caused by long-term zidovudine therapy. N Engl J Med 332:1098, 1990

DIMAURO S et al: Disorders of lipid metabolism in muscle. Muscle Nerve 3:369, 1980

ENGEL AG: Acid maltase deficiency, in *Myology*, AG Engel, BQ Banker (eds). New York, McGraw-Hill, 1986, vol. 2

GRIGGS RC, MOXLEY RT (eds): Metabolic myopathies. Semin Neurol 3:225, 1985

KOENIG M et al: Complete cloning of the Duchenne muscular dystrophy (DMD) cDNA and preliminary genomic organization of the DMD gene in normal and affected individuals. Cell 50:509, 1987

LACOMIS D et al: Myopathy in the elderly. Evaluation of the histopathologic spectrum and the accuracy of clinical diagnosis. Neurology 43:825, 1993

MATSAMURA K et al: Abnormal expression of dystrophin-associated proteins in Fukuyama-type congenital muscular dystrophy. Lancet 341:521, 1993

MORAES CT et al: Mitochondrial DNA deletions in progressive external ophthalmoplegia and Kearns-Sayre syndrome. N Engl J Med 320:1293, 1989

RIGGS JE (ed): *Muscle Disease,* in Neurologic Clinics, vol. 6. Philadelphia, Saunders, 1988

SIMPSON DM et al: Myopathies associated with human immunodeficiency virus and zidovudine. Can their effects be distinguished? Neurology 43:971, 1993

386   MYASTHENIA GRAVIS

DANIEL B. DRACHMAN

Myasthenia gravis (MG) is a neuromuscular disorder characterized by weakness and fatigability of skeletal muscles. The underlying defect is a decrease in the number of available acetylcholine receptors (AChRs) at neuromuscular junctions due to an antibody-mediated autoimmune attack. Treatment now available for MG is highly effective, although a specific cure has remained elusive.

PATHOPHYSIOLOGY   To diagnose and manage patients with MG, it is essential to understand the basic function of the neuromuscular junction and the changes that occur as a result of the disease process (see Fig. 386-1). Acetylcholine (ACh) is synthesized in the motor nerve terminal and stored in vesicles (quanta) containing approximately 10,000 molecules each. Quanta of ACh are released spontaneously, giving rise to miniature end-plate potentials. When an action potential reaches the nerve terminal, ACh from 150 to 200 vesicles is released and combines with AChRs that are densely packed at the peaks of postsynaptic folds. Channels in the AChRs are opened, permitting the rapid entry of cations, chiefly sodium, which produces depolarization at the end-plate region of the muscle fiber. If the depolarization is sufficiently large, it initiates an action potential that is propagated along the muscle fiber, triggering muscle contraction. This process is rapidly terminated by diffusion of ACh away from the receptor and hydrolysis of ACh by acetylcholinesterase (AChE).

In MG, the fundamental defect is a decrease in the number of available AChRs at the postsynaptic muscle membrane. In addition, the postsynaptic folds are flattened, or "simplified" (Fig. 386-1*B*). These changes result in decreased efficiency of neuromuscular transmission. Therefore, although ACh is released normally, it

produces small end-plate potentials which may fail to trigger muscle action potentials. Failure of transmission at many neuromuscular junctions results in weakness of muscle contraction.

The amount of ACh released per impulse *normally* declines on repeated activity (termed *presynaptic rundown*). In the myasthenic patient, decreased efficiency of neuromuscular transmission combined with the normal rundown results in the activation of fewer and fewer muscle fibers by successive nerve impulses and hence increasing weakness, or *myasthenic fatigue*. This mechanism also accounts for the decremental response to repetitive nerve stimulation seen on electrodiagnostic testing.

The neuromuscular abnormalities in MG are brought about by an autoimmune response mediated by specific anti-AChR antibodies. The anti-AChR antibodies reduce the number of available AChRs at neuromuscular junctions by three distinct mechanisms: (1) AChRs may be degraded at an accelerated rate by a mechanism involving cross-linking and rapid endocytosis of the receptors; (2) the active site of the AChR, i.e., the site that normally binds ACh, may be blocked by the antibodies; and (3) the postsynaptic muscle membrane may be damaged by the antibody in collaboration with complement.

How the autoimmune response is initiated and maintained in MG is not completely understood. However, the thymus appears to play a role in this process. The thymus is abnormal in approximately 75 percent of patients with MG; in about 65 percent of patients the thymus is "hyperplastic," with the presence of active germinal centers, while 10 percent of patients have thymic tumors (thymomas). Muscle-like cells within the thymus (myoid cells), which bear AChRs on their surface, may serve as a source of autoantigen and trigger the autoimmune reaction within the thymus gland.

CLINICAL FEATURES   Myasthenia gravis is not rare, with a prevalence rate of at least 1 in 10,000. It may affect individuals in any age group, but there are peaks of incidence in women in their twenties and thirties and in men in their fifties and sixties. Overall, women are affected more frequently than men, with a ratio of approximately 3:2. The cardinal features are *weakness* and *fatigability* of muscles. The weakness increases during repeated use (fatigue) and may improve following rest or sleep. The course of MG is often variable. Exacerbations and remissions may occur, particularly during the first few years after the onset of the disease. Remissions are rarely complete or permanent. Unrelated infections or systemic disorders often lead to increased myasthenic weakness and may precipitate so-called crisis (see below).

The distribution of muscle weakness has a characteristic pattern. The cranial muscles, particularly the lids and extraocular muscles, are often involved early, and diplopia and ptosis are common initial complaints. Facial weakness produces a "snarling" expression when the patient attempts to smile. Weakness in chewing is most noticeable after prolonged effort, as in chewing meat. Speech may have a nasal timbre caused by weakness of the palate or a dysarthric "mushy" quality due to tongue weakness. Difficulty in swallowing may occur as a result of weakness of the palate, tongue, or pharynx, giving rise to nasal regurgitation or aspiration of liquids or food. In approximately 85 percent of patients, the weakness becomes generalized, affecting the limb muscles as well. The limb weakness in MG is often proximal and may be asymmetric. Despite the muscle weakness, deep tendon reflexes are preserved. If weakness of respiration or swallowing becomes so severe as to require respiratory assistance or intubation, the patient is said to be in *crisis*.

DIAGNOSIS AND EVALUATION   The diagnosis is suspected on the basis of weakness and fatigability in the typical distribution described above, without loss of reflexes or impairment of sensation or other neurologic function. The suspected diagnosis should always be confirmed definitively before treatment is undertaken; this is essential because (1) other treatable conditions may closely resemble MG and (2) the treatment of MG may involve surgery and the prolonged use of drugs with adverse side effects.

Anticholinesterase test   Drugs that inhibit the enzyme AChE allow ACh to interact repeatedly with the limited number of AChRs,

FIGURE 386-1   Diagrams of (*A*) normal and (*B*) myasthenic neuromuscular junctions. V = vesicles; M = mitochondria. See text for description of normal neuromuscular transmission. The MG junction shows reduced number of AChRs (stippling); flattened, simplified postsynaptic folds; a widened synaptic space; and a normal nerve terminal.

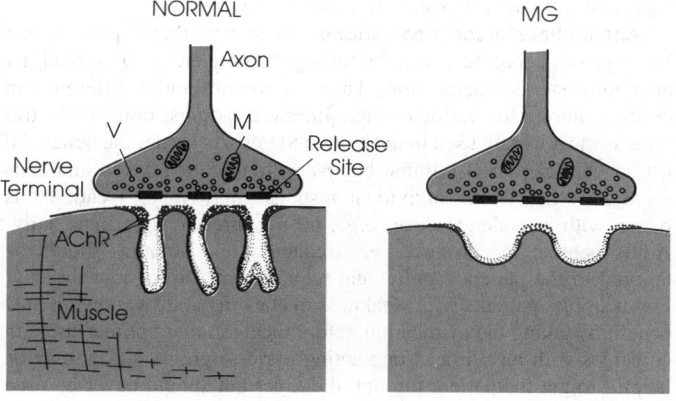

NORMAL   MG

Axon

V   M   Release Site

Nerve Terminal

AChR

Muscle

producing improvement in the strength of myasthenic muscles. Edrophonium is used most commonly, because of the rapid onset (30 s) and short duration (about 5 min) of its effect. It is essential that an objective endpoint be used to evaluate the effect of edrophonium. The examiner should focus on one or more unequivocally weak muscle groups and evaluate their strength objectively. For example, weakness of extraocular muscles, impairment of speech, or the length of time that the patient can maintain the arms in forward abduction may be useful measures. An initial dose of 2 mg edrophonium is given intravenously. If definite improvement occurs, the test is considered positive and terminated. If there is no change, the patient is given an additional 8 mg intravenously. The dose is administered in two parts because some patients react to edrophonium with unpleasant side effects such as nausea, diarrhea, salivation, fasciculations, and rarely syncope. Atropine (0.6 mg) should be at hand for intravenous administration if these symptoms become troublesome.

False-positive tests occur in occasional patients with other neurologic disorders, such as amyotrophic lateral sclerosis, and in placebo-reactors. False-negative or equivocal tests also may occur. In some cases it is helpful to use a longer-acting drug such as neostigmine, given orally, since this permits more time for detailed evaluation of strength. In virtually all instances, it is desirable to carry out further testing to establish the diagnosis of MG definitively.

Electrodiagnostic testing *Repetitive nerve stimulation* often provides helpful diagnostic evidence of MG. Anticholinesterase medication should be stopped at least 6 h prior to testing. It is best to test weak muscles or proximal muscle groups. Electric shocks are delivered at a rate of 2 or 3 per second to the appropriate nerves, and action potentials are recorded from the muscles. In normal individuals, the amplitude of the evoked muscle action potentials does not change at these rates of stimulation. However, in myasthenic patients there is a rapid reduction in the amplitude of the evoked responses of more than 10 to 15 percent. As a further test, a single dose of edrophonium may be given to prevent or diminish this decremental reaction.

Antiacetylcholine receptor antibody As noted above, anti-AChR antibodies are detectable in the serum of approximately 80 percent of all myasthenic patients, but in only about 50 percent of patients with weakness confined to the ocular muscles. The presence of anti-AChR antibodies is virtually diagnostic of MG, but a negative test does not exclude the disease. The measured level of anti-AChR antibody does not correspond well with the severity of MG in different patients. However, in an individual patient, a treatment-induced fall in the antibody level often correlates with clinical improvement.

Differential diagnosis Several other conditions that cause weakness of the cranial and/or somatic musculature must be considered in the differential diagnosis of MG; these include drug-induced myasthenia, Lambert-Eaton myasthenic syndrome, neurasthenia, hyperthyroidism, botulism, intracranial mass lesions, and progressive external ophthalmoplegia. Treatment with *penicillamine* (used for scleroderma or rheumatoid arthritis) may result in true MG, but the weakness is mild, and recovery occurs within weeks or months after discontinuing its use. Other drugs such as *aminoglycoside antibiotics* in very large doses and *procainamide* can cause neuromuscular weakness in normal individuals or exacerbation of weakness in myasthenic patients.

The *Lambert-Eaton myasthenic syndrome* is a presynaptic disorder of the neuromuscular junction that can cause weakness similar to that of MG. The proximal muscles of the lower limbs are most commonly affected, but other muscles may be involved as well. Cranial nerve findings, including ptosis of the eyelids and diplopia, occur in up to 70 percent of patients and resemble features of MG. However, the two conditions are readily distinguished, since patients with Lambert-Eaton syndrome have depressed or absent reflexes, autonomic changes such as dry mouth and impotence, and show incremental responses on repetitive nerve stimulation. It is now known that Lambert-Eaton syndrome is caused by an autoantibody directed against calcium channels on the motor nerve terminals, resulting in impaired release of ACh. A majority of patients with this syndrome have an associated malignancy, most commonly small cell carcinoma of the lung, which is thought to trigger the autoimmune response. The diagnosis of Lambert-Eaton syndrome may signal the presence of the tumor long before it would otherwise be detected, permitting early removal. Treatment of the neuromuscular disorder involves plasmapheresis and immunosuppression, as for MG.

Neurasthenia may present with weakness and fatigue, but muscle testing usually reveals the "jerky release" characteristic of nonorganic disorders, and the complaint of fatigue in these patients means tiredness or apathy rather than decreasing muscle power on repeated effort. *Hyperthyroidism* is readily diagnosed or excluded by tests of thyroid function, which should be carried out routinely in patients with suspected MG. It is worth noting that abnormalities of thyroid function (hyper- or hypothyroidism) may increase myasthenic weakness. *Botulism* can cause myasthenic-like weakness, but the pupils are often affected and repetitive nerve stimulation gives an *incremental*, rather than decremental, response. Diplopia that mimics the symptoms of MG may occasionally be due to *intracranial mass lesions* that compress nerves to the extraocular muscles (e.g., sphenoid ridge meningioma), but computed tomography (CT) or magnetic resonance imaging (MRI) scanning of the head and orbits usually reveals the lesion.

Progressive external ophthalmoplegia is a rare condition resulting in weakness of the extraocular muscles, which may be accompanied by weakness of the proximal muscles of the limbs, and a variety of other systemic features that are beyond the scope of this chapter. Most patients with this condition have mitochondrial disorders that can be detected on muscle biopsy (see Chap. 385).

Search for associated conditions Myasthenic patients have an increased incidence of several associated disorders. *Thymic abnormalities* occur in approximately 75 percent of patients, as noted above. Neoplastic change (thymoma) may produce enlargement of the thymus, which is best detected by CT or MRI scanning of the anterior mediastinum. Enlargement of the thymus in a patient over 40 years of age is highly suspicious of thymoma. *Hyperthyroidism* may occur in 3 to 8 percent of patients and may aggravate the myasthenic weakness. Tests of thyroid function should be obtained. Because of the *association with other autoimmune disorders*, blood tests for rheumatoid factor and antinuclear antibodies should be carried out in all patients. Chronic infection of any kind can exacerbate MG and should be sought carefully. Finally, measurements of *ventilatory function* are valuable because of the frequency and seriousness of respiratory impairment in myasthenic patients.

Because of the side effects of glucocorticoids and other immunosuppressive agents used in the treatment of MG, a thorough medical investigation should be made, searching specifically for evidence of chronic or latent infection (such as tuberculosis or hepatitis), hypertension, diabetes, renal impairment, and glaucoma.

MEDICAL AND SURGICAL THERAPY The prognosis has improved strikingly as a result of advances in treatment; virtually all myasthenic patients can be returned to full productive lives with proper therapy. The most important methods used in the treatment of myasthenia gravis include anticholinesterase medications, immunosuppressive agents, thymectomy, and plasmapheresis.

Anticholinesterase medications Most myasthenic patients can be improved, but few can be brought completely to normal by anticholinesterase medication. There is no substantial difference in efficacy among the various anticholinesterase drugs; oral pyridostigmine is most widely used in the United States. As a rule, the beneficial action of oral pyridostigmine begins within 15 to 30 min and lasts for 3 to 4 h, but the individual response may vary. Treatment is begun with a moderate dose, e.g., 60 mg three to five times daily. Adjustment of the dosage, i.e., frequency and amount, should be tailored to the patient's individual requirements throughout the day. For example, patients with weakness in chewing and swallowing may benefit by taking the medication before meals so that optimal strength coincides with mealtime. Long-acting pyridostigmine tablets may be helpful to get the patient through the night but should never be used for daytime medication because of their variable absorption. The maximum useful dose of pyridostigmine rarely exceeds 120 mg every 3 h during daytime. Overdosage with anticholinesterase medication may cause increased weakness and other side effects. In some patients, muscarinic side effects of the anticholinesterase medication (diarrhea, abdominal cramps, salivation, nausea) may limit the dosage tolerated. In these cases, propantheline bromide may be used to block the autonomic side effects without altering the beneficial effects on skeletal muscle. Loperamide is useful for the treatment of diarrhea.

Thymectomy Two separate issues should be distinguished: surgical removal of thymoma, and thymectomy as a treatment for myasthenia gravis. In the case of thymoma, surgical removal is necessary because of the possibility of local tumor spread, although most thymomas are benign. In the absence of a tumor, the available evidence suggests that up to 85 percent of patients improve after thymectomy, and of these, about 35 percent may achieve drug-free remission. However, the improvement is typically delayed for months to years. The advantage of thymectomy is that it offers the possibility of long-term benefit, in some cases diminishing or eliminating the need for continuing medical treatment. In view of these potential benefits and of the negligible risk in skilled hands, thymectomy has gained widespread acceptance in the treatment of MG. It is the consensus that thymectomy should be carried out in all patients with generalized MG between the ages of puberty and at least 55. Whether thymectomy should be recommended as a rule in children, in adults over 55 years of age, and in patients with weakness limited to the ocular muscles is still a matter of debate. Thymectomy must be carried out in a hospital where this procedure is performed regularly and where the staff is experienced in the pre- and postoperative management, anesthesia, and surgical techniques of total thymectomy.

Immunosuppression Immunosuppression using glucocorticoids, azathioprine, and other drugs is effective in nearly all patients with MG. The choice of which drugs to use should be guided by their relative benefits and risks for the individual patients. In general, clinical improvement begins somewhat more rapidly with steroid treatment than with the other immunosuppressive agents. The side effects of each drug may preclude its use in some patients, as indicated below.

STEROID THERAPY Glucocorticoids, when used properly, produce improvement in myasthenic weakness in the great majority of patients. The initial dose of prednisone should be relatively low (15 to 25 mg/d) to avoid the early weakening that occurs in about one-third of patients treated initially with a high-dose regimen. The dose is increased stepwise, as tolerated by the patient (usually 5 mg/d at 2- to 3-day intervals), until there is marked clinical improvement or the dose of 50 mg/d is reached. This dose is maintained for 1 to 3 months and then is gradually modified to an alternate-day regimen over the course of an additional 1 to 2 months, until the dosage of 100 mg on alternate days is reached. Generally, patients begin to improve within a few months after reaching the maximum dose, and improvement continues to progress for months or years. The prednisone dosage may gradually be reduced, but usually months or years may be needed to determine the minimum effective dose and close monitoring is required by patient and doctor. *Few patients are able to do without prednisone entirely.* Patients on long-term glucocorticoid therapy must be followed carefully to prevent or treat adverse side effects. The most common errors in the steroid treatment of myasthenic patients include:

1 Insufficient persistence; improvement may be delayed and gradual.
2 Too early, too rapid, or excessive tapering of steroid dosage.
3 Lack of attention to prevention and treatment of side effects.

The management of patients treated with glucocorticoids is discussed in Chap. 335.

OTHER IMMUNOSUPPRESSIVE DRUGS Azathioprine, cyclosporine (ciclosporin), or occasionally cyclophosphamide is effective in many patients, either alone or in combination with glucocorticoid therapy. Azathioprine is the most widely used because of its relative safety in most patients. Its therapeutic effect may add to that of glucocorticoids

and/or allow the steroid dose to be reduced. However, up to 10 percent of patients are unable to tolerate azathioprine because of idiosyncratic reactions consisting of flulike symptoms of fever and malaise, bone marrow depression, or abnormalities of liver function. An initial dose of 50 mg/d should be used to test for adverse side effects. If this is tolerated, the dose is gradually increased until the white blood count falls to approximately 3000. In patients who are concomitantly receiving steroids, leukocytosis precludes the use of this measure. A reduction of the lymphocyte count below 1000 per microliter and/or an increase of the mean corpuscular volume may be used as indications of adequacy of azathioprine dosage. The typical dosage range is 2 to 3 mg/kg total body weight. The beneficial effect of azathioprine takes at least 3 to 6 months to begin and even longer to reach a maximum level.

Cyclosporine is approximately as effective as azathioprine and is being used increasingly in the management of MG. Its beneficial effect occurs more rapidly than that of azathioprine. It may be used alone but is used most commonly as an adjunct to steroids, in order to reduce the steroid dosage required. The usual dose of cyclosporine is 4 to 5 mg/kg per day, given in two divided doses (so as to minimize side effects). Side effects of cyclosporine include hypertension and nephrotoxicity, which must be closely monitored. "Trough" blood levels of cyclosporine are measured 12 hours after the evening dose. The therapeutic range, as measured by radioimmunoassay, is 150 to 200 ng/L. Cyclophosphamide is reserved for patients refractory to the other drugs because of the relatively high risk of adverse side effects, including late development of malignancies.

Plasmapheresis In view of the antibody-mediated pathogenesis of MG, plasmapheresis has been used therapeutically. The plasma, which contains the pathogenic antibodies, is mechanically separated from the blood cells, which are returned to the patient in a suitable fluid medium. Plasmapheresis produces a short-term reduction in anti-AChR antibodies, with clinical improvement in many patients. Thus it is useful as a temporary expedient in seriously affected patients or to improve the patient's condition prior to surgery (e.g., thymectomy). The long-term treatment of myasthenic patients requires other methods of therapy outlined in this chapter.

Management of myasthenic crisis Myasthenic crisis is defined as an exacerbation of weakness sufficient to endanger life. The usual serious threats to life are respiratory failure, caused by diaphragmatic and intercostal weakness, and aspiration, secondary to pharyngeal weakness. Treatment should be carried out in an intensive care unit staffed with physicians experienced in the management of myasthenia gravis, respiratory insufficiency, infectious disease, and fluid and electrolyte therapy. The possibility that the deterioration could be due to excessive anti-ChE medication ("cholinergic crisis") is best excluded by temporarily stopping anti-ChE drugs. The most common cause of crisis is intercurrent infection. This should be treated immediately, because the mechanical and immunologic defenses of the patient can be assumed to be compromised. The myasthenic patient with fever and early infection should be treated like other immunocompromised patients. Early and effective antibiotic therapy, respiratory assistance, and pulmonary physiotherapy are essentials of the treatment program. As discussed above, plasmapheresis is frequently helpful in hastening recovery.

REFERENCES

ANDREWS PI et al: Acetylcholine receptor antibodies in juvenile myasthenia gravis. Neurology 43:977, 1993

DRACHMAN DB: Biology of myasthenia gravis. Ann Rev Neurosci 4:195, 1981

——— (ed): Myasthenia gravis: Biology and treatment. Ann NY Acad Sci 505:1, 1987

ENGEL AG et al: The motor endplate in myasthenia gravis and in experimental autoimmune myasthenia gravis: A quantitative ultrastructural study. Ann NY Acad Sci 274:60, 1976

FAMBROUGH DM et al: Neuromuscular junction in myasthenia gravis: Decreased acetylcholine receptors. Science 182:293, 1973

LINDSTROM J et al: Myasthenia gravis. Advances in Immunol 42:233, 1988

PENN AS et al (eds): Myasthenia gravis and related disorders: Experimental and clinical aspects. Ann NY Acad Sci 505:1, 1993

SOMNIER FE, TROJABORG W: Neurophysiological evaluation in myasthenia gravis—A comprehensive study of a complete patient population. Electroencephalogr Clin Neurophysiol 89:73, 1993

TOYKA KV et al: Myasthenia gravis: Study of humoral immune mechanisms by passive transfer to mice. N Engl J Med 296:125, 1977

387 PERIODIC PARALYSIS

LOUIS J. PTACEK / ROBERT C. GRIGGS

Disorders that cause patients of normal strength to become weak intermittently are not common. In contrast, the complaint of intermittent weakness is frequently encountered. The evaluation of such symptoms is challenging because the examination is often normal between attacks and because reliance on history is crucial for diagnosis. This chapter considers the primary periodic paralyses. Recent discoveries of the molecular defects in some of the periodic paralyses have provided insight into their pathogenesis and forms the basis for their classification. Other disorders that cause episodic weakness are considered elsewhere (see Chap. 23).

All primary periodic paralyses have some features in common. In most patients the disorders are inherited as autosomal dominant traits. Symptoms usually begin early in life and rarely commence after age 25. Attacks typically follow rest or sleep and almost never occur in the midst of vigorous activity, although antecedent exercise frequently provokes weakness. Patients remain alert during the attacks. Early in the course of these disorders interattack strength is normal but after years of attacks progressive weakness may develop. All forms of periodic paralysis are amenable to treatment and progressive weakness can be prevented and even reversed.

Diagnosis is based upon patient history and confirmed by appropriate evaluation of serum electrolytes during attacks and by evaluating the response of strength to provocative testing with glucose, insulin, potassium, and cold. Since the genetic defects of certain periodic paralyses have been defined, diagnosis will soon be possible by routine molecular DNA studies.

HYPOKALEMIC PERIODIC PARALYSIS This disorder occurs as an autosomal dominant condition in two-thirds of cases and as sporadic cases in one-third. Males are more frequently and more severely affected. Attacks of weakness characteristically begin in adolescence but may commence in the first decade. Onset after age 25 is rare; the new onset of episodic paralysis in older individuals is almost never due to periodic paralysis.

Attack frequency varies from daily to yearly. Attacks last from 3 to 4 h to as long as a day or more. Meals high in carbohydrate or high in sodium may provoke attacks. Paralysis involves limb muscles, usually proximal more than distal; rarely ocular, bulbar, or respiratory muscles are weakened, and bulbar and respiratory involvement may prove fatal. Reflexes become hypoactive, and cardiac arrhythmias may occur during attacks. Patients may develop persistent proximal weakness after years of attacks. Examination during attack-free intervals is otherwise normal except for the frequent presence of eyelid myotonia.

Diagnosis is established by demonstrating a low serum potassium during a paralytic attack and by excluding secondary causes of hypokalemia (Chap 23). Electrocardiograms during attacks show characteristic features of hypokalemia. Routine electromyography is not helpful in diagnosis, but muscle biopsy often shows the presence of single or multiple centrally placed vacuoles. Patients whose attacks are so infrequent as to preclude the study of a spontaneous attack require provocative testing with glucose and insulin administration. Such tests are potentially hazardous, and patients must be carefully monitored during their performance. Since these disorders are rare such testing is most appropriately carried out in referral centers.

Pathogenesis The pathogenesis of paralytic attacks is incom-pletely understood. There is evidence for an abnormality of muscle membrane. The contractile apparatus is normal. Distinctive abnormalities in potassium regulation occur in hypokalemic periodic paralysis. Patients with hypokalemic periodic paralysis often have a decrease in total body potassium but this may reflect muscle wasting. There is no increased excretion of potassium in the urine before or during attacks, but there is excessive flux of potassium from blood into muscle, possibly owing to an abnormality of muscle membrane that causes muscle to become electrically inexcitable. Muscle from these patients is abnormally sensitive to the effect of insulin on potassium uptake; the significance of this increased sensitivity is not known since weakness is often severe at levels of serum potassium that do not affect normal individuals. Moreover, attacks may occur when insulin levels are low. Therefore, factors other than hypokalemia per se are important in the induction of weakness.

Treatment ACUTE ATTACKS The acute paralysis improves following the administration of potassium salts. Oral KCl (0.2 to 0.4 mmol/kg) should be given to patients with severe weakness and repeated at 15 to 30 min intervals depending on the response of the ECG, serum potassium, and muscle strength. Milder attacks usually resolve spontaneously; resolution of weakness is hastened by exercising affected muscles. When patients are unable to swallow or are vomiting, intravenous therapy may be necessary. Small, repeated bolus therapy with KCl (0.1 mmol/kg) may be administered over 5 to 10 min with careful monitoring of the ECG and serum potassium. If potassium is administered as a dilute solution (20 to 40 mmol/L) in 5% glucose or in physiologic saline solution, serum potassium may decline, and weakness may worsen.

PREVENTION OF ATTACKS The goal of therapy is the elimination of attacks, which also prevents interattack weakness and may improve interattack weakness after it has developed. Prior to availability of effective means of attack prevention, chronic progressive interattack weakness frequently caused serious disability. Prophylactic administration of potassium salts, even in large dosage, does not prevent attacks but acetazolamide (125 to 1000 mg/d in divided dosage) abolishes attacks in the majority of cases. The mechanism of action of acetazolamide is not fully understood, but it may block the flux of potassium from blood into muscle. The metabolic acidosis that it produces may underlie its beneficial effect. Paradoxically, acetazolamide lowers serum potassium; to achieve an adequate response in some patients it may be necessary to give supplementary potassium along with acetazolamide and to avoid high-carbohydrate meals. Chronic acetazolamide treatment may be associated with renal calculi, and patients should be monitored for this complication. In occasional patients attacks may not respond to or may even be worsened by acetazolamide. In such patients triamterene (25 to 100 mg/d or spironolactone 25 to 100 mg/d) may prevent attacks.

THYROTOXIC PERIODIC PARALYSIS Attacks of hypokalemic periodic paralysis can occur in subjects with thyrotoxicosis, most commonly in Latin American or oriental men where up to 10 percent of thyrotoxic patients may have periodic paralysis. In many patients thyrotoxicosis has been overlooked for many months; periodic paralysis can occur with any cause of hyperthyroidism, including that induced by exogenous thyroid hormone administration. The usual age of onset of the disorder is that of thyrotoxicosis; otherwise the clinical features resemble familial hypokalemic periodic paralysis. Acute attacks respond to potassium administration. Treatment of underlying thyrotoxicosis abolishes attacks and β-adrenergic blocking agents reduce the frequency and severity of attacks while measures to control thyrotoxicosis are being instituted. Acetazolamide is not helpful in preventing attacks. The pathogenesis of thyrotoxic periodic paralysis is uncertain but there is evidence for a decrease in the activity of the calcium pump. The pathogenesis of thyrotoxic periodic paralysis may be different from that of nonthyrotoxic periodic paralysis since thyroid hormone does not worsen the latter.

PERIODIC PARALYSES CAUSED BY DISORDERS OF THE SKELETAL MUSCLE SODIUM CHANNEL These disorders differ from hypokalemic periodic paralysis in that attacks are usually brief

(1 to 2 h) and more frequent; clinical or electromyographic myotonia is often demonstrable. Disease onset is usually at an earlier age than for hypokalemic periodic paralysis; attacks of myotonia may be evident in the first year of life. The disorder is usually transmitted as an autosomal dominant defect; rare sporadic cases occur. Attacks are usually precipitated by fasting, potassium loading, muscle cooling, or by rest following exercise: the particular precipitant of the attacks allows clinical subclassification of these disorders into *hyperkalemic periodic paralysis*, *normokalemic periodic paralysis*, and *paramyotonia with periodic paralysis*. These three disorders were recognized historically as overlapping, but distinct, clinical entities and are now known to result from allelic defects in the skeletal-muscle sodium channel α subunit. Specific mutations have recently been defined; the correlation of site of sodium channel mutation with clinical phenotype is under study.

Hyper- and normokalemic periodic paralysis The name "hyperkalemic" is misleading since potassium levels are frequently normal in patients during attacks. The disorder is best defined by the fact that attacks are precipitated by potassium administration. "Potassium-sensitive" periodic paralysis is probably preferable terminology. Moreover, serum potassium is often slightly elevated when patients are not having attacks of weakness. Attacks are characterized by limb weakness. Only rarely are cranial and respiratory muscle involvement found. Cardiac arrhythmias occur occasionally. Paresthesias and muscle pain are frequently present during an attack.

Diagnosis of the hyperkalemic form is suggested by a modest elevation of serum potassium during attacks in nearly half of patients; at times, however, the serum potassium is normal or even low. Intravenous glucose-insulin loading does not precipitate weakness but potassium-loading tests (0.05 to 0.15 g/kg) will provoke weakness in such patients. Myotonia may be increased. Potassium-loading tests are potentially hazardous and are contraindicated in patients with renal disease and diabetes. Random serum potassium measurements may suggest the diagnosis since potassium elevations are frequent during attack-free intervals. Electromyographic evidence of myotonia and the finding of vacuoles on muscle biopsy provide supporting data.

Most subjects with periodic paralysis in whom potassium is normal during attacks behave like those with typical "hyperkalemic" periodic paralysis, since they are similarly sensitive to potassium administration. In fact, genetic linkage data suggest that the so-called hyperkalemic and normokalemic forms of this disorder are allelic disorders resulting from mutations of a single gene. Treatment is the same as for hyperkalemic periodic paralysis. Rare patients with episodic normokalemic paralysis are not potassium sensitive, but they usually

show evidence of muscle destruction or other features suggesting that they should not be classified as having a primary periodic paralysis.

Paramyotonia congenita with periodic paralysis Attacks of paralysis may occur in the paramyotonias, either provoked by cold or spontaneously. Paramyotonia congenita is characterized by paradoxical myotonia (i.e., worsening with activity), cold provocation, spontaneous attacks, and family history compatible with an autosomal dominant defect. The cold provocation of weakness and muscle stiffness distinguishes this disease from other periodic paralyses. A therapeutically useful subclassification of the paramyotonias has been proposed: (1) paramyotonia congenita in which spontaneous attacks of weakness are associated with a lowering of serum potassium and in which measures that decrease serum potassium provoke weakness; and (2) paralysis periodica paramyotonia in which spontaneous attacks may be associated with hyperkalemia and may be provoked by oral potassium administration. This potassium sensitivity has led in the past to the classification of this disorder as a variant of hyperkalemic or normokalemic periodic paralysis. Identification of mutations in these patients has demonstrated that these disorders are allelic defects in the adult skeletal muscle sodium channel α-subunit.

Clinical diagnosis depends upon the provocation of weakness and stiffness with cold. Glucose and insulin loading and potassium challenges aid in the subclassification of the disorder and provide assistance in the choice of medication for treatment. The molecular defect can be determined by appropriate studies of peripheral blood DNA.

Pathogenesis Patch-clamp recordings from cultured hyperkalemic periodic paralysis myotubes have demonstrated a defect in the voltage-dependent inactivation of a small fraction of sodium channels. Such abnormal inactivation in a subpopulation of channels may cause persistent membrane depolarization, inactivation of normal sodium channels and, ultimately, the membrane inexcitability known to be present in paralyzed patients. Recordings from muscle cells from patients with hyperkalemic and normokalemic periodic paralysis have shown abnormal regulation of skeletal muscle sodium channels. Two distinct sodium channel mutations have now been identified in hyperkalemic periodic paralysis patients (Fig. 387-1).

The two types of paramyotonia probably have different causes. In paramyotonia congenita, cooling of muscle results in an abnormal depolarization, leading first to myotonia and then to inexcitability. Sodium conductance becomes abnormal with cooling of muscle. Five distinct mutations have now been identified in patients with this form of the disorder (Fig. 387-1). It remains to be determined if the site

FIGURE 387-1 The sodium channel is depicted here as a molecule containing four homologous domains. Each domain contains six putative membrane spanning segments. The fourth segment of each domain is thought to act together as the "voltage sensor" for the channel and is cross-hatched in the figure. The tertiary structure of the protein in the membrane and the association of these segments is thought to form a pore through which ions could pass. Mutations that have been identified are shown along with the phenotype that they confer.

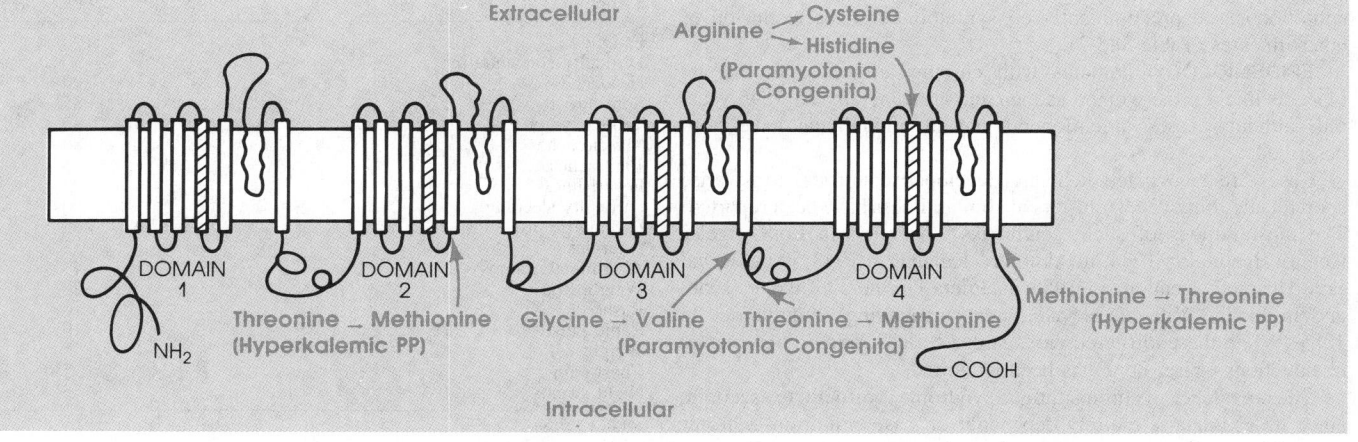

of the sodium channel mutations accounts for the clinical findings of the different forms of paramyotonia.

Treatment In hyperkalemic periodic paralysis, attacks of weakness are seldom severe enough to require emergency treatment and are never fatal. Oral glucose or other carbohydrate hastens recovery. Since interattack weakness may develop after repeated attacks, prophylactic treatment may be indicated. Remarkably, acetazolamide (125 to 1000 mg/d), the treatment of choice for hypokalemic periodic paralysis, was first found to be beneficial for hyperkalemic periodic paralysis, possibly because of its kaliopenic effect. Thiazide diuretics (e.g., chlorothiazide 250 to 1000 mg/d) are often effective and may have fewer side effects.

Spontaneous attacks of periodic paralysis in paramyotonia congenita are relatively infrequent. Many patients do not require prophylactic treatment for prevention. In the case of paramyotonia congenita, patients with severe and frequent attacks of weakness may respond to spironolactone, and subjects with paralysis periodica paramyotonica may respond to acetazolamide or thiazides. Acetazolamide may provoke weakness in paramyotonia congenita. Myotonia in both types of paramyotonia improves with mexiletine hydrochloride (150 to 900 mg/d). This antiarrhythmic agent may improve myotonia by blocking abnormal sodium channels; mexiletine also improves weakness and decreases the abnormal uptake of potassium by muscles.

REFERENCES

CANNON SC, STRITTMATTER SM: Functional expression of sodium channel mutations identified in families with periodic paralysis. Neuron 10:317, 1993

ENGEL AG: Periodic paralysis, in *Myology*, 2d ed, AG Engel, Franzini-Armstrong C (eds), New York, McGraw Hill, vol 2, 1994

FEERO WG et al: Hyperkalemic periodic paralysis—Rapid molecular diagnosis and relationship of genotype to phenotype in 12 families. Neurology 43:668, 1993

FONTAINE B et al: Hyperkalemic periodic paralysis and the adult muscle sodium channel gene. Science 250:1000, 1990

OBER KP: Thyrotoxic periodic paralysis in the United States: Report of 7 cases and review of the literature. Medicine 71:169, 1992

PTACEK LJ et al: Current concepts: Genetics of the myotonic muscle disorders. N Engl J Med 328:482, 1993

————: Mutations in an S4 segment of the adult skeletal muscle sodium channel cause paramyotonia congenita. Neuron 8:891, 1992

————: Sodium channel mutations in paramyotonia congenita and hyperkalemic periodic paralysis. Ann Neurol 33:300, 1993

RESNICK JS et al: Acetazolamide prophylaxis in hypokalemic periodic paralysis. N Engl J Med 278:582, 1968

ROJAS CV et al: A met-to-val mutation in the skeletal muscle Na+ channel α-subunit in hyperkalaemic periodic paralysis. Nature 354:387, 1991

STREIB EW: Paramyotonia congenita: Successful treatment with tocainide. Clinical and electrophysiological findings in seven patients. Muscle Nerve 10:155, 1987

section 3 Chronic fatigue syndrome

388 CHRONIC FATIGUE SYNDROME

STEPHEN E. STRAUS

DEFINITION *Chronic fatigue syndrome* is the current name for a disorder characterized by debilitating fatigue and a variety of associated physical, constitutional, and neuropsychological complaints (Table 388-1). The medical literature of the past three centuries informs us that this is not a new type of syndrome. Certain individuals who had been labeled in the past with diagnoses such as the vapors, neurasthenia, effort syndrome, hyperventilation syndrome, chronic brucellosis, epidemic neuromyasthenia, myalgic encephalomyelitis, hypoglycemia, multiple chemical sensitivity syndrome, chronic candidiasis, chronic mononucleosis, chronic Epstein-Barr virus infection, and postviral fatigue syndrome probably had what we are now calling chronic fatigue syndrome. For research purposes, the U.S. Centers for Disease Control and Prevention (CDC) has developed a case definition based predominantly on symptoms and the exclusion of other illnesses (Table 388-2).

EPIDEMIOLOGY Patients with chronic fatigue syndrome are twice as likely to be women as men and are generally 25 to 45 years old, although cases in childhood and in middle age have been described.

Cases are recognized in many developed countries. Most arise sporadically, but over 30 clusters of similar illness have been reported. The most famous of such "outbreaks" occurred in Los Angeles County Hospital in 1934; in Akureyri, Iceland, in 1948; in the Royal Free Hospital, London, in 1955; in Punta Gorda, Florida, in 1956; and in Incline Village, Nevada, and surrounding communities in 1985. While these clustered cases suggest a common environmental or infectious cause, none has been identified.

The prevalence of chronic fatigue syndrome is difficult to ascertain, since its estimate is entirely dependent on case definition. Chronic fatigue itself is a ubiquitous symptom, occurring in as many as 20 percent of patients attending a general medical clinic; the chronic fatigue syndrome is far less common. On the basis of one case definition for the syndrome, an estimate of 37 cases per 100,000 population was obtained in a survey of one rural Australian province. The CDC is currently studying the prevalence of illness meeting its case definition in four U.S. cities.

PATHOGENESIS The diverse names for the syndrome reflect the equally numerous and controversial hypotheses about its etiology. There are several common themes underlying attempts to understand the disorder: It is often postinfectious, it is associated with immunologic disturbances, and it is commonly accompanied by depression.

Some contemporary workers in the field espouse one or more of

TABLE 388-1 The approximate percentage of patients with the chronic fatigue syndrome reporting the indicated symptoms

Symptom	Percentage
Fatigue	100
Difficulty concentrating	90
Headache	90
Sore throat	85
Tender lymph nodes	80
Muscle aches	80
Joint aches	75
Feverishness	75
Difficulty sleeping	70
Psychiatric problems	65
Allergies	55
Abdominal cramps	40
Weight loss	20
Rash	10
Rapid pulse	10
Weight gain	5
Chest pain	5
Night sweats	5

SOURCE: *Straus.*

TABLE 388-2   Summary of the working definition of chronic fatigue syndrome

Both major criteria and either ≥6 minor symptom criteria plus ≥2 minor physical criteria or ≥8 symptom criteria must be present to fulfill the case definition.

Major criteria

1 Persistent or relapsing fatigue or easy fatigability that
  a Does not resolve with bed rest
  b Is severe enough to reduce average daily activity by ≥ 50%
2 Satisfactory exclusion of other chronic conditions, including preexisting psychiatric diseases

Minor criteria

Symptoms:

1 Mild fever (37.5–38.6°C oral if documented by the patient) or chills
2 Sore throat
3 Lymph node pain in anterior or posterior cervical or axillary chains
4 Unexplained generalized muscle weakness
5 Muscle discomfort, myalgia
6 Prolonged (≥24 h), generalized fatigue following previously tolerable levels of exercise
7 New, generalized headaches
8 Migratory noninflammatory arthralgia
9 Neuropsychological symptoms: photophobia, transient visual scotomata, forgetfulness, excessive irritability, confusion, difficulty thinking, inability to concentrate, or depression
10 Sleep disturbance
11 Patient's description of initial onset of symptoms as acute or subacute

Physical findings (documented by a physician on at least two occasions at least 1 month apart):

1 Low-grade fever (37.6–38.6°C oral or 37.8–38.8°C rectal)
2 Nonexudative pharyngitis
3 Palpable or tender anterior or posterior cervical or axillary lymph nodes (<2 cm in diameter)

SOURCE: *Adapted from GP Holmes, Rev Infect Dis 13(suppl 1):S53, 1991.*

several viruses as potential etiologic agents. Among these are lymphotropic herpesviruses, retroviruses, and enteroviruses. The data on which these presumptions rest are as follows: First, chronic fatigue syndrome can be precipitated by acute infections with Epstein-Barr virus, cytomegalovirus, and other agents. Some of these have the ability to persist in humans and cause chronic illness. Second, titers of antibodies to many infectious agents are elevated in patients with chronic fatigue. Included are antibodies to most herpesviruses, measles virus, rubella virus, and coxsackie virus B. Third, there are claims of increased levels of some viral antigens and nucleic acids in patients, but these assertions are not based on firm experimental evidence. While experience suggests that viruses can precipitate the syndrome, it is presently uncertain whether they actually contribute to its long-term features. Common, persisting viruses may simply have a greater likelihood to reactivate because of inadequate immune restraints on them, while causing no symptoms.

Numerous, subtle immunologic disturbances have been reported in patients with chronic fatigue syndrome. In addition to the elevated viral antibody titers mentioned above, there are also mild, nonspecific elevations in titers of antinuclear antibodies, modest immunoglobulin subclass reductions, mild deficiencies in mitogen-induced lymphocyte proliferation in vitro and in ensuing cytokine release, reduced natural killer cell activity, and shifts in lymphocyte phenotypes to greater than normal proportions of T cells expressing activation or differentiation markers. None of the immune findings appear in all patients, nor have any been correlated, as yet, with the severity of illness. None are specific for chronic fatigue syndrome; thus they remain nondiagnostic. An immune disturbance of some type, though, is in line with one favored theory that many of the symptoms of chronic fatigue syndrome derive from excessive cytokine release.

Recent controlled studies of patients with chronic fatigue syndrome documented abnormalities in endocrine function consistent with reduced production of corticotropin-releasing hormone in the hypothalamus. Mean serum cortisol concentrations were lower in patients than in controls; ACTH levels were correspondingly high. Hypothetically, these neuroendocrine abnormalities could contribute to the impaired energy and mood of patients. Whatever their importance, these changes further indicate the complex and multifactorial nature of chronic fatigue syndrome.

Mild to moderate depression is evident in about two-thirds of patients. Much of this depression may be reactive, but the prevalence exceeds that seen in other chronic medical illnesses. Thus some propose that chronic fatigue syndrome is fundamentally a psychiatric disorder and that the various neuroendocrine and immune disturbances arise secondarily.

MANIFESTATIONS   The typical case of chronic fatigue syndrome arises suddenly in a previously active individual. An otherwise unremarkable flulike illness or some other acute stress is recalled with great clarity as the triggering event. Unbearable exhaustion is left in the wake of this incident. Other symptoms, such as headache, sore throat, tender lymph nodes, muscle and joint aches, and frequent feverishness, lead to the belief that an infection persists, and medical attention is sought. Over several weeks, the impact of reassurances proffered during that initial evaluation fades as other features of the syndrome become evident—disturbed sleep, difficulty in concentration, and depression (see Table 388-1).

Depending on the dominant symptoms and the beliefs of the patient, additional consultations may be sought from allergists, rheumatologists, infectious disease specialists, psychiatrists, ecologic therapists, homeopaths, or other professionals, frequently with unsatisfactory results. Once the pattern of illness is established, the symptoms may fluctuate somewhat. Many patients report that diverse complaints are linked—that during periods of greatest fatigue they perceive the most pain and difficulty with concentration. Patients also commonly assert that excessive physical or emotional stress may exacerbate their symptoms.

Most patients remain capable of balancing their limited resources to accommodate the obligations of family, work, or community. The discretionary activities are abandoned first. Some feel unable to engage in any gainful employment. A minority of individuals require help with the activities of daily living.

Ultimately, isolation, pathetic resignation, and frustration can mark the protracted course of illness. Patients may become angry at physicians for failing to acknowledge or resolve their plight. Fortunately, the chronic fatigue syndrome does not appear to progress. On the contrary, many patients experience gradual improvement and eventual recovery.

DIAGNOSIS   Physical examination and routine laboratory tests are required to rule out other possible causes of the patient's symptoms. Prominent findings argue strongly in favor of other processes. No laboratory test, however esoteric or exotic, can diagnose this condition or measure its severity. Elaborate, expensive workups should therefore be avoided except in research settings. The great dilemma for patient and clinician alike is that chronic fatigue syndrome has no pathognomonic features and remains a constellation of symptoms and a diagnosis of exclusion. The case definition developed at the CDC for research purposes is cumbersome and imprecise (see Table 388-2). Nevertheless, it is increasingly used in the community for lack of suitable alternatives.

An important deficiency of the CDC case definition is its lack of clarity with regard to the impact of psychiatric illness on eligibility. As originally crafted, the criteria excluded any coexisting or past psychiatric problem. A modification was quickly proposed to allow mild to moderate current depression, recognizing that this condition could be situational. It remains uncertain as to whether an acute psychiatric problem long predating the onset of chronic fatigue should exclude the diagnosis.

MANAGEMENT   The primary responsibility of a physician confronted with a chronically fatigued patient is to address the cause by taking a thorough history, conducting a complete physical examination, judiciously using the laboratory, and, throughout this process, considering the differential diagnosis. If other illnesses are excluded, there are several points to address in the long-term care of a patient with chronic fatigue.

First, the patient should be informed about the illness and what is truly known of its pathogenesis; its potential impact on the physical, psychological, and social dimensions of life; and its prognosis. Patients are relieved when their complaints are taken seriously.

Second, periodic reassessment is appropriate to identify an underlying process that is late in declaring itself and to address intercurrent problems that must not be neglected as yet another subjective complaint.

Third, many symptoms of chronic fatigue syndrome respond to treatment. Nonsteroidal anti-inflammatory drugs alleviate headache, diffuse pain, and feverishness. Allergic rhinitis and sinusitis are common in patients with chronic fatigue syndrome; antihistamines or decongestants may be helpful. Although patients are often averse to psychiatric diagnoses, depression is a prominent symptom that should be confronted. Expert psychiatric assessment is sometimes advisable. Nonsedating antidepressants improve mood and disordered sleep and thereby attentuate the fatigue somewhat. Even modest improvements in symptoms can make an important difference in the patient's degree of self-sufficiency and ability to appreciate life's pleasures.

Fourth, practical advice should be given regarding lifestyle. The consumption of heavy meals with alcohol and caffeine at night can make it harder to sleep, compounding fatigue. Total rest is harmful. It leads to further deconditioning and the self-image of being an invalid. Exacerbation of exhaustion by strenuous exertion leads to total avoidance of exercise, so a moderate, carefully graded regimen needs to be encouraged.

Fifth, unproven treatments should be avoided. Controlled trials have established that acyclovir and intramuscular liver extract–folic acid–cyanocobalamin injections are of no value. There are conflicting claims regarding the efficacy of high-dose intravenous immunoglobulin therapy. One study documented no benefit; a second reported transient improvement in some patients. Given the considerable cost of this treatment and its side effects, there is little to recommend immunoglobulin therapy at this time. Countless anecdotes circulate regarding other traditional or nontraditional therapies. It is important to guide patients, flexibly, away from those therapeutic modalities which are most toxic, expensive, and unreasonable.

The physician should promote the patient's efforts toward improvement. A clinical trial in England showed behavioral therapy to be helpful. The therapy was aimed at dispelling cognitive distortions that lead to inactivity and despair. For chronic fatigue syndrome, as for many conditions, a comprehensive approach to physical, psychological, and social aspects is in order.

REFERENCES

ACHESON ED: The clinical syndrome variously called benign myalgic encephalomyelitis, Iceland disease and epidemic neuromyasthenia. Am J Med 26:569, 1959

HOLMES GP et al.: Chronic fatigue syndrome: A working case definition. Ann Intern Med 108:387, 1988

SCHLEUDERBERG A et al (eds): Considerations in the design of studies of chronic fatigue syndrome (monograph). Rev Infect Dis 13(suppl 1):S1, 1991

STRAUS SE: The chronic mononucleosis syndrome. J Infect Dis 157:405, 1988

———— et al.: Acyclovir treatment of the chronic fatigue syndrome: Lack of efficacy in a placebo-controlled trial. N Engl J Med 319:1692, 1988

section 4   Psychiatric disorders

389   MENTAL DISORDERS

LEWIS L. JUDD / KAREN THATCHER BRITTON / DAVID L. BRAFF

INTRODUCTION

Lewis L. Judd

Remarkable scientific progress in the understanding, accurate diagnosis, and successful treatment of the mental disorders has occurred in the last two decades. Fueled by the explosion of research emerging from modern neuroscience, it has been firmly established that the major mental disorders are diseases of the brain. Furthermore, there is unequivocal evidence that the mental disorders result from abnormal brain mechanisms that, with sophisticated neurobiologic techniques, can be characterized at cellular and molecular levels. The progressive unfolding of the pathophysiologic mechanisms in the brain that underlie the mental disorders has led to more rational, specific, and successful treatments for these disorders.

These rapidly accumulating discoveries, together with the development of a scientific, standardized, reliable, and clinically valid classification system for the mental disorders, the *Diagnostic, Statistical Manual of Mental Disorders,* Third Edition-Revised (DSM-III-R), has made it possible for clinicians to routinely identify and diagnose mental disorders that require treatment. Thus the focus of modern psychiatric clinical practice, like that of internal medicine, relies primarily on diagnosis, which in turn dictates the type of treatment prescribed and is highly predictive of clinical outcome.

The primary focus of this chapter is to highlight the most prevalent mental disorders that are of high relevance to the internal medicine and primary care physician. These are the mood and anxiety disorders, which at any one point in time, afflict about 10 percent of the U.S. population. Mood and anxiety disorders are central, or at least important, features in the clinical picture of approximately 25 percent of the patients who present in standard internal medicine practices. The last portion describes current understanding of the disease schizophrenia, which is included because of its prevalence in the general population and the highly disabling nature of its lifetime course. This aspect of the chapter focuses on issues of diagnoses, emphasizing the ability of the internist to differentiate the clinical features of schizophrenia from those of other brain diseases.

MOOD DISORDERS

Lewis L. Judd

The mood disorders are characterized by pervasive, prolonged, and disabling exaggerations of mood and affect that are associated with behavioral, physiologic, cognitive, neurochemical, and psychomotor dysfunctions. The major mood syndromes are *major depressive disorder* (also called unipolar disorder), *bipolar disorder* (also called manic depressive illness or bipolar depression), and *dysthymic disorder*. The classification of mood disorders into the unipolar and bipolar categories is useful clinically because these entities, although closely related mental disorders, are psychobiologically different with somewhat different clinical characteristics, disease patterns, and treatments.

EPIDEMIOLOGY OF MOOD DISORDERS AND RELEVANCE TO INTERNAL MEDICINE   Mood disorders are the second most common mental disorder, afflicting 5.1 percent of the U.S. population over 18 years of age at any one point in time (1-month prevalence). The 1-month prevalence for major depressive disorder is 2.2, for bipolar disorder 0.4, and for dysthymic disorder 3.3 percent. The 1-year prevalence for all mood disorders is 9.5 percent, making these diseases among the most common that people experience.

Clinical studies indicate that nonpsychiatric physicians frequently fail to accurately recognize or diagnose patients with mood disorders. Prevalence of mood disorders among primary care outpatients ranges from 4.8 to 8.6 percent for major depressive disorder, and 2.1 to 8.7 percent for dysthymic disorder. An additional 3.4 to 4.7 percent of patients who experience significant depressive symptoms do not reach the threshold criteria for a formal diagnosis of major depressive disorder or dysthymic disorder.

Therefore, 10.2 to 21 percent of primary care outpatients are suffering from clinically significant mood disorders. This is consistent with observations that patients with mood disorders are very high users of nonpsychiatric medical and primary care and emergency services. A presentation with depressive symptoms is the fourth most common complaint that patients report in primary care settings. The effective practice of internal medicine now requires that practitioners be thoroughly familiar with the accurate diagnosis of mood disorders in their patients. Mood disorders should always be a part of the differential diagnosis whenever patient complaints involve any symptoms in the depressive spectrum (e.g., low energy, difficulty with memory or concentration, impotence).

CLASSIFICATION Mood disorders are usually chronic in nature with a marked tendency to remission and exacerbation throughout the patient's lifetime. Remissions may last for weeks, months, or years (euthymia).

The diagnosis of a mood disorder should be based on the presence of signs and symptoms as defined in the DSM-III-R. Two general types of mood episodes may occur: major depressive episodes (sustained for at least 2 weeks) and manic episodes (sustained for at least 1 week). The diagnostic criteria for major depressive episodes and manic episodes are shown in Table 389-1 and 389-2.

Major depressive disorder may occur rarely as a single episode, but usually is recurrent (recurrent unipolar depression). Patients with the disorder manifest only a single extreme of pathologic mood, that of depression. In *bipolar disorder* both major depressive and manic episodes occur. Bipolar disorders are diagnosed as bipolar disorder, manic, if the current episode meets criteria for a manic episode and as bipolar disorder, depressed, if the episode meets criteria for a major depressive episode. Bipolar patients who have depressive and manic features simultaneously are classified as bipolar disorder, mixed.

Dysthymic disorder (dysthymia) is a chronic, less intense form of depression in which depressive symptoms persist for at least 2 years (see Table 389-3). Clinical studies have found that dysthymic disorder occurs together with major depressive disorder in about 25 percent of patients. This combined condition, called ''double-depression,'' has a much more grave prognosis with substantially higher risks for recurrence and resistance to treatment.

The signs and symptoms of *atypical depression* match those of major depressive disorder, but are distinguished from the latter by the following: reverse vegetative symptoms (e.g., overeating and hypersomnia), sensitivity to interpersonal rejection, a sense of ''leaden paralysis,'' the presence of a significant amount of pathologic anxiety, and/or unusual responsiveness to environmental changes. Distinguishing between atypical and typical major depressive disorder is useful because this disorder is often more responsive to monoamine oxidase (MAO) inhibitor antidepressants.

Other subgroups of mood disorders have been identified that are clinically less common and have less relevance to the internist. These include the following: *major depressive disorder, psychotic; major depressive disorder, melancholic; major depressive disorder, seasonal pattern; postpartum depression; brief recurrent depression; late luteal phase dysphoric disorder (premenstrual dysphoria);* and *cyclothymic*

TABLE 389-1 Diagnostic criteria for major depressive episode*

A At least five of the following symptoms have been present during the same 2-week period and represent a change from previous functioning; at least one of the symptoms is either (1) depressed mood, or (2) loss of interest or pleasure. (Do not include symptoms that are clearly due to a physical condition, mood-incongruent delusions or hallucinations, incoherence, or marked loosening of associations.)
  1 Depressed mood (or can be irritable mood in children and adolescents) most of the day, nearly every day, as indicated either by subjective account or observation by others
  2 Markedly diminished interest or pleasure in all, or almost all, activities most of the day, nearly every day (as indicated either by subjective account or observation by others of apathy most of the time)
  3 Significant weight loss or weight gain when not dieting (e.g., more than 5% of body weight in a month), or decrease or increase in appetite nearly every day (in children, consider failure to make expected weight gains)
  4 Insomnia or hypersomnia nearly every day
  5 Psychomotor agitation or retardation nearly every day (observable by others, not merely subjective feelings of restlessness or being slowed down)
  6 Fatigue or loss of energy nearly every day
  7 Feelings of worthlessness or excessive or inappropriate guilt (not merely self-reproach or guilt about being sick)
  8 Diminished ability to think or concentrate, or indecisiveness, nearly every day (either by subjective account or as observed by others)
  9 Recurrent thoughts of death (not just fear of dying), recurrent suicidal ideation without a specific plan, or a suicide attempt or a specific plan for committing suicide
B 1 It cannot be established that an organic factor initiated and maintained the disturbance.
  2 The disturbance is not a normal reaction to the death of a loved one (uncomplicated bereavement)†
C At no time during the disturbance have there been delusions or hallucinations for as long as 2 weeks in the absence of prominent mood symptoms (i.e., before the mood symptoms developed or after they have remitted).
D Not superimposed on schizophrenia or schizophreniform, delusional, or psychotic disorders.

* A major depressive syndrome is defined as criterion A above.
† Morbid preoccupation with worthlessness, suicidal ideation, marked functional impairment or psychomotor retardation, or prolonged duration suggest bereavement complicated by major depression.
SOURCE: Adapted from DSM-III-R.

TABLE 389-2 Diagnostic criteria for manic episode*

A A distinct period of abnormal and persistently elevated, expansive, or irritable mood.
B During the period of mood disturbance, at least three of the following symptoms have persisted (four if the mood is only irritable) and have been present to a significant degree:
  1 Inflated self-esteem or grandiosity
  2 Decreased need for sleep, e.g., feels rested after only 3 h of sleep
  3 More talkative than usual or pressure to keep talking
  4 Flight of ideas or subjective experience that thoughts are racing
  5 Distractibility, i.e., attention too easily drawn to unimportant or irrelevant external stimuli
  6 Increase in goal-directed activity (either socially, at work or school, or sexually) or psychomotor agitation
  7 Excessive involvement in pleasurable activities that have a high potential for painful consequences, e.g., the person engages in unrestrained buying sprees, sexual indiscretions, or foolish business investments
C Mood disturbance sufficiently severe to cause marked impairment in occupational functioning or in usual social activities or relationships with others, or to necessitate hospitalization to prevent harm to self or others.
D At no time during the disturbance have there been delusions or hallucinations for as long as 2 weeks in the absence of prominent mood symptoms (i.e., before the mood symptoms developed or after they have remitted).
E Not superimposed on schizophrenia or schizophreniform, delusional, or psychotic disorders.
F It cannot be established that an organic factor initiated and maintained the disturbance.†

* A manic syndrome is defined as including criteria A, B, and C above. A hypomanic syndrome is defined as including criteria A and B, but not C, i.e., no marked impairment.
† Somatic antidepressant treatment (e.g., drugs, electroconvulsive therapy) that apparently precipitates a mood disturbance should not be considered an etiologic organic factor.
SOURCE: Adapted from DSM-III-R.

TABLE 389-3 Diagnostic criteria for dysthmia

A Depressed mood (or can be irritable mood in children and adolescents)
   for most of the day, more days than not, as indicated either by subjective
   account or observation by others, for at least 2 years (1 year for children
   and adolescents).
B Presence, while depressed, of at least two of the following:
   1 Poor appetite or overeating
   2 Insomnia or hypersomnia
   3 Low energy or fatigue
   4 Low self-esteem
   5 Poor concentration or difficulty making decisions
   6 Feelings of hopelessness
C During a 2-year period (1 year for children and adolescents) of the disturbance, never without the symptoms in A for more than 2 months at a
   time.
D No evidence of an unequivocal major depressive episode during the first
   2 years (1 year for children and adolescents) of the disturbance.*
E Has never had a manic episode or an unequivocal hypomanic episode
   (see Table 389-2).
F Not superimposed on a chronic psychotic disorder, such as schizophrenia
   or delusional disorder.
G It cannot be established that an organic factor initiated and maintained
   the disturbance, e.g., prolonged administration of an antihypertensive
   medication.

---

* There may have been a previous major depressive episode, provided there was a full
remission (no significant signs or symptoms for 6 months) before development of the
dysthymia. In addition, after these 2 years (1 year in children and adolescents) of
dysthymia, there may be superimposed episodes of major depression, in which case
both diagnoses are given.
SOURCE: DSM-III-R.

disorder. The interested reader should refer to a standard textbook of
psychiatry for further information on these diagnostic subgroups.

COURSE OF ILLNESS Major depressive disorder Although
major depressive episodes can occur at any age, the peak age of onset
for the first episode is 25 years. Major depressive disorders occur
twice as frequently in women as in men. Symptoms may develop
over days, weeks, or occasionally months, and an untreated episode
lasts on average 10 to 12 months (range 6 to 24 months). Major
depressive disorder is a chronic disease with marked tendencies to
relapse and over 80 percent of patients have at least one more episode.
On average patients experience two to three episodes in their lifetime,
and 20 to 35 percent of patients manifest a chronic course with
considerable interepisode symptomatology and disability. Two-thirds
of the cases remit completely between episodes and functioning
returns to the premorbid level.

Bipolar disorder The age of risk for bipolar disorders is broad,
from 6 or 7 years to over 65 years; the peak age onset for a first
episode is 19 years. Bipolar disorders are slightly more frequent in
women than men (1.3 : 1). Men have more manic than depressive
episodes; women have more depressive episodes. Onset of symptoms
can be over hours but is usually over days or weeks and can begin
with either a manic or depressive episode. Over half of first episodes
are manic and approximately 60 percent of these patients have a
predominantly manic course, while the remaining one-third manifest
primarily depressive episodes. Clinical studies of untreated bipolar
patients show an average of 9 diagnosable manic and depressive
episodes during a lifetime (range 2 to more than 20). The typical
pattern is that the cycle length, which is measured from the onset of
one episode to the onset of the next, decreases and the number of
episodes increases over time. For example, in untreated bipolar
patients the time between the first and second episode averages from
3.5 to 4 years, between the second and third episodes about 2 years,
and between episodes three and four somewhere between 12 and 18
months. Untreated episode duration is from 4 to 13 months, and the
average is about 8.5 months, but may be shorter during manic phases
(i.e., the untreated illness tends to worsen over time, highlighting the
importance of intervention).

A small subgroup of bipolar patients manifest very rapid cycling
patterns, with from four episodes per year up to episodes every 24 h.
Eighty percent of rapid cyclers are women, and a relationship
to impaired thyroid function has been suggested. Although still

controversial, there is evidence that in some patients rapid cycling
may be related to previous treatment with tricyclic antidepressants
and that the condition can only be controlled effectively after tricyclics
are discontinued and treatment with thyroid supplement and lithium
is begun.

The life-long intensity of illness in all bipolar disorders is greater
than in major depressive disorder, recurrent; prior to the discovery of
lithium the long-term prognosis was very grim. Bipolar patients have
significantly more episodes of illness, require more hospitalizations,
spend more time in the hospital during their lifetimes, are more likely
to divorce, lose their jobs, and, if left untreated, are at significantly
higher risk for suicide.

Dysthymic disorder This disorder is characterized by chronic,
mild depressive symptoms manifested over many years. A significant
number of dysthymic disorders progress to a major depressive episode
within 1 year. Twenty percent or more develop double depression
(e.g., combined dysthymic disorder and major depressive disorder),
which is a much more malignant form of mood disorder.

MORBIDITY, MORTALITY, AND COMORBIDITY Morbidity
There is strong evidence that mood disorders have a major impact on
health status and quality of life. In a large sample of medical
outpatients (over 22,000 subjects) major depressive and dysthymic
disorders were shown to contribute greater disability in physical,
social, and occupational functioning than hypertension, diabetes,
chronic lung disease, or arthritis. Only patients with acute coronary
artery disease had more bed days during the previous month than
depressive disorders.

Mortality There are over 32,000 suicides each year in the United
States. Suicide is the eighth leading cause of death for adults in this
country. It has been estimated that 80 percent of the completed
suicides are related to mood disorders. Lifetime suicide attempt rate
in major depressive disorders is 14.3 percent and for dysthymic
disorders is 14.1 percent. Approximately 15 percent of patients with
recurrent major depressive disorders die by suicide.

Patients with bipolar disorders have increased death rate by suicide
amounting to 15 to 20 times that of the general population. Fifteen
to 20 percent of affected patients attempt suicide, more often women
than men, although men are more likely to succeed. Prior to lithium,
over 20 percent of manic patients died in the hospital, with about
two-thirds of these dying from "exhaustion."

Comorbidity with substance abuse disorders The high prevalence of mood disorders combined with a failure to recognize and
treat them probably contribute to the inordinately high rates at which
alcohol and/or drug abuse are concurrent with mood disorders. Thirty-
two percent of all mood disorder patients also are substance dependent
or substance abusers in their lifetime. Lifetime rates for this combination are 60.7 percent for bipolar disorder, 27.2 percent for major
depressive disorder, and 31.4 percent for dysthymic disorder. There
is growing evidence that concurrent substance abuse significantly
worsens the prognosis and treatability of mood disorders.

Comorbidity with medical conditions Many medical illnesses
may be associated with mood disorders, including autoimmune
disease, neurologic disease (stroke, demyelinative, degenerative,
traumatic disorders), metabolic disease, cardiovascular disease, endocrinopathies, and specific malignancies (pancreas, lung, kidney, G.I.,
brain). The clinical manifestations and the diagnosis of mood disorder
that is concurrent with medical disease are based on the same criteria
as the pure *primary* mood disorders.

Even though mood disorders may be associated with an extraordinarily large array of nonpsychiatric illnesses, several, because of their
importance, should be noted. For example, major depressive episodes
have been described in 25 to 55 percent of *poststroke* patients,
especially with strokes affecting the left anterior frontal lobe. These
episodes, if untreated, can persist for up to 12 months. Major
depressive disorder has been found to occur in 8.5 to 60 percent of
patients with *diabetes mellitus,* with the mean prevalence being about
30 percent.

About one quarter of patients with *malignancies* experience a clinically significant mood disorder, and 46 to 75 percent of patients with *chronic fatigue syndrome* are found to have a background of major depressive disorder. An even more substantial association between mood disorder and medical illness occurs in patients with *coronary artery disease*. Reports indicate that between 18 and 25 percent of patients after myocardial infarction experience a major depressive disorder that should be treated.

In addition, the chronic administration of the following medications may precipitate a major depressive episode: glucocorticoids, α-methyldopa, propranolol, benzodiazepines, reserpine derivatives, levodopa, neuroleptics, cimetidine, indomethacin, cycloserine, and anticancer drugs. Withdrawal from CNS stimulants such as amphetamines or drugs of abuse like cocaine may also be a precipitating factor.

It is important to recognize that these major depressive episodes occurring either in conjunction with a medical illness or the administration of a specific medication can often be the most important and disabling aspect of a patient's clinical picture and require immediate and specific treatment (e.g., some studies of transplant patients demonstrate the importance of treating depression before surgery to enhance postoperative recovery).

Two strategies can be used for treatment of a mood disorder concurrent with medical illness. First, if the symptoms are due to a primary "pure" mood disorder, the treatment should be initiated in a regimen identical to that used without a concomitant medical illness, unless the medical condition necessitates a modification, such as lowering the dosage because of impaired hepatic metabolism. When it is judged that the depressive symptoms are caused by the medical condition, it should be treated aggressively; at least one half of such patients show remission of depressive symptoms with effective treatment of the underlying medical illness. Often, however, treatment of the major depressive episode may need to be initiated in these patients to facilitate return to normal health.

ETIOLOGY AND PATHOPHYSIOLOGY OF THE MOOD DISORDERS Considerable scientific progress has been made in identifying and characterizing the etiologic factors in mood disorders. Several leads for focused scientific inquiry into the causes of these disorders have emerged; these leads have led to the development of more specific and effective treatments.

Genetic factors Mood disorders, like many other human diseases, result from complex interactions between the patient's genetic makeup and the environment. Genetic factors are particularly significant in bipolar disorders, although genetic components alone are probably insufficient to cause illness in the absence of environmental challenges. In general, the cause of a major mood episode can be conceptualized by two intersecting continua both with progressive intensities. One involves the patient's inherited constitutional vulnerability to develop mood disorder; this interacts with the second continuum of the environmental stresses and life events to which the patient is exposed. Some individuals with high genetic predisposition for mood disorder develop symptoms with minor precipitating events. Others with lower genetic vulnerability develop a mood disorder only when exposed to serious precipitating events and cumulative life stresses.

Data from numerous human genetic studies indicate significant genetic influences in the mood disorders, but as yet the mode of genetic transmission has not been established. The degree of genetic expression varies from one mood disorder to the other and from patient to patient. Twin studies of mood disorders report concordance rates among monozygotic (MZ) twins ranging from 33.3 to 75 percent, and for dizygotic (DZ) twins from 9 to 23 percent. This difference in concordance rates between MZ and DZ twins strongly suggests inherited genetic vulnerability. The concordance rate is highest for recurrent mood disorders (over three episodes). Although no definitive studies have been reported with identical twins reared apart, there are trends in such studies to suggest that adoptees have the higher incidence of affective illness of their biologic parents rather than of their adoptive parents.

Family studies of the mood disorders that include first-degree relatives show that the morbidity risk in relatives of bipolar patients is 2.8 to 17.7 percent and for major depressive disorders up to 22.4 percent. The first-degree relatives of major depressive disorder patients have a risk of 6.4 to 17.0 percent for major depressive episodes and of 0.3 to 29.0 percent for bipolar disorder. Thus bipolar patients have increased prevalence of both bipolar and major depressive disorders in their blood relatives, whereas major depressive disorder patients have increased prevalence of major depressive episodes, but not bipolar disorders, in their relatives.

There are several large ongoing studies combining careful diagnostic and family pedigree studies with molecular genetics in an attempt to identify linkage between specific gene(s) or DNA probes and mood disorder. Linkage on the X chromosome has been reported for bipolar disorder in an Israeli pedigree, as yet unconfirmed by others. In addition, a small subgroup of bipolar families has been found to have a linkage between protan-deutan (red-green) color blindness and glucose-6-phosphate dehydrogenase deficiency.

Neurotransmitter dysregulation The earliest investigations of etiologic mechanisms in the mood disorders involved studies of various neurotransmitter systems in the CNS. The *biogenic amine hypothesis* focused on the neurotransmitters norepinephrine, serotonin, and dopamine, attributing depression and mania, respectively, to the deficiency or excess of these neurotransmitters at important synaptic sites in the brain. This hypothesis continues as a subject of clinical research, and data both consistent and inconsistent with the hypothesis continue to emerge. Urinary and cerebrospinal fluid (CSF) studies of norepinephrine, its metabolite 3-methoxy-4-hydroxyphenethyleneglycol (MHPG), and the catalytic enzyme dopamine β-hydroxylase reported fluctuations in a predictable direction during major depressive and manic episodes. More recently, however, increases in norepinephrine have been described in *both* mania and depression. Studies have identified alterations in serotonin metabolism, with 5-hydroxyindoleacetic acid (5-HIAA), a metabolite, being reported to be reduced in the CSF of patients who make frequent impulsive, violent, and aggressive suicide attempts. However, this observation lacks specificity since similar changes have been observed in other mental disorders, including schizophrenia and antisocial personality disorders. Dopamine and gamma-aminobutyric acid (GABA) functions have also been reported to be abnormal in some patients with major depressive disorder; a cholinergic hypothesis which postulates increased central cholinergic tone in depression, decreased cholinergic tone in mania, and an imbalance between cholinergic and adrenergic neurotransmitter systems also has been proposed with inconclusive results.

More recently, with definition of receptor subtypes in the brain (see Chap. 364), there is growing interest in the possibility that postsynaptic receptor kinetics and activities may be altered during mood disorder episodes and that the psychotropic medications known to ameliorate these disorders may alter receptor functions. The role of postsynaptic receptor systems and especially the cascade of intraneuronal molecular and biochemical events in the postsynaptic neuron following the binding of the neurotransmitter to the receptor are currently under intensive study.

Environmental factors There are data on the type of stresses that are the most significant causes of major mood episodes. The data are inconsistent when efforts are made to relate early childhood loss and parental separation as predisposing factors for the development of a mood disorder. There is, not surprisingly, an overall temporal relationship between stressful and negative life events (e.g., spousal bereavement, a death of a child, job loss, marked change in social status, and severe assaults on self-esteem) and subsequent development of episodes of mood disorder. Research attempting to characterize qualitative differences in the impact of life stress have been disappointing.

Support for the idea of an influence of environmental events has been derived in experiments with subhuman primates. In these studies, phenomena that resemble or are analogous to depressive states in humans are seen in monkeys using mother/infant and peer separation paradigms. Interestingly, the monkey's "despair" response to the separation can be predictably altered (worsened or improved) by drugs known to specifically alter central concentrations and metabolites of several relevant CNS neurotransmitters (e.g., norepinephrine, dopamine), consistent with the view that psychosocial and CNS biochemical factors interact in the genesis of mood disorders.

Brain-environmental interactions One of the brain's most important and central functions is to receive incoming stimuli from the environment for purposes of storage, integration, and interpretation, which in turn provides the basis for an appropriate behavioral and cognitive response. Thus it should not be surprising to find that environmental events do exert consistent and powerful influences on brain function. Testable hypotheses are beginning to be developed. The learned helplessness paradigm of Seligman has been a very useful strategy in creating and studying depressive-like states in various animal models. These studies have been able to reduce brain 5-OH tryptamine (5HT) levels in response to behavioral stressors, which can be reversed by tricyclic antidepressants. Another exception is the CNS "kindling" hypothesis of Post and colleagues. From the data based in animal studies, including stimulant-induced behavioral sensitization and electrophysiologic kindling (increased sensitivity to electrically induced seizures), the suggestion has been made that a similar sensitization process may be involved in the recurrent episodes characteristic of the bipolar disorders. This hypothesis is consistent with the observations that spontaneous recurrences of affective episodes late in the progression of the illness seem, at times, to occur without precipitating factors; patients respond differently to pharmacotherapies at different stages of the disorder; there is frequently an increased sensitivity to anticonvulsant medications (i.e., carbamazepine combined with lithium) in some patients at late stages; and there is an increased rate of cycling as the disease progresses. One implication of this line of research is that prophylactic maintenance of pharmacotherapy may be justifiable early in the treatment of major depressive and bipolar mood disorders.

Biologic rhythms Major mood disorders show a marked tendency to periodic manifestation and to seasonal variation. This has stimulated hypotheses to explore dysregulation of biologic rhythms as a mechanism involved in the pathophysiology of some mood disorders. There are reports of desynchronization of circadian rhythms with some bipolar patients manifesting both rapid free-running circadian rhythms (e.g., 23- versus 24-h rhythms) and a phase delay in their rhythms.

There is also a special subgroup of patients with major depression in which the depressive episodes are manifested at specific seasons of the year. The most consistently studied groups are those with so-called "winter" depression (also called *seasonal affective disorder*). These patients, while residing in more northern latitudes, experience major depressive episodes during the winter when days are significantly shorter and periods of darkness more prolonged; conversely, there is a marked reduction or absence of depressive episodes in latitudes where the environmental light/dark cycles are not as extreme. Controlled treatment studies, using intense white light (>2000 lux) presented at a specified time during the day and for a precise period of time, have proven to be therapeutically effective in some patients with this syndrome. Finally, the consistent antidepressant effects of specific forms of sleep deprivation in major depressive disorders also provides support for this hypothesis.

BIOLOGIC CORRELATES AND LABORATORY STUDIES Neurohormonal correlates For a number of years, probes into the pathophysiologic mechanisms of the mood disorders have used various neurohormones whose secretion is regulated by one or more of the CNS neurotransmitter pathways (e.g., dopamine, norepinephrine, serotonin). One consistent finding from these studies has been that a significant subpopulation of patients with major depressive disorder hypersecrete cortisol and have abnormal cortisol circadian secretion patterns. Recent investigations with corticotropin-releasing hormone (CRH) stimulation have yielded blunted adrenocorticotropic hormone (ACTH) responses, suggesting that the corticosteroid abnormality is

of central origin. In addition, even though it is now controversial, the dexamethasone suppression test (DST) has been used in both diagnosis and monitoring of treatment in research settings. It has virtually no utility clinically because approximately 50 percent of patients with major depression do not have this abnormality. The standard DST used in psychiatry involves the administration of 1 mg of dexamethasone at 2300 hours with subsequent cortisol determinations at 1600 and 2300 hours the following day. The nonsuppression of cortisol is an abnormal or positive response [>140 nmol/L (>5 μg/dL) cortisol concentration in the 1600 or 2300 sample]. Initial studies reported that up to 50 percent of patients with serious major depressive episodes were nonsuppressors on the DST. Further investigations indicate that DST nonsuppression is a state marker, positive during the depressive episode, with return to normal after successful resolution of the episode. False-positives on the DST occur in patients with alcoholism, malnutrition, obesity, pregnancy, major physical illnesses, anticonvulsant use, excessive caffeine intake, and in patients over 65 years. This has eroded the usefulness of the test. In addition, more recently a number of studies have appeared in the literature reporting a much smaller percentage of DST nonsuppressors associated with major depressive episodes and an increased percentage in many other psychiatric illnesses. DST nonsuppression among depressed patients has now been reported as low as 10 to 15 percent, especially among depressed outpatients, making this test of no value as a screening test for depression. While the status of this diagnostic marker is still controversial, some clinicians advocate monitoring treatment efficacy in DST-positive depressives, since the DST response reverts to normal when the episode remits. Failure of DST to normalize despite apparent clinical recovery has, in some studies, been associated with suicide.

Other neuroendocrine markers have also been explored, but none as widely as the DST. In major depression, between 25 and 30 percent of patients respond to thyrotropin-releasing hormone (TRH) with blunted thyroid-stimulating hormone (TSH) responses. TSH blunting is not specific to depressive episodes, but an exaggerated TSH response is useful in identifying those refractory or rapid-cycling bipolar patients who would benefit from thyroid supplementation (e.g., T_3 or T_4). Small subgroups of depressed patients have manifested blunted growth hormone responses to the following challenge agents: clonidine, amphetamine, levodopa, 5-hydroxytryptophan, and hypoglycemia (insulin tolerance test). Even though 15 to 25 percent of depressed patients have blunted growth hormone responses, it has not been proved to be diagnostically useful. More recently, blunted prolactin responses to both TRH and opiate alkaloid challenges have also been reported in subpopulations of depressed patients; while these findings may be of interest in probing pathophysiologic mechanisms, they are not useful diagnostically.

Sleep studies The disruption of sleep patterns is present in virtually every patient with mood disorder, and polysomnographic studies of sleep in these patients have proved to be of importance. In approximately 60 percent of cases of major depressive disorder there is a significantly shortened time period between the onset of sleep and the appearance of the first rapid eye movement (REM) (i.e., *decreased REM latency*). In addition, the density of the REM epoch, measured by the number of eye movements, is increased; there is a tendency for the REM epoch to last longer, and there is a shift of REM activity to an earlier part of the night. *These findings from all-night EEG sleep recordings have remained among the most consistent biologic markers for major depressive episodes, although they lack specificity, since short REM latency has also been reported in anorexia nervosa, obsessive-compulsive disorders, sleep apnea, and narcolepsy.*

Neurotransmitter metabolites and enzymes The neurotransmitter hypotheses of mood disorders have stimulated a number of studies correlating biogenic amine metabolites with manic and depressive episodes. The data are inconclusive and have not been consistently useful either diagnostically or therapeutically. The one possible exception is MHPG, a metabolite of norepinephrine. Some workers have reported low MHPG excretion as predicting a positive therapeutic response to the "norepinephrine" antidepressants such as desipramine, and high MHPG excretion as predicting a response to serotoninergic agents like amitriptyline. While these data are of interest and with further study may result in the identification of biochemical subtypes in major depression, these findings have not been regularly replicated in other laboratories.

Investigators who have examined the levels of the enzyme MAO in platelets report it to be low in bipolar disorders and high in subjects with anxiety disorder. Further, ^{3}[H]imipramine-binding studies in platelets also have been found to be low in major depressives who were suicidal. Again, these findings, although of interest, lack specificity, since similar results have been reported in other psychiatric conditions such as alcoholism, anorexia and bulimia, and impulse control disorders.

GENERAL PRINCIPLES IN THE TREATMENT OF MOOD DISORDERS The prevalence of mood disorders is estimated to be as high as 20 percent in general medical and primary care settings. The first step in the treatment of any mood disorder is recognition. The primary care physician should be aware that a mood disorder may be present in patients exhibiting certain symptoms, although they may be somewhat vague, nonspecific, and of little consequence (e.g., low energy, easy fatigability, loss of interest in every day and pleasurable activities, dysphoria, insomnia, impotence). However, there are some clinical clues that should raise the index of suspicion, such as the presence of treatment for previous major depressive episodes, history of suicide attempts, family history of depression or of suicide attempts, or alcoholism or drug abuse.

Important advances have been made in the treatment of the mood disorders, and the vast majority of these patients can now be treated with a high degree of specificity and success. The most important discoveries have been made in the development of potent psychotropic medications for both major depression and bipolar disorders. The central therapeutic tools in the treatment of the major affective disorders are the antidepressants and lithium and to a lesser extent certain anticonvulsants (e.g., carbamazepine, sodium valproate) (see below).

Because mood disorders have strong tendencies for recurrence, an important aspect of the patient's treatment is the comprehensive education of patients and their families about the disorder. It should be emphasized to the patient that these are psychobiologic disorders that involve altered biochemical states in the brain, and that episodes can be triggered by adverse events and stresses in the environment but may occur spontaneously as well. As with any chronic disease, each patient should be urged to become an expert on his or her own disorder, concentrating on how it manifests itself and what early signs and symptoms may herald a manic or depressive episode. The patient and the family must be urged to take on the responsibility for the early recognition of the impending episode, since the earlier a patient presents for treatment, the easier it is to treat. The absolute necessity of medication compliance must be emphasized, and the patient must understand thoroughly the need to take the medications precisely as prescribed and to be aware of side effects and of the potential medical sequelae of the medications.

With the emergence of new evidence indicating that the mood disorders are chronic lifelong diseases, there has been an increasing emphasis on maintenance treatment strategies whose goals are to keep the patient free of symptoms throughout their lifetime. There is emerging support for the view that maintaining patients with recurrent major depressive disorder on an antidepressant medication at the same dosage that proved to be effective in the original acute episode may prevent relapse. There is an increasing acceptance that the disease model for treatment of the mood disorders more closely resembles diabetes mellitus than lobar pneumonia. The physician's therapeutic approach to patients who are suffering acute mood episodes is simple and straightforward. During the acute phase of these episodes, patients respond better to short (10 to 20 min) visits one to three times per week. During these visits the general focus is on monitoring the medication and side effects, but it is also essential that the physician be very informative, reassuring, and supportive.

Because patients are functioning essentially in an altered state secondary to the depressive or manic episode, the treatment must be sustained by the physician's optimism and knowledge that, with time, these episodes will abate if the proper medication and dose are prescribed. Virtually all the antidepressants and mood-stabilizing medications have a significant delay between when the drug is first taken and when full therapeutic benefits appear. It is during this time that supportive reassurance and encouragement from the physician is particularly important in sustaining the patient in treatment.

It bears repeating that there are approximately 32,000 suicides a year in this country, and clinical surveys indicate that approximately 80 percent of these patients have mood disorders. Suicidal ideation is one of the important symptoms that accompany major depressive episodes, in both bipolar and unipolar disorders; considerations of suicidal lethality are central in the management of these patients. Although it is not possible to distinguish precisely between patients who will attempt suicide and those who will not, there are some factors which should be considered. Generally speaking, it is agreed that patients who have developed a specific plan of suicide, who have concomitant alcoholism or drug abuse, and who are socially isolated with few (if any) social supports have a greater potential risk for suicide. The patient's level of hopefulness also tends to correlate with risk. In addition, elderly males and patients with terminal medical illnesses have a greater risk. Unfortunately, each of the above characteristics lacks specificity in the assessment of suicidal risk. Perhaps the most important of all risk factors is the presence of an undiagnosed and untreated mood disorder.

It is recommended that nonpsychiatric physicians rely primarily on the antidepressants or lithium (depending on the disorder treated) in combination with educational and supportive psychotherapeutic approaches in the management of patients with mood disorders. Specific psychotherapies (cognitive/behavioral psychotherapy and interpersonal psychotherapy of depression) can be used successfully in the treatment of mild to moderate major depressive episodes. It is, however, recommended that the nonpsychiatric physician not experiment with these techniques since competency in these forms of psychotherapy requires considerable training and experience to achieve results comparable to those obtained with the relatively simple administration of an appropriate antidepressant medication.

If the physician assesses the suicide risk to be high, the patient requires psychiatric consultation. High-risk patients may require a supervised environment such as a hospital, although in some instances involved family and friends may serve to monitor the patient.

Patients who have complicated psychiatric histories or fail to respond to the initial medication trial should be referred for psychiatric consultation. This may lead to medication combination (augmentations) or other sophisticated treatment such as electroconvulsive therapy (ECT). The latter remains a potent tool for refractory patients or those who cannot tolerate medication side effects.

ANTIDEPRESSANT MEDICATIONS An almost bewildering array of specific and effective antidepressant drugs is currently available, with new medications appearing with great frequency. The first-generation medications include the tricyclic (TCA) and the MAO inhibitor antidepressants. The main benefit of the newer antidepressants is that they have provided the physician with an expanded range of pharmacologic options for the treatment of patients who cannot tolerate or who do not respond to the older drugs. The MAO inhibitors are clinically effective, but the problems of drug-drug and drug-food interactions have made these a second-choice medication in the treatment of depressive disorders. However, the MAO inhibitors appear to be especially effective for depression accompanied by panic attacks or prominent anxiety. The TCAs imipramine and amitriptyline remain the standards for antidepressant efficacy, although newer drugs are equally effective with fewer side effects.

No antidepressant is ideal, and currently available drugs have at least one of the following undesirable characteristics: delayed onset of therapeutic action (7 to 28 days), significant anticholinergic side effects, sedation, agitation, cardiotoxicity, weight gain, the possible induction of manic or hypomanic episodes in patients with bipolar disorders, or other equally problematic adverse reactions. The search for new medications may yet yield a superior antidepressant, one with a consistently high rate of improvement, rapid onset of action, and fewer side effects.

Mechanisms of action   TCAs were originally hypothesized to increase synaptic concentrations of central nervous system monoaminergic neurotransmitter substances (e.g., norepinephrine, serotonin, and dopamine) by blocking their reuptake by presynaptic monoaminergic neurons. While this assumption is still valid, the focus now is on the regulation of postsynaptic receptor activity of monoaminergic neurons and the down-regulation of neurotransmitter receptors that have been associated with an antidepressant effect. These mechanisms have been hypothesized to account for the activity of most of the established antidepressants, but not some of the newer antidepressants. At present, therefore, there is a great deal of information available about how antidepressants may ameliorate the pathophysiologic processes associated with depressive disorders, but no precise central mechanism(s) has been identified by which all drugs with antidepressant properties work.

Clinical conditions for use   Antidepressants are very effective in treatment of the clinical syndrome of major depression but do not affect normal mood changes. Chronic low-grade depression or dysthymic disorders have generally not responded well to antidepressants alone, although more recent data indicate promising results from the newer selective serotoninergic antidepressants.

There is growing evidence that antidepressants are effective in the treatment of some anxiety disorders. TCAs and the MAO inhibitor antidepressants are the drugs of choice for agoraphobia and panic disorder. Patients with panic disorders have concomitant anxiety about the recurrence of these attacks; this ''anticipatory'' anxiety may not respond to antidepressants but may benefit from concomitant treatment with antianxiety medication or behavioral approaches such as desensitization. There is a definitive role for the antidepressants in the management of pure anxiety disorders and mixed depressed and anxious states.

Clinical use of antidepressants   Table 389-4 lists the more commonly used first-generation antidepressants and the oral doses needed for therapeutic efficacy in the typical patient. Currently imipramine and amitriptyline are the standards for antidepressant potency. Amitriptyline tends to have sedative effects, while imipramine is more energizing. Because of the undesirable side effects observed in these original TCAs, during the past decade growing numbers of experienced clinical psychopharmacologists have gradually selected the secondary tricyclic amines desipramine and nortriptyline as the antidepressant drugs of choice. Both desipramine and nortriptyline have fewer anticholinergic side effects and are less

sedating. Nortriptyline appears to have a clear relationship between plasma levels and clinical efficacy.

Before antidepressants are prescribed, a patient's physical health must be evaluated by a physical examination. The patient should show normal values on baseline complete blood count (CBC), urinalysis, liver function tests, and (if over 45 years) electrocardiogram (ECG). Patients are usually started on low doses (e.g., 25 mg desipramine qhs) and checked for side effects (e.g., postural hypotension). The dose is then raised over a few days to that needed for a full therapeutic response. The minimum daily dose for clinical response is the low figure in the ranges listed in Table 389-4, but often higher doses are needed. However, dose schedules in the elderly should be reduced 30 to 50 percent. Physicians inexperienced in psychopharmacology should not exceed the upper dosage limits listed in the table. Treatment from 7 to 28 days is required to achieve a full therapeutic effect. Changes in the depressive symptoms are often noted by friends and family before the patient reports feeling better. A therapeutic trial of an antidepressant requires at least 28 days at the upper end of the dose range. Patients are usually maintained on antidepressants for approximately 9 to 12 months after the depressive symptoms disappear, to reduce the possibility of relapse resulting from premature withdrawal of medication. Highest relapse rates occur during the first 2 months after medication is discontinued, and patients and clinicians should be especially watchful during this time period.

Medications can be given in a single dose an hour before bedtime once an appropriate dose has been established. This procedure improves medication compliance, and sedative side effects are likely to induce sleep in depressed patients, who are often insomniac. Further, if troublesome side effects occur, they do so while the patient is asleep. For patients who cannot tolerate the single bedtime dose, a daytime twice daily or thrice daily schedule is necessary. Tests for plasma levels of the tricyclic antidepressants are routinely available, but unfortunately the relationship of plasma levels to clinical response has been inconsistent. For imipramine, desipramine, and amitriptyline, the relationship is linear, but nortriptyline may have a curvilinear plasma level-response relationship, implying a therapeutic window. Plasma levels at steady state after 5 days of a given dose may be useful in treatment-resistant patients to evaluate compliance and to see if the dose is sufficient to maintain concentrations above the threshold necessary for response (e.g., imipramine, >180 ng/mL; desipramine, >125 ng/mL; amitriptyline, >95 ng/mL; and nortriptyline, 50 to 150 ng/mL).

After about 10 to 12 months of treatment with an antidepressant, the drug should be withdrawn gradually over a 3- to 4-week period rather than suddenly stopped. Should depressive symptoms reemerge, antidepressant treatment should be restored and maintained for several more months before the withdrawal attempt is repeated.

Side effects and interactions   Listed in Table 389-5 are some of the more common side effects from the tricyclic antidepressants. They include dry mouth, sedation, a fine tremor of the hands, and mild constipation. More serious are the effects on the cardiovascular system, of which tachycardia and postural hypotension are the most common. The TCAs, especially imipramine, have a quinidine-like action, can induce cardiac arrhythmias, and have been associated with sudden death in a few patients (see section below on overdose). For patients with preexisting cardiac illness, especially those with heart conduction defects, TCAs should be used cautiously; drugs with milder cardiac effects should be considered. In some instances, however, the quinidine-like effect can be used to advantage, i.e., to produce a significant antiarrhythmic effect with once-daily dosing. Imipramine has been used as a comparison drug for other type 1-A antiarrhythmics. The most bothersome symptoms are from the anticholinergic effects; while rarely serious, they do cause discomfort and compliance problems.

Some preexisting medical conditions increase the risks associated with using TCAs in certain depressed patients. Tricyclics can produce tachycardia, which may push some patients from asymptomatic congestive failure into symptomatic heart failure. TCAs also lower

TABLE 389-4 Commonly used first-generation antidepressants	
Antidepressant	Daily oral therapeutic dose range, mg
TRICYCLIC DERIVATIVES	
Amitriptyline	150–300
Nortriptyline	50–150
Imipramine	150–300
Desipramine	150–250
Doxepin	150–300
Trimipramine	100–250
MONOAMINE OXIDASE INHIBITORS	
Phenelzine	15–60
Tranylcypromine	20–30
Isocarboxazid	10–30

TABLE 389-5 Common side effects of tricyclic antidepressants

Anticholinergic (atropine-like) responses:
  Dry mouth
  Nausea and vomiting*
  Constipation
  Urinary retention
  Blurred vision (mydriasis and cycloplegia)
Cardiovascular effects:
  Postural hypotension*
  Tachycardia
  Cardiac conduction disturbances
Obstructive jaundice—more rare—is reversible when drug is removed
Drowsiness and sleepiness—may want to avoid driving a car until this
  diminishes*
Fine rapid tremor*
Dizziness, ataxia
Hematologic effects:
  Leukopenia
Endocrine effects:
  Syndrome of inappropriate ADH secretion

*Side effects seen most commonly

the seizure threshold and should be used cautiously in patients with seizures. The anticholinergic effects preclude TCA treatment in patients with narrow-angle glaucoma and pose a problem for men with mild to moderate prostatic hypertrophy, who may develop urinary retention. Finally, the use of tricyclic antidepressants in patients with bipolar disorders may shorten the cycle length between affective episodes, may induce an acute manic episode in some patients, and has been related to the phenomenon of rapid cycling.

The tricyclics, especially amitriptyline, imipramine, and doxepin, potentiate the effects of other CNS-depressant medications (e.g., ethanol, benzodiazepines), and patients should be cautioned about ethanol use while on antidepressants. Patients should either not drink or reduce their usual ethanol dose by one-half during tricyclic treatment. Cimetidine elevates tricyclic levels. Other drug interactions include the potentiation of other anticholinergic agents (e.g., antihistamines, antiparkinsonian agents), which can result in severe constipation, urinary retention, and even paralytic ileus. This combination in the elderly, which can produce a serious anticholinergic blockade (e.g., paralytic ileus, fecal impaction), often has been the cause of frank delirium and confusional states in geriatric patients; it is to be avoided in older patients.

Despite the problems, the risk-benefit ratio is overwhelmingly in favor of the antidepressants, and literally hundreds of thousands of patients have been treated with these compounds safely and effectively.

NEWER ANTIDEPRESSANTS Table 389-6 lists the more promising second-generation drugs for which evidence of antidepressant efficacy exists. Already they have expanded the physicians' therapeutic choices in the treatment of depressive disorders. These agents, particularly fluoxetine, bupropion, sertraline, and paroxetine offer significant advantages: no anticholinergic side effects, no weight gain, and no cardiac conduction effects.

Amoxapine is a tricyclic derivative with clinical efficacy equal to that of the original antidepressants. An early onset of action (within the first week) has been claimed by the manufacturer, although its clinical efficacy at the endpoint of treatment is identical to that of the

TABLE 389-6 Selected second-generation antidepressants

Antidepressant	Daily oral therapeutic dose range, mg
Fluoxetine	10–40
Bupropion	200–300
Paroxetine	20–40
Sertraline	50–200
Clomipramine	150–300
Amoxapine	150–300
Trazodone	100–600
Maprotiline	100–225

original TCAs. One of its metabolites (7-hydroxyamoxapine) is a neuroleptic, which accounts for the extrapyramidal side effects seen, including tardive dyskinesia and parkinsonism. The neuroleptic component, however, has made amoxapine a drug to be considered in depressed patients who show psychotic features. Other side effects appear to be similar to those of the original tricyclics, although a disproportionate number of seizures was found in some retrospective studies.

Clomipramine, a tricyclic that inhibits serotonin reuptake, commonly used worldwide, is now approved for use in the United States. It has been shown in controlled studies to be an effective drug in the treatment of depression and currently is the drug of choice in obsessive-compulsive disorder, which is frequently disabling and resistant to treatment.

Fluoxetine is a relatively selective serotonin-uptake inhibitor with antidepressant efficacy comparable to imipramine. Side effects similar to those observed with other serotonin-uptake blockers include nausea, diarrhea, tremor, headache, agitation, and weight loss, and range from mild to moderate severity. Administration may also be associated with akathisia, which may be related to controversial reports of suicidal ideas. Akathisia can be treated with a decreased dosage of benzodiazepines or with propranalol. The recommended dose of 20 mg/d is adequate for most patients, but both lower and higher doses may be needed (e.g., 10–40 mg/d). Fluoxetine is now available in elixir form for doses less than 20 mg/d. Patients show few signs of cardiac conduction effects. There are also reports of successful treatment of obsessive-compulsive disorder with fluoxetine in controlled studies. Fluoxetine is one of the first of a series of highly specific and potent serotonin-uptake inhibitors to be marketed in the United States. Sertraline is available in the United States. It is a potent serotonin receptor blocker that may cause less agitation than fluoxetine. It has a much shorter half-life (24 h) and no active metabolite as compared to fluoxetine (7 to 14 days). Paroxetine was approved for use in the United States in 1993. Others are still in clinical trial (e.g., fluroxamine, indalpine).

Maprotiline is a tetracyclic derivative that is equal in antidepressant potency to the original tricyclics and reportedly has fewer anticholinergic side effects. Originally it was offered as a promising drug for use in patients with cardiovascular problems, but this has not been established and it is not recommended for this purpose. It has been reported to cause seizures at two to four times the rate at which the TCAs induce seizures, and a lower dosage schedule is now recommended. Moreover, its use has been asssociated with more than the expected incidence of blood dyscrasia.

Trazodone is a triazolopyridine derivative originally introduced for use as an antidepressant. There remains controversy around whether it has significant antidepressant properties. The drug produces a high level of sedation and is useful as a hypnotic. It has few, if any, cardiotoxic effects but is associated with increased risk of priapism.

Bupropion was withdrawn from the market because it produced a high rate of seizures in a subpopulation of bulimic patients. It was subsequently re-released when the seizure rate was found to be no greater than that produced by the TCAs (estimated at about 0.4 percent) and is currently used for treating major depression. A role for bupropion in combination with lithium in stabilizing patients with rapid-cycling disorders has also been proposed. The mechanism of action may be related to dopamine-reuptake inhibition, although this is not fully established. Bupropion has energizing properties and consequently is less sedating, with mild side effects including headache, agitation, and some anticholinergic effects. It must be given in divided daytime dose to avoid increased seizure frequency.

TRICYCLIC OVERDOSAGE Antidepressants are the fourth most common cause of drug overdose seen in emergency departments in the United States and the third most frequent cause of drug-related death (after alcohol-drug combinations and heroin). Of the antidepressants, tricyclics are the most frequent cause of death. In a California study (Callaham and Kassel) the annual frequency of fatal tricyclic overdose was 1.3 per 100,000 population; more than two-thirds of the victims were women. Amitriptyline, desipramine, and nortriptyline were the most frequently implicated.

The first 6 h after an overdose of a tricyclic antidepressant are crucial. CNS depression and seizures, respiratory arrest, and cardiovascular arrhythmias are the principal causes of death. ECG changes showing QRS prolongation are early signs of toxicity, and ventricular fibrillation is a common complication. ECG changes are a more sensitive measure for monitoring patients than are blood levels of the drug.

LITHIUM AND OTHER MOOD-NORMALIZING MEDICATIONS

The most important psychotropic medication in this group is lithium. Although lithium possesses some antidepressant properties, it is not, strictly speaking, an antidepressant. Its effectiveness in treating patients with bipolar disorders and other disorders of mood has revolutionized the practice of psychiatry. Lithium's approval by the U.S. Food and Drug Administration in 1970 for the treatment of acute mania and in 1975 for the maintenance treatment of manic-depressive disorder generated an explosion of basic and clinical research focused on its pharmacologic mechanisms and clinical use.

Mechanism of action   The central mechanisms by which lithium exerts its clinical effects on extremes of mood are not fully understood. Lithium affects the brain's monoaminergic neurotransmitter concentrations at the synapse, has strong effects on biologic membranes, and intracellularly inhibits the conversion of inositol monophosphate to free inositol. This latter effect may, in turn, reduce neuronal excitability.

Clinical conditions for use   Lithium is the drug of choice for treating acute manic/hypomanic episodes and for prevention of recurrent episodes of mania and depression in bipolar illness. Recent studies suggest that the relapse rate among lithium-treated bipolar patients is about one-half that of control patients receiving a placebo. It may also be an effective agent in the prophylaxis of recurrent unipolar depressive disorders. Lithium also has antidepressant properties, especially in depressions seen in bipolar disorders; however, it is not a drug of choice for major depression per se. Lithium also is used to augment TCA and other antidepressants; i.e., to enhance response in nonresponders. It has also been successfully used in conjunction with neuroleptics in schizoaffective disorders; there may be a subpopulation of schizophrenics responsive to lithium, although most workers feel that such lithium responders are atypical bipolar patients and not schizophrenics. Finally, there are some reports that lithium may be useful in treating alcoholism, a possibility requiring further study.

Clinical use of lithium   Lithium is a very safe drug with an excellent risk-benefit ratio when it is used knowledgeably. The only genuine contraindication to lithium's use is seriously compromised renal function. The following baseline studies should be obtained before prescribing lithium: CBC, routine urinalysis with a concentration test, thyroxine (T_4), free T_4 index, thyroid-stimulating hormone (TSH), serum creatinine, electrolytes, and (for those over 40) an ECG.

Serum lithium levels peak 1 to 3 h after an oral dose, and the biologic half-life, which averages 24 h, varies with age. Elderly patients frequently have a drug half-life over 30 h, often requiring lower doses. Lithium is monitored by serum levels, which are most informative approximately 10 h after the last dose. Therapeutic efficacy in acute mania is achieved at levels between 0.8 and 1.4 mmol/L. Patients rarely require treatment at serum levels above 1.5 mmol/L. Lithium is always administered orally. Dose ranges are from 600 mg to 3000 mg daily, unless the patient is elderly. A general rule of thumb equates a 0.2 mmol/L rise in serum level with each additional 300-mg tablet of lithium. Unless sustained-release tablets are used, lithium is usually administered twice or three times daily, allowing for smooth, sustained 24-h serum levels. Because there is a 7- to 10-day delay in achieving full therapeutic effects, the addition of antipsychotic medications or clonazepam is often needed during the early phase of treating a manic patient. During acute manic

TABLE 389-7   Common lithium side effects

Severity	Side effect
SIDE EFFECTS COMMONLY SEEN	
Very mild	Thirst
	Nausea (particularly during first few days of treatment)
	Fine tremor of hand
Mild to moderate	Anorexia
	Vomiting
	Diarrhea
	"Upset stomach" or "abdominal pain"
	Polydipsia and/or polyuria
	Muscular weakness and fatigue
SIDE EFFECTS INDICATING TOXICITY	
	Muscle hyperirritability with twitching, muscle fasciculation, or chronic movements
	Sedation, sluggishness, languidness, drowsiness, giddiness
	Coarse tremor
	Ataxia
Moderate to severe	Hypertonic muscles
	Hyperactive deep tendon reflexes
	Hyperextension of arms and legs with grunts and gasping
	Chorea, athetotic movements
	Impairment of consciousness
	Somnolence, confusion, stupor
	Seizures
Very severe	Coma
	Complications of coma
	Death

episodes patients often tolerate relatively higher doses of lithium, but once the manic episode remits, it is necessary to reduce the dose.

The current maintenance treatment strategy is to prevent future recurrent episodes of mania and depression in patients with bipolar disorders. Clinicians are advised to seek the lowest possible serum levels in the range from 0.6 to 1.0 mmol/L that will prevent relapse. Lithium's excretion rate is very stable within each patient; as a result patients can be maintained on the same dose day in and day out, with relative certainty that stable levels are present. During maintenance patients are seen every 3 to 6 months, and serum lithium, sodium, potassium, T_4, free T_4 index, TSH, and creatinine are monitored along with urinalysis with a concentration test. The lithium excretion pattern is altered by conditions that change sodium concentrations, and patients on thiazide diuretics or low-salt diets should be warned and monitored more frequently.

Side effects and interactions   Lithium's side effects are listed in a continuum ranging from those seen relatively commonly to those indicating lithium toxicity (see Table 389-7). Many of these are minor side effects, which appear early and disappear as time passes, but some may persist throughout treatment. Because the rapid escalation of serum levels often induces side effects, especially those involving the gastrointestinal tract, smoother, more gradual serum lithium increases are desirable.

Some of the first signs of lithium toxicity are coarsening of tremor, increases in the deep tendon reflexes, and muscle fasciculations. Unusual degrees of sedation and cognitive disruption also may herald lithium toxicity. Lithium toxicity mimics barbiturate intoxication, and when death occurs it is secondary to respiratory depression and its complications. The treatment of lithium toxicity involves good supportive care and excellent hydration. Administration of normal saline is helpful in increasing lithium excretion. Since lithium's half-life is 24 h, this treatment sustains the patient until the kidneys eliminate the medication. Various methods to improve the treatment of lithium toxicity, such as increasing lithium excretion by aminophylline or alkalinizing the urine, have all been disappointing. For life-threatening cases, the last resort is renal dialysis, but toxicity does not commonly progress to the point where this intervention is needed.

There is some evidence that lithium is a teratogen, particularly when administered during the first trimester of pregnancy. Cardiovascular and valve abnormalities have been detected in 18-week-old fetuses. While there is little evidence for teratogenesis during the second and third trimesters other mood-stabilizing medications can be considered in pregnant women and weighed against the risk of untreated bipolar disorder.

Lithium's interactions with other drugs primarily involve its reciprocal relationship with the sodium ion. Diuretics, which increase sodium excretion, can increase lithium toxicity. There have also been reports that combined neuroleptic and lithium therapy has resulted in an irreversible neurotoxicity in a small number of middle-aged and older patients. Clinical observations indicate that this combination is safe and effective provided that both drugs are used in low to moderate doses, carefully monitored, and discontinued as soon as the lithium effect is sufficiently present for the patient to be managed without the neuroleptic.

Medical sequelae of lithium's use Several medical complications can develop during lithium treatment. Because of its effect on adenylate cyclase activity, lithium inhibits the thyroid gland's secretory function; nontoxic goiters and hypothyroidism can develop, which can be readily corrected during lithium therapy by thyroid supplement. Lithium may induce the following ECG changes especially in older patients: T-wave depression, sinus node dysfunctions, and, very rarely, sinoatrial block and ventricular irritability.

The most important sequelae are the renal complications. About 25 percent of patients develop some degree of vasopressin-resistant nephrogenic diabetes insipidus with polyuria and polydipsia. The lithium inhibition of adenylate cyclase activity is responsible for the disruption of renal tubular transport. These symptoms are usually completely reversible by lithium withdrawal and often can be ameliorated by a reduction in dosage. The most economic and accurate method of monitoring changes in renal function during lithium treatment is by the urine concentration test and serum creatinine level. Consistent urine concentration levels below a specific gravity of 1.025 indicate an early renal effect, and a creatinine clearance test should be obtained. If creatinine clearance is abnormal, the patient's clinical condition should be reevaluated and termination of the lithium treatment considered. There have been reports of renal focal necrosis and interstitial fibrosis in a few long-term lithium patients, and there is evidence, by biopsy, for an increased basal rate of renal pathology among patients with affective disorders. Nonetheless, this nonspecific renal lesion does appear more frequently in patients receiving long-term lithium.

Evidence has emerged linking the more serious renal complications to increased episodes of lithium toxicity and possibly to prolonged combined use of lithium and neuroleptics. While good clinical practice should obviate lithium toxicity, it may be equally important to avoid extremes of high and low serum lithium levels during the day. Despite these concerns, lithium remains one of the most important and effective psychotropic agents and its risk-benefit ratio is excellent.

Carbamazepine and valproic acid The anticonvulsant carbamazepine has, in controlled trials, been used successfully in the treatment of manic and, to a lesser extent, depressive episodes in bipolar patients. There is also growing evidence that some bipolar patients (15 to 60 percent) who do not respond to lithium benefit from carbamazepine treatment, and that the combination of lithium and carbamazepine may be therapeutically additive. The drug regimen for bipolar disorders is initiated with 200 mg bid administered orally, increasing to 600 to 1600 mg daily in divided doses and, although not well-correlated with therapeutic response, blood levels may range from 8 to 12 mg/dL.

Carbamazepine is not a completely benign drug; side effects include nausea, blurred vision, and ataxia, and more importantly there have been cases of fatal leukopenia and aplastic anemia reported (incidence ≤ 1 in 20,000). Patients treated with carbamazepine must be monitored for renal, liver, and bone marrow functions while they are on the medication. There are also reports of reversible CNS toxicity when this drug is combined with lithium. Therefore patients on this combination should be monitored carefully. Valproic acid, the drug of choice in certain seizure disorders, has also been reported to prevent recurrence of manic episodes in a number of bipolar patients. The development of this new class of psychotropic compounds is very promising and may herald the future development of a new and useful group of medications.

ANXIETY DISORDERS IN A MEDICAL SETTING
Karen Thatcher Britton

Anxiety symptoms are common in medically ill patients. Five to 20 percent of medical inpatients and 4 to 14 percent of general medical outpatients suffer from anxiety states. Patients with anxiety disorders are more likely to seek help for their emotional problems from general medical physicians than patients with other psychiatric disorders, and are more likely to use emergency room services. In a recent study, 29 percent of patients with panic disorder used an emergency service for treatment of emotional problems in the preceding year. Furthermore, antianxiety medications have consistently been among the most frequently prescribed medications in the United States over the past 15 years, and more than 80 percent of these prescriptions are written by primary care physicians. Anxiety may occur as a manifestation of a primary psychiatric disorder or secondarily to either the medical illness or the medications prescribed for treatment. It is important for the clinician to be familiar with the diagnosis of anxiety and the role it plays in the patient's illness.

Anxiety appears in several clinically recognizable forms. Distinctions are made between patients who complain of constant, unremitting nervousness, tension, and worry and patients who are relatively symptom free until an acute anxiety or panic attack arises. Further distinctions are made among patients with anxiety due to posttraumatic stress disorder, obsessive-compulsive disorder and the phobic disorders.

PANIC DISORDER   Definition and clinical manifestations The cardinal feature of panic disorder is the sudden, unexpected, and often overwhelming feeling of terror and apprehension accompanied by somatic symptoms in multiple organ systems such as dyspnea, palpitations, and faintness. The symptoms and signs of panic disorder are similar to those occurring during intense physical exertion or in a life-threatening situation.

A typical panic attack often begins abruptly and without warning when a patient is involved in a relatively nonthreatening and nonstressful activity, like entering a store, driving a car, or sitting at a desk working. The patient becomes lightheaded and sweaty and is overwhelmed by feelings of terror, apprehension, and impending doom. Dyspnea may occur with a subjective sense of choking or smothering, and palpitations or chest pain are often so severe that patients believe they are having a heart attack or are dying. The symptoms of panic attacks usually peak in less than 10 min and resolve in 20 to 30 min. Most frequently the first attack occurs away from home, often in a setting in which the person feels trapped or concerned about attracting attention. The usual response is to obtain help, sometimes going to a doctor's office or emergency room, but the fear has usually subsided by this time. Fatigue or exhaustion frequently follows a panic attack, and the patient may sleep. The DSM-III-R criteria for diagnosis of panic disorder are listed in Table 389-8.

Panic disorder is estimated to occur in 1 to 2 percent of the population and is a relapsing, remitting illness. The most frequent age of onset is the late teen years and early twenties. Panic disorders tend to be familial, and both panic disorders and affective disorders often coexist in the same family. If an individual has a diagnosed panic disorder, up to 18 percent of first-degree relatives also will have panic disorder. Furthermore, twin studies demonstrate a greater incidence in monozygotic twins, suggesting that panic anxiety may have a genetic basis.

Complications After repeated panic attacks, some patients develop anticipatory anxiety and try to avoid those situations that have

TABLE 389-8   Diagnosis of panic disorder

A At some time during the disturbance, one or more panic attacks (discrete periods of intense fear or discomfort) have occurred that were (*1*) unexpected and (*2*) not triggered by situations in which the person was the focus of others' attention.

B Either four attacks have occurred within a 4-week period or one or more attacks have been followed by a period of at least a month of persistent fear of having another attack.

C At least four of the following symptoms developed during at least one of the attacks.

  1 Shortness of breath (dyspnea) or smothering sensations
  2 Dizziness, unsteady feelings, or faintness
  3 Palpitations or accelerated heart rate
  4 Trembling or shaking
  5 Sweating
  6 Choking
  7 Nausea or abdominal distress
  8 Depersonalization or derealization
  9 Numbness or tingling sensations (paresthesias)
  10 Flushes or chills
  11 Chest pain or discomfort
  12 Fear of dying
  13 Fear of going crazy or of doing something uncontrolled

D During at least some of the attacks, at least four of the symptoms in *C* developed suddenly and increased in intensity within 10 min of the beginning of the first *C* symptom noticed in the attack.

E It cannot be established that an organic factor initiated and maintained the disturbance, e.g., amphetamine or caffeine intoxification or hyperthyroidism.

been paired with panic attacks in the past. Many patients, particularly females by a two to one ratio to men, develop *agoraphobia*—an irrational fear of being alone or in public places (see Table 389-9). Without effective treatment, the course of panic attacks and agoraphobia may lead to an increasingly restricted life-style marked by preoccupation with avoiding those situations that might trigger an attack. Patients often dramatically increase their use of health services when this complication develops, seeking help from multiple physicians with one or more frightening somatic complaints. Accurate diagnosis and treatment are important because cases of severe panic disorder with agoraphobia have been reported in which patients remain house-bound for one or more decades, convinced that leaving the house will induce an attack. Primary care physicians should ask whether the patient has begun to avoid any situations, especially social situations, since the attacks began, e.g., fear of crowds, public transportation, closed-in spaces like elevators, movie theaters, driving alone, etc. It is important to inquire whether the patient has become fearful of entering these situations *alone*, since many agoraphobic patients will enter fearful situations if accompanied by a spouse or friend.

Other complications of panic disorder are major depression and substance abuse. Approximately 60 to 90 percent of patients with panic disorder develop a major depression at some time in their lives, and 20 percent make a suicide attempt. Patients with panic disorder

TABLE 389-9   Panic disorder with agoraphobia

A Meets criteria for panic disorder

B Agoraphobia: Fear of being in places or situations from which escape might be difficult (or embarrassing) or in which help might not be available in the event of a panic attack. As a result of this fear, the person either restricts travel or endures agoraphobic situations despite intense anxiety. Common agoraphobic situations include being outside the home alone, being in a crowd or standing in line, being on a bridge, and traveling in a bus, train, or car.

Measuring severity of agoraphobic avoidance:

  Mild: Some avoidance (or endurance with distress), but relatively normal life-style.

  Moderate: Avoidance results in constricted life-style, e.g., the person is able to leave the house alone, but not to go more than a few miles unaccompanied.

  Severe: Avoidance results in being nearly or completely housebound or unable to leave the house unaccompanied.

may also attempt self-medication with alcohol and/or benzodiazepines. These agents have a short anxiolytic action, but the rapid drop in blood levels may then cause an exacerbation of anxiety. In addition, many of the symptoms of alcohol and drug withdrawal are similar to those of panic and therefore may present difficulty in differential diagnosis. Nearly 30 percent of patients with panic disorder experience, at some time in their lives, alcohol problems meeting DSM criteria for alcohol abuse. If alcohol or substance abuse is present, that disorder should be treated first and the patient reassessed after detoxification and treatment.

Differential diagnosis Once the presence of anxiety is established, the clinician must attempt to rule out an organic anxiety disorder. Medical disorders and medications known to be associated with anxiety are listed in Table 389-10. Thyroid dysfunction and cardiac disorders are the most common differential diagnoses to rule out. The patient's medical history and physical examination guide the clinician in this workup. For example, mitral valve prolapse should be investigated because there may be an increased prevalence of this condition in patients with panic disorder. Some studies have suggested an association between panic disorder and increased cardiovascular morbidity and mortality. Both pulmonary and gastrointestinal disorders also tend to evoke anxiety in many patients, and stress is often linked to exacerbations in these conditions. The physician must also review all pharmacologic agents that the patient is taking that could cause anxiety. For example, a patient with a toxic aminophylline level may have symptoms that mimic anxiety attacks.

Etiology, pathophysiology, and treatment The etiology of panic disorders is uncertain and involves an interplay of multiple psychological and biologic determinants.

Clinical and experimental evidence point to the involvement of noradrenergic neurons, particularly those projecting rostrally from the locus coeruleus in the upper brainstem in the pathophysiology of panic disorder. Three lines of evidence suggest that hyperactivity of noradrenergic pathways may play a role in the pathogenesis of panic. First, the clinical manifestations of panic attacks are similar to those induced by sudden, massive stimulations of beta-adrenergic receptors. Second, isoproterenol hydrochloride, a beta agonist, and yohimbine,

TABLE 389-10   Medical conditions and drugs associated with anxiety

MEDICAL CONDITIONS

Anemia	Hypothyroidism
Angina pectoralis	Insulinoma
Asthma	Menopausal symptoms
Carcinoid	Mitral valve prolapse
Cardiac arrhythmias	Mass lesion
Cardiomyopathies	Pheochromocytosis
Cushing's syndrome	Porphyria
Chronic obstructive pulmonary disease (COPD)	Pneumothorax
Electrolyte abnormalities	Pulmonary edema
Hyperparathyroidism	Pulmonary embolus
Hyperthyroidism	Temporal lobe epilepsy
Hypoglycemia	Vertigo

DRUGS

Alcohol	Glucocorticoids
Amphetamine	Hallucinogens
Aminophylline	Lidocaine
Anticholinergics	Methylphenidate
Antihistamines	Metrizamide
Antihypertensives	Monosodium glutamate
Antituberculous agents	Pentazocine
Bromocriptine	Phenylephrine
Caffeine	Pseudoephedrine
Cocaine	Salicylates
Digitalis (toxicity)	Sedative hypnotics (withdrawal)
Dopamine	Theophylline
Ephedrine	Thyroid agents
Epinephrine	

an alpha-adrenergic receptor antagonist that increases noradrenergic function, produce signs and symptoms that mimic panic attacks. Third, clinical studies support a role for noradrenergic beta blockers, such as propranolol, in successful treatment of pathologic anxiety.

Another avenue of investigation is based on the finding that infusions of sodium lactate into patients with a history of panic disorder often provoke a panic attack indistinguishable from a spontaneous one. Normal subjects without a history of panic disorder are unaffected. In addition, patients whose panic attacks are controlled by antidepressants are protected against lactate-induced panic attacks. Inhalation of CO_2 by susceptible persons also precipitates anxiety and panic. Although the mechanism of lactate's effect is unclear, the findings appear to have diagnostic usefulness and provide a good model of anxiety for further clinical investigation.

Overall, the evidence suggests that the main contribution to panic may be a genetic vulnerability to a biologic disease state. Over time, panic attacks may become associated with environmental events that by themselves are able to elicit symptoms. The particular constellation of environmental stimuli that precipitates panic attacks may be influenced by past experience or particular psychological conflicts. A full understanding of the etiology of anxiety probably will require knowledge of a combination of genetic, biologic, and psychological factors.

A comprehensive treatment program combines both pharmacologic and psychotherapeutic approaches. The first step is to block the attacks pharmacologically. Three classes of medication are effective for the treatment of panic disorder: TCAs, MAO inhibitors, and high-potency benzodiazepines (alprazolam or clonazepam). The usual first drug used is a tricyclic in low doses of 10 to 25 mg with increase in small (10- to 25-mg) increments to avoid precipitating panic. In some instances alprazolam or preferably clonazepam (which has a longer half-life) is used to cover panic episodes while a tricyclic is being increased over 1 to 2 weeks. These drugs are 80 to 90 percent effective in the treatment and prevention of spontaneous panic attacks. Beta blockers may block the peripheral manifestations of the panic attacks but have proved ineffective in preventing the psychic fear or panic. They also may predispose to or worsen depressive symptoms. Clonidine has been shown to block panic manifestations, but its efficacy is usually only transient. More recently, beneficial results have been reported for the serotonin uptake inhibitor fluoxetine.

For some patients with panic disorder, particularly those with debilitating agoraphobia, psychotherapy is indicated. The exact form of psychotherapy is controversial, but approaches that seek to understand the anxiety and encourage the patient to confront the feared situations are the most effective.

GENERALIZED ANXIETY DISORDER Unlike patients with panic disorder whose symptoms come on suddenly, patients with generalized anxiety disorder experience persistent diffuse anxiety without the specific symptoms that characterize phobic disorders, panic disorders, or obsessive-compulsive disorders. Although the symptoms and signs of anxiety vary from individual to individual, common signs are motor tension, autonomic hyperactivity, apprehensive expectation, and vigilance. Patients with generalized anxiety disorder do not report acute fluctuations in anxiety level and autonomic arousal characteristic of panic disorder.

The prevalence of generalized anxiety disorder has been estimated at 2 to 3 percent, but precise epidemiologic data are lacking because of variations in definition and case acquisition. In patients who seek professional help for anxiety, women outnumber men by two to one. There is no evidence to support the popular belief that anxiety is related to the stresses of modern society. In contrast to panic disorder, studies showing a familial or genetic basis for generalized anxiety disorder are inconclusive. Although generalized anxiety disorder tends to have a more favorable outcome than panic disorder, the symptoms are persistent and can lead to secondary depression and alcohol and drug abuse.

Etiology, pathophysiology, and treatment One approach to understanding the etiology of anxiety has been to delineate the mechanisms by which antianxiety drugs exert their effects. High-affinity, stereospecific receptors for benzodiazepines have been discovered which appear to be coupled to the receptor for the inhibitory neurotransmitter gamma-aminobutyric acid (GABA). Considerable evidence supports the hypothesis that the anxiolytic actions of the benzodiazepines are mediated through this receptor.

These findings have several implications. First, the characterization of a benzodiazepine receptor complex implies the existence of a natural (endogenous) ligand for the receptor. Conceivably, the levels of this substance might correlate with individual differences in anxiety or emotionality or tolerance to stress. Second, pharmacologic antagonists of this receptor block the effectiveness of benzodiazepines and may induce anxiety, a finding which implicates these mechanisms in pathologic anxiety. Third, new anxiolytic compounds that influence benzodiazepine receptor binding are being discovered that have fewer and potentially less serious side effects. The possibility exists that anxiogenic substances may also be found in the brain. Though major questions remain to be answered, these advances have opened new avenues for understanding the origins and management of anxiety.

Because feelings of anxiety are normal human emotions with adaptive value, a decision must be made before any treatment or medication is considered concerning whether or not the manifestations of anxiety are within the normal range. There is no justification for the use of anxiolytic drugs if anxiety is appropriate to the fear or threat. On the other hand if certain situations produce fear in which the feelings are disproportional to the threat, then treatment should be considered.

Once a decision is made to treat, consideration should be given first to modalities of nonpharmacologic intervention, including supportive or intensive psychotherapy. These approaches may modify maladaptive life-styles, cognition, and avoidance behaviors. Behavior therapy aims at teaching the patient practical techniques like relaxation training, biofeedback, and desensitization. These techniques are of at least temporary benefit for many people.

When generalized anxiety is severe enough to warrant treatment with drugs, benzodiazepines are the agents of choice. In many patients, short courses of anxiolytic drugs (5 to 7 days) are effective, following which the drug should be discontinued. Patients should be warned about the possibility of dependence with long-term use, and the physician should make regular assessments of the need for continuation of medications. Buspirone, a nonbenzodiazepine anxiolytic, may become a drug of first choice for these patients. Although it has a delayed onset of action of about one week, it lacks many of the problems associated with the benzodiazepines such as psychomotor impairment, physicial dependence, or withdrawal symptoms. (See also "Newer Anxiolytic Medications," below.)

POSTTRAUMATIC STRESS DISORDER The diagnostic criteria for posttraumatic stress disorders (PTSD) are listed in Table 389-11. PTSD is classified as either acute or chronic (or delayed). In the former, onset of symptoms begin within 6 months of the trauma, or the duration of the symptoms persist less than 6 months. In the latter, symptoms persist more than 6 months (chronic) or start more than 6 months after the trauma (delayed). Patients with PTSD have experienced a severe catastrophic event that is outside the range of normal human experience and would be distressing to anyone. The patient persistently reexperiences the event by having recurrent dreams or nightmares, or suddenly feels as if the event were recurring. In primary care, patients with PTSD are occasionally seen following trauma precipitated by automobile or industrial accidents or natural disasters such as flood, hurricane, or fire.

Etiology and treatment Whether or not PTSD develops appears to depend upon the nature of the trauma, the characteristics of the individual, and the context in which these events take place. The trauma can be anticipated or not, acute or chronic, constant or repetitive, or due to natural events or malevolence. PTSD can develop in individuals who were apparently healthy, successful, and well-adjusted prior to the traumatic experience. Among the factors which influence the development of PTSD are: (1) the extent to which the

TABLE 389-11   **Diagnosis of posttraumatic stress disorder**

A The person has experienced an event that is outside the range of usual human experience and that would be markedly distressing to almost anyone.

B The traumatic event is persistently reexperienced in at least one of the following ways.
  1 Recurrent and intrusive distressing recollections of the event
  2 Recurrent distressing dreams of the event
  3 Sudden acting or feeling as if the traumatic event were recurring
  4 Intense psychological distress at exposure to events that symbolize or resemble an aspect of the traumatic event

C Persistent avoidance of stimuli associated with the trauma or numbing of general responsiveness, as indicated by at least three of the following:
  1 Efforts to avoid thoughts or feelings associated with the trauma
  2 Efforts to avoid activities or situations that arouse recollections of the trauma
  3 Inability to recall an important aspect of the trauma
  4 Markedly diminished interest in significant activities
  5 Feeling of detachment or estrangement from others
  6 Restricted range of affect, e.g., unable to have loving feelings
  7 Sense of a foreshortened future, e.g., does not expect to have a career, marriage, children or a long life

D Persistent symptoms of increased arousal, as indicated by at least two of the following:
  1 Difficulty falling or staying asleep
  2 Irritability or outbursts of anger
  3 Difficulty concentrating
  4 Hypervigilance
  5 Exaggerated startle response
  6 Physiologic reactivity upon exposure to events that symbolize or resemble an aspect of the traumatic event

E Duration of the disturbance of at least 1 month (specify delayed onset if the onset of symptoms is at least 6 months after the trauma).

individual's life-space is affected; (2) the duration of the impact; (3) the extent to which the individual perceived human malevolence behind the traumatic event (e.g., a fire attributed to arson will probably be more traumatic than one attributed to lightning); and (4) social isolation. It is difficult to gauge the prevalence of PTSD following a traumatic event because studies that have been done often have followed subjects for only a short period of time, and the nature of the events is often very situation-specific. Following a major natural disaster, about 15 percent or more of the civilian population may experience mental distress severe enough to require treatment.

The treatment goals of PTSD are reduction of target symptoms, prevention of chronic disability, and occupational and social rehabilitation. Recent reports suggest both the TCAs and MAO inhibitors may be effective.

OBSESSIVE-COMPULSIVE DISORDER   Idiosyncratic rituals and odd personal habits are commonplace. Only when they cause marked anxiety and personal distress, occupy more than an hour a day, and cause significant social or vocational dysfunction do they indicate obsessive-compulsive disorder. The major characteristics of this disorder are recurrent *obsessions*, i.e., persistent, intrusive thoughts, impulses, or urges that are troublesome to the person. Typical examples are thoughts of violence or fears of germs or contamination. Obsessions produce a great amount of anxiety. *Compulsions* are repetitive behaviors performed in response to an obsession, according to specific rules or in a stereotyped fashion. They are designed to neutralize the occurrence of the dreaded or feared event. Typical examples are repetitive handwashing, checking an item repeatedly, or always counting a particular number. As with obsessions, compulsions are recognized by the individual with obsessive-compulsive disorder as being senseless. A consequence of this is that reassurance by a friend, physician, or therapist does not help reduce the behavior's occurrence.

Obsessive-compulsive disorders usually begin in adolescence or young adulthood with about 65 percent of cases beginning before age 25. They are seen less often in children. Clear precipitants are reported in up to 60 percent of cases. Long-term prognosis appears to be variable. Some patients, perhaps 10 percent, show a chronic, unremitting course, but the majority of patients show an episodic course with periods of incomplete remissions.

Etiology and treatment   The majority of individuals with obsessive-compulsive disorder are not recognized by primary care physicians because of the generally private nature of their rituals and because they are aware of the irrationality of their compulsions and are ashamed to admit their symptoms. The cause of obsessive-compulsive disorder is unknown, but there are associated changes in brain function. Positron-emission tomography studies have shown abnormalities in the prefrontal cortex that are reversed by chlorimipramine.

Clomipramine appears to be the most effective pharmacologic treatment for obsessive-compulsive disorder. The beneficial effects of clomipramine may be delayed 6 to 8 weeks, and it is most effective when specific compulsions are present. Recent reports suggest that fluoxetine, which has a similar effect on the serotoninergic neurotransmitter system, is also successful in the treatment of some patients with obsessive-compulsive disorder.

Obsessive-compulsive patients also may respond to psychotherapeutic intervention. However, in the absence of adequate studies of psychotherapy in obsessive-compulsive disorder, it is hard to make a valid generalization about its effectiveness. Behavioral therapy can be helpful in this disorder. Desensitization, flooding, implosion therapy, and aversive conditioning have all been used with variable success.

PHOBIC DISORDERS   Phobic disorders comprise a group of disorders having in common persistently recurring, irrational severe anxiety of specific objects, activities or situations with secondary avoidance of the phobic stimulus. Phobias are relatively commonplace, and the diagnosis of a phobic disorder is made only when fear or avoidance behavior is a significant source of distress to the individual or when it interferes with social or occupational functioning. Treatment, if required, is behavioral using relaxation therapy or systematic desensitization.

Agoraphobia, the fear of being alone or in public places, may occur rarely in the absence of panic disorder (see ''Panic Disorders,'' above).

Social phobias are persistent irrational fears and the need to avoid any situation where one might be exposed to scrutiny by others and potentially embarrassed or humiliated. Even the possibility of such a situation evokes anticipatory anxiety. The individual is aware that this fear is excessive. Common examples are excessive fear of public speaking, being unable to urinate in a public restroom, and anxiety induced by eating in restaurants or by any public performance. The resulting anxiety may actually impair performance and thereby potentiate the phobic disorder.

Simple phobias are persistent irrational fears and avoidance of specific objects or situations. Common examples include fear of heights (acrophobia), fear of closed spaces (claustrophobia), and fear of animals. Systematic desensitization and in vivo exposure are the most effective treatments for the simple phobias, and no real benefit has been shown from medication.

ANXIETY DISORDERS AND THEIR RELEVANCE TO INTERNAL MEDICINE   Unrecognized anxiety disorders are common in both outpatient and inpatient clinical practices. Panic disorder is a relatively new concept in medicine, and many physicians are unfamiliar with its diagnosis and natural history. Physicians in emergency room settings and cardiology clinics should be especially alert to the hidden patient with undiagnosed panic disorder.

A notable feature of many patients is an intense fear of having a heart attack during a panic episode. Because panic attacks often present with such alarming physical symptoms, it is usually the primary care physician who first sees these patients. The problem of chest pain in panic disorder warrants special mention. There is recent evidence that the presentation of chest pain in patients with panic attacks is leading to expensive cardiac workups. Several recent studies have found that 30 to 50 percent of chest pain patients with angiographically normal coronary arteries have panic disorder. In those with diseased coronary arteries, there is no higher than expected rate of panic disorder.

Although patients with panic disorder are frequently hypochondriacal about having heart disease and need reassurance, there is some evidence of increased cardiovascular morbidity and mortality associated with the disease. Higher rates of hypertension, hyperlipidemia, smoking, physical inactivity, and alcohol abuse have been reported in such patients. At this time there are no good guidelines to assist physicians in routine cardiovascular screening of panic disorder patients.

Anxiety also can play an important role in the clinical picture of a patient with documented medical illness and contribute to the distress experienced by the patient as well as influence the outcome of the disorder. Recognition of the presence of anxiety and its part in the symptoms will greatly improve the doctor's ability to provide comprehensive care for the patient. Anxiety can both increase vulnerability to exacerbations of some diseases and adversely affect the course of the disease process by increasing symptoms and impeding recovery. In spite of this, failure to recognize and treat anxiety disorders in the medically ill is common.

Anxiety and panic are frequently associated with pulmonary conditions such as COPD and asthma in an interactive way, thus worsening the attack. Similarly, heightened anxiety is a common response to myocardial infarction and bypass surgery, and has been negatively correlated with many postrecovery variables (e.g., return to work). Stress also has been implicated in the development of gastrointestinal disorders (irritable bowel syndrome, peptic ulcer, colitis), and subsequent anxiety has been linked to exacerbations of the condition. Psychiatric referral may be clinically beneficial in the management of such patients by reframing the medical illness as a condition that worsens with stress and providing treatment of maladaptive illness behavior.

There are a number of reasons why anxiety disorders are frequently unrecognized in the medical setting. A major obstacle is the overlapping of physical and psychological signs or symptoms. Nervousness, trembling, dizziness, tachycardia, chest pain and shortness of breath are symptoms of anxiety; however, each also may be produced by an enormous number of physical disorders and commonly used drugs (Table 389-10). Furthermore, even when anxiety symptoms are recognized by staff, they may be considered as relatively unimportant in comparison with profound medical illness or a natural reaction to illness (e.g., "anyone would feel anxious in his condition"). In addition, the demanding, irritable, hypervigilant nature of the patient with an anxiety symptom may be perceived by staff as negativistic and uncooperative and sometimes evoke anger.

MEDICAL TREATMENT OF ANXIETY DISORDERS

Lewis L. Judd

The development of the benzodiazepines has been a great advance in the pharmacologic management of anxiety. They have also replaced barbiturates as the sedative-hypnotic drugs of choice. The benzodiazepines, unlike the barbiturates, are partial CNS depressants and thus, even at high doses, are rarely associated with lethal respiratory depression or vasomotor collapse. In addition, depending upon the dose, benzodiazepines possess anticonvulsant and muscle relaxant properties.

MECHANISMS OF ACTION There is growing evidence that GABA plays a central role in the brain mechanism(s) of anxiety. Benzodiazepines selectively, but indirectly, enhance GABA neurotransmission, possibly by increasing neuronal receptor sensitivity to GABA. Also, a close interaction has been described between GABA and benzodiazepine receptor binding, leading to an increase in neuronal chloride conductance. Despite these observations, the specific mechanism by which benzodiazepines mediate their clinical effects is not completely understood.

CLINICAL CONDITIONS FOR USE The benzodiazepines are most effective in the management of relatively short-lived reactive states of tension and anxiety and are the drugs of choice in the treatment of generalized anxiety disorders. Although alprazolam at high doses (4 to 10 mg) can block panic attacks, the TCAs and MAO inhibitors are the drugs of choice for treating panic disorders. Recent studies have demonstrated that the MAO inhibitor phenelzine is effective in the treatment of social phobia. Furthermore, there is emerging evidence that short-acting, high-potency benzodiazepines such as clonazepam are also effective in this disorder. In addition, the benzodiazepines may have a role in the treatment of anticipatory anxiety, which is almost always present in patients with panic disorders. Sometimes, both a TCA and a benzodiazepine anxiolytic may be necessary in the treatment of panic disorder. The anxiolytics are also useful in treating anxiety symptoms that accompany phobic disorders.

CLINICAL USE OF ANTIANXIETY MEDICATIONS The benzodiazepines have been most frequently prescribed as anxiolytics. The shorter-acting benzodiazepines, however, are also effective sedative-hypnotics. The more commonly prescribed drugs are listed in Table 389-12 along with the usual oral dose ranges. The pharmacokinetic characteristics of many of the benzodiazepines are complicated by long drug elimination half-lives and the metabolic conversion of parent compounds to active metabolites (see Table 389-12). Diazepam is converted to the active metabolite desmethyldiazepam (nordiazepam) which, in turn, can be hydroxylated to yield oxazepam, also a potent benzodiazepine. This metabolic pathway extends the activity half-life of diazepam threefold. The hypnotic flurazepam is converted to active metabolite *N*-1-desalkylflurazepam, which has a half-life of more than 48 h; hence, repetitive daily doses given in excess of a week or two can result in the accumulation of the active metabolites of the drug. Prazepam has metabolic breakdown products identical to those of diazepam and has a similar drug elimination half-life. Oxazepam and lorazepam, both of which undergo glucuronide conugation, have no active metabolites and therefore have the advantage of a shorter half-life. The benzodiazepines temazepam, triazolam, and alprazolam also have the advantage of shorter half-lives and to date, no long-acting active metabolites have been identified. Triazolam, however, has such a short half-life that it has been known to produce rebound withdrawal anxiety. For this reason it should be used with caution and only for short intervals (less than 7 days).

Diazepam has been the standard against which all anxiolytic drugs are measured, and no other anxiolytics have demonstrated better antianxiety efficacy. The newly developed benzodiazepines appear equally effective and have eliminated certain of the undesirable side effects. Specifically, lorazepam, oxazepam, and alprazolam are without active metabolites and, with proper dosage, cumulative effects of daytime sedation are less noticeable.

TABLE 389-12 Commonly used benzodiazepines

Benzodiazepine	Daily oral dose range, mg	Half-life, h*
ANXIOLYTICS		
Chlordiazepoxide	20–100ᵈ	7–28*
Clonazepam	1–20	18–50
Diazepam	5–40ᵈ	20–90*
Lorazepam	1–10‡	10–12
Oxazepam	30–120‡	3–20
Prazepam	20–60ᵈ	40–70*
Alprazolam	0.75–10.0‡	12–15
SEDATIVE-HYPNOTICS		
Flurazepam	15–30ᵗ	24–100*
Temazepam	30ᵗ	8–10
Triazolam	0.125–0.5ᵗ	2–5

* Indicates long-acting active metabolites.
ᵈ Prescribed in a daily or twice daily regimen.
‡ Prescribed in a three or four times daily regimen.
ᵗ Prescribed in a daily or bedtime regimen.

Treatment regimens usually last 4 weeks or less, and medications are prescribed continually for 7 to 10 days followed by a 2- to 3-day drug holiday; then this sequence is repeated. This schedule helps avoid the development of tolerance to the anxiolytic effects. The shorter-acting medications (e.g., lorazepam, alprazolam, clonazepam) are prescribed in a three or four times daily regimen, and the longer-acting drugs (e.g., diazepam) are given in a single dose or a twice daily regimen. For example, it is common practice to prescribe one dose of diazepam at bedtime, since it will both promote sleep and reduce anxiety levels the following day.

In prescribing the anxiolytic benzodiazepines clinicians should avoid the possibility of habituating patients to chronic benzodiazepine use. One of the earliest signs is the development of tolerance in which the patient repeatedly requests escalations in drug dose. Since benzodiazepines do produce mild euphoria and a sense of well-being, anxious patients often want to preserve this feeling and request additional medication. However, clinical surveys of prescription practices have shown that clinicians are aware of the problems of benzodiazepine habituation and sometimes respond by being too cautious and by unnecessarily undertreating patients. The use of the drug holiday treatment regimen described above and the physician's resistance to repetitively increasing dosage will help to minimize the problem of drug habituation.

In addition to its role as an anxiolytic, diazepam is also the drug of choice in this class for muscle relaxation and for the treatment of alcohol withdrawal syndromes. It is the benzodiazepine of choice for intractable seizures. Oxazepam, because of the nonaccumulation of active metabolites, is a good choice for anxiolysis in the elderly.

Finally, the physician should be aware that during the last decade, there have been multiple controlled studies describing effective treatment strategies in the management of panic disorder. This common subtype of the anxiety disorders has proven to be amenable to treatment with tricyclic antidepressants, MAO inhibitor depressants, and high-potency, short-acting benzodiazepines (alprazolam, clonazepam, etc.). Further, there is now some indication that the selective serotonin reuptake inhibitor antidepressants (fluoxetine, sertraline, paroxetine, etc.) are also effective in panic disorder. However, longitudinal studies of medication treatment have identified high relapse rates (30 to 80 percent) when patients are removed from medications.

These observations have contributed significantly to our understanding of panic disorder; it is a chronic life-long illness which requires maintenance treatment. In addition, promising data are emerging from the empirical testing of a new type of psychotherapy, cognitive behavioral panic control, which has been designed specifically as a short-term, targeted disorder-specific psychotherapy. This type of psychotherapy shows promise in both the acute management of panic disorder and in the maintenance of therapeutic gains and significantly reduced relapse rates post treatment (10 percent or less). Evolving treatments promise new, more effective, and more lasting benefits in the management of panic disorder, which are likely to involve an integration of both medication and specific targeted psychotherapeutic techniques.

SIDE EFFECTS AND INTERACTIONS The most important adverse effect of the benzodiazepines is the discomfort caused by the withdrawal syndrome, which can occur after chronic treatment. There is little risk of debilitating addiction to these drugs when used appropriately. However, physical dependence does occur since withdrawal symptoms are seen in a high percentage of patients after cessation of chronic benzodiazepine treatment. Motivation to sustain mild feelings of well-being and avoid the discomfort of withdrawal symptoms may contribute to psychological dependence. Withdrawal symptoms include muscle aches, agitation, restlessness, insomnia, and generalized anxious dysphoria. In some patients, more commonly those taking short-acting benzodiazepines, more serious CNS withdrawal symptoms may appear, including confusional and delirium states and, more rarely, grand mal seizures. Rebound anxiety can also be seen in patients with anxiety disorders but is less prevalent

when benzodiazepines with long-acting metabolites are used and if medication is gradually discontinued. Risk for withdrawal symptoms increases with the length of treatment; they occur with much greater frequency (e.g., more than 90 percent) among patients who have been treated for 1 year or more. Withdrawal symptoms occur within the first 24 to 48 h after treatment with short-acting benzodiazepines ceases, but for those benzodiazepines with long-acting metabolites (e.g., diazepam, chlordiazepoxide) the withdrawal symptoms can occur 4 to 6 days and even longer after drug cessation. With the usual recommended dosage regimens and the gradual withdrawal technique (e.g., over 3 to 4 weeks), the appearance of a withdrawal syndrome in patients can be minimized significantly. While there is little true addiction potential, patients should be on these medications for only as long as necessary.

The most common minor side effects are daytime sedation, mild cognitive impairment, motor clumsiness, and (e.g., lorazepam, triazolam) specific memory decrements. Another rare but troublesome side effect from some benzodiazepines is paradoxical emotional responses, primarily manifested as aggressive and impulsive behavior.

Unlike barbiturates, the benzodiazepines do not noticeably induce hepatic microsomal enzyme activity and therefore do not affect the metabolism of other medications. The benzodiazepines potentiate the CNS depressant effects of other drugs including barbiturates, general anesthetics, and alcohol. The cross-tolerance with ethanol has made the benzodiazepines ideal medications for the treatment of alcohol withdrawal syndromes. Patients should be cautioned that ethanol's effects are potentiated by benzodiazepines and this combination should be avoided.

NEWER ANXIOLYTIC MEDICATIONS It has been established that certain beta-adrenergic blocking agents, such as *propranolol*, can dampen the peripheral physiologic symptoms of anxiety. Initially, it was felt that these drugs might be better nonsedative anxiolytic compounds, but this promise has not been fulfilled in controlled studies. While propranolol does attenuate somatic manifestations of anxiety (e.g., palpitations, tremor), it appears to have lesser effects on the psychological components (e.g., intense fearfulness). Although propranolol has been used for treating patients extremely fearful of speaking or performing in public (oral dose 40 to 320 mg daily), it is not a comprehensively effective anxiolytic. With additional study, other potentially peripheral blocking agents may prove to be more effective.

A new class of anxiolytic drugs, the azaspirodecanediones, which act on the serotoninergic system, has been developed. One of the first compounds studied clinically is *buspirone*, a compound that acts selectively on the serotonin$_{1A}$ receptor. It has no structural similarity to other anxiolytics or even to other psychotropics. It is not anticonvulsant, does not interact with the benzodiazepine receptor, is not cross-tolerant with other CNS depressants, and no abstinence syndrome has yet been described. In several controlled trials it has proved to be an effective anxiolytic with significantly less sedation and decrements in psychomotor performance, although it is not effective in panic disorder. Because of the near absence of sedation and motor impairment and the relatively long latency for anxiolytic effects to appear (i.e., days to weeks), patients occasionally report that the drug is ineffective. This is most common in individuals who have previously received benzodiazepines such as diazepam. Studies are currently being conducted with buspirone to determine possible side effects.

In addition to the efficacy of TCAs in panic and phobic disorders, there are controlled studies reporting that they are anxiolytics as effective as the benzodiazepines in generalized anxiety disorders. It is possible that continued investigations will identify a broader role for TCAs in the treatment of the full spectrum of anxiety disorders.

SCHIZOPHRENIC DISORDERS

David L. Braff

Schizophrenic disorders are serious mental illnesses characterized by hallucinations, delusions, and disorganized thought and behavior.

They last 6 months or more and cause significant social, vocational, and personal disability, and suffering. The schizophrenic patient may present to the emergency department in crisis with overtly bizarre and obviously psychotic complaints. Alternatively, schizophrenic patients may present more subtly to the primary care physician with strange complaints or ideas which, on close questioning, are related to delusions or thought disorder. Despite its frequently dramatic presentation, perhaps no other psychiatric disorder has proved as vexing and difficult to define, identify, and treat.

Schizophrenia has a lifetime prevalence rate of about 1 percent across all cultures. In the United States alone there are perhaps 2 million affected individuals who often become ill in their late teenage years and in the third decade of life. Poor outcome frequently leads to extensive and long-term disability, and schizophrenia accounts for an estimated 20 billion dollars or more per year of lost productivity. Most patients with schizophrenic disorders also cause major perturbations for family and social support systems, adding to the economic losses and the toll of human misery. Up to 25 percent of hospital beds in the United States may be occupied by schizophrenic patients at any one time. Cumulatively, these factors make schizophrenia one of the most costly and vexing health problems.

DEFINITION AND CLINICAL MANIFESTATIONS In 1919, Emil Kraepelin first made the distinction between dementia praecox, a psychotic illness with progressive deterioration, and manic depressive psychosis. Kraepelin noted, however, that about 13 percent of patients with dementia praecox did not have an inevitably deteriorating outcome, and the size of the group with a favorable outcome has significantly increased largely because of antipsychotic medications, discussed in detail in the section that follows. Eugene Bleuler concentrated on the putative underlying psychological splitting of personality functions in his classic work on the "group of schizophrenias." Bleuler's emphasis was on the "four A's" of schizophrenia: *a*utism, flattened *a*ffect, loose *a*ssociations, and *a*mbivalence. Other authors have focused on specific symptoms of schizophrenia such as the sense of being influenced by others and feelings of being controlled by outside forces. To date, research has yet to identify specific and inevitably pathognomonic signs or symptoms of the schizophrenic disorders since mania, drug-induced psychosis, and other states also present with prominent hallucinations, delusions, and agitated behavior.

According to the DSM-III-R, after the first and most central criterion of psychotic symptoms is met (see Table 389-13), the schizophrenic individual must show deterioration from a previous level of functioning in such areas as work, social relations, and self-care. The disorder is not attributable to other diagnoses such as mood disorder with psychotic features or organic-induced (e.g., drug-induced) syndromes. Finally, continuous signs of the illness should be present for 6 months at some point during the individual's life with some signs of illness at the time of diagnosis. There may be prodromal, active, and/or residual phases of the illness that are not always clearly demarcated. Prodromal or residual symptoms are somewhat nonspecific and may consist of isolation; marked psychosocial impairment; peculiar behavior; impaired personal hygiene and grooming; blunted, flat, or inappropriate affect; digressive, vague, overelaborate, circumstantial, or metaphorical speech; odd or bizarre ideation or magical thinking; and unusual perceptual experiences.

The DSM-III-R lists four major schizophrenic disorders:

1 Catatonic—stupor, rigidity, excitement, or posturing; relatively rare.

2 Disorganized—incoherence and flat or grossly disorganized affect.

3 Paranoid—preoccupation with suspiciousness and one or more systematized delusions.

4 Undifferentiated—prominent delusions, hallucinations, incoherence, or disorganized behavior, not meeting the criteria for the other three types (see DSM-III-R for more detailed descriptions).

This emphasis on subtypes carries forward Bleuler's notion of the "group of schizophrenias." There is moderate support for a paranoid/

TABLE 389-13 Diagnosis of schizophrenic disorders

A Presence of characteristic psychotic symptoms in active phase, either *1*, *2*, or *3* for at least 1 week (unless symptoms are successfully treated):
 1 Two of the following:
   Delusions
   Prominent hallucinations
   Incoherence or marked loosening of associations
   Catatonic behavior
   Flat or grossly inappropriate affect
 2 Bizarre delusions
 3 Prominent hallucinations of a voice with content having no apparent relation to depression or elation, or a voice keeping up a running commentary on the person's behavior or thoughts, or two or more voices conversing with each other
B During the course of disturbance, functioning in areas such as work, social relations, and self-care markedly below highest level achieved before onset of disturbance.
C Schizoaffective disorder and mood disorder with psychotic features have been ruled out.
D Continuous signs of disturbance for at least 6 months. This period must include an active phase (of at least 1 week, or less if symptoms have been successfully treated) during which they were psychotic symptoms characteristic of schizophrenia (see *A* above), with or without a prodromal or residual phase.
E It cannot be established that an organic factor initiated and maintained the disturbance.
F If a history of autistic disorder exists, the additional diagnosis of schizophrenia can be made only if prominent delusions or hallucinations are also present.

SOURCE: Adapted from DSM-III-R.

---

nonparanoid dichotomy as being important in schizophrenia. In an attempt to reduce diagnostic heterogeneity, researchers have identified as "type I" schizophrenic patients those with a predominance of "positive" symptoms (e.g., hallucinations, paranoid ideation), normal cerebral ventricular size, and symptoms that respond to the hypothesized dopaminergic blocking effects of antipsychotic drugs. In contrast, "type II" schizophrenic patients seem similar to Kraepelin's dementia praecox patients. Type II patients show a predominance of "negative" symptoms (e.g., anhedonia, social withdrawal, asociality), neuropsychological impairment, and possibly increased cerebral ventricular volume; they do not respond well to antipsychotic medications, but seem to display a "deficit" state. Their course of the illness is variable, from "in remission" to "chronic."

DIFFERENTIAL DIAGNOSIS Schizophrenic patients have no unique or pathognomonic signs and symptoms. At times, this makes the diagnosis difficult. DSM-III-R separates psychotic illnesses by a durational criterion into *brief reactive psychoses* lasting 2 weeks or less, *schizophreniform disorders* lasting between 2 weeks and 6 months, and *schizophrenic disorders* lasting more than 6 months. While these distinctions are practical, the scientific basis for such a durational criterion is poorly documented. In addition, an acute manic patient may be difficult to distinguish from the schizophrenic patient, especially on a cross-sectional as opposed to longitudinal basis. To complicate matters further, the initial clinical appearance of a patient intoxicated with phencyclidine (PCP) or amphetamines may be indistinguishable from that of the paranoid schizophrenic patient. It appears then that many functional and organic states may lead to a final common pathway of psychotic symptoms. The diagnosis can only be established reliably by a broad-based multifactorial approach utilizing neurobiologic data (e.g., toxicologic screens, genetic history) and psychosocial data (e.g., premorbid adjustment status) obtained both for the present and across time. Despite these problems, the DSM-III-R criteria for schizophrenic disorders have undergone extensive and successful field trials for reliability and validity. In general, clinicians using the DSM-III-R criteria can accurately and consistently diagnose schizophrenia.

PREDISPOSING, PRECIPITATING, AND SUSTAINING FACTORS These factors may be analyzed in terms of neuroanatomic, biochemical, neurophysiologic, psychophysiologic, intrapsychic, interpersonal, social, and socioeconomic contributors. In a complex, multifactorial disorder such as schizophrenia, neurobiologic and psychosocial factors should be seen as interactive rather than as competing or mutually exclusive. This approach is analogous to comprehensive analyses of diabetes mellitus or hypertension according to the contributions of genetics, receptor physiology, and physiologic, familial, psychosocial, and myriad other conceptually diverse factors. Within this context, predisposing factors are linked to etiologic variables, precipitating factors are related to onset of pathophysiology, and sustaining factors are linked to outcome variables.

ETIOLOGY   Genetic factors   It is clear from twin, family, and adoptive studies that schizophrenia has a significant genetic basis. Monozygotic twins have roughly a 65 percent or greater concordance rate for schizophrenia, whereas dizygotic twins have a 12 percent concordance rate. Other family studies show that the morbid risk for developing schizophrenia is 5 to 10 percent if one parent is schizophrenic. This figure rises to 46 percent or more if both parents are schizophrenics. Second-degree relatives of schizophrenics run a 2 to 4 percent risk of developing the illness compared to a risk of 1 to 2 percent in the general population.

Adoption studies reveal that these risk factors are largely genetically linked and are not primarily due to the "schizophrenogenic" psychosocial environment of certain families. Still, these genetic analyses are fraught with methodologic difficulties. For example, reflecting the probable complex mode of inheritance, 89 percent of schizophrenics do not have a parent who is schizophrenic. Eighty-one percent of schizophrenics do not have either a schizophrenic sibling or parent. The appropriate model with which to explain these figures is complex and may include a weighted polygenic model or other sophisticated interpretations of the available data. Most recently, there has been an explosion of new knowledge about the genetics of schizophrenia featuring molecular studies and linkages to chromosome 5 and possibly X (see the entire volume 15, no. 3, of *Schizophrenia Bulletin,* 1989, and Crow et al.).

The stress-diathesis model hypothesizes that there is a vulnerability which is inherited in schizophrenia-prone individuals. These vulnerable individuals are at high risk for developing schizophrenia under certain stressful circumstances. Studies of high-risk children with one or two schizophrenic parents indicate that such children may have a significantly increased incidence of morbidity in utero, at birth, and in the perinatal period. In addition, these infants and children may have psychophysiologic lability, attentional dysfunction, and specific motor disturbances. A number of human and animal model studies suggest that such labile attentional mechanisms may result partly or largely from instabilities and increased activity of the mesolimbic dopaminergic system and associated decreased frontal lobe activity (hypofrontality). The literature on neurophysiologically labile and vulnerable children seems to tie the genetic, dopaminergic, and attentional dysfunction hypotheses together.

According to the stress-diathesis model, a host of stressful factors may precipitate a psychotic state in a high-risk individual. These factors include intoxication with PCP or amphetamines as well as more nonspecific factors such as medical illnesses and psychosocial life events with concomitant general stress. Further, specific hallucinogens such as LSD may precipitate a rather long-lasting psychotic episode that is ultimately indistinguishable from a schizophrenic disorder. Lastly, there have been a dramatically increasing number of hypotheses that a viral vector or early developmental abnormalities may be important as etiologic agents in at least some cases of schizophrenic disorders.

Psychosocial factors   Empirical support for psychosocial hypotheses concerning the creation of a vulnerability to developing schizophrenia is variable, far from definitive, and interacts strongly with neurobiologic factors.

In the vulnerable individual, schizophrenia often has its onset in a critical developmental period. The teenager may attempt to leave home and separate from family members for school or work reasons. The onset is often, but not invariably, insidious. In terms of psychosocial approaches to schizophrenia, there is felt to be a developmental or intrapsychic deficit in the vulnerable individual.

Once set into motion, the disturbance passes through a series of stages leading to the final common pathway of a psychotic state.

Despite much theorizing, there is no inevitable schizophrenia-prone personality type, although at least a small but significant percentage of individuals with schizoid (withdrawn), paranoid (suspicious), and schizotypal (odd, eccentric) personality disorder do seem to be vulnerable to developing schizophrenic disorders. In the 1960s, a more family-systems–oriented view emerged. An example of this approach is the "double-bind" hypothesis of Bateson and coworkers (1956) who analyzed the formal communications patterns in "schizophrenogenic" families. In this view, communications content is less important than the frequently conflicting and self-contradictory form of communication style of schizophrenic patients' families. It remains unclear whether these familial factors are a cause or result of having a schizophrenic child in the family. As the importance of biologic factors in schizophrenia have become clearer, family psychosocial factors have been seen more as secondary or epiphenomenal factors.

Psychosocial researchers have also examined the importance of socioeconomic factors in schizophrenia. Lower socioeconomic status correlates with a higher incidence of schizophrenia. There are two possible interpretations of this data. First, there may be a "social drift" of vulnerable individuals to lower socioeconomic status. The second hypothesis is more etiologic, as socieconomic stressors may precipitate schizophrenic episodes, especially in vulnerable individuals.

PATHOPHYSIOLOGY   Neurotransmitters and neuropeptides   Neurobiologic factors have been correlated with schizophrenic episodes. The predominant neurotransmitter hypothesis involves dopaminergic overactivity. Evidence supporting this hypothesis comes from several sources. First, the potency of all traditional antipsychotic medications can be roughly predicted by their dopaminergic blocking capacity. Second, mesolimbic dopamine plays a role in attentional mechanisms and stimulus filtering. When stimulus filtering mechanisms break down, there is a collapse of the information processing capacity of the individual with resulting sensory inundation, cognitive fragmentation, and symptoms of thought disorder.

Despite this support, the dopamine hypothesis is fraught with difficulties when compared with the catecholamine theory of the affective disorders. Affective disorders hypothetically (and simplistically) reflect a decrease in norepinephrine tone in hypothalamic nuclei leading to a final common pathway of neurovegetative symptoms. In schizophrenia, there seems to be increased dopamine tone in critical subcortical pathways leading to cognitive fragmentation, thought disorder, and clinical symptoms that are quite complex and highly variable. In this framework, affective disorders may be seen as impinging on the diencephalic "core" of the brain, whereas schizophrenia is conceptualized as a disorder of the mesolimbic-frontal cortical mantle. It is doubtful if a "one neurotransmitter" or "one locus" theory can explain any psychiatric disorder, given the interactive complexity of neurobiologic and psychosocial systems, although such theories may be useful.

The hypothesis of dopamine overactivity in schizophrenia is generally characterized as a static theory. In reality, dopamine tone is related in a dynamic and variable manner to GABA, serotonin, and other neurotransmitters that are functionally arrayed in a cascade of important brain systems, such as the dorsolateral prefrontal cortex, mesial temporal cortex, nucleus accumbens, ventral pallidum, and the hippocampus. Longer-term correlates of schizophrenia may also involve alterations of neuropeptides, with their long latency and response effects on behavior. At an electrophysiologic level, it has been hypothesized that the initial disturbance in schizophrenia is an aberrant (perhaps excitotoxic-induced) temporal lobe focus that ultimately perturbs the homeostasis of the dopamine system. More recent evidence implicates a second trimester viremia as a possible early precursor of schizophrenia. According to this theory, the temporal lobes are damaged during fetal development and this deficit is "unmasked" in late adolescence by a failure to prune excess neurons or to down-regulate frontotemporal activity. All of these areas are receiving critical experimental scrutiny.

Neuropathologic factors The use of computed tomography (CT) and magnetic resonance imaging (MRI) has been widely employed in studies of schizophrenic patients. Initial reports indicated that a minority of schizophrenic patients have abnormally increased ventricular brain ratios, reflecting increased ventricular fluid volume associated with brain atrophy. Subsequent studies in identical twins discordant for schizophrenia have confirmed increased ventricular size and neuropsychologic deficits in schizophrenic patients and perhaps in their "unaffected" co-twin, supporting the contention that schizophrenia is accompanied by brain dysfunction. It is quite possible that type II patients have a disorder that is distinct and associated with poor medication response and poor clinical outcome. Positron emission tomography (PET) data reveal patterns of decreased frontal lobe activity in schizophrenia (hypofrontality) that seem important, especially in view of the close relationship of dopamine activity, frontal lobe function, and mesolimbic activity levels. Future PET studies utilizing new ligands will undoubtedly clarify the role of dopamine and other neurotransmitters in the schizophrenic disorders.

Psychophysiology and information processing Important insights into the pathophysiology of schizophrenia have also been generated by psychophysiologic and information processing studies. Individuals at high risk for developing schizophrenia and patients with a schizophrenic disorder are frequently psychophysiologically labile and vulnerable to being inundated by stimuli. The proposed mechanism for such vulnerability is an impairment in an individual's ability to screen out irrelevant stimuli and an associated inability to habituate to externally and internally generated cues. Ultimately, this dysfunction, which has been linked to dopamine overactivity in humans and animals, leads to an information processing overload. The affected person becomes inundated with stimuli and displays cognitive fragmentation and thought disorder. It is this fragmented thinking and lapses in speech which sometimes serve as an important clue to the primary care physician that the patient is experiencing serious psychiatric problems. Using attentional tasks, skin conductance habituation, and other measures, investigators have increasingly underscored the importance of these dysfunctions in the schizophrenic disorders. New techniques, such as magnetoencephalography (MEG) also offer exciting possibilities for specifying the possible frontal, temporal, and subcortical locus and type of brain disturbance characteristic of the various types of schizophrenic disorders.

TREATMENT AND OUTCOME **Neurobiologic factors** Five-year follow-up studies show that 60 percent of schizophrenic individuals have social recovery and half of those are employed. Some 30 percent are seriously and permanently handicapped, and 10 percent remain chronically hospitalized. This pattern of outcome seems still to be generally accurate across numerous studies. Which factors determine the outcome of the schizophrenic disorders are not clear. It is commonly stated that the outcome of schizophrenia is better when disorientation, affective symptoms, and acute onset are present. The outcome of schizophrenic disorders is thought to be poorer when the patient is well oriented and has fewer affective symptoms, and when the onset is insidious.

The outcome of schizophrenic disorders has been greatly improved by the use of potent and efficacious antipsychotic medications, such as the phenothiazines. Studies indicate that antipsychotic medications (often expressed in terms of chlorpromazine equivalents) act selectively against specific target symptoms that are similar to the "positive" symptoms of type I schizophrenia which include hallucinations and psychotic agitation. In contrast to these responsive target symptoms, antipsychotic medications may not necessarily improve "negative" symptoms such as anhedonia and social withdrawal. The primary modalities for treatment of the acute schizophrenic disorders are antipsychotic medication along with psychosocial therapies. The typical schizophrenic patient usually requires at least the equivalent of 600 to 800 mg/d of chlorpromazine administered for 4 to 6 weeks, although higher doses are frequently necessary. Maintenance doses

of antipsychotic medications in lower doses and given on a continuous or intermittent basis are often required to prevent relapse.

The primary care physician sees two main types of schizophrenic patients. First, there is the acute, psychotically agitated patient with poor behavioral control. These patients need to be referred to an emergency room or other acute care facility, often for rapid neuroleptic medication treatment on an out- or inpatient basis. It is quite important to determine if the psychotic state is of recent onset (which may need a careful differential diagnostic workup to rule out organic, drug-induced, or manic disorders, or an exacerbation of a chronic condition). The second type of schizophrenic patient has more subtle signs and symptoms of psychosis and, though not an emergency case, needs a rapid referral to a psychiatrist for appropriate care.

Antipsychotic medications alter dopaminergic-cholinergic balance in nigrostriatal structures (via dopamine blockade) so that acute extrapyramidal side effects are induced (e.g., dystonia, motor restlessness). These side effects can be treated with anticholinergic medications that restore dopaminergic-cholinergic balance. Aliphatic phenothiazines (such as chlorpromazine) with inherent anticholinergic properties cause fewer extrapyramidal side effects but induce more anticholinergic side effects such as hypotension or blurred vision. Additionally, blood dyscrasias, liver toxicity, and other idiosyncratic reactions occur. Also, the long-term use of antipsychotic medications may induce nigrostriatal damage and tardive dyskinesia, a long-lasting and potentially disabling motor syndrome (see Chap. 21). Thus, the search for new antipsychotic medications with more selective (i.e., nonnigrostriatal) sites of action is important for the pharmacologic treatment of schizophrenia. (See "Antipsychotic or Neuroleptic Medications," below.)

Psychosocial factors The outcome of schizophrenic patients can be divided into semi-independent axes of symptoms, social function, and vocational function. It is possible to treat the specific psychotic symptoms of a schizophrenic individual (affecting the symptomatic axis of outcome), but the patient may be left with major psychosocial deficits (the social axis of outcome). Antipsychotic medications should thus be combined with sensitive psychosocial management including, where appropriate, individual and group psychotherapy, family counseling, and vocational rehabilitation in order to maximize therapeutic outcome and to restore the patient to the premorbid level of adjustment. For example, returning an acutely treated schizophrenic patient to a home filled with hostility, criticisms, and emotional overinvolvement (the so-called high-expressed-emotion family) without the benefit of family education and therapy is poor psychosocial management and may lead to relapse. Along with appropriate use of antipsychotic medications, family counseling and education is often a critical determinant of therapeutic outcome in the schizophrenic disorders.

ANTIPSYCHOTIC OR NEUROLEPTIC MEDICATIONS
Lewis L. Judd

The antipsychotics have the capacity to sedate, tranquilize, blunt emotional expression, attenuate aggressive and impulsive behavior, and cause lack of initiative and loss of interest in the environment. Unique features of the drugs are that they leave higher intellectual functions relatively intact yet specifically ameliorate the agitation and bizarre behavior and thinking of psychotic patients. Unfortunately no antipsychotic medication currently available even approaches ideal in this respect. Virtually all have prominent anticholinergic side effects and produce a wide variety of dystonias and extrapyramidal symptoms. Of greater concern is the fact that long-term administration of these agents can cause tardive dyskinesia in some patients (see Chap. 21), a seriously disabling movement disorder that is often irreversible. Nonetheless, the antipsychotics, primarily used in schizophrenia, have helped to reduce enormously the patient populations in mental hospitals and have allowed chronic mentally ill patients who previously would have been lifelong residents of hospitals to live in the community.

MECHANISM OF ACTION With few exceptions, antipsychotic neuroleptics have notable effects on the brain's dopaminergic neurotransmitter system. Specifically, these medications antagonize the effects of the neurotransmitter dopamine in the basal ganglia and in the limbic portions of the forebrain. Since the central characteristic of neuroleptics is their capacity to block dopaminergic neurotransmission, this has led researchers to postulate that an abnormality in the CNS dopaminergic neurotransmitter system is one of the key pathophysiologic mechanisms in the etiology of schizophrenia. Many effects of antipsychotic medications on the brain have been well-described, but the underlying mechanism by which these drugs achieve their antipsychotic efficacy is not yet fully understood.

CLINICAL CONDITIONS FOR USE Because the overall risk of tardive dyskinesia is estimated at 20 to 40 percent with chronic treatment, antipsychotics should only be used when necessary and in those conditions for which they are the drug of choice: in treating schizophrenic disorders; in combination with lithium for acute manic episodes; and in combination with antidepressants for psychotic and agitated depressions. They are also used in treating Tourette's syndrome and Huntington's disease. Although the antipsychotics should be used with only a relatively narrow spectrum of mental disorders, patients with these disorders make up a significant majority of all patients with serious and chronic mental illness.

CLINICAL USE OF ANTIPSYCHOTICS The more commonly used antipsychotics from each pharmacologic class and their average daily oral doses are given in Table 389-14. Chlorpromazine, one of the first drugs of this class to be developed, is the prototypic antipsychotic drug and the potency standard for the others. Dose equivalence for an antipsychotic drug is calculated in comparison with the effect of 100 mg of chlorpromazine. For example, 5 mg of trifluoperazine or 2 mg of haloperidol is equivalent in potency to 100 mg of chlorpromazine. Using this ratio as a reference point, acutely psychotic patients usually require an accumulated dose of 500 to 800 mg orally of a chlorpromazine equivalent during the first 24 to 36 h. Following control of the acute agitation, the oral dose is increased over the next week to the chlorpromazine equivalent of between 600 and 1500 mg/d in divided doses. It is uncommon for therapeutic benefits to be measurably increased by exceeding the daily dose equivalent of 1500 mg of chlorpromazine, although it may be necessary to go to two and three times this level in some patients.

Because schizophrenia is a chronic disorder, patients need long-term maintenance on antipsychotics to prevent relapse. In controlled studies as many as 60 percent of schizophrenics relapse within 6 months after discontinuing drug therapy. Patients are maintained on the lowest dose possible that will prevent reemergence of symptoms. This is usually in the range of 20 percent of the peak dose level needed to ameliorate the acute phase of the psychotic symptoms. Compliance is difficult to achieve in this chronically disordered group of patients, and it is often therapeutically advantageous for the clinician to use parenteral long-acting fluphenazine enanthate or decanoate, which can be administered by injection every week or two. Previously it was recommended that drug holidays be used, but this practice has not prevented tardive dyskinesia, and there are few if any advantages to this technique, which is now rarely used.

SIDE EFFECTS AND INTERACTIONS Initially patients are sedated, lethargic, and drowsy, but within days they develop tolerance to these effects. All of the antipsychotics have anticholinergic action, which may produce dry mouth, cycloplegia, postural hypotension, constipation, and urinary retention. Obstructive jaundice, retinal pigmentation (thioridazine), lenticular opacities, skin pigmentation and hypersensitivity to sunlight, and male impotence are also side effects seen with antipsychotics.

The extrapyramidal side effects are the most troublesome, however. During the first five days of treatment, patients may develop acute muscular dystonic reactions but the extrapyramidal Parkinson-like syndrome is the most common. Both the dystonia and the parkinsonism respond well to antiparkinsonian medications (e.g., benztropine mesylate, 1 to 2 mg bid or tid; trihexyphenidyl, 2 to 5 mg bid or tid). Another common side effect is akathisia, a motor restlessness in which patients feel compelled to move their extremities and to move about. It is not uncommon to mistake akathisia for psychotic agitation and increase the antipsychotic dose, exacerbating the problem. Akathisia may respond to beta blockers and antiparkinsonian agents but more often requires decreasing the dose of the antipsychotic. It is rarely necessary to continue antiparkinsonian drug treatment beyond the first 3 months of antipsychotic maintenance.

The most serious side effect of the antipsychotics is tardive dyskinesia, which has been seen with virtually every neuroleptic. The specter of tardive dyskinesia has altered the risk-benefit ratio of the antipsychotics; they should only be used for those disorders in which they are clearly the drugs of choice. Usually the symptoms of tardive dyskinesia appear late in treatment and consist of involuntary, repetitive movements of the lips, tongue (e.g., tongue thrusting, lip smacking), and not infrequently of the extremities and trunk. Patients over 60 and those with preexisting CNS pathology are at a higher risk for this disorder (up to 70 percent), but other risk factors have not been confirmed. Although tardive dyskinesia cannot be prevented or reversed once it has developed, antipsychotic medications such as clozapine, which can attenuate some of the symptoms, may be substituted for the neuroleptic being used. However, it is too early to determine whether tardive dyskinesia is reduced with some of the newer antipsychotic medications.

The neuroleptic malignant syndrome, a rare complication of neuroleptic drugs, is discussed in Chap. 398.

NEWER ANTIPSYCHOTIC MEDICATIONS (ATYPICAL NEURO-LEPTICS) Although development of new antipsychotic medications has lagged significantly behind that of the antidepressants and anxiolytic drugs, some promising medications have appeared recently.

Clozapine is a dibenzodiazepine that binds to serotonin and alpha-adrenergic, histaminergic, and dopaminergic receptors. It has been approved by the FDA for use in treatment-refractory psychotic patients and in those who have intolerable side effects with their current medications. Its antipsychotic activity is comparable to the traditional neuroleptics, and it is also effective in attenuating anxiety and tension. Clozapine has proven effective in 30 to 40 percent of treatment-resistant schizophrenics. Often the full therapeutic effects of clozapine may not appear until at least 6 months of treatment. The drug produces some sedation and muscle relaxation but few extrapyramidal symptoms. It is not known to cause tardive dyskinesia and may, in high doses, attenuate it. Clozapine's side effects include orthostatic hypotension, sinus tachycardia, hypersalivation, temperature eleva-

TABLE 389-14   Some commonly used antipsychotic medications

	Average daily oral dose range, mg	Potency ratio compared to 100 mg of chlorpromazine
Phenothiazines		
Aliphatics:		
Chlorpromazine	400–800	1:1
Piperazines:		
Fluphenazine	4–20	1:50
Fluphenazine enanthate or decanoate	25–100*	
Perphenazine	8–32	1:10
Trifluoperazine	6–20	1:20
Piperidines:		
Thioridazine	200–600	1:1
Butyrophenones		
Haloperidol	8–32	1:50
Thioxanthenes		
Chlorprothixene	400–800	1:1 (approx)
Thiothixene	15–30	1:25
Oxoindoles		
Molindone	40–200	1:10
Dibenzoxazepines		
Loxapine	60–100	1:10

* For intramuscular injection only.

tion, lowered seizure threshold, and constipation. A 1 to 2 percent incidence of potentially fatal agranulocytosis has been reported but this may be considerably higher in eastern European and Jewish subpopulations. Frequent (e.g., weekly) CBCs should be obtained and medication discontinued if the WBC count begins to decrease.

Sulpiride, which is available in Europe, is a substituted benzamide that selectively binds to presynaptic, sodium-dependent, D-2 receptors. Its antipsychotic efficacy is comparable to traditional neuroleptics. Moreover, it may cause fewer cases of tardive dyskinesia and extrapyramidal syndrome. This novel structure may herald the development of new classes of safer and better antipsychotics.

The success of clozapine has fueled the search for new antipsychotic medications and there are a number of new compounds under active study (e.g., Remoxipride, respiridone, etc.).

REFERENCES

MICHAELS R, MARZUK PM: Progress in psychiatry (first of two parts). N Engl J Med 329:552, 1993

———, ———: Medical progress: Progress in psychiatry (second of two parts). N Engl J Med 329:628, 1993

Mood disorders

ALLEN JM et al: Depressive symptoms and family history in seasonal and nonseasonal mood disorders. Am J Psychiatry 150:443, 1993

BALDESSARINI RJ: Biological hypothesis in psychiatry, in *Chemotherapy in Psychiatry,* Cambridge, Mass, Harvard, 1985, pp 9–12

———: *Biomedical Aspects of Depression.* Washington, DC, APA Press, 1982, pp 1–83

BARON M, RISCH N: X-linkage and genetic heterogeneity in bipolar-related major affective illness: Reanalysis of linkage data. Ann Hum Genet 46 (pt 2):153, 1982

BURKE KC et al: Age at onset of selected mental disorders in five community populations. Arch Genl Psychiat, 47:511, 1990

CALLAHAM M, KASSEL D: Epidemiology of fatal tricyclic antidepressant ingestion: Implications for management. Ann Emerg Med 14:1, 1985

CARNEY RM et al: Major depressive disorder in coronary artery disease. Am J Cardiol 60(16):1273, 1987

CLAYTON PJ, BARRETT JE (eds): *Treatment of Depression: Old Controversies and New Approaches.* New York, Raven, 1983

DEVEAUGHGEISS J: Diagnosis and treatment of obsessive compulsive disorder. Annu Rev Med 44:53, 1993

Diagnostic and Statistical Manual of Mental Disorders, 3d ed. Washington, DC, American Psychiatric Association, 1980

Diagnostic and Statistical Manual of Mental Disorders, 3d ed, revised. Washington, DC, American Psychiatric Association, 1987

Drugs that cause psychiatric symptoms. Med Lett Drugs Ther 35:65, 1993

ELKIN I et al: National Institute of Mental Health Treatment of Depression Collaborative Research Program. General Effectiveness of Treatments. Arch Gen Psychiatry 46:971, 1989

FAEDDA GL et al: Seasonal mood disorders. Patterns of seasonal recurrrence in mania and depression. Arch Gen Psychiatry 50:17, 1993

FRANK E et al: Early recurrence in unipolar depression. Arch Gen Psychiatry 46:397, 1989

———: Conceptualization and rationale for consensus definitions of terms in major depressive disorder: Response, remission, recovery, relapse, and recurrence. Arch Gen Psychiatry 48(9):851, 1991

FRIIS R, NANJUNDAPPA G: Diabetes, depression, and employment status. Soc Sci Med 23(5):471, 1986

GOODWIN FK, JAMISON KR: *Manic-Depressive Illness.* New York, Oxford University Press, 1990

HARDMAN A et al: The recognition of psychiatric morbidity on a medical oncology ward. J Psychosom Res 33(2):235-9, 1989

KELSOE JR et al: Re-evaluation of the linkage relationship between chromosome 11p loci and the gene for bipolar affective disorder in the Old Order Amish. Nature 342:328, 1989

KLERMAN GL: History and development of modern concepts of affective illness, in *Neurobiology of Mood Disorders,* RM Post, RC Ballenger (eds). Baltimore, Williams & Wilkins, 1984, pp 1–19

MARTIN JB, REICHLIN S: *Clinical Neuroendocrinology,* 2d ed. Philadelphia, Davis 1987

OSSER DN: A systematic approach to the classification and pharmacotherapy of nonpsychotic major depression and dysthymia. J Clin Psychopharmacol 13:133, 1993

POST RM, BALLENGER JC (eds): *Neurobiology of Mood Disorders.* Baltimore, Williams & Wilkins, 1984, vol 1

———, WEISS SRB: Kindling and manic depressive illness, in *The Clinical Relevance of Kindling,* TB Bolwigm, MR Trimble (eds). Chichester, England, Wiley, 1989, pp 209–230

REGIER et al: Comorbidity of mental disorders with alcohol and other drug abuse. Results from the Epidemiologic Catchment Area (ECA) Study. JAMA 264(19):2511, 1990

———: One-month prevalence of mental disorders in the United States based on five Epidemiologic Catchment Area Sites. Arch Gen Psychiatry 45:977, 1988

ROBINSON RG et al: Two-year longitudinal study of poststroke mood disorders: Diagnosis and outcome at one and two years. Stroke 18(5):837, 1987

———, et al: Depression and diabetes. Diabetic Med 5(3):268, 1988

ROSENTHAL NE et al: Seasonal affective disorder: A description of the syndrome and preliminary findings with light therapy. Arch Gen Psychiatry 41:72, 1984

SELIGMAN MEP, BEAGLEY G: Learned helplessness in the rat. J Comp Physiol Psychol 88:534, 1975

STEWART AL et al: Functional status and well-being of patients with chronic conditions. Results from the Medical Outcomes Study. JAMA 262(7):907, 1989

WELLS KB et al: The functioning and well-being of depressed patients. Results from the Medical Outcomes Study. JAMA 262(7):914, 1989

WILLNER P: The validity of animal models of depression. Psychopharmacology 83:1, 1984

Anxiety disorders

AGRAS WS: The diagnosis and treatment of panic disorder. Annu Rev Med 44:39, 1993

CHARNEY DS et al: Noradrenergic function in panic anxiety. Arch Gen Psychiatry 41:75, 1984

——— et al: Psychobiologic mechanisms for posttraumatic stress disorder. Arch Gen Psychiatry 50:294, 1993

DIAMOND EL, GRAUER K: The spectrum of anxiety disorders in family practice. Am Fam Physician 36:167, 1987

GOLDBERG J et al: A twin study of the effects of the Vietnam war on posttraumatic stress disorder. JAMA 263:1227, 1990

HORWATH E et al: Epidemiology of panic disorder in African-Americans. Am J Psychiatry 150:465, 1993

KATON W: Panic disorder in the medical setting. Washington, DC, National Institute of Mental Health, Department of Health and Human Services publication (ADM), 1989

KECK PE et al: Valproate treatment of panic disorder and lactate-induced panic attacks. Biol Psychiatry 33:542, 1993

KELLER MB, HANKS DL: Course and outcome in panic disorder. Prog Neuropsychopharmacol Biol Psychiatry 17:551, 1993

KUSHNER MG et al: The relation between alcohol problems and anxiety disorders. Am J Psychiatry 47:685, 1990

McGLYNN TJ, METCALF HL (eds): *Diagnosis and Treatment of Anxiety Disorders: A Physicians Handbook.* Washington DC, American Psychiatric Press, 1989, pp 43–48

MARKOWITZ JS et al: Quality of life in panic disorder. Arch Gen Psychiatry 46:984, 1989

SHADER RI, GREENBLATT DJ: Drug therapy. Use of benzodiazepines in anxiety disorders. N Engl J Med 328:1398, 1993

YEHUDA R et al: Psychoneuroendocrine assessment of posttraumatic stress disorder. Current progress and new directions. Prog Neuropsychopharmacol Biol Psychiatry 17:541, 1993

Schizophrenic disorders

ALVIR JMJ et al: Clozapine-induced agranulocytosis. Incidence and risk factors in the United States. N Engl J Med 329:162, 1993

BRAFF DL: Attention, information processing, and habituation in psychiatric disorders. Psychiatry, III. Philadelphia, Lippincott, 1985

———, GEYER MA: Sensorimotor gating in schizophrenia. Arch Gen Psychiatry 47:181, 1990

BROWN GW et al: Influence of family life on the course of schizophrenic disorders: A replication. Br J Psychiatry 11:241, 1972

CARLSON G, GOODWIN F: The stages of mania. Arch Gen Psychiatry 28:221, 1973

CHRISTISON GW et al: The quantitative investigation of hippocampal pyramidal cell size, shape and variability of orientation in schizophrenia. Arch Gen Psychiatry 46:1027, 1989

CROW TJ: Molecular pathology of schizophrenia: More than one disease process? Br Med J 280:66, 1980

DOCHERTY JP et al: Stages of onset of schizophrenic psychosis. Am J Psychiatry 135:420, 1978

GERSON SL: Clozapine. Deciphering the risks. N Engl J Med 329:204, 1993

JESTE DV, LOHR JB: Hippocampal pathologic findings in schizophrenia. Arch Gen Psychiatry 46:1019, 1989

ROSENBAUM CP: *The Meaning of Madness.* New York, Science House, 1970

ROSENTHAL D, KETY S: *The Transmission of Schizophrenia.* New York, Pergamon, 1968

SHANER A et al: Unrecognized cocaine use among schizophrenic patients. Am J Psychiatry 150:758, 1993

SHENTON ME et al: Abnormalities of the left temporal lobe and thought disorder in schizophrenia. N Engl J Med 327:604, 1993

SIRIS SG et al: Histories of substance abuse, panic and suicidal ideation in schizophrenic patients with histories of post-psychotic depressions. Prog Neuropsychopharmacol Biol Psychiatry 17:609, 1993

Special Issue: Negative symptoms in schizophrenia. Schizophr Bull 11, 1985

Special Issue: Advances in the genetics of schizophrenia. Schizophr Bull 15(3), 1989

Special Issue: The cost of schizophrenia. Schizophr Bull 17, 1991

STRAUSS JS, CARPENTER WT: *Schizophrenia.* New York, Plenum, 1981

WALKER E et al: Environmental factors related to schizophrenia in psychophysiologically labile high-risk males. J Abnorm Psychol 90:313, 1981

WEINBERGER DR: Implications of normal brain development for the pathogenesis of schizophrenia. Arch Gen Psychiatry 44:660, 1987

WETZEL H, BENKERT O: Dopamine autoreceptor agonists in the treatment of schizophrenic disorders. Prog Neuropsychopharmacol Biol Psychiatry 17:525, 1993

WYSOWSKI DK, BAUM C: Antipsychotic drug use in the United States, 1976–1985. Arch Gen Psychiatry 46:929, 1989

section 5 Alcoholism and drug dependency

390 ALCOHOL AND ALCOHOLISM

MARC A. SCHUCKIT

Ninety percent of people drink alcohol, 40 to 50 percent of men have temporary alcohol-induced problems, and 10 percent of men and 3 to 5 percent of women develop pervasive and persistent alcohol-related problems (alcoholism). The usual alcoholic has a family and a job; only about 5 percent fit the skid row stereotype. Even light drinking may adversely interact with other medications, temporary heavier drinking can exacerbate most medical illnesses, and alcoholism can masquerade as many different medical disorders and psychiatric syndromes. The following sections describe the pharmacology and clinical effects of alcohol and identify circumstances where drinking may cause a major medical or psychiatric problem or exacerbate a preexisting disorder. While these comments apply to the hypothetical "average" person, there is considerable individual variability depending on genetic vulnerability, concomitant drug use, and prior unrelated pathology or disease.

PHARMACOLOGY OF ETHANOL: ABSORPTION AND METABO-LISM Ethanol is a weakly charged molecule that moves easily through cell membranes, rapidly equilibrating between blood and tissues. The effects of drinking depend in part on the amount of ethanol consumed per unit of body weight; the level of alcohol in the blood is expressed as milligrams or grams of ethanol per deciliter (e.g., 100 mg/dL or 0.1000 g/dL). In round figures, 340 mL (12 oz) of beer, 115 mL (4 oz) of nonfortified wine, and 43 mL (1.5 oz) (a shot) of 80-proof beverage each contain approximately 10 g of ethanol; 1 pint of 86-proof beverage contains approximately 160 g and 1 L of wine contains approximately 80 g of ethanol. Congeners found in alcohol beverages may contribute to body damage with heavy drinking; these include low-molecular-weight alcohols (e.g., methanol and butanol), aldehydes, esters, histamine, phenols, tannins, iron, lead, and cobalt.

Ethanol is a central nervous system (CNS) depressant that decreases activity of neurons, although some behavioral stimulation is observed at low blood levels. This drug has cross-tolerance and shares a similar pattern of behavioral problems with other brain depressants, including the benzodiazepines, barbiturates, and other sedatives and hypnotics. Alcohol is absorbed from mucous membranes of the mouth and esophagus (in very small amounts), from the stomach and large bowel (in modest amounts), and from the proximal portion of the small intestine (the major site). The rate of absorption *increases* with: rapid gastric emptying; the absence of proteins, fats, or carbohydrates (which interfere with absorption); the absence of congeners; dilution to a modest percentage of ethanol (maximum absorption is seen at about 20 percent by volume); and carbonation (champagne).

Between 2 percent (at low blood alcohol concentrations) and about 10 percent (at high blood alcohol concentrations) of ethanol is excreted directly through the lungs, urine, or sweat, but the greater part is metabolized to acetaldehyde in the liver. At least two metabolic routes, each with different optimal concentrations of ethanol (K_m), result in the metabolism of approximately one drink per hour. The *first* and clinically most important pathway occurs in the cell cytosol via alcohol dehydrogenase (ADH) with a K_m of about 2 mmol. This reaction produces acetaldehyde, which is then rapidly destroyed by aldehyde dehydrogenase (ALDH) in the cytosol and mitochondria.

Each of these steps requires nicotinamide adenine dinucleotide (NAD) as a cofactor, and it is the increased ratio of the reduced cofactor (NADH) to NAD (NADH:NAD) that is responsible for many of the metabolic derangements observed after drinking. *Second*, microsomes of the smooth endoplasmic reticulum (the microsomal ethanol-oxidizing system or MEOS) with a K_m of about 10 mmol may be responsible for 10 percent or more of ethanol oxidation at high blood alcohol concentrations. Increased activity of this system can be induced after repeated exposure to ethanol.

All pathways result in the production of acetaldehyde, which is oxidized to acetate. The specific clinical significance of acetaldehyde is not fully known, but low levels of this substance may cause stimulation and behavioral reinforcement. Accumulation of higher levels in liver, brain, or other body tissues may cause organ damage.

BEHAVIORAL EFFECTS, TOLERANCE, AND DEPENDENCE The behavioral and physiologic effects of any drug depend on the dose, its rate of increase in plasma, the concomitant presence of other drugs or medical problems, and the past experience with the agent. With alcohol, one also must consider whether observation is during rising (where the effects are more intense) or falling blood alcohol levels.

Even though "legal intoxication" requires a blood alcohol concentration of at least 80 to 100 mg/dL (0.1 g/dL), behavioral, psychomotor, and cognitive changes are seen at levels as low as 20 to 30 mg/dL (i.e., after one to two drinks). Narcosis or deep sleep is induced in many people at twice the legal intoxication level, and even in the absence of concomitant medications, death can occur with levels between 300 and 400 mg/dL. Ethanol, either alone or in combination with agents such as benzodiazepines, is probably responsible for more toxic overdose deaths than any other agent.

The mechanisms of action of ethanol on nervous tissues are not fully understood because even modest doses simultaneously change many neurotransmitters and increase the fluidity of neuronal cell membranes. After repeated exposure to the drug, the body compensates in at least three ways to tolerate higher ethanol levels. *First*, after 1 to 2 weeks of daily drinking the liver can increase the metabolic rate of ethanol by as much as 30 percent; i.e., there is *metabolic or pharmacokinetic tolerance*, an alteration that disappears almost as rapidly as it develops. *Second, cellular or pharmacodynamic tolerance* probably occurs through complex neurochemical changes in cell membranes with subsequent altered ion flow—adjustments that may contribute to physical dependence. *Third*, even at the same blood alcohol concentrations and neuronal adaptation, organisms can learn to adapt behavior and to function better than expected under drug influence (*behavioral tolerance*). For example, practicing driving while intoxicated might result in a psychomotor performance which (*while still impaired*) is better than that observed before practice.

Once the cells have adapted to chronic ethanol exposure, the structural or biochemical changes may not return to normal for several weeks or more. In the face of these adjustments, the neurons require ethanol to function optimally; i.e., the person is physically addicted or drug-dependent. This physical condition is distinct from psychological dependence, a poorly defined concept indicating that the person is psychologically uncomfortable without the drug.

NUTRITIONAL FACTORS One gram of ethanol has approximately 29.7 kJ (7.1 kcal), and a drink contains between 293.0 and 418.6 kJ (70 and 100 kcal) from ethanol and other carbohydrates. Therefore, 8 to 10 drinks can yield over 4186 kJ (1000 kcal) per day, but these are "empty" of nutrients such as minerals, proteins, and vitamins.

Any vitamin absorbed through the small intestine by active transport or stored in the liver may be deficient in alcoholics. These include folate (folacin or folic acid), pyridoxine (B_6), thiamine (B_1), nicotinic acid or niacin (B_3), and vitamin A. Thiamine deficiency causes Wernicke's and Korsakoff's syndromes (see Chap. 377).

Low blood potassium, magnesium, calcium, zinc, and phosphorus can occur as a consequence of dietary deficiency and acid-base imbalances during excess alcohol ingestion or withdrawal. Hypokalemia can lead to periodic muscle paralysis and areflexia. Deficiencies in magnesium can add to a clouded sensorium and other neurologic symptoms; hypocalcemia can cause tetany and weakness; low levels of zinc are speculated to contribute to gonadal dysfunction, anorexia, problems with wound healing, and immune deficiencies; and low phosphate levels can contribute to myocardial failure, brain dysfunction, weakness of muscles (including those of respiration), and white blood cell and platelet dysfunction.

An ethanol load in a fasting, healthy individual is likely to produce transient hypoglycemia within 6 to 36 h, secondary to the acute actions of ethanol on gluconeogenesis. This impairment is exacerbated by poor diet and by liver and pancreatic disease. As a result, glucose intolerance may be marked until the alcoholic has been abstinent for 2 to 4 weeks. Alcohol ketoacidosis, probably reflecting a decrease in fatty acid oxidation coupled with poor diet or recurrent vomiting, should not be misdiagnosed as diabetic ketosis. With the former, patients show an increase in serum ketones along with a mild increase in glucose but a large anion gap, a mild to moderate increase in serum lactate, and a β-hydroxybutyrate/lactate ratio of between 2:1 and 9:1 (with normal being 1:1).

THE EFFECTS OF ETHANOL ON BODY SYSTEMS

This overview of acute and chronic effects of alcohol on body systems outlines signs and symptoms that can aid in the recognition of the hidden alcoholic. It emphasizes the interactions between drinking and medications and the effects of alcohol on chronic medical conditions, factors that are also important in helping the clinician to understand the effects of alcohol on nonalcoholic patients.

CENTRAL NERVOUS SYSTEM In addition to acute behavioral effects, an evening of heavy drinking can result in an alcoholic *blackout*, i.e., an episode of forgetting all or part of what occurred during drinking. This problem is experienced by 30 to 40 percent of men in their late teens and early 20s, most of whom do not go on to develop more serious and pervasive alcohol-related problems. Even after only a few drinks, alcohol acutely decreases *sleep* latency (helping people to fall asleep) and depresses rapid eye movement (REM) sleep early in the night, sometimes followed by later REM rebound associated with bad dreams. The consequence is to "fragment" sleep, causing a more rapid than normal alternation between sleep stages and a deficiency in deep sleep. The overall effect is likely to be repeated awakenings and a sense of restless sleep.

Chronic intake of high doses of ethanol can cause *peripheral neuropathy* in 5 to 15 percent of alcoholics (see Chaps. 377 and 383). This syndrome probably results from both thiamine deficiency and direct effects of ethanol and/or acetaldehyde. Patients complain of bilateral limb numbness, tingling, and parasthesias, more pronounced distally than proximally. Although these symptoms can be incapacitating, more often the pain and numbness are mild to moderate in severity. The treatment is abstinence and thiamine supplementation.

Wernicke's and Korsakoff's syndromes are important problems in alcoholics (see Chap. 377). Thiamine deficiency is the major cause in vulnerable individuals (possibly interacting with a genetic transketolase deficiency). Classically, patients with Korsakoff's syndrome present with profound anterograde (unable to learn new material) and retrograde amnesia along with possible impairment in visuospatial, abstract, and conceptual reasoning but with a normal intelligence

quotient (IQ). In general, the level of recent memory loss is out of proportion to the global level of cognitive impairment. While most patients demonstrate an acute onset of Korsakoff's syndrome in association with the neurologic stigmata seen with Wernicke's syndrome (e.g., sixth nerve palsy and ataxia), some individuals may have a more gradual development of symptoms probably secondary to repeated bouts of thiamine deficiency. Wernicke's syndrome responds rapidly to oral thiamine replacement of 50 to 100 mg followed by 50 to 100 mg/d. However, only one-quarter of Korsakoff's patients are likely to achieve full recovery, one-half experience partial recovery, and one-quarter show no improvement with thiamine even after many months of supplementation.

About 1 percent of alcoholics with long histories of associated malnutrition develop *cerebellar degeneration*, a syndrome of progressive unsteady stance and gait often accompanied by mild nystagmus (see Chap. 377). Cerebellar atrophy is seen on CT scan or MRI, but the cerebrospinal fluid is usually normal. While ethanol or acetaldehyde may contribute to the problem, the major cause is probably nutritional, and identical symptoms can be seen with some forms of severe malnutrition alone. Treatment consists of abstinence and multiple vitamin supplementation, although improvement is often minimal.

Alcoholics can show severe *cognitive* problems and impairment in recent and remote memory for weeks to months after an alcoholic binge. Cortical functioning (e.g., psychomotor performance and short-term memory) tends to improve with abstinence, but long-term memory problems, perhaps reflecting subcortical damage, may persist. Increased size of the brain ventricles and cerebral sulci are seen in up to 50 percent of chronic alcoholics. These changes are partially reversible, returning toward normal after a year or more of abstinence. Permanent CNS impairment (*alcoholic dementia*) may supervene. Up to 20 percent of chronically demented patients may have had prior alcoholism. There is no single alcoholic dementia syndrome; rather, this label is used to describe patients who have apparently irreversible cognitive changes (possibly from diverse causes) in the midst of chronic alcoholism (see also Chap. 377).

Finally, to borrow a phrase from the past, alcohol could be termed "the great mimicker" because almost every psychiatric syndrome can be seen during heavy drinking or subsequent withdrawal. These include intense *sadness* lasting for days to weeks in the midst of heavy drinking, a problem that can be viewed as a "normal" effect of alcohol; severe *anxiety* during alcoholic withdrawal, often remaining for many months after cessation of drinking; *psychoses* during the severe form of the alcohol abstinence syndrome; and auditory *hallucinations* and/or *paranoid delusions* in the absence of any obvious signs of withdrawal—a state called *alcoholic hallucinosis* or *alcoholic paranoia*. Whatever the cause, the treatment of alcohol-induced psychopathology includes abstinence and supportive care, with the likelihood of full recovery within several days to 6 weeks. Alcohol intake is an important part of the differential diagnosis of *any* patient with one of these psychological symptoms. Another alcohol-related psychiatric syndrome is *pathologic intoxication* or alcohol idiosyncratic intoxication, a state of severe agitation, confusion, and violence lasting minutes to hours that is seen after a very low dose of ethanol (e.g., one to two drinks) and for which the individual is amnestic. This extremely rare phenomenon, seen almost exclusively in individuals with severe preexisting brain damage, is sometimes invoked erroneously for the purposes of legal defense.

THE GASTROINTESTINAL SYSTEM Esophagus and stomach Acute alcoholic intake can result in inflammation of the esophagus (possibly secondary to reflux of gastric contents) and stomach (resulting from damage to the gastric mucosal barrier). Esophagitis can cause epigastric distress, and gastritis, the most frequent cause of gastrointestinal bleeding in heavy drinkers, can present with anorexia and abdominal pain. Chronic heavy drinking, if associated with violent vomiting, can produce a longitudinal tear in the mucosa at the gastroesophageal junction—a Mallory-Weiss lesion. Although many gastrointestinal problems are reversible, two complications of chronic alcoholism, esophageal varices secondary to cirrhosis-induced portal hypertension and atrophy of gastric cells, may be irreversible (see Chaps. 251 and 253).

Small bowel The greater part of the ethanol is absorbed from the proximal small bowel, where it may interfere with absorption of B vitamins and other nutrients. Acutely, ethanol can cause hemorrhagic lesions of the duodenal villi and diarrhea secondary to increased small-bowel motility and decreased water and electrolyte absorption. Chronic alcoholism can contribute to diarrhea through its effects on the pancreas (see Chaps. 254 and 274).

Pancreas Alcoholics commonly develop acute or chronic pancreatitis (see Chap. 274).

Liver Ethanol absorbed from the small bowel is carried directly to the liver, where it becomes the preferred fuel; NADH accumulates and oxygen utilization escalates, gluconeogenesis is impaired (with a resulting fall in the amount of glucose produced from glycogen), lactate production increases, and there is a decreased oxidation of fatty acids in the citric cycle with an increase in fat accumulation within liver cells. In the healthy individual taking no medications, these changes are reversible, but with repeated exposure to ethanol more severe changes in liver functioning are likely to occur. These include, in overlapping stages, fatty accumulation, alcohol-induced hepatitis, and cirrhosis (see Chap. 268).

Increased cancer risk Cancer is the second leading cause of death in alcoholics (after cardiovascular disease), who have a rate of carcinoma 10 times higher than that expected in the general population. The sites with the greatest increase over expected rates include the head and neck, esophagus, cardia of the stomach, liver, pancreas, and, according to recent data, breast.

HEMATOPOIETIC SYSTEM Ethanol exerts multiple reversible acute and chronic effects on all blood cells. Alcohol alters acutely the production of red blood cells (RBC), and this reaches clinical significance after days to weeks of heavy drinking. The most common finding is an increase in RBC size (mean corpuscular volume, MCV) with a mild anemia. If this is accompanied by folic acid deficiency, there also can be hypersegmented neutrophils, reticulocytopenia, and hyperplastic bone marrow. Other forms of anemia, including sideroblastic changes, can occur concomitantly, especially in the presence of severe malnutrition.

Chronic heavy drinking also can decrease production of most white blood cells (WBC), decrease granulocyte mobility and adherence, and impair the delayed hypersensitivity response to new antigens (with a possible false-negative tuberculin skin test). While the changes in WBCs themselves are usually temporary, they may contribute to the risk of infections and liver damage and perhaps to the increased risk of cancers in alcoholics. Alcohol also can cause toxic granulocytosis.

Many alcoholics present with mild thrombocytopenia (rarely associated with hemorrhage) due to a decrease in platelet survival and altered function; hypersplenism may occur as a complication of cirrhosis. Alcohol may decrease platelet aggregation and inhibit release of thromboxane A_2. These problems usually return toward normal within a week of abstinence.

CARDIOVASCULAR SYSTEM Modest doses of alcohol can have both deleterious and beneficial effects in individuals with normal cardiovascular status who take no medications. Ethanol decreases myocardial contractility and causes peripheral vasodilatation, resulting in a mild drop in blood pressure and a compensatory increased heart rate and cardiac output. Exercise-induced increases in cardiac oxygen consumption are higher after alcohol. On the other hand, a maximum of one to two drinks per day over long periods may decrease the risk of cardiovascular death, perhaps through an increase in high-density lipoprotein (HDL) cholesterol or changes in clotting mechanisms.

Although ethanol in low doses causes a mild acute drop in blood pressure, the consumption of three or more drinks per day results in a dose-dependent increase in blood pressure which returns to normal within weeks of abstinence. As a result, heavy drinking is an important contributor to reversible causes of mild to moderate hypertension. Chronic heavy drinking can cause cardiomyopathy with symptoms ranging from unexplained arrhythmias in the presence of left ventricular impairment to heart failure with dilatation of all four heart chambers and hypocontractility of heart muscle. Mural thrombi can form in the left atrium or ventricle, while heart enlargement exceeding 25 percent can cause mitral regurgitation. Finally, there is an association between cerebrovascular accidents and alcoholism, especially within 24 h of heavy drinking. Atrial or ventricular arrhythmias, especially paroxysmal tachycardia, also can occur after a binge in individuals showing no other evidence of heart disease—a syndrome known as the "holiday heart."

GENITOURINARY SYSTEM CHANGES, SEXUAL FUNCTIONING, AND FETAL DEVELOPMENT Acutely, modest ethanol doses (e.g., blood alcohol concentrations of 100 mg/dL or even less) increase sexual drive in men. However, modest ethanol doses may simultaneously decrease erectile capacity. Even in the absence of liver impairment, a significant minority of chronic alcoholic men may show irreversible testicular atrophy with concomitant shrinkage of the seminiferous tubules and loss of sperm cells (see Chap. 339).

The repeated ingestion of high doses of ethanol by women can result in amenorrhea, a decrease in ovarian size, an absence of corpora lutea with associated infertility, and spontaneous abortions. Heavy drinking during pregnancy results in the rapid placental transfer of both ethanol and acetaldehyde, which may have serious consequences for fetal development. The *fetal alcohol syndrome* can include a mixture of any of the following: facial changes with epicanthal eye folds, poorly formed concha, and small teeth with faulty enamel; cardiac atrial or ventricular septal defects; an aberrant palmar crease and limitation in joint movement; and microcephaly with mental retardation (see Chap. 378). The specific amount of ethanol and/or specific time of vulnerability during pregnancy have not been defined, making it advisable for pregnant women to abstain completely.

OTHER EFFECTS OF ETHANOL Heavy drinking can produce an acute *alcoholic myopathy* characterized by painful and swollen muscles, high levels of serum creatine phosphokinase (CK), and, rarely, myoglobinemia and myoglobinuria. Effects on the *skeletal system* include alterations in calcium metabolism with an increased risk for fractures and osteonecrosis of the femoral head. *Hormonal* changes include an increase in cortisol levels, which can remain elevated during heavy drinking; inhibition of vasopressin secretion at rising blood alcohol concentrations and the opposite at falling blood alcohol concentrations, with the final result that most alcoholics are likely to be slightly overhydrated; a modest and reversible decrease in serum thyroxine (T_4); and a more marked decrease in serum triiodothyronine (T_3).

ALCOHOLISM (ALCOHOL DEPENDENCE)

Because many drinkers occasionally imbibe to excess, temporary alcohol-related pathology is common in nonalcoholics. The time of heaviest drinking is usually the late teens to the late twenties, when between one-third and one-half of male drinkers experience some isolated (although potentially dangerous) alcohol-related social, occupational, or driving difficulty. These include alcohol-related blackouts, a single drunk driving arrest, arguments with friends, and so on. This prevalent alcohol-related morbidity, however, is temporary and a separate problem from alcohol dependence. The following sections describe diagnostic criteria for alcoholism, offer suggestions for identifying the usual (i.e., middle-class) alcoholic in everyday medical practice, review evidence that alcoholism is a biologic and genetically influenced disorder, and offer advice on confrontation, detoxification, and rehabilitation of alcoholics.

DEFINITIONS AND EPIDEMIOLOGY The most recent revised version of the *Third Diagnostic and Statistical Manual* of the American Psychiatric Association (DSM-IIIR) divides alcoholism into alcohol abuse and alcohol dependence. *Alcohol abuse* indicates alcohol-related life impairment interfering with functioning. *Alcohol dependence* encompasses similar impairment *along with* evidence of a strong compulsion to use alcohol accompanied by increased ethanol tolerance or physical signs on withdrawal from alcohol. The dependence criteria require that three of nine items be met and describe what many clinicians would label alcoholism.

A modified approach to a definition of alcoholism is easier to apply in clinical settings. The diagnosis of *alcoholism* is made when an individual ignores the early warning signs that alcohol is causing problems in marriage and goes on to an alcohol-related marital separation or divorce; *or* when alcohol-related problems on the job actually result in the patient being fired or laid off; *or* when there are two or more arrests related to alcohol; *or* when there is physical evidence that alcohol has harmed health (e.g., cardiomyopathy, cirrhosis, alcoholic hepatitis), including signs of alcoholic withdrawal.

It is important to distinguish between *primary* and *secondary alcoholism.* For example, serious alcohol-related problems occurring during the course of mania or a preexisting antisocial personality disorder (i.e., secondary alcoholism) might be symptomatic of the primary diagnosis, and the course is likely to be that of the primary disorder, not alcoholism. The information on alcoholism offered in this chapter is relevant for *primary alcoholism.* This diagnosis applies to the majority of alcoholics (70 to 80 percent) who develop major life problems from alcohol *before* they fulfill criteria for any other major psychiatric illness.

Using this or similar criteria, the lifetime risk for primary alcoholism in most western countries is about 10 percent for men and 3 to 5 percent for women. When less stringent criteria are used, the rates are substantially higher, but the clinical syndrome is not likely to accurately predict future problems. Alcoholism is seen in all races, ethnic groups, and socioeconomic strata, and therefore, the average alcoholic (just as the average person) is a blue-collar or white-collar worker or housewife. The homeless or skid row alcoholic represents only 5 percent or less of alcoholics.

GENETICS OF ALCOHOLISM There is strong evidence that alcoholism is a multifactorial disorder in which biologic and genetic factors interact. The importance of genetic factors in alcoholism is supported by family, twin, and adoption studies. Close relatives of primary alcoholics have an approximately fourfold increased risk for the disorder but are not significantly more vulnerable for other psychiatric illnesses. The probability that the familial nature of the problem is in part a consequence of genetic factors is supported by twin research, where the risk for the identical twin of an alcoholic is much higher than for the fraternal twin of an alcohol abuser. Finally, adoption studies reveal that the fourfold increased risk for children of alcoholics is true even if they were adopted away at birth and raised without knowledge of the problems of their biologic parents.

The evidence supporting genetic influences in alcoholism has stimulated numerous studies of children of alcoholics. The goal is to identify possible trait markers of a vulnerability toward the disorder before alcoholism appears. For example, some studies suggest that these children become significantly less intoxicated at a given blood alcohol concentration than do controls, even before alcoholism develops. After modest alcohol doses, the sons of alcoholics report less intense subjective feelings of intoxication, show less alcohol-related impairment in cognitive and psychomotor tests, and have less intense changes in prolactin and cortisol secretion than do controls. These data may indicate that men at high future risk for alcoholism may be less able than controls to tell when they are beginning to become intoxicated. Taken as a whole, these data underscore the probability that alcoholism is biologically influenced and not related to a lack of "moral fiber." It is not surprising that the average alcoholic may continue to work, has a family, and may be difficult to identify if the physician persists with old stereotypes.

NATURAL HISTORY For the "average" alcoholic, the age of first drink and first minor problems (e.g., an argument with a friend while drunk or an alcoholic blackout) are similar to those in the general population. However, by the middle to late twenties, most men and women moderate their drinking (perhaps learning from minor problems), whereas difficulties for alcoholics are likely to escalate,

with the first major life problem from alcohol appearing in the late twenties to early forties. Once established, the course of alcoholism is likely to be one of exacerbations and remissions; the alcoholic becomes frightened when a problem develops and abstains for a period of days to months before experimenting with controlled drinking; this step almost inevitably results in escalation of drinking and problems. The course is not hopeless because a fifth or more achieve permanent abstinence without formal treatment or aid from self-help groups such as Alcoholics Anonymous (AA). However, should the alcoholic continue to drink, the life span is shortened by an average of 15 years, with the leading causes of death, in decreasing order, being heart disease, cancer, accidents, and suicide.

IDENTIFICATION AND CONFRONTATION OF THE ALCOHOLIC
The physician should recognize that any patient may have alcoholism and must therefore pay attention to physical findings and laboratory tests that are likely to be abnormal in the alcoholic. These include a high normal or slightly elevated MCV, γ-glutamyl transferase (GGT) (35 or more units), serum uric acid [greater than 416 μmol/L (7 mg/dL)], and triglycerides [2.0 mmol/L (180 mg/dL) or more]. Mild and fluctuating levels of hypertension (e.g., 140/95), repeated infections such as pneumonia, and otherwise unexplained cardiac arrhythmias all suggest that the patient might be an alcoholic. Certain specific clinical findings also should raise suspicions, including cancer of the head and neck, esophagus, or cardia of the stomach as well as cirrhosis, unexplained hepatitis, pancreatitis, bilateral parotid gland swelling, and peripheral neuropathy.

Once the likelihood of alcoholism is established, only a few moments are needed to gather the history of alcohol-related life problems. The patient *and spouse* should be asked about patterns of accidents, marital difficulties, problems on the job, and driving-related difficulties, after which the role played by alcohol should be identified. All physicians should be able to take the time needed to gather such information. In addition, a simple 25-item form to be answered by the patient, the Michigan Alcohol Screening Test (MAST), is available to aid in identifying the alcoholic. However, this is only a screening tool, and a careful face-to-face interview is still required for a meaningful diagnosis.

After an alcoholic is identified, he or she should be confronted with the diagnosis. The presenting complaint can be used as an entrée to the alcohol problem. For instance, the patient complaining of insomnia or hypertension could be told that these are clinically important symptoms and that laboratory tests and physical findings indicate that alcohol appears to have contributed to the complaints and is increasing the risk for further medical and psychological problems. The physician should share information about the course of alcoholism and explore possible avenues of attacking the problem.

The process of confrontation is rarely accomplished in one session. It is helpful to let patients know that they are responsible for their own actions and that the decision to quit drinking rests with them. For the person who refuses to stop drinking at the first confrontation, a logical step is to "keep the door open," establishing future meetings so that help is available as problems escalate. In the meantime the family may benefit from counseling or referral to self-help group such as Alanon (the Alcoholics Anonymous group for family members) and Alateen (for teenage children of alcoholics).

Those patients who refuse to stop but who want to "cut down" should be reminded that the average alcoholic successfully cuts back scores of times but that sooner or later drinking again escalates. The patient who refuses to stop might be offered a guideline of drinking no more than two drinks [115 mL (4 oz) of wine, 340 mL (12 oz) of beer, or 43 mL (1.5 oz) of 80-proof beverage amounts to one drink] in any 24-h period, but it is very unlikely that this will be effective for an extended period of time. This is another way of keeping the door open in the hope that the patient will return as drinking escalates.

TREATMENT OF THE ALCOHOL-RELATED WITHDRAWAL SYNDROME The clinical syndrome In the presence of ethanol-induced cellular tolerance, any sudden decrease in ethanol may lead to symptoms of withdrawal from the CNS depressant effects. As with most syndromes, most patients do not develop every symptom, and the usual clinical picture is mild. Features include a tremor of the hands (shakes or jitters); autonomic nervous system dysfunction such as increases in pulse, respiratory rate, and body temperature; insomnia, possibly accompanied by bad dreams; feelings of generalized anxiety or panic attacks; and gastrointestinal upset. Symptoms begin within 5 to 10 h of decreasing ethanol intake (addicted patients are likely to awaken in the morning with some signs of withdrawal), peak in intensity on day 2 or 3, and improve by day 4 or 5. Anxiety, insomnia, and mild levels of autonomic dysfunction may persist for 6 months or more as a protracted abstinence syndrome that may contribute to the tendency to return to drinking.

About 5 percent of alcoholics show evidence of severe withdrawal symptoms. These include a state of confusion sometimes accompanied by visual, tactile, or auditory hallucinations. These psychotic symptoms are likely to disappear as the mental state becomes clearer over a period of several days and are distinct from the chronic alcoholic auditory hallucinosis with a clear sensorium described earlier in this chapter. A small percentage of alcoholics also demonstrate one or two generalized seizures ("rum fits"), usually within 48 h of stopping drinking. These are rarely focal in nature (unless there is underlying neuropathology), and electroencephalographic abnormalities are mild and usually return to normal within several days. There is no evidence that withdrawal seizures represent "latent" epilepsy.

The diagnosis of delirium tremens (DTs) is made when the course progresses beyond the usual symptoms of withdrawal to include confusion (with associated delusions and hallucinations), severe agitation, and generalized seizures. The likelihood of developing severe withdrawal symptoms increases with concomitant infections or medical problems, a prior history of withdrawal seizures or DTs, and higher quantity and frequency of drinking. Most periods of severe withdrawal begin and end abruptly, rarely lasting longer than 3 to 5 days. The mortality risk for DTs is quite low but increases with preexisting medical illnesses or organ system failure.

Treatment of withdrawal   The *first* and most important step is to perform a *thorough* physical examination in all alcoholics who are considering stopping drinking and in those patients who might be undergoing withdrawal. It is necessary to evaluate organ systems likely to be impaired by heavy drinking, including searching for evidence of liver failure, gastrointestinal bleeding, cardiac arrhythmia, and glucose or electrolyte imbalance.

The *second* step in treating withdrawal is to give patients adequate nutrition and rest. All patients should be administered multiple B vitamins, including 50 to 100 mg of thiamine daily for a week or more. Most patients enter withdrawal with normal levels of body water or mild levels of overhydration, and intravenous fluids should be avoided unless there is evidence of hypotension or a history of recent excessive bleeding, vomiting, or diarrhea. Usually medications can be administered orally.

The *third* step in treatment is to recognize the CNS symptoms caused by removal of the brain-depressant effects of ethanol. Symptoms can be alleviated by administering another CNS depressant and gradually decreasing the levels of the drug over a 3- to 5-day period. While many CNS depressants are effective, the *benzodiazepines* have the highest margin of safety and are, therefore, the preferred class of drugs in the treatment of alcohol withdrawal. Benzodiazepines with short half-lives (see Chap. 389) are especially useful for patients with serious liver impairment or evidence of preexisting encephalopathy or brain damage. On the other hand, short-half-life benzodiazepines, e.g., oxazepam or lorazepam, result in rapidly changing drug blood levels; administration every 4 h is required to avoid abrupt fluctuations in blood levels that may increase the risk for seizures. Therefore, most clinicians use drugs with longer half-lives, such as diazepam or chlordiazepoxide. The goal is to administer sufficient drug on day 1 to alleviate most of the symptoms of withdrawal and then to decrease the dose by 20 percent on successive days over a period of 3 to 5 days. The dose is increased if signs of withdrawal escalate, and the medication is withheld if the patient is sleeping or shows signs of increasing orthostatic hypotension. The average patient requires 25 to 50 mg of chlordiazepoxide or 10 mg of diazepam given orally every 4 to 6 h on the first day.

The most effective treatment of *severe withdrawal* including delirium tremens remains controversial. Most clinicians use benzodiazepines, but despite as much as 300 mg or more per day of chlordiazepoxide, the patient may still remain awake and agitated. Since it is probable that the confused, agitated state will persist for 3 to 5 days regardless of the pharmacologic intervention used, drugs are given to control behavior rather than to change the course of the syndrome. Antipsychotic medications such as thioridazine or haloperidol are sometimes used for these delirium tremens (DTs), although they must be prescribed with care because they might lower the seizure threshold. The antipsychotic drugs, however, have no place in the treatment of mild withdrawal symptoms.

The generalized seizures or "rum fits" rarely require aggressive pharmacologic intervention beyond that given to the usual patient undergoing withdrawal, i.e., adequate doses of benzodiazepines. There is little evidence that phenytoin is effective in drug-withdrawal seizures, and the risk of seizures usually has passed by the time effective drug levels are reached. The rare patient with status epilepticus can be treated initially with intravenous diazepam. If anticonvulsants are used for alcohol-withdrawal seizures, they should be stopped within 5 to 7 days unless a cause for a persisting seizure disorder is documented.

While alcohol withdrawal is often treated in a hospital, efforts at reducing costs have resulted in experimentation with outpatient detoxification for alcoholics with mild abstinence syndromes. This outpatient approach is appropriate for patients in good physical condition who demonstrate mild signs of withdrawal despite low blood alcohol concentrations and for those without prior history of DTs or withdrawal seizures. Such individuals still require careful physical examination, evaluation of blood tests, and treatment with vitamin supplementation, and appropriate doses of benzodiazepines also might be used. The latter are given *in a 1- to 2-day supply* to be administered to the patient by a spouse four times a day. Patients are asked to *return daily* for evaluation of vital signs, and the patient's family or friends are told to bring him or her to the emergency room if signs and symptoms of withdrawal escalate.

THE TREATMENT OR REHABILITATION OF ALCOHOLICS

After completing alcoholic rehabilitation, 60 percent or more of middle-class alcoholics maintain abstinence for at least a year, many for a lifetime. There is no single best way to rehabilitate the alcoholic, and therapeutic approaches center on general supports that meet commonsense guidelines. Considering the lack of evidence for superiority of any specific treatment type, it is best to keep interventions as simple, safe, and inexpensive as possible.

Maneuvers in rehabilitation fall into two general categories. *First* are attempts to help the alcoholic achieve and maintain a high level of motivation toward abstinence. These include educating the patient about alcoholism, and teaching the family and/or friends to stop protecting the alcoholic from the problems caused by alcohol. The *second* series of maneuvers helps the patient to readjust to life without alcohol and to reestablish a functional lifestyle through personal counseling, vocational rehabilitation, family support, and sexual counseling.

There is no convincing evidence that inpatient rehabilitation is always more effective for the average primary alcoholic than is outpatient care. The decision to hospitalize can be made if (1) the patient has medical problems that are difficult to treat outside a hospital, (2) depression, confusion, or psychosis interfere with outpatient care, (3) the patient has such a severe life crisis that it is difficult to get his or her attention as an outpatient, (4) outpatient treatment has failed, or (5) the patient lives too far from the treatment center. If inpatient care is needed, free-standing treatment programs, units that are divisions of general hospitals, and those in psychiatric hospitals are equally effective. The characteristics of the patient predict outcome more than any specific attribute of the program.

Whether the treatment begins in an inpatient or an outpatient setting, subsequent contact should be maintained for a minimum of 6 months and preferably a full year after abstinence is achieved. Counseling with an individual physician or through groups focuses on day-to-day living—emphasizing areas of improved functioning in the absence of alcohol (i.e., why it is a good idea to continue to abstain) and helping the patient to deal with free time without alcohol, develop a nondrinking peer group, and handle stresses on the job without alcohol.

The physician serves an important role in identifying the alcoholic, treating medical or psychiatric syndromes associated with alcoholism, carrying out detoxification, referring to rehabilitation programs, and counseling alcoholics in an inpatient or outpatient setting. The physician also must regulate drug treatment during alcoholism rehabilitation. Once acute detoxification is complete (an average of 3 to 5 days), there is *no place* for hypnotics or antianxiety drugs in the treatment of most alcoholics. The patient has already demonstrated an inability to moderate the use of one brain depressant, alcohol, and is at considerable risk for abusing sleeping pills or tranquilizers. Anxiety and insomnia can be treated with behavior modification such as relaxation training, meditation, and exercise or through increased activity in hobbies or religion. For example, regarding insomnia, patients should be reassured that this is normal after alcohol withdrawal and will improve over the subsequent weeks and months. They should then follow a rigid bedtime and awakening schedule, avoiding any naps or use of caffeine in the evenings. The sleep pattern will improve rapidly.

One medication that has been used in alcohol rehabilitation is disulfiram, usually given as 250 mg/d. This drug inhibits aldehyde dehydrogenase, causing very high levels of acetaldehyde to accumulate after alcohol is consumed. The disulfiram-ethanol reaction includes tremor, hypertension or hypotension, nausea and possibly severe vomiting, and diarrhea. Disulfiram must not be given to persons for whom such a reaction could be dangerous, including patients with portal hypertension, diabetes mellitus, heart disease, or a history of stroke. All drugs have their dangers, and the physician is advised to read carefully about disulfiram and be fully aware of the potential, although rare, serious adverse reactions that can occur. Unfortunately, there is little convincing evidence from carefully controlled studies that the effectiveness of disulfiram is significantly greater than placebo. As result, this drug should not be routinely prescribed.

Finally, an inexpensive, readily available, and dedicated additional support for all alcoholics is available in almost every community. Alcoholics Anonymous is a self-help group of recovering alcoholics (men and women who have stopped drinking, perhaps many years ago) that offers an effective model showing that abstinence can be achieved, provides a sober peer group, and makes crisis intervention available when the drive to drink escalates. No matter what type of rehabilitation program is planned, the alcoholic should be offered the option of joining Alcoholics Anonymous.

REFERENCES

BLUM K et al: Allelic association of human dopamine D_2 receptor gene in alcoholism. JAMA 263:2055, 1990

CRIQUI MH: Alcohol consumption, blood pressure, lipids, and cardiovascular mortality. Alc Clin Exp Res 10:564, 1986

DONAHUE RP et al: Alcohol and hemorrhagic stroke. JAMA 255:2311, 1986

FULLER RK et al: Disulfiram treatment of alcoholism. JAMA 256:1449, 1986

GOODWIN DW, GUZE SB: *Psychiatric Diagnosis*, 4th ed. New York, Oxford University Press, 1989

GRANT I: Alcohol and the brain. JCCP 55:310, 1987

GREENSPON AJ, SCHAAL SF: The "holiday heart": Electrophysiologic studies of alcohol effects in alcoholics. Ann Intern Med 98:135, 1983

HARPER C et al: Are we drinking our neurones away? Br Med J 294:534, 1987

IRWIN M et al: Monitoring heavy drinking. Am J Psychiatry 145:595, 1988

ISHAK KG et al: Alcoholic liver disease: Pathologic, pathogenetic and clinical aspects. Alc Clin Exp Res 15:45, 1991

JERNIGAN TL et al: Reduced cerebral gray matter observed in alcoholics using magnetic resonance imaging. Alc Clin Exp Res 15:418, 1991

LIEBER C: *Metabolic Aspects of Alcoholism*. Lancaster, England, MTP Press, 1987

———: To drink (moderately) or not to drink? N Engl J Med 310:846, 1984

LISKOW BI, GOODWIN DW: Pharmacological treatment of alcohol intoxication, withdrawal, and dependence. J Stud Alcohol 48:356, 1987

LITTEN RZ et al: Pharmacotherapies for alcoholism. Alc Clin Exp Res 15:620, 1991

MAHESWARAN R et al: High blood pressure due to alcohol: A rapidly reversible effect. Hypertension 17:787, 1991

MEAGHER RC et al: Suppression of hematopoietic-progenitor-cell proliferation by ethanol and acetaldehyde. N Engl J Med 307:845, 1982

MELLO NK, BREE MP: Alcohol self-administration disrupts reproductive function in female macaque monkeys. Science 221:677, 1983

MENDELSON JH, MELLO NK: Biologic concomitants of alcoholism. N Engl J Med 301:912, 1979

MUKHREJEE AB et al: Transketolase abnormality in fibroblasts from chronic alcoholics. J Clin Invest 79:1039, 1987

ÖJEHAGEN A et al: Long-term use of aversive drugs in outpatient alcoholism treatment. Acta Psychiatr Scand 84:185, 1991

PFEFFERBAUM A et al: Brain CT changes in alcoholics. Alc Clin Exp Res 12:81, 1988

POTTER JF, BEEVERS DG: Pressor effect of alcohol in hypertension. Lancet 1:119, 1984

RUSSELL M et al: Measures of maternal alcohol use as predictors of development in early childhood. Alc Clin Exp Res 15:991, 1991

SCHUCKIT MA et al: A simultaneous evaluation of multiple markers of ethanol response in sons of alcoholics. Arch Gen Psychiatry 45:211, 1988

———: Genetic and clinical implications of alcoholism and affective disorder. Am J Psychiatry 143:140, 1986

———: *Drug and Alcohol Abuse: A Clinical Guide to Diagnosis and Treatment*, 3d ed. New York, Plenum, 1989

SCHUCKIT MA: *Alcohol Patterns and Problems*. New Brunswick, NJ, Rutgers Press, 1985

———: Genetics and the risk for alcoholism. JAMA 254:2614, 1985

SELLERS EM, KALANT H: Alcohol intoxication and withdrawal. N Engl J Med 294:757, 1976

VAILLANT GE: *The Natural History of Alcoholism*. Cambridge, Mass., Harvard University Press, 1983

VAN THIEL DH: Gastrointestinal and hepatic manifestations of chronic alcoholism. Gastroenterology 81:594, 1981

VICTOR M, ADAMS RD: *The Wernicke-Korsakoff Syndrome*, 2d ed. Philadelphia, Davis, 1989

WALSH DC et al: Treatment options for alcohol abusing workers. N Engl J Med 325:775, 1991

WALSH JK et al: Sedative effects of ethanol at night. J Stud Alcohol 52:597, 1991

391 OPIOID DRUG USE

MARC A. SCHUCKIT / DAVID S. SEGAL

The principal effects of the opioids (opiate-like drugs) are a significant damping of pain perception along with modest levels of sedation and euphoria. Drugs in this category range from heroin, morphine, and codeine to many nonsteroidal prescription analgesics and many antitussive agents. Thus comments made in this section have wide application in medicine and go far beyond the classical street addict.

Tolerance to any one opioid is likely to generalize to the others (i.e., cross-tolerance is likely), and all share a similar pattern of drug-related problems. Each of these substances is capable of producing physical addiction (and thus they all have some legal restrictions), and the abstinence syndrome from any one of the substances can be treated with administration of any of the others.

PHARMACOLOGY The prototypic opiates, morphine and codeine (3-methoxymorphine), are taken directly from the milky juice of the poppy, *Papaver somniferum*. The semisynthetic drugs produced from the morphine or thebane molecules include hydromorphone, codeine, diacetylmorphine (heroin), and oxycodone. The purely synthetic opioids, sharing many of the basic properties of opium and morphine, include meperidine, propoxyphene, diphenoxylate, buprenorphine, methadone, and pentazocine. Despite claims to the contrary, all these substances (including almost all prescription analgesics) are capable of producing euphoria as well as psychological and physical dependence when taken in high enough doses over prolonged periods of time.

The opioids produce their effects by binding to different types of opioid receptors throughout the body, including the central nervous system. Endogenous opioid peptides (i.e., enkephalins, endorphins, dynorphin, and others) have been identified that appear to be natural ligands for opioid receptors. These peptides have a distinct distribution in the CNS. Recent evidence suggests that the receptors with which opioid peptides interact may be differentially engaged in production of the various opiate effects such as analgesia, respiratory depression, constipation, and euphoria. Substances capable of antagonizing one or more of these actions include nalorphine, levallophan, cyclazocine, buprenorphine, and pentazocine, each of which has mixed agonist and antagonist properties, as well as naloxone and naltrexone, which are pure opiate antagonists. Mixed agonist-antagonist drugs (e.g., pentazocine), if administered to a patient addicted to other narcotics, may precipitate opiate withdrawal symptoms. The availability of relatively specific antagonists has helped identify different receptor subtypes, including the μ_1 and μ_2 subtypes, which affect some of the more classical opioid actions such as pain control and respirations; *kappa* receptors, with similar functions along with sedation and effects on hormones; *sigma* receptors, which have an impact on mood, hallucinations and delusions; and *delta* receptors, thought to respond preferentially to endogenous opiates.

Opiate tolerance, dependence, and withdrawal are considered to be related phenomena and may share some common underlying mechanisms. A number of neurochemical systems and psychological processes appear to be implicated in these effects that emerge with chronic administration of morphine or related opiates. Perhaps reflecting the actions of different classes of receptors, tolerance to various opiate actions may develop at different rates, and these same mechanisms may contribute to the diverse signs and symptoms characteristic of withdrawal. Other biochemical systems that may contribute to the development of tolerance and dependence include changes in intracellular modulators such as adenyl nucleotides, calcium, and related substances, as well as alterations in neurotransmitters, including acetylcholine, serotonin, and the catecholamines norepinephrine and dopamine. Evidence also implicates environmental and learning factors. For example, clinical observations suggest that classic conditioning plays a role in maintaining dependence in at least some addicts and that conditioning extinction procedures may be useful when integrated into a comprehensive treatment program for opioid addiction. Further research into these phenomena and efforts to elucidate neurochemical mechanisms could significantly facilitate the development of more effective approaches to treatment and prevention.

All the opioid drugs are easily absorbed from the gastrointestinal system, the lungs, and/or the muscles. The most rapid and pronounced effects occur following intravenous administration, with only slightly less efficient absorption after smoking or after inhaling the vapor ("chasing the dragon"), and the least intense actions are seen after absorption from the digestive tract, at least in part because some of the oral drug is metabolized before it passes into the general circulation. Most of the metabolism of opiates occurs in the liver, primarily through conjugation with glucuronic acid, and only small amounts are excreted directly in the urine or feces. The plasma half-lives of these drugs range from 2.5 to 3 h for morphine to more than 22 h for methadone and even longer for methadyl acetate.

Street heroin typically contains only 5 to 10 percent of the opiate. The remainder consists of materials such as lactose and fruit sugars, quinine, powdered milk, phenacetin, caffeine, antipyrine, and strychnine which are used to "cut" the drug and increase the margin of profit. Any marked unexpected increase in the purity of street drugs is likely to cause unintentional lethal overdoses in addicts expecting less effect from a "hit."

THE ACUTE AND CHRONIC EFFECTS OF OPIOID DRUGS ON BODY SYSTEMS With the exception of overdose conditions and changes associated with physical addiction, most opiate actions are relatively benign and rapidly reversible.

Effects on body systems Acute changes in the *gastrointestinal system* are the result of decreased GI motility with resulting constipation and anorexia. Chronic GI problems in opiate addicts typically occur as a consequence of impaired liver function resulting from concomitant administration of other drugs and from the development of hepatitis B from shared "dirty" needles.

The direct effects on opiate receptors in the *central nervous system* can result in nausea and vomiting (medulla), decreased pain perception (spinal cord, thalamus, and periaqueductal gray region), euphoria (limbic system), and sedation (reticular activating system and striatum). The adulterants added to street drugs may contribute to some of the more permanent nervous system damage, including peripheral neuropathy, amblyopia, myelopathy, and leukoencephalopathy, while use of contaminated needles can produce abscesses in the CNS and transmit AIDS. The latter has become a major health problem contributing significantly to the spread of this lethal disease among addicts and their sexual partners. Whether from the opiate, adulterants, or the consequences of dirty needles, at least one recent study revealed CNS defects in both cognition and CT evaluations of addicts. Acute opiate administration results in decreases in luteinizing hormone (LH), with a subsequent decrease in testosterone, which might contribute to the decreased sex drive reported by most opiate addicts. Other hormonal changes include a decrease in the release of thyrotropin as well as increases in prolactin and possibly in growth hormone (see Chap. 331).

Acute changes in the *respiratory system* include respiratory depression, which results from a decreased response of the brainstem to carbon dioxide tension, a component of the drug overdose syndrome described below. At even low drug doses, this effect can be clinically significant in individuals with compromised lung activity. *Cardiovascular* changes tend to be relatively mild, with no direct opiate effect on heart rhythm or myocardial contractility, but there is a potential problem from orthostatic hypotension, probably secondary to dilatation of peripheral vessels. Bacterial infections of both the lungs and heart valves can occur from contaminated needles, with the latter capable of producing emboli and a subsequent enhanced risk for stroke.

The toxic reaction or overdose syndrome High doses of opiates taken intentionally (in a suicide attempt) or by the street user who has misjudged the potency of the injected substance can result in a toxic reaction or overdose syndrome with a potentially lethal consequence. The typical syndrome, which occurs immediately with intravenous (IV) overdose, includes shallow respirations of two to four per minute, pupillary miosis (with mydriasis once brain anoxia develops), bradycardia, a decrease in body temperature, and a general absence of responsiveness to external stimulation. If this medical emergency is not treated rapidly, symptoms can progress to cyanosis, and death can ensue from respiratory depression and cardiorespiratory arrest. Postmortem examination reveals few specific changes except for diffuse cerebral edema. An "allergic-like" reaction, apparently at least in part related to adulterants, also can occur and is characterized by decreased alertness, a frothy pulmonary edema, and an elevation in the blood eosinophil count.

The first step in treating any overdose is to support the vital signs through a respirator and other emergency procedures. The preferred more definitive treatment for the typical opiate overdose is the narcotic antagonist naloxone given in an initial dose of 0.4 mg (1 mL) or 0.01 mg/kg intramuscularly (IM) or IV, which can be repeated in 3 to 10 min if no response occurs. Because the effects of this drug diminish within 2 to 3 h, it is important to monitor the individual for at least 24 h after a heroin overdose and 72 h after an overdose of longer-acting drugs such as methadone. Patients who are also physically addicted to an opioid are likely to experience a precipitous onset of an abstinence syndrome within 2 to 8 h after administration of the opioid antagonist, but aggressive treatment of this syndrome is not appropriate until all vital signs are relatively stable.

As with any drug overdose, treatment of either the typical or the "allergic" type of opiate toxic reaction often requires continued support of vital signs until the body detoxifies the substance. Patients may require a respirator (especially one using oxygen and positive-pressure breathing for the "allergic" type of overdose), IV fluids perhaps accompanied by pressor agents to support blood pressure, and gastric lavage to remove any remaining drug, with care taken to use a cuffed endotracheal tube to prevent aspiration if the patient is not alert. Cardiac arrhythmias and/or convulsions, especially likely to be seen with codeine, propoxyphene, or meperidine, also need to be treated.

THE OPIATE ABUSER   The medical abuser   Two groups of individuals are at high risk for abusing analgesics. First, evidence suggests that a majority of people with *chronic pain syndromes* (e.g., back, joint, and muscle disorders) may misuse their prescribed drugs at various times. If physical dependence is established, abstinence syndromes can then intensify the pain, promoting continued drug intake. A few precautions can help the physician to avoid contributing to physical dependence in chronic pain patients, particularly those who have demonstrated a history of misusing opioids: (1) the goal is to minimize the debilitating effects of pain with the understanding that discomfort may not be completely eliminated (see Chap. 11); (2) all possible efforts must be taken to reinforce the need for the patient to become actively involved in and committed to improvement; (3) analgesic medication should be only one component of treatment and limited to oral administration of the least potent analgesic required to take the "edge off" the pain (e.g., ibuprofen or, if needed, propoxyphene); all such drugs should be coordinated through one physician; (4) behavior modification techniques can include muscle relaxation and meditation, while carefully selected exercises can help increase function and decrease pain; and (5) nonmedicinal approaches including electrical transcutaneous neurostimulation for muscle and joint disease can be applied (see also Chap. 11).

The second group at high risk are *physicians*, *nurses*, and *pharmacists*, primarily because of their easy access to substances of abuse. Physicians may begin to use opiates to help them sleep or to reduce stress or physical aches and pains. While all physicians are at risk, a family history of substance abuse (including alcoholism) probably helps to identify the physician at exceptionally high risk. Because of the growing awareness of these problems, impaired physician programs have been established in many hospitals and by most state medical societies. These groups attempt to identify and aid substance-impaired physicians, giving them peer support and education so as to achieve abstinence before problems escalate to the point of licensure revocation. In general, doctors are advised never to prescribe opiates for themselves or for members of their family—physicians deserve the same level of care and protection from future problems as their patients.

The street abuser   Some opiate addicts satisfy criteria for the antisocial personality disorder as evidenced by serious antisocial problems in most life areas beginning prior to age 15 and before the first major life problem from drugs (see Chap. 389). However, the majority of opiate addicts have a relatively high level of premorbid functioning. The usual street abuser begins using opiates occasionally, often after experimenting with tobacco, then alcohol, then marijuana, and then brain depressants or stimulants. Occasional opiate use, or "chipping," might continue for some time, and some individuals probably never escalate their intake to the point of developing serious problems. Another pattern of temporary or intermittent abuse is represented by the experiences of Vietnam soldiers, most of whom had little or no prior experience with opiates and who found themselves in a situation of high stress and readily available drugs. Under these circumstances, as many as one-half tried opiates and, although many became physically addicted, those who had not misused drugs before Vietnam tended to return to drug-free status when back in their home communities.

Of course, opiate-addicted individuals are likely to continue to have experience with many other drugs. At least two of these often remain as problems during the course of opiate addiction. First, alcohol intake is classically used to moderate withdrawal problems, to enhance the opiate high, and as a substitute when the preferred drug is not readily available, including during methadone and other

treatments. This pattern of problematic drinking, often meeting criteria for alcohol dependence, is seen in the course of perhaps 50 percent of opiate addicts. The second drug, cocaine, appears to be taken for many of the same reasons as alcohol and is often administered IV concomitantly with the opiate in a mixture known as a "speedball." Dependence on these as well as other drugs must be addressed during opiate detoxification and rehabilitation.

Once persistent opiate use is established, the outcome is often extremely serious. At least 25 percent of such opiate abusers are likely to die within 10 to 20 years of active abuse, with death from suicide, homicide, accidents, and infectious diseases such as tuberculosis, serum hepatitis, or AIDS. The mortality rate has escalated in recent years in response to the epidemic of AIDS among IV drug abusers, with an estimated 60 percent of these men and women carrying the HIV virus (see Chap. 279). As many as 50 percent of male and 25 percent of female addicts turn to alcohol when their primary drug is not available, and many of these people meet the criteria for secondary alcohol abuse. The prevalence of alcohol misuse is higher in drug treatment dropouts than in those who stay with therapy, and abuse is more likely in individuals with a history of alcohol problems before they developed opiate-related difficulties.

PHYSICAL ADDICTION AND THE OPIATE ABSTINENCE SYNDROME   The symptoms of withdrawal   The time to onset as well as the intensity and duration of the acute abstinence syndrome are influenced by a number of factors, including the drug's half-life, its dose, and the chronicity of administration. The withdrawal symptoms tend to be opposite to the acute effects of the drug and include nausea and diarrhea, coughing, lacrimation, rhinorrhea, profuse sweating, twitching muscles, and piloerection, or "goose bumps"; mild elevations in body temperature, respiratory rate, and blood pressure are also observed. In addition, sensations of diffuse body pain, insomnia, and yawning occur with intense drug craving. Drugs with a short half-life, such as morphine or heroin, cause symptoms typically within 8 to 16 h of the last dose (thus many addicts awake in mild withdrawal every morning); peak symptom intensity is apparent within 36 to 72 h after discontinuation of the drug, and the acute syndrome disappears within 5 to 8 days. However, a protracted abstinence phase of mild symptoms (e.g., slight changes in pupillary size, autonomic dysfunction, changes in sleep pattern) may persist for 6 or more months. These lingering symptoms, which can be relieved by administering an opiate, probably contribute to relapse.

Treatment of the withdrawal syndrome   Patients *must* receive a thorough physical examination, which includes an assessment of liver and neurologic function as well as identification of local and systemic infections, especially abscesses. Proper nutrition and rest must be initiated as soon as possible.

Effective treatment of withdrawal, however, also requires readministration of sufficient opiate medication on day 1 to decrease symptoms, followed by a more gradual withdrawal of the drug, usually over 5 to 10 days. Any opiate will work (they all have some level of cross-tolerance), but for ease of administration, many physicians prefer to use a long-acting drug such as methadone. In estimating the first day's dose from the patient's history, 1 mg of methadone is approximately equivalent to 3 mg of morphine, 1 mg of heroin, or 20 mg of meperidine. Most patients require between 10 and 25 mg of methadone orally given twice on day 1, with higher doses given if prominent symptoms of withdrawal are not damped. After several days of a stabilized drug dose, the opiate is then decreased by 10 to 20 percent of the original day's dose each day.

Most states have restrictions on the prescription of opiates to addicts, and in the absence of special permits, detoxification with opiates is often proscribed or limited to 1 month or less. Thus pharmacologic treatments are often limited to symptomatic medication of diarrhea with kaopectate or a similar nonopiate, "sniffles" with decongestants, and pain with nonopiate analgesics (e.g., ibuprofen). Another relatively successful nonopiate approach to the treatment of withdrawal is the use of the alpha$_2$-adrenergic agonist clonidine, used in part to decrease sympathetic nervous system overactivity. Given at doses of approximately 5 μg/kg (up to 0.3 mg given two to four times a day), clonidine causes most patients undergoing opiate withdrawal to experience a decrease in autonomic nervous system dysfunction. Opiates, however, are more effective in relieving discomfort and pain, and clonidine is often not well tolerated because it produces high levels of sedation and orthostatic hypotension. Therefore, under most circumstances opiates are the treatment of choice.

A special case of opiate withdrawal is seen in the newborn passively addicted by the mother's drug misuse during pregnancy. Some level of addiction develops in 50 to 90 percent of children of heroin-dependent mothers, and the withdrawal syndrome carries a mortality of between 3 and 30 percent if not treated when prominent signs are apparent. In distinction to street addicts, as few as 25 percent of infants of methadone maintenance–addicted mothers show clinically relevant withdrawal symptoms. The syndrome consists of irritability, crying, a tremor (in 80 percent), increased reflexes, increased respiratory rate, diarrhea, hyperactivity (in 60 percent), vomiting (40 percent), and sneezing/yawning/hiccuping (in 30 percent). The child usually has a low birth weight but may be otherwise unremarkable until the second day, when symptoms are likely to begin.

The treatment follows the same general steps used in the treatment of the physically addicted adult. The child must be carefully evaluated to rule out medical problems such as hypoglycemia, hypocalcemia, infections, and trauma; general supports in a warm, quiet environment and regulation of electrolytes and glucose are also required. The infant with moderate to severe symptoms can be treated with any of the following: paregoric (0.2 mL orally every 3 to 4 h), methadone (0.1 to 0.5 mg/k per day), phenobarbital (8 mg/kg per day), or diazepam (1 to 2 mg/kg every 8 h). Medication should be given in decreasing levels for 10 to 20 days. It is also possible to help treat the addicted infants of mothers on methadone maintenance by having them breast feed while the mothers continue to take methadone.

REHABILITATION OF OPIATE ADDICTS   Despite some differences in demographics, the same general rules for rehabilitation apply to the opiate abuser and to the alcoholic. The basic strategy includes beginning detoxification and general family support. It is also important to establish realistic patient goals and a program of counseling and education to increase motivation toward abstinence. A long-term commitment to rebuilding a lifestyle without the substance is essential for preventing recidivism.

Identifying and confronting the patient   The first step in treatment requires identification of the opiate abuser—an especially difficult problem with the middle-class street abuser and the medical patient or physician with an iatrogenic addiction. An important step is to take the time with *every* patient, especially those with complaints of pain, to gather a clinical history that includes the patterns of opiate usage and the list of doctors and clinics from which they have received prescriptions. If the chronic use of opiates is suspected, gathering additional data from a resource person such as a spouse can be essential. Another indicator of an enhanced risk for opiate dependence is the history of pervasive antisocial problems beginning in the preteen years. Blood and urine screens can be used to identify opiates in patients in whom misuse is suspected, and clinicians should search for physical stigmata of misuse (e.g., needle marks). One potentially important diagnostic procedure (which should be used carefully because it can precipitate an intense withdrawal) is the opiate antagonist challenge. A 0.4-mg dose of naloxone is given subcutaneously or slowly IV over a 5-min period, and the patient is observed for signs of withdrawal over the next several hours. This challenge test should only be carried out in the presence of a physician, and it is important to be prepared to begin treating withdrawal if needed.

After identifying the opiate addict, the next step is confrontation. The need for active treatment of the abstinence syndrome can be presented, and the availability of help in establishing a drug-free lifestyle can be emphasized. The final decision, of course, rests with the

patient. Much of this approach of confrontation is presented in the chapter on alcoholism (see Chap. 390).

Rehabilitation   Most rehabilitation approaches have common elements. Patients are educated about their responsibility for improving their lives, and *motivation for abstinence* is increased by providing information about the medical and psychological problems that can be expected if addiction continues. Patients and families are helped to *establish an opiate-free lifestyle* by being educated about dealing with chronic pain and developing realistic vocational planning (e.g., this applies to pharmacists, physicians, and nurses). The addict also should be encouraged to establish a drug-free peer group and to participate in self-help groups such as Narcotics Anonymous. Much of this advice and counseling can be given by the physician, but many clinicians refer patients to more formal drug programs, including methadone maintenance clinics, programs using narcotic antagonists, and therapeutic communities. Long-term follow-up of treated patients shows that approximately one-third of addicts are completely drug free in the year before the follow-up interview and that a total of 60 percent are off opiates, although some may be abusing other substances. Individuals who stay in methadone maintenance or in therapeutic communities show significant decreases in police and social problems and increases in job functioning. In general, the best prognosis for rehabilitation is for those who are employed, who have higher levels of school completion, and who remain in treatment for at least 2 months. Addiction among health care deliverers, such as physicians, is treated with similar approaches. In addition, a closely supervised "diversion" procedure is usually instituted and carried out for 1 to 2 years or more.

METHADONE MAINTENANCE   Methadone and methadyl acetate maintenance should only be used along with education and counseling. It is important to note that drug maintenance is not aimed at "curing" opiate addiction; rather, it provides a substitute drug that is legally accessible, safer, can be taken orally, and has a long half-life so that it can be taken once a day. The goal is to help the addict who has repeatedly failed in drug-free programs to improve functioning within the family and job, to decrease legal problems, and to improve health.

Methadone is a long-acting opiate that possesses almost all the physiologic properties of heroin. The addict who has been carefully screened to rule out prior psychiatric disorders may be maintained on a relatively low dose (e.g., 30–40 mg/d); a better approach is to use a higher dosage schedule (100–120 mg/d), which may be more effective in blocking heroin-induced euphoria. Although the results are not definite, there is some evidence that the higher methadone doses may result in greater retention in treatment and consequently lower levels of arrest and readdiction to street drugs. Especially following the higher doses, three-quarters or more of addicts are likely to remain heroin-free for 6 months or longer. Methadone is administered in an oral liquid given once a day at the program center, with weekend portions taken by the patient at home. The longer-acting analogues, such as methadyl acetate, can be given in lower doses (e.g., 20–30 mg) two or three times a week, with levels increased to as high as 80 mg three times a week if needed. After a period of maintenance (usually 6 months to 1 year or longer), the clinician should work closely with the patient to regulate the rate of drug decrease (by about 5 percent per week).

In the past, the British have used heroin maintenance with similar goals and following similar guidelines as those used for methadone. There is no evidence that heroin maintenance has any advantages over methadone maintenance, but the heroin approach does add the risk that the drug will be sold on the streets. These factors have contributed to the virtual abandonment of the heroin maintenance approach. Treatment with mixed agonists-antagonists such as buprenorphine has been proposed, especially to help the individual who is also using cocaine. However, at present these must be considered experimental.

OPIATE ANTAGONISTS   The opiate antagonists (e.g., naloxone) compete with heroin and other opiates for opioid receptors, reducing the effects of the opiate agonists. Administered over long periods of time in order to block the "high" produced if the patient takes opiates, these drugs can be useful as part of an overall treatment approach that includes counseling and support. Cyclazocine was the first antagonist tested, but its blockade of receptors is incomplete, and the level of side effects (including an intoxicated feeling) is unacceptable. Naloxone is an excellent narcotic antagonist with no agonistic properties, but it has such a short period of action (2–3 h) that it is of little use in rehabilitation. The most widely used antagonist in rehabilitation is naltrexone, which is effective for about 24 h with few side effects. A dose of 50 mg of naltrexone per day will block 15 mg of heroin for 24 h, and higher doses (125–150 mg) are capable of blocking the effects of 25 mg of IV heroin for up to 3 days. Naltrexone is free of agonist properties, there are no known withdrawal symptoms when the medication is stopped, and side effects tend to be mild. Patients started on this antagonist should be free of opiates for a minimum of 5 days to avoid precipitating a withdrawal syndrome. In addition, they must be given a thorough physical examination and should be challenged with 0.4 or 0.8 mg of the shorter-acting naloxone to be certain that they are able to tolerate the long-acting antagonist. Following this procedure, a test dose of 10 mg of naltrexone can be given, with the expectation that any withdrawal symptoms will be seen in $\frac{1}{2}$ to 2 h. Several variations of this approach can be used with methadone maintenance, including a fairly rapid, medically supervised scheme. Over the next 10 days, the daily dose should be increased to about 100 mg on Mondays and Wednesdays and 150 mg on Fridays. Unfortunately, despite the apparent advantages of this treatment approach, patients demonstrate great resistance to continuing care. In one study, only about 60 percent of the patients completed 6 days of naltrexone induction, and only 10 percent remained in the program at the end of 6 months.

DRUG-FREE PROGRAMS   Most existing half-way houses and recovery centers for the opiate abuser utilize the therapeutic community approach. This is an exception to the general preference for short-term inpatient rehabilitation, since care lasts up to a year while the addict is taken out of the street culture and given a new life within the group. In this structure members, including addict leaders, frequently confront participants in an attempt to help them gain insights into more successful lifestyles for coping with problems.

As is true for treatments of all substance use disorders, it is likely that counseling, behavioral treatments, and relatively simple approaches at psychotherapy add significantly to a positive outcome. Most approaches focus on better handling of stress and enhanced understanding of personality attributes, improving cognitive styles, and addressing problems with interpersonal skills that might have contributed to either the initiation or progression of the substance-abuse problem. It appears as if the combination of these therapies with the approaches described above generates the best results.

Finally, a number of other nonpharmacologic approaches are being evaluated. These include some potentially promising results with acupuncture and transcranial electrostimulation. Efforts to help minimize consequences of opiate dependence, including syringe exchange schemes, are also of great potential importance but are beyond the scope of this chapter.

REFERENCES

BALL J, ROSS A: *The Effectiveness of Methadone Maintenance Treatments*. New York, Springer-Verlag, 1991

FINNEGAN L: Neonatal abstinence syndrome, in *Neonatal Therapy*, F Rubatelli (ed). New York, Elsevier, 1986

FRIEDLAND GH et al: Transmission of the human immunodeficiency virus. N Engl J Med 317:1125, 1987

JAFFE JH, MARTIN WR: Opiate analgesics and antagonists, in *Goodman and Gilman's The Pharmacological Basis of Therapeutics*, 7th ed, AG Gilman et al (eds). New York, Macmillan, 1985

JASINSKI D et al: Clonidine in morphine withdrawal. Arch Gen Psychiatry 42:1063, 1985

KAKU DA, LOWENSTEIN DH: Emergence of recreational drug abuse as a major risk factor for stroke in young adults. Ann Intern Med 113:821, 1990

KERR B et al: Concentration-related effects of morphine on cognition and motor control in human subjects. Neuropsychopharmacology 5:157, 1991

KLEBER HK, RIORDAN CE: The treatment of narcotic withdrawal: A historical review. J Clin Psychiatry 43:30, 1982

KOOB GF: Neural mechanisms of drug reinforcement. Ann NY Acad Sci 654:171, 1992

LEHMAN WEK et al: Alcohol use by heroin addicts 12 years after drug abuse treatment. J Stud Alcohol 51:233, 1990

LOIMER N et al: Similar efficacy of abrupt and gradual opiate detoxification. Am J Drug Alcohol Abuse 17:307, 1991

LONDON ED et al: Morphine-induced metabolic changes in human brain. Arch Gen Psychiatry 47:73, 1990

MCAULIFFE WE et al: Psychoactive drug use among physicians and medical students. N Engl J Med 315:805, 1986

MCKNIGHT AT, REES DC: Opioid receptors and their ligands. Neurotransmissions 7:1, 1991

O'BRIEN CP, WOODY GE: Long-term consequences of opiate dependence. N Engl J Med 304:1098, 1981

OLIVERIO A et al: Psychobiology of opioids. Int Rev Neurobiol 25:277, 1984

PASTERNAK GW: Multiple morphine and enkephalin receptors and the relief of pain. JAMA 259:1362, 1988

PHILIP P et al: Efficiency of transcranial electrostimulation on anxiety and insomnia symptoms during a washout period in depressed patients: A double-blind study. Biol Psychiatry 29:451, 1991

SAN L et al: Assessment and management of opioid withdrawal symptoms in buprenorphine-dependent subjects. Br J Addict 87:55, 1992

————: Follow-up after a six-month maintenance period on naltrexone versus placebo in heroin addicts. Br J Addiction 86:983, 1991

SCHUCKIT MA: *Drug and Alcohol Abuse: A Clinical Guide to Diagnosis and Treatment*, 3d ed. New York, Plenum, 1989

SIMPSON DD et al: Six-year follow-up of opioid addicts after admission to treatment. Arch Gen Psychiatry 39:1318, 1982

STIMSON GV et al: The pilot syringe-exchange project in England and Scotland: A summary of the evaluation. Br J Addiction 84:1283, 1989

STRANG J, GURLING H: Computerized tomography and neuropsychological assessment in long-term high-dose heroin addicts. Br J Addiction 84:1011, 1989

VAILLANT GE: A 20-year follow-up of New York narcotic addicts. Arch Gen Psychiatry 29:237, 1973

WALLOT H, LAMBERT J: Characteristics of physician addicts. Am J Drug Alcohol Abuse 10:53, 1984

392   COCAINE AND OTHER COMMONLY ABUSED DRUGS

JACK H. MENDELSON / NANCY K. MELLO

Although there has been a decline in the occurrence of drug abuse–related problems, particularly among youth, the prevalence of drug abuse in the United States remained at epidemic levels during the early 1990s and is believed to exceed that of other industrial nations. The primary data resources for assessing the scope and extent of drug abuse in the United States are the High School Senior Survey, The National Household Survey, and the Drug Abuse Warning Network (DAWN) supported by the National Institute on Drug Abuse (NIDA). During 1991, the High School Senior Survey involved 15,483 senior students from public and private schools, plus 18,000 eighth and 16,000 tenth grade students. The High School Survey revealed that 1.4 percent of students used cocaine within 30 days of their interview and that 0.9 percent of all students had used cocaine at least once in their life. The National Household Survey on drug abuse involved 32,594 randomly selected respondents throughout the United States and also included persons who lived in college dormitories and in homeless shelters. This survey revealed that marijuana continues to be the most commonly used illicit drug in the United States. During 1991, 5.3 million Americans used the drug on a weekly basis, and 3.1 million persons used marijuana daily. Approximately 0.9 percent of Americans over the age of 12 reported use of cocaine within 30 days of the survey interview. The Drug Abuse Warning Network revealed that drug-related emergency room episodes increased from 89,325 incidents in the fourth quarter of 1990 to 100,381 during the second quarter of 1991. Cocaine-related emergency room episodes increased from 19,381 during the fourth quarter of 1990 to 25,370 in the second quarter of 1991.

Chronic drug abuse may be associated with a number of adverse health consequences ranging from pulmonary disease to reproductive dysfunctions. Preexisting disorders such as hypertension and cardiac disease may be exacerbated by drug abuse, and the combined use of two or more drugs may accentuate medical complications associated with abuse of a single drug. The adverse health consequences of drug abuse are further complicated by AIDS, and drug abuse also increases the risk for HIV exposure. Drug abuse contributes to the recent AIDS epidemic through HIV infection transmitted by needle-sharing by intravenous drug users and by direct immunosuppressive and immuno-modulatory effects of abused drugs. In 1992 persons who self-administer drugs intravenously represented the largest single group with HIV infection in several major metropolitan areas in the United States as well as urban areas in Scotland, Italy, Spain, Thailand, and China. Over 30 countries throughout Europe, North America, South America, Asia, Australia, and Africa have reported AIDS or HIV infection among intravenous drug abusers.

The initiation and continuation of drug abuse is determined by a complex interaction of the pharmacologic properties and relative availability of each drug, the personality and expectancy of the user, and the environmental context in which the drug is used. Polydrug abuse, the concurrent use of several drugs with different pharmacologic effects, is increasingly common among individuals from all socioeconomic strata. There has been an alarming increase in a particularly dangerous form of polydrug abuse, the combined use of both heroin and cocaine intravenously, called "speedballing." There is no simple explanation for this change in polydrug use patterns. Sometimes drug abusers attempt to attenuate one drug effect with another, e.g., heroin or alcohol is used to modulate the cocaine high. Sometimes one drug is used to enhance the effects of another, as with benzodiazepines and methadone, or cocaine plus heroin in methadone-maintained patients. Toxic drug interactions associated with polydrug abuse also contribute to the adverse health consequences of drug abuse. This chapter discusses cocaine, marijuana, two hallucinogens (PCP and LSD), and polydrug abuse. Alcohol abuse is discussed in Chap. 390 and opioid abuse in Chap. 391.

COCAINE   Cocaine is a stimulant and a local anesthetic with potent vasoconstrictor properties. The leaves of the coca plant (*Erythroxylon coca*) contain approximately 0.5 to 1 percent cocaine. The drug produces physiologic and behavioral effects when administered orally, intranasally, intravenously, or via inhalation following pyrolysis (smoking). It is now recognized that cocaine has potent pharmacologic effects on dopamine, norepinephrine, and serotonin neurons in the central nervous system. These effects include alteration and blockade of cellular membrane transport and prevention of the reuptake of biogenic amines. It has been postulated that cocaine-induced euphoria is due to cocaine-induced blockade of dopamine reuptake, but chronic cocaine use may cause dopamine depletion and destruction of dopaminergic pathways in the brain.

Prevalence of cocaine use   Cocaine has become more widely available throughout the United States since its cost (relative to disposable income) has decreased considerably. Cocaine is no longer considered a "status" drug since cocaine abuse occurs in virtually all social and economic strata of society. The prevalence of cocaine abuse in the general population has also been associated with an increase in cocaine abuse by heroin-dependent persons, including those in methadone maintenance programs. Intravenous cocaine is often used concurrently with intravenous heroin (the speedball)—a combination that purportedly attenuates the postcocaine "crash" and substitutes a cocaine "high" for the heroin "high" blocked by methadone. Intravenous use of cocaine plus heroin may further increase risk for HIV infection, both through needle sharing and through the combined immunosuppressive effects of both drugs.

Acute and chronic cocaine intoxication   Although cocaine is commonly self-administered by inhalation (snorting), there has been a dramatic increase in both intravenous administration and inhalation of pyrolyzed material via smoking. Following intranasal administration, changes in mood and feeling states are perceived within 3 to 5 min and peak effects occur at 10 to 20 min. Duration of cocaine effects rarely exceed 1 h following intranasal administration. Inhalation of pyrolyzed materials include smoking coca paste, a product produced by extracting cocaine preparations with flammable solvents, and cocaine free-base smoking. Coca paste is frequently contaminated with toxic solvents used in its preparation. Cocaine free-base, including the free-base prepared with sodium bicarbonate (crack), is becoming increasingly popular because of the relative high potency of the compounds and their rapid onset of action (8 to 10 s following smoking).

Cocaine produces a brief, dose-related stimulation and enhancement of mood and dose-related increases in cardiac rate and blood pressure. Body temperature usually increases following cocaine administration, and high doses of cocaine may induce lethal pyrexia or hypertension. Because cocaine inhibits reuptake of catecholamines at adrenergic nerve endings, the drug potentiates sympathetic nervous system activity. Cocaine has a short plasma half-life of approximately 1 h. In humans, cocaine is primarily metabolized by plasma esterases, and cocaine metabolites are excreted in urine. The very short duration of euphorigenic effects of cocaine observed in chronic abusers is probably due to both acute and chronic tolerance. Frequent self-administration of the drug (two to three times per hour) is often reported by chronic cocaine abusers. Alcohol is used to modulate both the cocaine "high" and the dysphoria associated with the abrupt disappearance of cocaine's effects. A metabolite of cocaine, ethylcocaine, has been detected in blood and urine of persons who concurrently abuse alcohol and cocaine. Ethylcocaine induces changes in cardiovascular function similar to those of cocaine alone, and the pathophysiologic consequences of alcohol abuse plus cocaine abuse may be additive when both are self-administered together.

The prevalent assumption that cocaine use is relatively safe is challenged by reports of death from respiratory depression, cardiac arrhythmias, and convulsions after cocaine snorting and intravenous administration. Disorders of cerebral blood flow and perfusion in cocaine dependent persons have been detected with SPECT studies. These brain perfusion abnormalities are very similar to those which have been observed in patients with early HIV dementia. Severe pulmonary disease may develop in individuals who smoke coca paste; this is attributed both to the direct effects of cocaine and to residual solvent contaminants in the smoked material. Hepatic necrosis has also been reported to occur in coca paste smokers. Although men and women who abuse cocaine may report that the drug enhances libidinal drive, chronic cocaine use causes significant loss of libido and adversely affects reproductive function. Impotence and gynecomastia have been observed in male cocaine abusers, and these abnormalities often persist for long periods following drug abstinence. Women who abuse cocaine have reported major derangements in menstrual cycle function including galactorrhea, amenorrhea, and infertility. Chronic cocaine abuse may cause persistent hyperprolactinemia as a consequence of cocaine-induced disorders of dopaminergic regulation of prolactin secretion by the pituitary. Cocaine abuse also may adversely affect pregnancy. Infants exposed to cocaine in utero have an increased risk for congenital malformations as well as perinatal cardiovascular and cerebrovascular disease.

Numerous clinical reports, dating from the late nineteenth century, strongly suggest that protracted cocaine abuse may cause paranoid ideation and visual and auditory hallucinations, a state which resembles alcoholic hallucinosis. Psychological dependence upon cocaine, as manifested by inability to abstain from frequent compulsive use, also has been reported. Although occurrence of withdrawal syndromes involving psychomotor agitation and autonomic hyperactivity remains controversial, severe depression ("crashing") following cocaine intoxication may be a concomitant of drug withdrawal.

Treatment of cocaine intoxication and abuse   Treatment of cocaine overdose is a medical emergency that involves resuscitation in an intensive care unit. Cocaine toxicity produces hypertension, tachycardia, tonic-clonic seizures, dyspnea, and ventricular arrhythmias. Intravenous diazepam in doses up to 0.5 mg/kg administered over an 8-h period has been shown to be effective for control of seizures. The systemic concomitants of a hypermetabolic state produced by cocaine toxicity with concurrent ventricular arrhythmias have been managed successfully by administration of 0.5 to 1.0 mg of propranolol intravenously. Since many instances of cocaine-related mortality have also been associated with concurrent use of other illicit drugs (particularly heroin), the physician must be prepared to institute effective emergency treatment for multiple drug toxicity.

Treatment of chronic cocaine abuse requires combined efforts by family physicians, psychiatrists, and psychosocial care providers. Early abstinence from cocaine use is often complicated by symptoms of depression and guilt, insomnia, and anorexia, which may be as severe as those observed in major affective disorders. Individual and group psychotherapy, family therapy, and peer group assistance programs are often useful for inducing prolonged remission from drug use. Preliminary reports suggest that tricyclic antidepressant medication (desipramine) may be of value in the treatment of cocaine abuse, even when affective disorder or depression is not present. In fact, depressive illness does not appear to be a frequent antecedent of cocaine abuse.

MARIJUANA AND CANNABIS COMPOUNDS *Cannabis sativa* contains over 400 compounds in addition to the psychoactive substance, delta-9-tetrahydrocannabinol (THC). Marijuana cigarettes are prepared from the leaves and flowering tops of the plant, and a typical marijuana cigarette contains 0.5 to 1 g of plant material. Although the usual THC concentration varies between 5 and 20 mg, concentrations as high as 100 mg per cigarette have been detected. Hashish is prepared from concentrated resin of *Cannabis sativa* and contains a THC concentration of between 8 to 12 percent by weight. "Hash oil," a lipid-soluble plant extract, may contain a THC concentration of 25 to 60 percent, and it may be added to marijuana or hashish to enhance their THC concentration. Smoking is the most common mode of marijuana or hashish self-administration. During pyrolysis, over 150 compounds in addition to the THC are released in the smoke. Although most of these compounds do not have psychoactive properties, they do have potential physiologic effects.

THC is quickly absorbed from the lungs into blood and is then rapidly sequestered in tissues. It is metabolized primarily in the liver where it is converted to 11-hydroxy-THC, a psychoactive compound, and more than 20 other metabolites. Most THC metabolites are excreted through the feces at a rate of clearance that is relatively slow in comparison to that of most other psychoactive drugs.

Prevalence of marijuana use The National Institute on Drug Abuse's 1991 National Household Survey on Drug Abuse revealed that over one-third of all men and women surveyed had used marijuana or hashish at least once in their lifetime, and that 5 percent of the survey population reported using the drug at least once during the month prior to the survey. One encouraging datum is a continued trend in the decrease of marijuana use by high-school students. The annual use of marijuana decreased to 24 percent between 1990 and 1991 and was half the rate of marijuana use reported during 1980.

Acute and chronic marijuana intoxication Acute intoxication from marijuana and cannabis compounds is related to both the dose of THC and the route of administration. THC is absorbed more rapidly from marijuana smoking than from orally ingested *Cannabis* compounds. Acute marijuana intoxication usually consists of a subjective perception of relaxation and mild euphoria resembling mild to moderate alcohol intoxication. This condition is usually accompanied by some impairment in thinking, concentration, and perceptual and psychomotor functions. Higher doses of *Cannabis* may produce behavioral effects analogous to severe alcohol intoxication. Although the effects of acute marijuana intoxication are relatively benign in normal users, the drug can precipitate severe emotional disorders in individuals who have antecedent psychotic or neurotic problems. As with other psychoactive compounds, both set (user's

expectation) and setting (environmental context) are important determinants of the type and severity of behavioral intoxication.

As is true of alcoholics, chronic marijuana abusers may lose interest in common socially desirable goals and devote progressively more time to drug acquisition and use. However, it should be emphasized that THC does not cause a specific and unique "amotivational syndrome." The range of symptoms sometimes attributed to marijuana use are difficult to distinguish from mild depression and the maturational dysfunctions often associated with protracted adolescence. Chronic use of marijuana has also been reported to increase the probability of exacerbation of psychotic symptoms in individuals with a past history of schizophrenia.

Physical effects of marijuana Conjunctival injection and tachycardia are the most frequent immediate physical concomitants of smoking marijuana. Tolerance for marijuana-induced tachycardia develops rapidly among regular users; angina may be precipitated by marijuana smoking in persons with a history of coronary insufficiency. Exercise-induced angina may be increased after marijuana use to a greater extent than after tobacco cigarette smoking. Patients with cardiac disease should be strongly advised not to smoke marijuana or use *Cannabis* compounds.

Significant decrements in pulmonary vital capacity have been found in regular daily marijuana smokers. Because marijuana smoking typically involves deep inhalation and prolonged retention of marijuana smoke, marijuana smokers may develop pulmonary disease such as chronic bronchial irritation. Impairment of single-breath carbon monoxide diffusion capacity (DL_{co}) is greater in persons who smoke both marijuana and tobacco than in tobacco smokers. Despite the well-documented association between tobacco smoking and lung cancer, at present there is no direct evidence that marijuana smoking induces lung cancer. However, it should be emphasized that heavy marijuana use among Americans may be too recent to permit detection of this problem.

Although marijuana has also been associated with adverse effects on a number of other systems, many of these studies await replication and confirmation. For example, the reported correlation between marijuana use and decreased testosterone levels in males has not been confirmed. Decreased sperm count and motility and abnormalities of morphology of spermatozoa following marijuana use have also been reported. Administration of high doses of marijuana to female rhesus monkeys has revealed significant marijuana-induced suppression of pituitary gonadotropins and gonadal steroids. Carefully conducted prospective studies demonstrated a significant correlation between impaired fetal growth and development and heavy marijuana use during pregnancy. Marijuana also has been implicated in derangements of the immune response system, in chromosomal abnormalities, and in inhibition of DNA, RNA, and protein synthesis, but these findings have not been confirmed or related to any specific physiologic effect in humans. One report of *Cannabis*-induced brain atrophy in young adults has not been confirmed in computed tomography studies of young men who had documented histories of heavy marijuana smoking.

Tolerance and physical dependence Habitual marijuana users rapidly develop tolerance to the psychoactive effects of marijuana and often smoke more frequently and try to secure more potent *Cannabis* compounds. Tolerance for physiologic effects of marijuana develops at different rates; e.g., tolerance for marijuana-induced tachycardia develops rapidly, but tolerance for marijuana-induced conjunctival injection develops more slowly. Tolerance to both behavioral and physiologic effects of marijuana decreases rapidly upon cessation of marijuana use.

Withdrawal signs and symptoms have been reported in chronic *Cannabis* users, with severity of symptoms related to dosage and duration of use. These include tremor, nystagmus, sweating, nausea, vomiting, diarrhea, irritability, anorexia, and sleep disturbances. Withdrawal signs and symptoms observed in chronic marijuana users are usually relatively mild in comparison to those observed in heavy opiate or alcohol users and rarely require medical or pharmacologic intervention. Somewhat more severe and protracted abstinence syndromes may occur after sustained use of high-potency *Cannabis* compounds for long periods.

LYSERGIC ACID DIETHYLAMIDE (LSD)   The serendipitous discovery of psychedelic effects of LSD in 1947 culminated in an epidemic of LSD abuse during the 1960s. Imposition of stringent legal and regulatory constraints on the manufacture and distribution of LSD (classified as a Schedule I substance by the FDA), as well as public recognition that psychedelic experiences induced by LSD were a health hazard, has resulted in a significant reduction in LSD abuse. During 1991, relatively few instances of LSD abuse were reported, but the drug still retains some popularity among adolescents and young adults. Almost 2 percent of high school students reported using LSD within 30 days of the 1991 High School Survey. There are recent indications that the prevalence of LSD use among young persons has been accelerating in some communities in the United States.

LSD is a very potent drug; oral doses as low as 20 µg may induce profound psychological and physiologic effects. Tachycardia, hypertension, pupillary dilation, tremor, and hyperpyrexia occur within minutes following LSD in oral doses of 0.5 to 2 µg/kg. A variety of bizarre and often conflicting perceptual and mood changes, including visual illusions, synesthesias, and extreme lability of mood, usually occur within one-half hour after LSD intake. The action of LSD may persist for 12 to 18 h even though the half-life of the drug is only 3 h.

Tolerance develops rapidly for LSD-induced changes in psychological function when the drug is used one or more times per day over a course of 4 days or more. Abrupt abstinence following continued use does not produce withdrawal signs or symptoms. To date there have been no clinical reports of death caused by the direct effects of LSD.

The most frequent acute medical emergency associated with LSD use is panic episodes, which may persist up to 24 h (the ''bad trip''). Management of this problem is best accomplished by supportive reassurance (''talking down'') and, if necessary, administration of small doses of anxiolytic drugs. Adverse consequences of chronic LSD use include enhanced risk for schizophreniform psychosis and derangements in memory function, problem solving, and abstract thinking. Treatment of these disorders is best carried out in specialized psychiatric facilities.

PHENCYCLIDINE (PCP)   Phencyclidine, a cyclohexylamine derivative, is widely used in veterinary medicine to briefly immobilize large animals and is sometimes described as a dissociative anesthetic. PCP is easily synthesized and its abusers are primarily young people and polydrug users. The true extent of PCP abuse is unknown, but recent national surveys indicate an increase in frequency of use.

Phencyclidine is taken orally, by smoking, or by intravenous injection. It is also used as an adulterant in illicit sales of THC, LSD, amphetamine, or cocaine. The most common street preparation, ''angel dust,'' is a white granular powder which contains 50 to 100 percent of the drug. Low doses (5 mg) produce agitation, excitement, impaired motor coordination, dysarthria, and analgesia. Users may have horizontal or vertical nystagmus, flushing, diaphoresis, and hyperacusis. Behavioral changes include distortions of body image, disorganization of thinking, and feelings of estrangement. Higher doses of PCP (5 to 10 mg) may produce hypersalivation, vomiting, myoclonus, fever, stupor, or coma. PCP doses of 10 mg or more cause convulsions, opisthotonus, and decerebrate posturing which may be followed by prolonged coma.

The diagnosis of PCP overdose is difficult because the patient's initial symptoms may suggest an acute schizophrenic reaction. Confirmation of PCP use is possible by determination of PCP levels in serum or urine. PCP analysis is currently available at most toxicologic centers. Large quantities of PCP remain in urine for 1 to 5 days following high-dosage PCP intake.

PCP overdose requires prompt life support measures including treatment of coma, convulsions, and respiratory depression in a hospital intensive care unit. There is no specific antidote or antagonist for PCP. PCP excretion from the body can be enhanced by acidification of urine and gastric lavage. Death from PCP overdose may occur as a consequence of some combination of pharyngeal hypersecretion, hyperthermia, respiratory depression, severe hypertension, seizures, hypertensive encephalopathy, and intracerebral hemorrhage.

Acute psychosis associated with PCP use should be considered a psychiatric emergency since patients may be at high risk for suicide or extreme violence toward others. Phenothiazines should not be used for treatment of acute PCP psychosis because these drugs potentiate PCP's anticholinergic effects. Haloperidol (5 mg intramuscularly) has been administered on an hourly basis to induce suppression of psychotic behavior. PCP, like LSD and mescaline, produces vasospasm of cerebral arteries at relatively low doses. Chronic PCP use has been shown to induce insomnia, anorexia, severe social and behavioral changes, and, in some cases, chronic schizophrenia.

POLYDRUG ABUSE   Although drug abusers often report a preference for a particular drug, such as alcohol or opiates, the concurrent use of other drugs is common. Multiple drug use often involves substances which may have different pharmacologic effects from the preferred drug. Concurrent use of such dissimilar compounds as stimulants and opiates or stimulants and alcohol is not unusual. The diversity of reported drug use combinations suggests that achieving some perceptible change in state, rather than any particular direction of change (stimulation or sedation), may be the primary reinforcer in polydrug use and abuse. There is also evidence that intoxication with alcohol or opiates is associated with increased tobacco smoking, but marijuana smoking does not increase during alcohol intoxication. At present, there is relatively little systematic information available about drug interactions. However, it is known that the combined use of cocaine, heroin, and alcohol increases the risk for toxic effects and adverse medical consequences over risks associated with use of a single drug.

A practical determinant of polydrug use patterns is the relative availability and cost of the drugs. There are many examples of situationally determined drug use patterns, including the fact that soldiers who became dependent on heroin in Vietnam seldom continued heroin use after separation from military service. However, a significant number of men who were heroin addicts in Vietnam abused alcohol and became alcohol-dependent when they returned to the United States. Alcohol abuse, with its attendant medical complications, is one of the most serious problems encountered in former heroin addicts participating in methadone maintenance programs.

The physician must recognize that perpetuation of polydrug abuse and drug dependence is not necessarily a symptom of an underlying emotional disorder. Neither alleviation of anxiety nor reduction of depression accounts for initiation and perpetuation of polydrug abuse. Severe depression and anxiety are as frequently the consequences of polydrug abuse as they are the antecedents. There is also evidence that some of the most adverse consequences of drug use may be reinforcing and contribute to the continuation of polydrug abuse.

Adequate treatment of polydrug abuse, as well as other forms of drug abuse, requires innovative and eclectic programs of intervention. The first step in successful treatment is detoxification, a process which may be difficult because the patient has abused several drugs with different pharmacologic actions (e.g., alcohol, opiates, and cocaine). Since patients may not recall or may deny simultaneous multiple drug use, diagnostic evaluation should always include urinalysis for qualitative detection of psychoactive substances and their metabolites. Treatment of polydrug abuse requires hospitalization or inpatient residential care during detoxification and the initial phase of drug abstinence. When possible, specialized facilities for the care and treatment of chemically dependent persons should be used. Outpatient detoxification of polydrug abuse patients is likely to be ineffective and may be dangerous.

As in the treatment of alcohol abuse, no single therapeutic modality has been shown to be uniquely effective in inducing remission.

Polydrug abuse is a chronic disorder with an unpredictable pattern of remission and recrudescence. Therapeutic management of chronic disorders such as cardiac or neoplastic disease should serve as a model for helping the person with polydrug abuse problems. Even temporary remissions with attendant physical, social, and psychological improvements are preferable to the continuation or progressive acceleration of polydrug abuse and its related adverse medical and interpersonal consequences. In polydrug abuse, as in most chronic disorders, definitive ''cures'' rarely occur. The concerned physician should continue to assist polydrug abuse patients throughout the cyclic oscillations of this complex behavior disorder, recognizing that resumption of drug use may be the rule rather than the exception.

REFERENCES

CHO AK et al: A pharmacokinetic study of phenylcyclohexyldiethylamine—An analog of phencyclidine. Drug Metab Dispos 21:125, 1993

CREGLER LL, MARK H: Medical complications of cocaine abuse. N Engl J Med 315:1495, 1986

DAS G: Cocaine abuse in North America—A milestone in history. J Clin Pharmacol 33:296, 1993

GAWIN FH: Cocaine addiction: Psychology and neurophysiology. Science 251:1580, 1991

——, ELLINWOOD EH JR: Cocaine and other stimulants. Actions, abuse, and treatment. N Engl J Med 318:1173, 1988

——, ——: Cocaine dependence. Ann Rev Med 40:149, 1989

HOLMAN BL et al: Brain perfusion is abnormal in cocaine-dependent polydrug users: A study using Technetium-99m-HMPAO and ASPECT. J Nucl Med 32:1206, 1991

JAFFE JH: Drug addiction and drug abuse, in Goodman and Gilman's The Pharmacological Basis of Therapeutics, 8th ed., AG Gilman et al (eds). New York, Pergamon, 1990, p 522

JOHANSON CE, FISCHMAN MW: The pharmacology of cocaine related to its abuse. Pharmacol Rev 41:3, 1989

JONES RT: The pharmacology of cocaine smoking in humans, in Research Findings on Smoking of Abused Substances, NIDA Research Monograph vol. 99, CN Chiang, RL Hawks (eds). Washington, DC, U.S. Government Printing Office, 1990, pp 30–41

KREEK MJ: Multiple drug abuse patterns and medical consequences, in Psychopharmacology: The Third Generation of Progress, HY Meltzer (ed). New York, Raven Press, 1987, pp 1597–1604

MENDELSON JH: Marijuana, in Psychopharmacology: The Third Generation of Progress, HY Meltzer (ed). New York, Raven Press, 1987, pp 1565–1571

——, MELLO NK (eds): Medical Diagnosis and Treatment of Alcoholism. New York, McGraw-Hill, 1992

—— et al: Human studies on the biological basis of reinforcement, in Addictive States, CP O'Brien, JH Jaffe (eds). New York, Raven Press, 1992, pp 131–155

OM A et al: Management of cocaine-induced cardiovascular complications. Am Heart J 125:469, 1993

WEISS RD, MIRIN SM: Cocaine. Washington, American Psychiatric Press, 1987

WOODS JH, WINGER G: Phencyclidine and related substances, in Drug Abuse and Drug Abuse Research: The Third Triennial Report to Congress from the Secretary, Department of Health and Human Services. Washington, DC: U.S. Government Printing Office, 1991, p 145

393 NICOTINE ADDICTION

JOHN H. HOLBROOK

Cigarette smoking is the principal cause of preventable disease, disability, and premature death in the United States. Nonetheless, each year more than one million American children and teenagers start smoking, and most established smokers have great difficulty in quitting. The addictive effects of nicotine account for most of this persistent personal and public health dilemma. Recognition of tobacco use as an addiction and of nicotine as the addictive drug is essential for effective patient management.

The primary criteria for defining drug addiction are: compulsive use, psychoactive effects, and drug-reinforced behavior. Nicotine use fulfills these criteria because it produces a compelling urge to smoke, provides pleasurable alterations in mood, and motivates chronic tobacco-seeking and tobacco-using behavior. Tolerance and physical dependence, manifested by an abstinence-mediated withdrawal syn-

drome, contribute to the strong control exerted by nicotine on smoking behavior.

Smokers regulate their nicotine dose to obtain desired effects; these include both intrinsic positive effects, such as pleasure and enhanced performance, and avoidance of the withdrawal syndrome. This syndrome is characterized by anger, anxiety, craving for tobacco products, difficulty concentrating, hunger, impatience, and restlessness. Most of these symptoms peak in 1 to 2 days and return to baseline within 3 to 4 weeks of quitting; however, craving for tobacco products and hunger may persist for extended periods.

The use of tobacco products is a complex, learned behavior that is woven into the fiber of daily living and is linked to how the smoker deals with the world. Numerous daily activities, thoughts, and emotions serve as powerful cues to smoke. Such conditioned ties become paired with positive neuroregulatory effects of nicotine to reinforce the addictive process. Personal characteristics such as educational level, belief in one's ability to change, and coping skills are determinants of tobacco use. Similarly, environmental factors such as the level of acceptance of smoking in the home, peer group, workplace, and community norms influence smoking behavior.

PHYSICOCHEMICAL PROPERTIES OF CIGARETTE SMOKE
Cigarette smoke is a heterogeneous aerosol produced by incomplete combustion of the tobacco leaf. It is composed of a gas phase in which particulate matter is dispersed. Mainstream smoke emerges from the mouthpiece during puffing. Sidestream smoke is emitted between puffs at the burning cone and from the mouthpiece. The composition of the smoke is influenced by several factors including type of tobacco, temperature of combustion, length of the cigarette, porosity of the paper, additives, and filters. Cigarette temperatures vary greatly, from 30°C at the mouthpiece to 900°C at the burning cone. In the presence of intense heat some tobacco constituents undergo thermic decomposition (pyrolysis). Volatile substances are distilled directly into the smoke. Unstable molecules recombine to generate new compounds (pyrosynthesis). Concentration of smoke constituents occurs as the smoke is filtered by unburnt tobacco and is redistilled by the burning cone. Some substances found in tobacco pass unchanged into cigarette smoke.

Approximately 92 to 95 percent of the total weight of mainstream smoke is present in the gas phase. Nitrogen, oxygen, and carbon dioxide account for 85 percent of the smoke's weight. The remaining gases and particulate matter are the substances of medical importance (Table 393-1).

PHARMACOLOGY OF CIGARETTE SMOKE More than 4000 substances have been identified in cigarette smoke, including some that are pharmacologically active, antigenic, cytotoxic, mutagenic, and carcinogenic; these diverse biologic effects provide a framework for understanding the adverse consequences of smoking. A pack-a-day cigarette smoker puffs more than 70,000 times a year, and the membranes of the mouth, nose, pharynx, and tracheobronchial tree are exposed repetitively to tobacco smoke. Some constituents act directly on the membranes, while others are absorbed into the blood or are dissolved in saliva and swallowed.

Tissue and organ system responses to cigarette smoke inhalation are multiple and complex. Most studies in humans have dealt with exposure to whole smoke or to selected constituents thought to pose the greatest risk to health, such as nicotine and carbon monoxide. Relatively little is known about the individual effects and interactions of other potentially toxic smoke constituents that are present in low concentrations.

Nicotine is a highly toxic alkaloid that is both a ganglionic stimulant and depressant. Many of its complex effects are mediated by catecholamine release. Acute cardiovascular responses to nicotine observed in normal smokers include increases in systolic and diastolic blood pressure, heart rate, force of myocardial contraction, myocardial oxygen consumption, coronary artery blood flow, myocardial excitability, and peripheral vasoconstriction. Nicotine has also been shown to increase serum concentrations of glucose, cortisol, free fatty acids, vasopressin, and β-endorphin.

TABLE 393-1 Selected cigarette smoke constituents	
Substance	Effect(s)
PARTICULATE PHASE	
"Tar"*	Carcinogen
Polynuclear aromatic hydrocarbons	Carcinogens
Nicotine	Neuroendocrine stimulant and depressant; addicting drug
Phenol	Cocarcinogen and irritant
Cresol	Cocarcinogen and irritant
β-Naphthylamine	Carcinogen
N-Nitrosonornicotine	Carcinogen
Benzo[a]pyrene	Carcinogen
Trace metals (e.g., nickel, arsenic, polonium 210)	Carcinogens
Indole	Tumor accelerator
Carbazole	Tumor accelerator
Catechol	Cocarcinogen
GAS PHASE	
Carbon monoxide	Impairs oxygen transport and utilization
Hydrocyanic acid	Ciliotoxin and irritant
Acetaldehyde	Ciliotoxin and irritant
Acrolein	Ciliotoxin and irritant
Ammonia	Ciliotoxin and irritant
Formaldehyde	Ciliotoxin and irritant
Oxides of nitrogen	Ciliotoxin and irritant
Nitrosamines	Carcinogen
Hydrazine	Carcinogen
Vinyl chloride	Carcinogen

* The aggregate of particulate matter in cigarette smoke after subtracting nicotine and moisture.

Carbon monoxide is a toxic gas that interferes with oxygen transport and utilization. Because cigarette smoke contains 2 to 6 percent carbon monoxide, smokers inhale concentrations as high as 400 parts per million (ppm) and develop elevated carboxyhemoglobin (COHb) levels. The range of COHb found in smokers is 2 to 15 percent, while levels for nonsmokers are near 1 percent. The average COHb level of moderate cigarette smokers is 5 percent. Carbon monoxide produces its adverse effects by reducing the amount of available oxyhemoglobin and myoglobin, and by displacing the oxygen-hemoglobin dissociation curve to the left. Chronic, mild elevations of COHb due to smoking are a common cause of mild polycythemia and may produce subtle impairment of central nervous system function.

Cigarette smoke and its condensate are carcinogenic in several species of animals. The major identified carcinogens in cigarette smoke are polynuclear aromatic hydrocarbons, aromatic amines, and nitrosamines (Table 393-1). Cocarcinogens present in cigarette smoke, such as catechol, greatly enhance its carcinogenicity.

Potent pulmonary irritants and ciliotoxins are found in cigarette smoke (Table 393-1). These substances increase bronchial mucous secretion and mediate acute and chronic decreases in pulmonary and mucociliary function.

EPIDEMIOLOGY   Data from large prospective studies of populations in several countries have shown that cigarette-smoking men have 70 percent higher overall death rates than nonsmokers. The effect on mortality is proportionately greatest in younger age groups. The excess mortality of female smokers has been somewhat less than that of male smokers, but it has increased. Cigarette smoking is the largest single health risk in the United States and is responsible for an estimated 390,000 premature deaths each year; this is equivalent to more than one out of every six deaths. Coronary heart disease (CHD) and lung cancer are the chief contributors to smoking-related excess mortality. In the United States, cigarette smokers also experience more disability due to chronic illness and report significantly more days absent from work than do nonsmokers.

A strong dose-response relationship exists between cigarette smoking and excess mortality, as measured by the age at onset of smoking, the number of cigarettes smoked, the number of years of smoking, and the depth of inhalation. Cessation of smoking is associated with a decrease in the excess mortality. These observations together with clinical, experimental, and pathologic studies indicate that smoking, per se, causes the excess mortality.

CHARACTERISTICS OF SMOKERS   Demographic, anthropometric, physiologic, and laboratory features which distinguish cigarette smokers from nonsmokers are due both to baseline differences between these groups and to the effects of smoking. Smokers drink more alcohol, coffee, and tea than do nonsmokers. Their weight and blood pressure are slightly less and their heart rate is slightly faster than those of nonsmokers. In women the menopause comes earlier in smokers than in nonsmokers. Smokers have impaired maximum exercise performance and impaired immune systems compared to nonsmokers. A markedly increased number of pulmonary alveolar macrophages is present in smokers, and the function and metabolism of these cells are abnormal. When compared with nonsmokers, smokers show small increases in hematocrit, total white blood cell count, and platelet count, as well as small decreases in leukocyte vitamin C levels, serum uric acid, and albumin. In smokers, the ratio of high-density lipoprotein cholesterol to low-density lipoprotein cholesterol is reduced.

CLINICAL CORRELATIONS   Large population studies have shown a strong association between cigarette smoking and several diseases. Atherosclerotic cardiovascular disease, cancer, and chronic obstructive pulmonary disease account for most of the excess mortality and morbidity due to smoking.

Individual patient risks due to cigarette smoking vary widely. Factors which influence these risks include the duration, intensity, and type of smoke exposure; genetically mediated susceptibility; occupational and environmental exposures; use of medication; and coexisting risk factors and diseases.

Cardiovascular disease   Cigarette smoking is a major cause of coronary heart disease (CHD), and premature CHD is one of its most important medical consequences. Approximately 20 percent of the 500,000 CHD deaths occurring each year in the United States is attributable to smoking. Cigarette smoking, hypertension, and hypercholesterolemia are the three major CHD risk factors. Smoking acts both independently of and synergistically with these other CHD risk factors. Two risk factors may produce a fourfold increase in CHD risk and three risk factors may produce an eightfold increase in CHD risk. There is a dose-response relationship between CHD risk and cigarette smoking. CHD death rates are 60 to 70 percent greater in male smokers than nonsmokers. Sudden death may be the first manifestation of CHD, and it is two to four times more likely to occur in younger male cigarette smokers than in nonsmokers. Women cigarette smokers are also at greater risk of developing CHD than nonsmokers, and the use of both cigarettes and oral contraceptives increases this risk approximately tenfold. Those who continue to smoke after an acute myocardial infarction are more likely to die from CHD than are those who quit smoking. Smokers who undergo coronary artery bypass surgery have increased perioperative mortality compared to nonsmokers. Cigarette smoking contributes to both coronary atherosclerosis and acute ischemic, thrombotic, and arrhythmic coronary events. Cigarette smoking may interfere with the efficacy of medication used to treat CHD, such as propranolol.

Cigarette smoking is an important cause of cerebrovascular disease and accounts for an estimated 18 percent of the 150,000 stroke deaths that occur each year in the United States. Large epidemiologic studies in men and women have shown an increased risk of stroke among smokers compared to nonsmokers, a dose-response relationship between smoking and stroke risk, and a decrease in stroke risk with smoking cessation. Among women, subarachnoid hemorrhage is more likely to occur in smokers than nonsmokers, and the use of both cigarettes and oral contraceptives greatly increases this risk.

Cigarette smoking is the most powerful risk factor for arteriosclerosis obliterans and thromboangiitis obliterans. It also aggravates peripheral ischemia and may adversely affect peripheral bypass grafts. The mortality rate for atherosclerotic aortic aneurysm is greater in male smokers than nonsmokers.

Cigarette smoking is not a risk factor for the development of hypertension; however, hypertensives who smoke are at a greater risk to develop malignant hypertension and to die from hypertension. Because of the association with chronic obstructive pulmonary disease, cigarette smoking is an important factor leading to chronic pulmonary heart disease.

Cancer Cigarette smoking is the single most important cause of cancer mortality in the United States, accounting for 30 percent of all cancer deaths. In spite of the well-documented cause-and-effect relationship between cigarette smoking and lung cancer, more Americans continue to die from this cancer than from any other tumor (see Chap. 227). In 1991 an estimated 143,000 lung cancer deaths occurred in the United States; 85 percent of these deaths were attributable to cigarette smoking. The risk of developing lung cancer is quantitatively related to cigarette smoke exposure. Men who smoke one pack a day increase their risk tenfold compared with nonsmokers; men who smoke two packs a day may increase their risk more than 25 times compared with nonsmokers. Asbestos workers who smoke cigarettes are at especially high risk for developing lung cancer. Cigarette consumption by women increased rapidly in the United States during the past 50 years, and lung cancer mortality among smokers is currently increasing at a faster rate in women than in men. Lung cancer has become the leading cause of cancer death among American women.

Cigarette smoking is a cause of laryngeal, oral, esophageal, and bladder cancer in men and women. Cigarette smoking is an important contributory factor for the development of kidney and pancreatic cancer; it is also associated with cancer of the stomach and uterine cervix and with myelocytic leukemia.

Respiratory disease Cigarette smoking is the major cause of chronic obstructive pulmonary disease (COPD), that is, chronic bronchitis and emphysema (see Chap. 223). Of the estimated 70,000 deaths from COPD in the United States in 1988, 82 percent were attributable to smoking and many of these deaths were preceded by prolonged respiratory disability. There is a dose-response relationship between COPD death rates and cigarette smoking. Depending upon the extent of smoke exposure, male cigarette smokers experience from 4 to 25 times higher mortality secondary to COPD than do nonsmokers. Although the death rate from COPD among female smokers is somewhat lower than among male smokers, it is increasing much more rapidly in female than in male smokers. Chronic cough, sputum production, and breathlessness are much more common in smokers. Smokers are more likely than nonsmokers to show abnormalities in a number of pulmonary function tests including measurements of elastic recoil, airflow in large and small airways, and diffusing capacity. Mild airflow obstruction in small airways may be present even in teenage smokers.

Cigarette smoking has been associated with an increased incidence of respiratory infections and deaths from pneumonia and influenza. Postoperative respiratory complications and spontaneous pneumothorax are also more common in smokers. Because tobacco smoke may increase airway obstruction, asthmatics should be urged not to smoke. Chronic stomatitis and chronic laryngitis occur more frequently in smokers than in nonsmokers.

Pregnancy Smoking may delay conception, and smoking during pregnancy may affect the fetus adversely. Infants whose mothers smoked during pregnancy weigh, on average, 170 g less than infants whose mothers did not smoke. This effect probably results from impaired uteroplacental circulation. Maternal smoking during pregnancy increases the risk of spontaneous abortion, fetal death, neonatal death, and the sudden infant death syndrome. This increased risk may be much greater in pregnancies already at high risk due to other factors. Smoking during pregnancy may also adversely affect the long-term physical growth and intellectual development of the child.

Gastrointestinal disorders Gastric and duodenal ulcer disease is more prevalent in male and female cigarette smokers than in nonsmokers and causes more deaths in male smokers than in nonsmokers. Smoking impairs spontaneous and drug-induced healing of peptic ulcers, increases the likelihood of duodenal ulcer recurrence, inhibits pancreactic bicarbonate secretion, and decreases the pressure of esophageal and pyloric sphincters. Histamine-2-receptor antagonist inhibition of nocturnal gastric secretion is also prevented by smoking.

Depression Recent studies indicate that the prevalence of cigarette smoking is increased among those who have had a major depressive disorder. Furthermore, smoking cessation rates are lower among depressed smokers, compared to nondepressed smokers. What role antidepressants could play in such individuals who are attempting to quit smoking remains to be determined.

Involuntary smoke inhalation Indoor atmospheres and other confined spaces are often contaminated by tobacco smoke which is inhaled involuntarily by both smokers and nonsmokers. Most of the atmospheric pollutants arise from sidestream smoke. It contains greater concentrations of many smoke constituents than does mainstream smoke, but since sidestream smoke is diluted in a large volume of air, the smoke exposure from involuntary inhalation is less than that associated with smoking.

Initially, involuntary or passive smoking was thought to cause primarily an irritant effect such as ocular burning. It is now recognized as a cause of lung cancer in nonsmokers. Parental smoking in the home is associated with an increased risk of acute respiratory illnesses, middle-ear effusions, chronic respiratory symptoms, and slightly impaired lung function in children. Involuntary smoke inhalation may also cause coronary heart disease.

Drug effects Tobacco smoke constituents induce hepatic microsomal enzyme systems that are important in the metabolism of several drugs. For example, cigarette smoking increases the metabolism of propranolol, propoxyphene, and theophylline. Hence, changes in smoking behavior may cause significant alterations of serum drug levels that may result in either drug toxicity or failure of drug treatment.

TYPES OF SMOKING During the past 20 years the amount of tar and nicotine delivered by cigarettes made in the United States has decreased by more the 50 percent. Filter-tipped cigarettes and lower-tar and -nicotine cigarettes now account for more than 95 and 55 percent of sales, respectively. Lung cancer and laryngeal cancer are the only tobacco-related diseases for which the use of lower-tar and -nicotine cigarettes has been shown to result in risk reduction, compared with the use of higher-tar and -nicotine cigarettes; however, compared with not smoking or quitting, the benefits are minimal. Consumers who choose lower-tar and -nicotine cigarettes and then smoke a larger number of cigarettes or inhale more frequently or deeply may actually increase their exposure to harmful substances. There is also concern because unidentified flavoring agents are added to these cigarettes to enhance consumer acceptance.

Cigar and pipe smokers usually inhale less smoke than cigarette smokers, presumably because the alkaline pH of cigar and pipe tobacco makes it more irritating to the respiratory tract. The smoke exposure and overall mortality rates of pipe and cigar smokers in the United States are substantially less than those of cigarette smokers; however, death rates of cigarette, cigar, and pipe smokers are approximately equal for carcinoma of the oral cavity, larynx, and esophagus, sites where exposures to cigarette, cigar, and pipe smoke are similar. The mortality rates of most cigar and pipe smokers for cancer at other sites, CHD, and COPD are not greatly elevated above the rates of nonsmokers, but cigar and pipe smokers who inhale consistently may experience adverse health effects comparable with those of cigarette smokers.

The use of chewing tobacco and snuff may produce plasma nicotine levels comparable to those of cigarette smokers and lead to nicotine dependence or addiction. The use of such smokeless tobacco products also increases the risk for oral cancer.

CESSATION OF SMOKING   In the United States between 1965 and 1990, the prevalence of smoking in adults declined from 52 to 28 percent of men and 34 to 23 percent of women. In 1990 there were an estimated 45.8 million current adult smokers and 44.1 million former smokers; approximately one-half of living Americans who had ever smoked had successfully quit. In recent years, the smoking prevalence among senior high school students has leveled off at about 20 percent. The rate of decline in smoking prevalence among the least educated Americans lags behind other groups.

Benefits   Smoking cessation produces immediate and long-term physical, psychological, and economic benefits. Within days of quitting the sense of smell and taste may improve. One year after quitting there is a substantial decrease in risk for a myocardial infarction. When chronic smoking produces permanent damage, as it does in the case of emphysema, the benefits of cessation are more modest such as slowing of the rate of decline of pulmonary function. The U.S. Surgeon General recently summarized the major and immediate health benefits of cessation that are valid for men and women of all ages and for those with and without smoking-related disease. Former smokers live, on the average, longer than continuing smokers. For example those who quit prior to the age of 50 have one-half the risk of dying in the next 15 years, compared to continuing smokers. Cessation reduces the risk for tobacco-related cancers, myocardial infarction, cerebrovascular disease, and chronic obstructive pulmonary disease. Women who quit smoking prior to pregnancy, or during the first trimester, eliminate the risk of delivering a low birth weight baby. The health benefits of quitting smoking far exceed the risks of the average 5-pound weight gain or any adverse psychological effects that may occur after quitting.

Cessation process   Most American smokers would like to quit. 80 percent have attempted to stop smoking during their lifetime, and 30 percent have stopped for at least one day during the previous year. Most of these attempts to quit are only temporarily successful. Smoking cessation is a dynamic, cyclic process that leads to overcoming an addictive behavior. Smokers move through a series of stages in their attempts to quit including thinking about quitting, deciding to quit, attempting to quit, and maintaining the ex-smoker status. Most successful quitters relapse and recycle through these stages three or four times before attaining long-term abstinence. Less than 5 percent of smokers move directly to the confirmed ex-smoker status without experiencing relapses. Factors encouraging long-term cessation include decreased social acceptability of smoking, increased concern about the health consequences of active and passive smoking, and increased costs of tobacco products. Factors contributing to relapse include craving for nicotine, weight gain, social pressures, and attempts to cope with negative feelings and interpersonal conflicts.

Cessation methods   More than 90 percent of confirmed ex-smokers quit without formal assistance. Quitting "cold turkey" is the method used by more than 80 percent of successful ex-smokers. However, heavy smokers and those most addicted to nicotine may benefit from participation in a cessation program. Organized programs employ a variety of approaches including: self-help, physician advice and counseling, use of medication, group therapy, behavioral training, hypnosis, and acupuncture. With such methods 20 to 30 percent 1-year abstinence rates are commonly reported. Controlled trials have shown significantly greater cessation rates for smokers receiving interventions, compared to control groups. The most effective programs offer multiple treatment modalities, involvement of physician and nonphysician health personnel, and a clear nonsmoking message presented in a variety of formats over time.

Physician guidelines   Physicians have unique opportunities and effective tools to promote smoking cessation. Seventy percent of American smokers visit a physician at least once a year. Some of these visits occur when the patient is experiencing symptomatic illness. In such settings patients may be especially responsive to cessation messages, and quit rates may be substantially enhanced. Even brief, physician-delivered stop-smoking messages may double the spontaneous smoking cessation rate. Treatment of nicotine addic-

TABLE 393-2   Physician guidelines for managing nicotine addiction

Assessment
  A Smoking history
  B Level of nicotine addiction
  C Health status
  D Quitting experience
  E Interest in quitting
Intervention
  A Teach
    1 Benefits of cessation
    2 Cessation process
    3 Withdrawal syndrome
  B Advise to quit
    1 Personalized message
    2 Quit date
    3 "Cold turkey"
  C Select cessation method(s)
    1 Self-help
    2 Physician-assisted
    3 Nicotine replacement
    4 Behavioral training
    5 Group therapy
  D Implement method
  E Meet special needs
Follow-up
  A Measure progress
  B Provide support
  C Deal with relapse
  D Consider alternative methods
  E Consider referral

tion is at least as cost-effective as treating other common medical problems such as hypertension and hypercholesterolemia.

Nicotine addiction should be viewed as a chronic medical problem requiring long-term commitment and management skills. The primary goal for each clinic visit should be to assist the smoker to move one step closer to quitting. The three essential phases for physician management include assessment, intervention, and follow-up (Table 393-2). During the assessment phase data are collected on health status, nicotine addiction, quitting experience, and interest in quitting. If the patient doesn't want to stop smoking, the clinician should review the risks of smoking, recommend quitting, and defer further action until the next clinic visit. Most patients are interested in quitting and progress to the intervention phase. Smokers are taught about the benefits of quitting and the cyclical cessation process. The smoker is advised to choose a quit date and to go "cold turkey." A cessation method(s) is chosen and implemented. Physicians often provide educational material, counseling, and, recently, nicotine replacement therapy. Both nicotine chewing gum and transdermal patches improve cessation rates when used in combination with other interventions. The proper uses, contraindications, and side effects of these products should be understood. For example, nicotine replacement therapy should not be used when the patient is still smoking. The likelihood of success with any cessation method is enhanced when the clinician responds to individual concerns such as weight gain and helps the smoker to develop practical strategies to avoid relapse. The final phase, follow-up, involves assessing progress, providing support, and dealing with relapse. The last should not be viewed as failure but as part of the cyclic process leading to cessation. Follow-up discussions may focus on alternative cessation methods or referral to a smoking cessation specialist.

Political, social, and cultural forces play a critical role in the individual decision to start or stop smoking. For this reason, physicians should lead and support efforts to increase tobacco excise taxes, to eliminate all tobacco advertisements and promotional activities, and to ban smoking in public places.

PREVENTION   Ultimately, primary smoking prevention in the pediatric and adolescent age groups may be the most effective program. Young people who have been trained to resist social pressures, who understand the health consequences of smoking, and who appreciate the difficulty of quitting are less likely to start smoking.

REFERENCES

Fiore MC (ed): Cigarette smoking: A clinical guide to assessment and treatment. Med Clinic North Am 76:289, 1992

Lesmes GR (ed): The effects of cigarette smoking: A global perspective. Am J Med 93(1A):1S, 1992

U.S. Department of Health and Human Services: The health consequences of involuntary smoking. A report of the Surgeon General. DHHS(CDC) Publication no 87-8398, 1986

U.S. Department of Health and Human Services: The health consequences of smoking: Nicotine addiction. A report of the Surgeon General. DHHS(CDC) Publication no 88-8406, 1988

U.S. Department of Health and Human Services: Reducing the health consequences of smoking: 25 years of progress. A report of the Surgeon General. DHHS(CDC) Publication no 89-8411, 1989

U.S. Department of Health and Human Services: The health benefits of smoking cessation. A report of the Surgeon General. DHHS(CDC) Publication no 90-8416, 1990

PART FIFTEEN

ENVIRONMENTAL AND OCCUPATIONAL HAZARDS

394 PHYSICIANS AND HAZARDS OF THE ENVIRONMENT AND WORKPLACE

HOWARD HU / FRANK E. SPEIZER

The term *hazards* encompasses chemical hazards as well as other risks posed by the physical environment (changes in temperature or altitude/pressure, exposures to ionizing and nonionizing radiation) and selected natural phenomena (venoms and stings). Unless otherwise defined, *toxins* and *toxic exposures* are synonymous with *hazards*. These hazards may occur in the general environment or in the workplace. Strictly speaking, smoking, alcohol ingestion, poor nutrition, and infectious diseases also could be considered chemical or environmental hazards.

While the identification and control of hazards often lie in the domain of public health, there are a number of compelling reasons for all physicians to become acquainted with both the hazards themselves and the basic precepts of environmental/occupational medicine:

1 Millions of people are exposed to hazards at levels sufficient to result in demonstrable health problems. Public awareness of these hazards has grown, as has the expectation that physicians can diagnose and treat associated disorders.
2 Specialists in occupational/environmental health are few in number.
3 Many manifestations of exposure-related illnesses are nonspecific (e.g., dizziness, headache) or present as commonly encountered problems of general practice (e.g., myocardial infarction, cancer). The establishment of a connection with a hazard requires a high index of suspicion and application of fundamental concepts of environmental/occupational medicine.
4 Early recognition by physicians of unusual patterns of illness or asymptomatic exposure to toxins with low-level effects (e.g., an elevated blood lead level) can alert health officials to the need for control measures.
5 Physicians can contribute to toxicologic knowledge by reporting reactions to new chemicals (similar to the reporting of adverse drug effects). Case reports in the literature often prompt epidemiologic studies.
6 In many states and countries, the reporting by physicians of occupational/environmental diseases is mandatory. For instance, since 1992, physicians in Massachusetts have been required to report cases of pneumoconiosis, occupational asthma, carpal tunnel syndrome, carbon monoxide poisoning, and others.
7 Identification of an environmental/occupational etiology of an illness may have important economic ramifications for the patient (e.g., worker's compensation, which pays for medical bills as well as lost wages). Physicians are frequently asked to provide expert medical testimony on the causal relationship between toxic exposures and diseases during the course of litigation.

For any given physician, it is difficult to estimate the fraction of disease that is likely to be attributable to environmental and occupational factors. A summary of diagnoses based on referral visits to a clinic specializing in environmental/occupational disorders (Table 394-1) revealed a wide variety of disorders, asbestos-related pulmonary disorders being the most common. Whether recognized as hazard-associated illnesses or not, a similarly wide spectrum is probably seen by internists, although variations can be expected due to regional differences in hazardous exposures and referral patterns.

Clinical effects of chemical and environmental hazards are discussed in chapters devoted to the specifically involved organ (Chap. 219) or to specific exposures (Chaps. 395 to 401). To list the vast array of environmental hazard–disease relationships is beyond the scope of this chapter. Utilizing additional references (see "General References" at end of this chapter) is important when considering an environmental/occupational etiology.

THE ILL PATIENT: RECOGNIZING A CHEMICAL OR OTHER ENVIRONMENTAL ETIOLOGY

THE ENVIRONMENTAL/OCCUPATIONAL HISTORY Taking an appropriate environmental/occupational history as part of the medical workup is critical for recognizing these disorders. The level of detail that is called for depends on the clinical situation. *Always obtain information on the current and major past occupations for all patients seen.* When confronted by an illness of uncertain etiology or by an

TABLE 394-1 Most common disorders related to patient visits, 1987–1991[a]

Diagnoses	Average no. of visits per year[b]
Asbestos-related disease	
Pleural disease	220
Asbestosis	68
Mesothelioma	2
Lung cancer and heavy asbestos exposure	2
Unexplained pleural effusion	3
Pneumoconioses (other than asbestos)	3
Chemical bronchitis/tracheitis[c]	4
Occupational/environmental asthma	35
Chemical dermatitis	2
Low back strain	3
Carpal tunnel syndrome	6
Other cumulative trauma disorder	5
Toxic hepatitis[d]	4
Toxic encephalopathy[e]	9
Toxic peripheral neuropathy	5
Lead poisoning/over-exposure	7
Poisoning (miscellaneous)[f]	5
Multiple chemical sensitivity syndrome	5
Tight building syndrome	4
Symptoms, suspected but unproven link to occupational or environmental factors	41

[a] At the Harvard School of Public Health–affiliated Massachusetts Respiratory Hospital Center for Occupational/Environmental Medicine, Braintree, MA, between 1987 and 1991.
[b] Routine visits for screening exams have been excluded. Cases of contact dermatitis, low-back strain, and carpal tunnel syndrome are probably underrepresented because of referral bias.
[c] From welding fumes, chlorine vapors, and other irritants.
[d] Usually from exposure to solvents.
[e] Usually from solvents or carbon monoxide.
[f] From arsenic, mercury, vanadium, pesticides, PCBs, cyanide, ozone, carbon disulfide, etc.

illness for which an environmental/occupational source has not been entertained, these factors should be explored in detail, beginning with an environmental/occupational history.

The identification of potential chemical exposures can be difficult. Household products must list chemical ingredients on their labels. For workplace exposures, the Occupational Safety and Health Administration (OSHA) requires chemical suppliers to provide material safety data sheets (MSDS) with their products and requires employers to retain them and make them available to employees. They can be obtained by the physician or employee by a telephone or written request; failure of an employer to provide them within 30 days of such a request is a violation of OSHA regulations and punishable by fines. In addition to providing information on chemical ingredients and percent composition, the MSDS provides basic information on toxicity. This information is seldom adequate from a clinical perspective but may indicate the general type of toxicity that may be anticipated.

EVALUATING POSSIBLE CHEMICAL OR ENVIRONMENTAL HAZARDS   Given the wide variety of toxic exposures that may be uncovered during a workup, a clinician should routinely consult additional reference material to evaluate whether particular hazards may be associated with the illness at hand.

Many sources of information exist. Some regional poison control centers have extensive information on hazards that can be transmitted by telephone or facsimile. Other resources, depending on the area, may include county and state health departments, regional offices of the National Institute for Occupational Safety and Health (NIOSH) and the Environmental Protection Agency (EPA), the Centers for Disease Control and Prevention (CDC) in Atlanta, the Consumer Products Safety Commission (CPSC) in Washington, D.C., academic institutions, and individual toxicologists, occupational/environmental medicine specialists, or industrial hygienists.

Sophisticated computerized databases are also available, including detailed listings on CD-ROM information systems and MEDLARS, an electronic database maintained by the National Library of Medicine and accessible by modem. In addition to MEDLINE, the on-line bibliographic database familiar to many physicians, MEDLARS has other files that provide specific toxicity information on chemicals and that include toxicologic references not covered by MEDLINE.

As with any other illness, laboratory investigation may be crucial. For example, tests of carboxyhemoglobin level to document carbon monoxide exposure or of serum anticholinesterase level to document organophosphate pesticide absorption should be performed within hours of exposure. As with acute drug overdoses, it is useful to freeze urine and serum samples from any patient suspected of suffering from an acute chemical exposure; such specimens can be analyzed at a later date using sensitive methods of detection. Use of other tests must rely on knowledge of the specific hazard or illness in question.

SUSPICIOUS SCENARIOS   Some medical problems or clinical scenarios demand a particularly high degree of suspicion for occupational or environmental factors as causative or contributing agents of disease.

Respiratory disease   The contribution of occupational/environmental factors to respiratory disease is generally underrecognized, particularly among patients who smoke and the elderly (see Chap. 219). For instance, asthma related to chemical exposure may be treated without regard to cause or erroneously diagnosed as acute tracheobronchitis. Shortness of breath from asbestosis may be attributed to chronic obstructive pulmonary disease. Chemical pneumonitis may be misdiagnosed as a bacterial infection.

Cancer   Many cancers are thought to be causally related to occupational and environmental factors in addition to tobacco. Some are particularly likely to have a chemical or other environmental etiology, including cancers of the skin (solar radiation, arsenic, coal tar, soot), lung (asbestos, arsenic, nickel, radon), pleura (almost exclusively asbestos), nasal cavity and sinuses (chromium, nickel, wood and leather dusts), liver (arsenic, vinyl chloride), bone marrow (benzene, ionizing radiation), and bladder (aromatic amines).

Coronary disease   Carbon monoxide exposure is common, particularly in homes with malfunctioning furnaces or in workplaces close to motor vehicle exhaust. By reducing oxygen transport by hemoglobin and inhibiting mitochondrial metabolism, carbon monoxide can aggravate coronary disease. Methylene chloride, a solvent used in paint stripping, is converted to carbon monoxide and thus poses the same risk. Exposure to carbon disulfide, a chemical used in the production of rayon, accelerates the rate of atherosclerotic plaque formation.

Hepatitis/chronic liver disease   In the absence of evidence that a virus, alcohol ingestion, or drug is the main cause of hepatitis (see Chaps. 266 and 267), a toxin must be considered. Toxin-induced hepatic injury may be cytotoxic, cholestatic, or both. The list of hepatotoxic agents is long, but common ones include organic synthetic compounds such as carbon tetrachloride (used in solvents and cleaning fluids) and methylene diamine (a resin hardener), pesticides such as chlordecone (Kepone), metals, particularly arsenic (used in pesticides and paints and found in well water), and natural toxins such as the pyrrolidizine alkaloids.

Kidney disease   Many chemical and environmental factors can cause renal injury (see Chap. 236). The etiology of much chronic kidney disease, however, remains unknown. An increasing body of evidence now links chronic renal failure with hypertension to lead exposure. Some studies suggest that chronic exposure to hydrocarbons (e.g., gasoline, paints, solvents) may lead to various types of glomerulonephritis, including Goodpasture's syndrome.

Peripheral neuropathy   Organic solvents such as n-hexane, heavy metals such as lead and arsenic, and some organophosphate compounds can damage the axons of peripheral nerves. Dimethylaminopropionitrile (DMAPN), an industrial catalyst, causes bladder neuropathy. Nerve entrapment syndromes of the upper extremity, such as carpal tunnel syndrome, may be caused by jobs that involve repetitive motion, especially those which involve maintenance of awkward positions.

Neuropsychiatric symptoms   Fatigue, memory loss, difficulty in concentration, and emotional lability have been linked to chronic exposure to solvents such as toluene and perchlorethylene. Painters, metal degreasers, plastics workers, and cleaners are commonly exposed to solvents and develop these symptoms at a high rate. Characteristic patterns on formal neurobehavioral testing and stabilization of symptoms with gradual improvement following removal from exposure are among the features that distinguish these patients. Other substances associated with neurobehavioral dysfunction include metals, particularly lead, mercury, arsenic, and manganese; carbon monoxide; and pesticides, such as organophosphates and organochlorines.

Teratogenesis and reproductive problems   Toxins can impair successful reproduction at a variety of levels. Examples include insecticides and herbicides, PCBs and PBBs (polychlorinated and polybrominated biphenyls, see below), ethylene oxide (a sterilizing gas used in hospitals), metals (lead, arsenic, cadmium, mercury), and solvents. Dibromochloropropane (DBCP), a nematocide, suppresses spermatogenesis. Some toxins, such as PCBs, PBBs, and chlorinated pesticides, are concentrated in milk.

Immunosuppression, autoimmunity, and hypersensitivity   Evidence is increasing that exposures to some chemical agents can compromise the immune system, thereby leading to a generalized increased incidence of tumors (e.g., exposure to PBBs) or infections (e.g., respiratory infections after exposure to common air pollutants). Mercury, dieldrin, and methylcholanthrene are known to elicit autoimmune responses. Some chemicals are potent allergic sensitizers that cause dermal and respiratory problems (see Chaps. 53 and 219).

MANAGING A HAZARD-RELATED ILLNESS

Once a chemical or other environmental hazard has been identified as an important contributor to an illness, the next step is to prevent

TABLE 394-2   Environmental/occupational medicine: Examples of unsolved concerns for the 1990s

Topic	Summary of issues involved
Dioxin	(aka TCDD, or 2,3,7,8-tetrachlorodibenzo-*p*-dioxin) Chief ingredient of agent orange and a major contaminant of hazardous waste sites; potent animal carcinogen; most recent epidemiologic studies suggest that it conveys mild risk of soft tissue sarcomas in humans.
PCBs	(aka polychlorinated biphenyls, Arachlor) A mixture of synthetic compounds formerly used to insulate transformers and capacitors; potent animal liver carcinogen; consequences of human exposure unclear, but may involve cancer, reproductive, and neurologic effects.
Multiple chemical sensitivity	Nonspecific symptoms (e.g., headache, dizziness, fatigue, irritability, loss of memory or concentration) in relation to exposure to a wide variety of chemicals at extremely low levels (e.g., formaldehyde vapor from new carpets; solvents found in perfumes, glues, photocopy machines, dry-cleaned clothes); no laboratory abnormalities are found; incidence appears to be increasing; mechanism under investigation.
Hazardous waste	Exposure can occur through direct contact at abandoned or unsecured sites; volatilization or conversion to dust carried in air; seepage into groundwater used by wells; contamination of the food chain through marine organisms living in polluted waters and plants and animals living on contaminated soil; and dissemination by fire and explosion; nausea, headache, nose and throat irritation, and increased respiratory morbidity are common complaints of those residing near chemical waste dumps; the risk of cancer posed by exposure to part-per-billion concentrations of pollutants from such contamination is of continuing concern.
Global climatic change	Stratospheric depletion of ozone is leading to increased exposure to solar ultraviolet radiation (UVR); in addition to increasing the risk of skin cancers, UVR is a risk factor for cataractogenesis and may impair cellular immunity; global warming will lead to increased heat exposure and is also likely to have an indirect effect on health by altering the distribution of communicable disease vectors and exacerbating problems of crop growth and food availability.

further exposure. For chronic diseases such as cancer, this step is irrelevant; the illness remains when the exposure has come and gone. For others, the physician *must be willing to become an active advocate for the patient.* This may involve writing a letter stating that the patient should no longer be exposed to a hazard or should remain out of work, or it may involve contacting appropriate officials in government, industry, or labor or other advocates who can deal with a hazardous exposure. Treatment is dependent on the specific hazard.

In few areas of medicine does a physician deal with more scientific uncertainty. Comprehensive information on toxicants is available for only a small percentage of chemicals. In general, the physician should take a conservative approach (i.e., advise avoidance of a hazard if it is likely to have contributed to the illness) and to use common sense and up-to-date information to evaluate causal relationships.

LOW-LEVEL EXPOSURES AND THEIR EFFECTS

The subclinical effects of toxins that are widespread in our environment and workplaces are of increasing concern. Given the absence of any demonstrable effect threshold, low-level exposure to carcinogens should be avoided. Equally important are the noncarcinogenic effects of chronic low-level exposures such as lead.

Multiple pathways of exposure, including the combustion of leaded gasoline, the use of lead-based paints and solder, and the lead in cans containing food, have contributed to exposure of the entire population. Such low-level exposures can impair neurobehavioral development in infants and children (see Chap. 378) and raise blood pressure in adults. Furthermore, absorbed lead is stored in the skeleton and may reenter the circulation at times of heightened bone turnover (e.g., pregnancy, lactation, osteoporosis, hyperthyroidism).

Subclinical toxic effects can be prevented if chronic low-level exposure is detected early and curtailed. In the case of lead, this takes the form of a test of blood lead level, performed regularly in small children living in old neighborhoods, and as a precautionary measure in adults with a history of lead exposure.

UNSOLVED CONCERNS FOR THE 1990s

Examples of issues in this field, not mentioned elsewhere in this book, that are either of emerging concern or the sources of unresolved controversies are given in Table 394-2. The challenge is to remain abreast of developments in these areas, particularly when confronted by a relevant case.

SPECIFIC REFERENCES

Bailar J: How dangerous is dioxin? N Engl J Med 324:260, 1991
Fiedler N et al: Evaluation of chemically sensitive patients. J Occup Med 34:529, 1992
Freund E et al: Mandatory reporting of occupational diseases by clinicians. JAMA 262:3041, 1989
Goldman RH, Peters JM: The occupational and environmental health history. JAMA 246:2831, 1981
Haines A: Global warming and health. Br Med J 302:669, 1991
Himmelstein JS, Frumkin H: The right to know about toxic exposures: Implications for physicians. N Engl J Med 312:687, 1985
Paul M (ed): *Occupational/Environmental Hazards and Reproductive Health: A Guide for Clinicians.* Baltimore, Williams & Wilkens, 1992
White RF et al: Neurobehavioral effects of toxicity due to metals, solvents, and insecticides. Clin Neuropharmacol 13:392, 1990

GENERAL REFERENCES

Bezman Tarcher A (ed): *Principles and Practice of Environmental Medicine.* New York, Plenum, 1992
Cullen MR et al: Occupational medicine—Medical progress. N Engl J Med 322:594, 1990
LaDou J (ed): *Occupational Medicine.* Norwalk: Appleton & Lange, 1990
National Institute for Occupational Safety and Health: *Pocket Guide to Chemical Hazards.* Cincinnati, National Institute for Occupational Safety and Health, DHHS(NIOSH) Publ No 90-117, 1990.
Rom WN (ed): *Environmental and Occupational Medicine,* 2d ed. Boston, Little, Brown, 1992
Sullivan JB Jr, Krieger GR (eds): *Hazardous Materials Toxicology—Clinical Principles of Environmental Health.* Baltimore, Williams & Wilkins, 1992
Upton AC (ed): Environmental medicine. Med Clin North Am Volume 74: XXX, 1990

395   ACUTE POISON AND DRUG OVERDOSAGE

FREDERICK H. LOVEJOY, JR. / CHRISTOPHER H. LINDEN

A poison (toxin) is a substance capable of producing adverse effects in a living organism. Poisons may be divided into those intended for human use (foods and their additives, pharmaceuticals, toiletries, cosmetics) and those that are not (household products, industrial chemicals, nonfood nondrug botanicals). An overdose implies exposure to excessive amounts of the former and any amount of the latter; it may or may not result in harmful effects (poisoning).

Poisoning may be local (limited to the eyes, skin, lungs, or gastrointestinal tract), systemic, or both, depending on dose, absorption, distribution, potency, and host susceptibility. Absorption and distribution are influenced by properties of the chemical itself (molecular size, degree of ionization, lipid and water solubility, protein binding) and of the biologic barriers (membrane composition, pore size, chemical transport systems) through which it penetrates.

Local effects are due to nonspecific chemical reactions such as oxidation, protein denaturation, desiccation, and solvent activity. The severity and reversibility depend on the dose (concentration), contact time, potency of the chemical, and type and condition of the exposed surface. The nature, extent, severity, and reversibility of systemic effects depend on the dose, potency, and metabolic disposition of the chemical, the functional reserve of the individual, and the presence of secondary complications (shock, hypoxia). Other variables that influence toxicity include coexisting illnesses, previous chemical exposure (e.g., enzyme induction or inhibition, tolerance), and individual differences in biologic response, tissue concentration (pharmacodynamics), and/or absorption, distribution, metabolism, and elimination (pharmacokinetics). When compared with therapeutic dosing, effects of an overdose begin sooner, peak later, and last longer.

EPIDEMIOLOGY

In the United States, potential poisoning (exposures) result in an estimated 5 million requests for medical advice or treatment each year. The common routes of exposure are ingestion (79 percent), dermal (7 percent), ophthalmic (6 percent), inhalation (5 percent), bites and stings (3 percent), and parenteral injections (0.3 percent). Prescribed drugs are involved in 40 percent of exposures. Frequently involved substances include cleaning agents, analgesics, cosmetics, plants, cough and cold preparations, and hydrocarbons. Most exposures are acute, accidental, occur in the home, result in minor or no toxicity, and involve children under 6 years of age.

Accidental exposures can result from the improper use of chemicals at work or play, product mislabeling, label misreading, mistaken identification of unlabeled chemicals, uninformed self-medication, and dosing errors by nurses, parents, pharmacists, physicians, and the elderly. Excluding the recreational use of ethanol, attempted suicide is the most common reason for intentional exposure. Unintended poisonings may result from use of drugs for psychotropic effects (abuse) or excessive self-dosing (misuse).

Although only 4 percent of victims of chemical exposure require hospitalization, they account for roughly 5 percent of intensive care unit admissions and up to 30 percent of psychiatric admissions. Suicide attempts account for most (60 to 90 percent) serious or fatal poisonings. Deaths are most common from carbon monoxide poisoning and occur prior to arrival at a hospital. Antidepressants, analgesics, stimulants and street drugs, cardiovascular agents, sedative-hypnotics, and asthma medications are responsible for most drug-related fatalities. Nonpharmaceutical agents implicated in fatal poisoning include inorganic chemicals, alcohols and glycols, cleaning agents, and hydrocarbons.

DIAGNOSIS OF POISONING

Although poisoning can mimic other illnesses, the correct diagnosis usually can be established by the history, physical examination, routine and toxicologic laboratory evaluations, and clinical course. The history should include the time, route, duration, and circumstances (location, surrounding events, intent) of exposure; the name and amount of each drug, chemical, or ingredient involved; the time of onset, nature, and severity of symptoms; the time and type of first aid measures provided; and the past medical and psychiatric history.

In many cases the victim is confused, comatose, unaware of an exposure, or unable or unwilling to admit to one. Suspicious circumstances include unexplained illness in a previously healthy person; history of psychiatric problems (particularly depression); recent changes in health, economic status, or social relationships; and onset of illness while working with chemicals or after ingesting food, drink (especially ethanol), or medications. Patients who become ill soon after arriving from a foreign country or after arrest for criminal activity should be suspected of having illicit drugs concealed in body cavities (the gastrointestinal tract). Family, friends, paramedics, police, pharmacists, physicians, and employers may provide information regarding habits, hobbies, behavior changes, available medications, and antecedent events. A search of the clothes and place of discovery may reveal a suicide note or empty container of drugs or chemicals. The imprint code on pills and the label on chemical products may be used to identify the ingredients and potential toxicity of a suspected poison by consulting a reference text, a computerized chemical database, the manufacturer, or a regional poison information center.

The physical examination should initially focus on the vital signs and cardiopulmonary and neurologic status to assess the need for immediate supportive treatment. Since the clinical picture can usually be characterized by either physiologic stimulation or depression, these parameters also provide the most important diagnostic clues in poisoning of unknown etiology (Table 395-1). Examination of the eyes (for nystagmus, pupil size, and reactivity), abdomen (for bowel activity and bladder), and skin (for burns, bullae, color, warmth, moisture, pressure sores, and puncture marks) may narrow the diagnosis to a particular syndrome. Grading the severity of poisoning (Table 395-2) is useful for assessing prognosis and the clinical course.

The patient also should be examined for evidence of trauma and underlying illnesses. Except with carbon monoxide, theophylline, and drugs that cause hypoglycemia and hypoxia, seizures and neurologic dysfunction due to poisoning are almost never focal. Hence focal findings should prompt evaluation for a structural central nervous system (CNS) lesion. When the history is unclear, all orifices should be examined for the presence of chemical burns and drug packets. The odor of breath or vomitus and the color of nails, skin, or urine may provide diagnostic clues.

TABLE 395-1   Differential diagnosis of poisoning based on vital signs and CNS activity

Stimulant poisoning	Depressant poisoning
Sympathomimetic syndrome	**Sympatholytic syndrome**
Amphetamines	Adrenergic blockers
Caffeine	Antiarrhythmics
Cocaine	Antidepressants (tricyclic)
Decongestants	Antihypertensives
Ergot alkaloids	Calcium channel blockers
MAO inhibitors	Digoxin
Theophylline	**Cholinergic syndrome**
Anticholinergic syndrome	Bethanecol
Antidepressants (tricyclic)	Carbamate insecticides
Antihistamines	Organophosphate insecticides
Antiparkinsonian agents	Myasthenia gravis drugs
Antipsychotics	(e.g., pyridostigmine)
Antispasmodics (GI, GU)	Physostigmine
Belladonna alkaloids	**Narcotic syndrome**
Cyclobenzaprine	Analgesics
Mydriatics (topical)	Antispasmodics (GI)
Plants/mushrooms	**Sedative-hypnotic syndrome**
Hallucinogenic syndrome	Alcohol
LSD and synthetic analogues	Antiepileptics
Marijuana	Barbiturates
Mescaline and synthetic	Benzodiazepines
analogues	Ethchlorvynol
Phencyclidine	Hydrocarbons
Withdrawal syndrome	Glutethimide
Alcohol	Methyprylon
Antidepressants	
Beta-blockers	
Clonidine	
Narcotics	
Sedative-hypnotics	

TABLE 395-2   Severity of stimulant and depressant poisoning and drug withdrawal

Severity	Signs and symptoms
STIMULANT POISONING	
Grade 1	Diaphoresis, flushing, hyperreflexia, irritability, mydriasis, tremors
Grade 2	Confusion, fever, hyperactivity, hypertension, tachycardia, tachypnea
Grade 3	Delirium, mania, hyperpyrexia, tachyarrhythmias
Grade 4	Coma, convulsions, cardiovascular collapse
DEPRESSANT POISONING	
Grade 1	Lethargic but arousable; able to answer questions and follow commands
Grade 2	Comatose; withdraws from pain; brainstem and deep tendon reflexes intact
Grade 3	Comatose; no response to pain; most reflexes absent; respiratory depression
Grade 4	Comatose; no response to pain; reflexes absent; respiratory and cardiovascular depression

An anion gap metabolic acidosis is characteristic of methanol, ethylene glycol, and salicylate intoxication and may occur in any poisoning that results in hypoxia, hypotension, or seizures. The serum lactate concentration is low (less than the anion gap) in the former nd high (nearly equal to the anion gap) in the latter. An osmolal gap, the difference between the measured serum osmolality (freezing point depression, not the vapor pressure method) and the calculated osmolality (from the serum sodium, glucose, and BUN), of more than 10 mmol/L indicates the presence of a low-molecular-weight solute such as acetone, ethanol, ethylene glycol, isopropyl alcohol, or methanol or an unmeasured electrolyte (magnesium) or sugar (mannitol). An increased anion gap metabolic acidosis with respiratory alkalosis, ketosis, and tinnitus suggests salicylate poisoning; an increased osmolal gap accompanied by back pain, hypocalcemia, and crystalluria suggests ethylene glycol intoxication, and an increased osmolal gap accompanied by visual symptoms suggests methanol poisoning. Poisons that cause specific signs, symptoms, and other laboratory abnormalities are listed in the references cited.

Pulmonary edema (ARDS) can occur with carbon monoxide, cyanide, narcotic, paraquat, phencyclidine, sedative-hypnotic, and salicylate poisoning; inhalation of irritant gases, fumes, or vapors (ammonia, metal oxides, mercury); or prolonged anoxia, hyperthermia, or shock. Aspiration pneumonia is common in patients with coma, seizures, and petroleum distillate ingestion. Radiopaque densities may be visible on abdominal x-rays following the ingestion of calcium salts, chloral hydrate, chlorinated hydrocarbons, enteric-coated tablets, heavy metals, illicit drug packets, iodinated compounds, lithium, phenothiazines, and salicylates.

Bradycardia and AV block may occur in patients poisoned by antiarrhythmic agents, beta blockers, calcium channel blockers, cholinergic agents (carbamate and organophosphate insecticides), digitalis, lithium, phenylpropanolamine, and tricyclic antidepressants. QRS- and QT-interval prolongation may be caused by amantidine, antiarrhythmics, tricyclic antidepressants, fluorides, heavy metals (arsenic, thallium), lithium, magnesium, meperidine metabolites, neuroleptics, and potassium. Ventricular tachyarrhythmias may be seen in poisoning with sympathomimetics and agents that cause QRS and QT prolongation.

Analysis of urine and blood (and occasionally gastric contents and chemical samples) may be useful to confirm or rule out suspected poisoning. Interpretation of laboratory data requires knowledge of the tests used for screening and confirmation (thin-layer, gas-liquid, high-performance liquid chromatography; colorimetric and fluorometric assays; enzyme-multiplied and radioimmunoassays; gas chromatography; mass spectrometry), their sensitivity (limit of detection) and specificity, and the best type and time of sampling of biologic specimens for analysis. Personal communication with the laboratory is essential. A negative screen may mean the poison is not detectable by the test used or its concentration is too low for detection at the time of sampling. In the latter instance, repeating the test at a later time may yield positive results.

Since screening tests require 2 to 6 h for completion, immediate management must be based on the history, physical examination, and routine ancillary tests. When the patient is asymptomatic, or when the clinical picture is consistent with the reported history, qualitative screening is neither clinically useful nor cost-effective. It is of greatest value in patients with severe or unexplained toxicity such as coma, seizures, cardiovascular instability, metabolic or respiratory acidosis, and nonsinus cardiac rhythms. Quantitative analysis is useful for acetaminophen, acetone, alcohol (including ethylene glycol), antiarrhythmic, antiepileptic, barbiturate, digoxin, heavy metal, lithium, salicylate, and theophylline poisoning and in carboxyhemoglobinemia and methemoglobinemia. Results can often be available within an hour.

Response to antidotes also may be used for diagnostic purposes. Resolution of altered mental status and abnormal vital signs within minutes of intravenous dextrose, naloxone, or flumazenil administration is virtually diagnostic of hypoglycemia, narcotic poisoning, and benzodiazepine intoxication, respectively. The prompt reversal of acute dystonic (extrapyramidal) reactions following an intravenous dose of benztropine or diphenhydramine confirms the diagnosis of a drug etiology. *Vin rosé* urine color following a diagnostic dose of deferoxamine can be used to confirm iron poisoning when serum iron and total iron-binding capacity levels are not immediately available. Although reversal of both central and peripheral manifestations of anticholinergic poisoning by physostigmine is diagnostic, physostigmine may cause arousal in patients with CNS depression of any etiology.

The absence of signs and symptoms soon after an overdose does not rule out a poisoning. Common poisons whose effects are delayed in onset include acetaminophen, cancer chemotherapeutic agents, carbamazepine, carbon tetrachloride, colchicine, digoxin, disulfiram, ethylene glycol, heavy metals, lithium, methanol, monoamine oxidase inhibitors, mushrooms, some plants, narcotics, phenytoin, podophylline, salicylate, and enteric-coated, slow- or sustained-released medications.

TREATMENT

Treatment goals include support of vital signs, prevention of further poison absorption, enhancement of poison elimination, administration of specific antidotes, and prevention of reexposure (Table 395-3). Treatment depends on the identity of the poison, the route and amount of exposure, the time of presentation relative to the time of exposure, and the severity of poisoning. Knowledge of toxin pharmacokinetics and pharmacodynamics is essential.

For patients who present prior to the onset of manifestations (preclinical phase) decontamination is the highest priority, and treatment is based solely on the history. The maximum potential toxicity based on the greatest possible exposure should be assumed. When appropriate, gastrointestinal decontamination to minimize absorption and decrease the severity of toxicity is the first priority. Since decontamination is more effective the sooner performed, the history and physical examination should be brief. It is also advisable to establish intravenous access and initiate cardiac monitoring, particularly in patients with potentially serious ingestions or unclear histories. The choice of decontamination procedure depends on the predicted toxicity; the availability, efficacy, and contraindications of the procedure; and the nature, severity, and risk of complications. For the home management of patients with accidental ingestions, reliable histories, and mild predicted toxicity, emesis can be induced with ipecac syrup. For patients treated in medical facilities, activated

TABLE 395-3   Fundamentals of poisoning management

SUPPORTIVE CARE

A Airway protection
B Oxygenation/ventilation
C Treatment of arrhythmias
D Hemodynamic support
E Treatment of seizures
F Correction of temperature abnormalities
G Correction of metabolic derangements
H Prevention of secondary complications

PREVENTION OF FURTHER POISON ABSORPTION

A Gastrointestinal decontamination
   1 Syrup of ipecac–induced emesis
   2 Gastric lavage
   3 Activated charcoal
   4 Whole bowel irrigation
   5 Catharsis
   6 Dilution
   7 Endoscopic/surgical removal
B Decontamination of other sites
   1 Eye decontamination
   2 Skin decontamination
   3 Body cavity evacuation

ENHANCEMENT OF POISON ELIMINATION

A Multiple-dose activated charcoal
B Forced diuresis
C Alteration of urinary pH
D Chelation (see heavy metal section)
E Extracorporal removal
   1 Peritoneal dialysis
   2 Hemodialysis
   3 Hemoperfusion
   4 Hemofiltration
   5 Plasmapheresis
   6 Exchange transfusion
F Hyperbaric oxygenation

ADMINISTRATION OF ANTIDOTES

A Neutralization by antibodies
B Neutralization by chemical binding
C Metabolic antagonism
D Physiologic antagonism

PREVENTION OF REEXPOSURE

A Adult education
B Child-proofing
C Notification of regulatory agencies
D Psychiatric referral

charcoal has comparable or greater efficacy, fewer contraindications and complications, and is less invasive than ipecac or gastric lavage. Alternative methods should be used if the ingested agent is not well absorbed by activated charcoal. Unless there has been a witnessed ingestion of a potentially severe overdose, the use of a large-bore gastric lavage tube is rarely indicated in an asymptomatic patient, since serious complications (aspiration or esophageal perforation) may result from the forcible use of a lavage tube in an uncooperative patient.

When an accurate history is not obtainable and a poison causing delayed toxicity or irreversible damage is suspected, blood and urine should be sent for toxicologic screening and, if indicated, for quantitative analysis. Due to continuing absorption and distribution, blood levels may be greater than those in tissue and may not correlate with toxicity. However, high blood levels of agents whose metabolites are more toxic than the parent compound (acetaminophen, ethylene glycol, or methanol) may indicate the need for additional interventions (antidotes, dialysis).

After evaluation and decontamination, some patients may be sent home because the predicted toxicity is minimal or the time of expected maximal toxicity has passed without incident. Observation for at least

4 to 6 h after gastrointestinal tract decontamination ensures that most patients who remain asymptomatic can be discharged safely. However, patients ingesting agents that slow gastric emptying and intestinal motility (anticholinergics, narcotics, sedative hypnotics, salicylates), have slow dissolution and absorption characteristics (carbamazepine, phenytoin, enteric-coated tablets, lithium, salicylate, and sustained-release preparations), or tend to form bezoars or concretions (enteric-coated tablets, meprobamate, salicylate) may require longer observation. In such patients, documentation of a charcoal stool prior to discharge should prevent delayed absorption and subsequent toxicity.

From the time of onset of poisoning to the time of peak effects (the toxic phase), management is based primarily on clinical and laboratory findings. Resuscitation and stabilization are the first priority. All symptomatic patients should have an intravenous line, supplemental oxygen, cardiac monitoring, continuous observation, and baseline laboratory, ECG, and x-ray evaluation. Patients with altered mental status, particularly those with coma or seizures, should be given an intravenous bolus of glucose, naloxone, and thiamine and additional antidotes as indicated. Decontamination measures should be initiated as soon as possible. Further absorption of ingested poisons should be limited by administering activated charcoal or gastric lavage. Since aspiration is a hazard, ipecac syrup should be used with caution. Patients may be given charcoal by mouth or by a stomach tube. Administering a dose of charcoal both before and after gastric lavage may be more effective than giving charcoal only after lavage. An initial dose of charcoal can be given by small-bore (no. 18 French or less) nasogastric tube while monitoring and supportive measures are being initiated. Once the patient is stable, lavage with a large-bore orogastric tube can be followed with a second dose of charcoal. The rare patient who deteriorates after this regimen should be lavaged and given another dose of charcoal.

Measures that enhance poison elimination may shorten the duration of toxicity and lessen its severity. However, the risks must be weighed against the benefits. Diagnostic certainty (usually via laboratory confirmation) is generally a prerequisite. Intestinal dialysis using activated charcoal is safe and effective in enhancing the elimination of many poisons. Diuresis and chelation therapy are effective in enhancing the elimination of a relatively small number of poisons, and their use is associated with potential complications. Extracorporal methods are effective in removing many poisons, but the expense and risk make their use reasonable only in patients who would otherwise not have a favorable outcome.

Patients with severe poisoning (coma, respiratory depression, hypotension, cardiac conduction abnormalities, cardiac arrhythmias, hypothermia or hyperthermia, seizures), those needing close monitoring or antidotes or enhanced elimination therapy, those showing progressive clinical deterioration, and those with significant underlying medical problems should be admitted to an intensive care unit. Patients with mild to moderate toxicity can be managed on a general medical service, intermediate care unit, or emergency department observation area depending on the anticipated duration and level of monitoring needed (intermittent clinical observation versus continuous clinical, cardiac, and respiratory monitoring). Patients who have attempted suicide require continuous observation until they seem unlikely to make further attempts.

Between peak toxicity and full recovery (the resolution phase of poisoning), supportive care should continue until the patient is alert and laboratory and ECG abnormalities are resolved. Repeat charcoal dosing may prevent rebound toxicity when depressed gastrointestinal function improves and the poison still in the gut is absorbed or additional active metabolites are formed. Since poison is eliminated from the blood before tissues, blood levels are generally lower than tissue levels during this phase and once again may not correlate with toxicity. This is particularly true when extracorporal elimination procedures are used. Because of redistribution of poison, a rebound increase in blood level and clinical relapse may occur after the termination of such procedures. When a metabolite is responsible for toxic effects, continued treatment of an asymptomatic patient may be necessary because of a previous or present toxic blood level (acetaminophen, ethylene glycol, and methanol).

Prior to discharge, patients with accidental ingestions (and/or the caregivers) should be instructed about preventive measures, and suicidal patients should receive appropriate psychiatric assessment, disposition, and follow-up.

SUPPORTIVE CARE

The goal of supportive therapy is to maintain physiologic homeostasis until detoxification is accomplished and to prevent and treat secondary complications such as aspiration, bed sores, cerebral and pulmonary edema, pneumonia, rhabdomyolysis, sepsis, renal failure, and generalized organ dysfunction due to prolonged hypoxia or shock.

In addition to those needing urgent endotracheal intubation, many poisoned patients require semielective endotracheal intubation for protection of the airway against aspiration of gastrointestinal contents and of the poison itself. The gag reflex alone is not a reliable indicator of the need for intubation. Since patients may maintain airway patency while being stimulated but not if left unattended, those who cannot respond to voice or who are unable to sit and drink fluids without assistance are best managed by prophylactic intubation. Patients with severe excitation also may require intubation for airway protection (due to the risk or existence of seizures) and sedation or paralysis for control of agitation and prevention of hyperthermia, acidosis, and rhabdomyolysis. Since clinical assessment is often inaccurate, the need for oxygenation and ventilation is best determined by analyses of arterial blood gases.

Drug-induced pulmonary edema is usually noncardiac rather than cardiac in nature. Profound CNS depression and cardiac conduction abnormalities suggest the latter etiology. Measurement of pulmonary artery pressure may be necessary to establish etiology and direct appropriate therapy. Arrhythmias can result from direct cardiotoxicity, abnormal cardiovascular reflexes, or metabolic derangements. Supraventricular tachycardia associated with hypertension and CNS excitation is almost always due to sympathetic, anticholinergic, or hallucinogenic stimulation or to drug withdrawal (see Table 395-1). Most cases are mild or moderate in severity and require only observation or nonspecific sedation with a benzodiazepine. If severe or associated with hemodynamic instability, chest pain, or ECG evidence of ischemia, specific therapy is indicated. Hypoxia, hypoglycemia, and other metabolic causes of sympathetic stimulation also should be ruled out. For patients with sympathetic hyperactivity, treatment with a combined alpha and beta blocker (labetalol) or a combination of beta blocker and vasodilator (esmolol and nitroprusside) is preferred. For those with anticholinergic poisoning, physostigmine is the treatment of choice. Supraventricular tachycardia without hypertension is generally secondary to vasodilation or hypovolemia and responds to fluid administration.

Ventricular tachyarrhythmias may be caused by sympathetic stimulation, myocardial membrane destabilization, or metabolic derangements. Lidocaine and phenytoin are generally safe, but beta blockers can be hazardous unless the arrhythmia is clearly from sympathetic hyperactivity. In tricyclic antidepressant poisoning, quinidine and procainamide are contraindicated (because of similar electrophysiologic effects), but sodium bicarbonate may be therapeutic. Magnesium sulfate and overdrive pacing (by isoproterenol or a pacemaker) may be useful in patients with torsades de pointes and prolonged QT intervals. Magnesium and antidigoxin antibodies are used in patients with severe digitalis poisoning. Invasive (esophageal or intracardiac) ECG recording may sometimes be necessary to determine the origin (ventricular or supraventricular) of wide-complex tachycardias (see Chap. 198). If the patient is hemodynamically stable, however, it may be prudent to observe rather than to treat with a potentially harmful cardioactive agent. Arrhythmias may be resistant to drug therapy until underlying acid-base and electrolyte derangements, hypoxia, and hypothermia are corrected.

Bradyarrhythmias associated with hypotension generally should be treated as described in Chap 197. In beta blocker and calcium channel blocker poisoning, the administration of calcium and glucagon, respectively, may be effective. Antibody therapy may be indicated for digitalis poisoning. The management of hypotension is described in Chap. 34. If hypotension is unresponsive to volume expansion, norepinephrine or high-dose dopamine may be indicated.

Drug-induced seizures may be due to direct or indirect CNS neuroreceptor stimulation (or inhibition), neuronal membrane destabilization, ischemia, edema, or metabolic abnormalities. Seizures due to excessive stimulation of catecholamine receptors (sympathomimetic or hallucinogen poisoning and drug withdrawal) or decreased activity of gamma-aminobutyric acid (GABA) (isoniazid poisoning) or glycine (strychnine poisoning) are best treated with GABA agonists such as benzodiazepines or barbiturates. Seizures caused by isoniazid, which inhibits the synthesis of GABA, may not respond to agonist therapy until GABA synthesis is restored, because agonists act, at least partially, by promoting the release of GABA from presynaptic vesicles. High doses of pyridoxine, which is necessary for the synthesis of GABA, are often necessary to terminate such seizures. For poisons with central dopaminergic effects (phencyclidine), an agent with opposing activity, such as haloperidol, may be useful. Seizures resulting from membrane destabilization (beta blocker, cyclic antidepressant poisoning) may require a membrane-active agent such as phenytoin as well as a GABA agonist. In rare cases (anticholinergic or cyanide poisoning), specific antidotal therapy may be necessary.

The treatment of seizures secondary to ischemia, edema, or metabolic abnormalities should include correction of the underlying cause. Since prolonged convulsions can lead to rhabdomyolysis and severe acidosis, neuromuscular paralysis is indicated in refractory cases. EEG monitoring and continuing treatment of seizures are necessary to prevent permanent neurologic damage.

Invasive interventions, such as extracorporal membrane oxygenation, intraaortic balloon pump counterpulsation, and partial (femoral) cardiopulmonary bypass pump circulatory support, should be considered in severe but reversible poisoning. Temperature extremes; metabolic, hepatic, and renal abnormalities; and secondary complications should be treated by standard measures.

PREVENTION OF POISON ABSORPTION

GASTROINTESTINAL DECONTAMINATION *Syrup of ipecac* is administered orally in a dose of 30 mL for adults, 15 mL for children, and 10 mL for small infants. Clear liquids also should be given. Ipecac irritates the stomach and stimulates the central chemoreceptor trigger zone. Vomiting usually occurs approximately 22 min following administration. The dose may be repeated if vomiting does not occur. Experimentally, ipecac decreases chemical absorption by an average of 57 percent (range 28 to 73 percent) if given within 5 min of ingestion and about 30 percent (range 2 to 45 percent) if given within half an hour. Because there are no suitable control groups, its efficacy in overdose patients is not established. Side effects include lethargy in children (12 percent) and protracted vomiting (8 to 17 percent). Chronic ipecac use (by patients with anorexia nervosa or bulimia) may cause electrolyte and fluid abnormalities, cardiac toxicity, and myopathy. Except for aspiration, serious complications are rare. Isolated cases of gastric and esophageal tears and perforations and stroke have been reported. Ipecac is contraindicated in patients with recent gastrointestinal surgery, CNS depression, seizures, and ingestions of corrosives and rapidly acting CNS poisons (camphor, cyanide, tricyclic antidepressants, propoxyphene, strychnine).

Gastric lavage is performed using a no. 28 French orogastric tube in children and a no. 40 French tube in adults with volumes of about 5 mL fluid per kilogram of body weight. Except for infants, tap water is acceptable. The patient should be placed in Trendelenburg and left lateral decubitus positions to prevent aspiration (even if an endotracheal tube is in place). Experimentally, lavage decreases chemical absorption by an average of 69 percent (range 54 to 84 percent) if performed within 5 min of ingestion, 31 percent (range 26 to 38 percent) if performed at 30 min, and 11 percent (range 8 to 13 percent) if performed at 60 min. Its efficacy is similar to that of ipecac. Significant amounts of ingested drug are recovered in a tenth of patients. As with ipecac, its effect on the clinical outcome of poisoned patients is not known. Aspiration is a common complication (up to 10 percent), especially when lavage is improperly performed. Serious complications (tracheal lavage, esophageal and gastric perforation) occur in approximately 1 percent of patients. For this reason, only a physician should insert the lavage tube, and the patient must be restrained (with pharmacologic sedation if necessary) during the procedure. Gastric lavage is contraindicated in patients with ingestion of corrosives and petroleum distillate hydrocarbons because of the risk of aspiration-induced hydrocarbon pneumonia and gastroesophageal perforation.

Activated charcoal, as a suspension in water alone or with a cathartic, is given orally via a nippled bottle (for infants), cup, straw, or small-bore nasogastric tube (for uncooperative patients). The recommended dose is 1 to 2 g/kg of body weight, using 8 mL of diluent per gram of charcoal, if a premixed formulation is not available. Palatability may be increased by adding a sweetener (sorbitol) or a flavoring agent (cherry, chocolate, or cola syrup) to the suspension. Charcoal adsorbs ingested poisons within the gut lumen, allowing the charcoal-toxin complex to be evacuated with stool. The complex also can be removed from the stomach by induced emesis or lavage. In vitro, charcoal adsorbs 90 percent or more of most poisons when given in a ratio 10 times that of the toxin. Superactivated charcoal (SuperChar) is two to three times more effective than standard charcoal. Charged (ionized) chemicals such as mineral acids, alkalis, and highly dissociated salts of cyanide, fluoride, iron, lithium, and other inorganic compounds are not well adsorbed by charcoal. Experimentally, charcoal decreases the absorption of other chemicals by an average of 80 percent when given within 5 min of administration, 59 percent when given at 30 min, and 33 percent at 60 min. Charcoal is of equal or greater efficacy than ipecac syrup or gastric lavage. Lavage followed by charcoal is more effective than charcoal alone, and charcoal before and after lavage is more effective than charcoal alone or charcoal after lavage. In general, the clinical outcome after treatment with charcoal alone is more favorable than in those given ipecac followed by charcoal and those treated with lavage followed by charcoal. In comatose patients treated within 1 h of ingestion, however, the combination of lavage and charcoal may be more effective than charcoal alone. Side effects of charcoal include nausea, vomiting, and diarrhea or constipation. Charcoal also may prevent the absorption of orally administered therapeutic agents. Complications include mechanical obstruction of the airway, aspiration, vomiting, and bowel obstruction by inspissated charcoal. Charcoal is contraindicated in patients with corrosive ingestion because it obscures endoscopy.

Whole-bowel irrigation is performed by administering a bowel cleansing solution containing electrolytes and polyethylene glycol (Golytely, Colyte) orally or by gastric tube at a rate of up 0.5 L/h in children and 2.0 L/h in adults until rectal effluent is clear. The patient must be in a sitting position. Although data are limited, whole-bowel irrigation may be as or more effective than the previously discussed procedures, particularly in patients with foreign body, drug packet, and slow-release medication ingestions.

Cathartic salts (disodium phosphate, magnesium citrate and sulfate, sodium sulfate) or *saccharides* (mannitol, sorbitol) promote the rectal evacuation of gastrointestinal contents. The most effective cathartic is sorbitol in a dose of 1 to 2 g/kg of body weight. Alone, cathartics do not prevent poison absorption, except perhaps for the agents noted under whole-bowel irrigation. Their primary use is to prevent constipation following charcoal administration. Abdominal

cramps, nausea, and occasional vomiting are side effects. Complications of repeated dosing include hypermagnesemia and excessive diarrhea. The agents are contraindicated in patients who have ingested corrosives and in those with preexisting diarrhea. Magnesium-containing cathartics should not be used in patients with renal failure.

Dilution is accomplished by having the patient drink 5 mL/kg of body weight of water or other clear liquid as soon as possible after the ingestion of a corrosive (acids, alkali). Dilution also may be used as an adjunct to ipecac syrup. Otherwise, it is not indicated because it may increase the dissolution rate (and hence absorption) of capsules, tablets, and other solids.

Endoscopic or surgical removal of poisons may be useful in rare situations such as ingestion of a potentially toxic foreign body that fails to transit the gastrointestinal tract, a potentially lethal amount of a heavy metal (arsenic, iron, mercury, thallium), or large concretions of pills. Patients who ingest packets of drugs (cocaine) and then become toxic due to packet leakage or rupture require immediate surgical intervention.

DECONTAMINATION OF OTHER SITES Immediate copious flushing with water, saline, or other available clear drinkable liquid is the initial treatment of topical exposures (particularly with corrosives and solvents). Saline is preferred for eye irrigation. A triple wash (water then soap then more water) may be optimal for dermal decontamination. Inhalational exposures should be treated initially with fresh air or oxygen. The removal of liquid poisons from body cavities such as the vagina or rectum is best accomplished by irrigation. Solid poisons (drug packets, pills) should be manually removed with visual guidance.

ENHANCEMENT OF POISON ELIMINATION

Although the elimination of most poisons can be accelerated by therapeutic interventions, pharmacokinetic efficacy (removal of drug at a rate greater than that accomplished by intrinsic elimination) and the clinical benefits (shortened duration of toxicity, improved outcome) are often more theoretical than proven. Hence the decision to use a procedure should be based on the actual or predicted toxicity and the potential efficacy, cost, and risks of therapy.

MULTIPLE-DOSE ACTIVATED CHARCOAL Repeated oral dosing with charcoal (with sorbitol as needed to enhance gastrointestinal motility) enhances the elimination of some poisons. A dose of 1 g/kg of body weight every 2 to 4 h, adjusted downward to avoid regurgitation in patients with decreased gastrointestinal motility, is generally recommended. Experimentally, this treatment enhances the elimination of most drugs and chemicals tested (carbamazepine, dapsone, diazepam, digoxin, glutethimide, meprobamate, methotrexate, phenobarbital, phenytoin, salicylate, theophylline, valproic acid). Efficacy approaches that of hemodialysis for some agents (theophylline). Multiple-dose therapy is not effective in accelerating elimination of chlorpropamide, imipramine, or agents poorly adsorbed to charcoal.

FORCED DIURESIS AND ALTERATION OF URINARY pH Diuresis and ion trapping via alteration of urine pH may prevent the renal reabsorption of poisons that undergo excretion by glomerular filtration and active tubular secretion. Since membranes are more permeable to nonionized molecules than to their ionized counterparts, acidic (low pK_a) poisons are ionized and trapped in an alkaline urine, and basic poisons are ionized and trapped in an acid urine. Alkaline diuresis (a urine pH of 7.5 or greater and a urine output of 3 to 6 mL/kg of body weight per hour) enhances the elimination of chlorphenoxyacetic acid herbicides, chlorpropamide, diflunisal, fluoride, methotrexate, phenobarbital (and probably other long-acting barbiturates), and salicylates. Contraindications include congestive heart failure, renal failure, and cerebral edema. Acid-base, fluid, and electrolyte parameters should be carefully monitored. Saline diuresis may enhance the excretion of bromide, calcium, fluoride, lithium, meprobamate, potassium, and isoniazid. Acid diuresis enhances the renal elimination of amphetamines, chloroquine, cocaine, local anesthetics, phencyclidine, quinidine, quinine, sympathomimetics, strychnine, and tocainide. Its use, however, has been largely abandoned because risks are significant and clinical efficacy has not been established.

EXTRACORPORAL REMOVAL Peritoneal dialysis, hemodialysis, charcoal or resin hemoperfusion, hemofiltration, plasmapheresis, and exchange transfusion are capable of removing any toxin from the bloodstream. Toxins most amenable to enhanced elimination by dialysis have low molecular mass (<500 Da), high water solubility, low protein binding, small volumes of distribution (<1 L/kg of body weight), prolonged elimination (long half-life), and high dialysis clearance relative to total-body clearance. The efficacy of the other forms of extracorporal removal is not limited by molecular weight, water solubility, or protein binding. Dialysis should be considered in severe poisoning due to bromide, chloral hydrate, ethanol, ethylene glycol, isopropyl alcohol, lithium, methanol, salicylate, and possibly heavy metals. Although hemoperfusion may be more effective in removing some of these poisons, it does not correct associated acid-base and electrolyte abnormalities.

Hemoperfusion should be considered in severe poisoning due to chloramphenicol, disopyramide, and hypnotic-sedatives (barbiturates, ethchlorvynol, glutethimide, meprobamate, methaqualone, phenytoin, procainamide, and theophylline). Both techniques require central venous access and systemic anticoagulation and often result in transient hypotension. Hemoperfusion also may cause hemolysis, hypocalcemia, and thrombocytopenia. Peritoneal dialysis and exchange transfusion are less effective but may be used when other procedures are not available, are contraindicated, or are technically difficult (in infants). Exchange transfusion removes poisons affecting red blood cells (e.g., methemoglobinemia or arsine-induced hemolysis). The efficacy of other extracorporeal elimination procedures has not been defined.

Candidates for these invasive treatments include patients with severe toxicity who deteriorate despite aggressive supportive therapy; those with potentially prolonged, irreversible, or fatal toxicity; and those with dangerous blood levels of toxins, those who lack the capacity for self-detoxification because of liver or renal failure, and those with serious underlying illnesses or complications that adversely affect recovery.

OTHER TECHNIQUES The elimination of heavy metals can be enhanced by chelation and urinary excretion of the metal-chelator complex, and the elimination of carbon monoxide can be increased by hyperbaric oxygenation, as discussed with the specific poisons.

ADMINISTRATION OF ANTIDOTES

Antidotes counteract the effects of poisons by neutralizing them (antibody-antigen reactions, chelation, chemical binding) or by antagonizing their physiologic effects (activation of opposing nervous system activity, provision of competitive metabolic or receptor substrate). Antidotes can significantly reduce morbidity and mortality, but most antidotes are potentially toxic. Poisons or conditions with specific antidotes include acetaminophen, anticholinergic agents, anticoagulants, benzodiazepines, beta blockers, calcium channel blockers, carbon monoxide, cholinergic agents, cyanide, digitalis, drugs that cause dystonic reactions, ethylene glycol, fluoride, heavy metals, hydrogen sulfide, hypoglycemic agents, isoniazid, methemoglobinemia, narcotics, sympathomimetics, and vacor. Since the safe use of antidotes requires correct identification of a specific poisoning or syndrome, antidotal therapy is discussed with the conditions for which they are indicated.

PREVENTION OF REEXPOSURE

Poisoning is a preventable illness. Unfortunately, some adults and children are poison-prone, and recurrences are common. Adults with accidental exposures should be instructed regarding the safe use of medications and chemicals (according to labeling instructions). Confused patients may need assistance with the administration of medications. Errors in dosing by health care providers require special educational efforts. Patients should be advised to avoid circumstances that result in chemical exposure or poisoning. Appropriate agencies and health departments should be notified in cases of environmental or workplace exposure. The best approach with young children and patients with intentional overdose is to limit access to poisons. In households where children live or visit, alcoholic beverages, medications, household products (automotive, cleaning, fuel, pet-care, toiletry products), nonedible plants, and vitamins should be kept out of reach or in locked or child-proof cabinets. Depressed or psychotic patients should be given prescriptions for a limited supply of drugs and with a limited number of refills. All patients should be monitored for compliance and response to therapy.

SPECIFIC POISONS

The poisons discussed in this section are common, produce life-threatening toxicity, or require unique therapeutic interventions. Poisons not mentioned here are described in the referenced texts. Drug and alcohol abuse are discussed in Chaps. 390 to 392. Heavy metal poisoning is discussed in Chap. 396.

ACETAMINOPHEN At therapeutic doses, acetaminophen is metabolized to sulfate and glucuronide conjugates that are excreted in the urine. Minor amounts are excreted unchanged or as mercapturic acid after conjugation with hepatic glutathione. Following an acute overdose of 140 mg/kg of body weight or more, the sulfate and glucuronide pathways become saturated, resulting in an increased fraction of acetaminophen metabolized to mercapturic acid. Once hepatic glutathione is depleted, reactive metabolites are formed that bind covalently to hepatocytes and cause cell lysis. Acetaminophen is rapidly absorbed from the stomach and small bowel and has a volume of distribution of 1 L/kg of body weight. Plasma concentrations range from 160 to 660 μmol/L (0.5 to 2.0 mg/dL) following therapeutic doses. The plasma half-life is usually 2 to 4 h but may be prolonged following overdose.

Clinical toxicity Early manifestations of poisoning are nonspecific and not predictive of subsequent hepatotoxicity. Within 2 to 4 h of ingestion, nausea, vomiting, diaphoresis, and pallor develop. CNS depression is absent unless depressant drugs are coingested. Within 24 to 48 h, hepatotoxicity is evidenced by right upper quadrant tenderness and mild hepatomegaly and followed by the appearance of jaundice, clotting abnormalities, and hepatic encephalopathy. Renal function also may be impaired. Laboratory evidence of hepatic toxicity includes elevation in serum transaminase activity (AST, ALT). With severe poisoning, prolongation of the prothrombin time, elevation of serum bilirubin, and ultimately hyperammonemia may occur. A twofold prolongation of prothrombin time and/or serum bilirubin greater than 68 μmol/L (4 mg/dL) on the third to fifth day after ingestion indicate hepatotoxicity. Histologic evidence of liver damage varies from cytolysis to centrilobular necrosis. In patients who recover, liver function returns to normal within 1 week, and liver histology returns to normal within 3 months.

Diagnosis A serum acetaminophen level should be determined between 4 and 24 h after ingestion and compared against the Rumack-Matthew nomogram (Fig. 395-1). A level above the lower line on the nomogram indicates possible hepatotoxicity and the need for antidotal therapy.

Treatment In patients who present within 4 h of ingestion, initial treatment involves gastrointestinal decontamination. Activated charcoal should be administered. (Charcoal does not significantly interfere with acetylcysteine therapy.) In patients with a potentially toxic acetaminophen level, acetylcysteine is given at a loading dose of 140 mg/kg of body weight, followed by a maintenance dose of 70 mg/kg of body weight every 4 h for 17 doses. Treatment is most

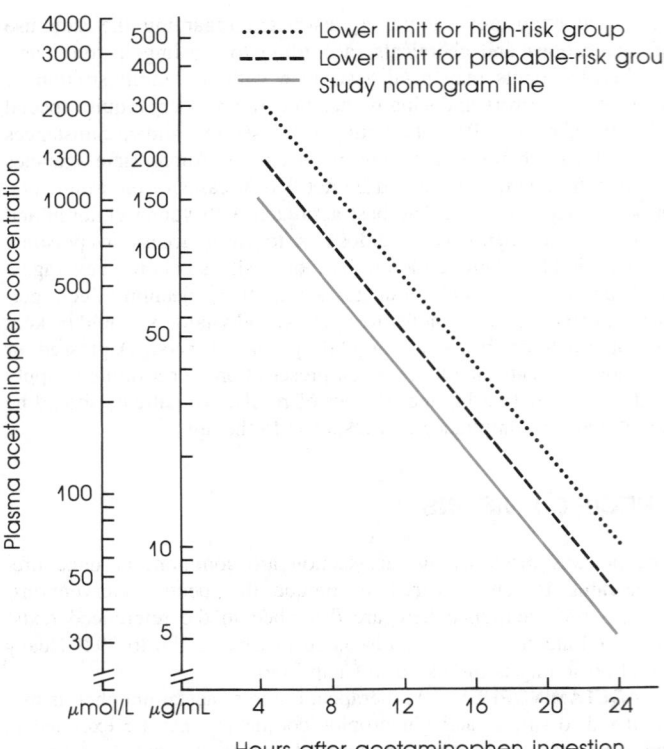

FIGURE 395-1 Nomogram to define risk according to initial plasma acetaminophen concentration. (*After BH Rumack, H Matthew, Pediatrics 55:871, 1975.*)

effective if started within 8 to 10 h but may have some benefit up to 24 h following ingestion. Side effects include nausea, vomiting, and epigastric discomfort. If treatment is started prior to availability of the serum level and if the level is subsequently shown to be below the toxic level, therapy may be discontinued.

ACIDS AND ALKALI   Common alkaline products include industrial-strength bleach, drain cleaners (sodium hydroxide), surface cleaners (ammonia, phosphates), laundry and dishwasher detergents (phosphates, carbonates), disk batteries, denture cleaners (borates, phosphates, carbonates), and Clinitest tablets (sodium hydroxides). Acids are used in toilet bowl cleaners (hydrofluoric, phosphoric, sulfuric acids), soldering fluxes (hydrochloric acid), antirust compounds (hydrofluoric, oxalic acids), automobile battery fluid (sulfuric acid), and slate cleaners (hydrofluoric acid).

Alkalies produce liquefactive necrosis with rapidly penetrating tissue burns and higher risk of perforation of the esophagus and stomach than do acids. Acids produce coagulative necrosis. Both burn the mouth, esophagus, and stomach. The lack of oral involvement does not rule out esophageal or gastric injury, however. Liquids tend to produce superficial, often circumferential burns over a larger surface area, while solids and tablets cause localized deeper burns. The severity of the burn relates to the contact time, amount ingested, and the pH (especially <2, >12) of the ingested product.

Clinical toxicity   Burns of the mouth result in excess salivation, pain, dysphonia, and dysphagia. Examination of the mouth shows erythema, edema, ulceration, and necrosis. Deep burns may destroy mucosal nerve endings and produce anesthesia. Esophageal symptoms and signs include drooling, painful swallowing, retrosternal pain, and neck tenderness. Vomiting of blood and mucus may occur. Perforation following alkali ingestion is suggested by increased severity of chest pain, often with respiratory distress. Epigastric pain, vomiting, and tenderness may occur with burns to the stomach. Aspiration of acids and alkalis results in fulminant tracheitis and bronchial pneumonia. In severe cases, hypotension, shock, metabolic acidosis, liver and renal dysfunction, hemolysis, and disseminated intravascular coagula-

tion may be seen. Edema, erythema, and ulceration of the esophagus may be followed by fibrosis with stricture formation and obstruction of the esophagus (in the case of alkalis) or of the gastric outlet (in the case of acids).

Diagnosis   A careful history will suggest the ingestion of an acid or an alkali. Endoscopy should be safe within 48 h (optimally 12 to 24 h) of the ingestion in all symptomatic patients. It will document the anatomic site and often the severity but not the depth of the injury. Residual effects of the ingestion can be assessed by barium swallow. Chest and abdominal x-rays and routine laboratory values should be obtained to evaluate for aspiration, perforation, and organ dysfunction.

Treatment   Treatment consists of immediate dilution. Weak acid or basic solutions should not be used because the heat of neutralization may cause thermal burns and increase tissue injury. Glucocorticoids have traditionally been used for alkali burns to prevent stricture formation. Controlled clinical data, however, have failed to show efficacy in preventing stricture formation following transmucosal (third-degree) injury, and first- and second-degree injuries do not result in stricture formation. Animal studies suggest that therapy should be initiated immediately on presentation. If used, a dose of 1 to 2 mg prednisone per kilogram every 4 to 6 h for at least 2 weeks is suggested. Prophylactic broad-spectrum antibiotic use is controversial. Glucocorticoids are not useful for acid burns. Antacids should be used for burns of the stomach. Esophageal stricture or gastric outlet obstruction may require subsequent dilation and bouginage or surgical reconstruction.

ANTIARRHYTHMIC DRUGS   Only drugs that act by blocking myocardial cell membrane sodium channels are discussed here. These agents can be divided into three subclasses: class IA (disopyramide, procainamide, quinidine, and moricizine), class IB (lidocaine, mexiletine, phenytoin, and tocainide), and class IC (encainide, ethmozine, propafanone, and flecainide). The pharmacology is presented in Chap. 198. Because of toxicity, some agents have been withdrawn from the market. These agents are rapidly absorbed (except for disopyramide and sustained-release formulations), have volumes of distribution ranging from 1 to 10 L/kg, have half-lives of 3 to 11 h, and are predominantly eliminated by hepatic metabolism.

Clinical toxicity   The acute ingestion of more than twice the usual daily dose is potentially toxic. Onset of toxicity occurs within 1 h, and peak effects are demonstrable within several hours. Toxicity also may develop during chronic therapeutic use. Manifestations include nausea, vomiting, and diarrhea, followed by lethargy, confusion, ataxia, bradycardia, hypotension, and cardiovascular collapse. Anticholinergic effects (blurred vision, dry mucosa) may be seen in disopyramide poisoning. Quinidine and class IB agents may cause agitation, dysphoria, and seizures. Nonspecific ECG findings include bradycardia with AV block and QRS-interval prolongation. Ventricular tachycardia, ventricular fibrillation (including the polymorphous form, torsades de pointes), and QT-interval prolongation are characteristics of poisoning due to class IA and IC drugs. Depressed myocardial contractility and arrhythmias may lead to decreased cardiac output and pulmonary edema. Hypoglycemia and mild hypokalemia may be seen with disopyramide and quinidine intoxication, respectively. Toxicology screening will detect most of these agents. Measurement of serum levels may confirm an overdose and indicate the need for monitoring.

Treatment   Treatment consists of gastrointestinal decontamination and supportive therapy. Hypotension, bradyarrhythmias, and seizures are treated with standard measures. Patients with persistent hypotension and bradycardia require monitoring of pulmonary arterial pressure. Cardiac pacing, intraaortic balloon pump counterpulsation, and cardiopulmonary bypass may be necessary. Ventricular tachyarrhythmias that cause hemodynamic instability should be treated with lidocaine, phenytoin, and bretylium. Sodium bicarbonate or sodium lactate (1 mmol/kg by intravenous bolus) may be effective for tachyarrhythmias due to class IA or IC agents. Mild hypokalemia may be protective, and potassium levels that do not fall below 3.0 mmol/L may be best treated by close monitoring. For torsades de pointes (polymorphous or atypical ventricular tachycardia), magnesium sulfate (4 g or 40 mL of a 10% solution intravenously as an initial dose) and overdrive pacing (with isoproterenol or electricity) may be effective. Hemodialysis and hemoperfusion may enhance the elimination of disopyramide, the active procainamide metabolite N-acetylprocainamide, and possibly other agents. However, clinical experience is inadequate to support routine use.

BARBITURATES Barbiturates are GABA receptor agonists and inhibit excitable cells of the CNS and other tissues. Long-acting barbiturates include mephobarbital, barbital, phenobarbital, and primidone. Short-acting agents include those with intermediate, short, and ultrashort durations of action such as amobarbital, aprobarbital, butabarbital, butalbital, pentobarbital, and secobarbital.

Barbiturates are well absorbed from the stomach and the small bowel. Peak plasma concentrations generally occur at a therapeutic dose within 1 to 4 h, with short-acting agents peaking earlier than long-acting ones. Barbiturates are weak acids with pK_a values ranging from 7.2 to 8.5, volumes of distribution of 0.8 to 1.5 L/kg of body weight, and 45 to 70 percent protein binding in the plasma. Most barbiturates are primarily eliminated by hepatic metabolism. Some long-acting agents are converted to active metabolites: mephobarbital to barbital and primidone to phenobarbital and phenylethylmalonanide (PEMA). In contrast to short-acting agents, long-acting ones also undergo significant renal excretion: 95 percent for barbital, 25 to 33 percent for phenobarbital, 15 to 42 percent for primidone, and 95 percent for PEMA. The half-life ranges from 1 to 6 days for long-acting agents and 3 to 48 h for short-acting ones.

Clinical toxicity Barbiturates cause CNS depression ranging from confusion and lethargy to deep coma. Hypothermia, hypotension, pulmonary edema, and cardiac arrest may occur in severe cases. Pupils are generally constricted but may dilate in terminal phases. Pressure sores can develop with prolonged coma. Bullous skin lesions are seen in severe barbiturate overdose. Signs of toxicity usually appear when serum concentrations of long-acting barbiturates exceed 170 μmol/L (4 mg/dL) and short-acting barbiturates exceed 88 μmol/L (2 mg/dL). Maximal toxicity occurs within 4 to 6 h after short-acting barbiturate but may be delayed 10 h or more after overdosage with long-acting barbiturates. Because of tolerance, the degree of CNS depression relative to ingested dose is dependent on prior exposure to the drug.

Treatment Initial management involves prompt gastrointestinal decontamination. Barbiturates are well adsorbed by activated charcoal. In the case of phenobarbital (and probably other long-acting barbiturate) poisoning, repetitive administration of activated charcoal every 2 to 4 h enhances elimination threefold and decreases half-life by approximately 50 percent. For all barbiturates, attention should be given to hemodynamic and respiratory support, correction of temperature and electrolyte derangements, and monitoring for pulmonary complications. Since short-acting barbiturates are predominantly metabolized by the liver, diuresis is ineffective. Renal elimination of phenobarbital (and probably other long-acting agents) is significantly enhanced by alkalinization of urine to a pH of 8 (by giving intravenous sodium bicarbonate) and by saline diuresis. Hemodialysis and hemoperfusion are effective in removing both long- and short-acting barbiturates, their use being reserved for severely intoxicated patients with high blood levels.

BENZODIAZEPINES Benzodiazepines potentiate the inhibitory effect of GABA on the CNS by binding to receptors at polysynaptic terminals where GABA is released, principally in the limbic system and the reticular formation of the midbrain.

Long-acting benzodiazepines include diazepam, chlordiazepoxide, clonazepam, flurazepam, clorazepate, quazepam, and prazepam. Short-acting agents include alprazolam, lorazepam, and oxazepam; ultra-short-acting agents include estrazolam, midazolam, temazepam, and triazolam. All benzodiazepines are well absorbed from the gastrointestinal tract, exhibit 85 to 99 percent protein binding in the plasma, are lipid soluble, and have an apparent volume of distribution of approximately 1.1 L/kg of body weight. They are weak acids with

pK_a values ranging from 1.3 to 6.2. Benzodiazepines are mainly eliminated by hepatic metabolism, and in the case of some (diazepam), the metabolites are pharmacologically active. Metabolites are generally excreted in the urine, whereas only a small amount of the parent compound is excreted unchanged by the kidneys. Long-acting benzodiazepines have half-lives of 1 to 8 days, short-acting agents have half-lives of 6 to 24 h, and ultra-short-acting agents have half-lives of 3 to 12 h.

Clinical toxicity Effects are evident within 30 min of an overdose and include weakness, ataxia, drowsiness, and in severe cases, coma and respiratory depression. Paradoxical excitation may occur early in the course of poisoning. Pupils are generally constricted. Ethanol enhances the absorption of benzodiazepine and potentiates the CNS depression. Confirmation of the diagnosis is made by identification of the metabolites in urine.

Treatment Initial management includes prompt gastrointestinal decontamination. Single-dose as well as repeated-dose activated charcoal is indicated. Respiratory support is rarely needed except in the case of ultra-short-acting agents, massive overdose, or the coingestion of other sedative drugs. Flumazenil, a competitive benzodiazepine receptor antagonist, can reverse CNS and respiratory depression and obviate the need for endotracheal intubation. It is administered intravenously in incremental doses of 0.2, 0.3, and 0.5 mg at 1-min intervals until the desired effect is achieved or a cumulative dose of 3 to 5 mg has been given. Since flumazenil has a relatively short duration of action, patients must be monitored carefully for relapse. Should this occur, treatment can be repeated (at intervals of 20 min with a maximum dose of 3 mg/h). Failure to respond to flumazenil suggests that benzodiazepines are not the cause of poisoning. Flumazenil can cause seizures in patients who have coingested stimulants and tricyclic antidepressants and should not be used in these situations. It also can cause seizures (withdrawal syndrome) in patients who are physically dependent on benzodiazepines as a result of chronic high-dose use. The lowest effective dose should be used in these patients. High protein binding of benzodiazepines limits efficacy of hemodialysis.

BETA-ADRENERGIC BLOCKING AGENTS Beta-adrenergic blocking agents include acebutolol, atenolol, betaxolol, carteolol, esmolol, labetalol, metoprolol, nadolol, penbutolol, pindolol, propranolol, sotalol, and timolol. These drugs act by competitively blocking beta-adrenergic neurohumoral receptors in the bronchial and vascular smooth muscle and myocardium. At therapeutic doses, some beta blockers act predominantly on $beta_1$ receptors and are "cardioselective" (acebutolol, atenolol, betaxolol, metoprolol), some have partial agonist or sympathomimetic activity (acebutolol, carteolol, pindolol, timolol, and possibly penbutol), and some have quinidine-like myocardial membrane stabilizing effects (acebutolol, metoprolol, pindolol, propranolol, sotalol, and possibly betaxolol). Antiarrhythmic effects are due to a reduction of sodium and calcium influx during membrane depolarization (phase 0) as a consequence of decreased production of cyclic AMP by adenylate cyclase. This activity defines beta blockers as class II antiarrhythmics. Beta blockers decrease cardiac contractility by directly inhibiting the release of calcium from sarcoplasmic reticulum. Following overdose, cardioselectivity is often lost, and all beta blockers may cause membrane depressant effects.

Beta blockers are rapidly and well absorbed, exhibit variable protein binding (5 to 93 percent), and have low water solubility and variable volumes of distribution (0.23 to 10.0 L/kg of body weight). Most beta blockers are eliminated predominantly by hepatic metabolism. Atenolol, carteolol, nadolol, and sotalol are primarily eliminated by renal excretion, and esmolol is metabolized by serum esterases.

Clinical toxicity Effects usually begin within 1/2 h following an overdose and become maximal within 2 h. Common findings include nausea, vomiting, and diarrhea, followed by bradycardia, hypotension, and CNS depression. However, agents with sympathomimetic activity can cause hypertension and tachycardia. CNS effects vary from lethargy and confusion to coma and seizures and tend to be more pronounced with highly lipophilic agents (acebutolol, metoprolol, pindolol, propranolol, and timolol). The skin is often pale and cool. Bronchospasm and pulmonary edema are uncommon unless there is a history of asthma, chronic obstructive pulmonary disease, or congestive heart failure. Metabolic abnormalities include hyperkalemia and hypoglycemia (as a direct result of beta-adrenergic receptor blockade) and metabolic acidosis (due to seizures, shock, or respiratory depression). ECG manifestations include all degrees of AV block, bundle branch block, prolonged QRS duration, and asystole. Sotalol poisoning also may cause QT-interval prolongation with ventricular tachycardia, ventricular fibrillation, and torsades de pointes. Patients with mild poisoning usually recover within 6 to 12 h, whereas those with severe poisoning may be symptomatic for 24 to 48 h. A toxicology screen may identify the presence of beta blockers, but blood levels are not generally available nor helpful in guiding therapy.

Treatment   Treatment includes gastrointestinal decontamination, nonspecific supportive measures, and the administration of calcium and glucagon. Because gastric emptying procedures may produce vagal stimulation and exacerbate bradyarrhythmias, monitoring should be instituted first. Treatment of bradycardia and hypotension should begin with atropine, isoproterenol, and vasopressors (dopamine, dobutamine, epinephrine, and norepinephrine have been used with variable success, alone or in combination). With severe poisoning, these agents may be ineffective, and glucagon, calcium, cardiac pacing (external or internal), and intraaortic balloon pump support may be necessary. Glucagon, which stimulates adenylate cyclase by a nonadrenergic mechanism, should be given at an initial dose of 5 to 10 mg for adults. Patients who respond favorably should then be given an infusion of 1 to 5 mg/h. Calcium, which may reverse nonadrenergic negative inotropic effects, should be given in the same initial dose as described for calcium channel blocker poisoning. Patients with altered mental status or abnormal vital signs also should be given an intravenous bolus of glucose. Bronchospasm may be treated with inhaled beta agonist, subcutaneous epinephrine, and intravenous aminophylline. Lidocaine, magnesium (as for antiarrhythmic poisoning), or overdrive pacing may be used for sotalol-induced ventricular tachyarrhythmias. Extracorporal elimination procedures are probably not of benefit, with the possible exceptions of atenolol, carteolol, metoprolol, nadolol, and sotalol.

BLEACH   Bleach (Clorox) solutions for home use generally contain 3 to 6% sodium hypochlorite, and industrial bleaches may have higher concentrations. These solutions have a pH or 10.5 to 11.0 and contain free chlorine, which gives the compound its characteristic odor.

Sodium hypochlorite decomposes to hypochloric acid on contact with moisture and is irritating but not caustic. Sodium hypochlorite mixed with acid releases chlorine gas and, when mixed with ammonia, produces chloramine gas. Both these gases are highly irritating.

Clinical toxicity   Sodium hypochlorite is irritating to the gastrointestinal mucosa and to mucous membranes of the lips, mouth, and eyes. Household bleach causes only superficial injury to the esophagus, but industrial bleaches cause deep burns of the esophagus with the potential for stricture formation. Chemical pneumonia and pulmonary edema may result from the aspiration of bleach or inhalation of chlorine and chloramine.

Treatment   Ingestion of small quantities of household bleach should be treated only by dilution. Large ingestions of sodium hypochlorite may require gastric lavage. When concentrated solutions have been ingested, therapy should be similar to that for acids and alkali. Neutralization is not necessary, and activated charcoal and cathartics are not indicated. Exposed skin and eyes also should be decontaminated. Treatment of pulmonary toxicity is symptomatic and supportive.

CALCIUM CHANNEL BLOCKERS   Calcium channel blocking agents include bepridil, felodipine, isradipine, diltiazem, nicardipine, nifedipine, nimodipine, and verapamil. These agents act by decreasing the influx of calcium across slow calcium channels in the membranes of myocardial and vascular smooth-muscle cells during phases 2

(plateau) and 4 (spontaneous depolarization) of the action potential. Electrophysiologic effects include decreased cardiac contractility, heart (SA nodal) rate, AV nodal conduction, and vascular tone. These actions define calcium channel blockers as class IV antiarrhythmics. Beprenil also has class I antiarrhythmic activity.

Calcium channel blockers are rapidly absorbed, exhibit high (80 to 99 percent) protein binding in the plasma, and have large volumes of distribution ranging from 0.6 to 10.0 L/kg of body weight. They are predominantly eliminated by hepatic metabolism, and their half-lives range from 1 to 24 h.

Clinical toxicity   Effects begin within 1/2 to 1 h of ingestion of amounts 5 to 10 times the usual therapeutic dose. Toxicity may be delayed following overdoses of sustained-release preparations. Clinical manifestations include bradycardia, hypotension, and CNS depression. Mental status changes range from confusion and drowsiness to coma and seizures and are due both to direct membrane effects and to cerebral hypoperfusion. Hypotension may precipitate myocardial ischemia, and depression of cardiac function may lead to pulmonary edema. ECG findings include all degrees of AV block, prolonged QRS and QT intervals (mainly with verapamil), evidence of ischemia or infarction, and asystole. Metabolic acidosis (secondary to shock) and hyperglycemia (resulting in the inhibition of insulin release) may be present. Serum calcium levels, however, remain normal.

Treatment   Gastrointestinal tract decontamination should be accomplished as soon as possible. Symptomatic bradycardia should be treated with atropine, calcium, isoproterenol, glucagon, and electrical (external or internal) pacing. Calcium, as the 10% chloride or gluconate salt solution, is given in a dose of 0.2 mL/kg of body weight (up to 10 mL) intravenously over 5 min. This dose may be repeated up to four times in patients with a partial, transient, or absent response, provided that serum calcium levels are monitored. A continuous calcium infusion (0.2 mL/kg of body weight per hour up to a maximum of 10 mL/h) may be appropriate when relapse occurs after an initial bolus. Although electrical pacing is often required, glucagon, in the same dose as for beta-blocker poisoning, should be tried first. Hypotension that persists despite resolution of bradycardia should be treated with fluids and vasopressors. Amrinone, dopamine, dobutamine, glucagon, and norepinephrine, alone or in combination, have been used. The benefit of restored perfusion is particularly important in patients with organ ischemia. Intraaortic balloon pump support should be used in patients unresponsive to the preceding measures. Patients with mild toxicity usually recover within a few hours, whereas those with severe toxicity or overdose with sustained-release preparations may remain symptomatic for 24 h or longer. Extracorporal removal techniques are unlikely to be of benefit.

CARBON MONOXIDE   Carbon monoxide is produced in large amounts in industry as well as by gasoline engines, home appliances, and the incomplete combustion of wood, natural gas, and tobacco products. In addition, methylene chloride, a solvent in paint removers, is metabolized to carbon monoxide.

Carbon monoxide is rapidly absorbed through the lungs and binds to hemoglobin (forming carboxyhemoglobin) with an affinity 210 times that of oxygen. This limits oxygen-carrying by hemoglobin and also decreases the release of oxygen to tissues (the oxygen dissociation curve shifts to the left). Carbon monoxide also binds to myoglobin, decreasing its oxygen-carrying capacity, and to mitochondrial cytochrome oxidase, thereby inhibiting cellular respiration. The net effect is profound tissue hypoxia, anaerobic metabolism, and lactic acidosis. Once carbon monoxide exposure is discontinued, dissociation of the hemoglobin–carbon monoxide complex occurs, and carbon monoxide is excreted through the lungs. In room air, the carbon monoxide half-life is 4 to 6 h; the half-life decreases to 40 to 80 min when breathing 100% oxygen and to 15 to 30 min with hyperbaric oxygen therapy. The apparent half-life after methylene chloride exposure is considerably longer.

Clinical toxicity   Manifestations of carbon monoxide poisoning include shortness of breath, dyspnea, tachypnea, headache, emotional lability, confusion, impaired judgment, clumsiness, and syncope. Nausea, vomiting, and diarrhea also may occur. Cerebral edema, coma, respiratory depression, and pulmonary edema occur with severe poisoning. Cardiovascular manifestations include ischemic chest pain, arrhythmias, heart failure, and hypotension. Blisters and bullae may develop over pressure points. Myoglobinuria secondary to muscle necrosis may result in renal failure. The "cherry red" color of skin and mucous membranes is rare, and cyanosis is usual. Visual field defects, blindness, and venous engorgement with papilledema or optic atrophy may be noted. Arterial blood gases reveal metabolic acidosis, a normal P_{O_2} decreased oxygen saturation (by direct CO-oximetry measurement rather than a calculated or pulse oximetry value), and normal or slightly decreased P_{CO_2}.

Traditionally, levels of 20 to 30 percent are associated with mild symptoms, 30 to 50 percent with moderate symptoms, 50 to 60 percent with severe symptoms, and levels above 60 percent are often fatal. While elevated carboxyhemoglobin levels document carbon monoxide exposure, they do not necessarily correlate with the severity of the poisoning. Serum creatine phosphokinase (CPK) and lactate dehydrogenase (LHD) levels may be elevated.

Up to the 30 percent of patients with loss of consciousness develop persistent neuropsychiatric sequelae evident 1 to 3 weeks after exposure. Manifestations vary from subtle personality changes and intellectual impairment to gross neurologic deficits such as blindness, deafness, incoordination, and parkinsonism.

Treatment The patients should be removed from the site of exposure. In conscious patients, oxygen (100%) should be administered by a non-rebreather mask at 10 L/min until carbon monoxide levels are less than 10 percent and all symptoms have resolved. Infants and pregnant women require treatment for several more hours because fetal hemoglobin has a high affinity for carbon monoxide. Endotracheal intubation and mechanical ventilation with 100% oxygen are indicated in patients with coma, significant CNS dysfunction, or cardiovascular instability. Hyperbaric oxygen at 2 to 3 atm decreases the half-life of carbon monoxide to 15 to 30 min and produces sufficient dissolved oxygen to prevent tissue hypoxia. Arrhythmias and hypotension are treated by usual measures. Patients with coma, syncope, or seizures and those with signs or symptoms of neurologic or cardiovascular dysfunction that do not resolve with oxygen and supportive therapy are candidates for hyperbaric oxygen therapy. Hyperbaric oxygenation shortens the duration of coma and may prevent delayed sequelae.

COCAINE See Chap. 392.

CYANIDE Hydrogen cyanide is used as a fumigant rodenticide and in chemical syntheses. Cyanide salts are used in photography, metallurgy, electroplating, metal cleaning, and ore refining. Organic cyanide compounds (nitriles) are used in the synthetic rubber industry, artificial nail removers, and rodenticides. Cyanogenic glycosides are present in the seeds of the chokeberry, cherry, plum, peach, apricot, pear, bean, apple, and crabapple.

Cyanide inhibits mitochondrial ferricytochrome oxidase and hence blocks electron transport, resulting in decreased oxidative metabolism and oxygen utilization. Lactic acidosis occurs as a consequence of anaerobic metabolism. Cyanide is rapidly absorbed from the stomach, lungs, mucosal surfaces, and unbroken skin. In the stomach it reacts with hydrochloric acid, liberating hydrocyanic acid, which is absorbed as cyanide ion. Cyanide is 60 percent protein-bound, is concentrated in red cells, and has a volume of distribution of 1.5 L/kg of body weight. Cyanide is metabolized by the mitochondrial enzyme rhodanase, which mediates the transfer of sulfur from thiosulfate to the cyanide ion producing thiocyanate, which in turn is excreted in the urine.

Clinical toxicity The lethal dose of potassium or sodium cyanide is 200 to 300 mg and of hydrocyanic acid is 50 mg. Effects begin within seconds of inhalation and within 30 min of ingestion. Initial manifestations of cyanide poisoning include headache, faintness, vertigo, excitement, anxiety, burning sensation in the mouth and throat, and dyspnea. Cardiovascular effects include tachycardia and

hypertension. Nausea, vomiting and diaphoresis are common. A bitter almond odor may be detected on the breath. Later effects include coma, convulsions, opisthotonus, trismus, paralysis, respiratory depression, pulmonary edema, arrhythmias, bradycardia, and hypotension. Variable correlation exists between blood cyanide levels and symptoms: Levels less than 8 μmol/L (0.02 mg/L) are associated with no symptoms, 20 to 40 μmol/L (0.05 to 0.1 mg/dL) with flushing and tachycardia, 40 to 100 μmol/L (0.1 to 0.25 mg/dL) with obtundation, 100 to 200 μmol/L (0.25 to 0.3 mg/dL) with coma and respiratory depression, and levels greater than 120 μmol/L (0.3 mg/dL) with death. Other laboratory abnormalities include lactic acidosis and narrowing of the arteriovenous oxygen saturation difference. ECG abnormalities include both tachyarrhythmias and bradyarrhythmias such as nodal or idioventricular rhythm, AV dissociation, and progressive slowing of heart rate.

Treatment Initial management involves general supportive measures and gastrointestinal decontamination. Since blood cyanide measurements are difficult to obtain, antidotal therapy using amyl nitrite, sodium nitrite, and sodium thiosulfate (the Lilly cyanide antidote kit) coupled with high-dose oxygen must be initiated on the basis of the history and clinical findings. Amyl nitrite is administered for 30 s of each minute. The ampule is broken between two pads of gauze and placed over the airway while the patient breathes spontaneously or is ventilated by a bag-mask unit. A new ampule should be used every 3 min. This process is continued while sodium nitrite is being prepared but may be omitted if endotracheal intubation has been performed or if sodium nitrite is available. Sodium nitrite is administered intravenously as a 3% solution at a rate of 2.5 to 5.0 mL/min up to a total dose of 10 to 15 mL (300 to 450 mg). The dose in children is 0.33 mL/kg of body weight (10 mg/kg of body weight). Sodium thiosulfate is then administered intravenously as a 25% solution at a dose of 50 mL (12.5 g) given over 1 to 2 min. The dose in children is 0.33 mL/kg of body weight (10 mg/kg of body weight). Sodium thiosulfate is then administered intravenously as a 25% solution at a dose of 50 mL (12.5 g) given over 1 to 2 min. The dose in children is 1.65 mL/kg of body weight (0.5 g/kg of body weight). With recurrent or persistent symptoms, half or full doses of both sodium nitrite and sodium thiosulfate are administered. The rationale for antidotal therapy is as follows: Nitrites induce methemoglobinemia; methemoglobin has a higher affinity for cyanide than does cytochrome oxidase, thereby promoting its dissociation from this enzyme; thiosulfate reacts with the cyanide that is slowly released from cyanomethemoglobin, forming the relatively nontoxic thiocyanate, which is excreted in the urine. Oxygen reverses the binding of cyanide to cytochrome oxidase sites and enhances the efficacy of sodium nitrite and sodium thiosulfate, in addition to acting as a substrate for metabolism. The value of hyperbaric oxygen therapy, however, has not been proven.

DIGOXIN Digitalis (cardiac glycoside) poisoning occurs most frequently as overdosage during therapeutic or suicidal use of digoxin and on occasion with plant (oleander) ingestion. Cardiac glycosides act by inhibiting the enzyme sodium-potassium ATPase, leading to increased intracellular Na^+ and Ca^{2+} and decreased K^+. Digoxin is slowly absorbed and slowly distributed. Serum levels may not correlate with pharmacologic effects for up to 8 h following a therapeutic oral dose. Digoxin is 25 to 30 percent protein-bound in the plasma, has a large volume of distribution of 5 to 6 L/kg of body weight, and is localized in skeletal muscle, liver, and heart. Elimination is primarily by renal excretion. The half-life ranges between 36 and 45 h, is prolonged in hepatic failure and in renal failure, and may be shortened in overdose. Approximately 60 percent of a dose is excreted unchanged by the kidneys, and the remainder is metabolized by the liver to inactive metabolites. The mean therapeutic serum concentration ranges from 0.6 to 2.5 nmol/L (0.5 to 2.0 ng/mL).

Clinical toxicity Symptoms of toxicity include vomiting, confusion, delirium, and occasionally hallucinations, blurred vision, photophobia, scotomata, and disturbed color perception. Cardiac manifestations include sinus arrhythmia, sinus bradycardia, and all degrees of atrioventricular block. Premature ventricular contractions, bigeminy, ventricular tachycardia, and fibrillation also occur. The combination of supraventricular tachyarrhythmia and AV block is highly suggestive of digitalis toxicity. While bradyarrhythmias and hypokalemia are common with chronic intoxication, tachyarrhythmias and hyperkalemia are generally seen with acute poisoning. Similarly, serum digoxin levels may be minimally elevated or even therapeutic in chronic toxicity, whereas they are usually markedly elevated following acute overdose. Clinical toxicity occurs with digoxin levels in excess of 3.8 to 6.4 nmol/L (3 to 5 ng/mL), and levels as high as 64 to 77 nmol/L (50 to 60 ng/mL) have been seen in the overdose setting. Levels measured sooner than 8 h after ingestion may not reflect complete tissue distribution.

Treatment Gastrointestinal decontamination should be accomplished as soon as possible, since emesis and gastric intubation may cause vagal stimulation, which may worsen existing conduction block. Activated charcoal is preferred. Repeated doses should be administered because this therapy also can enhance elimination of digoxin metabolites. Diuresis, hemodialysis, and hemoperfusion are ineffective, however. Potassium, magnesium, and calcium abnormalities should be corrected. Electrical pacing may be necessary when sinus bradycardia and second- and third-degree heart block result in hypotension and fail to respond to atropine and isoproterenol. Magnesium sulfate (as for antiarrhythmia poisoning), as well as phenytoin and lidocaine, may be useful in the treatment of ventricular tachyarrhythmias. Digoxin-specific Fab fragment antibodies are also available for the treatment of potentially life-threatening intoxication not immediately responsive to the above. Each 40-mg vial can neutralize 0.6 mg digoxin. Fab fragment antibodies are appropriate for patients with refractory arrhythmias and significantly elevated serum digoxin concentrations. Following their administration, cardiac arrhythmias and hyperkalemia are generally corrected within an hour; the antibodies are given intravenously over 30 min, unless cardiac arrest has occurred, in which case the solution is given as a bolus. The drug-antibody complex is excreted in the urine with a half-life of 16 to 20 h. In patients with renal failure, the drug-antibody complex is metabolized over a period of days to weeks. Although free digoxin levels rapidly decrease to zero following antibody administration, routine methods used to measure digoxin do not differentiate between bound and unbound drug and will have no correlation with toxicity after such therapy. Antibodies cross-react with other cardiac glycosides, but larger doses may be needed for toxicity not involving digoxin.

Formulas and tables for calculating the dose of antibody based on body weight and post-distribution serum digoxin level or the amount of drug acutely ingested are available in the package insert. Unfortunately, toxicity may occur before distribution is complete or before levels are available, the amount of an acute overdose may be unknown, the antibody is expensive, and calculated doses often exceed the effective dose. The following approach is therefore suggested. In patients with chronic digoxin intoxication, whose total-body drug load only slightly exceeds the therapeutic amount and who may be dependent on digoxin for its inotropic effects, begin with a dose of 1 to 2 vials. In acute digoxin overdose, begin with a dose of 5 to 10 vials. These doses may be repeated if necessary, but they will be effective in all but the most severe cases.

ETHANOL See Chap. 390.

ETHYLENE GLYCOL Ethylene glycol is a colorless, odorless, sweet-tasting, water-soluble liquid that is used as a solvent for paints, plastics, and pharmaceuticals and in the manufacture of explosives, fire extinguishers, foams, hydraulic fluids, windshield cleaners, radiator antifreeze, and de-icer preparations.

Ethylene glycol is rapidly absorbed. Peak levels occur approximately 2 h following ingestion. Ethylene glycol has a volume of distribution of 0.6 to 0.8 L/kg of body weight. It is oxidized by alcohol dehydrogenase to glycoaldehyde, which is then metabolized to glycolic acid, glyoxylic acid, and oxalic acid. As much as 20

percent is excreted unchanged in the urine. The half-life ranges from 3 to 8 h. Since alcohol dehydrogenase has a higher affinity for ethanol than ethylene glycol, ethanol is preferentially metabolized when both alcohols are present. Ethanol inhibits metabolism of ethylene glycol and prolongs its half-life to about 17 h. Ethylene glycol and its metabolites produce CNS depression in overdose. Ethylene glycol is more intoxicating than ethanol in this respect. Glycolic acid is responsible for decreased serum bicarbonate, metabolic acidosis, and increased anion gap, as well as for interstitial and tubular damage to the kidney. Glyoxylic acid is more toxic than glycolic acid, but because it is oxidized so rapidly to oxalic acid, glycolic acid contributes little to the toxicity of ethylene glycol. Oxalic acid may precipitate as calcium oxalate crystals in the brain, heart, kidney, lung, pancreas, and urine and may result in hypocalcemia.

Clinical toxicity As little as 120 mg/kg of body weight or 0.1 mL/kg of body weight (one swallow) of pure ethylene glycol can result in a potentially toxic blood concentration of 3 mmol/L (20 mg/dL). Effects begin 30 min following ingestion and include nausea, vomiting, slurred speech, ataxia, nystagmus, and lethargy. A faint, sweet aromatic odor may be detected on the breath. Coma, seizures, respiratory depression, cardiovascular collapse, and death may occur. Effects caused by metabolites begin 4 to 12 h following ingestion. At this stage the patient appears more ill than intoxicated. Manifestations include tachypnea, hypotension, agitation, confusion, lethargy, coma, and seizures. Hypocalcemia occurs in a third of patients. Leukocytosis is present in the majority. In severe cases, adult respiratory distress syndrome, cyanosis, pulmonary edema, and cardiomegaly may be seen. In this stage the diagnosis is suggested by metabolic acidosis, an increased anion gap (low bicarbonate and chloride), and an abnormal urinalysis (crystalluria). In patients who survive the early stages, acute tubular necrosis manifested by proteinuria, oliguria, and anuria ensues 12 to 24 h following ingestion. Renal failure may be permanent but typically lasts days to weeks. In early intoxication, osmolality is elevated. Later, an elevated anion gap and decreased serum bicarbonate and chloride are observed. Signs of alcohol-like intoxication suggest a serum ethylene glycol level greater than 8 to 16 mmol/L (50 to 100 mg/dL). Survival has been reported with levels as high as 100 mmol/L (650 mg/dL).

Diagnosis Diagnosis is suggested by a history of exposure to antifreeze in association with CNS depression, an elevated serum osmolality, and a large anion gap. Ethylene glycol and glycolic acid levels should be measured along with routine laboratory tests. Oxalate crystals in the urine suggest the diagnosis.

Treatment Gastrointestinal lavage and activated charcoal should be administered. Supportive measures include protection of the airway and ventilatory and circulatory support. Seizures should be treated with phenytoin, a short-acting barbiturate, or a benzodiazepine. Hypocalcemia is treated with intravenous calcium salts at a dose of 7 to 14 mL (a 10% solution diluted 10 to 1 with intravenous fluids and given at a rate of 1 mL/min). Metabolic acidosis should be corrected with sodium bicarbonate. Large doses are often required. Fluids and diuretics may reverse oliguria but do not enhance the elimination rate of ethylene glycol. Indications for ethanol therapy include a history or strong suspicion of ethylene glycol ingestion, an ethylene glycol concentration greater than 3 mmol/L (20 mg/dL), and acidosis regardless of the absolute ethylene glycol concentration. A serum ethanol level of at least 20 mmol/L (100 mg/dL) is required to inhibit alcohol dehydrogenase (higher levels may be needed with very high ethylene glycol concentrations). The loading and maintenance doses of ethanol are the same as for methanol poisoning. Serum ethanol and ethylene glycol concentrations should be monitored frequently. Hemodialysis reduces ethylene glycol half-life from 17 h on ethanol therapy to 3 h and enhances the elimination of toxic metabolites. Indications for hemodialysis include metabolic acidosis not readily correctable with bicarbonate and ethanol therapy, failure to improve despite treatment, ethylene glycol concentrations greater than 8 mmol/L (50 mg/dL), or renal failure. Supplemental thiamine and pyridoxine also may be beneficial.

HALLUCINOGENS (See also Chap. 392) Hallucinogens belong to three chemical classes, phenylalkylamines, tryptamines, and ergolines, with mescaline, psilocybin, and lysergic acid diethylamide (LSD) being the prototype for each. Large numbers of synthetic analogues exist in each class. Mescaline is a derivative of the peyote cactus which grows in the southwestern United States. Psilocybin is derived from mushrooms. Lysergic acid is found in the fungus *Claviceps purpurea*, which grows as a contaminant on rye and wheat and in morning glory seeds. Hallucinogens act by altering the function of the central (and peripheral) neurotransmitter serotonin.

Hallucinogens are well absorbed from the gastrointestinal tract. Mescaline is also rapidly absorbed through the nasal mucosa. Mescaline has an apparent volume of distribution of 2 to 3 L/kg of body weight and is eliminated by hepatic metabolism. Psilocybin itself is inactive but is converted to the active metabolite psilocin. LSD is rapidly absorbed by both the nasal mucosa and gastrointestinal tract. Peak levels of LSD are achieved within 1 to 2 h following ingestion. LSD is protein-bound (80 to 90 percent) and has an apparent volume of distribution of 0.8 L/kg of body weight and is metabolized to inactive metabolites with a half-life of 3 h.

Clinical toxicity Hallucinogens produce disordered thought, mood changes, and sensory misperceptions (auditory, gustatory, olfactory, and visual dysesthesias). The physiologic effects of LSD last for 4 to 6 h and include mydriasis, conjunctival injection, piloerection, hypertension, tachycardia, tachypnea, anorexia, tremors, and hyperreflexia. Psychological effects include loss of body image, visual illusions, and alteration of the senses. The psychological effects ("trip") generally last for 6 to 12 h and can be pleasant or alarming. The EEG may show paroxysmal discharges, and seizures may occur. Flashbacks or recurrences of visual images may appear up to 18 months after ingestion. The effects of mescaline include nausea, vomiting, and mild physiologic stimulation (see Table 395-2). Psilocybin has effects similar to those of LSD, with unique features including fever, hypotonia, and seizures.

Diagnosis Identification of LSD in serum is difficult because of its low concentration. In urine, LSD can be detected for up to 5 days following ingestion, and mescaline can be detected for up to 24 h. Psilocybin is not detected in the routine toxic screens.

Treatment Gastrointestinal decontamination is not useful once symptoms are present and may lead to further exacerbation of symptoms. The mainstay of therapy is prevention of physical injury by calming in a quiet room with low lights. Physical restraint may cause hyperthermia, rhabdomyolysis, and acute renal failure. Benzodiazepines are effective for acute panic reaction, and butyrephenones (haloperidol in particular) may be indicated for severe psychotic reactions (see Chap. 392).

HYDROCARBONS Hydrocarbons exist in a number of forms, including aromatic hydrocarbons, such as xylene and toluene, halogenated hydrocarbons, such as carbon tetrachloride and trichlorethane, and petroleum distillate hydrocarbons, such as gasoline, lacquer thinner, mineral seal oil, kerosene, and lighter fluid.

All hydrocarbons are CNS depressants. They are rapidly absorbed following inhalation or pulmonary aspiration. Aromatic and halogenated hydrocarbons are also absorbed following ingestion and are toxic to the gastrointestinal tract, heart, lung, liver, and kidneys. Aromatic hydrocarbons also can cause bone marrow suppression and skeletal muscle damage. Petroleum distillate hydrocarbons are poorly absorbed following ingestion but are toxic to the gastrointestinal tract, CNS and lungs. Lung involvement is predominantly due to aspiration pneumonitis.

Clinical toxicity Hydrocarbons produce excitation in low dose and depression of the CNS in high dose. Rarely, coma and seizures may occur. Psychosis, cerebral and cerebellar atrophy, encephalopathy, and peripheral neuropathy can result from chronic exposure. Other effects include nausea, vomiting, abdominal pain, hepatitis, renal tubular acidosis, acute hepatic or renal failure, and rhabdomyolysis. Sudden death due to myocardial irritability and ventricular fibrillation may occur following hydrocarbon sniffing. Petroleum distillate hydrocarbons cause burning of the mouth and throat with subsequent nausea, vomiting, and diarrhea. Respiratory effects include cough, dyspnea, tachypnea, wheezing, rhonchi, rales, hypoxia, and cyanosis. Lethargy is the most prominent CNS manifestation. Coma and convulsions are rare. Following aspiration, chest x-ray abnormalities include infiltrates, atelectasis, effusions, pneumothorax, and pneumatoceles. Metabolic acidosis with decreased serum calcium chloride phosphate and potassium may result from aromatic hydrocarbon poisoning. Laboratory diagnosis of aromatic, halogenated, or petroleum distillate hydrocarbon poisoning is not available at present.

Treatment The ingestion of aromatic and halogenated hydrocarbons requires prompt gastric lavage. Ipecac-induced emesis is contraindicated, and activated charcoal is ineffective. Supportive therapy includes oxygen, respiratory support, and monitoring of liver, renal, and myocardial function. In the case of petroleum distillate hydrocarbons, unless very large amounts (greater than 18 mL/kg of body weight) are ingested, gastric lavage and ipecac-induced emesis are contraindicated. Activated charcoal is both ineffective and hazardous because it may induce emesis. Pulmonary aspiration is treated by supportive therapy and by monitoring for superimposed bacterial infection. Glucocorticoids are ineffective. CNS effects are relatively short-lived and require careful monitoring and respiratory support.

HYDROGEN SULFIDE Hydrogen sulfide is a rapidly acting malodorous ("rotten eggs"), colorless, irritating gas that gains access to the blood through the mucous membranes of the tracheobronchial tree. It is encountered in the petroleum and mining industry, tanning of leather, vulcanization of rubber, production of synthetic fabrics, metal refining, production of heavy water for atomic reactors, and glue and felt manufacturing. It is also found in sewers, sulfur springs, the holds of fishing vessels, and as a by-product of manure storage.

The hydrogen sulfide anion inhibits electron transport in the cytochrome oxidase system, thereby inhibiting aerobic metabolism with resultant cellular anoxia and lactic acidosis. Hydrogen sulfide is detoxified to sulfate products that are principally excreted by the kidneys.

Clinical toxicity Hydrogen sulfide is highly irritating, resulting in rhinitis, conjunctivitis, and pharyngitis. Systemic effects include headache, vertigo, nausea, vomiting, confusion, seizures, and coma. It also produces hypoventilation, hypoxia, cyanosis, metabolic acidosis, pneumonia, and pulmonary edema. There is no readily available laboratory test, and the diagnosis is based on history and clinical features.

Treatment Treatment begins with prompt removal of the victim from the site of exposure. The airway should be cleared, ventilation should be assisted when indicated, and 100% oxygen should be administered. Nitrites (see "Cyanide" above) bind the sulfide ion by removing it from cytochrome oxidase sites, thereby forming a sulfide-methemoglobin complex (sulfmethemoglobin). They also enhance detoxification by acting as a catalyst for sulfide oxidation. Except for cardiac arrest, no clear-cut indications for nitrite administration exist. For optimal effectiveness, they must be utilized immediately in symptomatic patients (sulfide oxidation is so rapid that the amount of sulfide bound to cytochrome is minimal by the time the patient presents for treatment). The dosage schedule is the same as for cyanide poisoning (thiosulfate is not necessary). Hyperbaric oxygen should be considered in patients who do not respond to the preceding measures.

IRON Iron preparations contain ferrous salts that vary in elemental iron content (20 percent in the sulfate salt, 33 percent in the fumarate, and 12 percent in the gluconate). Ingestion of more than 20 mg/kg of body weight of elemental iron produces gastrointestinal toxicity and of more than 60 mg/kg of body weight results in systemic toxicity.

Ferrous iron is absorbed into mucosal cells of the duodenum and jejunum and is oxidized to ferric iron, where it is bound to ferritin. It is slowly released from ferritin into the plasma, where it is bound to transferrin, an iron-specific binding globulin, and transported to tissues for use in hemoglobin, cytochrome, and myoglobin synthesis. Approximately 70 percent of total-body iron is present as hemoglobin,

25 percent is stored in liver and spleen as ferritin and hemosiderin, and 5 percent is present in myoglobin and tissue enzymes. Iron bound to transferrin is nontoxic. Free iron that exceeds the iron-binding capacity and high ferritin levels are toxic to the vasculature and lead to the release of vasoactive substances such as serotonin and histamine. Increased capillary permeability, vasodilation, and fluid loss result in hypotension and metabolic acidosis. Free iron also injures mitochondria, causes lipid peroxidation, and results in renal, tubular, and hepatic necrosis and on occasion in myocardial and pulmonary injury. In overdose, iron is deposited in liver, spleen, and kidneys and causes fatty degeneration and necrosis in hepatocytes, renal tubules, and myocardial cells.

Clinical toxicity   Initial manifestations include vomiting and diarrhea (often bloody). X-rays may reveal iron tablets in the stomach or small bowel. A positive x-ray, fever above 101°F (38.5° C), hyperglycemia greater than 8.5 mmol/L (150 mg/dL), and leukocytosis white blood cell count (greater than 15,000 cells per cubic millimeter) are associated with serum iron levels above 50 μmol/L (300 μg/dL) and the potential for systemic toxicity. Systemic effects include lethargy, hypotension, and metabolic acidosis and, with severe poisoning, seizures, coma, pulmonary edema and vascular collapse. Jaundice, elevated hepatic enzymes, prolongation of prothrombin time, and hyperammonemia are indicative of liver injury. Proteinuria and cells in urine indicate renal injury. Pulmonary edema and hemorrhage are seen with severe overdose. In the recovering patient, gastric ulcerations and scars may cause outlet obstruction. Overgrowth of *Yersinia enterocolitica* with sepsis is a rare complication of iron overload.

Diagnosis   A serum iron concentration above the iron-binding capacity [a serum level generally greater than 50 μmol/L (300 μg/dL)] suggests serious poisoning. A positive urine deferoxamine provocative challenge test (a *vin rosé* color) indicating the presence of ferrioxamine (the complex of free iron bound to deferoxamine) is diagnostic and indicates an iron level greater than the iron-binding capacity.

Treatment   Removal of ingested iron is best accomplished with either ipecac-induced emesis or a large orogastric tube. An x-ray film following gastric lavage will define the success of the decontamination procedure. Whole-bowel irrigation, endoscopic removal, or gastrostomy may be necessary for concretion formation or large quantities of iron tablets. Activated charcoal is ineffective. Bicarbonate lavage (50 to 100 mL 1% solution) has been advocated in an effort to form insoluble ferrous carbonate salt. Oral deferoxamine is administered to complex iron remaining in the stomach into an insoluble, iron-deferoxamine complex (ferrioxamine). Since the amount of the deferoxamine required is large, and since iron is rapidly absorbed, these therapies are rarely used. Serum iron and total iron-binding capacity should be measured. Intravenous sodium bicarbonate should be used to correct metabolic acidosis. Hypotension may respond to volume expansion. Coagulation abnormalities should be treated with vitamin K or blood products.

When the serum iron level indicates potential systemic toxicity or exceeds the iron-binding capacity, parenteral deferoxamine should be administered. If levels are not immediately available, or if the patient has mild clinical toxicity, deferoxamine can be given intramuscularly in a challenge dose of 50 mg/kg up to 2 g. A *vin rosé* urine color indicates a positive test for free iron and the need for intravenous therapy. In those with a positive challenge test or with significant clinical toxicity, deferoxamine should be infused at a rate of 10 to 15 mg/kg per hour. Once the serum iron is less than the iron-binding capacity or the urine color has returned to normal, deferoxamine therapy can be discontinued. When iron levels exceed 180 μmol/L (1000 μg/dL), larger doses (up to 30 mg/kg per hour) of deferoxamine can be given. Exchange transfusion or plasmapheresis to remove the iron-desferal (ferrioxamine) complex should be reserved for patients with renal failure or for those who fail to respond to the preceding therapy.

ISONIAZID   Toxic doses of isoniazid decrease the synthesis of the inhibitory neurotransmitter GABA by inhibiting the pyridoxal phosphate–dependent enzyme glutamic acid decarboxylase. The consequence can be CNS stimulation or depression. Isoniazid is rapidly absorbed mainly from the small intestine. Peak serum concentrations occur within 1 to 2 h. The volume of distribution is approximately 0.6 L/kg of body weight. Serum protein binding is small. Isoniazid is primarily eliminated by acetylation to acetyl-isoniazid and then hydrolysis to isonicotinic acid. Approximately 15 percent of an ingested dose of isoniazid is excreted unchanged by the kidneys. The serum half-life of isoniazid in overdose is approximately 1 to 4 h.

Clinical toxicity   Effects begin within 30 min of ingestion of doses of greater than 20 mg/kg of body weight. Symptoms include nausea, vomiting, dizziness, slurred speech, lethargy, and confusion. The major manifestations include coma, respiratory depression, generalized seizures, and lactic acid acidosis. Seizures are protracted and relatively unresponsive to standard anticonvulsant therapy. Acidosis does not occur when seizures are prevented. Diagnosis is confirmed by identification of isoniazid in urine or blood. Toxicity occurs with concentrations as low as 15 μmol/L (2 mg/L). Significant symptoms are seen with serum concentrations greater than 30 to 35 μmol/L (4 to 5 mg/L).

Treatment   Initial therapy consists of prompt gastrointestinal decontamination and supportive measures. Ipecac-induced vomiting should be avoided because of the high incidence of seizures. Isoniazid is well adsorbed by activated charcoal. Seizures can sometimes be treated with benzodiazepines, barbiturates, and phenytoin but may be refractory to these agents. Pyridoxine (vitamin B6), however, is a cofactor for GABA synthesis and is efficacious in preventing and treating seizures. Diazepam is synergistic with pyridoxine. Bicarbonate may be necessary to correct acidosis. Pyridoxine should be given slowly intravenously in an amount equal to the ingested dose of isoniazid. When the ingested dose is not known, 5 g of pyridoxine should be administered. Pyridoxine should be given over 5 min to patients with seizures but over 30 min in the absence of seizures as a 5% to 10% concentration. Cessation of seizures and correction of metabolic acidosis are prompt. The dose may be repeated with partial response or when symptoms recur. Due to its low protein binding and small volume of distribution, isoniazid is efficiently removed by hemodialysis, but dialysis is rarely necessary because of the efficacy of pyridoxine.

ISOPROPYL ALCOHOL   Isopropyl alcohol is a component of rubbing alcohol, solvents, after-shave lotions, antifreeze, and window cleaners. Its metabolite, acetone, is found in cleaners, solvents, and nail polish removers.

Isopropyl alcohol and acetone are about twice as potent, as CNS depressants, as ethanol. Isopropyl alcohol is rapidly absorbed from the stomach and the lungs but only minimally through skin. It is distributed in body water and has a volume of distribution of 0.6 L/kg of body weight. Its half-life ranges from 3 to 6 h. Isopropyl alcohol is metabolized in the liver by the enzyme alcohol dehydrogenase to acetone, which is excreted by the kidneys and lungs with a half-life of 20 to 30 h. Up to 20 percent of isopropyl alcohol is excreted unchanged through the kidneys.

Clinical toxicity   Effects begin within 30 min of ingestion and include vomiting, abdominal discomfort, and hematemesis. A characteristic smell of rubbing alcohol may be noted. CNS manifestations include headache, dizziness, confusion, and excitation. With severe ingestion, obtundation, coma, respiratory depression, hypothermia, and hypotension may occur. Hypoglycemia may be seen. Isopropyl alcohol can cause a falsely elevated serum creatinine. A mild anion gap acidosis may be seen as well as an increase in the serum osmolality. Myopathy and hemolytic anemias are occasionally present. Concentrations of 8 to 17 mmol/L (50 to 100 mg/dL) produce lethargy, concentrations greater than 25 to 33 mmol/L (150 to 200 mg/dL) are associated with coma, and concentrations greater than 66 to 84 mmol/L (400 to 500 mg/dL) are potentially fatal.

Treatment Gastrointestinal decontamination must be instituted soon following ingestion. Activated charcoal is ineffective in significantly adsorbing isopropyl alcohol. The diagnosis is confirmed by elevated isopropyl alcohol (early) and acetone (late) levels. Supportive measures should include intravenous fluids and bicarbonate to correct dehydration, shock, and acidosis. Isopropyl alcohol and acetone are efficiently removed by hemodialysis. The procedure should be considered in patients with levels in the potentially lethal range [greater than 66 mmol/L (400 mg/dL)] or in patients inadequately managed by conservative therapy.

LITHIUM Lithium is most commonly available as the carbonate or the citrate salt. Lithium may substitute for cellular cations (K^+ and Na^+), thereby interfering with adenylate cyclase activation, inhibiting neurotransmitter (norepinephrine) release, and reducing sodium potassium ATPase activity.

The drug is rapidly absorbed from the gastrointestinal tract and reaches peak levels within 2 to 4 h of ingestion (later with overdosage and with sustained-release preparations). It has negligible plasma protein binding and a volume of distribution of approximately 0.6 L/kg of body weight. Removal from the body is primarily (95 percent) by glomerular filtration, with significant reabsorption (80 percent) by the proximal tubules. Lithium clearance is increased by alkalinization of the urine and decreased by hypovolemia and hyponatremia. Serum half-life ranges from 18 to 36 h; therapeutic levels range from 0.6 to 1.2 mmol/L.

Clinical toxicity Effects begin 1 to 4 h after ingestion. Gastrointestinal effects include nausea, vomiting, and diarrhea; neuromuscular effects include weakness, fasciculations, and twitching; CNS effects include ataxia, tremor, myoclonus, choreoathetosis, seizures, confusion, and coma; and cardiovascular effects include arrhythmias and hypotension. Hyperthermia may occur. Laboratory abnormalities include leukocytosis, hyperglycemia, albuminuria, glycosuria, and nephrogenic diabetes insipidus. ECG changes include sinus tachycardia or bradycardia, flattened or inverted T waves, atrioventricular block, and prolonged QT interval. In chronic intoxication, signs and symptoms occur at lower serum levels than with acute intoxication. In chronic poisoning, concentrations between 3 and 4 mmol/L may be associated with severe toxicity. In acute poisoning, serum levels may exceed 8 mmol/L despite minimal symptoms.

Treatment Within 2 to 4 h following ingestion, gastrointestinal decontamination is indicated. Lithium is poorly adsorbed by activated charcoal. Serial lithium levels should be measured until the peak level is achieved because both absorption and tissue distribution occur slowly in the overdose setting. Supportive therapy includes standard treatments for seizures, hypotension, and arrhythmias. Symptomatic patients with serum concentrations greater than 2 mmol/L require intravenous saline to correct dehydration and achieve a normal urine output. Diuresis and alkalinization of the urine are recommended to enhance renal excretion of lithium. Hemodialysis is indicated for severe intoxication and is frequently recommended in symptomatic patients with serum levels above 4.0 mmol/L. Hemodialysis may be indicated in chronic toxicity in patients with serum levels less than 4.0 mmol/L. It may need to be repeated or prolonged due to rebound in serum levels upon cessation of hemodialysis.

MONOAMINE OXIDASE (MAO) INHIBITORS MAO inhibitors include tranylcypromine, phenelzine, and isocarboxazid. These agents block monoamine oxidase, thus inhibiting a major pathway for catabolism of neurotransmitters such as dopamine, norepinephrine, and 5-hydroxytryptamine. Toxicity results from neurotransmitter accumulation and hence from potentiation of their actions.

MAO inhibitors are absorbed efficiently from the gastrointestinal tract. The volume of distribution is not known but is probably large. The drugs are eliminated predominantly by hepatic metabolism, and less than 5 percent is excreted unchanged in the urine. Plasma half-life of phenelzine and tranylcypromine at therapeutic doses is 24 h.

Clinical toxicity Effects may not begin until 6 to 12 h after ingestion and may not peak until 24 h following ingestion. Initial CNS effects include dilated pupils, hyperpyrexia, tachycardia, hypertension, and tachypnea (see Table 395-2). Nausea and vomiting also may occur. Agitation, hyperactivity, and confusion may be coupled with fasciculations, twitching, tremor, and rigidity. Cardiovascular collapse and CNS depression are late effects in severe poisoning. Toxic levels of MAO inhibitors have not been established, and no assay methods are commonly available.

Treatment Gastrointestinal decontamination should be performed as soon as possible. Hyperthermia should be treated with external cooling and sedation and in severe cases with neuromuscular paralysis. Dantrolene (2.5 mg/kg of body weight by mouth or intravenously every 6 h) may be effective for hyperthermia. Severe hypertension and tachycardia may require treatment with nitroprusside and propranolol, respectively. Hypotension should be treated with volume expanders, and pressor therapy should be administered with caution and at lower than normal initial doses because of the possibility of an exaggerated response. In fact, before any drug is given, potential adverse interactions should be investigated. Seizures and neuromuscular hyperactivity should be treated with benzodiazepines and barbiturates. Arrhythmias can be treated by usual measures. Diuresis, hemodialysis, and hemoperfusion are not effective. No specific antidote exists. Because of persistence of MAO inhibition, drug therapy and diet should be carefully controlled for 7 to 10 days after stopping the agents.

METHANOL Methanol is a component of shellacs, varnishes, paint removers, Sterno, windshield-washer solutions, and copy machine fluid. It is also a denaturant to make ethanol unfit for consumption.

Methanol, a slightly less potent CNS depressant than ethanol, is metabolized to formaldehyde and formic acid, which in turn causes metabolic acidosis and injury to the retina.

Methanol is rapidly and completely absorbed from the gastrointestinal tract, and peak levels occur within 1 to 2 h of ingestion. It is distributed throughout body water with a volume of distribution of 0.7 L/kg of body weight. Its protein binding is negligible. Elimination occurs predominantly by hepatic metabolism, with up to 10 percent excreted unchanged by the kidneys. Elimination follows first-order kinetics with a half-life of about 3 h at low serum levels (less than about 15 mmol/L or 50 mg/dL) and converts to zero-order kinetics with an elimination rate of 3 mmol/L per hour (8.5 mg/dL per hour) at higher levels. The rate of elimination at low overdose is approximately 14 to 20 h and at high overdose is 24 to 30 h. Inhibition of alcohol dehydrogenase by ethanol [20 to 30 mmol/L (100 to 150 mg/dL)] increases the elimination time to 30 to 35 h.

Clinical toxicity Onset is variable and may be delayed. Absence of signs and symptoms soon after ingestion should not be equated with absence of subsequent toxicity. Early manifestations are caused by methanol, and late manifestations are due to the metabolite formic acid. Methanol produces nausea, vomiting, abdominal pain, headache, vertigo, and confusion at low overdose. In large overdose [levels greater than 60 mmol/L (200 mg/dL)], obtundation, convulsions, coma, and an increased osmolal gap may be noted. Late manifestations include an increased anion gap, metabolic acidosis, and retinal injury and are due to acidosis secondary to accumulation of formic acid, lactic acid (the result of poor tissue perfusion), and ketones. Ophthalmologic manifestations occur 15 to 19 h or later following ingestion and include clouding and diminished vision, dancing and flashing spots, dilated or fixed pupils, hyperemia of the disk, retinal edema, and blindness. These changes are potentially reversible with prompt institution of therapy. With severe poisoning, myocardial depression, bradycardia, and shock may occur. Anuria predicts a poor prognosis.

Diagnosis Early diagnosis is suggested by ethanol-like signs of intoxication and an elevated serum osmolality and is confirmed by measurement of serum methanol [usually greater than 6 mmol/L (20 mg/dL)] 12 to 48 h following ingestion. The diagnosis of methanol-derived formic acidosis is suggested by a large anion gap, a low serum bicarbonate, an elevated serum formate level, and an elevated blood methanol. The diagnosis is confirmed by elevated serum methanol levels (early), elevated serum formate levels (late), or both.

Treatment Gastrointestinal decontamination is indicated soon after ingestion. Activated charcoal is not effective. Renal clearance is not increased by diuresis. Systemic acidosis should be corrected with sodium bicarbonate. Seizures should be treated with diazepam and phenytoin. Ethanol therapy is indicated in patients who are symptomatic or have a methanol level exceeding 6 to 9 mmol/L (20 to 30 mg/dL). The loading and maintenance doses of ethanol are as follows: loading dose—10 mL/kg of body weight of 10% ethanol intravenously or 1 mL/kg of body weight of 95% ethanol by mouth; maintenance dose—1.5 mL/kg of body weight per hour of 10% ethanol intravenously and 3.0 mL/kg of body weight per hour of 10% ethanol intravenously during dialysis. Therapy should be continued until the serum methanol level falls below 6 mmol/L (20 µg/dL) and all signs of toxicity are resolved. Hemodialysis is indicated when methanol levels exceed 15 mmol/L (50 mg/dL), for patients with visual signs, and when clinical or metabolic abnormalities are unresponsive to the preceding therapy. For patients seen late (12 to 24 h or more) after ingestion, ethanol should be used to block further conversion of methanol to formic acid, and sodium bicarbonate should be given to correct metabolic acidosis. Elimination of formic acid is enhanced by alkalization of the urine and by hemodialysis.

METHEMOGLOBINEMIA Methemoglobinemia results from exposure to chemicals that oxidize the iron in hemoglobin from its ferrous (Fe^{2+}) to its ferric (Fe^{3+}) state. Concomitant oxidation of hemoglobin protein may cause its precipitation (as Heinz bodies) and a hemolytic anemia (with bite cells seen on peripheral blood smear). Oxidizing agents include aniline and its derivates, aminophenols, aminophenones, chlorates, nitrites, nitrates, naphthalene, nitrobenzene and related chemicals, sulfonamides, phenazopyridine, dapsone, primaquine, lidocaine, and benzocaine.

Methemoglobin (ferric hemoglobin) cannot carry oxygen and results in a functional anemia, the shift of the oxygen dissociation curve to the left limiting the release of oxygen to tissues. Symptoms are due to hypoxia and anaerobic metabolism.

Various systems operate normally to keep methemoglobin at normal physiologic levels (1 percent of the total hemoglobin concentration). Oxidant inactivation systems include ascorbic acid and sulfhydryl agents such as glutathione, which combine with oxidizing agents and transform them to less toxic compounds. Mechanisms for reducing methemoglobin to oxyhemoglobin include NADH–methemoglobin reductase (responsible for 95 percent of activity), NADPH–methemoglobin reductase, reduced glutathione, methylene blue, and ascorbic acid.

Clinical toxicity Cyanosis, which is unresponsive to oxygen and may have a gray-brown hue, occurs with methemoglobin levels greater than 15 percent (15 g/L or 1.5 g/dL absolute methemoglobin). Patients are asymptomatic, however, until methemoglobin levels exceed 20 to 30 percent, at which point fatigue, headache, tachycardia, dizziness, and weakness develop. At levels greater than 55 percent, dyspnea, bradycardia, hypoxia, acidosis, seizures, coma, and cardiac arrhythmias may occur. Levels greater than 70 percent are rapidly fatal. Hemolytic anemia may cause hyperkalemia and renal failure within 1 to 3 days.

Diagnosis The diagnosis should be suspected in the presence of respiratory distress, brown or gray cyanosis unresponsive to oxygen, and absence of significant CNS depression. Arterial blood gases reveal a normal P_{O_2} and decreased oxygen saturation (measured by CO-oximeter rather than derived). Oxygen saturation by pulse oximetry may be falsely normal. Blood with high levels of methemoglobin is chocolate colored when placed on filter paper and compared with normal blood. The chocolate color does not revert to pink when oxygen is bubbled through a tube of blood but does return to normal when 10% potassium cyanide is added. Methemoglobin is identified by its absorption at a frequency of 630 nm on light spectrometry. Finally, the toxic screen on blood or urine may identify the drug or chemical that serves as the oxidizing agent.

Treatment The toxin, if recently ingested, should be removed by gastrointestinal decontamination. Most oxidizing agents are metabolized rapidly, making diuresis ineffective. Dialysis may be effective, depending on the specific compound. Methylene blue is indicated for methemoglobin levels above 30 g/L (cyanosis alone is not an indication for methylene blue therapy) or methemoglobinemia with hypoxia. In the patient with anemia or cardiovascular disease, methylene blue may be indicated at lower levels due to a greater risk from tissue hypoxia. Methylene blue is given at a dose of 1 to 2 mg/kg of body weight as a 1% solution over 5 min. If a clinical response is not observed within 1 h, the dose may be repeated. A methemoglobin level of 40 g/L can be expected to decrease by half in 1 to 2 h. As long as the oxidizing agent remains in the body, methemoglobin will be generated, and additional doses may be necessary. Side effects of methylene blue include precordial pain, dyspnea, restlessness, apprehension, and tremor; a transient blue color to the skin and urine; and the enhancement of methemoglobin levels at high doses (greater than 7 mg/kg of body weight). Methylene blue is contraindicated in patients with deficiency of glucose-6-phosphate dehydrogenase. Additional treatments include transfusion with packed red cells optimally to a hemoglobin of 150 g/L to increase oxygen-carrying capacity and administration of 100% oxygen or hyperbaric oxygen to enhance oxygen delivery to tissues. If the methemoglobin level is very high or the patient is deficient in glucose-6-phosphate dehydrogenase, exchange transfusion may be indicated.

MUSCLE RELAXANTS Muscle relaxants include orphenadrine, methocarbamol, baclofen, chlorphenesin, cyclobenzaprine, chlorzoxazone, and carisoprodol. Muscle relaxants exert some direct muscle activity but predominantly act as CNS depressants (see Table 395-2). They also depress spinal synaptic reflexes, prolong synaptic recovery time, and reduce repetitive discharges. Baclofen is a GABA agonist, and cyclobenzoprine and orphenadrine have anticholinergic activity. Muscle relaxants are rapidly and completely absorbed, and peak blood levels occur 1 to 2 h following ingestion. The half-lives are variable, with most between 2 and 6 h. The majority are metabolized by the liver to derivatives that are generally inactive and are excreted by the kidneys. Baclofen, an exception, is largely excreted unchanged in the urine.

Clinical toxicity Effects of carisoprodol, chlorphenesin, chlorzoxazone, and methocarbamol include nausea, vomiting, dizziness, headache, nystagmus, hypotonia, and central nervous system depression. Cyclobenzaprine and orphenadrine may cause agitation, hallucinations, tachycardia, mydriasis, hyperthermia, and dry skin and mucosa. Baclofen causes CNS depression, hypothermia, excitability, delirium, myoclonus, seizures, conduction abnormalities, tachycardia, bradycardia, and hypotension. The drugs may be identified in blood or urine by toxic screen.

Treatment Initial management includes prompt gastrointestinal decontamination. Muscle relaxants are well adsorbed by single-dose activated charcoal. Repetitive charcoal may be used for baclofen. Diuresis is ineffective. The efficacy of hemodialysis or hemoperfusion is not established. Physostigmine (1 to 2 mg intravenously over 2 to 5 min) will reverse the anticholinergic effects of orphenadrine and cyclobenzaprine but should be reserved for patients with severe hallucinations and hyperactivity.

NARCOTICS See Chaps. 391 and 392.

NONSTEROIDAL ANTI-INFLAMMATORY DRUGS Nonsteroidal anti-inflammatory drugs (NSAIDs) include diclofenac, diflunisal, fenoprofen, flurbiprofen, ibuprofen, indomethacin, ketoprofen, ketorolac, mefenamic acid, meclofenamate, naproxine, phenylbutazone, piroxicam, phenylbutazone, sulindac, and tolmetin. NSAIDs inhibit prostaglandin synthesis by blocking cyclooxygenase. They are rapidly absorbed, with peak blood concentrations achieved within 1 to 2 h following ingestion. They are highly bound (greater than 90 percent) to plasma protein and have volumes of distribution of less than 1.0 L/kg of body weight. The pK_a ranges from 3.5 to 6.3. They are predominantly metabolized by conjugation, oxidation, and hydroxylation. A small portion (1 to 15 percent) is eliminated unchanged by the kidneys. Half-lives vary from 1 to 16 h, with the exception of phenylbutazone, which has a half-life of 2 to 4 days.

Clinical toxicity Effects are usually mild and include nausea, vomiting, abdominal pain, drowsiness, headache, glycosuria, hematuria, and proteinuria. Acute renal failure and hepatitis are rare. Diflunisal may produce hyperventilation, tachycardia, and sweating. Ibuprofen can sometimes cause metabolic acidosis, coma, and seizures. Seizures are relatively common in mefanamic acid and phenylbutazone poisoning but rare with ketoprofen and naproxen. Coma, respiratory depression, and cardiovascular collapse or arrest may be caused by mefanamic acid and phenylbutazone. Metabolic acidosis occurs often in phenylbutazone poisoning and rarely with naproxen.

Diagnosis Toxicology testing will identify these drugs in the urine, but quantitative analysis is not useful.

Treatment Therapy for NSAID poisoning includes gastrointestinal decontamination and supportive care. Repeated doses of activated charcoal may be of benefit for indomethacin, phenylbutazone, and piroxicam. Renal excretion is not increased by diuresis, and protein binding limits efficacy of hemodialysis. Although experience is limited, hemoperfusion might be useful in patients with hepatic or renal failure and severe clinical toxicity.

ORGANOPHOSPHATE AND CARBAMATE INSECTICIDES Organophosphorus insecticides include malathion, parathion, dichlorvos, and diazinon. Carbamate insecticides include carbaryl, aldicarb, baygon, ficam, and propoxur. Ambenonium, neostigmine, physostigmine, and pyriodostigmine are related agents. Organophosphorus insecticides irreversibly inhibit acetylcholinesterase and cause accumulation of acetylcholine at muscarinic and nicotinic synapses. Carbamates reversibly inhibit this enzyme. The mechanism by which these insecticides affect the CNS is unclear. Organophosphates are absorbed through the skin, lungs, and gastrointestinal tract, are distributed widely in tissues, and are slowly eliminated by hepatic metabolism. The oxidative metabolites (paroxon, maloxone) are active. Subsequent hydrolysis produces inactive metabolites. Carbamates are rapidly eliminated by serum cholinesterases and by hepatic metabolism.

Clinical toxicity Organophosphorus compounds and carbamates produce muscarinic, nicotinic, and CNS effects. Manifestations occur 30 min to 2 h following exposure. Muscarinic effects include nausea, vomiting, abdominal cramps, urinary and fecal incontinence, increased bronchial secretions, cough, dyspnea, sweating, salivation, lacrimation, and urinary frequency and incontinence. Miosis is usual, and blurring of vision may occur. In severe poisoning, bradycardia, conduction block, hypotension, and pulmonary edema may occur. Nicotinic signs include twitching, fasciculations, weakness, hypertension, tachycardia, and in severe cases hypoventilation with respiratory failure. CNS effects include anxiety, restlessness, tremor, convulsions, confusion, weakness, and coma. Toxicity due to carbamates is shorter in duration and usually less severe than with organophosphates. Most patients recover within 24 to 48 h, but long-acting organophosphates may cause effects for weeks to months. Death is most often due to increased pulmonary secretions and inadequate ventilation.

In acute poisoning, cholinesterase activity in plasma and in red blood cells is reduced to less than 50 percent of normal. A reduction in red blood cell cholinesterase activity is more specific but less readily available, and some organophosphates may inhibit only one cholinesterase. Without treatment, blood cholinesterase activity returns to normal in 4 to 5 weeks.

With carbamate insecticides, depression in plasma or red blood cell cholinesterase levels is rare because of the rapid reversibility of the inhibition. Since cholinesterase assays are not routinely or rapidly available, the initial diagnosis is clinical. Insecticides may be identified in urine on toxic screen.

Treatment Contaminated clothing should be removed, and the skin should be washed with soap and water. The patient should be removed from the site of inhalation exposure, and in the case of ingestion, gastrointestinal decontamination should include activated charcoal. Atropine, a muscarinic receptor antagonist, should be administered for muscarinic effects. A dose of 0.5 to 2 mg atropine is given intravenously every 15 to 20 min until atropinization is adequate (drying of bronchial and mucous membrane secretions). Pupil size and heart rate cannot be used as end points. Repeated doses or a constant atropine drip may be necessary for several days. Atropine is less effective for CNS toxicity and ineffective for nicotinic effects. Pralidoxime (2-PAM), an oxime that reactivates cholinesterases, is indicated for nicotinic symptoms in organophosphate poisoning. The dose is 1 to 2 g intravenously over 5 to 20 minutes. The dose may be repeated every 4 to 6 h until nicotinic signs resolve. Like atropine, its ability to reverse CNS effects is less pronounced. In carbamate poisoning, controversy exists over the use of pralidoxime. It should probably not be used in carbaryl poisoning, and with other carbamates it should only be administered in conjunction with atropine.

PHENOTHIAZINE Phenothiazines include aliphatic (chlorpromazine, promethazine, promazine), piperidine (mesoridazine, thioridazine), and piperazine (perphenazine, fluphenazine, prochlorperazine, trifluoperazine) derivatives. Haloperidol, loxapine, pimozide, and thiothixene differ structurally but have similar pharmacologic activity. These agents block postsynaptic dopamine receptors, exhibit anticholinergic activity, and inhibit reuptake of norepinephrine and 5-hydroxytryptamine in the CNS. They also have peripheral alpha-adrenergic blocking and anticholinergic activity and lower the seizure threshold. Some phenothiazines have a quinidine-like effect on the heart. These agents are efficiently absorbed from the gastrointestinal tract, exhibit 90 to 95 percent protein binding, and have large apparent volumes of distribution (10 to 40 L/kg of body weight). They are slowly eliminated by hepatic metabolism with half-lives of 20 to 40 h. Only 1 percent is excreted unchanged in the urine. The majority of metabolites are inactive.

Clinical toxicity Effects begin within 30 to 60 min of ingestion and include lethargy, obtundation, respiratory depression, hypotension, hypothermia, and coma. Pupils are often constricted, and the skin is usually warm and dry. Cardiac effects include supraventricular tachycardia, atrioventricular block, and atrial and ventricular arrhythmias. Torsades de pointes, prolonged PR, QRS, and QT intervals, and U- and T-wave abnormalities may be seen, especially with thioridazine and its metabolite mesoridazine. The neuroleptic malignant syndrome rarely, if ever, occurs following acute overdose. The neuroleptic malignant syndrome is characterized by hyperthermia, extrapyramidal findings (rigidity, muscle spasms, posturing), autonomic instability (diaphoresis, incontinence, and bouts of hypertension, tachycardia, and tachypnea), altered mental status (confusion, delirium, coma), leukocytosis (white blood cell count >15,000 cells per milliliter), and an elevated creatinine kinase. In acute dystonic reactions, sustained muscle contractions may result in abnormal posturing of the eyes, face, tongue, jaw, neck, back, abdomen, and pelvis, but the patient remains alert. These reactions are idiosyncratic rather than dose-related. The diagnosis is established by toxic screen on blood and urine. Quantitative levels are not helpful.

Treatment Gastrointestinal decontamination should be accomplished as soon as possible. Treatment is supportive. Diuresis and dialysis are ineffective. Seizures should be treated with anticonvulsants, and hypotension should be managed with volume expanders and alpha agonists. Arrhythmias are treated by standard agents. Quinidine and procainanide, however, should be avoided. Sodium bicarbonate and magnesium may be useful for ventricular tachyarrhythmias associated with intraventricular conduction or repolarization abnormalities.

Dantrolene and bromocriptine may be useful in treatment of the neuroleptic malignant syndrome if symptoms cannot be controlled with benzodiazepines. In rare cases, neuromuscular paralysis may be indicated. Acute dystonic reactions respond rapidly to intravenous diphenhydramine (1 mg/kg of body weight) given over 2 min or benztropine (1 to 2 mg). Doses may be repeated in 20 min if the response is incomplete. Treatment is generally continued with an oral formulation for 2 to 3 days to prevent recurrence of symptoms.

SALICYLATES Salicylates increase the sensitivity of respiratory centers in the brain to changes in P_{O_2} and P_{CO_2} resulting in an increased rate and depth of respiration early in the course of poisoning. Later, salicylates uncouple oxidative phosphorylation and produce increases in metabolic rate, oxygen consumption, glucose utilization, and heat production. They also inhibit the Krebs tricarboxylic cycle and block carbohydrate and lipid metabolism, resulting in metabolic acidosis and ketonemia. Salicylates produce hepatocyte damage, resulting in increased plasma enzyme activity and prolongation of prothrombin time. Salicylates decrease platelet aggregation.

Salicylates are well absorbed both from the stomach and the small bowel, but absorption may continue for 24 h or longer following overdose. Therapeutic blood levels range from 0.7 to 1.4 mmol/L (10 to 20 mg/dL). In the plasma, 50 to 80 percent is bound to albumin. Because salicylate is a weak acid with a pK_a of 3, the unbound portion in the plasma exists mainly in an ionized state. It has a small volume of distribution (0.2 L/kg of body weight) which increases with chronic poisoning and with increasing doses. Acidosis increases distribution of salicylate into brain, liver, and other tissues. Salicylates are eliminated by both hepatic metabolism and renal excretion. The half-life is 2 to 3 h after a single therapeutic dose. Saturation of hepatic metabolic pathways results in a prolonged half-life (20 to 36 h) following overdose. By alkalinizing the urine to a pH of 8, the drug in the renal tubules is maintained in an ionized state, cannot be reabsorbed, and is excreted.

Clinical toxicity Manifestations of mild poisoning include vomiting, tachycardia, hyperpnea, fever, tinnitus, lethargy, confusion, respiratory alkalosis, and an alkaline urine (pH > 6). In severe poisoning, convulsions, coma, and respiratory and cardiovascular failure may occur. Vomiting, poor intake, and hyperventilation may cause severe dehydration, acute renal failure, and acidosis. An increased anion gap metabolic acidosis with an acidic urine (pH < 6) may be compounded by respiratory acidosis. Other complications include cerebral and pulmonary edema and myocardial or renal failure. An elevated hematocrit, white blood cell count, and platelet count; hypernatremia; hyperkalemia; and hypoglycemia may be seen. Respiratory alkalosis is commonly coupled with metabolic acidosis (40 to 50 percent), but respiratory alkalosis (20 percent), metabolic acidosis (20 percent), and mixed respiratory and metabolic acidosis (5 to 10 percent) also may be present. Lactic and other organic acids are responsible for an increased anion gap. Prothrombin time may be prolonged. Salicylates are identified by a positive ferric chloride test on either blood or urine. In the case of an acute single ingestion, a peak level less than 3 mmol/L (40 mg/dL) is associated with no symptoms, 3 to 7 mmol/L (40 to 100 mg/dL) with mild to moderate manifestations, and greater than 7 mmol/L (100 mg/dL) with severe toxicity. In chronic poisoning, symptoms may occur at levels only slightly above the therapeutic range.

Treatment Gastrointestinal decontamination is indicated if an ingested dose is greater than 150 mg/kg of body weight. Concretions may delay absorption, and decontamination may be helpful 12 to 24 h after ingestion. Elimination may be increased by repeated administration of activated charcoal. Parenteral fluids should be given to replace fluid losses and to produce a brisk urine flow. Supplemental glucose and oxygen should be given. Electrolyte and metabolic abnormalities should be corrected. Prolongation of prothrombin time should be corrected with intravenous vitamin K. Seizures should be controlled with intravenous phenobarbital or diazepam. Myocardial failure should be treated with standard therapy. Cerebral edema, pulmonary edema, and renal failure require fluid restriction and urgent hemodialysis. Sodium bicarbonate should be administered in the presence of acidosis and thus limit tissue distribution of salicylates. In patients without these complications, treatment should include saline diuresis and alkalinization of the urine to a pH of 8 to enhance urinary excretion. Depending on severity, one to three ampules (44 to 131 mmol) of bicarbonate and 20 to 60 mmol of potassium should be added to a liter of intravenous fluid containing dextrose and administered at a rate of 2 to 6 mL/kg per hour. Electrolytes, calcium,

acid-base status, urine pH, and fluid balance must be monitored carefully during such therapy. Salicylates are effectively removed by hemodialysis, which should be considered with severe overdose, cerebral edema, failure of conventional therapy, or compromised renal or hepatic function.

STIMULANTS Amphetamines, bronchodilators such as albuterol and metaproterenol, and decongestants such as ephedrine, pseudo-ephedrine, phenylephrine, and phenylpropanolamine stimulate receptors of the central and sympathetic nervous systems (see Table 395-1).

Amphetamines stimulate both alpha- and beta-adrenergic receptors, whereas bronchodilators are primarily beta agonists and decongestants are primarily alpha agonists. These agents are rapidly absorbed from the gastrointestinal tract, reaching peak levels 1 to 2 h following ingestion. They are weak bases with pK_a values ranging from 8 to 10 and a volume of distribution of 2 to 6 L/kg of body weight. These agents are eliminated by a combination of hepatic metabolism and renal excretion of unchanged drug. Excretion is enhanced in an acid urine and slowed in an alkaline urine. Half-lives range from 2 to 8 h to 6 to 34 h depending on urine flow and pH.

Clinical toxicity Effects are seen within 30 to 60 min following ingestion and include nausea, vomiting, diarrhea, and abdominal cramps. Talkativeness, irritability, confusion, delirium, headache, combativeness, auditory and visual hallucinations, tremors, tachycardia, palpitations, hypertension, and hyperreflexia are common. Other findings may include dilated pupils, dry mouth, pallor, flushing of the skin, and tachypnea. Hyperpyrexia, seizures, rhabdomyolysis, hypertensive crisis, intracranial hemorrhage, cardiac arrhythmias, and cardiovascular collapse may occur in severe overdose. Bronchodilators may cause hypotension as a result of beta-mediated vasodilatation, and decongestants may cause reflex bradycardia secondary to alpha-mediated hypertension. These agents may be identified in the urine by toxicology screening, but quantitative levels are not useful.

Treatment Gastrointestinal decontamination should be accomplished as soon as possible. Supportive care includes treatment of seizures with benzodiazepines, barbiturates, and phenytoin; hypertension with labetalol, nifedipine, or phentolamine; hyperpyrexia with cooling blankets, salicylates, and acetaminophen; and agitation with sedatives, and, if necessary, with paralyzing agents. Lidocaine and propranolol are preferred for the treatment of ventricular tachyarrhythmias. Although theoretically effective, acid diuresis is not recommended due to lack of documented efficacy and risks such as worsening acidosis and precipitation of myoglobinuric renal failure.

THEOPHYLLINE Theophylline causes the release of endogenous catecholamines and prolongs their effects by inhibiting the degradation of cyclic AMP by phosphodiesterase. Theophylline is rapidly absorbed from the stomach and upper small bowel. Following overdose, peak levels are achieved 1 to 2 h after ingestion of liquid preparations, by 2 to 4 h with tablets, and in 6 to 24 h with sustained-release preparations. Theophylline is approximately 60 percent bound to albumin and has a low volume of distribution (0.6 L/kg of body weight). Therapeutic serum levels are 55 to 110 μmol/L (10 to 20 mg/L). Theophylline is primarily eliminated by hepatic metabolism, which is saturable at levels in the high therapeutic range. The serum half-life, normally 4 to 6 h, is therefore prolonged in overdoses to 10 to 12 h. Only 5 percent of the theophylline is excreted unchanged by the kidneys. Theophylline elimination is also decreased with impaired liver function, congestive heart failure, viral infections, and concomitantly administered drugs such as cimetidine, erythromycin, and quinolone antibiotics.

Clinical toxicity Effects begin 30 min to 2 h following overdose and include nausea, vomiting, restlessness, irritability, agitation, tachypnea, tachycardia, and muscle tremors. Coma, hypotension, respiratory depression, generalized tonic-clonic and focal convulsions, and rhabdomyolysis may occur in severe poisoning. Convulsions are often protracted, repetitive, and resistant to therapy. Cardiovascular effects include atrial arrhythmias, multifocal premature ventricular contractions, idioventricular rhythms, ventricular tachycardia, and ventricular fibrillation. Metabolic abnormalities include ketosis, metabolic acidosis, increased serum amylase, hyperglycemia, and decreased serum potassium, calcium, and phosphorus. Toxicity occurs at lower theophylline levels with chronic than with acute poisoning. Mortality rates are higher after chronic ingestion. Cardiac arrhythmias and seizures occur following chronic ingestion at serum levels of 200 to 300 μmol/L (40 to 60 mg/L). Similar toxicity, along with hypotension, hypokalemia, and metabolic abnormalities, generally occurs at levels above 400 to 500 μmol/L (80 to 100 mg/L) following acute overdose. Serial levels should be measured to determine the peak concentration (serving as an important indicator for hemodialysis).

Treatment Initial therapy involves prompt gastrointestinal decontamination. Theophylline is well adsorbed by activated charcoal. With sustained-release forms, decontamination should be considered up to 12 to 24 h following ingestion. Repeated doses of charcoal shorten the serum half-life by approximately 50 percent. Metaclopramide is useful in controlling theophylline-induced vomiting. Extreme tachycardia should be treated with propranolol or esmolol, and hypotension is treated with volume expansion. Propranolol is also effective in reversing hypotension. Benzodiazepines and barbiturates are useful for convulsions and hyperactivity. Phenytoin is ineffective. Treatment of ventricular tachyarrhythmias should include propranolol as well as standard antiarrhythmics. Diuresis is ineffective for enhancing removal of theophylline. Hemodialysis and hemoperfusion are effective in removing theophylline and are indicated in patients with severe toxicity or after acute ingestion with a serum level greater than 440 μmol/L (80 mg/L). With chronic ingestion, hemodialysis or hemoperfusion is indicated with serum levels greater than 200 to 300 μmol/L (40 to 60 mg/L).

TRICYCLIC ANTIDEPRESSANTS Commonly available tricyclic compounds include amitriptyline, imipramine, chlomipramine, desipramine, doxepin, nortriptyline, protriptyline, and trimipramine. Related agents include amoxapine, bupropion, maprotiline, and trazodone. These agents block reuptake of synaptic transmitters such as norepinephrine, dopamine, and serotonin in the CNS. In addition, they have central and peripheral anticholinergic activity, peripheral alpha-blocking activity, and quinidine-like effects on the heart. Fluoxetine is unique in that it selectively inhibits the reuptake of serotonin.

Tricyclics are well absorbed from the gastrointestinal tract, and peak levels are reached within 2 to 6 h of overdose. In some cases, anticholinergic effects may predominate, resulting in prolonged absorption and delayed peak levels (6 to 12 h following ingestion). Tricyclics exhibit high protein binding in the plasma. They have large volumes of distribution in the range of 20 to 40 L/kg of body weight. Elimination is predominantly by hepatic metabolism with an initial demethylation generating pharmacologically active metabolites. These metabolites generally undergo enterohepatic circulation. Subsequent steps of metabolism result in increasing polarity of metabolites that are then excreted by the kidneys. Less than 5 percent of the parent compound is excreted unchanged in urine. The half-lives of tricyclics and their demethylated metabolites range from 25 to 30 h but may be longer in the overdose setting.

Clinical toxicity Effects generally develop within 30 min of overdose but may be delayed for up to 6 h. In low overdose, anticholinergic effects predominate and are manifest by agitation, myoclonus, mydriasis, urinary retention, confusion, hallucinations, mild fever, hypertension, and tachycardia. In high overdose, marked CNS depression is coupled with cardiotoxicity, seizures, and hypotension. Cardiovascular toxicity is not a feature of fluoxetine overdose, however. Ventricular tachyarrhythmias, atrioventricular and intraventricular conduction delays, terminal bradycardia, and decreased cardiac output occur with high overdose. Aspiration pneumonia and pulmonary edema also may develop. Death occurs usually within the first 2 to 6 h following ingestion. Prolongation of the QRS complex (greater than 100 ms) in severe overdose correlates with an increased risk of cardiac arrhythmias and seizures. Serum levels are diagnostic and generally correlate with severity. Metabolites as well as the parent

compound levels should be summed when estimating the total serum concentration. Levels less than about 1000 nmol/L (300 ng/mL) are therapeutic. Levels over 3300 nmol/L (1000 ng/mL) indicate serious poisoning and are associated with QRS complexes wider than 100 ms.

Treatment Ipecac-induced emesis is contraindicated with tricyclic ingestions. Gastric lavage is indicated for comatose patients with recent ingestions. Activated charcoal in single and repeated doses should be administered. Treatment includes support of respiration and volume expansion and norepinephrine or high-dose dopamine for hypotension. Hypertension is generally limited and does not require specific therapy. Seizures should be treated with phenytoin or diazepam. Treatment of ventricular tachyarrhythmias should include sodium bicarbonate (0.5 to 1 mmol/kg of body weight), lidocaine, and phenytoin. Beta-adrenergic blockers and class 1A antiarrhythmics (quinidine, procainamide, and disopyramide) should be avoided. Cardiac pacing may be necessary for the severely depressed myocardium and bradycardia. Correction of acidosis is an important component of the treatment of cardiac arrhythmias and seizures. Physostigmine (1 to 2 mg intravenously over 2 to 5 min) will reverse low-dose anticholinergic effects and may be administered in mild poisoning if deterioration has been excluded by a suitable period of observation. Physostigmine can cause asystole in severe poisoning and should not be used in this situation. Physostigmine is absolutely contraindicated in patients with arrhythmias or cardiac conduction disturbances.

REFERENCES

General aspects

AMDUR MO et al (eds): *Casarett and Doull's Toxicology: The Basic Science of Poisons,* 4th ed. New York, Pergamon Press, 1991

BRANCATA DJ, NELSON RC: Poisoning mortality in the United States 1980. Vet Hum Toxicol 26:273, 1984

LITOVITZ TL et al: 1987 Annual report of the American Association of Poison Control Centers National Data Collection System. Am J Emerg Med 6:479, 1988

McCARRON MM: Current trends in drug overdose. West J Med 141:98, 1984

Diagnosis

BRETT AS: Implication of discordance between clinical impression and toxicology analysis in drug overdose. Arch Intern Med 148:437, 1988

COUNCIL OF SCIENTIFIC AFFAIRS, AMERICAN MEDICAL ASSOCIATION: Scientific issues in drug testing. JAMA 257:3110, 1987

GLASSER L et al: Serum osmolality and its applicability to drug overdose. Am J Clin Pathol 60:695, 1973

HEPLER BR et al: Role of the toxicology lab in the treatment of acute poisoning. Med Toxicol 1:61, 1986

JAEGER RW et al: Radiopacity of drugs and plants in vivo—limited usefulness. Vet Hum Toxicol 23(Suppl 1):2, 1981

KELLERMANN AL et al: Impact of drug screening in suspected overdose. Ann Emerg Med 16:1206, 1987

OLSON KR et al: Physical assessment and differential diagnosis of the poisoned patient. Med Toxicol 2:52, 1987

OSTER JR et al: Use of the anion gap in clinical medicine. South Med J 81:229, 1988

ROBERTS JR et al: The body stuffer syndrome: A clandestine form of drug overdose. Am J Emerg Med 4:24, 1986

SCHERZ RG: The differential diagnosis of coma due to poisoning and exogenous toxins. Pediatrician 6:190, 1977

SMITHLINE N, GARDNER KD JR: Gaps—anionic and osmolal. JAMA 236:1594, 1976

Treatment

ALBERTSON TE et al: Superiority of activated charcoal alone compared with ipecac and activated charcoal in the treatment of acute toxic ingestions. Ann Emerg Med 18:56, 1989

BRETT AS et al: Predicting the clinical course of intentional drug overdose: Implications for utilization of the intensive care unit. Arch Intern Med 147:133, 1987

BURTON BT et al: Comparison of activated charcoal and gastric lavage in the prevention of aspirin absorption. J Emerg Med 1:411, 1984

CURTIS RA et al: Efficacy of ipecac and activated charcoal/cathartic: Prevention of salicylate absorption in a simulated overdose. Arch Intern Med 144:48, 1984

GARRETTSON LK, GELLER RJ: Acid and alkaline diuresis: When are they of value in the treatment of poisoning? Drug Safety 5:220, 1990

GOLDBERG MJ et al: An approach to the management of the poisoned patient. Arch Intern Med 146:1381, 1986

GOLDFRANK L et al: Newer antidotes and controversies in antidotal therapy, in *Emergency Medicine Annual,* DA Rund, BW Wolcott (eds). Norwalk, Conn, Appleton-Century-Crofts, 1984, vol 3, pp 223–266

KING WD: Syrup of ipecac: A drug review. Clin Toxicol 17:353, 1980

Kornberg AE, Dolgin J: Pediatric ingestions: Charcoal alone versus ipecac and charcoal. Ann Emerg Med 20:648, 1991

Krenzelok EP et al: Gastrointestinal transit times of carthartics combined with charcoal. Ann Emerg Med 14:1152, 1985

Kulig K et al: Management of acutely poisoned patients without gastric emptying. Ann Emerg Med 14:562, 1985

Litovitz TL: The anecdotal antidotes. Emerg Med Clin North Am 2:145, 1984

Manno BR, Manno JE: Toxicology of ipecac: A review. Clin Toxicol 10:221, 1977

McCarron MM, Wood JD: The cocaine "body packer" syndrome: Diagnosis and treatment. JAMA 250:1417, 1983

Merrigian KS et al: Prospective evaluation of gastric emptying in the self-poisoned patient. Am J Emerg Med 8:479, 1990

Minocha A, Spyker DA: Acute overdose with sustained-release drug formulations: Perspectives in treatment. Med Toxicol 1:300, 1986

Neuvonen PJ: Clinical pharmacokinetics of oral activated charcoal in acute intoxications. Clin Pharmacokinet 7:465, 1982

———, Olkkola KT: Oral activated charcoal in the treatment of intoxications: Role of single and repeated doses. Med Toxicol 3:33, 1988

Park GD et al: Expanded role of charcoal in the poisoned and overdosed patient. Arch Intern Med 146:969, 1986

Peterson RG, Peterson LN: Cleansing the blood: Hemodialysis, petitoneal dialysis, exchange transfusion, charcoal hemoperfusion, forced diuresis. Pediatr Clin North Am 33:675, 1986

Pond SM: Diuresis, dialysis and hemoperfusion: Indications and benefits. Emerg Med Clin North Am 2:29, 1984

Rosenberg J et al: Pharmacokinetics of drug overdose. Clin Pharmacokinet 6:161, 1981

Shannon M et al: Carthartics and laxatives: Do they still have a place in management of the poisoned patient? Med Toxicol 1:247, 1986

Spyker DA, Minocha A: Toxicodynamic approach to the management of the poisoned patient. J Emerg Med 6:117, 1988

Stead AH, Moffat AC: A collection of therapeutic, toxic and fatal blood drug concentrations in man. Hum Toxicol 3:437, 1983

Stewart JJ: Effects of emetic and cathartic agents on the gastrointestinal tract and the treatment of toxic ingestion. Clin Toxicol 20:199, 1983

Tenebein M: Whole bowel irrigation as a gastrointestinal decontamination procedure after acute poisoning. Med Toxicol 3:77, 1988

——— et al: Efficacy of ipecac-induced emesis, orogastric lavage, and activated charcoal for acute drug overdose. Ann Emerg Med 16:838, 1987

Wheeler-Usher DH et al: Gastric emptying: Risk versus benefit in the treatment of acute poisoning. Med Toxicol 1:142, 1986

Zaccara G et al: Clinical features, pathogenesis, and management of drug-induced seizures. Drug Safety 5:109, 1990

Reference texts

Arena JM, Drew RH: Poisoning: Toxicology, Symptoms, Treatments, 5th ed. Springfield, Ill, Charles C Thomas, 1986

Baset RC: Disposition of Toxic Drugs and Chemicals in Man, 2d ed. Davis, Calif, Biomedical Publications, 1982

Block JB: The Signs and Symptoms of Chemical Exposure. Springfield, Ill, Charles C Thomas, 1980

Bryson PD: Comprehensive Review in Toxicology. Rockville, Md, Aspen, 1989

Clayton GD, Clayton FE (eds): Patty's Industrial Hygiene and Toxicology, 3d ed. New York, Wiley, 1978

Dangaard J: Symptoms and Signs in Occupational Disease: A Practical Guide, Copenhagen, Year Book Medical Publishers, 1978

Ellenhorn MJ, Barceloux DG: Medical Toxicology: Diagnosis and Treatment of Human Poisoning. New York, Elsevier, 1988

Finkel AJ: Hamilton and Hardy's Industrial Toxicology, 4th ed. Boston, John Wright, 1983

Goldfrank LR et al (eds): Goldfrank's Toxicologic Emergencies, 3d ed. Norwalk, Conn, Appleton-Century-Crofts, 1986

Gosselin RE: Clinical Toxicology of Commercial Products: Acute Poisoning, 5th ed. Baltimore, Williams & Wilkins, 1984

Haddad LM, Winchester JF: Clinical Management of Poisoning and Drug Overdose 2d ed. Philadelphia, Saunders, 1990

Hayes WJ, Law ER: Handbook of Pesticide Toxicology. San Diego, Academic Press, 1991

Klassen CD et al (eds): Casarett and Doull's Toxicology: The Basic Science of Poisons, 3d ed. New York, Macmillan, 1986

Lampe KF, McCann MA (eds): AMA Handbook of Poisonous and Injurious Plants. Chicago, American Medical Association, 1985

Rumack BH (eds): Poisindex Information System (updated quarterly). Denver, Micromedex

Specific poisons

Acetaminophen

Flanagan RJ: The role of acetylcysteine in clinical toxicology. Med Toxicol 2:93, 1987

Prescott LF: Paracetamol overdose. Drugs 25:290, 1983

Smilkstein MJ et al: Efficacy of oral N-acetylcysteine in the treatment of acetaminophen overdose. N Engl J Med 319:1558, 1988

Acids and alkali

Anderson KD et al: Controlled trial of corticosteroids in children with corrosive injury of the esophagus. N Engl J Med 323:637, 1990

Friedman EM, Lovejoy FH Jr: The emergency management of caustic ingestions. Emerg Med Clin North Am 2:77, 1984

Howell JM et al: Steroids for the treatment of corrosive esophageal injury: A statistical analysis of past studies. Am J Emerg Med 10:421, 1992

Wason S: The emergency management of caustic ingestions. J Emerg Med 2:175, 1984

Antiarrhythmic drugs

Dunbar DN, Pentel PR: Antiarrhythmic drug toxicity, in Intensive Care Medicine, JM Rippe et al (eds). Boston, Little, Brown, 1991, p 1174

Freedman MD et al: Extracorporeal pump assistance—a novel treatment for acute lidocaine poisoning. Eur J Clin Pharmacol 22:129, 1982

Hruby K, Misslivetz J: Poisoning with oral antiarrhythmic drugs. Int J Clin Pharmacol 23:253, 1985

Stratman HG, Kennedy HL: Torsade de pointes associated with drugs and toxins: Recognition and management. Am Heart J 113:1470, 1987

Barbiturates

Boldy DAR et al: Treatment of phenobarbitone poisoning with repeat oral administration of activated charcoal. Q J Med 235:997, 1986

Matthew H: Barbiturates. Clin Toxicol 8(5):495, 1975

McCarron MM et al: Short-acting barbiturate overdosage: Correlation of intoxication score with serum barbiturate concentration. JAMA 248:55, 1982

Benzodiazepines

Divoll M et al: Benzodiazepine overdosage: Plasma concentrations and clinical outcome. Psycho Pharmacol 73:381, 1981

Greenblatt DJ et al: Acute overdosage with benzodiazepine derivatives. Clin Pharmacol Ther 21:497, 1977

Prischl F et al: Value of flumazenil in benzodiazepine self-poisoning. Med Toxicol 3:334, 1988

Beta blockers

Critchley JA, Ungar A: The management of acute poisoning due to beta-adrenoreceptor antagonists. Med Tox Adverse Drug Exp 4:32, 1989

Heath A: β-Adrenoceptor blocker toxicity: Clinical features and therapy. Am J Emerg Med 2:518, 1984

Weinstein RS: Recognition and management of poisoning with beta-adrenergic blocking agents. Ann Emerg Med 13:1123, 1984

Bleach

Gapay-Gapanavicuius M: Chloramine-induced pneumonitis from mixing household cleaning agents. Br Med J 288:1086, 1982

Gaudreault P et al: Predictability of esophageal injury from signs and symptoms. Pediatrics 71:767, 1983

Landau GD, Saunders WH: The effect of chlorine bleach on the esophagus. Arch Otolaryngol 80:174, 1964

Calcium channel blockers

Herrington DM et al: Nifedipine overdose. Am J Cardiol 81:344, 1986

McMillan R: Management of acute severe verapamil intoxication. J Emerg Med 6:193, 1988

Snover SW, Bocchino V: Massive diltiazem overdose. Ann Emerg Med 15:1221, 1986

Carbon monoxide

Dolan MC: Carbon monoxide poisoning. Can Med Assoc J 133:392, 1985 Symposium—carbon monoxide poisoning—mechanism of damage, late sequelae and therapy. Clin Toxicol 23:247, 1985

Mofenson HC et al: Carbon monoxide poisoning. Am J Emerg Med 2:254, 1984

Cyanide

Caraveti M, Litovitz T: Pediatric cyanide intoxication and death from acetonitrile-containing cosmetic. JAMA 260:3740, 1988

Graham DL et al: Acute cyanide poisoning complicated by lactic acidosis and pulmonary edema. Arch Intern Med 137:1051, 1977

Hall AH et al: Clinical toxicology of cyanide: North American clinical experiences, in Clinical and Experimental Toxicology of Cyanides, B Ballantyne, TC Marrs (eds). Bristol, Wright, 1987, p 312

Digoxin

Smith TW et al: Digitalis glycosides: Mechanisms and manifestations of toxicity. Prog Cardiovasc Dis 26:413, 1984 (part I); 26:495, 1984 (part II); 27:26, 1984 (part III).

——— et al: Treatment of life-threatening digitalis intoxication with digoxin-specific FAB antibody fragments. N Engl J Med 307:1357, 1982

Wanger TL et al: Treatment of 63 severely digitalis-toxic patients with digoxin-specific antibody fragments. J Am Coll Cardiol 5:118A, 1985

Ethanol

Gabow PA et al: Organic acids in ethylene glycol intoxication. Ann Intern Med 105:16, 1986

David DJ, Spyker DA: The acute toxicity of ethanol: Dosage and kinetic nomograms. Vet Hum Toxicol 21:272, 1979

Eckardt MJ et al: Health hazards associated with alcohol consumption. JAMA 246:648, 1981

Halperin ML et al: Metabolic acidosis in the alcoholic: A pathophysiologic approach. Metabolism 32:308, 1983

Ethylene glycol

JACOBSEN D, MCMARTIN KE: Methanol and ethylene glycol poisonings: Mechanism of toxicity, clinical course, diagnosis and treatment. Med Toxicol 1:309, 1986
PARRY MF, WALLACH R: Ethylene glycol poisoning. Am J Med 57:143, 1974

Hallucinogens

BROWN RT, BRADEN NJ: Hallucinogens. Pediatr Clin North Am 34:341, 1987
COHEN S: The hallucinogens and the inhalents. Psych Clin North Am 7:681, 1984

Hydrocarbons

ANAS N et al: Criteria for hospitalizing children who have ingested products containing hydrocarbons. JAMA 246:840, 1981
STREICHEN M et al: Syndromes of solvent sniffing in adults. Ann Intern Med 94:785, 1981
TRUEMPIER E et al: Clinical characteristics, pathophysiology and management of hydrocarbon ingestion: Case report and review of the literature. Pediatr Emerg Care 3:187, 1987

Hydrogen sulfide

HOIDAL CR et al: Hydrogen sulfide poisoning from toxic inhalations of roofing fumes. Ann Emerg Med 15:826, 1986
SMITH RP: Management of acute sulfide poisoning. Arch Environ Health 31:166, 1976
WHITECRAFT DD et al: Hydrogen sulfide poisoning treated with hyperbaric oxygen. J Emerg Med 3:23, 1985

Iron

BANNER W et al: Iron poisoning. Pediatr Clin North Am 33:393, 1986
PROUDFOOT AT et al: Management of acute iron poisoning. Med Toxicol 1:83, 1986
TENEBEIN M et al: Myocardial failure and shock in iron poisoning. Hum Toxicol 7:281, 1988

Isoniazid

ORLOWSKI JP et al: Treatment of potentially lethal dose isoniazid ingestion. Ann Emerg Med 17:73, 1988
WASON S et al: Single high-dose pyridoxine treatment for isoniazid overdose. JAMA 246:1102, 1981
YARBROUGH B, WOOD J: Isoniazid overdose treated with high-dose pyridoxine. Ann Emerg Med 12:303, 1983

Isopropyl alcohol

LACOUTURE PG et al: A review of acute isopropyl alcohol intoxication: Diagnosis and management. Am J Med 75:680, 1983
NATOWICZ M et al: Pharmacokinetic analysis of a case of isopropyl intoxication. Clin Chem 31:326, 1985

Lithium

AMDISEN A: Clinical features and management of lithium poisoning. Med Toxicol 3:18, 1988
DYSON EH et al: Self-poisoning and therapeutic intoxication with lithium. Human Toxicol 6:326, 1987

MAO inhibitors

KAPLAN RF et al: Phenelzine overdose treated with dantrolene sodium. JAMA 255:642, 1986
LINDEN CH: Monoamine oxidase inhibitor overdose. Ann Emerg Med 13:1137, 1984

Methanol

JACOBSEN D, MCMARTIN KE: Methanol and ethylene glycol poisoning: Mechanism of toxicity, clinical course, diagnosis and treatment. Med Toxicol 1:309, 1986
OSTERLOH JD et al: Serum formate concentrations in methanol intoxication as a criterion for hemodialysis. Ann Intern Med 104:200, 1986
SWARTZ RD et al: Epidemic methanol poisoning: Clinical and biochemical analysis of a recent episode. Medicine 60:373, 1981

Methemoglobinemia

CURRY S: Methemoglobinemia. Ann Emerg Med 11:214, 1982
HALL AH et al: Drug and chemical-induced methaemoglobinaemia. Med Toxicol 1:253, 1986
HARVEY JW, KEITT AS: Studies of the efficacy and potential hazards of methylene blue therapy in aniline-induced methaemoglobinaemia. Br J Haematol 53:29, 1983

Muscle relaxants

BAILEY DN: Meprobamate ingestion: A five-year review of cases with serum concentrations and clinical findings. Am J Clin Pathol 75:102, 1981
COHEN MD et al: Atropine in the treatment of baclofen overdose. Am J Emerg Med 4:552, 1986

Narcotics

CUDDY P: Management of acute opioid intoxication. Crit Care Q 4:65, 1982
FORD M et al: Opioids and designer drugs. Emerg Med Clin North Am 8:495, 1990
LAWSON AAH, NORTHRIDGE DB: Dextropropoxyphene overdose. Med Toxicol 2:430, 1987

Nonsteroidal anti-inflammatory drugs

COURT H, VOLANS GN: Poisoning after overdose with nonsteroidal anti-inflammatory drugs. Adverse Drug React Acute Poisoning Rev 3:1, 1984
HALL AH et al: Ibuprofen overdose: 126 cases. Ann Emerg Med 15:1308, 1986
VALE JA, MEREDITH TJ: Acute poisoning due to nonsteroidal anti-inflammatory drugs: Clinical features and management. Med Toxicol 1:11, 1986

Organophosphate and carbamate insecticides

MINTON NA, MURRAY VSG: A review of organophosphate poisoning. Med Toxicol 3:350, 1988
NAMBA T et al: Poisoning due to organophosphate insecticides. Am J Med 50:475, 1971
SENANAYAKE N, KARALLIEDDE L: Neurotoxic effects of organophosphorus insecticides: An intermediate syndrome. N Engl J Med 316:761, 1987

Phenothiazines

BARRY D et al: Phenothiazine poisoning: A review of 48 cases. Calif Med 118:1, 1983
BENOWITZ NL et al: Cardiopulmonary catastrophes in drug-overdosed patients. Med Clin North Am 63:267, 1979
BORYS DJ et al: Acute fluoxetine overdose: A report of 234 cases. Am J Emerg Med 10:115, 1992
LEE A: Treatment of drug-induced dystonic reactions. J Am Coll Emerg Phys 8:453, 1979
POPE HG et al: Frequency and presentation of neuroleptic malignant syndrome in a large psychiatric hospital. Am J Psychiatry 143:1227, 1986

Salicylates

BRENNER BE, SIMON RR: Management of salicylate intoxication. Drugs 24:335, 1987
GAUDREAULT P et al: The relative severity of acute vs chronic salicylate poisoning in children: A clinical comparison. Pediatrics 70:566, 1982
TEMPLE AR: Acute and chronic effects of aspirin toxicity and their treatment. Arch Intern Med 141:364, 1981
THISTED B et al: Acute salicylate poisoning in 177 consecutive patients treated in an ICU. Acta Anaesthesiol Scand 31:312, 1987

Stimulants

AARO CK: Sympathomimetics. Emerg Med Clin North Am 8:513, 1990
LINDEN CH et al: Amphetamines. Top Emerg Med 7:18, 1985
PENTEL P: Toxicity of over-the-counter stimulants. JAMA 252:1898, 1984

Theophylline

GAUDREAULT P, GUAY J: Theophylline poisoning. Med Toxicol 1:169, 1986
OLSON KR et al: Theophylline overdose: Acute single ingestion versus chronic repeated overmedication. Am J Emerg Med 3:386, 1985
PARK GD et al: Use of hemoperfusion for treatment of theophylline intoxication. Am J Med 74:961, 1983
SHANNON MW, LOVEJOY FH JR: The influence of age versus peak concentration on life-threatening events after chronic theophylline intoxication. Arch Intern Med 150:2045, 1990

Tricyclic antidepressants

BOEHNERT MT, LOVEJOY FH JR: Value of QRS duration versus the serum drug level in predicting seizures and ventricular arrhythmias after an acute overdose of tricyclic antidepressants. N Engl J Med 313:474, 1985
CROME P: Poisoning due to tricyclic antidepressant overdose. Med Toxicol 1:261, 1986
FROMMER DA et al: Tricyclic antidepressant overdose; A review. JAMA 257:521, 1987

396 HEAVY METAL POISONING

JOHN W. GRAEF

ARSENIC

SOURCE Inorganic arsenic compounds such as arsenic trioxide, arsenic pentoxide, and sodium and potassium arsenite and arsenate are found in insecticides, rodenticides, fungicides, wood preservatives, herbicides, and compounds used in glass manufacturing. Organic arsenic is widely distributed in the environment. Arsine gas is produced in the smelting and refining of metals, in galvanizing and etching, in lead plating, and in making silicon microchips. Historically, organic arsenical compounds have been used in the treatment of syphilis, epilepsy, psoriasis, and amebiasis. Currently, acute toxicity is encountered following accidental ingestion, industrial accidents, or suicidal or homicidal intoxications. Chronic exposures occur most commonly following low-dose exposure in industry or chronic consumption of contaminated food, water, or medications. Arsenic toxicity is a common cause of death in children after pesticide ingestion.

METABOLISM   Arsenic is absorbed through the skin, lungs, and gastrointestinal tract. Inorganic (trivalent) compounds are absorbed more readily than organic (pentavalent) forms, with greater than 80 percent of an ingested dose absorbed by the gastrointestinal tract. Arsine gas is absorbed through the lungs. Arsenic is distributed from blood to liver, kidney, lung, spleen, and intestine within 24 h of ingestion and to skin, hair, and bone within 2 weeks. Inorganic arsenic compounds are found in high concentrations in leukocytes. Inorganic arsenic does not cross the blood-brain barrier but does cross the placenta. Between 5 and 10 percent is excreted in feces, and 90 to 95 percent is excreted in the urine. Small amounts are recovered in bile, feces, saliva, and breast milk. Arsenic may be detected in urine for at least 10 days following an overdose and detected in the serum for a shorter period of time.

CLINICAL TOXICOLOGY   Arsine gas combines with the globin chain of hemoglobin in red blood cells to produce severe hemolysis with anemia, hemoglobinuria, and hematuria within 3 to 4 h of ingestion. Subsequent jaundice may be severe. Signs and symptoms of toxicity include nausea, vomiting and diarrhea, apprehension and malaise, tachycardia, and dyspnea. Acute renal failure is frequent and often fatal.

The reported lethal dose for arsenic ranges from 120 to 200 mg. As little as 2 mg/kg of body weight can be lethal for children. Manifestations of acute toxicity include for the gastrointestinal tract—burning in the throat, difficulty swallowing, nausea, vomiting, diarrhea, abdominal pain, and a garlic odor on the breath; for the cardiovascular system—cyanosis, difficulty breathing, and hypotension with myocardial depression and rare arrhythmias; for the central nervous system—delirium, coma, and seizures; for the kidneys—acute tubular necrosis and oliguria; and for the hematologic system—hemolysis, eosinophilia, and, rarely, bone marrow depression. Manifestations of chronic arsenic poisoning occur 2 to 8 weeks following ingestion and include for the skin and nails—erythroderma, hyperkeratosis, hyperpigmentation, exfoliative dermatitis, and Aldrich-Mees lines (transverse white striae of the fingernails); for the mucous membranes—laryngitis, tracheitis, and bronchitis; and for the peripheral nervous system—polyneuritis (sensory and motor). Basal cell carcinomas, squamous cell carcinomas, Bowen's disease of the skin (see Chap. 54), and lung carcinomas have been associated with chronic arsenic exposure. With chronic exposure, the risk of cancer of the bladder, kidney, and liver may be comparable to that for lung cancer in cigarette smokers.

Arsenic produces its toxicity by binding with tissue sulfhydryl groups. Arsenic also binds to enzymes in the Krebs tricarboxylic acid cycle, thereby interfering with oxidative phosphorylation. Other effects include capillary injury and direct toxic effects on large organs. Pathologic findings include necrosis of the stomach, small bowel, and vasculature and degenerative changes in the liver and kidneys.

LABORATORY FINDINGS   Arsenic is radiopaque and is seen on x-ray of the abdomen. It also may be detected in hair and nails for months following exposure. Specific organ effects include abnormal liver function tests; Q-T prolongation and T-wave inversion; anemia, leukocytosis, leukopenia, and hemoglobinemia; and proteinuria, hematuria, hemoglobinuria, and cellular casts in the urine. Urine arsenic (As) levels are normally less than 67 nmol/d (5 μg/d).

TREATMENT   Acute ingestion should be treated by inducing vomiting with ipecac syrup if the patient is alert. Gastric lavage is preferable if the patient is obtunded or the ingestion is severe. Activated charcoal and cathartics are of unclear benefit. Dimercaprol chelates arsenic by producing an insoluble complex that is excreted by the kidneys. For mild symptoms and elevated serum or urinary levels, 3 to 5 mg/kg of body weight per dose is given intramuscularly every 4 h for 24 h and then every 12 to 24 h for 7 to 10 days.

Adequacy of urinary mobilization of arsenic is confirmed and followed during treatment by measurement of serum and urinary levels. Treatment should be continued until 24-h urine As levels are less than 67 nmol/d (5 μg/d). Toxic manifestations of dimercaprol (increased blood pressure, tachycardia, nausea, vomiting, headache, burning sensation in the lips, mucous membrane irritation, coma, and convulsions) occur with increasing doses. The water-soluble analogue of dimercaprol, succimer (DMSA), may be more effective and is less toxic than dimercaprol.

Penicillamine has been used successfully in acute and chronic poisoning, administered orally at a dose of 100 mg/kg of body weight per day (the maximum dose not to exceed 1 g/d) in four divided doses for 5 days. Side effects of penicillamine include rash, leukopenia, thrombocytopenia, and nephrotoxicity. Hemodialysis removes arsenic (24 to 100 mg in 24 h) with a clearance of 80 to 90 mL/min and is indicated if renal failure occurs. Hemodialysis early in the clinical course in conjunction with dimercaprol may limit arsenic's distribution phase and enhance clearance of free and complexed arsenic.

Exchange transfusion is the preferred treatment for arsine gas poisoning. Dimercaprol affords no protection against red cell destruction.

CADMIUM

SOURCE   Exposure to cadmium is usually occupational or via pollution from mining or smelting operations. Cadmium is produced commercially as a by-product of copper and lead or zinc smelting and is used in the manufacture of batteries, in ceramics, in textiles, in soldering, in electroplating, and as a pigment in paints and plastics. In contaminated areas, high concentrations may be found in shellfish and foodstuffs.

METABOLISM   Absorption occurs via ingestion or inhalation. Normal daily oral intake is up to 200 μg, with an estimated mean of 20 to 40 μg/d. Only 5 to 10 percent of this is absorbed, although, like lead, absorption may be increased in the presence of calcium and iron deficiency. About 5 percent of inhaled cadmium is absorbed depending on particle size. Small, highly soluble particles are absorbed at a rate of 25 to 50 percent.

About 50 percent of absorbed cadmium is concentrated in the liver and kidneys. In erythrocytes and soft tissues, cadmium is bound to metallothionein, a low-molecular-weight polypeptide containing a large number of available sulfhydryl groups that exert a protective effect. With large single-dose cadmium exposures, saturation of the protein may result in loss of protective effect. Cadmium does not pass the placenta and gradually accumulates in the body with age. In limited studies, small amounts are found in breast milk. Biologic half-life has been estimated at more than 20 years, except in the presence of kidney damage, when urinary excretion is increased. In the kidney, metallothionein-bound cadmium is filtered at the glomerulus and is then reabsorbed by the proximal tubules. The urinary excretion rarely exceeds 5 nmol/d (0.5 μg/d).

CLINICAL TOXICOLOGY   Acute cadmium intoxication may occur after either ingestion or inhalation. Ingestion of water containing concentrations of 15 mg/L or foods containing as little as 30 mg cadmium can induce vomiting, abdominal pain, and severe diarrhea. Shock may ensue. Acute inhalation of cadmium dust produces dyspnea, weakness, chest pain, shortness of breath, and cough. A chemical pneumonitis produces pulmonary edema and respiratory failure. Clinical symptoms may occur with air exposure as low as 1 mg/m² of surface area over 8 h. During the same time period, inhalation of 5 mg/m² of surface area may be fatal. A latent period of 4 to 24 h from exposure to onset of symptoms may complicate accurate diagnosis. Death usually occurs in 5 to 10 days. Chemical pneumonitis may continue for several months, and pulmonary function can be abnormal for longer than 1 year after exposure.

Chronic intoxication usually occurs by industrial inhalation and produces emphysema and characteristic renal tubular damage with proteinuria and increased urinary excretion of beta$_2$ microglobulin. Cadmium's inhibitory effect on α_1-antitrypsin may be responsible for cadmium-induced emphysema. Relatively minor changes in liver function, a microcytic, hypochromic anemia unresponsive to iron therapy, and hypertension are associated findings. Chronic oral intake of contaminated rice and drinking water has produced a syndrome in Japan called *itai-itai* (ouch-ouch) disease with manifestations that include renal tubular damage and osteomalacia. Cadmium is probably a carcinogen for lung cancer, although a suggested association with cancer of the prostate has not been confirmed.

LABORATORY FINDINGS Measurement of blood cadmium levels is not useful. Urinary cadmium excretion exceeding 0.1 μmol/L (10 μg/L) is associated with renal tubular damage, especially when accompanied by elevated urinary beta$_2$ microglobulin and metallothionein levels. Kidney cadmium content obtained by renal biopsy can be assessed by neutron activation analysis. A renal cadmium concentration exceeding 2 μmol/g (200 μg/g) of wet weight is associated with renal disease.

TREATMENT Treatment is controversial. Although chelating agents bind cadmium, they may effectively shift cadmium to the kidney, where further damage can occur. In acute exposure, ethylenediaminetetraacetic acid (edetate) in a dose of 1.5 g/m^2 of surface area in a slow intravenous infusion daily can be beneficial. Dimercaprol is not effective. However, its water-soluble oral congener, succimer appears promising, although experience in cadmium poisoning is limited. Acute inhalation pneumonitis should be treated with glucocorticoids and diuretics. Itai-itai disease appears to respond to large doses of vitamin D. Long-term sequelae of chronic cadmium exposure include emphysema and chronic renal insufficiency.

LEAD

SOURCE Lead is a normal constituent of the earth's crust and is found throughout nature. The increased use of lead during the Industrial Revolution caused extensive disease among lead workers; the addition of lead salts to paints as coloring agents and stabilizers set the stage for the largest epidemic of lead poisoning in history, that of childhood plumbism. As many as 12 million preschool children in the United States may be affected annually by this syndrome, caused by ingestion of lead from paint, soil, household dust, and infrequently, drinking water. Evidence of permanent neurologic sequelae from levels of lead previously thought to be safe has raised fears of possible damage to the fetus and newborn as well. The nature of this epidemic has forced prohibition against the addition of organic lead salts to gasoline as well as extensive prohibitions against the use of lead in consumer products. These efforts have reduced the mean blood lead level in the United States from 0.8 μmol/L (16 μg/dL) in 1978 to less than 0.3 μmol/L (6 μg/dL) in 1990.

METABOLISM Inorganic lead salts are absorbed through ingestion or inhalation. Organic lead salts also may be absorbed through the skin. Generally, gastrointestinal absorption is about 10 percent of an ingested dose, but in children it may be as high as 50 percent. It is enhanced by deficiency of iron, calcium, and zinc. Absorption through the lung varies with tidal volume and particle size. Particles smaller than 1 μm may be absorbed if they reach the alveoli. Adults may ingest up to 0.5 μmol/d (100 μg/d) of lead from normal exposure to food and drinking water. Positive lead balance may occur at these levels, since renal excretion normally does not exceed 0.4 μmol/d (80 μg/d). In children, no more than 0.02 μmol/kg (5 μg/kg) of body weight is tolerated without increasing the body lead burden. Infants are a particular risk through consumption of formula reconstituted with contaminated tap water.

Under steady state conditions, 5 to 10 percent of ingested lead may be found in blood; 95 percent of that fraction is associated with the erythrocyte. In adults, up to 80 to 90 percent is taken up by bone and incorporated into hydroxyapatite crystals, where it is relatively inactive. The remainder is found in soft tissues, principally the kidneys and brain. The principal route of excretion is stool (80 to 90 percent), and the remainder is found in the urine (10 percent). Small amounts are excreted in hair, nails, sweat, and saliva. Lead passes the placenta and blood-brain barrier and may be found in human milk. The half-life of lead in blood and soft tissues is 24 to 40 days, and in bone, 10^4 days.

Lead is a poison of enzymes, binding to the sulfhydryl groups of proteins. It also interferes with Ca^{2+} transport, synthesis and release of neurotransmitters, and activation of protein kinase C. In high concentration, lead alters the tertiary structure of intracellular proteins, denaturing them and causing cell death and tissue inflammation.

CLINICAL TOXICOLOGY The toxic effects of lead differ between children and adults. The adult form is generally characterized by abdominal pain, anemia, renal disease, headache, peripheral neuropathy with demyelination of long neurons, ataxia, and memory loss. Symptoms are usually associated with prolonged elevation of lead levels above 4 to 5 μmol/L (80 to 100 μg/dL) of whole blood. A subclinical form in adults affects primarily the peripheral nervous system and the kidneys. A linear association between hypertension and elevated lead levels [i.e., greater than 1.5 μmol/L (30 μg/dL)] has been reported. Encephalopathy is rare in adults.

Childhood lead poisoning is manifested by abdominal pain and anemia, but the central nervous system effects are most important. As an enzymatic poison, lead affects developing tissues more than tissues with slow turnover. Hence subclinical lead poisoning is most dangerous to children because its effects emerge without associated symptoms that bring the victim to medical attention. In the acute clinical form, signs and symptoms reflect both the direct effect of high concentrations of lead [i.e., blood lead greater than 4 μmol/L (80 μg/dL)] and consequent severe alterations in porphyrin synthesis. Signs and symptoms include abdominal pain and irritability, followed by lethargy, anorexia, pallor (anemia), ataxia, and slurred speech. In severe cases, convulsions, coma, and death are usually due to severe generalized cerebral edema and renal failure. A history of "high-dose" exposure to lead (usually paint chips), pica (the ingestion of nonfood substances), and malnutrition (iron, calcium, and zinc deficiency) almost always is associated with this syndrome.

The subclinical form of childhood plumbism is associated with elevated blood lead with or without increased erythrocyte protoporphyrin when the blood lead level exceeds 1.5 μmol/L (30 μg/dL). However, no symptoms are usually detected. The syndrome is widespread, and its effects on the developing central nervous system are largely irreversible. These include mental retardation and selective deficits in language, cognitive functions, and behavior, depending on the age and duration of exposure. These latter factors are more important than the height of the lead level. Elevated lead levels at or about 2 years of age are predictive of neurodevelopmental outcome.

LABORATORY FINDINGS Laboratory abnormalities include blood lead levels greater than 0.5 μmol/L (10 μg/dL). Biochemical and neurodevelopmental abnormalities may occur in association with blood lead levels as low as 0.7 μmol/L (15 μg/dL), particularly in very young children. Although a hemolytic anemia is associated with acute plumbism, chronic plumbism is associated with iron deficiency. Other heme precursors are increased in plasma and urine (e.g., delta aminolevulinic acid).

Renal abnormalities include pyuria, the Fanconi syndrome, and azotemia. In plumbism, urinary excretion of lead exceeds 4 μmol/d (80 μg/d). In adults, demyelination of long nerves produces prolonged nerve conduction time and subsequent paralysis of extensor muscles with atrophy (wrist drop or foot drop). While slight prolongation of nerve conduction can be seen in children, it is clinically evident only in those with sickle cell disease. Abnormalities of cardiac, thyroid, and hepatic function occur in adults. In children, a characteristic finding is increased density at the metaphyseal plate of growing long bones, so-called lead lines. These are generally seen in association with levels greater than 2.4 μmol/L (50 μg/dL) of whole blood for a prolonged period. They are not seen in adults.

TREATMENT The *sine qua non* of treatment is removal of the source of exposure. Cases of industrial lead poisoning should be reported to the Occupational Safety Health Administration (OSHA). Cases of childhood plumbism should be reported to the local board of health to initiate examination of housing for sources of lead.

Reduction of the body burden of lead is accomplished by use of chelating agents, principally edetate calcium disodium (EDTA), dimercaprol, penicillamine, and succimer. The lead mobilization test may be used to determine the size of the "chelatable" pool of lead in patients with moderately elevated levels [i.e., 1.7 to 2.2 μmol/L (35 to 45 μg/dL)]. In this test, administration of a calculated dose of chelating agent, usually edetate, induces a lead diuresis that is then compared with the dose of chelating agent. The test is positive when greater than 2.5 nmol (0.5 μg) lead is excreted per milligram of chelating agent administered per 6 to 8 h. The use of x-ray fluorescence of bone to determine the lead burden is under investigation as an alternative to the lead mobilization test.

In acute encephalopathy, double therapy (dimercaprol and edetate) is used until blood lead levels are less than 2 μmol/L (40 μg/dL). Urine flow must be established, and even in the presence of cerebral edema, fluids must be sufficient to produce a lead diuresis. Cerebral edema should be managed in an intensive care setting, but removal of the metal is essential. In symptomatic adults and children, therapy with both dimercaprol and edetate should be used for 5 days at edetate doses of up to 1.5 g/m^2 of surface area daily and dimercaprol doses of 12 to 24 mg/kg of body weight per day. If further chelation is required, a minimum interval of 48 to 72 h should intervene between courses of therapy. The penicillamine dose is 20 to 40 mg/kg of body weight per day, not to exceed 1 g/d. Adverse effects, particularly allergy, may be reduced by beginning therapy with one-quarter of the total dose for 1 week and then doubling and redoubling the dose until full dose is reached. Penicillamine can be administered for 3 to 6 months until the body lead burden is depleted. Only penicillamine and, to a lesser extent, edetate remove lead directly from bone. If edetate is indicated, as many separate 5-day courses as are needed may be given provided that the total safe dose is not exceeded and proper intervals between courses are observed.

Succimer is licensed by the Food and Drug Administration for oral treatment of children with Pb levels of 2.2 μmol/L (45 μg/dL). Current recommendations for therapy are 5 days at 30 μg/kg per day in three divided doses, followed by 14 days at 20 μg/kg per day in two divided doses. Side effects include occasional vomiting and transient elevations in hepatic enzymes. "Rebound" in Pb levels as high as 80 percent of the original value necessitates repeat courses for effective reduction in lead burden.

MERCURY

SOURCE Humans may encounter mercury in an inorganic (elemental or mercuric salt) or an organic (usually methyl) form. All three are toxic, but organic mercury is most widespread and potentially dangerous. Elemental mercury is used in thermometers, sphygmomanometers, dental amalgams, and some disk batteries. It is volatile at room temperature and rapidly oxidizes to mercuric mercury when exposed to oxygen. Toxicity usually occurs from inhalation of mercury vapor during industrial exposure, although elevated mercury levels have been reported in neonates exposed to faulty mercury switches in incubators. Mercuric salts are found in topical medicines, in catalytic agents in the manufacture of plastics, in cathartics (e.g., Calomel), and in foodstuffs. Toxicity occurs usually as a result of gastrointestinal exposure. Organic mercury is found in paints, fungicides, seeds, foods, medicines, cosmetic agents, and wood preservatives. Large amounts of methyl mercury are formed by methylation of mercury salt wastes, as occurred in the mercury epidemic in Minamata Bay, Japan.

METABOLISM Elemental mercury is poorly absorbed by the gastrointestinal tract but is absorbed efficiently as vapor through the lungs, with 80 to 100 percent of inhaled mercury entering the bloodstream through the alveoli. Absorbed mercury vapor is lipid-soluble and readily crosses the blood-brain barrier and the placenta. It is rapidly oxidized to its mercuric form and combines with sulfhydryl groups. Excretion is via the urine and feces. The half-life of elemental mercury is approximately 60 days.

Inorganic mercury salts are absorbed through the gastrointestinal tract and skin. Large overdoses may produce corrosive effects on the gastrointestinal tract with consequent increased absorption. Normal uptake is less than 10 percent of an ingested dose. Ingestion of disk batteries with consequent decomposition in the gastrointestinal tract has resulted in elevated mercury levels without gastrointestinal symptoms. Mercuric salts accumulate primarily in the kidney but are distributed to the liver, erythrocytes, bone marrow, spleen, lung, intestine, and skin. Little, if any, crosses the blood-brain barrier. Excretion is via the urine and feces. The half-life of inorganic mercury is approximately 40 days.

Organic (methyl) mercury is readily absorbed through the intestines and the skin. Short-chain alkyl and methyl mercury penetrate the erythrocyte membrane and bind to hemoglobin. Because of its high lipid solubility, methyl mercury freely passes the placenta and blood-brain barrier and enters breast milk. Organic mercury also concentrates in the kidneys and the central nervous system. Metallothionein synthesis is induced by mercury, and the augmented concentration of the protein exerts a partial protective effect against tissue damage. Excretion is complex. About 1 percent of organic mercury is excreted in urine directly. Methyl mercury is acetylated in the liver or may be conjugated with cysteine or glutathione. The *N*-acetyl-homocysteine–methyl mercury complex then enters the enterohepatic circulation and is ultimately excreted in the urine. The half-life of organic mercury in humans is about 70 days. Phenyl mercuric compounds are excreted more rapidly.

CLINICAL TOXICOLOGY Acute metallic mercury (vapor) poisoning causes inflammation of large and small airways and interstitial pneumonitis. The rapid uptake of mercury vapor into the central nervous system produces tremor and increased excitability. Both acute and chronic mercury vapor poisoning primarily affects the central nervous system. Acute mercury vapor poisoning can cause acute inorganic mercury toxicity with consequent possibly irreversible neurologic sequelae. Initial symptoms include lassitude, anorexia, weight loss, and gastrointestinal disturbances. Increasing exposure produces the characteristic intention tremor of mercury poisoning and is accompanied by mercurial *erethism* (timidity, memory loss, insomnia, excitability, and, in severe cases, delirium). This neurologic picture in felt-hat workers exposed to mercury vapor and mercuric salts led to the phrase "mad as a hatter." Intravenous elemental mercury administration can produce symptomatic mercury granulomas in the lung but with little apparent consequence. A contribution of dental amalgams to toxicity has not been demonstrated.

Chronic inorganic mercury poisoning produces the preceding neurologic findings as well as excessive salivation, loosening of the teeth, gingivitis, and stomatitis. When applied to the skin, mercuric salts may cause hypersensitivity reactions ranging from mild erythema to exfoliative dermatitis. Acrodynia, or Pink's disease, occurs in young children and may be mistaken for Kawasaki's disease. Symptoms include generalized rash, irritability, photophobia, hypertrichosis, profuse perspiration, and swelling and desquamation of the feet and hands.

Acute inorganic mercury poisoning is characterized by corrosive effects on the gastrointestinal tract, including nausea, vomiting, hematemesis, and abdominal pain followed by tenesmus, bloody diarrhea, and necrosis of intestinal mucosa. Acute fluid redistribution in massive overdose can produce shock and death. Acute inorganic mercury poisoning causes acute tubular necrosis, while chronic inorganic mercury poisoning produces a nephrotic syndrome.

Acute and chronic organic mercury poisonings are indistinguishable. Prenatal poisoning produces cerebral palsy as a result of cortical and cerebellar atrophy. Postnatal poisoning causes paresthesias, headache, pain, visual, hearing, and speech disorders, neurasthenia, loss of memory, incoordination, erethism, spasticity, paralysis, stupor, and coma. These neurologic abnormalities are often permanent.

The daily intake of methyl mercury should not exceed 100 parts per billion. Blood mercury levels above 180 nmol/L (3.5 μg/dL) and urine mercury levels above 0.7 μmol/L (150 μg/L) are abnormal. Symptoms may be seen with blood mercury levels above 1 μmol/L (20 μg/dL) and urine mercury levels above 3 μmol/L (600 μg/L). Clinical findings may be associated with somewhat lower concentrations depending on when exposure occurred.

TREATMENT Treatment is aimed at reducing the absorption of mercury, protecting susceptible tissues, and enhancing elimination. In the case of ingestion of mercuric salts, initial treatment consists of removing mercury from the stomach by inducing emesis or by gastric lavage. Polythiol resins are effective in binding mercury in the gastrointestinal tract. Activated charcoal, however, does not bind metals.

Generally, chelation therapy is indicated when elevated urine or blood mercury levels are present. Chelating agents with active mono- or dithiol groups are most effective. These include dimercaprol and the oral chelators penicillamine and succimer.

In acute inorganic mercury poisoning, dimercaprol should be used at a dose not exceeding 24 mg/kg of body weight per 24 h, intramuscularly, in divided doses. Generally, therapy should not exceed 5 days at a time but can be reinstituted after a suitable rest period. Penicillamine can be used in the treatment of inorganic mercury poisoning but N-acetyl-DL-penicillamine is equally effective and less toxic. The dose is 30 mg/kg of body weight per day in two to three divided doses. Peritoneal dialysis and hemodialysis also have been used with some success, as has succimer in combination with extracorporeal regional complexing hemodialysis (ERCH) in patients with renal failure. Neither is as effective as chelation therapy, but they may be useful in the presence of renal failure, and neither has been shown to reverse the neurologic sequelae of inorganic mercury poisoning.

In chronic inorganic mercury poisoning, dimercaprol is ineffective. Penicillamine is the drug of choice. The investigational drug N-acetyl-DL-penicillamine is more effective than either dimercaprol or edetate. Succimer may enhance urinary mercury excretion without influencing clinical outcome.

THALLIUM

SOURCE Thallium is used as an insecticide, as a catalyst in fireworks, in manufacturing imitation jewelry and optical lenses, in industry as an alloy, and in cardiac perfusion imaging. It was banned in the United States as a rodenticide in 1972. Accidental as well as intentional ingestions of thallium occur. Epidemic poisoning has followed the ingestion of grain impregnated with thallium. Thallium is available as iodide, sulfate, acetate, carbonate, and nitrate salts.

METABOLISM Thallium is absorbed percutaneously, by inhalation, and by oral ingestion. It has a large volume of distribution of 4 to 6 L/kg of body weight with distribution to body organs including kidney, pancreas, spleen, liver, lung, muscles, and brain. It crosses the placenta. Thallium is bound to sulfhydryl groups on mitochondrial membranes at intracellular sites. The elimination half-life is variable, ranging from 3 to 15 days. The major pathway of elimination is in the urine; 3 percent of a dose is eliminated per day, or 75 mL/min total-body clearance.

Thallium is soluble at physiologic pH and interferes with oxidative phosphorylation by inhibition of ATPase. It substitutes for potassium in many physiologic reactions. Pathologic findings at postmortem include cerebral edema, loss of myelin in peripheral nerves, fatty infiltration of the liver, and degenerative changes in the myocardium.

CLINICAL TOXICOLOGY Severe poisoning occurs following a single ingested dose greater than 1 g or 8 mg/kg of body weight.

Death has occurred following an ingested dose of 15 mg/kg of body weight.

Immediate signs and symptoms (occurring within 3 to 4 h of ingestion) include nausea and vomiting, abdominal pain, diarrhea, hematemesis, and hematochezia. Intermediate manifestations (within 1 week of ingestion) include involvement of the central nervous system with confusion, psychosis, choreoathetosis, organic brain syndrome, convulsions, and coma. Peripheral neurologic involvement is both motor and sensory and includes paresthesias, myalgias, weakness, tremor, and ataxia. Autonomic manifestations are less common and include tachycardia, hypertension, and salivation. Ophthalmologic abnormalities are neuritis, ophthalmoplegia, ptosis, strabismus, and cranial nerve palsies. Late manifestations (occurring 2 to 4 weeks after ingestion) include diffuse hair loss (with sparing of pubic and body hair and the lateral one-third of the eyebrows) with regrowth occurring as body burden decreases over time. Residual effects include memory loss, ataxia, tremor, and foot drop.

LABORATORY FINDINGS Thallium is radiopaque and is evident on an abdominal x-ray. Thallium levels with severe ingestion range, in serum, from 1.5 to 30 μmol/L (30 to 600 μg/dL) and, in urine, from 0.05 to 600 μmol/d (10 to 120,000 μg/d). The electroencephalogram (EEG) is diffusely abnormal, and peripheral nerve conduction may be delayed.

TREATMENT Therapeutic modalities include gastrointestinal decontamination, enhanced renal excretion, and dialysis. Gastric lavage or ipecac syrup is indicated within 4 to 6 h of acute ingestion. Adequacy of removal of thallium can be documented by follow-up abdominal x-ray. Prussian blue absorbs thallium in the gastrointestinal tract by exchanging potassium for thallium on its crystal lattice network, thereby preventing absorption. The oral dose is 250 mg/kg of body weight, administered in three to four divided doses. Activated charcoal is as effective as Prussian blue in increasing fecal elimination by interrupting the enterohepatic circulation of thallium. Mannitol or magnesium citrate is used as a laxative to enhance gastrointestinal removal.

Forced diuresis is the oldest technique in use and increases urinary excretion by 50 to 100 percent. Potassium chloride promotes renal excretion of thallium through the exchange of potassium for thallium, thereby releasing thallium from tissue sites into blood and augmenting urinary excretion two- to threefold. This therapy shortens thallium half-life in humans but may aggravate neurologic symptoms by redistributing thallium into the brain. The amount of thallium removed as compared with the total ingested dose of potassium is small. Diuretics (furosemide) also increase urinary elimination of thallium. Peritoneal dialysis removes 15 to 20 mg thallium per day and hemodialysis 8 mg for each 8 h of dialysis. Prolonged hemodialysis can remove up to 25 mg thallium per day, the total amount removed being relatively small. Charcoal hemoperfusion achieves average blood clearance values of 100 mL/min at a blood flow rate of 300 mL/min. Thus the combination of forced diuresis, diuretic therapy, and hemoperfusion will most effectively enhance total-body clearance of thallium. This therapy should be combined with oral administration of Prussian blue or activated charcoal plus cathartics.

Ditiocarb has been advocated for early use in overdose because it leads to increased thallium blood levels and a two- to threefold increase in thallium excretion. However, ditiocarb-thallium complexes diffuse into the brain with subsequent clinical and EEG worsening; therefore, ditiocarb is contraindicated in thallium intoxication.

CHELATING AGENTS

Chelating agents are used to bind toxic metals in stable, cyclic compounds with relatively low toxicity and enhanced renal and fecal excretion.

DIMERCAPROL (BRITISH ANTI-LEWISITE, BAL) Dimercaprol was first developed as an antidote for the arsenical war gas lewisite; its chelating property is due to its four sulfhydryl groups which bind in a complex to polyvalent metal ions. Its affinity for metals is strong enough to reverse a significant portion of toxic metal enzyme binding. Dimercaprol diffuses into erythrocytes and enhances fecal as well as urinary metal excretion. It is given intramuscularly in peanut oil every 4 to 8 h in a dose of 12 to 24 mg/kg of body weight per 24 h. Toxicity includes mild febrile reactions, nausea, headache, lacrimation, conjunctivitis, salivation, and rhinorrhea. The drug emits a strong sulfide odor, and patients may complain of metallic taste. Contraindications to dimercaprol include glucose-6-phosphate dehydrogenase deficiency, allergy to peanut oil, and concurrent use of medicinal iron, which forms a toxic complex with dimercaprol.

EDETATE (EDTA)   Because the sodium salt of edetate can produce profound hypocalcemia, only the calcium disodium salt should be used in therapy of metal poisoning. Calcium edetate forms a complex with divalent cations, exchanging one atom of calcium for each metal ion. It enhances urinary excretion of lead 20- to 50-fold and also increases excretion of zinc and, to a lesser extent, other metals. It does not enter the erythrocyte but removes metals from the extracellular sites. Oral administration is contraindicated because it is variably absorbed and it enhances absorption of metals from the gastrointestinal tract. The drug is given parenterally either by constant intravenous infusion or intramuscular injection in a dose of 500 to 1000 mg/m^2 of surface area per day. The drug can be used safely in conjunction with other chelating agents. Toxicity increases after 4 to 5 days of administration with concomitant reduction in metal excretion; as a consequence, the drug is given for several "courses" of from 3 to 5 days each.

Toxicity is principally renal, dose-related, and usually reversible. It can be reduced by maintaining adequate urine flow. During treatment renal function should be carefully monitored.

SUCCIMER   Succimer (DMSA, di-mercapto-succinic acid) is a water-soluble oral congener of dimercaprol. It is licensed by the Food and Drug Administration for the treatment of children with blood lead levels exceeding 2.2 μmol/L (45 μg/dL) and is investigational for uses in children with lower lead levels and for treatment of arsenic and mercury poisoning. It is the only drug licensed exclusively for pediatric use to avoid its misuse in occupational exposures. Unlike D-penicillamine, it permits concomitant administration of iron when iron deficiency complicates childhood plumbism, as it often does. Enhancement of renal excretion appears to be comparable with that induced by parenteral edetate, but the relatively high "rebound" values usually necessitate multiple courses of administration. The current dosage regimen is 10 mg/kg of body weight tid for 5 days, followed by 10 mg/kg of body weight bid for 14 days. Rebound values should be measured within 2 weeks of therapy. Side effects include usually mild, apparently transient elevations in hepatic transaminases and cutaneous reactions, usually in adults receiving multiple courses. The drug has an unpleasant sulfurous odor, and vomiting of single doses is common. Because the dramatic but transient depression of blood lead can "mask" active ingestion of lead, its use should be deferred in children with ongoing exposure to lead hazards.

PENICILLAMINE   Penicillamine is the only commercially available oral chelating agent. Not presently approved by the Food and Drug Administration for treatment of lead poisoning, it is licensed for use in the treatment of rheumatoid arthritis, Wilson's disease, and cystinuria. Nevertheless, there is extensive experience in its use in chelation of other metals. The N-acetyl form is particularly helpful in the treatment of inorganic and organic mercury poisoning.

Penicillamine enhances excretion of heavy metals in the urine by an unclear mechanism. The drug is given orally in a dose of 40 mg/kg of body weight per day. By initiating therapy at low doses (usually 25 percent of the anticipated maximum dose) and gradually increasing the dose, the frequency of side effects can be reduced substantially.

Side effects may be seen in up to 20 to 30 percent of patients receiving penicillamine and resemble penicillin hypersensitivity, including rash, fever, thrombocytopenia, and leukopenia. Rare side effects include autoimmune hemolytic anemia and Stevens-Johnson

syndrome. Anorexia, nausea, sleep disturbances, and urinary frequency may be seen occasionally. Nephrotoxicity is reported in adults receiving large doses and in one case has been reported in a child. Patients receiving penicillamine should, therefore, be carefully monitored for signs of renal, hematologic, or allergic side effects.

REFERENCES

Arsenic

BATES MN et al: Arsenic ingestion and internal cancers: A review. Am J Epidemiol 135:462, 1992
ELLENHORN MJ, BARCELOUX DG: Medical Toxicology, New York, Elsevier, 1988
FESMIRE FM et al: Survival following massive arsenic ingestion. Am J Emerg Med 6:603, 1988
HUTTON JT et al: Arsenic poisoning. N Engl J Med 307:1080, 1982
MATHIES D et al: Massive arsenic poisoning: Effects of hemodialysis and dimercaprol on arsenic kinetics. Intensive Care Med 18(1):47, 1992

Cadmium

DUNPHY B: Acute occupational cadmium poisoning. J Occup Med 9:22, 1967
FRIBERG L et al: Cadmium in the Environment, 2d ed. Cleveland, CRC Press, 1974
LAUWERYS RR et al: Health risk assessment of long-term exposure to chemicals: Applications to cadmium and manganese. Arch Toxicol Suppl 15:97, 1992
WAALKES MP et al: Toxicological principles of metal carcinogenesis with special emphasis on cadmium. Crit Rev Toxicol 22(3–4):175, 1992

Lead

AGENCY FOR TOXIC SUBSTANCES DISEASE REGISTRY: The Nature and Extent of Lead Poisoning in Children in the United States: A Report to Congress. Washington, US Department of Health and Human Services, Public Health Service, July 1988
CARNOW B (ed): Health Effects of Occupational Lead and Arsenic Exposure: A Symposium. Washington, US Department of Health, Education, and Welfare, 1976
CENTERS FOR DISEASE CONTROL AND PREVENTION: Preventing Lead Poisoning in Young Children. Atlanta, CDCP, 1991
GRAEF J: Lead poisoning, parts I, II, and III. Clin Toxicol Rev 14(8, 9, 10), 1992
KEHOE RA: The metabolism of lead in man in health and disease. The Harben Lectures, 1960. J. Inst Public Health 24:101, 1961
SMITH MA et al: Lead Exposure and Childhood Development: An International Assessment for the Commission of the European Communities and the US Environmental Protection Agency. Norwell, MA, Kluwer Academic Publishers, 1989.

Mercury

ELHASSANI SB: The many faces of methylmercury poisoning. J Toxicol Clin Toxicol 19:875, 1982–83
GRAEF J: Mercury, parts I and II. Clin Toxicol Rev 2(7, 8), 1980
KOSTYNIAK PJ et al: Extracorporeal regional complexing hemodialysis treatment of acute inorganic mercury intoxication. Hum Exp Toxicol 9(3):137, 1990
NATIONAL ACADEMY OF SCIENCES: An Assessment of Mercury in the Environment. Washington, NAC, 1978
THORP JM JR et al: Elemental mercury exposure in early pregnancy. Obstet Gynecol 79(5):874, 1992

Thallium

DAVIS LE et al: Acute thallium poisoning: Toxicological and morphological studies of the nervous system. Ann Neurol 10(1):38, 1981
DEGROOT G: et al: The evaluation of the efficacy of charcoal hemoperfusion in the treatment of three cases of thallium poisoning. Arch Toxcicol 57:61, 1985
DESENCLOS JC et al: Thallium poisoning: An outbreak in Florida, 1988. South Med J 85(12):1203, 1992
LOVEJOY FH JR: Thallium. Clin Toxicol Rev 4(5), 1982
VILLANOVA E et al: Poisoning by thallium: A study of five cases. Drug Safety 5(5):384, 1990
WAINWRIGHT AP et al: Clinical features and therapy of acute thallium poisoning. Q J Med 69(258):939, 1988

Chelating Agents

APOSHIAN HV et al: Meso-2,3-dimercaptosuccinic acid: Chemical, pharmacological and toxicological properties of an orally effective metal chelating agent. Annu Rev Pharmacol Toxicol 30:279, 1990
CHISOLM JJ JR: The use of chelating agents in the treatment of acute and chronic lead intoxication in childhood. J Pediatr 73:1, 1968
GRAZIANO JH et al: Dose-response study of oral 2,3-dimercaptosuccinic acid in children with elevated blood level concentrations. J Pediatr 113:751, 1988
HRUBY R et al: 2,3-Dimercapto-1-propanesulphonate in heavy metal poisoning. Med Toxicol 2:317, 1987
SHANNON M et al: Efficacy and toxicity of D-penicillamine in low-level lead poisoning. J Pediatr 112:799, 1988
ZHENG W et al: Determination and metabolism of dithiol chelating agents: VII. Biliary excretion of dithiols and their interactions with cadmium and metallothionein. Fund Appl Toxicol 14(3):598, 1990

397 DISORDERS CAUSED BY VENOMS, BITES, AND STINGS

JAMES F. WALLACE

Humans come into contact with a great variety of venomous animals, including snakes, lizards, sea animals, spiders, scorpions, and numerous species of insects. In general three types of injuries result: infections, those due to the direct effect of venom on the victim, as exemplified in snakebite, and those due to indirect effects of the poison, as in hypersensitivity reaction to bee stings. Each year in the United States at least 50 persons die as the result of venomous injuries. Hymenopterous insects, snakes, and spiders account for over 90 percent of the fatalities. In addition, there is considerable morbidity and loss in economic productivity from the many nonfatal envenomations.

SNAKEBITE

EPIDEMIOLOGY   Fewer than one-tenth of the nearly 3500 known species of snakes are venomous. The poisonous varieties belong to five families: Elapidae (cobras, kraits, mambas, and coral snakes), found in all parts of the world except Europe; Viperidae, (true vipers) found in all parts of the world except the Americas; Hydrophidae (sea snakes); Crotalidae (pit vipers), found in Asia and the Americas; and Colubridae (broomslangs, bird snakes), of the African continent. The poisonous varieties of the United States, with the exception of the coral snake, are pit vipers and include rattlesnakes, the water moccasin, and the copperhead. Although this discussion centers around these species, most of the therapeutic measures are applicable to snakes in all parts of the world.

About 8000 individuals are bitten by poisonous snakes in the United States each year, with a large number occurring in the southeastern and Gulf states. Deaths number fewer than 20 per year, and most are due to rattlesnake bites. In many European countries, deaths from snakebite are unusual, but the annual deaths from snakebite throughout the world are between 30,000 and 40,000, with the largest number in Burma and Brazil, where 2000 deaths are estimated to occur each year.

ETIOLOGY   The *coral snake* is found in the southern states from Florida to Arizona. It is usually marked by alternating red and black bands separated by yellow rings; however, black and albino forms exist. Coral snakes are generally nocturnal in their activities, shy and elusive, and rarely bite humans. The fangs are short and permanently erect; the highly toxic venom is injected into multiple puncture wounds produced by a series of chewing movements.

The *pit vipers* are so named because of a small pit between the eye and the nostril. Large venom glands in the temporal regions give the head a triangular appearance. They are generally aggressive and likely to strike if disturbed. The fangs are long and hinged, folding posteriorly when the mouth is closed. Pit vipers strike suddenly with a forward thrust of the head. The instant that the erect fangs make contact, venom is expressed by sudden muscular contraction.

The *rattlesnakes*, recognized by the horny rattle on the tail which buzzes when the snake is disturbed, are widely distributed. The diamondbacks (*Crotalus adamanteus* in the Southeast and *C. atrox* in the Southwest) are the largest and most dangerous snakes in this country. Others include the prairie rattler (*C. confluentus*), the timber rattler (*C. horridus*), and the pigmy rattlers.

The *water moccasin* or cottonmouth (*Agkistrodon piscivorus*) is found in swampy areas or along the banks of streams. It is a strong swimmer and can bite under water. This snake is notorious for inflicting severe facial bites when disturbed in the branches of small trees. The copperhead or highland moccasin (*A. mokasen*) is a closely related species. Its bite is painful but rarely fatal.

PATHOGENESIS   **Snake venoms**   The venoms of most species contain mixtures of many toxic proteins and enzymes that have diversified and complicated pharmacologic effects. As an example, the venom of the Indian cobra (*Naja naja*) contains a neurotoxin, a hemolysin, a cardiotoxin, a cholinesterase, at least three phosphatases, a nucleotidase, and a potent inhibitor of cytochrome oxidase. Several venoms, including those of the pit vipers, contain hyaluronidase and proteolytic enzymes. Although the exact roles of these components in toxicity are incompletely understood, the venom of a given species is usually predominantly neurotoxic or necrotizing and is frequently associated with hemolysis, abnormalities of blood coagulation, changes in cardiac dynamics, and alterations in vascular resistance. Venoms of elapids, including the coral snake, are neurotoxic, and death results from respiratory paralysis due to central nervous system damage and interference with transmission at the neuromuscular junction. Venoms of crotalid snakes produce local tissue injury, hemorrhage, and hemolysis. Death is often preceded by circulatory collapse associated with a marked fall in circulating blood volume resulting from pooling of blood in the microcirculation and loss of plasma due to increased capillary permeability. Systemic absorption of venom occurs through the lymphatics, and therapeutic measures designed to reduce lymphatic function are helpful in controlling symptoms.

Factors affecting severity of snake bite   Several factors affect the outcome of snake bite:

1. The age, size, and health of the patient. A fatal outcome is more likely in children because a relatively large dose of poison is injected into a small victim.
2. Location of bite. Bites on extremities or into adipose tissue are less dangerous than those on the trunk or face or directly into a blood vessel. A direct strike of the fangs is more dangerous than a scratch, a glancing blow, or one hitting a bone. The discharge orifice of a fang is well above its tip so that the point of the fang can penetrate the skin without envenomation; even a thin layer of clothing may afford great protection. Because of the superficial nature of the wound, as many as one-fifth of patients bitten by venomous snakes have no evidence of envenomation, even though the fangs have penetrated the skin.
3. The size of the snake (a large pit viper can inject over 1000 mg of venom, six times a lethal dose for an adult), the extent of its anger or fear (if hurt, it may inject a larger amount of venom), the condition of the fangs (broken or recently renewed), and the state of the venom glands (recently discharged or full). Contrary to popular belief, the bite of a snake that has recently fed is not necessarily less venomous for humans; the snake usually does not exhaust its venom in a single bite.
4. The presence of various bacteria, particularly clostridia and other anaerobic organisms, in the mouth of the snake or on the skin of the victim. This may lead to serious infection in the necrotic tissues at the local site.
5. Exercise or exertion, such as running, immediately after the bite. This speeds systemic absorption of toxin.

MANIFESTATIONS   Following the bite of a pit viper, severe burning pain develops within a few minutes at the site of the wound. Local swelling develops rapidly and spreads in all directions, accompanied by the appearance of ecchymoses and bullae over the involved area. As the edema spreads, serosanguineous fluid oozes from the puncture wounds. Gangrene of the skin and subcutaneous tissues may develop. Systemic effects from the absorption of venom and local tissue destruction may include fever, nausea and vomiting, circulatory collapse, bleeding into the skin and from all body orifices, low-grade jaundice, muscle cramping, pupillary constriction, disorientation, delirium, and convulsions. Death may occur in 6 to 48 h. Survival may be attended by massive local tissue loss from gangrene or secondary infection or complicated by acute renal failure secondary to disseminated intravascular clotting and cortical necrosis or by tubular necrosis following circulatory collapse.

The bite of the coral snake causes little pain and local swelling. There are usually multiple fang marks. Within 10 to 15 min, numbness and weakness begin in the region of the bite, followed by ataxia, ptosis, pupillary dilatation, palatal and pharyngeal paralysis, slurring of speech, salivation, and occasionally nausea and vomiting. The patient becomes comatose, develops respiratory paralysis and seizures, and dies within 8 to 72 h.

Cobra bites are painful and are often accompanied by severe hemolysis, local necrosis, and sloughing in addition to their neurotoxic effects. There is little pain and no edema at the site of a sea snake bite. Symptoms of systemic envenomation follow a latent period which may vary from 15 min to 8 h. Although the venom is both myotoxic and neurotoxic, the injury to skeletal muscle is most prominent and is characterized by generalized muscle pain, weakness, and myoglobinuria. Hemorrhagic manifestations predominate following envenomation by colubrids (boomslangs and bird snakes) and many pit vipers, including certain species of rattlesnake.

LABORATORY ABNORMALITIES   Laboratory abnormalities may include progressive anemia, polymorphonuclear leukocytosis, thrombocytopenia, hypofibrinogenemia, disordered tests of coagulation, proteinuria, and azotemia.

TREATMENT   An attempt should be made to determine with certainty that the patient has been bitten by a poisonous snake. Absence of distinct fang punctures and failure of local pain, edema, numbness, or weakness to appear within 20 min are strong evidence against envenomation. The approximate size of the snake should be noted, since larger snakes usually cause more severe envenomation. If the species is not known, the offending snake should be killed to allow identification.

First aid   The victim should be reassured and calmed, measures should be instituted to retard the absorption of venom and to remove it from the tissues as quickly as possible after the bite, and arrangements should be made for transportation to the nearest hospital. The patient should be promptly placed at rest, and the bitten extremity should be immobilized to reduce the rate of spread of the venom. This is best achieved by splinting. If anatomically feasible, a wide constriction band should be placed a few centimeters above the bite and made tight enough to allow one finger to pass beneath with difficulty. The purpose is to impede lymph flow; it is not necessary to obstruct venous return. The band should be loosened and moved proximally when local swelling causes it to tighten. Since there is no evidence that incision and suction of the wound improve outcome in humans, and since incision in the field can cause secondary infection and traumatize tendons, nerves, and blood vessels, this procedure is no longer recommended.

To assess the severity of envenomation, the level of swelling should be marked on the skin every 15 min while the patient is being transported to a hospital. Ice packs relieve pain and slow lymphatic drainage but do not neutralize venom, and even a small amount of cooling may worsen damage to injured tissues by causing ischemia. For this reason, it is recommended that no form of cooling be used.

Immediate hospital care   This should include appropriate treatment for shock and respiratory difficulty, antivenin, measures to combat infection, and general supportive care. Initial laboratory studies in a patient with obvious crotalid envenomation should include blood typing and cross-matching, coagulation screening tests, and an electrocardiogram. None of these tests is particularly helpful in the initial evaluation of a patient with a coral snake bite.

Antivenin is the only specific treatment of snake venom poisoning, and its use in severe bites is vital. In the United States, polyvalent crotaline antivenin effective against all American pit vipers and antivenin for North American coral snake poisoning are commercially available. Both products are a lyophilized powder of refined horse serum. Kits contain antivenin powder (reconstituted by diluting with

water to 10 mL per vial), syringe, normal horse serum for prior sensitivity testing of the patient, and detailed instructions. Intravenously administered antivenin leads to the most rapid and effective response. It is not advisable to infiltrate antivenin at the local site. The initial dose should depend on an estimate of the amount of envenomation. For pit viper bites accompanied by progressive local swelling but no systemic symptoms, 5 vials (50 mL) are usually sufficient. When swelling has progressed beyond the site of the bite and mild systemic symptoms and/or hematologic and coagulation abnormalities are present, initial treatment should be 5 to 15 vials (50 to 150 mL). For severe poisonings associated with rapidly progressive and extensive local effects as well as systemic symptoms and evidence of hemolysis or coagulopathy, 15 to 20 vials (150 to 200 mL) or more should be administered. Up to 50 percent more antivenin should be given to children or small adults to neutralize the higher venom concentrations. Reconstituted antivenin is diluted in 500 mL of intravenous fluid and administered as rapidly as tolerated over 1 to 2 h. Additional infusions containing 5 to 10 vials (50 to 100 mL) should be repeated every 2 h until the progression of swelling in the bitten part ceases and systemic signs and symptoms disappear. When an adequate dose has been achieved, improvement in the clinical signs may be rapid.

If *any* evidence of envenomation appears within several hours following a coral snake bite, antivenin should be given without waiting for systemic manifestations. Four vials of antivenin should be given intravenously for bites associated with minimal swelling and/or local paresthesias. If evidence of a bite is more definitive, particularly if there was initial pain, 6 to 10 vials of antivenin should be given as soon as possible. Larger doses should be used in severe bites from large snakes, if the snake bite was prolonged for more than a few seconds, or if the victim is a child.

In the patient with severe envenomation who is allergic to horse serum, the relative risk of death from anaphylaxis rather than from venom poisoning should be weighed before undertaking desensitization with small doses of diluted horse serum.

No antivenin for other snakes is manufactured in the United States, but antiserum of various types is usually kept on hand at large zoos all over the world. A national antivenin index is maintained by the Oklahoma Poison Information Center in cooperation with the Oklahoma City Zoo [(405) 271-5454] and provides 24-h telephone consultation service for physicians needing advice in handling snakebite accidents.

Respiration should be maintained by mechanical or other means. In patients bitten by elapid snakes, respiratory failure is usually reversible. *Tetanus toxoid* or *tetanus immune globulin* of human origin should be given (see Chap. 106). If wound infections appear, antibiotics should be used with the knowledge that the predominant microorganisms in the mouths of snakes are gram-negative pathogens. Treatment should be preceded by appropriate aerobic and anaerobic cultures. *Fasciotomy* may be necessary to minimize ischemic injury to a massively swollen limb. Whenever possible, intracompartmental tissue pressures should be monitored, with surgical decompression undertaken only if pressure exceeds 30 to 40 mmHg. Vesicles and superficial necrotic tissue should be debrided surgically near the end of the first week following the bite. *Relief of pain* with salicylates or meperidine, moderate sedation, maintenance of fluid balance, measures to combat shock and hemorrhage, and appropriate management of coma or convulsions are all important.

Glucocorticoids do not prevent tissue damage or systemic intoxication but may be of value in the management of shock associated with envenomation and for allergic reactions, such as serum sickness, following the administration of antivenin.

PREVENTION   In snake-infested regions, long trousers, high shoes, boots, or leggings, and gloves should be worn. Most important of all is to look where one steps or reaches. A constriction band and antiseptic usually suffice for an emergency kit, but in inaccessible areas antivenin also should be carried.

POISONOUS LIZARD BITE

Only 2 of the nearly 3000 species of lizard in the world are venomous: the Gila monster (*Heloderma suspectum*) of the arid southwestern United States and the Mexican beaded lizard (*H. horridum*) of western Mexico. These reptiles are not aggressive, and virtually every instance of their attacking a human has resulted from teasing or handling the animals in captivity. The venom is elaborated in eight glands in the floor of the mouth and secreted directly into the oral cavity, where it bathes the teeth, which are grooved posteriorly. The lizard clings tenaciously and is often dislodged only after considerable effort; envenomation occurs by contamination of the wound. The venom contains a potent neurotoxin that rarely kills humans. Most often, bites in humans cause tissue injury, excruciating pain, massive edema, and erythema. Acute systemic symptoms may last for 3 to 4 days and include nausea, vomiting, hematemesis, blurred vision, dyspnea, dysphonia, and profound weakness. Intense hyperesthesia of the bitten extremity may persist for weeks. There is no antivenin available. Treatment should consist of constriction band, cooling of the bitten area, measures to prevent or combat infection, including tetanus, and supportive measures. Parenteral meperidine or infiltration of local anesthetic around the bite may be necessary to relieve pain.

SPIDER BITES

The bite of many spiders is locally irritating, and several species can cause severe, even fatal systemic poisoning in humans. In North America, two spiders are of medical importance: the widow spiders (*Latrodectus* species) and the recluse spiders (*Loxosceles* species).

WIDOW SPIDER BITE   The most numerous and important of the venomous spiders are members of the genus *Latrodectus*. In the United States and Canada, *L. mactans*, the black widow or show-button spider, causes a majority of clinical arachnidism. In Florida, *L. bishopi*, the red-legged widow spider, can cause similar effects.

It is the female *L. mactans*, the black widow, that bites humans. She is glossy black with a body 1 cm in diameter, a leg span of 5 cm, and a characteristic red hourglass mark on the abdomen. She spins her web in woodpiles, sheds, basements, or outdoor privies, is aggressive, and bites on slight provocation. The venom produces diffuse central and peripheral nervous excitement, autonomic activity, muscle spasm, hypertension, and vasoconstriction.

In the United States, most black widow bites occur between April and October. After a momentary sharp pain at the site, there is cramping pain that begins locally within 15 to 60 min and may spread to involve all extremities and the trunk. The abdomen is boardlike, and the waves of pain become excruciating, causing the patient to turn, toss, and cry out. Respirations are often labored and grunting. There are also nausea, vomiting, headache, sweating, salivation, hyperactive reflexes, twitching, tremor, paresthesias of the hands and feet, and occasionally, systolic hypertension. Leukocytosis is usual, and many patients have fever. After several hours, the pains subside, although mild recurrences for 2 or 3 days are common. It may be a week before well-being is restored. Deaths due to cardiac or respiratory failure have occurred, mostly in children and the aged.

Because the bite itself is not prominent, victims are often thought to have some abdominal catastrophe such as perforated ulcer, pancreatitis, or appendicitis. Renal colic, myocardial infarction, tetanus, strychnine poisoning, lead colic, and porphyria are other conditions to be ruled out. The abdomen is not tender to palpation in arachnidism, and pains in the extremities are not typical of most of these other disorders.

Treatment consists of pain relief and administration of antivenin. Initial treatment should include a hot tub bath which affords prompt, although temporary, relief. The administration of a vial (10 mL) of 10% calcium gluconate intravenously over 10 to 20 min usually produces transient cessation of cramps. The administration of 10%

methocarbamol intravenously also may relieve muscle spasms. Opiates are sometimes necessary. When symptoms are severe or when the patient is a small child or at special risk due to other associated medical problems, *Latrodectus* antivenin should be administered. An intravenous injection of 1 vial (2.5 mL) diluted in 50 mL of saline and administered over a 15-min period is usually effective within a few hours and can be repeated if symptoms recur. Since the antivenin is prepared from horse serum, appropriate testing for hypersensitivity should be undertaken prior to its administration.

***LOXOSCELES* SPIDER BITE**   Bites due to *Loxosceles* spiders can cause severe necrosis of tissue. Originally thought to be a problem only in the midwestern states and associated only with the brown recluse spider, necrotic arachnidism also occurs in the southern and southwestern states and in California and has been attributed to at least six species of *Loxosceles* spider. The bite of these spiders may initially produce only a mild stinging discomfort. In severe bites, intense local pain appears within 2 to 8 h, accompanied by bullae formation and erythema at the site of the wound. Subsequently, ischemic necrosis causes a deep ulcer with a necrotic base. The pathogenesis of the local reaction is not completely understood but is thought to involve complement-activated tissue damage. Some patients also experience a systemic reaction characterized by fever, myalgias, and a morbilliform rash 24 to 48 h after the bite. Intravascular hemolysis, hemoglobinuria, and acute renal failure may occur. Fatalities have been reported, mostly in children.

Treatment depends on the severity of the bite. If bullae formation, intense pain, and signs of rapidly progressing ischemic necrosis do not appear within the first 6 to 8 h, the bite is probably not severe, and treatment is unnecessary. When symptoms of more serious local reaction are present, the parenteral use of glucocorticoids within the first 24 h following a bite has been advocated by some to retard progression of the lesion. Dapsone and/or brown recluse antivenin have been reported to prevent extensive ulceration in rapidly progressing *Loxosceles* spider bites. However, use of these forms of therapy should be considered experimental. Other therapeutic measures consist mainly of local wound care, including cool compresses, elevation of the bitten extremity, timely surgical debridement, and treatment of secondary infection. The ulcer usually heals spontaneously, although skin grafting may be required. Patients with systemic loxoscelism should be hospitalized and monitored closely for hemolysis, disseminated intravascular coagulation, and acute renal failure. Although of unproven efficacy, systemic glucocorticoids are usually given for the duration of the acute phase of the illness, which lasts 2 to 4 days. The treatment of renal failure is described in Chap. 236.

SCORPION STING

Glands in the terminal segments of scorpions produce venom, which is injected into the victim by a stinger located on the tip of the tail. Scorpions often enter dwellings. During the day they retreat into crevices; emerging at night, they often get into shoes and clothing and even into bedding. They do not deliberately attack humans, but accidental contact results in a sting.

Of about 650 species, roughly 40 occur in the United States, distributed over three-fourths of the nation. The only dangerous species, *Centruroides exilicauda* (also known as *C. sculpturatus*), is limited to Arizona, New Mexico, southern California, parts of Texas, and northern Mexico. This species reaches a maximal length of about 7 cm. The sting may be fatal to young children or old people but seldom to a healthy adult.

Most of the nonlethal species of scorpions in the United States cause only minor reactions, like a bee sting. Some produce local edema and ecchymosis, with burning pain. In contrast, species whose venom has potentially lethal systemic effects, including the Arizona *Centruroides*, may evoke little or no visible reaction at the site of the sting. There is an immediate burning sensation, followed by local paresthesia ("pins and needles"), hyperesthesia, or numbness. These sensations spread to involve the whole extremity, followed within an hour or two by malaise, restlessness, neurologic hyperexcitability, lacrimation, rhinorrhea, salivation, perspiration, nausea, priapism, and vomiting.

The patient may pass from an agitated state with hyperactive reflexes into coma; convulsions follow, and pleocytosis of the cerebrospinal fluid may be present. Release of catecholamines may result in tachycardia, various arrhythmias, and hypertension. Myocarditis and pancreatitis also have been reported, and cardiomyopathy may be a late complication. Death may occur within 2 days of the sting.

TREATMENT   Despite the reputation for lethality associated with envenomation by *C. sculpturatus*, most often the pain and paresthesias last less than 4 h. These patients can be treated at home with cold compresses and mild analgesics. There is no clear consensus on the management of more severe envenomations. Although the use of constriction bands as in the treatment of snakebite has been recommended, the amount of venom is minute, produces no local necrotizing effect, and is absorbed very rapidly.

Specific antivenin, reconstituted from lyophilized goat serum, is available in some areas but is associated with toxicity and should be considered only if the victim develops signs of cranial nerve dysfunction and increased involuntary activity in skeletal muscles other than those innervated by cranial nerves. An intravenous injection of 1 or 2 vials (5.0 or 10.0 mL) administered over 15 to 30 min usually reverses the severe neurologic symptoms within minutes. Supportive therapy is directed at combating shock and dehydration. Diazepam or phenobarbital is useful in reducing restlessness, and adrenergic blockers may relieve symptoms secondary to catecholamine release. Cardiovascular manifestations can be controlled with channel blocking agents and peripheral vasodilators such as prazosin or isosorbide.

PREVENTION   This depends on alertness in avoiding contact with scorpions in infested areas. Clothing and shoes should be well shaken before being put on in the morning. Towels and bedclothes should be inspected. A house infested with scorpions can in time be rid of them by closing all obvious ways of ingress; picking up debris in the environment, such as piles of brush, logs, and stones; introducing a mixture of fuel oil or kerosene, containing a small amount of creosote, between the earth and the house foundation; and spraying with a mixture of 2% chlordane and 0.2% pyrethrins in an oil base.

HYMENOPTERA STINGS

Each year in the United States, nearly twice as many people die as a result of bites by hymenopterous insects (including bees, wasps, hornets, yellowjackets, and fire ants) as from poisonous snake bites. Occasionally, multiple stings in enormous numbers (500 to 1000) are the cause of death, but most systemic reactions and deaths are due to allergic reactions to the venoms.

Hymenoptera venoms contain many nonallergenic amines and peptides such as histamine and various kinins which contribute to the local sting reaction through their inflammatory and vasoactive properties. The allergenic venom proteins, which elicit an IgE antibody response in those who are stung, include phospholipases, hyaluronidases, acid phosphatases, and melittin. Venoms are distinctly different for each of the three genera capable of causing allergic sting reactions: Apidae (various species of bees), Vespidae (hornets, yellowjackets, and wasps), and *Solenopsis* (fire ants).

The usual reaction to a single bee or wasp sting is sharp pain, which lasts for several minutes, local wheal and erythema, followed by intense itching. All signs of the sting normally subside within a few hours. In the rare case when a bee is swallowed or inhaled, edema of the laryngopharynx or glottis may be life-threatening. A sting directly into a peripheral nerve can destroy its function for a time, and Bell's palsy can result from a sting into the trunk of the facial nerve. Unusual reactions such as optic neuritis, generalized polyneuropathy, and myasthenia gravis may follow a sting. The etiology of these reactions is unknown. Acute renal failure may occur following multiple bee stings, probably the consequence of venom-induced rhabdomyolysis and renal ischemia.

In hypersensitive individuals, the response to a single sting may vary from an exaggerated local reaction, unassociated with systemic symptoms, to anaphylaxis with urticaria, nausea, abdominal or uterine cramps, bronchospasm, edema of the face and glottis, dyspnea, cyanosis, hypotension, coma, and death. These symptoms usually appear within a few minutes of the sting. Other patients may experience delayed reactions of the serum-sickness type 10 to 14 days after envenomation. Sensitization is usually the result of previous stings. It has been estimated that 10 to 15 percent of the general population is allergic to hymenoptera venom. Those who have experienced a previous systemic allergic reaction to a sting, such as respiratory difficulty, hypotension, or generalized urticaria, are at greatest risk for serious reactions if stung again by the same type of insect.

Since being accidentally introduced into southern Brazil in 1957, Africanized bees have gradually spread through South and Central America and into Texas. Although widely touted as a human health problem, the actual risk is difficult to estimate because of a lack of reliable medical statistics. Africanized bee venom appears to be similar to that of European bees. The real danger from Africanized bees may be that they tend to be aggressive, and multiple stings are common.

Many species of ant can produce stinging bites with local redness and swelling. The most notorious of these are the fire ants (*Solenopsis*), particularly two "imported" South American species (*S. invicta* and *S. richteri*). The *invicta* species is found in many southern states and has largely supplanted other domestic species. In addition to being a major agricultural pest, fire ants, whose bites may result in extensive vesiculation and skin necrosis or cause serious hypersensitivity reactions, constitute a significant health hazard. Unlike other hymenoptera venoms, fire ant venom is mostly a simple insoluble alkaloid, but it may cause life-threatening allergic reactions of the type seen with IgE-mediated immediate hypersensitivity. There is limited cross-sensitivity between fire ant venom and the venoms of bees, wasps, hornets, and yellowjackets.

TREATMENT   The wound site should be examined for a stinger, which, if present, should be removed to prevent further envenomation from the attached gland. The local reaction is treated by local cool application and antipruritic lotions or oral antihistamines. Fire ant stings, which are frequently multiple, should be thoroughly cleaned with soap and water. Secondary bacterial infection is common and should be anticipated and treated promptly. Epinephrine, 0.3 to 0.5 mL of a 1:1000 aqueous solution subcutaneously repeated every 20 to 30 min, may be lifesaving in patients with an anaphylactic reaction to a sting. A tourniquet slows the absorption of venom, and ice packs may relieve pain. Oxygen, endotracheal intubation, vasopressors and other supportive measures should be used as needed. In addition, glucocorticoids should be employed in severe cases.

PREVENTION   Allergic persons should make every effort to avoid contact with these insects, including wearing shoes when outside and not wearing perfumes or bright colors which may attract them. In addition, such persons should keep epinephrine readily available for immediate use in case of a sting, without waiting for symptoms to develop. Sting kits containing premeasured doses of 1:1000 epinephrine in disposable syringes, tourniquets, and antihistamine tablets are available, and patients should be carefully instructed in their use.

IMMUNOTHERAPY   Desensitization by injection of venom of the specific insect has long been recommended for any person who has had a systemic or generalized reaction to hymenopterous insect stings. Purified hymenopterous venoms are used for the diagnosis of sting allergy by skin testing. In addition, venom immunotherapy stimulates production of circulating venom-specific IgG antibodies and provides protection against insect allergy. These venoms are the materials of choice for diagnosis and immunotherapy of high-risk patients, those who have had previous systemic sting reactions and who have positive venom skin tests. The optimal duration of immunotherapy remains to be defined.

TICK BITE

Although ticks may be vectors for such serious diseases as Rocky Mountain spotted fever, Q fever, tularemia, borreliosis, human babesiosis, and Lyme disease, the local reaction to the bite of a tick may be nothing more than an itching papule that subsides within a few days unless there is secondary bacterial infection. However, incomplete removal of a tick, with retention of the mouthparts, may result in the local formation of a pruritic nodule. The definitive treatment is surgical excision of the nodule. Histologically, the nodule is a granuloma, but the inflammatory response is sometimes so bizarre and changes in the overlying epithelium are so striking that, in the absence of a history of tick bite, a mistaken diagnosis of malignancy may be made.

Ticks should always be removed intact using gentle, steady traction. Fine tweezers or blunt forceps should be employed if possible. When fingers are used instead, they should be protected with facial tissue and washed afterwards. Application of a drop of oil, petrolatum, nail polish, or other organic solvent may facilitate removal without leaving embedded remnants. However, touching with a hot object such as a glowing cigarette should be discouraged because of the likelihood of injuring the patient.

TICK PARALYSIS A progressive, ascending, flaccid paralysis, acute ataxia, or a combination of both sometimes develops in humans while a tick is engorging on them. Human cases have most frequently been reported from the northwestern United States and western Canada, where the wood tick, *Dermacentor andersoni* Stiles, is responsible. *D. variabilis* Say, the dog tick, *Amblyomma americanum*, the Lone Star tick, *A. maculatum*, the Gulf Coast tick, and *Ixodes scapularis*, the black-legged deer tick, also have been incriminated.

This disorder is caused by a neurotoxin secreted in the saliva of the engorging tick which acts on spinal and bulbar nuclei, slowing motor nerve conduction without affecting neuromuscular transmission. The tick must feed for several days before symptoms develop.

Most human cases occur in children, generally in young girls. The tick is usually attached to the scalp and hidden by the hair but may be found on any part of the body, including the ear, axilla, groin, vulva, or popliteal region.

The patient may be irritable or restless for up to 24 h before frank motor involvement appears. Weakness usually is noted first in the distal muscles of the lower extremities, progressing over the next 24 to 48 h to flaccid paralysis, which may extend to involve the trunk, arms, neck, tongue, pharynx, and bulbar centers. Sensory changes are typically absent, and there is little or no fever unless a secondary infection is present. Results of routine laboratory tests, including cerebrospinal fluid examination, are normal. Nerve conduction studies may reveal decreased velocities and compound action potentials of nerves and their corresponding muscles.

Among diseases to be considered in the differential diagnosis are diphtheritic polyneuropathy, transverse myelitis, the Guillain-Barré syndrome, myasthenia gravis, the Eaton-Lambert syndrome, botulism, and poliomyelitis.

Definitive treatment requires removal of the tick, including any mouthparts retained in the skin. After this is done, there is striking improvement of motor function within a few hours and complete recovery within 48 h.

The patient should be observed until the recovery trend is established, because if other ticks or retained mouthparts are overlooked, the paralysis may progress. Bulbar or respiratory paralysis may cause death if the tick is not removed in time. The mortality rate is 10 percent; nearly all who die are children.

OTHER ARTHROPOD BITES AND ENVENOMATIONS

FLEA BITE Many fleas attack humans, including *Pulex irritans* and chicken fleas. In sensitive individuals, the salivary secretion of these bloodsuckers produces large, itching papules. Much of the papular urticaria of children is probably due to flea bites. Treatment is symptomatic. Elimination of fleas from the environment may be very difficult, but persistent treatment of animals and of premises with appropriate insecticides is usually successful.

CENTIPEDE BITE The giant desert centipede, which reaches 15 cm in length, is responsible for most centipede bites in the United States. It is capable of inflicting an intensely painful bite, associated with erythema, edema, and sometimes regional lymphangitis. Rhabdomyolysis and acute renal failure have occurred following the bite of this arthropod. Pain usually disappears within a few hours but may require oral or parenteral analgesics. The wound should be washed well with soap and water to help prevent secondary infection.

CATERPILLAR RASH Contact with the early larval or caterpillar stage of several species of moth produces irritation of skin and mucous membranes resulting in a pruritic, erythematous rash, occasionally accompanied by urticaria and bullae. Symptoms come on rapidly after direct contact with caterpillars, after handling cocoons, or on being exposed to windblown fuzz. The pathogenesis is thought to be due to the direct irritant effects of insect hairs or appendages, although other mechanisms, including intracutaneous injection of toxins or hypersensitivity to insect antigens, have been suggested. The symptoms usually subside within a few days. Local soaks and oral antihistamines are often indicated.

BEDBUG BITE Members of the genus *Cimex* inflict bites that leave reactions varying from a simple puncture to large urticarial lesions, apparently depending on the sensitivity of the bitten individual. There is no specific treatment.

KISSING BUG BITE Of the many species of true bugs, those in the family Reduviidae are relatively commonly associated with severe bite reactions. The most important reduviid bug in this country is the kissing bug (genus *Triatoma*), which is found throughout the southern crescent of the United States. The bites of this bug, which is a nocturnal feeder, are characteristically inflicted in multiple groups. Reactions are thought to be allergic in nature and may include intensely pruritic and painful papules with a central punctum, grouped vesicles with moderate swelling and redness but no central lesions, giant urticaria, generalized allergic reactions, including systemic anaphylaxis, and hemorrhagic nodular to bullous lesions on a hand or foot appearing several days after the bite. These may be confused with necrotizing spider bites or with erythema multiforme. However, the former are usually single lesions, and the latter rarely has a unilateral distribution. The possibility of kissing bug bites should be considered in patients who awaken in the middle of the night with intense itching, hives, and other signs of a systemic allergic reaction.

Treatment of the local reaction is symptomatic. More severe reactions should be managed similarly to other allergic sting reactions. Patients who have had accelerated reactions to reduviid bites should be provided with sting kits and instructions in their use. Immunotherapy with whole-body extracts of kissing bugs has been attempted but is unproven.

CHIGGERS OR REDBUGS These tiny mites are found in foliage or grass in many parts of the world. In the United States, the larval form of *Eutrobicula alfreddugesi* attacks the skin by secreting a substance that digests tissue, creating a red papule that itches intensely. The tiny reddish larva can be seen in the center of the lesion. Treatment is palliative and consists of antipruritic agents. The use of insect repellents, protective clothing, and prompt bathing after exposure reduce the risk of infestation.

BLOODSUCKING-FLY BITE Many species of flies, particularly the horsefly and the deerfly, attack and feed on warm-blooded animals, including humans. Transmission of diseases such as anthrax, tularemia, loiasis, and trypanosomiasis has been attributed to horseflies and deerflies. More commonly in North America, however, the bites are responsible for painful, intensely pruritic cutaneous lesions which may be followed by delayed localized allergic reactions characterized by erythema, edema, and urticaria. Treatment should include thorough cleaning of the bite sites, topical glucocorticoids, and oral antihistaminics for severe itching. Antibiotics may be necessary for secondary infections.

MARINE ANIMAL VENOM DISEASES

The venoms of certain marine animals can cause illness in humans after injection or inoculation under naturally occurring conditions. Information concerning these toxins is limited; most appear to be composed of proteins, peptides, and other substances. Although probably less complex than the venoms of reptiles, many marine animal venoms can cause several pathologic effects including neurotoxicity and local necrosis.

PORTUGUESE MAN-OF-WAR AND JELLYFISH STINGS The burning discomfort induced by contact with sea nettles or jellyfish is familiar to most surf bathers. Contact with the tentacles of the colorful Portuguese man-of-war (*Physalia* species), which is found mainly in or near the Gulf of Mexico, or the more toxic jellyfish (*Chiropsalmus* of the Indian Ocean and *Rhizostoma* of the Atlantic) is followed by burning pain, swelling, and erythema. Severe, generalized muscular cramps, nausea, vomiting, and pulmonary edema may occur. Victims can die as a result of jellyfish stings, sometimes within minutes after contact. In nonfatal cases, systemic symptoms usually subside within several hours. Treatment consists of bathing the wound in saltwater, taking care not to rub the area of the sting. Any tentacles still clinging to the skin should be scraped off after first inactivating any remaining nematocysts to prevent discharge of additional venom into the victim. This can be done by sprinkling baking soda over the wound to form a slurry for sea nettle stings or by bathing with vinegar for man-of-war stings. Rinsing with freshwater, isopropyl alcohol, or household ammonia or rubbing with sand are not recommended because these measures may actually cause nematocysts to discharge. Analgesics should be used for pain control, and antihistamines should be given for pruritus. Severe envenomations may require advanced life-support measures. Glucocorticoids may be helpful in these cases. An antivenin is available for treatment of stings by the highly lethal Australian sea wasp, *Chironex fleckeri*.

CORAL WOUNDS AND STINGS The colorful structures known as coral are composed of thousands of small marine animals of the coelenterate phylum surrounded by a stony exoskeleton of calcium carbonate. Several species, including the fire coral, contain microscopic nematocysts capable of producing painful stings similar to those caused by jellyfish. Often more serious are wounds resulting from abrasions and cuts by the sharp edges of the outer skeleton. These frequently contain small pieces of animal protein and skeletal material that act as foreign bodies and may lead to chronic, suppurative wound infections if not debrided promptly and adequately.

SEA ANEMONE STING ("SPONGE DIVER'S DISEASE") Contact with certain sea anemones (especially *Sargatia elegans*) in Mediterranean and African waters produces extensive dermatitis with chronic ulceration. Occasionally, especially during August and September, systemic symptoms include headache, sneezing, nausea, chills, fever, and collapse. Rare fatalities have occurred. Application of vinegar may inactivate nematocyst discharge. No other specific therapy is known; symptomatic treatment with topical steroids or oral antihistaminics may provide temporary relief.

CONE SHELL POISONING Many species of cone shells in the Pacific are venomous, a great danger to unwary hobbyists who pick them up. The poison, a neurotoxin, is delivered into a wound inflicted by pointed hollow teeth resembling darts in the long proboscis of the animal. Local manifestations include sudden intense pain, followed by swelling and numbness, which may persist for several days. Symptoms of serious poisoning include muscular incoordination and

weakness progressing to respiratory paralysis. Death may occur within 3 to 6 h, but recovery within 24 h is the rule. There is no specific therapy; recommended treatment is the use of tourniquet, incision, and suction and supportive measures which may include artificial respiration and administration of oxygen.

SPONGE DERMATITIS Direct contact with several species of sponge results in a painful dermatitis which may persist for several weeks. The lesions appear to be caused by mechanical irritation from the exoskeleton of the sponge as well as by toxins within its tissues. Delayed hypersensitivity reactions also may occur. Topical glucocorticoids or oral antihistamines may provide relief from the pruritus; dilute acetic acid ameliorates local pain, while alkali will intensify it. The lesions are self-limited.

SEA URCHIN WOUNDS AND STINGS Contact with the spines of some species of sea urchin results in painful erythema and ulceration, occasionally accompanied by neurotoxic symptoms of weakness and frank paralysis of lips, tongue, and face lasting for several hours. Treatment is purely symptomatic and supportive. The toxins isolated from sea urchins have produced paralysis in animals and are notably resistant to heat. Deaths from paralysis and drowning have been reported. Occasionally, fragments of sea urchin spines may remain in the skin, leading to granulomatous reactions, or they may migrate into a joint or lodge against a nerve, causing intractable pain. Treatment of these complications is surgical.

PARALYTIC AND NEUROTOXIC SHELLFISH POISONING Certain dinoflagellates, which make up part of the marine phytoplankton, elaborate a potent neurotoxin. Occasionally, conditions in coastal waters become favorable for the growth of excessive numbers of these organisms, causing the water to develop an amber appearance termed *red tide* and killing massive numbers of fish by exhausting their oxygen supply. When humans ingest shellfish which have themselves ingested toxic dinoflagellates, manifestations include paresthesias of the face and extremities, dysphonia, and generalized muscular weakness, often accompanied by nausea, vomiting, and diarrhea and occasionally by paralysis and respiratory arrest. The more severe syndrome, known as *paralytic shellfish poisoning*, is encountered along the Pacific northwest and New England coasts. A milder form, not associated with paralysis in humans, is seen along the Gulf and Atlantic coasts of Florida. Treatment should include induced emesis and purgation to remove unabsorbed toxin from the gastrointestinal tract and whatever additional supportive measures are necessary. Spontaneous recovery usually takes place within 24 h.

VENOMOUS FISH INJURIES The dorsal fins or spines of bullhead sharks, dogfish, and ratfish and the dorsal and other fins of the lionfish, weeverfish, toadfish, and catfish are grooved and contain venom glands at the base. Little is known of the venoms involved except that they contain proteins and are capable of causing toxic as well as allergic reactions.

Envenomation results in immediate, severe local pain and edema which, if untreated, reaches greatest intensity in 60 to 90 min and resolves within 8 to 12 h. Local necrosis may occur, particularly following lionfish and catfish stings. Systemic reactions, including cardiac arrhythmias, hypotension, muscular weakness, seizures, and paralysis, have been attributed to the effects of the venom.

Treatment should be immediate immersion of the wound in water as hot as the patient can stand for at least 1 h or until symptoms subside. The venoms are extremely heat labile, accounting for the usefulness of this procedure. Although rarely needed, an antivenin for patients with severe systemic reactions from stonefish envenomation can be obtained from the Health Services Department, Sea World of San Diego [(619) 222-0411]. Tetanus prophylaxis should be given as needed. Narcotics may be required to control pain. Secondary pyogenic infection is a frequent complication.

Probably the most frequent type of fish envenomation in the United States is that produced by the lashing tail of the stingray of the California coast (*Urobatis halleri*). The bony spine is encased in a sheath of epithelial cells containing venom which is expressed into the puncture wound. The wound may be several centimeters deep;

portions of the bony spine may break off in it, or more often, the integumentary sheath remains in the wound. The venom is a circulatory depressant in animals, but local injury predominates in humans. Severe pain and blanching are followed by erythema and edema. Symptoms due to systemic absorption of venom are infrequent but may include salivation, muscle cramps and weakness, cardiac arrhythmias, seizures, and death. Treatment consists of application of a constriction band (the vast majority of these injuries occur on the legs) and copious syringing of the wound with saltwater to remove fragments of sheath. Additional therapeutic measures are the same as for other fish envenomations, including immersion of the injured area in hot water for up to 1 h.

REFERENCES

Snake and lizard bites

GOLD BS, BARISH RA: Venomous snakebites: Current concepts in diagnosis, treatment, and management. Emerg Med Clin North Am 10:249, 1992

JURKOVICH GL et al: Complications of Crotalidae antivenin therapy. J Trauma 28:1032, 1988

KITCHENS CS, VAN MIEROP LHS: Envenomation by the eastern coral snake (Micrurus fulvius fulvius): A study of 39 victims. JAMA 258:1615, 1987

LOPRINZI CL et al: Snake antivenin administration in a patient allergic to horse serum. South Med J 76:501, 1983

MITRAKUL C, DHAMKROGN A: Clinical features of neurotoxic snake bite and response to antivenom in 47 children. Am J Trop Med Hyg 33:1258, 1984

RUSSELL FE: Snake Venom Poisoning. New York, Scholium International, 1983

——, BOGERT CM: Gila monster: Its biology, venom and bite: A review. Toxicon 19:341, 1981

WINGERT WA, CHAN L: Rattlesnake bites in southern California and rationale for recommended treatment. West J Med 148:37, 1988

Spider bite

ALLEN C: Arachnid envenomations. Emerg Med Clin North Am 10:269, 1992

CLARK RF et al: Clinical presentation and treatment of black widow spider envenomation review of 163 cases. Ann Emerg Med 21:782, 1992

FUTRELL JM: Loxoscelism. Am J Med Sci 304:261, 1992

WILSON DC, KING LE JR: Spiders and spider bites. Dermatol Clin 8:277, 1990

Scorpion sting

BERG RA, TARATINO MD: Envenomation by the scorpion Centruroides exilicauda (C. sculpturatus): Severe and unusual manifestations. Pediatrics 87:930, 1991

BOND GR: Antivenin administration for centruroides scorpion sting: Risks and benefits. Ann Emerg Med 21:788, 1992

GUERON M, SOFER S: Vasodilators and calcium blocking agents as treatment of cardiovascular manifestations of human scorpion envenomation. Toxicon 28:127, 1990

KUMAR EB et al: Scorpion venom cardiomyopathy. Am Heart J 123:725, 1992

Hymenoptera stings

DESHAZO RD et al: Reactions to the stings of the imported fire ant. N Engl J Med 323:462, 1990

ELGART GW: Ant, bee, and wasp stings: Dermatol Clin 8:229, 1990.

GOLDEN DBK et al: Discontinuing venom immunotherapy (VIT): Immunologic and clinical criteria. J Allergy Clin Immunol 79:126, 1987

MEJIA G et al: Acute renal failure due to multiple stings by Africanized bees. Ann Intern Med 104:210, 1986

REISMAN RE: Stinging insect allergy. Med Clin North Am 76:883, 1992

RHOADES RB et al: Survey of fatal anaphylactic reactions to imported fire ant stings. J Allergy Clin Immunol 84:159, 1989

TAYLOR OR JR: Health problems associated with African bees (editorial). Ann Intern Med 104:267, 1986

VALENTINE MD et al: The value of immunotherapy with venom in children with allergy to insect stings. N Engl J Med 323:1601, 1990

VAN DER LINDEN PWG et al: Insect-sting challenge in 138 patients: Relation between clinical severity of anaphylaxis and mast cell activation. J Allergy Clin Immunol 90:110, 1992

Tick bite and tick paralysis

GOTHE R et al: The mechanism of pathogenicity in the tick paralysis. J Med Entomol 16:357, 1979

KINCAID JC: Tick bite paralysis. Semin Neurol 10:32, 1990

NEEDHAM GR: Evaluation of 5 popular methods for tick removal. Pediatrics 75:997, 1985

SPIELMAN A: How to diagnose and treat tick and mite infestations. Drug Ther 11:77, 1981

Other arthropod bites and envenomations

FRAZIER CA: Insect Allergy: Allergic and Toxic Reactions to Insects and Other Arthropods. St. Louis, Grace, 1969

HUNT GR: Bites and stings of uncommon arthropods: Postgrad Med 70:107, 1981

LOGAN JL, OGDEN DA: Rhabdomyolysis and acute renal failure following the bite of the giant desert centiped Scolopendra heros. West J Med 142:549, 1985

PINSON RT, MORGAN JA: Envenomation by the puss caterpillar (Megalopyge opercularis). Ann Emerg Med 126:562, 1991

ROSEN T: Caterpillar dermatitis. Dermatol Clin 8:245, 1990

SHELLEY ED et al: The diagnostic challenge of non-burrowing mite bites. JAMA 251:2690, 1984

WIRTZ RA: Allergic and toxic reactions to non-stinging arthropods. Annu Rev Entomol 29:47, 1984

Marine animal venom diseases

AUERBACH PS, HALSTEAD BW: Hazardous marinelife, in Management of Wilderness and Environmental Emergencies, PS Auerbach, HR Gee (eds). New York, Macmillan, 1983

BROWN CK, SHEPHERD SM: Marine trauma, envenomations, and intoxications. Emerg Med Clin North Am 10:385, 1992

HUGHES JM, MERSON MH: Fish and shellfish poisoning. N Engl J Med 295:1117, 1976

McGOLDRICK J, MARX JA: Marine envenomations: 1. Vertebrates. J Emerg Med 9:497, 1991

——, ——: Marine envenomations: 2. Invertebrates. J Emerg Med 10:71, 1992

ROSSON CL, TOLLE SW: Management of marine stings and scrapes. West J Med 150:97, 1989

ZERMAN MG: Catfish stings: A report of 3 cases. Ann Emerg Med 18:211, 1989

---

398 HYPOTHERMIA AND HYPERTHERMIA

ROBERT G. PETERSDORF

CONTROL OF BODY TEMPERATURE

Normal body temperature in humans is maintained within a narrow range despite extremes in environmental conditions and physical activity. A common accompaniment of systemic illness is a disturbance in temperature regulation, usually an abnormal elevation, or *fever*. Even in the absence of a frank febrile response, interference with body temperature regulation by disease is evident. This may take the form of flushing, pallor, sweating, shivering, and abnormal sensations of cold or warmth, or it may consist of erratic fluctuations of body temperature. The pathogenesis, diagnosis, and treatment of fever are discussed in Chap. 16.

HEAT PRODUCTION The major sources of basal heat production are through thyroid hormone thermogenesis and the action of adenosine triphosphatase (ATPase) on the sodium pump of all membranes. The muscles are most important in promoting increased heat production through increased shivering. The quantity of heat production can be varied according to the need. This variation ranges from small increases and decreases of nerve impulses to the muscles with inapparent tensing or relaxing to shivering or even a generalized rigor. During digestion of food, gastrointestinal production of heat is significant.

HEAT LOSS Heat is lost from the body by *convection, conduction, radiation,* and *evaporation*. Small amounts are used in warming food or drink and in the evaporation of moisture from the respiratory tract. Heat loss by convection results from a temperature gradient between the body surface and the ambient air. Conduction heat loss occurs with direct contact of the body surface. The major loss occurs through radiation, defined as an exchange of electromagnetic energy between the body and the radiant environment. Evaporation is the fourth major mechanism for dissipating heat and is particularly important when the ambient temperature exceeds that of the body or when core temperatures are increased by vigorous exercise. The degree to which each of these four mechanisms contributes to heat loss depends on ambient temperature, wind, solar radiation, and body immersion.

The principal method of regulating heat loss is by varying the volume of blood flowing to the surface of the body. A rich circulation in the skin and subcutaneous tissues carries heat to the surface, where it can escape. In addition, sweating increases heat loss by providing water to be vaporized. The sweat, or eccrine, glands are under the control of cholinergic sympathetic nerves. Heat loss by sweating may be tremendous, and as much as 1 L/h of sweat may be evaporated. The amount of heat loss through sweating is also dependent on the humidity in the air. The greater the humidity, the less the ability to lose heat through sweat.

When there is need for conservation of heat, adrenergic autonomic stimuli cause a sharp reduction in the blood flow to the surface. This causes vasoconstriction and transforms the skin and subcutaneous tissue into layers of insulation.

HEAT TRANSFER WITHIN THE BODY This depends on conduction, i.e., the transfer of heat between adjacent organs, and on *circulatory convection*, which is governed by bulk movement of body fluids and which is responsible for the transfer of heat between the cells and the bloodstream. It is useful, although oversimplified, to visualize the body as a central core at uniform temperatures surrounded by an insulating shell. The role of the shell as a mediator for heat conservation and heat loss is determined in part by its blood supply and by vasoconstriction or vasodilatation. Although insulation is relatively uniform throughout the body, some parts, such as the digits, are particularly susceptible to cold because of the increased surface-to-volume ratio. Moreover, blood that reaches the digits has already been cooled on the way. Insulation may be enhanced by the addition of clothing.

NEURAL CONTROL OF TEMPERATURE The control of body temperature, integrating the various physical and chemical processes for heat production or heat loss, is a function of the hypothalamus. The temperature-regulating system is a negative feedback control system and possesses three elements essential to such a system: (1) receptors that sense the existing central temperatures, (2) effector mechanisms, consisting of the vasomotor, sudomotor, and metabolic effectors, and (3) integrative structures that determine whether the existing temperature is too high or too low and that activate the appropriate motor response. A rise in central temperature initiates mechanisms for losing heat, while a fall in central temperature activates mechanisms for heat production and heat conservation. The activation of these effector responses is governed by a central integrative mechanism that may be compared with a thermostat and that responds to a variety of stimuli, such as the sensory impulses engendered in flushing or sweating, behavioral impulses, exercise, endocrine influences, and probably the temperature of the blood circulating through the hypothalamic centers. In a sense, all these stimuli reset the thermostat, thereby activating compensatory heat loss or heat conservation mechanisms.

NORMAL BODY TEMPERATURE It is not practical to designate an exact upper level of normal body temperature because there are small differences among normal persons. There are rare individuals whose temperatures are always elevated slightly above accepted "normal" levels, and there is considerable variation in temperature in a given individual. In general, however, it is safe to regard an oral temperature above 37.7°C (99.9°F) in a person at bed rest as probable indication of disease. The temperature may be as low as 35.8°C (96.5°F) in healthy persons. Rectal temperature is usually 0.3 to 0.6°C (0.5 to 1.0°F) above oral temperature. In very hot weather, the body temperature may be elevated by the same amounts.

There is a distinct diurnal variation in body temperature in healthy human beings. Oral readings of 36.1°C (97°F) are relatively common on arising in the morning. Body temperature rises steadily through the day, reaches a peak of 37.2°C (99°F) or greater between 6 P.M. and 10 P.M., and then drops slowly to reach a minimum at 2 A.M. to 4 A.M. Although it has been postulated that this diurnal variation is dependent on increasing activity during the day and rest at night, the pattern is not reversed in individuals who work at night and sleep during the day. The variation is now attributed to a circadian rhythm driven by the hypothalamus (see Chap. 16). The febrile patterns of most human diseases also tend to follow this normal circadian variation. Fevers tend to be higher, i.e., to "spike," in the evening, and many patients with febrile disease have relatively normal temperatures in the early morning hours.

Body temperature is more labile in young children, and transient elevations after relatively slight exertion in warm weather are frequently observed.

Severe or prolonged exercise can produce considerable elevation in body temperature. For example, marathon runners may develop temperatures between 39 and 41°C (103.2 and 105.8°F). Although heat loss may be increased by cutaneous vasodilatation and by hyperventilation, these compensatory mechanisms may fail, leading to hyperpyrexia and, if uncontrolled, to heat stroke. Many of the adverse effects of long-distance running can be prevented by holding races only if the ambient temperature is below 27.8°C (82°F), preferably in the early morning or early evening, and by ensuring ample fluid intake both before and during a race.

DISORDERED THERMOREGULATION In exercise, there is a temporary imbalance between heat production and heat loss with prompt reestablishment of normal temperatures at rest due to continuing activation of heat loss mechanisms. In prolonged exercise cutaneous vasodilatation in response to an increase in central body temperature ceases in order to preserve central temperature. Less adaptation occurs in fever because once a stable body temperature is reached, heat production equals heat loss, but both are greater than in the basal state. Cutaneous blood flow plays a greater role in controlling heat production and heat loss in fever than does sweating. At the beginning of fever, the body temperature as sensed by the thermoreceptors is low, and the individual responds physiologically as if he or she were cold. *Heat production* is increased by shivering, and *heat loss* is decreased by vasoconstriction. These events explain the sensation of cold or chills that characterizes the beginning of fever. Conversely, when the cause of fever is removed, the temperature returns to normal, and the individual responds as if warm. Cutaneous vasodilation, sweating, and inhibition of shivering are the compensatory responses.

Deviations of ±3°C (approximately 5°F) from the normal body temperature do not interfere appreciably with most bodily functions. Convulsions are common at temperatures higher than 41.1°C (106°F) in children, and irreversible brain damage is common when temperatures of 42.2°C (108°F) are reached. Oral temperatures above 41.1°C (106°F) are relatively rare in humans. Conversely, when temperatures are lowered to 32.8°C (91°F) or below, confusion and loss of consciousness occur; at 30°C (86°F) and below, slow atrial fibrillation supervenes. Ventricular fibrillation occurs at extremely hypothermic temperatures and is often a terminal event.

Disease of the regulatory centers in the hypothalamus may affect body temperature. Destruction of the posterior hypothalamic centers controlling heat-conserving mechanisms results in hypothermia. Cerebral lesions also may cause hyperthermia; they include tumors, degenerative diseases, vascular accidents, particularly cerebral hemorrhage, or infections involving the hypothalamus, such as encephalitis. Central fever is accompanied by lack of a circadian variation, absence of sweating, resistance to antipyretic drugs, excessive response to external cooling, and loss of consciousness.

DISORDERS ASSOCIATED WITH HIGH TEMPERATURES

HEAT SYNDROMES Four clinical syndromes are associated with high environmental temperature: *heat cramps, heat exhaustion, exertional heat injury,* and *heat stroke.* Although each of these entities may be separated from the others on clinical grounds, there is considerable overlap between them, and they may be considered as a series of syndromes along a single spectrum. The incidence of heat syndromes is unknown, but during an ordinary summer about 200 cases of heat stroke are reported. During the heat wave of June 1984, there was a 35 percent increase in mortality in New York City almost exclusively due to a rise in deaths in elderly persons living at home. Heat syndromes occur primarily at elevated ambient temperatures [>32°C (>90°F)] and at high relative humidities (>60%) in elderly individuals, particularly those with mental illness or alcoholism or who receive antipsychotic drugs, diuretics, and anticholinergics, or those who reside in poorly ventilated places without air conditioning. Heat syndromes are especially prevalent during the first days of a heat wave before effective acclimatization can occur. Prophylaxis by augmenting fluid intake prior to exposure and by ensuring that susceptible individuals, particularly the elderly or the very young, wear light clothing, use fans, take frequent cool baths, remain in a cool environment, and avoid strenuous physical activity can help prevent the full-blown syndrome, especially heat stroke.

Acclimatization The mechanisms by which humans accommodate to excessive temperatures remain unclear. Acclimatization requires 7 to 14 days of exposure. Acclimatization lowers the threshold for sweating; i.e., sweating occurs at a lower core temperature. However, sweating is the most effective natural means of combating heat stress and can occur with little or no change in the core temperature of the body. As long as sweating continues, humans can withstand remarkably high temperatures, provided water and sodium chloride, the most important physiologic constituents of sweat, are replaced. The concentration of sodium chloride varies between very low concentrations and that of interstitial fluid. The sodium concentration in sweat may fall from 65 mEq/L to as low as 5 mEq/L after acclimatization, and the volume may increase from 1 L/h to as much as 4 L/h. Dilatation of the peripheral blood vessels in an attempt to dissipate heat is another major way for the body to acclimatize to hot temperatures. After acclimatization occurs, there is a decreased heart rate at a given temperature, and heat stress is accompanied by an increased stroke volume with no change in cardiac output. These changes occur because of a 10 to 25 percent increase in plasma volume. Other alterations include a decrease in renal blood flow and an increase of antidiuretic hormone (ADH), growth hormone, and aldosterone secretion. The hyperaldosteronism may result in potassium loss, which may be aggravated by replacement of sodium without concomitant repletion of potassium. As heat stress persists, venous return diminishes and cardiac output may fall. If environmental temperatures in excess of the body's temperature persist, heat is retained and hyperpyrexia develops.

Heat cramps Heat cramps are the most benign heat syndrome. They are characterized by brief, intermittent, and often excruciating cramping pain and usually follow strenuous exercise in the muscles that have been subjected to extensive work. They may develop in nonacclimatized laborers or in conditioned athletes. External temperatures do not usually exceed the body temperature, and direct exposure to the sun is not necessary. The body temperature is usually normal, and the victim sweats normally or excessively. Heat cramps may even be precipitated by strenuous exercise in cold environments in untrained persons who are heavily clothed. Muscles of the extremities bear the brunt of physical activity and hence show the highest incidence of cramps. Treatment consists of rest in a cool environment and replacement of sodium, potassium, and fluid. This syndrome may be prevented by liberal salting of food and ample intake of water. Salt tablets are gastric irritants and should not be given. Isotonic electrolyte solutions are recommended by some authors.

Heat exhaustion This is also called *heat prostration* or heat collapse and is probably the most common heat syndrome. Heat exhaustion occurs in two forms, one due to water depletion and the other due to salt depletion. The symptoms arise from a failure of cardiovascular responses to high external temperatures. Water depletion is common in elderly individuals who are receiving diuretics or in anyone who has inadequate water intake in a hot environment. Body temperature elevation is common. Salt depletion occurs with inadequate salt replacement, does not cause hyperthermia, and is accompanied by hyponatremia and hypochloremia. Both forms of heat exhaustion cause weakness, anxiety, fatigue, thirst, vertigo, headache, anorexia, nausea, vomiting, and the urge to defecate, and faintness may precede collapse. There may be hyperventilation, muscular incoordination, agitation, impaired judgment, and confusion. Heat collapse (heat syncope) occurs in both physically active and sedentary individuals. The onset is usually sudden and the duration of collapse brief. During the acute stage, the patient looks ashen-gray. The skin is cold and clammy. The pupils are dilated. Orthostatic hypotension is common, and the pulse rate is elevated. The duration of exposure and the extent to which sweat is lost determine the treatment, which consists of removing the patient to a cool area and placing him or her in the recumbent position. Spontaneous recovery then usually takes place. Intravenous administration of saline solution is sometimes recommended, administered slowly over 48 h, although oral replacement of water and electrolytes may be sufficient.

Heat stroke Heat stroke occurs when body thermal regulation is unable to dissipate adequate amounts of heat with rise in body temperature, often to greater than 41°C (106°F). This results in multiple organ system failure. Heat stroke often begins suddenly with central nervous system (CNS) signs, including headache, slurred speech, vertigo, faintness, hallucinations, seizures, confusion, delirium, or coma. Focal neurologic signs are unusual and should prompt aggressive evaluation of the patient for other causes of CNS abnormalities.

Heat stroke can be divided into *exertional* and *classic forms*. Exertional heat stroke occurs in healthy, young individuals and is usually sporadic. The patient sweats normally. Classic heat stroke occurs in older individuals in epidemic form during heat waves. Patients do not sweat normally. Many persons with classic heat stroke have preexisting chronic disease, including arteriosclerosis and congestive heart failure (particularly when such patients receive diuretics), diabetes mellitus, or alcoholism, or have received one of several drugs that interfere with heat loss. Excessive exertion leads initially to symptoms of headache, piloerection (gooseflesh), chills, hyperventilation, nausea, vomiting, muscle cramps, ataxia, unsteady gait, and incoherent speech. With progression, loss of consciousness may occur. Physical examination shows tachycardia, hypotension, and evidence of low peripheral resistance. Laboratory data show hemoconcentration, hypernatremia, abnormal liver and muscle enzymes, hypocalcemia, hypophosphatemia, and, in some instances, hypoglycemia. As the syndrome progresses after exertion, thrombocytopenia, hemolysis, disseminated intravascular coagulation, rhabdomyolysis, myoglobinuria, and acute tubular necrosis may ensue. Multiple organ failure may occur.

Exertional heat stroke can be prevented by (1) running races early in the morning when the temperature and humidity are likely to be low, (2) educating runners to enter a race well hydrated by drinking 300 mL of water 10 min before a race and 250 mL every 3 to 4 km (salt and glucose solutions should be avoided), (3) placing aid stations at 5-km intervals, (4) instructing runners not to increase their pace after most of the race has been run, and (5) avoiding alcohol before a race.

Classic heat stroke may develop rapidly with few premonitory symptoms, and loss of consciousness may be an early sign. Patients may complain of headache, vertigo, faintness, abdominal distress, confusion, or hyperpnea. Pyrexia and prostration are the most significant findings on physical examination. Rectal temperature greater than 41.1°C (106°F) is common, and internal body temperatures as high as 44.4°C (112 to 113°F) have been recorded. Skin is hot and dry, the pulse rate is rapid, and respirations are weak. The blood pressure is usually low. The muscles are flaccid, and tendon reflexes may be diminished. Lethargy, stupor, or coma, depending on the severity, is present. Shock is common in fatal cases. Coma, hypotension, disseminated intravascular coagulation, and the necessity for intubation are bad prognostic indicators.

Major organ system failure includes right-sided cardiac failure with tachycardia, elevated cardiac index, and elevated central venous pressure. Hepatic damage is common. Jaundice may occur 1 to 2 days after admission. Acute oliguric renal failure may occur. Urinalysis may reveal concentrated urine and proteinuria with granular casts and red blood cells. Rhabdomyolysis and myoglobinuria may contribute to renal failure. Any evidence of bleeding should suggest disseminated intravascular coagulation, which always carries a poor prognosis.

DIFFERENTIAL DIAGNOSIS   The presence of an extremely high core temperature (41°C or higher) with exposure to heat stress, CNS dysfunction, and elevation of liver enzymes are generally required to make the diagnosis of heat stroke. Other illnesses that may mimic the condition are cerebral malaria, meningitis, encephalitis, and rarely, stroke, particularly brainstem hemorrhage. Thyrotoxicosis, delirium tremens, anticholinergic poisoning, and a number of other systemic infectious diseases also may mimic heat stroke.

TREATMENT   Heat stroke is a medical emergency, and immediate heroic emergency measures are required. In hot climates, ambulances should be air-conditioned. Once the patient is in the emergency room, time is of the essence. All clothing should be removed. The patient should be wheeled into a shower on a gurney. At the same time, ice should be applied to the lateral aspects of the trunk while the patient is sprayed with tepid water from the shower. A fan should be directed on the patient to accelerate heat dissipation by convection. Intravenous solutions should be chilled before administration.

After immediate evaluation and measurement of vital signs, the temperature should be measured continuously with an equilibrated thermocouple. Immersion of the patient in an ice-water bath is a time-honored treatment, but it creates difficulties in medical care if resuscitation is required. It should only be used in centers with written protocols and experience with this form of treatment. Other adjunctive forms of cooling include cooling blankets and gastric and rectal lavage. Massage of the skin may be employed along with cooling because it may stimulate return of the cool peripheral blood to the brain and viscera.

Hydration should be done carefully because in most patients fluid requirement over the first 12 h is only 1000 to 1200 mL. If hypotension persists despite successful cooling, central venous pressure should be monitored and further intravenous therapy given. Establishment of a proper airway, avoidance of aspiration, treatment of convulsions, and watching for arrhythmias will lead to survival of most patients, particularly if they are young and were previously well. Unfortunately, the poor, ill, and elderly, who are often not discovered until heat hyperpyrexia has been present for some hours, have a much less favorable outcome.

MALIGNANT HYPERTHERMIA Etiology and epidemiology Malignant hyperthermia (MH) consists of a group of inherited disorders that are characterized by a rapid increase in temperature to 39 to 42°C (102.2 to 107.6°F) in response to inhalational anesthetics such as halothane, methoxyflurane, cyclopropane, and ethyl ether or muscle relaxants, notably succinylcholine. In one form of the disease in which the mechanism of inheritance is autosomal dominant, the individuals are normal between attacks, although some have an elevation in creatine phosphokinase (CPK), and in 90 percent of such cases, biopsied muscle from susceptible individuals contracts on exposure to caffeine or halothane at concentrations that do not alter normal muscle contraction.

Interval CPK screening is not useful in detection of susceptible patients. Muscle biopsy followed by the halothane-caffeine contraction reaction is accurate but tedious. A careful history from the patient, including questioning about abnormal reactions during surgery suggestive of MH in relatives, is the most accurate way to detect and prevent MH. The incidence of the autosomal dominant form is 1 in 50,000 to 1 in 100,000 persons. MH occurs in 1 in 40,000 adult and 1 in 15,000 pediatric surgical cases. A linkage to mutations in the skeletal muscle ryanodine receptor (RYR1) has been established in some families with the autosomal dominant disorder. However, not all families have mutations in RYR1.

A second, recessive, form occurs in young boys and, less commonly, girls with a number of congenital abnormalities, including short stature, undescended testes, lumbar lordosis, thoracic kyphosis, pectus carinatum, webbed neck, winged scapulae, small chin, low-set ears, and an antimongoloid obliquity of the palpebral fissures. This form is called the *King syndrome*. MH also has been described in several other myopathies, including myotonia congenita, central core disease, and Duchenne's muscular dystrophy, and in patients with osteogenesis imperfecta.

Pathogenesis   The triggering anesthetic releases calcium from the membrane of the muscle cell's sarcoplasmic reticulum, which is defective in storing this ion. The result is a sudden increase in myoplasmic calcium. The calcium activates myosin ATPase, which converts adenosine triphosphate to adenosine diphosphate, phosphate, and heat. There are also inhibition of troponin, uncoupling of oxidative phosphorylation, activation of phosphorylase kinase, and increased glycolysis. Muscular contraction occurs, and it, as well as the chemical events, leads to production of heat.

Manifestations   Existence of malignant hyperthermia can be suspected if diminished relaxation is noted during induction of anesthesia and muscle fasciculations become evident when succinylcholine is given. In some patients, trismus during intubation is the first sign of a muscle disorder. Although the elevation in temperature is the result of muscular contraction, it may rise very rapidly, and if the temperature is not monitored, the first signs may be a hot skin and tachycardia or a cardiac arrhythmia. During anesthesia, an increase in end-tidal CO_2, unexplained tachycardia, and an increase in core temperature provide early clues to the syndrome. In addition to the high fever, muscle rigidity, hypotension, and mottled cyanosis are present.

Early laboratory abnormalities include respiratory and metabolic acidosis, hyperkalemia and hypermagnesemia, and elevation in blood lactate and pyruvate. Late complications include massive skeletal muscle swelling, pulmonary edema, disseminated intravascular coagulation, acute renal failure, cerebral edema, and seizures.

Treatment   MH is a medical emergency. The treatment protocol prescribed by the American Society of Anesthesiologists should be followed. It includes prompt interruption of surgery, cessation of the inhalational anesthetic, changing rubber tubing on the anesthesia machine, and external cooling. One hundred percent oxygen should be given, along with sodium bicarbonate (1 to 2 mg/kg), to combat the severe metabolic acidosis. A diuresis should be induced with fluids and diuretics to reduce myoglobinemia and hyperkalemia. Specific treatment consists of dantrolene sodium, 1 mg/kg, by rapid intravenous infusion. The drug should be continued until symptoms have begun to subside or up to a maximum single dose of 10 mg/kg. The regimen can be repeated if symptoms recur. Drugs to combat arrhythmias should be administered under ECG monitoring (see Chap. 198).

Prevention   Because of the tendency of this syndrome to run in families, its detection is essential. This can be achieved by monitoring the temperature of all patients under anesthesia; the best way to avert it altogether is to take a thorough family history. However, up to 50 percent of affected patients give a history of prior uneventful anesthetic procedures. Examining patients preoperatively is often not helpful because between attacks persons susceptible to MH are usually entirely normal. In susceptible patients, dantrolene should be given prophylactically. The dose is 4 to 8 mg/kg by mouth for 1 to 2 days prior to surgery; the last dose should be administered 3 to 4 h prior to anesthesia. Some favor an additional dose of 2 to 5 mg/kg intravenously immediately prior to induction of anesthesia.

NEUROLEPTIC MALIGNANT SYNDROME (NMS)   This syndrome is characterized by autonomic dysfunction, extrapyramidal dysfunction, and hyperthermia. Autonomic dysfunction is characterized by tachycardia, labile blood pressure (range 40 to 180 mmHg systolic), profuse diaphoresis, dyspnea, and urinary incontinence. Extrapyramidal dysfunction is manifested by catatonic behavior, hystonia, generalized muscular rigidity, and pseudoparkinsonism (ptyalism, masked facies, tremors, and brady- or akinesia). The temperature may be as high as 41°C (106°F). Consciousness fluctuates from alertness to coma. Laboratory abnormalities consist of leukocytosis (15,000 to 30,000 per microliter) and elevation in CK. The syndrome occurs after use of potent neuroleptics in therapeutic doses. Most cases have been reported after use of haloperidol, thiothixene, or piperazine phenothiazines. Concomitant use of other psychotropic drugs, including lithium, antidepressants, and benzodiazepines, occurs in over half of reported cases of NMS. Young adult males with affective disorders predominate. The NMS lasts 5 to 10 days after administration of oral neuroleptics is discontinued and longer after depot injection. These drugs are not dialyzable, hence the long period necessary for their excretion. The overall mortality is 20 percent, and fatalities have occured as late as 30 days after onset and have been due to renal failure, arrhythmias, pulmonary emboli, or aspiration pneumonia.

The mechanism of action is presumed to be due to blockade of the dopaminic pathways in the basal ganglia and the hypothalamus. Because neuroleptic drugs block dopamine receptors, NMS is attributed to dopamine depletion, and this is the rationale for treatment with bromocriptine (a dopamine agonist) in dosage of 7.5 to 60 mg/d divided into 3 daily doses. Dantrolene sodium (as described above for oral prophylaxis of MH) has been successful occasionally, as has amantadine. Supportive measures, including cooling and drug withdrawal, are the *sine qua non* of treatment.

DISORDERS ASSOCIATED WITH LOW TEMPERATURES

HYPOTHERMIA *Hypothermia* is defined as a central or core temperature of 35°C (95°F) or lower. The central (core) temperature is maintained at the expense of the periphery. During cold weather, blood is shunted away from the skin and the extremities to preserve, protect, and maintain core temperatures. Although far less common than is elevation in temperature, hypothermia is of considerable importance because it can represent a medical emergency.

Accidental hypothermia This is a well-known complication of exposure to cold and has been reported frequently during the winter months. It usually occurs after prolonged exposure, not necessarily to excessively low external temperatures. The diagnosis of hypothermia may prove elusive because clinical thermometers do not record temperatures below 35°C (95°F). Whenever a patient presents with a temperature below this level, the true temperature should be determined with an incubator thermometer or a thermocouple. Accidental hypothermia has been found in association with sepsis, hypothyroidism, pituitary insufficiency, adrenal insufficiency, hypoglycemia, cerebrovascular disease, Wernicke's encephalopathy, myocardial infarction, cirrhosis, pancreatitis, and ingestion of drugs—most particularly alcohol. Alcohol increases heat loss by peripheral dilatation and interferes with thermogenesis by inhibiting shivering. From 1976 to 1985, 7450 deaths in the United States were caused by exposure to cold. Most had core temperatures <35°C (<95°F), and individuals older than age 60 were at greatest risk. In 428 cases reported from 13 emergency departments, there was a direct correlation between lower body temperatures and outcome.

These patients usually appear cold and pale and, when their temperatures are very low, give the appearance of having rigor mortis, so stiff is their musculature. Patients with temperatures less than 26.7°C (90°F) are usually unconscious. The pupils are usually miotic, respiration tends to be shallow and slow, there is bradycardia, and most patients are hypotensive. Generalized edema is often present. When the temperature falls below 25°C (77°F), coma, areflexia, and lack of pupillary response supervene.

Laboratory data tend to show hemoconcentration, mild azotemia, and metabolic acidosis. The acidosis is due to lactic acidemia, which in turn is a consequence of decreased perfusion and hypoxemia in peripheral tissues. At cold temperatures, the hemoglobin dissociation curve is shifted to the left, and there is decreased unloading of oxygen in the peripheral tissues. Some patients have hypoglycemia, while others have hyperglycemia. Thyroid function tests may give results typical of myxedema. Some patients have elevations in serum amylase, and a few show pancreatitis at autopsy. The electrocardiogram is distorted by muscular tremors and may show bradycardia or slow atrial fibrillation and a characteristic J wave (occurring at the junction of the QRS complex and ST segment). Other arrhythmias are common; ventricular fibrillation is usually a terminal event. The mortality rate is five times higher in people over age 75.

TREATMENT Hypothermia is a medical emergency, and therapy should be instituted at once. The following steps are indicated:

1 An airway must be established and maintained, and the patient should be well oxygenated. Warmed oxygen may be helpful. Tracheal intubation of these patients poses no undue risk.

2 Blood gases should be monitored.

3 Blood volume should be expanded with warmed glucose in saline. Maintenance of blood volume is necessary to prevent the infarctions which have been a hallmark in fatal cases and to avert "rewarming shock." If the patient has persistent hypotension, respiratory failure, or unexplained oliguria, hemodynamic monitoring with Swan-Ganz catheterization may be necessary.

4 Because of the tendency to arrhythmias, the serum potassium level should be monitored carefully; a transvenous pacemaker may be indicated.

5 Although external rewarming with heating blankets or placing the patient in a warm room is appropriate in patients with mild hypothermia, active external rewarming (AER) is the treatment of choice. A source of heat (warm blanket, heating pad, or radiant source) is applied to the thorax only. The extremities are left vasoconstricted to prevent sudden vasodilation and blood pressure fall, which may be accompanied by recirculation of accumulated lactic acid from the periphery to the core. Moderate to severe hypothermia should be treated with active core rewarming (ACR). Humidified warm air administered by endotracheal ventilation, peritoneal dialysis with warmed fluid, heated fluid irrigation of the stomach via gastric lavage, or cardiopulmonary bypass with externally warmed blood have been used. For patients with intractable ventricular fibrillation, mediastinal irrigation and direct mediastinal lavage via left thoracotomy may be the fastest method for rewarming the myocardium.

6 Many of these patients have systemic infections including sepsis (see Chap. 83); cultures of the blood, urine, and other suspected sites should be obtained and broad-spectrum antibiotic therapy initiated and continued until infection has been excluded. Sepsis should be considered strongly in patients on hemodynamic monitoring who are found to have a lowered systemic vascular resistance and elevated cardiac index.

7 Resuscitative efforts should be vigorous and prolonged despite the poor prognosis, which is related primarily to advanced age and associated debilitating disease. In younger individuals, some remarkable rescues have been recorded. Authorities agree that hypothermia victims without vital signs (prolonged asystole) should not be pronounced dead until they have been rewarmed to 36°C (96.8°F) and remain unresponsive to CPR at that temperature. "No one is dead until warm and dead." Mild hypothermia [above 32.2°C (90°F)] has a 25 percent mortality; in moderate hypothermia [26.6 to 32.2°C (80 to 90°F)], the mortality is 50 percent; and below 26.6°C (80°C), it is 60 percent.

Hypothermia secondary to acute illness There is a group of patients who develop moderate hypothermia in association with acute diseases, including congestive heart failure, uremia, diabetes mellitus, drug overdose, acute respiratory failure, and hypoglycemia. These patients are generally elderly and upon admission to the hospital are found to have temperatures of 33.3 to 34.4°C (92 to 93.9°F). They also have a severe metabolic acidosis, due to increased production of lactic acid, and cardiac arrhythmias. Most of these patients are comatose. This entity differs from accidental hypothermia only in the absence of exposure; these cases have all occurred at normal ambient temperatures. The mechanism appears to be an acute failure of thermoregulation; shivering did not occur in any of these patients. Usually these patients have been rewarmed within a few hours. Upon return to normal temperature, cardiac arrhythmias, which were present in most of these patients, responded to treatment, and the sensorium returned to normal. With the exception that core rewarming is established by external means, other facets of therapy should follow the steps outlined above. In addition, treatment of the underlying disease, such as diabetes with insulin, uremia with dialysis, or congestive heart failure with appropriate cardiac drugs and diuretics, is essential. The prognosis is good provided the syndrome is recognized early and treatment is instituted at once. In general, patients under age 60 have the most favorable outcome.

Immersion hypothermia   The treatment of immersion hypothermia is essentially identical to that of accidental hypothermia.

LOCAL COLD INJURIES Mechanisms of freezing injury These can be divided into phenomena that affect cells and extracellular fluids (direct effects) and those which disrupt the function of organized tissues and the integrity of the circulation (indirect effects).

When tissue freezes, ice crystals form and, concomitantly, solutes in the residual liquid become concentrated. The physical dislocation during slow freezing is extreme. Ice crystals many times the size of individual cells form but are confined to the extracellular spaces. Large ice crystals can develop between cells in soft tissue without producing irreversible injury as long as the percentage of water frozen does not exceed a critical amount. A major source of damage to living cells during freezing and thawing appears to be the strong salt solutions which develop during formation and dissolution of ice; changes in the proportions of lipids and phospholipids in the cell membrane are also of great importance.

The fulminating vascular reaction and stasis that supervene are associated with production of histamine-like substances which increase the permeability of the capillary bed. Within blood vessels, cellular elements aggregate. Irreversible occlusion of small blood vessels by cell masses has been demonstrated in thawed tissue following freezing injury. The damaged frozen tissue simulates tissue damage produced by burns.

Manifestations   The mildest form of cold injury is called *frostnip* and tends to occur in organs farthest removed from the core of the body such as the earlobes, nose, cheeks, fingers and toes, and hands and feet. Frostnip represents reversible damage that is characterized by discomfort and blanching of the skin and numbness. It can be prevented by warm clothing and treated with simple rewarming. More consequential local cold injuries may be divided into freezing (frostbite) and nonfreezing (immersion foot) injuries. The two types may be observed in the same extremity or in different extremities in the same individual. The diagnosis of freezing versus nonfreezing injury generally can be made on the basis of the history and clinical manifestations.

Immersion foot is an entity observed in shipwreck survivors or in soldiers (trench foot) whose feet have been wet but not freezing cold for prolonged periods. There is primarily injury to nerve and muscle tissue, but no gross or irreparable pathologic changes occur in the blood vessels and skin. Symptoms include numbness, painful paresthesias and leg cramping. The clinical picture reflects primary hypoxic trauma giving rise to three clearly recognizable states: (1) *ischemia*, denoted by a pale, pulseless extremity, (2) *hyperemia*, characterized by a bounding pulsatile circulation in red, swollen, painful feet, and (3) the *posthyperemic* or recovery period. The initial cold-induced vasoconstriction, increased blood viscosity, and impaired oxygen transport in the ischemic state are aggravated by such factors as malnutrition, general hypothermia, dehydration, and trauma from relatively fixed, pendant extremities. The problem of rewarming is critical in these patients during the stage of ischemia, when overheating of tissue may lead to gangrene. In the state of hyperemia, the red, swollen feet require judicious cooling. Severe cases may show muscular weakness, atrophy, ulceration, and gangrene of superficial areas. Sensitivity to cold and pain on weight bearing, which may cause discomfort for many years, are sequelae even of milder injuries.

Frostbite, in contrast to immersion foot, is primarily a vascular problem because the blood vessels may be severely and irreparably injured. The circulation of blood ceases, and the vascular bed of the frozen tissue is occluded by agglutinated cell aggregates and thrombi. The cutaneous injury consists in part of separation of the epidermal-dermal interface. Early the intravascular clumping is reversible. However, with the passage of time, clumped red blood cells within vessels in injured tissue lose their morphologic identity and take on the appearance of a homogeneous, hyalinaceous plug. It has been shown in some, but not all, experimental studies that much of the intravascular aggregation following freezing injury can be reversed and microcirculatory perfusion improved if low-molecular-weight dextran is given intravenously shortly after injury, but the data in humans are less convincing. Tissue damage can be aggravated by trauma to insensitive and friable limbs and by refreezing. Moreover, frostbitten tissues are often neglected and with thawing become macerated. It is important, therefore, not to walk, bear weight, or put excessive pressure on a thawed frostbitten area. Thawing followed by refreezing is particularly harmful. There are four degrees of frostbite. First degree is accompanied by erythema and edema; second degree, by vesiculation, blistering, and eschar formation; third degree, by hemorrhagic blistering and bluish gray discoloration; and fourth degree, by injury to subcutaneous tissue muscle, tendon, and bone leading to mottled, dry, black, and necrotic changes.

The method of rewarming has been a matter of controversy. It seems most rational to warm the core of the body before treating the local area of frostbite. Following restoration of the core temperature to normal, warming of a frostbitten limb should begin in water at 10 to 15°C (50 to 59°F), which is then increased 5°C (9°F) every 5 min to a maximum of 40°C (104°F). Once the frostbitten limb has been rewarmed, treatment of the areas of tissue damage should be conservative and consist of bed rest, elevation of the injured part, tetanus toxoid administration, and use of antibiotics if infection is present; aseptic early drainage of blebs and bullae; daily washes with chlorhexidine or an iodophor; and early institution of physiotherapy. Alcohol and cigarettes are strongly contraindicated. Parenteral analgesics and nonsteroidal anti-inflammatory drugs are usually required for pain. Except for compartment syndromes that may occur as a result of massive swelling in the early postthaw period and that may require surgical release, surgical amputation and reconstruction are usually not necessary. In fact, 3 to 6 months may be required to determine the true level of tissue loss, contraindicating aggressive surgery.

Some patients with frostbite have residua consisting of excessive sweating, pain, cold insensitivity, numbness, abnormal color, dry and cracking skin, arthralgias, and degenerative arthritis. The symptoms are generally worse in the winter and following exposure to cold. These patients also often show abnormal nails, discoloration and pigmentation, hyperhidrosis, and, by x-ray, osteoporosis and cystic defects near the joints. These abnormalities tend to be milder in patients who have had sympathetic blockade. Most cold injuries are preventable by graded exposure to cold, as well as by appropriate clothing in freezing temperatures.

REFERENCES

General

Mitchell D, LaBurn HP: Pathophysiology of temperature regulation. Physiologist 28:507, 1985

Mackowiak P et al: A critical appraisal of 98.6°F, the upper limit of the normal body temperature, and other legacies of Carl Reinhold August Wunderlich. JAMA 268:1578, 1992

Heat syndromes

Yarbrough B: Heat illness, in *Emergency Medicine: Concepts and Clinical Practice*, P Rosen (ed). St. Louis, Mosby, 1992, vol 1

———, HUBBARD R: Heat-related illnesses, in *Management of Wilderness and Environmental Emergencies*, P Auerbach, E Geehr (eds). St. Louis, Mosby, 1989

Malignant hyperthermia

HEIMAN-PATTERSON T: Malignant hyperthermia. Semin Neurol 11:3:220, 1991
LEVITT R: Prospects for the diagnosis of malignant hyperthermia susceptibility using molecular genetic approaches. Anesthesiology 76:1039, 1992
MacLENNAN D, PHILLIPS M: Malignant hyperthermia. Science 256:789, 1992

Neuroleptic malignant syndrome

ADDONIZIO G et al: Neuroleptic malignant syndrome: Review and analysis of 115 cases. Biol Psychol 22:1004, 1987
CAROFF S et al: Neuroleptic malignant syndrome. Med Clin North Am 77:185, 1993

Hypothermia

DANZL D: Accidental hypothermia, in *Emergency Medicine: Concepts and Clinical Practice*, P Rosen (ed). St. Louis, Mosby, 1992, vol 1
——— et al: Accidental hypothermia, in *Management of Wilderness and Environmental Emergencies*, P Auerbach, E Geehr (eds). St. Louis, Mosby, 1989
DELANEY KA et al: Assessment of acid-base disturbances in hypothermia and their physiologic consequences. Ann Emerg Med 18:72, 1989
JOLLY T et al: Accidental hypothermia. Emerg Med Clin North Am 10:311, 1992

Cold injury

DANZL D: Frostbite, in *Emergency Medicine: Concepts and Clinical Practice*, P Rosen (ed). St. Louis, Mosby, 1992, vol 1
SMITH D et al: Frostbite and other cold-induced injuries, in *Management of Wilderness and Environmental Emergencies*, P Auerbach, E Geehr (eds). St. Louis, Mosby, 1989

399 DROWNING AND NEAR-DROWNING

JEROME H. MODELL

It is an unexpected tragedy when a previously healthy person dies or is exposed to severe cerebral hypoxia and suffers permanent brain damage. For many years, drowning was considered a "fight for survival": a person who could not swim, arms flailing and screaming for help, struggled to remain on the surface of the water to reach safety. This situation is rarely reported by persons at the scene of aquatic emergencies. Thus no single set of circumstances comprises drowning or near-drowning. Furthermore, it may be a secondary event following such precursors as head or spinal trauma, hypoxic-induced unconsciousness, or unconsciousness due to preexisting cardiovascular disease, sudden cardiac death, or myocardial infarction. The initiating event is usually unknown, however, and the drowned or near-drowned victim must be treated based on probable physiologic effects of the near-drowning itself. If survival with normal brain function is to occur, a thorough understanding of the pathophysiology of drowning and an organized approach to therapy are imperative.

PATHOPHYSIOLOGY OF DROWNING Approximately 90 percent of drowning victims aspirate fluid into their lungs. In those who do not aspirate fluid, hypoxemia results simply from apnea. In those who do aspirate, the volume and the composition of the fluid determine the physiologic basis of the hypoxemia. Freshwater aspiration alters the surface tension properties of pulmonary surfactant and makes alveoli unstable, which causes a decreased ventilation/perfusion ratio. Some alveoli collapse and become atelectatic, which produces a true or absolute intrapulmonary shunt, while others are poorly ventilated and produce a relative shunt; in either case, significant pulmonary venous admixture occurs. Freshwater in the alveoli is hypotonic and is rapidly absorbed and redistributed throughout the body. While some have proposed that water continues to enter the lungs after death, at autopsy, the lungs of victims who died in the water frequently contain little water. These findings support the premise that active respiration determines the volume of water aspirated. Hypertonic seawater pulls additional fluid from the plasma into the lungs, and thus the alveoli are fluid-filled, but perfused, which causes substantial

pulmonary venous admixture. With both types of water, pulmonary edema may occur and add to the ventilation/perfusion abnormality.

Water that is grossly contaminated with particulate matter or bacteria may complicate the picture. Particulate matter can obstruct the smaller bronchi and respiratory bronchioles. Grossly contaminated water increases the risk of severe pulmonary infection. Neither problem is sufficiently common, however, to recommend specific routine therapy for all victims.

At least 85 percent of near-drowned victims are thought to aspirate 22 mL/kg of water or less, which does not significantly affect blood volume and serum electrolyte concentrations. After resuscitation, by the time blood is analyzed, serum electrolyte concentrations usually are normal or close to normal. Significant changes are documented in only approximately 15 percent of those who cannot be resuscitated and only rarely in those who are resuscitated. This suggests either a small amount of water was aspirated or fluid was rapidly redistributed. Therefore, electrolyte disturbance rarely needs treatment. When a large quantity of water is aspirated, seawater causes hypovolemia, which concentrates extracellular electrolytes, and freshwater causes acute hypervolemia. If enough water is aspirated that plasma becomes severely hypotonic and the patient is hypoxemic, red cell membranes can rupture and plasma hemoglobin and serum potassium concentrations increase significantly. However, this has been reported only on rare occasion. With rapid redistribution of fluid and development of pulmonary edema, even freshwater victims frequently demonstrate hypovolemia by the time they reach the hospital.

Hypercarbia, which is associated with apnea and/or hypoventilation, is less often documented by blood gas analysis than is hypoxemia. While hypoxemia due to pulmonary venous admixture persists in all near-drowned victims who aspirate water, hypercarbia is usually corrected sooner with artificial mechanical ventilation and improved minute ventilation, and thus is reported in a small percentage of victims evaluated at the hospital. Besides hypoxemia, metabolic acidosis also persists in the majority of patients. Abnormal cardiovascular function, usually ascribed to hypoxemia, is brief with effective, timely therapy. Abnormality in renal function is uncommon, but when it does occur, it too is secondary to hypoxemia, alterations in renal perfusion, or, in extremely rare circumstances, significant hemoglobinuria.

TREATMENT OF NEAR-DROWNING The first step is retrieving the victim from the water, and, if necessary, performing artificial ventilation and circulation. According to the American Heart Association recommendation an abdominal thrust should not be used routinely in victims of submersion but rather should be reserved for when the airway is obstructed with a foreign body or when the victim fails to respond to mouth-to-mouth ventilation. Furthermore, an abdominal thrust may lead to regurgitation and pulmonary aspiration of gastric contents and may delay ventilatory or circulatory resuscitation.

Because emergency services and intensive pulmonary and cardiovascular care have improved during the past two decades, central nervous system depression now presents the major therapeutic challenge. The rate of survival with normal cerebral function varies considerably in retrospective studies. Some factors that adversely influence survival are prolonged submersion, delay in initiation of effective cardiopulmonary resuscitation, severe metabolic acidosis (pH <7.1), asystole upon arrival to a medical facility, fixed dilated pupils, and low Glasgow coma score (<5). None of these predictors is absolute, however, and normal survivors have been reported in all of the above categories. In a comparison of outcomes between one institution that added brain preservation techniques to intensive pulmonary and circulatory treatment and another institution that did not add brain preservation techniques, outcome data did not differ significantly.

Hypothermia appears to be protective, but only if it occurs at the time of the accident. This permits the victim a greater chance of cerebral salvage after longer periods of acute hypoxia and cardiac arrest than might be expected with normothermia. The diving reflex produces bradycardia, breath-holding, and circulatory redistribution when the face is submerged in cold water. However, its protective effect in explaining cerebral recovery after prolonged immersion has not been specifically documented.

Significant pulmonary venous admixture usually persists even after successful resuscitation; therefore, supplemental oxygen should be administered until arterial blood gas analysis confirms that oxygen is no longer needed. Intravenous access should be established as soon as possible. Endotracheal intubation should be performed if required for airway maintenance or to facilitate mechanical ventilatory support. Electrocardiographic monitoring will facilitate prompt treatment of cardiac arrhythmias.

Victims should be transported to a hospital where they can receive definitive testing for adequacy of ventilation and blood gas exchange, cardiac activity, and effective circulating blood volume. Analysis of other parameters such as serum electrolyte concentrations, renal function, and cerebral status should be performed as indicated.

The single, most effective treatment for hypoxemia, regardless of its cause, is mechanical ventilatory support including continuous positive airway pressure (CPAP). After freshwater aspiration, improvement in ventilation/perfusion matching is more consistent when CPAP is combined with mechanical inflation of the lung than with spontaneous respiration. The application of CPAP with spontaneous respiration versus its combination with mechanical ventilation should be determined by whether the specific patient can perform the necessary work of breathing, adequately eliminate carbon dioxide, and adequately match ventilation/perfusion ratios. Positive airway pressure should be withdrawn gradually as the lungs stabilize and ventilation/perfusion ratio returns toward normal.

The pH in near-drowned victims is commonly significantly acidotic, which, in turn, can depress cardiac function. This should be corrected pharmacologically, although there is some disagreement on this point. With cardiovascular instability, cannulation of the pulmonary artery with a Swan Ganz catheter or evaluation of the patient with transesophageal echocardiography is indicated. Many patients will be hypovolemic from loss of fluid into the lung as pulmonary edema or from decreased venous return secondary to increased intrathoracic pressure during mechanical ventilatory support.

Body temperature should be taken into account before a decision is made to terminate therapy of individuals submerged under frigid conditions because recovery after long periods of such submersion has been reported. The body temperature of victims depends not only on the temperature of the water from which they are retrieved, but also on the degree of insulation they have from that temperature with body clothing. The volume of water actually aspirated is also important, because a large volume, if distributed before cardiac arrest occurs, can produce rapid central cooling. Thus, cold water can be protective when it produces total body hypothermia, which decreases metabolic oxygen requirement. On the other hand, cold water may also contribute to the accident if hypothermia occurs before total submersion, resulting in severe, or even fatal, cardiac arrhythmia. Several methods of rewarming hypothermic victims have been advocated, but any technique that increases oxygen utilization, such as shivering, should be avoided.

Regardless of the conditions surrounding a drowning or near-drowning, treatment should follow a sequence of priorities:

1 Remove the victim from the water as soon as possible and stabilize the patient's head and neck if trauma is suspected.
2 Immediately follow the ABCs of cardiopulmonary resuscitation—even in the water if this does not endanger the rescuer.
3 If the patient is unconscious, protect the airway as needed with endotracheal intubation.
4 Establish venous access as soon as possible.
5 Provide supplemental oxygen and ventilatory support until each is no longer needed. This can be judged from analysis of arterial blood for oxygen tension, carbon dioxide tension, and pH.
6 Monitor cardiac rhythm with an electrocardioscope as soon as possible.
7 Monitor body temperature and restore it to normal.
8 If the patient has persistent respiratory insufficiency, provide intensive pulmonary support with CPAP and mechanical ventilation therapy as necessary.
9 If the patient has cardiovascular instability, evaluate cardiac output and effective circulatory volume, by invasive monitoring, and measure serum electrolyte concentrations.
10 Renal function and cerebral status should be evaluated as indicated.

Monitoring of intracranial pressure, routine glucocorticoid therapy, and prophylactic antibiotic therapy are no longer recommended.

ACCIDENT PREVENTION   Because drowning begins as an accident that results in a medical problem, the definitive strategy is to prevent the accident. For those victims in whom the accident is secondary to a medical condition rather than the primary event, such as persons susceptible to syncope or seizure, the only way to prevent the accident is to identify those who ought to avoid the water or encourage them to use the buddy system. For young children, early swimming lessons, vigilant caretakers, and stringent laws governing pool enclosures are needed. Those who teach parenting classes should routinely warn parents about the risk of toddlers' drowning in such household fixtures as toilets, buckets of water, and even washing machines. Preventing accidents during boating, athletics, and other water-related recreational activities requires public education. Rules associated with these activities to maximize safety and judicious, responsible behavior should be portrayed as life-saving measures. Similarly, alcohol, a "ubiquitous catalyst" to drowning, should be portrayed as life-threatening whenever water is nearby.

REFERENCES

AMERICAN HEART ASSOCIATION: Guidelines for cardiopulmonary resuscitation and emergency cardiac care. JAMA 268:2171, 1992

BOHN DJ et al: Influence of hypothermia, barbiturate therapy, and intracranial pressure monitoring on morbidity and mortality after near-drowning. Crit Care Med 14:529, 1986

FULLER RH: The 1962 Welcome Prize Essay. Drowning and the postimmersion syndrome. A clinicopathologic study. Milit Med 128:22, 1963

GONZALEZ-ROTHI RJ: Near-drowning: Consensus and controversies in pulmonary and cerebral resuscitation. Heart Lung 16:474, 1987

MODELL JH: Drowning. N Engl J Med 328:253, 1993

———— : Pathophysiology and treatment of drowning and near-drowning. Springfield, IL, Charles C Thomas, 1971

————, CONN AW: Current neurological considerations in near-drowning, editorial. Can Anaesth Soc J 27:197, 1980

———— et al: Clinical course of 91 consecutive near-drowning victims. Chest 70:231, 1976

———— et al: Near-drowning: Correlation of level of consciousness and survival. Can Anaesth Soc J 27:211, 1980

ORNATO JP: The resuscitation of near-drowning victims. JAMA 256:75, 1986

400   ELECTRICAL INJURIES

ALAN R. DIMICK

EPIDEMIOLOGY   The exact incidence of electrical injury is unknown. Each year in the United States approximately 1000 deaths constituting roughly 1 percent of all accidental deaths are attributed to electric current. The prevalence of electrical technology in modern society has resulted in more people experiencing electrical injury. The current treatment of electrical injury has resulted in a low mortality, ranging from 3 to 15 percent, but the amputation rate remains high, and disfigurement due to extensive soft tissue destruction is frequent. More than 60 percent of the electricity-related fatalities occur in males, with the highest incidence among those 20 to 34 years of age. Approximately one-third of *high-voltage* injuries occur in electrical workers, one-third in construction workers, and the remainder from non-work-related events. One-half of *low-voltage* injuries occur at home, the majority of them to young children. Burn center referral is usually necessary for electrical burns.

PATHOPHYSIOLOGY Electrical burns result from the conversion of electrical energy into heat. Factors that determine the severity and distribution of injury include the type of current (direct or alternating), the quantity of the current (amperage), the potential of the current (voltage), the resistance offered by the body, the pathway of the current, and the duration of contact. These variables are interrelated, and their interactions produce the varied spectrum of injury seen clinically.

Direct and alternating current have different effects. At low voltages (less than 1000 V), the low-frequency (40 to 150 Hz) alternating current range, which is used almost exclusively for incandescent lighting and appliances, is three times more dangerous than direct current. Immediate death can result from ventricular fibrillation, central respiratory arrest, or asphyxia due to tetanic respiratory muscle contractions. Tetanic muscle spasms, which freeze the contact point to the power source, tend to increase the flow of current and the severity of injury. Cutaneous burns may be entirely absent or minimal. In contrast, at high voltages, high-frequency alternating current and direct current are equally lethal.

Survivals from electric shocks of greater than 100,000 V and deaths from as little as 50 V have occurred, which underscores the interplay of the variables already noted. Clinically, the severity of injury relates primarily to the voltage. Low-voltage contact, while potentially lethal, does not result in the magnitude of tissue necrosis seen with high-voltage injury. Tissue resistance is an important factor in determining both the initiation of current flow and its subsequent path. A person completing a circuit between two contact points has a resistance that is the sum of the skin resistances at both contact points plus the internal body resistance. If skin resistance is high, there will be considerable local tissue destruction. Conversely, if skin resistance is low, systemic effects such as those on the heart and brain predominate. Skin resistance varies widely according to the thickness, cleanliness, and wetness of the skin. The resistance of skin in water is only about 0.1 percent of the resistance of dry skin. The extent of tissue damage can be explained by the differing resistances of various tissues. Listed in the order of increasing magnitude of resistance are nerves, blood vessels, muscle, skin, tendon, fat, and bone.

All tissues and organs can be affected by electrical injury. The cutaneous burns are often limited, with variable deep tissue damage. Appreciation of this special property of electrical wounds is critical in their management. Skin wounds are typically leathery or charred areas of full-thickness skin loss. The entry and exit sites are usually depressed, giving the appearance that current exploded the tissues. The arc burn is produced by current coursing external to the body from contact to ground, favoring a path of least resistance. The flexor surfaces of the wrist, elbow, and axilla are most often involved, because the hand is the most commonly involved body part. After several days, the demarcation between viable and nonviable tissue becomes more obvious. Flame burns of the skin may result from ignition of clothing by electrical arcing and may be full-thickness burns because of the prolonged exposure of the dazed victim to the flame.

The most severe cardiopulmonary manifestations occur at the time of the injury. These include anoxia and ventricular fibrillation, which may cause immediate death due to respiratory or cardiac arrest. Major electrical injury is accompanied by a 3 to 15 percent incidence of acute renal failure, which is greater than the incidence after thermal burns.

Nervous tissue is highly susceptible to electrical injury because of its low resistance. Neurologic deficits can be seen up to 3 years after the initial injury, and neurologic aberrations are the most frequent nonfatal sequelae of electrical injury. Lesions of the central nervous system may cause varying levels of consciousness, respiratory, and motor paralysis, which are usually transient; recovery is the rule. If the effects are permanent, they often assume the character of cortical encephalopathy or hemiplegia with or without aphasia. Spinal cord damage is the most common permanent sequelae of electrical injury and is seldom complete. Many deficits seen initially resolve spontaneously; others may not develop until 6 to 9 months after the electrical injury. Permanent deficits may not be seen for days to months, are of gradual onset, and progress slowly. Often these disturbances are not noted until the rehabilitative phase of recovery, when gait abnormalities become evident. Peripheral nerves may be burned directly or may be compressed by surrounding edema or scar. Neuropathies also can develop in unburned limbs. Autonomic nervous system dysfunction may be seen in both the acute and recovery phases. Reflex sympathetic dystrophy or causalgia can occur. Late onset of burning pain, frequently associated with vasomotor, trophic, and dermal changes, is characteristic.

Cataracts characteristically occur following high-tension injuries. The incidence of these lesions, which are usually bilateral, may be as great as 30 percent when electrical contact is made above the clavicles, particularly when the entry wound is on the head. The latent period between the accident and the onset of blurred vision averages 6 months but ranges from a few weeks to 3 years.

Direct vascular injury is more common after electrical injury than after any other type of burn. The blood flow in large arteries and veins is usually sufficient to dissipate the heat generated by the electric current. However, smaller vessels may experience significant heat-related damage resulting in thrombosis. Direct vascular injury probably contributes to the high amputation rate after high-tension electrical injury. Delayed hemorrhage from mural necrosis of large blood vessels also may occur.

Associated injury in electrical accidents can be due to falls of considerable distance or to the explosive effects of the current. Fractures of the vertebrae and long bones and dislocations also may result from the violent tetanic muscle contractions.

TREATMENT At the scene of the accident, the patient must be separated immediately from the electric current, but rescuers must not touch or approach the patient until the current has been shut off to avoid injury to themselves. Flames should then be extinguished.

Cardiopulmonary support must be initiated if necessary and maintained during transport. Aggressive life support is essential because victims of high-voltage electrical injury may be resuscitated successfully without permanent neurologic damage even after a prolonged cessation of vital functions. Because blunt trauma and skeletal injury may both coexist, a thorough history and careful physical examination are essential. Accurate assessment of the extent and nature of the burns is essential to the determination of subsequent therapy. Neurologic status must be evaluated repeatedly during convalescence because it changes frequently.

Fluid replacement is essential in the initial management. Hypovolemia results from the rapid loss of fluid into damaged tissues. Small entry and exit wounds may lead to underestimation of the underlying injury, so fluid requirements may be grossly underestimated. Normal saline should be infused rapidly (0.5 to 1 mL/kg per hour) as necessary to correct hypovolemia and to maintain urinary output. Large volumes of fluid are necessary in high-voltage injury because the fluid and electrolyte needs are much greater than in patients with thermal burns of equivalent surface area. The adequacy of resuscitation is monitored, with urinary output being the single most reliable indicator of circulatory status. The presence of urinary hemoglobin and myoglobin may necessitate treatment with mannitol to prevent acute renal failure. When hemoglobinuria and/or myoglobinuria is present, the rate and volume of crystalloid infused must be sufficient to maintain a minimum urine output of 100 mL/h. This infusion is continued until the urine is grossly clear of pigment. Acute renal failure, if it occurs, is treated as described in Chap. 236. Red blood cell transfusion, plasma, dextran, or other plasma expanders are unnecessary during the acute resuscitative phase.

Low-voltage injury Injuries resulting from low-voltage current, such as those related to household appliances, are usually small and limited to the area of contact. These burns frequently involve the hands, feet, or, in children, the corners of the mouth, lips, and tongue. The evolution of tissue injury and vascular necrosis from the current itself are complete within 7 to 10 days. During this time, the wounds are allowed to slough and heal by contracture. Small but deep contact injuries on the trunk and extremities may be excised and grafted as necessary when the extent of the slough is evident. Early excision and local flap repair are rarely indicated. Delayed bleeding from the lip, seen in one-quarter of these injuries, is usually readily controlled by direct pressure.

High-voltage injury   High-voltage injuries with devitalized skin, fat, and muscle are fundamentally surgical problems. They usually involve a limited amount of the total body surface, have upper extremity contact points, and require amputation or other surgical procedures. They may affect any organ system. The ultimate treatment goals are stabilization of the patient, salvage of the limb, debridement of devitalized tissue, wound coverage, and rehabilitation. Prolonged expectant nonsurgical therapy only increases the risk of invasive infection.

The timing of surgical debridement and its aggressiveness are controversial issues. Opinions range from early total excision with primary wound closure to the now outmoded expectant nonsurgical approach. Most surgeons favor an intermediate approach, individualizing according to the amount of tissue destruction and location and type of injury. Major amputations and surgical debridement are usually performed 2 to 4 days following injury when the extent of necrosis is reasonably well defined but the risk of significant infection is small. High-voltage electrical burns frequently produce muscle compartment syndromes requiring fasciotomy. Circumferential deep limb burns due to associated flame or arc burns also may require escharotomy or fasciotomy. Indications for surgical decompression include loss of distal pulses, impaired capillary filling, paresthesia, and rigid muscle compartments.

Debridement   When possible, formal amputation and major debridement are delayed for 2 to 4 days following injury. During this interval, neurologic and cardiopulmonary abnormalities usually have stabilized or resolved, and demarcation between viable and nonviable tissues is more evident. Because these wounds are prone to anaerobic infection, particularly myonecrosis with clostridia, aqueous penicillin is given prophylactically from admission until debridement is complete. Antibiotic administration should be further guided by identification of infecting organisms. Local wound care is started immediately and includes mechanical cleansing followed by the application of topical antibacterial agents and cotton gauze dressings. Silver sulfadiazine cream has excellent antibacterial activity but penetrates only a few millimeters into the tissues. Sulfamylon, a burn cream containing mafenid (a carbonic anhydrase inhibitor which readily penetrates soft tissue), may be advantageous in deep injuries and, therefore, is the topical agent of choice in the prevention and/or treatment of deepseated infections. However, when absorbed, this drug causes a bicarbonate diuresis resulting in systemic acidosis.

Coverage of open wounds usually requires skin grafting. Deep electrical injuries frequently result in complex soft tissue wounds which may require skin flaps for coverage. Nutritional support is essential and should be instituted early. As with other types of burns, appropriate splints should be fashioned and applied, and an aggressive program of physical therapy should be formulated and instituted. Psychological counseling is usually beneficial for patients who require major amputation or other mutilating surgical procedures.

LIGHTNING INJURY

When the difference in potential between the undersurface of a cloud which progressively become more negative and the surface of the earth which is positive exceeds the insulator strength of air, electrical energy discharges as lightning. There are four mechanisms of lightning strike: direct strike, flashover phenomenon, side flash, and stride potential. Direct strike consists of a major current flow directly through the victim. It is the most serious type of strike and is facilitated by metal objects such as golf clubs, umbrellas, or tools carried during a thunderstorm. In flashover, the lightning travels on the outside of the body and is facilitated by wet garments and sweat. Side flash occurs when the current splashes from a building, tree, or other person and then travels to the victim. Stride potential occurs when the lightning strikes the ground close to a victim with one foot touching the ground closer to the point of the lightning strike. In this position there will be a potential electrical difference between the legs called *stride potential*. The lightning current may enter one leg and pass up through the victim's body and exit through the other leg. Stride potential and side-flash strikes can involve several individuals at once and may contribute to the multiple casualties often associated with lightning strike.

The pathophysiology of lightning injury is similar to that described for other electrical injuries. Lightning is direct current. The voltage of lightning may range from 3 million to 200 million volts and may carry a current of between 2000 and 3000 A. Lightning victims have a very short exposure to current because of the brief duration of lightning strike, which usually lasts only 1 to 100 ms. The majority of lightning current may flash over the outside of the body. In contrast, the duration of current contact with high-voltage electrical injuries may be prolonged, since the victim may become frozen to the current source. The resulting injuries with lightning strikes are similar to those with both direct current and alternating current, as described above. Thus treatment is essentially the same as for other types of electrical injury. The best form of treatment is prevention by avoiding dangerous situations during rainstorms and electrical storms, such as standing near tall structures and metal poles or beneath metal shelters. It is erroneous to assume that once lightning strikes it is safe to venture into the open, because another strike may occur in the same location. Many towers and churches have sustained multiple strikes.

REFERENCES

BOOZALIS GT et al: Ocular changes from electrical burn injuries. J Burn Care Rehabil 12:458, 1991

FONTANAROSA PB: Electrical shock and lightning strike. Ann Emerg Med 22:378, 1993

GRUBE BJ et al: Neurologic consequences of electrical burns. J Trauma 30:254, 1990

HAMMOND JS, WARD CG: High-voltage electrical injuries: Management and outcome of 60 cases. South Med J 81:1351, 1988

HANUMADASS ML et al: Acute electrical burns: A 10-year clinical experience. Burns 12:427, 1986

LEE RC, KOLODNEY MS: Electrical injury mechanisms: Electrical breakdown of cell membranes. Plast Reconstr Surg 80:672, 1987

LICHTENBERG R et al: Cardiovascular effects of lightning strikes. J Am Coll Cardiol 21:531, 1993

LIFSCHULTZ BD, DONOGHUE ER: Deaths caused by lightning. J Forensic Sci 38:353, 1993

ROSENBERG DB, NELSON M: Rehabilitation concerns in electrical burn patients: A review of the literature. J Trauma 28:808, 1988

401   RADIATION INJURY

STUART C. FINCH

Throughout life human beings are continuously exposed to many types of radiation, some harmless and some harmful. The most harmful is *ionizing radiation,* which damages tissue through the action of charged particles. More is known about the acute and late somatic, teratogenic, and genetic effects of ionizing radiation than about any other environmental, physical, or chemical agent or force, yet many gaps remain in our knowledge concerning its effects. Most important and least well understood are the late effects of chronic low-dose radiation exposure. There is little reliable direct information, based on studies for which there are good quantitative radiation dose estimates and high statistical power, so virtually all estimates of low-dose exposure risks are obtained by means of extrapolations from high-dose exposure results.

There are two types of ionizing radiation. The first consists of high-frequency electromagnetic waves of relatively short wavelength, such as naturally occurring gamma rays or machine-made x-rays. These waves are capable of deep tissue penetration and moderate ionization of the tissues along their pathways by indirect mechanisms. Their interactions with the atoms and molecules of tissue structures result in the release of orbital electrons and the formation of ions and reactive radicals that damage cell components and disrupt biologic processes. The second type of ionizing radiation consists of a variety of subatomic particles, the most important of which are electrically charged alpha particles, protons, electrons, and electrically uncharged neutrons. The charged particles densely ionize structures along their pathways in tissues. The depth of penetration is quite limited and varies as a function of mass, charge, and velocity. Tissue damage is due to the direct ionization of water, oxygen, and other molecules with the formation of free hydroxyl radicals and highly reactive oxygen species. Neutrons penetrate tissues much more deeply than charged particles of equivalent size (such as protons). They indirectly ionize through their interactions with the nuclei of atoms, resulting in the release of protons, alpha particles, and other nuclear fragments that damage other tissues.

The longer-wavelength waves of the electromagnetic spectrum do not ionize, but some may damage tissues by other mechanisms. For example, ultraviolet light penetrates very little, but repeated acute exposures induce photochemical cellular damage that is cumulative and irreversible, predisposing the development of melanomas, basal cell cancers, altered cell-mediated immunity, and other systemic effects. Infrared, radio, and microwave electromagnetic waves are capable of deep tissue penetration with the generation of heat, the effects of which are largely reversible. Weak, low frequency electromagnetic waves have been shown to modulate ion flow and to interfere with both RNA transcription and DNA synthesis at the cellular level. Reports of increased leukemia, brain tumors, and other neoplasms, especially in children, following prolonged exposure to various types of low-frequency electromagnetic waves remain to be confirmed. The controversial medical effects in humans of exposure to electromagnetic radiation are in sharp contrast to the well-established acute and late effects of exposure to ionizing radiation, which is the only subject considered in this chapter.

TERMINOLOGY AND DEFINITIONS Some familiarity with radiation terminology and units is essential for an understanding of the effects of ionizing radiation. An early term for the quantitation of exposure was the *roentgen* (R), which represents the amount of radiation-induced ionization in a standard volume of air. Much more important is the *rad* (radiation absorbed dose), which represents a unit of absorbed dose in tissue. One rad corresponds to the absorption of 100 ergs of energy (or about 1 R) in 1 g of tissue. Since the same dose in rads of different kinds of ionizing radiation can produce different biologic effects, the term *rem* (roentgen equivalent man) was introduced. It is the product of the rad multiplied by its relative biologic effectiveness (RBE), a factor that represents the biologic potency of one type of radiation as compared with another to produce the same biologic effect. The usual standard of comparison used for the RBE is 200-kV x-rays, which are similar in energy to gamma rays. Gamma radiation, therefore, has an RBE of about 1, and 1 rad of gamma exposure is roughly equal to 1 rem. Neutrons and some charged particles may have an RBE of 5 to 20 or greater. The terms *gray* (Gy), 1 unit of which is the equivalent of 100 rad, and *sievert* (Sv), 1 unit of which is equal to 100 rem, have been adopted to replace the terms *rad* and *rem,* respectively. One-thousandth of a gray is written as 10^{-3} Gy or 1 mGy, equivalent to 0.1 rad (10^{-1} rad) or 100 millirad (100 mrad). Similarly, one-thousandth of a sievert is written as 10^{-3} or 1 mSv, equivalent to 0.1 rem (10^{-1} rem) or 100 millirem (100 mrem).

The density of tissue ionization produced per unit length along the pathway of ionizing radiation is expressed as its *linear energy transfer* (LET). In general, electrically charged particles or particles of relatively high mass (alpha particles, protons, and neutrons) have a high energy transfer (high LET), resulting in relatively large amounts of tissue damage. In contrast, electromagnetic forms of ionizing radiation (gamma rays or x-rays) or charged particles of small mass (electrons) transfer less energy per unit length of travel (have low LET) and produce less tissue damage. There is quite a good correlation between LET and RBE.

The *threshold dose* for a specific biologic effects is the minimum radiation dose that will produce the effect. Radiation effects that vary in frequency with dose but not in severity are called *stochastic* effects. Examples of these are radiation-induced carcinogenic, mutagenic, and teratogenic effects. *Nonstochastic* effects vary in severity above a threshold dose depending on the number of cells injured. Examples of such effects are radiation-induced cataracts of the eye or fibrosis of the bone marrow. The interval of time between exposure and the occurrence of a radiation effect is identified as its *latent period.* The *maximum permissible* dose is that dose of ionizing radiation which, in the light of present knowledge, is not expected to cause any appreciable bodily injury to any person at any time during a lifetime. Recommended annual limits by most U.S. radiation regulatory agencies for absorbed whole-body radiation dose are 0.05 Sv for occupationally exposed persons and 0.001 Sv for the general public.

TYPES AND SOURCES OF IONIZING RADIATION Most of a person's lifetime radiation exposure is from low-dose background radiation. The average annual background dose for each person in the United States is quite variable but is estimated to be from 3 to 3.6 mSv. About 80 percent or four-fifths of this radiation is from natural sources, of which radon, cosmic rays, radionuclides in the earth, and radioactive elements in the body are the major contributors.

Radon now is believed to contribute about half of a person's total background radiation exposure. This represents about 1.5 to 2 mSv of exposure per year. Radon is a colorless, odorless, and tasteless alpha-particle-emitting radioactive gas which is derived from naturally occurring uranium deposits in the earth. It seeps up through soil into the air, where it and its decay products attach to dust, aerosols, or droplets that are inhaled and retained in bronchial epithelium and adjacent structures. The greatest exposures occur in certain indoor areas and mines where there are high adjacent rock concentrations of phosphates, granite, and black shale. Radon itself is not particularly harmful, but some of its alpha-emitting polonium radioactive decay products may heavily irradiate bronchial epithelial cells for many months or years.

Cosmic radiation accounts for about 0.3 mSv of background radiation per year at sea level. It is composed of protons, neutrons, and heavy nuclei from galactic sources and low-energy charged particles from the sun that interact with atmospheric nuclei to produce small secondary particles and electrons that enter the body and ionize tissue. The earth's atmosphere acts as a shield so that the dose is about doubled with every 1500 m of increase in altitude. Radioactive potassium and carbon and other radionuclides within the body contribute about another 0.3 to 0.4 mSv to the average person's annual background radiation exposure. Radioactive decay of thorium and uranium radionuclides in the earth's crust constitutes the major source of terrestrial radiation, which, in most areas, is about 0.3 mSv per year. Amounts of terrestrial radiation, however, may vary by a factor of 4 to 6 or more in different geographic locations.

The remaining background radiation exposure is from man-made sources. Diagnostic x-ray and nuclear medicine account for most of the average estimated annual total of from 0.4 to 1 mSv. Exposure from these sources has doubled in the United States and many other countries during the past 20 years. Contributions from nuclear explosions, nuclear power, and all other sources account for less than 1 percent of background radiation.

Most acute or intermittent excessive exposures to ionizing radiation occur in association with radiation diagnosis and therapy, nuclear weapon detonations, radiation device and nuclear reactor accidents, or improper use of radionuclides. Most of such exposures are to low-LET x-rays or gamma rays, but direct exposure to nuclear weapon detonations or fallout or the excessive ingestion, inhalation, or injection of certain radionuclides may result in significant exposures to neutrons, and alpha and beta particles, and high-LET gamma radiation.

PATHOGENESIS OF RADIATION INJURY   There are many types of cellular injury following exposure to ionizing radiation. Most important is damage to the genetic apparatus of the nucleus due to structural alterations of DNA and chromosomes.

Many types of DNA damage may occur, but most common with low-LET radiation are single-strand breaks and base alterations. High-LET radiation produces more double-strand breaks and more complex types of DNA base damage. In both instances, the free radicals generated by ionizing radiation are largely responsible for the DNA and chromosomal alterations. The extent to which damaged DNA will be responsible for cell death or will become a permanent mutation depends on the ability of the cells to repair the damage. Repair of DNA damage from low-LET radiation is much more efficient than it is from high-LET radiation. This is extremely important because most of the somatic mutational and late neoplastic effects in replicating cells probably are due to the persistence of radiation-induced unrepaired or misrepaired DNA bases.

Chromosomal damage of many types as a function of unrepaired DNA constitutes the other major type of radiation-induced injury to the genetic apparatus of the cell. Chromosomal breaks with rearrangements associated with loss of considerable amounts of chromosomal mass usually are responsible for cell death at the first or one of the first few postirradiation mitotic divisions. Consequently, the number of chromosomal aberrations present at any one time during the postirradiation period will depend on both the number induced and the rate of cell turnover. Unbalanced chromosomal rearrangements usually disappear rapidly. Balanced chromosomal rearrangements involving little loss of chromosomal material may persist as stable intracellular markers of radiation injury for many years. There is strong evidence that chromosomal rearrangements involving breaks near proto-oncogenes play an important role in the process of radiation-induced malignant transformation (see Chap. 63).

Repair of radiation-induced DNA and chromosomal damage is inversely related to the rate at which the radiation is absorbed. This is particularly true for low-LET radiation, where a high rate of radiation absorption may increase residual tissue damage by factors of 2 to 10 times that experienced with a low rate of radiation absorption. Thus a risk reduction factor of 2 or more may be applied to the estimation of risk of a biologic effect from exposure to low-LET radiation delivered at a low dose rate in comparison with the risk estimate for the same effect from similar radiation delivered at a high dose rate.

Large doses of radiation may produce direct cell death due to membrane or cytoplasmic structural damage. This type of interphase cell death of autonomic nerve cells, lymphocytes, and capillaries is responsible for most of the early severe clinical manifestations of partial- or whole-body high-dose acute radiation exposure. Direct cell killing from large radiation doses to localized areas also accounts for the late occurrence of tissue hypoplasia or fibrosis rather than the development of cancer.

HISTORY   Most of our knowledge concerning the *late* effects of ionizing radiation exposure for humans has been derived from a series of unfortunate accidents and errors during the past 75 years. In the early 1920s and 1930s, about 2000 luminous dial workers, mostly young women in the United States, inadvertently ingested large amounts of radium 226 by means of absorption from their tongues and lips. Many later developed carcinomas of the paranasal sinuses and osteosarcomas. In Germany in the mid-1940s, a number of children with bone tuberculosis and many adults with rheumatoid arthritis were injected with radium 224. Between 5 and 10 years later,

many of them also developed osteosarcomas. Increased mortality from leukemia and multiple myeloma was reported for radiologists during the early years of the use of medical x-ray equipment. In the 1930s and through the early 1950s, thorium dioxide (Thorotrast) was employed as a contrast medium in a number of medical clinics throughout the world. Many injected persons developed hepatic tumors, leukemia, or aplastic anemia in later years. Increased rates of thyroid cancer and leukemia have been reported in children treated with x-rays in the 1940s and 1950s for tinea capitis and presumed thymus enlargement. Radiation therapy between the years 1935 and 1954 to over 14,000 persons with ankylosing spondylitis in England and Northern Ireland resulted in increased leukemia and several other types of cancer. Survivors of the atomic bomb detonations in 1945 in Hiroshima and Nagasaki are most noted for the subsequent occurrence of leukemia and multiple-site malignant tumors. Fallout from weapons testing in the Marshall Islands in 1954 appears to have been responsible for a small number of cases of hypothyroidism, benign thyroid nodules, and thyroid cancer. An increased incidence of lung cancer has been recognized in uranium miners. Three incidents of industrial radioactive contamination in the Chelyabinsk region in Russia in the 1950s have resulted in an excess of leukemia. The late effects of the Chernobyl reactor accident in the Ukraine in 1986 are largely undetermined but appear to include increased thyroid cancer in exposed children.

Most information concerning the *acute effects* of excessive exposure to ionizing radiation derives from two sources: the many worldwide acute radiation accidents since 1901 and the atomic bomb explosions of 1945 in Japan. There were approximately 110,000 to 120,000 acute civilian deaths from the Japanese atomic bomb explosions, about one-third of which are believed to have been caused by radiation exposure. The Radiation Accident Registry at Oak Ridge, Tennessee, has identified 340 major worldwide radiation accidents between 1944 and 1991 involving 132,928 people. There were 3037 significant exposures and 116 fatalities (including the 32 at Chernobyl) due to either acute radiation effects or physical trauma.

The most extensive and reliable information concerning the *late effects* of excessive exposure to ionizing radiation orginate from three sources: the Japanese atomic bomb survivors and patients treated with radiation therapy for either cervical cancer or ankylosing spondylitis.

CLINICAL EFFECTS OF RADIATION EXPOSURE   *Acute* or *early clinical effects* are those which occur within the first few minutes and up to about 2 months following exposure to large amounts of ionizing radiation delivered over a short period of time. They are due to cell killing, impairment of cell function, inflammation, infection, and hemorrhage. *Intermediate effects* occur after the first few months and up to a few years following exposure. *Late effects* are the radiation-related diseases and disorders that develop anytime after the first few years following previous acute or chronic ionizing radiation exposure.

Acute radiation effects   The early systemic manifestations of acute exposure to excessive amounts of ionizing radiation constitute the *acute radiation syndrome*. Survivors of the complete syndrome will experience four classical clinical stages that vary considerably in time of onset, severity, and duration, depending on the quality, quantity, and extent of the radiation exposure. The earliest phase is the prodrome, which consists of anorexia, nausea, and vomiting but also may include diarrhea, increased salivation, abdominal cramps, and dehydration. It commences within minutes to hours of exposure and lasts from a few hours to 1 or 2 days. This phase usually is followed by a relatively asymptomatic second stage of a few days' to a few weeks' duration. The third stage usually begins during the second to fifth weeks following exposure with the abrupt onset of moderate to severe gastrointestinal tract disturbances and manifestations of bone marrow depression. The fourth stage involves recovery, which may take weeks to months.

Persons who receive whole-body radiation in the range of 50 Gy or more invariably will die within 24 to 48 h from complications associated with the *neurovascular syndrome*. This is characterized by the rapid onset of apathy, lethargy, and prostration, frequently followed by seizures ranging from muscle contractions to grand mal convulsions, ataxia, and death. The early occurrence of severe central nervous system problems frequently yields to manifestations of the *cardiovascular syndrome,* characterized by intractable hypotension, arrhythmias, and shock before death occurs.

A significant prodrome also develops rapidly in persons exposed to whole-body radiation in the range of 10 to 50 Gy. Following a latent period of a few days, the *gastrointestinal syndrome* develops as the result of intestinal tract ulceration, infection, and hemorrhage secondary to mucosal cell atrophy and bone marrow depression. Its clinical manifestations are associated with massive fluid, protein, and electrolyte loss. Death almost always supervenes within a few more days.

Whole-body exposures in the range of 2 to 10 Gy are characterized by manifestations of the *bone marrow syndrome* due to a loss of marrow stem cells. Following a prodrome of 1 to 3 days and a relatively asymptomatic period of 1 to 3 weeks, buccal and pharyngeal ulcerations, localized and systemic forms of infection, cutaneous petechiae, and possibly generalized bleeding may develop secondary to thrombocytopenia and agranulocytosis. Concomitant loss of gastrointestinal epithelium often results in persistent diarrhea, abdominal distention, dehydration, circulatory collapse, and death. Survivors will experience rapid clinical improvement following partial return of peripheral blood granulocytes and platelets in 6 to 8 weeks, but full recovery may take several months. Epilation usually commences 1 to 2 weeks following exposure and is greatest at 5 to 7 weeks. Regrowth of new hair may take 4 to 6 months or more.

Mild gastrointestinal symptoms are experienced by 25 to 75 percent of persons exposed to less than 2 Gy of whole-body radiation. Hematologic complications rarely develop, because there is only moderate depression of the formed blood elements. Complete recovery of almost everyone in this exposure category is expected within 2 to 5 weeks.

Peripheral blood lymphopenia invariably develops during the first 12 to 48 h following any significant exposure. The rate and magnitude of the drop in the lymphocyte counts are related to radiation exposures up to about 5 to 6 Gy. At higher levels of exposure, lymphopenia is extreme, so correlations with exposure dose are poor. Reduced lymphocyte levels usually persist for 6 to 8 weeks. There often is a modest increase in the number of peripheral blood granulocytes during the first 1 to 2 days in response to exposure of more than 2 Gy, followed by a continual decline to maximum granulocytopenia in 2 to 5 weeks. The rate of granulocyte decline and the severity of granulocytopenia are functions of the bone marrow exposure dose. The peripheral blood platelet count responses are similar to those of the granulocytes, except that early thrombocytosis is rare and rates of both decline and recovery usually are slower. Reversible dose-dependent reticulocytopenia and mild anemia may develop up to radiation doses of about 5 to 6 Gy. Higher exposures may result in variable amounts of irreversible bone marrow damage, although some stem cells may survive acute exposure of 10 Gy or more.

Early radiation-induced chromosomal aberrations observed in peripheral blood lymphocytes include dicentrics, rings, deletions, translocations, inversions, and other types of rearrangements. Several dose-related somatic mutations observed following acute or chronic exposure to ionizing radiation include the induction of hypoxanthine-guanine phosphoribosyl transferase (HPRT)–deficient lymphocytes, alteration of lymphocyte T cell antigen receptors (TCR), and loss of erythrocyte membrane glycophorin A. Ionizing radiation also may induce lymphocyte micronuclei and structural changes in bone and tooth enamel, resulting in dose-related alteration of electron spin resonance (ESR).

Reproductive system disturbances are other important early clinical sequelae of acute whole-body radiation exposure. Male oligospermia or aspermia usually is temporary for weeks or months following exposures of 1.5 to 4 Gy, but permanent sterility usually develops at exposures of 5 to 9 Gy or greater. Sterility may be temporary in females exposed to 1.5 to 6.5 Gy and permanent at higher levels.

Intermediate and late radiation effects   Bilateral posterior-central dotlike opacities with surrounding granules and vacuoles may develop in the *lens* of the eye within weeks or months following low-LET gamma radiation exposure. More heavily irradiated persons may have lateral extension of these tiny opacities with central clearing and anterior extension to the anterior surface of the lens. The lesions are defined as cataracts, but they rarely impair vision or progress over the years. Children are more prone to develop radiation-induced lenticular damage than are adults. The lenticular changes induced by radiation are nonstochastic, with a threshold dose of about 0.3 and 1 Gy for low-LET gamma radiation induction of minimal lesions and cataracts, respectively.

The most important *late effect* of exposure to ionizing radiation is an increased incidence of many different types of cancer. Reliable lifetime risk estimates for cancers due to low-dose radiation exposure are not available, but it is estimated that 3 to 5 percent of all human cancers are due to radiation from all sources. Risks usually are expressed in either *absolute* (additive) or *relative* (multiplicative) terms. The absolute risk is independent of natural incidence and represents the expected number of dose-related cancers above the baseline level. The relative risk represents the dose-related percentage increase above the natural or baseline level.

The earliest and most predictable type of cancer increased from excessive acute or chronic whole-body exposure to low-LET radiation is leukemia. An increased incidence first was observed in Japanese atomic bomb survivors within 2 to 3 years following exposure. Peak rates occurred about 7 to 8 years after the bombings. The types of leukemia which have demonstrated a significant relationship between incidence and radiation exposure dose are acute lymphocytic (ALL), acute myelogenous (AML), and chronic myelogenous (CML). The highest leukemia risks and shortest latent periods to maximum rates were in exposed children: CML for males and AML and ALL for both sexes. The initially high leukemia rates in exposed persons in most age groups have decreased in almost an exponential fashion to near baseline levels at the present time. The AML rate in the older exposed persons, however, has remained constant or has increased over the years. The overall male-to-female ratio for leukemia in exposed atomic bomb survivors was about 2:1. The leukemia response to radiation therapy in the other major worldwide experiences has been very similar to that of the Japanese except for a paucity of ALL in the spondylitis series and a virtual cessation of the leukemogenic response in the cervical irradiation series after 10 years. There is no evidence from any studies of human radiation effects that chronic lymphocytic leukemia is radiation-related. The excess number of deaths from leukemia from low-LET radiation exposure to the bone marrow from study of the atomic bomb survivors was 2.9 per 10^4 person-year-gray (Table 401-1). This risk was five to six times higher than that observed for the x-ray therapy–induced leukemias, probably due to the younger age of the atomic bomb survivors and their rapid rate of exposure. The dose-response curve for atomic bomb–induced leukemia is linear or linear-quadratic in configuration.

Increased incidence of thyroid cancer, benign thyroid adenomas, and hypothyroidism may occur following either external or internal exposure of the thyroid gland to ionizing radiation. The risk of developing thyroid cancer from external irradiation during childhood is about twice that for exposure during adulthood. The female-to-male ratio for radiation-induced thyroid cancer is uncertain and ranges from 4:1 to 1:1 in adults and children, respectively, with latent periods ranging from 4 to 30 years or longer. Persons of Jewish descent appear to be at higher risk than are those of other ethnic backgrounds who have been studied. The incidence of low-LET radiation-induced thyroid cancer is quite uncertain and depends on many factors. Reports range from 0.6 to 12.5 excess cases per 10^4 person-year-gray. The induction rate for benign adenomas is at least 30 to 50 percent greater than it is for thyroid cancer. Radioiodine therapy with thyroid gland doses greater than 40 to 50 Gy destroys parenchymal cells and almost invariably results in hypothyroidism rather than cancer. Radioiodine used for diagnostic thyroid studies increases the incidence of benign adenomas but does not increase the incidence of thyroid cancer.

A significant linear relationship between radiation exposure and the frequency of death from multiple myeloma and cancers of the female breast, esophagus, stomach, colon, lung, ovary, and urinary bladder has been reported in atomic bomb survivors (see Table 401-1). No increases in mortality with increased dose have been observed for lymphomas, bone tumors, and cancers of the larynx, upper respiratory track, rectum, gallbladder, pancreas, uterus, and prostate in this population. Atomic bomb and other studies of ionizing radiation from external sources also suggest radiation-related increases in the incidence of salivary and parathyroid gland tumors and possibly cancers of the skin, kidney, and central nervous system, other than brain. Most of the radiation-induced solid tumors have appeared at their usual ages of occurrence, with minimum latent periods ranging from 15 to 35 years, in marked contrast to the short latent period for leukemia. This suggests that the increased risk for cancer from radiation exposure lasts a lifetime. Children exposed under the age of 10 have shorter cancer latent periods and significantly higher cancer risks than do persons exposed at an older age. Excess deaths for radiation-induced non-sex-related solid tumors are about equal in males and females. The radiation response for the induction of tumors is believed to be stochastic, but organ-absorbed doses in the range of 0.2 to 0.49 Gy for leukemia, lung cancer, and several other cancers are the lowest levels for which a significant increase in cancer mortality has been observed in atomic bomb survivors (see Table 401-1). Excess deaths from low-LET radiation for cancers other than leukemia are estimated on the basis of atomic bomb survivor air dose information to be about 5.8 in males and 8.8 in females per 10^4 person-year-gray. Mortality on the basis of organ-exposed dose for sexes combined is 10.1 deaths per 10^4 person-year-gray (see Table 401-1).

Other late effects of whole-body exposure in atomic bomb survivors include accelerated decline in cell-mediated immunity with aging and an increased occurrence of hyperparathyroidism. On the other hand, the exposed populations have not experienced evidence of accelerated aging, increased infections, increased sterility, or consistent evidence of increased mortality from nonneoplastic diseases.

A radiation dose-response relationship for the occurrence of small head size has been observed in newborn infants following in utero exposure of the fetus to atomic bomb radiation during the first weeks of pregnancy. It has been observed in 40 to 50 percent of these infants following exposures of 1 Gy or more. A dose-related risk of mental retardation also has been observed in children following in utero exposure between the eighth and fifteenth weeks of gestation to greater than 0.4 Gy of low-LET radiation. A lower risk of mental retardation also exists for exposure between the sixteenth and twenty-fifth weeks of gestation with an apparent threshold at about 0.7 Gy. Exposure during the eighth to fifteenth weeks of gestation and, to a lesser extent, between the sixteenth and twenty-eighth weeks also is dose-related to an increased incidence of reduced school achievement, lower intelligence test scores, and unprovoked seizures later in life. Dose-related increased childhood cancer and leukemia have been related to in utero diagnostic x-ray exposure. In utero atomic bomb exposure studies, however, have not confirmed these relationships but have shown a dose-related increase in adult-type cancers with rates comparable with those of exposed children. Prenatal or early childhood whole-body atomic bomb radiation exposures in the range of 1 Gy or more also have resulted in slight reductions in maximum height.

No human studies to date have demonstrated a statistically significant genetic radiation risk in humans. It is believed, however, that there is a linear dose-response relationship without a threshold and that the overwhelming majority of induced mutations are damaging. Although atomic bomb survivor studies have failed to demonstrate a statistically significant increase in genetic effects in the children of exposed persons, the cumulative data from many measurements suggest that the amount of acute low-LET parental radiation required to double the spontaneous mutation rate (doubling dose) is about 2 Sv. The Japanese data also suggest a doubling dose for intermittent or long-term low-level parental radiation exposure between 3.4 and 4.5 Sv, in comparison with other estimates from mouse data ranging from 0.5 to 2.5 Sv. All these estimates have considerable uncertainty. Evidence suggesting that preconceptual parental radiation exposure increases childhood leukemia and possibly other cancers has not been confirmed in the large F_1 atomic bomb survivor populations.

The early radiation-induced dicentric and ring-form chromosomal aberrations in blood lymphocytes disappear with the first mitosis, so few remain in later years, but many of the radiation-induced balanced structural rearrangements persist as dose-related and age-independent biologic radiation markers throughout life. Reciprocal translocations and inversions predominate. The early radiation-induced dose-related structural alterations of glycophorin A in erythrocyte membranes and ESR of tooth enamel also persist for many years, but the lymphocyte micronuclei and other lymphocyte mutations (HPRT and TCR) disappear to virtually undetectable levels over a period of 1 to 5 years.

Many types of cancer and other late effects have been related to exposure to ionizing radiation from internally deposited radioisotopes (Table 401-2). The only clearly recognized late effect from radon exposure is lung cancer. The risk of death in the United States from indoor radon exposure is estimated to be about 0.4 percent. This would result in the development of 6000 to 25,000 lung cancers per year. The risks of radon exposure and smoking for lung cancer are at least additive and may be multiplicative.

TREATMENT   There is no specific therapy for tissue radiation injury, but much can be done to reduce morbidity and mortality for persons who have been acutely exposed to excessive amounts of whole-body ionizing radiation.

Persons with possible surface contamination from radioactive substances must be evacuated promptly, monitored for external contamination, and decontaminated if necessary. It is extremely important to estimate the dose of radiation exposure as early as possible for any acute exposure in order to determine the need for various types of therapy. This may be very difficult even under the best of circumstances. The most reliable early indicators of dose in the absence of an actual dosimeter measurement are the exposure history, the severity of clinical symptoms, and the frequency of

TABLE 401-1 Significant radiation-induced cancer information for atomic bomb survivors, 1950–1985 (radiation exposure expressed as organ-absorbed dose)

Type of cancer	Excess relative risk at 1 Gy*	Excess deaths per 10^4 person-year-gray	Minimum dose for increased mortality, Gy	Minimum latent period to death, years
Leukemia	5.2	2.9	0.2–0.5	3–5
Multiple myeloma	2.3	0.3	—	30–34
Ovary	1.3	0.7	0.2–0.3	25–29
Urinary tract	1.3	0.7	—	30–34
Female breast	1.2	1.2	0.5–1.0	20–24
Colon	0.9	0.8	1.0–1.9	30–34
Lung	0.6	1.7	0.2–0.5	20–24
Esophagus	0.6	0.5	—	—
All (except leukemia)	0.4	10.1	0.2–0.5	—
Stomach	0.3	2.4	0.5–1.0	15–19

* Rates from UNSCEAR and Radiation Effects Research Foundation reports have been rounded to the nearest tenth.

TABLE 401-2 Late effects of some common radionuclide exposures

Radionuclide	Route of administration	Late effects
[232]Thorium dioxide (Thorotrast)	Intravenous	Liver angiosarcoma, hemangioendothelioma, hepatic cell carcinoma and cirrhosis. Bile duct carcinoma, kidney cancer, leukemia, splenic atrophy and fibrosis, and aplastic anemia.
[224,226,227]Radium	Intravenous and oral	Osteosarcoma, chondroblastic sarcoma, cataracts, leukemia, and paranasal, mastoid, and colon cancers
[222]Radon	Inhalation	Lung cancer
[125,131]Iodine	External, oral and intravenous	Hypothyroidism, thyroid adenomas, and thyroid cancer.
[90]Strontium	Topical and inhalation	Anterior lenticular cataracts from eye applications, and beta skin burns with eventual scarring
[32]Phosphorous	Topical and intravenous	Beta skin burns with eventual scarring and leukemia

certain radiation-induced biologic markers in blood cells. The severity and rapidity of the development of lymphopenia may give some early index of exposure dose, but much more reliable is the radiation-induced frequency of dicentric chromosomal aberrations in mitogen-stimulated and spontaneously dividing peripheral blood lymphocytes. The rate of granulocyte decline also is a very reliable and practical early biologic radiation dosimeter, but it may take 3 to 5 days or more before the rate is determined accurately. Bone marrow aspirations have limited quantitative relationships to exposure, but if performed in various sites, they may indicate the extent of marrow damage. Reliable estimates of radiation dose by means of other biologic dosimeters such as ESR of tooth enamel, loss of lymphocyte T cell receptors, or quantitation of lymphocyte micronuclei may be very difficult to obtain on short notice for acute radiation exposures. These measurements, however, along with determination of the loss of HPRT in lymphocytes or glycophorin A in red cells, may be very useful for intermediate- or late-exposure dosimetry.

Persons with few symptoms probably are exposed to less than 2 Gy and will require little or no therapy but should be kept under close observation with at least daily blood counts for a few days. Persons with estimated exposures in the range of 2 to 5 or 6 Gy require hospitalization for vigorous supportive therapy. Intravenous fluids and broad-spectrum antibiotic coverage should be instituted if either bacterial infections or severe agranulocytosis develops. Other supportive measures may include the administration of immunoglobulin, antifungal and antiviral agents, and antibiotics for the reduction of intestinal tract bacterial flora. Platelet transfusions should be administered for either bleeding due to thrombocytopenia or platelet counts below 20×10^9 per liter. Blood transfusions may be administered if anemia is severe, but granulocyte transfusions are of no value. Bone marrow transfusions are not indicated for persons in this group, but the early and continuous administration of molecularly cloned hematopoietic growth factors, especially granulocyte-macrophage colony stimulating factor (GM-CSF) or granulocyte colony stimulating factor (GSF), may be important adjuncts to the other forms of supportive therapy.

If the level of granulocytes falls during the first week to 0.25×10^9 per liter or less and the level of platelets to less than 30×10^9 per liter in 10 days, the total-body exposure probably is in the range of 5 to 15 Gy. Survival of persons exposed to whole-body irradiation in the range of 7 to 10 or 12 Gy with supportive therapy alone usually is not possible, so the addition of bone marrow transplantation and the concomitant administration of molecularly cloned hematopoietic growth factors may offer the best hopes for survival (see Chap. 313). Bone marrow transplantations probably are most effective if performed within the first 3 to 5 days of exposure, so early radiation dose estimates are very important. Peripheral blood lymphocytes should be collected as early as possible for histocompatibility testing, since they disappear rapidly from circulation. Platelets and blood should be irradiated with about 20 Gy prior to transfusion to reduce recipient alloantigen sensitization. Preparatory immunosuppression probably is not advisable prior to bone marrow transfusion, since permanent engraftment may not be necessary. Furthermore, it will contribute considerably to the severity of the overall illness. Persons with acute exposure to more than 15 to 20 Gy should be admitted to the hospital for supportive therapy only.

It is recommended that persons exposed to fallout in contaminated areas be treated as early as possible with 130 mg/d of potassium iodide for 10 days in order to prevent the accumulation of radioiodine in the thyroid gland. Consumption of all local produce, especially milk and vegetables, should be avoided.

PROGNOSIS Prognosis for survival from acute whole-body exposure to ionizing radiation alone depends almost entirely on tissue dose and therapy. Mortality without any therapy is negligible at 1 Gy or less and is virtually 100 percent above 15 Gy despite optimal therapy. About 50 percent of persons exposed to between 2 and 3 Gy will succumb without therapy, but most will survive with vigorous support. The LD_{50} with optimal therapy is about 4.5 Gy. There is a very high probability of death, even with vigorous general support therapy, at exposures between 5 and 15 Gy, but it seems likely that some people exposed in the 7- to 10-Gy range will survive with bone marrow transplantation and other forms of supportive therapy. At levels of whole-body radiation exposure to 12 to 15 Gy or greater, bone marrow and other modalities of treatment are of little value because death ensues from extensive tissue damage of many other types. Prognosis at any level of exposure may be reduced if associated with thermal or radiation burns, trauma, or underlying illness.

There are no known forms of therapy for prevention of the late effects of ionizing radiation exposure. They are influenced by type of radiation, tissue dose, dose rate, extent of exposure, age at time of exposure, gender, inherent repair mechanisms, subsequent exposure to other carcinogens, and many other unknown constitutional and environmental factors. The clinical courses and responses to therapy of radiation-induced leukemias and solid tumors are not significantly different from those which are not radiation-related.

REFERENCES

BENGTSSON G, MOBERG L: What is a reasonable cost for protection against radiation and other risks. Health Phys 64:661, 1993

COMMITTEE ON THE BIOLOGICAL EFFECTS OF IONIZING RADIATION, NATIONAL RESEARCH COUNCIL: *Health Effects of Exposure to Low Levels of Ionizing Radiation* (BEIR V). Washington, D.C., National Academy Press, 1990

METTLER FA JR et al: The 1986 and 1988 UNSCEAR reports: Findings and implications. Health Phys 58:241, 1990

NEEL JV, SCHULL WJ: *The Children of Atomic Bomb Survivors: A Genetic Study.* Washington, D.C., National Academy Press, 1991

SHIMUZU Y et al: Studies of the mortality of A-bomb survivors: 9. Mortality, 1950–85, part 2: Cancer mortality based on the recently revised doses (DS 86). Radiat Res 121:120, 1990

UNITED NATIONS SCIENTIFIC COMMITTEES ON THE EFFECTS OF ATOMIC RADIATION: *Sources, Effects and Risks of Ionizing Radiation* (Report No. 88, IX, 7). New York, United Nations, 1988

LABORATORY VALUES OF CLINICAL IMPORTANCE

INTRODUCTORY COMMENTS

All laboratory appendices should be interpreted with caution because normal values differ widely among clinical laboratories. The values given in this appendix are meant primarily for use with this text. In preparing this Appendix, the editors have taken into account the fact the system of international units (SI, système international d'unités) is now used in most countries and in virtually all medical and scientific journals, including most in the United States.[1] However, most clinical laboratories in the United States continue to report values in traditional units. Therefore, a system has been adopted that utilizes both systems for this Appendix and for the text itself. Values in SI units appear first, and *traditional units appear in parentheses* after the SI units. This dual system is also used for the most part in the text. In those instances in which the numbers remain the same but only the terminology is changed (mmol/L for meq/L or IU/L for mIU/L, only the SI units are given. In all other instances in the text the SI unit is followed by the traditional unit in parentheses. The SI base units, SI derived units, other units of measure referred to in this Appendix and SI prefixes are listed in Tables A-1 to A-3 at the end of this Appendix. Conversions from one system to another can be made as follows:

$$mmol/L = \frac{mg/dL \times 10}{atomic\ weight}$$

$$mg/dL = \frac{mmol/L \times atomic\ weight}{10}$$

ASCITIC FLUID

See Chapter 43.

BODY FLUIDS AND OTHER MASS DATA

Body fluid, total volume: 50 percent (in obese) to 70 percent (lean) of body weight
  Intracellular: 0.3–0.4 of body weight
  Extracellular: 0.2–0.3 of body weight
Blood:
  Total volume:
    Males: 69 mL/kg of body weight
    Females: 65 mL/kg of body weight
  Plasma volume:
    Males: 39 mL/kg of body weight
    Females: 40 mL/kg of body weight
  Red blood cell volume:
    Males: 30 mL/kg of body weight (1.15–1.21 L/m² of body surface area)
    Females: 25 mL/kg of body weight (0.95–1.00 L/m² of body surface area)

[1] Young DS: Implementation of SI units for clinical laboratory data. Ann Intern Med 106:114–129, 1987

CEREBROSPINAL FLUID[2]

		Conversion Factor (CF) $C \times CF = SI$
Osmolarity	292–297 mmol/kg water (292–297 mOsmol/L)	—
Electrolytes:		
Sodium	137–145 mmol/L (137–145 meq/L)	—
Potassium	2.7–3.9 mmol/L (2.7–3.9 meq/L)	—
Calcium	1–1.5 mmol/L (2.1–3.0 meq/L)	0.5
Magnesium	1–1.2 mmol/L (2.0–2.5 meq/L)	0.5
Chloride	116–122 mmol/L (116–122 meq/L)	—
CO_2 content	20–24 mmol/L (20–24 meq/L)	—
P_{CO_2}	6–7 kPa (45–49 mmHg)	0.1333
pH	7.31–7.34	—
Glucose	2.2–3.9 mmol/L (40–70 mg/dL)	0.05551
Lactate	1–2 mmol/L (10–20 mg/dL)	0.1110
Total protein:	0.2–0.5 g/L (20–50 mg/dL)	0.01
Prealbumin	2–6 percent	—
Albumin	56–75 percent	—
Alpha₁ globulin	2–7 percent	—
Alpha₂ globulin	4–12 percent	—
Beta globulin	8–16 percent	—
Gamma globulin	3–12 percent	—
IgG	0.01–0.014 g/L (1–1.4 mg/dL)	0.01
IgG index[3]	<0.65	
IgA	0.001–0.003 g/L (0.1–0.3 mg/dL)	0.01
IgM	0.0001–0.00012 g/L (0.01–0.012 mg/dL)	0.01
Ammonia	15–47 μmol/L (25–80 μg/dL)	0.05872
Creatinine	44–168 μmol/L (0.5–1.9 mg/dL)	88.40
Myelin basic protein	<4 μg/L	—
CSF pressure	50–180 mmH₂O	—
CSF volume (adult)	100–160 mL	—
Leukocytes:		
Total	<4 per mL	
Differential:		
Lymphocytes	60–70 percent	

[2] Since cerebrospinal fluid concentrations are equilibrium values, measurements of the same parameters in blood plasma obtained at the same time is recommended. However, there is a time lag in attainment of equilibrium, and cerebrospinal levels of plasma constituents that can fluctuate rapidly (such as plasma glucose) may not achieve stable values until after a significant lag phase.

[3] $IgG\ index = \dfrac{CSF\ IgG\ (mg/dL) \times serum\ albumin\ (g/dL)}{Serum\ IgG\ (g/dL) \times CSF\ albumin\ (mg/dL)}$

		Conversion Factor (CF) $C \times CF = SI$
Monocytes	30–50 percent	—
Neutrophils	None	—

CHEMICAL CONSTITUENTS OF BLOOD

See also function tests, especially metabolic and endocrine.

	CF
Acetoacetate, plasma: <100 μmol/L (<1 mg/dL)	97.95
Albumin, serum: 35–55 g/L (3.5–5.5 g/dL)	10
Aldolase: 0–100 nkat/L (0–6 U/L)	16.67
Alpha$_1$ antitrypsin, serum: 0.8–2.1 g/L (85–213 mg/dL)	0.01
Alpha fetoprotein (adult), serum: <30 μg/L (<30 ng/mL)	—
Aminotransferases, serum:	
Aspartate (AST, SGOT): 0–0.58 μkat/L (0–35 U/L)	0.01667
Alanine (ALT, SGPT): 0–0.58 μkat/L (0–35 U/L)	0.01667
Ammonia, whole blood, venous: 47–65 μmol/L (80–110 μg/dL)	0.5872
Amylase, serum: 0.8–3.2 μkat/L; 60–180 U/L	0.01667
Arterial blood gases:	
[HCO$_3$$^-$]: 21–28 mmol/L (21–30 meq/L)	—
P$_{CO_2}$: 4.7–5.9 kPa (35–45 mmHg)	0.1333
pH: 7.38–7.44	—
P$_{O_2}$: 11–13 kPa (80–100 mmHg)	0.1333
Ascorbic acid (vitamin C), serum: 23–57 μmol/L (0.4–1.0 mg/dL)	56.78
Barbiturates, serum: normal, nondetectable	
Phenobarbital, "potentially fatal" level: approximately 390 μmol/L (9 mg/dL)	43.06
Most short-acting barbiturates, "potentially fatal" levels: approximately 150 μmol/L (35 mg/dL)	4.419
Base, total, serum: 145–155 mmol/L (145–155 meq/L)	—
β-Hydroxybutyrate, plasma: <300 μmol/L (<3 mg/dL)	96.05
Bilirubin, total, serum (Malloy-Evelyn): 5.1–17 μmol/L (0.3–1.0 mg/dL)	17.10
Direct, serum: 1.7–5.1 μmol/L (0.1–0.3 mg/dL)	17.10
Indirect, serum: 3.4–12 μmol/L (0.2–0.7 mg/dL)	17.10
Bromides, serum: nondetectable	
Toxic levels: >17 mmol/L (>17 meq/L)	—
Calciferols (vitamin D), plasma:	
1,25-Dihydroxyvitamin D [1,25(OH)$_2$D]: 40–160 pmol/L (16 to 65 pg/mL)	0.2400
25-Hydroxyvitamin D [25(OH)D]: 20–200 nmol/L (8–80 ng/mL)	2.496
Calcium, ionized: 1.1–1.4 mmol/L (4.5–5.6 mg/dL)	0.2495
Calcium, plasma: 2.2–2.6 mmol/L (9–10.5 mg/dL)	0.2495
Carbon dioxide content, plasma (sea level): 21–30 mmol/L (21–30 meq/L)	—
Carbon dioxide tension (P$_{CO_2}$), arterial blood (sea level): 4.7–6.0 kPa (35–45 mmHg)	0.1333
Carbon monoxide content, blood: symptoms with over 20 percent saturation of hemoglobin	
Carotenoids, serum: 0.9–5.6 μmol/L (50–300 μg/dL)	0.01863

	CF
Ceruloplasmin, serum: 270–370 mg/L (27–37 mg/dL)	10
Chlorides, serum (as Cl$^-$): 98–106 mmol/L (98–106 meq/L)	—
Cholesterol: see Table A-4	
Complement, serum:	
C3: 0.55–1.20 g/L (55–120 mg/dL)	0.01
C4: 0.20–0.50 g/L (20–50 mg/dL)	0.01
Copper, serum: 11–22 μmol/L (70–140 μg/dL)	0.1574
Creatine phosphokinase, serum (total):	
Females: 0.17–1.17 μkat/L (10–70 U/L)	0.01667
Males: 0.42–1.50 μkat/L (25–90 U/L)	0.01667
Creatinine, serum: <133 μmol/L (1.5 mg/dL)	88.40
Digoxin serum:	
Therapeutic level: 0.6–2.8 nmol/L (0.5–2.2 ng/mL)	1.281
Toxic level: >3.1 nmol/L (>2.4 ng/mL)	1.281
Ethanol, blood:	
Mild to moderate intoxication: 17–43 mmol/L (80–200 mg/dL)	0.2171
Marked intoxication: 54–87 mmol/L (250–400 mg/dL)	0.2171
Severe intoxication: >87 mmol/L (>400 mg/dL)	0.2171
Fatty acids, free (nonesterified), plasma: 180 mg/L (<18 mg/dL)	10
Ferritin, serum:	
Women: 10–200 μg/L (10–200 ng/ml)	—
Men: 15–400 μg/L (15–400 ng/ml)	
Fibrinogen, plasma: see "Hematologic Evaluations: Platelets and Coagulation"	—
Fibrinogen split products: see "Hematologic Evaluations: Platelets and Coagulation"	—
Folic acid, red cell: 340–1020 nmol/L cells (150–450 ng/mL cells)	2.266
Gastrin, serum: 40–200 ng/L (40–200 pg/mL)	—
Globulins, serum: 20–30 g/L (2.0–3.0 g/dL)	10
Glucose (fasting), plasma:	
Normal: 4.2–6.4 mmol/L (75–115 mg/dL)	0.05551
Diabetes mellitus: >7.8 mmol/L on more than one occasion (>140 mg dL)	0.05551
Glucose, 2 h postprandial, plasma:	
Normal: <7.8 mmol/L (<140 mg/dL)	0.05551
Impaired glucose tolerance: 7.8–11.1 mmol/L (140–200 mg/dL)	0.05551
Diabetes mellitus: >11.1 mmol/L on more than one occasion (>200 mg/dL)	0.05551
Hemoglobin, blood (sea level):	
Male: 140–180 g/L (14–18 g/dL)	10
Female: 120–160 g/L (12–16 g/dL)	10
Hemoglobin A$_{1c}$: up to 6 percent of total hemoglobin	—
Immunoglobulins, serum:	
IgA: 0.9–3.2 g/L (90–325 mg/dL)	0.01
IgD: 0–0.08 g/L (0–8 mg/dL)	0.01
IgE: <0.00025 g/L (<0.025 mg/dL)	0.01
IgG: 8.0–15.0 g/L (800–1500 mg/dL)	0.01
IgM: 0.45–1.5 g/L (45–150 mg/dL)	0.01
Iron, serum: 9–27 μmol/L (50–150 μg/dL)	0.01791
Iron-binding capacity, serum: 45–66 μmol/L (250–370 μg/dL)	0.01791
Saturation: 0.2–0.45 (20–45 percent)	
Lactate dehydrogenase, serum:	
200–450 units/mL (Wrobleski)	—
60–100 units/mL (Wacker)	—

	Conversion Factor (CF) C × CF = SI
0.4–1.7 μkat/L (25–100 units/L)	0.01667
Lactic dehydrogenase isoenzymes, serum (agarose):	
Fraction 1 (of total): 0.14–0.25 (14–26 percent)	0.01
Fraction 2: 0.29–0.39 (29–39 percent)	0.01
Fraction 3: 0.20–0.25 (20–26 percent)	0.01
Fraction 4: 0.08–0.16 (8–16 percent)	0.01
Fraction 5: 0.06–0.16 (6–16 percent)	0.01
Lactate, venous plasma: 0.6–1.7 mmol/L (5–15 mg/dL)	0.1110
Lead, serum: <1.0 μmol/L (<20 μg/dL)	0.04826
Lipids: see Table A-4	—
Lipids, triglyceride, serum: see "Triglycerides"	—
Lipoprotein: see Table A-4	—
Lithium, serum:	
Therapeutic level: 0.6–1.2 mmol/L (0.6–1.2 meq/L)	—
Toxic level: >2 mmol/L (2 meq/L)	—
Magnesium, serum: 0.8–1.2 mmol/L (2–3 mg/dL)	0.4114
Osmolality, plasma: 285–295 mmol/kg serum water (285–295 mosmol/kg serum water)	—
Oxygen content:	
Arterial blood (sea level): 17–21 volume percent	—
Venous blood, arm (sea level): 10–16 volume percent	—
Oxygen percent saturation (sea level):	
Arterial blood: 0.97 mol/mol (97 percent)	0.01
Venous blood, arm: 0.60–0.85 mol/mol (60–85 percent)	0.01
Oxygen tension (P_{O_2}) blood: 11–13 kPa (80–100 mmHg)	0.1333
pH, blood: 7.38–7.44	—
Phenytoin, plasma:	
Therapeutic level: 40–80 μmol/L (10–20 mg/L)	3.964
Toxic level: >120 μmol/L (>30 mg/L)	3.964
Phospatase, acid, serum: 0.90 nkat/L (0–5.5 U/L)	—
Phosphatase, alkaline, serum: 0.5–2.0 μkat/L (30–120 U/L)	—
Phosphorus, inorganic, serum: 1.0–1.4 mmol/L (3–4.5 mg/dL)	0.3229
Potassium, serum: 3.5–5.0 mmol/L (3.5–5.0 meq/L)	—
Proteins, total, serum: 55–80 g/L (5.5–8.0 g/dL)	10
Protein fractions, serum:	
Albumin: 35–55 g/L [3.5–5.5 g/dL (50–60 percent)]	10
Globulin: 20–35 g/L [2.0–3.5 g/dL (40–50 percent)]	10
Alpha₁: 2–4 g/L [0.2–0.4 g/dL (4.2–7.2 percent)]	10
Alpha₂: 5–9 g/L [0.5–0.9 g/dL (6.8–12 percent)]	10
Beta: 6–11 g/L [0.6–1.1 g/dL (9.3–15 percent)]	10
Gamma: 7–17 g/L [0.7–1.7 g/dL (13–23 percent)]	10
Pyruvate, venous, plasma: 60–170 μmol/L (0.5–1.5 mg/dL)	113.6
Quinidine, serum:	
Therapeutic range: 4.6–9.2 μmol/L (1.5–3 mg/L)	3.082
Toxic range: 15.4–18.5 μmol/L (5–6 mg/L)	3.082

	Conversion Factor (CF) C × CF = SI
Salicylate, plasma: 0 mmol/L	—
Therapeutic range: 1.4–1.8 mmol/L (20–25 mg/dL)	0.07240
Toxic range: >2.2 mmol/L (>30 mg/dL)	0.07240
Sodium, serum: 136–145 mmol/L (136–145 meq/L)	—
Steroids: see "Metabolic and Endocrine Tests"	—
Triglycerides: <1.8 mmol/L (<160 mg/dL)	0.01129
Urea nitrogen, serum: 3.6–7.1 mmol/L (10–20 mg/dL)	0.3570
Uric acid, serum:	
Men: 150–480 μmol/L (2.5–8.0 mg/dL)	59.48
Women: 90–360 μmol/L (1.5–6.0 mg/dL)	59.48
Vitamin A, serum: 0.7–3.5 μmol/L (20–100 μg/dL)	0.03491
Vitamin B₁₂, serum: 148–443 pmol/L (200–600 pg/mL)	0.7378
Zinc, serum: 11.5–18.5 μmol/L (75–120 μg/dL)	0.1530

CIRCULATION FUNCTION TESTS

Arteriovenous oxygen difference: 30–50 mL/L
Cardiac output (Fick): 2.5–3.6 L/m² of body surface area per minute
Contractility indexes:
Maximum left ventricular *dp/dt:* 1650 ± 300 mmHg/s
Maximum (*dp/dt*)/*p:* 44 ± 8.4 s⁻¹
(*dp/dt*)/DP at DP = 40 mmHg: 37.6 ± 12.2 s⁻¹ (DP = diastolic press.)
Mean normalized systolic ejection rate (angiography): 3.32 ± 0.84 end-diastolic volumes per second
Mean velocity of circumferential fiber shortening (angiography) 1.66 ± 0.42 circumferences per second
Ejection fraction, stroke volume/end-diastolic volume (SV/EDV):
Normal range: 0.55–0.78; average: 0.67
End-diastolic volume: 75 ± 15 mL/m²
End-systolic volume: 25 ± 8 mL/m²
Left ventricular work:
Stroke work index: 30–110 (g·m)/m²
Left ventricular minute work index: 1.8–6.6 [(kg·m)/m²]/min
Oxygen consumption index: 110–150 mL
Pulmonary vascular resistance: 20–120 (dyn·s)/cm⁵ (2–12 kPa·s/L)
Systemic vascular resistance: 770–1500 (dyn·s)/cm⁵ (77–150 kPa·s/L)

GASTROINTESTINAL TESTS

See also "Stool Analysis."

Absorption tests:
D-Xylose absorption test: After an overnight fast, 25 g xylose is given in aqueous solution by mouth. Urine collected for the following 5 h should contain 5–8 g (33–53 mmol) (or >20 percent of ingested dose). Serum xylose should be 25–40 mg/100 mL 1 h after the oral dose (1.7–2.7 mmol/L).
Vitamin A absorption test: A fasting blood specimen is obtained and 200,000 units of vitamin A in oil is given by mouth. Serum vitamin A levels should rise to twice fasting level in 3–5 h.
Bentiromide test (pancreatic function): 500 mg bentiromide (chymex) orally; *p*-aminobenzoic acid (PABA) measured in plasma and/or urine
Plasma: >3.6 (±1.1) μg/mL at 90 min
Urine: >50 percent recovered as PABA in 6 h
Gastric juice:
Volume:
24 h: 2–3 L
Nocturnal: 600–700 mL
Basal, fasting: 30–70 mL/h

	Conversion Factor (CF) C × CF = SI

Reaction:
  pH: 1.6–1.8
  Titratable acidity of fasting juice: 4–9 μmol/s (15–35 meq/h) — 0.261

Acid output:
  Basal:
    Females (mean ± 1 SD): 0.6 ± 0.5 μmol/s (2.0 ± 1.8 meq/h) — 0.2778
    Males (mean ± 1 SD): 0.8 ± 0.6 μmol/s (3.0 ± 2.0 meq/h) — 0.2778
    Maximal (after subcutaneous histamine acid phosphate 0.004 mg/kg body weight and preceded by 50 mg promethazine or after betazole 1.7 mg/kg body weight or pentagastrin 6 μg/kg body weight):
      Females (mean ± 1 SD): 4.4 ± 1.4 μmol/s (16 ± 5 meq/h) — 0.2778
      Males (mean ± 1 SD): 6.4 ± 1.4 μmol/s (23 ± 5 meq/h) — 0.2778
    Basal acid output/maximal acid output ratio: 0.6 or less

Gastrin, serum: 40–200 ng/L (40–200 pg/mL) — —

Secretin test (pancreatic exocrine function: 1 unit/kg of body weight, intravenously
  Volume (pancreatic juice): >2.0 mL/kg in 80 min — —
  Bicarbonate concentration: >80 mmol/L (80 meq/L) — —
  Bicarbonate output: >10 mmol in 30 min (10 meq in 30 min) — —

METABOLIC AND ENDOCRINE TESTS

Adrenocorticotropin (ACTH) plasma, 8 A.M.: <18 pmol/L (<80 pg/mL) — 0.2202
Adrenal cortex function tests: see Chap. 335 — —
Adrenal medulla function tests: see Chap 336 — —
Adrenal steroids, plasma:
  Aldosterone, 8 A.M.: <220 pmol/L (patient supine, 100 meq Na and 60–100 meq K intake) (<8 ng/dL) — 27.74
  Cortisol:
    8 A.M.: 140–690 nmol/L (5–25 μg/dL) — 27.59
    4 P.M.: 80–330 nmol/L (3–12 μg/dL) — 27.59
  Dehydroepiandrosterone (DHEA): 7–31 nmol/L (2–9 μg/L) — 3.467
  Dehydroepiandrosterone sulfate (DHEA sulfate): 1.3–6.7 μmol/L (500–2500 μg/L) — 0.002714
  11-Deoxycortisol (compound S): <30 nmol/L (<1 μg/dL) — 28.86
  17-Hydroxyprogesterone:
    Women: follicular phase, 0.6–3 nmol/L (0.20–1 μg/L); luteal phase, 1.5–10.6 nmol/L (0.5–3.5 μg/L) — 3.026
    Men: 0.2–9 nmol/L (0.06–3 μg L) — 3.026
Adrenal steroids, urinary excretion:
  Aldosterone: 14–53 nmol/d (5–19 μg/d) — 2.774
  Cortisol, free: 55–275 nmol/d (20–100 μg/d) — 2.759
  17-Hydroxycorticosteroids: 5.5–28 μmol/d (2–10 mg/d) — 2.759
  17-Ketosteroids:
    Men: 24–88 μmol/d (7–25 mg/d) — 3.467
    Women: 14–52 μmol/d (4–15 mg/d) — 3.467
Angiotensin II, plasma, 8 A.M.: 10–30 nmol/L (10–30 pg/mL) — —

	Conversion Factor (CF) C × CF = SI

Arginine vasopressin (AVP), plasma:
  Random fluid intake: 1.5–5.6 pmol/L (1.5–6 ng/L) — 0.92
Calcitonin, plasma: <50 ng/L (<50 pg/mL) — —
Catecholamines, urinary excretion:
  Free catecholamines: <590 nmol/d (<100 μg/d) — 5.911
  Epinephrine: <275 nmol/d (<50 μg/d) — 5.458
  Metanephrines: <7 μmol/d (<1.3 mg/d) — 5.458
  Vanillylmandelic acid (VMA): <40 μmol/d (<8 mg/d) — 5.046
Glucagon, plasma: 50–100 ng/L (50–100 pg/mL) — —
Gonadal function tests: see Chaps. 339 and 340 — —
Gonadal steroids, plasma:
  Androstenedione:
    Women: 3.5–7.0 nmol/L (1–2 ng/ml) — 3.492
    Men: 3.0–5.0 nmol/L (0.8–1.3 ng/ml) — 3.492
  Estradiol:
    Women: 70–220 pmol/L (20–60 pg/mL), higher at ovulation — 3.671
    Men: <180 pmol/L (<50 pg/mL) — 3.671
  Progesterone:
    Women: luteal peak >16 nmol/L (75 ng/mL) — 3.180
    Men, prepubertal girls, preovulatory women, and postmenopausal women: <6 nmol/L (<2 ng/mL) — 3.180
  Testosterone:
    Women: <3.5 nmol/L (<1 ng/mL) — 3.467
    Men: 10–35 nmol/L (3–10 ng/mL) — 3.467
    Prepubertal boys and girls: 0.17–0.7 nmol/L (0.05–0.2 ng/mL) — 3.467
Gonadotropins, plasma:
  Women, mature, premenopausal, except at ovulation:
    FSH: 5–20 IU/L (5–20 mIU/mL) — —
    LH: 5–25 IU/L (5–25 mIU/mL) — —
    Ovulatory surge:
      FSH: 12–30 IU/L (12–30 mIU/mL) — —
      LH: 25–100 IU/L (25–100 mIU/mL) — —
    Postmenopausal:
      FSH: 12–30 IU/L (12–30 mIU/mL) — —
      LH: >50 IU/L (>50 mIU/mL) — —
  Men, mature:
    FSH: 5–20 IU/L (5–20 mIU/mL) — —
    LH: 5–20 IU/L (5–20 mIU/mL) — —
  Children of both sexes, prepubertal:
    FSH: <5 IU/L (<5 mIU/mL) — —
Growth hormone, after 100 g glucose by mouth: <5 μg/L (<5 ng/mL) — —
Human chorionic gonadotropin, β subunit (β-hCG), plasma:
  Men and nonpregnant women: <3 IU/L (<3 mIU/mL) — —
Insulin, serum or plasma, fasting: 43–186 pmol/L (6–26 μU/mL) — 7.175
Insulin-like growth factor 1 (somatomedin C, IGF-1/SM-C): see Chap. 332 — —
Oxytocin: random 1–4 pmol/L (1.25–5 ng/L) — 0.80
  Ovulatory peak in women: 4–8 pmol/L (5–10 ng/L) — —
Pancreatic islet function tests: see Chap. 337 — —
Parathyroid function tests: see Chap. 357 — —
Pituitary function tests: see Chaps. 331 to 333 — —
Pregnancy tests: see Chap. 340 — —

	Conversion Factor (CF) C × CF = SI

Prolactin, serum: 2–15 μg/L (2–15 ng/mL) —
Renin-angiotensin function tests: see Chap. 335 —
Semen analysis: see Chap. 339 —
Thyroid function tests:
 Dynamic tests of thyroid function: see Chap. 334 —
 Radioactive iodine uptake, 24 h: 5–30 percent (range varies in different areas due to variations in iodine intake) —
 Resin T_3 uptake: 0.25–0.35 (25–35 percent) (varies among laboratories; for calculation of indexes of resin T_3 uptake, see Chap. 334) — 0.01
 Reverse triiodothyronine (rT_3), plasma: 0.15–0.61 nmol/L (10–40 ng/dL) — 0.01536
 Thyroid-stimulating hormone (TSH): 0.4–5 mU/L (0.4–5 μU/mL) —
 Thyroxine (T_4), serum radioimmunoassay: 64–154 nmol/L (5–12 μg/dL) — 12.86
 Triiodothyronine (T_3), plasma: 1.1–2.9 nmol/L (70–190 ng/dL) — 0.01536

PULMONARY FUNCTION TESTS

See Table A-7.

RENAL FUNCTION TESTS

Clearances (corrected to 1.72 m² of body surface area):
 Measures of glomerular filtration rate:
  Inulin clearance (C1):
   Males (mean ± 1 SD): 2.1 ± 0.4 mL/s (124 ± 25.8 mL/min) — 0.01667
   Females (mean ± 1 SD): 2.0 ± 0.2 mL/s (119 ± 12.8 mL/min) — 0.01667
  Endogenous creatinine clearance: 1.5–2.2 mL/s (91–130 mL/min) — 0.01667
  Urea: 1.0–1.7 mL/s (60–100 mL/min) — 0.01667
 Measures of effective renal plasma flow and tubular function:
  p-Aminohippuric acid clearance (Cl_{PAH}):
   Males (mean ± 1 SD): 10.9 ± 2.7 mL/s (654 ± 163 mL/min) — 0.01667
   Females (mean ± 1 SD): 9.9 ± 1.7 mL/s (594 ± 102 mL/min) — 0.01667
 Concentration and dilution test:
  Specific gravity of urine:
   After 12-h fluid restriction: 1.025 or more —
   After 12-h deliberate water intake: 1.003 or less —
 Protein excretion, urine: <0.15 g/d (<150 mg/d) — 0.01
  Males: 0–0.06 g/d (0–60 mg/d) — 0.01
  Females: 0–0.09 g/d (0–90 mg/d) — 0.01
 Specific gravity, maximal range: 1.002–1.028 —
 Tubular reabsorption, phosphorus: 79–94 percent of filtered load —

HEMATOLOGIC EVALUATIONS

See also "Chemical Constituents of Blood." —
Bone marrow   See Table A-6. —

	Conversion Factor (CF) C × CF = SI

Carboxyhemoglobin:
 Nonsmoker: 0–0.023 (0–2.3 percent) — 0.01
 Smoker: 0.021–0.042 (2.1–4.2 percent) — 0.01
Erythrocyte:
 Count: 4.15–4.90 × 10¹²/L (4.15–4.90 × 10⁶/mm³) —
 Distribution width (Coulter): 0.13–0.15 (13–15 percent) —
 Glucose-6-phosphate dehydrogenase: 12.1 ± 2 IU/gHb (WHO) —
 Life span:
  Normal survival: 120 days —
  Chromium-labeled, half-life ($t\frac{1}{2}$): 28 days —
 Mean corpuscular hemoglobin (MHC): 28–33 pg/cell (28–33 pg/cell) —
 Mean corpuscular hemoglobin concentration (MCHC): 320–360 g/L (32–36 g/dL) —
 Mean corpuscular volume (MCV): 86–98 fL (86–98 mm³) —
Ham's test (acid serum): negative —
Haptoglobin, serum: 0.5–2.2 g/L (50–220 mg/dL) — 0.01
Hematocrit:
 Males: 0.42–0.52 (42–52 percent) —
 Females: 0.37–0.48 (37–48 percent) —
Hemoglobin:
 Plasma: 0.6–3 μmol/L (1–5 mg/dL) — 0.6206
 Whole blood:
  Males: 8.1–11.2 mmol/L (13–18 g/dL) — 0.6206
  Females: 7.4–9.9 mmol/L (12–16 g/dL) — 0.6206
Hemoglobin A_2 (HbA_2): 0.015–0.035 (1.5–3.5 percent) — 0.01
Hemoglobin, fetal (HbF): <0.02 (<2 percent) — 0.01
Hemoglobin H prep: negative —
Leukocytes:
 Alkaline phosphatase (LAP): 0.2–1.6 μkat/L (13–100 U/L) —
 Count: 4.3–0.3X10⁹/L (4.3–10.8 × 10³/mm³) —
 Differential:
  Neutrophils: 0.45–0.74 (45–74 percent) —
  Bands: 0–0.04 (0–4 percent) —
  Lymphocytes: 0.16–0.45 (16–45 percent) —
  Monocytes: 0.04–0.10 (4–10 percent) —
  Eosinophils: 0–0.07 (0–7 percent) —
  Basophils: 0–0.02 (0–2 percent) —
Lysozyme (muramidase):
 Serum: 5–25 mg/L (5–25 μg/mL) —
 Urine: <2 mg/L (<2 μg/mL) —
Methemoglobin: <2 mg/L (<2 μg/mL) —
Osmotic fragility:
 Slight hemolysis: 0.45–0.39 percent —
 Complete hemolysis: 0.33–0.30 percent —
Plasma iron turnover: 20–42 mg/d or 0.45 mg/kg of body weight per day —
Platelets and coagulation parameters:
 Alpha₂ antiplasmin: 70–130 percent —
 Antithrombin III: 80–80–120 percent —
 Bleeding time:
  Duke method: <4 min —
  Simplate: <7 min —
 Clot retraction, qualitative: apparent in 60 min, complete <24 h, usually <6 h —
 Euglobulin lysis time: >2 h —
 Factor II: 60–100 percent —

	Conversion Factor (CF) C × CF = SI

Factor V: 60–100 percent
Factor VII: 60–100 percent
Factor IX: 60–100 percent
Factor X: 60–100 percent
Factor XI: 60–100 percent
Factor XII: 60–100 percent
Factor XIII: 60–100 percent
Fibrinogen: 200–400 mg/dL
Fibrin split products: <10 μg/mL
Plasminogen: 2.4–4.4 CTA U/mL
Protein C (antigenic assay): 58–148 percent
Protein S (antigenic assay): 58–148 percent
Partial thromboplastin time (activated PTT): comparable with control
Prothrombin time (quick one-stage): control ± 1 s
Protamine paracoagulation (3P) test: negative
Platelets: 130,000–400,000 per microliter
Thrombin time: control ± 3 s
von Willebrand's antigen: 60–150 percent

Protoporphyrin, free erythrocyte (FEP): 0.28–0.64 μmol/L of red blood cells (16–36 μg/dL of red blood cells) — 0.0177

Red cells: see "Erythrocytes"

Schilling test: 7–40 percent of orally administered vitamin B$_{12}$ excreted in urine

Sedimentation rate:
   Westergren, <50 years of age:
      Males: 0–15 mm/h
      Females: 0–20 mm/h
   Westergren, >50 years of age:
      Males: 0–20 mm/h
      Females: 0–30 mm/h

Sucrose hemolysis: negative

Viscosity
   Plasma: 1.7–2.1
   Serum: 1.4–1.8

White blood cells: see "Leukocytes"

URINE ANALYSIS

See also "Metabolic and Endocrine Tests"

	C × CF = SI
Acidity, titratable: 20–40 mmol/d (20–40 meq/d)	—
Ammonia: 30–50 mmol/d (30–50 meq/d)	—
Amylase: 35–260 Somogyi units/h	—
Amylase/creatinine clearance ratio [(Cl$_{am}$/Cl$_{cr}$) × 100]: 1–5	—
Bentiromide (pancreatic function): 50 percent excreted in 6 h as *p*-amino benzoic acid (PABA) after 500 mg oral bentiromide	—
Calcium (10 meq/d or 200-mg/d calcium diet): <3.8 mmol/d (<7.5 meq/d)	0.5
Catecholamines: <600 nmol/d (<100 μg/d)	5.911
Copper: 0–0.4 μmol/d (0–25 μg/d)	0.01574
Coproporphyrins (types I and III): 150–460 nmol/d (100–300 μg/d)	1.527
Creatine, as creatinine:	
Adult males: <380 pmol/d (<50 mg/d)	7.625
Adult females: <760 pmol/d (<100 mg/d)	7.625
Creatinine: 8.8–14 mmol/d (1.0–1.6 g/d)	8.840
Glucose, true (oxidase method): 0.3–1.7 mmol/d (50–300 mg/d)	0.5551
5-Hydroxyindoleacetic acid (5-HIAA): 10–47 μmol/d (2–9 mg/d)	5.230
Lead: <0.4 μmol/d (<80 μg/d)	0.004826
Protein: <0.15 g/d (<150 mg/d)	0.1
Porphobilinogen: none	—
Potassium: 25–100 mmol/d [25–100 meq/d (varies with intake)]	—
Sodium: 100–260 mmol/d [100–260 meq/d (varies with intake)]	—
Urobilinogen: 1.7–5.9 μmol/d (1–3.5 mg/d)	1.693
Vanillylmandelic acid (VMA): <40 μmol/d (<8 mg/d)	5.046
D-Xylose excretion: 5 to 8 g within 5 h after oral dose of 25 g	—

STOOL ANALYSIS

Bulk:	
Wet weight: <197.5 (115 ± 41) g/d	—
Dry weight: <66.4 (34 ± 15) g/d	—
Alpha$_1$ antitrypsin: 0.98 (±0.17) mg/g dry weight stool	—
Coproporphyrin: 600–1500 nmol/d (400–1000 μg/d)	1.527
Fat (on diet containing at least 50 g fat): <6.0 (4.0 ± 1.5) g/d when measured on a 3-day (or longer) collection	
Percent of dry weight: 0.30 (<30.4 percent)	0.01
Coefficient of fat absorption: >0.95 (>95 percent)	0.01
Fatty acid:	
Free: 0.01–0.10 (1–10 percent of dry matter)	0.01
Combined as soap: 0.005–0.12 (0.5–12 percent of dry matter)	0.01
Nitrogen: <1.7 (1.4 ± 0.2) g/d	—
Protein content: minimal	—
Urobilinogen: 68–470 μmol/d (40–280 mg/d)	1.693
Water: 0.65 (approximately 65 percent)	0.01

TABLE A-1 SI and other units

Quantity	Name of unit	Symbol for unit	Derivation of units
SI BASE UNITS			
Length	meter	m	
Mass	kilogram	kg	
Time	second	s	
Thermodynamic temperature	Kelvin	K	
Amount of substance	mole	mol	
SI DERIVED UNITS			
Area	square meter	m^2	
Force	newton	N	$(m \cdot kg)/s^2$
Pressure	pascal	Pa	$N \cdot m^2$
Work, energy	joule	J	$N \cdot m$
Celsius temperature	degree Celsius	°C	K
OTHER UNITS RETAINED FOR USE			
Time	minute	min	
	hour	h	
	day	d	
Volume	liter	L	

TABLE A-3 SI prefixes and their symbols

Factor	Prefix	Symbol for prefix
10^9	giga	G
10^6	mega	M
10^3	kilo	k
10^2	hecto	h
10^1	deka	da
10^{-1}	deci	d
10^{-2}	centi	c
10^{-3}	milli	m
10^{-6}	micro	μ
10^{-9}	nano	n
10^{-12}	pico	p
10^{-15}	femto	f
10^{-18}	alto	a

TABLE A-4 Classification of total cholesterol and LDL-cholesterol values

	Total plasma cholesterol	LDL-cholesterol	Conversion factor (C to SI)
Desirable	<5.20 mmol/L (<200 mg/dL)	<3.36 mmol/L (<130 mg/dL)	0.02586
Borderline high	5.20–6.18 mmol/L (200–239 mg/dL)	3.36–4.11 mmol/L (130–159 mg/dL)	0.02586
High	≥6.21 mmol/L (≥240 mg/dL)	≥4.14 mmol/L (≥160 mg/dL)	0.02586

SOURCE: The Expert Panel. Report of the National Cholesterol Education Program Expert Panel on Detection, Evaluation, and Treatment of High Blood Cholesterol in Adults. Arch Intern Med 148:36, 1988

TABLE A-2 Radiation derived units

Quantity	Old unit	SI unit	Name for SI unit (and abbreviation)	Conversion
Activity	curie (Ci)	Disintegrations per second (dps)	becquerel (Bq)	1 Ci = 3.7 × 10^{10} Bq 1 mCi = 37 mBq 1 μCi = 0.037 MBq or 37 GBq 1 Bq = 2.703 × 10^{-11} Ci
Absorbed dose	rad	joule per kilogram (J/kg)	gray (Gy)	1 Gy = 100 rad 1 rad = 0.01 Gy 1 mrad = 10^{-3} cGy
Exposure	roentgen (R)	coulomb per kilogram (C/kg)	—	1 C/kg = 3876 R 1 R = 2.58 × 10^{-4} C/kg 1 mR = 258 pC/kg
Dose equivalent	rem	joule per kilogram (J/kg)	sievert (Sv)	1 Sv = 100 rem 1 rem = 0.01 Sv 1 mrem = 10 μSv

TABLE A-5 Normal values of echocardiographic measurements in adults

	Range, cm	Mean, cm	Number of subjects
Age (years)	13 to 54	26	134
Body surface area (m^2)	1.45 to 2.22	1.8	130
RVD—flat	0.7 to 2.3	1.5	84
RVD—left lateral	0.9 to 2.6	1.7	83
LVID—flat	3.7 to 5.6	4.7	82
LVID—left lateral	3.5 to 5.7	4.7	81
Posterior LV wall thickness	0.6 to 1.1	0.9	137
Posterior LV wall amplitude	0.9 to 1.4	1.2	48
IVS wall thickness	0.6 to 1.1	0.9	137
Mid IVS amplitude	0.3 to 0.8	0.5	10
Apical IVS amplitude	0.5 to 1.2	0.7	38
Left atrial dimension	1.9 to 4.0	2.9	133
Aortic root dimension	2.0 to 3.7	2.7	121
Aortic cusps' separation	1.5 to 2.6	1.9	93
Percentage of fractional shortening‡	34 to 44%	36%	20
Mean rate of circumferential shortening (Vcf)‡, or mean normalized shortening velocity	1.02 to 1.94 circ/s	1.3 circ/s	38

* RVD = right ventricular dimension; LVID = left ventricular internal dimension; d = end diastole; s = end systole; LV = left ventricle; IVS = interventricular septum.

† $\dfrac{LVIDd - LVIDs}{LVIDd}$

‡ $\dfrac{LVIDd - LVIDs}{LVIDd \times ejection\ time}$

SOURCE: From H. Feigenbaum, Echocardiography, in *Heart Disease*, 4th ed, E Braunwald (ed). Philadelphia, Saunders, 1992.

TABLE A-6   Differential nucleated cell counts of bone marrow

	Normal, mean%*	Range, %[†]		Normal, mean%*	Range, %[†]
Myeloid:	56.7		Erythroid:	25.6	
Neutrophilic series:	53.6		Pronormoblasts	0.6	0.2–1.3
Myeloblast	0.9	0.2–1.5	Basophilic normoblasts	1.4	0.5–2.4
Promyelocyte	3.3	2.1–4.1	Polychromatophilic	21.6	17.9–29.2
Myelocyte	12.7	8.2–15.7	normoblasts		
Metamyelocyte	15.9	9.6–24.6	Orthochromatic normoblasts	2.0	0.4–4.6
Band	12.4	9.5–15.3	Megakaryocytes	<0.1	
Segmented			Lymphoreticular	17.8	
Eosinophilic series	3.1	1.2–5.3	Lymphocytes	16.2	11.1–23.2
Basophilic series	<0.1	0–0.2	Plasma cells	2.3	0.4–3.9
			Reticulum cells	0.3	0–0.9

* From MM Wintrobe et al, *Clinical Hematology*, 8th ed. Philadelphia, Lea & Febiger, 1981.
† Range observed in 12 healthy men.

TABLE A-7   Summary of values useful in pulmonary physiology

	Symbol	Typical values Men	Women

PULMONARY MECHANICS

	Symbol	Men	Women
Spirometry—volume-time curves:			
Forced vital capacity	FVC	≥4.0 L	≥3.0 L
Forced expiratory volume in 1 s	FEV_1	>3.0 L	>2.0 L
FEV_1/FVC	$FEV_1\%$	>60%	>70%
Maximal midexpiratory flow	MMF (FEF 25–27)	>2.0 L/s	>1.6 L/s
Maximal expiratory flow rate	MEFR (FEF 200–1200)	>3.5 L/s	>3.0 L/s
Spirometry—flow-volume curves:			
Maximal expiratory flow at 50% of expired vital capacity	V_{max} 50 (FEF 50%)	>2.5 L/s	>2.0 L/s
Maximal expiratory flow at 75% of expired vital capacity	V_{max} 75 (FEF 75%)	>1.5 L/s	>1.0 L/s
Resistance to airflow:			
Pulmonary resistance	RL (R_L)	<3.0 (cmH$_2$O/s)/L	
Airway resistance	Raw	<2.5 (cmH$_2$O/s)/L	
Specific conductance	SGaw	>0.13 cmH$_2$O/s	
Pulmonary compliance:			
Static recoil pressure at total lung capacity	Pst TLC	25 ± 5 cmH$_2$O	
Compliance of lungs (static)	CL	0.2 L/cmH$_2$O	
Compliance of lungs and thorax	C(L + T)	0.1 L/cmH$_2$O	
Dynamic compliance of 20 breaths per minute	C dyn 20	0.25 ± 0.05 L/cmH$_2$O	
Maximal static respiratory pressures:			
Maximal inspiratory pressure	MIP	>90 cmH$_2$O	>50 cmH$_2$O
Maximal expiratory pressure	MEP	>150 cmH$_2$O	>120 cmH$_2$O

LUNG VOLUMES

	Symbol	Men	Women
Total lung capacity	TLC	6–7 L	5–6 L
Functional residual capacity	FRC	2–3 L	2–3 L
Residual volume	RV	1–2 L	1–2 L
Inspiratory capacity	IC	2–4 L	2–4 L
Expiratory reserve volume	ERV	1–2 L	1–2 L
Vital capacity	VC	4–5 L	3–4 L

GAS EXCHANGE (SEA LEVEL)

	Symbol	
Arterial O$_2$ tension	Pa_{O_2}	12.7 ± 0.7 kPa (95 ± 5 mmHg)
Arterial CO$_2$ tension	Pa_{CO_2}	5.3 ± 0.3 kPa (40 ± 2 mmHg)
Arterial O$_2$ saturation	Sa_{O_2}	0.97 ± 0.02 (97 ± 2%)
Arterial blood pH	pH	7.40 ± 0.02
Arterial bicarbonate	HCO_3^-	24 + 2 meq/L
Base excess	BE	0 ± 2 meq/L
Diffusing capacity for carbon monoxide (single breath)	DL_{CO}	0.42 mLCO/s/mmHg (25 mL CO/min/mmHg)
Dead space volume	V_D	50 ± 25 mL
Physiologic dead space; dead space-tidal volume ratio	V_D/V_T	≤35% V_T
(rest)		
(exercise)		≤20% V_T
Alveolar-arterial difference for O$_2$	A-aD$_{O_2}$	≤2.7 kPa ≤20 kPa (≤20 mmHg)

INDEX

TOPICAL TABLE OF CONTENTS